Critical Care Medicine

Principles of Diagnosis and Management in the Adult

Critical Care Medicine

Principles of Diagnosis and Management in the Adult

Third Edition

Joseph E. Parrillo, MD
Professor of Medicine
University of Medicine and Dentistry of New Jersey-Robert
Wood Johnson Medical School
Chief, Department of Medicine
Edward D. Viner, MD, Chair, Department of Medicine
Director, Cooper Heart Institute
Cooper University Hospital
Camden, New Jersey

R. Phillip Dellinger, MD
Professor of Medicine
University of Medicine and Dentistry of New Jersey-Robert
Wood Johnson Medical School
Head, Division of Critical Care Medicine
Cooper University Hospital
Camden, New Jersey

MOSBY
ELSEVIER

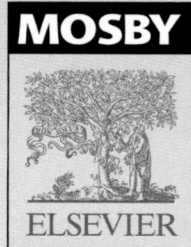

MOSBY
ELSEVIER

1600 John F. Kennedy Blvd.
Ste 1800
Philadelphia, PA 19103-2899

CRITICAL CARE MEDICINE: PRINCIPLES OF DIAGNOSIS AND MANAGEMENT IN THE ADULT ISBN: 978-0-323-04841-5

Notice

Knowledge and best practice in this field are constantly changing. As new research and experience broaden our knowledge, changes in practice, treatment, and drug therapy may become necessary or appropriate. Readers are advised to check the most current information provided (i) on procedures featured or (ii) by the manufacturer of each product to be administered, to verify the recommended dose or formula, the method and duration of administration, and contraindications. It is the responsibility of the practitioner, relying on his or her experience and knowledge of the patient, to make diagnoses, to determine dosages and the best treatment for each individual patient, and to take all appropriate safety precautions. To the fullest extent of the law, neither the Publisher nor the Editors assume any liability for any injury and/or damage to persons or property arising out of or related to any use of the material contained in this book.

The Publisher

Library of Congress Cataloging-in-Publication Data

Critical care medicine: principles of diagnosis and management in the adult / [edited by] Joseph E. Parrillo, R. Phillip Dellinger.—3rd ed.
p. ; cm.
Includes bibliographical references and index.
ISBN 978-0-323-04841-5
1. Critical care medicine. I. Parrillo, Joseph E. II. Dellinger, R. Phillip.
[DNLM: 1. Critical Care. 2. Intensive Care Units. WX 218 C9362 2008]
RC86.7.C744 2008 616′.028—dc22 2007015859

Executive Publisher: Natasha Andjelkovic
Developmental Editor: Pamela Hetherington
Publishing Services Manager: Frank Polizzano
Project Manager: Rachel Miller
Design Direction: Gene Harris

Printed in China.

Last digit is the print number: 9 8 7 6 5 4 3 2 1

DEDICATION

To Gale and Jennie

Contributors

Robert J. Anderson, MD
Meiklejohn Professor of Medicine and Chair, Department of Medicine, University of Colorado School of Medicine; Physician, University of Colorado Hospital, Denver, Colorado

Robert A. Balk, MD
Professor of Medicine, Rush Medical College; Director, Division of Pulmonary and Critical Care Medicine, Rush University Medical Center, Chicago, Illinois

Philip S. Barie, MD, MBA
Professor of Surgery and Public Health, Chief, Division of Critical Care and Trauma, Weill Cornell Medical College, New York; Director, Ann and Max A, Cohen Surgical Intensive Care Unit, Chief, Trauma Service, New York–Presbyterian Hospital, New York

Jeffrey F. Barletta, Pharm D
Adjunct Assistant Professor, Ferris State University College of Pharmacy; Clinical Specialist, Critical Care, Spectrum Health, Grand Rapids, Michigan

Richard G. Barton, MD
Associate Professor of Surgery, Director, Surgical Critical Care, Program Director, Surgical Critical Care Fellowship, University of Utah Health Sciences Center, Salt Lake City, Utah

Thaddeus Bartter, MD
Associate Professor of Medicine, UMDNJ–Robert Wood Johnson Medical School; Director, Diagnostic and Interventional Laboratories, Cooper University Hospital, Camden, New Jersey

C. Allen Bashour, MD
Assistant Medical Director, Cardiovascular Intensive Care Unit, Departments of Cardiothoracic Anesthesia and Outcomes Research, Division of Anesthesiology, Critical Care Medicine and Comprehensive Pain Management, Cleveland Clinic, Cleveland, Ohio

Richard Beale, MD
Head of Perioperative, Critical Care and Pain Services and Consultant Intensivist, Guy's and St. Thomas' Hospital, London, United Kingdom

Carolyn Bekes, MD
Professor of Medicine, UMDNJ–Robert Wood Johnson Medical School; Senior Vice President for Academic and Medical Affairs, Cooper University Hospital, Camden, New Jersey

Julian Bion, MD
Reader in Intensive Care Medicine, Department of Anesthesia and Intensive Care Medicine, University of Birmingham; Honorary Consultant in Intensive Care Medicine, University Hospital Birmingham NHS Foundation Trust, Birmingham, United Kingdom

Thomas P. Bleck, MD
Professor of Neurology, Neurological Surgery and Medicine, Division of Pulmonary and Critical Care Medicine, Vice-Chairman for Academic Programs, Department of Neurology, Northwestern University Feinberg School of Medicine, Chicago and Evanston, Illinois; Ruth Cain Ruggles Chairman, Department of Neurology, Evanston Northwestern Healthcare, Evanston, Illinois

Delia Borunda, MD
Professor, Public Health, Universidad la Salle, Mexico D.F.; Staff, Anesthesia and Critical Care Division, Instituto Nacional de Liencias Medicas y Nutricion "Salvador Zubiran," Mexico

Susan S. Braithwaite, MD
Clinical Professor of Medicine, Department of Medicine, Division of Endocrinology, University of North Carolina, Chapel Hill, North Carolina

William T. Browne, MD
Associate Professor of Medicine, Internal Medicine Residency Program Director, Department of Medicine, University of Minnesota Medical School, Minneapolis, Minnesota

John D. Buckley, MD
Director, Fellowship Program in Pulmonary and Critical Care Medicine, Henry Ford Hospital, Detroit, Michigan

Pietro Caironi, MD
Assistant Professor, Università Degli Studi di Milano; Staff Physician, Dipartimento di Anestesia e Rianimazione (Intensiva e Subintensiva) e Terapia del Dolore, Fondazione IRCCS—Ospedale Maggiore Policlinico, Mangiagalli, Regina Elena, Milan, Italy

Eleonora Carlesso, MSc
Istituto di Anestesiologia e Rianimazione, Università Degli Studi di Milano, Milan, Italy

John J. Caronna, MD
Professor of Clinical Neurology, Louis and Gertrude Feil Chair of Neurology, Weill Cornell Medical College; Attending Neurologist, New York–Presbyterian Hospital, New York

Michael Chansky, MD
Chairman, Department of Emergency Medicine, and Associate Professor of Emergency Medicine and Internal Medicine, UMDNJ–Robert Wood Johnson Medical School; Chief, Department of Emergency Medicine, Cooper University Hospital, Camden, New Jersey

Louis Chaptini, MD
Assistant Professor of Medicine, Department of Medicine, Division of Gastroenterology, Cooper University Hospital, UMDNJ–Robert Wood Johnson Medical School, Camden, New Jersey

Jonathan H. Cilley, Jr., MD
Associate Professor of Surgery, UMDNJ–Robert Wood Johnson Medical School; Acting Head, Division of Cardiothoracic Surgery, and Head, Section of Cardiac Surgery, Cooper University Hospital, Camden, New Jersey

Ismail Cinel, MD, PhD
Associate Professor, Department of Anesthesiology and Reanimation, Mersin University School of Medicine, Mersin, Turkey; Visiting Scientist, Cooper University Hospital, UMDNJ–Robert Wood Johnson Medical School, Camden, New Jersey

Christopher J. Crnich, MD
Assistant Professor of Medicine, University of Wisconsin School of Medicine and Public Health, Madison, Wisconsin

Brendan D. Curti, MD
Director, Genitourinary Oncology Research, Director, Biotherapy Program, Robert W. Franz Cancer Research Center, Earle A. Chiles Research Institute, Portland, Oregon

Marion Danis, MD
Chief, Ethics Consultation Service, National Institutes of Health Clinical Center, National Institutes of Health, Bethesda, Maryland

R. Phillip Dellinger, MD
Professor of Medicine, UMDNJ–Robert Wood Johnson Medical School; Head, Division of Critical Care Medicine, Cooper University Hospital, Camden, New Jersey

John W. Devlin, PharmD
Associate Professor, Northeastern University School of Pharmacy; Adjunct Associate Professor, Tufts University School of Medicine; Clinical Pharmacist, Medical Intensive Care Unit, Tufts–New England Medical Center, Boston, Massachusetts

Jack T. Dinh, MD
Fellow in Gastroenterology, UMDNJ–Robert Wood Johnson Medical School, Cooper University Hospital, Camden, New Jersey

Guillermo Domínguez-Cherit, MD
Professor, Critical Care Medicine, Universidad Nacional Autonoma de Mexico; Head, Critical Care Department, Instituto Nacional de Ciencias Medicas y Nutrición "Salvador Zubiran," Mexico

David J. Dries, MD
John F. Perry, Jr., Professor of Surgery, University of Minnesota; Assistant Medical Director for Surgical Care, Health Partners Medical Group, Minneapolis, Minnesota

Adam B. Elfant, MD
Associate Professor of Medicine, UMDNJ–Robert Wood Johnson Medical School; Associate Chief, Division of Gastroenterology and Hepatology, Associate Professor of Medicine, Cooper University Hospital, Camden, New Jersey

E. Wesley Ely, MD
Professor of Medicine, Vanderbilt University School of Medicine; Associate Director of Research GRECC, VA TN Valley Health Care System, Nashville, Tennessee

Ezekiel Emanuel, MD, PhD
Chair, Department of Bioethics, National Institutes of Health, Bethesda, Maryland

Ahmad Bilal Faridi, MD
Postdoctoral Fellow, Nephrology, UMDNJ–Robert Wood Johnson Medical School, Camden, New Jersey

J. Christopher Farmer, MD
Professor of Medicine, Associate Dean, Mayo School of Graduate Medical Education, Mayo Clinic College of Medicine; Consultant, Critical Care Medicine, Associate Chair for Education, Department of Medicine, Mayo Clinic, Rochester, Minnesota

Henry S. Fraimow, MD
Associate Professor of Medicine, Division of Infectious Diseases, UMDNJ–Robert Wood Johnson Medical School, Cooper University Hospital, Camden, New Jersey

Yaakov Friedman, MD
Associate Professor of Medicine, Rosalind Franklin University of Medicine and Science/The Chicago Medical School; Chairman, Department of Critical Care Medicine, Provident Hospital of Cook County, Chicago, Illinois

Susan Garwood, MD
Pulmonary/Critical Care Fellow, Medical University of South Carolina, Charleston, South Carolina

Luciano Gattinoni, MD
Professor, Università Degli Studi di Milano; Chief of Department, Dipartimento di Anestesia e Rianimazione (Intensiva e Subintensiva) e Terapia del Dolore, Fondazione IRCCS—Ospedale Maggiore Policlinico, Mangiagalli, Regina Elena, Milan, Italy

Nandan Gautam, MA
Consultant in Acute Medicine and Intensive Care Medicine, Associate Director of Clinical Skills and Simulation Training, University Hospital Birmingham NHS Foundation Trust, Birmingham, United Kingdom

Lawrence J. Gessman, MD
Associate Professor of Medicine, UMDNJ–Robert Wood Johnson Medical School, Cooper Heart Institute; Director, Electrophysiology, Cooper University Hospital, Camden, New Jersey

Fredric Ginsberg, MD
Assistant Professor of Medicine, UMDNJ–Robert Wood Johnson Medical School; Director, Heart Failure Program, Director, Nuclear Cardiology, Cooper University Hospital, Camden, New Jersey

John Godke, MD
Assistant Clinical Professor, Pulmonary and Critical Care Medicine, Louisiana State University School of Medicine, Earl K. Long Hospital, Department of Internal Medicine, Baton Rouge, Louisiana

H. Warren Goldman, MD, PhD
Professor of Neurosurgery, UMDNJ–Robert Wood Johnson School of Medicine; Chief, Department of Neurosurgery, Director, Cooper Neurological Institute, Cooper University Hospital, Camden, New Jersey

A. B. J. Groeneveld, MD, PhD
Professor of Intensive Care, Vrye University Faculty of Medicine; Director of Research and Vice Chairman, Residency Program, Vrye University Medical Center, Amsterdam, The Netherlands

Robin Gross, MD
Associate Professor of Medicine, Georgetown University School of Medicine; Attending Physician, Georgetown University Hospital, Washington, DC

David P. Gurka, MD, PhD
Assistant Professor of Medicine, Rush Medical College; Director, Section of Critical Care Medicine, and Director, Critical Care Services, Rush University Medical Center, Chicago, Illinois

Ghada Haddad, MD
Associate Professor of Medicine, UMDNJ–Robert Wood Johnson Medical School; Head, Division of Endocrinology, Cooper University Hospital, Camden, New Jersey

Marilyn T. Haupt, MD
Temple University School of Medicine, Philadelphia; Director, Pulmonary and Critical Care Services, Geisinger Health System, Danville, Pennsylvania

Michael J. Hockstein, MD
Medical Director, Surgical Intensive Care Unit, Washington Hospital Center, Washington, DC

Steven M. Hollenberg, MD
Professor of Medicine, UMDNJ–Robert Wood Johnson Medical School; Director, Coronary Care Unit, Cooper University Hospital, Camden, New Jersey

Leonard D. Hudson, MD
Professor of Medicine, Endowed Chair in Pulmonary Disease Research, University of Washington; Attending Physician, Pulmonary and Critical Care Medicine, Harborview Medical Center, Seattle, Washington

Gary W. Hunninghake, MD
Professor of Medicine, Department of Internal Medicine; Director, Division of Pulmonary Diseases, Critical Care, Occupational Medicine; Director, Institute for Clinical and Translational Science; Senior Associate Dean for Clinical and Translational Science, University of Iowa Carver College of Medicine, Iowa City, Iowa

James Jackson, PsyD
Assistant Professor of Medicine and Psychiatry, Vanderbilt University School of Medicine; Clinical Research Center of Excellence, VA TN Valley Health Care System, Nashville, Tennessee

C.A. Jamison, MBBCh, BAO
Anaesthetic and Intensive Care Specialist Registrar, Royal Victoria Hospital, Belfast, United Kingdom

Smith Jean, PhD
Researcher, Cooper University Hospital, UMDNJ–Robert Wood Johnson Medical School, Camden, New Jersey

Hani Jneid, MD
Instructor of Medicine, Harvard Medical School; Interventional Cardiology Fellow, Massachusetts General Hospital, Boston, Massachusetts

Robert G. Johnson, MD
C. Rollins Hanlon Professor and Chair, Department of Surgery, Saint Louis University School of Medicine; Chief of Surgery, Saint Louis University Hospital/Tenet, St. Louis, Missouri

Amal Jubran, MD
Professor of Medicine, Division of Pulmonary and Critical Care Medicine, Loyola University of Chicago Stritch School of Medicine, Maywood; Edward Hines, Jr. Veterans Affairs Hospital, Hines, Illinois

Nigel S. Kanagasundaram, MBChB, MRCP, MD
Honorary Clinical Lecturer, Department of Renal Medicine, Freeman Hospital; Consultant Nephrologist, Newcastle upon Tyne Hospitals–NHS Foundation Trust, Newcastle upon Tyne, United Kingdom

George Karam, MD
Paula Garvey Manship Professor of Medicine, Department of Internal Medicine, Louisiana State University School of Medicine, New Orleans, Louisiana; Head, Department of Internal Medicine, Earl K. Long Medical Center, Baton Rouge, Louisiana

Joseph A. Karam, MD
Assistant Professor of Surgery, Drexel University College of Medicine; Medical Director of Trauma and Surgical Critical Care, Hahnemann University Hospital, Philadelphia, Pennsylvania

Ankur A. Karnik, MD
Resident, Department of Medicine, Hospital of the University of Pennsylvania, Philadelphia, Pennsylvania

Ashok M. Karnik, MD
Professor of Clinical Medicine, Stony Brook School of Medicine, Stony Brook; Chief, Division of Pulmonary and Critical Care Medicine, Nassau University Medical Center, East Meadow, New York

M. Sean Kincaid, MD
Acting Assistant Professor, Department of Anesthesiology, University of Washington; Attending Physician, Anesthesiology and Critical Care Medicine, Harborview Medical Center, Seattle, Washington

Osman Samil Kozak, MD
Neurocritical Care Fellow, Department of Neurocritical Care, Mayo Clinic, Rochester, Minnesota

Anand Kumar, MD
Associate Professor of Medicine, Medical Microbiology and Pharmacology/Therapeutics, University of Manitoba Faculty of Medicine, Winnipeg, Manitoba, Canada; Associate Professor of Medicine, UMDNJ–Robert Wood Johnson Medical School, Camden, New Jersey; ICU Attending Physician, Health Sciences Center and St. Boniface Hospital, Winnipeg, Manitoba, Canada

Neil A. Lachant, MD
Professor of Medicine, UMDNJ–Robert Wood Johnson Medical School; Director, Thrombosis Program, Director, Hematologic Malignancy Program, Cooper Cancer Institute, Cooper University Hospital, Camden, New Jersey

Franco Laghi, MD
Professor of Medicine, Division of Pulmonary and Critical Care Medicine, Loyola University of Chicago Stritch School of Medicine, Maywood, Illinois; Professor of Medicine, Edward Hines, Jr., Veterans Administration Hospital, Hines, Illinois

Stephen E. Lapinsky, MB. Ch., MSc
Associate Professor of Medicine, University of Toronto; Site Director, Intensive Care Unit, Mount Sinai Hospital, Toronto, Ontario, Canada

G. G. Lavery, MD, MBBCh
Visiting Professor, University of Ulster Faculty of Life and Health Sciences; Director of Critical Care Services, Royal Hospitals, Belfast, United Kingdom

Dan L. Longo, MD
Scientific Director, National Institute on Aging, Intramural Research Program, Baltimore, Maryland

Ramya Lotano, MD
Assistant Professor of Medicine, UMDNJ–Robert Wood Johnson Medical School; Director, Pulmonary and Critical Care Fellowship Program, Cooper University Hospital, Camden, New Jersey

Vincent E. Lotano, MD
Assistant Professor of Surgery, Cooper University Hospital, UMDNJ–Robert Wood Johnson Medical School, Camden, New Jersey

John M. Luce, MD
Professor of Medicine and Anesthesia, University of California-San Francisco, San Francisco, California

Judith A. Luce, MD
Clinical Professor of Medicine, University of California, San Francisco; Director, Oncology Services, Division of Hematology/Oncology, San Francisco General Hospital, San Francisco, California

Dennis G. Maki, MD
Ovid O. Meyer Professor of Medicine, University of Wisconsin School of Medicine and Public Health; Attending Physician, Center for Trauma and Life Support, Hospital Epidemiologist, Department of Medicine, Infectious Diseases Section, University of Wisconsin Hospital and Clinics, Madison, Wisconsin

Robert J. March, MD
Associate Professor of Surgery, Cardiac and Vascular Surgery, Rush University Medical Center, Chicago, Illinois

Andrew O. Maree, MB, BCh, MSc
Lecturer in Medicine, Harvard Medical School; Attending, Division of Cardiology, Department of Medicine, Massachusetts General Hospital, Boston, Massachusetts

John Marini, MD
Professor of Medicine, University of Minnesota, Minneapolis, Minnesota; Director of Translational Research, Regions Hospital, St. Paul, Minnesota

John C. Marshall, MD
Professor of Surgery, University of Toronto Faculty of Medicine; Intensivist, Trauma, Critical Care and General Surgery, St. Michael's Hospital, Toronto, Ontario, Canada

Henry Masur, MD
Chief, Critical Care Medicine Department, Magnusson Clinical Center, National Institutes of Health, Bethesda, Maryland; Clinical Professor, George Washington School of Medicine and Public Health, Washington, DC

Christopher McFadden, MD
Assistant Professor of Medicine, UMDNJ–Robert Wood Johnson Medical School; Physician, Department of Nephrology, Cooper University Hospital, Camden, New Jersey

Philipp G. H. Metnitz, MD, PhD
Professor of Anesthesia and Critical Care Medicine, Medical Director, Intensive Care Unit, Department of Anesthesiology and General Intensive Care Medicine, Medical University of Vienna, Vienna, Austria

Thomas R. Mirsen, MD
Associate Professor of Neurology, UMDNJ–Robert Wood Johnson Medical School; Director, Stroke Program, Department of Medicine, Cooper University Hospital; Neurologist, Cooper University Hospital, Camden, New Jersey

Rui P. Moreno, MD, PhD
Director, Unidade de Cuidados Intensivos Polivalente, Centro Mospitalar de Lisboa Central, Lisboa, Portugal

Nick Murphy, MBBS
Honouree Senior Lecturer, University of Birmingham; Consultant Intensivist, Department of Critical Care and Hepatology, University Hospital Birmingham, Birmingham, United Kingdom

Michael J. Murray, MD, PhD
Professor, Department of Anesthesiology, Mayo Clinic College of Medicine, Rochester, Minnesota; Consultant, Department of Anesthesiology, Mayo Clinic, Scottsdale, Arizona

Sherif F. Nagueh, MD
Professor of Medicine, Weill Medical College of Cornell University, New York, New York; Associate Director, Echocardiography Laboratory, Methodist DeBakey Heart Center, The Methodist Hospital, Houston, Texas

Michael S. Niederman, MD
Professor and Vice-Chairman, Department of Medicine, Stony Brook School of Medicine, Stony Brook; Chairman, Department of Medicine, Winthrop-University Hospital, Mineola, New York

Luis Ostrosky-Zeichner, MD
Associate Professor of Medicine and Epidemiology, University of Texas Medical School at Houston; Medical Director for Epidemiology, Memorial Hermann Healthcare System, Houston, Texas

Daniel R. Ouellette, MS, MD
Associate Professor of Medicine, Wayne State University School of Medicine; Senior Staff Physician and Associate Director of Medical Critical Care, Henry Ford Hospital, Detroit, Michigan

Igor Ougorets, MD
Associate Professor of Neurology, Weill Medical College of Cornell University; Director, Neuroscience Intensive Care Unit of New York, Presbyterian Hospital/Cornell Medical Center, New York, New York

Lance J. Oyen, PharmD
Assistant Professor, Mayo Clinic College of Medicine, Pharmacy, Mayo Clinic; Clinical Pharmacist, Pharmacy, St. Mary's Hospital, Mayo Clinic, Rochester, Minnesota

Emil P. Paganini, MD
Head, Section of Dialysis and Extracorporeal Therapy, Department of Nephrology and Hypertension, Cleveland Clinic, Cleveland, Ohio

Igor F. Palacios, MD
Associate Professor of Medicine, Harvard Medical School; Director of Interventional Cardiology, Massachusetts General Hospital, Boston, Massachusetts

Pratik Pandharipande, MD
Assistant Professor, Anesthesiology and Critical Care, Vanderbilt University School of Medicine, Nashville, Tennessee

Joseph E. Parrillo, MD
Professor of Medicine, UMDNJ–Robert Wood Johnson Medical School; Chief, Department of Medicine; Edward D. Viner, MD, Chair, Department of Medicine; Director, Cooper Heart Institute, Cooper University Hospital, Camden, New Jersey

Amish Patel, MBBS
Specialist Registrar in Anaesthesia and Intensive Care Medicine, St. George's Hospital, London, United Kingdom

Steven Peikin, MD
Professor of Medicine, Department of Medicine, Head, Division of Gastroenterology, UMDNJ–Robert Wood Johnson Medical School, Cooper University Hospital, Camden, New Jersey

William Peruzzi, MD
Professor of Medicine, University of Texas Health Sciences Center; Chief Medical Officer, Memorial Hermann Hospital, Memorial Hermann Children's Hospital, Houston, Texas

Priscilla J. Peters, BA
Clinical Specialist in Echocardiography, Cooper University Hospital, Camden, New Jersey

John Popovich, Jr., MD
Professor (Clinician-Educator) FTA, Wayne State University School of Medicine; Chair, Department of Medicine, Henry Ford Health System, Detroit, Michigan

Juan Gabriel Posadas-Calleja, MD
Fellowship in Critical Care Medicine, Calgary University, Calgary, Alberta, Canada

Melvin R. Pratter, MD
Professor of Medicine, UMDNJ–Robert Wood Johnson School of Medicine; Head, Division of Pulmonary and Critical Care Medicine, Cooper University Hospital, Camden, New Jersey

S. Sujanthy Rajaram, MD
Assistant Professor of Medicine, UMDNJ–Robert Wood Johnson Medical School; Critical Care Intensivist, Division of Critical Care Medicine, Cooper University Hospital, Camden, New Jersey

Hannah Reay, MPhil
Research Fellow, Dept of Anaesthesia and Intensive Care Medicine, University of Birmingham; Registered Nurse, Selly Oak Critical Care, University Hospital Birmingham NHS Foundation Trust, Birmingham, United Kingdom

Annette C. Reboli, MD
Professor of Medicine, UMDNJ–Robert Wood Johnson Medical School; Head, Infectious Diseases Division, and Hospital Epidemiologist, Cooper University Hospital, Camden, New Jersey

John H. Rex, MD
Vice-President, Clinical Infection, AstraZeneca Pharmaceuticals, Macclesfield, United Kingdom

Andrew Rhodes, MBBS
Consultant in Intensive Care Medicine, St. George's Hospital, London, United Kingdom

Lewis J. Rubin, MD
Professor of Medicine, University of California, San Diego, School of Medicine, La Jolla, California

Maria Rudis, PharmD
Clinical Associate Professor, Department of Emergency Medicine, University of Southern California, Keck School of Medicine; Los Angeles County + University of Southern California Medical Center, Los Angeles, California

Nasia Safdar, MD
Assistant Professor, University of Wisconsin, Madison, Wisconsin

Jeffrey R. Saffle, MD
Professor of Surgery, University of Utah School of Medicine; Director, Burn-Trauma Intensive Care Unit, University of Utah Health Center, Salt Lake City, Utah

Steven A. Sahn, MD
Professor of Medicine and Director, Division of Pulmonary, Critical Care, Allergy, and Sleep Medicine, Medical University of South Carolina; Director, Pulmonary and Critical Care Medicine Training Program, and Attending Physician, MUSC Hospital and Charleston VA Hospital, Charleston, South Carolina

Gregory A. Schmidt, MD
Professor of Medicine, University of Iowa Carver College of Medicine; Director of Critical Care, University of Iowa Hospitals and Clinics, Iowa City, Iowa

Sam R. Sharar, MD
Professor, Department of Anesthesiology, University of Washington School of Medicine; Director, Harborview Anesthesiology Research Center, Attending Pediatric Anesthesiologist, Harborview Medical Center, Seattle, Washington

Henry Silverman, MD
Professor, University of Maryland School of Medicine, Baltimore, Maryland

Sabine Sobek, MD
Senior Attending Physician, Department of Critical Care Medicine, Provident Hospital of Cook County, Chicago, Illinois

Charlie Strange, MD
Professor of Medicine, Division of Pulmonary and Critical Care Medicine, Medical University of South Carolina, Charleston, South Carolina

Sanjay Subramanian, MD
Intensivist, The Everett Clinic, Everett, Washington

Wanchun Tang, MD
Clinical Professor of Medicine, University of Southern California Keck School of Medicine, Los Angeles; President, CEO, and CSO, Weil Institute of Critical Care Medicine, Rancho Mirage, California

Robert W. Taylor, MD
Clinical Professor, Saint Louis University School of Medicine; Director, Critical Care Training Program, St. John's Mercy Medical Center, St. Louis, Missouri

Boon Wee Teo, MBBCh
Assistant Professor, Department of Medicine, Yong Loo Lin School of Medicine, National University of Singapore; Associate Consultant, Department of Medicine, National University Hospital, Singapore

Martin J. Tobin, MD
Professor of Medicine and Anesthesiology, Loyola University Chicago Stritch School of Medicine, Maywood; Director, Division of Pulmonary and Critical Care Medicine, Edward Hines, Jr., Veterans Affairs Hospital, Hines; Attending Physician, RML Specialty Hospital, Hinsdale, Illinois

Sean Townsend, MD
Assistant Professor, Warren Alpert Medical School, Brown University; Associate Director, Medical Intensive Care Unit, Pulmonary and Critical Care Division, Rhode Island Hospital, Providence, Rhode Island

Richard Trohman, MD
Professor of Medicine, Grace DeForest and William Louis Veeck Professor of Cardiovascular Research, Rush Medical College of Rush University; Director, Electrophysiology, Arrhythmia and Pacemaker Services, Director, Heart Station, Associate Director, Section of Cardiology, Rush University Medical Center, Chicago, Illinois

Stephen Trzeciak, MD
Assistant Professor, UMDNJ–Robert Wood Johnson Medical School, Cooper University Hospital, Camden, New Jersey

Zoltan G. Turi, MD
Professor of Medicine, UMDNJ–Robert Wood Johnson Medical School; Director, Cooper Vascular Center, and Director, Cooper Structural Heart Disease Program, Cooper University Hospital, Camden, New Jersey

Alan R. Turtz, MD
Associate Professor of Surgery, UMDNJ–Robert Wood Johnson Medical School; Neurosurgeon, Cooper University Hospital, Camden, New Jersey

Jean-Louis Vincent, MD, PhD
Professor of Intensive Care, Free University of Brussels Faculty of Medicine; Head, Department of Intensive Care, Erasme University Hospital, Brussels, Belgium

Max Harry Weil, MD, PhD
Adjunct Professor of Medicine, Northwestern University Feinberg School of Medicine; Emeritus Clinical Professor, University of Southern California Keck School of Medicine, Los Angeles; Founding President and Honorary Chairman, Weil Institute of Critical Care Medicine, Rancho Mirage, California

Lawrence S. Weisberg, MD
Professor of Medicine, UMDNJ–Robert Wood Johnson Medical School; Head, Division of Neurology, Cooper University Hospital, Camden, New Jersey

Steven Werns, MD
Professor of Medicine, UMDNJ–Robert Wood Johnson Medical School; Director, Invasive Cardiovascular Services, Cooper University Hospital, Camden, New Jersey

Eelco F. M. Wijdicks, MD, PhD
Professor of Neurology; Head, Neurology Critical Care Division, Mayo Clinic, Rochester, Minnesota

Sergio L. Zanotti-Cavazzoni, MD
Assistant Professor, Department of Medicine, UMDNJ–Robert Wood Johnson Medical School; Attending Physician, Division of Critical Care Medicine, Cooper University Hospital, Camden, New Jersey

Janice L. Zimmerman, MD
Head, Critical Care Division, Director, Medical Intensive Care Unit, Methodist Hospital, Houston, Texas

Preface

Few fields in medicine have grown, evolved, and changed as rapidly as critical care medicine has during the past 30 years. From its origins in the postoperative recovery room and the coronary care unit, the modern intensive care unit (ICU) now represents the ultimate example of medicine's ability to supply the specialized personnel and technology necessary to sustain and restore seriously ill persons to productive lives. While the field continues to evolve rapidly, sufficient principles, knowledge, and experience have accumulated in the past few decades to warrant production of a textbook dedicated to adult critical care medicine. We chose to limit the subject matter of our book to critical care of *adult* patients, to allow production of a comprehensive textbook in a single volume.

This book was envisioned to be multidisciplinary and multiauthored by acknowledged leaders in the field but aimed primarily at practicing critical care physicians who spend the better part of their time caring for patients in an ICU. Thus, the book would be appropriate for critical care internists as well as for surgical or anesthesia critical care specialists. The goal was to produce the acknowledged "best practice" standard in critical care medicine.

The first edition of the textbook was published in 1995, co-edited by Joe Parrillo and Roger Bone. The book sold exceedingly well for a first edition text. After the untimely death of Roger Bone in 1997, Phil Dellinger joined Joe Parrillo as the co-editor for the second and now this third edition. As co-editors, we have labored to produce a highly readable text that can serve equally well for comprehensive review and as a reference source. We felt that it was important for usability and accessibility to keep the book to a single volume. This was a challenge, because critical care knowledge and technology have expanded significantly during the past decade. By placing emphasis on clear, concise writing and keeping the focus on critical care medicine in the adult, this goal was achieved.

Our view of critical care medicine is mirrored in the organization of the textbook. Modern critical care is a multidisciplinary specialty that includes much of the knowledge and technology contained in many disciplines represented by the classic organ-based subspecialties of medicine, as well as the specialties of surgery and anesthesiology. The book begins with a section consisting of chapters on the technology, procedures, and pharmacology that are essential to the practicing critical care physician. This section is followed by sections devoted to the critical care aspects of cardiovascular, pulmonary, infectious, renal, metabolic, neurologic, gastrointestinal, and hematologic-oncologic diseases. Subsequent chapters are devoted to important social, ethical, and other issues such as psychiatric disorders, severity of illness scoring systems, and administrative issues in the ICU. This third edition has significant content additions, including new chapters devoted to mechanical ventilation of obstructive airway disease (OAD) and acute respiratory distress syndrome (ARDS), as well as chapters on both general and cardiovascular postoperative care.

Each chapter is designed to provide a comprehensive review of pertinent clinical, diagnostic, and management issues. This is primarily a clinical text, so the emphasis is on considerations important to the practicing critical care physician; also presented, however, are the scientific (physiologic, biochemical, and molecular biologic) data pertinent to the pathophysiology and management issues. We have aimed for a textbook length that is comprehensive but manageable. Substantial references are provided for readers wishing to explore subjects in greater detail. We have identified key points and key references to highlight the most important issues within each chapter. New features of this third edition include a color-enhanced design and clinically useful management algorithms.

We have been fortunate to attract a truly exceptional group of authors to write the chapters for *Critical Care Medicine: Principles of Diagnosis and Management in the Adult.* For each chapter, we have chosen a seasoned clinician-scientist actively involved in critical care who is one of a handful of recognized experts in his or her chapter topic. With this edition, we have increased the international flavor of our authorship. To provide uniformity in content and style, one or both of us have edited and revised each chapter.

We wish to thank the highly dedicated people who provided us with the assistance needed to complete a venture of this magnitude. Our thanks go to Linda Rizzuto, who provided invaluable organizational and superb editorial input; to Noel Taylor, for her administrative assistance; and to the excellent editorial staff at Elsevier, including Natasha Andjelkovic, Pamela Hetherington, and Rachel Miller.

Joseph E. Parrillo
Camden, New Jersey
R. Phillip Dellinger
Camden, New Jersey

Contents

OVERVIEW

PART

I

CRITICAL CARE PROCEDURES, MONITORING, AND PHARMACOLOGY

Chapter 1

Cardiac Arrest and Cardiopulmonary Resuscitation

Wanchun Tang and Max Harry Weil

Each year, approximately 1 million individuals in the United States experience acute cardiac events. These events are predominantly caused by episodes of myocardial ischemia and account for the sudden death of approximately 500,000 individuals yearly. Of these victims, 350,000 die before they are admitted to the hospital and often before entry into the emergency medical system. More than 160,000 deaths occur in patients who are younger than 65 years old.

Sudden death that is predominantly due to coronary artery disease is the largest cause of fatalities, especially unexpected death, in the United States today.[1] Less frequently, unanticipated cardiac arrest occurs in settings of drowning, electrocution, suffocation, and drug intoxication.[2-4]

HISTORY

Cardiac arrest has been recognized since ancient times. The options for reversal of cardiac arrest, for practical purposes, have been developed only in the last 45 years, however. Cardiopulmonary resuscitation (CPR) is described in the Old Testament and provides a prime example of humanity's continued efforts to ward off death and even to revive those who have died.[5] Before the introduction of open-chest cardiac massage[6] and electrical reversal of ventricular fibrillation (VF),[7,8] resuscitation was successful primarily in victims of respiratory arrest.

The combined procedures of positive-pressure ventilation, closed-chest precordial compression, and electrical defibrillation were introduced into clinical practice in 1960 by a retired Johns Hopkins University Dean of Engineering, W. B. Kouwenhoven, who worked in collaboration with a surgical resident, J. R. Jude, and graduate student of biomedical engineering, G. G. Knickerbocker.[9,10] This ushered in the modern era of CPR.

ETIOLOGY

Cardiac arrest is characterized by abrupt cessation of mechanical activity of the heart and loss of spontaneous and effective circulation. The most common electrical mechanism of failure is VF, which accounts for 65% to 80% of episodes of cardiac arrest. Pulseless electrical activity (previously termed *electromechanical dissociation*) and asystole account for 20% to 30% of identifiable episodes. Since the 1980s, however, there has been a steady decline in the incidence of VF/ventricular tachycardia (VF/VT) as the first recorded rhythm. It is unknown whether this decline is related to an increased number of implantable defibrillators, or VF/VT becoming a shorter presenting rhythm after primary and secondary prevention strategies.[11-13]

In more than 80% of patients who present with cardiac arrest, underlying heart disease has been previously identified.[14] Especially in Western cultures, coronary atherosclerosis accounts for approximately 80% of fatal events resulting from heart disease. Only 50% of such patients have evidence of acute myocardial infarction, however.[15,16]

Cardiomyopathies account for an additional 10% to 15% of instances of cardiac death. Diverse etiologies include congenital heart disease, myocarditis, valvular disease, and electrophysiologic anomalies. Electrophysiologic abnormalities of special importance include preexcitation syndromes and prolonged QT interval. The events themselves may be triggered by transient ischemia, electrolyte and acid-base disturbances, proarrhythmic effects of drugs, and increased autonomic or endocrine stimulation accounting for disturbances in the electrophysiologic properties of the diseased heart.

Noncardiac causes account for approximately 20% of all cardiac arrests. These are predominantly due to failure of pulmonary gas exchange. Such events may be caused by pulmonary, central nervous system (CNS), voluntary muscle, or acute vascular defects. Cardiac arrest may supervene in cases of drowning, smoke inhalation, sedative or narcotic overdose, pulmonary embolism, cerebrovascular accidents, or CNS injury and neuromyopathies. In such instances, failure of ventilation typically ushers in cardiac arrest. Hypothermia terminates in cardiac arrest. Only a few cases are caused by electrocution.

CLINICAL FEATURES AND DIAGNOSIS

Cardiac arrest is characterized by loss of consciousness in which the victim is not aroused by vigorous stimulation and in the absence of palpable peripheral arterial pulses. Palpation of peripheral pulses may not be reliable, however.[17,18] CNS hypoxia may account for irregular respiration, including gasping.[19] The electrocardiogram (ECG) rhythm is typically such that there is little likelihood of effective circulation. The ECG most often confirms VF and less often VT, asystole, or agonal ventricular complexes. Pulseless supraventricular rhythms are more likely when circulatory shock is due to hypovolemia or mechanical defects of the circulation, such as pericardial tamponade, tension pneumothorax, or pulmonary embolism, rather than to primary heart disease.[20,21]

THERAPEUTIC APPROACH

Survival after cardiac arrest is contingent on a series of prompt interventions. The American Heart Association has introduced the concept *chain of survival* to highlight the sequence of critical actions. The chain includes four interdependent links: (1) early access, (2) early basic life support, (3) early defibrillation, and (4) early advanced cardiac care.[22]

Early access with presentation of cardiac arrest depends on early recognition of the urgency of the presenting symptoms and signs, including chest pain, shortness of breath, and syncope. Early recognition prompts early activation of the emergency medical system.

The second link, early basic life support, includes rescue breathing and precordial compression provided by one or two laypersons or by rescue personnel categorized as emergency medical technicians. Basic life support is for temporary support of ventilation and circulation to maintain cardiac and cerebral viability before more definitive care by professionally qualified medical, nursing, or paramedical personnel. The outcome of CPR is unequivocally improved if basic life support is maintained before the arrival of advanced life support providers.[23] The effectiveness of basic life support is relatively short-lived, however, and especially so in most patients with VF. For these patients, electrical defibrillation has the greatest promise.

Early electrical defibrillation, the third link in the chain of survival, is currently viewed as the most likely to improve the outcome of cardiac arrest. When defibrillation is instituted within 4 minutes, most victims of VF are resuscitated, and more than one third are discharged alive from the hospital.[24] When external countershock is delayed for more than 10 minutes, however, restoration of meaningful life such that the patient may be discharged from the hospital is very remote (Fig. 1-1). Defibrillation at the earliest time is the most critical intervention, and for many victims of cardiac arrest the only effective intervention, for successful resuscitation in conjunction with basic life support. The use of automated external defibrillators (AEDs) by lay providers in this setting has been strongly recommended by the American Heart Association, and the initial experiences have been encouraging.[25-27]

When initial defibrillation attempts fail, the likelihood that further countershocks will restore spontaneous circulation depends on the capability of the resuscitation interventions to generate cardiac output and peripheral resistance in amounts that would restore and maintain adequate flows of oxygenated blood to the myocardium. After myocardial blood flow is restored, defibrillation may be successful. Advanced cardiac life support is intended to fulfill this need and to increase the likelihood that spontaneous circulation will be restored. In addition to precordial compression and rescue breathing, advanced cardiac life support includes securing the airway and, specifically, endotracheal intubation, intravenous medication, and appropriate electrical methods for restoring a viable rhythm. In the United States, advanced cardiac life support is provided primarily by paramedics, nurses, and physicians.

In the hospital setting, advanced cardiac life support with prompt defibrillation is likely to be immediately available. Out-of-hospital management of cardiac arrest is contingent, however, on the location of the patient at the time of collapse and the immediate availability of appropriately trained laypersons or qualified rescue personnel with access to resuscitation equipment and supplies.[28,29]

Airway and Ventilation

In an unconscious patient, the normal muscle tone that typically maintains the jaw in an elevated position is lost. The tongue is likely to descend into the pharynx and align itself with the epiglottis, obstructing the airway.[30] When the lower jaw is physically lifted and displaced anteriorly, the tongue is lifted away from the pharynx, artificially restoring an open airway. These interventions are termed

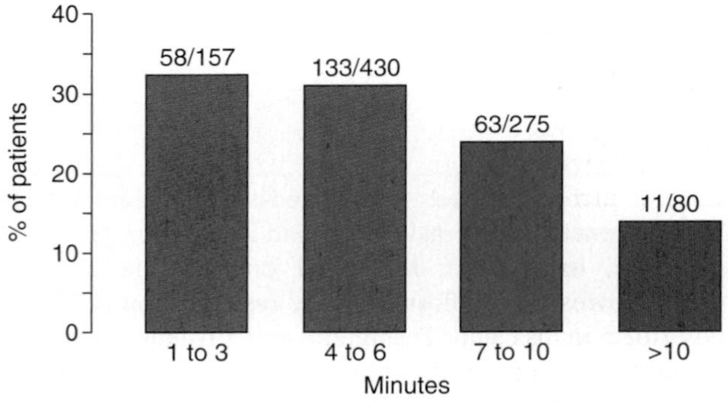

Figure 1-1. Relationship between the interval before attempted defibrillation and hospital discharge after out-of-hospital cardiac arrest. (Adapted from Weaver WD, Cobb LA, Hallstrom AP, et al: Factors influencing survival after out-of-hospital cardiac arrest. J Am Coll Cardiol 1986;7:752-757.)

head tilt–chin lift and *jaw thrust*. Airway adjuncts, specifically oropharyngeal and nasopharyngeal airways, may be used to preclude mechanical descent of the tongue over the airway.[31]

Early endotracheal intubation is generally preferred because it secures the patency of the airway and isolates it from the gastrointestinal tract. It reduces the risk of aspiration and greatly facilitates suctioning of the airways for removal of secretions or foreign material. Intubation also secures airtight closure when airway resistance is increased, and mechanical insufflation is required to deliver titrated tidal volumes under conditions when excesses of airway pressure must be avoided.[32] Devices that may be inserted without visualization of the trachea have gained some popularity, particularly the esophageal obturator airway,[33] the esophageal gastric tube airway,[34] the pharyngotracheal lumen airway,[35] the esophageal-tracheal tube,[36] and the laryngeal mask.[37] Current experience favors the laryngeal mask airway.[38]

These devices have not allowed for consistently effective positive-pressure ventilation, however, and their use in most instances has been associated with a large incidence of iatrogenic complications. Rescue breathing is accomplished by mouth-to-mouth, mouth-to-nose, or, occasionally, mouth-to-stoma breathing.[31,39] Alternatively, a barrier device may be used, which incorporates a facemask and shields.[40] Although early endotracheal intubation has remained the favored intervention,[41] there is increasing evidence that interruption of precordial compression and defibrillation for initial endotracheal intubation may compromise outcome. We recommend use of an oropharyngeal airway or, preferably, the laryngeal mask as a better option during the initial 5 to 7 minutes of CPR. Whatever barrier devices are used, they should be simple, well-fitting, made of transparent material to allow detection of gastric regurgitation, and inexpensive.

Barrier devices are reassuring to rescue personnel because of the perceived risks of transmission of human immunodeficiency virus or hepatitis B or C,[42] but there is no documented instance in which such viruses have been transmitted during the course of mouth-to-mouth or mouth-to-nose rescue breathing.[43] Bag-valve devices are ideal for the trained rescuer. These include a self-inflating bag with a nonrebreathing valve and a universal adapter. The adapter is used in conjunction with a facemask, laryngeal mask, or endotracheal tube. When a facemask is used, there is a serious risk of overenthusiastic "bagging." This causes gaseous distention of the stomach and proximal intestine, which compromises effective ventilation and greatly increases the risk of vomiting and aspiration. Finally, rescue breathing by trained rescuers in the field is effectively supplied by gas-powered, manually triggered positive-pressure devices and transport ventilators.[44]

Ventilation is conventionally maintained with 10 to 12 breaths per minute. There is increasing evidence, however, that frequency and tidal volumes may be substantially reduced without compromise of outcome.[45-47] The inspired gas mixture supplied by bag-valve devices or ventilators may be either room air or an oxygen mixture. Increases in fraction of inspired oxygen may be of substantial benefit. Objective evidence that early intermittent positive-pressure ventilation improves outcome is uncertain, however. These issues, together with the optimal oxygen concentrations of inspired gas mixture during CPR, are currently under active reinvestigation.[45-48] We caution against vigorous bag-valve ventilation. With greatly reduced pulmonary blood flow, tidal volumes that are one half of conventional values for anesthetized patients suffice.

Myocardial Perfusion

Re-establishment of myocardial blood flow is the most critical determinant of the restoration of spontaneous circulation by electrical defibrillation. Because there is maximal coronary vasodilation during global myocardial ischemia of cardiac arrest, myocardial blood flow becomes essentially pressure dependent.[49,50] A remarkably high correlation has been shown between myocardial blood flow and the pressure gradient between the aorta and the right atrium that represents the coronary perfusion pressure.[51] Coronary perfusion pressure has consistently been the best single predictor of cardiac resuscitability. In human patients, a coronary perfusion pressure of 15 mm Hg is the minimum threshold value that would predict successful cardiac resuscitation.[52] Increases in coronary perfusion pressure above this threshold level were accompanied by proportional increases in cardiac resuscitability. More than 80% of patients were successfully resuscitated when coronary perfusion pressure was increased by precordial compression to levels exceeding 25 mm Hg (Fig. 1-2).

Because of the pivotal role of myocardial perfusion for successful cardiac resuscitation, there is an appropriate focus on interventions by which coronary perfusion pressure may be maximally increased. This increase in coronary perfusion pressure is accomplished by increasing cardiac output and forward aortic blood flow or by increasing systemic vascular resistance (Fig. 1-3). Blood flow during conventional CPR is generated by closed-chest precordial compression, or alternatively by open-chest

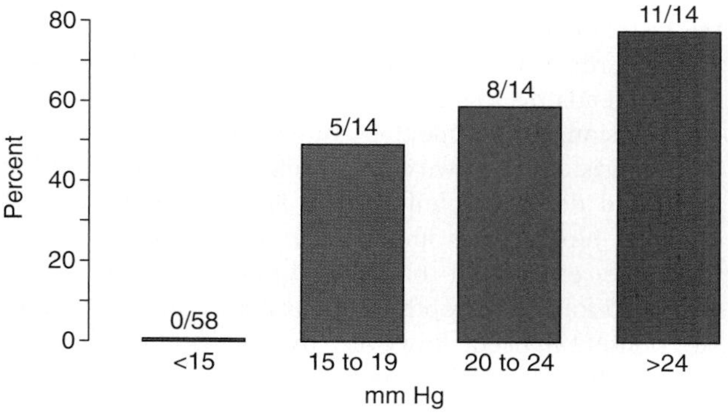

Figure 1-2. Relationship between cardiac resuscitability and maximum coronary perfusion pressure during cardiopulmonary resuscitation in human victims of out-of-hospital cardiac arrest. (Adapted from Paradis NA, Martin GB, Rivers EP, et al: Coronary perfusion pressure and the return of spontaneous circulation in human cardiopulmonary resuscitation. JAMA 1990;263:1106-1113.)

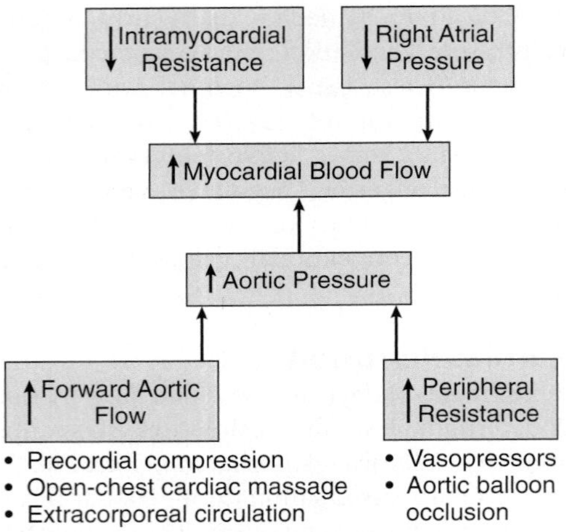

Figure 1-3. Effects of interventions by which myocardial blood flow is increased during cardiopulmonary resuscitation.

cardiac massage or extracorporeal circulation. The administration of vasopressor agents and especially catecholamines with predominantly α-adrenergic effects produces increases in peripheral resistance. This is at present the mainstay of pharmacologic interventions during CPR. Available vasoconstrictor drugs are discussed further in the next section on pharmacologic interventions. Alternative mechanical methods, as yet experimental, include methods by which systemic vascular resistance is increased with the aid of balloon occlusion of the ascending aorta[53] or the descending aorta.[54] The expansion of intravascular volume and augmentation of venous return to the heart also may increase aortic blood flow. This may be counterproductive, however, if it produces disproportional increases in right atrial pressure and reduces coronary perfusion pressure.[55]

Precordial Compression

Precordial compression includes repetitive and regularly timed applications of pressure over the lower half of the sternum. These compressions generate cardiac output and forward aortic blood flow as a result of a generalized increase in intrathoracic pressure or direct compression of the heart or both.[56,57]

The cardiac output generated by precordial compression depends on the depth, force, rate, and duration of compression. Experimental studies on animal models have consistently shown a linear relationship between the force and depth of compression and the magnitude of systemic blood flows and pressures generated.[58,59] The favorable effects on blood flow and pressures with increased force and depth of precordial compression may be counterbalanced, however, by the increased risk of injury to the rib cage, sternum, and intrathoracic or intra-abdominal organs.

The rate of compression also is important. When the rate of compression was increased from 60 to 120 per minute, significantly greater systemic blood flow and coronary perfusion pressures were observed.[60] Arterial pressure during chest compressions was maximum when duration of compression was 30% to 40% of the compression release cycle.[61] Current recommendations of the American Heart Association call for a compression rate of 100 per minute with a compression-to-ventilation ratio of 30:2.[22] Equal durations of compression and relaxation are presently regarded as optimal (i.e., a 50% duty cycle). The sternum should be depressed at its lower half for approximately 1.5 to 2 inches for a normal-sized adult. Simple manually operated and automatic chest compressors are commercially available. They may be used by trained personnel to increase consistency and to optimize compression force and depth. Mechanical chest compression has the advantage of reducing rescuer fatigue during prolonged CPR and facilitating physical transport of victims through tight spaces. Automatically triggered chest compressors have special advantages during transit in resuscitation vehicles and elevators.

The quantitative blood flow produced by precordial compression during experimental and clinical states of cardiac arrest is remarkably small. It may be only 10% of the normal cardiac output, and it rarely exceeds 40%. The hemodynamic efficacy of precordial compression also decreases over time.[62,63] This decrease in efficacy is explained, at least in part, by chest wall deformation. Elastic recoil decreases over time, and consequently there is less effective re-expansion of the chest when compression is released. Venous refill of the intrathoracic vascular pool is compromised. More recent experimental evidence indicates that progressive impairment of myocardial compliance is the primary mechanism that accounts for decreased efficacy of chest compression with prolongation of cardiac arrest.[64]

During precordial compression, systemic blood flow and especially cerebral blood flow occur during the interval of compression systole. Because there are essentially equal pressures in the aorta, right atrium, and ventricles during compression systole, there is no pressure gradient for myocardial blood flow during this interval. Myocardial blood flow occurs only during the interval of compression diastole and, more specifically, when the aortic pressure exceeds the pressure in the right atrium. Because myocardial blood flow during precordial compression rarely exceeds 20% to 30% of prearrest flow, it fails to do more than minimize progression of myocardial ischemia.[65] This may be sufficient, however, for successful defibrillation and restoration of spontaneous circulation.

Although myocardial blood flow is typically only 25% of normal during precordial compression, cerebral blood flow often exceeds 50% of normal.[63,66] Such levels are adequate to maintain cerebral blood flow at levels that maintain cerebral viability.[67,68] The cerebral circuit is autoregulating and protected.

The function of the venous valves at the superior thoracic inlet is regarded as important. These valves impede backflow into the cerebral circuit during precordial compression. A substantial pressure gradient favoring forward blood flow is maintained during compression systole and compression diastole. Since the 1980s, many new maneuvers have been proposed for augmenting intrathoracic pressure and the externally generated cardiac output. These include pneumatic vest CPR,[69] interposed abdominal compression,[70] active compression-decompression,[71] phased chest and abdominal compression-decompression, the so-called Lifestick resuscitation technique,[72] and use of an impedance threshold device.[73] There is experimental and preliminary clinical evidence that these maneuvers may augment systemic blood flow and coronary perfusion and improve initial success of resuscitation. More objective comparisons with conventional methods are needed, however, to establish whether these techniques improve the success of the initial resuscitation, neurologic outcome, and hospital discharge of victims.

The risk of traumatic injuries to thoracic and abdominal structures during precordial compression is 10% to 40%. At autopsy, approximately 30% of victims have rib fractures, and 20% have sternal fractures.[74,75] In a few instances, these account for mediastinal and pericardial hemorrhages or cardiac contusion or both. Potentially lethal complications of precordial compression include laceration of the atria, ventricles, or large vessels; lacerations of the liver and spleen; and gastroesophageal tears.[74,76] These risks are increased when less experienced operators apply pressure at unconventional sites or apply excessive pressure.[74] The incidence of these complications increases with increasing duration of the resuscitation procedure, especially in elderly patients.

Open-Chest Direct Cardiac Massage

Open-chest cardiac massage may provide near-normal perfusion of the brain and heart.[77-79] If it is used after a 15-minute interval of ineffective closed-chest CPR, it potentially improves outcome.[78] If direct cardiac massage is delayed for more than 20 minutes, however, there is no proof of improved outcome.[79] In a historically important study on 1200 victims of cardiac arrest, 29% of patients were successfully resuscitated and discharged from the hospital; this included numerous inpatients on surgical services.[6] The use of open-chest resuscitation declined strikingly in the early 1960s after the initial favorable reports on closed-chest precordial compression. Limitations in the training and experience of nonsurgical professionals for performing a thoracotomy, iatrogenic complications, and the substantial postresuscitation care required during recovery combined with the equivocal benefit constrained open-chest methods.[80] Nevertheless, direct cardiac massage is the appropriate intervention when cardiac arrest supervenes intraoperatively and especially during cardiac surgery; after traumatic injuries to the chest; in other settings in which there is likelihood of intrathoracic hemorrhage, pericardial tamponade, massive pulmonary thromboembolism; or when a chest deformity precludes successful closed-chest compression.

Extracorporeal Circulation

Extracorporeal circulation may sustain normal systemic, myocardial, and cerebral blood flows during cardiac arrest.[81-83] Experimental studies in animals and in human victims of cardiac arrest have documented its capability for re-establishment of spontaneous circulation after prolonged cardiac arrest and after failure of conventional CPR.[84-87] The clinical application of extracorporeal circulation is constrained by practical limitations, however. It is potentially feasible in the operating room, intensive care unit, or catheterization laboratory settings when trained personnel and ready-to-use, preferably preprimed, extracorporeal systems are immediately available. As yet, however, there are no persuasive data on human victims that provide a secure basis for the more general clinical application of extracorporeal techniques in other settings.

Defibrillation and Cardioversion

The success of cardiac defibrillation depends in part on the current delivered by the transthoracic electrical shock. Optimally, the current should be adequate for termination of VF without producing functional and morphologic myocardial damage.[88,89] The current delivered to the myocardium depends on the electrical power of the shock and on the electrical resistance (impedance) of the thorax. In human subjects, the resistance averages 75 ohms. Impedance increases with increasing chest circumference and decreases with optimal electrode skin contact and repetitive electrical shocks.[90,91]

Low-energy biphasic waveform defibrillation has been examined in experimental and clinical settings of VF as an alternative to conventional escalating energy monophasic waveform defibrillation. In animal studies, low-energy biphasic waveform shocks with energy levels between 120 J and 150 J were as effective as monophasic waveform shocks with escalating energy levels between 200 J and 360 J for initial resuscitation. After low-energy biphasic waveform defibrillation, significantly less severity of postresuscitation myocardial dysfunction was documented, however.[92,93] In a randomized clinical study, biphasic defibrillation waveform shocks with fixed energy of 150 J yielded significantly greater rates of successful defibrillation compared with conventional monophasic waveform shocks.[94] At the time of this writing, defibrillators manufactured in the United States use biphasic waveforms.

Because of the significant interruption of chest compression by the previously recommended three-stacked shock protocol and the high first-shock efficacy of the biphasic defibrillation waveforms, a one-shock protocol after every 2 minutes of chest compression is currently recommended.[22] The currently recommended electrical power for the biphasic defibrillation waveform depends on the specific waveforms—between 120 J and 200 J. The energy for monophasic waveform electrical countershock is 360 J. More recent studies have shown, however, that the severity of postresuscitation myocardial dysfunction and the duration of survival are closely related to the energy delivered during electrical defibrillation. This finding promoted a re-evaluation of current practice. The greater the delivered energy, the more severe was the postresuscitation myocardial dysfunction and the shorter was the duration of postresuscitation survival.[89]

After prolonged cardiac arrest (>4 to 5 minutes), the success of defibrillation is contingent on the restoration of myocardial blood flow. A 2- to 3-minute interval of CPR before defibrillation may improve the outcomes under these conditions.[95] Defibrillation and cardioversion may be performed with manual, automatic, or semiautomatic external defibrillators. Manual defibrillation is based on professional interpretation of the ECG rhythm. Automatic advisory, or semiautomatic, devices provide a computer-generated interpretation of the cardiac rhythm. With *semi-automatic* devices, the operator may or may not accept the interpretation and trigger defibrillation. In present *automated advisory* devices, the operator controls when the shock is delivered. In *fully automated* devices, the entire sequence proceeds without operator intervention; the device follows a decision sequence including interpretation, decision, and activation. Current AEDs provide verbal warnings to personnel, including "step back" so that bystanders will not be shocked. The effectiveness and safety of these devices have been shown. They are widely implemented for use by nonprofessional basic life support providers and emergency medical technicians in high-risk settings.[23]

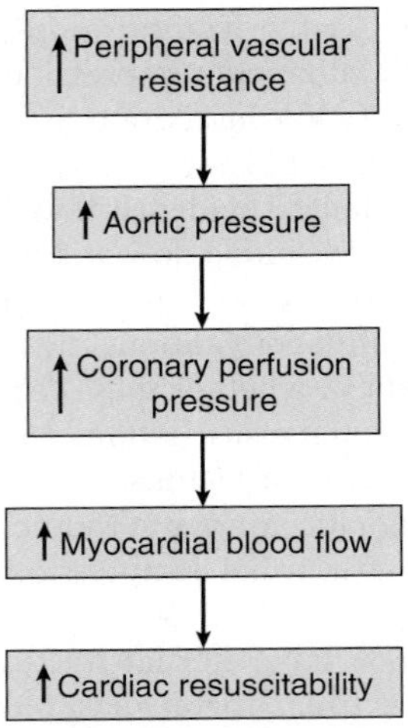

Figure 1-4. Mechanisms by which adrenergic vasopressor agents increase myocardial perfusion during cardiopulmonary resuscitation.

Pharmacologic Interventions

Site of Administration

Drugs are administered by the intravenous route during CPR. A proximal peripheral venous site—the antecubital, femoral, or external jugular vein—is selected. Peripheral vein cannulation typically precedes, but does not replace a central venous catheter. Precordial compression should not be interrupted for central venous cannulation because there is presently no conclusive evidence that this would improve initial outcome.[20] Lower peak drug levels and more prolonged circulation times are to be anticipated when the drug is injected into a peripheral vein, but this is not likely to affect outcomes. The drug is injected as a bolus, followed by a 20-mL flush. It may be helpful to elevate the extremity after the bolus injection.[96]

If attempts to gain prompt venous access fail, epinephrine may be administered through an endotracheal tube. Two to three times the intravenous dose, diluted in 10 mL of normal saline or distilled water, is advised.[97] Intraosseous administration of drugs is an effective alternative for pediatric patients.[20]

Vasopressor Agents

During cardiac arrest, there is maximal sympathoadrenal stimulation and maximal endogenous secretion of catecholamines. There is arterial vasoconstriction, especially in nonvital peripheral vascular beds. The scant flow generated by precordial compression is preferentially distributed to the coronary and cerebral circuits. Exogenously administered adrenergic vasopressor agents further increase peripheral vascular resistance and myocardial perfusion (Fig. 1-4). Epinephrine is still the preferred adrenergic agonist, even though it has substantial β-agonist actions.[97] There is evidence that its efficacy is selectively due to its α-adrenergic action.[98-100] The beneficial hemodynamic effects of epinephrine on myocardial and cerebral perfusion depend partly on dose.[101] Large doses (0.1 to 0.2 mg/kg) improve cerebral and myocardial perfusion and the outcome of resuscitation efforts in animal models. Several multicenter trials in human patients failed to show improved outcome after out-of-hospital cardiac arrest, however.[102,103] The appropriate intravenous dose of epinephrine for adult patients is 1 mg, preferably administered intravenously as a 10-mL bolus in a 1 : 10,000 solution. The dose may be repeated at intervals of 3 minutes.

Investigators also have become aware of potentially adverse effects of epinephrine. Although epinephrine produces increases in myocardial perfusion as a consequence of its α-adrenergic actions, it also increases myocardial oxygen requirements as a consequence of its β-adrenergic actions. Epinephrine may augment myocardial ischemia. Its role as an optimal vasopressor agent during advanced life support is challenged.[104] Epinephrine also may alter the distribution of pulmonary blood flow and provoke ventilation-perfusion abnormalities resulting in decreased oxygen content of systemic arterial blood and temporarily invalidate end-tidal pressure of carbon dioxide ($PetCO_2$) as a monitor.[105] Finally, epinephrine increases the risk of postresuscitation ventricular arrhythmias.[104]

Because of these potential side effects of epinephrine, the use of alternative and more selective α-adrenergic agents, which lack β-adrenergic activity, and even the concurrent administration of β-adrenergic blocking agents have been proposed.[106] Methoxamine (Vasoxyl) and phenylephrine (Neo-Synephrine) would serve as selective α_1-agonists. These considerations notwithstanding, no studies in human patients to date have shown the superiority of selective α_1-adrenergic agents or epinephrine with β-adrenergic blockade compared with epinephrine alone. There is promising research on newer selective α_2-adrenergic agents as alternatives to epinephrine.[107] In addition, experimental animal and human studies indicate that vasopressin may emerge as a useful alternative as a vasopressor agent in lieu of epinephrine.[108,109] A single dose of 40 U may be administered as a bolus by intravenous injection.[97]

Buffer Agents

The rationale for administration of alkalinizing agents and especially sodium bicarbonate during CPR was to reverse myocardial metabolic acidosis.[110] It was assumed that this would favor cardiac resuscitability. Studies on experimental animals failed to confirm, however, that the buffer agents altered myocardial pH during CPR, although the pH of systemic arterial and coronary venous blood was normalized.[111] Important adverse effects of the buffer agents were shown. These hypertonic solutions transiently decrease systemic vascular resistance and coronary perfusion pressure.[112] They also increase the affinity of hemoglobin for oxygen and compromise oxygen release to the tissues. When hypertonic buffers are administered in amounts that significantly increase serum osmolarity, potentially detrimental fluid shifts may exacerbate cerebral edema and global ischemic injury to the brain.[113] Finally, rapid shifts of hydrogen ion concentrations in blood may provoke ectopic ventricular arrhythmias and consequently recurrent VT and VF.[114] Because there is currently no proof that buffer agents improve outcome of CPR, the use of buffer agents is likely to be counterproductive. The routine use of sodium bicarbonate or alternative buffer agents during CPR is no longer recommended. Selective use of sodium bicarbonate in specific settings, including pre-existing metabolic acidosis, hyperkalemia, or tricyclic or phenobarbital overdose, is still supported.[22]

Antiarrhythmic Agents

If VF or VT is refractory to advanced cardiac life support interventions, or there is recurrent VT and VF, pharmacologic interventions with lidocaine, procainamide, and bretylium have been advised.[97] The benefits of these agents are not established with certainty, however. To the contrary, adverse proarrhythmic effects have been suspect. Electrical countershock remains the first option, and pharmacologic interventions with antiarrhythmic drugs are a second option only.

Amiodarone and lidocaine may be administered for treatment of recurrent ventricular ectopic rhythms and especially for recurrent VT and VF. The initial intravenous dose for amiodarone is 300 mg and for lidocaine is 1.5 mg/kg. Nevertheless, there is no persuasive evidence that these drugs improve outcomes.

Procainamide is an alternative. It is administered by intravenous infusion in amounts of 30 mg/min to a total dose of 17 mg/kg body weight to suppress ventricular ectopy.[115] There is no established proof of ultimate benefit.

Calcium, Magnesium, and Atropine

There is no secure evidence that the administration of *calcium* improves the outcome of CPR.[116] Its routine use is not advised. Selective use is recommended in settings of cardiac arrest associated with hyperkalemia, hypocalcemia, or intoxication by calcium entry channel blocking drugs. In these instances, a 10% solution of calcium chloride in a dose of 2 to 4 mg/kg is administered intravenously and may be repeated at 10-minute intervals.[117] *Magnesium* may be administered for management of recurrent VT and VF in settings that are suspicious for hypomagnesemia. A dose of 2 g of magnesium sulfate diluted in 100 mL of 5% dextrose in water is infused intravenously over an interval of 2 minutes.[118] *Atropine* may reverse extremes of bradycardia and even ventricular asystole after intense vagal stimulation, especially during anesthesia or surgical procedures.[119,120] In these instances, 1 mg of atropine sulfate is injected intravenously and repeated in 3 to 5 minutes if bradyarrhythmia persists. There is currently no indication, however, for its routine use during CPR. Atropine also has adverse effects, including atrioventricular conduction delay and supraventricular tachycardia.

MONITORING OF CARDIOPULMONARY RESUSCITATION

Current resuscitation methods are constrained in part by the lack of practical and reliable indicators of the efficacy of CPR. These are needed if clinicians are to have greater precision of management of patients during cardiac resuscitation.

Coronary perfusion pressure may be monitored if arterial and central venous lines are in place. This monitoring is not currently practical in out-of-hospital settings. In patients who have such catheters in place before cardiac arrest, however, the measurement of coronary perfusion pressure and even aortic diastolic pressure alone during CPR provides objective guides for resuscitation, including appropriate precordial compression and the effects of vasopressor drugs.[52]

$PetCO_2$ is a remarkably good correlate of pulmonary and systemic blood flow generated by precordial compression. It is also predictive of the success of cardiac resuscitation.[121] During cardiac arrest, $PetCO_2$ correlates well with coronary perfusion pressure.[122,123] End-tidal carbon dioxide has emerged as a relatively simple, continuous, and noninvasive monitor of the efficacy of CPR.[124] When $PetCO_2$ equals or exceeds 10 mm Hg, most patients are likely to be successfully resuscitated. If $PetCO_2$ is less than 10 mm Hg, however, the likelihood of successful resuscitation is remote.[125] In addition, $PetCO_2$ signals the return of spontaneous circulation with an increase in $PetCO_2$ to levels transiently exceeding prearrest values. $PetCO_2$ is transiently decreased after intravenous injection of epinephrine, which may indicate increased dead-space ventilation resulting from ventilation-perfusion abnormalities[105] and a decrease in the cardiac output, which is being generated by precordial compression.[126] End-tidal carbon dioxide is increased after injection of bicarbonate solution. We recommend routine monitoring of $PetCO_2$ by professional rescue personnel, who also are likely to use $PetCO_2$ measurements to confirm appropriate tracheal placement of endotracheal tubes.

Studies in human victims of cardiac arrest have established that the voltage of VF waveforms is predictive of the success of cardiac resuscitation.[127-129] Significantly greater VF voltages are associated with correspondingly greater success of initial resuscitation efforts and postresuscitation survival.[127] Current evidence supports the hypothesis that VF voltage is related to the hemodynamic efficacy of resuscitation efforts.[130] As yet unexplained is the influence of pharmacologic agents on the predictive value of VF voltage.

It was assumed that palpation of arterial pulses during precordial compression would indicate the adequacy of systemic perfusion. Palpation of carotid and femoral pulses had been the primary monitor of the efficacy of precordial compression.[131] Arterial pulses may at best represent transmission of the maximal intravascular pressure generated during each compression, however, which is poorly correlated with cardiac output.[17,18,20] This is now reflected in the guidelines for CPR,[22] which no longer view palpation of arterial pulses as a useful monitor of the efficacy of resuscitation attempts. The importance of $PetCO_2$ is underscored as a noninvasive monitor. We recognize the need, however, for additional simple methods of monitoring and anticipate prompt progress in this domain.

Arterial blood gas measurements also are of limited value for assessing the adequacy of systemic perfusion. A major arteriovenous carbon dioxide gradient is observed in animal models and human victims during cardiac arrest.[132,133] After sudden death, arterial blood gases measured during CPR typically show hypocarbic (respiratory) alkalosis. Depending on the oxygen concentration of inspired air, oxygen tension or hemoglobin saturation of arterial blood is normal or increased. Acidosis, especially metabolic acidosis resulting from other than pre-existing diseases, is observed only when there is protracted CPR. In venous blood, hypercarbic (respiratory) acidosis is predominant, with abnormally low oxygen tension and hemoglobin saturation reflecting low cardiac outputs generated during CPR.[134]

OUTCOME OF CARDIAC ARREST

A realistic assessment of the outcome of CPR indicates disappointing survival rates after in-hospital and out-of-hospital CPR. The pooled survival rate, defined as hospital discharge after out-of-hospital cardiac arrest in diverse communities, is 5% to 17%. It is greater—12% to 29%—when patients have VF when first monitored (Table 1-1).[23] In some metropolitan areas, such as Chicago, the survival rate is less than 2%,[135] and in rural communities without access to an emergency medical system, it may be even less.[23,136] The survival rates for in-hospital cardiac arrest between 1961 and 1989, based on 49 reports, ranged from 13% to 59% with an average of 39%. Only 15% (range 3% to 27%) of patients were discharged alive, however.[28,137] Among critically ill patients with advanced cardiorespiratory failure, and especially progressive circulatory shock, fewer than 1% were successfully resuscitated.[138] These statistics have not improved in the last 15 years. In a more recent report of a multicenter registry of in-hospital cardiac arrest, the rate of survival to hospital discharge was 18%.[139]

A beneficial outcome of CPR may be anticipated when the patient's collapse is witnessed, and basic life support is started promptly. Rapid response by defibrillation-qualified emergency medical technicians or paramedics secures the benefit of basic life support.[140]

Table 1-1. Estimates of Success of Cardiopulmonary Resuscitation Based on 31 Published Reports

	Hospital Discharge	
Intervention Categories	All Rhythms (%)	Ventricular Fibrillation (%)
BLS	5	12
BLS + defibrillation	10	16
ACLS	10	17
BLS + ACLS	17	26
BLS + defibrillation + ACLS	17	29

ACLS, advanced cardiac life support; BLS, basic life support.
Adapted from Cummins RO, Ornato JP, Thies WH, et al: Improving survival from sudden cardiac arrest: The "chain of survival" concept. Circulation 1991;83:1832-1847.

ETHICAL CONSIDERATIONS

The decision to initiate, or forego, CPR presents substantial ethical concerns for health care professionals, patients, and the families of patients. Patients or their surrogates may elect to forego resuscitation as a personal decision. This decision contrasts with "do not resuscitate" orders that may be entered by physicians on the basis of their medical judgment when no reasonable medical benefit, but only adverse effects of CPR are anticipated. Patients who are not likely to benefit from CPR include patients with metastatic disease or malignant invasion of vital organs, circulatory shock with lactic acidosis, sepsis with multiple organ failure, end-stage renal failure, pneumonia and bacteria unresponsive to treatment, end stages of chronic lung disease, and massive cerebral injuries resulting from vascular accidents or traumatic injuries.[141] If the medical judgment of physicians that CPR is of no value is challenged by the patient or the patient's surrogates, the physician's professional and ethical obligation to forego CPR is not diminished. It is also in the public interest that the physician has no duty to accede to an intervention that has no reasonable likelihood of success, but prejudices the care of patients with better chances of survival. In the rare instances in which the patient or family demands CPR, the patient and family should be offered additional consultation.[142] "Do not resuscitate" protocols for patients who sustain cardiac arrest outside the hospital and who are known to be terminally ill would allow rescuers to forego CPR attempts when they are futile.

Finally, when are we to cease the CPR procedure? Victims of cardiac arrest outside the hospital are not likely to benefit from continued interventions when the initial prehospital efforts have failed. Of 1445 patients in eight

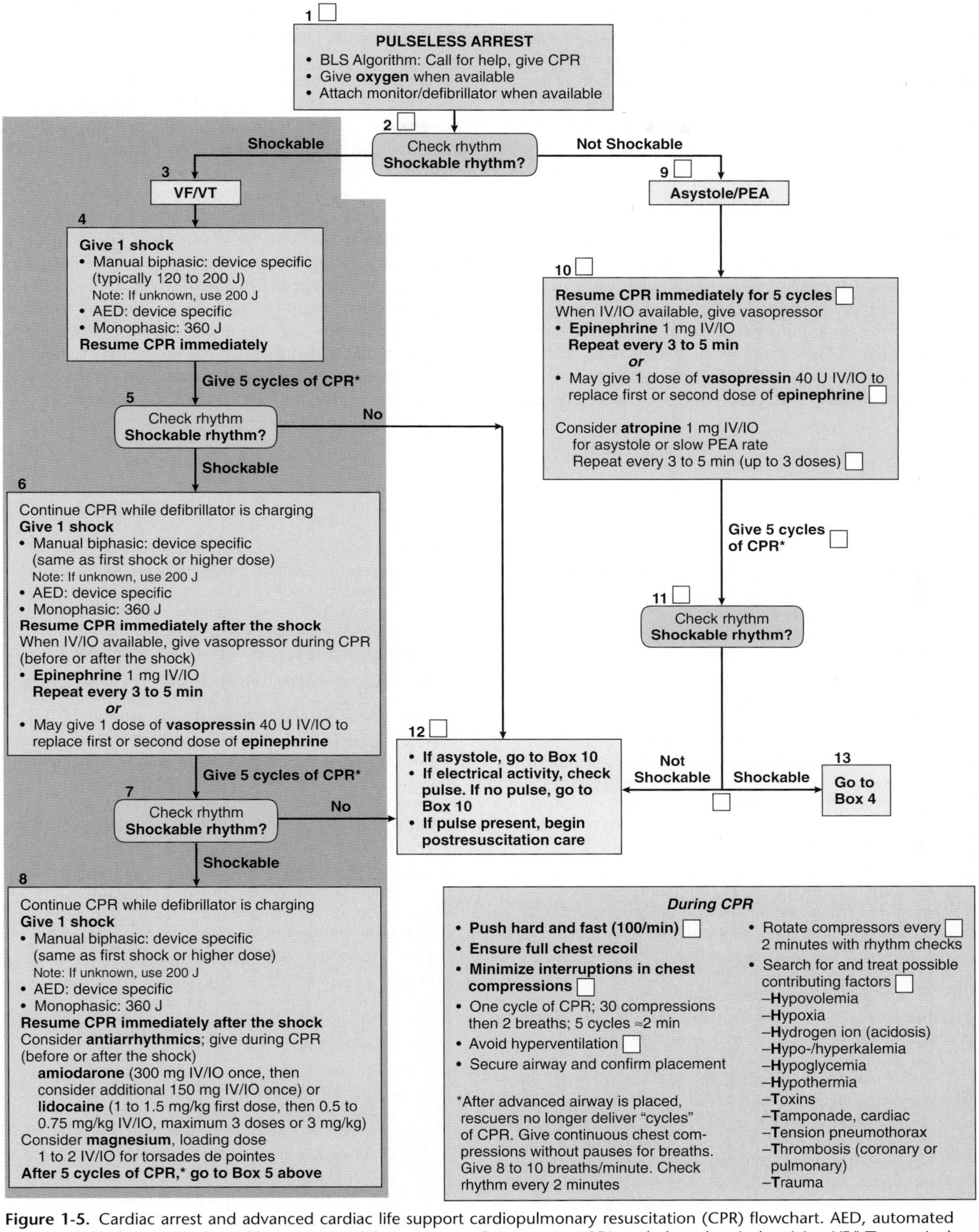

Figure 1-5. Cardiac arrest and advanced cardiac life support cardiopulmonary resuscitation (CPR) flowchart. AED, automated external defibrillator; BLS, basic life support; IV/IO, intravenous/intraosseous; PEA, pulseless electrical activity; VF/VT, ventricular fibrillation/ventricular tachycardia. (From Advanced Cardiovascular Life Support Provider Manual. American Heart Association, 2006.)

studies, only 10 (0.7%) survived to be discharged from the hospital.[143] Failure to increase $PetCO_2$ to exceed 8 mm Hg prognosticates almost certain failure of the resuscitation effort. When there is no significant response in the first 30 minutes, the risk of adverse effects of prolonged resuscitation efforts overrides a remote benefit. We advise termination of effort after 30 minutes.

ANTICIPATING THE FUTURE

After more than 45 years, during which time there has been widespread application of CPR, a re-evaluation of its benefits in terms of meaningful survival is urgently needed. CPR is recognized to be beneficial in only a few victims. The disappointing success rate is to a large extent a result of a delay in initiation of CPR and defibrillation. Communities should emphasize the value of early bystander-initiated CPR. AEDs operated by first responders or by laypersons are likely to be the key at this time for increasing the chances of survival (Fig. 1-5).

The hemodynamic efficacy of conventional techniques of precordial compression should be monitored. Methods for increasing the effectiveness of precordial compression or alternative options for mechanically restoring systemic blood flow and coronary and cerebral perfusion should be seriously investigated.

The choice and dose of vasopressor agents must be more critically defined, including the role of selective α_2-adrenergic or nonadrenergic vasopressor agents, such as vasopressin and angiotensin. The role of positive-pressure ventilation and oxygen enrichment of inspired air should be re-examined, together with the role of endotracheal intubation. Golden seconds are often lost, struggling to accomplish that which is least lifesaving. Finally, any ultimate measure of benefit must include not only survival, but also the quality and duration of *meaningful* life.

KEY POINTS

- When the duration of cardiac arrest is less than 4 minutes, early electrical defibrillation is currently viewed as the most likely intervention for improving the outcome of cardiac arrest. The recommended power for the electrical countershock is waveform specific. For biphasic waveforms, it is between 120 J and 200 J. The recommended power for monophasic waveform is 360 J.
- When the duration of cardiac arrest is prolonged (>4 to 5 minutes), the likelihood of restoring spontaneous circulation is contingent on the capability of the resuscitation interventions to generate cardiac output and increases in peripheral resistance being adequate for restoration of threshold blood flows to the myocardium. Under this condition, a 2- to 3-minute interval of chest compression before defibrillation may improve outcomes.
- Coronary perfusion pressure, represented by the pressure gradient between the aorta and the right atrium, has been consistently secured as a reliable predictor of cardiac resuscitability. The blood flow produced by precordial compression is usually only 25% of the normal cardiac output. Numerous new maneuvers, including pneumatic vest CPR, interposed abdominal compression, active compression-decompression, and use of an impedance threshold device, have been proposed for augmenting externally generated cardiac output. Direct cardiac massage is the appropriate intervention when cardiac arrest supervenes in the operating room; in association with cardiac surgery; after traumatic injuries to the chest; in other settings in which there is likelihood of intrathoracic hemorrhage, pericardial tamponade, or massive pulmonary thromboembolism; or when a chest deformity precludes successful closed-chest compression. Extracorporeal circulation is potentially feasible in the operating room, intensive care unit, or catheterization laboratory settings under conditions in which trained personnel and ready-to-use and, preferably, preprimed extracorporeal systems are immediately available.
- Epinephrine is still the mainstay of pharmacologic interventions during CPR. It increases systemic vascular resistance and coronary perfusion pressure. The dose of intravenous epinephrine for adult patients is 1 mg, and this is preferably administered intravenously as a 10-mL bolus of a 1:10,000 solution. Its β-adrenergic effects are detrimental, however, and we anticipate the introduction of alternative adrenergic and nonadrenergic vasoconstrictor drugs.
- End-tidal carbon dioxide is a remarkably good indicator of systemic blood flow generated by precordial compression. As a relatively simple, continuous, and noninvasive monitor of efficacy of CPR, we advise its routine employment for quality control in CPR.
- A realistic assessment of the outcome of CPR projects disappointing survival rates after in-hospital and out-of-hospital CPR. Pooled survival rates indicate hospital discharge rates range from 3% to 27%.
- The decision to initiate or forego CPR has prompted substantial ethical debate for health care professionals, patients, and the families of patients. Patients who are not likely to benefit from CPR include patients with metastatic disease or malignant invasion of vital organs, advanced circulatory shock with lactic acidosis, sepsis with multiple organ failure, irreversible renal failure, end-stage chronic lung disease, and massive cerebral injuries resulting from vascular accidents or trauma.

REFERENCES

1. Kuller LH: Sudden death: Definition and epidemiologic considerations. Prog Cardiovasc Dis 1980;23:1-12.
2. Althaus U, Aeberhard P, Schupbach P, et al: Management of profound accidental hypothermia with cardiorespiratory arrest. Ann Surg 1982;195:492-495.
3. Copass MK, Oreskovich MR, Bladergroen MR, et al: Prehospital cardiopulmonary resuscitation of the critically injured patient. Am J Surg 1984;148:20-26.
4. Fontanarosa PB: Electrical shock and lightning strike. Ann Emerg Med 1993;22:378-387.
5. Thangam S, Weil MH, Rackow EC: Cardiopulmonary resuscitation: A historical review. Acute Care 1986;12:63-94.
6. Stephenson HE Jr, Reid LC, Hinton JW: Some common denominators in 1,200 cases of cardiac arrest. Ann Surg 1953;137:731-744.
7. Beck CS, Pritchard WH, Feil HS: Ventricular fibrillation of long duration abolished by electric shock. JAMA 1947;135:985-986.
8. Zoll PM, Linenthal AJ, Gibson W, et al: Termination of ventricular fibrillation in man by externally applied electric countershock. N Engl J Med 1956;254:727-732.
9. Kouwenhoven WB, Jude JR, Knickerbocker GG: Closed-chest cardiac massage. JAMA 1960;173:1064-1067.
10. Jude JR, Kouwenhoven WB, Knickerbocker GG: Cardiac arrest: report of application of external cardiac massage on 118 patients. JAMA 1961;178:1063-1070.
11. Polentini MS., Pirrallo RG, McGill W: The changing incidence of ventricular fibrillation in Milwaukee, Wisconsin (1992-2002). Prehosp Emerg Care 2006;10:52-60.
12. Bunch TJ, White RD, Friedman PA, et al: Trends in treated ventricular fibrillation out-of-hospital cardiac arrest: A 17-year population-based study. Heart Rhythm 2004;1:255-259.
13. Bunch TJ, White RD: Trends in treated ventricular fibrillation in out-of-hospital cardiac arrest: Ischemic compared to non-ischemic heart disease. Resuscitation 2005;67:51-54.
14. Weaver DW, Lorch GS, Alvarez HA, et al: Angiographic findings and prognostic indicators in patients resuscitated from sudden cardiac death. Circulation 1976;54:895-900.
15. Cobb LA, Baum RS, Alvarez H III, et al: Resuscitation from out-of-hospital ventricular fibrillation: 4 years follow-up. Circulation 1975;52(Suppl 6):III-223-III-235.
16. Whitaker MP, Sheps DS: Prevalence of silent myocardial ischemia in survivors of cardiac arrest. Am J Cardiol 1989;64:591-593.
17. Weil MH, Gazmuri RJ, Rackow EC: The clinical rationale of cardiac resuscitation. Dis Mon 1990;36:426-468.
18. Ornato JP: Hemodynamic monitoring during CPR. Ann Emerg Med 1993;22:289-295.
19. Clark JJ, Larsen MP, Culley LL, et al: Incidence of agonal respirations in sudden cardiac arrest. Ann Emerg Med 1991;21:1464-1467.
20. Neimann JT: Cardiopulmonary resuscitation. N Engl J Med 1992;327:1075-1080.
21. Weil MH, von Planta M, Rackow EC: Acute circulatory failure (shock). In Braunwald E (ed): Heart Disease, 4th ed. Philadelphia, Saunders, 1992, pp 561-580.
22. Emergency Cardiac Care Committee and Subcommittees, American Heart Association: 2005 Guidelines for cardiopulmonary resuscitation and emergency cardiovascular care. Circulation 2005;112:IV-1-IV-211.
23. Cummins RO, Ornato JP, Thies WH, et al: Improving survival from sudden cardiac arrest: The "chain of survival" concept. Circulation 1991;83:1832-1847.
•24. Weaver WD, Cobb LA, Hallstrom AP, et al: Factors influencing survival after out-of-hospital cardiac arrest. J Am Coll Cardiol 1986;7:752-757.
25. Caffrey SL, Willoughby PJ, Pepe PE, et al: Public use of automated external defibrillators. N Engl J Med 2002;347:1242-1247.
26. Valenzuela TD, Roe DJ, Nichol G, et al: Outcomes of rapid defibrillation by security officers after cardiac arrest in casinos. N Engl J Med 2000;343:1206-1209.
27. White RD, Bunch TJ, Hankins DG: Evolution of a community-wide early defibrillation programme experience over 13 years using police/fire personnel and paramedics as responders. Resuscitation 2005;65:279-283.
28. McGrath RB: In-house cardiopulmonary resuscitation—after a quarter of a century. Ann Emerg Med 1987;16:1365-1368.
29. Eisenberg MS, Horwood BT, Cummins RO, et al: Cardiac arrest and resuscitation: A tale of 29 cities. Ann Emerg Med 1990;19:179-186.
30. Safar P, Escarraga LA, Chang F: Upper airway obstruction in the unconscious patient. J Appl Physiol 1959;14:760-764.
31. Safar P, Escarraga LA, Elam JO: A comparison of the mouth-to-mouth and mouth-to-airway methods of artificial respiration with the chest-pressure arm-lift methods. N Engl J Med 1958;258:671-677.
32. Pepe PE, Copass MK, Joyce TH: Prehospital endotracheal intubation: Rationale for training emergency medical personnel. Ann Emerg Med 1985;14:1085-1092.
33. Bryson TK, Benumof JL, Ward CF: The esophageal obturator airway: A clinical comparison to ventilation with a mask and oropharyngeal airway. Chest 1978;74:537-539.
34. Goldenberg IF, Campion BC, Siebold CM, et al: Esophageal gastric tube airway vs endotracheal tube in prehospital cardiopulmonary arrest. Chest 1986;90:90-96.
35. Niemann IT, Rosborough JP, Myers R, et al: The pharyngeotracheal lumen airway: Preliminary investigation of a new adjunct. Ann Emerg Med 1984;13:591-596.
36. Frass M, Frenzer R, Rauscha F, et al: Evaluation of the esophageal tracheal combitube in cardiopulmonary resuscitation. Crit Care Med 1987;15:609-611.
37. Janssens M, Lamy M: Laryngeal mask. Inten Care World 1993;10:99-102.
38. Levitan RM, Ochroch EA, Stuart S, et al: Use of the intubating laryngeal mask airway by medical and nonmedical personnel. Am J Emerg Med 2000;18:12-16.
39. Safar P: Ventilatory efficacy of mouth-to-mouth artificial respiration: airway obstruction during manual and mouth-to-mouth artificial respiration. JAMA 1958;167:335-341.
40. Safar P: Pocket mask for emergency artificial ventilation and oxygen inhalation. Crit Care Med 1974;2:273-276.
41. Pepe PE, Zachariah BS, Chandra NC: Invasive airway techniques in resuscitation. Ann Emerg Med 1993;22:393-403.
42. Centers for Disease Control: Guidelines for prevention of transmission of human immunodeficiency virus and hepatitis B virus to health-care and public-safety workers. MMWR Morb Mortal Wkly Rep 1989;38(Suppl 6):1.
43. Sande MA: Transmission of AIDS: The case against casual contagion. N Engl J Med 1986;314:380-382.
44. Osborn HH, Kayen D, Horne H, et al: Excess ventilation with oxygen-powered resuscitators. Am J Emerg Med 1984;2:408-413.
45. Tang W, Weil MH, Sun S, et al: Cardiopulmonary resuscitation by precordial compression but without mechanical ventilation. Am J Respir Crit Care Med 1994;150:1709-1713.
46. Berg R, Kern K, Sanders A, et al: Bystander cardiopulmonary resuscitation: Is ventilation necessary? Circulation 1993;88:1907-1915.
47. Noc M, Weil MH, Tang W, et al: Mechanical ventilation may not be essential for initial cardiopulmonary resuscitation. Chest 1995;108:821-827.
48. Chandra NC, Gruben KG, Tsitlik JE, et al: Observation of ventilation during resuscitation in a canine model. Circulation 1994;90:3070-3075.
49. Downey JM, Chargrasulis RW, Hemphill V: Quantitative study of intramyocardial compression in the fibrillating heart. Am J Physiol 1979;237:H191-H196.
50. Wolfe JA, Maier GW, Newton JR Jr, et al: Physiologic determinant of coronary blood flow during external cardiac massage. J Thorac Cardiovasc Surg 1988;95:523-532.
51. Ralston SH, Voorhees WD, Babbs CF: Intrapulmonary epinephrine during prolonged cardiopulmonary resuscitation: Improved regional blood flow and resuscitation in dogs. Ann Emerg Med 1984;13:79-86.
•52. Paradis NA, Martin GB, Rivers EP, et al: Coronary perfusion pressure and the return of spontaneous circulation in human

cardiopulmonary resuscitation. JAMA 1990;263:1106-1113.
53. Tang W, Weil MH, Noc M, et al: Augmented efficacy of external CPR by intermittent occlusion of the ascending aorta. Circulation 1993; 88:1916-1921.
54. Paradis NA, Rose MI, Pryor MA, et al: Selective aortic occlusion and oxygenation improves coronary perfusion pressure during CPR and advanced cardiac life support. Circulation 1992;86(Suppl 1):547 (Abstract).
55. Ditchey RV, Lindenfeld J: Potential adverse effects of volume loading on perfusion of vital organs during closed-chest resuscitation. Circulation 1984;69:181-189.
56. Rudikoff MT, Maughan WL, Effron M, et al: Mechanisms of blood flow during cardiopulmonary resuscitation. Circulation 1980;61:345-352.
57. Deshmukh HG, Weil MH, Gudipati CV, et al: Mechanism of blood flow generated by precordial compression during CPR: 1. Studies on closed chest precordial compression. Chest 1989;95:1092-1099.
58. Babbs CF, Voorhees WD, Fitzgerald KR, et al: Relationship of blood pressure and flow during CPR to chest compression amplitude: evidence for an effective compression threshold. Ann Emerg Med 1983;12: 527-532.
59. Halperin HR, Tsitlik JE, Guerci AD, et al: Determinants of blood flow to vital organs during cardiopulmonary resuscitation in dogs. Circulation 1986;73:539-550.
60. Swenson RD, Weaver WD, Niskanen RA, et al: Hemodynamics in humans during conventional and experimental methods of cardiopulmonary resuscitation. Circulation 1988;78:630-639.
61. Swart GL, Mateer JR, DeBehnke DJ, et al: The effect of compression duration on hemodynamics during mechanical high-impulse CPR. Acad Emerg Med 1994;1:430-437.
62. Sharff JA, Pantley G, Noel E: Effect of time on regional organ perfusion during two methods of cardiopulmonary resuscitation. Ann Emerg Med 1984;13:649-656.
63. Schleien CL, Dean JM, Koehler RC, et al: Effect of epinephrine on cerebral and myocardial perfusion in an infant animal preparation of cardiopulmonary resuscitation. Circulation 1986;73:809-817.
64. Klouche K, Weil MH, Sun S, et al: Stroke volumes generated by precordial compression during cardiac resuscitation. Crit Care Med 2002;30:2626-2631.
65. Ditchey RV, Horowitz LD: Metabolic evidence of inadequate coronary blood flow during closed-chest resuscitation in dogs. Cardiovasc Res 1985;19:419-425.
66. Voorhees WD, Babbs CF, Tacker WA Jr: Regional blood flow during cardiopulmonary resuscitation in dogs. Crit Care Med 1980;8: 134-136.
67. Sharbrough FW, Merssick JM Jr, Sundt TM Jr: Correlation of continuous electroencephalograms with cerebral blood flow measurements during carotid endarterectomy. Stroke 1973;4:674-683.
68. Branston NM, Symon L, Crockard HA, et al: Relationship between the cortical evoked potential and local cortical blood flow following acute middle cerebral artery occlusion in the baboon. Exp Neurol 1974;45: 195-208.
69. Halperin HR, Tsitlik JE, Gelfand M, et al: A preliminary study of cardiopulmonary resuscitation of circumferential compression of the chest with use of a pneumatic vest. N Engl J Med 1993;329:762-768.
70. Sack JB, Kesselbrenner MB, Bregman D: Survival from in-hospital cardiac arrest with interposed abdominal counterpulsation during cardiopulmonary resuscitation. JAMA 1992;267:379-385.
71. Plaisance P, Adnet F, Vicaut E, et al: Benefit of active compression-decompression cardiopulmonary resuscitation as a prehospital advanced cardiac life support: a randomized multicenter study. Circulation 1997;95:955-961.
72. Tang W, Weil MH, Schock RB, et al: Phased chest and abdominal compression-decompression: A new option for cardiopulmonary resuscitation. Circulation 1997;95: 1335-1340.
73. Aufderheide TP, Pirrallo RG, Provo TA, et al: Clinical evaluation of an inspiratory impedance threshold device during standard cardiopulmonary resuscitation in patients with out-of-hospital cardiac arrest. Crit Care Med 2005;33: 734-740.
74. Bedell SE, Fulton EJ: Unexpected findings and complications at autopsy after cardiopulmonary resuscitation (CPR). Arch Intern Med 1986;146: 1725-1728.
75. Krischer JP, Fine EG, Davis JH, et al: Complication of cardiac resuscitation. Chest 1987;92:287-291.
76. Adler SN, Klein RA, Pellecchia C, et al: Massive hepatic hemorrhage associated with cardiopulmonary resuscitation. Arch Intern Med 1983;143:813-814.
77. Sanders AB, Kern KB, Ewy GA, et al: Improved resuscitation from cardiac arrest with open-chest massage. Ann Emerg Med 1984;13:672-675.
78. Kern KB, Sanders AB, Badylak SF, et al: Long-term survival with open-chest cardiac massage after ineffective closed-chest compression in a canine model. Circulation 1987;75:498-503.
79. Kern KB, Sanders AB, Janas W, et al: Limitations of open-chest cardiac massage after prolonged, untreated cardiac arrest in dogs. Ann Emerg Med 1991;20:761-767.
80. Geehr EC, Lewis FR, Auerbach PS: Failure of open-heart massage to improve survival after prehospital nontraumatic cardiac arrest. N Engl J Med 1986;314:1189-1190.
81. Mattox KL, Beall AC Jr: Resuscitation of the moribund patient using portable cardiopulmonary bypass. Ann Thorac Surg 1976;22: 436-442.
82. Levine R, Gorayeb M, Safar P, et al: Cardiopulmonary bypass after cardiac arrest and prolonged closed-chest CPR in dogs. Ann Emerg Med 1987;16:620-627.
83. Pretto E, Safar P, Saito R, et al: Cardiopulmonary bypass after prolonged cardiac arrest in dogs. Ann Emerg Med 1987;16:611-619.
84. Reichman RT, Joyo CI, Dembitsky WP, et al: Improved patient survival after cardiac arrest using a cardiopulmonary support system. Ann Thorac Surg 1990;49:101-104.
85. Shawl FA, Domanski MJ, Wish MH, et al: Emergency cardiopulmonary bypass support in patients with cardiac arrest in the catheterization laboratory. Cathet Cardiovasc Diagn 1990;19:8-12.
86. Gazmuri RJ, Weil MH, von Planta M, et al: Cardiac resuscitation by extracorporeal circulation after failure of conventional CPR. J Lab Clin Med 1991;118:65-73.
87. Mooney MR, Arom KV, Joyce LD, et al: Emergency cardiopulmonary bypass support in patients with cardiac arrest. J Thorac Cardiovasc Surg 1991;101:450-454.
88. Dahl CF, Ewy GA, Warner ED, et al: Myocardial necrosis from direct current countershock. Circulation 1974;50:956-961.
89. Xie J, Weil MH, Sun SJ, et al: High energy defibrillation increases the severity of post-resuscitation myocardial dysfunction. Circulation 1997;96:683-688.
90. Kerber RE, Grayzel J, Hoyt R, et al: Transthoracic resistance in human defibrillation: Influence of body weight, chest size, serial shocks, paddle size, and paddle contact pressure. Circulation 1981;63: 676-682.
91. Sirna SJ, Ferguson DW, Charbonnier F, et al: Factors affecting transthoracic impedance during electrical cardioversion. Am J Cardiol 1988;62: 1048-1052.
92. Tang W, Weil MH, Sun SJ, et al: The effects of biphasic and conventional monophasic defibrillation on post resuscitation myocardial function. J Am Coll Cardiol 1999;34:815-822.
93. Tang W, Weil MH, Sun S, et al: A comparison of biphasic and monophasic waveform defibrillation after prolonged ventricular fibrillation. Chest 2001;120:948-954.
94. Schneider T, Martens P, Paschen HR, et al: Prospective, randomized trial demonstrating improved defibrillation and post-shock neurologic status after use of 150 J biphasic waveforms on cardiac arrest victims. Circulation 1999;100:I-315 (Abstract).
95. Wik L, Hansen TB, Fylling F, et al: Delaying defibrillation to give basic cardiopulmonary resuscitation to patients with out-of-hospital ventricular fibrillation: A randomized trial. JAMA 2003;289:1389-1395.
96. Kuhn GJ, White BC, Swetnam RE, et al: Peripheral vs central circulation times during CPR: A pilot study. Ann Emerg Med 1981;10:417-419.
•97. Emergency Cardiac Care Committee and Subcommittees, American Heart Association: Guidelines for

cardiopulmonary resuscitation and emergency cardiovascular care. Circulation 2000;102:I-86.
98. Redding JS, Pearson JW: Resuscitation from ventricular fibrillation: Drug therapy. JAMA 1968;203:255-260.
99. Yakaitis RW, Otto CW, Blitt CD: Relative importance of alpha and beta adrenergic receptors during resuscitation. Crit Care Med 1979;7: 293-296.
100. Otto C, Yakaitis RW, Blitt CD: Mechanism of action of epinephrine in resuscitation from asphyxial arrest. Crit Care Med 1981;9:364-365.
•101. Paradis NA, Koscove EM: Epinephrine in cardiac arrest: A critical review. Ann Emerg Med 1990;19:1288-1301.
102. Brown CG, Martin DR, Pepe PE, et al: A comparison of standard-dose and high dose epinephrine in cardiac arrest outside the hospital. N Engl J Med 1992;327:1051-1055.
103. Stiell IG, Hebert PC, Weitzman BN, et al: High-dose epinephrine in adult cardiac arrest. N Engl J Med 1992; 327:1045-1050.
104. Tang W, Weil MH, Sun SJ, et al: Epinephrine increases the severity of post-resuscitation myocardial dysfunction. Circulation 1995;92: 3089-3093.
105. Tang W, Weil MH, Gazmuri RJ, et al: Pulmonary ventilation/perfusion defects induced by epinephrine during cardiopulmonary resuscitation. Circulation 1991;84:2101-2107.
106. Ditchey RV, Goto Y, Lindenfeld J: Myocardial oxygen requirements during experimental cardiopulmonary resuscitation. Cardiovasc Res 1992;26:791-797.
107. Sun S, Weil MH, Tang W, et al: Alpha-methylnorepinephrine, a selective alpha$_2$-adrenergic agonist for cardiac resuscitation. J Am Coll Cardiol 2001;37:951-956.
108. Lindner KH, Prengel AW, Pfenninger EG, et al: Vasopressin improves vital organ blood flow during closed-chest cardiopulmonary resuscitation in pigs. Circulation 1995;91:215-221.
109. Lindner KH, Prengel AW, Brinkmann A, et al: Vasopressin administration in refractory cardiac arrest. Ann Intern Med 1996;124:1061-1064.
110. Stewart JS: Management of cardiac arrest with special reference to metabolic acidosis. BMJ 1964;5381: 476-479.
111. Kette F, Weil MH, von Planta M, et al: Buffer agents do not reverse intramyocardial acidosis during cardiac resuscitation. Circulation 1990;81:1660-1666.
112. Kette F, Weil MH, Gazmuri RJ: Buffer solution may compromise cardiac resuscitation by reducing coronary perfusion pressure. JAMA 1991;266: 2121-2126.
113. Mattar JA, Weil MH, Shubin H, et al: Cardiac arrest in the critically ill: Hyperosmolar states following cardiac arrest. Am J Med 1974;56: 162-168.
114. Lawson NW, Butler GH III, Ray CT: Alkalosis and cardiac arrhythmias. Anesth Analg 1973;52:951-964.
115. Giardina E-GV, Heissenbuttel RH, Bigger JT Jr: Intermittent intravenous procaine-amide to treat ventricular arrhythmias: Correlation of plasma concentration with effect on arrhythmia, electrocardiogram, and blood pressure. Ann Intern Med 1973;78:183-193.
116. Steuven H, Thompson BM, Aprahamian C, et al: Use of calcium in prehospital cardiac arrest. Ann Emerg Med 1983;12:136-139.
117. Thompson BM, Steuven HS, Tonsfeldt DJ, et al: Calcium: Limited indications, some danger. Circulation 1986;74(Suppl IV):90-93.
118. Ceremuzynski L, Jurgiel R, Kulakowski P, et al: Threatening arrhythmias in acute myocardial infarction are prevented by intravenous magnesium sulfate. Am Heart J 1989;118:1333-1334.
119. Meyers EF, Tomeldan SA: Glycopyrrolate compared with atropine in prevention of the oculocardiac reflex during eye muscle surgery. Anesthesiology 1979;51:350-352.
120. Sorensen O, Eriksen S, Hommelgaard P, et al: Thiopental-nitrous oxide-halothane anesthesia and repeated succinylcholine: Comparison of preoperative glycopyrrolate and atropine administration. Anesth Analg 1986;59:686-689.
121. Weil MH, Bisera J, Trevino RP, et al: Cardiac output and end-tidal carbon dioxide. Crit Care Med 1985;13:907-909.
122. Sanders AB, Atlas M, Ewy GA, et al: Expired PCO_2 as an index of coronary perfusion pressure. Am J Emerg Med 1985;3:147-149.
123. Duggal C, Weil MH, Gazmuri RJ, et al: Regional blood flow during closed chest cardiac resuscitation in rats. J Appl Physiol 1993;74:147-152.
•124. Falk JL, Rackow EC, Weil MH: End-tidal carbon dioxide concentration during cardiopulmonary resuscitation. N Engl J Med 1988;318:607-611.
125. Sanders AB, Kern KB, Otto CW, et al: End-tidal carbon dioxide monitoring during cardiopulmonary resuscitation: A prognostic indicator of survival. JAMA 1989;262:1347-1351.
126. Martin GB, Gentile NT, Paradis NA, et al: Effect of epinephrine on end-tidal carbon dioxide monitoring during CPR. Ann Emerg Med 1990;19:396-398.
127. Weaver DW, Cobb LA, Dennis D, et al: Amplitude of ventricular fibrillation waveform and outcome after cardiac arrest. Ann Intern Med 1985;102:53-55.
128. Stults KR, Brown DD, Kerber RE: Ventricular fibrillation amplitude predicts ability to defibrillate. J Am Coll Cardiol 1987;9:152A (Abstract).
129. Dalzell GW, Adgey AA: Determinants of successful transthoracic defibrillation and outcome in ventricular fibrillation. Br Heart J 1991;65:311-316.
130. Noc M, Weil MH, Tang W, et al: Electrocardiographic prediction of the success of cardiac resuscitation. Crit Care Med 1999;27:708-714.
131. Standards and guidelines for cardiopulmonary resuscitation (CPR) and emergency cardiac care (ECC). JAMA 1986;255:2905-2984.
132. Sanders AB, Ewy GA, Taft TV: Resuscitation and arterial blood gas abnormalities during prolonged cardiopulmonary resuscitation. Ann Emerg Med 1984;13:676-679.
133. Weil MH, Rackow EC, Trevino R, et al: Difference in acid-base state between venous and arterial blood during cardiopulmonary resuscitation. N Engl J Med 1986;315:153-156.
134. Grundler W, Weil MH, Rackow EC: Arteriovenous carbon dioxide and pH gradients during cardiac arrest. Circulation 1986;74:1071-1074.
135. Becker LB, Ostrander MP, Barrett J, et al: Outcome of CPR in a large metropolitan area: Where are the survivors? Ann Emerg Med 1991;20: 355-361.
136. Cobb LA, Eliastam M, Kerber RE, et al: Report of the American Heart Association Task Force on the Future of Cardiopulmonary Resuscitation. Circulation 1992;85:2346-2355.
•137. Jastremski MS: In-hospital cardiac arrest. Ann Emerg Med 1993;22: 113-117.
138. Camarata S, Weil MH, Hanashiro PK, et al: Cardiac arrest in the critically ill: I. A study of predisposing causes in 132 patients. Circulation 1971;44: 688-695.
139. Nadkarni VM, Larkin GL, Peberdy MA, et al: First documented rhythm and clinical outcome from in-hospital cardiac arrest among children and adults. JAMA 2006;295: 50-57.
140. Litwin PE, Eisenberg MS, Hallstrom AP, et al: The location of collapse and its effect on survival from cardiac arrest. Ann Emerg Med 1987;16:787-791.
141. Bedell SE, Delbanco TL, Cook EF, et al: Survival after cardiopulmonary resuscitation in the hospital. N Engl J Med 1983;309:569-576.
142. Fox M, Lipton HL: The decision to perform cardiopulmonary resuscitation. N Engl J Med 1983;309:607-608.
143. Kellermann AL, Staves DR, Hackman BB: In-hospital resuscitation following unsuccessful prehospital advanced cardiac life support: "Heroic efforts" or an exercise in futility? Ann Emerg Med 1988;17:589-594.

Chapter 2

Airway Management in the Critically Ill Adult

G. G. Lavery and C. A. Jamison

Appropriate management of the airway is the cornerstone of good resuscitation. It requires judgment (airway assessment), skill (airway maneuvers), and constant reassessment of the patient's condition. Although complex procedures sometimes are life-saving and always carry the potential to impress, the timely use of simple airway maneuvers often is very effective and may avoid the need for further intervention.

STRUCTURE AND FUNCTION OF THE NORMAL AIRWAY

Critical care staff require an understanding of structure and function in order to successfully manage the airway and the conditions that may affect it. The relevant information can be gained from a variety of sources.[1-5] The airway begins at the nose and oral cavity and continues as the pharynx and larynx, which lead to the trachea (beginning at the lower edge of the cricoid cartilage) and then the bronchial tree. The airway[1] provides a pathway for airflow between the atmosphere and the lungs[2]; facilitates filtering, humidification, and heating of ambient air before it reaches the lower airway[3]; prevents nongaseous material from entering the lower airway[6]; and allows phonation by controlling the flow of air through the larynx and oropharynx.[4]

The Nose

The nose has a midline septum separating two cavities that communicate externally via the external nares (nostrils). Each cavity has a roof formed by the nasal cartilages, frontal bones, cribriform plate, ethmoid, and body of sphenoid. Portions of the maxilla and palatine bones make up the nasal floor (which also forms part of the roof of the oral cavity). The medial wall of each nasal cavity is formed by the nasal septum, the vomer, and ethmoid bones. The lateral wall lies medial to the orbit, the ethmoid, and maxillary sinuses and has three horizontal bony projections—the superior, middle and inferior nasal conchae. These greatly increase the surface area, and the overlying mucosa is highly vascular, supplied by the maxillary arterial branch of the external carotid artery and the ethmoidal branch of the ophthalmic artery. The (nonolfactory) sensory innervation of the nasal mucosa is by two divisions of the trigeminal nerve.

The Oral Cavity

The teeth form the lateral wall of the oral cavity, while the floor is the tongue—a mass of horizontal, vertical, and transverse muscle bundles attached to the mandible and the hyoid bone. The sulcus terminalis, a V-shaped groove, divides the anterior two thirds of the tongue (sensory innervation from the lingual nerve and taste from the chordae tympani) from the posterior one third (sensory supply from the glossopharyngeal nerve). All intrinsic and extrinsic muscles of the tongue are supplied by the hypoglossal nerve, except the palatoglossus, which is supplied by the vagus nerve.

The Pharynx

The adult pharynx is a midline structure, running anterior to the cervical prevertebral fascia, from the base of the skull to the level of the sixth cervical vertebrae (approximately 14 cm), and continuing as the esophagus. It is a muscular tube with three portions: the nasopharynx, oropharynx, and laryngopharynx (or hypopharynx). It contains three groups of lymphoid tissue: the adenoids, the pharyngeal tonsil (on the posterior wall), and the palatine (lingual) tonsils and has the inner opening of the eustachian tube on each lateral wall. The vagus nerve supplies all but one of the pharyngeal muscles. Sensory supply is via branches of the glossopharyngeal and vagus nerves. The pharynx provides a common pathway for the upper alimentary and respiratory tracts and is concerned with swallowing and phonation.

The Larynx

The larynx sits anterior to the laryngopharynx and the fourth to the sixth cervical vertebrae and is posterior to the infrahyoid muscles, the deep cervical fascia, and the subcutaneous fat and skin that cover the front of the neck. Laterally lie the lobes of the thyroid gland and carotid sheath. The larynx acts as a sphincter at the upper end of the respiratory tract and is the organ of phonation. The epiglottis and the thyroid, cricoid, and paired arytenoid, cuneiform, and corniculate cartilages, together with the interconnecting ligaments, make up the skeleton of the larynx, which has a volume of 4 mL. Two pairs of parallel horizontal folds project into the lumen of the larynx—the false vocal cords (lying superiorly) and the true vocal cords (inferiorly). The opening between the true cords is called the glottis. The larynx communicates above with the (laryngo)pharynx and below with the trachea, which begins at the lower edge of the cricoid ring.

The superior aspect of the epiglottis is innervated by the glossopharyngeal nerve, whereas the vagus, via its superior laryngeal (SLN) and recurrent laryngeal (RLN) branches, innervates the larynx, including the inferior surface of the epiglottis. The external (motor) branch of the SLN supplies the cricothyroid muscle, and the internal branch is the sensory supply to the larynx down to the vocal cords. The RLN supplies all of the intrinsic laryngeal muscles and is the sensory supply to the larynx below the cords. Injury to the SLN causes hoarseness secondary to a loss of tension in the ipsilateral vocal cord. Complete unilateral RLN palsy inactivates both ipsilateral adductor and abductor muscles. Vocal cord adduction, however, is maintained by the unopposed SLN-innervated cricothyroid muscle. With bilateral RLN palsy, both cords are in adduction as a result of the unopposed action of the cricothyroid muscle. On inspiration, the adducted vocal cords then act like a Venturi device, generating a negative pressure that pulls the cords together, producing inspiratory stridor—the characteristic sign of upper airway obstruction. Laryngospasm, a severe form of airway obstruction, may be triggered by mechanical stimulation of the larynx or by cord irritation due to aspiration of oral secretions, blood, or vomitus.

In health, the laryngeal abductor muscles contract early in inspiration, separating the vocal cords and facilitating airflow into the tracheobronchial tree. Movements of the thyroid and arytenoid cartilages alter the length and tension of the vocal cords, while sliding and rotational movements of the arytenoid cartilages can alter the shape of the glottic opening between the vocal cords. Fine control of the muscles producing these movements allows vocalization as air passes between the vocal cords in expiration. The sound volume is increased by resonance in the sinuses of the face and skull.

The Tracheobronchial Tree

The trachea is a fibrous tube, 2 cm in diameter, running in the midline for 10 to 15 cm from the level of the sixth cervical vertebra to its bifurcation (carina) at the level of the fourth thoracic vertebra. The walls include 15 to 20 incomplete cartilaginous rings limited posteriorly by fibroelastic tissue and smooth muscle.

The cervical trachea lies anterior to the esophagus, with the recurrent laryngeal nerve in the groove between the two. Anteriorly lie the cervical fascia, infrahyoid muscles, isthmus of the thyroid, and the jugular venous arch. Laterally lie the lobes of the thyroid gland and the carotid sheath. In the thorax, the trachea is traversed anteriorly by the brachiocephalic artery and vein (which may be damaged or eroded by the tracheostomy tube). To the left are the common carotid and subclavian arteries and the aortic arch. To the right are the vagus nerve, the azygos vein, and the pleura. The carina lies anterior to the esophagus behind the bifurcation of the pulmonary trunk.

The bronchial tree is similar in structure to the trachea. Two main bronchi diverge from the carina. The right main bronchus is shorter, wider, and more vertical and runs close to the pulmonary artery and the azygos vein. The left main bronchus passes under the arch of the aorta, anterior to the esophagus, thoracic duct, and descending aorta.[7]

Overview of Airway Function

In the nose, inspired gas is filtered, humidified, and warmed before entering the lungs. Resistance to gas flow through the nose is twice that of the mouth, explaining the need to mouth-breathe during exercise when gas flows are high. Warming and humidification continue in the pharynx and tracheobronchial tree. Between the trachea and the alveolar sacs, airways divide 23 times. This increases the cross-sectional area for the gas exchange process but also reduces the velocity of gas flow. Hairs on the nasal mucosa filter inspired air, trapping particles greater than 10 μm in diameter. Many particles settle on the nasal epithelium. Particles 2 to 10 μm in diameter fall on the mucus-covered bronchial walls (as airflow slows), initiating reflex bronchoconstriction and coughing. Ciliated columnar epithelium lines the respiratory tract from the nose to the respiratory bronchioles (except at the vocal cords). The cilia beat at a frequency of 1000 to 1500 cycles per minute, enabling them to move particles away from the lungs at a rate of 16 mm per minute. Particles less than 2 μm in diameter may reach the alveoli, where they are ingested by macrophages. If ciliary motility is defective as a result of smoking or an inherited disorder (e.g., Kartagener's syndrome or another ciliary dysmotility syndrome), the "mucus escalator" does not work, so more particles are allowed to reach the alveoli, thereby predisposing the patient to chronic pulmonary inflammation.[8]

The larynx prevents food and other foreign bodies from entering the trachea. Reflex closure of the glottic inlet occurs during swallowing[6] and periods of increased intrathoracic (e.g., coughing, sneezing) or intra-abdominal (e.g., vomiting, micturition) pressure. In unconscious patients, these reflexes are lost, so glottic closure may not occur, with an increased risk of pulmonary aspiration.

ASSESSING ADEQUACY OF THE AIRWAY

Adequacy of the airway should be considered in four aspects:

- *Patency*. Partial or complete obstruction will compromise ventilation of the lungs and likewise gas exchange.
- *Protective reflexes*. These help maintain patency and prevent aspiration of material into the lower airways.
- *Inspired oxygen concentration*. Gas entering the pulmonary alveoli must have an appropriate oxygen concentration.
- *Respiratory drive*. A patent, secure airway is of little benefit without the movement of gas between the atmosphere and the pulmonary alveoli effected through the processes of inspiration and expiration.

Patency

Airway obstruction most frequently is due to reduced muscle tone, allowing the tongue to fall backwards against the postpharyngeal wall, thereby blocking the airway. Loss of patency by this mechanism often occurs in an obtunded or anesthetized patient lying supine. Other causes include the presence of blood, mucus, vomitus, or a foreign body in the lumen of the airway or edema, inflammation, swelling, or enlargement of the tissues lining or adjacent to the airway.

Upper airway obstruction has a characteristic presentation in the spontaneously breathing patient: noisy inspiration (stridor), poor expired airflow, intercostal retraction, increased respiratory distress, and paradoxical rocking movements of the thorax and abdomen.[9] These resolve quickly if the obstruction is removed. In total airway obstruction, sounds of breathing are absent entirely, owing to complete lack of airflow through the larynx. Airway obstruction may occur in patients with an endotracheal tube (ET) or tracheostomy tube in situ due to mucous plugging or kinking of the tube or the patient's biting down on a tube placed orally. If such patients are spontaneously breathing, they will have the same symptoms and signs as just described. Patients on assisted (positive-pressure) breathing modes will have high inflation pressures, decreased tidal and minute volumes, increased end-tidal carbon dioxide levels, and decreased arterial oxygen saturation.

Protective Reflexes

The upper airway shares a common pathway with the upper gastrointestinal tract.[6] Protective reflexes, which exist to safeguard airway patency and to prevent foreign material from entering the lower respiratory tract, involve the epiglottis, the vocal cords, and the sensory supply to the pharynx and larynx.[10] Patients who can swallow normally have intact airway reflexes, and normal speech makes absence of such reflexes unlikely. Patients with a decreased level of consciousness (LOC) should be assumed to have inadequate protective reflexes.

Inspired Oxygen Concentration

Oxygen demand is elevated by the increased work of breathing associated with respiratory distress[11] and by the increased metabolic demands in critically ill or injured patients. Often, higher inspired oxygen concentrations are required to satisfy tissue oxygen demand and to prevent critical desaturations during maneuvers for managing the airway. A cuffed ET, connected to a supply of oxygen, is a sealed system in which the delivered oxygen concentration also is the inspired concentration. A patient wearing a facemask, however, inspires gas from the mask and surrounding ambient air. Because the patient will generate an initial inspiratory flow in the region of 30 to 60 L per minute, and the fresh gas flow to a mask is on the order of 5 to 15 L per minute, much of the tidal inspiration will be "room air" entrained from around the mask. The entrained room air is likely to dilute the concentration of oxygen inspired to less than 50%, even when 100% oxygen is delivered to the mask.[12] This unwelcome reduction in inspired oxygen concentration can be combatted by (1) using a mask with a reservoir bag, (2) ensuring that the mask is fitted firmly to the patient's face, (3) using a high rate of oxygen flow to the mask (15 L per minute), and (4) supplying a higher oxygen concentration. Even if 100% oxygen is delivered to such a system, the patient may be inspiring significantly less than 50% oxygen.

Respiratory Drive

A patent, protected airway will not produce adequate oxygenation or excretion of carbon dioxide without adequate respiratory drive. Changing arterial carbon dioxide tension (P_{CO_2}), by changing H^+ concentration in cerebrospinal fluid (CSF), stimulates the respiratory center, which in turn controls minute volume and therefore arterial P_{CO_2} (negative feedback).[11,13] This assumes that increased respiratory drive can produce an increase in minute ventilation (increased respiratory rate or tidal volume, or both, per breath), which may not occur if respiratory mechanics are disturbed. Brain injury and drugs such as opioids, sedatives, and alcohol are direct-acting respiratory center depressants.

Ventilation can be assessed qualitatively by looking, listening, and feeling. In a spontaneously breathing patient, listening to (and feeling) air movement while looking at the extent, nature, and frequency of thoracic movement will give an impression of ventilation. These parameters may be misleading, however. Objective assessment of minute ventilation requires P_{CO_2} measurement in arterial blood or monitoring of end-tidal carbon dioxide, which can be used as a realtime measure of the adequacy of minute ventilation.[13] If respiratory drive or minute ventilation is inadequate, positive-pressure respiratory support may be required, and any underlying factors should be addressed if possible (e.g., depressant effect of sedatives or analgesics).

MANAGEMENT OF THE AIRWAY

The aims of airway management are to provide an adequate inspired oxygen concentration; to establish a patent, secure airway; and to support ventilation if required.

Providing an Adequate Inspired Oxygen Concentration

Although oxygen can be administered via nasal cannula, this method does not ensure delivery of more than 30% to 40% oxygen (at most). Other disadvantages include lack of humidification of gases, patient discomfort with use of flow rates greater than 4 to 6 L per minute, and predisposition to nasal mucosal irritation and potential bleeding.[14] Therefore, despite being more intrusive for patients, facemasks are superior for oxygen administration. The three main types of facemask are shown in Figure 2-1:

- Anesthesia-type facemask (mask A in Fig. 2-1)—a solid mask (with no vents) with a cushioned collar to provide a good seal. This is suitable for providing very high oxygen concentrations (approaching 100%) because entrainment is minimized and the anesthetic circuit normally includes a reservoir of gas. They become unacceptable for many *awake* patients within a few minutes, because of the association with heat, moisture, and claustrophobia.
- Simple facemask—a facemask with vents that allow heat or humidity out but that also entrain room air. These masks have no seal and are relatively loose-fitting. Such masks may have a reservoir bag (approximately 500 mL), sitting inferior to the mask (B2 in Fig. 2-1), or have no reservoir (B1 in Fig. 2-1). Without a reservoir bag, it is difficult to deliver an inspired oxygen concentration of 50% even with tight application.

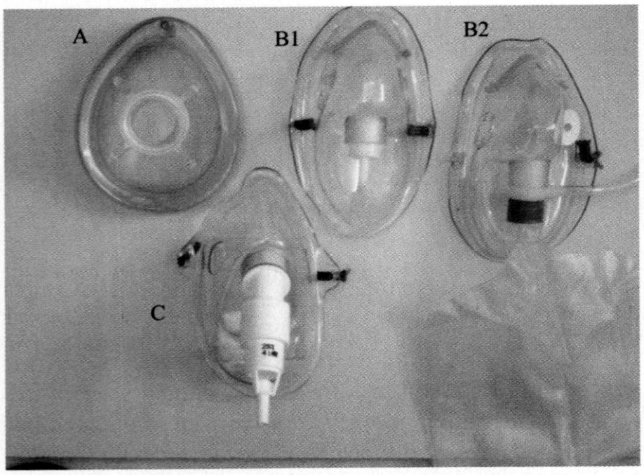

Figure 2-1. Facemasks: anesthesia mask (A); simple facemask (B1); simple facemask with reservoir bag (B2); Venturi mask (C).

- Venturi mask (C in Fig. 2-1)—a facemask with vents that entrain a known proportion of ambient air when a set flow of 100% oxygen passes through a Venturi device.[14] Thus, the inspired oxygen concentration (usually 24% to 35%) is known.

Establishing a Patent and Secure Airway

Establishing a patent and secure airway can be achieved using simple airway maneuvers, further airway adjuncts, tracheal intubation, or a surgical airway.

Airway Maneuvers

Simple airway maneuvers involve appropriate positioning, opening the airway, and keeping it open using artificial airways if needed.

Positioning for Airway Management

In the absence of any concerns about cervical spine stability (e.g., with trauma, rheumatoid arthritis, or severe osteoporosis), raising the patient's head slightly (5 to 10 cm) by means of a small pillow under the occiput can help in airway management. This adjustment extends the atlanto-occipital joint and moves the oral, pharyngeal, and laryngeal axes into better alignment, providing the best straight line to the glottis ("sniffing" position).[15,16]

Clearing the Airway

Acute airway obstruction in the obtunded patient often due to the tongue or extraneous material—liquid (saliva, blood, gastric contents) or solid (teeth, broken dentures, food) in the pharynx. In the supine position, secretions usually are cleared under direct vision using a laryngoscope and a rigid suction catheter.[17] In some cases, a flexible suction catheter, introduced through the nose and nasopharynx, may be the best means of clearing the airway. A finger sweep of the pharynx may be used to detect and remove larger solid material in unconscious patients without an intact gag reflex. During all airway interventions, if cervical spine instability cannot be ruled out, relative movement of the cervical vertebrae must be prevented—most often by manual in-line immobilization.[17,18]

Triple Airway Maneuver

The triple airway maneuver often is beneficial in obtunded patients if it is not contraindicated by concerns about cervical spine instability. As indicated by its name, this maneuver has three components: head tilt (neck extension), jaw thrust (pulling the mandible forward), and mouth opening.[19] The operator stands behind and above the patient's head. Then the maneuver is performed as follows:

- Extend the patient's neck with the operator's hands on both sides of the mandible.
- Elevate the mandible with the fingers of both hands, thereby lifting the base of the tongue away from the posterior pharyngeal wall.
- Open the mouth by pressing caudally on the anterior mandible with the thumbs or forefingers.

Artificial Airways

If the triple airway maneuver or any of its elements reduces airway obstruction, the benefit can be maintained for a prolonged period by introducing an artificial airway into the pharynx between the tongue and the posterior pharyngeal wall (Fig. 2-2).

The oropharyngeal airway (OPA) is the most commonly used artificial airway. Simple to insert, it is used temporarily to help facilitate oxygenation or ventilation before tracheal intubation. The OPA should be inserted with the convex side toward the tongue and then rotated through 180 degrees. Care must be taken to avoid pushing the tongue posteriorly, thereby worsening the obstruction. The nasopharyngeal airway (NPA) has the same indications as for the OPA but significantly more contraindications[20] (Box 2-1). It is better tolerated than the OPA, making it useful in semiconscious patients in whom the gag reflex is partially preserved. These artificial airways should be considered to be a temporary adjunct—to be replaced with a more secure airway if the patient fails to improve rapidly to the point at which an artificial airway no longer is needed. Such airways should not be used in association with *prolonged* positive-pressure ventilation.

Box 2-1

Contraindications to Insertion of Oropharyngeal and Nasopharyngeal Airways

Contraindications to Oropharyngeal Airways
- Inability to tolerate (gagging, vomiting)
- Airway swelling (burns, toxic gases, infection)
- Bleeding into the upper airway
- Absence of pharyngeal or laryngeal reflexes
- Impaired mouth opening (e.g., with trismus or temporomandibular joint dysfunction)

Contraindications to Nasopharyngeal Airways
- Narrow nasal airway in young children
- Blocked or narrow nasal passages in adults
- Airway swelling (burns, toxic gases, infection)
- Bleeding into the upper airway
- Absence of pharyngeal or laryngeal reflexes
- Fractures of the mid-face or base of skull
- Clinical scenarios in which nasal hemorrhage would be disastrous

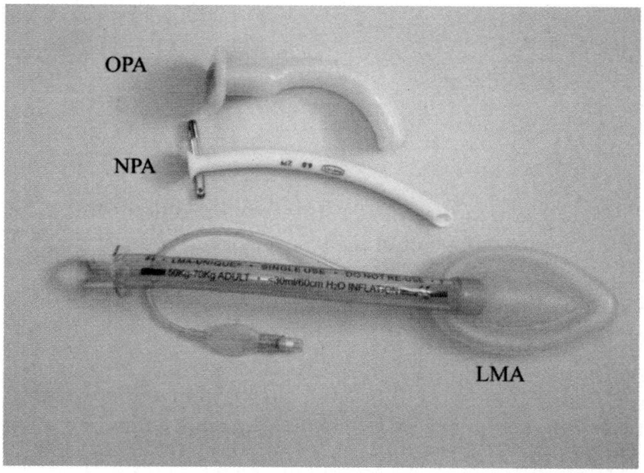

Figure 2-2. Artificial airways: oropharyngeal airway (OPA); nasopharyngeal airway (NPA,); laryngeal mask airway (LMA).

Advanced Airway Adjuncts

Advanced airway adjuncts fill the gap between simple airway maneuvers and the insertion of a tracheal tube or surgical airway. These devices can be used to facilitate safe reliable airway management and manual ventilation in the prehospital or emergency resuscitation setting, often without expert medical presence.

The laryngeal mask airway (LMA) is a small latex mask mounted on a hollow plastic tube.[121-126] It is placed "blindly" in the lower pharynx overlying the glottis. The inflatable cuff helps wedge the mask in the hypopharynx, sitting obliquely over the laryngeal inlet. Although the LMA produces a seal that will allow ventilation with gentle positive pressure, it does not definitively protect the airway from aspiration. Indications for use of the LMA in critical care are (1) as an alternative to other artificial airways, (2) the difficult airway, particularly the "can't intubate–can't ventilate" scenario, and (3) as a conduit for bronchoscopy. It is possible to pass a 6.0-mm ET through a standard LMA into the trachea, but the LMA must be left in situ. The intubating LMA (ILMA), which was developed specifically to aid intubation with a tracheal tube, has a shorter steel tube with a wider bore, a tighter curve, and a distal silicone laryngeal cuff.[27-30] A bar present near the laryngeal opening is designed to lift the epiglottis anteriorly. The ILMA allows the passage of a specially designed size 8.0 ET.

The Combitube (esophageal-tracheal double-lumen airway) is a combined esophageal obturator and tracheal tube, usually inserted blindly.[31-35] Whether the "tracheal" lumen is placed in the trachea or esophagus, the Combitube will allow ventilation of the lungs and give partial protection against aspiration. The Combitube also is a potential adjunct in the "cannot intubate–cannot ventilate" situation. Disadvantages include the inability to suction the trachea when the device is sitting in its commonest position (in the esophagus). Insertion also may cause trauma, and the Combitube is contraindicated in patients with known esophageal pathology or intact laryngeal reflexes and in persons who have ingested caustic substances.

Tracheal Intubation

If the foregoing interventions are not effective or are contraindicated, tracheal intubation is required. This modality will provide (1) a secure, potentially long-term airway; (2) a safe route to deliver positive-pressure ventilation if required; and (3) significant protection against pulmonary aspiration. *Orotracheal intubation* is the most widely used technique for clinicians practiced in direct laryngoscopy (indications and contraindications in Box 2-2). Normally, anesthesia with or without neuromuscular

Box 2-2

Orotracheal Intubation: Indications and Relative Contraindications

Indications

Long-term correction or prevention of airway obstruction
Securing the airway and protecting against pulmonary aspiration
Facilitating positive-pressure ventilation
Enabling bronchopulmonary toilet
Optimizing access to pharynx, face, or neck at surgery

Contraindications (Relative)

Possibility of cervical spine instability
Impaired mouth opening (e.g., trismus, temporomandibular joint dysfunction)
Potential difficult airway
Need for surgical immobilization of maxilla or mandible (wires, box frame)

blockade is necessary for this procedure, which is summarized in Box 2-3.

Tracheal intubation requires lack of patient awareness (as in the unconscious state or with general anesthesia) and the abolition of protective laryngeal and pharyngeal reflexes. The drugs commonly used to achieve these states are shown in Table 2-1. Anesthesia is achieved using an intravenous induction agent, although intravenous sedatives (e.g., midazolam) theoretically may be used. Opioids often are used in conjunction with induction agents because they may reduce the cardiovascular sequelae of laryngoscopy and intubation (tachycardia and hypertension) and also may contribute to the patient's unconsciousness.

Abolition of protective laryngeal and pharyngeal reflexes sometimes is achieved by inducing a deep level of unconsciousness using one or more of the aforementioned agents, followed by inhalation of high concentrations of a volatile anesthetic agent (e.g., sevoflurane, isoflurane). This technique sometimes is used in the difficult airway scenario to obtain conditions suitable for tracheal intubation in a patient who is still breathing spontaneously.

More usually, a muscle relaxant is used to abolish the protective reflexes, abduct the vocal cords, and facilitate tracheal intubation. In the elective situation, nondepolarizing neuromuscular blocking agents are used. These have the disadvantage of requiring several minutes to exert their effect, during which the patient must receive ventilation via a mask, thus allowing the possibility of gastric dilation and pulmonary aspiration. In patients at high risk of the latter (e.g., nonfasting patients), a depolarizing muscle relaxant (succinyl choline) is used because it produces suitable conditions for intubation within 15 to 20 seconds, and mask ventilation is not required. Succinylcholine has several side effects—among them hyperkalemia, muscle pains and (rarely) malignant hyperpyrexia.

Box 2-3

Procedure: Orotracheal Intubation

- Position patient and induce anesthesia ± neuromuscular blockade (if needed).
- Perform manual ventilation using triple airway maneuver and oropharyngela airway.
- Hold laryngoscope handle (left hand) near the junction with blade.
- Insert the blade along the right side of the tongue—moving tongue to the left.
- Advance tip of the blade in the midline between tongue and epiglottis.
- Pull upwards and along the line of the handle of the laryngoscope.
- Lift the epiglottis upward and visualize the vocal cords.
- Do *not* use the patient's teeth as a fulcrum when attempting to visualize the glottis.
- Pass tracheal tube through the vocal cords into the trachea (right hand).
- Stop advancing tube when cuff is 2 to 3 cm beyond the cords.
- Connect to a bag-valve system and pressurize it by squeezing bag.
- Inflate cuff until audible leak around tube stops.
- Check correct tube position (auscultation) and assess cuff pressure.
- Check end-tidal CO_2 trace.

Table 2-1. Drugs Used to Facilitate Tracheal Intubation

Drug	Dose (Intravenous)
Induction Agent	
Propofol	1-2.5 mg/kg
Opioids	
Fentanyl	1.0-1.5 μg/kg
Morphine	0.15 mg/kg
Nondepolarizing Agents	
Atracurium	0.4-0.5 mg/kg
Vecuronium	0.1 mg/kg
Rocuronium	0.45-0.6 mg/kg
Depolarizing Agent	
Succinylcholine (suxamethonium)	1.0-1.5 mg/kg

Nasotracheal intubation shares the problems and contraindications associated with the nasopharyngeal airway.[20] The technique usually is employed when there are relative contraindications to the oral route (e.g., anatomic abnormalities, cervical spine instability). Nasotracheal intubation may be achieved under direct vision or with use of a blind technique, either with the patient under general anesthesia or in the awake or lightly sedated patient with appropriate local anesthesia (Table 2-2). If orotracheal or nasotracheal intubation is required but cannot be achieved, then a surgical airway is required (see later).

Table 2-2. Procedure: Nasotracheal Intubation (Blind and under Direct Vision)

Prepare and Assess the Patient

1. Use a nasal decongestant such as phenylephrine to reduce bleeding
2. Provide local anaesthesia to nasal mucosa
3. Examine each nostril for patency and deformity
4. Choose the most patent nostril and choose appropriate sized ET
5. After induction of anaesthesia, position as for oral intubation

Blind Nasotracheal Intubation	Nasotracheal Intubation (Direct Vision)
Keep patient breathing spontaneously. Insert well-lubricated ET into the nostril (concavity forward, bevel lateral). While passing ET along nasal floor, listen for audible breathing through the tube. Advance ET, rotating as needed to maintain clear breath sounds. ET will pass through cords, and patient may cough. Technique takes time so it is not suitable for a desaturating patient. Do not force passage of ET because this could cause bleeding.	Patient may be apneic with or without relaxants. Gently advance ET through the nose. When ET tip is in oropharynx, perform laryngoscopy. Visualize ET in pharynx and advance toward glottis. Advance ET through cords into trachea, under direct vision if possible. Use Magill forceps if required to guide tip while advancing ET. Try to avoid damaging cuff if using forceps to help passage through cords.

With a need for isolation of one lung from another, a double-lumen tube (having one cuffed tracheal lumen and one cuffed bronchial lumen fused longitudinally) can be used.[36] The main indications are (1) to facilitate some pulmonary or thoracic surgical procedures; (2) to isolate a lung containing contaminated fluid (e.g., in lung abscess) or blood, thereby preventing contralateral spread; and (3) to enable differential or independent lung ventilation (ILV). ILV allows each lung to be treated separately—for example, to deliver positive-pressure ventilation with high positive end-expiratory pressure (PEEP) to one lung while applying low levels of continuous positive airway pressure (CPAP) only to the other. Such a strategy may be advantageous in cases of pulmonary air leak (bronchopleural fistula, bronchial tear, or severe lung trauma) or in severe unilateral lung disease requiring ventilatory support.[37,38]

Providing Ventilatory Support

If a patient has no (or inadequate) spontaneous ventilation, then a means of generating gas flow to the lower respiratory tract must be provided. Negative pressure, mimicking the actions of the respiratory muscles, occasionally is used in some patients who require long-term ventilation. In acute care, however, ventilation is achieved using positive pressure, which requires an unobstructed airway; in the nonintubated patient, this is best achieved by proper positioning, the triple airway maneuver, and use of an OPA or NPA. In a patient without an ET in place, particularly if some degree of airway obstruction exists, positive-pressure ventilation often will cause gastric distention and (potentially) regurgitation and pulmonary aspiration.

Bag-Valve-Mask Ventilation

Ventilation with a mask requires an (almost) airtight fit between mask and face. This is best achieved by firmly pressing the mask against the patient's face using the thumb and index finger (C-grip) while pulling the mandible upward toward the mask with the other three fingers. The other hand is used to squeeze the reservoir bag, generating positive pressure. Excessive pressure from the C-grip on the mask may lead to backward movement of the mandible with subsequent airway obstruction, or a tilt of the mask with leakage of gas. If a proper seal is difficult to attain, placing a hand on each side of the mask and mandible is advised, with a second person manually compressing the reservoir bag (four-handed ventilation). Bag-valve-mask systems have a self-reinflating bag, which springs back after compression, thereby drawing gas in through a port with a one-way valve. It is important to have a large reservoir bag with a continuous flow of oxygen attached to this port in order to ensure a high inspired oxygen concentration.[39,40] Bag-valve-mask ventilation usually is a short-term measure in urgent situations or is used in preparation for tracheal intubation.

Prolonged Ventilation Using a Sealed Tube in the Trachea

Ventilation of the lungs with a bag-valve-mask arrangement is difficult if required for more than a few minutes or if the patient needs to be transported. In these instances, ventilation through a sealed tube in the trachea is indicated. Orotracheal or nasotracheal intubation, surgical cricothyrotomy, and tracheostomy all achieve the same result: a cuffed tube in the trachea, allowing the use of positive-pressure ventilation and protecting the lungs from aspiration. Mechanical ventilation is discussed in Chapter 9.

Apneic Oxygenation

Apneic oxygenation is achieved using a narrow catheter that sits in the trachea and carries a flow of 100% oxygen. The catheter may be passed into the trachea via an ET or under direct vision through the larynx. This apparatus can be set up as a low-flow open system (gas flow rate of 5 to 8 L per minute) or as a high-pressure (jet ventilation) system[41] and can be used to maintain oxygenation with a difficult airway either at intubation or at extubation (see later).

PHYSIOLOGIC SEQUELAE AND COMPLICATIONS OF TRACHEAL INTUBATION

Laryngoscopy is a noxious stimulus that, in an awake or lightly sedated patient, would provoke coughing, retching, or vomiting and laryngospasm. In clinical practice, however, laryngoscopy and tracheal intubation usually are performed after induction of anesthesia, and in emergency situations, the patient often is hypoxic and hypercarbic, with increased sympathetic nervous system activity (SNA). Thus, the physiologic effects of laryngoscopy and tracheal intubation tend to be masked.

Laryngoscopy and intubation cause an increase in circulating catecholamines and increased SNA, leading to hypertension and tachycardia. This represents an increase in myocardial work and myocardial oxygen demand, which may provoke cardiac dysrhythmias and myocardial hypoxia or ischemia. Laryngoscopy increases cerebral blood flow and intracranial pressure—particularly in patients who are hypoxic or hypercarbic at the time of intubation.[42] This rise in intracranial pressure will be exaggerated if cerebral venous drainage is impeded by violent coughing, bucking, or breath-holding.

Coughing and laryngospasm occur frequently in patients undergoing laryngoscopy and intubation when muscle relaxation and anesthesia are inadequate. Increased bronchial smooth muscle tone, which increases airway resistance, may occur as a reflex response to laryngoscopy or may be due to the physical presence of the ET in the trachea; in its most severe form, termed bronchospasm, this increased tone causes audible wheeze and ventilatory difficulty. Increased resistance to gas flow will occur because the cross-sectional area of the ET is less than that of the airway. This difference usually is unimportant with positive-pressure ventilation but causes a significant increase in work of breathing in spontaneously breathing patients. Resistance is directly related to $1/r^4$ (where r is the radius of the ET) and will be minimized by use of a large-bore ET. Gas passing through an ET, bypassing the nasal cavity, also loses the beneficial effects of warming, humidification, and the addition of traces of nitric oxide (NO).[43]

The effects of intubation on functional residual capacity (FRC) are complex. In patients under anesthesia, a fall in FRC is well documented. This decrease may be due to the loss of respiratory muscle tone following induction of anesthesia and the relatively unopposed effect of the elastic recoil in the lungs.[43] The increased resistance to gas flow due to the presence of the ET may slow expiration, producing intrinsic PEEP (and therefore an increase in FRC) if the next inspiration begins before expiration is complete.

Laryngoscopy and intubation may cause bruising, abrasion, laceration, bleeding or displacement or dislocation of the structures in and near the airway (e.g., lips, teeth or dental prostheses, tongue, epiglottis, vocal cords, laryngeal cartilages). Dislodged structures such as teeth or dentures may be aspirated, blocking the airway more distally. Less common complications include perforation of the airway with the potential for the development of a retropharyngeal abscess or mediastinitis. Over time, erosions due to pressure and ischemia may develop on the lips or tongue (or external nares and anterior nose in patients with a nasotracheal tube) and in the larynx or upper trachea.[44] These lesions result in a breach of the mucosa with the potential for secondary infection. In the case of the lips and tongue, such lesions are (temporarily) disfiguring and painful and may inhibit attempts to talk or swallow.

The mucosa of the upper trachea (subglottic area) is subjected to the pressure of the cuff of the ET. This pressure reduces perfusion of the tracheal mucosa and, combined with the mechanical movement of the tube (from patient head movements, nursing procedures, or rhythmic flexion with action of the ventilator), tends to cause mucosal damage and increase the risk of superficial infection. These processes may lead to ulceration of the tracheal mucosa, fibrous scarring, contraction, and ultimately stenosis, which can be a life-limiting or life-threatening problem. Although irrefutable evidence is lacking, most clinicians believe that limiting the period of orotracheal or nasotracheal intubation and reducing cuff pressures may reduce the frequency of this complication.[44]

Any tube in the trachea has a significant effect on the mechanisms protecting the airway from aspiration and infection. The mucus escalator may be inhibited by mucosal injury and by the lack of warm humidified airflow over the respiratory epithelium.[45] The disruption of normal swallowing results in the pooling of saliva and other debris in the pharynx and larynx above the upper surface of the tube's inflatable cuff, which may become the source of respiratory infection if the secretions become colonized with microorganisms, or may pass beyond the cuff into the lower airways—that is, pulmonary aspiration (silent or overt).[46,47] The former may occur due to (1) colonization of the gastric secretions and the regurgitation of this material up the esophagus to the pharynx or (2) transmission of microorganisms from the health care environment to the pharynx via medical equipment or the hands of hospital staff or visitors (cross-infection).[45,47-50]

The presence of a tube traversing the larynx and sealing the trachea makes phonation impossible. The implications of this limitation for patients and their families often are ignored. If patients cannot tell caregivers about pain, nausea, or other concerns, they may become frustrated, agitated, or violent. This may result in the excessive use of sedative or psychoactive drugs, which prolong time on ventilation and stay in the intensive care unit (ICU), with the risk of infection increased accordingly.[51] The inability to communicate may therefore be a real threat to patient survival. Potential solutions involve the use of letter and picture boards, "speaking valves" (with tracheostomy), laryngeal microphones, or computer-based communication packages. The involvement and innovations of disciplines such as the speech and language center may be advantageous.

THE DIFFICULT AIRWAY

The difficult airway has been defined as "the clinical situation in which a conventionally trained anesthetist experiences difficulty with mask ventilation of the upper airway, tracheal intubation, or both."[52] It has been a commonly documented cause of adverse events including airway injury, hypoxic brain injury, and death under anesthesia.[53-59] The frequency of difficulty with mask ventilation has been estimated to be between 1.4% and 7.8%,[60-62] while tracheal intubation using direct laryngoscopy is difficult in 1.5% to 8.5% and impossible in up to 0.5% of general anesthetics.[58,63] The incidence of failed intubation is approximately 1:2000 in the nonobstetric population and 1:300 in the obstetric population.[64] In the critical care unit, up to 20% of all critical incidents are airway related,[65-67] and such incidents may occur at intubation, at extubation, or during the course of treatment (as with the acutely displaced or obstructed ET or tracheostomy tube).

Recognizing the Potentially Difficult Airway

Many conditions are associated with airway difficulty (Table 2-3), including anatomic abnormalities, which may result in an unusual appearance, thereby alerting the examiner. The goal is to identify the potentially difficult airway and develop a plan to secure it. Factors including age older than 55 years, body mass index greater than 26 kg/m^2, presence of a beard, lack of teeth, and a history of snoring have been identified as independent variables

Table 2-3. Conditions Associated with Difficult Airway

Causative Factor	Associated Conditions/Disorders
Abnormal facial anatomy/development	Small mouth and/or large tongue Dental abnormality Prognathia Obesity Advanced pregnancy Acromegaly Congenital syndromes*
Inability to open mouth	Masseter muscle spasm (dental abscess) Temporomandibular joint dysfunction Facial burns Postradiotherapy fibrosis Scleroderma
Cervical immobility/abnormality	Short neck/obesity Poor cervical mobility (e.g., ankylosing spondylitis) Previous cervical spine surgery Presence of cervical collar Postradiotherapy fibrosis
Pharyngeal or laryngeal abnormality	High or anterior larynx Deep vallecula: inability to reach base of epiglottis with blade of scope Anatomic abnormality of epiglottis or hypopharynx (e.g., tumor) Subglottic stenosis
Injury	Traumatic debris Obstructing foreign bodies Basilar skull fracture Bleeding into airway or adjacent swelling/hematoma Fractured maxilla/mandible Cervical spine instability (confirmed or potential) Laryngeal fracture or disruption
Infections	Epiglottitis Abscess Croup, brochiolitis Laryngeal papillomatosis Tetanus—trismus
Connective tissue/inflammatory	Rheumatoid arthritis—temporomandibular joint or cervical spine involvement, cricoarytenoid arthritis Ankylosing spondylitis Scleroderma Sarcoidosis
Endocrine disorders	Goiter: airway compression or deviation Hypothyroidism, acromegaly: large tongue

*Visit http://www.erlanger.org/craniofacial and http://www.faces-cranio.org for specific details.
Data from Criswell JC, Parr MJA, Nolan JP: Emergency airway management in patients with cervical spine injuries. Anaesthesia 1994;49:900-903; and Morikawa S, Safar P, DeCarlo J: Influence of head position upon upper airway patency. Anaesthesiology 1961;22:265.

predicting difficulty with mask ventilation—in turn associated with difficult tracheal intubation.[61,68]

Mallampati[69] developed a grading system (subsequently modified[64]) that predicted ease of tracheal intubation at direct laryngoscopy. The predictive value of the Mallampati system has been shown to be limited[70,71] because many factors that have no influence on the Mallampati classification—mobility of head and neck, mandibular or maxillary development, dentition, compliance of neck structures, and body shape—can influence laryngeal view.[53,66,72,73] A study of a complex system including some of these factors found the rate of difficult intubation to be 1.5%, but with a false-positive rate of 12%.[74] A risk index based on the Mallampati classification, a history of difficult intubation, and five other variables lacked sufficient sensitivity and specificity.[75] Airway management should be based on the fact that the difficult airway cannot be reliably predicted.[76,77] This is a particularly important consideration in the critical care environment.

The Obstructed Airway

Although the most common reason for an obstructed airway in the un-intubated patient is posterior displacement of the tongue in association with a depressed level of consciousness, it is the less common causes that provide the greatest challenges. It is important to elucidate the level at which the obstruction occurs and the nature of the obstructing lesion. This may be due to infection or edema (epiglottis, pharyngeal or tonsillar abscess, mediastinal abscess), neoplasm (primary malignant or benign tumor, metastastic spread, direct extension from nearby structures), thyroid enlargement, vascular lesions, trauma, or foreign body or impacted food.[14,78]

Airway lesions above the level of the vocal cords are considered to lie in the upper airway and commonly manifest with stridor.[79] If breathing is labored and associated with difficulties at night, rather than just noisy, then the narrowing probably is more than 50%. Patients with these lesions usually fall into one of two groups: (1) those who can be intubated, usually under inhalational induction, with the ENT surgeon immediately available to perform rigid bronchoscopy or tracheostomy if required, or (2) those who require a tracheostomy placed using local anesthesia. In patients with mid-tracheal obstruction, CT imaging usually is necessary to discover the exact level and nature of the obstruction and to allow planning of airway management for nonemergency clinical presentations.[79] Tracheostomy often is not beneficial because the tube may not be long enough to bypass the obstruction. In such instances, fiberoptic intubation often may be useful.[79] Lower tracheal obstruction often is due to space-occupying lesions in the mediastinum and necessitates multidisciplinary planning involving ENT, cardiothoracic surgery, anesthesia, and critical care.

Trauma and the Airway

Airway management in the trauma victim provides additional challenges because the victim often has other life-threatening conditions and preparation time for management of the difficult airway is limited. Approximately 15% of severely injured patients have maxillofacial involvement, and 5% to 10% of patients with blunt trauma have an associated cervical spine injury (often associated with head injury).[80]

Problems encountered in trauma patients include presence in the airway of debris or foreign bodies (e.g., teeth), vomitus, or regurgitated gastric contents; airway edema; tongue swelling; blood and bleeding; and fractures (maxilla and mandible). Patients must be assumed to have a full stomach (requiring bimanual cricoid pressure and a rapid-sequence induction for intubation) and many will have pulmonary aspiration before the airway in secured. An important consideration in most cases is the need to avoid movement of the cervical spine at laryngoscopy or intubation.[17,18] Direct injury to the larynx is rare but may result in laryngeal disruption, producing progressive hoarseness and subcutaneous emphysema. Tracheal intubation, if attempted, requires great care and skill because it may cause further laryngeal disruption. With Le Fort fractures, airway obstruction or compromised respiration requiring immediate airway control is present in 25% of cases.[81] Postoperative bleeding after operations to the neck (thyroid gland, carotid, larynx) may compress or displace the airway, leading to difficulty in intubation.

The Airway Practitioner and the Clinical Setting

Although airway difficulties often are due to anatomic factors as discussed, it is important to recognize that the inability to perform an airway maneuver also may be due to a practitioner's inexperience or lack of skill.[82-87] Expert opinion and clinical evidence also identify lack of skilled assistance as a factor in airway-related adverse events.[88-91] As might be expected, inexperience and lack of suitable help may contribute to failure in optimizing the conditions for laryngoscopy (Box 2-4). Airway and ventilatory management performed in the prehospital setting or in the hospital but outside an operating room (OR) carries a higher frequency of adverse events and a higher mortality rate when compared with anesthesia in an OR.[92-96] In the critical care unit, all invasive airway maneuvers are potentially difficult.[97] Positioning is more difficult on an ICU bed than on an OR table. The airway structures may be edematous after previous laryngoscopy or presence of an ET. Neck immobility, or the need to avoid movement in a

Box 2-4

Common Errors Compromising Successful Intubation

- Poor patient positioning
- Failure to ensure appropriate assistance
- Faulty light source in laryngoscope or no alternative scope
- Failure to use a longer blade in appropriate patients
- Use of inappropriate tracheal tube (size or shape)
- Lack of immediate availability of airway adjuncts

potentially unstable cervical spine, may be other contributing factors.[98-100] Poor gas exchange in ICU patients reduces the effectiveness of preoxygenation and increases the risk of significant hypoxia before the airway is secured.[101] Cardiovascular instability may produce hypotension or hypoperfusion, or may lead to misleading oximetry readings (including failure to record any value at all), a further confounding factor for the attending staff.[102,103]

Managing the Difficult Airway

Management of the difficult airway can be considered in the framework of three possible clinical scenarios with progressively increasing risks for the patient: (1) the anticipated difficult airway; (2) the unanticipated difficult airway; and (3) the difficult airway resulting in a "cannot intubate and cannot ventilate" situation.

Requirements for clinicians involved in airway management include the following:

- Expertise in recognition and assessment of the potentially difficult airway. This involves the use of the assessment techniques above and a "sixth sense."[76]
- The ability to formulate a plan (with alternatives).[52,53,104-106]
- Familiarity with algorithm(s) that outline a sequence of actions designed to maintain oxygenation, ventilation, and patient safety. The ASA guidelines[52] and the composite plan from the Difficult Airway Society (DAS)[104] are shown in Figures 2-3 and 2-4. The latter summarizes four airway plans (A-D), available from the DAS website (www.das.uk.com).
- The skills and experience to use a number of airway adjuncts, particularly those relevant to the unanticipated difficult airway.

The Anticipated Difficult Airway

The anticipated difficult airway is the "least lethal" of the three scenarios—with time to consider strategy, optimize patient status, and obtain appropriate adjuncts and personnel. The key questions are as follows:

1. Should the patient be kept awake or be anesthetized for intubation?
2. Which technique should be used for intubation?

Awake Intubation

Awake intubation is more time-consuming, requires experienced personnel, is less pleasant for the patient (compared with intubation under anesthesia), and may have to be abandoned as a result of the patient's inability or unwillingness to cooperate. Because spontaneous breathing and pharyngeal or laryngeal muscle tone is maintained, however, it is significantly safer. The techniques available are fiberoptic and retrograde intubation. It also may be used in patients judged to be at risk for a difficult airway, whereupon an initial direct laryngoscopic view allows intubation.

Fiberoptic Intubation Fiberoptic intubation is a technique in which a flexible endoscope with a tracheal tube loaded along its length is passed through the glottis. The tracheal tube is then pushed off the endoscope and into the trachea, and the endoscope is withdrawn. An informed patient, trained assistance, and adequate preparation time make fiberoptic intubation less stressful. The nasotracheal route is used most often and requires the use of nasal vasoconstrictors. Nebulized local anesthetic is delivered to the airway via facemask. Sedation may be given, but ideally the patient should remain breathing spontaneously and responsive to verbal commands. The procedure often is time-consuming and tends to be used in elective situations[107] (Box 2-5).

Box 2-5

Indications for Fiberoptic Intubation

- Anticipated difficult intubation
- Avoidance of dental damage in high-risk patient
- Direct laryngeal trauma
- Other need for awake intubation

Retrograde Intubation For retrograde intubation,[108,109] local anesthesia is provided and the cricothyroid membrane is punctured by a needle through which a wire or catheter is passed upward through the vocal cords. When it reaches the pharynx, the wire is visualized, brought out through the mouth, and then used to guide the ET through the vocal cords before it is withdrawn. This technique also can be used to guide a fiberoptic scope through the vocal cords. Owing to time constraints, it is not suitable for emergency airway access and is contraindicated in any patient with an expanding neck hematoma or coagulopathy.

Intubation under Anesthesia

It may be decided, in spite of the safety advantage of awake intubation, to anesthetize the patient before attempted intubation. Preparation of the patient, equipment, and staff is paramount (Box 2-6). Adjuncts such as those described later should be available, either to improve the chances of intubation or to provide a safe alternative airway if intubation cannot be achieved.

Unanticipated Airway Difficulty

The unanticipated difficult airway allows only a short period to solve the problem if significant hypoxemia, hypercarbia, and hemodynamic instability are to be avoided. The patient usually is anesthetized, may be apneic, and may have received muscle relaxants, and previous initial attempt(s) at intubation may have been unsuccessful. If appropriate equipment, assistance, and experience are not immediately to hand, little time is available to obtain them. Nevertheless, it is essential to maintain oxygenation and avoid hypercarbia if possible—commonly by mask ventilation with 100% oxygen. The four-handed technique often is used.

If the practitioner is inexperienced, if the patient has had no (or a relatively short-acting) muscle relaxant, and if ventilation is not a problem, it may be appropriate to let the patient recover consciousness. An awake intubation

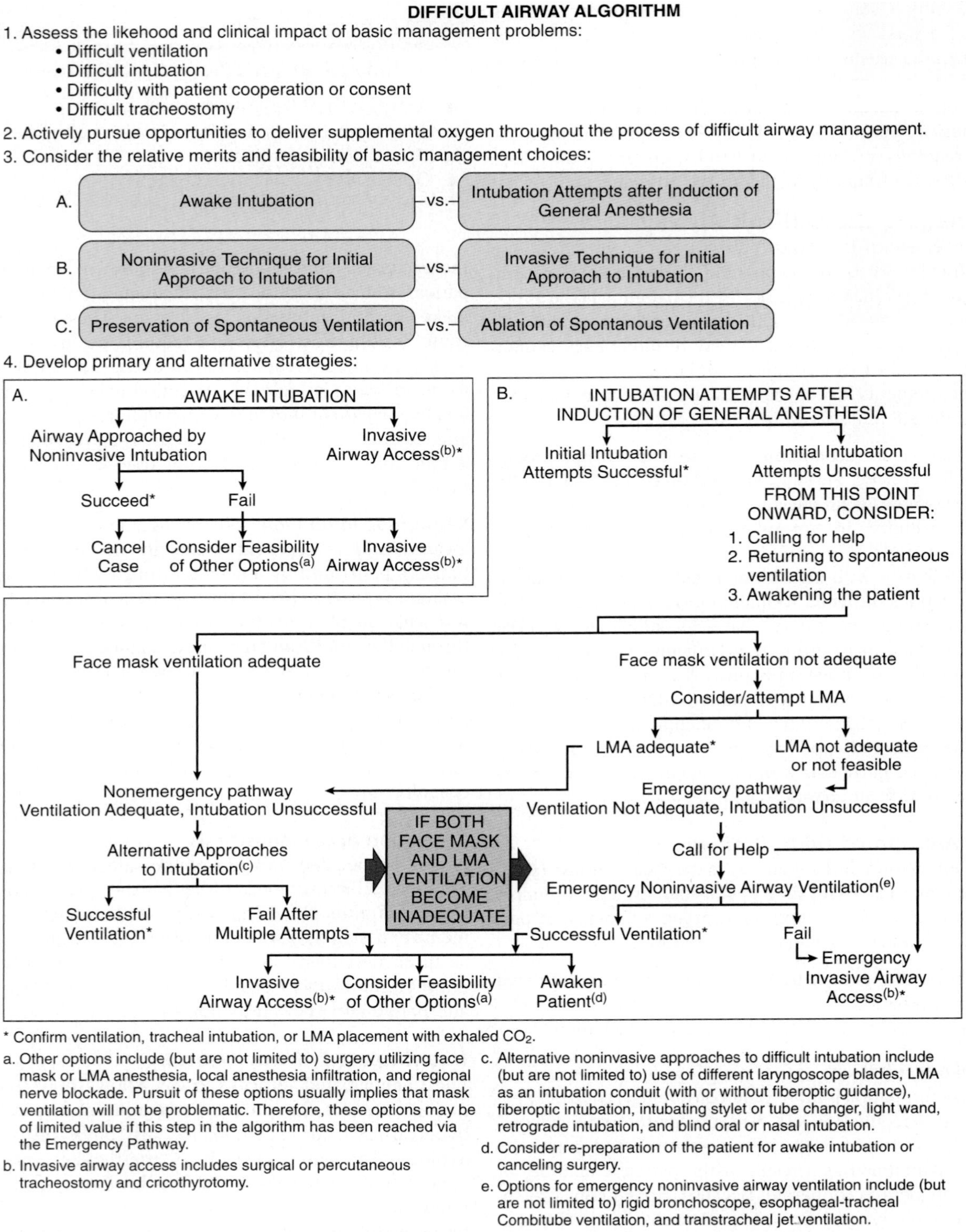
DIFFICULT AIRWAY ALGORITHM
1. Assess the likehood and clinical impact of basic management problems:
• Difficult ventilation
• Difficult intubation
• Difficulty with patient cooperation or consent
• Difficult tracheostomy
2. Actively pursue opportunities to deliver supplemental oxygen throughout the process of difficult airway management.
3. Consider the relative merits and feasibility of basic management choices:
A. Awake Intubation -vs.- Intubation Attempts after Induction of General Anesthesia
B. Noninvasive Technique for Initial Approach to Intubation -vs.- Invasive Technique for Initial Approach to Intubation
C. Preservation of Spontaneous Ventilation -vs.- Ablation of Spontanous Ventilation
4. Develop primary and alternative strategies:
A. AWAKE INTUBATION
Airway Approached by Noninvasive Intubation
Invasive Airway Access(b)*
Succeed*
Fail
Cancel Case
Consider Feasibility of Other Options(a)
Invasive Airway Access(b)*
B. INTUBATION ATTEMPTS AFTER INDUCTION OF GENERAL ANESTHESIA
Initial Intubation Attempts Successful*
Initial Intubation Attempts Unsuccessful
FROM THIS POINT ONWARD, CONSIDER:
1. Calling for help
2. Returning to spontaneous ventilation
3. Awakening the patient
Face mask ventilation adequate
Face mask ventilation not adequate
Consider/attempt LMA
LMA adequate*
LMA not adequate or not feasible
Nonemergency pathway
Ventilation Adequate, Intubation Unsuccessful
Emergency pathway
Ventilation Not Adequate, Intubation Unsuccessful
IF BOTH FACE MASK AND LMA VENTILATION BECOME INADEQUATE
Alternative Approaches to Intubation(c)
Call for Help
Emergency Noninvasive Airway Ventilation(e)
Successful Ventilation*
Fail After Multiple Attempts
Successful Ventilation*
Fail
Emergency Invasive Airway Access(b)*
Invasive Airway Access(b)*
Consider Feasibility of Other Options(a)
Awaken Patient(d)
* Confirm ventilation, tracheal intubation, or LMA placement with exhaled CO2.
a. Other options include (but are not limited to) surgery utilizing face mask or LMA anesthesia, local anesthesia infiltration, and regional nerve blockade. Pursuit of these options usually implies that mask ventilation will not be problematic. Therefore, these options may be of limited value if this step in the algorithm has been reached via the Emergency Pathway.
b. Invasive airway access includes surgical or percutaneous tracheostomy and cricothyrotomy.
c. Alternative noninvasive approaches to difficult intubation include (but are not limited to) use of different laryngoscope blades, LMA as an intubation conduit (with or without fiberoptic guidance), fiberoptic intubation, intubating stylet or tube changer, light wand, retrograde intubation, and blind oral or nasal intubation.
d. Consider re-preparation of the patient for awake intubation or canceling surgery.
e. Options for emergency noninvasive airway ventilation include (but are not limited to) rigid bronchoscope, esophageal-tracheal Combitube ventilation, and transtracheal jet ventilation.

Figure 2-3. Algorithm for managing the difficult airway. (Adapted from Practice guidelines for management of the difficult airway: An updated report by the American Society of Anesthesiologists Task Force on Management of the Difficult Airway. Anaesthesia 2003;98:1269.)

can then be planned either after a short period of recovery or on another occasion. With an experienced practitioner, it may be appropriate to continue, using techniques to improve the chances of visualizing and intubating the larynx. As discussed next, various adjuncts may be useful in this situation and also in the anticipated difficult airway when it has been decided to intubate with the patient under anesthesia.

Bimanual Laryngoscopy

Application of pressure on the cricoid area or the upper anterior tracheal wall, or both, by the laryngoscopist (a

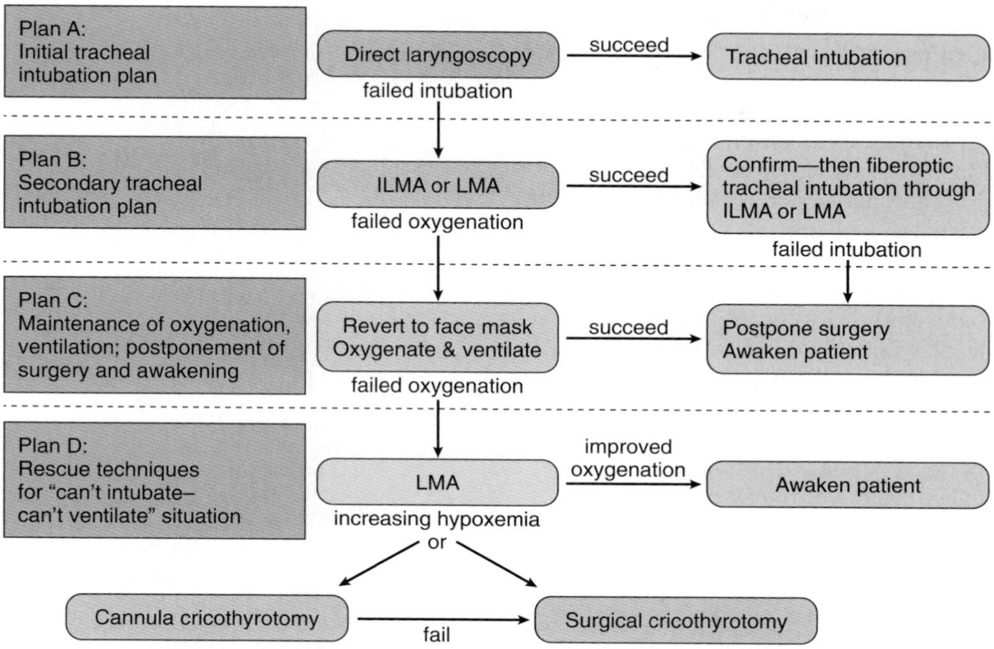

Figure 2-4. A four-component algorithm for managing the difficult airway. (From Difficult Airway Society: Difficult Airway Society Composite Plan. Anaesthesia 2004;59: 675-694.)

Box 2-6

Checklist for Anticipated Difficult Intubation of Patient under General Anesthesia

Prepare and assess the patient.
Prepare and test the equipment.
Ensure skilled assistance with knowledge of BURP/bimanual laryngoscopy.
Have available:

- A range of tracheal tubes lubricated and cuffs tested for patency (*women:* 7.0 to 7.5 mm in internal diameter; *men:* 7.5 to 9.0 mm in internal diameter).
- Endotracheal tube stylets
- Laryngeal mask airway (LMA)
- A range of laryngoscopes including specialized blades and handles

Check battery and bulb function.
Check functioning of suction devices.
Use optimal patient position.
Preoxygenation with 100% oxygen for 3 to 5 minutes if possible
Provide other equipment as desired:

- Gum elastic bougie*
- Lighted stylet*
- Combitube*
- Intubating LMA*
- Fiberoptic scope*

*Depending on choice of individual practitioner.
BURP, *b*ackward, *u*pward, and *r*ightward *p*ressure.

technique sometimes termed bimanual laryngoscopy) may improve laryngeal view.[110,111] When the view is optimized, an assistant maintains the pressure and thus the position of the larynx, freeing the hand of the laryngoscopist to perform the intubation. The use of "blind" cricoid pressure, or BURP (backward, upward, and rightward pressure), by an assistant may impair laryngeal visualization.[112-114]

Stylet ("Introducer") and Gum Elastic Bougie

The *stylet* is a smooth, malleable metal or plastic rod that is placed inside an ET to adjust the curvature—typically into a J or hockey-stick shape to allow the tip of the ET tube to be directed through a poorly visualized or unseen glottis.[115] The stylet must not project beyond the end of the ET, to avoid potential laceration or perforation of the airway.

The *gum elastic bougie* is a blunt-ended, malleable rod which at direct laryngoscopy may be passed through the poorly or nonvisualized larynx by putting a J-shaped bend at the tip and passing it blind in the mid-line upward beyond the base of the epiglottis. Then, keeping the laryngoscope in the same position in the pharynx, the ET can be "railroaded" over the bougie, which is then withdrawn. For many critical care practitioners, it is the first-choice adjunct in the difficult intubation situation.[111,116]

Different Laryngoscope or Blade

Greater than 50 types of curved and straight laryngoscope blades are available, the most commonly used being the curved Macintosh blade.[20] Using specific blades in certain circumstances has been both encouraged[117-119] and discouraged.[120] In patients with a large lower jaw or "deep pharynx," the view at laryngoscopy is often improved significantly, by using a size 4 Macintosh blade (rather than the more common adult size 3). This ensures the tip of the blade can reach the base of the vallecula to lift the epiglottis. Other blades, such as the McCoy, may be advantageous in specific situations.[121,122]

Lighted Stylet

A lighted stylet (light wand) is a malleable fiberoptic light source that can be passed along the lumen of an ET to facilitate blind intubation by transillumination. It allows the tracheal lumen to be distinguished from the (more posterior) esophagus on the basis of the greater intensity of light visible through anterior soft tissues of the neck as the ET passes beyond the vocal cords.[123] In elective anesthesia, the intubation time and failure rate with light wand–assisted intubation were similar to those with direct laryngoscopy,[124] and in a large North American survey, the light wand was the preferred alternative airway device in the difficult intubation scenario.[125] A potential disadvantage is the need for low ambient light, which may not be desirable (or easily achieved) in a critical care setting.

Fiberoptic Intubation

The fiberoptic bronchoscope can be used in the unanticipated difficult airway if it is readily available and the operator is skilled.[58,126,127] With an anesthetized patient, the technique may be more difficult. Loss of muscle tone will tend to allow the epiglottis and tongue to fall back against the pharyngeal wall. This can be counteracted by lifting the mandible.

Cannot Intubate–Cannot Ventilate

"Cannot intubate–cannot ventilate" is an uncommon but life-threatening situation best managed by adherence to an appropriate algorithm.[52,53,104] All personnel involved will be pressured (and motivated) by the potential for severe injury to the patient. Efficient teamwork will be more likely in an environment that is relatively calm. Although it may be difficult, shouting, impatience, anger, and panic should be avoided in such situations. Figure 2-5 presents a simple flow sheet summarizing the appropriate actions.[128]

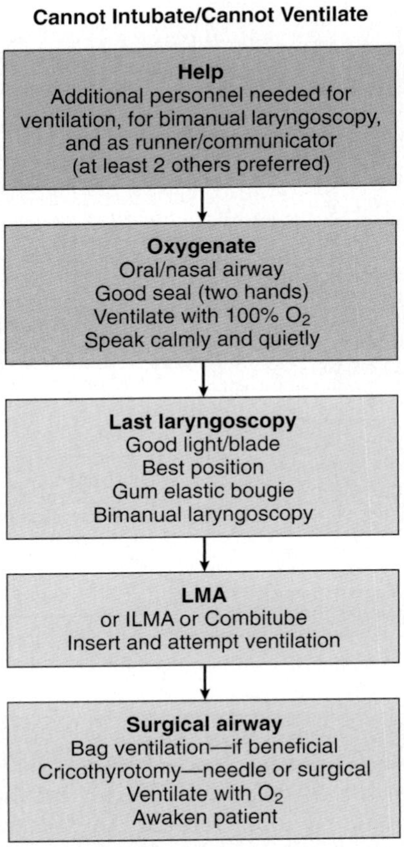

Cannot Intubate/Cannot Ventilate
Help
Additional personnel needed for ventilation, for bimanual laryngoscopy, and as runner/communicator (at least 2 others preferred)
Oxygenate
Oral/nasal airway
Good seal (two hands)
Ventilate with 100% O2
Speak calmly and quietly
Last laryngoscopy
Good light/blade
Best position
Gum elastic bougie
Bimanual laryngoscopy
LMA
or ILMA or Combitube
Insert and attempt ventilation
Surgical airway
Bag ventilation—if beneficial
Cricothyrotomy—needle or surgical
Ventilate with O2
Awaken patient

Figure 2-5. Flow chart for the cannot intubate–cannot ventilate scenario.

CONFIRMING TUBE POSITION IN THE TRACHEA

A critical factor in the difficult airway scenario, potentially leading to death or brain injury, is failure to recognize misplacement of the ET. Attempted intubation of the trachea may result in esophageal intubation. This alone is not life-threatening unless it goes unrecognized.[129] Thus, confirmation of ET placement in the trachea is essential.

Visualizing the ET as it passes between the vocal cords into the trachea is the definitive means of assessing correct tube positioning. This may not always be possible, however, owing to poor visualization. In addition, the laryngoscopist may be reluctant to accept that the ET is not in the trachea. Several clinical observations support the presence of the ET in the trachea.

Chest wall movement with positive-pressure ventilation (manual or mechanical) is usual but may be absent in patients with chronic obstructive pulmonary disease (COPD), obesity, or decreased compliance (e.g., in severe bronchospasm. Although condensation of water vapor in the ET suggests that the expired gas is from the lungs, this also may occur with esophageal intubation. The *absence of water vapor* usually is indicative of esophageal intubation. *Auscultation of breath sounds* (in both axillae) supports correct tube positioning but is not absolute confirmation.[130] Apparent inequality of breath sounds heard in the axillae may suggest intubation of a bronchus by an ET which has passed beyond the carina. Of note, after emergency intubation and clinical confirmation of the ET in the trachea, 15% of ETs may still be inappropriately close to the carina.[131]

The use of capnography to detect *end-tidal carbon dioxide* is the most reliable objective method of confirming tube position and is increasingly available in critical care.[132] False-positive results may be obtained initially when exhaled gases enter the esophagus during mask ventilation[133] or when the patient is generating carbon dioxide in the gastrointestinal tract (as with recent ingestion of carbonated beverages or bicarbonate-based antacids).[134] A false-negative result (ET in trachea but no carbon dioxide gas detected) may be obtained when pulmonary blood flow is minimal, as in cardiac arrest.[135] Visualizing the trachea or carina through a *fiberoptic bronchoscope,* which may be readily available in critical care, also will confirm correct placement of the ET.

SURGICAL AIRWAY

The indication for a surgical airway is inability to intubate the trachea in a patient who requires it, and the techniques available are cricothyrotomy and tracheostomy.

Cricothyrotomy

Cricothryotomy may be performed as a percutaneous (needle) or open surgical procedure (Table 2-4). The indication for both these techniques is the cannot intubate–cannot ventilate situation. Although needle cricothyrotomy is an emergency airway procedure, the technique is similar to that for "mini-tracheostomy," which is performed electively. Unlike the other surgical airway techniques, a needle cricothyrotomy does *not* create a definitive airway. It will not allow excretion of carbon dioxide but will produce satisfactory oxygenation for 30 to 40 minutes. It can be viewed as a form of apneic ventilation (see later on). There are several methods of connecting the intravenous cannula to a gas delivery circuit with the facility to ventilate, using equipment and connections readily available in the hospital. The appropriate method thus should be thought out in advance and available on the difficult airway trolley or bag. New commercial kits that come preassembled also are available.

A surgical cricothyrotomy allows a cuffed tube to be inserted through the cricothyroid membrane into the lower larynx or upper trachea. This allows positive-pressure ventilation for considerable periods and also protects against pulmonary aspiration.

Tracheostomy

A tracheostomy is an opening in the trachea—usually between the second and third tracheal rings or one space higher—that may be created surgically or made percutaneously.[136-140] The indications for and contraindications to tracheostomy are summarized in Box 2-7. In comparison with long-term orotracheal or nasotracheal intubation, tracheostomy often contributes to a patient who is less agitated, requires less sedation, and who may wean from ventilation more easily.[51,141] This increased ability to wean is sometimes attributed to reduced anatomic dead space. The potential reduction in sedation after tracheostomy, however, is a much greater advantage to weaning than the small reduction in dead space. The benefits and complications of tracheostomy are listed in Box 2-8. Percutaneous tracheostomy is becoming increasingly common and typically is carried out by medical staff in the ICU (Box 2-9).

Another technique involving retrograde (inside-out) intubation of the trachea has been developed: A specially designed tracheal tube is used to keep the neck tissues under tension until tube placement has been accomplished.[138] It is a more time-consuming technique that at present is not widely practiced.

Although no consensus exists on what defines prolonged tracheal intubation, or when tracheostomy should be performed,[142] most ICUs convert the intubated airway to a tracheostomy after 1 to 3 weeks, with earlier tracheostomy becoming increasingly favored.[141,142]

Conventional wisdom states that the tracheostomy procedure is more complex and time-consuming than a surgical cricothyrotomy and should be performed only by a surgeon.[143] Studies in the elective ICU situation suggest that cricothyrotomy is simpler and (at worst) has a similar complication rate.[144,145] Although needle cricothyrotomy has long been advocated as a life-saving emergency intervention,[146] recent work suggests that surgical

Table 2-4. Procedure: Needle and Surgical Cricothyrotomy

The cricothyroid membrane is diamond-shaped and lies between the thyroid and the cricoid cartilages. Inject subdermal lidocaine and adrenaline for local anesthesia.

Needle Cricothyrotomy	Surgical Cricothyrotomy
Identify the cricothyroid membrane and the midline.	Make a 1.5-cm skin incision over the cricothyroid membrane.
Insert a 14-gauge intravenous cannula and syringe through the skin and membrane.	Incise the superficial fascia and subcutaneous fat.
Continuously apply negative pressure until air enters the syringe.	Divide the cricothyroid membrane (short blade, blunt forceps, or the handle of a scapel often is used).
Stop at this point and push the cannula off the needle into the trachea.	Insert (6.0) cuffed tracheostomy tube through membrane between the thyroid and cricoid cartilages.
The insertion of the cannula into the trachea allows apneic (low-pressure) ventilation or jet (high-pressure) ventilation.	

Box 2-7

Tracheostomy: Indications and Contraindications

Indications for Tracheostomy

- Inability to maintain a patent airway
- Suspected cervical spine instability (percutaneous technique only)
- Prevention of damage to vocal cords and (possibly) subglottic stenosis
- Abnormal anatomy (percutaneous only)
- Upper airway obstruction
- High inotrope or ventilatory requirement (relative)
- Requirement for tracheobronchial toilet with suctioning
- Part of larger surgical procedure (e.g., laryngectomy)

Contraindications to Tracheostomy

- Prolonged orotracheal or nasotracheal intubation
- Local inflammation
- Failure to wean from ventilation
- Bleeding disorder (relative)
- Absence of protective airway reflexes
- Arterial bleeding in neck/upper thorax

Box 2-8

Tracheostomy: Benefits and Complications

Benefits
Comfort
Reduced need for sedation
Improved weaning from ventilation
Improved ability to suction trachea
Prevention of ulceration of lips and tongue or healing of such ulcers
Reduced upper airway injury
Potential for speech and oral nutrition

Complications
Misplacement of tube
Primary hemorrhage
Pneumothorax or tension pneumothorax; hemothorax
Surgical emphysema
Infection
Late hemorrhage—erosion of innominate (or other) vessels
Tracheoesophageal fistula

Box 2-9

Procedure: Bronchoscopy-Assisted Percutaneous Tracheostomy

- Withdraw ET until the cuff lies at or just below the cords.
- Pass a flexible bronchoscope down ET to distal end.
- Make a 1.5- to 2-cm transverse incision at midpoint between cricoid cartilage and suprasternal notch.
- Strip away tissue down to pretracheal fascia using blunt dissection (forceps).
- Under direct vision, use a 14-gauge cannula to puncture anterior tracheal wall (in midline).
- Advance cannula into trachea, aspirate air, and insert Seldinger guidewire.
- Dilate around guidewire using dilator(s) or special forceps.
- Pass tracheostomy tube over guidewire into trachea.
- Pass bronchoscope through tracheostomy to check position.

cricothyrotomy is the more advantageous procedure.[147] In patients with unfavorable anatomy, surgical cricothyrotomy is a viable alternative to elective tracheostomy.[144] Surgical cricothyrotomy has been viewed as a temporary airway that should be converted to tracheostomy within a few days, but it may be used successfully as a definitive (medium-term) airway,[148,149] thereby avoiding conversion from cricothyrotomy to tracheostomy, which can cause significant morbidity.[150,151]

EXTUBATION IN THE DIFFICULT AIRWAY PATIENT (DECANNULATION)

The patient with a difficult airway still poses a problem at extubation, because reintubation (if required) may be even more difficult than the original procedure. Between 4% and 12% of surgical ICU patients require reintubation[152] and may be hypoxic, distressed, and uncooperative at the time of reintubation. The presence of multiple risk factors for difficult intubation,[100] as well as acute factors such as airway edema and pharyngeal blood and secretions, makes reestablishing the airway in such patients challenging. Before extubation of any critical care patient, the critical care team should have formulated a strategy that includes a plan for reintubation.

Stylets (airway exchange catheters) that allow gas exchange either by jet ventilation or by insufflation of oxygen may be useful in the difficult extubation patient.[53,153,154] The stylet is placed through the ET, with care taken to ensure that the distal end has not reached as far as the carina. The ET can then be removed after a successful leak test. The stylet may remain in situ until the situation is judged to be stable.[100]

TUBE DISPLACEMENT IN THE CRITICAL CARE UNIT

Endotracheal Tube

ET displacement in the ICU is a life-threatening emergency that may result in significant morbidity.[155] Although tube dislodgement sometimes is viewed as unavoidable, often preventable factors are involved.[156-158] Changes in patient posture or head position cause significant movement of the tube within the trachea.[159,160] The frequency of tube displacement can be reduced by good medical and nursing practice,[161] attention to the arrangements and ergonomics around the bed, achieving appropriate sedation levels, and ensuring adequate ICU nurse staffing.[162,163] Experience and the ability to anticipate possible glitches constitute an important part of prevention. The management of ET displacement starts with an assessment of whether the patient can manage without the ET.[158] If replacement is required, preparations for a potentially difficult reintubation are indicated.

Tracheostomy Tube

Adverse events with tracheostomy tubes are quite common.[158,164] Displacement may be a life-threatening event,[165] especially if the tube has been in place less than 5 to 7 days[142] (before a well-defined tract between skin and trachea is formed) or if the procedure has been performed percutaneously (so that the external opening of the tract may not easily admit a new tube of the same size). The option to leave the patient without a tube should be considered, and if this option is pursued, the tracheostomy opening should be dressed to make it (to some degree) "airtight"—thus facilitating effective coughing. If the patient needs a tube but replacing the tracheostomy is not possible, then oral reintubation should be performed, after which the tracheostomy should be dressed. With a more mature tracheostomy (more than 7 days old), it usually is possible to insert a new tube through the mature tract between skin and trachea.[142]

Tracheostomy tubes may be displaced from the lumen of the trachea but appear to be normal when viewed externally. Difficulty with breathing, ventilation, or tracheal suctioning or the presence of a pneumothorax, pneumomediastinum, or surgical emphysema may be due to tracheostomy tube displacement. Fiberoptic assessment of the tube position and patency may be very useful. Assessing tracheostomy tube position on the chest x-ray film is of no value.

COMMON PROBLEMS IN AIRWAY MANAGEMENT

Problem 2-1 Ineffective (Spontaneous) Breathing despite Artificial Airway

Underlying Causes

1. Obstructed airway
2. Depressed respiratory drive (influence of drugs)
3. Inefficient respiratory effort (e.g., from fractured ribs or diaphragmatic injury)
4. Pulmonary pathologic process (pneumonitis, contusion, collapse, consolidation)

Action

Attempt to deliver 100% oxygen. Check airway. When airway obstruction has been corrected or ruled out, the patient's respiratory status should improve unless another underlying pathologic process is present. If no improvement is obtained, manually ventilate the patient. If respiratory status still fails to improve, proceed to tracheal intubation with manual or mechanical ventilation. Investigate and treat any underlying condition.

Problem 2-2 Ineffective Manual Ventilation despite Artificial Airway

Potential Causes

1. Obstructed airway
2. Poor seal or poor technique with mask or manual ventilation
3. Pulmonary pathologic process (pneumonitis, contusion, collapse, consolidation)

Action

Attempt to deliver 100% oxygen at 15 to 20 L/min. Check and readjust airway and patient head position. When airway obstruction has been corrected or ruled out, use a two-handed approach for mask and airway, with an assistant squeezing the bag. If no improvement is obtained, check for availability of someone with more airway experience. If no such person is available, proceed to tracheal intubation with manual or mechanical ventilation. Investigate and treat any underlying condition.

Problem 2-3 Unilateral Chest Movements in the Intubated Ventilated Patient

Potential Causes

1. Bronchial intubation
2. Bronchial obstruction
3. Lung collapse, pneumothorax
4. Hemothorax, pleural effusion
5. Consolidation, absent lung (pneumonectomy)

Action

If bronchial intubation is suspected, deflate the tracheal tube cuff and slowly withdraw the tube 1 to 2 cm. Reinflate the cuff and manually ventilate the patient while auscultating both sides of the chest. Is air entry present and equal on both sides? Be suspicious if the tube has to be withdrawn more than 3 to 4 cm or if the tube length at the teeth is much less than the expected correct length; another underlying cause may be involved. In an adult, the average distance from the vocal cords to the carina is 12 cm. The tip of an 8.0 (adult) tracheal tube typically is 6.5 cm below the upper surface of the balloon, which must sit below the vocal cords. Therefore, if the upper surface of a cuff is only 3 cm below the vocal cords, the tip will be within 2 to 3 cm of the carina. It is easy to inadvertently intubate a bronchus or leave the tip of the tube close enough to enter the bronchus with head movement or in moving the patient. In adults with normal bronchial anatomy, the tube tip usually will pass into the right main bronchus.

Problem 2-4 Sudden Airway or Ventilatory Compromise in Ventilated Patient with Orotracheal Tube

A ventilated patient with an orotracheal tube in place may suddenly develop dyspnea, hypoxemia, hypercarbia, and a see-saw respiratory pattern. The mechanical ventilator alarm will sound.

Potential Causes

1. Failure of oxygen or air supply to the ventilator
2. Ventilator disconnection or obstruction in ventilator circuit
3. Obstructed tracheal tube
   - Plugged by mucus or clot
   - Kink in tracheal tube
   - Biting on tube (previous biting may have narrowed the tube)
   - Obstruction of tube tip by side wall of lower airways or carina
4. Patient's fighting against ventilator
5. Respiratory fatigue (e.g., with weaning from mechanical support or new infection)
6. Pneumothorax or tension pneumothorax
7. Rapid development of large hemothorax or pleural effusion

Action

Disconnect the patient from the ventilator, and ventilate through the tracheal tube manually. Have the ventilator and circuit checked by another appropriate staff member. High resistance or inability to inflate the lungs suggests tube obstruction or an intrathoracic problem. The (recent) inability to pass a suction catheter down the lumen is suggestive of tube obstruction. If the patient's condition is stable or improving, a small fiberoptic bronchoscope or laryngoscope (if readily available) may be passed down the tube. An obstruction may be removed by suction catheter, or removal of the tube and use of mask ventilation (to reverse hypoxemia and hypercarbia), followed by reintubation, may be required. If no answer to the problem is found, consider whether the patient's condition could be due to a tension pneumothorax. If appropriate, use needle decompression. Otherwise, order emergency chest film and continue either manual or mechanical ventilation as appropriate.

Problem 2-5 Sudden Airway or Ventilatory Compromise in Ventilated Patient with Tracheostomy

A ventilated patient with a tracheostomy may suddenly develop dyspnea, hypoxemia, hypercarbia, and a see-saw respiratory pattern. The mechanical ventilator alarm will sound.

Potential Causes

Causes may include all those listed for Problem 2-4.

Action

Appropriate interventions are the same as for Problem 2-4, with an appreciation of the fact that tracheostomy tubes are shorter, more curved, and more rigid than tracheal tubes. They rarely kink but may become blocked with secretions or blood.[31,166] Suctioning the tube may resolve this. Double-skinned tracheostomy tubes may be unblocked by removing the inner tube (containing the obstruction) for washing, leaving the outer tube in place to maintain a clear airway. Such double-skinned tubes are safer for patients discharged to general wards. Tracheostomy tubes also may become obstructed when the distal opening is blocked by a mucosal flap, the side wall of the trachea, or (rarely) the carina.

KEY POINTS

- The difficult airway may be unanticipated despite expert preassessment. Airway practitioners must have plans to deal with this scenario.
- Use of the appropriate size and type of laryngoscope blade in conjunction with other adjuncts and techniques is an important element of successful tracheal intubation—particularly with the unanticipated difficult airway.
- Airway difficulty in critical care is common and may be precipitated long after intubation by acute events such as tube dislodgement or obstruction.
- Tube dislodgement in critical care is potentially avoidable and may be influenced by staffing levels, sedation policy, and other bedside factors.
- Surgical cricothyrotomy is a relatively simple procedure and may be used to establish a medium-term airway, avoiding the need for tracheostomy.
- In critical care, removal of a tracheal tube may precipitate an acute difficult airway scenario. A protocol for handling a difficult reintubation should always be in place.
- All critical care physicians should be familiar with one or more difficult airway algorithms and the practical skills they require.

REFERENCES

1. Finucane BT, Santora AH: Anatomy of the airway. In Principles of Airway Management, 2nd ed. St. Louis, Mosby–Year Book, 1996, pp 1-18.
2. Standring S (ed): Gray's Anatomy. The Anatomical Basis of Clinical Practice, 39th ed. London, Churchill-Livingstone, 2004.
3. Case Western Reserve University School of Medicine, Cleveland, Ohio: http://metrohealthanesthesia.com/edu/airway/anatomy1.htm
4. University of Virginia Health System: http://www.healthsystem.virginia.edu/Internet/Anesthesiology-Elective/airway/anatomy.cfm
5. Institute of Rehabilitation Research and Development, Ottawa, Ontario, Canada: http://www.irrd.ca/education/presentation.asp?refname22
6. Intellimed International Corporation: http://www.innerbody.com/anim/mouth.html
7. Intellimed International Corporation: http://www.innerbody.com/image/cardov.html
8. Cowan MJ, Gladwin MT, Shelhamer JH: Disorders of ciliary motility. Am J Med Sci 2001;321:3-10.
9. http://www.aafp.org/afp/991115ap/2289.html
10. Byron J, Bailey JB (eds): Head and Neck Surgery—Otolaryngology, 3rd ed. Philadelphia, Lippincott Williams & Wilkins, 1993, pp 485-491.
11. Hinds CJ, Watson D: Applied cardiovascular and respiratory physiology. In Hinds CJ, Watson D (eds): Intensive Care. A Concise Textbook, 2nd ed. London, WB Saunders, 1996, pp 19-39.
12. Sassoon CSH, McGovern GP: Oxygenation strategy. In Shoemaker WC, Ayres SM, Grenvik A, Holbrook PR (eds): Textbook of Critical Care, 4th ed. Philadelphia, WB Saunders, 1999, pp 1308-1323.
13. Burchardi H, Richter DW: Control of breathing. In Webb AR, Shapiro MJ, Singer M, Suter PM (eds): Oxford Textbook of Critical Care. Oxford, Oxford University Press, 1999, pp 45-47.
14. Hinds CJ, Watson D: Respiratory failure. In Hinds CJ, Watson D (eds): Intensive Care. A Concise Textbook, 2nd ed. London, WB Saunders, 1996, pp 125-159.
15. Civetta JM, Taylor RW, Kirby RR (eds): Critical Care, 3rd ed. Philadelphia, Lippincott-Raven, 1997, p. 760.
16. Stone DJ, Gal TJ: Airway management. In Miller RD (ed): Anesthesia, 5th ed, vol 1. Philadelphia, Churchill Livingstone, 2000.
17. Watson D: ABC of major trauma. Management of the upper airway. BMJ 1990;300:1388-1391.
18. Criswell JC, Parr MJA, Nolan JP: Emergency airway management in patients with cervical spine injuries. Anaesthesia 1994;49: 900-903.
19. Morikawa S, Safar P, DeCarlo J: Influence of head position upon upper airway patency. Anaesthesiology 1961;22:265.
20. Castello DA, Smith HS, Lumb PD: Conventional airway access. In Shoemaker WC, Ayres SM, Grenvik A, Holbrook PR (eds): Textbook of Critical Care,. 4th ed. Philadelphia, WB Saunders, 1999, pp 1232-1246.
21. Brain AI: The development of the laryngeal mask—a brief history of the invention, early clinical studies and experimental work from which the laryngeal mask evolved. Eur J Anaesthesiol Suppl 1991;4:5-17.
22. Maltby JR, Loken RG, Watson NC: The laryngeal mask airway: Clinical appraisal in 250 patients. Can J Anaesth 1990;37:509-513.
23. Pennant JH, White PF: The laryngeal mask airway. Its uses in anesthesiology. Anesthesiology 1993;79:144.
24. Ramachandran K, Kannan S: Laryngeal mask airway and the difficult airway.

Curr Opin Anaesthesiol 2004;17: 491-493.
25. Ezri T, Szmuk P, Warters RD, et al: Difficult airway management practice patterns among anesthesiologists practicing in the United States: Have we made any progress? J Clin Anesth 2003;15:418-422.
26. Parmet JL, Colonna-Romano P, Horrow JC, et al: The laryngeal mask airway reliably provides rescue ventilation in cases of unanticipated difficult tracheal intubation along with difficult mask ventilation. Anesth Analg 1998;87:661-665.
27. Brain AI, Verghese C, Addy EV, et al: The intubating laryngeal mask. II: A preliminary clinical report of a new means of intubating the trachea. Br J Anaesth 1997;79:699.
28. Joo HS, Kapoor S, Rose DK, et al: The intubating laryngeal mask airway after induction of general anesthesia versus awake fiberoptic intubation in patients with difficult airways. Anesth Analg 2001;92:1342-1346.
29. Combes X, Sauvat S, Leroux B, et al: Intubating laryngeal mask airway in morbidly obese and lean patients: A comparative study. Anesthesiology 2005;102:1106-1109.
30. Combes X, Le Roux B, Suen P, et al: Unanticipated difficult airway in anesthetized patients: Prospective validation of a management algorithm. Anesthesiology 2004;100:1146-1150.
31. Lavery GG, McCloskey B: Airway management. In Patient Centred Acute Care Training (PACT) 2003. European Society of Intensive Care Medicine, Brussels, 2003.
32. Krafft P, Schebesta K: Alternative management techniques for the difficult airway: Esophageal-tracheal Combitube. Curr Opin Anaesthesiol 2004;17:499-504.
33. Rabitsch W, Schellongowski P, Staudinger T, et al: Comparison of a conventional tracheal airway with the Combitube in an urban emergency medical services system run by physicians. Resuscitation 2003;57:27-32.
34. Mort TC: Laryngeal mask airway and bougie intubation failures: The Combitube as a secondary rescue device for in-hospital emergency airway management. Anesth Analg 2006;103:1264-1266.
35. Rumball CJ, MacDonald D: The PTL, Combitube, laryngeal mask, and oral airway: A randomized prehospital comparative study of ventilatory device effectiveness and cost-effectiveness in 470 cases of cardiorespiratory arrest. Prehosp Emerg Care 1997;1:1-10.
36. Campos JH: Which device should be considered the best for lung isolation: Double-lumen endotracheal tube versus bronchial blockers? Curr Opin Anaesthesiol 2007;20:27-31.
37. Wendt M, Hachenberg T, Winde G, Lawin P: Differential ventilation with low-flow CPAP and CPPV in the treatment of unilateral chest trauma. Intensive Care Med 1989;15:209-211, 1989.
38. Cheatham ML, Promes JT: Independent lung ventilation in the management of traumatic bronchopleural fistula. Am Surg 2006;72:530-533.
39. Bateman NT, Leach RM: ABC of oxygen. Acute oxygen therapy, BMJ 1998;317:798.
40. Campbell TP, Stewart RD, Kaplan RM, et al: Oxygen enrichment of bag-valve-mask units during positive-pressure ventilation: A comparison of various techniques. Ann Emerg Med 1988;17:22-25.
41. Hartmannsgruber MW, Loudermilk E, Stoltzfus D: Prolonged use of a Cook airway exchange catheter obviated the need for postoperative tracheostomy in an adult patient. J Clin Anesth 1997;9:496-498.
42. Turner BK, Wakim JH, Secrest J, et al: Neuroprotective effects of thiopental, propofol, and etomidate. AANA J 2005;73:297-302.
43. Hedenstierna G: Physiology of the intubated airway. In Webb AR, Shapiro MJ, Singer M, Suter PM (eds): Oxford Textbook of Critical Care. Oxford, Oxford University Press, 1999, pp 1293-1295.
44. Hinds CJ, Watson D: Respiratory support. In Intensive Care. A Concise Textbook, 2nd ed. London, WB Saunders, 1996, pp 161-192.
45. Levine SA, Niederman MS: The impact of tracheal intubation on host defenses and risks for nosocomial pneumonia. Clin Chest Med 1991;12:523-543.
46. Fleming CA, Balaguera HU, Craven DE: Risk factors for nosocomial pneumonia. Focus on prophylaxis. Med Clin North Am. 2001;85: 1545-1563.
47. Craven DE: Preventing ventilator-associated pneumonia in adults: Sowing seeds of change. Chest 2006;130:251-260.
48. Safdar N, Crnich CJ, Maki DG: The pathogenesis of ventilator-associated pneumonia: Its relevance to developing effective strategies for prevention. Respir Care 2003;50:725-739.
49. Crnich CJ, Safdar N, Maki DG: The role of the intensive care unit environment in the pathogenesis and prevention of ventilator-associated pneumonia. Respir Care 2005;50:813-836.
50. Lorente L, Lecuona M, Jimenez A, et al: Ventilator-associated pneumonia using a heated humidifier or a heat and moisture exchanger: A randomized controlled trial. Crit Care 2006;10:R116.
51. Lavery GG: Optimum sedation and analgesia in critical illness: we need to keep trying. Crit Care 2004;8:433-434. Epub 2004 Nov 3.
52. Practice guidelines for management of the difficult airway: an updated report by the American Society of Anesthesiologists Task Force on Management of the Difficult Airway. Anesthesiology 2003;98:1269-1277.
53. Benumof JL: Management of the difficult adult airway. With special emphasis on awake tracheal intubation. Anesthesiology 1991;75:1087-1110.
54. Rashkin MC, Davis T: Acute complications of endotracheal intubation Chest 1986;89:165-167.
55. Caplan RA, Posner KL, Ward RJ, et al: Adverse respiratory events in anaesthesia: A closed claims analysis. Anesthesiology 1990;72:828-833.
56. Rose DK, Cohen MM: The airway: problems and predictions in 18,500 patients. Can J Anaesth 1994;41:372-383.
57. Peterson GN, Domino KB, Caplan RA, et al: Management of the difficult airway: A closed claims analysis. Anesthesiology 2005;103:33-39.
58. Burkle CM, Walsh MT, Harrison BA, et al: Airway management after failure to intubate by direct laryngoscopy: Outcomes in a large teaching hospital. Can J Anaesth 2005;52:634-640.
59. Domino KB, Posner KL, Caplan RA, et al: Airway injury during anesthesia: A closed claims analysis. Anesthesiology 1999;91:1703-1711.
60. Kheterpal S, Han R, Tremper KK, et al: Incidence and predictors of difficult and impossible mask ventilation. Anesthesiology 2006;105:885-891.
61. Langeron O, Masso E, Huraux C, et al: Prediction of difficult mask ventilation. Anesthesiology 2000;92:1229.
62. Yildiz TS, Solak M, Toker K: The incidence and risk factors of difficult mask ventilation. J Anesth 2005;19:7-11.
63. Crosby ET, Cooper RM, Douglas MJ, et al: The unanticipated difficult airway with recommendations for management. Can J Anaesth 1998;45:757-776.
64. Samsoon GLT, Young JRB: Difficult tracheal intubation: A retrospective study. Anaesthesia 1987;42:487.
65. Needham DM, Thompson DA, Holzmueller CG, et al: A system factors analysis of airway events from the Intensive Care Unit Safety Reporting System (ICUSRS). Crit Care Med 2004;32:2227-2233.
66. Beckmann U, Baldwin I, Hart GK, et al: The Australian Incident Monitoring Study in Intensive Care: AIMS-ICU. An analysis of the first year of reporting. Anaesth Intensive Care 1996;24: 320-329.
67. Beckmann U, Baldwin I, Durie M, et al: Problems associated with nursing staff shortage: An analysis of the first 3600 incident reports submitted to the Australian Incident Monitoring Study (AIMS-ICU). Anaesth Intensive Care 1998;26:396-400.
68. Ezri T, Weisenberg M, Khazin V, et al: Difficult laryngoscopy: Incidence and predictors in patients undergoing coronary artery bypass surgery versus general surgery patients. J Cardiothorac Vasc Anesth 2003;17:321-324.
69. Mallampati SR, Gatt SP, Gugino LD, et al: A clinical sign to predict difficult tracheal intubation: A prospective study. Can Anaesth Soc J 1985; 32:429.
70. Cattano D, Panicucci E, Paolicchi A, et al: Risk factors assessment of the difficult airway: An Italian survey of 1956 patients. Anesth Analg 2004;99:1774-1779.
71. Lee A, Fan LT, Gin T, et al: A systematic review (meta-analysis) of the accuracy of the Mallampati tests to predict the difficult airway. Anesth Analg 2006;102:1867-1878.

72. Pilkington S, Carli F, Dakin MJ, et al: Increase in Mallampati score during pregnancy. Br J Anaesth 1995;74:638.
73. Benumof JL: Obesity, sleep apnea, the airway and anesthesia. Curr Opin Anaesthesiol 2004;17: 21-30, 2004.
74. Wilson ME, Spiegelhalter D, Robertson, JA, et al: Predicting difficult intubation. Br J Anaesth 1988;61:211.
75. El-Ganzouri AR, McCarthy RJ, Tuman KJ, et al: Preoperative airway assessment predictive value of a multivariate risk index. Anesth Analg 1996;82:1197.
76. Rosenblatt WH: Preoperative planning of airway management in critical care patients. Crit Care Med 2004;32: S186-S192.
77. Yentis SM: Predicting difficult intubation—worthwhile exercise or pointless ritual? Anaesthesia 2002;57:105-109.
78. Field JM, Baskett PJF: Basic airway management. In Webb AR, Shapiro MJ, Singer M, Suter PM (eds): Oxford Textbook of Critical Care. Oxford, Oxford University Press, 1999, pp 1-6.
79. Mason RA, Fielder CP: The obstructed airway in head and neck surgery. Anaesthesia 1999;54:625-628.
80. Morris CG, McCoy EP, Lavery GG: Spinal immobilisation for unconscious patients with multiple injuries. BMJ 2004;329:495-499.
81. Ardekian L, Rosen D, Klein Y, et al: Life threatening complications and irreversible damage following maxillofacial trauma. Injury 1998;29:253-256.
82. Awad Z, Pothier DD: Management of surgical airway emergencies by junior ENT staff: A telephone survey. J Laryngol Otol 2006;1-4 [Epub ahead of print].
83. Rosenstock C, Ostergaard D, Kristensen MS, et al: Residents lack knowledge and practical skills in handling the difficult airway. Acta Anaesthesiol Scand 2004;48: 1014-1018.
84. Schwid HA, Rooke GA, Carline J, et al: Evaluation of anesthesia residents using mannequin-based simulation: A multiinstitutional study. Anesthesiology 2002;97:1434-1444.
85. Sagarin MJ, Barton ED, Chang YM, et al: Airway management by US and Canadian emergency medicine residents: A multicenter analysis of more than 6,000 endotracheal intubation attempts. Ann Emerg Med 2005;46:328-336.
86. Kluger MT, Short TG: Aspiration during anaesthesia: A review of 133 cases from the Australian Anaesthetic Incident Monitoring Study (AIMS). Anaesthesia 1999;54:19-26.
87. Mayo PH, Hackney JE, Mueck JT, et al: Achieving house staff competence in emergency airway management: Results of a teaching program using a computerized patient simulator. Crit Care Med 2004;32:2422-2427.
88. Vickers MD: Anaesthetic team and the role of nurses—European perspective. Best Pract Res Clin Anaesthesiol 2002;16:409-421.
89. James MR, Milsom PL: Problems encountered when administering general anaesthetics in accident and emergency departments. Arch Emerg Med 1988;5:151-155.
90. Kluger MT, Bukofzer M, Bullock M, et al: Anaesthetic assistants: Their role in the development and resolution of anaesthetic incidents. Anaesth Intensive Care 1999;27:269-274.
91. Kluger MT, Bullock MF: Recovery room incidents: A review of 419 reports from the Anaesthetic Incident Monitoring Study (AIMS). Anaesthesia 2002;57:1060-1066.
92. Robbertze R, Posner KL, Domino KB: Closed claims review of anesthesia for procedures outside the operating room. Curr Opin Anaesthesiol 2006;19: 436-442.
93. Wang HE, Seitz SR, Hostler D, et al: DM. Defining the learning curve for paramedic student endotracheal intubation. Prehosp Emerg Care 005;2:156-162.
94. Wang HE, Kupas DF, Paris PM, et al: Multivariate predictors of failed prehospital endotracheal intubation. Acad Emerg Med 2003;10:717-724.
95. Krisanda TJ, Eitel DR, Hess D, et al: An analysis of invasive airway management in a suburban emergency medical services system. Prehospital Disaster Med 1992;7:121-126.
96. Wang HE, Sweeney TA, O'Connor RE, et al: Failed prehospital intubations: An analysis of emergency department courses and outcomes. Prehosp Emerg Care 2001;5:134-141.
97. Schwartz DE, Matthay MA, Cohen NH: Death and other complications of emergency airway management in critically ill adults. A prospective investigation of 297 tracheal intubations. Anesthesiology 1995;82:367-376.
98. Brimacombe J, Keller C, Kunzel KH, et al: Cervical spine motion during airway management: A cinefluoroscopic study of the posteriorly destabilized third cervical vertebrae in human cadavers. Anesth Analg 2000;91:1274-1278.
99. Waltl B, Melischek M, Schuschnig C, et al:.Tracheal intubation and cervical spine excursion: Direct laryngoscopy vs.intubating laryngeal mask. Anaesthesia 22001;56:221-226.
100. Loudermilk EP, Hartmannsgruber M, Stoltzfus DP, et al: A prospective study of the safety of tracheal extubation using a pediatric airway exchange catheter for patients with a known difficult airway. Chest 1997;111: 1660-1665.
101. Mort TC: Preoxygenation in critically ill patients requiring emergency tracheal intubation. Crit Care Med 2005;33:2672-2675.
102. Jensen LA, Onyskiw JE, Prasad NG: Meta-analysis of arterial oxygen saturation monitoring by pulse oximetry in adults. Heart Lung 1998;27:387-408.
103. Van de Louw A, Cracco C, Cerf C, et al: Accuracy of pulse oximetry in the intensive care unit. Intensive Care Med 2001;27:1606-1613.
104. Henderson JJ, Popat MT, Latto IP, et al: Difficult Airway Society guidelines for management of the unanticipated difficult intubation. Anaesthesia 2004;59:675-694.
105. Benumof JL: Laryngeal mask airway and the ASA difficult airway algorithm. Anaesthesiology 1996;84:686-699.
106. Heidegger T, Gerig HJ: Algorithms for management of the difficult airway. Curr Opin Anaesthesiol 2004;17: 483-484.
107. Cobley M, Vaughan RS: Recognition and management of difficult airway problems. Br J Anaesth 1992;68:90-97.
108. Gupta B, McDonald JS, Brooks JH, et al: Oral fiberoptic intubation over a retrograde guidewire. Anesth Analg 1989;68:517-519.
109. Finucane BT, Santora AH: Fibreoptic intubation in airway management. In Finucane BT, Santora AH (eds): Principles of Airway Management, 2nd ed. St. Louis, Mosby–Year Book, 1996, p 102.
110. Levitan RM, Mickler T, Hollander JE: Bimanual laryngoscopy: A videographic study of external laryngeal manipulation by novice intubators. Ann Emerg Med 2002;40:30-37.
111. Latto IP, Stacey M, Mecklenburgh J, et al: Survey of the use of the gum elastic bougie in clinical practice. Anaesthesia 2002;57:379-384.
112. Yentis SM: The effects of single-handed and bimanual cricoid pressure on the view at laryngoscopy. Anaesthesia 1997;52:332-335.
113. Snider DD, Clarke D, Finucane BT: The "BURP" maneuver worsens the glottic view when applied in combination with cricoid pressure. Can J Anaesth 2005;52:100-104.
114. Levitan RM, Kinkle WC, Levin WJ, et al: Laryngeal view during laryngoscopy: A randomized trial comparing cricoid pressure, backward-upward-rightward pressure, and bimanual laryngoscopy. Ann Emerg Med 2005;47:548-555. Epub 2006 Mar 14.
115. Finucane BT, Santora AH: Difficult intubation. In Principles of Airway Management. 2nd ed. St Louis: Mosby–Year Book, 1996, pp 187-226.
116. Bokhari A, Benham SW, Popat MT: Management of unanticipated difficult intubation: A survey of current practice in the Oxford region. Eur J Anaesthesiol 2004;21;123-127.
117. MacQuarrie K, Hung OR, Law JA: Tracheal intubation using Bullard laryngoscope for patients with a simulated difficult airway. Can J Anaesth 1999;46:760-765.
118. Yardeni IZ, Gefen A, Smolyarenko V, et al: Design evaluation of commonly used rigid and levering laryngoscope blades. Acta Anaesthesiol Scand 2002;1003-1009.
119. McIntyre JW: Laryngoscope design and the difficult adult tracheal intubation. Can J Anaesth 1989;36:94-98.
120. Sethuraman D, Darshane S, Guha A, et al: A randomised, crossover study of the Dorges, McCoy and Macintosh laryngoscope blades in a simulated difficult intubation scenario. Anaesthesia 1989;61:482-487.
121. Cook TM, Tuckey JP: A comparison between the Macintosh and the McCoy laryngoscope blades. Anaesthesia 1996;51:977-980.

122. Chisholm DG, Calder I: Experience with the McCoy laryngoscope in difficult laryngoscopy. Anaesthesia 1997;52:906-908.
123. Mehta S: Transtracheal illumination for optimal tracheal tube placement. A clinical study. Anaesthesia 1989;44:970-972.
124. Hung OR, Pytka S, Morris I: Clinical trial of a new lightwand device (Trachlight) to intubate the trachea. Anesthesiology 1995;83:509-514.
125. Wong DT, Lai K, Chung FF, et al: Cannot intubate-cannot ventilate and difficult intubation strategies: Results of a Canadian national survey. Anesth Analg 2005;100:1439-1446.
126. Morris IR: Continuing medical education: Fibreoptic intubation. Can J Anesthes 1994;41:996-1008.
127. Jolliet P, Chevrolet JC: Bronchoscopy in the intensive care unit. Intensive Care Med 1992;18:160-169.
128. Lavery GG, McCloskey BV: The difficult airway in the critical care unit. Crit Care Med (in press).
129. Schwartz DE, Matthay MA, Cohen NH: Death and other complications of emergency airway management in critically ill adults. A prospective investigation of 297 tracheal intubations. Anesthesiology 1995;82:367-376.
130. Birmingham PK, Cheney FW, Ward RJ: Esophageal intubation: A review of detection techniques. Anesth Analg 1986;65:886-891.
131. Schwartz DE, Lieberman JA, Cohen NH: Women are at greater risk than men for malpositioning of the endotracheal tube after emergent intubation. Crit Care Med 1994;22:1127-1131.
132. Erasmus PD: The use of end-tidal carbon dioxide monitoring to confirm endotracheal tube placement in adult and paediatric intensive care units in Australia and New Zealand. Anaesth Intensive Care 2004;32:672-675.
133. Linko K, Paloheimo M, Tammisto T: Capnography for detection of accidental oesophageal intubation. Acta Anaesthesiol Scand 1983;27: 199-202.
134. Sum Ping ST, Mehta MP, Symreng T: Reliability of capnography in identifying esophageal intubation with carbonated beverage or antacid in the stomach. Anesth Analg 1991;73:333.
135. Falk JL, Rackow EC, Weil MH: End-tidal carbon dioxide concentration during cardiopulmonary resuscitation. N Engl J Med 1988;318:607.
136. Moe KS, Stoeckli SJ, Schmid S, et al: Percutaneous tracheostomy: A comprehensive evaluation. Ann Otol Rhinol Laryngol 1999;108:384-391.
137. Powell DM, Price PD, Forrest LA: Review of percutaneous tracheostomy. Laryngoscope 1998;108:170-177.
138. Konopke R, Zimmermann T, Volk A, et al: Prospective evaluation of the retrograde percutaneous translaryngeal tracheostomy (Fantoni procedure) in a surgical intensive care unit: Technique and results of the Fantoni tracheostomy. Head Neck 2006;28: 355-359.
139. Westphal K, Byhahn C, Wilke HJ, et al: Percutaneous tracheostomy: A clinical comparison of dilatational (Ciaglia) and translaryngeal (Fantoni) techniques. Anesth Analg 1999;89: 938-943.
140. Groves DS, Durbin CG, Jr: Tracheostomy in the critically ill: Indications, timing and techniques. Curr Opin Crit Care 2007;13:90-97.
141. Schweikert WD, Gelbach BK, Pohlman AJ, et al: Daily interruption of sedative infusions and complications of critical illness in mechanically ventilated patients. Crit Care Med 2004;32: 1272-1276.
142. Hazard PB: Tracheostomy. In Webb AR, Shapiro MJ, Singer M, Suter PM (eds): Oxford Textbook of Critical Care. Oxford, Oxford University Press, 1999, pp 1305-1308.
143. Finucane BT, Santora AH: Surgical approaches to airway management. In Finucane BT, Santora AH (eds): Principles of Airway Management, 2nd ed. St. Louis: Mosby–Year Book, 1996, pp 251-284.
144. Rehm CG, Wanek SM, Gagnon EB, et al: Cricothyroidotomy for elective airway management in critically ill trauma patients with technically challenging neck anatomy. Crit Care 2002;6:531-535. Epub 2002 Sep 17.
145. Francois B, Clavel M, Desachy A, et al: Complications of tracheostomy performed in the ICU: Subthyroid tracheostomy vs surgical cricothyroidotomy. Chest 2003;123:151-158.
146. Smith RB, Schaer WB, Pfaeffle H: Percutaneous transtracheal ventilation for anaesthesia and resuscitation: A review and report of complications. Can Anaesth Soc J 1975;22:607-612.
147. Scrase I, Woollard M: Needle vs surgical cricothyroidotomy: A short cut to effective ventilation. Anaesthesia 2006;61: 921-923.
148. Brantigan CO, Grow JB: Cricothyroidotomy: Elective use in respiratory problems requiring tracheostomy. Thorac Cardiovasc Surg 2006;71:72-81.
149. Wright MJ, Greenberg DE, Hunt JP, et al: Surgical cricothyroidotomy in trauma patients. South Med J 2003;96:465-467.
150. DeLaurier GA, Hawkins ML, Treat RC, et al: Acute airway management. Role of cricothyroidotomy. Am Surg 1990; 56:12-15.
151. Altman KW, Waltonen JD, Kern RC: Urgent surgical airway intervention: A 3 year county hospital experience. Laryngoscope 2005;115:2101-2104.
152. Demling RH, Read T, Lind LJ, et al: Incidence and morbidity of extubation failure in surgical intensive care patients. Crit Care Med 1988;16: 573-577.
153. Bedger RC Jr, Chang JL: A jet-stylet endotracheal catheter for difficult intubation airway management. Anaesthesiology 1987;66:221-223.
154. Cooper RM: The use of an endotracheal ventilation catheter in the management of difficult extubations. Can J Anaesth 1996;43: 90-93.
155. Epstein SK, Nevins ML, Chung J: Effect of unplanned extubation on outcome of mechanical ventilation. Am J Respir Crit Care Med 2000;161:1912-1916.
156. Rothschild JM, Landrigan CP, Cronin JW, et al: The Critical Care Safety Study: The incidence and nature of adverse events and serious medical errors in intensive care. Crit Care Med 2005;33:1694-1700.
157. Beckmann U, Gillies DM: Factors associated with reintubation in intensive care: An analysis of causes and outcomes. Chest 2001;120:538-42.
158. Kapadia FN, Bajan KB, Raje KV: Airway accidents in intubated intensive care unit patients: An epidemiological study. Crit Care Med 2000;28:659.
159. Conrardy PA, Goodman LR, Lainge F, et al: Alteration of endotracheal tube position: Flexion and extension of the neck. Crit Care Med 1976;4:7.
160. Yap SJ, Morris RW, Pybus DA: Alterations in endotracheal tube position during general anaesthesia. Anaesth Intensive Care 1994;22: 586-88.
161. Birkett KM, Southerland KA, Leslie GD: Reporting unplanned extubation. Intensive Crit Care Nurs 2005;21: 65-75.
162. Morrison AL, Beckmann U, Durie M, et al: The effects of nursing staff inexperience (NSI) on the occurrence of adverse patient experiences in ICUs. Aust Crit Care 2001;14:116-121.
163. Chevron V, Menard JF, Richard JC, et al: Unplanned extubation: risk factors of development and predictive criteria for reintubation. Crit Care Med 1998;26:1049-1053.
164. Kapadia FN, Bajan KB, Singh S, et al: Changing patterns of airway accidents in intubated ICU patients. Intensive Care Med 2001;27:296-300.
165. Seay SJ, Gay SL, Strauss M: Tracheostomy emergencies. Am J Nurs 2002;102:59, 61-63.
166. Trottier SJ, Ritter S, Lakshmanan R, et al: Percutaneous tracheostomy tube obstruction: Warning. Chest 2002;122:1377-1381.

Chapter 3

Assessment of Cardiac Filling and Blood Flow

Amish Patel, Andrew Rhodes, and Richard Beale

Accurate assessment and manipulation of the circulatory system constitute an important goal in the management of critically ill patients. The principal objective of cardiorespiratory manipulation is to ensure optimal oxygen delivery. Physiologic metabolism, adequate delivery of substrates and pharmaceuticals, and eventual recovery of organs and tissues are possible only when this has been achieved. This chapter deals with the physiologic principles governing the cardiovascular system and discusses interpretation of hemodynamic data in given clinical context. With the increasing number of medical devices available to monitor the circulation, this chapter also outlines the principles underlying the design and function of these devices, as well as their uses and limitations (Boxes 3-1, 3-2, 3-3, and 3-4).

CARDIAC FILLING

Cardiac function is determined by a number of interplaying factors—preload, contractility, and afterload. An understanding of all of these factors is necessary to comprehend what is happening to the circulation in any critically ill patient.

The Frank-Starling mechanism states that within physiologic limits, the force of myocardial contraction is directly proportional to the end diastolic myocardial fiber length for any given level of intrinsic contractility or inotropy. Myocardial fiber length is related to the end diastolic ventricular volume (EDV). It is the Frank-Starling mechanism that matches stroke volume to venous return by equating the force of contraction to venous return within the physiologic range (Fig. 3-1). This occurs on a beat-to-beat basis, ensuring that whatever blood is returned to the heart is promptly and accurately ejected, thereby preventing acute cardiac dilation and failure. This stretch of the myocardial fibers or chambers is known as the cardiac preload and is one of the fundamental variables responsible for stroke volume and thus cardiac output. Preload is therefore of the utmost importance to clinicians who care for and treat critically ill patients with myocardial dysfunction or shock.

Preload

Preload is the tension developed by the stretch of the myocardial fibers. This is impossible to measure, so a number of surrogates are used to derive an estimate of this variable. These surrogates provide an estimate of either EDV or ventricular end diastolic pressure (EDP). The most commonly measured variable is the right atrial pressure (RAP), which is used as an estimate of the right ventricular EDP.

Cardiac filling pressures are monitored as an estimate of cardiac filling volumes, which in turn determine the stroke volumes of the right and left ventricles. Unfortunately, continuous monitoring of cardiac chamber volumes is an elusive goal in clinical practice. Accordingly, cardiac filling pressures are used as surrogates for estimating cardiac chamber volumes. The relationship between ventricular volume and filling pressure is dependent on ventricular compliance.

Determinants of preload include the following:

- Circulating blood volume.
- Venous tone. Sympathetic stimulation results in venoconstriction or reduction in venous capacitance and hence increased venous return.
- Posture. The Trendelenburg position (supine, head down) increases venous return. Clinically, passive leg raising may be used to assess volume responsiveness by autotransfusion of approximately 300 mL of blood from the lower limbs to the central circulation, simulating a rapid fluid bolus, thereby increasing preload, which should increase stroke volume.

Left ventricular end diastolic volume (LVEDV) corresponds to myocardial fiber length at the end of left ventricular filling and thus preload for the left ventricle (LV).

Box 3-1

Primary Measured Hemodynamic Data

Parameter/Formula	Normal Range
Arterial blood pressure (BP)	
Systolic (SBP)	90-140 mm Hg
Diastolic (DBP)	60-90 mm Hg
Mean arterial pressure (MAP): [SBP + (2 × DBP)]/3	70-105 mm Hg
Right atrial pressure (RAP)	2-6 mm Hg
Right ventricular pressure (RVP)	
Systolic (RVSP)	15-25 mm Hg
Diastolic (RVDP)	0-8 mm Hg
Pulmonary artery pressure (PAP)	
Systolic (PASP)	15-25 mm Hg
Diastolic (PADP)	8-15 mm Hg
Mean pulmonary artery pressure (MPAP): [PASP + (2 × PADP)]/3	10-20 mm Hg
Pulmonary artery occlusion pressure (PAOP)	6-12 mm Hg
Left atrial pressure (LAP)	6-12 mm Hg
Cardiac output (CO): HR × SV/1000	4.0-8.0 L/min

HR, heart rate; SV, stroke volume.

Box 3-2

Derived Hemodynamic Data

Derived Parameter/Formula	Normal Range
Cardiac index (CI): CO/BSA	2.5-4.0 L/min/m²
Stroke volume (SV): CO/HR × 1000	60-100 mL/beat
Stroke volume index (SVI): CI/HR × 1000	33-47 mL/m²/beat
Systemic vascular resistance (SVR): 80 × (MAP – RAP)/CO	1000-1500 dynes·s/cm⁵
Systemic vascular resistance index (SVRI): 80 × (MAP – RAP)/CI	1970-2390 dynes·s/cm⁵/m²
Pulmonary vascular resistance (PVR): 80 × (MPAP – PAOP)/CO	<250 dynes·s/cm⁵
Pulmonary vascular resistance index (PVRI): 80 × (MPAP – PAOP)/CI	255-285 dynes·s/cm⁵/m²

BSA, body surface area; CO, cardiac output; HR, heart rate; MAP, mean arterial pressure; MPAP, mean pulmonary artery pressure; RAP, right atical pressure; PAOP, pulmonary artery occlusion pressure.

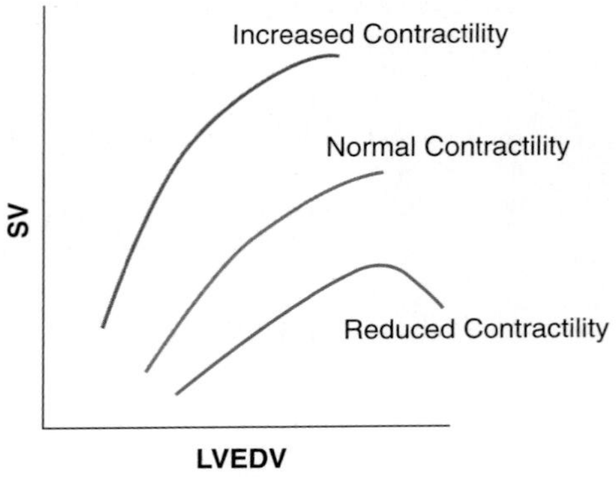

Figure 3-1. Graph to illustrate the Frank-Starling principle: The effect of preload on stroke volume in three different myocardial contractility states. LVEDV, left ventricular end diastolic volume; SV, stroke volume.

LVEDV is clinically difficult to assess, although an assessment can be made by means of echocardiography. Surrogate markers such as central venous pressure (CVP), right atrial pressure (RAP), pulmonary artery occlusion pressure (PAOP), pulmonary artery diastolic pressure (PADP), and left atrial pressure (LAP) often are used to estimate left ventricular end diastolic pressure (LVEDP), for which correlation with LVEDV is assumed. Of note, PAOP accurately reflects left cardiac function only when the patient's cardiopulmonary function meets certain criteria: Specifically, PAOP is accurate as a predictor of left ventricular end diastolic volume only if the vascular system between the catheter tip and the left ventricle is free from any pathologic condition that could influence the pressures detected by the catheter.

Instances in which PAOP *overestimates* LVEDP include maneuvers or conditions creating an interfering pressure gradient that does not represent the function of the left ventricle:

- Chronic mitral stenosis
- Positive end-expiratory pressure (PEEP)
- Left atrial myxoma
- Pulmonary hypertension

Instances in which PAOP *underestimates* LVEDP include conditions characterized by the increased pressure in the left ventricle, which the catheter tip cannot detect:

- Poorly compliant left ventricle
- LVEDP greater than 25 mm Hg

It should be borne in mind that the relationship between LVEDV and LVEDP is by definition dependent on LV compliance ($\Delta V/\Delta P$).

$$PAOP \rightarrow LAP \rightarrow LVEDP \approx LVEDV$$

CVP reflects RAP and often is used as a marker of RV preload, achieved by relating CVP to RVEDP and therefore RVEDV, and is reflective of LVEDV. In the presence of normal RV compliance and in the absence of pulmonary artery hypertension, right-sided heart pressures would be anticipated to be good. As with the LV, RV compliance is critical in the assumption that RVEDP reflects RVEDV. CVP does not accurately reflect LV preload and has been shown to poorly correlate with blood volume.[1-3] CVP is several steps away from LVEDP, and each approximation can be influenced by pathologic conditions—for example, tricuspid regurgitation, intrathoracic pressures, mitral valve disease, and LV compliance. The main clinical value of measuring CVP is to provide information about the right side of the heart, as in cases of RV failure or in assessing the RV response to pulmonary hypertension. A low CVP in the setting of tissue hypo-perfusion is likely to be predictive of benefit from fluid resuscitation.

Contractility

Contractility is defined as the force and velocity of cardiac contraction. It represents the systolic myocardial work done with a given preload and afterload. Clinically it is very difficult to measure. A number of factors can influence the contractile (inotropic) status of a patient.

The following factors *increase* myocardial contractility:

- Circulating catecholamines
- Inotropes
- Digoxin
- Calcium
- Sympathetic nervous system activity

The following factors *reduce* myocardial contractility:

- Hypoxia or hypercapnia
- Acidosis
- β-Adrenergic
- Myocardial ischemia or infarction
- Cardiomyopathy
- Hyperkalemia and hypocalcemia
- Parasympathetic nervous system

Afterload

The afterload of the heart may be considered as the ventricular wall tension required to eject the stroke volume during systole. Afterload relates to the mechanical resistance to shortening of the cardiac muscle fibers.

Afterload for the right and left ventricles is affected by various factors. For the *left* ventricle, afterload is increased by:

- Anatomic obstruction, e.g., aortic valve stenosis
- Raised systemic vascular resistance (SVR)
- Decreased elasticity of the aorta and great vessels
- Increased ventricular volume (greater tension is required to generate the necessary pressure for ejection—Laplace's law)

For the *right* ventricle, afterload is increased by:

- Anatomic obstruction, e.g., pulmonary valve stenosis
- Raised pulmonary vascular resistance (PVR), as in pulmonary hypertension, pulmonary emboli, hypoxia, and hypercarbia
- Increased ventricular volume

The *Anrep effect* describes an intrinsic regulatory mechanism of the heart in response to an acute increase in afterload, which results in an initial reduction in stroke volume followed by an increase in EDV, which restores the SV toward near-normal values.

In clinical practice, SVR and PVR are the most commonly used indices of afterload for the left and right ventricles, respectively. For reasons outlined later in the chapter, however, neither of these gives a reliable estimate of the actual variable and probably is best not used to guide and manipulate therapy.

Vascular resistance may be thought of as the mechanical property of the vascular system opposing the ejection and flow of blood into it. It has two components:

- *Flow component*—frictional opposition to flow in the vessels
- *Frequency-dependent component*—related to the compliance of the vessel walls and the inertia of the ejected blood

SVR, and likewise PVR, can be calculated from standard physiologic equations relating flow or cardiac output (CO), pressure (as mean arterial pressure [MAP]), and resistance.

$$SVR = 80 \times (MAP - RAP)/CO$$

In the same way, PVR may be calculated using the pressure differential across the pulmonary vasculature, between the mean pulmonary artery pressure (MPAP) and PAOP:

$$PVR = 80 \times (MPAP - PAOP)/CO$$

where PAOP is the pulmonary artery wedge pressure.

Clinical Limitations of the Systemic Vascular Resistance Variable

Although the concept of vascular resistance permits an intuitive understanding of the circulation, a number of limitations make it unwise to use the SVR variable to guide therapy. To begin with, SVR is a derived variable. Thus, although pressures and flow can be measured with some accuracy, when these numbers are combined in an equation, the errors in measurement are multiplied, making the derived number less accurate. An additional consideration is that an assumption with use of this equation is that the gradient of the line relating pressure to flow is both linear and intercepts both axes at zero. This is obviously untrue, because even with no flow, a pressure within the vasculature, known as the critical opening pressure, will be present. Accordingly, the gradient of the line will never be accurate unless these conditions are recognized (Fig. 3-2).

Clinical Interpretation of Filling Pressures[4,5]

Pulmonary artery catheterization is performed to measure hemodynamic variables in critical patients, including PAOP, PADP, CO, SVR, PVR, and mixed venous oxygen saturation ($M\text{v}O_2$). The pressure measurements are used to estimate left ventricular filling pressures, to help guide fluid and vasoactive or inotropic drug administration, when clinical signs or other monitored variables are

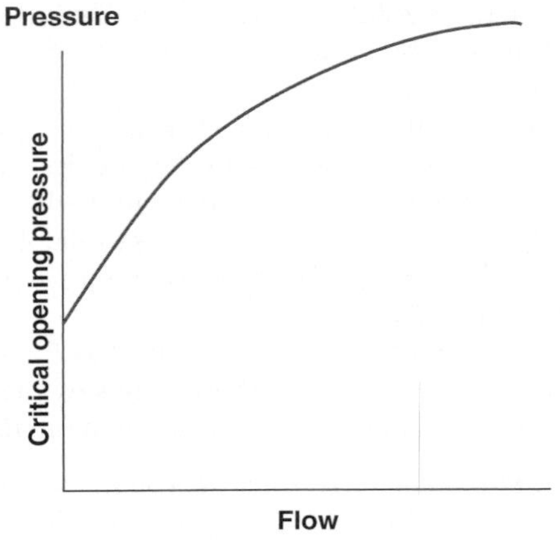

Figure 3-2. Relationship among pressure, flow, and resistance. The critical opening pressure reflects the pressure in the vasculature at zero flow. The important point to recognize is that this is not at the origin of the graph. This means that even when the flow is zero, a baseline pressure exists. Estimating systemic vascular resistance by calculating the gradient of pressure and flow for any given point will therefore be inaccurate, because the "line" is actually nonlinear and does not go through the zero origin.

believed to be inadequate or unreliable. When the pulmonary artery flotation catheter (PAFC) is wedged, blood flow ceases between the catheter tip and the distal pulmonary vein. A continuous static column of blood then connects the wedged PAFC tip to the blood in the pulmonary veins, near the left atrium. Because resistance to flow in the large pulmonary veins is negligible, PAOP provides an indirect measurement of both pulmonary venous pressure and LAP.

Interpretation of cardiac filling pressures requires an understanding of the underlying physiologic principles and an awareness of the clinical conditions under which the measurements have been performed. For example, how is a PAOP of 25 mm Hg interpreted?

According to the most common interpretation, the juxtacardiac pressure and ventricular compliance are assumed to be normal, suggesting the presence of hypervolemia, with an increased LVEDV causing an increased PAOP. However, if juxtacardiac pressure is increased, as in cardiac tamponade or constrictive pericarditis, then the same elevated PAOP may be associated with normal or reduced LVEDV. A third scenario is possible if ventricular compliance is reduced (e.g., diastolic dysfunction arising from myocardial ischemia), in which case again LVEDV may be normal or reduced despite elevated PAOP.

These problems delineate the basis of the arguments that are now made against use of the PAOP to detect either preload or the response to a fluid challenge.[4,5] Many studies have demonstrated that the PAOP bears little or no relationship to the subsequent response to a volume challenge.[4,5] It is important to realize, however, that pressure is one of the driving forces responsible for edema formation in the lungs. So although the PAOP is considered to have limited utility for predicting and guiding fluid challenges, it does have a role to play in determining how much volume should be administered to patients.[4-7] It should thus be regarded as more of a safety limit, rather than as a guide to therapy.

Relationship between Preload and Response to Volume

Although knowledge of the preload status of the heart is important because it provides information regarding one of the key parameters delineating cardiac function, in practice the utility of this information is limited. The key question that clinicians need to answer is whether or not the heart will respond to an increase in volume status (or preload)—whether the patient's cardiac output will increase in response to a volume challenge. This concept is known as *volume responsiveness*.[8,9] Intravascular volume expansion often is the first therapeutic maneuver in patients with circulatory failure. Only approximately 50% of patients given a fluid challenge will respond by increasing cardiac output. The ability to distinguish fluid-responsive patients from nonresponders is important, to avoid inappropriate and potentially harmful fluid challenges in nonresponder in whom inotropes or vasopressors should be preferentially used. Consequences of inappropriate fluid therapy include pulmonary edema, deterioration in gas exchange, and cardiac failure.

Conventional *static* markers of cardiac preload, such as CVP, PAOP, right ventricular end diastolic volume (RVEDV), and global end diastolic volume (GEDV) (the latter two measured by means of thermodilution), are poor predictors of fluid responsiveness. Both CVP and PAOP have been shown to overestimate transmural pressures in patients on external or intrinsic PEEP. It is the transmural and not the intracavitary pressures (CVP, PCWP) that are related to end diastolic volume through chamber compliance, and therefore it is not surprising that CVP and PCWP bear little relationship to fluid responsiveness. Starling's law of the heart (ventricular preload versus stroke volume) illustrates the dependence on cardiac systolic function—thus, for the same baseline preload, the increase in ventricular preload induced by a fluid challenge will result in an increased stroke volume significantly higher in patients with normal ventricular systolic function than in those with reduced ventricular systolic function (see Fig. 3-1). As a result, reliably predicting which patients will be fluid responsive is difficult, because it is not possible to know the position of an individual patient on his or her "personal" Starling curve. A patient may fail to respond to a fluid challenge because of high venous compliance or low ventricular compliance, or ventricular dysfunction.

Accordingly, a number of dynamic parameters have been described that allow the clinician at the bedside to predict with some accuracy which patients will or will not respond to a fluid challenge.[10-17] These parameters include the stroke volume variation (SVV), pulse pressure variation (PPV), and systolic pressure variation (SPV) during each respiratory cycle. In essence, these parameters detect changes in the arterial pressure tracing during mechanical ventilation. If the patient is volume responsive, then during a period of high intrathoracic pressure (positive mechanical inspiratory breath), the venous return will fall

Box 3-3

Hemodynamic Parameters—Adult

Parameter/Formula	Normal Range
Left ventricular stroke work (LVSW): SV × (MAP − PAOP) × 0.0136	58-104 g-m/beat
Left ventricular stroke work index (LVSWI): SVI × (AP − PAOP) × 0.0136	50-62 g-m/m^2/beat
Right ventricular stroke work (RVSW): SV × (MPAP − RAP) × 0.0136	8-16 g-m/beat
Right ventricular stroke work index (RVSWI): SVI × (MPAP − RAP) × 0.0136	5-10 g-m/m^2/beat
Coronary artery perfusion pressure (CPP): Diastolic BP − PAOP	60-80 mm Hg
Right ventricular end diastolic volume (RVEDV): SV/EF	100-160 mL
Right ventricular end systolic volume (RVESV): EDV − SV	50-100 mL
Right ventricular ejection fraction (RVEF): SV/EDV	40-60%

BP, blood pressure; CO, cardiac output; EF, ejection fraction; HR, heart rate; MAP, mean arterial pressure; MPAP, mean pulmonary artery pressure; PAOP, pulmonary artery occlusion pressure; RAP, right atrial pressure; SV, stroke volume; SVI, stroke volume index.

and therefore stroke volume will drop. This can be detected by changes in either the systolic pressure, pulse pressure or stroke volume. SPV, PPV, SVV variation greater than approximately 10% suggests that the patient will be volume responsive (Fig. 3-3). A caveat is that the patient must have a stable respiratory cycle (usually achieved using neuromuscular paralysis) and also a stable cardiac cycle (no arrhythmias).

Unfortunately, the critically ill patient rarely fulfills these conditions. For example, most of these patients are capable of some spontaneous respiratory efforts or demonstrate a number of atrial or ventricular ectopic beats. This makes interpretation of these variables difficult, and the value of such data often is limited. In these instances, production of a change in stroke volume by means of passive leg raising has been described to overcome some of these problems. Passive leg raising leads to an approximately 300-mL autotransfusion of blood to the central circulation that is by definition temporary. If the cardiac output increases in response to this maneuver, a similar response to a fluid challenge can be predicted.

It is important to recognize, however, that identification of a patient who is fluid responsive is not the same as saying that the patient should be given fluid without an

Box 3-4

Oxygenation Parameters—Adult

Parameter/Formula	Normal Range
Partial pressure of arterial oxygen (PaO_2)	80-100 mm Hg
Partial pressure of arterial carbon dioxide ($PaCO_2$)	35-45 mm Hg
Bicarbonate (HCO_3^-)	22-28 mEq/L
pH	7.38-7.42
Arterial oxygen saturation (SaO_2)	95-100%
Mixed venous oxygen saturation (SvO_2)	60-80%
Arterial oxygen content (CaO_2): $(0.0138 \times Hb \times SaO_2) + (0.0031 \times PaO_2)$	17-20 mL/dL
Venous oxygen content (CvO_2): $(0.0138 \times Hb \times SvO_2) + (0.0031 \times PvO_2)$	12-15 mL/dL
Arteriovenous oxygen content difference ($C(a-v)O_2$): $CaO_2 - CvO_2$	4-6 mL/dL
Oxygen delivery (DO_2): $CaO_2 \times CO \times 10$	950-1150 mL/min
Oxygen delivery index (DO_2I): $CaO_2 \times CI \times 10$	500-600 mL/min/m^2
Oxygen consumption (VO_2): $C(a-v)O_2 \times CO \times 10$	200-250 mL/min
Oxygen consumption index (VO_2I): $C(a-v)O_2 \times CI \times 10$	120-160 mL/min/m^2
Oxygen extraction ratio (O_2ER): $[(CaO_2 - CvO_2)/CaO_2] \times 100$	22-30%
Oxygen extraction index (O_2EI): $[(SaO_2 - SvO_2)/SaO_2] \times 100$	20-25%

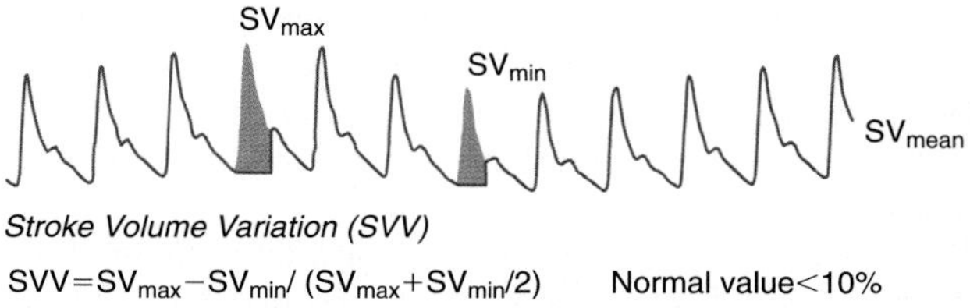

Figure 3-3. Stroke volume variation (SVV). The arterial pressure trace can be used to generate stroke volume (SV) on a beat-to-beat basis. The variation in stroke volume—stroke volume variation—with mechanical ventilation is a useful marker for identifying patients who are likely to respond to an increase in intravascular volume. This tracing demonstrates the fluctuations in stroke volume in a patient with an increased stroke volume variation.

appreciation of the clinical context. Most healthy patients will be volume responsive; however, few will benefit from volume challenges. In critically ill patients, other clinical factors need to be taken into account. Does the patient actually need a higher cardiac output? Or is cardiac output adequate, so that further increase may actually cause harm?

HEMODYNAMIC STATUS AND BLOOD FLOW

Cardiac output (or blood flow) is an important variable to be considered in a critically ill patient. Although arterial pressure has been used as the target for therapy, this focus is perhaps related more to convenience in measurement than to a sound physiologic rationale. When patients become critically ill, it is extremely difficult to predict cardiac output from routine clinical assessment, so sensible and logical use of vasoactive therapy requires monitoring of both pressure and flow. Arterial blood pressure often is mistakenly used as a surrogate marker for blood flow; however, no direct relationship between pressure and flow exists. Moreover, clinical estimation of cardiac output can be difficult and inaccurate, although clinical assessment must not be ignored. Clinical signs consistent with a low-cardiac-output state may include tachycardia with low volume pulse, pallor, diaphoresis, tachypnea, cool peripheries with a prolonged capillary refill time, increased core-peripheral temperature gradient, reduced level of consciousness, and oliguria. Often these signs constitute the only tool that a clinician may have to estimate a patient's hemodynamic status before admission to a critical care unit. At this stage the response of clinical assessment to simple therapeutic maneuvers can give important information. If, however, the patient fails to respond in a suitable fashion, monitoring of these variables becomes necessary in order to direct therapy.

Cardiac output is the volume of blood ejected by the left ventricle per minute. It is the product of heart rate and stroke volume. It should be borne in mind that excessive heart rates will reduce diastolic ventricular filling time, with a negative impact on stroke volume. Heart rhythm also is essential in determining cardiac output, and in general any rhythm other than sinus rhythm will result in a reduction in stroke volume. For example, the loss of atrial contribution to diastolic ventricular filling in atrial fibrillation results in a subsequent reduction in stroke volume and hence cardiac output.

Stroke volume is determined by cardiac *preload, contractility,* and *afterload.*

Cardiac output should not be considered in isolation from other relevant variables. The concept of oxygen delivery describes the relationship between cardiac output and arterial oxygen content.

$$\text{Oxygen delivery} = \text{arterial } O_2 \text{ content} \times \text{cardiac output}$$

This variable (oxygen delivery) has been used in many studies, especially in the high-risk surgical population, as a target for resuscitation.

Measurement of Cardiac Output

The ideal method of measuring cardiac output would be noninvasive, accurate, continuous, safe, easy to use, and operator independent; would provide rapid data acquisition; and would be cost effective. None of the cardiac output monitoring devices currently available possesses all of these properties. Conventional thermodilution remains the clinical gold standard for accuracy in cardiac output measurement; however, newer, less invasive monitoring methods that provide continuous cardiac output data are establishing a role in patients' hemo-dynamic management.[18]

The Fick Principle

Fick described the following relationship in the 19th century: $Q = M/(A - V)$. That is, the uptake or release of a substance (M) by an organ is the product of the blood flow (Q) through that organ and the arteriovenous concentration difference (A – V) of the substance in question.

Applying the Fick principle to cardiac output measurement of the pulmonary blood flow over 1 minute may be achieved by measuring the arteriovenous oxygen content difference across the lungs and the rate of oxygen uptake. Oxygen uptake may be determined using spirometry by measuring the expired gas volume over a known time and calculating the difference in oxygen concentration between the expired gas and that of inspired gas. Accurate collection of the gas is difficult unless the patient has an endotracheal tube, because of the leaks that occur around a facemask or mouthpiece. Analysis of the gas is straightforward if the inspired gas is air, but if it is oxygen-enriched air, two possible problems need to be taken into consideration: (1) the addition of oxygen may fluctuate, producing an error due to the non-constancy of the inspired oxygen concentration, and (2) measurement of small changes in oxygen concentration at the top end of the scale is difficult. Blood oxygen content is measured via blood gas analysis. In the absence of intrapulmonary or intracardiac shunts, the pulmonary blood flow is equal to the systemic blood flow and thus cardiac output.

The technique just described based on the Fick principle may thus be used as an accurate and reliable static measure of cardiac output, but remains a time-consuming and largely laboratory-based tool. Several variants of the basic method have been devised, but usually their accuracy is less good.

Thermodilution

As mentioned earlier, thermodilution from the pulmonary artery catheter (PAC) is considered to be the gold standard of cardiac output measurement for accuracy and acceptability in the clinical setting. Newer methods are routinely validated against the PAC thermodilution technique. A bolus of 5 to 10 mL of cold 0.9% NaCl or 5% dextrose is injected through the proximal port of a PAC into the right atrium. Temperature changes are measured by a distal thermistor in the pulmonary artery. A plot of temperature change against time gives a thermodilution curve from which cardiac output can be calculated from the Stewart-Hamilton equation (Fig. 3-4). Application of this equation assumes three major conditions: complete mixing of blood and indicator, no loss of indicator between place of injection and place of detection, and constant blood flow. For accurate results with this technique, it is important to ensure adherence to these conditions.

The degree of change in the temperature is inversely proportional to the cardiac output.

- Increased blood flow (and CO) = minimal temperature change
- Decreased blood flow (and CO) = pronounced temperature change

Modern PACs are able to provide a continuous reading of cardiac output. They contain an electric heating coil that sits in the right atrium, which heats up the blood in a semirandom binary fashion. The pulsed heating bursts can be detected by the thermistor in the pulmonary artery, which after autocorrelation with the inputting signal can provide continuous cardiac output.

Dye/Indicator Dilution

A number of techniques are available to measure cardiac output with the use of either a dye (indocyanine green) or an indicator (lithium).[19] The concept is exactly the same as that for thermodilution: injection of a substance into the right side of the heart and detection of the same substance distally, either in the pulmonary artery or in the aorta. A curve is generated, which is replotted semilogarithmically to correct for recirculation of the dye. CO is calculated from the injected dose, the area under the curve (AUC), and the duration of effect (short duration indicates high CO) from the Stewart-Hamilton equation, given below.

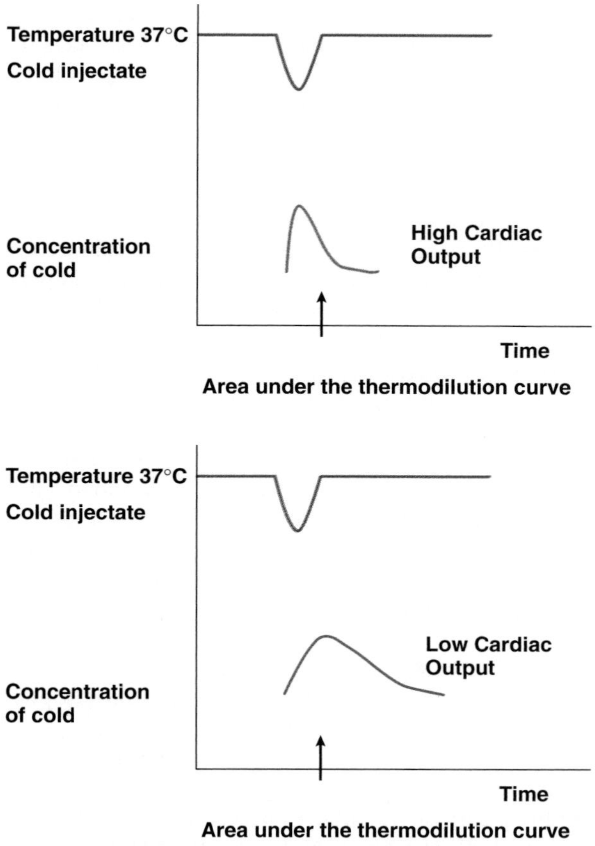

Figure 3-4. Thermodilution curves: A plot of temperature change versus time following a bolus of cold injectate. Cardiac output is inversely proportional to the area under the thermodilution curve. With a large cardiac output, the bolus is pumped rapidly past the thermistor, so the area is small.

$$\dot{Q} = \frac{V(T_B - T_I)K_1K_2}{T_B(t)dt}$$

$\dot{Q}$ = cardiac output
V = volume of injectate
T_B = blood temperature
T_I = injectate temperature
K_1K_2 = computer constants
$T_B(t)dt$ = change in blood temperature over time

Arterial Pulse Pressure Analysis[20,21]

Arterial pulse pressure analysis is a technique of measuring and monitoring stroke volume on a beat-to-beat basis from the arterial pulse pressure waveform. This newer technique has several advantages over existing technologies, including its essentially noninvasive nature, in that arterial access has already been established in most patients, and the ability to track changes in both stroke volume and cardiac output on an almost continuous basis.

The fluctuations of blood pressure around its mean value occur as a specific volume of blood—the stroke volume—is forced into the aorta by each cardiac contraction. The magnitude of this pressure change, the pulse pressure, is a function of the magnitude of the stroke volume. On a beat-to-beat basis, the only factor that determines changes in pulse pressure is change in stroke volume, owing to the relatively slow nature of reactive vascular changes. In order to translate the pressure waveform into an accurate stroke volume, however, an estimate of the arterial compliance and resistance must be made. The greater the compliance, the less will be the vascular resistance to the pulsatile increase in the arterial pressure, and the less will be the pressure required to distend the vessel to accommodate a given stroke volume.

The need to incorporate arterial compliance and resistance into the measurement system has hindered this technology for many years. The origins of the pulse contour method for estimation of beat-to-beat stroke volume are based on the Windkessel model described by Otto Frank in 1899. Only recently have methods been described that can compensate or correct for these compliance or resistance changes to provide an accurate determination of stroke volume. Different technologies address this by different methods. Both lithium dilution and thermodilution techniques have been validated to calibrate pulse pressure tracking systems. Newer devices are being marketed with the ability to self-calibrate after identifying vascular compliance and resistance directly from the pressure waveform, although trials of these devices are still under way.

Proprietary Systems

PiCCO System

The PiCCO system[20,22-25] (Pulsion Medical Systems, Munich, Germany) utilizes a pulse contour method of tracking arterial pressure to derive changes in stroke volume. This method identifies the systolic area by recognizing the dicrotic notch on the arterial waveform. The systolic area is by definition related to the stroke volume. It is converted to an absolute number by calibration with a transpulmonary thermodilution technique. In addition to tracking cardiac output and stroke volume, this technology also can provide the dynamic indicators of volume responsiveness (SVV, SPV, and PPV), as well as a number of volumetric markers of preload: global end diastolic volume, intrathoracic blood volume, and extravascular lung water.

LiDCOplus System

The LiDCOplus system[19,21,26] (LiDCO, Cambridge, UK) tracks the power of the arterial waveform, rather than the contour, in order to track changes in stroke volume. A theoretical advantage is that the effect of reflected waves is reduced because the device does not need to identify specific parts of the arterial waveform. Because the morphology is not assessed, this technology also decreases (but does not negate) the effects of damping on the pressure system. This system can be calibrated by any independent form of cardiac output monitoring device but is sold with the proprietary lithium dilution cardiac output modality. The LiDCOplus technology also tracks the dynamic parameters of preload: SVV, SPV, and PPV.

Flotrac

The Flotrac, or Vigileo, system (Edwards Lifesciences, Irvine, CA) is a new technology that assesses the variance of the arterial waveform in order to identify changes in stroke volume. This device does not need calibration because it assesses the compliance and resistance through a proprietary algorithm that analyzes changes in the shape of the arterial waveform in comparison with some specific demographic characteristics of the patient. This device currently is undergoing validation in a number of centers throughout the world.

Transesophageal Doppler

The Doppler technique for measuring flow has been used in medicine for many years. Currently, several companies market esophageal Doppler ultrasonography devices to measure cardiac output. The esophageal Doppler cardiac output monitor, described in the early 1970s, provides a safe and minimally invasive means of continuously monitoring the circulation. Initially, suprasternal transthoracic ultrasound or Doppler probes were used for determining cardiac output, but they were not widely adopted because probe position instability limited their use for repeated measures over extended periods. Esophageal probes were recognized to have two significant advantages over suprasternal probes: (1) The smooth muscle tone of the esophagus is a natural means of maintaining the probe in position for repeated measurements. (2) The esophagus is in close anatomic proximity to the aorta, hence signal interference from bone, soft tissue, and lung is minimized. The esophageal Doppler monitor measures blood flow velocity in the descending thoracic aorta using a flexible ultrasound probe. When these data are combined with the aortic cross-sectional area, other hemodynamic variables including stroke volume and cardiac output can be calculated. Aortic cross-sectional area is assumed (CardioQ, Deltex, Chichester, UK) or measured simultaneously with a two-dimensional echocardiogram (HemoSonic, ARROW, Middlesex, UK). With these minimally invasive techniques, aortic blood flow is measured, not cardiac output. However, a fixed relationship between aortic blood flow and cardiac output is assumed. Thus, CO can be calculated using this relationship.[27-29] Abrupt changes in cardiac output are much better followed with Doppler systems than with the PAC-based continuous cardiac output systems.

Despite several potential sources of error, good correlation has been observed between measures of cardiac output made simultaneously with the esophageal Doppler monitor and with conventional thermodilution.[27,28,30,31] Esophageal Doppler ultrasonography has been used for intravascular volume optimization both in the perioperative period and in the critical care setting.[29,32-35] One of the main advantages of the technique is the capability of rapid data acquisition after esophageal probe insertion.

Identification of the descending aortic waveform is essential for the correct use of the esophageal Doppler cardiac output monitor. Waveforms from other structures, such as the pulmonary artery, azygos vein, or celiac axis, may be encountered, leading to misinterpretation. After the characteristic descending aortic waveform is acquired, the signal is optimized before data acquisition by movement of the probe a centimeter up or down until the waveform indicates the best possible velocity and color intensities, followed by rotation of the probe to optimize the signal further if possible. The "Peak Velocity" display is used as a reference to the highest identified wave.

Esophageal Doppler waveform analysis has been increasingly evaluated as a method for determining optimum cardiac preload. The key preload parameter of interest is the flow time—the time required from the start of the waveform upstroke to return to baseline. Flow time represents the duration of left ventricular systole and makes up one third of the cardiac cycle (cycle time). Because the flow time (FT) is heart-rate dependent, it typically is corrected (FTc) to a rate of 60 beats per minute, to compensate for the change in duration of systole. The FTc reflects the afterload status of the circulation. Decreased levels commonly are seen in hypovolemic patients, but caution in interpretation is advised because this pattern also can be seen with profound vasoconstriction. A more sensible use of this device is in following the effects of a fluid challenge. Because stroke volume can be determined on a beat-to-beat basis, it is easy to see the effects on the circulation of a small fluid bolus. Diagrammatic representations of characteristic Doppler waveform patterns are shown in Figure 3-5.

Echocardiography

Transthoracic echocardiography (TTE) and transesophageal echocardiography (TEE) both are evolving tools in the critical care setting, and particularly TEE has become a standard of care for intraoperative monitoring in patients undergoing cardiac valvular replacement or repair. TEE has been used for a number of years for acute hemodynamic monitoring and diagnostic purposes in the cardiothoracic critical care setting and its use in the general critical care setting is now becoming commonplace.[36]

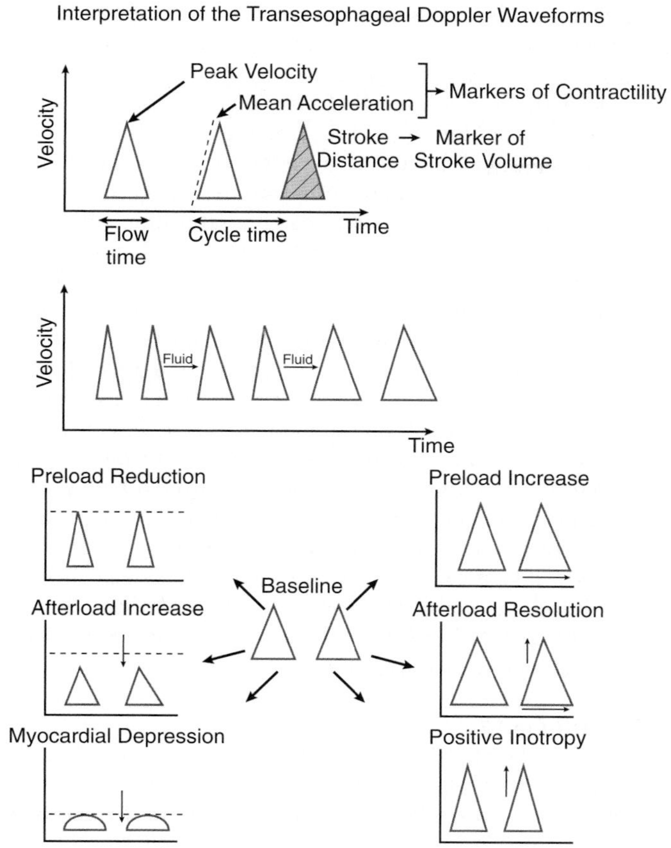

Figure 3-5. Diagrammatic representation of characteristic Doppler waveform patterns. The characteristic flow "triangles" generated in an esophageal Doppler study can be used to monitor cardiac output and stroke volume. The width of the base of the triangle (flow time) when corrected for heart rate provides an estimate of afterload. This diagram demonstrates the changes that are seen after a volume challenge in a variety of clinical conditions.

Echocardiography provides a dynamic assessment of cardiac function, allowing visualization of cardiac chamber dimensions, functional assessments such as estimation of ventricular ejection fractions, detection of regional and global wall motion abnormalities, detection of valvular abnormalities, and exclusion of pericardial effusion. It also can be used to derive cardiac output from measurement of blood flow velocity by recording the Doppler shift of ultrasound signals reflected from the red blood cells. The time-velocity integral, which is the integral of instantaneous blood flow velocities during one cardiac cycle, is obtained for the blood flow in the left ventricular outflow tract (other sites can be used). This is multiplied by the cross-sectional area and the heart rate to give cardiac output. The results for cardiac output measured by this device in skilled hands are comparable to those obtained with use of the PAC.

The main disadvantages of the method are that a skilled operator is needed, the probe is large and therefore heavy sedation or anesthesia is needed, the equipment is very expensive, and an expert user is needed to adjust the probe to give continuous cardiac output readings. Nonetheless, echocardiography has an important and established clinical role. The modality is covered in detail in Chapter 8.

Transthoracic Bioimpedance

Transthoracic bioimpedance is a technique initially developed as a noninvasive method of studying cardiovascular function during space flight. The underlying principle is the occurrence of changes in electrical impedance of the thoracic cavity with ejection of blood during systole.[37] In this model, the thorax is assumed to be a cylinder having electrical length between neck and xiphoid and has a basic impedance. A constant small current is passed between two outer electrodes, voltage change is sensed by two inner electrodes, and impedance is derived according to the equations described by Sramek and Bernstein.[38] Impedance is recognized to change with the cardiac cycle (related to changes in blood volume). The rate of change of impedance is a reflection of cardiac output. It is thought to be useful in estimating trends in cardiac output but not for absolute measurements. Contraction of the heart produces a cyclical change in transthoracic impedance of approximately 0.5%, unfortunately giving a rather low signal-to-noise ratio. Stroke volume and cardiac output can be measured continuously and at fixed intervals using this technique. Studies suggest that transthoracic bioimpedance is accurate in healthy volunteers, but its reliability decreases in critically ill patients, including those with sepsis or increased lung water, and in persons with pacemakers. The technique has not gained wide clinical acceptance to date.

Application of the Fick Principle

The NICO (Novametrix) system is a noninvasive device that applies Fick's principle on CO_2 and relies solely on airway gas measurement.[39] The method actually calculates effective lung perfusion—that part of the pulmonary capillary blood flow that has passed through the ventilated parts of the lung. The effects of unrecognized ventilation-perfusion inequality in patients may explain why the results with this method show a lack of agreement between thermodilution and CO_2-rebreathing cardiac output.[40]

Assessment of Adequacy of the Circulation

Resuscitation of critically ill patients is a complex process. The rationale for most resuscitation maneuvers is that the delivery of oxygen to the tissues is inadequate, resulting in tissue hypoxia. Resuscitation is therefore aimed at increasing the oxygen delivery to a level at which enough oxygen is brought to the tissues to ensure efficient metabolism, so that normal cellular processes can occur. Part of this process entails measuring cardiac output and then increasing this variable to an "adequate" level. Unfortunately, this strategy is complicated as a result of the fact that all patients' cardiac output requirements differ—no "normal" level of flow can be specified for any patient in any given situation. In order to assess adequacy of perfusion, therefore, a number of surrogate markers need to be assessed that give an estimate of the underlying metabolic status. The cardiac output then needs to be assessed in combination with these surrogate markers of metabolism in order to ensure that resuscitation is improving the clinical situation.

Mixed Venous Oxygenation

$M\text{vo}_2$ is the oxygen saturation of blood in the pulmonary artery. It reflects the overall venous saturation after the blood has been fully mixed in the right side of the heart. $M\text{vo}_2$ is related to the balance between oxygen delivery ($D\text{o}_2I$) and the ability to extract oxygen, or the oxygen extraction ratio (O_2ER). Under normal circumstances, oxygen consumption is independent of supply until oxygen delivery falls below the anerobic threshold. The normal O_2ER is approximately 25%, giving an $M\text{vo}_2$ of 75%. In the face of a reduction in oxygen delivery, the tissues maintain oxygen consumption by increasing oxygen extraction, so $M\text{vo}_2$ decreases. However, $M\text{vo}_2$ does not necessarily vary with cardiac output. Not all patients can increase their O_2ER if $D\text{o}_2I$ falls. Clinically, the response of MVO_2 to an increase in cardiac output or oxygen delivery can aid hemodynamic manipulation. $M\text{vo}_2$ can be measured by sampling blood from the distal lumen of a PAC and then measuring oxyhemoglobin saturation by means of co-oximetry, or by using an oximetric PAC that is able to continuously display $M\text{vo}_2$. A flow diagram of a published protocol using PAC-derived parameters is shown in Figure 3-6.

It has been suggested that $M\text{vo}_2$ should be monitored and the key variables manipulated to keep it within the normal range (65% to 75%).[41] In practice, this means ensuring that the hemoglobin concentration and arterial oxygen saturation are normal and then either increasing cardiac output or decreasing oxygen utilization (such as by sedation or cooling). Thus, $M\text{vo}_2$ monitoring provides a means of assessing the adequacy of cardiac output for a given patient. This strategy has been used with success in post–cardiac surgery patients and has been suggested for use in critically ill patients.

In patients without PACs in place, central venous oxygen saturation ($Sc\text{vo}_2$) may be measured by sampling from the distal lumen of a central venous line in the superior vena cava (SVC). This variable bears some relationship to the mixed venous oxygen saturation, although because the venous blood is not totally mixed in the SVC, the relationship should be considered as representing a guide rather than reflecting reality.[42] In practice, the central venous oxygen saturation should be used as a screening tool, rather than as an accurate marker of adequacy. If the level is very low, then the inference can be made that the circulation is inadequate; however, near-normal levels do not preclude underlying problems. The use of this variable in this fashion has proved highly successful in reducing mortality rates for early severe sepsis[43] and is recommended as a target for therapy by the Surviving Sepsis Campaign (an initiative of the European Society of Intensive Care Medicine, the International Sepsis Forum, and the Society of Critical Care Medicine; guidelines available at www.survivingsepsis.org).

Blood Lactate

Blood lactate levels represent the balance between lactate production and lactate metabolism. The liver is responsible for the major part of lactate metabolism. Inadequate oxygen delivery and tissue hypoxia, irrespective of the underlying etiology, results in increased lactate generation. In critically ill patients, high blood lactate levels develop from a combination of inadequate oxygen delivery secondary to poor perfusion (in terms of both perfusion pressure and flow), impaired cellular oxygen utilization from mitochondrial damage, and reduced hepatic clearance of lactate. A resolving lactic acidosis along with clinical signs of improved perfusion is an important indicator of improving perfusion after resuscitation.

GOAL-DIRECTED THERAPY

The concept of goal-directed therapy refers to the protocolized assessment and manipulation of hemodynamic variables in the resuscitation of critically ill patients. This approach became fashionable in the late 1980s and early 1990s, with a resurgence of interest in the early 2000s. Initially these protocols were relatively simple and consisted of measures to increase oxygen delivery and consumption to predefined targets. It was soon recognized that the same targets could not be used for every single group of patients undergoing different conditions and procedures, so protocols have now been refined for different patient populations.

Hemodynamic Optimization of the High-Risk Surgical Patient

Many different protocols have been used for the management of the high-risk surgical patient.[44-51] Initially all such protocols targeted an oxygen delivery index of 600 mL/min/m^2 with the use of fluids and positive inotropic agents. Measurement of cardiac output was performed through a PAC. Currently, many different protocols have been devised, some targeting oxygen delivery, some the mixed venous oxygen saturation, and some ensuring adequate volume loading by targeting a maximal stroke volume. The newer protocols reflect the newer monitoring technologies, so they typically involve less invasive strategies and techniques. Data suggesting one protocol over another are essentially lacking, so it is best to choose appropriate monitoring technologies and therapeutic end points in accordance with the particular characteristics of the patient group being treated, and depending on availability of appropriate devices and trained practitioners. Two protocols for optimization are shown in Figures 3-6 and 3-7.

Early Goal-Directed Therapy of Severe Sepsis

Resuscitation of patients with severe sepsis and septic shock has been studied with an early goal-directed approach[43] (Fig. 3-8).

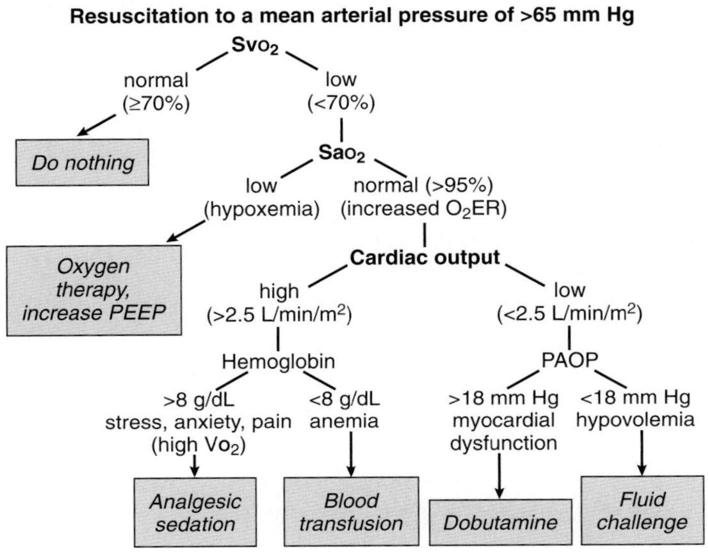

Figure 3-6. Flow chart for Pinsky-Vincent protocol. A diagnostic and treatment algorithm for the use of pulmonary artery catheter–derived variables. Sa_{O_2}, arterial oxygen saturation; O_2ER, oxygen extraction ratio; PAOP; pulmonary artery occlusion pressure; PEEP, positive end-expiratory pressure; V_{O_2}, oxygen consumption. (Adapted from Pinsky MR, Vincent JL: Let us use the PAC correctly and only when we need it. Crit Care Med 2005;33:1119-1122.)

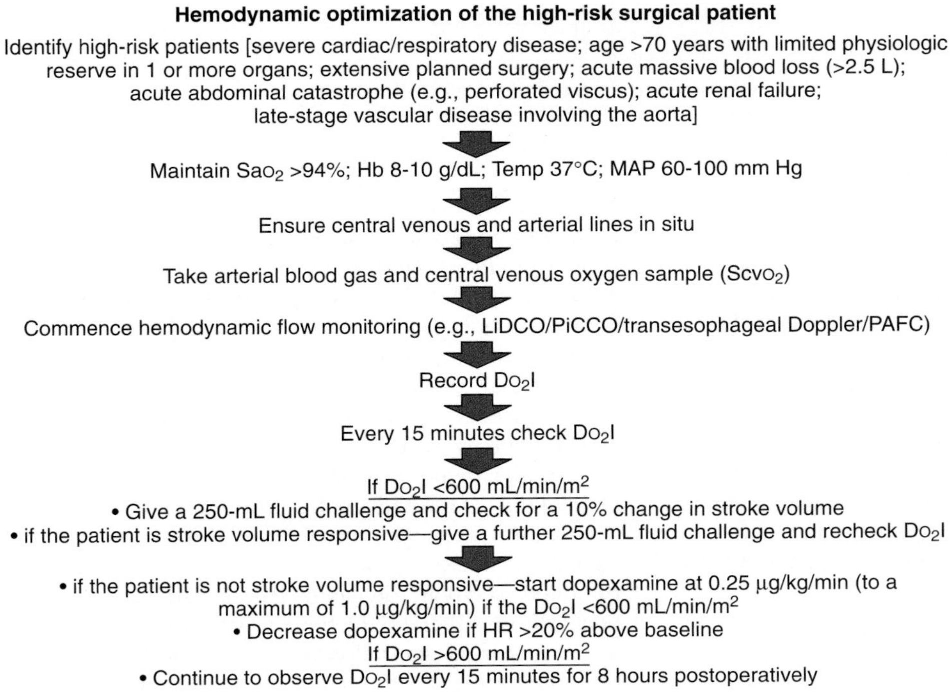
Hemodynamic optimization of the high-risk surgical patient
Identify high-risk patients [severe cardiac/respiratory disease; age >70 years with limited physiologic reserve in 1 or more organs; extensive planned surgery; acute massive blood loss (>2.5 L); acute abdominal catastrophe (e.g., perforated viscus); acute renal failure; late-stage vascular disease involving the aorta]
Maintain Sao2 >94%; Hb 8-10 g/dL; Temp 37°C; MAP 60-100 mm Hg
Ensure central venous and arterial lines in situ
Take arterial blood gas and central venous oxygen sample (Scvo2)
Commence hemodynamic flow monitoring (e.g., LiDCO/PiCCO/transesophageal Doppler/PAFC)
Record Do2I
Every 15 minutes check Do2I
If Do2I <600 mL/min/m2
• Give a 250-mL fluid challenge and check for a 10% change in stroke volume
• if the patient is stroke volume responsive—give a further 250-mL fluid challenge and recheck Do2I
• if the patient is not stroke volume responsive—start dopexamine at 0.25 μg/kg/min (to a maximum of 1.0 μg/kg/min) if the Do2I <600 mL/min/m2
• Decrease dopexamine if HR >20% above baseline
If Do2I >600 mL/min/m2
• Continue to observe Do2I every 15 minutes for 8 hours postoperatively

Figure 3-7. Pearse protocol for management of the high-risk surgical patient. $D_{O_2}I$, oxygen delivery index; Hb, hemoglobin concentration; HR, heart rate; LiDCO, lithium dilution cardiac output; MAP, mean arterial pressure; PAFC, pulmonary artery flotation catheter; PiCCO, pulse contour continuous cardiac output; Sa_{O_2}, arterial oxygen saturation; Scv_{O_2}, saturation central venous oxygen. (Adapted from Pearse RM, Dawson D, Fawcett J, et al: Early goal-directed therapy after major surgery reduces complications and duration of hospital stay. Crit Care 2005;9:687-693.)

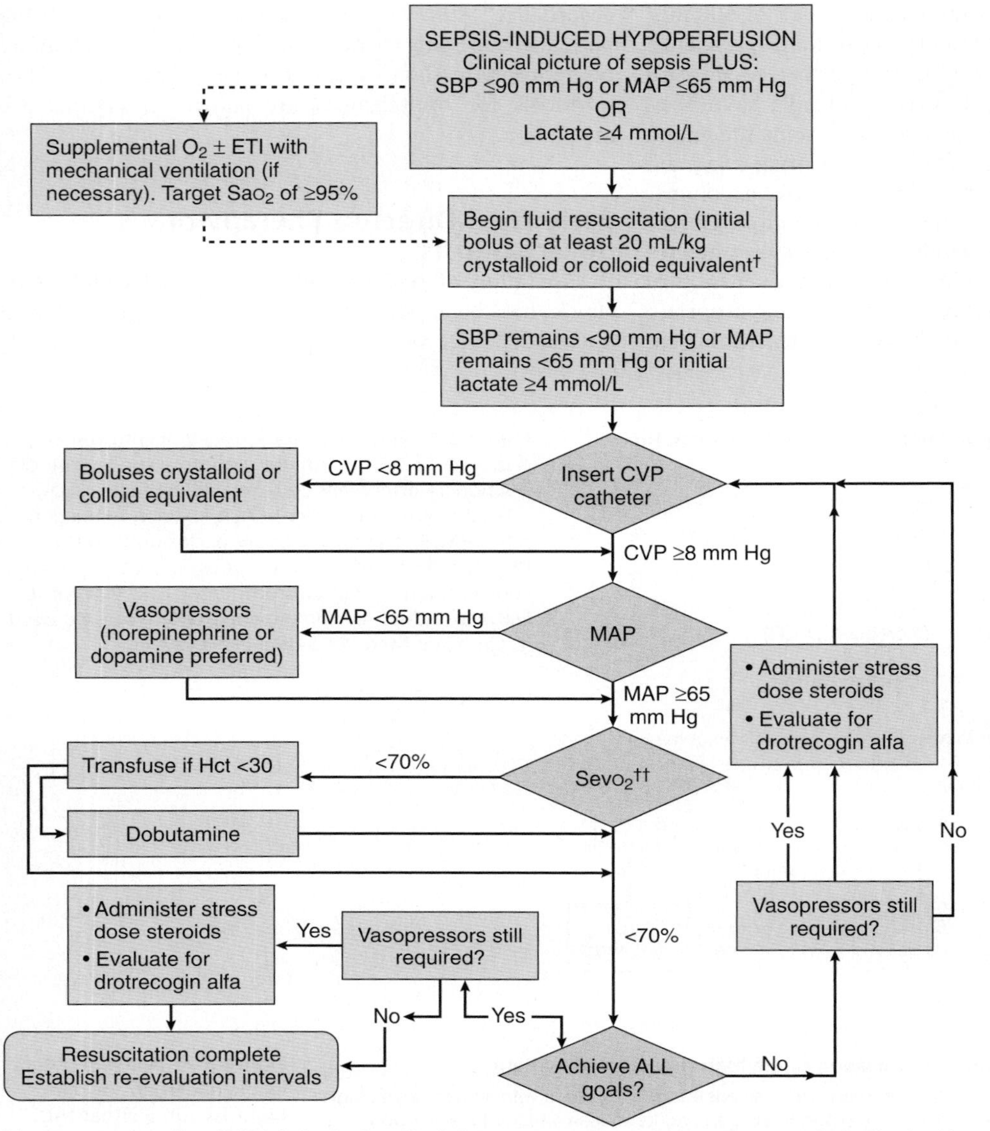

† In circumstances where MAP is judged to be critically low, vasopressors may be started at any point in this algorithm.
†† If pulmonary artery catheter is used, a mixed venous O_2 saturation is an acceptable surrogate and 65% would be the target.

Figure 3-8. Rivers protocol for hemodynamic management in severe sepsisor septic shock. This treatment algorithm provides a framework for the management of the hemodynamic disturbances associated with severe sepsis and septic shock. CVP, central venous pressure; ETI, endotracheal intubation; Hct, hematocrit; MAP, mean arterial pressure; SaO_2, arterial oxygen saturation; SBP, systolic blood pressure; $ScvO_2$, saturation central venous oxygen.

In this approach, cardiac output has not actually been measured; however, a number of surrogate markers of adequacy of the circulation have been targeted. Volume loading is instigated early in this protocol and then targeted against markers of lactate metabolism and central venous oxygen saturation. If these markers fail to fall, then oxygen utilization is decreased by sedation and mechanical ventilation, and oxygen delivery is increased with the use of red blood cell transfusion and a positive inotrope. It should be noticed that although different parameters are being used, this strategy is very similar in principle to that used in the high-risk surgical group of patients.

CONCLUSIONS

Resuscitation of critically ill patients is a complex process. Several simple steps need to be taken to ensure delivery of an appropriate level of resuscitation. First, the patient should attain an optimal level of preload. This is best achieved by identifying the group of patients who are likely to benefit from volume loading and then providing this intervention, while at the same time not giving excess intravascular volume to patients who are unlikely to benefit from it. If it is impossible to predict which patients will benefit, then the fluid should be given under tightly controlled circumstances in the form of a fluid challenge with close monitoring of the circulation. After appropriate volume resuscitation, the circulation of some patients will still be inadequate for their metabolic demands. These patients may then benefit from either a reduction in oxygen requirements or an increase in oxygen delivery. This approach necessitates the monitoring of the circulation and the metabolic status.

KEY POINTS

- Isolated measurements of either right atrial pressure or pulmonary artery pressure are not good markers for identifying patients who will respond to a fluid challenge.
- Dynamic measurements of pulse or stroke volume variation can predict volume responsiveness with a high degree of sensitivity and specificity.
- No "normal" cardiac output can be specified for any patient, so cardiac output must be compared with other markers of metabolic status.
- Cardiac output can be measured by a number of techniques. Less important than how it is measured is how this knowledge is applied.

REFERENCES

1. Osman D, Ridel C, Ray P, et al: Cardiac filling pressures are not appropriate to predict hemodynamic response to volume challenge. Crit Care Med 2007;35:1-5.
2. Kumar A, Anel R, Bunnell E, et al: Pulmonary artery occlusion pressure and central venous pressure fail to predict ventricular filling volume, cardiac performance, or the response to volume infusion in normal subjects. Crit Care Med 2004;32:691-699.
3. Lichtwarck-Aschoff M, Beale R, Pfeiffer UJ: Central venous pressure, pulmonary artery occlusion pressure, intrathoracic blood volume and right ventricular end diastolic volume as indicators of cardiac preload. J Crit Care 1996;11:180-188.
4. Pinsky MR: Clinical significance of pulmonary artery occlusion pressure. Intensive Care Med 2003;29:175-178.
5. Pinsky MR, Vincent JL: Let us use the pulmonary artery catheter correctly and only when we need it. Crit Care Med 2005;33:1119-1122.
6. Pinsky MR: Pulmonary artery occlusion pressure. Intensive Care Med 2003;29:19-22.
7. Dalen JE, Bone RC: Is it time to pull the pulmonary artery catheter? JAMA 1996;276:916-918.
8. Michard F, Teboul JL: Predicting fluid responsiveness in ICU patients. A critical analysis of the evidence. Chest 2002;121:2000-2008.
9. Bendjelid K, Romand JA: Fluid responsiveness in mechanically ventilated patients. A review of indices used in intensive care. Intensive Care Med 2003;29:352-360.
10. Tavernier B, Makhotine O, Lebuffe G, et al: Systolic pressure variation as a guide to fluid therapy in patients with sepsis-induced hypotension. Anaesthesiology 1998;89:1313-1321.
11. Parry-Jones AJD, Pittman JAL: Arterial pressure and stroke volume variability as measurements for cardiovascular optimisation. Int J Intensive Care 2003;10:67-72.
12. Reuter DA, Kirchner A, Felbinger TW, et al: Usefulness of left ventricular stroke volume variation to assess fluid responsiveness in patients with reduced cardiac function. Crit Care Med 2003;31:1399-1404.
13. Reuter DA, Felbinger TW, Schmidt C, et al: Stroke volume variations for assessment of cardiac responsiveness to volume loading in mechanically ventilated patients after cardiac surgery. Intensive Care Med 2002;28:393-398.
14. Berkenstadt H, Margalit N, Hadani M, et al: Stroke volume variation as a predictor of fluid responsiveness in patients undergoing brain surgery. Anesth Analg 2001;92:984-989.
15. Gunn SR, Pinsky MR: Implications of arterial pressure variation in patients in the intensive care unit. Crit Care 2001:7:212-217.
16. Michard F, Boussat S, Chemla D, et al: Relation between respiratory changes in arterial pulse pressure and fluid responsiveness in septic patients with acute circulatory failure. Am J Resp Crit Care Med 2000;162:134-138.
17. Kramer A, Zygun D, Hawes H, et al: Pulse pressure variation predicts fluid responsiveness following coronary artery bypass surgery. Chest 2004;126:1563-1568.
18. Allsager CM, Swanevelder J: Measuring cardiac output. Br J Anaesth CEPD Rev 2003;3:15.
19. Kurita T, Morita K, Kato S, et al: Comparison of the accuracy of the lithium dilution technique with the thermodilution technique for measurement of cardiac output. Br J Anaesth 1999;79:770-775.
20. Rodig G, Prasser C, Keyl C, et al: Continuous cardiac output measurement: Pulse contour versus thermodilution technique in cardiac surgical patients. Br J Anaesth 1999;50:52.
21. Pearse RM, Ikram K, Barry J: Equipment review: An appraisal of the LiDCOplus method of measuring cardiac output. Crit Care 2004;8:190-195.
22. Orme RML, Piggot DW, Mihm FG: Measurement of cardiac output by transpulmonary arterial thermodilution using a long radial artery catheter. A comparison with intermittent pulmonary artery thermodilution. Anaesthesia 2004;59:590-594.
23. Sakka SG, Ruhl CC, Pfeiffer UJ, et al: Assessment of cardiac preload and extravascular lung water by single transpulmonary thermodilution. Intensive Care Med 2000;26:180-187.
24. Michard F, Alaya S, Zarka V, et al: Global end-diastolic volume as an indicator of cardiac preload in patients with septic shock. Chest 2003;124:1900-1908.
25. Boussat S, Jacques T, Levy B, et al: Intravascular volume monitoring and extravascular lung water in septic patients with pulmonary edema. Intensive Care Med 2002;28:712-718.
26. Linton R, Band D, O'Brien T, et al: Lithium dilution cardiac output measurement: A comparison with thermodilution. Crit Care Med 1997;25:1796-1800.
27. Bein B, Worthmann F, Tonner PH, et al: A comparison of esophageal Doppler, pulse contour analysis and real time pulmonary artery thermodilution for the continuous measurement of cardiac output. J Cardiothorac Vasc Anesth 2004;18:185-189.
28. Freud PR: Modifications in the transesophageal Doppler: Comparison with thermodilution measurement of cardiac output in anaesthetized man. Anesthesiology 1996;65:A144.
29. Gan TJ, Arrowsmith J: The oesophageal Doppler monitor: A safe means of monitoring the circulation. BMJ 1997;315:893-894 (Editorial).
30. Gan TJ: The esophageal Doppler as an alternative to the pulmonary artery catheter. Curr Opin Crit Care 2000;6:214-221.
31. Marik PE: Pulmonary artery catheterization and esophageal Doppler monitoring in the ICU. Chest 1999;116:1085-1091.
32. Singer M, Clarke J, Bennett ED: Continuous hemodynamic monitoring by esophageal Doppler. Crit Care Med 1989;17:447-452.
33. Urrunaga JJ, Rivers E, Karriem-Norwood VA, et al: Hemodynamic evaluation of the critically ill in the emergency department: A comparison of clinical impression versus transesophageal Doppler measurement. Crit Care Med 1999;27(Suppl):A89.
34. Atlas G, Mort T: Placement of the esophageal Doppler ultrasound probe in awake patients. Chest 2001;119:319.
35. Roeck M, Jakob SM, Boehlen T, et al: Change in stroke volume in response to fluid challenge: Assessment using esophageal Doppler. Intensive Care Med 2003;29:1729.
36. Colreavy F, Donovan KD, Lee KY, Weekes JW: Transoesophageal echocardiography in critically ill patients. Crit Care Med 2002;30:989-996.
37. Bloch KE: Impedance and inductance monitoring of cardiac output. In Tobin MJ (ed): Principles and Practice of Intensive Care Monitoring. New York, McGraw-Hill, 1998, pp 915-930.
38. Van De Water JM, Miller TW, Vogel RL, et al: Impedence cardiography: The next vital sign technology? Chest 2003;123:2028-2033.
39. Van Heerden PV, Baker S, Lim SI, et al: Clinical evaluation of the non-invasive cardiac output (NICO) monitor in the intensive care unit. Anaesth Intensive Care 2000;28:427-430.
40. Nilsson LB, Eldrup N, Berthelsen PG: Lack of agreement between

thermodilution and carbon dioxide rebreathing cardiac output. Acta Anaesthesiol Scand 2001;45:680-685.
41. Pearse RM, Dawson D, Rhodes A, et al: Low central venous saturation predicts post-operative mortality. Intensive Care Med 2003;29:S15.
42. Edwards JD, Mayall RM: Importance of the sampling site for measurement of mixed venous oxygen saturation in shock. Crit Care Med 1998;26: 1356-1360.
43. Rivers E, Nguyen B, Havstad S, et al: Early goal directed therapy in the treatment of severe sepsis and septic shock. N Engl J Med 2001;345: 1368-1377.
44. Shoemaker WC, Appel PL, Kram HB, et al: Prospective trial of supranormal values of survivors as therapeutic goals in high-risk surgical patients. Chest 1988;94:1176-1186.
45. Pearse RM, Dawson D, Fawcett J, et al: Early goal-directed therapy after major surgery reduces complications and duration of hospital stay. Crit Care 2005;9:687-693.
46. Boyd O, Grounds RM, Bennett ED: A randomized clinical trial of the effect of deliberate perioperative increase of oxygen delivery on mortality in high risk surgical patients. JAMA 1993;270:2699-2707.
47. Gan TJ, Soppitt A, Maroof M, et al: Goal directed intraoperative fluid administration reduces length of hospital stay after major surgery. Anesthesiology 2002;97:820-826.
48. Gattinoni L, Brazzi L, Pelosi P, et al: A trial of goal-orientated hemodynamic therapy in critically ill patients. SvO_2 Collaborative Group. N Engl J Med 1995;333:1025-1032.
49. Lobo SM, Salgado PF, Castillo VG, et al: Effects of maximising oxygen delivery on morbidity and mortality in high risk surgical patients. Crit Care Med 2000;28:3396-3404.
50. Polonen P, Ruokonen E, Hippelainen M, et al: A prospective randomized study of goal-orientated hemodynamic therapy in cardiac surgical patients. Anesth Analg 2000;90:1052-1059.
51. Farrar D, Grocott MPW, Hamilton MA, et al: Optimal care of the higher risk surgical patient. Monograph prepared by the Centre for Anaesthesia, University College London, UK, for the October 2000 meeting on Optimization.

Chapter 4

Arterial, Central Venous, and Pulmonary Artery Catheters

Jean-Louis Vincent

ARTERIAL CATHETERS

What Do They Offer?

The placement of an arterial catheter permits (1) reliable and continuous monitoring of arterial pressure and (2) repeated blood sampling. Analysis of the arterial pulse pressure curve also may have other applications, including assessment of fluid responsiveness and estimation of cardiac output. The appearance of arterial pressure waves will vary according to the site at which the artery is sampled. As the arterial pressure wave is conducted away from the heart, three effects are observed: the wave appears narrower; the dicrotic notch becomes smaller; and the perceived systolic and pulse pressures rise and the perceived diastolic pressure falls.

Arterial Pressure Measurement

The optimal range of arterial pressure depends on individual patient characteristics, on underlying diseases, and also on treatment. Hence, it is impossible to give an optimal range of arterial pressure that is applicable in all patients. When arterial pressure needs to be evaluated accurately, oscillometric measurements become unreliable,[1] and insertion of an arterial catheter is indicated.

Four potential indications for insertion of an arterial catheter for measurement of arterial pressure are recognized:

1. *Hypotensive states associated with (a risk of) altered tissue perfusion.* Hypotension that is resistant to fluid administration requires the administration of vasopressor agents, and invasive measurement of arterial pressure then becomes absolutely necessary to titrate this form of therapy. Norepinephrine and dopamine are the vasopressor agents most commonly used in this setting. A mean arterial pressure of 65 to 70 mm Hg usually is targeted, but this level should be modified as indicated by the clinical scenario; in particular, elderly patients with atherosclerotic disease may require higher levels than young individuals with normal arteries.
2. *Vasodilator therapy*. Vasodilating therapy is a mainstay in the management of heart failure, because it can increase cardiac output. Nitrates and hydralazine usually are used for this purpose. Close monitoring of arterial pressure is essential to avoid excessive hypotension.
3. *Severely hypertensive states.* Extreme hypertension may result in organ impairment, especially of the brain and the heart. Sodium nitroprusside or calcium entry blockers usually are used to lower arterial pressure, and careful, accurate monitoring is essential to titrate the antihypertensive therapy.
4. *Induction of hypertension.* Hypertension sometimes is induced in patients with neurologic diseases. Severe cerebral edema with intracranial hypertension, in particular, requires vasopressor support to maintain cerebral perfusion pressure (the gradient between the mean arterial pressure and the intracranial pressure); likewise, hypertension may be used to treat or prevent the development of vasospasm secondary to subarachnoid hemorrhage, as part of the so-called triple-H therapy (hypertension, hypervolemia, hemodilution). Norepinephrine usually is used for this purpose.

Fluid Responsiveness

Variations in arterial pressure during positive-pressure ventilation have been used as a measure of fluid responsiveness. The transient increases in intrathoracic pressure influence venous return in patients who are likely to respond to fluid administration. This fluctuation in ventricular filling will translate into fluctuations in arterial

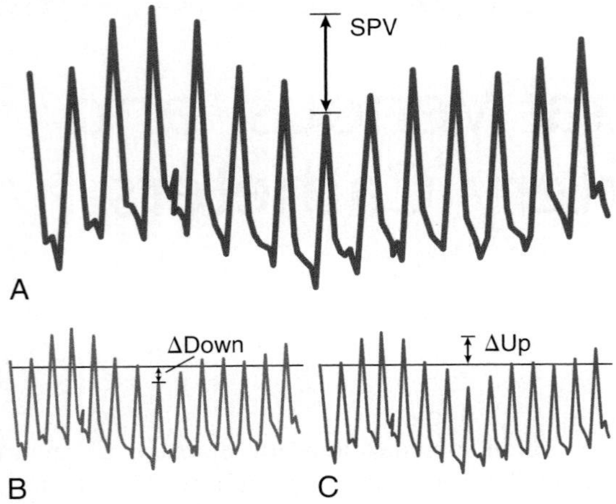

Figure 4-1. The systolic pressure variation (SPV) is the difference between the maximum and the minimum systolic blood pressures during one ventilatory cycle **(A).** The SPV is the sum of the ΔDown **(B)** and the ΔUp **(C).** (From Perel A, Pizov R, Cotev S: Systolic blood pressure variation is a sensitive indicator of hypovolemia in ventilated dogs subjected to graded hemorrhage. Anesthesiology 1987;67:498.)

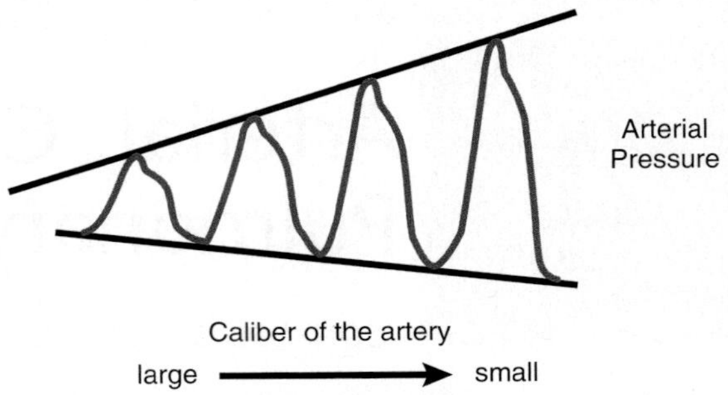

Figure 4-2. Schematic representation of an arterial pressure tracing showing that the pulse pressure increases as arterial size decreases.

pressure a few beats later. Accordingly, the greater the degree of systolic arterial pressure, or pulse pressure, variation during the respiratory cycle, the greater will be the increase in cardiac output in response to fluid administration (Fig. 4-1). However, this observation is valid primarily in patients without spontaneous respiratory movements and without significant arrhythmias, and only when a sufficient tidal volume is applied.[2,3]

Cardiac Output Assessment

The pulse contour analysis also can serve to estimate cardiac output less invasively than with the pulmonary artery catheter (PAC). Because the only determinants of arterial pressure are the stroke volume and the resistance and compliance factors of the blood and arteries, analysis of the pulse contour trace can help to monitor cardiac output over time. This can be done with regular calibrations whenever changes in vascular tone or blood volume occur, or even in the absence of calibration. These measurements are still approximations, so further technological developments can be expected to improve accuracy.

Blood Sampling

The presence of an arterial catheter can greatly facilitate blood sampling, especially in terms of enabling easy access to the circulation for regular monitoring of blood gases, such as may be required in severe respiratory failure or with acute metabolic alterations. Sensors can measure blood gases continuously, but widespread use of such sensors is limited by their cost.

Access

For placement of arterial catheters, usually the radial artery is used. The femoral artery can be easily cannulated and gives a better signal, but presence of a femoral catheter interferes more with patient mobility and warrants concern about infection.[4] Use of other sites, such as the brachial or the axillary artery or even the dorsalis pedis artery,[5] can be considered. An important point to keep in mind is that the pulse pressure increases from the core to the periphery. In other words, the systolic pressure is overestimated in smaller arteries (Fig. 4-2). Hence, it may be better to rely more on mean than on systolic or diastolic pressures.

Complications

The most feared complication with use of arterial catheters is ischemia. With any suspicion of ischemia, the catheter must be removed immediately. Allen's test, to determine occlusive arterial lesions distal to the wrist, is unreliable and is no longer widely used. The accidental disconnection of arterial lines can be associated with severe hemorrhage and even exsanguination. Infectious complications are rare.

CENTRAL VENOUS CATHETERS

What Do They Offer?

The central venous catheter can facilitate fluid administration. It also allows measurement of the central venous pressure (CVP) and enables access to central venous blood for sampling.

Fluid Administration

The large-bore central venous catheter allows fluids to be administered fast and reliably in the presence of acute hemorrhage. Placement of a central catheter is therefore essential in patients with hemorrhage due to polytrauma or with other forms of acute bleeding. It also allows irritating or hypertonic fluids to be administered, such as parenteral solutions, potassium-enriched solutions, and some therapeutic agents. Central venous lines also can be convenient in patients who need prolonged intravenous therapy when peripheral venous access becomes problematic.

Measurement of Central Venous Pressure

CVP is identical to right atrial pressure (RAP) (in the absence of vena cava obstruction) and to right ventricular (RV) end diastolic pressure (in the absence of tricuspid regurgitation). It is thus equivalent to the right-sided filling pressure. CVP is determined by the interaction of cardiac function and venous return, which is itself determined by the blood volume and the compliance characteristics of the venous system. Hence, an elevated CVP can reflect an increase in blood volume as well as an impairment in cardiac function. Because the CVP evaluates the right-sided filling pressures, CVP can be increased in the presence of pulmonary hypertension, even if left ventricular (LV) function is normal. The normal value in healthy persons is very low, not exceeding 5 mm Hg. Thus, the CVP value may not be much lower than normal in the presence of hypovolemia. In general, a CVP below 10 mm Hg can be considered to indicate that the patient is more likely to respond to fluid resuscitation, but exceptions to this rule exist. A high CVP suggests a certain blood volume but does not guarantee sufficient LV filling.

Clinically, CVP can be assessed by evaluation of the degree of jugular distention[6] or liver enlargement. A single CVP measurement is not very useful and is not a good indicator of a positive response to fluids; an increase in CVP without a concurrent increase in cardiac output is not only useless but also harmful, because it will lead to increased edema formation.

Access to Blood in Superior Vena Cava

Measuring the central venous oxygen saturation ($Scvo_2$) is a surrogate for measurement of the true mixed venous oxygen saturation (Svo_2). $Scvo_2$ can be obtained either intermittently (by withdrawal of blood samples) or continuously (with the use of a catheter equipped with fiberoptic fibers). This approach may be particularly helpful in the early resuscitation of the patient with severe sepsis and septic shock, as part of so-called "early goal-directed therapy."[7]

Trace Analysis

Analysis of the CVP waveform can provide some interesting information. In particular, a large y descent indicates a restrictive cardiac state, but not all restrictive patterns are associated with this finding.

Access

The central venous catheter generally is introduced via the internal jugular vein; the subclavian vein also can be used, although the risk of pneumothorax may be somewhat higher with this route. The introduction of a femoral catheter through the abdominal inferior vena cava to the right atrium can yield reliable CVP measurements.[8] The use of femoral catheters, however, is associated with a greater risk of infections and thrombophlebitis.[9]

Complications

Complications of central venous catheterization are related primarily to puncture of the central vein: Hemothorax can be life-threatening, especially in the presence of severe respiratory failure. In the presence of unilateral pathology, the catheter must be introduced on the affected side. Arterial puncture resulting in a local hematoma is not uncommon, but hematoma formation usually is without major consequences. Bedside ultrasonography can help guide the introduction of the catheter into the vein. Excessive advancement of a long catheter in a small patient can result in arrhythmias; such arrhythmias have been described with advancement of the catheter tip into the right ventricle, but this problem can be identified by the presence of an RV trace on the monitor display.

Catheter-related infections constitute the major long-term complication. Adherence to basic hygiene guidelines can decrease the incidence of catheter-related sepsis. Triple-lumen catheters may be associated with a higher incidence of catheter-related infection,[10] primarily as a result of increased catheter manipulation. The use of antimicrobial-coated catheters may decrease the risk of infections[11] but is associated with the threat of development of resistant organisms.[12] Routine replacement of catheters after 3 to 7 days is not recommended.[13]

PULMONARY ARTERY CATHETERS

What Do They Offer?

PACs allow collection of data on right atrial, pulmonary artery, and pulmonary artery occlusive pressures (Fig. 4-3); flow (cardiac output); and oxygenation (mixed venous oxygen saturation).

Pressures

Right Atrial Pressure

As indicated earlier, the RAP is identical to the CVP in the vast majority of cases.

Pulmonary Artery Occlusion Pressure

When the balloon on the catheter is inflated, it causes an obstruction (becomes wedged) in a small branch of the pulmonary artery, interrupting the flow of blood locally (but blood flow continues normally in the rest of the pulmonary circulation), so that (assuming the absence of an abnormal obstacle), a continuous column of blood is present between the tip of the PAC and the left atrium. This pulmonary artery occlusion pressure (PAOP), or pulmonary artery wedge pressure (PAWP), generally reflects the left atrial pressure well. Nevertheless, a number of steps must be taken to ensure the adequacy of the measurement.

A first question is whether the PAOP reflects the pressure in the pulmonary veins and not the alveolar pressure. The tip of the catheter should be in a West zone III position, where a continuous column of blood exists between the catheter tip and the left atrium (Fig. 4-4). These considerations are less important with fluid optimization and with today's lower positive end-expiratory pressures (PEEP).

To exclude a possible influence of airway pressure on PAOP readings, the changes in PAOP can simply be compared with the changes in pulmonary artery pressure (PAP) during the respiratory cycle. If PAOP reflects the

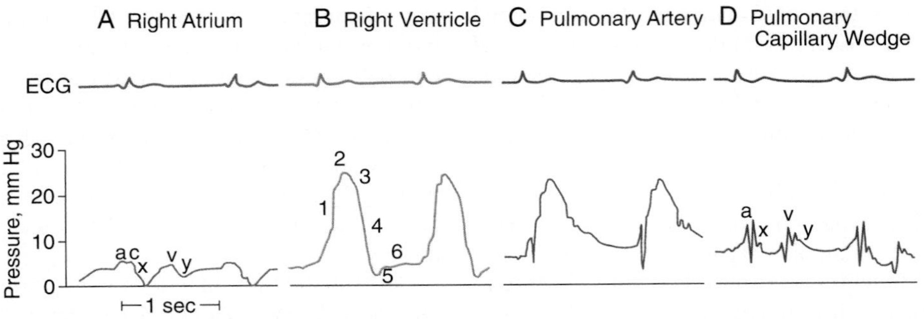

Figure 4-3. Pressure waveforms. **A,** The normal right atrial (RA) tracing. The a wave is the RA pressure rise resulting from atrial contraction and follows the P wave of the electrocardiogram (ECG). On simultaneous ECG and RA tracings it usually occurs at the beginning of the QRS complex. The c wave, caused by closure of the tricuspid valve, follows the a wave and is coincident with the beginning of ventricular systole. Atrial relaxation (x descent) is followed by a passive rise in RA pressure resulting from atrial filling during ventricular systole and occurs during the T wave of the simultaneously recorded ECG. The y descent reflects the opening of the tricuspid valve and passive atrial emptying. **B,** The normal right ventricular (RV) tracing. The sharp rise in RV pressure (1) is due to isometric contraction and is followed by a rapid pressure decrease (2) as blood is ejected through the pulmonary valve. This rapid ejection is followed by a phase of more reduced pressure decrease, which is often reflected in a small step in the downslope of the RV pressure waveform (3). The subsequent sharp decline in RV pressure (4) occurs as a result of isometric relaxation, and is noted once the RV pressure falls below the pulmonary artery (PA) pressure (with consequent closure of the pulmonary valve). As RV pressure falls below RA pressure, the tricuspid valve opens, and passive refilling (5) of the right ventricle occurs, followed by atrial contraction, causing a biphasic wave of ventricular filling to appear on the RV tracing (6). **C,** The normal pulmonary arterial waveform. A pulmonary artery systolic elevation is caused by ejection of blood from the right ventricle, followed by a decline in pressure as RV pressure falls. As RV pressure falls below pulmonary artery pressure, the pulmonary valve closes, which causes a momentary rise in the declining pulmonary artery pressure. This is the dicrotic notch characteristic of the pulmonary arterial (and also the systemic arterial) waveform. The pulmonary artery systolic wave usually occurs in synchrony with the T wave of the ECG. Pulmonary artery diastolic pressure (PADP) does not fall below RA pressure and therefore is higher than right ventricular end diastolic pressure (RVEDP): it is an approximation to left ventricular end diastolic pressure (LVEDP). **D,** The normal pulmonary artery occlusion pressure (PAOP) waveform. The waveform of the PCWP is subject to the same mechanical variables as the RA waveform, but because of the damping that occurs through the pulmonary circulation, the waves and descents often are less distinct. Similarly, the mechanical events are recorded later in the cardiac cycle, as seen on the ECG. Thus, the a wave is not seen until after the QRS complex, and the v wave occurs after the T wave of the ECG. The PCWP is a closer approximation to LVEDP than is PADP. (From Grossman W: Cardiac catheterization. In Braunwald E [ed]: Heart Disease: A Textbook of Cardiovascular Medicine, 3rd ed. Philadelphia, Saunders, 1992.)

pressure within the pulmonary veins, these changes should be identical, because the pulmonary artery and vein should be subjected to identical changes in intrathoracic pressures. If, on the other hand, the catheter tip is not in a West zone III, the changes in PAOP will be more significant than the changes in PAP. In these latter conditions, either fluid administration or some reduction in the PEEP level may abolish the differences.

The next question is whether the measured pressure is truly a transmural pressure—that is, the pressure difference between the vascular structures and the environmental structures. In other words, will changes in surrounding intrathoracic pressures influence the pressures measured? In the case of intrathoracic pressures, the changes in pleural pressure are particularly relevant. Hence, all measurements should be performed at end-expiration, when the pleural pressure is closest to zero. A marked fall in intrapleural pressure, as with a Mueller maneuver (forced inspiration against resistance), may dramatically increase the transmural pressures. A more common problem in the intensive care unit (ICU) is the increase in pleural pressure due to positive-pressure ventilation, sometimes with high PEEP levels.

One method of combating this problem could be to subtract the esophageal pressure from the measured PAOP, but this approach has a number of technologic limitations. Simple disconnection of the respirator to measure PAOP after obtaining an equilibration state is not recommended, because the measured PAOP will not represent the real value when PEEP is applied. A better method consists of measuring the lowest (nadir) PAOP within seconds after a very transient disconnection from the ventilator, to identify the true transmural pressure before a new equilibrium is reached.[14] Such a maneuver suppresses the high intrathoracic pressure and eliminates the influence of the extramural pressure, but the values obtained may not be valid in the presence of intrinsic PEEP. Other methods have been suggested, some relatively sophisticated[15] and others more simple, involving subtraction of approximately one third of the PEEP level from the measured PAOP, for example. The question is whether this is really so important, because absolute PAOP values are not very helpful.

In respiratory failure, PAOP does not represent true capillary pressure, which may be somewhat higher. The true capillary pressure may be estimated from the measurement of the intersection point of the rapid and slow pressure decay curves recorded after a rapid interruption of the blood flow; such measurements of capillary pressure are possible from the pressure trace. This pressure is well correlated with extravascular lung water in animal experiments. The need to know these values is question-

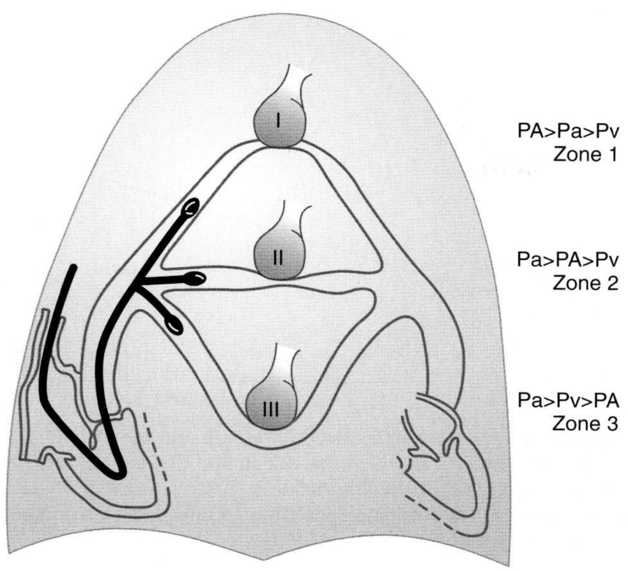

Figure 4-4. The position of the pulmonary artery catheter tip in relation to the zones of the theoretical lung model described by West. For pulmonary artery occlusion pressure (PAOP) to be a valid estimate of "left heart" filling pressure, a continuous column of blood must exist between the catheter tip and the left atrium. In zones I and II, pulmonary vasculature is either totally or partially compressed by the intra-alveolar pressure, and measurements of PAOP will be misleading. PA, alveolar pressure; Pa, pulmonary artery pressure; Pv, pulmonary venous pressure. (From Marini JJ: Respiratory Medicine and Intensive Care for the House Officer. Baltimore, Williams & Wilkins, 1991.)

able, however, because the primary goal remains to keep these hydrostatic pressures as low as possible while maintaining adequate cardiac output.

PAOP may not adequately reflect LV end diastolic pressure. It may be lower in patients with aortic regurgitation or higher in the presence of significant tachycardia or mitral valve disease. LV end diastolic pressure may not even accurately predict LV end diastolic volume. This was already demonstrated many years ago with radionuclide techniques.[16] Preload is more directly defined as the end diastolic volume. A stiff, noncompliant ventricle can result in a relatively high end diastolic pressure for a given end diastolic volume. An evaluation of end diastolic volumes can be obtained less invasively with echocardiographic techniques. Likewise, the use of transthoracic thermodilution techniques allows the estimation of intrathoracic blood volume and global end diastolic volumes. However, these assessments of end diastolic volumes do not give additional information about the likelihood of fluid responsiveness.

In sum, then, a given level of cardiac filling pressures does not provide much information about fluid responsiveness, but monitoring can be very helpful to guide a fluid challenge.[17] During fluid administration, the goal is to obtain a significant increase in cardiac output (by the Frank-Starling mechanism) with the least increment in cardiac filling pressures, in order to minimize the risk of edema formation. The goal is not to keep the cardiac filling pressures within predefined arbitrary limits; rather, PAOP is a direct determinant of edema formation in the lungs. The key principle is to keep the PAOP as low as possible, provided that all of the other organs are happy.

Pulmonary Artery Pressures

Normally the pulmonary vasculature is a low-resistance circuit, so that the diastolic PAP should be equal to or only slightly higher than the PAOP. An increased pressure gradient between the diastolic PAP and the PAOP indicates active primary pulmonary hypertension related to pulmonary vascular changes (hypoxia) or diseases (primary pulmonary artery hypertension). Pulmonary hypertension may result in RV dilation with septal shifts that may compromise LV function.

Cardiac Output

The reference method for measurement of cardiac output is use of the Fick equation; however, this is difficult to apply in practice. The indicator dilution technique has been used instead. Indocyanine green clearance has been used for many years, but this method is time-consuming and quite difficult to perform. The thermodilution technique developed by Ganz is a convenient technique which today allows the almost continuous measurement of cardiac output. The presence of tricuspid insufficiency is the major limitation to this technique.

More recently, other techniques, including the transpulmonary technique proposed by PiCCO (Munich, Germany) and the lithium dilution technique proposed by LiDCO (London), have been developed, but they are somewhat less precise.

The thermodilution technique estimates cardiac output over several cardiac cycles, whereas other techniques including those based on pulse contour analysis, may assess beat-to-beat variations. These may be useful to estimate the influence of changes in intrathoracic pressures on the stroke volume variation, an estimate of fluid responsiveness.

Right Ventricular Volumes

The use of a modified PAC equipped with a fast response thermistor also allows evaluation of the right ventricular ejection fraction (RVEF) (Fig. 4-5). With knowledge of the stroke volume, it becomes easy to calculate the end systolic and end diastolic volumes. This measurement can be particularly useful in the presence of RV failure, but this also is a situation in which the measurement is least reliable: tricuspid regurgitation secondary to pulmonary hypertension.

Mixed Venous Oxygen Saturation

SvO_2 represents the balance between oxygen consumption and oxygen supply. According to the Fick equation:

$$VO_2 = \text{cardiac output} \times (CaO_2 - CvO_2)$$

where VO_2 is oxygen uptake and CaO_2 and CvO_2 are the arterial and venous oxygen content, respectively. If the dissolved oxygen in the blood is neglected for the purposes of calculation, then

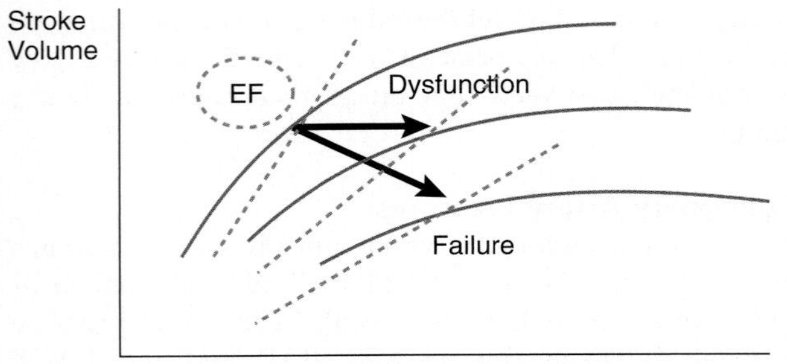

Figure 4-5. Ventricular function curve depicting the difference between ventricular dysfunction (decrease in the ventricular ejection fraction [EF] but preservation of stroke volume) and ventricular failure (defined as the inability of the heart to pump enough flow). The EF, the ratio between stroke volume and end diastolic volume, is represented by the *dashed lines;* it is decreased in all cases.

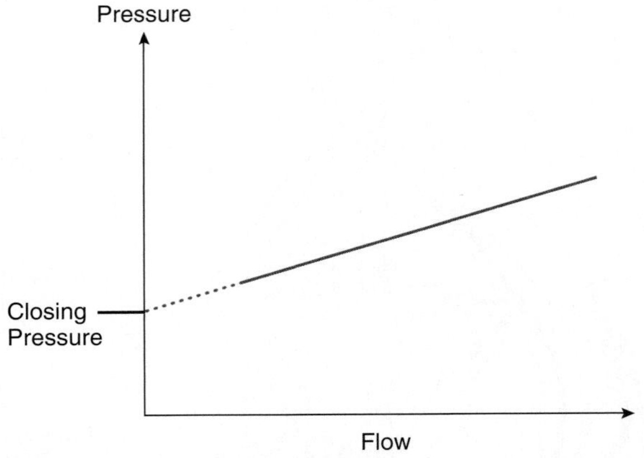

Figure 4-6. Relationship between pressure and blood flow, illustrating the limitations in the calculation of the vascular resistance. Note that the line defining that relationship does not go through the origin, since the pressure is not zero in the absence of blood flow.

$$Vo_2 = \text{cardiac output} \times Hb\ (Sao_2 - Svo_2) \times C$$

and

$$Svo_2 = Sao_2 - (Vo_2/\text{cardiac output} \times Hb \times C)$$

Accordingly, a decrease in Svo_2 can reflect either a decrease in Sao_2 (hypoxemia), anemia, or a relative inadequacy of cardiac output in relation to the oxygen demand of the tissues.

Svo_2 can be measured continuously using catheters equipped with fiberoptic fibers, and measurements are helpful to guide therapy. $Scvo_2$ has been proposed as a surrogate for Svo_2, but the relationship between $Scvo_2$ and Svo_2 is rather vague. Indeed, the $Scvo_2$ is lower than Svo_2 in healthy conditions (as a result of the low O_2 extraction by the kidneys) but is higher than Svo_2 in critically ill patients (because of relative increase in O_2 extraction in the kidneys and in the gut).[18] Moreover, O_2 extraction is high in the coronary circulation, and this is missed in the measurement of $Scvo_2$.

Derived Variables

Hemodynamic assessment can include a number of derived variables, including resistance, ventricular stroke work, oxygen transport, oxygen consumption, and venous admixture, as described next.

Resistance In steady-flow conditions, Ohm's law indicates that resistance is the ratio between the pressure drop and the flow in the system. In the pulmonary circulation, the inflow pressure would be the mean PAP and the outflow pressure would be PAOP; for the systemic circulation, these would be the MAP and the CVP, respectively. In either case, flow would be cardiac output. This approach is limited, however, by the fact that the extrapolated intercept of the PAP–cardiac output relationship represents the average closing pressure of the small pulmonary arterioles, and the slope represents the upstream arterial resistance. Accordingly, the increased PAP in pulmonary hypertension can be explained by both an increase in pulmonary vascular closing pressure and an increase in vascular tone, and pulmonary vascular resistance (PVR) is not a good reflection of vasomotor tone in the pulmonary vasculature. Pulmonary hemodynamics are therefore best assessed by altering blood flow to better evaluate this relationship (Fig. 4-6).

Calculation of systemic vascular resistance (SVR) is not very helpful either. It is better to base clinical decisions on primary variables. Simply stated, a relatively high cardiac output in relation to arterial pressure reflects a low SVR state, whereas a relatively low cardiac output reflects a high SVR state.

Ventricular Stroke Work The work developed by the ventricles is determined by the ventricular work as derived from the product of flow and the pressure generated. The relationship between stroke work and the respective filling pressure represents a better assessment of contractility than does the stroke volume. LV stroke work index (LVSWI) can be calculated using the equation

$$LVSWI = SI(MAP - PAOP) \times 0.0136$$

where SI represents the stroke work index.

Oxygen-Derived Variables Oxygen transport can be assessed as the product of cardiac output and the arterial oxygen content, according to the equation

$$\begin{aligned} Do_2 &= \text{cardiac output} \times Cao_2 \\ &= \text{cardiac output} \times ([Hb] \times Sao_2 \times 1.39) + 0.0031 \times Pao_2 \end{aligned}$$

Calculations of this variable benefit from combining measurements of cardiac output, Hb, and Sao_2 but have the limitation that the corresponding oxygen demand is unknown. Some studies suggested that maintaining supranormal Do_2 in the perioperative period or early after trauma may result in better outcomes.

Oxygen consumption also can be calculated from the product of cardiac output and the arteriovenous oxygen difference, according to the formula

$$Vo_2 = \text{cardiac output} \times (Cao_2 - Cvo_2)$$

where Cvo_2 is calculated in the same way as for Cao_2, using the Svo_2 instead of the Sao_2.

The difficulty is in evaluating the oxygen requirements (or the oxygen demand) of the body. VO_2 assessment may perhaps be useful to evaluate the caloric need of the critically ill patient.

The calculation of oxygen extraction is accomplished by determining the ratio of VO_2 to DO_2, or, in a simplified way:

$$
\begin{aligned}
O_2ER &= VO_2/DO_2 = (CaO_2 - CvO_2)/CaO_2 \\
&= (SaO_2 - SvO_2)Hb/SaO_2 \times Hb \\
&= (SaO_2 - SvO_2)/SaO_2
\end{aligned}
$$

Accordingly, when SaO_2 is close to 100%, in the absence of hypoxemia, O_2ER mirrors SvO_2. Its calculation can be useful in the presence of hypoxemia, when SaO_2 is decreased. Also, the relationship between cardiac output and O_2ER can be helpful to compare the central and the peripheral components of oxygen delivery (Fig. 4-7). This relationship is independent of Hb, so that it can be helpful to evaluate the cardiovascular status in the presence of anemia.[19]

Venous Admixture Venous admixture can be calculated by the Berggren equation:

$$
Qs/Qt = \frac{Cc'O_2 - CaO_2}{Cc'O_2 - CvO_2}
$$

in which Qs is shunt flow, Qt is total pulmonary blood flow, and $Cc'O_2$ represents the capillary oxygen content (assuming an oxygen saturation of 100%). This may help to assess the effects of various interventions (PEEP or other respiratory conditions, administration of vasoactive agents) on pulmonary hemodynamics.

Complications

Complications of pulmonary artery catheterization can be divided into seven categories as listed in Box 4-1. Many of these can be prevented, and most are relatively uncommon.

Complications of venous access are the same as for the insertion of a central venous catheter. Arrhythmias are common but usually are without major consequence, except in moribund patients. It has been suggested that lidocaine should be given prophylactically in predisposed patients, but this usually is not necessary. Likewise, complete atrioventricular block may develop in patients with left bundle branch block, but this is exceptional. Knot formation will be rare if the catheter is advanced carefully and if its presence in the pulmonary artery is confirmed before further advancement into the right ventricle. In particular, care should be taken not to advance the catheter by more than 30 to 35 cm into the right ventricle. Thrombotic complications have become rare with the development of heparin-coated catheters. The appearance of an infiltrate beyond the tip of the PAC on the chest film should suggest an evolving thrombotic event, which should lead to consideration of the withdrawal of the catheter. Endothelial lesions have been found at autopsy, but their clinical relevance is doubtful. Endocarditis is very rare. Valvular damage may occur as a result of improper handling of the catheter (in particular, its withdrawal with the balloon still inflated). Catheter-related infections remain a risk, but they do not seem to be any more common than with central venous catheters.

Pulmonary artery rupture is the most feared complication: Although it is exceptionally rare, it is associated with a high mortality rate. The usual cause is overinflating the balloon in the presence of resistance to inflation, particularly in the presence of preexisting PAH; other, less common causes are shown in Figure 4-8. The cardinal sign of rupture is the development of hemoptysis. The reaction to this event should not be to pull out the catheter entirely, but rather to withdraw it slightly and then inflate the balloon. If the hemorrhage does not stop, a thoracotomy may be necessary to repair the PA.

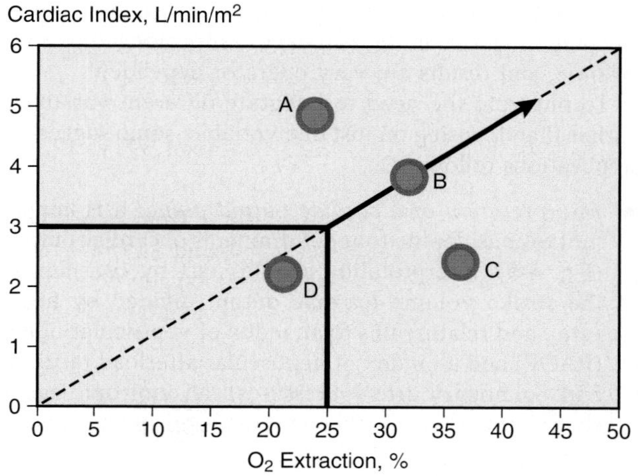

Figure 4-7. Diagram illustrating the relationship between cardiac index and O_2 extraction. Four typical examples are given: hyperkinetic state (A), anemia (B), low cardiac output state (C), and profound anesthesia (D).

Technical Limitations

Invasive measurements of pressures are based on fluid-filled systems with disposable transducers. The transducer includes a deformable membrane with a Wheatstone bridge modifying the electrical resistance and, correspondingly, the intensity of a current. Reliability is ensured by the excellent linearity between the pressure signal and the electrical signal generated by the transducer, in a

Box 4-1

Complications of Pulmonary Artery Catheter Insertion

- Complicated vascular access (pneumothorax, hematoma)
- Arrhythmias (e.g., heart block, ventricular tachycardia/fibrillation)
- Catheter knotting
- Pulmonary thrombosis and infarction
- Endothelial or valvular damage
- Colonization and bacteremia
- Pulmonary artery rupture

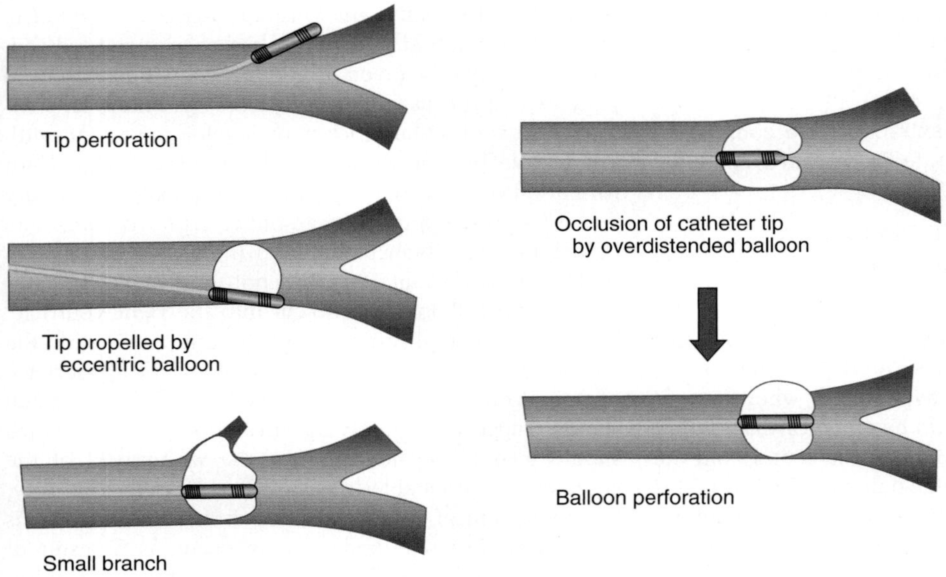

Figure 4-8. Possible mechanisms of pulmonary artery rupture (other than the most common cause, overinflating the balloon in the presence of resistance to inflation). (From Barash PG, Nardi D, Hammond G, et al: Catheter-induced pulmonary artery perforation. Mechanisms, management, and modifications. J Thorac Cardiovasc Surg 1981;82:5.)

range of frequency values largely exceeding the range of frequencies found in the human body.

Reliability is less secure in the intermediary system made of tubes and stopcocks along the extent of the pressure system. These can modify the morphology of the trace, resulting in damping. Motion artifacts can further complicate th e tracings. The presence of air bubbles also may alter the signal. Use of fluid-filled catheters to measure pressures provides reliable estimates of mean vascular pressures.

Three steps must be followed to guarantee reliable measurements:

1. The first step is appropriate zeroing. This is accomplished by opening the transducer to atmospheric pressure (taken as the zero value). All pressures must be measured with reference to an arbitrary reference point. This zero reference pressure level should ideally be where it is least influenced by location on the body. In humans, it is thought to be at the level of the right atrium, so the reference level usually is placed in the mid-chest (mid-axillary) position at the level of the fourth intercostal space. In healthy persons, the CVP referred to that region does not change with supine versus upright position. An alternative reference is 5 cm vertically below the sternal angle. Obviously, errors in zeroing are relatively more important for measurements of cardiac filling pressures than for arterial pressure measurements, because the errors are quantitatively identical but proportionally greater.
2. The second step is calibration, which is now done automatically by today's electronic systems.
3. The third step is ensuring the good quality of the trace. Shaking the catheter should result in large pressure variations on the screen. A damped system will underestimate systolic pressures. The liquid column should be continuous, without air bubbles in the system. Excessive tubing length, or multiple stopcocks and connectors, may decrease the resonant frequency, resulting in "whipped" traces. Likewise, the presence of bubbles must be carefully avoided. Transient flushing should be followed by an abrupt return of the pressure trace to its actual value.

Applications: Diagnosis versus Monitoring

Today the PAC is more useful in guiding therapy rather than in identifying abnormalities, this latter role having largely been taken over by noninvasive, mainly echocardiographic techniques (Table 4-1). In the past, analysis of waveforms was used—for example, the abnormal V waves of mitral regurgitation. Likewise, an increase of all pressures to identical levels should suggest pericardial tamponade. These findings should still alert the clinician to possible abnormalities, but echocardiographic techniques have largely replaced the use of the PAC for identifying valvular disease. The use of echocardiographic techniques for monitoring, however, is hampered by the difficulty of keeping the probe in the esophagus for prolonged periods of time, and results are very operator dependent.

To illustrate the need to integrate different variables, rather than focusing on just one variable, some suggested applications follow:

- *Interpretation of a cardiac output value:* It is important to consider the four determinants of cardiac output (Fig. 4-9). Interpretation should start by considering the stroke volume (cardiac output divided by heart rate), and relating this to an index of ventricular filling (PAOP) and an index of ventricular afterload (arterial and pulmonary artery pressures); an inotropic agent should be added only when preload and afterload have been optimized.
- *Fluid status:* Low cardiac filling pressures may be normal or reflect hypovolemia. It is the measurement of cardiac output and Sv_{O_2} that will help determine fluid needs. Indeed, hypovolemia typically is

Table 4-1. Pulmonary Artery (PA) Catheterization versus Echocardiographic Techniques for Management of Selected Disorders: Relative Value

	PA Catheterization		Echocardiography	
Disorder	Diagnosis	Monitoring	Diagnosis	Monitoring
Tamponade	+	++	+++	+
Hypovolemia	++	+++	++	+
Valvular disease	+	++	+++	+
Heart failure	++	+++	++	+
Right ventricular failure	++	+++	+++	++
Septic shock	+	+++	+	+

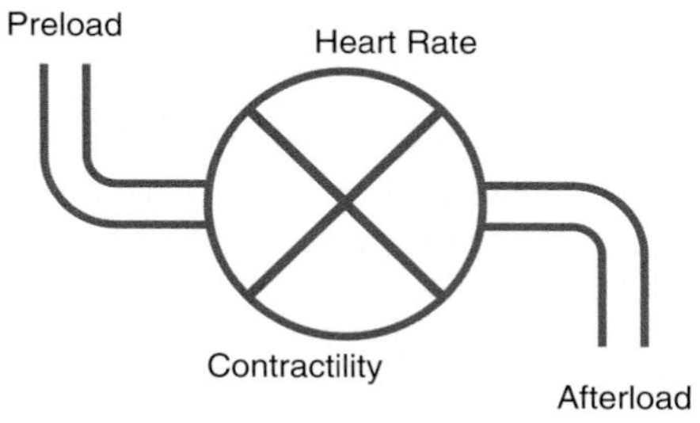

Figure 4-9. The four determinants of cardiac output.

associated with a low cardiac output and a low Svo_2 (Fig. 4-10). By contrast, hypervolemia in the presence of normal cardiac function will be manifested by high cardiac filling pressures associated with a relatively high cardiac output and normal or high Svo_2.

- *Hemodynamic versus nonhemodynamic pulmonary edema:* The distinction between hemodynamic and nonhemodynamic types of lung edema no longer requires pulmonary artery catheterization; the clinical history and less invasive (e.g., echocardiographic) measurements usually are sufficient to separate the two. Nevertheless, invasive hemodynamic monitoring can reveal that patients thought to meet only the acute lung injury/acute respiratory distress syndrome (ALI/ARDS) criteria sometimes have unexpectedly high PAOP.[20]
- *RV dysfunction versus failure:* A reverse gradient between RAP and PAOP (i.e., a higher RAP than PAOP) indicates RV dysfunction or failure and usually is secondary to pulmonary hypertension, as will be immediately apparent from the measurements of pulmonary artery pressures. RV dysfunction is manifested by RV dilation (and thus a decrease in RVEF) with no limitation on cardiac output. This is the most common situation in patients with ARDS, who usually maintain a hyper-kinetic state. Rather, RV failure refers to a state in which cardiac output is no longer sustained at adequate levels.[21] These different entities are illustrated in Figure 4-11.
- *LV dysfunction versus failure:* Here the gradient between PAOP and RAP will be higher than the typical 3 to 5 mm Hg. As with the right ventricle, in LV dysfunction the ventricular volumes may increase (so the

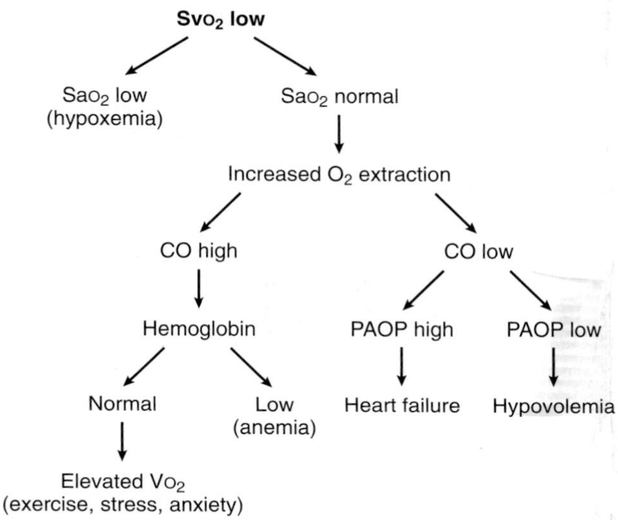

Figure 4-10. Interpretation of a low Svo_2 (mixed venous oxygen saturation). CO, cardiac output; PAOP, pulmonary artery occlusion pressure; Sao_2, arterial oxygen saturation; Vo_2, oxygen uptake.

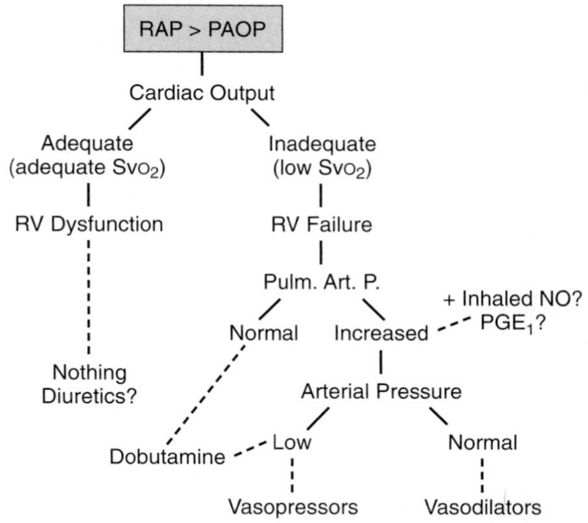

Figure 4-11. Interpretation of a reversed gradient between the right atrial pressure (RAP) and the pulmonary artery occlusion pressure (PAOP). NO, nitric oxide; PEG_1, prostaglandin E_1; RV, right ventricular; Svo_2, mixed venous oxygen saturation.

ejection fraction will decrease), but the cardiac output may be simultaneously preserved; such a situation may exist in septic shock. LV failure is more common and is manifested by a decrease in cardiac output and SvO_2.

Effects of Interventions

- *Fluid challenge:* A fluid challenge technique is indicated whenever the benefit of fluid administration is in doubt.[17] Ideally, fluid administration will result in increases in cardiac output and tissue perfusion without major increases in cardiac filling. An increase in PAOP in the absence of a significant change in cardiac output and SvO_2 indicates that fluid administration will only result in an increased risk of edema and should be discontinued.
- *Inotropic agents:* The use of inotropes aims to increase cardiac output and possibly decrease PAOP. Lack of an increase in cardiac output after administration of a β_1 inotropic agent indicates a desensitization of the β-adrenergic receptors and is associated with a worse prognosis.[22]
- *Vasopressors:* The use of pure vasoconstrictors is expected to increase arterial pressure but also cardiac filling pressures. An excessive increase in cardiac filling pressures with use of such an agent suggests the need for addition of an inotropic agent (e.g., dobutamine).
- *Vasodilators:* The administration of vasodilators may rapidly reduce arterial pressure, so that continuous arterial pressure monitoring is usually indicated. Moreover, a reduction in vascular tone in the presence of hypovolemia may reduce venous return and thus cardiac output.

Clinical Indications for Pulmonary Artery Catheter Insertion

The improvement in noninvasive diagnostic techniques means that today the PAC is used primarily for monitoring. Potential indications include the following:

- *Circulatory shock, including the need for vasopressor agents:* The PAC can be used to help guide fluid challenges and titrate inotropic agents. Shock due to hypovolemia (as in polytrauma or with other forms of massive bleeding) does not require insertion of a PAC, because management of such patients generally is quite straightforward.
- *RV failure:* The PAC can be used to monitor pulmonary artery pressures, the gradient between RAP and PAOP, cardiac output, and SvO_2.
- *Acute respiratory failure due to pulmonary edema:* Whether lung edema is hemodynamic or nonhemodynamic, the strategy should be to keep the hydrostatic pressures as low as possible, but this requires measurements of cardiac output and SvO_2 to make sure the systemic circulation is not compromised
- *Complex fluid management in the presence of impending renal failure:* Sometimes it is difficult to evaluate the fluid status in oliguric patients, in whom hypovolemia may compromise renal function but hypervolemia obviously must be avoided.
- *Dynamic assessment of cardiac function in specific conditions:* The best example is that of the patient who is difficult to wean from mechanical ventilation, possibly owing in part to cardiac dysfunction.

Pulmonary Artery Occlusion Pressure and Partial Occlusion

Partial occlusion of the pulmonary artery in the presence of pulmonary hypertension may be difficult to recognize and can lead to significant overestimation of the pulmonary artery occlusion pressure, denoted Ppao on Figure 4-12. A useful clue to partial occlusion is occurrence of a substantial increase in the Ppao without a concomitant change in the pulmonary artery diastolic pressure, denoted Ppad on the figure. If the Ppad – Ppao gradient is normal and the underlying disease process would predict increased pulmonary vascular resistance, partial occlusion should be suspected. Partial occlusion may occur if a catheter is either too proximal or too distal in the pulmonary artery, and appropriate repositioning may be corrective. The best Ppao may be obtained in some circumstances by further advancing the catheter with the balloon fully inflated and at other times by retracting the catheter to the original pulmonary artery position and attempting to occlude with 1.0 to 1.2 mL of air, instead of full inflation. It is imperative never to inflate against resistance. Figures 4-12 and 4-13 offer further information on diagnosis and management of partial occlusion.

Does the Use of a Pulmonary Artery Catheter Improve Outcome?

The use of the PAC has been challenged on the basis that it has not been shown to improve outcomes.[20,23-25] An improvement in outcome, however, has not been demonstrated with other monitoring techniques. Moreover, a number of studies have indicated that the use of the PAC can influence therapy.[26] If use of a PAC does not result in

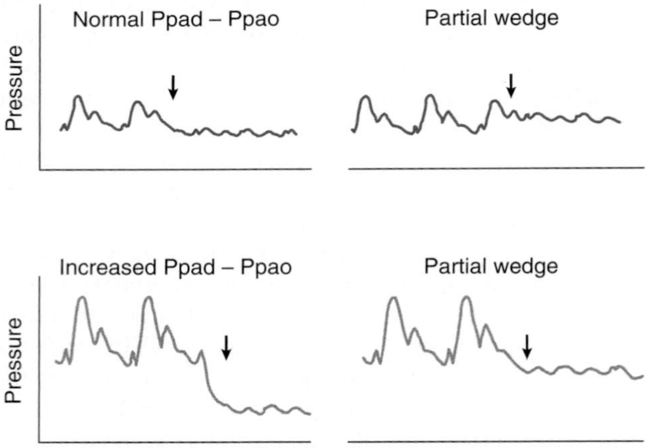

Figure 4-12. Schematic depiction of partial occlusion when the gradient between the pulmonary artery diastolic pressure (Ppad) and the pulmonary artery occlusion pressure (Ppao) is normal *(top)* or is increased *(bottom)*. *Arrow* denotes balloon inflation. (From Leatherman JW, Shapiro RS: Overestimation of pulmonary artery occlusion pressure in pulmonary hypertension due to partial occlusion. Crit Care Med 2003;31:93-97.)

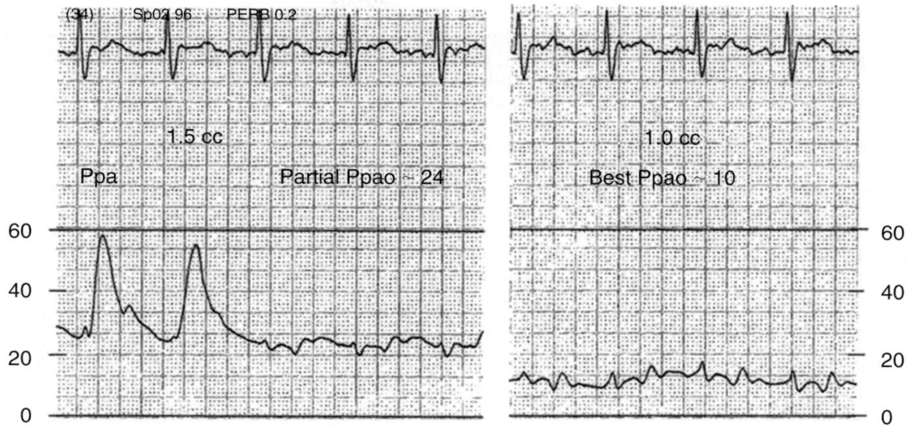

Figure 4-13. Partial pulmonary artery occlusion pressure (Ppao) measured when 1.5 cc of air was used to inflate the catheter balloon *(left graph);* a much lower Ppao was obtained with a 1.0-cc inflation *(right graph).* Review of the chest roentgenogram revealed that the catheter tip was too peripheral, so it was withdrawn to a more proximal location. Ppa, pulmonary artery pressure. See text for definition of partial and best Ppao values. Scale in mm Hg. (From Leatherman JW, Shapiro RS: Overestimation of pulmonary artery occlusion pressure in pulmonary hypertension due to partial occlusion. Crit Care Med 2003;31:93-97.)

Table 4-2. Components and Common Errors in Hemodynamic Monitoring

Component	Common Errors
1. Measure	■ Catheter misplacement ■ Errors in pressure measurements ■ No consideration of SvO_2
2. Interpret	■ Interpretation of cardiac output without consideration of SvO_2 ■ Neglect of PAP/PAOP gradient ■ Neglect of inversed RAP/PAOP gradient
3. Apply	■ Treating as if the data were not available ■ Giving diuretics for a high PAOP without other consideration

PAP, pulmonary artery pressure; PAOP, pulmonary artery occlusion pressure; RAP, right atrial pressure; SvO_2, mixed venous oxygen saturation.

better outcomes, important and challenging questions arise about the beneficial effects of many therapeutic interventions in the ICU. Some evidence suggests that the use of the PAC may improve outcomes in the most severely ill subsets of critically ill patients.[27,28] Errors in measurements from the PAC were identified many years ago,[29] and another consideration is the considerable interobserver variability in interpretation of PAC tracings.[30] In using a PAC, it is important to respect the three successive steps (Table 4-2): to take adequate and full measurements; to interpret the results correctly; and to apply the gathered information for the patient's benefit. Unfortunately, potential errors are associated with each step. Some of these issues can be addressed with better teaching and improved basic knowledge of hemodynamics and basic physiology.

KEY POINTS

- No simple guidelines for monitoring are available or applicable in all cases; monitoring should be tailored to each patient's needs.
- Each variable, taken individually, has limitations and is subject to error and difficulty in interpretation. Variables should be combined and integrated to provide a global picture of the clinical situation.
- A monitoring technique cannot improve outcome by itself; each of the three components of monitoring is important with any monitoring technique:
  Accurate collection of data
  Interpretation of the data
  Application of the information obtained
- Cardiac output is an adaptive value that must constantly adjust to the oxygen requirements of the organs.
- Separation of the four determinants of cardiac output—heart rate, contractility, preload, and afterload—is useful to consider the various interventions that can be used to increase it.
- Measurements of mixed venous oxygen saturation (i.e., SvO_2) are essential to interpret cardiac output measurements.
- The relationship between cardiac filling pressures and volumes is relatively weak. Pressure measurements are important, however, because pressures (rather than volumes) are the primary determinant of edema formation.
- The calculation of derived variables, such as vascular resistances, ventricular work, and oxygen-derived variables, is of limited usefulness.

REFERENCES

1. Bur A, Hirschl MM, Herkner H, et al: Accuracy of oscillometric blood pressure measurement according to the relation between cuff size and upper-arm circumference in critically ill patients. Crit Care Med 2000;28:371-376.
2. De Backer D, Heenen S, Piagnerelli M, et al: Pulse pressure variations to predict fluid responsiveness: Influence of tidal volume. Intensive Care Med 2005;31:517-523.
3. Heenen S, De Backer D, Vincent JL: How can the response to volume expansion in patients with spontaneous respiratory movements be predicted? Crit Care 2006;10:R102.
4. Lorente L, Santacreu R, Martin MM, et al: Arterial catheter-related infection of 2,949 catheters. Crit Care 2006;10:R83.
5. Martin C, Saux P, Papazian L, et al: Long-term arterial cannulation in ICU patients using the radial artery or dorsalis pedis artery. Chest 2001;119: 901-906.
6. Cook DJ, Simel DL: The rational clinical examination. Does this patient have abnormal central venous pressure? JAMA 1996;275:630-634.
7. Rivers E, Nguyen B, Havstad S, et al: Early goal-directed therapy in the treatment of severe sepsis and septic shock. N Engl J Med 2001;345: 1368-1377.
8. Joynt GM, Gomersall CD, Buckley TA, et al: Comparison of intrathoracic and intra-abdominal measurements of central venous pressure. Lancet 1996;347:1155-1157.
9. Merrer J, De Jonghe B, Golliot F, et al: Complications of femoral and subclavian venous catheterization in critically ill patients: A randomized controlled trial. JAMA 2001;286: 700-707.
10. Zurcher M, Tramer MR, Walder B: Colonization and bloodstream infection with single- versus multi-lumen central venous catheters: A quantitative systematic review. Anesth Analg 2004;99:177-182.
11. Darouiche RO, Raad II, Heard SO, et al: A comparison of two antimicrobial-impregnated central venous catheters. Catheter Study Group. N Engl J Med 1999;340:1-8.
12. Tambe SM, Sampath L, Modak SM: In vitro evaluation of the risk of developing bacterial resistance to antiseptics and antibiotics used in medical devices. J Antimicrob Chemother 2001;47: 589-598.
13. O'Grady NP, Alexander M, Dellinger EP, et al: Guidelines for the prevention of intravascular catheter–related infections. Infect Control Hosp Epidemiol 2002;23:759-769.
14. Pinsky MR, Vincent JL, De Smet JM: Estimating left ventricular filling pressure during positive end-expiratory pressure in humans. Am Rev Respir Dis 1991;143:25-31.
15. Teboul JL, Pinsky MR, Mercat A, et al: Estimating cardiac filling pressure in mechanically ventilated patients with hyperinflation. Crit Care Med 2000;28:3631-3636.
16. Calvin JE, Driedger AA, Sibbald WJ: Does the pulmonary capillary wedge pressure predict left ventricular preload in critically ill patients? Crit Care Med 1981;9:437-443.
17. Vincent JL, Weil MH: Fluid challenge revisited. Crit Care Med 2006;34: 1333-1337.
18. Varpula M, Karlsson S, Ruokonen E, et al: Mixed venous oxygen saturation cannot be estimated by central venous oxygen saturation in septic shock. Intensive Care Med 2006;32: 1336-1343.
19. Yalavatti GS, De Backer D, Vincent JL: The assessment of cardiac index in anemic patients. Chest 2000;118: 782-787.
20. Wheeler AP, Bernard GR, Thompson BT, et al: Pulmonary-artery versus central venous catheter to guide treatment of acute lung injury. N Engl J Med 2006;354:2213-2224.
21. Vincent JL: Is ARDS usually associated with right ventricular dysfunction or failure? Intensive Care Med 1995;21:195-196.
22. Rhodes A, Lamb FJ, Malagon I, et al: A prospective study of the use of a dobutamine stress test to identify outcome in patients with sepsis, severe sepsis, or septic shock. Crit Care Med 1999;27:2361-2366.
23. Sakr Y, Vincent JL, Reinhart K, et al: Use of the pulmonary artery catheter is not associated with worse outcome in the intensive care unit. Chest 2005;128: 2722-2731.
24. Harvey S, Harrison DA, Singer M, et al: Assessment of the clinical effectiveness of pulmonary artery catheters in management of patients in intensive care (PAC-Man): A randomised controlled trial. Lancet 2005;366: 472-477.
25. Rhodes A, Cusack RJ, Newman PJ, et al: A randomised, controlled trial of the pulmonary artery catheter in critically ill patients. Intensive Care Med 2002;28:256-264.
26. Mimoz O, Rauss A, Rekik N, et al: Pulmonary artery catheterization in critically ill patients: A prospective analysis of outcome changes associated with catheter-prompted changes in therapy. Crit Care Med 1994;22: 573-579.
27. Chittock DR, Dhingra VK, Ronco JJ, et al: Severity of illness and risk of death associated with pulmonary artery catheter use. Crit Care Med 2004;32: 911-915.
28. Friese RS, Shafi S, Gentilello LM: Pulmonary artery catheter use is associated with reduced mortality in severely injured patients: A National Trauma Data Bank analysis of 53,312 patients. Crit Care Med 2006;34: 1597-1601.
29. Morris AH, Chapman RH, Gardner RM: Frequency of wedge pressure errors in the ICU. Crit Care Med 1985;13: 705-708.
30. Al Kharrat T, Zarich S, Amoateng-Adjepong Y, et al: Analysis of observer variability in measurement of pulmonary artery occlusion pressures. Am J Respir Crit Care Med 1999;160: 415-420.

Chapter 5

Temporary Cardiac Pacing

Lawrence J. Gessman and Joseph E. Parrillo

Temporary cardiac pacing involves insertion of a pacemaker electrode into the heart, usually under emergency or semiemergency conditions, or semielectively during or after cardiac surgery, to treat transient bradyarrhythmias or tachyarrhythmias. The indications for temporary pacing are slightly different than the indications for permanent pacing. The techniques for insertion of temporary pacemakers also are quite different from techniques for insertion of permanent pacemakers. This chapter reviews indications for temporary pacing, various methods of temporary pacing (including transvenous, transesophageal, epicardial, and transcutaneous), various modes of temporary pacing (including VVI, DVI, VDD, AAI, and DDD), and postinsertion care and complications of temporary pacing. Emphasis is on practical aspects of temporary pacing in the emergency department and intensive care unit (ICU).

INDICATIONS FOR TEMPORARY PACING

Any indication for permanent pacing is an indication for temporary pacing, if permanent pacing cannot be established in a timely manner. In some situations, avoidance of temporary pacing and expeditious insertion of a permanent pacemaker is advisable because it avoids two procedures and may reduce complications. Temporary pacing before permanent pacing is a risk factor for infection of the permanent pacemaker.[1,2] In general, temporary pacing is used for emergency treatment of bradyarrhythmias or tachyarrhythmias that occur suddenly causing severe hemodynamic compromise. Temporary pacing also is indicated for bradycardias or tachycardias that result from an acute and reversible cause that would not likely require permanent pacing.

Reversible Causes of Sinus Dysfunction or Heart Block

Reversible causes of sinus dysfunction or heart block include injury to the conduction system during open heart surgery; Lyme disease; toxic or metabolic electrolyte abnormalities; drug toxicities, such as hyperkalemia, digitalis toxicity, β-blocker or calcium blocker sensitivity or overdose, and antiarrhythmic drug sensitivity or overdose; some neurologic diseases; subacute bacterial endocarditis with aortic valve abscess damaging the His conduction system; and catheter-induced or other cardiac trauma. Swan-Ganz catheter insertion into the right heart in patients who already have a left bundle-branch block (LBBB) infrequently can cause the development of temporary heart block.[3,4] It is advisable to anticipate this and have an external temporary pacer available.

The complications of emergency transvenous pacing are described later in the chapter. The risks and benefits of transvenous pacing must be considered against the ease, but less certain establishment, of transcutaneous pacing in many situations. Transcutaneous pacing can be established more rapidly, but is associated with significant pain. It is important to distinguish bradycardias that are likely to be very transient and short-lived, for which transcutaneous pacing is more appropriate, from bradycardias likely ultimately to need permanent pacing, where temporary transvenous pacing as a bridge to permanent pacing is more appropriate. Once transcutaneous pacing is established, high-risk patients should be switched from transcutaneous to transvenous temporary pacing. Recommendations for transvenous and transcutaneous pacing are part of guidelines from the American Heart Association and American College of Cardiology (Box 5-1).[5]

Temporary Bradycardia Pacing in Myocardial Infarction

Temporary bradycardia pacing may be needed in acute myocardial infarction in situations in which permanent pacing is not anticipated (Fig. 5-1). Permanent pacing is rarely needed after acute inferior myocardial infarction, but often is required after acute anterior infarction with new conduction deficits. Indications for temporary pacing in acute myocardial infarction are described in guidelines from the American Heart Association and American College of Cardiology (Box 5-2).[5,6] Indications include asystole, symptomatic sinus bradycardia not responsive to atropine, Mobitz type II second-degree or transient complete heart block, bilateral or alternating bundle-branch block (BBB), new right bundle-branch block (RBBB) with left anterior hemiblock, left posterior hemiblock, new BBB with first-degree block, and old RBBB with first-degree and new fascicular block. Bradycardia in the setting of myocardial infarction may decrease coronary blood flow, myocardial perfusion, and myocardial output. Thrombolytics and antiplatelet drugs, often used to treat infarction, may increase the risk of bleeding, however, from transvenous insertion of temporary pacing catheters. The risks and benefits of temporary transvenous pacing must be weighed against the use of standby external pacers in these situations. The recommendations for placement of transcutaneous patches and active demand transcutaneous pacing are listed in Box 5-3.

Temporary Overdrive Pacing to Terminate Supraventricular Tachycardia and Ventricular Tachycardia

Temporary overdrive atrial and ventricular pacing, at a rate slightly faster than the tachycardia rate, often can be used to terminate tachycardia.[7-9] This technique is useful in patients who have implanted temporary pacing leads or wires for bradycardias or who have frequently recurring tachycardias not responsive to antiarrhythmic drugs. Overdrive atrial pacing is often used to treat postoperative atrial flutter.[10] Atrial flutter can be terminated by pacing the atrium at a rate slightly greater than the flutter rate at high output for several seconds, ensuring capture of the atrium by the pacer. Pacing is then suddenly shut off. If

Box 5-1

Recommendations for Temporary Transvenous Pacing*

Class I

1. Asystole
2. Symptomatic bradycardia (includes sinus bradycardia with hypotension and type 1 second-degree AV with hypotension not responsive to atropine)
3. Bilateral BBB (alternating BBB, or RBBB with alternating LAFB/LPFB) (any age)
4. New or indeterminate age bifascicular block (RBBB with LAFB or LPFB, or LBBB)
5. Mobitz type II second-degree AV block

Class IIa

See also indications for transcutaneous pacing.

1. RBBB and LAFB or LPFB (new or indeterminate)
2. RBBB with first-degree AV block
3. LBBB, new or indeterminate
4. Incessant VT, for atrial or ventricular overdrive pacing
5. Recurrent sinus pauses (>3 seconds) not responsive to atropine

Class IIb

1. Bifascicular block of indeterminate age
2. New or age-determinate isolated RBBB

Class III

1. First-degree heart block
2. Type 1 second-degree AV block with normal hemodynamics
3. Accelerated idioventricular rhythm
4. BBB known to exist before acute myocardial infarction

American College of Cardiology/American Heart Association Classification

Class I—conditions for which there is evidence or general agreement or both that a given procedure or treatment is useful and effective
Class II—conditions for which there is conflicting evidence or a divergence of opinion or both about the usefulness and efficacy of a procedure or treatment
Class IIa—weight of evidence and opinion in favor of usefulness and efficacy
Class IIb—usefulness and efficacy less well established by evidence and opinion
Class III—conditions for which there is evidence or general agreement or both that the procedure or treatment is not useful and in some cases may be harmful

*In choosing an intravenous pacemaker system, patients with substantially depressed ventricular performance, including right ventricular infarction, may respond better to atrial AV sequential pacing than ventricular pacing.
AV, atrioventricular; BBB, bundle-branch block; LAFB, left anterior fascicular block; LBBB, left bundle-branch block; LPFB, left posterior fascicular block; RBBB, right bundle-branch block; VT, ventricular tachycardia.
Adapted from Ryan TJ, Anderson JL, Antman EM, et al: ACC/AHA guidelines for the management of patients with acute myocardial infarction. A report of the American College of Cardiology/American Heart Association Task Force on Practice Guidelines (Committee on Management of Acute Myocardial Infarction). J Am Coll Cardiol 1996;28:1328.

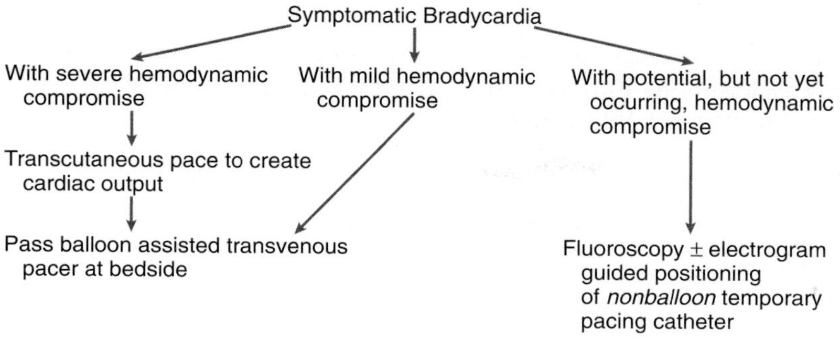

Figure 5-1. Approach to administering temporary pacing in patients with symptomatic bradycardia.

Box 5-2

Recommendations for Temporary Transvenous Pacing in Acute Myocardial Infarction*

Class I

1. Asystole
2. Symptomatic bradycardia (includes sinus bradycardia with hypotension and type 1 second-degree AV block with hypotension not responsive to atropine)
3. Bilateral BBB (alternating BBB or RBBB with alternating LAFB/LPFB) (any age)
4. New or indeterminate-age bifascicular block (RBBB with LAFB or LPFB, or LBBB)
5. Mobitz type II second-degree AV block

Class IIa

See also indications for transcutaneous pacing.

1. RBBB and LAFB or LPFB (new or indeterminate)
2. RBBB with first-degree AV block
3. LBBB, new or indeterminate
4. Incessant VT, for atrial or ventricular overdrive pacing
5. Recurrent sinus pauses (>3 seconds) not responsive to atropine

Class IIb

1. Bifascicular block of indeterminate age
2. New or age-determinate isolated RBBB

Class III

1. First-degree heart block
2. Type 1 second-degree AV block with normal hemodynamics
3. Accelerated idioventricular rhythm
4. BBB or fascicular block known to exist before acute myocardial infarction

American College of Cardiology/American Heart Association Classification

Class I—conditions for which there is evidence or general agreement or both that a given procedure or treatment is useful and effective

Class II—conditions for which there is conflicting evidence or a divergence of opinion or both about the usefulness and efficacy of a procedure or treatment

Class IIa—weight of evidence and opinion in favor of usefulness and efficacy

Class IIb—usefulness and efficacy less well established by evidence and opinion

Class III—conditions for which there is evidence or general agreement or both that the procedure or treatment is not useful and in some cases may be harmful

*In choosing an intravenous pacemaker system, patients with substantially depressed ventricular performance, including right ventricular infarction, may respond better to atrial AV sequential pacing than ventricular pacing.

AV, atrioventricular; BBB, bundle-branch block; LAFB, left anterior fascicular block; LBBB, left bundle-branch block; LPFB, left posterior fascicular block; RBBB, right bundle-branch block; VT, ventricular tachycardia.

Adapted from Ryan TJ, Anderson JL, Antman EM, et al: ACC/AHA guidelines for the management of patients with acute myocardial infarction. A report of the American College of Cardiology/American Heart Association Task Force on Practice Guidelines (Committee on Management of Acute Myocardial Infarction). J Am Coll Cardiol 1996;28:1328.

the flutter is not terminated, the process is repeated at a slightly faster pacing rate. If atrial flutter cannot be terminated cleanly by this method, it is often useful to convert the atrial flutter purposely to atrial fibrillation by a very rapid burst of high output atrial pacing or ramp (decremental burst) atrial pacing. The ventricular response to atrial flutter is often more rapid than the ventricular response to atrial fibrillation because of the phenomenon of concealed conduction caused by atrial fibrillation on the atrioventricular (AV) node. The atrial fibrillation induced also may be short lived, spontaneously converting to sinus rhythm.

Transvenous or transesophageal pacing also can terminate atrial arrhythmias in medical patients. The conversion rate for atrial flutter is lower in medical than surgical patients (47% versus 95% in one study).[11] Antiarrhythmic drug therapy or electrical cardioversion is generally tried first. AV nodal re-entrant tachycardia and AV re-entrant tachycardia caused by concealed or overt bypass tracts in Wolff-Parkinson-White syndrome and some atrial tachycardias are responsive to adenosine (6 to 18 mg intravenous bolus). If frequently recurrent, overdrive pacing to prevent or frequently to treat these arrhythmias may be useful until long-acting

Box 5-3

Recommendations for Placement of Transcutaneous Patches* and (Demand) Transcutaneous Pacing in Myocardial Infarction

Class I

1. Sinus bradycardia (rate <50 beats per minute) with symptoms of hypotension (systolic blood pressure <80 mm Hg) unresponsive to drug therapy†
2. Mobitz type II second-degree AV block†
3. Third-degree heart block†
4. Bilateral BBB (alternating BBB, or RBBB and alternating LAFB/LPFB) (regardless of time of onset)
5. Newly acquired or age-indeterminate LBBB, LBBB and LAFB, RBBB and LPFB
6. RBBB or LBBB and first-degree AV block

Class IIa

1. Stable bradycardia (systolic blood pressure >90 mm Hg, no hemodynamic compromise, or compromise responsive to initial drug therapy)
2. Newly acquired or age-indeterminate RBBB*

Class IIb

1. Newly acquired or age-indeterminate first-degree AV block*

Class III

1. Uncomplicated acute myocardial infarction without evidence of conduction system disease

American College of Cardiology/American Heart Association Classification

Class I—conditions for which there is evidence or general agreement or both that a given procedure or treatment is useful or effective

Class II—conditions for which there is conflicting evidence or a divergence of opinion or both about the usefulness and efficacy of a procedure or treatment

Class IIa—weight of evidence and opinion in favor of usefulness and efficacy

Class IIb—usefulness and efficacy less well established by evidence and opinion

Class III—conditions for which there is evidence or general agreement or both that the procedure or treatment is not useful and in some cases may be harmful

*Apply patches and attach system; system is in either active or standby mode to allow immediate use on demand as required. In facilities where transvenous pacing or expertise to place an intravenous system is unavailable, consideration should be given to transporting the patient to a facility equipped and competent in placing transvenous systems.

†Transcutaneous patches may be attached and activated within a brief time if needed. Transcutaneous pacing may be helpful as an urgent expedient. Because it is associated with significant pain, high-risk patients likely to require pacing should receive a temporary pacemaker.

AV, atrioventricular; BBB, bundle-branch block; LAFB, left anterior fascicular block; LBBB, left bundle-branch block; LPFB, left posterior fascicular block; RBBB, right bundle-branch block.

Adapted from Ryan TJ, Anderson JL, Antman EM, et al: ACC/AHA guidelines for the management of patients with acute myocardial infarction. A report of the American College of Cardiology/American Heart Association Task Force on Practice Guidelines (Committee on Management of Acute Myocardial Infarction). J Am Coll Cardiol 1996;28:1328.

antiarrhythmic drug therapy or radiofrequency ablation therapy can be instituted.

Monomorphic ventricular tachycardia (VT), especially when less than 180 beats per minute, usually also can be overdrive pace terminated by rapid ventricular pacing with a success rate of 80%.[12] Fast VT (>188 beats per minute) can be pace terminated 75% of the time.[13] The technique is to start ventricular pacing at a rate 10 to 20 beats per minute faster than the VT rate. Pacing is applied for 3 to 10 seconds and abruptly stopped. If VT persists, pacing at a faster rate is tried, up to 250 beats per minute. Pacing rates greater than 250 beats per minute often accelerate VT or cause ventricular fibrillation (VF). A defibrillator should be present when this is tried because overdrive ventricular pacing often results in conversion of monomorphic VT to polymorphic VT, a faster monomorphic VT that cannot be pace terminated, or VF. Many external temporary pacers cannot deliver pacing at these high rates. Depending on the external pacemaker generator used, a rate multiplier function may be needed. Programmed stimulators from the electrophysiology laboratory can always deliver these high external pacing rates. Also, explanted permanent pacemakers or implantable cardioverter defibrillators (appropriately cleaned to prevent infection) with remaining battery power can be used as temporary monitors and automatic overdrive pace terminating devices, if connected properly to external pacing electrodes.[14] β-blockers followed by intravenous amiodarone or lidocaine are first-line therapy for a VT electrical storm. Pace termination of drug-refractory monomorphic VT is useful in this situation and is preferred over repeated external DC countershocks.

Temporary Pacing to Prevent Arrhythmias

In patients with bradycardia-tachycardia syndrome who have sinus bradycardia alternating with periods of paroxysmal atrial fibrillation, pacing the atrium at a rate slightly faster than the sinus rate may prevent atrial fibrillation (ADOPT trial).[15] Overdrive atrial pacing is often used after cardiac surgery to prevent atrial fibrillation. In one study,[16] 96 postoperative patients not treated with antiarrhythmic drugs were randomly assigned to sinus rhythm or overdrive atrial pacing to prevent postoperative atrial fibrillation. Overdrive pacing for 24 hours reduced the incidence of atrial fibrillation from 27% in the control group to 10% in the atrial paced group.[17] Pretreatment with and maintenance of β-blockers and amiodarone or procainamide are first-choice therapy, however, to prevent postoperative atrial fibrillation. Polymorphic VT resulting from genetic or antiarrhythmic drug–induced long QT syndrome often can be prevented by pacing at a rate slightly greater than sinus rate. Atrial or ventricular pacing at rates of 90 to 110 beats per minute can shorten the QT interval and sometimes prevent the premature ventricular contractions causing long-short RR intervals that induce torsades de pointes VT. Magnesium and β-blocker therapy and discontinuation of QT interval–prolonging drugs are first-choice therapy for preventing torsades de pointes VT.[18,19]

Temporary Dual and Biventricular Pacing to Improve Hemodynamics

Temporary AV sequential or biventricular pacing may be useful for hemodynamic benefit in patients with poor left ventricular (LV) function secondary to acute myocardial infarction with right ventricular (RV) involvement, in patients after cardiac surgery, or in patients with cardiomyopathy.[20] RV pacing can cause septal dyskinesis, which may be useful in decreasing the intraventricular gradient in patients with hypertrophic cardiomyopathy with LV outflow tract gradient. In most situations, RV pacing can be harmful to cardiac output, however, by causing septal to lateral wall dyssynergy owing to the artificial RV pacing induced LBBB in patients with poor LV function. In this situation, temporary LV only or biventricular pacing may be more useful. Temporary biventricular pacing with a transvenous catheter placed in the coronary sinus may provide short-term benefit to selected patients in cardiogenic shock.[21] A successful response to therapy may indicate the subsequent use of permanent biventricular pacing.

Prophylactic Pacing before Cardiac Surgery

Pacing before noncardiac surgery is rarely needed. Bradycardias frequently occur after cardiac surgery, so prophylactic insertion of epicardial pacing wires is usually done at the end of the operative procedure, with wires typically left in place until postoperative day 3 or 4. Atrial pacing is often used postoperatively to maximize cardiac output, typically by pacing at rates of 80 to 100 beats per minute, and to suppress atrial fibrillation and the premature atrial contractions and premature ventricular contractions that often initiate arrhythmias. An improvement in cardiac output of 30% often can be achieved by atrial pacing with intact AV conduction or AV pacing compared with ventricular pacing alone.[22] AV block occurs in approximately 2% of bypass graft surgeries[23] and is much more frequent after valve replacement or congenital heart surgery.[24] AV block is most common after aortic valve replacement surgery and is often transient, lasting 4 to 5 days. If complete heart block lasts longer, a permanent pacer is often indicated. If first-degree heart block or BBB remains after complete heart block resolves, a predischarge His conduction electrophysiologic study is often recommended to check the conduction system and ensure a permanent pacer is not needed before hospital discharge.

METHODS OF TEMPORARY PACING

Temporary pacing can be performed with the following:

1. Transvenous or endocardial leads
2. Conversion of an existing hollow or fluid-filled (i.e., Swan-Ganz) catheter into a pacer via insertion of a pacing guidewire
3. Atrial or ventricular epicardial leads or both placed at the time of surgery
4. An esophageal pill or catheter electrode, primarily used for atrial recording and overdrive atrial pacing to terminate atrial arrhythmias
5. External transcutaneous patches
6. Transthoracic insertion via a needle into the heart placed directly through the chest wall

All of these techniques are discussed in more detail subsequently. Before implantation of a temporary pacer, knowledge about normal and abnormal anatomy and ability to distinguish atrial from ventricular and normal from abnormal electrograms is required. An American College of Physicians/American College of Cardiology/American Heart Association task force and other expert authors[25-28] recommend that a physician needs to place 25 Swan-Ganz catheters and 10 ventricular temporary pacemaker implants to gain initial independent privileges and at least 2 per year to maintain skills. Temporary pacemaker lead access and insertion skill are discussed subsequently.

All of the techniques require that the temporary electrode be inserted into a temporary pacemaker generator. Several types of pulse generators are available that permit single and dual chamber pacing. Most temporary pacer generators have all of the available features of a permanent pacemaker, including programmable atrial and ventricular sensitivity and output settings, programmable AV delays, and programmable pacing modes. Typical modes used include V00 (ventricular pacing with no sensing), VVI (ventricular pacing inhibited by natural QRS or R waves), A00 (atrial pacing with no sensing), AAI (atrial pacing inhibited by natural P waves), DVI (atrial and ventricular pacing inhibited by natural R waves, which is useful when atrial sensing is unreliable), and DDD (atrial and ventricular pacing inhibited by natural P and R waves). Some temporary pacemaker generators pace with constant current with programmable outputs typically 1 to 20 mA. Some temporary pacemaker generators are programmable, similar to permanent pacemakers, with outputs programmable by changing the output voltage (typically 1 to 10 volts) or output pulse duration (typically 0.1 to 2.0 mV). Esophageal pacing is best and least painfully accomplished by initially programming wide 10-ms pacing pulse widths and adjusting the voltage upward until capture of the atrium is obtained.[29] Special generators are often needed that have high output and pulse width settings to accomplish esophageal pacing. Typically, at initial implant, one should expect to have an R wave of greater than 5 mV and a ventricular pacing threshold of less than 1 to 2 mA, or less than 1 to 2 volts and 0.5-ms pulse width. If the R wave or thresholds are not this good, and time and safety permit, another lead location should be chosen in the ventricle. Typical good initial values for atrial pacing are P waves greater than 1 mV and atrial pacing threshold less than 1 to 2 mA, or 1 to 2 volts at 0.5-ms pulse width. To ensure a proper safety margin for capture, the outputs on the temporary pacer should be set at twice the threshold for non–pacer-dependent individuals and three times threshold for pacer-dependent individuals. Sensing should be set at one third the R or P wave amplitude: If the R wave measures 9 mV, the ventricular sensitivity setting should be set at 3 mV.

Transvenous or Endocardial Temporary Pacing

Various types of transvenous electrode catheters are available from many manufacturers (Fig. 5-2). Some are stiff, and others are floppy with balloon tips for easier insertion. A balloon-tipped catheter is useful when the patient has an underlying rhythm and blood flows to pull the balloon across the tricuspid valve into the right ventricle, where the balloon is deflated. When circulation is inadequate, a stiffer catheter without a balloon tip is preferred. These come with various preformed curves, including preformed J-shaped curves at the tip for atrial pacing. They come in various French sizes from 2F to 7F. Electrophysiology catheters also can be used as temporary pacing catheters. Stiffer catheters maintain better stability. They may cause higher incidence of perforation, however. Medtronic (Minneapolis, MN) makes an active fixation screw-in temporary pacemaker lead. Permanent screw-in atrial leads from all manufacturers can be used for temporary atrial pacing, but are expensive. Active screw-in leads must be unscrewed before removal. Selection of type of electrode catheter is based on operator's experience, hospital inventory, urgency, availability of fluoroscopy, degree of pacer dependency, and expected duration of temporary pacing. Few data are available to help in this selection. In a randomized comparison of insertion of standard semirigid versus balloon-tipped temporary pacemaker catheters positioned using fluoroscopy guidance, the balloon-tipped catheters were quicker to insert (4.4 minutes versus 9 minutes) and more likely to be positioned in the RV apex.[30] There was no difference in incidence of dislodgment, but the average observation time in this study was only 36 hours. In other observational studies, 6F or 7F semirigid catheters were less likely to dislodge.[31]

The best access for temporary transvenous pacing is via the left subclavian vein or right internal jugular vein. The femoral vein approach is often used during catheterization laboratory or fluoroscopic guided insertion, but is not recommended for long-term use because of the risk of infection and deep vein thrombosis, and it is less stable when moving the patient. The femoral and external jugular veins may be the preferred route in patients receiving thrombolytic agents[32] because these areas are compressible for hemostasis in case bleeding occurs. The advantages of the subclavian vein approach are stable attachment to the patient and more freedom of patient movement if long-term temporary pacing is required. The disadvantage is the 1% to 2% risk of pneumothorax. Another disadvantage is that a permanent pacemaker cannot be placed in this location, which is the usual location performed by right-handed patients, if this site is taken by temporary pacing. The right internal jugular approach eliminates the risk of pneumothorax, but is less comfortable for the patient.

The Seldinger insertion technique is usually used. A needle is inserted into the access vein, a floppy-tipped guidewire is inserted through the needle, and the needle is removed leaving the guidewire in the vein. A peel-away or side port sheath is placed over the guidewire into the vein, and the guidewire and sheath introducer are removed leaving the hollow sheath in the vein. The side port is backflushed to remove trapped air and connected to a flushing intravenous line. The lead is placed through a sterile con-

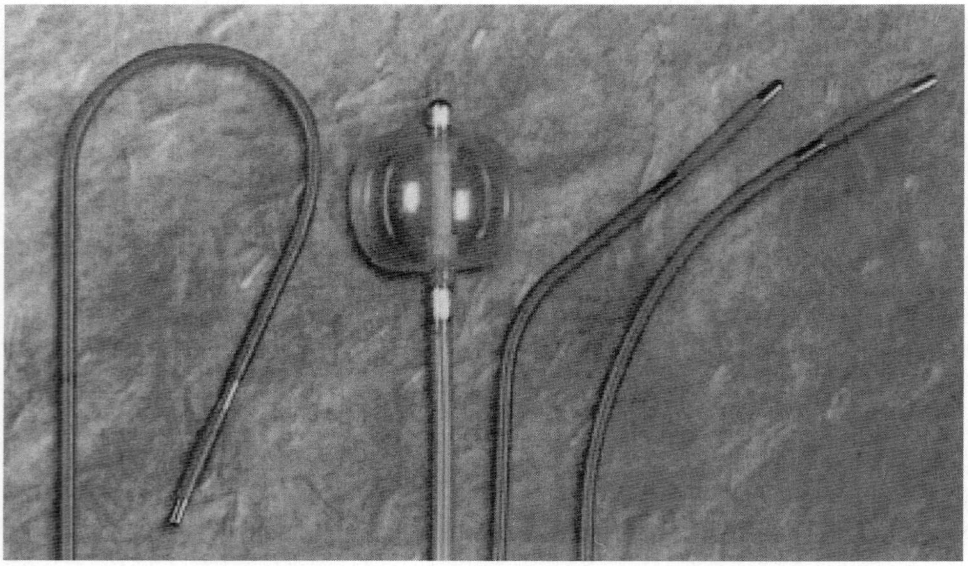

Figure 5-2. Temporary bipolar pacing catheters. *From left to right,* atrial J, semifloating balloon-tipped, and two ventricular catheters with different curves. (Courtesy of Daig Corporation/St. Jude Medical, Minneapolis, MN.)

nector accordion covering through the sheath into the heart. The connector covering allows the lead to be moved or repositioned, if needed, maintaining sterility. Either the sheath or the connector covering should have an O-ring seal, which is opened while inserting the lead, but which can be closed to tighten on the lead to prevent back-bleeding and movement of the lead when in final position.

The lead can be positioned into the heart via fluoroscopy or without fluoroscopy using bedside electrocardiogram (ECG) or electrogram guidance.[33-35] A pacing balloon-tipped or Swan-Ganz catheter is less stable and should be less relied on in a pacer-dependent patient. The technique of insertion via electrogram guidance is shown in Figure 5-3, with each step described in detail in the figure legend. When the lead is placed in the right ventricle, there should be slight forward tension placed on the lead, and the lead should be locked in place by an O-ring seal or Tuey-Borst seal connected to the introducer sheath to prevent lead dislodgment. The lead should be sutured to the skin in at least two spots, one of which maintains the excess lead in a coiled tension loop so that this tension loop absorbs tension mistakenly applied to the connector cables, which might otherwise dislodge the lead. Antibiotic ointment should be applied at the skin entry site

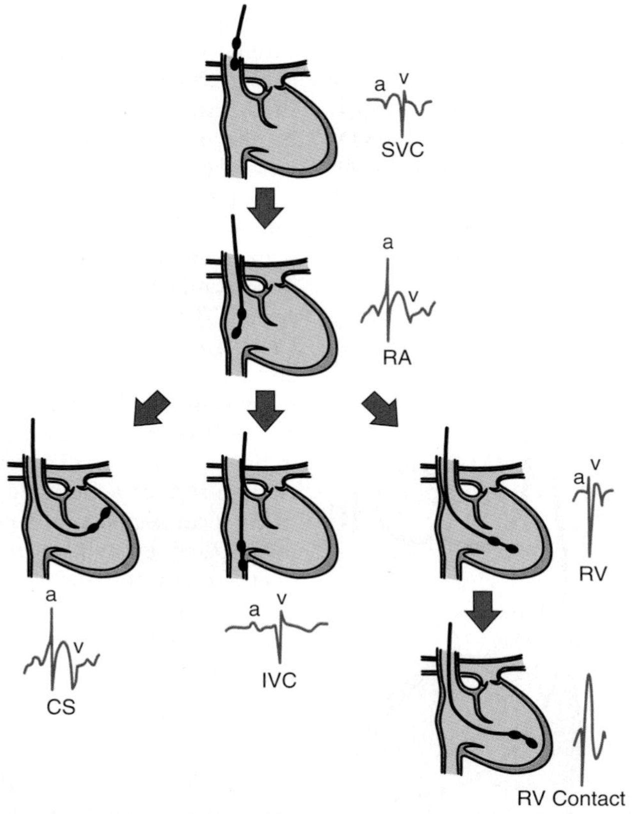

Figure 5-3. The technique of electrogram guidance to place a temporary ventricular pacemaker. It is useful to use a balloon-tipped catheter if there is some blood flow, and first to position the catheter over the patient's chest wall and mark the distance from catheter entry to right ventricle (RV) apex. The end of the electrode catheter is connected to an electrocardiogram (ECG) monitor to guide intracardiac placement. The preferred approach to placement of a temporary transvenous pacemaker electrode catheter is to enter the circulation via the left subclavian vein or right internal jugular vein using Seldinger technique. When the sheath is in place, the electrode catheter is advanced into the superior vena cava (SVC), while watching the electrogram configuration, which should show an a wave and a deep v wave (see electrogram labeled *SVC*). The catheter is advanced to the right atrium (RA), where it inscribes a tall a wave and slightly smaller v wave as shown in the electrogram labeled *RA*. The catheter is advanced with a goal of entering the RV. The electrogram changes from large a, small v, to small or no a and very large v wave. When the catheter is advanced further into the RV wall, the RV contact electrogram shows injury current or ST elevation. The catheter should be disconnected from the ECG monitor and connected to a temporary pacemaker generator, and pacing thresholds should be determined. Starting from the RA location, the electrode catheter may advance into the inferior vena cava (IVC) instead of the RV, whereupon the electrogram suddenly loses the a wave amplitude and suddenly grows a v wave greater than the a wave, as shown in the electrogram labeled *IVC*. The catheter should be pulled back to the RA, getting a more equal a and v wave and readvanced with different torque on the catheter to try to cross the tricuspid valve. It also is possible that the catheter would be advanced from the RA into the coronary sinus (CS), whereupon a tall a and moderate v would be recorded as per the electrogram labeled *CS*. The catheter should be withdrawn back into the RA, torqued differently, and advanced until an RV electrogram is obtained. From the RA position, advancement of the catheter also can cause coiling in the RA, maintaining the RA electrogram despite advancement. The catheter should be withdrawn to the SVC position, and the process is started again.

of the temporary pacing system, and the entry site and coiled excess lead should be covered in 4 × 4 cm sterile bandages, which should be re-dressed daily to prevent infection.

Typically, this temporary transvenous RV pacing system should last 5 to 7 days without significant infection risk. After this time, if pacing is still required, a permanent pacemaker or new transvenous temporary system should be inserted. Pacing sensing and pacing thresholds should be checked daily and charted. Pacing outputs should be adjusted to maintain the two to three times safety margin for capture and appropriate sensing. If bipolar pacing thresholds are too high, the bipolar pacing system can be converted to a unipolar pacing system by replacing the ring electrode by a skin ground (a self-adhesive defibrillator electrode could serve as a good unipolar ground) (Fig. 5-4). The distal tip electrode should be connected to the negative pace generator port. In bipolar pacing, the ring is connected to the positive port. In unipolar pacing, the skin ground is connected to the positive port. Unipolar thresholds sometimes may be better than bipolar thresholds. Unipolar pacing spikes are larger and easier to see on monitors than bipolar spikes. Large unipolar spikes can be used, instead of variable QRS complexes, to time intra-aortic balloon pumps.

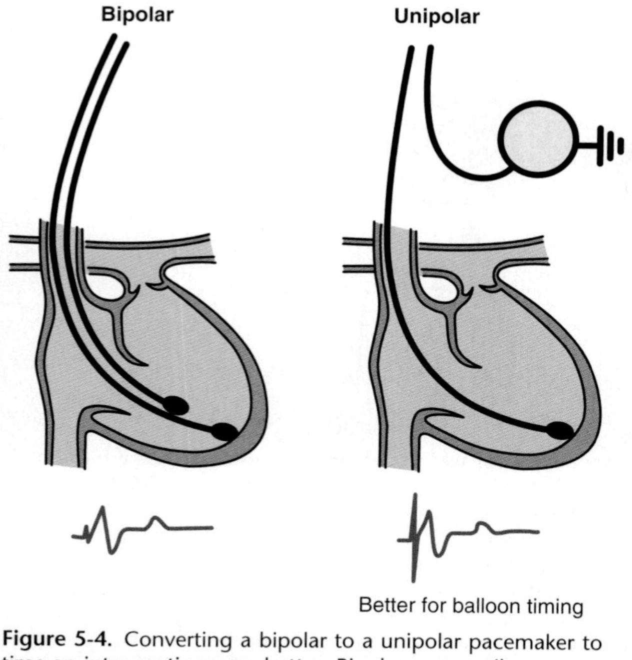

Figure 5-4. Converting a bipolar to a unipolar pacemaker to time an intra-aortic pump better. Bipolar pacer spikes are usually much lower amplitude than unipolar spikes. This patient had a low amplitude surface QRS complex. Instead of using the QRS as a balloon trigger, a large unipolar pacing spike was created to be used as the balloon pump trigger. The tip electrode of the temporary pacer catheter was connected to the negative pacer port, referenced to a large surface area defibrillator electrode serving as a unipolar ground inserted into the positive port. The pacer generator output was increased until the unipolar spike was now larger than the QRS complex. The unipolar spike, rather than QRS, now served as a stable balloon pump trigger.

Conversion of a Cardiac Catheter into an Emergency Transvenous Pacemaker

The method of converting a fluid-filled hollow cardiac catheter into a pacemaker was described by Gessman and colleagues[36] and is the principal idea behind the current PacePort Swan-Ganz catheter design (Edwards, Irvine, CA). This method of emergency pacing is particularly useful in the ICU, where patients often have Swan-Ganz pulmonary arterial pressure monitoring catheters already in place before their bradycardia emergency. The method also is useful in the cardiac catheterization laboratory where x ray contrast injection can cause sinus arrest and sinus bradycardia, and where catheter manipulation can cause heart block (especially right heart catheterization–induced RBBB in a patient with pre-existing LBBB, causing temporary complete heart block). Because the cardiac catheter in the catheterization laboratory that caused the bradycardia emergency is already in place in the heart, it can be rapidly converted into a pacemaker by the method described by Gessman and colleagues[36] and repeated here.

A unipolar guidewire pacing electrode is prepared by removing the Teflon insulation (scrape it off with a sterile scapula blade) from 5 mm at each end of a standard Teflon-coated 170-cm, 0.018-inch diameter, flexible-tip spring. The wire is passed through an O-ring seal of a Y-connector, which can be interposed between the catheter and its pressure transducer connecting tubing or simply passed directly through the catheter. The guidewire is now an insulated unipolar pacer wire and should be connected to the negative port of a temporary pacemaker generator. A large surface adhesive defibrillator or other skin electrode is connected to the positive port to serve as a unipolar pacer ground. Using this method, average right ventricular pacing thresholds in 10 patients were 1.52 ± 0.4 mA, and left ventricular thresholds in 4 patients were 1.33 ± 0.1 mA.[36] Commercially available pacer guidewire PacePort electrodes are available from Edwards. Several methods of conversion of a fluid-filled catheter to a pacemaker exist, which are described next.

Conversion of the Distal Swan-Ganz Pressure Port into an Emergency Right Ventricular Pacer

A pulmonary artery Swan-Ganz catheter is withdrawn under pressure control until a pulmonary artery-to-right ventricular pressure transition is observed (Fig. 5-5A). The distal Swan-Ganz catheter tip is now located in the right ventricle. The flexible tip of the homemade or commercially available guidewire or PacePort electrode is advanced through the pulmonary artery catheter lumen until the electrode tip contacts the RV endocardium. Pulse generator output is increased until pacing capture is achieved. (The Swan-Ganz catheter is no longer usable for pulmonary arterial pressure monitoring.) If there is complete asystole, and no pressure guidance is possible, an alternative method is to advance the pacing guidewire into the distal Swan port now located in the pulmonary artery. If the length of the guidewire is known or premeasured compared with the length of the catheter, the tip should be advanced so that it is exiting the tip of the

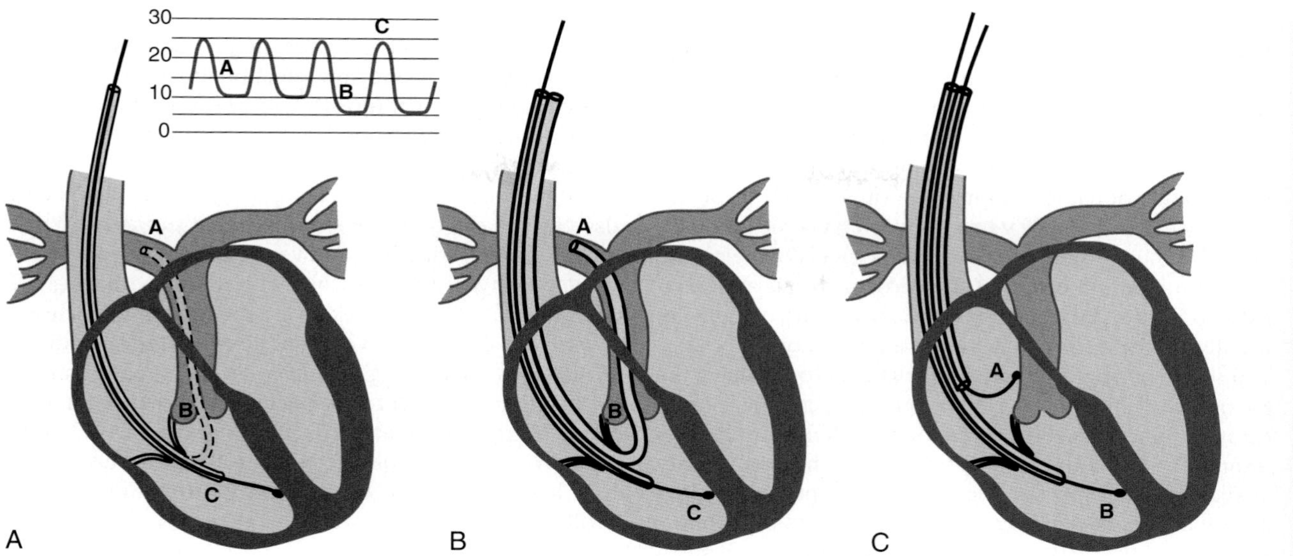

Figure 5-5. Emergency conversion of a Swan-Ganz pulmonary artery catheter to a pacemaker. **A,** A preinserted Swan-Ganz catheter can have its distal tip pulled back from the pulmonary artery to the right ventricles using pressure waveforms as a guide (from position *A* via *B* to *C*). When the tip of the catheter is in the right ventricle, a pacing guidewire already connected to a temporary pacing generator set at high output can be inserted through a Tohy-Borst Y-connector with O-ring seal into the distal port of the catheter and advanced until its tip exits the catheter and touches the right ventricle. This is confirmed by seeing ventricular pacing capture by electrocardiogram monitoring. **B,** Alternatively, the thermodilution injection port of the Swan-Ganz catheter can be connected to a fluid pressure sensor with the Swan-Ganz catheter distal tip left in the pulmonary artery for continued pulmonary arterial pressure monitoring. The fluid injection port of the catheter may already be in the right ventricle, or by slight advancement or slight retraction, the catheter can be placed in the right ventricle as confirmed by right ventricular pressure waveform monitoring. Then the pacing guidewire can be inserted via the injection port to obtain right ventricular pacing without sacrificing pulmonary arterial pressure monitoring. **C,** Temporary atrioventricular sequential pacing can be achieved by placing the catheter tip in the right ventricle by pressure monitoring and passing a pacing guidewire to the right ventricle via the distal port to pace the right ventricle. Then, by positioning the injection port in the right ventricle via pressure monitoring, a second pacing guidewire is passed via the injection port, contacting the right atrium for atrial pacing. Precurling the tip of the pacing guidewire is often helpful to allow it to coil in the right atrium as it exits the injection port.

pulmonary artery catheter by several centimeters. The guidewire is locked in place by tightening the O-ring seal. With pacer output set to maximum, the pulmonary artery catheter is slowly withdrawn until the tip with pacing guidewire falls into and contacts the endocardial wall of the right ventricle, effecting capture.

Conversion of the Injection Port of the Swan-Ganz Catheter to Achieve Right Ventricular Pacing

The injection port of the Swan-Ganz catheter is connected to a pressure monitor and either slightly advanced or withdrawn until right atrium–to–right ventricle transition is seen (see Fig. 5-5B). With the port still in the right ventricle, the guidewire pacer is advanced through the injection port, maintaining high output pacing until capture of the right ventricle is achieved. In some patients, pulmonary artery monitoring is still possible using this configuration.

Conversion of a Swan-Ganz Catheter to an Atrioventricular Sequential Temporary Pacer

The above-described methods are combined (see Fig. 5-5C). The pulmonary artery catheter is withdrawn to the right ventricle via pressure monitoring, and the distance from the skin entry point is noted. The injection port is connected to pressure monitoring, and the catheter is advanced or withdrawn to find the pressure transition from right atrium to right ventricle, and the distance from the skin entry point is noted. The atrial and ventricular guidewire pacers are advanced into the right ventricle and right atrium by positioning the appropriate port in the appropriate chamber (pulmonary artery port in right ventricle and injection port in right atrium).

Conversion of a Left Heart Catheter into an Emergency Left Ventricular Pacer

If sinus arrest or complete heart block occurs during left heart catheterization during a ventriculogram or right conus artery injection, the pigtail or right coronary catheter can be fluoroscopically positioned in the LV cavity. The guidewire pacer is passed through the left heart catheter with pacer output set to maximum until the LV endocardium is contacted and LV pacing begins. LV pacing typically gives a paced RBBB complex compared with RV pacing, which gives a paced LBBB complex on 12-lead surface ECG.

Temporary Guidewire Biventricular Pacing

During a right and left heart catheterization, combining the above-described methods or inserting a standard RV temporary pacer via the right femoral vein, combined with temporary LV pacing by the above-mentioned guidewire method, can effect temporary biventricular pacing. This method might be useful in desperate, cardiogenic shock situations during emergency catheterizations during acute myocardial infarctions, until the patient is stabilized further by intra-aortic balloon, inotropic drug support, or more conventional temporary or permanent biventricular pacing via the coronary veins. LV pacing via the coronary veins is time-consuming and requires special expertise to engage the mouth or OS of the coronary sinus and navigate to posterolateral coronary sinus veins, which are usually the best for resynchronization therapy.

If future pacing needs are anticipated before placing the Swan-Ganz pulmonary artery monitoring catheter, a specially designed PacePort Swan-Ganz catheter can be preinserted for hemodynamic monitoring with ports already available in the proper location to accept future right atrium and right ventricle guidewire pacemakers. In our experience, this catheter is rarely used because, if need for pacing was anticipated, a standard transvenous pacing catheter would already have been inserted. In semielective situations, a standard Swan-Ganz catheter can be exchanged or replaced by the PacePort Swan-Ganz catheter. (Go to *www.Baxter.com* for information on the Model 931 RV PacePort, 991 A-V PacePort, and model 100 and 500 "Guidewire" pacing probes.)

Temporary Epicardial Pacing after Open Heart Surgery

Bradycardias and tachycardias commonly occur after cardiac surgery. Complications of AV block occur in approximately 2% of coronary artery bypass graft surgeries[37] and more commonly post–valvular heart surgery.[38] AV block is usually transient, lasting 1 to 5 days, but sometimes remains complete. Permanent pacing is needed more often in patients who develop complete heart block after aortic valve replacement surgery[39] and after repeat surgery.[40] For these reasons, epicardial pacing is routinely used postoperatively in our institution. Patients undergoing coronary artery bypass grafting with good preoperative ejection fractions usually receive epicardial temporary ventricular pacing wires only. Patients undergoing valve replacement and all patients with low ejection fraction receive epicardial ventricular and atrial temporary wires to enable temporary AV sequential pacing to improve cardiac output if necessary postoperatively. These patients also have a higher incidence of developing atrial and ventricular arrhythmias, which can be diagnosed and, in some cases, treated by overdrive pacing.

In addition to treating heart block, epicardial temporary pacing is frequently used to increase the rate and cardiac output of relatively bradycardic patients by atrial pacing 80 to 90 beats per minute. Sometimes, sequential atrial or AV pacing 100 to 110 beats per minute is necessary to optimize cardiac output. Increases in cardiac output of 30% can be achieved by atrial pacing or AV sequential pacing compared with ventricular pacing at the same rate.[41] If AV conduction is intact, it is best to use atrial pacing rather than AV or V pacing to increase heart rate and cardiac output. A natural QRS creates a more effective ejection fraction than an RV paced QRS, which usually creates intraventricular dyssynchrony. In patients with pre-existing LBBB and low ejection fraction preoperatively, it may be expeditious to place temporary LV pacing wires in the lateral LV free wall and right ventricle. This could enable temporary postoperative biventricular pacing to optimize cardiac output. Temporary higher rate pacing also can be used to suppress rate-related supraventricular ectopy, atrial fibrillation, and ventricular ectopy and ventricular tachycardia, especially in patients with long QT intervals. Although β-blockers are the treatment of choice to prevent postoperative atrial fibrillation, a study of 96 patients undergoing coronary artery bypass grafting showed that atrial overdrive pacing could reduce the incidence of atrial fibrillation on postoperative day 2 from 27% to 10%.[42] Prophylactic biatrial epicardial pacing also has been used to prevent postoperative atrial fibrillation.[43]

Technique of Epicardial Temporary Pacing

Epicardial pacing is accomplished by placing one or two Teflon-coated stainless steel wires on the right or left ventricle or right atrium at the end of the open heart operation. For bipolar pacing, two wires must be attached to each chamber. For unipolar pacing, one wire is attached to the right atrium, and one wire is attached to the left ventricle or right ventricle, with both referenced to a single or double skin ground sewn to the chest wall. In our institution, by convention, atrial bipolar and unipolar wires are brought through the right subcostal area, and RV or LV wires are brought through the left subcostal area. Initially, epicardial wires usually have good thresholds. Thresholds rapidly deteriorate over 3 to 5 days, however, making them unreliable for long-term temporary pacing. With older temporary epicardial wire products, AV sequential pacing at 20 mA maximal pacing output was possible in less than 40% of patients by postoperative day 5.[44] Newer epicardial pacer wires have better performance.[45]

Thresholds should be checked daily to increase the output of the pacer generator as needed to maintain a twofold to threefold safety margin for pacing and adequate safety margin for sensing. When not in use, the pins on the end of the pacing wires should be capped or kept insulated. Otherwise, these wires could cause stray leakage currents in the ICU or coronary care unit to pass directly to the heart, resulting in heart burns or arrhythmias. When the clinician approaches an ICU patient with two temporary epicardial wires exiting the left chest wall, he or she can tell if the wires are configured as a unipolar or bipolar ventricular pacing system by carefully removing the bandage covering the wire entry into the skin and examining the insulation on the wires as they pass through the skin. In bipolar pacing systems, both wires are insulated and cleanly pass through the skin, and both attach to atrium or ventricle. In unipolar pacing systems, only one of two insulated wires cleanly passes through the skin and is attached to the atrium or ventricle. The other wire is stripped of insulation as it enters the skin, with bare conductor wire exposed and sewn to skin. This wire is the ground for unipolar pacing and should be plugged into the positive pacer generator port, with the active wire plugged into the negative pacing port. The polarity of connecting bipolar wires to the generator does not matter.

Conversion of a Bipolar Epicardial to Unipolar Epicardial Temporary Pacing System

If a bipolar pacing system is deteriorating, it is possible that only one of the two wires in the bipolar system is responsible for the threshold deterioration, and that the system can be retrieved by converting to a unipolar pacing system (Fig. 5-6). In this example, a bipolar atrial pacemaker is converted to a unipolar atrial pacemaker. The ventricular pacemaker is unipolar. A skin ground is created by sewing an epicardial wire to the skin or applying a large surface adhesive defibrillation electrode to the skin. Next, each of the two active atrial wires in the bipolar system is individually tested as the active pacing lead

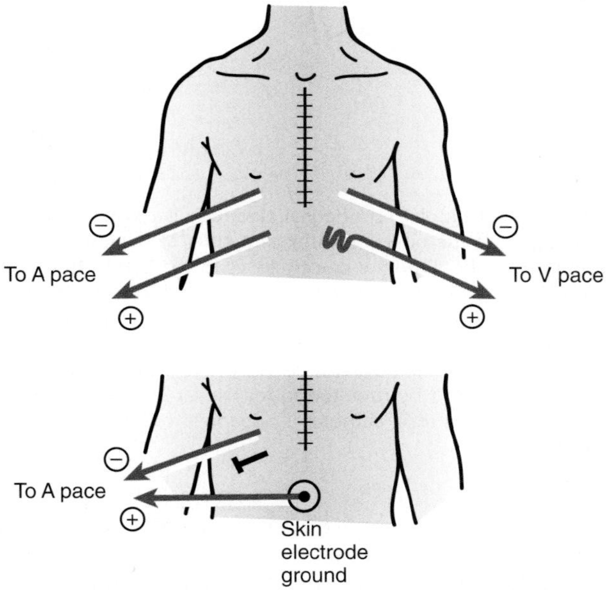

Figure 5-6. Conversion of a temporary epicardial bipolar pacemaker to a unipolar pacemaker. The figure shows a post–coronary artery bypass grafting patient who has two epicardial atrial temporary pacing wires, both sewn into the atrium and exiting the right chest, and one epicardial ventricular wire sewn into the ventricle and exiting the left chest. The atrial wires are inserted into the positive and negative port of the generator supporting bipolar atrial pacing. The active ventricular wire is inserted into the negative pacer port and is referenced to a skin ground (diagrammed as a curly wire sewn into the skin) plugged into the positive pacer port supporting unipolar ventricular pacing. Because of increasing bipolar atrial pacing threshold on postoperative day 3, unipolar thresholds were determined on each of the atrial wires referenced to a skin ground. (An adhesive defibrillator electrode or a new wire sewn into the skin can serve as the new unipolar ground.) The atrial electrode with the lower pacing threshold is chosen as the new pacer cathode and inserted into the negative pacer generator port, referenced to a large surface area skin patch plugged into the positive pacer generator port serving as a unipolar ground. The higher threshold atrial electrode is abandoned and capped.

plugged into the negative port of the pacemaker generator referenced to the skin ground lead plugged into the positive port. In this example, the atrial bipolar threshold was 15 mA. One of the two wires, when unipolarized, had a threshold of 5 mA; the other, 15 mA. A knot can be tied in the least effective pacing wire, and the wire can be capped and abandoned. The better 5 mA threshold wire is left connected to the negative pacing port, referenced to the skin ground, providing unipolar atrial pacing at 5 mA. This is now a sufficient safety margin possibly to last several more days, without having to upgrade to a transvenous temporary pacing system while awaiting conduction system recovery.

Use of Epicardial Wires to Diagnose Postoperative Arrhythmias

As always, the key to diagnosing most arrhythmias is the ability to see the P wave clearly and its relation to the QRS complex. When P waves cannot be seen on surface ECGs, they still may be present buried within the surface QRS or T wave. Epicardial pacing wires can be used to provide atrial electrograms displayed simultaneously with surface ECGs to discern P waves easily during tachyarrhythmias and bradyarrhythmias. The technique of using atrial wires to provide an atrial electrogram is described here and shown in Figure 5-7. Unipolar atrial electrograms can be recorded by connecting the pin of the atrial wire to the V1 lead of a 12-lead ECG. The limb leads are connected to the patient in the usual manner. V1, now a unipolar atrial electrogram, can be displayed simultaneously with two other surface leads in most ECG machines to discern the P wave and QRS relationships better. If bipolar atrial wires are present, they can be connected to the right atrial and left atrial connections, or lead 1 of a 12-lead ECG or monitor, and simultaneously be displayed with other surface ECG leads to accomplish the same goal.

Use of Epicardial Wires to Treat Postoperative Arrhythmias

The most common postoperative arrhythmias are atrial fibrillation and atrial flutter. Overdrive pacing at a rate slightly faster than the atrial flutter rate can be used to pace terminate this arrhythmia. The specific technique is to start pacing the atrium at 10 to 20 beats per minute faster than the atrial flutter rate for 10 to 30 seconds and then to turn off atrial pacing abruptly. If ineffective, the pacing rate can be increased to 120% to 130% faster than the atrial flutter rate for 30 seconds. In some cases, atrial flutter, if not terminable, can be converted to atrial fibrillation purposely by aggressive, very rapid, high output or ramp (continuous atrial overdrive burst pacing with slowly increasing rate) atrial stimulation protocols. The ventricular response to atrial flutter is typically 2:1 block or 150 beats per minute. The ventricular response to purposely induced atrial fibrillation is usually slower and more easily further slowed by AV nodal blocking drugs. Patients with atrial tachycardia and 1:1 conduction to the ventricle often can be atrial paced at a rate faster than the tachycardia rate to achieve 2:1 block to the ventricle,

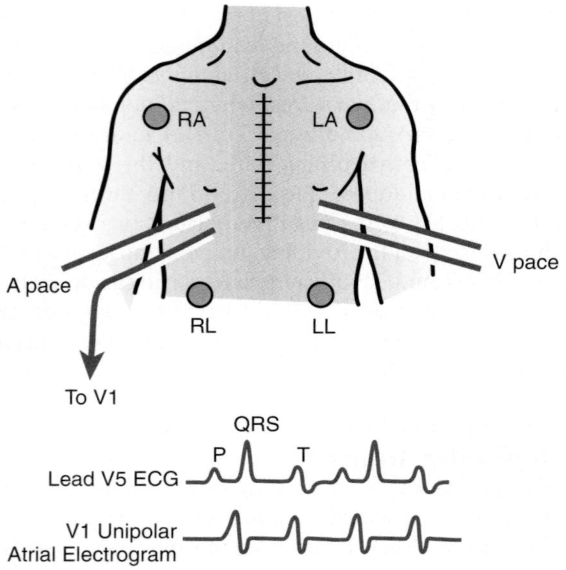

Figure 5-7. Using a temporary atrial pacing wire to create an atrial electrogram for atrial arrhythmia diagnosis. The figure shows a post–coronary artery bypass grafting patient who has bipolar atrial and ventricular temporary pacing wires. The patient develops a narrow complex, 150 beats per minute arrhythmia that may be supraventricular tachycardia or atrial flutter with 2:1 block. P waves cannot be seen clearly on the surface electrogram. One of the two atrial wires is disconnected from the temporary atrial pacer generator and alligator clipped to lead V1 on a standard electrocardiogram (ECG) machine. The unipolar atrial electrogram now appears on lead V1 referenced to surface lead V5, clearly showing two P waves for every QRS, with an atrial rate of 300 beats per minute and a ventricular rate of 150 beats per minute, indicating atrial flutter with 2:1 block. The atrial leads are connected to a pacemaker generator capable of pacing at high rates. Atrial pacing at 320 beats per minute overdrive pace terminates atrial flutter to normal sinus rhythm.

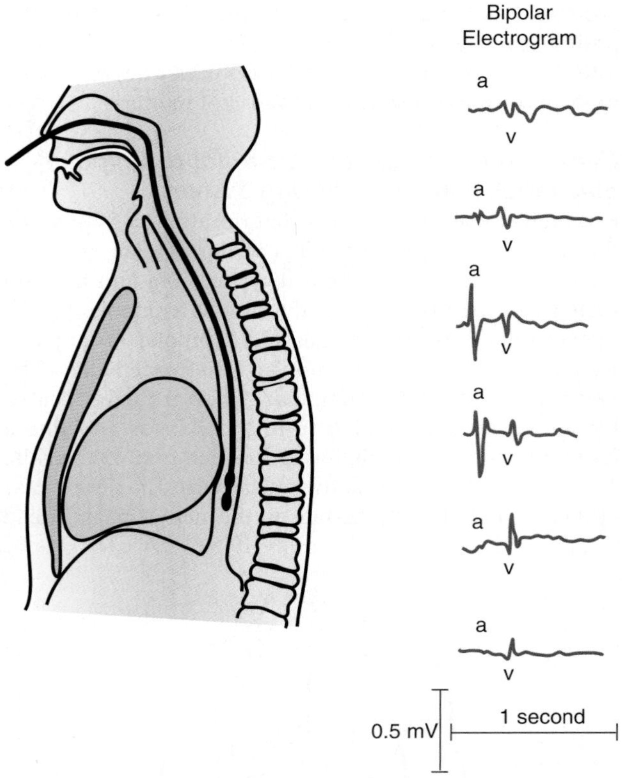

Figure 5-8. A bipolar esophageal electrode is passed into the esophagus via the nose in a similar manner to passing a nasogastric tube. Optimal placement is found by electrogram mapping. The distal esophageal electrode is connected to the V lead of a 12-lead electrocardiogram, and electrograms are recorded. When above or below the left atrial indentation of the esophagus, small a waves are seen. The esophageal lead is optimally placed by monitoring for the largest possible a wave, or the electrode catheter is advanced gently or withdrawn.

temporarily slowing the ventricular rate until pharmacologic control of atrial tachycardia is achieved.[46]

Overdrive ventricular pacing can terminate monomorphic VT by similar burst pacing techniques as described previously. The more aggressive the stimulation protocol, the more likely it is to induce VF inadvertently. A backup defibrillator should be available to terminate VF immediately or terminate VT if overdrive pacing is ineffective. Rarely, timed single, double, or triple extra stimuli delivered via an electrophysiologic laboratory–programmed stimulator can effectively terminate monomorphic VT with less risk of inducing VT than burst or ramp pacing. Most temporary external pacer generators do not deliver timed pacing or programmed stimulation. The programmed stimulator can be borrowed from the electrophysiologic laboratory and connected as a temporary pacer to the epicardial wire ventricular electrodes, if repeated terminations of VT are required, until intravenous amiodarone or other pharmacologic control is achieved. Alternatively, an old, explanted permanent pacemaker or implantable cardioverter defibrillator generator with remaining battery power can be connected to the epicardial ventricular pacing wires, with the device preprogrammed to detect and automatically terminate VT with single, double, or triple burst or ramp pacing techniques. This latter method should be employed by consulting an electrophysiologist skilled in programming implantable cardioverter defibrillators.[14]

Esophageal Recording and Temporary Pacing

Esophageal atrial pacing and recording can be achieved by placing an electrode catheter via the mouth or nose into the esophagus and positioning it at a point where it is closest to the left atrium, which usually indents the esophagus in its midportion. Various catheters have been specifically designed for this purpose or adapted for this purpose. An esophageal "pill" electrode for recording esophageal atrial electrograms also is available. The technique for insertion of esophageal electrodes is shown in Figure 5-8 and described in the figure legend. Esophageal atrial pacing is painful and is rarely used except to terminate atrial arrhythmias, for which only brief pacing is required. Usually, to capture the left atrium via the esophagus, high current (typically 15 to 20 mA), wide pulse width (typically 10 ms) pacing is required. Pain can be minimized, but not eliminated using 10-ms, rather than 1- to 2-ms, pulse width pacing. Pulse widths wider than 1 to 2 ms are usually unavailable on standard external pacemaker generators. A special generator, or an electrophysiologic laboratory–programmed stimulator, may be required for wider pulse width and high current pacing. Also, less painful and more effective capture can be achieved using wider bipolar electrode spacing at the esophageal electrode tip.

Esophageal atrial recording is a more useful, relatively painless (same pain as passing a nasogastric tube) technique for diagnosing arrhythmias when surface ECG P waves cannot be seen. Figure 5-9 illustrates an example where a 120-beat-per-minute, wide-complex tachycardia is seen on surface ECG, but P waves are not easily seen. The differential diagnosis of this ECG is VT versus supraventricular tachycardia with aberration versus supraventricular tachycardia with pre-existing BBB. Because the patient was stable, and time existed to make a proper diagnosis, and because treatment would differ depending on diagnosis, an esophageal electrode was placed. The esophageal recording displayed simultaneously with surface ECG shows slow atrial flutter or atrial tachycardia, with an atrial rate 240 beats per minute with 2:1 block. In addition to making the diagnosis, the arrhythmia was easily overdrive pace terminated through the esophageal lead using high current, wide pulse width, burst overdrive atrial pacing.

External Transcutaneous Pacing

Many external defibrillators have external pacing capability. Large, self-adhesive, low-impedance patches are used for defibrillation. Higher impedance patches are more ideal for external pacing. External pacing is best achieved by placing the electrodes in an anteroposterior position, more fully described subsequently, rather than the standard position used for defibrillation.[47] External pacing usually causes significant pain and should be used only on temporarily unconscious or sedated patients in emergency bradycardia situations until transvenous temporary pacing can be established. External pacing has been used as emergency treatment for asystolic arrest and as prophylaxis during right heart catheterization in patients with pre-existing LBBB or in patients with transient, brief, and reversible bradycardias, serving as potentially standby pacing in case invasive temporary pacing might be needed. It also is used as standby therapy for patients at high risk for developing bradycardias, such as patients with sick sinus syndrome requiring antiarrhythmic drugs or with acute myocardial infarction who have a conduction abnormality that might result in a serious bradycardia. External pacing can be used to deliver overdrive pacing to terminate tachycardias, although it is rarely used for this purpose.

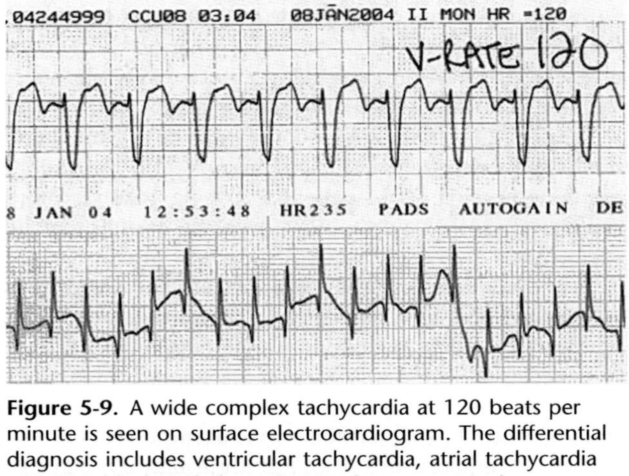

Figure 5-9. A wide complex tachycardia at 120 beats per minute is seen on surface electrocardiogram. The differential diagnosis includes ventricular tachycardia, atrial tachycardia with 2:1 block and aberration, and supraventricular tachycardia with aberration or pre-existing bundle-branch block. The esophageal atrial electrogram clearly shows an atrial rate of 240 beats per minute with 2:1 block to the ventricle, establishing the diagnosis of atrial tachycardia or slow atrial fibrillation with 2:1 block.

Technique of External Pacing

The skin should be cleansed with alcohol, but not shaved. Two sets of electrodes are applied (standard ECG electrodes for monitoring and large surface area, typically 8-cm diameter electrodes for adult external pacing). One pacing patch is placed over the mid-dorsal spine along the left paravertebral line, serving as ground or anode. The other patch electrode is placed over the palpable cardiac impulse or centered over the usual position of lead V3.[48] The external pacer generator is turned on at low output, and current is increased until capture is observed. In stable patients, thresholds for external pacing are typically 40 to 80 mA. Higher thresholds, up to 140 mA, can be observed after prolonged asystole. Usually, only ventricular capture can be achieved by external, transcutaneous pacing. Transcutaneous pacing pulses are approximately $^1/_{1000}$ that of defibrillation energy and do not pose a risk to hospital staff caring for the patient. Chest compressions during cardiopulmonary resuscitation can be administered directly over the pacing electrodes while pacing with no adverse consequences to the rescuer.

It is often difficult to determine if ventricular capture is occurring because the pacing artifact is often larger and obscures the paced QRS complex. Capture should be confirmed by taking the patient's pulse manually, by Doppler ultrasound, or by observing a pressure waveform if an arterial or Swan-Ganz catheter is already in place that matches the set external pacer generator rate.

Transthoracic Insertion of a Needle into the Heart, with Subsequent Insertion of a Guidewire Temporary Pacemaker through the Needle

This technique is now obsolete because it has been replaced by external transcutaneous pacing as described previously. The technique is described here for historical purposes. The technique still may be useful in emergency department situations to treat asystolic arrest if transcutaneous pacing is unavailable or ineffective. In our opinion, this is the most rapid and reliable method of obtaining pacing in extreme emergencies when death is otherwise imminent in minutes. Recovery from asystolic arrest is unlikely, even if emergency pacing can be rapidly established. Transthoracic emergency pacer kits were previously sold by Elecath Corporation (Rahway, NJ), but are no longer commercially available. A transthoracic emergency kit can be constructed as described by Gessman and associates.[49] The construction of a transthoracic needle pacemaker is similar to the construction of a guidewire pacemaker shown in Figure 5-4 except that the fluid-filled catheter is now replaced by a long, 19-gauge spinal or side-holed needle (see Gessman and colleagues[49] for details of construction and use).

COMPLICATIONS

The complications of temporary pacing are frequent, but usually minor. The complications largely depend on the insertion technique used and the experience of the temporary implantor.[49,50-55] Serious complications are rare and include lead dislodgment and disconnection,[56] perforation,[57,58] pericardial tamponade,[59] VF,[60] thrombophlebitis,[61] pneumothorax, local infection,[59] sepsis,[53] bleeding, pulmonary embolus,[61] catheter knotting,[62] subdiaphragmatic stimulation, central venous air embolization,[63] and inadvertent dislodgment of permanent lead on removal.[64]

Electromagnetic interference causing inhibition of temporary pacing from cellular phones and walkie-talkies has been reported.[65] Temporary DDD pacemakers are subject to causing pacemaker-mediated tachycardias and cross-talk resulting in failure to pace a patient with complete heart block if not properly programmed (see section on sophisticated DDD programming).

POSTINSERTION CARE OF TEMPORARY PACEMAKERS

Temporary pacing is a basically unreliable method of pacing, with failure to capture or sense properly occurring in 9%[56] to 37%[57] of patients. After initial placement, pacing capture and sensing thresholds should be measured and charted, and a posteranterior and lateral (if possible) chest x-ray should be obtained for localization of initial position. If the position looks mechanically unstable in a pacemaker-dependent patient, another temporary pacer should be inserted, or the original should be moved under fluoroscopic guidance. There are some ECG clues as to the location of the pacing lead tip. Paced QRS complexes arising from the RV apex usually show a LBBB QRS pattern with a superior axis (upright QRS in leads 1 and avL).[66,67] Pacing from the RV outflow tract gives an LBBB pattern in V leads and strongly positive complexes in leads 2, 3, and avF (inferior axis). Pacing the left ventricle usually gives a RBBB QRS pattern. Pacing from the coronary sinus usually requires high output for ventricular capture and gives simultaneous A and V capture, with V capture showing an RBBB QRS complex. Lower outputs often capture the atrium, but fail to capture the ventricle. An electrogram recorded from a lead placed in the coronary sinus shows large a and v waves.

The pacing, sensing, and capture thresholds should be checked and charted daily. A rising threshold, especially if near the maximal output of the temporary pacemaker generator, should warrant plans for elective wire repositioning or replacement. The wire exit site should be checked daily for infection and should be cleansed daily with iodine solution, with application of an antibiotic ointment and a dry, sterile occlusive dressing.[59] A physical examination also should be performed daily to evaluate for a pericardial friction rub, which might indicate perforation; for the presence of decreased or absent breath sounds in the lung on the side of a subclavian implanted temporary pacer, indicating pneumothorax; and for hypotension and elevation of jugular veins, indicating possible tamponade.

Temporary pacing catheters should be removed as soon as stable recovery heart rhythm is ensured, or immediately after insertion of a permanent pacer. Removal of the temporary pacer after permanent pacer insertion should be performed using fluoroscopic guidance to avoid dislodging the newly implanted permanent leads. Before removal of a temporary pacer, it may be wise to program backup VVI 40 pacing and observe the patient on telemetry for 24 hours to ensure that the conduction system recovery is complete and durable. A bedside electrophysiologic study including sinus node recovery time, Wenckebach point, AV interval times, and ventricular atrial (VA) conduction time can be performed to assess further if recovery is complete, or incomplete but tolerable without need for further backup temporary pacing. A more detailed discussion of bedside electrophysiologic studies via the temporary pacemaker follows in the next section. If a patient develops a fever, blood cultures should be obtained, antibiotics that include antistaphylococcal coverage should be started, and the wire should be changed if wire infection is suspected.

Bedside Electrophysiologic Study to Determine Recovery, or Lack of Recovery, of the Conduction System

The simplest bedside maneuver to determine if sinus node function or AV node conduction has returned is to program the temporary pacer to VVI 40. If the patient takes over with sinus rhythm at a acceptable rate, or atrial fibrillation with adequate ventricular response, a period of 24 to 48 hours of observation on ECG telemetry with the pacer left at VVI 30 to 40 is tried. If there is no use of the pacer in the next 24 to 48 hours, recovery can be assumed, and the temporary pacemaker can be removed. If the patient has a temporary AV sequential pacing system, more sophisticated electrophysiologic bedside testing can be performed.

If normal sinus rhythm with natural conduction is observed at VVI 40, a sinus node recovery time test can be performed to assess sinus node automaticity. Atrial A00 or AAI pacing at 100 beats per minute is performed for 1 minute, with abrupt termination of pacing. If sinus node recovery after pacing termination is prompt (sinus recovery time in milliseconds from last atrial paced P wave to first sinus recovery P wave minus the sinus recovery stable cycle length ≤550 ms), sinus node automaticity is normal. AV node conduction can be assessed during atrial pacing at 100 beats per minute, 120 beats per minute, and 150 beats per minute for 15 seconds each. If AV node conduction is 1 : 1 at atrial paced rates of 100 beats per minute and 120 beats per minute with normal PR interval (<200 ms), and Wenckebach occurs at equal to or greater than 150 beats per minute, AV node conduction is normal. If Wenckebach, 2 : 1 or higher degrees of AV block occur at atrially paced rates of 100 to 120 beats per minute, AV node or distal His conduction is abnormal.

Minor degrees of abnormality of sinus node or AV node function may be tolerated, and temporary pacing may be discontinued. Moderate degrees of abnormality should prompt an electrophysiologic consultation, if the safety of discontinuation of temporary pacing is uncertain. High-degree AV block, long pauses on sinus node recovery time testing, very slow sinus rate, or very slow ventricular response to atrial fibrillation should prompt continuation of temporary pacing. The presence or absence of VA conduction can be determined by bedside electrophysiologic testing by pacing the ventricle at a rate slightly faster than the intrinsic sinus rate and recording from the atrial wires. If the P waves walk through the ventricular-paced rhythm uninterrupted, there is no VA conduction. If the atrial rate is entrained by ventricular pacing with a fixed VA interval between paced QRS and retrograde P wave, VA conduction is present.

The patient's blood pressure and cardiac output can be seriously compromised by VA conduction. During ventricular pacing, the mitral and tricuspid AV valves are shut. The retrograde P wave caused by VA conduction causes atrial contraction against closed AV valves, pushing blood backward up the neck causing observable v waves in the jugular pulse. Blood pressure during intrinsic sinus rate and ventricular pacing at a rate slightly faster than sinus rate should be determined. If there is a major decline in blood pressure (or Swan-Ganz catheter–measured cardiac output) with ventricular pacing with positive VA conduction, "pacemaker syndrome" is present, and the patient should receive continued AAI or AV sequential pacing, rather than VVI pacing, if needed. If permanent pacing is ultimately needed, a permanent DDD rather than VVI pacemaker is indicated.

Sophisticated Temporary DDD Pacemaker Programming

Pacemaker-mediated tachycardia can occur in patients with positive VA conduction during temporary or permanent DDD pacing. The paced ventricular beat causes retrograde conduction to the atrium. The retrograde P wave is sensed by the atrial lead of the DDD pacemaker as a "sinus" P wave and tracked. When retrograde A sensing occurs, an AV interval is timed out, and the ventricle is paced again. If the VA interval is 200 ms, and the DDD pacer is programmed to an AV interval of 200 ms, a pacemaker-mediated tachycardia of 400 ms cycle length or 150 beats per minute ensues. The tachycardia cycle length is determined by the sum of the programmed AV interval and retrograde VA interval and can be faster or slower than 150 beats per minute used in the earlier example. The post–ventricular atrial refractory period (PVARP) on the temporary or permanent pacer should be set greater than the measured VA interval to prevent pacemaker-mediated tachycardia. Also, a maximum tracking rate of 120 beats per minute or 130 beats per minute should be programmed "ON" in external temporary DDD pacemakers to limit the ventricular response of potential pacemaker-mediated tachycardias, episodes of tracked atrial fibrillation or flutter, or other atrial tachycardias.

Crosstalk on Temporary and Permanent DDD Pacemakers

Crosstalk is a phenomenon in which the atrial pacing spike is sensed by the ventricular amplifier as a "QRS complex," inhibiting ventricular pacing in a DDD pacemaker. This is a potentially fatal complication of pacing if the patient has complete heart block. Crosstalk is most likely to occur using unipolar temporary pacing when the atrial output is set high because of high atrial pacing threshold, and the ventricular sensitivity is set nominal or low (to sense low amplitude QRS complexes). The high amplitude unipolar pacing spike is sensed by the sensitive setting on the ventricular amplifier as a QRS complex, and the ventricular pacing output is inhibited. Crosstalk can be eliminated by programming a higher ventricular sensitivity, a lower atrial pacing output, or programming from DDD to D00 pacing.

TROUBLESHOOTING TEMPORARY PACEMAKER DYSFUNCTION

The simplest way to troubleshoot a temporary DDD pacing system is to break the system down into its simplest parts by reprogramming to VVI or V00 first, then AAI or A00 if AV conduction is intact, and then DDD (Fig. 5-10).

Failure to Pace or Capture

Most temporary pacemaker generators have blinking lights or other indicators that indicate a paced or sensed event. In the VVI mode, if there is failure to pace the ventricle at the highest programmed output, the clinician first should look to see if the pacer indicator is flashing at the programmed rate. If flashing but no pacing spike or ventricular capture is seen on ECG, there is a disconnect between the generator and the patient. The clinician should check the wires that connect the generator to the temporary pacemaker electrode, and check that the electrode is still in the body or the heart. If a spike with no capture is seen on ECG, the pacemaker electrode may have developed a high threshold, be fractured, or be dislodged from the heart. The clinician should try reversing polarity, or converting a bipolar temporary pacemaker to a unipolar pacemaker by the methods described earlier and shown in Figure 5-4. The lead can be replaced if these measures locate the problem to the lead, and the lead cannot be fixed by converting to unipolar. If no flashing indicator, no spike, and no capture are seen, the generator battery may be low or the generator faulty. The clinician should replace the battery or the generator.

If instead of the pacing indicator blinking at the programmed rate, a sensing indicator is blinking at double the natural QRS rate, T wave oversensing may be present and

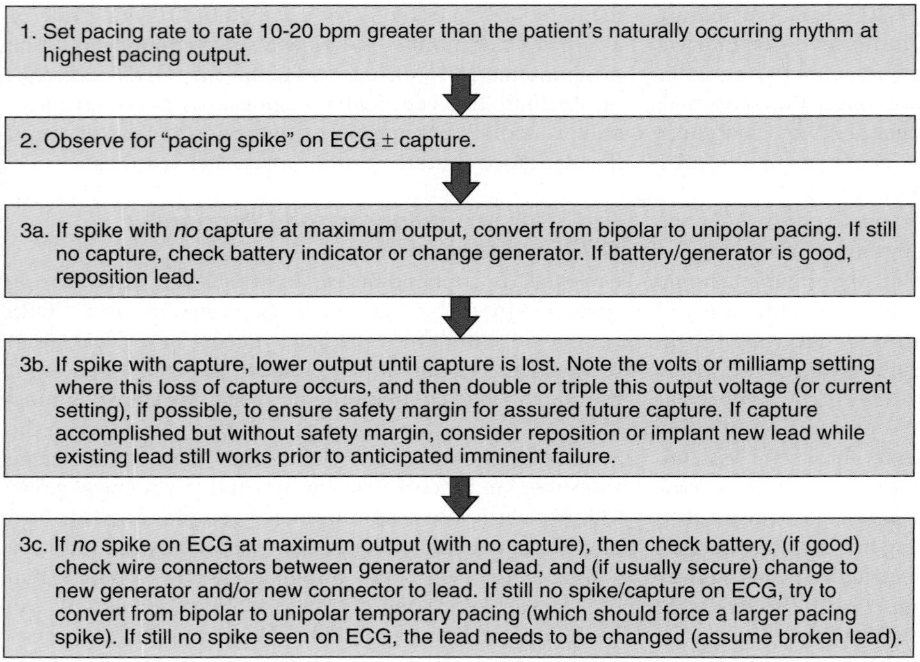

1. Set pacing rate to rate 10-20 bpm greater than the patient's naturally occurring rhythm at highest pacing output.
2. Observe for "pacing spike" on ECG ± capture.
3a. If spike with *no* capture at maximum output, convert from bipolar to unipolar pacing. If still no capture, check battery indicator or change generator. If battery/generator is good, reposition lead.
3b. If spike with capture, lower output until capture is lost. Note the volts or milliamp setting where this loss of capture occurs, and then double or triple this output voltage (or current setting), if possible, to ensure safety margin for assured future capture. If capture accomplished but without safety margin, consider reposition or implant new lead while existing lead still works prior to anticipated imminent failure.
3c. If *no* spike on ECG at maximum output (with no capture), then check battery, (if good) check wire connectors between generator and lead, and (if usually secure) change to new generator and/or new connector to lead. If still no spike/capture on ECG, try to convert from bipolar to unipolar temporary pacing (which should force a larger pacing spike). If still no spike seen on ECG, the lead needs to be changed (assume broken lead).

Figure 5-10. Approach to troubleshooting and fixing a previously implanted ventricular temporary pacing electrode catheter that is not capturing.

inhibiting pacing. If random higher frequency sense indicator blinking is present, 60 cycle or random noise or noise from electromagnetic interference or loose lead connection may be inhibiting the pacer if in VVI mode. The clinician should program to V00 mode and see if pacing ensues. If so, the clinician needs to troubleshoot the source of oversensing. If the patient has a stable escape rhythm, the pacemaker electrode can be disconnected from the temporary generator and connected to an ECG machine, as described in Figures 5-6 and 5-7, to record a ventricular bipolar electrogram with the patient coughing or taking a deep breath, or rolling from right to left side, or moving from supine to sitting posture. If there is noise on the bipolar ventricular electrogram, the clinician should create a ground referenced unipolar electrogram and individually check each of the two bipolar wires to locate which one (or both) may be causing the oversensing problem. Converting from bipolar to unipolar sensing by abandoning the noisy lead may solve the oversensing problem. Failure to pace ventricularly also can be caused by crosstalk (especially with high output unipolar atrial pacing and ventricular sensitivity set low or nominal). See the discussion on crosstalk.

Testing for Ventricular Pacing and Sensing Thresholds

To check for ventricular pacing threshold, the VVI mode is set at a rate greater than the patient's intrinsic rate and maximal output. The output is lowered until ventricular capture is lost. This value is doubled or tripled for 200% to 300% safety margin for capture. To check for ventricular sensing, the device is set at VVI at a rate lower than the patient's intrinsic ventricular rate at maximal, or lowest sensitivity setting. The temporary pacemaker should remain inhibited with sense indicator blinking, and no pacer spikes or capture should be seen on ECG. The clinician should slowly raise the sensitivity level until the ventricular pacing indicator blinks, or paced spikes or ventricular beats are seen on ECG, or both. This point measures the R wave amplitude of the patient's natural QRS escape rhythm. The clinician should lower the sensitivity setting to one third to one half of this value for stable ventricular sensing.

Testing for Atrial Pacing and Sensing Thresholds

If the patient has an escape rhythm with no heart block, programming to AAI or A00 mode or both can be used to troubleshoot the atrial lead in a similar process to that described for the ventricular lead. One does not have to see P waves (which are often difficult to see on single-lead bedside monitors) to check for atrial capture if the patient has intact AV conduction. The device is set to AAI or A00 mode at maximal output at a rate greater than the patient's intrinsic a and v rates. The clinician looks for 1:1 P wave capture, or if difficult to see, 1:1 natural QRS beats at a rate equal to the programmed atrial pacing rate. The clinician should lower atrial output until P waves are lost, or 1:1 natural QRS tracking of the programmed rate is lost. This point is the atrial pacing capture threshold. If complete heart block is present, the atrial lead must be checked in a DDD, DVI, or D00 mode. The clinician should set the temporary pacemaker generator to maximal atrial output and to DVI mode (ventricular inhibited dual chamber pacing) at a rate greater than the patient's natural atrial rate. Captured P waves should be observed before each paced QRS complex. The clinician should lower the atrial output until P capture is lost, and then double or triple the output from this point to have a 200% to 300% safety margin for capture.

Atrial sensing can be checked by setting the temporary pacer generator to DDD mode at a rate lower than the patient's intrinsic atrial rate, at most sensitive (lowest mV number) sensitivity. Despite programming a low rate, the pacer tracks the P waves at the patient's natural rate, time-out, and AV delay and paces the ventricle if atrial sensing is occurring, and one indicator blinks per natural P wave. The clinician should raise the atrial sensitivity setting until the atrial blink is no longer seen, and the ventricular paced rate suddenly falls from the patient's natural P wave rate to the programmed lower rate. This is the atrial sensing threshold, or P wave amplitude. This value is lowered to one third to one half for final atrial sensitivity setting.

Inappropriately High Rate Ventricular Pacing

Inappropriately high rate ventricular pacing can be caused by tracking noise, atrial tachyarrhythmias, or pacemaker-mediated tachycardia. If the patient is set to DDD mode and atrial fibrillation or flutter occurs, the DDD pacemaker may track the flutter or some of the atrial fibrillation waves at a high ventricular paced rate, limited only by the programmed maximum tracking rate of the DDD pacemaker. The atrial indicator lamp would be blinking at a high rate. The maximal tracking rate should be lowered to 100 to 110 beats per minute to prevent excessive ventricular pacing rates if atrial fibrillation should occur. The pacer should be reprogrammed to VVI mode if atrial fibrillation is persistent. If atrial fibrillation or flutter waves are undersensed by the atrial lead, the pacer appears to DDD pace at the programmed lower rate with no atrial capture after the atrial spike. The pacer should be reprogrammed to VVI mode if atrial fibrillation is persistent. The etiology of pacemaker-mediated tachycardia is discussed in a previous section. This tachycardia initially appears as an inappropriately rapid ventricular paced rhythm. Because it is due to sensing retrograde P waves, the arrhythmia can be stopped by programming to any pacer mode that does not sense P waves, such as VVI, DVI, or D00 modes. This immediately stops a pacemaker-mediated tachycardia. To solve this problem permanently while remaining in DDD mode, the clinician can check for VA conduction, set post–ventricular atrial refractory period (PVARP) longer than the measured VA interval, and reset the pacemaker to DDD mode.

CONCLUSION

This chapter is not meant to be all-inclusive on pacemaker mode selection, programming, and troubleshooting. The reader is urged to consult a standard permanent pacemaker textbook for more details if required. Also, refer to Chapter 4 in this textbook for more details on Seldinger insertion technique and Swan-Ganz pressure waveforms used to position guidewire pacer electrodes.

KEY POINTS

- Temporary pacing is indicated in patients with systematic or potentially life-threatening bradycardias that are expected to be transient.
- Transcutaneous pacing can serve as an emergency bridge to more stable temporary transvenous pacing.
- A pre-existing Swan-Ganz catheter can be rapidly converted into a transvenous temporary pacemaker in emergency situations.
- Temporary pacemakers can be used to diagnose and overdrive pace terminate some atrial and ventricular tachycardias.
- Temporary epicardial wires are valuable in diagnosing and treating of postoperative arrhythmias.
- Patients with temporary transvenous or epicardial electrodes need daily evaluations to check for infection, pacing threshold, and lead integrity and stability.
- Bedside electrophysiologic studies to check for sinus node and AV node function can be accomplished via a temporary AV sequential pacing system.
- Programming modes of temporary pacing stimulation and troubleshooting of a temporary pacemaker system are similar to permanent pacemakers.

REFERENCES

1. Winner S, Boon N: Clinical problems with temporary pacemaker prior to permanent pacing. J R Coll Physicians Lond 1989;23:161.
2. Aggarwal RK, Connelly DT, Ray SG, et al: Early complications of permanent pacemaker implantation: No difference between dual and single chamber systems. Br Heart J 1995;73:571.
3. DeGuzman M, Rahimtoola SH: What is the role of pacemakers in patients with coronary artery disease and conduction abnormalities. Cardiovasc Clin 1983;13:191.
4. Gilchrist IC, Caeron A: Chronic bundle branch block and use of temporary transvenous pacemakers during coronary arteriography. Cathet Cardiovasc Diagn 1988;15:229.
5. Ryan TJ, Antman EM, Crooks NH, et al: 1999 update: ACC/AHA guidelines for the management of patients with acute myocardial infarction: Executive summary and recommendations. A report of the American College of Cardiology/American Heart Association Task Force on Practice Guidelines (Committee on Management of Acute Myocardial Infarction). Circulation 1999;100:1016.
6. Ryan TJ, Anderson JL, Antman EM, et al: ACC/AHA guidelines for the management of patients with acute myocardial infarction. A report of the American College of Cardiology/American Heart Association Task Force on Practice Guidelines (Committee on Management of Acute Myocardial Infarction). J Am Coll Cardiol 1996;28:1328.
7. Gillette PC: Antitachycardia pacing. Pacing Clin Electrophysiol 1997;20(8 Pt 2):2121.
8. Obel IW, Scott Millar RN: Temporary transvenous atrial pacing for the control of supraventricular tachycardia in the coronary care unit. Crit Care Med 1983;11:313.
9. Waldo AL, Wells JL Jr, Cooper TB, et al: Temporary cardiac pacing: applications and techniques in the treatment of cardiac arrhythmias. Prog Cardiovasc Dis 1981;23:451.
10. Greenberg ML, Kelly TA, Lerman BB, et al: Atrial pacing for conversion of atrial flutter. Am J Cardiol 1986;58:95.

11. Peters RW, Shorofsky SR, Pelini M, et al: Overdrive atrial pacing for conversion of atrial flutter: Comparison of postoperative and nonpostoperative patients. Am Heart J 1999;137:100.
12. Oldroyd KG, Rankin AC, Rai AP, et al: Pacing termination of spontaneous ventricular tachycardia in the coronary care unit. Int J Cardiol 1992; 36:223.
13. Wathen MS, Sweeney MO, DeGroot PJ, et al: Shock reduction using antitachycardia pacing for spontaneous rapid ventricular tachycardia in patients with coronary artery disease. Circulation 2001;104:796.
14. Ahern TS, Nydegger C, Greenspon AJ, et al: Programmable external automatic antitachycardia pacing as a bridge to definitive therapy in patients with recurrent sustained ventricular tachycardia. Pacing Clin Electrophysiol 1992;15:1258.
15. Carlson MD, Ip J, Messenger J, et al: A new pacemaker algorithm for the treatment of atrial fibrillation: Results of the Atrial Dynamic Overdrive Pacing Trial (ADOPT). J Am Coll Cardiol 2003;42:627.
16. Daubert JC, Mabo P: Atrial pacing for the prevention of postoperative atrial fibrillation: How and where to pace? J Am Coll Cardiol 2000;35:1423.
17. Blommaert D, Gonzalez M, Mucumbitsi J, et al: Effective prevention of atrial fibrillation by continous atrial overdrive pacing after coronary artery bypass surgery. J Am Coll Cardiol 2000;35:1411.
18. Viskin S: Long QT syndromes and torsade de pointes. Lancet 1999;354:1625.
19. Banai S, Tzivoni D: Drug therapy for torsade de pointes. J Cardiovasc Electrophysiol 1993;4:206.
20. O'Rourke RA: Cardiac pacing: An alternative treatment for selected patients with hypertrophic cardiomyopathy and adjunctive therapy for certain patients with dilated cardiomyopathy. Circulation 1999;100:786-788.
21. Guo H, Hahn D, Olshansky B: Temporary biventricular pacing in a patient with subacute myocardial infarction, cardiogenic shock, and third degree AV block. Heart Rhythm 2005;2:112.
22. Curtis J, Wall J, Boley T, et al: Influence of atrioventricular synchrony on hemodynamics in patients with normal and low ejection fractions following open heart surgery. Am Surg 1986;52:93.
23. Pires LA, Wagshal AB, Lancey R, et al: Arrhythmias and conduction disturbances after coronary artery bypass graft surgery: Epidemiology, management, and prognosis. Am Heart J 1995;129:799.
24. Keefe DL, Griffin JC, Harrison DC, et al: Atrioventricular conduction abnormalities in patients undergoing isolated aortic or mitral valve replacement. Pacing Clin Electophysiol 1985;8(3 Pt 1):393.
25. Clinical competence in insertion of a temporary transvenous ventricular pacemaker. ACP/ACC/AHA Task Force on Clinical Privileges in Cardiology. J Am Coll Cardiol 1994;23:1254.
26. Francis GS, Williams SV, Archolr JL, et al: Clinical competence in insertion of a temporary transvenous ventricular pacemaker: A statement for physicians from the ACP/ACC/AHA Task Force on Clinical Privileges in Cardiology. Circulation 1994;89:1913.
27. Krueger SK, Rakes S, Wilkerson J, et al: Temporary pacemaking by general internists. Arch Intern Med 1983;143:1531.
28. Murphy JJ, Frain JP: Training and supervision of temporary transvenous pacemaker insertion. Br J Clin Pract 1995;49:126.
29. Verbeet T, Castro J, Decoodt P: Transesophageal pacing: A versatile diagnostic and therapeutic tool. Ind Pacing Electrophysiol J 2003;3:202
30. Ferguson JD, Banning AP, Bashir Y: Randomised trial of temporary cardiac pacing with semirigid and balloon-flotation electrode catheters. Lancet 1997;349:1983.
31. Jowett NI, Thompson DR, Pohl JEF: Temporary transvenous cardiac pacing: 6 years experience in one coronary care unit. Postgrad Med J 1989;65:211.
32. Choice of route of insertion of temporary pacing wires: Recommendations of the Medical Practice Committee and Council of the British Cardiac Society. Br Heart J 1993;70:592.
33. Bing OH, McDowell JW, Hantman J, et al: Pacemaker placement by electrocardiographic monitoring. N Engl J Med 1972;287:651.
34. Brown CH, Hutchins GM, Gurley HT, et al: Placement accuracy of percutaneous transthoracic pacemakers. Am J Emerg Med 1985;3:193.
35. Evans GL, Glasser SP: Intracavitary electocardiography as a guide to pacemaker positioning. JAMA 1971;216:483.
36. Gessman LJ, Gallagher JD, MacMillan R, et al: Emergency guide wire pacing: New methods for rapid conversion of a cardiac catheter into a pacemaker. Pacing Clin Electrophysiol 1984;7:917.
37. Pires LA, Wagshal AB, Lancey R, et al: Arrhythmias and conduction disturbances after coronary artery bypass graft surgery: Epidemiology, management, and prognosis. Am Heart J 1995;129:799.
38. Keefe DL, Griffin JC, Harrison DC, et al: Atrioventricular conduction abnormalities in patients undergoing isolated aortic or mitral valve replacement. Pacing Clin Electrophysiol 1985;8(3 Pt 1):393.
39. Del Rizzo DF, Nishimura S, Lau C, et al: Cardiac pacing following surgery for acquired heart disease. J Card Surg 1996;11:332.
40. Jaeger FJ, Trohman RG, Brener S, et al: Permanent pacing following repeat cardiac valve surgery. Am J Cardiol 1994;74:505.
41. Curtis J, Walls J, Boley T, et al: Influence of atriventricular synchrony on hemodynamics in patients with normal and low ejection fractions following open heart surgery. Am Surg 1986;52:93.
42. Blommaert D, Gonsalez M, Mucumbitsi J, et al: Effective prevention of atrial fibrillation by continuous atrial overdrive pacing after coronary artery bypass surgery. J Am Coll Cardiol 2000;35: 1411.
43. Daubert JC, Mabo P: Atrial pacing for the prevention of postoperative atrial fibrillation: How and where to pace. J Am Coll Cardiol 2000;35: 1423.
44. Kosmas CE, Ryder RG, Poon MJ, et al: Time-limited efficacy of pacing electrodes following open heart surgery. Ind Heart J 1996;48:681.
45. Kallis P, Batrick N, Bindi F, et al: Pacing thresholds of temporary epicardial electrodes: Variation with electrode type, time, and epicardial position. Ann Thorac Surg 1994;57:623.
46. Baciewicz FA, Leighton RF, Davis JT: Use of rapid atrial pacing to induce 2:1 atrioventricular block with marked improvement in hemodynamics. Int J Cardiol 1987;17:327.
47. Luck JC, Markel ML: Clinical applications of external pacing: A renaissance? Pacing Clin Electophysiol 1991;14:1299.
48. Falk RH, Ngai ST: External cardiac pacing: Influence of electrode placement on pacing threshold. Crit Care Med 1986;14:931.
49. Gessman LJ, Wertheimer JH, Davison J: A new device and method for rapid emergency pacing: Clinical use in 10 patients. Pacing Clin Electrophysiol 1982;5:929-933.
50. Rubenfire M, Melean J, Conrad E: Pseudoarrhythmia caused by temporary transvenous pacemaker. JAMA 1976;235:842.
51. Austin JL, Preis LK, Crampton RS, et al: Analysis of pacemaker malfunction and complications of temporary pacing in the coronary care unit. Am J Cardiol 1982;49:301.
52. Hill PE: Complications of permanent transvenous cardiac pacing: A 14 year review of all tranvenous pacemakers inserted at one community hospital. Pacing Clin Electrophysiol 1987;10:564.
53. Murphy JJ: Current practice: complications of temporary transvenous cardiac pacing. BMJ 1996;312:1134.
54. Nolewajka aJ, Goddard MD, Brown TC: Temporary transvenous pacing and femoral vein thrombosis. Circulation 1980;62:646.
55. McLeod AA, Jokhi PP: Pacemaker induced ventricular fibrillation in coronary care units. BMJ 2004;328:1249.
56. Austin JL, Preis L, Crampton RS, et al: Analysis of pacemaker malfunction and complications of temporary pacing in the coronary care unit. Am J Cardiol 1982;49:301.
57. Abinader KEG, Sharig D, Malouf S, et al: Temporary transvenous pacing: Analysis of indications, complications, and malfunctions in acute myocardial infarction versus noninfarction settings. Isr J Med Sci 1987;23:877.
58. Winner S, Boon N: Clinical problems with temporary pacemaker prior to permanent pacing. J R Coll Physicians Lond 1989;23:161.
59. Berry TA, Baas L, Hickey CS: Infection precautions with temporary pacing leads: A descriptive study. Heart Lung 1996;25:182.

60. Sclarovsky S, Safrir N, Strasberg KB, et al: Ventricular fibrillation complicating temporary pacing in acute myocardial infarction: Significance of right ventricular infarction. Am J Cardiol 1981;48:1160.
61. Pandian NG, Kosowsky BD, Burewich V: Transfemoral temporary pacing and deep venous thrombosis. Am Heart J 1980;100(6 Pt):847.
62. Katyal I: Complication of temporary endocardial pacing: Knotting of catheter. N Y State J Med 1978;78:94.
63. Fitchet A, Fitzpatrick AP: Central venous air embolism causing pulmonary edema mimicking left ventricular failure. BMJ 1998;316:604.
64. Jaeger HJ, Mathioa K, Neise M, et al: Lead dislodgement of a permanent pacemaker due to removal of a temporary pacing electrode. Pacing Clin Electrophysiol 1994;17:1565.
65. Trigano AJ, Asoulay A, Rochdi M, et al: Electromagnetic interference of external pacemakers by walkie-talkies and digital cellular phones: Experimental study. Pacing Clin Electrophysiol 1999;22:588.
66. Ezeugwu CO, Oropello MJ, Pasik AS, et al: Position of temporary transvenous pacemaker after insertion. J Cardiothorac Vasc Anesth 1994;8:367.
67. Goldberger J, Kruse J, Ehlert FA, et al: Temporary transvenous pacemaker placement: What criteria constitute an adequate pacing site. Am Hear J 1993;126:488.

Chapter 6

Pericardial Tamponade: Clinical Presentation, Diagnosis, and Catheter-Based Therapies

Hani Jneid, Andrew O. Maree, and Igor F. Palacios

Pericardial diseases have variable clinical presentations, including acute pericarditis, asymptomatic pericardial effusion, and pericardial tamponade. Although pericarditis is often a self-limiting disorder responsive to nonsteroidal anti-inflammatory drugs or steroid therapy, pericardial tamponade is a life-threatening condition and requires immediate therapy. Echocardiography and cardiac catheterization are important diagnostic tools and help in guiding therapies. Percutaneous catheter-based therapies, including pericardiocentesis and percutaneous balloon pericardiotomy, are safe and effective therapeutic modalities. Percutaneous balloon pericardiotomy is a relatively novel catheter-based technique that is gradually replacing the more invasive surgical pericardial window procedures. Pericardiectomy remains the definitive therapy for certain conditions, such as constrictive pericardial disease.

ETIOLOGY OF PERICARDIAL EFFUSION AND TAMPONADE

Pericarditis or pericardial effusion or both may result from an infectious, metabolic, inflammatory, autoimmune, or a neoplastic process (Box 6-1).[1-3] The frequency of specific etiologies depends on the geographic location, time period, and characteristics of the populations studied. In one European series of patients presenting with moderate and severe pericardial effusions, acute idiopathic pericarditis and iatrogenic causes accounted for most cases.[1] In a smaller series in the United States comprising patients presenting to a tertiary medical center with large pericardial effusions, malignancy was the most common etiology.[4] Pericardial effusions occurring after radiation therapy, myocardial infarction, and surgical and interventional cardiac procedures are increasing in incidence. Uremia and hypothyroidism remain important etiologies, but are seen less frequently given the prompt diagnosis and treatment of these disorders.

Pericardial fluid can be either a transudate or an exudate. Although transudative effusions typically occur in patients with congestive heart failure, exudative effusions may occur with most types of pericarditis and are characterized by a high concentration of proteins and fibrin. Pericardial effusions may be serous (or serosanguineous), suppurative, or hemorrhagic. Although the presence of suppurative effusion is pathognomonic for an acute infectious etiology, usually bacterial, hemorrhagic pericardial effusion is commonly related to chronic infections, with tuberculosis a classic example, particularly in developing countries. In developed countries, hemorrhagic pericardial effusions are likely to be iatrogenic or malignant in etiology. In a retrospective analysis of 150 patients in the United States who underwent pericardiocentesis for relieving cardiac tamponade, 64% of patients had a hemorrhagic pericardial effusion (with iatrogenic causes and malignancy accounting for most cases).[5]

CLINICAL PRESENTATION

The clinical presentation of patients with pericardial effusion varies. Some patients are completely asymptomatic, whereas others develop pericardial tamponade and cardiovascular collapse.

The normal pericardium is a fibroelastic sac composed of visceral and parietal layers separated by the pericardial cavity and containing a thin layer (20 to 50 mL) of straw-colored fluid surrounding the heart.[3] The normal pericardium has a steep pressure-volume curve: It is distensible when the intrapericardial volume is small, but becomes gradually inextensible when the volume increases. In the presence of pericardial effusion, the intrapericardial pressure depends on the relationship between the absolute

Box 6-1

Etiology of Pericardial Effusion and Tamponade

- Idiopathic
- Infectious
  - Viral
  - Bacterial
  - Fungal
  - Others
- Metabolic
  - Uremia
  - Myxedema
- Collagen and other autoimmune disorders
  - Systemic lupus erythematosus
  - Rheumatoid arthritis
  - Rheumatic fever
  - Dressler's syndrome
  - Others
- Neoplastic
  - Primary
  - Pericardial metastasis
  - Local invasion
- Volume overload
  - Chronic heart failure
- Miscellaneous
  - Chest wall irradiation
  - Cardiotomy or thoracic surgery
  - Adverse drug reaction
  - Aortic dissection
  - Post–myocardial infarction
  - Traumatic

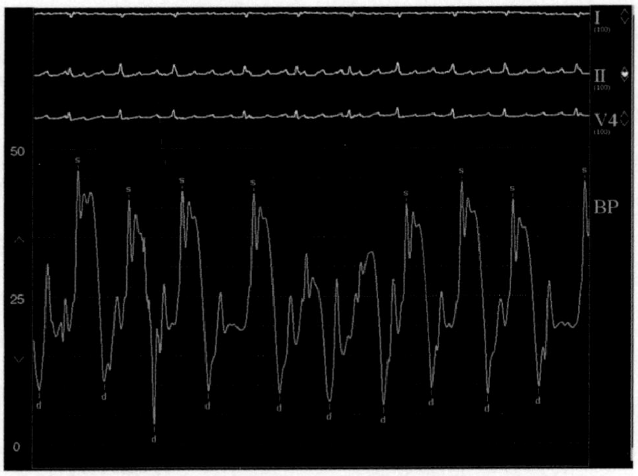

Figure 6-1. The patient is a 61-year-old woman with recent tricuspid valve repair presenting with increased dyspnea, orthopnea, and presyncope. She was hypotensive and had distended jugular veins and distant heart sounds on physical examination. The hemodynamic trace depicts elevated right ventricular pressure with exaggerated respiratory variation consistent with pericardial tamponade.

volume of the effusion, the speed of fluid accumulation, and pericardial elasticity. Although the rapid accumulation of small amounts of fluid (150 to 200 mL) can result in cardiac tamponade, the slow accumulation of larger effusions (>1 L, as in uremic pericardial effusions) is usually well tolerated.[6,7] The clinical presentation is not only related to the size of the effusion, but also, and more importantly, to the rapidity of fluid accumulation.

Pericardial tamponade is a clinical syndrome with defined hemodynamic and echocardiographic abnormalities, which result from the accumulation of intrapericardial fluid and impairment of ventricular diastolic filling.[7,8] The ultimate mechanism of hemodynamic compromise is the compression of cardiac chambers secondary to increased intrapericardial pressure.[8] Pericardial tamponade is usually a clinical diagnosis, with patients showing elevated systemic venous pressure, tachycardia, dyspnea, arterial pulsus paradoxus, muffled heart sounds, and evidence of electrical alternans on electrocardiogram (ECG).[3] Pulsus paradoxus, which describes the exaggerated inspiratory decline in arterial blood pressure (>10 mm Hg), is largely attributed to interventricular dependence within the confined pericardial space. Although its diagnostic utility was recognized many decades earlier,[9] various conditions may lead to its absence in patients with cardiac tamponade (e.g., in patients with concomitant aortic regurgitation, atrial septal defects, severe left ventricular dysfunction, aortic regurgitation, severe hypotension, pericardial adhesions, pulmonary artery obstruction, or positive-pressure ventilation).[8]

The ECG shows sinus tachycardia and low voltage. Electrical alternans, which describes the beat-to-beat alterations in the QRS complex reflecting cardiac swinging in the pericardial fluid, is a relatively specific sign for tamponade and is rarely seen with very large pericardial effusions alone.[10] Patients with pericardial effusions have an enlarged cardiac silhouette with clear lung fields on chest radiograph. The pericardial effusion has to reach 200 mL in volume to appear on the chest radiograph, which occurs usually in slowly accumulating pericardial effusions (which are less likely to cause tamponade).[11] Rapidly accumulating small pericardial effusions may cause tamponade and have a normal chest radiograph.

The diagnosis of pericardial tamponade is best confirmed by a two-dimensional echocardiogram that shows a pericardial effusion, right atrial compression, and abnormal respiratory variations in the right and left ventricular dimensions and in the tricuspid and mitral valve flow velocities (Fig. 6-1).[12] The classic hemodynamic findings of pericardial tamponade include arterial pulsus paradoxus, elevation and diastolic equalization of right and left ventricular diastolic pressures with pericardial pressure, and depression of cardiac output.[8] Because patients with critical tamponade operate on the steep portion of the pericardial pressure-volume curve, drainage of even small pericardial volume causes a drastic reduction in intrapericardial pressure and rapid clinical and hemodynamic improvement (by shifting the stretched pericardium back to the flat portion of the pericardium pressure-volume curve).[8]

DIAGNOSTIC ROLE OF ECHOCARDIOGRAPHY

Echocardiography is recognized as a particularly useful imaging modality for pericardial disease.[13,14] Currently, two-dimensional echocardiography has become the gold standard diagnostic modality because it provides a highly sensitive and specific noninvasive imaging technique for pericardial pathology.[12,15] It is also an important tool for the longitudinal follow-up of pericardial effusions over time (given a class IIa recommendation in the American Heart Association/American College of Cardiology guidelines for the clinical application of echocardiography).[12] Classically, a persistent echo-free space throughout the cardiac cycle between the parietal pericardium and the epicardium is pathognomonic for pericardial effusion by M-mode echocardiography.[13]

Two-dimensional echocardiography allows delineation of the size and distribution of the effusion, including loculated effusions, and helps assess the success of pericardiocentesis. The echocardiogram also can provide a reasonable estimate of the total volume of the effusion.[15] Circumferential effusion greater than 1 cm in width is considered large (>500 mL). Moderate effusions (100 to 500 mL) are usually circumferential but ≤ 1 cm, whereas small effusions (<100 mL) are usually localized posterior to the left ventricle and measure less than 1 cm. Classification criteria differ significantly among various echocardiographers and institutions. The typical echocardiographic signs of pericardial tamponade are listed in Box 6-2.

The nature of the pericardial fluid is difficult to identify by echocardiography. Increased echogenicity is suspicious, however, for the presence of proteins or cells or both in the pericardial fluid. Fibrin deposits localized in the epicardial surface can be identified as echogenic masses. In one study of 42 patients with tuberculous and viral or idiopathic pericardial effusions, intrapericardial echocardiogram abnormalities, such as a greater degree of pericardial thickening, frequency and thickness of exudative coating or deposits, and strands crossing the pericardial space, were useful criteria in the diagnosis of tuberculous pericardial effusion and in differentiating it from chronic idiopathic pericardial effusion.[16]

The classic echocardiographic signs of cardiac tamponade are right atrial and right ventricular diastolic collapse. The right atrium and right ventricle are compliant structures. As a result, increased intrapericardial pressure leads to their collapse when intracavitary pressures are only slightly exceeded by those in the pericardium. At end-diastole (i.e., during atrial relaxation), right atrial volume is minimal, but pericardial pressure is maximal, causing the right atrium to buckle. Right atrial collapse, especially when it persists for more than one third of the cardiac cycle, is a highly sensitive, but less specific sign for tamponade. Early diastolic collapse of the right ventricle (usually occurs in early diastole when the ventricular volume is still low) is present when the intrapericardial pressure exceeds the right ventricular pressure and is a highly specific sign for tamponade. Right ventricular collapse may not occur when the right ventricle is hypertrophied, or its diastolic pressure is greatly elevated. Left atrial collapse is seen in nearly 25% of patients and is specific for tamponade. Left ventricular collapse is less common because the wall of the left ventricle is more muscular. Dilation of the inferior vena cava with lack of inspiratory collapse (usually <50% reduction in its diameter) and swinging of the heart also are seen in patients with pericardial tamponade. Doppler echocardiography provides direct assessment of the ventricular filling patterns in pericardial tamponade.[11,12,17,18] Patients with pericardial tamponade have a marked increase in tricuspid and pulmonic flow velocities and a marked decrease in mitral and aortic valve flow velocities during inspiration compared with normal subjects and patients with effusions but not tamponade. Changes in left atrial inflow pattern and exaggerated respiratory variations in pulmonary venous flow velocity also are observed. In one study aiming to correlate clinical and echocardiographic findings prospectively, the highest specificity (98%) was seen in patients with right atrial and right ventricular collapse plus abnormal venous flow.[19] The sensitivity and specificity of any chamber collapse were 90% and 65%.[19]

In addition to echocardiography, computed tomography and magnetic resonance imaging are useful techniques in the evaluation of patients with pericardial disease. Their high resolution is useful in the assessment of pericardial thickness (particularly important in constrictive-effusive pericarditis) and in the detection of pericardial effusion, masses, and cysts.

Box 6-2

Echocardiographic Findings

1. Abnormal inspiratory increase of right ventricular dimensions and abnormal inspiratory decrease of left ventricular dimensions
2. Right atrium collapse (>30% of cardiac cycle)
3. Right ventricular early diastolic collapse
4. Abnormal inspiratory increase in blood flow velocity through tricuspid and pulmonic valves and abnormal inspiratory decrease of mitral and aortic valves flow velocity
5. Respiratory variations of pulmonary and hepatic venous flow
6. Dilated inferior vena cava with lack of inspiratory collapse
7. Swinging heart

CATHETER-BASED DIAGNOSTIC AND THERAPEUTIC STRATEGIES

Cardiac catheterization historically has been the standard diagnostic modality for cardiac tamponade. Right heart catheterization can confirm the significance of a pericardial effusion and allows evaluation of hemodynamic changes occurring after pericardiocentesis. It usually shows two major findings in patients with pericardial tamponade: (1) elevation and equilibration of intracardiac

Box 6-3

Cardiac Catheterization Findings

1. Elevated filling pressures
2. Diastolic equalization of pressures
3. Absence or blunted Y descent in the right atrium pressure tracing
4. Absence or blunted early diastolic dip in the right ventricular pressure tracing
5. Arterial pulsus paradoxus

diastolic pressures (usually 10 to 30 mm Hg) and (2) inspiratory increase in right-sided pressures and reduction in left-sided pressures (ventricular disconcordance), which are responsible for the presence of a pulsus paradoxus (Box 6-3).[8] With equalization of intrapericardial pressures, the mean right atrial, left atrial, diastolic pulmonary artery, and right and left ventricular end diastolic pressures all are within 5 mm Hg of each other. In addition to producing elevation in the central venous pressure, cardiac tamponade produces characteristic changes in the waveforms of the hemodynamic tracings. With increasing severity of cardiac tamponade, the "Y descent" and the early diastolic dip in the ventricular pressure tracings are gradually obliterated and eventually disappear. The absence of the Y descent in the right atrial tracing is an important finding in pericardial tamponade. As pericardial fluid is removed, the intrapericardial pressure usually returns to the intrapleural pressure level, and the right atrial waveform normalizes with reappearance of the diastolic Y descent. If the right atrial pressure remains elevated after the pericardiocentesis, however, and a prominent Y descent appears, the diagnosis of effusive-constrictive disease must be considered.[20] Although the latter condition is infrequent, it may be missed in some patients presenting with tamponade in whom it usually causes significant morbidity until they undergo surgical epicardiectomy. Pulsus paradoxus is another hallmark of pericardial tamponade; however, it may be absent in many conditions, or alternatively may be present in patients without cardiac tamponade, as previously stated.

PERICARDIOCENTESIS

Indications

Pericardiocentesis is the technique of catheter-based aspiration of pericardial fluid. It is a diagnostic and therapeutic modality in patients with pericarditis with pericardial effusion, pericardial effusion with pericardial tamponade, and effusive-constrictive pericarditis.

When the diagnosis of pericardial effusion has been made, it is important to determine whether the effusion is creating significant hemodynamic compromise. Many asymptomatic patients with large effusions do not require pericardiocentesis if they have no hemodynamic compromise, unless there is a need for fluid analysis for diagnostic purposes. In a prospective long-term follow-up of large idiopathic chronic pericardial effusion (up to 20 years), Sagrista-Sauleda and colleagues[21] concluded that large idiopathic chronic pericardial effusions were usually well tolerated for long periods in most patients with severe tamponade; however, they may develop unexpectedly at any time. Although pericardiocentesis was effective in resolving these effusions, recurrences were common, prompting the authors to recommend referral of these patients for pericardiectomy when recurrence occurs.[21] When cardiac tamponade occurs, the emergency drainage of pericardial fluid by pericardiocentesis is a lifesaving therapy in a patient who would otherwise develop pulseless electrical activity and cardiac arrest.

When performed, pericardiocentesis should achieve several objectives, as follows: (1) relief of tamponade, when present; (2) obtaining fluid for appropriate analyses; and (3) assessment of hemodynamics after pericardial fluid evacuation to exclude effusive-constrictive pericardial effusion. Elective pericardiocentesis is contraindicated in patients receiving anticoagulation and in patients with bleeding disorders or thrombocytopenia (platelet count <50,000/mm^3). Pericardiocentesis also is ill advised when the presence of pericardial fluid is not confirmed, and when the effusion is very small or loculated. When pericardial tamponade occurs complicating acute aortic dissection, pericardiocentesis is contraindicated because of the risk of increased dP/dt and further hemorrhage and extension of the dissection. The patient instead should undergo direct aortic repair together with pericardial drainage in the operating room.

Technique

Pericardiocentesis is most commonly performed via a subxiphoid approach under ECG and fluoroscopy guidance (Fig. 6-2A). Traditionally, pericardiocentesis has been performed in the cardiac catheterization laboratory with arterial and right heart pressure monitoring. Today the procedure also is performed in the noninvasive laboratory, intensive care units, or even at the bedside under echocardiographic guidance.[22,23] Whichever modality is used, it is a safe procedure when performed by appropriately trained personnel.

Pericardiocentesis is a procedure based on the Seldinger technique of percutaneous catheter insertion. After the administration of local anesthesia (1% to 2% lidocaine) to the skin and deeper tissues of the left xiphocostal area, the pericardial needle is connected to an ECG lead. The needle is advanced from the left of the subxiphoid area while aiming toward the left shoulder (usually under fluoroscopic or echocardiographic guidance; however, blinded procedures are undertaken in cases of extreme emergencies). Often, a discrete pop is felt as the needle enters the pericardial space. ST segment elevation is seen on the ECG lead tracing when the needle touches the epicardium and helps confirm the needle position (see Fig. 6-2B). The needle should be withdrawn slightly until the ST segment elevation disappears. When the pericardial space is entered, a stiff guidewire is introduced into the pericardial space through the needle, which is thereafter

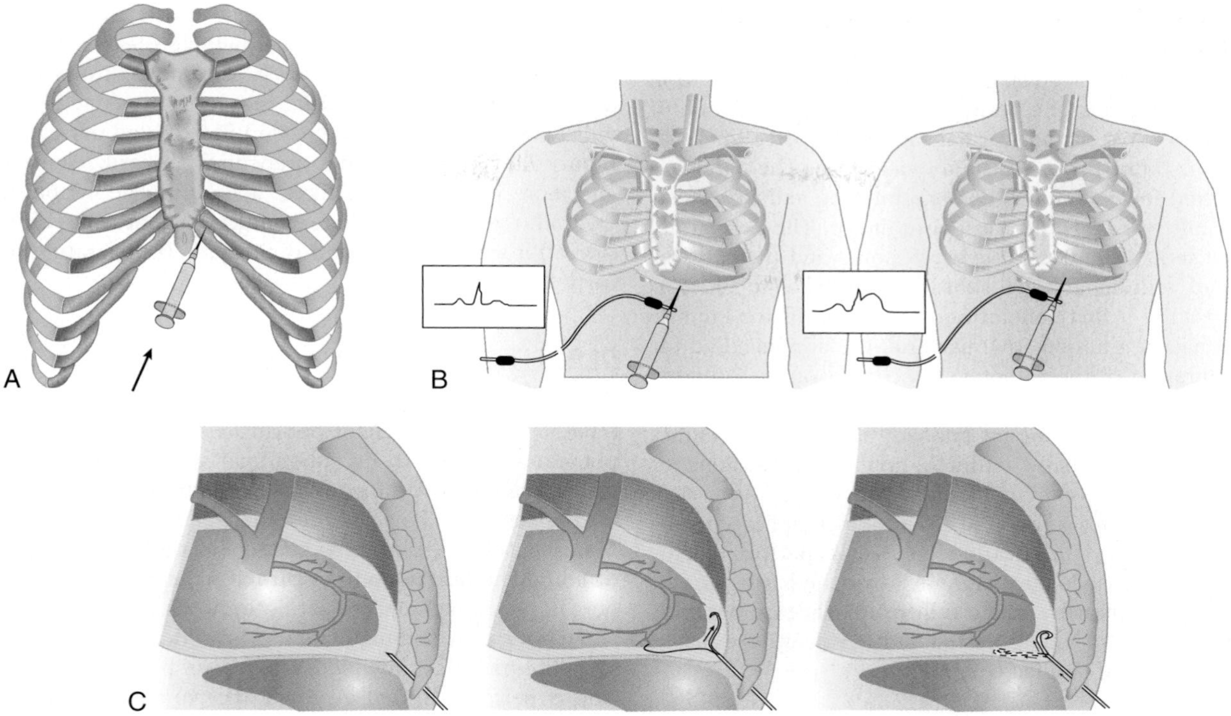

Figure 6-2. **A,** Diagrammatic representation of a pericardiocentesis procedure using the subxiphoid approach. **B,** The pericardial needle is connected to an ECG lead. The needle is advanced from the left of the subxiphoid area aiming toward the left shoulder. ST segment elevation is seen on the ECG lead tracing when the needle touches the epicardium. The needle should be retracted slightly until the ST segment elevation disappears. **C,** After the pericardial space is entered with the pericardial needle, a guidewire is introduced in the pericardial space through the needle. The needle is removed, and a catheter is inserted in the pericardial sac over the guidewire (either anteriorly or inferiorly in the pericardial sac).

removed, and a catheter is inserted into the pericardial sac over the guidewire (see Fig. 6-2C). The drainage catheter used (often a pigtail catheter, denoting its shape) has an end hole and multiple side holes. Intrapericardial pressure is measured by connecting a pressure transducer system to the intrapericardial catheter. Pericardial fluid is then removed. Samples of pericardial fluid should be sent for appropriate biochemical, cytologic, bacteriologic, and immunologic analyses to assist in the diagnosis of the etiology of the effusion (the first sample is usually reserved for microbiologic studies).

In the presence of pericardial tamponade, aspiration of fluid should be continued until clinical and hemodynamic improvement occurs. The catheter is frequently left in place for continuous drainage and as a route to instill sclerosing or chemotherapeutic agents if needed. The catheter is secured to the skin with sterile sutures and covered with a sterile dressing. The success rate of pericardiocentesis increases and the incidence of complications decreases with the increasing size of the effusion.

Complications

The potential complications of pericardiocentesis include the laceration of the heart or a coronary vessel, sometimes causing fatal consequences. Puncture of the right atrium or the right ventricle with hemopericardial fluid accumulation, arrhythmias, air embolism, pneumothorax, and puncture of the peritoneal cavity or abdominal viscera all have been reported. Acute pulmonary edema may infrequently occur when the pericardial tamponade is decompressed too rapidly.

Other approaches of pericardiocentesis include the right xiphocostal, apical, right-sided, and parasternal approaches. Although these approaches may be useful under certain circumstances, they are associated with greater incidence of complications. The right xiphocostal approach is associated with higher incidence of right atrium and inferior vena cava injury. Puncture of the left pleura and the lingula is more frequent with the apical approach, and puncture of the left anterior descending and the internal mammary artery is more frequent with the parasternal approach.

Echocardiographically guided pericardiocentesis is a safe and effective technique.[23,24] In a series of 1127 therapeutic echocardiographically guided pericardiocenteses performed in 977 patients at the Mayo Clinic between 1979 and 1998, the procedural success rate was 97% overall, with a total complication rate of 4.7%.[24] Echocardiography allows identification of the ideal site of needle entry and trajectory and is especially useful in patients with loculated effusions. In contrast to pericardiocenteses performed in the cardiac catheterization laboratory, the left chest wall, rather than the subcostal, approach is often used with echocardiographically guided pericardiocenteses.

Management after Pericardiocentesis

Pericardiocentesis does not completely evacuate the effusion in most cases, given particularly that active secretion and bleeding into the pericardial space may continue. It is best to leave the pericardial catheter in place for 24 to 72 hours after the initial fluid evacuation. The patient is admitted for continuous ECG monitoring and for assessment of the rate of pericardial drainage. The pericardial space should be drained every 8 hours and the catheter flushed with heparinized solution, and systemic antibiotics (usually a first-generation cephalosporin for empiric coverage of gram-positive bacteria) are administered for the duration of the catheter stay. Based on the etiology of the effusion, the patient's clinical and hemodynamic condition, and the amount drained, the pericardial catheter is removed usually within 72 hours, and decisions for additional therapy are contemplated.

No special care is required after an uncomplicated pericardiocentesis. If pericardiocentesis is performed for cardiac tamponade, the patient is watched for signs of recurrent tamponade, and a follow-up echocardiogram is useful to monitor the resolution of the pericardial effusion and for signs of cardiac compression.

Prevention of Recurrent Tamponade

For many patients with pericardial effusion and tamponade, standard percutaneous pericardial drainage with an indwelling pericardial catheter is sufficient to avoid recurrence of pericardial effusion and tamponade. Patients who continue to drain more than 100 mL per 24 hours 3 days after standard catheter drainage should be considered for more aggressive therapy. Reaccumulation of the pericardial fluid is particularly common in patients with malignant pericardial effusions. Additional therapeutic approaches are available to prevent pericardial fluid reaccumulation, including intrapericardial instillation of sclerosing agents, use of chemotherapy, radiotherapy, percutaneous balloon pericardial window, and surgical intervention.[25-28] Reaccumulation of fluid with recurrence of cardiac tamponade has been considered a definitive indication for an open surgical pericardial window or for percutaneous balloon pericardiotomy.[29]

OPEN SURGICAL PERICARDIAL WINDOW

Surgical procedures for creating a pericardial window range from a simple subxiphoid pericardial incision (pericardiotomy) to the removal of a variable portion of the pericardium (pericardiectomy). Although recurrence is higher with the pericardiotomy procedure, pericardiectomy often requires an anterior thoracotomy or sternotomy, rather than a subxiphoid approach, and is associated with a higher postoperative complication rate. Many physicians advocate the performance of subxiphoid pericardiotomy in critically ill patients with limited life expectancy, reserving pericardiectomy for patients with a relatively better prognosis.

Subxiphoid pericardiotomy allows for an adequate evacuation of the pericardial contents, direct inspection of the pericardial space to break down loculations, and the performance of pericardial biopsies and fluid sampling for diagnostic purposes. The procedure can be done safely and quickly under local anesthesia and provides prompt and long-term relief. Subxiphoid pericardiotomy alleviates the need for repeated pericardiocentesis and more invasive and difficult open drainage methods. Overall, the symptomatic recurrence of pericardial effusion after surgical window is reported in the literature to be 5%.

PERCUTANEOUS BALLOON PERICARDIOTOMY

Patients with a malignant pericardial effusion and tamponade are likely to be suboptimal surgical candidates because of their overall poor health conditions and limited life expectancies. Palacios and colleagues[29,30] pioneered at Massachusetts General Hospital in Boston the technique of percutaneous balloon pericardial window (also called percutaneous balloon pericardiotomy) as an alternative and less invasive technique to surgical pericardial window. With this modality, adequate drainage of pericardial effusion is performed, and a pericardial window is created percutaneously under fluoroscopic guidance using a balloon-dilation catheter. The technique of percutaneous pericardial window is relatively simple and safe and is performed in the catheterization laboratory under local anesthesia with minimal discomfort. Conscious sedation with intravenous narcotics and a short-acting benzodiazepine is generally used.

Percutaneous Balloon Pericardiotomy Technique

Percutaneous balloon pericardial window is offered as an alternative technique to the surgical pericardial window procedure for patients with persistent drainage from their indwelling intrapericardial catheter (≥3 days of >100 mL/24 hours drainage) or as primary therapy at the time of initial pericardiocentesis. The subxiphoid area around the indwelling pigtail pericardial catheter is infiltrated with local anesthesia (1% to 2% lidocaine). A small amount (5 to 10 mL) of iodinated contrast agent is injected in the pericardial space to help outline the parietal pericardium (Fig. 6-3A). A 0.038-inch stiff guidewire with a preshaped curve at the tip is advanced through the pigtail catheter into the pericardial space. The catheter is removed, leaving the guidewire in the pericardial space. After predilation of the skin and subcutaneous tissue along the track of the wire using a 10F dilator, a 20-mm-diameter × 3-cm-long balloon-dilation catheter (Boston Scientific, Watertown, MA) is advanced over the guidewire and positioned to straddle the parietal pericardium. Care should be taken to advance the proximal end of the balloon beyond the skin and the subcutaneous tissue to avoid dilation of the skin and subcutaneous tissue (and the resultant formation of a pericardial-cutaneous fistula) (see Fig. 6-3B). The balloon is inflated manually until the waist produced by the parietal pericardium disappears (see Fig. 6-3C). Biplane fluoroscopy is helpful to ascertain the correct

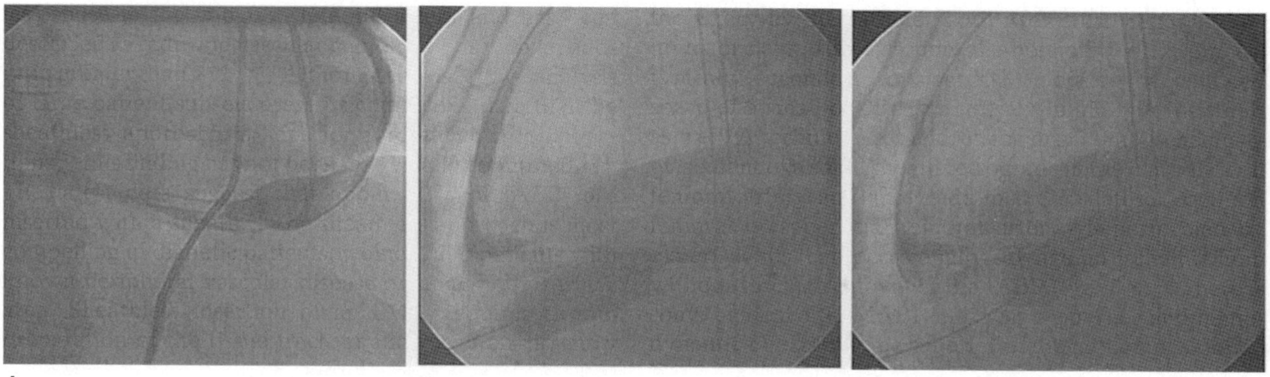
A B C

Figure 6-3. Diagrammatic representation of a percutaneous balloon pericardiotomy procedure. **A,** Injection of a small amount of iodinated contrast material confirms the intrapericardial location of the catheter. **B,** A left lateral projection showed an inflated dilating balloon catheter without a waist, indicating the need to reposition the balloon catheter to straddle the parietal pericardium. **C,** The balloon catheter is in the correct position and appears straddling the parietal pericardium in the left lateral projection.

position of the balloon straddling the parietal pericardium with the left lateral projection being particularly useful (see Fig. 6-3B and C). Two to three inflations are usually performed to have adequate opening of the parietal pericardium. The balloon-dilation catheter is removed, leaving the stiff guidewire in the pericardial space, where a new pigtail catheter is advanced over it and left indwelling in the pericardial space.

Patients are admitted to a regular medical ward unit after a percutaneous balloon pericardiotomy procedure and do not require a coronary unit admission. The pericardial catheter is aspirated every 6 to 8 hours and flushed with heparinized solution (5 mL, 100 U/mL). Pericardial drainage volumes are recorded, and the catheter is removed when there is less than 50 to 75 mL of pericardial drainage in 24 hours. Chest radiographs are obtained to check for the development of pleural effusion resulting from drainage of the pericardial fluid.

Outcome Data after Percutaneous Balloon Pericardiotomy

Palacios and colleagues[29] reported the first human experience with the technique of percutaneous balloon pericardiotomy in eight patients with malignant pericardial effusion and tamponade. The technique was successful in all patients with no immediate or late procedure-related complications. The mean time to radiologic development of a new or a significantly increased pleural effusion was 2.9 ± 0.4 days (range 2 to 5 days). No patient developed recurrence of the pericardial effusion or tamponade at a mean follow-up of 6 ± 2 months (range 1 to 11 months). Five patients died from their primary malignancy at 1, 4, 9, 10, and 11 months. A success rate of 87% was reported in the multicenter percutaneous balloon pericardial window registry, which enrolled 130 patients between 1987 and 1994 in 16 centers.[31,32] In this registry, three patients sustained pericardial bleeding and were considered to have a failed procedure and ended up undergoing surgical window procedures. Eight patients had recurrence of pericardial effusion (mean time to recurrence 54 ± 65 days), of whom seven ended up having surgical window procedures (with recurrence occurring in four of those patients).

Complications

Minor complications occurred in 13% of the patients.[31,32] The development of a large pleural effusion remains the major concern after percutaneous balloon pericardial window. Most patients develop a left pleural effusion within 24 to 48 hours of the procedure, which in most cases resolves spontaneously (presumably owing to the greater resorption capacity of the pleural surface). Thoracocentesis or chest tube placement was required in 15% of patients with pre-existing pleural effusions compared with 9% of patients without pre-existing pleural effusions.[31,32] It is desirable to aspirate most of the pericardial fluid before creating the window to limit the potential volume of fluid that can immediately leak to the pleural space. When the preprocedure chest radiograph reveals a large pleural effusion, the chance of requiring thoracentesis subsequent to the percutaneous pericardial window is higher, and the procedure should be performed only when its benefits outweigh the risks of thoracentesis or chest tube placement or both. It is not advised to perform the procedure in patients with marginal pulmonary reserve, as in postpneumonectomy patients, because the development of a pleural effusion may significantly compromise their respiratory function. Finally, an increased risk of bleeding from the pericardiotomy site occurs in patients with platelet or coagulation abnormalities. In these patients, a surgical procedure under direct visualization may be safer. Thoracoscopic techniques were developed to create a larger pericardial window with low morbidity compared with open surgical techniques.[33] This technique allows adequate long-term drainage and the ability to obtain specimens for pathologic analysis.[33]

KEY POINTS

- Patients with pericardial effusion have a variable clinical presentation; some are completely asymptomatic, whereas others develop tamponade and cardiovascular collapse.
- Pericardial tamponade is a clinical syndrome with defined hemodynamic and echocardiographic abnormalities, which result from the accumulation of intrapericardial fluid and impairment of ventricular diastolic filling.
- Two-dimensional echocardiography allows delineation of the size and distribution of the pericardial effusion, provides a reasonable estimate of its total volume, and helps assess the success of pericardiocentesis.
- Pericardiocentesis is the technique of catheter-based aspiration of pericardial fluid and is a diagnostic and therapeutic modality.
- Pericardiocentesis is most commonly performed via the subxiphoid approach under ECG and fluoroscopy guidance in the cardiac catheterization laboratory with arterial and right heart pressure monitoring. It also can be performed in the noninvasive laboratory or at the bedside using echocardiographic guidance.
- Percutaneous balloon pericardiotomy is an effective therapy for recurrent malignant pericardial effusion and is a less invasive alternative to surgical pericardial window.
- Surgical pericardiectomy is the definitive therapy for patients with constrictive pericardial disease.

REFERENCES

1. Sagrista-Sauleda J, Merce J, Permanyer-Miralda G, et al: Clinical clues to the causes of large pericardial effusions. Am J Med 2000;109:95-101.
2. Troughton RW, Asher CR, Klein AL: Pericarditis. Lancet 2004;363:717-727.
3. Lange RA, Hillis LD: Clinical practice: Acute pericarditis. N Engl J Med 2004;351:2195-2202.
4. Corey GR, Campbell PT, Van Trigt P, et al: Etiology of large pericardial effusions. Am J Med 1993;95:209-213.
5. Atar S, Chiu J, Forrester JS, et al: Bloody pericardial effusion in patients with cardiac tamponade: Is the cause cancerous, tuberculous, or iatrogenic in the 1990s? Chest 1999;116:1564-1569, 1999.
6. Spodick DH: Pathophysiology of cardiac tamponade. Chest 1998;113: 1372-1378.
7. Fowler NO: Cardiac tamponade: A clinical or an echocardiographic diagnosis? Circulation 1993;87: 1738-1741.
8. Spodick DH: Acute cardiac tamponade. N Engl J Med 2003;349:684-690.
9. Shabetai R, Fowler NO, Fenton JC, et al: Pulsus paradoxus. J Clin Invest 1965;44: 1882-1898.
10. Bruch C, Schmermund A, Dagres N, et al: Changes in QRS voltage in cardiac tamponade and pericardial effusion: Reversibility after pericardiocentesis and after anti-inflammatory drug treatment. J Am Coll Cardiol 2001;38:219-226.
11. Maisch B, Seferovic PM, Ristic AD, et al: Guidelines on the diagnosis and management of pericardial diseases: Executive summary. The Task Force on the Diagnosis and Management of Pericardial Diseases of the European Society of Cardiology. Eur Heart J 2004;25:587-610.
12. Cheitlin MD, Armstrong WF, Aurigemma GP, et al: ACC/AHA/ASE 2003 guideline update for the clinical application of echocardiography: Summary article: A report of the American College of Cardiology/ American Heart Association Task Force on Practice Guidelines (ACC/AHA/ASE Committee to Update the 1997 Guidelines for the Clinical Application of Echocardiography). Circulation 2003;108:1146-1162.
13. Feigenbaum H, Waldhausen JA, Hyde LP: Ultrasound diagnosis of pericardial effusion. JAMA 1965;191:711-714.
14. Moss AJ, Bruhn F: The echocardiogram: An ultrasound technic for the detection of pericardial effusion. N Engl J Med 1966;274:380-384.
15. Prakash AM, Sun Y, Chiaramida SA, et al: Quantitative assessment of pericardial effusion volume by two-dimensional echocardiography. J Am Soc Echocardiogr 2003;16:147-153.
16. George S, Salama AL, Uthaman B, et al: Echocardiography in differentiating tuberculous from chronic idiopathic pericardial effusion. Heart 2004;90: 1338-1339.
17. Appleton CP, Hatle LK, Popp RL: Cardiac tamponade and pericardial effusion: Respiratory variation in transvalvular flow velocities studied by Doppler echocardiography. J Am Coll Cardiol 1988;11:1020-1030.
18. Schutzman JJ, Obarski TP, Pearce GL, et al: Comparison of Doppler and two-dimensional echocardiography for assessment of pericardial effusion. Am J Cardiol 1992;70:1353-1357.
19. Merce J, Sagrista-Sauleda J, Permanyer-Miralda G, et al: Correlation between clinical and Doppler echocardiographic findings in patients with moderate and large pericardial effusion: Implications for the diagnosis of cardiac tamponade. Am Heart J 1999;138:759-764.
20. Sagrista-Sauleda J, Angel J, Sanchez A, et al: Effusive-constrictive pericarditis. N Engl J Med 2004;350:469-475.
21. Sagrista-Sauleda J, Angel J, Permanyer-Miralda G, et al: Long-term follow-up of idiopathic chronic pericardial effusion. N Engl J Med 1999;341:2054-2059.
22. Ristic AD, Seferovic PM, Maisch B: Management of pericardial effusion the role of echocardiography in establishing the indications and the selection of the approach for drainage. Herz 2005;30: 144-150.
23. Lindenberger M, Kjellberg M, Karlsson E, et al: Pericardiocentesis guided by 2-D echocardiography: The method of choice for treatment of pericardial effusion. J Intern Med 2003;253: 411-417.
24. Tsang TS, Enriquez-Sarano M, Freeman WK, et al: Consecutive 1127 therapeutic echocardiographically guided pericardiocenteses: Clinical profile, practice patterns, and outcomes spanning 21 years. Mayo Clin Proc 2002;77:429-436.
25. Shepherd FA, Morgan C, Evans WK, et al: Medical management of malignant pericardial effusion by tetracycline sclerosis. Am J Cardiol 1987;60:1161-1166.
26. Davis S, Sharma SM, Blumberg ED, et al: Intrapericardial tetracycline for the management of cardiac tamponade secondary to malignant pericardial effusion. N Engl J Med 1978;299: 1113-1114.
27. Vaitkus PT, Herrmann HC, LeWinter MM: Treatment of malignant pericardial effusion. JAMA 1994;272:59-64.
28. Palatianos GM, Thurer RJ, Kaiser GA: Comparison of effectiveness and safety of operations on the pericardium. Chest 1985;88:30-33.
29. Palacios IF, Tuzcu EM, Ziskind AA, et al: Percutaneous balloon pericardial window for patients with malignant pericardial effusion and tamponade. Cathet Cardiovasc Diagn 1991;22: 244-249.
30. Ziskind AA, Pearce AC, Lemmon CC, et al: Percutaneous balloon pericardiotomy for the treatment of cardiac tamponade and large pericardial effusions: Description of technique and report of the first 50 cases. J Am Coll Cardiol 1993;21:1-5.
31. Ziskind AA: Final report of the percutaneous balloon pericardiotomy registry for the treatment of effusive pericardial disease. Circulation 1994;90: I-121.
32. Ziskind AA, Rodriguez S, Lemmon C, et al: Percutaneous pericardial biopsy as an adjunctive technique for the diagnosis of pericardial disease. Am J Cardiol 1994;74:288-291.
33. Ozuner G, Davidson PG, Isenberg JS, et al: Creation of a pericardial window using thoracoscopic techniques. Surg Gynecol Obstet 1992;175:69-71.

Chapter 7

Intra-aortic Balloon Counterpulsation

Zoltan G. Turi

The first and most widely used of the percutaneously placed cardiac assist devices, the intra-aortic balloon pump (IABP) displaces blood from the descending aorta during diastole, resulting in altered myocardial mechanics during systole. By raising diastolic perfusion pressure, the IABP has the potential to augment coronary flow. Unlike the majority of more recently developed and generally mechanically more complex devices, the IABP provides auxiliary rather than independent support of cardiac output. Although it uses complex software algorithms, it is the simplest of the invasive devices mechanically, is the lowest in profile, and is associated with relatively low failure rates. Its advantages include the feasibility of allowing insertion in the cardiac catheterization laboratory or operating room or at the bedside, as well as a relatively small footprint allowing placement in the vasculature with less morbidity than other devices in its class. The indications, complications, and relative effectiveness of the IABP have been studied extensively for nearly four decades. National Center for Health Statistics data show that 37,000 intra-aortic balloons were placed in the United States in 2004.[1] The primary hospital location where IABPs are placed varies according to patient acuity and types of procedures performed in individual institutions, but the cardiac catheterization laboratory has become the primary site,[2,3] and the rate of bedside placement in critical care units has declined to low single-digit percentages.

HISTORY

Initial experiments aimed at altering the timing of phases of the cardiac cycle originated with animal experiments conducted by Adrian Kantrowitz in the early 1950s in the laboratory of Carl Wiggers at Western Reserve Medical School.[4] The focus was initially oriented toward improving coronary blood flow rather than augmentation of cardiac output. With the appreciation that coronary flow (particularly in the left coronary circulation) occurs primarily in diastole, the concept was to delay the peak systolic pressure pulse to the diastolic phase of the cardiac cycle.[5] During the subsequent decade, this approach was followed by animal experiments attempting to use the diaphragm to provide the power for diastolic augmentation by wrapping it around the distal thoracic aorta.[6] Clauss and colleagues[7] effectuated counterpulsation by withdrawing blood from the circulation during systole and restoring it during diastole, but it was the work of Moulopoulos and associates[8] that introduced counterpulsation with a carbon dioxide (CO_2)–filled tube synchronized to the electrocardiogram in canines. Kantrowitz subsequently changed the gas to helium, which is used in modern IABPs because it has only 5% of the density of CO_2 and allows faster inflation-deflation cycles and greater precision in timing. In addition, helium is inert, although it is less soluble and potentially more toxic in case of gas leak in the circulation. The IABP was introduced in humans in 1967 (Fig. 7-1). Initial favorable experience with intra-aortic counterpulsation in critically ill patients in cardiogenic shock[9,10] led to the first major multicenter trial. The trial demonstrated significant hemodynamic benefit but only a 17% survival to discharge.[11] A number of incremental improvements over the next four decades resulted in introduction of a percutaneous approach,[12] a second lumen for guidewire support of balloon advancement through the circulation,[13] increasing automation of the control consoles, and prefolded and progressively lower-profile balloons.[14]

PHYSIOLOGY

The classic concept of intra-aortic balloon counterpulsation involves inflation in synchrony with aortic valve closure, at the onset of isovolumic diastole and the appearance of the dicrotic notch, displacing blood comparable to the balloon's volume into the peripheral circulation during diastole. To accomplish further unloading, and to prevent interference with left ventricular (LV) ejection, balloon deflation has traditionally begun before opening of the aortic valve and the beginning of LV ejection, although as discussed subsequently, this may not be the optimal algorithm. An example of the effects of balloon counterpulsation on systolic and diastolic pressure is seen in Figure 7-2. The hemodynamic response to institution of an IABP is quite variable and depends on a complex array consisting of the patient's intrinsic blood pressure, heart rate, heart rhythm, aortic compliance, overall peripheral vascular resistance, intravascular volume status, cardiac function, adjunctive pharmacotherapy, disease state of the coronary vasculature, and degree of preservation of coronary flow autoregulation. In addition, the exact location of the IABP in the vasculature, the volume of the balloon, the frequency of inflation (frequencies from 1:1 to 1:8 are available, depending on manufacturer), and timing of inflation and deflation all play important roles. Thus, the "classic" response consisting of the lowering of systolic blood pressure and augmentation of diastolic pressure may not be seen; this classic response is based on the

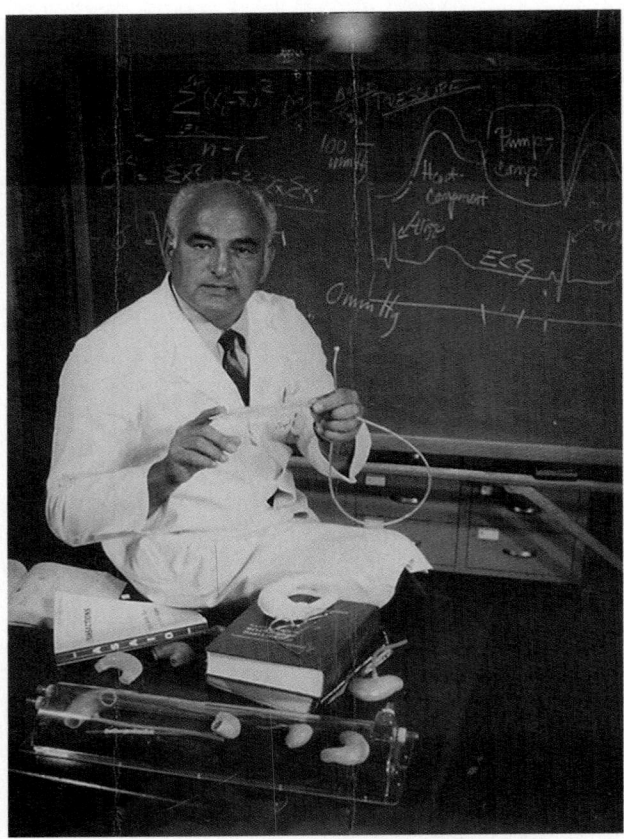

Figure 7-1. Adrian Kantrowitz with early model of working intra-aortic balloon pump used in patients circa 1967, the year of the initial human experience with the device.

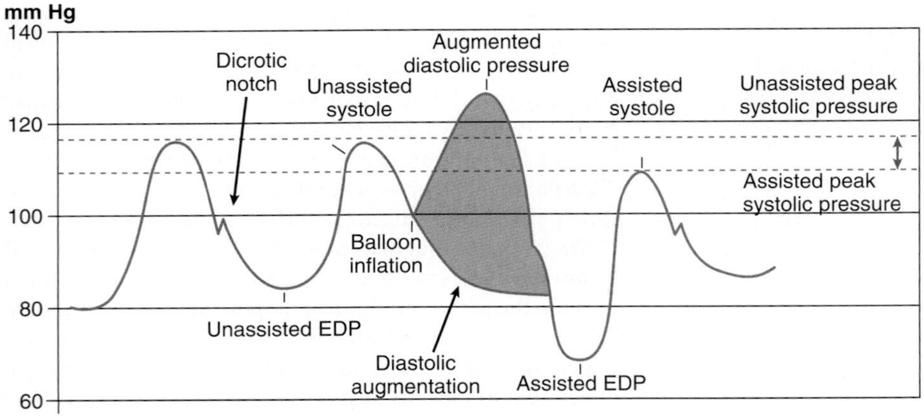

Figure 7-2. Systemic pressure response to an intra-aortic balloon pump. The console is set to trigger at 1:2, hence both unassisted and assisted systole and diastole are seen. Note decrease in systolic pressure with balloon counterpulsation (*double arrow*) and augmentation of diastolic pressure (area under curve in *blue*), thus decreasing afterload and increasing inflow pressure to the coronary and other vascular beds during diastole. EDP, end-diastolic pressure.

initial experience in cardiogenic shock, which led to a 20% drop in systolic pressure and a 30% rise in diastolic pressure.[11] In fact, systolic pressure can increase secondary to improved cardiac output, can decrease, or can be unchanged, as can coronary blood flow. An important characteristic of the IABP, in contrast to most mechanical assist devices, is that it contributes to pulsatile flow, with theoretical benefits to end-organ perfusion beyond any actual change in mean flow or pressures.

Diastole and Coronary Blood Flow

Because the majority of coronary flow occurs in diastole, an increase in diastolic pressure has the potential to augment coronary flow as well as flow to other end organs. Diastolic pressure may in fact be augmented substantially, in part because balloon inflation is rapid, yielding an abrupt increase in volume and affecting a rapid rise on the pressure-volume curve. A variety of physical and biologic parameters, including compliance characteristics of the aorta and vascular bed, affect the degree of augmentation.[15] The extent of peak pressure rise has been reported in a range from minimal to near doubling of diastolic pressure.[16,17] However, increase in diastolic pressure and hence coronary perfusion pressure may not result in an increase in coronary flow because autoregulation modulates this potential and because in normal patients, end organs capable of autoregulation maintain flow without significant change.

Despite both several decades of experimentation in animal models and attempts to assess coronary flow in a variety of clinical settings in humans, the effect of the IABP on coronary flow remains incompletely defined. Experimental and clinical data fail to show change in flow in native coronary arteries[18,19] or in bypass grafts[20] regardless of the severity of coronary stenosis.[21] Although total coronary blood flow may not increase, coronary blood flow velocity has consistently been demonstrated to rise.[16,22,23] In turn, data from a thrombolysis in myocardial infarction model suggest that the pulsatile waveform generated by the IABP during diastole may contribute to improved time to coronary reperfusion without concomitant increase in coronary blood flow[24]; in all likelihood this improvement reflects the enhancement in peak flow velocity that may also help prevent reocclusion.[22] In general, augmentation of blood flow appears most likely to occur in patients in profound shock.[16,23,25] Thus, most of the benefits of the IABP are related to improvement in hemodynamics with secondary relief of ischemia. Amelioration of ischemia may in turn result in better LV function and additional improvement in hemodynamics.

Systole and Myocardial Mechanics

Although the IABP is generally described as both improving myocardial oxygen supply and lowering myocardial oxygen demand, the predominant effect is the latter. This is based on decreased afterload and wall stress with increased stroke volume and cardiac output, in particular in patients with low-output states. In general, the magnitude of hemodynamic response is proportional to the extent of depression of cardiac function.[15] Because stroke volume improves, heart rate stays the same or tends to decrease even as cardiac output rises. Reduction in LV end diastolic pressure and improved cardiac output is associated with lower left heart filling and pulmonary arterial pressures, whereas systolic pressure typically decreases and mean blood pressure stays the same in hemodynamically stable patients. In patients in shock, mean blood pressure rises, and systolic pressure may increase as well. When IABP placement results in improved end-organ perfusion, as evidenced by signs such as better urine output, the overall prognosis is generally improved.[11] Reduction in left heart filling and pulmonary artery pressures also leads to reduced right ventricular (RV) afterload; thus, IABP insertion may be helpful in some patients with right heart failure.[26] Although ejection phase indices tend to improve with unloading, the extent of augmentation of cardiac output is limited by the overall reserve in LV systolic function. Thus, at the extremes of ventricular dysfunction, even with excellent positioning of the balloon and timing and large IABP volumes, the IABP may not provide sufficient augmentation of cardiac output in some patients.

Effects on Organs Other Than the Heart

The effect of IABPs on flow to end organs other than the heart is also incompletely characterized. In the cranial circulation as in the heart, net flow does not appear to increase in patients with a stable hemodynamic state. Further, with balloon deflation, there is some evidence for transient reversal of blood flow as well,[27] although this may be a consequence of early deflation (see section on timing). Similarly, overall carotid flow is not changed in this setting.[28] During hypothermia while patients are under cardiopulmonary bypass, pulsatile augmentation as obtained by the IABP does appear to improve cerebral oxygenation.[29] Indirect evidence again suggests additional benefit in the setting of shock, with better cerebral blood flow, a setting in which there is modest clinical experience with using IABPs in patients with refractory cerebral vasospasm.[30] Even in the setting of cardiogenic shock, despite improvement in cardiac output with the IABP, gastric tonometry has not shown improvement in the splanchnic circulation,[31] and renal vein thermodilution has failed to show improvement in overall renal blood flow.[32]

THE IABP APPARATUS

With the introduction of a separate guidewire lumen in the early 1980s,[13] the safety of IABP placement improved significantly. Previously, bulky 12F or larger devices were placed via a surgical approach through an end-to-side graft to the femoral artery, with substantial associated morbidity. The device was then advanced through the femoral and iliac systems without a guidewire, frequently at the bedside with no fluoroscopic guidance. This led to a high rate of major vascular complications, in particular iliac artery dissection but also aortic perforation and IABP malposition. The introduction of the percutaneous approach did not alleviate these problems until a guidewire lumen was added.[13]

There were conflicting demands on balloon design: first, to minimize the central lumen size as part of reducing overall profile, and second, at the same time to maintain a large enough lumen both for guidewires that could provide safe passage through the circulation as well as sufficient diameter for high-fidelity hemodynamic recordings. One solution to the latter has been the introduction of a line of catheters with a fiberoptic pressure measurement sensor.[33] In general, the guidewire lumens are designed to accommodate guidewires in the 0.025-inch to 0.030-inch range. The gas exchange lumen is concentrically placed around the guidewire lumen. Improvements in technology allowed for the introduction of tightly folded balloons prewrapped around the central lumen (Fig. 7-3); previously, a cumbersome process that sometimes led to device failure required the operator to wrap the balloon just before insertion.

Balloon Dimensions

The available IABP catheters range in gas volume from 25 to 50 mL and in shaft lengths from approximately 60 to 72 cm. The actual length of the balloon segment varies by manufacturer and balloon volume: Commercial balloon lengths range from 17 to 26 cm. Although balloon volume does affect the extent of diastolic augmentation[34] and cardiac output[35] and may be particularly important in patients with severe, refractory cardiogenic shock, little difference was found in IABP effectiveness between 32-mL and 40-mL balloons in one study,[36] and risk to the patient is significantly higher if inflated balloon diameter approximates or exceeds aortic diameter (see "Complications"). Thus the decision for IABP size is typically based on patient size and severity of hemodynamic compromise, with the 40-mL balloon used in approximately three fourths of patients.[37] A special consideration for balloon volumes is patient air transport; rapid changes in altitude leads to increased (during ascent) or decreased (with descent) volume, requiring monitoring to ensure that appropriate balloon volume is maintained.[38]

Because it is essential to locate the balloon below the origin of the left subclavian artery at the upper margin and above the renal arteries at the lower (a "safe zone"; Fig. 7-4), the tolerances are relatively low. Studies looking at the length of this segment in Japanese patients found a range of 21 to 25 cm, with good correlation between patient height and length of this segment (although in the relatively short Japanese population, the balloon lengths commonly exceeded the "safe zone" length for individual patients).[39] Recommendations vary by manufacturer: A 50-mL size is generally recommended for patients taller than 6 feet (183 cm), and the 25-mL for patients shorter than 5 feet (152 cm). Early balloon models were designed to be occlusive during inflation, and experimental data have demonstrated optimal augmentation with 100% occlusion of the aorta.[34,35] Such full occlusion is generally avoided because of potential trauma to the aorta, ischemia to the spinal circulation, or abrasion of the balloon, which might contribute to a risk of rupture. The generally accepted value for ratio of balloon to aorta size is 80% to 90%; in the study by Igari[39] in Japanese patients, the range of commercially available balloon diameters was noted to be 14 to 15 mm, whereas aortic diameter mean at the level of the renal arteries was 17.5±3.2 mm, within the accepted 80% to 90% range, although at least one 50-mL balloon has an expanded diameter of 18 mm (Arrow International, Inc., Reading, PA). In an earlier study in Americans, 90% of midthoracic aortas were larger than 19 mm.[40] Balloons are typically made of polyurethane or polyethylene, with materials chosen to allow rapid inflation-deflation cycles and tolerate the average of 100,000 to 150,000 cycles per day. Experimental materials with heparin and hydrophilic coating have been developed to address thrombosis risk and trauma to the vasculature during device passage[41,42] but are not commercially available.

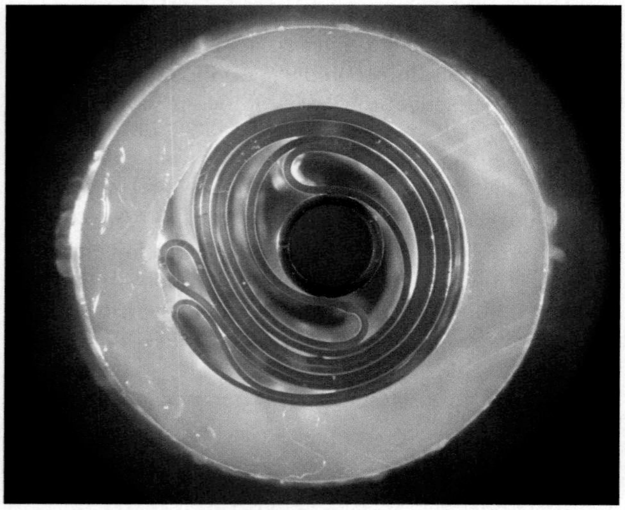

Figure 7-3. Magnified cross-sectional view of prefolded intra-aortic balloon (a 7.5 French wrap). The prefolding was a significant advance in technology in the early 1980s because it eliminated folding at the bedside, a process that occasionally led to tearing of the balloon membrane, and substantially reduced the overall profile of the device at insertion. *Red arrows* point to membrane folds, *yellow arrow* to the central pressure and guidewire lumen. (Courtesy of Datascope, Montvale, NJ.)

Balloon Console

IABPs are driven by complexly engineered consoles with extensive artificial intelligence designed to recognize electrocardiogram (ECG) rhythms and hemodynamics, with the ability to trigger balloon inflation either from the ECG (including paced rhythms) or from pressure waveforms, although in some settings, such as during cardiopulmonary bypass, an automatic trigger at a preset rate can be

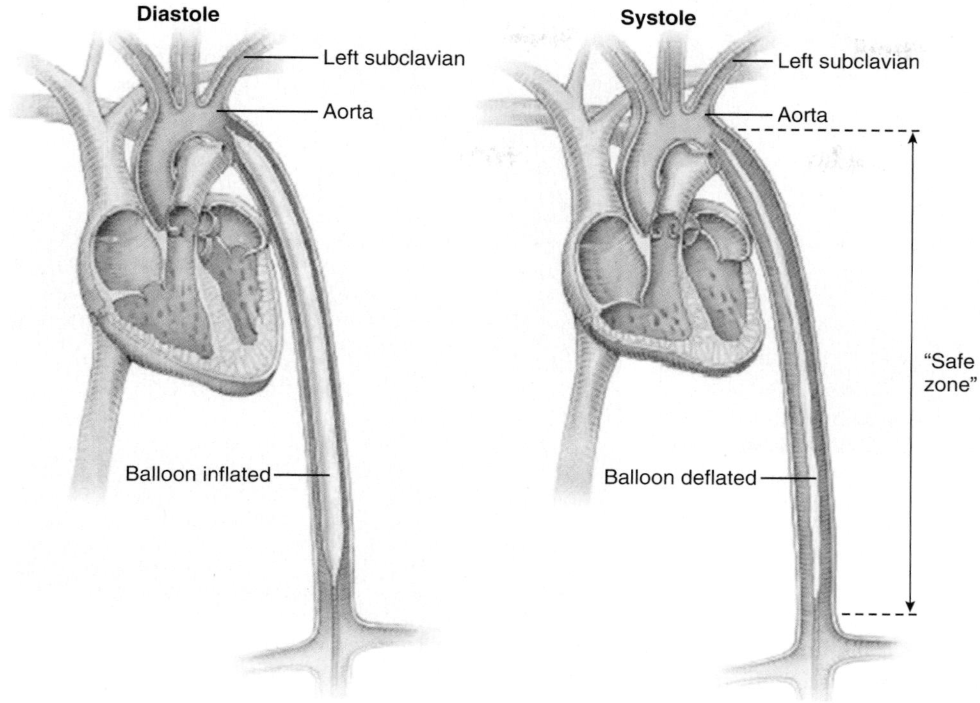

Figure 7-4. Location of intra-aortic balloon during inflation and deflation. Ideally the tip should be a few centimeters distal to the origin of the left subclavian artery and the proximal portion above the origins of the renal arteries, the "safe zone." (Adapted from figure provided by Arrow International, Reading, PA.)

used. Tachyarrhythmias and irregular rhythms have substantial influence on the effectiveness of the IABP, the former in part because of the disproportionately shorter diastolic filling periods and the latter because of difficulties predicting the timing of occurrence of the dicrotic notch, although improved algorithms have been incorporated.[43] The central lumen of the balloon is typically connected to a transducer and separate ECG leads are connected to the console. A series of alarms identify leaks in the IABP circuit, high or low pressure, loss of trigger signals, blood in the gas line, low battery and other anomalies that foreshadow or indicate impending or existing system failures. (Figure 7-5 demonstrates the control panel of a modern IABP console.)

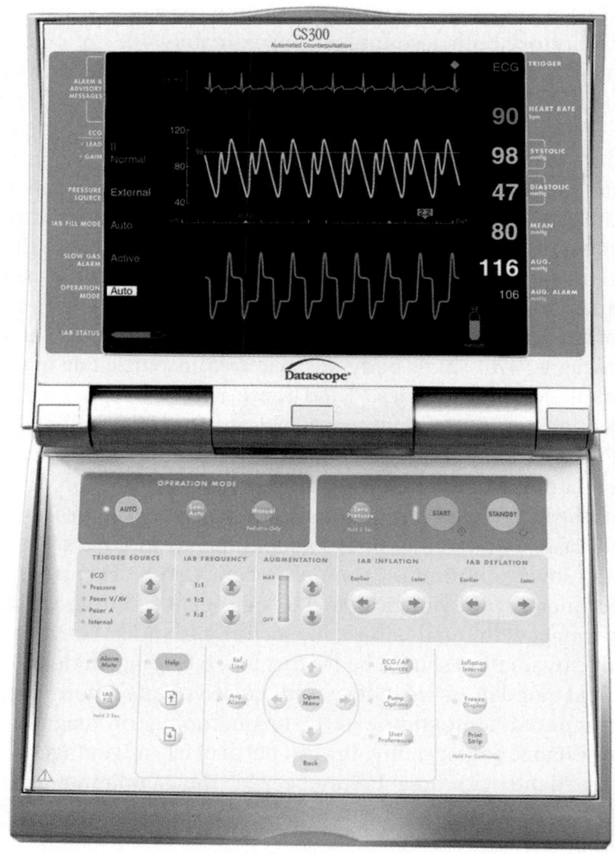

Figure 7-5. Intra-aortic balloon console showing electrocardiogram, systemic pressure (note diastolic augmentation), and balloon inflation volumes. (Courtesy of Datascope, Montvale, NJ.)

PREPARATION

Balloon preparation requires establishing a vacuum in the gas lumen by drawing back on a large volume syringe, and also flushing the central guidewire lumen (Fig. 7-6). If the procedure is to be done at the bedside without fluoroscopy, measuring the approximate distance along the course of the femoral and iliac arteries and then up the descending aorta is essential prior to IABP placement. The approximate depth to which it needs to be inserted should be noted on the shaft prior to beginning insertion. The ECG leads should be connected to the IABP console prior to introducing the catheter if ECG triggering is to be performed.

BALLOON INSERTION

On the basis of data from the Benchmark Registry, nearly two thirds of IABP insertions in the United States occur

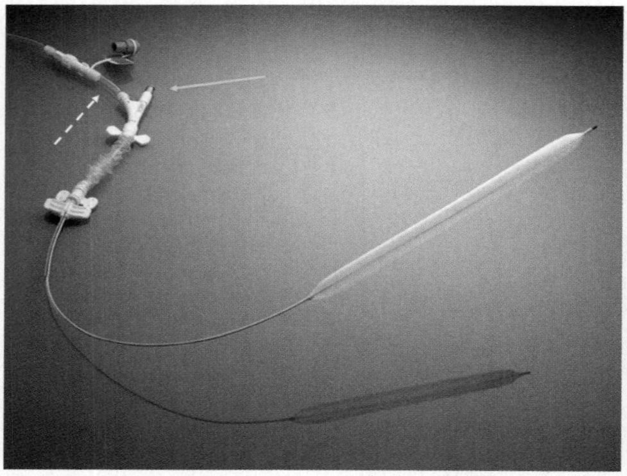

Figure 7-6. A modern intra-aortic balloon. Central lumen (*yellow arrow*) and gas lumen (*dashed white arrow*) are highlighted. This model is designed to be introduced through an 8F sheath. (Adapted from image courtesy of Arrow International, Reading, PA.)

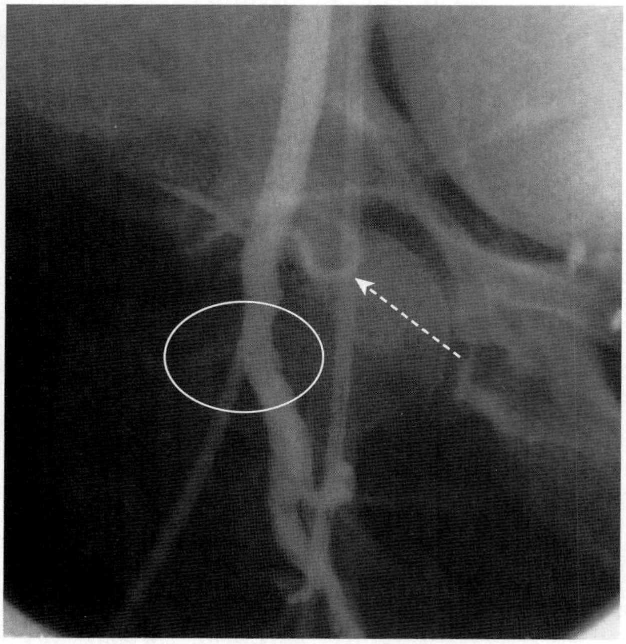

Figure 7-7. Optimal access for placement of an intra-aortic balloon pump, right femoral artery, left anterior oblique view. The sheath entry is above the femoral bifurcation near the center line of the femoral head *(circle)*. Note the location of the inferior epigastric artery (IEA; *arrow*). The lowest inflection of the IEA lies just above the inguinal ligament; punctures below this point have a lower likelihood of subsequent retroperitoneal hemorrhage.

in the cardiac catheterization laboratory, one fourth in the operating room, and the remainder at the bedside in a variety of hospital locations. In contrast, outside the United States, the operating room and the catheterization laboratory both account for approximately 40% of placements, with the remaining 20% performed at the bedside.[3]

The modern IABP is designed to be introduced percutaneously through the common femoral artery, which is the method used in 95% to 98% of cases, two thirds via the right common femoral artery.[37,44] A variety of disease states affect the ability to freely pass the device to the central aorta, in particular atherosclerosis, but also spasm and congenitally small vessels. Pre-procedure assessment of the vascular tree is important: Diabetics, women, and patients with small body surface area in particular have small femoral arteries,[45] and there is a correspondingly higher rate of vascular complications in these patients.[46] Pulses at the common femoral artery and below must be carefully documented before catheter insertion, and if there is suspected or confirmed peripheral vascular disease, angiography of the abdominal aorta, iliac artery, and lower extremities should be considered. This step is frequently not practical in the emergency setting or in patients with renal failure; in elective situations, noninvasive evaluation should be performed, including ankle brachial blood pressure indices with pulse volume recordings, computed tomography (CT) angiography, or magnetic resonance angiography, the last particularly advantageous in patients with renal failure because the gadolinium used for contrast has low nephrotoxicity.

Femoral Access

Every effort should be made to ensure that femoral puncture is above the femoral bifurcation and below the inguinal ligament (Fig. 7-7). An excellent practice is to place a short 5F or 6F pilot sheath in the femoral artery and to perform angiography of the common femoral artery to confirm sheath entry below the inferior excursion of the inferior epigastric artery; punctures above this landmark correlate strongly with retroperitoneal hemorrhage.[47] Puncture below the femoral head drastically increases the likelihood of puncture into the femoral bifurcation vessels (77% of femoral bifurcations are at or below the inferior margin of the femoral head[45]), which in turn is associated with acute leg ischemia due to vascular obstruction, and pseudoaneurysm formation upon balloon removal is more likely because of lack of the anvil of the femoral head against which to perform manual compression. If the pilot sheath is found to have entered outside the common femoral artery on femoral angiography, consideration should be given to switching to the contralateral side. Using fluoroscopy to aid in puncturing the common femoral artery at a point over the lower half of the femoral head is a recommended technique to ensure proper sheath placement.

Sheathless Insertion

The use of a sheathless insertion technique has been recommended to reduce complications.[48] Sheaths typically add between 0.6 and 0.8 mm to the overall diameter required to place a device, so the sheath for an 8F balloon approximates 10F in outer diameter. "Going sheathless" therefore has the advantage of having the device occupy less space in the common femoral artery and has been described as reducing vascular complications with an odds ratio greater than 2 : 1.[49,50] Although retrospective analysis of large patient subsets presents compelling data that the sheathless approach is superior for reducing complications,[51] this finding has not been universally confirmed.[46,52] The latest data suggest that about 80% of IABPs are inserted with a sheath.[37] The sheathless approach is most compelling in diabetic patients, women, and patients with known peripheral vascular disease or small body surface area. Sheathless insertion of an IABP requires careful preparation of the tissue track to allow atraumatic entry of the balloon tip into the artery directly through the skin over a wire. Spreading of tissue and predilation with a dilator are essential. Fibrosed tissue tracks or thickened/calcified arterial walls frequently resist sheathless entry. In some cases, a stiff guidewire provides an adequate rail along which to slide the naked balloon catheter into the vessel.

Balloon Advancement and Positioning

Once suitable access is gained, guidewire passage to the aortic arch is ideally performed under fluoroscopic guidance. Without fluoroscopy at the bedside, approximating the distance from the femoral puncture to a point near the top of the descending aorta is imprecise and adds to the risk of trauma/ischemia to head and neck vessels, the aorta, or the renal arteries. In the critical care setting, transesophageal echocardiography is a suitable alternative to fluoroscopy for enabling precise balloon placement.[53] If fluoroscopy is not used, prompt postprocedure radiography to confirm location is imperative.

If guidewire passage meets resistance, alternative approaches include use of guidewires that are hydrophilic, steerable, or both.[54] If significant iliac stenosis is noted, balloon dilation or stenting of the iliac artery is an accepted practice with high success rate both for achieving passage of the IABP and as an adjunct to preventing distal ischemia.[55,56] As more cardiologists become skilled in endovascular intervention, the ability to perform combined iliac stenting and IABP placement is expanding.[57]

Once the balloon has been advanced to a point 1 to 2 cm inferior to the left subclavian artery origin (see Fig. 7-4)—typically near the top of the descending aorta—the guidewire is withdrawn and the central lumen flushed. The vacuum port (minus its one-way valve) is connected to gas line tubing that in turn is connected to the console, and the dead space is purged and then filled with helium. The central catheter lumen is connected to a transducer on the console. After triggering is initiated, typically on every other beat, fluoroscopy should be used to confirm balloon location and filling, and pressure contours should be evaluated for appropriateness of timing (see later). Once the timing is considered satisfactory, continuous pumping can be initiated. The balloon should be repositioned with the console turned to standby to avoid trauma to the aorta.

The distal circulation should be assessed carefully after IABP placement. Distal ischemia is relatively common. The most likely cause of acute ischemia is obstruction of the artery by the catheter shaft itself. If ischemia occurs hours or days after insertion, the possibility of thrombus, typically secondary to stagnant blood in the confined space of a small or diseased vessel, should be considered as well. A technique for addressing distal limb ischemia—placement of a small sheath retrograde in the contralateral femoral artery and antegrade in the ipsilateral common femoral or superficial femoral artery—if performed by expert hands, can occasionally salvage an ischemic limb without forcing removal of the IABP (Fig. 7-8).[58] There is some evidence that IABP inflation properties and hemodynamic effects may be superior in the patient positioned horizontally than in the patient tilted at a 30-degree angle.[59] Postprocedure and subsequent monitoring of left arm pressures can lead to early diagnosis of inadvertent balloon advancement that obstructs left subclavian artery inflow, a phenomenon to which the restless patient who flexes the thigh is predisposed.

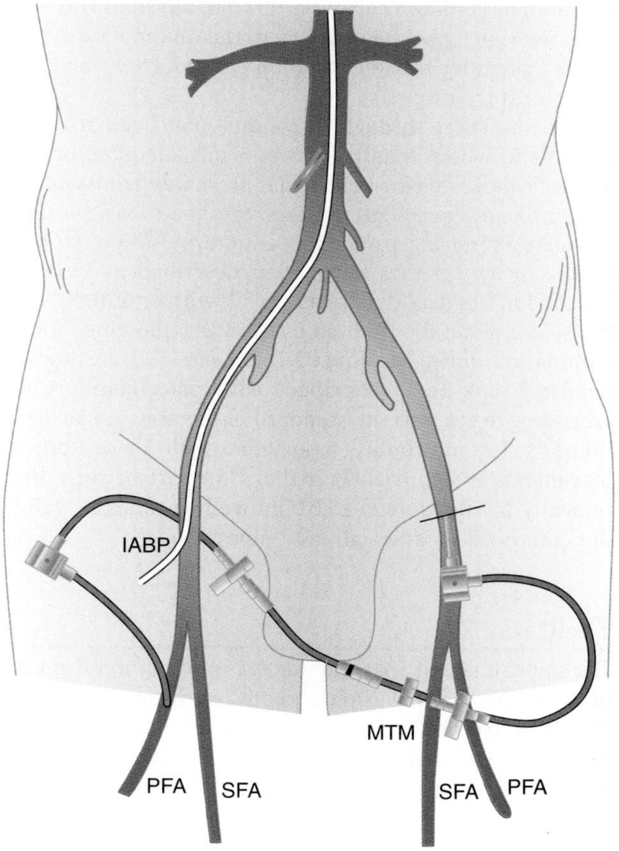

Figure 7-8. Percutaneous external femoral-femoral shunt for a patient with critical leg ischemia after placement of an intra-aortic balloon pump (IABP) in the right common femoral artery. The patient had an occluded right superficial femoral artery (SFA), so distal circulation depended on profunda femoris to superficial femoral collateral vessels. The antegrade sheath is placed directly into the profunda femoris. MTM, male-to-male adapter; PFA, profunda femoris artery. (From Merhi WM, Turi ZG, Dixon S, et al: Percutaneous ex-vivo femoral arterial bypass: A novel approach for treatment of acute limb ischemia as a complication of femoral arterial catheterization. Catheter Cardiovasc Interv 2006;68:435-440.)

Alternate Access Routes

Multiple alternatives to percutaneous femoral access have been described, all associated with higher complication rates. In part, this difference in rates is selection related: Patients with severe peripheral vascular disease have multiple comorbidities that affect IABP complications. In addition, introduction of a balloon into a peripheral vessel smaller than the common femoral artery, or into a large central vessel through surgical approaches of necessity creates hazards associated with the introduction, maintenance, and withdrawal of the IABP.

Approaches described to date include the brachial, subclavian, axillary, iliac, transthoracic and translumbar. Although the brachial approach has been successful in isolated cases[60,61] and sheathless entry reduces the overall diameter of lumen encroachment to less than 3 mm, the potential for complications is substantial. They include not only vascular injury and ischemia of the hand but also potential neurologic consequences from formation of thrombus on an indwelling catheter underneath the origin of the right common carotid artery (as the shaft traverses from the right subclavian artery to the innominate artery) as well as under the left common carotid artery and subclavian artery origin.[62]

Iliac insertion through a conduit has been used for patients in whom femoral access is not adequate or who are not candidates for ventricular assist devices: With retroperitoneal placement, patients can be at least partially ambulatory during prolonged counterpulsation.[63] Other routes of access that have been described are via the subclavian[64] and axillary arteries,[65,66] with or without conduits, and generally with an eye toward allowing modest ambulation during prolonged IABP use. A transthoracic approach has been described, with placement via the ascending aorta into the standard descending aortic location.[67,68] The morbidity associated with these surgical placements is significantly higher,[69] in part because they typically involve longer IABP indwelling times as well as the comorbidity issues already mentioned.

TIMING

The importance of IABP timing was understood from the time of the original Moulopolous study in 1962.[8] The timing of balloon inflation and deflation is designed to optimize afterload reduction and enhancement of diastolic pressure without interfering with ventricular ejection. Classically, it was considered optimal to inflate at the dicrotic notch, as soon as aortic valve closure occurred, and to deflate near the onset of ventricular depolarization, anticipating the beginning of mechanical systole (Fig. 7-9). In fact, significant enhancements to IABP efficiency can be obtained with refinements to these concepts.

Late Inflation and Early Deflation

Gross errors in inflation and deflation lead to failure to obtain benefit from an IABP and occasionally to significant hemodynamic compromise. Early in the history of IABP deployment, it was appreciated that inflation throughout the period from closure of the aortic valve to its subsequent opening was necessary for optimal hemodynamic effect.[15] Both late inflation and early deflation reduce augmented LV stroke volume and result in decreased peak diastolic coronary velocity[22]; the latter is demonstrated with transthoracic Doppler ultrasound, a tool that can potentially be used to optimize timing. An additional concern exists with early deflation: The abrupt decrease in IABP volume during diastole can lead to reversal of both coronary and other end-organ (e.g., cerebral) flow back into the aorta, shunting blood from vital end organs.[27]

Early Inflation

Early inflation results in increased afterload late in LV ejection with consequent impairment of LV systolic function. The ejection phase is shortened, LV end systolic pressure rises and stroke volume decreases; inflation, in the range of 130 to 190 msec before the dicrotic notch, results in a 20% decrease in stroke volume.[70] This effect may not be seen if early balloon inflation is less pronounced; no hemodynamic effect was noted when IABP inflation occurred 50 msec before the dicrotic notch. Regardless, although early inflation theoretically lengthens diastole and allows for a longer period of diastolic augmentation, the net effect does not appear to be salutary. In addition, early inflation carries theoretical risks associated with the increased afterload and wall stress, including aneurysm formation and rupture in the perimyocardial infarction period.

Late Deflation

Similarly, late balloon deflation could be expected to interfere with ventricular ejection and decrease stroke volume. In fact, somewhat counterintuitively, a similar 110- to 180-msec delay in IABP deflation appears to have salutary effects and is associated with a stroke volume increase of 18%,[70] which apparently results from both an increase in diastolic filling period and an augmented decrease in afterload later in the cycle. This finding confirms a prior observation by Kern and associates[71] and suggests that in general, most operators have timed deflation too early. The beneficial effect occurs with timing deflation to be simultaneous with LV ejection; delaying deflation beyond the range described, however, raises concerns similar to those described for early inflation.

Electrocardiogram Triggering

When the ECG is used as the trigger, the descending slope of the T wave correlates best with the onset of diastole[34] and is the usual timing for balloon inflation. Deflation is typically timed to the R wave, which denotes a short time delay after the onset of electrical systole. Algorithms were developed early to effect prompt deflation and prevent inflation in the setting of ectopy, and IABP software recognizes pacemaker spikes in contrast to QRS complexes as well. As in the findings described previously,[70,71] deflation timed to the J point, with adjustment for the delay between onset of isovolumic systole and aortic valve opening, and perhaps slightly later, was shown early in the IABP literature to improve stroke volume.[34]

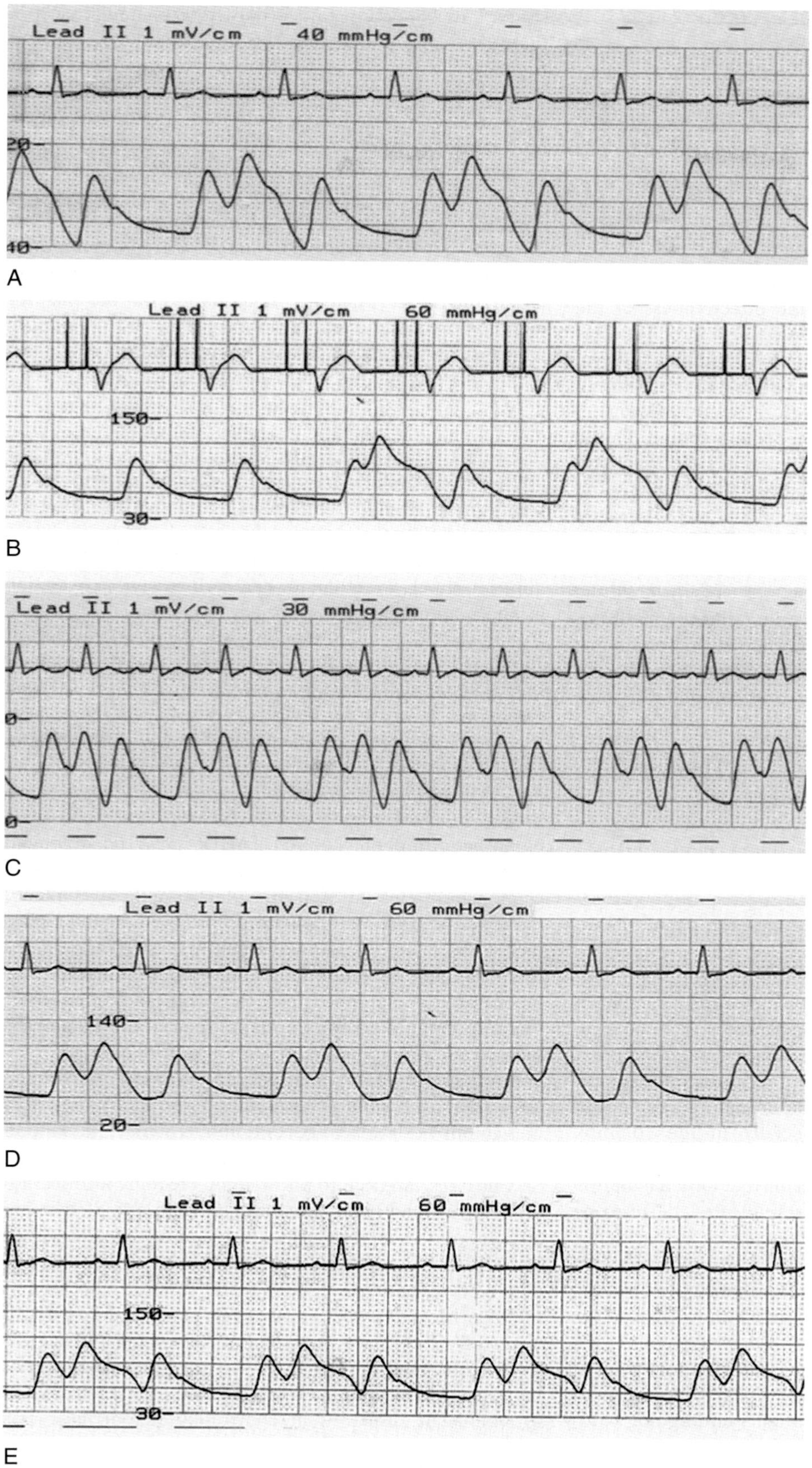

Figure 7-9. Examples of timing of intra-aortic balloon pump inflation and deflation with 1:2 balloon pumping. **(A)**, Optimal timing results in mild lowering of systolic pressure with diastolic augmentation. Also shown are examples of early inflation before the dicrotic notch **(B)**, late inflation **(C)**, early deflation **(D)**, and late deflation **(E)**.

Other Considerations

A common problem has been proper timing in patients with underlying arrhythmias. Atrial fibrillation has been particularly vexing, with unpredictable beat-to-beat intervals. An algorithm to predict the occurrence of the distance between the QRS and the dicrotic notch was developed in the mid-1990s.[72] Newer dicrotic notch prediction algorithms using high-fidelity micromanometer pressure sensors have been described.[43] However, atrial fibrillation poses difficulties beyond timing alone; rapid ventricular rates result in a disproportionate decrease in the diastolic interval and limit the effectiveness of the IABP because of the inherently short period of counterpulsation,[73] including subtraction of the fixed time interval required for shuttling helium into and out of the balloon. Operating at 1:2 rates may be required in this setting.

Lack of augmentation despite proper timing should result in troubleshooting the IABP console, checking with fluoroscopy to visualize inflation of the balloon and confirm the level of balloon placement, and excluding kinking of the gas line or other mechanical failures. Apparently normal IABP function with absence of hemodynamic improvement should raise a suspicion that the patient has a baseline hemodynamic state that will not benefit from LV unloading, in particular hypovolemia, sepsis, or profound hemodynamic collapse as well as a number of conditions described subsequently (see "Contraindications").

Overall, timing of the IABP should result in diastolic pressure augmentation and lowering of assisted peak systolic pressure when possible, with the former a generally used end point for patients with shock and the latter the primary goal in patients with more stable hemodynamics at the time of IABP insertion.

ADJUNCTIVE PHARMACOTHERAPY

Adjunctive pharmacotherapy typically includes heparinization. There are two theoretical reasons for anticoagulation: First, in patients receiving less than 1:1 counterpulsation, there is concern regarding clot formation on the balloon apparatus, and second, stagnant blood around the catheter shaft, especially in the common femoral artery, has been thought to raise the risk of thrombosis. The general consensus remains that anticoagulation should be administered if not contraindicated, despite one randomized comparison that failed to show any evidence of thrombosis in unanticoagulated patients followed for a relatively short course of IABP use, with a higher bleeding risk in patients given heparin.[74] The balloons themselves have a thrombogenic surface,[41] and occlusion of vessels requiring thromboembolectomy has been reported to be one of the most common complications, with a rate of nearly 3% in one series of 911 patients undergoing coronary artery bypass grafting (CABG).[49]

A second adjunctive pharmacotherapy issue is the use of prophylactic antibiotics. Although fever, bacteremia, and sepsis were reported to be common (occurring at rates of 47%, 15%, and 12%, respectively) in one small study,[75] the infection rate in larger series has been less than 1%,[49] and the consensus is that the evidence base is too thin and the public health implications too unfavorable to recommend routine antibiotic use unless otherwise clinically warranted.[76] A third medication issue relates to sedation. Continuous bed rest in a critical care setting is frequently associated with disorientation or agitation. Balloon migration from leg bending and patient movement risks significant trauma to the aorta, renal arteries, and head and neck vessels. Careful sedation is essential. Finally, antiarrhythmic agents to slow and regularize the heart rate can have important benefits for lengthening diastole and optimizing balloon timing, both of which in turn enhance IABP augmentation.

BALLOON REMOVAL

Removal of the IABP poses several challenges. First, the ability to maintain hemodynamic stability without counterpulsation must be confirmed as part of the weaning process. Although cardiac output is disproportionately decreased with lowering of pumping ratios, such lowering appears superior to decreasing volumes as a weaning method, an approach confirmed by one small retrospective evaluation.[77] The balloon should not be turned off completely until the activated clotting time value confirms that anticoagulation has been effectively discontinued and the patient is ready for balloon removal, because thrombosis on the balloon surface occurs rapidly.[41] Most operators run the IABP at a low cycle rate, 1:3 to as low as 1:8 (depending on manufacturer), until anticoagulation has worn off sufficiently and the balloon can be removed. Nonfunctioning or stopped IABPs must be removed promptly, preferably within 20 minutes or less. A second challenge relates to the size of the deflated balloon. Because the balloon is delivered prefolded by the manufacturer (see Fig. 7-3), it passes readily through its delivery sheath during insertion. Once inflated, it will not refold when vacuum is applied, and the profile is too large for retrieval without bringing both the sheath and the balloon out of the body together.

Removing the balloon, especially after long indwelling times (mean indwelling time is 53 to 77 hours[37,44]), requires meticulous attention to several details. First, the balloon gas line should be aspirated to reduce the balloon profile. Second, it is essential to allow some bleeding after catheter removal and prior to compression to avoid stripping any clot off the balloon inside the common femoral artery. Because these are relatively large catheters, frequently deployed in patients with vascular disease who have a tenuous hemodynamic status even at the time of IABP removal, patients may not tolerate prolonged and aggressive compression of the groin. Recent discontinuation of heparin combined with a large arteriotomy size can result in significant difficulty in controlling hemorrhage and achieving hemostasis.

Surgical closure is sometimes preferable, particularly with severely obese patients, after very long indwelling times, with uncorrectable anticoagulation status, or with low or high punctures.[78] Vascular closure devices have been used successfully in small series[79,80] but require extreme caution; significant mortality is associated with infections related to vascular closure devices,[81] and ensuring sterility at the time of IABP removal is difficult. When use of a closure device is required, I typically place a 0.018-inch stiff guidewire inside the lumen after extensive efforts to achieve sterility of both the field and the device, withdraw the IABP, and place our closure device over the wire; we cannot recommend this off-label approach, however, until a better evidence base is available. Finally, it is important to continue to monitor patients for adverse events because nearly 25% of IABP-related complications have been reported to occur *after* IABP removal.[82]

INDICATIONS

As with the original patients in 1968,[9] cardiogenic shock remained the most common indication for several decades, although later data suggest that circulatory support for percutaneous intervention has replaced hemodynamic instability in the acute myocardial infarction (MI) setting as the primary indication for IABP insertion.[37] Other common indications are perioperative support for patients undergoing cardiac surgery, weaning from cardiopulmonary bypass, management of unstable angina, severe congestive heart failure, and, with less evidence base, refractory ventricular arrhythmias or angina after MI as well as a host of miscellaneous settings largely defined by case reports (Box 7-1).

In general, indications can be divided into several categories: prophylactic versus therapeutic; hemodynamic support versus improved end-organ flow; and preoperative, intraoperative, or postoperative management. The rate of prophylactic use, defined as IABP insertion prior to percutaneous or surgical intervention, rose from 17.3% in 1992 to 31.3% in 2001 as a proportion of IABP use in the United States according to the Benchmark Registry.[3] The management and particularly the complications associated with these subcategories are substantially different. Box 7-1 lists indications for IABP use. The class I indications include cardiogenic shock if not quickly reversible with pharmacologic therapy, acute mitral insufficiency or ventricular septal rupture, recurrent ischemia or infarction, hypotension that does not respond to other interventions, and a low-output state.

In general, use of an IABP identifies a high-risk population, with in-hospital mortality exceeding 20% among more than 22,000 patients (Fig. 7-10).[3,44,83] The Benchmark Registry examined the use of IABPs in more than 5000 patients with acute MI; this represented 24% of all IABP placements at the 250 participating medical centers. Twenty-seven percent of the patients were in cardiogenic shock, an additional 12% needed support because of acute ventricular septal rupture or severe mitral insufficiency, and 5% underwent IABP placement for refractory LV failure. Thus, nearly half the patients with IABP placements and MI had hemodynamic settings in which balloon support was likely life sustaining.[44]

Despite a strong evidence base for its utility in salvaging myocardium and decreasing mortality, and despite a significant associated complication rate, there are no separate American College of Cardiology/American Heart Association guidelines for placing an IABP.[84] However, indications for IABP use are included in the Guidelines for ST-Segment Elevation Myocardial Infaction.[85] It is important to note that severe hemodynamic deterioration, including cardiogenic shock, occurs in some patients with acute MI without ST segment elevation.[86]

Cardiogenic Shock

The classic understanding of cardiogenic shock has been stunning or irreversible loss of a large amount of myocardium (≥40%) with resultant low output and compensatory elevated systemic vascular resistance to maintain central organ perfusion pressure. The definition of cardiogenic shock (CS) has varied, although the essential elements are a low cardiac index and elevated left heart filling pressure. The most common current definition is hypotension (blood

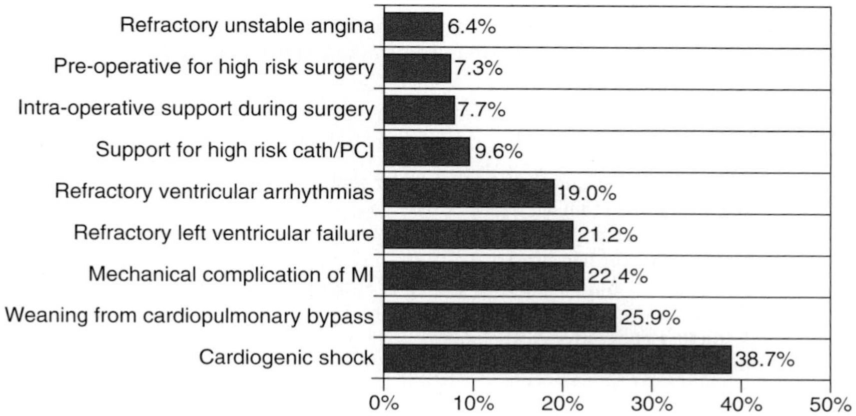

Figure 7-10. In-hospital mortality in 5495 patients with acute myocardial infarction (MI) enrolled in the Benchmark Registry. Note the threefold higher mortality among patients with rescue placement of intra-aortic balloon pumps (IABPs) compared with those in whom IABPs were inserted preoperatively for high-risk surgery, and the continuing high mortality for patients with cardiogenic shock. Cath, cardiac catheterization; PCI, percutaneous coronary intervention. (Adapted from Stone GW, Ohman EM, Miller MF, et al: Contemporary utilization and outcomes of intra-aortic balloon counterpulsation in acute myocardial infarction: The Benchmark Registry. J Am Coll Cardiol 2003;41:1940-1945.)

Box 7-1

Indications for Use of an Intra-aortic Balloon Pump

Acute ST Elevation Myocardial Infarction (STEMI)*

Class I indications

Cardiogenic shock not promptly reversed with pharmacologic therapy
Acute mitral regurgitation
Ventricular septal rupture
Recurrent ischemia and infarction
Hypotension not responding to other interventions
Low-output state

Class II indications

IIa: Refractory polymorphic ventricular tachycardia
IIb: Refractory pulmonary congestion

Additional recommendations

In patients with cardiogenic shock after STEMI who are not candidates for revascularization.
As a short- or long-term mechanical support as bridge to recovery or heart transplant.

Other Settings†

Percutaneous intervention

- High-risk coronary angioplasty
  - Acute coronary syndrome with hemodynamic instability
  - Severe left ventricular (LV) dysfunction
  - Unprotected left main or single remaining vessel intervention
- Hemodynamic support for decompensated patients undergoing structural heart disease interventions

Cardiac surgery

- Preoperative use
  - Severe LV dysfunction
  - Left main disease
  - Acute coronary syndrome
  - Repeat thoracotomy
- Perioperative or postoperative use
  - Hemodynamic deterioration
  - Inability to wean from bypass

Unstable angina

Uncomplicated myocardial infarction‡

Congestive heart failure

- Fulminant myocarditis
- Decompensated aortic stenosis‡
- Drug toxicity‡
- Thyrotoxicosis‡
- Multiple sclerosis‡
- Lightning strike‡
- Right ventricular (RV) failure‡
  - RV infarction
  - After heart transplantation
  - Bridge to transplantation

Miscellaneous

- Cardiopulmonary resuscitation‡
- Noncardiac surgery
  - Recent MI
  - Left ventricular failure
  - Unrevascularized myocardium
  - Emergency surgery

*Based on Antman EM, Anbe DT, Armstrong PW, et al: ACC/AHA guidelines for the management of patients with ST-elevation myocardial infarction: A report of the American College of Cardiology/American Heart Association Task Force on Practice Guidelines (Committee to Revise the 1999 Guidelines for the management of patients with acute myocardial infarction). J Am Coll Cardiol 2004;44:E1-E211.
†Based on available literature (cited in text) without formal guidelines.
‡Minimal or inconsistent evidence base for indication.
Class I, conditions for which there is evidence for or general agreement that the procedure is benefical, useful, and effective; Class II, conditions for which there is conflicting evidence or a divergence of opinion about the usefulness or efficacy of a procedure.

Distribution of Indications from the Benchmark Registry[37]

Cardiogenic shock	18.8%
Acute mitral regurgitation or ventricular septal defect	5.5%
Refractory arrhythmia	1.7%
High-risk percutaneous intervention	20.6%
Preoperative cardiac surgery	13.0%
Perioperative and postoperative cardiac surgery	16.1%
Unstable angina (including post-MI)	12.3%
Refractory congestive heart failure	6.5%
Miscellaneous or information missing	5.5%

pressure <90 mm Hg systolic), with cardiac index less than 2.2 l/min/m^2 and pulmonary artery wedge pressure greater than 15 mm Hg. Data from the SHOCK (SHould we emergently revascularize OCcluded coronaries in cardiogenic shocK?) trial have called several classic assumptions into question,[87] in part because some of the patients in this trial with CS had relatively preserved ejection fractions whereas other patients with apparently a much larger amount of dysfunctional or nonfunctional heart muscle were hemodynamically compensated.

Although the incidence of CS has declined,[88] it remains significant; the most recent estimates are that it is seen in approximately 6% of acute MIs. Mortality, once described as high as 80% (though variable in the literature, primarily because of the multiple definitions used), has declined in part because of better interventional tools,[89] because patients with coronary artery disease are receiving better long-term medical therapy, which in turn helps limit infarct size, and because the pharmacotherapy for CS itself has improved. Mortality remains high, however, with a nearly 40% in-hospital death rate being reported in the Benchmark Registry.[44]

IABP use in cardiogenic shock dates to the beginning of the IABP experience, and it results in predictable hemodynamic improvement in the majority of patients. Figure 7-11 provides an algorithm for CS management; it is notable that the IABP is at the center of the algorithm, and part of early management in all patients except those with rapid response to initial pharmacologic interventions. In general, use of an IABP as an adjunct to coronary intervention in cardiogenic shock improves outcomes,[90] including a nearly 60% reduction in the rate of major adverse events (ventricular fibrillation, cardiopulmonary resuscitation, prolonged hypotension) in the cardiac catheterization laboratory (odds ratio 2:1) after IABP insertion.[91] A trend toward lower 30-day and 1-year all-cause mortality has been demonstrated in patients in whom IABPs have been inserted within 1 day of presentation with CS,[92] albeit with a higher associated complication rate. Stabilization of patients with IABPs and thrombolytic therapy and subsequent transfer for coronary intervention also appear to have favorable effects on survival,[93] mimicking animal data showing that reperfusion combined with an IABP is superior to reperfusion alone in salvaging heart muscle.[94] IABP plus mechanical ventilation may also have incremental benefit in CS management.[95]

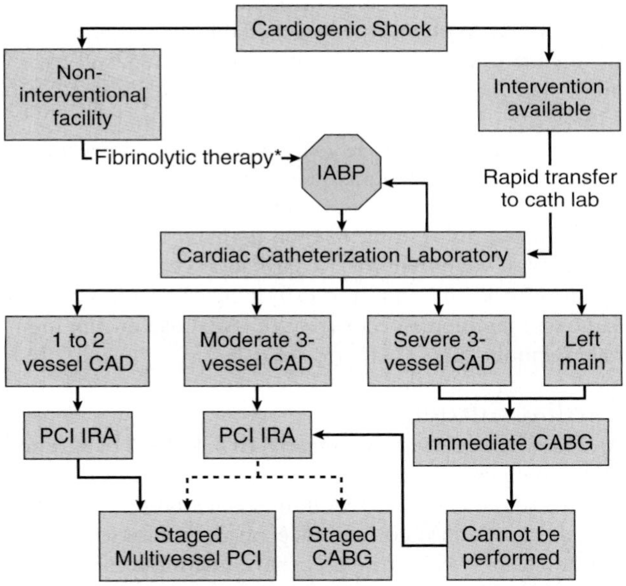

Figure 7-11. Algorithm for management of cardiogenic shock based on the SHOCK trial. Central to the treatment algorithm is rapid institution of intra-aortic balloon pump (IABP) treatment. For patients admitted to a hospital without interventional capacity, fibrinolytic therapy and IABP placement (if available) should be followed by rapid transfer to an interventional facility; if IABP treatment is unavailable, it can be started on the patient's arrival in the catheterization laboratory (cath lab) at an intervention-capable institution. *Fibrinolytic therapy should be given if there is more than a 90-minute delay until percutaneous coronary intervention (PCI) is available, less than 3 hours have passed since onset of infarction, and fibrinolysis is not contraindicated. CABG, coronary artery bypass grafting; CAD, coronary artery disease; IRA, infarct-related artery. (Adapted and modified from Hochman JS: Cardiogenic shock complicating acute myocardial infarction: expanding the paradigm. Circulation 2003;107:2998-3002, by permission of the American Heart Association.)

IABPs have been shown to be beneficial in the setting of acute MI and CS when patients are *not* treated with percutaneous coronary intervention. The National Registry of Myocardial Infarction (NRMI) 2 compared results in patients with CS who received adjunctive IABPs and those who did not.[96] Alhough mortality was not affected in patients undergoing primary angioplasty, those receiving only thrombolytic therapy had a significantly higher mortality (67% without IABP vs. 49% with IABP). Similar findings were shown in the SHOCK trial.[97] However, statistical analyses do not clarify whether selection bias may have influenced the association. A small and underpowered, randomized trial also suggested that patients with Killip class III or IV heart failure after MI have lower mortality when treated with fibrinolysis combined with IABP than when treated with fibrinolysis alone.[98] There is some basis for these findings in animal data, which suggest improved reperfusion when thrombolysis without other intervention is combined with IABP use.[24] An important consideration for the use of the IABP in shock is that the etiology should not be hypovolemia. Similarly, patients with shock and preserved systolic function are unlikely to benefit; settings such as vigorous ejection fraction in patients who have volume-depleted hypertrophic left ventricles may lead to deterioration with IABP placement, even without outflow obstruction, whereas use of the device with dynamic outflow obstruction can lead to hemodynamic collapse.

Finally, consideration has been given to the use of the IABP in RV infarction; isolated RV failure occurs in approximately 3% of patients with CS.[99] In this setting, patients commonly have severe hemodynamic decompensation and their overall prognosis is poor[100]; within the cohort of patients with CS, however, RV dysfunction is associated with inferior MI and a relatively better prognosis than CS based on LV dysfunction alone.[101] IABP use does not reliably result in hemodynamic improvement with RV infarction, and a variety of RV assist devices have been investigated, including pulmonary artery counterpulsation[102] and a right atrium–pulmonary artery bypass pump.[102,103] An occasional consideration in RV infarction is right-to-left shunting across a patent foramen ovale because of acute elevation in right heart filling pressures, which result in a gradient that drives right-to-left atrial flow. Unloading of the left ventricle with an IABP can potentially exacerbate such shunting.[104]

Mechanical Complications of Acute Myocardial Infarction

Afterload reduction has significant hemodynamic benefits in patients with abnormal unloading of the left ventricle into the right ventricle (RV) (ventricular septal rupture) or left atrium (severe mitral regurgitation).[105] The theoretical effect of counterpulsation in lowering afterload is in improving the ratio of forward flow through the aortic valve. The physiologic benefit in acute mitral insufficiency (MR) is widely accepted, resulting in a higher percentage of patients with severe MR and CS receiving IABP support than patients with CS alone.[106] The mechanism of benefit appears to be lowered aortic impedance with consequent improvement in cardiac output and a modest decrease in regurgitant fraction.[107] The IABP is used in nearly all (98%) patients in this setting undergoing mitral valve repair, compared with less than half (43%) of those treated without surgery, a difference also influenced by selection issues. As with acute MR, the vast majority (75%) of ventricular septal rupture patients in the SHOCK registry underwent IABP placement.[108] Although systolic pressure did rise (from a median 81 mm Hg to 102 mm Hg) with institution of IABPs in patients with ventricular septal rupture, mortality was dismal in both groups. In-hospital survival was only 13% with ventricular septal rupture, compared with 45% with severe MR. Nevertheless, IABP use is an essential element of intervention in acute ventricular septal rupture, and one goal of therapy has been stabilization before closure of the defect is undertaken.[109]

Acute Myocardial Infarction without Shock

IABP use for uncomplicated acute MI is controversial. As with many modalities that lower myocardial oxygen demand, the IABP theoretically helps decrease infarct size even when reperfusion does not take place.[94] However, a number of older trials and two randomized trials from the past decade did not demonstrate compelling risk-to-benefit ratios with routine IABP use in acute MI patients undergoing percutaneous coronary intervention (PCI).[110,111] Economic analysis did not demonstrate significant increase in hospital costs in patients randomly assigned to undergo routine IABP insertion in this setting.[112] The potential benefit of the IABP in maintaining patency has been demonstrated in two randomized studies showing that an open artery is more likely at 5 days[113] and at 3 weeks[114] in patients randomly assigned to IABP placement.

The IABP has been used to manage recurrent ischemia and malignant ventricular arrhythmias in the peri-infarction setting, although the evidence base for these indications is less compelling, and both are class II indications (see Box 7-1) in patients with ST elevation myocardial infarction.[85]

Unstable Angina

IABP use in unstable angina dates from an era in which the available alternatives were medical therapy and coronary bypass surgery, and IABPs were used to stabilize patients before they were taken to the operating room. In certain settings, such as severe left main coronary artery disease discovered in the cardiac catheterization laboratory or in unstable angina with attendant hemodynamic instability, this approach is still appropriate.[115] Reducing myocardial oxygen demand frequently stabilizes these patients, and the IABP may have additional benefits during subsequent revascularization in the cardiac catheterization laboratory or operating room, as discussed later.

Prophylactic Use for Coronary Intervention

Prophylactic use of an IABP prior to PCI appears to be a sound strategy for high-risk patients, typically defined as having acute coronary syndrome with hemodynamic instability, severe LV dysfunction, or undergoing unprotected left main artery intervention. Prophylactic IABP insertion in this setting had substantially better outcomes than rescue IABP placement according to retrospective multivariate analysis,[116] including evaluation of high-risk patients with severely depressed LV ejection fraction[117] undergoing angioplasty and patients undergoing unprotected left main PCI.[118]

A misconception is that IABP use during high-risk angioplasty provides adequate protection to allow prolonged ischemia in a critical vascular bed during coronary intervention. With total occlusion of flow to a large amount of myocardium, such as with unprotected left main angioplasty or angioplasty of a sole remaining vessel, hemodynamics may be preserved during the procedure, and ischemia and necrosis may be limited by lowering of myocardial oxygen demand effectuated by the IABP. However, because cardiac output remains dependent on LV ejection, myocardial oxygen demand is substantially higher than when temporary cardiac or cardiopulmonary bypass is used, and significant stunning or necrosis or both of heart muscle can occur despite IABP use during high-risk angioplasty.

Cardiac Surgery

An IABP is used in approximately 10% to 15% of patients undergoing cardiac surgery, with a substantial rise in the rate in the past decade.[119] A number of studies have demonstrated a favorable influence on outcomes, including mortality.[120-122] Nevertheless, there is considerable variability in use among centers, reflecting a lack of consensus about indications for perioperative IABP use.[119,123] The vast majority of IABP insertions occur preoperatively.[119] The effectiveness of this approach has been controversial. One small randomized trial of high-risk patients demonstrated lower mortality, higher postoperative cardiac index, and shorter intubation time, ICU stay, and hospitalization in patients with preoperative IABP placement.[115] In contrast, results of a propensity analysis suggested excess mortality in nearly 2000 patients receiving preoperative IABP insertion compared with 28,000 who did not.[124] Because of the limitations of propensity analysis, it is possible that selection bias determined the unfavorable outcomes associated with preoperative IABP use. Patients most likely to benefit from preoperative IABP insertion are those with depressed LV function, unstable angina, or left main artery disease or who are undergoing repeat thoracotomy.

Several mechanisms can be postulated for superior outcomes with preoperative IABP insertion. Counterpulsation can provide hemodynamic support during anesthesia induction and during the stress of surgery before cardiopulmonary bypass is begun.[122,125] Use of an IABP during cardiopulmonary bypass also appears to have favorable effects on end-organ perfusion,[126,127] with protection of both coronary and cerebral blood flow.[128] IABP insertion can also be used to assess prognosis; requirement for catecholamine support and overall hemodynamics 1 hour after institution of perioperative balloon pump insertion is highly predictive of overall outcome.[129]

Although studies have reported mortality in high-risk patients treated with an IABP as high as 53%, preoperative placement of an IABP was associated with substantially lower morbidity and mortality (24%), while postoperative insertion, in this case creating bias toward late insertion in situations with bad outcomes, was associated with a 63% mortality.[130] Similarly, a nonrandomized study of patients with an ejection fraction of 25% or less compared patients who were treated with a preoperative IABP with those who were not. Mortality was 2.7% in the former group compared with 11.9% in the latter group, despite the presence of New York Heart Association (NYHA) class III or IV heart failure in 92% of the former group and only 55% of the latter group.[120] Several other post hoc analyses have found results consistent with advantages of preoperative IABP use.[131,132]

Outcomes in addition to mortality that were superior in patients undergoing preoperative IABP insertion were duration of IABP support required, length of hospital stay, and postoperative LV ejection fraction in a randomized study of high-risk patients with ejection fraction of 30% or less.[133] Similarly, preoperative use of an IABP in high-risk off-pump CABG appears to be favorable.[134,135] Thus, although the evidence base is incomplete, the overall preoperative use of IABPs is growing.[119] Cost analysis appears to be favorable; combining high-risk cohorts randomly assigned to receive preoperative IABP placement or not,[115,125] costs were 36% less in patients with preoperative IABP insertion because of shorter IABP treatment time, shorter hospitalizations, and less use of critical care facilities.[136]

Congestive Heart Failure

The IABP has been used successfully in a variety of settings that result in acute congestive heart failure, including fulminant myocarditis[137] and severe decompensated aortic stenosis.[138] On the basis of case reports, the device has also been helpful as adjunctive therapy for myocardial depression secondary to drug toxicity,[139,140] myocardial contusion,[141] anaphylaxis,[142] thyrotoxicosis,[143] multiple sclerosis,[144] and even lightning strike.[145] Animal data suggest some benefit in the setting of RV failure[146]; the mechanism appears to be lowered pulmonary vascular resistance with consequent improvement in RV ejection.[26] IABP insertion has also improved outcomes in patients with acute RV failure after heart transplantation.[147]

Finally, the IABP has been used as a bridge to transplantation, typically with placement in the axillary or external iliac arteries to allow ambulation during prolonged counterpulsation.[148] With development of a range of LV assist devices designed for longer-term implantation, the use of IABP for this indication has waned.[149]

Miscellaneous Indications

Limited data suggest that IABP placement during cardiopulmonary resuscitation has favorable effects.[150,151] The device has been used in pregnancy in patients undergoing heart surgery with an eye toward preserving uterine and fetal flow during cardiopulmonary bypass.[152] In patients at high risk for cardiac events during noncardiac surgery (e.g., recent myocardial infarction, LV failure, unrevascularized ischemic myocardium),[153,154] the IABP has been shown to have significant benefits for outcome,[155] although the evidence base consists largely of case reports[156,157]; a randomized trial has not been performed. Prophylactic IABP insertion seems particularly appropriate in high-risk patients undergoing emergency noncardiac surgery.[157]

Use of the Intra-aortic Balloon Pump

Overall, the existing data suggest that the IABP is underused. In more than 23,000 patients in cardiogenic shock reported by NRMI 2, only 31% were treated with IABP. As is the case for a number of other interventions, women were less likely to undergo IABP placement; there was an age and race difference as well, with lower rates in nonwhites and older patients.[158] A number of studies from the 1990s demonstrated less than 25% use of IABPs in CS[92,159]; this figure contrasts with 86% use in the SHOCK trial.[90] Although some exclusion criteria in the latter may have improved suitability for IABP placement in the cohort enrolled in the study, the threefold higher use of the device in the SHOCK trial is consistent with wide underuse in clinical practice, similar to findings for a variety of pharmacologic and invasive interventions in acute MI.[84]

CONTRAINDICATIONS

The classic absolute contraindication to IABP use is aortic insufficiency (Table 7-1). Because the acute hemodynamic effects are so deleterious, animal and clinical investigations all date to the 1970s.[160] Increased volume displacement retrograde into the left ventricle during diastole greatly exacerbates wall stress, with greater potential for hemodynamic decompensation as well as LV pseudoaneurysm formation and LV rupture in the post-MI setting. The amount of aortic insufficiency that constitutes an absolute contraindication has no objective basis, but most operators use a threshold of trivial to mild. Similarly, the presence of aortic dissection or aortic aneurysm is considered an absolute contraindication because of the risk of extending dissection or causing aneurysmal rupture. Patent ductus arteriosus, like aortic insufficiency, theoretically has deleterious results from shunting of blood flow from the aorta with IABP induction, in this case increas-

Table 7-1. Contraindications to the Use of the Intra-aortic Balloon Pump

Absolute contraindications	Aortic insufficiency* Aortic dissection Aortic aneurysm Patent ductus arteriosus Comorbidity with minimal survival expectancy Brain death
Relative contraindications	Hypovolemia Severe peripheral vascular disease Hypertrophic obstructive cardiomyopathy Sepsis† Bilateral femoral-popliteal bypass grafts[194]

*No evidence base exists for a minimal level of aortic insufficiency constituting an absolute contraindication.
†The evidence base does not suggest significant hemodynamic benefit for patients with septic shock.[195]

ing left-to-right flow into the pulmonary artery. Generally, patients who have severe comorbidities at end of life or who exhibit brain death are considered to have contraindications to IABP placement.

Relative contraindications include placement of an indwelling foreign body into a patient with active infection including sepsis, severe peripheral vascular disease likely to result in limb ischemia, bleeding diathesis (although in practice, many patients who have low fibrinogen levels or are receiving aggressive anticoagulant or antiplatelet treatment undergo IABP placement), and contraindications to afterload reduction, such as dynamic LV outflow obstruction,[161] a condition that has on occasion been unmasked by institution of counterpulsation.[162] Patients with shock due to severe hypovolemia will not benefit from insertion of an IABP and may deteriorate with IABP-induced afterload reduction.

COMPLICATIONS

From the initial experiences with IABPs in the 1960s, the significant complication rate has been the single largest drawback to its use (Table 7-2). The predominant complications have related to the access site, with bleeding and limb ischemia being the most common, but they also include infection, thrombocytopenia, stroke, device failure, and a variety of vascular misadventures. Table 7-2 describes complications of IABPs from multiple registries, trials, and case reports. The complication rate associated with IABPs is affected by the insertion of indwelling, typically 7F to 10F devices into the femoral arteries of patients with a high prevalence of diabetes, peripheral vascular disease, and other major comorbidities. As would be expected, duration of IABP use correlates with risk of complications overall,[163,164] including sepsis.[165,166] Thus, frequent reevaluation of the patient to confirm ongoing need for an IABP is prudent. Death due to IABPs has been relatively uncommon, with the rate typically less than 0.3% to as low as 0.05%,[37] and this fact should be weighed against its considerable survival benefits.

The influence of procedure volume on outcomes has been demonstrated in a wide variety of cardiac procedures. Chen and associates[84] looked at data from NRMI 2 and found a significant correlation after multivariate analysis between number of IABP implantations per year and cardiogenic shock mortality.[84] The study did not address complications related directly to IABPs as a function of procedure volume for individual hospitals or operators.

Comparing overall complication rates among different series is hindered by lack of uniform definitions, variable demographics, comorbidities, duration of data collection, years when the data were collected (during which significant changes in technology may have occurred), and indications for IABP insertion. Major complications have been reported to be in the 2% to nearly 50% range. However, the early data, which included surgical insertion, lack of a guidewire lumen for safer passage through the iliac arteries and aorta, and larger catheter and sheath sizes, were much worse than those in more recent series, with same center analyses describing as much as a fivefold decrease in major complications.[167] Thus, Kantrowitz and co-workers[168] reported a 47% complication rate over the first 15 years of IABP experience, and Alderman and colleagues[169] described a 42% rate of limb ischemia alone in their mid-1980s study. With improvements in technology, periprocedure pharmacology, patient selection, and management, the overall complication rates have declined to 15% in a large single hospital review published in 2000[46] and 6.5% in the Benchmark Registry, which incorporates the largest experience to date.[170] Although the series use variable definitions, the trend is unequivocal.

In general, diabetic patients and women have a higher complication rate,[168] coincident with the finding that these two populations also have significantly smaller femoral arteries.[45] A review of the existing literature on IABP complications shows peripheral vascular disease and female gender as nearly uniform markers of higher complication risk, with age, diabetes, size of catheter inserted, and smaller body surface area common but somewhat less consistent markers on multivariate analyses.[37,46]

Vascular Complications

Vascular complications including limb ischemia are the most common serious adverse events related to IABP insertion. Amputation is rare (0.1%),[37] but major limb ischemia, defined in the Benchmark Registry as "loss of pulse or sensation, or abnormal limb temperature or pallor requiring surgical intervention," occurred in 1.3% of cases.[170] Minor limb ischemia, defined as not requiring surgery and improving with balloon removal, occurred in another 1.2% in the same series. These numbers are consistent with steady improvement over the past decade: A smaller but still substantial earlier series from India involving 911 patients (with a much higher proportion of diabetic patients and likely significantly smaller body surface area) reported a 5.9% incidence of major vascular

Table 7-2. Complications of the Use of the Intra-aortic Balloon Pump (IABP) from the Benchmark Registry

Study	All Benchmark Patients†	Patients with Myocardial Infarction Only‡
Year published	2001	2003
Total patients	16,909	5495
All complications:	7.0%	8.1%
Major*	2.8%	2.7%
Minor*	4.2%	5.4%
Vascular complications:		
Limb ischemia	2.9%	2.3%
Major*	0.9%	0.5%
Vascular surgery	—	0.7%
Amputation	0.1%	0.1%
Hematologic complications:		
Bleeding	2.4%	4.3%
Severe*	0.8%	1.4%
Infection	—	0.1%
Neurologic complications:		
Stroke	—	0.1%
Death		
Due to IABP	0.05%	0.05%
Due to underlying morbidities	21.2%	20.0%
Others		
Deep vein thrombosis,	—	0.1%
Bowel, renal, or spinal cord infarction	—	0.1%
Equipment malfunction	2.6%	2.3%
Balloon leak	1.0%	0.8%

**Major complications* are major limb ischemia, severe bleeding, balloon leak or death attributable to IABP insertion or failure; *major limb ischemia* consists of loss of pulse, loss of sensation, abnormal limb temperature or pallor requiring intervention, arterial repair, or amputation; *severe bleeding* is defined as bleeding that requires transfusion or surgical intervention or results in hemodynamic compromise. Independent risk factors for major complications: female gender, peripheral vascular disease, body surface area <1.65 m^2, and age ≥75 years.
†Based on data from Ferguson JJ III, Cohen M, Freedman RJ Jr, et al: The current practice of intra-aortic balloon counterpulsation: results from the Benchmark Registry. J Am Coll Cardiol 2001;38:1456-1462.
‡Based on data from Stone GW, Ohman EM, Miller MF, et al: Contemporary utilization and outcomes of intra-aortic balloon counterpulsation in acute myocardial infarction: The Benchmark Registry. J Am Coll Cardiol 2003;41:1940-1945.

complications and 5.8% rate of minor vascular complications.[49] This series used a 9.5F shaft IABP, which has been shown to have higher vascular complication rates than the 8F shaft balloons that have been available for the past decade.[171] Vascular complications, likely in part because of comorbidities, are associated with a much higher overall mortality—as much as a twofold increase.[82]

Trauma to the aorta has been reported, with paraplegia caused by spinal necrosis due to subadventitial hematoma,[172] cholesterol embolization to spinal and mesenteric arteries,[173] and aortic dissection[174] as well as no obvious cause in some patients. The presence of friable atheroma in the descending aorta has been associated with embolization.[175] IABP use has been identified as an independent predictor for neurologic complications of percutaneous intervention, although whether this feature is due to embolic phenomena or confounding variables has not been established.[176]

A complication particular to IABP is thrombocytopenia, occurring presumably because of destruction of platelets that adhere to the IABP surface, although the mechanism remains unclear. Patients receiving critical care who have IABPs and are undergoing heparin therapy have a 7:1 odds ratio of a 50% drop in platelet count compared with patients without IABPs who are undergoing heparin therapy at similar doses,[177] lowering the likelihood that heparin-induced thrombocytopenia is the etiologic factor.

Mechanical Failure

Several complications of mechanical failure of the balloon or console have serious consequences. Rupture of the balloon was more common early in the IABP era, with an incidence reported to range from 1.7%[178] to 5.2%.[179] Typically the diagnosis was made from the appearance of blood in the gas lumen, with triggering of alarms. The usual site of rupture has been at a point where the aorta is at its nadir in diameter along the course of the IABP. Small vessel size is associated with abrasion of the IABP (thus the observation that it is more common in women[180] likely correlates with their smaller body surface area); similar concerns arise for larger balloon sizes. Rupture of the balloon with a major gas leak, a rare event, has been reported to cause stroke secondary to gas embolization.[181] Experimental hydrophilically coated balloons hold some promise for further reducing the risk of rupture through potentially decreasing abrasion of the balloon surface.[42] Fracturing of the IABP can occur with entrapment, including separation and migration of part of the device.[182] Clot may also form in the gas lumen after loss of balloon integrity and has been reported to interfere with balloon deflation, requiring use of a thrombolytic agent in the gas line to allow deflation and removal of the balloon.[183]

Treating Complications Related to The Intra-aortic Balloon Pump

Several approaches to managing IABP-related complications have been proposed. Limb ischemia has traditionally been most successfully treated by removal of the IABP,[49,184] even in patients wholly dependent on the balloon, in order to avoid loss of limb. This situation has occasionally forced physicians and families to choose between loss of limb and patient survival. Surgical femoral-femoral shunting performed at the bedside with exteriorization of the graft has been described as one potential approach.[185] As previously mentioned, we have performed percutaneous nonsurgical external femoral-femoral shunting to effectively address limb ischemia by placing one sheath retrograde into the femoral artery contralateral to the IABP and another antegrade in the ipsilateral vessel, connecting the two sheaths with tubing and a flow regulator (see Fig. 7-5).[58] Infusion of prostaglandin E_1 through the balloon central lumen has been shown to relieve lower limb ischemia in a small series, presumably through increase in caliber of collateral vessels or relief of spasm in the common femoral or iliac system.[186]

FUTURE CONSIDERATIONS

Kantrowitz, who began this work more than a half century ago, continues to develop a permanently implantable IABP. Initial results of a pilot trial demonstrate substantial improvement in hemodynamics. The ability to use the device intermittently rather than continuously, theoretically without thromboembolic risk once the device is fully endothelialized, and its location downstream from the head and neck vessels differentiate it from other ventricular assist devices.[187]

A number of other percutaneous extracorporeal ventricular assist devices have been developed, although they lack the flexibility of bedside insertion and the low profile of the IABP (Fig. 7-12). These devices are inserted in the cardiac catheterization laboratory and provide temporary cardiac output support. These have been used to support high-risk angioplasty, including the left atrial to femoral bypass TandemHeart device (CardiacAssist, Inc., Pittsburgh, PA) and the retrogradely placed transaortic valve Impella rotary pump (Abiomed, Danvers, MA). A small randomized trial has been performed comparing the TandemHeart with the IABP in patients with cardiogenic shock, demonstrating superior hemodynamics with the TandemHeart device.[188] However, the latter requires transseptal puncture, institution of cardiac bypass with much larger arterial cannulas than the IABP, and in general is far more complex with greater risk of complications, as shown in a study comparing it with IABP in

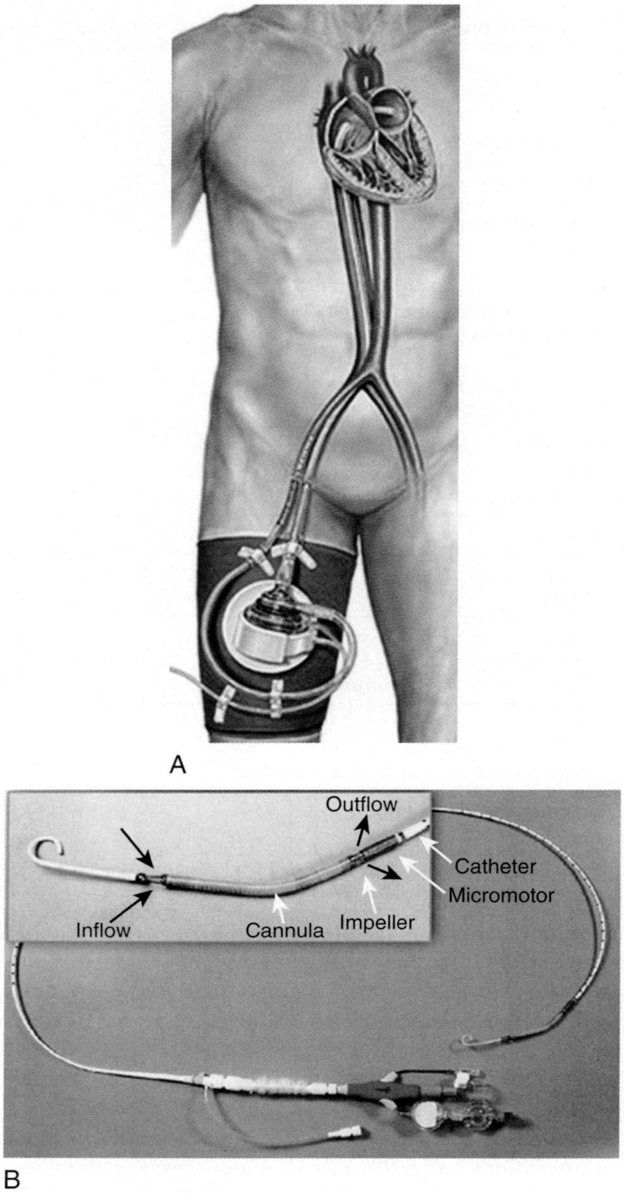

Figure 7-12. The TandemHeart device **(A)** draws oxygenated blood from a left atrial catheter placed across the interatrial septum and provides arterial return via a cannula placed into the femoral artery. The Impella catheter **(B)** draws blood from the left ventricle via a pigtail catheter placed retrograde across the aortic valve and pumps blood into the aorta. Although both devices actively provide systemic flow independent of left ventricular ejection, neither delivers pulsatile flow and both require significantly larger arterial punctures than an intra-aortic balloon pump.

patients presenting with CS who were being considered for percutaneous coronary intervention.[189] It also cannot be shut off temporarily and requires far more aggressive monitoring than balloon counterpulsation.

The Impella device is a 12F catheter–based system that uses a miniature rotary pump to unload the left ventricle, pumping blood into the aorta through a pigtail catheter placed retrogradely across the aortic valve.[190] Unlike the TandemHeart, it does not require transseptal puncture or extracorporeal circulation with the attendant complexity and risks. Both devices appear promising for circulatory support in a variety of settings but do not provide pulsatile flow and currently lack a significant evidence base.[191] Unlike the IABP, neither the TandemHeart nor the Impella catheter should be used in post-MI ventricular septal rupture: both could theoretically trigger severe right-to-left shunting because of low LV pressure as a result of substantial volume extraction from the left heart circulation.

A vast array of other ventricular assist devices and alternative counterpulsation technologies are under development. The use of the IABP in conjunction with assist devices that do not provide pulsatile flow may provide symbiotic preservation of end-organ circulation.[192,193]

KEY POINTS

- The IABP is the most widely used cardiac assist device, featuring modest though significant risk, straightforward percutaneous insertion, and excellent hemodynamic support.
- There is a wide range of indications for IABP use, from prophylactic support prior to percutaneous or surgical intervention, to stabilization in the setting of cardiogenic shock.
- Unlike more complex ventricular assist devices, the IABP does not independently generate systemic output; thus, it provides auxiliary support of cardiac function.
- The primary benefit of the IABP is decrease in afterload and secondary improvement in hemodynamics; diastolic perfusion pressure is augmented but end-organ total flow is usually not increased directly.
- Timing of IABP inflation and deflation, absence of arrhythmia, and length of diastole all contribute to the effectiveness of an IABP.
- A small but significant complication rate remains associated with IABP use, in particular vascular compromise and bleeding.

REFERENCES

1. Kozak LJ, DeFrances CJ, Hall MJ: National Hospital Discharge Survey: 2004 annual summary with detailed diagnosis and procedure data. National Center for Health Statistics. Vital Health Stat 13 2006; (162):1-209. Available at: http://www.cdc.gov/nchs/data/series/sr_13/sr13_162.pdf/
2. Torchiana DF, Hirsch G, Buckley MJ, et al: Intraaortic balloon pumping for cardiac support: Trends in practice and outcome, 1968 to 1995. J Thorac Cardiovasc Surg 1997;113:758-764.
3. Cohen M, Urban P, Christenson JT, et al: Intra-aortic balloon counterpulsation in US and non-US centres: Results of the Benchmark Registry. Eur Heart J 2003;24: 1763-1770.
4. Kantrowitz A: Experimental augmentation of coronary flow by retardation of the arterial pressure pulse. Surgery 1953;34:678-687.
5. Kantrowitz A: Moments in history: Introduction of left ventricular assistance. ASAIO Trans 1987; 33:39-48.
6. Kantrowitz A, McKinnon WM: The experimental use of the diaphragm as an auxiliary myocardium. Surg Forum 1958;9:266-268.
7. Clauss RH, Birtwell WC, Albertal G, et al: Assisted circulation. I: The arterial counterpulsator. J Thorac Cardiovasc Surg 1961;41:447-458.
8. Moulopoulos SD, Topaz S, Kolff WJ: Diastolic balloon pumping (with carbon dioxide) in the aorta—a mechanical assistance to the failing circulation. Am Heart J 1962;63: 669-675.
9. Kantrowitz A, Tjonneland S, Freed PS, et al: Initial clinical experience with intraaortic balloon pumping in cardiogenic shock. JAMA 1968;203:113-118.
10. Kantrowitz A, Tjonneland S, Krakauer JS, et al: Mechanical intraaortic cardiac assistance in cardiogenic shock: Hemodynamic effects. Arch Surg 1968;97:1000-1004.
11. Scheidt S, Wilner G, Mueller H, et al: Intra-aortic balloon counterpulsation in cardiogenic shock: Report of a co-operative clinical trial. N Engl J Med 1973;288:979-984.
12. Bregman D, Casarella WJ: Percutaneous intraaortic balloon pumping: Initial clinical experience. Ann Thorac Surg 1980;29:153-155.
13. Merav AD, Solomon N, Montefusco CM, et al: A new guidable double lumen percutaneous intra-aortic balloon. Trans Am Soc Artif Intern Organs 1981;27:593-597.
14. Wolvek S: The development of a safe and highly durable balloon catheter for the IAB. Artif Organs 1993;17:891-892.
15. Weber KT, Janicki JS: Intraaortic balloon counterpulsation: A review of physiological principles, clinical results, and device safety. Ann Thorac Surg 1974;17:602-636.
16. Kern MJ, Aguirre FV, Tatineni S, et al: Enhanced coronary blood flow velocity during intraaortic balloon counterpulsation in critically ill patients. J Am Coll Cardiol 1993;21: 359-368.
17. Stefanadis C, Dernellis J, Tsiamis E, et al: Aortic function in patients during intra-aortic balloon pumping determined by the pressure-diameter relation. J Thorac Cardiovasc Surg 1998;116:1052-1059.
18. Anderson RD, Gurbel PA: The effect of intra-aortic balloon counterpulsation on coronary blood flow velocity distal to coronary artery stenoses. Cardiology 1996;87:306-312.
19. Toyota E, Songfang L, Kimura A, et al: Evaluation of intramyocardial coronary blood flow waveform during intraaortic balloon pumping in the absence or presence of coronary stenosis. Artif Organs 1996;20: 166-168.
20. Gitter R, Cate CM, Smart K, et al: Influence of ascending versus descending balloon counterpulsation on bypass graft blood flow. Ann Thorac Surg 1998;65:365-370.
21. Kimura A, Toyota E, Lu S, et al: Effects of intraaortic balloon pumping on septal arterial blood flow velocity waveform during severe left main coronary artery stenosis. J Am Coll Cardiol 1996;27:810-816.
22. Takeuchi M, Nohtomi Y, Yoshitani H, et al: Enhanced coronary flow velocity during intra-aortic balloon pumping assessed by transthoracic Doppler echocardiography. J Am Coll Cardiol 2004;43:368-376.
23. Zehetgruber M, Mundigler G, Christ G, et al: Relation of hemodynamic variables to augmentation of left anterior descending coronary flow by intraaortic balloon pulsation in coronary artery disease. Am J Cardiol 1997;80:951-955.
24. Gurbel PA, Anderson RD, MacCord CS, et al: Arterial diastolic pressure augmentation by intra-aortic balloon counterpulsation enhances the onset of coronary artery reperfusion by thrombolytic therapy. Circulation 1994;89:361-365.

25. Kveim M, Cappelen C Jr, Frooysaker T, et al: Intra-aortic balloon pumping in the treatment of cardiogenic shock following open-heart surgery. Scand J Thorac Cardiovasc Surg 1976;10: 231-235.
26. Nordhaug D, Steensrud T, Muller S, et al: Intraaortic balloon pumping improves hemodynamics and right ventricular efficiency in acute ischemic right ventricular failure. Ann Thorac Surg 2004;78:1426-1432.
27. Schachtrupp A, Wrigge H, Busch T, et al: Influence of intra-aortic balloon pumping on cerebral blood flow pattern in patients after cardiac surgery. Eur J Anaesthesiol 2005;22:165-170.
28. Applebaum RM, Wun HH, Katz ES, et al: Effects of intraaortic balloon counterpulsation on carotid artery blood flow. Am Heart J 1998;135: 850-854.
29. Hashimoto K, Onoguchi K, Takakura H, et al: Beneficial effect of balloon-induced pulsatility on brain oxygenation in hypothermic cardiopulmonary bypass. J Cardiovasc Surg (Torino) 2001;42:587-593.
30. Rosen CL, Sekhar LN, Duong DH: Use of intra-aortic balloon pump counterpulsation for refractory symptomatic vasospasm. Acta Neurochir (Wien) 2000;142:25-32.
31. Janssens U, Graf J, Koch KC, et al: Gastric tonometry in patients with cardiogenic shock and intra-aortic balloon counterpulsation. Crit Care Med 2000;28:3449-3455.
32. Haywood GA, Keeling PJ, Parker DJ, et al: Short-term effects of intra-aortic balloon pumping on renal blood flow and renal oxygen consumption in cardiogenic shock. J Card Fail 1995;1: 217-222.
33. Reesink KD, van der NT, Bovelander J, et al: Feasibility study of a fiber-optic system for invasive blood pressure measurements. Cathet Cardiovasc Interv 2002;57:272-276.
34. Weber KT, Janicki JS, Walker AA: Intra-aortic balloon pumping: An analysis of several variables affecting balloon performance. Trans Am Soc Artif Intern Organs 1972;18:486-492.
35. Stamatelopoulos SF, Nanas JN, Saridakis NS, et al: Treating severe cardiogenic shock by large counterpulsation volumes. Ann Thorac Surg 1996;62:1110-1117.
36. Cohen M, Fasseas P, Singh VP, et al: Impact of intra-aortic balloon counterpulsation with different balloon volumes on cardiac performance in humans. Catheter Cardiovasc Interv 2002;57:199-204.
37. Ferguson JJ III, Cohen M, Freedman RJ Jr, et al: The current practice of intra-aortic balloon counterpulsation: Results from the Benchmark Registry. J Am Coll Cardiol 2001;38:1456-1462.
38. Hatlestad DC, Van Horn J: Air transport of the IABP patient. Intra-Aortic Balloon Pump. Air Med J 2002;21: 42-48.
39. Igari T: The length of the aorta from the subclavian artery to the renal artery based on computed tomographic measurements in Japanese adults. J Artif Organs 2006;9:267-270.
40. Weikel AM, Jones RT, Dinsmore R, et al: Size limits and pumping effectiveness of intraaortic balloons. Ann Thorac Surg 1971;12:45-53.
41. Mueller XM, Tevaearai HT, Hayoz D, et al: Thrombogenicity of deflated intraaortic balloon: impact of heparin coating. Artif Organs 1999;23: 195-198.
42. Winters KJ, Smith SC, Cohen M, et al: Reduction in ischemic vascular complications with a hydrophilic-coated intra-aortic balloon catheter. Catheter Cardiovasc Interv 1999;46: 357-362.
43. Schreuder JJ, Castiglioni A, Donelli A, et al: Automatic intraaortic balloon pump timing using an intrabeat dicrotic notch prediction algorithm. Ann Thorac Surg 2005;79:1017-1022.
44. Stone GW, Ohman EM, Miller MF, et al: Contemporary utilization and outcomes of intra-aortic balloon counterpulsation in acute myocardial infarction: The Benchmark Registry. J Am Coll Cardiol 2003;41:1940-1945.
45. Schnyder G, Sawhney N, Whisenant B, et al: Common femoral artery anatomy is influenced by demographics and comorbidity: Implications for cardiac and peripheral invasive studies. Catheter Cardiovasc Interv 2001;53:289-295.
46. Cohen M, Dawson MS, Kopistansky C, et al: Sex and other predictors of intra-aortic balloon counterpulsation-related complications: prospective study of 1119 consecutive patients. Am Heart J 2000;139:282-287.
47. Ellis SG, Bhatt D, Kapadia S, et al: Correlates and outcomes of retroperitoneal hemorrhage complicating percutaneous coronary intervention. Catheter Cardiovasc Interv 2006;67:541-545.
48. Meisel S, Shochat M, Sheikha SA, et al: Utilization of low-profile intra-aortic balloon catheters inserted by the sheathless technique in acute cardiac patients: Clinical efficacy with a very low complication rate. Clin Cardiol 2004;27:600-604.
49. Meharwal ZS, Trehan N: Vascular complications of intra-aortic balloon insertion in patients undergoing coronary revascularization: analysis of 911 cases. Eur J Cardiothorac Surg 2002;21:741-747.
50. Menon P, Totaro P, Youhana A, et al: Reduced vascular complication after IABP insertion using smaller sized catheter and sheathless technique. Eur J Cardiothorac Surg 2002;22:491-492.
51. Erdogan HB, Goksedef D, Erentug V, et al: In which patients should sheathless IABP be used? An analysis of vascular complications in 1211 cases. J Card Surg 2006;21:342-346.
52. Patel JJ, Kopisyansky C, Boston B, et al: Prospective evaluation of complications associated with percutaneous intraaortic balloon counterpulsation. Am J Cardiol 1995;76:1205-1207.
53. Tatar H, Cicek S, Demirkilic U, et al: Exact positioning of intra-aortic balloon catheter. Eur J Cardiothorac Surg 1993;7:52-53.
54. Corcos T, Guerin Y, Favereau X: Stiff hydrophilic glidewire: A useful tool for percutaneous insertion of intraaortic balloon counterpulsation catheters. Catheter Cardiovasc Interv 1999; 46:497.
55. Colyer WR Jr, Burket MW, Ansel GM, et al: Intra-aortic balloon pump placement following aorto-iliac angioplasty and stent placement. Catheter Cardiovasc Interv 2002; 55:163-168.
56. Lewis BE, Sumida C, Hwang MH, et al: New approach to management of intraaortic balloon pumps in patients with peripheral vascular disease: Case reports of four patients requiring urgent IABP insertion. Cathet Cardiovasc Diagn 1992;26:295-299.
57. Turi ZG: Vascular turf wars: Getting a leg up on iliac artery disease during intraaortic balloon pumping. Cathet Cardiovasc Diagn 1997;42:7.
58. Merhi WM, Turi ZG, Dixon S, et al: Percutaneous ex-vivo femoral arterial bypass: A novel approach for treatment of acute limb ischemia as a complication of femoral arterial catheterization. Catheter Cardiovasc Interv 2006;68:435-440.
59. Khir AW, Price S, Hale C, et al: Intra-aortic balloon pumping: Does posture matter? Artif Organs 2005;29:36-40.
60. Noel BM, Gleeton O, Barbeau GR: Transbrachial insertion of an intra-aortic balloon pump for complex coronary angioplasty. Catheter Cardiovasc Interv 2003;60:36-39.
61. Onorati F, Bilotta M, Pezzo F, et al: Transbrachial insertion of a 7.5-Fr intra-aortic balloon pump in a severely atherosclerotic patient. Crit Care Med 2006;34:2231-2233.
62. Werns SW: Should the transbrachial route be used for intra-aortic balloon pumps? Almost never! Crit Care Med 2006;34:2259-2261.
63. Patel MR, Buchanan SA, Bergin JD, et al: As originally published in 1994: Ambulatory intraaortic balloon counterpulsation. Updated in 2001. Ann Thorac Surg 2001;72:975.
64. Rubenstein RB, Karhade NV: Supraclavicular subclavian technique of intra-aortic balloon insertion. J Vasc Surg 1984;1:577-578.
65. Cochran RP, Starkey TD, Panos AL, et al: Ambulatory intraaortic balloon pump use as bridge to heart transplant. Ann Thorac Surg 2002;74: 746-751.
66. H'Doubler PB Jr, H'Doubler WZ, Bien RC, et al: A novel technique for intraaortic balloon pump placement via the left axillary artery in patients awaiting cardiac transplantation. Cardiovasc Surg 2000;8:463-465.
67. Arafa OE, Geiran OR, Svennevig JL: Transthoracic intra-aortic balloon pump in open heart operations: Techniques and outcome. Scand Cardiovasc J 2001;35:40-44.
68. Santini F, Mazzucco A: Transthoracic intraaortic counterpulsation: A simple method for balloon catheter positioning. Ann Thorac Surg 1997;64:859-860.
69. Mueller DK, Stout M, Blakeman BM: Morbidity and mortality of intra-aortic balloon pumps placed through the aortic arch. Chest 1998;114:85-88.
70. Schreuder JJ, Maisano F, Donelli A, et al: Beat-to-beat effects of intraaortic balloon pump timing on left

ventricular performance in patients with low ejection fraction. Ann Thorac Surg 2005;79:872-880.
71. Kern MJ, Aguirre FV, Caracciolo EA, et al: Hemodynamic effects of new intra-aortic balloon counterpulsation timing methods in patients: a multicenter evaluation. Am Heart J 1999;137:1129-1136.
72. Sakamoto T, Arai H, Maruyama T, et al: New algorithm of intra aortic balloon pumping in patients with atrial fibrillation. ASAIO J 1995;41: 79-83.
73. Papaioannou TG, Terrovitis J, Kanakakis J, et al: Heart rate effect on hemodynamics during mechanical assistance by the intra-aortic balloon pump. Int J Artif Organs 2002;25:1160-1165.
74. Jiang CY, Zhao LL, Wang JA, et al: Anticoagulation therapy in intra-aortic balloon counterpulsation: Does IABP really need anti-coagulation? J Zhejiang Univ Sci 2003;4:607-611.
75. Crystal E, Borer A, Gilad J, et al: Incidence and clinical significance of bacteremia and sepsis among cardiac patients treated with intra-aortic balloon counterpulsation pump. Am J Cardiol 2000;86:1281-1284, A9.
76. Niederhauser U, Vogt M, Vogt P, et al: Cardiac surgery in a high-risk group of patients: Is prolonged postoperative antibiotic prophylaxis effective? J Thorac Cardiovasc Surg 1997;114: 162-168.
77. Lewis PA, Mullany DV, Courtney M, et al: Australasian trends in intra-aortic balloon counterpulsation weaning: Results of a postal survey. Crit Care Resusc 2006;8:361-367.
78. Manord JD, Garrard CL, Mehra MR, et al: Implications for the vascular surgeon with prolonged (3 to 89 days) intraaortic balloon pump counterpulsation. J Vasc Surg 1997;26: 511-515.
79. Chadow HL, Hauptman RE, Strizik B, et al: Vasoseal after intra-aortic balloon pump removal: A pilot study. Catheter Cardiovasc Interv 2000;50:495-497.
80. Kato K, Sato N, Yamamoto T, et al: Initial experiences of removal of intra-aortic balloon pumps with the Angio-Seal. J Invasive Cardiol 2006;18:130-132.
81. Sohail MR, Khan AH, Holmes DR Jr, et al: Infectious complications of percutaneous vascular closure devices. Mayo Clin Proc 2005;80:1011-1015.
82. Busch T, Sirbu H, Zenker D, et al: Vascular complications related to intraaortic balloon counterpulsation: An analysis of ten years experience. Thorac Cardiovasc Surg 1997;45: 55-59.
83. Urban PM, Freedman RJ, Ohman EM, et al: In-hospital mortality associated with the use of intra-aortic balloon counterpulsation. Am J Cardiol 2004;94:181-185.
84. Chen EW, Canto JG, Parsons LS, et al: Relation between hospital intra-aortic balloon counterpulsation volume and mortality in acute myocardial infarction complicated by cardiogenic shock. Circulation 2003;108:951-957.
85. Antman EM, Anbe DT, Armstrong PW, et al: ACC/AHA guidelines for the management of patients with ST-elevation myocardial infarction: A report of the American College of Cardiology/American Heart Association Task Force on Practice Guidelines (Committee to Revise the 1999 Guidelines for the Management of patients with acute myocardial infarction). J Am Coll Cardiol 2004;44: E1-E211.
86. Holmes DR Jr, Berger PB, Hochman JS, et al: Cardiogenic shock in patients with acute ischemic syndromes with and without ST-segment elevation. Circulation 1999;100:2067-2073.
87. Hochman JS: Cardiogenic shock complicating acute myocardial infarction: Expanding the paradigm. Circulation 2003;107:2998-3002.
88. Goldberg RJ, Gore JM, Thompson CA, et al: Recent magnitude of and temporal trends (1994-1997) in the incidence and hospital death rates of cardiogenic shock complicating acute myocardial infarction: The Second National Registry of Myocardial Infarction. Am Heart J 2001;141: 65-72.
89. Dauerman HL, Goldberg RJ, White K, et al: Revascularization, stenting, and outcomes of patients with acute myocardial infarction complicated by cardiogenic shock. Am J Cardiol 2002;90:838-842.
90. Hochman JS, Sleeper LA, Webb JG, et al: Early revascularization in acute myocardial infarction complicated by cardiogenic shock. SHOCK Investigators. SHould we emergently revascularize OCcluded coronaries for cardiogenic shocK? N Engl J Med 1999;341:625-634.
91. Brodie BR, Stuckey TD, Hansen C, et al: Intra-aortic balloon counterpulsation before primary percutaneous transluminal coronary angioplasty reduces catheterization laboratory events in high-risk patients with acute myocardial infarction. Am J Cardiol 1999;84:18-23.
92. Anderson RD, Ohman EM, Holmes DR Jr, et al: Use of intraaortic balloon counterpulsation in patients presenting with cardiogenic shock: Observations from the GUSTO-I Study. Global Utilization of Streptokinase and TPA for Occluded Coronary Arteries. J Am Coll Cardiol 1997;30:708-715.
93. Kovack PJ, Rasak MA, Bates ER, et al: Thrombolysis plus aortic counterpulsation: Improved survival in patients who present to community hospitals with cardiogenic shock. J Am Coll Cardiol 1997;29:1454-1458.
94. Nanas JN, Nanas SN, Kontoyannis DA, et al: Myocardial salvage by the use of reperfusion and intraaortic balloon pump: Experimental study. Ann Thorac Surg 1996;61:629-634.
95. Kontoyannis DA, Nanas JN, Kontoyannis SA, et al: Mechanical ventilation in conjunction with the intra-aortic balloon pump improves the outcome of patients in profound cardiogenic shock. Intensive Care Med 1999;25:835-838.
96. Barron HV, Every NR, Parsons LS, et al: The use of intra-aortic balloon counterpulsation in patients with cardiogenic shock complicating acute myocardial infarction: Data from the National Registry of Myocardial Infarction 2. Am Heart J 2001;141: 933-939.
97. Sanborn TA, Sleeper LA, Bates ER, et al: Impact of thrombolysis, intra-aortic balloon pump counterpulsation, and their combination in cardiogenic shock complicating acute myocardial infarction: a report from the SHOCK Trial Registry. SHould we emergently revascularize OCcluded coronaries for cardiogenic shocK? J Am Coll Cardiol 2000;36:1123-1129.
98. Ohman EM, Nanas J, Stomel RJ, et al: Thrombolysis and counterpulsation to improve survival in myocardial infarction complicated by hypotension and suspected cardiogenic shock or heart failure: Results of the TACTICS Trial. J Thromb Thrombolysis 2005;19: 33-39.
99. Hochman JS, Buller CE, Sleeper LA, et al: Cardiogenic shock complicating acute myocardial infarction—etiologies, management and outcome: A report from the SHOCK Trial Registry. SHould we emergently revascularize Occluded Coronaries for cardiogenic shocK? J Am Coll Cardiol 2000;36:1063-1070.
100. Jacobs AK, Leopold JA, Bates E, et al: Cardiogenic shock caused by right ventricular infarction: a report from the SHOCK registry. J Am Coll Cardiol 2003;41:1273-1279.
101. Mendes LA, Picard MH, Sleeper LA, et al: Cardiogenic shock: Predictors of outcome based on right and left ventricular size and function at presentation. Coron Artery Dis 2005;16:209-215.
102. Skillington PD, Couper GS, Peigh PS, et al: Pulmonary artery balloon counterpulsation for intraoperative right ventricular failure. Ann Thorac Surg 1991;51:658-660.
103. Giesler GM, Gomez JS, Letsou G, et al: Initial report of percutaneous right ventricular assist for right ventricular shock secondary to right ventricular infarction. Catheter Cardiovasc Interv 2006;68:263-266.
104. Hasan RI, Deiranyia AK, Yonan NA: Effect of intra-aortic balloon counterpulsation on right-left shunt following right ventricular infarction. Int J Cardiol 1991;33:439-442.
105. Liuzzo JP, Shin YT, Choi C, et al: Simultaneous papillary muscle avulsion and free wall rupture during acute myocardial infarction: Intra-aortic balloon pump: A bridge to survival. J Invasive Cardiol 2006;18:135-140.
106. Thompson CR, Buller CE, Sleeper LA, et al: Cardiogenic shock due to acute severe mitral regurgitation complicating acute myocardial infarction: A report from the SHOCK Trial Registry. SHould we use emergently revascularize Occluded Coronaries in cardiogenic shocK? J Am Coll Cardiol 2000;36:1104-1109.
107. Dekker AL, Reesink KD, van der Veen FH, et al: Intra-aortic balloon pumping in acute mitral regurgitation reduces aortic impedance and regurgitant fraction. Shock 2003;19:334-338.
108. Menon V, Webb JG, Hillis LD, et al: Outcome and profile of ventricular septal rupture with cardiogenic shock after myocardial infarction: A report from the SHOCK Trial Registry. Should

we emergently revascularize Occluded Coronaries in cardiogenic shocK? J Am Coll Cardiol 2000;36:1110-1116.

109. Thiele H, Lauer B, Hambrecht R, et al: Short- and long-term hemodynamic effects of intra-aortic balloon support in ventricular septal defect complicating acute myocardial infarction. Am J Cardiol 2003;92:450-454.
110. Stone GW, Marsalese D, Brodie BR, et al: A prospective, randomized evaluation of prophylactic intraaortic balloon counterpulsation in high risk patients with acute myocardial infarction treated with primary angioplasty. Second Primary Angioplasty in Myocardial Infarction (PAMI-II) Trial Investigators. J Am Coll Cardiol 1997;29:1459-1467.
111. 't Hof AW, Liem AL, de Boer MJ, et al: A randomized comparison of intra-aortic balloon pumping after primary coronary angioplasty in high risk patients with acute myocardial infarction. Eur Heart J 1999;20:659-665.
112. Talley JD, Ohman EM, Mark DB, et al: Economic implications of the prophylactic use of intraaortic balloon counterpulsation in the setting of acute myocardial infarction. The Randomized IABP Study Group: Intraaortic Balloon Pump. Am J Cardiol 1997;79:590-594.
113. Ohman EM, George BS, White CJ, et al: Use of aortic counterpulsation to improve sustained coronary artery patency during acute myocardial infarction: Results of a randomized trial. The Randomized IABP Study Group. Circulation 1994;90:792-799.
114. Kono T, Morita H, Nishina T, et al: Aortic counterpulsation may improve late patency of the occluded coronary artery in patients with early failure of thrombolytic therapy. J Am Coll Cardiol 1996;28:876-881.
115. Christenson JT, Simonet F, Badel P, et al: Optimal timing of preoperative intraaortic balloon pump support in high-risk coronary patients. Ann Thorac Surg 1999;68:934-939.
116. Mishra S, Chu WW, Torguson R, et al: Role of prophylactic intra-aortic balloon pump in high-risk patients undergoing percutaneous coronary intervention. Am J Cardiol 2006;98:608-612.
117. Briguori C, Sarais C, Pagnotta P, et al: Elective versus provisional intra-aortic balloon pumping in high-risk percutaneous transluminal coronary angioplasty. Am Heart J 2003;145:700-707.
118. Briguori C, Airoldi F, Chieffo A, et al: Elective versus provisional intraaortic balloon pumping in unprotected left main stenting. Am Heart J 2006;152:565-572.
119. Baskett RJ, O'Connor GT, Hirsch GM, et al: A multicenter comparison of intraaortic balloon pump utilization in isolated coronary artery bypass graft surgery. Ann Thorac Surg 2003;76:1988-1992.
120. Dietl CA, Berkheimer MD, Woods EL, et al: Efficacy and cost-effectiveness of preoperative IABP in patients with ejection fraction of 0.25 or less. Ann Thorac Surg 1996;62:401-408.
121. Craver JM, Murrah CP: Elective intraaortic balloon counterpulsation for high-risk off-pump coronary artery bypass operations. Ann Thorac Surg 2001;71:1220-1223.
122. Gutfinger DE, Ott RA, Miller M, et al: Aggressive preoperative use of intraaortic balloon pump in elderly patients undergoing coronary artery bypass grafting. Ann Thorac Surg 1999;67:610-613.
123. Ghali WA, Ash AS, Hall RE, et al: Variation in hospital rates of intraaortic balloon pump use in coronary artery bypass operations. Ann Thorac Surg 1999;67:441-445.
124. Baskett RJ, O'Connor GT, Hirsch GM, et al: The preoperative intraaortic balloon pump in coronary bypass surgery: A lack of evidence of effectiveness. Am Heart J 2005;150:1122-1127.
125. Christenson JT, Badel P, Simonet F, et al: Preoperative intraaortic balloon pump enhances cardiac performance and improves the outcome of redo CABG. Ann Thorac Surg 1997;64:1237-1244.
126. Onorati F, Cristodoro L, Bilotta M, et al: Intraaortic balloon pumping during cardioplegic arrest preserves lung function in patients with chronic obstructive pulmonary disease. Ann Thorac Surg 2006;82:35-43.
127. Onorati F, Cristodoro L, Mastroroberto P, et al: Should we discontinue intraaortic balloon during cardioplegic arrest? Splanchnic function results of a prospective randomized trial. Ann Thorac Surg 2005;80:2221-2228.
128. Geppert A, Frey B, Gabriel H, et al: Effects of intraaortic balloon pumping on coronary and carotid flow during percutaneous cardiopulmonary support. Ann Thorac Surg 1996;61:1539-1541.
129. Hausmann H, Potapov EV, Koster A, et al: Predictors of survival 1 hour after implantation of an intra-aortic balloon pump in cardiac surgery. J Card Surg 2001;16:72-77.
130. Arafa OE, Pedersen TH, Svennevig JL, et al: Intraaortic balloon pump in open heart operations: 10-year follow-up with risk analysis. Ann Thorac Surg 1998;65:741-747.
131. Fasseas P, Cohen M, Kopistansky C, et al: Pre-operative intra-aortic balloon counterpulsation in stable patients with left main coronary disease. J Invasive Cardiol 2001;13:679-683.
132. Pfeiffer S, Frisch P, Weyand M, et al: The use of preoperative intra-aortic balloon pump in open heart surgery. J Cardiovasc Surg (Torino) 2005;46:55-60.
133. Marra C, De Santo LS, Amarelli C, et al: Coronary artery bypass grafting in patients with severe left ventricular dysfunction: A prospective randomized study on the timing of perioperative intraaortic balloon pump support. Int J Artif Organs 2002;25:141-146.
134. Vohra HA, Dimitri WR: Elective intraaortic balloon counterpulsation in high-risk off-pump coronary artery bypass grafting. J Card Surg 2006;21:1-5.
135. Christenson JT, Licker M, Kalangos A: The role of intra-aortic counterpulsation in high-risk OPCAB surgery: A prospective randomized study. J Card Surg 2003;18:286-294.
136. Christenson JT, Simonet F, Schmuziger M: Economic impact of preoperative intraaortic balloon pump therapy in high-risk coronary patients. Ann Thorac Surg 2000;70:510-515.
137. Ahmar W, Leet A, Morton J: Diagnostic dilemmas and management of fulminant myocarditis. Anaesth Intensive Care 2007;35:117-120.
138. Gu YL, Jessurun GA, van den Merkhof LF, et al: Intra-aortic balloon counterpulsation for complex aortic stenosis in hybrid strategy. Int J Cardiol 2007;117:e46-e48.
139. Timperley J, Mitchell AR, Brown PD, et al: Flecainide overdose—support using an intra-aortic balloon pump. BMC Emerg Med 2005;5:10.
140. David JS, Gueugniaud PY, Hepp A, et al: Severe heart failure secondary to 5-fluorouracil and low-doses of folinic acid: Usefulness of an intra-aortic balloon pump. Crit Care Med 2000;28:3558-3560.
141. Penney DJ, Bannon PG, Parr MJ: Intra-aortic balloon counterpulsation for cardiogenic shock due to cardiac contusion in an elderly trauma patient. Resuscitation 2002;55:337-340.
142. Yeguiayan JM, Ravisy J, Lenfant F, et al: Anaphylactic shock: The advantages of intra-aortic balloon counter pulsation for the treatment of heart failure. Resuscitation 2007;72:493-495.
143. Ngo AS, Lung T: Thyrotoxic heart disease. Resuscitation 2006;70: 287-290.
144. Uriel N, Kaluski E, Hendler A, et al: Cardiogenic shock in a young female with multiple sclerosis. Resuscitation 2006;70:153-157.
145. Rivera J, Romero KA, Gonzalez-Chon O, et al: Severe stunned myocardium after lightning strike. Crit Care Med 2007;35:280-285.
146. Darrah WC, Sharpe MD, Guiraudon GM, et al: Intraaortic balloon counterpulsation improves right ventricular failure resulting from pressure overload. Ann Thorac Surg 1997;64:1718-1723.
147. Arafa OE, Geiran OR, Andersen K, et al: Intraaortic balloon pumping for predominantly right ventricular failure after heart transplantation. Ann Thorac Surg 2000;70:1587-1593.
148. Boehmer JP, Popjes E: Cardiac failure: Mechanical support strategies. Crit Care Med 2006;34:S268-S277.
149. Mather PJ, Konstam MA: Percutaneous mechanical devices in the management of decompensated heart failure. Curr Heart Fail Rep 2007;4: 43-47.
150. Emerman CL, Pinchak AC, Hagen JF, et al: Hemodynamic effects of the intra-aortic balloon pump during experimental cardiac arrest. Am J Emerg Med 1989;7:378-383.
151. Lurie KG: Recent advances in mechanical methods of cardiopulmonary resuscitation. Acta Anaesthesiol Scand Suppl 1997;111: 49-52.
152. Willcox TW, Stone P, Milsom FP, et al: Cardiopulmonary bypass in pregnancy: Possible new role for the intra-aortic balloon pump. J Extra Corpor Technol 2005;37:189-191.

153. Georgeson S, Coombs AT, Eckman MH: Prophylactic use of the intra-aortic balloon pump in high-risk cardiac patients undergoing noncardiac surgery: A decision analytic view. Am J Med 1992;92:665-678.
154. Browner WS, Li J, Mangano DT: In-hospital and long-term mortality in male veterans following noncardiac surgery. The Study of Perioperative Ischemia Research Group. JAMA 1992;268:228-232.
155. Jafary FH: Preoperative use of intra-aortic balloon counterpulsation in very high-risk patients prior to urgent noncardiac surgery. Acta Cardiol 2005;60:557-560.
156. Masaki E, Takinami M, Kurata Y, et al: Anesthetic management of high-risk cardiac patients undergoing noncardiac surgery under the support of intraaortic balloon pump. J Clin Anesth 1999;11:342-345.
157. Shayani V, Watson WC, Mansour MA, et al: Intra-aortic balloon counterpulsation in patients with severe cardiac dysfunction undergoing abdominal operations. Arch Surg 1998;133:632-635.
158. Goldberg RJ, Gore JM, Alpert JS, et al: Cardiogenic shock after acute myocardial infarction: Incidence and mortality from a community-wide perspective, 1975 to 1988. N Engl J Med 1991;325:1117-1122.
159. Hasdai D, Holmes DR Jr, Topol EJ, et al: Frequency and clinical outcome of cardiogenic shock during acute myocardial infarction among patients receiving reteplase or alteplase: Results from GUSTO-III. Global Use of Strategies to Open Occluded Coronary Arteries. Eur Heart J 1999;20:128-135.
160. Yellin E, Levy L, Bregman D, et al: Hemodynamic effects of intra-aortic balloon pumping in dogs with aortic incompetence. Trans Am Soc Artif Intern Organs 1973;19:389-394.
161. Tse RW, Masindet S, Stavola T, et al: Acute myocardial infarction with dynamic outflow obstruction precipitated by intra-aortic balloon counterpulsation. Cathet Cardiovasc Diagn 1996;39:62-66.
162. Cohen R, Rivagorda J, Elhadad S: Asymmetric septal hypertrophy complicated by dynamic left ventricular obstruction after intra-aortic balloon counterpulsation placement in the setting of anterior myocardial infarction. J Invasive Cardiol 2006;18:E207-E208.
163. Scholz KH, Ragab S, von zur MF, et al: Complications of intra-aortic balloon counterpulsation: The role of catheter size and duration of support in a multivariate analysis of risk. Eur Heart J 1998;19:458-465.
164. Cook L, Pillar B, McCord G, et al: Intra-aortic balloon pump complications: A five-year retrospective study of 283 patients. Heart Lung 1999;28:195-202.
165. Arafa OE, Pedersen TH, Svennevig JL, et al: Vascular complications of the intraaortic balloon pump in patients undergoing open heart operations: 15-year experience. Ann Thorac Surg 1999;67:645-651.
166. Pawar M, Mehta Y, Ansari A, et al: Nosocomial infections and balloon counterpulsation: Risk factors and outcome. Asian Cardiovasc Thorac Ann 2005;13:316-320.
167. Elahi MM, Chetty GK, Kirke R, et al: Complications related to intra-aortic balloon pump in cardiac surgery: A decade later. Eur J Vasc Endovasc Surg 2005;29:591-594.
168. Kantrowitz A, Wasfie T, Freed PS, et al: Intraaortic balloon pumping 1967 through 1982: Analysis of complications in 733 patients. Am J Cardiol 1986;57:976-983.
169. Alderman JD, Gabliani GI, McCabe CH, et al: Incidence and management of limb ischemia with percutaneous wire-guided intraaortic balloon catheters. J Am Coll Cardiol 1987;9:524-530.
170. Christenson JT, Cohen M, Ferguson JJ, III, et al: Trends in intraaortic balloon counterpulsation complications and outcomes in cardiac surgery. Ann Thorac Surg 2002;74:1086-1090.
171. Cohen M, Ferguson JJ III, Freedman RJ Jr, et al: Comparison of outcomes after 8 vs. 9.5 French size intra-aortic balloon counterpulsation catheters based on 9,332 patients in the prospective Benchmark registry. Catheter Cardiovasc Interv 2002;56:200-206.
172. Tyras DH, Willman VL: Paraplegia following intraaortic balloon assistance. Ann Thorac Surg 1978;25:164-166.
173. Harris RE, Reimer KA, Crain BJ, et al: Spinal cord infarction following intraaortic balloon support. Ann Thorac Surg 1986;42:206-207.
174. Beholz S, Braun J, Ansorge K, et al: Paraplegia caused by aortic dissection after intraaortic balloon pump assist. Ann Thorac Surg 1998;65:603-604.
175. Karalis DG, Quinn V, Victor MF, et al: Risk of catheter-related emboli in patients with atherosclerotic debris in the thoracic aorta. Am Heart J 1996;131:1149-1155.
176. Wong SC, Minutello R, Hong MK: Neurological complications following percutaneous coronary interventions (a report from the 2000-2001 New York State Angioplasty Registry). Am J Cardiol 2005;96:1248-1250.
177. Vonderheide RH, Thadhani R, Kuter DJ: Association of thrombocytopenia with the use of intra-aortic balloon pumps. Am J Med 1998;105:27-32.
178. Nishida H, Koyanagi H, Abe T, et al: Comparative study of five types of IABP balloons in terms of incidence of balloon rupture and other complications: A multi-institutional study. Artif Organs 1994;18:746-751.
179. Patel JJ, Kopistansky C, Boston B, et al: Prospective evaluation of factors associated with intraaortic balloon rupture. ASAIO J 1996;42:37-40.
180. Sutter FP, Joyce DH, Bailey BM, et al: Events associated with rupture of intra-aortic balloon counterpulsation devices. ASAIO Trans 1991;37:38-40.
181. Cruz-Flores S, Diamond AL, Leira EC: Cerebral air embolism secondary to intra-aortic balloon pump rupture. Neurocrit Care 2005;2:49-50.
182. Totaro P, Degno N, Smith J, et al: The missing intra-aortic balloon pump catheter. Ital Heart J 2005;6:361-362.
183. Fukushima Y, Yoshioka M, Hirayama N, et al: Management of intraaortic balloon entrapment. Ann Thorac Surg 1995;60:1109-1111.
184. Barnett MG, Swartz MT, Peterson GJ, et al: Vascular complications from intraaortic balloons: Risk analysis. J Vasc Surg 1994;19:81-87.
185. Dosluoglu HH, Dryjski ML: External femorofemoral bypass to relieve acute leg ischemia during circulatory assist. Vascular 2004;12:198-201.
186. Nakano T, Tominaga R, Shiraishi K, et al: Prostaglandin E1 from the tip of an intraaortic balloon catheter for lower limb ischemia. Ann Thorac Surg 1998;65:1158-1160.
187. Jeevanandam V, Jayakar D, Anderson AS, et al: Circulatory assistance with a permanent implantable IABP: Initial human experience. Circulation 2002;106:I183-I188.
188. Burkhoff D, Cohen H, Brunckhorst C, et al: A randomized multicenter clinical study to evaluate the safety and efficacy of the TandemHeart percutaneous ventricular assist device versus conventional therapy with intraaortic balloon pumping for treatment of cardiogenic shock. Am Heart J 2006;152:469;e1-8.
189. Thiele H, Sick P, Boudriot E, et al: Randomized comparison of intra-aortic balloon support with a percutaneous left ventricular assist device in patients with revascularized acute myocardial infarction complicated by cardiogenic shock. Eur Heart J 2005;26:1276-1283.
190. Henriques JP, Remmelink M, Baan J Jr, et al: Safety and feasibility of elective high-risk percutaneous coronary intervention procedures with left ventricular support of the Impella Recover LP 2.5. Am J Cardiol 2006;97:990-992.
191. Lee MS, Makkar RR: Percutaneous left ventricular support devices. Cardiol Clin 2006;24:265-275, vii.
192. Collart F, Kerbaul F, Mekkaoui C, et al: Balloon-pump-induced pulsatility improves coronary and carotid flows in an experimental model of BioMedicus left ventricular assistance. Artif Organs 2004;28:743-746.
193. Drakos SG, Charitos CE, Ntalianis A, et al: Comparison of pulsatile with nonpulsatile mechanical support in a porcine model of profound cardiogenic shock. ASAIO J 2005;51:26-29.
194. Trost JC, Hillis LD: Intra-aortic balloon counterpulsation. Am J Cardiol 2006;97:1391-1398.
195. Engoren M, Habib RH: Effects of intraaortic balloon augmentation in a porcine model of endotoxemic shock. Resuscitation 2004;60:319-326.

Chapter 8

Echocardiography

Sherif F. Nagueh and Priscilla J. Peters

Echocardiography has become an invaluable tool in the management of critically ill patients. Its safety, accuracy, and portability allow for expeditious use at the bedside, providing detailed information regarding myocardial, pericardial, and valvular function. In the intensive care unit (ICU), close collaboration between the echocardiographer and the intensivist facilitates focused examinations that can be interpreted in the correct clinical context. In addition to confirming a clinical suspicion, echocardiography can alert the clinician to an unsuspected diagnosis and can direct therapy appropriately; echocardiography also can reliably exclude cardiovascular disease as a cause of hemodynamic instability (Box 8-1).

COMPONENTS OF THE ECHOCARDIOGRAPHIC EXAMINATION

Echocardiography uses ultrasound (i.e., sound above the audible range) to evaluate the heart and proximal great vessels and typically combines two modalities: tissue imaging and blood flow detection with velocity determination (Doppler). Tissue imaging is based on the transmission of ultrasound into the chest and its reflection by intrathoracic structures, which is determined by their acoustic properties. The two imaging modalities in general clinical use are M-mode and two-dimensional imaging.

M-mode uses a single scan line or beam to produce what is known as the "ice-pick" or one-dimensional view through intracardiac structures along the path of the ultrasound beam. It has the advantage of an extremely high sampling rate (1000 to 3000 Hz compared with 20 to 60 Hz for traditional two-dimensional imaging) because only a single beam path is interrogated. M-mode is useful for measuring linear dimensions (e.g., chamber dimensions) and for appreciating high-frequency motion (i.e., the vibration of a torn leaflet) and has utility for timing of events, especially valve opening and closing. M-mode provides a limited field of view, however, and is now primarily used as an adjunct to two-dimensional imaging.

Two-dimensional images are obtained from multiple sequential scan lines generated electronically (phased array) and processed to create a tomographic imaging plane with an expanded field of view. The time required to obtain all necessary scan lines reduces the frame rate to the range of 30 to 60 frames per second. Current ultrasound systems use fundamental and harmonic imaging. Harmonic imaging transmits sound at a particular frequency (the *fundamental frequency*), but creates the image from sound reflected at twice the fundamental frequency, called the *second harmonic,* which improves image quality because the stronger harmonic signal undergoes considerably less distortion. This is particularly useful for endocardial border definition. Multiple two-dimensional images from different projections are needed to provide a complete view of the heart, and images are generally obtained from parasternal, apical, subxiphoid, and suprasternal positions, manipulating the probe to provide long-axis and short-axis images of each structure interrogated.[1-3]

Doppler echocardiography uses ultrasound to determine blood flow velocity and direction within the heart. The Doppler principle states that the ultrasound frequency is changed when it is reflected by a moving object and that the resultant frequency shift (Δf) can be used to determine the velocity of the reflecting object. The Doppler shift equation is:

$$\Delta f = 2f_0(V)\cos\theta/c$$

Where f_0 = frequency of the transmitted ultrasound, θ = the angle of incidence of the ultrasound beam relative to the moving object, and c = speed of ultrasound in biologic

Box 8-1

Use of Echocardiography in the Intensive Care Setting

General
Determine presence of occult cardiac disease
Source of murmur
Source of embolus
Integrity of the aorta
Procedural guidance (especially pericardiocentesis)

Hemodynamics
Hypotension
Pericardial effusion/tamponade
Assess volume status
Left ventricular function
- Regional wall motion abnormalities
- Global dysfunction
- Transient dysfunction (sepsis, ischemic/catecholamine stunning)

Right ventricular function
Outflow tract obstruction
Valvular stenosis/insufficiency

Hypoxia
Right ventricular function
Right ventricular pressure
Intracardiac/extracardiac shunting
Pulmonary embolus

Infections
Bacterial endocarditis

Box 8-2

Use of Spectral and Color Flow Doppler

Quantify normal flow
- Stroke volume/cardiac output

Detect and quantify abnormal flow
- Valve regurgitation (color/spectral)
- Intracardiac shunts (color/spectral)

Blood flow velocity
- Pressure gradients
- Valve areas
- Right heart pressure

Evaluation of ventricular filling dynamics
- Primary myocardial disease
- Pericardial constraint

tissues (1540 m/s). An important consequence of the Doppler shift equation is that the angle of incidence of the Doppler beam must be as close to zero as possible to ensure that the value of $\cos\theta$ is close to 1, to avoid underestimation of the velocity.

Two principal types of spectral Doppler techniques are used, termed *continuous wave* and *pulsed wave*. Continuous wave uses two separate transducer crystals, one continuously transmitting and one continuously receiving the ultrasound signal. The high sampling rate of continuous wave allows it to measure high velocities, but the source of any specific velocity measurement along the interrogated path cannot be differentiated *(range ambiguity)*. Pulsed wave uses one crystal, which alternates between sending and receiving a discrete pulse of ultrasound. The principal advantage of this technique is that signals arise only from the area of interrogation, called the *sample volume (range resolution)*. Because the same crystal is used for sending and receiving the signal, however, a new pulse of ultrasound cannot be transmitted until the previous returning signal has been detected. This "pulsed" process results in too low a sampling rate to quantitate high velocities. Pulsed wave and continuous wave Doppler are complementary, with pulsed wave localizing the source of a signal and continuous wave allowing for the unambiguous measurement of high velocities.[4] Doppler recordings can be obtained with a two-dimensional ("steerable") imaging probe or with a stand-alone (Pedoff) nonimaging probe that records only spectral Doppler velocities. This nonimaging probe has a very small footprint, making it ideally suited for small acoustic windows, such as intercostal spaces. The Pedoff probe has a higher signal-to-noise ratio than the steerable probe, which enables it to localize the highest velocity of flow from a particular window. The Pedoff probe is particularly useful in evaluating the high-velocity, low-volume flow of critical obstruction, such as aortic stenosis. A high degree of operator skill is necessary to use this probe effectively.

In addition to the evaluation of high-velocity blood flow, pulsed Doppler can evaluate the velocity of moving myocardium, which produces a signal of low velocity, but high amplitude. Called Doppler tissue imaging, systolic and diastolic velocities within the myocardium and at the corners of mitral annulus can be recorded. Mitral annular velocities as measured by Doppler tissue imaging are commonly used to evaluate diastolic function.[5]

Color flow imaging is a form of two-dimensional Doppler in which pulsed Doppler information is coded with colors and superimposed on a two-dimensional ultrasound image. Black and white identifies anatomic structures, and color identifies blood flow velocities (Box 8-2). Color has shown great utility in the evaluation of valvular regurgitant lesions and intracardiac shunts (Fig. 8-1).

TRANSESOPHAGEAL ECHOCARDIOGRAPHY

In any context in which standard transthoracic echocardiography (TTE) image quality is suboptimal, including situations in which the patient is obese, has significant lung disease, is unable to cooperate by changing position, is ventilated, or has bandages or drainage tubes that obscure the standard access windows, transesophageal echocardiography (TEE) may be beneficial.[6,7] TEE involves insertion into the esophagus of an endoscope-like probe with an ultrasound transducer on its tip. Image resolution is improved with TEE because the ultrasound beam is

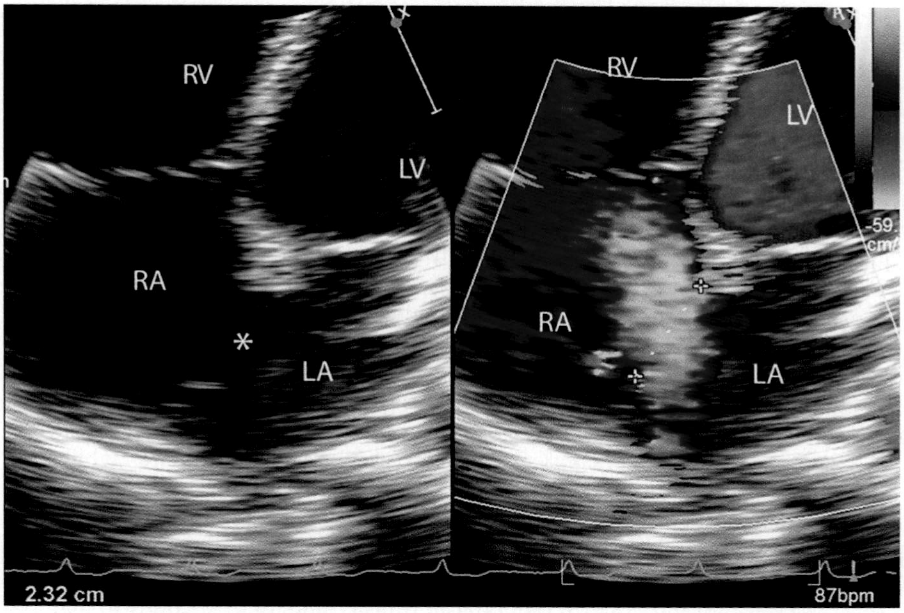

A B

Figure 8-1. Color flow of secundum atrial septal defect. **A,** Apical image of dilated right-sided structures. *Asterisk* indicates atrial septal defect. **B,** Color flow *(orange)* from left atrium through defect. LA, left atrium; LV, left ventricle; RA, right atrium; RV, right ventricle.

unimpeded by bone and air, and because proximity to the heart enables use of high-frequency (7 MHz) probes.

TEE can be performed easily at the bedside. Active esophageal pathology is the major contraindication. A topical oral anesthetic spray and an agent for conscious sedation are administered. TEE can be done with a nasogastric tube in place, but the nasogastric tube should be removed if there are any difficulties with passing the probe or in acquiring the images. Patients require blood pressure, respiratory, oxygen saturation, and heart rate monitoring during the procedure. A comprehensive transesophageal examination typically takes about 20 minutes for imaging, then requires a period of recovery time (Box 8-3).

Intravascular and Intracardiac Ultrasound

Intravascular ultrasound uses ultraminiaturized transducers mounted on modified intracoronary catheters to provide radial anatomic imaging of intracoronary calcification and plaque formation. Intracoronary ultrasound is performed in the catheterization laboratory by an invasive cardiologist and is usually used to determine optimal intracoronary stent deployment.[8] *Intracardiac echocardiography* uses a single-plane, high-frequency transducer (7.5 to 10 MHz) on the tip of a steerable intravascular catheter. The catheter is typically 9F to 13F, can be steered and flexed, and can provide two-dimensional images and spectral and color Doppler. Intracardiac echocardiography is used only in the catheterization laboratory, but offers substantial anatomic and hemodynamic information during procedures such as atrial septal defect or patent foramen ovale closure (transseptal puncture, device placement), percutaneous balloon valvuloplasty (transseptal puncture, balloon placement, mitral regurgitation [MR] after balloon inflation), and isolation of pulmonary veins for ablation in the setting of atrial fibrillation.[9-11]

Box 8-3

Indications for Transesophageal Imaging

- Evaluate suspected aortic dissection or trauma
- Evaluate prosthetic valves, especially mitral
- Investigate persistent hypoxemia
- Determine presence of valvular vegetations and complications of infective endocarditis
  - Abscesses
  - Leaflet perforation
  - Pseudoaneurysm formation
- Identify cardiac source of systemic embolus
  - Intracardiac thrombus, especially left atrium and left atrial appendage
  - Patent foramen ovale/atrial septal aneurysm
  - Atheromatous debris of the aorta
- Identify pulmonary embolus-in-transit
- Define intracardiac tumors
- Characterize intracardiac shunts
  - Atrial septal defect
  - Ventricular septal defect
  - Anomalous pulmonary venous connections
- Guide invasive procedures
  - Shunt closure
  - Percutaneous balloon valvuloplasty
- Intraoperative
  - Monitor left ventricular function in noncardiac surgery
  - Assess efficacy of valve repair surgery
- Evaluate ventricular function
- Inadequate transthoracic echocardiography

Three-Dimensional Echocardiography

Early three-dimensional echocardiography was hindered by the prolonged and tedious nature of data acquisition and the necessary offline analysis. Contemporary real-time three-dimensional echocardiography can eliminate the labor-intensive offline reconstruction and analysis. Current ultrasound systems offer transducers that are equipped with a rectangular ultrasound array of send/receive crystals that allow for acquisition of pyramidal image data sets (so-called volume-rendered images). These three-dimensional "volumes" can be promptly processed and displayed. Studies have determined that three-dimensional calculated left ventricular (LV) volumes, ejection fractions, and LV mass are comparable to those obtained with nuclear imaging and magnetic resonance imaging (MRI). The technique is subject to the same technical considerations of standard two-dimensional imaging, however, and not all patients produce adequate real-time three-dimensional echocardiography images. Nonetheless, this technology is a major advance in the assessment of patients with structural abnormalities, and the expectation is that further refinements in acquisition and analysis will make it useful to most patients with heart disease.[12-16]

Contrast Echocardiography

Echocardiographic contrast agents are substances that enhance the reflected ultrasound signal. Simple agitated saline can be used as contrast material to detect intracardiac shunts, commonly at the atrial level. Commercially available contrast agents, specifically formulated to survive pulmonary transit, can be used to opacify intracardiac chambers to enhance endocardial border definition. In addition, newer contrast agents, designed for continuous intravenous infusion in association with specific ultrasound imaging protocols, can provide information about myocardial microperfusion.

To detect an intracardiac shunt, a contrast study can be done with agitated saline. In this technique, 10 mL of normal saline is connected to a second 10-mL syringe via a three-way stopcock. Brisk exchange of the saline between the syringes creates microbubbles, which are rapidly injected as an intravenous bolus, resulting in opacification of the right heart chambers. These bubbles are too large to pass through the pulmonary capillaries, but may appear in the left atrium and left ventricle as a result of passage across an intracardiac (atrial septal defect or patent foramen ovale) or intrapulmonary communication; occasionally, a cough or Valsalva maneuver may transiently increase right heart pressures and facilitate right-to-left crossover of bubbles. This is a useful undertaking in a critical care patient with unexplained persistent hypoxemia.[17] Pulmonary arteriovenous malformations show contrast in the left atrium after a delay of 5 to 15 beats, which represents the typical transit time of the contrast material through the pulmonary bed and the arteriovenous malformation into the pulmonary veins (Fig. 8-2).

Commercial contrast agents have generated substantial interest because of bubble stability, uniform size, and the ability to survive pulmonary transit to facilitate opacification of left heart chambers and the myocardium. When activated, contrast agents yield perfluorocarbon microbubbles encapsulated in a lipid or albumin shell, which exhibit lower acoustic impedance than blood and enhance the intrinsic backscatter of blood. These agents are useful in improving image quality in technically difficult echocardiograms and can provide additional diagnostic information, especially regarding the presence of LV wall

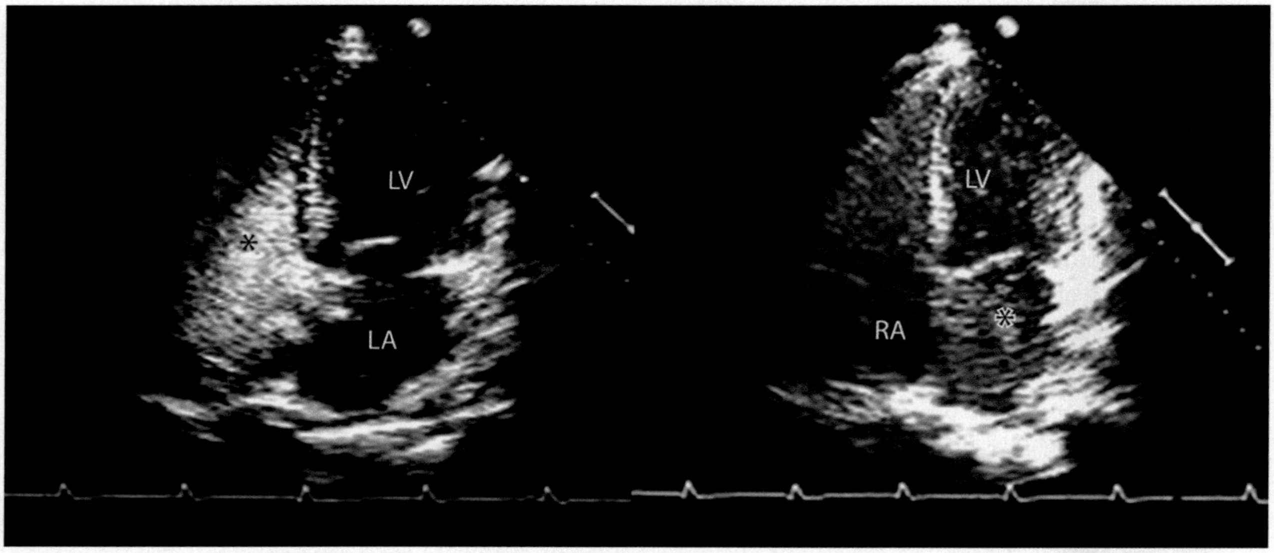

A B

Figure 8-2. Young patient with hypoxia who had a saline contrast injection to rule out patent foramen ovale. **A,** Saline (*) enters right heart, and there is little right-to-left transit in the first three beats. **B,** As the right heart is emptied of saline, there is delayed and persistent opacification (*) of the left heart, strongly suggesting a pulmonary arteriovenous malformation. LA, left atrium; LV, left ventricle; RA, right atrium.

motion abnormalities. Because the increment of additional useful information is substantial, the threshold should be low for the use of contrast agents in critical care patients.[18-20] Substantial work has shown that contrast agents can facilitate the detection of myocardial perfusion abnormalities and predict coronary stenoses before the development of ventricular dysfunction.[21-23] Additional progress in the development of site-targeted microbubbles offers the possibility of using contrast agents as the delivery mechanism for either drug or gene therapy.[24-28]

Hand-Carried Cardiac Ultrasound

Hand-held ultrasound devices (small ultrasound machines typically weighing <6 lb) are now widely available and can provide two-dimensional and Doppler images. Early concerns that unskilled users would obtain and subsequently misinterpret poor-quality data have largely been ameliorated, and several reasonable studies suggest that non–cardiology-trained intensivists can successfully perform and correctly interpret goal-directed TTE with a hand-held device. "Goal-directed" two-dimensional imaging is typically limited to the assessment of overall myocardial contractility, LV size and function, and presence or absence of pericardial effusion. Because it seems that the device is technically adequate to evaluate major cardiac pathology, it is reasonable to conclude that a focused two-dimensional study done by a trained individual with only a hand-held device has great potential for rapid triage of patients in the emergency department or ICU.[29-34]

Assessment of Global Left Ventricular Systolic Function

Numerous reasonably accurate methods are available to assess global LV systolic properties, including indices of pump performance as stroke work (stroke volume × mean arterial pressure), systolic function (as fractional shortening and ejection fraction), LV chamber contractility as maximal systolic elastance, and myocardial contractility as midwall fractional shortening and its relation to LV systolic wall stress. For practical purposes, LV ejection fraction using two-dimensional images (and more recently three-dimensional imaging) is most frequently used.[15,35] Ejection fraction can be quantified online using border detection algorithms, assessed visually (usually as a range or qualitative assessment of mild, moderate, or severe depression), or offline in the laboratory (Fig. 8-3) using one of several methods (most accurate being biplane multiple discs method, shown in Box 8-4). Visual assessment

Box 8-4

Quantification of Left Ventricular Volumes and Ejection Fraction

Area-length method: $V = 0.85\ (A^2/L)$
Method of multiple discs (modified Simpson's)
Multiple diameter method
Three-dimensional methods

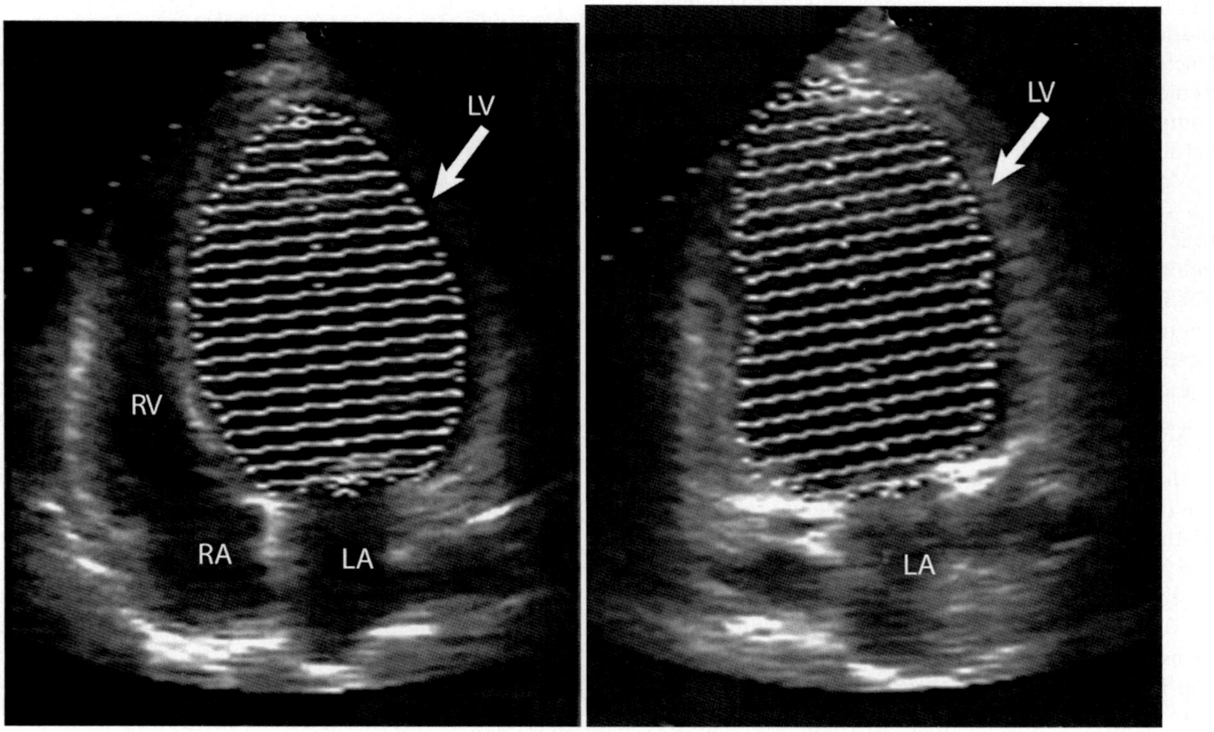

A B

Figure 8-3. Left ventricular volumes and ejection fraction calculated using method of discs *(arrow)*. **A,** Diastole. **B,** Systole. End-diastolic volume = 214 mL; end-systolic volume = 158 mL; stroke volume = 56 mL; and ejection fraction = 0.26. LA, left atrium; LV, left ventricle; RA, right atrium; RV, right ventricle.

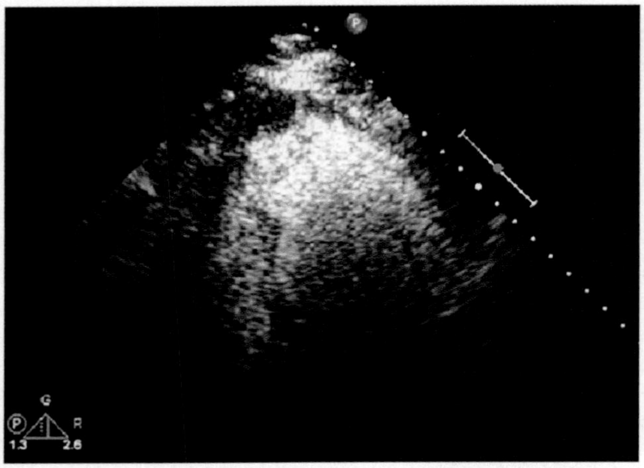

Figure 8-4. Apical four-chamber view with contrast enhancement showing a filling defect in the left ventricular apex, typical of thrombus.

is most reliable when technically adequate images are evaluated by experienced echocardiographers. Ejection fraction (end diastolic volume – end systolic volume/end diastolic volume) depends not only on intrinsic contractility but also on LV preload and afterload. Both factors should be considered when drawing inferences about LV systolic function. Even when quantification is applied, technically adequate images and experience are still essential to avoid erroneous calculations.

In the presence of regional dysfunction, ejection fraction from multiple views and not fractional shortening should be applied given the presence of segmental wall motion abnormalities. To improve the accuracy of ejection fraction calculation by echocardiography, it is essential to avoid foreshortened apical views and to use intravenous contrast agents (Fig. 8-4) when needed to enhance endocardial border definition.

Many other potentially useful methods exist to assess LV systolic function, including Doppler-derived LV systolic function (dP/dt), from the spectral continuous wave velocity profile of MR, when an adequate signal is present. The instantaneous pressure gradient, ΔP, between the left ventricle and left atrium throughout systole can be calculated from the MR velocity, v, by the modified Bernoulli equation:

$$\Delta P = 4v^2$$

In this approach, it is assumed that the rate of increase in the LV–left atrial (LA) pressure gradient is representative of the rate of increase in LV pressure or dP/dt. dP/dt can be estimated by measuring the time interval taken for the MR velocity to increase from 1 to 3 m/s (a change of 32 mm Hg). Although it can correlate well with invasively derived dP/dt, it also is dependent on preload, and its accuracy can be limited in cases in which MR is not present or its jet by continuous wave is incomplete.[36-38]

More recently tissue Doppler–derived measurements (Box 8-5) have been used to assess global LV systolic properties.[39] This approach is dependent on tissue Doppler technology to record mitral annulus and myocardial signals, which can be acquired from any area of the heart. Because of their dependence on Doppler principles, however, they are of no or limited value when proper alignment cannot be achieved between the ultrasound beam and the plane of cardiac motion. The measurements include peak annular or myocardial velocities measured during isovolumic contraction or systolic ejection (Fig. 8-5). Also, it is possible to measure the rate of acceleration of the isovolumic contraction velocity. The clinical utility of the latter measurement is not well established, however, and in one report, it was heavily affected by preload such that it did not identify real changes in myocardial function with induction of ischemia.[40] Velocity measurements are affected by translation and tethering, and parameters of regional deformation can provide a more accurate assessment of LV systolic function (Fig. 8-6).

Box 8-5

Tissue Doppler for Assessment of Left Ventricular Systolic Function

Mitral annulus systolic velocity during ejection
Mitral annulus systolic velocity during isovolumic contraction
Isovolumic acceleration rate
Systolic strain rate
Systolic strain

Studies have verified the aforementioned premise in animal and human models, although strain rate and strain measurements have their highest utility as indices of regional performance.[41] In addition, they are heavily affected by preload and afterload. An alternative approach to measuring regional velocity and deformation is based on speckle tracking. This approach is not angle dependent and has been validated against sonomicrometry and cardiac MR studies in many promising early reports.[42]

Aside from measurements of systolic function, it is possible to use two-dimensional echocardiography to obtain reliable measurements of LV dimensions, wall thickness, volumes, and mass and LA volumes, and to calculate end systolic and diastolic wall stress in several planes.[35] Although it is feasible to measure meridional, circumferential, and radial wall stress, these measurements may not be needed in many patients in the ICU. Rather, a reliable assessment of LV dimensions and ejection fraction, particularly when combined with knowledge of filling pressures, can be used to guide and assess the response to therapeutic measures of volume infusion or intravenous administration of inotropic/vasodilator or vasopressor drugs.

Evaluation of Regional Left Ventricular Systolic Function

Echocardiographic assessment of regional function can be useful in the ICU when the diagnosis of ischemia or infarction is entertained. Adequate images, particularly

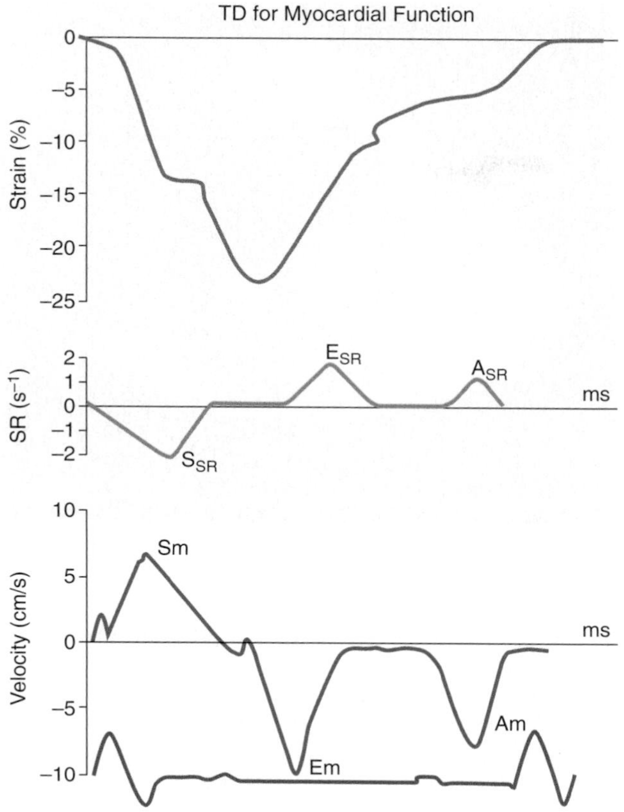

Figure 8-5. Tissue Doppler (TD) data obtained from the apical position. *Blue* (top signal), strain; *green* (second signal), strain rate; *violet* (third signal), myocardial velocities; *red* (bottom signal), ECG. By convention, systolic cardiac velocity toward the apex (and transducer) is shown as a positive deflection (Sm) above the baseline. The recoil velocities in early (Em) and late diastole (Am) away from the transducer are shown as signals below the baseline. For strain and strain rate, compression in systole is displayed as a negative signal, whereas expansion is a positive deflection when the transducer is in an apical position. The rate of deformation is strain rate, and is measured in s^{-1}, whereas strain is a dimensionless parameter (strain is defined as change in length relative to baseline length). A_{SR}, late diastolic strain rate; E_{SR}, early diastolic strain rate; S_{SR}, systolic strain rate.

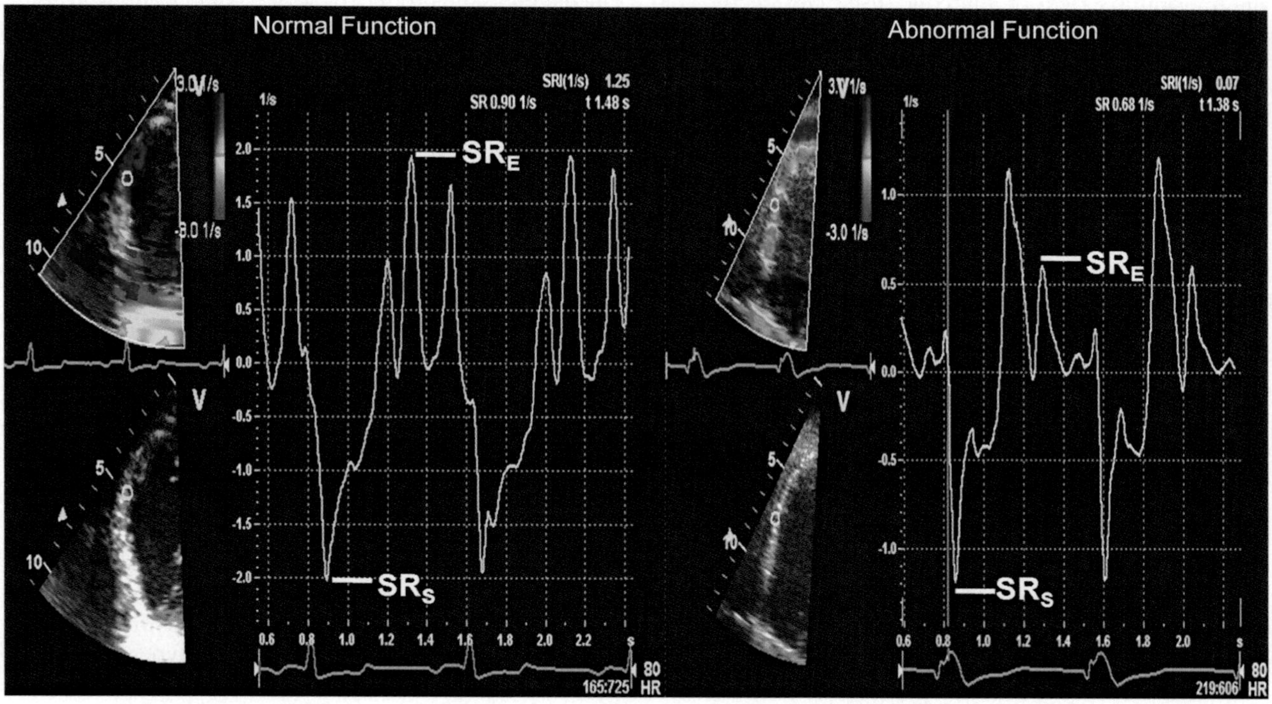

A

B

Figure 8-6. Evaluation of normal **(A)** and abnormal **(B)** myocardial strain rate. **A,** In the patient with normal cardiac function, systolic (SR_S) and early diastolic (SR_E) strain rates are 2 s^{-1}. **B,** The patient with abnormal function has reduced systolic (SR_S) at 1.38 s^{-1}, and early diastolic (SR_E) strain rate at 0.68 s^{-1}.

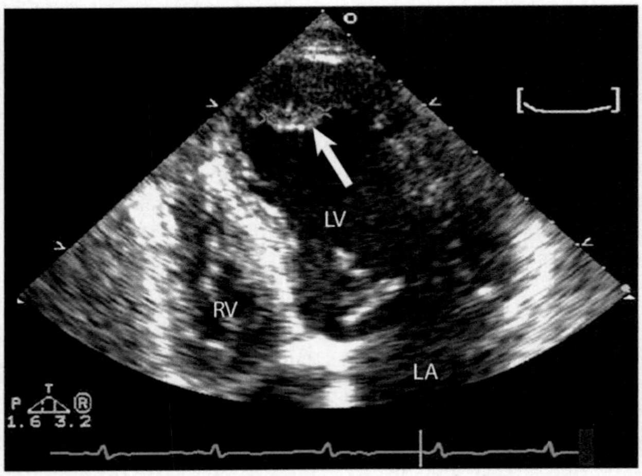

Figure 8-7. Four-chamber view of the left ventricle (LV) showing apical thrombus *(arrow)*. LA, left atrium; RV, right ventricle.

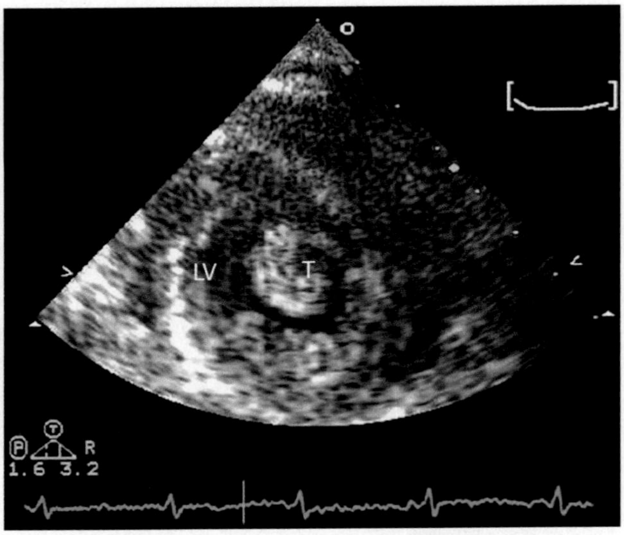

Figure 8-8. Short-axis view of the same patient in Figure 8-7 showing thrombus (T). LV, left ventricle.

when combined with harmonics and intravenous contrast material, can provide comparable information to that obtained by TEE.[18,19] Serial assessment of regional function is possible after the administration of antianginal or thrombolytic drugs or percutaneous revascularization.

In addition to technical quality, interpretation by an experienced echocardiographer is essential for achieving the highest accuracy. Regional function is determined by examining endocardial motion and local thickening. As described previously, regional velocity and particularly strain rate and strain also can be performed. Early reports have shown that measurements of local deformation can provide insight into the transmural extent of infarction, using MRI as the gold standard. In general, abnormal function is ascertained when the dysfunction is observed in more than one plane. In addition to epicardial coronary artery disease, myocarditis, dilated cardiomyopathy, and abnormal conduction patterns (particularly right ventricular [RV] pacing and left bundle branch block) can result in regional dysfunction. Final conclusions regarding the etiology should be drawn only after a thorough evaluation of clinical findings.

In the setting of acute myocardial infarction, numerous studies have substantiated the prognostic power of echocardiography, particularly LV ejection fraction and the global wall motion score index.[43] Regional function is most reflective of long-term outcome when imaging is performed after recovery of myocardial stunning (usually 7 to 10 days after presentation). In the acute setting, echocardiography may be obtained to help establish the diagnosis of an acute ischemic syndrome; determine the extent of myocardium at risk; identify apical clots (Figs. 8-7 and 8-8); and detect the presence of mechanical complications, such as ventricular septal defect (Fig. 8-9), MR, pericardial effusion, RV infarction, and cardiac rupture (Fig. 8-10).

Calculation of Flow by Doppler

It is possible to calculate blood flow at several levels in the heart and aorta using Doppler echocardiography.[44] These measurements of flow can be useful in the ICU to derive LV stroke volume, cardiac output, regurgitant volumes of MR and aortic regurgitation (AR), flow across an atrial septal defect or ventricular septal defect, valve areas (by continuity principle), response to therapeutic measures such as intravenous administration of inotropic drugs, or the effect of an intra-aortic balloon pump on systemic output.

Stroke volume (in mL or cm^3) is calculated as the product of the cross-sectional area (cm^2) of the LV outflow tract and the time velocity integral (cm) by pulsed wave Doppler (Fig. 8-11) at this site.[45,46] Cardiac output can be calculated as the product of stroke volume and heart rate. Many studies have shown good accuracy of Doppler echocardiography when compared with measurements derived by thermodilution, including data obtained from patients in the ICU. Doppler-derived stroke volume can provide important clues in situations of reduced output (whether due to volume depletion or LV systolic dysfunction) and cases of high-output states, such as sepsis and liver failure.

Evaluation of Left Ventricular Diastolic Function

LV diastolic dysfunction in the ICU may be present as a result of cardiac and systemic disorders that can affect cardiac function (e.g., diabetes mellitus, sarcoidosis, and rheumatologic disorders). A careful assessment of LV diastolic function can contribute essential information for the management of these patients. Echocardiography can provide unique information in this regard.[47-49] The availability of numerous methods makes it possible to determine LV filling pressures with reasonable accuracy. Aside from identifying diastolic dysfunction in the setting of hypertension, coronary artery disease, hypertrophic cardiomyopathy, or restrictive cardiomyopathy, other lesions that result in increased LV filling pressures (e.g., mitral stenosis or regurgitation) can be readily diagnosed.

In general, LV diastolic function refers to LV relaxation (measured as the rate of decay of LV systolic pressure

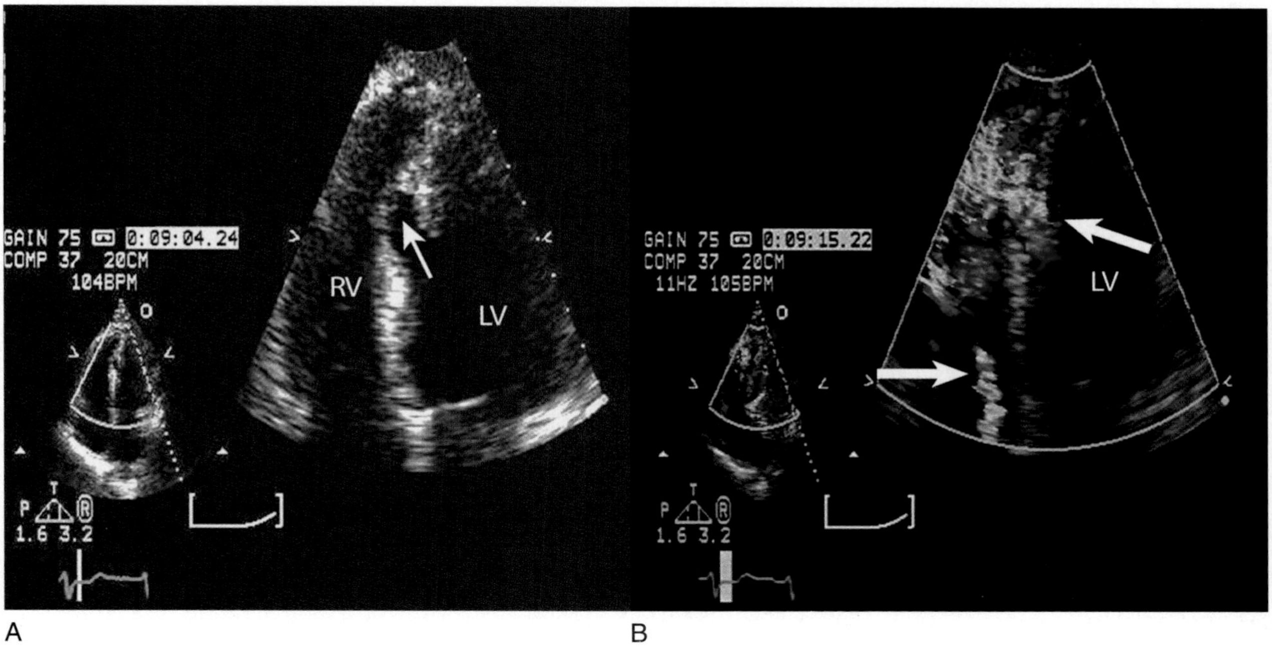

Figure 8-9. A, Four-chamber view showing postinfarct ventricular septal defect *(arrow)*. **B,** Color flow showing left-to-right shunting across ventricular septal defect *(upper arrow)* and tricuspid regurgitation *(lower arrow)*. LV, left ventricle; RV, right ventricle.

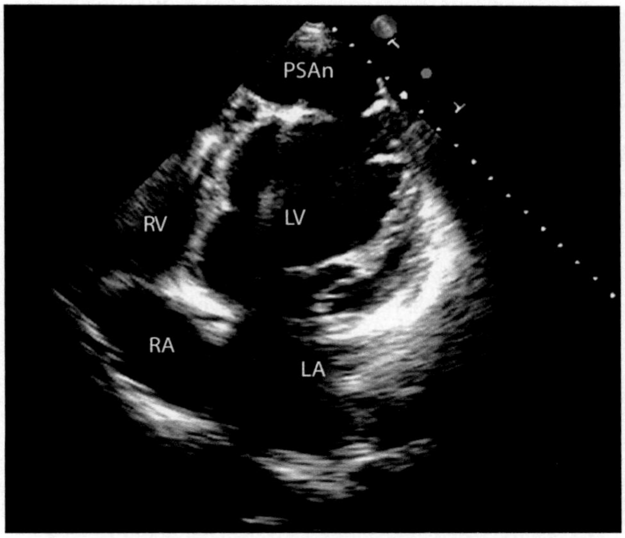

Figure 8-10. Pseudoaneurysm (PSAn) of the left ventricular apex. LA, left atrium; LV, left ventricle; RA, right atrium; RV, right ventricle.

during the isovolumic relaxation period) and LV chamber stiffness. Chamber stiffness is calculated using measurements of LV volume and pressure during the diastolic filling period. There are Doppler parameters that relate best to each of these two variables. Prediction of LV filling pressures integrates the effects of the aforementioned hemodynamic variables and other factors such as RV filling, pericardial constraint, and LA function on LV diastolic function, however.

Our clinical approach (Box 8-6) begins with the two-dimensional examination to determine LV dimensions and volumes and the presence and extent of LV hypertrophy, using standard American Society of Echocardiography criteria.[35] Patients with a depressed ejection fraction or LV hypertrophy or both have impaired LV relaxation. Even in the absence of any corroborating Doppler information, one can still conclude that LV relaxation is impaired in these patients. This information can be combined with the mitral inflow pattern to predict filling pressures. It also is important to measure LA volume using apical four-chamber and two-chamber views because LA volume is related to the extent of diastolic dysfunction, whereby LA volume increases in parallel with the deterioration of LV diastolic function.[50]

Box 8-6

Echocardiographic Assessment of Left Ventricular Diastolic Function

- Two-dimensional echocardiography
- Mitral inflow
- Tricuspid regurgitation jet and pulmonary artery systolic pressure
- Pulmonic regurgitation jet and pulmonary artery diastolic pressure
- Pulmonary venous flow
- Tissue Doppler of mitral annulus
- Flow propagation velocity

Mitral inflow is successfully recorded in most patients referred for echocardiographic evaluation. Using pulsed Doppler, a 1- to 2-mm sample volume is placed at the level of the mitral valve annulus and tips to record the mitral

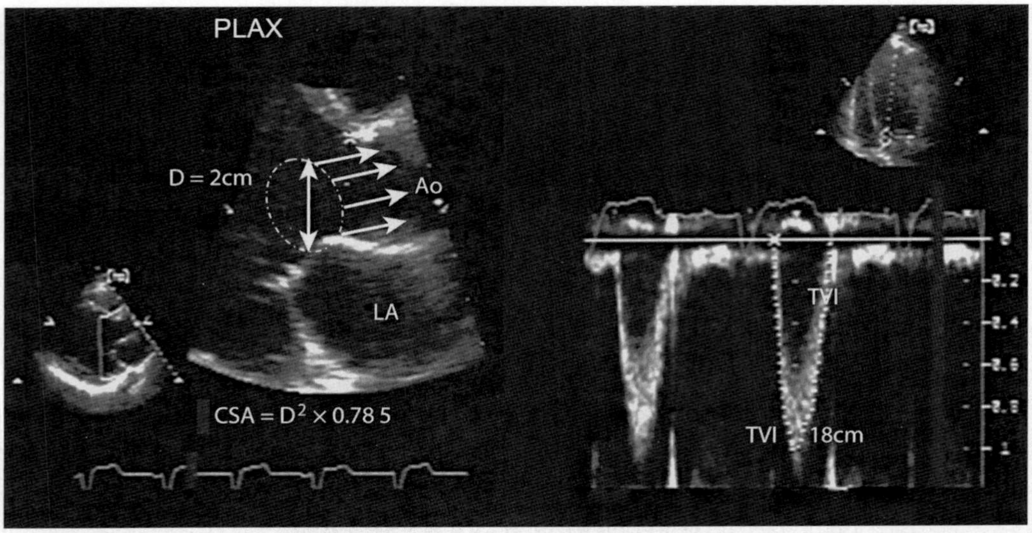

Figure 8-11. Method for stroke volume (SV) calculation using aortic annulus and aortic time velocity integral (TVI). SV = CSA × TVI. Ao, aorta; CSA, cross-sectional area; LA, left atrium; PLAX, parasternal long-axis view.

inflow signals at each of these two sites.[51] Early diastolic flow and velocity (*E* velocity) occur in response to a positive-pressure gradient between the left atrium and the left ventricle, owing to a rapidly decreasing LV pressure secondary to LV relaxation and early diastolic suction. In late diastole, LA contraction leads to another positive-pressure gradient and late diastolic flow (*A* velocity). With normal LV relaxation, early diastolic flow predominates, and the E/A ratio is greater than 1. When LV relaxation is impaired, however, LV diastolic pressure is elevated, and a reduced E velocity is observed; this leads to a higher LA preload and contraction velocity. The E/A ratio decreases in the presence of impaired LV relaxation. Because LA pressure usually increases to maintain forward stroke volume, early diastolic transmitral pressure gradient increases leading to a higher E velocity and E/A ratio. Because of the simulation to normal mitral inflow, this pattern is referred to as a "pseudonormal mitral inflow pattern." In more advanced disease with markedly elevated LA pressure, the E velocity increases further, resulting in a "restrictive" inflow pattern, where E/A ratio is equal to or greater than 2. Nevertheless, it is possible to unmask the presence of impaired LV relaxation in these cases by performing a Valsalva maneuver. The decrease in venous return during the strain phase of the Valsalva maneuver results in a decrease in LA pressure and E/A ratio.[52-54]

Pulmonary venous flow also can be analyzed to predict LV filling pressures. Pulmonary venous flow signals are readily recorded in most patients seen in the outpatient laboratory, but can be challenging in the ICU. Antegrade forward flow from the pulmonary vein into the left atrium occurs during systole (S) and early and mid diastole (D). After atrial contraction, retrograde flow (Ar) from the left atrium into the pulmonary vein occurs. At the earlier stages of diastolic dysfunction when LV end diastolic pressure is increased, the peak velocity and duration of Ar (velocity <30 cm/s and Ar-A duration 35 ms) become more prominent.[54,55] Later on, with the increase in mean LA pressure, antegrade systolic flow decreases, whereas the D velocity increases with a shortening of its deceleration time.

Assessment of pulmonary arterial systolic and diastolic pressures (see later) can provide helpful corroborating evidence of the status of LV filling pressures. In the absence of pulmonary parenchymal and vascular disease, and in the presence of significant cardiac valvular disease or cardiomyopathy or both, one can reasonably infer that pulmonary arterial pressures are increased as a result of an elevated LA pressure.

The opposite effects of preload and relaxation on mitral velocities and time intervals have led to the search for other noninvasive, load-independent indices of LV relaxation. These include the early diastolic color flow propagation velocity (Vp)[56] and early diastolic (Ea) myocardial velocities by tissue Doppler.[57] Vp is affected by LV relaxation and end systolic volume, such that Vp is higher in the presence of faster LV relaxation and smaller LV end systolic volume. Vp may appear normal, however, despite impaired LV relaxation in the presence of normal ejection fraction and LV volumes.[57]

Tissue Doppler–derived Ea can be recorded by numerous techniques, including pulsed wave Doppler from the mitral annulus and the individual myocardial segments. Many studies support its utility as a marker of LV relaxation that is independent of preload in the presence of myocardial disease. These include its decline with age and its inverse relation with the time constant of LV relaxation in murine, canine, and human studies.[58] Data also exist relating it to the extent of interstitial fibrosis, β-adrenergic receptor density,[59] and myocardial gene expression of tumor necrosis factor-α and inducible nitric oxide synthase.[60]

An example of normal Doppler signals is shown in Figure 8-12, impaired relaxation is shown in Figure 8-13, and restrictive LV filling is shown in Figure 8-14. In patients with LV systolic dysfunction, mitral inflow has

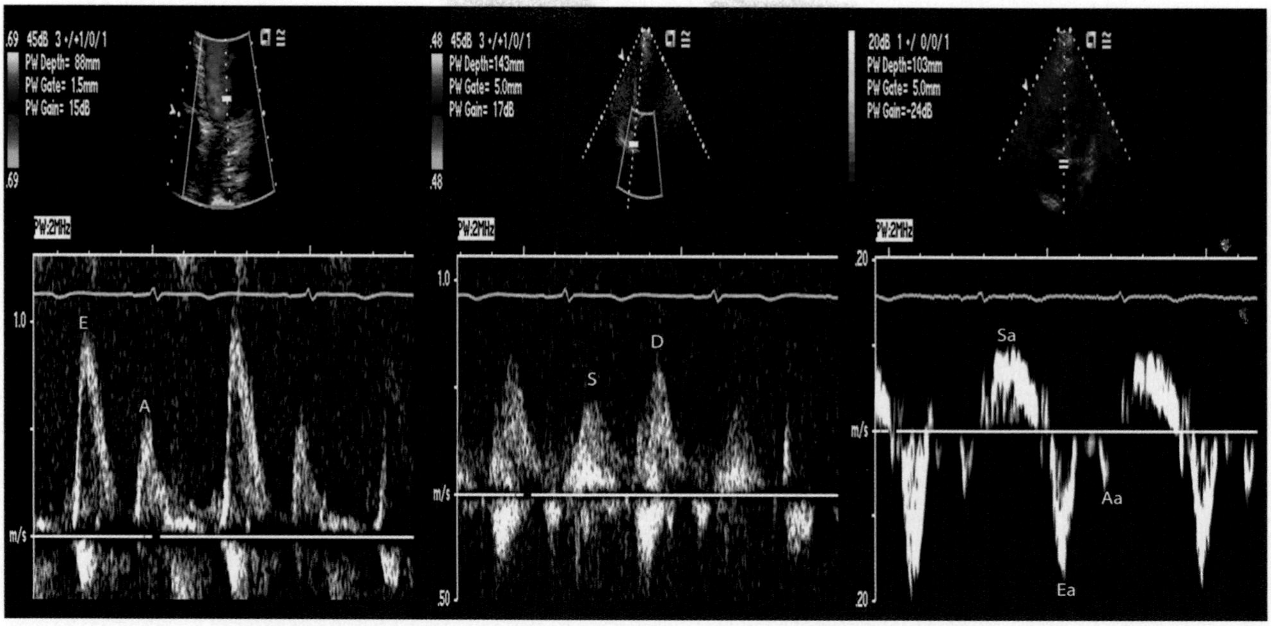

A B C

Figure 8-12. Doppler signals in normal diastolic function. **A,** Mitral inflow with normal E/A and predominant early diastolic flow. **B,** Pulmonary venous flow. **C,** Normal septal annular tissue Doppler.

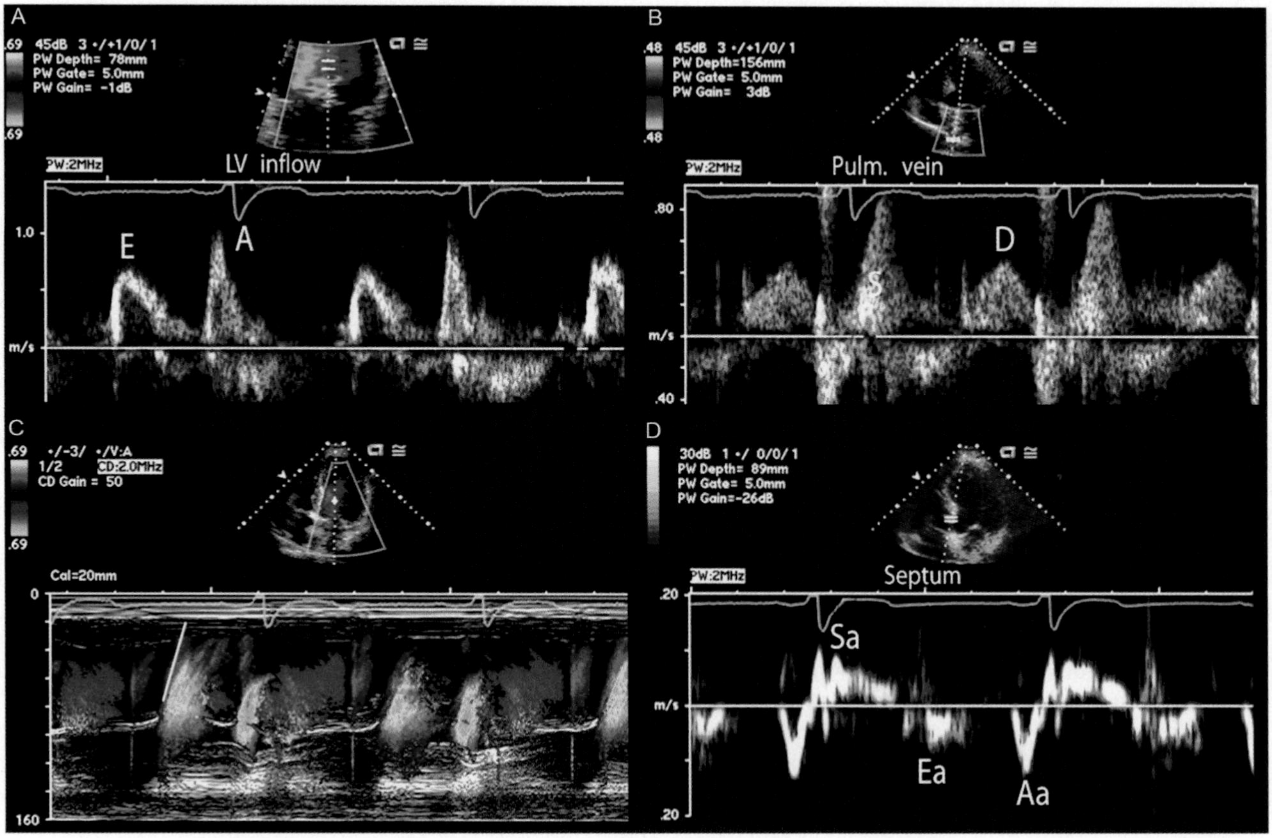

Figure 8-13. Doppler filling pattern of impaired relaxation. **A,** Mitral inflow E/A < 1 with prolonged deceleration time. **B,** Predominant systolic flow of pulmonary veins. **C,** Reduced flow propagation velocity (note measure of slope on left). **D,** Tissue Doppler (TD) Ea velocity reduced.

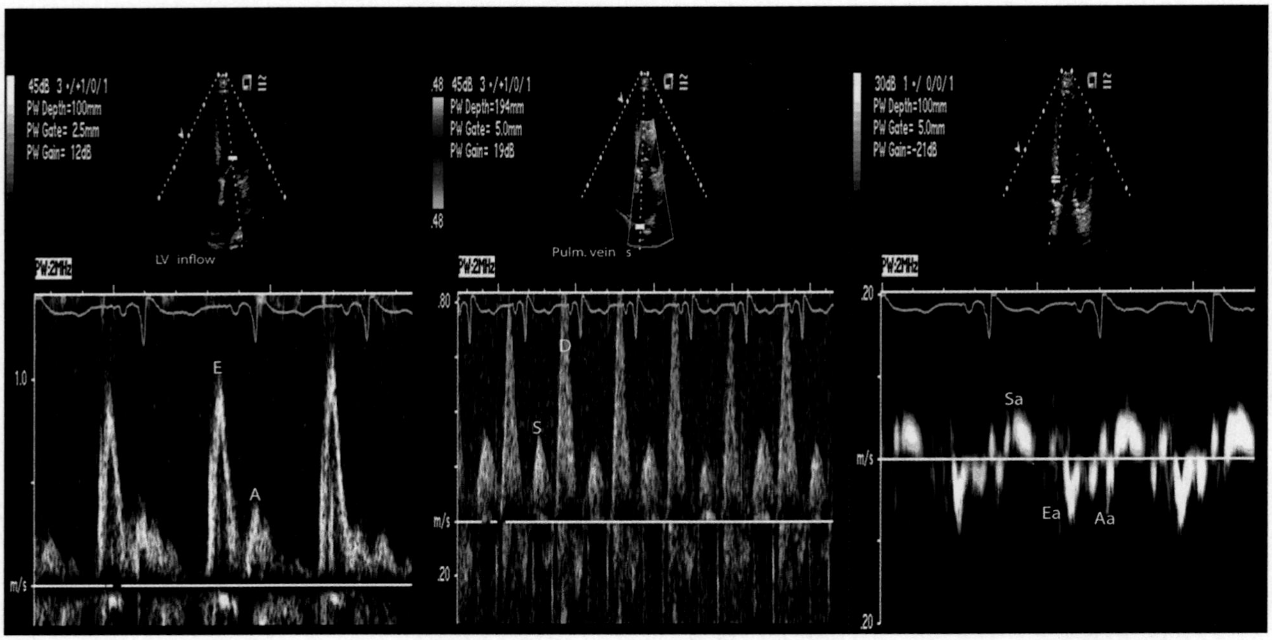

A B C

Figure 8-14. The filling patterns of restrictive physiology. **A,** Mitral inflow with tall E wave and markedly reduced A wave (E/A >3) with shortened deceleration time. **B,** Pulmonary vein pattern showing predominantly diastolic flow with rapid diastolic deceleration. **C,** Diminished tissue Doppler (TD) Ea wave.

reasonable accuracy in determining LV filling pressures and following the response to interventions such as diuresis or inotropic drugs. It has limited accuracy in patients with normal ejection fraction.[57] In these patients, clinical and echocardiographic data are needed to arrive at reliable estimates of filling pressures. Figure 8-15 is an algorithm that can be useful in these patients.

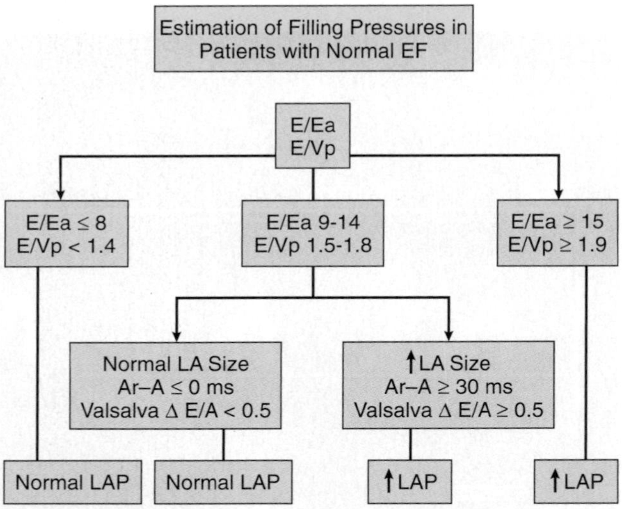

Figure 8-15. Algorithm for estimation of filling pressures in patients with normal ejection fraction. LA, left atrium; LAP, left atrial pressure.

Estimation of Pulmonary Arterial Pressures and Vascular Resistance

Peak pulmonary arterial systolic pressure is determined from the peak Doppler velocity (*v*) of tricuspid regurgitation (TR) by continuous wave (Fig. 8-16A). Using the modified Bernoulli equation, the peak systolic gradient (ΔP, in mm Hg) between the right ventricle and right atrium is given by $4v^2$ (where v is in m/s). An estimate of right atrial (RA) pressure is added to ΔP to estimate peak RV systolic pressure and, in the absence of pulmonic stenosis, peak pulmonary arterial systolic pressure.[61]

RA pressure can be estimated from the change in inferior vena cava diameter with spontaneous breathing, as recorded from subcostal views. Normal variation or collapse of the inferior vena cava with breathing implies normal RA pressure (0 to 5 mm Hg). Partial collapse is generally estimated at 5 to 10 mm Hg, whereas no (or only minimal) change in inferior vena cava diameter implies a RA pressure of 15 mm Hg or more. When available, RA pressure can be obtained directly from a central venous pressure tracing or estimated from the level of jugular venous distention. In addition, hepatic venous flow may be used, particularly in patients on mechanical ventilation. Similar to pulmonary venous flow, a high RA pressure is associated with decreased RA filling from the hepatic veins during systole (see Fig. 8-16C). This measurement has been shown to have a good correlation with invasively measured RA pressure.[62] When it is impossible to image the inferior vena cava and hepatic veins, tricuspid peak E velocity to tricuspid annulus Ea velocity may be used, provided that velocities are measured at end-expiratory apnea or as the average of five consecutive respiratory cycles.[63]

Mean pulmonary arterial pressure can be estimated from the acceleration time of the pulmonary arterial Doppler signal. The acceleration time is the time from

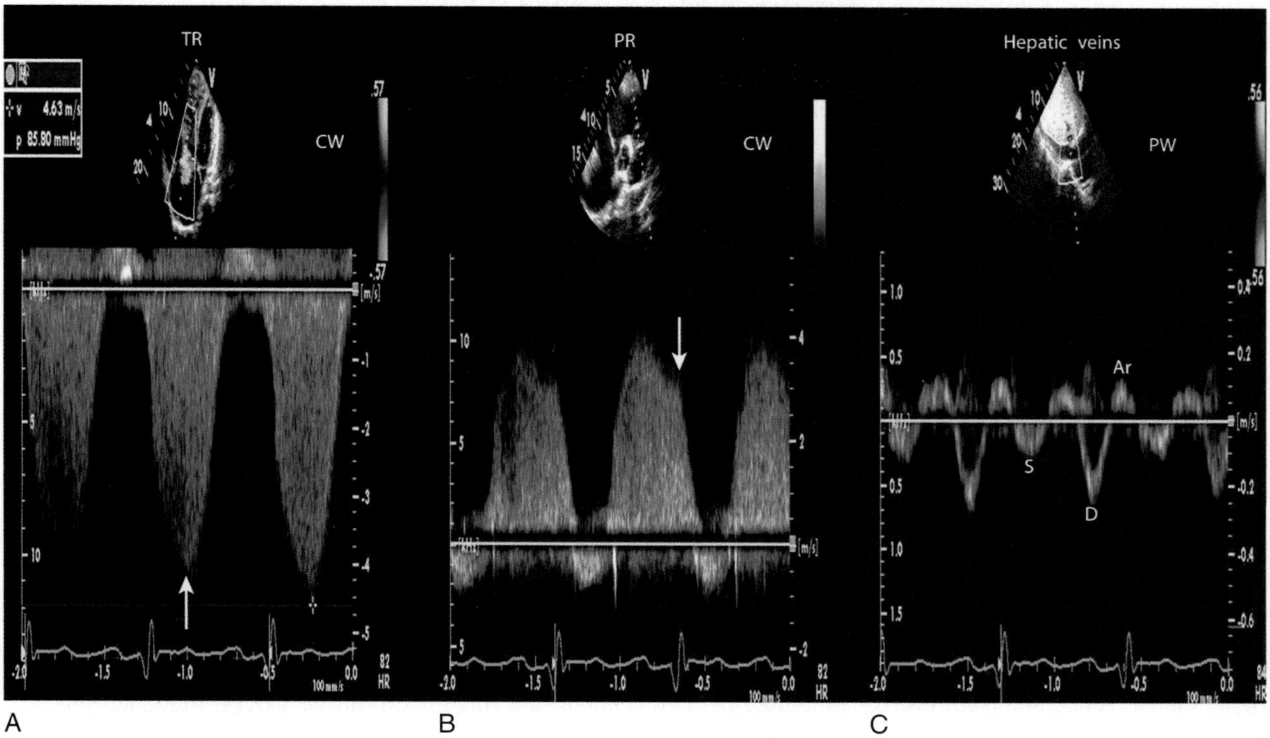

Figure 8-16. Assessment of pulmonary artery systolic pressure in a patient with primary pulmonary hypertension (PPH). **A,** Peak tricuspid regurgitation (TR) velocity *(arrow)* of 4.6 m/s yields RV – RA gradient of 86 mm Hg. **B,** Pulmonary regurgitation (PR) signal showing end-diastolic velocity of 3.1 m/s, yielding calculated gradient of 38 mm Hg. In this patient, the elevated pulmonary arterial diastolic pressure is due to PPH, not elevated left atrial pressure. **C,** Predominant diastolic hepatic vein flow consistent with elevation of right atrial pressure. CW, continuous wave Doppler; PW, pulsed wave Doppler.

onset to the peak of pulmonary arterial flow and is inversely proportional to mean pulmonary arterial pressure.[64] Acceleration time less than 100 ms usually indicates elevated mean pulmonary arterial pressure. Alternatively, the jet of pulmonic regurgitation (PR) can be used. With PR, mean pulmonary arterial pressure is given by $4\ v^2$ (where v is peak velocity of PR, measured in m/s).[65]

Pulmonary arterial end diastolic pressure is calculated again using the modified Bernoulli equation with the Doppler spectrum of PR to obtain the gradient between the pulmonary artery and right ventricle at end diastole (see Fig. 8-16B). The end diastolic gradient (ΔP, in mm Hg) between the pulmonary artery and right ventricle is given by $4v^2$ (where v is the end diastolic velocity of PR, measured in m/s). An estimate of RA pressure (see earlier) is added to ΔP to estimate pulmonary arterial end diastolic pressure.[66] Many patients in the ICU have an adequate PR signal for this calculation. This signal can be enhanced using intravenous contrast material, which may be indicated for other reasons (e.g., LV cavity opacification).

The ratio of peak tricuspid regurgitant velocity (in m/s) to RV outflow tract time velocity integral was shown to relate well with pulmonary vascular resistance.[67] It may be used to monitor noninvasively the effect of medical therapy in patients with pulmonary hypertension.

Assessment of Right Ventricular Function

Echocardiographic assessment of RV function is challenging because of its complex shape. It is possible to integrate information from multiple views, however, to reach reasonably accurate conclusions on RV size and function. The inflow area of the right ventricle is imaged from the parasternal position, the muscular portion from the apical transducer position, and the outflow tract from the parasternal short-axis and subcostal views. In the parasternal short-axis view, the right ventricle appears crescent-shaped, whereas in the apical four-chamber view, it is triangular with its base along the tricuspid valve. Several two-dimensional–based geometric models have been validated, but are seldom needed for routine clinical application. The assessment of RV size is usually done visually by comparing the RV with LV dimensions. In general, the RV dimensions are one third of the LV dimensions. As the right ventricle dilates, its free wall bulges, and in patients with moderate enlargement, the RV dimensions are almost equal to LV dimensions.

RV size is larger than LV size in patients with severe enlargement, with the right ventricle forming the cardiac apex. It is possible to measure RV end diastolic and end systolic dimensions and area in the apical four-chamber view. Caution should be exercised, however, to avoid tangential and foreshortened views. Normal RV dimension at the midventricular level in the apical four-chamber view is 2.7 to 3.3 cm. RV wall thickness is normally less than 0.5 cm and is most reliably measured by two-dimensional echocardiography in subcostal views at the level of the tricuspid valve chordae tendineae.[35] If needed, contrast enhancement may be used. During TEE, RV size can be assessed in the midesophageal four-chamber view.

RV systolic function is estimated qualitatively in clinical practice as normal or mildly, moderately, or severely depressed function. It also is possible to obtain a quantitative measurement of RV systolic function by measuring RV fractional area change (end diastolic area – end systolic area/end diastolic area) in the apical four-chamber view. This is a simple method with reasonable reproducibility and accuracy, and normal values range from 32% to 60%.[35] RV Tei index (TR duration – duration of systolic flow through the RV outflow tract/duration of systolic flow through the RV outflow tract) can be calculated as well, but it provides a combined assessment of RV systolic and diastolic function.[68] The tricuspid annulus motion can provide useful information in patients with suboptimal visualization of RV free wall. Normally, the tricuspid annulus descent is 1.5 to 2 cm. Additional information may be obtained by tissue Doppler–derived tricuspid annulus systolic velocity[69] and the acceleration rate of the systolic signal obtained during isovolumic contraction. More recently, strain and strain rate[70] measurements have been applied in many diseases that affect the right ventricle, such as congenital heart disease, pulmonary embolism, and idiopathic pulmonary hypertension. Their clinical application awaits additional improvements in the technique, however, to enhance its reproducibility and to show the incremental information provided over two-dimensional imaging and myocardial velocities.

Conditions of RV volume overload (e.g., atrial septal defect, severe TR or pulmonic regurgitation) result in diastolic flattening of the interventricular septum, which becomes rounded in systole. RV pressure overload (e.g., primary pulmonary hypertension, acute or chronic thromboembolic disease, cor pulmonale) results in systolic and diastolic flattening of the interventricular septum ("D" shape in systole and diastole) (Fig. 8-17).[71] Acute RV dilation can reduce LV filling through an increase in intrapericardial pressure, which reduces LV transmural filling pressure.[72] An acute decline in RV function is usually accompanied by RV dilation and decrease in RV systolic function in the presence of normal wall thickness. In the setting of an acute coronary syndrome, this may happen as a result of RV ischemia or infarction or both. The presence of normal or reduced pulmonary arterial pressures along with regional dysfunction can help identify these patients. Patients with chronic RV pressure overload (e.g., idiopathic pulmonary hypertension) often exhibit a dilated right ventricle with reduced contractility and increased wall thickness (Fig. 8-18) in the presence of increased pulmonary arterial pressures and vascular resistance.[73]

EVALUATION OF VALVULAR HEART DISEASE

Echocardiography provides important anatomic and physiologic information on cardiac valves. Valve morphology can be reliably assessed using two-dimensional and three-dimensional imaging. The presence of thickening and calcification of aortic valves and the presence of prolapse or flail (Fig. 8-19) or rheumatic deformity of the mitral valve can be readily identified. Secondary changes, such as chamber enlargement and left ventricular or right ventricular function, can be followed serially, enabling timely decisions with respect to surgery or percutaneous interventions. Using two-dimensional images and pulsed wave, continuous wave, or color Doppler, it is possible to assess

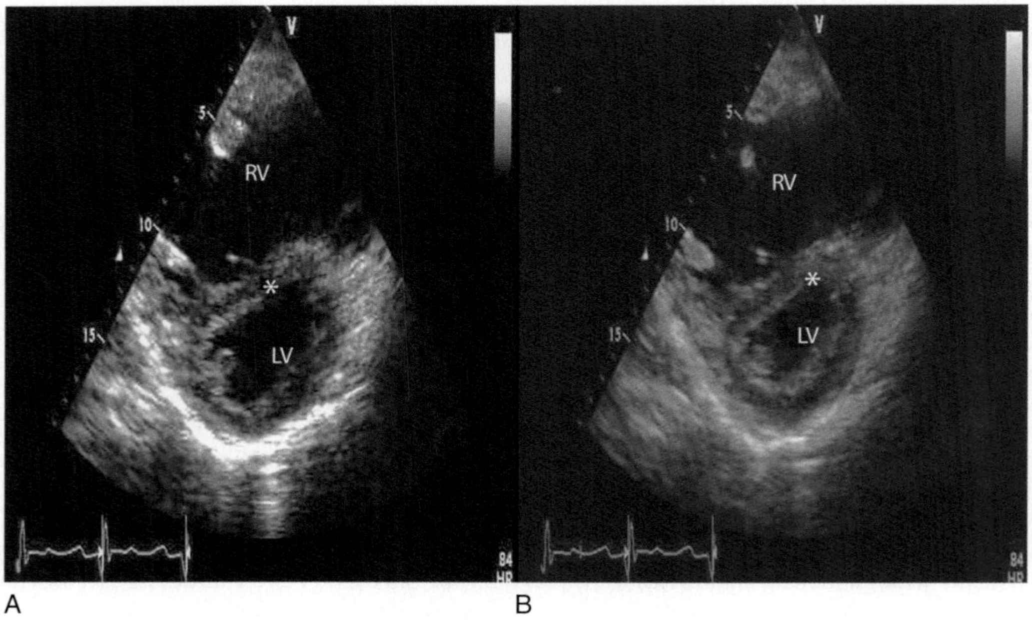

Figure 8-17. Short-axis view of the left ventricle showing D-shaped septum (*) at end diastole **(A)** and end systole **(B)** in a patient with pulmonary hypertension. LV, left ventricle; RV, right ventricle.

the severity of valvular stenosis or regurgitation and to calculate pulmonary arterial pressures. If needed, the hemodynamic data also can be obtained during exercise. The following sections address only the diagnostic applications of echocardiography in valvular heart disease; the reader is referred to other chapters for additional details on management issues. Many of the key points are summarized in Tables 8-1, 8-2, and 8-3.

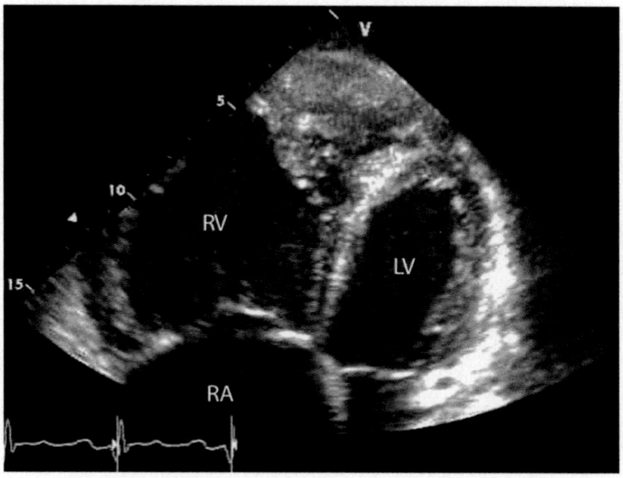

Figure 8-18. The right ventricle (RV) as imaged from the apex. Note markedly increased right ventricular size and significant right ventricular hypertrophy in a patient with pulmonary hypertension. Note relative reduced size of left ventricle (LV). RA, right atrium.

Evaluation of Mitral, Tricuspid, and Aortic Regurgitation

Similar principles apply to the assessment of MR, TR, and AR. Pulsed wave, continuous wave, and color Doppler are effective in identifying MR, TR, and AR and assessing their severity.[74] Color Doppler has a very high sensitivity in detecting physiologic lesions that have no clinical consequences; these lesions are not discussed any further. A standard examination includes the display of color-coded velocity maps in parasternal and apical views. Using these images, it is possible to identify the direction

Table 8-1. Assessment of Aortic Regurgitation Severity

	Mild	Moderate	Severe
Central jets: jet width by color Doppler/LVOT	<25%	25-64%	≥65%
Vena contracta	<0.3 cm	0.3-0.6 cm	>0.6 cm
Pressure half-time	>500 ms	200-500 ms	<200 ms
LV end-diastolic dimension	Normal	5-6 cm	>6 cm
Regurgitant volume	<30 mL	30-59 mL	≥60 mL
Regurgitant fraction	<30%	30-49%	≥50%
Regurgitant orifice area	<0.1 cm^2	0.1-0.29 cm^2	≥0.3 cm^2

LV, left ventricular; LVOT, left ventricular outflow tract.

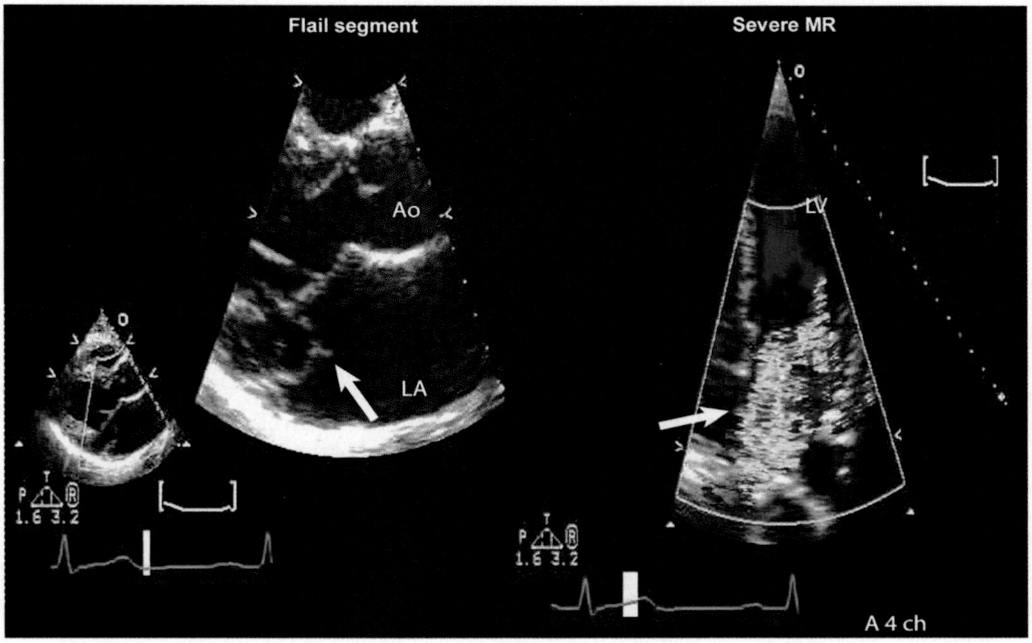

Figure 8-19. A, Parasternal long-axis view of flail posterior mitral leaflet *(arrow)*. **B,** Apical four-chamber view (A4ch) in the same patient showing severe eccentric mitral regurgitation (MR) *(arrow)*. The jet is directed anteromedially. *Note:* Color always moves in the direction *opposite* the affected leaflet. Ao, aorta; LA, left atrium; LV, left ventricle.

Table 8-2. Assessment of Mitral Regurgitation Severity

	Mild	Moderate	Severe
Central jets: jet area by color Doppler/LA area	<20%	20-39%	>40%
Vena contracta	<0.3 cm	0.3-0.69 cm	≥0.7 cm
Pulmonary veins	Predominant systolic	Blunted systolic	Systolic reversal
LA size	Normal	Normal or dilated	Dilated
LV size	Normal	Normal or dilated	Dilated
Regurgitant volume	<30 mL	30-59 mL	≥60 mL
Regurgitant fraction	<30%	30-49%	≥50%
Regurgitant orifice area	<0.2 cm^2	0.2-0.39 cm^2	≥0.4 cm^2

LA, left atrial.

Table 8-3. Assessment of Tricuspid Regurgitation Severity

	Mild	Moderate	Severe
Central jets: jet area by color Doppler	<5 cm^2	5-10 cm^2	>10 cm^2
Vena contracta	Not defined	Not defined, but <0.7 cm	>0.7 cm
PISA radius	≤0.5 cm	0.6-0.9 cm	>0.9 cm
RA size	Normal	Normal or dilated	Dilated
RV size	Normal	Normal or dilated	Dilated
Jet density	Soft	Dense	Dense
Jet contour	Parabolic	Variable	Triangular with early peak
Hepatic veins	Predominant systolic	Blunted systolic	Systolic reversal

PISA, proximal isovelocity surface area; RA, right atrial; RV, right ventricular.

and size of regurgitant jets. Color Doppler can have reasonable accuracy in assessing the severity of MR, TR, or AR when such jets have a central location. The severity of eccentric jets that spread along a given wall, rather than the middle of the receiving chamber, can be underestimated. In addition, several technical and physiologic factors can affect the size of the jet, regardless of the regurgitant volume, including color gain, pulse repetition frequency, filter settings, and atrial (or aortic) and ventricular pressures. It is important to record the systemic and pulmonary arterial pressures at the time of the echocardiographic examination. For MR and TR, the ratio of the jet area to LA or RA area has been used in clinical and research studies to assess these lesions. The method has reasonable accuracy in central (but not eccentric) jets when one pays attention to the aforementioned details. For AR, the width of the jet at its origin is related to that of the LV outflow tract to arrive at a ratio that expresses the severity of AR (Fig. 8-20). It is also possible to measure the cross-sectional area of the regurgitant jet by planimetry and relate that to the corresponding area of the LV outflow tract in the short-axis views.

The "vena contracta" of the regurgitant jet can be readily imaged and measured. This is the narrowest area of the jet that occurs at the orifice.[75] As the regurgitant volume increases, vena contracta width increases (Fig. 8-21), and clinical studies have shown it to be a useful parameter of the severity of regurgitant lesions. The flow convergence method is a quantitative approach that can measure the regurgitant volume and the regurgitant orifice area. Color flow mapping enables the visualization of the concentric hemispheres of flow as they approach the regurgitant orifice area. The regurgitant orifice area is calculated as:

$$6.28 \times r^2 \times V_a/V_{peak}$$

Where V_a is the aliasing velocity, r is the maximal radius of the proximal isovelocity surface area, and V_{peak} is the peak velocity of the regurgitant signal by continuous wave Doppler (Fig. 8-22). This method is most reliable when jets are centrally located, and the regurgitant orifice is adequately visualized.[76]

Aside from identifying the peak velocity of MR, TR, or AR, the continuous wave signal can provide potentially useful information because the brightness of these signals—compared with antegrade flow—increases with increasing severity of regurgitation. For patients with MR or TR, who have severe lesions and a rapid increase in LA or RA pressure resulting in large regurgitant "V" wave, early systolic peaking is seen (Fig. 8-23). For AR,

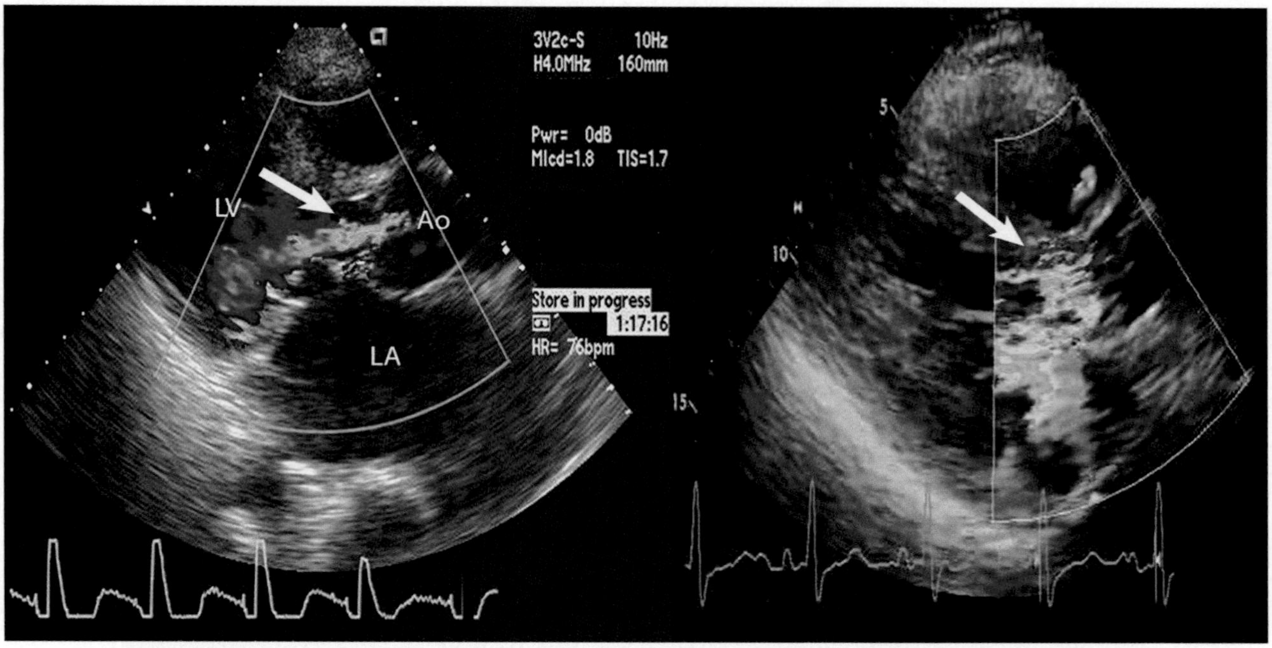

A B

Figure 8-20. A, Long-axis view of mild central aortic regurgitation (AR) *(arrow)*. **B,** Long-axis view of severe aortic regurgitation *(arrow)*, which fills the outflow tract. Ao, aorta; LA, left atrium; LV, left ventricle.

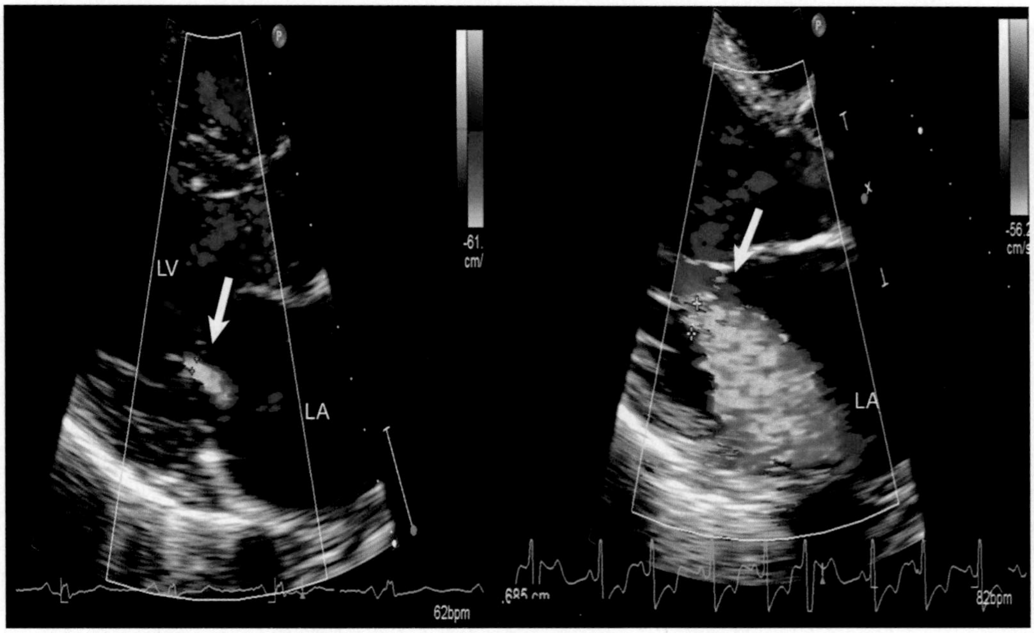

A B

Figure 8-21. Vena contracta measurements *(arrows)* of mild **(A)** and severe mitral regurgitation **(B).** LA, left atrium; LV, left ventricle.

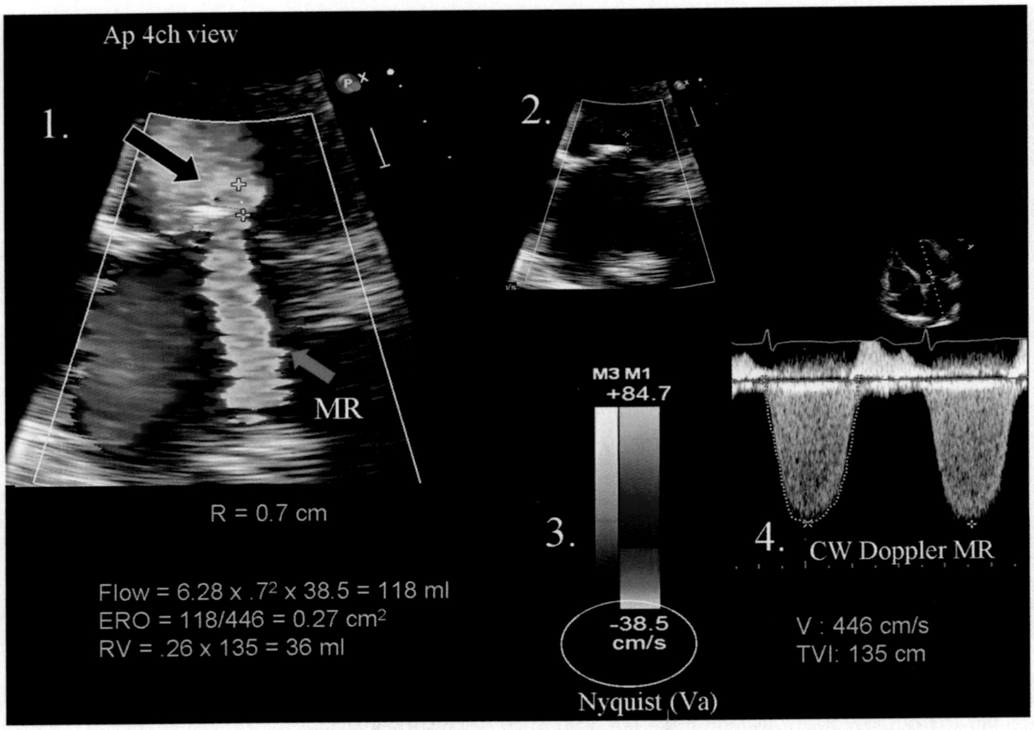

Figure 8-22. Moderate mitral regurgitation (MR) as calculated by the proximal isovelocity surface area method. *1,* Isolation and measurement of proximal color radius *(black arrow)*. *2,* Confirmation of caliper placement without color. *3,* Nyquist (Va) velocity. *4,* Continuous wave (CW) Doppler of MR velocity and time velocity integral (TVI). *Red arrow* indicates MR jet.

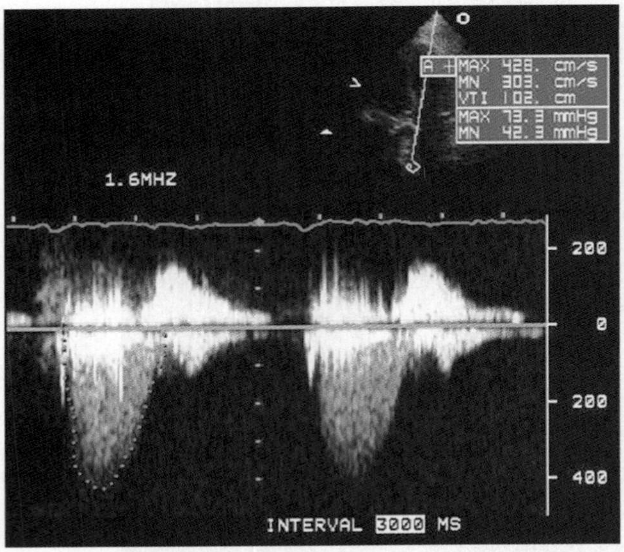

Figure 8-23. Spectral Doppler of severe mitral regurgitation. Note relatively low velocity, early peaking, and rapid fall-off of flow, consistent with marked elevation of left atrial pressure (big "V" wave).

the deceleration time (and pressure half-time spectral Doppler signal (Fig. 8-24) is related to the rate at which aortic and LV pressures equilibrate in diastole, such that patients with hemodynamically significant lesions exhibit a rapid increase in LV diastolic pressure, leading to steep deceleration of AR velocity signal. The pressure half-time is most reliable in cases with acute AR (Fig. 8-25) and may be prolonged in patients with chronic severe AR resulting from a concomitant increase in LV compliance.

Pulsed wave Doppler provides useful clues to assess the severity of regurgitant lesions. For MR and TR, peak early diastolic filling velocity (E velocity) is increased in the setting of significant regurgitation because of the increased transvalvular flow generated by the regurgitant volume. In severe MR, a peak E velocity greater than 1.2 m/s is usually present. In addition, pulmonary and hepatic venous flows show abnormalities in cases of severe MR (pulmonary flow) and TR (hepatic flow). The most reliable observation is systolic reversal of flow (Figs. 8-26 and 8-27), corresponding to the large regurgitant "V" wave in atrial pressure. Many patients may show only reduced (rather than reversal) antegrade systolic flow, however. The latter observation is nonspecific because it may be seen in cases of increased LA pressure or reduced LA compliance or both.

For AR, diastolic flow reversal is noticed in the descending aorta (see Fig. 8-25C). Normally, no brief flow reversal (or only a minimal amount) is seen in the descending aorta in early diastole. In patients with severe AR, holodiastolic flow reversal is observed.

Using pulsed wave spectral recordings, MR regurgitant volume can be calculated by subtracting aortic (or pulmonic) systolic flow from mitral diastolic inflow (see earlier section for flow calculation by Doppler). The difference between the two is the regurgitant volume, which can be divided by mitral diastolic flow to calculate

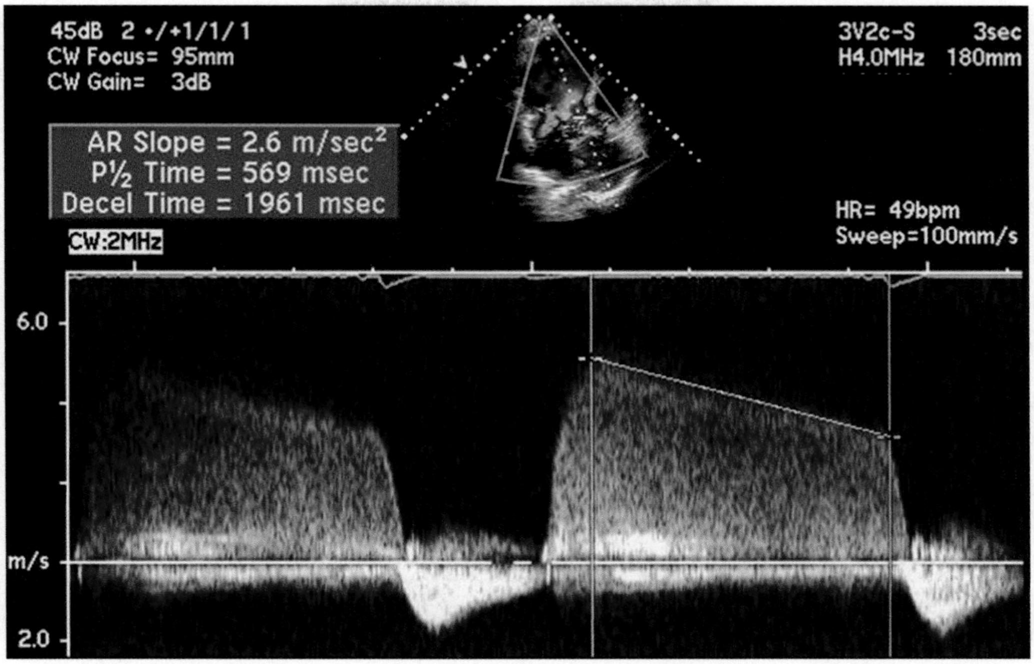

Figure 8-24. Example of online measurement of pressure half-time ($P^{1}/_{2}$ time) of continuous wave spectral Doppler of aortic regurgitation.

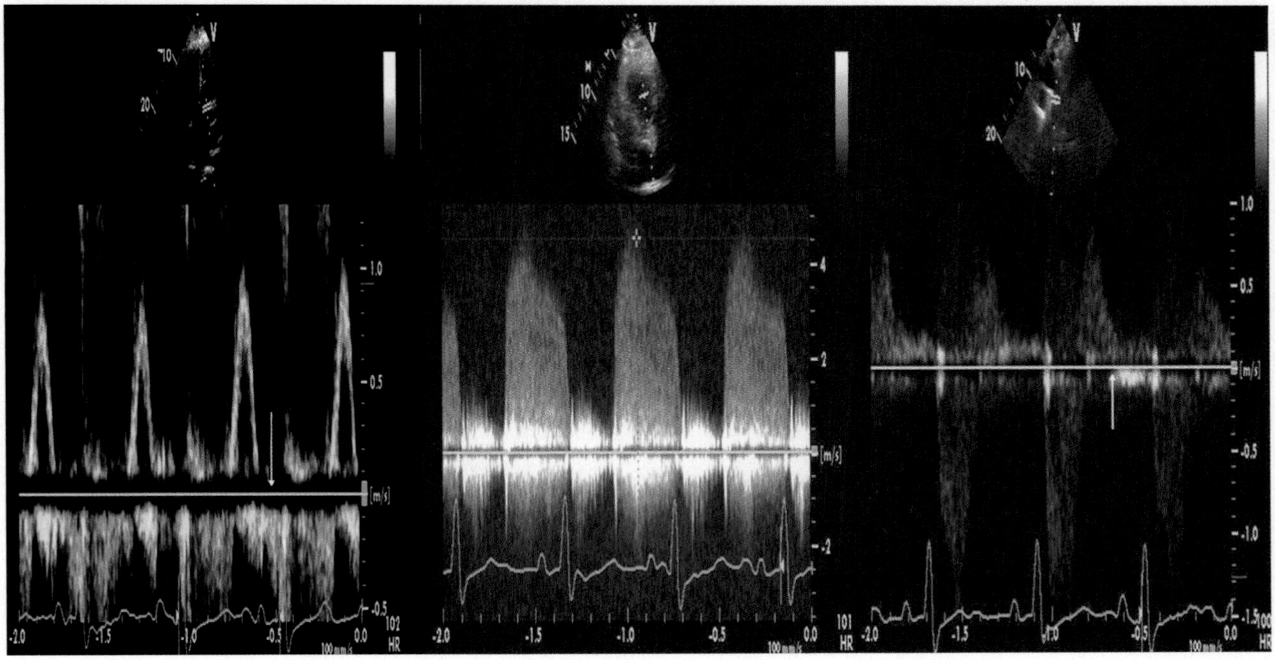

Figure 8-25. Acute aortic regurgitation secondary to infective endocarditis. **A,** Pulsed wave Doppler of mitral inflow (E/A waves merge owing to tachycardia) shows early termination of flow and diastolic mitral regurgitation *(arrow)*. **B,** Continuous wave Doppler of aortic regurgitation shows shortened pressure half-time secondary to elevated left ventricular end-diastolic pressure. **C,** Holodiastolic flow reversal *(arrow)* in the descending thoracic aorta.

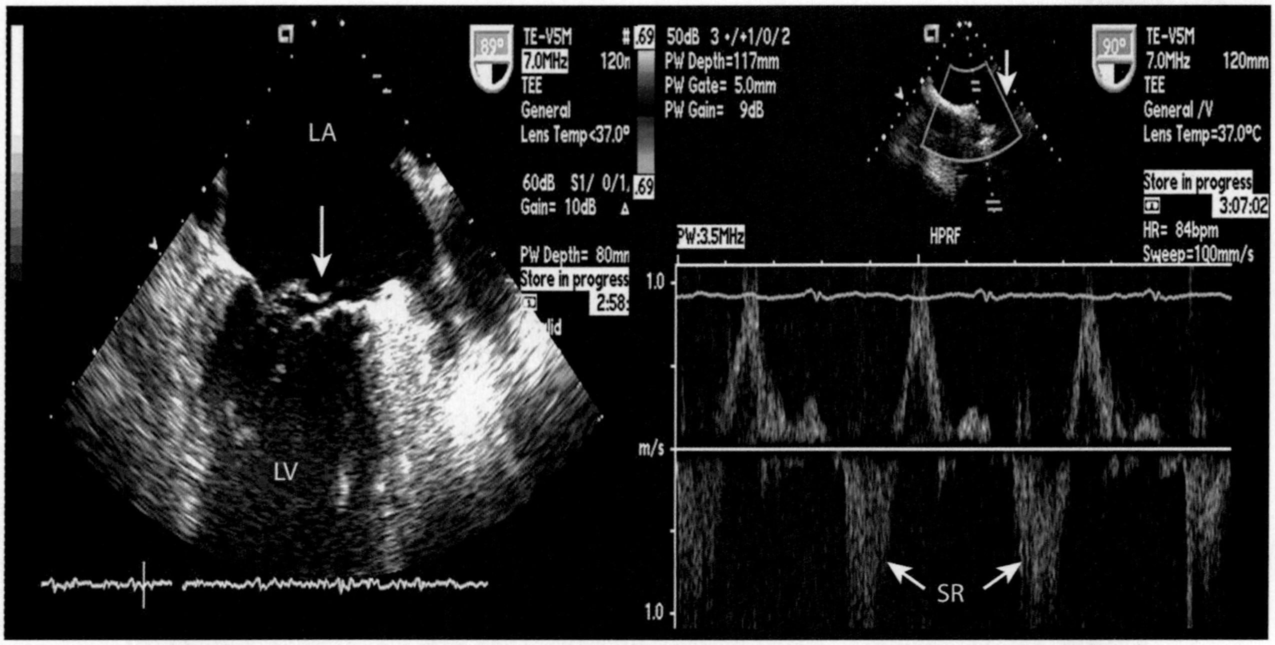

A B

Figure 8-26. **A,** Transesophageal image of flail posterior mitral leaflet *(arrow)*. **B,** Systolic flow reversal (SR) of left upper pulmonary vein. LA, left atrium; LV, left ventricle.

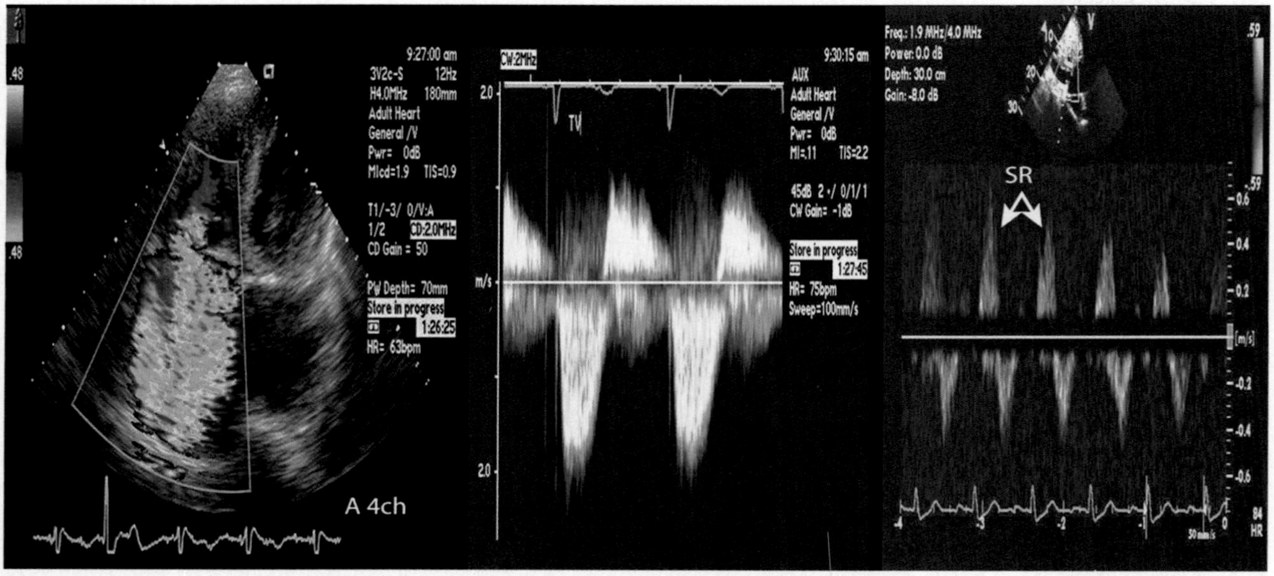

A B C

Figure 8-27. **A,** Color flow of severe tricuspid regurgitation (TR). **B,** Continuous wave Doppler (CW) signal of TR. Note comparable antegrade/retrograde densities of CW signal and the low velocity (2 m/s), early peaking, and rapid fall-off, all consistent with increased right atrial pressure. **C,** Systolic reversal (SR) of hepatic vein flow. A4ch, apical four-chamber view.

MR regurgitant fraction (Fig. 8-28). Similarly, it is possible to compute AR regurgitant volume by subtracting mitral (or pulmonic) flow from aortic systolic flow (Fig. 8-29). This method is most accurate, however, when applied by experienced echocardiographers, and failure to measure the annulus diameter correctly or failure to trace the modal velocity in the pulsed wave spectral tracing correctly may lead to major errors in quantification.

In arriving at the final conclusions, it is important to integrate all of the findings obtained by two-dimensional and Doppler echocardiography.[74] Patients with chronic severe regurgitant lesions usually have dilation of the cardiac chambers (for MR, left atrium and left ventricle; for TR, right atrium and right ventricle; for AR, left ventricle) along with a large regurgitant volume. Unless one is dealing with a case of acute regurgitation, normal

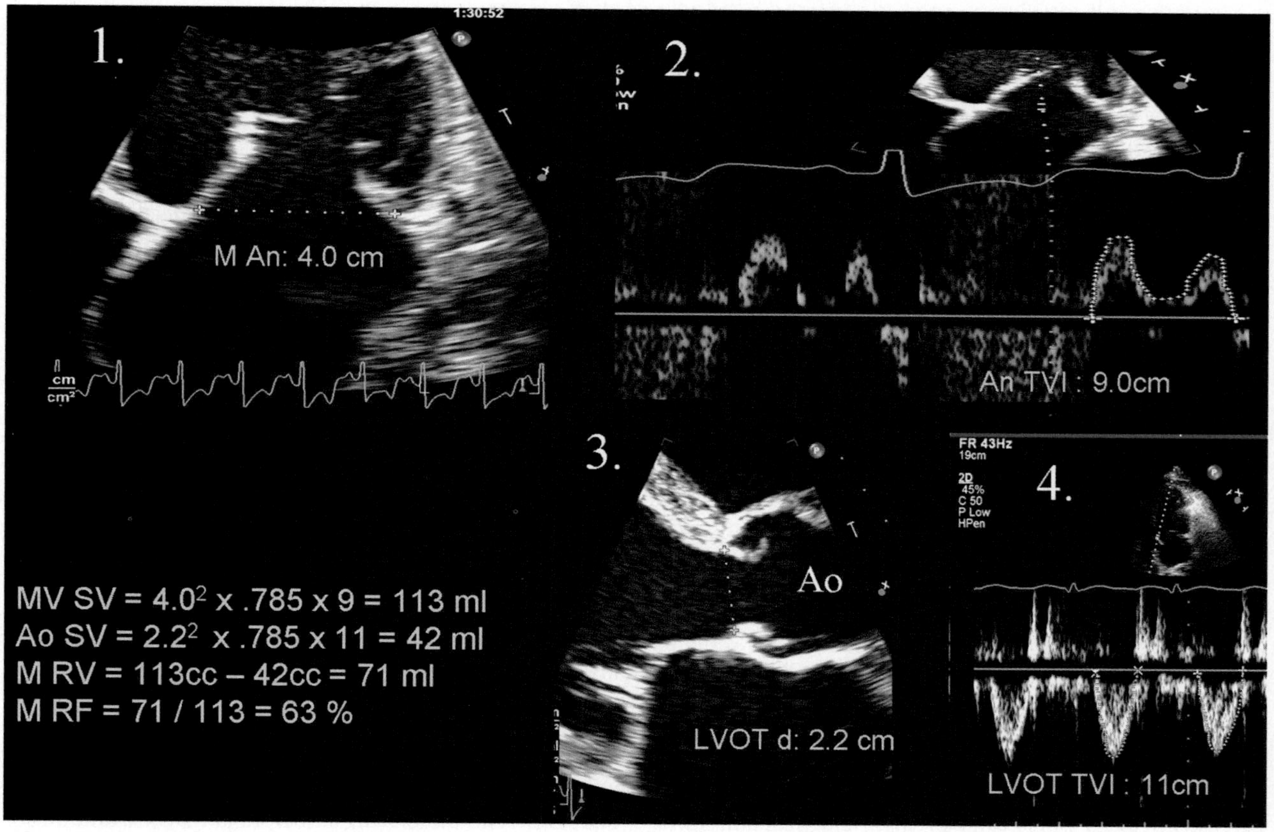

Figure 8-28. Calculation of mitral regurgitant fraction in a patient with severe mitral regurgitation. *1,* Measurement of mitral annulus from apical four-chamber view. *2,* Time velocity integral (TVI) of annular flow. *3,* Measurement of left ventricular outflow tract (LVOT) diameter. *4,* TVI of LVOT. RF, regurgitant fraction; RV, regurgitant volume.

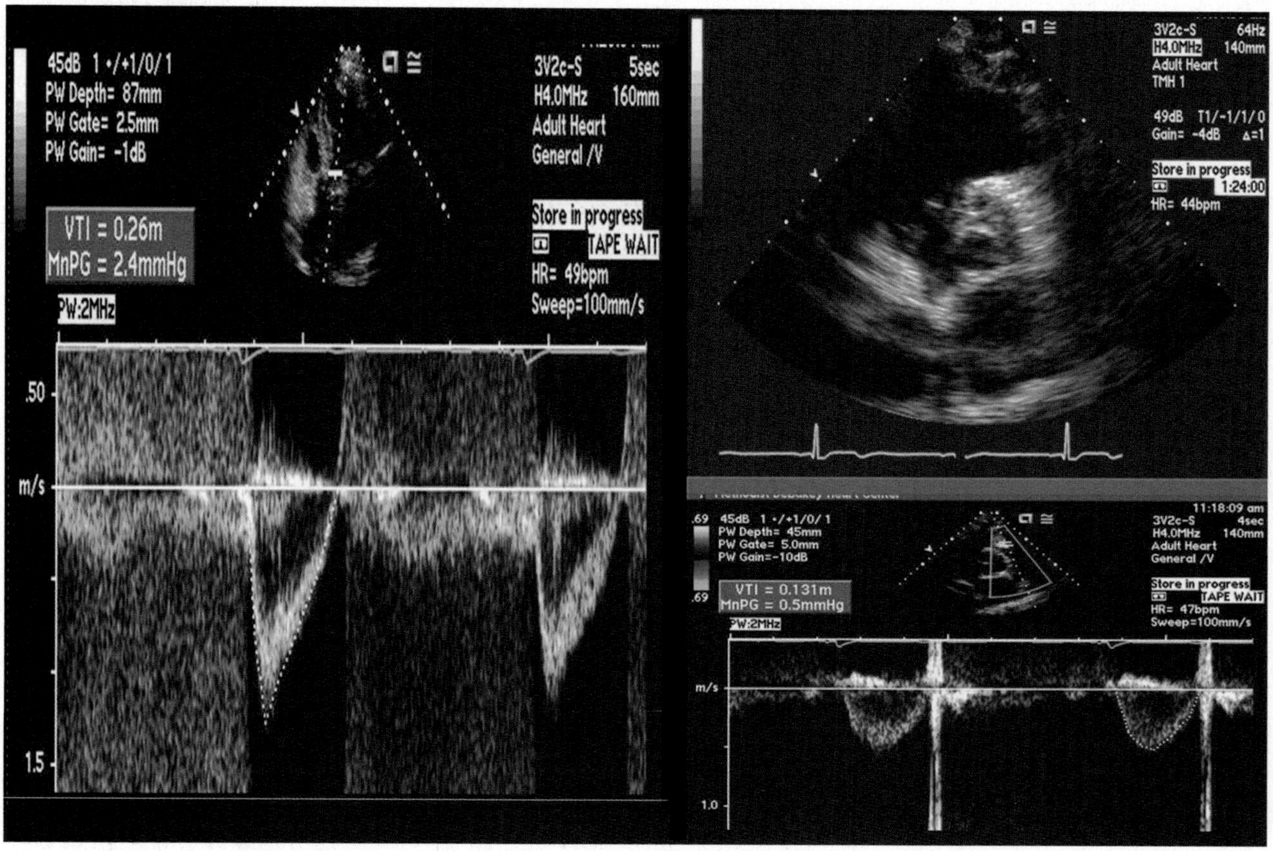

Figure 8-29. Calculation of aortic regurgitant volume in a patient with moderate aortic regurgitation (AR), using aortic and pulmonary forward flow. Calculation of left ventricular stroke volume: $3.14 \times 26 = 82$ mL. Calculation of right ventricular stroke volume: $4.15 \times 13.1 = 54$ mL. Calculation of regurgitant volume and regurgitant fraction (RF): 82 cc − 54 cc = 28 cc; 28/82 = 34%. Conclusion: AR Vol = 28 mL; RF = 34%.

chamber dimensions should negate the diagnosis of a severe lesion.

If the quality of the transthoracic images precludes the assessment of valvular pathology or the severity of MR or AR, it is reasonable to proceed to TEE. Given the anterior location of the tricuspid valve, TEE is seldom needed for the evaluation of TR. All of the aforementioned methods can be applied to quantify regurgitant lesions imaged by TEE. With respect to MR assessment by TEE, given the proximity of the TEE probe to the left atrium, MR jet area can be larger than that acquired by transthoracic imaging. To avoid overestimation of MR severity, it is advisable to consider only the high-velocity signals in the MR jet for planimetry. In addition, TEE can provide unique information that is essential for successful mitral valve repair.

Evaluation of Aortic Stenosis

Patients with aortic stenosis have abnormally thickened or calcified (or both) valve leaflets along with reduced leaflet excursion seen by two-dimensional echocardiography, including TEE. Some patients have the disease as part of progressive valvular degeneration with age, and most of these patients have three cusps. Aortic stenosis and AR also can develop in patients with bicuspid aortic valves, however, which can be readily diagnosed in short-axis views of the aortic valve during systole. In addition to morphologic changes of the aortic valve, two-dimensional imaging is needed to determine LV dimensions, wall thickness, and ejection fraction. These data are essential to assess the impact of aortic stenosis on LV function, which is needed as part of the routine evaluation of patients with this disease.

Aortic stenosis severity is assessed most reliably by the mean transvalvular systolic pressure gradient across the aortic valve and valve area, both of which are measured by Doppler echocardiography. Using the modified Bernoulli equation ($\Delta P = 4v^2$), the peak and mean gradients across the aortic valve can be calculated from the continuous wave Doppler signal. An excellent correlation was observed between invasive and Doppler measurements of mean gradient when both measurements were simultaneously obtained.[77] Technical requirements to achieve these results include proper alignment of the ultrasound beam with aortic flow, which necessitates the use of the stand-alone (Pedoff) continuous wave transducer, multiple imaging windows (apical, right parasternal, subcostal, and suprasternal), and intravenous contrast agents when weak Doppler signals are recorded (Fig. 8-30). Patients with a mild degree of aortic stenosis may develop increased velocity and gradient when the transvalvular flow rate is increased because of AR or the development of a hyperdynamic state. Likewise, patients with severe aortic stenosis may have lower than expected gradients with intravascular volume depletion or severely depressed ejection fraction. It is important to calculate the aortic valve area.

Aortic valve area is calculated using the continuity equation. The underlying principle is that the amount of blood flow through the LV outflow tract and aortic valve would be the same because they are in continuity.[78] Aortic valve area (in cm^2) is given by systolic flow through LV outflow tract/time velocity integral of aortic stenosis signal by continuous wave (LV outflow tract diameter^2 × 0.785 × LV outflow tract time velocity integral/aortic time velocity integral). The main source of error in this calcula-

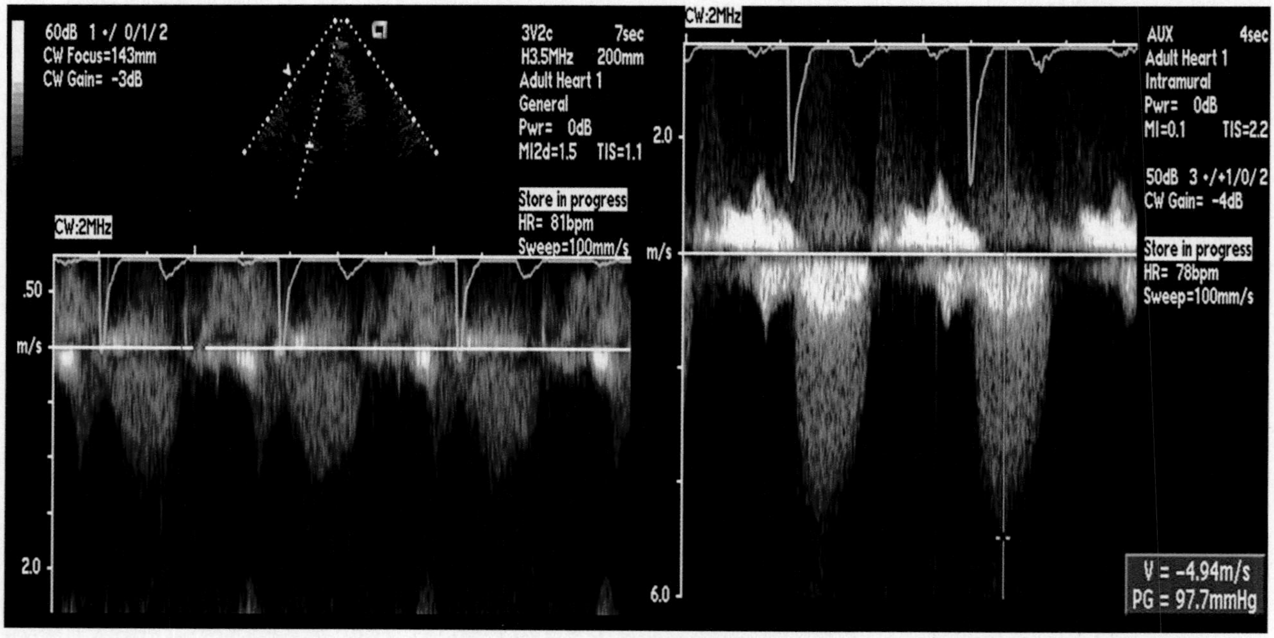

A B

Figure 8-30. Weak continuous wave Doppler signals across the aortic valve **(A).** After injection of contrast material to visualize the left ventricle better, markedly increased velocities (peak gradient 98 mm Hg) across the aortic valve were identified **(B).**

tion is in the measurement of the LV outflow tract diameter. When there is doubt, and in the absence of other significant valvular lesions, it is possible to use systolic flow through the RV outflow tract or diastolic mitral inflow in the numerator. Alternatively, LV stroke volume measured by two-dimensional echocardiography (difference between end diastolic and end systolic volumes) may be used, provided that adequate two-dimensional images are present.

Some patients with severely depressed ejection fraction have only mildly or modestly elevated transvalvular gradients across the aortic valve, but tight aortic stenosis when the valve area is calculated (typically <1 cm^2) (Fig. 8-31). It is reasonable to proceed to low-dose (≤20 μg/kg/min) dobutamine echocardiography in these patients to assess not only LV contractile reserve, but also the effect of increased transvalvular flow on the calculated aortic valve area.[79] Patients with dobutamine-induced increase in aortic valve area (>1 cm^2) are unlikely to have real aortic stenosis, but their reduced valve area is largely the result of reduced flow rate. When there is an increase in gradient, but still a severely reduced aortic valve area, valvular surgery should be considered because LV function and clinical status are likely to improve after valve replacement.

Evaluation of Mitral Stenosis

In patients with rheumatic mitral stenosis, two-dimensional imaging shows the presence of valvular thickening and calcification along with abnormal leaflet mobility, such that there is doming of the anterior mitral leaflet along with reduced mobility of the posterior leaflet. The anterior leaflet has a classic "hockey-stick" deformity when viewed in the parasternal long-axis view (Fig. 8-32A), and variable degrees of subvalvular pathology are usually present (Fig. 8-32B). Direct planimetry of mitral valve area is feasible in cases in which the mitral valve orifice is well visualized in the parasternal short-axis view. This measurement can be inaccurate, however, when there is extensive calcification of valve leaflets, and when the short-axis plane is not positioned correctly at the level of valve tips. Color Doppler shows the proximal isovelocity surface area hemispheres on the LA side of the mitral valve during diastole (Fig. 8-33).

Doppler echocardiography can provide a reliable measurement of the transmitral pressure gradient and mitral valve area in most patients with mitral stenosis (Fig. 8-34). Current ultrasound systems have the capability to measure online peak and mean transvalvular gradients, using the modified Bernoulli equation (see earlier). Doppler-derived gradients have been shown to have excellent reproducibility and accuracy compared with the simultaneously obtained LA-LV pressure gradient by cardiac catheterization. The transmitral pressure gradient depends on many variables, however, other than the valve area. The mean gradient can be increased with high transvalvular flow rate (owing to a hyperdynamic flow state or MR) or short R-R interval, even though mitral stenosis is only of a mild degree.

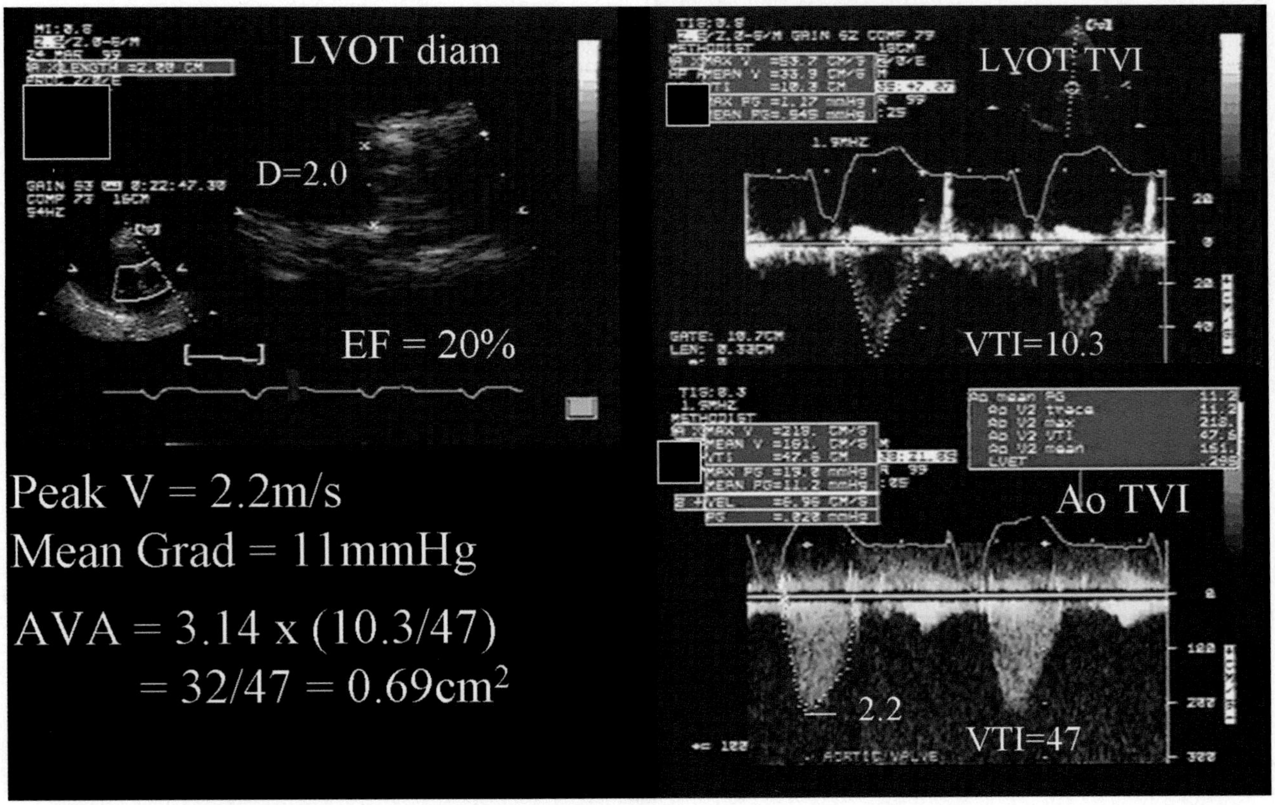

Figure 8-31. Assessment of aortic stenosis in a patient in class III heart failure. Although the mean gradient is only 11 mm Hg, the calculated valve area is 0.69 cm^2. In this setting, the use of dobutamine may be useful. Ao, aorta; AVA, aortic valve area; EF, ejection fraction; LVOT, left ventricular outflow tract; TVI, time velocity integral.

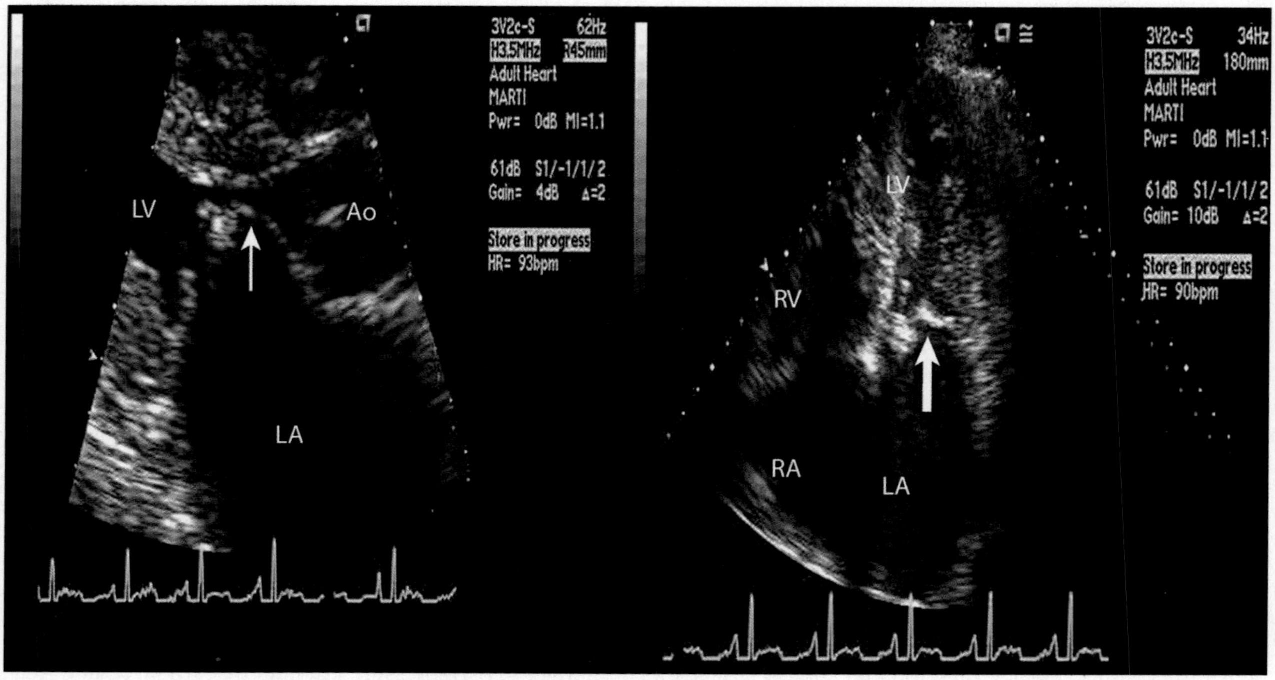

Figure 8-32. **A,** Typical rheumatic deformity of the mitral valve, showing "hockey-stick" appearance of anterior leaflet and relatively immobile posterior leaflet. **B,** Calcium involves the mitral leaflets as seen from the apex *(arrow)*. Ao, aorta; LA, left atrium; LV, left ventricle; RA, right atrium; RV, right ventricle.

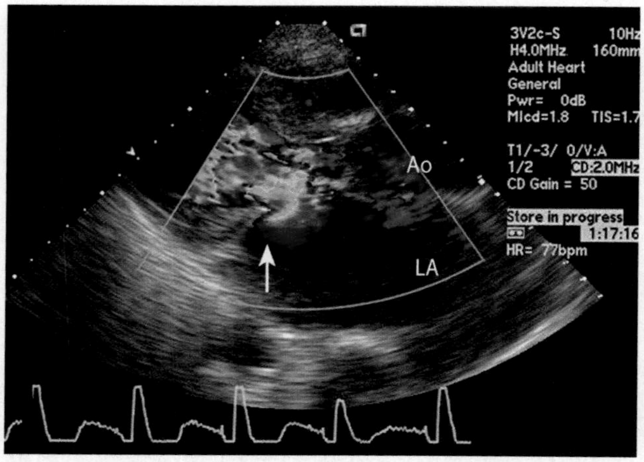

Figure 8-33. Parasternal long-axis view of a stenotic mitral valve showing flow acceleration by color (proximal isovelocity surface area [PISA]) on the atrial side of the valve *(arrow)*. Ao, aorta; LA, left atrium.

Mitral valve area is most easily calculated by Doppler, using the pressure half-time method. This method originally was conceived in the cardiac catheterization laboratory.[80] In essence, the severity of the stenosis is judged based on the time needed for the transmitral pressure gradient to decrease by 50% from its initial value in early diastole. This time increases with the severity of the stenosis and mitral valve area (in cm^2) and can be derived as 220/pressure half-time (in ms). Although simple and highly reproducible, its accuracy is limited in patients with abnormal LA or LV compliance (or both) and patients with significant AR.[81] The continuity equation is an additional method that is applicable in cases without significant AR and MR. In this method, the mitral valve area is given by systolic flow through the LV outflow tract/time velocity integral of mitral stenosis jet by continuous wave.

In cases in which there is a discrepancy between symptoms and echocardiographic findings at rest, it is reasonable to perform stress echocardiography using a supine bike protocol to determine the transmitral pressure gradient and the pulmonary arterial systolic pressure with exercise. Patients with an exercise-induced increase in transvalvular pressure gradient (>15 mm Hg) and pulmonary arterial systolic pressure (>60 mm Hg) can be referred to percutaneous or surgical interventions.

Evaluation of Prosthetic Valves

Echocardiography is the test of choice to assess prosthetic valve function.[82,83] From transthoracic windows, it is possible to identify the type of the prosthetic valve—tissue or mechanical. In some cases, large vegetations or thrombi may be visualized. In many situations, the size of these and the image resolution is such that TEE is needed. Reliable recording of transvalvular gradients is possible by Doppler in almost all cases, provided that the ultrasound beam is parallel to the direction of flow (Fig. 8-35). Prosthetic valve gradients should be interpreted with the knowledge of the valve type, size, and position because mean values vary depending on these variables. Consideration should be given to transvalvular flow

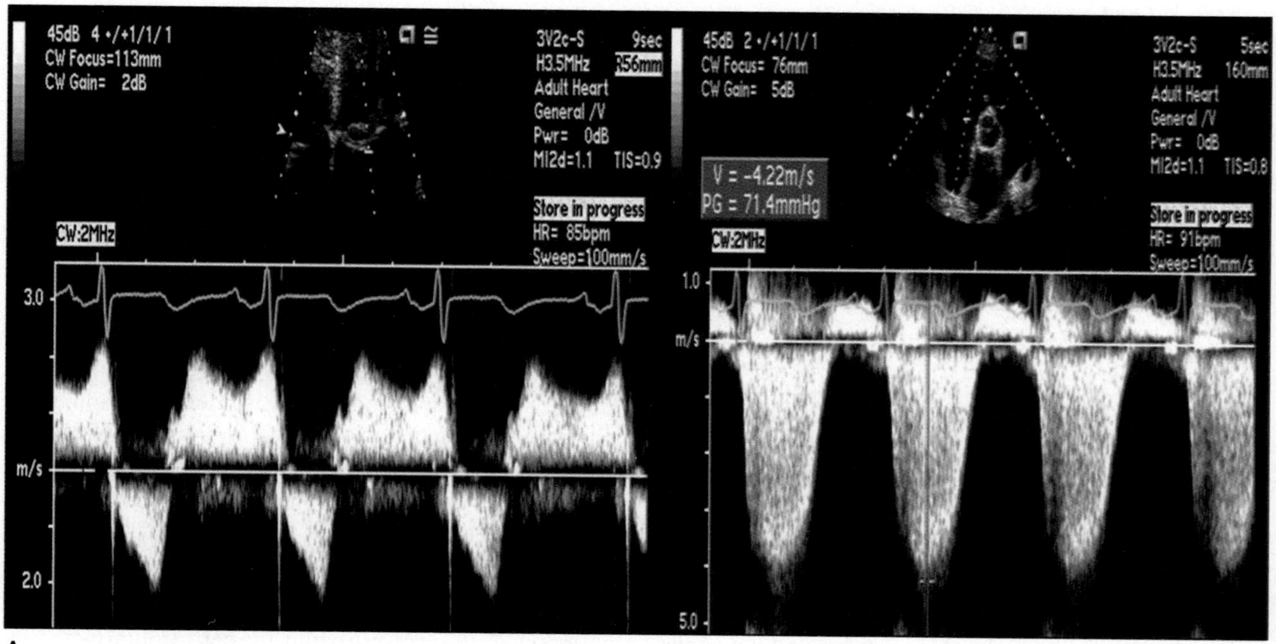

A B

Figure 8-34. **A,** Continuous wave (CW) Doppler display of mitral stenosis. Peak velocity is 2.2 m/s; time velocity integral, 67 cm; mean gradient, 11 mm Hg; and mitral valve area, 1.3 cm^2, at a heart rate of 85 beats/minute. **B,** Tricuspid regurgitant signal from same patient showing secondary pulmonary hypertension and a calculated right ventricular systolic pressure (RVSP) of at least 81 mm Hg, assuming a right atrial pressure of at least 10 mm Hg. TR, tricuspid regurgitation.

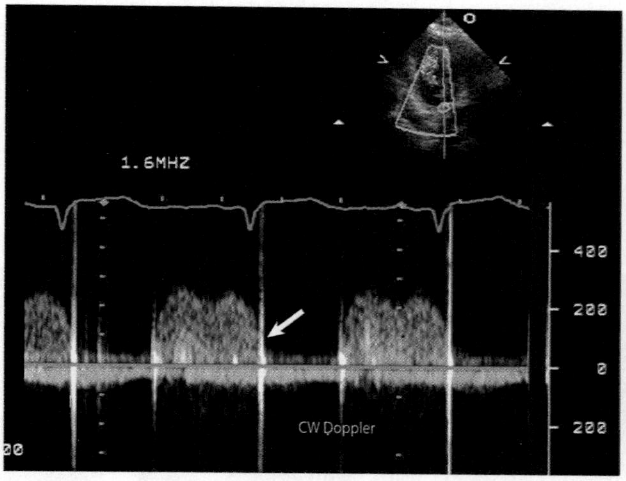

Figure 8-35. Continuous wave (CW) Doppler of an obstructed mechanical mitral valve prosthesis. Peak velocity is 2.5 m/s; time velocity integral, 80 cm; mean gradient, 18 mm Hg; heart rate, 93 beats/minute. *Arrow* indicates mitral closing click.

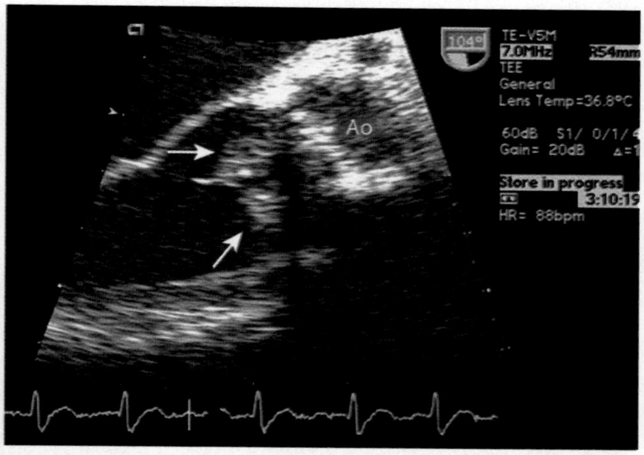

Figure 8-36. Transesophageal echocardiography image of vegetations *(arrows)* on prosthetic aortic valve. Ao, aorta.

rate and R-R interval when conclusions are drawn about prosthetic valve function. It is useful to compare Doppler-derived gradients with previous results (taking into consideration flow and heart rates) in detecting possible changes in prosthetic valve function over time. For prosthetic aortic valves, the Doppler velocity index is calculated as peak velocity in LV outflow tract/ peak velocity across the valve by continuous wave Doppler. Patients with normal function have a ratio ≥0.25. This ratio is particularly helpful in patients with increased transvalvular flow rate leading to increased mean gradient because they also would have an increased flow velocity in the LV outflow tract and a normal Doppler velocity index.[84]

When there is doubt about structural or functional abnormalities of prosthetic valves, TEE should be considered because it is possible with TEE to visualize small-sized thrombi or vegetations (Fig. 8-36) and to assess leaflet thickening and mobility. A pannus or thrombus may result in reduced or absent leaflet motion and prosthetic valve stenosis. Depending on the thrombus burden and the clinical status of a patient, TTE and TEE may be used to guide and follow the response to intravenous thrombolytic therapy. Although the severity and etiology of prosthetic valve regurgitation may not be easily determined by TTE because of acoustic shadowing, TEE is extremely useful in evaluating the degree of regurgitation and in identifying the site of origin and direction of perivalvular leaks. In contrast to prosthetic mitral valves, adequate visualization and Doppler interrogation of prosthetic aortic valves can be challenging by TEE. If doubt remains, one should consider biplane fluoroscopy to assess the mobility of aortic valve discs.

ECHOCARDIOGRAPHY IN DISEASES OF THE PERICARDIUM

The detection of pericardial effusion generated much of the early interest in ultrasound as a useful cardiac diagnostic tool.[85] Echocardiography is routinely used today to diagnose and manage pericardial disease. Pericardial effusion, tamponade, and, to a lesser extent, pericardial constriction can be readily and reliably assessed with echocardiography.

On two-dimensional echocardiography, findings of pericardial effusion include an echo-free space adjacent to the heart and absence of pericardial motion. Effusions are termed small, moderate, and large based on the visually estimated volume of fluid, its location (posterior only or circumferential), and the size of the heart relative to the size of the fluid space (Fig. 8-37). Particularly large free-flowing effusions occasionally may result in "swinging" of the heart within the pericardial space, a phenomenon that correlates with the electrical alternans noted on the ECG.[86] Loculated pericardial effusions can be identified in post–cardiac surgery patients and in patients who sustain trauma to the chest. In these circumstances, the effusion is localized (typically by adhesions) to a single area of the pericardial space. Although loculated effusions may appear to be small in volume, it is important to identify these accumulations because an opportunistic small volume of fluid in a critical location may rapidly result in hemodynamic compromise. Localized organizing hematoma in postoperative or post-trauma patients can create a compressive effect similar to that of free-flowing fluid (Figs. 8-38 and 8-39).

Pericardial tamponade occurs when, in the presence of fluid* accumulating in the pericardial space, the pressure in the pericardium exceeds the pressure in the cardiac chambers, resulting in impaired filling and reduction of stroke volume and cardiac output, eventuating in tachycardia, hypotension, and jugular venous distention.[87] The physiologic consequences depend on the amount of fluid, the rate of accumulation, the distensibility of the pericardium, and the compliance of cardiac chambers.[88]

There are several echocardiographic features of pericardial tamponade. Pericardial effusion, usually at least moderate in volume, must be present (rarely does tamponade physiology result from pneumopericardium or mediastinal mass). As the pressure within the pericardium increases, cardiac chamber collapse ensues.[89] Impairment of filling is sequential: The atria collapse before the higher pressure ventricles.[90] The compressive effect of fluid is seen when the pressure is lowest in the chamber; RA collapse begins in late ventricular diastole (before or at the P wave) and should persist through at least one third of ventricular systole (see Fig. 8-37). RA collapse occurs early in the course of tamponade, but is a less specific marker than collapse of the right ventricle because the thin-walled

*Tamponade may result from accumulation of fluid, pus, blood, clots, or gas within the pericardium.

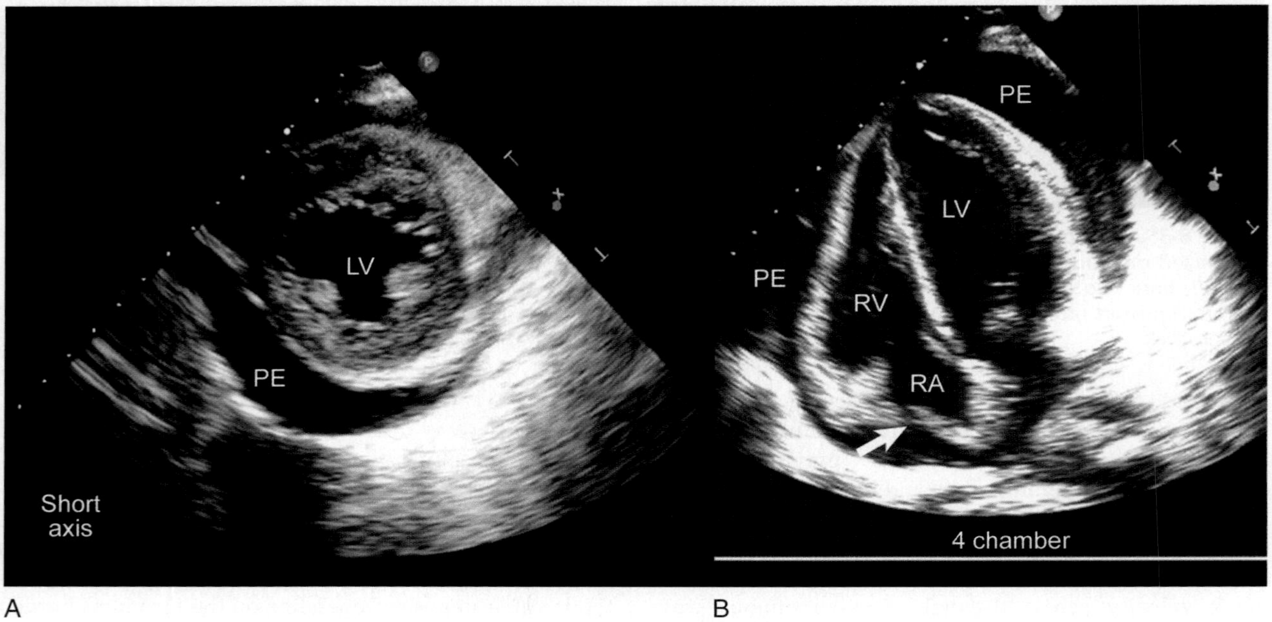

Figure 8-37. Large pericardial effusion from the short axis **(A)** and the apex **(B)**. Note right atrial collapse *(arrow)*. LV, left ventricle; PE, pericardial effusion; RA, right atrium; RV, right ventricle.

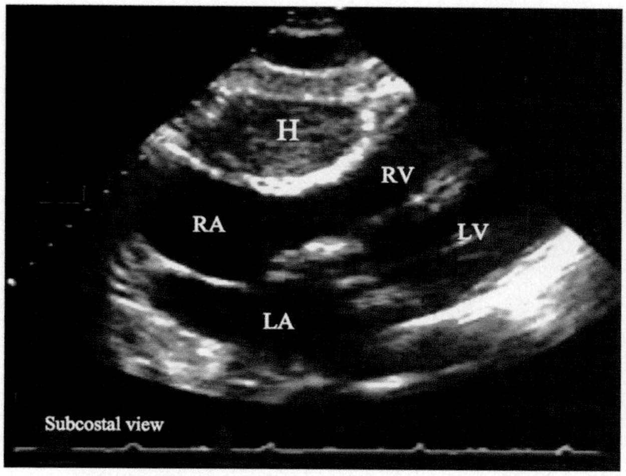

Figure 8-38. Subcostal image of a post-traumatic *pericardial* hematoma (H). LA, left atrium; LV, left ventricle; RA, right atrium; RV, right ventricle.

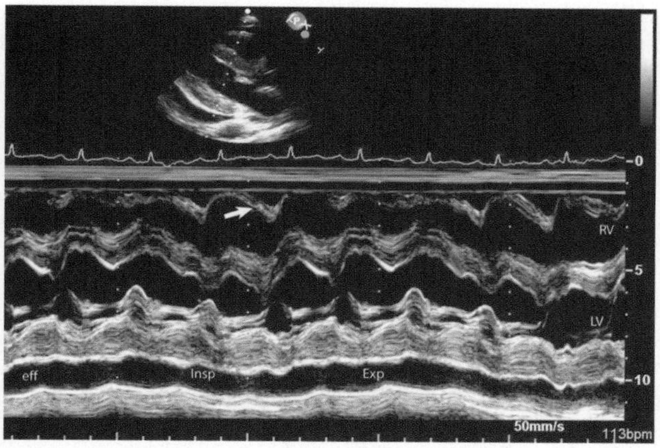

Figure 8-40. M-mode of left and right ventricles in pericardial tamponade. Note right ventricular diastolic collapse *(arrow)*. eff, effusion; Exp, expiration; Insp, inspiration; LV, left ventricle; RV, right ventricle.

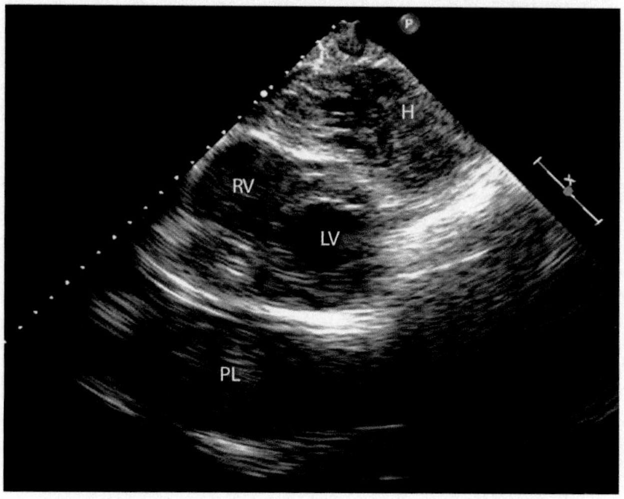

Figure 8-39. Short-axis view of a post-traumatic *mediastinal* hematoma (H). This patient with hematoma and the patient with hematoma in Figure 8-38 had tamponade physiology. It may be difficult to distinguish a pericardial from a mediastinal process with echocardiography alone. LV, left ventricle; PL, pleural effusion; RV, right ventricle.

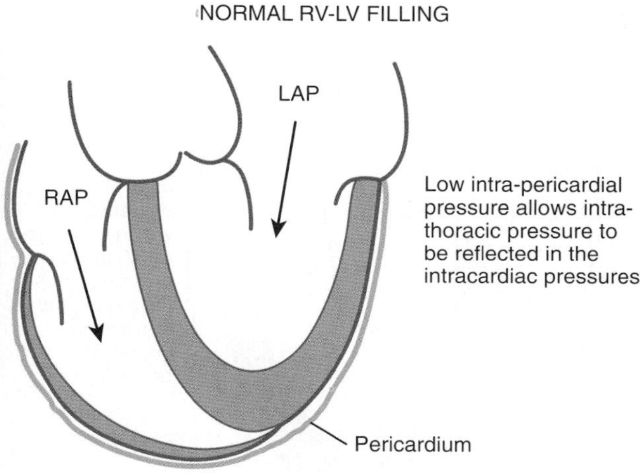

Figure 8-41. Diagram of normal ventricular filling. LAP, left atrial pressure; RAP, right atrial pressure; RV-LV, right ventricle–left ventricle. (Courtesy of Miguel Quinones, MD, Methodist DeBakey Heart Center.)

right atrium can invert in the absence of tamponade when there is intravascular volume depletion. RV collapse occurs in early diastole.[91] This finding manifests later in the continuum, but is probably more specific for significant hemodynamic compromise.[92] RV collapse is best appreciated when the ultrasound beam is perpendicular to the RV outflow tract from a subcostal or parasternal short-axis view (Fig. 8-40). Timing of the onset and duration of collapse can be appreciated with M-mode. Right heart chamber collapse may be absent when tamponade occurs in the setting of severely elevated right heart filling pressures, left-to-right shunting, or RV ischemia.[93] In this setting, additional hemodynamic assessment may be needed. When the effusion is loculated behind the left ventricle in the setting of reduced LV volumes, as might be seen in postoperative patients, diastolic collapse of the left ventricle may be the only indicator of hemodynamic compromise.

Reciprocal respiratory changes in RV and LV volumes become evident in tamponade, and increased right heart filling occurs at the expense of left heart filling in a process mediated by the pericardium. RV volume increases with inspiration, shifting the septum toward the left ventricle in diastole and toward the right ventricle in systole. RV volume decreases with expiration, normalizing septal motion as LV filling increases (Figs. 8-41, 8-42, and 8-43). These findings correspond to the clinical finding of pulsus paradoxus. Transvalvular Doppler flow velocities show respirophasic changes in tamponade as well.[94] Initial transmitral velocities are enhanced with expiration and diminished (>25%) with inspiration in tamponade; transtricuspid flow augments with inspiration and diminishes with expiration. Correspondingly, the RV outflow time velocity integral increases with inspiration, whereas the

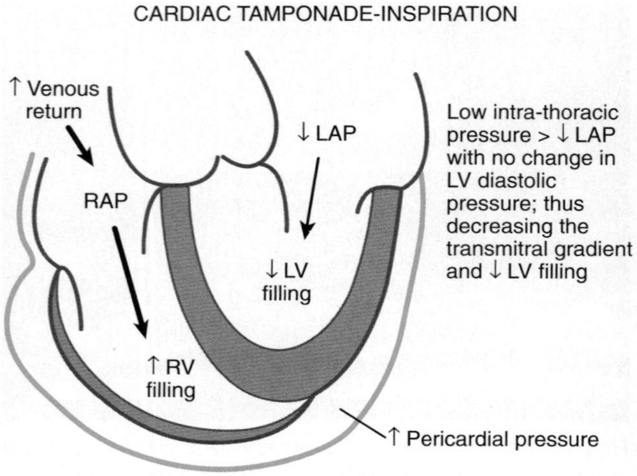

Figure 8-42. Alterations in left ventricular and right ventricular filling with inspiration in pericardial tamponade. LAP, left atrial pressure; LV, left ventricle; RAP, right atrial pressure; RV, right ventricle. (Courtesy of Miguel Quinones, MD, Methodist DeBakey Heart Center.)

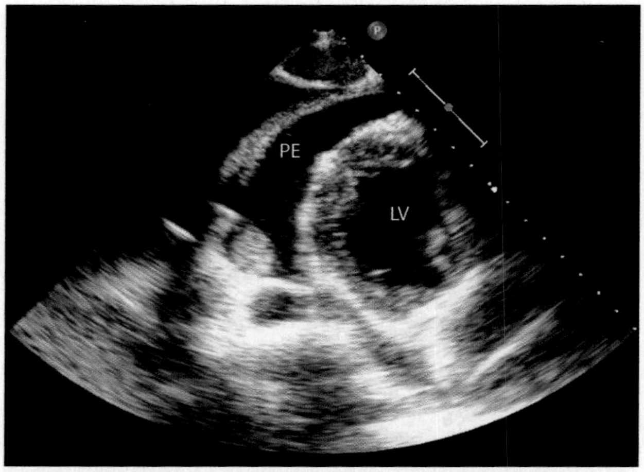

Figure 8-44. Echocardiogram during pericardiocentesis, before injection of saline. LV, left ventricle; PE, pericardial effusion.

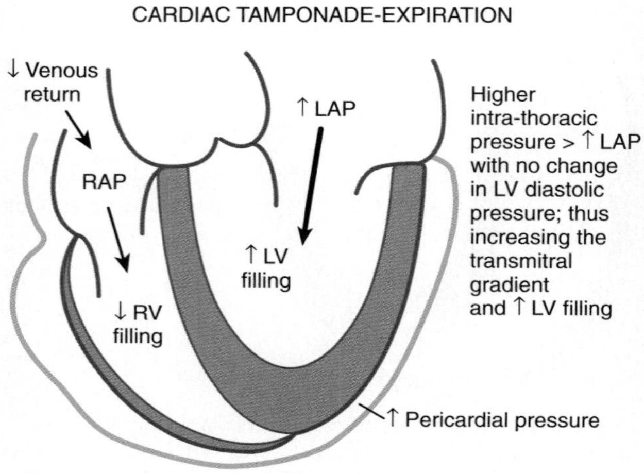

Figure 8-43. Ventricular filling pattern in cardiac tamponade during expiration. LAP, left atrial pressure; LV, left ventricle; RAP, right atrial pressure; RV, right ventricle. (Courtesy of Miguel Quinones, MD, Methodist DeBakey Heart Center.)

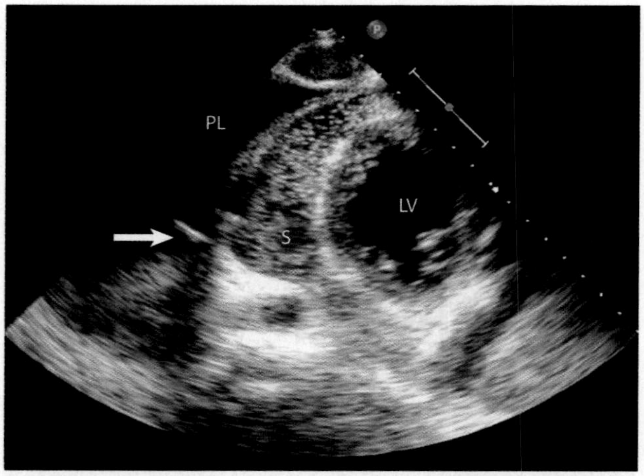

Figure 8-45. Echocardiogram in the same patient from Figure 8-44 after injection of saline to confirm location of needle *(arrow)* in pericardial space. LV, left ventricle; PL, pleural space; S, saline.

LV outflow time velocity integral decreases. These are useful findings, but can be difficult to show with precision in an acutely ill patient.

As in pulsus paradoxus, conditions other than tamponade can cause prominent respirophasic changes in transvalvular flow velocities, including obstructive airway disease and constrictive pericarditis. These entities are distinguished from tamponade by the absence of a pericardial effusion. As noted, Doppler evidence for tamponade can be absent in patients with atrial septal defects when RV and LV filling are equal.

Echocardiography has been used to guide the percutaneous drainage of pericardial fluid.[95] Subcostal imaging is valuable in showing the amount of inferior fluid in the typical location accessed by the subxiphoid needle approach and determining the optimal site of puncture. Imaging from the cardiac apex in patients with large circumferential effusions can aid in determining needle position and guide advancement, although identifying the needle tip occasionally can be problematic. When needle position is deemed appropriate, and the initial aspirate is obtained, an injection of a small amount of agitated saline confirms correct needle position within the pericardium[96]; this is an especially important maneuver to distinguish intracardiac from intrapericardial positioning when the fluid is sanguineous (Figs. 8-44 and 8-45). Echocardiography also confirms resolution or persistence of pericardial fluid.

Constrictive physiology is operant when the visceral and parietal layers of the pericardium become adherent and fibrotic, resulting in marked impairment of LV filling. Chronic constrictive pericarditis is usually not associated with free pericardial fluid. The echocardiographic findings in constriction include a thickened pericardium (pericardial thickening may not be uniform), normal LV size, abrupt termination of ventricular filling in early diastole (best seen on M-mode), interventricular septal motion showing a diastolic inward "bounce" in early diastole, and dilation of the inferior vena cava. In addition, there is Doppler flow evidence of ventricular interaction with exaggerated respirophasic changes in transvalvular velocities, similar to the changes noted in tamponade (Fig. 8-46).

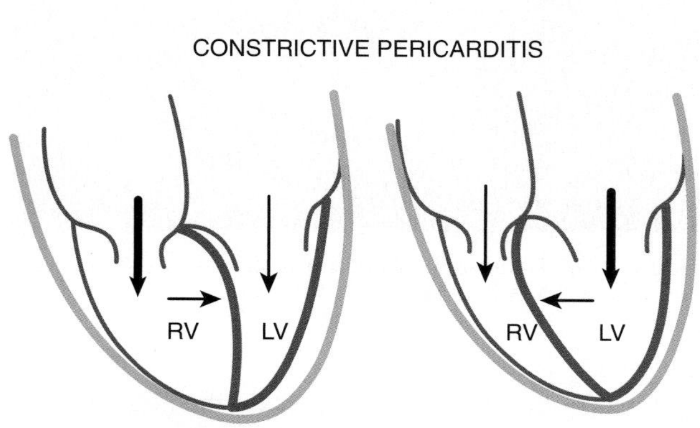

Figure 8-46. Ventricular interdependence in constrictive pericarditis. LV, left ventricle; RV, right ventricle. (Courtesy of Miguel Quinones, MD, Methodist DeBakey Heart Center.)

Tissue Doppler evaluation of diastolic filling is useful in distinguishing between pericardial constriction and restrictive cardiomyopathy because there is commonly substantial overlap of spectral Doppler findings in these entities because both share features of limited or restrictive ventricular diastolic filling. Data suggest that the mitral annulus early diastolic velocity (Ea) by tissue Doppler is usually higher in patients with constrictive pericarditis (Fig. 8-47) than in patients with primary restrictive cardiomyopathy because the rate of LV relaxation is impaired in patients with restrictive cardiomyopathy.[97,98]

Evaluation of Aortic Trauma and Dissection

Although TEE is the preferred method for evaluating the aorta, transthoracic imaging can visualize the proximal ascending aorta and occasionally can identify an intimal flap, either from the parasternal views or from the suprasternal notch. In addition, TTE can evaluate the integrity of the aortic valve and quantify the degree of AR, can recognize any LV wall motion abnormalities (but in this setting TTE cannot distinguish between primary ischemia and ischemia secondary to coronary extension of the dissecting flap), and can identify any associated pericardial effusion. The sensitivity of TTE for the diagnosis of dissec-

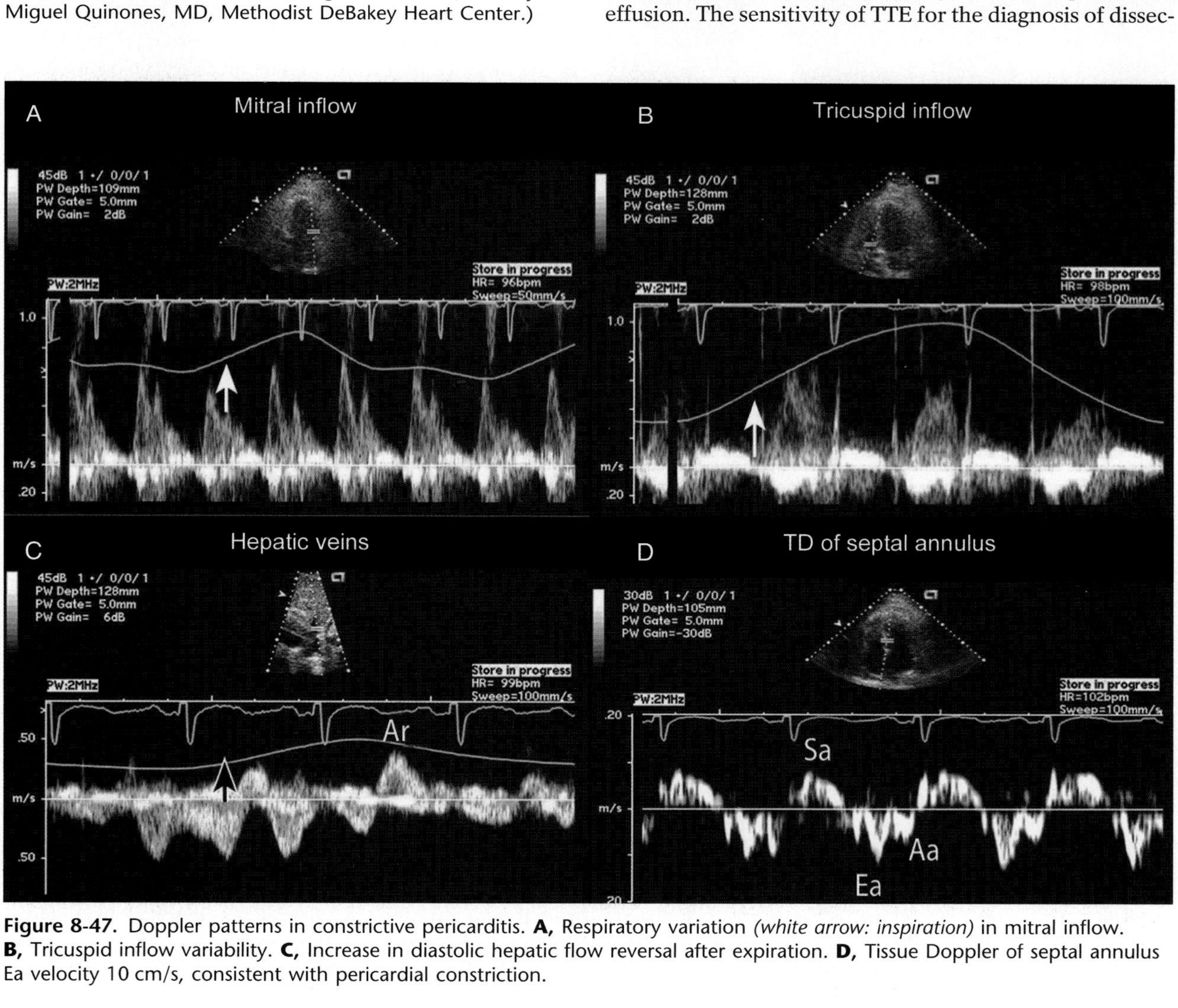

Figure 8-47. Doppler patterns in constrictive pericarditis. **A,** Respiratory variation *(white arrow: inspiration)* in mitral inflow. **B,** Tricuspid inflow variability. **C,** Increase in diastolic hepatic flow reversal after expiration. **D,** Tissue Doppler of septal annulus Ea velocity 10 cm/s, consistent with pericardial constriction.

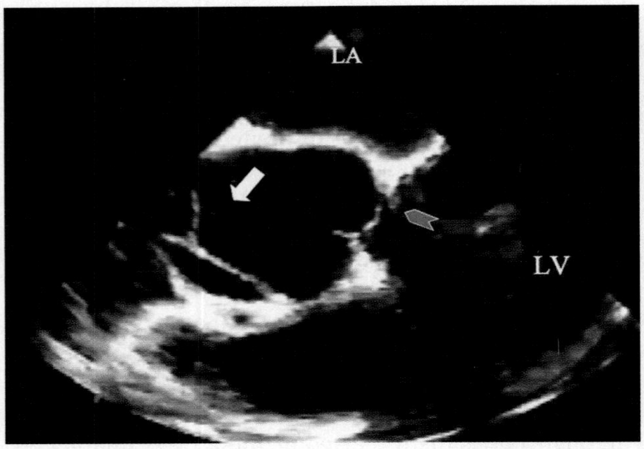

Figure 8-48. Transesophageal echocardiography image of discrete intimal flap of proximal aortic dissection *(arrow)*. *Red arrow* indicates aortic valve. LA, left atrium; LV, left ventricle.

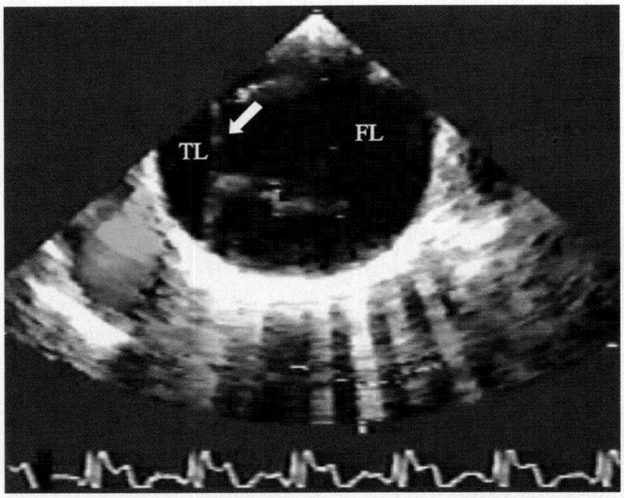

Figure 8-49. Transesophageal echocardiography of flap of aortic dissection *(arrow)* showing entry sites with color flow from true (TL) to false lumen (FL).

tion is quite low, however, and a negative transthoracic study does not exclude dissection.

The close proximity of the esophagus to the aorta makes TEE the superior modality for the evaluation of aortic dissection, with sensitivity and specificity of 98%.[99-103] The ascending aorta, aortic arch, and descending thoracic aorta can be visualized with excellent resolution. TEE can be performed rapidly and safely at the bedside. Particular attention must be given to ensuring adequate sedation to avoid hypertension, tachycardia, or gagging in patients with suspected dissection. Common features of dissection on TEE imaging include the following:

- An intimal flap that moves toward the false lumen in systole (Fig. 8-48)
- Color Doppler flow in the true lumen and the false lumen
- Color flow identification of entry and exit sites (Fig. 8-49)

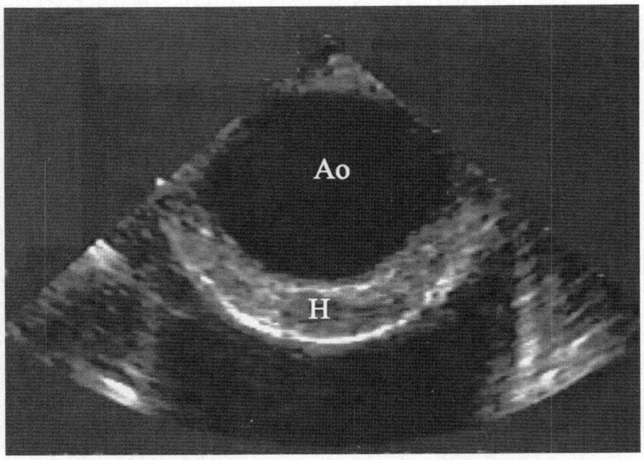

Figure 8-50. Transesophageal echocardiography of intramural hematoma (H). Ao, aorta.

- Stasis or thrombosis or both within the false lumen
- Intramural hematoma (Fig. 8-50)

Intramural hematoma, originally described as bleeding into the outer layers of the aortic media caused by rupture of the vasa vasorum without a primary tear, appears as crescentic thickening of the aortic wall greater than 0.7 cm in the absence of a frank dissection flap.[104] Considered a variant of overt aortic dissection, intramural hematoma is an important diagnosis to make. Data from the International Registry of Aortic Dissection suggest intramural hematoma is a lethal condition when it involves the ascending aorta, and 16% of patients with intramural hematoma have evidence of evolution to classic aortic dissection on serial imaging.[105,106]

TEE also is useful in the evaluation of the aorta after blunt injury, usually a result of high-speed deceleration accidents.[107,108] Traumatic disruption of the aorta usually involves the region of the aortic isthmus, the aortic segment between the left subclavian and the first intercostal arteries. Blunt injuries that can be identified by TEE include more minor localized hematoma, limited intimal flaps, and mural thrombus, injuries not requiring surgical intervention, and significant subadventitial rupture or complete transsection, injuries that require urgent surgical intervention. Subadventitial disruption commonly shows a localized "thick medial flap" on TEE in association with significant change in the contour of the isthmus, or complete rupture with pseudoaneurysm formation can be seen.

Cardiac Source of Systemic Emboli

Seventeen percent to 25% of all strokes are cardioembolic in origin.[109] Echocardiography, particularly TEE, is commonly used to search for potential cardiac sources of arterial emboli (Figs. 8-51 and 8-52), among the most significant of which are atrial fibrillation with LA and LA appendage thrombus, atheromatous disease of the aorta, and patent foramen ovale with or without atrial septal aneurysm (Box 8-7).[110,111] Although color Doppler occasionally may show a right-to-left shunt at the atrial level,

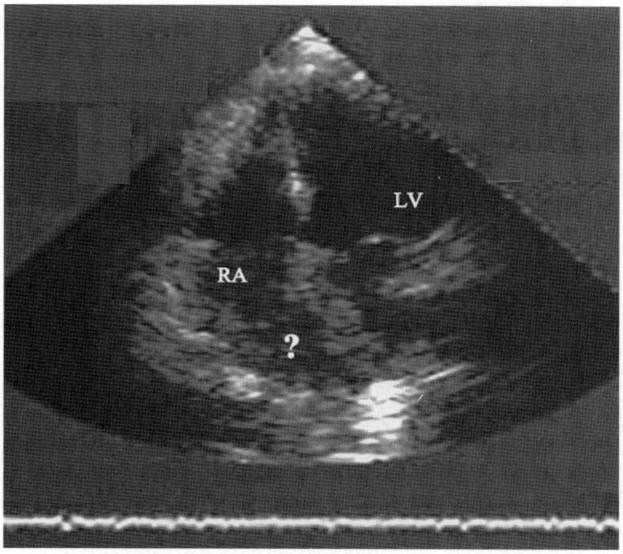

Figure 8-51. Marginal quality transthoracic apical image from a patient who presented with upper extremity emboli. *Question mark* indicates a questionable mass. LV, left ventricle; RA, right atrium.

Box 8-7

Echocardiographic Evaluation of Cardiac Source of Embolus

Intracardiac thrombus
- Ventricular (apex)
- Atrial (body of left atrium, left atrial appendage)
- Prosthetic material (valves, monitoring lines, pacer wires)
- Spontaneous contrast

Valvular vegetations
Patent foramen ovale with or without atrial septal defect
Atrial septal aneurysm
Intracardiac tumors
- Primary—myxoma, fibroelastoma
- Metastatic (lung, breast)

Mitral valve prolapse
Mitral annular calcification
Aortic annular calcium
Atheromatous debris of the aorta

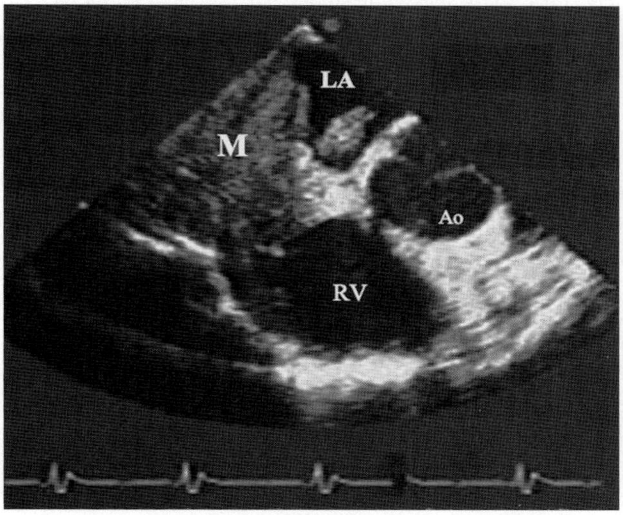

Figure 8-52. Transesophageal echocardiography from the same patient in Figure 8-51 done 2 hours later, showing a large mass invading both atria. The patient was determined to have metastatic lung cancer. Ao, aorta; LA, left atrium; M, mass; RV, right ventricle.

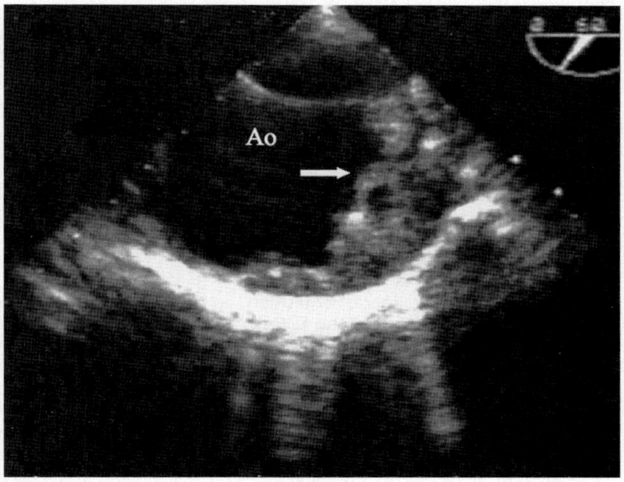

Figure 8-53. Transesophageal echocardiography image of dense protruding atheromatous debris of the aorta with mobile segment *(arrow)*. Ao, aorta.

injection of agitated saline in this setting is particularly useful in determining right-to-left bubble crossover.

Atrial fibrillation predisposes to thrombus formation in the body of the left atrium and in the LA appendage. Although TTE can identify abnormalities that predispose to atrial fibrillation, such as mitral stenosis, TEE is necessary for a thorough assessment of the body of the left atrium and of the LA appendage, which is the most common site of thrombus formation in atrial fibrillation.[112,113]

A significant association exists between aortic atheroma and stroke.[114] TEE reliably identifies aortic debris and can determine location, morphologic characteristics, and mobility of identified lesions (Fig. 8-53).[112,113,115]

KEY POINTS

- Echocardiography is a valuable diagnostic tool in the ICU, but data must be acquired and interpreted with knowledge of the patient's clinical status.
- TEE should be used to provide more detailed or more comprehensive information when transthoracic images are inadequate. TEE may be considered for the evaluation of the aorta, for the assessment of native and prosthetic valves, and for the evaluation of intracardiac shunting. Commercially available contrast agents can now salvage many otherwise uninterpretable transthoracic studies.
- Echocardiography offers numerous reasonably accurate methods to assess global LV systolic properties, including ejection fraction using two-dimensional imaging, Doppler-derived dP/dt, and tissue Doppler–derived measurements such as parameters of regional deformation as assessed by strain and strain rate imaging. Cardiac output also can be reliably determined in most patients.
- Echocardiography now offers numerous methods to determine LV filling pressures with reasonable accuracy. A reliable assessment of LV dimensions and ejection fraction, when combined with knowledge of filling pressures, can be used to guide and assess the response to therapeutic measures.
- Pulmonary artery systolic and diastolic pressures can be calculated with confidence in most patients in the ICU.
- Mechanical complications of myocardial infarction, including acute MR, ventricular septal defect, pseudoaneurysm formation, and LV thrombus, are readily evaluated with echocardiography.
- Although the echocardiographic assessment of the right ventricle is still challenging because of its complex shape, it is possible to integrate information from multiple views to reach reasonably accurate conclusions regarding RV size and function, particularly in the setting of RV pressure or volume overload.
- Echocardiography is particularly well suited to the evaluation of cardiac valve anatomy, morphology, and motion. The integration of two-dimensional anatomy with spectral and color Doppler methods of quantifying obstructive and regurgitant lesions provides a comprehensive assessment of valvular pathology. TEE may be needed to evaluate prosthetic valves.
- Pericardial effusion can be localized and quantified and its hemodynamic impact can be assessed with thoughtful application of imaging and Doppler techniques. In the setting of trauma and the post–cardiac surgical state, opportunistic loculated effusions must be identified.

REFERENCES

1. Physics and instrumentation. In Feigenbaum H, Armstrong W, Ryan T (eds): Feingenbaum's Echocardiography, 6th ed. Philadelphia, Lippincott Williams & Wilkins, 2005, pp 11-44.
2. Otto C: Principles of echocardiographic image acquisition and doppler analysis. In Otto C (ed): Textbook of Clinical Echocardiography, 3rd ed. Philadelphia, Elsevier, 2004, pp 1-29.
3. Christensen AE, Tobiassen M, Jensen TK, et al: Cross sectional echocardiographic examination. In Weyman AE (ed): Principles and Practice of Echocardiography, 2nd ed. Philadelphia, Lippincott Williams & Wilkins, 1994, pp 75-123.
4. Ultrasound physics. In Edelman SK (ed): Understanding Ultrasound Physics, 3rd ed. Houston, ESP Inc, 2004, pp 16-47.
5. Donovan CL, Armstrong WF, Bach DS: Quantitative Doppler tissue imaging of the left ventricular myocardium: Validation in normal subjects. Am Heart J 1995;130:100-104.
6. Huttemann E: Transoesophageal echocardiography in critical care. Minerva Anestesiol 2006;72:891-913.
7. Beaulieu Y, Marik P: Bedside ultrasonography in the ICU. Part 1 and Part 2. Chest 2005;128:881-895 (Part 1), 2005;128:1766-1781 (Part 2).
8. Escolar E, Weigold G, Fuisz A, et al: New imaging techniques for diagnosing coronary artery disease. Can Med Assoc J 2006;174:487-495.
9. Bruce CJ, Friedman PA: Intracardiac echocardiography. Minerva Cardioangiol 2002;50:487-495.
10. Earing MG, Cabalka AK, Seward JB, et al: Intracardiac echocardiographic guidance during transcatheter device closure of atrial septal defect and patent foramen ovale. Mayo Clin Proc 2004;79:24-34.
11. Maloney JD, Burnett JM, Dala-Krishna P, et al: New directions in intracardiac echocardiography. J Interv Card Electrophysiol 2005;13(Suppl 1):23-29.
12. Spicer D, Marwick T: Three-dimensional echocardiography: Research toy or clinical tool? Heart Lung Circ 2000;9:98-107.
13. Belohlavek M, Tanabe K, Jakrapanichakul D, et al: Rapid three-dimensional echocardiography: Clinically feasible alternative for precise and accurate measurement of left ventricular volumes. Circulation 2001;103:2882-2884.
14. Krenning BJ, Voormolen NM, Roelandt J: Assessment of left ventricular function by three-dimensional echocardiography. Cardiovasc Ultrasound 2003;1:12-17.
15. Corsi C, Lang RM, Veronesi F, et al: Volumetric quantification of global and regional left ventricular function from real-time three-dimensional echocardiographic images. Circulation 2005;112:1161-1170.
16. Sugeng L, Coon P, Weinert L, et al: Use of real-time 3-dimensional transthoracic echocardiography in the evaluation of mitral valve disease. J Am Soc Echocardiogr 2006;19: 413-421.
17. Yeh YL, Liu CK, Chang WK, et al: Detection of right to left shunt by transesophageal echocardiography in a patient with post-operative hypoxemia. J Formos Med Assoc 2006;105:418-421.
18. Reilly JP, Tunick P, Timmermans RJ, et al: Contrast echocardiography clarifies uninterpretable wall motion in intensive care unit patients. J Am Coll Cardiol 2000;35:485-490.
19. Yong Y, Fernandes V, Wu D, et al: Diagnostic accuracy and cost-effectiveness of contrast echocardiography on evaluation of cardiac function in technically very difficult patients in the intensive care unit. Am J Cardiol 2002;89: 711-718.
20. Costa JM, Tsutsui JM, Nozawa E, et al: Contrast echocardiography can save nondiagnostic exams in mechanically ventilated patients. Echocardiography 2005;22:389-394.
21. Lepper W, Belcik T, Wei K, et al: Myocardial contrast echocardiography. Circulation 2004;109:3132-3135
22. Wei K, Tong KL, Belcik T, et al: Detection of coronary stenoses at rest with myocardial contrast echocardiography. Circulation 2005;112:1154-1160.
23. Lindner J: Evolving applications for contrast ultrasound. Am J Cardiol 2002;90:72J-80J.
24. Behm CZ, Lindner JR: Cellular and molecular imaging with targeted contrast ultrasound. Ultrasound Q 2006;22:67-72.
25. Bekeredjian R, Grayburn PA, Shohet RV: Use of contrast agents for gene or drug delivery in cardiovascular

medicine. J Am Coll Cardiol 2005;45: 329-335.
26. Weyman AE: The year in echocardiography. J Am Coll Cardiol 2006;47:856-863.
27. Lindner J: Contrast echocardiography: Clinical utility for the evaluation of left ventricular systolic function. Am Heart Hosp J 2004;2:16-20.
28. Kaufmann BA, Wei K, Lindner J: Contrast echocardiography. Curr Probl Cardiol 2007;32:51-96.
29. Seward JB, Douglas PS, Erbel R, et al: Hand-carried cardiac ultrasound (HCU) device: Recommendations regarding new technology: A report from the Echocardiography Task Force on New Technology of the Nomenclature and Standards Committee of the American Society of Echocardiography. J Am Soc Echocardiogr 2002;15:369-373.
30. Spevack DM, Tunick PA, Kronzon I: Hand carried echocardiography in the critical care setting. Echocardiography 2003;20:455-461.
31. de Groot-de Laat LE, ten Cate FJ, Vourvouri EC, et al: Impact of hand-carried cardiac ultrasound on diagnosis and management during cardiac consultation rounds. Eur J Echocardiogr 2005;6:196-201.
32. Hellmann DB, Whiting-O'Keefe Q, Shapiro EP, et al: The rate at which residents learn to use hand-held echocardiography at the bedside. Am J Med 2005;118:1010-1018.
33. Spurney CF, Sable CA, Berger JT, et al: Use of a hand-carried ultrasound device by critical care physicians for the diagnosis of pericardial effusions, decreased cardiac function, and left ventricular enlargement in pediatric patients. J Am Soc Echocardiogr 2005;18:313-319.
34. Manasia AR, Nagaraj HM, Kodali RB, et al: Feasibility and potential clinical utility of goal-directed transthoracic echocardiography performed by noncardiologist intensivists using a small hand-carried device in critically ill patients. J Cardiothorac Vasc Anesth 2005;19:155-159.
35. Lang RM, Bierig M, Devereux RB, et al: Recommendations for chamber quantification: a report from the American Society of Echocardiography's Guidelines and Standards Committee and the Chamber Quantification Writing Group, developed in conjunction with the European Association of Echocardiography, a branch of the European Society of Cardiology. J Am Soc Echocardiogr 2005;18: 1440-1463.
36. Chen C, Rodriguez L, Guerrero JL, et al: Noninvasive estimation of the instantaneous first derivative of left ventricular pressure using continuous wave Doppler echocardiography. Circulation 1991;83:2101-2110.
37. Chen C, Rodriguez L, Lethor JP, et al: Continuous wave Doppler echocardiography for noninvasive assessment of left ventricular dP/dt and relaxation time constant from mitral regurgitant spectra in patients. J Am Coll Cardiol 1994;23:970-976.
38. Garcia-Lledo A, Moya JL, Balaguer J, et al: Sensitivity of the Doppler rate of pressure rise to changes in the inotropic state: An experimental comparison with invasively obtained dP/dt. Eur J Echocardiogr 2000;1: 271-276.
39. Ruan Q, Nagueh SF: Usefulness of isovolumic and systolic ejection signals by tissue Doppler for the assessment of left ventricular systolic function in ischemic or idiopathic dilated cardiomyopathy. Am J Cardiol 2006;97:872-875.
40. Lyseggen E, Rabben SI, Skulstad H, et al: Myocardial acceleration during isovolumic contraction: Relationship to contractility. Circulation 2005;111: 1362-1369.
41. Hoffmann R, Altiok E, Nowak B, et al: Strain rate measurement by Doppler echocardiography allows improved assessment of myocardial viability in patients with depressed left ventricular function. J Am Coll Cardiol 2002;39: 443-449.
42. Amundsen BH, Helle-Valle T, Edvardsen T, et al: Noninvasive myocardial strain measurement by speckle tracking echocardiography: Validation against sonomicrometry and tagged magnetic resonance imaging. J Am Coll Cardiol 2006;47:789-793.
43. Armstrong WF, Pellikka P, Ryan T, et al: Stress echocardiography: Recommendations for performance and interpretation of stress echocardiography. J Am Soc Echocardiogr 1998;11:97-104.
44. Valdes-Cruz LM, Horowitz S, Mesel E, et al: A pulsed Doppler echocardiographic method for calculating pulmonary and systemic blood flow. Circulation 1984;69:80.
45. Lewis JF, Lawrence CK, Nelson JG, et al: Pulsed Doppler echocardiogrpahic determination of stroke volume and cardiac output: clinical validation of two new methods using the apical window. Circulation 1984;70:425.
46. Huntsman LL, Stewart DK, Barnes SR, et al: Noninvasive Doppler determination of cardiac output in man: Clinical validation. Circulation 1983;67:593-602.
47. Nishimura RA, Tajik AJ: Evaluation of diastolic filling of the left ventricle in health and disease: Doppler echocardiography is the clinician's Rosetta Stone. J Am Coll Cardiol 1997;30:8-1897.
48. Oh JK: Echocardiography as a noninvasive Swan-Ganz catheter. Circulation 2005;111:3192-3194.
49. Oh JK, Appleton CP, Hatle L, et al: The noninvasive assessment of left ventricular diastolic function with two-dimensional and Doppler echocardiography. J Am Soc Echocardiogr 1997;10:246-270.
50. Abhayaratna WP, Seward JB, Appleton CP, et al: Left atrial size: Physiologic determinants and clinical applications. J Am Coll Cardiol 2006;47:2357-2363.
51. Appleton CP, Jensen J, Hatle L, et al: Doppler evaluation of left and right ventricular diastolic function: A technical guide for obtaining optimal flow velocity recordings. J Am Soc Echocardiogr 1997;10:271-291.
52. Khouri A, Maly G, Suh DD, et al: A practical approach to the echocardiographic evaluation of diastolic function. J Am Soc Echocardiogr 2004;17:290-297.
53. Nagueh SF: Estimation of left ventricular filling pressures by Doppler echocardiography. ACC Curr J Review 2001;Jan/Feb:41-45.
54. Ommen SR: Echocardiographic assessment of diastolic function. Curr Opin Cardiol 2001;16:240-245.
55. Ommen SR, Nishimura RA, Appleton CP, et al: Clinical utility of Doppler echocardiography and tissue Doppler imaging in the estimation of left ventricular filling pressures: A comparative simultaneous Doppler-catheterization study. Circulation 2000;102:1788-1794.
56. Garcia MJ, Ares MA, Asher C, et al: Color M-mode flow velocity propagation: An index of early left ventricular filling that combined with pulsed Doppler peak E velocity may predict capillary wedge pressure. J Am Coll Cardiol 1997;29:448-454.
57. Rivas-Gotz C, Khoury DS, Manolios M, et al: Time interval between onset of mitral inflow and onset of early diastolic velocity by tissue Doppler: A novel index of left ventricular relaxation: Experimental studies and clinical application. J Am Coll Cardiol 2003;42:1463-1470.
58. Naqvi T: Diastolic function assessment incorporating new techniques in Doppler echocardiography. Rev Cardiovasc Med 2003;4:81-99.
59. Shan K, Bick RJ, Poindexter BJ, et al: Relation of tissue Doppler derived myocardial velocities to myocardial structure and beta-adrenergic receptor density in humans. J Am Coll Cardiol 2000;36:89-96.
60. Kalra DK, Ramchandani M, Zhu X, et al: Relation of tissue Doppler derived myocardial velocities to serum levels and myocardial gene expression of tumor necrosis factor-alpha and inducible nitric oxide synthase in patients with ischemic cardiomyopathy having coronary artery bypass grafting. Am J Cardiol 2002;90: 708-712.
61. Quinones MA, Otto CM, Stoddard M, et al: Recommendations for quantification of Doppler echocardiography: A report from the Doppler Quantification Task Force of the Nomenclature and Standards Committee of the American Society of Echocardiography. J Am Soc Echocardiogr 2002;15:167-184.
62. Nagueh SF, Kopelen HA, Zoghbi WA: Relation of mean right atrial pressure to echocardiographic and Doppler parameters of right atrial and right ventricular function. Circulation 1996;93:1160-1169.
63. Nageh MF, Kopelen HA, Zoghbi WA, et al: Estimation of mean right atrial pressure using tissue Doppler imaging. Am J Cardiol 1999;84:1448-1451.
64. Mahan G, Dabestani A, Gardin J, et al: Estimation of pulmonary artery pressure by pulsed Doppler echocardiography. Circulation 1983;68(Suppl 3):III-367 (Abstract).
65. Masuyama T, Kodama K, Kitabatake A, et al: Continuous wave Doppler echocardiographic detection of

pulmonary regurgitation and its application to noninvasive estimation of pulmonary artery pressure. Circulation 1986;74:484-492.
66. Lee RT, Lord CP, Plappert T, et al: Prospective Doppler echocardiographic evaluation of pulmonary artery diastolic pressure in the medical intensive care unit. Am J Cardiol 1989;64:1366.
67. Abbas AE, Fortuin FD, Schiller NB, et al: A simple method for noninvasive estimation of pulmonary vascular resistance. J Am Coll Cardiol 2003;41:1021-1027.
68. Tei C, Dujardin KS, Hodge DO, et al: Doppler echocardiographic index for assessment of global right ventricular function. J Am Soc Echocardiogr 1996;9:838-847.
69. Alam M, Wardell J, Andersson E, et al: Right ventricular function in patients with first inferior myocardial infarction: Assessment by tricuspid annular motion and tricuspid annular velocity. Am Heart J 2000;139:710-715.
70. Kjaergaard J, Snyder EM, Hassager C, et al: Impact of preload and afterload on global and regional right ventricular function and pressure: A quantitative echocardiographic study. J Am Soc Echocardiogr 2006;19:515-521.
71. Ryan T, Petrovic O, Dillon JC, et al: An echocardiographic index for separation of right ventricular volume and pressure overload. J Am Coll Cardiol 1985;5:918.
72. Louie EK, Rick S, Levitsky S, et al: Doppler echocardiographic demonstration of the differential effects of right ventricular pressure and volume overload on left ventricular geometry and filling. J Am Coll Cardiol 1992;19:84.
73. Hinderliter AL, Willis PW, Barst RJ, et al: Effects of longterm infusion of prostacyclin (epoprostenol) on echocardiographic measures of right ventricular structure and function in idiopathic pulmonary hypertension. Idiopathic Pulmonary Hypertension Study Group. Circulation 1997;95:1479-1486.
74. Zoghbi WA, Enriquez-Sarano M, Foster E, et al: Recommendations for evaluation of the severity of native valvular regurgitation with two dimensional and Doppler echocardiography: A report from the American Society of Echocardiography Nomenclature and Standards Committee and the Task Force on Valvular Regurgitation, developed in conjunction with the ACC Echocardiography Committee, the Cardiac Imaging Committee Council on Clinical Cardiology, the American Heart Association, and the European Society of Cardiology. J Am Soc Echocardiogr 2003;16:777-802.
75. Hall SA, Brickner ME, Willett DL, et al: Assessment of mitral regurgitant severity by Doppler color flow mapping of the vena contracta. Circulation 1997;95:636-642.
76. Bargiggia GS, Tronconi L, Sahn DJ, et al: A new method for quantification of mitral regurgitation based on color flow Doppler imaging of flow convergence proximal to the regurgitant orifice. Circulation 1991;84:1481-1489.
77. Currie PJ, Seward JB, Reeder G, et al: Continuous wave Doppler assessment of severity of calcific aortic stenosis: A simultaneous Doppler-catheter correlative study in 100 adult patients. Circulation 1985;71:1162-1169.
78. Otto CM, Pearlman AS, Comess KA, et al: Determination of the stenotic aortic valve area in adults using Doppler echocardiography. J Am Coll Cardiol 1986;7:509-517.
79. deFilippi CR, Willet DL, Brickner ME, et al: Usefulness of dobutamine echocardiography in distinguishing severe from nonsevere valvular aortic stenosis in patients with depressed left ventricular systolic function and low transvalvular gradients. Am J Cardiol 1995;75:191-194.
80. Hatle L, Brubakk A, Tromsdal A, et al: Noninvasive assessment of pressure drop in mitral stenosis by Doppler ultrasound. Br Heart J 1978;40:131-140.
81. Nakatani S, Masuyama T, Kodama K, et al: Value and limitations of Doppler echocardiography in the quantitation of stenotic mitral valve area: comparison of pressure half-time and continuity equation methods. Circulation 1988;77:78-85.
82. Rosenhek R, Binder T, Maurer G, et al: Normal values for Doppler echocardiographic assessment of heart valve prostheses. J Am Soc Echocardiogr 2003;16:1116-1127.
83. Van den Brink RB: Evaluation of prosthetic heart valves by transesophageal echocardiography: Problems, pitfalls, and timing of echocardiography. Semin Cardiothorac Vasc Anesth 2006;10:89-100.
84. Barbetseas J, Zoghbi WA: Evaluation of prosthetic valve function and associated complications. Cardiol Clin 1998;16:505-530.
85. Feigenbaum H, Waldhausen JA, Hyde LP: Ultrasound diagnosis of pericardial effusion. JAMA 1965;191:711-714.
86. Tsang T, Oh JK, Seward JB, et al: Diagnostic value of echocardiography in cardiac tamponade. Herz 2000;25:734-740.
87. Spodick DH: Acute cardiac tamponade. N Engl J Med 2003;349:684-690.
88. Little WC, Freeman G: Pericardial disease. Circulation 2006;113:1622-1632.
89. Singh S, Wann S, Schuchard GH, et al: Right ventricular and right atrial collapse in patients with cardiac tamponade: A combined echocardiographic and hemodynamic study. Circulation 1984;70:966-971.
90. Gillam LD, Guyer DE, Gibson TC, et al: Hemodynamic compression of the right atrium: An echocardiographic sign of cardiac tamponade. Circulation 1983;68:294-301.
91. Reydel B, Spodick DH: Frequency and significance of chamber collapses during cardiac tamponade. Am Heart J 1990;199:1160-1163.
92. Armstrong WF, Schilt BF, Helper DJ, et al: Diastolic collapse of the right ventricle with cardiac tamponade: an echocardiographic study. Circulation 1982;65:1491-1496.
93. Joffe II, Douglas PS: Cardiac tamponade in association with an atrial septal defect: Echocardiographic and hemodynamic observations. J Am Soc Echocardiogr 1996;9:909-914.
94. Appleton CP, Hatle LK, Popp RL: Cardiac tamponade and pericardial effusion: Respiratory variation in transvalvular flow velocities by Doppler echocardiography. J Am Coll Cardiol 1988;11:1020-1030.
95. Callahan JA, Seward JB, Nishimura RA, et al: Two-dimensional echocardiographically guided pericardiocentesis: Experience in 117 consecutive patients. Am J Cardiol 1985;55:476.
96. Chandraratna PAN, Reid CL, Nimalasuriya A, et al: Application of 2-dimensional contrast studies during pericardiocentesis. Am J Cardiol 1983;52:1120.
97. Rajagopalan N, Garcia MJ, Rodriguez L, et al: Comparison of new Doppler echocardiographic methods to differentiate constrictive pericardial disease and restrictive cardiomyopathy. Am J Cardiol 2001;87:86-94.
98. Ha JW, Ommen SR, Tajik AJ, et al: Differentiation of constrictive pericarditis from restrictive cardiomyopathy using mitral annular velocity by tissue Doppler echocardiography. Am J Cardiol 2004;94:316-319.
99. Nienaber CA, Spielman RP, von Kodolitsch Y, et al: Diagnosis of thoracic aortic dissection: Magnetic resonance imaging versus transesophageal echocardiography. Circulation 1992;85:434-447.
100. Cigarroa JE, Isselbacher EM, DeSanctis RW, et al: Diagnostic imaging in the evaluation of suspected aortic dissection: old standards and new directions. N Engl J Med 1993;328:35-43.
101. Nienaber CA, von Kodolitsch Y, Nicolas V, et al: The diagnosis of thoracic aortic dissection by noninvasive imaging procedures. N Engl J Med 1993;328:1-9.
102. Willens HJ, Kessler KM: Transesophageal echocardiography in the diagnosis of diseases of the thoracic aorta: Part 1. Aortic dissection, aortic intramural hematoma, and penetrating atherosclerotic ulcer of the aorta. Chest 1999;116:1772-1779.
103. Nienaber CA, Eagle KA: Aortic dissection: New frontiers in diagnosis and management. Part 1: From etiology to diagnostic strategies. Part 2: Therapeutic management and follow-up. Circulation 2003;108:628 (Part 1), 2003;108:772-778 (Part 2).
104. Song JK, Kim HS, Kang DH, et al: Different clinical features of aortic intramural hematoma versus dissection involving the ascending aorta. J Am Coll Cardiol 2001;37:1604-1610.
105. von Kodolitsch Y, Csosz SK, Koschyk DH, et al: Intramural hematoma of the aorta: Predictors of progression to dissection and rupture. Circulation 2003;107:1158-1163.

106. Evangelista A, Mukherjee D, Mehta RH, et al: Acute intramural hematoma of the aorta: A mystery in evolution. Circulation 2005;111:1063-1070.
107. Vignon P, Gueret P, Vedrinne JM, et al: Role of transesophageal echocardiography in the diagnosis and management of traumatic aortic disruption. Circulation 1995;92:2959-2968.
108. Vignon P, Martaille JF, Francois B, et al: Transesophageal echocardiography and therapeutic management of blunt aortic injuries. J Trauma 2005;58:1150-1158.
109. Cerebral Embolism Task Force: Cardiogenic brain embolism. The second report of the Cerebral Embolism Task Force. Arch Neurol 1989;46:727-743.
110. Horton SC, Bunch TJ: Patent foramen ovale and stroke. Mayo Clin Proc 2004;79:79-88.
111. Mas JL, Arquizan C, Lamy C, et al: Recurrent cerebrovascular events associated with patent foramen ovale, atrial septal aneurysm, or both. N Engl J Med 2001;345:1740-1746.
112. Reynolds H, Tunick P, Kronzon I: Role of transesophageal echocardiography in the evaluation of patients with stroke. Curr Opin Cardiol 2003;18:340-345.
113. Woods T: Transesophageal echocardiography and stroke. Curr Atheroscler Rep 2005;7:255-262.
114. Vitebskiy S, Fox K, Hoit BD: Routine transesophageal echocardiography for the evaluation of cerebral emboli in elderly patients. Echocardiography 2005;22:770-774.
115. Tunick PA, Kronzon I: Embolism from the aorta: atheroemboli and thromboemboli. Curr Treat Options Cardiovasc Med 2001;3:181-186.

Chapter 9

General Principles of Mechanical Ventilation

Ismail Cinel, Smith Jean, and R. Phillip Dellinger

Mechanical ventilation is often the focal point of the care rendered in the intensive care unit (ICU) because respiratory failure is the most common diagnosis requiring treatment in the ICU.[1] Modifying the variables of mechanical ventilation can result in more appropriate therapy with less risk of trauma to the lungs and fewer negative interactions with other organ systems. In this chapter, we explore the basic general principles of mechanical ventilation, features of ventilators, acute complications of mechanical ventilation, newer forms of mechanical ventilation, and adjuncts to mechanical ventilation.

HISTORY

The concept behind mechanical ventilation dates back centuries. In the first form of mechanical ventilation, Paracelsus (1493-1541) used "fire bellows" connected to a tube inserted into a patient's mouth as a device for assisted ventilation. The first known mechanical device designed specifically to provide ventilation for the patient was the foot pump developed by Fell O'Dwyer in 1888.

The first generation of mechanical ventilators focused primarily on the intermittent delivery of a bulk volume of gas to the patient with limited monitoring. Because gas flow requires a pressure gradient, a mechanical ventilator must produce a pressure gradient between the airway opening and the alveoli in order to produce inspiratory flow and volume delivery. Negative-pressure ventilation creates a pressure gradient (called transairway pressure gradient) by decreasing the alveolar pressures to a level below the airway opening pressure. Two classic devices that provide negative-pressure ventilation are the "iron lung" and the chest cuirass or chest shell. Iron lungs were widely used during the poliomyelitis epidemics of the 1930s and 1940s. These devices encased the patient from the neck down and applied negative pressure around the patient to expand the lungs. The chest cuirass or chest shell was intended to alleviate the problems of patient access and tank shock that occur secondary to venous pooling in the lower abdomen during the application of negative pressure associated with iron lungs.[2] Although the chest shell improves patient access and decreases the potential for tank shock, ventilation with this device may be limited by the difficulties in maintaining an airtight seal between the shell and the patient's chest wall.

In the 1950s this type of ventilation was generally abandoned for intermittent positive-pressure ventilation via a cuffed tracheostomy tube to prevent gross aspiration in patients unable to protect their airways. These crude devices initiated the era of mechanical ventilators, and over the years, they have evolved into sophisticated machines undreamed-of by their early pioneers. The improvements in mechanical ventilators came about as understanding was gained in manipulating variables of flow and pressure for patient benefit. Technical evolution of ventilators included advances such as intermittent mandatory ventilation, synchronous intermittent mandatory ventilation (SIMV), and the introduction of positive end-expiratory pressure (PEEP). Monitoring capabilities were better than those of the first-generation ventilators, and with these later machines, the practitioner was able to alter inspiratory flow as well as pressure through different flow patterns.

The present-day machines boast microprocessors that serve both in the operating mechanism of the device and in the monitoring systems and also enable automatic adjustment of most aspects of the mechanical breath being delivered. Important improvements include (1) the ability to monitor the patient's interaction with the ventilator, thus allowing modes that use continuous feedback, and (2) self-regulation by the mechanical ventilator itself.

INDICATIONS FOR MECHANICAL VENTILATION

Mechanical ventilation should be instituted when the patient cannot maintain spontaneous ventilation to provide adequate oxygenation and/or carbon dioxide removal. Mechanical assistance may also be needed to maintain pH, decrease the work of breathing, or reduce cardiac workload in the presence of a compromised cardiovascular system (Table 9-1). Acute ventilatory failure, impending ventilatory failure, severe hypoxemia, and prophylactic ventilatory support are the clinical conditions leading to mechanical ventilation. Clinical indicators such as tachycardia, arrhythmias, hypertension, and tachypnea, use of accessory respiratory muscles, diaphoresis, and cyanosis are used to diagnose respiratory distress.

Blood pH is generally a better indicator than $P\text{CO}_2$ for adjusting minute ventilation. Hypercapnia should not prompt aggressive intervention if pH remains acceptable and the patient remains alert. The physiologic consequences of altered pH are still debated and clearly depend on the underlying pathophysiology and comorbidities. However, a sustained pH of 7.65 or greater or 7.10 or less is often considered sufficiently dangerous in itself to require control of minute ventilation by mechanical ventilation. Within these extremes, the threshold for initiating support varies with the clinical setting, guided by trends in pH, arterial blood gas values, mental status, respiratory pattern, hemodynamic stability, and response to therapy.

Supplementing $F\text{IO}_2$ (fraction of inspired oxygen), adding PEEP, or changing the pattern of ventilation to increase mean airway pressure and, consequently, mean alveolar pressure are the mechanisms by which mechanical ventilation improves oxygenation. A better balance between oxygen delivery and consumption may be achieved when ventilation is controlled, thereby freeing needed oxygen for other organ systems. Observations demonstrate the importance of minimizing the ventilatory

Table 9-1. Indications for Mechanical Ventilation

Physiologic Mechanisms	Clinical Indicators	Normal Range	Values Supporting Need for Mechanical Ventilation
Inadequate alveolar ventilation	$Pa\text{CO}_2$ (mm Hg)	36-44*	Acute increase from normal or from patient's baseline
Inadequate lung expansion	VT (mL/kg)	5-8	<4-5
	VC (mL/kg)	60-75	<10-15
	Respiratory rate (breaths/min)	12-20	≥35
Ventilatory muscle weakness	MIP (cm H_2O)	80-100	<20-30
	MVV (L/min)	120-180	<2×resting VE requirement
	VC (mL/kg)	60-75	<10-15
Excessive work of breathing	VE required to keep $Pa\text{CO}_2$ normal (L/min)	5-10	>15-20
	VD/VT (%)	25-40	>60
		—	—
Hypoxemia	$P(A-a)O_2$ difference on $F\text{IO}_2=1.0$ (mm Hg)	25-65	>350
	$Pa\text{O}_2/F\text{IO}_2$ ratio (mm Hg)	350-400	<200

$F\text{IO}_2$, inspired oxygen fraction; MIP, maximum inspiratory pressure; MVV, maximum voluntary ventilation; $P(A-a)O_2$, alveolar to arterial $P\text{O}_2$ difference; VC, vital capacity; VD, dead space ventilation; VE, minute ventilation; VT, tidal volume.
*Normal values at sea level.
Adapted from Pierson DJ, Kacmarek R: Foundations of Respiratory Care. New York, Churchill Livingstone, 1992.

O_2 requirement during cardiac insufficiency or ischemia by allowing diaphragmatic blood flow to be redirected to the vital organs. Additionally, reducing ventilatory effort to overcome the excessive respiratory workload may reduce afterload to the left ventricle. Patients with metabolic acidosis may need ventilatory support to avoid decompensation.

PHYSIOLOGIC EFFECTS OF MECHANICAL VENTILATION

Ventilators currently employed in adult care use positive pressure to inflate the lungs. Although positive pressure is responsible for the beneficial effects of mechanical ventilation, it is also responsible for many deleterious side effects. Mechanical ventilation can affect nearly every organ system of the body due to the homeostatic interactions between the lungs and the other organ systems.

During normal spontaneous breathing, diaphragm and other respiratory muscles create gas flow by lowering pleural, alveolar, and airway pressures. Alveolar pressure is normally atmospheric at end-inspiration and end-expiration. Diaphragmatic and intercostal muscle activation during normal inspiration expands the chest and decreases intrapleural pressure from –5 cm H_2O to –8 cm H_2O. Alveolar pressure fluctuates from +1 cm H_2O during exhalation to –1 cm H_2O during inhalation. Intrathoracic pressure decreases during exhalation, and venous return is greatest.

Shunt refers to the condition in which areas of the lung that are perfused but not ventilated. The shunt may be intracardiac (anatomic) or intrapulmonary (capillary). Normal intrapulmonary shunt fractions are about 2% to 5%. Mechanical ventilation may increase the shunt fraction to approximately 10% in the normal individual. Mechanical ventilation usually decreases shunt in acute infiltrative lung disease, improving the distribution of ventilation especially in previously underventilated lung areas. Pressures greater than alveolar opening and closing pressures expand the collapsed alveolus and prevent its collapse, respectively. However, if positive-pressure ventilation produces overdistention, redistribution of pulmonary blood flow to unventilated regions may occur, resulting in hypoxemia.[3] With mechanical ventilation, a rise in alveolar pressure increases pulmonary vascular resistance, thereby impeding flow through the lungs. *Mean airway pressure*—the average pressure within the airway during one complete respiratory cycle—is directly related to inspiratory time, respiratory rate, peak inspiratory pressure, and positive end-expiratory pressure. It should be kept as low as possible if an anatomic right-to-left shunt is present.

Dead space refers to an area of lung that is ventilated but not perfused. *Anatomic dead space* is the volume of the conducting airways of the lungs, about 150 mL. *Alveolar dead space* refers to alveoli that are overventilated relative to perfusion; it is enlarged by any condition that reduces pulmonary blood flow. *Mechanical dead space* refers to the rebreathed volume of the ventilator circuit; this volume behaves like an extension of the anatomic dead space. Mechanical ventilation can also increase anatomic dead space by distending nonconducting airways.

An increased dead space fraction requires a greater minute ventilation to maintain alveolar ventilation and $Pa{CO_2}$. Hyperventilation lowers $Pa{CO_2}$, an effect that may be desirable when intracranial pressure is elevated but otherwise should be avoided because of the injurious effects of overdistention. Hypoventilation raises $Pa{CO_2}$; a modest elevation (50-70 mm Hg) is probably not by itself injurious and reduces pH. It has become increasingly recognized that hypercapnia during mechanical ventilation may not be harmful.

Positive-pressure ventilation may decrease cardiac output, resulting in hypotension and potential tissue hypoxia. Higher pulmonary vascular resistance results in greater right ventricular afterload and, if severe, produces ventricular septal shift and compromise of left ventricular function. Urine output can decrease because of lower renal perfusion associated with reduced cardiac output or the elevation in plasma antidiuretic hormone and reduction in atrial natriuretic peptide that occur with mechanical ventilation. By increasing pleural and therefore juxtacardiac pressure, however, positive-pressure ventilation assists left ventricular ejection and may be of utility in the presence of severe left ventricular dysfunction.

In patients with head injury, positive-pressure ventilation may decrease cerebral blood flow via two mechanisms: (1) decrease in cardiac output due to decrease in venous return and (2) increase in jugular vein pressure.

Mechanical ventilation is also one of the risk factors for development of stress ulcers.

MECHANICAL BREATH GENERATION

A *mode* of mechanical ventilation refers to the program by which the ventilator interacts with the patient, the relationship between the possible types of breaths allowed by the ventilator, and the variables (trigger, limit, and cycle) that define inspiration (Table 9-2). Each mechanical respiratory cycle can be broken down into the following four phases:

Inspiration is the point at which the ventilator causes the exhalation valve to close and channels fresh gas under pressure into the thorax.

Cycling is the changeover from inspiration to expiration. Cycling can occur in response to elapsed time, delivered volume, or a predetermined decrement in flow rate. After cycling occurs, the exhalation valve opens, inspiration ends, and passive exhalation occurs.

Expiration begins when the main ventilator flow is stopped or interrupted and the exhalation circuit is opened to allow gas to escape from the lungs. Exhalation continues until the next inspiration begins. It is not predicated on the return to a specific lung volume.

Table 9-2. Overview of Features of Selected Modes of Mechanical Ventilation

Ventilator Mode	Control	Trigger	Limit	Cycling	Inspiratory Flow
Controlled mechanical ventilation (CMV)	Ventilator	Time	Flow/volume or pressure	Volume or time	Selected or decelerating
Assist volume control (AVC)	Assist	Patient or time	Flow, volume	Volume	Square, decelerating, or sinusoidal
Assist pressure control (APC)	Assist	Patient or time	Pressure, inspiratory time	Time	Decelerating
Synchronized intermittent mandatory ventilation (SIMV)	Assist	Patient or time	None for patient breaths Flow/volume (VC) or pressure (PC) for ventilator breaths	Flow for spontaneous breaths Volume or time for ventilator breaths	Decelerating for spontaneous breath Square (VC), decelerating (VC or PC), or sinusoidal (VC) for ventilator breaths
Pressure-regulated volume control (PRVC)	Assist	Patient or time	Pressure (may vary from breath to breath)	Time	Decelerating
Pressure-support ventilation (PSV)	Assist	Patient	None	Flow	Decelerating

Triggering is the changeover from expiration to inspiration.

All mechanical ventilators require some signal from the patient (except in control mode, in which the patient does not interact with the ventilator) to determine when inhalation should begin. In the absence of patient interaction with the ventilation, breaths are delivered on the basis of elapsed time. This is called an *unassisted breath,* because it is delivered in controlled ventilation. When the patient is allowed to trigger the breath (*assisted breath*), triggering results from a perturbation in either the airway pressure or gas flow in the inspiratory limb of ventilation. According to these definitions, two ventilator breath types are possible, full ventilator control (mandatory) and partial ventilator control (assist).

Ventilator-Controlled Ventilation

In *controlled mechanical ventilation* (CMV), there is no patient triggering; rather, all breaths are triggered, limited, and cycled by the ventilator. With currently available ventilators, a CMV mode cannot be selected. This mode is achieved when the patient is unable to interact with the ventilator, such as with neuromuscular paralysis.

Partial Ventilator-Controlled (Assist) Ventilation

In *assist volume control* (AVC) *ventilation* or *assist pressure control* (APC) *ventilation,* the clinician sets a minimum rate and either tidal volume or pressure, respectively. The patient can trigger the ventilator at a more rapid rate and will receive the set volume each time. In *intermittent mandatory ventilation* (IMV), ventilator-limited (i.e., by volume or pressure) breaths are similarly delivered at a set (minimum) rate, but the patient can breathe spontaneously by triggering a demand valve between machine-limited breaths. With current ventilators, IMV is modified to *synchronized IMV* (SIMV), in which the ventilator synchronizes the timing of machine breaths with patient effort. In *pressure support ventilation* (PSV), flow delivery is determined by the pressure support settings and the patient may trigger all the breaths without ventilatory assistance.

TRIGGERING MECHANISM

Triggering may be accomplished by reducing airway pressure in the proximal circuit (near the ventilator) to a threshold below the set circuit pressure (atmospheric unless PEEP is present). When the patient makes an inspiratory effort, the drop in pressure is sensed by the ventilator, and when the preset threshold (usually referred to as the *sensitivity*) level is reached, inspiration is triggered (the exhalation valve closes, and pressurization of the inspiration circuit occurs). The threshold for triggering a breath (i.e., the set sensitivity) can be altered according to the clinical setting; however, the greatest challenge in mechanical ventilation is determining the level at which sensitivity pressure should be set (usually at −1 to −2 cm H_2O). If sensitivity is set too low, the ventilator will be triggered by any process that causes the airway pressure to drop below the set threshold. Such processes include patient motion, external compression, gastric suctioning, and air leaks in the circuit or in the chest tubes. Conversely, if the threshold is set too high, the work of breathing increases; that is, to trigger every breath, the patient must make a significant effort to overcome the threshold limit for inspiratory flow to occur.

Flow sensing was developed as an alternative to pressure triggering to reduce the delay in response time between signal generation by the patient and delivery of

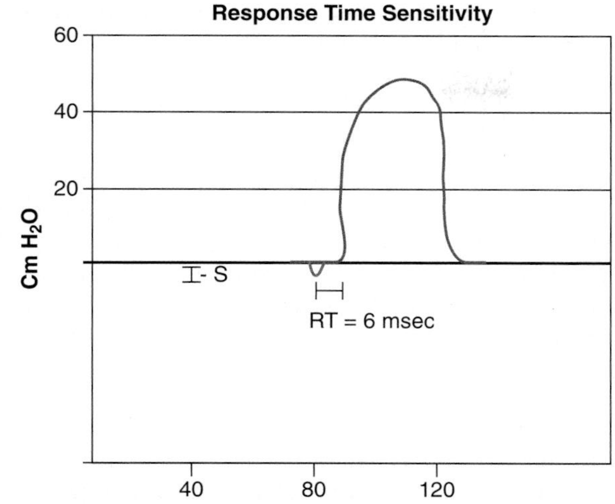

Figure 9-1. Pressure wave showing time relationship between patient inspiratory effort and ventilator response (RT).

gas volume by the ventilator.[4,5] Whereas pressure triggering requires a direct effect of a pressure drop on the inspiratory sensor, flow triggering requires pressure drop–induced disruption in a constant stream of air flow in the inspiratory circuit maintained during expiration and has been demonstrated to decrease work of breathing compared with pressure triggering.[6] Refinement and improvement in pressure triggering, however, make these two mechanisms of triggering similar to the work of breathing.[7]

In recent years much attention has been directed at shortening the time between patient effort and initiation of the ventilator breath, thus minimizing patient effort. This inherent delay, although greatly reduced, between signal and delivery of gas can lead to significant patient-ventilator dyssynchrony and may increase the work of breathing for the patient (Fig. 9-1). Although a direct cause-and-effect relationship is unlikely, trigger asynchrony has been demonstrated to be associated with worsened outcome.[8] Ongoing research looks to define new triggers, such as esophageal pressure, inspiratory muscle signals, and direct central nervous system signals, to further reduce the delay in delivering inspiratory gas flow.

LIMITING PARAMETERS DURING INSPIRATION

Three parameters can be programmed on ventilators in the ICU to limit inspiration: volume, pressure, and flow. In volume control mode, the limiting parameter is volume, and although this mode ensures a preselected volume, excessive inspiratory pressures may result if the patient's lung compliance decreases or airway resistance increases. In pressure-limited breaths, as in APC ventilation, gas flows until pressure in the patient equals pressure in the ventilator or preset inspiratory time is reached. Although this mechanism allows limitation of pressure in the lung at end-inspiration, tidal volume and minute ventilation will decrease if the patient's lung compliance diminishes, potentially leading to significant alveolar hypoventilation. In flow-limited breaths, as in traditional AVC, the ventilator-delivered breath during inspiration will not exceed the preset flow rate value.

Cycling Mechanisms

The changeover from inspiration to expiration cycling can occur in response to elapsed time, delivered volume (volume-cycled), elapsed time (pressure control), or a predetermined decrement in flow rate (pressure support). After cycling occurs, the exhalation valve opens, inspiration ends, and passive exhalation occurs.

Volume-Cycled Breaths

With volume cycling, the ventilator continues to deliver fresh gas until a preselected volume of gas is delivered. In a closed ventilator circuit, the rise of pressure is directly proportional to the volume of gas delivered, airway resistance, and lung/chest wall compliance. Volume-cycled ventilators potentially deliver a predetermined volume regardless of the airway pressure needed to deliver the volume. For this reason, these devices almost always include a pressure relief ("pop-off") valve to protect the patient against excessive inhalation pressures during the tidal volume delivery. The pop-off pressure is selected through use of the pressure limit alarm. Under these circumstances, after the preset pressure limit is reached, the inspiratory cycle is prematurely terminated, and exhalation is allowed to proceed. This process continues until either the cause of the increased impedance is corrected or a new preset pressure limit is provided by the operator. During this period of pressure limiting, the preset volume is not being delivered, and significant alveolar hypoventilation can occur.

Time-Cycled Breaths

With time-cycled breaths (pressure-control breaths), inspiration continues for a preset interval. Cycling is therefore time dependent. Exhalation begins when this period has elapsed, regardless of whether or not the desired volume has been delivered or the preset ventilator system pressure has been achieved in the airspace. With time-cycled ventilation, the end of inspiration does not depend on the patient's lung characteristics or even on whether the ventilator is attached to the patient. As in flow-cycled breaths (pressure-support breaths, discussed later), pressure is preset in the ventilator and maintained at that constant level throughout inspiration[9,10]; this yields a square pressure-over-time waveform. Assuming respiratory rate is controlled, inspiration time can be set to give a precise inhalation-to-expiration (I:E) ratio. This ratio can be adjusted, for example, from 3:1 to 1:5, depending on the needs of the patient.

The inspiratory flow during this type of breath is initially high and then tapers as the alveolar pressures rises. The delivered tidal volume at any point is not guaranteed to be maintained and increases or decreases with changes in airway resistance or lung elastance. The development of automatic positive end-expiratory pressure (auto-PEEP, see Chapter 10) further reduces the delivery of the tidal volume as *end-expiration pressure*—the downstream gradient for flow over the fixed inspiratory time—increases. Potential benefits from this type of breath are that airway pressures may be limited and that the greatest part of inspiratory volume is achieved earlier in the respiratory cycling, allowing for more uniform distribution of the tidal volume during the latter part of inspiration. As in flow-cycled breaths (discussed later), tidal volume may vary with changes in patient effort or in lung compliance and airways resistance. This mode, therefore, is not recommended in situations in which lung mechanics are rapidly changing, and monitoring of expired gas volumes over time is crucial to ensure adequate alveolar ventilation.

Flow-Cycled Breaths

With flow cycling (pressure-support breaths), when a predetermined decrement of flow is achieved (typically, a drop to 25% of initial flow), inspiration is terminated. As in pressure control, flow is achieved across a pressure gradient between a rapidly achieved ventilator system pressure and the patient. Breaths may also be terminated when excessive airway pressure is detected (e.g., coughing during inspiration) or after a preset time interval, the latter as a safety factor in case leaks in the system (such as cuff leaks) prevent proper cycling. Both time-cycled and flow-cycled breaths are "pressure-limited." Because flow rate decreases dramatically as patient inspiratory effort decreases and then ceases, the patient exerts control not only of initiation of breath but also of its termination. Strength and duration of patient inspiratory effort influence tidal volume. This type of ventilator breath may be used as a mode of mechanical ventilation (stand-alone PSV), with SIMV to augment spontaneous breaths or with continuous positive airway pressure (CPAP), as discussed later, to overcome endotracheal tube resistance during a weaning trial.

INSPIRATORY FLOW PATTERNS

Inspiratory flow patterns may be automatically determined by the mode selection or can be selected and variable with some modes. Many mechanical ventilators allow selection of one of three different types of inspiratory flow patterns when volume-cycled breaths are used with volume control mode of ventilation or SIMV with volume limited breaths (versus selection of pressure limited breaths) (Fig. 9-2). These are as follows:

- A *square wave* (constant flow), in which the inspiratory flow rises rapidly to a preset level and then stays at that level until cycling occurs
- A *sinusoidal flow wave* pattern, in which the flow first increases and then decreases during inspiration
- A *descending ramp wave,* in which the flow increases rapidly to a maximum level and then decreases gradually until the end of inhalation

Of the three, the sinusoidal flow wave pattern mimics the normal inspiratory pattern most closely. The inspiratory flow pattern in pressure control and pressure support modes of mechanical ventilation are always the descending ramp because flow decreases over time as the pressure gradient between the constant ventilation pressure and the patient narrows as the pressure in the lungs rises throughout interaction.

When heterogeneous abnormality exists in the lung parenchyma or airways, there is a tendency for inhomogeneous ventilation to occur (i.e., patent areas are overventilated and obstructed areas are underventilated). Studies have demonstrated that prolonging the inspiratory time can lead to more homogeneous distribution of ventilation within abnormal lungs.[11,12] Techniques for improving the distribution of air to severely obstructed portions of the respiratory tree include adding an inspiratory pause and varying the inspiratory flow pattern. In lung models, the distribution of ventilation can be quite different when the flow pattern changes. A decelerative flow pattern, such as the descending ramp, yields the most even distribution under most abnormal airway conditions.[13] Studies have also demonstrated that a decelerating flow pattern improves the geographical distribution of lung vibration as a presumed surrogate of airflow.[14] The sinusoidal pattern usually results in a prolongation of inspiration because it requires the longest period to deliver a given tidal volume at a specific set peak inspiratory flow rate. When the demand for ventilation is very high, it is difficult to deliver large minute ventilation with sufficient expiratory time unless one uses a square wave pattern of inspiratory gas flow. The receptors in the airways may react adversely to the high flow rates, and at times this reaction can provoke spasmodic coughing. The square wave pattern is also associated with the highest peak airway pressure. However, this peak is offset by a shorter inspiratory time and a longer expiratory time, allowing amelioration of hyperinflation and auto-PEEP. The square waveform is therefore preferred in patients with severe obstruction to minimize auto-PEEP. As previously stated, theoretical results have demonstrated that prolongation of inspiration at low flows in a decelerating wave pattern would result in the most homogeneous distribution of gas and may be the preferred pattern for inspiratory flow in patients with nonobstructive lung disorders. The end-inspiratory alveolar pressure, as measured

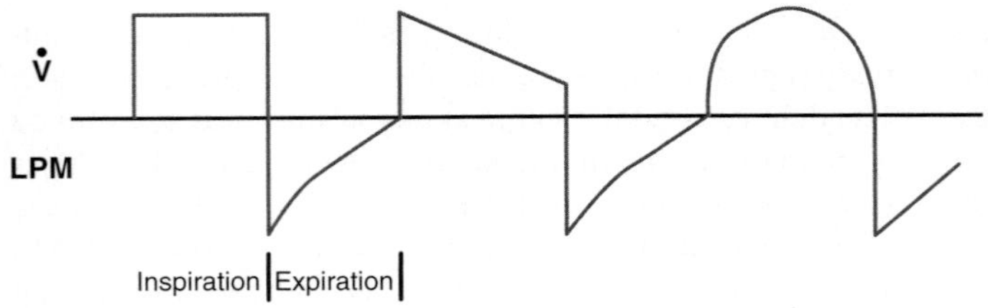

Figure 9-2. Depicted are (left to right) square, decelerating, and sine inspiratory flow waveforms as options for delivery of volume ventilation. Note that the square waveform produces the shortest inspiratory time and that the decelerating waveform does not return to zero flow at end-inspiration. LPM, liters per minute; V̇, flow.

by an end-inspiratory hold, is the same for a given tidal volume regardless of type of inspiratory flow pattern and associated peak inspiratory pressure.

COMMONLY USED MODES OF MECHANICAL VENTILATION

Modes of mechanical ventilation that are commonly used are AVC, APC, SIMV, pressure-regulated volume control, and PSV. CMV is less commonly used. Table 9-2 summarizes the features of these modes, and Table 9-3 lists their advantages and disadvantages.

Assist Volume Control

The AVC mode of ventilation delivers volume-limited breaths triggered by the patient or ventilator. All of the breaths are ventilator-delivered with a preset tidal volume (volume-cycled). The assist modes allow the patient to determine the number and frequency of mechanical ventilator breaths. Breaths may be assisted, unassisted, or a combination. Assisted breaths are triggered by a change in airway pressure or flow (Fig. 9-3B). In the assist modes, a backup rate is set to ensure a minimal number of ventilator breaths in case the patient's respiratory rate drops below the preset rate. If the patient breathes more often than the set rate, additional ventilator breaths are delivered. An inspiratory hold can be performed to obtain the plateau pressure that approximates the alveolar pressure (Fig. 9-4). This maneuver is performed to approximate the static compliance of the lungs.

In most circumstances, ventilation using assist modes results in a marked diminution in the work of breathing, which in some circumstances can approximate zero. With an assisted breath, however, certain patients continue to exert significant effort throughout inspiration.[15] Such patients can perform a considerable amount of ventilatory work in this mode. Although it is not exactly clear why this undesirable situation occurs, the reason may be the inherent delay between the triggering and onset of pressurization and volume flow through the airways by the mechanical ventilator (see Fig. 9-1). Because the respiratory drive for a given ventilation is determined by the lung mechanics and demand of the previous breath during the first 100 ms, a delay of this magnitude can result in the patient's failure to sense that the ventilator will deliver a satisfactory tidal volume. Under these circumstances, the patient's inspiratory effort continues despite adequate ventilation from the device. Evaluating the pressure-time curves of each breath may yield subtle hints that this situation is occurring (i.e., change in the shape of the inspiratory rise—the greater the patient effort, the more concave the inspiratory rise in pressure).

Assist Pressure Control

APC ventilation is a partial ventilator-controlled mode similar to AVC ventilation, in that it is an assist mode based on patient or automatic triggering and all of the breaths are ventilator-delivered. This mode provides pressure-limited, time-cycled breaths on the basis of set applied pressure limits and inspiratory time, allowing limitation of peak inspiratory pressures (see Fig. 9-3C). The tidal volumes delivered can vary according to the set pressure, the compliance of the lungs and chest wall, and patient effort. Although this mode may be better tolerated by the patient, greater monitoring is necessary because changes in lung compliance may lead to hyperventilation or hypoventilation.

Table 9-3. Potential Advantages and Disadvantages of Selected Modes of Mechanical Ventilation

Mode	Advantages	Disadvantages
Controlled mechanical ventilation (CMV)	Rests muscles of respiration	Requires use of sedation/neuromuscular blockade
Assist volume control (AVC)	Reduced work of breathing Guarantees delivery of set tidal volume (unless peak pressure limit alarm is exceeded)	Potential adverse hemodynamic effects May lead to inappropriate hyperventilation and excessive inspiration pressures
Assist pressure control (APC)	Allows limitation of peak inspiratory pressures	Same as AVC Potential hyperventilation or hypoventilation with lung resistance/compliance changes
Synchronized intermittent mandatory ventilation (SIMV)	Less interference with normal cardiovascular function	Increased work of breathing compared with assist control Patient may find it difficult to adjust to two different ventilation breaths
Pressure-regulated volume control (PRVC)	Maintains similar tidal volumes with varying resistance and compliance	Same as AVC Inspiratory pressures may vary
Pressure-support ventilation (PSV)	Patient comfort Improved patient-ventilator interaction Decreased work of breathing	Apnea alarm is only backup Variable patient tolerance

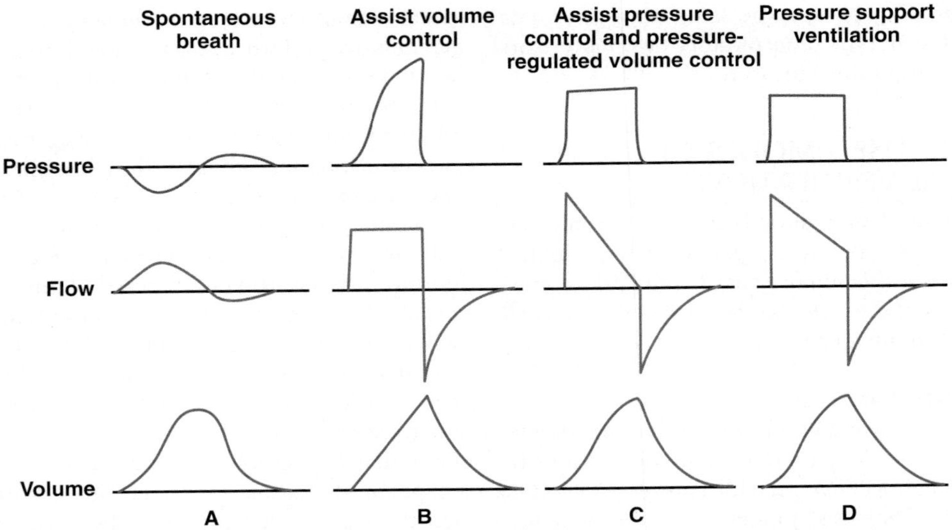

Figure 9-3. Characteristic pressure-flow waveforms with breathing spontaneously and various types of ventilation. **A,** Spontaneous breath. Such breaths are spontaneous, and inspiratory flow is achieved by the negative pressure generated by the respiratory muscles. Expiration occurs as these muscles relax. The combination of mandatory ventilator breaths (B or C) with spontaneous breaths (with or without pressure support) is called synchronized intermittent mandatory ventilation (SIMV). **B,** Assist volume control (AVC) ventilation. The flow is constant and pressure increases throughout inspiration. **C,** Assist pressure control (APC) ventilation or pressure-regulated volume control (PRVC). The pressure is constant and flow decreases throughout inspiration. In PRVC, the level of applied pressure may vary from one breath to the next. **D,** Pressure support ventilation. The pressure is constant and flow decreases throughout inspiration. When the flow reaches one fourth of its initial value, inspiration ends (flow-cycled). The flow and respiratory time are determined by patient effort and level of pressure support applied. The tidal volume varies from one breath to the next.

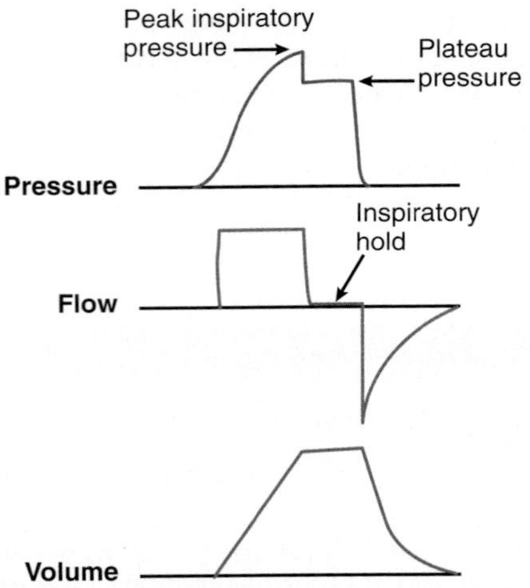

Figure 9-4. A plateau pressure measurement can be obtained in assist volume control mode by the performance of an inspiratory hold to better estimate the pressure in the lungs.

Synchronized Intermittent Mandatory Ventilation

SIMV permits the patient to breathe spontaneously (see Fig. 9-3A) from a fresh gas source without ventilator assistance in between mechanical breaths delivered at predetermined intervals (see Fig. 9-3B or C). Some studies have shown that SIMV may reduce the need for sedation or analgesic agents, thus facilitating weaning from mechanical ventilation.[16] This mode of ventilation was specifically created to allow the weaning of patients from mechanical ventilation when the only other modes that existed were CMV and assist control. Because SIMV is typically associated with lower intrathoracic pressure than the other modes, it has been advocated by some writers to enhance cardiac performance.[17]

The combination of PSV and SIMV allows spontaneous breaths to be increased to an acceptable tidal volume not achieved with spontaneous effort alone.[18] A very low level of PSV may also be selected to compensate for the inherent impedances of the ventilator circuit and endotracheal tube, enabling the patient to establish a more natural breathing pattern and to have the sensation of breathing spontaneously without an endotracheal tube in place. Higher levels can be selected when respiration muscle strength or lung disease makes spontaneous breaths inadequate. A potential advantage of stand-alone PSV (discussed previously) is that all breaths are partially supported to the same degree, whereas with SIMV plus PSV, the patient receives a totally supported mechanical breath followed by one or more less supported breaths. In this regard, the patient's inherent neurologic mechanisms may find the alternating pattern disturbing.

A potential difficulty associated with the SIMV mode is the higher level of work the patient must perform to obtain a spontaneous breath. The spontaneous respiration's work is increased because the patient must overcome the impedance of the ventilatory circuit and the endotracheal tube. It is unusual for SIMV to be used without some level of pressure support to offset this increased work of breathing. Some newer ventilators automatically apply endotracheal tube compensation in the form of pressure support based on breath-by-breath estimation of airway resistance. When SIMV is used as a weaning mode, evaluation for extubation typically occurs with an SIMV rate of 4 to 6 breaths per minute.

Pressure-Regulated Volume Control

Pressure-regulated volume control mode is a variant on APC ventilation whereby the pressure is allowed to go up or down within set limits to achieve a targeted tidal volume (see Fig. 9-3C). This is achieved by adjusting the ventilator system pressure up or down (within preset limits) to achieve the desired tidal volume. This mode allows use of a pressure control breath and associated decelerating flow pattern while limiting the disadvantage of changing tidal volumes in response to changes in airways resistance or lung compliance.

Pressure Support Ventilation

PSV (flow-cycled breaths) was introduced in the mid-1980s to reduce the work of spontaneous breathing in the SIMV mode. It is now commonly used as the sole method of ventilation support. With PSV, as the patient inhales, the ventilator automatically adjusts the flow to provide and maintain a preset inspiratory support pressure. The ventilator's pressure support mechanism provides a variable flow but a constant pressure, allowing the patient to participate in selecting inspiratory flow rates and VT that are in tune with the inherent problem and respiratory muscle status (see Fig. 9-3D). Pressure support levels are now available up to 100 cm H_2O, depending on the ventilator model. Most ventilators also offer adjustment of the inspiratory rise in the pressure, which allows more synchrony in patients with either high or low inspiratory demands.

For weaning a patient off ventilator support, pressure support is gradually diminished—2 to 5 cm H_2O at a time—until the patient is tolerating 5 cm H_2O of PSV, at which point extubation can be undertaken. Patients intubated with smaller endotracheal tubes, even if ready to be weaned, may not tolerate pressure support of 5 cm H_2O and may require 7 or 10 cm H_2O.

Because PSV depends on an intact ventilatory drive, it cannot be used in patients with respiratory drive suppression.[19,20] It is not ideal for patients with bronchospasm or excessive bronchial secretions because of the frequently changing airway resistance and lung compliance in these patients. A consequence of a preset pressure delivered to the patient is that any change in either airway impedance or lung compliance will result in a concomitant change in the volume the patient is able to obtain with a given level of pressure support.

Controlled Mechanical Ventilation

With CMV, the patient has no influence on mechanical ventilation, including no ability to initiate breaths or to determine characteristics of a breath. It is predominantly used for stabilizing patients with the severest respiratory compromise during the initial phase of mechanical ventilation support. After stabilization by this mode of ventilation, patients are switched to an alternative mode in which nonsupported spontaneous ventilation or partially supported spontaneous ventilation can be maintained by the patients themselves. The duration of CMV can vary from hours to days to weeks, or even to months, depending on the nature of the lung injury. Current ventilators do not have a CMV setting; this mode is achieved by selecting the AVC (see Fig. 9-3B) or APC (see Fig. 9-3C) mode and instituting heavy sedation or paralysis so there is no patient interaction with the ventilator.

OTHER MODES OF MECHANICAL VENTILATION

The majority of patients supported on mechanical ventilation initially receive AVC. Less frequently used modes of mechanical ventilation are bilevel ventilation, proportional assist ventilation, volume-assisted pressure support ventilation, high-frequency ventilation, and inverse ratio ventilation.

Bilevel Ventilation

Bilevel ventilation is characterized by ventilating, over time, from two system pressures, one higher (P_{high}) and one lower (P_{low}). This mode was introduced in 1987 as *airway pressure release ventilation* (APRV).[21] It initially targeted paralyzed patients with acute respiratory distress syndrome (ARDS) with no spontaneous ventilation capability, featuring brief periods of P_{low} to clear CO_2. This mode of mechanical ventilation has evolved into one that allows not only spontaneous ventilation but also application of pressure support to spontaneous breaths. It is now also known as APRV with spontaneous breathing as well as *bilevel positive airway pressure* (BiPAP) (not to be confused with the brand name BiPAP ventilation by Respironics, one of many commercially available ventilators made for noninvasive ventilation).[22]

Bilevel ventilation can be used with two different conceptual applications and settings. In both circumstances the P_{high} is targeted to maintain an open lung in patients with ARDS through application of an upper pressure below the upper deflection zone (area of overinflation) of the pressure volume curve but yet high enough to open the majority of alveoli that can be recruited. In one application (APRV with spontaneous breathing), P_{low} is set at a level at which significant expiratory flow is still occurring but prior to the point of significant end-expiratory alveolar closure. In this circumstance the time at the low system pressure setting (T_{low}) is brief and is not associated with capability for spontaneous breathing but is long enough to allow adequate full expiration (Fig. 9-5A).[23] Spontaneous breathing occurs on P_{high} with the second application (BiPAP); the P_{low} is set above the lower inflection point and may be maintained for a time (T_{low}) that allows spontaneous breathing during both P_{high} and P_{low} (see Fig. 9-5B). Therefore, the ratio of T_{high} to T_{low} tends to be around 6:1 for APRV with spontaneous breathing and 1:2 for BiPAP. In both cases, the drop from P_{high} to P_{low} is intended to allow CO_2 elimination and spontaneous breathing from either P_{high} alone or, in the case of BiPAP, both P_{high} and P_{low}. This modality is intended to elicit diaphragm activity and increase dependent lung ventilation and therefore oxygen-

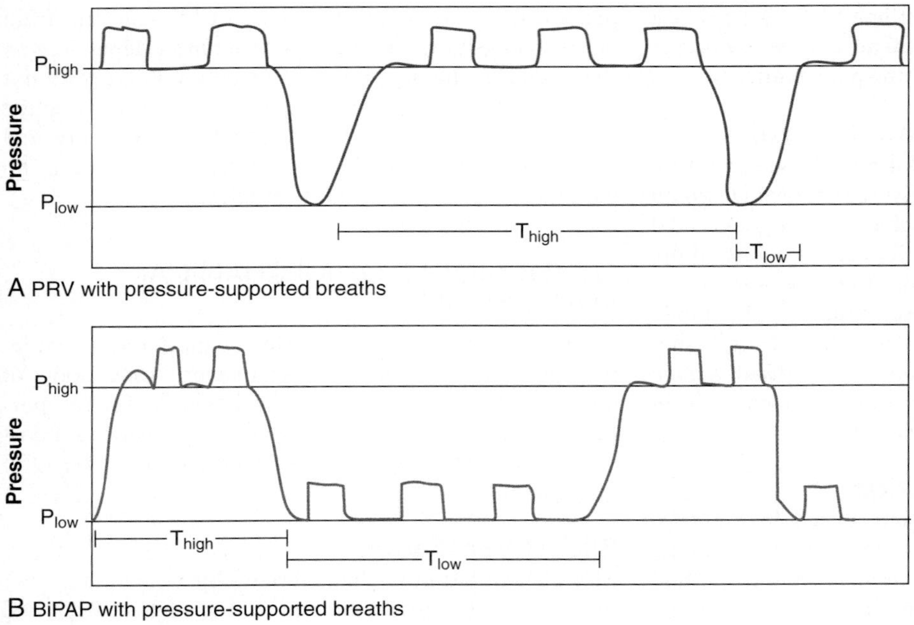

Figure 9-5. Pressure-time waveforms showing the use of airway pressure release ventilation (PRV) to normalize airway pressure at the end of each breath. **A,** PRV with pressure-supported breaths. **B,** Bilevel positive airway pressure (BiPAP) with pressure-supported breaths.

ation in the area where shunt and low $\dot{V}/\dot{Q}$ is marked.[24] Although the application of pressure support may increase tidal volume during spontaneous breathing, it might also decrease diaphragm activity. In addition, the work of breathing at high lung pressure (P_{high}) is less if the P_{high} is associated with lung recruitment and improved compliance. Finally, setting P_{high} at a target consistent with lung protection strategy (30 cm H_2O or less) does not factor in the additional increase in transalveolar pressure associated with the negative intrathoracic pressure generated by spontaneous breathing. It has been shown that bilevel ventilation can decrease inspiratory work of breathing more than CPAP can alone.[25] Bilevel ventilation may be used for maintenance ventilatory support of patients with ARDS to facilitate the weaning process.[26-29]

Proportional Assist Ventilation

One of the shortcomings of traditional mechanical ventilation is that the ventilator cannot adjust from breath to breath to accommodate the patient's change in demand for ventilation. Normal individuals do not breathe spontaneously with the same inspiratory flow and V_T with each inspiratory effort. Varied respiratory patterns are likely a patient preference.

Proportional assist ventilation varies inspiratory support with each mechanical breath on the basis of a patient's inspiratory effort.[30] After measurement of inspiratory resistance and lung compliance, constants are entered into the device, which then facilitate variable amplifications of the patient's effort. As the patient's demand increases, the assist from the mechanical ventilator augments proportionately; likewise, when the patient's demand decreases, the patient is assisted less by the mechanical ventilator. This type of ventilator-patient coupling may allow the patient to feel more comfortable with mechanical ventilation.

During the course of the illness, compliance and resistance of the patient's airways will change, requiring reentry of the constants used to facilitate inspiratory augmentation. Proportional assist ventilation is based on the assumption that the patient will respond in an appropriate manner to determine the optimal type of inspiratory effort, rate, and frequency that should be employed. This assumption may not always be true.

Volume-Assisted Pressure Support

Pressure support ventilation can be delivered by volume-assisted pressure support.[31] This form of ventilation ensures a minimum PSV-delivered tidal volume. It is achieved by having two ventilators, working in parallel, within one device. If the V_T falls below a preset limit, the secondary ventilator then cycles in concert to deliver the additional volume necessary to achieve the target preset V_T. This form of mechanical ventilation has been demonstrated to be well tolerated, although studies are not available to document whether it offers any clinical outcome benefit.[16]

High-Frequency Ventilation

High-frequency ventilation (HFV) employs positive-pressure ventilation with V_T smaller than or equal to the anatomic dead space (V_D) of the lung at typical respiratory frequencies of 60 to 150 breaths per minute or more. Ventilators that employ respiratory frequencies of between 240 and 660 breaths per minute have been designated as ultrahigh-frequency jet ventilators. High-frequency oscillatory ventilation (HFOV) uses a piston, diaphragm, or high-fidelity speaker and generates frequencies in the range of 180 to 900 breaths per minute, with V_T in the range of about 5 to 80 mL. In high-frequency percussive ventilation (HFPV), gas is delivered as a pressure-limited conventional breath with oscillations superimposed on the breath. The most common approach to high-frequency ventilation used today is high-frequency oscillation.

Breaths delivered from these ventilators are time-cycled, positive-pressure breaths in which both inspiration and exhalation are actively generated by the ventilator. The method of breath delivery can be a reciprocating pump, diaphragm, or high-fidelity speaker, depending on the device. Adequacy of ventilation depends on the bias flow that is generated and passed in front of the pump or speaker, which propels the gas into the endotracheal tube. This bias flow is also used to flush out CO_2 during the active expiratory phase. A significant component of bulk convection distributes gases through the large airways, at which point the distribution of gas throughout the rest of the respiratory tree is based on other physical properties. *Pendelluft,* or the movement of gas from fast-filling and fast-emptying units of the lung into slower ones, probably plays a significant role in distributing the gas within the alveoli. *Taylor dispersion* is the radial diffusion of gases associated with a convective process that allows molecules in the central zones, where axial velocities are higher, to diffuse into the lateral zones, where axial velocities are lower. In a theoretical model, Fredburg[32] demonstrated that at these frequencies and velocities, augmented diffusion would play a significant role in achieving gas transport and that gas molecules enhanced with greater energy would move down concentration gradients with greater speed. Gas exchange would be better matched to perfusion because the gases are relying on concentration gradients rather than pressure gradient. The major advantage of delivering small tidal volumes is that it can be done at relatively low pressures, potentially reducing the risk of barotraumas. However, it has not been shown to be superior to conventional ventilation.

Inverse Ratio Ventilation

Typical I:E ratios for the spectrum of mechanically ventilated patients range from 1:2 to 1:5, lower ratios being used for patients with obstructive airways disease. Inverse ratio ventilation (IRV), positive-pressure ventilation with an I:E greater than 1, has been advocated by some for use in patients with severe ARDS (see Chapter 11).[33] IRV can be achieved with either volume-cycled or time-cycled ventilation and has been shown to effectively increase oxygenation in patients with ARDS.[34,35] Extending the inspiratory time while holding tidal volume constant increases the mean airway pressure without raising the peak alveolar pressure. IRV therefore also allows achievement of the same mean airway pressure with a lower inspiratory plateau pressure (IPP). Theoretically this has a potential advantage for patients with severe ARDS. Evidence supports a benefit to limiting IPP.[36]

The most common application of IRV is with the use of pressure-controlled (time-cycled) ventilation. Figure 9-6 displays pressure and flow waveforms during application of IRV. The peak airway pressure remains the same, whereas inspiratory time is lengthened. In this way, mean airway pressure rises but peak inspiratory pressure, as a reflection of peak alveolar pressure, does not. Oxygenation may therefore be improved while limiting peak alveolar pressure. The bulk of the oxygenation improvement seen can be obtained at I:E ratios of 1:1, and further increases in I:E: ratios are not usually efficacious. Patients with significant airflow obstruction should not be treated with this mode of ventilation. Prolonged I:E ratios may raise the rate of pneumothorax, as the shortened expiratory time may not allow for complete expiration, resulting in auto-positive end-expiratory pressure (auto-PEEP).

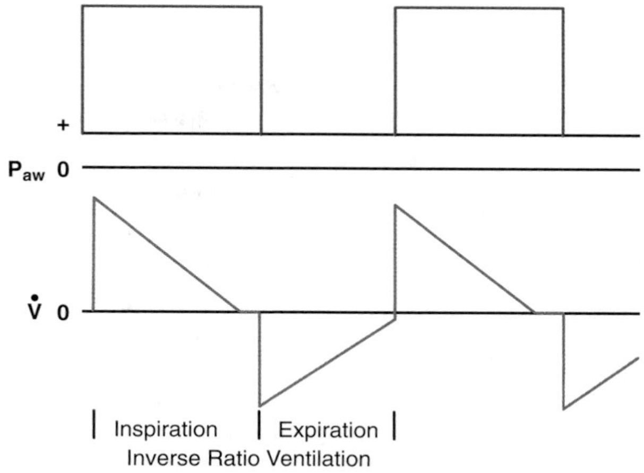

Figure 9-6. Characteristic pressure-flow waveform in a patient undergoing inverse ratio ventilation (the inspiration-to-expiration [I:E] ratio is approximately 1.2:1.0). *Upper panel,* The pressure (P_{aw}) waveform is square, indicating that time-cycled (pressure-control) ventilation is in place. *Lower panel,* The characteristic decelerating inspiratory flow ($\dot{V}$) waveform. The inspiratory flow waveform returns to baseline (zero flow state) before the end of inspiration, signifying that the set inspiratory time is long enough to allow equilibration of pressures between the ventilator and the patient before the end of inspiration. Further prolongation of inspiratory time will therefore not increase tidal volume. Also note that the end-expiratory flow does not return to baseline, making the diagnosis of auto–positive end-expiratory pressure (auto-PEEP).

IRV remains controversial but should be considered when conventional ventilation modes leave the patient with ARDS in persistent severe hypoxemia,[37] particularly in the presence of an IPP greater than 30 cm H_2O.

Continuous Positive Airway Pressure and Positive End-Expiratory Pressure

The CPAP system uses a high-pressure reservoir and a constant flow of gas that exceeds the patient's inspiratory peak flow demands. Consequently, the patient initiates inspiration from a pressure that is constantly above ambient (Fig. 9-7). CPAP is not a mode of mechanical ventilation because no positive pressure above baseline system pressure is applied during inspiration. Used alone or with low levels of PSV, it provides a supply of fresh gas during weaning trials; used alone or in combination with modes of mechanical ventilation, CPAP allows application of PEEP. Typically the terms CPAP and PEEP are used interchangeably. The presence of PEEP without CPAP would imply that patient inspiratory effort (either spontaneous or to trigger a ventilator breath) is dropping ventilation system pressure below zero. This scenario

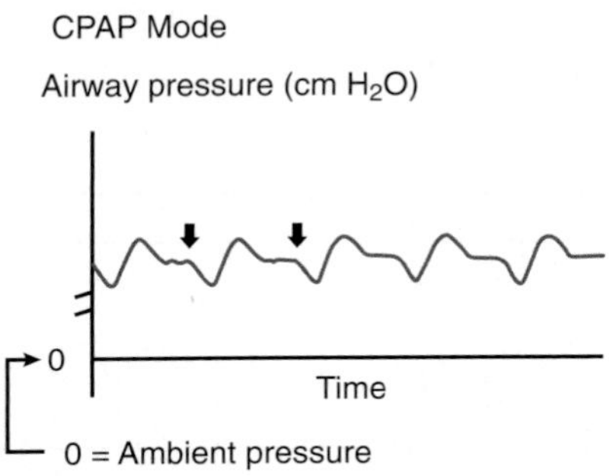

Figure 9-7. A pressure-time waveform in a patient with continuous positive airway pressure (CPAP) without application of pressure support ventilation is demonstrated. The patient is breathing spontaneously at an elevated baseline system pressure. With initiation of inspiration (*arrows*), pressure becomes more negative (but remains positive) and with the expiration pressure becomes more positive. Note that this figure demonstrates the application of both CPAP and positive end-expiratory pressure (PEEP). The only mechanism by which PEEP could be present without CPAP in this patient would be if the initial inspiratory drop in pressure went below 0 cm H_2O, which is not desirable.

would be difficult to achieve and, if achieved, would be associated with significantly and undesirably high work of breathing for the patient.

PEEP ventilation provides a pressure above atmospheric at end-expiration, preventing destabilized alveoli in patients with acute lung injury from collapsing at the end of the respiratory cycle. By preventing alveolar collapse at end-expiration in such patients, PEEP prevents atelectasis, increases functional residual capacity (FRC), and improves oxygenation. When PEEP is applied, the mean airway pressure is increased in proportion to the level of PEEP. PEEP can be set on most ventilators from 2 to 45 cm H_2O, although it is most commonly employed in the range of 5 to 20 cm H_2O. When the patient is started on PEEP ventilation, the pressure-triggering thresholds on the ventilators are also set to this new elevated end-expiratory pressure. The operator then titrates PEEP in increments of 2 to 3 cm H_2O until an adequate arterial oxygen tension is achieved at an acceptable level of inspired oxygen concentration. Although high sustained IPP recruits previously atelectatic lung, adequate PEEP is needed to prevent derecruitment. When calculating dynamic and static compliance of a ventilator patient receiving PEEP ventilation, one has to remember to subtract the PEEP value from the peak and plateau pressures to obtain accurate measurements.

POTENTIAL FUTURE MODES

Greater knowledge of the mechanisms that determine respiratory failure has led to the development of new technologies aimed at improving ventilatory treatment. The main difference between modes is essentially the manner in which positive pressure is applied to the airway, and therefore, a "new" mode generally introduces a novel approach to support delivery. As long as the patient's respiratory centers, phrenic nerves, and neuromuscular junctions are intact and his or her ventilatory drive is not suppressed by drugs, the amount of support provided should instantaneously correspond to the ventilatory demand, irrespective of variations in muscle length or contractility. Neurally adjusted ventilatory assist (NAVA) has been designed with the goal of improving patient-ventilator interaction by matching the ventilator support with the neural output of the respiratory centers.[38]

Neurally Adjusted Ventilatory Assist

Neurally adjusted ventilatory assist is an experimental mode in which the ventilator assistance is titrated in proportion to the electrical activity of the diaphragm (EAdi) during assisted ventilation, assessed by means of an esophageal electrode. Detection and quantification of the electrical activity of the crural diaphragm (EAdi) by means of an esophageal array of bipolar electrodes have been validated in humans.[39,40] Crural EAdi has been shown to accurately express global diaphragm activation in healthy subjects[41] and in patients with either chronic[42] or acute respiratory failure (ARF).[43] The array of bipolar electrodes can be mounted on a feeding tube, which is routinely introduced in critically ill patients. For accurate measurement purposes, the active region of the diaphragm is determined through cross-correlation of the signals obtained along the electrode array.[39] The processed signal is then transferred to the ventilator unit to regulate the ventilatory support, which is therefore instantaneously applied in relation to EAdi. The amount of ventilatory assistance for a given level of EAdi depends on a user-adjustable proportionality factor that determines how much pressure will be delivered for a given EAdi amplitude.[38] Because the ventilator is triggered directly by EAdi, the synchrony between neural and mechanical inspiratory time is guaranteed both at the onset and at the end of inspiration, regardless of PEEP, air leaks, and respiratory mechanics. The use of neural control of mechanical ventilation has the capability to dramatically enhance the coordination between mechanical ventilation and respiratory muscle activity, thereby improving patient comfort.

Biologically Variable (or Fractal) Ventilation

Controlled modes of mechanical ventilation may be responsible for alveolar collapse, increased shunt fraction, and deterioration in arterial oxygenation, even in healthy subjects during prolonged general anesthesia.[44] It has been hypothesized that the loss of the physiologic variability of the breathing pattern may contribute to the deterioration in respiratory mechanics and gas exchange abnormalities observed over time with controlled mechanical ventilation.[45] Biologically variable ventilation is a mode that mimics spontaneous breath-to-breath variability, incorporating natural variable noise into a volume-targeted, controlled mode.[46] The ventilator is programmed to modulate respiratory rate and tidal volume while maintaining a fixed minute ventilation on the basis of a previously generated data file. Respiratory rate and tidal volume vary reciprocally, and minute ventilation remains constant at each breath.[47] The results obtained in animal models support the validity of the mathematical model that assumes a positive effect (especially improvement in oxygenation and shunt fraction) of adding random breath-to-breath variability to mechanical ventilation.[48]

INSTITUTING MECHANICAL VENTILATION

Decisions about ventilatory support are usually made under emergency conditions. Yet adequate patient preparation is necessary to ensure that the mechanical ventilation experience will be as minimally traumatic and as effective as possible. The goals of mechanical ventilation in ARF are to maintain adequate alveolar ventilation and reverse hypoxemia while minimizing complications.

Preparing the Patient for Mechanical Ventilation

After the decision to initiate ventilation is made, the ventilator should be prepared and tested in the department with the proper patient circuit, and brought to the bedside. At the bedside, the ventilator should be reevaluated for operation and preset to initial parameters to minimize any delay between intubation and onset of mechanical ventilation. Box 9-1 suggests guidelines for setting basic operating parameters in a mechanical ventilator.

After mechanical ventilation is instituted, the lungs should be auscultated to ensure that there is appropriate exchange of gas bilaterally. Inspiratory and expiratory volumes should be compared to ensure that there are no leaks in the patient's circuit and that the patient is not becoming hyperinflated because of excessive volumes or air trapping. Careful observation of patient effort and delivery of the ventilator breaths is necessary to optimize patient-ventilator synchrony. One should pay particular attention to the inspiratory gas flow rate, because underestimating or overestimating it is one of the leading causes of patient discomfort. Excessive inspiratory gas flow causes the patient to cough with each ventilator cycle, and inspiratory flows that are too low cause significant air hunger and create a very uncomfortable sensation. To determine the latter, the clinician should observe the airway pressure manometer. When demand exceeds flow, the pressure indicator needle does not rise smoothly but exhibits a ratcheting type of pattern during inflation. This same information may be obtained by evaluating the pressure-time curves on the ventilator's graphic display.

In addition to inspiratory and expiratory volumes, the I:E ratio should be evaluated. An adequate I:E ratio allows ample time for exhalation, therefore preventing hyperinflation and auto-PEEP (see Chapter 10).

In most patients, the initial F_{IO_2} value should be 0.95 to 1.0. This approach alleviates hypoxemia quickly and safeguards against complications of intubation that may have worsened oxygenation. An F_{IO_2} value of 0.95 is recommended by some experts from concern that pure oxygen may result in an increased right-to-left shunt because of absorptive atelectasis.

After mechanical ventilation is established, arterial blood gas levels should be measured to ascertain the adequacy of alveolar ventilation. Oxygenation can be monitored quite nicely in the vast majority of patients through pulse oximetry. In most patients it is best to wait approximately 30 minutes after a ventilator change before measuring arterial blood gas values to ensure that adequate equilibration has occurred between alveolar ventilation and the arterial blood. If the Pa_{CO_2} is too high (more than 50 mm Hg in the patient who was normocapnic before admission), alveolar ventilation is increased by changing either the VT or the respiratory rate. The new respiratory frequency can usually be determined by the following equation:

$$\text{Desired Respiratory Rate} = \text{Prior Rate} \times (\text{Prior } Pa_{CO_2}/Pa_{CO_2})$$

In a patient who is chronically hypercapnic, it is wise to adjust the ventilator to keep him or her in a similar hypercapnic state as at the baseline; otherwise, bicarbon-

Box 9-1

Guidelines for the Initiation of Mechanical Ventilation

1. Choose the ventilator mode with which you are most familiar. The primary goals of ventilatory support are adequate oxygenation/ventilation, reduced work of breathing, synchrony between the patient and ventilator, and avoidance of high end-inspiration alveolar pressures.
2. The initial F_{IO_2} (fraction of inspired oxygen) value should be 1.0. The F_{IO_2} thereafter can be titrated downward to maintain the Sp_{O_2} (oxyhemoglobin saturation) at 92% to 94%. In severe acute respiratory distress syndrome (ARDS) ≥88% Sp_{O_2} may be acceptable to minimize complications of mechanical ventilation.
3. Initial tidal volume (VT) should be 8-10 mL/kg. Patients with acute renal failure (ARF) from neuromuscular disease often require VT of 10-12 mL/kg to satisfy air hunger. In patients with ARDS, it is recommended to use a VT of 6 mL/kg and to keep inspiratory plateau pressure (IPP) 30 cm H_2O or greater.
4. Choose a respiratory rate and minute ventilation appropriate for the particular clinical requirements. Target pH, not Pa_{CO_2}. Initial respiratory rate is typically 10-12 breaths/min.
5. Use positive end-expiratory pressure (PEEP) in diffuse lung injury to support oxygenation and reduce the F_{IO_2}.
6. In COPD patients, avoid choosing settings that limit expiratory time and cause or worsen auto-PEEP.
7. When poor oxygenation, inadequate ventilation, or excessively high peak inspiration pressures are thought to be related to patient intolerance of ventilator settings and are not corrected by ventilator adjustment, consider initiating or increasing sedation or analgesia.

Adapted from Fundamental Critical Care Support, Des Plaines, IL, 2007, Society of Critical Care Medicine.

ate stores will be lost and subsequent weaning of the patient will result in a significant elevation in CO_2 in the arterial blood, and a respiratory acidosis will ensue. It should also be noted that increased CO_2 production has been demonstrated to be the main cause of greater ventilatory demand in mechanically ventilated patients in the ICU.[49]

Monitoring Mechanical Ventilatory Support

Monitoring airway pressures can be helpful both in deciding when a patient's acute lung injury is healing and in determining when problems have developed in the mechanical ventilator circuit. For example, peak inspiratory pressure is a function of both airway resistance and lung compliance, whereas the plateau pressure, obtained by placing an inspiratory pause at the end of inhalation, is a function only of the elastic recoil of the lung. The difference between the peak and plateau pressures, therefore, represents the pressure necessary to overcome the resistance of the airways. When there is a change in the compliance of the lung, the peak and plateau pressures rise together. This occurs in situations such as ARDS, increases in lung fluid secondary to congestive heart failure, pneumothorax (both tension and nontension), and right and left mainstem bronchial intubation. If the peak inspiratory pressure rises but the plateau pressure does not change or increases only a small amount, an increase in airway resistance has usually occurred. Such an increase can result from bronchospasm, mucus secretions, kinking of the endotracheal tube, or some other obstruction in the ventilator circuit.

Oxygenation is usually monitored by measuring either the alveolar-arterial pressure gradient or the alveolar-to arterial pressure (A : a) ratio. If the FiO_2 is changed often, it is probably better to use A : a ratio because it varies less with changes in FiO_2 than the alveolar-arterial gradient.

The Importance of Sedation and Analgesia in Mechanically Ventilated Patients

Sedation therapy is a paradigm of the multidisciplinary nature of critical care that demands collaboration among nursing and medical professionals. Critically ill patients who are mechanically ventilated often require sedative and analgesic drugs such as benzodiazepines, propofol, and opiates.[50-52] The ideal sedative and analgesic regimen would provide adequate sedation and pain control, rapid onset of action, rapid recovery after discontinuation, minimal systemic accumulation, and minimal adverse effects—without raising health care costs.[50] The primary aim of these medications is to reduce the physiologic stress of respiratory failure and to improve the tolerance of mechanical ventilation. Previous studies have reported pain and anxiety as common experiences for patients during ICU stay, especially after invasive procedures such as endotracheal suctioning.[53] Many patients requiring mechanical ventilation suffer from impaired gas exchange and cardiovascular instability. Sedatives and analgesics have been shown to reduce oxygen consumption and autonomic hyperactivity, helping oxygen delivery and consumption balance.[54] The critical state of the patient in ICU creates a difficult balance between maintaining adequate levels of sedation and analgesia and avoiding the potential adverse effects of these therapies.

Even with studies that show that sedation protocols lead to improved patient outcomes, defining adequate sedation is difficult. Several reliable instruments for assessing level of sedation, such as the Ramsey Scale, the Sedation Agitation Scale, the Richmond Agitation-Sedation Scale, and the Adaptation to Intensive Care Environment instrument, are available.[55-57] Because of changes in the sedative dose-response relationship in critically ill patients, the individual level of sedation is important, and those scales have been tested extensively for validity and reliability in measuring consciousness and tolerance domains of patients. Moreover, it has been suggested that multiple-domain sedation scales (i.e., two behavioral domains, including level of consciousness and spontaneous motor activity) that have a few ordered levels more accurately characterize sedated patients than a single-domain scale with numerous levels.[58,59]

Sedatives are administered by either continuous intravenous infusion or intermittent boluses. The latter is preferable, especially when targeted to dosing for effect. Continuous infusion can maintain a more consistent level of sedation, but for the prevention of oversedation, monitoring is necessary. Intermittent bolus techniques may reduce the total amount of drug given; however, a potential of reduced patient comfort and greater burdens on bedside clinicians are the issues that must be addressed. With protocols, frequent assessments of patient needs and goal-directed titration of analgesics and sedatives are possible. Daily interruption of sedative infusions or holding back an intermittent administration order allows patients to spend some of their ICU time awake and interactive, potentially reducing the amount of sedative and opiate given as well as decreasing the need for diagnostic studies (e.g., brain computed tomography scan) to evaluate unexplained alterations in mental status. In addition, it allows assessment for readiness for extubation. Studies have found that protocol directed by bedside nurses or a routine of daily interruption of sedative infusions improved outcomes such as duration of mechanical ventilation, length of ICU and hospital stays, and the need for tracheostomy.[60,61] There is an inverse relationship between sedation intensity and spontaneous motor activity.[57,62] Studies show that increasing wakefulness during mechanical ventilation is associated with improved ICU and post-ICU outcomes.[61,63,64] Allowing more (but noninjurious) spontaneous movement during mechanical ventilation may prevent loss of muscle mass and joint function.[62]

Secretion Clearance and Positioning

Secretion clearance is impaired in the mechanically ventilated patient owing to decreased mucociliary activity and inability to cough effectively. The presence of an artificial airway, airway trauma due to suctioning, high FiO_2 values, and inadequate humidification all contribute to impairment of mucociliary activity. The presence of an artificial airway and depressed neurologic status due to sedation and, often, the underlying disease process impair cough effectiveness. Methods commonly used to improve secretion clearance in intubated patients include suctioning, inhaled β-agonists, postural drainage therapy with or without percussion, positioning, and bronchoscopy.

Suctioning is an important aspect of airway care. Turning the patient's head to the opposite side, lateral positioning, and use of curved-tip catheters facilitate selective endobronchial suctioning. Closed suction prevents both alveolar derecruitment during suctioning and contamination of clinicians during the suction procedure. Hypoxemia, atelectasis, airway trauma, cardiac arrhythmias, contamination, increased intracranial pressure, coughing, and bronchospasm are the complications of suctioning. Saline instillation was often used in the past to facilitate secretion removal; because more saline is instilled than is removed, however, this policy may be problematic. It may be useful for selected patients with tenacious secretions but should not be a routine procedure. Manual hyperinflation therapy is of little benefit and potentially dangerous in acutely ill patients who are producing little sputum. Preoxygenation with an FIO_2 value of 1.0, a closed-suction system, proper catheter size (one-half to one-third the internal diameter of the airway), gentle technique, least amount of vacuum necessary to evacuate secretions (<150 mm Hg), and limiting the time of each suction attempt to less than 15 seconds with suctioning applied only during withdrawal of the catheter are techniques that avoid suctioning-related complications. Fiberoptic bronchoscopy should be used for secretion management only when lobar or larger-area atelectasis persists despite conservative methods.

FEATURES OF VENTILATORS

Alarms and Safety Features

Current ventilators are equipped with monitors that constantly or periodically assess the ventilator's operation and the patient's status. These monitors are usually associated with alarms that visually or audibly notify the operator of any variation from the preset norm. Although different ventilators have different alarm systems, the following alarms should be basic to any ventilator: low exhaled volume alarm, low inspiratory pressure alarm, high inspiratory pressure alarm, apnea alarm, high respiratory rate alarm, and FIO_2 alarm. Typical monitoring and alarm systems are shown in Figure 9-8. The alarms should be backed up by a battery source to prevent malfunction in the event of electrical failure. As sophisticated as these

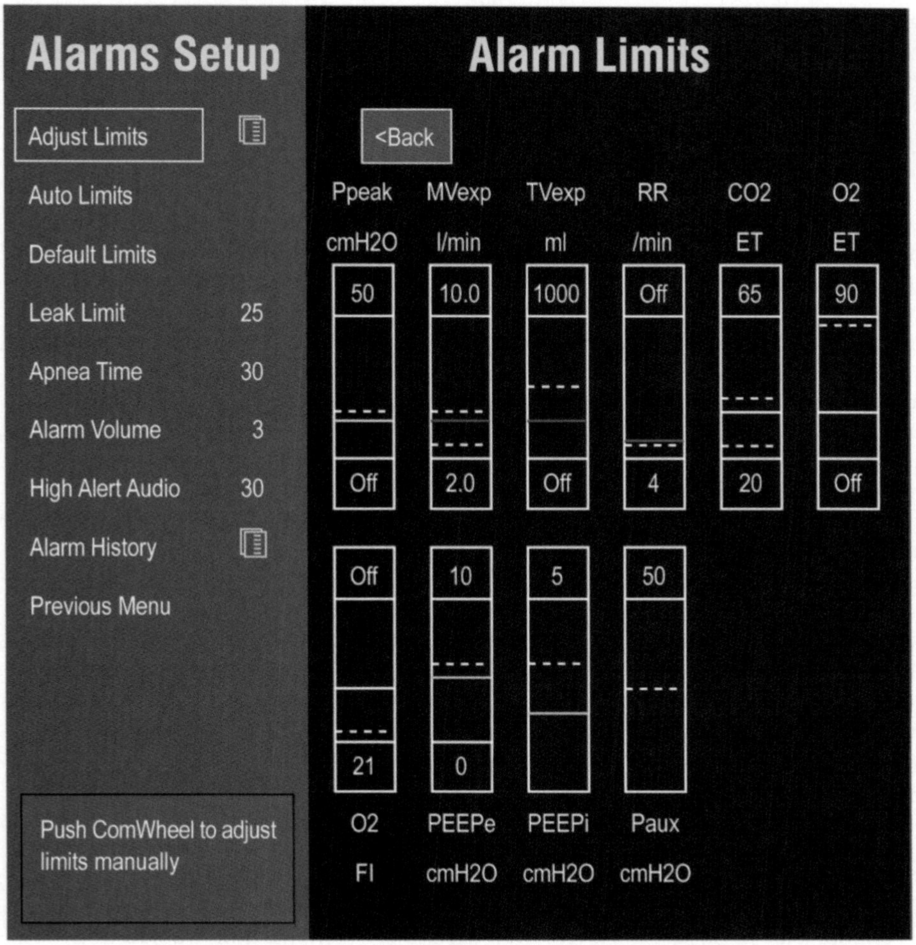

Figure 9-8. The alarm panel of a Draeger Evita 4 ventilator showing the alarms typically used on current ventilators. (Reproduced with permission from Draeger Medical, Inc., Lübeck, Germany.)

monitors may appear, however, they are not infallible and in fact often switch off when nothing is wrong (i.e., false alarms). One study has estimated that 64% of all activated alarms are false.[65] The frequency of false alarms is extremely disruptive in the critical care unit, and the high number of false alarms may lead to an alarm's being ignored. Obviously we cannot condone this practice, but it reminds us that monitors can never be a substitute for close patient observation by qualified health care workers.

Heated Humidifier and Respiratory Circuit

In the body, inspired gases are conditioned in the airway just before the carina so that they are fully saturated with water at body temperature by the time they reach the alveoli (37°C, 100% relative humidity, 44 mg/L absolute humidity, 47 mm Hg water vapor pressure). This portion of the airway acts as a heat and moisture exchanger. Under normal conditions, about 250 mL of water is lost from the lungs each day to humidify the inspired gases.

Gases delivered from mechanical ventilators are typically dry, and the upper airways of patients being ventilated are functionally bypassed by artificial airways, necessitating the use of external humidifying apparatus in the breathing circuit. Because the upper airway is bypassed during mechanical ventilation, the inspired gas temperature should be kept close to the body temperature. Inspired gases that bypass the upper respiratory tract through endotracheal tubes or tracheostomy tubes should be heated to at least 32° to 34°C at 95% to 100% relative humidity. The temperature probe for the heated humidifier should be placed inside the inspiratory limb of the ventilator circuit as close to the patient as possible. Moisture loss and subsequent dehydration of the respiratory tract result in epithelial damage.

A heat and moisture exchanger (HME), which is placed between the artificial airway and the ventilator circuit, may be used to replace the traditional heated humidifier. During exhalation, moisture and heat from the patient are absorbed into the honeycomb structure of the exchanger and are transferred back to the patient during the next inhalation. Ventilator circuits with bacterial-viral filtering heat and moisture exchangers cost less to maintain and are less likely to colonize bacteria than those with heated humidifiers.[66,67] Contraindications for use of a heat and moisture exchanger are thick or large amounts of secretions, minute volume exceeding 10 L/min, body temperature less than 32°C, and need for aerolized medications.[68]

Ventilator circuits are compliant and expand during a positive-pressure breath. The amount of circuit expansion results in a volume that does not reach the patient but is recorded as a part of the expired tidal volume. This volume lost in the ventilator circuit, called the *circuit compressible volume,* may be calculated.[69] Once the circuit compressible volume is known, the patient's corrected tidal volume can be calculated by subtracting the circuit compressible volume from the expired tidal volume. The tidal volume actually delivered to the patient's lungs is usually lower than the ventilator-delivered tidal volume. The reasons are circuit compressible volume loss, gas leakage in the ventilator circuitry, and endotracheal tube cuff leak. Minor gas leakage and circuit compressible volume loss can be compensated by using a larger tidal volume. Some ventilators automatically compensate for the compressible volume loss and thus maintain a stable tidal volume. Others measure the volume delivered to the patient at the airway opening, allowing detection of significant volume loss due to circuit compression factor or gas leakage.

Automatic Tube Compensation

Traditionally, most clinicians applied some amount of preselected pressure support to compensate for the increased work of breathing during expiration related to endotracheal tube resistance. The amount of PSV needed to counterbalance this resistance depended not only on the internal diameter of the endotracheal tube but also on flow, bend of the tube, and mucus buildup in the tube, so this was an imprecise estimate only.

Automatic tube compensation (ATC) compensates for endotracheal tube resistance via closed-loop control of calculated tracheal pressure. A ventilator with ATC compensates for the pressure drop across the endotracheal tube during inspiration by increasing the airway pressure and during expiration by decreasing airway pressure according to actual gas flow.[70,71] This technique uses a continuous calculation of the flow-dependent drop in pressure across the endotracheal tube. ATC is similar to PSV, but the pressure applied by the ventilator varies as a function of endotracheal tube resistance and flow demand. Most of the interest in ATC revolves around eliminating the imposed work of breathing during inspiration. During expiration, however, ATC may also compensate for that flow resistance by lowering the pressure in the expiratory circuit limb transiently from its PEEP setting, helping reduce effective expiratory resistance and auto-PEEP.[72] In addition to overcoming the work of breathing imposed by the artificial airway, ATC may improve patient-ventilator synchrony by varying the flow commensurate with demand and may reduce air trapping by compensating for imposed expiratory resistance. During weaning trials, this technique may allow a more reliable prediction of patient performance when the tube is removed.

COMPLICATIONS OF MECHANICAL VENTILATION

Complications of mechanical ventilation can be grouped into two broad categories, those caused by the cyclical pressure inflation of the lung and those associated with the state of being treated with a mechanical ventilator. The conditions associated with cyclical pulmonary inflation are pneumothorax, pneumomediastinum, pneumoperitoneum, subcutaneous emphysema, pulmonary interstitial emphysema, hyperinflation injury (volutrauma), shear stress injury from collapse and reopening of airspaces with each cycle, and the adverse reaction of the elevated mean airway pressure on cardiac function. Other well-described complications associated with mechanical ventilation are the loss of upper airway defenses against invasion by the omnipresent bacteria in the ICU; problems associated with the immobility of the patient, such as the development of deep venous thrombosis and pulmonary emboli; the stress of receiving mechanical ventilation, such as gastritis and ulcer formation; the changes associated with intravascular volume regulation, resulting in electrolyte imbalance and renal insufficiency; and the complications associated with intubation with a cuffed endotracheal tube or the need for a tracheostomy.

Decreased Cardiac Output

Reduced cardiac output associated with positive-pressure ventilation is a not-uncommon and potentially serious complication of mechanical ventilation. There are multiple contributing factors. Mechanical ventilation, by raising intrathoracic pressure, decreases venous return to the heart. The rise in intrathoracic pressure also results in a concomitant increase in right atrial and right ventricular pressures. The result may be a shift of the intraventricular septum from its normal position to a position impinging on the left ventricular cavity, decreasing diastolic filling. Positive pressure in the lung surrounding the left and right ventricles also reduces diastolic filling by lowering the transmural filling pressure. PEEP (set PEEP or auto-PEEP) or using IRV is particularly problematic in that it causes a decrease in cardiac output. Careful bedside evaluation for signs and symptoms of reduction in cardiac output in the patient at risk is crucial to adequately maintaining such a patient. Strategies for maintaining patients with acute lung injury who are undergoing mechanical ventilation should revolve around keeping the lowest mean airway pressure that will support adequate oxygenation at a favorable FIO_2. The effect of increasing intrathoracic pressure on cardiac output is influenced significantly by intravascular volume, with lower intravascular volume facilitating the effect.

Barotrauma

Elevated peak inspiratory pressures and mean airway pressures have been implicated as being traumatic to the lung parenchyma. High peak inspiratory pressures are associated with pneumothorax, whereas elevated mean airway pressures are associated with pneumothorax and reduction in cardiac output.[73] It is not clear whether high peak inspiratory pressures are a primary or secondary phenomenon associated with the generation of pneumothorax. It is possible that nonhomogeneous lung ventilation (areas of poorly ventilated and well-ventilated alveoli in close proximity) results in pressure gradients across the interstitium and alveoli and the potential for rupture. However, it is a common clinical strategy to try to limit peak inspiratory pressure and mean airway pressure as much as possible. Animal studies have demonstrated in normal lungs that higher volume per respiration is associated with greater transudation of fluid across the pulmonary capillary membrane. Originally it was believed to be the result of the difference in pressure, but studies in animal models have now shown that it is not the pressure that causes edema genesis but the change in gas volume.[74] As a precaution, strategies have been developed to lower the peak inspiratory pressure in the hope of reducing complications secondary to mechanical ventilation.

Barotrauma is the most commonly associated complication of mechanical ventilation, with the literature suggesting an incidence of between 7% and 25%.[75] Much of the difference depends on the case mix in a particular study as well as the definition of barotrauma used. Some investigators identify only patients with overt bronchopleural fistula requiring chest tube drainage as having barotrauma, and include the presence of interstitial air in the definition. There also appears to be an association between higher incidence of pneumothorax and greater peak inspiratory pressures. Interestingly, however, investigators demonstrated equal incidences of pneumothorax for high-frequency ventilation and standard mechanical ventilation.[76,77] The patients in the studies had significantly low peak inspiratory pressure, but the incidence of pneumothorax remained the same. The conclusion of the two investigating teams was that the incidence of pneumothorax is more closely related to the underlying disease than to the level of peak inspiratory pressure. Patients who have necrotizing processes within the lung have a tendency to have a higher rate of pneumothorax than patients who do not. Additionally, in other studies, patients in whom hyperinflation resulted from severe airway obstruction had a marked tendency to have pneumothorax.[78,79]

At present, many investigators believe that pneumothorax is secondary to inhomogeneous ventilation, regardless of the underlying disease in the lung. Necrotizing lung processes, however, result in rupture of alveolar sacs with lower airway pressures than nonnecrotizing processes.

Barotrauma is usually evidenced by a sudden increase in peak inspiratory pressure on the ventilator pressure manometer. If the barotrauma results in a tension pneumothorax, there is usually significant hemodynamic compromise, with an increase in heart rate and a decrease in blood pressure. A reduction in arterial saturation is usually noted in these patients as well. Such patients must be attended to very rapidly. Auscultation of the chest should demonstrate reduced breath sounds on the side of the pneumothorax. A shift of the mediastinum away from a tension pneumothorax is usually evident as well (Fig. 9-9). Under these circumstances, the insertion of a needle into the second intercostal space in the midclavicular line on the appropriate side is indicated to relieve the intrathoracic pressure and restore hemodynamic function.

In the event that the patient is not hemodynamically compromised and a simple pneumothorax is suspected, a chest radiograph should be obtained immediately, and a chest tube should then be placed under more controlled circumstances. Even when the pneumothorax is small, it is probably not prudent for it to be left undrained in a patient who is receiving positive-pressure ventilation. When a large pneumothorax develops and chest tubes are inserted, a large percentage of the V_T generated by the

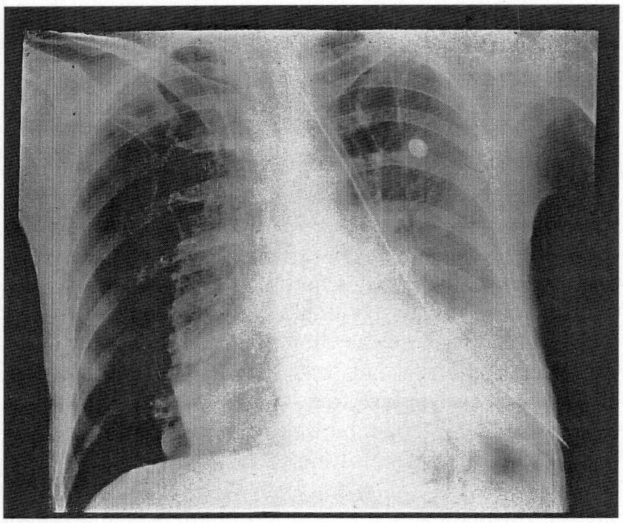

Figure 9-9. Chest radiograph showing right lower lobe infiltrate and right-sided tension pneumothorax with shift of the right heart border past the midline.

ventilator may be exhausted through the chest tube drainage, resulting in significant alveolar hypoventilation. This occurs because there is less resistance for the gas to move across the chest tube than to enter the lung. Some studies have shown that under these circumstances, high-frequency jet ventilation may result in a more uniform distribution of gas because of the smaller VT employed.[80] There are no data yet to suggest that the smaller VT with less leakage across the thoracostomy tube results in earlier closure of pneumothorax after it occurs. Currently, several high-frequency ventilators are available, and anecdotal data have suggested better outcomes in patients without good response to conventional ventilation.

Barotrauma may also manifest as rupture toward the mediastinal surface of the lungs. The earliest sign on the chest radiograph is mediastinal air or air shadows in the pericardial or pleural mediastinal planes. Subcutaneous emphysema is often palpated in these circumstances and can become quite extensive, with air migrating through the tissue planes up to the head, down through the abdomen into the groin, and even into the lower extremities. Cosmetically this migration is very unattractive, although from a clinical standpoint subcutaneous emphysema does not appear to have any significant adverse effects on the patient. There is no way to drain subcutaneous emphysema; however, after the air leak stops, the migrated air is usually quickly reabsorbed, and the subcutaneous emphysema dissipates on its own.

Nosocomial Infection

Virtually all patients in the ICU who are intubated become colonized with the prevalent organisms within 48 hours. It is well established that these organisms, in a significant percentage of patients, lead to ventilator-acquired pneumonia (VAP). Each day of mechanical ventilation raises the risk of VAP. The morbidity and mortality associated with these infections are considerable. Mortality rates can be significantly reduced by appropriate antibiotic selection and aggressive therapy. It is important to recognize the causative organism, because when VAP is treated aggressively, risk of death can be markedly decreased.

Differentiating colonization from infection is not always easy in patients receiving intensive care. Such patients may have fevers for other reasons, and their white blood cell counts may be elevated from other inflammatory processes. Their chest radiographs are usually abnormal and difficult to interpret. For these reasons, a large percentage of patients who do not have bacterial pneumonia are exposed to expensive and ineffective antibiotic therapy with increased risk for potential toxicities and colonization by resistant organisms.

Microscopic evaluation of secretions aspirated from the colonized tracheas of patients undergoing ventilator therapy are inaccurate and can be misleading in directing the selection of antibiotics. Trying to distinguish patients who have colonization from those who have nosocomial infection has resulted in attempts to use quantitative cultures from protected bronchoscopy brush techniques and bronchoalveolar lavage (BAL) to sample tracheobronchial secretions without contamination from the upper airways. The use of bronchoalveolar lavage and protective brush techniques along with specific colony counts may be helpful in improving the specificity and sensitivity of the evaluation of secretions from peripheral airways of the lung.

Recognizing and treating appropriate nosocomial respiratory infections in the patient who is mechanically ventilated remain among the most difficult and frustrating aspects of intensive care medicine. (See also Chapter 51.)

Gastrointestinal Bleeding

A large percentage of patients receiving mechanical ventilation have either occult or overt upper gastrointestinal bleeding. Gastrointestinal blood loss may range from trivial to requiring surgical intervention. It has been demonstrated that potential gastrointestinal bleeding can be reduced with prophylactic measures, including histamine H_2 blocker, sucralfate, and proton pump inhibitor therapy.

Pulmonary Embolism

Pulmonary embolism may be a serious and potentially fatal complication in mechanically ventilated patients. Appropriate therapy for pulmonary emboli can significantly reduce morbidity and mortality; however, the diagnosis is difficult to make in a patient with baseline acute lung injury or another cause of hypoxemia. Low-dose heparin and intermittent pneumatic compression devices have been demonstrated to decrease the incidence of pulmonary embolism in mechanically ventilated patients. Intermittent pneumatic compression devices are recommended in patients for whom heparin treatment poses a high risk.

Pulmonary emboli in the patient receiving mechanical ventilation can be suspected from a sudden increase in minute ventilation without a change in partial pressure of CO_2, indicating an increase in physiologic dead space ventilation, or from a reduction in blood pressure or arterial PO_2. Spiral (helical) CT scanning in combination with leg ultrasonography and a portable single-view perfusion scan is useful in diagnosis. (See also Chapter 45.)

NONINVASIVE POSITIVE-PRESSURE VENTILATION

Noninvasive positive-pressure ventilation (NPPV) offers the potential to provide ventilatory assistance without an invasive artificial airway. NPPV may be accomplished using a facemask or nasal mask fitted to the face and connected through standard ventilator tubing to either a standard mechanical ventilator or smaller ventilators made specifically to deliver noninvasive mechanical ventilation. With the growing availability of improved interfaces and efficient valving mechanisms, the option of applying ventilatory support by suitable mask, in a quick manner without the risk and discomfort of intubation, is now widely exercised. NPPV allows the patient to communicate, and with the mask temporarily removed, to expectorate and eat. Additionally, brief intervals without the mask every several hours may help patients tolerate ventilation better.

The advantages of ventilators specifically designed for NPPV are small size, portability, and ease of use. Such devices that use a common inspiratory and expiratory line can cause rebreathing of exhaled gas and a rise in $PaCO_2$. Expiratory positive airway pressure settings of 3 cm H_2O or higher will likely prevent this situation. Use of standard ventilators for NPPV allows the delivery of precisely measured inspired oxygen concentrations and the use of sophisticated ventilator monitors or an alarm. Any mode can be used, but PSV may be better tolerated. Although variable from patient to patient, the nasal mask is usually better tolerated than the facemask; however, the nasal mask is less effective in mouth breathers and edentulous patients. To reduce air leak through the mouth, patients are coached to keep the mouth shut, chin straps are used, or a full-face mask may be tried. NPPV is not recommended for patients with swallowing dysfunction or difficulty clearing secretions. It should not be used in patients with hypotension, uncontrolled arrhythmias, acute cardiac ischemia, or acute gastrointestinal hemorrhage.

NPPV seems to be particularly helpful when implemented at an early stage in patients with rapidly reversible diseases such as congestive heart failure and exacerbated chronic airflow obstruction and in patients for whom intubation is not an acceptable option. The worth of NPPV for patients with acute pulmonary edema is now proven.[81] NPPV reduced the need for intubation and mortality in patients with acute cardiogenic pulmonary edema, acute exacerbation of chronic obstructive pulmonary disease (COPD),[82] and hypoxemic ARF.[83] However, during NPPV up to 40% of patients may require endotracheal intubation and invasive mechanical ventilation, primarily because of poor patient tolerance and the severity of underlying disease.[84] Although NPPV has been used for a variety of causes of ARF, success is more likely in hypercapnic respiratory failure resulting from chronic COPD. In this circumstance, it is a temporizing measure until bronchodilator and anti-inflammatory therapy lead to improvement. NPPV may also be useful when postextubation acute hypercapnia develops after extubation in a patient with COPD.[85]

Success is less likely in patients with pneumonia, in whom high levels of ventilatory requirements may exist, reduced lung compliance requires higher pressure levels, and the ability to adequately clear secretions (especially with a facemask in place) may be compromised. Although it offers utility as a method for delivery of PEEP to potentially improve hypoxemia in patients with diffuse lung infiltrates, the primary utility of NPPV is for inspiratory assistance in the presence of respiratory muscle fatigue. For marginally compensated patients, NPPV may prove especially helpful at night, when sleep impairs ventilatory drive. It has been suggested that nocturnal support may allow the sleep quality needed to preserve adequate ventilatory drive and muscle strength. The decision to apply facemask or nasal mask NPPV in patients with ARDS should be tempered by the potential for delaying intubation until it must be performed with the patient in respiratory arrest and by the higher risk of aspiration if emesis occurs. Furthermore, NPPV may lead to gastric distention and further risk of aspiration.

Many factors have the potential to influence the effectiveness of NPPV. One way of reducing the need for premature termination of NPPV could be to use a different interface to limit the chances of pressure necrosis of the skin, air leaks, and discomfort. A plastic "helmet" that covers the patient's whole head, originally used to deliver an air mixture during hyperbaric oxygen therapy, has now been developed for NPPV.[86,87] The helmet makes no contact with the head, so it should be more comfortable than the face mask, although it may be more likely to produce a sense of claustrophobia. In patients with acute hypoxemic respiratory failure and cardiogenic pulmonary edema, the helmet was found to improve gas exchange like the facemask but was more comfortable and permitted longer continuous application.[88] One of the most important drawbacks of the helmet, because of its larger inner volume compared with the facemask (i.e., a dead space volume of 8 to 12 L), is carbon dioxide rebreathing, which could limit the efficacy of NPPV.[89] Two studies in humans that evaluated the helmet and facemask in healthy subjects during PSV found a similar breathing pattern, but the helmet required greater inspiratory muscle effort and took a longer time to reach the selected level of airway pressure.[86,90] It was also shown that by increasing the level of pressure support or PEEP, the helmet significantly diminished the delay times and pressure-time product.[91] A practical clinical conclusion from these studies related to NPPV vis a helmet is that the physician should set higher levels of PEEP and pressure support to reduce inspiratory muscle effort, much as is done with the facemask.[92]

Two prospective epidemiologic surveys found that NPPV was used in 5% to 15% of patients with respiratory failure[84,93]; however, the percentage of patients treated with NPPV significantly differed among centers, ranging from none in eight ICUs to 67% in a ninth.[84] Among the most important elements of success in addition to patient selection are rigorous training of support personnel, early intervention, and efforts to encourage the patient to accept noninvasive ventilation in the first few hours of its application.

General recommendations for NPPV are as follows:

1. For pressure-cycled ventilation, it is best to start at lower inspiratory pressures and gradually increase to target level.
2. Gastric distention is unlikely to occur with peak inspiratory pressure less than 25 cm H_2O.
3. Do not use NPPV in patients with rapidly deteriorating ventilatory status who are at risk for sudden respiratory arrest.
4. NPPV should not be used unless the physician or the respiratory therapist is familiar with the technical operation and fitting of the device.
5. Consider NPPV primarily in alert, oriented, hemodynamically stable, and cooperative patients with respiratory failure, especially hypercapnic respiratory failure, and more especially hypercapnic respiratory failure resulting from COPD (see Chapter 10).
6. For hypoxemic and hypercapnic respiratory failure, initially choose PSV mode with applied inspiratory pressure set 5 to 10 cm H_2O above expiratory positive airway pressure (EPAP) or PEEP. The potential positive-pressure boost to inspiration is directly correlated with the difference between inspiratory pressure and end-expiratory pressure levels. For hypercapnic respiratory failure, choose an initial expiratory pressure level of 3 cm H_2O. For hypoxemic respiratory failure, choose an initial expiratory pressure of 5 cm H_2O and then titrate up for best PEEP effect, if appropriate.
7. For hypercapnic respiratory failure, increase inspiratory pressure in increments of 2 cm H_2O titrated to achieve an acceptable pH level.
8. For hypoxemic respiratory failure, when titrating end-expiration pressure, increase inspiratory pressure and expiratory pressure in increments of 2 cm H_2O to preserve inspiratory support.
9. Applied NPPV may be very effective in patients with cardiogenic pulmonary edema because it exerts the following four potential beneficial effects:
   a. EPAP (PEEP) improves both functional residual capacity (lung recruitment) and oxygenation.
   b. Applied inspiratory improves ventilation and reduces the work of breathing.
   c. Increased intrathoracic pressure decreases preload.
   d. Increased intrathoracic pressure decreases afterload.
10. Supplemental oxygen may be added directly into the pressure tubing at the mask and titrated to maintain adequate oxygenation with machines made specifically for NPPV.
11. Follow the patient's vital signs, clinical appearance, and arterial blood gas levels. If a downward trend is not immediately reversed, proceed to intubation. The inability of NPPV to improve patient status within several hours also makes its success unlikely.
12. Restrict oral intake until the effectiveness of NPPV in reversing acute ventilatory failure is confirmed.
13. Patients receiving NPPV for ARF must be monitored as closely as any other patient with acute respiratory deterioration and should be treated in an ICU or respiratory care unit setting. Continuous pulse oximetry and cardiac monitoring are desirable.

KEY POINTS

- There are three parts to a ventilator breath: triggering, inspiration, and cycling. Triggering is the means by which the ventilator senses when to begin inspiration. Inspiration involves the creation of a pressure or flow gradient for gas to enter the endotracheal tube. Cycling is the change from inspiration to exhalation and can be related to a particular pressure, flow, time, or volume.
- During pressure limiting with volume-cycled ventilation, the preset volume is not being delivered, and significant alveolar hypoventilation can occur.
- With time-cycled breaths, the delivered tidal volume at any point in time is not guaranteed to be maintained and increases or decreases with changes in airway resistance or lung elastance.
- Because flow rate drops dramatically as patient inspiratory effort decreases and then ceases with PSV, the patient exerts control not only on initiation but also on termination of breaths.
- In most circumstances, assist control ventilation results in a marked diminution in the work of breathing, and in some circumstances, the work of breathing can approximate zero. Certain patients undergoing assisted breath ventilation, however, continue to exert significant effort throughout inspiration.
- The combination of PSV and SIMV allows spontaneous breaths to be increased to an acceptable tidal volume not achievable with spontaneous effort alone.
- No large controlled studies have been performed that compare inverse I:E ratio with more conventional forms of mechanical ventilation in patients with ARDS; however, the studies that are available have demonstrated only modest improvements in arterial P_{O_2} in comparison with conventional ventilation at similar mean airway pressures.
- On the basis of the results of the ARDS network trial, we recommend the use of a tidal volume of 6 mL per kg

predicted body weight in patients with ARDS, targeted to keep the IPP less than 30 cm H_2O.

- The diagnosis of pulmonary emboli in the patient undergoing mechanical ventilation can be suspected from a sudden increase in minute ventilation without a change in partial pressure of CO_2, indicating an increase in physiologic dead space ventilation, or from a reduction in blood pressure or arterial PO_2.
- Consider NPPV primarily in alert, oriented, hemodynamically stable, and cooperative patients with respiratory failure, especially hypercapnic respiratory failure, and more especially hypercapnic respiratory failure resulting from chronic obstructive pulmonary disease.
- Patients receiving NPPV for newly diagnosed ARF must be monitored as closely as any other patient with acute respiratory deterioration and should be treated in an ICU or respiratory care unit setting. Continuous pulse oximetry and cardiac monitoring are desirable.

REFERENCES

1. Esteban A, Anzueto A, Alia I, et al, for the Mechanical Ventilation International Study Group: How is mechanical ventilation employed in the intensive care unit? Am J Respir Crit Care Med 2000;161:1450.
2. Linton DM: Cuirass ventilation: A review and update. Crit Care Resusc 2005;7:22.
3. Guyton AC, Hall JE: Textbook of Medical Physiology, 11th ed. Philadelphia, Elsevier-Saunders, 2006.
4. Aslanian P, Atrous SE, Isabey D, et al: Effects of flow triggering on breathing effort during partial ventilatory support. Am J Respir Crit Care Med 1998;157:135.
•5. Fabry B, Guttman J, Eberhard L, et al: An analysis of desynchronization between the spontaneously breathing patient and ventilator during inspiratory pressure support. Chest 1995;107:1387.
6. Branson RD, Campbell RS, Davis K, et al: Comparison of pressure and flow triggering systems during continuous positive airway pressure. Chest 1994;106:540.
7. Tutuncu A, Cakar N, Camci E, et al: Comparison of pressure- and flow-triggered pressure-support ventilation on weaning parameters in patients recovering from acute respiratory failure. Crit Care Med 1997;25:756.
8. Chao DC, Scheinhorn D, Stearn-Hassenpflug M: Patient-ventilator trigger asynchrony in prolonged mechanical ventilation. Chest 1997;112:1592.
9. Blanch PB, Jones M, Layon AJ, et al: Pressure-preset ventilation. Part 1: Physiologic and mechanical considerations. Chest 1993:104:590.
10. Blanch PB, Jones M, Layon AJ, et al: Pressure-preset ventilation. Part 2: Mechanics and safety. Chest 1993;104:904.
11. Kimball WR, Leith DE, Robins AG: Dynamic hyperinflation and ventilator dependence in chronic obstructive pulmonary disease. Am Rev Respir Dis 1982;126:991.
12. Ravencraft SA, Burke WC, Marini JJ: Volume cycled deceleration flow: An alternative form of mechanical ventilation. Chest 1992;101:1342.
13. Davis K, Branson RD, Campbell RS, et al: Comparison of volume control and pressure control ventilation: Is flow waveform the difference? J Trauma 1996;41:808.
14. Dellinger RP, Jean S, Cinel I, et al: Regional distribution of acoustic-based lung vibration as a function of mechanical ventilation mode. Critical Care 2007;11:R26.
15. Marini JJ, Rodriguez RM, Lamb VJ: The inspiratory workload of patient initiated ventilation. Am Rev Respir Dis 1986;89:56.
•16. Groeger JS, Levinson MR, Carlon GC: Assist control versus synchronized intermittent mandatory ventilation during acute respiratory failure. Crit Care Med 1989;17:607.
17. Zobel G, Dacar D, Rodl S: Hemodynamic effects of different modes of mechanical ventilation in acute cardiac and pulmonary failure: An experimental study. Crit Care Med 1994;22:1624.
18. Jounieaux V, Duran A, Levi-Valensi P: Synchronized intermittent mandatory ventilation with and without pressure support ventilation in weaning patients with COPD from mechanical ventilation. Chest 1994;105:1204.
19. Stewart KG: Clinical evaluation of pressure support ventilation. Br J Anaesth 1989;63:362.
20. Hess DR: Ventilator waveforms and the physiology of pressure support ventilation. Respir Care 2005;50:166.
21. Downs JB, Stock MC: Airway pressure release ventilation: A new concept in ventilatory support. Crit Care Med 1987;15:459.
22. Hormann C, Baum M, Putensen C, et al: Biphasic positive airway pressure (BIPAP)—a new mode of ventilatory support. Eur J Anaesthesiol 1994; 11:37.
23. Neumann P, Golisch W, Strohmeyer A, et al: Influence of different release times on spontaneous breathing pattern during airway pressure release ventilation. Intensive Care Med 2002;28:1742.
24. Henzler D, Dembinski R, Bensberg R, et al: Ventilation with biphasic positive airway pressure in experimental lung injury: Influence of transpulmonary pressure on gas exchange and haemodynamics. Intensive Care Med 2004;30:935.
25. Chadda K, Annane D, Hart N, et al: Cardiac and respiratory effects of continuous positive airway pressure and noninvasive ventilation in acute cardiac pulmonary edema. Crit Care Med 2002;30:2457.
26. Hedenstierna G, Lichtwarck-Aschoff M: Interfacing spontaneous breathing and mechanical ventilation: New insights. Minerva Anestesiol 2006;72:183.
27. Putensen C, Zech S, Wrigge H, et al: Long-term effects of spontaneous breathing during ventilatory support in patients with acute lung injury. Am J Respir Crit Care Med 2001;164:43.
28. Neumann P, Wrigge H, Zinserling J, et al: Spontaneous breathing affects the spatial ventilation and perfusion distribution during mechanical ventilatory support. Crit Care Med 2005;33:1090.
29. Wrigge H, Zinserling J, Neumann P, et al: Spontaneous breathing with airway pressure release ventilation favors ventilation in dependent lung regions and counters cyclic alveolar collapse in oleic-acid-induced lung injury: A randomized controlled computed tomography trial. Crit Care 2005;9:R780.
30. Younces M, Roberts D, Light RB, et al: Proportional assist ventilation: A new approach to ventilatory support. Am Rev Respir Dis 1989;139:A363.
31. Amato MD, Barbas CS, Bonassa J, et al: Volume assured pressure support ventilation (VAPSV): A new approach for reducing muscle workload during acute respiratory failure. Chest 1992;102:1225.
32. Fredburg JJ: Augmented diffusion in the airways can support pulmonary gas exchange. J Appl Physiol 1980; 49:232.
33. Abraham E, Yoshihara G: Cardiorespiratory effects of pressure controlled inverse ratio ventilation in severe respiratory failure. Chest 1989;96:1356.
34. Tharratt RS, Allen RP, Albertson TE: Pressure controlled inverse ratio ventilation in severe adult respiratory failure. Chest 1988;94:755.
35. Armstrong BW, MacIntyre NR: Pressure-controlled, inverse ratio ventilation that avoids air trapping in the adult respiratory distress syndrome. Crit Care Med 1995; 23:279.
•36. Lain DC, DiBenedetto R, Morris SL, et al: Pressure control inverse ratio ventilation as a method to reduce peak inspiratory pressure and provide

adequate ventilation and oxygenation. Chest 1989;95:1081.
37. Shanholtz C, Brower R: Should inverse ratio ventilation be used in adult respiratory distress syndrome? Am J Respir Crit Care Med 1994;149:1354.
38. Sinderby C, Navalesi P, Beck J, et al: Neural control of mechanical ventilation in respiratory failure. Nat Med 1999;5:1433.
39. Beck J, Sinderby C, Lindström L, et al: Influence of bipolar esophageal electrode positioning on measurements of human crural diaphragm EMG. J Appl Physiol 1996,81:1434.
40. Sinderby C, Beck J, Lindström L, et al: Enhancement of signal quality in esophageal recordings of diaphragm EMG. J Appl Physiol 1997;82:1370.
41. Beck J, Sinderby C, Lindström L, et al: Effects of lung volume on diaphragm EMG signal strength during voluntary contractions. J Appl Physiol 1998; 85:1123.
42. Sinderby C, Beck J, Weinberg J, et al: Voluntary activation of the human diaphragm in health and disease. J Appl Physiol 1998;85:2146.
43. Beck J, Gottfried SB, Navalesi P, et al: Electrical activity of the diaphragm during pressure support ventilation in acute respiratory failure. Am J Resp Crit Care Med 2001;164:419.
44. Hedenstierna G, Tokics L, Strandberg A, et al: Correlation of gas exchange impairment to the development of atelectasis during anaesthesia and muscle paralysis. Acta Anaesthesiol Scand 1986;30:183.
45. Lefevre GR, Kowalski SE, Girling LG, et al: Improved arterial oxygenation after oleic acid lung injury in the pig using a computer-controlled mechanical ventilator. Am J Respir Crit Care Med 1996;154:1567.
46. Navalesi P, Costa R: New modes of mechanical ventilation: Proportional assist ventilation, neurally adjusted ventilatory assist, and fractal ventilation. Curr Opin Crit Care 2003;9:51.
47. Mutch WAC, Harms S, Graham MR, et al: Biologically variable or naturally noisy mechanical ventilation recruits atelectatic lung. Am J Respir Crit Care Med 2000;162:319.
48. Boker A, Graham MR, Walley KR, et al: Improved arterial oxygenation with biologically variable or fractal ventilation using low tidal volumes in a porcine model of acute respiratory distress syndrome. Am J Respir Crit Care Med 2002;165:456.
49. Kiiski R, Takala J: Hypermetabolism and efficiency of CO2 removal in acute respiratory failure. Chest 1994;105:1198.
50. Osterman M, Keenan S, Sieferling R, et al: Sedation in the intensive care unit. JAMA 2000;283:1451.
51. Jacobi J, Fraser GL, Coursin DB, et al: Clinical practice guidelines for the sustained use of sedatives and analgesics in the critically ill adult. Crit Care Med 2002;30:119.
52. Kress JP, Hall JP: Sedation in the mechanically ventilated patient. Crit Care Med 2006;34:2541.
53. Turner JS, Briggs SJ, Springhorn HE, et al: Patients' recollection of intensive care unit experience. Crit Care Med 1990;18:966.
54. Kress JP, O'Connor MF, Pohlman AS, et al: Sedation of critically ill patients during mechanical ventilation: A comparison of propofol and midazolam. Am J Respir Crit Care Med 1996;153:1012.
55. Riker RR, Picard JT, Fraser GL: Prospective evaluation of the Sedation-Agitation Scale for adult critically ill patients. Crit Care Med 1999;27:1325.
56. Sessler CN, Gosnell MS, Grap MJ, et al: The Richmond Agitation-Sedation Scale: Validity and reliability in adult intensive care unit patients. Am J Respir Crit Care Med 2002;166:1338.
57. Ely EW, Truman B, Shintani A, et al: Monitoring sedation status over time in ICU patients: Reliability and validity of the Richmond Agitation-Sedation Scale (RASS). JAMA 2003;289:2983.
58. De Jonghe B, Cook D, Griffith L, et al: Adaptation to the Intensive Care Environment (ATICE): Development and validation of a new sedation assessment instrument. Crit Care Med 2003;31:2344.
59. de Lemos J, Tweeddale M, Chittock D: Measuring quality of sedation in adult mechanically ventilated critically ill patients: The Vancouver Interaction and Calmness Scale. Sedation Focus Group. J Clin Epidemiol 2000;53:908.
60. Brook AD, Ahrens TS, Schaiff R, et al: Effect of a nursing-implemented sedation protocol on the duration of mechanical ventilation. Crit Care Med 1999;27:2609.
61. Kress JP, Pohlman A, O'Connor MF, et al: Daily interruption of sedative infusions in critically ill patients undergoing mechanical ventilation. N Engl J Med 2000;342:1471.
62. Weinert CR, Calvin AD: Epidemiology of sedation and sedation adequacy for mechanically ventilated patients in a medical and surgical intensive care unit. Crit Care Med 2007;35:393.
63. De Jonghe B, Bastuji-Garin S, Fangio P, et al: Sedation algorithm in critically ill patients without acute brain injury. Crit Care Med 2005;33:120.
64. Kress J, Gehlbach B, Lacy M, et al: The long-term psychological effects of daily sedative interruption on critically ill patients. Am Respir J Crit Care Med 2003;168:1457.
65. Eubanks D, Bone RC: Mechanical ventilation. In Comprehensive Respiratory Care: A Learning System, 2nd ed. St. Louis, Mosby, 1990.
66. Boots RJ, Howe S, George N, et al: Clinical utility of hygroscopic heat and moisture exchangers in intensive care patients. Crit Care Med 1997;25:1707.
67. Kirton OC, DeHaven B, Morgan J, et al: Prospective, randomized comparison of an in-line heat moisture exchange filter and heated wire humidifiers: Rates of ventilator-associated early-onset (community-acquired) or late-onset (hospital-acquired) pneumonia and incidence of endotracheal tube occlusion. Chest 1997;112:1055.
68. Kacmarek RM, Dimas S, Mack CW: Aerosol and humidity therapy. In The Essentials of Respiratory Care, 4th ed. St. Louis, Mosby, 2005.
69. Hess DR, Kacmarek RM: Humidification and the ventilator circuit. In Essentials of Mechanical Ventilation, 2nd ed. New York, McGraw-Hill, 2002.
70. Mols G, Rohr E, Benzing A, et al: Breathing pattern associated with respiratory comfort during automatic tube compensation and pressure support ventilation in normal subjects. Acta Anaesthesiol Scand 2000;44:223.
71. Haberthur C, Elsasser S, Eberhard L, et al: Total versus tube-related additional work of breathing in ventilator-dependent patients. Acta Anaesthesiol Scand 2000; 44:749.
72. Marini JJ, Wheeler AP: Indications and options for mechanical ventilation. In Critical Care Medicine, 3rd ed. Philadelphia, Lippincott Williams & Wilkins, 2006.
73. Bone RC: Pulmonary barotrauma complicating mechanical ventilation. Am Rev Respir Dis 1976;113(Suppl): 1988.
74. Hernandez LA, Peevy AA, Parker JC: Chest wall restriction limits high airway pressure induced lung injury in young rabbits. J Appl Physiol 1989;66:2364.
75. Haake R, Schlichtig R, Ulstad DR, et al: Barotrauma: Pathophysiology, risk factors, and prevention. Chest 1987; 91:608.
76. Carlon GC, Howland WS, Groeger JS, et al: High frequency jet ventilation: A prospective randomized evaluation. Chest 1983;84:551.
77. Gluck EH, Heard S, Patel C, et al: Use of ultra high frequency ventilation in patients with ARDS. Chest 1993; 103:1413.
78. Leatherman J, Ravenscraft SA, Iber C, et al: High peak inflation pressures do not predict barotrauma during mechanical ventilation of status asthmaticus. Am Rev Respir Dis 1989;139:A154.
79. Kolobow T, Moretti MP, Fumagalli R, et al: Severe impairment of lung function induced by high peak airway pressure during mechanical ventilation. Am Rev Respir Dis 1987;135:312.
80. Orlando R, Gluck EH, Cohen M, Mesologites C: Ultra high frequency jet ventilation in a bronchopleural fistula model. Arch Surg 1988;123: 591.
81. Masip J, Roque M, Sanchez B, et al: Noninvasive ventilation in acute cardiogenic pulmonary edema: Systematic review and meta-analysis. JAMA 2005;294:3124.
82. Lightowler JV, Wedzicha JA, Elliott MW, et al: Non-invasive positive pressure ventilation to treat respiratory failure resulting from exacerbations of chronic obstructive pulmonary disease: Cochrane systematic review and meta-analysis. BMJ 2003;326:185.
83. Antonelli M, Conti G, Rocco M, et al: A comparison of noninvasive positive-pressure ventilation and conventional mechanical ventilation in patient with acute respiratory failure. N Engl J Med 1998;339:429.
84. Carlucci A, Richard JC, Wysocki M, et al: Noninvasive versus conventional mechanical ventilation: An

epidemiologic survey. Am J Respir Crit Care Med 2001;163:874.
•85. Hilbert G, Gruson D, Portel L, et al: Noninvasive pressure support ventilation in COPD patients with postextubation hypercapnic respiratory insufficiency. Eur Respir J 1998;11: 1349.
86. Chiumello D, Pelosi P, Gattinoni L, et al: Noninvasive positive pressure ventilation delivered by helmet vs. standard face mask. Intensive Care Med 2003;29:1671.
87. Costa R, Navalesi P, Antonelli M, et al: Physiologic evaluation of different levels of assistance during noninvasive ventilation delivered through a helmet. Chest 2005;128:2984.
88. Tonnelier JM, Prat G, Nowak E, et al: Noninvasive continuous positive airway pressure ventilation using a new helmet interface: A case-control prospective pilot study. Intensive Care Med 2003;29:2077.
89. Taccone P, Hess D, Bigatello LM, et al: Continuous positive airway pressure delivered with a "helmet": Effects on carbon dioxide rebreathing. Crit Care Med 2004;32,2090.
90. Rocca F, Appendin L, Ranieri M, et al: Effectiveness of mask and helmet interfaces to deliver non-invasive ventilation in a human model of resistive breathing. J Appl Physiol 2005;99:1262.
91. Moerer O, Fisher S, Quintel M, et al: Influence of two interfaces for noninvasive ventilation compared to invasive ventilation on the mechanical properties and performance of a respiratory system: A lung model study. Chest 2006; 129,1424.
92. Chiumello D: Is the helmet different than the face mask in delivering noninvasive ventilation? Chest 2006;129:1402.
93. Esteban A, Anzueto A, Frutos F, et al: Characteristics and outcomes in adult patients receiving mechanical ventilation: A 28-day international study. JAMA 2002;287:345.

Chapter 10

Ventilatory Management of Obstructive Airway Disease

John Marini

Positive pressure ventilators have been in widespread clinical use for more than 4 decades. Our understanding of respiratory muscle function and ventilatory failure has undergone major revision over that period, helping to gear equipment and treatment strategies more effectively to patient requirements. Some of the more important advances in this area concern the interactions of patients with obstructive pulmonary disease (airflow obstruction [AO]) with the mechanical ventilator. Others concern physiologic principles important in withdrawing machine support from ventilator-dependent patients, many of whom have chronic obstructive pulmonary disease (COPD) or asthma. With these advances in mind, the purpose of this chapter is to provide an updated physiologic background for understanding mechanical ventilation in patients with AO, as well as to review selected aspects of this problem that are frequently overlooked and, though noteworthy, may be unfamiliar to many practitioners.

SPECIAL CHALLENGES OF PATIENTS WITH SEVERE AIRFLOW OBSTRUCTION

By assuming a major portion of the ventilatory workload, mechanical ventilation affords the opportunity to rest the respiratory muscles while maintaining pH homeostasis and oxygenation, thereby averting progressive ventilatory failure or respiratory arrest, or both. Unfortunately, these benefits are not cost free—mechanical ventilation is expensive, uncomfortable, and inherently hazardous; few would dispute the desirability of avoiding the need for its implementation or of accelerating the process of its withdrawal. Although deceptively simple in concept, the management of patients with airflow obstruction who require mechanical support is a rather complex clinical undertaking. To manage respiratory failure effectively in patients with severe airflow obstruction, it is important to understand their distinctive problems. Patients with severe airflow obstruction can be characterized by a number of salient clinical features. Paramount among these are increased work of breathing and compromise of the ventilatory pump that must contend with it. Such patients are also distinguished by their susceptibility to the hazards of machine support.

Increased Work of Breathing

The mechanical breathing workload during passive ventilation can be quantified as the product of mean inflation pressure and minute ventilation. The mean inflation pressure (Pm) is approximated in a modification of the equation of motion of the respiratory system:

$$Pm = R\ (flow) + Vt/2C + PEEPi$$

In this equation R = resistance; Vt is tidal volume; C is respiratory system compliance; and PEEPi is auto-PEEP, the positive end-expiratory alveolar pressure in excess of set PEEP because of dynamic hyperinflation (Fig. 10-1).

Increased resistance to airflow is responsible (directly or indirectly) for many of the physiologic disturbances that typify this disease. Flow resistance, an important determinant of Pm, is increased by structural and functional narrowing of the airway. Structural changes include a reduced number of airway channels, as well as narrowed cross-sectional airway caliber. In this already narrowed system of tubes, the additional reduction of airway caliber caused by mucosal edema, functional compression, increased bronchomotor tone, or secretion accumulation noticeably increases the work of breathing because resistance relates linearly to the airway length but inversely to the fourth power of airway radius. For similar reasons, resistance within these critically narrowed airways is highly volume dependent, so loss of lung volume is accompanied by loss of elastic recoil tension, reduction of cross-sectional area, and major increases in the frictional workload.[1,2]

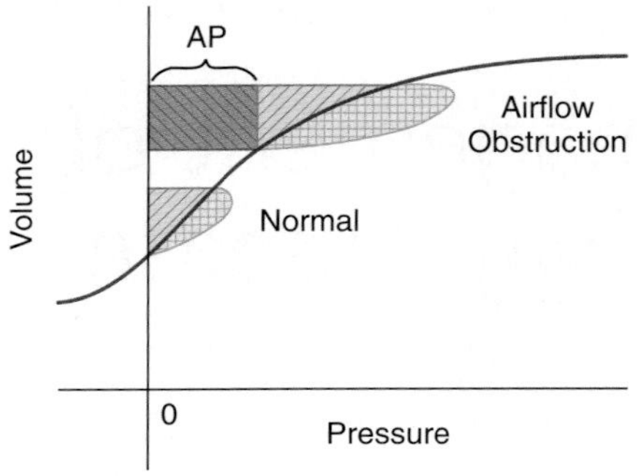

Figure 10-1. Depiction of the elements of the inspiratory equation of motion and their associated work of breathing. Stippled area is resistive work, and striped areas represent the elastic work associated with tidal volume and auto–positive end-expiratory pressure, respectively.

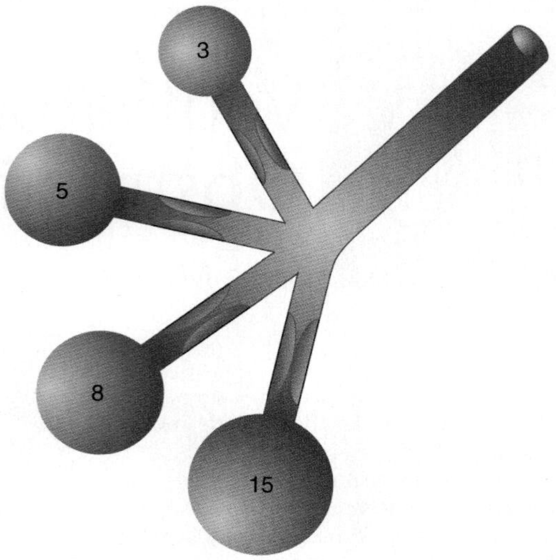

Figure 10-2. The auto–positive end-expiratory pressure (PEEP) effect. Auto-PEEP is the positive flow driving the difference between alveolar and airway opening pressures at end expiration. As depicted here, it can vary widely from site to site within the lung.

Although each factor just enumerated contributes to airflow obstruction, functional compression of the airway during exhalation is of overriding importance in many patients with components of emphysema or vigorous expiratory effort. Loss of elastic recoil encourages collapse of these narrowed bronchi as their transluminal distending pressure gradients decline (or reverse) during the course of exhalation. In most patients who require mechanical ventilatory support, dynamic airway collapse occurs even during tidal breathing, so the average expiratory resistance is often several times higher during the exhalation phase than during the inspiratory phase of ventilation. This compressive mechanism underlies the phenomenon of air trapping and such hyperinflation-related consequences as loss of inspiratory power and reduced compliance of the respiratory system.

Dynamic Hyperinflation (Air Trapping)

Expiration is normally a passive process that uses elastic energy stored during inflation to drive expiratory airflow. If the energy potential developed during inflation is insufficient to return the system to a relaxed equilibrium before the next inspiration begins, flow continues throughout expiration and alveolar pressure remains positive at end-expiration, exceeding the clinician-selected PEEP value (Fig. 10-2).[3-7] This positive distending pressure within the alveoli increases the driving pressure for expiratory airflow and increases lung volume, thereby helping to overcome airflow resistance. Unfortunately, such hyperinflation also places the expiratory musculature at a mechanical disadvantage. Furthermore, because this end-expiratory alveolar pressure (auto-PEEP, or intrinsic PEEP, PEEPi) is expiratory in nature, it must first be counterbalanced by positive pressure applied to the central airway or by negative pleural pressure before inspiration can begin.[8,9] Thus PEEPi adds to the other components of the equation of motion to elevate the mean inflation pressure and inspiratory work of breathing. The process of air trapping contributes to an increase in the respiratory work of breathing in at least two other ways. Hyperinflation drives the respiratory system upward toward the least compliant portion of the pressure volume relationship, incurring increased elastic work per liter of ventilation (see Fig. 10-1). Furthermore, at these higher volumes the lung approaches its elastic limit as the recoil tension of the distended rib cage becomes *expiratory* rather than inspiratory in nature. Finally, hyperinflation tends to convert more of the well-perfused ("zone 3") lung into less well perfused tissue, thereby increasing ventilatory deadspace and the minute ventilation requirement.

Generally, resistance in patients with chronic airflow obstruction and many of those with severe asthma concentrates within small airways.[1] Yet for certain asthmatic patients, the central airways and larynx contribute to resistance, accounting for the helpfulness of helium-oxygen (heliox) mixtures in some (but not all) patients during exacer-bated asthma.[10] According to some reports, heliox helps to reduce air trapping in patients with COPD as well. Although there is some concern regarding the generalizability and accuracy of such observations, several mechanisms can be evoked, even if the *primary* site of expiratory obstruction is too peripheral for helium to reduce resistance there. These include reduced inspiratory turbulence, faster expiratory flow in non–flow-limited channels and increased wave speed, modestly decreased CO_2 production caused by these aforementioned factors and improved comfort, and perhaps less gas trapping and less compromise of respiratory muscle efficiency.

Of note, dynamically positive end-expiratory alveolar pressure can also exist without hyperinflation, provided that airway collapse does not occur. In these instances expiratory muscle contraction increases pleural pressure, alveolar pressure, and the speed of expiratory airflow, obviating the need for hyperinflation to complete exhalation in the allotted time. Such mechanisms are employed by normal subjects during heavy exercise or when faced with major expiratory loads. Indeed, many uncoached and untrained normal subjects expire to positions below the equilibrium point of the chest when exposed to PEEP. In this way the respiratory muscles can begin contraction from a mechanically advantageous position, and the expiratory muscles can share in the ventilatory burden. Using this strategy, PEEP actually provides a boost to *inspiration,* experienced early in the cycle when the *expiratory* muscles relax. This "work-sharing" strategy, although effective for a normal individual, cannot be implemented by patients who experience dynamic airway collapse during tidal breathing. Because forceful expiratory efforts succeed not only in raising alveolar pressure but also in intensifying dynamic airway collapse, flow rate is determined strictly by lung volume and is not accelerated by expiratory muscle activity.

When dynamic collapse occurs during tidal respiration and breathing requirements are high, there is little alternative to hyperinflation or CO_2 retention, or both. At the chosen level of minute ventilation, maintenance of the lower lung volume may be either too energy costly or physically impossible. For this reason, many patients with severe obstruction do not or cannot decrease their lung volumes when recumbent. Such considerations may help to explain the extreme dyspnea experienced by most patients with severe airflow obstruction on assuming horizontal positions. For the same recumbent angle, the lateral position allows more decompression than does the supine position.[11] The distribution of gas trapping varies regionally throughout the lung depending on the local mechanical properties of the airways. Therefore at the end of the expiratory cycle some regions are continuously gas trapped, some remain patent, and some have sealed much earlier in the expiratory cycle (see Fig. 10-2). The end-expiratory value of auto-PEEP detected at the airway opening may not reflect the intensity of gas trapping.[12] During volume-controlled ventilation, plateau pressure tracks hyperinflation more reliably.

In some patients, especially those who passively receive ventilatory support, the problems presented by air trapping and dynamic hyperinflation are as much cardiovascular as pulmonary in nature. A relatively high fraction of the positive alveolar pressure is transmitted to the pleural space, where it impedes venous return and confuses interpretation of hemodynamic pressure measurements (Fig. 10-3). Lung distention also adds to pulmonary vascular resistance, exacerbating the tendency of patients with cor pulmonale toward low cardiac output and hypotension. Marked respiratory variation of systolic and pulse pressures during passive inflation indicates phasically adverse cardiac loading and strongly implies the possibility of dynamic hyperinflation (Fig. 10-4).

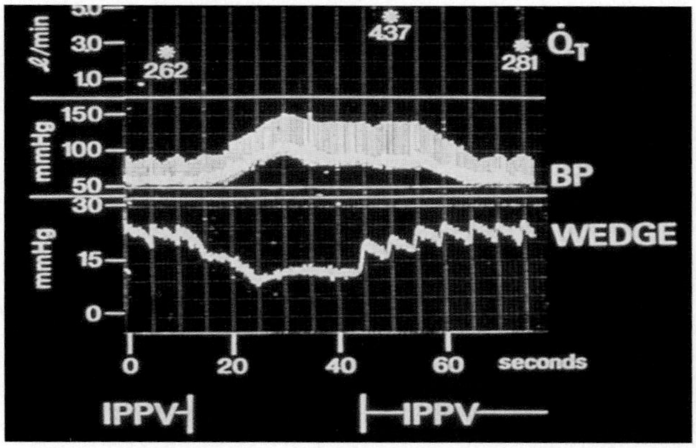

Figure 10-3. The hemodynamic impact of auto-PEEP in a passively ventilated patient with severe airflow obstruction. A 40-second disconnection of the ventilator was associated with rising blood pressure and cardiac output despite a falling pulmonary artery wedge pressure.

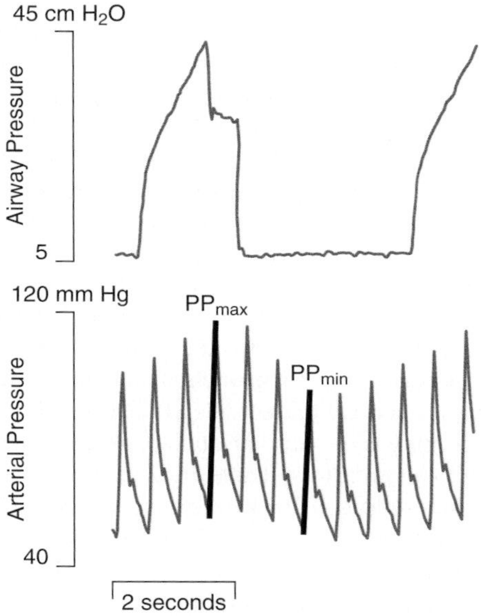

Figure 10-4. Marked respiratory variation of systemic arterial blood pressure, indicative of the relative variation in cardiac loading conditions associated with dynamic hyperinflation. PP, pulse pressure. (From Michard F, Teboul J-L: Using heart-lung interactions to assess fluid responsiveness during mechanical ventilation. Crit Care 2000;4:282-289.)

Increased Minute Ventilation Requirement

Ventilation-perfusion mismatching is widespread in patients with severe airflow obstruction, reducing the efficiency of carbon dioxide elimination.[1] It is not uncommon for the resting minute ventilation requirement to exceed 12 L per minute (twice the normal value) in patients with asthma or extensive emphysema and preserved chemical drives to breathe. Not only do such increases in ventilation requirement act as a linear cofactor in the work of breathing equation already discussed, but the high minute ventilation requirement itself increases most components of inspiratory pressure: flow, elastance (the reciprocal of compliance), tidal volume, and auto-PEEP. It is not surprising, therefore, that enormous increases in the oxygen consumption rate of the ventilatory muscles have been observed in patients with obstructive lung disease. During exacerbations, the oxygen consumed by ventilation and metabolic demands associated with heightened vigilance, agitation, or anxiety may double the total body oxygen consumption observed during fully supported breathing.

Reduced Mechanical Efficiency

In patients with exacerbated COPD or decompensated asthma, the oxygen consumption dedicated to the ventilatory task is disproportionate to the amount of mechanical work actually performed. The muscles of the hyperinflated ventilatory system are inefficiently aligned, force-length relationships of the shortened end-inspiratory fibers are suboptimal, and normally efficient coordination among the various muscles of the ventilatory group is often disrupted.[12,13] The energy cost of breathing, therefore, is greatly increased for the pressure and mechanical work actually generated by the breathing effort.

PROBLEMS AND HAZARDS OF VENTILATION WITH POSITIVE PRESSURE

Patients with AO who require mechanical ventilation present special challenges to the clinician for yet another reason: an unusual predisposition to its adverse consequences that are only loosely related to the airflow resistance. For reasons that are not entirely clear, patients with COPD have been reported to have an increased incidence of gastrointestinal ulceration and bleeding, especially during stress periods. This tendency is accentuated to an important degree by poor nutrition, stress, and the therapeutic use of high-dose corticosteroids. In modern intensive care unit practice, the incidence of ulceration has been greatly attenuated by the use of proton pump inhibitors and other means of acid suppression.

Even when able to cough with maximal force, patients with severe airflow obstruction have difficulty in clearing contaminated secretions from the central and peripheral airways, predisposing to bronchial and lung infections. This tendency is accentuated when the airway is intubated or when noninvasive ventilation is provided with poorly humidified gas mixtures. These interventions accentuate the impediment to coughing efficiency and assist entry of contaminated secretions from the upper airway. In conjunction with mucus plugging, air trapping, and the tendency toward parenchymal infections, markedly inhomogeneous ventilation predisposes the ventilated patient with severe airflow obstruction to the varied forms of barotrauma—pneumomediastinum, subcutaneous emphysema, and tension pneumothorax. Because the lungs cannot collapse, even a small pneumothorax in a ventilated patient with severe airflow obstruction can rapidly develop a tension component, leading to ventilatory and circulatory compromise.

The hemodynamic sensitivity to positive pressure ventilation of patients with airflow obstruction arises for several reasons. The overexpanded lungs press outward on the chest wall, raising intrapleural pressure. When breathing efforts are silenced, as they are immediately after sedation and intubation, mean intrathoracic pressure abruptly changes from modestly negative to markedly positive. Increased pleural pressure raises the right atrial backpressure to venous return. Simultaneously, increased peripheral vascular capacitance (caused in part by drug effects and the loss of muscular tone) and reduced peripheral vascular tone limit the rise in mean systemic pressure, the upstream driver of venous return. Blood pressure routinely falls, and cardiac output falls disproportionately to oxygen demand. Measured central vascular pressures (CVP and wedge) are misleadingly high and do not reflect intravascular filling and preload adequacy.[5] Marked respiratory variation of systolic and pulse pressures with the ventilatory cycle ("paradox") is a hemodynamic marker of relative hypovolemia caused by such mechanisms (see Fig. 10-4). Depending on choice of tidal volume, backup frequency, and set (and auto) PEEP, the afterload to right ventricular ejection may rise with any further lung expansion, whereas the tendency for alveolar dead-space creation is accentuated. Consequently, great care must be taken not to ventilate excessively and to provide adequate intravenous fluid support during this period. This advice pertains especially to patients with AO who require cardiac resuscitation.

Interactions of Pressure-Targeted Modes with Auto-PEEP

Pressure-targeted modes of ventilation, exemplified by pressure control and pressure support, have become increasingly popular to employ in the care of intubated patients, as well as those receiving noninvasive ventilation by facemask. Because the development of auto-PEEP reduces the pressure difference between airway opening and alveolus that drives inspiration, it has a powerful influence on ventilation efficacy (Fig. 10-5). As already described, auto-PEEP varies not only with airway mechanics but also with the pattern of breathing and minute ventilation. For a fixed value of applied airway pressure, inspiratory tidal volume in patients with airflow obstruction will be more sensitive to the frequency and the inspiratory time fraction (an expression of the I:E ratio) than are normal subjects or those with restrictive disease[14] (Fig. 10-6). Faster breathing frequencies, for example, allow auto-PEEP to build, and this auto-PEEP must first be

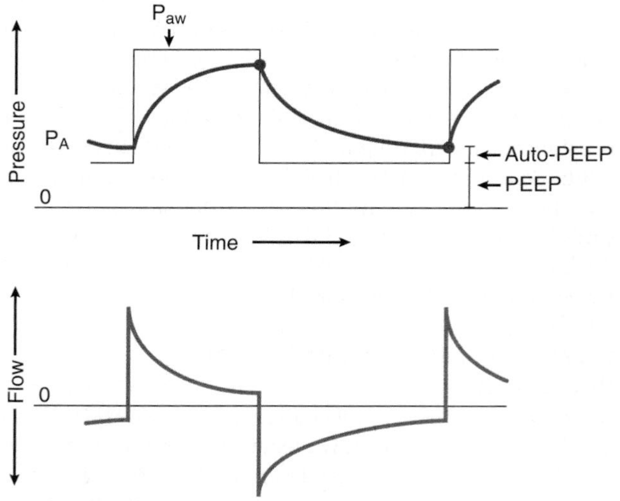

Figure 10-5. Interaction of alveolar *(red line)* and applied airway *(fine line)* pressures in a patient ventilated with pressure-targeted ventilation. Auto-PEEP diminishes the driving pressure of the subsequent ventilatory cycle.

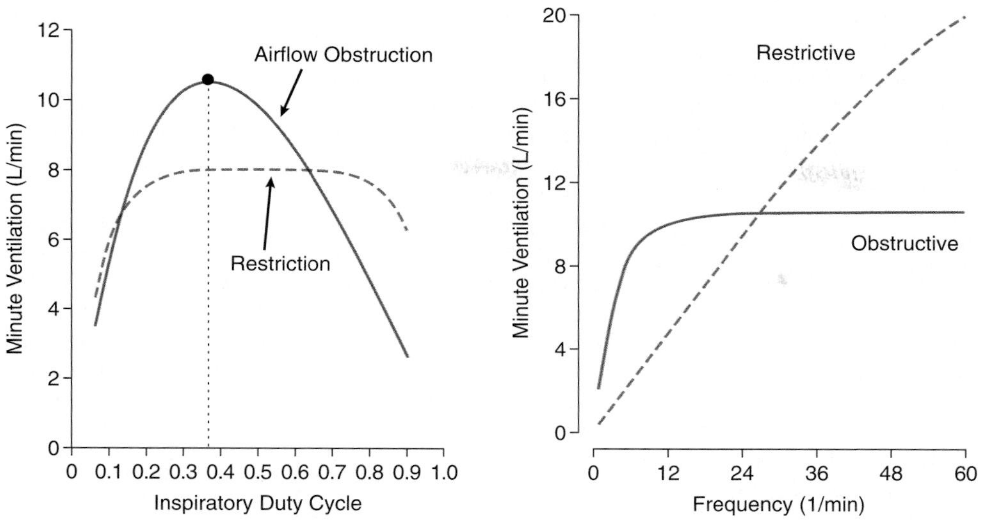

Figure 10-6. Relative sensitivity of patients with airflow obstruction to the settings of frequency and inspiratory time fraction for a fixed pressure target in pressure-controlled ventilation. This sensitivity is induced primarily by the impact of these settings on auto-PEEP.

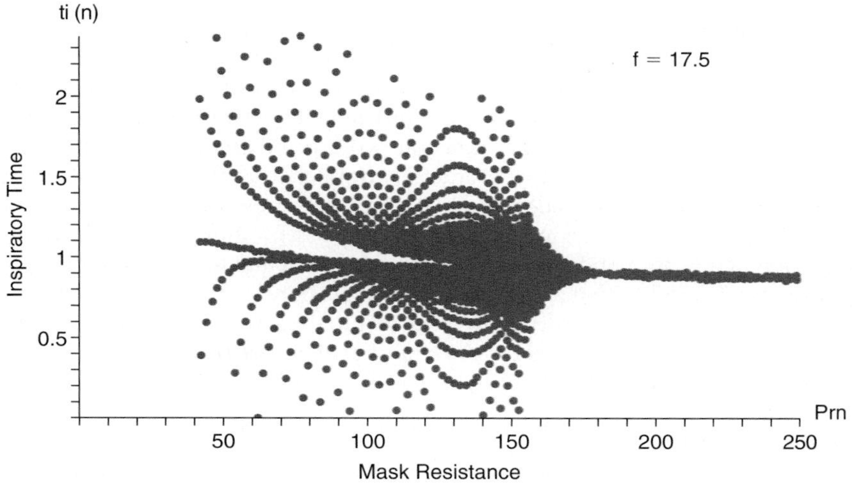

Figure 10-7. Theoretical behavior of tidal volume in response to pressure support by mask ventilation in a patient experiencing auto-PEEP. At a certain critical value of mask leak, there is wide cycle-to-cycle variation in tidal volume despite unchanging levels of pressure support and patient effort. Near "chaotic" behavior is a consequence of auto-PEEP. (From Hotchkiss JR, Adams AB, Dries DJ, et al: Dynamic behavior during noninvasive ventilation. Chaotic support? Am J Resp Crit Care Med 2001;163:374-378.)

counterbalanced for inspiratory airflow to begin. If the patient is passive or the amount of inspiratory muscle force remains constant, delivered tidal volume falls as the auto-PEEP builds.

This auto-PEEP/driving pressure interaction may result in an intriguing phenomenon resembling chaotic respiration during noninvasive ventilation with a leaky mask interface.[13] The coupled PEEPi and V_T form a "feed forward" system in which a building auto-PEEP of one cycle adversely influences the tidal volume of the next one. But this smaller tidal volume also reduces the auto-PEEP of that restricted cycle, which allows the breath that follows it—the third in the cycle—to have a larger effective driving pressure and tidal volume, and the cycling continues. This may account for some of the wide variability in breathing rhythm often observed in these patients.[15] If the mask leak volume is a function of the I:E ratio, it can be shown mathematically and experimentally that fractal and chaotic tidal volume delivery may occur, even when the patient's effort and mechanics remain unchanged (Fig. 10-7).[16] The consequences for comfort and sleep efficiency are likely to be significant, but clinical data are lacking on these issues at this time.

PRINCIPLES OF MANAGING THE VENTILATED PATIENT WITH SEVERE AIRFLOW OBSTRUCTION

Most patients hospitalized with exacerbations of asthma or COPD can be managed effectively by regimens that incorporate aggressive secretion clearance techniques, antibiotics, corticosteroids, intensified bronchodilators, hydration, cardiovascular support, and supplemental oxygen. Noninvasive ventilation is often helpful as a temporizing measure for those with disease of *mild-moderate* severity, especially when cough is adequate to clear airway secretions and the patient is fully alert and accepting of a full face mask.[17-22] Only a minority of such patients treated in this way need translaryngeal intubation and institution of mechanical ventilatory support. When mechanical ventilation is required, however, the rationale underlying certain key management principles can easily be understood against a background of the physiologic derangements already described. These principles are (1) provide adequate support for muscle rest at adequate PaO_2 and pH; (2) do not overventilate; (3) minimize the minute ventilation requirement; (4) minimize risk of barotrauma; (5) maintain adequate bronchial hygiene; (6) prevent panic reactions; (7) establish appropriate nutrition.

Principle 1: Provide adequate support to rest the ventilatory muscles, while avoiding hypoxemia and profound acidemia.

Poised on the edge of decompensation, the ventilatory muscles must be rested adequately before withdrawal of machine support can be considered. Rest may allow recovery of the energy reserves and restore the balance between ventilatory capability and demand. Indeed, benefits may accrue to muscle rest, even when it occurs intermittently on a chronic basis. Sufficient oxygen and mechanical support must be provided to achieve this goal and to avoid significant hypoxemia (arterial oxygen saturation <85%) and acidemia (pH < 7.2)—derangements that increase pulmonary vascular resistance; stimulate vigorous breathing; and inhibit mental, cardiac, and skeletal muscle functions.

Principle 2: Do not overventilate.

Although it is important to provide adequate ventilation, overventilation is detrimental on several counts. Rapid reduction in the alveolar CO_2 tension tends to cause bronchoconstriction and impair neuromuscular and cardiovascular function. Furthermore, excess ventilation exacerbates dynamic hyperinflation and auto-PEEP, whereas moderate $Paco_2$ elevations are generally well tolerated.[23] Generally it is a mistake to depress the $Paco_2$ below the level that the patient chronically maintains. Such a strategy may temporarily reset chemical drives, effectively increasing respiratory workload intensity. If $Paco_2$ falls sufficiently, the patient will not maintain unassisted breathing without intolerable effort.

Principle 3: Minimize minute ventilation requirement.

Because hyperinflation, mean inflation pressure, and the adverse cardiovascular consequences of mechanical ventilation are intimately linked to the minute ventilation requirement, ventilatory deadspace and CO_2 output must be minimized and metabolic acidosis avoided.

Principle 4: Minimize the risk of barotrauma.

The predisposition of patients with severe airflow obstruction to barotrauma must be combated by intelligent choices for tidal volume, ventilation frequency, PEEP, and machine settings of trigger sensitivity and flow. Reduction of the minute ventilation requirement decreases the mean or peak alveolar pressures, or both, reducing the incidence of barotrauma. The relative contributions of mean alveolar pressure, PEEP, dynamic cycling pressure, and peak static (plateau) ventilatory pressure to the risk of barotrauma are not clear. Based on epidemiologic evidence, however, peak inflation pressures should be kept below 40 cm H_2O wherever possible. Selecting a tidal volume at the low end of the recommended range (6 to 8 mL per kilogram of ideal body weight) is probably best. The question of optimal flow setting is of no small importance: auto-PEEP and mean alveolar pressure are reduced by selection of relatively rapid flow settings when minute ventilation is high. Overall ventilation-perfusion matching may improve as well. Higher peak dynamic airway pressures are not entirely without risk, however; units served by low resistance pathways are in jeopardy from overdistention. For the same inspiratory time, a constant ("square") flow waveform often serves better than a decelerating one. The risk of barotrauma can also be minimized by maintaining the lungs free of infection and the airways clear of secretions.

Principle 5: Maintain effective bronchial hygiene.

Secretion retention may dramatically increase airflow resistance and effectively seal off banks of alveoli, preventing their participation in ventilation. Thickened central airway secretions are a particular risk during mechanical ventilation, whether invasive or noninvasive (Fig. 10-8).[24] Apart from raising the end-inspiratory pressure, the resulting dynamic hyperinflation can detrimentally affect cardiovascular function, work of breathing, and ventilatory capability. In addition to effective suctioning, bronchodilators, adequate hydration, corticosteroids, mucolytics and infection control, frequent repositioning, mobilization, and physiotherapy are fundamental to secretion management. Tracheotomies not only reduce resistance and provide improved access to the lower airway but also limit the direct connection between the pharynx and trachea established by tracheal intubation.

Principle 6: Prevent panic reactions.

In patients susceptible to dynamic airway collapse, an abrupt need to augment ventilation often precipitates a downward spiral in which the capability of the patient is overwhelmed by the imposed workload. Not only is minute ventilation increased during such episodes, but the resulting increase of dynamic hyperinflation impairs muscle strength and endurance. Respiratory acidosis, dyspnea, and anxiety result in an imbalance in the demand/capability relationship that creates a need for aggressive intervention. Anxiolytics, although hazardous to employ, may be extremely helpful in carefully selected circumstances.

Principle 7: Maintain appropriate nutrition and prevent obstipation.

In stressed and often malnourished patients, the nature and quantity of nutritional support can make the difference between eventual compensation and continued ventilatory insufficiency. Although reasonable caution is advisable, an adequate number of calories should be provided, via the enteral route whenever possible. Care must be taken to ensure that bowel motility is normal; patients with AO frequently develop breathing discomfort because of abdominal distention within a compartment bounded by a hyperinflation-depressed diaphragm.

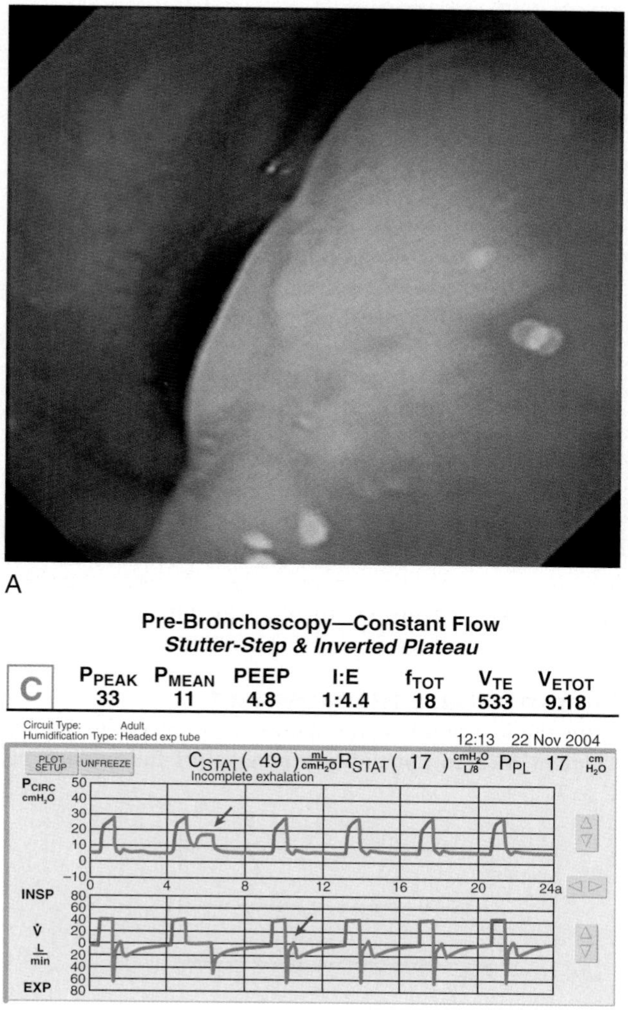

Figure 10-8. **A,** Central airway mucus retained in a ventilated patient with severe airflow obstruction. **B,** The resulting inverted plateau and stutter step deformations of the airway pressure and flow tracings during controlled, volume-cycled ventilation. (From Zamanian M, Marini JJ: Pressure-flow signatures of central-airway mucus plugging. Crit Care Med 2006;34:223-226.)

PRACTICAL MANAGEMENT OF THE VENTILATED PATIENT

Intubation

An understandable reluctance to initiate mechanical ventilation in patients with COPD or perennial asthma exists because many such individuals are so chronically disabled as to be miserable or despondent at home—even when everything is going as well as possible from a physiologic viewpoint. The development of comfortable noninvasive systems, coupled with emerging experience, has given rise to the initial use of mask ventilation in those who are alert and can tolerate it. However, the most severely affected patients, especially those with copious or thick secretions, claustrophobia, anxiety, cardiovascular decompensation, or somnolence, continue to require intubation to stabilize their deteriorating conditions.[25]

A mounting load of secretions audibly retained within the central airways generally indicates a patient too weak or breathless to expectorate and often portends an imminent crisis. Hence when this sign arises in a compatible clinical setting, most physicians consider it to be strong evidence favoring intubation for secretion management and ventilation support. Overt disorganization of the breathing rhythm and gasping or ataxic respirations strongly suggest approaching exhaustion.

Initial Support

Postintubation Problems

The first 24-hour period following tracheal intubation and initiation of positive pressure ventilation is a highly dynamic one for the patient with AO. Many of these individuals have depleted intravascular volume and impaired cardiovascular reflexes—features that prepare them poorly to compensate for the suddenly increased pleural pressure and impediment to venous return that usually accompany initiation of mechanical support. In this postintubation phase there is an understandable but unfortunate tendency for the physician to intentionally overventilate the patient, and many patients cough vigorously or fight against the rhythm imposed by the machine.

One reason for the agitation that some patients experience is a sudden buildup of positive intrathoracic pressure through the process of dynamic hyperinflation. When these intubated patients are deeply sedated and paralyzed, respiratory efforts cease and vasodilation occurs related to hypercapnia and sedative drugs. The consequent rise of intrathoracic pressure, coupled with a fall in mean systemic pressure, almost routinely depresses venous return and cardiac output (see Fig. 10-3). Therefore the physician is well advised to remain alert to the predictable development of cardiovascular depression and hypotension following intubation or sedation and be prepared to intervene to reduce ventilation or to support the circulation at the initially selected level, or both. A catastrophic error is to misinterpret the development of sudden hypotension as the uncloaking of tension pneumothorax and then to undertake needle puncture of the chest wall. In such individuals it is also wise to remember the potential contribution of auto-PEEP to hypotension during CPR resuscitation attempts.

Shortly after intubation there may be agitation, coughing, and retching related to tube insertion. When this interferes with comfort or ventilation, many lightly sedated patients benefit from 3 to 5 mL of 1% to 2% lidocaine instilled through the endotracheal tube. Instillation may be repeated one or two times, but care should be exercised, as lidocaine absorption easily occurs via the lung. Fortunately, intolerance of tube placement gradually abates with sedation and the passage of time.

Machine Settings

As a general rule, ventilation should be supported during this initial phase, but it is better to underventilate cautiously than to overventilate the patient. One reasonable approach is to use assisted mechanical ventilation, delivered with a square wave profile, with the backup rate set to provide about two thirds of the estimated minute ventilation requirement. Although the flow setting is adjusted empirically to coordinate the cycle lengths of the patient and the ventilator, an initial peak flow setting of approximately five to six times the minute ventilation requirement usually suffices to meet expiratory time requirements and minimize auto-PEEP without imposing undue risks that attend extraordinarily high peak cycling pressures. For increasing airflow carries a high pressure and work cost, a constant flow setting of about 60 L per minute is usually appropriate. This yields an I:E ratio of 1:4, which is considerably shorter than customary in a patient with normal mechanics who breathes at this level of minute ventilation. In patients with such severe airflow obstruction, increasing airflow carries a high pressure and work cost, so a constant inspiratory flow is preferable to a decelerating one when flow-controlled, volume-cycled ventilation is in use. Pressure-targeted ventilation is a sensible choice only if it is monitored closely or adjusted automatically by the ventilator to maintain tidal volume in response to changing airflow impedance.

The triggering threshold of the ventilator is set to be as sensitive as possible, and the auto-PEEP level is estimated when feasible to do so. (This generally requires passive inflation to allow predictable occlusion of the circuit at end-expiration.) If auto-PEEP exceeds 5 cm of water and expiratory flow is limited during tidal breathing (which is almost invariably the case during the initial phase), an uncomfortable patient who makes spontaneous breathing efforts may benefit from the addition of a low level of end-expiratory pressure to counterbalance auto-PEEP and reduce the breathing workload (Fig. 10-9). PEEP levels in excess of 15 cm water may be necessary in some instances to reestablish patency of some air channels.

The plateau pressure is a better guide to the degree of hyperinflation than is the measured level of auto-PEEP, for reasons already given. First, most machines do not allow estimation of auto-PEEP in a patient who is spontaneously triggering the ventilator and varies the length of the respiratory cycle. On the other hand, a plateau pressure estimate is usually recordable during triggered, as well as during controlled, volume-cycled breathing. Just as importantly, the auto-PEEP estimated by central airway occlusion is simply the volume-weighted average of those airways that remain open at end-expiration, which generally have shorter time constants and better mechanical properties than those that seal earlier in the expiratory period at higher pressure (see Fig. 10-2).

The flow tracing gives some indication of the underlying presence of gas trapping but does not indicate its severity. For example, a severely obstructed airway may be totally occluded and therefore unable to transmit its high pressure to the pressure sensor located within the machine. Similarly, a narrow airway may give rise to an almost imperceptible flow at end-expiration. Several features of the flow tracing are of value: High-frequency variations of the flow tracing suggest the presence of retained airway secretions or water in the external tubing. An abrupt transition between the earliest part of expiration and what follows ("hockey sticking") indicates a flow limitation during tidal breathing and the potential value of added PEEP if flow persists to the onset of the next breathing cycle (Fig. 10-10). Quite recently, several signs have been reported that appear to be signatures of partial central airway occlusion, as by mucus plugging (see Fig. 10-8).[24]

Support Phase Management

After the first hours of ventilatory support, rational management focuses not only on reversal of the underlying

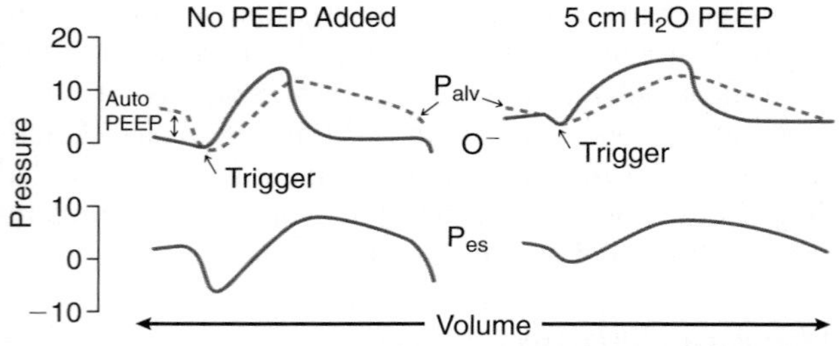

Figure 10-9. Work of breathing and ventilatory effort are improved in patients with tidal flow limitation by the addition of PEEP marginally less than the original value of auto-PEEP. Airway pressure *(top)* and intrapleural pressure *(bottom)*. P_{alv}, alveolar pressure; P_{es}, esophageal pressure.

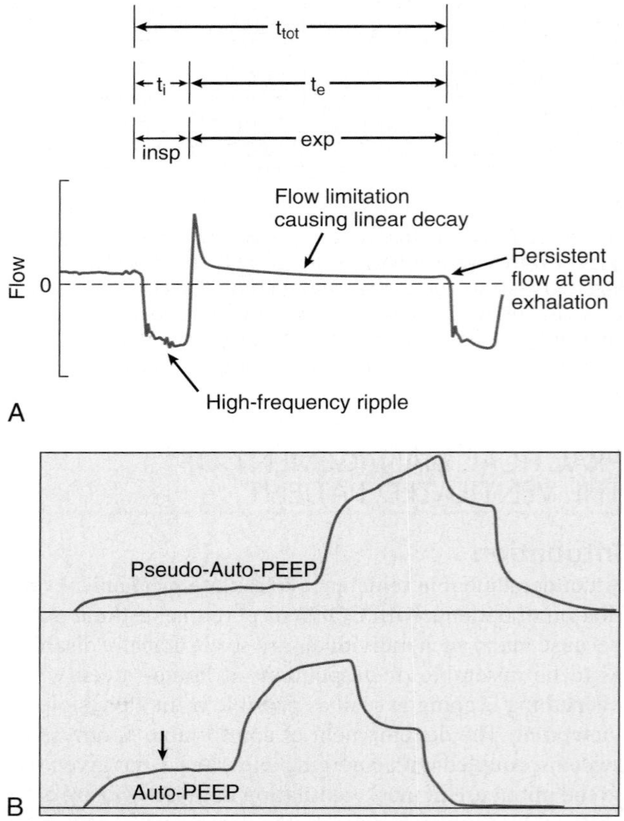

Figure 10-10. A, Typical flow tracing of a patient demonstrating flow limitation during tidal breathing. **B,** High-frequency ripple suggests secretions or circuit fluid, whereas "hockey sticking" and linear flow decay during expiration characterize flow limitation.

problems of infection, bronchospasm, secretion retention, and cardiac insufficiency but also on replenishing spent nutritional reserves and building endurance. It makes sense to support ventilation fully in patients intubated for ventilatory failure while fundamental pathologic processes and precipitating causes are being addressed—at least for the initial 24 to 48 hours. Because it is not known what intensity of ventilatory effort is best for patients with AO to undertake during the support phase of the illness, controversy exists as to the optimal mode of ventilation. During the support phase, the major objective should be to provide sufficient breathing assistance to alleviate discomfort yet not risk deconditioning of the ventilatory muscles. To this end, it is reasonable to use volume- or pressure-targeted assist-control (assisted mechanical ventilation) or synchronized intermittent mandatory ventilation (SIMV). In patients who are not deeply sedated and who breathe chaotically, the latter mode applied with pressure support sufficient to replicate the tidal volume of the mandated breaths may reduce the number of dyssynchronous "collisions" between the rhythms of patient and machine. Adequate sedation must be provided so as to assure comfort and reduce the minute ventilation requirement as other fundamental elements of ventilatory therapeutics are addressed (e.g., antibiotics, corticosteroids, regulation of intravascular volume, secretion extraction, cardiovascular support). Adequate oxygenation, ventilatory muscle rest, and restorative sleep deserve emphasis. Deep sedation and muscle relaxants, although occasionally necessary in achieving therapeutic objectives early in the ventilatory process, may prove detrimental when their use is prolonged unnecessarily. Not only does sedation present risks of muscle deconditioning and even neuromyopathy, but secretions tend to pool in dependent areas when breathing efforts and coughs are suppressed. As a general rule, deep sedation and paralysis should not be continued for longer than 40 to 72 hours after intubation.

Apart from improving expiratory resistance and reducing the minute ventilation requirement, another intervention aimed at reducing mean alveolar pressure and auto-PEEP is to modestly lengthen expiratory time (e.g., by increasing inspiratory flow rate). Flow rate should initially be set at approximately four to five times the minute ventilation requirement when using a constant inspiratory flow profile. Extending the expiratory time further is usually fruitless, unless minute ventilation is simultaneously reduced. Decelerating flow profiles are often poorly tolerated by the patient with severe airflow obstruction who makes spontaneous efforts because the latter half of the inspiratory period may require higher flows than imposed by the tightly regulated and stereotyped flow waveform of the ventilator. Adjustments to the flow that triggers expiration can help manage this problem during pressure-supported ventilation (Fig. 10-11).

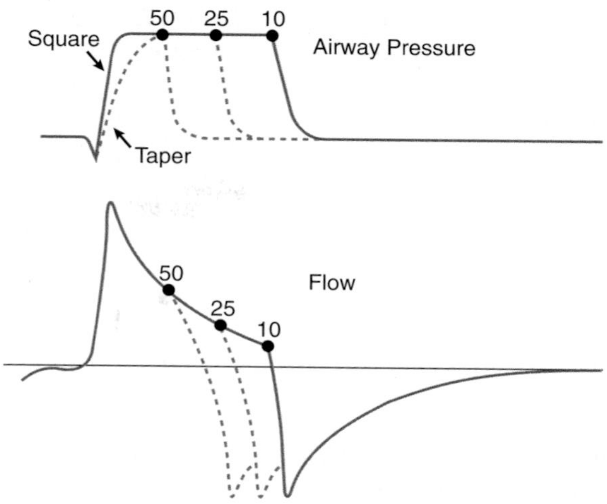

Figure 10-11. Adjustment of the expiratory flow trigger during pressure support can help to compensate for a slowly decelerating inspiratory flow profile that typifies patients with severe airflow obstruction. The appropriate adjustment in this schematic drawing might be from 25% to 50%.

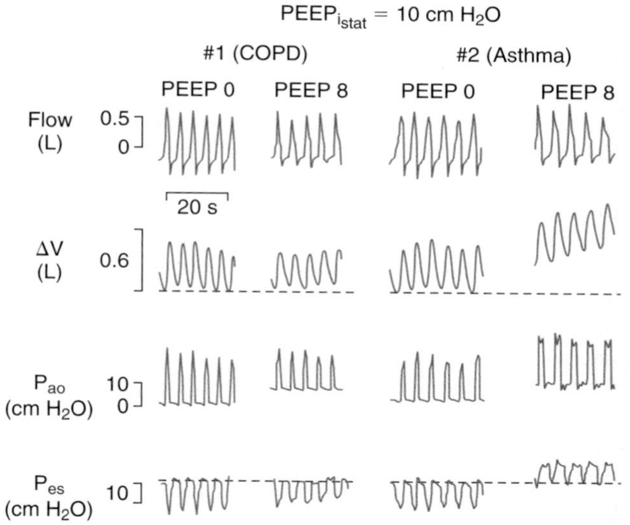

Figure 10-12. Differing responses of a flow-limited patient with chronic obstructive pulmonary disease (COPD) and a non–flow-limited patient with asthma to the application of PEEP. The rises of lung volume (V) and airway opening pressure (Pao) in asthma and the absence of these features in the patient with COPD are demonstrated. (From Ranieri VM, Giuliani R, Cinnella G, et al: Physiologic effects of positive end-expiratory pressure in patients with chronic obstructive pulmonary disease during acute ventilatory failure and controlled mechanical ventilation. Am Rev Respir Dis 1993;147:5-13.)

PEEP and CPAP in Severe Airflow Obstruction

The deliberate use of PEEP in patients with AO has historically been considered undesirable, but there is now ample reason to believe that most of these patients benefit from the application of low levels of PEEP or continuous positive airway pressure (CPAP).[6,8,9] When applied downstream of airways that collapse dynamically during the exhalation phase of tidal breathing, PEEP helps to improve the effective triggering responsiveness of the machine without significantly increasing the alveolar pressure or hyperinflation (Fig. 10-12). Most benefit is provided to patients who do not experience proportionate increases of peak static or peak dynamic cycling pressures after PEEP application.[9,26] When using a fixed level of targeted pressure (pressure control or pressure support), tidal volume may increase after PEEP is applied. This occurs because the added PEEP counterbalances auto-PEEP to allow the applied inspiratory pressure to more effectively drive inspiratory flow. In effect, PEEP improves the driving pressure for *inspiratory* flow. Applied PEEP may also help to keep airways more widely patent, and thereby improve secretion clearance. Finally, the application of the external PEEP may help to even the distribution of ventilation among multiple units with heterogeneous time constants (Fig. 10-13).

Newer Modes of Ventilation in Airflow Obstruction

The majority of ventilatory support of AO is still currently provided with modes of ventilation that are now decades old—flow-controlled, volume-cycled ventilation ("assist-control"); pressure control (PCV); pressure support (PSV); and SIMV. When combined with PEEP/CPAP and an attentive provider, these time-tested options suffice for the majority of patients. Increasingly, however, practitioners have recognized the need to offload responsibility for minute-by-minute and even intra-breath adjustment of settings for flow and pressure delivery in response to changing conditions of mechanics or ventilatory demand. Patients with dyspnea generally need faster rise of pressure and flows to their target values, unimpeded inspiratory flow, and precise termination of the ventilator's inspiratory phase so as to avoid collisions between the patient's and the ventilator's cycling rhythms. Once set, however, a specified flow pattern regulates the ventilator's contribution, and once set, the pressure provided by the ventilator is capped at the targeted value. Time-cycled assist control (whether flow or pressure regulated) disregards the duty cycle rhythm variations of the patient's own drive center. In either case the *relative* power contribution of the machine declines as effort increases and rises as patient effort declines. Moment by moment intra-cycle adjustment of flow or pressure is not an option with these "traditional" modes of ventilation. Logic dictates that better synchrony between patient and machine would require continuously monitored feedback and flexibility to adjust to the vagaries of patient need.

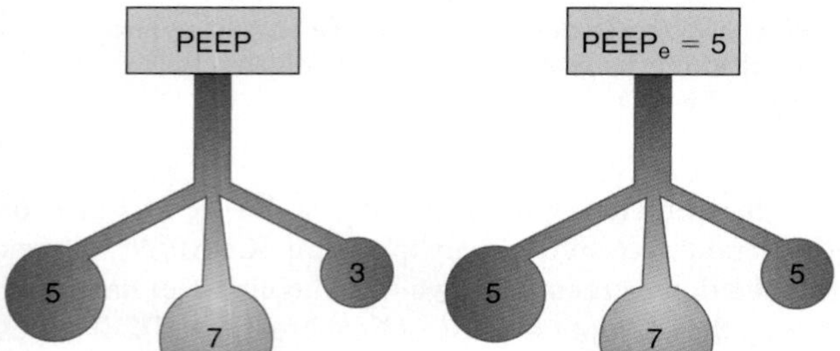

Figure 10-13. PEEP evens the flow distribution by counterbalancing auto-PEEP in flow-limited channels with differing levels of gas trapping.

Of the newer modes of ventilation, five that have implications for AO have garnered considerable attention and have been incorporated into some of the latest equipment:

High-Frequency Oscillation

Designed for problems of edema and parenchymal disease, high-frequency oscillation (HFO) offers no significant advantage over more conventional modes for patients with AO and runs the risk of significantly increased gas trapping and attendant hemodynamic compromise.

Airway Pressure Release Ventilation and Bi-level

As with HFO, these modes were not intended for patients with lengthy expiratory time constants. Airway pressure release ventilation does not take full advantage of its release phase in patients with lengthy expiratory time constants and therefore ineffectively ventilates unless the release frequency is high. The machine's inspiratory phase pressure is generally higher than that encountered during conventional ventilation, introducing the problems associated with sustained hyperinflation in patients with relatively flexible lungs.

Proportional Assist

Proportional assist, a mode based on the equation of motion of the respiratory system that regulates delivered pressure in proportion to externally sensed inspiratory flow and volume demands, effectively mimics the actions of an auxiliary muscle in patients without gas trapping.[27,28] Quite unlike pressure support, which targets the same pressure for every breath, PAV is meant to provide help in proportion to effort (Fig. 10-14). Unfortunately, a considerable fraction of inspiratory muscle effort is spent in counterbalancing auto-PEEP, an event that precedes the onset of inspiratory flow. Given the strong dependence of dynamic hyperinflation on minute volume (V_E) and the expiratory time constant, PAV cannot easily fulfill its intended

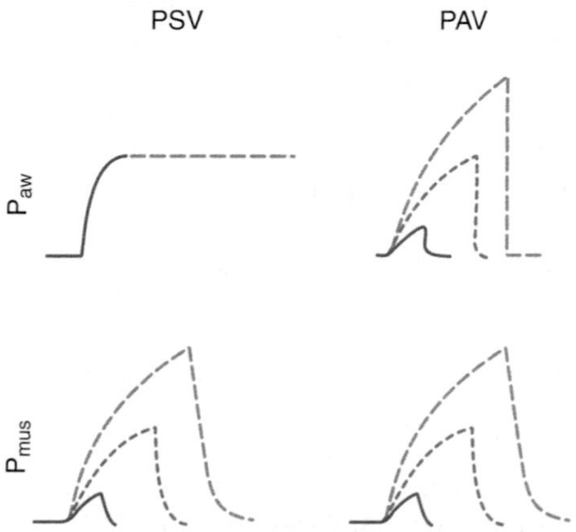

Figure 10-14. Comparison of pressure support (PSV) and proportional assist (PAV) in response to muscular efforts of varying intensity. The machine pressure mirrors the patient's muscular effort during PAV but not during PSV. (From Younes M: Proportional assist ventilation, a new approach to ventilatory support. Theory. Am Rev Respir Dis 1992;145: 114-120.)

function in patients with severe OA and changing mechanics or minute ventilation needs. Despite these theoretical disadvantages, PAV has shown at least equivalent comfort in patient trials, as well as no greater missed triggering events and greater tidal volume variability than pressure support, both in invasive and noninvasive settings.[29] That said, however, no outcome advantage over PSV has yet been convincingly demonstrated in any setting.

Neurally Adjusted Ventilatory Assist

Neurally adjusted ventilatory assist (NAVA) is similar in concept to PAV in that it attempts to regulate the machine's power support moment by moment by sensing inspiratory effort from the patient.[30] The difference is that the diaphragmatic electromyogram (EMG) provides the signal, so the traffic from the phrenic nerve regulates the amplitude of the pressure delivered, not the lung's mechanical response. A thin, multielectrode esophageal catheter is used to pick up the strength of the EMG signal, and failure to detect it has not been a major problem. The dynamic hyperinflation drawbacks of PAV in patients with airflow obstruction are theoretically nullified by placing the "effort detector" closer to the respiratory drive controller—inspiratory efforts related to auto-PEEP are tracked and supported well before inspiratory flow actually begins. Inherent protective reflexes are believed to help the patient avoid overdistention, even if the machine's power boost factor is set inappropriately high. Despite its intuitive appeal, NAVA is still too new to the clinical arena to allow a firm advantage to be declared.

Adaptive Support Ventilation

Adaptive support ventilation (ASV) is a mode that regulates machine output with pressure-targeted breaths delivered at a variable frequency and with variable pressure in accordance with breathing pattern feedback from the patient (Fig. 10-15). Its intent is to minimize the work of breathing and auto-PEEP, and it does this by optimizing the tidal volume and frequency combination that comprises minute ventilation. As such, ASV is one step closer to closed loop ventilation, in which clinical goals are set, monitored, and accomplished automatically. Once the clinician has determined the PEEP, FiO_2, and cycling triggers for pressure support, he or she must input the patient's ideal body weight (from which the series deadspace is estimated) and the fraction of estimated "normal" minute ventilation the machine should provide. It then varies the mandatory breath number and the pressure targets of a pressure-regulated SIMV algorithm. All the while, the machine tries to nudge the patient toward the ventilatory pattern optimum that *should* minimize deadspace, work of breathing, and auto-PEEP.

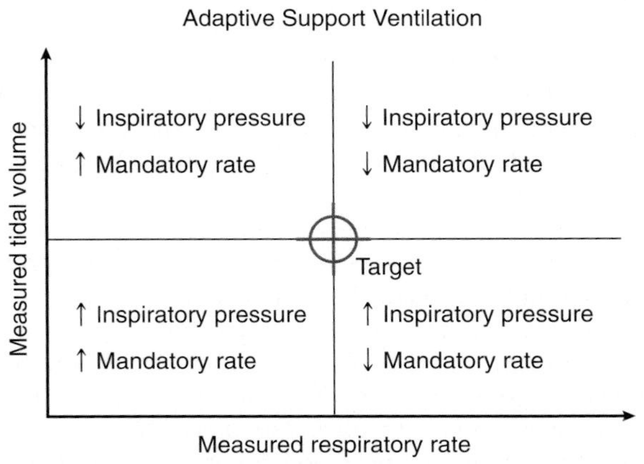

Figure 10-15. Regulation of ventilation by adaptive support. By changing the number of mandated pressure-controlled breaths and by regulating the pressure support rendered to each triggered cycle, adaptive support aims to keep breathing frequency and tidal volume within acceptable physiologic ranges (see text).

In observational studies ASV appears to regulate tidal volume and total breathing frequency effectively, without the need for clinician intervention. As with all advanced modes, however, its performance in severe stress settings has not been validated and no outcome benefit has yet been reported. As currently implemented, ASV lacks gas exchange feedback, does not calculate total physiologic deadspace, does not account for adjustment to the ideal optimum breathing pattern incurred by disease or deformity, and requires the clinician to specify what percentage of the ideal minute ventilation to shoot for. Nonetheless, it is a promising approach that modifies machine output in response to changing need and may prove to reduce the gas trapping that dysfunctional patterns of AO engender.

Weaning ("Liberation") Phase

Protracted ventilator dependence is perhaps the most feared consequence of intubating patients with exacerbated COPD and perennial asthma. Not only are breathing workloads high, but the ability of the patient to sustain them is compromised by muscle weakness, hyperinflation, disadvantageous thoracic geometry, blunted ventilatory drive, and abnormal cardiovascular function. Rational management of the weaning patient with airflow obstruction includes provision of adequate rest and nutritional support, enhancement of neuromuscular and cardiovascular function, and minimization of the breathing workload. Maintenance of positive mental attitude can greatly speed the weaning process.

Patients may fail to wean from mechanical ventilation for a wide variety of reasons. Among these are hypoxemia, cardiac arrhythmias or cardiovascular instability, and psychological dependence. However, imbalance between ventilatory capability and demand is perhaps the most common reason for failure to wean in patients with ventilatory failure.[31]

Predicting Readiness for Spontaneous Breathing

In clinical practice a panel of indices has long been used to predict the outcome of the weaning trial. Most individual elements of these panels can be classified as indicators of either ventilatory capability or demand, but not both. Some capability indicators depend on patient effort as well. Thus a maximal inspiratory pressure measurement exceeding 30 cm H_2O and a minute ventilation requirement of less than 10 L/minute are standard components of the traditional predictive battery. Although minute ventilation has been criticized as unreliable, it is still a highly useful observation, particularly when referenced to blood gas measurements. A high degree of variation of minute ventilation suggests some degree of ventilatory reserve.[32] Because the product of minute ventilation and the average inspiratory pressure per breath are the main components of the breathing workload, minute ventilation must not be disregarded, even when more integrative indices are in use, such as the frequency-to–tidal volume ratio (rapid shallow breathing index, RSBI).[31]

Numerous other weaning outcome indices have been suggested over the years, but none stands alone as infallible, including the RSBI. The most successful of these indicators reliably relate power requirement to the ability of the patient to sustain it. Certain physiologic measurements such as the $P_{0.1}$ (a measurable indicator of ventilatory drive) have predictive appeal but are not universally available and cannot be relied on in all cases. Because many factors may limit the patient's ability to be removed from the ventilator, more than one single indicator is usually necessary to observe. Alertness, degree of cardiovascular compensation, clinical trajectory over the preceding days, oxygenation status, secretion load, upper airway patency, coughing efficiency and psychologic well-being are as important as any single predictive measure based on mechanics and muscle strength.

Repeated failure to wean is often explained by cardiovascular factors such as ischemia and diastolic dysfunction. Clues may appear in the form of cardiac dysrhythmias and an unfavorable excess of fluid intake over output. In part for such reasons, weaning protocols must be constructed carefully; failure to meet weaning criteria must be considered a cue to undertake a careful review of all potential factors that prevent success, not necessarily an indication to allow a bit more time with unchanging therapy.[33]

Weaning Approaches

Preparations

Preparations for ventilator withdrawal should include ensuring adequate nocturnal rest with fully supported breathing, adequate nutrition, good circulatory reserve, avoidance of excessive intravascular volume and edema, treatment of infection, appropriate body positioning, and judicious sedation.[31] Obstipation, urinary retention, pleural effusions, gastric distention, musculoskeletal pain, severe anemia, and chemical imbalances must be avoided or reversed. During the full support phase of ventilation, care must be taken not to allow sedatives to accumulate or secretions to collect within the airways. Withdrawal of sedatives should be attempted on a daily basis in an attempt to prevent oversedation, especially when the sedating drug is continuously infused. The patient must not depend on high levels of PEEP for either oxygenation or ventilatory comfort. It must be remembered that PEEP and CPAP aid ventilation in patients with flow-limited auto-PEEP.

The use of propofol as the sedative of choice in the hours prior to spontaneous breathing trials and weaning attempts has helped to avoid the common problem of benzodiazepine hangover. Dexmedetomidine (Precedex), a sedative agent with relatively little hypnotic action, has proved helpful in some cases in which calm alertness is desired but difficult to otherwise achieve. When benzodiazepines are given for lengthy periods, lingering sedative effects can persist for up to a week after the last dose is given. In well-selected cases, alertness-enhancing drugs such as modafinil (Provigil) or atomoxetine (Strattera) have been helpful.

Specific Modes

Considerable effort has gone into the delineation of the optimal weaning technique. It is generally true that the majority of patients do not need a lengthy period of gradual machine withdrawal once the primary problems that brought the patient to medical attention have been addressed. It is also true that a distinct subset of these patients with underlying airflow obstruction cannot tolerate abrupt transitions to spontaneous breathing. More graded reloading is sometimes necessary because of fragile cardiovascular status, neuromuscular weakness, or psychologic factors. Pressure support ventilation is generally to be preferred to SIMV, as the reloading process tends to be less sudden and more predictable. Intermittent T-piece weaning makes little sense to employ in patients like this; each transition to fully spontaneous breathing abruptly imposes a full stress workload. All patients, however, should be *tested* with low-level pressure support or T-piece breathing before any gradual withdrawal of support is undertaken, as the latter may not be necessary.[34] Once the patient is breathing on low level of pressure support or from an oxygenated T-piece, observation should be continued at least 30 minutes, but generally less than 2 hours before decannulation of the airway is attempted. During the attempt at spontaneous breathing, the patient must be watched carefully and not allowed to fatigue because recovery from that condition may require more than a day to restore energy reserve.[35]

Periextubation Phase

In intubated patients suspected of upper airway obstruction, a cuff deflation test should be conducted before decannulating the airway. This is performed by elevating PEEP to 10 to 20 cm H_2O in advance of deflation. An audible leak should be heard if the glottic space is not prohibitively tight. In questionable cases, advance preparations should be made for urgent intervention, should that prove necessary after tube extraction.

The postextubation phase should be as carefully managed as the ventilated one. The first 24 hours off the ventilator are often difficult and tenuous, but in successful cases there should be progressive improvement. Coughing, deep breathing, adequate oxygenation, avoidance of arrhythmias, adequate bronchodilation and airstream hydration, maintenance of a clear central airway, and a mechanically efficient posture are crucial. Oral refeeding must be undertaken with extreme caution because swallowing difficulty in chronic dysfunction can persist days to weeks postextubation in patients who have been ventilated for lengthy periods. Although CPAP and noninvasive ventilation may be helpful in selected patients,[36] mask ventilation generally impedes secretion clearance, dries oral secretions, and encourages displacement of oral secretions into the central airway. Therefore it is common for patients who receive mask ventilation postextubation to require reintubation for clearance of thickened airway mucus.

KEY POINTS

- By assuming a major portion of the ventilatory workload, mechanical ventilation affords the opportunity to rest the respiratory muscles while maintaining pH homeostasis and oxygenation, thereby averting progressive ventilatory failure or respiratory arrest, or both.
- Increased resistance to airflow is responsible (directly or indirectly) for many of the physiologic disturbances that typify AO.
- When dynamic collapse occurs during tidal respiration and breathing requirements are high, there is little alternative to hyperinflation or CO_2 retention, or both.
- Ventilation-perfusion mismatching is widespread in patients with severe airflow obstruction, reducing the efficiency of carbon dioxide elimination.
- Pressure-targeted modes of ventilation, exemplified by pressure control and pressure support, have become increasingly popular in the care of intubated patients, as well as those receiving noninvasive ventilation by facemask.
- Most patients hospitalized with exacerbations of asthma or COPD can be managed effectively by regimens that incorporate aggressive secretion clearance techniques, antibiotics, corticosteroids, intensified bronchodilators, hydration, cardiovascular support, and supplemental oxygen.
- The first 24-hour period following tracheal intubation and initiation of positive pressure ventilation is a highly dynamic one for the patient with AO.
- The majority of ventilatory support of AO is still currently provided with modes of ventilation that are now decades old—flow-controlled, volume-cycled ventilation ("assist-control"); PCV; PSV; and SIMV.
- The postextubation phase should be as carefully managed as the ventilated one. The first 24 hours off the ventilator are often difficult and tenuous, but in successful cases there should be progressive improvement.

REFERENCES

1. Hogg JC: Pathophysiology of airflow limitation in chronic obstructive pulmonary disease. Lancet 2004;364:709-721.
2. Rossi A, Poggi R, Roca J: Physiologic factors predisposing to chronic respiratory failure. Respir Care Clin North Am 2002;8:379-404.
3. Kimball WR, Leith DE, Robins AG: Dynamic hyperinflation and ventilator dependence in chronic obstructive pulmonary disease. Am Rev Respir Dis 1982;126:991-995.
4. Calverley PM, Koulouris NG: Flow limitation and dynamic hyperinflation: key concepts in modern respiratory physiology. Eur Respir J 2005;25:186-199.
5. Pepe PE, Marini JJ: Occult positive end-expiratory pressure in mechanically ventilated patients with airflow obstruction: The auto-PEEP effect. Am Rev Respir Dis 1982;126:166-170.
6. Rossi A, Polese G, Brandi G, Conti G: Intrinsic positive end-expiratory pressure (PEEPi). Intensive Care Med 1995;21:522-536.
7. Rossi A, Gottfried SB, Zocchi L, et al: Measurement of static compliance of the total respiratory system in patients with acute respiratory failure during mechanical ventilation. The effect of intrinsic positive end-expiratory pressure. Am Rev Respir Dis 1985;131:672-677.
8. Marini JJ: Should PEEP be used in airflow obstruction? Am Rev Respir Dis 1989;140:1-3.
9. Smith TC, Marini JJ: Impact of PEEP on lung mechanics and work of breathing in severe airflow obstruction. J Appl Physiol 1988;65:1488-1499.
10. Marini JJ: Heliox in chronic obstructive pulmonary disease . . . time to lighten up? Crit Care Med August 2000;28:3086-3087.
11. Marini JJ, Tyler ML, Hudson LD, et al: Influence of head-dependent positions on lung volume and oxygen saturation in chronic airflow obstruction. Am Rev Respir Dis 1984;129:101-105.
12. Leatherman JW: Mechanical ventilation in obstructive lung disease. Clin Chest Med 1996;17:577-590.
13. Similowski T, Yan S, Gauthier AP, et al: Contractile properties of the human diaphragm during chronic hyperinflation. N Engl J Med 1991;325:917-923.
14. Marini JJ, Crooke PS, Truwit JD: Determinants and limits of pressure preset ventilation: A mathematical model of pressure control. J Appl Physiol 1989;67:1081-1092.
15. Hotchkiss JR, Adams AB, Dries DJ, et al: Dynamic behavior during noninvasive ventilation. Chaotic support? Am J Resp Crit Care Med 2001;163:374-378.
16. Jubran A, Van de Graaff WB, Tobin MJ: Variability of patient-ventilator interaction with pressure support ventilation in patients with chronic obstructive pulmonary disease. Am J Respir Crit Care Med 1995;152:129-136.
17. Brochard L, Mancebo J, Wysocki M, et al: Noninvasive ventilation for acute exacerbations of chronic obstructive pulmonary disease. N Engl J Med 1995;333:817-822.
18. Brochard L, Isabey D, Piquet J, et al: Reversal of acute exacerbations of chronic obstructive lung disease by inspiratory assistance with a face mask. N Engl J Med 1990;323:1523-1530.
19. Lightowler JV, Wedzicha JA, Elliott MW, Ram FS: Non-invasive positive pressure ventilation to treat respiratory failure resulting from exacerbations of chronic obstructive pulmonary disease: Cochrane Systematic Review and Meta-analysis. BMJ 2003;326:185.
20. British Thoracic Society Standards of Care Committee: Non-invasive ventilation in acute respiratory failure. Thorax 2002;57:192-211.
21. Nava S, Ceriana P: Causes of failure of noninvasive mechanical ventilation. Respir Care 2004;49:295-303.
22. Ambrosino N, Foglio K, Rubini F, et al: Non-invasive mechanical ventilation in acute respiratory failure due to chronic obstructive pulmonary disease: Correlates for success. Thorax 1995;50:755-757.
23. Feihl F, Perret C: Permissive hypercapnia. How permissive should we be? Am J Respir Crit Care Med 1994;150:1722-1737.
24. Zamanian M, Marini JJ: Pressure-flow signatures of central-airway mucus plugging. Crit Care Med 2006;34:223-226.

25. Celli BR, MacNee W: ATS/ERS Task Force. Standards for the diagnosis and treatment of patients with COPD: A summary of the ATS/ERS position paper. Eur Respir J 2004;23:932-946.
26. Ranieri VM, Giuliani R, Cinnella G, et al: Physiologic effects of positive end-expiratory pressure in patients with chronic obstructive pulmonary disease during acute ventilatory failure and controlled mechanical ventilation. Am Rev Respir Dis 1993;147:5-13.
27. Younes M: Proportional assist ventilation, a new approach to ventilatory support. Theory. Am Rev Respir Dis 1992;145:114-120.
28. Giannouli E, Webster K, Roberts D, Younes M: Response of ventilator-dependent patients to different levels of pressure support and proportional assist. Am J Respir Crit Care Med 1999;159:1716-1725.
29. Navalesi P, Hernandez P, Wongsa A, et al: Proportional assist ventilation in acute respiratory failure: Effects on breathing pattern and inspiratory effort. Am J Respir Crit Care Med 1996;154: 1330-1338.
30. Sinderby C, Navalesi P, Beck J, et al: Neural control of mechanical ventilation in respiratory failure. Nat Med 1999;5:1433-1436.
31. Marini JJ: Weaning from mechanical ventilation. N Engl J Med 1991;324: 1496-1498.
32. Wysocki M, Cracco C, Teixeira A, et al: Reduced breathing variability as a predictor of unsuccessful patient separation from mechanical ventilation. Crit Care Med 2006;34:2076-2083.
33. Hill NS: Following protocol: weaning difficult-to-wean patients with chronic obstructive pulmonary disease. Am J Respir Crit Care Med 2001;164: 186-187.
34. Esteban A, Frutos F, Tobin MJ, et al: A comparison of four methods of weaning patients from mechanical ventilation. Spanish Lung Failure Collaborative Group. N Engl J Med 1995;332: 345-350.
35. Laghi F, D'Alfonso N, Tobin MJ: Pattern of recovery from diaphragmatic fatigue over 24 hours. J Appl Physiol 1995;79: 539-546.
36. Esteban A, Frutos-Vivar F, Ferguson ND, et al: Noninvasive positive-pressure ventilation for respiratory failure after extubation. N Engl J Med 2004;350: 2452-2460.

Chapter 11

Mechanical Ventilation in Acute Respiratory Distress Syndrome

Luciano Gattinoni, Eleonora Carlesso, and Pietro Caironi

Since the first description of acute respiratory distress syndrome (ARDS) in 1967,[1] mechanical ventilation has been the primary "buying time" treatment for acute lung injury (ALI). Mechanical ventilation is not a "gas exchanger," but instead replaces, totally or partially, the force normally generated by the respiratory muscles to promote ventilation, providing muscle rest. The effects of mechanical ventilation on gas exchange are indirect and include (1) better clearance of carbon dioxide (CO_2) by the power of the mechanical ventilator to expand the diseased and collapsed lung; (2) improvement in oxygenation by preventing alveolar hypoxia caused by hypoventilation; (3) improvement in oxygenation by increasing inspiratory oxygen fraction, which affects alveolar partial pressure of oxygen (P_{AO_2}); (4) improvement in oxygenation by opening lung regions otherwise collapsed (alveolar recruitment); and (5) improving oxygenation by maintaining positive end-expiratory pressure (PEEP), preventing the collapse of the lung regions previously recruited during the inspiratory phase.

The negative effects of mechanical ventilation are interwoven with its positive effects. First, the driving force applied by the ventilator, if excessive, may alter, in different ways, the lung parenchyma and produce ventilator-induced lung injury (VILI). Second, the positive-pressure ventilation unavoidably turns the physiologically negative intrathoracic pressures into positive pressures. In consideration of this, the guiding principle of mechanical ventilation of ARDS patients should be that, whenever one manipulates the ventilator settings, one should refer to one polar star: The new setting is less harmful to the lung structure than the previous one.

HISTORY

Extensive reviews on the history of mechanical ventilation of ARDS can be found elsewhere.[2,3] In the 1970s, mechanical ventilation was recommended and performed with low PEEP and high tidal volume: ". . . larger tidal volumes (10 to 15 per kilogram) are preferable, having been used in several thousand ventilated patients with no evidence of development of pulmonary damage."[4] Today, this advice seems inconceivable. At that time, the main concerns were the putative harm of high inspiratory oxygen fraction and the hemodynamic impairment. It was later recognized in experimental and clinical settings[5-7] that high-volume/high-pressure mechanical ventilation could severely damage the lung parenchyma. Such lesions, primarily attributed to the excessive airway pressure, were collectively classified as *barotrauma.* In the same period, Suter and colleagues[8] published a report that, for the first time, systematically described the interaction between PEEP, lung mechanics, gas exchange, and hemodynamics.

In the 1980s, based on the work of Dreyfuss,[9,10] the focus progressively shifted from the potential harm of pressure to the harm of volume (overdistention), a concept that was popularized as *volutrauma.*[11] In the mid 1980s, the application of computed tomography (CT)[12,13] and the quantitative approach to CT analysis[14] led to the concept of *baby lung,*[15,16] which accounted for most of the previous observations on respiratory mechanics, gas exchange functionality, and potential harm of mechanical ventilation. The premise of this line of thought is that high pressure or excessive distention applied to a small fraction of the lung parenchyma (with a size similar to the lung of a baby) unavoidably leads to structural lesions of the lung regions open to ventilation. Total *lung rest* was achievable with the use of extracorporeal CO_2 removal, targeted to prevent the damages of high pressure/volume ventilation.[17-19] The target of mechanical ventilation shifted toward lung protection, rather than normal gas exchange functionality. Hickling and associates[20] proposed the "permissive hypercapnia" strategy for ARDS, providing "gentle treatment" of the portion of the lung that remains open to ventilation (the baby lung) through less aggressive mechanical ventilation, at the acceptable price of an abnormally higher arterial partial pressure of carbon dioxide ($PaCO_2$).

A large amount of experimental and clinical data over the years has supported the approach of a *lung protective strategy*.[21-25] Low tidal volume prevents the excessive global stress and strain of the baby lung, whereas higher PEEP prevents the regional excessive stress and strain by avoiding alveolar collapse and reopening during mechanical ventilation.[26] These mechanical events are associated with an inflammatory reaction of the epithelial and endothelial lung cells *(biotrauma/atelectrauma)* as shown by the seminal study of Tremblay and colleagues[27] (see also references 11, 28). The literature to date supports that the harm of mechanical ventilation is due to excessive global or regional stress and strain.[29] This leads to two results—a physical rupture of the lung and a mechanically induced inflammation of the lung parenchyma, constituting VILI. The best "mechanical ventilation" would provide adequate gas exchange with the lowest amount of VILI.

PHYSIOLOGIC BASIS OF MECHANICAL VENTILATION

Driving Force

To ventilate the respiratory system, force is required. The driving force for ventilation under normal circumstances is provided by the respiratory muscles. During spontaneous breathing, the thoracic cage expands. This causes a decrease in intrathoracic pressure (pleural pressure, P_{pl}) relative to the atmosphere (in normal conditions approximately 2 mm Hg of ΔP_{pl} is sufficient to expand the thoracic cage by 0.5 L). Because the lungs are connected in series with the thoracic cage, their volume is expanded to a near equal extent (not considering the blood shift[30]). The force that distends the lung is the pressure difference between the alveoli and the pleural cavity (the transpulmonary pressure, P_L). As the lung expands, the alveolar pressure becomes subatmospheric, and gas flow is generated *(inspiration)*. When the respiratory muscles relax, the potential energy accumulated in the respiratory system (lung and chest wall) returns the chest wall and the lung parenchyma to the resting position *(expiration)*. In spontaneously breathing subjects, the driving force (muscular pressure, ΔP_{musc},) is spent partly to expand the chest wall (ΔP_{pl}), partly to expand the lung (ΔP_L), and partly to overcome the resistances to the gas flow. In *quasistatic* conditions, in which the resistances to gas flow are negligible:

$$\Delta P_{musc} = \Delta P_{pl} + \Delta P_L$$

During positive-pressure mechanical ventilation, the rules are exactly the same, with the exception that ΔP_{musc} is substituted by the force provided by the ventilator, and the force is applied to the lung parenchyma and not to the chest wall. The driving pressure, which coincides with the airway pressure at plateau during an end inspiratory pause (in quasistatic conditions), is spent first to expand the lung and second to expand the chest wall:

$$\Delta P_{aw} = \Delta P_L + \Delta P_{pl}$$

In spontaneous breathing and during positive-pressure mechanical ventilation, the distending force of the lung is the transpulmonary pressure. During spontaneous breathing, pleural pressure is negative (facilitating venous return), however, whereas during mechanical ventilation it is positive (impairing venous return). What matters from the pulmonary perspective is the distending force (i.e., the transpulmonary pressure [ΔP_L]), whereas what matters from the hemodynamic perspective is the pleural pressure (ΔP_{pl}).

Transpulmonary Pressure

At the same driving force applied to the whole respiratory system (lung and chest wall), the resulting transpulmonary pressure, ΔP_L, may be extremely variable. If the lung is relatively "stiff," and the chest wall is relatively "soft" (e.g., during pulmonary fibrosis or ARDS of pulmonary origin), a greater fraction of the driving pressure is spent to distend the lung (high transpulmonary pressure). In contrast, if the lung is relatively soft, but the chest wall is relatively stiff (e.g., during an abdominal disease or severe obesity), most of the driving force is spent to move the chest wall (high pleural pressure).

To express this phenomenon quantitatively, it is convenient to consider the concept of *elastance*. The elastance of the whole respiratory system is the driving force (ΔP_{aw}) required to increase the lung and the chest wall 1 L above their resting position ($E_{TOT} = \Delta P_{aw}/1$ L). Part of this driving force is spent to increase the lung volume of 1 L ($E_L = \Delta P_L/1L$), and part is spent to increase the chest wall by the same amount ($E_{CW} = \Delta P_{pl}/1$ L). Transpulmonary pressure (ΔP_L) can be expressed as the driving force times the ratio between lung elastance and total elastance of the respiratory system:

$$\Delta P_L = \Delta P_{aw} \times E_L/E_{TOT}$$

The transpulmonary pressure for a given driving pressure uniquely depends on the ratio of lung elastance to respiratory system elastance. In normal subjects E_L/E_{TOT} is approximately 0.5, whereas in patients with ARDS it may range from 0.2 (e.g., in obese patients or in patients with high intra-abdominal pressure) to 0.8 (e.g., in patients with a very small baby lung and a normal chest wall elastance). This variability implies that for the same driving force applied and read on the ventilator display (e.g., 30 cm H_2O), the resulting transpulmonary pressure may range from 6 to 24 cm H_2O (Fig. 11-1).

Force-Bearing Structure of Lung Parenchyma

The transpulmonary pressure is applied to the force-bearing structure of lung parenchyma, the extracellular matrix, which constitutes the *lung skeleton*.[31] The lung

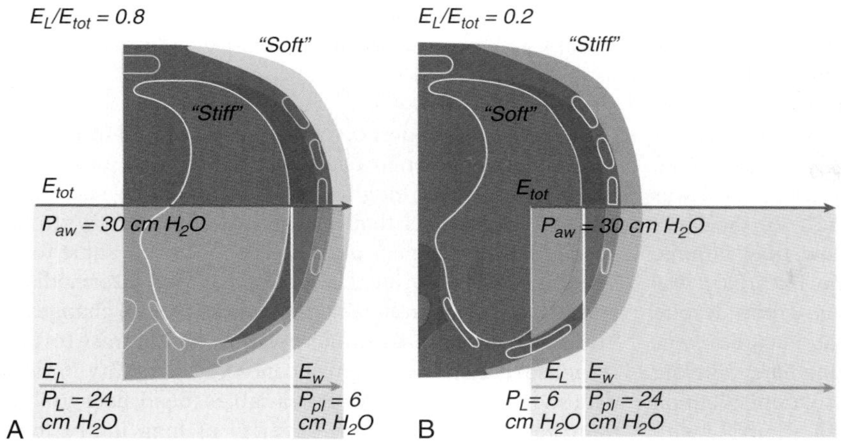

Figure 11-1. Two examples of E_L/E_{TOT} variability in patients with acute lung injury/acute respiratory distress syndrome. **A,** $E_L/E_{TOT} = 0.2$. **B,** $E_L/E_{TOT} = 0.8$. This variability implies that for the same airway pressure applied (e.g., 30 cm H_2O), the resulting transpulmonary pressure (P_L) may range from 6 to 24 cm H_2O.

skeleton is a complex and metabolically active structure that includes a network of several components—elastin, collagen, and proteoglycans. All these molecules are involved in determining the mechanical characteristics of the respiratory system. The elastin may be considered as an elastic spring, whereas the unextensible collagen, which is folded at end expiration and completely unfolded at a lung volume equal to total lung capacity, acts as a stop-length fiber.[32,33] The proteoglycans stabilize the collagen-elastin network, contributing to lung elasticity and alveolar stability at low and medium lung volumes.[34]

The matrix of elastin, collagen, and proteoglycans is arranged in two main fiber systems: (1) the *axial* system, which originates from the pulmonary hilum and runs deeply into the lung parenchyma down to the alveolar level, where it joins (2) the *peripheral* system, which originates from the visceral pleura and runs centripetally within the lung parenchyma.[31] The lung skeleton may be considered as a continuous elastic structure that reaches its extension limits at total lung capacity, a lung volume equal to about threefold the lung resting volume. At this level of alveolar distention, the collagen is completely unfolded, and further expansion is prevented. The epithelial and endothelial cells do not directly bear the applied forces because they are anchored to the extracellular matrix by a series of structural proteins (integrins), which are connected to the cytoskeleton. During lung expansion, the epithelial and the endothelial cells modify their shape.

It is well documented that mechanically induced cellular deformation activates a series of mechanosensors with the production of several inflammatory mediators, such as cytokines interleukin-6, tumor necrosis factor-α, and interferon-γ,[27,35] metalloproteinases (enzymes involved in the remodeling of the matrix),[36] leukotrienes,[37] and interleukin-8,[38-40] the most powerful attractor of neutrophils.[41] Gross barotrauma (e.g., pneumothorax) is due to the stress at rupture of the lung skeleton, whereas intrapulmonary inflammation is primarily due to the excessive strain of the epithelial and endothelial cells.

Concept of Stress and Strain

Stress is the applied force, and strain is the linear deformation of material. In the whole lung, the rough approximation of stress is the transpulmonary pressure, whereas the approximation of the average strain is the change in volume relative to the lung resting volume. The ratio between alveolar stress and strain is defined as *lung-specific elastance* (E_{spec}), which is mathematically defined as:

$$\Delta P_L = E_{spec} \times \Delta V/V_0$$

where ΔV is the volume variation applied to the lung (i.e., the tidal volume), and V_0 is the lung resting volume (i.e., the functional residual capacity at atmospheric pressure [without any application of PEEP]). The lung-specific elastance is the transpulmonary pressure required to double the lung resting volume (i.e., the ΔP_L when $\Delta V/V_0$ is equal to 1). In ALI/ARDS, lung-specific elastance is similar to normal,[16,42] reinforcing the concept of the baby lung (lung is small and not stiff), and questions the use of normalizing the tidal volume to the ideal body weight. The same tidal volume per kilogram may result in completely different strain according to the size of the baby lung (the V_0 of the previous equation). For example, a 70-kg man with ARDS may have, according to the severity of the lung injury, a residual baby lung equal to 60%, 40%, or 20% of his normal lung size. If the ventilator is set to deliver 10 mL/kg, the actual delivered tidal volume would generate an alveolar strain, which would result from the application, in normal lung, of a tidal volume equal to 17 mL/kg, 25 mL/kg, and 50 mL/kg, values associated with a significant lung injury in laboratory studies.[11,29]

PATIENT CHARACTERIZATION

Setting the least harmful mechanical ventilation requires a preliminary knowledge of the main pathophysiologic characteristics of the patient. The most relevant characteristics are the kind and amount of the lung injury, the chest wall elastance, and the lung recruitability.

Gas Exchange

Oxygen

$Pa{O_2}$, $Pa{O_2}$-to-fraction of inspired oxygen ratio ($Pa{O_2}/F{I}{O_2}$), and Riley's shunt fraction[43] are the most commonly used variables to assess the severity of lung injury. In particular, the PaO_2/FIO_2 thresholds of 300 and 200 are used to define ALI (300) and ARDS (200).[44] Consequently, the PaO_2/FIO_2 ratio is perceived as a key variable by most intensive care unit (ICU) physicians: The lower the PaO_2/FIO_2, the greater the lung injury. This equivalence is highly questionable. First, in most large studies on ARDS, no association was found between hypoxemia and outcome.[45] In the large study showing a better outcome with low tidal volume compared with higher tidal volume, the PaO_2/FIO_2 was significantly lower in the low tidal volume group despite ending with better outcome.[25] Finally, the PaO_2/FIO_2 was not different in patients with early, intermediate, and late ARDS, suggesting that oxygenation was not dependent on the structural changes of lung parenchyma occurring with time.[46] In a study[47] in which the lung severity was assessed by CT scan (and defined as a fraction of the gasless tissue), we did not find significant changes of PaO_2/FIO_2 over a wide range of nonaerated tissue (Fig. 11-2), and PaO_2/FIO_2 was not associated with outcome.

Most data suggest that PaO_2/FIO_2 is a weak indicator of the overall lung severity, with compensatory rearrangement of perfusion during ARDS limiting the deterioration of oxygenation. The same limits apply when PaO_2/FIO_2 changes are used to assess lung recruitment. Because this maneuver is unavoidably associated with changes of perfusion (global or regional), the increase of PaO_2/FIO_2 may be partly due to decrease of perfusion, as shown in the 1980s.[48-50] Most data suggest that the use of oxygenation variables alone to assess lung severity is misleading.

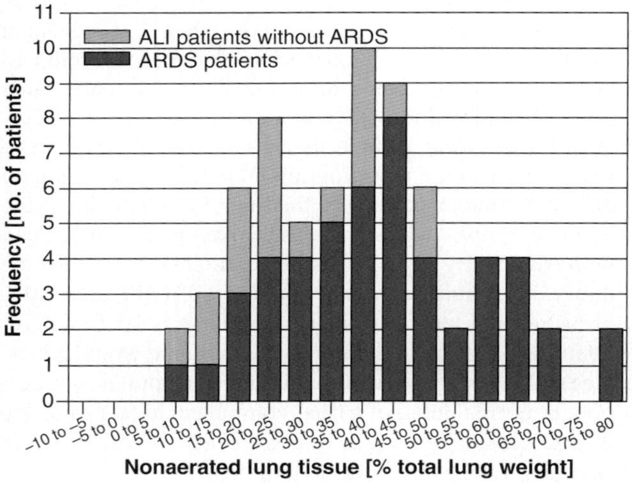

Figure 11-2. Frequency distribution of nonaerated lung tissue, expressed as a proportion of the total lung weight, recorded at 5 cm H_2O positive end-expiratory pressure in 68 patients with acute lung injury/acute respiratory distress syndrome (ALI/ARDS). *Green columns* represent patients with PaO_2/FIO_2 less than 300 (ALI without ARDS), whereas *gray columns* represent patients with PaO_2/FIO_2 less than 200 (ARDS). The nonaerated lung tissue was defined as the lung tissue having a physical density at CT scan image analysis between +100 houndsfield units (HU) and −100 HU, representing the portion of lung parenchyma that is consolidated or collapsed or both (i.e., the lung injury severity). (With permission from Gattinoni L, Caironi P, Cressoni M, et al: Lung recruitment in patients with the acute respiratory distress syndrome. N Engl J Med 2006;354:1775-1786.)

Carbon Dioxide

Although less considered, the variables derived from CO_2, as the total or alveolar deadspace, seem to be of greater value in assessing lung severity. It has been shown in ALI/ARDS patients that deadspace at entry is a strong predictor of outcome,[51] and that $PaCO_2$ for the same total ventilation steadily increases from early to intermediate and to late ARDS, reflecting the lung structural changes.[46] The PCO_2 response to prone position (in contrast to PO_2 response) is a strong prognostic index of mortality.[52] Most data suggest that CO_2-related variables (deadspace), more than PaO_2/FIO_2, reflect the severity of lung injury (and associated mortality) at the time of presentation and the structural changes of lung parenchyma occurring with time (fibrosis, *Pneumocystis*, and possibly perfusion defects).

Respiratory Mechanics, Chest Wall Elastance, and Lung Volume

In the original description of ARDS,[1] the low compliance (i.e., high elastance) of the respiratory system was a landmark of the syndrome. The respiratory system compliance is not considered in the current definition of ARDS, however.[44] For years, the low compliance was attributed uniquely to the lung component (lung stiffness and lack of surfactant). Quantitative CT shows, however, that the respiratory system compliance primarily reflects the size of lung open to gases (the baby lung[14,16]), suggesting that the intrinsic functioning lung elasticity in ARDS is close to normal (the lung is "small" rather than "stiff"). More than gas exchange, the respiratory system compliance indirectly assesses the lung injury severity (the smaller baby lung, the greater lung injury),[53] as confirmed in animal experiments.[54] Another variable also must be taken into account—the elastance of the chest wall. It has been shown in a significant portion of ALI/ARDS patients that the chest wall elastance is greater than normal because of increased intra-abdominal pressure, obesity, or severe edema.[55] In patients with extrapulmonary ARDS[56] and in obese patients,[57] the high elastance of the respiratory system may be due to the chest wall and to the lung derangement. Measurement of intra-abdominal pressure should be considered when selecting mechanical ventilator settings.

Severity of Lung Injury and Lung Recruitability

CT can be used to assess the severity of lung injury by measuring the fraction of nonaerated lung tissue at end expiration (end expiration pause at 5 cm H_2O). This fraction includes the lung tissue that is "consolidated" (i.e., not openable at 45 cm H_2O airway pressure) and the tissue that is collapsed but openable at 45 cm H_2O. These values were chosen to produce a minimal risk during the maneuver and because this is the most frequently used in the literature for recruitment maneuver.[47] In patients with elevated chest wall elastance, the resulting transpulmonary pressure could be insufficient, however, to overcome the opening pressure of some pulmonary units.

The total fraction of nonaerated lung tissue (consolidated plus recruitable) and the recruitable tissue alone (tissue that regains aeration at 45 cm H_2O airway pressure) are strongly associated with mortality. The data of Figure 11-2 show the inadequacy of the term *ALI/ARDS,* as currently defined, to describe the lung injury.[47] The data refer to a population of ALI/ARDS patients, classified according to the American-European Consensus Conference on ARDS,[44] in which a CT-based quantitative analysis of the whole lung parenchyma at 5 cm H_2O PEEP was performed. As shown in Figure 11-3, the fraction of the nonaerated lung tissue (consolidated or collapsed or both) may range from 5% to 70% of the entire lung parenchyma. Patients meeting ALI/ARDS criteria may have a baby lung size very close to that of normal subjects, or a baby lung that is just a small fraction of the expected normal lung. When the distending force is applied to the lungs by the mechanical ventilator, previously collapsed lung regions may open. Lung recruitability may be expressed as the amount of lung tissue regaining aeration when increasing the applied driving force from 5 to 45 cm H_2O. As shown in Figure 11-3, in some patients, lung recruitability was almost negligible, whereas in others was equal to 25% to 35% of the entire lung parenchyma. Lung recruitability was strongly associated with the fraction of nonaerated tissue, suggesting that the greater the inflammatory edema, the greater the lung collapse. It seems that the best way to assess the overall lung severity and the related lung recruitability, both strongly associated with mortality, is the CT scan analysis. Physiologic variables are poor indicators of the severity of the lung injury. This is shown in Figure 11-4—for a large variation of lung injury, ranging from 20% to 60% of the lung parenchyma, the values of PaO_2/FIO_2, lung compliance, and $PaCO_2$ greatly overlap.

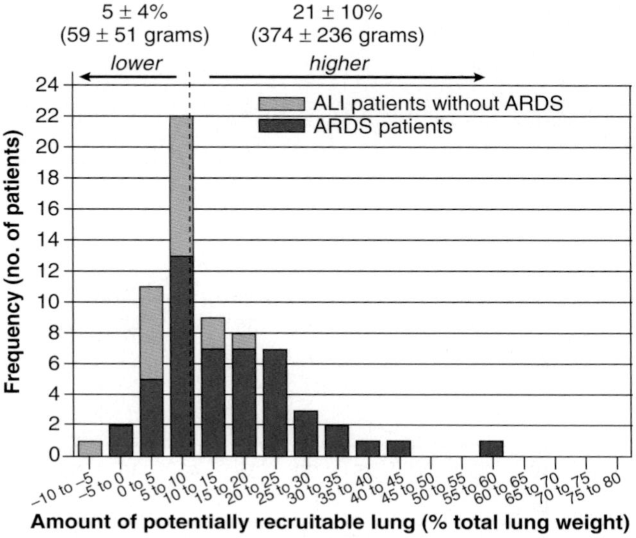

Figure 11-3. Frequency distribution of 68 patients with acute lung injury/acute respiratory distress syndrome (ALI/ARDS) according to the percentage of potentially recruitable lung, expressed as the percentage of total lung weight. ALI without ARDS was defined by a PaO_2/FIO_2 less than 300, but not less than 200; ARDS was defined by a PaO_2/FIO_2 less than 200. The percentage of potentially recruitable lung was defined as the proportion of lung tissue in which aeration was restored at airway pressures between 5 and 45 cm H_2O. (With permission from Gattinoni L, Caironi P, Cressoni M, et al: Lung recruitment in patients with the acute respiratory distress syndrome. N Engl J Med 2006;354:1775-1786.)

MECHANICAL VENTILATION IN ACUTE RESPIRATORY DISTRESS SYNDROME: AVAILABLE EVIDENCE

Setting Tidal Volume

The main results of several outcome studies specifically designed to compare different tidal volumes are summarized in Table 11-1. A survival benefit was found in the study comparing 6 mL/kg tidal volume versus 12 mL/kg, the highest tidal volume range tested,[25] whereas no survival differences were found in the other studies, which compared intermediate values of tidal volumes.[21,23,24] As previously discussed, the tidal volume per ideal body

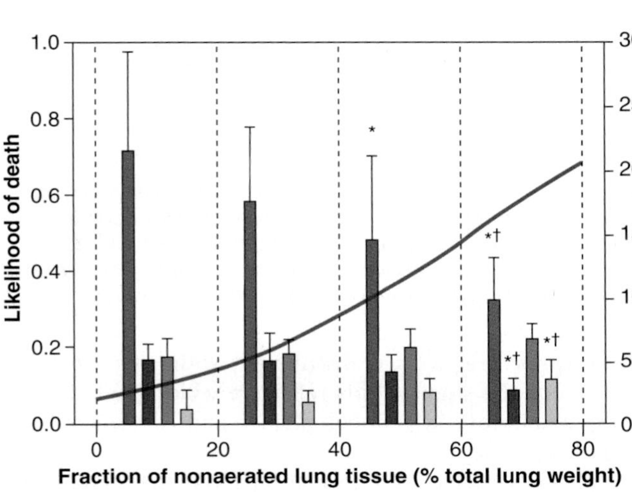

Figure 11-4. Mean ± standard deviation values of respiratory variables of a population of 68 patients with acute lung injury/acute respiratory distress syndrome. *Blue columns* represent PaO_2/FIO_2 at positive end-expiratory pressure (PEEP) 5 cm H_2O (mm Hg), *red columns* represent respiratory system compliance at PEEP 5 cm H_2O (mL/cm H_2O), *green columns* represent deadspace fraction (%), and *gold columns* represent alveolar deadspace fraction (%). *$P < .05$ versus patients with a fraction of nonaerated tissue recorded at 5 cm H_2O PEEP less than 0.2. †$P < .05$ versus patients with a fraction of nonaerated tissue recorded at 5 cm H_2O PEEP ranging from 0.2 to 0.4. The *continuous black line* represents the likelihood of death predicted by the fraction of nonaerated lung tissue recorded at 5 cm H_2O PEEP ($P = .015$).

Table 11-1. Different Tidal Volumes per Ideal Weight and Airway Plateau Pressures Investigated in Other Studies

Study	Group	No.	Tidal Volume (mL/kg)	Plateau Pressure (cm H_2O)	Mortality (%)	*P* (Outcome)
Acute Respiratory Distress Syndrome Network[25]	Control	429	11.8 ± 0.8	33 ± 9	39.8	.007
	Treatment	432	6.2 ± 0.9	25 ± 7	31	
Brochard et al[23]	Control	58	10.3 ± 1.7	31.7 ± 6.6	37.9	NS
	Treatment	58	7.1 ± 1.3	25.7 ± 5	46.6	
Stewart et al[21]	Control	60	10.7 ± 1.4	26.8 ± 6.7	47	NS
	Treatment	60	7 ± 0.7	22.3 ± 5.4	50	
Brower et al[24]	Control	26	10.2 ± 0.1	30.6 ± 0.8	46	NS
	Treatment	26	7.3 ± 0.1	24.9 ± 0.8	50	
Amato et al[22]	Control	24	12 (768 ± 13 mL)*	36.8 ± 0.9	71	<.001
	Treatment	29	<6 (348 ± 6 mL)*	30.1 ± 0.7	38	

*Mean ± standard error values of tidal volume (mL/kg) were not provided in the paper of Amato et al. The value set by the physician and the mean ± standard error values of tidal volume in mL (first 36 hrs) have been provided.

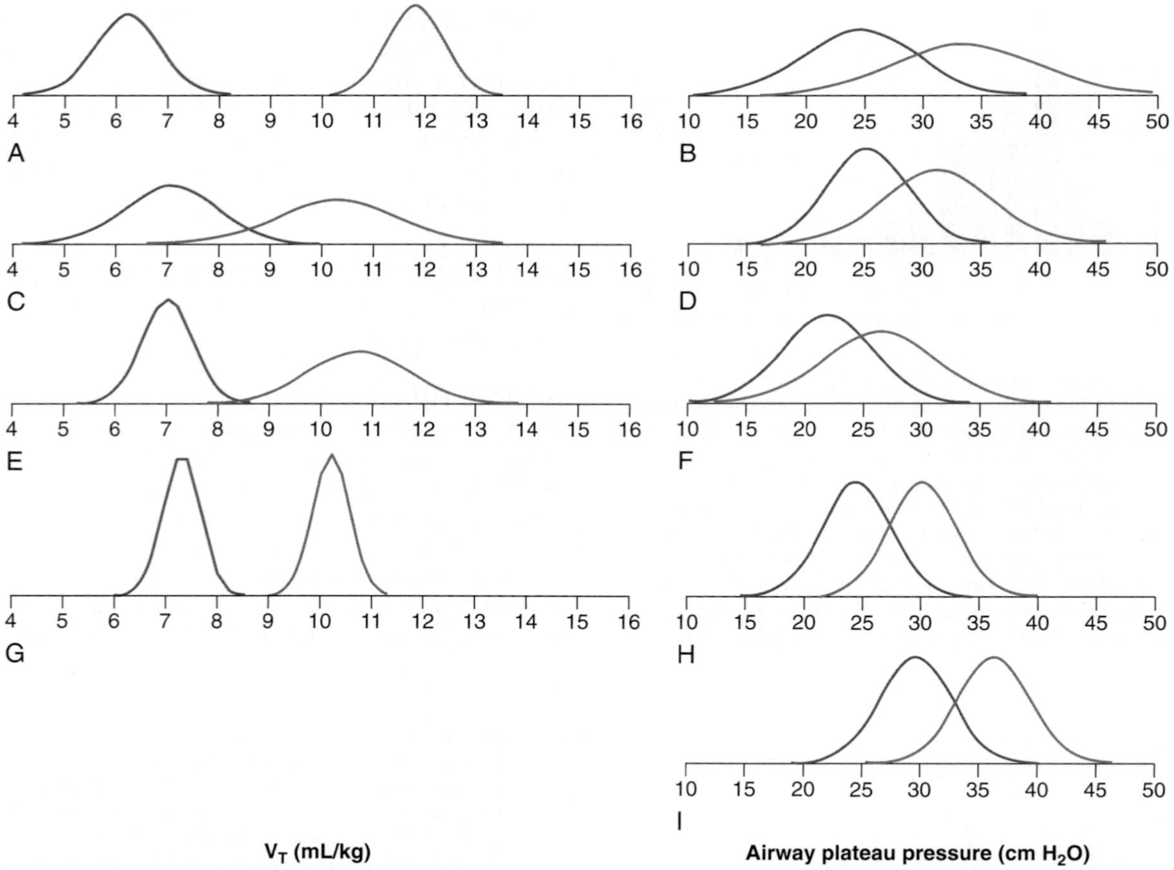

Figure 11-5. Distribution of tidal volume (V_T) per ideal body weight *(left column)* and of plateau pressure *(right column)* (*red line* = treated group; *blue line* = controls) in five randomized trials (computed from the reported mean ± standard deviation assuming a gaussian distribution). **A** and **B,** Acute Respiratory Distress Syndrome Network.[25] **C** and **D,** Brochard et al.[23] **E** and **F,** Stewart et al.[21] **G** and **H,** Brower et al.[24] **I,** Amato et al.[22] (With permission from Gattinoni L, Carlesso E, Cadringher P, et al: Physical and biological triggers of ventilator-induced lung injury and its prevention. Eur Respir J Suppl 2003;47:15s-25s.)

weight is a poor surrogate of strain because ARDS patients with similar body weight may have completely different lung sizes and consequently different strain at equal tidal volume. This is confirmed by the plateau pressures measured in these different studies (Fig. 11-5). As shown for the same tidal volume per ideal body weight, the plateau pressures are widely distributed with huge overlap between the studies. This reflects a wide distribution of the respiratory system compliance and consequently of the lung size.

Despite the lack of information about stress and strain in each individual patient, most available data strongly suggest that a gentle ventilation is safer than the application of high volumes and pressures. This evidence does not mean that 6 mL/kg ideal body weight represents the ideal tidal volume. In a patient with a very small baby lung, it still may be harmful, inducing excessive strain, whereas if applied to a lung characterized by a large ventilatable area, it may be low. There is little doubt, however, that 12 mL/kg ideal body weight is excessively high and unnecessary. It is evident that low tidal volume ventilation, decreasing the global alveolar stress and strain, is advantageous compared with high tidal volume ventilation in different patient.

It has been suggested that a plateau pressure of 30 cm H_2O represents the safe limit for plateau pressure.[58] In a retrospective analysis, such a safe limit has been challenged, however.[59] This is understandable if we consider that the airway plateau pressure is a poor surrogate of stress owing to the high variability of the chest wall compliance. The same plateau pressure, 30 cm H_2O, may result in completely different stress values in different patients.

Setting Positive End-Expiratory Pressure

The available evidence on the effects of higher versus lower levels of PEEP in ALI/ARDS patients is summarized in Table 11-2. As shown, the largest studies comparing higher versus lower PEEP levels in unselected ALI/ARDS patients were unable to find any difference in outcome.[60] Two of the studies presented in Table 11-2 are unpublished at the time of this writing, but results showing no differences between higher or lower PEEP levels are available (see Table 11-1).[61,62] In contrast, the study by Amato and colleagues[22] and the study by Villar and associates[63] reported differences in outcome. The Amato study, in an unselected population, also was characterized by large differences in tidal volume, making it more difficult to discriminate the effects of higher PEEP from the effects of lower tidal volume.[22] In contrast, the Villar study was performed in a *selected* group of ALI/ARDS patients: They were enrolled in the study after a 24-hour treatment period only if they still manifested severe ALI/ARDS criteria.[63] This led to a selection of patients with a more severe lung injury compared with previous studies. The data in this study suggest that the application of a higher PEEP level may be effective in selected patients with severe ARDS.

The putative beneficial effect of PEEP on survival is related to the prevention of excessive regional stress and strain by keeping open lung regions that would otherwise collapse.[26,64] It is tempting to speculate that PEEP is effective only in patients with extensive areas of the lungs collapsed. When we studied lung recruitability in an unselected ALI/ARDS population, we found that it varied from 0% to more than 50% of the whole lung.[47] We found that severity of lung injury was associated with higher lung recruitability and more severe hypoxemia, greater deadspace, and lower compliance of the respiratory system. By arbitrarily dividing the study population into patients with higher or lower lung recruitability, we first observed that in the latter, the amount of recruitable lung was almost negligible, amounting to about 50 g of tissue

Table 11-2. Summary of Available Evidence on the Effects of Higher PEEP in ALI/ARDS Patients

Study	Population	Group	No.	PEEP (cm H_2O)	Tidal Volume (mL/kg)	Plateau Pressure (cm H_2O)	Mortality (%)	*P* (Outcome)
Brower et al[60]	Unselected	Lower PEEP	273	8.9 ± 3.5 (first day)	6.1 ± 0.8 (first day)	24 ± 7 (first day)	24.9 (hospital discharge)	NS
		Higher PEEP	276	14.7 ± 3.5 (first day)	6 ± 0.9 (first day)	27 ± 6 (first day)	27.5 (hospital discharge)	
LOVS (unpublished data)*	Unselected	Control	983	9.4 ± 2.8	6	<30	40.4 (hospital discharge)	NS
		LOVS Group	983	13.5 ± 3.5	6	<40	36.4 (hospital discharge)	NS
ExPress (unpublished data)†	Unselected	Minimal distention	382	7.1 ± 1.8	6.1 ± 0.4	21.1 ± 4.7	31.2 (28 day)	NS
		Maximal recruitment	385	14.6 ± 3.2	6.1 ± 0.3	27.5 ± 2.4	27.8 (28 day)	NS
Villar et al[63]	Selected	Control	45	9 ± 2.7 (first day)	10.2 ± 1.2 (first day)	32.6 ± 6.2 (first day)	55.5 (hospital discharge)	.41
		P flex	50	14.1 ± 2.8 (first day)	7.3 ± 0.9 (first day)	30.6 ± 6 (first day)	34 (hospital discharge)	

*Comparison of two strategies for setting positive end-expiratory pressure in ALI/ARDs (ExPress Study).
†Canadian/Australian/Saudi Arabian Lung Open Ventilation Study (LOVS).
ALI/ARDS, acute lung injury/acute respiratory distress syndrome; NS, not significant; PEEP, positive end-expiratory pressure; P flex, lower inflection point of the pressure volume curve of the respiratory system.

weight. The response to the application of higher levels of PEEP was minimal and much lower than that observed in patients with higher lung recruitability. Based on these findings, we speculate that, in an unselected ALI/ARDS population, the random application of lower or higher PEEP is not associated with differences in survival because beneficial effects of higher PEEP in patients with greater lung recruitability are offset by negative effects in patients with lower lung recruitability in whom global alveolar stress and strain are increased. These observations may help to explain the results of Villar and associates[63] because the more severe patients (i.e., the patients enrolled in this study) represent a group with greater lung recruitability. Although further studies are necessary to prove this hypothesis, it is evident that a random application of higher or lower PEEP in an unselected population does not have any physiologic or clinical rationale.

Setting Respiratory Rate

Although extensive work has been devoted to understanding better how to set tidal volume and PEEP in ARDS, the potential importance of respiratory rate in the development of VILI has been scarcely investigated. Technology allows the use of respiratory rate from near zero breaths per minute using extracorporeal techniques to remove CO_2 to 2000 to 3000 breaths per minute, by employing high-frequency oscillation. Each tidal volume delivered may be considered as a stress cycle. Increasing the number of stress cycles may increase the lung damage. In experimental ARDS models, it has been observed that decreasing the respiratory rate decreases edema formation in isolated rabbit lung,[65] whereas an increase in respiratory rate, during spontaneous breathing, leads to an increase in edema formation.[66] It is conceivable that the respiratory rate may play a role in the pathogenesis of VILI when associated with a harmful tidal volume or inadequate PEEP. A different issue is the use of very high respiratory frequencies in association with very low tidal volumes and adequate PEEP. In experimental models, gas exchange functionality and respiratory mechanics were similar after a ventilation with frequencies equal to 15 breaths per minute, 120 breaths per minute, or 1000 breaths per minute.[67] The possible harmful role of respiratory frequency, at least in the range clinically employed (10 to 45 breaths per minute), is at the moment only putative. In the presence of stress or strain, however, the greater the breaths per minute, one can assume the greater the lung injury.

Setting Inspiratory-to-Expiratory Ratio

Mechanical ventilators provide a wide range of inspiratory-to-expiratory (I:E) ratios. Setting an adequate I:E ratio may be of great importance when ventilating patients with structural alterations of lung parenchyma, such as chronic obstructive pulmonary disease and emphysema, and during asthmatic exacerbation. In these conditions characterized by a time constant of the respiratory system greater than normal, a longer expiratory time must be provided to allow deflation of gas from the lungs before the next respiratory cycle, avoiding dynamic hyperinflation and intrinsic PEEP.[68] During ALI/ARDS, no convincing evidence has been provided for the advantages of setting a I:E ratio different from 1:1.

In the past, inverse ratio ventilation[69] was advocated as a tool to improve the effects of mechanical ventilation in ARDS.[70-72] Studies primarily showed an improvement of arterial oxygenation. Increased mean airway pressure, intrinsic PEEP, and a decrease in cardiac output were problematic.[73] Extreme forms of manipulating I:E ratio are not recommended; an I:E ratio in ALI/ARDS of 0.5 to 1.5 is appropriate.

INDIVIDUALIZING MECHANICAL VENTILATION IN PATIENTS WITH ACUTE RESPIRATORY DISTRESS SYNDROME

General principles underlying the application of mechanical ventilation in ALI/ARDS patients have been discussed. We now present the sequence of interventions that we believe are most appropriate for tailoring mechanical ventilation in an individual patient.[74]

The first intervention after admission to the ICU is to determine whether the patient has the criteria for ARDS diagnosis, keeping in mind that this syndrome consists of diffuse inflammatory lung edema. Patient history (research for possible etiology leading to ARDS) and clinical observation (cyanosis, higher respiratory rate, use of accessory respiratory muscles, inspiratory crackles at lung auscultation mainly in the dependent lung regions) may suggest a possible lung inflammatory edema. Blood gas analysis and chest x-rays may confirm the initial diagnosis of the syndrome. The choice between an attempt of noninvasive respiratory support (facemask continuous positive airway pressure or noninvasive ventilation) or endotracheal intubation should be made on a clinical basis, according to the severity of illness, and whether the patient is stable or deteriorating. We pay particular attention to the improvement of Pa_{O_2} after oxygen administration and to Pa_{CO_2}. The lack of remarkable response in oxygenation to increased F_{IO_2} indicates a remarkable fraction of right-to-left intrapulmonary shunt, which is typical of ARDS. Low Pa_{CO_2} suggests that the respiratory muscles of the patient are still able to deal with the decreased compliance of the respiratory system (i.e., sustaining the increased respiratory effort), whereas normal or high levels of Pa_{CO_2} suggest a near exhaustion of the respiratory muscles and need of immediate ventilatory support.

Clinicians should be aware of the immediate possible consequences of intubation and initiation of mechanical ventilation. Sedation, either by itself or in association with muscle paralysis, produces a loss of respiratory muscle tone and a cranial shift of the diaphragm, promoting further lung collapse with immediate consequences in gas exchange. Mechanical ventilation produces an increase in intrathoracic pressure and decreased venous return. The intravascular volume status of the patient should be assessed before intubation, and hypovolemia should be corrected. The rate and the amount of fluid replacement should be decided for each individual patient. Inadequate fluid replacement may lead to a severe hemodynamic impairment immediately after beginning positive-pressure ventilation. An excessive fluid replacement in an inflamed lung with leaking capillaries may result in a dramatic increase of pulmonary edema with devastating consequences on gas exchange. For these reasons, we prefer to tailor fluid replacement according to the results of a fluid challenge test. Echocardiography also may be helpful in assessing the volumetric status.[75]

After endotracheal intubation, the initial ventilatory setting employed is blind because the pathophysiologic characteristics of the patient have not yet been assessed. We usually set the ventilator (volume controlled) with a tidal volume equal to 6 to 8 mL/kg ideal body weight, F_{IO_2} equal to 0.7, and a respiratory rate of 15 breaths per minute, with an I : E ratio of 1 : 1. As soon as hemodynamic stability is obtained, a PEEP trial (preceded by a recruitment maneuver) is performed by applying in a random sequence of 5 to 15 cm H_2O PEEP with the patient under sedation and, sometimes, muscle paralysis. At each level of PEEP, we maintain tidal volume, respiratory rate, F_{IO_2}, and I : E ratio constant for about 20 minutes, after which we measure (1) arterial oxygenation, (2) respiratory system compliance, and (3) alveolar deadspace. Patients who, after the application of higher PEEP, improve at least two of these three parameters have a greater likelihood of having a higher lung recruitability. Alternatively, it is possible to target a specific saturation on the basis of pulse oximetry, if available, aiming at a hemoglobin oxygen saturation of 90%.

The improvement in arterial oxygenation alone, although commonly employed, may be misleading for the assessment of lung recruitment because it may be the result of a slight decrease in cardiac output or a modification of regional distribution of pulmonary blood flow or both. It has been shown that improvement in respiratory physiologic variables from a PEEP trial has low sensitivity (71%) and specificity (59%) in assessing lung recruitability[47]; we prefer to obtain whole lung CT scanning. In the CT scan facility, while maintaining the baseline ventilator setting, whole lung CT scanning is performed at 5 cm H_2O PEEP at end expiration and 45 cm H_2O at end inspiration. The subsequent quantitative analysis of the CT scans allows us to obtain a precise assessment of lung recruitability. In patients with higher recruitability we apply PEEP greater than 15 cm H_2O, up to 20 cm H_2O and exceptionally greater than 20 but not exceeding 25 cm H_2O, whereas in patients with lower lung recruitability we apply a PEEP level not greater than 10 cm H_2O.

If CT scan is unavailable, and only the PEEP trial has been performed, we assign to the high-recruitment group patients with either a baseline Pa_{O_2}/F_{IO_2} less than 150 when measured at 5 cm H_2O PEEP or patients who respond to 15 cm H_2O PEEP compared with 5 cm H_2O with a positive response of two of the following three variables: increased Pa_{O_2}, decreased alveolar deadspace, or increased compliance of the respiratory system.

We attempt to keep the plateau pressure less than 30 cm H_2O by modifying tidal volume and respiratory rate. As discussed earlier, however, tidal volume and plateau pressure are inadequate surrogates for alveolar stress and strain. We now measure, in each severe ARDS patient, the transpulmonary pressure by helium dilution technique, by employing an esophageal balloon (lung resting volume of 0 cm H_2O or 5 cm H_2O PEEP). With mechanical ventilation, a global pulmonary strain greater than about 1.8 (strain is dimensionless because it is the ratio of two volumes), or an end inspiratory transpulmonary pressure greater than 25 cm H_2O, may cause VILI, with irreversible respiratory failure to follow.[11,29] These values of alveolar stress and strain are the ones at which the residual ventilatable lung reaches its near-total lung capacity, with a full extension of the collagen fibers of the lung skeleton.

In some patients, we have observed that a tidal volume of 8 to 10 mL/kg per ideal body weight determines a lung strain value less than 1 and a transpulmonary pressure value less than 14 cm H_2O. In these patients, we employ a tidal volume greater than 6 mL/kg per ideal body weight, avoiding excessive hypercapnia or need for sedation. In contrast, in the most severe patients, in which the baby lung is extremely small, even a ventilation with 6 mL/kg ideal body weight may result in values of alveolar stress and strain higher than those required to reach total lung capacity. Evidence from the literature and physiologic reasoning strongly indicate that for these patients a safe form of mechanical ventilation does not exist.[76] We reserve to them the use of extracorporeal support. We acknowledge that measuring alveolar stress and strain may seem to be a physiologic curiosity or a research tool. Nonetheless, we have introduced them in our clinical practice as the most logical approach for VILI prevention.

Some authors advocate the use of different forms of mechanical ventilation in patients with ARDS, such as high-frequency ventilatory oscillation[77] or an early application of pressure support ventilation.[78,79] The rationale of the latter proposal relies on the possibility of decreasing the need for sedation, preserving the contribution of spontaneous breathing, with possible advantages on gas and flow pulmonary distribution. During the full-blown phase of the illness, we prefer to keep the patient well sedated. This approach may help to reduce energy requirement and oxygen consumption and CO_2 production.

The onset of recovery is characterized by the control or reversal, or both, of the cause of ARDS. An increase of systemic oxygenation and respiratory system compliance follows. When a Pa_{O_2} value greater than 80 mm Hg is obtained at F_{IO_2} of 0.4, we start the weaning from PEEP application, decreasing the PEEP level no more than 1 cm H_2O every 4 to 6 hours, and suspending the process if the oxygenation consistently deteriorates. Subsequently, after an appropriate adjustment of sedation, we shift from pressure-controlled or volume-controlled to pressure-support ventilation, initially setting the support at the same inspiratory pressure used during controlled ventilation. According to the patient's response, pressure-support level is progressively decreased, and the final phase of weaning is initiated at pressure support of 5 to 10 cm H_2O, F_{IO_2} lower than 0.4, and PEEP level equal to 5 cm H_2O.

POSSIBLE ADJUNCTS TO MECHANICAL VENTILATION

Prone Position

Prone positioning, first proposed in 1974[80] and first applied in ARDS patients in 1976,[81] results in improved arterial oxygenation in most patients. After the introduction of CT scanning, showing lung consolidation located in the dependent lung regions and the aerated baby lung in the nondependent lung regions,[12,16] we integrated prone positioning as standard practice in clinical treatment of ARDS patients to improve systemic oxygenation.[82] The initial hypothesis was that better perfusion of the baby lung, located in the dependent lung regions after prone positioning, would provide advantages in gas exchange. The picture observed was quite different, however. We did observe an improvement in arterial oxygenation, but the mechanism was likely different because CT scans taken in the prone position showed a density redistribution toward the dependent lung areas.[83]

This observation led to our introduction of the "sponge model" as our pathophysiologic understanding of ARDS.[84] Whatever the position of the patient, the increased weight of the nondependent lung tissue squeezes the gas out of the dependent regions of the lung.[42] The mechanisms of improved gas exchange were different from that first hypothesized. It is not the aim of this chapter to discuss the possible physiologic mechanisms of prone positioning, which may be found elsewhere.[85-89] Taken together, all of the studies, including small and large series of patients, consistently showed that in 70% of the patients systemic oxygenation improves in prone compared with supine positioning,[89,90] without any change in the applied airway pressure. There is no doubt that in life-threatening severe hypoxemia a trial in the prone position is indicated.

A different issue is the effectiveness of the prone position in improving ARDS outcome. Is mechanical ventilation in ARDS less harmful in the prone compared with the supine position? Does mechanical ventilation induce less alveolar stress and strain in the prone position? There is a consistent physiologic rationale to believe that this is the case. In experimental settings[91-94] and in normal subjects and patients affected by ARDS, CT scan shows a more homogeneous distribution of gas throughout the lung parenchyma in the prone compared with the supine position.[89] This observation strongly suggests that the distribution of alveolar stress and strain is more homogeneous in the prone position. In experimental models of ARDS, there is evidence that prone positioning prevents or significantly delays the development of VILI.[94,95] Two large randomized studies on prone positioning were unable to show a significant benefit on outcome[88,96]; however, prone positioning was applied for only about a quarter of the day, and mechanical ventilation was not controlled. In a more recent trial,[97] in which prone positioning was applied for 20 hours per day and mechanical ventilation was strictly controlled, a positive benefit was found for the patients treated with prone positioning. We believe that prone positioning is not harmful and should be used in patients with moderate to severe ARDS and no contraindication to use, such as spinal fractures and hemodynamic instability (see Suter et al[8] for reference).

Extracorporeal Support

Extracorporeal support of ARDS was first applied in 1972.[98] The first randomized trial ever performed in ALI/ARDS showed that patients treated with extracorporeal support or with conventional ventilation had similar mortality, equal to about 90%.[99] In the 1980s, our center introduced extracorporeal CO_2 removal in ARDS, aiming at lung rest with a suggestion of benefit.[100,101] A randomized study performed in 1994 did not show any survival benefit with extracorporeal CO_2 removal support.[102] The results of this trial may have been significantly influenced by bleeding complications in patients undergoing extracorporeal CO_2 removal.

This technology has since been greatly improved, and there are increasing numbers of reports describing simple forms of extracorporeal support, primarily aiming at CO_2 removal.[103] The problem of alveolar stress and strain is mainly associated with the need of ventilation, which may be greatly reduced by extracorporeal supports. Extracorporeal techniques should be applied only in experienced institutions and should be reserved for patients for whom a "safe" mechanical ventilation does not exist. With greater experience and more sophisticated technology, the indications for extracorporeal support may be enlarged, and this approach might be employed with the same simplicity we have in the application of continuous venovenous hemofiltration for renal support.

Ultrasonography also may be of potential benefit in assessing the volumetric status. In general, during the clinical course, a conservative strategy of fluid management is preferable compared with a liberal fluid strategy because it has been convincingly shown that a conservative fluid strategy may be advantageous in reaching better oxygenation parameters and in decreasing the length of stay in the ICU.[104]

KEY POINTS

- The targets of mechanical ventilation in ARDS have shifted from providing normal gas exchange to protecting the lung from VILI.
- Mechanical ventilation replaces the action of the respiratory muscles. The driving force of mechanical ventilation (airway pressure displayed on the ventilator) is spent partly to overcome the resistances to flow, partly to inflate the lung and partly to inflate the chest wall.
- The distending force of the lung (the trigger of VILI) is the transpulmonary pressure (P_L)—the difference between the airway pressure (P_{aw}) and the pleural pressure. For the same driving force, in normal conditions, the transpulmonary pressure equals the

driving force multiplied by the ratio between the lung elastance and the respiratory system elastance (lung elastance + chest wall elastance): $P_L = P_{aw} \times E_L/E_{TOT}$. In normal subjects, this ratio is approximately 0.5; in ALI/ARDS patients, it may be 0.2 to 0.8. Consequently, the airway pressure alone may be misleading to assess the transpulmonary pressure imposed on the lung by mechanical ventilation (i.e., to assess the stress). We used airway pressure to indicate end inspiratory pressure.

- The delivered tidal volume increases the lung volume and in the process produces strain on the lung. The ratio of change in lung volume over resting lung volume ($\Delta V/V_0$) is a rough approximation of the strain. Excessive strain causes shape changes of endothelial and epithelial cells inducing an inflammatory reaction. Because the resting volume (V_0, the baby lung) may vary largely in ARDS, the same tidal volume per ideal body weight may induce largely different strain values.
- Stress and strain, the triggers of VILI, are linked by a constant, specific lung elastance (E_{spec}), accounting for the following relationship: P_L (stress) = $E_{spec} * \Delta V/V_0$ (strain). The specific lung elastance is similar in normal subjects and in ARDS patients.
- Physiologic variables are generally poor indicators of the severity of lung injury, with the alveolar deadspace being the only variable associated with outcome. The severity of lung injury may be assessed by CT scan. The fraction of nonaerated lung tissue is strongly associated with mortality. The greater the lung injury, the smaller the baby lung, and the greater the stress-strain induced by mechanical ventilation.
- Among outcome studies testing different tidal volumes, only the study comparing the two extreme values tested (6 mL/kg versus 12 mL/kg) showed a significant benefit of lower tidal volume. Data from clinical studies and rationale from physiologic studies are strongly in favor of using the lowest tidal volume possible, likely associated with lower stress and strain, accepting hypercapnia as a side effect.
- All studies comparing lower versus higher PEEP randomly applied to *unselected* ARDS populations failed to show benefits on survival. In contrast, benefits of higher PEEP were found in more severe *selected* ARDS patients.
- The lung recruitability may vary greatly within the ALI/ARDS population (5% to 50% of the lung parenchyma) and is correlated with the overall lung injury severity. Higher PEEP possibly should be reserved only for patients with higher recruitability.
- When treating patients with ALI/ARDS, individual characteristics (lung injury severity, gas exchange, lung mechanics, abdominal pressure) should be assessed to tailor the least harmful mechanical ventilation according to the available evidence and physiologic rationale, providing the lowest stress and strain possible.

REFERENCES

1. Ashbaugh DG, Bigelow DB, Petty TL, et al: Acute respiratory distress in adults. Lancet 1967;2:319-323.
2. Bernard GR: Acute respiratory distress syndrome: A historical perspective. Am J Respir Crit Care Med 2005;172:798-806.
3. Ware LB, Matthay MA: The acute respiratory distress syndrome. N Engl J Med 2000;342:1334-1349.
4. Pontoppidan H, Geffin B, Lowenstein E: Acute respiratory failure in the adult, 3. N Engl J Med 1972;287:799-806.
5. Webb HH, Tierney DF: Experimental pulmonary edema due to intermittent positive pressure ventilation with high inflation pressures: Protection by positive end-expiratory pressure. Am Rev Respir Dis 1974;110:556-565.
6. Kumar A, Falke KJ, Geffin B, et al: Continuous positive-pressure ventilation in acute respiratory failure. N Engl J Med 1970;283:1430-1436.
7. Baeza OR, Wagner RB, Lowery BD: Pulmonary hyperinflation: A form of barotrauma during mechanical ventilation. J Thorac Cardiovasc Surg 1975;70:790-805.
8. Suter PM, Fairley B, Isenberg MD: Optimum end-expiratory airway pressure in patients with acute pulmonary failure. N Engl J Med 1975;292:284-289.
9. Dreyfuss D, Basset G, Soler P, et al: Intermittent positive-pressure hyperventilation with high inflation pressures produces pulmonary microvascular injury in rats. Am Rev Respir Dis 1985;132:880-884.
10. Dreyfuss D, Soler P, Basset G, et al: High inflation pressure pulmonary edema: Respective effects of high airway pressure, high tidal volume, and positive end-expiratory pressure. Am Rev Respir Dis 1988;137:1159-1164.
11. Dreyfuss D, Saumon G: Ventilator-induced lung injury: Lessons from experimental studies. Am J Respir Crit Care Med 1998;157:294-323.
12. Gattinoni L, Mascheroni D, Torresin A, et al: Morphological response to positive end expiratory pressure in acute respiratory failure: Computerized tomography study. Intensive Care Med 1986;12:137-142.
13. Maunder RJ, Shuman WP, McHugh JW, et al: Preservation of normal lung regions in the adult respiratory distress syndrome: Analysis by computed tomography. JAMA 1986;255:2463-2465.
14. Gattinoni L, Pesenti A, Avalli L, et al: Pressure-volume curve of total respiratory system in acute respiratory failure: Computed tomographic scan study. Am Rev Respir Dis 1987;136:730-736.
15. Gattinoni L, Pesenti A: ARDS: The non-homogeneous lung; facts and hypothesis. Intensive Crit Care Digest 1987;6:1-4.
16. Gattinoni L, Pesenti A: The concept of "baby lung." Intensive Care Med 2005;31:776-784.
17. Kolobow T, Gattinoni L, Tomlinson TA, et al: Control of breathing using an extracorporeal membrane lung. Anesthesiology 1977;46:138-141.
18. Kolobow T, Gattinoni L, Tomlinson T, et al: An alternative to breathing. J Thorac Cardiovasc Surg 1978;75:261-266.
19. Gattinoni L, Kolobow T, Tomlinson T, et al: Control of intermittent positive pressure breathing (IPPB) by extracorporeal removal of carbon dioxide. Br J Anaesth 1978;50:753-758.
20. Hickling KG, Henderson SJ, Jackson R: Low mortality associated with low volume pressure limited ventilation with permissive hypercapnia in severe adult respiratory distress syndrome. Intensive Care Med 1990;16:372-377.
21. Stewart TE, Meade MO, Cook DJ, et al: Evaluation of a ventilation strategy to prevent barotrauma in patients at high risk for acute respiratory distress syndrome. Pressure- and Volume-Limited Ventilation Strategy Group. N Engl J Med 1998;338:355-361.
22. Amato MB, Barbas CS, Medeiros DM, et al: Effect of a protective-ventilation strategy on mortality in the acute respiratory distress syndrome. N Engl J Med 1998;338:347-354.
23. Brochard L, Roudot-Thoraval F, Roupie E, et al: Tidal volume reduction for prevention of ventilator-induced lung injury in acute respiratory distress syndrome. The Multicenter Trial Group on Tidal Volume Reduction in ARDS.

Am J Respir Crit Care Med 1998;158:1831-1838.

24. Brower RG, Shanholtz CB, Fessler HE, et al: Prospective, randomized, controlled clinical trial comparing traditional versus reduced tidal volume ventilation in acute respiratory distress syndrome patients. Crit Care Med 1999;27:1492-1498.
25. Ventilation with lower tidal volumes as compared with traditional tidal volumes for acute lung injury and the acute respiratory distress syndrome. The Acute Respiratory Distress Syndrome Network. N Engl J Med 2000;342:1301-1308.
26. Lachmann B: Open up the lung and keep the lung open. Intensive Care Med 1992;18:319-321.
27. Tremblay L, Valenza F, Ribeiro SP, et al: Injurious ventilatory strategies increase cytokines and c-fos m-RNA expression in an isolated rat lung model. J Clin Invest 1997;99:944-952.
28. Tremblay LN, Slutsky AS: Ventilator-induced lung injury: From the bench to the bedside. Intensive Care Med 2006;32:24-33.
29. Gattinoni L, Carlesso E, Cadringher P, et al: Physical and biological triggers of ventilator-induced lung injury and its prevention. Eur Respir J Suppl 2003;47:15s-25s.
30. Aliverti A, Dellaca R, Pelosi P, et al: Optoelectronic plethysmography in intensive care patients. Am J Respir Crit Care Med 2000;161:1546-1552.
31. Weibel ER: Functional morphology of lung parenchyma. In American Psychological Society (ed): Handbook of Physiology: A Critical, Comprehensive Presentation of Physiological Knowledge and Concepts. Baltimore, Waverly Press, 1986, pp 83-111.
32. Maksym GN, Bates JH: A distributed nonlinear model of lung tissue elasticity. J Appl Physiol 1997;82: 32-41.
33. Maksym GN, Fredberg JJ, Bates JH: Force heterogeneity in a two-dimensional network model of lung tissue elasticity. J Appl Physiol 1998;85:1223-1229.
34. Souza-Fernandes AB, Pelosi P, Rocco PR: Bench-to-bedside review: The role of glycosaminoglycans in respiratory disease. Crit Care 2006;10:237.
35. Dos Santos CC, Slutsky AS: Invited review: Mechanisms of ventilator-induced lung injury: A perspective. J Appl Physiol 2000;89:1645-1655.
36. Haseneen NA, Vaday GG, Zucker S, et al: Mechanical stretch induces MMP-2 release and activation in lung endothelium: Role of EMMPRIN. Am J Physiol Lung Cell Mol Physiol 2003;284:L541-L547.
37. Caironi P, Ichinose F, Liu R, et al: 5-Lipoxygenase deficiency prevents respiratory failure during ventilator-induced lung injury. Am J Respir Crit Care Med 2005;172:334-343.
38. Pugin J, Dunn I, Jolliet P, et al: Activation of human macrophages by mechanical ventilation in vitro. Am J Physiol 1998;275:L1040-L1050.
39. Yamamoto H, Teramoto H, Uetani K, et al: Cyclic stretch upregulates interleukin-8 and transforming growth factor-beta1 production through a protein kinase C-dependent pathway in alveolar epithelial cells. Respirology 2002;7:103-109.
40. Vlahakis NE, Schroeder MA, Limper AH, et al: Stretch induces cytokine release by alveolar epithelial cells in vitro. Am J Physiol 1999;277: L167-L173.
41. Belperio JA, Keane MP, Burdick MD, et al: Critical role for CXCR2 and CXCR2 ligands during the pathogenesis of ventilator-induced lung injury. J Clin Invest 2002;110:1703-1716.
42. Gattinoni L, D'Andrea L, Pelosi P, et al: Regional effects and mechanism of positive end-expiratory pressure in early adult respiratory distress syndrome. JAMA 1993;269: 2122-2127.
43. Riley RL, Cournand A: "Ideal" alveolar air and the analysis of ventilation-perfusion relationships in the lungs. J Appl Physiol 1949;1:827-847.
44. Bernard GR, Artigas A, Brigham KL, et al: The American-European Consensus Conference on ARDS. Definitions, mechanisms, relevant outcomes, and clinical trial coordination. Am J Respir Crit Care Med 1994;149:818-824.
45. Luhr OR, Karlsson M, Thorsteinsson A, et al: The impact of respiratory variables on mortality in non-ARDS and ARDS patients requiring mechanical ventilation. Intensive Care Med 2000;26:508-517.
46. Gattinoni L, Bombino M, Pelosi P, et al: Lung structure and function in different stages of severe adult respiratory distress syndrome. JAMA 1994;271:1772-1779.
47. Gattinoni L, Caironi P, Cressoni M, et al: Lung recruitment in patients with the acute respiratory distress syndrome. N Engl J Med 2006;354:1775-1786.
48. Dantzker DR, Brook CJ, Dehart P, et al: Ventilation-perfusion distributions in the adult respiratory distress syndrome. Am Rev Respir Dis 1979;120:1039-1052.
49. Dantzker DR, Lynch JP, Weg JG: Depression of cardiac output is a mechanism of shunt reduction in the therapy of acute respiratory failure. Chest 1980;77:636-642.
50. Matamis D, Lemaire F, Harf A, et al: Redistribution of pulmonary blood flow induced by positive end-expiratory pressure and dopamine infusion in acute respiratory failure. Am Rev Respir Dis 1984;129:39-44.
51. Nuckton TJ, Alonso JA, Kallet RH, et al: Pulmonary dead-space fraction as a risk factor for death in the acute respiratory distress syndrome. N Engl J Med 2002;346:1281-1286.
52. Gattinoni L, Vagginelli F, Carlesso E, et al: Decrease in $PaCO_2$ with prone position is predictive of improved outcome in acute respiratory distress syndrome. Crit Care Med 2003;31: 2727-2733.
53. Gattinoni L, Pesenti A, Baglioni S, et al: Inflammatory pulmonary edema and positive end-expiratory pressure: Correlations between imaging and physiologic studies. J Thorac Imaging 1988;3:59-64.
54. Henzler D, Pelosi P, Dembinski R, et al: Respiratory compliance but not gas exchange correlates with changes in lung aeration after a recruitment maneuver: An experimental study in pigs with saline lavage lung injury. Crit Care 2005;9:R471-R482.
55. Malbrain ML, Chiumello D, Pelosi P, et al: Prevalence of intra-abdominal hypertension in critically ill patients: A multicentre epidemiological study. Intensive Care Med 2004;30:822-829.
56. Gattinoni L, Pelosi P, Suter PM, et al: Acute respiratory distress syndrome caused by pulmonary and extrapulmonary disease: Different syndromes? Am J Respir Crit Care Med 1998;158:3-11.
57. Pelosi P, Croci M, Ravagnan I, et al: Total respiratory system, lung, and chest wall mechanics in sedated-paralyzed postoperative morbidly obese patients. Chest 1996;109: 144-151.
58. Tobin MJ: Culmination of an era in research on the acute respiratory distress syndrome. N Engl J Med 2000;342:1360-1361.
59. Hager DN, Krishnan JA, Hayden DL, et al: Tidal volume reduction in patients with acute lung injury when plateau pressures are not high. Am J Respir Crit Care Med 2005;172:1241-1245.
60. Brower RG, Lanken PN, MacIntyre N, et al: Higher versus lower positive end-expiratory pressures in patients with the acute respiratory distress syndrome. N Engl J Med 2004;351:327-336.
61. Meade MO, Cook DJ, Arabi Y, et al: A multinational RCT of lung open ventilation strategy in ALI/ARDS—preliminary results. Am J Respir Crit Care Med 2007;175(abstract issue): A507.
62. Mercat A, Richard SC, Brochard L, et al: Comparison of two strategies for setting PEEP in ALI/ARDS (ExPress Study). Am J Respir Crit Care Med 2007;175(abstract issue):A507.
63. Villar J, Kacmarek RM, Perez-Mendez L, et al: A high positive end-expiratory pressure, low tidal volume ventilatory strategy improves outcome in persistent acute respiratory distress syndrome: A randomized, controlled trial. Crit Care Med 2006;34: 1311-1318.
64. Mead J, Takishima T, Leith D: Stress distribution in lungs: A model of pulmonary elasticity. J Appl Physiol 1970;28:596-608.
65. Hotchkiss JR Jr, Blanch L, Murias G, et al: Effects of decreased respiratory frequency on ventilator-induced lung injury. Am J Respir Crit Care Med 2000;161:463-468.
66. Mascheroni D, Kolobow T, Fumagalli R, et al: Acute respiratory failure following pharmacologically induced hyperventilation: An experimental animal study. Intensive Care Med 1988;15:8-14.
67. Sedeek KA, Takeuchi M, Suchodolski K, et al: Open-lung protective ventilation with pressure control ventilation, high-frequency oscillation, and intratracheal pulmonary ventilation results in similar gas exchange, hemodynamics, and lung mechanics. Anesthesiology 2003;99:1102-1111.

68. Pepe PE, Marini JJ: Occult positive end-expiratory pressure in mechanically ventilated patients with airflow obstruction: The auto-PEEP effect. Am Rev Respir Dis 1982;126:166-170.
69. Lachmann B, Haendly B, Schulz H, et al: Improved arterial oxygenation, CO_2 elimination, compliance and decreased barotrauma following changes of volume generated PEEP ventilation with inspiratory/expiratory (I/E) ratio of 1/2 to pressure generated ventilation with I/E ratio of 4:1 in patients with severe adult respiratory distress syndrome (ARDS). Intensive Care Med 1980;6:64.
70. Lessard MR, Guerot E, Lorino H, et al: Effects of pressure-controlled with different I:E ratios versus volume-controlled ventilation on respiratory mechanics, gas exchange, and hemodynamics in patients with adult respiratory distress syndrome. Anesthesiology 1994;80:983-991.
71. Mercat A, Titiriga M, Anguel N, et al: Inverse ratio ventilation (I/E = 2/1) in acute respiratory distress syndrome: A six-hour controlled study. Am J Respir Crit Care Med 1997;155:1637-1642.
72. Zavala E, Ferrer M, Polese G, et al: Effect of inverse I:E ratio ventilation on pulmonary gas exchange in acute respiratory distress syndrome. Anesthesiology 1998;88:35-42.
73. Mang H, Kacmarek RM, Ritz R, et al: Cardiorespiratory effects of volume- and pressure-controlled ventilation at various I/E ratios in an acute lung injury model. Am J Respir Crit Care Med 1995;151:731-736.
74. Marini JJ, Gattinoni L: Ventilatory management of acute respiratory distress syndrome: A consensus of two. Crit Care Med 2004;32:250-255.
75. Vignon P: Hemodynamic assessment of critically ill patients using echocardiography Doppler. Curr Opin Crit Care 2005;11:227-234.
76. Terragni PP, Rosboch G, Tealdi A, et al: Tidal hyperinflation during low tidal volume ventilation in acute respiratory distress syndrome. Am J Respir Crit Care Med 2007;175:160-166.
77. Rimensberger PC: Allowing for spontaneous breathing during high-frequency oscillation: The key for final success? Crit Care 2006;10:155.
78. Cereda M, Foti G, Marcora B, et al: Pressure support ventilation in patients with acute lung injury. Crit Care Med 2000;28:1269-1275.
79. Henzler D, Pelosi P, Bensberg R, et al: Effects of partial ventilatory support modalities on respiratory function in severe hypoxemic lung injury. Crit Care Med 2006;34:1738-1745.
80. Bryan AC: Conference on the scientific basis of respiratory therapy: Pulmonary physiotherapy in the pediatric age group: Comments of a devil's advocate. Am Rev Respir Dis 1974;110:143-144.
81. Piehl MA, Brown RS: Use of extreme position changes in acute respiratory failure. Crit Care Med 1976;4:13-14.
82. Langer M, Mascheroni D, Marcolin R, et al: The prone position in ARDS patients: A clinical study. Chest 1988;94:103-107.
83. Gattinoni L, Pelosi P, Vitale G, et al: Body position changes redistribute lung computed-tomographic density in patients with acute respiratory failure. Anesthesiology 1991;74:15-23.
84. Bone RC: The ARDS lung: New insights from computed tomography. JAMA 1993;269:2134-2135.
85. Lamm WJ, Graham MM, Albert RK: Mechanism by which the prone position improves oxygenation in acute lung injury. Am J Respir Crit Care Med 1994;150:184-193.
86. Lee DL, Chiang HT, Lin SL, et al: Prone-position ventilation induces sustained improvement in oxygenation in patients with acute respiratory distress syndrome who have a large shunt. Crit Care Med 2002;30: 1446-1452.
87. Pelosi P, Tubiolo D, Mascheroni D, et al: Effects of the prone position on respiratory mechanics and gas exchange during acute lung injury. Am J Respir Crit Care Med 1998;157:387-393.
88. Albert RK: Prone position in ARDS: What do we know, and what do we need to know? Crit Care Med 1999;27:2574-2575.
89. Gattinoni L, Valenza F, Pelosi P, et al: Prone positioning in acute respiratory failure. In Tobin MJ (eds): Principles and Practice of Mechanical Ventilation, 2nd ed. New York, McGraw-Hill, 2006, pp 1081-1092.
90. Gattinoni L, Tognoni G, Pesenti A, et al: Effect of prone positioning on the survival of patients with acute respiratory failure. N Engl J Med 2001;345:568-573.
91. Du HL, Yamada Y, Orii R, et al: Beneficial effects of the prone position on the incidence of barotrauma in oleic acid-induced lung injury under continuous positive pressure ventilation. Acta Anaesthesiol.Scand 1997;41:701-707.
92. Nishimura M, Honda O, Tomiyama N, et al: Body position does not influence the location of ventilator-induced lung injury. Intensive Care Med 2000;26: 1664-1669.
93. Johansson MJ, Wiklund A, Flatebo T, et al: Positive end-expiratory pressure affects regional redistribution of ventilation differently in prone and supine sheep. Crit Care Med 2004;32:2039-2044.
94. Valenza F, Guglielmi M, Maffioletti M, et al: Prone position delays the progression of ventilator-induced lung injury in rats: Does lung strain distribution play a role? Crit Care Med 2005;33:361-367.
95. Broccard A, Shapiro RS, Schmitz LL, et al: Prone positioning attenuates and redistributes ventilator-induced lung injury in dogs. Crit Care Med 2000;28:295-303.
96. Guerin C, Gaillard S, Lemasson S, et al: Effects of systematic prone positioning in hypoxemic acute respiratory failure: A randomized controlled trial. JAMA 2004;292:2379-2387.
97. Mancebo J, Fernandez R, Blanch L, et al: A multicenter trial of prolonged prone ventilation in severe acute respiratory distress syndrome. Am J Respir Crit Care Med 2006;173: 1233-1239.
98. Hill JD, O'Brien TG, Murray JJ, et al: Prolonged extracorporeal oxygenation for acute post-traumatic respiratory failure (shock-lung syndrome): Use of the Bramson membrane lung. N Engl J Med 1972;286:629-634.
99. Zapol WM, Snider MT, Hill JD, et al: Extracorporeal membrane oxygenation in severe acute respiratory failure: A randomized prospective study. JAMA 1979;242:2193-2196.
100. Gattinoni L, Agostoni A, Pesenti A, et al: Treatment of acute respiratory failure with low-frequency positive-pressure ventilation and extracorporeal removal of CO_2. Lancet 1980;2: 292-294.
101. Gattinoni L, Pesenti A, Mascheroni D, et al: Low-frequency positive-pressure ventilation with extracorporeal CO_2 removal in severe acute respiratory failure. JAMA 1986;256:881-886.
102. Morris AH, Wallace CJ, Menlove RL, et al: Randomized clinical trial of pressure-controlled inverse ratio ventilation and extracorporeal CO_2 removal for adult respiratory distress syndrome. Am J Respir Crit Care Med 1994;149:295-305.
103. Bein T, Prasser C, Philipp A, et al: [Pumpless extracorporeal lung assist using arterio-venous shunt in severe ARDS: Experience with 30 cases]. Anaesthesist 2004;53:813-819.
104. ARDS Clinical Trials Network, Wiedemann HP, Wheeler AP, et al: Comparison of two fluid-management strategies in acute lung injury. N Engl J Med 2006;354:2564-2575.

Chapter 12

Bronchoscopy and Lung Biopsy in Critically Ill Patients

Thaddeus Bartter and Melvin R. Pratter

Bronchoscopy plays an important role in the care of critically ill patients. Since the introduction of the flexible fiberoptic bronchoscope in 1968, flexible bronchoscopy has slowly gained importance as a diagnostic and a therapeutic tool. It has largely replaced rigid bronchoscopy in the intensive care unit (ICU) because of the lack of need for complete anesthesia, the ease of use, and the fact that with a flexible bronchoscope one can perform procedures on a critically ill ventilated patient through an endotracheal tube or tracheostomy tube.

Lung biopsy is a procedure of last resort in a critically ill patient with lung disease not responding to therapy. Most such patients are on mechanical ventilation, and the potential benefits of biopsy need to outweigh the potential risks. Data have accumulated that show a reasonable benefit-to-risk ratio when this is the scenario.

This chapter reviews bronchoscopy and lung biopsy in critically ill patients. By definition, a critically ill patient has one or more organs that are under stress and have limited reserve. Stresses that are tolerated by less ill individuals might have serious sequelae for a patient in the ICU. This chapter reviews first the physiologic stresses induced by bronchoscopy. It then reviews specific diagnostic and therapeutic indications of bronchoscopy in the ICU, ending with a review of bronchoscopic and nonbronchoscopic approaches to lung biopsy.

PHYSIOLOGY OF BRONCHOSCOPY

Cannulation of the airway for any reason is not a physiologically neutral event. Changes occur in hemodynamics and in pulmonary function. Passage through the larynx results in about a 30% increase in mean arterial pressure and cardiac index, a 40% increase in heart rate, and an 86% increase in pulmonary arterial occlusion pressure in patients even after sedation and topical anesthesia with lidocaine.[1] The response seems to represent a reflex. A significant hemodynamic response occurs even when patients are anesthetized and paralyzed before tracheal cannulation, with conflicting data as to whether there is a difference in hemodynamic response between the nasal and the oral routes.[2,3] Topical lidocaine anesthesia of the upper airway attenuates (but does not ablate) the cardiovascular responses.[3,4]

Apart from the initial airway cannulation, the stimulus with the greatest cardiovascular response is suctioning; the profile is similar to that of airway entry.[1] The cardiovascular reflex responses are not unique to bronchoscopy. Intubation and suctioning of the airway through an endotracheal tube cause similar cardiovascular changes.[5]

The major significance of these cardiovascular changes with bronchoscopy lies in their impact on two end organs—the heart and the brain. The increase in rate pressure product has the potential to cause cardiac ischemia in patients with limited cardiac perfusion. In one careful physiologic study, 3 of 10 monitored patients, all of whom were 55 years old or older, developed electrocardiogram changes of ischemia.[5] In another study designed specifically to look at ischemia in older patients, the incidence of ischemia was 17%.[6] These impressively high numbers have not been associated with high rates of death owing to ischemic complications; in series of bronchoscopies ranging from 10 to 48,000 procedures, the rate of death from ischemic events ranged from 0% to approximately 0.01%.[5-11]

A second potential cardiac complication of bronchoscopy is the triggering of arrhythmias. A study looking specifically for arrhythmias during bronchoscopy found a high incidence of "major arrhythmias"—11%.[12] Similar to ischemia, however, large studies of complications of bronchoscopy have documented a 0.04% or less incidence of arrhythmias deemed serious, with related mortality in 0% to 0.04% of cases.[7,9]

With respect to the brain, bronchoscopy and endotracheal suctioning cause a significant increase in intracranial pressure.[5,13] Mean arterial pressure and intracerebral pressure increase roughly in parallel; there is little change in cerebral perfusion pressure.[5,13] This may mitigate the increase in intracerebral pressure, and no adverse intracerebral sequelae have been reported.[13] Close attention to intracerebral pressure in brain-injured individuals undergoing bronchoscopy is warranted, however.

Bronchoscopy changes work of breathing, pressures, and volumes within the lung. Transnasal cannulation of the trachea leads to a decrease in inspiratory and expiratory flow, a decrease in vital capacity, and an increase in functional residual capacity.[14] Bronchoscopy through an endotracheal tube in a sedated, but not ventilated patient leads to a significant further decrease in flows and vital capacity and a marked increase in the work of breathing.[14,15]

Bronchoscopy and Ventilated Patients

Bronchoscopy of patients on ventilators adds significant complexity to the physiologic sequelae of bronchoscopy. The details were elegantly explored by Lindholm and colleagues.[15] The first notable change is a dramatic increase in upper airway resistance. The airway narrowing of endotracheal tube insertion by itself introduces an increase in airway resistance, and the introduction of a bronchoscope through the endotracheal tube greatly increases that resistance, with specifics related to the area of the lumen of the endotracheal tube and the cross-sectional area of the bronchoscope being inserted.[15] The resulting pressure gradient has implications for ventilator gas delivery. With a volume-cycled mode, pressures escalate near the end of the inspiratory cycle. The set volume may not be delivered owing to a pressure pop-off set in the alarm/safety parameters of the ventilator. Although peak pressures of 60 to 80 cm H_2O could be reached, the pressure gradient limits the pressure delivered distal to the endotracheal tube.[15] With a pressure-cycled mode of mechanical ventilation, the volume delivered per breath decreases on bronchoscopic cannulation as a result of the increase in upper airway resistance, rather than a pressure pop-off, with degree of decrease related to endotracheal tube lumen and bronchoscope cross-sectional area.

The upper airway narrowing caused by introduction of the bronchoscope also causes expiratory airflow resistance. Sequential delivered volumes are incompletely exhaled (the major driving force being the passive recoil of the lungs), and there is a slow buildup of intrathoracic volume and positive end-expiratory pressure (PEEP). Lindholm and colleagues[15] documented several cases of PEEP greater than 18 cm H_2O; one patient being bronchoscoped through an endotracheal tube with an internal diameter of 7 mm developed a PEEP of 35 cm H_2O.

Suctioning adds one more layer to the complexity. In addition to the hemodynamic changes stimulated by suctioning already mentioned, suctioning changes lung pressures and volumes. The PEEP induced during bronchoscopy can be eliminated, and with prolonged suctioning, a negative intratracheal pressure can be created.[15] This can lead to significant decreases in functional residual capacity, tidal volume, and minute ventilation, with a potential for alveolar collapse, hypercarbia, and hypoxemia.

Hypoxemia

That bronchoscopy can cause hypoxemia is not questioned, but the degree of hypoxemia and the mechanisms responsible have been variably reported. The administration of benzodiazepines and narcotics can cause hypoxemia and respiratory depression in normal volunteers,[16] and one study showed a 35% incidence of desaturation after sedation and before bronchoscopy.[17] The desaturation may not be completely due to central nervous system depression; Chhajed and coworkers[18] showed that hypoxemia during bronchoscopy could be corrected in most of their lung transplant patients by the insertion of a nasopharyngeal tube, which illustrated in their population that upper airway collapse was a major cause of hypoxemia. Apart from the sedation given, the process of bronchoscopy itself also can cause hypoxemia, with suctioning and its impact on functional residual capacity probably a major factor.[19-22] Higher incidences of hypoxemia in some cases have been shown to correlate with degree of prebronchoscopy pulmonary impairment, suctioning, and bronchoalveolar lavage.[20-25] The hypoxemia induced by bronchoscopy does not resolve immediately on removal of the bronchoscope and sometimes can persist for more than 2 hours.[17,23,25] Hypoxemia could contribute to any organ impairment caused by the tachycardia and hypertension often associated with bronchoscopy; hypoxemia may play a contributory role in cardiac ischemia and arrhythmias associated with bronchoscopy.[1]

Bronchoscopy through the endotracheal tube of a patient on a ventilator has been reported to cause an increase in PAO_2 with an increase in PCO_2 and a decrease in PAO_2 with no change in PCO_2.[14,15] The seemingly contradictory differences in findings probably reflect differences in suctioning.

Summary

In summary, bronchoscopy almost always triggers a reflex response that includes tachycardia and an increase in blood pressure. Bronchoscopy frequently causes hypoxemia, which may be of prolonged duration. For patients on ventilators, disparate physiologies can be created based on the size of the endotracheal tube, the size of the bronchoscope, the duration of suctioning, and the flow rate that the suction channel of the bronchoscope is able to attain. Bronchoscopy can cause significant physiologic stress, and the critically ill patient may be less able to tolerate that stress than an otherwise healthy individual.

AIRWAY EVALUATION AND MANAGEMENT

Intubation and Endotracheal Tube Management

The flexible fiberoptic bronchoscope can be an asset in the insertion and management of endotracheal tubes.[26,27] For cases anticipated to be difficult, an endotracheal tube can be inserted over the bronchoscope and slid into the trachea after the bronchoscope has been guided into it. A similar technique can be used for changing the endotracheal tube in a tenuous patient, with a switch from nasal to oral or oral to nasal the simplest.[26] Bronchoscopy is valuable in the placement of tubes for single-lung ventilation or placement of double-lumen tubes.[27] Bronchoscopy also allows the bronchoscopist to place the tip of an endotracheal tube at a point approximately 2.5 cm above the carina under direct visualization or, when there is a process such as tumor compression of the trachea, to place the tube wherever it is needed for optimal ventilation.[26]

Percutaneous Dilational Tracheostomy

Percutaneous dilational tracheostomy (PDT) has emerged as a tracheostomy technique of value in ICU patients. It has a lower incidence of overall complications than does open surgical tracheostomy, and it can be performed at the bedside, avoiding the risks of transport of a critically ill patient.[28-30] It also is more cost-effective.[28] PDT can be performed not only by surgeons, but also by trained intensivists and pulmonologists; it has become a standard intensivist procedure in many institutions.[31,32] Although its overall safety profile is better than for open surgical tracheostomy, PDT does have a higher risk of posterior tracheal wall injury and false passage.[33] Bronchoscopy offers the opportunity for direct observation of the insertion and the tracheal walls and has been suggested by several authors to be a safety factor in the procedure,[30,33-38] although its use is not universally practiced.[32,39] Direct visualization is a protection against inadvertent tracheal injury and a means of assessing injury for intervention should injury occur.[33,35-38] The most logical approach to PDT is a team approach with at least two principal operators—one managing the bronchoscope and the endotracheal tube and the second working at the neck to insert the tracheostomy tube.[30,33,37] The risk of bronchoscopy during PDT is that of hypoventilation because the patient is being ventilated through the endotracheal tube during the procedure.[36] This can be obviated with the use of a pediatric bronchoscope for guidance; a large working channel is not needed for this application.

Airway Obstruction and Atelectasis

The upper airway can become obstructed for several reasons. Bronchoscopy is valuable in diagnosing all of them. When an endotracheal tube is inserted, it becomes part of the airway; kinking of the endotracheal tube or luminal blockage owing to hardened secretions causes the same physiologic problems as a primary tracheal process. Granulation tissue at the distal end of a tracheostomy tube can cause obstruction and difficulty with inflation or deflation of the lungs. (This is much less common with endotracheal tubes than with tracheostomy tubes because of Murphy's eye, the distal side port, on endotracheal tubes.) Benign or malignant processes can cause strictures or compression of the trachea. Finally, edema of the vocal cords and periglottic structures can lead to upper airway obstruction not evident with an endotracheal tube in place, but marked by repeated respiratory failure after extubation; extubation over a bronchoscope with evaluation of the upper airway as the endotracheal tube is withdrawn can lead to diagnosis of this problem.[26]

Foreign bodies can cause obstruction at various points in the airways. This is one diagnosis for which rigid bronchoscopy is the traditional tool, with its capacity for airway control and rapid passage of and removal of tools larger than the tools that can be used through a flexible bronchoscope.[40] Flexible bronchoscopes are the only choice, however, in an intubated patient, and the combination of larger channels (2.8 mm) for the passage of instruments and of different baskets and grasping tools makes flexible fiberoptic bronchoscopy a viable option in many cases.[27,40,41] A flexible bronchoscope through a rigid bronchoscope sometimes is an optimal approach.[40]

Atelectasis is a common ICU problem, and bronchoscopy for atelectasis has been one of the most common uses of bronchoscopy in ICUs.[42,43] The argument is obvious: if suctioning is routine and useful, why not use suctioning under visualization for local airway obstruction often due to secretions? One key study done by Marini and coworkers[44] challenged the assumption that bronchoscopy is an optimal approach to atelectasis. In their study of patients with atelectasis, a regimen of initial bronchoscopy followed by regular chest physiotherapy was given to one group, while a second group received regular chest physiotherapy alone followed by delayed bronchoscopy at 48 hours if atelectasis persisted. The authors showed no difference in rate or degree of improvement between the two groups and noted that bronchoscopy could lead to more significant decreases in oxygenation.[44] They also looked at the presence or absence of air bronchograms, postulating that patients with air bronchograms had more distal consolidation (as opposed to proximal obstruction causing atelectasis) and would be more refractory to any attempts to re-expand consolidated lung. Their results strongly supported their postulate.[44]

These data are valuable and should lead to initial trials of chest physiotherapy in most cases of atelectasis, but they do not apply universally in clinical medicine. Some patients with chest trauma or spinal cord injury are not candidates for chest physiotherapy.[45] Some patients have atelectasis and a severe refractory hypoxemia as a result of shunting of blood through the atelectatic lung. In these patients, a 24-hour wait may be inappropriate, and bronchoscopy sometimes leads to marked improvement. Judicious use of bronchoscopy for atelectasis is a clinical decision involving the art of medicine.[45] For patients who have a bronchoscope inserted for atelectasis, one technique that has been moderately successful is that of isolated segmental inflation; the bronchoscope or a ballooned catheter is wedged into the atelectatic segment, and pressure is applied through the bronchoscope or catheter at a pressure of at least 30 mm H_2O to open that specific segment.[43,45] This focal approach is more rational for focal atelectasis than recruitment maneuvers applied to the whole chest because such maneuvers are more likely to overdistend compliant alveoli than to open atelectatic ones.[43]

Trauma

The value of bronchoscopy for the evaluation of chest trauma was defined in a landmark paper by Hara and

Prakash.[46] The authors looked at 53 cases of blunt trauma to the chest or neck or both in which bronchoscopy was performed within 3 days of injury. Bronchoscopy was believed to be of clinical value in 53% of the 53 cases. They documented injury and tears of the upper and lower airways, contusion or hemorrhage, aspirated material, and plugging or secretions. Only one of eight major tracheal injuries was not completely diagnosed. The data are compelling evidence for visual bronchoscopic evaluation of the bronchial tree in all cases of significant blunt chest trauma.

Smoke Inhalation

Inhalation injury is an entirely different form of trauma to the bronchial tree. Most inhalation injuries are due not to heat alone, but to the deposition in the bronchial tree of soot, which is a vector for various products of combustion.[47] Early ventilatory support and aggressive pulmonary toilet probably improve outcomes for inhalation injury,[48,49] but the severity of inhalation injury may not become manifest for a maximum of 5 days (usually 3 days).[48] Bronchoscopy has been advocated in the evaluation of patients with possible inhalation injury.[48-50] Some patients have mucosal injuries obvious to even an inexperienced bronchoscopist, but in some patients with significant injury, the bronchoscopic appearance may be minimally abnormal. For patients who have relatively normal-looking mucosae, biopsy specimens of segmental or subsegmental carinae can yield pathologic information that is predictive of degree of inhalation injury (or lack thereof) and can be used to guide aggressiveness of management.[48,49] Another tool for evaluation of inhalation injury is the ventilation-perfusion scan,[47,50] but the objectivity and reproducibility of bronchoscopic endobronchial biopsy could lead one to argue that this is the new standard of care for the diagnosis of possible inhalation injury.

Hemoptysis

Hemoptysis can run the gamut from scant to massive. There are several definitions of massive hemoptysis with varying quantities of blood specified over different intervals. The best definition of massive hemoptysis is functional: Massive hemoptysis is hemoptysis in quantities that threaten to cause death by asphyxiation owing to filling of the bronchial tree with blood.[51,52] Patients with massive hemoptysis are admitted to the ICU.

Bronchoscopy plays two roles in massive hemoptysis—diagnostic and therapeutic. Most authors recommend bronchoscopy as soon as possible to localize the site of bleeding.[51-53] Rigid bronchoscopy and flexible bronchoscopy have their advocates. The argument for rigid bronchoscopy is that it allows better visualization of the major airways, more aggressive suctioning, removal of clots, and local tamponade with packing materials.[53,54] The argument for flexible bronchoscopy is that it does not require the operating room or general anesthesia, it allows more thorough evaluation of the bronchial tree, and it allows directed intubation.[52,53] Intubation may be with a regular endotracheal tube in the trachea or in the left lung or with a double-lumen tube. (The right upper lobe takeoff is too early in the right bronchial tree to allow selective right main bronchus intubation.) If bleeding is too great, flexible bronchoscopy is inhibited because of the small lens, which must remain clear for guidance to be possible.[52] For massive hemoptysis, the goals of bronchoscopy are to identify the bleeding site and to stabilize the patient enough for arterial embolization, surgery, or a sequence of the two; embolization and surgery are the two most effective options. Several temporizing endobronchial therapies have been advocated: iced saline lavage, topical 1 : 20,000 epinephrine, endobronchial tamponade with packing or a Fogarty catheter, and endobronchial laser therapy.[51-53]

DIAGNOSIS OF INFECTION

Bronchoscopy is a powerful tool for the diagnosis of pulmonary infection in a critically ill patient. A variety of organisms, including *Mycobacterium tuberculosis, Pneumocystis jiroveci* (formerly *P. carinii*), fungi, viruses, and bacteria, are capable of causing severe pneumonia in critically ill patients. Given the broad differential diagnosis, it makes sense to cast a broad net in terms of diagnostic studies. Bronchoscopy offers access to lower airway secretions, which can lead to accurate diagnosis, focused therapy, and sometimes the withdrawing of unnecessary therapy. Bronchoalveolar lavage (BAL) is the most useful diagnostic modality. BAL can be performed in a patient who cannot or will not produce expectorated sputum or who is intubated, and it samples alveoli more reliably than induced sputum. BAL fluid also is helpful for a broader range of diagnoses than induced sputum. In some cases, BAL recovery of organisms is not adequate alone, and biopsy is needed to confirm tissue invasion.

For BAL, the bronchoscope is wedged into a peripheral airway, and aliquots of sterile saline totaling at least 120 mL are instilled to ensure that alveolar spaces are reached. Box 12-1 summarizes the method for BAL. Fluid retrieved via suctioning is sent for diagnostic studies. The BAL technique samples about 1 million alveoli, or 1% of the lung.[55] For some infections, the presence of an organism in the lung is diagnostic of active infection, whereas for others quantitative cultures are needed to rule out upper airway contamination.

M. tuberculosis is a cause of pneumonia that should not be forgotten in critical care medicine. BAL is a sensitive tool for the diagnosis of *M. tuberculosis,* one of the organisms for which the presence of the organism is per se diagnostic of infection.[60,61] BAL is more sensitive than gastric washings for the diagnosis of tuberculosis.[62] BAL or protected specimen brushings are often positive in patients who have pulmonary tuberculosis but negative sputum smears,[60,63,64] and BAL is more sensitive for diagnosis than transbronchial biopsies for tuberculous pneumonia.[65] For miliary tuberculosis, biopsy is of great value.[66] The addition of molecular techniques, such as polymerase chain reaction (PCR), can increase further the sensitivity of BAL for *M. tuberculosis.*[67]

P. jiroveci is a pathogen of immunocompromised individuals that became widely known only in the 1980s with

Box 12-1

Bronchoalveolar Lavage

Wedge the bronchoscope into a peripheral area of whatever segment is most suspect radiologically. If there is no such segment, wedge into an upper lobe segment if *Pneumocystis* pneumonia is suspected or into a posterior lower lobe segment otherwise.

Instill 30- to 60-mL aliquots of sterile nonbacteriostatic saline through the wedged bronchoscope until some fluid can be retrieved using suction. Discard approximately the first 20 mL of fluid.

Attach a sterile specimen cup in line with the suction tubing, and instill further aliquots until at least 120 mL have been instilled and at least several milliliters of fluid have been obtained.

Bilateral lavage has a higher yield than unilateral lavage.

Have the fluid divided into two aliquots. One is plated using quantitative techniques; the second is centrifuged, stained, and examined for intracellular organisms and other diagnostic findings.

Time from obtaining bronchoalveolar lavage fluid to plating of quantitative specimen should be <4 hours.

Data from references 55-59.

the emergence of acquired immunodeficiency syndrome (AIDS); in the 1960s and 1970s, only about 100 cases had been diagnosed per year in the United States.[68] In the 1980s, thousands of cases were diagnosed.[68] Because the organism cannot be cultured, its diagnosis depends on identification in respiratory secretions. BAL greatly increases the yield for *Pneumocystis* pneumonia over bronchial washings and brushings and is the diagnostic procedure of choice.[65,69,70] As with *M. tuberculosis, P. jiroveci* is an organism that can sometimes be difficult to find on smears, especially in patients with *Pneumocystis* pneumonia who do not have AIDS or who have AIDS but have received inhaled pentamidine.[71,72] PCR can increase the sensitivity of fluid examination with the caveat that some patients can have *Pneumocystis* colonization with-out infection, and the PCR method is sensitive enough to detect those cases.[73,74] In patients without AIDS or patients with AIDS receiving inhaled pentamidine, transbronchial biopsy adds to the yield.[72,75]

The diagnosis of fungal pulmonary infection is more problematic; some fungi can colonize the bronchial tree without being a cause of active infection. Fungal infection is a major issue in the immunocompromised host, but can occur in immunocompetent individuals and can be community-acquired.[76] *Candida* species often colonize the respiratory tract in critically ill patients; their isolation from BAL fluid alone is not diagnostic of tissue invasion.[76,77] *Aspergillus* runs the gamut of possibilities; it can colonize the upper airways without infection, and it can be difficult to detect sometimes when it is the cause of deep tissue infection. In the appropriate clinical and radiologic setting, a positive BAL for *Aspergillus* would be a reasonable criterion for starting therapy, but a negative BAL for *Aspergillus* is inadequate to rule out fungal infection.[78] PCR would seem promising to increase sensitivity for *Aspergillus,* but published results have been variable, and it is not a standard tool.[79-81] Because of the possibility of colonization with *Aspergillus* and *Candida* species, lung biopsy showing tissue invasion is needed to show active infection by these fungi.[77,79] In contrast, *Cryptococcus neoformans* is a ubiquitous fungus that does not routinely colonize the respiratory tract, and its detection in samples of lung fluid is strong presumptive evidence for an active role in pulmonary infection.[82,83]

The endemic fungi, *Histoplasma capsulatum, Blastomyces dermatitidis,* and *Coccidioides immitis,* are capable of causing fulminant infection and cannot be ignored as diagnostic possibilities for pneumonia in patients who live in or travel through endemic areas.[84-87] Diagnosis is sometimes problematic, although the organism may be more plentiful and easier to identify in pulmonary secretions of patients who have fulminant disease. BAL fluid has a much higher yield than sputum.[88] If organisms are not seen, fungal cultures take weeks, an unacceptable interval for seriously ill patients. For *H. capsulatum,* an antigen can be detected in bodily fluids (including BAL) and is of clinical value.[86] The other two endemic fungi have been more problematic when not demonstrable on staining of fluids or biopsy material, but promising techniques with antigen detection, DNA probes, and PCR are in evolution and should become clinically available soon.[85,87,89,90]

Similar to fungi, viral pneumonias occur more frequently in immunocompromised hosts, but viruses play a role in community-acquired pneumonias as well.[91-93] In a multinational study, viruses alone were identified in 9% of community-acquired pneumonias, and viruses as copathogens were identified in an additional 9% of community-acquired pneumonias.[93] Viral pneumonia is relevant to the critical care setting; in the multinational study, 8% of patients with pure viral pneumonia were admitted to the ICU owing to severity of disease.[93] In another study using the most sensitive available virus detection technique, reverse transcriptase PCR, viruses were present as pathogens or copathogens in 23% of patients hospitalized for community-acquired pneumonia.[92] Just as has been shown with atypical pneumonias, no clinical characteristics reliably differentiate viral from bacterial pneumonia.[92-94]

The virology of viral pneumonia is different for pneumonia in the immunocompetent and immunocompromised host. For immunocompetent individuals, the most common viruses are influenza A and B, parainfluenza, respiratory syncytial virus, and adenovirus.[94] For immunocompromised patients, the herpesviruses—herpes simplex, varicella zoster, and cytomegalovirus—are most common, with adenovirus, respiratory syncytial virus, and measles also occurring.[94,95] BAL is useful in the diagnosis of viral pneumonia; BAL fluid is an ideal substrate for most studies done to detect viral infection.[96,97] For all but herpes simplex virus and cytomegalovirus, the presence of the virus is diagnostic of infection.[97,98] Cytomegalovirus and herpes simplex virus can be present in BAL fluid in the absence of pneumonia; proof of tissue invasion is far more diagnostic of active infection.[97,98] Viruses sometimes are difficult to diagnose or take days to weeks to culture; the most useful diagnostic techniques emphasize sensitivity, with reverse transcriptase PCR the newest and most sensitive tool.[99]

BAL is a major tool in the diagnosis of bacterial pneumonias. It has long been recognized that patients in the ICU often have colonization of the upper airways by several potentially pathogenic organisms, and that culture of upper airway secretions cannot be used to diagnose infections of the lower airways. The combination of obtaining secretions from the lower airways and of using quantitative cultures to be able to ignore probable upper airway contaminants has led to the emergence of BAL as a major diagnostic tool. An alternative to BAL is the protected specimen brush (PSB). BAL allows the sampling of a much larger area of lung than does the PSB and logically would be a better diagnostic modality. Although the two modalities are equally accurate in some studies, for several reasons BAL has become the diagnostic procedure of choice for bacterial pneumonia (Box 12-2).[55,56] A third technique, the blind passage of a protected brush into the airways without bronchoscopic guidance, has been described.[100] This technique has a relatively low sensitivity, which probably depends on which lobe is most involved with infection; it cannot be passed into the upper lungs.[55,100] For this reason and the reasons cited in Box 12-2, BAL has evolved as the procedure of choice.[56]

Two methods of quantitation of bacteria obtained by BAL have been described. The first is a simple log count; any bacteria present in greater than or equal to 10^4 colonies by quantitative methods is a pathogen unless proven otherwise.[55] (If PSB is used, a smaller area of lung is sampled and a concentration of $>10^3$ colonies is considered diagnostic of infection.[55]) The second, called the bacterial index, was described by Johanson and colleagues.[101] This method recognizes the fact that in careful studies numerous patients with pneumonia have more than one infecting organism.[24,93,101,102] For the bacterial index, the log numbers of each cultured organism are summed (10^4 *Staphylococcus aureus* + 10^3 *Pseudomonas aeruginosa* = bacterial index of 7). With this system, a bacterial index greater than 6 was a sign of moderate to severe pneumonia.[101] Although the bacterial index system is more rational, single-organism quantitation has gained precedence in current clinical practice.

Reinforcing the value of BAL for clinical management of bacterial infection is a study by Rodriguez and associates.[103] The authors performed quantitative cultures on BAL fluid and PSB from 32 ventilated patients not suspected to have pneumonia. There were six "false-positives," with quantitative cultures in the pneumonia range. Four of the six patients subsequently developed clinical pneumonia.

If a patient with suspected bacterial pneumonia has already been given antibiotics, the quantitative culture of distal airway secretions loses sensitivity.[104,105] A decrease in recovered organisms becomes significant within 12 hours of initiation of antimicrobial therapy and reaches 50% between 24 and 48 hours.[106] This is not surprising because even quantitative cultures of lung tissue have a dramatic loss of sensitivity and specificity for patients who have received prior antibiotic therapy.[107] Despite this loss in sensitivity, BAL may make sense in the evaluation of critically ill patients with lung infiltrates who are receiving antibiotics when these limitations have been acknowledged; BAL could recover organisms not being covered by any current antibiotic regimen, and BAL could help to define nonbacterial infectious agents or other processes responsible for the clinical presentation.

When discussing the diagnostic utility of bronchoscopy for the diagnosis of severe lung infection, it is important to mention diagnoses that may be missed with the techniques already discussed. The atypical pneumonias—principally *Legionella pneumophila, Mycoplasma pneumoniae,* and *Chlamydia pneumoniae* and *C. psittaci*—can be community-acquired. The myth that "atypical" and "typical" pneumonias can be distinguished clinically has been abolished. *Legionella* is particularly capable of causing severe disease, and the other organisms can be coinfectants in severe disease.[108-110] *Legionella* is not typically visible on Gram stain, does not grow on standard bacterial culture, and requires about 1 week to grow on special media when it is present. BAL material in a patient being evaluated for severe community-acquired pneumonia should be sent for direct fluorescent antibody staining for *Legionella* and for culture.[111] The direct fluorescent antibody staining is reasonably sensitive and very specific for *Legionella,*[108] and direct fluorescent antibody staining of pulmonary secretions and of urine are

Box 12-2

Reasons to Use Bronchoalveolar Lavage (BAL) over Protected Specimen Brush for the Diagnosis of Lung Infiltrates

- BAL has a higher sensitivity
- BAL is less expensive
- BAL has a lower complication rate (pneumothorax or bleeding with protected specimen brush)
- BAL allows Gram stain of concentrated smear to look for extracellular organisms
- BAL offers the opportunity to evaluate cells for intracellular organisms, additional proof of active infection
- BAL is a tool for the diagnosis of infections other than bacterial infections
- BAL yields specimens that can be used for probe techniques such as polymerase chain reaction
- BAL is a tool for the diagnosis of other infiltrative processes (e.g., alveolar bleeding) that can mimic infection radiologically

Data from references 55, 56, and 101.

the most rapid diagnostic tools available. The direct fluorescent antibody of pulmonary secretions remains positive for at least 48 hours after institution of appropriate therapy.[111]

There is an importance to negative findings of bronchoscopy for quantitative bacterial culture. A prospective study comparing management using invasive diagnostic techniques (BAL or PSB) with clinical management showed that the patients whose therapy was started or withheld based on quantitative bacterial studies had less antibiotic use, lower mortality, and less sepsis-related organ failure.[112] The importance of negative bacterial studies lies not only in the capacity to withhold or discontinue treatment for bacterial pneumonia, but also in the implication that other types of pulmonary infection or injury should be sought, and that, in some cases, extrapulmonary sources of bacterial infection should be sought.[55,112] The implications for a critically ill patient extend beyond the lungs.

The bronchoscopic diagnosis of pulmonary infection is a valuable tool in intensive care medicine. BAL is the most valuable single tool, with the diagnostic implications dependent on the organism being evaluated. It is important to remember the spectrum of infections that can cause pneumonia in critically ill patients and to evaluate for all that may be present and not simply for typical bacteria.[113] When BAL fluid has been obtained, the diagnostic techniques of greatest value vary dramatically. For some infecting organisms, detection can be difficult even in the presence of severe infection, and extremely sensitive assays such as PCR help in the rapid specific diagnosis of an etiologic agent and allow rapid tailored therapy. In other cases, such as bacterial infection, organisms abound, and it can be difficult to separate colonization from infection; in these cases, quantitative cultures are of greatest value. For other organisms, tissue samples are needed for definitive diagnosis. Table 12-1 summarizes diagnostic methods relevant to different lung infections. BAL fluid is the optimal substrate for almost every listed study with the exception of titers and biopsy material.

LUNG BIOPSY—SURGICAL AND TRANSBRONCHIAL

The decision of when or whether to perform an open lung biopsy is difficult and a matter of debate. Open lung biopsy is the gold standard for the diagnosis of severe cryptogenic disease.[114,115] There are promising data concerning open lung biopsy. When performed, it has a diagnostic accuracy of close to 100%; rarely, an autopsy changes the diagnosis.[114] Open lung biopsy is useful not only in the diagnosis of infection (particularly infections for which tissue invasion is essential to diagnose clinical relevance), but also in the diagnosis of primary lung involvement by disease such as malignancy, of nonspecific inflammatory lung disease, and of lung-related toxicities of therapeutic interventions. Box 12-3 contains a sampling of diagnoses reached with open lung biopsy after other negative diagnostic studies and shows the breadth of possibilities.

Box 12-3

Diagnoses with Open Lung Biopsy after Other Studies Are Negative

- Infection
  - Fungal infection
  - Mycobacterial infection
  - Pyogenic bacteria
  - Cytomegalovirus pneumonia
- Malignancy
  - Leukemia
  - Lymphoma
  - Angiosarcoma
  - Adenocarcinoma
  - Histiocytosis
  - Choriocarcinoma
- Cryptogenic organizing pneumonia
- Vasculitis
- Drug toxicity
- Interstitial fibrosis
- Diffuse alveolar damage
- Pulmonary embolism
- Wegener's granulomatosis
- Pulmonary alveolar proteinosis
- Idiopathic pulmonary fibrosis
- Interstitial pneumonitis
- Sarcoidosis
- Diffuse panbronchiolitis

Data from references 115-118.

Open lung biopsy leads to a change in therapy in 57% to 75% of cases in which it is performed.[114-118] Open lung biopsy can be performed in patients with respiratory distress and patients on ventilators with a reasonable rate of perioperative complications; death attributed to the biopsy procedure itself is rare, and complications, such as persistent air leak, resolve over time.[114,116,118] Complication rates have been reported to be the same with video-assisted thoracic surgery as with thoracotomy.[117] Open lung biopsy has several serious drawbacks, however.

First, authors who separated open lung biopsy results into "specific" (allowing focused therapy thought or known to have some efficacy) and "nonspecific" (a pattern of injury such as diffuse lung damage with no clear cause and no documented effective therapy) found that 38% to 46% of patients had nonspecific injury and no specific therapeutic benefit.[114,117] Second, mortality is extremely high in this group despite diagnoses and the above mentioned changes in therapy, particularly if the patients have respiratory compromise; for those patients, the short-term mortality ranges from 52% to 70%.[116-118] Short-term mortality is believed by most authors to be related far more to the underlying disease than to the open lung biopsy procedure.[116-118] Third, most patients already have received appropriate therapy; in most cases, the change in therapy would be discontinuation of unnecessary drugs. In some, the benefit of open lung biopsy would be acknowledgment of end-stage disease

Table 12-1. Diagnostic Techniques for Important Potentially Severe Pulmonary Infections

Organism Important	Presence in BAL Diagnostic?	Culture	Serology	Detection with Antibodies	Gene Amplification	Cytology/Pathology/Other
M. tuberculosis	Yes	Usually positive—slow			PCR	Necrotizing granulomas
Legionella	Yes	Special media, slow	≥1:256 or 4-fold increase	IF of sputum or BAL	PCR +/–	DFA of urine or pleural fluid
"Typical" bacteria	No	BAL $>10^4$ PSB $>10^3$ BI >6				DFA—urinary pneumococcal antigen
Influenza (A, B, and C)	Yes	Positive—slow	4-fold increase	IF ELISA (A and B)	PCR	Hemadsorption testing
Herpes simplex	No	Cell culture—cytopathic effects		IF ELISA		Nuclear inclusions (Cowdry A bodies)
Cytomegalovirus	No	Cell culture—cytopathic effects		ELISA		Nuclear inclusions ("owl's eye")
Varicella-zoster	Yes	Cell culture—cytopathic effects				Nuclear inclusions (Cowdry A bodies) Typical rash helpful—Tzanck preparation
Respiratory syncytial virus (rare)	Yes	Cell culture—cytopathic effects		IF	PCR	Eosinophilic cytoplasmic inclusions
Parainfluenza (1-4)	Yes	Cell culture—cytopathic effects		IF	PCR	Hemadsorption testing Small eosinophilic cytoplasmic inclusions
Adenovirus	Yes	Cell culture—cytopathic effects		IF	PCR	Variable inclusion pattern
Cryptococcus	Yes	Slow				Antigen—serum Tissue invasion
Aspergillus	No					Tissue invasion
Candida	No					Tissue invasion
Coccidioides	Yes		High or increasing			
Histoplasma	Yes		≥1:64 or 4-fold increase	ELISA (cross-reacts with *Blastomyces*)		Can be hard to find even with culture Antigen—urine or serum Tissue invasion
Blastomyces	Yes			ELISA (cross-reacts with *Histoplasma*)		

BAL, bronchoalveolar lavage; BI, bacterial index; DFA, direct fluorescent antibody; ELISA, enzyme-linked immunosorbent assay; IF, immunofluorescence testing (direct or indirect); PCR, polymerase chain reaction; PSB, protected specimen brush.
Data from references 84, 89, 92, 94, 96, 111, and 113.

and withdrawal of all therapy. Cases in which a new therapeutic intervention was started and may have been effective are extremely rare.[114,116,118] In 1988, Warner and colleagues[118] discussed open lung biopsy in patients with respiratory compromise and said, "any complications of a procedure of unknown benefit is of concern." Some authors hold this opinion to this day. Most patients have received anti-infectives or steroids or both before open lung biopsy is considered, and one could argue that most patients who could respond would have responded before open lung biopsy. That the controversy is alive and well is illustrated by a quote from Chuang and associates[115]: "[I]t is not ethical to avoid open lung biopsy in patients with unclear diagnoses, as open lung biopsy is known to be the most sensitive and specific test available at this time."

Given the controversies and the available data, a few principles would seem appropriate in considering whether or not open lung biopsy should be performed. First, in most cases, BAL (and perhaps transbronchial biopsy; see later) should be performed before open lung biopsy is considered. Second, patients who have more than three organs failing (lung plus two more) probably should not undergo biopsy; the prognosis is too poor.[114] Third, decisions about open lung biopsy should be based more on the prior condition of the patient and the potential utility of the study than on the degree of ventilatory distress or compromise of the patient; short-term mortality from the procedure is acceptable. Open lung biopsy in a critically ill patient with undiagnosed pulmonary infiltrates remains a valuable tool that is uncommonly indicated but that would occasionally provide a diagnosis that results in lifesaving therapy.

Bronchoscopic transbronchial lung biopsy may fill the gap between "nontissue" procedures such as BAL and open lung biopsy with its large amount of tissue for pathology and culture. Open lung biopsy by definition requires anesthesia and by definition results in chest tube placement, with many patients having air leaks after the procedure.[116-118] Transbronchial lung biopsy requires only conscious sedation and would require chest tube placement only if a complication occurred, not as a matter of routine. As noted earlier in the discussion of infection, some diagnoses, such as invasive aspergillosis, *Candida* pneumonia, and cytomegalovirus pneumonia, require tissue samples showing tissue invasion. Tissue samples can increase the diagnostic yield for other organisms, such as *M. tuberculosis* and *P. jiroveci*.[119] Diagnoses such as cryptogenic organizing pneumonia and several others listed in Box 12-3 cannot be made without tissue. Transbronchial lung biopsy would be reasonable with BAL or after a negative BAL in compromised patients with infiltrates of unknown etiology.[119-121] It was formerly thought that to perform transbronchial lung biopsy in a patient on a ventilator carried too high a risk of complications to be warranted.[122] The available data challenge this concept. Two early studies[123,124] and several more recent studies[121,125-127] have evaluated the yield and complications of transbronchial lung biopsy in ventilated patients. All of these studies showed high yields similar to the yields for open lung biopsy. The pneumothorax rates varied from 0% to 24%. Bleeding was considered to be significant in 6% to 20%, with all cases self-limited. No fatalities occurred. When transbronchial lung biopsy in ventilated patients is compared with open lung biopsy, for which general anesthesia, incisions, violation of the visceral pleura, and a chest tube are requisites, it is apparent that transbronchial lung biopsy is underused in this population; it has a favorable risk-to-benefit ratio.

SPECIAL SITUATIONS

Immunocompromised Host

Immunocompromise is a recognized risk factor for respiratory infection. Years of elegant work have helped to define classic types of immunocompromise and patterns of infection that are more typical for the different types.[128-130] Long-recognized diseases causing immunocompromise include solid tumors on chemotherapy, hematologic malignancies, organ transplantation, chronic diseases for which cytotoxic or steroid therapy is given, HIV infection, and other less common acquired or congenital diseases.[122,128] Although the classification of immunocompromise definitely includes the above-mentioned diseases, it has no clear boundaries. Patients with chronic insulin-dependent diabetes, alcoholics, patients with severe malnutrition, and patients on drugs such as infliximab, a tumor necrosis factor antagonist, almost certainly have degrees of immunocompromise that affect their susceptibility to infection.[131-135] The stresses of critical illness and organ dysfunction coupled with the broaching of natural defense systems (skin by central lines, lungs by intubation, urinary tract by catheters) put critically ill patients at increased risk for infection.

Many chronic illnesses probably also carry an increased risk for infection. Shelhamer and colleagues[128] recognized the difficulty with this issue and defined immunocompromise as "any condition, congenital or acquired, temporary or chronic, in which the response of the host to a foreign antigen is subnormal." For patients with classic known forms of immunocompromise, special diagnostic attention has to be paid to the possibility of *Pneumocystis* pneumonia, invasive fungal infection, infection with the herpesviruses, and tuberculosis. Three factors make this a gray area rather than black-and-white: (1) Lack of knowledge that a patient is immunocompromised does not rule out immunocompromise, (2) degrees of immunocompromise exist, and (3) most of the pathogens discussed are capable of causing disease in "normal" hosts. For these reasons, some specific issues related to immunocompromise have been mentioned throughout this chapter, but in the clinical approach to a patient with severe respiratory disease, it makes sense to assume that any patient might be immunocompromised; the diagnostic work-up should, as mentioned, cast a wide net.

Thrombocytopenia

Thrombocytopenia is an obvious risk factor for bleeding from invasive procedures. BAL has been shown to be safe and clinically useful in thrombocytopenic patients.[136]

Bronchoscopic procedures and open lung biopsies have been performed safely in patients with thrombocytopenia.[117,137] Historically, procedures have been limited to BAL, or platelets have been given before bronchoscopic or surgical procedures.[117,137]

COMPLICATIONS AND DEATH

As with the issue of immunocompromise, many procedure-related complications have already been mentioned. The true incidence of complications of bronchoscopy in the ICU has not been well defined. Most reviews of the topic[26,34,138-141] cite several older studies of bronchoscopy in general,[7,8,10,11,142] not specifically in critically ill patients. The two largest and most-cited reports are by Credle and colleagues[11] and Suratt and coworkers[7] and reviewed 24,521 (Credle) and "approximately 48,000" (Suratt) procedures. These were retrospective reports based on mailed questionnaires. Death rates were 0.01% and 0.03%.[7,11]

The next largest study was a retrospective single-institution study of 4273 bronchoscopies, which reported 0% mortality and a 0.5% frequency of major complications (pneumothorax, bleeding, respiratory failure requiring intubation).[9] Three prospective studies reported on 205 to 1146 flexible bronchoscopies and reported mortality rates of 0%,[10] 0.1%,[142] and 0.5%.[8] The highest reported mortality rate came out of a study from a consortium of expert bronchoscopists studying autofluorescence.[143] The study included the requisite of at least two endobronchial biopsies, and in a series of 300 cases the immediate post-bronchoscopic mortality was 0.7%. Two retrospective studies[42,144] and one prospective study[125] reviewed bronchoscopies performed specifically on patients in the ICU. No procedure-related mortality was reported. Throughout these studies, only death rates are consistently noted; major and minor complications are variably defined.

Several principles emerge from the above-cited studies. The complication rates depend on the invasiveness of the procedure. The highest incidence of complications occurs with lung biopsy and then, in descending order, with brushings, lavage, and simple observation. On review of studies of the patients one would expect to have the highest complication rate—patients on ventilators undergoing transbronchial biopsies—there is a pneumothorax rate of 24%, but no fatalities have been reported.[121,123-127] None of those studies involved large numbers of patients; it is inevitable that fatalities would occur in this subset of high-risk cases. Nevertheless, many years of experience with flexible fiberoptic bronchoscopy have led to the conclusion that its benefits outweigh its risks. No bronchoscopy should be done on a critically ill patient without a reason, but when a reason is present, bronchoscopy is often the unique or the safest method known of obtaining data that may affect care.

SUMMARY

Since its inception in 1968, flexible fiberoptic bronchoscopy has evolved into a major tool in the evaluation and management of critically ill patients. The bronchoscope allows evaluation of and sometimes management of airway problems. The bronchoscope follows the most natural pathway into the lung—the airway—and allows sampling of secretions and tissues from the alveolar level. The basic techniques have been defined for many years. What has been refined is understanding of their utility and testing methodologies; increasing sensitivities and specificities over the years have greatly enhanced our capacities, particularly in the diagnosis of lung infections. Some lung infections require lung tissue for definitive diagnosis, as do several diagnoses that can cause diffuse lung disease and can sometimes mimic infection. Open lung biopsy is a time-honored approach with high diagnostic accuracy that may sometimes be an optimal approach. Transbronchial lung biopsy, even in a ventilated patient, has a clinical impact similar to that of open lung biopsy and is probably underused in critically ill patients with diffuse infiltrates who are failing empiric therapies. It is clear that the more ill the patient, the higher the risk of any invasive procedure, but the literature points the risk-to-benefit ratio of bronchoscopy in favor of performing bronchoscopy for the indications outlined in this chapter.

KEY POINTS

- Bronchoscopy has become a major tool in the evaluation of the airways and lung parenchyma of critically ill patients.
- Bronchoscopy stimulates a series of reflexes affecting blood pressure, heart rate, and intracerebral pressure, but this is true for any invasion of the upper airway (e.g., suctioning), and bronchoscopy for the evaluation of lung problems in critically ill patients has a favorable risk-to-benefit ratio.
- Inserting a bronchoscope through an endotracheal tube causes upper airway obstruction and can cause hypoventilation or hyperinflation or both; the physiologic changes caused by the bronchoscope need to be understood and possibly compensated for.
- Bronchoscopy is a valuable tool for the diagnosis and management (especially intubation and percutaneous tracheostomy) of upper airway problems.
- Bronchoscopy with BAL is the most effective and accurate clinical tool currently available for the diagnosis of pulmonary infection in critically ill patients.
- The potential of bronchoscopy for the diagnosis of infection is being advanced at present not by bronchoscopic techniques, but by the development and clinical application of extremely sensitive tools such as PCR assays.
- Critically ill patients with undiagnosed infiltrates occasionally benefit from lung biopsy; the results often affect management, but rarely affect outcome. Available data suggest that bronchoscopic transbronchial lung biopsy has yields similar to those for open lung biopsy with a more favorable risk-to-benefit ratio.

REFERENCES

1. Lundgren R, Haggmark S, Reiz S: Hemodynamic effects of flexible fiberoptic bronchoscopy performed under topical anesthesia. Chest 1982;82:295-299.
2. Staender S, Marsch SC, Schumacher P, et al: Haemodynamic response to fibreoptic versus laryngoscopic nasotracheal intubation under total intravenous anaesthesia. Eur J Anaesthesiol 1994;11:175-179.
3. Kaplan JD, Schuster DP: Physiologic consequences of tracheal intubation. Clin Chest Med 1991;12:425-432.
4. Stoelting RK: Circulatory changes during direct laryngoscopy and tracheal intubation: Influence of duration of laryngoscopy with or without prior lidocaine. Anesthesiology 1977;47:381-384.
5. Rudy EB, Turner BS, Baun M, et al: Endotracheal suctioning in adults with head injury. Heart Lung 1991;20:667-674.
6. Matot I, Kramer MR, Glantz L, et al: Myocardial ischemia in sedated patients undergoing fiberoptic bronchoscopy. Chest 1997;112:1454-1458.
7. Suratt PM, Smiddy JF, Gruber B: Deaths and complications associated with fiberoptic bronchoscopy. Chest 1976;69:747-751.
8. Dreisin RB, Albert RK, Talley PA, et al: Flexible fiberoptic bronchoscopy in the teaching hospital: Yield and complications. Chest 1978;74:144-149.
9. Pue CA, Pacht ER: Complications of fiberoptic bronchoscopy at a university hospital. Chest 1995;107:430-432.
10. Lukomsky GI, Ovchinnikov AA, Bilal A: Complications of bronchoscopy: Comparison of rigid bronchoscopy under general anesthesia and flexible fiberoptic bronchoscopy under topical anesthesia. Chest 1981;79:316-321.
11. Credle WF Jr, Smiddy JF, Elliott RC: Complications of fiberoptic bronchoscopy. Am Rev Respir Dis 1974;109:67-72.
12. Shrader DL, Lakshminarayan S: The effect of fiberoptic bronchoscopy on cardiac rhythm. Chest 1978;73:821-824.
13. Kerwin AJ, Croce MA, Timmons SD, et al: Effects of fiberoptic bronchoscopy on intracranial pressure in patients with brain injury: A prospective clinical study. J Trauma 2000;48:878-882.
14. Matsushima Y, Jones RL, King EG, et al: Alterations in pulmonary mechanics and gas exchange during routine fiberoptic bronchoscopy. Chest 1984;86:184-188.
15. Lindholm CE, Ollman B, Snyder JV, et al: Cardiorespiratory effects of flexible fiberoptic bronchoscopy in critically ill patients. Chest 1978;74:362-368.
16. Bailey PL, Pace NL, Ashburn MA, et al: Frequent hypoxemia and apnea after sedation with midazolam and fentanyl. Anesthesiology 1990;73:826-830.
17. Kristensen MS, Milman N, Jarnvig IL: Pulse oximetry at fibre-optic bronchoscopy in local anaesthesia: Indication for postbronchoscopy oxygen supplementation? Respir Med 1998;92:432-437.
18. Chhajed PN, Aboyoun C, Malouf MA, et al: Management of acute hypoxemia during flexible bronchoscopy with insertion of a nasopharyngeal tube in lung transplant recipients. Chest 2002;121:1350-1354.
19. Albertini RE, Harrell JH, Kurihara N, et al: Arterial hypoxemia induced by fiberoptic bronchoscopy. JAMA 1974;230:1666-1667.
20. Shinagawa N, Yamazaki K, Kinoshita I, et al: Susceptibility to oxygen desaturation during bronchoscopy in elderly patients with pulmonary fibrosis. Respiration 2006;73:90-94.
21. Jones AM, O'Driscoll R: Do all patients require supplemental oxygen during flexible bronchoscopy? Chest 2001; 119:1906-1909.
22. Petersen GM, Pierson DJ, Hunter PM: Arterial oxygen saturation during nasotracheal suctioning. Chest 1979; 76:283-287.
23. Sharma SK, Pande JN, Sarkar R: Effect of routine fiberoptic bronchoscopy and bronchoalveolar lavage on arterial blood gases. Indian J Chest Dis Allied Sci 1993;35:3-8.
24. Guerra LF, Baughman RP: Use of bronchoalveolar lavage to diagnose bacterial pneumonia in mechanically ventilated patients. Crit Care Med 1990;18:169-173.
25. Montravers P, Gauzit R, Dombret MC, et al: Cardiopulmonary effects of bronchoalveolar lavage in critically ill patients. Chest 1993;104:1541-1547.
26. Dellinger RP, Bandi V: Fiberoptic bronchoscopy in the intensive care unit. Crit Care Clin 1992;8:755-772.
27. Dellinger RP: Fiberoptic bronchoscopy in adult airway management. Crit Care Med 1990;18:882-887.
28. Freeman BD, Isabella K, Lin N, et al: A meta-analysis of prospective trials comparing percutaneous and surgical tracheostomy in critically ill patients. Chest 2000;118:1412-1418.
29. Freeman BD, Isabella K, Cobb JP, et al: A prospective, randomized study comparing percutaneous with surgical tracheostomy in critically ill patients. Crit Care Med 2001;29:926-930.
30. Melloni G, Muttini S, Gallioli G, et al: Surgical tracheostomy versus percutaneous dilatational tracheostomy: A prospective-randomized study with long-term follow-up. J Cardiovasc Surg (Torino) 2002;43:113-121.
31. Polderman KH, Spijkstra JJ, de Bree R, et al: Percutaneous dilatational tracheostomy in the ICU: Optimal organization, low complication rates, and description of a new complication. Chest 2003;123: 1595-1602.
32. Ernst A, Silvestri GA, Johnstone D: Interventional pulmonary procedures: Guidelines from the American College of Chest Physicians. Chest 2003;123: 1693-1717.
33. Barba CA, Angood PB, Kauder DR, et al: Bronchoscopic guidance makes percutaneous tracheostomy a safe, cost-effective, and easy-to-teach procedure. Surgery 1995;118:879-883.
34. Shennib H, Baslaim G: Bronchoscopy in the intensive care unit. Chest Surg Clin N Am 1996;6:349-361.
35. Marx WH, Ciaglia P, Graniero KD: Some important details in the technique of percutaneous dilatational tracheostomy via the modified Seldinger technique. Chest 1996;110: 762-766.
36. Grundling M, Pavlovic D, Kuhn SO, et al: Is the method of modified percutaneous tracheostomy without bronchoscopic guidance really simple and safe? Chest 2005;128:3774-3775.
37. Polderman KH, Spijkstra JJ, de Bree R, et al: Percutaneous tracheostomy in the intensive care unit: Which safety precautions? Crit Care Med 2001;29: 221-223.
38. deBoisblanc BP, Deblieux P: Percutaneous dilational tracheostomy. Clin Pulm Med 2002;9:109-112.
39. Kearney PA, Griffen MM, Ochoa JB, et al: A single-center 8-year experience with percutaneous dilational tracheostomy. Ann Surg 2000;231:701-709.
40. Swanson KL: Airway foreign bodies: What's new? Semin Respir Crit Care Med 2004;25:405-411.
41. Cunanan OS: The flexible fiberoptic bronchoscope in foreign body removal: Experience in 300 cases. Chest 1978;73(5 Suppl):725-726.
42. Olopade CO, Prakash UB: Bronchoscopy in the critical-care unit. Mayo Clin Proc 1989;64:1255-1263.
43. Kreider ME, Lipson DA: Bronchoscopy for atelectasis in the ICU: A case report and review of the literature. Chest 2003;124:344-350.
44. Marini JJ, Pierson DJ, Hudson LD: Acute lobar atelectasis: A prospective comparison of fiberoptic bronchoscopy and respiratory therapy. Am Rev Respir Dis 1979;119:971-978.
45. Tsao TC, Tsai YH, Lan RS, et al: Treatment for collapsed lung in critically ill patients: Selective intrabronchial air insufflation using the fiberoptic bronchoscope. Chest 1990;97:435-438.
46. Hara KS, Prakash UB: Fiberoptic bronchoscopy in the evaluation of acute chest and upper airway trauma. Chest 1989;96:627-630.
47. Pruitt BA Jr, Cioffi WG: Diagnosis and treatment of smoke inhalation. J Intensive Care Med 1995;10:117-127.
48. Masanes MJ, Legendre C, Lioret N, et al: Using bronchoscopy and biopsy to diagnose early inhalation injury: Macroscopic and histologic findings. Chest 1995;107:1365-1369.
49. Chou SH, Lin SD, Chuang HY, et al: Fiber-optic bronchoscopic classification of inhalation injury: Prediction of acute lung injury. Surg Endosc 2004;18: 1377-1379.
50. American Burn Association: Inhalation injury: Diagnosis. J Am Coll Surg 2003;196:307-312.
51. Lenner R, Schilero GJ, Lesser M: Hemoptysis: Diagnosis and management. Compr Ther 2002;28: 7-14.
52. Cahill BC, Ingbar DH: Massive hemoptysis: Assessment and

management. Clin Chest Med 1994;15:147-167.
53. Thompson AB, Teschler H, Rennard SI: Pathogenesis, evaluation, and therapy for massive hemoptysis. Clin Chest Med 1992;13:69-82.
54. Knott-Craig CJ, Oostuizen JG, Rossouw G, et al: Management and prognosis of massive hemoptysis: Recent experience with 120 patients. J Thorac Cardiovasc Surg 1993;105:394-397.
55. Chastre J, Combes A, Luyt CE: The invasive (quantitative) diagnosis of ventilator-associated pneumonia. Respir Care 2005;50:797-807.
56. Fagon JY: Diagnosis and treatment of ventilator-associated pneumonia: Fiberoptic bronchoscopy with bronchoalveolar lavage is essential. Semin Respir Crit Care Med 2006;27:34-44.
57. Meduri GU, Stover DE, Greeno RA, et al: Bilateral bronchoalveolar lavage in the diagnosis of opportunistic pulmonary infections. Chest 1991; 100:1272-1276.
58. Baughman RP, Dohn MN, Shipley R, et al: Increased *Pneumocystis carinii* recovery from the upper lobes in *Pneumocystis* pneumonia: The effect of aerosol pentamidine prophylaxis. Chest 1993;103:426-432.
59. Meduri GU, Reddy RC, Stanley T, et al: Pneumonia in acute respiratory distress syndrome: A prospective evaluation of bilateral bronchoscopic sampling. Am J Respir Crit Care Med 1998;158: 870-875.
60. de Gracia J, Curull V, Vidal R, et al: Diagnostic value of bronchoalveolar lavage in suspected pulmonary tuberculosis. Chest 1988;93:329-332.
61. Miro AM, Gibilara E, Powell S, et al: The role of fiberoptic bronchoscopy for diagnosis of pulmonary tuberculosis in patients at risk for AIDS. Chest 1992;101:1211-1214.
62. Dickson SJ, Brent A, Davidson RN, et al: Comparison of bronchoscopy and gastric washings in the investigation of smear-negative pulmonary tuberculosis. Clin Infect Dis 2003;37:1649-1653.
63. Willcox PA, Benatar SR, Potgieter PD: Use of the flexible fibreoptic bronchoscope in diagnosis of sputum-negative pulmonary tuberculosis. Thorax 1982;37:598-601.
64. Jett JR, Cortese DA, Dines DE: The value of bronchoscopy in the diagnosis of mycobacterial disease: A five-year experience. Chest 1981;80: 575-578.
65. Stover DE, Zaman MB, Hajdu SI, et al: Bronchoalveolar lavage in the diagnosis of diffuse pulmonary infiltrates in the immunosuppressed host. Ann Intern Med 1984;101:1-7.
66. Willcox PA, Potgieter PD, Bateman ED, et al: Rapid diagnosis of sputum negative miliary tuberculosis using the flexible fibreoptic bronchoscope. Thorax 1986;41:681-684.
67. Tueller C, Chhajed PN, Buitrago-Tellez C, et al: Value of smear and PCR in bronchoalveolar lavage fluid in culture positive pulmonary tuberculosis. Eur Respir J 2005;26:767-772.
68. Schliep TC, Yarrish RL: *Pneumocystis carinii* pneumonia. Semin Respir Infect 1999;14:333-343.
69. Turner D, Schwarz Y, Yust I: Induced sputum for diagnosing *Pneumocystis carinii* pneumonia in HIV patients: New data, new issues. Eur Respir J 2003;21:204-208.
70. Roblot F, Le Moal G, Godet C, et al: *Pneumocystis carinii* pneumonia in patients with hematologic malignancies: A descriptive study. J Infect 2003;47:19-27.
71. Zahar JR, Robin M, Azoulay E, et al: *Pneumocystis carinii* pneumonia in critically ill patients with malignancy: A descriptive study. Clin Infect Dis 2002;35:929-934.
72. Edelstein H, McCabe RE: Atypical presentations of *Pneumocystis carinii* pneumonia in patients receiving inhaled pentamidine prophylaxis. Chest 1990;98:1366-1369.
73. Olsson M, Elvin K, Lofdahl S, et al: Detection of *Pneumocystis carinii* DNA in sputum and bronchoalveolar lavage samples by polymerase chain reaction. J Clin Microbiol 1996;34:2052.
74. Elvin K, Olsson M, Lidman C, et al: Detection of asymptomatic *Pneumocystis carinii* infection by polymerase chain reaction: Predictive for subsequent pneumonia. AIDS 1996;10:1296-1297.
75. Rodriguez M, Fishman JA: Prevention of infection due to *Pneumocystis* spp. in human immunodeficiency virus-negative immunocompromised patients. Clin Microbiol Rev 2004;17: 770-782.
76. Chen KY, Ko SC, Hsueh PR, et al: Pulmonary fungal infection: Emphasis on microbiological spectra, patient outcome, and prognostic factors. Chest 2001;120:177-184.
77. el Ebiary M, Torres A, Fabregas N, et al: Significance of the isolation of *Candida* species from respiratory samples in critically ill, non-neutropenic patients: An immediate postmortem histologic study. Am J Respir Crit Care Med 1997; 156(2 Pt 1):583-590.
78. Cordonnier C, Escudier E, Verra F, et al: Bronchoalveolar lavage during neutropenic episodes: Diagnostic yield and cellular pattern. Eur Respir J 1994;7:114-120.
79. Reichenberger F, Habicht JM, Gratwohl A, et al: Diagnosis and treatment of invasive pulmonary aspergillosis in neutropenic patients. Eur Respir J 2002;19:743-755.
80. Bart-Delabesse E, Marmorat-Khuong A, Costa JM, et al: Detection of *Aspergillus* DNA in bronchoalveolar lavage fluid of AIDS patients by the polymerase chain reaction. Eur J Clin Microbiol Infect Dis 1997;16:24-25.
81. Bretagne S, Costa JM, Marmorat-Khuong A, et al: Detection of *Aspergillus* species DNA in bronchoalveolar lavage samples by competitive PCR. J Clin Microbiol 1995;33:1164-1168.
82. Nadrous HF, Antonios VS, Terrell CL, et al: Pulmonary cryptococcosis in nonimmunocompromised patients. Chest 2003;124:2143-2147.
83. Bottone EJ, Sindone M, Caraballo V: Value of assessing cryptococcal antigen in bronchoalveolar lavage and sputum specimens from patients with AIDS. Mt Sinai J Med 1998;65:422-425.
84. McAdams HP, Rosado-de-Christenson ML, Lesar M, et al: Thoracic mycoses from endemic fungi: Radiologic-pathologic correlation. Radiographics 1995;15:255-270.
85. Valdivia L, Nix D, Wright M, et al: Coccidioidomycosis as a common cause of community-acquired pneumonia. Emerg Infect Dis 2006;12:958-962.
86. Wheat LJ, Kauffman CA: Histoplasmosis. Infect Dis Clin North Am 2003;17:1-19.
87. Martynowicz MA, Prakash UB: Pulmonary blastomycosis: An appraisal of diagnostic techniques. Chest 2002;121:768-773.
88. Baughman RP, Dohn MN, Loudon RG, et al: Bronchoscopy with bronchoalveolar lavage in tuberculosis and fungal infections. Chest 1991;99:92-97.
89. Hage CA, Davis TE, Egan L, et al: Diagnosis of pulmonary histoplasmosis and blastomycosis by detection of antigen in bronchoalveolar lavage fluid using an improved second-generation enzyme-linked immunoassay. Respir Med 2007;101:43-47.
90. Bialek R, Gonzalez GM, Begerow D, et al: Coccidioidomycosis and blastomycosis: Advances in molecular diagnosis. FEMS Immunol Med Microbiol 2005;45:355-360.
91. Bartlett JG, Mundy LM: Community-acquired pneumonia. N Engl J Med 1995;333:1618-1624.
92. Angeles MM, Camps M, Pumarola T, et al: The role of viruses in the aetiology of community-acquired pneumonia in adults. Antivir Ther 2006;11:351-359.
93. de Roux A, Marcos MA, Garcia E, et al: Viral community-acquired pneumonia in nonimmunocompromised adults. Chest 2004;125:1343-1351.
94. Greenberg SB: Viral pneumonia. Infect Dis Clin N Am 1991;5:603-621.
95. Chien JW, Johnson JL: Viral pneumonias: Infection in the immunocompromised host. Postgrad Med 2000;107:67-74.
96. Leland DS, Emanuel D: Laboratory diagnosis of viral infections of the lung. Semin Respir Infect 1995;10: 189-198.
97. Connolly MG Jr, Baughman RP, Dohn MN, et al: Recovery of viruses other than cytomegalovirus from bronchoalveolar lavage fluid. Chest 1994;105:1775-1781.
98. Ruutu P, Ruutu T, Volin L, et al: Cytomegalovirus is frequently isolated in bronchoalveolar lavage fluid of bone marrow transplant recipients without pneumonia. Ann Intern Med 1990;112:913-916.
99. Osiowy C: Direct detection of respiratory syncytial virus, parainfluenza virus, and adenovirus in clinical respiratory specimens by a multiplex reverse transcription-PCR assay. J Clin Microbiol 1998;36: 3149-3154.
100. Casetta M, Blot F, Antoun S, et al: Diagnosis of nosocomial pneumonia in cancer patients undergoing mechanical ventilation: A prospective comparison of the plugged telescoping catheter with the

protected specimen brush. Chest 1999;115:1641-1645.
101. Johanson WG Jr, Seidenfeld JJ, Gomez P, et al: Bacteriologic diagnosis of nosocomial pneumonia following prolonged mechanical ventilation. Am Rev Respir Dis 1988;137:259-264.
102. Chastre J, Viau F, Brun P, et al: Prospective evaluation of the protected specimen brush for the diagnosis of pulmonary infections in ventilated patients. Am Rev Respir Dis 1984;130:924-929.
103. Rodriguez DC, Sole J, Elcuaz R: Quantitative cultures of protected brush specimens and bronchoalveolar lavage in ventilated patients without suspected pneumonia. Am J Respir Crit Care Med 1994;149(2 Pt 1):320-323.
104. Montravers P, Fagon JY, Chastre J, et al: Follow-up protected specimen brushes to assess treatment in nosocomial pneumonia. Am Rev Respir Dis 1993;147:38-44.
105. Gracia JD, Miravitlles M, Mayordomo C, et al: Empiric treatments impair the diagnostic yield of BAL in HIV-positive patients. Chest 1997;111:1180-1186.
106. Prats E, Dorca J, Pujol M, et al: Effects of antibiotics on protected specimen brush sampling in ventilator-associated pneumonia. Eur Respir J 2002;19:944-951.
107. Torres A, el Ebiary M, Padro L, et al: Validation of different techniques for the diagnosis of ventilator-associated pneumonia: Comparison with immediate postmortem pulmonary biopsy. Am J Respir Crit Care Med 1994;149(2 Pt 1):324-331.
108. Falco V, Fernandez DS, Alegre J, et al: *Legionella pneumophila*: A cause of severe community-acquired pneumonia. Chest 1991;100:1007-1011.
109. Stout JE, Yu VL: Legionellosis. N Engl J Med 1997;337:682-687.
110. Lieberman D, Schlaeffer F, Boldur I, et al: Multiple pathogens in adult patients admitted with community-acquired pneumonia: A one year prospective study of 346 consecutive patients. Thorax 1996;51:179-184.
111. Kohorst WR, Schonfeld SA, Macklin JE, et al: Rapid diagnosis of Legionnaires' disease by bronchoalveolar lavage. Chest 1983;84:186-190.
112. Fagon JY, Chastre J, Wolff M, et al: Invasive and noninvasive strategies for management of suspected ventilator-associated pneumonia: A randomized trial. Ann Intern Med 2000;132:621-630.
113. Chien JW, Johnson JL: Viral pneumonias: Multifaceted approach to an elusive diagnosis. Postgrad Med 2000;107:67-72.
114. Flabouris A, Myburgh J: The utility of open lung biopsy in patients requiring mechanical ventilation. Chest 1999;115:811-817.
115. Chuang ML, Lin IF, Tsai YH, et al: The utility of open lung biopsy in patients with diffuse pulmonary infiltrates as related to respiratory distress, its impact on decision making by urgent intervention, and the diagnostic accuracy based on the biopsy location. J Intensive Care Med 2003;18:21-28.
116. Canver CC, Mentzer RM Jr: The role of open lung biopsy in early and late survival of ventilator-dependent patients with diffuse idiopathic lung disease. J Cardiovasc Surg (Torino) 1994;35:151-155.
117. White DA, Wong PW, Downey R: The utility of open lung biopsy in patients with hematologic malignancies. Am J Respir Crit Care Med 2000;161(3 Pt 1):723-729.
118. Warner DO, Warner MA, Divertie MB: Open lung biopsy in patients with diffuse pulmonary infiltrates and acute respiratory failure. Am Rev Respir Dis 1988;137:90-94.
119. Cazzadori A, Di Perri G, Todeschini G, et al: Transbronchial biopsy in the diagnosis of pulmonary infiltrates in immunocompromised patients. Chest 1995;107:101-106.
120. Jain P, Sandur S, Meli Y, et al: Role of flexible bronchoscopy in immunocompromised patients with lung infiltrates. Chest 2004;125:712-722.
121. Martin C, Papazian L, Payan MJ, et al: Pulmonary fibrosis correlates with outcome in adult respiratory distress syndrome: A study in mechanically ventilated patients. Chest 1995;107:196-200.
122. Williams D, Yungbluth M, Adams G, et al: The role of fiberoptic bronchoscopy in the evaluation of immunocompromised hosts with diffuse pulmonary infiltrates. Am Rev Respir Dis 1985;131:880-885.
123. Pincus PS, Kallenbach JM, Hurwitz MD, et al: Transbronchial biopsy during mechanical ventilation. Crit Care Med 1987;15:1136-1139.
124. Papin TA, Grum CM, Weg JG: Transbronchial biopsy during mechanical ventilation. Chest 1986;89:168-170.
125. Turner JS, Willcox PA, Hayhurst MD, et al: Fiberoptic bronchoscopy in the intensive care unit—a prospective study of 147 procedures in 107 patients. Crit Care Med 1994;22:259-264.
126. O'Brien JD, Ettinger NA, Shevlin D, et al: Safety and yield of transbronchial biopsy in mechanically ventilated patients. Crit Care Med 1997;25:440-446.
127. Bulpa PA, Dive AM, Mertens L, et al: Combined bronchoalveolar lavage and transbronchial lung biopsy: Safety and yield in ventilated patients. Eur Respir J 2003;21:489-494.
128. Shelhamer JH, Toews GB, Masur H, et al: NIH conference. Respiratory disease in the immunosuppressed patient. Ann Intern Med 1992;117:415-431.
129. Sharma S, Nadrous HF, Peters SG, et al: Pulmonary complications in adult blood and marrow transplant recipients: Autopsy findings. Chest 2005;128:1385-1392.
130. Rolston KV: The spectrum of pulmonary infections in cancer patients. Curr Opin Oncol 2001;13:218-223.
131. Happel KI, Nelson S: Alcohol, immunosuppression, and the lung. Proc Am Thorac Soc 2005;2:428-432.
132. Kristan SS, Kern I, Music E: Invasive pulmonary aspergillosis. Respiration 2002;69:521-525.
133. Imaizumi K, Sugishita M, Usui M, et al: Pulmonary infectious complications associated with anti-TNFalpha therapy (infliximab) for rheumatoid arthritis. Intern Med 2006;45:685-688.
134. Hage CA, Wood KL, Winer-Muram HT, et al: Pulmonary cryptococcosis after initiation of anti-tumor necrosis factor-alpha therapy. Chest 2003;124:2395-2397.
135. Wood KL, Hage CA, Knox KS, et al: Histoplasmosis after treatment with anti-tumor necrosis factor-alpha therapy. Am J Respir Crit Care Med 2003;167:1279-1282.
136. Weiss SM, Hert RC, Gianola FJ, et al: Complications of fiberoptic bronchoscopy in thrombocytopenic patients. Chest 1993;104:1025-1028.
137. Cordasco EM Jr, Mehta AC, Ahmad M: Bronchoscopically induced bleeding: A summary of nine years' Cleveland clinic experience and review of the literature. Chest 1991;100:1141-1147.
138. Feldman NT, Huber GL: Fiberoptic bronchoscopy in the intensive care unit. Int Anesthesiol Clin 1976;14:31-42.
139. Jolliet P, Chevrolet JC: Bronchoscopy in the intensive care unit. Intensive Care Med 1992;18:160-169.
140. Anzueto A, Levine SM, Jenkinson SG: The technique of fiberoptic bronchoscopy: Diagnostic and therapeutic uses in intubated, ventilated patients. J Crit Illness 1992;7:1657-1664.
141. Brandstetter RD, Croce SA, Schiaffino E, et al: Flexible fiberoptic bronchoscopy in the elderly. N Y State J Med 1984;84:546-548.
142. Pereira W Jr, Kovnat DM, Snider GL: A prospective cooperative study of complications following flexible fiberoptic bronchoscopy. Chest 1978;73:813-816.
143. Bechara R, Beamis J, Simoff M, et al: Practice and complications of flexible bronchoscopy with biopsy procedures. J Bronchol 2005;12:139-142.
144. Lindholm CE, Ollman B, Snyder J, et al: Flexible fiberoptic bronchoscopy in critical care medicine: Diagnosis, therapy and complications. Crit Care Med 1974;2:250-261.

Chapter 13

Noninvasive Respiratory Monitoring

Amal Jubran and Martin J. Tobin

Various devices are available for effective and noninvasive monitoring of the patient's gas exchange function, respiratory neuromuscular capacity, and respiratory mechanics. Such measurements are helpful in characterizing the pathophysiology of an underlying respiratory disorder, tracking the course of illness and the effects of treatment, minimizing the risk of complications, and determining the patient's readiness for the withdrawal of therapeutic interventions and support devices.

Advances in respiratory monitoring continue to occur in terms of technological improvements and in enhancing current understanding of the pathophysiology of respiratory failure.[1] It is estimated that 20% to 40% of patients in intensive care units (ICUs) are admitted solely for the purposes of monitoring and do not receive any treatment that is unique to the ICU.[2]

GAS EXCHANGE

The human eye is poor at recognizing hypoxemia.[3,4] With the availability of pulse oximetry, episodic hypoxemia has been found to be more common than was previously suspected, with an incidence ranging from 20% to 82%.[5] Patients experiencing hypoxemia have a three-fold higher risk of death compared with patients who do not display desaturations.[6] Whether earlier detection and treatment of episodic hypoxemia can affect patient outcome is not known.

Pulse Oximetry

Pulse oximeters determine oxygen (O_2) saturation by measuring light absorption of arterial blood at two specific wavelengths, 660 nm (red) and 940 nm (infrared).[5,7] The ratio of absorbencies at these two wavelengths is calibrated empirically against direct measurements of arterial blood oxygen saturation (Sa_{O_2}), and the resulting calibration algorithm is used to generate the pulse oximeter's estimate of arterial saturation (Sp_{O_2}).[7] In addition to the digital readout of O_2 saturation, most pulse oximeters display a plethysmographic waveform, which can help clinicians distinguish an artifactual signal from the true signal[8] (Fig. 13-1).

Accuracy

The accuracy of commercially available oximeters in critically ill patients has been validated in several studies.[9] Compared with the measurement standard (multiwavelength oximeter), pulse oximeters have a mean difference (bias) of less than 1% and a standard deviation (precision) of less than 2% when Sa_{O_2} is 90% or above.[8] Although pulse oximetry is accurate in reflecting one-point measurements of Sa_{O_2}, it does not reliably predict changes in Sa_{O_2}. In 1085 simultaneous measurements of Sa_{O_2} and Sp_{O_2} in 41 ICU patients, changes in Sa_{O_2} correlated moderately with changes in Sp_{O_2} ($r = 0.6$), and the pulse oximeter tended to overestimate actual changes in Sa_{O_2}.[10]

The accuracy of pulse oximeters deteriorates when Sa_{O_2} falls to 80% or less[11] (Fig. 13-2). In critically ill patients, poor agreement between the oximeter and a CO-oximeter was observed, with bias ranging from −12% to 18%; and oximetry tended to systematically underestimate Sa_{O_2} when it was less than 80%.[12]

Limitations

Oximeters have a number of limitations that may lead to inaccurate readings (Box 13-1). Pulse oximeters measure Sa_{O_2}, which is physiologically related to arterial oxygen tension (Pa_{O_2}) according to the O_2 dissociation curve. Because the dissociation curve has a sigmoid shape, oximetry is relatively insensitive in detecting hypoxemia in patients with high baseline levels of Pa_{O_2}.[8,13]

Pulse oximeters use only two wavelengths of light; accordingly, they can discriminiate only two substances, oxyhemoglobin and reduced hemoglobin. Elevated carboxyhemoglobin and methemoglobin levels can

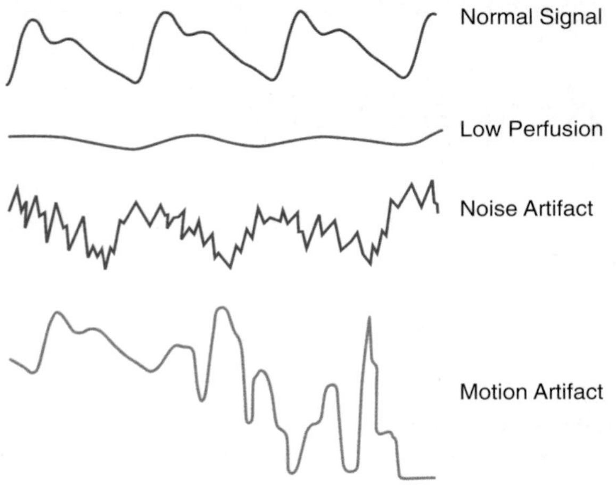

Figure 13-1. Common pulsatile signals on a pulse oximeter. *Top tracing,* Normal signal showing the sharp waveform with a clear dicrotic notch. *Second tracing,* Pulsatile signal during low perfusion showing a typical sine wave. *Third tracing,* Pulsatile signal with superimposed noise artifact giving a jagged appearance. *Bottom tracing,* Pulsatile signal during motion artifact showing an erratic waveform. (From Jubran A: Pulse oximetry. In Tobin MJ [ed]: Principles and Practice of Intensive Care Monitoring. New York, McGraw-Hill, 1998, pp 261-287.)

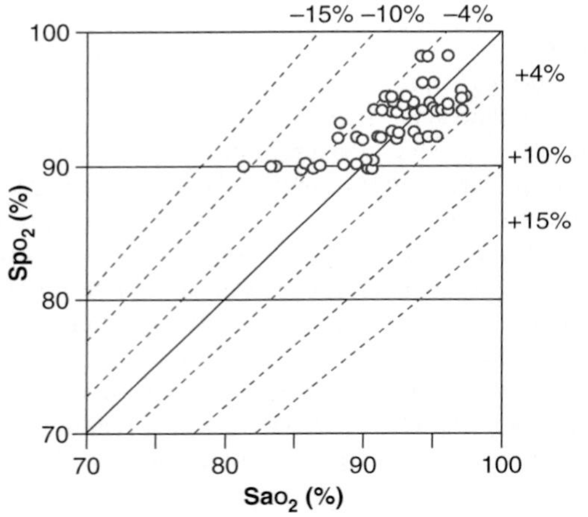

Figure 13-2. Arterial oxygen saturation (SaO_2) versus oxygen saturation measured by pulse oximetry (SpO_2) in patients receiving mechanical ventilation. The *solid line* is the line of identity and the *dashed lines* are isopleths of different levels of bias. Accuracy of pulse oximetry deteriorates when SaO_2 is less than 90%. (From Jubran A, Tobin MJ: Reliability of pulse oximetry in titrating supplemental oxygen therapy in ventilator-dependent patients. Chest 1990;97:1420-1425, with permission.)

therefore cause inaccurate oximetry readings.[14-17] Anemia does not appear to affect the accuracy of pulse oximetry.[18,19]

Intravenous dyes such as methylene blue, indocyanine green, and indigo carmine can cause falsely low SpO_2 readings, an effect that persists for up to 20 minutes.[20] Nail polish, if blue, green, or black, causes inaccurate SpO_2 readings,[21,22] although acrylic nails do not interfere with readings.[23] Falsely low and falsely high SpO_2 readings occur with fluorescent and xenon arc surgical lamps.[24]

Box 13-1

Limitations of Pulse Oximetry

Physiologic limitations
- Shape of oxyhemoglobin dissociation curve

Interference from substances
- Dyshemoglobins: carboxyhemoglobin, methemoglobin
- Dyes
- Nail polish
- Ambient light
- Skin pigmentation

Limitation in signal processing
- Low-perfusion state
- Motion artifact
- False alarms

Limitation in knowledge of the technique

Skin pigmentation can affect the accuracy of pulse oximetry.[25,26] In critically ill patients,[11] bias plus precision was greater in black patients, 3.3 + 2.7%, than in white patients, 2.2 + 1.8%; also, a bias greater than 4% occurred more frequently in black patients (27%) than in the white patients (11%).

Low-perfusion states, such as low cardiac output, vasoconstriction, and hypothermia, may impair peripheral perfusion, making it difficult for a sensor to distinguish a true signal from background noise. In patients experiencing hypothermia and poor perfusion during cardiac surgery, only 2 of 20 oximeters (Criticare CSI 503, Datex Satlite, Helsinki, Finland) provided measurements within +4% of the CO-oximeter value.[27] Measurements of SpO_2 with a Biox 3700 oximeter had an associated bias greater than ±4% in 37% of patients receiving vasoactive therapy.[28]

Motion artifact is a frustrating problem, and it results in inaccurate readings and false alarms. Patient motion is a common reason for temporary or definitive abandonment of pulse oximetry in a particular patient. An innovative technological approach, termed Masimo Signal Extraction Technology (SET), was introduced to extract the true signal from artifact secondary to noise and low perfusion[29] (Fig. 13-3). In 18 healthy volunteers, investigators recently compared the latest generation of pulse oximeters—Masimo SET (Irvine, Calif), Nellcor OxismartXL (Pleasanton, Calif), Philips Medical Systems FAST-SpO_2 (Andover, Mass), Respironics Novametrix MARSpO_2 (Wallingford, Conn), and Siemens Oxisure (Danvers, Mass)—with an older model, Nellcor N-200, under conditions of low perfusion and motion.[9] Of the five new-generation oximeters, Masimo SET and Nellcor OxismartXL outperformed the other three devices in reducing nuisance alarms and ensuring alarm reliability. These two oximeters also were found to have better protection against light interference than the other three devices.

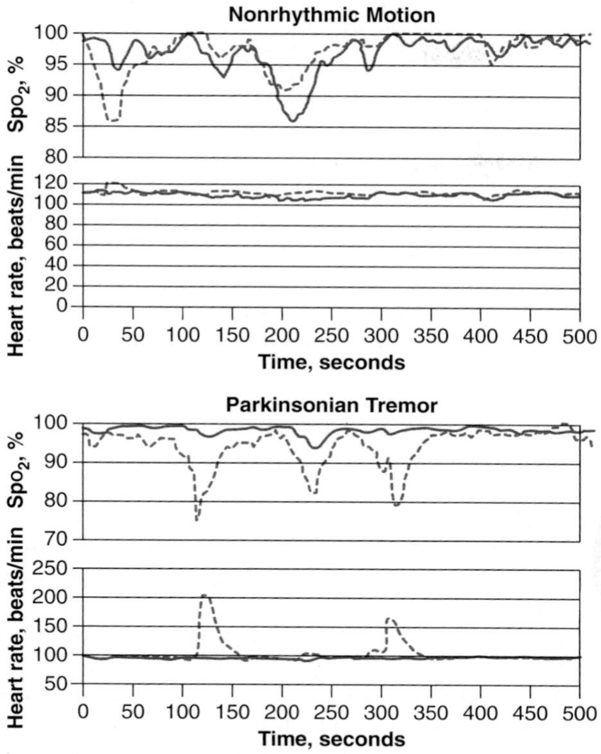

Figure 13-3. Pulse oximetry signals with motion artifact: *top panel,* recorded during nonrhythmic motion (i.e., gross arm motion); *lower panel,* recorded during Parkinsonian tremor. *Red line* denotes Masimo Signal Extraction Technology (SET), aimed at minimizing spurious pulse oximetry readings due to motion artifact; *blue line* denotes conventional pulse oximetry. Spurious changes in measured oxygen saturation (Spo_2) were less with Masimo SET than with conventional pulse oximetry. (From Dumas C, Wahr JA, Tremper KK: Clinical evaluation of a prototype motion artifact resistant pulse oximeter in the recovery room. Anesth Analg 1996;83:269-272.)

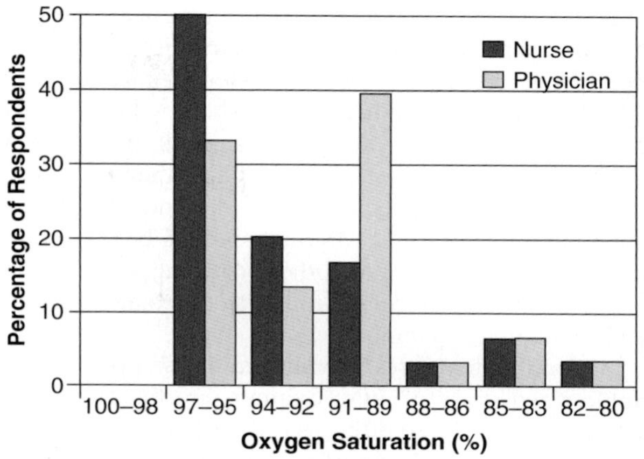

Figure 13-4. The lowest values for O_2 saturation measured by pulse oximetry (Spo_2) considered acceptable in a fit adult by a group of physicians and nurses. Spo_2 values less than 88% (equivalent to Pao_2 of less than 55 mm Hg) were considered acceptable by 27% of the respondents. The percentages represented by *bars* for each of the respondent groups add up to 100%. (Modified from Stoneham MD, Saville GM, Wilson IH: Knowledge about pulse oximetry among medical and nursing staff. Lancet 1994;344:1339-1342, with permission).

Despite their popularity for continuous monitoring of O_2 saturation, pulse oximeters fail to provide valid data in a variety of settings.[30-32] In a prospective study in ICU patients, Spo_2 signals accounted for almost half of a total of 2525 false alarms.[33] In 235 surgical ICU patients, a recent study revealed that false alarms from the pulse oximeter were secondary to low perfusion (21%), cardiac arrhythmias (9%), motion artifacts (8.4%), shivering (1.7%), and extubation (1.7%).[34]

An underrecognized and worrisome problem with pulse oximetry is that many users have a limited understanding of how the oximeter functions and the implications of the measurements obtained. One survey revealed that 30% of physicians and 93% of nurses thought that the oximeter measured Pao_2. Some clinicians did not recognize that Spo_2 values in the high 80s represent seriously low values of Pao_2. Of special concern was the observation that some doctors and nurses were not especially worried about patients with Spo_2 values as low as 80% (equivalent to Pao_2 less than 45 mm Hg)[35] (Fig. 13-4). A more recent audit also demonstrated a deficit in knowledge about the limitation of the technique. Although a majority of trained nurses and physicians were able to identify that shock and hypothermia can alter oximetry readings, less than 50% of nurses and physicians were able to identify that motion artifact, arrhythmias, and nail polish can affect the accuracy of pulse oximetry.[36]

Clinical Applications

With the introduction of pulse oximetry, hypoxemia (defined as an Spo_2 value less than 90%) is now detected more often in critically ill patients.[37] Changes in Spo_2 may not accurately reflect changes in Pao_2. Accordingly, caution is required in clinical decision making in critically ill patients based solely on pulse oximetry. Although pulse oximetry is a suitable way of measuring arterial oxygenation, it does not assess ventilation. Indeed, measurements of Spo_2 have been shown to be inaccurate in assessing abnormal pulmonary gas exchange, defined as an elevated alveolar-arterial O_2 difference.[5]

Pulse oximetry can assist with titration of fractional inspired oxygen concentration (F_IO_2) in ventilator-dependent patients, although the appropriate Spo_2 target depends on a patient's pigmentation.[11] The Spo_2 target value that predicts a satisfactory level of oxygenation is 92% in white patients and 95% in black patients.

Pulse oximetry has been evaluated as a means of screening for respiratory failure in patients with severe asthma.[38] Respiratory failure was unlikely in patients with Spo_2 greater than 92%. Of interest, this threshold value of 92% is the same target value that reliably predicted a satisfactory level of oxygenation during titration of F_IO_2 in ventilator-dependent patients.[11]

The use of pulse oximetry compared with other vital signs in predicting hospital complications from pulmonary embolus has been investigated.[39] In 207 patients with documented pulmonary embolism, a room-air Spo_2 value obtained in the emergency department was the most important predictor of death: The mortality rate was 2% in patients with Spo_2 95% or greater, versus 20% with Spo_2 less than 95%. When the threshold value was prospectively evaluated in 119 patients, in 10 of whom hospital complications developed, Spo_2 less than 95% had a sensitivity of 90%, specificity of 64%, and overall diagnostic accuracy of 67%. Although the number of patients with complications was low, these data suggest that pulse oximetry may be useful in predicting outcome in patients with pulmonary embolus.

Moller and associates[40] conducted the first prospective, randomized study of pulse oximetry on the outcome of anesthesia care in 20,802 surgical patients. Detection of hypoxemia (defined as an Spo_2 less than 90%) was 19-fold higher in the oximeter group than in the control group. Myocardial ischemia was more common in the control group than in the oximetry group, occurring in 26 and 12 patients, respectively. Pulse oximetry, however, did not decrease the rate of postoperative complications or mortality.

The lack of proven efficacy of pulse oximetry in the study of Moller and associates[40] was related to the sample size. These investigators concluded that it would take at least 500,000 patients to show a reduction in a rare event such as myocardial infarction, and 1,900,000 patients to show a reduction in anesthesia-related deaths. When anesthesiologists in the study were surveyed,[41] 80% of them reported feeling more secure when they used a pulse oximeter. Of 104 anesthesiologists, 19 believed that the pulse oximeter helped them avoid serious complications (such as esophageal intubation, tracheal tube disconnection or displacement, anesthesia machine failure, and respiratory problems immediately after extubation). It is this mindset that has established pulse oximetry as an essential component of the standard of care despite a failure to achieve a level of proven efficacy with a P value of less than .05. The lack of concurrence between randomized trial proof of efficacy of pulse oximetry and its requirement as part of the standard of care has major ramifications for all monitoring techniques.[1]

Cost-Effectiveness

Studies evaluating the cost-effectiveness of pulse oximetry have reported that fewer arterial blood gas (ABG) samples were obtained if Spo_2 data were available to the caregivers.[42-44] The effect of implementing pulse oximetry in an ICU without any specific plan for its appropriate use was examined in 148 patients before the implementation of oximetry and 141 patients after its implementation.[45] The number of ABG samples decreased from 7.2 to 6.4 per patient per day—a reduction of only 10.3%, compared with average reductions of 39% in the previous studies.[5] This suggests that without explicit guidelines, the pulse oximeter was used in addition to, rather than instead of, blood gas sampling.

Pulse oximetry probably constitutes one of the most important advances in respiratory monitoring. The major challenge facing pulse oximetry is whether this technology can be incorporated effectively into diagnostic and management algorithms that improve the efficiency of clinical management in the ICU.

Transcutaneous Blood Gas Monitoring

Transcutaneous measurements of O_2 tension ($Ptco_2$) are made by placing a heated Clark polarographic electrode directly on the skin and measuring the O_2 that diffuses from the blood to the skin.[46] This technique more commonly is used by neonatologists because neonatal skin is thin, so $Ptco_2$ values approximate Pao_2 values. In a multicenter study including 251 patients of various ages (range, 4 weeks to 60 years), $Ptco_2/Pao_2$ ratio was 1.05 in neonates and 0.93 in older patients when Pao_2 was less than 80 mm Hg. This ratio, however, decreased to 0.88 in neonates and 0.74 in older patients when the Pao_2 was greater than 80 mm Hg.[47] During low-perfusion states, $Ptco_2$ measurements do not reflect changes in Pao_2. In critically ill patients, the $Ptco_2/Pao_2$ ratio decreased from 0.79 ± 0.12 (SD) when cardiac index was greater than 2.2 L/min/m^2 to 0.12 ± 12 when cardiac index was less than 1.5 L/min/m^2.[48]

Transcutaneous monitoring of the partial pressure of carbon dioxide ($Ptcco_2$) can be performed using a modified Severinghaus electrode. The underlying skin is heated to 44°C to enhance CO_2 diffusion through the skin. Heating also increases the local production of CO_2, with the result that transcutaneous Pco_2 values usually are higher than arterial Pco_2 ($Paco_2$) values.[48] Because of greater diffusibility of CO_2 compared with O_2 through the skin, the correlation of $Ptcco_2$ with $Paco_2$ usually is good: $r = 0.93$.[47]

The accuracy of $Ptcco_2$ as a surrogate measure for $Paco_2$ was recently evaluated in 50 critically ill patients in a medical ICU.[49] Of the 189 paired measures of Pco_2 obtained, 21 were excluded from analysis because of profound skin vasoconstriction. Of the available 168 measurements, mean difference between $Paco_2$ and $Ptcco_2$ was -0.2 ± 4.6 mm Hg; correlation between two measurements was 0.92. A strong correlation was observed between changes in $Paco_2$ and $Ptcco_2$ ($R^2 = 0.78$) (Fig. 13-5). These data suggest that transcutaneous Pco_2 may be reliable in monitoring changes in arterial Pco_2, provided that no major vasoconstriction is present.

Capnography

The carbon dioxide concentration at the end of a tidal breath—end-tidal CO_2—can be employed as a continuous, indirect measure of $Paco_2$ (Fig. 13-6). In intubated patients with respiratory failure, correlation between end-tidal CO_2 and $Paco_2$ was good ($r = 0.78$).[50] The correlation between changes in end-tidal CO_2 and changes in $Paco_2$ from baseline, however, was considerably weaker ($r = 0.58$). Change in end-tidal CO_2 incorrectly indicated the direction of change in $Paco_2$ in 43% of patients being weaned from mechanical ventilation after cardiac surgery.[51]

Capnometry commonly is used in detecting esophageal intubation.[52-54] When the trachea of a patient with an intact pulmonary circulation is intubated, end-tidal CO_2 is recorded. When, however, the endotracheal tube is

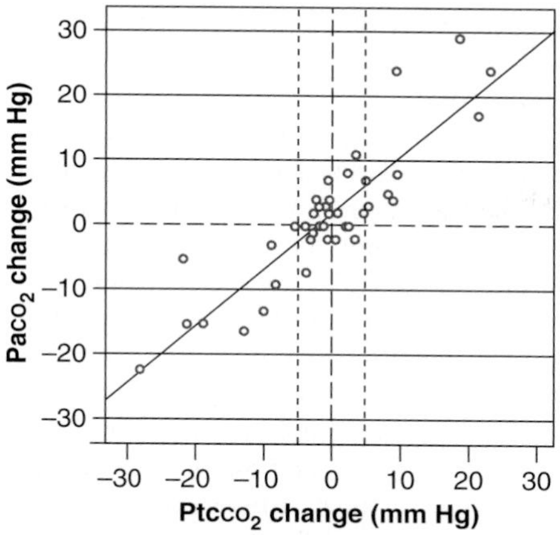

Figure 13-5. Change in transcutaneous P_{CO_2} ($Ptcco_2$) versus change in arterial P_{CO_2} ($Paco_2$) in 40 samples. The *solid line* represents the linear regression equation ($R^2 = 0.78$); *broken lines* represent $Ptcco_2$ values at 0, +5, and −5 mm Hg. Note that a mismatch between changes in $Ptcco_2$ and $Paco_2$ (transcutaneous changes were positive while arterial changes were negative, or vice versa) occurred in 8 of the 40 values (22%). (Modified from Rodriguez P, Lellouche F, Aboab J, et al: Transcutaneous arterial carbon dioxide pressure monitoring in critically ill adult patients. Intensive Care Med 2006;32:309-312, with permission.)

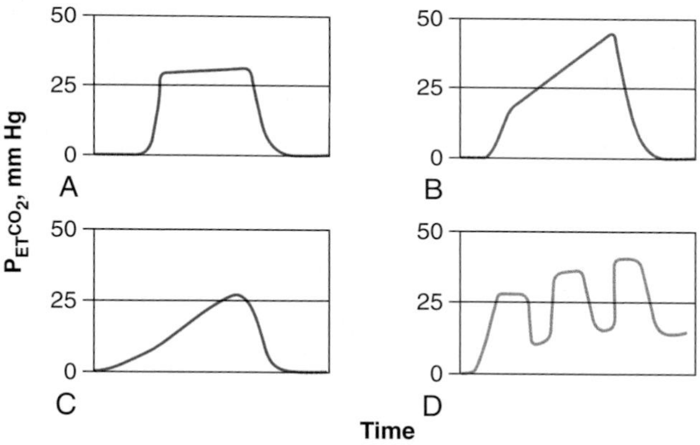

Figure 13-6. A, Normal capnograph. During inspiration, the CO_2 level is 0 mm Hg. The P_{CO_2} rises sharply during expiration to reach a smooth plateau. The P_{CO_2} at the end of the plateau is the end-tidal P_{CO_2} ($P_{ET}CO_2$). **B,** The capnograph in a patient with airflow obstruction demonstrating the lack of a plateau. **C,** The capnograph in a patient with an obstructed endotracheal tube, exhibiting a gradual increase in $Paco_2$ during expiration while the end-tidal P_{CO_2} ($P_{ET}CO_2$) value remains unaffected. **D,** The capnograph in a patient who is rebreathing previously expired gas; note the increase in both inspired and expired P_{CO_2}. (From Jubran A, Tobin MJ: Monitoring gas exchange during mechanical ventilation. In Tobin MJ [ed]: Principles and Practice of Mechanical Ventilation. New York, McGraw-Hill, 1994, p 919.)

erroneously placed in the esophagus, end-tidal CO_2 will be zero. Monitoring of end-tidal CO_2 has been compared with three other methods—auscultation, negative-pressure testing using a self-inflating bulb, and transillumination—for verifying tracheal tube placement.[55] Monitoring of end-tidal CO_2 was found to be the most reliable.

RESPIRATORY NEUROMUSCULAR FUNCTION

Airway Occlusion Pressure

Measuring airway pressure 0.1 second after initiation of an inspiratory effort against airway occlusion ($P_{0.1}$) provides a measure of respiratory drive. In ventilator-dependent patients, $P_{0.1}$ has been shown to correlate significantly with work of breathing during pressure-support ventilation ($r = 0.87$).[56] By taking advantage of the decrease in airway pressure to open the demand valve during triggering, investigators have demonstrated that commercially available ventilators can measure $P_{0.1}$ accurately.[57] Several studies[57-59] have indicated that an elevated $P_{0.1}$ predicted weaning failure, but the threshold separating success from failure differed among the studies.[60]

Maximal Inspiratory Airway Pressure

Maximum inspiratory pressure (PImax), a global measure of inspiratory muscle strength, is measured using a one-way valve that allows exhalation but prevents inhalation.[61,62] PImax is one of the standard measurements employed to determine a need for the continuation of mechanical ventilation. Values that are more negative than −30 cm H_2O are considered to predict weaning success; values that are less negative than −20 cm H_2O are predictive of weaning failure. These criteria, however, frequently are falsely positive and falsely negative.[63]

Breathing Pattern

Rapid shallow breathing is a common respiratory pattern in patients who fail a trial of weaning from mechanical ventilation,[64] and this can be quantitated in terms of the frequency–to–tidal volume ratio (f/V_T). The higher the f/V_T, the more pronounced the rapid, shallow breathing and the greater the likelihood of unsuccessful weaning. An f/V_T above 100 breaths per minute per liter suggests that a trial of weaning is unlikely to be successful.[63] When prospectively evaluated, f/V_T was found to be superior to nine other weaning predictors: sensitivity was 0.97, specificity 0.64, positive predictive value 0.78, and negative predictive value 0.95.[60]

The usefulness of f/V_T in predicting weaning outcome was recently challenged. Using a meta-analysis, an American College of Chest Physicians (ACCP) Task Force concluded that f/V_T was unreliable.[65,66] In their evaluation of published reports on f/V_T, the Task Force ignored the important influence of pre-test probability on the interpretation of a test results. The implications of pre-test probability are greater for weaning than for many clinical situations because weaning involves a sequence of three diagnostic tests: measurement of predictors, followed by a weaning trial, followed by an extubation trial. The undertaking of three diagnostic tests in a sequential manner poses an enormous risk for the occurrence of test referral and spectrum bias. The introductions of such biases, will, in turn, increase the pre-test probability.[67,68] Indeed, the mean pre-test probability of weaning success was 75% in the studies included in the meta-analysis.

When data from studies included in the Task Force meta-analysis were entered into a bayesian model with pre-test probability as the operating point, the observed post-test probabilities were closely correlated with the values predicted by the original study on f/V_T: $r = 0.86$ for positive predictive value and $r = 0.82$ for negative predictive value.[69]

It has been suggested that measurements of f/V_T at 30 minutes into a weaning trial more accurately predict outcome than measurements in the first minute.[70,71] Although it is true that including data for the first 30 seconds or so may be unrepresentative, this does not mean that it takes 30 minutes to establish a steady state.

Jubran and colleagues[72] studied the time required for f/V_T to reach a point of equilibration in 17 "weaning failure" and 14 "weaning success" patients. The median time (plus interquartile range) to reach +10% of the final value of f/V_T was 2 (1 to 2) minutes in both the weaning success and the weaning failure patients (Fig. 13-7). Within 2 minutes of the onset of the T-tube trial, 77% of the weaning failure patients and 73% of the weaning success patients had reached +10% of the final value of f/V_T. As indicated by these data, a reasonable strategy is to commence measurement of f/V_T at 60 seconds after removal of the ventilator and then continue the measurement for another 60 seconds.

Continuous recording of breathing pattern provides an important approach for assessing the ability of the respiratory controller to maintain or adjust its response over time. Simple measurements, such as coefficients of variation, indicate that healthy subjects display considerable variation in tidal volume and respiratory cycle time from one breath to the next.[73] Signal analysis techniques reveal that this variability is composed of random and nonrandom fractions.[74-79] The predominantly random character of the variability makes it possible for the respiratory system to engage in tasks other than gas exchange. A smaller fraction of variability is nonrandom; moreover, tidal volume and respiratory cycle time of one breath are significantly related to those of the preceding breath.[74,75,77,78] When healthy subjects are faced with external chemical or mechanical loads, however, the random fraction decreases significantly.[75,77,78] This decrease in random variability may lessen the freedom of the respiratory system to undertake behavioral tasks.[77,78,80]

Using autocorrelation analysis and fast-Fourier transformation, Brack and associates[81] showed that patients with restrictive lung disease display a marked decrease in breath-to-breath variability of breathing. The random fraction of variability was approximately $\frac{1}{27}$ of that found in healthy subjects, and the nonrandom correlated fraction was as much as 3 times higher in the patients. Slight variations from the average resting tidal volume caused large increases in dyspnea in the patients, but not in the healthy subjects[81] (Fig. 13-8). In patients undergoing a weaning

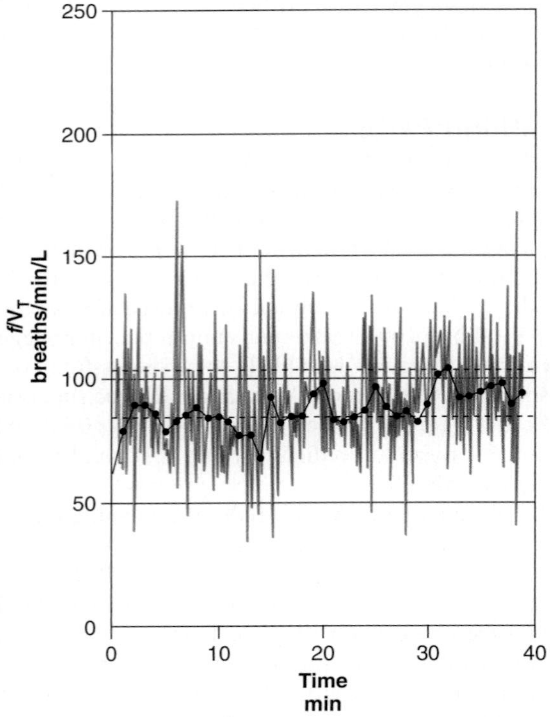

Figure 13-7. Time-series plot of frequency–to–tidal volume ratio (f/V_T) during a T-tube trial of spontaneous breathing in a weaning failure patient. *Black dots* represent 1-minute averages. The *solid line* indicates the average value of f/V_T of the final minute of the trial. The *dashed horizontal lines* indicate +10% of the final minute values of f/V_T. The time taken to reach +10% of the final value of f/V_T was 2 minutes. (From Jubran A, Grant BJ, Laghi F, et al: Weaning prediction: Esophageal pressure monitoring complements readiness testing. Am J Respir Crit Care Med 2005;171:1252-1259, with permission).

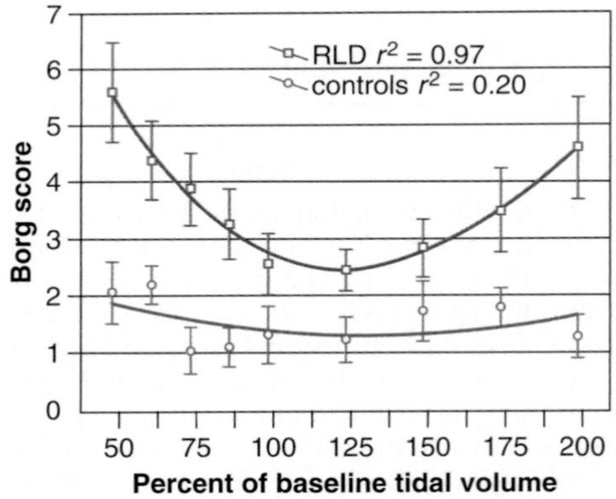

Figure 13-8. The relationship between variation in tidal volume and dyspnea (Borg score) in patients with restrictive lung disease (RLD) and in control subjects. Dyspnea scores were higher in the patients than in the control subjects ($P < .01$, ANOVA); dyspnea varied with tracked volume in the patients ($P < .05$, ANOVA) but not in the control group. The regression between dyspnea and tidal volume was parabolic in the patients ($y = 10.3 - 0.12x + 0.0005x^2$; $P < .0001$), but not in the control subjects ($y = 2.76 - 0.02x + 0.00008x^2$; $P = .5$). *Bars* represent ± SEM. ANOVA, analysis of variance; SEM, standard error of the mean. (From Brack T, Jubran A, Tobin MJ: Dyspnea and decreased variability of breathing in patients with restrictive lung disease. Am J Respir Crit Care Med 2002;165:1260-1264, with permission.)

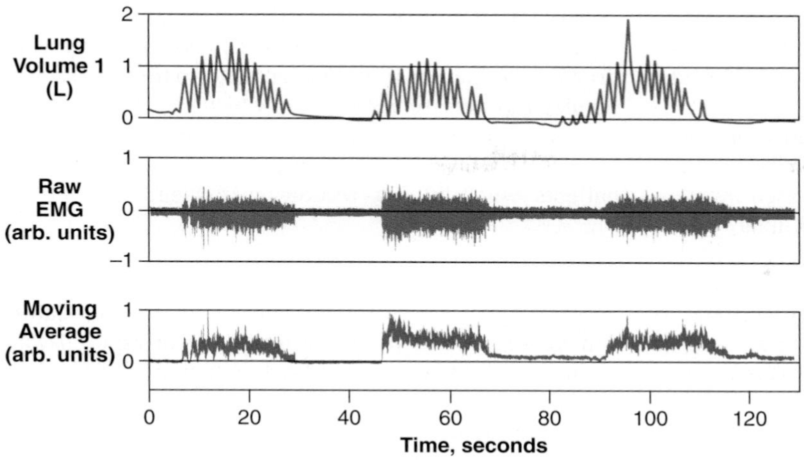

Figure 13-9. Changes in lung volume measured by inductive plethysmography *(top tracing),* raw electromyographic signal of scalene muscle activity (EMG) *(middle tracing),* and moving time average *(bottom, integrated signal)* during three consecutive cycles of Cheyne-Stokes breathing in a representative patient. Note the repeated increases in end-expiratory lung volume with each hyperpnea. (From Brack T, Jubran A, Laghi F, Tobin MJ: Fluctuations in end-expiratory lung volume during Cheyne-Stokes respiration. Am J Respir Crit Care Med 2005;17(112):1408-1413, with permission.)

trial, Wysocki and coworkers[82] recently noted a higher gross variability of breathing (quantitated in terms of coefficient of variation) in patients who were successfully weaned than in patients who failed the trial. These data suggest that an increase in the ability to vary breathing may be associated with a favorable weaning outcome.[83]

Changes in End-Expiratory Lung Volume

Alterations in the end-expiratory level of signal from an inductive plethysmograph can provide a measurement of the change in functional residual capacity provided that motion artifact is absent[84,85] (Fig. 13-9). Inductive plethysmography has been used to estimate a patient's level of auto-PEEP.[50] By noting the level of external PEEP at which end-expiratory lung volume increased, a close estimate of the patient's original level of auto-PEEP can be obtained. An attractive feature of this technique is that it does not disturb expiration, unlike the occlusive technique, in which foreshortening of expiratory time is unavoidable.[86]

RESPIRATORY MECHANICS

Measurements of respiratory mechanics in a relaxed ventilator-dependent patient can be obtained using the technique of rapid airway occlusion during constant-flow inflation.[87] Rapid airway occlusion at the end of a passive inflation produces an immediate drop in both airway pressure (P_{aw}) and transpulmonary pressure (P_L) from a peak value (P_{peak}) to a lower initial value (P_{init}), followed by a gradual decrease until a plateau (P_{plat}) is achieved after 3 to 5 seconds[88,89] (Fig. 13-10). P_{plat} on the Paw, P_L, and Pes tracings represents the static end-inspiratory recoil pressure of the total respiratory system, lung, and chest wall, respectively.

Elastance (Compliance)

The end-inspiratory airway occlusion method is used clinically to measure the static compliance, or its reciprocal, elastance, of the respiratory system ($E_{st,rs}$) according to the following equation[90]:

$$E_{st,rs} = P_{plat} - PEEP_{tot}/V_T$$

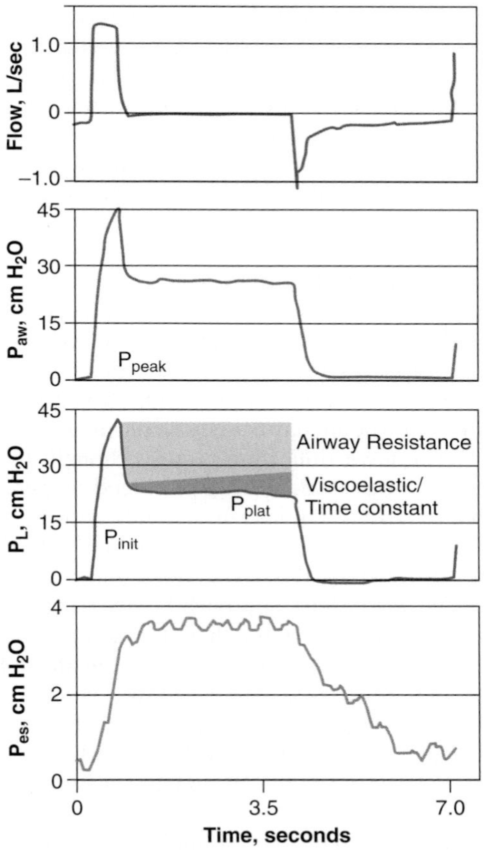

Figure 13-10. Flow (inspiration upward), airway pressure (P_{aw}), transpulmonary pressure (P_L), and esophageal pressure (P_{es}) tracings in a representative patient during passive ventilation. An end-inspiratory occlusion produced a rapid decline in both P_{aw} and P_L from a peak value (P_{peak}) to a lower initial pressure (P_{init}), followed by gradual decrease to a plateau pressure (P_{plat}). P_{plat} on the P_{aw}, P_L, and P_{es} tracings represents the static end-inspiratory recoil pressures of the total respiratory system, lung, and chest wall, respectively. Using this technique, total resistance can be partitioned into ohmic airway resistance and tissue resistance, which reflects the viscoelastic properties (stress relaxation) and time-constant inhomogeneities within the respiratory tissues. (Modified from Jubran A, Tobin MJ: Passive mechanics of lung and chest wall in patients who failed and succeeded in trials of weaning. Am J Respir Crit Care Med 1997;155:916-921, with permission.)

where P_{plat} is plateau pressure obtained after occlusion of the airway, $PEEP_{tot}$ is the sum of external and intrinsic positive end-expiratory pressures if present, and VT is tidal volume (see Fig. 13-10).

Mechanical ventilation in itself can produce or aggravate lung injury in patients with acute respiratory distress syndrome (ARDS).[91-93] Injury may be decreased by minimizing alveolar overdistention. To avoid lung injury, ideally the alveolar volume should be monitored, but that is not possible. Alveolar volume is reflected by peak alveolar pressure, which can be assessed indirectly by measuring the plateau pressure during an end-inspiratory hold maneuver. It has been recommended that plateau pressure not exceed 32 cm H_2O.[94,95]

A new era of ventilatory management began in 1990, when a report demonstrated that lowering tidal volume caused a 60% decrease in the expected mortality rate among patients with ARDS.[96] Subsequently, randomized trials were undertaken.[97-100] In 861 patients, the ARDS Network investigators reported a 22% difference in mortality rates with use of a tidal volume of 6 mL/kg versus 12 mL/kg.[101] It is now generally accepted that the use of high tidal volumes in patients with ARDS is associated with high mortality rates.[94,102] Whether the use of low tidal volumes infers a survival advantage is controversial.[102-104]

Pressure-Volume Curves

A pressure-volume curve of the respiratory system in a paralyzed patient can be constructed by measuring the airway pressure as the lungs are progressively inflated with a 1.5- to 2-L syringe. A lower inflection point and an upper inflection point may be seen on the pressure-volume curve.[105] The lower inflection point is thought to reflect the point at which small airways or alveoli reopen, corresponding to closing volume. In patients with acute lung injury, investigators have recommended that PEEP be set at a pressure slightly above the lower inflection point.[106]

When an "open-lung approach," consisting of use of a lower tidal volume (less than 6 mL/kg) with PEEP individually titrated to be consistently above the inflection point on the pressure-volume curve, was compared with a conventional approach, consisting of use of tidal volume of 12 mL/kg and a low PEEP level, the mortality rate was significantly reduced in the group managed with the new approach.[107,108]

An NIH-sponsored trial of high versus low PEEP, however, failed to demonstrate a significant survival advantage for patients randomized to the high PEEP group.[109] Several methodologic considerations cast doubt on the conclusions of the investigators.[110] First, baseline characteristics of the two groups were not balanced; the low PEEP group patients had higher PaO_2/F_IO_2 ratios and were younger than patients in the high PEEP group. Second, PEEP-induced recruitment was estimated by improvement in oxygenation. It is well known that changes in oxygenation depend not only on recruitment but also on cardiac output.[111] Thus, oxygenation may have improved without any lung recruitment. Third, recruitment potential was not stratified, so that patients who were not likely to benefit were assigned to both groups.[112]

The importance of individualizing PEEP in ventilator management in patients with ARDS was recently confirmed in a Spanish trial. One group of patients was randomized to a treatment group in which PEEP was titrated to 2 cm H_2O above the lower inflection point. The mortality rate was lower in these patients than in control group patients who did not receive customized titration of PEEP.[113]

Resistance

Airway resistance can be measured in ventilator-dependent patients using the technique of rapid airway occlusion during constant-flow inflation[87,88,90,114] (see Fig. 13-10).

Measurements of airway resistance are helpful in assessing the response of patients to bronchodilator therapy. In a study in ventilator-dependent patients with COPD, a significant decrease in airway resistance occurred after giving 4 puffs, with no additional effect after the addition of 8 and 16 puffs (cumulative doses of 12 and 28 puffs).[115,116]

Intrinsic Positive End-Expiratory Pressure

The static recoil pressure of the respiratory system at end-expiration may be elevated in patients receiving mechanical ventilation.[90] This positive recoil pressure, or intrinsic PEEP (static $PEEP_i$), can be quantified in relaxed patients using an end-expiratory hold maneuver on a mechanical ventilator immediately before the onset of the next breath[117] (Fig. 13-11), or as a change in P_{aw} required to reduce expiratory flow to zero and initiate lung inflation

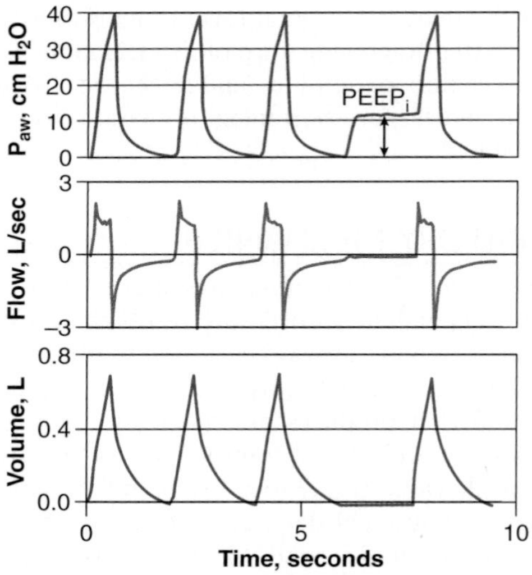

Figure 13-11. Recordings of airway pressure (P_{aw}), flow, and volume in a patient receiving controlled mechanical ventilation. After the third breath, the airway was occluded at end-expiration using the end-expiratory hold function on the ventilator. During the period of zero flow, pressure in the alveoli and in the ventilator circuit equilibrates, and the plateau pressure reflects auto- or intrinsic positive end-expiratory pressure ($PEEP_i$), indicated by the *arrow.* (From Tobin MJ, Van de Graaff WB: Monitoring of lung mechanics and work of breathing. In Tobin MJ [ed]: Principles and Practice of Mechanical Ventilation. New York, McGraw-Hill, 1994, pp 967-1003.

by the ventilator (dynamic $PEEP_i$). In patients with COPD, dynamic $PEEP_i$ is lower than static $PEEP_i$; this discrepancy is attributed to the presence of time-constant inequalities.[118,119]

$PEEP_i$ poses a significant inspiratory threshold load that has to be fully counterbalanced by increasing inspiratory muscle effort in order to generate a negative pressure in the central airway and trigger the ventilator. Thus, $PEEP_i$ adds to the triggering pressure such that the total inspiratory effort needed to trigger the ventilator is the set trigger sensitivity plus the level of $PEEP_i$. This is one of the factors that may account for the not infrequent observation of a patient who is unable to trigger a ventilator despite obvious respiratory effort[120-122] (Fig. 13-12).

In a study of ventilator-dependent patients, Leung and colleagues[122] reported that ineffective triggering occurred with all assisted modes of mechanical ventilation. The ineffective or wasted efforts were significantly related to resistance ($r = 0.85$), elastance ($r = -0.61$) and static $PEEP_i$ ($r = 0.77$). A decrease in the magnitude of inspiratory effort at a given level of assistance was not the cause—indeed, effort was 38% higher during nontriggering attempts than during the triggering phase of attempts that successfully opened the inspiratory valve. Significant differences, however, were observed in the breaths before the triggering and nontriggering attempts. Breaths before nontriggering attempts were associated with shorter respiratory cycle time and expiratory time and higher static $PEEP_i$ compared with the breaths before triggered attempts. These findings suggest that ineffective triggering resulted not from a decrease in the magnitude of effort but rather from inspiratory efforts that were premature and insufficient to overcome the elevated elastic recoil pressure associated with dynamic hyperinflation.

Airway Pressure Profile

A continuous recording of airway pressure provides helpful information about the amount of respiratory work being performed by a patient receiving ventilator assistance. Ideally the waveform should show a smooth rise with a convex appearance during inspiration.[1] By contrast, a prolonged negative phase with excessive scalloping of the tracing reflects increased inspiratory effort; this pattern indicates unsatisfactory sensitivity and inappropriate flow settings (Fig. 13-13). A "bump" on the airway pressure tracing observed while the ventilator is still pumping gas in the patient may reflect recruitment of expiratory muscles (Fig. 13-14).

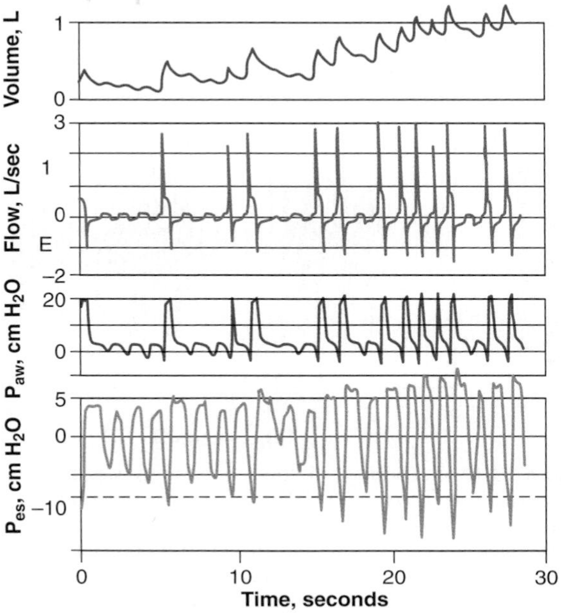

Figure 13-12. Recordings of tidal volume, flow, airway pressure (P_{aw}), and esophageal pressure (P_{es}) in a patient with chronic obstructive pulmonary disease receiving pressure support ventilation. Approximately half of the patient's inspiratory efforts do not succeed in triggering the ventilator. Triggering occurred only when the patient generated a P_{es} less than 8 cm H_2O (indicated by the *dashed line*), which was equal in magnitude to the opposing elastic recoil pressure. (From Tobin MJ, Jubran A: Pathophysiology of failure to wean from mechanical ventilation. Schweiz Med Wochenschr 1994;124:2139-2145.)

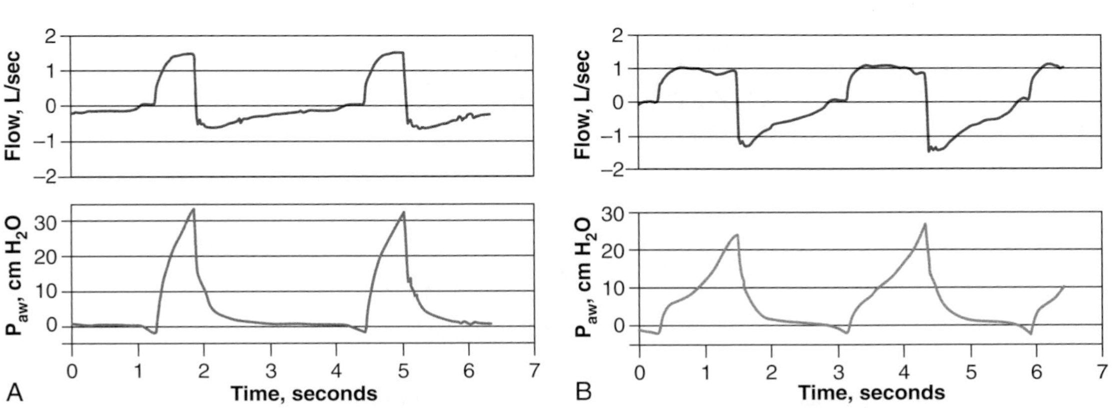

Figure 13-13. Flow and airway pressure (P_{aw}) during assist-control ventilation at different flow rates: 60 L/min **(A)** and 30 L/min **(B).** In **A,** the small negative phase coupled with the smooth rise and convex appearance of the P_{aw} waveform indicates that the patient is making a slight inspiratory effort to breathe. In **B,** the more pronounced negative phase together with excessive scalloping of the P_{aw} waveform indicates that the patient is making a strenuous effort to breathe as a result of the inadequate flow setting. (From Jubran A, Tobin MJ: Monitoring during mechanical ventilation. In Tobin MJ [ed]: Principles and Practice of Mechanical Ventilation. New York, McGraw-Hill, 2006, p 1051, with permission.)

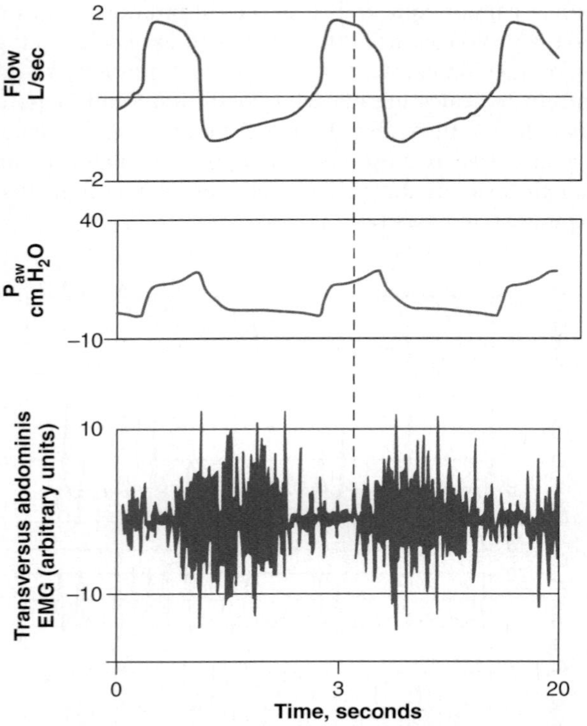

Figure 13-14. Recordings of flow (*top*) and airway pressure (P_{aw}; *middle*) and transversus abdominis electromyogram (EMG; *bottom*) in a critically ill patient with chronic obstructive pulmonary disease receiving pressure support of 20 cm H_2O. The onset of expiratory muscle activity *(vertical dotted line)* occurred when mechanical inflation was only partly completed. (From Parthasarathy S, Jubran A, Tobin MJ: Cycling of inspiratory and expiratory muscle groups with the ventilator in airflow limitation. Am J Respir Crit Care Med 1998;58:1471-1478, with permission.)

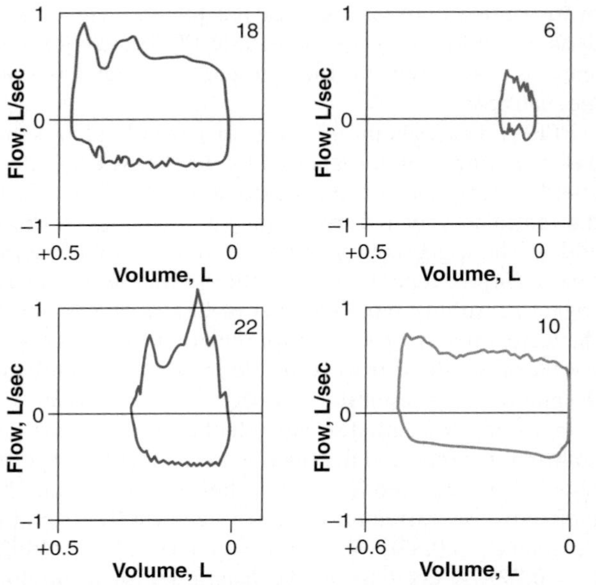

Figure 13-16. Flow-volume curves obtained in four patients with secretions. Note the presence of a sawtooth pattern on both the inspiratory and expiratory flow-volume curves. (The numbers to the *upper right* in each grid are the original patient numbers.) (From Jubran A, Tobin MJ: Use of flow-volume curves in detecting secretions in ventilator-dependent patients. Am J Respir Crit Care Med 1994;150:766-769.)

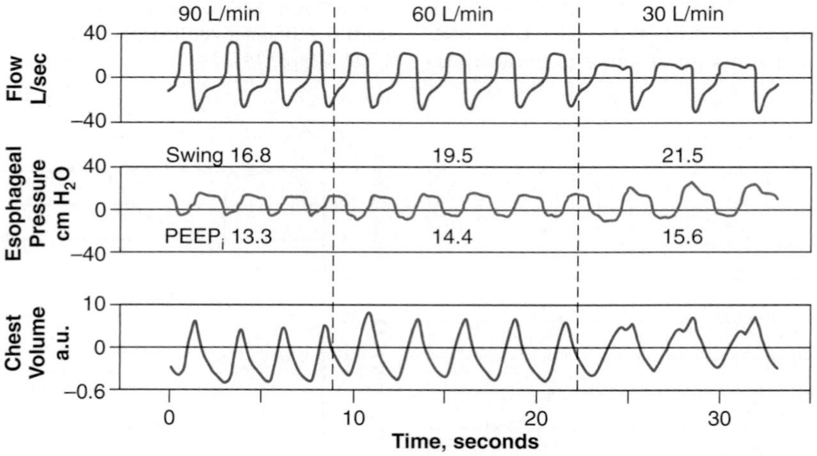

Figure 13-15. Continuous recordings of flow, esophageal pressure (P_{es}), and the sum of rib cage and abdominal motion in a patient with chronic obstructive pulmonary disease receiving assist-control ventilation at a constant tidal volume. As flow increased from 30 L/min to 60 and 90 L/min (from *right* to *left*), frequency increased (from 18 breaths per minute to 23 and 26 breaths per minute, respectively), $PEEP_i$ decreased (from 15.6 cm H_2O to 14.4 and 13.3 cm H_2O, respectively), and end-expiratory lung volume also fell. Increases in flow from 30 L/min to 60 and 90 L/min also led to decreases in the swings in P_{es} from 21.5 cm H_2O to 19.5 and 16.8 cm H_2O, respectively. a.u., arbitrary units; $PEEP_i$, intrinsic positive end-expiratory pressure. (From Laghi F, Segal J, Choe WK, Tobin MJ: Effect of imposed inflation time on respiratory frequency and hyperinflation in patients with chronic obstructive pulmonary disease. Am J Respir Crit Care Med 2001;163:1365, with permission.)

Use of a flow setting that does not meet a patient's ventilatory demands will cause inspiratory effort to increase. Sometimes the flow is increased to shorten the inspiratory time and increase the expiratory time. An increase in flow, however, can cause immediate and persistent tachypnea; if this happens, the resulting decrease in expiratory time may lead to intrinsic PEEP ($PEEP_i$).[123,124] In general, however, an increase in inspiratory flow does not lead to an increase in $PEEP_i$[124] (Fig. 13-15).

Flow-Volume Curves

Flow-volume curves also may be helpful in indicating a need for endotracheal suctioning. In 50 intubated patients, Jubran and Tobin[125] found that the presence of a sawtooth pattern strongly suggested the presence of secretions (positive predictive value, 94%), and the absence of this pattern suggested that secretions are unlikely to be present (negative predictive value, 77%) (Fig. 13-16). Clinical examination had much higher false-positive and false-negative rates (42% and 43%, respectively) than the flow-volume curves (12% and 14%, respectively). The usefulness of a sawtooth pattern for detecting secretions was confirmed by Guglielminotti and colleagues[126] in a study of 62 patients who were receiving pressure support or assist-control ventilation.

KEY POINTS

- Some 20% to 40% of patients in an ICU are admitted mainly for the purpose of monitoring.
- Pulse oximetry can accurately measure oxygen saturation at levels of 90% or above; its accuracy deteriorates when the saturation falls to 80% or less.
- Inaccurate readings from pulse oximetry can occur as a result of interference from substances or from problems in signal processing.
- Hypoxemia is detected more frequently in patients monitored with pulse oximetry than in patients in whom this modality is not used.
- Transcutaneous monitoring of P_{CO_2} may be reliable in monitoring changes in arterial P_{CO_2} in the absence of major vasoconstriction.
- Measuring airway pressure at 0.1 second after initiating an inspiratory effort against an occluded airway is closely associated with increased work of breathing during mechanical ventilation.
- One-time measurements of breathing pattern (frequency and tidal volume) are helpful in predicting weaning outcome; continuous measurements of breathing pattern can provide information about the function of the respiratory controller.
- Measurements of respiratory mechanics in a ventilator-dependent patient can be easily performed at the bedside using the rapid airway occlusion technique.
- Continuous recordings of airway pressure can provide useful information about the respiratory work performed by a patient receiving mechanical ventilation.
- Flow-volume curves may be helpful in indicating a need for endotracheal suctioning.

REFERENCES

1. Jubran A, Tobin MJ: Monitoring during mechanical ventilation. In Tobin MJ (ed): Principles and Practice of Mechanical Ventilation. New York, McGraw-Hill, 2006, pp 1051-1080.
2. Henning RJ, McClish D, Daly B, et al: Clinical characteristics and resource utilization of ICU patients: Implications for organization of intensive care. Crit Care Med 1987;15:264-269.
3. Comroe JH, Bothello S: The unreliability of cyanosis in the recognition of arterial anoxemia. Am J Med Sci 1947;214:1-9.
4. Mower WR, Sachs C, Nicklin EL, et al: Effect of routine emergency department triage pulse oximetry screening on medical management. Chest 1995;108:1297-1302.
5. Jubran A: Pulse oximetry. In: Tobin MJ (ed): Principles and Practice of Intensive Care Monitoring. New York, McGraw-Hill, 1998, pp 261-287.
6. Bowton DL, Scuderi PE, Haponik EF: The incidence and effect on outcome of hypoxemia in hospitalized medical patients. Am J Med 1994;97:38-46.
7. Wukitisch MW, Peterson MT, Tobler DR, Pologe JA: Pulse oximetry: Analysis of theory, technology, and practice. J Clin Monit 1988;4:290-301.
8. Jubran A: Pulse oximetry. Intensive Care Med 2004;30:2017-2020.
9. Emergency Care Research Institute: Next-generation pulse oximetry. Health Devices 2003;32:49-103.
10. Perkins GD, McAuley DF, Giles S, et al: Do changes in pulse oximeter oxygen saturation predict equivalent changes in arterial oxygen saturation? Crit Care 2003;7:R67-R71.
11. Jubran A, Tobin MJ: Reliability of pulse oximetry in titrating supplemental oxygen therapy in ventilator-dependent patients. Chest 1990;97:1420-1425.
12. Van de Louw A, Cracco C, Cerf C, et al: Accuracy of pulse oximetry in the intensive care unit. Intensive Care Medicine 2001;27:1606-1613.
13. Webb RK, Ralston AC, Runciman WB: Potential errors in pulse oximetry. II—Effects of changes in saturation and signal quality. Anaesthesia 1991;96:207-212.
14. Barker SJ, Tremper KK: The effect of carbon monoxide inhalation on pulse oximeter signal detection. Anesthesiology 1987;67:599-603.
15. Tawaklna MT, Greville HW: The effect of carboxyhemoglobin on the accuracy of pulse oximetry in ambulatory care patients. Chest 1991;143:A72.
16. Hampson NB: Pulse oximetry in severe carbon monoxide poisoning (see comments). Chest 1998;114:1036-1041.
17. Barker SJ, Tremper KK, Hyatt J: Effects of methemoglobinemia on pulse oximetry and mixed-venous oximetry. Anesthesiology 1989;70:112-117.
18. Jay GD, Hughes L, Renzi FP: Pulse oximetry is accurate in acute anemia from hemorrhage. Ann Emerg Med 1994;24:32-35.
19. Ortiz FO, Aldrich TK, Nagel RL, et al: Accuracy of pulse oximetry in sickle cell disease. Am J Respir Crit Care Med 1999;159:447-451.
20. Saito S, Fukura H, Shimada H, Fujita T: Prolonged interference of blue dye "patent blue" with pulse oximetry readings. Acta Anaesthesiol Scand 1995;89:268-269.
21. Cote CJ, Goldstein EA, Fuchsman WH, Hoaglin DC: The effect of nail polish on pulse oximetry. Anesth Analg 1989;67:683-686.
22. Hinkelbein J, Genzwuerker HV, Sogl R, Fiedler F: Effect of nail polish on oxygen saturation determined by

pulse oximetry in critically ill patients. Resuscitation 2007;72:82-91.
23. Edelist G: Acrylic nails and pulse oximetry [Letter]. Anesth Analg 1995;81:882-891.
24. Amar D, Neidzwski J, Wald A, Finck AD: Fluorescent light interferes with pulse oximetry. J Clin Monit 1989;5:135-136.
25. Jubran A: Advances in respiratory monitoring during mechanical ventilation. Chest 1999;116: 1416-1425.
26. Zeballos RJ, Weisman IM: Reliability of noninvasive oximetry in black subjects during exercise and hypoxia. Am Rev Respir Dis 1991;144:1240-1244.
27. Clayton D, Webb RK, Ralston AC, et al: Pulse oximeter probes: A comparison between finger, nose, ear, and forehead probes under conditions of poor perfusion. Anaesthesia 1991;46:260-265.
28. Ibanez J, Velasco J, Raurich JM: The accuracy of the Biox 3700 pulse oximeter in patients receiving vasoactive therapy. Intensive Care Med 1991;17:484-486.
29. Dumas C, Wahr JA, Tremper KK: Clinical evaluation of a prototype motion artifact resistant pulse oximeter in the recovery room. Anesth Analg 1996;83:269-272.
30. Reich DL, Timcenko A, Bodian CA, et al: Predictors of pulse oximetry data failure. Anesthesiology 1996;84: 859-864.
31. Moller JT, Hohannessen NW, Berg H, et al: Hypoxaemia during anesthesia—an observer study. Br J Anaesth 1991;66:437-444.
32. Lawless ST: Crying wolf: False alarms in a pediatric intensive care unit. Crit Care Med 1994;22:981-985.
33. Tsien CL, Fackler JC: Poor prognosis for existing monitors in the intensive care unit. Crit Care Med 1997;25:614-619.
34. Lutter NO, Urankar S, Kroeber S: False alarm rates of three third-generation pulse oximeters in PACU, ICU and IABP patients. Anesth Analg 2002;94: S69-S75.
35. Stoneham MD, Saville GM, Wilson IH: Knowledge about pulse oximetry among medical and nursing staff. Lancet 1994;344:1339-1342.
36. Howell M: Pulse oximetry: An audit of nursing and medical staff understanding. Br J Nurs 2002;11: 191-197.
37. Bowton DL, Scuderi PE, Harris L, et al: Pulse oximetry monitoring outside the intensive care unit: Progress or problem? Ann Intern Med 1991;115:450-454.
38. Carruthers DM, Harrison BDW: Arterial blood gas analysis or oxygen saturation in the assessment of acute asthma. Thorax 1995;50:186-188.
39. Kline JA, Hernandez-Nino J, Newgard CD, et al: Use of pulse oximetry to predict in-hospital complications in normotensive patients with pulmonary embolism. Am J Med 2003;115:203-208.
40. Moller JT, Pedersen T, Rasmussen LS, et al: Randomized evaluation of pulse oximetry in 20,802 patients: I—Design, demography, pulse oximetry failure rate and overall complication rate. Anesthesiology 1993;78:436-444.
41. Moller JT, Johannessen NW, Espersen K, et al: Randomized evaluation of pulse oximetry in 20,802 patients: II—Perioperative events and postoperative complications. Anesthesiology 1993;78:445-453.
42. Bierman MI, Stein KL, Snyder JV: Pulse oximetry in postoperative care of cardiac surgical patients: a randomized controlled trial. Chest 1992;102: 1367-1370.
43. Le Bourdelles G, Estagnasie P, Lenoir F, et al: Use of a pulse oximeter in an adult emergency department: Impact on the number of arterial blood gas analyses ordered. Chest 1998;113: 1042-1047.
44. Solsona JF, Marrugat J, Vazquez A, et al: Effect of pulse oximetry on clinical practice in the intensive care unit. Lancet 1993;342:311-312.
45. Inman KJ, Sibbald WJ, Rutledge FS, et al: Does implementing pulse oximetry in a critical care unit result in substantial arterial blood gas savings? Chest 1993;104:542-546.
46. Hutchison DCS, Gray BJ: Transcutaneous and transconjunctival oxygen monitoring. In Tobin MJ (ed): Principles and Practice of Intensive Care Monitoring. New York, McGraw-Hill, 1998, pp 289-302.
47. Palmisano BW, Severinghaus JW: Transcutaneous P_{CO_2} and P_{O_2}: A multicenter study of accuracy. J Clin Monit 1990;6:189-195.
48. Tremper KK, Shoemaker WC: Transcutaneous oxygen monitoring of critically ill adults, with and without low flow shock. Crit Care Med 1981;9:706-709.
49. Rodriguez P, Lellouche F, Aboab J, et al: Transcutaneous arterial carbon dioxide pressure monitoring in critically ill adult patients. Intensive Care Med 2006;32: 309-312.
50. Hoffman RA, Ershowsky PF, Krieger BP: Determination of auto-PEEP during spontaneous and controlled ventilation by monitoring changes in end-expiratory thoracic gas volume. Chest 1989;96:613-616.
51. Hess D, Schlottag A, Levin B, et al: An evaluation of the usefulness of end-tidal Pco2 to aid weaning from mechanical ventilation following cardiac surgery. Respir Care 1991;36:837-843.
52. Birmingham PK, Cheney FW, Ward RJ: Esophageal intubation: A review of detection techniques. Anesth Analg 1986;65:886-891.
53. Vaghadia H, Jenkins LC, Ford RW: Comparison of end-tidal carbon dioxide, oxygen saturation and clinical signs for the detection of oesophageal intubation. Can J Anaesth 1989;36: 560-564.
54. Linko K, Paloheimo M, Tammisto T: Capnography for detection of accidental oesophageal intubation. Acta Anaesthesiol Scand 1983;27: 199-202.
55. Knapp S, Kofler J, Stoiser B, et al: The assessment of four different methods to verify tracheal tube placement in the critical care setting. Anesth Analg 1999;88:766-770.
56. Alberti A, Gallo F, Fongaro A, et al: P0.1 is a useful parameter in setting the level of pressure support ventilation. Intensive Care Med 1995;21:547-553.
57. Conti G, Cinnella G, Barboni E, et al: Estimation of occlusion pressure during assisted ventilation in patients with intrinsic PEEP. Am J Respir Crit Care Med 1996;154:907-912.
58. Capdevila XJ, Perrigault PF, Perey PJ, et al: Occlusion pressure and its ratio to maximum inspiratory pressure are useful predictors for successful extubation following T-piece weaning trial. Chest 1995;108:482-489.
59. Sassoon CSH, Mahutte CK: Airway occlusion pressure and breathing pattern as predictors of weaning outcome. Am Rev Respir Dis 1993;148:860-866.
60. Tobin MJ, Jubran A: Weaning from mechanical ventilation. In Tobin MJ (ed): Principles and Practice of Mechanical Ventilation. New York, McGraw-Hill, 2006, pp 1185-1220.
61. Marini JJ, Smith TC, Lamb V: Estimation of inspiratory muscle strength in mechanically ventilated patients: The measurement of maximal inspiratory pressure. J Crit Care 1986;1:32-38.
62. Multz AS, Aldrich TK, Prezant DJ, et al: Maximal inspiratory pressure is not a reliable test of inspiratory muscle strength in mechanically ventilated patients. Am Rev Respir Dis 1990;142: 529-532.
63. Yang K, Tobin MJ: A prospective study of indexes predicting outcome of trials of weaning from mechanical ventilation. N Engl J Med 1991;324: 1445-1450.
64. Tobin MJ, Guenther SM, Perez W, et al: The pattern of breathing during successful and unsuccessful trials of weaning from mechanical ventilation. Am Rev Respir Dis 1986;134:1111-1118.
65. Meade M, Guyatt G, Cook D, et al: Predicting success in weaning from mechanical ventilation. Chest 2001;120(6 Suppl):400S-424S.
66. MacIntyre NR, Cook DJ, Ely EW Jr, et al: Evidence-based guidelines for weaning and discontinuing ventilatory support: A collective task force facilitated by the American College of Chest Physicians; the American Association for Respiratory Care; and the American College of Critical Care Medicine. Chest 2001;120(6 Suppl):375S-395S.
67. Feinstein AR: Clinical Epidemiology: The Architecture of Clinical Research. Philadelphia, WB Saunders, 1985.
68. Sox HCJ, Clatt MA, Higgins MC, Marton KI: Medical Decision Making. Boston, Butterworths, 1988.
69. Tobin MJ, Jubran A: Variable performance of weaning-predictor tests: Role of Bayes' theorem and spectrum and test-referral bias. Intensive Care Med 2006;32: 2002-2012.
70. Jacob B, Chatila W, Manthous CA: The unassisted respiratory rate/tidal volume ratio accurately predicts weaning outcome in postoperative patients. Crit Care Med 1997;25:253-257.

71. Chatila W, Jacob B, Guaglionone D, Manthous CA: The unassisted respiratory rate–tidal volume ratio accurately predicts weaning outcome. Am J Med 1996;101:61-67.
72. Jubran A, Grant BJ, Laghi F, et al: Weaning prediction: Esophageal pressure monitoring complements readiness testing. Am J Respir Crit Care Med 2005;171:1252-1259.
73. Tobin MJ, Mador MJ, Guenther SM, et al: Variability of resting respiratory drive and timing in healthy subjects. J Appl Physiol 1988;65:309-317.
74. Tobin MJ, Yang KL, Jubran A, Lodato RF: Interrelationship of breath components in neighboring breaths of normal eupneic subjects. Am J Respir Crit Care Med 1995;152:1967-1976.
75. Jubran A, Grant BJB, Tobin MJ: Effect of hyperoxic hypercapnia on variational activity of breathing. Am J Respir Crit Care Med 1997;156:1129-1139.
76. Preas HL, Jubran A, Vandivier RW, et al: Effect of cyclooxygenase inhibition on ventilatory responses to human experimental endotoxemia. Am J Respir Crit Care Med 2001;164:620-626.
77. Brack T, Jubran A, Tobin MJ: Effect of elastic loading on variational activity of breathing. Am J Respir Crit Care Med 1997;155:1341-1348.
78. Brack T, Jubran A, Tobin MJ: Effect of resistive loading on variational activity of breathing. Am J Respir Crit Care Med 1998;157:1756-1763.
79. Jubran A, Tobin MJ: Effect of isocapnic hypoxia on variational activity of breathing. Am J Respir Crit Care Med 2000;162:1202-1209.
80. Goldberger AL: Non-linear dynamics for clinicians: Chaos theory, fractals, and complexity at the bedside. Lancet 1996;347:1312-1314.
81. Brack T, Jubran A, Tobin MJ: Dyspnea and decreased variability of breathing in patients with restrictive lung disease. Am J Respir Crit Care Med 2002;165:1260-1264.
82. Wysocki M, Cracco C, Teixeira A, et al: Reduced breathing variability as a predictor of unsuccessful patient separation from mechanical ventilation. Crit Care Med 2006;34:2076-2083.
83. Marini JJ: Breathing patterns as integrative weaning predictors: Variations on a theme. Crit Care Med 2006;34:2241-2243.
84. Brack T, Jubran A, Laghi F, Tobin MJ: Fluctuations in end-expiratory lung volume during Cheyne-Stokes respiration. Am J Respir Crit Care Med 2005;171:1408-1413.
85. Jubran A, Tobin MJ: The effect of hyperinflation on rib cage-abdominal motion. Am Rev Respir Dis 1992;146:1378-1382.
86. Tobin MJ: Noninvasive monitoring of ventilation. In Tobin MJ (ed): Principles and Practice of Intensive Care Monitoring. New York, McGraw-Hill, 1998 pp 465-495.
87. Bates JHT, Rossi A, Milic-Emili J: Analysis of the behaviour of the respiratory system with constant inspiratory flow. J Appl Physiol 1985;58:1840-1848.
88. Jubran A, Tobin MJ: Passive mechanics of lung and chest wall in patients who failed and succeeded in trials of weaning. Am J Respir Crit Care Med 1997;155:916-921.
89. Polese G, Rossi A, Appendini L, et al: Partitioning of respiratory mechanics in mechanically ventilated patients. J Appl Physiol 1991;71:2425-2433.
90. Rossi A, Polese G, Milic-Emili J: Monitoring respiratory mechanics in ventilator-dependent patients. In Tobin MJ (ed): Principles and Practice of Intensive Care Monitoring. New York, McGraw-Hill, 1998, pp 553-596.
91. Dreyfuss D, Soler P, Basset G, Saumon G: High inflation pressure pulmonary edema: Respective effects of high airway pressure, high tidal volume, and positive end-expiratory pressure. Am Rev Respir Dis 1988;137:1159-1164.
92. Dreyfuss D, Saumon G: Ventilator-induced injury. In Tobin MJ (ed): Principles and Practice of Mechanical Ventilation. New York, McGraw-Hill, 1994, pp 793-811.
93. Muscedere JG, Muller JBM, Gan K, et al: Tidal volume at low airway pressures can augment lung injury. Am J Respir Crit Care Med 1994;149:1327-1334.
94. Tobin MJ: Culmination of an era in research on the acute respiratory distress syndrome (Editorial; comment). N Engl J Med 2000;342:1360-1361.
95. Tobin MJ: Advances in mechanical ventilation. N Engl J Med 2001;344:1986-1996.
96. Hickling KG, Henderson SJ, Jackson R: Low mortality associated with low volume pressure limited ventilation with permissive hypercapnia in severe adult respiratory distress syndrome. Intensive Care Med 1990;16:372-377.
97. Amato MB, Barbas CS, Medeiros DM, et al: Effect of a protective-ventilation strategy on mortality in the acute respiratory distress syndrome. N Engl J Med 1998;338:347-354.
98. Brochard L, Roudot-Thoraval F, Roupie E, et al: Tidal volume reduction for prevention of ventilator-induced lung injury in acute respiratory distress syndrome. Am J Respir Crit Care Med 1998;158:1831-1838.
99. Brower RG, Shanholtz CB, Fessler HE, et al: Prospective, randomized, controlled clinical trial comparing traditional versus reduced tidal volume ventilation in acute respiratory distress syndrome patients (See comments). Crit Care Med 1999;27:1492-1498.
100. Stewart TEM, Meade MO, Cook DJ, et al: Evaluation of a ventilation strategy to prevent barotrauma in patients at high risk for acute respiratory distress syndrome. N Engl J Med 1998;338:355-361.
101. Ventilation with lower tidal volumes as compared with traditional tidal volumes for acute lung injury and the acute respiratory distress syndrome. The Acute Respiratory Distress Syndrome Network. N Engl J Med 2000;342:1301-1308.
102. Eichacker PQ, Gerstenberger EP, Banks SM, et al: Meta-analysis of acute lung injury and acute respiratory distress syndrome trials testing low tidal volumes. Am J Respir Crit Care Med 2002;166:1510-1514.
103. Deans KJ, Minneci PC, Cui X, et al: Mechanical ventilation in ARDS: One size does not fit all. Crit Care Med 2005;33:1141-1143.
104. Kallet RH, Jasmer RM, Pittet JF, et al: Clinical implementation of the ARDS network protocol is associated with reduced hospital mortality compared with historical controls. Crit Care Med 2005;33:925-929.
105. Brochard L: Respiratory pressure-volume curves. In Tobin MJ (ed): Principles and Practice of Intensive Care Monitoring. New York, McGraw-Hill, 1998, pp 597-616.
106. Matamis D, Lemaire F, Harf A, et al: Total respiratory pressure-volume curves in the adult respiratory distress syndrome. Chest 1984;86:58-66.
107. Amato MBP, Barbas CSV, Medeiros D, et al: Effect of a protective-ventilation strategy on mortality in the acute respiratory distress syndrome. N Engl J Med 1998;338:347-354.
108. Amato MBP, Barbas CSV, Medeiros DM, et al: Beneficial effects of the "open lung approach" with low distending pressures in acute respiratory distress syndrome: A prospective randomized study on mechanical ventilation. Am J Respir Crit Care Med 1995;152:1835-1846.
109. Brower RG, Lanken PN, MacIntyre N, et al: Higher versus lower positive end-expiratory pressures in patients with the acute respiratory distress syndrome. N Engl J Med 2004;351:327-336.
110. Marini JJ: Mechanical ventilation in the acute respiratory distress syndrome. In Tobin MJ (ed): Principles and Practice of Mechanical Ventilation. New York, McGraw Hill, 2006, pp 625-648.
111. Navalesi P, Maggiore SM. Positive end-expiratory pressure. In Tobin MJ (ed): Principles and Practice of Mechanical Ventilation. New York, McGraw Hill, 2006, pp 273-326.
112. Grasso S, Fanelli V, Cafarelli A, et al: Effects of high versus low positive end-expiratory pressures in acute respiratory distress syndrome. Am J Respir Crit Care Med 2005;171:1002-1008.
113. Villar J, Kacmarek RM, Perez-Mendez L, Aguirre-Jaime A: A high positive end-expiratory pressure, low tidal volume ventilatory strategy improves outcome in persistent acute respiratory distress syndrome: A randomized, controlled trial. Crit Care Med 2006;34:1311-1318.
114. Jubran A, Laghi F, Mazur M, et al: Partitioning of lung and chest wall mechanics before and after lung volume reduction surgery. Am J Respir Crit Care Med 1998;158:306-310.
115. Dhand R, Duarte AG, Jubran A, et al: Dose response to bronchodilator delivered by metered-dose inhaler in ventilator-supported patients. Am J Respir Crit Care Med 1996;154:388-393.
116. Dhand R, Jubran A, Tobin MJ: Efficacy of bronchodilator delivered by metered-dose inhaler in ventilator-supported patients with COPD. Am J Respir Crit Care Med 1995;152:129-136.

117. Tobin MJ, Van de Graaff WB: Monitoring of lung mechanics and work of breathing. In Tobin MJ (ed): Principles and Practice of Mechanical Ventilation. New York, McGraw-Hill, 1994, pp 967-1003.
118. Petrof BJ, Legaré M, Goldberg P, et al: Continuous positive airway pressure reduces work of breathing and dyspnea during weaning from mechanical ventilation in severe chronic obstructive pulmonary disease. Am Rev Respir Dis 1990;141:281-289.
119. Maltais F, Reissmann H, Navalesi P, et al: Comparison of static and dynamic measurements of intrinsic PEEP in mechanically ventilated patients. Am J Respir Crit Care Med 1994;150: 1318-1324.
120. Nava S, Bruschi C, Rubini F, et al: Respiratory response and inspiratory effort during pressure support ventilation in COPD patients. Intensive Care Med 1995;21:871-879.
121. Parthasarathy S, Jubran A, Tobin MJ: Cycling of inspiratory and expiratory muscle groups with the ventilator in airflow limitation. Am J Respir Crit Care Med 1998;158:1471-1478.
122. Leung P, Jubran A, Tobin MJ: Comparison of assisted ventilator modes on triggering, patient effort, and dyspnea. Am J Respir Crit Care Med 1997;155:1940-1948.
123. Puddy A, Younes M: Effect of inspiratory flow rate on respiratory output in normal subjects. Am Rev Respir Dis 1992;146:787-789.
124. Laghi F, Segal J, Choe WK, Tobin MJ: Effect of imposed inflation time on respiratory frequency and hyperinflation in patients with chronic obstructive pulmonary disease. Am J Respir Crit Care Med 2001;163: 1365-1370.
125. Jubran A, Tobin MJ: Use of flow-volume curves in detecting secretions in ventilator- dependent patients. Am J Respir Crit Care Med 1994;150: 766-769.
126. Guglielminotti J, Alzieu M, Maury E, et al: Bedside detection of retained tracheobronchial secretions in patients receiving mechanical ventilation: Is it time for tracheal suctioning? Chest 2000;118: 1095-1099.

Chapter 14

Arterial Blood Gas Measurements

Robin Gross and William Peruzzi

The basic electrochemical methods necessary to analyze blood gases were first described in the 1890s.[1] Arterial blood gases (ABGs) became clinically applicable in the 1950s with the invention of the arterial oxygen tension (Pa_{O_2}) electrode by Clark[2] and the arterial carbon dioxide tension (Pa_{CO_2}) electrode by Stow and Severinghaus.[3] In the 1960s, physicians considered ABGs the most valuable laboratory test available.[4] Today, ABGs are the most frequently ordered test in the intensive care unit (ICU),[5] so it has become essential for the intensivist to master ABG interpretation completely. This chapter discusses ABG measurement for supporting ventilation, oxygenation, and acid-base imbalance in critically ill patients.

TECHNICAL CONSIDERATIONS

A *clinical analyzer* requires removal of body fluid or tissue to perform a measurement and allows a single device to serve multiple patients.[6] Standards have been developed for the collection[7] and processing[8] of ABG samples. Scheduled proficiency testing of ABG analyzers is performed within laboratories.[9] Routine calibration is rarely necessary because modern ABG analyzers now have microprocessors that self-calibrate before analysis of every sample. The major clinical disadvantages of ABG analyzers are that (1) they provide intermittent data, (2) there is often considerable delay in obtaining results secondary to time involved in sample transport and result transmission, and (3) the frequency of measurements is limited because there is permanent blood loss associated with the testing.[10] These instruments function reliably outside the traditional laboratory setting and are now routinely available in ICUs, eliminating the delay between drawing the sample and obtaining results from a central laboratory.

ARTERIAL BLOOD GAS SPECIMENS

The ABG sample is subject to preanalytic errors,[11] including intrasubject variability[12] (particularly in the setting of hyperventilation[13]) and inconsistency in methods for aspirating[14,15] and transporting[16] samples. Sample handling is particularly important because higher storage temperatures produce alterations in values (higher Pa_{CO_2}, lower pH and Pa_{O_2}),[16] particularly in the setting of high leukocyte counts.[17] Although ABGs also provide immediate results regarding electrolytes (potassium, calcium) and hemoglobin, errors may occur, particularly with regard to potassium.[18] Verification of results in a central laboratory is recommended before initiating treatment.

Because transport of carbon dioxide (CO_2) and oxygen (O_2) involves gases in solution that are affected by temperature variation, a blood sample of given O_2 and CO_2 contents manifests different gas tensions when analyzed at various temperatures. The ABG analyzer's pH, P_{CO_2}, and P_{O_2} electrodes are encased in a constant 37° C environment to which the blood sample chamber also is exposed. Independent of the patient's temperature, the pH, P_{CO_2}, and P_{O_2} are analyzed in a closed system at 37° C. *Temperature correction* applies mathematical adjustments to the measured 37° C values for the purpose of obtaining a "truer" reflection of the in vivo gas tensions.[19] This adjustment is not routinely necessary[20-22] because pH and oxygen consumption vary predictably with temperature. Although pH and Pa_{O_2} measured at 37° C probably reflect accurate in vivo acid-base imbalance[23] and oxygenation status, temperature correction may be useful in a patient with profound temperature deviation from 37° C.

Other issues with regard to ABG sampling include the complications of ABG aspiration, such as pain,[24] vasospasm,[13] and tissue damage. Frequent ABG sampling may require the placement of an arterial line, which also permits continuous blood pressure monitoring. This device is not free of complications because it may cause thrombosis[25] and lead to more frequent (and possibly unnecessary) blood sampling.[5]

Because this gold standard technology provides challenges for the individuals obtaining clinically vital information, the physician must decide when the ABG is required, and when alternative data would suffice. A normotensive patient with an asthma exacerbation may be monitored with pulse oximetry, whereas a hypotensive patient with poor perfusion and additional metabolic derangements would require an ABG. The same asthma patient in acute respiratory failure would require multiple ABGs to assess the need for intubation and adjustments in the ventilator settings. Daily ABGs would add little clinically useful information, however, in a patient with static ventilator settings and a stable medical condition. The physician first must determine whether the ABG is clinically warranted by asking whether the information obtained from the ABG would alter the treatment plan.

RESPIRATORY HOMEOSTASIS

Respiration is the diffusion of O_2 and CO_2 molecules across semipermeable membranes. Respiratory homeostasis encompasses all physiologic mechanisms acting to balance O_2 and CO_2 exchange at the lung and cellular levels. Critically ill patients often require therapeutic and supportive interventions to maintain respiratory homeostasis. Such clinical decisions depend, to a major degree, on the availability and interpretation of ABG values. Accepted normal blood gas value ranges are pH 7.35 to 7.45, Pa_{CO_2} 35 to 45 mm Hg, Pa_{O_2} 75 to 100 mm Hg, HCO_3^- 22 to 26 mmol/L, standard base excess (BE) 0 ± 3 mmol/L, and O_2 saturation 95% to 100%.

ASSESSMENT OF PHYSIOLOGIC VENTILATION

Ventilation is gas movement in and out of the pulmonary system and is most readily measured in critically ill patients as the gas volume exhaled in 1 minute, known as the minute ventilation (V_E), expressed as:

$$V_E = f \times V_T$$

where f is the respiratory rate and V_T is the tidal volume (the volume of air per breath). The V_E portion that results in gas exchange (i.e., CO_2 removal from the blood and transfer of O_2 into the blood) is referred to as *alveolar ventilation* (V_A); the portion of the V_E that does not result in gas exchange is designated as *deadspace ventilation* (V_D).

Arterial Carbon Dioxide Tension Reflects Alveolar Ventilation

Respiratory acid-base balance depends on the ability of homeostatic systems to maintain a balance between CO_2 production (V_{CO_2}), determined by the metabolic rate, and excretion, determined by cardiopulmonary function. This relationship is expressed as:

$$V_A = K \cdot V_{CO_2}/P_{ACO_2}$$

where K = 0.863 (a unit conversion factor) and P_{ACO_2} is the *alveolar* partial pressure of CO_2, the major determinant of CO_2 excretion; this value varies to some degree among the millions of individual alveoli. The arterial P_{CO_2} (Pa_{CO_2}) usually reflects the mean P_{ACO_2} because of the high diffusibility[26] of CO_2 across the alveolar-endothelial interface. In the absence of significant ventilation-perfusion ($\dot{V}/\dot{Q}$) mismatch,[27] Pa_{CO_2} may be substituted for P_{ACO_2} in the previous equation.

It is imperative that significantly abnormal CO_2 production be identified when interpreting the Pa_{CO_2} because the rate of CO_2 production affects the intracellular P_{CO_2}, which influences the rate of CO_2 diffusion into the venous blood. Common circumstances of abnormal CO_2 production are temperature deviation (which alters CO_2 production by approximately 10% for every degree Celsius change in temperature), excessive muscular activity (e.g., rigors), physiologic stress responses, the systemic inflammatory response syndrome, and excessive carbohydrate load.[28]

CO_2 stores influence the Pa_{CO_2}. This rarely becomes an issue with tissue stores of oxygen,[29] which is consumed immediately, or nitrogen, which exists in equilibrium. Alterations in P_{ACO_2} immediately alter central CO_2 stores, but not peripheral stores. This is because CO_2 is produced in cells, and peripheral stores in bone and fat change slowly over days. The stores in skeletal muscle and organ tissue may change in hours (muscle tissue) and minutes (organ tissue). Peripheral stores may be increased as a compensatory mechanism for CO_2 retention to maintain respiratory homeostasis. Peripheral stores also may be depleted when CO_2 excretion exceeds CO_2 production for significant periods, as occurs in patients with hyperventilation associated with significant central nervous system injury. Skeletal muscle depletion of CO_2 stores occurs in a few hours,[30] whereas bone depletion takes several days.[31] For these reasons, changes in minute ventilation may not immediately be reflected in the ABG $Pa{CO_2}$ and a delay in the ABG draw after a change in VE is recommended; this period should be extended in patients with known elevations in peripheral CO_2 stores.

Deadspace Ventilation

Ventilation is the sum of alveolar and deadspace components:

$$V_E = V_A + V_D$$

Increases in VD require an increase in VE to maintain a consistent VA. Anatomic and alveolar deadspace constitute the physiologic deadspace, which is calculated by the Bohr equation:

$$V_D/V_T = [P_{ACO_2} - P_{ECO_2}]/P_{ACO_2}$$

where P_{ECO_2} is expired CO_2. Deadspace is increased by conditions that impede the transfer of gas across the alveolar-capillary interface or increase the distance air must travel to participate in gas exchange at the alveolar-capillary interface. This includes diseases that decrease perfusion, such as acutely diminished cardiac output or pulmonary emboli. Positive-pressure ventilation favors redistribution of ventilation to nondependent (less perfused) lung regions,[32,33] may cause vascular compression from overdistention of alveoli, and may add to anatomic deadspace (usually comprising the conducting airways) owing to increased endotracheal tube length.

Minute Ventilation–Arterial Carbon Dioxide Tension Disparity

In normal exercising humans, the VE increases in proportion to the metabolic rate and cardiac output[34]; the $Pa{CO_2}$ remains the same or decreases to a small degree.[35] In contrast, a normal subject undergoing positive-pressure ventilation requires a greater than normal VE to maintain a normal $Pa{CO_2}$, an effect generally attributed to an increase in VD.[36,37] Clinical observation that VE is increased *without* an appropriate decrease in $Pa{CO_2}$ raises the possibility of increased VD. Table 14-1 assumes a CO_2 production of 200 mL/min and shows the ideal relationship between VE, VA, and $Pa{CO_2}$ when the VE is doubled, redoubled, and halved. In general:

1. When the VE is associated with a $Pa{CO_2}$ significantly greater than predicted and an increased CO_2 production can be reasonably excluded, increased VD is the most likely explanation.
2. When the VE is associated with a $Pa{CO_2}$ significantly less than predicted, diminished CO_2 production or depleted CO_2 stores should be suspected.

Table 14-1. Ideal Minute Ventilation (VE), Alveolar Ventilation (VA), and Arterial Carbon Dioxide Tension ($Pa{CO_2}$) Relationships

VE (L)	VA (L)	$Pa{CO_2}$ (mm Hg)
3	2	80
6	4	40
12	8	30
24	16	20

EVALUATING ACID-BASE ABNORMALITIES

Before attempting to assess acid-base status (Fig. 14-1), the physician should verify the internal consistency of the data. The $Pa{CO_2}$ from the ABG and the HCO_3^- from the metabolic panel should be used to predict the hydrogen ion concentration ($[H^+]$) of the ABG sample using a modified version of the Henderson-Hasselbalch equation (Table 14-2):[38]

$$[H^+] = 24 \cdot ([Pa{CO_2}]/[HCO_3^-])$$

where 24 is a constant that combines the pK′ and CO_2 solubility coefficient. A calculated pH that diverges significantly from the measured pH warrants additional sampling and reanalysis of the ABG and metabolic panel.

Traditional Respiratory Acid-Base Balance

Table 14-3 lists the ventilatory and acid-base nomenclature used in this chapter and the criteria for using each term. Experience in critical care medicine has revealed that clinical judgments are rarely influenced by minor variations from the normal ranges of arterial CO_2 or pH measurements. Broader, "clinically acceptable" ranges for arterial pH and $P{CO_2}$ have emerged. Table 14-4 lists the criteria for the traditional nomenclature of respiratory acidosis and respiratory alkalosis.[39,40]

Respiratory Acidosis

As the $Pa{CO_2}$ increases acutely, the plasma carbonic acid concentration correspondingly increases, resulting in an increased free hydrogen ion concentration (decreased pH) in the plasma (Fig. 14-2):

$$CO_2 + H_2O \rightarrow H_2CO_3 \rightarrow H^+ + HCO_3^-$$

This relationship is linear,[41] and the expected changes from normal values are:

$$\Delta pH = -0.008 \cdot (\Delta Pa{CO_2})$$

Table 14-2. Predicting pH from Hydrogen Ion Concentration

$[H^+]$ (nmol/L)	pH (unit)
60	7.20
50	7.30
40	7.40
30	7.50
20	7.60

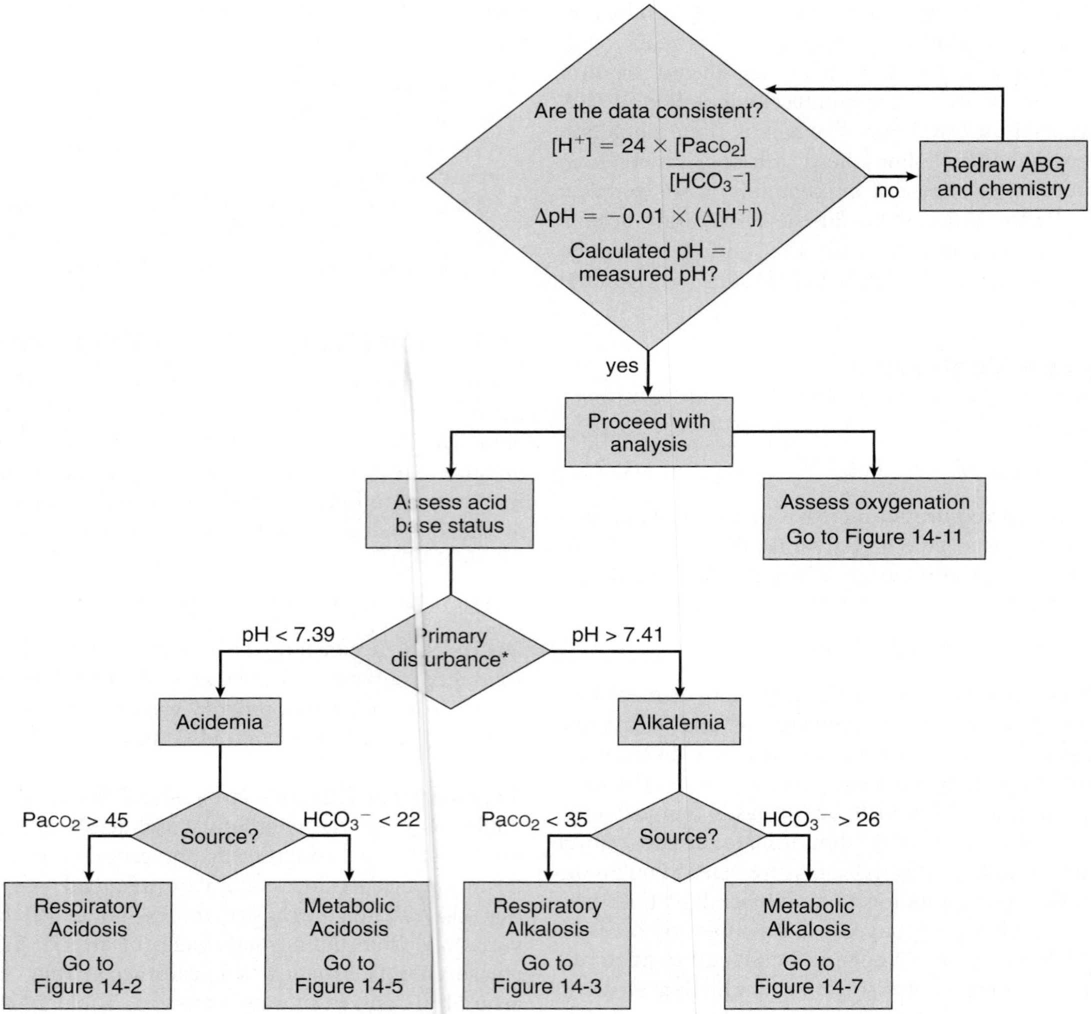

*Although within "normal" range, a minor deviation from 7.40 should reflect the underlying problem.

Figure 14-1. Algorithm for approach to arterial blood gas interpretation.

Initial compensatory mechanisms are cellular, occurring primarily in erythrocytes. The renal response to an increased hydrogen ion concentration, usually functional within 3 to 5 days of the acute insult, is the excretion of more hydrogen ions and increased reabsorption of bicarbonate ions into the blood. Given time, this renal mechanism corrects the pH to near-normal. The interrelationship of the pulmonary and renal response to acid-base imbalance is predictable such that for a chronic respiratory acidosis, the expected changes are:

$$\Delta pH = -0.003 \cdot (\Delta Pa_{CO_2})$$

A measured pH that falls between the values calculated in the previous equations indicates the presence of a combined acute and chronic respiratory acidosis.

Ventilatory Failure (Acute Respiratory Acidosis)

Traditional physiology considers the need to excrete CO_2 in terms of respiratory acid-base balance, inferring that the biologic insult of CO_2 accumulation is the chemically associated accumulation of free hydrogen ions. Ventilation is primarily controlled by the medulla in response to pH changes sensed by the carotid bodies.[42,43] An acidotic cerebrospinal fluid pH triggers neuronal output and stimulates peripheral receptors in the lungs and respiratory muscles to augment ventilation. This system is dysfunctional in *ventilatory failure*, a diagnosis made on the basis of ABG analysis. It is shown by an abnormally high Pa_{CO_2} in the setting of an acute decrease in pH. The etiology of ventilatory failure may be central (narcotic overdose, neurologic injury), pulmonary (acute respiratory distress syndrome, pneumonia, interstitial disease), peripheral (neuromuscular disease, mitochondrial dysfunction), or detrimental work of breathing (WOB) resulting from excessive demands on the patient's cardiopulmonary reserves (failing compensation for metabolic acidosis). Nevertheless, from a clinical viewpoint, the accumulation of CO_2 represents the pulmonary system's failure to excrete adequately the waste product of metabolism, and treatment is directed toward decreasing the WOB to support CO_2 elimination.

The signs and symptoms of detrimental breathing include dyspnea, tachypnea, tachycardia, hypertension, intercostal retraction, use of accessory muscles of ventilation, diaphoresis, and mental status changes. A patient with these signs and symptoms who has a normal Pa_{CO_2} has *impending ventilatory failure*, a clinical diagnosis. Metabolic acidemia or hypoxemia is common in these patients and can be reversed rapidly when appropriate ventilatory assistance and hemodynamic support are instituted. The *progressive* nature of these clinical signs and symptoms is important in diagnosing detrimental WOB because it indicates exhaustion of cardiopulmonary reserves and the gradual fatigue of the respiratory muscles, often the final step in respiratory failure.[44] When clinically significant acute ventilatory failure is present, the following factors must be immediately considered: the need for and adequacy of ventilatory assistance, tissue hypoxia, and concomitant acute metabolic acidosis resulting from inadequate O_2 supply or use or both.

Table 14-3. Nomenclature and Criteria for Clinical Interpretation of Blood Gases

Clinical Terminology	Criteria
Ventilatory failure (respiratory acidosis)	Pa_{CO_2} >45 mm Hg
Alveolar hypoventilation (respiratory acidosis)	Pa_{CO_2} >35 mm Hg
Acute ventilatory failure (respiratory acidosis)	Pa_{CO_2} >45 mm Hg; pH <7.35
Chronic ventilatory failure (respiratory acidosis)	Pa_{CO_2} >45 mm Hg; pH 7.36-7.44
Acute alveolar hyperventilation (respiratory alkalosis)	Pa_{CO_2} <35 mm Hg; pH >7.45
Chronic alveolar hyperventilation (respiratory alkalosis)	Pa_{CO_2} <35 mm Hg; pH 7.36-7.44
Acidemia	pH <7.35
Alkalemia	pH >7.45
Acidosis	HCO_3^- <20 mmol/L BD >5 mmol/L
Alkalosis	HCO_3^- >28 mmol/L BE >5 mmol/L

BD, base deficit; BE, base excess.

Chronic Respiratory Acidosis

Chronic hypercapnia (Pa_{CO_2} >45 mm Hg; pH >7.35) is seen in patients with chronic obstructive pulmonary disease, morbid obesity (pickwickian syndrome), rare central nervous system disorders, and, less commonly, chronic restrictive pulmonary disease. The increased peripheral CO_2 stores allow for the maintenance of CO_2 homeostasis (lung excretion equal to cellular production),

Table 14-4. Traditional Respiratory Acid-Base Nomenclature

Nomenclature	pH	P_{CO_2}	$[HCO_3^-]$	BE
Respiratory Acidosis				
Uncompensated (acute)	↓*	↑	N	N
Partly compensated (subacute)	↓	↑	↑	↑
Compensated (chronic)	N	↑	↑	↑
Respiratory Alkalosis				
Uncompensated (acute)	↑	↓	N	N
Partly compensated (subacute)	↑	↓	↓	↓
Compensated (chronic)	N	↓	↓	↓

*Arrows indicate depressed (↓) or elevated (↑) levels.
BE, base excess; N, normal.

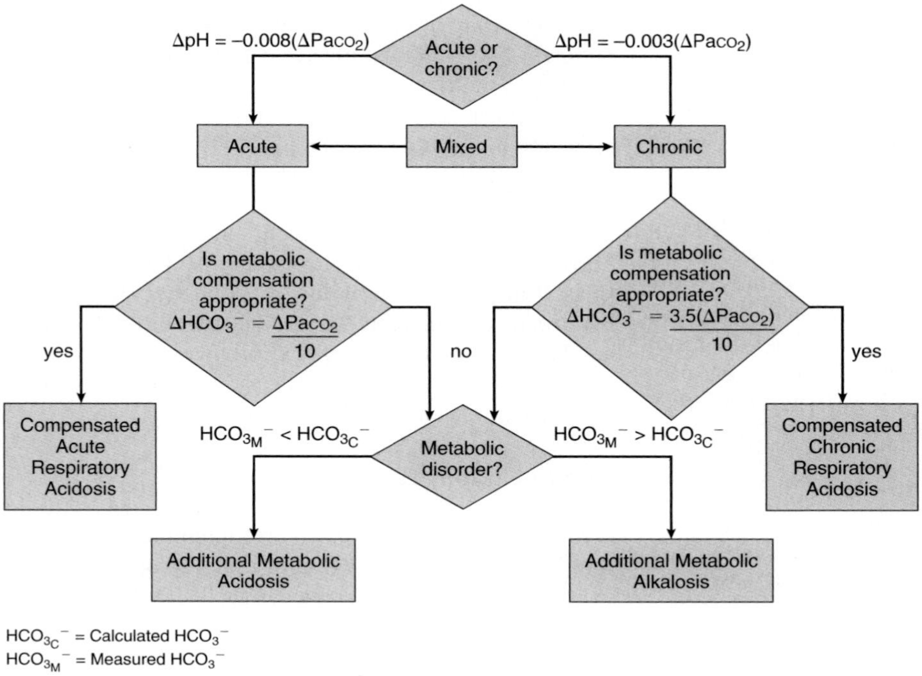

Figure 14-2. Algorithm for respiratory acidosis.

while maintaining an increased P_{ACO_2}. Because inspired gas is essentially void of CO_2, in any steady-state circumstance, a smaller V_E is required to maintain an increased P_{ACO_2} than to maintain a normal P_{ACO_2}.

Chronic hypercapnia (chronic ventilatory failure) involves intracellular adaptation to an increased cellular P_{CO_2} despite intracellular acidosis and significantly diminished oxygen delivery. Extracellular acid-base balance is maintained by accumulating an increased bicarbonate ion concentration in concert with a chloride ion deficiency. These patients often have a slightly greater extracellular pH than normal individuals.[45] This is not explained by diuretic use, but is primarily the result of water and chloride ion shifts between intracellular and extracellular spaces.[45,46]

Patients with chronic hypercapnia have a limited capability to increase cardiopulmonary work in response to stress. Although most do not hypoventilate, some patients become significantly more hypercapnic in response to excessive oxygen administration.[47] This is believed to be secondary to the loss of hypoxic vasoconstriction resulting in $\dot{V}/\dot{Q}$ mismatching,[48,49] with an additional increase in alveolar deadspace.[50]

Chronic Hypercapnia and Acute Ventilatory Failure

In chronic hypercapnia and acute ventilatory failure, typical room air blood gas is pH less than 7.35, P_{CO_2} greater than 60 mm Hg, and P_{O_2} less than 45 mm Hg. The severity of this condition must be judged by the degree of acute acidemia. Regardless of the P_{CO_2} level, a pH greater than 7.30 usually denotes a tolerable change from baseline. If the pH decreases to less than 7.20, evaluation for ventilatory assistance is mandatory. The intensivist should have a low threshold for instituting noninvasive positive-pressure ventilation to decrease WOB.[51] Lactic acidosis is common in these patients, and sodium bicarbonate administration is relatively contraindicated before supporting ventilation.

Chronic Hypercapnia and Acute Hyperventilation

In chronic hypercapnia and acute hyperventilation, typical room air blood gas is pH greater than 7.45, P_{CO_2} greater than 40 mm Hg, and P_{O_2} less than 50 mm Hg. These blood gas values should be interpreted initially as a partly compensated metabolic alkalosis with significant hypoxemia; however, diseases causing metabolic alkalemia rarely cause significant hypoxemia. When presented with these blood gas values, the physician should consider the probability that a patient with chronic hypercapnia may respond transiently to an acute stress by hyperventilating, "unmasking" the pre-existing base excess.

Permissive Hypercapnia

The concept of *permissive hypercapnia* is based on the assumption that low V_T and lung protective ventilatory strategies avoid alveolar overdistention and iatrogenic lung injury, termed *volutrauma*.[52-55] When lung protective strategies result in an increased Pa_{CO_2}, the hypercapnia is accepted; most authors agree that an arterial pH equal to or greater than 7.25 is usually well tolerated by patients without preexisting cardiac disease. Relative contraindications are intracerebral injury because hypercapnia causes vasodilation and increased intracranial pressure that may result in seizures. In pregnancy, CO_2 crosses the placenta and causes fetal acidosis and a rightward shift of the oxygen dissociation curve, resulting in hemoglobin oxygen unloading.[56] The use of permissive hypercapnia in pregnancy is limited. Finally, permissive hypercapnia may result in pulmonary vasoconstriction or increased shunt, although Pa_{O_2} is generally preserved.[57]

The acidemia caused by permissive hypercapnia may be corrected with bicarbonate administration.[55] Some evidence suggests, however, that this acidosis might be "protective" by exerting anti-inflammatory effects.[58] This is controversial,[59] and studies are ongoing.

Respiratory Alkalosis

Acute Respiratory Alkalosis

Acute respiratory alkalosis (Pa_{CO_2} <30 mm Hg; pH >7.50) represents *acute alveolar hyperventilation* and usually indicates the presence of increased WOB (Fig. 14-3). Three common causes of acute alveolar hyperventilation in critically ill patients are (1) homeostatic response to arterial hypoxemia, (2) homeostatic response to metabolic acidosis, and (3) response to central nervous system (brain) dysfunction or injury. The latter two are seldom concomitant with arterial hypoxemia; acute respiratory alkalosis *without hypoxemia* is most commonly secondary to intracranial pathology, anxiety, or pain. Severe anemia, carbon monoxide poisoning, and methemoglobinemia should be excluded as contributory factors, however. The expected ABG change is:

$$\Delta pH = -0.008 \cdot (\Delta Pa_{CO_2})$$

Acute Respiratory Alkalosis with Hypoxemia

Acute respiratory alkalosis with hypoxemia is a blood gas anomaly that is almost always attributable to cardiopulmonary pathology. Acute hypocapnia blunts the ventilatory response to hypoxemia, whereas the response is augmented in acute hypercapnia.[60] When the hypoxemia is the result of a pulmonary process that is *responsive* to oxygen therapy ($\dot{V}/\dot{Q}$ mismatch), oxygen administration should improve oxygen content and oxygen delivery, decrease the WOB, and normalize the Pa_{CO_2} and vital signs. When hypoxemia is due to a pulmonary process that is *refractory* to oxygen therapy (shunt), the ABG values and WOB do not change significantly with oxygen administration because there is little or no enhancement of oxygen content or oxygen delivery.

Chronic Respiratory Alkalosis

Chronic respiratory alkalosis occurs with high altitude; liver disease, particularly with portopulmonary hypertension[61]; pregnancy; cerebral injury; and idiopathic hyperventilation (not usually an issue in the ICU). The expected ABG change is:

$$\Delta pH = -0.017 \cdot (\Delta Pa_{CO_2})$$

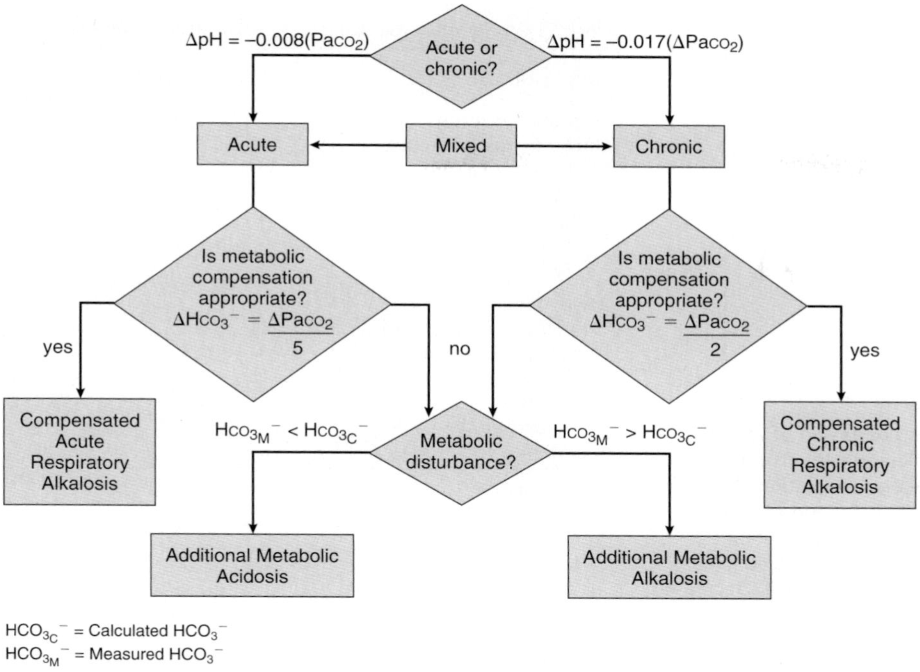

Figure 14-3. Algorithm for respiratory alkalosis.

Iatrogenic Hyperventilation

Most ABG analysis focuses on the pH, rather than the Pa_{CO_2}. The one exception occurs in the setting of intracranial hypertension. Pa_{CO_2} becomes important here because hyperventilation reduces intracerebral CO_2, causing vasoconstriction and a decrease in the intracranial pressure. This therapeutic intervention is effective only for 24 hours, and a very low Pa_{CO_2} or prolonged hyperventilation would result in cerebral ischemia.[62]

Another instance in which hyperventilation may be harmful is cardiac arrest.[63] Severe alkalosis (usually mixed) is associated with increased morbidity and mortality.[64] Hyperventilation in patients with severe chronic obstructive pulmonary disease may be detrimental for two reasons. A high $\dot{V}_E$ can augment instrinsic positive end-expiratory pressure (PEEP), leading to decreased venous return and hemodynamic instability,[65] and hyperventilation in a chronic CO_2 retainer may result in alkalosis and renal excretion of bicarbonate. This loss of buffering capacity may become problematic when an attempt is made to liberate the patient with CO_2 retention from the ventilator.

Respiratory Compensation for Metabolic Disturbances

In the presence of a metabolic acidosis, there is compensatory hyperventilation. The expected Pa_{CO_2} may be calculated with Winter's formula:[66]

$$Pa_{CO_2} = 1.5 \cdot [HCO_3^-] + 8 \pm 2$$

A respiratory disturbance exists if the calculated Pa_{CO_2} does not match the measured Pa_{CO_2}. For metabolic alkalosis, hypoventilation occurs (decreased $\dot{V}_E$); the expected Pa_{CO_2} is:

$$Pa_{CO_2} = 0.9[HCO_3^-] \pm 15$$

SURROGATE MEASURES OF ARTERIAL CARBON DIOXIDE TENSION

End-tidal Carbon Dioxide

End-tidal CO_2 pressure (P_{ETCO_2}) monitors are used routinely to ensure adequate endotracheal tube placement. Generally, the P_{ETCO_2} is several millimeters of mercury less than the Pa_{CO_2}. As shown in Figure 14-4, the two major factors that alter this gradient are (1) lung disease and (2) changes in cardiac output. Because the $P(A\text{-}ET)CO_2$ gradient is a function of V_D, in the absence of significant pulmonary disease, an acute change in the $P(a\text{-}ET)CO_2$ gradient without capnographic confirmation indicates a decrease in cardiac output.[67] P_{ETCO_2} may abruptly decrease with a pulmonary embolism and increase with treatment.[68] P_{ETCO_2} also may be helpful in assessing the adequacy of rescuscitation attempts because successful cardiopulmonary resuscitation (CPR) is associated with an increase in P_{ETCO_2}.[69] Because exhaled gas measurements reflect the in vivo (temperature-corrected) Pa_{CO_2}, the ABG Pa_{CO_2} must be temperature-corrected to ensure that the two values are being considered at the same temperature.[70]

Transcutaneous Carbon Dioxide

Transcutaneous partial pressure of CO_2 (Ptc_{CO_2}) monitors have been available for years, but are not used routinely in the ICU. This is a skin electrode that must be warmed. Results correlate with Pa_{CO_2}, but depend on factors such as hemoglobin affinity and skin perfusion.[71] There may be a delay between the time of Pa_{CO_2} change and registration of the Ptc_{CO_2} sensor, which may be problematic in patients with rapidly changing ventilatory conditions. Also, results may not be reliable when the Pa_{CO_2} is elevated.[72] Finally, increased skin thickness in adults may

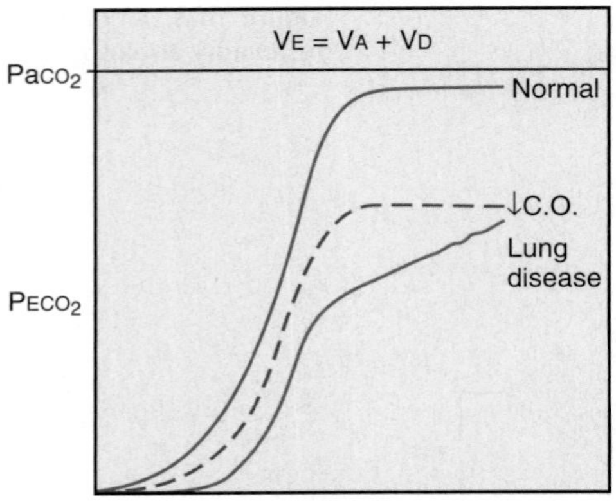

Figure 14-4. Total ventilation (VE) is composed of alveolar ventilation (VA) and deadspace ventilation (VD). The $PaCO_2$ is considered the best reflection of alveolar ventilation. The end-tidal PCO_2 is the expired PCO_2 ($PECO_2$) at the end of the plateau. An increased VE manifests as an increased $PETCO_2$ gradient. The two most common causes of increased VD are decreased cardiac output (↓C.O.) and lung disease. Decreased pulmonary perfusion *(dashed curve)* results in more alveoli having lower PCO_2; the net result is a decreased expired PCO_2, but no change in lung emptying pattern. Lung disease involves changing emptying patterns and a change in the shape of the curve. (From Shapiro BA, Peruzzi WT, Templin R: Clinical Application of Blood Gases, 5th ed. St. Louis, Mosby, 1994.)

alter transcutaneous readings, although they can be used in infants.[72]

Other Measures of Carbon Dioxide

Gastric mucosal PCO_2 is a measure of tissue hypoxia because local PCO_2 levels increase with hypoperfusion,[73] particularly in the gut mucosa. The PCO_2 gap is the difference between the tonometric PCO_2 the (measured by gastric balloon) and the $PaCO_2$ and may be predictive of mortality.[74] The mucosal pH is no longer used.[75] Because of the expense and technological considerations associated with the device, tonometry is not routinely used.

Sublingual capnometry has an optode with a fiberoptic sensor that indirectly senses PCO_2 (the $slCO_2$) by measuring pH. The $PslCO_2$-$PaCO_2$ gap may be predictive of survival,[76,77] and studies are ongoing.

The venous-arterial PCO_2 gradient, or $P(v{-}a)CO_2$, similar to the previously mentioned indices, reflects O_2 use. The gradient increases as cardiac output decreases[78] and deadspace[79] increases. This is because of the inability of tissues to unload CO_2 and the inability of the lungs to eliminate CO_2. The $P(v{-}a)CO_2$ declines with improvement in cardiac output.[80]

METABOLIC ACID-BASE IMBALANCE

The clinical form of the Henderson-Hasselbalch equation allows for the calculation of plasma bicarbonate (HCO_3^-) concentration when pH and PCO_2 are known (pK [dissociation constant] is 6.1 and S [solubility coefficient] is 0.0301):

Table 14-5. Traditional Metabolic Acid-Base Nomenclature

Nomenclature	pH	PCO_2	$[HCO_3^-]$	BE
Metabolic Acidosis				
Uncompensated (acute)	↓*	N	↓	↓ (–)
Partly compensated (subacute)	↓	↓	↓	↓ (–)
Completely compensated (chronic)	N	↓	↓	↓ (–)
Metabolic Alkalosis				
Uncompensated (acute)	↑	N	↑	↑ (+)
Partly compensated (subacute)	↑	↑	↑	↑ (+)
Completely compensated (chronic)	N	↑	↑	↑ (+)

*Arrows indicate depressed (↓) or elevated (↑) levels.
BE, base excess; N, normal.

$$pH = \frac{pK + \log[HCO_3^-]}{(s)(PCO_2)}$$

The terms *acidosis* and *alkalosis* refer to states of abnormal acid-base balance in which either an acid or a base milieu is dominant, but the pH need not be abnormal. Essentially, metabolic acidosis and alkalosis are determined by the calculation of the HCO_3^- concentration. In contrast, blood pH measurement determines *acidemia* and *alkalemia*—an excess or deficit of free hydrogen ion (H^+) activity. Table 14-5 lists the traditional nomenclature in regard to metabolic acid-base imbalance.

EVALUATING METABOLIC ACID-BASE ABNORMALITIES

In the absence of blood gas and pH measurements, metabolic acid-base imbalances can be detected and estimated to a limited degree from routine clinical chemistry studies. There are three generally accepted approaches to nonrespiratory acid-base balance: (1) anion gap, (2) base excess, and (3) strong ion difference. Selection of the appropriate process has produced significant debate and controversy for decades,[81] but these historical concerns should not confuse our clinical ability to interpret ABG values properly.[82] All three methods are appropriate and result in clinically acceptable accuracy.[83]

Anion Gap

The need for electrochemical neutrality dictates that significant differences in plasma cation and anion concentrations cannot exist. The anion gap (Fig. 14-5) is an artificial disparity between the routinely measured major plasma cations and anions—Na^+, Cl^-, and HCO_3^-. Minor plasma cations include calcium (Ca^{++}) and magnesium (Mg^{++}), whereas minor plasma anions include phosphates ($PO_4^{=}$), sulfates ($SO_4^{=}$), and organic anions such as proteins. Potassium (K^+), a minor cation, is occasionally used in the equation. The anion gap is calculated by subtracting the

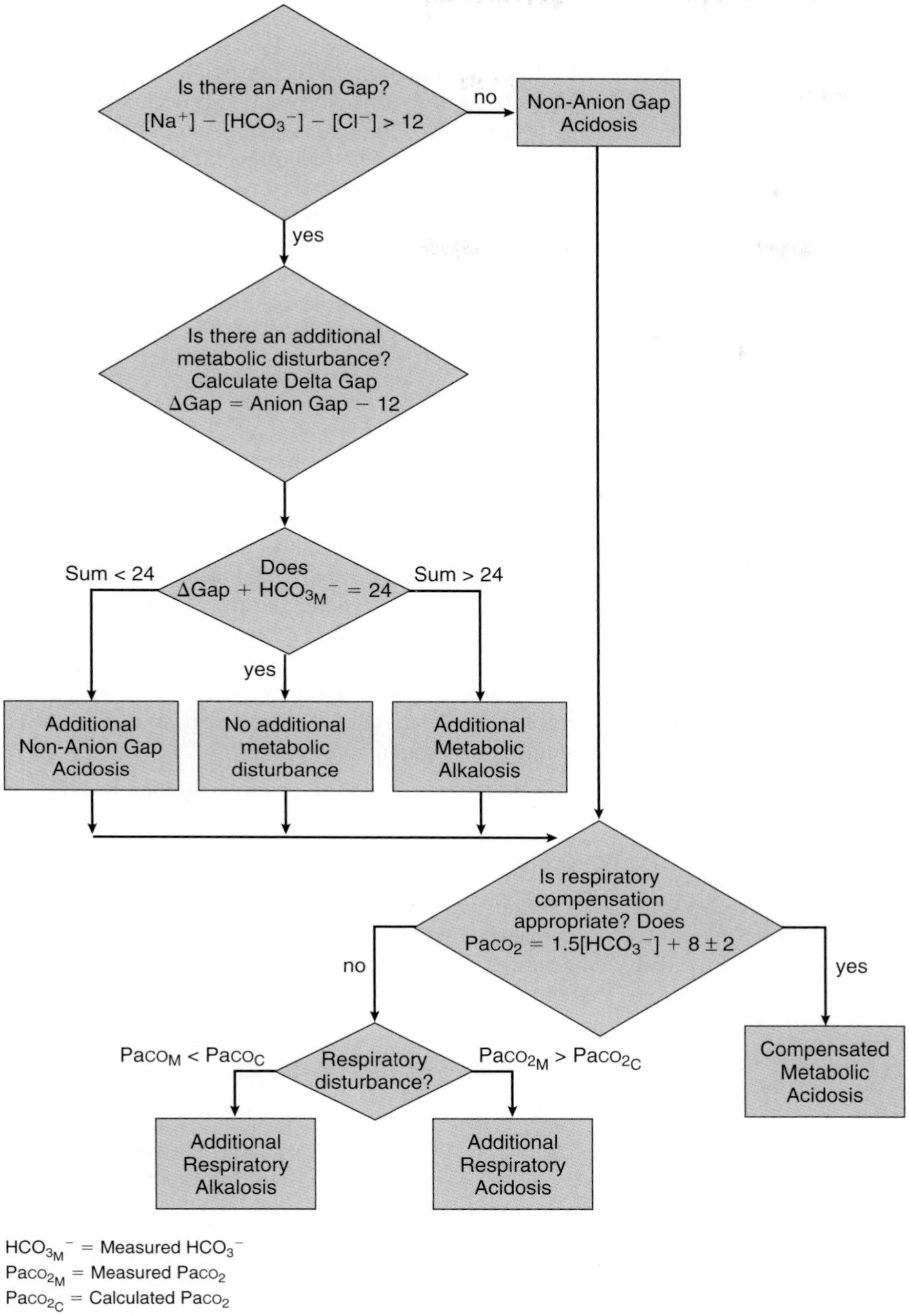

Figure 14-5. Algorithm for metabolic acidosis.

sum of the major anions from the major cations, as follows:

$$\text{Anion gap} = [Na^+ + (K^+)] - ([Cl^-] + [HCO_3^-])$$

The normal anion gap is 8 to 16 mmol/L when potassium is excluded from the calculation and 12 to 20 mmol/L when potassium is included as a major cation. Minor anions, such as phosphate and albumin, may influence the anion gap. Plasma albumin normally accounts for approximately 11 mmol/L of the anion gap[84]; a decreased anion gap is commonly the result of either hypoalbuminemia or severe hemodilution. The recommended correction for a low albumin (g/L) is[85]:

$$\text{Adjusted anion gap} = \text{observed anion gap} + 2.5 \times ([\text{normal albumin}] - [\text{measured albumin}])$$

Less commonly, a decreased anion gap is the result of an increase in the nonmajor cations, as is encountered with lithium toxicity, hypercalcemia,[86] hypermagnesemia, and bromide toxicity.

Anion Gap Acidosis

Any process that increases minor anions should create an anion gap and metabolic acidosis, as seen with lactic acidosis, ketoacidosis, renal failure (increased sulfates and phosphates), excessive electrolyte administration (i.e., sodium chloride, sodium acetate, carbenicillin, high-dose penicillin), and dehydration. Ingestion of salicylates, methanol, ethylene glycol, and other such agents causes accumulation of nonvolatile organic acids, including acetic acid. Rarely, an anion gap may result from decreased minor cation (i.e., calcium and magnesium) concentrations, which results in increased sodium concentration.

Non–Anion Gap Acidosis

A metabolic acidosis without an increased anion gap is typically associated with an increased plasma Cl^- that has replaced depleted plasma HCO_3^-. Such hyperchloremic acidosis is most commonly the result of gastrointestinal loss of HCO_3^- (diarrhea), loss from ureteral drains, renal wasting of HCO_3^- (renal tubular acidosis),[87] or excessive chloride administration,[88,89] often the result of large volume resuscitation.

Lactic Acidosis

Although it has traditionally been assumed that a non–anion gap metabolic acidosis reliably excludes hyperlactatemia,[84,90] more than half of critically ill patients with mild to moderate hyperlactatemia show a non–anion gap metabolic acidosis.[91,92] This is most likely because of preexisting hypoalbuminemia, hyperchloremia, and mixed acid-base disorders in this population.[93-96]

Because lactate is the end product of anaerobic glucose metabolism (Fig. 14-6), hyperlactatemia is a credible clinical indicator of tissue hypoxia. The cellular production of lactic acid is unreliably reflected, however, in arterial or central venous blood because specific organ system perfusion and hepatic function (i.e., clearance) vary. Anaerobic metabolism may be present despite a normal lactic acid level; conversely, a mild impairment in tissue oxygenation with a severely injured liver would result in an extremely high lactate level.

Lactate accumulation also is present in situations where the metabolic process is poisoned. This occurs when electron transport is inhibited, such as in the presence of cyanide toxicity and elevated nitric oxide levels associated with the systemic inflammatory response syndrome.[97-100] Correlation of hyperlactatemia with mortality in critically ill patients is well established.[101-104] In light of these factors, lactate levels should be measured where the clinical suspicion of lactic acidosis exists, and this is specifically recommended in early goal-directed therapy for patients with sepsis.[105]

Base Excess

Blood normally has an enormous buffering capacity that allows notable changes in acid content with little change in free H^+ concentration (pH). The concept of base excess (BE) or deficit is founded on the premise that the degree of deviation from the normal total buffer base availability can be calculated independent of compensatory $P\text{CO}_2$ changes.[106] A negative BE is referred to as a base deficit. The BE or base deficit is the amount of buffer needed to return pH to 7.40 if $Pa\text{CO}_2$ is 40 mm Hg. Most ABG analyzers report the BE or standard base excess (SBE) (assuming hemoglobin = 50 g/dL):[107,108]

$$BE = \{[HCO_3^-] - 24.4 + (2.3 \cdot \text{hemoglobin} + 7.7) \cdot (pH - 7.4)\} \cdot (1 - 0.023 \cdot \text{hemoglobin})$$

$$SBE = 0.93 \cdot \{[HCO_3^-] + 14.84 \cdot (pH - 7.4) - 24.4\}$$

Another method to calculate BE uses the predictable relationship between $Pa\text{CO}_2$ and pH. Under normal circumstances, a 10 mmol/L variance from the normal buffer baseline represents a pH change of approximately 0.15

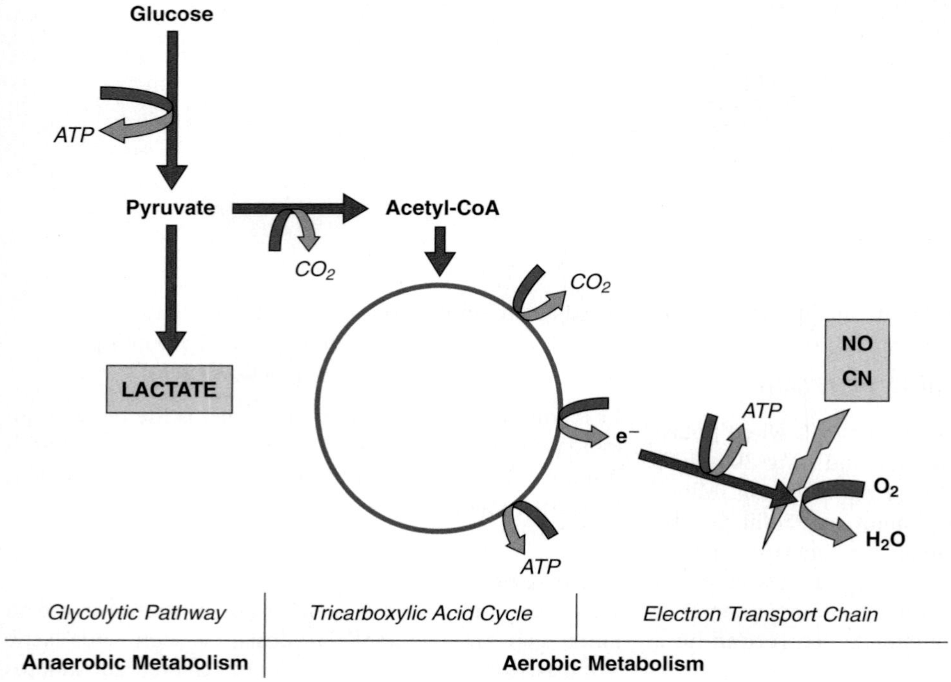

Figure 14-6. Schematic diagram of the relationship between anaerobic and aerobic metabolism. The reactions are not stoichiometrically balanced, but illustrate the key points of energy (adenosine triphosphate [ATP] production, CO_2 production, and O_2 consumption). Accumulation of lactate occurs when electron transport is blocked by agents such as nitric oxide (NO) or cyanide (CN). Lactate also accumulates in situations where O_2 is unavailable to act as the terminal electron acceptor. (From Shapiro BA, Peruzzi WT, Templin R: Clinical Application of Blood Gases, 5th ed. St. Louis, Mosby, 1994.)

units. If one moves the pH decimal point two places to the right, a two thirds relationship (i.e., 10 : 15) results. This can be used to estimate the BE or base deficit as outlined in Box 14-1.

An abnormal pH with a BE or base deficit ± 3 mmol/L denotes a normal metabolic acid-base status. A BE or base deficit ± 5 mmol/L denotes a relatively balanced clinical metabolic acid-base status. An abnormal pH with a BE or base deficit ± 10 mmol/L denotes a clinically significant metabolic acid-base imbalance that may be life-threatening.

Strong Ion Difference

The Stewart approach[109] states that the basic principles of acid-base balance are as follows: (1) strong ions are those that completely (or nearly so) dissociate in solution; (2) there is an absolute need to maintain intracellular and extracellular electrical neutrality; and (3) pH (i.e., the H^+ ion concentration) and HCO_3^- are dependent variables that change in response to changes in three key independent variables: the strong ion difference (SID), P_{CO_2}, and the total weak acid concentration (A^-).[110]

The various strong ionic species that affect the acid-base balance are primarily Na^+, K^+, Mg^{++}, and Ca^{++} on the cationic side and Cl^- and $lactate^-$ on the anionic side, such that[110]:

$$\text{SID (mEq/L)} = [Na^+] + [K^+] + [Ca^{++}] + [Mg^{++}] - [Cl^-] \pm [lactate^-]$$

These strong ions are completely dissociated in solution, and their respective concentrations (ionic activity) determine the equilibrium position of H^+ with respect to water ($H_2O \rightarrow H^+ + OH^-$) and that of bicarbonate ($H_2CO_3 \rightarrow H^+ + HCO_3^-$). In hyperchloremic acidosis from intraoperative rescuscitation with 0.9% NaCl (saline),[88] the calculation of the serum HCO_3^- concentration via the Henderson-Hasselbalch equation or the SID approach yields equivalent results. In this setting, it may be wise to use SID calculations rather than the anion gap because the SID of crystalloid is known to be zero (equal Na^+ and Cl^-),[111] whereas the albumin dilution[89] from saline rescuscitation would unpredictably decrease the anion gap. It is probably the decrease in SID, rather than the increased chloride, that explains this "hyperchloremic acidosis."[112]

Factors that decrease the SID (i.e., hyperchloremia or hyponatremia) cause a metabolic acidosis, and factors that increase the SID (i.e., hypochloremia or hypernatremia) result in a metabolic alkalosis. As expected, factors that increase the A^- (primarily albumin and phosphate) cause a metabolic acidosis, and factors that decrease the A^- produce a metabolic alkalosis.

Box 14-1

Steps for Determining Base Excess or Deficit

1. Determine P_{CO_2} Variance

Calculate the difference between measured P_{CO_2} and 40

Move the decimal point two places to the left

2. Determine Predicted pH

If P_{CO_2} is >40, subtract half of the P_{CO_2} variance from 7.40

If P_{CO_2} is <40, add the full P_{CO_2} variance to 7.40

3. Estimate Base Excess/Deficit

Determine difference between measured and predicted pH

Move decimal point two places to the right

Multiply by two thirds

A *base excess* is present if the measured pH is greater than predicted pH. A *base deficit* is present if the measured pH is less than predicted pH and is frequently represented as a negative base excess (i.e., base excess of −15 mm/L).

Metabolic Alkalosis

Metabolic alkalosis (Fig. 14-7) is most frequently seen in an ICU patient with a contraction alkalosis from severe dehydration, from diuretic use, or as compensation for a metabolic acidosis. These disease states are divided into chloride-responsive and chloride-unresponsive states and are discussed further in Chapter 58.

Mixed Acid-Base Abnormalities

The term *mixed acid-base abnormality* refers to circumstances in which respiratory and metabolic imbalances or two metabolic disturbances coexist. Examples include sepsis (decreased CO_2 production, increased minute ventilation[113] with lactic acid production) and salicylate toxicity (stimulation of the respiratory center with uncoupling of oxidative phosphorylation), both of which have combined anion gap acidosis and respiratory alkalosis. Patients with cirrhosis may have a lactic acidosis from decreased lactate clearance, combined with a respiratory alkalosis (possibly secondary to $\dot{V}/\dot{Q}$ mismatch or hormones).[114] Patients with diabetic or alcoholic ketoacidosis usually have a mixed anion gap acidosis and contraction metabolic alkalosis. Treatment with normal saline subsequently produces a non–anion gap acidosis. Because of these coexisting problems, a severe mixed acid-base disturbance might easily be overlooked. One simple way of determining whether a patient with an anion gap acidosis has an associated metabolic disturbance is to calculate the "delta gap":

$$\Delta\text{gap} = \text{anion gap} - \text{normal anion gap}$$

This number, added to the measured bicarbonate in the chemistry sample, should equal 24. A deviation from 24 signifies either a coexisting non–anion gap acidosis (<24) or a metabolic alkalosis (>24).

METABOLIC COMPENSATION FOR RESPIRATORY DISTURBANCES

For acute respiratory acidosis and alkalosis, buffering first occurs at the cellular level and then through renal mechanisms.[115]

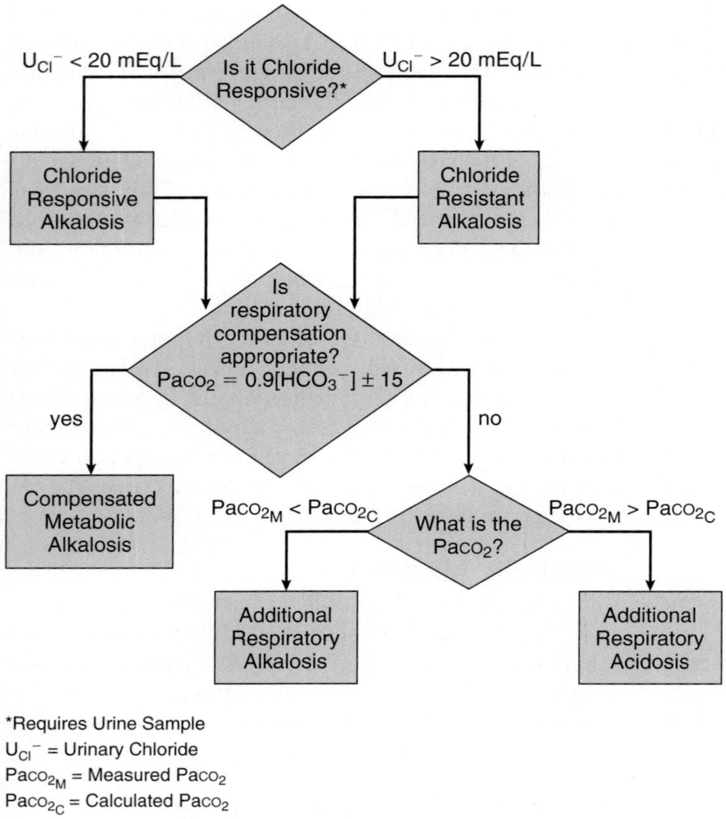

Figure 14-7. Algorithm for metabolic alkalosis.

Respiratory Acidosis

For acute respiratory acidosis, the predicted change in bicarbonate is:

$$\Delta[HCO_3^-] = \frac{\Delta PaCO_2}{10}$$

For chronic hypercapnia, bicarbonate changes as follows:

$$\Delta[HCO_3^-] = 3.5 \cdot \frac{\Delta PaCO_2}{10}$$

Respiratory Alkalosis

For acute respiratory alkalosis:

$$\Delta[HCO_3^-] = 2 \cdot \frac{\Delta PaCO_2}{10}$$

For chronic respiratory alkalosis:

$$\Delta[HCO_3^-] = 5 \cdot \frac{\Delta PaCO_2}{10}$$

Bicarbonate levels that differ from expected results indicate the presence of a mixed respiratory and metabolic disorder.

ADMINISTRATION OF BUFFER SOLUTIONS

Sodium Bicarbonate

Intravenous sodium bicarbonate ($NaHCO_3$) solution is an appropriate intervention for reversing metabolic acidemia, provided that lung and cardiac function are adequate. $NaHCO_3$ solution adds HCO_3^- to the blood only after the CO_2 load inherent in the $NaHCO_3$ solution is eliminated by the lungs. When $NaHCO_3$ solution is administered to a patient with acute ventilatory failure (respiratory acidosis), the $PaCO_2$ usually increases, and pH decreases because the CO_2 load cannot be eliminated. As illustrated in Figure 14-8, low cardiac output may be a limiting factor in CO_2 excretion. When $NaHCO_3$ solution is administered to a patient with very poor cardiac output, the venous blood shows a paradoxical respiratory acidosis.

When $NaHCO_3$ is administered intravenously to correct severe metabolic acidemia, it is essential to quantify the abnormality as a guide to therapy. A simple way to calculate the amount of bicarbonate to administer is:

$$\text{mmol } HCO_3^- = \text{base deficit (mmol/L)} \times \text{ideal weight (kg)} \times 0.25 \text{ (L/kg)}$$

where 0.25 represents the volume of distribution of the bicarbonate. It is generally prudent to administer one half to one third of the calculated deficit, obtain another ABG sample in 5 minutes, and re-evaluate.

Other Buffers

Other buffers include tris(hydroxymethyl)-aminomethane (tromethamine [THAM]), which binds protons directly, and Carbicarb, which contains equal parts of $NaHCO_3$ and sodium carbonate (Na_2CO_3); neither buffer solution produces CO_2 in the buffering process.[116-118] Tribonat is a combination of THAM, sodium bicarbonate, acetate, and phosphate. It reportedly does not have many of the side

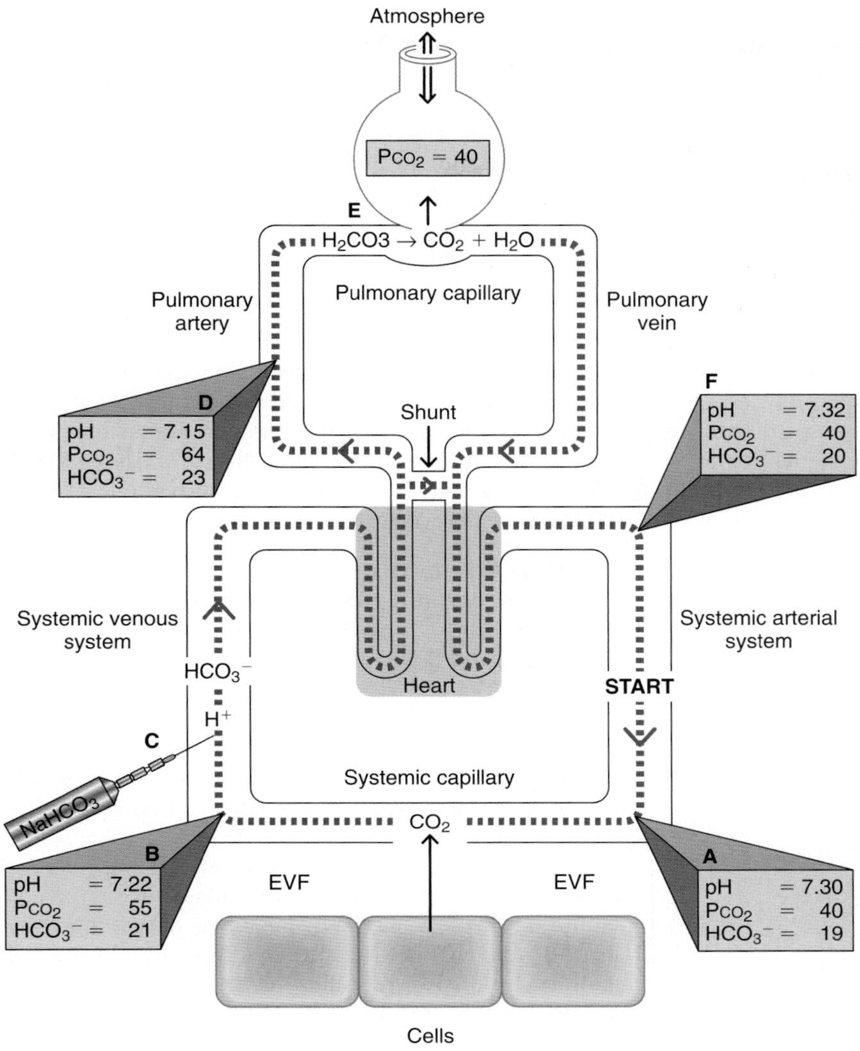

Figure 14-8. Schematic illustration of a single circulation time showing the effect of intravenous sodium bicarbonate ($NaHCO_3$) administration when a metabolic acidemia is present secondary to a low cardiac output (hypoperfusion and lactic acidemia). The diminished cardiac output is represented by the *broken circulation line.* The schema begins in the systemic arterial system *(START). Box A* represents the original arterial blood pH 7.30, Pco_2 40 mm Hg, and HCO_3^- 19 mmol/L. *Box B* represents the systemic venous system blood pH 7.22, Pco_2 55 mm Hg, and HCO_3^- 21 mmol/L before intravenous $NaHCO_3$ administration. *Box C* represents the site of intravenous $NaHCO_3$ injection, adding carbonic acid to the blood (essentially a hydrogen ion [H^+] and a bicarbonate ion [HCO_3^-]. *Box D* represents the mixed venous blood pH 7.15, Pco_2 64 mm Hg, and HCO_3^- 23 mmol/L after intravenous $NaHCO_3$ administration. *Box E* represents alveolar CO_2 excretion for the diminished blood flow per unit time. *Box F* represents the resultant arterial blood pH 7.32, Pco_2 40 mm Hg, and HCO_3^- 20 mmol/L. Note the relatively unchanged values between *A* and *F,* whereas the venous blood is significantly hypercapnic and acidemic as a result of the $NaHCO_3$ administration. EVF, extravascular fluid. (From Shapiro BA, Peruzzi WT, Templin R: Clinical Application of Blood Gases, 5th ed. St. Louis, Mosby, 1994.)

effects (hypoglycemia, changes in sodium, hypokalemia) of other buffers.[119] These agents are not routinely used in the clinical setting.

SURROGATE MEASURES OF ARTERIAL BLOOD GAS FOR METABOLIC ABNORMALITIES

Central venous blood gas measurement usually reflects ABG pH and Pco_2[120,121] and may identify acidemia before ABGs[122] in patients with shock. Peripheral venous blood gases correlate with ABGs[123]; usually the pH is slightly lower and the Pco_2 is slightly higher. This relationship can be predicted.[124] Venous blood gases are less invasive and may guide therapy when ABGs would not normally be obtained, such as in diabetic ketoacidosis.[125]

ASSESSMENT OF OXYGENATION

The status of tissue oxygenation is a global concept that cannot be directly measured and often requires ABGs.

Oxygen Content and Delivery

Because of the allosteric properties of hemoglobin,[126] most of the oxygen in the blood exists in chemical combination with hemoglobin, and less than 5% is dissolved in the plasma. The quantity of oxygen that moves into, or out of, the blood depends on three factors: (1) the amount of dissolved oxygen (Po_2); (2) the amount of oxygen combined with hemoglobin (% $HgbO_2$); and (3) the strength with which the hemoglobin binds oxygen (hemoglobin-O_2 affinity). The volume (milliliters) of oxygen contained in 100 mL (1 dL) of blood is defined as the *arterial oxygen content* (Cao_2), calculated:

$$Cao_2\ (mL/dL) = 1.34 \cdot \text{hemoglobin (g/dL)} \cdot O_2\ \text{saturation}\ (\%) + [Pao_2\ (mm\ Hg) \cdot 0.003]$$

Where 1.34 (to 1.39) is the amount of oxygen bound to each gram of hemoglobin and Pao_2 times 0.003 represents the dissolved hemoglobin in the blood. For the assessment of Cao_2 at normal ambient atmospheric pressure, the amount of dissolved oxygen is very small and often ignored. Under certain hyperbaric conditions (e.g., treatment for carbon monoxide poisoning), the amount of dissolved oxygen can be significant, however, and for brief periods can supplant the need for hemoglobin. *Oxygen delivery* ($\dot{D}O_2$) is the volume of oxygen presented to the tissues in 1 minute, expressed as:

$$\dot{D}O_2\ (mL/min/M^2) = CaO_2\ (mL/dL) \cdot CO\ (L/min)$$

where CO is cardiac output.

Several factors influence hemoglobin affinity for oxygen secondary to the Bohr effect (Fig. 14-9),[127] including acid-base status, PCO_2, temperature, and 2,3-diphosphoglycerate levels. A decrease in hemoglobin-O_2 affinity results in a diminished oxygen content that may limit oxygen delivery despite increased oxygen unloading, whereas an increase in hemoglobin-O_2 affinity increases the oxygen content, but inhibits oxygen unloading to the tissues.

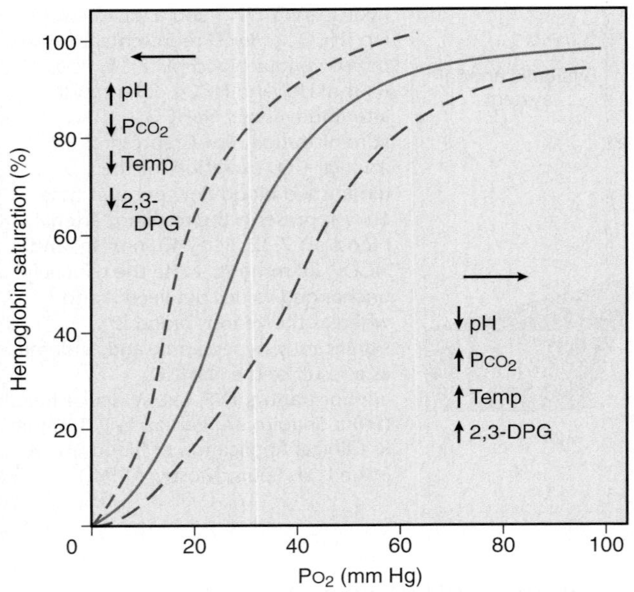

Figure 14-9. The oxyhemoglobin saturation curve and factors that alter hemoglobin affinity for oxygen. *Solid line* represents the normal curve. *Dashed lines* represent changes in affinity of hemoglobin for oxygen, and the factors listed beside the lines represent the causes of respective shifts in affinity. A shift to the left indicates an increase in hemoglobin affinity for oxygen, whereas a shift to the right represents a decrease in hemoglobin affinity for oxygen. 2, 3-DPG, 2, 3-diphosphoglycerate.

Oxygen-hemoglobin binding also is affected by abnormal hemoglobin moieties, such as methemoglobin, which cannot bind to oxygen because of the reduced state of iron (Fe^{3+}). Carboxyhemoglobin has a 300× higher affinity for oxygen, and the curve is shifted to the left, decreasing oxygen unloading to tissues.[128]

Oxygen consumption ($\dot{V}O_2$) is defined as the volume of oxygen consumed in 1 minute and may be calculated by the Fick principle:

$$\dot{V}O_2\ (mL\ O_2/min) = CO\ (L/min) \cdot [CaO_2 - CvO_2\ (mL\ O_2/100\ mL)]$$

Where $C\bar{v}O_2$ is the oxygen content of mixed venous blood and $CaO_2 - C\bar{v}O_2$, also expressed as $C_{(a\text{-}\bar{v})}O_2$, is the *arteriovenous oxygen difference*. It is generally agreed that when $\dot{D}O_2$ is three to four times greater than $\dot{V}O_2$, tissue oxygen needs are reasonably satisfied in patients without systemic inflammatory processes.[129]

Oxygen Extraction

Oxygen extraction represents the oxygen transferred to the tissues from 100 mL (or 1 dL) of blood. The *oxygen extraction ratio* (OER) is:

$$OER = C_{(a\text{-}\bar{v})}O_2/CaO_2$$

When the $\dot{V}O_2$ is constant, the $C_{(a\text{-}\bar{v})}O_2$ varies inversely with the cardiac output. Table 14-6 shows expected changes in $C_{(a\text{-}v)}O_2$ as cardiac reserves become increasingly inadequate in response to stress.[130]

The relationship between oxygen supply and oxygen demand also can be reflected in the mixed venous oxygen saturation ($S\bar{v}O_2$) when the hemoglobin content is greater than 10 g/dL.[131] The $S\bar{v}O_2$ represents the composite oxygen saturation of blood returning to the heart. Early goal-directed therapy recommends continuous monitoring of the $S\bar{v}O_2$ or $C\bar{v}O_2$,[105] which is slightly higher. The hyperdynamic response of sepsis involves a decreased oxygen extraction [$C(a\text{-}\bar{v}O_2)$], however, which is most likely secondary to decreased oxidative metabolism[113,132] and abnormal intracellular use, possibly mediated by nitric oxide interference with electron transport (see Fig. 14-6). The result is an increase in $S\bar{v}O_2$ and a seemingly improved arterial oxygenation status.

Oxygenation Deficits

As depicted in Figure 14-10, correction of arterial hypoxemia depends greatly on delineation of the degree to

Table 14-6. Predicted Oxygenation Values in Health and Disease for Pulmonary Arterial Blood

	$P\bar{v}O_2$ (%)		$S\bar{v}O_2$ (%)		$[C(a\text{-}\bar{v})O_2]$ (mL O_2/100 mL)	
Condition	**Range**	**Average**	**Range**	**Average**	**Range**	**Average**
Healthy resting human volunteer	37-43	40	70-76	75	4.5-6	5
Critically ill patient with good cardiovascular reserves	35-40	37	68-75	70	2.5-4.5	3.5
Critically ill patient with stable but limited cardiovascular reserves	30-35	32	56-68	60	4.5-6	5
Critically ill patient with cardiovascular disease	<30	<30	<56	56	>6	>6

$C(a\text{-}\bar{v})O_2$, arteriovenous oxygen difference; $P\bar{v}O_2$, peripheral venous oxygen saturation; $S\bar{v}O_2$, mixed venous oxygen saturation.

which each of three essential functions are contributing to the hypoxemia: (1) oxygen transfer across the lungs, (2) cardiac output, and (3) oxygen consumption.

Arterial Hypoxemia

Definition of Hypoxemia

Deficiencies in arterial oxygen content that demand increased cardiac work to ensure adequate $\dot{D}O_2$ are considered significant arterial oxygenation deficits (Fig. 14-11). There is no set cutoff for defining arterial hypoxemia because an adequate PaO_2 is relative to metabolic requirement. Most authors would agree that hypoxemia becomes clinically significant at a PaO_2 of 60 mm Hg or less, corresponding to an $HgbO_2$ less than 90% (see Fig. 14-9). When the PaO_2 is greater than 60 mm Hg (>90% $HgbO_2$), the blood oxygen content is close to the maximum for that hemoglobin content, and $\dot{D}O_2$ depends primarily on cardiac output and capillary perfusion; there is little to gain by increasing the PaO_2 further. A PaO_2 of 40 to 60 mm Hg may seriously threaten tissue oxygenation and result in end-organ damage if cardiac output or total hemoglobin is insufficient to compensate for the diminished oxygen content. An arterial PO_2 less than 40 mm Hg (most often associated with an $HbgO_2$ <75%) reflects not only severely decreased oxygen content, but also hemoglobin molecules less able to release oxygen to tissues; this usually results in tissue *hypoxia* despite increases in cardiac output. Also, at this steep point on the oxygen-hemoglobin dissociation curve, very small changes in PaO_2 alter hemoglobin unloading of oxygen to tissues.

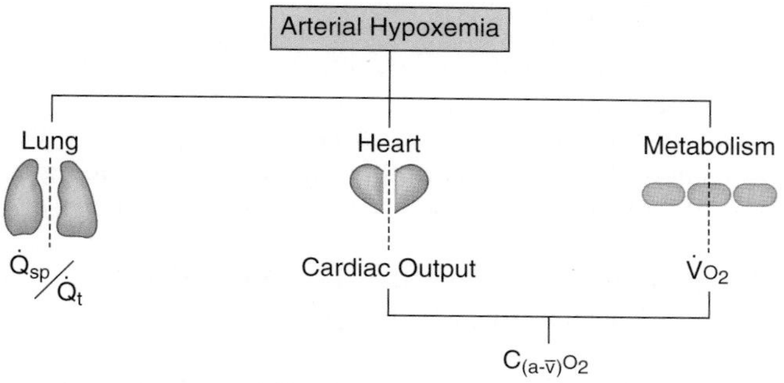

Figure 14-10. Arterial hypoxemia is attributable to some alteration in (1) lung function, (2) cardiac function, (3) metabolic function, or (4) combinations of these factors. Measurement of systemic and pulmonary arterial blood gases allows for calculation of the intrapulmonary shunt fraction ($\dot{Q}sp/\dot{Q}t$), which reliably quantifies changes in the lung's oxygen transfer capability. Measurement of systemic and pulmonary arterial blood gases allows for calculation of the arterial to mixed venous oxygen content difference ($C_{(a-\bar{v})}O_2$), which reliably reflects the relationship between the cardiac output and the oxygen consumption. $\dot{V}O_2$ is the volume of oxygen consumed in 1 minute. (From Shapiro BA, Peruzzi WT, Templin R: Clinical Application of Blood Gases, 5th ed. St. Louis, Mosby, 1994.)

Causes of Hypoxemia

Many factors causing hypoxemia occur simultaneously in critically ill patients. When an elevated $PaCO_2$ is present, the alveolar-arterial oxygenation difference ($AaDO_2$) may (1) help determine whether hypoventilation alone is the cause of hypoxemia and (2) give an indication as to the severity of the oxygenation problem:

$$AaDO_2 = PAO_2 - PaO_2$$

$$PAO_2 = FIO_2\,(PB - PH_2O) - PaCO_2/R$$

where PB is barometric pressure, PH_2O is the atmospheric pressure of water (usually 47 mm Hg), and R is the respi-

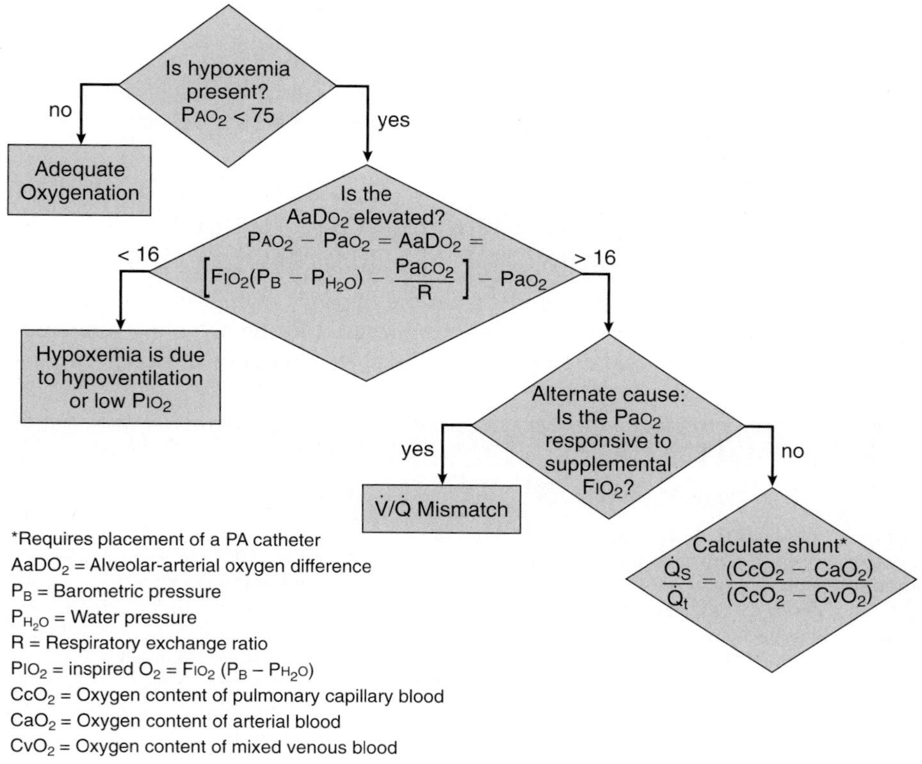

Figure 14-11. Assessment of oxygenation.

ratory exchange ratio; this is increased by conditions that increase CO_2 production: $R = \dot{V}CO_2/\dot{V}O_2$.

When the $AaDO_2$ is greater than normal (3 to 16 mm, with age-related increases),[133] hypoventilation[134] (or low fraction of inspired oxygen [FIO_2]) is not the likely cause of hypoxemia, and another cause must be sought. Rarely is a diffusion abnormality the cause of hypoxemia. The most common cause of hypoxemia is a $\dot{V}/\dot{Q}$ mismatch (Fig. 14-12).[135] Diseases that decrease perfusion (i.e., increase deadspace) result in high $\dot{V}/\dot{Q}$ ratios; complete vascular obstruction results in a unit with an infinite $\dot{V}/\dot{Q}$ ratio, whereas pulmonary hypertension causes a high $\dot{V}/\dot{Q}$ ratio. Obstructive lung disease or the incomplete filling of alveoli from pneumonia or pulmonary edema produce alveolar capillary units with low $\dot{V}/\dot{Q}$ ratios. $\dot{V}/\dot{Q}$ mismatch typically responds to oxygen administration. A complete alveolar filling process, such as acute respiratory distress syndrome, produces an intrapulmonary shunt (zero $\dot{V}/\dot{Q}$ ratio). An intracardiac shunt is produced when blood traverses the right to the left heart without contacting alveolar gas; hypoxemia results if the volume of shunted blood is significant (usually >10%). The degree of hypoxemia that results is a function of the amount (i.e., volume) of shunted blood and the oxyhemoglobin saturation of the shunted and nonshunted blood. Arterial hypoxemia occurs because the amount of oxygen dissolved in the plasma of the well-saturated (nonshunted) blood is insufficient to saturate fully the hemoglobin of the shunted blood. This results in a total hemoglobin saturation that is below normal and results in a low PaO_2 as shown by the oxyhemoglobin dissociation curve (see Fig. 14-9). This is pronounced in disease states with more than one component, such as acute respiratory distress syndrome, where shunt and $\dot{V}/\dot{Q}$ mismatch coexist.[136]

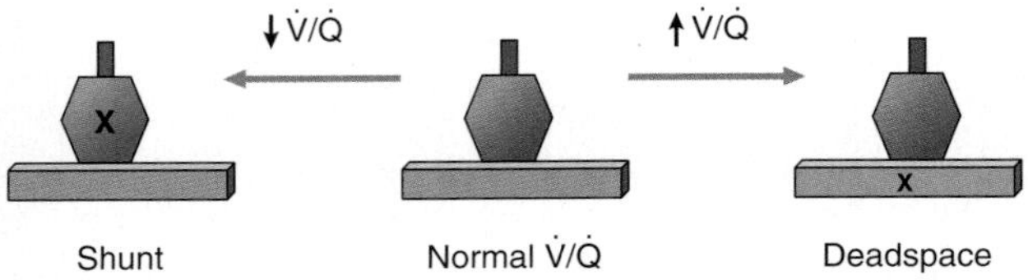

Figure 14-12. Ventilation-perfusion relationships. In acute respiratory distress syndrome, a shunt ($\dot{V}/\dot{Q} = 0$) produces blood that is not oxygenated and is refractory to increases in FIO_2. A large pulmonary embolus creates deadspace ($\dot{V}/\dot{Q} = \infty$). In between are varying degrees of $\dot{V}/\dot{Q}$ mismatch.

INTRAPULMONARY SHUNT NOMENCLATURE

Intrapulmonary shunt nomenclature is controversial and arbitrary. The sum of anatomic and capillary shunts is most commonly termed *zero* $\dot{V}/\dot{Q}$, or *true shunt,* often simply referred to as *shunt. Venous admixture* is often referred to as *low* $\dot{V}/\dot{Q}$, *$\dot{V}/\dot{Q}$ inequity,* or *shunt effect.* Shunt nomenclature is defined further in Table 14-7. The total shunt can be quantified by the shunt equation as follows[131]:

$$\dot{Q}sp/\dot{Q}t = \frac{Cc O_2 - CaO_2}{CcO_2 - C\bar{v}O_2}$$

CcO_2 is the ideal end pulmonary capillary oxygen content, calculated using the ideal alveolar gas equation to determine the ideal PO_2. The shunt equation calculates the portion of the cardiac output that traverses from the right heart to the left heart without increasing oxygen content.

Alternatives to the Shunt Calculation

Shunt calculations require analysis of pulmonary artery blood. *Oxygen tension*–based indices, such as $P(A\text{-}a)O_2$, PAO_2/PaO_2, and PaO_2/FIO_2, do not require mixed venous oxygen analysis, but have important limitations in their ability to reflect shunt fractions in critically ill patients reliably.[137]

When pulmonary arterial blood gases are unavailable, it makes physiologic and clinical sense to use an oxygen content index rather than an oxygen tension index. The most widely used oxygen content index, the estimated shunt, is derived by mathematical manipulation of the shunt equation that places the $C(a\text{-}\bar{v})O_2$ in the denominator.[138] In critically ill patients, the $C(a\text{-}\bar{v})O_2$ is approximately 35 mL/L or 3.5 volume percent:[139]

$$\text{EST}\,\dot{Q}sp/\dot{Q}t = \frac{CcO_2 - CaO_2}{[CcO_2 - CaO_2] - C(a - \bar{v})O_2} = \frac{CcO_2 - CaO_2}{[CcO_2 - CaO_2] + 3.5}$$

As shown in Table 14-8, the estimated shunt is far superior to all oxygen tension–based indices in reflecting changes in the $\dot{Q}sp/\dot{Q}t$.[140]

HYPOXEMIA, OXYGEN THERAPY, AND TIMING OF ARTERIAL BLOOD GASES

PAO_2 results from the dynamic equilibrium between the oxygen molecules delivered to the alveolus (ventilation and FIO_2) and the oxygen molecules diffusing into the

Table 14-7. Shunt Nomenclature

Classic Shunt: $\dot{Q}s/\dot{Q}t$	Physiologic Shunt: $\dot{Q}sp/\dot{Q}t$	Venous Admixture: $\dot{Q}va/\dot{Q}t$
Calculation of intrapulmonary shunt while breathing 100% inspired oxygen concentrations. Most commonly referred to as "the shunt" because this was originally believed to represent only the zero $\dot{V}/\dot{Q}$ and not venous admixture.	Calculation of intrapulmonary shunt at <100% inspired oxygen concentrations. In a normal person breathing room air, this is a measurement of the normal intrapulmonary shunt. When applied to patients with diseased lungs, it represents the severity of diminishment of the lung as an oxygenator.	Calculation of intrapulmonary shunt at <100% inspired oxygen concentrations. Exactly the same as the physiologic shunt. Preferred by some to avoid the term *physiologic* in a pathologic circumstance.

Table 14-8. Comparison of Gas Exchange Indices

Variable	Range		
	Mean (± SD)	Minimum-Maximum	R Value
$\dot{Q}sp/\dot{Q}t$	22.3 (11.2)	3-53	—
Estimated shunt	27.6 (11.3)	2.7-62.3	+0.94
RI*	3.1 (2.6)	0.3-14	+0.74
PAO_2/PaO_2	0.3 (0.2)	0.06-0.77	−0.72
PAO_2/FIO_2	1.8 (0.9)	0.1-4.3	−0.71
$P(A\text{-}a)O_2$	222.8 (141.7)	32-611	+0.62

*Respiratory index, $P(A\text{-}a)O_2/PaO_2$.

pulmonary capillary blood. All other factors remaining constant, increasing the FIO_2 increases the delivery of oxygen molecules to the alveolus and increases the PAO_2. Whether arterial hypoxemia is responsive or refractory to increased oxygen administration depends on the degree of $\dot{V}/\dot{Q}$ mismatch.

As mentioned, there are no O_2 stores to affect PaO_2. Although adjustments in PEEP may take time, changes in FIO_2 are reflected relatively quickly (within minutes) in the PaO_2.[141,142] There is evidence in animal models[143] that the timing of ABGs within the respiratory cycle has significant effects on the PaO_2 because tidal recruitment (atelectasis with expiration and alveolar expansion with inhalation) results in variation in the shunt fraction; this produces high PaO_2 during inspiration and significantly lower PaO_2 at expiration.[143]

Permissive Hypoxemia

Patients with severe lung disease often present the dilemma of what level of hypoxemia to accept. Most experts agree that an arterial PO_2 of 60 mm Hg is adequate for oxygenation in most patients, and few would argue with the acceptance of a PaO_2 in the 50s to avoid a deleterious FIO_2 or PEEP level, provided that cardiovascular function and hemoglobin content are adequate. Permissive hypoxemia is accepted as a balance of risk and benefit between the deleterious effects of advancing therapy and the deleterious effects of hypoxia.

Surrogate Measures of Arterial Oxygen Tension

Pulse oximetry measures the arterial hemoglobin saturation (SpO_2) by sensing red and infrared light emitted through oxyhemoglobin and reduced hemoglobin. States of poor perfusion[144] may be problematic. Also there may be a delay of the ability of the device to sense desaturations from digits in hypothermic patients.[145] In this setting, a forehead sensor may perform more effectively. With regard to abnormal hemoglobin moieties, carboxyhemoglobin is sensed as oxyhemoglobin, and methemoglobin significantly alters SpO_2 readings. New pulse oximeters have the ability to detect more than two wavelengths and may be able to detect these substances[146]; currently ABG analysis by co-oximeter is required.

Transcutaneous Oxygen

Similar to the $PtcCO_2$, the $PtcO_2$ is subject to variability[147] secondary to hemoglobin oxygen affinity and concentration and skin thickness and perfusion.[71] Also, monitors must be moved frequently to prevent skin damage. In shock, $PtcO_2$ is thought to reflect oxygen delivery, and it may be particularly helpful because vasoconstriction of the skin occurs before other organs. In this setting, the $PtcO_2$ response to administered FIO_2 may predict survival.[148]

ARTERIAL BLOOD GASES AND ACID-BASE BALANCE DURING CARDIOPULMONARY RESUSCITATION

Lung function normally determines CO_2 excretion and maintains a venous-arterial PCO_2 gradient of approximately 8 mm Hg. Pulmonary blood flow becomes the limiting factor determining CO_2 excretion with CPR, however, when $P(\bar{v}\text{-}a)CO_2$ may increase 3-fold to 10-fold.[149] Generally, venous hypercapnia occurs in conjunction with arterial hypocapnia.[150]

Inadequate tissue perfusion inevitably leads to anaerobic metabolism and lactic acid production. Plasma bicarbonate depletion resulting from lactic acid accumulation is seldom present, however, in the first 10 to 15 minutes of CPR,[151] probably because the liver has preserved oxygenation and metabolizes lactate to CO_2, contributing further to venous hypercapnia.

CPR generally includes an FIO_2 approaching 1.0, so arterial hypoxemia must be attributable to zero $\dot{V}/\dot{Q}$ mechanisms in the lungs. A $\dot{Q}sp/\dot{Q}t$ greater than 25% is associated with hypoxemia during CPR despite a high FIO_2. As the $P(\bar{v}\text{-}a)CO_2$ increases during CPR, blood traveling from the right heart to the left heart without exchanging with alveolar gas (true shunt or zero $\dot{V}/\dot{Q}$) has a significantly higher PCO_2 despite an adequate V_E.

Mixed venous pH is always less than the arterial pH. During CPR, an arterial pH of less than 7.2 reflects severe tissue acidosis and is a poor prognostic sign.[152] An alkalemic arterial pH during CPR is almost always the result of a low $PaCO_2$ and does not reflect the tissue acid-base state.[153] A bicarbonate deficiency (metabolic acidosis) does not produce a significant disparity between the arterial and venous blood despite differing levels of PCO_2. The degree of metabolic acidosis in arterial blood can be considered reflective of total body metabolic acidosis.

ARTERIAL BLOOD GAS MONITORS

An ABG *monitor* is a patient-dedicated device that measures arterial pH, PCO_2, and PO_2 with miniaturized sensors, or optodes,[154,155] which detect changes in fluorescence. To avoid the interface problems[156] encountered with intra-arterial placement of the optodes,[157,158] extra-arterial ABG monitoring systems have been developed. Although these devices provide *intermittent* ABG values, the measurements can be made every 3 minutes and provide routine and urgent ABGs at the bedside.[158] ABG monitors do not require the removal of blood from the patient, resulting in blood conservation in critically ill patients,[159-162] less chance of infection from line manipulation, and less blood exposure to clinical personnel. Problems with accuracy secondary to artifact[163] and wall effect (combined reading of blood and endovascular Po_2) limit their use, however.[164]

It has been suggested that combining an ABG monitor with capnography and transcutaneous oxygen measurements may allow trending of changes in cardiac output and intrapulmonary shunting.[155] Although it seems appealing to use a combination of newer and less invasive techniques to assess hemodynamic status and oxygenation, pulmonary arterial and ABG sampling remain the gold standard.

KEY POINTS

- Common circumstances that increase deadspace are acutely diminished cardiac output, acute pulmonary emboli, acute pulmonary hypertension, severe acute lung injury, and positive-pressure ventilation.
- An acute change in the $P(a\text{-ET})CO_2$ gradient without a simultaneous change in capnographic configuration indicates a change in cardiac output.
- It is important to verify the internal consistency of the ABG and blood chemistry data before proceeding with ABG interpretation.
- A decreased anion gap is commonly due to either hypoalbuminemia or severe hemodilution.
- Lactic acidosis may be present despite a normal anion gap.
- Factors that decrease the SID (i.e., hyperchloremia or hyponatremia) result in a metabolic acidosis and factors that increase the SID cause a metabolic alkalosis.
- It is generally agreed that when $\dot{D}O_2$ is three to four times greater than $\dot{V}O_2$, tissue oxygen needs are reasonably satisfied in patients without systemic inflammatory processes.
- The relationship between oxygen supply and oxygen demand also can be reflected in the $S\bar{v}O_2$ when the hemoglobin content is greater than 10 g/dL.
- The hypoxemia caused by true intrapulmonary shunting (zero $\dot{V}/\dot{Q}$) is relatively *refractory* to increased FIO_2 because the nonshunted blood is well oxygenated, so increasing the PAO_2 adds insignificant quantities of oxygen to the pulmonary capillary blood. Hypoxemia secondary to low $\dot{V}/\dot{Q}$ mechanisms is due to a diminished PAO_2; the arterial hypoxemia is *responsive* to an increased FIO_2.

REFERENCES

1. Severinghaus JW, Astrup PB: History of blood gas analysis. Int Anesthesiol Clin 1987;25:1-224.
2. Clark LC Jr: Measurement of oxygen tension: An historical perspective. Crit Care Med 1981;9:690-692.
3. Severinghaus JW, Bradley AF: Electrodes for PO_2 and PCO_2 determination. J Appl Physiol 1958;13:515-520.
4. Severinghaus JW: First electrodes for blood PO_2 and PCO_2 determination. J Appl Physiol 2004;97:1599-1600.
5. Muakkassa FF, Rutledge R, Fakhry SM, et al: ABGs and arterial lines: The relationship to unnecessarily drawn arterial blood gas samples. J Trauma 1990;30:1087-1095.
6. Shapiro BA: In-vivo monitoring of arterial blood gases and pH. Respir Care 1992;37:165.
7. International Federation of Clinical Chemistry (IFCC): Approved IFCC recommendations on whole blood sampling, transport and storage for simultaneous determination of pH, blood gases and electrolytes. Eur J Clin Chem Clin Biochem 1995;33:247-253.
8. Medicare, Medicaid and CLIA Programs: Laboratory requirements relating to quality systems and certain personnel qualifications: Final rule 68. Fed Reg 2003;3639:1022.
9. Minty BD, Nunn JF: Regional quality control survey of blood-gas analysis. Ann Clin Biochem 1977;14:245-253.
10. Peruzzi WT, Parker MA, Lichtenthal PR, et al: A clinical evaluation of a blood conservation device in medical intensive care unit patients. Crit Care Med 1993;21:501-506.
11. Walton JR, Shapiro BA, Wine C: Pre-analytic error in arterial blood gas measurement. Respir Care 1981;21:1136 (Abstract).
12. Sasse SA, Chen PA, Mahutte CK: Variability of arterial blood gases over time in stable medical ICU patients. Chest 1994;106:187-193.
13. AARC clinical practice guideline: Sampling for arterial blood gas analysis. Respir Care 1992;37:913-917.
14. Adams AP, Morgan-Hughes JO, Sykes MK: pH and blood-gas analysis: Methods of measurement and sources of error using electrode systems. Anaesthesia 1967;22:575-597.
15. Severinghaus JW, Stupfel M, Bradley AF: Accuracy of blood pH and PCO_2 determinations. J Appl Physiol 1956;9:189-196.
16. Madiedo G, Sciacca R, Hause L: Air bubbles and temperature effect on blood gas analysis. J Clin Pathol 1980;30:864-867.
17. Schmidt C, Müller-Plathe O: Stability of PO_2, PCO_2 and pH in heparinized whole blood samples: Influence of storage temperature with regard to leukocyte count and syringe material. Eur J Clin Chem Clin Biochem 1992;30:767-773.
18. Johnston HLM, Murphy R: Agreement between an arterial blood gas analyzer and a venous blood analyzer in the measurement of potassium in patients in cardiac arrest. Emerg Med J 2005; 22:269-271.
19. Ashwood ER, Kost G, Kenny M: Temperature correction of blood gas and pH measurement. Clin Chem 1983;29:1877-1885.
20. Shapiro BA: Temperature correction of blood gas values. Respir Care Clin N Am 1995;1:69-76.
21. Crapo RO, Jensen RL, Hegewald M, et al: Arterial blood gas reference values for sea level and an altitude of 1,400 meters. Am J Respir Crit Care Med 1999;160:1525-1531.
22. Shapiro BA, Harrison RA, Cane RD, et al: Clinical Application of Blood Gases, 4th ed. Chicago, Year Book Medical Publishers, 1989.
23. Rahn H, Reeves RB, Howell BJ: Hydrogen ion regulation, temperature and evaluation. Am Rev Respir Dis 1975;112:165-172.
24. Giner J, Casan P, Belda J, et al: Pain during arterial puncture. Chest 1996;110:1443-1445.
25. Davis FM, Stewart JM: Radial artery cannulation: A prospective study in patients undergoing cardiothoracic surgery. Br J Anaesth 1980;52:41-47.
26. Riley RL, Cournand A: "Ideal" alveolar air and the analysis of ventilation-perfusion relationships in the lungs. J Appl Physiol 1949;1:825-847.
27. Weinberger SE, Schwartzstein RM, Weiss JW: Hypercapnia. N Engl J Med 1989;321:1223-1231.
28. Grant JP: Nutrition care of patients with acute and chronic respiratory failure. Nutr Clin Pract 1994;9:11-17.
29. Farhi LE, Rahn H: Gas stores of body and unsteady states. J Appl Physiol 1955;7:472-484.

30. Ward SA, Whipp BJ, Koyal S, et al: Influence of body CO_2 stores on ventilatory dynamics during exercise. J Appl Physiol 1983;55:742-749.
31. Bolot JR, Berstein S, Guerin MA, et al: Iliac crest bone CO_2 and CO_2/C_a ratio in man during respiratory failure. Bull Eur Physiopathol Respir 1976;12: 39-47.
32. Wulff KE, Aulin I: The regional lung function in the lateral decubitus position during anesthesia and operation. Acta Anaesthesiol Scand 1972;16:195-205.
33. Rehder K, Wenthe FM, Sessler AD: Function of each lung during mechanical ventilation with ZEEP and with PEEP in man anesthetized with thiopental-meperidine. Anesthesiology 1973;39:597-606.
34. Higgs BE, Clode M, McHardy GJR, et al: Changes in ventilation, gas exchange and circulation during exercise in normal subjects. Clin Sci 1967;32:329-337.
35. Jones NL, McHardy GJR, Naimark A: Physiological deadspace and alveolar-arterial gas pressure differences during exercise. Clin Sci 1966;31:19-29.
36. Bergman NA: Effect of varying respiratory wave forms on distribution of inspired gas during artificial ventilation. Am Rev Respir Dis 1969;100:518-525.
37. Hedenstierna G, McCarthy G: Mechanics of breathing, gas distribution and functional residual capacity at different frequencies of respiration during spontaneous and artificial ventilation. Br J Anaesth 1975;47:706-712.
38. Kassirer JP, Bleich HL: Rapid estimation of plasma carbon dioxide tension from pH and total carbon dioxide content. N Engl J Med 1965;272:1067-1068.
39. Winters RW: Terminology of acid-base disorders. Ann Intern Med 1965;63: 873-884.
40. Bartels H, DeJours P, Kellogg RH, et al: Glossary on respiration and gas exchange. J Appl Physiol 1973;34: 549-558.
41. Brackett NC, Cohen JJ, Schwartz WB: Carbon dioxide titration curve of normal man. N Engl J Med 1965;272: 6-12.
42. Pappenheimer JR: Cerebral HCO_3^- transport and control of breathing. Fed Proc 1966;25:884-886.
43. Lahiri S, Forster RE: CO_2/H+ sensing: Peripheral and central chemoreception. Int J Biochem Cell Biol 2003;35:1413-1435.
44. Pratter MR, Corwin RW, Irwin RS: An integrated analysis of lung and respiratory muscle dysfunction in the pathogenesis of hypercapnic respiratory failure. Respir Care 1982;27:55-61.
45. Robin ED: Abnormalities of acid-base regulation in chronic pulmonary disease, with special reference to hypercapnia and extracellular alkalosis. N Engl J Med 1963;268:917-922.
46. Boddy K, Davies DL, Howie AD, et al: Total body and exchangeable potassium in chronic airways obstruction: A controversial area? Thorax 1978;33:62-66.
47. Milic-Emili J, Aubier M: Some recent advances in the study of the control of breathing in patients with chronic obstructive lung disease. Anesth Analg 1980;59:865-873.
48. Aubier M, Murciano D, Milic-Emili J, et al: Effects of the administration of O_2 on ventilation and blood gases in patients with chronic obstructive pulmonary disease during acute respiratory failure. Am Rev Respir Dis 1980;122:747-754.
49. West JB: Causes of carbon dioxide retention in lung disease. N Engl J Med 1971;284:1232-1236.
50. Robinson TD, Freiberg DB, Regnis JA, et al: The role of hypoventilation and ventilation-perfusion redistribution in oxygen-induced hypercapnia during acute exacerbations of chronic obstructive pulmonary disease. Am J Respir Crit Care Med 2000;161: 1524-1529.
51. Keenan SP, Sinuff T, Cook DJ, et al: Which patients with acute exacerbation of chronic obstructive pulmonary disease benefit from noninvasive positive-pressure ventilation: a systematic review of the literature. Ann Intern Med 2003;138:861-870.
52. Tsuno K, Miura K, Takeya M, et al: Histopathologic pulmonary changes from mechanical ventilation at high peak airway pressures. Am Rev Respir Dis 1991;143:1115-1120.
53. Parker JC, Hernandez LA, Peevy KJ: Mechanisms of ventilator-induced lung injury. Crit Care Med 1993;21: 131-143.
54. Hickling KG: Low volume ventilation with permissive hypercapnia in the adult respiratory distress syndrome. Clin Intensive Care 1992;3:67-78.
55. Acute Respiratory Distress Syndrome Network: Ventilation with lower tidal volumes as compared with traditional tidal volumes for acute lung injury and the acute respiratory distress syndrome. N Engl J Med 2000;342:1301-1308.
56. Campbell LA, Klocke RA: Implications for the pregnant patient. Am J Respir Crit Care Med 2001;163:1051-1054.
57. Pfeiffer B, Hachenberg T, Wendt M, et al: Mechanical ventilation with permissive hypercapnia increases intrapulmonary shunt in septic and nonseptic patients with acute respiratory distress syndrome. Crit Care Med 2002;30:285-289.
58. Laffey JG, Tanaka M, Engelberts D, et al: Therapeutic hypercapnia reduces pulmonary and systemic injury following in vivo lung reperfusion. Am J Respir Crit Care Med 2000;162: 2287-2294.
59. O'Croinin DF, Hopkins HO, Moore MM, et al: Hypercapnic acidosis does not modulate the severity of bacterial pneumonia-induced lung injury. Crit Care Med 2005;33:2606-2612.
60. Weil JV, Byrne-Quinn E, Sodal IE, et al: Hypoxic ventilatory drive in normal man. J Clin Invest 1970;49:1061-1072.
61. Kuo PC, Plotkin JS, Johnson LB, et al: Distinctive clinical features of portopulmonary hypertension. Chest 1997;112:980-986.
62. Brain Trauma Foundation, American Association of Neurological Surgeons, Joint Section on Neurotrauma and Critical Care: Guidelines for Management of Severe Head Injury. New York, Brain Trauma Foundation, 1995.
63. Aufderheide TP, Lurie KG: Death by hyperventilation: A common and life threatening problem during cardiopulmonary resuscitation. Crit Care Med 2004;32:S345-S351.
64. Wilson RF, Gibson D, Percinel AK, et al: Severe alkalosis in critically ill surgical patients. Arch Surg 1972;105: 197-203.
65. Marini JJ, Culver BH, Butler J: Mechanical effect of lung distension with positive pressure on cardiac function. Am Rev Respir Dis 1981; 124:382-386.
66. Albert MD, Dell RB, Winters RW: Quantitative displacement of acid-base equilibrium in metabolic acidosis. Ann Intern Med 1967;66:312-322.
67. Anderson CT, Breen PH: Carbon dioxide kinetics and capnography during critical care. Crit Care 2000;4: 207-215.
68. Weigand UK, Kurowski V, Giannitsis E, et al: Effectiveness of end-tidal carbon dioxide tension for monitoring thrombolytic therapy in acute pulmonary embolism. Crit Care Med 2000;28:3588-3592.
69. Cantineau JP, Lambert Y, Merckx P, et al: End-tidal carbon dioxide during cardiopulmonary resuscitation in humans presenting mostly with asystole: A predictor of outcome. Crit Care Med 1996;24:279-796.
70. Smallhout B, Kalenda Z: An Atlas of Capnography. Zeist, Netherlands, Kerckebosch. 1975.
71. Burki NK, Albert RK: Noninvasive monitoring of arterial blood gases: A report of the ACCP section on respiratory pathophysiology. Chest 1983;83:666-670.
72. Tobias JD, Meyer DJ: Noninvasive monitoring of carbon dioxide during respiratory failure in toddlers and infants: End-tidal versus transcutaneous carbon dioxide. Anesth Analg 1997;85:55-58.
73. Maynard N, Bihari D, Beale R, et al: Assessment of splanchnic oxygenation by gastric tonometry in patients with acute circulatory failure. JAMA 1993;270:1203-1210.
74. Levy B, Gawalkiewicz P, Vallet B, et al: Gastric capnometry with air-automated tonometry predicts outcome in critically ill patients. Crit Care Med 2003;31:474-480.
75. Schlichtig R, Mehta N, Gayowski TJ: Tissue-arterial PCO_2 difference is a better marker of ischemia than intramural pH (pHi) or arterial pH-pHi difference. J Crit Care 1996;11:51-56.
76. Rackow EC, O'Neil P, Astiz ME, et al: Sublingual capnometry and indexes of tissue perfusion in patients with circulatory failure. Chest 2001;120:1633-1638.
77. Marik PE, Bankov A: Sublingual capnometry versus traditional markers of tissue oxygenation in critically ill patients. Crit Care Med 2003;31:818-822.
78. Groeneveld ABJ: Interpreting the venous-arterial PCO_2 difference. Crit Care Med 1998;26:979-980.
79. Bakker J, Vincent JL, Gris P, et al: Veno-arterial carbon dioxide gradient in

human septic shock. Chest 1992;101:509-515.
80. Teboul JL, Mercat A, Lenique F, et al: Value of the venous-arterial PCO_2 gradient to reflect the oxygen supply to demand in humans: Effects of dobutamine. Crit Care Med 1998;26:1007-1010.
81. Severinghaus JW: Acid-base balance controversy. J Clin Monit 1991;7: 274-275.
82. Fagan T: Base excess and inappropriate bicarbonate. J Clin Monit 1993;9:67-68 (Letter and reply).
83. Dubin A, Menises MM, Masevicius FD, et al: Comparison of three different methods of evaluation of metabolic acid-base disorders. Crit Care Med 2007;35:1-6.
84. Emmett M, Narins RG: Clinical use of the anion gap. Medicine 1977;56:38-54.
85. Figge J, Jabor A, Kazda A, et al: Anion gap and hypoalbuminemia. Crit Care Med 1998;26:1807-1810.
86. Oster JR, Gutierrez R, Schlessinger FB, et al: Effect of hypercalcemia on the anion gap. Nephron 1990;55: 164-169.
87. Koch SM, Taylor RW: Chloride ion in intensive care medicine. Crit Care Med 1992;20:227-240.
88. Scheingraber S, Rehm M, Sehmisch C, et al: Rapid saline infusion produces hyperchloremic acidosis in patients undergoing gynecologic surgery. Anesthesiology 1999;90:1265-1270.
89. Prough DS: Hyperchloremic metabolic acidosis is a predictable consequence of intraoperative infusion of 0.9% saline. Anesthesiol 1999;90:1247-1249 (Editorial).
90. Oh MS, Carroll HJ: The anion gap. N Engl J Med 1977;297:814-817.
91. Iberti TJ, Leibowitz AB, Papadakos PJ, et al: Low sensitivity of the anion gap as a screen to detect hyperlactatemia in critically ill patients. Crit Care Med 1990;18:275-27790.
92. Mehta K, Kruse JA, Carlson RW: The relationship between anion gap and elevated lactate. Crit Care Med 1986;14:405 (Abstract).
93. Mizock BA: Controversies in lactic acidosis: Implications in critically ill patients. JAMA 1987;258:497-501.
94. Madias NE, Cohen JJ, Adrogue HJ: Influence of acute and chronic respiratory alkalosis on preexisting chronic metabolic alkalosis. Am J Physiol 1990;258:479.
95. Neary RH, Edwards JD: Metabolic alkalosis and hyperlactatemia. BMJ 1987;294:1462.
96. Kruse JA, Carlson RW: Lactate metabolism. Crit Care Clin 1987;3:725-746.
97. Leist M, Single B, Naumann H, et al: Inhibition of mitochondrial ATP generation by nitric oxide switches apoptosis to necrosis. Exp Cell Res 1999;249:396-403.
98. Nishikawa M, Sato EF, Kuroki T, et al: Macrophage-derived nitric oxide induces apoptosis of rat hepatoma cells in vivo. Hepatology 1998;28: 1474-1480.
99. Hurst RD, Clark JB: Nitric oxide-induced blood-brain barrier dysfunction is not mediated by inhibition of mitochondrial respiratory chain activity and/or energy depletion. Nitric Oxide 1997;1:121-129.
100. Okada S, Takehara Y, Yabuki M, et al: Nitric oxide, a physiologic modulator of mitochondrial function. Physiol Chem Phys Med NMR 1996;28:69-82.
101. Broder G, Weil MH: Excess lactate: An index of reversibility of shock in human patients. Science 1964;143:1457-1459.
102. Peretz DI, Scott HM, Duff J, et al: The significance of lactic acidemia in the shock syndrome. Ann N Y Acad Sci 1965;119:1133-1141.
103. Luft D, Deichel G, Schmulling RM, et al: Definition of clinically relevant lactic acidosis in patients with internal diseases. Am J Clin Pathol 1983;80:484-489.
104. Husain FA, Martin MJ, Mullenix PS, et al: Serum lactate and base deficit as predictors of mortality and morbidity. Am J Surg 2003;185:485-491.
105. Rivers E, Havstad S, Ressler J, et al: Early goal-directed therapy in the treatment of severe sepsis and septic shock. N Engl J Med 2001;345: 1368-1377.
106. Morgan TJ, Clark C, Endre ZH: Accuracy of base excess: An in vitro evaluation of the Van Slyke equation. Crit Care Med 2000;28: 2932-2936.
107. Siggaard-Anderson O: The Van Slyke equation. Scand J Clin Lab Invest 1977;37(Suppl 146):15-19.
108. Severinghaus JW: Acid-base balance nomogram—a Boston-Copenhagen détente. Anesthesiology 1976;45: 539-541.
109. Stewart PA: Modern quantitative acid-base chemistry. Can J Physiol Pharmacol 1983;51:1444-1461.
110. Kellum JA: Determinants of plasma acid-base balance. Crit Care Clin 2005;21:329-346.
111. Morgan TJ: Clinical review: The meaning of acid-base abnormalities in the intensive care unit—effects of fluid administration. Crit Care 2005;9: 204-211.
112. Story DA, Morimatsu H, Bellomo R: Hyperchloremic acidosis in the critically ill: One of the strong-ion acidosis? Crit Care Trauma 2006;103: 144-148.
113. Nishijima H, Weil MH, Shubin H, et al: Hemodynamic and metabolic studies on shock associated with gram negative bacteremia. Medicine 1973; 52:287-294.
114. Lustik SJ, Chibber AK, Kolano JW, et al. The hyperventilation of cirrhosis: Progesterone and estradiol effects. Hepatology 1997;25:55-58.
115. Narins RG, Emmett M: Simple and mixed acid-base disorders: A practical approach. Medicine 1980;59:161-187.
116. Adrogue HJ, Madias NE: Medical progress: Management of life-threatening acid-base disorders, first of two parts. N Engl J Med 1998;338:26-34.
117. Arieff AI: Efficacy of buffers in the management of cardiac arrest. Crit Care Med 1998;26:1311-1313.
118. Bar-Joseph G, Weinberger T, Castel T, et al: Comparison of sodium bicarbonate, Carbicarb, and THAM during cardiopulmonary resuscitation in dogs. Crit Care Med 1998;26:1397-1408.
119. Bjerneroth G: Tribonat—a comprehensive summary of its properties. Crit Care Med 1999;27:1009-1013.
120. Phillips B, Peretz DI: A comparison of central venous and arterial blood gas values in the critically ill. Ann Intern Med 1969;10:745-749.
121. Malinoski DJ, Todd SR, Slone S, et al: Correlation of central venous and arterial blood gas measurements in mechanically ventilated trauma patients. Arch Surg 2005;140: 1122-1125.
122. Benjamin E, Paluch TA, Berger SR, et al: Venous hypercarbia in canine hemorrhagic shock. Crit Care Med 1987;15:516-518.
123. Yildizdas D, Yaicioglu H, Yilmas HK, et al: Correlation of simultaneously obtained capillary, venous and arterial blood gases of patients in a pediatric intensive care unit. Arch Dis Child 2004;89:176-180.
124. Chu YC, Chen CZ, Lee CH: Prediction of arterial blood gas values from venous blood gas values in patients with acute respiratory failure receiving mechanical ventilation. J Formos Med Assoc 2003;102:539-543.
125. Ma OJ, Rush MD, Godfrey MM, et al: Arterial blood gas results rarely influence emergency physician management of patients with suspected diabetic ketoacidosis. Acad Emerg Med 2003;10:836-841.
126. Perutz M: Stereochemistry of cooperative effects in hemoglobin. Nature 1970;228:726-734.
127. Bock AV, Field H, Adair GS: Oxygen and carbon dioxide dissociation curves of human blood. J Biol Chem 1924; 59:353-378.
128. Collier CR: Oxygen affinity of human blood in the presence of carbon monoxide. J Appl Physiol 1976;40: 487-490.
129. Shoemaker WC, Appel PL, Waxman K, et al: Clinical trial of survivors' cardiorespiratory patterns as therapeutic goals in critically ill postoperative patients. Crit Care Med 1982;10:398-403.
130. Harrison RA, Davison R, Shapiro BA, et al: Reassessment of the assumed A-V oxygen content difference in the shunt calculation. Anesth Analg 1975;54:198-202.
131. Hess D, Maxwell C, Shefet D: Determination of intrapulmonary shunt: Comparison of an estimated shunt equation and a modified shunt equation with the classic equation. Respir Care 1987;32:268.
132. Fink MP: Cytopathic hypoxia: Mitochondrial dysfunction as a mechanism contributing to organ dysfunction in sepsis. Crit Care Clin 2001;17:219-237.
133. Kanber GJ, King FW, Eshchar YR, et al: The alveolar-arterial oxygen gradient in young and elderly men during air and oxygen breathing. Am Rev Respir Dis 1968;9:376-381.
134. Farhi LE, Rahn H: Theoretical analysis of the alveolar-arterial O_2 difference with special reference to the distribution effect. J Appl Physiol 1955;7:699-703.

135. Gowda M, Klocke R: Variability of indices of hypoxemia in adult respiratory distress syndrome. Crit Care Med 1997;25:41-45.
136. Dantzker DR, Brook CJ, Dehart P, et al: Ventilation-perfusion distributions in the adult respiratory distress syndrome. Am Rev Respir Dis 1979;120:1039-1052.
137. Foex P, Prys-Roberts C, Hahn CEW, et al: Comparison of oxygen content of blood measured directly with values derived from measurements of oxygen tension. Br J Anaesth 1970;42: 803-804.
138. Bendixen HH, Egbert LD, Hedley-Whyte J, et al: Respiratory Care. St. Louis, Mosby, 1965.
139. Harrison RA, Davison R, Shapiro BA, et al: Reassessment of the assumed A-V oxygen content difference in the shunt calculation. Anesth Analg 1975;54:198-202.
140. Cane RD, Shapiro BA, Templin R, et al: The unreliability of oxygen tension based indices in reflecting intrapulmonary shunting in critically ill patients. Crit Care Med 1988;16: 1243-1245.
141. Gilbert R, Keighley JF: The arterial/alveolar oxygen tension ratio: An index of gas exchange applicable to varying inspiratory oxygen concentrations. Am Rev Respir Dis 1974;109:142-145.
142. Hess D, Good C, Didyoung R, et al: The validity of assessing arterial blood gases 10 minutes after an FIO_2 change in mechanically ventilated patients without chronic pulmonary disease. Respir Care 1985;30: 1037-1041.
143. Pfeiffer B, Syring RS, Markstaller K, et al: The implications of arterial PO_2 oscillations for conventional arterial blood gas analysis. Anesth Analg 2006;102:1758-1764.
144. Reich DL, Timcenko A, Bodian CA, et al: Predictors of pulse oximetry data failure. Anesthesiology 1996;84:859-864.
145. MacLeod DB, Cortinez LI, Keifer JC, et al: The desaturation response time of finger pulse oximeters during mild hypothermia. Anaesthesia 2005;60: 65-71.
146. Barker SJ, Curry J, Redford D, et al: Measurement of carboxyhemoglobin and methemoglobin by pulse oximetry: A human volunteer study. Anesthesiology 2006;105:892-897.
147. Green GE, Hassell KT, Mahutte CK: Comparison of arterial blood gas with continuous intra-arterial and transcutaneous PaO_2 sensors in adult critically ill patients. Crit Care Med 1987;15:491-494.
148. Yu M, Morita SY, Daniel SR, et al: Transcutaneous pressure of oxygen: A noninvasive and early detector of peripheral shock and outcome. Shock 2006;26:450-456.
149. Benjamin E, Paluch TA, Berger SR, et al: Venous hypercarbia in canine hemorrhagic shock. Crit Care Med 1987;15:516-518.
150. Weil MH, Rackow EC, Trevino R, et al: Difference in acid-base state between venous and arterial blood during cardiopulmonary resuscitation. N Engl J Med 1986;315:153-156.
151. Sanders AB, Ewy GA, Taft TV: Resuscitation and arterial blood gas abnormalities during prolonged cardiopulmonary resuscitation. Ann Emerg Med 1984;13:676.
152. Suljaga-Pechtel K, Goldberg E, Strickon P, et al: Cardiopulmonary resuscitation in a hospitalized population: Prospective study of factors associated with outcome. Resuscitation 1984;12: 77-95.
153. Ornato JP, Gonzalez ER, Coyne MR, et al: Arterial pH in out of hospital cardiac arrest: Response time as a determinant of acidosis. Am J Emerg Med 1985;3:498-502.
154. Optiz N, Lubbers DW: Theory and development of fluorescence-based optochemical oxygen sensors: Oxygen optodes. Int Anesthesiol Clin 1987; 25:177-197.
155. Shapiro BA, Cane RD, Chomka CM, et al: Preliminary evaluation of an intra-arterial blood gas system in dogs and humans. Crit Care Med 1989; 17:455-460.
156. Mahutte CK, Sassoon CSH, Muro JR, et al: Progress in the development of a fluorescent intravascular blood gas system in man. J Clin Monit 1990;6:147-157.
157. Greene GE, Hassell KT, Mahutte CK: Comparison of arterial blood gas with continuous intra-arterial and transcutaneous PO_2 sensors in adult critically ill patients. Crit Care Med 1987;15:491-494.
158. Shapiro BA, Mahutte CK, Cane RD, et al: Clinical performance of a blood gas monitor: A prospective, multicenter trial. Crit Care Med 1993;121:487-494.
159. Shapiro BA: Quality improvement standards for intensive care unit monitors: We must be informed and involved. Crit Care Med 1992;20: 1629-1930.
160. Medicare, Medicaid and CLIA programs: Regulations implementing the clinical laboratory improvement amendments of (CLIA '88). Fed Reg 1992;57:7008.
161. Salem B, Chernow B, Burke R: Bedside diagnostic testing: Its accuracy, rapidity, and utility in blood conservation. JAMA 1991;266: 382-389.
162. Chernow B, Salem M, Stacey J: Blood conservation—a critical imperative. Crit Care Med 1991;19: 313-314.
163. Coule LW, Truemper EJ, Steinhart CM, et al: Accuracy and utility of a continuous intra-arterial blood gas monitoring system in pediatric patients. Crit Care Med 2001;29: 420-426.
164. Zimmerman JL, Dellinger RP: Initial evaluation of a new intra-arterial blood gas system in humans. Crit Care Med 1993;21:495-500.

Chapter 15

Tracheostomy

Yaakov Friedman and Sabine Sobek

HISTORY

Most medications, devices, and surgical techniques employed in today's intensive care unit (ICU) have resulted from 20th century medical advances. However, one of the most common surgical procedures, tracheostomy, has been described for nearly 6000 years. The terms *tracheostomy* and *tracheotomy* are derived from the Greek word *tracheia arteria,* translated "rough artery" and referring to the trachea being the vital conduit of air.[1] Tracheostomy means permanent opening (*stoma,* Greek for "mouth"), to be distinguished from the temporary nature of a tracheotomy (*tome,* "to cut"). Today the terms are used interchangeably for any artificial airway created in the trachea, with tracheostomy used more commonly.

In the seminal historical article on tracheostomy, Frost noted the procedure actually preceded the Greeks.[2] The first written reference to tracheostomy is in the sacred book of Hindu medicine, the *Rig Veda,* dated between 2000 BCE and 1000 BCE, and describes "the bountiful one, who without a ligature, can cause the windpipe to reunite when the cervical cartilages are cut across."[2,3] The earliest depictions of a tracheostomy being performed date back to about 3600 BCE and show two Egyptian kings undergoing a tracheostomy.[4,5] In 124 BCE, Asclepiades of Prusa referred to the tracheostomy as being practiced by the ancients, and he probably performed one himself. None of the existing fragments of his writing confirm this, however, and the operation is credited to him only through the writing of Galen and Aretaeus.

The next successful tracheostomy was performed in the 2nd century CE by Antyllus. He is quoted in a text 400 years later by Paul of Aegina:[6]

> In cases of cynache [today known as "Croup"] we entirely disapprove of this operation, because . . . the lungs are affected; but in [cases] which obstruct the mouth of the windpipe, and the trachea is unaffected, it will be proper to have recourse to pharyngotomy in order to avoid the risk of suffocation. When, therefore, we engage in the operation we slit open a part of the arteria aspera (for it is dangerous to divide the whole) below the top of the windpipe, about the third or fourth ring. . . . Wherefore bending the patient's head backwards, so as to bring the windpipe better into view, we are to make a transverse incision between two of the rings, so that it may not be the cartilage which is divided, but the membrane connecting the cartilages. . . . We judge the windpipe has been opened from the air rushing through it with a whizzing noise and from the voice having been lost.

Mention of tracheostomy can be found in the Roman and Arabic literature, although during the Dark Ages of medicine and science the technique of tracheostomy (and virtually all other surgeries) was forgotten for nearly 1000 years.[5,7] During the Renaissance, European physicians experimented with tracheostomy for trauma, aspirated foreign bodies, drowning, and Ludwig's angina, although the procedure was still viewed with considerable skepticism and fear. Fabricius of Aquapendente tells us that this timidity was due partly to "lack of knowledge of anatomy, partly to fear of a loss of reputation [infamiae metus], should the patient die after the operation." In his day, the tracheostomy was known as the "scandal of surgery." About the same time, in 1546, the first clear account of a successful tracheotomy was recorded by Antonius Brasavola, who "told of opening the windpipe and saving the life of a patient near death from angina and an abscess which was obstructing the canalis pulmonis."[1,7] Over the next 2 centuries, opposition to tracheostomy diminished because of the interest in anatomy and autopsy, as evidenced by the drawings and writings of Leonardo da Vinci, Julius Casserius, and others.[5,8-10]

In Western Europe in the 18th and 19th centuries, the clinical importance of tracheostomy became evident during sporadic diphtheria epidemics, and multiple publications of successful tracheostomies can be found in many European countries after 1620.[7] In 1730, Scottish surgeon George Martine treated upper airway obstruction resulting from diphtheria with tracheostomy. He also recommended the use of an inner cannula for ease of care and recognized that tracheal wounds heal spontaneously without the need for surgical repair.[7,11] In America, fear of tracheostomy was still quite prevalent, as evidenced in the well-known controversy surrounding the death of George Washington in 1799, when bloodletting won over relieving an epiglottitis-related upper airway obstruction with a tracheostomy.[5,12] Until 1825, during these first several thousand years in the history of tracheostomy, only 28 tracheostomies are verifiable.

After Napoleon Bonaparte's "son" died of diphtheria in 1807, a grand prize was offered for new insights into this disease and its treatment. Based on subsequent research especially by Bretonneau and his pupil Trousseau, tracheostomy became a relatively established procedure, particularly for croup and diphtheria. Before Bretonneau, tracheostomy had been known under many different names (e.g., bronchotomy, laryngotomy, pharyngotomy, sectio epiglottis, scisio cannae, incisio cannae pulmonis). In 1718 Heister had introduced the term *tracheotomy* and recommended that all other terms be discarded, but it was not until Bretonneau used this term in a paper describing a successful operation in 1825 for diphtheria that it gained widespread acceptance.[7,13] Trousseau described a series of 200 French children, most dying of diphtheria, in whom he reduced mortality from nearly 100% to 75% with tracheostomy.[14] American surgeon Thomas Shastid published an account of performing tracheostomies on children in the 1890s in a small Illinois town during a diphtheria epidemic.[15,16]

In the mid 1800s, Snow and Trendelenburg advocated tracheostomy for administration of inhaled anesthetics,[2,17] but endotracheal intubation, performed by MacEwan in 1878[18] and O'Dwyer in 1880[19] and popularized by Bartholomay and Dufor in 1907 and Kelly in 1912, soon replaced tracheostomy as the route for delivering general anesthesia.[2,20] This put the performance of tracheostomy squarely in the hands of surgeons experienced in upper airway problems, most notably Chevalier Jackson, whose name became virtually synonymous with tracheostomy. In his hands, mortality attributable to tracheostomy decreased from 25% to less than 5%.[21]

The current era of tracheostomy began in the last half of the 20th century, heralded by a revolutionary shift in the indications for the procedure and major advances in the technique. Two major causes of upper airway obstruction (severe croup and diphtheria), which was virtually the only indication for tracheostomy, practically disappeared as a result of the development of antibiotics and immunization. In the 1950s, with the poliomyelitis epidemic in Europe and North America, the need for positive-pressure ventilation (PPV) and tracheobronchial suctioning created new indications for tracheostomy.[22] At present, these are still the major indications for tracheostomy in the ICU, and they caused the number of tracheostomies performed at Massachusetts General Hospital to increase from fewer than 10 in 1947 to more than 150 in 1959. Before 1958, not a single tracheostomy was performed there for the sole purpose of providing PPV.[23]

The exponential increase in tracheostomy in the 1950s and 1960s revived older controversies. In 1921, Chevalier Jackson discussed proper technique and complications.[24] He condemned the use of high tracheostomy, believing it caused laryngeal stenosis, and that, if done, it should be immediately converted to a low tracheostomy. For 50 years, this was the prevailing wisdom of neck surgery and airway maintenance. Jackson drew his conclusions, however, primarily from unsterile emergency tracheostomies performed by inexpert practitioners.[24] Laryngeal stenosis probably resulted from factors other than the site of incision, especially when performed with preexistent laryngeal pathology.[25,26] Jackson's reputation made surgeons reluctant to perform high tracheostomies until the advent of cardiac surgery made them necessary to avoid contaminating median sternotomy incisions. In 1976, two cardiac surgeons, Brantigan and Grow, published the first large series of high tracheostomies and found few complications.[27] Acceptance of high tracheostomy permitted reintroduction of percutaneous tracheostomy, a technique described 20 years earlier.

As previously described, when ICUs were developed, tracheostomy became one of the most frequently performed procedures in critically ill patients.[28] This situation created a need for a safe, cost-effective bedside procedure that would eliminate the necessity for transport of the patient from the ICU to the operating room, with its attendant risks, which are discussed subsequently.

In 1955, Shelden and colleagues[29] described the first percutaneous tracheostomy using a slotted needle to guide a cutting trochar into the trachea. This technique was abandoned after fatalities resulted from trocar lacerations of vital structures adjacent to the airway.[30,31] In 1969, Toye and Weinstein[32] described a modified Seldinger technique in which a splitting needle was inserted into the trachea, and through this a guidewire was placed. A single lead dilator was passed over the guidewire, the needle split away, and the tracheostomy tube placed. This technique had a 1% incidence of perioperative death and a 6% incidence of paratracheal insertion, which ultimately caused it also to be abandoned.[33]

In 1985, Ciaglia and coworkers,[34] drawing from experience with cricothyroidotomy, described a true Seldinger technique for quick and easy bedside tracheostomy, percutaneous dilational tracheostomy (PDT). In this technique, multiple curved dilators of gradually increasing size are placed over a guidewire, creating an opening for a tracheostomy tube.

Subsequently, several different versions of percutaneous tracheostomy have been described. In 1988, Hazard and associates[35] had few complications using only three straight instead of Ciaglia's seven curved dilators. In 1989, Schachner and colleagues[36] reported a dilating forceps technique (Rapitrac), which is no longer available for use because of its high incidence of complications. In 1990, Griggs and coworkers[37] described passing a blunt-tipped modified Kelly forceps over a guidewire to allow dilation of an aperture adequate to place a tracheostomy tube (GWDF). This technique is similar to the Rapitrac, but with a lower incidence of complications. In 1999, Ciaglia developed a tapered dilator (Blue Rhino; Cook Critical Care, Inc., Bloomington, IN), in which stomal creation occurs in a single-step dilation.[38] This replaced the multiple dilations necessary in Ciaglia's original kit, theoretically reducing complications and the time necessary to perform PDT. Fantoni's translaryngeal tracheotomy technique was introduced in 1993 and modified in 1996.[39] A guidewire is directed retrograde from the trachea to the mouth over which a cuffed cone-cannula is placed. The cannula is drawn through the neck, and a cuffed tube is placed in the trachea over the cannula as it is removed. The PercuTwist, developed in 2002, uses a dilator with a threaded screw to allow the insertion of a 9-mm tracheostomy tube.[40]

ARTIFICIAL AIRWAYS

In critical care medicine, regardless of the patient's diagnosis, there are four indications for placement of an artificial airway (either an endotracheal tube or tracheostomy): (1) relieving airway obstruction, (2) providing PPV or continuous positive airway pressure (CPAP), (3) preventing aspiration in an unprotected airway, and (4) facilitating suctioning of secretions for ineffective cough.[41,42]

Intubation and tracheostomies are performed not because of a specific disease, but because an indication is present as a result of disease. Patients do not need intubation because they have chronic obstructive pulmonary disease or have taken a drug overdose; rather, they need PPV or cannot protect their airway. In examining the rationale for intubation or tracheostomy, clinicians working in the ICU should identify the patient as having an indication for an artificial airway, and before the airway is removed, the indication must no longer exist.

Although tracheostomy previously was considered the emergency airway of choice, endotracheal intubation is now preferred for initial airway management because more practitioners are familiar with endotracheal intubation (which requires less specialized equipment and training), and studies indicate that in the emergency setting, endotracheal intubation has fewer life-threatening complications.[43-45] The trachea, situated deep in the neck, is surrounded by blood vessels capable of significant and life-threatening hemorrhage. The incidence of bleeding, essentially negligible in endotracheal intubation, is about 5% in tracheostomies. Pneumothorax is seen in 5% of tracheostomies, but rarely in endotracheal intubation. Independent of esophageal placement, mortality from endotracheal intubation is 0.05%, but ranges from 1% to 2% for emergency tracheostomy.[28] Tracheostomy should be considered an elective or semielective procedure when the airway is already secured.

Occasionally, endotracheal intubation under direct laryngoscopic visualization is not the initial airway management of choice because of massive facial trauma, tracheal obstruction, or anomalous anatomy.[46,47] In such cases, endotracheal intubation sometimes can be facilitated through fiberoptic bronchoscopy.[48] When intubation is impossible, even with bronchoscopy, or when bronchoscopy is unavailable, the preferred emergency airway procedure is cricothyroidotomy.[49,50] The primary role of tracheostomy is long-term airway care for patients who initially were treated with endotracheal tubes or cricothyroidotomies, although case reports of percutaneous tracheostomy performed in an emergency setting have been published.[51-53]

CONVERTING ENDOTRACHEAL TUBES TO TRACHEOSTOMIES

The question as to when to replace an endotracheal tube with a tracheostomy tube is a subject of much discussion and remains highly controversial and is independent of technique. Beatrous[41] stated in 1968 that, "Timing is an aspect of tracheostomy that deserves much more emphasis than it is apparently receiving. Delay defeats the purpose of the operation."

Three more recent studies from different European countries document the use of tracheostomies. The results vary from early tracheostomies within the first week, nearly all of them performed through a percutaneous technique in Spain and England, to late procedures mostly done surgically in France.[54-56]

The debate as to when to replace an endotracheal tube with a tracheostomy tube centers on the advantages and disadvantages of the tracheostomy tube, as listed in Table 15-1.

Until more recently, the debate as to when to perform a tracheostomy in a patient on long-term ventilation was more often based on personal preference than on data. For patients with an unresectable airway obstruction, tracheostomy is the treatment of choice because it is the only airway that can remain long-term.[109-110] In most other situations, the decision is not as straightforward because ultimately only approximately 10% to 20% of patients on mechanical ventilation require placement of a tracheostomy tube. Although the need for tracheostomy sometimes can be predicted early (e.g., in a neurosurgical patient with a low Glasgow Coma Scale score[98]), in most situations this is not the case. Finding early clinical predictors to identify patients who would require a tracheostomy is most problematic in patients receiving PPV.[111-114] Many studies from the early and mid 1990s attempted to establish criteria to satisfy the recommendations of the Consensus Conference on Artificial Airways in Patients Receiving Mechanical Ventilation from 1989. At the Consensus Conference it was stated, "the decision to convert to tracheotomy should be made as early as possible . . . to minimize the duration of translaryngeal intubation. Once the decision is made, the procedure should be done without undue delay."[115]

In the surgical patient population, two out of three studies showed a decreased ICU length of stay with early tracheostomy.[71,88,98] The investigation by Sugerman and colleagues[71] showed no differences in any of the measured outcomes (ICU length of stay, death, pneumonia), but was significantly limited by incomplete data collection and physician bias. Until more recently, the benefits of early tracheostomy were not proven for the medical patient.

Table 15-1. Advantages and Disadvantages of Tracheostomy

Advantages	Disadvantages
Protection from laryngeal injury[57-73]	Tracheal complications[28,68,70,73,101,102]
Security of airway[68,72-76]	Procedural risk[28,41,44,45,72,73,93,102-107]
Facilitation of weaning[73,77-91]	Risk of stoma infection[41,45,73,93,105]
Improved patient comfort and psychological well-being[73,92,93]	Risk of cannula displacement[28,45,73,105]
Earlier oral nutrition[94]	Delay in weaning and decannulation[84,108]
Possibility of speech[72,94-97]	Delay in ICU discharge[99]
Easier nursing care (mouth care, tracheal suctioning)[72,73,95-97]	Increased risk of pneumonia[28,73,108]
Improved patient mobility[72,73]	Poor stoma healing after decannulation[45,101]
Decreased sedation requirements[93]	Poor cosmetic results after decannulation[45,107]
Decreased risk of sinusitis and pneumonia[72,73,84,86,88]	
Earlier ICU discharge[85,86,88,90,91,98]	
Earlier hospital discharge[88]	
Improved survival[86,87,90,99,100]	

ICU, intensive care unit.

Multiple publications address the question of timing of tracheostomy in a variety of patient populations.[84-91,116] Most are retrospective reviews of ICU databases, and timing of tracheostomy is retrospectively correlated with multiple outcomes. In these studies, the definition of "early" may range from 3 to 21 days, and "late" may range from 7 to more than 21 days, but it is hard to draw any firm conclusions. It seems clear from these studies, however, that the procedural and short-term complications of tracheostomy are low, and that in general the outcome of patients with tracheostomy is at least no worse than that of patients managed with prolonged translaryngeal endotracheal intubation. Some studies show a decrease in mortality in patients with tracheostomy[99,100]; nevertheless, one has to question if this difference is partly explained by the fact that patients with anticipated high mortality are not offered a tracheostomy. A frequently seen result is that placement of a tracheostomy reduces time on mechanical ventilation,[85,86,88-91] but even this is not a consistent finding. No change in time of mechanical ventilation is seen,[84,116] or occasionally even markedly prolonged times are seen.[99] This possibly reflects a less aggressive approach to weaning after a potentially permanent airway has been placed or shows a selection bias reflecting a higher early mortality in the patients not receiving a tracheostomy.

To date, only one randomized controlled study comparing early PDT with prolonged intubation has been done. In 2004, Rumbak and associates[86] showed that in critically ill medical patients early tracheostomy decreased time on mechanical ventilation, ICU length of stay, and ventilator-associated pneumonia. Additionally, early tracheostomy decreased mortality by 50% despite well-matched baseline characteristics. Rumbak and associates[86] also evaluated the patients for the most feared complication of tracheostomy, tracheal stenosis, during the hospital course and at 10 weeks. No significant differences in the incidence or severity of stenosis were seen, although there was a trend favoring early tracheostomy. These findings conflict with the findings of Stauffer and colleagues,[68] which are frequently quoted as an argument for prolonged translaryngeal intubation. These investigators found significantly more complications, usually judged more severe, in patients who underwent tracheostomy compared with patients with translaryngeal intubation. Most notably, the incidence of tracheal stenosis after tracheostomy was significantly higher (65% versus 19%). Nonetheless, Stauffer and colleagues[68] also found that patients treated with prolonged translaryngeal intubation followed by tracheostomy had significantly more laryngeal injury and an increased frequency of tracheal stenosis compared with patients who underwent tracheostomy after a short period of translaryngeal intubation.

Conclusions from these more recent studies indicate that a tracheostomy should be offered only to patients anticipated to survive and who require secure, long-term airway access. The timing of tracheostomy tube placement should be individualized and depends on three factors: (1) underlying disease, (2) indication for artificial airway, and (3) expected ultimate outcome. Taking older and more recent studies into account and with the emergence of bedside percutaneous tracheostomy, a recommendation for earlier tracheostomy seems appropriate because the early complication rate in experienced hands is low and is far outweighed by the likely benefits. Figures 15-1 through 15-3 provide suggested algorithms regarding the timing of tracheostomy placement based on whether the patient's pathologic condition is primarily pulmonary, neuromuscular, or upper airway obstruction.

Upper Airway Obstruction

For airway obstruction, the timing of tracheostomy depends on three factors: (1) the type of obstruction, (2)

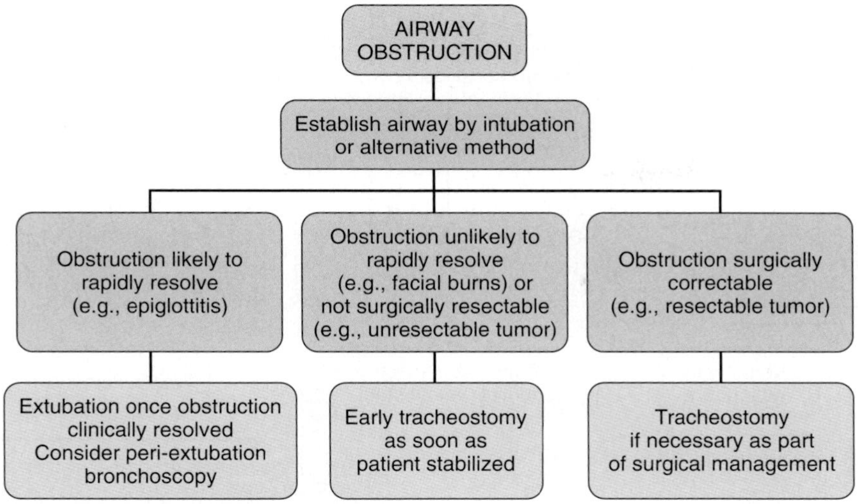

Figure 15-1. Timing of tracheostomy in airway obstruction.

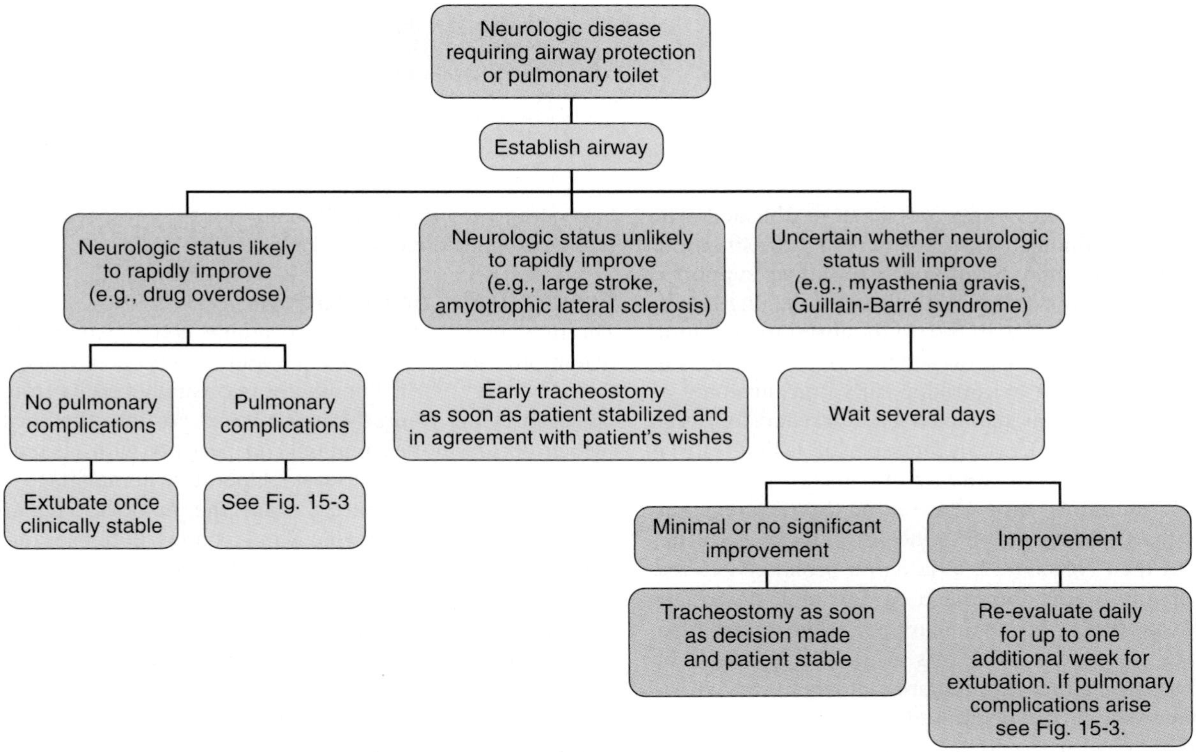

Figure 15-2. Timing of tracheostomy in neurologic disease.

the likelihood of rapid resolution, and (3) whether the obstruction can be surgically relieved.

Neuromuscular Conditions (Airway Protection and Tracheobronchial Toilet)

Many ICU patients intubated because of stupor, coma, or neuromuscular weakness are susceptible to aspiration, and many weak patients cannot generate an effective cough because their forced vital capacity is not at least triple their tidal volume.[117] In most patients, the duration of the pathologic condition is predictable—either short (e.g., drug overdose) or long (e.g., large stroke, amyotrophic lateral sclerosis).[118-123] In some cases of postoperative weakness, cerebrovascular accident, and peripheral neuromuscular weakness (e.g., Guillain-Barré syndrome, myasthenia gravis), the course is uncertain.[117,124-127] A second factor involved in the decision to perform tracheostomy is coexistence of complicating pulmonary complications, such as atelectasis, pneumonia, or aspiration (see Fig. 15-2).

Pulmonary Conditions (Positive-Pressure Ventilation or Continuous Positive Airway Pressure)

The spectrum of diseases for patients intubated because they require PPV or CPAP is so broad that firm rules

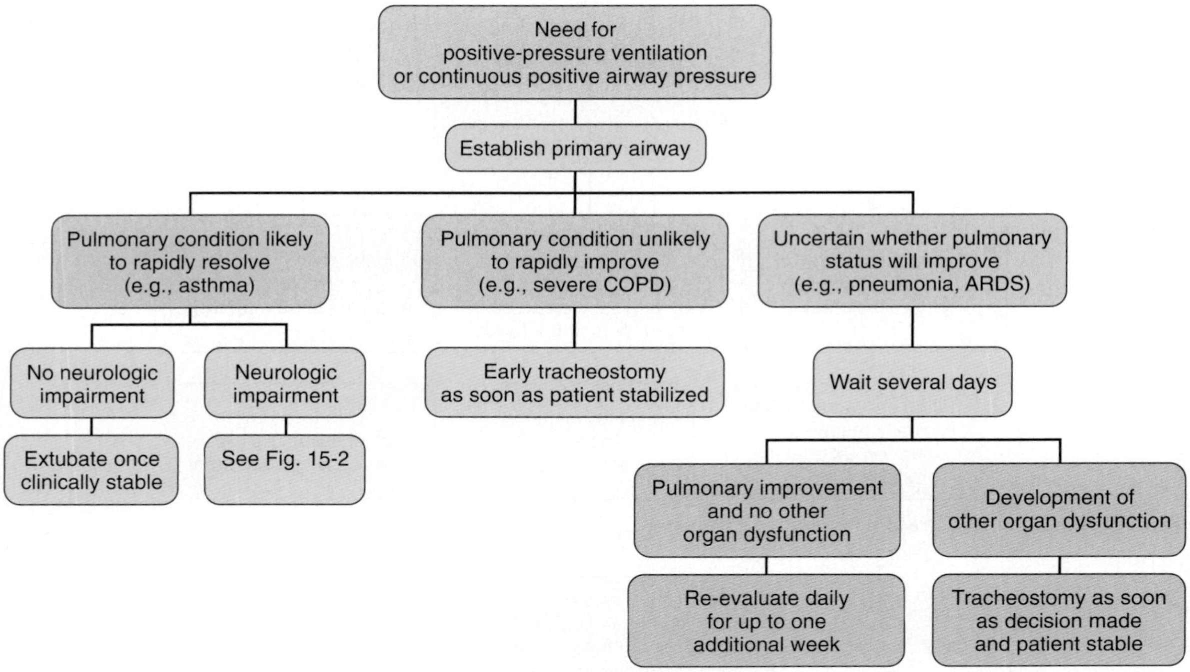

Figure 15-3. Timing of tracheostomy in pulmonary disease. ARDS, adult respiratory distress syndrome; COPD, chronic obstructive pulmonary disease.

regarding tracheostomy have not been established. The approach to the timing of tracheostomy in these situations is difficult because the duration of ventilatory support is frequently hard to predict. With the encouraging results of more recent studies with regard to mortality and duration of mechanical ventilation and improved patient well-being, it is advisable to consider early tracheostomy as soon as the patient has stabilized and a tracheostomy can be performed safely. Current thinking still is that translaryngeal intubation is the airway of choice for the first 3 weeks of ventilatory support based on the recommendations of the Consensus Conference in 1989.[116] A tracheostomy is then considered, although a prolonged course was probably predictable much earlier, and the patient might have benefited from an earlier tracheostomy. Also, the overall short-term prognosis of the patient has to be taken into consideration. A patient unlikely to survive the acute illness should not be offered a tracheostomy. A flexible and anticipatory approach is particularly required in patients with pulmonary conditions, with the recommendation for earlier tracheostomy based on more recent studies (see Fig. 15-3).

COMPLICATIONS OF TRACHEOSTOMIES

Throughout the history of tracheostorny, complications have been the most scrutinized aspect. Studies have been organized according to whether complications occurred during performance of the tracheostomy (procedural), while the tube was in the patient's airway (in situ), or after tube removal (late).[28,101,105] Combined, the major complication rate is approximately 15% (range 6% to 66%), and mortality is approximately 1.5% (range 0% to 5%).[28,44,45,68,70,101-106,128] In recent years, several studies have shown lower morbidity and mortality, especially in tracheostomies done since 1985.[129-131]

Procedural Complications

The most common serious procedural complications are pneumothorax (0.9% to 5%) and severe hemorrhage (5%).[41,44,45,70,102,104,128] Pneumothorax usually results from violation of the pleural space as it ascends into the neck (which occurs more commonly in patients with chronic obstructive pulmonary disease). Operative hemorrhage is usually venous, originating from the anterior jugular venous system or the thyroid gland isthmus. Other serious but rare complications (<1%) include tube misplacement, tracheoesophageal perforation, aspiration, thyroid laceration, and cardiopulmonary arrest.[28,45,128,129] Less serious complications are subcutaneous emphysema (owing to excessive cervical dissection or overenthusiastic closure of the tracheostomy incision), hypotension, desaturation, and minor hemorrhage.[129-131]

In Situ Complications

After a tracheostomy tube is placed, it is susceptible to obstruction and/or displacement, which may be potentially life-threatening.[28,45,105] Tube displacement may result from poor tracheostomy tube selection, excessive patient motion, or careless reinsertion after dislodgment. Obstruction is often caused by tenacious secretions. Use of a double-cannula tube with a disposable inner cannula protects against occlusion by encrusted secretions.[7,132]

Tube displacement is especially dangerous in the first days after tracheostomy placement because the fistulous tract permitting tube reinsertion is not yet developed. Obstruction and displacement may be indicated by increases in peak airway pressure during mechanical ventilation, difficulty during manual bag ventilation, or when it is difficult or impossible to pass a suction catheter down the tracheostomy tube. Providing adequate humidity, adhering to suctioning and tracheostomy care protocols, and minimizing tube manipulation help avert obstruction and displacement.[45,105,128]

Another common in situ tracheostomy complication is infection. Stomal infection (cellulitis or significant purulence at the stoma site) occurs in 36% of all tracheostomies.[68] Trivial stomal infection can be managed locally.[45] However, wound infection can extend into the mediastinum, causing mediastinitis and life-threatening sepsis that necessitate administration of broad-spectrum antibiotics.[133]

Significant airway aspiration of gastric contents occurs in 1% to 8% of cases.[44,45,68] Some degree of tracheitis, manifesting as purulent secretions, is unavoidable, but severity can be minimized through meticulous asepsis and frequent irrigation and suctioning.[45] Many patients (50% to 66%) develop nosocomial pneumonia, varying from trivial to life-threatening.[28,102,109] Patients with tracheostomies are especially prone to bacterial colonization with *Pseudomonas* and other enteric gram-negative organisms that antibiotic therapy often fails to eradicate.[109,134] Patients who are persistently colonized are especially susceptible to develop nosocomial pneumonia.[134]

In contrast to intraprocedural venous hemorrhage, hemorrhage after tracheostomy placement usually results from the tracheostomy tube tip eroding into a major artery (0.2% to 4%).[28,68] The involvement of the innominate artery results in a tracheoinnominate fistula that may provoke massive lethal hemorrhage, either by airway compromise or by exsanguination. Bleeding may be heralded by prominent pulsation of the tracheostomy tube or tracheal aspiration of arterial blood, but massive hemorrhage can appear without warning. Treatment consists of immediate tamponade and operative ligation. As an interim step, some authors advocate removing and replacing the tracheostomy tube with an endotracheal tube.[28,45,135]

A vexing problem arises when excessive cuff pressure is required in an unsuccessful attempt to seal the airway (0% to 23%).[68,136] Occasionally, the air leak around the cuff is severe enough to compromise the delivery of adequate tidal volumes. No technique proposed to treat this issue has proven absolutely effective.[137,138] Other in situ complications include mucosal ulceration, tracheal erosion, and tracheoesophageal fistula.[45,68,105,139,140]

Late Complications

The most important late complication of tracheostomy placement is tracheal stenosis either at the site of the stoma or the cuff.[28,68,70,73,102] There is disagreement over which site is more common. Defined as reduction in the transverse tracheal air column of greater than 10%, tracheal stenosis has been documented by tomograms in 65% of patients after tracheostomy (compared with a 19% incidence of tracheal stenosis after endotracheal intubation alone).[68] A still asymptomatic but more advanced degree of stenosis (25% reduction in air column diameter) may occur in 25% to 45[illegible] early months after decannulation.[23,68,101]

Most patients with tracheal stenosis remain asymptomatic and require no treatment.[73] Symptoms tend to occur when tracheal lumen diameter is reduced by either 75% relatively or to less than 5 mm absolutely.[102] Because history taking, physical examination, and flow-volume curves are insensitive in detecting tracheal injury, tomograms are essential to forming an accurate profile of tracheal stenosis.[141,142] Some authors recommend routine laryngotracheal tomograms within 3 months of decannulation in all patients.[68] Surgical repair is necessary in severe symptomatic stenosis.[143-145] Stomal and cuff stenosis (the most common tracheostomy injuries) generally can be repaired more easily than can subglottic stenosis (the most common intubation injury).

Studies suggest that tracheal stenosis is more common in patients with tracheostomies than in patients with endotracheal tubes,[68] but confounding variables make it impossible to predict whether a specific patient would experience tracheal injury with either airway. Factors cited as contributing to late airway injury include duration of intubation, cuff inflation pressure, age and sex of the patient, size of the tube relative to the trachea, tube movement, patient movement, steroid use, hypotension, diabetes, infection, and tracheostomy technique.[63,68,139,146-149] Because many of these variables cannot be controlled, most authorities recommend meticulous monitoring of the one controllable variable, cuff inflation pressure, with a goal of keeping pressures less than 20 to 25 mm Hg.[150-152] Even this may not prevent tracheal injury because lateral wall pressure varies widely, is unmeasurable, and may compromise local tracheal blood supply.[138,153] Other late complications, which occur infrequently, include tracheomalacia, tracheal granulomas, vocal cord dysfunction, and cosmetic deformities.[101,129,154]

Risks of Patient Transport

A further risk for patients who are having a tracheostomy performed is not related to the procedure itself, but is related to transporting patients to the operating room. Several articles indicate the potential for harmful events in 33% to 68% of patients during transport,[155,156] with Waddell[157] reporting that "one patient a month suffered major cardiorespiratory collapse or death as a direct result of movement." To address this issue and to perform tracheostomies with fewer complications, Ciaglia developed the technique of PDT in 1985.[34]

PERCUTANEOUS TRACHEOSTOMY

There have been many descriptive series examining short-term and long-term complications of PDT[103,158-167] and prospective comparisons of PDT with surgical tracheostomy.[168-175] By virtue of these studies, PDT has become an integral part of the care of critically ill patients. In many institutions, it is the procedure of choice when a tracheostomy is needed for a patient in the ICU.[176]

Questions that need to be answered when discussing percutaneous tracheostomy are as follows: What

…d be per- … tracheostomy …e) be performed rather … (Discussed later.) One needs …T techniques are percutaneous tra- …but not all percutaneous tracheostomies are …chniques.

Most of the reports in the literature describe the use of the Ciaglia dilational technique (PDT).[129,103,161] Also, the Ciaglia PDT kit is the most widely sold equipment throughout the world used for percutaneous tracheostomy (Cook Critical Care, personal communication, July 2006). Confusion with respect to the different techniques of percutaneous tracheostomy is evident, however, as seen in an article on surgical airway management in the ICU in which the description of PDT is given that "sequential dilators are used to enlarge a tract," but the picture of the commercial kit that "has the necessary instruments" for the procedure is one of the single-dilator Blue Rhino.[178]

Confusion also is created in the literature when publications describe percutaneous tracheostomy performed using the kit made by Portex (Keene, NH), but fail to clarify which of the two kits that Portex makes for percutaneous tracheostomy was used. One kit is manufactured in the United States and is made for the Ciaglia PDT technique, using the modification by Hazard and colleagues[35] of three straight dilators. The other kit is made in Europe and is made for the Griggs guidewire dilator forceps technique.[37]

Each of these techniques has nuances with respect to performance and specific complication rates. When comparing percutaneous tracheostomy with surgical tracheostomy, each technique must be compared individually. This was not done in the meta-analysis by Dulguerov and coworkers,[129] significantly affecting the conclusions.[179]

Based on the fact that most reports of percutaneous tracheostomy refer to Ciaglia's dilational technique, predominantly using curved dilators, the most popular technique of percutaneous tracheostomy seems to be PDT. Eight of 10 prospective studies that compared percutaneous tracheostomy with surgical tracheostomy used Ciaglia's technique.[168-175] One of the 10 compared translaryngeal tracheostomy versus surgical tracheostomy,[180] and the other compared Griggs versus surgical tracheostomy.[181]

More recent reports by van Heerden and colleagues[182] and Nates and associates[183] have compared short-term outcomes using the Griggs GWDF technique versus PDT. van Heerden and colleagues[182] showed no difference in complications, but Nates and associates[183] showed a significantly higher incidence of bleeding using the Griggs technique. Cantais and coworkers[184] compared GWDF with translaryngeal tracheostomy, finding a higher rate of serious complications in the translaryngeal tracheostomy group.

In an attempt to reduce the chance of injury to the posterior tracheal wall, and to speed up the procedure, Ciaglia developed the gradually tapered soft Blue Rhino dilator in 1999.[38] Two randomized comparisons of multiple-dilator PDT with the single-dilator Blue Rhino PDT[38,185] showed a shorter procedure duration for the single-dilator PDT. Also, no intervention was required despite a statistically higher incidence of tracheal ring fracture in the single-dilator group in one study.[38] In the multiple-dilator group, there were two injuries to the posterior tracheal wall and one pneumothorax.[38] From the widespread usage and acceptance of PDT and the many articles regarding its use in the literature, it seems that the Ciaglia PDT, either as a multiple-dilator technique or as a single-dilator technique, has become the benchmark against which all other techniques of percutaneous tracheostomy are to be compared in terms of efficacy and complications.

Technique

The technique of PDT is not complicated, although it carries the hazards associated with any airway procedure. PDT can be learned by attending a training course or observing the procedure, followed by initially assisting and then performing 10 to 20 procedures.[175] The operator's initial efforts should be performed under supervision of an experienced operator using bronchoscopic guidance.[130] Usually an elective procedure, PDT performed early in the operator's practice should be done only in an already intubated patient. An emergent PDT to establish an airway should be done only by practitioners with significant experience in the procedure.

Initially, PDT was thought to be contraindicated in emergencies, in children, in obese patients, in patients who had a previous tracheostomy, and in patients with uncorrectable coagulopathies or severe anatomic neck deformities,[34] but its performance has been described in all of these groups except children younger than 14 years old.[51,53,158,159,162,186] We believe PDT remains absolutely contraindicated in young children, patients with certain severe anatomic neck deformities (e.g., fused, anterior flexed neck, overlying possibly malignant neck mass), and in emergencies if performed by inexperienced operators.

Before performing PDT, the patient is given glycopyrrolate, intravenous sedation, and usually a paralytic agent. Fraction of inspired oxygen is increased to 100% to prevent hypoxemia. The patient is placed supine with the neck hyperextended. The first or second tracheal interspace is identified, and the endotracheal tube is positioned so that the end of the tube, while still in the trachea, is just proximal to the intended tracheostomy site.

The endotracheal tube is usually positioned in one of two ways. One method backs the tube by approximation to just below the vocal cords.[34] It is helpful to palpate the endotracheal tube cuff to identify the tube position.[187] Alternatively, the tube is positioned using bronchoscopic guidance.[103,160,188] Besides facilitating proper tube positioning, using the bronchoscope allows direct visualization of needle insertion, ensuring midline placement and intratracheal insertion of the tracheostomy tube.[103] Marx and colleagues,[189] who originally recommended nonendoscopic endotracheal tube positioning, now recommend use of bronchoscopy because of the aforementioned reasons.

After the skin is anesthetized (1% lidocaine with epinephrine to prevent bleeding), a 22-gauge needle is introduced into the tracheal lumen, and 3 to 5 mL of lidocaine is injected into the trachea. If a bronchoscope is not used, the endotracheal tube should be gently rotated and oscillated to ensure that the needle did not impale it. To guarantee midline placement of the tracheostomy, the head must remain midline and the trachea immobilized during each step of the procedure.

When it is established that the 22-gauge needle has not pierced the endotracheal tube, a 15-gauge needle is inserted, a guidewire is passed through it, and the needle is removed. A 1-cm midline vertical incision is made. An 11F punch dilator is inserted to enlarge the tract from skin to trachea. An 8F plastic guiding catheter is placed over the guidewire to stiffen it and remains in place for the duration of the procedure. The tract is progressively dilated until a size 6 or size 8 double-cannula tracheostomy tube (with the inner cannula removed) previously loaded on a curved obturator can be inserted. The dilators should be inserted at a right angle to the patient's neck. Resistance is felt initially as the dilator is inserted, and a "pop" is felt when the trachea is entered. If straight dilators are used, they should be angled caudally after the trachea has been entered (Figs. 15-4 to 15-6). The dilations may be performed with multiple curved dilators,[34] three straight dilators,[35,187] or a single tapered dilator (Blue Rhino).[38] The obturator, guidewire, and guiding catheter are removed; the inner cannula is inserted; and the cuff is inflated. Breath sounds, returned tidal volume, and cuff pressure must be checked before the tracheostomy is secured. A chest film should be obtained to verify tube position and the absence of complications. In experienced hands, the procedure can be performed in less than 10 minutes.

Most PDT complications are minor, ranging from transient hypoxemia or hypotension during the procedure to minor postoperative bleeding, local wound infection, or subcutaneous emphysema.[103,154,159,161,162] The most serious morbidity, paratracheal tube insertion (in <1% of cases), generally occurs as a result of operator inexperience, or when the procedure is performed in a patient with a short, thick neck. It usually can be prevented if the procedure is performed under bronchoscopic guidance.[130] If paratracheal insertion is suspected, as indicated by a significant decrease in oxygen saturation or marked resistance to ventilation, the tube should be removed immediately and replaced under bronchoscopic guidance or in an open surgical procedure after translaryngeal reintubation.

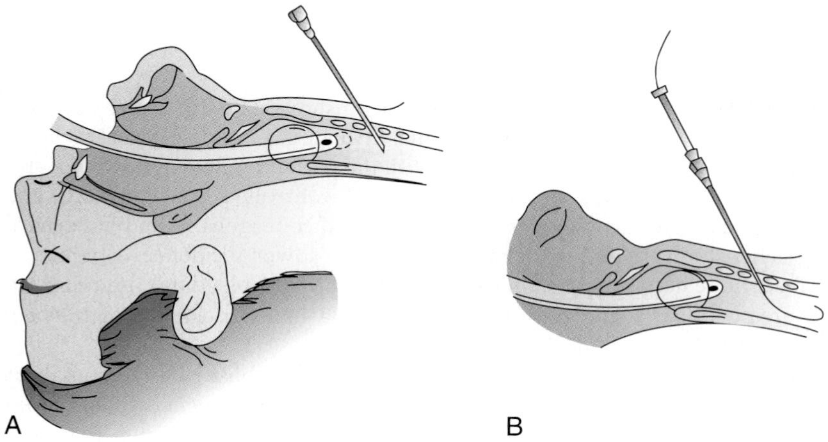

Figure 15-4. A, Insertion of a 15-gauge needle into the trachea. **B,** Guidewire is inserted through the needle into the trachea. (From Friedman Y, Franklin C: The technique of percutaneous tracheostomy. J Crit Illness 1993;8:289. Copyright Margulies Medical Art, Miami, Fla.)

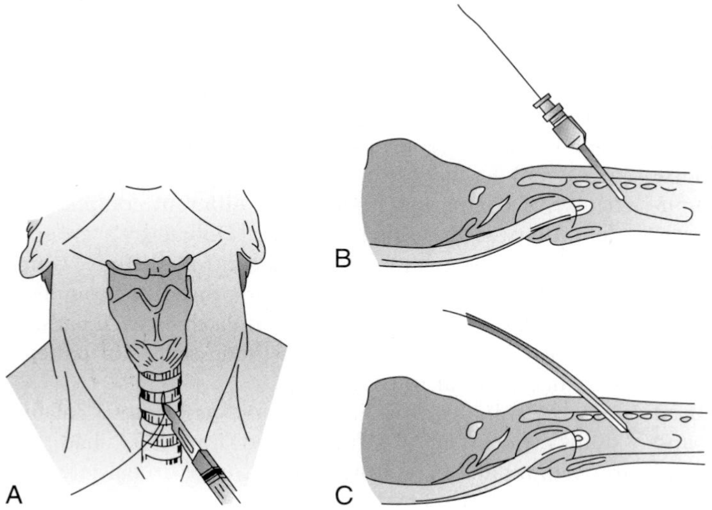

Figure 15-5. A, A vertical incision is made in the skin. **B,** An 11F punch dilator is inserted. **C,** An 8F plastic guiding catheter is introduced over the guidewire. (From Friedman Y, Franklin C: The technique of percutaneous tracheostomy. J Crit Illness 1993;8:289. Copyright Margulies Medical Art, Miami, Fla.)

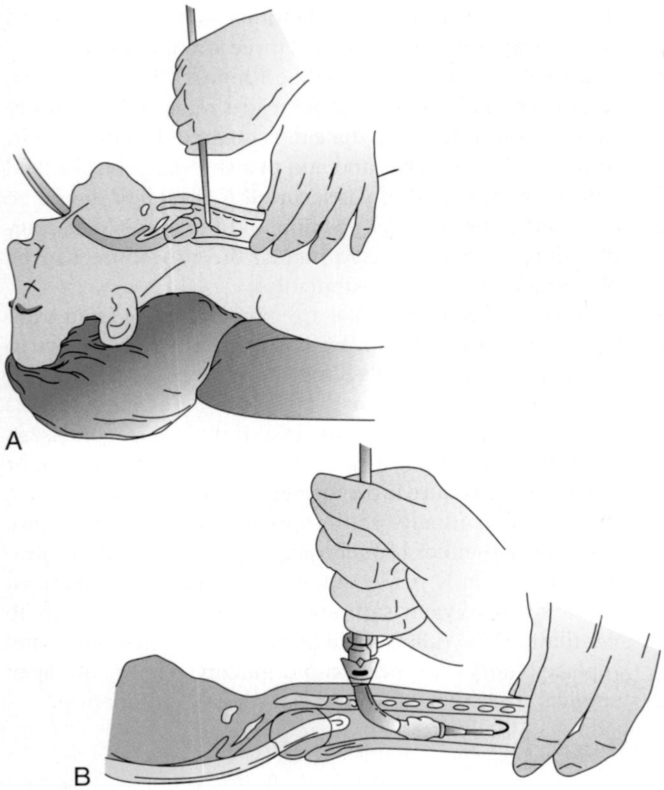

Figure 15-6. **A,** The dilator is inserted over the guidewire-guiding catheter assembly. **B,** Placement of the tracheostomy tube obturator assembly. (From Friedman Y, Franklin C: The technique of percutaneous tracheostomy. J Crit Illness 1993;8:289. Copyright Margulies Medical Art, Miami, Fla.)

Percutaneous Dilational Tracheostomy versus Surgical Tracheostomy

As mentioned previously, from the widespread use of PDT it seems that the Ciaglia PDT, either as a multiple-dilator technique or as a single-dilator technique, has become the benchmark for percutaneous tracheostomy. Although other techniques have been described, none has been as widely accepted,[32,36,37,39,40] and some are no longer available.[32,36] Kits currently available to perform PDT contain a single tapered dilator or three straight dilators. The original kit containing multiple curved dilators is no longer being produced. At this point in the history of percutaneous tracheostomy, PDT is the technique that should be the focus of discussion.

Nonrandomized, observational studies of PDT show short-term and long-term complication rates (e.g., mortality, paratracheal insertion, bleeding, infection, tracheal stenosis),[34,35,103,130,158-167] that are comparable to or lower than those in similar reports of surgical tracheostomy complication rates.[41,44,68,70,73,101-105,107,108] Attempting to use these data to say that PDT has the same or fewer complications as surgical tracheostomy is not good science, however. The articles are from different generations with corresponding improvement in techniques or equipment or both. Also, the authors may have defined their complications differently and selected different complications for study. It is important to examine the eight prospective trials,[168-175] which presumably used the same definitions and procedures in both groups, and the two meta-analyses[129,190] of PDT versus surgical tracheostomy.

Crofts and colleagues[170] showed no difference in procedural complications between PDT and surgical tracheostomy. Compared with the remaining seven, however, this was not a randomized, controlled trial. Hazard and coworkers,[168] Friedman and colleagues,[169] and Holdgaard and associates[171] showed a lower incidence of minor in situ complications (infection and bleeding), and Hazard and coworkers[168] showed a lower incidence of tracheal stenosis in PDT.

Dulguerov and colleagues[129] published a meta-analysis comparing complications of surgical tracheostomy before 1985, surgical tracheostomy after 1985 (when PDT was described), and percutaneous tracheostomy. They concluded that percutaneous tracheostomy had a higher procedural complication rate than surgical tracheostomy. This article, besides having the issues associated with all meta-analyses,[191] had significant methodologic problems. Many different techniques of percutaneous tracheostomy were included in the analysis, complications such as cardiac arrest and death were counted twice, and there is the difficulty of comparing studies with different complication definitions as described earlier.[179] Dulguerov's group[172] published their own randomized controlled study, which showed significantly higher minor procedural complications and more difficulty with cannula changes in patients who had PDT and more "unesthetic scars" in patients who had surgical tracheostomy.

A meta-analysis by Freeman and associates[190] of five studies (including Croft) showed that PDT had less procedural and in situ bleeding, a lower stomal infection rate, and lower overall postoperative complications.

Freeman and colleagues' own randomized study[173] showed no difference in complication rates, but a lower cost for PDT.

Silvester and coworkers[174] published the largest prospective, randomized controlled study, looking at short-term and long-term end points, to try to resolve the continuing controversy related to PDT versus surgical tracheostomy. They found no difference in the complication rates between the groups. There was a shorter interval from the time of the decision to perform a tracheostomy until the procedure for patients having PDT, however, as was found in the only other study that looked at this variable.[169] This may enable faster weaning and may allow for earlier transfer from the ICU, a significant cost-containment factor.

PDT has been shown to be a faster procedure than surgical tracheostomy.[168,169] It eliminates the need for use of the operating room, reducing morbidity of transport. PDT has been shown to be more cost-effective than surgical tracheostomy.[173]

Although the complication rate of PDT cannot be conclusively shown to be lower than that of surgical tracheostomy, it is at least as low and may be lower. The convenience and ease of performing PDT afford flexibility in managing patients receiving ventilatory support for weaning and long-term care. We believe PDT offers the advantage of avoiding the inherent morbidity of patient transport to the operating room and the prospect of reduction in costly operating room time and hospital stay. Although there will always be some indications for surgical tracheostomy, either at bedside or in the operating room, PDT seems to be a reasonable alternative that intensivists, anesthesiologists, and surgeons can and should learn to perform.

KEY POINTS

- Artificial airways are placed for one of the following indications: relieving obstruction, providing PPV or CPAP, preventing aspiration, or tracheobronchial toilet.
- Tracheostomy usually acts as a replacement for a previously established airway. Whenever possible, tracheostomy should be performed in a controlled setting with an artificial airway already in place.
- As a long-term airway, a tracheostomy has several advantages over an endotracheal tube (e.g., protection from laryngeal injury, airway security, patient comfort and mobility, and easier nursing care). More data are needed to determine the degree to which tracheostomy facilitates weaning, allows earlier ICU discharge, or has fewer long-term complications.
- Patients who require a tracheostomy must be identified as early as possible, and the procedure must be performed without delay to minimize the duration of translaryngeal intubation.
- Complications from tracheostomies can be procedural, in situ, or late and range from 6% to 66% (serious complications range from 5% to 15%). The mortality rate for tracheostomy is roughly 1.5% (range 0% to 5%).
- PDT is an alternative to surgical tracheostomy. Complications, morbidity, and mortality rates are comparable with those of surgical tracheostomy. As more practitioners become familiar with PDT, it may become the procedure of choice for ICU patients.
- Several significantly different techniques of percutaneous tracheostomy have been described with varying complication rates. Practitioners need to be clear about which technique of percutaneous tracheostomy is being used or discussed.

REFERENCES

1. Nelson TG: Tracheotomy: A clinical and experimental study. Am Surgeon 1957;23:660-694.
2. Frost EAM: Tracing the tracheostomy. Ann Otol Rhinol Laryngol 1976;85: 618-624.
3. Wright J: A History of Laryngology and Rhinology. Philadelphia, Lea & Febiger, 1914.
4. Pahor AL: Ear nose and throat in ancient Egypt. J Laryngol Otol 1992;106:773-779.
5. Guerrier Y, Mounier-Kuhn P: Histoire de maladies de l'oreille, du nez et la gorge. Paris, Les Editions Roger Dacosta, 1980.
6. Wright J: The Nose and Throat in Medical History. St. Louis, Matthews, 1898.
7. Goodall EW: The story of tracheostomy. Br J Child Dis 1934;31:167-176, 253-272.
8. Stevenson RS: A History of Oto-laryngology, Edinburgh, Livingstone, 1949.
9. Garrison FH: An Introduction to the History of Medicine. Philadelphia, Saunders, 1929.
10. Casserius J (trans): The larynx, organ of voice. Acta Otolaryngol Suppl 1969;261:1-36.
11. Guthrie D: Early records of tracheotomy. Bull Hist Med 1947;15: 59-64.
12. Morens DM: Death of a president. N Engl J Med 1999;341:1845-1849.
13. Bretonneau M: Sporadic tracheal diphtherite. In Semple RH (ed): Memoirs on Diphtheria. London, The New Sydenham Society, 1859, pp 59-71
14. Trousseau A: In Cormack JR (trans): Tracheostomy in diphtheria. In Lectures on Clinical Medicine, vol 2. London, The New Sydenham Society, 1869, pp 594-617.
15. Shastid TH: My Second Life, Ann Arbor, University of Michigan Press, 1944.
16. Shorter E: Primary care. In Porter R (ed): Cambridge Illustrated History of Medicine. Melbourne, Cambridge University Press, 1996, pp 118-153.
17. Alberti PW: Tracheostomy versus intubation. Ann Otol Rhinol Laryngol 93:333-337, 1984.
18. MacEwen W: Clinical observations on the introduction of tracheal tubes by the mouth instead of performing tracheotomy or laryngotomy. BMJ 1880;2:122-124, 163-165.
19. O'Dwyer J: Intubation of the larynx. N Y Med J 1885;4:145-157.
20. Stoller JK: The history of intubation, tracheotomy, and airway appliances. Respir Care 1999;44:595-601.
21. Jackson C: Tracheotomy. Laryngoscope 1909;19:285-290.
22. Hilberman M: The evolution of the intensive care unit. Crit Care Med 1975;3:159-165.
23. Head JM: Tracheostomy in the management of respiratory problems. N Engl J Med 1961;264:587-591.
24. Jackson C: High tracheotomy and other errors the chief cause of

laryngeal stenosis. Surg Gynecol Obstet 1921;32:392-398.
25. DeLaurier GA, Hawkins ML, Treat RC, et al: Acute airway management. Am Surg 1990;56:12-15.
26. Brantigan CO, Grow JB Sr: Subglottic stenosis after cricothyroidotomy. Surgery 1982;91:217-221.
27. Brantigan CO, Grow JB Sr: Cricothyroidotomy: Elective use in respiratory problems requiring tracheotomy. J Thorac Cardiovasc Surg 1976;71:72-81.
28. Heffner JE, Miller KS, Sahn SA: Tracheostomy in the intensive care unit: Part 1. Indications, technique, management. Part 2. Complications. Chest 1986;90:269-274 (Part 1), 1986;90:430-436 (Part 2).
29. Shelden CH, Pudenz RH, Freshwater DB, et al: A new method for tracheostomy. J Neurosurg 1955;12: 428-431.
30. Smith VM: Perforation of trachea during tracheostomy performed with Sheldon tracheostome. JAMA 1957; 165:2074-2076.
31. Hamilton RD: Fatal hemorrhage during tracheostomy. JAMA 1960;174: 530-531.
32. Toye FJ, Weinstein JD: A percutaneous tracheostomy device. Surgery 1969; 65:384-389.
33. Toye FJ, Weinstein JD: Clinical experience with percutaneous tracheostomy and cricothyroidotomy in 100 patients. J Trauma 1986;6: 1034-1040.
34. Ciaglia P, Firsching R, Syniec C: Elective percutaneous dilatational tracheostomy. Chest 1985;87: 715-719.
35. Hazard PB, Garrett HE, Adams JW: Bedside percutaneous tracheostomy: Experience with 55 elective procedures. Ann Thorac Surg 1988;46:63-67.
36. Schachner A, Ovil Y, Sidi J, et al: Percutaneous tracheostomy—a new method. Crit Care Med 1989;17: 1052-1056.
37. Griggs WM, Worthley LIG, Gilligan JE, et al: A simple percutaneous tracheostomy technique. Surg Gynecol Obstet 1990;170:543-545.
38. Byhahn C, Wilke HJ, Halbig S, et al: Percutaneous tracheostomy: Ciaglia Blue Rhino versus the basic Ciaglia technique of percutaneous dilational tracheostomy. Anesth Analg 2000;91: 882-886.
39. Fantoni A, Ripamonte D: A non-derivative, non-surgical tracheostomy: The translaryngeal method. Intensiv Care Med 1997;23:386-392.
40. Frova G, Quintel M: A new simple method for percutaneous tracheostomy: Controlled rotating dilation—a preliminary report. Intensive Care Med 2002;28:229-232.
41. Beatrous WP: Tracheostomy: Its expanded indications and its present status. Laryngoscope 1968;78:3-55.
42. Shapiro BA, Harrison RA, Kacmarek, RM, et al (eds): The artificial airway. In: Clinical Application of Respiratory Care, 3rd ed. Chicago, Year Book Medical Publishers, 1985, pp 213-241.
43. Stauffer JL: Medical management of the airway. Clin Chest Med 1991;12: 449-482.
44. Skaggs JA, Cogbill CL: Tracheostomy: Management, mortality and complications. Am Surg 1969;35: 393-396.
45. Chew JY, Cantrell RW: Tracheostomy: Complications and their management. Arch Otolaryngol 1972;96:538-545.
46. Schwartz DE, Wiener-Kronish JP: Management of the difficult airway. Clin Chest Med 1991;12:483-495.
47. Latto IP, Vaughn RS: Difficulties in Tracheal Intubation, 2nd ed. London, Saunders, 1997.
48. Weiss YG, Deutschman CS: The role of fiberoptic bronchoscopy in airway management of the critically ill patient. Crit Care Clin 2000;16: 445-451.
49. American College of Surgeons Committee on Trauma: Advanced Trauma Life Support Course for Physicians, Instructor's Manual. Chicago, The College, 1985.
50. Burkey B, Escalamado R, Morganroth M: The role of cricothyroidotomy in airway management. Clin Chest Med 1991;12:561-571.
51. Myles PS, Venema HR, Lindholm DE: Trauma patient managed with the laryngeal mask airway and percutaneous tracheostomy after failed intubation. Med J Aust 1994;161:640.
52. Griggs WM, Myburgh JA, Worthley LIG: Urgent airway access—an indication for percutaneous tracheostomy? Anaesth Intensive Care 1991:19:586-587.
53. Dob DP, McLure HA, Soni N: Failed intubation and emergency percutaneous tracheostomy. Anaesthesioloy 1998;53:69-78.
54. Blot F, Melot C: Indications, timing, and techniques of tracheostomy in 152 French ICUs. Chest 2005;127: 1347-1352.
55. Anon JM, Escuela MP, Gomez V, et al: Use of percutaneous tracheostomy in intensive care units in Spain: Results of a national survey. Intensive Care Med 2004;30:1212-1215.
56. Krishnan K, Elliot SC, Mallick A: The current practice of tracheostomy in the United Kingdom: A postal survey. Anaesthesia 2005;60:360-364.
57. Lindholm CE: Prolonged endotracheal intubation. Acta Anaesth Scand Suppl 1969;33:1-131.
58. Weymuller E, Bishop MJ, Fink BR, et al: Quantification of intralaryngeal pressure exerted by endotracheal tubes. Ann Otol Rhinol Laryngol 1983;92:444-447.
59. Steen JA, Lindholm CE, Brdlik GC, et al: Tracheal tube forces on the posterior larynx. Crit Care Med 1982;10:186-189.
60. Supance JS, Reilly JS, Doyle WJ, et al: Acquired subglottic stenosis following prolonged endotracheal intubation. Arch Otolaryngol 1982;108:727-731.
61. Santos PM, Afrassiabi A, Weymuller EA: Risk factors associated with prolonged intubation and laryngeal injury. Otolaryngol Head Neck Surg 1994;111:453-459.
62. Peppard SB, Dickens JH: Laryngeal inury following short term intubation. Ann Otol Rhinol Laryngol 1983;90:327-330.
63. Gaynor EB, Greenberg SB: Untoward sequelae of prolonged intubation. Laryngoscope 1985;95:1461-1467.
64. Donnelly WH: Histopathology of endotracheal intubation. Arch Pathol 1969;88:511-520.
65. Whited RE: A prospective study of laryngotracheal sequelae in long-term intubation. Laryngoscope 1984;94: 367-377.
66. Bishop MJ, Weymuller EA, Fink BR: Laryngeal effects of prolonged intubation. Anesth Analg 1984;63: 335-342.
67. Benjamin B: Laryngeal trauma from intubation: Endoscopic evaluation and classification. In Cummings CW, Fredrickson JM, Harker LA, et al (eds): Otolaryngology Head and Neck Surgery, 3rd ed. St. Louis, Mosby, 1998, pp 2013-2035.
68. Stauffer JL, Olson DE, Petty TL: Complications and consequences of endotracheal intubation and tracheotomy. Am J Med 1981;70: 65-76.
69. Bishop M: Mechanisms of laryngotracheal injury following prolonged tracheal intubation. Chest 1989;96:185-186.
70. Marsh HM, Gillespie DJ, Baumgartner AE: Timing of tracheostomy in the critically ill patient. Chest 1989;96: 190-193.
71. Sugerman HJ, Wolfe L, Pasquale MD, et al: Multicenter, randomized, prospective trial of early tracheostomy. J Trauma 1997;43:741-747.
72. Heffner JE: Tracheotomy: Indications and timing. Respir Care 1999;44: 807-815.
73. Heffner JE: Timing of tracheotomy in ventilator-dependent patients. Clin Chest Med 1991;12: 611-625.
74. Coppolo DP, May JJ: Self-extubations. Chest 1990;98:165-169.
75. Campbell RS: Extubation and the consequences of reintubation. Respir Care 1999;44:799-803.
76. Torres A, Gatell JM, Aznar E, et al: Re-intubation increases the risk of nosocomial pneumonia in patients needing mechanical ventilation. Am J Respir Crit Care Med 1995;152: 137-141.
77. Davis K, Campbell RS, Johannigman JA, et al: Changes in respiratory mechanics after tracheostomy. Arch Surg 1999;134:59-62.
78. Heffner JE: The role of trachestomy in weaning. Chest 2001;120: 477S-481S.
79. Villafane MC, Cinella G, Lofaso F, et al: Gradual reduction of endotracheal tube diameter during mechanical ventilation via different humidification devices. Anesthesia 1996;85: 1341-1349.
80. Lin MC, Huang CC, Yang CT, et al: Pulmonary mechanics in patients with prolonged mechanical ventilation requiring tracheostomy. Anaesth Intensive Care 1999;27: 581-585.
81. Diehl JL, El Atrous S, Touchard D, et al: Changes in the work of breathing induced by tracheostomy in ventilator-dependent patients. Am J Respir Crit Care Med 1999;159: 383-388.

82. Wright PE, Marini JJ, Bernard GR: In vitro versus in vivo comparison of endotracheal airflow resistance. Am Rev Respir Dis 1989;140:10-16.
83. Bersten AD, Rutten AJ, Vedig AE: Additional work of breathing imposed by endotracheal tubes, breathing circuits, and intensive care ventilators. Crit Care Med 1989;17:671-677.
84. Boynton JH, Hawkins K, Eastridge BJ, et al: Tracheostomy timing and the duration of weaning in patients with acute respiratory failure. Crit Care 2004;8:R261-R267.
85. Arabi Y, Haddad S, Shirawi N, et al: Early tracheostomy in intensive care trauma patients improves resource utilization: A cohort study and literature review. Crit Care 2004;8: R347-R352.
86. Rumbak MJ, Newton M, Truncale T, et al: A prospective, randomized, study comparing early percutaneous tracheotomy to prolonged translaryngeal intubation (delayed tracheotomy) in critically ill medical patients. Crit Care Med 2004;32:1689-1694.
87. Hsu CL, Chen KY, Chang CH, et al: Timing of tracheostomy as a determinant of weaning success in critically ill patients: A retrospective study. Crit Care 2005;9:R46-R52.
88. Rodriguez JL, Steinberg SM, Luchetti FA, et al: Early tracheostomy for primary airway management in the surgical critical care setting. Surgery 1990;108:655-659.
89. Bouderka MA, Fakhir B, Bouggad A, et al: Early tracheostomy versus prolonged endotracheal intubation in severe head trauma. J Trauma 2004;57:251-254.
90. Flaatten H, Gjerde S, Heimdal JH, et al: The effect of tracheostomy on outcome in intensive care unit patients. Acta Anaesthesiol Scand 2006;50:92-98.
91. Griffith J, Barber VS, Morgan L, et al: Systematic review and meta-analysis of studies of the timing of tracheostomy in adult patients undergoing artificial ventilation. BMJ 2005;330:1243-1246.
92. McGeehin WH, Scoma R, Igidbashian L, et al: Tracheostomy versus endotracheal intubation: the ICU nurse's perspective. Crit Care Med 1990;18:S224.
93. Astrachan DI, Kirchner JC, Goodwin WJ: Prolonged intubation vs. tracheotomy: Complications, practical and psychological considerations. Laryngoscope 1988;98:1165-1169.
94. Heffner JE, Hess D: Tracheostomy management in the chronically ventilated patient. Clin Chest Med 2001;22:55-69.
95. Kluin KJ, Maynard F, Bogdasarian RS: The patient requiring mechanical ventilatory support: Use of the cuffed tracheostomy "talk" tube to establish phonation. Otolaryngol Head Neck Surg 1984;92:625-627.
96. Manzano JL, Lubillo S, Henriquez D, et al: Verbal communication of ventilator-dependent patients. Crit Care Med 1993;21:512-517.
97. Bergbom-Engbert I, Haljamae H: Assessment of patient's experience of discomforts during respirator therapy. Crit Care Med 1989;17:1068-1072.
98. Koh WY, Lew TWK, Chin NM, et al: Tracheostomy in a neuro-intensive care setting: Indications and timing. Anaesth Intensive Care 1997;25: 365-368.
99. Kollef MH, Ahrens TS, Shannon W: Clinical predictors and outcomes for patients requiring tracheostomy in the intensive care unit. Crit Care Med 1999;27:1714-1720.
100. Freeman BD, Borecki IB, Coopersmith CM, et al: Relationship between tracheostomy timing and duration of mechanical ventilation in critically ill patients. Crit Care Med 2005;33: 2513-2520.
101. Wood DE, Mathisen DJ: Late complications of tracheotomy. Clin Chest Med 1991;12:597-609.
102. Lewis RJ: Tracheostomies—indications, timing, and complications. Clin Chest Med 1992;13:137-149.
103. Kost KM: Endoscopic percutaneous dilatational tracheotomy: A prospective evaluation of 500 consecutive cases. Laryngoscope 2005;115:1-30.
104. Goldstein SI, Breda SD, Schneider KL: Surgical complications of bedside tracheotomy in an otolaryngology residency program. Laryngosope 1987;97:1407-1409.
105. Myers EN, Carrau MR: Early complications of tracheotomy. Clin Chest Med 1991;12:589-595.
106. Rosenbower TJ, Morris JA, Eddy VA, et al: The long-term complications of percutaneous tracheostomy. Am Surg 1998;64:82-86.
107. Davis HS, Kretchmer HE, Bryce-Smith R: Advantages and complications of tracheotomy. JAMA 1953;153: 1156-1159.
108. El-Naggar M, Sadagopan S, Levine H, et al: Factors influencing choice between tracheostomy and prolonged translaryngeal intubation in acute respiratory failure: A prospective study. Anesth Analg 1976;55:195-201.
109. Heffner JE: Medical indications for tracheotomy. Chest 1989;96: 186-190.
110. Wenig BL, Applebaum EL: Indications for and techniques of tracheotomy. Clin Chest Med 1991;12:545-553.
111. HeffnerJE, Zamora CA: Clinical predictors of prolonged translaryngeal intubation in patients with the adult respiratory distress syndrome. Chest 1990;97:447-451.
112. Johnson SB, Kearney PA, Barker DE: Early criteria predictive of prolonged mechanical ventilation. J Trauma 1992;33:95-99.
113. Heffner JE, Brown LK, Barbieri CA, et al: Prospective validation of an acute respiratory distress syndrome predictive score. Am J Crit Care Med 1995;152:1518-1526.
114. Seneff MG, Zimmerman JE, Knaus WA, et al: Predicting the duration of mechanical ventilation. Chest 1996;110:469-479.
115. Plummer AL, Gracey DR: Consensus conference on artificial airways in patients receiving mechanical ventilation. Chest 1989;96:178-180.
116. Saffle JR, Morris SE, Edelman L: Early tracheostomy does not improve outcome in burn patients. J Burn Care Rehab 2002;23:431-438.
117. Bella I, Chad DA: Neuromuscular disorders and acute respiratory failure. Neurol Clin North Am 1998;16:391-417.
118. Steiner T, Mendoza G, De Georgia M, et al: Prognosis of stroke patients requiring mechanical ventilation in a neurological critical care unit. Stroke 1997;28:711-715.
119. Grotta J, Pasteur W, Khwaja G, et al: Elective intubation for neurologic deterioration after stroke. Neurology 1995;45:640-644.
120. Gujjar AR, Deibert E, Manno EM, et al: Mechanical ventilation for ischemic stroke and intracerebral hemorrhage: indications, timing, and outcome. Neurology 1998;512: 447-451.
121. Wijdicks EF, Scott JP: Outcome in patients with acute basilar artery occlusion requiring mechanical ventilation. Stroke 1996;27: 1301-1303.
122. Tandan R, Bradley WG: Amyotrophic lateral sclerosis: Part 1. Clinical features, pathology, and ethical issues in management. Ann Neurol 1985;18:271-280.
123. Braun SR: Respiratory system in amyotrophic lateral sclerosis. Neurol Clin 1987;5:9-31.
124. Gracey DR, McMichan JC, Divertie MB, et al: Respiratory failure in Guillain-Barré syndrome. Mayo Clin Proc 1982;57:742-746.
125. Ropper AH, Kehne SM: Guillain-Barré syndrome: Management of respiratory failure. Neurology 1985;35: 1662-1665.
126. Borel CO, Guy J: Ventilatory management in critical neurologic illness. Neurol Clin 1995;13: 627-644.
127. Gracey DR, Divertie MB, Howard FM: Mechanical ventilation for respiratory failure in myasthenia gravis. Mayo Clin Proc 1983;58:597-602.
128. Stock MC, Woodward CG, Shapiro B, et al: Perioperative complications of elective tracheostomy in critically ill patients. Crit Care Med 1986;14: 861-863.
129. Dulguerov P, Gysin C, Perneger TV, et al: Percutaneous or surgical tracheostomy: A meta-analysis. Crit Care Med 1999;27:1617-1625.
130. Zeitouni A, Kost K: Tracheostomy: A retrospective review of 281 patients. J Otolaryngol 1994;23:61-66.
131. Goldenberg D, Golz A, Netzer A, et al: Tracheostomy: Changing indications and a review of 1130 cases. J Otolaryngol 2002;31:211-215.
132. Johnson JT: Wagner RL, Sigler BA: Disposable inner cannula tracheotomy tube: A prospective trial. Otolaryngol Head Neck Surg 1988;99:83-84.
133. Snow N, Richardson JD, Flint LM: Management of necrotizing tracheostomy infections. J Thorac Cardiovasc Surg 1986;82:341-344.
134. Niederman NS, Ferranti RD, Ziegler A, et al: Respiratory infection complicating long-term tracheostomy: The implication of persistent gram-negative tracheobronchial colonization. Chest 1984;85:39-44.

135. Jones JW, Reynolds M, Hewitt RL, et al: Tracheoinnominate artery erosion: Successful surgical management of a devastating complication. Ann Surg 1977;184:194-204.
136. King K, Mandava B, Kamen J: Tracheal tube cuffs and tracheal dilatation. Chest 1975;67:458-462.
137. Jaeger JM, Wells NC, Kirby RR, et al: Mechanical ventilation of a patient with decreased lung compliance and tracheal dilatation. J Clin Anesthesiol 1992;4:147-152.
138. Lee TS: Routine monitoring of intracuff pressure. Chest 1992;102:1309.
139. Dane TEB, King EG: A prospective study of complications after tracheostomy for assisted ventilation. Chest 1975;67:398-404.
140. Grillo HC: Post-intubation tracheoesophageal fistula. In Grillo HC, Eschapasse H (ed): International Trends in General Thoracic Surgery, vol 2, Major Challenges. Philadelphia, Saunders, 1987, pp 61-68.
141. James AE Jr, MacMillan AS Jr, Eaton SB, et al: Roentgenology of tracheal stenosis resulting from cuffed tracheostomy tubes. AJR Am J Roentgenol 1970;109:455-466.
142. Weber AL, Grillo HC: Tracheal stenosis: An analysis of 151 cases. Radiol Clin North Am 1978;16:291-308.
143. Grillo HC: Surgical treatment of post-intubation tracheal injuries. J Thorac Cardiovasc Surg 1979;78:860-873.
144. Grillo HC: Acquired tracheal stenosis. In Grillo HC, Austen WG, Wilkins EW, et al (eds): Current Therapy in Cardiothoracic Surgery. Toronto, Decker, 1989, pp 57-61.
145. Cooper JD: Complications of tracheostomy: Pathogenesis, treatment, and prevention. In Grillo HC, Eschapasse H (eds): International Trends in General Thoracic Surgery, vol 2, Major Challenges. Philadelphia, Saunders, 1987, pp 21-28.
146. Andrews MJ, Pearson FG: Incidence and pathogenesis of tracheal injury following cuffed tube tracheostomy with assisted ventilation: Analysis of a two-year prospective study. Ann Surg 1971;173:249-263.
147. Grillo HC, Cooper JD, Geffin B, et al: A low-pressure cuff for tracheostomy to minimize tracheal injury: A comparative clinical trial. J Thorac Cardiovasc Surg 1971;62:898-906.
148. Pearson FG, Goldberg M, daSilva AJ: Tracheal stenosis complicating tracheostomy with cuffed tubes: Clinical experience and observation from a prospective study. Arch Surg 1968;97:380-392.
149. Crawley BE, Cross DE: Tracheal cuffs: A review and dynamic pressure study. Anaesthesia 1975;30:4-11.
150. Lewis FR Jr, Schlobohm RM, Thomas AN: Prevention of complications from prolonged tracheal intubation. Am J Surg 1978;135:452-457.
151. Ching N, Ayres S, Paegle R, et al: The contribution of cuff volume and pressure in tracheostomy tube damage. J Thorac Cardiovasc Surg 1971;62:402-408.
152. Guyton D, Banner MJ, Kirby RR: High volume, low-pressure? Chest 1991; 100:1076-1081.
153. Black AMS, Seegobin RD: Pressures on endotracheal tube cuffs. Anaesthesia 1981;36:498-511.
154. Friedman Y: Indications, timing, techniques, and complications of tracheostomy in the critically ill patient. Curr Opin Crit Care 1996;2:47-53.
155. Smith I, Fleming S, Cernaianu A: Mishaps during transport from the intensive care unit. Crit Care Med 1990;18:278-281.
156. Indeck M, Peterson S, Brotman S: Risk, cost and benefit of transporting patients from the ICU for special studies. Crit Care Med 1987;15:350.
157. Waddell G: Movement of critically ill patients within hospital. BMJ 1975;2:417-419.
158. Friedman Y, Mayer AD: Bedside percutaneous tracheostomy in critically ill patients. Chest 1993;104:532-535.
159. Toursarkissian B, Zweng TN, Kearney PA: Percutaneous dilational tracheostomy: Report of 141 cases. Ann Thorac Surg 1994;57:862-867.
160. Winkler WB, Karnik R, Seelman O, et al: Bedside percutaneous dilational tracheostomy with endoscopic guidance: Experience with 71 ICU patients. Intensive Care Med 1994;20:476-479.
161. Powell DM, Price PD, Forrest LA: Review of percutaneous tracheostomy. Laryngoscope 1998;108:170-177.
162. Hill BB, Zweng TN, Maley RH, et al: Percutaneous dilational tracheostomy: Report of 356 cases. J Trauma 1996;40:238-244.
163. Walz MK, Peitgen K, Thurauf N, et al: Percutaneous dilational tracheostomy—early results and long-term outcome of 326 critically ill patients. Intensive Care Med 1998;24:685-690.
164. Ciaglia P, Graniero KD: Percutaneous dilatational tracheostomy: Results and long-term follow-up. Chest 1992;101: 464-467.
165. Thompson EC, Fernandez LG, Norwood S, et al: Percutaneous dilatational tracheostomy in a community hospital setting. South Med J 2001;94:208-211.
166. van Heurn LWE, Goei R, de Ploeg I, et al: Late complications of percutaneous dilatational tracheostomy. Chest 1996;110: 1572-1576.
167. Law RC, Carney AS, Manara AR: Long-term outcome after percutaneous dilational tracheostomy: Endoscopic and spirometry findings. Anaesthesia 1997;52:51-56.
168. Hazard P, Jones C, Benitone J: Comparative clinical trial of standard operative tracheostomy with percutaneous tracheostomy. Crit Care Med 1991;19:1018-1024.
169. Friedman Y, Fildes J, Mizock B, et al: Comparison of percutaneous and surgical tracheostomies. Chest 1996;110:480-485.
170. Crofts SL, Alzeer A, McGuire GP, et al: A comparison of percutaneous and operative tracheostomies in intensive carepatients. Can J Anaesth 1995;42: 775-779.
171. Holdgaard HO, Pederson J, Jensen RA, et al: Percutaneous dilatational tracheostomy versus conventional surgical tracheostomy: A clinical randomized study. Acta Anaesthesiol Scand 1998;42:545-550.
172. Gysin C, Dulguerov P, Guyot JP, et al: Percutaneous versus surgical tracheostomy: A double-blind randomized trial. Ann Surg 1998;230:708-714.
173. Freeman BD, Isabella K, Cobb JP, et al: A prospective, randomized study comparing percutaneous with surgical tracheostomy in critically ill patients. Crit Care Med 2001;29:926-930.
174. Silvester W, Goldsmith D, Uchino S, et al: Percutaneous versus surgical tracheostomy: A randomized controlled study with long-term follow-up. Crit Care Med 2006;34: 2145-2152.
175. Massick DD, Yao S, Powell DM, et al: Bedside tracheostomy in the intensive care unit: A prospective randomized trial comparing open surgical tracheostomy with endoscopically guided percutaneous dilatational tracheostomy. Laryngoscope 2001;111:494-500.
176. Cooper RM: Use and safety of percutaneous tracheostomy in intensive care: Report of a postal survey of ICU practice. Anaesthesia 1998;53:1209-1227.
177. Friedman Y: Percutaneous tracheostomy: What technique is it? Crit Care Med 2001;29:1289-1290.
178. Pryor JP, Reilly PM, Shapiro MB: Surgical airway management in the intensive care unit. Crit Care Clin 2000;16:473-488.
179. Friedman Y, Mizock BA: Percutaneous versus surgical tracheostomy: Procedure of choice or choice of procedure? Crit Care Med 1999;27: 1684-1685.
180. Antonelli M, Michetti V, Di Palma A, et al: Percutaneous translaryngeal versus surgical tracheostomy: A randomized trial with 1-yr double-blind follow-up. Crit Care Med 2005;33:1015-1020.
181. Heikkinen M, Aarnio P, Hannukainen J: Percutaneous dilational tracheostomy or conventional surgical tracheostomy. Crit Care Med 2000;28:1399-1402.
182. van Heerden PV, Webb SAR, Power BM, et al: Percutaneous dilational tracheostomy—a clinical study evaluating two systems. Anaesth Intensive Care 1996;24:56-59.
183. Nates JL, Cooper DJ, Myles PS, et al: Percutaneous tracheostomy in critically ill patients: A prospective, randomized comparison of two techniques. Crit Care Med 2000;28:3734-3739.
184. Cantais E, Kaiser E, Le-Goff Y, et al: Percutaneous tracheostomy: Prospective comparison of the translaryngeal technique versus the forceps-dilational technique in 100 critically ill adults. Crit Care Med 2002;30:815-819.
185. Johnson JJ, Cheatem ML, Sagraves SG, et al: Percutaneous dilatational tracheostomy: A comparison of single vs. multiple dilator techniques. Crit Care Med 2001;29:1251-1254.
186. Guzman J, Bander J, Weinmann MD: Percutaneous diational tracheostomy: A safe technique in patients at risk for

bleeding. Am J Respir Crit Care Med 1995;151:A489.
187. Friedman Y, Franklin C: The technique of percutaneous tracheostomy. J Crit Illness 1993;8:289-297.
188. Barba CA, Angood PB, Kauder DR, et al: Bronchoscopic guidance makes percutaneous tracheostomy easy to teach, safe, and cost effective. Surgery 1995;118:879-883.
189. Marx WH, Ciaglia P, Graniero KD: Some important details in the technique of percutaneous dilatational tracheostomy via the modified Seldinger technique. Chest 1996;110:762-766.
190. Freeman BD, Isabella K, Lin N, et al: A meta-analysis of prospective trials comparing percutaneous and surgical tracheostomy in critically ill patients. Chest 2000;118:1412-1418.
191. Eysenck HJ: Meta-analysis and its problems. BMJ 1994;309:789-792.

Chapter 16

Chest Tube Thoracostomy

Vincent E. Lotano

Chest thoracostomy chest tubes can be lifesaving. Decisions regarding chest tubes can be confusing, however, and chest tubes can be dangerous if placed when not indicated or by inexperienced personnel without proper supervision. The technique, indications, and potential complications of chest tubes should be well known to health care personnel working in the intensive care unit (ICU), as should management after placement. A nonfunctioning or malpositioned chest tube provides misleading information to the managing clinicians.

HISTORY

Hippocrates drained an empyema using a metal tube.[1] Playfair developed underwater seal drainage of chest tubes in 1875.[2] Credit for the invention of the chest tube is usually given to Hewett,[3] who in 1876 devised a system of continuous drainage of the empyema cavity using a rubber catheter that drained into a glass jar filled with a weakly antiseptic solution.[4] Use of the chest tube was not widely adopted, however, until the 1917 influenza epidemic.[5] Closed tube thoracostomy drainage of the pleural space after thoracotomy was first reported by Lilienthal in 1922.[6]

ANATOMY AND PHYSIOLOGY OF THE PLEURAL SPACE

The pleural space is the interface between the chest wall and the lung and represents a critical component of pulmonary function. The visceral and parietal pleurae are composed of a single layer of mesothelium. The blood supply of the parietal pleura is of systemic origin (intercostal vessels), whereas the blood supply of the visceral pleura is of pulmonary origin (pulmonary artery and veins). The bronchial arteries may contribute significantly to the blood supply of the visceral surface.[7]

Both pleural surfaces are lined by an extensive lymphatic network that ultimately drains into the thoracic duct via the mediastinal (visceral) and intercostal (parietal) lymph nodes. There are extensive communications between lymphatics above and below the diaphragm.

Pleural fluid may originate from three sources—parietal capillaries, visceral capillaries, or interstitium. Starling's law of transcapillary exchange governs the movement of fluid across the pleural space. The pressure in the capillaries of the visceral pleura is less than that in the parietal capillaries because it drains into the pulmonary venous bed. The net hydrostatic pressure (35 cm H_2O) favors movement of fluid from the parietal pleura to the pleural space (Fig. 16-1). This pressure is derived from the subtraction of −5 cm H_2O (pleural pressure) from 30 cm H_2O (parietal hydrostatic pressure). This net hydrostatic pressure is opposed by the net oncotic pressure (29 cm H_2O), which is derived from the subtraction of 5 cm H_2O (pleural oncotic pressure) from 34 cm H_2O (plasma oncotic pressure). There is a gradient of 6 cm H_2O (34 − 29 cm H_2O) favoring pleural fluid formation.[8] The pleural lymphatics prevent the accumulation of this pleural fluid. Stomas, unique to the parietal pleura, facilitate communication between the pleural space and the capillaries. It is estimated that this mechanism allows clearance of 20 mL/h/hemithorax of pleural fluid in a 70-kg human.[9,10] The lymphatic network clears protein from the pleural space; smaller molecules can be directly absorbed by the pleural capillaries. Intercostal and diaphragmatic muscle activity influence the rate of lymphatic flow. Hypoventilation and anesthesia reduce lymphatic flow and the rate of absorption of protein.[11]

DRAINAGE SYSTEMS

The original three-bottle system has been compartmentalized into a plastic unit that is easily transportable and readily pressure-adjustable, consisting of a trap bottle, a water-seal bottle, and a manometer bottle (Fig. 16-2). The trap bottle collects the pleural fluid. The water-seal bottle prevents air from returning to the pleural space during the negative pleural pressure phase on inspiration. The manometer bottle uses the distance below its fluid line to generate a negative pressure when suction is applied. For example, 20 cm of water generates a −20 cm H_2O pressure.[12] Modern collection and suction systems use a single compartmentalized system (Fig. 16-3).

INDICATIONS AND CONTRAINDICATIONS

Simple Pneumothorax

Pneumothorax is defined as air that has entered the pleural space, either spontaneously or as a result of traumatic tears in the pleura after chest injury or after invasive procedures. Treatment of pneumothorax entails removing air from the pleural space, re-expanding the underlying lung, and preventing recurrence.[13] If the patient is clinically stable, the treatment depends on the size of the pneumothorax and whether or not the patient is mechanically ventilated. If the pneumothorax is small, and the patient is not mechanically ventilated, the pneumothorax can be observed. If the pneumothorax is large, or the patient is mechanically ventilated, a chest tube should be placed.[14] A large pneumothorax is defined as being greater than 15% to 20%.[15]

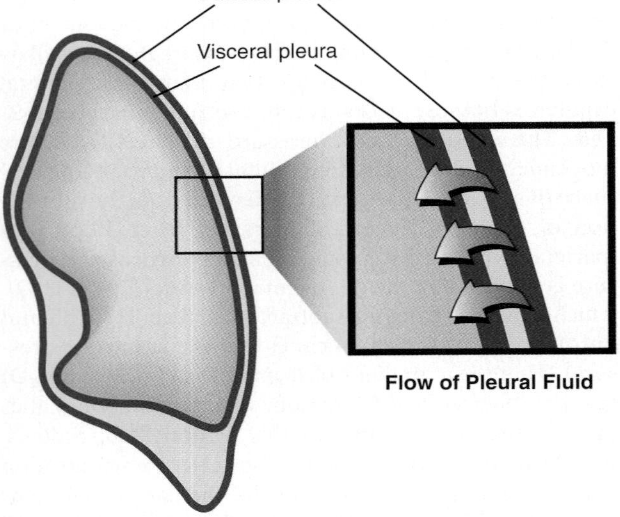

Figure 16-1. The direction of fluid movement across the pleural space is shown, moving from the parietal through the visceral pleural surface where transport into the lymphatic system occurs.

Tension Pneumothorax

Tension pneumothorax is a life-threatening clinical situation that requires emergent and immediate treatment (Fig. 16-4). Air collects and builds up pressure in the chest cavity through a tear in the lung or bronchial tree. Air enters the chest with each mechanical or spontaneous breath, with no route for escape. Initially, the affected lung simply collapses, but as tension increases, the diaphragm flattens, and the mediastinum is shifted toward the contralateral side.[16] The contralateral lung is compressed, further decreasing effective ventilation. The great vessels also are compressed, and venous return is drastically reduced. This reduction in venous return results in rapid and disastrous cardiopulmonary collapse.[17] The diagnosis is ideally made on a clinical basis, and treatment is initiated without waiting for radiographic confirmation. Any tension pneumothorax should have immediate large-bore needle decompression. A readily available large-bore angiocatheter is preferentially inserted in the second intercostal space at the midclavicular line. A rush of pleural air under pressure confirms the diagnosis and location. After decompression (conversion to a simple pneumothorax), the catheter is left in until a tube thoracostomy has been placed.[18]

Pleural Effusions

Pleural effusions, both transudative and exudative, are frequently seen in the ICU. The incidence of pleural effusions in the ICU varies with screening methods, from approximately 8% for physical examination to more than 60% for routine ultrasound.[19,20] Several factors contribute to the occurrence of pleural effusions in ICU patients. Large amounts of intravenous fluid are often administered during the first few days to patients admitted for shock. Pneumonia also is common as a reason for ICU admission and as a complication of mechanical ventilation. Heart failure, atelectasis, hypoalbuminemia, and liver disease are present in many ICU patients. In surgical ICUs, cardiac or abdominal surgery is often followed by specific, large, protracted pleural effusion; in multiple-injury patients, hemothorax is possible.[21] The criteria of Light and colleagues,[22] which are based on the ratio of protein or lactate dehydrogenase levels in the pleural fluid and blood, differentiate exudates from transudates with a

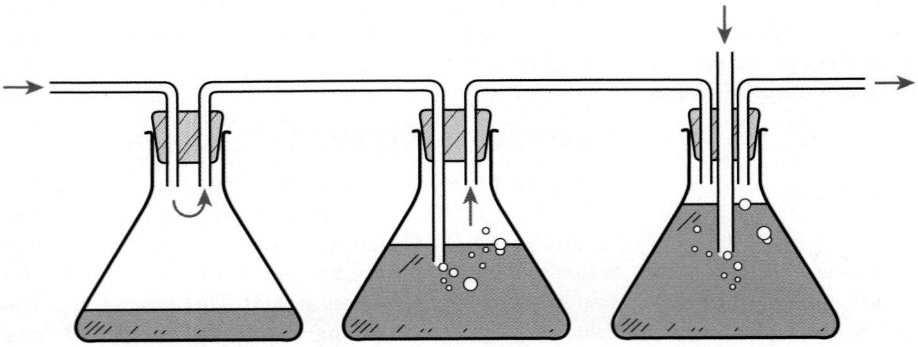

Figure 16-2. Three-bottle system consisting of from *left to right* trap bottle, water-seal bottle, and manometer bottle.

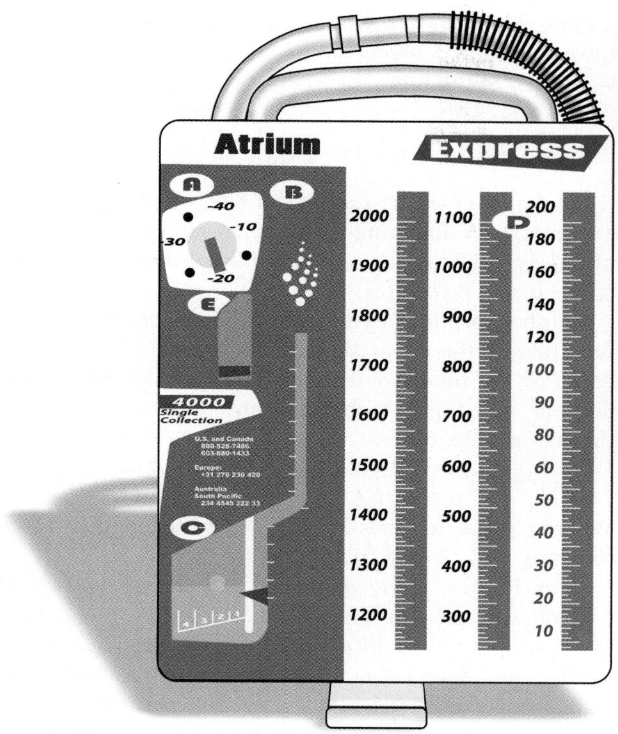

Figure 16-3. Modern drainage system.

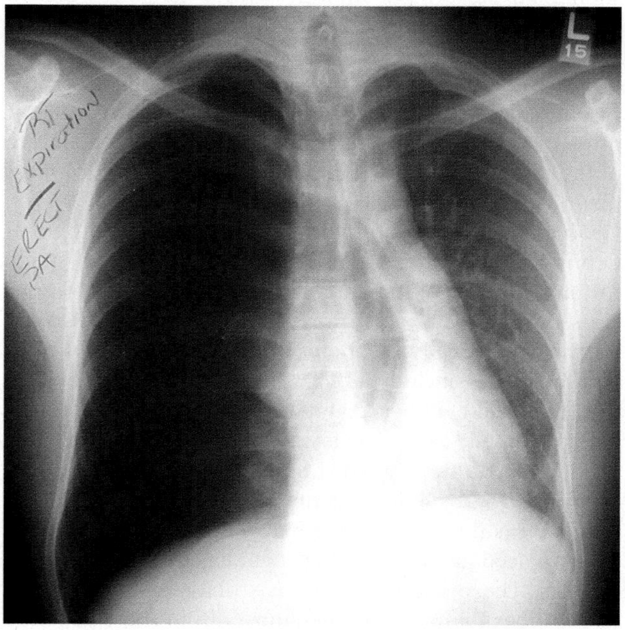

Figure 16-4. Chest radiograph shows a left-sided tension pneumothorax with mediastinal shift to the right.

negative predictive value of 96% and a sensitivity of 98%.[23]

Provided that basic rules are followed, thoracentesis is safe in ICU patients.[24] A chest tube may be placed for large or symptomatic pleural effusions. The optimal drainage duration for uninfected pleural effusions has not been established. A reasonable approach may be to remove the chest tubes when drainage decreases to <200 mL/d.[25]

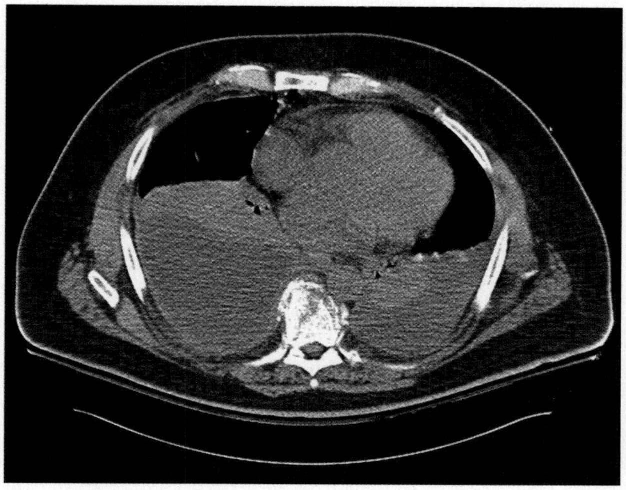

Figure 16-5. An empyema is shown in the right pleural space. Note the thickened pleura surrounding the collection, characteristic of this diagnosis.

In the evaluation of a parapneumonic effusion or empyema, if the thickness of the pleural fluid is more than 10 mm on a decubitus radiograph, or if the pleural fluid is of similar depth and loculated, the pleural fluid should be examined to determine the stage of the effusion. Drainage of an infected pleural space is required to achieve source control as a key component of treatment (Fig. 16-5). If the fluid is removed completely and does not reaccumulate, no additional therapy need be directed toward the effusion. At the time of the initial therapeutic thoracentesis, the pleural fluid should be sent for Gram stain and culture and analysis of leukocyte, lactate dehydrogenase, glucose, and pH levels. Indicators of a poor prognosis from the pleural fluid include positive Gram stain or culture, glucose less than 60 mg/dL, lactate dehydrogenase more than three times the upper limits of normal for serum, or pH less than 7.20.

If the therapeutic thoracentesis removes all of the pleural fluid and the fluid recurs, the next step is guided by the initial pleural fluid findings. If none of the poor prognostic indicators is present, no invasive procedures are indicated if the patient is doing well clinically. If any of the poor prognostic indicators were present at the initial thoracentesis, a second therapeutic thoracentesis should be performed, and the pleural fluid should be reanalyzed. If the pleural fluid accumulates a third time, a small chest tube should be inserted into the pleural space, unless none of the poor prognostic factors was present at the time of the second thoracentesis.[26] If the patient shows signs of systemic infection, and fluids have been inadequately drained, an open thoracotomy and drainage may be required.[27,28]

When a hemothorax is suspected, the essential management, along with appropriate resuscitation, is intercostal drainage. This achieves two objectives: first, to drain the pleural space allowing expansion of the lung and, second, to allow assessment of rates of continuing blood loss.

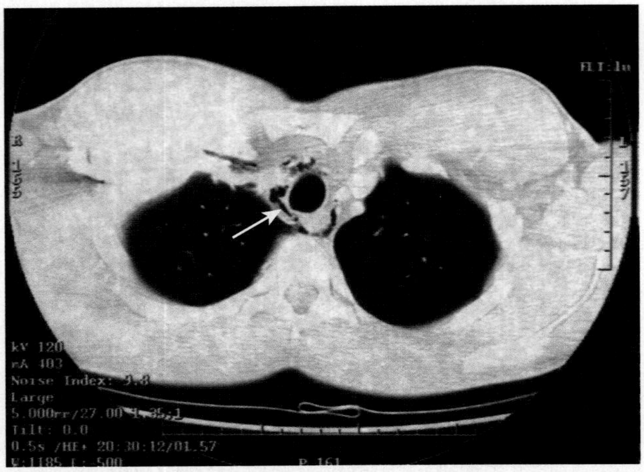

Figure 16-6. Pneumomediastinum *(arrow)*. The pneumomediastinum occurred during a forceful singing period.

After satisfactory resolution of hemothorax managed with intercostal drainage alone, the drain should not be removed too promptly. Other circumstances permitting, the patient should be mobilized fully with adequate thoracic physiotherapy. These measures should allow optimal drainage of the pleural cavity.[29] Complete drainage of blood also prevents empyema and fibrothorax.

Pneumomediastinum is usually a self-limited entity (Fig. 16-6). It follows alveolar rupture into the pulmonary interstitium and is produced by an acute episode of high intrathoracic pressure. The differential diagnosis includes cardiac, pulmonary, musculoskeletal, and esophageal causes. Spontaneous pneumomediastinum is usually a self-limited clinical entity.[30] Coupled with positive-pressure ventilation or subcutaneous emphysema, however, cautious observation is recommended owing to the possibility of a pneumothorax leading to tension pneumothorax.

There is no good evidence to support prophylactic chest tubes with high levels of positive end-expiratory pressure. These tubes may be difficult to place and may create more issues. A patient on high positive end-expiratory pressure should be closely observed for any evidence of pneumothorax. If this should occur, a chest tube should be placed at that time.

Contraindications to chest tube placement are mainly relative. The most common would be coagulopathy. If the draining indication is less than urgent and can be delayed until the coagulopathy can be corrected, the procedure should be postponed. If chest tube placement is emergently needed, one must proceed with caution and actively correct the coagulation issues while proceeding with the tube thoracostomy.

CHEST TUBE SIZE

There is some difference of expert opinion as to optimal chest tube size for various indications. Medicine in general is always moving in the direction of less invasive, smaller, more focused and direct treatments for issues that require some type of intervention. Chest drainage is no different. In an effort to determine the best size tube, two laws are quoted. The first is Poiseuille's law, which states that flow through a tube depends on the internal diameter (D) and length (L) of the tube, the viscosity of the liquid (η), and the pressure difference between its ends (ΔP):

$$\text{Flow rate} = (\pi/128)\ (D^4\ \Delta P/\eta L)$$

If the diameter of the tube is doubled, flow increases by a factor of 16, implying that a small increase in the size of the drainage tubes would result in substantial improvements in the flow rates.[31]

Another formula key to chest tube size selection is the flow rate of the air or the liquid that can be accommodated by the tube. The Fanning equation determines the flow of moist gas with turbulent flow characteristics through a chest tube:

$$v = p^2 r^5 P/fl$$

Where v is the flow, r is the radius, l is the length, P is the pressure, and f is the friction factor).[32-35]

In an in vitro study, Park and coworkers[36] measured flow rates of different viscosity fluids (serous, blood, pus) through catheters of different diameters, ranging from 6F to 18F, and found that flow rates increased for larger catheters as predicted by Poiseuille's law. At catheter sizes larger than 7F, however, the differences were small.

Reports on drainage techniques suggest that before drainage of a collection, diagnostic needle aspiration should be performed, initially with a 22-gauge needle and, if this is unsuccessful, subsequently with a 20-gauge or 18-gauge cannula.[37] It has been postulated that if pus can be aspirated by such a needle, it should be drainable through a catheter twice the size (i.e., ≥6F).[38] As such, if drain patency can be maintained, the maximum flow rate of the catheter is unlikely to be the limiting factor for most pleural collections.[39]

Given the variety of liquids and accompanying pleural debris that may be drained by a chest tube, no single formula for flow of these many materials exists. The principal determinants of airflow through a tube, bore and length, are logically key determinants of flow for various pleural liquids, including blood and pus. Chest tube selection must take into account not only what material is being drained, but also its rate of formation. Ongoing production of more viscous fluids requires a larger bore tube than for a similar volume of air produced.[40]

In our institution, we have had good success with small tubes placed under radiologic guidance into empyema cavities. These small catheters also have complemented larger tubes that have drained most of the chest but have left small residual pockets, which would be difficult to access blindly with large, less flexible tubes.

TECHNIQUE OF INSERTION

When inserting a chest drain for the first time, regardless of the technique, the procedure should be proctored by an experienced supervisor whenever possible. The procedure can be life-saving or life-threatening depending on how it is done. Many things should be verified before any skin incision or needle stick is performed. The patient should be well informed as to what is going to happen and why and give consent. The chest radiograph should be present at the procedure, and the date, patient's name, and affected side should be confirmed by the operator and one other health care professional. Next, all instruments should be confirmed to be present at the procedure. Someone should be available to get additional items needed during the procedure and to reassure the patient during the procedure.

Mild sedation or anxiolysis is typically needed before the procedure, and intravenous access is essential for the ability to give intravenous pain medication. If the procedure is done carefully and with good local anesthesia, there is usually minimal to no need for intravenous sedation. Coagulation parameters (i.e., prothrombin time, partial thromboplastin, and platelets) should be confirmed to be normal or, if abnormal, adequate for coagulation (typically platelet count 50,000/μL and international normalized ratio ≤1.5 IU). Most hospitals have closed tube thoracostomy trays premade; however, the components that should be available are as follows[41]:

1. Skin antiseptic solution
2. Sterile drapes
3. Syringes—10 mL × 3
4. Needles—21-gauge, 23-gauge, 25-gauge
5. Local anesthesia—1% or 2% 10 mL lidocaine
6. Scalpel—No. 11 or 15 blade
7. Sutures—2-0 silk (to anchor tube) and 3-0 nylon (to close site when tube is removed if desired)
8. Heavy scissors
9. Drain sponge dressings and 4 × 4 dressings
10. Curved hemostat clamps
11. Clamp for chest tube
12. Underwater seal collection system
13. Sterile chest tube—sizes 24F and 32F (depending on what is found to be drained; blood or pus should be 32F, air or fluid can be 24F)
14. Syringes or specimen cups for culture

The patient should be positioned supine with the head of the bed elevated to 30 degrees and the arm held behind the head or abducted to 90 degrees if placement behind the head is impossible. Mark the site of insertion with indelible marker so it is not removed with the skin preparation.

Insertion should be in the "safe triangle" illustrated in Figure 16-7. This is the triangle bordered by the anterior border of the latissimus dorsi, the lateral border of the pectoralis major muscle, a line superior to the horizontal level of the nipple, and an apex below the axilla. The most common position for chest tube insertion is in the midaxillary line, through the safe triangle. This position minimizes risk to underlying structures such as the internal mammary artery and avoids damage to muscle and breast tissue resulting in scarring. A more posterior position may be chosen if suggested by the presence of a loculus, although this site is more uncomfortable for the patient, and there is a risk of the drain kinking.[42]

The patient should be prepared and draped in sterile fashion with a wide field (Fig. 16-8), and the operator should be wearing sterile gown, gloves, hat, and mask. Local anesthesia should be instilled with a 23-gauge or 25-gauge needle making a skin wheal and allowing 2 to

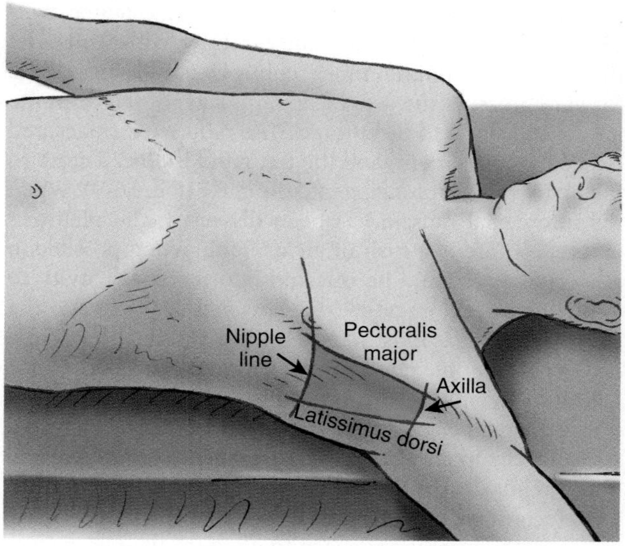

Figure 16-7. Position of patient and safe triangle for identification of injection site.

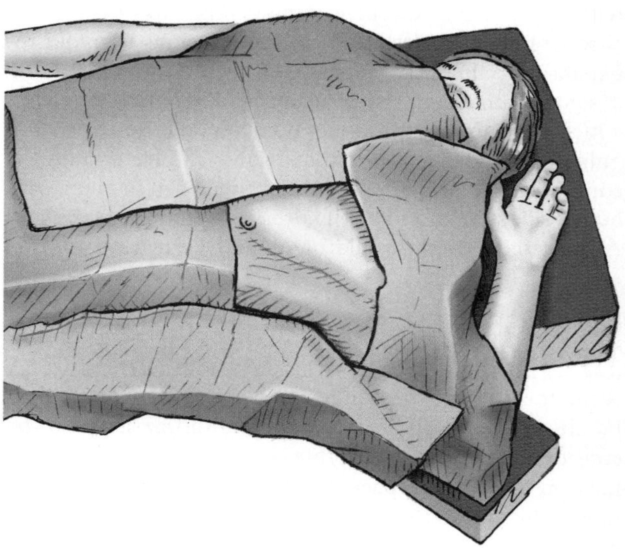

Figure 16-8. Prepared field for chest tube placement.

5 minutes for anesthetic to take effect. Deeper infiltration follows with a 21-gauge needle to the intercostal muscles, the area over the rib, periosteum, and parietal pleura (when air or fluid is aspirated, withdraw the needle slightly and reinfiltrate to ensure anesthetizing the pleura).[41]

A 1- to 1.5-cm incision is made parallel to the rib and down to the subcutaneous fat at the lower border of the rib space to allow for a small tunnel or tract to prevent air from being drawn around the tube and to close the incision when the tube is removed. A vertical or horizontal mattress suture is placed through the incision tying a knot at the free ends of the suture. This can be used later when the chest tube is removed to close the skin incision. A tract is created using a small curved hemostat by inserting it closed into the incision and gently spreading. It should be removed and reinserted with each spreading maneuver.[43] This needs to be done slowly and carefully to prevent pain; this is done multiple times continuously using gentle forward pressure toward the upper border of the rib at the intercostal space to be entered. The right hand opens and closes the instrument, and the left hand is placed close to the tip to prevent plunging into the chest (Fig. 16-9). When the intercostal muscle has been dissected, the pleura is entered. There is a rush of air or fluid. When possible, a gloved finger should be inserted into the chest cavity to ensure there are no adhesions between the lung and the chest wall. This is most important if the patient has had a history of multiple chest tubes or thoracic surgery.

Before beginning the procedure, the tube should be prepared and placed on the sterile field within easy reach. A closed clamp may be passed through the distal hole and out the end of the tube to facilitate placement (Fig. 16-10). This technique may be easier than trying to open the clamp in the intercostal space to advance the chest tube. When placed, the tube should be clamped at the distal end to prevent leakage. The tube should be connected to the tubing in a sterile fashion. The clamp can then be removed. Re-expansion of a long-standing pneumothorax may be painful, and re-expansion should be done slowly with use of intermittent clamping. This also is true for chronic pneumothorax and pleural effusions to avoid re-expansion pulmonary edema. Onset of coughing may be a sign of onset of re-expansion pulmonary edema, at which point the clamp should be reapplied. Re-expansion pulmonary edema is discussed later in the section on complications. The tube should be anchored in place with heavy silk suture, and sterile dressings should be applied. A chest radiograph should be obtained and reviewed.

MANAGEMENT OF THORACOSTOMY TUBES

A malfunctioning chest tube can be more dangerous than no chest tube at all. Tension pneumothorax may not be considered as a cause of hypotension if a drainage catheter is in the pleural space; however, if the catheter is not functioning properly, a tension pneumothorax may still be present. In the ICU, especially in the presence of positive-pressure ventilation, a chest tube should be assessed as frequently as any vital sign, ensuring that the tube is patent and draining. If a moderate or large air leak suddenly stops, the tube should be assessed immediately to ensure the tube is not kinked or plugged.

When a thoracic drain has been placed, a chest radiograph should be obtained immediately and reviewed. This is done to confirm placement and assess success of intervention. The amount and character of the drainage or air leak or both should be assessed. A chest radiograph should be done every day for as long as the tube is in place.[44,45] The question as to whether to place a tube to water seal or suction when an air leak is present is an ongoing debate. In two studies of postoperative patients, it was shown that water seal was superior to suction in stopping air leak.[46,47] In the presence of a large air leak, however, if the pneumothorax increases or a subcutaneous emphysema develops, the tube should be placed back to suction (usually 20 cm H_2O), and a chest radiograph should be immediately obtained. If there is no air leak for 24 hours, and the drainage is less than 2 mL/kg/d, it is safe to remove the tube.[48] One protocolized option begins with thoracostomy tubes placed to 20 cm H_2O suction immediately after insertion.[44] Tubes are usually assessed for air leak and drainage. Suction is continued if an air leak is present, or if the drainage is greater than or equal to 200 mL in 24 hours. If these criteria are not met, the tubes are placed to water seal. Chest radiographs are not obtained routinely on water seal or before removal. If no air leak is present after 6 hours on water seal, the tube is removed.[49] If a tube is nonfunctioning, it should be removed. If one chooses to place the tube to water seal before removal, a chest radiograph obtained 3 hours after water seal excludes development of a clinically significant pneumothorax.[50]

Clamping a chest drain before removal is necessary. If an air leak is small and intermittent, clamping followed by chest film may help determine if the patient is likely to develop a pneumothorax after removal. The house staff

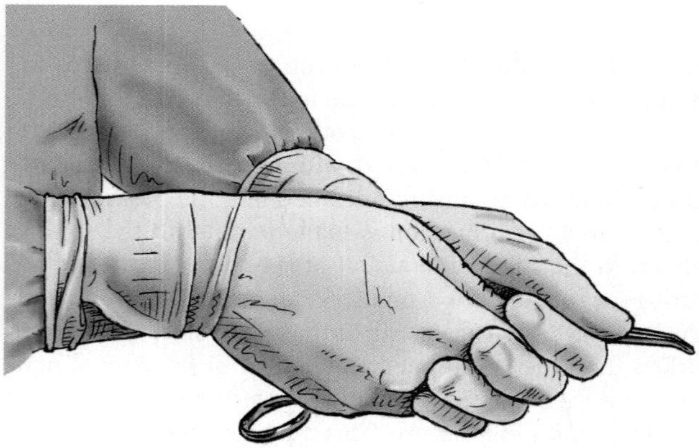

Figure 16-9. Position of hands on Hemostat or clamp to minimize iatrogenic injury.

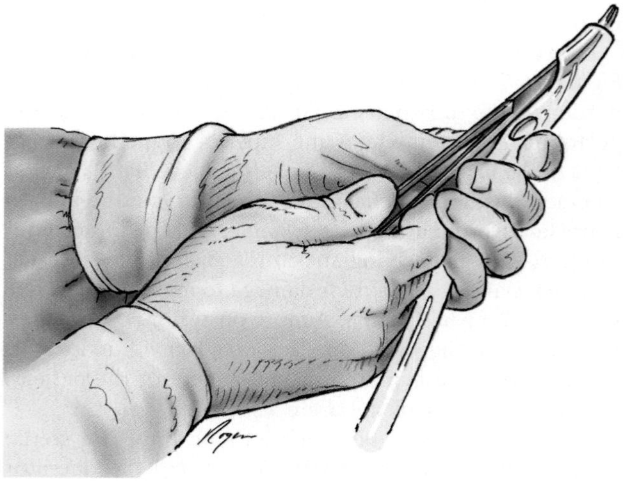

Figure 16-10. Insertion of clamp through distal hole of chest tube to facilitate proper placement of chest tube.

and nursing staff must be fully informed, however, so the tube can be immediately unclamped if these is any respiratory difficulty. Clamping of the chest tube in the face of massive hemothorax (1500 mL on placement) also has been advocated; however, in a study creating hemothorax spontaneously in piglets, chest tube clamping did not decrease hemorrhage or mortality, but worsened gas exchange without improving hypotension.[51]

There are no data to support prophylactic antibiotic use for chest tube placement in the ICU in nontrauma patients. In traumatic hemothorax, multiple factors, including the condition under which the tube is inserted (emergent or urgent), the mechanism of injury, retained hemothorax, and ventilator care, contribute to development of pleural space infection. The incidence of empyema ranges between 0% and 18% and is decreased with the use of prophylactic antibiotics. Administration of antibiotics for longer than 24 hours does not reduce this risk further.[52]

Obtaining a chest film after removal of a chest tube has been standard practice at most institutions. Timing usually ranges from 6 to 24 hours after the tube is removed. Two retrospective studies concluded that it is unnecessary to obtain routine chest radiographs after chest tube removal.[53,54] Other authors, in light of no prospective randomly assigned clinical studies, advocate obtaining a single upright chest radiograph 24 hours after chest tube removal to evaluate for recurrence of hemothorax or pneumothorax.[54] In a mechanically ventilated patient, a chest film should be obtained after chest drain removal. A study by Pizano and colleagues[55] of 214 patients undergoing positive-pressure ventilation concluded that the number of clinically significant pneumothoraces after chest tube removal seems to be small. The concern persists, however, regarding expansion of a small pneumothorax into a tension pneumothorax. Failure to diagnose a large and expanding pneumothorax could lead to a life-threatening situation. Pizano and colleagues[55] supported obtaining a chest film within 3 hours after chest tube removal. It also seemed safe to remove a chest tube from patients undergoing positive-pressure ventilation if standard removal criteria were met.[55]

Routine milking and stripping of chest tubes is performed primarily in postoperative cardiac surgical patients. The data do not support routine milking and stripping unless there is clot in the tubing. A significant negative pressure can be generated in the chest during the procedure, which could be detrimental. Few such complications are cited in the literature, however.[56]

Postplacement chest radiograph may raise the question of placement in the fissure of the lung, potentially compromising function. This may lead to manipulation to change position. Chest tubes appearing to be in the pleural fissure on plain radiograph function as effectively, however, as tubes located elsewhere in the pleural space.[57]

The positioning of the tubing connecting the chest tube to the drainage system is important. In one study, three tubing positions were studied: straight, coiled, and dependent loop (allowing fluid to collect in a dependent loop with loop left alone in some, and periodically lifted and drained at 15-minute intervals in others). It was found that the dependent loop left alone did not drain adequately. The straight and coiled positions were optimal for drainage of fluid. If the dependent loop cannot be avoided, lifting and draining it every 15 minutes would maintain adequate drainage.[58]

Removal of a chest tube is associated with pain. In one study, 4 mg of intravenous morphine was given 20 minutes before removal versus 30 mg of intravenous ketorolac given 60 minutes before removal. Either of these regimens was found to reduce pain substantially during chest tube removal without causing adverse sedative effects.[59] Another study compared topical lidocaine-prilocaine cream (EMLA) versus intravenous morphine. The investigators found that topical EMLA cream was more effective, but it had to be applied 3 hours before chest tube removal.[60]

Removal of the chest tube must be timed with the breathing pattern of the patient. Some authors advocate removal at end inspiration, whereas others recommend removal at end expiration. The reason some advocate end inspiration is that when the tube is removed the patient may gasp from the pain and may be more likely to suck in air through the site. In one study, a similar rate of postremoval pneumothorax was found. Both methods were found to be safe.[61] There are two ways to close the sites after the tube has been removed. If sutures were placed, they are tied down. If no sutures were placed, an occlusive dressing must be made with 4 × 4 dressings and tape and petroleum jelly gauze.

COMPLICATIONS

Complications of chest tube placement include improper positioning, bleeding, nerve damage, injury to diaphragm or abdominal organs, mechanical problems, pain, and bronchopleural fistula. Any structure or organ in the chest or upper abdomen can be damaged or perforated with chest tube insertion. The heart, lung, aorta, vena cava, pulmonary artery, nerves, liver, spleen, and stomach all are vulnerable. Damage is more likely to occur with the use of a trocar, but can occur if the clamp dissecting through the intercostal space is not controlled by the operator. A sudden thrust into the chest, especially in a small chest, can easily reach the mediastinum.

Re-expansion pulmonary edema is a rare and potentially lethal complication of tube placement for pneumothorax, pleural effusion, and severe atalectasis (Fig. 16-11).[62] The estimated mortality is 20%.[63] Onset of symptoms is often immediate, but can be delayed 24 hours.[64] Severe coughing heralds the development of pulmonary edema. The patient becomes tachypneic and tachycardic as hypoxia increases. The patient does not respond to oxygen therapy because blood is shunted past fluid-filled alveoli. Rarely, bilateral or contralateral edema develops.[65] The pathophysiology is complex. Multiple factors contribute to a capillary bed with increased permeability. An inflammatory response occurs when the lung re-expands. This response is believed to be secondary to expansion-related mechanical injury to the alveolar-capillary membrane and reperfusion injury as blood flow returns to the now fully expanded lung.[66] Patients 20 to

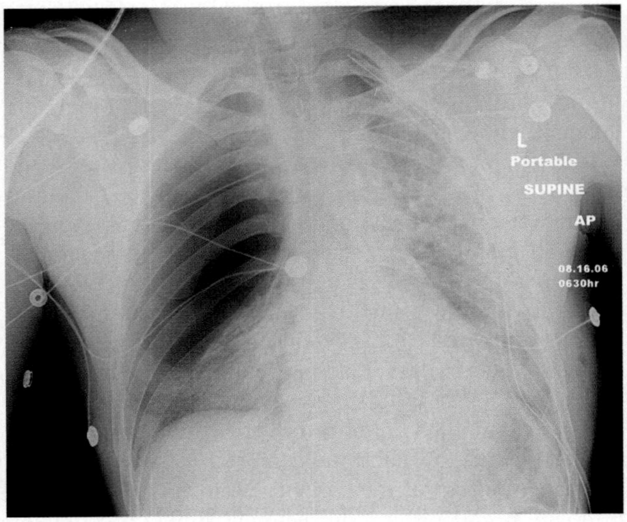

Figure 16-11. Chest radiograph shows re-expansion pulmonary edema on left and giant blebs on right.

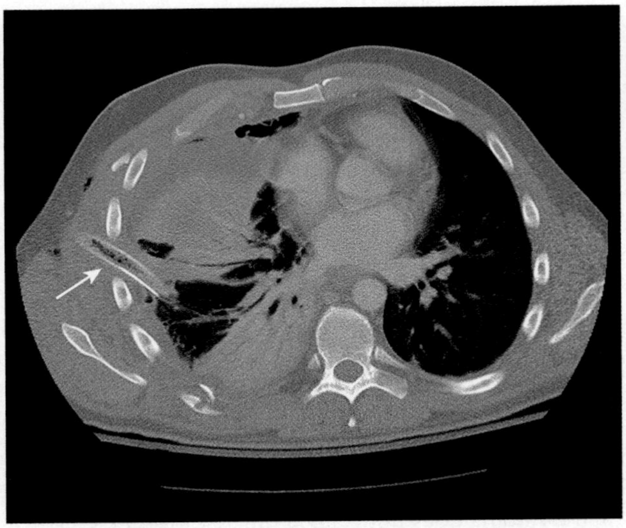

Figure 16-12. CT scan shows a loculated pleural effusion with chest tube location indicated by *arrow*.

39 years old are more susceptible.[67] The duration of pneumothorax also has been implicated in the incidence of re-expansion pulmonary edema.[68] Early case series found that spontaneous pneumothorax was present an average of 14 days with a minimum of 3 days before edema would develop.[69] The severity of the pneumothorax may be more predictive than its duration in developing pulmonary edema. In the series by Matsuura and coworkers,[67] no patient with a pneumothorax less than 30% of the lung field developed pulmonary edema. Seventeen percent of patients with total collapse and 44% of patients with tension pneumothorax had this complication. Some authors support slow re-expansion by lower negative pressure as beneficial, whereas others support the idea that it is not so much the degree of negative pressure as the rate of re-expansion that is important.[70] In clinically stable patients with a large (30% of the lung field) primary pneumothorax, the American College of Chest Physicians recommends either small-bore (≤14F) catheter or 16F to 22F chest tube placement.[14] Connection to a Heimlich valve or a water-seal device is recommended. If the lung fails to re-expand, suction is deemed appropriate.

The mainstay of therapy remains oxygenation, a low threshold for mechanical ventilation with positive end-expiratory pressure, diuresis if it can be tolerated, and hemodynamic support. Re-expansion pulmonary edema usually resolves in 24 to 72 hours.[66]

IMAGING

Areas in the chest that require chest tube drainage may be loculated owing to adhesions from pneumonias or multiple chest tube placements, making it difficult and dangerous to place a drain blindly into the chest. The use of ultrasound or computed tomography (CT) guidance can be invaluable.[71] Ultrasound and CT also can be used to verify location of tubes previously placed. In one study, 51 pigtail catheters placed under radiologic guidance (CT or ultrasound) were reviewed, with an overall success rate of 88%. The specific success rates were 92%, 85%, and 91% for loculated pleural effusion, pneumothorax, and empyema. Complications were few and minor.[72]

A chest radiograph should be performed immediately after chest drain placement, but the position of the tube may still be in question. CT has proved to be useful when this occurs (Fig. 16-12). Placements such as intraparenchymal, intrafissural, mediastinal, chest wall, and abdominal may be identified.[73] In a study in which CT revealed 28 malpositioned chest tubes among 76 tubes placed in 54 patients, frontal chest radiograph revealed only 6 of the 28.[74]

KEY POINTS

- Chest tube selection must take into account not only what material is being drained, but also its rate of formation.
- When inserting a chest drain for the first time, the procedure should be proctored by an experienced supervisor.
- The chest radiograph should be present at the procedure, and the date, patient's name, and affected side should be confirmed by the operator and one other health care professional.
- Insertion should be in the "safe triangle."
- In the ICU, especially in the presence of positive-pressure ventilation, a chest tube should be assessed as frequently as any other vital sign.
- There are no data to support prophylactic antibiotic use for chest tube placement in the ICU in nontrauma patients.
- The mainstay in therapy for re-expansion pulmonary edema remains oxygenation, a low threshold for mechanical ventilation, diuresis (if tolerated), and hemodynamic support.
- CT has proved to be extremely accurate in evaluating the position of a chest tube.

REFERENCES

1. Hippocrates: Genuine Works, vol 2 (trans by Francis Adams). New York, William Wood & Company, 1886.
2. Playfair GE: Case of empyema treated by aspiration and subsequently by drainage: Recovery. BMJ 1875;1:45.
3. Hewett C: Drainage for empyema. BMJ 1876;1:317.
4. Hewett C: Thoracentesis: The plan for continuous aspiration. BMJ 1876;1:317.
5. Graham EA, Bell RD: Open pneumothorax: Its relation to the treatment of empyema: War medicine. Am J Med Sci 1918;156:839.
6. Lilienthal H: Pulmonary resection for bronchiectasis. Ann Surg 1922;75:257.
7. Albertine KH, Wiener-Kronish JP, Roos PJ, et al: Structure, blood supply, and lymphatic vessels of the sheep's visceral pleura. Am J Anat 1982;165:277.
8. Miserocchi G, Agostini E: Pleural liquid and surface pressures at various lung volumes. Respir Physiol 1980;39: 315.
9. Broaddus VC, Staub NC: Pleural liquid protein turnover in health and disease. Semin Respir Med 1987;9:7.
10. Broaddus VC, Weiner-Kronish JP, Berthiauma Y, et al: Removal of pleural liquid and protein by lymphatics in awake sheep. J Appl Physiol 1988;64: 384.
11. Kinasewitz GT, Fishman AP: Influence of alterations in Starling forces of visceral pleural fluid movement. J Appl Physiol 1981;51:671.
12. Miller KS, Sahn FA: Chest tubes: Indication, technique, management and complications. Chest 1987;91:258.
13. Jenkinson SG: Pneumothorax. Clin Chest Med 1985;6:153-161.
14. Baumann MH, Strange C, Heffner JE, et al: Management of spontaneous pneumothorax. American College of Chest Physicians Delphi Consensus Statement. Chest 2001;119:590-602.
15. Putukian M: Pneumothorax and pneumomediastinum. Clin Sports Med 2004;23:443-454.
16. Sabiston DC, Spencer FC: Gibbon's Surgery of the Chest, 3rd ed. Philadelphia, Saunders, 1975.
17. Vulkich DJ: Pneumothorax, hemothorax, and other abnormalities of the pleural space. Emerg Med Clin N Am 1983;1: 431-448.
18. Gilbert TB, McGrath BJ, Soberman M: Chest tubes: Indications, placement, management, and complications. J Intensive Care Med 1993;8:73-86.
19. Fartoukh M, Azoula E, Galliot R, et al: Clinically documented pleural effusions in medical ICU patients: How useful is routine thoracentesis. Chest 2002;121:178-184.
20. Mattison LE, Coppage L, Alderman DF, et al: Pleural effusions in the medical ICU: Prevalence, causes, and clinical implications. Chest 1997;111: 1018-1023.
21. Azoulay Elie: Pleural effusions in the intensive care unit. Curr Opin Pulm Med 2003;9:291-297.
22. Light RW, Macgregor MI, Luchsinger PC, et al: Pleural effusions: The diagnostic separation of transudates and exudates. Ann Intern Med 1972;77:507-513.
23. Azoulay E: Pleural effusions in the intensive care unit. Curr Opin Pulm Med 2003;9:291-297.
24. Fartoukh M, Azoula E, Galliot R, et al: Clinically documented pleural effusions in medical ICU patients: How useful is routine thoracentesis? Chest 2002;121:178-184.
25. Younes RN, Gross JL, Aguiar S, et al: When to remove a chest tube? A randomized study with subsequent prospective consecutive validation. J Am Coll Surg 2002;195:658-662.
26. Light RW: The management of parapneumonic effusions and empyema. Curr Opin Pulm Med 1998;4:227-229.
27. Roper WH, Waring JJ: Primary serofibrinous pleural effusion in military personnel. Am Rev Tuberc 1955;71: 616-635.
28. Pablo A, Villena V, Echave-Sustaeta J, et al: Are pleural fluid parameters related to the development of residual pleural thickening in tuberculosis? Chest 1997;112:1293-1297.
29. Perry GW: Management of haemothorax. Ann R Coll Surg Engl 1996;78:325-326.
30. Koullias GJ, Korkolis DP, Wang XJ, et al: Current assessment and management of spontaneous pneumomediastinum: Experience in 24 adult patients. Eur J Cardiothorac Surg 2004;25:852-855.
31. Tattersall DJ, Traill ZC, Gleeson FV: Chest drains: Does size matter? Clin Radiol 2000;55:415-421.
32. Baumann MH, Strange C: Treatment of spontaneous pneumothorax: A more aggressive approach? Chest 1997;112: 789-804.
33. Batchelder TL, Morris KA: Critical factors in determining adequate pleural drainage in both the operated and nonoperated chest. Am Surg 1962;28:296-302.
34. Miller KS, Sahn SA: Chest tubes, indications, technique, management and complications. Chest 1987;91: 258-264.
35. Swenson EW, Birath G, Ahbeck A: Resistance to air flow in bronchospirometric catheters. J Thorac Surg 1957;33:275-281.
36. Park JK, Kraus FC, Haaga JR: Fluid flow during percutaneous drainage procedures: An in vitro study of the effects of fluid viscosity, catheter size, and adjunctive urokinase. AJR Am J Roentgenol 1993;160:165-169.
37. van Sonnenberg E, Ferruci JT, Mueller PR, et al: Percutaneous drainage of abscesses and fluid collections: Technique, results and applications. Radiology 1982;142:1-10.
38. Meuller PR, van Sonnenberg E, Ferruci JT: Percutaneous drainage of 250 abdominal abscesses and fluid collections: Part II. Current procedural concepts. Radiology 1984;151:343-347.
39. Tattersall DJ, Traill ZC, Gleeson FV: Chest drains: Does size matter? Clin Radiol 2000;55:415-421.
40. Baumann MH: What size chest tube? What drainage system is ideal? And other chest tube management questions. Curr Opin Pulm Med 2003;9:276-281.
41. Tomlinson MA, Treasure T: Insertion of a chest drain: How to do it. Br J Hosp Med 1997;58:248-252.
42. Laws D, Neville E, Duffy J; on behalf of the British Thoracic Society Pleural Disease Group, a subgroup of the British Thoracic Society Standards of Care Committee: BTS guidelines for the insertion of a chest tube. Thorax 2003;58(suppl II):ii-53-ii-59.
43. Parmar JM: How to insert a chest drain. Br J Hosp Med 1989;42:231-233.
44. Martino K, Merrit S, Boyakye K, et al: Prospective randomized trial of thoracostomy removal algorithms. J Trauma 1999;46:369.
45. Mattox KL: Perhospital care of the patient with an injured chest. Surg Clin North Am 1989;69:21.
46. Cerfolio RJ, Tummala RP, Holman WL, et al: A prospective algorithm for the management of air leaks after pulmonary resection. Ann Thorac Surg 1998;66:1726-1731.
47. Cerfolio RJ, Bass C, Katholi CR: Prospective randomized trial compares suction versus water seal for air leaks. Ann Thorac Surg 2001;71: 1613-1617.
48. Davis JW, Mackersie RC, Hoyt DB, et al: Randomized study of algorithms for discontinuing tube thoracostomy drainage. J Am Coll Surg 1994; 179:553.
49. Adrales G, Huynh T, Broering B, et al: A thoracostomy tube guideline improves management efficiency in trauma patients. J Trauma Injury Infection Crit Care 2002;52:210-216.
50. Schulman CI, Cohn SM, Blackbourne L, et al: How long should you wait for a chest radiograph after placing a chest tube on water seal? A prospective study. J Trauma Injury Infection Crit Care 2005;59:92-95.
51. Ali J, Qi W: Effectiveness of chest tube clamping in massive hemothorax. J Trauma Injury Infection Crit Care 1995;38:59-63.
52. Luchette FA, Barrie PS, Oswanski MF, et al: Practice management guidelines for prophylactic antibiotic use in tube thoracostomy for traumatic hemopneumothorax: The EAST Practice Management Guidelines Work Group. Eastern Association for Trauma. J Trauma Injury Infection Crit Care 2000;48:753-757.
53. Palesty JA, McKelvey AA, Dudrick SJ: The efficacy of x-rays after chest tube removal. Am J Surg 2000;179: 13-16.
54. Pacanowski JP, Waack ML, Daley BJ, et al: Is routine roentgenography needed after closed tube thoracostomy removal? J Trauma Injury Infection Crit Care 2000;48:684-688.
55. Pizano LR, Houghton DE, Cohn SM, et al: When should a chest radiograph be obtained after chest tube removal in mechanically ventilated patients? A prospective study. J Trauma Injury Infection Crit Care 2002;53: 1073-1077.
56. Teplitz L: Update: are milking and stripping chest tubes necessary? Focus Crit Care 1991;18:506-511.
57. Curtin JJ, Goodman LR, Quebbeman EJ, et al: Thoracostomy tubes after acute

chest injury: Relationship between location in a pleural fissure and function. AJR Am J Roentgenol 1994;163:1339-1342.

58. Schmelz JO, Johnson D, Norton JM, et al: Effects of position of chest drainage tube on volume drained and pressure. Am J Crit Care 1999;8:319-323.
59. Puntillo K, Ley SJ: Appropriately timed analgesics control pain due to chest tube removal. Am J Crit Care 2004;13:292-304.
60. Valenzuela RC, Rosen DA: Topical lidocaine-prilocaine cream (EMLA) for thoracostomy tube removal. Anesth Analg 1999;88:1107-1108.
61. Bell RL, Ovadia P, Abdullah F, et al: Chest tube removal: End-inspiration or end-expiration? J Trauma Injury Infection Crit Care 2001;50: 674-677.
62. Sherman SC: Reexpansion pulmonary edema: A case report and review of the current literature. J Emerg Med 2003;24:23-27.
63. Mahfood S, Hix WR, Aaron BL, et al: Reexpansion pulmonary edema. Ann Thorac Surg 1988;45:340-345.
64. Mahfood S, Hix WR, Aaron BL, et al: Reexpansion pulmonary edema. Ann Thorac Surg 1988;45:340-345.
65. Heller B, Grathwohl M: Contralateral reexpansion pulmonary edema. South Med J 2000;93:828-831.
66. Trachiotis GD, Vricella LA, Aaron BL, et al: Reexpansion pulmonary edema: Updated in 1997. Ann Thorac Surg 1997;63:1206-1207.
67. Matsuura Y, Nomimura T, Murakami H, et al: Clinical analysis of reexpansion pulmonary edema. Chest 1991;100: 1562-1566.
68. Murphy K, Tomlanovich MC: Unilateral pulmonary edema after drainage of a spontaneous pneumothorax: Case report and review of the world literature. J Emerg Med 1983;1: 29-36.
69. Kassis E, Philipsen E, Clausen K: Unilateral pulmonary edema following spontaneous pneumothorax. Eur J Respir Dis 1981;62:102-106.
70. Murphy K, Tomlanovich MC: Unilateral pulmonary edema after drainage of a spontaneous pneumothorax: Case report and review of the world literature. J Emerg Med 1983;1:29-36.
71. Iberti TJ, Stern PM: Chest tube thoracostomy. Crit Care Clin 1992;8:879-895.
72. Cantin L: Chest tube drainage under radiological guidance for pleural effusion and pneumothorax in a tertiary care university teaching hospital: Review of 51 cases. Can Respir J 2005;12:29-33.
73. Gayer G, Rozenman J, Hoffmann C, et al: CT diagnosis of malpositioned chest tubes. Br J Radiol 2000;73:786-790.
74. Lim KE, Tai SC, Chan CY, et al: Diagnosis of malpositioned chest tubes after emergency tube thoracostomy: Is computed tomography more accurate than chest radiograph? Clin Imaging 2005;29:401-405.

Chapter 17

Intracranial Monitoring

Alan R. Turtz

In general, chapters on intracranial monitoring focus on intracranial pressure (ICP). This chapter expands the scope of discussion to include the intracranial monitoring of pressure, cerebral blood flow (CBF), and brain tissue oxygenation.

INTRACRANIAL PRESSURE MONITORING

The history of ICP monitoring dates to 1891, when Quincke measured the cerebrospinal fluid (CSF) pressure via a lumbar puncture.[1] Soon afterward, Cushing showed that as ICP increases and approaches systemic arterial pressure in an animal model, hypertension, bradycardia, and respiratory changes become evident.[2] The use of continuous ICP monitoring was first described by Guillaume and Janny[3] using an intraventricular catheter in 1951. Nine years later, Lundberg[4] published the first systematic observations of ICP and its response to medical and physiologic interventions. Using ventricular catheters, he showed the clinical value of direct ICP monitoring and described pressure waveforms, of which the Lundberg A wave has the most practical importance in the intensive care unit (ICU). These A, or plateau, waves are characterized by a steep increase in ICP to 60 to 80 mm Hg lasting 2 to 5 minutes or longer, followed by a rapid decrease to near initial baseline pressures. This represents a pathologic response to decompensation of pressure controlling mechanisms.[4,5,6] Since these early investigations, CSF pressure and ICP measurement have been developed and refined further.

An ICP monitor is an invaluable research and clinical tool, contributing to the understanding of intracranial pathologic conditions and the assessment of therapeutic interventions. ICP monitoring can be used for patients with intracerebral hemorrhage, Reye's syndrome, hepatic encephalopathy, encephalitis, stroke, hydrocephalus, near-drowning, and subarachnoid hemorrhage, but most of the clinical experience with ICP monitoring involves traumatic brain injury (TBI). In severe TBI, it is important to know if ICP is elevated. Early signs and symptoms of increased ICP include headache, lethargy, nausea, and vomiting. In critically ill patients, these clinical signs may be nonspecific and unreliable.[6] In addition, the positive trend toward early intubation and sedation, if not pharmacologic paralysis, eliminates the neurologic assessment of a patient with the exception of pupils. Even papilledema, a hard physical sign of increased ICP, is rarely seen acutely in patients with TBI.[7] Computed tomography (CT) is arguably the most useful diagnostic tool in patients with TBI, but may not reliably determine the ICP.

ICP monitoring in severe TBI has become routine because it facilitates rational management, provides prognostic information, and improves outcomes.[8-10] ICP monitoring can provide crucial information relative to cerebral perfusion pressure (CPP); detect the development or enlargement of a mass lesion, such as contusion or hematoma; facilitate the estimation of intracranial compliance, and be the only parameter to follow in a pharmacologically paralyzed patient, apart from the pupillary examination. It is rarely justifiable to treat a patient for intracranial hypertension empirically without a mechanism for measuring the effect of treatment, such as a clinical examination or ICP.

There are well-defined guidelines for the use of ICP monitoring in TBI, which include patients with an abnormal CT scan and a Glasgow Coma Scale score of 8 or less after cardiopulmonary resuscitation. An abnormal CT scan is defined as one that reveals hematomas, contusion, edema, or compressed cisterns. It also is recommended to consider monitoring head-injured patients with a Glasgow Coma Scale score of 8 or less even if the head CT scan is negative if two of the following three criteria are met on admission: age older than 40, systolic blood pressure less than 90 mm Hg, or signs of posturing (Fig. 17-1).[11]

Although ICP monitoring can be a useful tool in the ICU, this technology has limitations. It is crucial not to assign undue weight to a normal ICP if other clinical information suggests otherwise. ICP does not always increase in the presence of midline shift.[12,13] More specifically, a temporal lobe mass can herniate over the tentorial edge and cause brainstem compression without a concomitant increase in ICP.[14,15] Likewise, there is not good correlation between supratentorial and infratentorial pressures,[16] so it is imperative to remember that patients

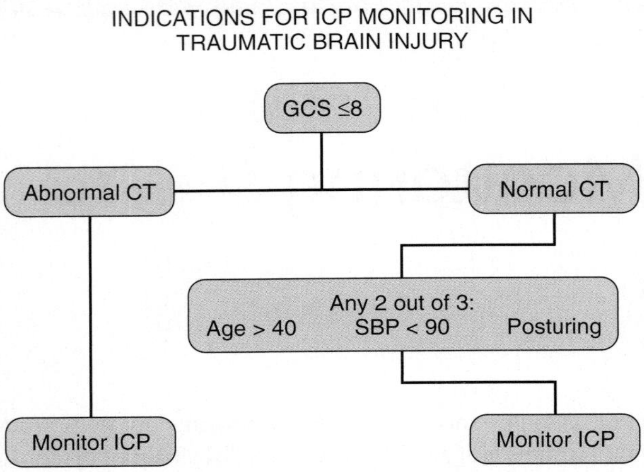

Figure 17-1. Indications for intracranial pressure (ICP) monitoring. CT, computed tomography; GCS, Glasgow Coma Scale; SBP, systolic blood pressure. (From Brain Trauma Foundation, American Association of Neurological Surgeons, Joint Section on Neurotrauma and Critical Care: Management and prognosis of severe traumatic brain injury: Part I. Guidelines for the management of severe traumatic brain injury. J Neurotrauma 2000;17:47-69.)

with a posterior fossa mass can deteriorate rapidly without a significant increase in ICP measured in the supratentorial compartment.[6]

ICP waveform analysis includes systolic and diastolic pressures with superimposed respiratory variation; however, the mean pressure is of practical importance. A normal adult mean ICP is 10 mm Hg or less with transient physiologic elevations above this value seen in a head-down position or during a Valsalva maneuver (see discussion of secondary injury in Chapter 67).[6] The Association for the Advancement of Medical Instrumentation developed standards for ICP monitoring devices that require a pressure range from 0 to 100 mm Hg, an accuracy of ±2 mm Hg in the range of 0 to 20 mm Hg, and a maximal error of 10% between 20 mm Hg and 100 mm Hg.[17] There are four basic types of clinically useful monitoring systems: ventricular catheter, subarachnoid bolt, fiberoptic device, and catheter tip strain gauge.

Ventricular Catheter

A ventriculostomy is the gold standard for ICP monitoring. It can be inserted through a twist drill craniostomy at the bedside and can also be used to drain CSF or for the estimation of intracranial compliance. The catheter is connected to a fluid-filled system, which is connected to an external transducer. The transducer converts the measured pressure to an electrical signal, which provides a waveform and numerical value displayed on a monitor through a signal processor. A three-way stopcock is used to divert CSF from the monitor to a drainage bag if needed. This setup allows the catheter to be zeroed as frequently as necessary with the transducer positioned at the level of the center of the brain, which generally corresponds to the external auditory meatus. This system has the potential to be opened and contaminated and infected. The most significant risk of a ventriculostomy is infection; rates of 27% have been cited,[10,18,20,21] although most reported rates are in the 1% to 10% range.[20,22-25] Infection rates are similar regardless of procedure location (ICU or the operating room).[19,20,26] Tunneling the catheter subcutaneously to a distant skin exit site seems to reduce the infection risk. Other risk factors for infection include irrigation of the catheter or drainage system and the presence of intraventricular blood.[19,20,27] Duration of monitoring also may be a risk factor for infection. Some studies have found an increase in infection rates when ventriculostomies were left in for longer than 5 days,[19,20,24] but more recent data reveal no significant reduction in infection rates when catheters were replaced before the fifth day.[28] Likewise, other investigators have found no significant relationship between duration of monitoring and rate of daily infection for 2 weeks.[29] The role of prophylactic antibiotics during external CSF drainage is unclear.[19,25,27,30] Our practice is to give a single dose of periprocedural antibiotics and monitor the CSF as clinically indicated; we do not routinely replace the catheter unless we suspect infection.

Hemorrhage at the time of placement occurs about 1% to 2% of the time and only rarely needs to be surgically evacuated.[6,24,31] A more common problem with placement is difficulty in accessing small, compressed, or shifted ventricles, resulting in malposition and a poor waveform. Although a ventriculostomy is generally considered to be the most precise and accurate method of measuring ICP,[32] malfunction occurs if the ventriculostomy becomes clogged with air, blood, or debris, or if the ventricles are collapsed around the fenestrations in the catheter tip.

In addition to its primary use as an ICP monitor, a ventriculostomy is commonly used in the ICU as a drain for patients with TBI or hydrocephalus. Common causes of acute hydrocephalus in an adult ICU include cerebellar stroke or hemorrhage, intraventricular hemorrhage, and aneurysmal subarachnoid hemorrhage. A common and often debated concern regarding CSF drainage with a ventriculostomy is that it can cause subfalcine herniation in the presence of a hemispheric mass or upward herniation of the cerebellum in the presence of an infratentorial lesion.[33] Under these circumstances, we believe that surgical decompression of the primary mass also should be considered. Another potential risk of ventricular catheter insertion is aneurysmal rebleeding[34] after an acute subarachnoid hemorrhage. Our group's opinion is that the benefit of treating hydrocephalus with high ICP far outweighs the small, potential risk of aneurysmal rebleeding, and we have a low threshold for placing a ventriculostomy in these patients.

If a ventriculostomy is primarily used for drainage of CSF, adequate spontaneous CSF resorption must be restored before the catheter can be safely removed. CSF resorptive capacity must be gauged according to the CSF drainage rate. Adjusting the height of the drainage system drip chamber controls the rate of external CSF drainage and the ICP that must be exceeded before drainage occurs. It can be assumed that 1 cm of CSF equals 1 cm H_2O. The height of the drip chamber is measured from the same external anatomic landmark as the ICP transducer, ranging from 0 to 20 cm (approximately 15 mm Hg) above the external auditory meatus in usual circumstances.

To reduce the amount of external CSF drainage, the drip chamber is usually raised by incremental amounts every 12 to 24 hours. As this is done, CSF resorptive mechanisms are gradually challenged. If CSF resorption is insufficient, most of the CSF continues to drain through the ventriculostomy, but if CSF resorption is sufficient, little CSF drains externally. When CSF resorption seems to be sufficient, CSF drainage is stopped, and ICP is monitored for 24 hours or more to confirm that spontaneous CSF resorption is adequate and ICP will not increase to dangerous levels.

We generally manage ventriculostomies for hydrocephalus by leaving the reservoir open to drain at a specific height above the ear and close it every hour for an ICP reading. In hydrocephalus, the ICP should never be significantly higher than the gradient which the patient is draining against (i.e., the height of the drip chamber). We also specify our drainage gradient in millimeters of mercury to correlate the drip chamber to the monitor and manually correlate the height of the CSF column in the drainage system with the monitor as a system check at least daily. A typical order may read: "leave ventriculostomy open to drain at 15 mm Hg (20 cm CSF) above the ear and monitor ICP every hour." ICP readings with the drain open are inaccurate, and the drainage port needs to be temporarily clamped when measuring an ICP. Likewise, the drain should be clamped and placed to monitor when changing position or during transport to avoid overdrainage, which may cause ventricular collapse and possibly subdural bleeding.

Subarachnoid Bolt

The subarachnoid bolt technique for ICP monitoring was developed because of concern about the infection rate associated with ventriculostomies, and because small ventricular size after head trauma often makes catheter insertion difficult.[35] A subarachnoid bolt is a self-tapping metal or plastic tube that is screwed into a twist drill craniostomy at the bedside. The dura at the base of the bolt is perforated with a spinal needle to allow CSF to fill the bolt, which is connected to pressure tubing filled with preservative-free (nonbacteriostatic) saline that leads to an external transducer leveled to the ear. In contrast to a ventriculostomy, the subarachnoid bolt is only a monitoring instrument; CSF is not withdrawn from it. It usually provides a reliable ICP waveform and pressure reading, but is susceptible to error if the dural perforations become obstructed with blood or debris, or if brain swelling obliterates communication with CSF. Uncapping the bolt to flush debris with 0.2 mL of preservative-free saline solution can restore accurate ICP readings and is unlikely to cause dangerous ICP elevation.[36] The subarachnoid bolt tends to underestimate ICP, particularly when ICP is elevated.[36,37] Because the subarachnoid bolt measures the local ICP at the surface of the hemisphere, it can be inaccurate if a pressure gradient is present between the left and right supratentorial compartments.[18] The existence of compartmental pressure differences has been debated, but such gradients can occur between the left and right hemispheres or the supratentorial and infratentorial compartments and sometimes are only transient.[18,38-40] This is an important phenomenon to consider, and if a discrepancy exists between an apparently normal ICP and the patient's clinical condition or CT scan or both, treatment of elevated ICP may be warranted.

The infection risk for subarachnoid bolts is extremely low, and infections are nearly always superficial and rarely involve the brain or meninges.[19] No local or systemic infection was reported with the use of subarachnoid bolts in 124 comatose children.[41] Risk of subarachnoid bolt infection is increased when the bolt is opened and flushed to improve the waveform.[19] Subarachnoid bolts are rarely associated with brain injury; however, intracerebral hematoma may occur[42] if there is a mishap with the drill, or if the needle used to puncture the dura is passed too deeply. Since the introduction of fiberoptic catheters, subarachnoid bolts are being used less often.

Fiberoptic Intracranial Pressure Monitors

Fiberoptic ICP monitors use miniature transducers that are coupled via fiberoptic cables to an external instrument. These monitors can be placed at the bedside through a standard twist drill craniostomy or through a smaller opening made with a 2.71-mm bit (Fig. 17-2). The transducer is incorporated into the end of a tube and can be used alone or in combination with a ventriculostomy. Fiberoptic systems operate by projecting light through an

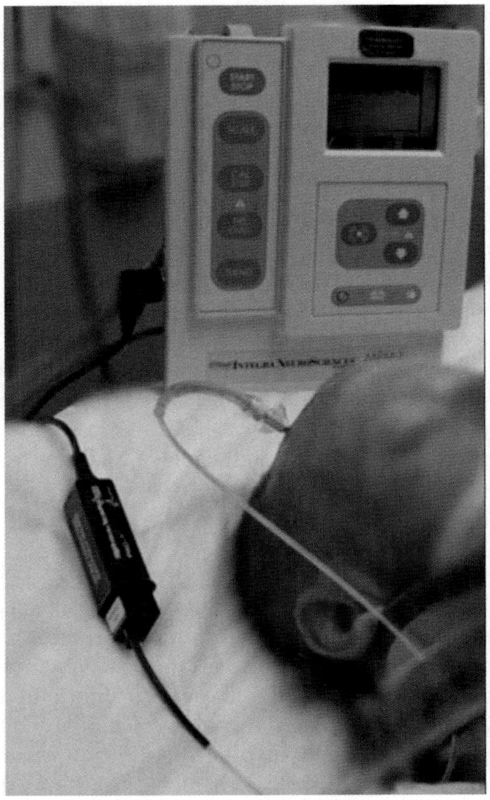

Figure 17-2. Fiberoptic intraparenchymal intracranial pressure (ICP) monitor.

optic fiber to a miniature, displaceable mirror in the catheter tip.[43] The amount of light reflected to a collecting optic fiber depends on the mechanical displacement of the mirror, which is a function of ICP. Fiberoptic devices can be inserted into the lateral ventricle, the brain parenchyma, or the subdural space. The greatest advantage of fiberoptic catheters is that they do not require fluid coupling for pressure transduction, which avoids the problems of waveform dampening and artifacts from poor coupling. Because they do not require fluid coupling, there also is less opportunity for contamination. The mechanism that does the actual pressure transduction is what is inserted into the patient; the system functions independent of head position, and the monitor is zeroed once before it is placed. This feature also is a disadvantage because the transducer cannot be recalibrated to zero after insertion. System accuracy compared with a ventriculostomy has been shown in the subdural space, brain parenchyma, and ventricles, although the parenchymal fiberoptic pressures may consistently exceed ventriculostomy pressures by nearly 10 mm Hg.[44-46] The fiberoptic device has an average daily drift of ±0.6 mm Hg. Over a 5-day period, there is an average drift of 2.1 mm Hg with a maximal drift of ±6 mm Hg. This drift over time may be enough to necessitate replacement if ICP monitoring is required for more than 5 days.[6,46,47]

Complications with the use of fiberoptic catheters relating to hemorrhage[48,49] and infection[48] have been reported, but our experience is that clinically relevant problems are unusual, particularly with intraparenchymal monitors. We do exercise caution, however, in patients with coagulopathy.

Catheter Tip Strain Gauge

The catheter tip strain gauge consists of a miniaturized solid-state pressure sensor mounted in a titanium case at the tip of a long, thin, flexible nylon tube. The transducer tip contains a silicon microchip with diffuse piezoresistive strain gauges that connect to tiny wires that travel the length of the tube. This is a small wire with a diameter of 1.2 mm that can be placed at the bedside. It can be incorporated into a ventricular catheter and used in any intracranial space. This device is accurate with a low daily drift range between −0.125 mm Hg and +0.110 mm Hg. It shares many of the advantages and disadvantages of fiberoptic devices,[6,50,51] but we have found it more cumbersome to place and secure through a bedside twist drill craniostomy.

CEREBRAL BLOOD FLOW MONITORING

The primary objective concerning the ICU management of brain-injured patients is the prevention and management of secondary injury in an effort to prevent ischemia. We typically monitor ICP and mean arterial blood pressure continuously, which allows us to calculate CPP. Under normal circumstances, knowing the CPP allows a good estimation of CBF, which is a more direct measure of blood supply to the brain. In head injury, the relationship between CPP and CBF is less predictable. An ideal intracranial monitor would provide direct, continuous measurements of regional and global CBF at the bedside.

Measuring CBF outside of the ICU began with Kety and Schmidt in 1948 and more recently has been done with xenon-enhanced CT,[52,53] but these methods only give snapshots of CBF and do not allow for continuous monitoring at the bedside.[54] Continuous monitoring techniques in the ICU are classified as direct or indirect. Direct and continuous monitoring of CBF at the bedside includes laser Doppler flowmetry and thermal diffusion.

The laser Doppler flow sensor (1.5 mm diameter), which emits a monochromatic light, is placed into the white matter through a burr hole. The sensor measures the volume or concentration of red blood cells and their velocity and generates a flow signal. Although laser Doppler flow does allow continuous measurements of perfusion, the sample volume is small (1 mm^3), and only relative changes can be determined. Laser Doppler flow provides a qualitative estimate of regional CBF displayed in arbitrary units.[55] A quantitative estimate of regional CBF can be acquired with the thermal diffusion method.[56] With this technique, a probe with two small thermistors is inserted into the brain to measure the tissue's ability to dissipate heat, and a microprocessor converts this into CBF displayed in the standard units of mL/100 g/min.[54]

An indirect method for measuring blood flow at the bedside is transcranial Doppler ultrasound, which measures mean blood flow velocity in the basal cerebral vessels.[57] While not equivalent to volume flow, changes in CBF can be inferred from changes in blood flow velocity.[58] Continuous transcranial Doppler monitoring is still cumbersome, however, because of problems of probe fixation to the head and computer interfacing.[54] Another indirect way of continuously monitoring CBF at the bedside is by measuring jugular venous bulb oxygenation.

Normal mean CBF is 50 to 60 mL/100 g/min with higher flow in the gray matter and lower flow in the white matter. When hemoglobin is fully saturated with oxygen, arterial blood carries approximately 20 mL of oxygen per deciliter to the brain. The oxygen content of venous blood draining the brain varies and depends primarily on how much oxygen the brain extracts. Normal internal jugular hemoglobin oxygen saturation ranges from 55% to 69%, and the normal difference between the arterial and jugular venous oxygen content (arteriojugular difference [$AJDO_2$]) is 6.3 ± 2.4 mL/dL. Stated differently, under normal circumstances, the brain extracts 6.3 ± 2.4 mL/dL of oxygen from the arterial blood to meet the metabolic needs of the brain.

Normally, the cerebral metabolic rate of oxygen ($CMRO_2$) is coupled to CBF; as demand increases, supply increases, and vice versa. In head injury, there may be a problem with supply (i.e., CBF may be compromised). If there is inadequate CBF to meet the metabolic demands of the brain, more oxygen is extracted from the available blood. Under this circumstance, the difference between blood going into the brain and blood coming out of the brain increases; $AJDO_2$ increases as the oxygen saturation in the jugular vein decreases.

$AJDO_2$ is proportional to $CMRO_2$ or inversely proportional to CBF or both.[59-62] Assuming that the $CMRO_2$ is constant, an increase in the amount of oxygen extraction as reflected by a decrease in jugular oxygen saturation (increased $AJDO_2$) implies that CBF has been compromised. Conversely, if $AJDO_2$ decreases, and metabolism remains constant, we can infer an increase in CBF (i.e., hyperemia). Measuring jugular bulb oxygen can be a useful way to monitor a patient who requires hyperventilation for ICP control (see Chapter 67). Hyperventilation is a powerful tool for reducing ICP and enhancing CPP, but at the expense of increasing cerebrovascular resistance, with the consequent reduction of blood in the brain. The goal of treatment is to prevent ischemia, the ultimate and proximate cause of secondary injury. There is an obvious conflict when attempting to prevent ischemia by reducing the amount of blood delivered to the brain. $AJDO_2$ is sensitive to changes in cerebrovascular resistance; jugular vein monitoring may reveal inappropriate reductions of CBF as a result of hyperventilation.[59]

Most of the data concerning jugular bulb monitoring comes from the trauma literature. In a prospective study of 353 patients with severe TBI, Cruz[63] found that outcome at 6 months was significantly better in the patients who had monitoring and management of cerebral extraction of oxygen along with CPP compared with the patients undergoing monitoring and management of CPP alone.

Increased $AJDO_2$ also can be detected during the early phases of head injury when CBF is pathologically reduced. Typically, the patient is being rescued at the scene, transported, and triaged during this early phase of injury, when CBF is low and ventilation is not carefully titrated. Hyperventilation is frequently used during this vulnerable period, often empirically and sometimes inadvertently.[59,64] Complicating this scenario is superimposed hypotension and hypoxia, which can occur during the early phases of resuscitation and later in the ICU.[65-67] Despite its usefulness, there are significant limitations to this monitoring technique. Measurements can be done by intermittent sampling, which is accurate but is limited by intermittent information, or continuous monitoring of oxygen saturation using fiberoptic catheters, which require careful maintenance and have reliability issues.[60,68]

It is easier to use the oxygen saturation of the venous blood in the jugular, rather than direct measurements of oxygen content, but because the percentage of oxygen saturation in the jugular bulb depends on hemoglobin concentration, it cannot be used independently for estimating the relationship between $CMRO_2$ and CBF. If the patient is anemic, more oxygen may be extracted from the available blood, even under conditions of normal CBF. When measuring oxygen saturation, $AJDO_2$ needs to be calculated, taking the hemoglobin concentration into consideration. Also, $AJDO_2$ is an overall estimate of the global relationship between CBF and $CMRO_2$ and cannot differentiate focal abnormalities. In addition, there is a limit to how much oxygen can be extracted from the available blood. If maximal extraction is reached, and CBF continues to deteriorate, the $AJDO_2$ does not continue to increase. Under this circumstance, $AJDO_2$ appears stable despite a progressively worsening situation. Other pitfalls in monitoring $AJDO_2$ are observed under conditions in which oxygen extraction itself is impaired, such as in cases of mitochondrial dysfunction, or a large stroke where oxygen is not extracted at all.[59]

Several important technical factors are associated with $AJDO_2$ monitoring. The side chosen (right or left jugular bulb) is important and can be affected by the side of the brain with the most injury and whether or not it is the side of dominant venous drainage.[69-71] How high the tip of the catheter is positioned is another consideration and requires x-ray confirmation.[72] The speed at which samples are drawn also may affect the results.[73] Complications are uncommon and include carotid puncture[60,74] and subclinical internal jugular vein thrombosis.[74]

Ultimately, jugular bulb monitoring is geared toward the assessment of global CBF and cerebral oxygenation and can be useful in guiding therapeutic hyperventilation.[75,76] In severe TBI, there is enough evidence to recommend its use for titrating the level of hyperventilation[77]; however, some clinicians find jugular bulb monitoring to be cumbersome, to be prone to artifact, and to have other potential problems with poor data quality.[78-80] Because of all of the problems involved with this technique, monitoring of $AJDO_2$ has not been universally accepted as a useful tool in the routine management of head-injured patients. There remain strong arguments for and against the use of jugular bulb monitoring.[63,81]

BRAIN TISSUE OXYGENATION MONITORING

Oxygen tension in brain tissue is as close to a gold standard of cerebral oxygenation as we have at the bedside. Brain tissue oxygen tension can be directly measured using a small flexible microcatheter (<0.5 mm in diameter) that is usually inserted into the frontal white matter and fixed onto a special bolt. The normal brain tissue oxygen tension is approximately 40 mm Hg.[82-86] Cerebral oxygen tension is generally reflective of CBF and local oxygen extraction. In this sense, brain tissue oxygen tension may represent the "pool of oxygen" in brain tissue.[54,87,88] Changes in brain tissue oxygen tension can be used to monitor evolving disturbances of tissue metabolism.[78,89-91]

Ischemic damage seems to correlate to a brain tissue oxygen tension less than 8 to 10 mm Hg as measured by a Licox catheter (Integra Neuroscience, Plainsboro, NJ).[78] A meta-analysis of three studies including 158 patients with severe TBI found overall cerebral hypoxia, defined as a monitored brain tissue oxygen tension less than 10 mm Hg, was associated with worse outcome and increased mortality.[92] Another study treated 70 severe head injury patients with management directed to maintaining brain tissue oxygenation greater than 25 mm Hg in addition to conventional ICP and CPP management. The results were compared with 53 matched, historical controls treated with conventional management only. The mean daily ICP and CPP and the frequency of episodes of ICP greater than 20 mm Hg and CPP less than

60 mm Hg were similar in both groups. Forty percent of patients with management guided by only ICP and CPP had a favorable outcome compared with 70% of patients with management guided by brain tissue oxygenation.[93]

Local cerebral hypoxia in the presence of normal ICP, CPP, and mean blood pressure may be caused by insufficient arterial oxygenation,[89] a mismatch between supply (CBF) and demand ($CMRO_2$),[94] or hyperventilation-induced hypocapnia.[89,95] Hyperventilation can decrease brain tissue oxygen tension because of decreased CBF, which can negate the perceived benefit of improving ICP and CPP.[78,90,95-101] Hyperventilation has a particular risk of causing cerebral hypoxia when P_{CO_2} is less than or equal to 30 mm Hg, or within the first 24 hours[97,98] because of a further reduction of an already reduced CBF.[102] Brain tissue oxygen tension has been shown not to be independently influenced by increases in CPP greater than 60 mm Hg,[80,90,101] which supports more recent evidence suggesting that maintaining a CPP greater than 60 mm Hg is more appropriate than the previously recommended threshold of 70 mm Hg.[103,104]

When strategically placed, these monitors are very sensitive in detecting local tissue hypoxia at the tip of the probe. An inherent problem with this technique (as with all focal monitors) is that placement of the probe into the area of interest becomes imperative.[54] There are rational arguments as to the best region to monitor. Brain tissue oxygen tension values close to a contusion are smaller relative to a region that looks normal on a CT scan.[105] Some authors recommend monitoring the zone surrounding a contusion because of its high risk of tissue death. Other authors place the probes in uninjured brain with the idea being that a reduction in the brain tissue oxygen tension in the uninjured hemisphere is reflecting a diffuse decrease in arterial oxygenation, an increase in ICP, a decrease in CPP, overaggressive hyperventilation, or some other global event.[78]

SUMMARY

Most intracranial monitoring techniques are employed for circumstances involving increased ICP, and ICP monitoring has proved to be useful, reliable, and straightforward. As such, ICP monitoring has become a standard of care and is widely used. It is much more difficult to obtain continuous, clinically useful information with CBF monitoring methods, and these methods have found limited use outside of academic institutions. Brain tissue oxygen monitoring is a relatively new technique with mounting evidence to justify continued use, with the hope of providing additional information to the clinician charged with managing the complicated, dynamic pathophysiologic processes of brain-injured patients.

KEY POINTS

- The primary objective concerning ICU management of brain-injured patients is the prevention and management of secondary injury in an effort to prevent ischemia.
- ICP monitoring should be considered for patients with TBI with a Glasgow Coma Scale score of 8 or less.
- ICP monitoring in severe TBI has become routine because it facilitates rational management, provides prognostic information, and improves outcomes.
- It is crucial not to assign undue weight to a normal ICP if other clinical information suggests otherwise.
- A normal adult mean ICP is 10 mm Hg or less with transient physiologic elevations above this value, and normal CPP is generally 60 to 80 mm Hg.
- Ventriculostomies and fiberoptic intraparenchymal monitors are the mainstays of ICP monitoring devices.
- Oxygen tension in brain tissue is as close to a gold standard of cerebral oxygenation as we have at the bedside.
- Local cerebral hypoxia in the presence of normal ICP, CPP, and mean blood pressure may be caused by insufficient arterial oxygenation, a mismatch between supply (CBF) and demand ($CMRO_2$), or hyperventilation-induced hypocapnia.
- Hyperventilation has a particular risk of causing cerebral hypoxia when P_{CO_2} is less than or equal to 30 mm Hg, or within the first 24 hours.
- Maintaining CPP greater than 60 mm Hg is more appropriate than the previously recommended threshold of 70 mm Hg.

REFERENCES

1. Quincke H: Die Lumbarpunktion des Hydrocephalus. Klin Wochenschr 1891;28:965.
2. Cushing H: Some experimental observations concerning states of increased intracranial tension. Ann J Med Sci 1902;124:375.
3. Guillaume J, Janny P: Manometrie intracranienne continue: interet de la methode et premiers resultants. Rev Neurol 1951;84:131.
4. Lundberg N: Continuous recording and control of ventricular fluid pressure in neurosurgical practice. Acta Psychiatr Neurol Scand 1960;36:1.
5. Lundberg N, Troupp H, Lorin H: Continuous recording of the ventricular-fluid pressure in patients with severe acute traumatic brain injury: A preliminary report. J Neurosurg 1965;22:581-590
6. Feldman Z, Narayan RK: Intracranial pressure monitoring: Techniques and pitfalls. In Cooper PR, Golfinos JG (eds): Head Injury, 4th ed. New York, McGraw-Hill, 2000, pp 265-292.
7. Selhorst JB, Gudeman SK, Butterworth JF: Papilledema after acute head injury. Neurosurgery 1985;16:357-363.
8. Gopez JJ, Meagher RJ, Narayan RK: When and how should I monitor intracranial pressure? In Valadka AB, Andrews BT (eds): Neurotrauma. New York, Thieme, 2005, pp 53-57.
9. Marmarou A, Anderson RL, Ward JD, et al: Impact of ICP instability and hypotension on outcome in patients with severe head injury. J Neurosurg 1991;75:S59-S66.
10. Rosner MJ, Rosner SD, Johnson AH: Cerebral perfusion pressure: Management protocol and clinical results. J Neurosurg 1995;83:949-962.

11. Brain Trauma Foundation, American Association of Neurological Surgeons, Joint Section on Neurotrauma and Critical Care: Management and prognosis of severe traumatic brain injury: Part I. Guidelines for the management of severe traumatic brain injury. Indications for intracranial pressure monitoring. J Neurotrauma 2000;17:47-69.
12. Galbraith S, Teasdale GM: Predicting the need for operation in patients with an occult traumatic intracranial hematoma. J Neurosurg 1981;55: 75-81.
13. Murphy A, Teasdale E, Matheson M, et al: Relationship between CT indices of brain swelling and intracranial pressure after head injury. In Ishii S, Nagai H, Brock M (eds): Intracranial Pressure, 5th ed. Berlin, Springer-Verlag, 1983, pp 562-566.
14. Andrews BT, Chiles BW, Olsen WL: The effect of intracerebral hematoma location on the risk of brainstem compression and on clinical outcome. J Neurosurg 1988;69:518-522.
15. Solonik D, Pitts LH, Lovely M: Traumatic intracerebral hematomas: Timing of appearance and indications for operative removal. J Trauma 1986;26:787-794.
16. Rosenwasser RH, Kleiner LI, Krzeminski JP: Intracranial pressure monitoring in the posterior fossa: A preliminary report. J Neurosurg 1989;71:503-505.
17. Brown E: Intracranial Pressure Monitoring Devices. Arlington, VA, Association for the Advancement of Medical Instrumentation, 1988.
18. Ohrstrom JK, Skou JK, Ejlertsen T, et al: Infected ventriculostomy: Bacteriology and treatment. Acta Neurochir 1989;100:67.
19. Aucoin PJ, Kotilainen HR, Gantz NM, et al: Intracranial pressure monitors: Epidemiologic study of risk factors and infections. Am J Med 1986;80: 369-376.
20. Mayhall CG, Archer NH, Lamb VA, et al: Ventriculostomy-related infections: A prospective epidemiologic study. N Engl J Med 1984;310:553-559.
21. Smith RW, Alksne JF: Infections complicating the use of external ventriculostomy. J Neurosurg 1976;44:567.
22. Clark CW, Muhlbauer MS, Lowery R, et al: Complications of intracranial pressure monitoring in trauma patients. Neurosurgery 1989;25: 20-24.
23. Kanter RK, Weiner LB: Ventriculostomy-related infection. N Engl J Med 1984;311:987.
24. Narayan RK, Kishore PRS, Becker DP, et al: Intracranial pressure: To monitor or not to monitor? J Neurosurg 1982; 56:650-659.
25. Rosner MJ, Becker DP: ICP monitoring: Complications and associated factors. Clin Neurosurg 1976;23:494-519.
26. Friedman WA, Vries JK: Percutaneous tunnel ventriculostomy: Summary of 100 procedures. J Neurosurg 1980; 53:662.
27. Wyler AR, Kelly WA: Use of antibiotics with external ventriculostomies. J Neurosurg 1972;37:185.
28. Holloway KL, Barnes T, Choi S, et al: Ventriculosomy infection: The effect of monitoring duration and catheter exchange in 584 patients. J Neurosurg 1996;85:419-424.
29. Winfield JA, Rosenthal P, Kantner RK, et al: Duration of intracranial pressure monitoring does not predict daily risk of infectious complications. Neurosurgery 1993;33:424-431.
30. Poon WS, Ng S, Wai S: CSF antibiotic prophylaxis for neurosurgical patients with ventriculostomy: A randomised study. Acta Neurochir Suppl 1998; 71:146.
31. Paramore CG, Turner DA: Relative risk of ventriculostomy infection and morbidity. Acta Neurochir (Wien) 1994;127:79-84.
32. Brain Trauma Foundation: Recommendations for intracranial pressure monitoring technology. J Neurotrauma 1996;13:685.
33. Cuneo RA, Caronna JJ, Pitts L, et al: Upward transtentorial herniation: Seven cases and a literature review. Arch Neurol 1979;36:618.
34. Pare L, Delfino R, Leblanc R: The relationship of ventricular drainage to aneurysmal rebleeding. J Neurosurg 1992;76:422.
35. Vries JK, Becker DP, Young HF: A subarachnoid screw for monitoring intracranial pressure: Technical note. J Neurosurg 1973;39:416.
36. Dearden NM, McDowall DG, Gibson RM: Assessment of Leeds device for monitoring intracranial pressure. J Neurosurg 1984;60:123.
37. Mendelow AD, Rowan JO, Murray L, et al: A clinical comparison of subdural screw pressure measurements with ventricular pressure. J Neurosurg 1983;58:45.
38. Gambardella G, d'Avella D, Tomasello F: Monitoring of brain tissue pressure with a fiberoptic device. Neurosurgery 1992;31:918.
39. Johnston IH, Rowan JO: Raised intracranial pressure and cerebral blood flow: 4. Intracranial pressure gradients and regional cerebral blood flow. J Neurol Neurosurg Psychiatry 1974;37:585.
40. Yano M, Ikeda Y, Kobayashi S, et al: Intracranial pressure in head-injured patients with various intracranial lesions is identical throughout the supratentorial intracranial compartment. Neurosurgery 1987;21:688.
41. Nussbaum E, Maggi JC: Intracranial pressure monitoring by subarachnoid bolt in comatose children. Clin Pediatr 1985;24:329.
42. Bobo H, Miller JD, Evans OB, et al: Delayed intracerebral hematoma at the site of a subarachnoid bolt pressure monitor: Case report. J Neurosurg 1986;64:673.
43. Barnett G, Chapman P: Insertion and care of intracranial pressure monitoring devices. In Ropper A, Kennedy S (eds): Neurological and Neurosurgical Intensive Care. Rockville, MD, Aspen, 1988.
44. Crutchfield JS, Narayan RK, Robertson CS, et al: Evaluation of a fiberoptic intracranial pressure monitor. J Neurosurg 1990;72:482.
45. Ostrup RC, Luerssen TG, Marshall LF, et al: Continuous monitoring of intracranial pressure with a miniaturized fiberoptic device. J Neurosurg 1987;67:206.
46. Chambers IR, Mendelow AD, Sinar EJ, et al: A clinical evaluation of the Camino subdural screw and ventricular monitoring kits. Neurosurgery 1990;26:421.
47. Price DJ, Van Hille PT, Mason J: Evaluation of a fiber-optic system for monitoring vantricular pressure. In Hoff JT, Betz AL (eds): Intracranial Pressure, 7th ed. Berlin, Springer-Verlag, 1989, pp 52-54.
48. Bekar A, Goren S, Korfali E, et al: Complications of brain tissue pressure monitoring with a fiberoptic device. Neurosurg Rev 1998;21:254.
49. Blei AT, Olafsson S, Webster S, et al: Complications of intracranial pressure monitoring in fulminant hepatic failure. Lancet 1993;341:157.
50. Gopinath SP, Robertson CS, Contant CF, et al: Clincal evaluation of a miniature strain-gauge transducer for monitoring intracranial pressure. Neurosurgery 1995;36:1137-1141.
51. Gray WP, Palmer JD, Gill J, et al: A clinical study of parenchymal and subdural miniature strain gauge transducer for monitoring intracranial pressure. Neurosurgery 1996;39: 927-931.
52. Kety SS, Schmidt CF: The nitrous oxide method for the quantitative determination of cerebral blood flow in man: Theory, procedure, and normal values. J Clin Invest 1948;27: 476-483.
53. Yonas H, Johnson D, Pindzola RR: Xenon-enhanced CT of cerebral blood flow. Sci Am Sci Med 1995;2:58-67.
54. De Georgia MA, Deogaonkar A: Multimodal monitoring in the neurological intensive care unit. Neurologist 2005;11:45-54.
55. Bolognese P, Miller JI, Heger IM, et al: Laser Doppler flowmetry in neurosurgery. J Neurosurg Anesthesiol 1993;5:151-158.
56. Carter LP, Weinand ME, Oommen KJ: Cerebral blood flow (CBF) monitoring in intensive care by thermal diffusion. Acta Neurochirurg Suppl 1993;59: 43-46.
57. Aaslid R: Cerebral hemodynamics. In Newell DW, Aaslid R (eds): Transcranial Doppler. New York, Raven Press, 1992, pp 49-58.
58. Kontos HA: Validity of cerebral arterial blood calculations from velocity measurements. Stroke 1989;20:1-3.
59. Stocchetti N: Should I monitor jugular venous oxygen saturation? In Valadka AB, Andrews BT (eds): Neurotrauma. New York, Thieme, 2005, pp 58-61.
60. Macmillan CS, Andrews PJ: Cerebrovenous oxygen saturation monitoring: practical considerations and clinical relevance. Intensive Care Med 2000;26:1028-1036.
61. Robertson CS, Narayan RK, Gokaslan ZL, et al: Cerebral arteriovenous oxygen difference as an estimate of cerebral blood flow in comatose patients. J Neurosurg 1989;70: 222-230.
62. Obrist WD, Langfitt TW, Jaggi JL, et al: Cerebral blood flow and metabolism in comatose patients with acute head injury: Relationship to intracranial hypertension. J Neurosurg 1984;61:241-253.
63. Cruz J: The first decade of continuous monitoring of jugular bulb

oxyhemoglobin saturation: Management strategies and clinical outcome. Crit Care Med 1998;26: 344-351.
64. Schneider GH, von Helden A, Lanksch WR, et al: Continuous monitoring of jugular bulb oxygen saturation in comatose patients: therapeutic implications. Acta Neurochir (Wien) 1995;134:71-75.
65. Vespa P: Should I monitor cerebral blood flow after traumatic brain injury? In Valadka AB, Andrews BT (eds): Neurotrauma. New York, Thieme, 2005, pp 68-72.
66. Chestnut RM, Marshall LF, Klauber MR, et al: The role of secondary brain injury in determining outcome from severe head injury. J Trauma 1993;34:216-222.
67. Stocchetti N, Furlan A, Volta F: Hypoxemia and arterial hypotension as the accident scene in head injury. J Trauma 1996;40:764-767.
68. Rossi S, Cormio M, Marmarou A: Internal jugular vein oxygen saturation: clinical usefulness and limitations in the management of head-injured patients. Crit Rev Neurosurg 1996;6:202-208.
69. Dearden NM: Jugular bulb venous oxygen saturation in the management of severe head injury. Curr Opin Anaesthesiol 1991;4: 279-286.
70. Stocchetti N, Paparella A, Bridelli F, et al: Cerebral venous oxygenation saturation studied with bilateral samples in the internal jugular veins. Neurosurgery 1994;34:38-44.
71. Metz C, Holzschuh M, Bein T, et al: Monitoring of cerebral oxygen metabolism in the jugular bulb: Reliability of unilateral measurments in severe head injury. J Cereb Blood Flow Metab 1998;18:332-343.
72. Bankier AA, Fleisschmann D, Windisch A, et al: Position of jugular oxygen saturation catheter in patients with head trauma: assessment by use of plain films. AJR Am J Roentgenol 1995;164:437-441.
73. Matta BF, Lam AM: The rate of blood withdrawal affects the accuracy of jugular venous bulb: oxygen saturation measurements. Anesthesiology 1997;86:806-808.
74. Coplin WM, O'Keefe GE, Grady MS, et al: Thrombotic, infectious, and procedural complications of the jugular bulb catheter in the intensive care unit. Neurosurgery 1997;41: 101-109.
75. Sheinberg M, Kantner MJ, Robertson CS, et al: Continuous monitoring of jugular venous oxygen saturation in head-injured patients. J Neurosurg 1992;76:212-217.
76. Fandino J, Stocker R, Prokop S, et al: Cerebral oxygenation and systemic trauma related factors determining neurologic outcome after brain injury. J Clin Neurosci 2000;7: 226-233.
77. Brain Trauma Foundation, American Association of Neurological Surgeons, Joint Section on Neurotrauma and Critical Care: Guidelines for the management of severe traumatic brain injury: Hyperventilation. J Neurotrauma 2000;17:513-520.
78. Kiening KL, Sarrafzadeh AS, Stover JF, et al: Should I monitor brain tissue PO2? In Valadka AB, Andrews BT (eds): Neurotrauma. New York, Thieme, 2005, pp 62-67.
79. Deardon NM, Midgley S: Technical considerations in continuous jugular venous oxygen saturation measurement. Acta Neurochir Suppl (Wien) 1993;59:91-97.
80. Kiening KL, Unterberg AW, Bardt TF, et al: Monitoring of cerebral oxygenation in patients with severe head injuries: Brain tissue PO2 versus jugular vein oxygen saturation. J Neurosurg 1996;85:751-757.
81. Latronico N, Beindorf AE, Rasulo FA, et al: Limits of intermittent jugular bulb oxygen saturation monitoring in the management of severe head trauma patients. Neurosurgery 2000;46:1131-1139.
82. Maas AI, Fleckenstein W, de Jong DA, et al: Monitoring cerebral oxygenation: Experimental studies and preliminary clinical results of continuous monitoring of cerebrospinal fluid and brain tissue oxygen tension. Acta Neurochirurg Suppl 1993;59:50-57.
83. Meixensberger J, Dings J, Kuhnigk H, et al: Studies of tissue PO2 in normal and pathological human brain cortex. Acta Neurochirurg Suppl 1993;59: 58-63.
84. van den Brink WA, Haitsma IK, Avezaat CJ, et al: Brain parenchyma/pO_2 catheter interface: A histopathological study in the rat. J Neurotrauma 1998;15:813-824.
85. Leniger-Follert E: Oxygen supply and microcirculation of the brain cortex. Adv Exp Med Biol 1985;191: 3-19.
86. Hoffman WE, Charbel FT, Edelman G, et al: Brain tissue oxygen pressure, carbon dioxide pressure and pH during ischemia. Neurol Res 1996;18: 54-56.
87. Hemphill JC 3rd, Knudson MM, Derugin N, et al: Carbon dioxide reactivity and pressure autoregulation of brain tissue oxygen. Neurosurgery 2001;48:377-383.
88. Scheufler KM, Rohrborn HJ, Zentner J: Does tissue oxygen-tension reliably reflect cerebral oxygen delivery and consumption? Anesth Analg 2002;95: 1042-1048.
89. Gopinath SP, Valadka AB, Uzura M, et al: Comparison of jugular venous oxygen saturation and brain tissue PO2 as monitors of cerebral ischemia after head injury. Crit Care Med 1999;27:2337-2345.
90. Kiening KL, Hartl R, Unterberg AW, et al: Brain tissue PO2-monitoring in comatose patients: Implications for therapy. Neurol Res 1997;19:223-240.
91. Manley GT, Pitts LH, Morabito D, et al: Brain tissue oxygenation during hemorrhagic shock, resuscitation, and alterations in ventilation. J Trauma 1999;46:261-267.
92. Maloney Wilensky E, Gracias V, Christian S, et al: Brain tissue oxygen and outcome after severe traumatic brain injury: A meta-analysis. Digital Poster 584,Congress of Neurological Surgeons 55th Annual Meeting, 2005, Boston.
93. Spiotta AM, Stiefel MF, Gracias VH, et al: Brain tissue oxygen directed management improves outcome after severe traumatic brain injury. Oral Poster 41, Congress of Neurological Surgeons 55th Annual Meeting, 2005, Boston.
94. Grohn OH, Kauppinen RA: Assessment of brain tissue viability in acute ischemic stroke by BOLD MRI. NMR Biomed 2001;14:432-440.
95. Imberti R, Bellinzona G, Langer M: Cerebral tissue PO2 and SjvO2 changes during moderate hyperventilation in patients with severe traumatic brain injury. J Neurosurg 2002;96:97-102.
96. Zhi DS, Zhang S, Zhou LG: Continuous monitoring of brain tissue oxygen pressure in patients with severe head injury during moderate hypothermia. Surg Neurol 1999;52:393-396.
97. Carmona Suazo JA, Maas AI, van den Brink WA, et al: CO2 reactivity and brain oxygen pressure monitoring in severe head injury. Crit Care Med 2000;28:3268-3274.
98. Dings J, Meixensberger J, Amschler J, et al: Brain tissue PO2 in relation to cerebral perfusion pressure, TCD findings and TCD-CO2-reactivity after severe head injury. Acta Neurochir (Wien) 1996;138:425-434.
99. Dings J, Meixensberger J, Amschler J, et al: Continuous monitoring of brain tissue PO2: A new tool to minimize the risk of ischemia caused by hyperventilation therapy. Zentralbl Neurochir 1996;57:177-183.
100. Schneider GH, Sarrafzadeh AS, Kiening KL, et al: Influence of hyperventilation on brain tissue PO2, PCO2, and pH in patients with intracranial hypertension. Acta Neurochir Suppl (Wien) 1998;71:62-65.
101. Unterberg AW, Kiening KL, Hartl R, et al: Multimodal monitoring in patients with head injury: Evaluation of the effects of treatment on cerebral oxygenation. J Trauma 1997;42: S32-S37.
102. Bouma GJ, Muizelaar JP, Stringer WA, et al: Ultra-early evaluation of regional cerebral blood flow in severely head-injured patients using xenon-enhanced computerized tomography. J Neurosurg 1992;77:360-368.
103. Brain Trauma Foundation, American Association of Neurological Surgeons, Joint Section on Neurotrauma and Critical Care: Guidelines for the management of severe traumatic brain injury. J Neurotrauma 2000;17: 507-511.
104. Brain Trauma Foundation, American Association of Neurological Surgeons, Congress of Neurological Surgeons, Joint Section on Neurotrauma and Critical Care: Update Notice: Guidelines for the Management of severe Traumatic Brain Injury. Cerebral Perfusion Pressure. New York, Brain Trauma Foundation/American Association of Neurological Surgeons, 2000. Updated CPP Guidelines approved by the AANS on March 14, 2003, pp 1-14.
105. Sarrafzadeh AS, Kiening KL, Bardt TF, et al: Cerebral oxygenation in contusioned vs. nonlesioned brain tissue: monitoring of $BtiO_2$ with Licox and Paratrend. Acta Neurochir Suppl (Wien) 1998;71:186-189.

Chapter 18

Gastrointestinal Endoscopy

Jack T. Dinh and Adam B. Elfant

HISTORY

The first documented endoscopic foray into the human body was performed by Bozinni in the early 1800s, when he used a speculum fitted with a candle and mirror to examine the urinary tract.[1] The first gastroscopy was performed in 1868 by German physician Kussmaul. His gastroscope was a rigid metal tube passed carefully down the patient's esophagus to the stomach. In 1932, Schindler, in collaboration with a German engineer, Wolff, developed a semiflexible instrument with a rigid proximal and flexible distal shaft. This device was hailed as the first safe workable gastroscope.[2] Limitations included incomplete visualization of the esophagus and stomach, patient discomfort, absence of photographic documentation, and a deficiency of adequately trained gastroscopists.[2] The first fiberoptic endoscope was constructed in 1957 by Hirschowitz. The 1960s and 1970s saw tremendous advancements with development of fiberoptic endoscopes with longer length, improved visualization, and greater control. Video cameras and monitors were subsequently incorporated into endoscopic technology, allowing others to view what was previously available only to the endoscopist.

Early experience with rigid and semiflexible proctosigmoidoscopes and colonoscopes was disappointing because of the tortuous nature of the sigmoid and colon. Early fiberoptic instruments fared no better. Oberholt made adjustments in torque and control to develop a prototype flexible fiberoptic instrument in 1963.[3] Further refinements were carried out in England, the United States, and Japan, and the first polypectomy was performed in 1969.[4] Shortly thereafter, colonoscopy became a standard procedure performed not only by gastroenterologists, but also by other health care providers.

Endoscopic cannulation of the duodenal ampulla was accomplished by McCune and colleagues[5] in 1968 and is considered the first reported case of endoscopic retrograde cholangiopancreatography (ERCP). Sphincterotomy was performed in 1974,[6] ushering in a new era of therapeutic pancreaticobiliary endoscopy. Today, ERCP remains an invaluable procedure in evaluating and treating diseases of the pancreas and biliary tract.

The first ultrasound examination within the gastrointestinal (GI) lumen was performed by Wild and Reid in 1956, when they developed the transrectal ultrasound probe.[7] The incorporation of ultrasound into a standard endoscope occurred in 1976, when Lutz and Rosch passed an ultrasound probe through an accessory port of an endoscope. Further improvements were achieved by Strohm and colleagues and DiMagno and coworkers, who introduced their own prototype echoendoscopes in 1980. The first endoscopic ultrasound (EUS)–guided fine-needle aspiration was performed on submucosal lesions of the stomach in 1991 by Caletti and colleagues.[8]

The introduction of wireless capsule technology to clinical practice has revolutionized the evaluation of the small bowel. The wireless capsule was first used on a human subject in 1999 after a decade of research and development.[9] Clinical trials subsequently were carried out in 2000, and U.S. Food and Drug Administration approval was granted later that same year.

ENDOSCOPIC EQUIPMENT

Fiberoptics have greatly advanced the technology of the endoscope. Thousands of individual glass fibers capable of transmitting light are grouped to form bundles. A typical endoscope bundle has a diameter between 0.5 mm and 3 mm with approximately 5000 to 40,000 individual fibers.[10] The more fibers and bundles present, the better the image quality. The fiberoptic images can be transmitted directly to an eyepiece at the end of the endoscope or to a video monitor by a charge-coupled device.[11]

Four-way deflection of the distal endoscope tip is performed through manipulation of the proximal angulation control knobs, which are attached to a series of wires that run the length of the endoscope. The endoscope has controls for suction, insufflation, and water. Channel ports distal to the hand controls allow for passage of various accessories. The distal end of the endoscope, either forward viewing (i.e., endoscope, colonoscope) or side viewing (duodenoscope), contains lenses for illumination and imaging and channel openings for air, water, suction, and passage of instruments.

The EUS equipment differs from the standard endoscope in that an ultrasound transducer is incorporated into the distal end. The transducer emits sound waves, which are directed into adjacent tissues and deflected back to the transducer. Individual tissues have different acoustic qualities. Radial and linear echoendoscopes are available. Interventional procedures, such as fine-needle aspiration and injections, may be performed safely with the latter echoendoscope.[12]

The wireless video capsule is a small disposable unit containing a small chip camera, short focal length lens, light source, two batteries, and a radio telemetry transmitter.[13] The capsule is activated by removal from a magnetic holder, and battery life is approximately 8 hours. Two frames per second are captured by the camera and transmitted to a data recorder that is carried by the patient. Data are downloaded from the recorder to a personal computer and interpreted.

ANESTHESIA

Before any endoscopic procedure, informed consent should be obtained, and the method of sedation should be assessed. Informed consent is obtained from the patient or by the power of attorney if the patient's decision-making capabilities are impaired. Informed consent should clearly explain the procedure to be performed, the reason the procedure is being performed, expected benefits, potential risks, and possible alternatives.[14]

The choice of anesthesia is based on the patient profile, the endoscopic procedure, and preference of the endoscopist. Essential patient information includes prior adverse events from anesthesia, current medications, pertinent medical history, cardiopulmonary status, age, allergies, body habitus, and social history. Patients with alcohol or narcotic dependency may require high doses of opiates and benzodiazepines. Agents such as propofol may facilitate their sedation. Pregnancy should be excluded in any woman of childbearing age. The endoscopic procedure also may determine the level of sedation required. Flexible sigmoidoscopy and esophagogastroduodenoscopy (EGD) may require minimal or moderate sedation, whereas more complex and lengthier procedures, such as ERCP and EUS, may require deep or general anesthesia.

The American Society of Anesthesiologists Task Force defined the different depths of sedation.[15] Minimal sedation is considered a form of anxiolysis, with normal patient response to verbal stimuli. There is no effect on airway, ventilation, or cardiovascular function. Moderate or conscious sedation is defined as a level at which the patient is able to make a purposeful response to verbal or tactile stimuli with preserved cardiovascular and ventilatory status. Deep sedation occurs when a purposeful response is made only to repeated or painful stimuli, and airway support may be needed. Patients under general anesthesia are unarousable, even to painful stimuli, and may require cardiopulmonary support.

Regardless of the type of sedation, cardiopulmonary status should be monitored at all times. A prospective study reported the cardiopulmonary complication rate for EGD to be 0.005% and for colonoscopy to be 0.01%.[16] Standard equipment should include a pulse oximeter, continuous electrocardiogram, and cyclical blood pressure monitoring. Personnel trained in airway support should always be present.

Four drug types are commonly used in GI endoscopies: pharyngeal anesthesia, benzodiazepines, opiates, and propofol. Pharyngeal anesthetics, such as lidocaine, benzocaine, and tetracaine, are used to suppress the gag reflex during upper GI tract procedures. These agents, applied by spray or gargling, are active for approximately 1 hour. A study by Soma and coworkers[17] showed topical agents to be more beneficial in patients younger than 40 years old or undergoing endoscopy for the first time. Potential risks include aspiration owing to loss of gag reflex and, rarely, methemoglobinemia.[18]

Benzodiazepines are used to induce relaxation and amnesia by binding to receptors of the postsynaptic γ-aminobutyric acid neuron. Two agents, midazolam and diazepam, are commonly used. Both have similar properties, with the latter possessing a longer half-life and milder amnestic properties.[19] Onset of action occurs in 1 to 2.5 minutes with intravenous midazolam and 8 minutes with diazepam.[20] Adverse reactions include respiratory depression and hypotension. Overdoses can be reversed with flumazenil, although caution should be used because seizures secondary to acute withdrawal may occur.

Opiates such as fentanyl and meperidine can be given to provide analgesia and sedation. A synergistic effect occurs when opiates are given concurrently with intravenous benzodiazepines. Fentanyl has a rapid onset (1.5 minutes) with a short duration of action (0.5 to 1 hour), whereas meperidine has an onset of 5 minutes and lasts 3 to 5 hours.[20] Common adverse reactions include respiratory depression, hypotension, constipation, and nausea and vomiting. Overdosage can be reversed with naloxone, an opioid antagonist. Long-term opiate users may experience acute withdrawal symptoms with naloxone, however. Serotonin syndrome may occur if monoamine oxidase inhibitors are used with meperidine.

Propofol, an ultra-short-acting anesthetic agent, has been increasingly used in recent years.[21] Propofol has a rapid onset of action, deeper levels of sedation, and faster recovery time compared with narcotics and benzodiazepines.[22] A meta-analysis by Qadeer and associates[23] showed that propofol use during colonoscopy had a lower risk of cardiopulmonary complications compared with traditional agents. Current controversies exist as to its cost-effectiveness and whether the agent should be administered exclusively by an anesthesiologist.

ESOPHAGOGASTRODUODENOSCOPY

EGD, or upper endoscopy, is one of the most commonly performed procedures in the world and has become the primary tool for evaluating the esophagus, stomach, and proximal portion of the duodenum. Upper endoscopy is performed for a wide variety of indications and has a diagnostic and therapeutic role (Table 18-1). There are relatively few contraindications to upper endoscopy (Table 18-2).

EGD is a safe procedure. Perforation occurs in approximately 0.05% to 0.70%,[24] with the higher incidence in patients undergoing therapeutic intervention (i.e., biopsy, dilation, mucosal resection). Bleeding also may occur as a result of Mallory-Weiss tears, cautery injury, sclerotherapy injection, and after biopsy or polypectomy.

Preparation for EGD is straightforward. Patients should be fasting for at least 3 to 6 hours in elective cases. Motility agents, such as erythromycin, may be beneficial in clearing the stomach of blood or food.[25] In situations of possible airway compromise, the patient may need to be intubated before endoscopy. One prospective study by Lipper and colleagues[26] showed a 20% incidence of aspiration pneumonia after emergent EGD for upper GI bleed. A retrospective study of 220 patients failed, however, to show any significant difference in post-EGD pulmonary infiltrates, witnessed aspiration, cardiopulmonary complications, or in-hospital mortality.[27] Nevertheless, because of a lack of a conclusive double-blinded randomized trial, endotracheal intubation may be appropriate in patients with massive active hematemesis, altered mental status, unstable cardiopulmonary function, or agitation. Alternatives to intubation may include pre-endoscopy lavage, overtube placement, or the use of large-caliber endoscopes for suction.

Before administration of anesthesia, patients should be in the left lateral position, with the head elevated and supported by a pillow. Monitoring devices for vital signs, electrocardiogram, and pulse oximetry are attached, supplemental oxygen should be administered, and a bite guard should be placed in the mouth.

In addition to diagnostic capabilities, therapeutic interventions can be performed during upper endoscopy, particularly in the setting of GI hemorrhage. Several modalities are available for treating GI bleeding, including thermal cautery, electrocautery, needle injection, rubber band ligation, mechanical clips, laser therapy, argon plasma coagulation, and tissue adhesives.

Thermal cautery probes deliver predetermined pulses of heat (250°C) to an endoscopic catheter tip, which is

Table 18-1. Indications for Esophagogastroduodenoscopy

Persistent upper abdominal symptoms despite appropriate therapy
Upper abdominal symptoms associated with signs or symptoms suggesting serious organic disease (anorexia, weight loss) or in patients >45 years old
Dysphagia or odynophagia
Esophageal reflux symptoms (persistent or recurrent despite appropriate therapy)
Persistent vomiting of unknown cause
Familial adenomatous polyposis syndromes
Confirmation and specific histologic diagnosis of radiologically shown lesions Suspected neoplastic lesions Gastric or esophageal ulcer Upper tract stricture or obstruction
Gastrointestinal bleeding Active or recent bleed Suspected bleed (chronic blood loss and iron deficiency anemia)
Sampling of tissue or fluid
Document or treat varices (banding, sclerotherapy)
Assess acute injury after caustic ingestion
Treatment of bleeding lesions such as ulcers, tumors, vascular abnormalities (electrocoagulation, heater probe, laser photocoagulation, injection therapy)
Removal of foreign bodies
Removal of selected polypoid lesions
Dilation of stenotic lesions
Placement of feeding or drainage tubes (percutaneous endoscopic gastrostomy, percutaneous endoscopic jejunostomy)
Management of achalasia (botulinum toxin, balloon dilation)
Palliative treatment of neoplasms (laser, multipolar electrocoagulation, stent placement)
Surveillance for malignancy in patients with premalignant conditions (Barrett's esophagus)

Adapted from Appropriate use of gastrointestinal endoscopy. American Society of Gastrointestinal Endoscopy. Gastrointest Endos 2000;52:831-837.

Table 18-2. Contraindications for Esophagogastroduodenoscopy
Risk to patient's health or life judged to outweigh most favorable benefits of procedure
Adequate patient cooperation or consent cannot be obtained
Perforated viscus known or suspected
Adapted from Appropriate use of gastrointestinal endoscopy. American Society of Gastrointestinal Endoscopy. Gastrointest Endos 2000;52:831-837.

transferred to tissue on contact.[28] Thermal probe coagulation can be applied to peptic ulcers, vascular lesions, and Mallory-Weiss tears. Perforation is a rare but potential complication.

Another option for contact thermal coagulation is monopolar or bipolar electrocautery. With electrocautery, electrical current flows from electrode tip through contacted tissue. Monopolar cautery requires attaching an electrical ground to the patient and may cause extensive burn injuries and tissue stickiness. Monopolar cautery is typically not used for hemostasis, but serves a role in snare polypectomy. Bipolar cautery consists of two active electrodes incorporated into a single catheter probe, allowing electrical current to pass from one electrode through the tissue and back to the other electrode. Consequently, bipolar cauterization is more confined, allowing control of coagulation depth.

Injection therapy for nonvariceal and variceal bleeding is done with sclerotherapy injector needles. Solutions commonly employed are epinephrine in saline (1:10,000) and sclerosing agents, such as polidocanol, ethanol, and ethanolamine. Epinephrine reduces bleeding by vasoconstriction, vessel tamponade, and platelet aggregation.[29,30] The potential exists for systemic side effects from submucosal injections because plasma epinephrine levels can transiently increase four to five times above basal levels.[31] To date, only a single case of hypertension and ventricular tachycardia after epinephrine injection has been reported.[32] Sclerosing agents achieve hemostasis through inflammation and sclerosis and have been employed in peptic ulcer hemorrhage and variceal bleeding. Mediastinitis, perforation, stricture formation, and infection are among the reported complications.[33]

Injector needles also are used in nonbleeding situations. Polyps can be raised with submucosal injections of saline or epinephrine before polypectomy. This technique reduces the likelihood of postpolypectomy bleed or perforation.[34] Superficial gastric tumors can be removed by mucosectomy after submucosal injection. Lesions requiring surgery can be tattooed with ink for easy future localization by the surgeon.

Rubber band ligation is an effective tool for hemostasis. The delivery system is loaded onto the endoscope tip, and current models allow for multiple deployments of rubber bands before reloading. For variceal bleeding, endoscopic variceal ligation has become the treatment of choice, with superiority to endoscopic sclerotherapy in speed of variceal eradication, decreased risk of recurrent bleeding, and fewer complications.[35] Other uses of banding include gastric varices, peptic ulcers, Dieulafoy's lesions, postpolypectomy bleeding, and internal hemorrhoids.

Metal clips, or endoclips, have been used successfully for GI bleeding,[36] closure of perforations,[37] anastomotic leaks,[38] and prevention of postpolypectomy bleeding.[39] The potential for significant tissue injury is small because only the mucosal and submucosal layers are involved in the grasping.[40] The procedure is technically difficult if massive bleeding is present, or the angle of approach is tangential to the lesion.[41]

Laser therapy, such as neodymium : yttrium-aluminum-garnet (YAG) and argon, is delivered through probes passed via the endoscope to treat bleeding lesions and for tumor ablation. Neodymium : YAG and argon differ in the width and depth of tissue effect, with the former having the greater effect.[42] Advantages of laser therapy include improved accuracy and not requiring direct contact with the desired target.

Argon plasma coagulation is a new noncontact method of hemostasis that delivers argon gas through a catheter probe. The argon gas is ionized, delivering thermal energy to the adjacent target tissue. Large areas and tissue not in direct view, owing to the tangential arcing nature of the argon gas, can be treated rapidly. Clinical uses include adjunctive ablative therapy after piecemeal resection of colonic polyps, radiation proctopathy, GI vascular lesions, bleeding peptic ulcers, Barrett's esophagus ablation, and palliation of GI malignancies.[43,44]

Tissue adhesives constitute a newer class of agents for GI hemostasis. The major types of tissue adhesives are fibrin sealants and cyanoacrylate. Fibrin sealants form a coagulum through the interaction of fibrinogen, factor XIII, and thrombin.[45] Extensively used in the surgical fields for tissue adhesion, hemostasis, and wound care, fibrin sealants also have been used endoscopically in bleeding peptic ulcers,[46] variceal bleeding,[47] and GI fistulas.[48] Cyanoacrylate is synthetic glue that rapidly polymerizes into a solid complex when in contact with water or blood.[49] Cyanoacrylate has been used with success for esophageal and gastric varices.[50,51] A serious complication of tissue adhesives is embolization and infarction.[52]

In addition to hemostasis, upper endoscopy is routinely employed for other therapeutic situations. Foreign object ingestion and food bolus impaction occur commonly. Although most foreign bodies pass spontaneously, 10% to 20% of cases may require endoscopic intervention.[53] Various types of endoscopy, ranging from rigid to flexible, and equipment (Table 18-3) are available for foreign body retrieval. An overtube is available for airway protection and frequent esophageal intubations. Retrieval should be performed within 24 hours or more urgently if the ingested object is sharp, a disc battery, or is causing the patient pain or difficulty in handling secretions.[54] If unable to remove endoscopically and the object size is less than 2.5 cm, the object can be gently maneuvered into the stomach, from which spontaneous passage usually occurs.[55] Unsuccessful removal or obstruction requires surgical evaluation.

Esophageal narrowing is a common reason for recurrent food impaction. Narrowing may occur from benign condi-

Table 18-3. Devices Used for Foreign Body Retrieval
Overtube
Pronged forceps
Tooth forceps
Nets
Baskets
Retrieval loops
Magnetic extractors
Adapted from Nelson DB, Bosco JJ, Curtis WD, et al: The ASGE technology status evaluation report: Endoscopic retrieval devices. February 1999. American Society for Gastrointestinal Endoscopy. Gastrointest Endosc 1999;50:932-934.

Table 18-4. Causes of Esophageal Narrowing
Peptic stricture
Schatzki's ring
Radiation-induced stricture
Caustic injury
Anastomotic stricture
Pill-induced injury
Infectious esophagitis
Sclerotherapy-induced injury
Photodynamic therapy–induced injury
Eosinophilic esophagitis
Malignancy

tions, such as peptic strictures and Schatzki's rings, or malignancy compressing the lumen (Table 18-4). Endoscopic dilation can be performed on anatomic narrowings of the esophagus and pyloric and anastomotic strictures. Four types of dilators are currently available: tip-weighted push bougies (Maloney or Hurst), wire-guided dilators (Savary-Gilliard or American), through-the-scope dilating balloons, and clear optical dilators that allow direct endoscopic visualization. Dilation also is indicated in patients with achalasia, although recurrence is common, and clinical efficacy is decreased with subsequent dilations.[56] In general, endoscopic dilation increases the risk of perforation, with reported rates between 0.1% and 0.4%.[57]

Endoscopic stenting with endoprosthesis can be performed in a wide variety of clinical scenarios. Stenting is performed for fistulas, anastomotic leaks,[58] and malignant and nonmalignant perforations.[59,60] In addition, malignant obstructive lesions of the esophagus, stomach, duodenum, and colon can be stented for palliation. Stents vary in size, in material (plastic or metal mesh), and by the presence or absence of a covering. Complications include increased reflux if the gastroesophageal junction is involved, bleeding, perforation, and stent migration.

Photodynamic therapy involves pretreatment of a desired target lesion with an injected photosensitizing agent, which is subsequently activated by the application of a light source. The activated photosensitizer achieves an excited state with reactive oxygen radicals that result in cellular injury.[61] In addition to high-grade dysplasia of Barrett's esophagus and esophageal cancer, photodynamic therapy has been employed for neoplasms throughout the GI tract, including the stomach, bile duct, pancreas, and colon.[62]

Percutaneous endoscopic gastrostomy (PEG) tube placement is a common procedure for gastroenterologists. The purpose of PEG placement is to improve quality of life, shorten hospitalization, prevent aspiration, improve nutritional and functional status, and prolong survival.[63] Controversy exists as to whether PEG placement is beneficial in patients with terminal anorexia-cachexia syndromes or in permanent vegetative states.[64,65] In addition to providing nutritional support, PEG placement has been used for long-term gastric decompression and recurrent gastric volvulus management. Placement is contraindicated if the anterior abdominal wall cannot be brought into contact with the anterior gastric wall, such as in morbid obesity and significant ascites. Complications, although infrequent, include wound infection, necrotizing fasciitis, peritonitis, septicemia, peristomal leakage, device dislodgment, bowel perforation, and fistula formation.[65] Possible implantation metastasis in patients with head and neck cancer also has been reported.[66] Pneumoperitoneum is seen in 40% of cases, but most are asymptomatic and eventually resolve.[67]

ENTEROSCOPY

A limitation of upper endoscopy is that only a portion of the proximal small bowel is visualized. When the remaining small bowel requires evaluation, a longer endoscope is needed. The enteroscope is used to evaluate the distal duodenum, the jejunum, and occasionally the ileum. In general, direct visualization provides a higher yield, especially for obscure bleeding, in the small bowel compared with barium studies.[68] In addition to evaluating GI hemorrhage and other lesions in the small bowel, the enteroscope may be used for percutaneous endoscopic jejunostomy and nasojejunal tube placement.

Currently, three variations of the enteroscope are available. The push enteroscope is a long endoscope (≥210 cm) that typically reaches the midjejunum. Specially manufactured push enteroscopes are available, but a thin-diameter adult colonoscope or pediatric colonoscope is occasionally substituted. The reach of the enteroscope can be extended with the incorporation of a stiffening overtube, which helps limit small bowel looping. With the overtube, an evaluation can be made 125 cm beyond the ligament of Treitz.[69] Mucosal stripping and perforation have been reported with the use of an overtube during push enteroscopy.[70] If a distal portion of the small bowel beyond the reach of a push enteroscope needs to be evaluated, several options are available. A retrograde approach through the colon, with ileocecal intubation, into the ileum can be performed. Another alternative is intraoperative enteroscopy, when a laparotomy is performed, and the enteroscope is guided through the small bowel by direct manipulation of the surgeon.

The Sonde endoscope is a long enteroscope (250 to 400 cm) with a balloon attached to the tip. After transnasal or oral intubation, the balloon is inflated, and peristalsis carries the enteroscope passively to the distal small bowel. Evaluation is subsequently done during withdrawal. The advantage of this procedure is the ability to visualize most of the small bowel. The disadvantage is the long examination time required (typically 6 to 8 hours) and the lack of accessory channels to perform biopsies or therapeutic interventions. Complications apart from perforation may include nasal discomfort and epistaxis.

The double-balloon enteroscope is a relatively new instrument. Employing two balloons located on the endoscope with an overtube, and performed with a push-pull method, the double-balloon enteroscope is designed to visualize the entire small intestine. Antegrade (oral) and retrograde (anal) approaches are performed. Early studies have shown the double-balloon enteroscope to be safe and effective,[71,72] but success rates for total small bowel evaluation vary (0% to 86%).[73,74] This wide variation can be attributed to the steep learning curve required. Double-balloon enteroscopy is promising, however, because of the potential to eliminate intraoperative enteroscopy as the gold standard for therapeutic intervention of the entire small bowel.

WIRELESS CAPSULE ENDOSCOPY

Wireless video capsule endoscopy (VCE) is a safe, noninvasive alternative for visualizing the entire small bowel. The capsule examination typically is performed in an ambulatory setting. Preparation involves an overnight fast. A bowel preparation may be used, although the data are conflicting.[75,76] Metoclopramide also may be beneficial in ensuring a complete small bowel evaluation before expiration of the battery life.[77] After swallowing the pill, the patient can leave the outpatient office, resume nonstrenuous daily activity, and eat 4 hours later. The data recorder is returned after 8 hours.

Common indications for VCE are evaluating obscure GI bleeding, suspected Crohn's disease, small intestinal tumors and polyps, diarrhea, malabsorption disorders, and abdominal pain.[78,79] A meta-analysis by Treister and colleagues[80] found VCE to be superior to push enteroscopy and small bowel barium radiography in detecting sources of obscure GI bleeding. Superiority also was shown when VCE was compared with double-balloon enteroscopy.[81] A major limitation of VCE is the inability to perform therapeutic interventions.

In general, VCE is a safe procedure. Contraindications for VCE include swallowing disorders, known or suspected GI obstruction, stricture, fistula, pregnancy, and possibly cardiac pacemakers or implantable defibrillators. (Although listed as a contraindication by the manufacturer, more recent studies have shown no interference with cardiac pacemakers and implantable defibrillators by VCE.[82,83]) Capsule retention occurs in 1.9% of all examinations, usually secondary to an anatomic abnormality, and may require endoscopic or surgical removal.[84] A patency system similar in size to a video capsule, but dissolvable if retained in the body, may be useful in screening high-risk patients for possible small bowel stenosis.[85] Patients with swallowing disorders or delayed gastric emptying can have the capsule placed in the small bowel by endoscopy.

A variation of the small bowel video capsule exists to evaluate the esophagus. Although similar in design to the small bowel capsule, the esophageal video capsule incorporates a camera at each end, with each camera taking 7 frames per second for a total of 14 frames per second.[13] Fasting time is only 2 hours, and the examination time is less than 1 hour. The patient ingests the pill in a supine position and is gradually raised to an upright position at 2-minute intervals. The esophageal video capsule can be used to evaluate for Barrett's disease, esophageal varices, and gastroesophageal reflux disease.

COLONOSCOPY

The colonoscope is used by general practitioners, surgeons, and gastroenterologists to evaluate the colon and distal ileum, if indicated. A shorter version, the flexible sigmoidoscope, is available for sigmoid examination. The standard colonoscope has essentially replaced the sigmoidoscope and barium studies, however, as the gold standard for large bowel evaluation. Indications range from colorectal screening and evaluation of anemia to therapeutic interventions such as polypectomy and palliative stenting (Table 18-5). Relative contraindications to colonoscopy are recent myocardial infarction, acute diverticulitis, and suspected perforation.

Before colonoscopy, the patient should be on a clear liquid diet and fasting after bowel preparation. Several bowel preparations are commercially available, including polyethylene glycol, low-volume polyethylene glycol with bisacodyl, aqueous sodium phosphate, and tablet sodium phosphate.[86] Nausea, vomiting, and abdominal discomfort are common side effects among all bowel preparations. Sodium phosphate, owing to inducement of rapid volume changes, is contraindicated in patients with serum electrolyte abnormalities, advanced hepatic dysfunction, renal failure, recent myocardial infarction, unstable angina, congestive heart failure, ileus, malabsorption, and ascites.[86] Inadequate bowel preparation has been attributed to failure to follow preparation instructions; later colonoscopy start time; inpatient status; procedural indication of constipation; use of tricyclic antidepressants; male gender; and history of cirrhosis, stroke, or dementia.[87] Patients undergoing flexible sigmoidoscopy usually do not require complete bowel purgation. An enema before the procedure usually is sufficient to clear the distal colon.

Complete colonoscopic examination is achieved in approximately 94% of patients.[88] Advanced age, female gender, body mass index less than 25 kg/m,[2] diverticular disease in women, and a history of constipation or reported laxative abuse in men are predictors of a technically difficult colonoscopy.[89] In general, complications from diagnostic colonoscopy are rare. Hemorrhage and perfora-

Table 18-5. Indications for Colonoscopy

Evaluation of abnormal imaging study
Evaluation of unexplained gastrointestinal bleeding Hematochezia Melena Presence of fecal occult blood
Unexplained iron deficiency anemia
Screening and surveillance for colonic neoplasia
Chronic inflammatory bowel disease
Clinically significant diarrhea of unexplained origin
Intraoperative identification of a lesion not apparent at surgery (polypectomy site, location of a bleeding site)
Treatment of bleeding from lesions such as vascular malformations, ulceration, neoplasia, and postpolypectomy site (electrocoagulation, heater probe, laser, or injection therapy)
Foreign body removal
Excision of polyp
Decompression of acute megacolon or sigmoid volvulus
Balloon dilation of stenotic lesions
Palliative treatment of stenosing or bleeding neoplasms (laser, electrocoagulation, stenting)
Marking a neoplasm for localization during surgery

Adapted from Appropriate use of gastrointestinal endoscopy. American Society of Gastrointestinal Endoscopy. Gastrointest Endos 2000;52:831-837.

Table 18-6. Role of Endoscopic Retrograde Cholangiopancreatography

Treatment of choledocholithiasis
Treatment of biliary pancreatitis
Evaluation and treatment of recurrent pancreatitis
Evaluation and treatment of ascending cholangitis
Tissue sampling of suspected biliary and pancreatic malignancies
Diagnosis of ampullary tumors
Malignant and benign biliary stricture management (sphincterotomy, dilation, stent placement)
Photodynamic therapy
Diagnosis and treatment of biliary and pancreatic duct injury and leak
Pancreatic pseudocyst (stent)
Stent removal
Biliary manometry
Endoscopic sphincterotomy in type I sphincter of Oddi dysfunction
Endoscopic sphincterotomy in type II sphincter of Oddi dysfunction if manometry confirmed pressure >40 mm Hg

Adapted from Adler DG, Baron TH, Davila RE, et al: ASGE guideline: The role of ERCP in diseases of the biliary tract and pancreas. American Society of Gastrointestinal Endoscopy. Gastrointest Endosc 2005;62:1-8.

tion occur in 0.001% to 0.008% and 0.005% to 0.14%.[90,91] Interventional procedures, such as polypectomy, can increase the risk of bleeding and perforation to 2% and 0.3%.[92] There is a theoretical risk of colonic explosion during cautery from accumulation of colonic gases, usually as a result of a carbohydrate-based bowel preparation such as mannitol.[93]

Polypectomy is one of the most common interventions during colonoscopy. Pedunculated or sessile polyps may be removed with biopsy forceps, snare cautery, or argon plasma coagulation. As noted earlier, complications may be reduced with submucosal injection of saline or epinephrine.

Common causes of colonic hemorrhage include diverticulosis, postpolypectomy bleeding, vascular malformations, and hemorrhoids. Diverticular and postpolypectomy bleeding may be controlled with epinephrine injection, heater probe, electrocautery, or metallic clips. Band ligation also may be effective in hemostasis of postpolypectomy bleeds. Vascular malformations may be ablated with heater probe, electrocautery, laser, argon plasma coagulation, and metallic clips. Hemorrhoidal bleeds are effectively controlled with elastic band ligation, either with a rigid proctoscope or with a flexible videoendoscope.[94]

Anastomotic strictures may occur from inflammatory bowel disease or postsurgical resection. These strictures can be dilated with balloon dilators or managed with self-expanding metallic stents.[95] Endoluminal stenting may be used as palliation or as a bridge to surgery for near obstructive malignant lesions.[96] Laser therapy is another option for tumor ablation.[97]

Colonic decompression and placement of temporary rectal tubes is indicated in patients with sigmoid or cecal volvulus and acute pseudo-obstruction. Foreign objects also may be removed endoscopically.

ENDOSCOPIC RETROGRADE CHOLANGIOPANCREATOGRAPHY

ERCP is used to evaluate and treat diseases of the pancreas, bile ducts, gallbladder, and liver. With the advent of highly diagnostic alternative modalities, such as magnetic resonance imaging and EUS, the role of ERCP has slowly evolved into a therapeutic rather than diagnostic tool (Table 18-6).[98] The procedure is performed under anesthesia with the patient lying on the left side or prone. Significant coagulopathy should be corrected if sphincterotomy is to be performed. Antibiotic prophylaxis is indicated in cases of suspected biliary obstruction, known pancreatic pseudocyst, or ductal leaks.[99] Patients with iodine dye allergy should be premedicated with steroids and antihistamines. Glucagon may be beneficial to reduce peristalsis of the small bowel, facilitating cannulation of the bile duct.

After oral intubation, the side-viewing duodenoscope is advanced into the second portion of the duodenum, where the papilla of Vater is located. The papilla is subsequently cannulated. Visualization of the common bile duct or pancreatic duct is achieved with injection of contrast dye and radiographic fluoroscopy. Biliary obstruction, usually secondary to choledocholithiasis, may be treated with ERCP. Stone extraction is successful in 90% of cases.[100] Techniques for stone extraction involve biliary sphincterotomy or balloon sphincteroplasty, followed by stone removal by soft balloon or wire basket. Large stones may be fragmented before removal with mechanical, laser, or electrohydraulic lithotripsy. Inadequate bile drainage may require biliary stenting to prevent ascending cholangitis.

Bile duct stenting is used to alleviate obstruction caused by malignant and benign pathology and to treat bile duct injuries and leaks.[101] Pancreatic stents are used for pancreatic duct disruptions[102] and pseudocysts that communicate with the pancreatic duct.[103] Stents vary in diameter, length, material (plastic, metallic, and biodegradable), and occlusion rates.

Malignant and benign strictures may be dilated with hydrostatic balloons. ERCP also is used to obtain brush cytology, fine-needle aspiration, or biopsy specimens of a suspected malignancy. Sensitivity is typically low, ranging from 30% with brushings to 60% with all three methods combined.[104] Reports of photodynamic therapy for nonresectable cholangiocarcinoma have been described.[105] Manometry, the measurement of biliary and pancreatic sphincter pressures, may be used to evaluate sphincter of Oddi dysfunction, postcholecystectomy pain, and idiopathic pancreatitis.

Choledochoscopes and pancreatoscopes, often referred to as "mother-daughter scopes," are small endoscopes that can be passed through a duodenoscope channel port into the common bile duct or pancreatic duct. This allows direct visualization of the duct lumen. Direct visualization of vasculature within a biliary stricture may help differentiate benign from malignant lesions.[106]

ERCP carries a substantial morbidity risk. Pancreatitis is the most common complication, occurring in 7% of cases.[107] Although the benefits of prophylactic administration of gabexate mesylate are controversial,[108,109] pancreatic stenting of high-risk patients seems to be efficacious.[110] Stenting decreases papillary hindrance to pancreatic duct drainage. Other reported complications include hemorrhage, cholangitis, and perforation.[111]

ENDOSCOPIC ULTRASOUND

EUS, a combination of endoscopy and ultrasonography, is used for evaluation of luminal walls and structures adjacent to the GI tract. Dedicated ultrasound endoscopes with linear array or radial viewing can be used. In addition, high-frequency ultrasound probes that can be passed through the channel port of standard endoscopes are commercially available.[112]

A common application of EUS is to evaluate benign and malignant mucosal and submucosal lesions. EUS is employed routinely for detection and staging of esophageal, gastric, ampullary, pancreaticobiliary, colorectal, and lung neoplasms. EUS also is used to evaluate chronic pancreatitis and biliary pathologies, such as calculi. In general, EUS is an extremely sensitive tool and often superior to computed tomography or magnetic resonance imaging for diagnosis and staging of neoplasia.[113] An advantage of EUS over these noninvasive modalities is the ability to perform therapeutic interventions when needed. Fine-needle aspiration can be done with EUS, which also can be used for pseudocyst drainage, celiac plexus blocks, cholangiography, pancreatography, and tumor ablation.[114] Endoscopic mucosal resection also has been reported,[115] as has the diagnosis and management of GI bleeding.[116]

Preparation of the patient is similar to standard endoscopy. Complications from instrumentation vary depending on the clinical scenario. Perforation rates, usually cervical esophageal in origin, occur in 0.03%.[117] Despite the low risk of bacteremia after EUS fine-needle aspiration, prophylactic antibiotics are recommended for pancreatic cystic lesions and perhaps the perirectal space.[118] Pancreatitis, hemorrhage, and bile peritonitis also have been reported.[118]

FUTURE OF ENDOSCOPY

In the field of GI endoscopy, new innovative instruments and techniques are constantly being developed to aid the endoscopist. Enhanced imaging is one such potential tool. Chromoendoscopy, in conjunction with high magnification and resolution endoscopes, can detect lesions easily missed by conventional endoscopy. Dyes such as methylene blue, Lugol's iodine solution, and indigo carmine have been applied to tissue to identify preneoplastic and neoplastic lesions. Chromoendoscopy has been used with success in detecting Barrett's esophagus[119] and early colorectal neoplasm[120] and differentiating adenomatous from nonadenomatous polyps.[121] Other novel imaging techniques being studied involve spectroscopy, laser scanning microscopy, narrow band imaging, fluorescence, and photosensitizers.[122] Computed tomographic colonography, a noninvasive imaging test of the colon, is promising. Data to date are conflicting, however, on the rate of polyp detection, especially diminutive lesions, compared with optical colonoscopy.[123,124] Limitations for use include lack of therapeutic and interventional capabilities.

Endoscopic sewing and stapling devices have been developed to control GI bleeding,[125] place pH probes in the esophagus, and serve as an alternative to surgical fundoplication for gastroesophageal reflux disease. In addition, computer-assisted colonoscopy with three-dimensional imaging and self-propulsion is under development.

Natural Orifice Transluminal Endoscopy Surgery (NOTES) is a controversial, experimental technique whereby an endoscope is passed into the peritoneal cavity after an internal incision is made through the stomach, colon, or bladder wall. Surgical procedures such as cholecystectomy, appendectomy, and tubal ligation are then subsequently carried out. Potential advantages of NOTES include faster recovery time and lack of external scars, although at present, there is minimal clinical experience in human beings.

The future of endoscopy promises to introduce a plethora of new tools to evaluate the human body. With improved imaging, miniaturizations, and refinement of technique, the endoscopist and, more importantly, the patient will benefit.

KEY POINTS

- Endoscopy serves a diagnostic and a therapeutic role in the management of patients.
- Informed consent must be obtained before any elective endoscopic procedure.
- Perforation and bleeding are the major complications of endoscopy. Although standard endoscopy is generally low risk, interventional procedures increase the rate of complications. A benefit versus risk analysis must be done before any procedure.
- Cardiopulmonary decompensation is a possible complication of anesthesia.
- Endoscopy is the most effective technique to identify and control GI hemorrhage.
- Endoscopy plays a crucial role in the palliative care of patients with GI tract malignancy.
- ERCP has evolved into a therapeutic tool for treating pancreaticobiliary disease.
- Advances in technology are rapidly changing the landscape of endoscopy.

REFERENCES

1. Edmonson JM: History of the instruments for gastrointestinal endoscopy. Gastrointest Endosc 1991;37:S27-S56.
2. Haubrich WS, Edmonson JM: History of endoscopy. In Sivak MV (ed): Gastroenterologic Endoscopy, 2nd ed. Philadelphia, Saunders, 2000, pp 2-15.
3. Edmonson JM: Focus on fiberoptic colonoscope. Gastrointest Endosc 2000;52:17A-20A.
4. Sivak MV: Polypectomy: Looking back. Gastrointest Endosc 2004;60:977-982.
5. McCune WS, Shorb PE, Moscovitz H: Endoscopic cannulation of the ampulla of Vater: A preliminary report. Ann Surg 1968;167:752-756.
6. Kawai K, Akasaka Y, Murakami K, et al: Endoscopic sphincterotomy of the ampulla of Vater. Gastrointest Endosc 1974;20:148-151.
7. Edmonson JM: Endoscopic ultrasound. Gastrointest Endosc 2000;52:13A-14A.
8. Yamao K, Sawaki A, Mizuno N, et al: Endoscopic ultrasound-guided fine-needle aspiration biopsy (EUS-FNAB: past, present, and future). J Gastroenterol 2005;40:1013-1023.
9. Iddan GJ, Swain CP: History and development of capsule endoscopy. Gastrointest Endosc Clin N Am 2004;14:1-9.
10. Kawahara I, Ichikawa H: Flexible endoscope technology: The fiberoptic endoscope. In Sivak MV (ed): Gastroenterologic Endoscopy, 2nd ed. Philadelphia, Saunders, 2000, pp 16-28.
11. Barlow DE: Flexible endoscope technology: The video image endoscope. In Sivak MK (ed): Gastroenterologic Endoscopy, 2nd ed. Philadelphia, Saunders, 2000, pp 29-49.
12. Roesch T: Endoscopic ultrasonography: Equipment and technique. Gastrointest Endosc Clin N Am 2005;15:13-31.
13. Mishkin DS, Chuttani R, Croffie J, et al: ASGE technology status evaluation: Wireless capsule endoscopy. Gastrointest Endosc 2006;63:539-545.
14. Plumeri PA: Informed consent for gastrointestinal endoscopy in the 90's and beyond. Gastrointest Endosc 1994;40:379.
15. American Society of Anesthesiologists Task Force: Practice guidelines for sedation and analgesia by non-anesthesiologists. Anesthesiology 2002;96:1004-1017.
16. Sieg A, Hachmoeller-Eisenbach U, Eisenbach T: Prospective evaluation of complications in outpatient GI endoscopy: A survey among German gastroenterologists. Gastrointest Endosc 2001;53:620-627.
17. Soma Y, Saito H, Kishibe T, et al: Evaluation of topical pharyngeal anesthesia for upper endoscopy including factors associated with patient tolerance. Gastrointest Endosc 2001;53:14-18.
18. Gunaratnam NT, Vazquez-Sequeiros E, Gostout CJ, et al: Methemoglobinemia related to topical benzocaine use: Is it time to reconsider the empiric use of topical anesthesia before sedated EGD? Gastrointest Endosc 2000;52:692-693.
19. Waring JP, Baron TH, Hirota WK, et al: Guidelines for conscious sedation and monitoring during gastrointestinal endoscopy. Gastrointest Endosc 2003;58:317-322.
20. Horn E, Nesbit SA: Pharmacology and pharmokinetics of sedatives and analgesics. Gastrointest Endosc Clin N Am 2004;14:247-268.
21. Rex D: The science and politics of propofol. Am J Gastroenterol 2004;99:2080-2083.
22. Ulmer BJ, Hansen JJ, Overley CA, et al: Propofol versus midazolam/fentanyl for outpatient colonoscopy: Administration by nurses supervised by endoscopists. Clin Gastroenterol Hepatol 2003;1:425-432.
23. Qadeer MA, Vargo JJ, Khandwaa F, et al: Propofol versus traditional sedative agents for gastrointestinal endoscopy: A meta-analysis. Clin Gastroenterol Hepatol 2005;3:1049-1056.
24. Wolfsen HC, Hemminger LL, Achem SR, et al: Complications of endoscopy of the upper gastrointestinal tract. Mayo Clin Proc 2004;79:1264-1267.
25. Coffin B, Pocard M, Panis Y, et al: Erythromycin improves the quality of EGD in patients with acute upper GI bleeding: A randomized controlled study. Gastrointest Endosc 2002;56:174-179.
26. Lipper B, Simon D, Cerrone F: Pulmonary aspiration during emergency endoscopy in patients with upper gastrointestinal hemorrhage. Crit Care Med 1991;19:330-333.
27. Rudolf SJ, Landsverk BK, Freeman ML: Endotracheal intubation for airway protection during endoscopy for severe upper GI hemorrhage. Gastrointest Endosc 2003;57:58-61.
28. Jensen DM: Thermal contact methods for endoscopic hemostasis. In Sivak MV (ed): Gastroenterologic Endoscopy, 2nd ed. Philadelphia, Saunders, 2000, pp 317-329.
29. Chung SCS, Leung FW, Leung JWC: Is vasoconstriction the mechanism of hemostasis in bleeding ulcers with adrenalin? A study using reflectance spectrophotometry. Gastrointest Endosc 1998;34:A174.
30. O'Brien JR: Some effects of adrenaline and anti-adrenaline compounds on platelets in vitro and in vivo. Nature 1963;200:763-764.
31. Sung JY, Chung SC, Low LM, et al: Systemic absorption of epinephrine after endoscopic submucosal injection in patients with bleeding peptic ulcers. Gastrointest Endosc 1993;39:20-22.
32. Stevens PD, Lebwohl O: Hypertensive emergency and ventricular tachycardia after endoscopic epinephrine injection of a Mallory Weiss tear. Gastrointest Endosc 1994;40:77-78.
33. Truesdale RA, Wong RK: Complications of esophageal variceal sclerotherapy. Gastroenterol Clin North Am 1991;20:859-870.
34. Shirai M, Nakamura T, Matsuura A, et al: Safer colonoscopic polypectomy with local submucosal injection of hypertonic saline-epinephrine solution. Am J Gastroenterol 1994;89:334-338.
35. Qureshi W, Adler DG, Davila R, et al: ASGE guideline: The role of endoscopy in the management of variceal hemorrhage, updated July 2005. Gastrointest Endosc 2005;62:651-655.
36. Binmoeller KF, Thonke F, Soehendra N: Endoscopic hemoclip treatment for gastrointestinal bleeding. Endoscopy 1993;25:167-170.
37. Minami S, Gotoda T, Ono H, et al: Complete endoscopic closure of gastric perforation induced by endoscopic resection of early gastric cancer using endoclips can prevent surgery (with video). Gastrointest Endosc 2006;63:596-601.

38. Rodella L, Laterza E, De Manzoni G, et al: Endoscopic clipping of anastomotic leakages in esophagogastric surgery. Endoscopy 1998;30:453-456.
39. Iida Y, Miura S, Munemoto Y, et al: Endoscopic resection of large colorectal polyps using a clipping method. Dis Colon Rectum 1994;37:179-180.
40. Devereaux CE, Binmoeller KF: Endoclip: closing the surgical gap. Gastrointest Endosc 1999;50: 440-442.
41. Lo CC, Hsu PI, Lo GH, et al: Comparison of hemostatic efficacy for epinephrine injection alone and injection combined with hemoclip therapy in treating high-risk bleeding ulcers. Gastrointest Endosc 2006;63: 767-773.
42. Swain CP: Laser therapy. In Sivak MV (ed): Gastroenterologic Endoscopy, 2nd ed. Philadelphia, Saunders, 2000, pp 330-344.
43. Barr H, Stone N, Rembacken B: Endoscopy therapy for Barrett's oesophagus. Gut 2005;54:875-884.
44. Vargo JJ: Clinical applications of the argon plasma coagulator. Gastrointest Endosc 2004;59:8 1-88.
45. Albala DM: Fibrin sealants in clinical practice. Cardiovasc Surg 2003;11: 5-11.
46. Pescatore P, Jornod P, Borovicka J, et al: Epinephrine versus epinephrine plus fibrin glue injection in peptic ulcer bleeding: A prospective randomized trial. Gastrointest Endosc 2002;55:348-353.
47. Heneghan MA, Byrne A, Harrison PM: An open pilot study of the effects of a human fibrin glue for endoscopic treatment of patients with acute bleeding from gastric varices. Gastrointest Endosc 2002;56:422-426.
48. Huang CS, Hess DT, Lichtenstein DR: Successful endoscopic management of postoperative GI fistula with fibrin glue injection: Report of two cases. Gastrointest Endosc 2004;60:460-463.
49. Seewald S, Sriram PV, Naga M, et al: Cyanoacrylate glue in gastric variceal bleeding. Endoscopy 2002;34: 926-932.
50. Maluf-Filho F, Sakai P, Ishioka S, et al: Endoscopic sclerosis versus cyanoacrylate endoscopic injection for the first episode of variceal bleeding: A prospective, controlled and randomized study in Child-Pugh class C patients. Endoscopy 2001;22: 421-427.
51. Lo GH, Lai KH, Cheng JS, et al: A prospective, randomized trial of butyl cyanoacrylate injection versus band ligation in the management of bleeding gastric varices. Hepatology 2001;33:1060-1064.
52. Petersen B, Barkun A, Carpenter S, et al: Tissue adhesives and fibrin glues: Technology status evaluation report. Gastrointest Endosc 2004;60:327-333.
53. Web WA: Management of foreign bodies. Gastrointest Endosc 1995;41:39-51.
54. Ginsberg GG: Management of ingested foreign bodies and food bolus impactions. Gastrointest Endosc 1995;41:33-38.
55. Eisen GM, Baron TH, Dominitz JA, et al: Guideline for the management of ingested foreign bodies. Gastrointest Endosc 2002;55:802-806.
56. Karamanolis G, Sgouros S, Karatzias G, et al: Long-term outcome of pneumatic dilation in the treatment of achalasia. Am J Gastroenterol 2005;100:270-274.
57. Egan JV, Baron TH, Adler DG, et al: Esophageal dilation. Gastrointest Endosc 2006;63:755-760.
58. Siersema PD: Treatment of esophageal perforations and anastomotic leaks: The endoscopist is stepping into the arena. Gastrointest Endosc 2005;61:897-900.
59. Ferri L, Lee JK, Law S, et al: Management of spontaneous perforation of esophageal cancer with covered self expanding metallic stents. Dis Esophagus 2005;18:67-69.
60. Siersema PD, Homs MY, Haringsma J, et al: Use of large diameter metallic stents to seal traumatic nonmalignant perforations of the esophagus. Gastrointest Endosc 2003;58:356-361.
61. Dougherty JJ, Gomer CT, Henderson BW, et al: Photodynamic therapy. J Natl Cancer Inst 1998;90:889-905.
62. Wolfsen HC: Uses of photodynamic therapy in premalignant and malignant lesions of the gastrointestinal tract beyond the esophagus. J Clin Gastroenterol 2005;39:653-664.
63. Niv Y, Abuksis G: Indications for percutaneous endoscopic gastrostomy insertion: Ethical aspects. Dig Dis 2002;20:253-256.
64. Rabeneck L, McCullough LB, Wray NP: Ethically justified, clinically comprehensive guidelines for percutaneous endoscopic gastrostomy tube placement. Lancet 1997;349: 496-498.
65. Nicholson FB, Korman MG, Richardson MA: Percutaneous endoscopic gastrostomy: A review of indications, complications, and outcomes. J Gastroenterol Hepatol 2000;15: 21-25.
66. Cruz I, Mamel JJ, Brady PG, et al: Incidence of abdominal wall metastasis complicating PEG tube placement in untreated head and neck cancer. Gastrointest Endosc 2005;62: 708-711.
67. Gottfried EB, Plummer AB, Clair MR: Pneumoperitoneum following percutaneous endoscopic gastrostomy: A prospective study. Gastrointest Endosc 1986;32:397-399.
68. Lewis BS: Radiology versus endoscopy of the small bowel. Gastrointest Endosc Clin N Am 1999;9:13-27.
69. Taylor AC, Chen RY, Desmond PV: Use of an overtube for enteroscopy—does it increase depth of insertion? A prospective study of enteroscopy with and without an overtube. Endoscopy 2001;33:227-230.
70. Wayne JD: Enteroscopy. Gastrointest Endosc 1997;46:247-256.
71. Heine GD, Hadithi M, Groenen MJ, et al: Double balloon endoscopy: Indications, diagnostic yields and complications in a series of 275 patients with suspected small bowel disease. Endoscopy 2006;38:42-48.
72. DiCaro S, May A, Heine DG, et al: The European experience with double balloon enteroscopy: Indications, methodology, safety, and clinical impact. Gastrointest Endosc 2006;62:545-550.
73. Kaffes AJ, Koo JH, Meredith C: Double balloon enteroscopy in the diagnosis and management of small bowel disease: An initial experience in 40 patients. Gastrointest Endosc 2006;63:81-86.
74. Yamamoto H, Sekine Y, Sato Y, et al: Clinical outcomes of double balloon endoscopy for diagnosis and treatment of small bowel disease. Clin Gastroenterol Hepatol 2004;11: 1010-1016.
75. Ben-Soussan E, Savoye G, Antonietti M, et al: Is a 2-liter PEG preparation useful before capsule endoscopy? J Clin Gastroenterol 2005;39:381-384.
76. Dai N, Gubler C, Hengstler P, et al: Improved capsule endoscopy after bowel preparation. Gastrointest Endosc 2005;61:28-31.
77. Selby W: Complete small-bowel transit in patients undergoing capsule endoscopy: Determining factors and improvement with metoclopramide. Gastrointest Endosc 2005;61:80-85.
78. Sturniolo GC, Leo VC, Vettorato MG, et al: Small bowel exploration by wireless capsule endoscopy: Results from 314 procedures. Am J Med 2006;119:341-347.
79. Tatar EL, Shen EH, Palance AL, et al: Clinical utility of wireless capsule endoscopy: Experience of 200 cases. J Clin Gastroenterol 2006;40: 140-144.
80. Treister SL, Leighton JA, Leontiadis GI, et al: A meta-analysis of the yield of capsule endoscopy compared to other diagnostic modalities in patients with obscure gastrointestinal bleeding. Am J Gastroenterol 2005;100:2407-2418.
81. Hadithi M, Heine GD, Jacobs MA, et al: A prospective study comparing video capsule endoscopy with double-balloon enteroscopy in patients with obscure gastrointestinal bleeding. Am J Gastroenterol 2006;101:52-57.
82. Payeras G, Piqueras J, Moreno VJ, et al: Effects of capsule endoscopy on cardiac pacemakers. Endoscopy 2005;37:1181-1185.
83. Leighton JA, Srivathsan K, Carey EJ, et al: Safety of wireless capsule endoscopy in patients with implantable cardiac defibrillators. Am J Gastroenterol 2005;100:1732-1735.
84. Rondonotti E, Herrerias JM, Pennazio M, et al: Complications, limitations, and failures of capsule endoscopy: A review of 733 cases. Gastrointest Endosc 2005;62:712-716.
85. Signorelli C, Rondonotti E, Villa F, et al: Use of the Given Patency System for the screening of patients at high risk for capsule retention. Dig Liver Dis 2006;38:326-330.
86. Wexner SD, Beck DE, Baron TH, et al: A consensus document on bowel preparation before colonoscopy: Prepared by a task force from the American Society of Colon and Rectal Surgeons (ASCRS), the American Society for Gastrointestinal Endoscopy (ASGE), and the Society of American Gastrointestinal and Endoscopic

Surgeons (SAGES). Dis Colon Rectum 2006;49:1-18.
87. Ness RM, Manam R, Hoen H, et al: Predictors of inadequate bowel preparation for colonoscopy. Am J Gastroenterol 2001;96:1797-1802.
88. Church JM: Complete colonoscopy: How often? And if not, why? Am J Gastroenterol 1994;89:556-560.
89. Anderson JC, Messing CR, Cohn W, et al: Factors predictive of difficult colonoscopy. Gastrointest Endosc 2001;54:558-562.
90. Fruhmorgen P, Demling L: Complications of diagnostic and therapeutic colonoscopy in the Federal Republic of Germany: Results of an inquiry. Endoscopy 1979;11:146-150.
91. Sieg A, Hachmoeller-Eisenbach U, Eisenbach T: Prospective evaluation of complications in outpatient GI endoscopy: A survey among German gastroenterologists. Gastrointest Endosc 2001;53:620-627.
92. Waye JD, Lewis BS, Yessayan S: Colonoscopy: A prospective report of complications. J Clin Gastroenterol 1992;15:347-351.
93. Bigard MA, Gaucher P, Lassalle C: Fatal colonic explosion during colonoscopic polypectomy. Gastroenterology 1979;77:1307-1310.
94. Wehrmann T, Riphaus A, Feinstein J, et al: Hemorrhoidal elastic band ligation with flexible videoendoscopes: A prospective, randomized comparison with the conventional techniqued that uses rigid proctoscopes. Gastrointest Endosc 2004;60:191-195.
95. Forshaw MJ, Sankararajah D, Stewart M, et al: Self-expanding metallic stents in the treatment of benign colorectal disease: Indications and outcomes. Colorect Dis 2006;8:102-111.
96. Baron TH: Colonic stenting: technique, technology, and outcomes for malignant and benign disease. Gastrointest Endosc Clin N Am 2005;15:757-771.
97. Wood JW, Innes JW: Tumor ablation by endoscopic Nd : YAG laser. Am J Gastroenterol 1985;80:715-718.
98. Cohen S, Bacon BR, Berlin JA, et al: National Institutes of Health State-of-the-Science Conference Statement: ERCP for diagnosis and therapy, January 14-16, 2002. Gastrointest Endosc 2002;56:803-809.
99. Hirota WK, Petersen K, Baron TH, et al: Guidelines for antibiotic prophylaxis for GI endoscopy. Gastrointest Endosc 2003;58:475-482.
100. Carr-Locke DL: Therapeutic role of ERCP in the management of suspected common bile duct stones. Gastrointest Endosc 2002;56:S170-S174.
101. Katsinelos P, Kountouras J, Paroutoglou G, et al: The role of endoscopic treatment in postoperative bile leaks. Hepatogastroenterology 2006;53:166-170.
102. Cay A, Imamoglu M, Ozdemir O, et al: Nonoperative treatment of traumatic pancreatic duct disruption in children with an endoscopically placed stent. J Pediatr Surg 2005;40:9-12.
103. Sharma SS, Bhargawa N, Govil A: Endoscopic management of pancreatic pseudocyst: A long-term follow-up. Endoscopy 2002;34:203-207.
104. Jailwala J: Triple tissue sampling at ERCP in malignant biliary obstruction. Gastrointest Endosc 2000;51:383-390.
105. Ortner MA, Liebetruth J, Schrieber SJ, et al: Photodynamic therapy of non-resectable cholangiocarcinoma. Gastroenterology 1998;114:536-542.
106. Kim HJ, Kim MH, Lee SK, et al: Tumor vessel: A valuable cholangioscopic clue of malignant biliary stricture. Gastrointest Endosc 2000;52:635-638.
107. Mallery SJ, Baron TH, Dominitz JA, et al: Complications of ERCP. Gastrointest Endosc 2003;57:633-638.
108. Cavallini G, Tittobello A, Frulloni L, et al: Gabexate for the prevention of pancreatic damage related to endoscopic retrograde cholangiopancreatography. N Engl J Med 1996;335:919-923.
109. Andriulli A, Clemente R, Solmi L, et al: Gabexate or somatostatin administration before ERCP in patients with high risk for post-ERCP pancreatitis: A multicenter placebo-controlled randomized clinical trial. Gastrointest Endosc 2002;56:488-495.
110. Testoni PA: Preventing post-ERCP pancreatitis: Where are we? J Pancreas 2003;4:22-32.
111. Masci E, Toto G, Mariani A, et al: Complications of diagnostic and therapeutic ERCP: A prospective multicenter study. Am J Gastroenterol 2001;96:417-423.
112. Carpenter S, Chuttani R, Croffie J, et al: Endoscopic ultrasound probes. Gastrointest Endosc 2006;63:751-754.
113. Lowe AS, Kay CL: Noninvasive competition for endoscopic ultrasound. Gastrointest Endoscopy Clin N Am 2005;15:209-224.
114. Shami VM, Waxman I: Technology insight: Current status of endoscopic ultrasonography. Nat Clin Pract Gastroenterol Hepatol 2005;2:38-45.
115. Wehrmann T, Martchenko K, Nakamura M, et al: Endoscopic resection of submucosal esophageal tumors: A prospective case series. Endoscopy 2004;36:802-807.
116. Folvik G, Nesje LB, Berstad A, et al: Endosonography-guided endoscopic band ligation of Dieulafoy's malformation: A case report. Endoscopy 2001;33:636-638.
117. Das A, Sivak MV, Chak A: Cervical esophageal perforation during EUS: A national survey. Gastrointest Endosc 2001;53:599-602.
118. Adler DG, Davila RE, Hirota WK, et al: ASGE guideline: complications of EUS. Gastrointest Endosc 2005;61:8-12.
119. Olliver JR, Wild CP, Sahay P, et al: Chromoendoscopy with methylene blue and associated DNA damage in Barrett's oesophagus. Lancet 2003;362:373-374.
120. Hurlstone DP, Fujii T: Practical uses of chromoendoscopy and magnification at colonoscopy. Gastrointest Endosc Clin N Am 2005;15:687-702.
121. Eisen GM, Kim CY, Fleischer DE, et al: High resolution chromoendoscopy for classifying colonic polyps: A multicenter study. Gastrointest Endosc 2002;55:687-694.
122. Dekker E, Fockens P: Advances in colonic imaging: New endoscopic imaging methods. Eur J Gastroenterol Hepatol 2005;17:803-808.
123. Pickhart PJ, Choi JR, Hwang I, et al: Computed tomographic virtual colonoscopy to screen for colorectal neoplasia in asymptomatic adults. N Engl J Med 2003;349:2191-2200.
124. Cotton PB, Durkalski VL, Pineau BL, et al: Computed tomographic colonography (virtual colonoscopy): A multicenter comparison with standard colonoscopy for detection of colorectal neoplasms. JAMA 2004;291:1713-1719.
125. Hu B, Chung SC, Sun LC, et al: Developing an animal model of massive ulcer bleeding for assessing endoscopic hemostatic devices. Endoscopy 2005;37:847-851.

Chapter 19

Continuous Renal Replacement Therapy

Boon Wee Teo, Nigel S. Kanagasundaram, and Emil P. Paganini

Although the kidney is often only one of numerous failing organ systems in a critically ill patient, the presence of acute renal failure (ARF) confers a disproportionate disadvantage in terms of survival[1,2] and leads to an increased risk of developing "nonrenal" complications such as bleeding and sepsis.[1] Although the high mortality rate of at least 50% for dialysis-requiring intensive care unit (ICU) patients with ARF remains unchanged, the presentation of a sicker patient population[3,4] suggests that we are gaining ground overall. Advances in the care of critically ill patients include specific developments in the provision of renal replacement therapy to critically ill patients with ARF.

Renal replacement therapy, although initially mirroring dialytic practice in the long-term dialysis population, has evolved to treat a very different patient population with different therapeutic goals. One result of this evolution has been the establishment of continuous renal replacement therapy (CRRT) as part of routine ICU nephrology practice in many parts of the world. Theoretical consideration of continuous dialytic support in ARF patients was reported in 1960,[5] although advances in materials and technology to allow for its widespread clinical application did not occur until later.[6,7]

Intuitively, CRRT might be seen as the modality of choice in a critically ill ICU patient, with suggested advantages including maintenance of hemodynamic stability, enhancing fluid removal and hyperalimentation, and improvements in the delivered dialysis dose (gauged by clearance of marker solutes such as urea). So far, such presumed superiority over intermittent dialytic modalities has failed to translate into clear improvements in patient outcome.[8]

This chapter first reviews theoretical considerations behind the multifaceted aspect of CRRT before moving onto technical and therapeutic considerations. We also discuss possible explanations for the failure to detect clear survival advantages for CRRT (including possible deleterious effects) and "nonrenal" uses of the modality.

THEORETICAL CONSIDERATIONS

Mechanistically, extracorporeal renal replacement therapy relies on two processes—*convection* and *diffusion*—either in isolation or in combination. The process of *convection* involves the movement of a solution en bloc. Solute is transferred by *solvent drag* and is limited only by the pore size or electrostatic charge of any semipermeable membrane that is applied across the passage of the solution. Convective removal of plasma water from blood across a large-pore, semipermeable membrane should result in an *ultrafiltrate* with a solute composition equivalent to plasma water.

The process of *diffusion* involves the net movement of solute down a concentration gradient until equilibrium is reached. There is no net movement of solvent. Any semipermeable membrane that might be applied across the path of the concentration gradient would affect solute transfer as dictated by membrane surface area, thickness, pore size, and electrostatic charge.

Beyond these two physical processes lies a wider nomenclature, specific to renal replacement therapy (Table 19-1). Fluid removal is termed *ultrafiltration* (UF). When used in extracorporeal therapy, UF relies on hydrostatic pressure applied across a semipermeable membrane. Convective removal of solute is involved, but its impact on blood clearance depends on the fluid volume removed. It may be applied in isolation (in volumes usually <5 L/d) or in combination with other blood clearance techniques.

Dialysis is a diffusive process that also requires a semipermeable membrane to separate blood from an aqueous solution (called *dialysate*). This semipermeable membrane

Table 19-1. Commonly Used Forms of Extracorporeal Renal Replacement Therapy

Therapy	Definition	Use	Access	Abbreviation
Ultrafiltration (UF)	Plasma water removal Usually <5 L/d	Fluid overload High delivery in CRF ARF CHF	AV/VV continuous VV continuous AV/VV intermittent	SCUF CVVUF IUF
Hemodialysis (HD)	Diffusion-based process using dialysate and semipermeable membrane	Azotemia Acid-base disturbance Electrolyte balance Volume control	AV continuous VV continuous AV/VV intermittent	CAVHD CVVHD IHD SLED
Hemofiltration (H)	Convective-based process using plasma water exchange methods across semipermeable membrane	Azotemia Acid-base disturbance Electrolyte balance Volume control Cytokine removal ARDS, ARF, CHF, MOF	AV continuous VV continuous AV/VV intermittent	CAVH CVVH IH
Hemodiafiltration (HDF)	Combining diffusion and convection (10-L exchanges) for small and middle molecular loss	Azotemia Volume control Cytokine removal ARDS, ARF, CHF, MOF	AV continuous VV continuous AV/VV intermittent	CAVHDF CVVHDF IHDF

ARDS, acute respiratory distress syndrome; ARF, acute renal failure; AV, arteriovenous; CHF, congestive heart failure; CRF, chronic renal failure; MOF, multiple organ failure; SCUF, slow continuous ultrafiltration; SLED, sustained low-efficiency dialysis; VV, venovenous.

may be artificial (the *dialyzer* in extracorporeal *hemodialysis* [HD]) or living (the peritoneal membrane in peritoneal dialysis). Solute diffusion depends on the dialyzer membrane composition and surface area and on the concentration gradient. In HD, blood and dialysate usually flow *countercurrent* to each other to maintain the concentration gradient. UF is usually applied to allow fluid removal from a hypervolemic patient, although convective solute removal is not a major component of overall blood clearance.

Hemofiltration relies on convective removal of plasma solute, in high fluid volumes, across a semipermeable membrane—the *hemofilter* (the terms *filter* and *membrane* loosely cover dialyzers and hemofilters). Transmembrane hydrostatic pressure is applied as a positive pressure on the blood side of the membrane or a negative pressure on the fluid collection *(hemofiltrate)* side or both. Fluid lost through this process is replaced with hemofiltration replacement fluid in either a predilutional mode (before the hemofilter) or a postdilutional mode (after the hemofilter) and in volumes appropriate to achieve patient euvolemia. The hemofiltrate composition created by this system of plasma water exchange depends on the membrane *sieving coefficient* for that particular solute and that particular semipermeable membrane and is a function of membrane thickness, pore size, and electrostatic charge. It is expressed in terms of the ratio of the solute concentrations of hemofiltrate to plasma (Fig. 19-1). Figure 19-2 illustrates the differences in clearance between dialytic and filtrative modalities in terms of solute molecular weight. Hemofiltration is less efficient in clearing low-molecular-weight compounds, but more so for larger solutes. The end product of hemofiltration depends on the differing solute concentrations in the fluid removed and the fluid replaced.

Finally, *hemodiafiltration* (HDF) combines diffusive and (major) convective solute removal and allows efficient

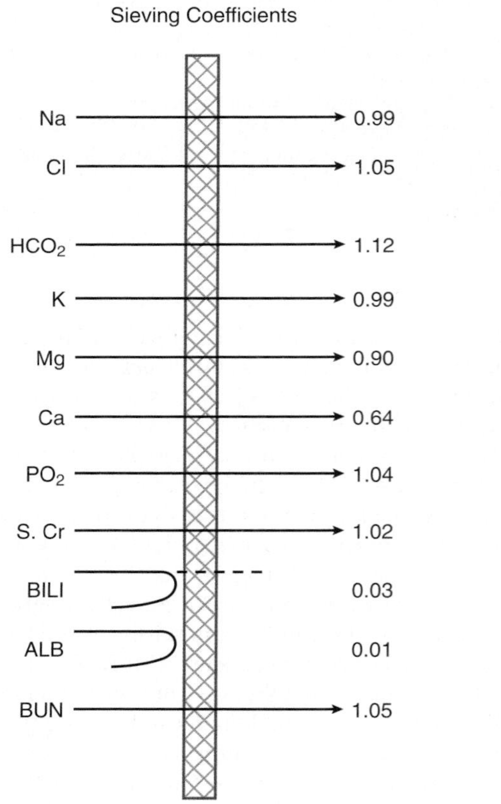

Figure 19-1. In vivo measured sieving coefficients for various elements during hemofiltration with a noncuprophane membrane.

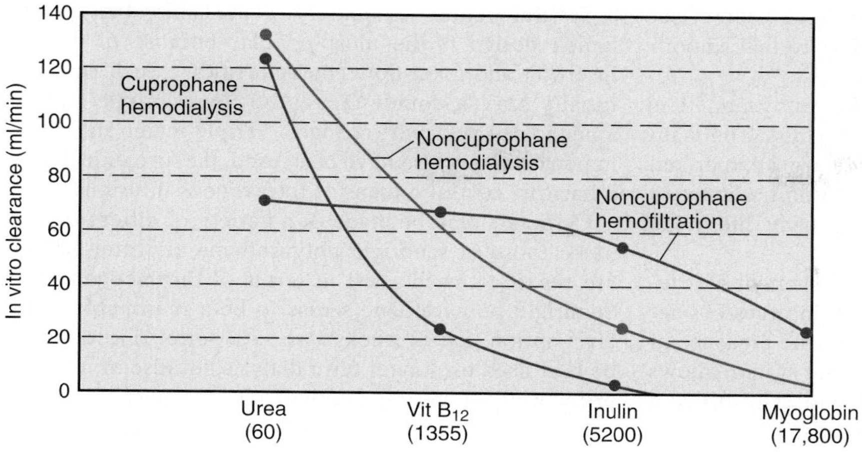

Figure 19-2. In vitro clearance differences between hemodialysis and hemofiltration. Note the effect of modality, membrane type, and molecular weight.

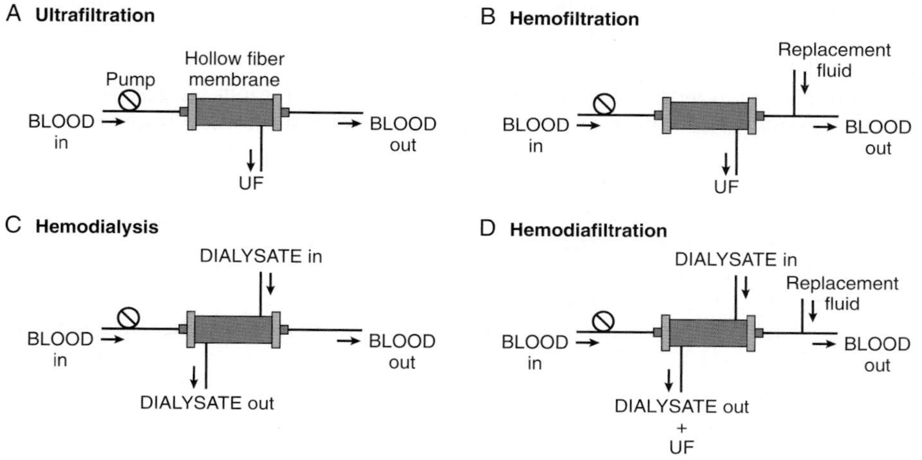

Figure 19-3. Commonly used extracorporeal renal replacement techniques. **A,** Ultrafiltration. **B,** Hemofiltration (replacement fluid infusion may be predilutional or, as in this figure, postdilutional). **C,** Hemodialysis. **D,** Hemodiafiltration. Continuous arteriovenous techniques are generally pumpless. UF, ultrafiltration.

low-molecular and enhanced middle-molecular clearances. Technical improvements in hardware have eased its use for circumstances such as sepsis[9-11] and multiple organ failure,[12,13] where removal of mediator substances is thought to be important.

Figure 19-3 illustrates the mechanics of each of these modalities, which may be performed on an intermittent (I) or a continuous (C) basis (see Table 19-1). Vascular access may be either arteriovenous (AV) or venovenous (VV). In intermittent techniques, AV and VV treatments (through AV fistulas or grafts for AV access and central venous catheters for VV access) require pumps in the blood circuitry. In continuous techniques, although VV modalities require blood pumps, the AV designation generally implies that the blood circuit is pumpless (systemic arterial pressure providing the driving force for blood flow). As an additional point of dialysis nomenclature, the afferent limb of the blood circuitry is termed "arterial" regardless of whether this is truly arterial blood (AV) or not (VV). The returning, efferent limb is termed "venous."

Any given modality may be described according to its frequency (intermittent versus continuous) and technique (hemofiltration, HD, HDF, or stand-alone UF) as shown in Table 19-1. Continuous techniques are additionally described according to their vascular access. Adherence to this descriptive system is important in understanding exactly what type of therapy a given patient has received.

TECHNICAL CONSIDERATIONS

Circuits and Material

Access

Early in the evolution of CRRT, the most important consideration, vascular access, dictated the form of therapy used. In patients who had a usable arterial system, pumpless AV therapy was preferred because of its technical simplicity, ease of implementation, and intrinsic feedback quality. The low systemic arterial blood pressures inherent in many critically ill patients translated into poor blood circuit flows and poor efficacy. This problem, coupled with other complications associated with maintaining arterial access (e.g., thrombosis, local or generalized infections, hemorrhage, cholesterol embolization),[14] has led to increasing usage of VV access, such that most continuous therapy is now provided using pumped VV methods.[14] Not only may this technique be more efficacious,[15] but also technical complexities have been offset by improvements in hardware and software that smooth the interface with the bedside nurse.

Despite this shift in emphasis in recent years, it is still worthwhile examining AV vascular access. The main differences between AV and VV access are summarized in Table 19-2. AV therapies remain a useful adjunct to ICU nephrology practice and may be truly lifesaving in instances of civil disaster relief.

The choice of catheter is an important element of arterial access. Nontapered catheters without intravessel side-hole blood entry should be used because the presence of a single, end-hole opening into the arterial system allows accurate placement of the catheter tip and helps prevent arterial bleeding. Nontapered polyurethane 8F catheters are recommended for arterial and venous entry for AV therapies because this allows transmission of systemic arterial blood pressure through the dialyzer to the venous system.[16] In patients with lower systemic arterial pressures, a more central arterial access may be necessary.[17] Percutaneous catheterization of the femoral artery is most frequently used; surgically placed AV shunts seem to provide lower blood flows[18] and, at least in one report, show a tendency toward reduced circuit life span.[19]

Adding a blood pump to the circuit eliminates the need for arterial puncture, although VV systems are still catheter-dependent. A prospective study of intermittent dialysis in the ICU noted catheter failure to be the most frequently noted cause of therapy underdelivery.[20] System clotting and resistance to blood flow were cited as the most frequent manifestations of catheter failure. This same experience also has been seen with continuous VV techniques.

Several venous catheters are available; the double-lumen design is the most popular because of ease of insertion and good flow characteristics.[21] Such catheters usually have a double-D cross-sectional profile and are amenable to guidewire changes.[18] Triple-lumen and single-lumen catheters also have been used, the former including a narrow, central lumen for intravenous infusions.

Catheters may be made of a variety of different polymers; those of semirigid polyurethane or softer silicone are regarded as the best in terms of thrombogenicity.[14] Semirigid polyurethane seems to be a reasonable short-term option (for <2 weeks), whereas softer silicone might be best used for longer term dialysis because of its lower propensity for causing endovascular trauma.[14]

Despite potential for vessel stenosis with repeated acute access, the most frequently placed venous access remains the subclavian catheter, with femoral and internal jugular approaches also used. Femoral access requires the patient to remain in bed with no more than a 30-degree bend between trunk and leg. Other sites of access allow for mobilization, but carry with them the risk of accidental pneumothorax or other intrathoracic trauma—potentially fatal in a critically ill patient with acute pulmonary disease. Femoral catheters shorter than 20 cm from hub to tip are associated with higher degrees of access recirculation.[22,23] Catheters at least 24 cm in length may produce improved flow rates,[22] presumably because their tip reaches the inferior vena cava. Because of the risks of femoral vein thrombosis, some researchers recommend the removal and replacement of catheters at least weekly.[22] More recent studies on routine changes of catheters (every 3 to 7 days) to prevent infection suggest that catheters

Table 19-2. Access for Continuous Renal Replacement Therapy

	Placement	Location	Contraindications: Relative	Contraindications: Absolute	Complications (% Frequency)
Arterial Access	Percutaneous (single-lumen catheter)	Femoral	Inexperience	Arterial bypass graft	Bleeding
					Hematoma (10%)
		Brachial	Uncooperative patient	Severe stenosis	Retroperitoneal (1%)
		Axillary		Advanced atherosclerosis	Infection
					AV malfunction (<0.5%)
	Surgical (AV shunt)	Brachial	Prior surgery	Positive Allen test (1-2%)	Thrombosis (>1-2%)
		Femoral	Poor distal pulses		Compromised arterial flow
			Future AVF site		Cholesterol embolization
Venous Access	Percutaneous	Subclavian	Uncooperative patient	Prior surgery	Bleeding
					Mild (8%)
		Femoral			Severe (2%)
		Internal jugular			
					Infection (3-6%)
					Stenosis (5-10%)
	Surgical (usually tunnelled)	Subclavian	Prior surgery	Venous stenosis	Pneumothorax (1-2%)
					Hemopneumothorax (<0.5%)
		Internal jugular	Internal jugular graft		

AV, arteriovenous; AVF, arteriovenous fistula.

should be changed only when clinically indicated; guidelines from the Centers for Disease Control and Prevention do not recommend routine changes of central venous catheters.[24,25] The supposed benefit of a reduced risk of infection with routine changes is outweighed by the increase in complications associated with the catheterization procedure, such as bleeding, pneumothorax, peripheral ischemia, arterial atheroemboli, aneurysms, and catheter dysfunction. Use of the subclavian approach, in addition to encompassing the caveats associated with any upper body central venous access, also includes the long-term risk of subclavian venous stenosis. Although such stenoses may occur elsewhere, here it is potentially important as the vein drains a future upper limb AV access. Subclavian access should be minimized in patients who are likely to progress to end-stage renal disease.

The internal jugular approach may be associated with a lower incidence of accidental pneumothorax[22] and long-term stenosis[26] compared with subclavian access and may be the preferred upper body access. Infection may be more common, however, especially in patients with tracheostomies.[14] For an average adult, upper body catheters should be about 20 cm long on the right and 24 cm long on the left[14] to ensure safe positioning of the catheter tip in the lower superior vena cava.

The incorporation of a VV system in parallel with either ventricular assist devices or extracorporeal oxygenators is a frequently used adaptation. These systems use the prepump blood tubing (low pressure) as the venous return of the VV blood circuit and the postpump tubing (high pressure) as the arterial access. Although this design might lend itself to recirculation of dialyzed blood straight back into the dialysis circuit, the relative blood flows in the two parallel circuits keep the percentage of recirculation at less than 15%. One must be sure—especially with the use of ventricular assist devices—that all air is purged from the dialysis membrane before connection to avoid the risk of air embolism. Alternatively, the venous return may be directed into the venous system (usually the femoral vein). This not only avoids access recirculation, but also acts as a safeguard against arterial embolic events.[27,28]

Tubing

Longer blood lines translate into an increased exposure of blood to nonbiologic surfaces, with increased blood cooling and an increased risk of clotting. The interposition of sampling ports, entry ports, and stopcocks creates undue blood turbulence and should be minimized. The air-blood interface in the postdialyzer venous bubble trap increases the risk of clotting and is regarded as the "Achilles heel" of the circuit. At present, it seems to be a necessary evil (although see later section on anticoagulation): Negative preblood pump pressures can easily introduce air into the circuit from a dysfunctional afferent limb of a catheter and would carry the risk of air embolism were it not for the presence of an air trap in the efferent limb of the circuit.

Membrane

It is beyond the scope of this book to cover more than the basics of membrane technology, but the two concepts of filter design and membrane composition are discussed. Generally, of the two types of filter design used in CRRT—hollow-fiber and plate—the former is now more commonly used. Each design consists of a blood compartment and a dialysate compartment, with respective inflow and outflow ports, separated by a semipermeable membrane. Ultimately, they differ only in the way that the blood-dialysate interface is maximized. In hemofiltration or isolated UF, rather than dialysate, the corresponding compartment is filled with generated ultrafiltrate and does not require an inlet.

The hollow-fiber dialyzer constitutes a tubular casing containing thousands of narrow capillary fibers through which blood flows between the arterial and venous header—two small spaces at either end of the filter where blood collects before and after running through the capillary fiber bundle. The capillaries, whose walls constitute the semipermeable membrane, are bathed in dialysate fluid, usually running in countercurrent fashion to blood flow.

In the plate dialyzer, the semipermeable membrane is laid out in a stack of sheets with blood and dialysate running in alternate spaces between these sheets. Blood flows in a more tortuous route—between and around the ends of these sheets—than in the hollow-fiber filter.

Each design has various mechanical pros and cons. The more direct pathway for blood flow afforded by the hollow-fiber design is needed for AV therapy to prevent undue dissipation of systemic blood pressure. The formation of clots at the arterial header has a large impact, however, with a much greater surface area of membrane unavailable for use than with similar clots in the plate filter, which can simply be bypassed. The larger blood channels of the plate design also reduce the risk of clotting, but may detract from the diffusive process because of a comparatively higher blood volume-to-surface area ratio.

The second important technological concept is membrane material, of which there are four broad categories: (1) cellulose (e.g., cuprophane), (2) substituted cellulose (the free hydroxyl groups of cellulose, thought to activate complement, are bound to other substances, e.g., acetate in cellulose acetate membranes), (3) cellulosynthetic (synthetic material incorporated with the cellulose polymer, e.g., Hemophan), and (4) synthetic (made of noncellulosic materials, e.g., polysulfone, polyacrylonitrile [PAN], polyamide, and polymethyl methacrylate). The biocompatibility of each of these materials is a measure of its propensity to activate complement, the coagulation cascade, and leukocytes,[29] with cellulosic membranes considered the least biocompatible (i.e., most bioincompatible) and synthetic the most biocompatible, with modified cellulose composites somewhere in between.

Sequelae of the effects of bioincompatibility relevant to ARF patients are thought to include prolongation of renal damage[30]; a greater tendency to filter clotting; and the potential for impairment of pulmonary gas exchange, cardiovascular instability, hypercatabolism, and an increased risk of infection[29]—although many of these observations are extrapolated from in vitro, animal, or long-term dialysis settings.[29] Prospective, randomized, clinical studies in intermittent hemodialysis (IHD)–treated ARF have not uniformly corroborated the benefits of increased membrane biocompatibility, with some studies finding improvements in patient survival[31,32] and renal recovery,[31,32] and others not finding improvements.[33,34]

An editorial review of available data by Vanholder and Lameire[35] highlighted problems with patient selection and matching for illness severity. There were additional concerns about corrections for the delivered dialysis dose.[36] Two studies compared the more biocompatible substituted cellulose type of filter with synthetic filters in terms of clinical outcome[37] and cellular responses[38] in ARF patients receiving IHD. No differences were found. Although prospective, randomized data comparing membranes of varying biocompatibility in CRRT are lacking, extrapolation of current evidence suggests the use of either substituted cellulose or synthetic materials and the avoidance of cellulose filters.

The variety of synthetic membranes represents a heterogeneous group of materials that may differ in terms of filter longevity[39,40] and cardiovascular stability.[41,42] A final caveat for the use of the PAN filter is the concurrent use of angiotensin-converting enzyme inhibitors; the highly negatively charged membrane tends to bind and activate Hageman factor XII, with subsequent generation of bradykinin—a potential cause for anaphylactic reactions during long-term IHD with PAN.[29] Administration of angiotensin-converting enzyme inhibitors may compound the problem because of their propensity to increase bradykinin production.

The last component of filter choice is modality. The asymmetric design of the polyamide membrane is well suited for UF and hemofiltration, but not for diffusion. PAN and cellulose acetate may have a better structure for diffusive therapies. Convective therapies also rely on the use of membranes with high hydraulic permeability and are indicated as the UF coefficient, K_{Uf}, a marker of water permeability and a function of membrane thickness and pore size.

Fluid

When hemofiltration is performed, replacement fluid composition dictates the resultant end point of therapy. Understanding what fluid type is lost helps in choosing the appropriate replacement solution. The sieving coefficients for relevant electrolytes and blood components are listed in Figure 19-1. Elements with a negative charge that are small enough to cross the membrane do so at greater than unity. This apparent active transport is actually accomplished through a dynamic process similar to the Gibbs-Donnan effect seen in stagnant fluid balance. Because negatively charged proteins are unable to cross the membrane, chloride and bicarbonate move against a concentration gradient to maintain electrical neutrality. The exaggerated loss of these elements must be reflected in the replacement solution used.

For short periods, lactated Ringer's solution or 0.9% saline solution can be substituted. The latter is frequently used when there is a metabolic alkalosis, and bicarbonate removal is the treatment goal. Care should be taken in giving an appropriate balance of solutions in any hemofiltrative therapy. Patients frequently develop a sodium deficit if all infusion solutions are not converted to normal saline. Patients receiving parenteral nutrition also should have the sodium concentration of the solution increased. Calcium and magnesium levels should be monitored closely, and replacement should be initiated at an early stage. Because therapy is effective in removing phosphate, deficiencies develop, requiring some sort of supplementation.

As a general rule, to avoid undue hemoconcentration, the filtration rate for postdilutional hemofiltration should be no more than 15% of plasma flow through the filter. A 30% filtration fraction may be allowed in predilutional techniques.

Hemodialysate fluids tend to be less varied, but a clear understanding of the desired therapy end point is still an important determinant of choice. One vital role of replacement and dialysate fluids is the replacement of endogenous bicarbonate lost in buffering acid and across the membrane (especially in filtrative modalities). A variety of strategies have been employed to this end, involving the use of bicarbonate or a bicarbonate generator—acetate, lactate, or citrate—in the fluid. Citrate plays a dual role as bicarbonate donor and anticoagulant when used as replacement solution[43] (for more detail see the section on anticoagulation). Acetate-based and lactate-based fluids are more stable than bicarbonate, and commercial versions are readily available as IHD or peritoneal dialysis formulations.

Acetate, although previously used extensively in long-term HD, may give rise to respiratory and vascular complications resulting from the supraphysiologic load of the buffer received during therapy.[44] The potential for vasodilation, myocardial depression, and increased oxygen consumption[45] suggests that its use should be avoided in CRRT for critically ill patients. Additionally, the use of lactate buffer in continuous venovenous hemofiltration (CVVH) has been shown to produce a significantly higher serum bicarbonate level and pH than does acetate.[46]

Lactate undergoes hepatic conversion to bicarbonate on an equimolar basis. Although more stable than bicarbonate, there are numerous theoretical disadvantages to its use in CRRT. Although bicarbonate-based and lactate-based solutions can correct acidosis, bicarbonate is preferred because lactate-buffered fluids may require intravenous bicarbonate supplementation to achieve the same bicarbonate level.[47] The metabolism of exogenous lactate may be impaired in critical illness, with accumulation giving rise to a paradoxic metabolic acidosis.[48] Hyperlactatemia carries with it potential negative hemodynamic effects[49] and metabolic complications, including increased protein catabolism and reduced adenosine triphosphate regeneration.[44] Complications of lactate overload are more likely to develop in patients with liver impairment and poor peripheral perfusion, particularly with high-volume treatment.[50] Lactate intolerance is defined arbitrarily as a greater than 5 mmol/L increase in lactate levels during therapy. Lactate solutions developed for use in peritoneal dialysis carry significant glucose loads (the osmotic agent used to drive transperitoneal UF). The use of fluids with glucose concentrations greater than 1.5% should be avoided to minimize glucose loading.

Bicarbonate, although the more physiologic anion, also has specific drawbacks. It exists in solution with other ions in a state of equilibrium under specific physical conditions of temperature and pressure: $CO_2 + H_2O \leftrightarrow H_2CO_3 \leftrightarrow H^+ + HCO_3^-$. When CO_2 outgassing from the solution occurs (e.g., delivering bicarbonate using an open-top container), overall bicarbonate concentration may be reduced. Additionally, calcium and magnesium can precipitate out as insoluble carbonate compounds when sterilized with the buffer. Many bicarbonate-based solutions are produced with lower concentrations of both cations to help ameliorate this problem, with final mixing of the electrolyte and bicarbonate solutions just before use. A novel adaptation has electrolyte and bicarbonate solutions housed and sterilized in separate chambers of the same bag. A connecting valve is broken just before use to mix the two fluids. A final caveat to the use of bicarbonate is its apparent predilection to bacterial growth—at least in liquid bicarbonate concentrates used in long-term dialysis[51,52]—although microbial contamination is not confined to this particular base.[53]

There is a paucity of comparative studies examining the impact of base in patients undergoing CRRT. One prospective, randomized study comparing lactate (44.5 mmol/L)–buffered and bicarbonate (40 mmol/L)–buffered CVVH found equivalent degrees of correction of acidosis at 24-hour follow-up without differences in hemodynamics or oxygen transport characteristics.[54] Lactate levels were significantly higher in the lactate-buffered group. There were no subjects with a primary diagnosis of hepatic failure, however. A longer term, randomized, crossover study in CVVH also compared lactate (44.5 mmol/L) with bicarbonate (34.5 mmol/L).[55] Patients with hepatic failure were excluded. There were no differences in hemodynamics, "azotemic control," ammonia, glucose, pH, or base excess. Nitrogen excretion was increased in the first 4 days of therapy by lactate buffer (suggesting increased protein catabolism), however, and lactate levels were significantly higher during lactate-buffered therapy (although still remaining within normal limits and showing an overall decline in both groups). Bicarbonate levels were significantly higher in lactate-buffered therapy, probably as a result of the higher provision of bicarbonate substrate in this group. A subsequent study[56] of the effects of 40 mmol/L of bicarbonate found higher patient bicarbonate levels than had been achieved in the earlier comparison, although it was unclear what format the later study took in terms of control and patient population. The authors speculated that apparent lactate tolerance may have resulted from a lower rate of exposure despite an overall lactate load equivalent to that in IHD, where overt hyperlactatemia may develop, especially in the presence of hepatic failure.[49]

A large retrospective analysis examined patients with progressive lactic acidosis or lactate intolerance after receiving lactate-buffered CVVH.[57] Commencement or substitution of bicarbonate-based CVVH never failed to restore and maintain normal arterial pH and base deficit. A small pediatric series of continuous arteriovenous hemodialysis (CAVHD) treatments showed that substitution of bicarbonate successfully increased pH and bicarbonate levels in metabolic acidosis unresponsive to acetate-buffered or lactate-buffered therapy.[58] Although these studies usually compare only the biochemical effects of the fluids, it also has been noted that bicarbonate-based fluids, compared with lactate-based fluids, reduce hypotensive events (systolic blood pressure <70 mm Hg) in critically ill patients on CVVH, with a trend toward a survival advantage in patients with a history of cardiac failure.[59]

From the limited data available, although it seems that lactate-based substitution or dialysate fluids may be used safely in many patients, they should be avoided in patients with lactic acidosis or hyperlactatemia and in patients with hepatic failure. Bicarbonate-buffered solutions should be used in these cases. The complexity of preparation of bicarbonate fluids, commercially or in the hospital pharmacy, adds significantly to the overall running costs of CRRT. Sterility must be the primary concern for bicarbonate *replacement* fluid, but at the Cleveland Clinic we have been producing bicarbonate *dialysate* for continuous venovenous hemodialysis (CVVHD) since 1993.[60] Briefly, reverse osmosis–treated water from the long-term dialysis unit is mixed with bicarbonate and acid concentrates within a single-pass, proportioning dialysis machine (Althin 1000; Althin CD Medical Inc, Miami, Fla). The resulting custom solution is ultrafiltered through an F80 polysulfone dialyzer (Fresenius AG, Bad Homburg, Germany) and collected in sterile plastic bags. The solution can be kept safely for 72 hours without precipitation or bacterial growth and comes at a fraction of the price of commercial or pharmacy-manufactured preparations.

Anticoagulation

Circuit clotting is the most frequent cause of therapy interruption in CRRT. In addition to the hypercoagulable state of a critically ill patient with ARF,[61] the technical factors discussed subsequently may promote system clotting within the extracorporeal circuit (Fig. 19-4).

Vascular access may create nonlaminar or turbulent flow, especially with the use of tapered, narrow-diameter devices and perhaps also in devices with double-D as opposed to double-O cross-sectional aspects. Disruption of laminar flow predisposes to circuit clotting and may be exacerbated by kinked or narrow blood tubing and the "sawtooth" pressure profile produced by the near-ubiquitous occlusive or partially occlusive roller-type pump.[61] The development of a nonocclusive bellows-type pump may ameliorate this problem.[61] The bioincompatible membrane and the air-blood interface of the venous bubble trap are two further foci for circuit clotting. Infusion of fluid directly into the bubble trap may help reduce the air-blood interface.[62] Substitution of the bubble trap with an air-porous plastic diaphragm may prove to be a more technically satisfying solution.[61] Finally, the hemoconcentration induced by high UF volumes in CVVH/continuous

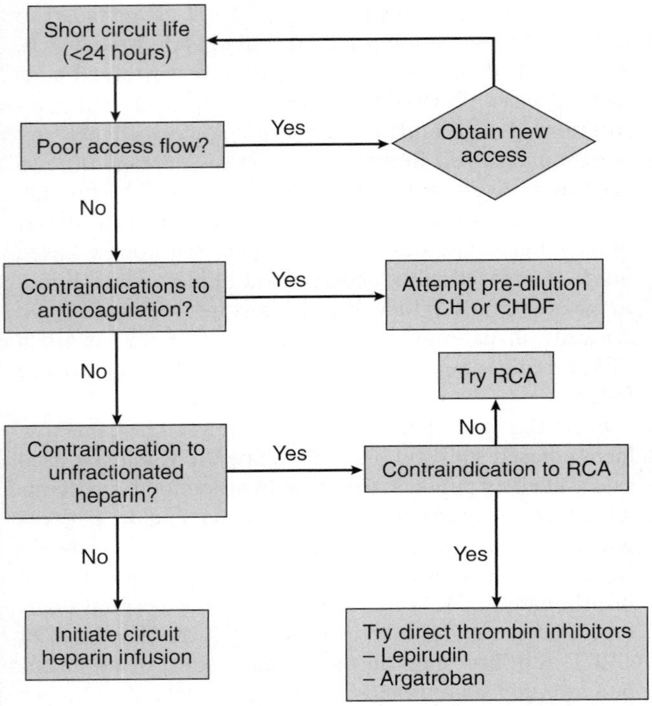

Figure 19-4. Algorithm for managing circuit longevity. CH, continuous hemofiltration; CHDF, continuous hemodiafiltration; RCA, regional citrate anticoagulation. (Adapted from Bartlett RH, Bosch J, Geronemus R, et al: Continuous arteriovenous hemofiltration for acute renal failure. ASAIO Trans 1988;34:67-77.)

venovenous hemodiafiltration (CVVHDF) promotes clotting, but may be minimized by predilutional fluid replacement (see later). This comes at the price, however, of the inefficiency of ultrafiltering a mixture of just-infused replacement fluid and plasma, the proportions of which are important considerations in the CRRT prescription.

Efforts to reduce extracorporeal circuit clotting traditionally have relied on the use of infusions of unfractionated heparin into its arterial limb. Unfractionated heparin should be administered postpump, if applicable, avoiding the danger of drawing excess anticoagulant into the circuit through high, negative, prepump pressures. Concerns about exacerbating existing bleeding tendencies in this critically ill population have led to the development of a variety of different schedules and alternatives (Box 19-1), none of which has gained widespread acceptance.[63]

Heparin, unfractionated and low-molecular-weight, is not effectively cleared by CRRT.[64] The most appropriate dose of the standard prefilter heparin infusion is still unclear and probably represents a balance between maintenance of the CRRT circuit and the perceived risks of bleeding in the individual patient. Different groups support different approaches to heparin therapy with dosing either guided by the activated partial thromboplastin time (APTT) or administered at a standard rate, without regular APTT-guided adjustments.

One retrospective study found no differences in filter survival between patients receiving a low dose of heparin (100 to 700 IU/h) and patients receiving a high, cumulative dose (>700 IU/h).[65] The high-dose group included patients receiving systemic heparin for non–CRRT-related indications and patients whose prefilter dose had been increased because of frequent clotting. The inference from this study is that increasing heparin dose is efficacious in prolonging circuit life in patients who are frequent clotters. No clear differences were found in terms of bleeding complications, but patients were not matched between each group, and patients perceived to be at high risk of bleeding would not have been included in either. Subsequent to this study, it has been observed that in patients for whom the only circuit-maintenance strategy was regular saline flushes, the patients receiving systemic heparin for non–CRRT-related indications were at lower risk of circuit clotting.[65]

Other retrospective work has looked at the effects of activated partial thromboplastin time (APTT)-targeted prefilter therapy in predilutional continuous arteriovenous hemofiltration (CAVH) or continuous AV HDF.[39] In this study, the systemic APTT was checked every 6 hours, and heparin infusion was adjusted to maintain values in the 40- to 50-second range. In comparing therapies with achieved APTTs of 15 to 35 seconds with therapies with values of 45 to 55 seconds, there were significant differences in the crude incidence of filter clotting (17.7/1000 hours versus 9/1000 hours) and of patient hemorrhage (2.9/1000 hours versus 7.4/1000 hours). For every 10-second increase in APTT, the risk of filter clotting decreased by 25%, but the risk of patient hemorrhage increased by 50%. There was no correlation between either end point and the administered dose of heparin. The authors believed that safety and efficacy were optimal at an APTT of 35 to 45 seconds, although they noted that there was no threshold value below which heparin was safe. The predilutional mode of fluid replacement might have produced results that could be quite different with other techniques. Incidentally, the administration of coumarin derivatives seemed to decrease the incidence of filter clotting twofold, without increasing the crude incidence of hemorrhage, raising interesting questions as to

Box 19-1

Current Strategies to Prevent Continuous Renal Replacement Therapy Circuit Clotting

- Heparin
  - Standard, prefilter
  - Regional
  - Low dose, prefilter
  - Systemic
- Low-molecular-weight heparin
- Citrate
- Prostacyclin
- Hirudin
- Heparin bonding
- Serine protease inhibitors
- No anticoagulation
  - Saline solution flushes
  - No intervention

the role of the extrinsic coagulation pathway in extracorporeal circuit clotting.

Modifications of the standard prefilter heparin infusion have included regional heparinization,[19,66] in which postfilter protamine administration is intended to reverse prefilter anticoagulation. Such an improvement may provide improvements in filter survival over low-dose heparinization (500 IU/h), but without any clear benefits in terms of hemorrhagic complications.[19] Difficulties in maintaining an appropriate balance between heparin and protamine administration may lead to ineffective heparin reversal or protamine-induced anticoagulation. An adequate mean filter survival of 31.4 hours with prefilter infusion of 500 IU/h heparin in CVVHDF seems to justify preferential use of the low-dose method over the complex regional technique.[19]

Low-molecular-weight heparins have good antithrombotic activity and a reduced risk of bleeding compared with unfractionated heparin, at least in long-term dialysis (see references 8 and 9 in de Pont and colleagues[67]). Dalteparin, enoxaparin, and nadroparin were used in five studies.[68] Dalteparin probably can be used as a bolus of about 20 U/kg followed by an infusion of 10 IU/kg/h for adequate anticoagulation without an excess of bleeding in CVVHDF.[69] In patients with heparin-induced thrombocytopenia, there is likely cross-reactivity with unfractionated heparin, and low-molecular-weight heparins probably should not be used; also, prostacyclin was reported unhelpful.[70] In a study with CVVHD, a dalteparin dose of 35 IU/kg bolus followed by 13 IU/kg/h had good filter patency rates, but there were bleeding episodes.[71] At a lower dose of 8 IU/kg bolus and infusion of 5 IU/kg/h, however, circuit life was poor. Enoxaparin and nadroparin also may be used, but the experience is limited.[67,72] Lower dose dalteparin (8 IU/kg bolus and 5 IU/kg/h) may lead to more marked clotting and reduced clearances in CVVHD.[71] The type of low-molecular-weight heparin seems not to be important.[67]

Prostacyclin (prostaglandin I_2) is a potent, short-acting, endogenous inhibitor of platelet aggregation whose anticoagulant properties leave the intrinsic coagulation system intact. A half-life of 2 minutes and antiaggregatory properties lasting only 30 minutes[73] make it potentially useful in patients at risk of bleeding. Drawbacks include its expense and systemic vasodilatory properties, which could limit its use in critically ill patients. Although prostacyclin binds to albumin and platelet surface membranes, 30% may be cleared during CRRT techniques.[74]

With these considerations in mind, a prospective, randomized, controlled trial compared anticoagulation with the use of prostacyclin alone (7.7 ng/kg/min), with heparin alone (6 IU/kg/h), and with prostacyclin plus heparin (6.4 ng/kg/min and 5 IU/kg/h) in CVVH.[75] All were administered prefilter. The prostacyclin-alone group showed significant reductions in mean arterial pressure and systemic and pulmonary vascular resistance. Hemodynamics remained stable in the other two groups. Mean hemofilter duration was longest in the prostacyclin plus heparin group. No major or clinically important bleeding occurred in any study group. Because heparin may be insufficient to inhibit platelet aggregation and could actually induce it (see references 10 and 14 in the Langenecker and coworkers study[75]), the authors speculated on the additive role of prostacyclin.

A combination of prostacyclin (4 ng/kg/min) and low-molecular-weight heparin (enoxaparin, 25 μg/kg/h) preserved CVVH hemofilter function better than unfractionated heparin (9 IU/kg/h) without inducing bleeding or hypotension.[76] A comparison of prostacyclin (starting systemically at 2 ng/kg/min, increasing to 5 ng/kg/min, then switching to prefilter) and unfractionated heparin (maintaining thrombotest at 100 to 160 seconds) found better filter survival with the former in pumpless AV techniques and equivalence in pump-assisted modes.[77] This patient population, with combined acute renal and hepatic failure and abnormal baseline coagulation, showed more clinically important bleeding with heparin. Systemic infusion of prostacyclin caused hemodynamic instability and increased intracranial pressure, but these were not sustained after switching to prefilter administration.

Combined prefilter administration of prostaglandin E_1 and unfractionated heparin can significantly prolong hemofilter life without compromising hemodynamics or causing clinically important bleeding.[78] With its half-life of less than 1 minute, prostaglandin E_1 may provide a suitable alternative to prostacyclin, although comparative studies have yet to be performed in CRRT.

Regional citrate anticoagulation provides the second alternative to heparin therapy. Regional citrate anticoagulation may be performed using 4% trisodium citrate or with ACD-A solution (Anticoagulant Citrate Dextrose Form A) containing 3% combined trisodium citrate (2.2 g/100 mL), citric acid (0.73 g/100 mL), and dextrose (2.45 g/100 mL) (Baxter-Fenwal Healthcare Corp, Deerfield, Ill). ACD-A is preferred over trisodium citrate for routine regional citrate anticoagulation because it is less hypertonic and commercially prepared, potentially reducing mixing errors and the complications associated with overinfusion. Regional citrate anticoagulation protocols differ in the type of citrate preparation used, the mode of dialysis, and the ability to customize dialysis solutions.[43,79-85] The anticoagulant effect is neutralized when returning citrated, extracorporeal blood dilutes in the central venous pool, and any degree of ionized hypocalcemia is returned to normal via a separate, central venous infusion.[43,79] The technique requires frequent monitoring of the serum ionized calcium to titrate citrate dose within a therapeutic range. The major complications of regional citrate anticoagulation are hypocalcemia and metabolic alkalosis from citrate toxicity, particularly in patients with liver dysfunction,[86,87] and long-term regional citrate anticoagulation for CRRT may mask the immobilization hypercalcemia of critically ill patients causing a decrease in calcium infusion requirements and subsequent excessive bone resorption resulting in fractures.[88]

Hepatic, renal, and skeletal muscle metabolism of citrate to bicarbonate returns levels to normal within 30 minutes of stopping the infusion.[89] Use of this technique can minimize[89] or prevent bleeding complications, while achieving a mean filter survival of 30 hours to 4 days.[43,79,89]

Disadvantages include the need for regular monitoring of ionized calcium and a separate central venous access for calcium infusion, the risk of metabolic alkalosis (corrected by hydrogen chloride infusion[79]), and the need for special low-sodium dialysate and replacement fluids without alkali buffer or calcium. Citrate also is extensively cleared through the filter, especially with dialytic techniques, and may be poorly metabolized in patients with severe hepatic failure and lactic acidosis.[90]

Other anticoagulative methods that have been used in CRRT include the direct thrombin inhibitors recombinant hirudin (lepirudin)[91] and argatroban and the serine protease inhibitor nafamostat.[92] Lepirudin is mainly eliminated by the kidneys, and the dose is adjusted according to residual renal and dialysis clearance. It is administered as a continuous infusion or in repeated boluses with typical doses of 0.005 to 0.025 mg/kg/body weight per hour. The anticoagulative effect is monitored by measuring APTT, aiming to keep it at about 1.5 to 2 times normal.[88,93] After more than 5 days of lepirudin use, antilepirudin antibodies may develop, and these enhance the effects of lepirudin such that a dose reduction is required to decrease the risk of bleeding.[94] Daily APTT measurements are recommended during prolonged therapy. Argatroban is eliminated predominantly by liver metabolism and biliary secretion.[95] It is initiated at 0.5 to 1 μg/kg/min, using lower doses in patients with hepatic dysfunction. The anticoagulation effect also is monitored by measuring APTT. Bleeding resulting from overdosage of lepirudin or argatroban may be treated with the administration of fresh frozen plasma. Hemofiltration with high-flux dialyzers also can reduce the plasma levels of hirudin.

Heparin-bonded filters and other nonthrombogenic materials have been investigated for use in long-term dialysis. Their precise role in CRRT is unclear, although one group used a lower technology approach by temporarily adsorbing heparin to polysulfone and Hemophan membranes by recirculating heparinized saline solution through them before use.[62]

The final approach to preventing clotting in the extracorporeal circuit is that of no anticoagulation, with or without regular flushes with saline solution.[96] Since our institution changed its practice to CVVHD, no-heparin, no-flush circuit maintenance has been sustained with a rigorous preventive strategy performed by renal technical staff: Individual components of the extracorporeal circuit are changed at the first signs of clotting and before the circuit as a whole shuts down. Overall therapy downtime is minimized, and near-continuity of the system is achieved. Others, in a randomized, controlled trial, have looked at different schedules of prescribed blood flow and saline flush frequency during CVVHD[65] and found that 100-mL hourly saline solution flushes at a blood flow of 125 mL/min sustained filter survival as effectively as a more intense flush and flow schedule (blood flow rates of 200 to 250 mL/min and 100-mL saline flushes twice hourly). Mean filter survival was 23 hours. Although the advantages of saline flush techniques seem clear, disadvantages include the need for increased UF, the risk of dialyzer fiber rupture, and the extra nursing workload.

Our current approach at the Cleveland Clinic is to start all CVVHD patients on prefilter, unfractionated heparin at 250 IU/h, checking the APTT after 6 hours and then daily to ensure values stay below two to three times normal. In patients with contraindications or who are systemically anticoagulated, a no-heparin, no-flush approach is used.

Thrombocytopenia may develop during heparin therapy in two separate manifestations.[70] In the first, termed *heparin-induced thrombocytopenia type I*, the reduction in platelet count is often time-dependent and dose-dependent and responds to a simple dose reduction. In the second, heparin-induced thrombocytopenia type II, platelet aggregation and activation may occur in 1% of patients receiving porcine heparin.[70,97] This is usually associated with the development of heparin-associated antibodies to the heparin–platelet factor 4 complex 5 to 12 days after starting heparin therapy.[70] Paradoxic thrombosis and hemorrhage may occur. Platelet aggregation studies are highly specific, but lack sensitivity, so if they and heparin-induced platelet activation tests yield negative results, an enzyme-linked immunosorbent assay should be performed.[70,97] If heparin-induced thrombocytopenia type II is confirmed, heparin therapy should be discontinued. Prostacyclin[97] and synthetic heparinoids[70] may be useful substitutes for heparin, although occasional antibody cross-reactivity with the latter[98] may be problematic.

Regional citrate anticoagulation offers a third alternative, although our approach is to adopt a no-anticoagulant approach. Frequent cross-reactivity with low-molecular-weight heparins[98] may preclude their use in heparin-induced thrombocytopenia type II. See Chapter 79 for further discussion of heparin-induced thrombocytopenia.

THERAPEUTIC CONSIDERATIONS

In assessing the need for CRRT, one should consider renal and nonrenal conditions. The systemic effects of the various forms of continuous renal therapies should be evaluated as a therapeutic end and a possible cause of further compromise. Although there may be one overriding need at one particular time in the course of a patient's disease, that need may change rapidly, and the form of applied therapy should respond to that change. Although the following descriptions are formulated on the "pure" state, such an entity rarely exists in ICU patients. Combination therapies are usual among ICU patients with complicated and uncomplicated status.

Ultrafiltration

Fluid removal or control is the most frequently requested application for dialytic intervention and is considered the simplest form of continuous therapy. Fluid is drawn from the blood space across a relatively tight semipermeable membrane and so has the characteristics of plasma water. With knowledge of the sieving coefficients of a particular membrane for various solutes, the ultrafiltrate can be used to determine the composition of serum and can help avoid an excessive number of blood draws.

In prescribing UF, a specific volume of fluid loss should be determined, with the UF rate (Q_F) set to achieve that loss in a desired time frame. It cannot be overemphasized that this form of therapy is by nature *slow*. The steady, constant loss of fluid at a rate that does not exceed the plasma-refilling rate gives this form of therapy its stability. If extremely rapid UF in a short time frame is the therapeutic intent, intermittent forms of pump-driven UF are the treatment of choice.

The artificial membranes usually employed have a high UF coefficient (K_{Uf}), allowing water to pass quite freely. Any pressure difference between the blood side and the ultrafiltrate side of the filter results in fluid passage. Higher pressures in the blood compartment of the filter, in pumped and pumpless techniques, result in net fluid flow from the blood to the ultrafiltrate compartment. This flow is enhanced by applying negative pressures to the ultrafiltrate compartment through gravity (by altering the vertical distance between filter and drainage bag) or by pumped mechanical suction. This pressure should be held constant and not be subject to rapid variations. It is recommended that a peristaltic–type IV infusion pump be used in an effort to avoid the rapid fluid withdrawal that accompanies syringe-type pumps. The high transmembrane pressures that result may lead to membrane rupture and blood loss.

Common UF rates range from 100 to 400 mL/h. Larger amounts may be obtained if there is a need for rapid fluid removal. Automated continuous machines control UF through a volume-driven system, establishing a fixed loss of some determined amount of fluid from the system over a given period (usually on an hourly basis). These systems are much more accurate in their measurements than the infusion-pump systems described earlier. When using these infusion pumps, a secondary, direct measure of UF volume should be set in place to serve as a check on actual volume removed.

The blood flow rate (Q_B) has a significant effect on any UF system. During either spontaneous (AV) or pumped (VV) therapy, some measurement of plasma flow needs to be established. This is easily determined and regulated with a blood pump by knowing the stroke volume (SV) of the pump segment and multiplying this value by the number of revolutions per minute (rpm):

$$Q_B = SV \times rpm$$

During AV treatments, this value can only be estimated. Given a fixed rate of UF in milliliters per minute (Q_F) and having determined the hematocrit immediately before (Hct_i) and after (Hct_o) the filter during UF, then:

$$Q_B = (Q_F \times Hct_o)/(Hct_i - Hct_o)$$

When performed in the clinical arena, there may be large variations in the hematocrit level that frequently lead to fallacious readings. For this reason, several simultaneous draws should be made at each site, and the *average* hematocrit level used in the formula. Plasma flow (Q_P) can now be determined:

$$Q_P = Q_B - Hct_i$$

and ultimately the filtration fraction (FF) at which the system is operating can be calculated:

$$FF = Q_F/Q_P$$

Careful attention should be given to the amount of access recirculation. Rates greater than 15% are associated with a greater incidence of clotting. This tendency is more evident at higher UF rates (>300 mL/h), at which the returning blood tends to be more inspissated, creating a more viscous, afferent blood flow. As was noted earlier, the system should be kept below a filtration fraction of 15% in postdilution and 30% in predilution hemofiltration for efficient operation and a lower risk of clotting.

Hemofiltration

When the rate of fluid removal is increased such that replacement fluid infusions are required, one has begun the process of hemofiltration or plasma water exchange. Fluid replacement can be delivered into the blood circuit either prefilter, before UF has occurred (predilutional hemofiltration), or after fluid has been removed by the filter (postdilutional hemofiltration).

With the predilutional format, ultrafiltrated fluid reflects the mixture of blood and replacement solution. To use ultrafiltrate as a surrogate for blood sampling (see previous discussion) would be problematic because correction has to be made for the degree of dilution and for the electrolytic composition of the replacement fluid. Because the oncotic pressure of blood would be much reduced within the filter, a greater rate of fluid removal is possible at the same transmembrane hydrostatic pressure. This increased rate of fluid removal is offset by dilution of plasma solute, such that overall mass transfer of uremic toxins is reduced, and higher rates of fluid exchange are required to compensate. It is common to have exchange rates of 30 to 40 L/d, with transmembrane pressure gradients usually being augmented with the help of a filtrate pump (see earlier discussion).

Some authors[27,99] have advocated this predilutional technique for patients with low AV flow rates or for patients with high hematocrit levels in an effort to reduce clotting episodes. We have not been able to substantiate a clinically significant reduction in system clotting compared with the more easily managed postdilutional method.

Postdilutional fluid replacement has the advantage of being easier to perform with lower rates of fluid exchange compared with the predilutional system. Because solute transport is predominantly achieved by convection, the solute flux across the membrane is proportional to the UF rate (Q_F) and the sieving coefficient of that particular molecule, so:

$$Cl = Q_F \times S_{coef}$$

If clearance by hemofiltration is standardized to the clearance of urea (which has a sieving coefficient of 1), the fluid exchange rate and urea clearance are equal. In a postdilutional system, Q_F equals hemofiltrative clearance.

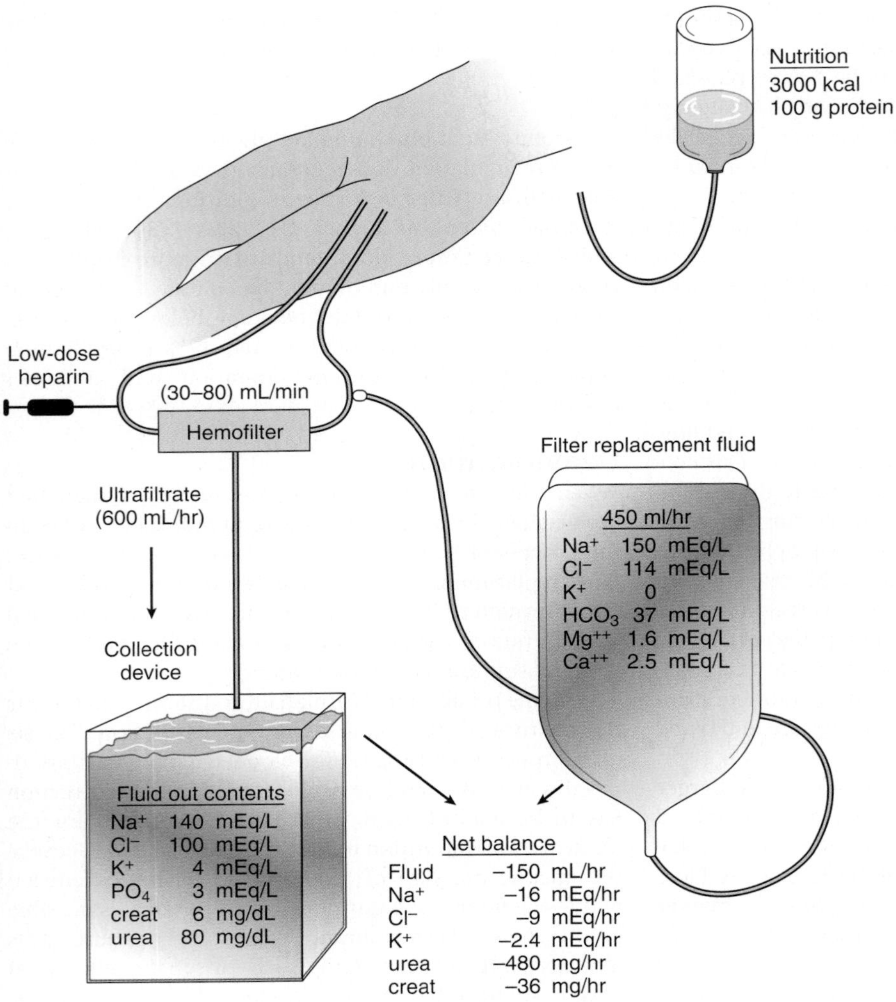

Figure 19-5. Net balance of fluid, electrolytes, and waste products during a typical hemofiltration process. (Adapted from Bartlett RH, Bosch J, Geronemus R, et al: Continuous arteriovenous hemofiltration for acute renal failure. ASAIO Trans 1988;34:67-77.)

One problem with this form of replacement is the increased oncotic pressures noted at the venous end of the filter. With high rates of exchange or high degrees of access recirculation, blood viscosity may be increased to the extent that clotting may occur. Fluid exchange rates may ultimately be dictated by such factors as hematocrit, blood flow, and access recirculation.

In terms of solute clearances, the end point of hemofiltrative therapy is dictated by the balance between elements removed with the ultrafiltrate and the elements replaced with the substitution fluid. Figure 19-5 shows the interplay between various elements in a postdilutional CAVH system.[100] The addition of a blood pump to the circuit has the advantage of increasing the blood flow, allowing higher filtration rates. The use of infusion pumps for the delivery of replacement solution and for control of UF rates allows for precise prospective balancing of fluid and solute.

Hemodialysis

Maintaining the same basic blood flow circuit but using the filter in a different manner, diffusion dialysis can be performed. The flow of dialysate should be countercurrent to that of blood to maximize transmembrane concentration differences across all blood concentrations and at all levels of the kidney. Blood flow (100 to 300 mL/min) is maintained well above the usual dialysate flow rates (15 to 30 mL/min), in contradistinction to IHD, where blood rather than dialysate flow is the limiting factor in diffusive clearance. Clearance of low-molecular-weight substances (e.g., urea, creatinine) is "flow-dependent" because there is little resistance to transmembrane movement posed by the porous membrane itself. Substances of larger molecular weight (e.g., β_2-microglobulin, vitamin B_{12}) are relatively slow in crossing the dialyzer membrane and are "membrane-dependent" molecules. Using the high-flux membrane characteristics generally employed with continuous therapies, substances with molecular weights of 20,000 to 30,000 daltons (D) are transferred at rates that bear an inverse relationship to their molecular weights. This relationship may not be as marked as in other dialytic techniques, which often use membranes of tighter pore size.

Electrolytes, urea, and creatinine easily cross membranes at a rate that is directly proportional to membrane surface area, temperature, and concentration difference, and inversely proportional to viscosity, distance from the membrane, and molecular size. Changing the concentration of various elements in the dialysate alters solute balance. Balance is achieved, however, only between transferable particles. Bound elements do not play a role in creating the concentration differences that drive molecular movement, whereas the free elements are the key players in this transfer. This concept is the basis for altered drug kinetics when patients are subjected to continuous supportive therapy (see later).

Dialysate flow rates remain the most influential factor determining urea clearance.[101] Dialysate usually is delivered via infusion pumps at rates of 15 to 30 mL/min. Given adequate blood flow through the circuit, one can see why the limiting factor for flow-dependent transfer is the relatively low dialysate flow rate. Differing kidney geometry, altering blood flow, or changing membrane type would have only limited effects on the diffusion of molecules compared with the potential of dialysate flow changes.

Dialysate delivery systems consisting of infusion pumps in parallel can be set to deliver 2000 mL/h or more to the dialysate inflow port of the artificial kidney. The dialysate outflow also must be controlled. By setting the outflow rate higher than dialysate inflow rates, one can create a negative transmembrane pressure promoting UF across the dialysis membrane. This difference in flow is used to establish the rate of UF. An increase or decrease in this flow difference would increase or decrease the rate of fluid loss. There also are dramatic differences among commercially available continuous therapy delivery machines. Although some alter the UF rate by changing the outflow rate (Q_{DO}) against a fixed inflow rate (Q_{DI}) to achieve the required UF, others keep the outflow rate fixed and alter the dialysate inflow rate. The fixed outflow rate sees no change in the clearance rates with increasing or decreasing UF rates used, but the variable outflow rates change the system clearances as they change the UF rates (see later). Because dialysate flow is external to and independent of blood flow, one may see continued dialysate flow in a system with virtually no blood flow. This difference is frequently not appreciated by the bedside personnel who may equate dialysate flow to hemofiltrative fluid exchanges. The former relates to dialysate compartment flows only, whereas the latter depends on blood flow. Although decreases in hemofiltration flow rate may herald system clotting, dialysate flow rate changes have no predictive value for clotting and may continue despite total blood-side occlusion.

Understanding the delivered dose of therapy has been a focus of extensive discussion. The continuous nature of this technique offers advantages over the more traditional intermittent delivery systems; when comparison of kinetics (and clearances) is attempted, differences occur. In continuous dialysis, dialyzer urea clearance (K_D) can be calculated as:

$$K_D = Q_{DO} \times (C_{DO}/C_P)$$

where Q_{DO} is dialysate outflow rate, C_{DO} is dialysate outlet urea concentration, and C_P is plasma urea concentration. During the life span of a continuous treatment, the urea kinetic relationship can be seen as a single pool. Modeling of CVVHD may follow a simplistic formulation: Using the steady-state blood urea concentration (equivalent to the time averaged concentration of urea [TAC_{UREA}]), the clearance of the CVVHD system, and the residual renal clearance, urea generation can be determined, providing an insight into the state of catabolism of the patient. This approach does not equate to dialysis dose delivery because the urea volume of distribution also must be known. Further confounders include therapy interruptions, hyperalimentation, and changes in its prescription.

In terms of delivered dose, a specific dose-outcome relationship has yet to be fully determined for CRRT. A retrospective analysis showing an improved survival with increased delivered dialysis[102] has been confirmed in a prospective trial with hemofiltration.[103] A statistical improvement in outcome was observed among patients randomly assigned to hemofiltrative clearances of 35 to 45 mL/kg dry body weight per hour versus the more usual 20 mL/kg/h. Increased dose and individualization of dose seem to be important.

Continuous Renal Replacement Therapy versus Intermittent Therapy

There are many theoretical benefits that may favor the use of CRRT over intermittent forms of therapy, such as improved hemodynamic stability and increased dialysis dose delivery. Clinical trials that would allow an evidence-based assessment of these potential advantages are lacking. This section critically examines perceived advantages of CRRT in terms of hemodynamics, dose delivery, and outcome and includes a brief discourse on the use of severity scoring systems in ARF. (A more detailed analysis of dosing precedes this section, and a critique of the role of CRRT in cytokine removal is provided in the section on nonrenal application of continuous therapies.)

Hemodynamic stability may be the sine qua non for the use of CRRT over intermittent modalities. Slower removal of solute and fluid from the intravascular space by continuous techniques should allow adequate time for refilling from the interstitium and intracellular space, theoretically minimizing therapy-induced hypotension. This theory seems to have been borne out by studies that have shown IHD-resistant fluid overload in ARF can respond well to slow continuous ultrafiltration (SCUF), allowing enhanced nutrition and drug delivery,[104] and that cardiac index may be improved by fluid removal during CAVH.[105] There are longer term implications for renal recovery, with IHD-related hemodynamic instability potentially predisposing to recurrent renal injury.[106] The data from rigorous, comparative studies seem to lead to varying conclusions, however.

Perhaps the most convincing work in favor of CRRT comes from Davenport and colleagues,[107] who, confirming earlier findings,[108] showed better hemodynamic tolerance during the first 5 hours of CAVH/CAVHD than in 4-hour IHD sessions in unstable patients with combined acute renal and hepatic failure. Oxygen delivery and consumption also were better maintained in the CRRT group. This study, although prospective, was not fully randomized, with patients with increased intracranial pressure being diverted to the continuous therapy arm (although this should have biased results against CRRT).

Other data have failed to bear out these findings. Misset and coworkers,[109] in a randomized crossover study, compared hemodynamic tolerance during 24-hour periods of CAVH and 24-hour periods encompassing a 4-hour IHD treatment. Each period was separated by a 24-hour washout. There were no differences in any of the hemodynamic variables measured, although a 31% dropout rate (mostly early deaths) could potentially have selected out patients who might have shown a modality-specific response. In addition, discrete hypotensive episodes were not reported and may have been missed if not picked up in the course of regular hemodynamic monitoring. Other comparative studies, although showing greater hemodynamic instability with intermittent therapies, have been hampered by their retrospective and nonrandomized nature.[110,111]

Noncomparative data have been published that may support the improved hemodynamic tolerability of modern IHD techniques. A prospective, single-center analysis of all intermittent treatments for ARF showed that of the 7.9% of sessions terminated prematurely, only half of these were because of hypotension.[112] The authors concluded that modern intermittent methods could provide excellent hemodynamic stability, although there was no indication of the incidence of discrete episodes of intradialytic hypotension that did not require discontinuation of therapy.

At present, concrete evidence confirming the hemodynamic superiority of continuous techniques over intermittent techniques is lacking, although intuition sways toward this position. The development of complementary technologies, such as sodium and UF profiling and online optical hematocrit monitoring of plasma volume, may enhance further the tolerability of intermittent therapy.[113]

Assessment of dose delivery is covered in detail elsewhere in this chapter, but it is worthwhile noting that theoretical comparisons of actual solute removal—the gold standard for dialysis dosing—show continuous techniques can deliver a given dose with greater ease.[8] Intermittent therapy may have to be provided at a high frequency to produce equivalent levels of solute removal.[114] Such theoretical considerations do not take into account interruptions to continuous therapy, however, which would reduce delivered dialysis dose. In practice, none of the numerous published comparative articles on acute dialysis modality has adequately corrected for delivered dose. Comparisons of absolute blood solute levels[110,115,116] may fail to account for interindividual and intraindividual variations in solute generation[117] or solute volume of distribution,[118] which may be large in the critically ill patient population.

Jakob and associates[119] examined patient outcome in an extensive review of studies dealing with CRRT. Of the 67 published studies that were available at the time (1996), only 15 were comparative. In only three of these[107,108,120] were both modality groups studied prospectively, with only one study[120] showing a significantly lower mortality rate with CRRT. No study had complete randomization. Small numbers hampered many studies. Incomplete descriptions of patient populations and dialysis therapy were widespread. In the 12 studies in which filter type was recorded, none applied the same filter across modalities: Biocompatible membranes tended to be used in CRRT, and bioincompatible membranes tended to be used in intermittent therapies. Two of the 15 comparative studies[115,116] used a "conventional dialysis" group as historical controls and included patients receiving peritoneal dialysis and adjunctive SCUF, making it difficult to draw valid conclusions. Renal recovery was addressed in only two of the studies, with no definite conclusions being drawn. While acknowledging their methodologic problems, the authors combined all 15 comparative studies for further analysis. No clear benefit of CRRT could be found despite adjustment for comorbidities. In meta-analyses, one study did not show an advantage of CRRT over IHD, but another showed a small survival advantage with CRRT over IHD.[121,122] It has been suggested, however, that CRRT may improve renal recovery from ARF.[123]

At this point, it is worthwhile examining severity scoring systems and their role in ICU ARF. General severity scoring systems, such as APACHE (Acute Physiology, Age, and Chronic Health Evaluation) II, can underestimate risk of death when used in the context of ARF.[2,124] The development of a variety of ARF-specific risk models has generally led to a much closer fit between predicted and actual mortality.[2] This increased predictive accuracy may be explained in two ways: First, it may reflect prognostic factors brought into play in the presence of ARF that are not completely represented in general ICU models[2]; second, certain general models designed for use in the first 24 hours after admission to the ICU may be less valid than models designed to follow subjects throughout their ICU stay, especially models used from the time of first dialysis.[2] van Bommel and coworkers[125] suggested that the APACHE II score around the time of dialysis initiation may be more predictive of outcome than the same score, taken conventionally, at the time of ICU admission. Even then, the score performed suboptimally. We have found the APACHE II at dialysis initiation not to predict outcome.[102] The van Bommel group also found that the ratio of APACHE II at the time of dialysis initiation to that at ICU admission (AP_2/AP_1) was highly predictive of death.[125]

ARF-specific models may not be the panacea that first appearances might suggest, however. Even models with good performance within their own institution may perform suboptimally outside of it,[102,124] suggesting that they describe patient groups, rather than the individual outcome expectation.[102]

Definitive data to support many of the suspected advantages of CRRT are still lacking. Interpretation of much of the published data has been hampered by retrospective analysis, the use of historical controls, incomplete randomization, incomplete descriptions of patient populations and dialysis dose delivery, and study group–control group heterogeneity.

Box 19-2

Indications for Renal Support

- Fluid control
- Electrolyte balance
  - Hyperkalemia
  - Hyponatremia
  - Hyperphosphatemia
  - Hypermagnesemia
- Acid-base control
  - Metabolic acidosis
  - Mixed acidosis/alkalosis
  - Severe metabolic alkalosis
- Azotemia
- Uremic symptoms
  - Gastrointestinal upset
  - Obtundation
- Uremic signs
  - Pericarditis
  - Neuropathy
- Other
  - Toxin removal

Table 19-3. Clinical Considerations in Choice of Continuous or Intermittent Forms of Renal Support in the Intensive Care Unit

	Method of Delivery	
Condition	**Intermittent**	**Continuous**
Hemodynamic instability	No/yes	Yes
High fluid requirements	No/yes	Yes
High potassium generation	Yes	No
High catabolism	Yes	Yes/no
Peripheral vascular disease	Yes	Yes/no*
Global cardiac dysfunction	No/yes	Yes
Septic shock	No/yes	Yes
APACHE II >25	No/yes	Yes

*Arteriovenous may be contraindicated.

Table 19-4. Clinical Contraindications to the Use of Continuous Renal Replacement Therapy

	Arteriovenous Therapy	Venovenous Therapy
Relative		
Patient mobility	Yes	Yes/no
Short duration	Yes	No
Inexperience	Yes/no	Yes/no
Infrequent use	Yes/no	Yes/no
Bleeding tendency	Yes	No
Hypercatabolism	No	No
Absolute		
Severe atherosclerosis	Yes/no	No
Bypass graft (new)	Yes	No
Ischemic limb	Yes	No

As practicing clinicians, we make choices based on the best available evidence, but to build on undoubted progress in the acute dialysis field, it seems essential to establish common denominators, such as *who* (with valid severity scoring systems) and *what* (in terms of dose delivered) we are comparing. A large-scale multicenter study to describe a more global ICU ARF experience is needed. Validated ICU ARF patient severity scores and unifying dosing methodologies seem pivotal to any such approach.

In the absence of a solid evidence base, how should one decide between prescribing continuous or intermittent therapy? The basic indications for delivering renal support remain fairly constant (Box 19-2) and range from the most frequent request for fluid balance to more esoteric requirements such as toxin removal. Common considerations in choosing to apply intermittent or continuous support are listed in Table 19-3, being mindful of numerous relative and absolute contraindications to CRRT (Table 19-4).

We have used a more mechanistic approach in deciding which therapy to apply. In calculating the ratio of the APACHE II at renal consultation (A2) to that at ICU admission (A1)—A2 : A1—a value less than 1 suggests that a patient may be placed on intermittent therapy. With values greater than this, strong consideration is given to CRRT. An absolute APACHE score greater than 25 usually points toward the use of CRRT.

Continuous Hemodialysis versus Continuous Hemofiltration

When the decision has been made to proceed with continuous therapy, the next consideration is the particular form. Rate of catabolism, mean arterial pressure with resultant blood flow rates, UF rates required or desired, and access choice all influence this selection. The primary diagnosis also may have some influence on therapy type, especially in light of more recent data suggesting an improved outcome with the use of hemofiltration in some patients with multiple organ failure. Therapy effect on such vastly differing substances as urea and creatinine, molecules of "middle" molecular weight (β_2-microglobulin, vitamin B_{12}), cytokines (tumor necrosis factor-α, interleukins), or hormones (endothelin, angiotensin) is the subject of intense research on potential differences in therapy choice and its influence on patient outcome.[13,126]

Comparative data looking at relative efficiencies of the various forms of continuous therapies have been reported.[127-129] Figure 19-6 compares the theoretical urea clearance (in L/d) for hemofiltration, HD, and HDF, with AV and VV access.[130] Assuming a flawless period of therapy delivered by all forms, these rates would have a great influence on therapy choice. Circuit variations, anticoagulation, "downtime" of the differing techniques,

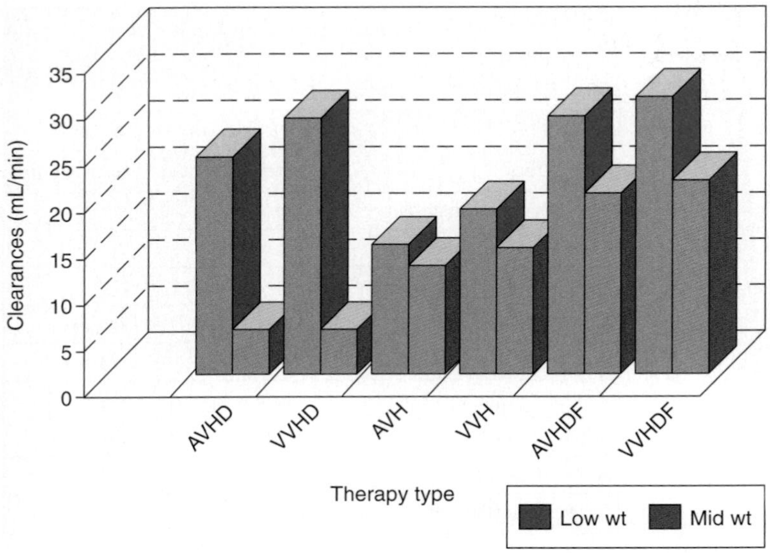

Figure 19-6. Comparative clearance rates of low-molecular-weight *(Low wt)* and middle-molecular-weight *(Mid wt)* substances with various forms of continuous renal support: arteriovenous and venovenous hemodialysis (AVHD and VVHD), arteriovenous and venovenous hemofiltration (AVH and VVH), and arteriovenous and venovenous hemodiafiltration (AVHDF and VVHDF). (Adapted from Sigler M, Teehan BP: Solute transport in slow continuous arteriovenous hemodialysis: An improved method for treating acute renal failure. Proceedings of the Third International Symposium on Acute Continuous Renal Replacement Therapy, Fort Lauderdale, Fla, 1987.)

clotting frequency, and blood and dialysate flow rates all should be considered in the choice, however. HD often exhibits a higher frequency of clotting than hemofiltration; VV techniques may do so more than AV modes. Such interruptions to therapy decrease overall treatment effectiveness.

Blood urea nitrogen and creatinine are frequently used as indicators of the need for renal support. Urea or creatinine appearance rates can be used as a gauge of the *quantity* of therapy required. "Galloping azotemia" (blood urea nitrogen increase ≥30 mg/dL/24 h; serum creatinine increase ≥3 mg/dL/24 h) may require diffusive rather than convective treatment for maintenance of a reasonable steady state. Patients with high urea generation rates should receive HD. When coupled with the need for large fluid losses, the choice becomes even more apparent. Because the only influence on urea removal in hemofiltration is fluid *exchange* rates, the increased need for fluid removal carries with it a need for greater differences in fluid exchanges, limiting the replacement volume. Given a maximal UF rate dictated by the system's blood flow rate (maximal filtration fraction) and by the patient's hematocrit level, solute clearances are restricted and may be inadequate for that particular patient's needs. Selection of HD allows for the UF rates needed without compromising solute clearance because dialysate flow rates are generally not as limited.

The influence of the dialysate rate on dialyzer clearance is depicted in Figure 19-7.[101] The higher the rate, the more effective the urea clearance, until one reaches a rate approximating the effective plasma flow of the system. With AV access systems, the maximal urea clearance expected would not generally exceed 28 ± 4 mL/min. Switching to a pump-driven system with the possibility of higher blood flows, one can effectively arrive at much higher values because the blood and the dialysate flow rates can be increased. One should realize, however, that the stability of continuous therapies lies in their low rates of exchange over a longer period. The increase in clearance rates must be balanced against the desire to provide stable therapy. If one desired a high rate of removal in a short time, the obvious choice would be some form of intermittent therapy.

A drawback to diffusive methods of delivery is the relatively low removal rates of the higher molecular weight substances. As noted earlier, convection provides greater clearance for substances 5000 to 20,000 D. HD may have limitations when the goal of therapy is targeted toward these larger molecules. This may be the basis for the early reports of improved outcome with patients who were subjected to HDF techniques. The removal of cytokines, the influence on endotoxin adsorption, and the ability to avoid the negative effect of backdiffusion of Limulus Amebacyte lystate-positive material during dialysis also are listed as possible advantages of HDF therapy.

Pharmacokinetics during Continuous Renal Replacement Therapy

Altered drug kinetics is another therapeutically important aspect of CRRT management, with some agents being cleared in significant quantities. Depending on membrane pore size, the passage of substances with molecular weights of 20,000 to 30,000 D is possible and should easily accommodate most drugs. Because only the free, non–protein-bound fraction of a drug is cleared, however, the degree of plasma protein binding dictates whether dialysis or filtration would result in significant removal. Pharmacokinetics also is highly dependent on the drug's volume of distribution. A final consideration is the contribution of alternative elimination pathways to overall drug clearance—if large, the clinical relevance of extracorporeal removal may be minimal.[131] To be considered significant, a regional clearance (e.g., extracorporeal clearance) must exceed 30% of total body clearance.[132]

A drug with low protein binding, a low volume of distribution, and low clearance by alternative pathways is one that would be cleared significantly by CRRT. Vancomycin and the aminoglycosides are good examples, and

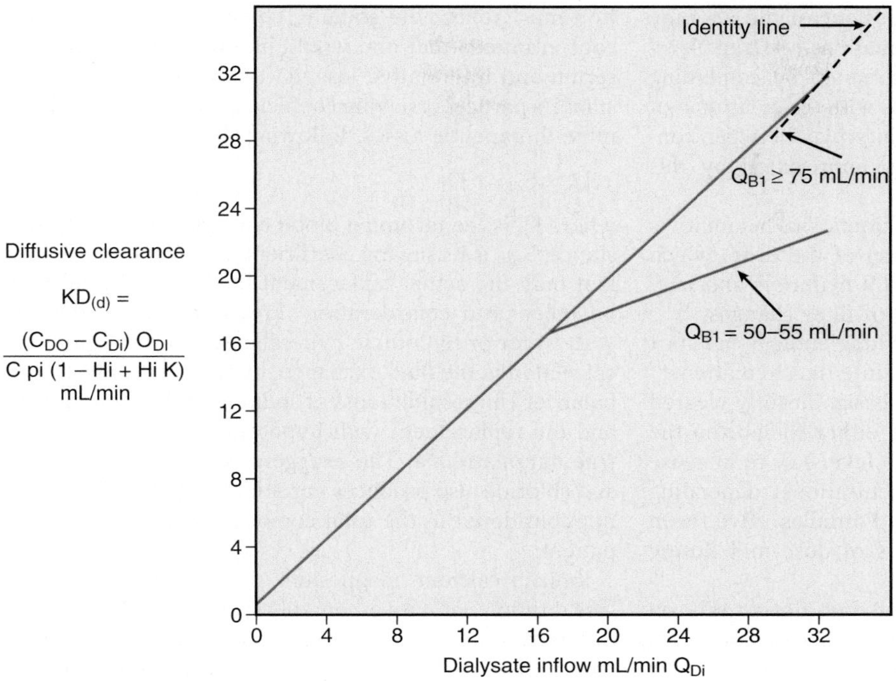

Figure 19-7. Relationship of blood flow rates (Q_{BI}), dialysate flow rates (Q_{DI}), and diffusive clearance ($K_{D(d)}$) during continuous hemodialysis. (Adapted from Sigler M, Teehan BP: Solute transport in slow continuous arteriovenous hemodialysis: An improved method for treating acute renal failure. Proceedings of the Third International Symposium on Acute Continuous Renal Replacement Therapy, Fort Lauderdale, Fla, 1987.)

such agents require dosage adjustments if administered during continuous therapy.

If published data are unavailable, the following concepts may be helpful in guiding drug dosing. The sieving coefficient (S_{coef}) of a drug is defined as the amount of substance transferred across the membrane into the ultrafiltrate ($[\,]_{UF}$) compared with the available drug concentrations at the arterial ($[\,]_A$) and the venous ($[\,]_V$) ends of the artificial kidney, following the formula:

$$S_{coef} = 2[\,]_{UF}/[\,]_A - [\,]_V$$

For postdilutional CAVH/CVVH or SCUF, the clearance (Cl) of a substance can be estimated from:

$$Cl = S_{coef} \times Q_F$$

where Q_F is the UF rate. For predilutional CAVH/CVVH, the dilutional effect must be factored into this equation:

$$Cl = S_{coef} \times Q_F \times (Q_B/[Q_B + Q_R])$$

where Q_B is the blood flow rate, and Q_R is the rate of predilutional fluid replacement.

Table 19-5 lists the sieving coefficients of some medications commonly used in the ICU. (Golper and Marx[132] provide a more exhaustive list.) If the sieving coefficient for the substance is unknown or cannot easily be calculated, knowledge of the degree of protein binding can be used to estimate filtrative clearances.[131] S_{coef} seems to correlate reasonably well with the free fraction of many drugs.[132] For postdilutional therapy or SCUF:

$$Cl = Q_F \times (1 - \text{protein bound fraction})$$

and for predilutional replacement:

$$Cl = Q_F \times (Q_B/[Q_B + Q_B]) \times (1 - \text{protein bound fraction})$$

Table 19-5. Sieving Coefficients for Selected Drugs during Continuous Arteriovenous Hemofiltration

Drug	Sieving Coefficient
Digoxin	0.96
Gentamicin	0.81
Tobramycin	0.78
Vancomycin	0.69
Ampicillin	0.69
Amphotericin	0.40
Phenytoin	0.45
Procainamide	0.86
Theophylline	0.87

Body clearance of drugs without significant tubular secretion or reabsorption is a linear function of creatinine clearance. Individualized drug dosing may be possible in these circumstances using a total creatinine clearance approach[133]; this is achieved with knowledge of filtrative and residual renal creatinine clearance and published pharmacokinetic data on drug clearances in anuric patients and in patients with normal renal function.

Estimation of drug clearance by dialytic modalities is a more complex proposition and has to take account of dialysate and blood flow rates; the molecular weight of the drug; and membrane surface area, thickness, and composition. Nomograms used in the prediction of dialytic drug clearance may be used,[131] but these provide only a general guideline. The impact of molecular weight differs between dialytic techniques and may be lower in CVVHD, which usually uses high flux membranes at a low dialysate flow rate (Q_D). Under these circumstances, the Q_D may approximate Q_F in the previous equations.[132] Drug clearance during CVVHDF may be estimated by combining calculations of filtrative removal with calculations of dialytic removal, but the complex interplay between convection and diffusion is not fully appreciated by this approach.

A final confounder of pharmacokinetic predictability is the impact of membrane adsorption of the drug, which may be substantial with PAN/AN69 materials and may vary depending on the frequency of filter changes.[131,132] Such filters that remain in situ for long enough can start to release their adsorbed drug back into the circulation.[132] In adjusting dosing of a drug that is significantly cleared by CRRT, a choice must be made either to shorten the dosing interval (to maintain plasma levels) or to increase the dose (to optimize peak concentrations) depending on that agent's mode of action. Formulas have been developed to estimate adjustments of dose and dosing interval.[131-133]

The above-described concepts of drug dosing rely on specific knowledge of extracorporeal renal clearance. This requirement may be bypassed by a final approach to drug kinetics that estimates total body clearance without having to know its individual components.[132] Peak and trough plasma levels are repeated until a clear pattern is established, with the supplemental dose (SD) calculated as follows[132]:

$$SD = \text{difference level} \times V_D \times \text{body weight (kg)}$$

where the difference level equals the desired drug level minus current drug level, and V_D is the drug's volume of distribution. Estimates of V_D may vary significantly from actual values,[132] and although this approach theoretically self-corrects with repeated sampling, actual V_D (not to mention endogenous clearances and the extracorporeal prescription) may vary over the course of the patient's hospital stay, resulting in a process of "catch-up." Although published data do exist to help guide drug dosing during CRRT,[134] the multiplicity of combinations of drugs and CRRT prescriptions, coupled with the heterogeneity of critically ill patients, means that the use of aids to dose estimation, such as those detailed previously, is required.

Therapy-Related Complications

Therapy-specific differences correlate with potential complications. The simplicity of pumpless, continuous techniques may lead to a less than attentive approach to the particulars of its delivery. Even with contemporary CRRT hardware, the capacity of each therapy variation may be underestimated by the uninformed or inexperienced prescriber. Although there are specific areas that require more attention than others, the basic concept of total patient care management is crucial in patients who are subjected to continuous extracorporeal therapy techniques.

Perhaps the most frequent problems encountered are electrolyte derangements. With the use of hemofiltration, as we have seen earlier, the replacement solution determines the final electrolyte outcome. The replacement solution must reflect the sodium, chloride, and bicarbonate concentrations that one would like to achieve in patient serum and the relative loss via the hemofilter. The substance's particular sieving coefficient can be used to determine therapeutic losses, following the formula:

$$[\,]_s \times S_{coef} \times Q_F$$

where $[\,]_s$ is the incoming blood concentration of the substance, S_{coef} is its sieving coefficient, and Q_F is the UF rate. Not only the actual replacement fluid, but *all* fluid must be taken into consideration. Frequently, drug vehicles with water or hypotonic hyperalimentation solutions are calculated in the fluid exchange, but not in the electrolyte balance. The resultant loss of sodium (in the hemofiltrate) and the replacement with hypotonic solution produce a true hyponatremia. The exaggerated loss of bicarbonate and chloride also produces variations if these balances are not considered in the total composition delivered to the patient.

Ionized calcium, magnesium, and phosphate also are lost during continuous hemofiltration and HD. This is a different situation from that of intermittent therapies, where these substances are usually retained and need to be subject to a limited intake. It is not unusual for patients to require the addition of magnesium, calcium, and phosphate to cover therapeutic losses and establish normal plasma levels. Serum levels should be checked every 2 days, and replacement should be calculated as noted earlier.

Continuous HD procedures also require frequent electrolyte monitoring. Serum values generally reflect the dialysate concentration of that particular solute. Establishing a potassium floor of 4 mEq/L merely requires that the dialysate concentration of potassium also be set at 4 mEq/L. When using 1.5% Dianeal solution (peritoneal dialysate solution) as the dialysate for continuous dialysis, other aspects of the patient's needs must be considered. This lactate-based solution may be associated with lactate intolerance and acidosis in patients with severely compromised peripheral perfusion or liver disease. Although glucose loading is not usually a problem, a simple switch of concentration from 1.5% to higher glucose dialysate loads (e.g., 2.5%, 4.25%) would result in significant glucose influx and severe hyperglycemia. The cause of this glucose intolerance may be missed in an acutely ill patient in the ICU. The low sodium concentrations in this dialysate (132 mEq/L) may be problematic and could be compounded by dialysate glucose-mediated osmotic drag pulling water into the dialysate compartment. This dilution would reduce the effective dialysate sodium to around 128 mEq/L, generating hyponatremia over time. It is beneficial to add sodium chloride to the dialysate, increasing the baseline sodium concentration to 140 to 145 mEq/L. Common electrolyte problems seen in patients receiving continuous therapies are listed in Table 19-6. Box 19-3 lists other possible complications.

In several balance studies,[117,135,136] concomitant administration of hyperalimentation in the form of amino acid solutions, fat, and carbohydrate formulas may be associated with a markedly positive balance compared with

Table 19-6. Common Electrolyte Problems during Continuous Renal Replacement Therapy with Their Solutions

Problem	Solutions
↓ Na	1. Change all fluid infusions to 0.9% saline or equivalent 2. Increase dialysate sodium (add NaCl) 3. Ensure adequate Na delivery in replacement solution
↓ HCO_3^-	1. Ensure adequate HCO_3^- concentration in dialysate/replacement 2. If lactate-based solution, consider change to HCO_3^- base (especially in liver failure or shock) 3. Increase HCO_3^- in TPN
↓ Ca^{++}	1. Increase Ca^{++} in TPN 2. Add Ca^{++} to dialysate/replacement (if HCO_3^- base, may need to add elsewhere) 3. Ensure adequate oral Ca^{++} intake if appropriate
↓ PO_4^{2-}	1. Close attention to antacid use (acts as gastrointestinal PO_4^{2-} binder; may need to be stopped) 2. Increase PO_4^{2-} in TPN
↓ Mg^{++}	1. Increase Mg^{++} in TPN 2. Add Mg^{++} to dialysate/replacement (if HCO_3^- base, may need to add elsewhere) 3. Supplement as MgCl or $MgSO_4$
↑/↓ K^+	1. Avoid repeated bolus therapy if ↓ K^+ 2. Adjust K^+ in dialysate/replacement 3. If ↑ K^+ uncontrolled, add intermittent therapy 4. May need addition or discontinuation of K^+ binder therapy

TPN, total parenteral nutrition.

Box 19-3

Possible Complications of Continuous Renal Replacement Therapy

- Access
  - Distal arterial insufficiency
  - Embolism (air, thrombus, foreign body)
  - Early
    - Early thrombosis
    - Infection
    - Hematoma (local/retroperitoneal)
  - Late
    - Angiocutaneous fistula
    - Stenosis
    - Aneurysm (pseudo/real)
    - Loss of potential long-term intermittent hemodialysis arteriovenous fistula/graft site
- Blood pump
  - Air embolism
  - Blood loss
- Lines
  - Disconnection/hemorrhage
  - Infection
  - Thrombosis
  - Kinking
- Kidney
  - Clotting
  - Membrane rupture
  - Backdiffusion of pyrogens from contaminated dialysate
  - Membrane hypersensitivity reaction
- Therapy
  - Overanticoagulation/citrate intoxication
  - Electrolyte abnormalities (see Table 19-6)
  - Amino acid losses
  - Fluid imbalance
  - Hypothermia

losses induced by the therapy itself. Use of infused protein seems to be improved in patients with a lower nonprotein calorie-to-nitrogen ratio, and energy expenditure seems to be well predicted by a modified Harris-Benedict formula. When continuous therapy is delivered for a prolonged period (>48 hours) and the patient is not receiving adequate intake of these same substances, an amino acid loss occurs, however, that must be covered. Table 19-7 lists the various sieving coefficients for the most common amino acids. Knowledge of a particular serum amino acid level allows for calculation of a patient's specific amino acid loss through therapy.

Renal Recovery

Recovery of endogenous renal function may manifest quite differently, depending on whether the patient was supported with intermittent or continuous techniques. Although the daily doubling of urine production has been thought to be one of the early signs of renal recovery, these data have been generated from patients subjected to intermittent therapy. Because of the manner of fluid balance with continuous therapies, these patients are generally much closer to their ideal fluid content and so may not show this sign of recovery. A decrease in the baseline serum creatinine without a change in the CRRT prescription may herald renal improvement in these patients. Urine creatinine and sodium may be more helpful in assessing patients receiving continuous rather than intermittent therapy. Recognizing these differences helps avoid extending therapy beyond what is needed and aids in hastening recovery when it has begun (Table 19-8).

Nonrenal Application of Continuous Therapies

The hemodynamic stability of continuous renal therapies has contributed to their use in situations in which fluid loss is desired, but patient status has restricted more standard dialytic or other therapeutic interventions. The ability to manipulate a continuous extracorporeal blood circuit also has opened wide opportunities to assess a variety of different nonrenal applications (Fig. 19-8). The basic circuit has been incorporated into liver assist devices (currently undergoing clinical testing), and the ability to either warm or cool circulating blood has applications in clinical and experimental medicine. The adsorptive nature of different membrane types and structures also has been the focus for potential therapeutic interventions.

Perhaps the most frequently cited area of use has been isolated UF for the treatment of congestive heart failure. Several studies have described the utility of UF for the removal of extravascular lung water in models subjected to pulmonary damage[137] or fluid overload.[138] These observations paralleled reports of improved pulmonary and cardiac function in HD patients with congestive heart failure after fluid removal with isolated UF.[139,140] Coraim and colleagues[141] noted an improvement in patients who were difficult to wean from cardiopulmonary bypass after they had been subjected to hemofiltration and postulated the removal of a mediator substance (or substances) with therapy. Reports of improved pulmonary compliance and enhanced function with hemofiltration in patients with acute respiratory distress syndrome began to surface, first as clinical vignettes[142] and later in more formal clinical studies.[12,143]

Application of UF techniques to various other circuits has seen some moderate success in the dewatering of patients and in improved outcome. Extending the process of "hemoconcentration" to the cardiopulmonary bypass system, especially in children, has been shown to reduce weight, limit blood loss, improve left ventricular systolic and diastolic function, decrease pulmonary vascular resistance, and improve oxygenation. When larger exchange volumes are attempted (high-volume hemofiltration), there has been further improvement, thought to result from a dampened inflammatory response.

Severe, intractable congestive heart failure has been the focus of more recent clinical studies resulting in marked, albeit short-lived, improvement in cardiac function.[144,145]

Table 19-7. Sieving Coefficients of Essential Amino Acids during Continuous Arteriovenous Hemofiltration

Amino Acid	Sieving Coefficient
Valine	1.069
Cystine	1.047
Methionine	1.000
Isoleucine	1.010
Leucine	1.014
Tyrosine	1.089
Phenylalanine	1.078
Lysine	1.080
Histidine	1.109
Threonine	1.236

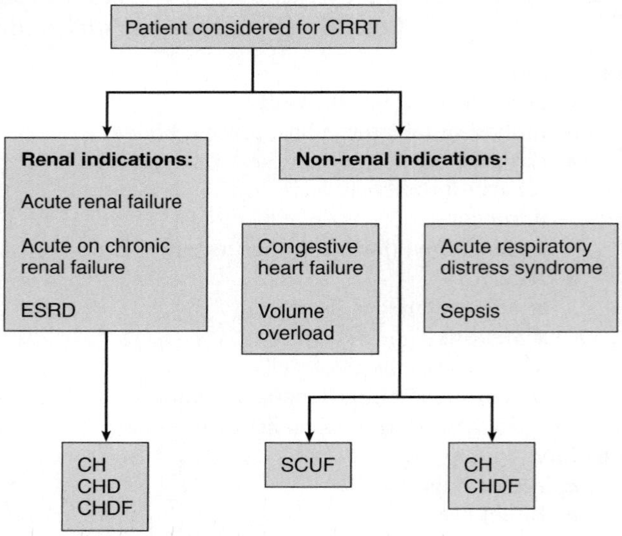

Figure 19-8. Algorithm for the choice of modality in continuous renal replacement therapy (CRRT). CH, continuous hemofiltration; CHD, continuous hemodialysis; CHDF, continuous hemodiafiltration; ESRD, end-stage renal disease; SCUF, slow continuous ultrafiltration.

Table 19-8. Clinical Hints of Renal Recovery in Patients Supported with Intermittent or Continuous Renal Therapies

	Intermittent	Continuous
Serum creatinine	Lower rate of increase between sessions	Decreases without changing therapy
Urine creatinine	Not helpful	Increased
Urine volume	Dramatic increase (the "daily increase double")	May not see increase
Urine sodium	Not helpful	May see decrease

Whether this is the result of a pure hemodynamic effect or the removal of some depressant factor is debatable. Data showing the effectiveness of ongoing therapy with isolated UF hemofiltration have heightened interest in these forms of therapy in cardiac patients.[107,146-149]

The sieving and adsorptive qualities of the continuous extracorporeal circuit have found their way into the manipulation and eventual management of patients with sepsis or systemic inflammatory response syndrome. Numerous experimental studies have touted the ability of various membranes either to remove or to adsorb various cytokines. Tumor necrosis factor-α, interleukin-1, interleukin-6, and interleukin-8 have been the most studied, but endothelin, lipopolysaccharide fragments, and C3a and C5a also have been identified. High-volume zero-balance hemofiltration has been the focus of several animal experiments, in which control of systemic inflammatory response syndrome has been noted.

Clinical translation of this approach has failed to confirm consistently bench findings for many reasons.[150] First, extracorporeal removal of inflammatory mediators may be negligible in relation to endogenous turnover. Second, extracorporeal treatment was usually initiated within a short time frame after induction of experimental sepsis—a scenario at odds with the clinical milieu, where sepsis may be well established by the time therapy is instituted. Third, potentially beneficial substances, such as interleukin-10, water-soluble vitamins (especially vitamin E), and elements such as zinc or selenium, also may be cleared. As a result, clinical application of these techniques has been viewed with some caution. Current clinical technology also restricts adoption of these high-exchange therapies because the volumes employed (at rates >150 mL/kg/h) may be prohibitive.

High-volume hemofiltration (HVHF) has been applied as a blood purification therapy in various clinical situations.[151-153] HVHF can be defined as UF rate greater than 50 to 60 mL/kg/h (60 L/d including net UF) according to previous studies. Based on the humoral theory of sepsis, HVHF (>6 L/h or >80 to 100 mL/kg/h) has been used to remove inflammatory and anti-inflammatory mediators involved in the sepsis syndrome and multiple organ dysfunction syndrome.[154] Studies in animal models of septic shock showed improvements in right ventricular function, blood pressure, cardiac output, immune cell hyporesponsiveness, and reduced mortality.[11,103,155-157] More recently, human studies showed similar findings.[152,153,158] Rather than continuously using a high rate of UF throughout the day, many of these studies used short periods (4 to 8 hours) of high-volume filtration, followed by hemofiltration at the standard 35 mL/kg/h—this method being termed "pulse" HVHF.[154] To minimize technical difficulties and improve the success of delivering this form of therapy, good vascular access is required. It is desirable to have catheter blood flows of at least 300 mL/min to keep the filtration fraction less than 15% to 20% to minimize clotting. Other considerations include using a large (1.8 to 2 m^2 in a 70-kg patient) biocompatible membrane with a high permeability coefficient of at least 30 to 40 mL/h/mm Hg to achieve the UF rates required and applying predilution instead of (or in addition to) postdilution replacement fluids. Unresolved questions of this technique before it can be routinely applied include the timing of initiating HVHF and the lack of large randomized controlled studies with mortality as the primary outcome. Nonetheless, there seems to be some evidence that hemodynamically compromised septic patients optimized with traditional measures may benefit from HVHF.

The adsorptive qualities of specific membranes (AN-69, PAN) have been the most accepted mode of clinical attempts at cytokine control. Although early data seem to point to an impact in lowering blood cytokine levels, a cumbersome and costly exchange of circuit filters, with saturation seen at 2 to 4 hours, brings into question the practicality of this approach.

Hybrid Therapies

Hybrid therapies that combine CRRT and IHD techniques are described in the literature as extended daily dialysis, sustained low efficiency dialysis, or prolonged daily intermittent renal replacement therapy.[159-161] These therapies use standard IHD equipment to apply lower solute clearances and UF rates for prolonged periods (Table 19-9) and aim to combine the desirable features of each modality—reduced rate of UF for improved hemodynamic stability, low efficiency solute removal to minimize solute dysequilibrium, longer treatment duration to achieve prescribed dialysis dose, and intermittency for the convenience of diagnostic and therapeutic procedures during scheduled downtime.[162]

Sustained low efficiency dialysis is typically performed with low blood flows of about 200 mL/min and dialysate flows of 100 to 300 mL/min.[159] Clearance is predominantly diffusive, although there are also reports on hybrid therapy that combines diffusive and convective clearance via HDF using systems with online replacement fluid.[161,163] These systems are fully monitored and have computerized volumetric UF control. Dialysate flows and urea clearances are higher during this form of dialysis compared with CRRT. Overall, hybrid therapy provides a high dose of dialysis with minimal urea dysequilibrium and good control of electrolytes, with survival similar to that predicted by a variety of illness severity scores.[160,164,165]

SUMMARY

The use of continuous extracorporeal therapies in the management of ARF has added another therapeutic option to the armamentarium of clinicians caring for an increasingly complicated ICU population. The heterogeneity of the ICU ARF experience warrants the availability and use of the appropriate form of renal support as dictated by the individual patient's condition, allowing the patient to derive the greatest potential benefit.

Although pumped VV therapies have largely superseded low-technology AV modalities, to attempt to point to one approach as being better than another is missing the point of having multiple choices for support. What

Table 19-9. Comparison of Hybrid Therapies

	Medical School Hospital, Hannover, Germany[166]	Middlemore Hospital, New Zealand[163,164,167]	University of California Davis, U.S.[159]	University of Parma, Italy[168]
Hemodialysis machine	Fresenius Genius	Fresenius 4008S ArRT-Plus	Fresenius 2008H	Gambro AK200S Ultra
Hemodialyzer	Fresenius F60S	Fresenius AV600S	Toray 1.0	Fresenius F7HPS
Composition	Polysulfone	Polysulfone	Polymethyl methacrylate	Polysulfone
Area	1.25 m^2	1.4 m^2	1 m^2	1.6 m^2
Flux	High	High	High	Low
Duration (h)	8-18	8-10	8	8-9
Time of day	Nocturnal	Nocturnal/diurnal	Diurnal	Diurnal
Frequency	Daily	Daily/5-6 d/wk	Daily/6 d/wk	Daily/6 d/wk
Q_B (mL/min)	70	200-350	150-200	200
Q_D (mL/min)	70	200	300	100
QF (mL/min)	0	100	0	0
Dialysate	Bicarbonate	Bicarbonate	Bicarbonate	Bicarbonate

may be best in one situation would not be so in another. What works well in one ICU may not yield similar outcomes in another. Just as all patients cannot be treated with a generic approach to a specific condition, so too all patients with ARF cannot be approached in the same way. We are all learning during the process of treatment evaluation about the strengths and the limitations of our tools. Applying these various tools in a rational and cost-effective manner is the true challenge for physicians who practice intensive care medicine.

KEY POINTS

- CRRT holds many theoretical advantages over intermittent modalities, including maintenance of hemodynamic stability, enhanced fluid removal and hyperalimentation, and increased dialysis dose delivery. Despite these benefits, there has yet to be a clear outcome advantage with this form of therapy.
- Pumped continuous VV therapies have largely superseded pumpless AV modes. Improvements in CRRT hardware have smoothed the interface with the bedside and dialysis staff.
- Membranes are evolving into semiporous and adsorptive species. The characteristics of the various membranes are expected to become an important aspect of care in a variety of specific entities. The role of therapy application (diffusion versus convection) may be decided less on the character of the therapy and more on the potential for membrane clearance. The addition of a cellular component to create a bioartificial membrane may add an interactive component that is currently missing.
- Replacement solutions and dialysate are thought best to be sterile. A variety of bicarbonate-based and lactate-based solutions are available commercially. Close evaluation of the various components helps identify the appropriate composition for the particular patient need. There are efforts to have this solution generated at the bedside by the continuous machines, eliminating the need for additional solution delivery.
- Many different strategies currently are available to help prevent clotting of the extracorporeal circuit, although none has gained universal acceptance. In deciding the appropriate approach, the physician must make an individualized assessment of the risk of bleeding, weighing the importance of optimal therapy delivery against the potential gravity of induced hemorrhage.
- The influence of dose and method of delivery is under active investigation. The use of high-volume hemofiltration in pulse or continuous format for patients with septic shock is being actively studied, and research with extracorporeal cytokine alteration is ongoing.
- CRRT affects the pharmacokinetics of many drugs prescribed in critical care practice. Knowledge of the extracorporeal prescription and individual properties of the drug helps determine appropriate dosing during ongoing continuous treatment.
- The potential for nonrenal applications of extracorporeal therapy continues to receive attention in conditions as diverse as congestive heart failure, acute respiratory distress syndrome, and severe sepsis. The precise role of these adjunctive extracorporeal therapies remains to be clearly defined.

REFERENCES

1. Levy EM, Viscoli CM, Horwitz RI: The effect of acute renal failure on mortality: A cohort analysis. JAMA 1996;275:1489-1494.
2. Douma CE, Redekop WK, van der Meulen JH, et al: Predicting mortality in intensive care patients with acute renal failure treated with dialysis. J Am Soc Nephrol 1997;8:111-117.
3. Turney JH, Marshall DH, Brownjohn AM, et al: The evolution of acute renal failure, 1956-1988. QJM 1990;74:83-104.
4. McCarthy JT: Prognosis of patients with acute renal failure in the intensive-care unit: A tale of two eras. Mayo Clin Proc 1996;71:117-126.
5. Scribner BH, Buri R, Caner JE, et al: The treatment of chronic uremia by means of intermittent hemodialysis: A preliminary report. 1960. J Am Soc Nephrol 1998; 9:719-726.
6. Kramer P, Wigger W, Rieger J, et al: [Arteriovenous haemofiltration: A new and simple method for treatment of over-hydrated patients resistant to diuretics]. Klin Wochenschr 1977;55:1121-1122.
7. Paganini EP, Nakamoto S: Continuous slow ultrafiltration in oliguric acute renal failure. ASAIO Trans 1980;26:201-204.
8. Kanagasundaram NS, Paganini EP: Critical care dialysis—a Gordian knot (but is untying the right approach?). Nephrol Dial Transplant 1999;14:2590-2594.
9. Stein B, Pfenninger E, Grunert A, et al: Influence of continuous haemofiltration on haemodynamics and central blood volume in experimental endotoxic shock. Intensive Care Med 1990;16:494-499.
10. Gomez A, Wang R, Unruh H, et al: Hemofiltration reverses left ventricular dysfunction during sepsis in dogs. Anesthesiology 1990;73:671-685.
11. Grootendorst AF, van Bommel EF, van der Hoven B, et al: High volume hemofiltration improves right ventricular function in endotoxin-induced shock in the pig. Intensive Care Med 1992;18:235-240.
12. Barzilay E, Kessler D, Berlot G, et al: Use of extracorporeal supportive techniques as additional treatment for septic-induced multiple organ failure patients. Crit Care Med 1989;17:634-637.
13. Hirasawa H, Sugai T, Ohtake Y, et al: Continuous hemofiltration and hemodiafiltration in the management of multiple organ failure. Contrib Nephrol 1991;93:42-46.
14. Canaud B, Leray-Moragues H, Leblanc M, et al: Temporary vascular access for extracorporeal renal replacement therapies in acute renal failure patients. Kidney Int Suppl 1998;66: S142-S150.
15. Storck M, Hartl WH, Zimmerer E, et al: Comparison of pump-driven and spontaneous continuous haemofiltration in postoperative acute renal failure. Lancet 1991;337:452-455.
16. Jenkins R, Funk J, Chen BD, et al: Effects of access catheter dimensions on bloodflow in continuous arteriovenous hemofiltration. Contrib Nephrol 1991;93:171-174.
17. Lauer A, Saccaggi A, Ronco C, et al: Continuous arteriovenous hemofiltration in the critically ill patient: Clinical use and operational characteristics. Ann Intern Med 1983;99:455-460.
18. Uldall R: Vascular access for continuous renal replacement therapy. Semin Dial 1996;9:93-97.
19. Bellomo R, Teede H, Boyce N: Anticoagulant regimens in acute continuous hemodiafiltration: A comparative study. Intensive Care Med 1993;19:329-332.
20. Paganini E, Pudelski B, Bednarz D: Dialysis delivery in the ICU: Are patients receiving the prescribed dialysis dose? J Am Soc Nephrol 1992;3:384.
21. Tapson JS, Hoenich NA, Wilkinson R, et al: Dual lumen subclavian catheters for haemodialysis. Int J Artif Organs 1985;8:195-200.
22. Kelber J, Delmez JA, Windus DW: Factors affecting delivery of high-efficiency dialysis using temporary vascular access. Am J Kidney Dis 1993;22:24-29.
23. Leblanc M, Fedak S, Mokris G, et al: Blood recirculation in temporary central catheters for acute hemodialysis. Clin Nephrol 1996;45:315-319.
24. O'Grady NP, Alexander M, Dellinger EP, et al: Guidelines for the prevention of intravascular catheter-related infections. MMWR Morb Mortal Wkly Rep 2002;51(RR 10):1-26.
25. Wester JP, de Koning EJ, Geers AB, et al: Catheter replacement in continuous arteriovenous hemodiafiltration: The balance between infectious and mechanical complications. Crit Care Med 2002;30:1261-1266.
26. Cimochowski GE, Worley E, Rutherford WE, et al: Superiority of the internal jugular over the subclavian access for temporary dialysis. Nephron 1990;54:154-161.
27. Macris MP, Barcenas CG, Parnis SM, et al: Simplified method of hemofiltration in ventricular assist device patients. ASAIO Trans 1988;34:708-711.
28. Paganini EP, Suhoza K, Swann S, et al: Continuous renal replacement therapy in patients with acute renal dysfunction undergoing intraaortic balloon pump and/or left ventricular device support. ASAIO Trans 1986;32:414-417.
29. Jones CH: Continuous renal replacement therapy in acute renal failure: Membranes for CRRT. Artif Organs 1998;22:2-7.
30. Schulman G, Fogo A, Gung A, et al: Complement activation retards resolution of acute ischemic renal failure in the rat. Kidney Int 1991;40:1069-1074.
31. Schiffl H, Lang SM, Konig A, et al: Biocompatible membranes in acute renal failure: Prospective case-controlled study. Lancet 1994;344:570-572.
32. Hakim RM, Wingard RL, Parker RA: Effect of the dialysis membrane in the treatment of patients with acute renal failure. N Engl J Med 1994;331:1338-1342.
33. Kurtal H, von Herrath D, Schaefer K: Is the choice of membrane important for patients with acute renal failure requiring hemodialysis? Artif Organs 1995;19:391-394.
34. Jorres A, Gahl GM, Dobis C, et al: Haemodialysis-membrane biocompatibility and mortality of patients with dialysis-dependent acute renal failure: A prospective randomised multicentre trial. International Multicentre Study Group. Lancet 1999;354:1337-1341.
35. Vanholder R, Lameire N: Does biocompatibility of dialysis membranes affect recovery of renal function and survival? Lancet 1999;354:1316-1318.
36. Kanagasundaram NS, Sakiewicz PG, Liangos O, et al: Biocompatibility and acute renal failure. Lancet 2000;355:313.
37. Gastaldello K, Melot C, Kahn RJ, et al: Comparison of cellulose diacetate and polysulfone membranes in the outcome of acute renal failure: A prospective randomized study. Nephrol Dial Transplant 2000;15:224-230.
38. Jaber BL, Cendoroglo M, Balakrishnan VS, et al: Impact of dialyzer membrane selection on cellular responses in acute renal failure: A crossover study. Kidney Int 2000;57:2107-2116.
39. van de Wetering J, Westendorp RG, van der Hoeven JG, et al: Heparin use in continuous renal replacement procedures: The struggle between filter coagulation and patient hemorrhage. J Am Soc Nephrol 1996;7:145-150.
40. Martin PY, Chevrolet JC, Suter P, et al: Anticoagulation in patients treated by continuous venovenous hemofiltration: A retrospective study. Am J Kidney Dis 1994;24:806-812.
41. Davenport A, Davison AM, Will EJ: Membrane biocompatibility: Effects on cardiovascular stability in patients on hemofiltration. Kidney Int Suppl 1993;41:S230-S234.
42. Jones CH, Goutcher E, Newstead CG, et al: Hemodynamics and survival of patients with acute renal failure treated by continuous dialysis with two synthetic membranes. Artif Organs 1998;22:638-643.
43. Palsson R, Niles JL: Regional citrate anticoagulation in continuous venovenous hemofiltration in critically ill patients with a high risk of bleeding. Kidney Int 1999;55:1991-1997.
44. Veech RL: The untoward effects of the anions of dialysis fluids. Kidney Int 1988;34:587-597.
45. Feriani M, Dell'Aquila R: Acid-base balance and replacement solutions in continuous renal replacement therapies. Kidney Int Suppl 1998;66: S156-S159.
46. Morgera S, Heering P, Szentandrasi T, et al: Comparison of a lactate-versus acetate-based hemofiltration replacement fluid in patients with acute renal failure. Ren Fail 1997;19:155-164.

47. McLean AG, Davenport A, Cox D, et al: Effects of lactate-buffered and lactate-free dialysate in CAVHD patients with and without liver dysfunction. Kidney Int 2000;58:1765-1772.
48. Davenport A, Will EJ, Davison AM: Hyperlactataemia and metabolic acidosis during haemofiltration using lactate-buffered fluids. Nephron 1991;59:461-465.
49. Davenport A, Will EJ, Davison AM: The effect of lactate-buffered solutions on the acid-base status of patients with renal failure. Nephrol Dial Transplant 1989;4:800-804.
50. Murphy ND, Kodakat SK, Wendon JA, et al: Liver and intestinal lactate metabolism in patients with acute hepatic failure undergoing liver transplantation. Crit Care Med 2001;29:2111-2118.
51. Ebben JP, Hirsch DN, Luehmann DA, et al: Microbiologic contamination of liquid bicarbonate concentrate for hemodialysis. ASAIO Trans 1987;33:269-273.
52. Man NK, Ciancioni C, Faivre JM, et al: Dialysis-associated adverse reactions with high-flux membranes and microbial contamination of liquid bicarbonate concentrate. Contrib Nephrol 1988;62:24-34.
53. Bambauer R, Schauer M, Jung WK, et al: Contamination of dialysis water and dialysate: A survey of 30 centers. ASAIO J 1994;40:1012-1016.
54. Thomas AN, Guy JM, Kishen R, et al: Comparison of lactate and bicarbonate buffered haemofiltration fluids: Use in critically ill patients. Nephrol Dial Transplant 1997;12:1212-1217.
55. Kierdorf H, Leue C, Heintz B, et al: Continuous venovenous hemofiltration in acute renal failure: Is a bicarbonate- or lactate-buffered substitution better? Contrib Nephrol 1995;116:38-47.
56. Kierdorf HP, Leue C, Arns S: Lactate- or bicarbonate-buffered solutions in continuous extracorporeal renal replacement therapies. Kidney Int Suppl 1999;72:S32-S36.
57. Hilton PJ, Taylor J, Forni LG, et al: Bicarbonate-based haemofiltration in the management of acute renal failure with lactic acidosis. QJM 1998;91:279-283.
58. Jenkins RD, Jackson E, Kuhn R, et al: Benefit of bicarbonate dialysis during CAVHD. ASAIO Trans 1990;36: M465-M466.
59. Barenbrock M, Hausberg M, Matzkies F, et al: Effects of bicarbonate- and lactate-buffered replacement fluids on cardiovascular outcome in CVVH patients. Kidney Int 2000;58:1751-1757.
60. Leblanc M, Moreno L, Robinson OP, et al: Bicarbonate dialysate for continuous renal replacement therapy in intensive care unit patients with acute renal failure. Am J Kidney Dis 1995;26:910-917.
61. Davenport A: The coagulation system in the critically ill patient with acute renal failure and the effect of an extracorporeal circuit. Am J Kidney Dis 1997;30:S20-S27.
62. Gretz N, Quintel M, Ragaller M, et al: Low-dose heparinization for anticoagulation in intensive care patients on continuous hemofiltration. Contrib Nephrol 1995;116:130-135.
63. Mehta RL: Anticoagulation strategies for continuous renal replacement therapies: What works? Am J Kidney Dis 1996;5:8.
64. Singer M, McNally T, Screaton G, et al: Heparin clearance during continuous veno-venous haemofiltration. Intensive Care Med 1994;20:212-215.
65. Ramesh Prasad GV, Palevsky PM, Burr R, et al: Factors affecting system clotting in continuous renal replacement therapy: Results of a randomized, controlled trial. Clin Nephrol 2000;53:55-60.
66. Kaplan AA, Petrillo R: Regional heparinization for continuous arterio-venous hemofiltration (CAVH). ASAIO Trans 1987;33:312-315.
67. de Pont AC, Oudemans-van Straaten HM, Roozendaal KJ, et al: Nadroparin versus dalteparin anticoagulation in high-volume, continuous venovenous hemofiltration: A double-blind, randomized, crossover study. Crit Care Med 2000;28:421-425.
68. Sagedal S, Hartmann A: Low molecular weight heparins as thromboprophylaxis in patients undergoing hemodialysis/ hemofiltration or continuous renal replacement therapies. Eur J Med Res 2004;9:125-130.
69. Reeves JH, Cumming AR, Gallagher L, et al: A controlled trial of low-molecular-weight heparin (dalteparin) versus unfractionated heparin as anticoagulant during continuous venovenous hemodialysis with filtration. Crit Care Med 1999;27:2224-2228.
70. Davenport A: Management of heparin-induced thrombocytopenia during continuous renal replacement therapy. Am J Kidney Dis 1998;32:E3.
71. Jeffrey RF, Khan AA, Douglas JT, et al: Anticoagulation with low molecular weight heparin (Fragmin) during continuous hemodialysis in the intensive care unit. Artif Organs 1993;17:717-720.
72. Wynckel A, Bernieh B, Toupance O, et al: Guidelines to the use of enoxaparin in slow continuous hemodialysis. Contrib Nephrol 1991;93:221-224.
73. Ponikvar R, Kandus A, Buturovic J, et al: Use of prostacyclin as the only anticoagulant during continuous venovenous hemofiltration. Contrib Nephrol 1991;93:218-220.
74. Zobel G, Trop M, Muntean W, et al: Anticoagulation for continuous arteriovenous hemofiltration in children. Blood Purif 1988;6:90-95.
75. Langenecker SA, Felfernig M, Werba A, et al: Anticoagulation with prostacyclin and heparin during continuous venovenous hemofiltration. Crit Care Med 1994;22:1774-1781.
76. Journois D, Chanu D, Pouard P, et al: Assessment of standardized ultrafiltrate production rate using prostacyclin in continuous venovenous hemofiltration. Contrib Nephrol 1991;93:202-204.
77. Davenport A, Will EJ, Davison AM: Comparison of the use of standard heparin and prostacyclin anticoagulation in spontaneous and pump-driven extracorporeal circuits in patients with combined acute renal and hepatic failure. Nephron 1994;66:431-437.
78. Kozek-Langenecker SA, Kettner SC, Oismueller C, et al: Anticoagulation with prostaglandin E1 and unfractionated heparin during continuous venovenous hemofiltration. Crit Care Med 1998;26:1208-1212.
79. Mehta RL, McDonald BR, Aguilar MM, et al: Regional citrate anticoagulation for continuous arteriovenous hemodialysis in critically ill patients. Kidney Int 1990;38:976-981.
80. Tolwani AJ, Campbell RC, Schenk MB, et al: Simplified citrate anticoagulation for continuous renal replacement therapy. Kidney Int 2001;60:370-374.
81. Hofmann RM, Maloney C, Ward DM, et al: A novel method for regional citrate anticoagulation in continuous venovenous hemofiltration (CVVHF). Ren Fail 2002;24:325-335.
82. Tobe SW, Aujla P, Walele AA, et al: A novel regional citrate anticoagulation protocol for CRRT using only commercially available solutions. J Crit Care 2003;18:121-129.
83. Mitchell A, Daul AE, Beiderlinden M, et al: A new system for regional citrate anticoagulation in continuous venovenous hemodialysis (CVVHD). Clin Nephrol 2003;59:106-114.
84. Swartz R, Pasko D, O'Toole J, et al: Improving the delivery of continuous renal replacement therapy using regional citrate anticoagulation. Clin Nephrol 2004;61:134-143.
85. Gupta M, Wadhwa NK, Bukovsky R: Regional citrate anticoagulation for continuous venovenous hemodiafiltration using calcium-containing dialysate. Am J Kidney Dis 2004;43:67-73.
86. Meier-Kriesche HU, Gitomer J, Finkel K, et al: Increased total to ionized calcium ratio during continuous venovenous hemodialysis with regional citrate anticoagulation. Crit Care Med 2001;29:748-752.
87. Meier-Kriesche HU, Finkel KW, Gitomer JJ, et al: Unexpected severe hypocalcemia during continuous venovenous hemodialysis with regional citrate anticoagulation. Am J Kidney Dis 1999;33:e8.
88. Fischer KG, van de Loo A, Bohler J: Recombinant hirudin (lepirudin) as anticoagulant in intensive care patients treated with continuous hemodialysis. Kidney Int Suppl 1999;72:S46-S50.
89. Kutsogiannis DJ, Mayers I, Chin WD, et al: Regional citrate anticoagulation in continuous venovenous hemodiafiltration. Am J Kidney Dis 2000;35:802-811.
90. Kirschbaum B, Galishoff M, Reines HD: Lactic acidosis treated with continuous hemodiafiltration and regional citrate anticoagulation. Crit Care Med 1992;20:349-353.
91. Fischer KG, van de Loo A, Bohler J: Recombinant hirudin (lepirudin) as anticoagulant in intensive care patients treated with continuous hemodialysis. Kidney Int Suppl 1999;72:S46-S50.
92. Ohtake Y, Hirasawa H, Sugai T, et al: Nafamostat mesylate as anticoagulant in continuous hemofiltration and continuous hemodiafiltration. Contrib Nephrol 1991;93:215-217.

93. Dager WE, White RH: Argatroban for heparin-induced thrombocytopenia in hepato-renal failure and CVVHD. Ann Pharmacother 2003;37:1232-1236.
94. Eichler P, Friesen HJ, Lubenow N, et al: Antihirudin antibodies in patients with heparin-induced thrombocytopenia treated with lepirudin: Incidence, effects on aPTT, and clinical relevance. Blood 2000;96:2373-2378.
95. Tang IY, Cox DS, Patel K, et al: Argatroban and renal replacement therapy in patients with heparin-induced thrombocytopenia. Ann Pharmacother 2005;39:231-236.
96. Uchino S, Fealy N, Baldwin I, et al: Continuous venovenous hemofiltration without anticoagulation. ASAIO J 2004;50:76-80.
97. Samuelsson O, Amiral J, Attman PO, et al: Heparin-induced thrombocytopenia during continuous haemofiltration. Nephrol Dial Transplant 1995;10:1768-1771.
98. Vun CM, Evans S, Chong BH: Cross-reactivity study of low molecular weight heparins and heparinoid in heparin-induced thrombocytopenia. Thromb Res 1996;81:525-532.
99. Kaplan AA, Longnecker RE, Folkert VW: Suction-assisted continuous arteriovenous hemofiltration. ASAIO Trans 1983;29:408-413.
100. Bartlett RH, Bosch J, Geronemus R, et al: Continuous arteriovenous hemofiltration for acute renal failure. ASAIO Trans 1988;34:67-77.
101. Sigler MH, Teehan BP: Solute transport in continuous hemodialysis: A new treatment for acute renal failure. Kidney Int 1987;32:562-571.
102. Paganini EP, Tapolyai M, Goormastic M: Establishing a dialysis therapy/patient outcome link in intensive care unit acute dialysis for patients with acute renal failure. Am J Kidney Dis 1996;28:S81-S89.
103. Ronco C, Bellomo R, Homel P, et al: Effects of different doses in continuous veno-venous haemofiltration on outcomes of acute renal failure: A prospective randomised trial. Lancet 2000;356:26-30.
104. Paganini EP, O'Hara P, Nakamoto S: Slow continuous ultrafiltration in hemodialysis resistant oliguric acute renal failure patients. ASAIO Trans 1984;30:173-178.
105. Lauer A, Alvis R, Avram M: Hemodynamic consequences of continuous arteriovenous hemofiltration. Am J Kidney Dis 1988;12:110-115.
106. Conger JD: Does hemodialysis delay recovery from acute renal failure? Semin Dial 1990;3:146.
107. Davenport A, Will EJ, Davidson AM: Improved cardiovascular stability during continuous modes of renal replacement therapy in critically ill patients with acute hepatic and renal failure. Crit Care Med 1993;21:328-338.
108. Davenport A, Will EJ, Davison AM: Continuous vs. intermittent forms of haemofiltration and/or dialysis in the management of acute renal failure in patients with defective cerebral autoregulation at risk of cerebral oedema. Contrib Nephrol 1991;93:225-233.
109. Misset B, Timsit JF, Chevret S, et al: A randomized cross-over comparison of the hemodynamic response to intermittent hemodialysis and continuous hemofiltration in ICU patients with acute renal failure. Intensive Care Med 1996;22:742-746.
110. van Bommel E, Bouvy ND, So KL, et al: Acute dialytic support for the critically ill: Intermittent hemodialysis versus continuous arteriovenous hemodiafiltration. Am J Nephrol 1995;15:192-200.
111. Paganini EP: Slow continuous hemofiltration and slow continuous ultrafiltration. ASAIO Trans 1988;34:63-66.
112. Sandroni S, Arora N, Powell B: Performance characteristics of contemporary hemodialysis and venovenous hemofiltration in acute renal failure. Ren Fail 1992;14:571-574.
113. Paganini EP, Sandy D, Moreno L, et al: The effect of sodium and ultrafiltration modelling on plasma volume changes and haemodynamic stability in intensive care patients receiving haemodialysis for acute renal failure: A prospective, stratified, randomized, cross-over study. Nephrol Dial Transplant 1996;11(Suppl 8):32-37.
114. Clark WR, Mueller BA, Alaka KJ, et al: A comparison of metabolic control by continuous and intermittent therapies in acute renal failure. J Am Soc Nephrol 1994;4:1413-1420.
115. Bellomo R, Boyce N: Continuous venovenous hemodiafiltration compared with conventional dialysis in critically ill patients with acute renal failure. ASAIO J 1993;39:M794-M797.
116. Bellomo R, Mansfield D, Rumble S, et al: A comparison of conventional dialytic therapy and acute continuous hemodiafiltration in the management of acute renal failure in the critically ill. Ren Fail 1993;15:595-602.
117. Chima CS, Meyer L, Hummell AC, et al: Protein catabolic rate in patients with acute renal failure on continuous arteriovenous hemofiltration and total parenteral nutrition. J Am Soc Nephrol 1993;3:1516-1521.
118. Clark WR, Murphy MH, Alaka KJ, et al: Urea kinetics during continuous hemofiltration. ASAIO J 1992;38:M664-M667.
119. Jakob SM, Frey FJ, Uehlinger DE: Does continuous renal replacement therapy favourably influence the outcome of the patients? Nephrol Dial Transplant 1996;11:1250-1255.
120. Bastien O, Saroul C, Hercule C, et al: Continuous venovenous hemodialysis after cardiac surgery. Contrib Nephrol 1991;93:76-78.
121. Tonelli M, Manns B, Feller-Kopman D: Acute renal failure in the intensive care unit: A systematic review of the impact of dialytic modality on mortality and renal recovery. Am J Kidney Dis 2002;40:875-885.
122. Kellum JA, Angus DC, Johnson JP, et al: Continuous versus intermittent renal replacement therapy: A meta-analysis. Intensive Care Med 2002;28:29-37.
123. Jacka MJ, Ivancinova X, Gibney RT: Continuous renal replacement therapy improves renal recovery from acute renal failure. Can J Anaesth 2005;52:327-332.
124. Halstenberg WK, Goormastic M, Paganini EP: Validity of four models for predicting outcome in critically ill acute renal failure patients. Clin Nephrol 1997;47:81-86.
125. van Bommel EF, Bouvy ND, Hop WC, et al: Use of APACHE II classification to evaluate outcome and response to therapy in acute renal failure patients in a surgical intensive care unit. Ren Fail 1995;17:731-742.
126. Bellomo R, Tipping P, Boyce N: Tumor necrosis factor clearances during veno-venous hemodiafiltration in the critically ill. ASAIO Trans 1991;37:M322-M323.
127. Ifediora OC, Teehan BP, Sigler MH: Solute clearance in continuous venovenous hemodialysis: A comparison of cuprophane, polyacrylonitrile, and polysulfone membranes. ASAIO J 1992;38:M697-M701.
128. Relton S, Greenberg A, Palevsky PM: Dialysate and blood flow dependence of diffusive solute clearance during CVVHD. ASAIO J 1992;38:M691-M696.
129. Paganini EP: Acute Continuous Renal Replacement Therapy. Boston, M. Nijhoff, 1986.
130. Ronco C: Continuous renal replacement therapies for the treatment of acute renal failure in intensive care patients. Clin Nephrol 1993;40:187-198.
131. Bohler J, Donauer J, Keller F: Pharmacokinetic principles during continuous renal replacement therapy: Drugs and dosage. Kidney Int Suppl 1999;72:S24-S28.
132. Golper TA, Marx MA: Drug dosing adjustments during continuous renal replacement therapies. Kidney Int Suppl 1998;66:S165-S168.
133. Keller F, Bohler J, Czock D, et al: Individualized drug dosage in patients treated with continuous hemofiltration. Kidney Int Suppl 1999;72:S29-S31.
134. Schetz M, Ferdinande P, Van den Berghe G, et al: Pharmacokinetics of continuous renal replacement therapy. Intensive Care Med 1995;21:612-620.
135. Mault JR, Bartlett RH, Dechert RE, et al: Starvation: A major contribution to mortality in acute renal failure? ASAIO Trans 1983;29:390-395.
136. Paganini EP, Flaque J, Whitman G, et al: Amino acid balance in patients with oliguric acute renal failure undergoing slow continuous ultrafiltration (SCUF). ASAIO Trans 1982;28:615-620.
137. Sivak ED, Tita J, Meden G, et al: Effects of furosemide versus isolated ultrafiltration on extravascular lung water in oleic acid-induced pulmonary edema. Crit Care Med 1986;14:48-51.
138. Magilligan DJ Jr: Indications for ultrafiltration in the cardiac surgical patient. J Thorac Cardiovasc Surg 1985;89:183-189.
139. Chen WT, Chaignon M, Omvik P, et al: Hemodynamic studies in chronic hemodialysis patients with hemofiltration/ultrafiltration. ASAIO Trans 1978;24:682-686.
140. Paganini EP, Fouad F, Tarazi RC, et al: Hemodynamics of isolated

ultrafiltration in chronic hemodialysis patients. ASAIO Trans 1979;25:422-425.
141. Coraim FJ, Coraim HP, Ebermann R, et al: Acute respiratory failure after cardiac surgery: Clinical experience with the application of continuous arteriovenous hemofiltration. Crit Care Med 1986;14:714-718.
142. Gotloib L, Barzilay E, Shustak A, et al: Sequential hemofiltration in nonoliguric high capillary permeability pulmonary edema of severe sepsis: Preliminary report. Crit Care Med 1984;12:997-1000.
143. Cosentino F, Paganini E, Lockrem J, et al: Continuous arteriovenous hemofiltration in the adult respiratory distress syndrome: A randomized trial. Contrib Nephrol 1991;93:94-97.
144. Levine B, Kalman J, Mayer L, et al: Elevated circulating levels of tumor necrosis factor in severe chronic heart failure. N Engl J Med 1990;323:236-241.
145. Rimondini A, Cipolla CM, Della Bella P, et al: Hemofiltration as short-term treatment for refractory congestive heart failure. Am J Med 1987;83:43-48.
146. Susini G, Zucchetti M, Bortone F, et al: Isolated ultrafiltration in cardiogenic pulmonary edema. Crit Care Med 1990;18:14-17.
147. L'Abbate A, Emdin M, Piacenti M, et al: Ultrafiltration: A rational treatment for heart failure. Cardiology 1989;76:384-390.
148. Biasioli S, Barbaresi F, Barbiero M, et al: Intermittent venovenous hemofiltration as a chronic treatment for refractory and intractable heart failure. ASAIO J 1992;38:M658-M663.
149. Canaud B, Cristol JP, Klouche K, et al: Slow continuous ultrafiltration: A means of unmasking myocardial functional reserve in end-stage cardiac disease. Contrib Nephrol 1991;93:79-85.
150. De Vriese AS, Vanholder RC, De Sutter JH, et al: Continuous renal replacement therapies in sepsis: Where are the data? Nephrol Dial Transplant 1998;13:1362-1364.
151. Journois D, Israel-Biet D, Pouard P, et al: High-volume, zero-balanced hemofiltration to reduce delayed inflammatory response to cardiopulmonary bypass in children. Anesthesiology 1996;85:965-976.
152. Cole L, Bellomo R, Journois D, et al: High-volume haemofiltration in human septic shock. Intensive Care Med 2001;27:978-986.
153. Honore PM, Jamez J, Wauthier M, et al: Prospective evaluation of short-term, high-volume isovolemic hemofiltration on the hemodynamic course and outcome in patients with intractable circulatory failure resulting from septic shock. Crit Care Med 2000;28:3581-3587.
154. Ratanarat R, Brendolan A, Ricci Z, et al: Pulse high-volume hemofiltration in critically ill patients: A new approach for patients with septic shock. Semin Dial 2006;19:69-74.
155. Grootendorst AF, van Bommel EF, van Leengoed LA, et al: High volume hemofiltration improves hemodynamics and survival of pigs exposed to gut ischemia and reperfusion. Shock 1994;2:72-78.
156. Rogiers P, Zhang H, Smail N, et al: Continuous venovenous hemofiltration improves cardiac performance by mechanisms other than tumor necrosis factor-alpha attenuation during endotoxic shock. Crit Care Med 1999;27:1848-1855.
157. Yekebas EF, Eisenberger CF, Ohnesorge H, et al: Attenuation of sepsis-related immunoparalysis by continuous veno-venous hemofiltration in experimental porcine pancreatitis. Crit Care Med 2001;29:1423-1430.
158. Ratanarat R, Brendolan A, Piccinni P, et al: Pulse high-volume haemofiltration for treatment of severe sepsis: Effects on hemodynamics and survival. Crit Care 2005;9:R294-R302.
159. Kumar VA, Craig M, Depner TA, et al: Extended daily dialysis: A new approach to renal replacement for acute renal failure in the intensive care unit. Am J Kidney Dis 2000;36:294-300.
160. Marshall MR, Golper TA, Shaver MJ, et al: Sustained low-efficiency dialysis for critically ill patients requiring renal replacement therapy. Kidney Int 2001;60:777-785.
161. Naka T, Baldwin I, Bellomo R, et al: Prolonged daily intermittent renal replacement therapy in ICU patients by ICU nurses and ICU physicians. Int J Artif Organs 2004;27:380-387.
162. Fliser D, Kielstein JT: Technology insight: Treatment of renal failure in the intensive care unit with extended dialysis. Natl Clin Pract Nephrol 2006;2:32-39.
163. Marshall MR, Ma T, Galler D, et al: Sustained low-efficiency daily diafiltration (SLEDD-f) for critically ill patients requiring renal replacement therapy: Towards an adequate therapy. Nephrol Dial Transplant 2004;19:877-884.
164. Marshall MR, Golper TA, Shaver MJ, et al: Urea kinetics during sustained low-efficiency dialysis in critically ill patients requiring renal replacement therapy. Am J Kidney Dis 2002;39:556-570.
165. Kielstein JT, Kretschmer U, Ernst T, et al: Efficacy and cardiovascular tolerability of extended dialysis in critically ill patients: A randomized controlled study. Am J Kidney Dis 2004;43:342-349.
166. Lonnemann G, Floege J, Kliem V, et al: Extended daily veno-venous high-flux haemodialysis in patients with acute renal failure and multiple organ dysfunction syndrome using a single path batch dialysis system. Nephrol Dial Transplant 2000;15:1189-1193.
167. Marshall MR, Ma TM, Eggleton K, et al: Regional citrate anticoagulation during simulated treatments of sustained low efficiency diafiltration. Nephrology (Carlton) 2003;8:302-310.
168. Fiaccadori E, Maggiore U, Rotelli C, et al: Removal of linezolid by conventional intermittent hemodialysis, sustained low-efficiency dialysis, or continuous venovenous hemofiltration in patients with acute renal failure. Crit Care Med 2004;32:2437-2442.

Chapter 20

Use of Sedatives, Analgesics, and Neuromuscular Blockers

Michael J. Murray, Lance J. Oyen, and William T. Browne

Patients who are critically ill are frequently anxious, uncomfortable, and in pain. Even if they are unconscious and not experiencing any of these sensations or perceptions, they may be agitated and at risk of injuring themselves or others (Box 20-1). If physicians are unsuccessful in providing improved anxiolysis and analgesia for patients, the therapy for anxiety and pain is likely to become part of quality assurance activities, surveys of health care plan members' perceptions of care, and quality improvement measures. Aside from these considerations, physicians are ethically obliged to provide compassionate care, the kind of care they would want for themselves or their family members, and independent of any regulations or laws, important physiologic reasons exist for treating patients' anxiety and pain.

Maintaining an optimal level of comfort and safety through the use of anxiolytics, analgesics, and neuromuscular blocking agents (NMBAs) is a universal goal of intensive care unit (ICU) practitioners. The aim is to decrease patients' adverse perceptions and experiences, increase their sense of well-being and comfort, and improve their clinical outcomes. Surveys have repeatedly shown that hospitalized patients worry about receiving relief from anxiety and pain.[1-3] These concerns are well founded; many health care providers have misconceptions regarding the use of anxiolytics, opioids, and NMBAs.[4,5] These misconceptions are surprising because the necessary knowledge, techniques, and therapies to provide effective anxiolysis and analgesia are available. The Joint Commission on Accreditation of Healthcare Organizations (JCAHO) announced its new goals and requirements in its 2007 Hospital/Critical Access Hospital National Patient Safety Goals.* Patients' families would most likely be quite vocal about the safety of an agitated ICU patient, and a hospital's lack of a formal program to address the safety of such patients would affect its JCAHO accreditation. Similarly, the Center for Medicare and Medicaid Services† has initiated its Hospital Quality Measures (Pay for Performance), which include acute myocardial infarction, heart failure, pneumonia, and surgical infection prevention goals. In 2007, patient perspectives on hospital care were expected to be included. Adverse experience in the ICU (Box 20-2) related to anxiety and pain could affect patients' perspectives of their care.

ANXIETY

Etiology

All physicians have experienced and intuitively understand anxiety. Anxious patients describe a sense of uncertainty, heightened awareness, and apprehension (with or without apparent stimulus) and frequently report physiologic changes, such as sweating, tachycardia, and dry mouth. Anxiety can lead to agitation, neuroses, delirium, or frank psychosis. Teleologically, anxiety is a stimulus or precursor to the fight-or-flight response described by Cannon in the 1920s,[6] which focuses an individual's attention on avoiding injury or if already injured on avoiding further injury. This focusing of attention has been studied by Berns and colleagues,[7] who examined 32 volunteers using functional magnetic resonance imaging to assess the neurologic effects of a cutaneous shock. They showed how powerful a motivator anxiety is; individuals chose an electrical shock rather than experience anxiety. In the study, subjects dreaded an *anticipated* electrical shock so much so that they would opt for a higher voltage shock immediately rather than wait for a lower voltage shock just so that they could be finished with the experiment. The prolonged anxiety and fear and the cost of maintaining "attentiveness" to the anticipated shock were the reasons postulated for why these volunteers would select a more painful shock.[7] Sedatives reduce the stress of

*http://www.jointcommission.org/PatientSafety/NationalPatientSafetyGoals

†http://www.cms.hhs.gov/HospitalqualityInits/downloads/HospitalHQA2004_2007200512.pdf

Box 20-1

Definitions

Agitation: Increased motor activity that includes writhing in bed; moaning; trying to get out of bed; and removal of catheters, monitoring devices, or tubes. Associated with signs of autonomic hyperactivity.

Analgesia: The relief of pain.

Anxiety: Feelings of nervousness, apprehension, or fear.

Cognitive dysfunction: Decreasing memory and analytical skills, confusion, and impaired judgment.

Delirium: An acute change in mental status with inattention, confusion, disorganized thinking or speech, and altered level of consciousness.

Hypnosis: A sleeplike state.

Pain: An unpleasant sensory and emotional experience associated with actual or potential tissue damage.

Sedation (anxiolysis): Decrease in anxiety and agitation; induction of a calm state.

Box 20-2

Adverse Experiences of Patients in the Intensive Care Unit

- Pain
- Anxiety
- Dyspnea
- Insomnia
- Trouble speaking
- Thirst
- Procedures
- Not being in control
- Difficulty swallowing
- Noise
- Depressed
- Fearful
- Restrained
- Missing spouse or friends
- Feeling something bad will happen
- Awakening in the middle of the night
- Feeling lonely
- Thoughts of death or dying
- Nightmares

anxiety and may help patients to cope better in the ICU.[8]

Many factors influence a patient's perception of anxiety. Admission to a hospital or to an ICU provokes anxiety. Concerns about personal welfare, family, job, and the underlying reason for hospitalization; loss of autonomy; feelings of helplessness or depression or both; and concerns about survival all contribute to the perception of anxiety. Other experiences act to increase levels of anxiety (Table 20-1). The discomfort that a patient experiences in

Table 20-1. Stimuli to Patient's Anxieties in an Intensive Care Unit

Pain
Not sleeping/insomnia
Noise/alarms
Room temperature
Physiotherapy
Tracheal suctioning
Movement
Monitors/machines
Disability
Loss of loved ones
Death

a strange environment and frequently uncomfortable bed increases anxiety. Pain, either from a surgical incision or from an underlying disease process such as myocardial infarction or pancreatitis, also heightens the patient's sense of anxiety. Anxiety and pain are frequently concomitant on a continuum, and each increases the perception of the other. Anxiety also can lead to insomnia, and similarly, sleep deprivation can lead to an increased perception of anxiety.[9] Sleep deprivation can occur secondary to pain, anxiety, noise levels in an ICU, the extremes of temperature found in some ICU rooms, and ambient light levels.[10] Other factors in an ICU also can increase the perception of anxiety, pain, discomfort, and sleep deprivation. Noise levels in present-day ICUs have reached levels that were unimaginable 20 or 30 years ago.[11] The combination of machines, alarms, therapeutic interventions, and inconsiderate hospital personnel increases noise that heightens a patient's anxiety and pain perception. Patients who require prolonged mechanical ventilation often have recollections of being intubated, ventilated, or suctioned. If patients could remember such events, they recalled them as being moderately to extremely stressful. Their recollections were associated with feelings of terror, nervousness, and insomnia.[12] Age also may have an effect on perception of anxiety because as we age, our "brain" reserve decreases. Depending on comorbidities, underlying illness, and psychotropic medications, older patients are more at risk of cognitive dysfunction,[13] which may increase agitation and delirium.[14]

Agitation and Delirium

Box 20-1 provides definitions of the disorders discussed in this chapter. There is increasing recognition and concern that anxiety may lead to agitation and agitation to delirium, or anxiety may lead directly to delirium. Delirium may be the first manifestation of abnormal neuropsychiatric functioning in a critically ill patient (Fig. 20-1).

Agitated patients are more likely to injure their caregivers and themselves.[15] Woods and colleagues[15] conducted a prospective study of their 18-bed medical ICU over a 4-month period and identified 145 patients who were agitated, as defined using the Motor Activity Assessment Scale (MAAS), which scores patients from 0 (unresponsive, does not move to noxious stimuli) to 6

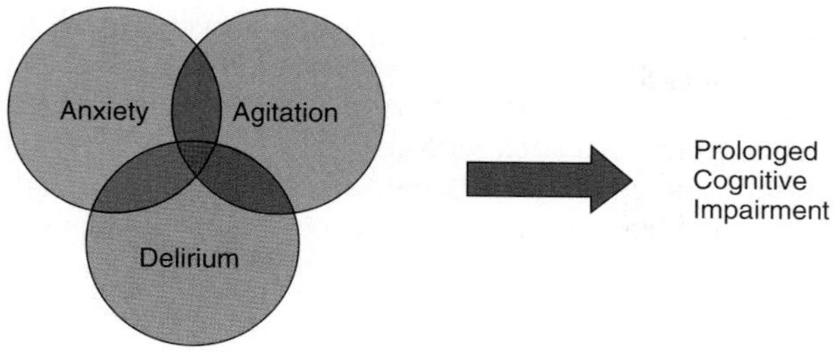

Figure 20-1. There is overlap among anxiety, agitation, and delirium, and all may lead to prolonged cognitive impairment.

(dangerously agitated). Agitated patients were younger and more frequently had a widened alveolar-arterial gradient. Their length of stay in the medical ICU and the number of ventilator days were increased compared with patients who did not become agitated. Agitated patients were more likely to self-extubate themselves and were more likely to receive benzodiazepines, opioids, and NMBAs. Agitated patients were not more likely to receive specific therapy targeted at delirium (haloperidol). The authors concluded that in their patient population, 16% of patients became agitated, which was associated with adverse events and prolonged ICU and hospital stays.

Other authors have found an even higher incidence of agitation. Chase and colleagues[16] in New Zealand found that 71% of their sedated adult patients became agitated. In their study, they used the Riker Sedation-Agitation Scale (SAS). In the MAAS and SAS agitation scores, patient movement is the primary, if not the entire, means by which patients are assessed. The patient's movement of arms or legs can injure health care providers, and movement of arms, legs, and head enables a patient to inflict self-injury through self-extubation or removal of chest tubes and intravenous or intra-arterial devices. As stated in Woods' study,[15] such patients are more likely to receive a combination of benzodiazepines and opioids, which in and of itself can lead to increased length of mechanical ventilation and duration of ICU and hospital stay.

Woods and colleagues[17] also noted that agitation was more common in young patients, whereas other investigators have noted that delirium is more common in older patients. Agitation is characterized by an increase in motor activity, whereas delirium is characterized more by cognitive impairment, although there are subtypes of delirium in which patients are hyperactive or hypoactive, and a mixed type has been identified.

Delirium is an acute, fluctuating change in mental status with inattention and altered levels of consciousness.[18] Development of delirium in critically ill patients predicts post-ICU length of stay and is associated with a threefold increase in mortality at 6 months.[19] Ely and coworkers[19] speculated that delirium is a marker of end-organ dysfunction or damage just as a decreased fraction of inspired oxygen ratio is a marker of lung injury, both of which not only may be a marker of multiple organ dysfunction syndrome, but also a promoter of the inflammatory cascade and of systemic inflammatory response syndrome.

Of equal concern is that delirium is associated with prolonged cognitive impairment at 6 months after hospital discharge. In a society that places a premium on independent living, maintenance of autonomy and preservation of cognitive abilities leading to an acceptable quality of life for individuals who survive an ICU stay are of paramount importance. In the guidelines, "Surviving Intensive Care: A Report from the 2002 Brussels Roundtable," the participants reviewed the literature on neurocognitive impairment among patients who survive an ICU stay; agitation and delirium can lead to increased pulmonary dysfunction, prolonged mechanical ventilation, and self-injury.[20]

To treat delirium, it is imperative that an ICU have methods to detect it. In a survey of health care providers, few physicians and nurses monitor for delirium, while admitting that it is underdiagnosed.[21] A relatively simple tool of diagnosing delirium that has been validated in several clinical and research environments is the Confusion Assessment Method (CAM) and the CAM for the ICU (CAM-ICU).[22] The criteria for delirium include (1) acute mental status change, (2) inattention, (3) disorganized thinking, and (4) altered level of consciousness. Other investigators have developed a Delirium Detection Score, which also has been reported to have excellent sensitivity and specificity.[23] For this evaluation, points are scored for disorientation, agitation, anxiousness, hallucinations, seizures, tremors, sweating, or altered sleep-wake cycles. Patients are rated as having no delirium, mild delirium (can be managed with words[24] and bolus medication), moderate delirium (in which the patient is given continuous infusion of medications), and severe delirium (in which the patient cannot be managed despite treatment with a combination of drugs and is at high risk of self-injury).

In terms of medications administered to patients with delirium, practitioners use haloperidol (66%), lorazepam (12%), and atypical antipsychotics (5%).[21] Lorazepam is an inappropriate treatment for delirium and is an independent risk factor for transitioning to delirium. Whether or not this is a cause and effect or merely an association is debatable.[25] Of equal concern, as mentioned earlier, is the association between delirium and cognitive decline, a concern that is highlighted by the fact that many survivors (perhaps one in three critically ill patients with delirium) developed prolonged cognitive impairment as measured by neuropsychiatric tests at 6 months.[26] As recommended in the 2002 consensus conference, additional investigations into the relationship between anxiety, agitation, delirium, and post-ICU stay cognitive impairment are crucial for managing patients surviving an ICU stay.[20]

The anatomic basis for anxiety probably lies in the limbic system, including the preferential cortex, thalamus, amygdala, hypothalamus, and periaqueductal gray substance.[27] Patients with panic disorder (a relatively common anxiety disorder) have increased blood flow within the hippocampus during a panic attack, as measured by positron emission tomography.[28] Increased serum catecholamines are associated with an increase in anxiety,[29] but most likely are only mediators that stimulate the physiologic changes that accompany anxiety. Activity in the hippocampus stimulates the release of catecholamines, and catecholamines are responsible for many of the physiologic sequelae that accompany anxiety, such as tachycardia, sweating, and tachypnea.

Alternatively, other evidence suggests that neurons in the hypothalamus and brainstem may provide the anatomic basis for stress.[30] When activated, they innervate and increase activity in the sympathetic outflow systems, as occurs in the fight-or-flight response.

Another endogenous compound thought to be involved in the perception of anxiety, γ-aminobutyric acid (GABA), is released in one third of synapses in the central nervous system.[31] Activation of postsynaptic $GABA_A$ receptors increases chloride conductance, resulting in increased intracellular chloride and a fast inhibitory postsynaptic potential.[32] Activation of $GABA_B$ receptors opens potassium channels that produce more chronic inhibition.[33] Any agent or event that increases GABA activity (e.g., benzodiazepines) produces postsynaptic inhibition and decreases excitability.[34] Conversely, any inhibition of GABA activity increases the excitability of neurons and leads to an increased perception of anxiety.

Pathophysiology

Independent of how anxiety arises or of any beneficial effects thereof, untreated anxiety can be pathologic. Anxiety levels are predictive of hypertension[35] and correlate with decreases in myocardial blood flow in regions with normal coronary anatomy.[36] Anxiety interferes with sleep[37] and leads to an increased perception of pain. Patients with unmitigated anxiety are more likely to experience psychiatric manifestations, and anxiety per se has been implicated in the development of ICU delirium, or the ICU syndrome.[38] Respiratory failure is a common reason for admission to the ICU or for extending patients' length of stay. Rosenkranz and associates[39] exposed six volunteers with mild allergic asthma to an inhalation challenge with subject-specific allergens. Patients showed a small decrease in forced expiratory volume in 1 second (FEV_1) and an increase in sputum eosinophilia, both of which correlated with an increase in activity as measured by functional magnetic resonance imaging of the insula and anterior cingulated cortex, the same areas responsible for panic attacks. The brain changes occurred before the secondary phase decrease in FEV_1, suggesting that emotion-initiating areas of the brain play a role in the subsequent airway obstruction.[39] The implications for patients who are critically ill are self-evident.

Anxiety can lead to agitation, which can lead to injury—from patients removing their monitoring and therapeutic devices (i.e., self-extubation or decannulation of arterial and central venous lines); from patients trying to get out of bed, increasing the incidence of falls; by compromising surgical anastomoses; by decreasing patient compliance with therapeutic maneuvers (e.g., chest physiotherapy); and by increasing oxygen consumption. An increase in oxygen consumption may lead to myocardial ischemia with an increase in myocardial events, such as arrhythmias and myocardial ischemia or infarction. An unfavorable balance between oxygen delivery and oxygen consumption correlates with a worse outcome.[40] A decrease in oxygen requirements can be achieved through the use of anxiolysis or analgesia[41] or, if all other maneuvers fail, through paralysis with NMBAs.[42]

Treatment

Nonpharmacologic Interventions

The cost of pharmacologic therapy of anxiety in the ICU is high in terms of dollars[43] and side effects.[44] In the 2002 Brussels Roundtable report, the authors recommended greater study in this area.[20] It is clear that we need greater focus on nonpharmacologic therapy. The level of environmental stress for any patient in the ICU must be reduced as much as possible. This requires awareness by and commitment of health care providers to the provision of a more compassionate caring milieu. Over the last 30 years, the level of environmental stress with respect to noise, interventions, and interruptions has consistently increased in ICUs.[10] Efforts to attenuate these environmental stimuli are paramount in providing effective patient comfort and increasing patients' amount of sleep and rest. As a general rule, noise levels in an ICU must be kept at a minimum. Nighttime interventions, such as routine chest x-rays, blood draws, and chest physiotherapy, also should be kept at a minimum. Doors of patient rooms should be closed as much as possible during the night to facilitate the patients' redevelopment of normal nocturnal sleep patterns. There is evidence that a liberal visitation policy can decrease cardiovascular complications, possibly through decreased anxiety, which is manifested by more favorable hormonal and cytokine levels in ICU patients.[45] Early tracheotomy in mechanically ventilated patients also decreases anxiety.[46]

Pharmacologic Interventions

Despite the best efforts of health care personnel, ICU patients may continue to experience anxiety, agitation, and delirium with all of their attendant problems. Most patients in the ICU require medication to treat anxiety, agitation, and delirium and to provide analgesia.

Most patients in the ICU can be managed with a level of sedation in which they are sleepy but arousable. Deeper sedation should be reserved for select patients, such as patients receiving NMBAs, patients who are extremely agitated, or patients with critical oxygenation difficulties. Patients receiving NMBAs experience pain and anxiety just as other patients do, so it is imperative that they be adequately sedated.

Not all studies show a benefit to sedation, and although these studies have limitations, they do raise important points. Using a matched-case controlled approach, Rodrigues and Gomes do Amaral[47] studied 307 patients, matching 97 with sedation and 97 without sedation. The sedated patients had increased mortality, increased length of stay, and more complications, which the authors attributed to the greater immobility in the sedated patients. The

Table 20-2. Dosage and Mode of Administration of Drugs Commonly Used in Sedation

Drug	Route	Bolus	Infusion
Benzodiazepines			
Midazolam	IV	1 mg repeated to effect	0.04-0.2 mg/kg/h
Diazepam	IV	2-5 mg IV push q1-4h	NA
Lorazepam	IV, IM	1-4 mg q4-6h	0.01-0.05 mg/kg/h
Propofol	IV	0.3-0.7 mg IV push	10-100 μg/kg/min
Dexmedetomidine	IV	10 μg/kg	0.2-0.7 μg/kg/h
Ketamine	IV	1-2 mg/kg IV push	0.5-4.5 μg/kg/h
Barbiturates			
Pentobarbital	IV	3-5 mg/kg	1-3 mg/kg/h
Thiopental	IV	3-5 mg/kg	2-5 mg/kg/h
Butyrophenones			
Haldol	IV, IM	0.5-5 mg, repeat doses every 30-45 min	

IM, intramuscular; IV, intravascular; NA, not applicable.

authors acknowledged, however, that even though patients were matched for severity of disease, the tools for assessing severity of disease are imperfect, and they have identified an association, not a cause and effect. A balanced approach, adopted by many ICUs, is to assess on a daily basis the need for sedative-analgesic medications.

Commonly used sedative and hypnotic drugs include the benzodiazepines, propofol, butyrophenones, α-agonists (dexmedetomidine), and barbiturates (Table 20-2). Sedative-hypnotics do not have analgesic properties, so they can provide pain relief only when obtundation of consciousness or anesthesia occurs. Opioids, in addition to their analgesic attributes, provide a certain amount of sedation.

Box 20-3

Criteria for Sedation Scale

- Multidisciplinary development
- Ease of administration
- Easy to recall
- Easy to interpret
- Well-defined, discrete criteria
- Sufficient choices to titrate medication effectively
- Assessment of agitation
- Reproducibility
- Validity

Monitoring of Sedation

There are several subjective and objective techniques for monitoring sedation, but none is ideal. The ICU practitioner should be familiar with at least one or two methodologies for monitoring sedation and should use one of them in managing patients who require anxiolysis. Ideally, the monitoring method chosen should be simple to use and document and should describe accurately the degree of anxiety or agitation and the level of sedation that is achieved (Box 20-3). The Ramsa scale (Table 20-3) has been used for decades and has an acceptable reliability, but there is little ability to grade levels of sedation.[48,49] The SAS also has been proven reliable in ICU patients.[50] The MAAS is an extension of the Riker SAS and has been used in ICU patients to quantify agitation.[51] Ely and colleagues[52] favor the Richmond Agitation-Sedation Scale for anxious or delirious patients because it quantifies changes in status over the time continuum, and the score correlates with sedative and analgesic medications. There is also a Vancouver Interaction and Calmness scale that has been used in ICUs, and for children, the COMFORT scale has been widely evaluated and used (Table 20-4).[53,54]

Table 20-3. Ramsay Level of Sedation

Level	Characteristic
1	Patient anxious and agitated, restless, or both
2	Patient cooperative, oriented, and tranquil
3	Patient asleep, responds to commands only
4	Patient asleep, has a brisk response to a light glabellar tap
5	Patient asleep, has a sluggish response to a light glabellar tap
6	No response

Reprinted with permission from Murray MJ: Use of sedatives, analgesics, and neuromuscular blocking drugs. In Parrillo JE (ed): Current Therapy in Critical Care Medicine, 3rd ed. St. Louis, Mosby, 1997, pp 66-71.

All of these assessment tools are subjective, but many ICU practitioners would prefer an objective measure of sedation. Heart rate and blood pressure are neither specific nor sensitive indicators of the level of sedation and cannot be recommended. The electroencephalogram is influenced by sedation, but it is costly to monitor and difficult to interpret. There have been many attempts to manipulate the electroencephalogram using computer algorithms that simplify monitoring and interpretation. The bispectral index has been extensively tested in the operating room and is increasingly being used in ICU

Table 20-4. Sedation Scales

MSAT	Minnesota Sedation Assessment Tool
ATICE	Adaptation to the Intensive Care Environment
VICS	Vancouver Interactive and Calmness Scale
SAS	Sedation Agitation Scale
RASS	Richmond Agitation Sedation Scale

patients. In ICU situations in which it has been tested, there are limitations.[55,56] The bispectral index varies among patients, and one study indicates that the subjective scales have more reproducibility, especially at lower levels of sedation.[57] In patients who are receiving NMBAs, the bispectral index may have utility, but it has not yet been validated for these patients. In addition to monitoring the depth of sedation, one should consider daily interruption of all sedative infusions.[58]

Benzodiazepines

The benzodiazepines are the most commonly used sedative-hypnotic medications in the ICU. They have anxiolytic, sedative-hypnotic, muscle relaxant, and anticonvulsive properties. Benzodiazepines also provide anterograde amnesia, but retrograde amnesia varies. They do not have analgesic action, but do have synergy with opioids. They act by engaging benzodiazepine receptors (modulator subunits of the $GABA_A$ receptors) in the limbic system of the brain, enhancing the effects of GABA in a dose-dependent fashion.[59] Benzodiazepines can be titrated to produce effects ranging from light sedation to coma. Respiratory depression is dose-dependent and is much more likely to occur in elderly patients and patients receiving opioids.

Most benzodiazepines are metabolized in the liver, and the metabolites are excreted by the kidneys. In critically ill patients, especially elderly patients and patients with liver failure, these drugs have prolonged half-lives, and accumulation of the drugs and their metabolites is possible.[60] Benzodiazepines are not effectively removed with hemodialysis. Overdosage results in amplification of the therapeutic effects, but serious sequelae are uncommon in a monitored setting. Benzodiazepines and opioids act synergistically to produce deeper sedation (and depression of cardiopulmonary function) than they would be expected to produce additively.

Diazepam is the best-known benzodiazepine. It can be given orally or intravenously. It is an effective sedative-hypnotic with amnestic effects. Diazepam is considered a long-acting benzodiazepine because it has a prolonged elimination half-life (50 hours) with active metabolites that also have hypnotic effects.

Midazolam is a short-acting benzodiazepine that, on intravenous administration, causes no pain or venous thrombosis, and its potency is two to four times that of diazepam. Midazolam is readily redistributed in tissues and is rapidly cleared by the liver and kidneys. The clinical effects of midazolam are short-lived owing to an elimination half-life of 1.5 to 3.5 hours. These properties make midazolam a suitable drug for continuous infusion because it has a rapid onset of effects, it is potent, and patients generally awaken rapidly after discontinuation of the infusion. Midazolam elimination may be decreased, however, in critically ill patients with low albumin, decreased renal function, or obesity, leading to prolonged sedation. An active metabolite, α-hydroxymidazolam, also contributes to prolongation of effect with prolonged infusions.[61] Continuous infusions of midazolam are ideally used on a short-term basis for sedation, anxiolysis, and amnesia in critically ill patients. A loading dose may be used in 1-mg increments until the desired affect is achieved, followed by a continuous infusion of 2 to 5 mg/h.

Lorazepam has less effect than other benzodiazepines on cardiovascular and respiratory centers and fewer potential drug interactions, owing to metabolism via glucuronidization. Lorazepam is recommended for ICU patients requiring sedation for greater than 24 hours. It should be initiated using intermittent intravenous boluses to achieve the desired level of sedation, followed by an infusion for maintenance (0.5 to 2 mg/h). The solvent in the 2 mg/mL product contains polyethylene glycol 400 and propylene glycol and, with prolonged or high dosage, has been reported to produce acute tubular necrosis, lactic acidosis, and hyperosmolar state.

Flumazenil, a highly specific benzodiazepine antagonist, reverses all known central nervous system effects of the benzodiazepines.[62] It reaches maximal concentration in the brain within 5 to 10 minutes after intravenous administration. The mean terminal half-life of flumazenil is approximately 1 hour. It is completely metabolized to free carboxylic acid and glucuronide, both of which are inactive metabolites and renally excreted. It is helpful in reversing respiratory depression resulting from high dosages of benzodiazepines. Reversal of the effects of therapeutic doses of benzodiazepines can be achieved with the intravenous administration of 0.1 to 1 mg of flumazenil. Higher doses of flumazenil may be given, but the antagonist effect may make immediate resedation difficult.

Propofol

Propofol (di-isopropylphenol) is an intravenous anesthetic agent, chemically unrelated to other anesthetics, that has sedative and hypnotic characteristics at lower doses. The original formulation of this drug with Cremophor EL was associated with a high risk of anaphylaxis. It is now formulated in a lipid emulsion (Intralipid 10%) either with ethylenediaminetetraacetic acid or with bisulfite as preservatives to decrease the incidence of bacterial overgrowth. Hypertriglyceridemia may result from high-dose infusions, which may increase morbidity associated with its use. Propofol is short-acting and rapidly metabolized, making it a suitable drug for continuous infusion. It has no analgesic properties.

Propofol should be administered in a dedicated intravenous catheter because of the potential for drug incompatibility and to decrease the chances of nosocomial infection (increased because of the lipid emulsion). Given the potential for long-term use and contamination in

ICUs, aseptic technique is imperative, and infusion lines and bottles should be changed at regular intervals. When used for sedation, an initial dose of 0.3 to 0.7 mg/kg should be used, followed by an infusion at approximately 10 to 100 μg/kg/min. The infusion rate should be titrated to the desired level of sedation. Recovery usually occurs within 15 to 20 minutes of the discontinuation of the infusion.

Many studies have compared propofol with midazolam for sedation in the ICU, but most of the trials are flawed by inadequate study design. From a clinical perspective, propofol and midazolam have similar recovery times. For sedation lasting greater than 72 hours, propofol may have a more rapid and reliable awakening profile,[63] although even this is controversial.[64]

Propofol may cause a decrease in mean arterial pressure, probably as a result of peripheral vasodilation and not direct myocardial depression. There have been reports of sudden death from metabolic acidosis in patients receiving propofol (propofol infusion syndrome); most cases have involved children.[65] Myoclonic activity versus frank seizures have been observed in patients after discontinuation of propofol. Propofol also has been used to treat status epilepticus and to treat increased intracranial pressure.

Butyrophenones

Butyrophenones induce a state of apathy and mental detachment in patients with dysharmonious brain function. They inhibit dopamine-mediated neurotransmission in the cerebrum and basal ganglia. The result is a decrease is abnormal thought patterns, but the patient is so detached from his or her environment that he or she has a characteristic flat affect. Butyrophenones inhibit the chemoreceptor trigger zone in the medulla and are effective antiemetics.

Of the butyrophenones, haloperidol is the most useful drug for treatment of delirium in ICU patients. The drug has a wide therapeutic margin of safety, with little effect on heart rate and blood pressure and no effect on ventilation; reported cases of hypotension after administration of haloperidol virtually always occur in hypovolemic patients. The initial dose of haloperidol should be 0.5 to 5 mg administered parenterally. Higher doses should be reserved for young, severely agitated patients. The onset of sedation is delayed, with a peak pharmacologic response in 30 minutes. To allow for this delayed onset, repeat doses should be staggered by 30 to 45 minutes. If a patient tolerates the initial dose, but does not display adequate sedation, the dose may be doubled for the next bolus. Recurrence of agitation should be the indication for further doses. When the patient has returned to baseline mental clarity, small nighttime doses for a few days help prevent nighttime delirium, or "sundowning." Patients may develop extrapyramidal side effects, probably owing to an active metabolite, but less so when given intravenously than when given intramuscularly.[66] As with all neuroleptics, tardive dyskinesia and neuroleptic malignant syndrome are rare but serious side effects that may occur even with the modest doses prescribed in the ICU.

Haloperidol and any of the butyrophenones also may induce a dose-dependent prolongation of the QT interval leading to ventricular arrhythmias and torsades de pointes.[67] Patients with cardiac disease are at greater risk of this complication. It is recommended that ICU patients receiving haloperidol be monitored for ECG changes as well as for extrapyramidal side effects.

Dexmedetomidine

Dexmedetomidine is a new sedative agent that acts by binding to α_{2A}-adrenoreceptors located in the locus caeruleus with an affinity of 1620 : 1 compared with its affinity to the α_1-receptor. At this site, it releases norepinephrine and decreases sympathetic activity.[68] It has sedative, analgesic, and amnestic properties,[69] but is most notable because of its unique mechanism of action. By decreasing sympathetic activity, patients appear sedated, but can be easily aroused. Dexmedetomidine is increasingly being used to sedate patients after coronary artery bypass graft surgery[70] as a safe drug that decreases the use of opioids, β-blockers, and antiemetics. Dexmedetomidine is particularly useful in fast-tracking patients after cardiac surgery. Whether it is superior to currently used sedative agents in the ICU is unknown.[71] Because of its α_2 mechanisms, it decreases blood pressure and heart rate (which is often beneficial in ICU patients), and so far there are few case reports of any complications, although cardiac arrest has been reported,[72] and there is concern that if continued for greater than 24 hours and then stopped abruptly, it could precipitate a hyperdynamic state similar to what happens when clonidine that has been used long-term is stopped abruptly.[73] Whether dexmedetomidine turns out to be a drug with properties that would extend its use in the recovery room and postanesthesia care unit is yet to be determined.[74]

Barbiturates

Barbiturates are one of the oldest classes of sedative-hypnotic agents. They have significant depressive cardiovascular and respiratory effects, however, and have been largely replaced in the ICU by the benzodiazepines, propofol, butyrophenones, and other newer agents. Barbiturates are occasionally used for deep sedation or anesthesia in mechanically ventilated patients with status epilepticus and in patients with elevated intracranial pressure (barbiturate coma). In patients with closed-head injury and increased intracranial pressure refractory to conventional therapies, survival has been improved by adding high-dose barbiturates to conventional therapy.

Opioids

As mentioned previously, opioids also have sedative effects in addition to their analgesic effects. They are discussed later.

PAIN

Etiology

The anatomic substrate for pain is better understood than is the substrate for anxiety. Pain most frequently arises in the periphery, usually secondary to tissue damage that results in increased levels of biochemicals such as histamine, serotonin, and prostaglandins. These substances activate nerve terminals that result in neuroelectric activity in C and A delta nerve fibers. These fibers synapse in the spinal cord, activating other neurons whose axons terminate in the reticular activating system in the diencephalon. Positron emission tomography scans have shown that activity in the anterior cingulate cortex is associated with the unpleasant perception of pain,[75] implicating this area of the brain in the linkage between anxiety and pain. As already mentioned, anxious and sleep-deprived patients experience greater levels of pain and require more analgesics to control their pain than anxiety-free, well-rested patients.

Pathophysiology

Similar to anxiety, uncontrolled pain results in numerous sequelae. Pain has a beneficial role in that it stimulates avoidance of further injury and conservation of resources used for healing. Pain can have adverse effects, however, by increasing levels of catecholamines that lead to an increase in sympathetic activity, in demands on the cardiovascular system, and in oxygen requirements,[7] all of which critically ill patients tolerate poorly. Associated with these adverse sequelae of the stress response is hyper-metabolism, which, if unabated, may lead to excessive catabolism, decreased immune function, and delayed wound healing. Pain causes a delay in mobilization and activity with a possible increased incidence of deep venous thrombosis and pulmonary embolism. Nociceptive stimuli may cause ileus, nausea, and vomiting. All of these effects increase discomfort and morbidity, prolong hospital stay, and may increase mortality. Treatment of anxiety and pain is an integral part of good patient care.

Treatment

Nonpharmacologic Interventions

Transcutaneous electrical nerve stimulation, cryoanalgesia, acupuncture, nerve blocks, local anesthetics (epidural and intrapleural), and neurolytic agents all have roles in the management of patients in the ICU who experience pain. It is beyond the scope of this chapter to discuss these, but an intensivist managing ICU patients must be aware of these modalities, individualizing them to patients with unique analgesic requirements. Most patients require parenteral or enteral medications to control their pain, however.

Pharmacologic Interventions

Nonopioid Analgesics

The nonopioid analgesics include salicylates, acetaminophen, and other nonsteroidal anti-inflammatory drugs (NSAIDs) (Table 20-5). Release of prostaglandins and leukotrienes leads to inflammation and sensitization of nociceptors, resulting in hyperalgesia that is characterized by a decrease in the pain threshold. The origin of pain could be at the site of injury, owing to biochemical changes in the surrounding area, but the pain signal also could be amplified or modified in the spinal cord secondary to the action of prostaglandins.[76] Salicylates and NSAIDs inhibit cyclooxygenase, reducing concentrations of prostaglandins and other inflammatory mediators.

In postoperative patients, many clinical studies have shown that, compared with placebo, NSAIDs significantly reduce pain intensity and opioid requirements. Oral ibuprofen has been compared with intravenous fentanyl; the patients taking ibuprofen and fentanyl were more comfortable in the postoperative period than the patients who received fentanyl alone. Ketorolac tromethamine is currently the only available intravenous agent. Its parenteral administration is advantageous in the postoperative period if the patient is unable to take oral medication. Ketorolac tromethamine is comparable to intramuscular morphine for the relief of moderate to severe postoperative pain. The requirements for intravenous morphine also are significantly reduced when ketorolac is administered concomitantly.

Ketorolac and the other NSAIDs have unwanted side effects, including an increased incidence of gastrointestinal bleeding (bleeding secondary to platelet inhibition and renal insufficiency). Elderly patients and patients with hypotension or hypovolemia are more susceptible to NSAID-induced renal injury.[77] Ketorolac use for greater than 5 days has been associated with an increased inci-

Table 20-5. Dosage and Mode of Administration of Common Nonopioid Analgesics

Drug	Route	Dose (mg)	Frequency
Ibuprofen	PO	200-400	q4-6h
Ketorolac	IM	30-60 initially	Repeat 15-30 q4-6h
Indomethacin (Indocin)	PO, PR*	25 (PO), 50 (PR)	q6-8h
Naproxen (Naprosyn)	PO	250-500	q12h
Acetaminophen	PO, PR	500-1000†	q4-6h
Aspirin	PO, PR*	300-1000	q4-6h

*Parenteral preparation is available.
†Maximum dose is 4000 mg/d.
IM, intramuscular; PO, by mouth; PR, per rectum.

dence of gastrointestinal and wound bleeding.[78] Patients without renal dysfunction or risk of gastrointestinal bleeding can be given ketorolac intramuscularly at an initial bolus of 15 to 30 mg followed by a dose of 15 mg intramuscularly every 6 hours. Ketorolac should be limited to fewer than 5 days of use during the postoperative period because of concerns about adverse events.

NSAIDs neither cause respiratory depression nor decrease the level of consciousness. They do not interfere with intestinal and bile duct motility, and compared with opioids, they have less nausea, vomiting, and adynamic ileus associated with their use. Their combination with opiates enables smaller dosages of the latter, achieving good pain control with fewer side effects. The main side effects of therapeutic doses of NSAIDs are gastric irritation and inhibition of platelet and renal function. The role of more selective cyclooxygenase-2 inhibitors in ICU patients has not been studied yet. Their dosage and administration should be individualized to each patient.

Opioid Analgesics

Opioids are the mainstay of postoperative analgesic treatment. Traditionally, they have been administered orally, intramuscularly, or intravenously, but over the last 15 years, epidural, intrathecal, transdermal, and transmucosal delivery systems have been developed.

Opioids produce analgesia and sedation through their agonist effects on opiate receptors in the central nervous system. They are best used for acute pain and at equivalent dosages are equally potent. Commonly used opioids are summarized in Table 20-6. Morphine, fentanyl, and hydromorphone are the most frequently used opioids for postoperative pain relief in the ICU.

The intramuscular route is the time-honored and most common technique for administration of opioids. These drugs can be given at discrete time intervals (every 3 to 6 hours) or on an as-needed basis. This simple practice is universally applicable. Absorption of the drug is gradual, giving rise to potentially therapeutic levels for longer duration. Greater than 70% of patients describe adequate analgesia after an intramuscular injection with fewer side effects, such as cardiorespiratory depression, than patients receiving an equivalent dose of opioids intravenously.[79] This is not to say that intramuscular opioids are free of side effects. Patients receiving opioids intramuscularly can exhibit an abdominal respiratory pattern to their breathing, oxygen desaturation, and apnea. Local pain and increased creatine kinase levels are associated with the needle stick; the former is unpleasant and the latter could be mistaken for myocardial necrosis.

Several other problems have been noted when using the intramuscular route. There is a large variation among patients' needs for analgesics. A "standard dose" may be optimal only for a small portion of patients, and a "safe" dose is often inadequate. Serum opioid levels required to produce analgesia in different patients also vary fourfold.

Given intravenously as a bolus, opioids provide high blood levels for a short duration. From the time a patient requests pain relief until analgesia is achieved is similar, however, between intravenous and intramuscular routes. The intravenous administration of opioids is associated with a higher risk of respiratory depression, sometimes of life-threatening severity. There also is a greater reduction in sympathetic tone and enhancement of vagal and parasympathetic tone, which may lead to bradycardia and hypotension. Intravenous opioids are given in small dose increments that avoid wide fluctuations in plasma concentrations and allow near-optimal levels of analgesia, less sedation, less drug use, and fewer adverse events.

To individualize therapy better, a technique of patient-controlled analgesia was developed in the late 1960s.[80] Using patient-controlled analgesia, patients self-administer small doses of opioids when they experience pain. Patients titrate opioids to their own needs within guidelines deemed safe (Table 20-7). Patient-controlled devices have been used for the administration of other drugs, including midazolam and propofol.

Oral opioids can be administered as soon as oral intake is possible. In appropriate doses, they may be remarkably effective, and patients can choose the dose and frequency of administration best suited to their needs. Although most patients in the ICU do not tolerate oral opioids, for the patients who do, analgesia can be effectively provided via the oral route.

Table 20-6. Standard Equivalents of Selected Opioid Analgesics

Drug	Oral Dose (mg)*	Parenteral Dose (mg)*
Alphaprodine HCl (Nisentil)	—	45
Codeine	200	130
Fentanyl (Sublimaze)	—	0.1
Hydromorphone HCl (Dilaudid)	7.5	1.5
Meperidine HCl (Demerol)	200	50
Methadone HCl (Dolophine HCl)	10	8.8
Morphine sulfate	60	10
Oxycodone HCl (Roxicodone)	30	15
Oxymorphone HCl (Numorphan)	—	1.5
Pentazocine (Talwin)	—	60

*70-kg adult.

Table 20-7. Acceptable Drugs, Intravenous Drugs, and Lockout Intervals for Use with Postoperative Patient-Controlled Analgesia Pump

Drug	Dose (mg)	Lockout Interval (min)
Morphine sulfate	0.2-3	5-20
Meperidine HCl (Demerol)	2-30	5-15
Fentanyl (Sublimaze)	0.02-0.1	3-10
Hydromorphone HCl (Dilaudid)	0.02-0.5	5-15

Compared with intramuscular or intravenous morphine, many studies have consistently shown that patients receiving opioids epidurally report superior analgesia, have fewer pulmonary complications, have earlier return of bowel function, and ambulate sooner.[81] Epidural opioids are effective for the pain associated with thoracotomies, intra-abdominal procedures, and genitourinary and lower limb operations. They do not cause sympathetic or motor block or hypotension. Patients can use patient-controlled analgesia pumps to self-administer epidural opioids (patient-controlled epidural analgesia) as needed.

The main side effects of epidural opioids are respiratory depression, pruritus, urinary retention, nausea, and vomiting. Respiratory depression is observed in 1% to 5% of patients and is associated with advanced age, concomitant use of systemic opioids or other central nervous system depressants, extensive surgery, and higher dosages. Patients receiving epidural opioids need to be under surveillance with respiratory monitoring. Pruritus sometimes can be relieved by antihistamines (diphenhydramine hydrochloride) or by placing a transdermal scopolamine patch. Urinary retention is more common in men and at times requires bladder catheterization.

Administration of naloxone reverses the side effects of epidural opioids and, in proper doses, allows effective analgesia. Naloxone is a short-acting drug, however, and recurrence of side effects should be anticipated unless the naloxone is administered repeatedly or by a continuous intravenous infusion at 2 to 5 µg/kg/h.

Agents

Fentanyl, a synthetic opioid, is 50 to 100 times more potent than morphine for pain relief. *Remifentanil* is a synthetic opioid with a very short half-life because of its unique mode of metabolism whose context-sensitive half-life does not change, regardless of duration of infusion. It has been used for analgesia-based sedation in the ICU with good results.[82,83]

Ketamine, a potent analgesic chemically related to the hallucinogen phencyclidine, produces a unique anesthetic condition, described as "dissociative" anesthesia. Ketamine and a benzodiazepine are frequently used for sedation in children. In the ICU, ketamine can be given before airway intubation of hypovolemic patients, dressing changes, laceration repair, abscess incision and drainage, and orthopedic manipulations. In addition, this drug can be given to anesthetize patients for surgical procedures performed in the ICU (e.g., for a chest tube placement or tracheostomy). General anesthesia with ketamine is characterized by a hyperdynamic circulatory response and maintenance of protective airway reflexes and of minute ventilation. Ketamine has no detrimental effects on hepatic or renal function. Although ketamine is a safe anesthetic for most critically ill patients, it has been associated with hallucinations and emergence reactions, with hypoxia, and with hypotension and hypertension.

Ketamine can be given orally, rectally, intramuscularly, or intravenously. Intravenous doses of 0.2 to 0.3 mg/kg of ketamine produce analgesia with little loss of consciousness, whereas intravenous doses of 1 to 2 mg/kg induce general anesthesia. Because ketamine is marketed in three concentrations (10, 50, or 100 mg/mL), clinicians must read the medication label carefully before administration to avoid dosing errors.

Although ketamine is a direct myocardial depressant, it inhibits reuptake of catecholamines and produces mild to moderate increases in mean arterial pressure, heart rate, and cardiac output. These cardiostimulatory effects could be detrimental to patients with coronary artery disease or hypertensive emergencies. In addition, patients with impaired myocardial reserve or depleted endogenous catecholamine stores may have a hypotensive response to ketamine caused by direct myocardial depression. Ketamine increases pulmonary arterial pressures and may exacerbate pulmonary hypertension. Nevertheless, because other anesthetics (e.g., barbiturates) may produce severe cardiovascular instability in hypovolemic patients, ketamine is frequently chosen by anesthesiologists for induction of patients with hemorrhagic shock. Ketamine is not proarrhythmic and can be used to provide anesthesia for cardioversion.

Ketamine is a bronchodilator and has been used in the treatment of status asthmaticus. Tracheal intubation is almost never necessary with ketamine anesthesia because this drug produces only mild dose-related respiratory depression. It does not depress protective airway reflexes such as coughing. Salivary and tracheobronchial secretions are increased by ketamine, and a prophylactic antisialagogue (e.g., glycopyrrolate 0.2 mg intravenously) is recommended if there are no contraindications. Cases of aspiration, laryngospasm, and prolonged apnea are rare, but have been reported in association with large, rapid bolus doses, in head-injured patients, and in neonates. Cases of laryngospasm have been attributed to stimulation of hypersensitized laryngeal reflexes, respiratory infection, and hypersalivation.

The effects of a single injection of ketamine generally last less than 30 minutes, although coadministration of drugs that are metabolized by the liver (e.g., benzodiazepines) can increase the half-life of ketamine. During recovery, ketamine-induced ataxia and dysequilibrium can prevent patients from walking until these symptoms resolve (usually within 1 to 4 hours). During emergence from ketamine, patients may have vivid dreams (pleasing and unpleasant) or hallucinations or both. Benzodiazepines, such as midazolam, are effective at preventing these psychic phenomena. Although tolerance after repeated administration of ketamine has been reported, increased doses have not been associated with an increased incidence of adverse effects or physical dependence.

Unless contraindicated, a benzodiazepine (to reduce psychic emergence phenomena) and an anticholinergic (to reduce airway secretions) should be given in conjunction with ketamine. Ketamine is no different from other anesthetics in that clinicians should be prepared to provide artificial ventilation, airway intubation, and resuscitation to treat the unusual complications of airway obstruction, apnea, or cardiovascular instability should they arise.

Gabapentin is an anticonvulsant, a drug with GABA activity. It is increasingly being used for neuropathic and perioperative pain and may find its way into ICU practice.[84]

NEUROMUSCULAR BLOCKING AGENTS

Patients in an ICU occasionally remain agitated despite the administration of what should be effective anxiolysis and analgesia. Sometimes the therapeutic window for these medications is so small that effective anxiolytic or analgesic therapy cannot be administered safely because of their side effects, which include hemodynamic compromise (i.e., hypotension). In addition, restlessness may be so severe that sedatives and analgesics are inadequate to control the agitation. Patients with closed-head injuries, tetanus, or acute lung injury requiring mechanical ventilation occasionally require chemical paralysis with NMBAs. Before resorting to muscle paralysis, health care providers must ascertain that all other modalities and interventions have been exhausted (Box 20-4).

Indications

Indications for the use of NMBAs in the ICU include mechanically ventilated patients with severe obstruction or acute respiratory distress syndrome (ARDS) that would not allow controlled ventilation without NMBAs, patients who have sustained a closed-head injury and have elevated intracranial pressure, and patients with tetanus. Other situations may arise that require NMBAs, but they are uncommon.

Newer modes of mechanical ventilation (e.g., reverse I/E ratio) and permissive hypercapnia in the management of ARDS often require paralysis.[85] The use of NMBAs in patients with ARDS can improve gas exchange.[86] These patients, if agitated and hemodynamically unstable, may have decreased mixed venous oxygen saturation, below a critical level. They frequently do not tolerate combinations of sedatives and analgesics because of hemodynamic compromise, and in some circumstances, even if hemodynamics allow these agents, their mixed venous oxygen saturation is still low (usually 50% to 60%). Under these circumstances, the use of NMBAs improves gas exchange, as documented in patients with ARDS.[86]

Box 20-4

Goals of Sedation and Analgesia in Patients Undergoing Neuromuscular Blockade for Mechanical Ventilation

- Careful patient evaluation
- Medication based on patient's specific factors
- Treatment goals delineated and reassessed daily
- Titrate medications based on objective sedation scales
- Peripheral nerve stimulator
- Intermittent versus continuous therapy
- Daily drug "holidays"
- Discontinue medication therapy as soon as possible

Monitoring

Traditionally, patients requiring muscle paralysis through the use of NMBAs have been followed clinically, assessing skeletal muscle movement or evidence of respiratory effort. The use of clinical judgment is frequently insufficient, however, and patients can be overdosed with NMBAs. Monitoring the depth of block may allow the lowest NMBA dose and may decrease complications,[87] but not all studies have shown that it makes a difference.[88] Some type of electronic assessment of the depth of block in ICU patients is recommended. Monitoring the degree of neuromuscular block with a neuromuscular twitch stimulator, usually with facile assessment of a train-of-four ratio, allows for more appropriate dosing of NMBAs. A peripheral nerve stimulator, a device capable of delivering electrical current transcutaneously, is required (Box 20-5). After cleaning the skin at the wrist, two silver chloride electrodes are attached approximately 5 cm apart along the course of the ulnar nerve. The stimulator is connected to the electrodes, and holding the thumb in abduction, the train-of-four button on the stimulator is activated. If there is no response, the amperage on the device is increased in 10-mA increments from 20 to 100 mA or greater. The response to stimulation is assessed with each increase in amperage until a response occurs. In an unparalyzed patient who is receiving no NMBAs, four serial abductions are typically seen in the thumb using 20 to 40 mA. In a patient receiving NMBAs, an adequate level of block would be defined as one to two responses (train-of-four of one to two). This correlates with approximately 90% to 95% of the neuromuscular receptors being blocked. Patients who have 0 twitches are usually overdosed (or it could be related to difficulty with the electrodes, such as caused by sweating, skin thickness, or hypoperfusion of extremities) and would require stopping or decreasing the dose of NMBA. Many patients maintain a single twitch and yet still develop prolonged neuromuscular block after the NMBA is discontinued (acute quadriparetic myopathy syndrome [AQMS]).[89] With two to four twitches, it still may be possible to ventilate the patient adequately, but with a decreased incidence of AQMS. If the therapeutic goal is achieved with more than one to two twitches, that is optimal.

Complications

AQMS is a serious complication of NMBA administration, significantly prolonging the requirement for mechanical ventilation, ICU stay, and hospitalization. This complication is one of the reasons that the indiscriminate use of NMBAs is discouraged. AQMS is manifested by diffuse weakness that persists long (days) after the NMBA is discontinued and drug metabolites have been eliminated. On examination, the patient has a significant motor deficit in the upper and lower extremities along with depressed deep tendon reflexes. Ocular muscle function is usually preserved, as is sensory function. On electromyography, there are low-amplitude compound motor action potentials and muscle fibrillations. Modest creatine kinase increases are observed in approximately 50% of patients.

Box 20-5

Protocol for Monitoring the Degree of Neuromuscular Block Using a Nerve Stimulator and Assessment of the Train-of-Four Twitch

Purpose

To describe the process of using a nerve stimulator to stimulate the ulnar nerve, usually with tactile assessment of a neuromuscular twitch (usually tactile assessment of an abducted thumb) to assess the degree of neuromuscular block.

Definitions

Neuromuscular block: The process by which the postsynaptic acetylcholine receptor is depressed and variably responds to release of acetylcholine in the neuromuscular junction cleft.

Peripheral nerve stimulation: Electrical stimulation, usually 40 to 120 mA at a peripheral nerve (usually the ulnar, either at the elbow or at the wrist).

Train-of-four: A specific kind of nerve stimulation in which the nerve stimulator delivers an electrical stimulus to the nerve lasting 10 ms and repeated every 500 ms for a total of four stimuli.

Equipment

1. Peripheral nerve stimulator
2. Two electrode pads (electrocardiogram pads may be used)

Procedure

1. Clean the area where the electrode pads will be placed with alcohol to remove any skin oils. This reduces the resistance at the skin and decreases the amount of current needed to stimulate the nerve. If the resistance of the skin is still high, an abrasive compound can be used to remove dead skin.
2. Place two electrodes over the ulnar nerve, usually 3 to 5 cm apart.
3. Attach electrodes to the leads, usually the positive electrode proximally.
4. Cover the fingers and abduct the thumb. Increase the amperage of the stimulator until four twitches of the thumb are palpated by tactile assessment. Stimuli should not be delivered more frequently than every 20 seconds. After four twitches are palpated, a supramaximal stimulus can be delivered by increasing the amperage 10% to 30% over the amperage required to palpate four twitches.

Goals

1. To achieve a level of train-of-four of two to four. If with three or four twitches the patient either spontaneously triggers the ventilator or exhibits muscular activity that adversely affects oxygenation or airway or intracranial pressure, increased neuromuscular block is required.
2. A train-of-four of one to zero indicates that the degree of neuromuscular block is too great, and the dosage of neuromuscular blocking agent should be decreased.

Although AQMS develops in patients receiving NMBAs alone, it is strongly associated with the use of corticosteroids. Thirty percent of patients who receive NMBAs for greater than 24 to 48 hours and corticosteroids at a dose of greater than 1000 mg methylprednisolone are at significant risk of developing AQMS with associated type II muscle fiber atrophy, vacuolization and disordered sarcomeric architecture, and extensive loss of myosin on muscle biopsy specimen.

AQMS has been reported most commonly with the aminosteroidal blocking drugs, especially vecuronium and pancuronium, but also has been reported after use of the benzylisoquinolinium compounds (doxacurium, atracurium, cisatracurium). Because of these concerns, every effort should be made to discontinue NMBAs as soon as possible, especially in patients receiving corticosteroids. Whether a drug-free period every day decreases the incidence of AQMS is unknown.

Pharmacology

Aminosteroidal Compounds

Pancuronium

Pancuronium, one of the original NMBAs used in ICUs, is a long-acting, nondepolarizing compound that after a bolus dose of 0.06 to 0.08 mg/kg is effective for 90 minutes. Although it is commonly given as an intravenous bolus, it can be used as a continuous infusion, titrating the dose to the degree of NMBA that is desired. Pancuronium is vagolytic, which limits its use in patients who would not tolerate an increase in heart rate. In patients with renal failure or cirrhosis, the neuromuscular blocking effects of pancuronium are prolonged because of the increased elimination half-life of the agent and its 3-hydroxypancuronium metabolite, which has one third to one half the activity of pancuronium.

Vecuronium

Vecuronium is an intermediate-acting NMBA that is a structural analogue of pancuronium, but is not vagolytic. An intravenous bolus dose of 0.08 to 0.10 mg/kg produces block within 2.5 to 3 minutes, which typically lasts 25 to 30 minutes. After a bolus dose, it can be given as a continuous infusion of 1 to 2 µg/kg/min, titrating the rate to the degree of block desired. The 3-desacetylvecuronium metabolite has 50% of the pharmacologic activity of the parent compound,[90] so patients with hepatic dysfunction may have increased plasma concentrations of the parent compound and the active metabolite, causing prolonged block. Vecuronium is associated with AQMS in patients receiving corticosteroids. Vecuronium is being used with decreased frequency in ICU patients.

Rocuronium

Rocuronium is a newer nondepolarizing NMBA with a monoquaternary steroidal chemistry, with an intermediate duration of action and a very rapid onset. When given as a bolus of 0.6 to 0.1 mg/kg, block is almost always achieved within 2 minutes, with maximal block occurring within 3 minutes; continuous infusions are begun at 10 µg/kg/min.[91] Rocuronium's metabolite, 17-desacetylrocuronium, has only 5% to 10% activity compared with the parent compound. Renal failure should not have an effect on duration of action, but hepatic failure may prolong NMBA action.

Benzylisoquinolinium Compounds

Atracurium

Atracurium is an intermediate-acting NMBA with minimal cardiovascular side effects, but is associated with histamine release at higher doses. It is inactivated in plasma by ester hydrolysis and by Hofmann elimination so that renal or hepatic dysfunction does not affect duration of block. Atracurium can be administered to various critically ill patients, including patients with liver failure, renal failure, or multiple organ dysfunction syndrome, to facilitate mechanical ventilation. Atracurium has been associated with persistent neuromuscular weakness, as has been reported with other NMBAs.

Cisatracurium

Cisatracurium, an isomer of atracurium, is an intermediate-acting benzylisoquinolinium NMBA that is increasingly used in lieu of atracurium. It produces few, if any, cardiovascular effects and has less of a tendency to produce mast cell degranulation than atracurium. Bolus doses with 0.10 to 0.2 mg/kg result in paralysis in an average of 2.5 minutes, and recovery begins at approximately 25 minutes; maintenance infusion rates should be started at 2.5 to 3 µg/kg/min. Cisatracurium also is metabolized by ester hydrolysis and Hofmann elimination, so duration of block should not be affected by renal or hepatic dysfunction. There have not yet been reports of significantly prolonged recovery associated with cisatracurium. The mean peak plasma laudanosine concentrations are lower in patients receiving cisatracurium compared with patients receiving clinically equivalent doses of atracurium.

Other Concerns

Because multiple complications have been associated with the use of NMBAs whenever any of these compounds are used, other factors must be considered. Because loss of airway produces an immediate emergency situation, individuals present in the ICU who are skilled in airway and ventilator management are fundamental to the success of using these compounds. When using these compounds, one also must be aware of interactions that increase the degree of neuromuscular block. Antibiotics such as neomycin, streptomycin, lincomycin, and tetracycline all have been implicated in prolonging the action of NMBAs. Cardiovascular drugs such as antiarrhythmics also may prolong neuromuscular block. Any compound, including local and inhalation anesthetic agents, that affects cell membranes would produce prolonged block. Electrolytes also play an important role; hypermagnesemia, hypokalemia, hypocalcemia, and lithium prolong neuromuscular block. Acidosis and hypothermia also prolong neuromuscular block. In addition, patients with certain disease states or conditions are likely to develop prolonged block if they receive NMBAs, including patients with any sort of neuromuscular disease, such as myasthenia gravis; patients at the extremes of age (i.e., neonates or elderly); and patients with hepatic or renal dysfunction.

Patients receiving NMBAs must receive concomitant sedation or analgesia or both. NMBAs have neither sedative nor analgesic properties; patients must *not* be paralyzed and conscious.[92] Patients who are paralyzed also are at risk of developing keratitis and corneal abrasion. Ophthalmic ointment or drops and taping eyelids closed with or without eye patches is recommended. Patients in ICUs are at risk of deep venous thrombosis, especially patients receiving NMBAs. They should receive appropriate prophylaxis.

CONCLUSION

Critically ill patients frequently experience anxiety and pain and occasionally experience severe agitation. These factors may have significant effects on the patient's sense of well-being and, perhaps equally important, on the patient's outcome. It is incumbent on health care providers to maintain a stress-free and comfortable environment to minimize these perceptions. If these environmental interventions are unsuccessful in controlling a patient's symptoms, pharmacologic interventions must be initiated. Sedation and analgesia and rarely muscle relaxation should be implemented when appropriate with the goal of improving patient satisfaction and outcome.

KEY POINTS

- Patients admitted to an ICU experience fear, anxiety, and pain; this activates the stress response with the release of numerous endogenous mediators that may adversely affect outcome.
- Activation of the limbic system is associated with anxiety; adrenergic mechanisms underlie the physiologic sequelae of anxiety.
- Tissue destruction releases biochemicals that stimulate peripheral pain receptors. Delta and C fibers carry the pain signal to the spinal cord where second-order neurons carry the signal to third-order neurons in the telencephalon and diencephalon. Modulation of the signal in the spinal cord occurs secondary to the action of other centrally acting neurotransmitters.

- Pain and anxiety are treated to provide patient comfort with the understanding that effective treatment may decrease morbidity and improve survival.
- Treatment of pain and anxiety is given most effectively in a compassionate, caring, and quiet environment, allowing the patient uninterrupted rest and sleep.
- Benzodiazepines, butyrophenones, barbiturates, propofol, opioids, dexmedetomidine, and occasionally ketamines can be used for anxiolysis.
- Benzodiazepines, by stimulating GABA receptors, inhibit central neurotransmission with a decrease in anxiety.
- Many nontraditional modalities, including cryotherapy, transcutaneous nerve stimulation, and peripheral nerve blocks, provide effective analgesia in subgroups of patients.
- In some patients, NSAIDs provide as effective analgesia as more commonly used opioids. NSAIDs are associated with several side effects, including gastric irritation, gastrointestinal bleeds, renal failure, and inhibition of platelet function.
- Opioids are the time-tested therapy most commonly used to provide analgesia. Oral, intramuscular, and intravenous routes are effective modes of administration that must be tailored to patient needs. Patient-controlled use of these modalities improves patients' acceptance and benefit from opioids.
- Opioid administration through the epidural, intrathecal, or transdermal route may have a role in unique patient groups.
- NMBAs occasionally must be used to manage agitated patients, but only when other modalities have been tried without success.
- Commonly used NMBAs include pancuronium and cisatracurium, each with associated benefits and side effects.
- When using NMBAs, we must guarantee that patients are adequately sedated, pain-free, and mechanically ventilated. Appropriate safeguards must be used to protect against accidental extubations or ventilator disconnects and against eye injury and deep venous thrombosis.
- AQMS is a serious side effect of the use of NMBAs.

REFERENCES

1. Carroll KC, Atkins PJ, Herold GR, et al: Pain assessment and management in critically ill postoperative and trauma patients: A multisite study. Am J Crit Care 1999;8:105-117.
2. Novaes MA, Knobel E, Bork AM, et al: Stressors in the ICU: Perception of the patient, relatives and health care team. Intensive Care Med 1999;25:1421-1426.
3. Ferguson J, Gilroy D, Puntillo K: Dimensions of pain and analgesic administration associated with coronary artery bypass in an Australian intensive care unit. J Adv Nursing 1997;26:1065-1072.
4. Loper KA, Butler S, Nessly M, et al: Paralyzed with pain: The need for education. Pain 1989;37:315-316.
5. Whipple JK, Lewis KS, Quebbeman EJ, et al: Analysis of pain management in critically ill patients. Pharmacotherapy 1995;15:592-599.
6. Cannon WB: Bodily Changes in Pain, Hunger, Fear, and Rage: An Account of Recent Researches into the Function of Emotional Excitement. New York, Appleton & Company, 1915.
7. Berns GS, Chappelow J, Cekic M, et al: Neurobiological substrates of dread. Science 2006;312:754-758.
8. Cohen D, Horiuchi K, Kemper M, et al: Modulating effects of propofol on metabolic and cardiopulmonary responses to stressful intensive care unit procedures. Crit Care Med 1996;24:612-617.
9. Treggiari-Venzi M, Borgeat A, Fuchs-Buder T, et al: Overnight sedation with midazolam or propofol in the ICU: Effects on sleep quality, anxiety and depression. Intensive Care Med 1996;22:1186-1190.
10. Meyer TJ, Eveloff SE, Bauer MS, et al: Adverse environmental conditions in the respiratory and medical ICU settings. Chest 1994;105:1211-1216.
11. Grumet GW: Pandemonium in the modern hospital. N Engl J Med 1993;328:433-437.
12. Rotondi A, Lakshmipathi C, Sirio C, et al: Patients' recollections of stressful experiences while receiving prolonged mechanical ventilation in an intensive care unit. Crit Care Med 2002;30:746-752.
13. Fong HK, Sands LP, Leung JM: The role of postoperative analgesia in delirium and cognitive decline in elderly patients: a systematic review. Anesth Analg 2006;102:1255-1266.
14. Vaurio L, Sands LP, Wang Y, et al: Postoperative delirium: The importance of pain and pain management. Anesth Analg 2006;102:1267-1273.
15. Woods JC, Mion LC, Connor JT, et al: Severe agitation among ventilated medical intensive care unit patients: Frequency, characteristics and outcomes. Intensive Care Med 2004;30:1066-1072.
16. Chase JG, Agogue F, Starfinger C, et al: Quantifying agitation in sedated ICU patients using digital imaging. Comput Methods Programs Biomed 2004;76:131-141.
17. Peterson JF, Pun BT, Dittus RS, et al: Delirium and its motoric subtypes: A study of 614 critically ill patients. J Am Geriatr Soc 2006;54:479-484.
18. Pandharipande P, Jackson J, Ely EW: Delirium: Acute cognitive dysfunction in the critically ill. Curr Opin Crit Care 2005;11:360-368.
19. Ely EW, Shintani A, Truman B, et al: Delirium as a predictor of mortality in mechanically ventilated patients in the intensive care unit. JAMA 2004;291:1753-1762.
20. Angus DC, Carlet J, 2002 Brussels Roundtable Participants: Surviving intensive care: A report from the 2002 Brussels Roundtable. Intensive Care Med 2003;29:368-277.
21. Ely EW, Stephens RK, Jackson JC, et al: Current opinions regarding the importance, diagnosis, and management of delirium in the intensive care unit: A survey of 912 healthcare professionals. Crit Care Med 2004;32:106-112.
22. McNicoll L, Pisani MA, Ely EW, et al: Detection of delirium in the intensive care unit: Comparison of confusion assessment method for the intensive care unit with confusion assessment method ratings. J Am Geriatr Soc 2005;53:495-500.
23. Otter H, Martin J, Bäsell K, et al: Validity and reliability of the DDS for severity of delirium in the ICU. Neurocrit Care 2005;2:150-158.
24. Alasad J, Ahmad M: Communication with critically ill patients. J Adv Nursing 2005;50:356-362.
25. Pandharipande P, Shintani A, Peterson J, et al: Lorazepam is an independent risk factor for transitioning to delirium in intensive care unit patients. Anesthesiology 2006;104:21-26.
26. Jackson JC, Gordon SM, Hart RP, et al: The association between delirium and cognitive decline: A review of the empirical literature. Neuropsychol Rev 2004;14:87-98.
27. Gorman JM, Kent JM, Sullivan GM, et al: Neuroanatomical hypothesis of panic disorder, revised. Am J Psychiatry 2000;157:493-505.
28. Reiman EM, Raichle ME, Robins E, et al: The application of positron emission tomography to the study of panic disorder. Am J Psychiatry 1986;143:469-477.

29. Starkman MN, Zelnik TC, Nesse RM, et al: Anxiety in patients with pheochromocytomas. Arch Intern Med 1985;145:248-252.
30. Jansen AS, Nguyen XV, Karpitskiy V, et al: Central command neurons of the sympathetic nervous system: Basis of the fight-or-flight response. Science 1995;270:644-646.
31. Bloom FE, Iversen LL: Localizing ^{3}H-GABA in nerve terminals of rat cerebral cortex by electron microscopic autoradiography. Nature 1971; 229:628-630.
32. Olsen RW, Tobin AJ: Molecular biology of $GABA_A$ receptors. FASEB J 1990;4:1469-1480.
33. Bowery N: $GABA_B$ receptors and their significance in mammalian pharmacology. Trends Pharmacol Sci 1989;10:401-407.
34. Guidotti A, Toffano G, Costa E: An endogenous protein modulates the affinity of GABA and benzodiazepine receptors in rat brain. Nature 1978; 275:553-555.
35. Markovitz JH, Matthews KA, Kannel WB, et al: Psychological predictors of hypertension in the Framingham study: Is there tension in hypertension? JAMA 1993;270:2439-2443.
36. Arrighi JA, Burg M, Cohen IS, et al: Myocardial blood-flow response during mental stress in patients with coronary artery disease. Lancet 2000;356: 310-311.
37. Parthasarathy S, Tobin MJ: Sleep in the intensive care unit. Intensive Care Med 2004;30:197-206.
38. Vinik HR, Kissin I: Sedation in the ICU. Intensive Care Med 1991;17:S20-S23.
39. Rosenkranz MA, Busse WW, Johnstone T, et al: Neural circuitry underlying the interaction between emotion and asthma symptom exacerbation. Proc Natl Acad Sci U S A 2005;102: 13319-13324.
40. Shoemaker WC, Appel PL, Kram HB: Role of oxygen debt in the development of organ failure sepsis, and death in high-risk surgical patients. Chest 1992;102:208-215.
41. Bruder N, Dumont JC, Francois G: Evolution of energy expenditure and nitrogen excretion in severe head-injured patients. Crit Care Med 1991;19:43-48.
42. Coggeshall JW, Marini JJ, Newman JH: Improved oxygenation after muscle relaxation in adult respiratory distress syndrome. Arch Intern Med 1985;145:1718-1720.
43. Al-Haddad M, Hayward I, Walsh TS: A prospective audit of cost sedation, analgesia and neuromuscular blockade in a large British ICU. Anaesthesia 2004;59:1121-1125.
44. Riker RR, Fraser GL: Adverse events associated with sedatives, analgesics, and other drugs that provide patient comfort in the intensive care unit. Pharmacotherapy 2005;25:8S-18S.
45. Fumagalli S, Boncinelli L, Lo Nostro A, et al: Reduced cardiocirculatory complications with unrestrictive visiting policy in an intensive care unit: Results from a pilot, randomized trial. Circulation 2006;113:946-952.
46. Nieszkowska A, Combes A, Luyt C-E, et al: Impact of tracheotomy on sedative administration, sedation level, and comfort of mechanically ventilated intensive care unit patients. Crit Care Med 2005;33:2527-2533.
47. Rodrigues GR Jr, Gomes do Amaral JL: Influence of sedation on morbidity and mortality in the intensive care unit. Sao Paulo Med J 2004;122:8-11.
48. Ramsay MA, Savege TM, Simpson BRJ, et al: Controlled sedation with alphaxalone/alphadolone. BMJ 1974;2:656-659.
49. Hansen-Flaschen J, Cowen J, Polomano RC: Beyond the Ramsay scale: need for a validated measure of sedating drug efficacy in the intensive care unit. Crit Care Med 1994;22:732-733.
50. Riker RR, Picard JT, Fraser GL: Prospective evaluation of the sedation-agitation scale for adult critically ill patients. Crit Care Med 1999;27: 1325-1329.
51. Devlin JW, Boleski G, Mlynarek M, et al: Motor activity assessment scale: A valid reliable sedation scale for use with mechanically ventilated patients in an adult surgical intensive care unit. Crit Care Med 1999;27:1271-1275.
52. Ely EW, Truman B, Shintani A, et al: Monitoring sedation status over time in ICU patients: Reliability and validity of the Richmond Agitation-Sedation Scale (RASS). JAMA 2003;289:2983-2991.
53. de Lemos J, Tweeddale M, Chittock DR: Measuring quality of sedation in adult mechanically ventilated critically ill patients: The Vancouver interaction and calmness scale. J Clin Epidemiol 2000;53:908-919.
54. Ambuel B, Hamlett KW, Marx CM, et al: Assessing distress in pediatric intensive care environments: The COMFORT scale. J Pediatr Psychol 1992;17:95-109.
55. Tonner PH, Wei C, Bein B, et al: Comparison of two bispectral index algorithms in monitoring sedation in postoperative intensive care patients. Crit Care Med 2005;33:580-584.
56. Fraser GL, Riker RR: Bispectral index monitoring in the intensive care unit provides more signal than noise. Pharmacotherapy 2005;25:19S-27S.
57. Liu J, Singh H, White PF: Electroencephalogram bispectral analysis predicts the depth of midazolam-induced sedation. Anesthesiology 1996;84:64-69.
58. Schweicker WD, Gahlbach BK, Pohlman AS, et al: Daily interruption of sedative infusions and complications of critical illness in mechanically ventilated patients. Crit Care Med 2004;32: 1272-1276.
59. Cassem EH, Lake CR, Boyer WF: Psychopharmacology in the ICU. In Chernow B (ed): The Pharmacologic Approach to the Critically Ill Patient, ed 3. Baltimore, Williams & Wilkins, 1994, pp 651-665.
60. Hammerlein A, Derendorf H, Lowenthal DT: Pharmacokinetic and pharmacodynamic changes in the elderly. Clin Pharmacokinet 1998;35:49-64.
61. Boulieu R, Lehmann B, Salord F, et al: Pharmacokinetics of midazolam and its main metabolite 1-hydroxymidazolam in intensive care patients. Eur J Drug Metab Pharmacokinet 1998;23: 255-258.
62. Weintraub M, Standish R: Flumazenil (Ro 15-1788): A benzodiazepine antagonist. Hosp Formul 1988;23: 332-341.
63. Kress JP, O'Connor MF, Pohlman AS, et al: Sedation of critically ill patients during mechanical ventilation: A comparison of propofol and midazolam. Am J Resp Crit Care Med 1996;153:1012-1018.
64. Walder B, Elia N, Henzi I, et al: A lack of evidence of superiority of propofol versus midazolam for sedation in mechanically ventilated critically ill patients: A qualitative and quantitative systematic review. Anesth Analg 2001;92:975-983.
65. Parke TJ, Stevens JE, Rice ASC, et al: Metabolic acidosis and fatal myocardial failure after propofol infusion in children: Five case reports. BMJ 1992;305:613-616.
66. Menza MA, Murray GB, Holmes VF, et al: Decreased extrapyramidal symptoms with intravenous haloperidol. J Clin Psychiatry 1987;48:278-280.
67. Sharma ND, Rosman HS, Padhi D, et al: Torsades de pointes associated with intravenous haloperidol in critically ill patients. Am J Cardiol 1998;81: 238-240.
68. Maze M, Scarfini C, Cavaliere F: New agents for sedation in the intensive care unit. Crit Care Clin 2001;17:881-897.
69. Hall JE, Uhrich TD, Barney JA, et al: Sedative, amnestic, and analgesic properties of small-dose dexmedetomidine infusions. Anesth Analg 2000;90:699-705.
70. Herr DL, Sum-Ping J, England M: ICU sedation after coronary artery bypass graft surgery: Dexmedetomidine-based versus propofol-based sedation regimens. J Cardiothorac Vasc Anesth 2003;17:576-584.
71. Mallow Corbett S, Rebuck JA, Greene CM, et al: Dexmedetomidine does not improve patient satisfaction when compared with propofol during mechanical ventilation. Crit Care Med 2005;33:940-945.
72. Videira RLR, Ferreira RM: Dexmedetomidine and asystole. Anesthesiology 2004;101:1479.
73. Shehabi Y, Ruettimann U, Adamson H, et al: Dexmedetomidine infusion for more than 24 hours in critically ill patients: Sedative and cardiovascular effects. Intensive Care Med 2004;30: 2188-2196.
74. Shelly MP: Dexmedetomidine: A real innovation or more of the same? Br J Anaesth 2001;87:677-678.
75. Rainville P, Duncan GH, Price DD, et al: Pain affect encoded in human anterior cingulate but not somatosensory cortex. Science 1997;277:968-971.
76. Malmberg AB, Yaksh TL: Hyperalgesia mediated by spinal glutamate or substance P receptor blocked by spinal cyclooxygenase inhibition. Science 1992;257:1276-1279.
77. Feldman HI, Kinman JL, Berlin JA, et al: Parenteral ketorolac: The risk for acute renal failure. Ann Intern Med 1997;126: 193-199.
78. Strom BL, Berlin JA, Kinman JL, et al: Parenteral ketorolac and risk of gastrointestinal and operative site bleeding: A postmarketing surveillance study. JAMA 1996;275:376-382.

79. Tammisto T: Analgesics in postoperative pain relief. Acta Anaesth Scand 1978;70:47-50.
80. Sechzer PH: Objective measurements of pain. Anesthesiology 1968;29:209-210.
81. de Leon-Casasola OA, Lema MJ: Postoperative epidural opioid analgesia: What are the choices? Anesth Analg 1996;83:867-875.
82. Kuhlen R, Putensen C: Remifentanil for analgesia-based sedation in the intensive care unit. Crit Care 2004;8:13-14.
83. Karabinis A, Mandragos K, Stergiopoulos S, et al: Safety and efficacy of analgesia-based sedation with remifentanil versus standard hypnotic-based regimens in intensive care unit patients with brain injuries: a randomized, controlled trial [ISRCTN50308308]. Crit Care 2004;8: R268-R280.
84. Wiffen PJ, McQuay HJ, Edwards JE, et al: Gabapentin for acute and chronic pain. Cochrane Database Syst Rev 2005;3: CD005452.
85. Sessler CN: Sedation, analgesia, and neuromuscular blockade for high-frequency oscillatory ventilation. Crit Care Med 2005;33:S209-S216.
86. Gainnier M, Roch A, Forel J-M, et al: Effect of neuromuscular blocking agents on gas exchange in patients presenting with acute respiratory distress syndrome. Crit Care Med 2004;32:113-119.
87. Murray MJ, Cowen J, DeBlock H, et al: Clinical practice guidelines for sustained neuromuscular blockade in the adult critically ill patient. Crit Care Med 2002;30:142-156.
88. Baumann MH, McAlpin W, Brown K, et al: A prospective randomized comparison of train-of-four monitoring and clinical assessment during continuous ICU cisatracurium paralysis. Chest 2004;126:1267-1273.
89. Murray MJ, Brull SJ, Bolton C: Brief review: Nondepolarizing neuromuscular blocking drugs and critical illness myopathy. Can J Anaesth 2006;53: 1148-1156.
90. Segredo V, Caldwell JE, Matthay MA, et al: Persistent paralysis in critically ill patients after long-term administration of vecuronium. N Engl J Med 1992; 327:524-528.
91. Khuenl-Brady KS, Sparr H, Pühringer F, et al: Rocuronium bromide in the ICU: Dose finding and pharmacokinetics. Eur J Anesth 1995;12:79-80.
92. Ballard N, Robley L, Barrett D, et al: Patients' recollections of therapeutic paralysis in the intensive care unit. Am J Crit Care 2006;15:86-95.

Chapter 21

Principles of Drug Dosing in Critically Ill Patients

John W. Devlin and Jeffrey F. Barletta

Drug therapy plays a key role in improving the care of critically ill patients. With patients admitted to the intensive care unit (ICU) receiving on average more than 30 different medications throughout their admission, ICU clinicians are faced with making many important drug dosing decisions each day.[1] Even when the correct medication is chosen, a dosing regimen or route of administration that is not optimal can result in therapeutic failure or drug toxicity. Most dosing regimens employed in the ICU are extrapolated from clinical trials completed in non-ICU patients, or even healthy patients, and usually do not account for the substantial pharmacokinetic and pharmacodynamic variability seen in this patient population.[2-5]

The alterations in volume status, plasma protein binding, and end-organ function that occur during critical illness may affect drug bioavailability, volume of distribution (Vd), and clearance.[6] Many factors may compromise drug bioavailability in critically ill patients when drugs are administered by nonintravenous routes (e.g., enteral, subcutaneous, transdermal, or endotracheal). Failure to account for these alterations when establishing medication dosing regimens may lead to unpredictable drug effects, undesirable clinical outcomes, and increased drug toxicity.[2]

Numerous factors may affect the pharmacodynamic response to medications in the ICU, including altered postreceptor binding, downregulation of receptors, and a host of different physiologic alterations.[6] These principles have led to many changes in the way dosing regimens are designed and drugs are administered (e.g., the use of continuous infusions of β-lactam antibiotics). Knowledge regarding the role that genetics plays in medication response has grown substantially and is expected to influence medication selection and dosing increasingly in the ICU.[7]

This chapter reviews current pharmacokinetic and pharmacodynamic principles that guide the development of dosing regimens. Unique factors that alter drug pharmacokinetic and pharmacodynamic parameters are increasingly being found in the ICU (e.g., renal failure, hepatic failure, obesity, elderly age, pregnancy, or burn injury). Important dosing considerations in these special populations are reviewed. Principles of therapeutic drug monitoring (TDM) that may or may not involve the use of serum drug concentrations are discussed along with the use of alternative routes of drug administration. It is important to note that this chapter is not a drug pharmacopeia or a review of therapeutics for any particular disease state. For specific therapeutic recommendations, clinicians are referred to the corresponding chapter in this textbook. For information regarding dosing, precautions, adverse effects, drug interactions, or monitoring parameters, clinicians are encouraged to refer to package inserts, personal digital assistants (PDAs), or online, or print reference sources, or consult with an ICU clinical pharmacist.

GENERAL PHARMACOKINETIC PRINCIPLES

Pharmacokinetics is the quantitative study of how drugs enter the body, distribute within various organ systems, and are eliminated.[8] Familiarity with pharmacokinetic parameters, such as bioavailability, Vd, elimination half-life, and clearance, greatly enhances the clinician's ability to select the appropriate drug and dosage regimen to achieve the desired therapeutic goal, while minimizing adverse effects (Fig. 21-1). The term that describes the amount of drug that reaches the bloodstream is *bioavailability*. Bioavailability is always 100% after intravenous (IV) drug administration, but may be substantially less when administration occurs via the oral, enteral, subcutaneous, transdermal, or endotracheal route.[6] Many disease states (e.g., liver disease) can alter bioavailability.

Vd is a mathematical concept that reflects the nonphysiologic compartments into which the drug disperses.[8] It describes the relationship between the amount of drug in the body and the concentration in the plasma after absorption and distribution are completed. Vd may be affected by body size, physicochemical characteristics of the drug, tissue binding, plasma protein binding, and regional blood flow.[8] For a drug that remains in the vasculature (i.e., is not distributed to other tissues), the serum drug concentration can be estimated by dividing the dose that is administered by the vascular volume. Most drugs distribute to tissues outside of the vasculature, however, and accumulate in body tissues at far higher concentrations than those seen in serum. Drugs that are hydrophilic (i.e., do not penetrate fat well) remain within the plasma (e.g., aminoglycosides) and have a low Vd (<0.6 L/kg), whereas drugs that are lipophilic and sequestered outside the circulation (e.g., midazolam, digoxin) have a much higher Vd.

Although initial loading doses are estimated based on Vd, maintenance doses depend on clearance. The term *clearance* is based on the concept of the whole body acting as a drug-eliminating system, but most clearance occurs through the liver or kidneys or both. As a drug is removed from a compartment (i.e., the vascular space or otherwise), there is a rate constant (k) that describes the rate at which the drug is eliminated from that compartment. The clearance of a drug from a compartment can be calculated as follows: clearance = k × Vd. Half-life refers to the time required for drug concentrations to decrease by 50% in a particular compartment. Rate constants can be determined for drug distribution from one compartment (e.g., vascular) to another (e.g., soft tissues) or for drug excretion from the body (e.g., elimination rate constant).

Although some medications follow a one-compartment model where drug concentrations are confined within one space (i.e., vascular), most follow a more complex two-compartment or three-compartment model.[8] In these situations, the administration of a drug by IV bolus initially results in a peak increase in the plasma (central compartment), but a portion of the dose distributes into a second peripheral compartment, leading to a subsequent decrease in the plasma concentration. Peripheral compartments are usually a specific physiologic space (e.g., the intracellular volume), rather than an isolated anatomic space or organ, and are usually the place where the drug exerts its primary effect. Ultimately, drug is redistributed back to the central compartment from the peripheral compartment and terminally eliminated from the body (rate = elimination rate constant). For many agents, this multiple compartment model results in a prolonged drug effect, even when the drug has a short half-life (e.g., midazolam), that is more pronounced after extended therapy.[9]

PHARMACOKINETIC ALTERATIONS IN CRITICALLY ILL PATIENTS

Many factors may affect drug absorption, distribution, and clearance in critically ill patients.[2,6] Failure to appreciate these various pharmacokinetic alterations when establishing drug therapy regimens may result in unpredictable serum concentrations that can lead to therapeutic failure or drug toxicity. Factors that can alter drug absorption in critically ill patients include (1) gut wall edema or stasis; (2) alterations in gastric or intestinal blood flow; (3) concurrent therapy with an anticholinergic agent, narcotic

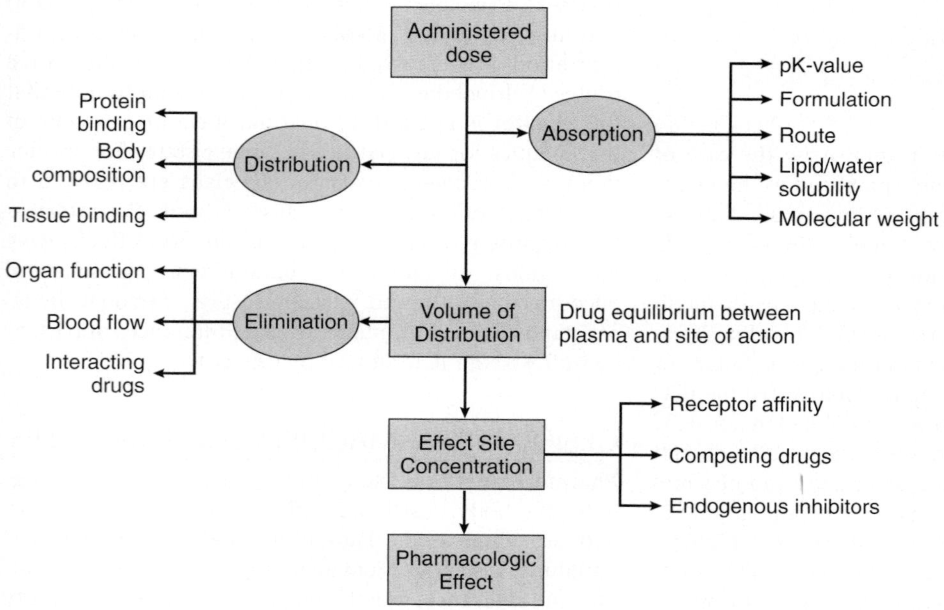

Figure 21-1. Drug pharmacokinetic and pharmacodynamic factors can alter the intensity of the pharmacologic response. Factors that affect absorption, distribution, elimination, and effect site concentration are presented. (Adapted with permission from Devlin JW, Zarowitz BJ: Alterations in drug disposition in the elderly. In Grenvik A, Ayres SM, Holbrook PR, et al [eds]: Textbook of Critical Care. Philadelphia, Saunders, 2000, pp 991-1000.)

analgesic, antacid, or enteral nutrition; and (4) incomplete oral medication disintegration or dissolution.[10-12]

The fluid shifts and the protein binding changes that occur during critical illness may alter drug distribution.[2,6,13] Increases in total body water, particularly after fluid resuscitation, may result in lower plasma concentrations for drugs having a low Vd (e.g., aminoglycosides) and usually necessitate the use of larger doses in these patients (Fig. 21-2).[14] Mechanical ventilation reduces cardiac output by increasing intrathoracic pressure and raises Vd by increasing intravascular and extravascular water distribution. Hypoalbuminemia potentiates these changes as

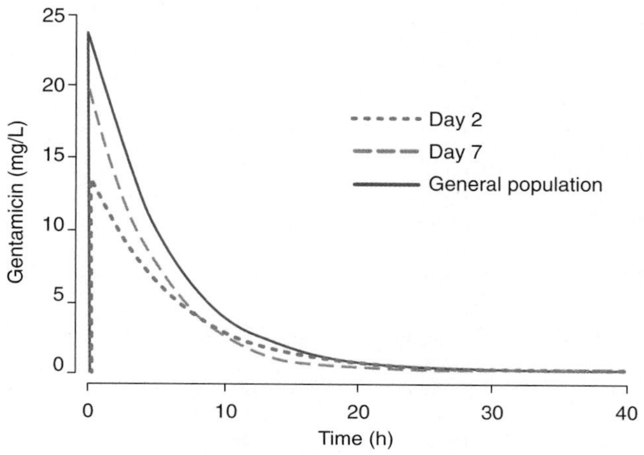

Figure 21-2. Simulation of a single dose of gentamicin, 6 mg/kg infused over 20 minutes, in intensive care unit patients on days 2 and 7 after admission compared with a general population of non–critically ill patients. (Adapted with permission from Power BM, Forbes AM, van Heerden PV, Ilett KF: Pharmacokinetics of drugs used in critically ill adults. Clin Pharmacokinet 1998;34:25-56.)

the central compartment fluid volume contracts and the extracellular and total body water increases. When establishing loading doses of medications, particularly drugs with a low Vd, clinicians should estimate fluid status by monitoring fluid input and output, central venous pressure, and serum albumin, and for evidence of pulmonary or subcutaneous edema. The effects of volume status, particularly hypovolemia, on the pharmacokinetics of certain agents are shown in Figure 21-3.

Plasma protein concentrations may change dramatically during critical illness and affect Vd by altering the amount of the pharmacologically active unbound or free drug.[2,6] Three major plasma proteins affect protein binding—albumin, α_1-acid glycoprotein, and lipoproteins (Table 21-1).[8] Albumin concentrations often decrease in patients with burns, liver disease, sepsis, uremia, and trauma. The resulting reduction in drug-protein binding leads to an increase in the unbound (and active) fraction of acidic agents, such as phenytoin, theophylline, and warfarin.[15] Protein binding is reduced for other reasons, including the accumulation of endogenous binding inhibitors, qualitative changes on binding sites, and the competition for binding by other substances.[8] Basic drugs, such as morphine, are primarily bound to the acute-phase reactant, α_1-acid glycoprotein, which is often increased in patients with renal failure, burns, infections, myocardial infarctions, and recent surgery. In these situations, protein binding of basic drugs is elevated, decreasing their clinical effects and often necessitating dosage increases.[6]

Metabolic clearance by the liver is the predominant route for drug detoxification and elimination. With hepatic dysfunction present in more than half of critically ill patients, drug clearance may be reduced because of lower hepatic blood flow, decreased hepatocellular enzyme activity, or lower bile flow.[16] With shock resulting in a

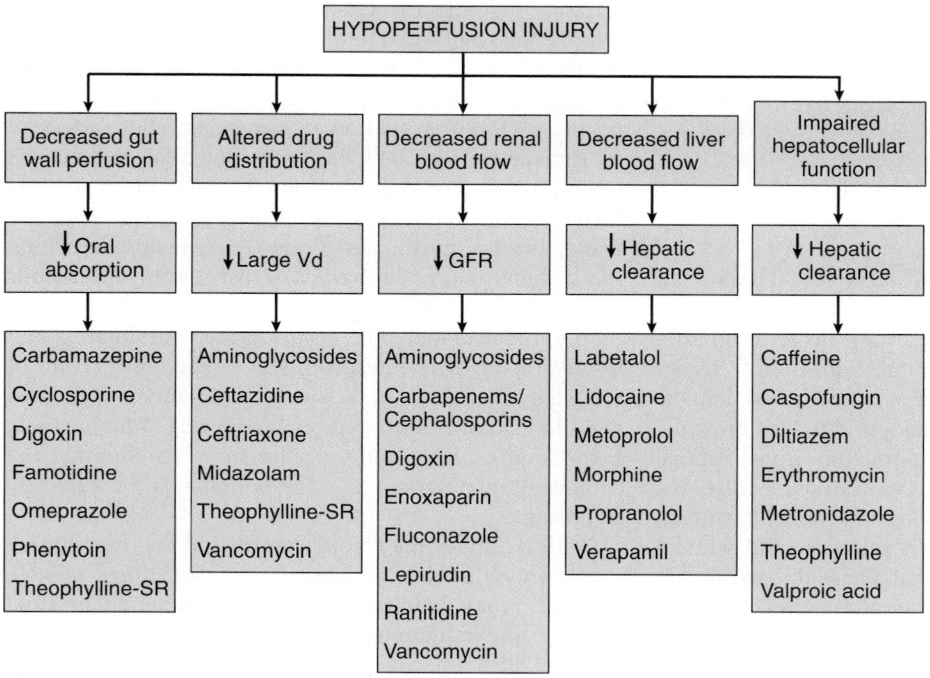

Figure 21-3. Hypoperfusion-induced changes in blood flow and organ system function may result in decreased absorption, altered distribution, impaired renal excretion, and decreased hepatic metabolism of clinically important drugs. GFR, glomerular filtration rate. (Adapted with permission from Devlin JW, Zarowitz BJ: Alterations in drug disposition in the elderly. In Grenvik A, Ayres SM, Holbrook PR, et al [eds]: Textbook of Critical Care. Philadelphia, Saunders, 2000, pp 991-1000.)

Table 21-1. Commonly Administered Drugs in the Intensive Care Unit and Their Predominant Binding Proteins*

Albumin
Ceftriaxone
Clindamycin
Dexamethasone
Diazepam
Ibuprofen
Nafcillin
Naproxen
Oxacillin
Phenytoin
Valproic acid
Warfarin
Albumin and AAG
Carbamazepine
Erythromycin
Lidocaine
Meperidine
Methadone
Verapamil
Albumin and Lipoproteins
Cyclosporine
Albumin, AAG, and Lipoproteins
Amitriptyline
Bupivacaine
Chlorpromazine
Diltiazem
Propranolol
Quinidine

*Medications included are those that are >70% protein bound.
AAG, α1-acid glycoprotein.
Adapted from Bauer LA: Clinical pharmacokinetics and pharmacodynamics. In DiPiro JT, Talbert RL, Yee GC, et al (eds): Pharmacotherapy: A Pathophysiologic Approach, ed 6. New York: McGraw-Hill, 2005, pp 51-73.

Table 21-2. Important Relationships Between Drugs That Are Commonly Administered in the Intensive Care Unit and Cytochrome P-450 (CYP) Enzymes

	Drug Substrates	Inhibitors	Inducers
CYP1A2	Sertraline Theophylline	Cimetidine Ciprofloxacin Ticlopidine	Omeprazole Tobacco
CYP2C9	Diclofenac Ibuprofen Losartan Phenytoin Warfarin	Fluconazole Fluvastatin	Rifampin
CYP2C19	Diazepam Lansoprazole Omeprazole Pantoprazole Voriconazole	Cimetidine Fluvoxamine Isoniazid	Rifampin
CYP2D6	Codeine Haloperidol Metoprolol Propafenone Propranolol Risperidone	Amiodarone Cimetidine Fluoxetine Haloperidol Quinidine Ritonavir	—
CYP3A4	Clarithromycin Cyclosporine Diltiazem Erythromycin Fentanyl Midazolam Nimodipine Quinidine Sildenafil Tacrolimus Ziprasidone	Amiodarone Clarithromycin Erythromycin Fluconazole Grapefruit juice Itraconazole Ritonavir Isoniazid	Barbiturates Carbamazepine Phenytoin Rifampin

From Drug Interactions. Med Lett Drugs Therap 2003;45:44-48.

threefold decrease in liver blood flow, the clearance of medications that rely on flow-dependent hepatic clearance (i.e., high extraction drugs) may be reduced substantially (e.g., labetalol, morphine, lidocaine).[2,6] Drugs dependent on enzymatic function rather than hepatic blood flow for clearance (e.g., haloperidol, lansoprazole, phenytoin) are considered low extraction drugs. Animal models of traumatic injury have shown differential decreases in phase I (e.g., oxidation, reduction, hydrolysis) and phase II (e.g., glucuronidation, sulfation, and acetylation) biotransformation.[6] In general, phase II reactions are less affected by critical illness than phase I reactions.

Critical illness may compromise the cytochrome P-450 (CYP-450) system, a common pathway for drug metabolism, by decreasing hepatic blood flow, intracellular oxygen tension, and cofactor availability (Table 21-2).[6] Hepatic hypoxemia results in a reduction in the amount of hepatic enzymes produced and the efficiency of the enzymes produced. With the number of medications metabolized by the CYP-450 system ever increasing, clinicians need to remain vigilant in identifying potential interactions with coadministered drugs. These interactions may occur through drugs that cause enzyme inhibition (e.g., ketoconazole, erythromycin, cimetidine) or enzyme induction (e.g., phenytoin, phenobarbital).[17] Erythromycin inhibits CYP3A4 and may reduce the clearance of warfarin, methyprednisolone, and cyclosporine. Although a full discussion of drug interactions is beyond the scope of this chapter, the clinician is urged to refer to numerous web-based and PDA-based references (e.g., Micromedex, Lexi-Comp) or consult a pharmacist to identify the drug-drug interactions with the potential to be clinically significant.

Critical illness may compromise kidney function in many ways, including reduced perfusion (e.g., shock), intrinsic renal damage secondary to ischemia or drug toxicity, and immunologic injury.[18] A decrease in the glomerular filtration rate (GFR) would increase the half-life of medications that are renally cleared and may result in drug or metabolite accumulation. Drug toxicity would be most pronounced in kidney dysfunction when drug metabolites are renally cleared and active, and the parent drug has a narrow therapeutic window. For example, the pharmacologically active metabolite of midazolam, α-hydroxymidazolam, has been shown to accumulate in the presence of renal failure and lead to prolonged sedation.[9] In addition to affecting the renal clearance of medications, severe kidney failure can reduce nonrenal clearance, although the degree to which this occurs depends on whether the patient has end-stage renal disease or acute renal failure. Studies examining the clearance of vancomycin and imipenem in patients with renal failure show that the non-renal component of clearance is substantially greater in patients with acute renal failure than in patients with end-stage renal disease.[19]

PHARMACODYNAMIC PRINCIPLES

Pharmacokinetics characterizes the absorption, distribution, metabolism, and elimination of a drug (i.e., what the body does to the drug), whereas pharmacodynamics describes the relationship between the concentration of drug at the site of action and the observed clinical response (i.e., what the drug does to the body) (Fig. 21-4).[8] Pharmacodynamic response can be categorized as being either direct or indirect and either reversible or irreversible. Adrenergic vasopressors (e.g., phenylephrine) are an example of a class of medications that elicit a direct response because increases in dose lead to increases in α_1-adrenergic receptor binding, thus greater blood pressure effect is observed.[5] Warfarin elicits an indirect response because its anticoagulant effect is potentiated through the inhibition of new vitamin K clotting factor production as opposed to a dose-related destruction in circulating clotting factors. Although most drugs are considered reversible (i.e., pharmacologic effect subsides as drug concentrations decline), some agents are classified as irreversible (e.g., bactericidal antibiotics, antineoplastic agents) because the pharmacologic response continues well after the drug has been eliminated from the body. A review of the numerous pharmacodynamic models that have been developed to relate effect site concentration with pharmacologic response is beyond the scope of this chapter.[8]

Because of the numerous barriers to conducting pharmacodynamic studies in humans, especially in a heterogeneous population such as critically ill patients, pharmacodynamic data often must be extrapolated from animal or in vitro models. In recent years, knowledge of how pharmacodynamic values can be used to optimize drug dosing to improve patient outcome has increased substantially. Although pharmacodynamic knowledge theoretically can be used to optimize dosing regimens for all medications that are used in the ICU, it has been most investigated with antibiotics.

Antibiotics are typically categorized as having either concentration-dependent or time-dependent killing (Table 21-3).[20] The activity of concentration-dependent antibiotics increases as the peak serum concentrations of drug increase, and these antibiotics include aminoglycosides,

Table 21-3. Pharmacokinetic and Pharmacodynamic Parameters of Anti-Infective Drugs in the Intensive Care Unit

Concentration Dependent		Time Dependent	
Renal Elimination	**Hepatic Elimination**	**Renal Elimination**	**Hepatic Elimination**
Amikacin	Caspofungin	Acyclovir	Ceftriaxone
Ciprofloxacin	Metronidazole	Ampicillin	Clindamycin
Daptomycin	Micafungin	Aztreonam	Linezolid
Gentamicin	Moxifloxacin	Cefazolin	Nafcillin
Levofloxacin		Cefepime	Oxacillin
Tobramycin		Cefotaxime	
		Ertapenem	
		Fluconazole	
		Imipenem	
		Meropenem	
		Piperacillin	
		Ticarcillin	
		Vancomycin	
		Voriconazole	

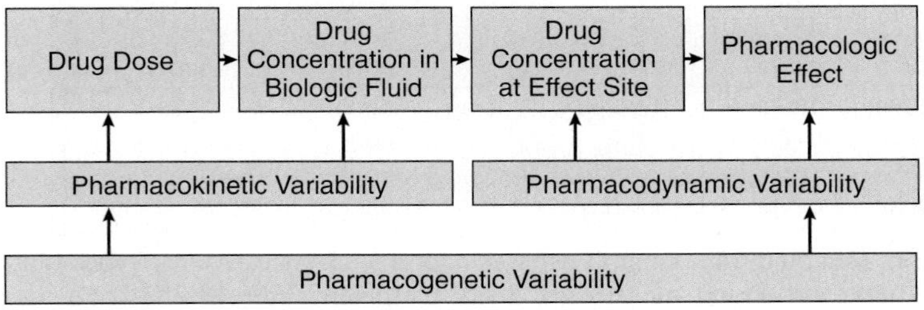

Figure 21-4. Pharmacokinetics, pharmacodynamics, and pharmacogenetics as determinants of the dose-response relationship. (Adapted from Bauer LA: Clinical pharmacokinetics and pharmacodynamics. In DiPiro JT, Talbert RL, Yee GC, et al [eds]: Pharmacotherapy: A Pathophysiologic Approach, ed 6. New York, McGraw-Hill, 2005, pp 51-73.)

fluoroquinolones, and daptomycin. In contrast, time-dependent antibiotics, such as β-lactams, kill at the same rate regardless of the peak serum concentration that is attained above the minimum inhibitory concentration (MIC) (Fig. 21-5). The primary concern when using time-dependent antibiotics is to ensure that the antibiotic reaches a serum concentration that is above the MIC throughout most or all of the dosing interval.

The pharmacodynamic parameters that most closely approximate the activity of concentration-dependent antibiotics are the ratio of the maximum serum antibiotic concentration (Cmax) to MIC and the ratio of the area-under-the-concentration-time curve over 24 hours (AUC) to the MIC (Fig. 21-6).[8] The ratio of AUC to MIC also is referred to as the area-under-the-inhibitory curve (AUIC). A higher AUIC correlates with a greater rate and extent of bactericidal activity. The AUIC can be used to predict effectiveness and can be used as a parameter when comparing dosing regimens for different concentration-dependent antibiotics. An infection caused by *Pseudomonas aeruginosa* with MIC to gentamicin of 4 μg/mL and MIC to tobramycin of 2 μg/mL would be expected to have a better response to tobramycin because a higher AUIC can be achieved using the same dose. In contrast, an increase in dose generally is not associated with improved outcome for time-dependent antibiotics. Instead, clinicians should focus on increasing the dosing frequency, which may include the use of a continuous infusion.[21]

Another important concept surrounding the pharmacodynamic optimization of antibiotics is postantibiotic effect (PAE). PAE refers to the continued suppression of bacterial growth despite a drug concentration that falls below

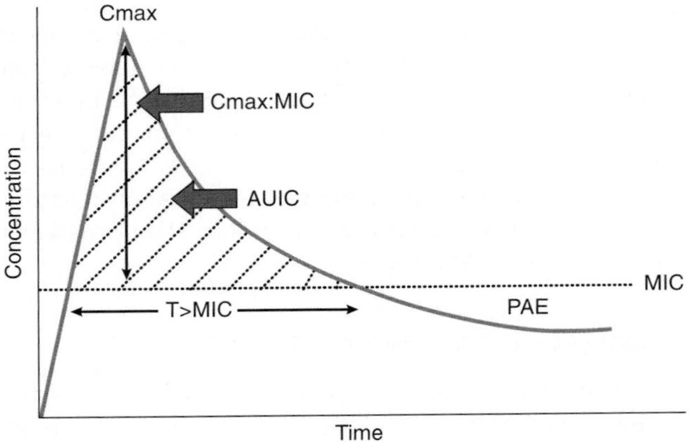

Figure 21-5. Pharmacokinetic and pharmacodynamic parameters considered when developing antimicrobial dosing regimens. AUIC, area-under-the-inhibitory curve; MIC, minimum inhibitory concentration; PAE, postantibiotic effect.

Vancomycin Dosing Nomogram									
Actual weight (kg)	Creatinine Clearance (mL/min)								
	30	40	50	60	70	80	90	100	≥110
50	500mg q24hr	500mg q24hr	500mg q12hr	500mg q12hr	500mg q12hr	500mg q12hr	500mg q12hr	500mg q8hr	500mg q8hr
55	500mg q24hr	500mg g24hr	500mg q12hr	500mg q12hr	500mg q12hr	500mg q12hr	500mg q12hr	500mg q8hr	500mg q8hr
60	500mg q24hr	500mg q24hr	500mg q12hr	500mg q12hr	1000mg q12hr	1000mg q12hr	1000mg q12hr	500mg q8hr	500mg q8hr
65	1000mg q24hr	1000mg q24hr	1000mg q24hr	1000mg q12hr	1000mg q12hr	1000mg q12hr	1000mg q12hr	1000mg q12hr	1000mg q8hr
70	1000mg q24hr	1000mg q24hr	1000mg q24hr	1000mg q12hr	1000mg q12hr	1000mg q12hr	1000mg q12hr	1000mg q8hr	1000mg q8hr
75	1000mg q24hr	1000mg q24hr	1000mg q24hr	1000mg q12hr	1000mg q12hr	1000mg q12hr	1000mg q12hr	1000mg q8hr	1000mg q8hr
80	1000mg q24hr	1000mg q24hr	1000mg q24hr	1000mg q12hr	1000mg q12hr	1000mg q12hr	1000mg q12hr	1000mg q8hr	1000mg q8hr
85	1000mg q24hr	1000mg q24hr	1000mg q24hr	1000mg q12hr	1000mg q12hr	1000mg q12hr	1000mg q8hr	1000mg q8hr	1000mg q8hr
90	1000mg q24hr	1000mg q24hr	1000mg q12hr	1000mg q12hr	1000mg q12hr	1000mg q8hr	1000mg q8hr	1000mg q8hr	1000mg q8hr
95	1000mg q24hr	1000mg q24hr	1000mg q12hr	1000mg q12hr	1000mg q12hr	1000mg q8hr	1000mg q8hr	1000mg q8hr	1000mg q8hr
100	1000mg q24hr	1000mg q24hr	1000mg q12hr	1000mg q12hr	1000mg q12hr	1000mg q8hr	1000mg q8hr	1000mg q8hr	1000mg q8hr
105	1000mg q24hr	1000mg q24hr	1000mg q12hr	1000mg q12hr	1000mg q12hr	1000mg q8hr	1000mg q8hr	1000mg q8hr	1000mg q8hr
≥110	1000mg q24hr	1000mg q24hr	1000mg q12hr	1000mg q12hr	1000mg q12hr	1000mg q8hr	1000mg q8hr	1000mg q8hr	1000mg q8hr

Figure 21-6. Nomogram for initial doses of vancomycin. (Adapted from Karam CM, McKinnon PS, Neuhauser MM, Rybak MJ: Outcome assessment of minimizing vancomycin monitoring and dosing adjustments. Pharmacotherapy 1999;19:257-266.)

the MIC of the bacteria. Although the PAE was first described with penicillin against gram-positive organisms in the 1940s, β-lactams have only a modest PAE against gram-positive organisms and little to no PAE against gram-negative organisms.[22] One exception is carbapenems (e.g., imipenem, meropenem), which have a more prolonged PAE, particularly against *P. aeruginosa*.[22] The agents where PAE is most prominent are those that inhibit protein synthesis (i.e., aminoglycosides, fluoroquinolones, and macrolides). With the duration of the PAE correlating with the Cmax that is reached, the PAE properties of aminoglycosides are a major rationale for using a high-peak, extended-interval dosing strategy. In this instance, suppression of bacterial growth would continue after serum concentrations become undetectable.[20]

USING PHARMACOKINETIC AND PHARMACODYNAMIC PRINCIPLES TO OPTIMIZE DRUG DOSING IN CRITICALLY ILL PATIENTS

The primary goal of drug therapy in the ICU is to maximize clinical efficacy, while minimizing toxicity. Pharmacokinetic principles should be used to ensure adequate drug concentrations are reached at the site of action, while optimizing elimination characteristics to minimize adverse effects. Pharmacodynamic principles can be used to ensure that the drug concentration that is achieved results in the best possible therapeutic response. Knowledge of how to apply these pharmacokinetic and pharmacodynamic principles in the clinical setting has grown substantially in recent years. Optimization of drug dosing using pharmacokinetic and pharmacodynamic parameters and TDM would help achieve the best possible therapeutic outcomes among heterogeneous, critically ill patients.

Anti-infectives

β-Lactams

The efficacy of β-lactam agents correlates best with the percentage of time the drug concentration exceeds the MIC, but the time above the MIC (T > MIC) does not need to reach 100% to optimize therapy fully.[20] The recommended T > MIC values in non-neutropenic hosts vary by organism (i.e., gram-positive versus gram-negative). Animal models in the non-neutropenic host have shown a bacteriostatic effect against gram-negative organisms when serum concentrations exceed the MIC for only 40% of the dosing interval and the maximal killing that were achieved with a T > MIC was 70%.[22] Animal studies evaluating *Streptococcus pneumoniae* have shown survival to reach 100% with a T > MIC of 50%. In the neutropenic host, the T > MIC ideally should be longer with a T > MIC that exceeds 60% for agents with PAE and a T > MIC that exceeds 90% for agents without PAE.[21,22]

Pharmacodynamic differences exist among agents within the β-lactam class. In general, T > MIC values in non-neutropenic patients should be 50% to 60% for penicillins, 60% to 70% for cephalosporins, and 40% to 50% for carbapenems.[20,23] This observed variability in the T > MIC among β-lactams is likely a reflection of differences in the rate of killing among agents in the β-lactam class (i.e., fastest for carbapenems; slowest for cephalosporins).[22]

The pharmacodynamic profile of β-lactams has led some authors to investigate their administration as a continuous infusion.[24-28] Although pharmacodynamic modeling using Monte Carlo simulations predicted continuous infusions to be superior, clinical studies comparing continuous and intermittent dosing strategies yielded mixed results.[29-31] One study comparing intermittent and continuous piperacillin-tazobactam dosing strategies in patients with pneumonia revealed faster temperature normalization in patients receiving the continuous infusion, but clinical and microbiologic cures were similar.[26] A second study reported an improvement in clinical cure rate when meropenem was administered by continuous infusion in a cohort of ICU patients with ventilator-associated pneumonia.[27] In this study, differences in cure rates were most profound with organisms having an MIC of 0.5 or greater. Equivalent outcomes have been reported in studies evaluating a continuous infusion dosing strategy for other β-lactams including ceftazidime, cefuroxime, and cefepime.[24,25,28] The lack of superiority with continuous infusions in the clinical trials completed to date is likely attributable to the fact that the intermittent dosing regimen yielded a T > MIC that was adequate to kill the pathogen. Administration of β-lactams by continuous infusion may be most useful for pathogens having MICs with borderline susceptibility, in patients with compromised immunity, or for agents with a short half-life (i.e., penicillin).[21,23]

The duration of time drug concentrations remaining above the MIC can be calculated for β-lactams administered intravenously by the following formula:

$$T > MIC\ (\%) = \ln[\text{dose}/(Vd * MIC)] * [T_{1/2}/0.693] * [100/DI]$$

where ln is natural log, dose is dose in milligrams, Vd is volume of distribution in liters, MIC is MIC in mg/L, $T_{1/2}$ is half life in hours, and DI is dosing interval in hours.[23] This formula can be used to ensure that the individualized dosing regimen achieves the desired pharmacodynamic goal, particularly for pathogens with a borderline susceptibility. When a regimen with a suboptimal T > MIC is identified, clinicians should consider increasing the dose, using combination therapy, or selecting an agent with a more optimal T > MIC.

Vancomycin

Vancomycin is increasingly being used in the ICU to treat *Staphylococcus aureus* infections because of high resistance rates to methicillin.[32] Vancomycin shows slow bactericidal killing activity that is time-dependent. The pharmacodynamic parameter associated with clinical outcome is unclear, but seems to approximate most closely the AUIC.[32] Vancomycin has a PAE lasting 3 hours when used to treat staphylococcal infections. Vancomycin's large molecular size leads to a low penetration into many organs and body cavities (e.g., lung, cerebrospinal fluid) that could compromise outcome for infections in these sites. Vancomycin distribution into the pulmonary epithelial lining fluid of critically ill patients has been shown to be only approximately 20% of the concentrations achieved in the serum.[33] The very poor penetration of vancomycin into the cerebrospinal fluid often necessitates intrathecal or intrashunt administration.

The nephrotoxic potential of vancomycin remains controversial, but is certainly far less than previously thought. In one study of 1750 patients, an incidence of vancomycin nephrotoxicity of only 1.4% was reported.[32] Cases of nephrotoxicity and ototoxicity historically associated with vancomycin are now believed to have been secondary to impurities in the early formulation of the drug, rather than exposure to larger doses or longer durations of therapy. The risk for nephrotoxicity does seem to be elevated, however, when vancomycin is used concomitantly with an aminoglycoside.[32]

Although the role for therapeutic drug monitoring (TDM) with vancomycin remains controversial, it is suggested that trough (rather than peak) concentrations should be used with the primary goal of TDM to ensure efficacy (i.e., maintenance of adequate serum concentrations over the dosing interval), rather than to prevent toxicity. In general, the trough serum vancomycin concentration should be maintained at approximately four to five times the MIC of the pathogen.[34] If vancomycin is being used to treat a bacteremia with an organism having an MIC of 1 μg/mL, the trough level should be maintained greater than 5 μg/mL. This therapeutic range has been elevated at some institutions, however, where antibiogram data reveal higher staphylococcal MICs. More recent guidelines for the treatment of hospital-acquired, ventilator-associated, and health care–associated pneumonia suggest obtaining a target vancomycin trough concentration of 15 to 20 μg/mL because of the poor penetration of vancomycin into lung tissue.[35] These recommendations are based on pharmacodynamic evidence suggesting that an AUIC of 400 is associated with improved outcomes in patients with methicillin-resistant *S. aureus* pneumonia, rather than clinical evidence linking improved outcome with attainment of trough concentrations of 15 μg/mL.[20] In the ICU, clinicians should consider drawing vancomycin trough concentrations when patients (1) are receiving concomitant aminoglycoside therapy, (2) are being treated for pneumonia but have an inadequate response, (3) have rapidly changing kidney function, (4) are undergoing renal replacement therapy, or (5) are obese.[32] Studies are needed to determine the optimal vancomycin therapeutic range for various disease states and whether vancomycin TDM improves outcome.

The primary factors to consider when establishing a vancomycin dosing regimen include the predicted or known MIC of the gram-positive organism, the site of infection, the patient's weight, and the patient's kidney function. With vancomycin's relatively large Vd (0.7 L/kg), actual body weight should be used in all dosing calculations. Vancomycin clearance occurs primarily through glomerular filtration, so dosing adjustments are necessary in patients with renal insufficiency. Validated dosing nomograms can be used to establish initial vancomycin dosing regimens. If the goal of therapy is to maintain a trough concentration of 15 mg/mL, however, larger doses than those recommended in the nomogram may be required (see Fig. 21-6).[34]

Aminoglycosides

With early clinical studies showing that the achievement of higher peak aminoglycoside levels leads to better clinical outcomes, the ratio of Cmax to MIC is the pharmacodynamic parameter that clinicians should focus on optimizing.[36,37] Patients who respond to aminoglycoside therapy have been shown to have higher Cmax-to-MIC ratio (8.5 ± 5) than patients who do not (5.5 ± 3.6; $P < .001$).[38] Kashuba and colleagues[39] evaluated the impact of pharmacodynamic parameters on therapeutic response in a cohort of patients with nosocomial pneumonia. In this study, a Cmax-to-MIC ratio of 10 predicted a 90% probability of temperature and leukocyte resolution. Doses that provide a Cmax-to-MIC ratio of 12 should be avoided, however, because efficacy has not been shown to improve with ratios greater than 12, and the risk for nephrotoxicity increases.[40]

The pharmacodynamic characteristics of aminoglycosides support the use of a high peak, extended-interval dosing regimen (also known as once-daily dosing) in some patients. Administration of a larger dose less frequently maximizes the Cmax-to-MIC ratio, increasing the rate and extent of bactericidal activity. PAE maintains bacterial suppression at the end of the dosing interval and allows for undetectable trough values. With aminoglycoside accumulation in the renal tubule being a saturable process, overall drug exposure to the kidney is less with high-dose, extended-interval dosing. In addition, a drug-free period at the end of the dosing interval decreases the development of adaptive resistance, a transient decrease in bactericidal activity when bacteria are exposed to low drug concentrations. Finally, a reduction in health care costs may be realized as a result of decreased monitoring and administration costs. It should be noted, however, that although the clinical trials evaluating high-peak, extended-interval dosing regimens have shown them to be safe and efficacious, none has been shown superior over conventional dosing regimens.[41-44] In addition, few comparative studies have included large numbers of critically ill patients with ventilator-associated pneumonia.[45]

High-peak, extended-interval dosing seems to work best in middle-aged patients whose estimated creatinine clearance (CrCl) is 40 to 100 mL/min. In these patients, the targeted Cmax-to-MIC ratio should be 10. Many empiric dosing regimens are designed to obtain a target Cmax of 20 μg/mL, based on the assumption that *P. aeruginosa* is the most prominent pathogen and has an MIC no greater than 2 μg/mL.[41] Other authors have individualized dosing regimens using patient-specific target serum concentrations and infection type.[42,43] For example, target Cmax values when treating pulmonary infections were 16 to 20 μg/mL for gentamicin and tobramycin and 60 to 80 μg/mL for amikacin. For nonpulmonary infections, smaller Cmax values were targeted, but in all cases, the Cmax-to-MIC ratio of 10:1 was maintained. Institutions should consider local aminoglycoside resistance patterns when establishing Cmax target goals.

Patients with an estimated CrCl of less than 40 mL/min generally are not candidates for high-peak, extended-interval therapy and should receive a traditional dosing regimen. A traditional dosing strategy also should be used for patients with very high predicted aminoglycoside clearance (e.g., patients with cystic fibrosis or burn injuries) because of concerns that a daily dosing regimen in this population would result in a prolonged drug-free interval. This interval would be of greatest concern if the aminoglycoside is the sole agent providing gram-negative coverage.

Aminoglycosides are the prototypical drugs for which TDM can be employed to individualize therapy, particularly in the ICU, where substantial variability in aminoglycoside pharmacokinetic parameters exist.[46] Critically ill patients can have a Vd that is substantially greater than 0.25 L/kg owing to increases in the extracellular fluid volume. Aminoglycoside clearance has been shown to increase in hypermetabolic critically ill patients who have increased oxygen consumption, cardiac output, and renal perfusion.[47]

Goal serum concentration ranges have been established for traditional and high-peak, extended-interval dosing regimens in an effort to optimize clinical response and minimize toxicity (Table 21-4). Many factors need to be considered when establishing a dose, including: the site of infection, the MIC of the suspected or identified pathogen, and concomitant drug therapy. Critically ill patients who are started on a high-peak, extended-interval dosing regimen should have two random serum concentrations drawn at least 4 hours apart (e.g., 2 hours and 8 hours) after the administration of the first dose to allow for calculation of the appropriate pharmacokinetic parameters (i.e., Cmax, minimum serum antibiotic concentration [Cmin], Vd, k, and half-life). TDM after the first dose not only allows clinicians to confirm that adequate peak serum concentrations are being obtained, but also helps identify patients at high risk for aminoglycoside accumulation and nephrotoxicity. Patients who have a Cmin of 0.25 mg/dL for gentamicin or tobramycin or 1 mg/dL for amikacin generally should be converted to traditional dosing regimens or to a high-peak regimen that would achieve an acceptable Cmin value.[43]

Fluoroquinolones

The pharmacodynamic parameters that best correlate with clinical outcome for fluoroquinolones are the Cmax-to-MIC ratio and the AUIC. One trial that evaluated ciprofloxacin pharmacodynamics in a cohort of critically ill patients with predominantly gram-negative infections found that a higher AUIC improves clinical outcome.[13] In patients in whom an AUIC less than 125 was achieved, clinical and microbiologic cures were only 42% and 26%. When AUIC values exceeded 125, clinical and microbiologic cure rates exceeded 80% ($P < .001$). The median time to bacterial eradication for AUIC less than 125, AUIC between 125 and 250, and AUIC greater than 250 were 32 days, 7 days, and 1.9 days ($P < .005$). In a second trial that prospectively evaluated levofloxacin pharmacodynamics in patients with respiratory, skin, or urinary tract infections, Cmax-to-MIC ratio rather than the AUIC was found to be a stronger predictor of outcome.[48] The Cmax-to-MIC ratio and AUIC were strongly correlated, however ($r = .942$). In this trial, clinical and microbiologic cure rates were improved if the Cmax-to-MIC ratio was greater than 12. Studies evaluating the pharmacodynamics of levofloxacin and grepafloxacin during acute exacerbations of chronic bronchitis have found that an AUIC greater than 75 resulted in clinical and microbiologic cures, but bacterial eradication was most optimal when AUIC was greater than 175.[49,50]

Several in vitro models have shown that AUIC thresholds are lower when treating gram-positive infections.[51-53] One trial in patients with community-acquired respiratory

Table 21-4. Target Aminoglycoside Serum Concentrations for High Peak Extended Interval and Traditional Dosing Regimens

High-Peak, Extended Interval Dosing				
	Gentamicin/Tobramycin		Amikacin	
Disease State	Peak (mg/L)	Estimated Dose (Based on IBW)	Peak (mg/L)	Estimated Dose (Based on IBW)
Cystitis/gram-positive synergy	6-8	2-3 mg/kg q24h	30-40	10-15 mg/kg q24h
Pneumonia	16-20	5-7 mg/kg q24h	60-80	20-25 mg/kg q24h
All other infections	12-16	4-5 mg/kg q24h	50-70	20 mg/kg q24h

Traditional Dosing		
	Gentamicin/Tobramycin	Amikacin
Disease State	Peak (mg/L)	Peak (mg/L)
Cystitis/gram-positive synergy	3-4	15-20
Pneumonia	8-10	30-45
All other infections	6-8	25-30

IBW, ideal body weight.

tract infections caused by *S. pneumoniae* identified an AUIC of 34 as the threshold that was associated with a higher probability of bacterial eradication (64% versus 100%; $P < .01$).[54]

The AUIC also has been shown to predict the development of bacterial resistance. In a study of patients with lower respiratory tract infections, an inverse relationship was noted between the AUIC and the probability of developing resistance (defined as the isolation of a bacterial strain that was initially susceptible to the treatment regimen, but later tested resistant).[55] When the AUIC was 100, only 9% of susceptible pathogens became resistant. In contrast, when the AUIC was less than 100, 82% of patients developed an infection with a resistant organism within 20 days. When the pharmacodynamics of ciprofloxacin were evaluated during monotherapy for infections caused by *P. aeruginosa,* 100% of the patients developed resistance when the AUIC was less than 100 compared with 25% when the AUIC was 100. Monotherapy with a fluoroquinolone for infections caused by *Pseudomonas* should be discouraged when the pharmacodynamic properties are not optimal.

Although strong evidence exists to support pharmacodynamic optimization of fluoroquinolone therapy, it may not be practical to calculate these values at the bedside. Table 21-5 lists the relationship between pharmacokinetic and pharmacodynamic characteristics for the individual fluoroquinolones and the MIC threshold where the pharmacodynamic properties would be less than ideal, specifically an AUIC less than 125. These thresholds may vary from the MIC breakpoints established by the Clinical and Laboratory Standards Institute. For example, the established breakpoint for levofloxacin is 2 μg/mL. Using a dose of 500 mg daily, optimal pharmacodynamic activity would be achieved only for organisms with an MIC less than 0.53. This has led to an increase in the dosages now recommended for serious infections for IV levofloxacin (750 mg daily) and ciprofloxacin (400 mg every 8 hours).[21] Pathogens with MICs above this threshold might still be reported as susceptible, but the use of dosing regimens with these suboptimal pharmacodynamic parameters may lead to treatment failure. It is important for clinicians to consider these pharmacokinetic and pharmacodynamic concepts to optimize outcomes and prevent the emergence of resistant organisms with use.

Antifungals

Similar to the antibacterial medications, antifungal agents are classified as having either concentration-dependent or time-dependent activity. Concentration-dependent antifungal agents include the polyenes (e.g., amphotericin B) and the echinocandins (e.g., caspofungin, micafungin, anidulafungin).[56,57] The antifungal agents with time-dependent activity include the triazoles (e.g., fluconazole, voriconazole) and flucytosine. The categorization of antifungal agents as being fungicidal or fungistatic varies among antifungal agents within the same class and depends on the pathogen being treated (e.g., yeast versus mold).[56,57] Voriconazole is fungistatic against *Candida,* but has fungicidal activity against *Aspergillus.* In contrast, the echinocandins are fungicidal against *Candida,* but fungistatic against *Aspergillus.* The clinical significance of an agent having fungistatic versus fungicidal activity has yet to be determined.

Most of the current antifungal pharmacodynamic data surround the treatment of *Candida* rather than *Aspergillus* infections.[56,57] The pharmacodynamic properties of antifungal agents commonly used in the ICU are listed in Table 21-3. With susceptibility testing of antifungal organisms becoming more common, these pharmacodynamic properties will be more clinically relevant because clinicians will be able to choose the drug regimen that is most appropriate based on the patient-specific pharmacodynamic properties, rather than non–patient-specific surveillance reports or in vitro data.

Anticonvulsants

With anticonvulsant toxicity generally attributable to excessive peak concentrations, the primary goal of therapy is to maintain the lowest effective dose, and thus the trough level is used most frequently to monitor therapy.[58] Because of their physicochemical and pharmacokinetic properties, however, anticonvulsants as a group are particularly prone to fluctuations in drug concentrations, potentially leading to unexpected changes in seizure control or the development of drug toxicity. Challenges that face clinicians when designing dosing regimens for anticonvulsants include narrow therapeutic ranges (e.g., phenytoin, carbamazepine), saturable hepatic elimination (e.g., phenytoin), saturable protein binding (e.g., phenytoin, valproic acid) and numerous drug-drug interactions (e.g., phenytoin, carbamazepine, valproic acid).

Table 21-5. Relationship between Fluoroquinolone Pharmacokinetics and Pharmacodynamics

Drug	Dosage	AUC (μg/hr/mL)	MIC Threshold for Optimal Pharmacodynamics
Ciprofloxacin	400 mg IV q8h	40*	0.32
Levofloxacin	500 mg IV q24h	66.1†	0.53
Gatifloxacin	400 mg IV q24h	39.5†	0.32
Moxifloxacin	400 mg IV q24h	36.9*	0.30
Ofloxacin	400 mg IV q12h	87*	0.70

*AUC in healthy volunteers with normal renal function.
†AUC in critically ill patients with normal renal function
AUC, area under the curve; IV, intravenous; MIC, minimum inhibitory concentration.
Data from references 13, 85, 200, and 201.

Phenytoin remains the most commonly used anticonvulsant in the ICU and can be difficult to dose appropriately because of its capacity (i.e., saturable) liver metabolism.[6] Because of capacity-limited metabolism, a small change in the dose or bioavailability can produce a dramatic change in the average steady-state concentration. At serum concentrations greater than 4 μg/mL, alterations in the administered dose do not produce proportional changes in serum concentrations, and small dosage increases may result in phenytoin levels greater than the generally accepted range of 10 to 20 μg/mL.[58] Consequently, maintenance doses generally should not be increased by greater than 100 mg/d.

Phenytoin loading doses can be estimated using phenytoin's average Vd of 0.7 L/kg; this is particularly useful for patients whose weight is outside of the normal range. For example, the estimated phenytoin loading dose for a 50-kg patient to achieve a concentration of approximately 15 mg/dL would be only 500 mg. Loading doses should be administered with each dosing increase and can be calculated using the following equation:

$$\text{IV dose (mg/kg)} = 0.7\ (\text{concentration desired} - \text{concentration observed})$$

Patients with head injuries may require higher than average doses of phenytoin to maintain therapeutic concentrations because of the increased clearance that has been reported in these patients.[59]

Phenytoin, carbamazepine, and valproic acid are highly bound to serum proteins. When serum albumin concentrations fall below the normal range, which is commonly observed in many critically ill populations, the free (and active) fraction of these agents increases. The free (or unbound) fraction is what should be used to guide therapy and is available for phenytoin, but not carbamazepine or valproic acid. If free phenytoin levels are unavailable at the clinician's institution, the total level can be adjusted for the serum albumin using the following equation:

$$\text{Adjusted concentration} = \text{measured total concentration}/[(0.2 \times \text{albumin}) + 0.1]$$

In the presence of renal failure (CrCl less than 10 mL/min), adjustments for serum albumin in patients with renal failure can be made using the following equation:

$$\text{Adjusted concentration} = \text{measured total concentration}/[(0.1 \times \text{albumin}) + 0.1]$$

Sedatives and Analgesics

Critically ill patients often require prolonged sedation and analgesia therapy.[60] Pharmacokinetic data derived from short-term sedative and analgesia administration studies are often not predictive of the pharmacokinetic parameters that are seen after longer term infusions because of the multicompartment behavior of the parent drug and its metabolites.[4] In addition, time-related changes in hepatic metabolism and Vd may complicate steady-state concentrations.[6]

Differences in the clinical response to benzodiazepines are related to pharmacokinetic and pharmacodynamic variability and are most pronounced when these agents are administered to critically ill patients as continuous infusions.[60] Important differences between midazolam and lorazepam account for the higher likelihood that midazolam will result in prolonged sedation after long-term use.[9,61] The higher lipid solubility of midazolam has been associated with prolonged sedation in obese patients. Although lorazepam's metabolites are not active, midazolam has an active metabolite that accumulates in patients with renal failure. In patients with liver failure, the metabolism of midazolam (hydroxylation) is much more likely to be compromised than the metabolism of lorazepam (glucuronidation). Potential limitations with the use of lorazepam compared with midazolam include its slower onset of action, its decreased solubility in IV solutions, and the risk for propylene glycol toxicity with high doses.[60]

Metabolism of propofol does not seem to be altered significantly by hepatic or renal disease, although in critical care populations clearance is generally slower than in the general population because of decreases in hepatic blood flow.[4,6] Elderly patients have decreased clearance and a prolonged half-life, and maintenance infusions generally should be reduced in an age-related fashion.

Many important pharmacokinetic and pharmacodynamic considerations exist with the use of opioids in critically ill patients.[4,6] Use of morphine and meperidine should be avoided in patients with renal insufficiency because each has active metabolites that accumulate and cause prolonged analgesia. Accumulation of meperidine's active metabolite normeperidine in renal insufficiency also may cause myoclonus, tremors, and seizures that are not reversible with naloxone.[62,63] Although the Vd and half-life of fentanyl, a highly lipid-soluble opioid, have been shown to be elevated in critical illness, its clearance remains normal. The pharmacokinetics of remifentanil have not been shown to be affected by liver disease or critical illness.[4]

Cardiac Agents

In general, antiarrhythmics are dosed to effect, with acceptable serum concentrations being those that suppress the arrhythmia without causing side effects. Although the use of antiarrhythmics for which serum concentration monitoring is available, such as digoxin, procainamide, and lidocaine, continues to decrease, many important pharmacokinetic considerations remain with their use.

Digoxin represents a challenge for clinicians to optimize because of its large Vd, long half-life, renal elimination, and lack of consensus regarding the most appropriate serum concentration goal. Loading doses generally should be given when initiating digoxin therapy to achieve serum concentrations of 1 to 2 ng/mL for ventricular rate control and 0.5 to 1.2 ng/mL for inotropy, although the correlation between any particular serum digoxin concentration and clinical outcome in patients with heart failure is poor.[64] Because digoxin has a prolonged distribution phase, serum concentrations should be drawn at least 6 hours after the dose is administered. With the risk for adverse effects increasing dramatically when the steady-state serum concentration exceeds 2 ng/mL, serum levels should be monitored in the following situations: decreasing kidney function, use of concomitant medications shown to reduce digoxin clearance (e.g., verapamil), electrolyte disturbances (e.g., hypokalemia), and electrocardiogram changes consistent with digoxin toxicity (e.g., peaked T waves).

Procainamide therapy is challenging to optimize in the ICU because of its narrow therapeutic window, and the fact that one of its metabolites, N-acetyl procainamide (NAPA), has class III anti-arrhythmic properties of its own. Continuous infusions of procainamide should be dosed to maintain serum concentrations between 4 μg/mL and 10 μg/mL.[65] NAPA is approximately one third to one sixth as potent as procainamide, and therapeutic concentrations of NAPA are approximately 10 to 30 μg/mL. Procainamide dosing can be problematic in patients with renal failure and is typically characterized by subtherapeutic procainamide concentrations with supratherapeutic NAPA concentrations.

Maintenance infusions of lidocaine should be dosed to maintain a serum level of 2 to 6 μg/mL. Clearance of lidocaine is decreased in patients with heart failure, shock, or liver disease, and smaller doses are usually required in these patients. As with all antiarrhythmics, electrocardiogram findings should be used in conjunction with serum levels to guide therapy.

Although amiodarone serum concentrations are not routinely monitored in clinical practice, there are some important pharmacokinetic principles for the clinician to consider. Amiodarone has a tremendously large Vd (approximately 70 to 150 L/kg), which indicates extensive tissue distribution, particularly to fat tissue. In the ICU, amiodarone is administered intravenously in three distinct phases—a rapid loading phase, a slow loading phase, and a maintenance infusion phase. Despite an aggressive IV loading dose, it may take several weeks before peak plasma concentrations are achieved.[66] Amiodarone serum concentrations of 1 to 2.5 mg/L are considered therapeutic, but are considered a poor measure of myocardial concentrations, which tend to be 10 to 50 times higher.[65] The elimination half-life for amiodarone ranges from 20 to 120 days.

Antithrombotics

Anticoagulants such as unfractionated heparin (UFH), low-molecular-weight heparins (LMWHs), and direct thrombin inhibitors are frequently used in the ICU to treat many different thrombus-mediated conditions (e.g., venous thromboembolism, myocardial infarction, acute arterial occlusion) or to prevent thrombus formation during procedures that use extracorporeal membranes (e.g., renal replacement therapy) or angiography (e.g., percutaneous coronary intervention).

Although the activated partial thromboplastin time (APTT) remains the primary test that is used to measure the anticoagulant effect of UFH, it often produces highly variable and inconsistent results.[67] Factors shown to affect the APTT assay include the reagent used, the instrument used to determine the test result, the source of the collection tube, and the volume of blood collected. APTT therapeutic ranges differ among institutions. Each laboratory completing APTT testing must develop a reagent-specific APTT therapeutic range in seconds that is calibrated to correspond with a heparin serum concentration of 0.2 to 0.4 U/mL by protamine titration or an anti–factor Xa activity of 0.3 to 0.7 U/mL.[68] Although there are many potential advantages for the use of point-of-care devices to measure the APTT in the ICU (e.g., quicker result, smaller sample of blood, reduced sampling and handling errors), the inherent inaccuracy of the APTT assay itself remains, and these tests have not yet enjoyed widespread use.[68]

The activated clotting time (ACT) is most frequently used to monitor high-dose UFH in patients undergoing invasive procedures, such as valve replacement surgery or percutaneous coronary intervention, in patients who are receiving therapy with a device having an extracorporeal circuit (e.g., cardiopulmonary bypass or renal replacement therapy). For renal replacement therapy, an ACT of 170 to 220 seconds has been recommended.[67] During percutaneous coronary intervention, the desired ACT range varies depending on the ACT instrument and the presence or absence of concomitant antiplatelet therapy. In the absence of a glycoprotein IIb/IIIa inhibitor, the American College of Chest Physicians Consensus Guidelines recommend a goal ACT of 250 to 350 seconds.[67] If glycoprotein IIb/IIIa is used, the goal ACT is greater than 200 seconds.[67] Warfarin, glycoprotein IIb/IIIa antagonists, and aprotinin all have been shown to prolong the ACT.

Another method for monitoring anticoagulation therapy is thromboelastography. Thromboelastography is a single test that provides information on platelet function, coagulation, and fibrinolysis. Specifically, thromboelastography can reveal the time to initial fibrin formation, speed of clot strengthening, maximal clot strength, and rate of clot lysis.[69,70] Thromboelastography has been primarily studied in liver transplant and cardiac surgery. Barriers to the widespread application of thromboelastography to other critical care situations include its poor correlation to standard blood tests and the need for tests to be evaluated by a trained expert.[71]

LMWHs have a more predictable anticoagulant effect than UFH because of their greater anti–factor Xa activity and lower anti–factor IIa activity. Although LMWHs can be easily and accurately dosed in most critically ill populations, there are several instances in ICU practice where the dose-response effects of LMWHs may be unpredictable, or safety concerns exist. These situations include patients with extremes of body weight, kidney dysfunction, or pregnancy. In these circumstances, individual monitoring is warranted. In contrast to with UFH, APTT or ACT cannot be used to monitor the anticoagulation effect of LMWHs. Anti–factor Xa activity monitoring has evolved as a means to measure the LMWH pharmacodynamic response for patients in whom the pharmacokinetic response to LMWHs may be altered (e.g., renal insufficiency, morbid obesity).[67]

Many controversies are associated with the use of anti–factor Xa activity monitoring, including the optimal draw time in relation to LMWH administration, the method of testing (i.e., amidolytic versus chromogenic), and the desired therapeutic range. Current recommendations suggest that an anti–factor Xa activity level be drawn 4 hours after the LMWH dose and no sooner than 2 days after the start of therapy.[67] For patients receiving therapeutic twice-daily LMWH therapy, anti–factor Xa activity should be maintained in the range of 0.4 to 1.1 IU/mL; for once-daily therapy, 1 to 2 IU/mL.[72] It should be noted that these recommended anti–factor Xa activity therapeutic ranges have never been correlated to clinical outcomes (e.g., bleeding) in large, prospective studies. Numerous additional factors exist that can affect the reliability of anti–factor Xa activity testing, including the test employed, the reagent manufacturer, the LMWH studied, and the lot of LMWH used.[67] Patients with multiple organ dysfunction, with excessive body weight, or receiving vasopressor therapy have been shown to have lower than expected anti–factor Xa activity, although it remains unclear if higher LMWH doses are warranted in these patients.[73]

DRUG DOSING CONSIDERATIONS FOR SPECIFIC CONDITIONS

Ventilator-Associated Pneumonia

Optimizing antibiotic therapy for patients with ventilator-associated pneumonia requires consideration of several different factors.[45] For empiric therapy, the clinician should consult ICU-specific antibiogram data (as opposed to institution-specific) to determine antimicrobial MIC breakpoints for the common pathogens that cause ventilator-associated pneumonia in his or her institution. In instances where a pathogen has been isolated, the MIC for each antimicrobial tested against the organism must be reviewed with appreciation of the patient-specific pharmacokinetic and pharmacodynamic parameters for that agent (see earlier sections on pharmacokinetics and pharmacodynamics). In all cases, the effects of renal or hepatic insufficiency on these dosing regimens need to be considered.

Lastly, it is important to consider the degree to which the antibiotic penetrates into the lung by being familiar with reported serum concentrations in the lung. Antibiotic lung penetration may be determined by measuring antibiotic concentrations in lung tissue samples, epithelial lining fluid, or alveolar macrophages, and by using intrapulmonary microdialysis. The degree to which antibiotics penetrate the lung varies substantially among agents.[45] Fluoroquinolones and linezolid equal or exceed their serum concentrations in bronchial secretions, whereas many β-lactam antibiotics achieve less than 50% of their serum concentrations in the lung.[45] The lung penetration of some antibiotics, such as aminoglycosides and vancomycin, is poor, and larger than usual doses are recommended when these agents are used for pneumonia.[20]

Meningitis

Bacterial eradication from the central nervous system is the primary goal of antibiotic therapy for meningitis.[74] Factors that affect the clinical response to therapy include the penetration of the antibiotic into the cerebrospinal fluid, the activity of the antibiotic within purulent cerebrospinal fluid, the mode of antibiotic administration, whether the antibiotic is bactericidal or bacteriostatic, and its in vitro susceptibility.[74] The degree of meningeal inflammation is the most important patient-related factor that affects antibiotic penetration. Any process that decreases inflammation (e.g., dexamethasone administration) would lower absorption across the blood-brain barrier. Antibiotic penetration is greatest if the drug (1) has a low molecular weight, (2) has a low degree of ionization, (3) is highly lipophilic, (4) has a low degree of protein binding, and (5) is not susceptible to removal from the cerebrospinal fluid by an active transport system (e.g., penicillin) (Table 21-6). It is more important to evaluate antibiotic penetration into the cerebrospinal fluid in the context that the principal determinant of antibiotic effectiveness is the relationship between antibiotic concentrations in cerebrospinal fluid and the minimum bactericidal concentration for the infecting organism, rather than the absolute percentage of antibiotic that is delivered.[75] Although the penetration of β-lactams is seldom greater than 10%, therapeutic concentrations can be readily achieved in the cerebrospinal fluid because large doses can be administered systemically without toxicity.

The degree of cerebrospinal fluid purulence affects antibiotic activity.[74] In an experimental rabbit model of

Table 21-6. Variables Affecting Antibiotic Concentrations in the Cerebrospinal Fluid

Variable	Example	Result
Drug lipophilicity	Fluoroquinolones	Rapid entry into CSF
High degree of ionization	β-lactam antibiotics	Poor penetration through BBB
High serum protein binding	Ceftriaxone	Delayed CSF entry; long CSF and serum half-life
Active transport system	Penicillin	Short duration of effective CSF concentration
Infecting organism	*Listeria, Haemophilus* *Escherichia coli, Streptococcus pneumoniae*	Greater antibiotic penetration Lesser antibiotic penetration

BBB, blood-brain barrier; CSF, cerebrospinal fluid.
From Lutsar I, McCracken GH Jr, Friedland IR: Antibiotic pharmacodynamics in cerebrospinal fluid. Clin Infect Dis 1998;27:1117-1127.

Proteus mirabilis meningitis, the acidic conditions of the cerebrospinal fluid (largely as a result of lactate accumulation) were shown to inhibit aminoglycoside activity.[76] Bactericidal activity also may be modified by the so-called inoculum effect, in which the MIC of an antibiotic increases dramatically as the bacteria inoculum size increases. Lastly, purulent cerebrospinal fluid has been shown to lead to antagonism when a bactericidal agent is coadministered with a bacteriostatic agent.[76] With host immunity being impaired in the cerebrospinal fluid, rapid bacterial killing during meningitis is observed only when cerebrospinal fluid concentrations of β-lactams or aminoglycosides exceed the minimum bactericidal concentration by 10-fold to 20-fold. The pharmacodynamic properties associated with clinical response should be used when optimizing antibiotic dosing regimens (see earlier section on using pharmacokinetic and pharmacodynamic principles to optimize drug dosing).

Pancreatitis

The effectiveness of antibiotic therapy for pancreatic and pancreas-related infections depends on the degree of antibiotic penetration into the pancreatic tissue and ducts.[77,78] Studies measuring the concentration of antibiotics into pancreatic tissue have shown substantial variability in antibiotic penetration. Antibiotics that yield low pancreatic tissue concentrations and concentrations that are well below the MIC for the bacteria found in pancreatic infections include aminoglycosides, ampicillin, cefazolin, cefotaxime, piperacillin, and vancomycin. Antibiotics showing high pancreatic tissue levels and high bactericidal activity against common pancreatic pathogens include fluoroquinolones (e.g., ciprofloxacin), imipenem, meropenem, metronidazole, and fluconazole. Limitations with these data include the varied methodology that was used in the studies and the lack of correlation to clinical outcomes. Few data exist regarding the pancreatic penetration for most newer anti-infectives.

PRINCIPLES OF THERAPEUTIC DRUG MONITORING

The art and science of TDM is the ability to use multiple static data to assess an ever-changing clinical situation.[8] With pharmacokinetic and pharmacodynamic parameters often changing in critically ill patients, TDM is frequently employed in the ICU. Patient-specific pharmacokinetic parameters derived from strategically obtained serum drug concentrations can be used to individualize doses for patients with variable distribution volumes and elimination characteristics. The goal of TDM in the ICU is to help maximize clinical outcomes, minimize toxicity, and ensure that cost-effective drug therapy is provided. Criteria have been proposed to help define the situations in which TDM should be considered (Table 21-7).[79] Drugs that frequently produce toxicity at dosages close to those required for therapeutic effects (e.g., phenytoin) are the medications most commonly monitored and for which commercial assays are usually available. With such drugs, the "target" serum concentration is usually narrow, necessitating a precise selection of drug dosage and schedule. The therapeutic range for most drugs is the range of drug concentrations where the probability of reaching the desired clinical response is relatively high, and the probability of unacceptable toxicity is relatively low. An important consideration when using TDM to optimize drug therapy in the ICU is that most of the target drug concentration ranges used to guide therapy have been validated in only small cohorts of healthy patients.

Table 21-7. Seven Criteria for the Use of Therapeutic Drug Monitoring

1. An appropriate drug assay is available (satisfactory accuracy and precision, minimal cost, short analysis time, small sample volume requirements, and high assay specificity)
2. There is documented and significant interindividual variability in drug absorption, elimination, and distribution
3. Adequate pharmacokinetic data concerning the drug are available
4. The pharmacologic effect is proportional to the plasma drug concentration
5. A narrow range exists between the efficacious and toxic drug concentrations
6. A constant pharmacologic effect over an extended period exists
7. Clinical study exists that defines the therapeutic and toxic ranges of the drug

From Spector R, Park GD, Johnson GF, et al: Therapeutic drug monitoring. Clin Pharmacol Ther 1988;43:345-353.

Clinicians should employ a systematic approach to TDM; otherwise, drug concentrations may be uninterpretable, unhelpful, or potentially harmful.[79] Numerous drug, host, logistical, and analytical variables may influence the interpretation of drug concentration data. These include the time, duration, and route of drug administration; the dose administered; the time blood samples are drawn; the handling and storage conditions of samples; the precision and accuracy of the analytical method employed; the validity of the pharmacokinetics model; the impact of concurrent drug therapy; and the patient's disease and biologic tolerance to drug therapy. The impact of these latter variables, each of which can influence individual responsiveness to drug therapy, is why drug concentrations should be considered only an intermediate end point when evaluating therapeutic response and not a replacement for measurable clinical outcomes.

The ideal time at which to monitor serum drug concentrations in relation to the time of dose administration (i.e., trough versus peak) depends on the particular agent being monitored (see previous section on pharmacokinetics and pharmacodynamics). Unless drug toxicity is suspected, clinicians generally should wait until a new steady-state concentration is reached (i.e., four to five drug half-lives) after any dose change before re-evaluating serum drug concentrations. End-organ dysfunction prolongs half-life, increasing the time required for a steady-state concentration to be achieved.

BIOAVAILABILITY ISSUES WITH MEDICATIONS NOT ADMINISTERED BY THE INTRAVENOUS ROUTE

Medications are frequently administered to critically ill patients by routes other than the IV route for many reasons, including (1) the lack of an available IV formulation, (2) to prolong the duration of drug effect, (3) to decrease monitoring requirements, (4) to facilitate ICU discharge, and (5) to decrease drug costs. In general, bioavailability is nearly always lower when drugs are administered by non-IV routes. In critically ill patients, these differences can be substantial, and numerous important factors should be considered when administering medications orally, enterally, subcutaneously, transdermally, or endotracheally.

Oral and Enteral

Intestinal function is significantly altered in critical illnesses, particularly in patients with trauma, burns, or sepsis, and this may affect drug and nutrient absorption.[80] The alterations in gastrointestinal physiology seen in many critically ill patients are the result of numerous complex, interacting factors, including a decrease in mucosal blood flow (i.e., splanchnic hypoperfusion); inadequate luminal nutrient delivery; alterations in mucosal immunity; and changes in neural, hormonal, and inflammatory mediators.[81]

Critically ill patients often have pharmacologically mediated or disease-induced decreases in gastric acid secretion.[82] An increase in the gastric pH may decrease the absorption of weak bases (e.g., ketoconazole, itraconazole) and alter the release characteristics of enteric-coated formulations (e.g., proton-pump inhibitors, mesalamine). Delayed gastric emptying, occurring in 60% of mechanically ventilated patients and in 80% of head-injured patients, may decrease drug absorption.[83] This may be an important consideration for patients in whom the nasogastric tube is clamped after drug administration. If the drug has not emptied into the small intestine by the time nasogastric suction is re-established, the drug is removed from the body and not absorbed. Patients who are hemodynamically unstable, particularly patients receiving vasopressor therapy, are likely to have splanchnic hypoperfusion and altered intestinal permeability. Owing to the numerous structural and physiologic alterations in the gastrointestinal tract of these patients, IV drug therapy should be employed whenever possible because drug absorption is likely to be impaired.[11]

Sequential IV-to-oral therapy is increasingly being promoted in the ICU because it facilitates earlier hospital discharge, may lead to fewer administration-related adverse drug events, and can decrease health care costs.[84] Drugs with a proven high bioavailability in healthy patients (e.g., fluoroquinolone antibiotics, fluconazole, and proton-pump inhibitors) are ideally suited for sequential therapy. The numerous physiologic and end-organ changes seen in critically ill patients preclude, however, extrapolation of data from the pharmacokinetic studies that have evaluated oral bioavailability in healthy volunteers to critically ill patients.[6]

There is a paucity of high-quality studies evaluating nasogastric tube bioavailability in critically ill patients for medications that exhibit high oral bioavailability in healthy patients. One prospective, randomized, single-dose, two-way, crossover study in 16 critically ill patients (APACHE [Acute Physiology, Age, and Chronic Health Evaluation] II score 16) found that gatifloxacin administered by gastric tube does not consistently yield a high bioavailability, with the absolute bioavailability found to be less than 70% in 3 patients.[85] The clinical implications of this and other studies can be explored by evaluating the impact of this pharmacokinetic variability on established pharmacodynamic variables. Assuming the MIC for gatifloxacin is less than 1 μg/mL for most organisms, the gatifloxacin AUIC values that were observed in some patients after gastric administration were 20 μg/mL/h. The resulting AUIC of 20 is far lower than the generally accepted AUIC breakpoint of 125 that has been established for the treatment of gram-negative organisms.[86] Further research is needed to identify critically ill patients who are predisposed to reduced bioavailability after gastric administration and for whom an empiric dosage increase should be considered.

Administration of medication via the gastric tube requires that a tablet be crushed, dissolved, and administered using an oral syringe through the nasogastric, orogastric, or gastronomy tube. These added administration steps compound the risk that residual drug may be left behind in the receptacle in which the tablet was crushed and reconstituted, in the syringe used for administration, or in the actual gastric tube.[87] The bioavailability of several medications (e.g., phenytoin, ciprofloxacin) has been shown to decrease by 80% when concomitantly administered with enteral nutrition formulations.[88,89] The mechanism for this decrease in biovailability varies with each drug. Lower phenytoin absorption is attributable to enteral nutrition–induced increases in gastrointestinal transit, whereas ciprofloxacin binds directly to the cations in the enteral formulation. It is unclear why studies evaluating the concomitant administration of other fluoroquinolone products (e.g., gatifloxacin, levofloxacin) with enteral nutrients have not shown this same interaction.[85] To resolve this problem, enteral nutrition can be held for 1 to 2 hours before and after each dose. Food may impair the absorption of proton-pump inhibitors, and the manufacturer of omeprazole immediate release in bicarbonate suspension recommends that enteral continuous gastric feedings be suspended for 1 hour before and 3 hours after the administration of each dose via a nasogastric tube. When enteral feedings are being held for drug administration, clinicians should adjust the tube feeding rate so that the entire daily enteral nutrition prescription is delivered.

Subcutaneous

Medications that are administered subcutaneously may yield lower serum concentrations in critically ill patients because of the frequent presence of factors shown to result in poor or erratic drug absorption, including low cardiac output, peripheral edema (e.g., sepsis), and vasopressor-induced peripheral blood vessel vasoconstriction. Numerous studies have compared the anti–factor Xa activity profile after subcutaneous administration of LMWHs among various populations of critically ill patients (e.g., medical, burn, and trauma) and general ward medical patients.[90-92] One study that compared anti–factor Xa activity after daily enoxaparin 40 mg subcutaneous dosing between 16 critically ill patients (13 of whom who were receiving vasopressor therapy) and 13 noncritically ill patients found the peak anti–factor Xa activity (3 hours after administration) and the AUC at 0 to 12 hours to be substantially lower in ICU patients (2.6 ± 1 U/mL^{-1}/hr^{-1} versus 4.2 ± 1.7 U/mL^{-1}/hr^{-1}; $P = .008$).

Another study evaluated the impact of peripheral edema on LMWH absorption in patients with multiple trauma by comparing anti–factor Xa activity between edematous (10 kg weight gain from admission) and nonedematous patients after the administration of subcutaneous enoxaparin. The investigators found that 7 of the 10 edematous patients had barely quantifiable anti–factor Xa activity results. The clinical implications of this study are profound when one considers that the incidence of venous thrombosis in patients with multiple trauma is only 6.3% when the anti–factor Xa factor activity is greater than 0.1 IU/mL, but 18.8% when anti–factor Xa activity is 0.05 IU/mL.[93] The investigators in the study questioned whether enoxaparin 30 mg subcutaneous dosing twice daily should be the standard recommended dose for prophylaxis against venous thrombosis in patients with multiple trauma, particularly patients with significant peripheral edema. Further studies are necessary to identify the proper dosage and route of administration of LMWHs to provide effective deep venous thrombosis prophylaxis.

Transdermal

Although transdermal drug administration is sometimes an alternative to parenteral drug administration in a patient being kept NPO (nothing by mouth) (e.g., fentanyl patch), there are many important limitations associated with this dosage form in the ICU. Transdermal drug absorption and delivery may be compromised in patients with alterations in blood flow to subcutaneous tissues (e.g., shock). The slow onset for initial drug effect (usually 8 to 12 hours) is often inappropriate in the ICU where an immediate drug effect is desired. Finally, the inability to titrate transdermal medications (i.e., a prolonged drug effect is observed for 6 to 12 hours after patch removal) may present safety concerns in some situations. Transdermal administration should be discouraged in the ICU if other methods of drug delivery are available (i.e., enteral, oral, or IV).

Aerosolized

Patients who are mechanically ventilated routinely require pharmacologic agents by aerosol form, including β_2-agonists and anticholinergics. Prostacyclins and antibiotics may also be administered. The choice exists of nebulizer versus metered-dose inhaler (MDI) use. Administration using an MDI offers several advantages over a nebulizer, including a lower cost, dosing that is more reliable and simpler, and a low risk for drug contamination.[94] When an MDI is chosen, there are many in vitro variables in mechanically ventilated patients that affect the amount of drug delivered into the lung, including the ventilator mode and settings, the heat and humidification of the inspired gas, the density of the inhaled gas, the endotracheal tube size, and the method by which the MDI is connected to the ventilatory circuit.[95] To account for the ventilator circuit, MDI doses generally should be at least twice what would be administered to a patient who is not mechanically ventilated.[96] Studies have evaluated the use of locally instilled or aerosolized antibiotics (particularly aminoglycosides for the treatment of ventilator-associated pneumonia) to enhance antibiotic penetration into the lung and minimize toxicity.[97,98] One side effect of aerosolized antibiotics is bronchospasm, which can be induced by the antibiotic or the diluent by which it is administered.[99]

PHARMACOGENETICS

It is now well established that many of the genes that encode proteins dictating drug metabolism, transport, and pharmacodynamic action display genetic polymorphism. It has been estimated that genetics accounts for half of the variability in response that is observed in patients.[100] Pharmacogenetics is the study of the role of inheritance in the individual variation in drug response. Pharmacogenomics uses genome-wide approaches to identify genetic polymorphisms that govern an individual's response to a particular drug. It is expected that as knowledge about pharmacogenetics increases, and the ability to diagnose patients' genetic predisposition to drug therapy improves, these tools will be used routinely to optimize drug therapy in the ICU.[7]

Although pharmacogenetics can influence drug absorption, distribution, and elimination, most knowledge pertains to the effect of genetic variants on drug metabolism. Significant genetic variation has been noted with phase I reactions (i.e., hydrolysis, oxidation, and reduction) and phase II conjugation reactions (i.e., acetylation, glucuronidation, sulfation, and methylation). Of the phase I reactions, CYP-450 enzymes are the most important, and the most studied enzyme is CYP2D6. Other well-studied CYP-450 subsets include CYP2C9 and CYP2C19 (Table 21-8).

Proton-pump inhibitors, predominantly metabolized through CYP2C19, are an example of a class of medications that are commonly used in the ICU that display pharmacogenetic variability. The prevalence of CYP2C19 mutations, resulting in slower drug metabolism, is nearly four times greater in Asians (23%) than whites of European or North American descent (6%).[101] Given that slow drug metabolizers have a longer elimination half-life and a greater area-under-the-plasma concentration time curve, it is not surprising that slow metabolizers have been shown to have a greater response to proton-pump inhibitor therapy.[102] One meta-analysis of studies evaluating

Table 21-8. Pharmacogenetics of Drug Metabolism

Drug Metabolizing Enzyme	Approximate Frequency of Poor-Metabolism Phenotype	Drugs Metabolized	Result of Polymorphism
Phase I Drug Metabolism			
CYP2D6	6.8% in Sweden 1% in China	Nortriptyline Codeine	Increased drug effect Decreased drug effect
CYP2C9	3% in England (homozygous for the *2 and *3 alleles)	Warfarin Phenytoin	Increased drug effect
CYP2C19	2.7% among white Americans 14.6% in China 18% in Japan	Omeprazole	Increased drug effect
Butyrylcholinesterase (pseudocholinesterase)	1 in 3500 Europeans	Succinylcholine	Increased drug effect
Phase II Drug Metabolism			
N-acetyltransferase 2	52% among white Americans 17% in Japan	Isoniazid Hydralazine Procainamide	Increased drug effect
Thiopurine S-methyltransferase	1 in 300 whites 1 in 2500 Asians	Mercaptopurine Azathioprine	Increased drug effect (toxicity)

From Weinshilboum R: Inheritance and drug response. N Engl J Med 2003;348:529-537.

proton-pump inhibitor therapy for peptic ulcer bleeding that stratified studies between those completed in Asian ($n = 7$) and non-Asian ($n = 16$) countries found that the effects of proton-pump inhibitors on gastric rebleeding and need for surgery were quantitatively greater in Asian patients. Thirty-day all-cause mortality was significantly lower in Asian (odds ratio 0.35; 95% confidence interval 0.16 to 0.74) but not in non-Asian (odds ratio 1.36; 95% confidence interval 0.94 to 1.96) patients.[102]

It is hoped that as understanding of pharmacogenetic and pharmacodynamic variability increases, clinicians will be able to conduct assessments before initiating drug therapy. Genetic variability could be characterized, and patients who would experience the desired therapeutic outcome or in some cases potentially unwanted toxic effects could be identified. Clinicians could optimize therapy with that particular agent or choose an alternative drug. The pharmacogenetic literature is growing rapidly with the most knowledge currently available for cardiovascular, hormone/hormone modifier, and psychotropic drugs.[103] Although a test for detecting genotype polymorphisms to CYP2D6 and CYP2C19 is currently approved, it remains unclear how this test should be used in routine clinical practice in the ICU.

DRUG DOSING IN SPECIAL CRITICAL CARE POPULATIONS

Kidney Failure

Kidney dysfunction is common in the ICU, with acute renal failure (the most severe form of acute kidney dysfunction) occurring in 25% of patients in some ICUs.[18] Approximately two thirds of patients with acute renal failure require some form of renal replacement therapy, and continuous renal replacement therapy (CRRT) is the most commonly used modality. Despite the many advances made in critical care medicine, the overall mortality for acute renal failure is approximately 60%.[18] Because most medications used in the ICU are eliminated by the kidney, it is imperative that the clinician have a thorough understanding of the principles of drug dosing in kidney failure and renal replacement therapies.

Formulas to Calculate Creatinine Clearance

Equations exist to estimate the GFR or CrCl and are commonly used to assess kidney function in the ICU. Many different formulas exist to calculate CrCl in various hospitalized populations, including patients with liver disease, obesity, and unstable renal function (Table 21-9). These formulas typically use serum creatinine and other patient variables, such as age, weight, and gender. The use of these serum creatinine–based formulas in the ICU has been questioned, however, because of non–steady-state serum creatinine pharmacokinetics that result when kidney function is rapidly changing, the variability in serum creatinine produced in critically ill patients, and the fact that the formulas do not account for tubular secretion of creatinine, which may represent a greater proportion of total clearance at low GFR values.[104] Increases in serum creatinine usually lag behind decreases in kidney function, and formulas estimating CrCl may not detect declining kidney status until a significant portion of kidney function is lost. A formula estimating the GFR has yet to be validated for use in critically ill patients.

The most common formula used to estimate CrCl in clinical practice is the Cockcroft-Gault equation.[105] Studies evaluating the Cockcroft-Gault equation in critically ill patients have shown a poor correlation with estimated CrCl and measured CrCl or inulin clearance or both.[106,107]

Table 21-9. Equations for the Estimation of Creatinine Clearance

Adult Patients with Stable Renal Function[105,109,110,202-204]	
Cockcroft/Gault—standard measurement of CrCl for drug dosing	CrCl (mL/min) = [(140 − age) × IBW]/[72 × SCr] × (multiply by 0.85 if patient is female)
Jelliffe—alternative to Cockcroft/Gault	CrCl (mL/min) = [114 − (0.8 × age)]/SCr × (multiply by 0.9 if patient is female)
MDRD—patients with CKD and GFR <90 mL/min	CrCl (mL/min/1.73m^2) = 170 × (SCr)$^{-0.999}$ × (Age)$^{-0.176}$ × (0.762 if patient is female) × (1.180 if patient is black) × (BUN)$^{-0.170}$ × (Albumin)$^{+0.318}$
Modified MDRD—patients with CKD and GFR <90	CrCl (mL/min/1.73m^2) = 186 × (SCr)$^{-1.154}$ × (Age)$^{-0.203}$ × (0.742 if patient is female) × (1.210 if patient is black)
Salazar-Corcoran—patients with obesity	Men: CrCl (mL/min) = [(137 − age)] × [(0.285 × TBW) + (12.1 × height^2)]/[51 × SCr] Women: CrCl (mL/min) = [(146 − age)] × [(0.287 × TBW) + (9.74 × height^2)]/[60 × SCr]
Nix—patients with end-stage liver disease	CrCl (mL/min) = (80/SCr) × (TBW/70)$^{0.75}$ × (multiply by 0.661 if patient is female)
Adult Patients with Unstable Renal Function[206,207]	
Jelliffe	**Men*** E^{ss} = weight [29.3 − 0.203(Age)] E^{ss}corr = E^{ss}[1.035 − 0.0337(SCr)] E = E^{ss}corr − [4 weight(SCr_2 − SCr_1)]/(Δt day) CrCl (mL/min/1.73 m^2) = E/14.4(SCr) **Women*** E^{ss} = weight [25.1 − 0.175(Age)] E^{ss}corr = E^{ss}[1.035 − 0.0337(SCr)] E = E^{ss}corr − [4 weight(SCr_2 − SCr_1)]/(Δt day) CrCl (mL/min/1.73 m^2) = E/14.4(SCr)
Brater	CrCl (mL/min/70 kg) = [[293 − 2.03(Age)] × [1.035 − 0.01685(SCr_1 + SCr_2)]/(SCr_1 + SCr_2)] + [[49 (SCr_1 − SCr_2)]/(SCr_1 + SCr_2)(Δt day)] × (multiply by 0.86 if patient is female)

All measurements for weight (i.e., TBW, IBW) are in kg; height, in meters; age, in years.
*Use IBW if weight >30% above IBW.
CKD, chronic kidney disease; CrCl, creatinine clearance; E, creatinine excretion; E^{ss}, steady-state creatinine excretion; E^{ss}corr, corrected steady-state creatinine excretion; GFR, glomerular filtration rate; IBW, ideal body weight; MDRD, modification of diet in renal disease; SCr, serum creatinine; TBW, total body weight.

Robert and associates[107] found the Cockcroft-Gault formula to be more accurate when modified to use the lower of ideal body weight (IBW) or total body weight (TBW) along with the use of a minimal serum creatinine value of 1 mg/dL when the serum creatinine is less than 1 mg/dL in 20 medical ICU patients (mean SCr 1.8 mg/dL). Pesola and colleagues[108] found the Cockcroft-Gault formula to be accurate when measured CrCl values exceeded 100 mL/min. When CrCl was less than 100 mL/min, estimated clearance was overestimated by the Cockcroft-Gault formula. The degree of overestimation was reduced when lean body weight (LBW) was substituted for TBW.[104]

Other formulas exist to estimate CrCl, but have limitations that are similar to the limitations of the Cockcroft-Gault method. Formulas proposed by Jelliffe and Hull have been shown consistently to underestimate CrCl. In an attempt to improve on CrCl estimates, Levey and coworkers[109] proposed a series of equations to estimate GFR derived from patients enrolled in the MDRD (Modification of Diet in Renal Disease) Study.[109] Two variations of this formula are used in clinical practice—the original equation using six variables and a modified version using four variables.[109,110] The six-variable equation has been shown to provide a more accurate estimate of GFR than the Cockcroft-Gault equation in patients with stable kidney function and an estimated GFR less than 90 mL/min/1.73 m^2.[109] Guidelines from the National Kidney Foundation/Kidney Disease Outcome Quality Initiative recommend that the modified version of the MDRD equation should be used in patients with chronic kidney disease and who have a GFR less than 90 mL/min/1.73 m^2.[111] Limited data exist regarding the validity of using the MDRD equation to estimate GFR in patients with rapidly changing kidney function.

Given the limitations with many of the formulas that are available to predict kidney function in critically ill patients, the completion of timed, urine creatinine collection studies has been advocated as a better means to estimate CrCl. Classically, a 24-hour urine collection has been recommended because of the temporal variations that might occur in volume status or hemodynamic parameters that may affect CrCl estimates. In many cases, however, waiting 24 hours for a urine collection to be completed and analyzed is not practical, and some investigators have investigated shorter collection periods.[112,113] One study in critically ill surgical and trauma patients compared a 24-hour collection period with 2-hour, 6-hour, 8-hour, and 16-hour collections.[112] A poor correlation was shown for urine collections less than 8 hours ($r^2 < .8$), and a minimum collection time of 8 hours was recommended. Similarly, a second study observed clearance values from 8-hour and 12-hour collections to be within 20% of the 24-hour clearance value.[113] Although this degree of variability is unlikely to be clinically significant for patients with a higher CrCl, caution must be emphasized in patients with marginal kidney function, particularly when dosing regimens are being established for medications that have a narrow therapeutic window.

Practical Considerations When Dosing Medications in Renal Failure

Many considerations exist when establishing the optimal dosing regimen for critically ill patients with kidney dysfunction. Along with estimating the GFR, the contribution of kidney clearance to the total body clearance of a drug must be considered. For most medications, when kidney clearance accounts for less than 30% of the total body clearance, kidney dysfunction has a negligible effect on total drug removal, and dosing adjustments are unnecessary.[114] A second consideration requires the clinician to balance the need for aggressive therapy with the adverse effect profile of the individual agent. It is not always acceptable to choose the lower end of the dosing range, particularly with agents that are considered relatively safe (e.g., penicillins, cephalosporins) in critically ill patients, given the severity of disease and the pharmacokinetic alterations that occur in critical illness. Use of a dose that is too small may result in a suboptimal pharmacodynamic response and ultimately treatment failure. Finally, the pharmacodynamic properties of the medication, particularly with antibiotics, should be considered. Adjustments to doses of antibiotics with concentration-dependent activity typically should be made by prolonging the dosing interval to optimize the AUC or peak-to-MIC ratio. Conversely, antibiotics with time-dependent activity should be adjusted by decreasing the dose, but maintaining the same dosing interval to optimize the time above the MIC (Fig. 21-7). Several references, including PDA or web-based programs, exist to aid critical care clinicians when making drug dosing decisions at the bedside for patients with renal failure.

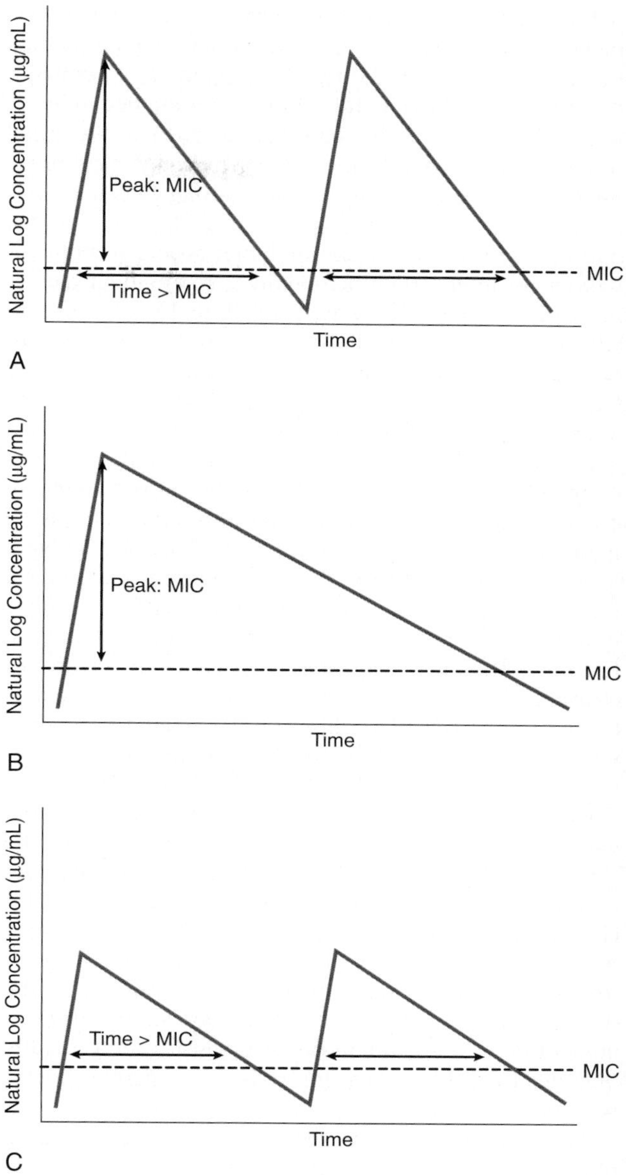

Figure 21-7. Pharmacodynamic considerations for dosage adjustments in renal failure. **A,** Plasma concentration curves for a patient with normal renal function. **B,** Dosage adjustment for renal failure using the same dose but a prolonged interval (preferred for concentration-dependent antimicrobials). **C,** Dosage adjustment for renal failure using a smaller dose but the same interval (preferred for time-dependent antimicrobials). MIC, minimum inhibitory concentration.

Renal Replacement Therapy

Drug Dosing in Hemodialysis

Generally, the impact of hemodialysis on drug removal depends on three main factors: drug characteristics, dialysis filter characteristics, and the dialysis prescription used.[115] The predominant mechanism by which drugs are removed by hemodialysis is diffusion. Factors related to drug removal through diffusion are the drug's Vd, protein binding, water solubility, and molecular weight.[114-116] Another mode of dialysis uses convection, which is characterized by the fluid transport of dissolved solutes across a membrane. Techniques to maximize drug removal via convection include increasing the hydrostatic pressure gradient across the dialysis membrane and using a more permeable dialysis filter.

Drugs with the following characteristics are more likely to be removed by hemodialysis: (1) small Vd, (2) not highly protein bound, (3) water-soluble, and (4) low molecular weight.[114-116] Conventional dialysis filters (e.g., filters composed of cellulose, cellulose acetate, regenerated cellulose, or cuprophane) are generally impermeable to drugs with a molecular weight greater than 1000 D. Newer, "high-flux" dialysis filters (e.g., filters composed of polysulfone, cellulose triacetate, or polymethyl methacrylate) have greater pore sizes and allow for passage of drugs that have a molecular weight of 20,000 D. Vancomycin, with a molecular weight of approximately 1450 D, is typically considered to be a drug with one of the largest molecular weights. Vancomycin is not removed via a conventional dialysis filter, but is removed with dialysis using a high-flux filter.

Drug Dosing in Continuous Renal Replacement Therapy

Optimizing drug dosing in patients receiving CRRT for acute renal failure can be particularly challenging because of the lack of pharmacokinetic studies that have been completed in these patients and the numerous confounders that have been shown to affect drug removal. A complete description of these CRRT dosing recommendations is beyond the scope of this chapter, and clinicians are urged to consult published dosing guidelines or a clinical pharmacist. When interpreting available dosing guidelines, it is essential that ICU clinicians recognize their limitations, particularly in terms of extrapolating dosing recommendations for intermittent hemodialysis to a patient receiving CRRT. Typically, recommendations for drug dosing with intermittent hemodialysis are based on studies conducted in healthy patients with chronic kidney failure treated with older, low-flux dialysis filters. They do not account for the fact that nonrenal clearance is increased in patients with acute renal failure. Published dosing recommendations specific to CRRT may be outdated in many cases owing to the facts that ultrafiltration rates have increased and that dialysis filter technology has evolved. When extrapolating these recommendations into clinical practice, careful consideration must be given to the filter type and the flow rates used in the referenced studies. Finally, differences may exist based on the method of clearance used—convection (i.e., continuous venovenous hemofiltration [CVVH]), diffusion (i.e., continuous venovenous hemodialysis [CVVHD]) or combined (i.e., continuous venovenous hemodiafiltration [CVVHDF]).

Drug removal during CVVH occurs through convection, which is influenced by the ultrafiltration rate and the sieving coefficient. The sieving coefficient is the measure of a solute's ability to cross the dialysis membrane and is calculated as the ultrafiltrate solute concentration divided by the simultaneous arterial solute concentration. Because sieving coefficients may not be readily available to the bedside clinician, the unbound fraction of the drug (1 minus the percent protein bound), which can be readily obtained from the package insert, is an acceptable alternative for most drugs.[116]

Although sieving coefficients are used to calculate drug removal during CVVH, saturation coefficients are used to calculate drug removal during CVVHD. Drug removal during CVVHD is based on diffusion principles in which the saturation coefficient is equal to the dialysate solute concentration divided by the simultaneous arterial solute concentration. With low-volume CRRT, it is safe to assume that the saturation coefficient is equal to the sieving coefficient, but with high-volume CRRT this may not be accurate.[19] Because diffusion is inversely related to molecular size, the difference noted between saturation coefficients and sieving coefficients is more substantial for larger sized molecules.

Many ICUs use a combination of diffusive and convective clearance mechanisms (i.e., CVVHDF), which present the most challenging scenarios to clinicians when optimizing drug dosing. In general, diffusion is more efficient at removing small particles, whereas convection is more efficient at removing midsized to larger sized molecules. The simultaneous combination of the two methods can result in less solute removal than what would be expected from the sum of each individual method alone. In one study, the clearance of small solutes (i.e., urea, creatinine) via CVVHDF was similar to the sum of the clearances when CVVH and CVVHD were performed separately.[117] The clearance of large solutes (i.e., β-microglobulin), on the other hand, was markedly different because the addition of diffusion did not increase clearance beyond that achieved with convection alone. This may have considerable impact when adjusting doses of medications with larger molecular weights, such as vancomycin and daptomycin, during CVVHDF.[19] Unfortunately, there is a paucity of data to guide clinicians when making dosing adjustments in patients who are receiving CRRT that uses both convective and diffusive methods.

Along with the mode of clearance used during CRRT, drug clearance also can be affected by the dialysis prescription used within each mode.[19,114,116,118] Changes in blood flow rate seem to have minimal effect on drug clearance regardless of the method of clearance (diffusive or convective). In CVVH, clearance is directly proportional to ultrafiltration rate. In CVVHD, clearance is affected by dialysate flow rate, but also is influenced by the drug's molecular weight (Fig. 21-8). Increasing the dialysate flow rate has a more profound effect on the clearance of smaller sized molecules than larger ones. Furthermore, drug clearance varies based on the individual filter that is used. In a study by Joy and colleagues,[119] vancomycin clearance obtained through CVVHD with a polymethyl methacrylate filter was significantly greater than the clearance obtained with acrylonitrile copolymer 0.6 m^2 (AN69) and polysulfone filters when dialysate flow rates exceeded 25 mL/min. Vancomycin clearance obtained through CVVH was not significantly affected by filter type.

The method by which replacement fluids are administered during CVVH or CVVHDF also can influence drug removal. It is common practice in the United States for replacement fluids to be administered proximal to the filter, whereas elsewhere in the world replacement fluids

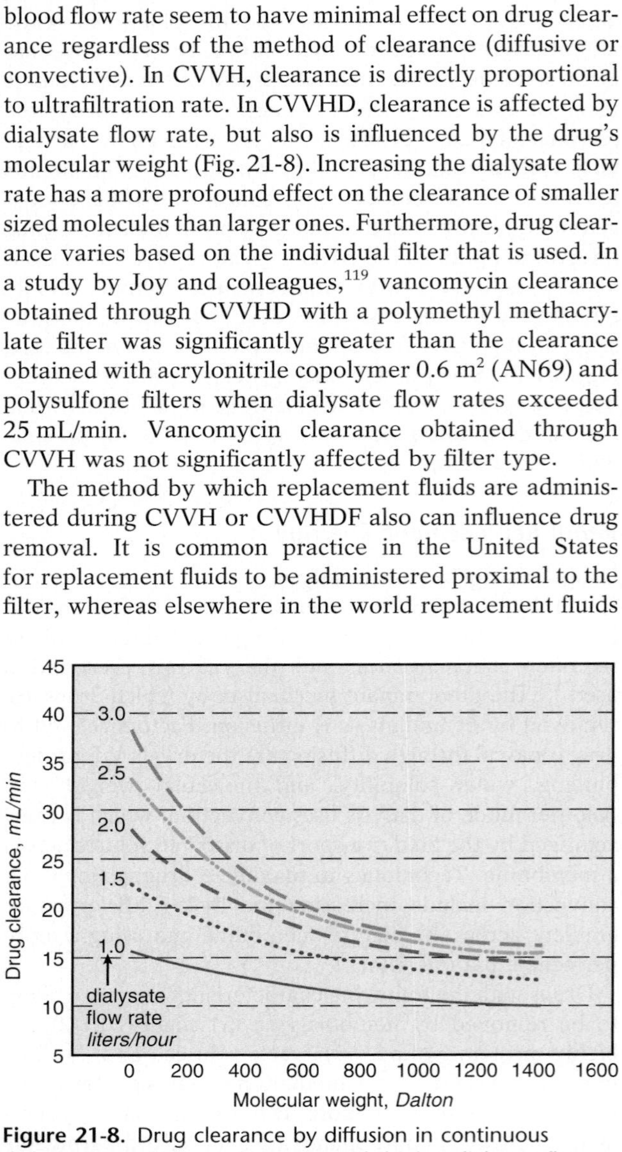

Figure 21-8. Drug clearance by diffusion in continuous dialysis. Drug clearance increases with higher dialysate flow rates, but clearance of larger molecules benefits less from higher dialysate flow rates. (Adapted with permission from Bohler J, Donauer J, Keller F: Pharmacokinetic principles during continuous renal replacement therapy: drugs and dosage. Kidney Int Suppl 1999;72:S24-S28.)

are administered distally. Administration of replacement fluids prefilter dilutes the concentrations of solutes in the blood and can decrease clearance by approximately 15%.[117] This usually can be overcome through the use of additional ultrafiltration volume.

Vd is another drug-specific factor that can significantly influence clearance with CRRT.[114] Drugs that have a smaller Vd (i.e., <0.6 L/kg) are removed more effectively by CRRT than drugs with a larger Vd. Patients with acute renal failure are often fluid overloaded, which in and of itself increases the Vd of water-soluble drugs, such as aminoglycoside antibiotics.[19] Removal of this extra fluid through CRRT can rapidly change the Vd and alter drug clearance. Figure 21-9 describes the pharmacokinetic principles of drug removal through CRRT.[19] Only solutes present in the plasma, which in pharmacokinetic terms is known as the *central compartment,* are removed by CRRT. Drugs with a small Vd generally preside in the central compartment, but drugs with a large Vd tend to distribute into deeper tissues. As drugs are rapidly cleared from the central compartment during CRRT, equilibration or "rebound" may occur as drug is transferred from a deeper, auxiliary compartment into the central compartment. For drugs with a large Vd, the rate-limiting step for high-dose CRRT becomes the rate at which drug can transfer from these auxiliary compartments into the central compartment.

Two basic strategies can be used to individualize drug dosing during CRRT. The first method starts by using the dosing recommendation for patients with normal renal function and adjusts the dose downward, and the second method begins with the dosing recommendation for patients with chronic kidney disease and adjusts the dose upward.[120,121] The first method seems more accurate than the second, especially for drugs with higher sieving coefficients.[19] Using this method, the dose is reduced in proportion to the reduction in total body clearance. During CRRT, total body clearance represents clearance obtained through CRRT, residual renal clearance, and nonrenal clearance. Several resources exist listing CRRT clearance and total body clearance values of selected drugs.[115,118,122] The relationship between CrCl and total body clearance also is described in Table 21-10. This relationship can be used to calculate total body clearance (in a patient with normal renal function) or residual renal clearance (in a patient with acute renal failure). The dosage adjustment factor would be equal to total body clearance while on CRRT divided by total body clearance with normal renal function. Pharmacodynamic principles should be considered to determine whether the dose should be decreased or the interval prolonged according to the calculated dosage adjustment factor.

Hepatic Failure

Drug dosing in hepatic failure can be particularly challenging because a simple method to quantify liver function does not exist. Although liver function tests are frequently evaluated to detect hepatocellular changes (e.g., alanine aminotransferase) and evaluate synthetic function (e.g., international normalized ratio), currently available tests do not reflect the ability of the liver to metabolize drugs. For some medications, dosing adjustments in patients with liver failure are based on the Child-Pugh score. For example, in patients with a Child-Pugh score of 7, the dose of caspofungin should be decreased from 50 mg to 35 mg daily.

The pharmacokinetic changes that occur with hepatic dysfunction have been described previously and include alterations in absorption, distribution, and hepatic clearance.[123] These changes are related to reductions in drug metabolism, plasma protein synthesis, and liver blood flow. Pharmacokinetic alterations depend on individual drug characteristics, such as degree of hepatic extraction and protein binding. Drugs that have high hepatic

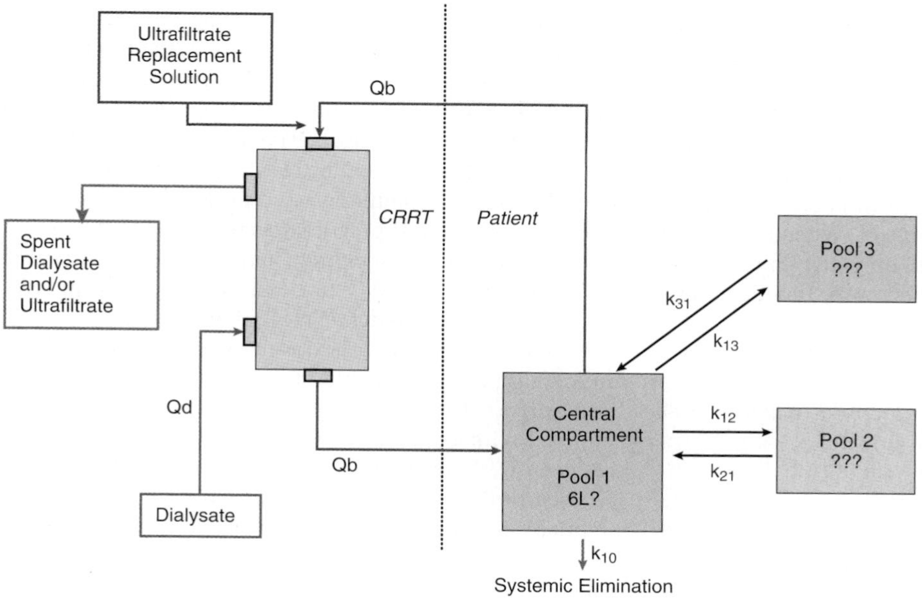

Figure 21-9. Pharmacokinetic principles of drug removal through continuous renal replacement therapy (CRRT). (Adapted with permission from Mueller BA, Pasko DA, Sowinski KM: Higher renal replacement therapy dose delivery influences on drug therapy. Artif Organs 2003;27:808-814.)

Table 21-10. Relationship between Creatinine Clearance and Total Body Clearance for Selected Drugs

Drug	Total Body Clearance
Acyclovir	3.37 (CrCl) + 0.41
Amikacin	0.6 (CrCl) + 9.6
Aztreonam	0.8 (CrCl) + 26.6
Cefepime	0.96 (CrCl) + 10.9
Ceftazidime	1.15 (CrCl) + 10.6
Ciprofloxacin	2.83 (CrCl) + 363
Digoxin	0.88 (CrCl) + 23
Gentamicin	0.983 (CrCl)
Lithium	0.235 (CrCl)
Ofloxacin	1.04 (CrCl) + 38.7
Penicillin G	3.35 (CrCl) + 35.5
Piperacillin	1.36 (CrCl) + 1.5
Teicoplanin	7.09 (CrCl) – 16.2
Tobramycin	0.801 (CrCl)
Vancomycin	0.69 (CrCl) + 3.7

CrCl, creatinine clearance.
Data from references 115 and 122.

extraction are expected to have increased bioavailability with decreased clearance. With drugs with low hepatic extraction, bioavailability is not altered, but clearance is decreased.[123]

Less is known about the pharmacodynamic alterations that occur in liver failure, but patients are often more sensitive to medication effects, particularly agents with central nervous system effects (e.g., benzodiazepines).[16,123] Renal failure secondary to nonsteroidal anti-inflammatory drugs has been reported in patients with cirrhosis and ascites. Doses of loop diuretics, on the other hand, may need to be increased in patients with liver failure owing to decreased sensitivity to the drug effects.[123]

When developing a drug therapy plan for patients with liver failure, it is best to choose agents not extensively metabolized by the liver (e.g., cisatracurium rather than vecuronium). If this is impossible, an agent with a shorter duration of action is preferred (e.g., lorazepam rather than diazepam). For drugs that have high hepatic extraction and are administered orally (e.g., propranolol), initial and maintenance doses should be reduced. When these drugs are administered intravenously, only the maintenance dose should be reduced. It is unnecessary to adjust initial doses of drugs that have a low hepatic extraction regardless of the route of administration, but maintenance doses should be reduced. It is difficult to predict the magnitude of dose reduction, but generally a decrease of at least 50% is recommended.

Obese Patients

As obesity has become a major epidemic in the United States, the prevalence of obese patients in the ICU has increased. Approximately 9% to 26% of ICU patients can be categorized as being obese, with 1.4% to 7% being morbidly obese.[124] Morbid obesity has been shown to be an independent risk factor for mortality among surgical critically ill patients, with death being 7.4 times more likely in obese patients.[125] This presents a major challenge for clinicians attempting to optimize drug dosing in obese, critically ill patients because pharmacokinetic properties can be a crucial determinant for drug success.

Issues that the ICU clinician must consider when selecting a dosing regimen are the most appropriate weight to use (for medications requiring weight-based dosing), the pharmacokinetic alterations that occur with obesity, and the therapeutic index that exists for a specific agent. Because of the lack of published literature or evidence-based recommendations for obese, critically ill patients, a thorough understanding of the pharmacokinetic and pharmacodynamic properties of an agent and how this might relate to obesity when making decisions on drug dosing is required.

Definitions and Terminology

Confusion exists regarding the best way to characterize body weight when estimating drug doses. Several definitions exist using various cutoffs that are based on some measure of the patient's height and weight (e.g., body mass index [BMI], lean body weight [LBW], ideal body weight [IBW], adjusted body weight [AdjBW], and total body weight [TBW]). Equations used to estimate these values are provided in Table 21-11.

BMI is the parameter used to characterize obesity by the World Health Organization.[126] A BMI between 25 kg/m^2 and 29.9 kg/m^2 is classified as overweight; a BMI between 30 kg/m^2 and 34.9 kg/m^2, moderate obesity; a BMI between 35 kg/m^2 and 39.9 kg/m^2, severe obesity; and a BMI 40 kg/m^2 or greater, morbid obesity. Although BMI is a good indicator for adiposity and is becoming the standard for defining obesity, it is not commonly used in the clinical setting for medication dosing.

LBW, which accounts for nonfat cell mass and intercellular connective tissue, can be a useful predictor of pharmacokinetic behavior of drugs that are highly water-soluble. Most pharmacokinetic studies in obese patients have used IBW, however, rather than LBW. IBW is often used as a surrogate for LBW when estimating drug distribution into nonadipose tissue because LBW determinations are not practical in the clinical setting. The equation for estimating IBW that is most commonly used in the pharmacokinetic literature and clinical practice was proposed by Devine[127] (see Table 21-11). Most pharmacokinetic studies have used IBW greater than 120% to define obesity and an IBW greater than 200% to define morbid obesity.[128]

AdjBW is often used for dosing medications that have an increased Vd that results from increased weight (i.e., into adipose tissue). This increased distribution is presumed to range from 20% to 50% of the difference between TBW and IBW. The correction factor that should be used in the ICU to account for obesity can vary substantially and depends on factors such as fluid balance, frequency of surgical procedures, and serum albumin concentrations.

Table 21-11. Equations Used to Estimate Size	
Size Descriptor	**Equation**
Body mass index (kg/m^2)	TBW/height $(m)^2$
Body surface area (m^2) (DuBois)	$TBW^{0.425} \times$ height $(cm)^{0.725} \times 0.007184$
Body surface area (m^2) (Mosteller)	$\sqrt{[\text{height (cm)} \times \text{TBW}/3600]}$
Ideal body weight (kg) (Devine)	Men: 50 kg + 2.3 kg/inch for height >5 ft Women: 45 kg + 2.3 kg/inch for height >5 ft
Ideal body weight (kg) (Robinson)	Men: 50 kg + 1.9 kg/inch for height >5 ft Women: 49 kg + 1.7 kg/inch for height >5 ft
Lean body weight (kg) (James)	Men: $[1.1 \times \text{TBW}] - 120[\text{TBW/height (cm)}]^2$ Women: $[1.07 \times \text{TBW}] - 148[\text{TBW/height (cm)}]^2$
Adjusted body weight (kg)	CF [TBW − IBW] + IBW

CF, correction factor (most commonly equal to 0.4); IBW, ideal body weight; TBW, total body weight.
Data from references 127 and 208-211.

Pharmacokinetic Alterations in Obese Patients

Morbid obesity can have profound implications on the pharmacokinetic principles of medications used in the ICU because of the degree to which organ system derangements can occur (Table 21-12). Although drug absorption seems to be minimally affected, drug distribution can be markedly altered.[129] Several factors can influence drug distribution, including body composition, regional blood flow, and binding to plasma proteins. Obese patients have an increased fat and lean body mass compared with nonobese patients of the same age, height, and sex. This increase in mass is predominantly fat mass, however, because the percentage of LBW calculated per kg of TBW is reduced, whereas that of fat is doubled.[130]

Obesity-induced changes in hemodynamic status and regional blood flow also can affect distribution. Blood flow is substantially reduced to fat (5%) compared with lean tissue (22%) or viscera (73%).[130] In morbidly obese individuals, blood flow per gram of fat is significantly lower than in obese or normal-weight individuals.[131] In addition, the reduction in cardiac function caused by obesity itself may reduce perfusion. The effect of obesity on protein binding is unclear. Although drug binding to albumin is unaffected by obesity, drug binding to α_1-acid glycoprotein may be altered.[129] This may be due in part to increased levels of other binding substances, such as triglycerides, cholesterol, free fatty acids, and lipoproteins.

Studies evaluating the effect of obesity on renal clearance have provided conflicting results.[129,130,132] Although some studies have shown an increase in the GFR in obese patients, most likely because of increased renal blood flow and increased kidney weight, others have shown no significant change in renal clearance between obese and nonobese individuals. Formulas to estimate kidney function have been shown to be inaccurate in their ability to predict CrCl.[131,132] The inaccuracies can be linked to the value used for weight in these calculations. When TBW was used in the various equations, CrCl was markedly overestimated. In contrast, when IBW was used, CrCl was underestimated. A measured CrCl should be considered in obese patients with renal failure, particularly when establishing dosing regimens for medications with a narrow therapeutic index.

Table 21-12. Major Organ System Derangements in Obesity	
Organ System	**Pathology**
Respiratory	↑ FEV_1/FVC ↓ FRC, TLC, VC, IC, ERV
Cardiovascular	↑ Blood volume ↑ Vascular tone ↓ Ventricular contractility
Renal	↑ Clearance of renally excreted drugs Hypertensive and diabetic nephropathy
Hematologic	↑ Fibrinogen ↑ PAI-1 ↓ AT-III
Gastrointestinal	↑ Gastric secretion volume ↓ Gastric pH Hiatal hernia
Metabolic/endocrine	↑ Resting energy expenditure ↑ Proteolysis Insulin resistance
Immunologic	↑ TNF-α ↑ IL-6 Impaired neutrophil function

AT-III, antithrombin III; ERV, expiratory reserve volume; FEV_1/FVC, ratio of forced expiratory volume in 1 second to forced vital capacity; FRC, functional residual capacity; IC, inspiratory capacity; IL-6, interleukin-6; PAI-1, plasminogen activator inhibitor-1; TLC, total lung capacity; TNF-α, tumor necrosis factor-α; VC, vital capacity.
From Pieracci FM, Barie PS, Pomp A: Critical care of the bariatric patient. Crit Care Med 2006;34:1796-1804.

Factors to Consider When Making Dosing Recommendations in Obese Patients

Because of the lack of consistent pharmacokinetic data in obesity for medications commonly administered in the ICU, there are several points the ICU clinician must consider when making dosing decisions in this population. The first is the adverse effect profile for a particular therapy. When dealing with agents that are generally considered safe, with a wide therapeutic index (e.g., β-lactam antibiotics), a more aggressive approach could be sought. Conversely, with medications that have severe adverse effects associated with their use, particularly in high doses (e.g., sedatives and narcotics), a more conservative approach would be appropriate. A second consideration is the administration schedule for the dosing regimen. With some medications (e.g., sedatives, opioids), it may be preferable to use a series of smaller medication doses with immediate assessment of effect, rather than a single, large bolus dose. Such strategies are often used with procedural (i.e., moderate) sedation. A final consideration is the ability to monitor the dosing regimen using laboratory markers or clinical assessment. Doses of anticoagulants, such as heparin, lepirudin, or argatroban, are adjusted based on APTT values, and neuromuscular blocking agents can be adjusted using peripheral nerve stimulation. This ability to monitor and adjust therapy may allow the clinician to choose a more conservative dosing approach given the fact the dose can be titrated upward should the initial response not meet the established goal of therapy. Table 21-13 provides recommendations for the most appropriate weight to use when establishing doses for medications that are commonly administered in the ICU.

Table 21-13. Dosing Recommendations for Selected Agents in Morbidly Obese Patients

Medication	Calculate Dose Based on
Anticoagulants	
Heparin	AdjBW or TBW with dose capping strategy
LMWH	TBW with dose capping strategy
Antimicrobials	
AG	AdjBW = IBW + [0.4(TBW − IBW)]
Vancomycin	TBW
β-lactams	Use upper end of dosing range with consideration for adverse effect profile of given agent
Quinolones	Use upper end of dosing range with consideration for adverse effect profile of given agent. If weight-based, use AdjBW = IBW + [0.45(TBW − IBW)]
Linezolid	Standard dosing
β-blockers	IBW
Corticosteroids	IBW or AdjBW or TBW with dose capping strategy
Digoxin	IBW
Drotrecogin alfa (activated)	TBW
NMBA	
Succinylcholine	TBW
Vecuronium	IBW
Atracurium	IBW or TBW
Cisatracurium	IBW
Rocuronium	IBW
Opioid analgesics	IBW
Phenytoin	AdjBW = IBW + 1.33(TBW − IBW). Total loading dose should not exceed 2 g Maintenance dose: IBW
Sedatives	
Benzodiazepines	IBW
Propofol	IBW
Thrombolytics	Use dosing regimen used in clinical trials or IBW with dose capping strategy

AdjBW, adjusted body weight; AG, aminoglycosides; IBW, ideal body weight; LMWH, low-molecular-weight heparin; NMBA, neuromuscular blocking agent; TBW, total body weight.

Dosing Recommendations for Specific Classes of Drugs

Although opioid analgesics are highly lipophilic compounds, IBW is the most appropriate weight measurement for dosing calculations. Studies with fentanyl have indicated that dosing based on TBW may lead to excessive dosing in obese patients.[133,134] Egan and coworkers[135] found remifentanil pharmacokinetics to be more closely related to LBM than to TBM. In a study by Schwartz and associates,[136] sufentanil Vd was positively correlated with the degree of obesity, but clearance was prolonged in obese patients. This study has led some authors to advocate using TBW for loading doses and IBW for maintenance doses.[131,137] In all cases, the degree of underlying pain, the age of the patient, the presence of ventilatory support, and the likelihood that tolerance is occurring should be used to guide therapy.

Benzodiazepines are highly lipophilic compounds, and pharmacokinetic studies have shown significant increases in Vd and elimination half-life with obesity.[131] In one study, midazolam Vd and elimination half-life were nearly three times greater in obese compared with nonobese volunteers.[138] IBW should be used when calculating dosages for continuous infusions given the prolonged clearance in obese patients. For single doses, it has been suggested that TBW be used (because of increased Vd), but it may be safer to use IBW or administer a series of smaller IV doses until the desired effect is obtained.

The pharmacokinetics of propofol do not seem to be affected by obesity, based on one study that found the Vd and elimination half-life to be similar between obese and nonobese populations.[139] Nevertheless, given the hemodynamic concerns with large IV doses of propofol, and the fact that propofol can rapidly be titrated to effect, IBW should be used for initial dosing calculations.

Most neuromuscular blocking agents are polar, hydrophilic compounds, which would suggest that distribution into adipose tissue is limited. This suggestion was confirmed in several pharmacokinetic studies evaluating the neuromuscular blocking agents vecuronium, rocuronium, and cisatracurium; a longer duration of action was noted when doses were calculated based on TBW.[140-142] In contrast, one study of atracurium found Vd, clearance, and recovery time to be similar between obese and nonobese individuals.[143] Although this study recommended TBW be used for dosing calculations, clinicians still may want to dose these agents based on IBW given the fact that they are usually dosed to clinical effect and train-of-four end points.[128] Succinylcholine, on the other hand, should be dosed based on TBW because pseudocholinesterase activity correlates with BMI in obese patients. Studies have indicated that dosing based on IBW rather than TBW more frequently leads to intubating conditions that are considered poor.[144,145]

Phenytoin loading doses should be calculated using an AdjBW, which is calculated as follows:

$$\text{AdjBW} = \text{IBW} + 1.33(\text{TBW} - \text{IBW})$$

Loading doses should not exceed 2 g. This recommendation is based on the results of one study that compared the pharmacokinetics of phenytoin between obese (TBW of 124 kg, or 178% of IBW) and nonobese healthy volunteers and found the Vd to be significantly higher in the obese patients (80.5 ± 7.2 L versus 39.8 ± 1.9 L; $P < .001$).[146] This Vd, when corrected for TBW, also correlated with percent IBW ($r = .45$; $P < .05$), suggesting a disproportionate distribution of phenytoin into fat. Phenytoin maintenance doses should be calculated using IBW, however, and optimized through TDM.

Propranolol pharmacokinetics have been evaluated in several studies comparing obese and nonobese individuals.[147,148] Despite the high lipophilicity of propranolol, no differences in serum concentrations or Vd were noted. One study reported decreased Vd in obese patients (208.9 ± 71.9 L versus 318.6 ± 91.8 L; $P < .01$).[149] Collectively, this implies that IBW should be used for weight-based calculations. Although the pharmacokinetics of esmolol have not been evaluated in obese individuals, it is suggested that IBW be used when dosing this agent. Despite the large Vd of digoxin, its distribution into adipose tissue is limited. IBW should be used for dosing calculations.[150]

Dosing of anticoagulants such as UFH, LMWHs, and direct thrombin inhibitors is challenging in obese patients given the potentially deleterious sequelae of administering a dose that is too small and the increased bleeding that may occur with the administration of doses that are too large. Although nomograms (e.g., Raschke nomogram) that are based on TBW are commonly employed for the initial dosing and adjustment of UFH, none has been validated for use in obese populations.[151] With UFH having a Vd that is similar to the blood volume, and given that the blood volume of adipose tissue is substantially less than that of lean tissue, the use of the TBW to guide UFH dosing in obese patients may lead to supratherapeutic APTT values and increased bleeding.

Although some studies that have evaluated the pharmacokinetics of UFH in obesity have concluded that TBW should be used when dosing, definitions for obesity have been inconsistent, and few patients have had a TBW greater than 100 kg.[152-154] Given the limited data on direct UFH dosing in obesity, the variability in response that is frequently observed in patients receiving UFH therapy and the availability of APTT monitoring to guide therapy, either AdjBW or TBW with a dose-capping strategy should be used.

Although several studies have evaluated the impact of obesity on LMWH dosing, a clear correlation between weight and anti–factor Xa activity has not been established.[155-160] In a subgroup analysis of obese patients from the ESSENCE and TIMI 11B trials, there was no difference in clinical outcomes compared with nonobese patients.[161] The maximal weight for patients included in these trials was 159 kg. Given that LMWHs do not seem to be affected by obesity, TBW should be used when seeking therapeutic levels of anticoagulation. The largest weight reported in the literature is 190 kg (using dalteparin); it seems prudent to implement a dose cap at that point.[159] Anti–factor Xa activity monitoring can be considered in obese patients, although its utility has not been firmly established. When used for prophylaxis against venous thrombosis, larger doses of LMWHs should be used based on the results of one study in bariatric surgery patients, which showed a lower incidence of deep venous thrombosis but no difference in bleeding when a dose of enoxaparin 40 mg twice daily subcutaneously was used, rather than 30 mg twice daily subcutaneously.[162,163] The effect of obesity on the pharmacokinetics of thrombolytic agents has not been studied; clinicians should follow the dosing regimens used in clinical trials. A maximal dose was used in these trials, so no adjustment for obesity can be recommended.

TBW should be used when dosing vancomycin because vancomycin Vd and clearance correlate with TBW, and vancomycin clearance is 2.5 times higher in obese patients.[164] Given vancomycin's time-dependent bactericidal activity, for obese patients requiring large daily doses of vancomycin it may be preferable to administer smaller doses more frequently, rather than larger doses less frequently. TDM for vancomycin, despite the controversy surrounding its routine use to guide therapy, should be considered in obese patients.

AdjBW should be used to dose aminoglycosides in obese patients given their hydrophilic structure and their variable distribution into adipose tissue (AdjBW = 0.4[TBW − IBW]).[164] Aminoglycosides are a particular challenge to dose in the subgroup of obese patients who are morbidly obese given the importance that high peak concentrations play in optimizing therapy, particularly when used for the treatment of pneumonia. Even with aggressive TDM, optimal peak concentrations may not be obtained for several days. For this reason, aminoglycosides are generally considered a second-line therapy for the treatment of gram-negative infections in morbidly obese patients. If aminoglycosides are used in these patients, a high-peak, extended-interval dosing regimen may produce doses above the comfort level of most clinicians (i.e., gentamicin or tobramycin doses >1 g). In these scenarios, either a traditional dosing regimen or a dose-capping strategy should be used.

Relatively few studies have evaluated other classes of antibiotics, such as β-lactams and quinolones, in morbidly obese patients.[164,165] Although the dose of these agents is typically determined using an established range (e.g., 1 to 2 g per dose for most cephalosporins) and not calculated on a milligram-per-kilogram basis, their pharmacokinetics are often still affected by obesity. The Vd for nafcillin was found to be greater in obese patients receiving it to treat endocarditis.[166] The Vd of cefotaxime is 50% greater in patients who weigh more than twice their IBW.[167] One study found the Vd of ciprofloxacin to be 23% greater in obesity and recommended a weight-based dosage using AdjBW for dosing calculations.[168] Using this recommendation, one case report described a 226-kg patient who received ciprofloxacin 800 mg intravenously every 12 hours and achieved a peak serum concentration within the desired therapeutic range.[169] Given the benign adverse effect profile for most of these agents, and the need to achieve high serum concentrations in critically ill patients, the higher end of the dosing range should generally be employed. For agents where adverse effects may be a concern with the administration of larger doses (e.g., seizures with imipenem), alternative agents with a better safety profile should be considered (e.g., piperacillin-tazobactam).

One study evaluated the pharmacokinetics of linezolid in seven obese patients (>150% IBW) with cellulitis.[170] In this study, mean linezolid serum concentrations were lower than in nonobese healthy volunteers, but still provided inhibitory activity against common pathogens associated with skin and soft tissue infections. Based on minimal data, standard dosing for linezolid seems adequate, but caution should be advised for organisms that may have a higher MIC, or when the patient response is inadequate.

The Vd of methylprednisolone in patients with spinal cord injury is not altered in obesity, suggesting that the IBW should be used for dosing calculations.[171] In the NASCIS III trial, methylprednisolone was administered based on TBW, but patients weighing more than 109 kg were excluded.[172] Given this discrepancy between current pharmacokinetic data and the dosing schedule used in clinical trials, it would seem reasonable to use TBW for patients who weigh up to 109 kg and IBW, AdjBW, or TBW with a dose-capping strategy for patients who weigh more.

The PROWESS trial used a drotrecogin alfa (activated) dose of 24 μg/kg/h based on TBW, but patients weighing greater than 135 kg were excluded.[173] Prior pharmacokinetic studies have shown that drotrecogin alfa (activated) clearance increases proportionally with body weight.[174] This was confirmed in a study that compared drotrecogin alfa (activated) plasma concentrations between patients who weighed 135 kg and patients who weighed greater than 135 kg.[175] Twenty patients with a mean weight of 158 kg (range 137-227 kg) were compared with 32 patients with a mean weight of 93 kg (range 59-133 kg; $P < .001$). No difference was noted in steady-state plasma concentrations between the two groups, indicating that dosing requirements should be based on TBW in all situations.

Elderly Patients

In the next 30 years, with the population older than 65 years expected to double and the population older than 80 years expected to triple, the proportion of elderly patients admitted to the ICU will grow substantially.[176] Critically ill elderly patients are at significantly greater risk than younger patients for experiencing adverse drug reactions because of the large number of prehospital medications that they take, their lower BMI, their age-related organ dysfunction, and a longer history of prior drug reactions.[177] One analysis of prescribing errors in a large hospitalized cohort found advanced age to be the most common pathophysiologic factor not appropriately accounted for when the initial selection of a drug dose was made.[178]

The fact that biologic age is not synonymous with chronologic age leads to a great deal of heterogeneity among elderly critically ill patients. Various age-related physiologic changes (e.g., impairment of baseline organ function) usually are complicated further by the critical illness these patients develop. A major limitation to predicting an elderly patient's response to drug therapy is the paucity of comparative drug trials that include elderly patients. Only since 1990 has the U.S. Food and Drug Administration (FDA) required drugs intended for use in elderly patients to undergo testing in this population and to be labeled with prescribing information for patients older than 65 years.[179] At present, prescribing decisions are often made through the extrapolation of drug study results involving younger, healthier patients, who may respond differently to therapy. There is a substantial need for well-designed postmarketing surveillance studies in elderly patients.

A thorough understanding of the physiologic changes that occur in elderly critically ill patients, coupled with an awareness of the pharmacokinetic and pharmacodynamic profiles of drugs commonly used in these patients, allows the ICU clinician to optimize therapeutic efficacy and to avoid adverse drug reactions. Many age-related changes affect drug bioavailability, Vd, and clearance. The reduced gastric acidity and impaired gastrointestinal motility in elderly patients may slow the rate of dissolution and absorption after oral or nasogastric tube drug administration, and the IV route should be the primary route of medication administration. In elderly patients, lean body mass decreases by 10%, but total body mass changes little because of increases in adipose tissue.[180] Because of these changes, hydrophilic drugs (e.g., aminoglycosides) have a lower Vd, and lipophilic drugs (e.g., anesthetics, benzodiazepines) have a higher Vd. Lipophilic drugs have a longer half-life because the drug is redistributed more slowly from fat back to the bloodstream before being cleared from the body.

With hepatic blood decreasing by about 30% between ages 30 and 75 years, older patients are particularly sensitive to the impairments in hepatic perfusion and hepatocellular function commonly seen in critically ill patients with shock, congestive heart failure, and sepsis. The clearance of high intrinsic clearance drugs (e.g., labetalol, morphine, lidocaine), whose elimination depends primarily on liver blood flow, is reduced in states of hepatic hypoperfusion. Medications that undergo phase I reactions (e.g., diazepam) are more affected by age and acuity of illness than medications that undergo phase II reactions (e.g., lorazepam).[181]

Reduced renal elimination of medications is a factor that complicates pharmacotherapy in elderly critically ill patients. After the age of 25, the GFR progressively declines at a rate of approximately 0.5 to 1 mL/min per 70 kg/y, and by age 80, GFR has decreased by about 40%.[182] These changes are secondary to age-related decreases in renal mass, loss of functional nephrons, and diminished renal artery perfusion. Critical illness may impair kidney function further in the elderly because of reduced perfusion (e.g., with shock) and intrinsic renal damage secondary to ischemia, drugs, toxins, and immunologic injury. Elderly patients, many of whom are immobile and malnourished, frequently have low serum creatinine concentrations that mask the ability to detect a reduction in the GFR via serial serum creatinine concentrations. Although the Cockcroft-Gault equation, used to estimate the GFR by calculating a CrCl, is age-adjusted, it should be used with caution in elderly patients to estimate GFR. Dosage regimens for many drugs used in elderly ICU patients may be modified using linear regression equations and empiric recommendations.

Elderly critically ill patients, because of multiple organ dysfunction and impaired homeostatic responses, may have an increased sensitivity to drug effects. This increased sensitivity is usually manifested as either an increased therapeutic response or a dose-related adverse effect. In clinical practice, increased responsiveness or excess effect is frequently shown in the elderly for drugs having neurologic, cardiovascular, gastrointestinal, and anti-infective effects. Age-related pharmacodynamic changes have been shown in controlled clinical trials for only a few drugs, however, including opioid analgesics and warfarin.

Elderly patients are more sensitive to benzodiazepines because of a combination of pharmacokinetic and pharmacodynamic factors. Of the benzodiazepines, lorazepam is least likely to accumulate in elderly patients because it is cleared primarily by glucuronidation and, in contrast to midazolam and diazepam, is not oxidatively metabolized to active metabolites. Haloperidol, sometimes required to manage delirium-related agitation, should be started at a low dose to avoid hypotension and prolonged corrected QT interval–related effects.

Altered blood pressure homeostasis may lead to increased responsiveness to vasodilators and calcium channel blockers. Age-related declines in β-adrenoreceptor function may be associated with decreased responsiveness to β-adrenergic agonists and higher circulating plasma norepinephrine concentrations. The clinical relevance of these changes may be minor, however, because most agents used in the ICU that act on β-receptors (e.g., albuterol, dopamine) are titrated to clinical effect.[183] Several drugs with cardiovascular mechanisms should be prescribed and monitored carefully when used in elderly ICU patients. The bradyarrhythmic and blood pressure–related effects may be exaggerated because of underlying age-related changes (e.g., decreased baroreceptor responsiveness, a lower baseline heart rate, and β-adrenoreceptor functional impairment).[184]

Age-related decreases in the clearance of antiarrhythmic drugs (particularly quinidine, procainamide, and lidocaine) may increase the incidence of adverse effects, such as proarrhythmias. The advanced cardiac life support guidelines recommend that for elderly patients, doses of lidocaine maintenance infusions be decreased by 50%, and that high-dose epinephrine boluses be avoided.[185] Elderly patients are at a particularly high risk for experiencing medication-induced tachyarrhythmias, and albuterol, dobutamine, theophylline, erythromycin, and haloperidol therapy should be carefully monitored. Although heparin dose requirements have not been shown to be affected by age, bleeding complications and the incidence of heparin-induced thrombocytopenia have been reported to occur more frequently in elderly patients.[186] Critically ill elderly patients tend to have lower dosage requirements and a higher incidence of warfarin-related bleeding. This may result from decreased hepatic function, reduced vitamin K intake, and concomitant administration of drugs that inhibit warfarin metabolism (e.g., amiodarone) or induce hypoprothrombinemia (e.g., cefotetan).[187] Metoclopramide, used in the ICU for its prokinetic properties, has been shown in elderly patients to increase arginine vasopressin release, an effect that may exacerbate hyponatremia and lead to a higher incidence of extrapyramidal effects. Increasing age also places patients at higher risk for erythromycin-induced corrected QT interval prolongation. Age-related and critical illness–related decreases in renal function require appropriate dose reductions for renally excreted anti-infective agents, such as β-lactams, vancomycin, and aminoglycosides. Elderly patients are at increased risk for trimethoprim-sulfamethoxazole–induced hyperkalemia and antibiotic-associated pseudomembranous colitis.

Although age-related changes in drug disposition are usually aligned with known age-related physiologic changes, many questions remain regarding the pharmacokinetic parameters that are altered with age, and their subsequent effects on pharmacodynamic response. There is an urgent need for more pharmacokinetic and pharmacodynamic studies in elderly patients of drugs commonly used in the ICU. Lastly, the ICU clinician should be careful not to withhold potentially lifesaving drug therapy on the grounds of age alone. One analysis of old elderly patients (>75 years old) who received drotrecogin alfa (activated) for severe sepsis found its safety, efficacy, and cost-effectiveness to be the same in old elderly patients compared with the overall population.[188]

In elderly critically ill patients, drugs with the best risk-benefit profile and drugs likely to induce the fewest adverse effects should be considered first-line options. Therapy should be initiated at a low dose and carefully titrated until the lowest effective dose is achieved, especially in patients known to have compromised organ function, concomitant disease, or altered homeostasis. Drug therapy that does not result in a beneficial effect or that is suspected of inducing an adverse effect should be stopped.

Pregnant Patients

Pregnant women when admitted to the ICU present many challenges to the ICU clinician because of their unique physiology and the specific medical disorders that occur during pregnancy and the postpartum period.[189] Pregnancy induces physiologic changes in virtually every organ system, and drug absorption, distribution, and clearance may be affected. The clinical significance for many of these alterations has not been fully elucidated, however, and the need for an alteration in drug dosing is not clearly established in many situations.[190]

During pregnancy, drug absorption may be decreased because of reduced gastrointestinal motility and increased gastric pH. With the blood volume of pregnant women being 50% greater than in nonpregnant women, the resulting increase in Vd, particularly for hydrophilic medications, often necessitates the use of larger doses. Serum albumin declines by 25% to 30% because of volume expansion. The resulting decrease in serum albumin binding capacity results in increased fractions of unbound phenytoin and other drugs that are highly bound to albumin. The maternal hormones progesterone and estradiol have been shown to affect hepatic drug metabolism—enhancing elimination of some drugs (e.g., phenytoin) and inhibiting the metabolism of others (e.g., theophylline).[190] Limited data suggest that the metabolism of drugs catalyzed by the CYP-450 isoenzymes CYP3A4, CYP2D6, and CYP2C9 are increased during pregnancy, and the doses of medications predominantly metabolized by these isoenzymes may need to be increased during pregnancy to avoid loss of efficacy (see Table 21-2). Renal plasma flow and GFR increase by 80% in the first half of pregnancy, and the upper limit of normal for serum creatinine during pregnancy is 0.8 mg/dL.

Heparin remains the antithrombotic of choice for pregnant patients in the ICU because of its titratability, ability to be accurately monitored, and large molecular size that ensures it will not cross the placenta and induce fetal hemorrhage or teratogenesis. The bleeding risk to pregnant women treated with heparin seems to be comparable to the risk of nonpregnant patients treated with heparin or warfarin. Pregnant patients may require doses of heparin two times the normal weight–based dose because of the increased circulating levels of heparin-binding proteins, increased plasma volume, increased renal clearance owing to increased GFR, and increased heparin degradation in the placenta.[191] Although LMWHs, similar to UFH, do not cross the placenta, they are less titratable, and dosing has been shown to be less predictable in this population. LMWH dosing requirements, although shown to be higher during pregnancy, are unpredictable, and anti–factor Xa activity monitoring has been advocated.[191,192]

One of the greatest concerns regarding the use of medications in pregnant women in the ICU relates to the risk of affecting fetal development. Although some drugs have the potential to cause teratogenic effects (FDA category X), most medications required by critically ill pregnant women can be used safely. The most commonly used system to evaluate teratogen risk, the FDA category system, ranks very few drugs as being safe during pregnancy (category A) because of the requirement for a controlled trial to establish safety. Most drugs, although ranked B or C, are safe to use, particularly in a critically ill obstetric patient who often has a life-threatening requirement for the medication.[193]

Burn Injury

Burn injuries exceeding 15% of total body surface area give rise to numerous physiologic alterations, including changes in organ blood flow, protein binding, and hepatic and renal function, that lead to substantial pharmacokinetic and pharmacodynamic alterations for many medications.[194] In pharmacokinetic terms, the physiologic changes that occur during burn injury may be divided into two broad phases—the acute phase lasting up to 48 hours after injury and the hypermetabolic or recovery phase (>48 hours after injury). In the acute phase, protein-rich fluid is lost from the vascular space, resulting in hypovolemia that lowers cardiac output and decreases hepatic and renal perfusion. During the subsequent hypermetabolic phase, assuming adequate fluid resuscitation has been delivered, the cardiac output is elevated leading to increased hepatic and renal perfusion.

Providing clinicians with specific dosing recommendations for this population is challenging because the burn population shows significant interpatient and intrapatient variability. There is a paucity of information in the literature to support dosing recommendations for many medications. Of the pharmacokinetic reports that are available, most are small and frequently not standardized to the variables that are most likely to affect drug handling. Table 21-14 summarizes the pharmacokinetic alterations that may occur as a result of the physiologic changes that occur after burn injury.

Although information is limited regarding the effects of burn injury on drug absorption, the profound alterations in gastrointestinal physiology, including delayed gastric emptying, alterations in intestinal transit, and increased intestinal permeability, suggest that changes in drug absorption are likely to occur. It would be expected that medications that exhibit gastric emptying rate-limited absorption, such as acetaminophen or loop diuretics, might have a delayed effect if administered orally or enterally.

Major alterations in drug Vd may be seen after burn injury because of the alterations that occur in extracellular fluid volume. Changes in Vd are most clinically important for hydrophilic drugs having a small Vd. Studies of

Table 21-14. Patient-Specific Factors That Affect Drug Pharmacokinetics after Burn Injury
Size of burn
Depth of burn
Age
Time since burn injury
Creatinine clearance
Hydration status
Serum protein levels
Presence of sepsis

aminoglycoside dosing in burn patients have shown that some patients require gentamicin doses of 16.8 mg/kg/d to maintain dosing concentrations within the desired therapeutic range. Substantial variation in individual dosing requirements exist, however, and no single factor (e.g., age, burn size, or renal function) correlates with altered aminoglycoside dosing requirements.[195] Evaluation of high-peak, extended-interval aminoglycoside dosing strategies in this patient population has revealed that patients may have undetectable drug concentrations 8 hours after dose administration, giving a drug-free period of more than 12 hours.[196] Burn injury patients with normal renal function may need to receive larger doses more frequently than every 24 hours or be converted to a traditional dosing regimen with careful TDM that is optimized using standard pharmacokinetic principles.

Burn injury also causes considerable changes in plasma protein levels. During burn injury, albumin and total plasma protein concentrations are markedly diminished for prolonged periods, and free fractions of agents bound to albumin (e.g., diazepam, phenytoin) are increased. In contrast, the concentrations of the acute-phase proteins (e.g., α_1-acid glycoprotein) increase over time after burn injury, resulting in a decrease in the free fraction of drugs bound to α_1-acid glycoprotein (e.g., lidocaine, meperidine, propranolol). Clinicians should be careful not to assume that a total drug concentration within the normal therapeutic range represents an appropriate drug dose and to draw unbound or free concentrations whenever possible.

Burn injury affects drug clearance via many mechanisms, including renal function, metabolism, protein binding, and increased elimination through the skin. For these subpopulations of burn patients who eliminate drugs extremely rapidly, a concern exists over the adequacy of antibiotic dosing. Time since injury affects the hepatic clearance of high extraction drugs such as lidocaine. Immediately after a burn injury, the resultant hypovolemia, depressed myocardial function, and release of vasoactive substances lead to decreased cardiac output and may decrease hepatic blood flow by 50%.[194] During the subsequent hypermetabolic phase, during which blood flow to organs and tissues is increased, the clearance of high extraction drugs subsequently increases. The limited data that exist regarding the effects of burn injury on drug clearance via the CYP-450 system reveal that effects are quite variable (i.e., increasing some, decreasing others, or having no affect on others).

Burn injury influences renal function and the elimination of renally excreted drugs in many ways. Initially, renal dysfunction, as a result of acute tubular necrosis, may occur secondary to hypovolemia, myoglobinura, or hypotension. Within 2 to 3 days of injury, however, GFR is increased (CrCl increases on average to 170 mL/min), whereas tubular function is impaired. Although vancomycin dosing requirements have been shown to be higher in burn patients, dosing requirements in other renally cleared drugs such as fluconazole or imipenem have not been shown to be altered, although in each study significant interpatient variability was noted.[197,198] For renally cleared medications that are not titrated to clinical effect or where serum drug monitoring is not an option, clinicians should consider using doses in the maximal range to ensure a therapeutic response, particularly when the therapeutic window for the medication is wide.[199]

Numerous pharmacodynamic alterations may occur in postburn patients. High concentrations of circulating catecholamines may lead to a diminished responsiveness to β-blockers. After burn injury, the membranes of myocytes become supersensitive to usual doses of acetylcholine or succinylcholine, and thus succinylcholine administration should be avoided in burn injury patients because the intense repeated muscle contractions that may ensue may cause large amounts of potassium to leak out from the motor end plates, leading to potential cardiac arrest. Although nondepolarizing blockers (e.g., vecuronium) are not associated with hyperkalemia, larger doses (often 2.5-fold to 5-fold) are needed in patients with burn injuries.[194]

CONCLUSION

Many important principles guide medication dosing and monitoring in critically ill patients. Clinicians should be familiar with the unique pharmacokinetic and pharmacodynamic alterations that can occur in critical illness because they often have an impact on therapeutic outcomes. Patient populations with unique characteristics affecting drug dosing requirements are often admitted to the ICU, including patients with kidney dysfunction or hepatic failure and patients who are elderly, are pregnant, or have burn injuries. Critical care clinicians should be familiar with many important considerations when administering medication via nonintravenous routes. All dosing regimens in the ICU should be individualized and consider patient-specific pharmacokinetic alterations, currently available pharmacodynamic and pharmacogenetic data, and the optimal route for administration, and all regimens should incorporate available TDM tools. Application of these principles leads to drug therapy that maximizes therapeutic outcomes, while minimizing toxicity.

KEY POINTS

- Most dosing regimens employed in the ICU are extrapolated from clinical trials completed in non-ICU patients, or even healthy patients, and usually do not account for the substantial pharmacokinetic and pharmacodynamic variability seen in this patient population.
- Failure to appreciate the physiologic changes in critically ill patients that may lead to pharmacokinetic alterations (e.g., alterations in volume status, plasma protein binding, and end-organ function) when establishing drug therapy regimens may result in unpredictable serum concentrations, which can lead to therapeutic failure or drug toxicity.

- Numerous factors may compromise drug bioavailability in critically ill patients when drugs are administered by nonintravenous routes (e.g., enteral, subcutaneous, transdermal, or endotracheal).
- Numerous factors may affect the pharmacodynamic response to medications in ICU patients, including altered postreceptor binding, downregulation of receptors, and a host of different physiologic alterations.
- Antibiotics are typically categorized as having either concentration-dependent or time-dependent killing, with the activity of concentration-dependent antibiotics increasing as the peak serum concentrations of drug increases, whereas time-dependent antibiotics kill at the same rate regardless of the peak serum concentration that is attained above the MIC.
- Patients with unique factors that alter drug pharmacokinetic, pharmacodynamic, and pharmacogenetic parameters are increasingly being admitted to the ICU (e.g., patients with renal replacement therapy, obese patients, elderly patients, pregnant patients, and patients with burn injury).
- TDM (i.e., the use of patient-specific pharmacokinetic parameters derived from strategically obtained serum drug concentrations) can be used to individualize doses for patients and maximize clinical outcomes, minimize toxicity, and ensure that cost-effective drug therapy is provided.

REFERENCES

1. Cullen DJ, Sweitzer BJ, Bates DW, et al: Preventable adverse drug events in hospitalized patients: A comparative study of intensive care and general care units. Crit Care Med 1997;25:1289-1297.
2. Power BM, Forbes AM, van Heerden PV, et al: Pharmacokinetics of drugs used in critically ill adults. Clin Pharmacokinet 1998;34:25-56.
3. Belzberg H, Zhu J, Cornwell EE 3rd, et al: Imipenem levels are not predictable in the critically ill patient. J Trauma 2004;56:111-117.
4. Wagner BK, O'Hara DA: Pharmacokinetics and pharmacodynamics of sedatives and analgesics in the treatment of agitated critically ill patients. Clin Pharmacokinet 1997;33:426-453.
5. Johnston AJ, Steiner LA, O'Connell M, et al: Pharmacokinetics and pharmacodynamics of dopamine and norepinephrine in critically ill head-injured patients. Intensive Care Med 2004;30:45-50.
6. Bodenham A, Shelly MP, Park GR: The altered pharmacokinetics and pharmacodynamics of drugs commonly used in critically ill patients. Clin Pharmacokinet 1988;14:347-373.
7. Cariou A, Chiche JD, Charpentier J, et al: The era of genomics: Impact on sepsis clinical trial design. Crit Care Med 2002;30(5 Suppl):S341-S348.
8. Bauer LA: Clinical pharmacokinetics and pharmacodynamics. In DiPiro JT, Talbert RL, Yee GC, et al (eds): Pharmacotherapy: A Pathophysiologic Approach, ed 6. New York, McGraw-Hill, 2005, pp 51-73.
9. Bauer TM, Ritz R, Haberthur C, et al: Prolonged sedation due to accumulation of conjugated metabolites of midazolam. Lancet 1995;346:145-147.
10. Ritz MA, Fraser R, Tam W, et al: Impacts and patterns of disturbed gastrointestinal function in critically ill patients. Am J Gastroenterol 2000;95:3044-3052.
11. Ceppa EP, Fuh KC, Bulkley GB: Mesenteric hemodynamic response to circulatory shock. Curr Opin Crit Care 2003;9:127-132.
12. Schmidt H, Martindale R: The gastrointestinal tract in critical illness. Curr Opin Clin Nutr Metab Care 2001;4:547-551.
13. Forrest A, Nix DE, Ballow CH, et al: Pharmacodynamics of intravenous ciprofloxacin in seriously ill patients. Antimicrob Agents Chemother 1993;37:1073-1081.
14. Dasta JF, Armstrong DK: Variability in aminoglycoside pharmacokinetics in critically ill surgical patients. Crit Care Med 1988;16:327-330.
15. Boucher BA, Kuhl DA, Fabian TC, et al: Effect of neurotrauma on hepatic drug clearance. Clin Pharmacol Ther 1991;50(5 Pt 1):487-497.
16. Rodighiero V: Effects of liver disease on pharmacokinetics: An update. Clin Pharmacokinet 1999;37:399-431.
17. Drug interactions. Med Lett Drugs Therap 2003;45:44-48.
18. Uchino S, Kellum JA, Bellomo R, et al: Acute renal failure in critically ill patients: A multinational, multicenter study. JAMA 2005;294:813-818.
19. Mueller BA, Pasko DA, Sowinski KM: Higher renal replacement therapy dose delivery influences on drug therapy. Artif Organs 2003;27:808-814.
20. McKinnon PS, Davis SL: Pharmacokinetic and pharmacodynamic issues in the treatment of bacterial infectious diseases. Eur J Clin Microbiol Infect Dis 2004;23:271-288.
21. Rodvold KA: Pharmacodynamics of antiinfective therapy: Taking what we know to the patient's bedside. Pharmacotherapy 2001;21(11 Pt 2):319S-330S.
22. Craig WA: Pharmacokinetic/pharmacodynamic parameters: Rationale for antibacterial dosing of mice and men. Clin Infect Dis 1998;26:1-10.
23. Turnidge JD: The pharmacodynamics of beta-lactams. Clin Infect Dis 1998;27:10-22.
24. Ambrose PG, Quintiliani R, Nightingale CH, et al: Continuous versus intermittent infusion of cefuroxime for the treatment of community-acquired pneumonia. Infect Dis Clin Pract 1998;7:463-470.
25. Georges B, Conil JM, Cougot P, et al: Cefepime in critically ill patients: Continuous infusion vs. an intermittent dosing regimen. Int J Clin Pharmacol Ther 2005;43:360-369.
26. Grant EM, Kuti JL, Nicolau DP, et al: Clinical efficacy and pharmacoeconomics of a continuous-infusion piperacillin-tazobactam program in a large community teaching hospital. Pharmacotherapy 2002;22:471-483.
27. Lorente L, Lorenzo L, Martin MM, et al: Meropenem by continuous versus intermittent infusion in ventilator-associated pneumonia due to gram-negative bacilli. Ann Pharmacother 2006;40:219-223.
28. Nicolau DP, McNabb J, Lacy MK, et al: Continuous versus intermittent administration of ceftazidime in intensive care unit patients with nosocomial pneumonia. Int J Antimicrob Agents 2001;17:497-504.
29. Krueger WA, Bulitta J, Kinzig-Schippers M, et al: Evaluation by Monte Carlo simulation of the pharmacokinetics of two doses of meropenem administered intermittently or as a continuous infusion in healthy volunteers. Antimicrob Agents Chemother 2005;49:1881-1889.
30. Kuti JL, Dandekar PK, Nightingale CH, et al: Use of Monte Carlo simulation to design an optimized pharmacodynamic dosing strategy for meropenem. J Clin Pharmacol 2003;43:1116-1123.
31. Tam VH, Louie A, Lomaestro BM, et al: Integration of population pharmacokinetics, a pharmacodynamic target, and microbiologic surveillance data to generate a rational empiric dosing strategy for cefepime against *Pseudomonas aeruginosa*. Pharmacotherapy 2003;23:291-295.
32. Rybak MJ: The pharmacokinetic and pharmacodynamic properties of vancomycin. Clin Infect Dis 2006;42(Suppl 1):S35-S39.
33. Lamer C, de Beco V, Soler P, et al: Analysis of vancomycin entry into pulmonary lining fluid by bronchoalveolar lavage in critically ill patients. Antimicrob Agents Chemother 1993;37:281-286.
34. Karam CM, McKinnon PS, Neuhauser MM, et al: Outcome assessment of minimizing vancomycin monitoring

and dosing adjustments. Pharmacotherapy 1999;19:257-266.
35. Guidelines for the management of adults with hospital-acquired, ventilator-associated, and healthcare-associated pneumonia. Am J Respir Crit Care Med 2005;171:388-416.
36. Moore RD, Smith CR, Lietman PS: Association of aminoglycoside plasma levels with therapeutic outcome in gram-negative pneumonia. Am J Med 1984;77:657-662.
37. Moore RD, Smith CR, Lietman PS: The association of aminoglycoside plasma levels with mortality in patients with gram-negative bacteremia. J Infect Dis 1984;149:443-448.
38. Moore RD, Lietman PS, Smith CR: Clinical response to aminoglycoside therapy: Importance of the ratio of peak concentration to minimal inhibitory concentration. J Infect Dis 1987;155:93-99.
39. Kashuba AD, Nafziger AN, Drusano GL, et al: Optimizing aminoglycoside therapy for nosocomial pneumonia caused by gram-negative bacteria. Antimicrob Agents Chemother 1999;43:623-629.
40. Rotschafer JC, Rybak MJ: Single daily dosing of aminoglycosides: A commentary. Ann Pharmacother 1994;28:797-801.
41. Nicolau DP, Freeman CD, Belliveau PP, et al: Experience with a once-daily aminoglycoside program administered to 2,184 adult patients. Antimicrob Agents Chemother 1995;39:650-655.
42. Rybak MJ, Abate BJ, Kang SL, et al: Prospective evaluation of the effect of an aminoglycoside dosing regimen on rates of observed nephrotoxicity and ototoxicity. Antimicrob Agents Chemother 1999;43:1549-1555.
43. Murry KR, McKinnon PS, Mitrzyk B, et al: Pharmacodynamic characterization of nephrotoxicity associated with once-daily aminoglycoside. Pharmacotherapy 1999;19:1252-1260.
44. Olsen KM, Rudis MI, Rebuck JA, et al: Effect of once-daily dosing vs. multiple daily dosing of tobramycin on enzyme markers of nephrotoxicity. Crit Care Med 2004;32:1678-1682.
45. Micek ST, Heuring TJ, Hollands JM, et al: Optimizing antibiotic treatment for ventilator-associated pneumonia. Pharmacotherapy 2006;26:204-213.
46. Barletta JF, Johnson SB, Nix DE, et al: Population pharmacokinetics of aminoglycosides in critically ill trauma patients on once-daily regimens. J Trauma 2000;49:869-872.
47. Tholl DA, Shikuma LR, Miller TQ, et al: Physiologic response of stress and aminoglycoside clearance in critically ill patients. Crit Care Med 1993;21:248-251.
48. Preston SL, Drusano GL, Berman AL, et al: Pharmacodynamics of levofloxacin: A new paradigm for early clinical trials. JAMA 1998;279:125-129.
49. Cazzola M, Matera MG, Donnarumma G, et al: Pharmacodynamics of levofloxacin in patients with acute exacerbation of chronic bronchitis. Chest 2005;128:2093-2098.
50. Forrest A, Chodosh S, Amantea MA, et al: Pharmacokinetics and pharmacodynamics of oral grepafloxacin in patients with acute bacterial exacerbations of chronic bronchitis. J Antimicrob Chemother 1997;40(Suppl A):45-57.
51. Lister PD: Pharmacodynamics of gatifloxacin against *Streptococcus pneumoniae* in an in vitro pharmacokinetic model: Impact of area under the curve/MIC ratios on eradication. Antimicrob Agents Chemother 2002;46:69-74.
52. Lister PD, Sanders CC: Pharmacodynamics of trovafloxacin, ofloxacin, and ciprofloxacin against *Streptococcus pneumoniae* in an in vitro pharmacokinetic model. Antimicrob Agents Chemother 1999;43: 1118-1123.
53. Zhanel GG, Walters M, Laing N, et al: In vitro pharmacodynamic modelling simulating free serum concentrations of fluoroquinolones against multidrug-resistant *Streptococcus pneumoniae.* J Antimicrob Chemother 2001;47: 435-440.
54. Ambrose PG, Grasela DM, Grasela TH, et al: Pharmacodynamics of fluoroquinolones against *Streptococcus pneumoniae* in patients with community-acquired respiratory tract infections. Antimicrob Agents Chemother 2001;45:2793-2797.
55. Thomas JK, Forrest A, Bhavnani SM, et al: Pharmacodynamic evaluation of factors associated with the development of bacterial resistance in acutely ill patients during therapy. Antimicrob Agents Chemother 1998;42:521-527.
56. Andes D: Clinical pharmacodynamics of antifungals. Infect Dis Clin North Am 2003;17:635-649.
57. Theuretzbacher U: Pharmacokinetics/pharmacodynamics of echinocandins. Eur J Clin Microbiol Infect Dis 2004;23:805-812.
58. Winter WE, Tozer TT: Phenytoin. In Burton ME, Shaw LM, Schentag JJ, et al (eds): Applied Pharmacokinetics and Pharmacodynamics. Philadelphia, Lippincott Williams & Wilkins, 2006, pp 463-490.
59. Boucher BA, Rodman JH, Jaresko GS, et al: Phenytoin pharmacokinetics in critically ill trauma patients. Clin Pharmacol Ther 1988;44:675-683.
60. Jacobi J, Fraser GL, Coursin DB, et al: Clinical practice guidelines for the sustained use of sedatives and analgesics in the critically ill adult. Crit Care Med 2002;30:119-141.
61. Shelly MP, Mendel L, Park GR: Failure of critically ill patients to metabolise midazolam. Anaesthesia 1987;42:619-626.
62. Armstrong PJ, Bersten A: Normeperidine toxicity. Anesth Analg 1986;65:536-538.
63. Milne RW, Nation RL, Somogyi AA, et al: The influence of renal function on the renal clearance of morphine and its glucuronide metabolites in intensive-care patients. Br J Clin Pharmacol 1992;34:53-59.
64. Terra SG, Washam JB, Dunham GD, et al: Therapeutic range of digoxin's efficacy in heart failure: What is the evidence? Pharmacotherapy 1999;19:1123-1126.
65. Bauman JL, Dekker-Schoen M: Arrhythmias. In DiPiro JT, Talbert RL, Yee GC, et al (eds): Pharmacotherapy: A Pathophysiologic Approach, ed 6. New York, McGraw-Hill, 2005, pp 321-356.
66. Tsikouris JP, Cox CD: A review of class III antiarrhythmic agents for atrial fibrillation: Maintenance of normal sinus rhythm. Pharmacotherapy 2001;21:1514-1529.
67. Hirsh J, Raschke R: Heparin and low-molecular-weight heparin: The Seventh ACCP Conference on Antithrombotic and Thrombolytic Therapy. Chest 2004;126(3 Suppl):188S-203S.
68. Spinler SA, Wittkowsky AK, Nutescu EA, et al: Anticoagulation monitoring, part 2: Unfractionated heparin and low-molecular-weight heparin. Ann Pharmacother 2005;39:1275-1285.
69. Srinivasa V, Gilbertson LI, Bhavani-Shankar K: Thromboelastography: Where is it and where is it heading? Int Anesthesiol Clin 2001;39:35-49.
70. Luddington RJ: Thrombelastography/thromboelastometry. Clin Lab Haematol 2005;27:81-90.
71. Salooja N, Perry DJ: Thrombelastography. Blood Coagul Fibrinol 2001;12:327-337.
72. Laposata M, Green D, Van Cott EM, et al: College of American Pathologists Conference XXXI on laboratory monitoring of anticoagulant therapy: The clinical use and laboratory monitoring of low-molecular-weight heparin, danaparoid, hirudin, and related compounds, and argatroban. Arch Pathol Lab Med 1998;122: 799-807.
73. Mayr AJ, Dunser M, Jochberger S, et al: Antifactor Xa activity in intensive care patients receiving thromboembolic prophylaxis with standard doses of enoxaparin. Thromb Res 2002;105:201-204.
74. Chowdhury MH, Tunkel AR: Antibacterial agents in infections of the central nervous system. Infect Dis Clin North Am 2000;14:391-408.
75. Lutsar I, McCracken GH Jr, Friedland IR: Antibiotic pharmacodynamics in cerebrospinal fluid. Clin Infect Dis 1998;27:1117-1127.
76. Schmidt T, Tauber MG: Pharmacodynamics of antibiotics in the therapy of meningitis: Infection model observations. J Antimicrob Chemother 1993;31(Suppl D):61-70.
77. Buchler M, Malfertheiner P, Friess H, et al: Human pancreatic tissue concentration of bactericidal antibiotics. Gastroenterology 1992;103:1902-1908.
78. Shrikhande S, Friess H, Issenegger C, et al: Fluconazole penetration into the pancreas. Antimicrob Agents Chemother 2000;44:2569-2571.
79. Spector R, Park GD, Johnson GF, et al: Therapeutic drug monitoring. Clin Pharmacol Ther 1988;43:345-353.
80. Mutlu GM, Mutlu EA, Factor P. GI complications in patients receiving mechanical ventilation. Chest 2001;119:1222-1241.
81. Schmidt T, Martindale R: The gastrointestinal tract in critical illness. Curr Opin Clin Nutr Metab Care 2001;4:547-551.
82. Martin LF, Booth FV, Karlstadt RG, et al: Continuous intravenous cimetidine decreases stress-related

upper gastrointestinal hemorrhage without promoting pneumonia. Crit Care Med 1993;21:19-30.
83. Dive A, Moulart M, Jonard P, et al: Gastroduodenal motility in mechanically ventilated critically ill patients: A manometric study. Crit Care Med 1994;22:441-447.
84. Laing RB, Mackenzie AR, Shaw H, et al: The effect of intravenous-to-oral switch guidelines on the use of parenteral antimicrobials in medical wards. J Antimicrob Chemother 1998;42:107-111.
85. Kanji S, McKinnon PS, Barletta JF, et al: Bioavailability of gatifloxacin by gastric tube administration with and without concomitant enteral feeding in critically ill patients. Crit Care Med 2003;31:1347-1352.
86. Madaras-Kelly KJ, Larsson AJ, Rotschafer JC: A pharmacodynamic evaluation of ciprofloxacin and ofloxacin against two strains of *Pseudomonas aeruginosa.* J Antimicrob Chemother 1996;37:703-710.
87. Engle KK, Hannawa TE: Techniques for administering oral medications to critical care patients receiving continuous enteral nutrition. Am J Health Syst Pharm 1999;56: 1441-1444.
88. Mimoz O, Binter V, Jacolot A, et al: Pharmacokinetics and absolute bioavailability of ciprofloxacin administered through a nasogastric tube with continuous enteral feeding to critically ill patients. Intensive Care Med 1998;24:1047-1051.
89. Rosemurgy AS, Markowsky S, Goode SE, et al: Bioavailability of fluconazole in surgical intensive care unit patients: A study comparing routes of administration. J Trauma 1995;39:445-447.
90. Haas CE, Nelsen JL, Raghavendran K, et al: Pharmacokinetics and pharmacodynamics of enoxaparin in multiple trauma patients. J Trauma 2005;59:1336-1343.
91. Dorffler-Melly J, deJonge E, Pont AC, et al: Bioavailability of subcutaneous low-molecular-weight heparin to patients on vasopressors. Lancet 2002;359:849-850.
92. Priglinger U, Delle Karth G, Geppert A, et al: Prophylactic anticoagulation with enoxaparin: Is the subcutaneous route appropriate in the critically ill? Crit Care Med 2003;31:1405-1409.
93. Levine MN, Planes A, Hirsh J, et al: The relationship between anti-factor Xa level and clinical outcome in patients receiving enoxaparine low molecular weight heparin to prevent deep vein thrombosis after hip replacement. Thromb Haemost 1989;62:940-944.
94. Summer W, Elston R, Tharpe L, et al: Aerosol bronchodilator delivery methods: Relative impact on pulmonary function and cost of respiratory care. Arch Intern Med 1989;149:618-623.
95. Fink JB, Dhand R, Duarte AG, et al: Aerosol delivery from a metered-dose inhaler during mechanical ventilation: An in vitro model. Am J Respir Crit Care Med 1996;154(2 Pt 1):382-387.
96. Fuller HD, Dolovich MB, Posmituck G, et al: Pressurized aerosol versus jet aerosol delivery to mechanically ventilated patients: comparison of dose to the lungs. Am Rev Respir Dis 1990;141:440-444.
97. Palmer LB, Smaldone GC, Simon SR, et al: Aerosolized antibiotics in mechanically ventilated patients: delivery and response. Crit Care Med 1998;26:31-39.
98. Wood GC, Boucher BA, Croce MA, et al: Aerosolized ceftazidime for prevention of ventilator-associated pneumonia and drug effects on the proinflammatory response in critically ill trauma patients. Pharmacotherapy 2002;22:972-982.
99. Hamer DH: Treatment of nosocomial pneumonia and tracheobronchitis caused by multidrug-resistant *Pseudomonas aeruginosa* with aerosolized colistin. Am J Respir Crit Care Med 2000;162:328-330.
100. Weinshilboum R: Inheritance and drug response. N Engl J Med 2003;348:529-537.
101. Furuta T, Ohashi K, Kosuge K, et al: CYP2C19 genotype status and effect of omeprazole on intragastric pH in humans. Clin Pharmacol Ther 1999;65:552-561.
102. Leontiadis GI, Sharma VK, Howden CW: Systematic review and meta-analysis: Enhanced efficacy of proton-pump inhibitor therapy for peptic ulcer bleeding in Asia—a post hoc analysis from the Cochrane Collaboration. Aliment Pharmacol Ther 2005;21:1055-1061.
103. Zineh I, Pebanco GD, Aquilante CL, et al: Discordance between availability of pharmacogenetics studies and pharmacogenetics-based prescribing information for the top 200 drugs. Ann Pharmacother 2006;40: 639-644.
104. Robert S, Zarowitz BJ: Is there a reliable index of glomerular filtration rate in critically ill patients? Drug Intell Clin Pharm 1991;25:169-178.
105. Cockcroft DW, Gault MH: Prediction of creatinine clearance from serum creatinine. Nephron 1976;16:31-41.
106. Martin C, Alaya M, Bras J, et al: Assessment of creatinine clearance in intensive care patients. Crit Care Med 1990;18:1224-1226.
107. Robert S, Zarowitz BJ, Peterson EL, et al: Predictability of creatinine clearance estimates in critically ill patients. Crit Care Med 1993;21:1487-1495.
108. Pesola GR, Akhavan I, Madu A, et al: Prediction equation estimates of creatinine clearance in the intensive care unit. Intensive Care Med 1993;19:39-43.
109. Levey AS, Bosch JP, Lewis JB, et al: A more accurate method to estimate glomerular filtration rate from serum creatinine: A new prediction equation. Modification of Diet in Renal Disease Study Group. Ann Intern Med 1999;130:461-470.
110. Levey AS, Greene T, Kusek JW, et al: A simplified equation to predict glomerular filtration rate from serum creatinine. J Am Soc Nephrol 2000;11:155A.
111. K/DOQI clinical practice guidelines for chronic kidney disease: Evaluation, classification, and stratification. Am J Kidney Dis 2002;39(2 Suppl 1): S1-S266.
112. Cherry RA, Eachempati SR, Hydo L, et al: Accuracy of short-duration creatinine clearance determinations in predicting 24-hour creatinine clearance in critically ill and injured patients. J Trauma 2002;53:267-271.
113. Baumann TJ, Staddon JE, Horst HM, et al: Minimum urine collection periods for accurate determination of creatinine clearance in critically ill patients. Clin Pharm 1987;6: 393-398.
114. Bugge JF: Influence of renal replacement therapy on pharmacokinetics in critically ill patients. Best Pract Res Clin Anaesthesiol 2004;18:175-187.
115. Matzke GR, Comstock TJ: Influence of renal function and dialysis on drug disposition. In Burton ME, Shaw LM, Schentag JJ, et al (eds): Applied Pharmacokinetics and Pharmacodynamics. Philadelphia, Lippincott Williams & Wilkins, 2006, pp 187-212.
116. Golper TA, Marx MA: Drug dosing adjustments during continuous renal replacement therapies. Kidney Int Suppl 1998;66:S165-S168.
117. Brunet S, Leblanc M, Geadah D, et al: Diffusive and convective solute clearances during continuous renal replacement therapy at various dialysate and ultrafiltration flow r ates. Am J Kidney Dis 1999;34: 486-492.
118. Joy MS, Matzke GR, Armstrong DK, et al: A primer on continuous renal replacement therapy for critically ill patients. Ann Pharmacother 1998;32:362-375.
119. Joy MS, Matzke GR, Frye RF, et al: Determinants of vancomycin clearance by continuous venovenous hemofiltration and continuous venovenous hemodialysis. Am J Kidney Dis 1998;31:1019-1027.
120. Bugge JF: Pharmacokinetics and drug dosing adjustments during continuous venovenous hemofiltration or hemodiafiltration in critically ill patients. Acta Anaesthesiol Scand 2001;45:929-934.
121. Reetze-Bonorden P, Bohler J, Keller E: Drug dosage in patients during continuous renal replacement therapy: Pharmacokinetic and therapeutic considerations. Clin Pharmacokinet 1993;24:362-379.
122. Frye RF, Matzke GR: Drug therapy individualization for patients with renal insufficiency. In DiPiro JT, Talbert RL, Yee GC, et al (eds): Pharmacotherapy: A Pathophysiologic Approach, ed 6. New York, McGraw-Hill, 2005, pp 919-935.
123. Delco F, Tchambaz L, Schlienger R, et al: Dose adjustment in patients with liver disease. Drug Saf 2005;28:529-545.
124. Pieracci FM, Barie PS, Pomp A: Critical care of the bariatric patient. Crit Care Med 2006;34:1796-1804.
125. Nasraway SA Jr, Albert M, Donnelly AM, et al: Morbid obesity is an independent determinant of death among surgical critically ill patients. Crit Care Med 2006;34:964-970.

126. World Health Organization: Report of a WHO Consultation on Obesity: Obesity: Preventing and Managing the Global Epidemic. Geneva, World Health Organization, 1998.
127. Devine BJ: Case number 25: Gentamicin therapy. Drug Intell Clin Pharm 1974;8:650-655.
128. Erstad BL: Dosing of medications in morbidly obese patients in the intensive care unit setting. Intensive Care Med 2004;30:18-32.
129. Blouin RA, Warren GW: Pharmacokinetic considerations in obesity. J Pharm Sci 1999;88:1-7.
130. Cheymol G: Effects of obesity on pharmacokinetics implications for drug therapy. Clin Pharmacokinet 2000;39:215-231.
131. Casati A, Putzu M: Anesthesia in the obese patient: Pharmacokinetic considerations. J Clin Anesth 2005;17:134-145.
132. Erstad BL: Which weight for weight-based dosage regimens in obese patients? Am J Health Syst Pharm 2002;59:2105-2110.
133. Shibutani K, Inchiosa MA Jr, Sawada K, et al: Accuracy of pharmacokinetic models for predicting plasma fentanyl concentrations in lean and obese surgical patients: Derivation of dosing weight ("pharmacokinetic mass"). Anesthesiology 2004;101:603-613.
134. Shibutani K, Inchiosa MA Jr, Sawada K, et al: Pharmacokinetic mass of fentanyl for postoperative analgesia in lean and obese patients. Br J Anaesth 2005;95:377-383.
135. Egan TD, Huizinga B, Gupta SK, et al: Remifentanil pharmacokinetics in obese versus lean patients. Anesthesiology 1998;89:562-573.
136. Schwartz AE, Matteo RS, Ornstein E, et al: Pharmacokinetics of sufentanil in obese patients. Anesth Analg 1991;73:790-793.
137. Brunette DD: Resuscitation of the morbidly obese patient. Am J Emerg Med 2004;22:40-47.
138. Greenblatt DJ, Abernethy DR, Locniskar A, et al: Effect of age, gender, and obesity on midazolam kinetics. Anesthesiology 1984;61:27-35.
139. Servin F, Farinotti R, Haberer JP, et al: Propofol infusion for maintenance of anesthesia in morbidly obese patients receiving nitrous oxide: A clinical and pharmacokinetic study. Anesthesiology 1993;78:657-665.
140. Leykin Y, Pellis T, Lucca M, et al: The effects of cisatracurium on morbidly obese women. Anesth Analg 2004;99:1090-1094.
141. Leykin Y, Pellis T, Lucca M, et al: The pharmacodynamic effects of rocuronium when dosed according to real body weight or ideal body weight in morbidly obese patients. Anesth Analg 2004;99:1086-1089.
142. Schwartz AE, Matteo RS, Ornstein E, et al: Pharmacokinetics and pharmacodynamics of vecuronium in the obese surgical patient. Anesth Analg 1992;74:515-518.
143. Varin F, Ducharme J, Theoret Y, et al: Influence of extreme obesity on the body disposition and neuromuscular blocking effect of atracurium. Clin Pharmacol Ther 1990;48:18-25.
144. Bentley JB, Borel JD, Vaughan RW, et al: Weight, pseudocholinesterase activity, and succinylcholine requirement. Anesthesiology 1982;57:48-49.
145. Lemmens HJ, Brodsky JB: The dose of succinylcholine in morbid obesity. Anesth Analg 2006;102:438-442.
146. Abernethy DR, Greenblatt DJ: Phenytoin disposition in obesity: Determination of loading dose. Arch Neurol 1985;42:468-471.
147. Cheymol G, Poirier JM, Carrupt PA, et al: Pharmacokinetics of beta-adrenoceptor blockers in obese and normal volunteers. Br J Clin Pharmacol 1997;43:563-570.
148. Wojcicki J, Jaroszynska M, Drozdzik M, et al: Comparative pharmacokinetics and pharmacodynamics of propranolol and atenolol in normolipaemic and hyperlipidaemic obese subjects. Biopharm Drug Dispos 2003;24:211-218.
149. Cheymol G, Poirier JM, Barre J, et al: Comparative pharmacokinetics of intravenous propranolol in obese and normal volunteers. J Clin Pharmacol 1987;27:874-879.
150. Abernethy DR, Greenblatt DJ, Smith TW: Digoxin disposition in obesity: Clinical pharmacokinetic investigation. Am Heart J 1981;102:740-744.
151. Raschke RA, Reilly BM, Guidry JR, et al: The weight-based heparin dosing nomogram compared with a "standard care" nomogram: A randomized controlled trial. Ann Intern Med 1993;119:874-881.
152. Ellison MJ, Sawyer WT, Mills TC: Calculation of heparin dosage in a morbidly obese woman. Clin Pharm 1989;8:65-68.
153. Spruill WJ, Wade WE, Huckaby WG, et al: Achievement of anticoagulation by using a weight-based heparin dosing protocol for obese and nonobese patients. Am J Health Syst Pharm 2001;58:2143-2146.
154. Yee WP, Norton LL: Optimal weight base for a weight-based heparin dosing protocol. Am J Health Syst Pharm 1998;55:159-162.
155. Al-Yaseen E, Wells PS, Anderson J, et al: The safety of dosing dalteparin based on actual body weight for the treatment of acute venous thromboembolism in obese patients. J Thromb Haemost 2005;3: 100-102.
156. Hainer JW, Barrett JS, Assaid CA, et al: Dosing in heavy-weight/obese patients with the LMWH, tinzaparin: A pharmacodynamic study. Thromb Haemost 2002;87:817-823.
157. Sanderink GJ, Le Liboux A, Jariwala N, et al: The pharmacokinetics and pharmacodynamics of enoxaparin in obese volunteers. Clin Pharmacol Ther 2002;72:308-318.
158. Smith J, Canton EM: Weight-based administration of dalteparin in obese patients. Am J Health Syst Pharm 2003;60:683-687.
159. Wilson SJ, Wilbur K, Burton E, et al: Effect of patient weight on the anticoagulant response to adjusted therapeutic dosage of low-molecular-weight heparin for the treatment of venous thromboembolism. Haemostasis 2001;31:42-48.
160. Yee JY, Duffull SB: The effect of body weight on dalteparin pharmacokinetics: A preliminary study. Eur J Clin Pharmacol 2000;56:293-297.
161. Spinler SA, Inverso SM, Cohen M, et al: Safety and efficacy of unfractionated heparin versus enoxaparin in patients who are obese and patients with severe renal impairment: Analysis from the ESSENCE and TIMI 11B studies. Am Heart J 2003;146:33-41.
162. Geerts W, Selby R: Prevention of venous thromboembolism in the ICU. Chest 2003;124(6 Suppl): 357S-363S.
163. Scholten DJ, Hoedema RM, Scholten SE: A comparison of two different prophylactic dose regimens of low molecular weight heparin in bariatric surgery. Obes Surg 2002;12:19-24.
164. Bearden DT, Rodvold KA: Dosage adjustments for antibacterials in obese patients: Applying clinical pharmacokinetics. Clin Pharmacokinet 2000;38:415-426.
165. Wurtz R, Itokazu G, Rodvold K: Antimicrobial dosing in obese patients. Clin Infect Dis 1997;25:112-118.
166. Yuk J, Nightingale CH, Sweeney K, et al: Pharmacokinetics of nafcillin in obesity. J Infect Dis 1988;157:1088-1089.
167. Yost RL, Derendorf H: Disposition of cefotaxime and its desacetyl metabolite in morbidly obese male and female subjects. Ther Drug Monit 1986;8:189-194.
168. Allard S, Kinzig M, Boivin G, et al: Intravenous ciprofloxacin disposition in obesity. Clin Pharmacol Ther 1993;54:368-373.
169. Caldwell JB, Nilsen AK: Intravenous ciprofloxacin dosing in a morbidly obese patient. Ann Pharmacother 1994;28:806.
170. Stein GE, Schooley SL, Peloquin CA, et al: Pharmacokinetics and pharmacodynamics of linezolid in obese patients with cellulitis. Ann Pharmacother 2005;39:427-432.
171. Dunn TE, Ludwig EA, Slaughter RL, et al: Pharmacokinetics and pharmacodynamics of methylprednisolone in obesity. Clin Pharmacol Ther 1991;49:536-549.
172. Bracken MB, Shepard MJ, Holford TR, et al: Administration of methylprednisolone for 24 or 48 hours or tirilazad mesylate for 48 hours in the treatment of acute spinal cord injury: Results of the Third National Acute Spinal Cord Injury Randomized Controlled Trial. National Acute Spinal Cord Injury Study. JAMA 1997;277:1597-1604.
173. Bernard GR, Vincent JL, Laterre PF, et al: Efficacy and safety of recombinant human activated protein C for severe sepsis. N Engl J Med 2001;344:699-709.
174. Macias WL, Dhainaut JF, Yan SC, et al: Pharmacokinetic-pharmacodynamic analysis of drotrecogin alfa (activated) in patients with severe sepsis. Clin Pharmacol Ther 2002;72:391-402.
175. Levy H, Small D, Heiselman DE, et al: Obesity does not alter the pharmacokinetics of drotrecogin alfa

(activated) in severe sepsis. Ann Pharmacother 2005;39:262-267.
176. Somme D, Maillet JM, Gisselbrecht M, et al: Critically ill old and the oldest-old patients in intensive care: Short- and long-term outcomes. Intensive Care Med 2003;29:2137-2143.
177. Montamat SC, Cusack BJ, Vestal RE: Management of drug therapy in the elderly. N Engl J Med 1989;321:303-309.
178. Lesar TS, Lomaestro BM, Pohl H: Medication-prescribing errors in a teaching hospital: A 9-year experience. Arch Intern Med 1997;157: 1569-1576.
179. FDA: Guideline for the study of drugs likely to be used in the elderly. Rockville, Md, Food and Drug Admininstration. Center for Surgical Evaluation and Research, 1989, p 16.
180. Novak LP: Aging, total body potassium, fat-free mass, and cell mass in males and females between ages 18 and 85 years. J Gerontol 1972;27: 438-443.
181. Greenblatt DJ, Harmatz JS, Shader RI: Clinical pharmacokinetics of anxiolytics and hypnotics in the elderly: Therapeutic considerations (part II). Clin Pharmacokinet 1991;21:262-273.
182. Sokoll LJ, Russell RM, Sadowski JA, et al: Establishment of creatinine clearance reference values for older women. Clin Chem 1994;40: 2276-2281.
183. Scarpace PJ, Tumer N, Mader SL: Beta-adrenergic function in aging: Basic mechanisms and clinical implications. Drugs Aging 1991;1:116-129.
184. Stolarek I, Scott PJ, Caird FI: Physiological changes due to age: Implications for cardiovascular drug therapy. Drugs Aging 1991;1:467-476.
185. 1997-1999 Emergency Cardiovascular Care Programs, Advanced Cardiac Life Support. Chicago, American Heart Association, 1997.
186. Campbell NR, Hull RD, Brant R, et al: Aging and heparin-related bleeding. Arch Intern Med 1996;156:857-860.
187. Redwood M, Taylor C, Bain BJ, et al: The association of age with dosage requirement for warfarin. Age Ageing 1991;20:217-220.
188. Alexander SL, Ernst FR: Use of drotrecogin alfa (activated) in older patients with severe sepsis. Pharmacotherapy 2006;26: 533-538.
189. Anderson GD: Pregnancy-induced changes in pharmacokinetics: A mechanistic-based approach. Clin Pharmacokinet 2005;44:989-1008.
190. Loebstein R, Koren G: Clinical relevance of therapeutic drug monitoring during pregnancy. Ther Drug Monit 2002;24:15-22.
191. Bates SM, Ginsberg JS: How we manage venous thromboembolism during pregnancy. Blood 2002;100:3470-3478.
192. Ensom MH, Stephenson MD: Pharmacokinetics of low molecular weight heparin and unfractionated heparin in pregnancy. J Soc Gynecol Invest 2004;11:377-383.
193. Koren G, Pastuszak A, Ito S: Drugs in pregnancy. N Engl J Med 1998;338:1128-1137.
194. Weinbren MJ: Pharmacokinetics of antibiotics in burn patients. J Antimicrob Chemother 1999;44:319-327.
195. Zaske DE, Sawchuk RJ, Gerding DN, et al: Increased dosage requirements of gentamicin in burn patients. J Trauma 1976;16:824-828.
196. Hoey LL, Tschida SJ, Rotschafer JC, et al: Wide variation in single, daily-dose aminoglycoside pharmacokinetics in patients with burn injuries. J Burn Care Rehab 1997;18:116-124.
197. Rybak MJ, Albrecht LM, Berman JR, et al: Vancomycin pharmacokinetics in burn patients and intravenous drug abusers. Antimicrob Agents Chemother 1990;34:792-795.
198. Boucher BA, King SR, Wandschneider HL, et al: Fluconazole pharmacokinetics in burn patients. Antimicrob Agents Chemother 1998;42:930-933.
199. Bonate PL: Pathophysiology and pharmacokinetics following burn injury. Clin Pharmacokinet 1990;18:118-130.
200. Pickerill KE, Paladino JA, Schentag JJ: Comparison of the fluoroquinolones based on pharmacokinetic and pharmacodynamic parameters. Pharmacotherapy 2000;20:417-428.
201. Rebuck JA, Fish DN, Abraham E: Pharmacokinetics of intravenous and oral levofloxacin in critically ill adults in a medical intensive care unit. Pharmacotherapy 2002;22:1216-1225.
202. Jelliffe RW: Creatinine clearance: Bedside estimate. Ann Intern Med 1973;79:604-605 (Letter).
203. Nix DE, Erstad BL, Nakazato PZ, et al: Estimation of creatinine clearance in end-stage liver disease. Ann Pharmacother 2006;40:900-908.
204. Salazar DE, Corcoran GB: Predicting creatinine clearance and renal drug clearance in obese patients from estimated fat-free body mass. Am J Med 1988;84:1053-1060.
205. Magee LA, Cham C, Waterman EJ, et al: Hydralazine for treatment of severe hypertension in pregnancy: Meta-analysis. BMJ 2003;327:955-960.
206. Brater DC: Drug Use in Renal Disease. Balgowlah, Australia, ADIS Health Science Press, 1983.
207. Jelliffe R: Estimation of creatinine clearance in patients with unstable renal function, without a urine specimen. Am J Nephrol 2002;22:320-324.
208. DuBois D, DuBois EF: Clinical calorimetry. Tenth paper: A formula to estimate the approximate surface area if height and weight be known. Arch Intern Med 1916;17:863.
209. James WP: Research on Obesity. London, Her Majesty's Stationery Office, 1976.
210. Mosteller RD: Simplified calculation of body-surface area. N Engl J Med 1987;317:1098.
211. Robinson JD, Lupkiewicz SM, Palenik L, et al: Determination of ideal body weight for drug dosage calculations. Am J Hosp Pharm 1983;40: 1016-1019.
212. Devlin JW, Zarowitz BJ: Alterations in drug disposition in the elderly. In Grenvik A, Ayres SM, Holbrook PR, et al (eds): Textbook of Critical Care. Philadelphia, Saunders, 2000, pp 991-1000.
213. Bohler J, Donauer J, Keller F: Pharmacokinetic principles during continuous renal replacement therapy: drugs and dosage. Kidney Int Suppl 1999;72:S24-S28.

PART

II

CRITICAL CARE CARDIOVASCULAR DISEASE

Chapter 22

Shock: Classification, Pathophysiology, and Approach to Management

Anand Kumar and Joseph E. Parrillo

The syndrome of shock in humans is often the final pathway through which a variety of pathologic processes lead to cardiovascular failure and death. Shock is perhaps the most common and important problem with which critical care physicians contend. The importance of shock as a medical problem can be appreciated by the prominence of its three dominant forms. Cardiogenic shock related to pump failure is a major component of the mortality associated with cardiovascular disease, the leading cause of death in the United States with almost 700,000 deaths annually.[1,2] Similarly, hypovolemic shock remains a major contributor to early mortality from trauma, the most common cause of death in individuals younger than 45 years old (approximately 100,000 cases annually).[1,3,4] Finally, despite improving medical and surgical therapy, overall mortality coded as septicemia has increased since the 1990s from the 13th to the 10th most frequent cause of death in the United States.[1,5-7] Current estimates suggest more than 100,000 cases of septic shock annually in the United States alone.[8,9] In addition, all forms of shock increase the probability of other major comorbidities, such as serious infection, acute respiratory distress syndrome (ARDS), and multiple organ dysfunction syndrome (MODS).

This chapter provides an overview of circulatory shock with an emphasis on the common elements and important differences in the pathophysiology and pathogenesis of the various forms of the syndrome. This focus on common elements of different forms of shock continues through sections on systemic shock hemodynamics, microvascular dysfunction, mechanisms of cellular injury, oxygen supply dependency, compensatory responses, diagnostic approach and evaluation, and management and therapy.

HISTORY

Despite recognition of a post-traumatic syndrome by Greek physicians such as Hippocrates and Galen, the origin of the term *shock* is generally credited to the French surgeon Le Dran, who in his 1737 "A Treatise of Reflections Drawn from Experience with Gunshot Wounds," coined the term *choc* to indicate a severe impact or jolt.[10] In 1743, an inappropriate translation by the English physician Clarke led to the introduction of the word *shock* to the English language to indicate the sudden deterioration of a patient's condition with major trauma.[10] Moses[11] began to popularize the term, using it in his 1867 "A Practical Treatise on Shock after Operations and Injuries." He defined shock as "a peculiar effect on the animal system, produced by violent injuries from any cause, or from violent mental emotions." Before this definition, the rarely used term *shock* referred in a nonspecific sense to the immediate and devastating effects of trauma, not a specific post-trauma syndrome. Although not entirely accurate by today's standards, Moses' definition was one of the first to separate the syndrome involving the body's response to massive trauma from the immediate, direct manifestations of trauma itself.

By the late 1800s, two theories of traumatic shock physiology dominated. Fischer proposed the first, based on observations by Bernard, Charcot, Goltz, and others, in 1870.[12-14] He suggested that traumatic shock was caused by generalized "vasomotor paralysis" resulting in splanchnic blood pooling. The corollary was that total circulating blood volume is preserved in shock. The second dominant theory, articulated by Mapother[15] in 1879, suggested that decreased cardiac output in traumatic shock is caused by intravascular volume loss secondary to extrusion of plasma through the vessel wall from the intravascular space to the interstitium. He proposed that this was a consequence of the failure of "vasodilator nerves" in traumatic shock and subsequent generalized arteriolar vasoconstriction. With the 1899 publication of "An Experimental Research into Surgical Shock" (perhaps the first experimental studies of shock), Crile[16] provided scientific data supporting a variation of the vasomotor paralysis theory. After documenting the importance of decreased central venous pressure (CVP) and venous return in experimental shock secondary to hemorrhage and showing the potential for intravascular volume replacement as therapy, he proposed that traumatic shock was caused by exhaustion of the overstimulated "vasomotor center" and subsequent generalized relaxation of large vessels (veins) leading to decreased ventricular filling and cardiac output.

Further advances in shock research were substantially driven by military concerns. During World War I, Cannon and other physiologists and physicians studied the early clinical response to battlefield trauma. Their work eventually led to the publication of the classic monograph "Traumatic Shock" in 1923.[17] Cannon and colleagues were the first to relate trauma-associated hypotension in a large group of patients to a decrease in blood volume, loss of bicarbonate, and accumulation of organic acids. Others, using dye dilution techniques, showed that severity of shock was directly related to the decrease in intravascular volume.[18] Clinical data from war casualties also suggested the importance of reduced blood flow (independent of blood pressure) in shock.[19] The observation that blood in the capillaries of victims of massive trauma was hemoconcentrated compared with venous blood led to the practice of resuscitating trauma patients with dried pooled plasma rather than whole blood in the early part of World War II.[20]

Although work originating from the battlefields of World War I clearly linked traumatic shock associated with substantial, obvious bleeding to a loss of circulating blood volume, the origin of traumatic shock in the absence of defined hemorrhage was unclear. The accepted explanation for this phenomenon remained a variation of the vasomotor paralysis theory of shock. It was postulated that nonhemorrhagic, post-traumatic shock ("wound shock") was caused by the liberation of "wound toxins" (histamine and other substances), which resulted in "neurogenic" vasodilation and peripheral blood pooling. After World War I, Blalock[21] and others showed in animal models, however, that nonhemorrhagic traumatic shock was due to the loss of blood and fluids into injured tissue, rather than circulating toxins resulting in stasis of blood within the circulation.

Additional advances occurred during World War II. Using injured subjects from the European front, Beecher and coworkers[22] confirmed that hemorrhage and fluid loss leading to metabolic acidosis was a major cause of shock. In the first use of indicator dye techniques in humans for studying blood flow, Cournand and associates,[23] in 1943, showed that cardiac output was typically reduced in shock. They also reinforced Blalock's findings regarding nonhemorrhagic "wound shock" in trauma patients by showing that circulating blood volume was reduced in such patients through loss of fluid into damaged tissues. The importance of maintaining intravascular volume in traumatic and hemorrhagic shock was supported by the well-known cardiovascular physiologist Wiggers,[24] who published a landmark series of studies in the 1940s using a standardized animal model that showed prolonged hypovolemic shock resulted in a resuscitation-resistant state, which he termed *irreversible shock*. Wiggers defined it as a condition resulting from "a depression of many functions but in which reduction of the effective circulating blood volume is of basic importance and in which impairment of the circulation steadily progresses until it eventuates in a state of irreversible circulatory failure." Aggressive fluid support became the standard of resuscitation for trauma and shock.

Subsequently, the Korean War fueled the research that showed the relationship of acute tubular necrosis (ATN) and acute renal failure to circulatory shock.[25] In addition, studies of battlefield casualties showed the relationship between early resuscitation and survival.[25] During the Vietnamese conflict, with the widespread use of ventilator technology, the dominant research concern became post-shock infection and "shock lung" (ARDS), a concern that has evolved to the present interest in shock-related MODS.

DEFINITIONS AND CATEGORIZATION OF SHOCK

The definition of shock has evolved in parallel with understanding of the phenomenon. As noted, until the late 1800s, the term *shock* was used to indicate the immediate response to massive trauma, without regard to a specific post-trauma syndrome. The definition consisted of descriptions of its obvious clinical signs. In 1895, Warren[26] referred to shock as "a momentary pause in the act of death," which was characterized by an "imperceptible" or "weak, thread-like" peripheral pulse and a "cold, clammy sweat."

Subsequently, with the introduction of noninvasive blood pressure monitoring devices, most clinical definitions of shock added the requirement for arterial hypotension. In 1930, Blalock[12] included arterial hypotension as one of the required manifestations of shock when he defined it as "peripheral circulatory failure resulting from a discrepancy in the size of the vascular bed and the volume of the intravascular fluid." In 1964, Simeone[27] suggested that shock exists when "the cardiac output is insufficient to fill the arterial tree with blood under sufficient pressure to provide organs and tissues with adequate blood flow."

Current technology, which allows assessment of perfusion independent of arterial pressure, has shown that hypotension does not define shock. The emphasis in defining shock is now on tissue perfusion in relation to cellular function. According to Fink,[28] shock is "a syndrome precipitated by a systemic derangement of perfusion leading to widespread cellular hypoxia and vital organ dysfunction." Cerra[29] emphasized supply/demand mismatch in his definition: "a disordered response of organisms to an inappropriate balance of substrate supply and demand at a cellular level."

The appropriate definition of shock varies with the context of its use. For paramedical personnel, a definition that incorporates the typical clinical signs of shock (arterial hypotension, tachypnea, tachycardia, altered mental status, and decreased urine output) may suffice. For physiologists, shock may be defined by specific hemodynamic criteria involving alterations of ventricular filling pressures, venous pressures, arterial pressures, cardiac output, and systemic vascular resistance (SVR). Similarly, in the appropriate context, shock also could be defined by alterations of biochemical and bioenergetic pathways or intracellular gene expression. For physicians, we find the most appropriate definition to be "the state in which profound and widespread reduction of *effective* tissue perfusion leads first to reversible, and then, if prolonged, to irreversible cellular injury."

"Effective" tissue perfusion, as opposed to tissue perfusion per se, is an important issue. Effective tissue perfusion may be reduced by a global reduction of systemic perfusion (cardiac output) or by increased ineffective tissue perfusion resulting from a maldistribution of blood flow or a defect of substrate use at the subcellular level (Box 22-1).

Box 22-1

Determinants of Effective Tissue Perfusion in Shock

Cardiovascular Performance (Total Systemic Perfusion/Cardiac Output)

- Cardiac function
  - Preload
  - Afterload
  - Contractility
  - Heart rate
- Venous return
  - Right atrial pressure (dependent on cardiac function)
  - Mean circulatory pressure
    - Stressed vascular volume
    - Mean vascular compliance
    - Venous vascular resistance
    - Distribution of blood flow

Distribution of Cardiac Output

- Intrinsic regulatory systems (local tissue factors)
- Extrinsic regulatory systems (sympathetic/adrenal activity)
- Anatomic vascular disease
- Exogenous vasoactive agents (inotropes, vasopressors, vasodilators)

Microvascular Function

- Precapillary and postcapillary sphincter function
- Capillary endothelial integrity
- Microvascular obstruction (fibrin, platelets, white blood cells, red blood cells)

Local Oxygen Unloading and Diffusion

- Oxyhemoglobin affinity
- Red blood cell 2,3-diphosphoglycerate
- Blood pH
- Temperature

Cellular Energy Generation and Usage Capability

- Citric acid (Kreb's) cycle
- Oxidative phosphorylation pathway
- Other energy metabolism pathways (e.g., adenosine triphosphate use)

CLASSIFICATION

Although hypovolemic shock associated with trauma was the first form of shock to be recognized and studied, by the early 1900s it became broadly recognized that other clinical conditions could result in a similar constellation of signs and symptoms. Sepsis as a distinct cause of shock was initially proposed by Laennec[30] in 1831 and subsequently supported by Boise[31] in 1897. In 1934, Fishberg and colleagues[32] introduced the concept of primary cardiogenic shock secondary to myocardial infarction. Later the same year, Blalock[33] developed the precursor of the most commonly used classification systems of the present. He subdivided shock into four etiologic categories: hematogenic or oligemic (hypovolemic), cardiogenic, neurogenic (e.g., shock after spinal injury), and vasogenic (primarily septic shock). In 1967, Weil[34] proposed the additional etiologic categories of hypersensitivity (i.e., anaphylactic), bacteremic (i.e., septic), obstructive, and endocrinologic shock.

As the hemodynamic profiles of the different forms of shock were uncovered, however, a classification based on cardiovascular characteristics, initially proposed in 1972 by Hinshaw and Cox,[35] came to be accepted by most clinicians. The categories include (1) hypovolemic shock, owing to a decreased circulating blood volume in relation to the total vascular capacity and characterized by a reduction of diastolic filling pressures and volumes; (2) cardiogenic shock, related to cardiac pump failure owing to loss of myocardial contractility and functional myocardium or structural and mechanical failure of the cardiac anatomy and characterized by elevations of diastolic filling pressures and volumes; (3) extracardiac obstructive shock, involving obstruction to flow in the cardiovascular circuit and characterized by either impairment of diastolic filling or excessive afterload; and (4) distributive shock, caused by loss of vasomotor control resulting in arteriolar and venular dilation and (after resuscitation with fluids) characterized by increased cardiac output with decreased SVR. We have adapted these categories into an etiologic/

physiologic classification of shock that is summarized in Figure 22-1 and Box 22-2. This classification represents our current understanding of the causes and typical hemodynamic features of different forms of shock.

Despite this hemodynamically based categorization system, it is important to note the mixed nature of most forms of clinical shock. Septic shock is nominally considered a form of distributive shock. Before resuscitation with fluids, however, a substantial hypovolemic component may exist owing to venodilation and third spacing. In addition, depression of the myocardium in human septic shock is well documented (see Fig. 22-1).[36-38] Similarly, hemorrhagic shock in experimental models has been linked to myocardial depression[39,40] and vascular dysfunction (see Fig. 22-1).[41,42] Cardiogenic shock typically manifests with increased ventricular filling pressures. Many patients have been aggressively diuresed before the onset of shock, however, and may have a relative hypovolemic component. Finally, shock from any cause may cause a deterioration of the coronary perfusion pressure, the difference between mean arterial pressure (MAP) and the higher of left ventricular diastolic pressure or right atrial pressure, resulting in some degree of myocardial ischemia and myocardial dysfunction.[43] Although four categories of shock exist based on hemodynamic profile, clinical shock states tend to combine components of each.

Hypovolemic Shock

Hypovolemic shock may be related to dehydration, internal or external hemorrhage, gastrointestinal fluid losses (diarrhea or vomiting), urinary losses secondary to either diuretics or kidney dysfunction, or loss of intravascular volume to the interstitium as a result of decrease of vascular permeability (in response to sepsis or trauma). In addition, venodilation secondary to many causes (sepsis, spinal injury, and various drugs and toxins) may result in a relative hypovolemic state (see Box 22-2 and Fig. 22-1). Hemodynamically, hypovolemic shock is characterized by a decrease in ventricular preload resulting in decreased ventricular diastolic pressures and volumes (Table 22-1). Cardiac index (CI) and stroke volume index are typically reduced. In addition to hypotension, a decreased pulse pressure may be noted. Because of a decreased output and unchanged or increased metabolic demand, mixed venous oxygen saturation ($S\bar{v}O_2$) may be decreased, and the arteriovenous oxygen content difference may be widened. Clinical characteristics include pale, cool, clammy skin (often mottled); tachycardia (or, if severe shock, bradycardia)[11,44]; tachypnea; flat, nondistended peripheral veins; decreased jugular venous pulse; decreased urine output; and altered mental status.

Numerous factors may influence the development and hemodynamic characteristics of hypovolemic shock in humans. Studies in animals and humans have shown a clear relationship between the degree of circulating blood volume loss and clinical response.[45-48] Acute loss of 10% of the circulating blood volume is well tolerated with tachycardia the only obvious sign. CI may be minimally decreased despite a compensatory increase in myocardial contractility. SVR typically increases slightly, particularly if sympathetic stimulation augments MAP. Compensatory mechanisms begin to fail with a 20% to 25% volume loss. Mild-to-moderate hypotension and decreased CI may be present. Orthostasis (with a blood pressure decrease of 10 mm Hg and increased heart rate of 20 to 30 beats per minute) may become apparent. There is a marked elevation in SVR, and serum lactate may begin to increase. With decreases of the circulating volume of 40% or more,

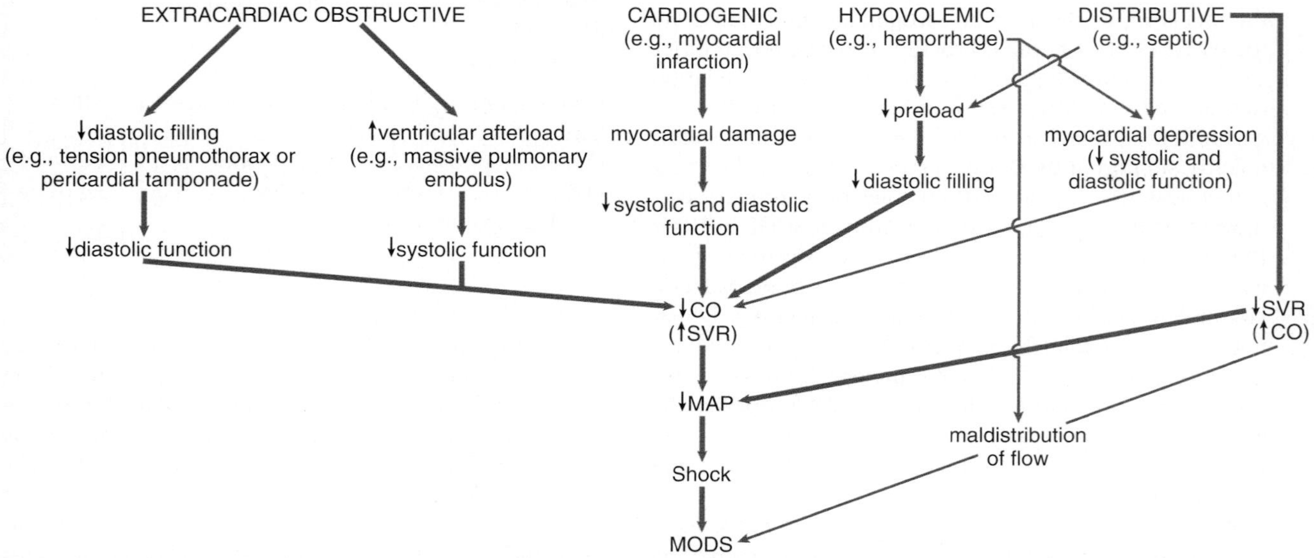

Figure 22-1. The inter-relationships between different forms of shock. For cardiogenic, hypovolemic, and obstructive shock, hypotension is primarily due to decreased cardiac output (CO) with systemic vascular resistance (SVR) increasing secondarily. With distributive (and particularly septic) shock, hypotension is primarily due to a decrease in SVR with a secondary increase of CO. In many forms of shock, the hemodynamic characteristics are influenced by elements of hypovolemia, myocardial depression (ischemic or otherwise), and vascular dysfunction (which may affect afterload). Dominant pathophysiologic pathways are denoted by *heavier lines.* MAP, mean arterial blood pressure; MODS, multiple organ dysfunction syndrome.

Box 22-2

Classification of Shock

Hypovolemic (Oligemic)
- Hemorrhagic
  - Trauma
  - Gastrointestinal
  - Retroperitoneal
- Fluid depletion (nonhemorrhagic)
  - External fluid loss
    - Dehydration
    - Vomiting
    - Diarrhea
    - Polyurea
  - Interstitial fluid redistribution
    - Thermal injury
    - Trauma
    - Anaphylaxis
- Increased vascular capacitance (venodilation)
  - Sepsis
  - Anaphylaxis
  - Toxins/drugs

Cardiogenic
- Myopathic
  - Myocardial infarction
    - Left ventricle
    - Right ventricle
  - Myocardial contusion (trauma)
  - Myocarditis
  - Cardiomyopathy
  - Post–ischemic myocardial stunning
  - Septic myocardial depression
  - Pharmacologic
    - Anthracycline cardiotoxicity
    - Calcium channel blockers
- Mechanical
  - Valvular failure (stenotic or regurgitant)
  - Hypertrophic cardiomyopathy
  - Ventricular septal defect
- Arrhythmic
  - Bradycardia
    - Sinus (e.g., vagal syncope)
    - Atrioventricular blocks
  - Tachycardia
    - Supraventricular
    - Ventricular

Extracardiac Obstructive
- Impaired diastolic filling (decreased ventricular preload)
  - Direct venous obstruction (vena cava)
    - Intrathoracic obstructive tumors
  - Increased intrathoracic pressure (decreased transmural pressure gradient)
    - Tension pneumothorax
    - Mechanical ventilation (with positive end-expiratory pressure or volume depletion)
  - Decreased cardiac compliance
    - Constrictive pericarditis
    - Cardiac tamponade
      - Acute
        - Post–myocardial infarction free wall rupture
        - Traumatic
        - Hemorrhagic (anticoagulation)
      - Chronic
        - Malignant
        - Uremic
        - Idiopathic
- Impaired systolic contraction (increased ventricular afterload)
  - Right ventricle
    - Pulmonary embolus (massive)
    - Acute pulmonary hypertension
  - Left ventricle
    - Saddle embolus
    - Aortic dissection

Distributive
- Septic (bacterial, fungal, viral, rickettsial)
- Toxic shock syndrome
- Anaphylactic, anaphylactoid
- Neurogenic (spinal shock)
- Endocrinologic
  - Adrenal crisis
- Thyroid storm
- Toxic (e.g., nitroprusside, bretyllium)

marked hypotension with clinical signs of shock is noted. CI and tissue perfusion may decrease to less than half of normal. Lactic acidosis is usually present and predicts a poor outcome.[49,50]

The rate of loss of intravascular volume and the preexisting cardiac reserve is of substantial importance in the development of hypovolemic shock. Although an acute blood loss of 1 L in a healthy adult may result in mild-to-moderate hypotension with a reduced pulmonary wedge pressure (PWP) and CVP,[46] the same loss over a longer time may be well tolerated because of compensatory responses, such as tachycardia, increased myocardial contractility, increased red blood cell 2,3-diphosphoglycerate, and increased fluid retention. A similar slow blood loss may lead to substantial hemodynamic compromise, however, in an individual with a limited cardiac reserve even while the PWP and CVP remain elevated.

Hypovolemic shock represents more than a simple mechanical response to loss of circulating volume. It is a dynamic process involving competing adaptive (compensatory) and maladaptive responses at each stage of development. Although intravascular volume replacement is always a necessary component of resuscitation from hypovolemia or hypovolemic shock, the biologic responses to

Table 22-1. Hemodynamic Profiles of Shock*

Diagnosis	CO	SVR	PWP	CVP	$S\bar{v}O_2$	Comments
Cardiogenic shock						
Caused by myocardial dysfunction	↓↓	↑	↑↑	↑↑	↓	Usually occurs with evidence of extensive myocardial infarction (>40% of left ventricular myocardium nonfunctional), severe cardiomyopathy, or myocarditis
Caused by a mechanical defect						
Acute ventricular septal defect	LVCO ↓↓ RVCO > LVCO	↑	nl or ↑	↑↑	↑ or ↑↑	If shunt is left-to-right, pulmonary blood flow is greater than systemic blood flow; oxygen saturation "step-up" (≥5%) occurs at right ventricular level; ↑ $S\bar{v}O_2$ is caused by left to right shunt
Acute mitral regurgitation	Forward CO ↓↓	↑	↑↑	↑ or ↑↑	↓	Large V waves (≥10 mm Hg) in pulmonary wedge pressure tracing
Right ventricular infarction	↓↓	↑	nl or ↑	↑↑	↓	Elevated right atrial and right ventricular filling pressures with low or normal pulmonary wedge pressures
Extracardiac obstructive shock						
Pericardial tamponade	↓ or ↓↓	↑	↑↑	↑↑	↓	Dip and plateau in right and left ventricular pressure tracings. The right atrial mean, right ventricular end-diastolic, pulmonary artery end-diastolic, and pulmonary wedge pressures are within 5 mm Hg of each other
Massive pulmonary emboli	↓↓	↑	nl or ↓	↑↑	↓	Usual finding is elevated right-sided heart pressures with low or normal pulmonary wedge pressure
Hypovolemic shock	↓↓	↑	↓↓	↓↓	↓	Filling pressures may appear normal if hypovolemia occurs in the setting of baseline myocardial compromise
Distributive shock						
Septic shock	↑↑ or nl, rarely ↓	↓ or ↓↓	↓ or nl	↓ or nl	↑ or ↑↑	The hyperdynamic circulatory state (↑ CO, ↓ SVR) associated with distributive forms of shock usually depends on resuscitation with fluids; before such resuscitation, a hypodynamic circulation is typical
Anaphylaxis	↑↑ or nl, rarely ↓	↓ or ↓↓	↓ or nl	↓ or nl	↑ or ↑↑	

*The hemodynamic profiles summarized in this table refer to patients with the diagnosis listed in the left column who are also in shock (mean arterial blood pressure <60-65 mm Hg).
CO, cardiac output; *CVP*, central venous pressure; *LV*, left ventricular; *nl*, normal; *PWP*, pulmonary wedge pressure; *SVR*, systemic vascular resistance; $S\bar{v}O_2$, mixed venous oxygen saturation; ↑↑ or ↓, mild-to-moderate increase or decrease; ↑↑ or ↓ ↓, moderate-to-severe increase or decrease.
Modified from Parrillo JE: Septic shock: Clinical manifestations, pathogenesis, hemodynamics, and management in a critical care unit. In Parrillo JE, Ayers SM (eds): *Major Issues in Critical Care Medicine.* Baltimore, Williams & Wilkins, 1984.

the insult may progress to the point where such resuscitation is insufficient to reverse the progression of the shock syndrome. Patients who have sustained a greater than 40% loss of blood volume for 2 hours or more may be unable to be effectively resuscitated.[41,45,48] A series of inflammatory mediator, cardiovascular, and organ responses to shock is initiated, which supersede the importance of the initial insult in driving further injury.

Cardiogenic Shock

Cardiogenic shock results from the failure of the heart as a pump (see Box 22-2 and Fig. 22-1). It is the most common cause of in-hospital mortality in patients with Q wave myocardial infarction.[51,52] Hemodynamically, cardiogenic shock is characterized by increased ventricular preload (increased ventricular volumes, PWP, and CVP) (see Table 22-1). Otherwise, hemodynamic characteristics are similar to those for hypovolemic shock (see Table 22-1). In particular, both involve reduced CI, stroke volume index, and ventricular stroke work index with increased SVR. Because of inadequate tissue perfusion, the $S\bar{v}O_2$ is substantially reduced, and the arteriovenous oxygen content difference is increased. The degree of lactic acidosis may predict mortality.[53] Clinically, the specific signs of shock are similar. Signs of congestive heart failure (volume overload) are typically present in cardiogenic shock, however. The jugular and peripheral veins may be distended. An S_3 and evidence of pulmonary edema are usually found.

Cardiogenic shock is most commonly due to ischemic myocardial injury with a total of 40% of the myocardium nonfunctional.[52,54-56] Such damage may involve a single large myocardial infarction or may involve accumulation of damage from multiple infarctions. In addition, viable but dysfunctional "stunned" myocardium may contribute temporarily to cardiogenic shock postinfarction. Cardiogenic shock usually involves an anterior myocardial infarction with left main or proximal left anterior descending artery occlusion. Historically, the incidence of cardiogenic shock secondary to Q wave infarction has ranged from 8% to 20%.[51,57,58] Although more recent, large studies show lower incidence rates (4% to 7%) when patients receive thrombolytic interventions,[58-62] retrospective community studies suggest no overall decrease in incidence of postinfarction cardiogenic shock over the last 2 decades.[51] No trials have shown that thrombolytic therapy reduces mortality rates in patients with established cardiogenic shock.[62,63] In contrast, two major studies (one prospective) suggest that mortality of infarction-related cardiogenic shock may be improved by emergent angioplasty.[62,64,65] Despite the availability of thrombolytics and emergent angioplasty, however, the overall mortality for cardiogenic shock has remained unchanged (70% to 90%).[51]

Mortality is better for cardiogenic shock secondary to surgically remediable cardiac lesions. Mitral valve failure may be associated with rupture or dysfunction of chordae or papillary muscles owing to myocardial ischemia or infarction, endocarditis, blunt chest trauma, or prosthetic valve deterioration and is characterized by v waves of greater than 10 mm Hg on a PWP tracing. Ischemic papillary muscle rupture frequently occurs 3 to 7 days after an infarct in left anterior descending coronary artery territory and may be preceded by the onset of a mitral regurgitant murmur.[66] Mortality is high in the absence of surgical therapy.[66] Acute aortic valve failure is most commonly due to endocarditis, but may involve mechanical failure of prosthetic valves or aortic dissection. Ventricular septal defects caused by myocardial infarction also may result in the abrupt onset of cardiogenic shock and can be diagnosed by a 5% step up in hemoglobin oxygen saturation between the right atrium and the pulmonary artery (owing to left-to-right shunting of blood through the septum).[67] As with ischemic papillary muscle rupture, rupture of the intraventricular septum is seen most frequently with occlusions of the left anterior descending artery, a few days after infarction.[67]

The pathophysiology of cardiogenic shock secondary to a right ventricular infarction and failure is different than other forms of cardiogenic shock. Although some degree of right ventricular involvement is seen in half of inferior myocardial infarctions, only the largest 10% to 20% result in right ventricular failure and cardiogenic shock.[68] These infarctions usually involve part of the left ventricular wall as well. Isolated infarctions of the right ventricle are rare.[68,69]

Because therapy of this form of shock requires fluid resuscitation and inotropes (rather than vasopressors), differentiation from other causes of cardiogenic shock is crucial. Conditions compromising right ventricular function, such as cardiac tamponade, restrictive cardiomyopathy, constrictive pericarditis, and pulmonary embolus, also are included in the differential diagnosis. Each of these conditions may manifest with some of the typical clinical and hemodynamic findings of right ventricular infarction, including Kussmaul's sign and pulsus paradoxus with elevation and equalization of CVP, right ventricular systolic pressure, pulmonary artery diastolic pressure, and PWP. Prognosis in this form of cardiogenic shock is distinctly better than that of cardiogenic shock resulting from left ventricular infarction[70,71]; however, an inferior infarction with right ventricular injury has a substantially worse prognosis than such an infarction without significant right-sided involvement.[72]

As with hypovolemic shock, many interactions may complicate the development of cardiogenic shock. Optimal cardiac performance in patients with impaired myocardial contractility may occur at substantially higher than normal PWP (20 to 24 mm Hg). Yet patients who develop cardiogenic shock frequently are initially treated with diuretics and may have a degree of hypovolemia (relative to their optimal requirements). Patients should not be diagnosed with cardiogenic shock unless hypotension (MAP $<$ 65 mm Hg) and reduced cardiac output (CI $<$ 2.2 L/min/m^2) coexist with a PWP of greater than 18 mm Hg.[73] Cautious fluid challenge may be required (in the absence of overt pulmonary edema) to increase the PWP to an optimal range. Other interactions include increased right ventricular ischemia owing to decreased right coronary perfusion pressure (MAP decreased, while right ventricular end diastolic pressure is increased) and increased right ventricular afterload owing to pulmonary hypertension. Right ventricular ischemia also may lead to right ventricular dilation, septal shift, and impairment of left ventricular function. Other causes of cardiogenic shock include acute myocarditis, end-stage cardiomyopathy, bradyarrhythmias or tachyarrhythmias, hypertrophic cardiomyopathy with obstruction, and traumatic myocardial contusion (see Box 22-2).

Obstructive Shock

Extracardiac obstructive shock results from an obstruction to flow in the cardiovascular circuit (see Box 22-2 and

Fig. 22-1). Pericardial tamponade and constrictive pericarditis directly impair diastolic filling of the right ventricle. Tension pneumothorax and intrathoracic tumors indirectly impair right ventricular filling by obstructing venous return. Massive pulmonary emboli (two or more lobar arteries with >50% of the vascular bed occluded), nonembolic acute pulmonary hypertension, large systemic emboli (e.g., saddle embolus), and aortic dissection may result in shock owing to increased ventricular afterload.

The characteristic hemodynamic and metabolic patterns are, in most ways, similar to other low output shock states (see Table 22-1). CI, stroke volume index, and stroke work indices are usually decreased. Because tissue perfusion is decreased, the $S\bar{v}O_2$ is low, the arteriovenous oxygen content difference is increased, and serum lactate frequently is elevated. Other hemodynamic parameters depend on the site of the obstruction. Tension pneumothorax and mediastinal tumors may obstruct the great thoracic veins resulting in a hemodynamic pattern (decreased CI and elevated SVR) similar to hypovolemia (although distended jugular and peripheral veins may be seen). Cardiac tamponade typically causes increased and equalized right and left heart ventricular diastolic pressures, pulmonary artery diastolic pressure, CVP, and PWP. In constrictive pericarditis, right and left ventricular diastolic pressures are elevated and within 5 mm Hg of each other. Mean right and left atrial pressures may or may not be equal as well. Massive pulmonary embolus results in right ventricular failure with elevated pulmonary artery and right heart pressures while PWP remains normal. A systemic saddle embolus or aortic occlusion secondary to dissection causes peripheral hypotension and signs of left ventricular failure, including elevated PWP. Clinical signs similarly depend on the site of the obstruction.

As with other forms of shock, the time course of development of the insult has a substantial impact on the clinical response. Ischemic rupture of the left ventricular free wall (usually 3 to 7 days after myocardial infarction) leads to immediate cardiac tamponade and shock with 150 mL blood in the pericardium.[74-76] Survival requires emergency surgery.[75,76] Similar situations may develop with bleeding into the pericardium after blunt chest trauma or thrombolytic therapy. Pericardial tamponade secondary to malignant or inflammatory pericardial effusions usually develops much more slowly. Although shock may still develop, it usually requires substantially more pericardial fluid (1 to 2 L) to cause critical failure of right ventricular diastolic filling.[74] Similarly, in patients without preexisting cardiopulmonary disease, a massive embolus involving two or more lobar arteries and 50% to 60% of the vascular bed[77,78] may result in obstructive shock. If recurrent smaller pulmonary emboli result in right ventricular hypertrophy, however, a substantially larger total occlusion of the pulmonary vascular bed may be required to cause right ventricular decompensation. More recent analyses have suggested that the presence of shock secondary to pulmonary embolus (regardless of underlying chronic cardiopulmonary dysfunction) indicates a threefold to sevenfold increase in mortality risk with most deaths occurring within 1 hour of presentation. Shock secondary to pulmonary embolism is an indication for urgent thrombolysis.[79,80]

Distributive Shock

The defining feature of distributive shock is loss of peripheral resistance. Septic shock is the most common form and has the greatest impact on intensive care unit (ICU) morbidity and mortality.

Hemodynamically, distributive shock is characterized by an overall decrease in SVR (see Table 22-1). Resistance in any specific organ bed or tissue may be decreased, increased, or unchanged, however. Initially, CI may be depressed, and ventricular filling pressures may be decreased. After fluid resuscitation, when filling pressures are normalized or increased, CI is usually elevated. As a result of hypotension, left and right ventricular stroke work indices are normally decreased. $S\bar{v}O_2$ is increased above normal. Concomitantly, arteriovenous oxygen content difference is narrowed despite the fact that oxygen demand is usually increased (particularly in sepsis). The basis of these phenomena may be that although total body perfusion (CI) is increased, perfusion is ineffective in that either it does not reach the necessary tissues or the tissues cannot use the substrates presented. As a reflection of this inadequate "effective" tissue perfusion, lactic acidosis may ensue. In contrast to the other forms of shock, clinical characteristics of resuscitated distributive shock include warm, well-perfused extremities, a decreased diastolic blood pressure, and an increased pulse pressure. Nonspecific signs of shock include tachycardia, tachypnea, decreased urine output, and altered mentation. In addition, evidence of the primary insult may exist (urticaria for anaphylaxis, spinal injury for neurogenic shock, and evidence of infection in septic shock).

Septic shock, the leading cause of ICU mortality,[81] is caused by the systemic activation of the inflammatory cascade (see Box 22-2). Numerous mediators, including cytokines, kinins, complement, coagulation factors, and eicosanoids, are activated or systemically released, resulting in profound disturbances of cardiovascular and organ system function.[81] These mediators, particularly tumor necrosis factor (TNF)-α, interleukin (IL)-1, platelet-activating factor (PAF), and prostaglandins, are thought to mediate reduced peripheral vascular resistance seen in septic shock.

Loss of vascular autoregulatory control may explain some of the typical metabolic findings of sepsis and septic shock. An early theory postulated the existence of microanatomic shunts between the arterial and venous circulations. During sepsis, these shunts were said to result in decreased SVR and increased $S\bar{v}O_2$.[82] Although microanatomic shunting has been noted in localized areas of inflammation, however, systemic evidence of this phenomenon in sepsis and septic shock is lacking.[82-86] "Functional" shunting as a result of defects of microcirculatory regulation in sepsis also has been suggested.[87,88] Overperfusion of tissues with low metabolic requirements would result in increased $S\bar{v}O_2$ and narrowing of the arteriovenous oxygen content difference. Relative vasoconstriction of vessels supplying more metabolically active tissues would result in tissue hypoxia and lactate production owing to anaerobic metabolism. Observations that some capillary beds may be occluded by platelet microaggregates, leukocytes, fibrin deposits, and endothelial damage support this theory.[83,87,89] Additional support comes from studies that show evidence of oxygen supply–dependent oxygen consumption in sepsis.[90-94] A third theory suggests that circulating mediators cause an intracellular metabolic defect involving substrate use, which results in bioenergetic failure (decreased high-energy phosphate production) and lactate production.[95,96] Increased $S\bar{v}O_2$ could be explained by perfusion, which is increased in excess of tissue oxygen use capability. More recent animal studies using nuclear magnetic resonance spectroscopy show, however, that high-energy phosphates are not depleted in septic animals, as is expected in all of these theories.[97-99] According to these and other studies, cellular ischemia is not the dominant factor in metabolic dysfunction in sepsis.[97-103] Rather, circulating mediators may result in cellular dysfunction, aerobic glycolysis, and lactate production in the absence of global ischemia.[98] This position is weakened by data suggesting that increased lactate in septic shock also is associated with decreased pH (which would not be expected in aerobic glycolysis)[98] and, to some extent, by studies that support the existence of oxygen supply–dependent oxygen consumption in sepsis.[91-94]

The trigger for systemic activation of the inflammatory cascade is gram-negative bacilli in 50% to 75% of cases of septic shock. Gram-positive bacteria account for most of the remainder, but infection with fungi, protozoa, and viruses also can result in septic shock.[104-106] More recent investigations suggest a surprising commonality of signaling mechanisms in septic shock via Toll-like receptors from a broad range of etiologic agents.[107-111] Despite aggressive supportive care and antibiotic treatment, mortality is 50% overall and may exceed 70% for gram-negative septic shock.[104] Of deaths due to septic shock, approximately 75% are early deaths (within 1 week of shock), primarily as a result of hyperdynamic circulatory failure.[112] Late mortality is usually due to MODS.[112]

More than any other form of shock, distributive, particularly septic, shock involves substantial elements of the hemodynamic characteristics of other shock categories (see Fig. 22-1 and Table 22-1). As noted, all forms of distributive shock involve decreased mean peripheral vascular resistance. Before fluid resuscitation, distributive shock also involves a relative hypovolemic component. The first element of this relative hypovolemia is an increase of the vascular capacitance owing to venodilation. This phenomenon has been directly supported in animal models of sepsis[113-117] and is reinforced by the fact that clinical hypodynamic septic shock (low cardiac output) usually can be converted to hyperdynamic shock (high cardiac output) with adequate fluid resuscitation.[112,118,119] Relaxation of vascular smooth muscle is attributed to many of the mediators known to circulate during sepsis. These same mediators also contribute to the second cause of hypovolemia in sepsis, third spacing of fluid to the interstitium owing to loss of endothelial integrity. In addition, numerous studies have shown that human septic shock is characterized by myocardial depression (biventricular dilation and decreased ejection fraction).[36-38] Circulating substances such as TNF-α, IL-1, PAF, leukotrienes, and, most recently, IL-6 have been implicated in this process.[120-127]

Anaphylactic shock is a form of distributive shock caused by release of mediators from tissue mast cells and circulating basophils. Anaphylaxis, an immediate hypersensitivity reaction, is mediated by the interaction of IgE antibodies on the surface of mast cells and basophils with the appropriate antigen. Antigen binding results in release of the primary mediators of anaphylaxis contained in the basophilic granules of mast cells and basophils. These include histamine, serotonin, eosinophil chemotactic factor, and various proteolytic enzymes.[128] Subsequently, many secondary lipid mediators are synthesized and released, including PAF, bradykinin prostaglandins, and leukotrienes (slow reacting substance of anaphylaxis).[128] An anaphylactoid reaction (clinically indistinguishable from anaphylaxis) results from direct, nonimmunologic release of mediators from mast cells and basophils and can lead to shock.

Anaphylaxis is triggered by insect envenomations (Hymenoptera [bees, hornets, and wasps]) and certain drugs, especially antibiotics (β-lactams, cephalosporins, sulfonamides, and vancomycin).[128] In addition, less frequently, heterologous serum (e.g., tetanus antitoxin, snake antitoxin, antilymphocyte antisera), blood transfusion, immunoglobulin (particularly in IgA-deficient patients), and egg-based vaccine products have been implicated.[128] Anaphylactoid reactions can be caused by a wide range of medical agents, including ionic contrast media, protamine, opiates, polysaccharide volume expanders such as dextran and hydroxyethyl starch, muscle relaxants, and anesthetics.[128]

The hemodynamic features of anaphylactic shock are similar to septic shock and include elements of hypovolemia (owing to interstitial edema and venodilation) and myocardial depression.[129-133] Cardiac output and ventricular filling pressures may be reduced until patients are fluid resuscitated.[133,134] In addition to typical findings of shock, patients may have urticaria, angioedema, laryngeal edema, and severe bronchospasm.

Neurogenic shock involves loss of peripheral vasomotor control secondary to dysfunction or injury of the nervous system. The classic example is shock associated with spinal injury. A similar phenomenon is active in vasovagal syncope and spinal anesthesia, but such conditions are self-limited and transient. The major cause of shock in spinal injury seems to be loss of venous tone resulting in increased venous capacitance. Arteriolar tone also may be affected resulting in increased cardiac output after fluid resuscitation.

Adrenal crisis (see also Chapter 60) is an uncommon cause of shock that can be difficult to diagnose because it occurs in patients with other active disease processes, and the clinical features may mimic infection. It is a life-threatening emergency that requires prompt diagnosis and management. Adrenal crisis is caused by a deficiency of adrenal production of mineralocorticoids and glucocorticoids. It may occur de novo in patients with critical illness or may occur against a background of occult adrenal insufficiency. In the critical care setting, the most common cause of de novo acute adrenal insufficiency is bilateral adrenal hemorrhage in association with overwhelming infections (classically meningococcal, but frequently gram-negative bacteria), human immunodeficiency virus infection, or anticoagulation.[135,136] In addition, fungal infections, such as histoplasmosis, blastomycosis, and coccidioidomycosis, and malignant infiltration of the adrenals may cause acute adrenal insufficiency in ICU patients.[136] In some patients, steroid production remains adequate for the baseline state despite adrenal disease. When stressed, however, adrenal response is inadequate, leading to decompensation and adrenal crisis. Stressors may be relatively innocuous or may be severe. A febrile illness, infection, trauma, surgery, dehydration, or any other intercurrent illness may trigger the crisis. Abrupt cessation of glucocorticoid therapy or replacement also may result in adrenal crisis.

Symptoms are generally nonspecific and may include anorexia, nausea, vomiting, diarrhea, abdominal pain, myalgia, joint pains, headache, weakness, confusion, and agitation or delirium.[136,137] Fever (often out of proportion to any minor infection) is almost always present, and hypotension, initially caused by hypovolemia, is frequent.[136] The initial hemodynamic pattern may resemble hypovolemic shock (if shock is due only to adrenal crisis). With volume resuscitation, a high-output, vasopressor-refractory shock may become apparent.[138,139]

Shock secondary to adrenal crisis may be masked by or contribute to shock resulting from other concomitant critical illness, particularly septic shock. If vasopressor-refractory shock occurs in patients potentially predisposed to adrenal insufficiency, a cortisol level and rapid adrenocorticotropic hormone stimulation test must be performed, and the patient must be given glucocorticoids and other therapy.

More recently, an unrecognized "relative" adrenal insufficiency has been implicated in the pathogenesis of human septic shock.[140-144] In this circumstance, sepsis is associated with a suboptimal adrenal response with an improvement in cardiovascular parameters or outcome or both with "stress dose" corticosteroid administration.[140,142,143,145,146] One randomized controlled trial suggested that prospective stress dose therapy with a combination of hydrocortisone (50 mg intravenously every 6 hours) and fludrocortisone (50 μg orally or via nasogastric tube daily) for 7 days improved outcome in nonresponders to corticotropin challenge.[147,148] In another study of severe community-acquired pneumonia, hydrocortisone infusion was shown to be associated with reduced hospital length of stay.[148] However, the ideal test for determination of adrenal insufficiency has yet to be determined.[141,144]

PATHOGENESIS AND PATHOPHYSIOLOGY

The inability of cells to obtain or use oxygen in sufficient quantity optimally to meet their metabolic requirements has classically been considered to be the pathophysiologic basis of all forms of shock. In the first half of the 20th century, the study of shock focused on the relatively distinct hemodynamic physiology that characterizes the different forms of shock. Since then, evidence has accumulated that the various types of clinical shock have significant overlap in their hemodynamic characteristics. In parallel, shock of most etiologies has been shown to involve similar biochemical and metabolic pathways. This section reviews the pathophysiology and pathogenesis of shock from the hemodynamic to the molecular level.

Hemodynamic Basis of Shock

From a hemodynamic perspective, shock is the failure of cardiovascular adaptation to systemic dyshomeostasis induced by trauma, infection, or other insult such that cardiac output or blood pressure or both are compromised. This failure is manifested by inadequate organ and tissue perfusion. Although effective perfusion also depends on microcirculatory and intracellular factors (see Box 22-1), the hemodynamic aspects of shock can be described in part by the contributions of cardiac and arterial vascular function to blood pressure and cardiac output.

Arterial Pressure

Although cardiac output may be expressed as a function of MAP and vascular resistance (CO = [MAP − CVP]/SVR), cardiac output is not directly dependent on MAP in most physiologic states. Instead, blood pressure typically depends on cardiac output and vascular resistance. Blood pressure does provide a mechanism, however, to sense cardiac output and global perfusion perturbations indirectly for autoregulatory purposes.

The ability of all organ vascular beds to support normal blood flow depends on maintenance of blood pressure within the defined range for that organ (Fig. 22-2).[149] Vital organs, such as the brain and heart in particular, are able to autoregulate blood flow over a wide range of blood pressures. Failure to maintain the minimal MAP and perfusion pressure required for autoregulation during hypodynamic circulatory shock indicates a severe reduction in

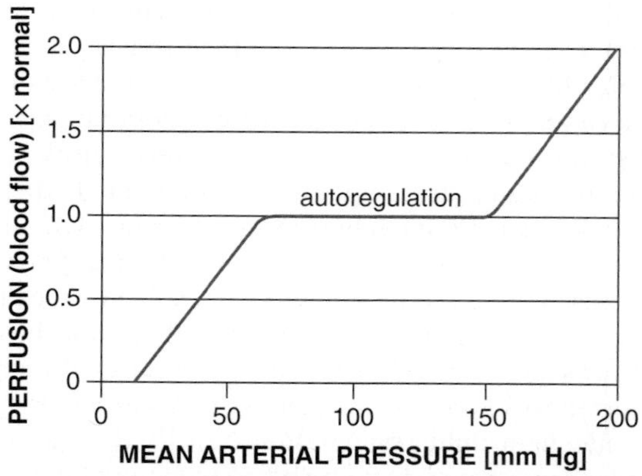

Figure 22-2. Idealized representation of blood flow autoregulation. Within the autoregulatory range of blood pressure for a tissue or organ, perfusion can be held relatively constant. Outside this range, autoregulation fails, and perfusion becomes a function of mean arterial pressure.

cardiac output. Pharmacologic support of blood pressure in such situations (with α-adrenergic agonists) usually results in decreased total systemic perfusion as sensitive vascular beds constrict, and overall vascular resistance increases. Because of their strong autoregulatory capacity, however, vital organs maintain increased perfusion under these conditions.

In addition to sufficient cardiac output, effective perfusion requires appropriate distribution of blood flow. Failure to maintain blood pressure within the autoregulatory range results in distribution of blood flow that is strictly dependent on the passive mechanical properties of the vasculature.[150] Inappropriate distribution of perfusion between and within tissues and organs may result. Late hemorrhagic shock has been shown to be characterized by abnormal microvascular flow with dilation of precapillary sphincters.[41]

Cardiac Output

The fact that total systemic perfusion is defined by cardiac output underlies its importance in shock. The product of heart rate and stroke volume determines cardiac output ($CO = HR \times SV$). Stroke volume (a measure of myocardial performance) depends on preload, afterload, and contractility.

Preload represents the extent of precontraction myocardial fiber (or sarcomere) stretch. In vivo, preload is the end diastolic ventricular volume. Because measurement of such volumes in the clinical context is difficult, intracardiac pressures, which can be determined more easily, are frequently substituted. There are difficulties with this approach. The relationship of ventricular end diastolic volume (preload) to end diastolic pressure is nonlinear. Alterations of myocardial compliance render CVP and PWP unreliable as estimates of preload in critically ill patients.[151]

Preload depends on circulating volume, venous tone, atrial contraction, and intrathoracic pressure among other factors.[149,152] Atrial contraction is particularly important in patients with impaired ventricular function. Although accounting for only 5% to 10% of cardiac output in healthy humans, synchronized atrial contraction contributes 40% to 50% of the cardiac output in patients with severe left ventricular dysfunction.[152] Increased intrathoracic pressure or increased venous capacitance affect preload by reducing venous return.[149,153] Nitrovasodilators such as nitroglycerin may decrease cardiac output despite arteriolar vasodilation owing to their venodilatory (decreased preload) effects. Conversely, the earliest increases in cardiac output seen with sympathetic stimulation and exogenous catecholamine infusion are related to venoconstriction-induced increases of venous return and preload.[154] Cardiogenic and some forms of obstructive shock are typically characterized by increased preload. Preresuscitation distributive shock and hypovolemic shock are uniformly associated with decreased preload.

Afterload refers to the total resistance to ejection of blood from the ventricle during contraction. Increasing afterload results in decreased extent and velocity of myocardial contraction. Excessive afterload (aortic dissection, pulmonary embolus) causes some forms of obstructive shock. Ex vivo, afterload can be easily defined as a resistive force applied to an isolated papillary muscle. Because the heart does not displace a fixed mass, but rather rhythmically moves a viscous, non-newtonian fluid through branching viscoelastic conduits, the definition of afterload in vivo is difficult.

Afterload has been suggested to be equivalent to systolic myocardial wall stress. This definition suggests that afterload is substantially dependent on intrinsic cardiac mechanical and functional properties.[155] An alternative approach equates left ventricular afterload with the mechanical properties of the arterial side of the circulatory system. Aortic input impedance, which represents the total resistance to flow from outside the left ventricle, is determined by the inertial and viscous properties of blood and the resistive and viscoelastic properties of the arterial system. The term is inclusive of SVR, heart rate effects, and pulse wave reflections in the arterial tree.[155] Although an accurate measure of afterload in pulsatile systems, assessment of impedance is technically difficult requiring continuous harmonic analysis of rhythmic variations of aortic pressure and flow. SVR is a limited approximation of aortic input impedance based on a model that assumes nonpulsatile flow. At a heart rate of 0, SVR and aortic input impedance are equivalent. From a clinical point of view, SVR is the most practical way of assessing afterload.

Afterload is increased in pathologic conditions such as aortic stenosis, systemic embolism, and hypertension. Vasopressors, including α-agonists (e.g., phenylephrine, norepinephrine) and vasopressin, also increase afterload, whereas nitrates and other vasodilator agents decrease it. Increased intrathoracic pressure owing to mechanical ventilation and positive end-expiratory pressure decrease left ventricular afterload, while increasing right ventricular afterload. Hypodynamic shock and hyperdynamic shock usually are characterized by increased and decreased afterload.

Contractility refers to the intrinsic ability of myocardial fibers to shorten under given loading conditions. Under normal conditions, determinants of contractility include myocardial mass and sympathoadrenal activation state. In pathologic states (e.g., shock), hypoperfusion-ischemia, myocardial cell injury (e.g., reperfusion injury, myocarditis), acidosis, and circulating myocardial depressant substances (such as seen in sepsis) depress cardiac contractility (Fig. 22-3).

As with preload and afterload, the ex vivo/in vitro assessment of contractility is straightforward. Assessment of in vivo contractility (even in experimental animals) is substantially more difficult because of intrinsic lability of preload and afterload. Relatively load-independent variables, such as peak systolic pressure–to–end systolic volume ratio, may be the most clinically useful measures of contractility.[156] Many of these variables can be obtained echocardiographically.

Venous Function in Shock

Given that the cardiovascular circuit is a closed system, and cardiac output cannot exceed the rate of return of

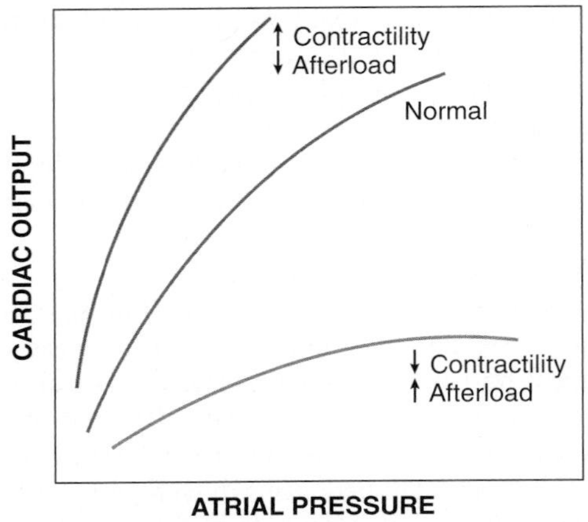

Figure 22-3. Cardiac function curve showing the effect of variations of preload (atrial pressure), contractility, and afterload on cardiac performance.

blood to the right ventricle, venous return can be considered a fundamental determinant of cardiac performance. Although preload is a related variable, it primarily reflects ventricular properties related to compliance and heart rate, whereas venous return is substantially dependent on the extracardiac properties of the systemic venous circulation. Maximal venous return is described by the equation:

$$(Pmc - Pa)/Rv \qquad \text{(Equation 1)}$$

where Pmc is the mean circulatory pressure (the upstream driving pressure of the systemic venous circulation, i.e., the intravascular pressure measured when the heart is stopped), Pa is the right atrial pressure (the downstream pressure, which opposes flow to the right ventricle), and Rv is the venous resistance (resistance of the conduit to flow). Pmc equals the stressed volume or Vs (portion of the vascular volume that contributes to venous pressure) divided by the mean vascular compliance (C):

$$Pmc = Vs/C \qquad \text{(Equation 2)}$$

Stressed volume depends on total vascular volume (Vt) and the state of venous tone (i.e., venoconstriction). It is defined as the difference between Vt and the unstressed vascular volume (Vo), the intravascular volume that remains when the vascular circuit is equalized to atmospheric pressure (i.e., the volume remaining after passive exsanguinations). Data show that stressed volume is approximately 30% of total blood volume in humans and in experimental animals.[157-159] Compliance refers to the total elastic properties of the entire cardiovascular circuit including the heart and vasculature.

As can be seen in Equation 1, the only direct role the heart plays in venous return is by altering right atrial pressure (Pa). MAP has no direct effect at all despite the fact that it is closely related to cardiac output in the systemic circulation ($MAP - CVP = CO \times SVR$).

Rapid alterations of venous return typically are mediated by changes of Pmc or Rv. Pmc is acutely influenced by changes of Vs, either directly through alterations of venous capacitance, which primarily involves changes of small vein and venular tone (exogenous vasopressors or vasodilators, sympathetic stimulation), or indirectly by changes of Vt (volume depletion or infusion). Compliance is substantially a passive mechanical property of the vasculature and does not cause acute alterations of Pmc or venous return. Venous resistance (Rv) to flow is acutely altered by changes of the caliber of large-diameter veins, particularly the vena cava and great veins of the thorax. Although resistance resides primarily in large veins and the vena cava, and venous capacitance resides primarily in small veins and venules, all veins contribute to resistance and capacitance to some extent. Alterations of venous tone (either pharmacologic or physiologic) tend to induce opposing changes in Pmc and Rv with respect to venous return. Vasodilation decreases Pmc by decreasing stressed volume, but also decreases Rv. Vasoconstriction results in increases of Pmc and Rv. Only alterations in Vt alter Pmc without affecting Rv.

The venous return relationship is shown in Figure 22-4.[149,160,161] Because the systemic venous bed comprises the bulk of venous capacitance, the systemic venous vasculature dominates the physiology of venous return. Venous return is linearly related to Pa (right atrial pressure) down to 0 cm H_2O (= atmospheric pressure), at which point intermittent collapse of the great veins results in limitation of return producing the plateau.[149,162] The slope of the line representing venous return is the inverse of the resistance (1/Rv). The ordinate intercept denotes the right atrial pressure (Pa) at which venous return is zero. According to Equation 1, venous return is zero only when right atrial pressure (Pa) equals the Pmc. The intercept of the atrial pressure axis represents Pmc. Changes of Pmc shift the curve to the left or right without changing the slope of the line (see Fig. 22-4, line *a* to line *b* and *c*). Changes of Rv change the slope of the line without changing the Pmc (see Fig. 22-4, line *a* to line *d* and *e*).

Graphic Analysis of Venous-Cardiac Interactions during Shock

In a closed system, cardiac output as determined by heart rate, preload, afterload, and contractility must equal venous return as determined by mean circulatory pressure, right atrial pressure, and venous resistance. Cardiac output is not strictly a product of cardiac or vascular function, but depends on their interaction. Because venous return and cardiac output are equal and depend on atrial pressure, the right heart Starling function curves can be superimposed on the systemic venous return curves using the same graphic parameters. The intersection of the two curves defines cardiac output and venous return for any given set of conditions involving the right heart and the systemic venous circulation. The circulatory physiology of shock can be described by the interaction of cardiac function and venous return curves.

Cardiogenic shock and obstructive shock secondary to increased afterload of the right or left ventricle result in a common change of the right ventricular Starling function curves. In the case of primary left ventricular loading or damage, this occurs because increased left ventricular filling pressures are passively transmitted to the right

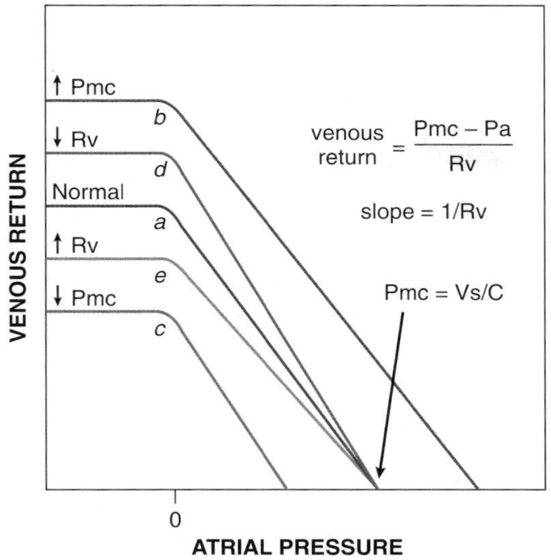

Figure 22-4. Graphic representation of venous return with varying atrial pressures (Pa), mean circulatory pressures (Pmc), and venous resistance (Rv). Altering mean circulatory pressure displaces the line representing venous return (line *a* to line *b* or *c*) without changing the slope (which represents venous resistance to flow). Altering venous resistance changes the slope of the venous return curve (line *a* to line *d* or *e*) without changing the intercept point of the venous return line with the ordinate (which defines mean circulatory pressure). See text for details.

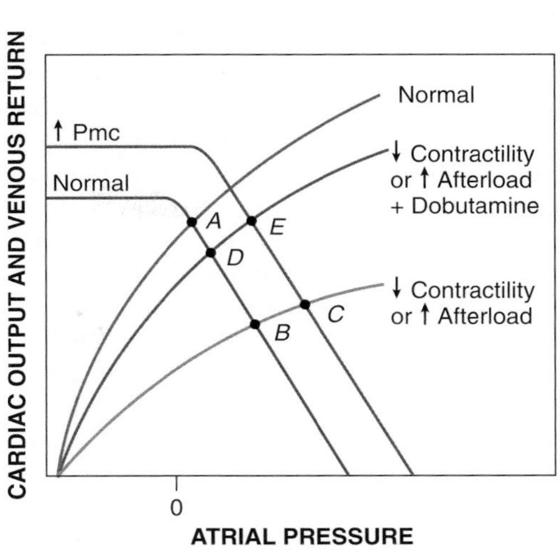

Figure 22-5. Graphic representation of systemic venous return–right heart performance interactions during cardiogenic shock (point *A* to *B*) and therapy (see text for details).

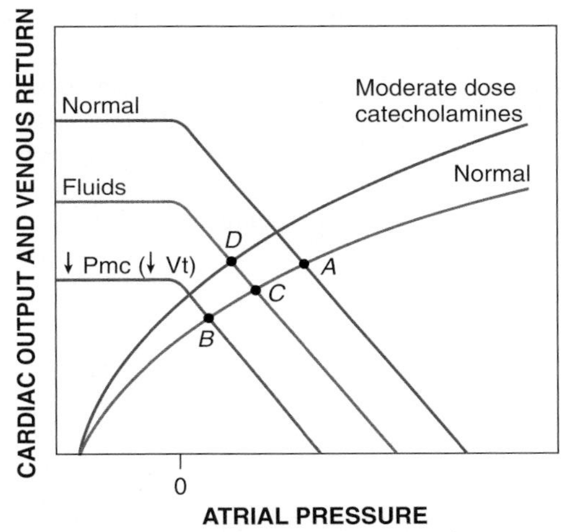

Figure 22-6. Graphic representation of systemic venous return–right heart performance interactions during hypovolemic shock (point *A* to *B*) and therapy (see text for details).

ventricle. The Starling curves are shifted downward and to the right (flatter) (Fig. 22-5, point *A* to *B*) resulting in decreased cardiac output at increased atrial pressures. Therapy can consist of fluid resuscitation (increased Vt and Pmc), which may result in only modest augmentation of cardiac output despite significant increases of atrial pressures and ventricular filling pressures (point *C*); dobutamine, a β_1- and β_2-agonist that increases cardiac output by increasing contractility (point *D*); and fluids and dobutamine (point *E*). Other catecholamines, such as dopamine and norepinephrine, which increase myocardial contractility and reduce venous capacitance, also increase afterload and have variable effects on cardiac output and venous return depending on which effect is dominant. Resistance to therapy may be noted if myocardial damage is sufficiently severe to flatten the Starling function curve to the point that increasing Pmc has little effect on increasing venous return and cardiac output, and insufficient functional myocardium remains to respond to inotropes with increased contractility (a steeper Starling relationship).

Hypovolemic shock results from decreased Vt, Vs, and Pmc (Fig. 22-6, point *A* to *B*). The venous return curve is shifted downward and to the left resulting in a reduced venous return and cardiac output at lower right atrial pressures. Although late depression of myocardial contractility with shift of the Starling function curve downward and to the right (analogous to myocardial depression during cardiogenic shock) has been noted in experimental hemorrhagic shock,[39,40] this phenomenon is not considered here. Volume therapy, whether with crystalloid or colloid, tends to correct Pmc and venous return toward the original value (point *C*). Although optimal therapy of hypovolemic shock involves volume resuscitation, low-dose catecholamines exert similar hemodynamic effects; Pmc and venous return are augmented by an increase of the stressed volume (Vs), whereas the total (reduced from baseline) circulating volume (Vt) is unchanged (also point *C*).[161,163,164] These changes outweigh any deleterious effect on increasing venous resistance (Rv). Cardiac contractility and vascular resistance are minimally affected at these doses. At moderate infusion rates (and with sympathetic stimulation), cardiac contractility also is augmented (point *D*). With higher catecholamine infusion rates, venous resistance and afterload may increase to the point of decreasing cardiac output and venous return (not shown). For that reason, vasopressors must be used with great caution in hypovolemic shock.

Septic shock is especially complicated. Sepsis may involve elements of hypovolemia, myocardial depression, and altered distribution of cardiac output. Total circulating volume (Vt) and stressed volume (Vs) are decreased owing to loss of fluids to the interstitium (third spacing) and owing to insensible losses. Stressed circulating volume (Vs) is decreased further because of active dilation of small venules and veins resulting in increased venous capacitance. This increase in unstressed volume (Vt) and decrease in stressed volume (Vs) has been confirmed in experimental animal models of canine and porcine endotoxemia.[117,165] In unresuscitated septic shock, Pmc is almost universally decreased resulting in reduced venous return and cardiac output (Fig. 22-7, point *A* to *B*). Sepsis also is associated with dilation of large veins and shunting of arterial blood flow to low-resistance (fast time constant) vascular beds, both of which decrease venous resistance and tend to augment venous return. Decreased venous resistance does not fully compensate, however, for decreased Pmc in unresuscitated septic shock. Cardiac output remains depressed (point *B* to *C*). With fluid resuscitation, Pmc may be corrected back toward normal allowing the decreased Rv to be manifested by supernormal cardiac output and venous return (point *D*).[117] Patients with septic shock also develop myocardial depression, which is typically masked by the overall increase in cardiac output (point *E*). In about a fifth of patients, myocardial depression is sufficiently severe, however, that venous return and cardiac output remain depressed even after resuscitation (point *F*).

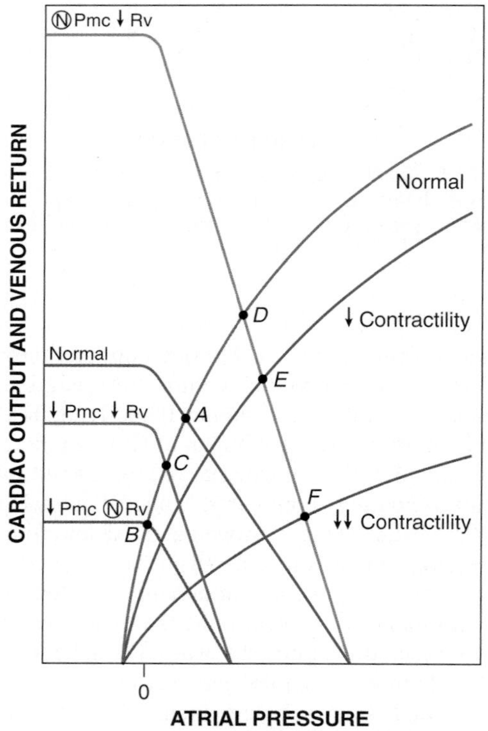

Figure 22-7. Graphic representation of systemic venous return–right heart performance interactions during septic shock (point *A* to *B*) and therapy (see text for details).

More recent human data suggest that sepsis is associated with a decrease of total vascular compliance.[166,167] It is unclear, however, whether this represents a primary septic phenomenon or a neurohumorally mediated compensatory response.[166,168,169] After fluid resuscitation, therapy of septic shock primarily involves catecholamines, such as norepinephrine and dopamine. These affect the venous and cardiac function curves as specified earlier, although some data suggest that vascular and myocardial responsiveness to sympathomimetics may be reduced. In addition, they may affect vascular compliance similar to the potential compensatory neurohumoral effects described previously.

Ventricular function of each distinct form of shock also can be examined by using end-systolic and end-diastolic pressure-volume analysis. Such analysis can be shown graphically using ventricular pressure-volume loops. Changes in stroke volume and ventricular contractility can be examined with respect to ventricular volume and pressure alterations in circulatory shock states. Although this represents a useful approach to the study of circulatory shock physiology, a review of the subject is beyond the scope of this chapter. The interested reader is referred to cogent reviews.[170-172]

Microvascular Function in Shock

Preserved microvascular (vessels <100 to 150 μM diameter) function is a critical determinant of appropriate tissue perfusion during shock. Although adequate cardiac output at sufficient blood pressure is required for appropriate global perfusion and systemic hemodynamics, effective tissue perfusion also requires intact local and systemic microvascular function.

Distribution of cardiac output is a complicated process involving local intrinsic autoregulation and extrinsic regulation mediated by autonomic tone and humoral factors. Blood flow to individual organs may be affected by system-wide changes in microarteriolar tone or by local alterations in metabolic activity. Blood flow within organs also requires microvascular regulation to match blood flow to areas of highest metabolic activity.

Intrinsic control (autoregulation) of blood flow is thought to occur through two mechanisms. Rapid alterations of microvascular tone are mediated through endothelial stretch receptors so that sudden changes in perfusion pressure can be compensated by opposing changes in vascular resistance to maintain perfusion.[173] In addition, increases in metabolic activity within tissues and organs are thought to cause local elevation of various metabolites (e.g., carbon dioxide [CO_2], H^+) resulting in vasodilation and increased perfusion to match substrate demand.[173]

Extrinsic control of vascular tone is exerted primarily through the autonomic nervous system. Parasympathetic release of acetylcholine to blood vessels results in nitric oxide and cyclic guanosine monophosphate (cGMP) generation in endothelial cells and vascular smooth muscle leading to vascular relaxation. Increases of sympathetic tone cause local norepinephrine release, activation of vascular α-adrenoreceptors, and increased vascular tone. Under stress, epinephrine and norepinephrine can be released systemically by sympathetic stimulation of the adrenal medulla. Basal control of blood pressure and flow resides in the activity of the renin-angiotensin system.

Alterations in microvascular function are effected through precapillary and postcapillary sphincters that are sensitive to intrinsic and extrinsic control mechanisms. Because exchange of CO_2, oxygen, and other substrates/metabolites and compartmental regulation of fluids occur at the capillary level, alteration of tone of either sphincter may have varying effects. Opening of non-nutrient capillary sphincters (microanatomic shunts)[82] or increased flow to hypometabolic tissues (functional shunts)[83] results in suboptimal distribution of substrate supply with increased $S\bar{v}O_2$. Failure to dilate sphincters supplying metabolically active tissues may result in ischemia and anaerobic metabolism with lactate production. Increased precapillary tone as seen with sympathetic stimulation results in increased blood pressure systemically and decreased hydrostatic pressure locally. This decreased hydrostatic pressure favors redistribution of volume from the interstitium to the circulation. Increased postcapillary tone (relative to precapillary) results in vascular pooling of blood and loss of fluid to interstitium (owing to increased hydrostatic pressure).

Organ blood flow changes are well characterized in shock states. Autoregulation of blood flow depends on maintenance of blood pressure within a defined range that varies between organs. The autoregulatory capacity of various organs can be determined by mechanically altering blood pressure in the organ vascular bed. With isolated local hypotension, the brain exhibits dominant autoregulatory capability with the ability to maintain blood flow over a wide range of pressures (30 to 200 mm Hg in dogs).[150] Coronary perfusion also is substantially autoregulated between 40 and 100 mm Hg. In contrast, mesenteric and renal blood flow becomes pressure dependent below about 60 mm Hg, whereas the vascular bed of skeletal muscle behaves in a passive manner at pressures outside 50 and 100 mm Hg. Human data suggest that, overall, good autoregulation of blood flow exists in humans between pressures of 60 and 100 mm Hg.[150] In the context of normal physiology, blood flow is not effectively autoregulated outside this range. Without local adaptation, this would result in mismatching of blood flow and metabolic demands, producing organ failure and the metabolic correlates of shock. Extrinsic adaptive mechanisms to protect the most vital organs come into play, however.

During hypovolemia and other hypodynamic forms of shock, extrinsic blood flow regulatory mechanisms overwhelm the autoregulatory response of most vascular beds. Blood flow to the heart and brain is well preserved because of dominant local autoregulation of flow. Blood flow to other organs is reduced relative to the decrease in total cardiac output as organ vascular resistance increases to maintain blood pressure.[174] This effect is mediated partly by sympathetic neural activity and adrenal release of catecholamines.[150,174] This adaptive mechanism maintains perfusion to vital organs at mild-to-moderate levels of reduced cardiac output. If the insult is sufficiently severe or prolonged, organ ischemia and subsequent organ failure may develop. Even if resuscitation restores systemic circulatory hemodynamics, microvascular perfusion abnormalities persist for days.[175] Experimental data suggest that perfusion of brain, kidneys, liver, and other splanchnic organs remains impaired after resuscitation from hemorrhagic shock.[175] Persistence of inadequate matching of tissue substrate demand and delivery after resuscitation of shock can lead to continued ischemia-hypoxia of some tissues. This may explain why hemorrhagic shock–related tissue injury can be irreversible if the duration and severity is excessive. Animal models suggest this irreversible phase severe hemorrhagic shock is characterized by vasodilation of precapillary sphincters.[41]

During sepsis and septic shock, organ blood flow is disturbed at higher MAP, suggesting a primary defect of microvascular function. Cerebral blood flow to the brain in humans has been shown to be depressed even before the onset of septic shock in patients with systemic inflammatory response syndrome.[176] This pathologic vasoconstriction (apparently a unique response of the cerebral circulation to sepsis) does not seem to be the cause of septic encephalopathy. Cerebral autoregulation remains intact during sepsis.[177] The greater decrease in coronary vascular resistance than SVR during human septic shock may suggest that myocardial autoregulation also remains intact despite the fact that, in contrast to the brain, myocardial perfusion is often increased during septic shock.[178,179]

Animal models show that all other vascular beds (splanchnic, renal, skeletal, cutaneous) exhibit decreased vascular resistance, with flow in these beds becoming increasingly dependent on cardiac output. This suggests an active vasodilatory process and failure of extrinsic control of blood flow.[150] Inappropriate levels of splanchnic and skeletal muscle perfusion also are observed in humans during sepsis.[85] Other experimental data suggest that sepsis and septic shock also are associated with aberrant distribution of flow within organs.[83] In sepsis, vasodilation and autoregulatory failure of the microvasculature may be responsible for mismatches of oxygen delivery and demand resulting in anaerobic glycolysis with lactate production despite increased $S\bar{v}O_2$.

During irreversible hemorrhagic shock and septic shock, peripheral vascular failure results in worsened matching of tissue demand and substrate supply, leading to failure of all organs and death. The potential responsible mechanisms include (1) tissue acidosis,[180] (2) catecholamine depletion and mediator-related vascular resistance to catecholamines,[181] (3) release of vasodilating and vasoconstricting arachidonic acid metabolites,[182] (4) decreased sympathetic tone owing to altered central nervous system perfusion,[183] and (5) pathologic generation of nitric oxide by vascular smooth muscle cells (Fig. 22-8).[42,184]

In addition to vasomotor dysfunction, shock is associated with other microvascular pathology. Prime among these is disruption of endothelial cell barrier integrity. The endothelial layer is responsible for maintaining oncotic proteins (mostly albumin) within the circulatory space. During shock, capillary permeability is increased resulting

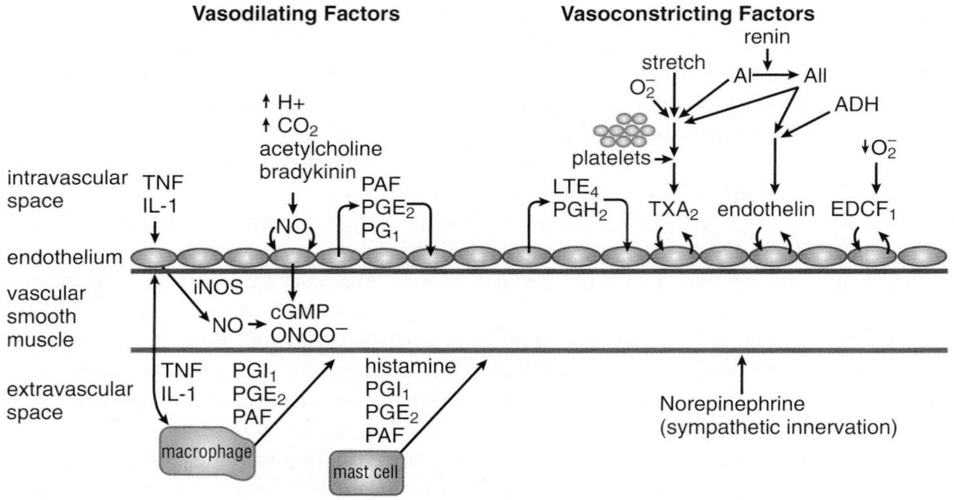

Figure 22-8. Physiologic and pathophysiologic vasoactive factors. ADH, antidiuretic hormone (vasopressin); AI, angiotensin I; AII, angiotensin II; cGMP, cyclic guanosine monophosphate; $EDCF_1$, endothelium-derived contracting factor; IL-1, interleukin-1β; iNOS, inducible nitric oxide synthetase; LTE_4, leukotriene E_4; NO, nitric oxide; O_2^-, superoxide anion; $ONOO^-$, peroxynitrite; PAF, platelet-activating factor; PGE_2, prostaglandin E_2; PGI_2, prostacyclin; PGH_2, prostaglandin H_2; TNF, tumor necrosis factor-α; TXA_2, thromboxane A_2.

in loss of plasma proteins into the interstitium. Endothelial injury, through the action of neutrophil-generated free radicals[185] and nitric oxide/peroxynitrite generation,[186,187] may account for this phenomenon. Release of vasoactive intermediaries, such as histamine, bradykinin, PAF, leukotrienes, and TNF-α, seem to drive this pathologic process. Injury is initiated by leukocyte–endothelial cell interactions via adhesion molecules (integrins, selectins) that allow emigration of neutrophils to the tissues. Blockade of such activity or depletion of neutrophils attenuates tissue injury in animal models of shock.[188] With the loss of plasma proteins, the plasma oncotic pressure decreases, interstitial edema develops, and circulating volume decreases.

There also is evidence of intravascular hemagglutination of red blood cells, white blood cells, and platelets in almost all shock syndromes.[83,189] This may be due to primary microvascular clotting leading to microthrombi. Alternatively, clotting may occur as a consequence of primary endothelial damage secondary to circulating cytokines, free radicals produced by reperfusion and neutrophils, or complement activation. In any case, the result may be further endothelial cell injury, microvascular abnormalities, and inadequate distribution of perfusion within tissues. Decreased deformability of erythrocytes secondary to membrane free radical injury also may play a role in microcirculatory alterations in hemorrhagic and septic shock.[190]

Mechanisms of Cellular Injury in Shock

Shock of all forms involves common cellular metabolic processes that typically end in cell injury, organ failure, and death. The pathogenesis of cellular dysfunction and organ failure as a consequence of shock seems to involve multiple, interrelated factors, including (1) cellular ischemia, (2) circulating or local inflammatory mediators, and (3) free radical injury (Fig. 22-9).

Cellular ischemia and reduced oxygen consumption relative to requirements plays a pivotal role in all hypodynamic shock states and may play a significant role in hyperdynamic shock associated with hypermetabolism. During the stressed, preshock phase of injury, physiologic adaptive mechanisms seem to compensate so that tissue perfusion is unaffected.

During circulatory shock, adaptation is inadequate, and progressive defects of mitochondrial metabolism and adenosine triphosphate (ATP) generation occur. As circulatory inadequacy progresses, and the oxygen supply becomes deficient for tissue metabolic requirements, mitochondrial oxidation of pyruvate (citric acid cycle) is inhibited. This blocks aerobic energy production with resulting anaerobic production of ATP through the cytoplasmic pyruvate-lactate shunt pathway. Anaerobic metabolism yields just 5% of the energy of the aerobic pathway, however, and results in accumulation of lactate (see Fig. 22-10). Acidosis results as available ATP is hydrolyzed with limited resynthesis. When cardiac output cannot be maintained, and tissue perfusion of nonvital, followed by vital, organs is compromised, increasing dependence on anaerobic glycolysis for cellular energy requirements becomes manifest. Intracellular lactate increases, and pH decreases. Essential ATP-dependent intracellular metabolic processes that may be adversely affected include maintenance of transmembrane electrical potential (sodium and potassium transport),[191] mitochondrial function,[192] carbohydrate metabolism,[193] and energy-dependent enzyme reactions. Some vital organs, such as the liver and kidneys, are particularly sensitive, and ATP-dependent processes are rapidly impaired.[191,194-197] Eventually, other organs, including skeletal muscle,

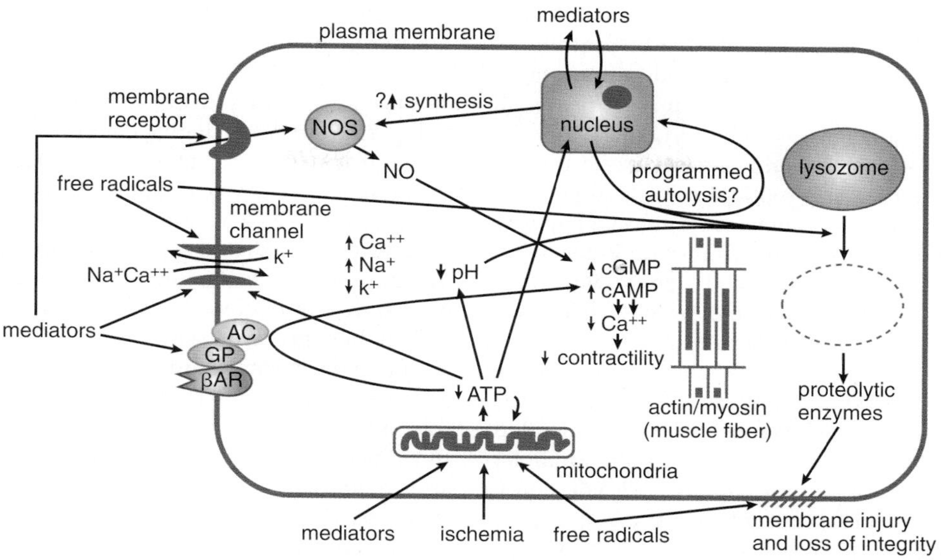

Figure 22-9. Mechanisms of cellular dysfunction and injury in shock. Cell injury is mediated by multiple mechanisms during shock. Tissue ischemia may result in limitation of aerobic adenosine triphosphate (ATP) generation. This results in further mitochondrial impairment owing to deficits of mitochondrial membrane function, altered signal transduction including decreased muscle contractility (ATP is the precursor of cyclic adenosine monophosphate [cAMP]), impaired energy-dependent maintenance of transmembrane potential and ion gradients, increased intracellular pH owing to anaerobic metabolism, and possible initiation of autolytic mechanisms. Free radicals may result in broad injury to cellular membranes causing impaired maintenance of transmembrane potential and ion gradients, mitochondrial generation of ATP, and activation of autolytic pathways involving DNA degradation and lysosomal rupture (apoptosis). Various circulating mediators (including cytokines, kinins, eicosanoids, and complement components) may result in mitochondrial dysfunction, signal transduction abnormalities, membrane protein channel alterations, and possibly alterations of gene expression. Any of these may lead to cell death through metabolic failure and lysozymal enzyme release. βAR, β-adrenergic receptor; cGMP, cyclic guanosine monophosphate; GP, G proteins; NO, nitric oxide; NOS, nitric oxide synthetase.

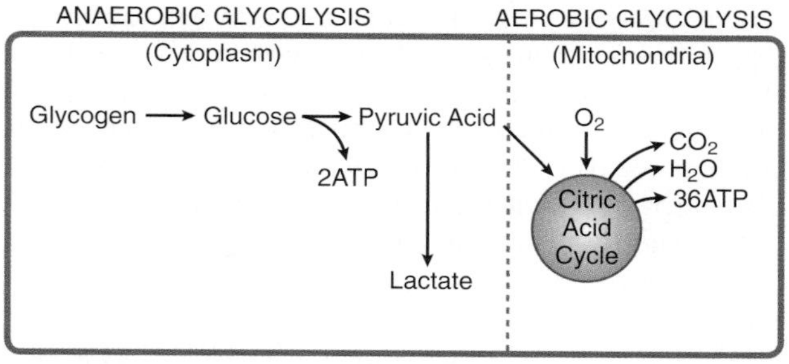

Figure 22-10. Aerobic and anaerobic glucose metabolism. Under anaerobic conditions, pyruvic acid cannot enter the citric acid cycle in the mitochondria (to produce adenosine triphosphate [ATP] optimally) and is shunted to lactate in the cytoplasm. This produces less high-energy phosphates per mole of glucose metabolized. Hydrolysis of ATP molecules in an anaerobic environment results in production of H^+ ions, which cannot be metabolized or cleared resulting in intracellular acidosis. (Adapted from Mizock BA, Falk JL: Lactic acidosis in critical illness. Crit Care Med 1992;20:80.)

become involved. Ultrastructural deterioration of mitochondria becomes apparent.[198] Worsening of shock, organ failure, and death ensue.

In sepsis, tissue ATP levels may initially remain normal, and mitochondrial function may be unaffected. This may suggest that ischemia does not contribute to early septic organ dysfunction.[99,102] Overall normal levels of ATP do not rule out the possibility, however, of patchy, focal deficits within tissues related to inadequately distributed perfusion. Inflammatory microthrombi in the microvasculature may mechanically obstruct microcirculatory flow. This could result in cellular dysfunction owing to persistent focal ischemic areas. Evidence to support ischemia as a contributor to cell dysfunction in sepsis includes evidence of oxygen supply–dependent oxygen consumption, washout of organic acids (from ischemic tissues) into the circulation in patients with sepsis and MODS after treatment with vasodilators, and elevated ATP degradation products with decreased acetoacetate-to-hydroxybutyrate ratio (suggesting altered hepatic mitochondrial redox potential). Based on the totality of evidence, however, the question of whether ischemia plays a role in sepsis pathophysiology remains open. Some newer trends in therapy of septic shock and related states are predicated, however, on concepts developed through this work.[199]

Inflammatory mediator effects on cellular metabolism are of prime importance in organ dysfunction caused by sepsis and septic shock. Circulating inflammatory mediators also may play a substantial role in other forms of shock, including hemorrhagic shock associated with extensive tissue trauma.[200,201] Sepsis and trauma are associated with generalized, systemic activation of the inflammatory response. Resulting cell injury and hypermetabolism may culminate in organ failure. Numerous triggers can result in activation of the inflammatory cascade. The best studied is endotoxin from gram-negative bacteria, but other bacterial antigens and cell injury itself also can initiate the cascade. Macrophage production of cytokines such as TNF-α, IL-1β, and IL-6 seems to be central.

TNF-α is a 51-kD trimeric peptide produced by macrophages in response to a variety of inflammatory stimuli, including bacterial antigens and other cytokines. Circulating levels of TNF-α are transiently elevated soon after the onset of shock (particularly septic shock).[202] Administration of TNF-α to animals or humans results in a hyperdynamic circulatory state (with or without dose-dependent hypotension) similar to untreated sepsis and septic shock.[123] Although clinical trials to date have yielded disappointing results, anti-TNF-α strategies protect animals from experimental endotoxic and septic shock.[203] Among the many effects of TNF-α are release of IL-1, IL-6, IL-8, PAF, leukotrienes, thromboxanes, and prostaglandins; stimulation of production and activity of polymorphonuclear leukocytes; promotion of immune cell adhesion to endothelium; activation of coagulation and complement systems; direct endothelial cell cytotoxicity; depression of myocardial contractility; and fever production by the hypothalamus.[123,204] TNF-α causes alterations of skeletal transmembrane electrical potential similar to those described in hemorrhagic and septic shock.[205] These membrane effects precede hemodynamic alterations, suggesting that TNF-α exerts a primary effect on cell metabolism independent of perfusion alterations. Although TNF-α seems to be of central importance in the pathogenesis of septic shock, it also is known to be elevated in congestive heart failure[206] and hemorrhagic shock.[200]

Other substances are involved in the inflammatory process. These include IL-1β, which can potentiate the in vivo effects of TNF-α; IL-2, which can cause hemodynamic abnormalities in humans; IL-6, which is involved in the acute-phase response and has been implicated in septic myocardial depression; interferon-γ, which promotes the release of other cytokines, enhances adhesion of immune cells, and promotes macrophage activation; IL-10, which is an anti-inflammatory cytokine that limits macrophage generation of proinflammatory cytokines; transforming growth factor-β which is another anti-inflammatory cytokine that, in addition to limiting macrophage proinflammatory responses, blocks the effects of proinflammatory cytokines on target cells; endothelin-1, a cytokine that strongly promotes vasoconstriction, particularly in the renal vascular bed, possibly resulting in renal hypoperfusion and decreased glomerular filtration rate; PAF, which stimulates TNF-α, thromboxane, and leukotriene release, stimulates free radical formation, and alters microvascular permeability; leukotrienes, which release other arachidonic acid metabolites, alter vascular endothelial permeability, and may mediate vascular and myocardial depression in shock; thromboxanes, which may contribute to altered microvascular vasomotor and permeability function; prostaglandins, which produce fever, induce vasodilation, and inhibit thrombus formation; and complement fragments C3a and C5a, which constrict vascular smooth muscle, release histamine, and promote chemotaxis (Table 22-2).[127,204,207]

In recent years, several newly recognized mediators have been shown to have important roles in shock, particularly septic shock. These include most notably macrophage migration inhibitory factor (MIF) and high mobility group 1 protein (HMG-1). MIF has been shown to be produced by monocytes and macrophages after exposure to bacterial toxins, including endotoxin, toxic shock syndrome toxin 1, and streptococcal pyrogenic toxin A, and to proinflammatory cytokines, including TNF-α and interferon-γ.[208] MIF results in expression of other proinflammatory mediators by monocytes/macrophages and activation of T cells. Increased MIF concentrations have been shown in the blood of mice subjected to peritonitis and in humans with septic shock.[209] Injection of MIF during experimental murine *Escherichia coli* peritonitis increases mortality.[209] HMG-1 also seems to have a key role in the pathogenesis of gram-negative sepsis.[210] Mice show increased levels of HMG-1 in serum 8 to 32 hours after endotoxin administration. Patients dying of septic shock also show increased serum HMG-1 levels.[210] Administration of HMG-1 to normal and endotoxin-resistant mice induces dose-dependent mortality with signs consistent with endotoxic shock.[210]

Two other sepsis mediators warrant special mention. A circulating myocardial depressant substance is present in the blood of patients with septic shock who exhibit myocardial depression with biventricular dilation and reduced ventricular ejection fractions.[211] Similar substances have been shown to be present in animal models of hemorrhagic shock.[212] Other data suggest canine myocardial infarction[213] and human cardiogenic shock[214] also may be associated with circulating myocardial depressant substances. Serum from appropriate septic patients or animal models depresses myocardial tissue in vitro.[36,211] Myocardial depressant substances from septic and hemorrhagic shock seem to be dependent on calcium.[215] The substance implicated in human sepsis may represent a synergistic combination of TNF-α and IL-1β that produces depression by inducing myocardial nitric oxide production.[211,216,217] TNF-α and IL-1β are elevated in shock and cause similar depression of myocardial tissue.[216,218] Other data suggest that IL-6 may have a central role.[127,207]

Another important mediator, nitric oxide, has a vital role in normal intracellular signal transduction.[219] Of particular importance to shock, nitric oxide is the mediator through which endothelial cells normally cause relaxation of adjacent smooth muscle.[219] Endothelial cells, through a constitutive nitric oxide synthetase, produce picomolar quantities of nitric oxide in response to numerous vasodilatory mediators, such as acetylcholine and bradykinin. This nitric oxide diffuses to adjacent smooth muscle and activates guanylate cyclase to produce cGMP, which effects vascular relaxation. Nitrovasodilators bypass nitric oxide synthetase to relax smooth muscle directly through the guanylate cyclase pathway. During septic shock, an inducible nitric oxide synthetase capable of producing nanomolar quantities of nitric oxide is generated in vascular smooth muscle.[184,219] Studies also have implicated nitric oxide in late vascular dysfunction seen in hemorrhagic shock.[42] Nitric oxide–mediated generation of cGMP may explain the profound loss of arterial vascular tone and venodilation seen in septic shock[184,220] and may partly

Table 22-2. Inflammatory Mediators in Sepsis and Septic Shock

Mediator	Major Reported Effects
TNF-α	Stimulates release of IL-1β, IL-6, IL-8, platelet-activating factor, leukotrienes, thromboxane A_2, and prostaglandins; may be able to stimulate macrophages directly to promote its own release Stimulates production of polymorphonuclear cells by bone marrow; enhances phagocytic activity of polymorphonuclear cells Promotes adhesion of endothelial cells, polymorphonuclear cells, eosinophils, basophils, monocytes, and occasionally lymphocytes by inducing increased expression of adhesion molecules Activates common pathway of coagulation and complement system Directly toxic to vascular endothelial cells; increases microvascular permeability Acts directly on hypothalamus to produce fever Reduces transmembrane potential of muscle cells and depresses cardiac myocyte contractility Decreases arterial pressure, systemic vascular resistance, and ventricular ejection fraction; increases cardiac output
Interleukins	
IL-1β	Stimulates release of TNF-α, IL-6, IL-8, platelet-activating factor, leukotrienes, thromboxane A_2, and prostaglandins; also may be capable of stimulating its own production Activates resting T cells to produce lymphocytes and other products; supports B cell proliferation and antibody production; is cytotoxic for insulin-producing B cells Promotes adhesion of endothelial cells, polymorphonuclear cells, eosinophils, basophils, monocytes, and occasionally lymphocytes by inducing increased expression of adhesion molecules Promotes polymorphonuclear cell activation and accumulation Increases endothelial procoagulant activity Acts synergistically with TNF-α; enhances tissue cell sensitivity to TNF-α Depresses cardiac myocyte contractility Acts directly on hypothalamus to produce fever
IL-2	May promote release of TNF-α and interferon-γ Decreases arterial pressure, systemic vascular resistance, ejection fraction; increases cardiac output
IL-4	Enhances lymphocyte adhesion to endothelial cells Induces antigen expression on macrophages Synergistically increases TNF-α–induced or IL-1β–induced antigen expression on endothelial cells, but inhibits increased expression of adhesion molecules by TNF-α, IL-1β, or interferon-γ
IL-6	Induces hepatic acute-phase protein response Induces myelomonocytic and terminal B lymphocyte differentiation; activates T cells/thymocytes Possible role in septic myocardial depression Inhibits TNF-α production
IL-8	Chemotactic for neutrophils and lymphocytes; induces tissue infiltration of both Inhibits endothelial-leukocyte adhesion; decreases hyperadhesion induced by those molecules
Interferon-γ	Promotes release of TNF-α, IL-1β, and IL-6 (possibly due to its ability to augment effects of endotoxin on macrophages); augments production of adhesion molecules May act synergistically with TNF-α to produce cytotoxic and cytostatic activity; interacts with other cytokines in variable ways Encourages polymorphonuclear cell activation and accumulation; enhances phagocytic activity of polymorphonuclear cells Promotes macrophage activation, macrophage microbicidal function, and expression of cellular receptors for TNF-α
Endothelin-1	Strongly promotes vasoconstriction
Platelet-activating factor	Stimulates release of TNF-α leukotrienes, thromboxane A_2 Promotes leukocyte activation and subsequent free radical formation Encourages platelet aggregation leading to thrombosis Markedly alters microvascular permeability, promoting microvascular fluid loss Exerts negative inotropic effect on the heart; lowers arterial blood pressure
Leukotrienes	Promote neutrophil chemotaxis and adhesion of neutrophils to endothelium (neutrophils have specific receptors for leukotriene B_4) Increase vascular permeability, either directly or through interaction of neutrophils and endothelial cells Decrease coronary blood flow and myocardial contractility

Continued

Table 22-2. Inflammatory Mediators in Sepsis and Septic Shock—cont'd

Mediator	Major Reported Effects
Thromboxane A_2	Produces vasoconstriction of vascular beds; secondarily promotes release of endothelium-derived relaxing factor and may stimulate prostacyclin production Causes platelet aggregation and neutrophil accumulation Increases vascular permeability; enhances permeability of single-unit and double-unit membranes Produces pulmonary bronchoconstriction
Prostaglandins	
Prostaglandin E_2	Inhibits IL-1β production Stimulates TNF-α release in low concentrations; higher concentrations suppress TNF-α production at dose-dependent level Causes vasodilation and increased blood flow Has beneficial effect on tissue perfusion and may decrease severity of tissue damage Acts synergistically with prostacyclin to increase effects of serotonin and bradykinin on vascular permeability
Prostacyclin (prostaglandin I_2)	Inhibits platelet aggregation and adhesion Causes vasodilation and increased blood flow; in early sepsis, exerts a beneficial effect on tissue perfusion Produces smooth muscle relaxation
Phospholipase A_2	Releases arachidonic acid (precursor of eicosanoids such as leukotrienes, prostaglandins, and thromboxanes) Decreases arterial pressure, systemic vascular resistance, and ventricular ejection fraction; increases cardiac output
Complement fragments	
C3a	Causes mast cell degranulation and vasodilatory mediator release
C5a	Causes smooth muscle contraction and mucus secretion Causes mast cells to degranulate and release vasodilatory mediators Promotes TNF-α release Enhances polymorphonuclear cell activation, migration, adherence, and aggregation Induces capillary leakage May decrease systemic vascular resistance and produce hypotension

IL, interleukin; TNF, tumor necrosis factor.
Adapted from Bone RC: The pathogenesis of sepsis. Ann Intern Med 1991;115:457.

explain irreversible vascular collapse seen late in hemorrhagic shock.[42] A potential role for nitric oxide in inflammation-associated edema and third spacing during shock also has been suggested.[186] The in vitro myocardial depressant effects of TNF-α, IL-1, and serum from septic humans may be mediated by a similar nitric oxide–dependent and cGMP-dependent pathway.[123,216]

In 1990, Beckman and colleagues[221] described an alternative pathway by which nitric oxide may play a role in the cardiovascular pathophysiology of shock and sepsis. Peroxynitrite ($ONOO^-$), a highly reactive oxidant, is produced from the interaction of superoxide (OH^-) and nitric oxide (NO^-). It is known to react rapidly with proteins, lipids, and DNA during sepsis and shock states.[222-225] Lipids may be peroxidized, and proteins may be oxidized, nitrated, or nitrosated, the last-mentioned resulting in nitrotyrosine residues.[221,226,227] Peroxynitrite inactivates mitochondrial aconitase disrupting the Krebs cycle and otherwise interferes with ATP production and usage,[228-233] an activity similar to that described for nitric oxide.[234-236] It also generates DNA strand breaks leading to poly-ADP ribose synthetase activation, which may itself have significant pathophysiologic effects.[237,238] Peroxynitrite, similar to NO, also activates guanylate cyclase in vascular tissues.[239,240] In the periphery, the result may be cellular energetic failure, vascular contractile dysfunction (vasodilation), and reperfusion injury.[237,241-243] Many other molecular targets of NO relevant to the cardiovascular system exist and are well reviewed elsewhere.[226,244]

As part of the release of inflammatory mediators, immune cells, including macrophages, polymorphonuclear leukocytes, and lymphocytes, also may be activated in some forms of hypodynamic shock (e.g., hemorrhagic shock) resulting in a self-perpetuating, systemic inflammatory response (similar to that seen in sepsis). This response can contribute to vascular and parenchymal injury and culminate in MODS.

Free radical injury induced by reperfusion or neutrophil activity is another mechanism of organ injury during hemorrhagic and septic shock, burns, and myocardial infarction.[245] During tissue ischemia, oxygen deficiency leads to accumulation of ATP degradation products, including adenosine, inosine, and hypoxanthine (Fig. 22-11).[246] With resuscitation and reperfusion of ischemic areas, oxygen drives the generation of superoxide (O_2^-), the most common precursor of reactive oxidants, by xanthine oxidase, in endothelial cells. Most of the superoxide is converted spontaneously or through superoxide dismutase to hydrogen peroxide ($H_2O_2^-$). This further reacts to produce tissue-damaging hydroxyl radicals (or other highly reactive free radicals).[245] These radicals interact with critical cell targets, such as the plasma membrane,

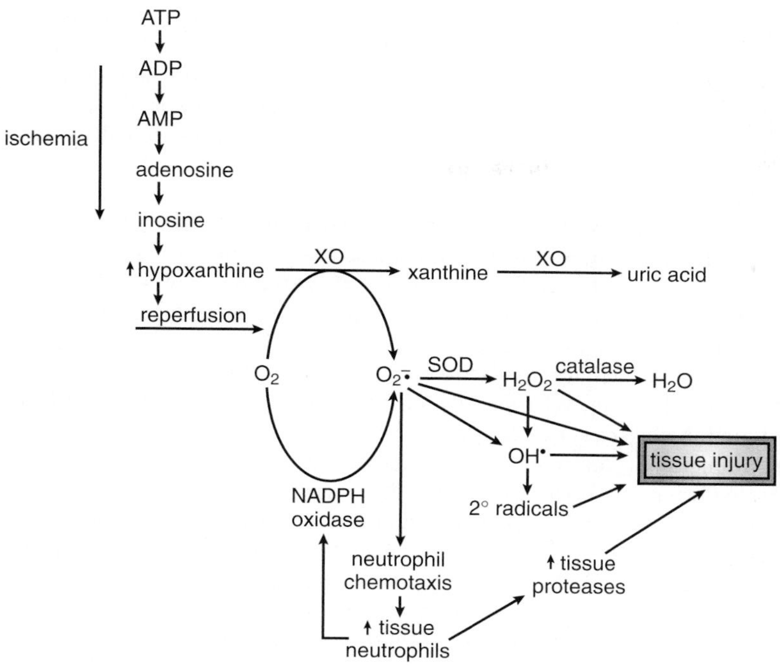

Figure 22-11. Free radical–mediated tissue injury. Superoxide (O_2^-) is primarily produced in shock from hypoxanthine (a metabolite of adenosine triphosphate [ATP] degradation) by xanthine oxidase (XO) during reperfusion postischemia. Superoxide can be converted to hydrogen peroxide (H_2O_2) by superoxide dismutase (SOD) and then to H_2O or may be converted to the highly reactive hydroxyl ($OH^•$), which mediates tissue injury. Free radical tissue injury may be amplified by superoxide recruitment of neutrophils, which secondarily produce additional superoxide through reduced nicotinamide adenine dinucleotide phosphate (NADPH) oxidase. ADP, adenosine diphosphate; AMP, adenosine monophosphate. (Adapted from Calandra T, Baumgartner J, Grau GE, et al: Prognostic values of tumor necrosis factor/cachectin, interleukin-1, and interferon-γ in the serum of patients with septic shock. J Infect Dis 1990;161:982.)

lipid membranes of organelles, and various enzymes, resulting in cell lysis and tissue injury. Oxidant activity, directly and through endothelial damage, attracts and activates neutrophils resulting in amplification of superoxide generation by a neutrophil reduced nicotinamide adenine dinucleotide phosphate (NADPH) oxidase and in further tissue damage owing to neutrophil protease release.[245] Injured tissue may release xanthine oxidase into the circulation resulting in systemic microvascular injury.[247]

A parallel process is found during reperfusion of ischemic myocardium after myocardial infarction.[248] Thrombolytic therapy or balloon angioplasty results in sudden delivery of oxygen to ischemic myocardium. Although substantial salvage of myocardial function results, free oxygen radical–mediated reperfusion injury can contribute to myocardial "stunning."[249] Cardiogenic shock during this phase may resolve as the reperfusion injury settles. Free radical damage likely also plays a role in tissue damage during sepsis and septic shock. After activation by inflammatory mediators and during phagocytosis, polymorphonuclear leukocytes undergo a respiratory burst during which they consume oxygen and generate superoxide and hydrogen peroxide through a membrane-associated NADPH oxidase.[245] Macrophages similarly produce oxygen radicals on activation. Activation also enhances adhesion and tissue migration of leukocytes so that vascular endothelial and parenchymal tissue damage may result. Free radical injury may play an important role in the development of organ failure after shock.[250]

A notable result of cellular injury in shock involves cellular membrane function. Movement of most solutes through cells depends partly on active transport through the plasma cell membrane. During hemorrhagic and septic shock, marked changes of plasma membrane function occur. Normal gradients of sodium, chloride, potassium, and calcium are not maintained. Changes of intracellular electrolytes and pH may affect sensitive intracellular enzyme systems and impair cell metabolism further. Impairment of membrane function is reflected by reversible changes in transmembrane electrical potential in skeletal muscle and liver. Because maintenance of membrane transport functions and electrochemical gradient is an energy-dependent process, decreased production of ATP during shock has been proposed as the cause of this defect.[195] Alterations of liver and skeletal muscle transmembrane potential occur early in shock, however, before the decrease in levels of high-energy phosphates and onset of hypotension. The membrane defect is not prevented by administration of membrane permeable forms of high-energy phosphates, such as ATP-$MgCl_2$.[251]

Variations in stress response genes between individuals and alteration of gene expression in immune, endothelial, muscle, and organ parenchymal cells are another important aspect of cellular dysfunction and injury in circulatory shock. Although shock can be present immediately after injury (massive trauma, hemorrhage, or endotoxin infusion), before the onset of substantial alterations of gene expression, its evolution depends on a combination of the ongoing nature of the insult, the genetically passive compensatory physiologic/metabolic response, the underlying genotype with respect to stress response elements, and stress-related modulation of gene expression in a variety of cells.

The clinical presentation of shock, progression of the syndrome, and final outcome may be substantially controlled by genetic factors.[252] Genetic factors have been best studied in septic shock. Studies have shown that the human TNF-α promoter polymorphism, TNF2, imparts an increased susceptibility to and mortality from septic shock.[253] Other studies suggest increased TNF-α generation, severity of sepsis, and mortality with another human TNF-α gene polymorphism.[254] A specific locus on chromosome 12 in mice has been shown to be associated with resistance to mortality owing to TNF-α-induced shock.[255] A human IL-1 receptor antagonist gene polymorphism has been linked to increased susceptibility to sepsis.[256] Several additional linked polymorphisms have been described in recent years.[257] It seems likely that gene polymorphisms also may play similar roles in other forms of shock.

Beyond the role of gene alleles in the development and clinical response to shock, the progression of irreversible circulatory shock and MODS may have its basis in genetically driven vascular or parenchymal responses. Production of cytokines by macrophages during shock requires acute expression of the genes coding for TNF-α, IL-1β, and other proinflammatory cytokines. The production of adhesion molecules by endothelial cells and inducible nitric oxide synthetase by vascular smooth muscle during shock requires active upregulation of gene expression. Both events are thought to be key to the development of MODS after shock in humans. In addition, human and animal research indicates that apoptosis, a genetically programmed process of cell autolysis, occurs in a variety of organs during shock and subsequent organ failure.[258,259] Data suggest that a variety of transcription factors may be activated in models of sepsis in association with the process.[260] Further research should elucidate the important link between irreversible shock, refractory shock, and shock-associated MODS and genetically programmed cell responses to inflammatory stimulation or injury or both.

Whatever the initiating event or events, progressive cell metabolic failure occurs. Mitochondrial activity continues to deteriorate, subcellular organelles are damaged, and intracellular (and possibly systemic) release of lysosome hydrolytic enzymes occurs, accelerating cell death and organ failure (see Fig. 22-9).

Compensatory Responses to Shock

Shock is usually not a discrete condition occuring abruptly after injury or infection. With the onset of hemodynamic stress, homeostatic compensatory mechanisms engage to maintain effective tissue perfusion. At this time, subtle clinical evidence of hemodynamic stress may be apparent (tachycardia, decreased urine output), but overt evidence of shock (hypotension, altered sensorium, metabolic acidosis) may not. Therapeutic interventions have a high probability of preventing ischemic tissue injury and initiation of systemic inflammatory cascades during this early compensated stage. Adaptive compensatory mechanisms fail, and organ injury ensues if the injury that initiates shock is too extensive or progresses despite therapy. As the duration of established shock increases, therapy is less likely to be effective in preventing organ failure and death.

Various sensing mechanisms involved in physiologic compensatory responses exist to recognize hemodynamic and metabolic dyshomeostasis (Fig. 22-12). Low-pressure right atrial and pulmonary artery stretch receptors sense volume changes. A decrease in circulating volume (or

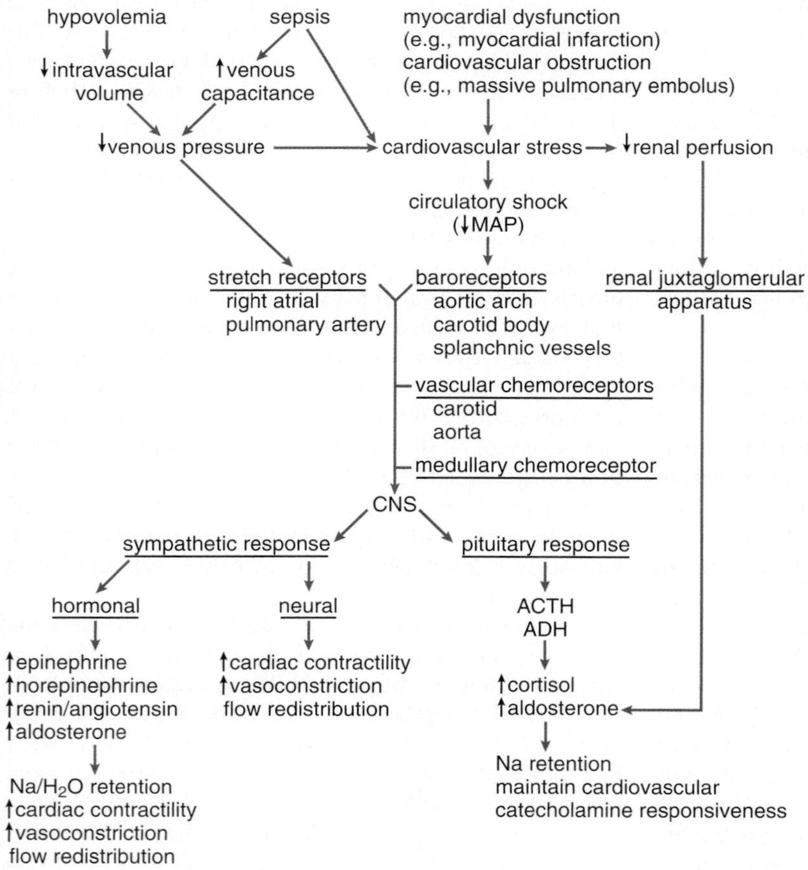

Figure 22-12. Neurohormonal response to shock. During early cardiovascular stress, the neurohormonal response may be limited to increased activity of the juxtaglomerular apparatus and stimulation of right atrial and pulmonary artery low-pressure mechanoreceptors. With further hypotension, high-pressure vascular baroreceptors, vascular chemoreceptors, and the medullary chemoreceptor are sequentially stimulated, resulting in augmented neurohormonal activity with increased pituitary hormone (adrenocorticotropic hormone [ACTH] and antidiuretic hormone [ADH]) release and increased sympathetic outflow from the central nervous system (CNS). Volume retention, increased venous tone, increased cardiac contractility, and blood flow redistribution to vital organs result. MAP, mean arterial pressure.

increase of venous capacitance) results in an increase in sympathetic discharge from the medullary vasomotor center.[149,261,262] Aortic arch, carotid, and splanchnic high-pressure baroreceptors sense early blood pressure changes close to the physiologic range.[149,261,262] An increase of sympathetic discharge from the medullary vasomotor center results from a small to moderate decrease in blood pressure associated with early shock. When MAP falls below about 80 to 90 mm Hg, however, aortic baroreceptor activity is absent. Subsequently, carotid baroreceptor response is eliminated as MAP decreases to less than 60 mm Hg. As blood pressure continues to decrease, carotid and aortic chemoreceptors, sensitive to decreased PO_2, increased PCO_2, and increased hydrogen ion concentrations (decreased pH), dominate the response. These receptor complexes, active only when MAP is less than approximately 80 mm Hg, are of minimal relevance during physiologic states.[149] During shock, they make a substantial contribution to increases of sympathetic tone.

During severe shock, the most powerful stimulus to sympathetic tone is the central nervous system ischemic response.[149] The lower medullary chemoreceptors for this response (thought to be sensitive to increased CO_2 associated with decreased cerebral perfusion) become active when MAP decreases to less than 60 mm Hg. Sympathetic stimulation provided by these receptors peaks at MAP of 15 to 20 mm Hg and results in maximal stimulation of the cardiovascular system.[149] The Cushing response to increased intracranial pressure is an example of activation of this reflex under different circumstances.

Other mechanisms also play a role in the compensatory response to shock. Vasopressin release is regulated by alterations of serum osmolality. During effective hypovolemia secondary to intravascular volume loss or increased vascular capacitance, low-pressure right atrial stretch receptors can override osmolar control of vasopressin response to effect retention of body water.[149,263] Similarly, during hypovolemia and shock, the juxtaglomerular apparatus in the kidneys responds to decreased perfusion pressure by renin release.[149]

All compensatory responses to shock, whether hemodynamic, metabolic, or biochemical, support oxygen delivery to vital organs. These responses are similar (to varying extents) for different classes of shock and can be broken down into four components: (1) maintenance of mean circulatory pressure, a measure of venous pressure, by maintaining total intravascular volume or increasing stressed volume (i.e., increasing venous tone); (2) optimizing cardiac performance; (3) redistributing perfusion to vital organs; and (4) optimizing unloading of oxygen at the tissues (Box 22-3; see Fig. 22-4).

Mean circulatory pressure and venous return are sustained in early shock by numerous mechanisms. Acutely, total intravascular volume is supported by alterations of capillary hydrostatic pressure as described by Starling.[264] Sympathetic activation results in precapillary vasoconstriction. In combination with initial hypotension, this results in decreased capillary hydrostatic pressure.[264] A decrease in capillary hydrostatic pressure enhances intravascular fluid shift owing to maintained plasma oncotic pressures. Transcapillary fluid influx after removal of 500 to 1000 mL blood volumes in humans can be 2 mL/min with full correction of intravascular volume by 24 to 48 hours.[265] The intravascular volume also may be supported by the osmotic activity of glucose generated by glycogenolysis. Increased extracellular osmolarity results in fluid redistribution from the intracellular to the extracellular space.

Intravascular volume also is conserved by decreasing renal fluid losses. Renal compensatory mechanisms are of limited value in acute shock, but can have more impact in the subacute phase. Decreased renal perfusion associated with reduced cardiac output and afferent arteriolar constriction results in a decrease in glomerular filtration rate and urine output. In addition, decreased renal perfusion pressure, sympathetic stimulation, and compositional changes in tubular fluid[149] result in renin release from the juxtaglomerular apparatus. Renin release leads to adrenal cortical release of aldosterone (via angiotensin II), which increases sodium reabsorption in the distal tubules of the kidney in exchange for potassium or hydrogen ion.[149]

Box 22-3

Cardiovascular and Metabolic Compensatory Responses to Shock

Maintain Mean Circulatory Pressure (Venous Pressure)
- Volume
  - Fluid redistribution to vascular space (increased total vascular volume)
    - From interstitium (Starling effect)
    - From intracellular space (osmotic)
  - Decreased renal fluid losses
    - Decreased glomerular filtration rate
    - Increased aldosterone
    - Increased vasopressin
- Pressure
  - Decreased venous capacitance (increased stressed volume)
    - Increased sympathetic activity
    - Increased circulating (adrenal) epinephrine
    - Increased angiotensin
    - Increased vasopressin

Maximize Cardiac Performance
- Increase contractility
  - Sympathetic stimulation
  - Adrenal stimulation

Redistribute Perfusion
- Extrinsic regulation of systemic arterial tone
- Dominant autoregulation of vital organs (heart, brain)

Optimize Oxygen Unloading
- Increased red blood cell 2,3-diphosphoglycerate
- Tissue acidosis
- Pyrexia
- Decreased tissue PO_2

Angiotensin II also exerts a powerful direct vasoconstricting effect (particularly on mesenteric vessels), while increasing sympathetic outflow and adrenal epinephrine release. As noted, vasopressin (antidiuretic hormone) release occurs through activation of right atrial low pressure. Angiotensin II augments this release by increasing sympathetic outflow. The release of vasopressin from the posterior pituitary results in water retention at the expense of osmolarity. Hyponatremia can result. Vasopressin, similar to angiotensin II, also results in vasoconstriction, particularly of the splanchnic circulation.

Finally, increased sympathetic activity and release of adrenal epinephrine results in systemic venoconstriction, particularly of the venous capacitance vessels of the splanchnic circulation. This supports mean circulatory pressure and venous return by increasing stressed volume.

Increased sympathetic nervous system activity accounts for most of the enhancement of cardiac performance during shock. Local release of norepinephrine by sympathetic nerves and systemic release of epinephrine result in stimulation of cardiac α-adrenergic and β-adrenergic receptors, resulting in increases of heart rate and contractility that optimize cardiac output and support blood pressure. Angiotensin II also may exert direct and indirect (sympathetic stimulation) inotropic effects on myocardium. Improved cardiac function also results in decreased right atrial pressure, which tends to increase venous return.

Redistribution of blood flow during shock already has been discussed. Increased sympathetic vasoconstrictor tone, systemic release of epinephrine from the adrenals, vasopressin, endothelin, and angiotensin II cause vasoconstriction in all sensitive vascular beds, including skin, skeletal muscle, kidneys, and splanchnic organs.[150] Dominant autoregulatory control of blood flow spares brain and heart blood work from these effects. Redistribution of flow to these vital organs is the effective result.

The effects of decreased delivery of oxygen to the tissues during shock can be attenuated by local adaptive responses. Hypoperfusion and tissue ischemia result in local acidosis owing to decreased clearance of CO_2 and anaerobic metabolism. Local acidosis results in decreased affinity between oxygen and hemoglobin at the capillary level.[149] The resultant rightward shift of the oxyhemoglobin dissociation curve allows greater unloading of oxygen from hemoglobin for a given PO_2. Tissue ischemia also is accompanied by decreased tissue PO_2 (relative to normal), which further augments unloading of oxygen. Pyrexia associated with sepsis also may contribute to a rightward shift of the oxyhemoglobin dissociation curve, whereas hypothermia is associated with a leftward shift. For that reason, maintenance of normothermia during resuscitation from shock is helpful in optimizing oxygen unloading.

Organ System Dysfunction Resulting from Shock

Table 22-3 summarizes organ system dysfunction resulting from shock.

Table 22-3. Organ System Dysfunction in Shock

Central nervous system	Encephalopathy (ischemic or septic) Cortical necrosis
Heart	Tachycardia, bradycardia Supraventricular tachycardia Ventricular ectopy Myocardial ischemia Myocardial depression
Respiratory	Acute respiratory failure Adult respiratory distress syndrome
Kidney	Prerenal failure Acute tubular necrosis
Gastrointestinal	Ileus Erosive gastritis Pancreatitis Acalculous cholecystitis Colonic submucosal hemorrhage Transluminal translocation of bacteria/antigens
Liver	Ischemic hepatits "Shock" liver Intrahepatic cholestasis
Hematologic	Disseminated intravascular coagulation Dilutional thrombocytopenia
Metabolic	Hyperglycemia Glycogenolysis Gluconeogenesis Hypoglycemia (late) Hypertriglyceridemia
Immune system	Gut barrier function depression Cellular immune depression Humoral immune depression

Central Nervous System

Central nervous system neurons are extremely sensitive to ischemia. The central nervous system vascular supply is highly resistant to extrinsic regulatory mechanisms. Although cerebral perfusion is impaired in shock, flow remains relatively well preserved until the later stages.[266,267] In the absence of primary cerebrovascular impairment, cerebral function is well supported until MAP decreases to less than approximately 50 to 60 mm Hg.[268] Eventually, irreversible ischemic injury may occur to the most sensitive areas of the brain (cerebral cortex). Before this fixed injury, an altered level of consciousness, varying from confusion to unconsciousness, may be seen depending on the degree of perfusion deficit. Disturbances of acid-base and electrolytes also may contribute. Electroencephalographic recordings show nonspecific changes compatible with encephalopathy. Sepsis-related encephalopathy may occur at higher blood pressures (owing partly to the effects of circulating inflammatory mediators) and is associated with increased mortality.[269]

Heart

The major clinically apparent manifestations of shock on the heart are due to sympathoadrenal stimulation.

Increased heart rate, in the absence of disturbances of cardiac conduction, is almost universally present. Vagally mediated paradoxical bradycardia may be seen occasionally in severe hemorrhage.[44] In patients predisposed to myocardial ischemia or irritability, catecholamine-driven supraventricular tachycardias and ventricular ectopy with ischemic electrocardiogram changes are uncommon. Similar to the brain, the blood supply to the heart is autoregulated. This autoregulation, in combination with the resilient nature of myocardial tissue, renders it resistant to sympathetically driven vasoconstriction and shock-related hypoperfusion injury. Overt necrosis typically does not occur, although evidence of cellular injury may be present.

Most forms of shock are associated with increased contractility of healthy myocardium. Despite this, shock has a substantial impact on myocardial contractility and compliance. Hypotension during cardiogenic shock (and other forms of shock) is associated with decreased coronary artery perfusion pressure. In patients with coronary artery disease or increased filling pressures or both, decreased coronary artery perfusion pressure may lead to overt ischemia. Circulating myocardial depressant substances contribute to myocardial depression in septic[211] and hemorrhagic[212] shock. This has been linked to decreased β-adrenoreceptor affinity and density and potential defects of intracellular signal transduction involving nitric oxide, G proteins, cyclic adenosine monophosphate (cAMP), and cGMP.[123] Circulating depressant substances also may be present during cardiogenic shock.[214]

Respiratory

Early alterations of pulmonary function seen during acute circulatory shock are primarily related to changes in central drive or muscle fatigue. Increased minute volume occurs as a result of augmented respiratory drive secondary to peripheral stimulation of pulmonary J receptors and carotid body chemoreceptors and hypoperfusion of the medullary respiratory center. This results in hypocapnia and primary respiratory alkalosis.[149,270] With increased minute volume and decreased cardiac output, the ventilation-perfusion ratio is increased. Unless arterial hypoxemia complicates shock, pulmonary resistance is initially unchanged or minimally increased. Coupled with an increased workload, respiratory and diaphragmatic muscle impairment owing to hypoperfusion (manifested by decreased transmembrane electrical potential) may lead to early respiratory failure.[271] ARDS resulting from inflammatory or free radical injury to the alveolocapillary cell layers after established shock may develop as a late cause of respiratory failure.

Kidney

Acute renal failure is a major complication of circulatory shock with associated mortality rates between 35% and 80%.[272] Although initial injury manifested by decreased urine output occurs, other clinical manifestations of renal dysfunction (increased creatinine, urea, and potassium) may not be noted for 1 to 3 days. When hemodynamic stabilization has been achieved, it becomes apparent that urine output does not immediately improve, and serum creatinine and urea continue to increase. The most common cause of acute renal failure is renal hypoperfusion resulting in ATN. The most frequent cause of renal hypoperfusion is hemodynamic compromise from septic shock, hemorrhage, hypovolemia, trauma, and major operative procedures. ATN that occurs in the setting of circulatory shock is associated with a higher mortality than in other situations.

Part of the reason for the kidney's sensitivity to hypoperfusion has to do with the nature of its vascular supply. The renal vascular bed is moderately autoregulated. Increases of efferent arteriolar tone initially can maintain glomerular perfusion despite compromise of renal flow.[273] Renal hypoperfusion does not become critical until relatively late in shock when maximal vasoconstriction of renal preglomerular arterioles[273] results in cortical, then medullary, ischemic injury.

Decreased urine output in shock can pose a diagnostic dilemma because it can be associated with oliguric ATN and hypoperfusion-related prerenal failure without ATN. Indices suggestive of the latter include a benign urine sediment, urine sodium concentration less than 20 mEq/L, fractional urine sodium excretion less than 1%, urine osmolality greater than 450 mOsm/L, and urine-to-plasma creatinine ratio greater than 40. Useful markers of acute renal failure caused by ATN include hematuria and heme granular casts, urine sodium concentration greater than 40 mEq/mL, fractional excretion of urine sodium greater than 2%, urine osmolarity less than 350 mOsm/L, and urine-to-plasma creatinine ratio less than 20.[274] ATN caused by circulatory shock may be associated with urine sodium less than 20 mEq/L and fractional excretion less than 1% if the acute renal injury is superimposed on chronic effective volume depletion, as may be seen with cirrhosis and congestive heart failure.[275]

Gastrointestinal

The gut is relatively sensitive to circulatory failure. The splanchnic vasculature is highly responsive to sympathetic vasoconstriction. Typical clinical gut manifestations of hypoperfusion, sympathetic stimulation, and inflammatory injury associated with shock include ileus, erosive gastritis, pancreatitis, acalculous cholecystitis, and colonic submucosal hemorrhage. Enteric ischemia produced by circulatory shock and free radical injury with resuscitation may breach gut barrier integrity with translocation of enteric bacteria and antigens (notably endotoxin) from the gut lumen to the systemic circulation resulting in propagation and amplification of shock and MODS.[276,277]

Liver

Similar to the gut, the liver is highly sensitive to hypotension and hypoperfusion injury. "Shock liver," associated with massive ischemic necrosis and major elevations of transaminases, is atypical in the absence of extensive hepatocellular disease or very severe insult.[278] Centrilobular injury with mild increases of transaminases and lactate dehydrogenase is more typical. Transaminases usually peak within 1 to 3 days of the insult and resolve over 3 to 10 days. In either case, early increases in bilirubin and alkaline phosphatase are modest. Despite the production of acute-phase reactants in early circulatory shock, synthetic functions may be impaired with decreased generation of prealbumin, albumin, and hepatic coagulation factors. After hemodynamic resolution of shock, evidence of biliary stasis with increased bilirubin and alkaline phosphatase can develop even though the patient is otherwise improving. Postshock MODS involves similar hepatic pathology.

Hematologic

Hematologic manifestations of circulatory shock tend to depend on the nature of shock. Disseminated intravascular coagulation, characterized by microangiopathic hemolysis, consumptive thrombocytopenia, consumptive coagulopathy, and microthrombi with tissue injury, is most commonly seen in association with septic shock. Because it is due to simultaneous systemic activation of coagulation and fibrinolysis cascades, it can be differentiated from the coagulopathy of liver failure by determination of endothelial cell–produced factor VIII (normal or increased with hepatic dysfunction). In the absence of extensive tissue injury or trauma, hemorrhagic shock is rarely associated with disseminated intravascular coagulation.[279] Dilutional thrombocytopenia is the most common cause of coagulation deficits after resuscitation for hemorrhage.[280]

Metabolic

Metabolic alterations associated with shock occur in a predictable pattern. Early in shock, when hemodynamic instability triggers compensatory responses, sympathoadrenal activity is enhanced. Increased release of adrenocorticotropic hormone, glucocorticoids, and glucagon and decreased release of insulin result in glycogenolysis, gluconeogenesis, and hyperglycemia.[263,281] Increased release of epinephrine results in skeletal muscle insulin resistance, sparing glucose for use by glucose-dependent organs (heart and brain). Late in shock, hypoglycemia may develop, possibly as a result of glycogen depletion or failure of hepatic glucose synthesis. Fatty acids are increased early in shock, but decrease later as hypoperfusion of adipose-containing peripheral tissue progresses. Hypertriglyceridemia is often seen during shock as a consequence of catecholamine stimulation and reduced lipoprotein lipase expression induced by circulating TNF-α.[281] Increased catecholamines, glucocorticoids, and glucagon also increase protein catabolism, resulting in a negative nitrogen balance.[281]

Immune System

Immune dysfunction, frequent during and after circulatory shock and trauma, rarely has immediate adverse effects, but likely contributes to late mortality. Underlying mechanisms of immune dysfunction include ischemic injury to barrier mucosa (particularly of the gut) leading to anatomic breaches (colonic ulceration) and potential mucosal translocation of bacteria and bacterial products; parenchymal tissue injury secondary to associated trauma, inflammation, ischemia, or free radical injury; and direct ischemic or mediator-induced (immunosuppressant cytokines, corticosteroids, prostaglandins, catecholamines, or endorphins) dysfunction of cellular and humoral immune system.[282,283] In particular, macrophage function is adversely affected during trauma and circulatory shock. A decrease in antigen presenting ability impairs the activation of T and B lymphocytes. Associated with this defect are a decrease in Ia antigen expression, a decrease in membrane IL-1 receptors, and the presence of suppressor macrophages. Phagocytic activity of the reticuloendothelial system also is compromised, partially as a result of an acute decrease in fibronectin levels. Suppression of T lymphocyte immune function is manifested by decreased responsiveness to antigenic stimulation and a decreased helper-to-suppressor ratio. Decreased production of IgG and IgM suggests B cell suppression. Nonspecific immune suppression is expressed as decreased neutrophil bactericidal function, chemotaxis, opsonization, and phagocytosis.

Resuscitation agents used in shock also may substantially depress immune function. Dopamine, used for hemodynamic support in shock, has been shown to suppress pituitary production of prolactin (required for optimal immune function), resulting in suppression of T cell proliferative responses.[284] Dopamine may contribute, along with stress-induced increases in immunosuppressive glucocorticoids, to T cell anergy seen in critically ill patients.

All of these factors may contribute to the propensity of critically ill patients to develop ongoing organ system dysfunction and a variety of infections during the postshock phase. One third to one half of patients with shock die late in their course after resolution of the acute shock phase.

DIAGNOSTIC APPROACH AND EVALUATION

Shock is always a life-threatening emergency. Diagnosis, evaluation, and management often must occur virtually simultaneously. The diagnosis must be made as early as possible while shock is well compensated. When marked hypotension and hypoperfusion are present, mortality is increased. Because early recognition and treatment are key to survival, the diagnosis is primarily a clinical one. Laboratory and imaging studies are useful for confirmation of the diagnosis and determination of the specific shock etiology. Therapy of shock should never be delayed, however, to accommodate these studies. The initial diagnosis of shock can and should be made strictly based on clinical signs and symptoms. Because shock is the common end point of a variety of insults, evaluation and management for all forms of shock involves a common approach (Box 22-4).

Clinical Evaluation

Impending shock is characterized by the typical compensatory response to cardiovascular stress. Tachycardia, tachypnea, and oliguria (<0.5 mL/kg/h) are usually

Box 22-4

General Approach to Shock: Initial Diagnosis and Evaluation

Clinical (Primary Diagnosis)

Tachycardia, tachypnea, cyanosis, oliguria, encephalopathy (confusion), peripheral hypoperfusion (mottled extremities), hypotension (systolic blood pressure <90 mm Hg)

Laboratory (Confirmatory)

Hemoglobin, white blood cell count, platelets
Prothrombin time/partial thromboplastin time
Electrolytes, arterial blood gases
Calcium, magnesium
Blood urea nitrogen, creatinine
ECG

Monitoring

Continuous ECG and respiratory monitors
Arterial pressure catheter
Central venous pressure monitor (uncomplicated shock) ± central venous oximetry
Pulmonary artery flotation catheter
- Cardiac output
- Pulmonary wedge pressure
- Mixed venous oxygen saturation (intermittent or continuous)*
- Oxygen delivery ($\dot{D}O_2$) and oxygen consumption ($\dot{V}O_2$)*

Oximetry*
Echocardiogram (functional assessment)*

Imaging

Chest radiograph
Abdominal radiographs*
CT scan of abdomen or chest*
Echocardiogram (anatomic assessment)*
Pulmonary perfusion scan*

*Optional.
CT, computed tomography; ECG, electrocardiogram.

present. Cool extremities are seen in hypodynamic shock. The blood pressure may be elevated or normal with maximal sympathetic stimulation. With progression, however, blood pressure decreases, while pulse pressure narrows (except in the case of distributive shock). Frank hypotension (MAP < 60 to 65 mm Hg in adults) may ensue. The chronic level of blood pressure must be considered. Normotension in a normally hypertensive patient may denote a critical degree of hypoperfusion. With further progression, anuria may develop, extremities may become mottled and dusky (except in distributive shock), and the sensorium may become clouded. Clinical parameters can underestimate initial resuscitative requirements in critically ill patients, including patients with septic shock.[285-288]

Other clinical manifestations of shock are useful in attempting to differentiate the etiology. Hypovolemic shock is characterized by decreased jugular venous pressure. Cardiogenic shock is characterized by elevated jugular venous pressure with hepatojugular reflux, an S_3, an S_4, and regurgitant heart murmurs. Obstructive shock signs usually depend on the nature of the obstruction. Pulmonary embolus may be characterized by dyspnea and right-sided evidence of heart failure. Cardiac tamponade may be characterized by Kussmaul's sign, pulsus paradoxus, and distant heart sounds. Septic shock in the absence of neutropenia usually exhibits a focus of infection along with fever, chills, and warm extremities. Patients with septic shock and neutropenia often have no clinically apparent focus. Elderly patients may present with little more than unexplained hyperventilation and hypotension.

Laboratory Studies

Laboratory data are used to confirm the diagnosis of shock and to help clarify the etiology. Leukocyte count frequently is elevated early in shock owing to demargination of neutrophils. Leukopenia may be found in sepsis and late shock. Hemoglobin concentration is variably affected depending on the etiology of shock. Nonhemorrhagic hypovolemic shock and septic shock with extravasation of intravascular water to the interstitium may result in an apparent erythrocytosis. Platelet count increases acutely with the stress of circulatory shock, but with progression of sepsis or resuscitation of massive hemorrhage, thrombocytopenia may occur. Arterial blood gases and electrolytes may show a non–anion gap acidosis if hypovolemic shock is associated with excessive diarrhea and metabolic alkalosis if associated with vomiting. An anion gap acidosis, often caused by elevated levels of lactic acid, usually reflects prolonged inadequate tissue perfusion. Blood urea nitrogen and creatinine are rarely changed after the acute onset of shock even if renal injury is present. An isolated increased blood urea nitrogen with anemia and normal creatinine may suggest gastrointestinal bleeding. An arterial blood gas helps to determine the adequacy of oxygenation and gives evidence of acid-base disturbances. An electrocardiogram is crucial for diagnosis of ischemic cardiac injury as a primary cause of cardiogenic shock or secondary to hypotension associated with shock of another etiology.

Lactate levels (particularly serial determinations) are useful in assessment of prognosis. Substantial data suggest that lactate levels, as a marker of tissue oxygen debt and supply-dependent oxygen consumption, can predict outcome in shock.[49,50,289-293] The utility of lactate assessment is limited by the fact that it is a relatively late marker of tissue hypoperfusion.[294,295] Significant tissue ischemia and injury are present by the time it is elevated. In addition, lactate is cleared by the liver. Liver failure may markedly increase elevated lactate levels during hypoperfusion. Conversely, normal hepatic clearance may obscure limited lactate production by ischemic tissues. Glycolysis and alkalosis also nonspecifically increase lactate levels.[296,297] Because in the appropriate setting, arterial lactate levels greater than 2 mEq/L are associated with increased mortality,[50,53,291,292,298] however, such levels should be considered to represent tissue ischemia in the absence of another clearly defined etiology. The adequacy of resuscitation of shock can be assessed using serial changes of systemic lactate.[293,298] Resolution of elevated lactate may lag, however, after implementation of effective resuscitation.[299]

Imaging

A chest radiograph is useful in ruling out pneumonia as a source of septic shock and pulmonary edema as a manifestation of cardiogenic shock, tension pneumothorax, or pericardial tamponade. Although abdominal views occasionally may be helpful, intra-abdominal processes resulting in shock are usually clinically apparent. Computed tomography may be helpful in directing management in specific instances (e.g., occult internal hemorrhage, aortic dissection, pulmonary embolus). Similarly, transthoracic and transesophageal echocardiography can diagnose specific repairable cardiac or aortic lesions associated with shock with great accuracy and can be highly suggestive of other important diagnoses, including hemodynamically significant pulmonary embolus. Pulmonary perfusion scans are useful to confirm massive pulmonary embolism. Other imaging modalities have less of a role in the evaluation of acute shock.

Invasive Hemodynamic Monitoring

All patients suspected to have circulatory shock should have an indwelling arterial pressure catheter placed. Blood pressure assessment by manual sphygmomanometry or automated noninvasive oscillometric techniques may be inaccurate during shock owing to marked peripheral vasoconstriction.[300] In addition, neither technique supplies continuous monitoring of the rapidly changing hemodynamic status of unstable patients. An arterial catheter allows ready access for arterial blood gas samples and other laboratory tests. In most cases, a peripheral site, such as the radial artery, is used. Given the potential for disparity of pressures between central and peripheral sites,[301] however, if marked peripheral vasoconstriction owing to either sympathetic stimulation or exogenous catecholamines obscures the peripheral pulses, a central site, such as the femoral artery, may be preferred.

CVP monitoring is frequently used during the perioperative period to assess intravascular volume status in patients without critical illness. Because of the relatively stable hemodynamic status of these patients and the questionable benefit of pulmonary artery catheterization in such patients, such an approach is adequate. Similarly, CVP monitoring for otherwise healthy patients being resuscitated for hypovolemic shock may provide useful data. In the appropriate clinical context, CVP monitoring also occasionally may be useful in differentiating between different forms of shock (e.g., low CVP in hypovolemic shock, high CVP in cardiac tamponade). As a rule, however, CVP monitoring is inadequate for the hemodynamic assessment of critically ill patients, particularly patients with shock. Numerous studies have conclusively shown that CVP does not accurately estimate left ventricular preload in critically ill patients.[302,303]

The use of flow-directed, balloon-tipped pulmonary artery catheters with thermodilution cardiac output determination capability has been the standard of practice for the hemodynamic assessment of circulatory shock. Their use is supported by many studies, which show that experienced physicians cannot accurately determine cardiac filling pressures or cardiac output based on clinical evaluation alone.[304,305] In addition to cardiac output determination, pulmonary artery catheters provide continuous monitoring of central venous and pulmonary artery waveforms and pressures. PWP (as an estimate of left ventricular end diastolic pressure and volume) and waveform can be obtained intermittently. Waveform analysis may be useful in cardiovascular diagnoses of cardiac tamponade, restrictive cardiomyopathy, congestive heart failure, ventricular hypertrophy, and mitral or tricuspid regurgitation. These devices also allow withdrawal of blood from the pulmonary artery enabling determination of $S\bar{v}O_2$ to verify sufficient oxygen delivery during hypodynamic shock. In addition, they can show evidence of right heart and pulmonary artery oxygen saturation "stepups" for the diagnosis of left-to-right shunts associated with cardiac anatomic abnormalities, such as ventricular septal defect. In shock, a flow-directed, balloon-tipped pulmonary artery catheter is useful for etiologic classification, to determine optimal management, and to follow the response to therapy. Typical hemodynamic profiles of different forms of shock are described in Table 22-1.

The utility of pulmonary artery catheterization has been questioned in a case-matched study that suggested increased resource use and mortality associated with the use of pulmonary artery catheters in the ICU.[306] A series of randomized studies performed since then have reported on the role of the pulmonary artery catheter in settings of major noncardiac surgery, congestive heart failure, sepsis, and ARDS and in the general ICU.[307-309] In the perioperative management of patients undergoing major noncardiac surgery, the use of pulmonary artery catheters did not affect mortality and was associated with a greater incidence of pulmonary embolism.[308] In critically ill patients diagnosed with congestive heart failure, management directed with the use of a pulmonary artery catheter did not influence mortality, but resulted in more in-hospital adverse events.[310] A large trial evaluating the role of the pulmonary artery catheter in the management of patients with ARDS secondary to sepsis also found no significant differences in mortality if a pulmonary artery catheter was used or not.[309] Two randomized studies of general ICU patients similarly concluded that the use of pulmonary artery catheters among critically ill patients neither increased nor decreased mortality.[307,311] Meta-analyses have yielded conflicting results.[312-314] Despite these data, no studies have examined the use of pulmonary artery catheters in cases of shock specifically.

One parameter that a pulmonary artery catheter uniquely provides is $S\bar{v}O_2$. This measure may provide an assessment of adequacy of resuscitation of low output states before the presence of anaerobic metabolism (as signified by increased lactate). $S\bar{v}O_2$ increases with elevations of perfusion above requirements and decreases, with increasing oxygen extraction ratio, as perfusion becomes inadequate (Fig. 22-13). Normal $S\bar{v}O_2$ falls within the 65% to 75% range. During myocardial infarction, $S\bar{v}O_2$ values of less than 60% are found with congestive heart failure, and values less than 40% are found with cardiogenic shock.[315] Lactate accumulation and supply-dependent oxygen consumption begin to appear as saturation levels decrease to less than 30% to 40%.[316,317] $S\bar{v}O_2$ is especially useful in determining whether low cardiac outputs indicate supply-dependent oxygen consumption ($S\bar{v}O_2$ low) or normally depressed metabolic demands (normal $S\bar{v}O_2$). As a result of the maldistribution of perfusion in distributive shock (or substrate usage defect in septic shock) and left-to-right shunting in cardiogenic shock associated with ventricular septal defects, $S\bar{v}O_2$ is not useful in assessment in those conditions. Central venous oxygen saturation has been proposed as an alternative way to examine adequacy of resuscitation with excellent clinical results.[199,288]

Oxygen delivery and oxygen consumption variables also can be determined using pulmonary artery catheter–derived data. Although such global perfusion data seem

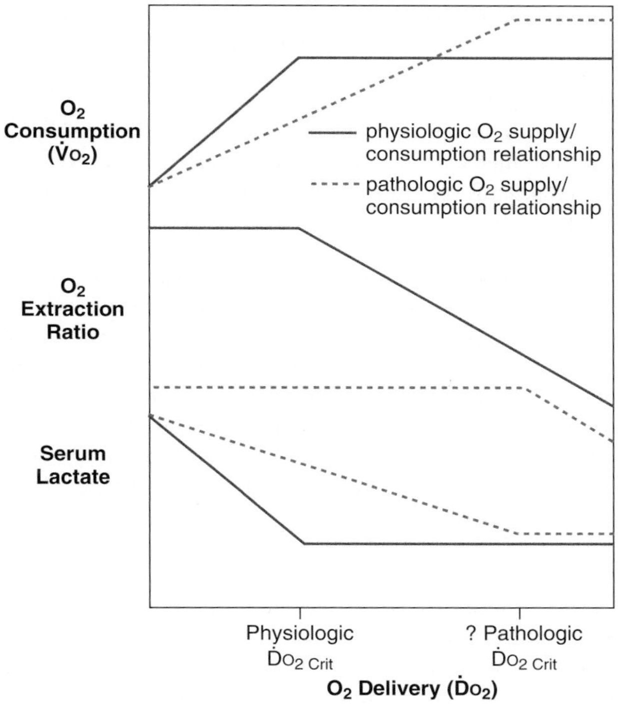

Figure 22-13. Oxygen supply–dependent oxygen consumption in shock. Physiologic supply-dependent oxygen consumption is characterized by a biphasic relationship between oxygen delivery ($\dot{D}O_2$) and oxygen consumption ($\dot{V}O_2$). The inflection point defines the physiologic critical oxygen delivery ($\dot{D}O_{2crit}$). Below this $\dot{D}O_{2crit}$, $\dot{V}O_2$ is linearly dependent on $\dot{D}O_2$, the oxygen extraction ratio is maximal, and lactate (indicating anaerobic metabolism) is produced. Above the physiologic $\dot{D}O_{2crit}$, $\dot{V}O_2$ is independent of $\dot{D}O_2$, the oxygen extraction ratio varies to maintain a constant $\dot{V}O_2$, and lactate is not produced. Pathologic oxygen supply dependency exists when oxygen consumption depends on $\dot{D}O_2$ over a much wider range of $\dot{D}O_2$ values. $\dot{D}O_{2crit}$, if one exists, is shifted to the right, the oxygen extraction ratio varies throughout a wide range of $\dot{D}O_2$ values, and lactate is produced with higher than normal $\dot{D}O_2$.

to have prognostic significance for large groups of critically ill patients, their utility is controversial when applied to individual patients.

Modifications to the standard pulmonary artery flotation catheter allow continuous monitoring of $S\bar{v}O_2$ or determination of right ventricular ejection fractions and volumes. Although both innovations have been used for clinical research purposes, and each theoretically offers unique insights into shock, they have no defined role at this time in clinical shock management.

Ancillary Monitoring Techniques

Oximetry

Because oxygen delivery depends on arterial oxygen saturation, pulse oximetry should, in theory, provide useful data during circulatory shock. Limitations of the technique include the fact that ambient light sources, dyshemoglobinemias (methemoglobin, carboxyhemoglobin), lipemia, and hypothermia can affect results.[318] Motion artifact may generate a false signal.[319] Shock-associated vasoconstriction also impairs signal acquisition. One study has shown that a CI less than 2.4 L/min/m^2 is associated with signal loss.[320] Although these problems limit the utility of pulse oximetry in the acute management of circulatory shock, the technique may be more helpful during postresuscitation monitoring. At this time, sequential arterial blood gases provide more reliable data during acute shock.

Transcutaneous and Transconjunctival Oxygen Tension

Transcutaneous and transconjunctival oxygen tension measurements are newer, noninvasive techniques for determination of tissue oxygen tension that show some promise in the management of patients at risk for or after the resuscitation of circulatory shock. In the absence of shock, transcutaneous probes reflect arterial oxygenation.[321] Numerous studies have suggested, however, that if arterial oxygen tension is stable, the devices may be useful in assessing global or regional changes in perfusion and oxygen metabolism.[322-325] Global hypoperfusion caused by low output shock (and local vasoconstriction) results in decreased transcutaneous oxygen tension and a decreased ratio of transcutaneous to arterial oxygen tension.[323] Decreased transcutaneous oxygen tension, seen early in hemorrhagic shock, may precede hypotension.[324,325] Decreases in transconjunctival oxygen tension predict hemodynamic collapse in perioperative patients[322] and death in patients with cardiogenic shock.[325] Transcutaneous and transconjunctival measurement of oxygen tension also may be useful in assessing adequacy of tissue perfusion during resuscitation from hypodynamic shock.[326,327]

Gastric Intramucosal pH

Because anaerobic glycolysis with lactate generation is paralleled by the production of hydrogen ions during hypodynamic shock, noninvasive measurement of tissue pH may provide an attractive, metabolism-based assessment of adequacy of tissue oxygenation and perfusion. Because the stomach is easily accessible and may reflect overall splanchnic perfusion during shock,[328] and splanchnic perfusion is known to be altered early in shock,[329] most clinical work has focused on gastric mucosal pH. Studies suggest that gastric intramucosal pH correlates closely with systemic and organ oxygen consumption, organ failure, and outcome in critically ill humans.[330,331] Normalization of gastric mucosal pH has been suggested as one appropriate target during resuscitation of circulatory shock.[332] Limited evidence suggests such an approach may be associated with improved survival.[333] Further supportive studies are required, however, before this can be accepted as an appropriate therapeutic target.

Near-Infrared Spectroscopy

Near-infrared spectroscopy is an innovative technique able to monitor noninvasively regional tissue blood flow, oxygen delivery, and oxygen use. Although several investigators have claimed the ability to examine mitochondrial oxidation state (particularly the redox state of cytochrome aa_3, the terminal portion of the electron transport chain), these measurements may reflect only tissue oxygenation. Normal tissue oxygenation is the ultimate expression of normal cardiopulmonary function. Any major perturbation of cardiopulmonary status, including incipient shock, should ultimately be expressed as decreased tissue oxygenation. Because peripheral tissue perfusion is, as part of normal compensatory mechanisms, one of the first mechanisms to become restricted during cardiovascular stress, peripheral tissue oxygenation may serve as an excellent marker of cardiovascular stress. Near-infrared light is known to pass through biologic tissues, such as skin and muscles. By illuminating a tissue with a known amount of incident light, the amount recovered depends on the degree of absorption by chromophores within the tissue and amount of scattering. Only three chromophores are known to absorb light in the near-infrared wavelength spectrum—hemoglobin, myoglobin, and cytochrome aa_3. All three are known to vary their absorption of near-infrared light depending on whether they are in an oxygenated or deoxygenated/reduced state. By monitoring these parameters, near-infrared spectroscopy is a unique tool that allows for real-time assessment of the adequacy of tissue perfusion during the resuscitation and ongoing management of patients with shock. Studies in animals and humans have suggested potential utility of this technique in assessing shock, including hypovolemic and traumatic shock[334-339] and septic shock.[340,341]

Echocardiography

The application of advanced echocardiography techniques in the ICU as intermittent monitoring tools may represent one of the most exciting developments in critical care management. Numerous factors have hastened this development. These include questions regarding the safety and efficacy of routine pulmonary artery catheter use; the availability of relatively inexpensive, portable echocardiography systems; the application of advanced software algorithms to analysis of data; and the development of new, high-resolution echocardiographic techniques, including transesophageal and contrast echocardiography. The confluence of these factors has resulted in a substantial increase in use of echocardiography in the ICU to assess hemodynamic instability and shock. In addition to its long recognized ability to detect anatomic lesions (pericardial tamponade, pericardial effusion, septal defects, valvular disease, aortic dissection), new techniques allow direct measurement of cardiac output, stroke volume, preload (ventricular volumes), systolic contractility (ejection fraction), diastolic function, and regional motion abnormalities at baseline and under stressed conditions.[342] Utility for diagnosis of hemodynamically significant pulmonary embolism also has been established.[343] The widespread dissemination of echocardiographic skills among the next generation of intensivists may allow for a substantial reduction in use of invasive monitoring techniques, including pulmonary artery catheterization.

MANAGEMENT AND THERAPY

Patients suspected to be in circulatory shock should be managed in an ICU with continuous electrocardiogram monitoring and close nursing support. Patients whose etiologic diagnosis is in doubt, whose hemodynamic instability does not quickly resolve with intravenous fluids, or who are medically complicated should undergo invasive hemodynamic monitoring with arterial and pulmonary artery catheters. Laboratory tests as mentioned earlier should be performed at or before admission.

Management of shock can be divided into specific therapy for the triggering injury and general therapy of the shock syndrome. Examples of specific therapy include antibiotics and drotrecogin alfa (activated) for treatment of septic shock, blood transfusion for hemorrhagic shock, thrombolysis for acute myocardial infarction or massive pulmonary embolus, and pericardial aspiration for pericardial tamponade. Specific therapy for different etiologies of shock is discussed in separate chapters.

Aims

Because the shock syndrome shares many characteristics across different etiologies, the general management of shock is similar in all cases. The basic goal of circulatory shock therapy is the rapid restoration of effective perfusion to vital organs and tissues before the onset of cellular injury. Because effective tissue perfusion depends on sufficient cardiac output and adequate driving pressure, therapy of shock requires maintenance of an appropriate CI and mean blood pressure (Box 22-5). Because, for brief periods, marked hypoperfusion is better tolerated than severe hypotension, however, the first specific resuscitative aim, support of blood pressure (>60 to 65 mm Hg in a baseline normotensive patient), may initially take priority over the second specific aim, maintenance of CI. Finally, maintaining perfusion sufficiently high that arterial lactate concentration remains less than 2.2 mmol/L is a generally accepted approach to avoiding anaerobic metabolism and ischemic tissue injury (see Box 22-5). The

Box 22-5

General Approach to Shock: Immediate Goals

Hemodynamic

Mean arterial pressure >60-65 mm Hg (higher in the presence of coronary artery disease)

Pulmonary wedge pressure 15-18 mm Hg (may be higher for cardiogenic shock)

Cardiac index >2.1 L/min/m^2 for cardiogenic and obstructive shock

Cardiac index >4-4.5 L/min/m^2 for septic and resuscitated traumatic/hemorrhagic shock

Optimization of Oxygen Delivery

Hemoglobin >9 g/dL (>7 g/L postshock is sufficient)

Arterial saturation >92%

Mixed venous oxygen saturation >60%, $sCVO_2$>70%

Normalization of serum lactate (to <2.2 mM/L)

Reverse Organ System Dysfunction

Reverse encephalopathy

Maintain urine output >0.5 mL/kg/h

$sCVO_2$, central venous oxygen saturation.

practice of targeting oxygen delivery to specified supranormal oxygen delivery goals or to evidence of supply-independent oxygen consumption in the ICU has been substantially discredited by clinical studies.[344-347] Early (<6 hours after presentation) resuscitation to a central venous oxygen saturation of greater than 70% using a defined protocol with fluids, blood transfusion, and dobutamine support has been shown, however, to improve outcome in severe sepsis and septic shock.[199] This approach has not been validated in other forms of shock.

A major achievement in shock therapy since the 1990s has been the recognition that speed of implementation of supportive and specific therapies may be crucial to improvement in outcomes. This concept of a "golden hour" has long been recognized in the context of specific and resuscitative therapy of trauma-induced hypovolemic shock with blood products and surgical management[348] and then cardiogenic shock secondary to myocardial infarction with emergent primary angioplasty or thrombolysis.[349] In recent years, a similar rapid treatment paradigm has been established for thrombolytic therapy for obstructive shock secondary to massive pulmonary embolus.[79,80] Similarly, rapid fluid resuscitation (<6 hours),[199] antimicrobial therapy (<1 hour),[104] and drotrecogin alfa (activated) (<24 hours)[350] all have been shown to be key to maximizing survival in severe sepsis and septic shock. The importance of early aggressive resuscitative and specific therapy of all shock states cannot be sufficiently emphasized.

Resuscitation

The universal basics of resuscitation underlie the initial management of circulatory shock. Because many patients with circulatory shock may have accompanying trauma or decreased level of consciousness or both, the ventilatory status of the patient must be secured. This may involve tracheal intubation or mechanical ventilation or both, if necessary. Oxygen should be provided at a sufficiently high concentration to provide an arterial oxygen saturation of greater than 90% to 92%. In unintubated patients, high flow (30 to 45 L/min) or rebreathing oxygen delivery systems may be required because many patients have unusually high minute ventilation volumes. Intubated patients should initially receive full ventilatory support to decrease systemic oxygen demand. Given that pulmonary infiltrates (aspiration, pneumonia, or ARDS) are common, positive end-expiratory pressure may be necessary to ensure adequate oxygenation. Potential adverse hemodynamic effects from positive-pressure ventilation (related primarily to decreased venous return) may be seen, but can be minimized by fluid loading so that the patient is euvolemic or modestly hypervolemic.

Depending on the clinical situation, pain management may be necessary. Potential adverse hemodynamic effects may be seen if intravascular volume is inadequate because all measures result in some degree of venodilation either directly or by decreasing sympathetic tone. Boluses of morphine, 2 to 4 mg intravenously, are recommended. During circulatory shock, clearance of morphine by the liver may be impaired owing to hepatic hypoperfusion. Besides relieving pain, analgesia also should decrease systemic oxygen consumption.

Management of lactic acidosis developing during circulatory shock is problematic. Bicarbonate therapy may have adverse effects on intracellular pH even while improving the pH of the extracellular fluid. Even when pH is extremely low, bicarbonate therapy does not improve systemic hemodynamics in shock associated with acidosis.[351] In addition, increasing serum pH may adversely affect the oxyhemoglobin dissociation relationship. The optimal approach to the management of lactic acidosis is to improve organ and systemic perfusion so that anaerobic metabolism is limited, and the liver and, to a lesser extent, kidneys can clear the accumulated lactate. If this is ineffective, restricting the use of sodium bicarbonate to situations in which pH is less than 7.1 to 7.15 may be appropriate.

Fluids

Initial management of circulatory shock almost always should include a crystalloid fluid challenge. In the absence of invasive monitoring with a pulmonary artery catheter, the only practical exception is if clinical evidence strongly suggests ventricular filling pressures are already elevated. This is usually limited to clinical situations involving cardiogenic shock and marked pulmonary edema. Even then, if pulmonary edema is manageable, crystalloid challenge may be appropriate. The volume of the challenge varies. Large volumes, on the order of 1 to 2 L given rapidly (0.5 to 1 L every 10 to 15 minutes), are frequently used in hemorrhagic and septic shock. During cardiogenic shock, 100- to 200-mL boluses may be used. If shock does not resolve promptly after the initial fluid challenge, patients should have a balloon-tipped pulmonary artery catheter placed immediately. A PWP of 15 to 18 mm Hg optimizes cardiac performance in most patients with circulatory shock without causing formation of pulmonary edema. Cardiac patients with low ventricular compliance may require an even higher PWP (≥20 mm Hg). Some studies have suggested patients with altered vascular permeability (distributive shock, especially septic shock) may avoid noncardiogenic pulmonary edema with lower pressures (12 to 15 mm Hg),[302] and that patients with ARDS similarly may achieve improved outcomes.[352]

Substantial controversy exists regarding the appropriate use of crystalloid and colloid fluids after initial resuscitation attempts. The basis of this controversy is the differing oncotic properties of the fluids. Crystalloid fluids (e.g., normal saline and lactated Ringer's solution) contain sodium chloride in a quantity that closely matches extracellular fluid. No large molecules are present. Such fluids distribute into the extracellular space. In addition, colloids contain albumin or large osmotically active carbohydrates (hydroxyethyl starch, dextran), which may be held within the intravascular space resulting in an increase of the plasma oncotic pressure. It has been proposed that colloids may provide better outcomes in the resuscitation of shock owing to the rapidity and persistence of volume expansion compared with crystalloid infusion.[45,353] Clinical studies of hypovolemic, traumatic, and septic shock have not supported this contention, however.[354-356] A meta-analysis of randomized, controlled studies examining the effect of fluid administration in critically ill patients with burn injury, hypovolemia, or hypoalbuminemia suggested increased mortality in patients treated with colloids.[357] Other studies have proposed that in shock associated with microvascular changes of permeability (e.g., sepsis), colloid fluids remain in the intravascular space leading to decreased tissue edema and noncardiogenic pulmonary edema.[354] Limited human studies suggest that although radiographic infiltrates may appear more severe with crystalloid resuscitation of sepsis, gas exchange is comparable to colloid resuscitation.[45] In a large, randomized study of albumin versus normal saline, a trend toward improved outcomes with albumin in severe sepsis and saline in trauma failed to reach significance.[358] Given the much higher costs of colloids, resuscitation of shock generally should focus on crystalloid solutions, unless speed of resuscitation is paramount (i.e., acute major trauma or massive hemorrhage). In those settings, colloidal solutions may be initially favored until blood is available.

With respect to hemoglobin, one randomized trial has suggested that a hemoglobin level of 70 g/L is sufficient for most patients in the ICU (other than patients with high severity of illness or acute coronary syndrome[359,360]). Although several other studies have pointed out the potential risks associated with blood transfusion in the ICU,[361-364] no study has directly examined hemoglobin requirements during shock. The only study (indirectly) to examine blood transfusion in shock suggested that early augmentation of hematocrit to greater than 30% during septic shock as part of a protocol to drive central venous oxygen saturation to greater than 70% was associated with improved survival.[199] We continue to recommend that a hemoglobin level of 90 to 100 g/L be maintained during acute shock.

Vasopressors/Inotropes

When intravascular volume is optimized, the next line of therapy of circulatory shock usually involves inotropes and vasopressors. Alternatively, vasopressors occasionally may be required for brief periods of blood pressure support in extremely hypotensive patients before initiation of fluid infusion.

Four major classes of agents are used clinically for inotropic or vasopressor support: sympathomimetics, phosphodiesterase inhibitors, cardiac glycosides, and vasopressin (antidiuretic hormone) (Table 22-4). Sympathomimetics (catecholamines) may activate cardiac β_1-adrenoreceptors and α-adrenoreceptors, peripheral vascular α-receptors or β_2-receptors, and vascular dopaminergic receptors. Cardiac β_1-adrenoreceptors augment heart rate and myocardial contractility by increasing activity of adenylate cyclase resulting in increased generation of cAMP.[365] α-Receptors act through phospholipase C production of inositol triphosphate and diacylglycerol.[366-368] Peripheral vascular α-receptors cause vasoconstriction, whereas peripheral β_2-adrenoreceptors induce a mild vasodilation. Cardiac α-adrenoreceptors contribute to increased contractility (but not heart rate) when stimulated.[366,368] Dopaminergic adrenoreceptors, mediating dilation, are found in the arterial vessels supplying vital organs (including the heart, brain, kidneys, and splanchnic organs).[369] Phosphodiesterase inhibitors, such as amrinone and milrinone, augment cardiac contractility by inhibition of cAMP degradation. They also relax vascular smooth muscle.[370] Despite a long history of digitalis use in the management of congestive heart failure and more recent data suggesting hemodynamic benefit in sepsis,[371] cardiac glycosides are rarely used for the acute management of circulatory shock owing to their narrow therapeutic index and long half-life. Uncontrolled studies have shown that endogenous vasopressin concentrations may be relatively deficient in shock states, and that infusion of vasopressin (which has little effect in healthy, normotensive subjects) can have a profound pressor effect during vasodilatory shock.[372-375]

Dopamine typically is the initial vasopressor used for all types of circulatory shock. A central and peripheral nervous system neurotransmitter and the biologic precursor of norepinephrine, it stimulates three different receptors—vascular dopaminergic, cardiac β_1, and vascular α. The effects of stimulation of each of these receptors have been suggested to dominate the overall hemodynamic response at different infusion rates (Fig. 22-14).[369] In addition, part of its myocardial effects are mediated by release of endogenous norepinephrine. At infusion rates of less than 4 to 5 μg/kg/min, dopaminergic effects dominate. Vascular dopamine-2-receptors vasodilate the renal, mesenteric, myocardial, and cerebral vascular beds. In addition, renal dopamine-1-receptors mediate a mild natriuresis.[376] "Low" or "renal" dose dopamine may be useful in maintaining renal perfusion (while only minimally increasing cardiac contractility) during low output states or in combination with more powerful vasopressors, such as norepinephrine.[377,378] Its use to optimize renal perfusion during critical illness with renal impairment is

Table 22-4. Relative Potency of Intravenously Administered Vasopressors/Inotropes Used in Shock*

		Cardiac		Peripheral Vasculature			
	Dose	Heart Rate	Contractility	Vasoconstriction	Vasodilation	Dopaminergic	Typical Clinical Use
Dopamine	1-4 μg/kg/min 5-10 μg/kg/min 11-20 μg/kg/min	1+ 2+ 2+	1-2+ 2+ 2+	0 1-2+ 2-3+	1+ 1+ 1+	4+ 4+ 4+	All shock
Norepinephrine	2-20 μg/min	2+	2+	4+	0	0	Refractory shock
Dobutamine	1-20 μg/kg/min	1-2+	3+	1+	2+	0	CHF; cardiogenic, obstructive and septic shock
Dopexamine[†]	0.5-6 μg/kg/min	2+	1+	0	3-4+	4+	CHF; cardiogenic shock
Epinephrine	1-8 μg/min	4+	4+	4+	3+	0	Refractory shock or anaphylactic shock
Phenylephrine	20-200 μg/min	0	1+	4+	0	0	Neurogenic or septic shock
Isoproterenol	1-8 μg/min	4+	4+	0	4+	0	Cardiogenic shock (bradyarrhythmia), torsade des pointes, ventricular tachycardia
Vasopressin	0.04-0.10 U/min (start 0.01-0.04 U/min; titrate up 0.02-0.04 U/min every 20-30 min)	0	0	4+	0	0	Vasodilatory (e.g., septic) shock
Milrinone	37.5-75 μg/kg bolus over 10 min; 0.375-0.75 μg/kg/min infusion	1+	3+	0	2+	0	CHF; cardiogenic shock

*The 1-4+ scoring system represents an arbitrary quantitation of the comparative potency of different vasopressors/inotropes.
[†]Not clinically released in the United States.
CHF, congestive heart failure.

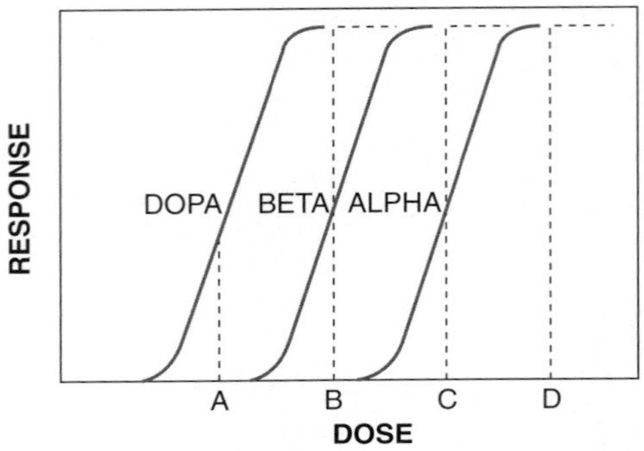

Figure 22-14. Idealized receptor dose response to dopamine. Dopaminergic (DOPA) effects dominate at lower doses *(A)*; β-adrenergic effects (BETA) dominate at moderate doses *(B)* despite near-maximal dopaminergic activity; α-adrenergic effects dominate (ALPHA) at higher doses *(C)* even though dopaminergic and β-adrenergic activity are maximal. At point *D,* dopaminergic activity, β-adrenergic activity, and α-adrenergic activity all are maximal. No data exist to substantiate clear separation of these curves. (Adapted from Breslow MF, Ligier B: Hyperadrenergic states. Crit Care Med 1991;19:1566.)

unproven. At infusion rates of 5 to 10 μg/kg/min, cardiac output is augmented by increased myocardial contractility (cardiac β-adrenoreceptors) and increased venous tone and return (vascular α-adrenoreceptors). At infusion rates greater than 10 μg/kg/min, vascular α-adrenoreceptor effects become more pronounced with increasing blood pressure and smaller increases in cardiac output. Dopaminergic and cardiac adrenergic effects are not suppressed at higher doses, but rather additional effects are seen (see Fig. 22-14). In addition, there is substantial interindividual variation in response, with some patients showing substantial vasopressor or inotropic responses at low infusion rates. For management of circulatory shock, dopamine should be started at 5 μg/kg/min and increased rapidly (5 μg/kg/min every 2 or 3 minutes) to a maximum of 20 μg/kg/min until the target blood pressure is reached. If vasopressor effects are inadequate at these infusion rates, norepinephrine infusion is begun.

Norepinephrine, another endogenous catecholamine, exerts powerful inotropic (cardiac α-adrenoreceptors and β_1-adrenoreceptors) and peripheral vasoconstriction effects (α-adrenoreceptors). It can be used for persistent hypotension despite high-dose dopamine during septic and obstructive shock. It generally should be used only transiently in cardiogenic shock because it may drastically reduce forward flow. Similarly, it should not be required during hemorrhagic shock except for extremely brief periods of blood pressure support pending volume infusion. Infusion rates of 2 to 20 μg/min are commonly used, but if necessary higher infusion rates may be tried. Limited evidence suggests that the concomitant use of low-dose dopamine may result in relative sparing of renal perfusion.[377]

Dobutamine, which is structurally derived from isoproterenol, is a racemic mixture of two synthetic stereoisomers. In combination, the stereoisomers result in increased myocardial contractility through α and β_1 cardiac adrenoreceptors.[379,380] Weak arteriolar vasodilatory effects are mediated through dominance of β_2-adrenoreceptor–mediated vascular relaxation over α-adrenoreceptor–mediated vasoconstriction in the arterial circulation. Evidence suggesting dobutamine induces vasoconstriction in the systemic venous bed (resulting in increased mean circulatory pressure and augmentation of venous return and cardiac output) implies that α-adrenoreceptor–mediated effects may be dominant in small capacitance vessels.[163,379,380]

Although its hemodynamic effects are otherwise similar to those of isoproterenol, dobutamine has been reputed to exert minimal chronotropic effects.[380,381] This attribute has been questioned in more recent studies[382] and may have been based on the selection of congestive heart failure patients with β-adrenoreceptor downregulation and other potential alterations of adrenoreceptor signal transduction.[381,383] Dobutamine's powerful inotropic effect is due to a combination of its direct effect on myocardial contractility, its afterload-reducing effect, and α-adrenoreceptor–mediated venoconstriction.[380,381] In contrast to dopamine, it causes a reduction in filling pressures and a greater increase in cardiac output at equivalent doses.[384,385] In addition, although it increases myocardial oxygen demand (similar to dopamine), myocardial perfusion also is augmented (in contrast to dopamine).[386] The most well-accepted use of dobutamine in circulatory shock relates to cardiac etiologies.[380,381] When blood pressure is corrected, dobutamine may be used to increase cardiac performance and decrease elevated ventricular filling pressures associated with cardiogenic pulmonary edema. In this setting, dobutamine may increase blood pressure. Alternatively, if myocardial damage is extensive, vasodilatory properties may dominate, resulting in hypotension. Dobutamine also may be useful in obstructive shock pending definitive intervention, and more recently it has been used for augmentation of oxygen delivery in septic shock.[387,388] In the latter context, infusion rates far above standard maximums have been used occasionally. Our own experience suggests that maintenance of a PWP of at least 15 mm Hg is required during dobutamine infusion to avoid hypotension in patients with septic shock.

Epinephrine is occasionally used when other inotropes/vasopressors have failed to support blood pressure or cardiac output or both in circulatory shock. It is the first-line agent for management of anaphylactic shock. In addition, it is used to support myocardial contractility after cardiopulmonary bypass.[389] Epinephrine stimulation of α-receptors, β_1-receptors, and β_2-receptors results in increases of myocardial contractility that are more pronounced than with any other inotrope. Epinephrine ng/kg/min infusion rates result in significant increases in cardiac output.[389] Epinephrine also frequently is used in septic shock refractory to other inotropes/vasopressors. Effects attributable to impaired myocardial perfusion (chest pain, arrhythmias, ST-segment depression) in patients with known coronary artery disease are usually limited to patients receiving more than 120 ng/kg/min.[390] Although the usual infusion rate is 1 to 8 μg/min, higher rates can be used, with the potential for increasing toxicity.

Milrinone, a bipyridine phosphodiesterase inhibitor, increases intracellular concentrations of cAMP by blocking cAMP breakdown.[370] Although some controversy has existed regarding the relative contributions of increased myocardial contractility and decreased vascular tone with respect to the apparent inotropic properties of phosphodiesterase inhibitors, more recent data confirm the presence of substantial increases of myocardial contractility[391]; these agents also produce substantial vasodilation. The most accepted use for milrinone in the ICU is in the management of congestive heart failure, cardiogenic shock, and post–cardiopulmonary bypass myocardial dysfunction.[370] Experimental animal studies suggest phosphodiesterase inhibitors may exert beneficial hemodynamic effects in sepsis by augmenting cardiac output and increasing oxygen delivery without increasing consumption.[392] Occasional clinical reports suggest a potential management role in catecholamine-refractory septic shock.[393]

Phenylephrine is a synthetic catecholamine that is unique in its almost pure α-adrenergic agonist effects. Its most common uses are intraoperatively to counteract the vasodilatory effects of anesthetics and in septic shock, where its lack of β-adrenergic activity may help limit deleterious increases in heart rate seen with other agents. Isoproterenol is another synthetic catecholamine with dominant β_1 and β_2 activity. Its previous indications for use have largely been supplanted by dobutamine. Because of its powerful chronotropic effects, it can be useful in the management of bradyarrhythmias and torsades de pointes ventricular tachycardia (for overdrive pacing), but otherwise it has no specific role in the management of circulatory shock.

In recent years, vasopressin levels in septic shock have been shown to be significantly suppressed.[372] Further data have suggested that intravenous infusion of vasopressin into patients with septic shock results in a profound pressor response.[373] This profound pressor response occurs despite the absence of such an effect with even larger amounts of vasopressin in normotensive patients. Investigators also have documented efficacy in other vasodilatory shock states with refractory hypotension, including milrinone-induced shock in severe heart failure,[394] postcardiotomy vasodilatory shock,[395] unstable brain-dead organ donors,[396] and late-phase hemorrhagic shock.[375] Vasopressin (0.1 to 1 U/mL in normal saline or 5% dextrose in water) may be initiated at 0.01 to 0.04 U/min and titrated up every 20 to 30 minutes to a maximum of 0.1 U/min. Few patients respond with higher doses. Because of the limited experience with this compound and the relatively longer half-life of the drug, vasopressin should be used only after hemodynamic stabilization with standard agents (catecholamines) has been attempted. In large doses, vasopressin may produce bradycardia, minor arrhythmias, premature atrial contraction, heart block, peripheral vascular constriction or collapse, coronary insufficiency, decreased cardiac output, myocardial ischemia, and myocardial infarction. In patients with vascular disease (especially of the coronary arteries), even small doses of the drug can precipitate angina. Coronary vasodilators (e.g., amyl nitrite or nitroglycerin) may be used to treat angina if it occurs. At the upper end of dosing, a significant subset of patients may develop digital, mesenteric, or myocardial ischemia, so it is imperative to use the minimal amount of vasopressin possible to achieve desired blood pressure goals. Published data suggest vasopressin can be used for 4 to 6 days if necessary. A randomized, blinded study of vasopressin has more recently been completed. The use of vasodilators and mechanical cardiac support devices is limited mainly to the management of cardiogenic shock and is discussed in Chapter 23.

CONCLUSION

Although the syndrome of shock ultimately involves common late pathologic elements, the early pathophysiologic processes underlying different conditions resulting in circulatory shock are diverse and complex. Concepts of shock, which previously focused on broad cardiovascular physiologic mechanisms, more recently have centered on issues of microvascular function and cellular metabolism. In the future, this focus may evolve toward questions of altered cellular gene expression in a variety of tissues. Advances in therapy have developed in parallel to these changes in understanding of shock pathophysiology. Early work on therapy of shock concentrated on correction of hemodynamic derangements through the use of vasopressors and inotropes. Clinical trials since the 1990s have centered on anticytokines such as anti-TNF-α, novel resuscitative compounds such as diaspirin-linked hemoglobin, metabolic modulators such as dichloracetate, and arachidonic acid metabolite inhibitors such as ibuprofen. The most advanced experimental therapies being examined today involve direct manipulation of gene expression via antisense oligonucleotides and transcription factor inhibitors. Despite these advances, however, many questions remain; only ongoing basic research and clinical trials can answer them.

KEY POINTS

- Shock is the final pathway through which a variety of pathologic processes lead to cardiovascular failure and death.
- Shock is the state in which profound and widespread reduction of effective tissue perfusion leads to cellular injury. The inability of cells to obtain or use oxygen in sufficient quantity optimally to meet their metabolic requirements is common to all forms of shock. Hypotension alone does not define shock.
- Based on hemodynamic characteristics, shock is categorized as hypovolemic, cardiogenic, extracardiac obstructive, or distributive.

- Although one hemodynamic categorization dominates, most forms of clinical shock involve some cardiovascular characteristics of several categories.
- The clinical picture of shock depends on the etiology, the magnitude of the injury or insult, and the degree of physiologic compensation. Physiologic compensation is determined by the time course of development of shock and the pre-existing cardiovascular reserve.
- The systemic hemodynamic aspects of shock can be described by the interactive contributions of cardiac and vascular function to blood pressure and cardiac output.
- Physiologically, blood pressure depends on cardiac output and vascular resistance; cardiac output does not depend on blood pressure.
- Failure to maintain the blood pressure required for autoregulation during hypodynamic circulatory shock indicates a severe reduction in cardiac output.
- In a closed cardiovascular circuit, cardiac output, as determined by heart rate, preload, afterload, and contractility, equals venous return, as determined by venous pressure (mean circulatory pressure), right atrial pressure, and venous resistance. Total systemic perfusion depends on cardiac-vascular interactions.
- In addition to sufficient cardiac output at sufficient pressure, effective perfusion requires normal local and systemic microvascular function resulting in appropriate distribution of cardiac output.
- During hypovolemic and other forms of hypodynamic shock, extrinsic blood flow regulatory mechanisms overwhelm the autoregulatory response of most vascular beds. Blood flow to vital organs such as the heart and brain is relatively well preserved owing to dominant autoregulatory control.
- During distributive shock, particularly septic shock, organ blood flow is disturbed at higher MAP, suggesting a primary defect of microvascular function.
- Cellular dysfunction and organ failure in shock involves the interactions of cellular ischemia, circulating or local inflammatory mediators, and free radical injury.
- All compensatory responses to shock support oxygen delivery to vital tissues. The mechanisms include support of venous pressure, maximization of cardiac function, redistribution of perfusion to vital organs, and optimization of oxygen unloading.
- Circulatory shock may be associated with encephalopathy, ARDS, ATN, ischemic hepatitis or intrahepatic cholestasis, thrombocytopenia, immunosuppression, and MODS.
- Because early recognition and treatment is key to improved survival, the diagnosis of shock is primarily based on clinical criteria. Laboratory and radiologic data are used to confirm the diagnosis and to help clarify etiology.
- Clinically, shock is characterized by physiologic compensatory responses, including tachycardia, tachypnea, and oliguria, and by signs of physiologic decompensation, particularly hypotension.
- Shock should be managed in an ICU with continuous monitoring and close nursing support. Patients whose etiologic diagnosis is in doubt, whose hemodynamic instability does not quickly resolve with intravenous fluids, or who are medically complicated should undergo invasive hemodynamic monitoring with arterial and, possibly, pulmonary artery catheters.
- The basic goal of therapy of circulatory shock is the restoration of effective perfusion to vital organs and tissues before the onset of cellular injury.
- The specific aims of resuscitation of shock include support of mean blood pressure greater than 60 to 65 mm Hg, maintenance of CI greater than 2.1 L/min/m^2 for cardiogenic and obstructive shock or greater than 4 to 4.5 L/min/m^2 for septic and post-traumatic hemorrhagic shock, and restriction of arterial lactate concentrations to less than 2.2 mmol/L.

REFERENCES

1. Heath Statistics 2003. National Center for Health Statistics, CDC, 2003.
2. National Center for Health Statistics. Health, United States, 1986. DHHS pub no (PHS) 87-1232. Washington, DC, Government Printing Office, 1986.
3. Committee on Trauma Research: Injury in America. Washington, DC, National Academy Press, 1985.
4. Eastman AB, West JG: Field triage. In Moore EE, Mattox KL, Feliciano DV (eds): Trauma. Norwalk, CT, Appleton & Lange, 1991, pp 67-79.
5. Finland M: Changing ecology of bacterial infections as related to antibacterial therapy. J Infect Dis 1970;122:419-431.
6. Increase in National Hospital Discharge Survey rates for septicemia in the United States, 1979-1987. JAMA 1990;263:937.
7. Centers for Disease Control and Prevention: National Center for Health Statistics. Mortality patterns—United States, 1990. Monthly Vital Statistics Report 1993;41:5.
8. Dellinger RP: Cardiovascular management of septic shock. Crit Care Med 2003;31(3):946-955.
9. Martin GS, Mannino DM, Eaton S, et al: The epidemiology of sepsis in the United States from 1979 through 2000. N Engl J Med 2003;348(16): 1546-1554.
10. Clarke J: Translation from the French original of H.F. Le Dran (1737). A Treatise, or Reflections Drawn from Practice on Gun-Shot Wounds. London, 1743.
11. Morris EA: A Practical Treatise on Shock after Operations and Injuries. London, 1867.
12. Blalock A: Acute circulatory failure as exemplified by shock and hemorrhage. Surg Gynecol Obstet 1934;58: 551-566.
13. Fischer H: Ueber den Shock. Samml klin Vortr No 10, 1870.
14. Goltz FR: Ueber den Tonus der Gerfaesse und seine Bedeutung fuer die Blutbewegung. Arch F Path Anat U Physiol 1864;29:394-417.
15. Mapother ED: Shock: Its nature, duration, and mode of treatment. BMJ 1879;2:1023-1042.
16. Crile GW: An Experimental Research into Surgical Shock. Philadelphia, Lippincott, 1899.
17. Cannon WB: Traumatic Shock. New York, Appleton, 1923.
18. Keith NM: Blood Volume Changes in Wound Shock and Primary Hemorrhage (Special Report Series No. 27). London, Medical Research Council, 1919.
19. Archibald EW, McLean WS: Observations upon shock, with particular reference to the condition as seen in war surgery. Trans Am Surg Assoc Phila 1917;35:522-532.
20. Simeone FA: Foreword. In Clowes GHA (ed): Trauma, Sepsis, and Shock: The

Physiological Basis of Therapy. New York, Dekker, 1988, pp iii-iv.
21. Blalock A: Experimental shock: Cause of low blood pressure produced by muscle injury. Arch Surg 1930;20:959-996.
22. Beecher HK, Simeone FA, Burnett CH, et al: The internal state of the severely wounded man on entry to the most forward hospital. Surgery 1947;22:672-711.
23. Cournand A, Riley RL, Bradley SE, et al: Studies of the circulation in clinical shock. Surgery 1943;13:964-995.
24. Wiggers CJ: The Physiology of Shock. Cambridge, Mass, Harvard University Press, 1950.
25. Battle Casualties in Korea: Surgical Research Team in Korea, Vol 1. Washington, DC, Army Medical Graduate School, Walter Reed Medical Center, 1954.
26. Warren JC: Surgical Pathology and Therapeutics. Philadelphia, Saunders, 1895.
27. Simeone FA: Shock. In: Davis L, editor. Christopher's Textbook of Surgery. Philadelphia: Saunders, 1964:58.
28. Fink MP: Shock: An overview. In Rippe JM, Irwin RS, Alpert JS, et al (eds): Intensive Care Medicine. Boston, Little, Brown, 1991, pp 1417-1435.
29. Cerra FB: Shock. In Burke JF (ed): Surgical Physiology. Philadelphia, Saunders, 1983, p 497.
30. Laennec RTH: Traite de L'uscultation Mediate et des Maladies des Poumons et du Coeur. Paris, JS Chaude, 1831.
31. Boise E: The differential diagnosis of shock, hemorrhage, and sepsis. Trans Am Assoc Obstet 1897;9:433-438.
32. Fishberg AM, Hitzig WM, King FH: Circulatory dynamics in myocardial infarction. Arch Intern Med 1934;54:997-1019.
33. Blalock A: Shock: Further studies with particular reference to the effects of hemorrhage. Arch Surg 1937;29:837-857.
34. Weil MH: Bacterial shock. In Weil MH, Shubin H (eds): Diagnosis and Treatment of Shock. Baltimore, Williams & Wilkins, 1967, p 10.
35. Hinshaw LB, Cox BG: The Fundamental Mechanisms of Shock. New York, Plenum Press, 1972.
36. Reilly JM, Cunnion RE, Burch-Whitman C, et al: A circulating myocardial depressant substance is associated with cardiac dysfunction and peripheral hypoperfusion (lactic acidemia) in patients with septic shock. Chest 1989;95:1072-1080.
37. Ognibene FP, Parker MM, Natanson C, et al: Depressed left ventricular performance: Response to volume infusion in patients with sepsis and septic shock. Chest 1988;93:903-910.
38. Parker MM, Shelhamer JH, Bacharach SL, et al: Profound but reversible myocardial depression in patients with septic shock. Ann Intern Med 1984;100:483-490.
39. Walley KR, Cooper DJ: Diastolic stiffness impairs left ventricular function during hypovolemic shock in pigs. Am J Physiol 1991;260: H702-H712.
40. Alyono D, Ring WS, Chao RYN, et al: Character of ventricular function in severe hemorrhagic shock. Surgery 1983;94:250-258.
41. Bond RF, Johnson GI: Vascular adrenergic interactions during hemorrhagic shock. Fed Proc 1985;44:281-289.
42. Thiemermann C, Szabö C, Mitchell JA, et al: Vascular hyporeactivity to vasoconstrictor agents and hemodynamic decompensation in hemorrhagic shock is mediated by nitric oxide. Proc Natl Acad Sci U S A 1993;90:267-271.
43. Sarnoff SJ, Case RB, Waitag PE, et al: Insufficient coronary flow and myocardial failure as a complicating factor in late hemorrhagic shock. Am J Physiol 1954;176:439-444.
44. Sander-Jenson K, Secher NH, Bie P, et al: Vagal slowing of the heart during hemorrhage: Observations from twenty consecutive hypotensive patients. BMJ 1986;295:364-366.
45. Rackow EC, Falk JL, Fein IA, et al: Fluid resuscitation in circulatory shock: A comparison of the cardiorespiratory effects of albumin, hetastarch, and saline solutions in patients with hypovolemic and septic shock. Crit Care Med 1983;11:839-850.
46. Shenkin HA, Cheney RH, Govons SR, et al: On the diagnosis of hemorrhage in man: A study in volunteers bled large amounts. Am J Med Sci 1944;208:421-436.
47. Knopp R, Claypool R, Leonardt D: Use of the tilt test in measuring acute blood loss. Ann Emerg Med 1980;9:72-75.
48. Rush BF: Irreversibility in post-transfusion phase of hemorrhagic shock. Adv Exp Med Biol 1971;23:215-234.
49. Dunham C, Siegel J, Weireter L: Oxygen debt and metabolic acidemia as quantitative predictors of mortality and the severity of the ischemia insult in hemorrhagic shock. Crit Care Med 1991;19:231-243.
50. Viteck V, Cowley R: Blood lactate in the prognosis of various forms of shock. Ann Surg 1971;173:308-313.
51. Goldberg RJ, Gore JM, Alpert JS, et al: Cardiogenic shock after acute myocardial infarction: Incidence and mortality from a community-wide perspective. N Engl J Med 1991;325:1117-1122.
52. Wackers FJ, Lie KI, Becker AE: Coronary artery disease in patients dying from cardiogenic shock or congestive heart failure in the setting of acute myocardial infarction. Br Heart J 1976;38:906-910.
53. Afifi AA, Chang PC, Liu VY, et al: Prognostic indexes in acute myocardial infarction complicated by shock. Am J Cardiol 1974;33:826-832.
54. Page DL, Caulfield JB, Kastor JA: Myocardial changes associated with cardiogenic shock. N Engl J Med 1971;285:133-137.
55. Alonso DR, Scheidt S, Post M, et al: Pathophysiology of cardiogenic shock: Quantification of myocardial necrosis: Clinical, pathologic, and electrocardiographic correlation. Circulation 1973;48:588-596.
56. Weber KT, Ratshin RA, Janicki JS: Left ventricular dysfunction following acute myocardial infarction: A clinicopathologic and hemodynamic profile of shock and failure. Am J Med 1973;54:697-705.
57. Scheidt S, Ascheim R, Killip T: Shock after acute myocardial infarction: A clinical and hemodynamic profile. Am J Cardiol 1970;26:556-564.
58. Simoons ML, Vander Brand M, DeZwaan M: Improved survival after early thrombolysis in acute myocardial infarction. Lancet 1985;578-581.
59. Chesebro JH, Knatterud G, Roberts R, et al: Thrombolysis in Myocardial Infarction (TIMI) Trial, Phase I: A comparison between intravenous tissue plasminogen activator and intravenous streptokinase: Clinical findings through hospital discharge. Circulation 1987;76:142-154.
60. Kennedy JW, Ritchie JL, Davis KB, et al: Western Washington randomized trial of intracoronary streptokinase in acute myocardial infarction. N Engl J Med 1983;309:1477-1482.
61. The Gusto Investigators: An international randomized trial comparing four thrombolytic strategies for acute myocardial infarction. N Engl J Med 1993;329:673-682.
62. Hollenberg SM, Kavinsky CJ, Parrillo JE: Cardiogenic shock. Ann Intern Med 1999;131:47-59.
63. Gruppo Italiano per lo Studio della Streptochinasi nell'Infarto Miocardico (GISSI): Effectiveness of intravenous thrombolytic treatment in acute myocardial infarction. Lancet 1986;1:397-402.
64. Hochman JS, Sleeper LA, Webb JG, et al: Early revascularization in acute myocardial infarction complicated by cardiogenic shock. SHOCK Investigators. Should We Emergently Revascularize Occluded Coronaries for Cardiogenic Shock? N Engl J Med 1999;341:625-634.
65. Berger PB, Holmes DR Jr, Stebbins AL, et al: Impact of an aggressive invasive catheterization and revascularization strategy on mortality in patients with cardiogenic shock in the Global Utilization of Streptokinase and Tissue Plasminogen Activator for Occluded Coronary Arteries (GUSTO-1) trial: An observational study. Circulation 1997;96:122-127.
66. Wei HY, Hutchins GM, Bulkley BH: Papillary muscle rupture in fatal acute myocardial infarction: A potentially treatable form of cardiogenic shock. Ann Intern Med 1979;90:149-152.
67. Felix SB, Baumann G, Hashemi T, et al: Characterization of cardiovascular events mediated by platelet activating factor during systemic anaphylaxis. J Cardiovasc Pharmacol 1990;15:987-997.
68. Cohn JN, Guiha NH, Broder MI, et al: Right ventricular infarction: Clinical and hemodynamic features. Am J Cardiol 1974;33:209-214.
69. Roberts N, Harrison DG, Reimer KA, et al: Right ventricular infarction with shock but without significant left ventricular infarction: A new clinical syndrome. Am Heart J 1985;110:1047-1053.
70. Leinbach RC: Right ventricular infarction. J Cardiovasc Med 1980;5:499-509.

71. Lloyd EA, Gersh BJ, Kennelly BM: Hemodynamic spectrum of "dominant" right ventricular infarction in 19 patients. Am J Cardiol 1981;48:1016-1022.
72. Zehender M, Kasper W, Kauder E, et al: Right ventricular infarction as an independent predictor of prognosis after acute inferior myocardial infarction. N Engl J Med 1993;328:981-988.
73. Da Luz P, Weil MH, Shubin H: Plasma volume prior to and following volume loading during shock complicating acute myocardial infarction. Circulation 1974;49:98-105.
74. Reddy PS, Curtiss EI, O'Toole JD, et al: Cardiac tamponade: Hemodynamic observations in man. Circulation 1978;58:265-272.
75. London RE, London SB: Rupture of the heart: A critical analysis of 47 consecutive autopsy cases. Circulation 1965;31:202-208.
76. McMullen MH, Kilgore TL, Dear HD, et al: Sudden blowout rupture of the myocardium after infarction: Urgent management. J Thorac Cardiovasc Surg 1985;89:259-263.
77. Sharma GVRK, McIntyre KM, Sharma S, et al: Clinical and hemodynamic correlates in pulmonary embolism. Clin Chest Med 1984;5:421-437.
78. McIntyre KM, Sasahara AA: The hemodynamic response to pulmonary embolism in patients without prior cardiopulmonary disease. Am J Cardiol 1971;28:288-294.
79. Wood KE: The presence of shock defines the threshold to initiate thrombolytic therapy in patients with pulmonary embolism. Intensive Care Med 2002;28:1537-1546.
80. Wood KE: Major pulmonary embolism: Review of a pathophysiologic approach to the golden hour of hemodynamically significant pulmonary embolism. Chest 2002;121:877-905.
81. Parrillo JE: Pathogenetic mechanisms of septic shock. N Engl J Med 1993;328:1471-1477.
82. Cohn JD, Greenspan M, Goldstein CR, et al: Arteriovenous shunting in high cardiac output shock syndromes. Surg Gynecol Obstet 1968;127: 282-288.
83. Thijs LG, Groenveld ABJ: Peripheral circulation in septic shock. Appl Cardiopulm Pathol 1988;2:203-214.
84. Wright CJ, Duff JH, McLean APH, et al: Regional capillary blood flow and oxygen uptake in severe sepsis. Surg Gynecol Obstet 1971;132:637-644.
85. Finley RJ, Duff JH, Holliday RL, et al: Capillary muscle blood flow in human sepsis. Surgery 1975;78:87-94.
86. Cronenwett JL, Lindenauer SM: Direct measurement of arteriovenous anastomic blood flow in the septic canine hindlimb. Surgery 1979;85:275-282.
87. Dantzker D: Oxygen delivery and utilization in sepsis. Crit Care Clin 1989;5:81-98.
88. Wolf YG, Cotev S, Perel A, et al: Dependence of oxygen consumption on cardiac output in sepsis. Crit Care Med 1987;15:198-203.
89. Shoemaker WC, Chang P, Czer L, et al: Cardiorespiratory monitoring in postoperative patients: I. Prediction of outcome and severity of illness. Crit Care Med 1979;7:237-242.
90. Haupt MT, Gilbert EM, Carlson RW: Fluid loading increases oxygen consumption in septic patients with lactic acidosis. Am Rev Respir Dis 1985;131:912-916.
91. Samsel RW, Nelson DP, Sanders WM, et al: Effect of endotoxin on systemic and skeletal muscle oxygen extraction. J Appl Physiol 1988;65:1377-1382.
92. Vincent JL, Roman A, DeBacker D, et al: Oxygen uptake/supply dependency: Effects of short-term dobutamine infusion. Am Rev Respir Dis 1990;142:2-8.
93. Fenwick JC, Dodek PM, Ronco JJ, et al: Increased concentrations of plasma lactate predict pathological dependence of oxygen consumption on oxygen delivery in patients with adult respiratory distress syndrome. J Crit Care 1990;5:81-87.
94. Gutierrez G, Pohil RJ: Oxygen consumption is linearly related to oxygen supply in critically ill patients. J Crit Care 1986;1:45-53.
95. Astiz M, Rackow EC, Weil MH, et al: Early impairment of oxidative metabolism and energy production in severe sepsis. Circ Shock 1988;26:311-320.
96. Mizock B: Septic shock: A metabolic perspective. Arch Intern Med 1984;144:579-585.
97. Song SK, Hotchkiss RS, Karl IE, et al: Concurrent quantification of tissue metabolism and blood flow via 2H/31P NMR in vivo: III. Alterations of muscle blood flow and metabolism during sepsis. Magn Reson Med 1992;25:67-77.
98. Hotchkiss RS, Karl IE: Reevaluation of the role of cellular hypoxia and bioenergetic failure in sepsis. JAMA 1992;267:1503-1510.
99. Solomon MA, Correa R, Alexander HR, et al: Myocardial energy metabolism and morphology in a canine model of sepsis. Am J Physiol 1994;266: H757-H768.
100. Hotchkiss RS, Rust RS, Dence CS, et al: Evaluation of the role of cellular hypoxia in sepsis by the hypoxic marker [18F] fluoromisonidazole. Am J Physiol 1991;261:R965-R972.
101. Hotchkiss RS, Song SK, Neil JJ, et al: Sepsis does not impair tricarboxylic acid cycle in the heart. Am J Physiol 1991;260:C50-C57.
102. Chaudry IH, Wichterman KA, Baue AE: Effect of sepsis on tissue adenine nucleotide levels. Surgery 1979;85:205-211.
103. Geller ER, Tankauskas S, Kirpatrick JR: Mitochondrial death in sepsis: A failed concept. J Surg Res 1986;40:514-517.
104. Kumar A, Roberts D, Wood KE, et al: Duration of hypotension before initiation of effective antimicrobial therapy is the critical determinant of survival in human septic shock. Crit Care Med 2006;34:1589-1596.
105. The Veterans Administration Systemic Sepsis Cooperative Study Group: The effect of high dose glucocorticoid therapy on mortality in patients with clinical signs of systemic sepsis. N Engl J Med 1987;317:659-665.
106. Ziegler EJ, Fisher CJ Jr, Sprung C, et al: Treatment of gram-negative bacteremia and septic shock with HA-1A human monoclonal antibody against endotoxin. N Engl J Med 1991;324:429-436.
107. Bauer S, Kirschning CJ, Hacker H, et al: Human TLR9 confers responsiveness to bacterial DNA via species-specific CpG motif recognition. Proc Natl Acad Sci U S A 2001;98:9237-9242.
108. Dziarski R, Wang Q, Miyake K, et al: MD-2 enables Toll-like receptor 2 (TLR2)-mediated responses to lipopolysaccharide and enhances TLR2-mediated responses to gram-positive and gram-negative bacteria and their cell wall components. J Immunol 2001;166:1938-1944.
109. Yang RB, Mark MR, Gray A, et al: Toll-like receptor-2 mediates lipopolysaccharide-induced cellular signalling. Nature 1998;395:284-288.
110. Lien E, Sellati TJ, Yoshimura A, et al: Toll-like receptor 2 functions as a pattern recognition receptor for diverse bacterial products. J Biol Chem 1999;274:33419-33425.
111. Schwandner R, Dziarski R, Wesche H, et al: Peptidoglycan- and lipoteichoic acid-induced cell activation is mediated by toll-like receptor 2. J Biol Chem 1999;274:17406-17409.
112. Parker MM, Shelhamer JH, Natanson C, et al: Serial cardiovascular variables in survivors and nonsurvivors of human septic shock: Heart rate as an early predictor of prognosis. Crit Care Med 1987;15:923-929.
113. Teule GJJ, Van Lingen A, Verweij-van Vught MA, et al: Role of peripheral pooling in porcine *Escherichia coli* sepsis. Circ Shock 1984;12:115-123.
114. Natanson C, Fink MP, Ballantyne HK, et al: Gram-negative bacteremia produces both severe systolic and diastolic cardiac dysfunction in a canine model that simulates human septic shock. J Clin Invest 1986;78:259-270.
115. Carroll GC, Snyder JV: Hyperdynamic severe intravascular sepsis depends on fluid administration in cynomolgus monkey. Am J Physiol 1982;243: 131-141.
116. Teule GJJ, Den Hollander W, Bronsveld W, et al: Effect of volume loading and dopamine on hemodynamics and red cell distribution in canine endotoxic shock. Circ Shock 1983;10:41-50.
117. Magder S, Vanelli G: Circuit factors in the high cardiac output of sepsis. J Crit Care 1996;11:155-166.
118. Donnino M, Nguyen HB, Rivers EP: A hemodynamic comparison of early and late phase severe sepsis and septic shock. Chest 2002;122:4S.
119. MacLean LD, Mulligan WG, McLean APH, et al: Patterns of septic shock in man: A detailed study of 56 patients. Ann Surg 1967;166:543-562.
120. Eichenholz PW, Eichacker PQ, Hoffman WD, et al: Tumor necrosis factor challenges in canines: Patterns of cardiovascular dysfunction. Am J Physiol 1992;263:H668-H675.
121. Vincent JL, Bakker J, Marecaux G, et al: Administration of anti-TNF antibody improves left ventricular function in septic shock patients: Results of a pilot study. Chest 1992;101:810-815.

122. Hosenpud JD, Campbell SM, Mendelson DJ: Interleukin-1-induced myocardial depression in an isolated beating heart preparation. J Heart Transplant 1989;8:460-464.
123. Kumar A, Krieger A, Symeoneides S, et al: Myocardial dysfunction in septic shock: Part II. Role of cytokines and nitric oxide. J Cardiovasc Thorac Anesth 2001;15:485-511.
124. Massey CV, Kohout TR, Gaa ST, et al: Molecular and cellular actions of platelet-activating factor in rat heart cells. J Clin Invest 1991;88:2106-2116.
125. Schutzer KM, Haglund U, Falk A: Cardiopulmonary dysfunction in a feline septic model: Possible role of leukotrienes. Circ Shock 1989;29:13-25.
126. Werdan K, Muller U, Reithmann C: "Negative inotropic cascades" in cardiomyocytes triggered by substances relevant to sepsis. In Schlag G, Redl H (eds): Pathophysiology of Shock, Sepsis and Organ Failure. Berlin, Springer-Verlag, 1993, pp 787-834.
127. Pathan N, Hemingway CA, Alizadeh AA, et al: Role of interleukin 6 in myocardial dysfunction of meningococcal septic shock. Lancet 2004;363:203-209.
128. Bochner BS, Lichtenstein LM: Anaphylaxis. N Engl J Med 1991;324:1785-1790.
129. Chrusch C, Sharma S, Unruh H, et al: Histamine H3 receptor blockade improves cardiac function in canine anaphylaxis. Am J Respir Crit Care Med 1999;160:1142-1149.
130. Parrillo JE: Cardiovascular dysfunction in human septic shock. Prog Clin Biol Res 1989;308:191-199.
131. Otero E, Onufer JR, Reiss CK, et al: Anaphylaxis-induced myocardial depression treated with amrinone. Lancet 1991;337:682.
132. Raper RF, Fisher MMD: Profound reversible myocardial depression after anaphylaxis. Lancet 1988;1:386-388.
133. Silverman HJ, Van Hook C, Haponik EF: Hemodynamic changes in human anaphylaxis. Am J Med 1984;77: 341-344.
134. Smith PL, Kagey-Sobotka A, Bleecker ER, et al: Physiologic manifestations of human anaphylaxis. J Clin Invest 1980;66:1072-1080.
135. Rao RH, Vagnucci AH, Amico JH: Bilateral massive adrenal hemorrhage: Early recognition and treatment. Ann Intern Med 1989;110:227-235.
136. Chin R: Adrenal crisis. Crit Care Clin 1991;7:23-42.
137. Burke CW: Adrenocortical insufficiency. Clin Endocrinol Metab 1985;14: 948-976.
138. Claussen MS, Landercasper J, Cogbill TH: Acute adrenal insufficiency presenting as shock after trauma and surgery: Three cases and review of the literature. J Trauma 1992;32:94-100.
139. Dorin RI, Kearns PJ: High output circulatory failure in acute adrenal insufficiency. Crit Care Med 1988;16:296-297.
140. Annane D, Bellissant E, Sebille V, et al: Impaired pressor sensitivity to noradrenaline in septic shock patients with and without impaired adrenal function reserve. Br J Clin Pharmacol 1998;46:589-597.
141. Annane D, Sebille V, Troche G, et al: A 3-level prognostic classification in septic shock based on cortisol levels and cortisol response to corticotropin. JAMA 2000;283:1038-1045.
142. Rothwell PM, Udwadia ZF, Lawler PG: Cortisol response to corticotropin and survival in septic shock. Lancet 1991;337:582-583f.
143. Soni A, Pepper M, Wyrwinski PM, et al: Adrenal insufficiency occurring during septic shock: Incidence, outcome, and relationship to peripheral cytokine levels. Am J Med 1995;28:266-271.
144. Marik PE, Zaloga GP: Adrenal insufficiency during septic shock. Crit Care Med 2003;31:141-145.
145. Bollaert PE, Charpentier C, Levy B, et al: Reversal of late septic shock with supraphysiologic doses of hydrocortisone. Crit Care Med 1998;26:645-650.
146. Briegel J, Forst H, Haller M, et al: Stress doses of hydrocortisone reverse hyperdynamic septic shock: A prospective randomized, double-blind, single-center study. Crit Care Med 1999;27:723-732.
147. Annane D, Sebille V, Charpentier C, et al: Effect of treatment with low doses of hydrocortisone and fludrocortisone on mortality in patients with septic shock. JAMA 2002;288:862-871.
148. Confalonieri M, Urbino R, Potena A, et al: Hydrocortisone infusion for severe community-acquired pneumonia: A preliminary randomized study. Am J Respir Crit Care Med 2005;171:242-248.
149. Guyton AC: Textbook of Medical Physiology, 8th ed. Philadelphia, Saunders, 1991.
150. Bond RF: Peripheral macro- and microcirculation. In Schlag G, Redl H (eds): Pathophysiology of Shock, Sepsis and Organ Failure. Berlin, Springer-Verlag, 1993, pp 893-907.
151. Calvin JE, Driedger AA, Sibbald WJ: Does the pulmonary wedge pressure predict left ventricular preload in critically ill patients? Crit Care Med 1981;9:437-443.
152. Braunwald E, Frahm CJ: Studies on Starling's law of the heart: IV. Observations on hemodynamic functions of the left atrium in man. Circulation 1961;24:633-642.
153. Sylvester JT, Goldberg HS, Permutt S: The role of the vasculature in the regulation of cardiac output. Clin Chest Med 1983;4:111-126.
154. Bressack MA, Raffin TA: Importance of venous return, venous resistance, and mean circulatory pressure in the physiology and management of shock. Chest 1987;92:906-912.
155. Milnor WR: Arterial impedance as ventricular afterload. Circ Res 1975;36:565-570.
156. Carabello BA, Spann JF: The uses and limitations of end-systolic indices of left ventricular function. Circulation 1984;69:1058-1064.
157. Magder S, De Verennes B: Clinical death and the measurement of stressed vascular volume. Crit Care Med 1998;26:1061-1064.
158. Deschamps A, Magder S: Baroreflex control of regional capacitance and blood flow distribution with or without alpha adrenergic blockade. Am J Physiol 1992;262: H1755-H1763.
159. Deschamps A, Magder S: Effects of heat stress on vascular capacitance. Am J Physiol 1994;266:H2122-H2129.
160. Rothe CF: Reflex control of veins and vascular capacitance. Physiol Rev 1983;63:1281-1295.
161. Guyton AC, Jones CE, Coleman TG: Circulatory Physiology: Cardiac Output and Its Regulation, 2nd ed. Philadelphia, Saunders, 1973.
162. Permutt S, Riley S: Hemodynamics of collapsible vessels with tone: The vascular waterfall. J Appl Physiol 1963;18:924-932.
163. Brinkley PF, Murray KD, Watson KM, et al: Dobutamine increases cardiac output of the total artificial heart. Circulation 1991;84:1210-1215.
164. Marino RJ, Romagnoli A, Keats AS: Selective venoconstriction by dopamine in comparison with isoproterenol and phenylephrine. Anesthesiology 1975;43:570-572.
165. Pinsky MR, Matushek M: Hemodynamic changes in endotoxic shock. J Crit Care 1986;1:18-31.
166. Stephan F, Novara A, Tournier B, et al: Determination of total effective vascular compliance in patients with sepsis syndrome. Am J Respir Crit Care Med 1998;157:50-56.
167. Astiz ME, Tilly E, Rackow EC, et al: Peripheral vascular tone in sepsis. Chest 1991;99:1072-1075.
168. Bressack MA, Morton NS, Hortop J: Group B streptococcal sepsis in the piglet: Effects of fluid therapy on venous return, organ edema, and organ blood flow. Circ Res 1987;61:659.
169. Schumacker PT: Peripheral vascular responses in septic shock: Direct or reflex effects? Chest 1991;99: 1057-1058.
170. Calvin JE, Sibbald WJ: Applied cardiovascular physiology in the critically ill with special reference to diastole and ventricular interaction. In Shoemaker WC, Ayres S, Grenvik A, et al (eds): Textbook of Critical Care. Philadelphia, Saunders, 1989, pp 312-325.
171. Suga H, Sagawa K: Instantaneous pressure-volume relationships and their ratio in the excised, supported canine left ventricle. Circ Res 1974;35:117-126.
172. Katz AM: Influence of altered inotropy and lusitropy on ventricular pressure-volume loops. J Am Coll Cardiol 1988;11:438-445.
173. Johnson PC: Autoregulation of blood flow. Circ Res 1986;59:483-495.
174. Gutteriez G, Brown SD: Response of the macrocirculation. In Schlag R, Redl H (eds): Pathophysiology of Shock, Sepsis and Organ Failure. Berlin, Springer-Verlag, 1993, pp 215-229.
175. Wang P, Hauptman JG, Chaudry IH: Hemorrhage produces depression in microvascular blood flow which persists despite fluid resuscitation. Circ Shock 1990;32:307-318.
176. Bowton DL, Bertels NH, Prough DS, et al: Cerebral blood flow is reduced

in patients with sepsis syndrome. Crit Care Med 1989;17:399-403.
177. Ekstrom-Jodal B, Haggendal E, Larsson LE: Cerebral blood flow and oxygen uptake in endotoxic shock: An experimental study in dogs. Acta Anaesthesiol Scand 1982;26:163-170.
178. Cunnion RE, Schaer GL, Parker MM, et al: The coronary circulation in human septic shock. Circulation 1986;73:637-644.
179. Dhainaut JF, Huyghebaert MF, Monsallier JF, et al: Coronary hemodynamics and myocardial metabolism of lactate, free fatty acids, glucose, and ketones in patients with septic shock. Circulation 1987;75:533-541.
180. Cryer HM, Kaebrick H, Harris PD, et al: Effect of tissue acidosis on skeletal muscle microcirculatory responses to hemorrhagic shock in unanesthetized rats. J Surg Res 1985;39:59-67.
181. Coleman B, Glaviano VV: Tissue levels of norepinephrine in hemorrhagic shock. Science 1963;139:54.
182. Chernow B, Roth BL: Pharmacologic manipulation of the peripheral vasculature in shock: Clinical and experimental approaches. Circ Shock 1986;18:141-155.
183. Koyama S, Aibiki M, Kanai K, et al: Role of the central nervous system in renal nerve activity during prolonged hemorrhagic shock in dogs. Am J Physiol 1988;254:R761-R769.
184. Lorente JA, Landin L, Renes E, et al: Role of nitric oxide in the hemodynamic changes of sepsis. Crit Care Med 1993;21:759-767.
185. Carden DI, Smith JK, Zimmerman BJ, et al: Reperfusion injury following circulatory collapse: The role of reactive oxygen metabolites. J Crit Care 1989;4:294-300.
186. Kubes P: Nitric oxide modulates microvascular permeability. Am J Physiol 1992;262:H611-H615.
187. Wang LF, Patel M, Razavi HM, et al: Role of inducible nitric oxide synthase in pulmonary microvascular protein leak in murine sepsis. Am J Respir Crit Care Med 2002;165:1634-1639.
188. Redl H, Schlag G, Kneidinger R, et al: Activation/adherence phenomena of leukocytes and endothelial cells in trauma and sepsis. In Redl H, Schlag G (eds): Pathophysiology of Shock, Sepsis and Organ Failure. Berlin, Springer-Verlag, 1993, pp 549-563.
189. Shah DM, Dutton RE, Newell JC, et al: Vascular autoregulatory failure following trauma and shock. Surg Forum 1977;28:11-13.
190. Hurd TC, Dasmahapatra KS, Rush BF Jr, et al: Red blood cell deformability in human and experimental sepsis. Arch Surg 1988;123:217-220.
191. Van Rossum GD: The relation of sodium and potassium ion transport to respiration and adenine nucleotide content of liver slices treated with inhibitors of respiration. Biochem J 1972;129:427-438.
192. Vogt MT, Fraber E: The effects of ethionine treatment on the metabolims of liver mitochondria. Arch Biochem Biophys 1970;141: 162-173.
193. Chaudry IH: Cellular mechanisms in shock and ischemia and their correction. Am J Physiol 1983;245: R117-R134.
194. Horpacsy G, Schnells G: Metabolism of adenine nucleotides in the kidney during hemorrhagic hypotension and after recovery. J Surg Res 1980;29:11-17.
195. Chaudry IH, Sayeed MM, Baue AE: Alteration in high-energy phosphates in hemorrhagic shock as related to tissue and organ function. Surgery 1976;79:666-668.
196. Chaudry IH, Sayeed MM, Baue AE: Effect of adenosine triphosphate-magnesium chloride administration in shock. Surgery 1974;75:220-227.
197. Chaudry IH, Sayeed MM, Baue AE: Effect of hemorrhagic shock on tissue adenine nucleotides in conscious rats. Can J Physiol Pharmacol 1974;52: 131-137.
198. Chaudry IH, Ohkawa M, Clemens MG, et al: Alterations in electron transport and cellular metabolism with shock and trauma. Prog Clin Biol Res 1983;111:67-88.
199. Rivers E, Nguyen B, Havstad S, et al: Early goal-directed therapy in the treatment of severe sepsis and septic shock. N Engl J Med 2001;345: 1368-1377.
200. Ayala A, Perrin MM, Meldrum DR, et al: Hemorrhage induces an increase in serum TNF which is not associated with elevated levels of endotoxin. Cytokine 1990;2:170-174.
201. Calandra T, Baumgartner J, Grau GE, et al: Prognostic values of tumor necrosis factor/cachectin, interleukin-1, and interferon-γ in the serum of patients with septic shock. J Infect Dis 1990;161:982-987.
202. Girardin E, Grau GE, Dayer JM, et al: Plasma tumor necrosis factor and interleukin-1 in the serum of children with severe infectious purpura. N Engl J Med 1989;319:397-400.
203. Zanotti S, Kumar A, Kumar A: Cytokine modulation in sepsis and septic shock. Expert Opinion Invest Drugs 2002;11:1061-1075.
204. Bone RC: The pathogenesis of sepsis. Ann Intern Med 1991;115:457-469.
205. Tracey KJ, Lowry SF, Beutler B, et al: Cachectin/tumor necrosis factor mediates changes of skeletal muscle plasma membrane potential. J Exp Med 1986;164:1368-1373.
206. Levine B, Kalman J, Mayer L, et al: Elevated circulating levels of tumor necrosis factor in severe chronic heart failure. N Engl J Med 1990;323: 236-241.
207. Pathan N, Sandiford C, Harding SE, et al: Characterization of a myocardial depressant factor in meningococcal septicemia. Crit Care Med 2002;30:2191-2198.
208. Calandra T, Echtenacher B, Roy DL, et al: Protection from septic shock by neutralization of macrophage migration inhibitory factor. Nat Med 2000;6:164-170.
209. Calandra T, Glauser MP: Immunocompromised animal models for the study of antibiotic combinations. Am J Med 1986;80:45-52.
210. Wang H, Yang H, Czura CJ, et al: HMGB1 as a late mediator of lethal systemic inflammation. Am J Respir Crit Care Med 2001;164(10 Pt 1):1768-1773.
211. Parrillo JE, Burch C, Shelhamer JH, et al: A circulating myocardial depressant substance in humans with septic shock: Septic shock patients with a reduced ejection fraction have a circulating factor that depresses in vitro myocardial cell performance. J Clin Invest 1985;76:1539-1553.
212. Hallstrom S, Vogl C, Redl H, et al: Net inotropic plasma activity in canine hypovolemic traumatic shock: Low molecular weight plasma fraction after prolonged hypotension depresses cardiac muscle performance in-vitro. Circ Shock 1990;30:129-144.
213. Brar R, Kumar A, Schaer GL, et al: Myocardial infarction and reperfusion produces soluble myocardial depressant activity that correlates with infarct size. Crit Care Med 1996;24: A30.
214. Coraim F, Trubel W, Ebermann R, et al: Isolation of low molecular weight peptides in hemofiltrated patients with cardiogenic shock: A new aspect of myocardial depressant substances. Contrib Nephrol 1991;93:237-240.
215. Hallstrom S, Koidl B, Muller U, et al: A cardiodepressant factor isolated from blood blocks Ca^{2+} current in cardiomyocytes. Am J Physiol 1991;260:H869-H876.
216. Kumar A, Thota V, Dee L, et al: Tumor necrosis factor-alpha and interleukin-1 beta are responsible for depression of in vitro myocardial cell contractility induced by serum from humans with septic shock. J Exp Med 1996;183: 949-958.
217. Kumar A, Brar R, Wang P, et al: The role of nitric oxide and cyclic GMP in human septic serum-induced depression of cardiac myocyte contractility. Am J Physiol 1999;276: R265-R276.
218. Cain BS, Meldrum DR, Dinarello CA, et al: Tumor necrosis factor-α and interleukin-1β synergistically depress human myocardial function. Crit Care Med 1999;27:1309-1318.
219. Nathan C: Nitric oxide as a secretory product of mammalian cells. FASEB J 1992;6:3051-3064.
220. Kilbourn RG, Gross SS, Jubran A, et al: N-methyl-L-arginine inhibits tumor necrosis factor-induced hypotension: Implications for the involvement of nitric oxide. Proc Natl Acad Sci U S A 1990;87:3629-3623.
221. Beckman JS, Beckman TW, Chen J, et al: Apparent hydroxyl radical production by peroxynitrite: Implications for endothelial injury from nitric oxide and superoxide. Proc Natl Acad Sci U S A 1990;87:1620-1624.
222. Szabo C, Salzman AL, Ischiropoulos H: Endotoxin triggers the expression of an inducible isoform of nitric oxide synthase and the formation of peroxynitrite in the rat aorta in vivo. FEBS Lett 1995;363:235-238.
223. Brovkovych V, Patton S, Brovkovych S, et al: In situ measurement of nitric oxide, superoxide and peroxynitrite during endotoxemia. J Physiol Pharmacol 1997;48:633-644.
224. Pryor WA, Squadrito GL: The chemistry of peroxynitrite: A product from the reaction of nitric oxide with

superoxide. Am J Physiol 1995;268(5 Pt 1):L699-L722.
225. Wizemann TM, Gardner CR, Laskin JD, et al: Production of nitric oxide and peroxynitrite in the lung during acute endotoxemia. J Leukoc Biol 1994;56:759-768.
226. Balligand JL, Cannon PJ: Nitric oxide synthases and cardiac muscle: Autocrine and paracrine influences. Arterioscl Thromb Vasc Biol 1997;17:1846-1858.
227. Crow JP, Beckman JS: Reactions between nitric oxide, superoxide, and peroxynitrite: Footprints of peroxynitrite in vivo. Adv Pharmacol (New York) 1995;34:17-43.
228. Hausladen A, Fridovich I: Superoxide and peroxynitrite inactivate aconitases, nitric oxide does not. J Biol Chem 1994;269:29405-29408.
229. Szabo C, Salzman AL: Endogenous peroxynitrite is involved in the inhibition of mitochondrial respiration in immuno-stimulated J774.2 macrophages. Biochem Biophys Res Commun 1995;209:739-743.
230. Bolanos JP, Heales SJ, Land JM, et al: Effect of peroxynitrite on the mitochondrial respiratory chain: Differential susceptibility of neurones and astrocytes in primary culture. J Neurochem 1995;64:1965-1972.
231. Zingarelli B, Day BJ, Crapo JD, et al: The potential role of peroxynitrite in the vascular contractile and cellular energetic failure in endotoxic shock. Br J Pharmacol 1997;120:259-267.
232. Radi R, Rodriguez M, Castro L, et al: Inhibition of mitochondrial electron transport by peroxynitrite. Arch Biochem Biophys 1994;308:89-95.
233. Zingarelli B, Hasko G, Salzman AL, et al: Effects of a novel guanylyl cyclase inhibitor on the vascular actions of nitric oxide and peroxynitrite in immunostimulated smooth muscle cells and in endotoxic shock. Crit Care Med 1999;27:1701-1707.
234. Shen W, Xu X, Ochoa M, et al: Role of nitric oxide in regulation of oxygen consumption in conscious dogs. Circ Res 1994;75:1086-1095.
235. Shen W, Hintze TH, Wolin MS: Nitric oxide: an important singaling mechanism between vascular endothelium and parenchymal cells in the regulation of oxygen consumption. Circulation 1995;92:3503-3508.
236. Poderoso JJ, Peralta JG, Lisdero CL, et al: Nitric oxide regulates oxygen uptake and hydrogen peroxide release by the isolated beating rat heart. Am J Physiol 1998;274(1 Pt 1):C112-C119.
237. Szabo C, Zingarelli B, Salzman AL: Role of poly-ADP ribosyltransferase activation in the vascular contractile and energetic failure elicited by exogenous and endogenous nitric oxide peroxynitrite. Circ Res 1996;78:1051-1063.
238. Stoclet JC, Muller B, Gyorgy K, et al: The inducible nitric oxide synthase in vascular and cardiac tissue. Eur J Pharmacol 1999;375:139-155.
239. Tarpey MM, Beckman JS, Ischiropoulos H, et al: Peroxynitrite stimulates vascular smooth muscle cell cyclic GMP synthesis. FEBS Lett 1995;364:314-318.
240. Mayer B, Schrammel A, Klatt P, et al: Peroxynitrite-induced accumulation of cyclic GMP in endothelial cells and stimulation of purified soluble guanylyl cyclase: Dependence on glutathione and possible role of S-nitrosation. J Biol Chem 1995;270:17355-17360.
241. Iesaki T, Gupte SA, Kaminski PM, et al: Inhibition of guanylate cyclase stimulation by NO and bovine arterial relaxation to peroxynitrite and H2O2. Am J Physiol 1999;277(3 Pt 2): H978-H985.
242. Ma XL, Lopez BL, Liu GL, et al: Peroxynitrite aggravates myocardial reperfusion injury in the isolated perfused rat heart. Cardiovasc Res 1997;36:195-204.
243. Szabo C: The pathophysiological role of peroxynitrite in shock, inflammation, and ischemia-reperfusion injury. Shock 1996;6:79-88.
244. Liaudet L, Soriano FG, Szabo C: Biology of nitric oxide signaling. Crit Care Med 2000;28(Suppl):N37-N52.
245. McCord JM: Oxygen-derived free radicals. New Horiz 1993;1:70-76.
246. Saugstad OD, Ostrem T: Hypoxanthine and urate levels of plasma during and after hemorrhagic hypotension in dogs. Eur Surg Res 1977;9:48-56.
247. Yokoyama Y, Parks DA: Circulating xanthine oxidase: Release of xanthine oxidase from isolated rat liver. Gastroenterology 1988;94:607-611.
248. Jolly SR, Kane WJ, Bailie MB, et al: Canine myocardial reperfusion injury: Its reduction by the combined administration of superoxide dismutase and catalase. Circ Res 1984;54:277-285.
249. Przyklenk K, Kloner RA: Superoxide dismutase plus catalase improve contractile function in the canine model of the "stunned myocardium." Circ Res 1986;58:148-156.
250. Granger DN, Rutili G, McCord JM: Superoxide radicals in feline intestinal ischemia. Gastroenterology 1981;81:22-29.
251. Peitzman AB, Shires GTI, Illner H, et al: Effect of intravenous ATP-MgCl2 on cellular function in liver and muscle in hemorrhagic shock. Curr Surg 1981;38:300.
252. Murphy K, Haudek SB, Thompson M, et al: Molecular biology of septic shock. New Horiz 1998;6:181-193.
253. Mira J, Cariou A, Grall F, et al: Susceptibility to and mortality of septic shock are associated with TNF2, a TNF-alpha promotor polymorphism: A multicenter study. JAMA 1999;282:561-568.
254. Stuber F, Petersen M, Bokelmann F, et al: A genomic polymorphism within the tumor necrosis factor locus influences plasma tumor necrosis factor-alpha concentrations and outcome of patients with severe sepsis. Crit Care Med 1996;24:381-384.
255. Libert C, Wielockx B, Hammond GL, et al: Identification of a locus on distal mouse chromosome 12 that controls resistance to tumor necrosis factor-induced lethal shock. Genomics 1999;55:284-289.
256. Fang XM, Schroder S, Hoeft A, et al: Comparison of two polymorphisms of the interleukin-1 gene family: Interleukin-1 receptor antagonist polymorphism contributes to susceptibility to severe sepsis. Crit Care Med 1999;27:1330-1334.
257. Holmes CL, Russell JA, Walley KR: Genetic polymorphisms in sepsis and septic shock: Role in prognosis and potential for therapy. Chest 2003;124:1103-1115.
258. Lightfoot EJ, Horton JW, Maass DL, et al: Major burn trauma in rats promotes cardiac and gastrointestinal apoptosis. Shock 1999;11:29-34.
259. Xu YX, Wichmann MW, Ayala A, et al: Trauma-hemorrhage induces increased thymic apoptosis while decreasing IL-3 release and increasing GM-CSF. J Surg Res 1997;68:24-30.
260. Kumar A, Kumar A, Michael P, et al: Human serum from patients with septic shock activates transcription factors STAT1, IRF1 and NFkB and induces apoptosis in human cardiac myocytes. J Biol Chem 2005;280: 42619-42626.
261. Chien S: Role of the sympathetic nervous system in hemorrhage. Physiol Rev 1967;47:214-288.
262. Bond RF, Green HD: Cardiac output redistribution durng bilateral common carotid artery occlusion. Am J Physiol 1969;216:393-403.
263. Woolf PD: Endocrinology of shock. Ann Emerg Med 1986;15:1401-1405.
264. Haupt MT: The use of crystalloidal and colloidal solution for volume replacement in hypovolemic shock. CRC Crit Rev Clin Lab Sci 1989;27:1-23.
265. Skillman JJ, Awwad HK, Moore FD: Plasma protein kinetics of the early transcapillary refill after hemorrhage in man. Surg Gynecol Obstet 1967;125:983-996.
266. Forsyth RP, Hoffbrand BI, Melmon KL: Redistribution of cardiac output during hemorrhage in the unanesthetized monkey. Circ Res 1970;27:311-320.
267. Kaihara S, Rutherford RB, Schwentker EP, et al: Distribution of cardiac output in experimental hemorrhagic shock in dogs. J Appl Physiol 1969;27:218-222.
268. Harper AM: Autoregulation of cerebral blood flow: Influence of the arterial blood pressure on the blood flow though the cerebral cortex. J Neurol Neurosurg Psychiatry 1966;29: 398-403.
269. Sprung CL, Peduzzi PN, Shatney CH, et al: Impact of encephalopathy on mortality in the sepsis syndrome. The Veterans Administration Systemic Sepsis Cooperative Study Group. Crit Care Med 1990;18:801-806.
270. Douglas ME, Downs JB, Dannemiller FB, et al: Acute respiratory failure and intravascular coagulation. Surg Gynecol Obstet 1976;143:555-560.
271. Roussos C, Macklem PT: The respiratory muscles. N Engl J Med 1982;307:786-797.
272. Hou SH, Bushinsky DA, Wish JB, et al: Hospital acquired renal insufficiency: A prospective study. Am J Med 1983;74:243-248.
273. Myer B, Moran S: Hemodynamically mediated acute renal failure. N Engl J Med 1986;314:97-105.
274. Rose BD: Meaning and application of urine chemistries. In: Clinical Physiology of Acid-Base and Electrolyte

Disorders. New York, McGraw-Hill, 1984, pp 271-278.
275. Diamond JR, Yoburn DC: Nonoliguric acute renal failure associated with a low fractional excretion of sodium. Ann Intern Med 1982;96:597-600.
276. Mainous MR, Deitch EA: Bacterial translocation. In Schlag G, Redl H (eds): Pathophysiology of Shock, Sepsis and Organ Failure. Berlin, Springer-Verlag, 1993, pp 265-278.
277. Lillehei RC, MacLean LD: The intestinal factor in irreversible endotoxin shock. Ann Surg 1958;148:513-519.
278. Champion HR, Jones RT, Trump BF, et al: A clinicopathologic study of hepatic dysfunction following shock. Surg Gynecol Obstet 1976;142:657-663.
279. Garcia-Barreno P, Balibrea JL, Aparicio P: Blood coagulation changes in shock. Surg Gynecol Obstet 1978;147:6-12.
280. Counts HB, Haisch C, Simon TL, et al: Hemostasis in massively transfused trauma patients. Ann Surg 1979;190:91-99.
281. Arnold J, Leinhardt D, Little RA: Metabolic response to trauma. In Schlag G, Redl H (eds): Pathophysiology of Shock Sepsis and Organ Failure. Berlin, Springer-Verlag, 1993, pp 145-160.
282. Hoyt DB, Junger WG, Ozkan AN: Humoral mechanisms. In Schlag G, Redl H (eds): Pathophysiology of Shock Sepsis and Organ Failure. Berlin, Springer-Verlag, 1993, pp 111-130.
283. Stephan R, Ayala A, Chaudry IH: Monocyte and lymphocyte responses following trauma. In Schlag G, Redl H (eds): Pathophysiology of Shock Sepsis and Organ Failure. Berlin, Springer-Verlag, 1993, pp 131-144.
284. Devins SS, Miller A, Herndon BL, et al: The effects of dopamine on T-cell proliferative response and serum prolactin in critically ill patients. Crit Care Med 1992;20:1644-1649.
285. Oud L, Haupt MT: Persistent gastric intramucosal ischemia in patients with sepsis following resuscitation from shock. Chest 1999;115:1390-1396.
286. Wo CC, Shoemaker WC, Appel PL, et al: Unreliability of blood pressure and heart rate to evaluate cardiac output in emergency resuscitation and critical illness. Crit Care Med 1993;21:218-223.
287. Ward KR, Ivantury RR, Barbee WR: Endpoints of resuscitation for the victim of trauma. J Intensive Care Med 2001;16:55-75.
288. Rady MY, Rivers EP, Nowak RM: Resuscitation of the critically ill in the ED: Responses of blood pressure, heart rate, shock index, central venous oxygen saturation, and lactate. Am J Emerg Med 1996;14:218-225.
289. Gilbert EM, Haupt MT, Mandanas RY, et al: The effect of fluid loading, blood transfusion, and catecholamine infusion on oxygen delivery and consumption in patients with sepsis. Am Rev Respir Dis 1986;134:873-878.
290. Bakker J, Coffemils M, Leon M, et al: Blood lactate levels are superior to oxygen-derived variables in predicting outcome in human septic shock. Chest 1992;99:956-962.
291. Weil MH, Afifi AA: Experimental and clinical studies on lactate and pyruvate as indicators of the severity of acute circulatory failure (shock). Circulation 1970;41:989-1001.
292. Henning RJ, Weil MH, Weiner F: Blood lactate as a prognostic indicator of survival in patients with acute myocardial infarction. Circ Shock 1982;9:307-315.
293. Vincent JL, Roman A, Kahn RJ: Dobutamine administration in septic shock: Addition to a standard protocol. Crit Care Med 1990;18: 689-693.
294. Cain SM: Oxygen delivery and uptake in dogs during anemic and hypoxic hypoxia. J Appl Physiol 1977;42: 228-234.
295. Cilley R, Scharenberg A, Bongiorno P, et al: Low oxygen delivery produced by anemia, hypoxia, and low cardiac output. J Surg Res 1991;51:425-433.
296. Madias NE: Lactic acidosis. Kidney Int 1986;29:752-774.
297. Eldridge F, Sulzer J: Effect of respiratory alkalosis on blood lactate and pyruvate in humans. J Appl Physiol 1967;22: 461-468.
298. Waxman K, Nolan LS, Shoemaker WC: Sequential perioperative lactate determination: Physiological and clinical implications. Crit Care Med 1982;10:96-99.
299. James JH, Luchette FA, McCarter FD, et al: Lactate is an unreliable indicator of tissue hypoxia in injury or sepsis. Lancet 1999;354:505-508.
300. Cohn JN: Blood pressure measurement in shock: Mechanism of inaccuracy in auscultatory and palpatory methods. JAMA 1967;199:118-122.
301. Pauca AL, Wallenhaupt SL, Kon ND, et al: Does radial artery pressure accurately reflect aortic pressure? Chest 1992;102:1193-1198.
302. Packman MI, Rackow EC: Optimum left heart filling pressure during fluid resuscitation of patients with hypovolemic and septic shock. Crit Care Med 1983;11:165-169.
303. Weisul RD, Vito L, Dennis RC, et al: Myocardial depression during sepsis. Am J Surg 1977;133:512-521.
304. Connors AF Jr, McCaffree DR, Gray BA: Evaluation of right-heart catheterization in the critically ill patient without acute myocardial infarction. N Engl J Med 1983;308:263-267.
305. Connors AF Jr, Dawson NV, McCaffree DR, et al: Assessing hemodynamic status in critically ill patients: Do physicians use clinical information optimally? J Crit Care 1987;2:174-180.
306. Connors AF Jr, Speroff T, Dawson NV, et al: The effectiveness of right heart catheterization in the initial care of critically ill patients. JAMA 1996;276:889-897.
307. Rhodes A, Cusack RJ, Newman PJ, et al: A randomised, controlled trial of the pulmonary artery catheter in critically ill patients. Intensive Care Med 2002;28:256-264.
308. Sandham JD, Hull RD, Brant RF, et al: A randomized, controlled trial of the use of pulmonary-artery catheters in high-risk surgical patients. N Engl J Med 2003;348:5-14.
309. Richard C, Warszawski J, Anguel N, et al: Early use of the pulmonary artery catheter and outcomes in patients with shock and acute respiratory distress syndrome: A randomized controlled trial. JAMA 2003;290: 2713-2720.
310. Binanay C, Califf RM, Hasselblad V, et al: Evaluation study of congestive heart failure and pulmonary artery catheterization effectiveness: The ESCAPE trial. JAMA 2005;294: 1625-1633.
311. Harvey S, Harrison DA, Singer M, et al: Assessment of the clinical effectiveness of pulmonary artery catheters in management of patients in intensive care (PAC-Man): A randomised controlled trial. Lancet. 2005;366:472-477.
312. Shahid M, Rodger IW: Enhancement of amrinone-induced positive inotropy in rabbit papillary muscles with depressed contractile function: Effects on cyclic nucleotide levels and phosphodiesterase isoenzymes. J Pharm Pharmacol 1991;43:88-94.
313. Ivanov R, Allen J, Calvin JE: The incidence of major morbidity in critically ill patients managed with pulmonary artery catheters: A meta-analysis. Crit Care Med 2000;28:615-619.
314. Friese RS, Shafi S, Gentilello LM, et al: Pulmonary artery catheter use is associated with reduced mortality in severely injured patients: A National Trauma Data Bank analysis of 53,312 patients. Crit Care Med 2006;34:1597-1601.
315. Goldman RH, Klughaupt M, Metcalf T, et al: Measurement of central venous oxygen saturation in patients with myocardial infarction. Circulation 1968;38:941-946.
316. Weber K, Janicki J, Muskin C: Pathophysiology of cardiac failure. Am J Cardiol 1985;56:3B-7B.
317. Simmons D, Alpas A, Tashkin D, et al: Hyperlactatemia due to arterial hypoxemia or reduced cardiac output or both. J Appl Physiol 1978;45:195-202.
318. Ralston AC, Webb RK, Runciman WB: Potential errors in pulse oximetry: III. Effects of interferences, dyes, dyshaemoglobins and other pigments. Anaesthesia 1991;46:291-295.
319. Norley I: Erroneous actuation of the pulse oximeter. Anaesthesia 1987;42:1116.
320. Palve H, Vuori A: Pulse oximetry during low cardiac output and hypothermia states immediately after open heart surgery. Crit Care Med 1989;17:66-69.
321. Abraham E, Smith M, Silver L: Continuous monitoring of critically ill patients with transcutaneous oxygen and carbon dioxide, and conjunctival oxygen sensors. Ann Emerg Med 1984;13:1021-1026.
322. Nolan LS, Shoemaker WC: Transcutaneous O_2 and CO_2 monitoring of high risk surgical patients during the perioperative period. Crit Care Med 1982;10:762-764.
323. Tremper KK, Shoemaker WC: Transcutaneous oxygen monitoring of critically ill adults, with and without low flow shock. Crit Care Med 1981;9:706-709.

324. Abraham E, Oye R, Smith M: Detection of blood volume deficits through conjunctival oxygen tension monitoring. Crit Care Med 1984;12:931-934.
325. Tremper KK, Keenan B, Applebaum R, et al: Clinical and experimental monitoring with transcutaneous PO2 during hypoxia, shock, cardiac arrest, and CPR. J Clin Invest 1981;6:149.
326. Waxman K, Sulder R, Eisner M: Transcutaneous oxygen monitoring of emergency department patients. Am J Surg 1983;146:35-38.
327. Abraham E, Smith M, Silver S: Conjunctival and transcutaneous oxygen monitoring during cardiac arrest and cardiopulmonary resuscitation. Crit Care Med 1984;12:419-421.
328. Montgomery A, Hartmann M, Jonsson K, et al: Intramucosal pH measurement with tonometers for detecting gastrointestinal ischemia in porcine hemorrhagic shock. Circ Shock 1989;29:319-327.
329. Nelson DP, Samsel RW, Wood LD, et al: Pathological supply dependency of systemic and intestinal O2 uptake during endotoxemia. J Appl Physiol 1988;64:2410-2419.
330. Gutierrez G, Bismar H, Dantzker D, et al: Comparison of gastric intramucosal pH with measures of oxygen transport and consumption in critically ill patients. Crit Care Med 1992;20:451-457.
331. Maynard N, Bihari D, Beal R, et al: Assessment of splanchnic oxygenation by gastric tonometry in patients with acute circulatory failure. JAMA 1993;270:1203-1210.
332. Fiddian-Green RG, Haglund U, Gutierrez G, et al: Goals for the resuscitation of shock. Crit Care Med 1993;21:S25-S31.
333. Gutierrez G, Palizas F, Poglia G, et al: Gastric intramucosal pH as a therapeutic index of tissue oxygenation in critically ill patients. Lancet 1992;339:195-199.
334. Cohn SM, Varela JE, Giannotti G, et al: Splanchnic perfusion evaluation during hemorrhage and resuscitation with gastric near-infrared spectroscopy. J Trauma Inj Infect Crit Care 2001;50:629-634.
335. Beilman GJ, Groehler KE, Lazaron V, et al: Near-infrared spectroscopy measurement of regional tissue oxyhemoglobin saturation during hemorrhagic shock. Shock 1999;12:196-200.
336. McKinley BA, Marvin RG, Cocanour CS, et al: Tissue hemoglobin O_2 saturation during resuscitation of traumatic shock monitored using near infrared spectrometry. J Trauma Inj Infect Crit Care 2000;48:637-642.
337. Rhee P, Langdale L, Mock C, et al: Near-infrared spectroscopy: Continuous measurement of cytochrome oxidation during hemorrhagic shock. Crit Care Med 1997;25:166-170.
338. Cairns CB, Moore FA, Haenel JB, et al: Evidence for early supply independent mitochondrial dysfunction in patients developing multiple organ failure after trauma. J Trauma Inj Infect Crit Care 1997;42:532-536.
339. Puyana JC, Soller BR, Zhang S, et al: Continuous measurement of gut pH with near-infrared spectroscopy during hemorrhagic shock. J Trauma Inj Infect Crit Care 1999;46:9-15.
340. Griebel JA, Moore FA, Piantadosi CA: In-vivo responses of mitochondrial redox levels to *Escherichia coli* bacteremia in primates. J Crit Care 1990;5:1-9.
341. Ogata H, Mishio M, Luo XX, et al: Significance of elevated cytochrome aa3 in a state of endotoxemia in dogs. Resuscitation 1996;33:63-68.
342. Porembka DT: Transesophageal echocardiography. Crit Care Clin 1996;12:875-918.
343. ten Wolde M, Sohne M, Quak E, et al: Prognostic value of echocardiographically assessed right ventricular dysfunction in patients with pulmonary embolism. Arch Intern Med 2004;164:1685-1689.
344. Gattinoni L, SVO_2 Collaborative Group: A trial of goal-oriented hemodynamic therapy in critically ill patients. N Engl J Med 1995;333:1025-1032.
345. Hayes MA, Timmins AC, Yau EHS, et al: Elevation of systemic oxygen delivery in the treatment of critically ill patients. N Engl J Med 1994;330:1717-1722.
346. Durham RM, Neunaber K, Mazuski JE, et al: The use of oxygen consumption and delivery as endpoints for resuscitation in critically ill patients. J Trauma 1996;41:32-40.
347. Yu M, Takanishi D, Myers SA, et al: Frequency of mortality and myocardial infarction during maximizing oxygen delivery: A prospective, randomized trial. Crit Care Med 1995;23:1025-1032.
348. Blow O, Magliore L, Claridge JA, et al: The golden hour and the silver day: Detection and correction of occult hypoperfusion within 24 hours improves outcome from major trauma. J Trauma Inj Infect Crit Care 1999;47:964-969.
349. Boersma E, Maas AC, Deckers JW, et al: Early thrombolytic treatment in acute myocardial infarction: Reappraisal of the golden hour. Lancet 1996;348:771-775.
350. Vincent JL, Bernard GR, Beale R, et al: Drotrecogin alfa (activated) treatment in severe sepsis from the global open-label trial ENHANCE: Further evidence for survival and safety and implications for early treatment. Crit Care Med 2005;33:2266-2277.
351. Cooper DJ, Walley KR, Wiggs BR, et al: Bicarbonate does not improve hemodynamics in critically ill patients who have lactic acidosis: A prospective, controlled clinical study. Ann Intern Med 1990;112:492-498.
352. Humphrey H, Hall J, Sznajder I, et al: Improved survival in ARDS patients associated with a reduction in pulmonary capillary wedge pressure. Chest 1990;97:1176-1180.
353. Lillehei RC, MacLean LD: The intestinal factor in irreversible hemorrhagic shock. Surgery 1958;42:1043-1054.
354. Haupt MT, Kaufman BS, Carlson RW: Fluid resuscitation in patients with increased vascular permeability. Crit Care Clin 1992;8:341-353.
355. Bissoni RS, Holtgrave DR, Lawler R, et al: Colloids versus crystalloids in fluid resuscitation: An analysis of randomized control trials. J Fam Pract 1991;32:387-393.
356. Velanovich V: Crystalloid versus colloid fluid resuscitation: A meta-analysis of mortality. Surgery 1989;105:65-71.
357. Human albumin administration in critically ill patients: Systematic review of randomised controlled trials. Cochrane Injuries Group Albumin Reviewers. BMJ 1998;317:235-240.
358. Finfer S, Bellomo R, Boyce N, et al: A comparison of albumin and saline for fluid resuscitation in the intensive care unit. N Engl J Med 2004;350:2247-2256.
359. Hebert PC, Wells G, Blajchman MA, et al: A multicenter, randomized, controlled clinical trial of transfusion requirements in critical care. Transfusion Requirements in Critical Care Investigators, Canadian Critical Care Trials Group. N Engl J Med 1999;340:409-417.
360. Hebert PC, Yetisir E, Martin C, et al: Is a low transfusion threshold safe in critically ill patients with cardiovascular diseases? Crit Care Med 2001;29:227-234.
361. Hebert PC, Fergusson D, Blajchman MA, et al: Clinical outcomes following institution of the Canadian universal leukoreduction program for red blood cell transfusions. JAMA. 2003;289:1941-1949.
362. Shorr AF, Duh MS, Kelly KM, et al: Red blood cell transfusion and ventilator-associated pneumonia: A potential link? Crit Care Med 2004;32:666-674.
363. Shorr AF, Jackson WL, Kelly KM, et al: Transfusion practice and blood stream infections in critically ill patients. Chest 2005;127:1722-1728.
364. Jackson WL Jr, Shorr AF, Jackson WLJ, et al: Blood transfusion and the development of acute respiratory distress syndrome: More evidence that blood transfusion in the intensive care unit may not be benign. Crit Care Med 2005;33:1420-1421.
365. Levitski A: From epinephrine to cyclic AMP. Science 1988;241:800-806.
366. Fedida D, Braun AP, Giles WR: Alpha-1 adrenoreceptors in myocardium: Functional aspects and transmembrane signalling mechanisms. Physiol Rev 1993;73:469-487.
367. Ruffolo RR, Nichols AJ, Stadel JM, et al: Structure and function of alpha-adrenoreceptors. Pharmacol Rev 1991;43:475-505.
368. Landzberg JS, Parker JD, Gauthier DF, et al: Effects of myocardial alpha-1 adrenergic receptor stimulation and blockade on contractility in humans. Circulation 1991;84:1608-1614.
369. Goldberg LI: Dopamine: Clinical uses of an endogenous catecholamine. N Engl J Med 1974;291:707.
370. Colucci WS, Wright RF, Braunwald E: New positive inotropic agents in the treatment of heart failure: Mechanisms of action and recent clinical developments, II. N Engl J Med 1986;314:349-358.
371. Nasraway SA, Rackow EC, Astiz ME, et al: Inotropic response to digoxin and dopamine in patients with severe sepsis, cardiac failure, and systemic

hypoperfusion. Chest 1989;95:612-615.
372. Landry DW, Levin HR, Gallant EM, et al: Vasopressin deficiency contributes to the vasodilatation of septic shock. Circulation 1997;95:1122-1125.
373. Landry DW, Levin HR, Gallant EM, et al: Vasopressin pressor sensitivity in vasodilatory septic shock. Crit Care Med 1997;25:1279-1282.
374. Malay MB, Ashton RC Jr, Landry DW, et al: Low-dose vasopressin in the treatment of vasodilatory septic shock. J Trauma Inj Infect Crit Care 1999;47:699-703.
375. Morales D, Madigan J, Cullinane S, et al: Reversal by vasopressin of intractable hypotension in the late phase of hemorrhagic shock. Circulation 1999;100:226-229.
376. Hilberman M, Maseda J, Stinson EB, et al: The diuretic properties of dopamine in patients after open-heart operations. Anesthesiology 1984;61:489-494.
377. Schaer GL, Fink MP, Parrillo JE: Norepinephrine alone versus norepinephrine plus low-dose dopamine: Enhanced renal blood flow with combination pressor therapy. Crit Care Med 1985;13:492-496.
378. Breckenridge A, Orme M, Dollery CT: The effect of dopamine on renal blood flow in man. Eur J Clin Pharm 1971;3:131-136.
379. Kenakin TP: An in-vitro quantitative analysis of the alpha-adrenoreceptor partial agonist activity of dobutamine and its relevance to inotropic selectivity. J Pharmacol Exp Ther 1981;216:210-219.
380. Ruffolo RR Jr: The pharmacology of dobutamine. Am J Med Sci 1987;294:244-248.
381. Akhtar N, Mikulic E, Cohn JN, et al: Hemodynamic effects of dobutamine in patients with severe heart failure. Am J Cardiol 1975;36:202-205.
382. Butterworth JF, Strickland RA, Mark LJ, et al: Dobutamine increases heart rate more than epinephrine in patients recovering from aortocoronary bypass surgery. J Cardiothorac Vasc Anesth 1992;6:535-541.
383. Ligget SB: Desensitization of the beta-adrenergic receptor: Distinct molecular determinants of phosphorylation by specific kinases. Pharmacol Res 1991;24:29-41.
384. Shoemaker WC, Appel PL, Kram HB, et al: Comparison of hemodynamic and oxygen transport effects of dopamine and dobutamine in critically ill surgical patients. Chest 1989;96:120-126.
385. DiSesa VJ, Brown D, Mudge GH, et al: Hemodynamic comparison of dopamine and dobutamine in the postoperative volume-loaded, pressure-loaded, and normal ventricle. J Thorac Cardiovasc Surg 1982;83:256-263.
386. Fowler MB, Alderman EL, Oesterle SN, et al: Dobutamine and dopamine after cardiac surgery: Greater augmentation of myocardial blood flow with dopamine. Circulation 1984;70(Suppl I):I-103-I-111.
387. Tuchschmidt J, Fried J, Astiz M, et al: Elevation of cardiac output and oxygen delivery improves outcome in septic shock. Chest 1992;102: 216-220.
388. Edwards JD, Brown GCS, Nightingale P, et al: Use of survivors cardiorespiratory values as therapeutic goals in septic shock. Crit Care Med 1989;17:1098-1103.
389. Royster RL, Butterworth JF, Prielipp RC, et al: A randomized, blinded, placebo-controlled evaluation of calcium chloride and epinephrine for inotropic support after emergence from cardiopulmonary bypass. Anesth Analg 1992;74:3-13.
390. Sung BH, Robinson C, Thadani U, et al: Effects of 1-epinephrine on hemodynamics and cardiac function in coronary disease: Dose response studies. Clin Pharmacol Ther 1988;43:308-316.
391. Konstram MA, Cohen SR, Weiland DS, et al: Relative contribution of inotropic and vasodilator effects to amrinone-induced hemodynamic improvement in congestive heart failure. Am J Cardiol 1986;57:242-248.
392. Hermiller JB, Mehegan JP, Nadkarni VM, et al: Amrinone during porcine intraperitoneal sepsis. Circ Shock 1991;34:247-251.
393. Hoffman P, Schockenhoff B: Amrinone in catecholamine-refractory cardiac failure in septic shock. Anaesthetist 1985;34:663-669.
394. Gold J, Cullinane S, Chen J, et al: Vasopressin in the treatment of milrinone-induced hypotension in severe heart failure. Am J Cardiol 2000;85:506-508.
395. Morales DL, Gregg D, Helman DN, et al: Arginine vasopressin in the treatment of 50 patients with postcardiotomy vasodilatory shock. Ann Thorac Surg 2000;69:102-106.
396. Chen JM, Cullinane S, Spanier TB, et al: Vasopressin deficiency and pressor hypersensitivity in hemodynamically unstable organ donors. Circulation 1999;100(19 Suppl):II-244-II-246.

Chapter 23

Cardiogenic Shock

Steven M. Hollenberg and Joseph E. Parrillo

Cardiogenic shock is a state of inadequate tissue perfusion as a result of cardiac dysfunction. Acute myocardial infarction (MI) is the leading cause of cardiogenic shock.[1,2] Rapid evaluation and prompt initiation of supportive measures and definitive therapy in patients with cardiogenic shock may improve early and long-term outcomes.

DEFINITION

The clinical definition of cardiogenic shock includes decreased cardiac output and evidence of tissue hypoxia in the presence of adequate intravascular volume. The diagnosis of circulatory shock (Box 23-1) is made at the bedside by the presence of hypotension and a combination of clinical signs indicative of poor tissue perfusion, including oliguria, clouded sensorium, and cool, mottled extremities. Hemodynamic criteria include sustained hypotension (systolic blood pressure <90 mm Hg for at least 30 minutes) and a reduced cardiac index (<2.2 L/min/m^2) in the presence of elevated pulmonary capillary occlusion pressure (>15 mm Hg).[3] Cardiogenic shock is diagnosed after documentation of myocardial dysfunction and exclusion or correction of factors such as hypovolemia, hypoxia, and acidosis.

HISTORY AND INCIDENCE

History

Pump failure secondary to cardiogenic shock has long been known to carry a high mortality. The seminal article outlining prognosis after MI was a single-center series of 250 patients reported by Killip and Kimball in 1967.[3] Killip and Kimball divided patients into four classes as follows:

Killip class I—no evidence of congestive heart failure
Killip class II—presence of S_3 gallop or bibasilar rales or both
Killip class III—pulmonary edema (rales greater than halfway up the lung fields)
Killip class IV—cardiogenic shock

Of the 250 patients in Killip's series, 19% were in class IV at presentation, and their mortality was 81%.[3]

With the advent of right heart catheterization, Forrester and colleagues[4] defined hemodynamic subsets after MI analogous to the clinical subsets outlined by Killip. Subset I consisted of patients with normal pulmonary capillary wedge pressure and cardiac output, subset II consisted of patients with elevated pulmonary capillary wedge pressure and normal cardiac output, subset III consisted of patients with normal pulmonary capillary wedge pressure and decreased cardiac output, and subset IV consisted of patients with elevated pulmonary capillary wedge pressure and decreased cardiac output.[4]

Despite advances in management of heart failure and acute MI, the mortality of patients with cardiogenic shock has remained high.[2,5-7] Data suggest an increase in survival in the 1990s, coincident with the use of reperfusion strategies.[6-8] Cardiogenic shock remains the most common cause of death, however, in hospitalized patients with acute MI.

Incidence

Accurate determination of the precise incidence of cardiogenic shock is difficult because patients who die as a

Box 23-1

Diagnosis of Cardiogenic Shock

Clinical Signs
Hypotension
Oliguria
Clouded sensorium
Cool and mottled extremities

Hemodynamic Criteria
Systolic blood pressure <90 mm Hg for >30 minutes
Cardiac index <2.2 L/min/m^2
Pulmonary artery occlusion pressure >15 mm Hg

Box 23-2

Causes of Cardiogenic Shock

Acute Myocardial Infarction
- Pump failure
  - Large infarction
  - Smaller infarction with pre-existing left ventricular dysfunction
  - Infarct extension
  - Reinfarction
  - Infarct expansion
- Mechanical complications
  - Acute mitral regurgitation secondary to papillary muscle rupture
  - Ventricular septal defect
  - Free wall rupture
  - Pericardial tamponade
- Right ventricular infarction

Other Conditions
- End-stage cardiomyopathy
- Myocarditis
- Myocardial contusion
- Prolonged cardiopulmonary bypass
- Septic shock with severe myocardial depression
- Left ventricular outflow tract obstruction
  - Aortic stenosis
  - Hypertrophic obstructive cardiomyopathy
- Obstruction to left ventricular filling
  - Mitral stenosis
  - Left atrial myxoma
- Acute mitral regurgitation (chordal rupture)
- Acute aortic insufficiency

result of MI before reaching the hospital generally do not receive this diagnosis.[5,9-12] Nonetheless, estimates from a variety of sources have been fairly consistent. The Worcester Heart Attack Study,[5] a community-wide analysis, found an incidence of cardiogenic shock of 7.5%. This incidence has remained fairly stable from 1975 to 1997.[5,8] In the GUSTO (Global Utilization of Streptokinase and Tissue Plasminogen Activator for Occluded Coronary Arteries) trial,[13] the incidence of cardiogenic shock was 7.2%, a rate similar to that found in other multicenter thrombolytic trials.[9-11] The incidence in patients with ST segment elevation MI in the National Registry of Myocardial Infarction (NRMI) database from 1995 to 2004 was 8.6%.[6] A report of National Hospital Discharge Survey data found an incidence of cardiogenic shock of 3.9% in 1979 and 1.7% in 2003; this report may not be directly comparable to the other reports because it included ST segment elevation and non–ST segment elevation MI and because with the introduction of troponin to define infarction, patients with less severe infarctions were likely included in the database.[7]

ETIOLOGY AND EPIDEMIOLOGY

The most common cause of cardiogenic shock is left ventricular failure in the setting of an extensive acute MI, although a smaller infarction in a patient with previously compromised left ventricular function also may precipitate shock. Shock that has a delayed onset may result from infarct extension, reocclusion of a previously patent infarct artery, or decompensation of myocardial function in the noninfarct zone owing to metabolic abnormalities. Large areas of nonfunctional but viable myocardium also can cause or contribute to the development of cardiogenic shock in patients after MI.

Cardiogenic shock also can be caused by mechanical complications, such as acute mitral regurgitation, rupture of the interventricular septum, or rupture of the free wall, or by large right ventricular infarctions. Other causes of cardiogenic shock include myocarditis, end-stage cardiomyopathy, myocardial contusion, septic shock with severe myocardial depression, myocardial dysfunction after prolonged cardiopulmonary bypass, valvular heart disease, and hypertrophic obstructive cardiomyopathy (Box 23-2). In a report of the SHOCK (SHould we emergently revascularize Occluded Coronaries for shocK) trial registry of 1160 patients with cardiogenic shock,[2] 74.5% of patients had predominant left ventricular failure, 8.3% had acute mitral regurgitation, 4.6% had ventricular septal rupture, 3.4% had isolated right ventricular shock, 1.7% had tamponade or cardiac rupture, and 8% had shock resulting from other causes.

Patients may have cardiogenic shock at initial presentation, but most do not; shock usually evolves over several hours,[14,15] suggesting that early treatment potentially may prevent shock. More recent data indicate that early thrombolytic therapy may decrease the incidence of cardiogenic shock.[16] In the SHOCK trial registry, 75% of patients developed cardiogenic shock within 24 hours after presentation, with a median delay of 7 hours.[2] Results from the GUSTO trial were similar[12]; among patients with shock, 11% were in shock on arrival, and 89% developed shock after admission.

Risk factors for the development of cardiogenic shock in MI generally parallel the risk factors for left ventricular dysfunction and the severity of coronary artery disease.

Shock is more likely to develop in patients who are elderly, are diabetic, and have anterior infarction.[4,14,17,18] Patients with cardiogenic shock also are more likely to have histories of previous infarction, peripheral vascular disease, and cerebrovascular disease.[17,18] Decreased ejection fractions and larger infarctions (as evidenced by higher cardiac enzymes) also are predictors of the development of cardiogenic shock.[17,18] Analysis from the GUSTO-3 trial has identified age, lower systolic blood pressure, heart rate, and Killip class as significant predictors of the risk for development of cardiogenic shock after presentation with acute MI.[19] Use of a predictive scoring system derived from this study may be helpful in identifying patients at high risk for the development of cardiogenic shock and targeting such patients for closer monitoring.

Cardiogenic shock is most often associated with anterior MI. In the SHOCK trial registry, 55% of infarctions were anterior, 46% were inferior, 21% were posterior, and 50% were in multiple locations.[2] These findings were consistent with the findings in other series.[20] Angiographic evidence most often shows multivessel coronary disease (left main occlusion in 20% of patients, three-vessel disease in 64%, two-vessel disease in 23%, and one-vessel disease in 13% of patients).[21] The high prevalence of multivessel coronary artery disease is important because compensatory hyperkinesis normally develops in myocardial segments that are not involved in an acute MI, and this response helps maintain cardiac output. Failure to develop such a response, because of previous infarction or high-grade coronary stenoses, is an important risk factor for cardiogenic shock and death.[15,22]

PATHOGENESIS

Systemic Effects

Cardiac dysfunction in patients with cardiogenic shock is usually initiated by MI or ischemia. The myocardial dysfunction resulting from ischemia worsens that ischemia, creating a downward spiral (Fig. 23-1).[23] When a critical mass of left ventricular myocardium is ischemic or necrotic and fails to pump, stroke volume and cardiac output decrease. Myocardial perfusion, which depends on the pressure gradient between the coronary arterial system and the left ventricle and on the duration of diastole, is compromised by hypotension and tachycardia, exacerbating ischemia. The increased ventricular diastolic pressures caused by pump failure reduce coronary perfusion pressure further, and the additional wall stress elevates myocardial oxygen requirements, worsening ischemia further. Decreased cardiac output also compromises systemic perfusion, which can lead to lactic acidosis and further compromise of systolic performance.

When myocardial function is depressed, several compensatory mechanisms are activated, including sympathetic stimulation to increase heart rate and contractility and renal fluid retention to increase preload. These compensatory mechanisms may become maladaptive and can

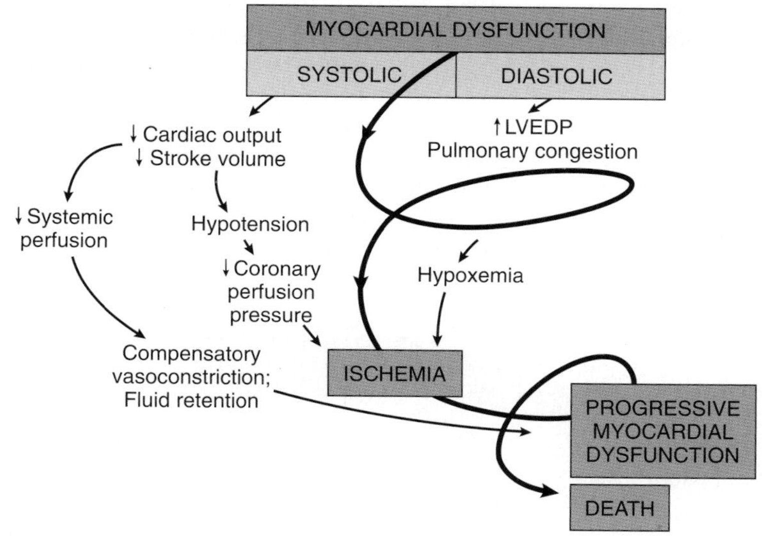

Figure 23-1. The "downward spiral" in cardiogenic shock. Cardiac dysfunction is usually initiated by myocardial infarction or ischemia. When a critical mass of left ventricular myocardium fails to pump, stroke volume and cardiac output decrease. Myocardial perfusion is compromised by hypotension and tachycardia, exacerbating ischemia. The increased ventricular diastolic pressures that result from pump failure reduce coronary perfusion pressure further, and the additional wall stress elevates myocardial oxygen requirements, also worsening ischemia. Decreased cardiac output also compromises systemic perfusion, which can lead to lactic acidosis and further compromise of systolic performance. When myocardial function is depressed, several compensatory mechanisms are activated, including sympathetic stimulation to increase heart rate and contractility and renal fluid retention to increase preload. These compensatory mechanisms may become dysfunctional and can worsen the situation when cardiogenic shock develops by increasing myocardial oxygen demand and afterload. Myocardial dysfunction resulting from ischemia worsens the ischemia, setting up a vicious cycle that must be interrupted to prevent the patient's death. LVEDP, left ventricular end-diastolic pressure. (Modified from Hollenberg SM, Kavinsky CJ, Parrillo JE: Cardiogenic shock. Ann Intern Med 1999;131:49.)

worsen the situation when cardiogenic shock develops. Increased heart rate and contractility increase myocardial oxygen demand and exacerbate ischemia. Fluid retention and impaired diastolic filling caused by tachycardia and ischemia may result in pulmonary congestion and hypoxia. Vasoconstriction to maintain blood pressure increases myocardial afterload, impairing cardiac performance further and increasing myocardial oxygen demand. This increased demand, in the face of inadequate perfusion, worsens ischemia and begins a vicious cycle that ends in death if not interrupted (see Fig. 23-1). The interruption of this cycle of myocardial dysfunction and ischemia forms the basis for the therapeutic regimens for cardiogenic shock.

Data suggest that not all patients fit into this classic paradigm. In the SHOCK trial, the average systemic vascular resistance was not elevated, and the range of values was wide, suggesting that compensatory vasoconstriction is not universal. Some patients had fever and elevated white blood cell counts along with decreased systemic vascular resistance, suggesting a systemic inflammatory response syndrome.[24] These data have led to an expansion of the classic paradigm to include the possibility of the contribution of inflammatory responses to vasodilation and myocardial stunning, leading clinically to persistence of shock (Fig. 23-2).[24] Supporting this notion is the fact that the mean ejection fraction in the SHOCK trial was only moderately decreased (30%), suggesting that mechanisms other than pump failure were operative.[24] Immune activation seems to be common to many different forms of shock. Activation of inducible nitric oxide synthase with production of nitric oxide and peroxynitrite has been proposed as one potential mechanism.

Myocardial Pathology

Cardiogenic shock is characterized by systolic and diastolic myocardial dysfunction.[15,25] Progressive myocardial necrosis has been observed consistently in clinical and pathologic studies of patients with cardiogenic shock.[15,26] Patients who develop shock after admission often have evidence of infarct extension, which can result from reocclusion of a transiently patent infarct artery, propagation of intracoronary thrombus, or a combination of decreased coronary perfusion pressure and increased myocardial oxygen demand.[17,18] Myocytes at the border zone of an infarction are more susceptible to additional ischemic episodes; these adjacent segments are at particular risk.[27] Mechanical infarct expansion, which is seen most dramatically after extensive anterior MI, also can contribute to late development of cardiogenic shock.[17,28]

Ischemia remote from the infarct zone may be particularly important in producing systolic dysfunction in patients with cardiogenic shock.[22,29] Patients with cardiogenic shock usually have multivessel coronary artery disease,[2,15] with limited vasodilator reserve, impaired autoregulation, and consequent pressure-dependent coronary flow in several perfusion territories.[30] Hypotension and metabolic derangements have the potential to impair the contractility of noninfarcted myocardium in patients with shock.[31] This can limit hyperkinesis of uninvolved segments, a compensatory mechanism typically seen early after MI.[22,29]

Myocardial diastolic function also is impaired in patients with cardiogenic shock. Myocardial ischemia causes decreased compliance, increasing the left ventricular filling pressure at a given end-diastolic volume.[32,33] Compensatory increases in left ventricular volumes to maintain stroke volume increase filling pressures further. Elevation of left ventricular pressures can lead to pulmonary edema and hypoxemia (see Fig. 23-1).

In addition to abnormalities in myocardial performance, valvular abnormalities can contribute to increased pulmonary congestion. Papillary muscle dysfunction caused by ischemia is common and can lead to substantial increases in left atrial pressure; the degree of mitral regurgitation may be lessened by afterload reduction. This mechanism is distinct from complete rupture of the papillary muscle, a mechanical complication that manifests dramatically, with pulmonary edema and cardiogenic shock.

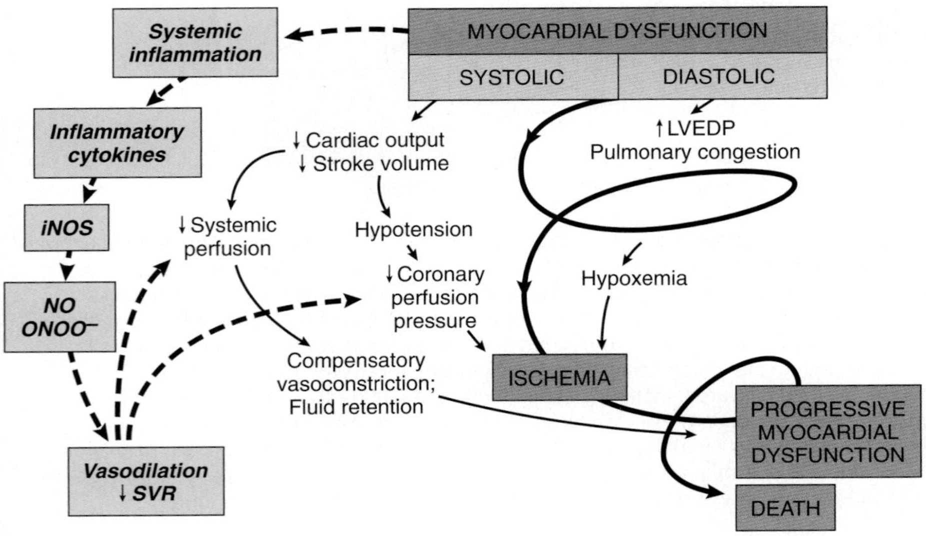

Figure 23-2. Expansion of the pathophysiologic paradigm of cardiogenic shock to include the potential contribution of inflammatory mediators. LVEDP, left ventricular end-diastolic pressure; NO, nitric oxide; iNOS, inducible nitric oxide synthase; $ONOO^-$, peroxynitrite; SVR, systemic vascular resistance. (From Hochman JS: Cardiogenic shock. Ann Intern Med 1999;131:47.)

Cellular Pathology

Tissue hypoperfusion and consequent cellular hypoxia lead to anaerobic glycolysis, with depletion of adenosine triphosphate and intracellular energy reserves. Anaerobic glycolysis also causes accumulation of lactic acid and resultant intracellular acidosis. Failure of energy-dependent ion transport pumps decreases transmembrane potential, causing intracellular accumulation of sodium and calcium and myocyte swelling.[34] Cellular ischemia and intracellular calcium accumulation can activate intracellular proteases.[35] If the ischemia is severe and prolonged enough, myocardial cellular injury can become irreversible, with the classic pattern of myonecrosis—mitochondrial swelling; accumulation of denatured proteins and chromatin in the cytoplasm; lysosomal breakdown; and fracture of the mitochondria, nuclear envelope, and plasma membrane.[34,35]

Accumulating evidence indicates that apoptosis (programmed cell death) also may contribute to myocyte loss in MI.[27,35,36] Although myonecrosis clearly outweighs apoptosis in the core of an infarcted area, evidence for apoptosis has been found consistently in the border zone of infarcts after ischemia and reperfusion and sporadically in areas remote from the ischemia area.[27,36] Activation of inflammatory cascades, oxidative stress, and stretching of myocytes have been proposed as mechanisms that activate the apoptotic pathways.[35,36] Although the magnitude of apoptotic cell loss in MI remains uncertain, inhibitors of apoptosis have been found to attenuate myocardial injury in animal models of postischemic reperfusion; these inhibitors also may have therapeutic potential for myocyte salvage after large infarctions.[36]

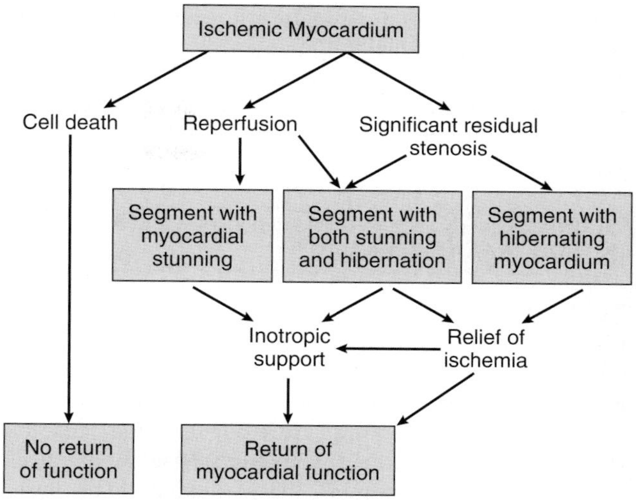

Figure 23-3. Possible outcomes after myocardial ischemia. After myocardial ischemia, either necrosis or reversible dysfunction may occur. Myocardial stunning represents postischemic dysfunction that persists despite restoration of normal flow. These segments respond to inotropes and recover function if supported. Hibernating myocardium is a state of persistently impaired myocardial function at rest resulting from residual stenosis; function can be restored to normal by relieving ischemia. Repetitive episodes of stunning can coexist with or mimic myocardial hibernation, or both. The concept that stunned or hibernating segments can recover contractile function emphasizes the importance of measures to support hemodynamics in patients with cardiogenic shock. (Modified with permission from Hollenberg SM, Kavinsky CJ, Parrillo JE: Cardiogenic shock. Ann Intern Med 1999;131:50.)

Reversible Myocardial Dysfunction

A key to understanding the pathophysiology and treatment of cardiogenic shock is to realize that large areas of nonfunctional but viable myocardium also can cause or contribute to the development of cardiogenic shock in patients after MI (Fig. 23-3). This reversible dysfunction can be described in two main categories—stunning and hibernation.

Myocardial stunning represents postischemic dysfunction that persists despite restoration of normal blood flow; eventually, however, myocardial performance recovers completely.[37] Originally defined in animal models of ischemia and reperfusion,[38] stunning has been recognized in the clinical arena.[37,39] Direct evidence for myocardial stunning in humans has been found using positron emission tomography in patients with persistent wall motion abnormalities after angioplasty for acute coronary syndromes; perfusion measured by ^{13}N-ammonia was normal in the presence of persistent contractile dysfunction.[40] The pathogenesis of stunning has not been conclusively established, but seems to involve a combination of oxidative stress,[41] perturbation of calcium homeostasis, and decreased myofilament responsiveness to calcium.[37,42,43] In addition to these direct effects, data from studies in isolated cardiac myocytes suggest that circulating myocardial depressant substances may contribute to contractile dysfunction in myocardial stunning.[44] The intensity of stunning is determined primarily by the severity of the antecedent ischemic insult.[37]

Myocardial hibernation comprises segments with persistently impaired function at rest as a result of severely reduced coronary blood flow; inherent in the definition of hibernating myocardium is the notion that function can be normalized by improving blood flow.[45-47] Hibernation can be seen as an adaptive response to reduce contractile function of hypoperfused myocardium and restore equilibrium between flow and function, minimizing the potential for ischemia or necrosis.[48] Revascularization of hibernating myocardium can lead to improved myocardial function,[49] and improved function seems to translate into improved prognosis.[50,51]

Although hibernation is conceptually and pathophysiologically different from myocardial stunning, the two conditions are difficult to distinguish in the clinical setting and may coexist.[37,51] Repetitive episodes of myocardial stunning can coexist with or mimic myocardial hibernation.[37,45,52] Consideration of myocardial stunning and hibernation is vital in patients with cardiogenic shock because of their therapeutic implications. Hibernating myocardium improves with revascularization, and stunned myocardium retains inotropic reserve and can respond to inotropic stimulation.[37] In addition, the fact that the severity of the antecedent ischemic insult determines the intensity of stunning[37] provides a rationale for re-establishment of patency of occluded coronary arteries in patients with cardiogenic shock. Finally, the notion that some myocardial tissue may recover function emphasizes the importance of measures to support hemodynamics and minimize myocardial necrosis in patients with shock.

CLINICAL ASSESSMENT AND INITIAL MANAGEMENT

Evaluation

Cardiogenic shock is an emergency. The clinician must initiate therapy before shock irreversibly damages vital organs; at the same time, he or she must perform the clinical assessment required to understand the cause of shock and to target therapy to that cause. A practical approach is to make a rapid initial evaluation on the basis of a limited history, physical examination, and specific diagnostic procedures (Fig. 23-4).[23] Cardiogenic shock is diagnosed after documentation of myocardial dysfunction and exclusion of alternative causes of hypotension, such as hypovolemia, hemorrhage, sepsis, pulmonary embolism, tamponade, aortic dissection, and pre-existing valvular disease.

Patients with shock are usually ashen or cyanotic and can have cool skin and mottled extremities. Cerebral hypoperfusion may cloud the sensorium. Pulses are rapid and faint and may be irregular in the presence of arrhythmias. Jugular venous distention and pulmonary rales are usually present, although their absence does not exclude the diagnosis. A precordial heave resulting from left ventricular dyskinesis may be palpable. The heart sounds may be distant, and S_3 or S_4 or both are usually present. A systolic murmur of mitral regurgitation or ventricular septal defect may be heard, but these complications may occur without an audible murmur.

An electrocardiogram should be performed immediately. Other initial diagnostic tests usually include a chest radiograph and measurement of arterial blood gas, electrolytes, complete blood count, and cardiac enzymes.

Echocardiography is an excellent initial tool for confirming the diagnosis of cardiogenic shock and ruling out other causes of shock (Box 23-3); early echocardiography should be routine. Echocardiography provides information on overall and regional systolic function and can

Box 23-3

Role of Echocardiography in Diagnosing Cardiogenic Shock

Evaluate overall systolic performance
Delineate regional wall motion abnormalities
Rule out mechanical causes of shock
Papillary muscle rupture
Ventricular septal rupture
Free wall rupture
Tamponade
Diagnose right ventricular infarction

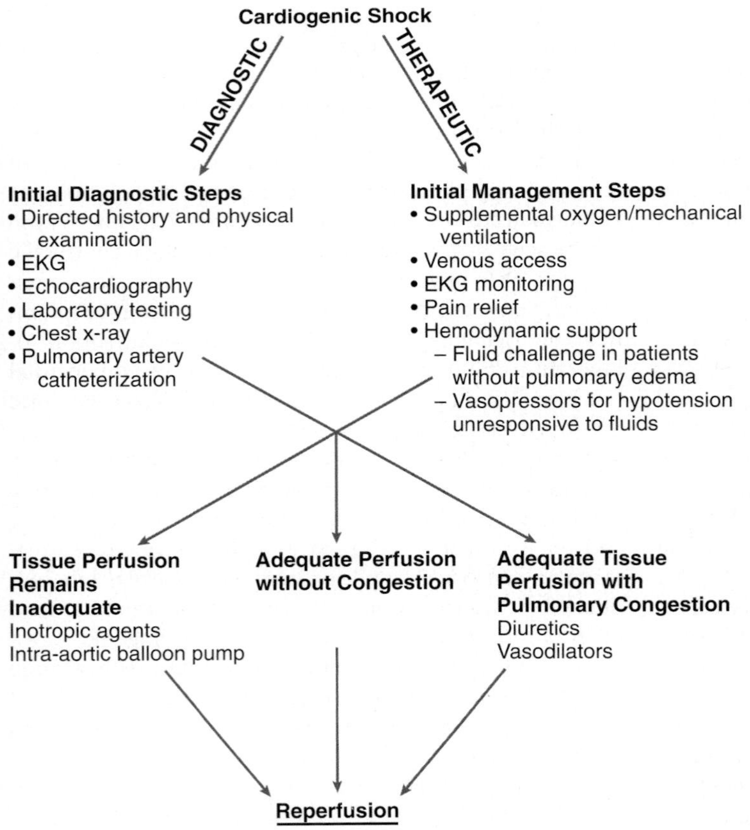

Figure 23-4. Approach to the diagnosis and treatment of cardiogenic shock caused by myocardial infarction. Right ventricular infarction and mechanical complications are discussed in the text. (Modified with permission from Hollenberg SM, Kavinsky CJ, Parrillo JE: Cardiogenic shock. Ann Intern Med 1999;131:51.)

rapidly diagnose mechanical causes of shock, such as papillary muscle rupture and acute mitral regurgitation, acute ventricular septal defect, and free wall rupture and tamponade.[53,54] Unsuspected severe mitral regurgitation is common. In some cases, echocardiography may reveal findings compatible with right ventricular infarction.

Invasive hemodynamic monitoring can be quite useful to exclude volume depletion, right ventricular infarction, and mechanical complications.[15,34] The hemodynamic profile of cardiogenic shock includes a pulmonary capillary occlusion pressure greater than 15 mm Hg and a cardiac index less than 2.2 L/min/m^2.[2] Optimal filling pressures may be greater than 15 mm Hg in individual patients as a result of left ventricular diastolic dysfunction. Right heart catheterization may reveal an oxygen step-up diagnostic of ventricular septal rupture or a large v wave that suggests severe mitral regurgitation. The hemodynamic profile of right ventricular infarction includes high right-sided filling pressures in the presence of normal or low occlusion pressures.[55,56]

Coronary angiography is usually performed as a precedent to revascularization. It is discussed in a later section.

Initial Management

Maintenance of adequate oxygenation and ventilation is crucial; intubation and mechanical ventilation are often required, if only to reduce the work of breathing and facilitate sedation and stabilization before cardiac catheterization. Central venous and arterial access, bladder catheterization, and pulse oximetry are routine. Electrolyte abnormalities should be corrected. Hypokalemia and hypomagnesemia are predisposing factors to ventricular arrhythmias, and acidosis can decrease contractile function. Relief of pain and anxiety with morphine sulfate (or fentanyl if systolic pressure is compromised) can reduce excessive sympathetic activity and decrease oxygen demand, preload, and afterload. Arrhythmias and heart block may have major effects on cardiac output and should be corrected promptly with antiarrhythmic drugs, cardioversion, or pacing. Cardiology consultation has been shown to be associated with improved outcomes in patients with MI and is strongly indicated in cardiogenic shock.[57] In addition, measures proven to improve outcome after MI, such as nitrates, β-blockers, and angiotensin-converting enzyme inhibitors,[58] have the potential to exacerbate hypotension in cardiogenic shock and should be stopped until the patient stabilizes.

After initial stabilization and restoration of adequate blood pressure, tissue perfusion should be assessed (see Fig. 23-4). If tissue perfusion remains inadequate, inotropic support or intra-aortic balloon pumping (IABP) should be initiated. If tissue perfusion is adequate, but significant pulmonary congestion remains, diuretics may be employed. Vasodilators also can be considered, depending on the blood pressure.

The initial approach to a hypotensive patient should include fluid resuscitation, unless frank pulmonary edema is present. Patients are commonly diaphoretic, and relative hypovolemia may be present. In the original description of hemodynamic subsets in MI, approximately 20% of patients had low cardiac index and low pulmonary capillary wedge pressure; most had reduced stroke volume and compensatory tachycardia.[59] Some of these patients would be expected to respond to fluid infusion with an increase in stroke volume, although the magnitude of such a response depends on the degree of ischemia and cardiac reserve.

Fluid infusion is best initiated with predetermined boluses titrated to clinical end points of heart rate, urine output, and blood pressure.[60] Ischemia produces diastolic and systolic dysfunction, and elevated filling pressures may be necessary to maintain stroke volume in patients with cardiogenic shock. Patients who do not respond rapidly to initial fluid boluses or patients with poor physiologic reserve should be considered for invasive hemodynamic monitoring. Optimal filling pressures vary among patients; hemodynamic monitoring can be used to construct a Starling curve at the bedside, identifying the filling pressure at which cardiac output is maximized. Maintenance of adequate preload is particularly important in patients with right ventricular infarction.

When arterial pressure remains inadequate, therapy with vasopressor agents may be required to maintain coronary perfusion pressure. Maintenance of adequate blood pressure is essential to break the vicious cycle of progressive hypotension with further myocardial ischemia. Dopamine increases blood pressure and cardiac output and is usually the first choice in patients with systolic pressures less than 90 mm Hg. When hypotension remains refractory, norepinephrine may be necessary to maintain organ perfusion pressure.[61,62] Phenylephrine, a selective α_1-adrenergic agonist, may be employed to support blood pressure when tachyarrhythmias limit therapy with other vasopressors, although it does not improve cardiac output.

In patients with inadequate tissue perfusion and adequate intravascular volume, cardiovascular support with inotropic agents should be initiated. Dobutamine, a selective β_1-adrenergic receptor agonist, can improve myocardial contractility and increase cardiac output without markedly changing heart rate or systemic vascular resistance; it is the initial agent of choice in patients with systolic pressures greater than 80 mm Hg.[63-65] Dobutamine may exacerbate hypotension in some patients and can precipitate tachyarrhythmias. Dopamine acts directly on myocardial β_1-adrenergic receptors and acts indirectly by releasing norepinephrine. It has inotropic and vasopressor effects, and its use is preferable in the presence of systolic pressures less than 80 mm Hg.[30,66,67] Tachycardia and increased peripheral resistance with dopamine administration may exacerbate myocardial ischemia. In some situations, a combination of dopamine and dobutamine can be more effective than either agent alone.[68]

Phosphodiesterase inhibitors such as milrinone increase intracellular cyclic adenosine monophosphate by mechanisms not involving adrenergic receptors, producing positive inotropic and vasodilatory actions. Milrinone has fewer chronotropic and arrhythmogenic effects than catecholamines.[69] In addition, because milrinone does not stimulate adrenergic receptors directly, its effects may be additive to the effects of the catecholamines.[70] Milrinone has the potential to cause hypotension, however, and has a long half-life; in patients with tenuous clinical status, its use is often reserved for situations in which other agents have proved ineffective.[15] Standard administration of milrinone calls for a bolus loading dose followed by an infusion, but many clinicians eschew the loading dose (or halve it) in patients with marginal blood pressure.

Infusions of vasoactive agents need to be titrated carefully in patients with cardiogenic shock to maximize coronary perfusion pressure with the least possible increase in myocardial oxygen demand. Invasive hemodynamic monitoring can be extremely useful in allowing optimization of therapy in these unstable patients because clinical estimates of filling pressure can be unreliable[71]; in addition, changes in myocardial performance and compliance and therapeutic interventions can change cardiac output and filling pressures precipitously. Optimization of filling pressures and serial measurements of cardiac output (and other parameters such as mixed venous oxygen saturation) allow for titration of the dosage of inotropic agents and vasopressors to the minimal dosage required to achieve the chosen therapeutic goals. This minimizes the increases in myocardial oxygen demand and arrhythmogenic potential.[60,72]

Diuretics should be used to treat pulmonary congestion and enhance oxygenation. Vasodilators should be used with extreme caution in the acute setting because of the risk of precipitating further hypotension and decreasing coronary blood flow. After blood pressure has been stabilized, however, vasodilator therapy can decrease preload and afterload. Sodium nitroprusside is a balanced arterial and venous vasodilator that decreases filling pressures and can increase stroke volume in patients with heart failure by reducing afterload.[73] Nitroglycerin is an effective venodilator that reduces the pulmonary capillary occlusion pressure and can decrease ischemia by reducing left ventricular filling pressure and redistributing coronary blood flow to the ischemic zone.[74] Both agents may cause acute and rapid decreases in blood pressure, and dosages must be titrated carefully; invasive hemodynamic monitoring can be useful in optimizing filling pressures when these agents are used.

THROMBOLYTIC THERAPY

Although it has been shown convincingly that thrombolytic therapy reduces mortality rates in patients with acute MI,[9,75-77] the benefits of this therapy in patients with cardiogenic shock are less certain. It is clear that thrombolytic therapy can reduce the likelihood of subsequent development of shock after initial presentation.[13,75,76,78] This is important because most patients develop cardiogenic shock more than 6 hours after hospital presentation.[2,13]

Nonetheless, no trials have shown that thrombolytic therapy reduces mortality in patients with established cardiogenic shock. The numbers of patients are small because most thrombolytic trials have excluded patients who have cardiogenic shock at presentation.[79] In the GISSI (Gruppo Italiano per lo Studio Della Streptochinasi Nell'Infarto Miocardico) trial,[9,79] 30-day mortality rates were 69.9% in 146 patients with cardiogenic shock who received streptokinase and 70.1% in 134 patients receiving placebo. The International Study Group reported a mortality rate of 65% in 93 patients with shock treated with streptokinase and a mortality rate of 78% in 80 patients treated with recombinant tissue plasminogen activator.[11] In the GUSTO trial,[12] 315 patients had shock on arrival; mortality was 56% in patients treated with streptokinase and 59% in patients treated with recombinant tissue plasminogen activator.[13,80]

The failure of thrombolytic therapy to improve survival in patients with cardiogenic shock may seem paradoxical in light of evidence that the absolute reduction in mortality with thrombolytics is greatest in patients at highest risk at presentation. The meta-analysis performed by the Fibrinolytic Therapy Trialists Collaborative Group showed a reduction in mortality rate from 36.1% to 29.7% when thrombolytic therapy was used in patients with initial systolic blood pressures less than 100 mm Hg. In patients with initial heart rates greater than 100 beats/min, the mortality rate decreased from 23.8% to 18.9%.[81] Most patients in these subgroups did not meet criteria for cardiogenic shock, however.

Consideration of the efficacy of thrombolytic therapy when cardiogenic shock has been established makes the disappointing results in this subgroup of patients easier to understand. The degree of reperfusion correlates with outcome,[78,82] and reperfusion has been shown to be less likely for patients in cardiogenic shock.[20,82,83] When reperfusion is successful, mortality has been shown to be significantly reduced.[20] The lower rates of reperfusion in patients with shock may explain some of the disappointing results in this subgroup in the thrombolytic trials.

The reasons for decreased thrombolytic efficacy in patients with cardiogenic shock are not fully understood, but probably include hemodynamic, mechanical, and metabolic factors. Decreased arterial pressure limits the penetration of thrombolytic agents into a thrombus.[84] Passive collapse of the infarct artery in hypotension also can contribute to decreased thrombolytic efficacy, as can acidosis, which inhibits the conversion of plasminogen to plasmin.[84] Two small studies support the notion that vasopressor therapy to increase aortic pressure improves thrombolytic efficacy.[85,86] The use of IABP in conjunction with thrombolytics is discussed subsequently.

INTRA-AORTIC BALLOON PUMPING

IABP reduces systolic afterload and augments diastolic perfusion pressure, increasing cardiac output and improving coronary blood flow.[87,88] These beneficial effects, in contrast to the effects of inotropic or vasopressor agents, occur without an increase in oxygen demand. IABP is efficacious for initial stabilization of patients with cardiogenic shock.[89,90] Small randomized trials in the prethrombolytic era failed to show that IABP alone increases survival, however.[91,92] IABP alone does not substantially improve blood flow distal to a critical coronary stenosis.[93]

IABP is probably not best used as an independent modality to treat cardiogenic shock. It may be an essential support mechanism, however, to allow definitive therapeutic measures to be undertaken. In the GUSTO trial, patients who presented with shock and had early IABP placement showed a trend toward lower mortality, even after exclusion of patients who underwent revascularization.[12,94] A similar trend was seen in the SHOCK trial registry, although it did not persist after adjustment for age and catheterization.[2] Several observational studies also have suggested that IABP can improve outcome in patients with shock, although revascularization procedures are a confounding factor in these studies.[95-98] IABP has been shown to decrease reocclusion and cardiac events after emergency angioplasty for acute MI.[99,100] The TACTICS trial randomly assigned 57 patients with MI complicated by hypotension or cardiogenic shock to IABP or placebo in conjunction with fibrinolysis; the trial was terminated early because of difficulties with enrollment and was underpowered.[101] Although there was no difference in the primary end point of 6-month mortality (34% versus 43%; $P = .23$), patients presenting in Killip class III or IV heart failure showed a trend toward benefit with IABP (39% versus 80%; $P = .05$).[101]

The role of direct angioplasty in the therapy of cardiogenic shock is discussed subsequently. In hospitals without direct angioplasty capability, stabilization with IABP and thrombolysis followed by transfer to a tertiary care facility may be the best management option. IABP may be a useful adjunct to thrombolysis in this setting by increasing drug delivery to the thrombus, improving coronary flow to other regions, preventing hypotensive events, or supporting ventricular function until areas of stunned myocardium can recover.[102] Two retrospective studies showed that patients with cardiogenic shock who were treated in the community hospital with IABP placement followed by thrombolysis had improved in-hospital survival and improved outcomes after subsequent transfer for revascularization, although selection bias is a confounding factor.[97,98] The role of IABP as an adjunct to thrombolytic agents in the community hospital needs to be addressed in clinical trials.

REVASCULARIZATION

Pathophysiologic considerations and extensive retrospective data favor aggressive mechanical revascularization for patients with cardiogenic shock resulting from MI. Emergency percutaneous revascularization is the only intervention to date that has been shown consistently to reduce mortality rates in patients with cardiogenic shock.

Direct Coronary Angioplasty

Re-establishment of brisk (TIMI [Thrombolysis In Myocardial Infarction] grade 3) flow in the infarct-related artery is an important determinant of left ventricular function and survival after MI.[78] Direct percutaneous transluminal coronary angioplasty (PTCA) can achieve TIMI grade 3 flow in 80% to 90% of patients with MI[103-105] compared with rates of 50% to 60% 90 minutes after thrombolytic therapy.[78,106] In addition to improving wall motion in the infarct territory, increased perfusion of the infarct zone has been associated with augmented contraction of remote myocardium, possibly as a result of recruitment of collateral blood flow.[22]

Use of angioplasty in patients with cardiogenic shock grew out of its use as primary therapy in patients with MI. An analysis of the first 1000 patients treated with primary angioplasty at the Mid America Heart Institute showed a mortality of 44% in the subgroup of 79 patients presenting with cardiogenic shock, substantially lower than the mortality in historical controls, which was 80% to 90%.[107] Most other reported case series also showed results with percutaneous intervention superior to the results with either fibrinolytic therapy or conservative medical management, with mortality rates of approximately 40% to 50%.[20,108-117] Observational studies from registries of randomized trials also have reported improved outcomes in patients with cardiogenic shock selected for revascularization. Notable among these are the GUSTO-1 trial. In a subgroup analysis of the 2972 patients with cardiogenic shock in this trial, 30-day mortality was significantly lower in patients who had angioplasty (43% compared with 61% for patients with shock on arrival and 32% compared with 61% for patients who developed shock).[13] In this trial, patients treated with an "aggressive" strategy (coronary angiography performed within 24 hours of shock onset with revascularization by PTCA or bypass surgery) had significantly lower mortality (38% compared with 62%).[83] This benefit was present even after adjustment for baseline characteristics[83] and persisted out to 1 year.[118]

Reports from NRMI-2 (National Registry of Myocardial Infarction-2), which collected 26,280 shock patients with cardiogenic shock in MI between 1994 and 1997, similarly supported the association between revascularization and survival.[119] Improved short-term mortality was noted in patients who then underwent revascularization during the reference hospitalization, via either PTCA (mortality 12.8% versus 43.9%) or coronary artery bypass grafting (mortality 6.5% versus 23.9%).[119] These data complement the GUSTO-1 substudy data and are important not only because of the sheer number of patients from whom these values are derived, but also because NRMI-2 was a national cross-sectional study, which more closely represents general clinical practice than carefully selected trial populations.

Coronary Artery Bypass Surgery

Several trials have reported favorable outcomes for patients with cardiogenic shock who undergo coronary artery bypass surgery.[31,95,120,121] Left main and three-vessel coronary disease are common in patients with cardiogenic shock,[2,21,78] and the potential contribution of ischemia in the noninfarct zone to myocardial dysfunction in patients with shock would argue for complete revascularization. Nonetheless, the logistic and time considerations involved in mobilizing an operating team, the high operative morbidity and mortality, and the generally favorable results of percutaneous interventions all militate against routine bypass surgery for these patients. In the series reported by DeWood and colleagues,[95] IABP support was used successfully as a bridge to coronary artery bypass surgery. The roles of other supportive measures, such as emergency cardiopulmonary bypass[122] or placement of percutaneous assist devices,[123] remain to be defined.

Randomized Studies

These studies of revascularization in patients with cardiogenic shock were retrospective and uncontrolled. Selection bias is present in that patients selected for revascularization tend to be younger, less critically ill, and more likely to receive IABP support; they also tend to have less comorbidity.[2,13,83] In addition, patients who deteriorate before planned revascularization is performed are counted in the nonrevascularized group. In the SHOCK trial registry, not only was mortality in patients selected for cardiac catheterization lower than in patients not selected (51% compared with 85%), but also mortality was lower (58%) in catheterized patients who did not undergo revascularization.[2]

A small randomized study, the SMASH (Swiss Multicenter evaluation of early Angioplasty for SHock) trial,[124] showed no significant difference in mortality rate between patients randomly assigned to angioplasty and patients randomly assigned to medical treatment (69% compared with 78%), although the trial was stopped early because of difficulties in patient recruitment. The landmark SHOCK study[21,125] was a randomized, multicenter international trial that assigned patients with cardiogenic shock to receive optimal medical management—including IABP and thrombolytic therapy—or cardiac catheterization with revascularization using PTCA or coronary artery bypass grafting.[21] The trial enrolled 302 patients and was powered to detect a 20% absolute decrease in 30-day all-cause mortality rates. Mortality at 30 days was 46.7% in patients treated with early intervention and 56% in patients treated with initial medical stabilization, but this difference did not reach statistical significance (P = .11).[21] The control group (patients who received medical management) had a lower mortality rate than that reported in previous studies; this may reflect the aggressive use of thrombolytic therapy (64%) and IABP (86%) in these controls. These data provide indirect evidence that the combination of thrombolysis and IABP may produce the best outcomes when cardiac catheterization is not immediately available. At 6 months, mortality in the SHOCK trial was reduced significantly (50.3% compared with 63.1%; P = .027),[21] and this risk reduction was maintained at 12 months (mortality 54.3% versus 66.4%; P < .03) (Fig. 23-5).[125] This 12% absolute improvement in survival remained stable at 3 and 6 years of follow-up.[126] In addition, most survivors have good functional status.[127]

Subgroup analysis showed a substantial improvement in mortality rates in patients younger than 75 years old at 30 days (41.4% versus 56.8%; P = .01) and 6 months

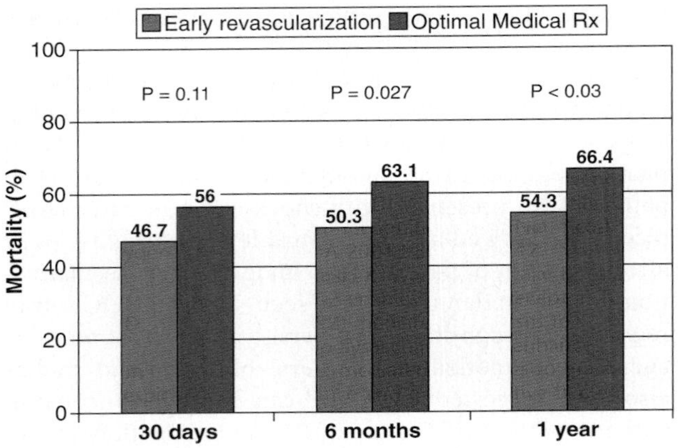

Figure 23-5. Mortality in the randomized SHOCK trial at 30 days, 6 months, and 1 year in the early revascularization and optimal medical management groups. (Data from Hochman JS, Sleeper LA, Webb JG, et al: Early revascularization in acute myocardial infarction complicated by cardiogenic shock. N Engl J Med 1999;341:625-634; and Hochman JS, Sleeper LA, White HD, et al: One-year survival following early revascularization for cardiogenic shock. JAMA 2001;285:190-192.)

(44.9% versus 65%; P = .003).[21] For patients older than 75, no benefit of revascularization was shown in the SHOCK trial, although this was a small subgroup, and further analysis suggested baseline differences so that the elderly patients randomly assigned to medical therapy seemed to have been a lower risk group.[128] In the SHOCK trial registry, elderly patients treated with early revascularization had better outcomes than the patients treated medically, suggesting that it is possible to select elderly patients who would benefit from aggressive treatment.[129]

The SMASH trial was independently conceived and had a similar design, although a more rigid definition of cardiogenic shock resulted in enrollment of sicker patients and a higher mortality.[124] The trial was terminated early because of difficulties in patient recruitment, for two different reasons: Early on, several centers declined to participate because it was thought that it would not be ethical to undertake early invasive evaluation in such extremely ill patients, and then, after publication of several encouraging studies documenting the superiority of PCI over thrombolysis for acute MI, many centers thought that it had become unethical *not* to proceed to early evaluation and revascularization.[130] In the SMASH trial, an absolute reduction in 30-day mortality similar to that seen in the SHOCK trial was observed (mortality 69% in the invasive group versus 78% in the medically managed group; relative risk [RR] 0.88, 95% confidence interval [CI] 0.6 to 1.2; P = not significant).[124] This benefit also was maintained at 1 year.

When the results of the SHOCK and SMASH trials are put into perspective with results from other randomized, controlled trials of patients with acute MI, an important point emerges: Despite the moderate *relative* risk reduction (for the SHOCK trial, RR 0.72, CI 0.54-0.95; for the SMASH trial, RR 0.88, CI 0.60-1.20) the *absolute* benefit is important, with 9 lives saved for 100 patients treated at 30 days in both trials, and 13.2 lives saved for 100 patients treated at 1 year in the SHOCK trial. This latter figure corresponds to a number needed to treat of 7.6, one of the lowest figures ever observed in a randomized, controlled trial of cardiovascular disease. In our judgment, these data strongly support the superiority of a strategy of early revascularization in most patients with cardiogenic shock (see Fig. 23-4). In the latest American College of Cardiology/American Heart Association guidelines for the management of acute MI, primary coronary intervention was given a class I indication for patients younger than 75 and a class IIa indication for patients older than 75.[58]

OTHER CAUSES OF CARDIOGENIC SHOCK

Right Ventricular Infarction

Right ventricular infarction occurs in 30% of patients with inferior infarction and is clinically significant in 10%.[131] Patients present with hypotension, elevated neck veins, and clear lung fields. Diagnosis is made by identifying ST segment elevation in right precordial leads or by characteristic hemodynamic findings on right heart catheterization (elevated right atrial and right ventricular end-diastolic pressures with normal to low pulmonary artery occlusion pressure and low cardiac output). Echocardiography can show depressed right ventricular contractility.[56] Patients with cardiogenic shock on the basis of right ventricular infarction have a better prognosis than patients with left-sided pump failure.[131] This may be due in part to the fact that right ventricular function tends to return to normal over time with supportive therapy,[132] although such therapy may need to be prolonged.

Supportive therapy for patients with right ventricular infarction begins with maintenance of right ventricular preload with fluid administration. In some cases, fluid resuscitation may increase pulmonary capillary occlusion pressure, but may not increase cardiac output, however, and overdilation of the right ventricle can compromise left ventricular filling and cardiac output.[132] Inotropic therapy with dobutamine may be more effective in increasing cardiac output in some patients, and monitoring with serial echocardiograms also may be useful to detect right ventricular overdistention.[132] Maintenance of atrioventricular synchrony also is important in these patients to optimize right ventricular filling.[56] For patients with continued hemodynamic instability, IABP may be useful, particularly because elevated right ventricular pressures and volumes increase wall stress and oxygen consumption and decrease right coronary perfusion pressure, exacerbating right ventricular ischemia.

Reperfusion of the occluded coronary artery also is crucial. A study using direct angioplasty showed that restoration of normal flow resulted in dramatic recovery of right ventricular function and a mortality rate of only 2%, whereas unsuccessful reperfusion was associated with persistent hemodynamic compromise and a mortality of 58%.[133]

Acute Mitral Regurgitation

Ischemic mitral regurgitation is usually associated with inferior MI and ischemia or infarction of the posterior papillary muscle, which has a single blood supply, usually from the posterior descending branch of a dominant right coronary artery.[134] Papillary muscle rupture typically occurs 2 to 7 days after acute MI and manifests dramatically with pulmonary edema, hypotension, and cardiogenic shock. When a papillary muscle ruptures, the murmur of acute mitral regurgitation may be limited to early systole because of rapid equalization of pressures in the left atrium and left ventricle. More importantly, the murmur may be soft or inaudible, especially when cardiac output is low.[135]

Echocardiography is extremely useful in the differential diagnosis, which includes free wall rupture, ventricular septal rupture, and infarct extension with pump failure. Hemodynamic monitoring with pulmonary artery catheterization also may be helpful. Management includes afterload reduction with nitroprusside and IABP as temporizing measures. Inotropic or vasopressor therapy also may be needed to support cardiac output and blood pressure. Definitive therapy is surgical valve repair or replacement, however, which should be undertaken as soon as possible because clinical deterioration can be sudden.[135,136]

Ventricular Septal Rupture

Patients who have ventricular septal rupture have severe heart failure or cardiogenic shock, with a pansystolic murmur and a parasternal thrill. The hallmark finding is a left-to-right intracardiac shunt ("step-up" in oxygen saturation from right atrium to right ventricle). On pulmonary artery catheter tracing, it can be difficult to distinguish ventricular septal rupture from mitral regurgitation because both can produce dramatic v waves. The diagnosis is most easily made with echocardiography.

Rapid stabilization—using IABP and pharmacologic measures followed by operative repair, is the only viable option for long-term survival. The timing of surgery is controversial, but most authorities now suggest that operative repair should be undertaken early, within 48 hours of the rupture.[136-138]

Free Wall Rupture

Ventricular free wall rupture usually occurs during the first week after MI; the classic patient is elderly, female, and hypertensive. The early use of thrombolytic therapy reduces the incidence of cardiac rupture, but late use may increase the risk, particularly in older patients.[139] Free wall rupture manifests as a catastrophic event with a pulseless rhythm. Salvage is possible with prompt recognition, pericardiocentesis to relieve acute tamponade, and thoracotomy with repair.[140]

Myocardial Dysfunction after Cardiopulmonary Bypass

Transient depression of ventricular contractility is common after cardiopulmonary bypass and can represent a significant clinical problem. The differential diagnosis includes inadequate operation, cardiac tamponade (which may be localized and difficult to detect), and increased right ventricular afterload, but most cases likely result from myocardial stunning. The heart is rendered globally ischemic during aortic cross-clamping and then reperfused, and because demonstrable myocardial necrosis is rare, stunning can be implicated. Stunning after bypass has been documented in a study in which an ultrasound probe was left on the epicardial surface for 2 to 3 days in 31 patients after bypass surgery; left ventricular wall thickening decreased after surgery, reached a nadir at 2 to 6 hours, and subsequently improved, usually returning to baseline by 24 to 48 hours.[141]

The degree of myocardial dysfunction after cardiac surgery varies and may depend on the cardioplegia solution, the method of administration (antegrade or retrograde), the mode of administration (continuous or intermittent), and the temperature of the solution and of the patient during surgery.[37] In the clinical setting, transient depression of ventricular contractility is common and usually reversible within 24 to 48 hours. The depression of contractility can be severe enough to cause cardiogenic shock. In this event, therapy with inotropic agents, vasodilators, and IABP is necessary. Occasionally, a left ventricular assist device may be employed.[39] Better understanding of the mechanisms of post–cardiopulmonary bypass myocardial dysfunction may lead to better preventive and therapeutic approaches.

Myocarditis

Acute myocarditis can be benign and self-limited or fulminant, with severe congestive heart failure or atrial and ventricular arrhythmias, or both heart failure and arrhythmias. After acute myocarditis, patients can recover completely, or they can have severe left ventricular dysfunction. In some patients with acute inflammatory myocarditis, an aberrant immune response occurs, with continuing inflammation, and this can result in the eventual development of a dilated cardiomyopathy.

Evidence exists that some patients with myocarditis would benefit from immunosuppressive therapy, but how to identify which patients should be treated is controversial. A trial initiated at the National Institutes of Health randomly assigned 102 patients with dilated cardiomyopathy, no significant coronary artery disease, and ejection fraction less than 35% to oral prednisone or placebo.[142] The prospectively defined end point, an increase in radionuclide-measured ejection fraction of more than 5 percentage points, was observed in 53% of patients treated with prednisone compared with only 27% of controls at 3 months ($P < .05$), but the improvement did not persist at 9 months when patients were switched to alternate-day prednisone therapy.[142] Another clinical trial of immunosuppressive therapy for myocarditis showed no improvement in mean ejection fraction with immunosuppression, although the admission criteria in this trial were quite restrictive, the therapeutic regimens were heterogeneous, and the incidence of definitive myocarditis was uncertain.[143]

Although it might seem that patients with fulminant myocarditis might be the best candidates for immunosuppressive therapy, one series confounds this notion by reporting excellent long-term survival in patients with myocarditis and a fulminant course.[144] Patients with acute myocarditis without a fulminant course had a much worse prognosis in this series,[144] emphasizing the need for further research to identify subgroups of patients with dilated cardiomyopathy who may benefit from adjunctive therapies.

In patients with potentially reversible causes of myocardial dysfunction, aggressive cardiovascular support with a combination of inotropic agents and intra-aortic balloon counterpulsation may be required for hours or days to allow sufficient time for recovery. If these measures fail, mechanical circulatory support with left ventricular assist devices can be considered.[145] These devices can be used as a bridge to cardiac transplantation in eligible patients or as a bridge to myocardial recovery; functional improvement with such support can be dramatic.[123,146]

CONCLUSION

Mortality rates in patients with cardiogenic shock have improved, but remain high. The pathophysiology involves a downward spiral in which ischemia causes myocardial dysfunction, which worsens ischemia. Areas of nonfunctional but viable myocardium also can cause or contribute to the development of cardiogenic shock. The key to achieving a good outcome is an organized approach with rapid diagnosis and prompt initiation of therapy to maintain blood pressure and cardiac output. Expeditious coronary revascularization is crucial. When available, emergent cardiac catheterization and revascularization with angioplasty or coronary surgery seems to improve survival and represents standard therapy at this time. In hospitals without direct angioplasty capability, stabilization with IABP and thrombolysis followed by transfer to a tertiary care facility may be the best option. The SHOCK multicenter randomized trial[21] provides important data that help clarify the appropriate role and timing of revascularization in patients with cardiogenic shock.

KEY POINTS

- Cardiogenic shock is a state of inadequate tissue perfusion resulting from cardiac dysfunction. Acute MI is the leading cause.
- The pathogenesis of cardiogenic shock is a "downward spiral" in which MI or ischemia causes myocardial dysfunction and compromised myocardial perfusion, exacerbating ischemia.
- Large areas of nonfunctional but viable myocardium (stunned, hibernating, or both) also can cause or contribute to the development of cardiogenic shock in patients after MI.
- The challenge in initial management of cardiogenic shock is that evaluation and therapy must begin simultaneously. The clinician must perform the clinical

assessment required to understand the cause of shock while initiating supportive therapy before shock causes irreversible damages.

- Thrombolytic therapy alone has less efficacy in patients with cardiogenic shock than in other settings; this is due to a combination of hemodynamic, mechanical, and metabolic factors.
- IABP alone has not been shown to decrease mortality in cardiogenic shock, but may be an essential support mechanism to allow definitive therapeutic measures to be undertaken.
- Pathophysiologic considerations and extensive retrospective data favor aggressive mechanical revascularization for patients with cardiogenic shock secondary to MI. Results of SHOCK support a strategy of early revascularization in most patients with cardiogenic shock.
- Other acute mechanical causes of low cardiac output must be excluded. If present, urgent surgery may be required.
- In patients with potentially reversible causes of myocardial dysfunction (including severe myocarditis), aggressive cardiovascular support with a combination of inotropic agents and intra-aortic balloon counterpulsation may be required for hours or days to allow sufficient time for recovery.

REFERENCES

1. Hollenberg SM: Recognition and treatment of cardiogenic shock. Semin Respir Crit Care Med 2004;25:661-671.
2. Hochman JS, Boland J, Sleeper LA, et al: Current spectrum of cardiogenic shock and effect of early revascularization on mortality: Results of an International Registry. Circulation 1995;91:873-881.
3. Killip T, Kimball JT: Treatment of myocardial infarction in a coronary care unit: A two year experience with 250 patients. Am J Cardiol 1967;20:457-464.
4. Forrester JS, Diamond G, Chatterjee K, et al: Medical therapy of acute myocardial infarction by application of hemodynamic subsets. N Engl J Med 1976;295:1356-1362.
5. Goldberg RJ, Gore JM, Alpert JS, et al: Cardiogenic shock after acute myocardial infarction: Incidence and mortality from a community-wide perspective, 1975 to 1988. N Engl J Med 1991;325:1117-1122.
6. Babaev A, Frederick PD, Pasta DJ, et al: Trends in management and outcomes of patients with acute myocardial infarction complicated by cardiogenic shock. JAMA 2005;294:448-454.
7. Fang J, Mensah GA, Alderman MH, et al: Trends in acute myocardial infarction complicated by cardiogenic shock, 1979-2003, United States. Am Heart J 2006;152:1035-1041.
8. Goldberg RJ, Samad NA, Yarzebski J, et al: Temporal trends in cardiogenic shock complicating acute myocardial infarction. N Engl J Med 1999;340: 1162-1168.
9. Gruppo Italiano per lo Studio Della Streptochinasi Nell'Infarto Miocardico (GISSI): Effectiveness of intravenous thrombolytic treatment in acute myocardial infarction. Lancet 1986;2:397-402.
10. ISIS-3 (Third International Study of Infarct Survival) Collaborative Group: ISIS-3: A randomised comparison of streptokinase vs tissue plasminogen activator vs anistreplase and of aspirin plus heparin vs aspirin alone among 41,299 cases of suspected acute myocardial infarction. Lancet 1992;339:753-770.
11. International Study Group: In-hospital mortality and clinical course of 20,891 patients with suspected acute myocardial infarction randomised between alteplase and streptokinase with or without heparin. Lancet 1990;336:71-75.
12. GUSTO Investigators: An international randomized trial comparing four thrombolytic strategies for acute myocardial infarction. N Engl J Med 1993;329:673-682.
13. Holmes DR Jr, Bates ER, Kleiman NS, et al: Contemporary reperfusion therapy for cardiogenic shock: The GUSTO-I trial experience. The GUSTO-I Investigators. Global Utilization of Streptokinase and Tissue Plasminogen Activator for Occluded Coronary Arteries. J Am Coll Cardiol 1995;26:668-674.
14. Scheidt S, Ascheim R, Killip T: Shock after acute myocardial infarction: A clinical and hemodynamic profile. Am J Cardiol 1970;26:556-564.
15. Califf RM, Bengtson JR: Cardiogenic shock. N Engl J Med 1994;330: 1724-1730.
16. Bonnefoy E, Lapostolle F, Leizorovicz A, et al: Primary angioplasty versus prehospital fibrinolysis in acute myocardial infarction: A randomised study. Lancet 2002;360:825-829.
17. Hands ME, Rutherford JD, Muller JE, et al: The in-hospital development of cardiogenic shock after myocardial infarction: Incidence, predictors of occurrence, outcome and prognostic factors. The MILIS Study Group. J Am Coll Cardiol 1989;14:40-46.
18. Leor J, Goldbourt U, Reicher-Reiss H, et al: Cardiogenic shock complicating acute myocardial infarction in patients without heart failure on admission: incidence, risk factors, and outcome. SPRINT Study Group. Am J Med 1993;94:265-273.
19. Hasdai D, Califf RM, Thompson TD, et al: Predictors of cardiogenic shock after thrombolytic therapy for acute myocardial infarction. J Am Coll Cardiol 2000;35:136-143.
20. Bengtson JR, Kaplan AJ, Pieper KS, et al: Prognosis in cardiogenic shock after acute myocardial infarction in the interventional era. J Am Coll Cardiol 1992;20:1482-1489.
21. Hochman JS, Sleeper LA, Webb JG, et al: Early revascularization in acute myocardial infarction complicated by cardiogenic shock. N Engl J Med 1999;341:625-634.
22. Grines CL, Topol EJ, Califf RM, et al: Prognostic implications and predictors of enhanced regional wall motion of the noninfarct zone after thrombolysis and angioplasty therapy of acute myocardial infarction. The TAMI Study Groups. Circulation 1989;80:245-253.
23. Hollenberg SM, Kavinsky CJ, Parrillo JE: Cardiogenic shock. Ann Intern Med 1999;131:47-59.
24. Hochman JS: Cardiogenic shock complicating acute myocardial infarction: Expanding the paradigm. Circulation 2003;107:2998-3002.
25. Greenberg MA, Menegus MA: Ischemia-induced diastolic dysfunction: New observations, new questions. J Am Coll Cardiol 1989;13:1071-1072.
26. Page DL, Caulfield JB, Kaster JA, et al: Myocardial changes associated with cardiogenic shock. N Engl J Med 1971;285:133-137.
27. Olivetti G, Quaini F, Sala R, et al: Acute myocardial infarction in humans is associated with activation of programmed myocyte cell death in the surviving portion of the heart. J Mol Cell Cardiol 1994;28:2005-2016.
28. Weisman HF, Healy B: Myocardial infarct expansion, infarct extension, and reinfarction: pathophysiologic concepts. Prog Cardiovasc Dis 1987;30:73-110.
29. Widimsky P, Gregor P, Cervenka V, et al: Severe diffuse hypokinesis of the remote myocardium—the main cause of cardiogenic shock? An echocardiographic study of 75 patients with extremely large myocardial infarctions. Cor Vasa 1988;30:27-34.
30. McGhie AI, Golstein RA: Pathogenesis and management of acute heart failure and cardiogenic shock: Role of inotropic therapy. Chest 1992;102:626S-632S.
31. Webb JG: Interventional management of cardiogenic shock. Can J Cardiol 1998;14:233-244.
32. Harizi RC, Bianco JA, Alpert JS: Diastolic function of the heart in clinical cardiology. Arch Intern Med 1988;148:99-109.

33. Oh JK, Hatle L, Tajik AJ, et al: Diastolic heart failure can be diagnosed by comprehensive two-dimensional and Doppler echocardiography. J Am Coll Cardiol 2006;47:500-506.
34. Hollenberg SM, Parrillo JE: Shock. In Fauci AS, Braunwald E, Isselbacher KJ, et al (eds): Harrison's Principles of Internal Medicine, 14th ed. New York, McGraw-Hill, 1997, pp 214-222.
35. Okuda M: A multidisciplinary overview of cardiogenic shock. Shock 2006;25:557-570.
36. Bartling B, Holtz J, Darmer D: Contribution of myocyte apoptosis to myocardial infarction? Basic Res Cardiol 1998;93:71-84.
37. Bolli R: Basic and clinical aspects of myocardial stunning. Prog Cardiovasc Dis 1998;40:477-516.
38. Arnold JM, Braunwald E, Sandor T, et al: Inotropic stimulation of reperfused myocardium with dopamine: Effects on infarct size and myocardial function. J Am Coll Cardiol 1985;6:1026-1034.
39. Ballantyne CM, Verani MS, Short HD, et al: Delayed recovery of severely "stunned" myocardium with the support of a left ventricular assist device after coronary artery bypass graft surgery. J Am Coll Cardiol 1987;10:710-712.
40. Gerber BL, Wijns W, Vanoverschelde JL, et al: Myocardial perfusion and oxygen consumption in reperfused noninfarcted dysfunctional myocardium after unstable angina: Direct evidence for myocardial stunning in humans. J Am Coll Cardiol 1999;34:1939-1946.
41. Jeroudi MO, Hartley CJ, Bolli R: Myocardial reperfusion injury: Role of oxygen radicals and potential therapy with antioxidants. Am J Cardiol 1994;73:2B-7B.
42. Gao WD, Liu Y, Mellgren R, et al: Intrinsic myofilament alterations underlying the decreased contractility of stunned myocardium: A consequence of Ca2+-dependent proteolysis? Circ Res 1996;78:455-465.
43. Atar D, Gao WD, Marban E: Alterations of excitation-contraction coupling in stunned myocardium and in failing myocardium. J Mol Cell Cardiol 1995;27:783-791.
44. Brar R, Kumar A, Schaer GL, et al: Release of soluble myocardial depressant activity by reperfused myocardium. J Am Coll Cardiol 1996;27:386A (Abstract).
45. Wijns W, Vatner SF, Camici PG: Hibernating myocardium. N Engl J Med 1998;339:173-181.
46. Kloner RA, Jennings RB: Consequences of brief ischemia: Stunning, preconditioning, and their clinical implications, part 1. Circulation 2001;104:2981-2989.
47. Bito V, Heinzel FR, Weidemann F, et al: Cellular mechanisms of contractile dysfunction in hibernating myocardium. Circ Res 2004;94:794-801.
48. Marban E: Myocardial stunning and hibernation: The physiology behind the colloquialisms. Circulation 1991;83:681-688.
49. Topol EJ, Weiss JL, Guzman PA, et al: Immediate improvement of dysfunctional myocardial segments after coronary revascularization: Detection by intraoperative transesophageal echocardiography. J Am Coll Cardiol 1984;4:1123-1134.
50. Tillisch J, Brunken R, Marshall R, et al: Reversibility of cardiac wall-motion abnormalities predicted by positron tomography. N Engl J Med 1986;314:884-888.
51. Wu KC, Lima JA: Noninvasive imaging of myocardial viability: Current techniques and future developments. Circ Res 2003;93:1146-1158.
52. Kim SJ, Peppas A, Hong SK, et al: Persistent stunning induces myocardial hibernation and protection: Flow/function and metabolic mechanisms. Circ Res 2003;92:1233-1239.
53. Nishimura RA, Tajik AJ, Shub C, et al: Role of two-dimensional echocardiography in the prediction of in-hospital complications after acute myocardial infarction. J Am Coll Cardiol 1984;4:1080-1087.
54. Berkowitz MJ, Picard MH, Harkness S, et al: Echocardiographic and angiographic correlations in patients with cardiogenic shock secondary to acute myocardial infarction. Am J Cardiol 2006;98:1004-1008.
55. Kinch JW, Ryan TJ: Right ventricular infarction. N Engl J Med 1994;330:1211-1217.
56. Nedeljkovic ZS, Ryan TJ: Right ventricular infarction. In Hollenberg SM, Bates ER (eds): Cardiogenic Shock. Armonk, NY: Futura Publishing Company, 2002, pp 161-186.
57. Jollis JG, DeLong ER, Peterson ED, et al: Outcome of acute myocardial infarction according to the specialty of the admitting physician. N Engl J Med 1996;335:1880-1887.
58. Antman EM, Anbe DT, Armstrong PW, et al: ACC/AHA guidelines for the management of patients with ST-elevation myocardial infarction—executive summary: a report of the American College of Cardiology/American Heart Association Task Force on Practice Guidelines. Circulation 2004;110:588-636.
59. Forrester JS, Diamond G, Chatterjee K, et al: Medical therapy of acute myocardial infarction by application of hemodynamic subsets. N Engl J Med 1976;295:1404-1413.
60. Hollenberg SM, Ahrens TS, Annane D, et al: Practice parameters for hemodynamic support of sepsis in adult patients: 2004 update. Crit Care Med 2004;32:1928-1948.
61. Hollenberg SM, Parrillo JE: Pharmacologic circulatory support. In Shires GT, Barie PL (eds): Surgical Critical Care. New York, Little Brown, 1993, pp 417-451.
62. Moyer J, Skelton J, Mills L: Norepinephrine: Effect in normal subjects; use in treatment of shock unresponsive to other measures. Am J Med 1953;15:330-343.
63. Tuttle RR, Mills J: Dobutamine: Development of a new catecholamine to selectively increase cardiac contractility. Circ Res 1975;36:185-196.
64. Gillespie TA, Ambos HD, Sobel BE, et al: Effects of dobutamine in patients with acute myocardial infarction. Am J Cardiol 1977;39:588-594.
65. Keung EC, Siskind SJ, Sonneblick EH, et al: Dobutamine therapy in acute myocardial infarction. JAMA 1981;245:144-146.
66. Holzer J, Karliner JS, O'Rourke RA, et al: Effectiveness of dopamine in patients with cardiogenic shock. Am J Cardiol 1973;32:79-84.
67. Goldberg LI, Hsieh YY, Resnekov L: Newer catecholamines for treatment of heart failure and shock: An update on dopamine and a first look at dobutamine. Prog Cardiovasc Dis 1977;17:327-340.
68. Richard C, Ricome JL, Rimailho A, et al: Combined hemodynamic effects of dopamine and dobutamine in cardiogenic shock. Circulation 1983;67:620-626.
69. Benotti JR, Grossman W, Braunwald E, et al: Effects of amrinone on myocardial energy metabolism and hemodynamics in patients with severe congestive heart failure due to coronary artery disease. Circulation 1980;62:28-34.
70. Gage J, Rutman H, Lucido D, et al: Additive effects of dobutamine and amrinone on myocardial contractility and ventricular performance in patients with severe heart failure. Circulation 1986;74:367-374.
71. Hansen RM, Viquerat CE, Matthay MA, et al: Poor correlation between pulmonary arterial wedge pressure and left ventricular end-diastolic volume after coronary artery bypass graft surgery. Anesthesiology 1986;64:764-770.
72. Hollenberg SM, Hoyt JW: Pulmonary artery catheters in cardiovascular disease. New Horiz 1997;5:207-213.
73. Cohn JN, Burke LP: Nitroprusside. Ann Intern Med 1979;91:752-757.
74. Flaherty JT, Becker LC, Bulkley BH, et al: A randomized trial of intravenous nitroglycerin in patients with acute myocardial infarction. Circulation 1983;68:576-588.
75. Wilcox RG, von der Lippe G, Olsson CG, et al: Trial of tissue plasminogen activator for mortality reduction in acute myocardial infarction. Anglo-Scandinavian Study of Early Thrombolysis (ASSET). Lancet 1988;2:525-530.
76. AIMS Trial Study Group: Effect of intravenous APSAC on mortality after acute myocardial infarction: Preliminary report of a placebo-controlled clinical trial. Lancet 1988;1:545-549.
77. ISIS-2 Collaborative Group: Randomised trial of intravenous streptokinase, oral aspirin, both, or neither among 17,187 cases of suspected acute myocardial infarction: ISIS-2. Lancet 1988;2:349-360.
78. GUSTO Angiographic Investigators: The effects of tissue plasminogen activator, streptokinase, or both on coronary-artery patency, ventricular function, and survival after acute myocardial infarction. N Engl J Med 1993;329:1615-1622.
79. Col NF, Gurwitz JH, Alpert JS, et al: Frequency of inclusion of patients with cardiogenic shock in trials of

thrombolytic therapy. Am J Cardiol 1994;73:149-157.
80. Bates ER, Moscucci M: Post-myocardial infarction cardiogenic shock. In Brown DL (ed): Cardiac Intensive Care. Philadelphia, Saunders, 1998, pp 215-228.
81. Fibrinolytic Therapy Trialists' (FTT) Collaborative Group: Indications for fibrinolytic therapy in suspected acute myocardial infarction: Collaborative overview of early mortality and major morbidity results from all randomised trials of more than 1000 patients. Lancet 1994;343:311-322.
82. Kennedy HL, Whitlock JA, Sprague MK, et al: Long-term follow-up of asymptomatic healthy subjects with frequent and complex ventricular ectopy. N Engl J Med 1985;312: 193-197.
83. Berger PB, Holmes DR Jr, Stebbins AL, et al: Impact of an aggressive invasive catheterization and revascularization strategy on mortality in patients with cardiogenic shock in the Global Utilization of Streptokinase and Tissue Plasminogen Activator for Occluded Coronary Arteries (GUSTO-I) trial: An observational study. Circulation 1997;96:122-127.
84. Becker RC: Hemodynamic, mechanical, and metabolic determinants of thrombolytic efficacy: A theoretic framework for assessing the limitations of thrombolysis in patients with cardiogenic shock. Am Heart J 1993;125:919-929.
85. Garber PJ, Mathieson AL, Ducas J, et al: Thrombolytic therapy in cardiogenic shock: Effect of increased aortic pressure and rapid tPA administration. Can J Cardiol 1995;11:30-36.
86. Prewitt RM, Gu S, Garber PJ, et al: Marked systemic hypotension depresses coronary thrombolysis induced by intracoronary administration of recombinant tissue-type plasminogen activator. J Am Coll Cardiol 1992;20:1626-1633.
87. Mueller H, Ayres SM, Giannelli SJ, et al: Effect of isoproterenol, l-norepinephrine, and intraaortic counterpulsation on hemodynamics and myocardial metabolism in shock following acute myocardial infarction. Circulation 1972;45:335-351.
88. Santa-Cruz RA, Cohen MG, Ohman EM: Aortic counterpulsation: A review of the hemodynamic effects and indications for use. Cathet Cardiovasc Interv 2006;67:68-77.
89. Willerson JT, Curry GC, Watson JT, et al: Intraaortic balloon counterpulsation in patients in cardiogenic shock, medically refractory left ventricular failure and/or recurrent ventricular tachycardia. Am J Med 1975;58: 183-191.
90. Trost JC, Hillis LD: Intra-aortic balloon counterpulsation. Am J Cardiol 2006;97:1391-1398.
91. O'Rourke MF, Norris RM, Campbell TJ, et al: Randomized controlled trial of intraaortic balloon counterpulsation in early myocardial infarction with acute heart failure. Am J Cardiol 1981;47:815-820.
92. Flaherty JT, Becker LC, Weiss JL, et al: Results of a randomized prospective trial of intraaortic balloon counterpulsation and intravenous nitroglycerin in patients with acute myocardial infarction. J Am Coll Cardiol 1985;6:434-446.
93. Kern MJ, Aguirre F, Bach R, et al: Augmentation of coronary blood flow by intra-aortic balloon pumping in patients after coronary angioplasty. Circulation 1993;87:500-511.
94. Anderson RD, Ohman EM, Holmes DR Jr, et al: Use of intraaortic balloon counterpulsation in patients presenting with cardiogenic shock: observations from the GUSTO-I Study. Global Utilization of Streptokinase and TPA for Occluded Coronary Arteries. J Am Coll Cardiol 1997;30:708-715.
95. DeWood MA, Notske RN, Hensley GR, et al: Intraaortic balloon counterpulsation with and without reperfusion for myocardial infarction shock. Circulation 1980;61: 1105-1112.
96. Waksman R, Weiss AT, Gotsman MS, et al: Intra-aortic balloon counterpulsation improves survival in cardiogenic shock complicating acute myocardial infarction. Eur Heart J 1993;14:71-74.
97. Stomel RJ, Rasak M, Bates ER: Treatment strategies for acute myocardial infarction complicated by cardiogenic shock in a community hospital. Chest 1994;105:997-1002.
98. Kovack PJ, Rasak MA, Bates ER, et al: Thrombolysis plus aortic counterpulsation: Improved survival in patients who present to community hospitals with cardiogenic shock. J Am Coll Cardiol 1997;29:1454-1458.
99. Ishihara M, Sato H, Tateishi H, et al: Intraaortic balloon pumping as the postangioplasty strategy in acute myocardial infarction. Am Heart J 1991;122:385-389.
100. Ohman EM, George BS, White CJ, et al: Use of aortic counterpulsation to improve sustained coronary artery patency during acute myocardial infarction: Results of a randomized trial. Circulation 1994;90:792-799.
101. Ohman EM, Nanas J, Stomel RJ, et al: Thrombolysis and counterpulsation to improve survival in myocardial infarction complicated by hypotension and suspected cardiogenic shock or heart failure: results of the TACTICS Trial. J Thromb Thrombolysis 2005;19:33-39.
102. Bates ER, Stomel RJ, Hochman JS, et al: The use of intraaortic balloon counterpulsation as an adjunct to reperfusion therapy in cardiogenic shock. Int J Cardiol 1998;65(Suppl 1): S37-S42.
103. Grines CL, Browne KF, Marco J, et al: A comparison of immediate angioplasty with thrombolytic therapy for acute myocardial infarction. N Engl J Med 1993;328:673-679.
104. Zijlstra F, de Boer MJ, Hoorntje JC, et al: A comparison of immediate coronary angioplasty with intravenous streptokinase in acute myocardial infarction. N Engl J Med 1993;328:680-684.
105. Gibbons RJ, Holmes DR, Reeder GS, et al: Immediate angioplasty compared with the administration of a thrombolytic agent followed by conservative treatment for myocardial infarction. N Engl J Med 1993;328:685-691.
106. TIMI Study Group: The Thrombolysis In Myocardial Infarction (TIMI) trial: Phase I findings. N Engl J Med 1985;312:932-936.
107. O'Keefe JH Jr, Bailey WL, Rutherford BD, et al: Primary angioplasty for acute myocardial infarction in 1,000 consecutive patients: Results in an unselected population and high-risk subgroups. Am J Cardiol 1993;72:107G-115G.
108. O'Neill W, Erbel R, Laufer N, et al: Coronary angioplasty therapy of cardiogenic shock complicating acute myocardial infarction. Circulation 1985;72(Suppl II):309 (Abstract).
109. Lee L, Bates ER, Pitt B, et al: Percutaneous transluminal coronary angioplasty improves survival in acute myocardial infarction complicated by cardiogenic shock. Circulation 1988;78:1345-1351.
110. Lee L, Erbel R, Brown TM, et al: Multicenter registry of angioplasty therapy of cardiogenic shock: Initial and long-term survival. J Am Coll Cardiol 1991;17:599-603.
111. Gacioch GM, Ellis SG, Lee L, et al: Cardiogenic shock complicating acute myocardial infarction: The use of coronary angioplasty and the integration of the new support devices into patient management. J Am Coll Cardiol 1992;19:647-653.
112. Hibbard MD, Holmes DR Jr, Bailey KR, et al: Percutaneous transluminal coronary angioplasty in patients with cardiogenic shock. J Am Coll Cardiol 1992;19:639-646.
113. Moosvi AR, Khaja F, Villanueva L, et al: Early revascularization improves survival in cardiogenic shock complicating acute myocardial infarction. J Am Coll Cardiol 1992;19:907-914.
114. Seydoux C, Goy JJ, Beuret P, et al: Effectiveness of percutaneous transluminal coronary angioplasty in cardiogenic shock during acute myocardial infarction. Am J Cardiol 1992;69:968-969.
115. Eltchaninoff H, Simpfendorfer C, Franco I, et al: Early and 1-year survival rates in acute myocardial infarction complicated by cardiogenic shock: A retrospective study comparing coronary angioplasty with medical treatment. Am Heart J 1995;130:459-464.
116. Vogt A, Niederer W, Pfafferott C, et al: Direct percutaneous transluminal coronary angioplasty in acute myocardial infarction: Predictors of short-term outcome and the impact of coronary stenting. Study Group of the Arbeitsgemeinschaft Leitender Kardiologischer Krankenhausarzte (ALKK). Eur Heart J 1998;19:917-921.
117. Antoniucci D, Santoro GM, Bolognese L, et al: A clinical trial comparing primary stenting of the infarct-related artery with optimal primary angioplasty for acute myocardial infarction: Results from the Florence Randomized Elective Stenting in Acute Coronary Occlusions (FRESCO) trial. J Am Coll Cardiol 1998;31:1234-1239.

118. Berger PB, Tuttle RH, Holmes DR Jr, et al: One-year survival among patients with acute myocardial infarction complicated by cardiogenic shock, and its relation to early revascularization: Results from the GUSTO-I trial. Circulation 1999; 99:873-878.
119. Rogers WJ, Canto JG, Lambrew CT, et al: Temporal trends in the treatment of over 1.5 million patients with myocardial infarction in the US from 1990 through 1999: The National Registry of Myocardial Infarction 1, 2 and 3. J Am Coll Cardiol 2000;36: 2056-2063.
120. Laks H, Rosenkranz E, Buckberg GD: Surgical treatment of cardiogenic shock after myocardial infarction. Circulation 1986;74(Suppl III):11-16.
121. Subramanian VA, Roberts AJ, Zema MJ, et al: Cardiogenic shock following acute myocardial infarction: Late functional results after emergency cardiac surgery. N Y State J Med 1980;80:947-952.
122. Matsuwaka R, Sakakibara T, Shintani H, et al: Emergency cardiopulmonary bypass support in patients with severe cardiogenic shock after acute myocardial infarction. Heart Vessels 1996;11:27-29.
123. Burkhoff D, Cohen H, Brunckhorst C, et al: A randomized multicenter clinical study to evaluate the safety and efficacy of the TandemHeart percutaneous ventricular assist device versus conventional therapy with intraaortic balloon pumping for treatment of cardiogenic shock. Am Heart J 2006;152:e461-e468.
124. Urban P, Stauffer JC, Bleed D, et al: A randomized evaluation of early revascularization to treat shock complicating acute myocardial infarction. The (Swiss) Multicenter Trial of Angioplasty for Shock—(S)MASH. Eur Heart J 1999;20: 1030-1038.
125. Hochman JS, Sleeper LA, White HD, et al: One-year survival following early revascularization for cardiogenic shock. JAMA 2001;285:190-192.
126. Hochman JS, Sleeper LA, Webb JG, et al: Early revascularization and long-term survival in cardiogenic shock complicating acute myocardial infarction. JAMA 2006;295:2511-2515.
127. Sleeper LA, Ramanathan K, Picard MH, et al: Functional status and quality of life after emergency revascularization for cardiogenic shock complicating acute myocardial infarction. J Am Coll Cardiol 2005;46:266-273.
128. Dzavik V, Sleeper LA, Picard MH, et al: Outcome of patients aged > or = 75 years in the SHould we emergently revascularize Occluded Coronaries in cardiogenic shocK (SHOCK) trial: Do elderly patients with acute myocardial infarction complicated by cardiogenic shock respond differently to emergent revascularization? Am Heart J 2005;149:1128-1134.
129. Dzavik V, Sleeper LA, Cocke TP, et al: Early revascularization is associated with improved survival in elderly patients with acute myocardial infarction complicated by cardiogenic shock: A report from the SHOCK Trial Registry. Eur Heart J 2003;24:828-837.
130. Urban P, Stauffer J-C: Randomized trials of revascularization therapy for cardiogenic shock. In Hollenberg SM, Bates ER (eds): Cardiogenic Shock. Armonk, NY, Futura Publishing Company, 2002, pp 135-144.
131. Zehender M, Kasper W, Kauder E, et al: Right ventricular infarction as an independent predictor of prognosis after acute inferior myocardial infarction. N Engl J Med 1993;328:981-988.
132. Dell'Italia LJ, Starling MR, Blumhardt R, et al: Comparative effects of volume loading, dobutamine, and nitroprusside in patients with predominant right ventricular infarction. Circulation 1985;72:1327-1335.
133. Bowers TR, O'Neill WW, Grines C, et al: Effect of reperfusion on biventricular function and survival after right ventricular infarction. N Engl J Med 1998;338:933-940.
134. Voci P, Bilotta F, Caretta Q, et al: Papillary muscle perfusion pattern: A hypothesis for ischemic papillary muscle dysfunction. Circulation 1995;91:1714-1718.
135. Khan SS, Gray RJ: Valvular emergencies. Cardiol Clin 1991;9: 689-709.
136. Bolooki H: Emergency cardiac procedures in patients in cardiogenic shock due to complications of coronary artery disease. Circulation 1989;79:I-137-I-148.
137. Chaux A, Blanche C, Matloff JM, et al: Postinfarction ventricular septal defect. Semin Thorac Cardiovasc Surg 1998;10:93-99.
138. Killen DA, Piehler JM, Borkon AM, et al: Early repair of postinfarction ventricular septal rupture. Ann Thorac Surg 1997;63:138-142.
139. Bueno H, Martinez-Selles M, Perez-David E, et al: Effect of thrombolytic therapy on the risk of cardiac rupture and mortality in older patients with first acute myocardial infarction. Eur Heart J 2005;26: 1705-1711.
140. Reardon MJ, Carr CL, Diamond A, et al: Ischemic left ventricular free wall rupture: Prediction, diagnosis, and treatment. Ann Thorac Surg 1997;64:1509-1513.
141. Bolli R, Hartley CJ, Chelly JE, et al: An accurate nontraumatic ultrasonic method to monitor myocardial wall thickening in patients undergoing cardial surgery. J Am Coll Cardiol 1990;15:1055-1065.
142. Parrillo JE, Cunnion RE, Epstein SE, et al: A prospective, randomized, controlled trial of prednisone for dilated cardiomyopathy. N Engl J Med 1989;321:1061-1068.
143. Mason JW, O'Connell JB, Herskowitz A, et al: A clinical trial of immunosuppressive therapy for myocarditis. N Engl J Med 1995;333: 269-275.
144. McCarthy RE 3rd, Boehmer JP, Hruban RH, et al: Long-term outcome of fulminant myocarditis as compared with acute (nonfulminant) myocarditis. N Engl J Med 2000;342: 690-695.
145. Hunt SA, Abraham WT, Chin MH, et al: ACC/AHA 2005 guideline update for the diagnosis and management of chronic heart failure in the adult—summary article. J Am Coll Cardiol 2005;46:1116-1143.
146. Hunt SA, Frazier OH: Mechanical circulatory support and cardiac transplantation. Circulation 1999;97:2079-2090.

Chapter 24

Septic Shock

Stephen Trzeciak, R. Phillip Dellinger, and Joseph E. Parrillo

HISTORICAL PERSPECTIVE

The word *sepsis* came from the Greek language. *Sepsis* was synonymous with putrefaction and pertained to the bacterial-mediated decomposition of organic matter.[1] The term persisted for more than 2700 years with essentially unchanged meaning.[2] In the 20th century, our modern understanding of the term *sepsis* became rooted in a clinical disease in which the constellation of clinical findings that characterize this disorder was attributed to severe infection and the release of pathogenic bacterial products into the bloodstream.[3,4]

The term *shock* comes from the French word "choquer," meaning "to collide with." This appears to be particularly appropriate terminology given our modern understanding of the pathophysiology of septic shock, in which the body's host defenses essentially collide with the invading microorganism, triggering a profound proinflammatory response.[1]

CONTEMPORARY DEFINITIONS

Shock is defined as failure of the cardiovascular system to maintain effective tissue perfusion. If effective tissue perfusion is not promptly restored, cellular dysfunction and acute organ failure may occur and may become irreversible, leading to acute organ system failure. When shock develops because of a systemic inflammatory response to infection, it is termed *septic shock*. The American College of Chest Physicians (ACCP) and the Society of Critical Care Medicine (SCCM) first published consensus conference definitions for sepsis syndromes in 1992,[5] and these definitions were revisited and further developed by international consensus in 2003.[6] *Septic shock* was defined as sepsis-induced hypotension (systolic blood pressure <90 mm Hg [or a drop of >40 mm Hg]) with signs of tissue hypoperfusion despite adequate fluid resuscitation. The overarching purpose and major impact of the efforts to establish these contemporary definitions was the promotion of uniformity in inclusion criteria for sepsis clinical trials.[7]

EPIDEMIOLOGY

Severe sepsis (sepsis plus acute organ system dysfunction) is a common and deadly disease with major public health implications. Although heterogeneity of definitions of sepsis has historically made the incidence of severe sepsis and septic shock difficult to measure precisely, estimates of the incidence have been possible. Using the International Classification of Diseases (ICD)-9 codes for infection and organ dysfunction, Angus and colleagues[8] estimated that 751,000 cases of severe sepsis occur in the United States each year. Figure 24-1 displays the incidence of severe sepsis in the United States in 2002 compared with other common diseases. The incidence of severe sepsis currently exceeds the incidence of lung and colon cancer, venous thromboembolic disease, and acquired immunodeficiency syndrome (AIDS),[8-11] and the incidence is projected to increase by 1.5% per year, resulting in more than 1 million cases of severe sepsis annually by the year 2020.[8] The incidence of sepsis and septic shock is known to be increasing because of a longer lifespan for patients with severe chronic medical conditions that predispose them to acquiring sepsis. This includes an increase in the numbers of immunocompromised patients and infections caused by resistant organisms, increased use of intravascular catheters, and aging of the population.[8]

Sepsis is the leading cause of death in critically ill patients[12] and is responsible for as many deaths annually in the United States as acute myocardial infarction.[8] In

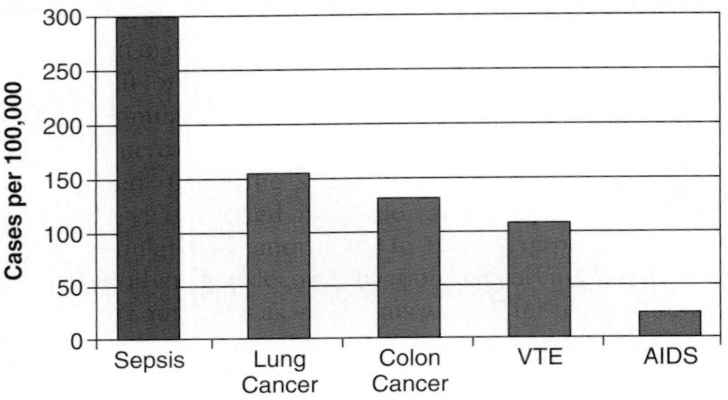

Figure 24-1. Incidence (cases per 100,000 population) of severe sepsis in the United States compared with four high-profile diseases. AIDS, acquired immunodeficiency syndrome; VTE, venous thromboembolic disease. (Data from references 8, 9, 10, 11.)

recent septic shock clinical trials the control arm mortality rates have ranged from 33% to 87%.[1] These control arm mortality rates are displayed in Figure 24-2. Overall, severe sepsis ranks as the tenth leading cause of death in the United States, with 215,000 deaths annually and a 30% in-hospital mortality rate.[8,13] Figure 24-3 displays the mortality rate for severe sepsis compared with three high-profile diseases that may require critical care (stroke, acute myocardial infarction, and trauma).[8,14-16] The apparent disparity in mortality rates across these diseases may be explained in part by differences in the conventional approach to treatment because acute stroke, myocardial infarction, and trauma are all typically treated with aggressive interventions in a time-sensitive fashion. Similar to the "golden hour" concept for trauma care that was first recognized more than 30 years ago,[17] experts are now beginning to understand that early aggressive interventions for sepsis (particularly early aggressive hemodynamic support) can also have a profound impact on outcome. Sepsis remains a major problem of public health disparities because patients from minority groups have higher mortality.[18]

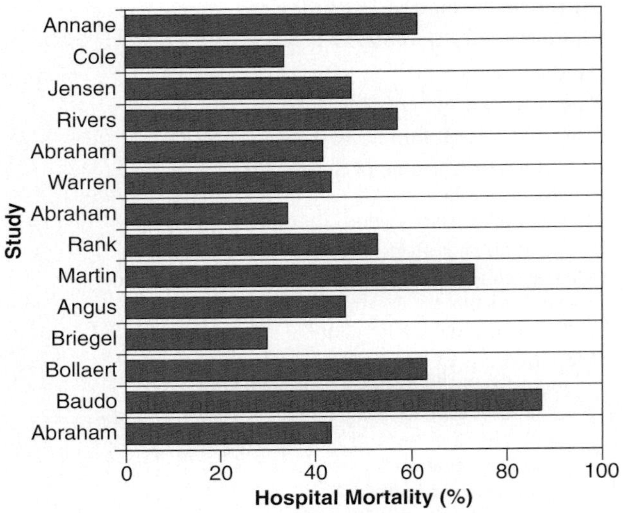

Figure 24-2. A compilation of septic shock mortality rates taken from the placebo arms of sepsis clinical trials published over the past decade (listed by first author). (Data from Dellinger RP: Cardiovascular management of septic shock. Crit Care Med 2003;31:946-955.)

PATHOGENESIS

Septic shock results when infectious microorganisms in the bloodstream induce a profound inflammatory response causing hemodynamic decompensation. The pathogenesis involves a complex response of cellular activation that triggers the release of a multitude of proinflammatory mediators. This inflammatory response causes activation of leukocytes and endothelial cells, as well as activation of the coagulation system. The excessive inflammatory response that characterizes septic shock is driven primarily by the cytokines tumor necrosis factor alpha (TNF-α) and interleukin-1 (IL-1), which are produced by monocytes in response to an infection. Although TNF and IL-1 are central to the pathophysiology of septic shock and act synergistically to induce hypotension in experimental models, a number of other vital mediators are also known to play a major role including high-mobility group box 1 (HMGB1) protein.[19] Another important recent advance in our understanding of septic shock pathophysiology has been identification of the close link that exists between the proinflammatory response of septic shock and activation of the coagulation system.[20] Although the systemic inflammatory response of sepsis triggers profound macrocirculatory and microcirculatory changes that impair tissue perfusion, another important mechanism playing a role in the development of acute organ dysfunction in septic shock is apoptosis (programmed cell death). Accelerated

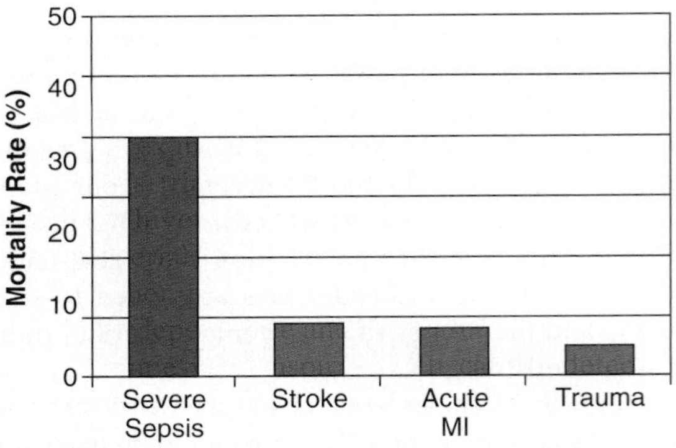

Figure 24-3. Mortality rate of severe sepsis in the United States compared with three diseases that are treated aggressively with time-sensitive interventions. MI, myocardial infarction. (Data from references 8, 14, 15, 16.)

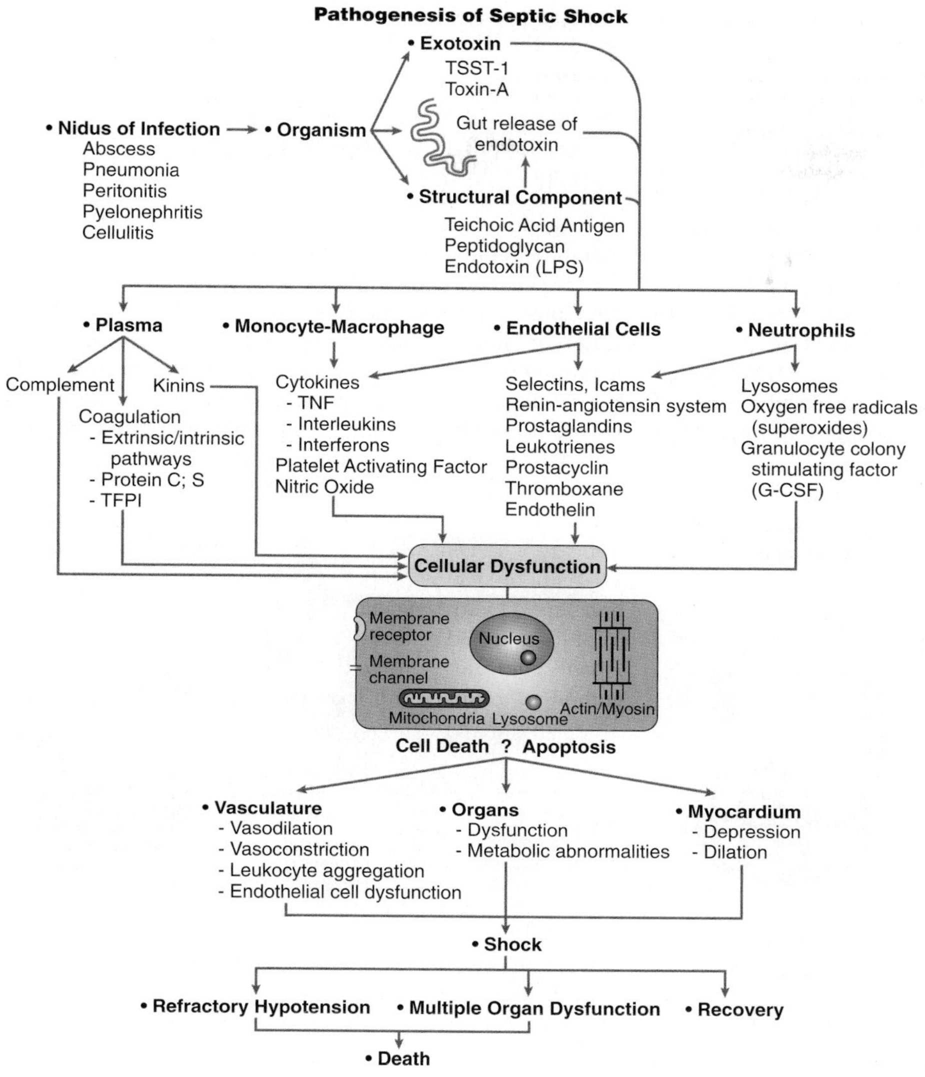

Figure 24-4. Pathogenetic sequence of the events in septic shock. TSST-1 denotes toxic shock syndrome toxin 1. Toxin A is *Pseudomonas aeruginosa* toxin A. LPS, lipopolysaccharide; TFPI, tissue factor pathway inhibitor; TNF, tumor necrosis factor. (Data from Parrillo JE: Pathogenetic mechanisms of septic shock. N Engl J Med 1993;328:1471-1477.)

apoptosis is a pivotal pathogenic event in this disease. In addition, certain genetic polymorphisms are becoming recognized as major determinants of susceptibility to infection, as well as risk of death from septic shock. Key steps in the pathogenesis of septic shock are shown in Figure 24-4.

CLINICAL PRESENTATION

Patients with septic shock will typically manifest signs of systemic inflammation including fever, tachycardia, tachypnea, and elevation of the white blood cell count. Although the absence of arterial hypotension does not necessarily exclude the possibility of subclinical tissue hypoperfusion,[21] the hallmark of septic shock is arterial hypotension despite adequate volume resuscitation requiring vasoactive drugs for hemodynamic support. Other signs of potential tissue hypoperfusion may include lactic acidosis, oliguria, encephalopathy, or diminished capillary refill in the extremities. Patients with septic shock typically have multiple organ system dysfunctions; clinical evidence of other organ system dysfunction may range from subtle abnormalities to overt organ failure. Multiorgan system involvement in sepsis may include cardiovascular, respiratory, renal, central nervous system, hepatic, metabolic, or hematologic dysfunction. Respiratory system dysfunction manifests as acute lung injury or, in extreme cases, the acute respiratory distress syndrome (ARDS). Sepsis-induced renal dysfunction typically manifests with oliguria and may progress to acute renal failure requiring dialysis. Central nervous system dysfunction will manifest as encephalopathy, which may range from mild cognitive impairment to overt coma. Cholestasis is a common manifestation of hepatic dysfunction in sepsis, but in the presence of severe shock, ischemic hepatitis ("shock liver") may occur. Metabolic derangements of septic shock include a loss of glycemic control (both hyperglycemia and hypoglycemia) and metabolic acidosis. Septic shock is commonly associated with a consumptive coagulopathy, which is likely present in almost all patients at least subclinically[22] but may also manifest clinically with thrombocytopenia; prolongation of the prothrombin time; or, in the most severe cases, disseminated intravascular coagulation.

The multiple organ dysfunction associated with septic shock is not only a critical event in the pathogenesis of this disease but is also closely linked with mortality.[8,18,23] An approximate 20% increase in septic shock mortality occurs with each additional organ system that fails.[8] *Early* evidence of organ failure is an especially strong predictor of mortality.[23,24] Early improvement in organ function (e.g., 0- to 24-hour improvement in the Sequential Organ Failure Assessment [SOFA] score[25,26]) is closely related to sepsis survival, whereas later improvement after the first 24 hours has little predictive value.[24] These data, garnered largely from observational studies and placebo arms of interventional trials, support the concept that aggressive therapy for sepsis and modulation of organ system failure within the first 24 hours is a critical determinant of outcome.

HEMODYNAMIC PROFILE OF SEPTIC SHOCK

The hemodynamic profile of septic shock is the most complex hemodynamic profile of all shock etiologies (Fig. 24-5). What sets septic shock apart from other causes of circulatory shock is the fact that there may be multiple different mechanisms of circulatory shock occurring simultaneously.[1,27] Septic shock may have features of (1) hypovolemic shock (poor cardiac filling secondary to severe systemic capillary leak) and increased venous

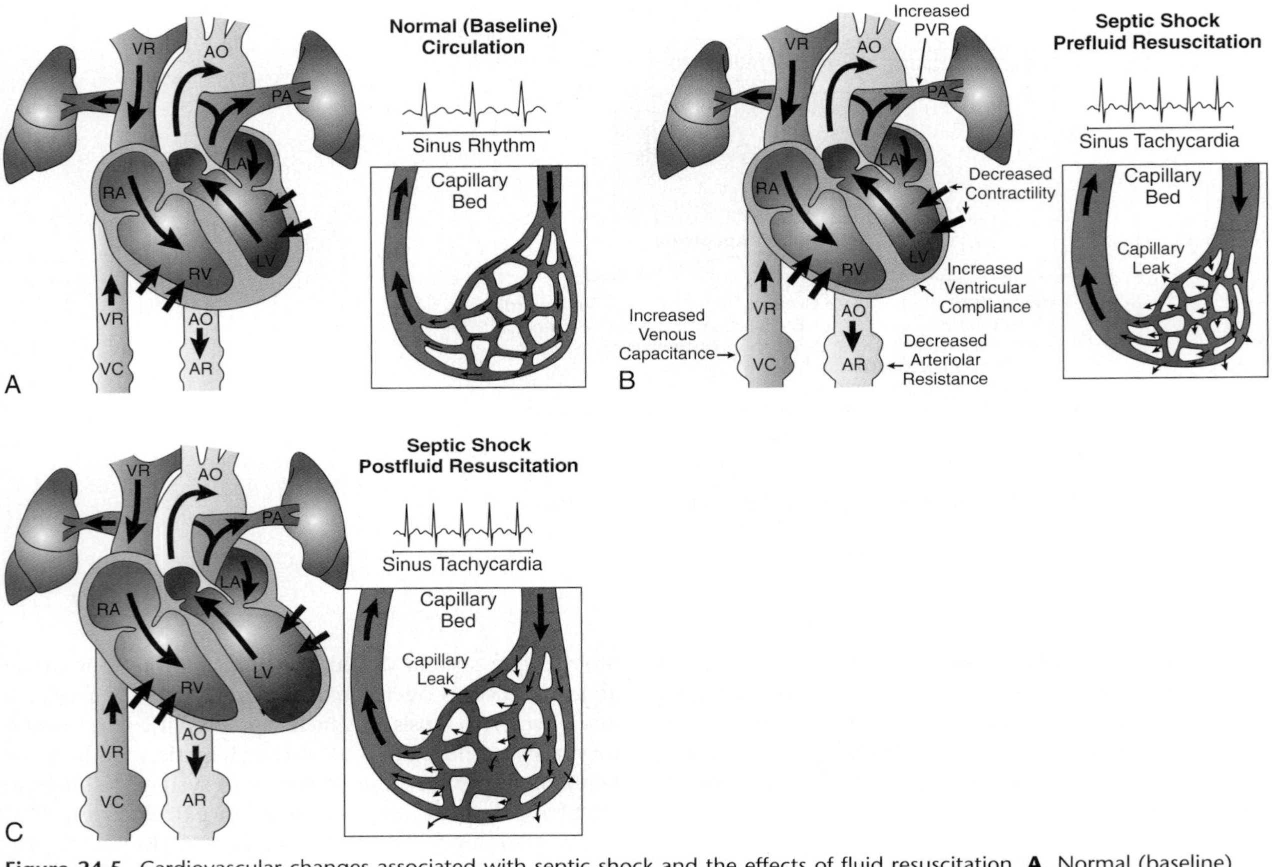

Figure 24-5. Cardiovascular changes associated with septic shock and the effects of fluid resuscitation. **A,** Normal (baseline) state. **B,** In septic shock, left ventricular blood return is reduced because of a combination of capillary leak (inset), increased venous capacitance (VC), and increased pulmonary vascular resistance. The stroke volume is further compromised by a sepsis-induced decrease in left and right ventricular (RV) contractility. Tachycardia and increased left ventricular compliance serve as countermeasures to combat low cardiac output, the latter by increasing left ventricular preload. However, cardiac output remains low to normal. Finally, a decrease in arteriolar (systemic vascular) resistance allows a higher stroke volume at any given contractility and left ventricular filling state, but also the potential for severe hypotension despite restoration of adequate left ventricular filling. **C,** Aggressive fluid resuscitation compensates for capillary leak, increased venous capacitance, and increased pulmonary vascular resistance by re-establishing adequate left ventricular blood return. Decreased arteriolar resistance (AR), tachycardia, and increased left ventricular compliance compensate for decreased ejection fraction. Ejection fraction increases as left ventricular filling increases. The net result is that after adequate volume resuscitation, most patients with severe sepsis have a high cardiac output and low systemic vascular resistance state. Blood flow (cardiac output) is indicated by *single arrows;* contractility is indicated by *double arrows.* AO, aorta; LA, left atrium; LV, left ventricle; PA, pulmonary artery; PVR, peripheral vascular resistance; RA, right atrium; VR, venous return. (From Dellinger RP: Cardiovascular management of septic shock. Crit Care Med 2003;31:946-955.)

capacitance; (2) cardiogenic shock (severe sepsis-induced myocardial depression); and (3) distributive shock (tissue hypoperfusion in the face of an adequate cardiac output).[1]

Hypovolemia

As proinflammatory mediators are released into the circulation, this causes injury to the integrity of the endothelial cell surface throughout the systemic microvasculature, resulting in severe capillary leak and extravasation of fluid into tissues. Venodilation also compromises venous return. These are major factors in producing hypovolemia in the patient with septic shock. The septic shock patient may have a markedly decreased cardiac preload, especially in the initial phase of therapy. Aggressive resuscitation with intravenous volume expansion modulates the hemodynamic profile of septic shock and allows the patient to achieve a hyperdynamic (i.e., high cardiac output) state.[1] The combination of a decreased preload and myocardial depression means that in the early phase of sepsis resuscitation, patients may initially be hypodynamic (i.e., have low cardiac output) prior to receiving adequate volume resuscitation. Capillary leak is an ongoing process in the course of septic shock therapy, and therefore hypovolemia may reoccur later in the course of the disease, even after adequate cardiac filling has been initially achieved. Fluid balance (input of intravenous fluids and output of urine) is often an unreliable parameter for assessing adequacy of fluid resuscitation in septic shock.

Myocardial Dysfunction

Septic shock is associated with depression of biventricular function with a decrease in the ejection fraction. Ventricular dilation occurs as a compensatory mechanism and raises end-diastolic volume so that stroke volume can be preserved, taking advantage of the Starling principle. When myocardial dysfunction occurs, a high cardiac output can still be achieved in many circumstances because of biventricular dilation, tachycardia, and arteriolar dilation, as long as the patient is adequately volume resuscitated and does not have a preexisting cardiomyopathy or severe cardiac suppression.[27] The most important inflammatory mediators that induce myocardial depression are TNF-α, IL-1, and perhaps nitric oxide.[28,29] Coronary blood flow is typically normal or increased in septic shock.[30] Although coronary blood flow can be diminished by severe arterial hypotension that compromises coronary perfusion pressure (especially if there is preexisting coronary artery disease), myocardial ischemia does not appear to be the causative factor of the depression in myocardial performance. Reportedly, nearly half of patients with septic shock will have echocardiographic evidence of depressed systolic function, even in the absence of preexisting cardiac disease.[31] However, myocardial depression is typically not judged to be the predominant feature of the septic shock hemodynamic profile.[27] For the majority of patients, aggressive volume resuscitation to restore adequate cardiac filling pressures will be enough to achieve a reasonable cardiac output.

Distributive Shock

Septic shock is characterized by peripheral maldistribution of blood flow to tissues so that tissue hypoperfusion abnormalities can still persist despite a normal or high cardiac output. This is called "distributive shock."[27] This maldistribution of blood flow may occur at both microcirculatory and macrocirculatory levels. The role of microcirculatory dysfunction is discussed in detail in the next section of this chapter. At the level of the macrocirculation, the autoregulation of blood flow within any single organ system in a normal host can typically maintain effective tissue perfusion over a wide range of systemic pressures (usually ranging from a mean arterial pressure [MAP] of 50 mm Hg to 150 mm Hg). However, there is heterogeneity of blood flow distribution throughout the body in septic shock because of preferential shunting of blood flow to "vital" organs (e.g., brain, myocardium). The gastrointestinal tract may be the earliest organ system to experience tissue hypoperfusion in septic shock, as blood is shunted away from the splanchnic circulation in order to preserve blood flow elsewhere. Ischemic injury to the gastrointestinal tract may be a source of ongoing systemic inflammation in septic shock.

The three components of the hemodynamic profile of septic shock are displayed in Figure 24-6.

MICROCIRCULATORY AND MITOCHONDRIAL DYSFUNCTION

After restoration of adequate cardiac filling pressures and achievement of optimal cardiac output in patients with septic shock, tissue dysoxia may still occur via a number of pathogenic mechanisms. These mechanisms of tissue dysoxia in the face of a normal or a supranormal cardiac output may be caused by either (1) microcirculatory failure or (2) mitochondrial dysfunction. These pathogenic mechanisms impair the way in which individual cells can either receive or utilize oxygen, respectively.

Microcirculatory Dysfunction

Microcirculatory dysfunction is a pivotal element of the pathogenesis of septic shock.[32-35] Although the macrocirculation (heart and large arteries) regulate the global distribution of blood flow throughout the body, it is the microcirculation that controls the delivery of blood flow to tissues. Using intravital videomicroscopy, experimental models of sepsis have demonstrated impaired microcirculatory flow velocity, "stopped-flow" microvessels, increased heterogeneity of regional perfusion, and low density of perfused capillaries.[36-39] These derangements can cause marked alterations of oxygen transport including impaired tissue oxygen extraction.[40] With the advent of new investigational videomicroscopy techniques, it is now possible to study the microcirculatory network in human subjects with septic shock. Microcirculatory "failure" appears to be one of the critical pathogenic events in sepsis that is associated with acute multiorgan dysfunction and mortality.[32-35] As these alterations of microcirculatory flow in sepsis can occur in the *absence*

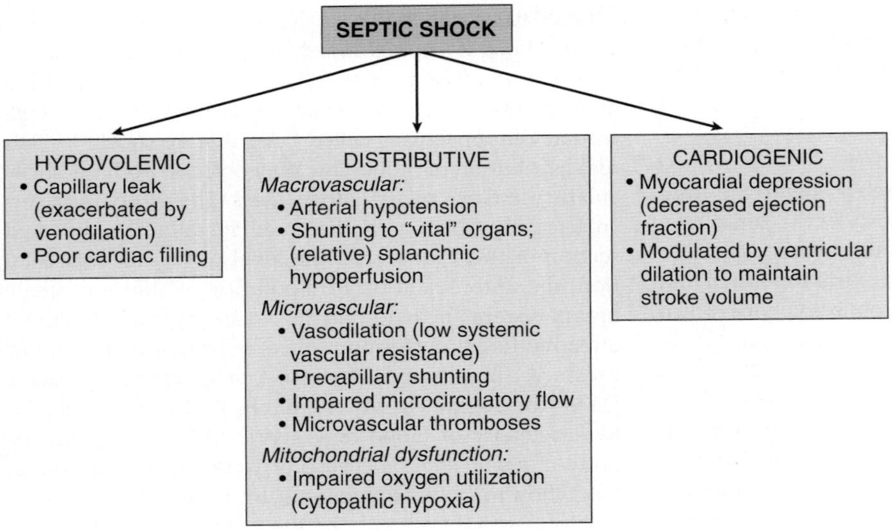

Figure 24-6. Major components of the hemodynamic profile in septic shock. (From Trzeciak S, Parrillo JE: Septic shock. In Society of Critical Care Medicine 8th Adult Critical Care Refresher Course. Chicago, Society of Critical Care Medicine, 2004.)

of global hemodynamic perturbations (i.e., absence of low arterial pressure and/or low cardiac output),[33,39,41] derangements of small vessel perfusion are largely a function of intrinsic events in the microcirculation.

The causes of microcirculatory flow alterations in sepsis (Fig. 24-7) are multifactorial: endothelial cell dysfunction, increased leukocyte adhesion, microthrombi formation, rheologic abnormalities, altered local perfusion pressures because of regional redistribution of blood flow, and functional shunting.[36,42] The proinflammatory cytokines released in sepsis cause diffuse endothelial cell activation, which is associated with neutrophil activation, expression of endothelial adhesion molecules (i.e., integrins and selectins), and localization of white blood cells to areas of microvascular injury. Pan-endothelial cell injury increases microvascular permeability with the influx of proinflammatory cells into the tissues; this is hypothesized to be an important pathogenic step in the development of acute system organ dysfunction in sepsis. Leukocyte adhesion of white blood cells to the microvessel endothelial surface (primarily in the postcapillary venule) further impedes microcirculatory blood flow. The endothelial injury also triggers the activation of the coagulation cascade via expression of tissue factor on the microvascular endothelium, resulting in fibrin deposition and microvascular thrombosis that may further impair microcirculatory flow. All of these mechanisms collectively contribute to microcirculatory "failure" in septic shock.[34,36]

Although septic shock research has classically been focused on macrocirculatory hemodynamic parameters that reflect the distribution of blood flow globally throughout the body, a functional microcirculation is another critical component of the cardiovascular system that is necessary for *effective* blood flow to tissues. This conceptual framework is depicted in Figure 24-8. Although a shift of research focus from global hemodynamic parameters to indices of microvascular perfusion could potentially be viewed as a major change of direction for septic shock research, the microcirculation likely represents a logical next frontier in the evolution of our understanding of

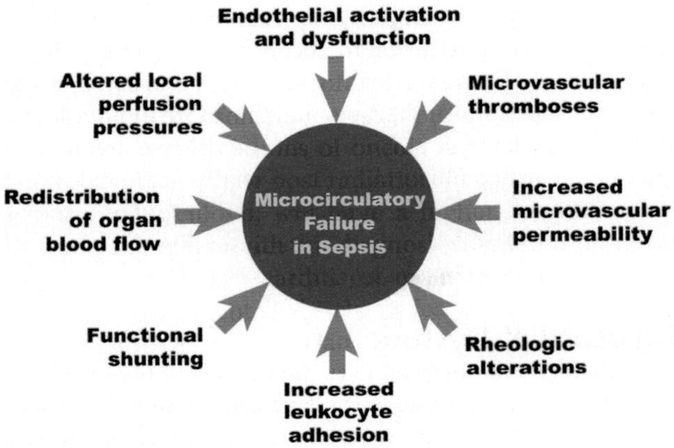

Figure 24-7. Causes of microcirculatory failure in sepsis. (Adapted from Spronk PE, Zandstra DF, Ince C: Bench-to-bedside review: Sepsis is a disease of the microcirculation. Crit Care 2004;8:462-468.)

circulatory failure in shock states.[34,43] Although there are currently no therapies to specifically target microcirculatory dysfunction in sepsis, going beyond optimization of macrocirculatory hemodynamics and developing innovative strategies to reverse microcirculatory failure could (in the future) potentially represent a cutting edge method to augment tissue perfusion in sepsis.

Mitochondrial Dysfunction

Strong evidence indicates that cellular utilization of oxygen can be markedly impaired in septic shock.[44] Bioenergetic failure can occur even after effective restoration of blood flow to tissues has been achieved, and this has been termed *cytopathic hypoxia*. Despite the current absence of therapies to reverse cytopathic hypoxia, this phenomenon does have some relevance for clinical practice because impaired cellular utilization of oxygen can manifest clinically with supranormal values for mixed venous oxygen saturation (SvO_2). Cytopathic hypoxia may also be an important determinant of acute organ

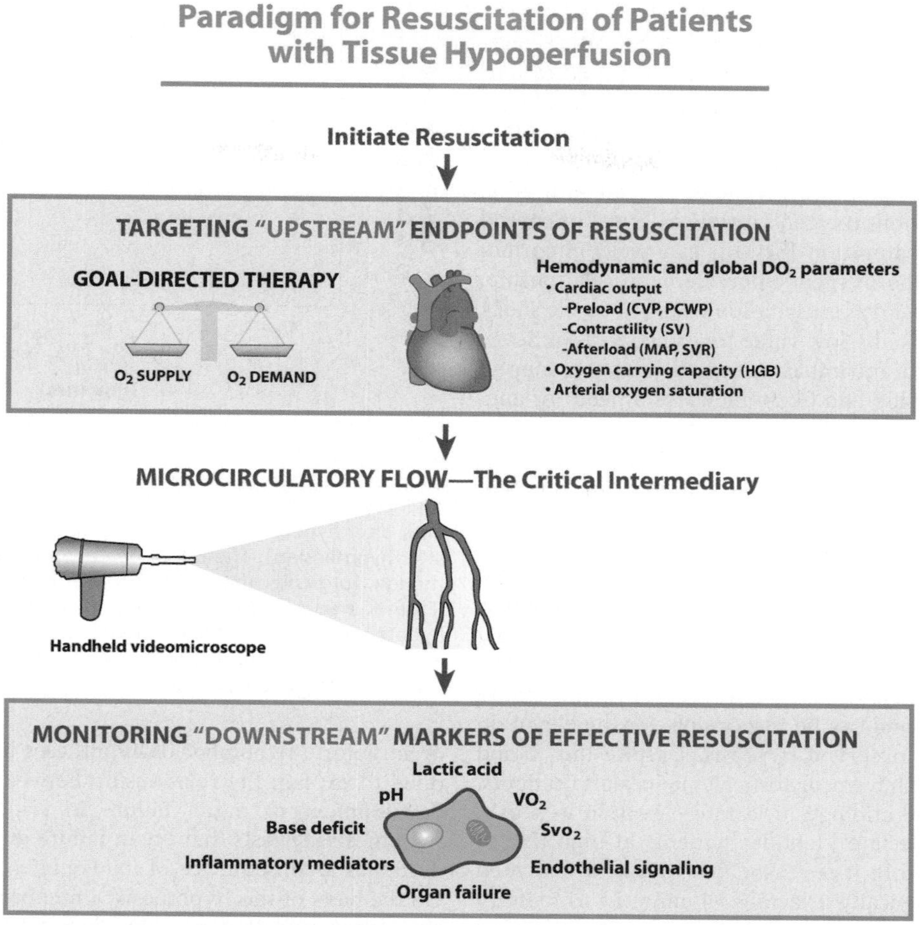

Figure 24-8. New paradigm of the cardiovascular profile of septic shock featuring the importance of microcirculation. Conventional resuscitation targets the optimization of macrocirculatory (i.e., "upstream") hemodynamic parameters, with the monitoring of "downstream" surrogates of tissue perfusion to determine the effectiveness of resuscitation. The microcirculation is the critical intermediary. Although the macrocirculation (heart and large arteries) regulates the global distribution of blood flow throughout the body, an intact and functional microcirculation is necessary for the effective delivery of blood flow to tissues. Intrinsic microcirculatory dysfunction can be a pivotal pathogenic event in the development of sepsis-associated tissue hypoperfusion. Using new videomicroscopy techniques, microcirculatory flow can now be studied in human subjects with septic shock. CVP, central venous pressure; DO_2, oxygen delivery; HGB, hemoglobin; MAP, mean arterial pressure; PCWP, pulmonary capillary wedge pressure; SV, stroke volume; Svo_2, mixed venous oxygen saturation; SVR, systemic vascular resistance; VO_2, oxygen consumption.

dysfunction, but the extent to which this occurs has not yet been elucidated.

Microcirculatory and mitochondrial dysfunction likely coexist in septic shock. Both of these pathogenic mechanisms can impair tissue oxygen delivery and utilization, but the relative contribution of either mechanism is difficult to discern.

MANAGEMENT OF SEPTIC SHOCK

Overview and Management Guidelines

In 2004 the Surviving Sepsis Campaign (SSC) published the first comprehensive international consensus guidelines for sepsis management.[45,46] These guidelines were endorsed by 11 medical professional societies. The SSC guidelines will continue to be updated over time as the best evidence for sepsis management continues to evolve. The critical care practitioner should be familiar with the full scope of content included in the SSC guidelines and is referred to the most recent executive summary for a comprehensive review.[47] The following specific treatment points are based on the SSC guidelines.

General Principles

The patient with septic shock should be brought to a critical care area as quickly as possible to assist rapid resuscitation and optimal hemodynamic support. Continuous electrocardiographic monitoring and pulse oximetry are useful tools in the management of critically ill patients with sepsis.[48,49] In addition, a variety of more invasive devices may be of utility. The arterial catheter has two important functions: (1) It allows for frequent blood sampling, and (2) it is useful for continuous assessment of arterial pressure. The pulmonary artery catheter (PAC) will provide such data as cardiac filling pressures, cardiac index, and systemic vascular resistance. The data gathered from the PAC are often indispensable for titrating vasoactive medications in septic shock. Although indications for PAC utilization are controversial and often debated, it is important to recognize that the PAC represents a tool for guiding therapy rather than being a therapeutic intervention in itself. Monitoring venous oxygen saturation (either mixed venous oxygen saturation [SvO_2] or central venous oxygen saturation [$ScvO_2$]) can yield important information on the oxygen supply/demand relationship, especially in the early resuscitation phase of septic shock therapy.[21] A markedly low value for either SvO_2 or $ScvO_2$ indicates a significant imbalance in the oxygen supply/demand relationship and likely indicates a need for augmenting global oxygen delivery.

Metabolic parameters to monitor the effectiveness of resuscitation and cardiovascular support are limited; however, measurement of blood lactate can provide important clinical information. In 1964 Broder and Weil[50] first proposed the utilization of blood lactate levels as a surrogate of adequacy of tissue perfusion. Importantly, however, elevation of blood lactate does not necessarily indicate ineffective tissue perfusion because metabolic derangements and altered cellular metabolism may cause hyperlactatemia and can be responsible for the elevation of blood lactate observed in sepsis. Despite this, blood lactate levels still have prognostic value in septic patients. Regardless of the etiology of lactate elevation in sepsis, elevated blood lactate identifies patients at high risk of death.[51-55] Therefore it is reasonable to use an elevated blood lactate (typically a lactate >4 mmol/L) to identify patients at high risk of death who warrant aggressive therapy.

Antibiotic Therapy and Source Control

Early administration of empirical antibiotic therapy and expeditious source control to eliminate any nidus of infection are imperative in the management of septic shock. Appropriate antibiotics given early may substantially improve the likelihood of survival.[56,57] A choice of antibiotics is usually empirical because the organism is not yet identified when antibiotics must be delivered. Failure to include antibiotic coverage for what is later identified to be the offending organism has been associated with increased mortality[58]; therefore broad-spectrum antibiotics are necessary as soon as septic shock is identified. Recently, Kumar and colleagues[59] performed a large-scale multicenter retrospective analysis of registry data for patients with septic shock. The authors reported a linear relationship between the duration of hypotension prior to first dose of antibiotic administration and risk of death (Fig. 24-9). In summary, early effective antibiotic administration is imperative in septic shock, and delays in antibiotic administration are clearly deleterious with respect to outcome.

Early Resuscitation

One of the principal goals in the early management of a patient with septic shock is aggressive resuscitation to restore effective tissue perfusion and decrease the risk of organ injury. A number of hypotheses have been developed to explain the relationship between shock and the development of organ failure in critical illness. One hypothesis suggests that organ failure during critical care occurs as a consequence of inadequate oxygen delivery. On the basis of this hypothesis, a number of investigators have suggested that patients should be resuscitated to supranormal goals of systemic oxygen delivery in an attempt to prevent organ failure and improve outcome. The concept of supranormal oxygen delivery refers to the use of fluid resuscitation and inotropic drugs to drive up the oxygen delivery to achieve a predefined target. Several studies have examined this concept. The earliest clinical trials in perioperative high-risk surgery patients demonstrated an outcome benefit.[60,61] Subsequently, however, numerous trials of supranormal oxygen delivery in critically ill patients failed to demonstrate any benefit. In the largest of these studies, Gattinoni and colleagues[62] found no difference in survival or organ failure in a large number of critically ill patients when comparing patients resuscitated with supranormal endpoints to those receiving standard care. In a study by Hayes and colleagues,[63] increasing oxygen delivery to supranormal levels with the use of high-dose dobutamine was associated with a reduction in survival. A meta-analysis concluded that supranormal oxygen delivery in critically ill patients was not beneficial,[64] and this concept largely fell out of favor in the 1990s.

For goal-oriented hemodynamic optimization to be beneficial, it has become clear that *timing* is critical. In contrast to the trials in perioperative high-risk surgery patients, subjects in the Gattinoni and colleagues[62] study were randomized much later, up to 72 hours after initial presentation. In a meta-analysis that stratified studies by severity and the timing of interventions (early versus late),

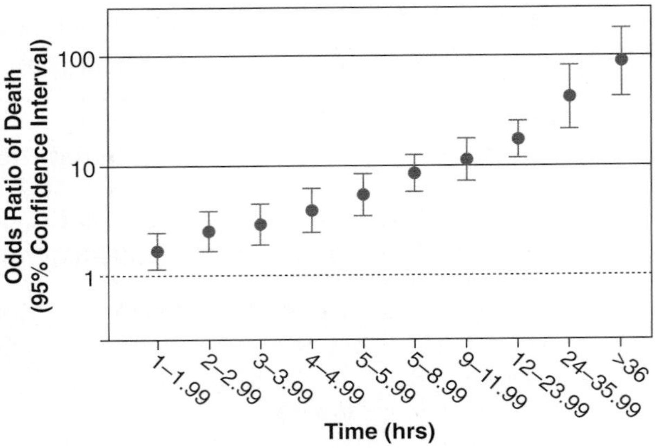

Figure 24-9. Mortality risk (expressed as adjusted odds ratio of death) with increasing delays in initiation of effective antimicrobial therapy. Bars represent 95% confidence interval. An increased risk of death is already present by the second hour after hypotension onset (compared with the first hour after hypotension). The risk of death continues to climb, though, to greater than 36 hours after hypotension onset. (From Kumar A, Roberts D, Wood KE, et al: Duration of hypotension before initiation of effective antimicrobial therapy is the critical determinant of survival in human septic shock. Crit Care Med 2006;34:1589-1596.)

an outcome benefit was identified in the subset of patients with a high severity of illness and early initiation of interventions.[65] These data suggest that hemodynamic optimization can be beneficial—in the right patient.

This early intervention concept was the rationale behind the landmark study of early goal-directed therapy (EGDT) for severe sepsis and septic shock by Rivers and colleagues.[21] Early goal-directed therapy refers to rapid protocol-directed hemodynamic optimization in the earliest stage of septic shock therapy. In a randomized controlled trial of 263 emergency department (ED) patients with severe sepsis and septic shock, Rivers and colleagues[21] targeted predefined endpoints of resuscitation including central venous pressure (CVP) 8 to 12 mm Hg, MAP greater than 65 mm Hg, and central venous oxygen saturation ($ScvO_2$) greater than 70%. They employed therapeutic interventions in a stepwise manner to achieve these target values within an hour from initial presentation. The EGDT protocol was associated with a 16% absolute risk reduction for mortality (30.5% vs. 46.5%). Although it is not possible to determine which component of the protocol was most responsible for the mortality benefit, this study showed that the early resuscitation phase of therapy can impact clinically significant long-term endpoints including 28-day mortality. Although EGDT was originally described in the ED setting, the concept can also be broadly applied to the early resuscitation of patients who develop septic shock in the hospital. In a recent randomized controlled trial of 224 ICU patients with septic shock, Lin and colleagues[66] demonstrated that a modified, goal-directed resuscitation protocol initiated in the ICU setting was associated with a more rapid resolution of shock and a 17.9% absolute risk reduction for mortality (53.7% vs. 71.6%). To date, these trials of early goal-directed resuscitation collectively represent the two largest mortality benefits demonstrated in sepsis randomized controlled trials. Although the optimal endpoints of goal-directed resuscitation remain controversial, it is generally accepted that the earlier the therapeutic interventions are delivered, the greater the capacity for benefit. Therefore the resuscitation phase of therapy appears to be the greatest window of opportunity for impact on outcome.

A treatment algorithm for the provision of early goal-directed resuscitation is shown in Figure 24-10.[67] This algorithm from the authors' institution is an adaptation of the original EGDT protocol by Rivers and colleagues.[21]

Cardiovascular Support

The main goal of cardiovascular support in septic shock is to use intravascular volume expansion and vasoactive agents to help restore and maintain effective tissue perfusion. The main components of cardiovascular support in septic shock can be grouped into three separate and distinct categories: volume resuscitation, vasopressor therapy, and inotropic support. The goal of volume resuscitation is to optimize cardiac filling in order to augment cardiac output. Although many vasoactive drugs have both vasopressor and inotropic activity, this distinction is made on the basis of intended goals of therapy. Vasopressor activity primarily raises the arterial pressure, whereas inotropic activity augments myocardial contractility and raises cardiac output.

Volume Resuscitation

Aggressive intravascular volume expansion is a cornerstone of septic shock therapy and is the best initial therapy for the cardiovascular instability of sepsis. The initial hypotension observed in many patients with sepsis-induced cardiovascular instability may be reversed with volume infusion alone. A reasonable approach to initial volume resuscitation in the adult patient is the rapid administration of 2 to 3 L of crystalloid solution (e.g., 0.9% NaCl or lactated Ringer's solution). If (after initial volume infusion) the hemodynamic instability has resolved, further aggressive resuscitation may be unnecessary and the patient may be relegated to a somewhat higher maintenance fluid regimen. Because there is no demonstrable benefit of colloid therapy over crystalloids,[68] we recommend initiating volume resuscitation with crystalloid in most patients (exceptions may include patients with a serum albumin level less than 2 g/dL and when crystalloid resuscitation is judged to be ineffective).

If a pulmonary artery catheter is in place, the target for pulmonary capillary wedge pressure in a patient without preexisting cardiopulmonary disease is likely in the range of 12 to 15 mm Hg[69]; however, it is imperative to remember that the "optimal" cardiac filling pressure may vary widely from patient to patient. One prudent strategy of volume resuscitation (rather than targeting a predefined cardiac filling pressure) would be to continue fluid bolus administration until the cardiac index fails to rise with additional intravascular volume expansion, indicating optimization of cardiac preload. An extremely high left ventricular filling pressure should be avoided because it could contribute to pulmonary capillary leak and cause impairment of oxygenation if the patient has concomitant acute lung injury. In the absence of a PAC to guide therapy, and if a patient has persistent hypotension refractory to an initial 20 to 30 mL/kg crystalloid intravascular volume infusion, it would be prudent to continue administering fluid boluses in attempts to raise the arterial pressure (unless the patient is manifesting clinical signs that pulmonary edema is developing, e.g., increasing supplemental oxygen requirement).[70]

Vasopressor Therapy

In addition to fluid administration, pharmacologic support of blood pressure is frequently necessary in both the initial resuscitation and subsequent support of patients with septic shock. These are, after fluids, the next most important interventions for the initial management of the hemodynamically unstable patient. Restoration of adequate arterial pressure is the endpoint of vasopressor therapy. However, blood pressure does not always equate to systemic blood flow, and the precise MAP to target may not necessarily be the same for all patients. Traditional recommendations to maintain a MAP greater than 65 mm Hg were based on data that organ systems capable of circulatory autoregulation (e.g., brain, kidney) need a MAP greater than 65 mm Hg to reliably maintain adequate per-

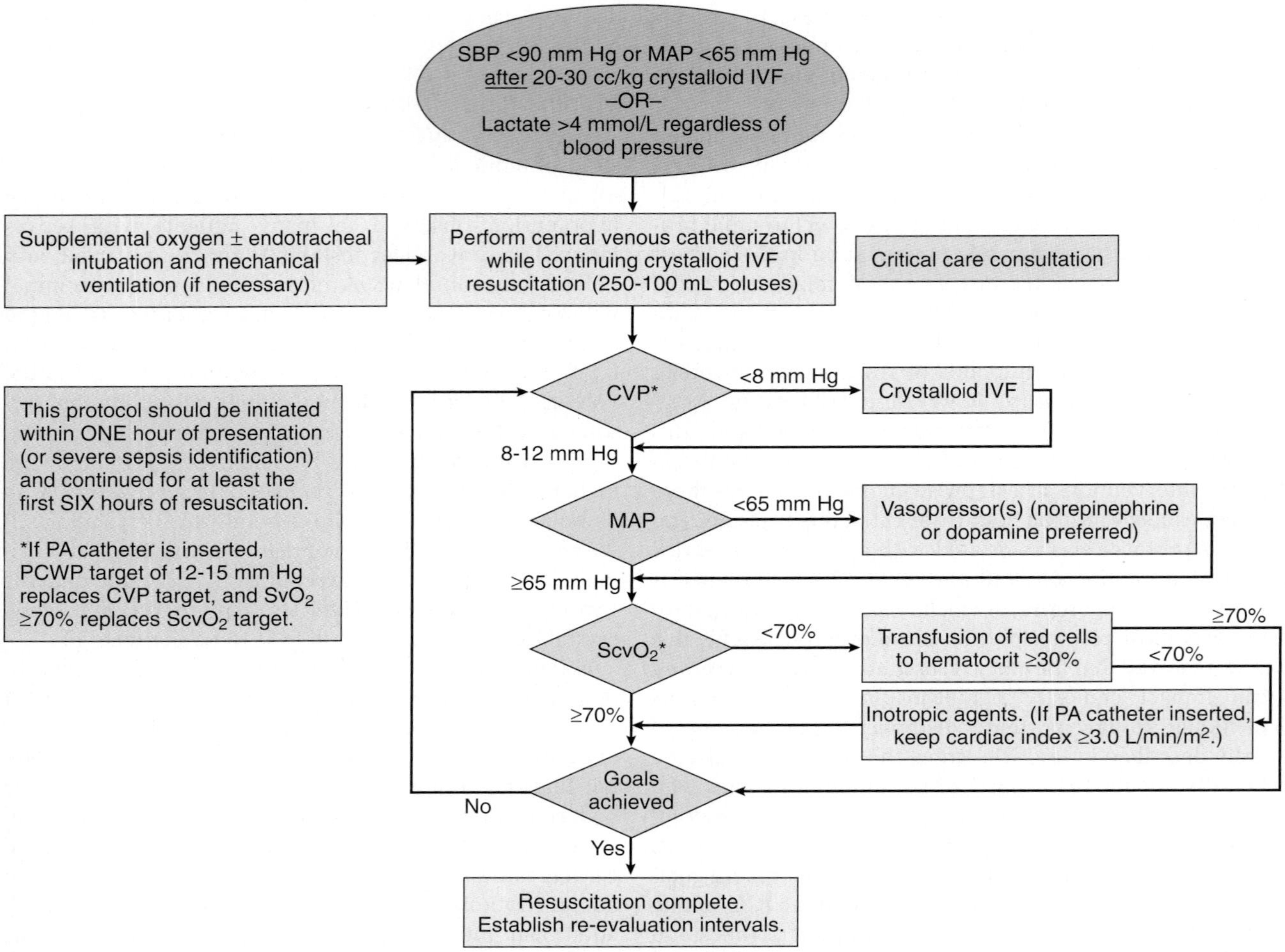

Figure 24-10. A clinical algorithm (from the authors' institution) for cardiovascular support in the resuscitation of patients with sepsis. This is an adaptation of the early goal-directed therapy protocol from Rivers and colleagues.[21] Choice of monitoring techniques (central venous catheter versus pulmonary artery catheter) is based on individual clinician preference and may depend on location of the patient when the protocol is initiated (i.e., non-ICU vs. ICU). If a pulmonary artery (PA) catheter is inserted, a pulmonary capillary occlusion pressure target of 12 to 15 mm Hg replaces CVP target, and mixed venous oxygen saturation greater than 70% replaces the target for $ScvO_2$. CVP, central venous pressure; IVF, intravenous fluids; MAP, mean arterial pressure; PA, pulmonary artery; SBP, systolic blood pressure; $ScvO_2$, central venous oxygen saturation; SvO_2, mixed venous oxygen saturation. (From Trzeciak S, Dellinger RP, Abate NL, et al: Translating research to clinical practice: A one-year experience with implementing early goal-directed therapy for septic shock in the emergency department. Chest 2006;129:225-232.)

fusion. Although a MAP less than 60 mm Hg can be reliably expected to cause tissue hypoperfusion, driving up the MAP has not been associated with a meaningful impact in tissue perfusion indices.[71] Of note is that a MAP of 65 mm Hg may be inadequate for a patient with preexisting poorly controlled essential hypertension and associated vascular disease. Similarly, it should be recognized that in select patients it might be possible to have arterial pressures lower than 65 mm Hg without tissue hypoperfusion. Hypotension in the presence of tissue hypoperfusion merits therapy with vasopressor agents. Endpoints of resuscitation such as arterial pressure should be combined with assessment of regional and global perfusion. Other bedside indicators of persistent tissue hypoperfusion (besides hypotension) include oliguria, encephalopathy, poor capillary refill, and acidosis.

The appropriate use of vasopressors may require accurate assessment of a patient's cardiovascular status with invasive hemodynamic monitoring. However, in the earliest stage of therapy, it is not uncommon to institute vasopressor therapy when invasive monitoring data are not immediately available if a patient remains hypotensive despite adequate intravascular volume expansion. If the MAP remains low (e.g., <60 to 65 mm Hg) despite adequate fluid resuscitation, vasopressor therapy is indicated.

Individual Vasoactive Agents

Norepinephrine, dopamine, epinephrine, phenylephrine, and vasopressin can effectively achieve arterial pressure goals in the management of patients with septic shock. The different catecholamine agents have different effects on α- and β-adrenergic receptors. The hemodynamic actions of these receptors are well described: α-adrenergic receptors promote vasoconstriction, whereas β-1 adrenergic receptors increase heart rate and myocardial contractility and β-2 adrenergic receptors cause peripheral vasodilation. Given the differential effects of vasopressor drugs on adrenergic receptors, these different agents have different effects on arterial pressure and systemic blood flow. In this context the quintessential question as to which catecholamine is the best initial choice for treating septic shock is best framed as a question of which agent is most appropriate for a given therapeutic strategy in an individual patient and depends largely on that individual patient's hemodynamic status. Rather than a "one-size-fits-all" strategy, vasoactive agents should be selected carefully on the basis of the intended goals of therapy.

Vasoactive agents are summarized in Table 24-1. Most intensivists use either dopamine or norepinephrine as their initial choice for a vasoactive drug in septic shock. The selection of one of these drugs over the other as a first-line agent is a controversial and an often-debated subject in the field of critical care medicine. Both dopamine and norepinephrine will effectively raise the blood pressure and cardiac index, but the rise in cardiac index will be greater with dopamine. Dopamine, however, may cause or exacerbate tachycardia. Norepinephrine is a more potent drug than dopamine in achieving a target MAP.[1]

One observational study has reported a survival benefit with norepinephrine compared with other vasoactive agents.[72] In the only randomized trial comparing vasopressor agents in septic shock, 32 volume-resuscitated septic shock patients were treated with dopamine versus norepinephrine with a primary outcome of normalization of arterial pressure and oxygen transport parameters over 6 hours. Norepinephrine infusion was successful in a higher proportion of subjects (93% vs. 31%, $P<0.001$). Of the dopamine nonresponders, 10 of 11 responded when norepinephrine was added. Norepinephrine administration was also associated with a decrease in blood lactate levels, perhaps suggesting an improvement in tissue oxygenation.[73] Currently, in the absence of strong data in favor of one agent over the other, either dopamine or norepinephrine is a reasonable first choice in patients with septic shock.

Phenylephrine is a pure vasoconstrictor with α-adrenergic effects alone. Although one advantage of using phenylephrine is that it will not cause or exacerbate tachycardia, the increase in peripheral resistance may be deleterious to a patient who already has a low cardiac output. Phenylephrine may be useful in patients with severe dysrhythmias associated with catecholamine infusion because it has no β-adrenergic effects, as well as in patients with hypotension in the presence of a high cardiac output.

Epinephrine is a potent α- and β-adrenergic agent that increases MAP by vasoconstriction and also increases the cardiac index. Although epinephrine is a potent agent in raising the arterial pressure, the chief concern with the use of epinephrine has been the potential for impaired splanchnic perfusion.[74-76] Recently a large-scale randomized controlled trial comparing epinephrine to norepinephrine plus dobutamine reported no difference in vasopressor withdrawal, organ failure, and mortality. No difference occurred in the rates of serious adverse events, either. The authors concluded that there is no difference in efficacy and safety for epinephrine versus norepinephrine plus dobutamine in the management of septic shock.[77]

The agent vasopressin has both vasoconstrictive and antidiuretic properties. Vasopressin constricts vascular smooth muscle directly via V-1 receptors and may also increase the responsiveness of the vasculature to endogenous or exogenous catecholamines.[78,79] Normally, endogenous vasopressin levels are low and there is essentially no vasoconstriction effect in a normal host. However, in septic shock vasopressin levels are initially extremely elevated. In prolonged septic shock, a relative vasopressin deficiency can develop. It has been postulated that this relative vasopressin deficiency may result from depletion of the pituitary stores or the downregulation of vasopressin production by the pituitary via the effects of nitric oxide.[78] Exogenous administration of low-dose vasopressin can have a dramatic hemodynamic response in this scenario, rapidly restoring arterial pressure.[80,81] Recently a large randomized clinical trial was completed that compared vasopressin with norepinephrine in 776 subjects with vasopressor-dependent septic shock. Patients were randomized to vasopressin (0.03 U/minute) or norepinephrine (15 μg/minute). For the group as a whole (intent-to-treat analysis) there was no difference in the primary endpoint of 28-day mortality. Apparently, vasopressin (up to 0.03 U/minute) may be equally as safe and effective as norepinephrine in patients with septic shock after fluid resuscitation.[82] Doses of vasopressin higher than 0.04 U/min are not recommended because of concerns of coronary, digital, and mesenteric ischemia.

Inotropic Support

Inotropic support may be required for patients with septic shock. In the context of severe sepsis-induced myocardial

Table 24-1. Vasopressor Agents for Hemodynamic Support in Sepsis

Agent	Typical Dose	Chronotropic Effects	Inotropic Effects	Vasoconstriction
Dopamine	6-20 μg/kg/min	++	++	+ or ++ (dose-dependent)
Epinephrine	1-10 μg/min	++	++	++
Norepinephrine	2-30 μg/min	+	+	++
Phenylephrine	20-200 μg/min	—	—	++
Vasopressin	0.01-.03 U/min		—	++

From Trzeciak S, Parrillo JE: Septic shock. In Society of Critical Care Medicine 8th Adult Critical Care Refresher Course. Chicago, Society of Critical Care Medicine, 2004.

depression or if the patient has severe preexisting myocardial dysfunction, an inotrope may be necessary to augment cardiac output. We recommend that dobutamine be the inotrope selected; however, dopamine could have an inotropic effect and raise arterial pressure at the same time, if that is desired. We recommend that inotropic therapy be guided by measurements of cardiac index. A reasonable goal for inotropic therapy would be a cardiac index greater than or equal to 3 L/minute/m^2.

Novel Therapies for Septic Shock

Historically, there have been numerous anti-inflammatory and other novel therapies for sepsis tested in randomized controlled trials. Only one novel agent (recombinant human activated protein C [rhAPC]) is currently approved by the U.S. Food and Drug Administration for sepsis therapy. For a specific discussion of the history of novel agents for sepsis (and specifically rhAPC), see Chapter 26.

Corticosteroids

Administering high doses of steroids (30 mg/kg of methylprednisolone) failed to show an outcome benefit in septic shock in large-scale randomized controlled trials in the 1980s.[83,84] These studies used large doses of steroids over a short time period in an attempt to blunt the proinflammatory response of sepsis. In contrast, an alternative strategy of administering low-dose (i.e., "stress" or "physiologic" dose) steroids appeared to be promising in multiple small studies in the 1990s.[85,86] Despite the fact that septic shock patients typically have elevated serum cortisol levels, it was identified that some patients with septic shock have "relative adrenal insufficiency," as evidenced by failure to mount a significant elevation of serum cortisol in response to intravenous adrenocorticotropic hormone (ACTH) stimulation.

In 2000 Annane and colleagues[87] performed an observational study focusing on the ability to respond to an ACTH stimulation test in septic shock. The highest 28-day mortality (75%) was observed in patients whose serum cortisol level did not increase greater than 9 μg/dL. Being a "nonresponder" was a better predictor of death than an initially low cortisol value. In 2002, in a randomized controlled trial by the same investigators, 300 severely ill (persistent hypotension despite fluid resuscitation and vasopressor initiation) septic shock patients were randomized to 7 days of hydrocortisone plus fludrocortisone versus placebo.[88] The study found that in the 229 nonresponders, administration of low-dose steroids was associated with an improvement in time to shock reversal and mortality. Patients who responded appropriately to the ACTH stimulation test did not demonstrate a benefit with low-dose steroids.

The concept of low-dose steroid administration was further tested in a multicenter randomized controlled trial (CORTICUS) that was recently completed.[89] This study found no difference in the primary outcome measure of mortality between those treated with steroids compared with placebo. However, it is notable that (1) in contrast to the Annane and colleagues study in which all subjects had vasopressor-refractory septic shock, the CORTICUS study tested a more diverse patient population with overall lower severity; and (2) randomization in the Annane study occurred within 8 hours of developing shock as opposed to CORTICUS, which randomized subjects up to 72 hours after shock onset. Despite the fact that low-dose steroids do not appear to improve outcome in diverse populations of patients with sepsis, patients with vasopressor-unresponsive septic shock are suggested to benefit (especially in the absence of an appropriate response to an ACTH stimulation test). In summary, although steroid therapy should not be used in all patients with septic shock, it should be used in those with persistent hypotension despite vasopressor agents.

SUMMARY

Successful management of the patient with septic shock continues to be a major clinical and public health challenge, as evidenced by persistently high mortality rates associated with this disease. The principal goals of sepsis therapy remain early identification, early empiric antibiotic therapy and source control, aggressive resuscitation, and effective cardiovascular support. The hemodynamic profile of septic shock is the most complex of all shock profiles and may be characterized by simultaneous hypovolemia, myocardial depression, and peripheral vascular dysfunction. Clinicians should define goals and endpoints of hemodynamic support in individual patients, titrate therapies to those endpoints, and evaluate the effectiveness of their interventions based on improving indices of tissue perfusion.

KEY POINTS

- Septic shock is a clinical syndrome that results from a systemic infection that triggers an excessive inflammatory response and produces cardiovascular instability.
- The initial management of the patient with septical shock remains aggressive resuscitation and cardiovascular support, as well as early empiric administration of broad-spectrum antibiotics.
- Initial cardiovascular support is achieved with aggressive intravascular volume expansion.
- Vasopressors are administered to patients who remain hypotensive despite fluid administration. Although the selection of vasopressors must be individualized, either norepinephrine or dopamine are useful first-line agents.
- Endpoints of resuscitation should be physiologic values that reflect adequacy of regional and global perfusion. Clinicians should define goals and endpoints of hemodynamic support, titrate therapies to those endpoints, and evaluate the results of their interventions on improving indices of tissue perfusion.

REFERENCES

1. Dellinger RP: Cardiovascular management of septic shock. Crit Care Med 2003;31:946-955.
2. Geroulanos S, Douka ET: Historical perspective of the word "sepsis." Intensive Care Med 2006;32:2077.
3. Schottmueller H: Wesen und Behandlung der Sepsis. Inn Med 1914;31:257-280.
4. Vincent JL, Abraham E: The last 100 years of sepsis. Am J Respir Crit Care Med 2006;173:256-263.
5. American College of Chest Physicians/Society of Critical Care Medicine Consensus Conference: Definitions for sepsis and organ failure and guidelines for the use of innovative therapies in sepsis. Crit Care Med 1992;20:864-874.
6. Levy MM, Fink MP, Marshall JC, et al: 2001 SCCM/ESICM/ACCP/ATS/SIS International Sepsis Definitions Conference. Crit Care Med 2003;31:1250-1256.
7. Trzeciak S, Zanotti-Cavazzoni S, Parrillo JE, Dellinger RP: Inclusion criteria for clinical trials in sepsis: Did the American College of Chest Physicians/Society of Critical Care Medicine consensus conference definitions of sepsis have an impact? Chest 2005;127:242-245.
8. Angus DC, Linde-Zwirble WT, Lidicker J, et al: Epidemiology of severe sepsis in the United States: Analysis of incidence, outcome, and associated costs of care. Crit Care Med 2001;29:1303-1310.
9. American Heart Association: Heart disease and stroke statistics—2004 update. Dallas, AHA, 2004.
10. Centers for Disease Control and Prevention: Cases of HIV infection and AIDS in the United States by race/ethnicity, 1998-2002. Rockville, Md, CDC, 2003.
11. American Cancer Society: Cancer facts and figures 2003. Atlanta, ACA, 2003.
12. Hotchkiss RS, Karl IE: The pathophysiology and treatment of sepsis. N Engl J Med 2003;348:138-150.
13. Kochanek KD, Smith B: National Vital Statistics Report. Deaths: Preliminary data for 2002. Hyattsville, Md, CDC, 2004.
14. Lee KL, Woodlief LH, Topol EJ, et al: Predictors of 30-day mortality in the era of reperfusion for acute myocardial infarction. Results from an international trial of 41,021 patients. GUSTO-I Investigators. Circulation 1995;91:1659-1668.
15. Rosamond WD, Folsom AR, Chambless LE, et al: Stroke incidence and survival among middle-aged adults: 9-year follow-up of the Atherosclerosis Risk in Communities (ARIC) cohort. Stroke 1999;30:736-743.
16. American College of Surgeons: National Trauma Data Bank Report 2006. Chicago, ACS, 2006.
17. Cowley RA: Trauma center. A new concept for the delivery of critical care. J Med Soc N J 1977;74:979-987.
18. Martin GS, Mannino DM, Eaton S, Moss M: The epidemiology of sepsis in the United States from 1979 through 2000. N Engl J Med 2003;348:1546-1554.
19. Sama AE, D'Amore J, Ward MF, et al: Bench to bedside: HMGB1—a novel proinflammatory cytokine and potential therapeutic target for septic patients in the emergency department. Acad Emerg Med 2004;11:867-873.
20. Dellinger RP: Inflammation and coagulation: Implications for the septic patient. Clin Infect Dis 2003;36:1259-1265.
21. Rivers E, Nguyen B, Havstad S, et al: Early goal-directed therapy in the treatment of severe sepsis and septic shock. N Engl J Med 2001;345:1368-1377.
22. Yan SB, Helterbrand JD, Hartman DL, et al: Low levels of protein C are associated with poor outcome in severe sepsis. Chest 2001;120:915-922.
23. Shapiro N, Howell MD, Bates DW, et al: The association of sepsis syndrome and organ dysfunction with mortality in emergency department patients with suspected infection. Ann Emerg Med 2006;48:583-590.
24. Levy MM, Macias WL, Vincent JL, et al: Early changes in organ function predict eventual survival in severe sepsis. Crit Care Med 2005;33:2194-2201.
25. Ferreira FL, Bota DP, Bross A, et al: Serial evaluation of the SOFA score to predict outcome in critically ill patients. JAMA 2001;286:1754-1758.
26. Vincent JL, Moreno R, Takala J, et al: The SOFA (Sepsis-related Organ Failure Assessment) score to describe organ dysfunction/failure. On behalf of the Working Group on Sepsis-Related Problems of the European Society of Intensive Care Medicine. Intensive Care Med 1996;22:707-710.
27. Parrillo JE: Pathogenetic mechanisms of septic shock. N Engl J Med 1993;328:1471-1477.
28. Kumar A, Haery C, Parrillo JE: Myocardial dysfunction in septic shock. Crit Care Clin 2000;16:251-287.
29. Kumar A, Short J, Parrillo JE: Genetic factors in septic shock. JAMA 1999;282:579-581.
30. Cunnion RE, Schaer GL, Parker MM, et al: The coronary circulation in human septic shock. Circulation 1986;73:637-644.
31. Charpentier J, Luyt CE, Fulla Y, et al: Brain natriuretic peptide: A marker of myocardial dysfunction and prognosis during severe sepsis. Crit Care Med 2004;32:660-665.
32. De Backer D, Creteur J, Preiser JC, et al: Microvascular blood flow is altered in patients with sepsis. Am J Respir Crit Care Med 2002;166:98-104.
33. Sakr YL, Dubois MJ, De Backer D, et al: Persistent microcirculatory alterations are associated with organ failure and death in septic shock (abstract). Intensive Care Med 2003;29:S66.
34. Spronk PE, Zandstra DF, Ince C: Bench-to-bedside review: Sepsis is a disease of the microcirculation. Crit Care Dec 2004;8:462-468.
35. Trzeciak S, Dellinger RP, Parrillo JE, et al: Early microcirculatory perfusion derangements in patients with severe sepsis and septic shock: Relationship to hemodynamics, oxygen transport, and survival. Ann Emerg Med 2007;49:88-98.
36. Bateman RM, Sharpe MD, Ellis CG: Bench-to-bedside review: Microvascular dysfunction in sepsis—hemodynamics, oxygen transport, and nitric oxide. Crit Care 2003;7:359-373.
37. Farquhar I, Martin CM, Lam C, et al: Decreased capillary density in vivo in bowel mucosa of rats with normotensive sepsis. J Surg Res 1996;61:190-196.
38. Fries M, Weil MH, Sun S, et al: Increases in tissue Pco2 during circulatory shock reflect selective decreases in capillary blood flow. Crit Care Med 2006;34:446-452.
39. Lam C, Tyml K, Martin C, Sibbald W: Microvascular perfusion is impaired in a rat model of normotensive sepsis. J Clin Invest 1994;94:2077-2083.
40. Ellis CG, Bateman RM, Sharpe MD, et al: Effect of a maldistribution of microvascular blood flow on capillary O_2 extraction in sepsis. Am J Physiol Heart Circ Physiol 2002;282:H156-164.
41. Trzeciak S, Rivers EP: Clinical manifestations of disordered microcirculatory perfusion in severe sepsis. Crit Care 2005;9(Suppl 4):S20-26.
42. Ince C, Sinaasappel M: Microcirculatory oxygenation and shunting in sepsis and shock. Crit Care Med 1999;27:1369-1377.
43. Abate NL, Trzeciak S: Is impaired capillary perfusion a marker of tissue hypoxia and a hallmark of incipient circulatory shock? Crit Care Med 2006;34:566-567.
44. Fink MP: Cytopathic hypoxia. Mitochondrial dysfunction as mechanism contributing to organ dysfunction in sepsis. Crit Care Clin 2001;17:219-237.
45. Dellinger RP, Carlet JM, Masur H, et al: Surviving sepsis campaign guidelines for management of severe sepsis and septic shock. Crit Care Med 2004;32:858-873.
46. Dellinger RP, Carlet JM, Masur H, et al: Surviving sepsis campaign guidelines for management of severe sepsis and septic shock. Intensive Care Med 2004;30:536-555.
47. The Surviving Sepsis Campaign (website): Available at http://www.survivingsepsis.com/ Accessed March 2007.
48. Wiedemann HP, Matthay MA, Matthay RA: Cardiovascular-pulmonary monitoring in the intensive care unit (part 2). Chest 1984;85:656-668.
49. Wiedemann HP, Matthay MA, Matthay RA: Cardiovascular-pulmonary monitoring in the intensive care unit (Part 1). Chest 1984;85:537-549.
50. Broder G, Weil MH: Excess lactate: An index of reversibility of shock in human patients. Science 1964;143:1457-1459.
51. Aduen J, Bernstein WK, Khastgir T, et al: The use and clinical importance of a substrate-specific electrode for rapid determination of blood lactate concentrations. JAMA 1994;272:1678-1685.
52. Bakker J, Coffernils M, Leon M, et al: Blood lactate levels are superior to oxygen-derived variables in predicting outcome in human septic shock. Chest 1991;99:956-962.
53. Bakker J, Gris P, Coffernils M, et al: Serial blood lactate levels can predict

the development of multiple organ failure following septic shock. Am J Surg 1996;171:221-226.
54. Shapiro NI, Howell MD, Talmor D, et al: Serum lactate as a predictor of mortality in emergency department patients with infection. Ann Emerg Med 2005;45: 524-528.
55. Trzeciak S, Dellinger RP, Chansky ME, et al: Serum lactate as a predictor of mortality in patients with infection. Intensive Care Medicine 2007;33: 970-977.
56. Kreger BE, Craven DE, McCabe WR: Gram-negative bacteremia. IV. Re-evaluation of clinical features and treatment in 612 patients. Am J Med 1980;68:344-355.
57. Natanson C, Danner RL, Reilly JM, et al: Antibiotics versus cardiovascular support in a canine model of human septic shock. Am J Physiol 1990;259(5 Pt 2): H1440-1447.
58. Kollef MH, Sherman G, Ward S, Fraser VJ: Inadequate antimicrobial treatment of infections: A risk factor for hospital mortality among critically ill patients. Chest 1999;115:462-474.
59. Kumar A, Roberts D, Wood KE, et al: Duration of hypotension before initiation of effective antimicrobial therapy is the critical determinant of survival in human septic shock. Crit Care Med 2006;34:1589-1596.
60. Boyd O, Grounds RM, Bennett ED: A randomized clinical trial of the effect of deliberate perioperative increase of oxygen delivery on mortality in high-risk surgical patients. JAMA 1993;270: 2699-2707.
61. Shoemaker WC, Appel PL, Kram HB, et al: Prospective trial of supranormal values of survivors as therapeutic goals in high-risk surgical patients. Chest 1988;94:1176-1186.
62. Gattinoni L, Brazzi L, Pelosi P, et al: A trial of goal-oriented hemodynamic therapy in critically ill patients. SvO2 Collaborative Group. N Engl J Med 1995;333:1025-1032.
63. Hayes MA, Timmins AC, Yau EH, et al: Elevation of systemic oxygen delivery in the treatment of critically ill patients. N Engl J Med 1994;330: 1717-1722.
64. Heyland DK, Cook DJ, King D, et al: Maximizing oxygen delivery in critically ill patients: A methodologic appraisal of the evidence. Crit Care Med 1996; 24:517-524.
65. Kern JW, Shoemaker WC: Meta-analysis of hemodynamic optimization in high-risk patients. Crit Care Med 2002;30: 1686-1692.
66. Lin SM, Huang CD, Lin HC, et al: A modified goal-directed protocol improves clinical outcomes in intensive care unit patients with septic shock: A randomized controlled trial. Shock 2006;26:551-557.
67. Trzeciak S, Dellinger RP, Abate NL, et al: Translating research to clinical practice: A 1-year experience with implementing early goal-directed therapy for septic shock in the emergency department. Chest 2006;129:225-232.
68. Choi PT, Yip G, Quinonez LG, Cook DJ: Crystalloids vs. colloids in fluid resuscitation: A systematic review. Crit Care Med 1999;27:200-210.
69. Packman MI, Rackow EC: Optimum left heart filling pressure during fluid resuscitation of patients with hypovolemic and septic shock. Crit Care Med 1983;11:165-169.
70. Vincent JL, Weil MH: Fluid challenge revisited. Crit Care Med 2006;34:1333-1337.
71. LeDoux D, Astiz ME, Carpati CM, Rackow EC: Effects of perfusion pressure on tissue perfusion in septic shock. Crit Care Med 2000;28:2729-2732.
72. Martin C, Viviand X, Leone M, Thirion X: Effect of norepinephrine on the outcome of septic shock. Crit Care Med 2000;28:2758-2765.
73. Martin C, Papazian L, Perrin G, et al: Norepinephrine or dopamine for the treatment of hyperdynamic septic shock? Chest 1993;103:1826-1831.
74. Levy B, Bollaert PE, Charpentier C, et al: Comparison of norepinephrine and dobutamine to epinephrine for hemodynamics, lactate metabolism, and gastric tonometric variables in septic shock: A prospective, randomized study. Intensive Care Med 1997;23: 282-287.
75. Martikainen TJ, Tenhunen JJ, Giovannini I, et al: Epinephrine induces tissue perfusion deficit in porcine endotoxin shock: Evaluation by regional CO(2) content gradients and lactate-to-pyruvate ratios. Am J Physiol Gastrointest Liver Physiol 2005;288: G586-592.
76. Meier-Hellmann A, Reinhart K, Bredle DL, et al: Epinephrine impairs splanchnic perfusion in septic shock. Crit Care Med 1997;25:399-404.
77. Martin C: Norepinephrine plus dobutamine versus epinephrine alone for the management of septic shock. Barcelona, Spain, European Society of Intensive Care Medicine, 2006.
78. Holmes CL, Patel BM, Russell JA, Walley KR: Physiology of vasopressin relevant to management of septic shock. Chest 2001;120:989-1002.
79. Landry DW, Oliver JA: The pathogenesis of vasodilatory shock. N Engl J Med 2001;345:588-595.
80. Landry DW, Levin HR, Gallant EM, et al: Vasopressin deficiency contributes to the vasodilation of septic shock. Circulation 1997;95:1122-1125.
81. Landry DW, Levin HR, Gallant EM, et al: Vasopressin pressor hypersensitivity in vasodilatory septic shock. Crit Care Med 1997;25:1279-1282.
82. Russell JA, Walley K: Vasopressin and Septic Shock Trial (VASST): Study results. Barcelona, Spain, European Society of Intensive Care Medicine, 2006.
83. Bone RC, Fisher CJ Jr, Clemmer TP, et al: A controlled clinical trial of high-dose methylprednisolone in the treatment of severe sepsis and septic shock. N Engl J Med 1987;317: 653-658.
84. Sprung CL, Caralis PV, Marcial EH, et al: The effects of high-dose corticosteroids in patients with septic shock. A prospective, controlled study. N Engl J Med 1984;311:1137-1143.
85. Bollaert PE, Charpentier C, Levy B, et al: Reversal of late septic shock with supraphysiologic doses of hydrocortisone. Crit Care Med 1998;26:645-650.
86. Briegel J, Forst H, Haller M, et al: Stress doses of hydrocortisone reverse hyperdynamic septic shock: A prospective, randomized, double-blind, single-center study. Crit Care Med 1999;27:723-732.
87. Annane D, Sebille V, Troche G, et al: A three-level prognostic classification in septic shock based on cortisol levels and cortisol response to corticotropin. JAMA 2000;283:1038-1045.
88. Annane D, Sebille V, Charpentier C, et al: Effect of treatment with low doses of hydrocortisone and fludrocortisone on mortality in patients with septic shock. JAMA 2002;288:862-871.
89. Sprung CL: CORTICUS trial: Study results. Orlando, Fla, Society of Critical Care Medicine, 2007.

Chapter 25

Cardiac Tamponade

Zoltan G. Turi

FUNDAMENTALS OF TAMPONADE

Cardiac tamponade is a condition characterized by increase in pressure external to the heart resulting in impaired filling of the cardiac chambers. In the typical scenario, as fluid in the pericardium accumulates, cardiac output falls. The diagnosis represents a continuum from mild tamponade with subtle diagnostic findings to a critical clinical setting with imminent mortality.[1] The variability in presentation, including diagnostic findings and course, and the morbidity and mortality associated with treatment make this a particularly challenging clinical problem in critical care medicine.

Pericardial Anatomy

The pericardium consists of a visceral and a parietal pericardial segment, the former being composed of a single layer of cells that adhere to the cardiac epicardial surface.[2,3] The parietal pericardium is the structure responsible for the clinically relevant features of tamponade; it is a relatively noncompliant structure composed of collagen and elastin and normally is less than 2 mm thick. The mechanical properties of the pericardium—in particular, those reflected by its pressure-volume curve (Fig. 25-1)—are responsible for the clinical features seen in cardiac tamponade.

The pericardium extends from the lower third of the superior vena cava to the apex of the heart. It is attached to the sternum, the diaphragm, and the great vessels. Because it extends beyond the heart border, trauma to not only the heart but also the great vessels approaching the heart borders can lead to cardiac tamponade.[4]

Physiology

Cardiac tamponade is a result of increased transmural pressure, typically from accumulation of fluid in the pericardial space (Fig. 25-2). Other causes of "tamponade-like physiology" are related to extrinsic compression of the heart,[5] although these pathologic processes should be separated from those causing constriction rather than true tamponade. Differentiating these two distinct physiologic entities, constriction and tamponade, is essential to diagnosis and management.

The fluid accumulating in the pericardial space can be blood, serous fluid, purulent material, clot, or rarely gas. As fluid accumulates, the pericardium stretches, until it reaches a point (see Fig. 25-1) at which its degree of compliance is exhausted, so that it has become largely inelastic. At this point, any further increase in intrapericardial fluid is associated with a decrease in intracardiac chamber volume, because the total volume of pericardial fluid, heart muscle, and the cardiac chambers becomes fixed by pericardium no longer able to stretch. This in turn results in decreased filling of the heart and consequently decreased stroke volume. To maintain cardiac output, an early compensatory mechanism is an increase in heart rate. Subsequent adaptations to maintain blood flow to central end organs (heart, brain, kidneys) are venous pressure rise, peripheral vasoconstriction, increase in ejection fraction, and selective shunting of blood to preserve flow to the essential end organs. Venous pressure increase is accomplished by fluid retention and peripheral venoconstriction. In severe tamponade, equalization of right atrial, right ventricular diastolic, pulmonary diastolic, pulmonary artery wedge, and intrapericardial pressures occurs. Tamponade is a continuum, ranging from a primarily echocardiographic finding of right-sided chamber collapse to shock and pulseless electrical activity.

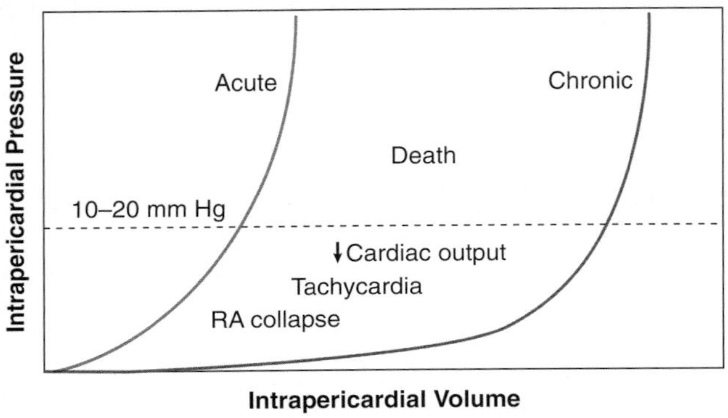

Figure 25-1. Pressure-volume curves for normal pericardium on the *left* and compliant pericardium on the *right*. In the setting of rapid onset of effusion in the normal pericardium, low volumes, typically rising from less than 50 mL, lead to a rise in pressure that exceeds the limit of pericardial stretch, with early onset of tamponade physiology. With more compliant pericardium, a result of chronic stretching, critical extramural pressures do not result until substantially higher volumes are achieved, in some cases more than 1 L.

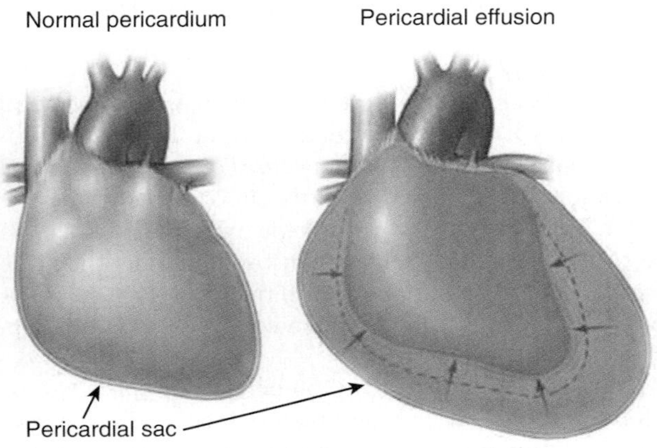

Figure 25-2. The pericardium surrounding the heart in a normal physiologic setting and in tamponade. The pericardium can be seen to extend to the proximal great vessels. Note the large amount of effusion in the image on the *right,* consistent with chronic pericardial stretch, which leads more slowly to tamponade. (Courtesy of the Mayo Foundation for Medical Education.)

Pericardial Pressure

The normal pericardium contains a small amount of fluid, typically in a range of 20 to 50 mL, resulting in no more than 5 mm of separation between the visceral and the parietal pericardial surfaces. Pressure in the normal pericardium reflects intrathoracic pressure, which in turn reflects atmospheric pressure, with variation influenced by respiration. During inspiration, the pressure falls a few millimeters below atmospheric pressure (by convention, 0 mm Hg); during expiration, a few millimeters above. The difference between intracardiac and intrapericardial pressures, the transmural pressure, in turn distends or compresses the cardiac chambers. Because intrapericardial mean pressure in patients breathing unassisted typically is the same as atmospheric pressure, while right atrial pressure is normally in the range of 2 to 8 mm Hg, the latter is the typical range of net right atrial transmural pressure. When intrapericardial pressure rises to the level of right atrial pressure, the right atrium collapses, a typical feature of early cardiac tamponade, though this nonspecific finding can be seen with hypovolemia alone.

The normal parietal pericardium, because of its limited compliance, functions to limit abrupt expansion of the heart as a whole.[6] Thus, in the setting of right ventricular infarction, for example, acute dilation of the right ventricle is at the cost of left ventricular volume decrease—a ventricular interdependence phenomenon similar to that illustrated in Figure 25-3. Acute chamber enlargement due to other etiologic conditions or disorders, such as abrupt volume loading or sudden onset of severe valvular regurgitation, is impeded by the constraint of pericardium that has reached the limits of its intrinsic elasticity. Because right-sided heart filling occurs preferentially with inspiration, when negative intrathoracic pressures result in increased venous return and higher right-sided chamber volume, left ventricular stroke volume and hence systolic blood pressure tend to fall as left atrial and left ventricular volumes are decreased. This exaggerates the normal respiratory variation, and systemic pressure falls with inspiration to a level at which pulsus paradoxus, defined by convention as a greater than 10 mm Hg decrease in systolic pressure, is seen. In addition, decreased intrathoracic pressure has a disproportionate effect on the pulmonary venous circulation, which is not exposed to the high pericardial pressures; hence, a disproportionate fall during inspiration in the pulmonary vein to left atrial gradient further exacerbates the decrease in left atrial filling.[7] The fall in systolic pressure is not in fact a paradox but rather an exaggeration of normal respiratory variation of approximately 3%[8] with associated inspiratory decrease in left ventricular stroke volume. With severe tamponade, total elimination of pulse pressure can be seen with individual heart beats, as in the example in Figure 25-4.

The inability to dilate further means that additional volume beyond the intrinsic stretch limit of the pericardium, such as from bleeding into the pericardial sac, results in increasing compression of heart chambers as volume expands in the pericardial space. Because the right-sided chambers have the lowest intracardiac pressures, in particular the right atrium, those are the first chambers showing collapse, in particular in diastole, when the tricuspid valve is open and the right atrium can decompress into the right ventricle. With progressive increase in intrapericardial pressure, compression of the right ventricle in diastole occurs during pressure equalization with the right atrium. Eventually, as intrapericardial pressure continues to rise, compression of the left-sided chambers ensues.

In contrast with acute tamponade physiology, in which hemodynamic decompensation may occur after only a modest accumulation of fluid, generally in the range of 100 to 200 mL, chronic pericardial effusion results in gradual increase in distensibility of the pericardium. With increasing compliance, large amounts of fluid can accumulate at low pressure without increasing transmural

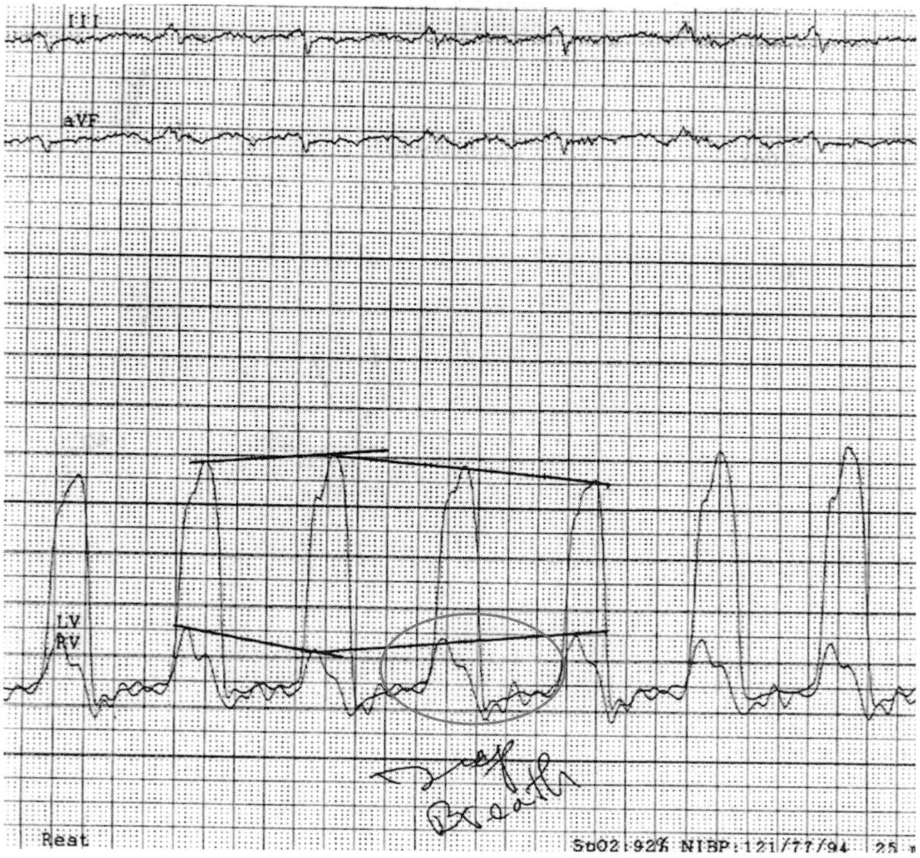

Figure 25-3. Hemodynamic tracings from a patient with ventricular interdependence (200 mm Hg scale). With inspiration, left ventricle (LV) systolic pressure falls as right ventricle (RV) systolic pressure increases. Because of ventricular interdependence, the right ventricular and left ventricular systolic pressures trend in opposite directions (lines connecting peak systolic pressures diverge during phases of the respiratory cycle). Diastolic pressures in both ventricles are essentially identical *(green oval)*. Absence of pulsus paradoxus and preserved systolic pressure make this physiology consistent with constriction rather than tamponade. The patient had a clot in the pericardial space after prior cardiac trauma.

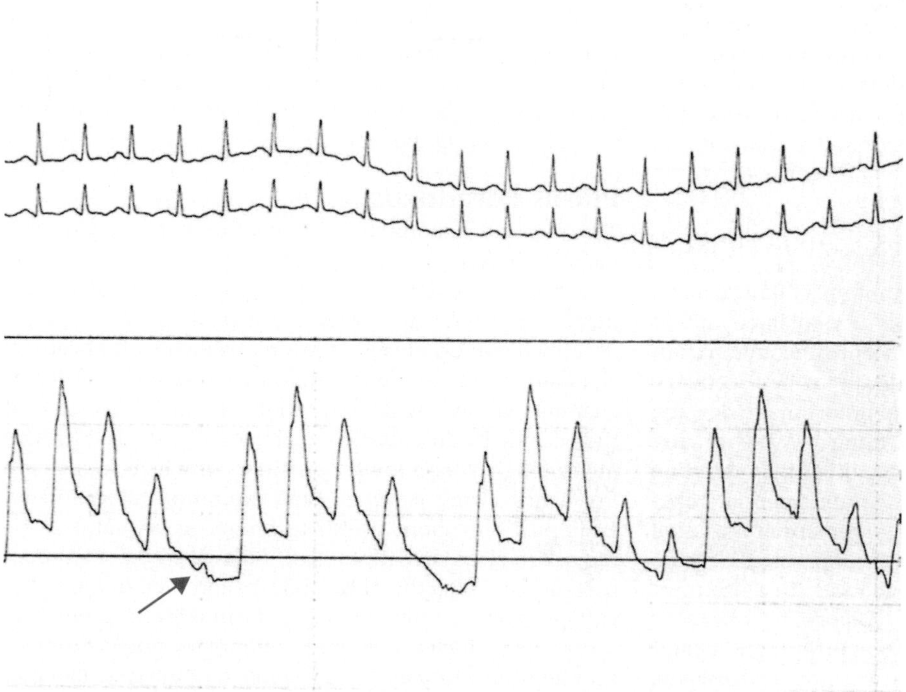

Figure 25-4. Hemodynamic tracing of systemic pressure in cardiac tamponade, 100 mm Hg scale. Systolic pressure variation is nearly 40 mm Hg, and pulse pressure is markedly reduced during inspiration. Note the complete obliteration of the systemic pressure during deep inspiration in the beat highlighted by the *arrow.* Because of low stroke volume, cardiac output is being maintained to some extent by a high heart rate (146 beats per minute).

pressure or compressing the cardiac chambers (see Fig. 25-1). Even in chronic low pressure–high volume tamponade, a limit of distensibility is eventually reached that results in similar pathophysiology as with acute tamponade, in some cases only after a liter or more of fluid has accumulated. Once the steep portion of the pressure-volume curve is reached, it is important to appreciate that with accumulation of another 50 to 100 mL of pericardial fluid, hemodynamic decompensation can occur rapidly, with similar outcomes as in patients who suffer from acute tamponade, such as is seen with penetrating trauma, coronary artery perforation, or cardiac rupture.

Etiology

Pericardial effusions generally can be characterized as transudate or exudate, infectious or bloody, with tamponade occurring with variable frequency depending both on the rapidity of fluid accumulation and, to a somewhat lesser degree, on characteristics of the effusion and physiology determined by its etiology. Transudates are characteristic of congestive heart failure; exudates, of infections and malignancy (see Chapter 6). Conditions predisposing to slow accumulation such as heart failure, myxedema, chronic renal failure, and connective tissue disorders in general are less likely to cause acute tamponade, whereas those associated with rapid development, such as malignancy, infection, or particularly hemorrhage, commonly result in abrupt hemodynamic deterioration. The effect of inflammation in decreasing compliance of the pericardium exacerbates the hemodynamic effects of effusions associated with pericarditis.[9] The potential etiologic disorders are highly variable, with significant influence of demographics and geography, so that tamponade secondary to tuberculous pericardial effusion in immune compromised patients is a not uncommon presentation in Africa,[10] whereas in industrialized nations malignant effusions are a far more common cause.[11] The most common etiologic disorders are listed in Table 25-1; more detailed discussion of the various causes is presented later in the chapter, organized by the hospital setting in which presentation typically is seen.

Table 25-1. Etiology of Cardiac Tamponade

Causative Disorder/Condition	Frequency (%)
Most common*	
Idiopathic	23
Malignancy	22
Iatrogenic	18
Acute myocardial infarction	8
Purulent (including tuberculous)	8
Renal failure	3
Miscellaneous	18
Aortic dissection	
Myxedema	
Trauma	
Connective tissue disorders	
Radiation therapy	

*Frequency of common etiologies of tamponade is based on 119 cases in Barcelona, Spain. Other relatively common causes of effusion include congestive heart failure, hypoalbuminemia, coagulopathy, and post-cardiotomy and Dressler's syndromes. Etiologies of tamponade will be dependent on geography and patient demographics and also will be strongly influenced by the presence of oncology, trauma, or dialysis units. For a comprehensive list of tamponade etiologies based on prior data, see Box 6-1.

Data from Sagrista-Sauleda J, Merce J, Permanyer-Miralda G, et al: Clinical clues to the causes of large pericardial effusions. Am J Med 2000;109:95-101.

HISTORY AND PHYSICAL EXAMINATION

Dyspnea is the most common symptom of tamponade, although its etiology sometimes is unexplained and it usually is not associated with significant concomitant pulmonary vascular congestion. It is likely to be secondary to decreased cardiac output and encroachment on lung volume by the expanding pericardium as well as any simultaneous pleural effusions. The patient may describe a sensation of fullness in the chest or abdomen and dysphagia, associated with venous engorgement and passive congestion, stretching of the richly innervated pericardium and occasionally vagal stimulation.[12] Because most patients with tamponade have comorbid conditions accounting for their effusion, additional signs and symptoms are likely to be related to pericarditis, malignancy, or other concomitant conditions.

The hallmarks of cardiac tamponade on physical examination relate to features associated with venous hypertension, low cardiac output, and effects of the layer of fluid between the heart and the chest wall. In patents with tamponade, the general appearance changes substantially during progressive increase in pericardial pressure. Because tamponade represents a continuum, some patients with early tamponade physiology look well, whereas patients with more advanced tamponade show features of a low-output state, with clinical manifestations reflecting the high catecholamine levels required to maintain cardiac output. They become progressively more anxious and agitated and less communicative and may be struggling to breathe.

Pulsus Paradoxus

The physical examination in significant tamponade can include Beck's triad, described in 1935 by the surgeon C. S. Beck.[13] This entity features jugular venous distention, decreased arterial pressure, and a small, quiet heart. As described earlier, pulsus paradoxus is the result of cardiac chamber interdependence and decrease in left ventricular chamber volume with inspiration. It can be detected at the bedside by auscultation of Korotkoff sounds, identifying the highest and lowest pressures at which sounds are first heard during inspiration and expiration; alternatively, a simpler and more useful technique is to palpate the radial artery pulse with the cuff inflated to the maximum pressure at which the pulse appears and then to lower the cuff pressure in increments of 10 mm Hg to detect the pressure at which pulses are continuously noted throughout the respiratory cycle. It is important to recognize that although pulsus paradoxus is a classic feature of severe tamponade, as a diagnostic feature it is of limited sensitivity and specificity.

Various thresholds other than the relatively arbitrary 10 mm Hg threshold have been proposed to increase specificity, including a 10% decrease, rather than 10 mm Hg fall.[14] A drop in *systolic* pressure greater than 50% of the *pulse* pressure also has been proposed.[1] Use of a 15 or 20 mm Hg fall in pressure by physical examination is a less sensitive but far more specific finding for tamponade but may result in later diagnosis. Pulsus paradoxus may be present in other conditions that result in exaggerated decrease in systolic pressure with inspiration, such as massive pulmonary embolism, severe chronic obstructive pulmonary disease (which also can feature constrictive physiology because of limited expansion of the heart in the setting of hyperexpanded lungs),[14] and right ventricular infarction.[15] Furthermore, other features of the systemic blood pressure and pulse are important to consider. With progressive decrease in cardiac filling overall, a decline in systemic pressure (regardless of phase of the respiratory cycle) as well as a decrease in pulse pressure (the difference between systolic and diastolic pressures) occurs, reflecting decreasing stroke volume and decreasing cardiac output. Thus, it may be impossible to palpate radial artery pulsations; with severe tamponade, the patient is likely to feel cool and clammy, a finding consistent with severe peripheral vasoconstriction.

Tachycardia is almost invariable, except for comorbid conditions associated with a decrease in heart rate, such as electrical conduction disturbances, severe hypothyroidism, or aggressive β-blockade. Tachycardia is a compensatory mechanism for decreased stroke volume, also is caused by high catecholamine levels, and may result from pericardial irritation of the sinus node that stimulates a higher heart rate. On occasion, acute bradycardia may be seen in tamponade, sometimes the first finding after hemorrhage into the pericardial sac. Although a well-preserved systolic pressure and a wide pulse pressure are uncommon in tamponade, neither low pressure or a narrow pulse pressure is totally specific.

The pulsus paradoxus may be absent in conditions in which ventricular interdependence is masked[16] (Table 25-2), such as a nonrestrictive atrial septal defect, in which inspiration also increases left atrial filling, or aortic insufficiency, in which left ventricular filling in diastole is increased by regurgitation from a high-pressure source: the aorta. Localized tamponade may have some general tamponade features (such as decreased stroke volume) but may not result in ventricular interdependence—hence, the clinical picture may be that of a sick patient with tamponade but without pulsus paradoxus. Markedly elevated left-sided heart diastolic pressures in severe left ventricular hypertrophy and other disease states may exceed the elevated right atrial and intrapericardial pressures in tamponade, decreasing the effect of inspiration on interdependence of right and left sides of the heart. An example in which both pulse pressure and pulsus paradoxus would be insensitive markers of tamponade is aortic dissection that combines aortic insufficiency with tamponade, in which a wide pulse pressure may be seen in some patients with partial compensation, and in which pulsus paradoxus, as discussed, may be masked. By contrast, conditions resulting in impaired right ventricular filling, such as right ventricular hypertrophy in severe pulmonary hypertension, also may result in absence of a pulsus paradoxus[17]; furthermore, in settings such as cor pulmonale, the dramatic elevation in right-sided diastolic pressures will delay onset of the otherwise highly sensitive and early finding of right atrial and right ventricular diastolic collapse until tamponade is severe.[18] A substantial number of case reports describe physiologic conditions in which the classic findings for tamponade are not seen or are attributable to other etiologic disorders.[19]

Table 25-2. Tamponade Settings in Which Pulsus Paradoxus May Not Be Present
■ Non-restrictive (large) atrial septal defect
■ Severe aortic insufficiency
■ Loculated effusion
■ Left ventricular hypertrophy and other causes of elevated LV diastolic pressure
■ Shock due to hypovolemia, or profound circulatory collapse with tamponade
■ Severe left ventricular dysfunction
■ Low-pressure tamponade
■ Right ventricular hypertrophy or other cause of impaired RV filling.
■ Positive-pressure ventilation
■ Arrhythmias
LV, left ventricular; RV, right ventricular.

Venous Pressure

Because impairment of right-sided filling is usually the first manifestation of increasing pericardial pressure, high jugular venous pressure manifested by prominent venous pulsations may be the earliest finding on physical examination, occurring with increasing intrapericardial and right atrial pressures. Jugular venous distention may, however, be simultaneously absent because venoconstriction, a common finding with acute tamponade, makes detection of elevated venous pressures difficult. It also will be masked by low-volume tamponade, including volume-depleted states such as trauma, when, in addition to hemorrhage into the pericardium, significant blood loss has occurred. Other settings in which venous distention may not be observed are post-dialysis in patients with uremic pericardial effusions, and excessive diuresis, sometimes as part of treatment for symptoms of congestive heart failure when the cause of elevated filling pressures has not been appreciated.[20] In general, lack of venous engorgement in tamponade, particularly when the latter is acute, is not uncommon. Thus, prominent jugular venous distention may suggest an alternative diagnosis, such as severe right-sided heart failure. Increased venous pressure with inspiration, Kussmaul's sign, is a feature of constriction, reflecting increased venous return to the thorax without increased right atrial filling, because the latter is constricted by the pericardium. This is in contrast with tamponade, in which negative intrathoracic pressure is transmitted through the pericardial effusion, and results in increased right-sided heart filling with decrease in venous pressure. Because these findings are difficult to differentiate in most acutely ill patients, much of the subsequent description about right atrial pressure is based on catheter-based hemodynamic findings rather than the physical examination.

The Y descent, in contrast with pericardial constriction, in which it is prominent, typically is limited or absent (Fig. 25-5). Unlike in pericardial constriction, filling of the right ventricle (and hence emptying of the right atrium) is impaired throughout the cardiac cycle, because extrinsic compression by pericardial fluid results in elevated diastolic pressures in the right ventricle when rapid filling would otherwise occur. Because the pericardium allows additional atrial expansion during ventricular ejection (when ventricular volume decreases), the X descent is typically the more prominent negative pressure wave seen. The classic square root sign seen in the right ventricular pressure tracing in constriction is absent in tamponade.

In contrast with acute tamponade, with chronic effusion persistent elevation in pericardial pressure leads to parallel rise in central and peripheral venous pressure, as well as fluid retention with elevated intravascular volume. Venous congestion as well as peripheral edema and end-organ signs of chronic venous hypertension, such as passive congestion of the liver, become more common in this setting.

Cardiac and Chest Examination

The quiet heart in Beck's triad relates to several features that tend to muffle the intensity of heart sounds. First, the insulating effects of pericardial fluid on sound waves tend to decrease the sound volume transmitted to the chest wall. Second, low stroke and filling volumes tend to decrease the forces that cause the sounds generated by heart valve closure, with low pulse pressure in both the aortic and the pulmonary arteries. Because the S3 gallop is created by rapid ventricular filling, a phenomenon absent in tamponade, it would not be expected, nor would an S4, because the hemodynamic characteristics of late diastolic atrial emptying that causes the fourth heart sound are not seen.[1] A pericardial friction rub, if pericarditis is involved, may be heard. Except in severe tamponade, the pericardium around the apex of the heart may contain relatively little fluid, and left ventricular contraction typically is vigorous unless underlying left ventricular dysfunction also is present. Hence, a palpable point of maximal impulse may be felt.

A particular feature that differentiates tamponade from decompensated congestive heart failure is the typical presence of clear lungs in the case of the former. Although both right and left atrial pressures are markedly elevated, flow into the pulmonary circulation is limited, and the pressure-volume curve for the pulmonary vascular system is not affected.

DIAGNOSTIC TESTS

Echocardiography

The hallmarks of pericardial tamponade have been discussed earlier, and examples are presented in Chapter 8. In general, echocardiography is the most sensitive, specific, and accurate of diagnostic modalities for evaluation of tamponade.[21] Besides evaluating presence and degree of chamber collapse, the echocardiogram is useful for assessing the amount and location of effusion in the pericardial space, for characterizing the fluid, and for judging

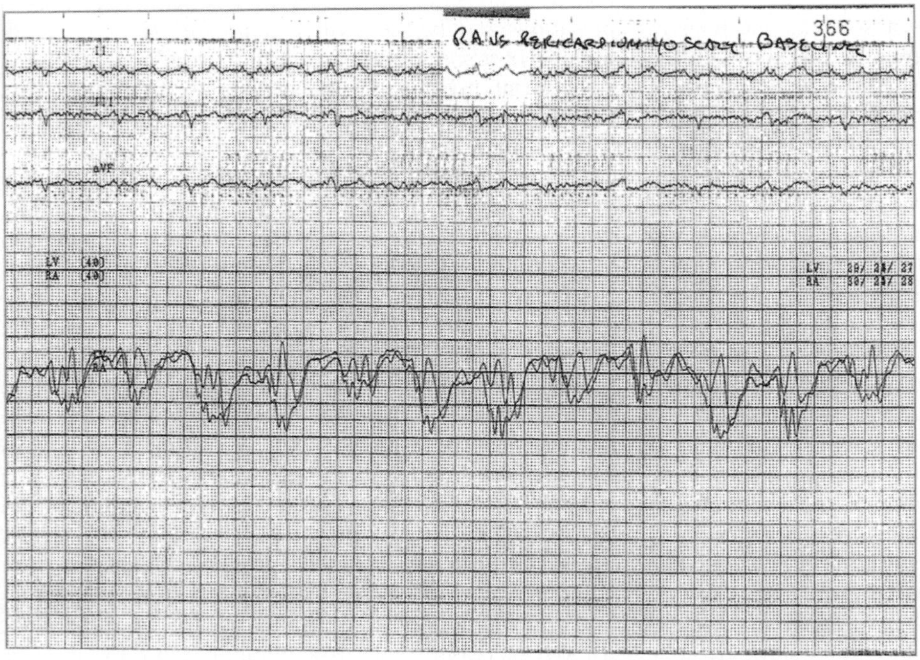

Figure 25-5. Hemodynamic tracings showing right atrial (RA) and intrapericardial pressures (incorrectly labeled LV) on 40 mm Hg scale. Note the equivalence of pressures as well as the high mean pressure, 27 mm Hg, consistent with tamponade and hemodynamic decompensation. The Y descent is nearly absent.

the hemodynamic effects of tamponade, including ventricular interdependence.[22] In general, prolonged collapse along the free wall of the right ventricle in diastole is a relatively specific finding for tamponade[2] (whereas right atrial collapse can be seen with hypovolemia alone), especially with variations in mitral and tricuspid inflow velocities, pulmonary and hepatic vein Doppler findings, and sustained dilation of the vena cava as described in Chapter 8.[23] Portable echocardiography at the bedside, in the emergency department, or in critical care units is a simple and highly reliable modality,[24] although adequate training is essential because misdiagnosis, such as confusing an epicardial fat pad with pericardial effusion, has been described,[25] and pleural effusions, mediastinal masses, and atelectasis can confound the diagnosis as well.[26] It is important to assess loculation; presence of clot, masses, or fibrinous material; and compression from outside the pericardium, all of which will influence management decisions. Typically, patients are recumbent, and until tamponade reaches the moderate to severe category, fluid may be shifted by gravity to a location primarily posterior to the heart (Fig. 25-6).

X-Ray Studies

The classic "water bottle" configuration of the heart is due to a large pericardial effusion and therefore occurs only if the pressure-volume curve has altered sufficiently through chronic accumulation to allow significant increase in pericardial volume. It is a misconception that a normal-sized heart excludes tamponade; in acute tamponade the heart size can be expected to appear normal or minimally enlarged. With marked enlargement of the cardiac silhouette, the finding is nonspecific and not readily distinguishable from cardiomegaly, although in tamponade pulmonary vascular congestion is usually not seen, while prominence of the vena cava may be noted. Other modalities such as CT scanning and magnetic resonance imaging show large effusions and can demonstrate chamber collapse. In addition, characterization of pericardial thickness and of the pericardial fluid to differentiate between blood and fluid of different densities can be useful. Although CT and MR show primarily anatomy rather than physiology, besides chamber collapse, reflux into the azygos vein is a useful sign of tamponade.[27]

Electrocardiography

The classic electrocardiographic features include low voltage, a result of poor transmission of electrical activity across the fluid in the pericardial space, and electrical alternans, an insensitive but relatively specific finding for tamponade generated by swinging of the heart in the fluid-filled chamber (Fig. 25-7). Electrical alternans typically is seen only with large effusions in the later stages of tamponade, although the finding is related more to fluid volume and the ability of the heart to swing within the pericardial space. It may involve alternans of both QRS complexes and P waves. Thus, tamponade with adhesions (Fig. 25-8), loculation, or masses that restrict heart motion may not manifest the alternans phenomenon.

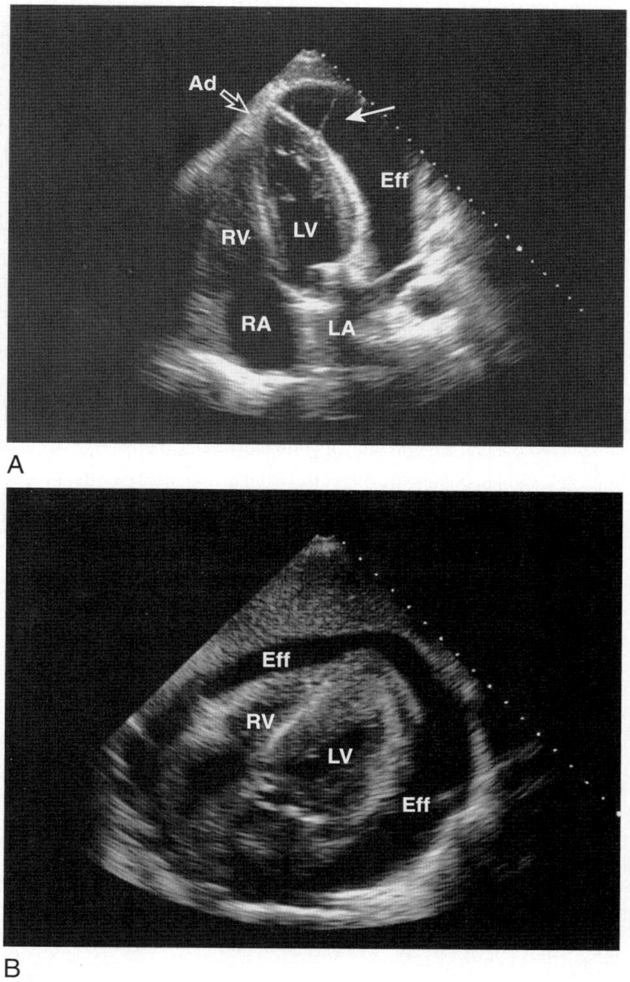

Figure 25-6. Echocardiographic images of two types of pericardial effusions. **A,** A large posterior pericardial effusion, with relatively little fluid anterior to the heart or at the apex. The apex is adherent to the pericardial surface. The *arrow* points to a fibrous strand. This is a fairly typical appearance of a chronic post-cardiotomy effusion. Needle access would be problematic. **B,** By contrast, this effusion is circumferential, with somewhat more fluid behind the left ventricle, a largely gravitational effect. Leaning the patient forward 20 to 30 degrees would facilitate pericardiocentesis, although the patient was not significantly hemodynamically compromised. Ad, adhesion; Eff, effusion; LA, left atrium; LV, left ventricle; RA, right atrium; RV, right ventricle.

OVERALL ASSESSMENT

In general, the severity of tamponade can be judged by the extent of hypotension, tachycardia, and pulsus paradoxus on physical examination and confirmed by findings on echocardiography.[28] Mild tamponade features no hypotension or tachycardia, and no pulsus, with mild RV collapse by echo. Patients with moderate tamponade have preservation of systemic pressure, but have tachycardia, some degree of pulsus paradoxus, and clear RV collapse on echo. Severe pulsus is associated with tachycardia, shock, profound pulsus paradoxus, and chamber collapse with a swinging heart on ultrasound.[15] Hemodynamic findings correlate with increasing pericardial pressure at

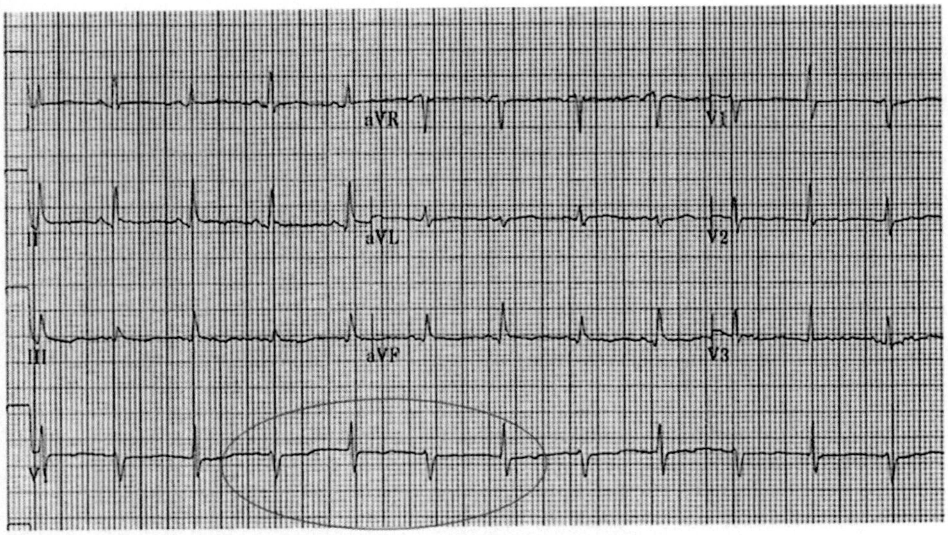

Figure 25-7. Electrocardiogram demonstrating classic electrical alternans in a patient with pericardial tamponade. Note the change in amplitude of the R wave in lead V1 *(red oval).* Similar findings are seen throughout the limb and precordial leads shown.

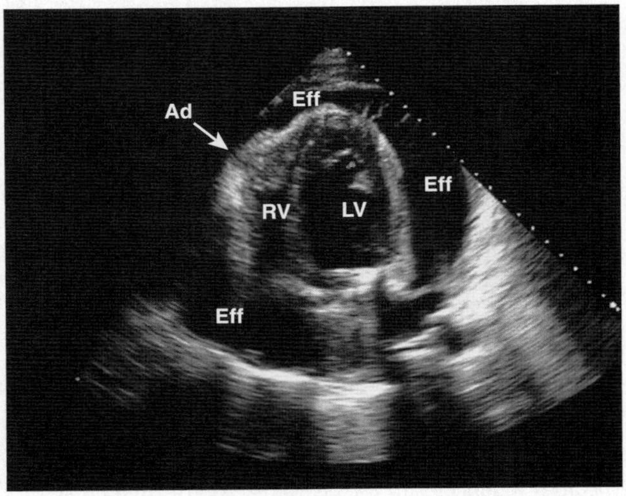

Figure 25-8. Echocardiogram showing pericardial tamponade with right-sided collapse, adhesion of the right ventricle to the pericardium *(arrow),* and fibrous strands of early adhesions seen at the 1 o'clock position near the apex of the left ventricle. Even if the effusion accumulates further, electrical alternans would be less likely because of lack of mobility of the heart. Ad, adhesion; Eff, effusion; LV, left ventricle; RV, right ventricle.

each stage of tamponade,[29] initially less than right atrial or pulmonary wedge pressure, then equilibrating with right but less than left atrial pressure, and in severe tamponade equilibrating with both.

SPECIAL SYNDROMES IN TAMPONADE

Although most cases of tamponade have at least some of the classic features, there are several important variants. Loculated effusions that compress the heart primarily in one region are typically post surgical, although they may be due to neoplasms or a number of other etiologies; they are discussed in the section on post cardiac surgery cases that follows. There are also a number of conditions where pulsus paradoxus does not occur or is masked, summarized in Table 25-2.

Effusive Constrictive Disease

This phenomenon is an important to recognize condition occurring in less than 10% of patients with tamponade,[30] but up to 40% in some series. Hospitals with disproportionately high populations of oncology patients, because of tumor metastases or post radiation pericardial involvement, or tuberculosis, will have a higher percentage of tamponade patients with this diagnosis. The syndrome can occur after acute pericarditis of multiple etiologies and may even be transient.[31] The classic features of tamponade are seen on presentation, and a history of malignancy should increase the suspicion pre-pericardiocentesis.

Effusive constrictive disease is a setting in which careful hemodynamic monitoring is very helpful for accurate diagnosis. Monitoring of intrapericardial and right atrial or wedge pressure during pericardiocentesis demonstrates findings as seen in Figure 25-9. In general, with relief of tamponade intrapericardial hypertension resolves, and classic respiratory variation is seen in most patients, while right atrial pressure remains elevated though lower than prior to the pericardiocentesis. The Y descent becomes prominent because of the elimination of high transmural pressures that restrict filling during early diastole in tamponade, unmasking classic constrictive physiology. Figure 25-10 shows echocardiographic images in a typical patient with this syndrome.

Low- and High-Pressure Tamponade

Low pressure tamponade has been defined as featuring hypotension secondary to pericardial effusion but with low venous and intrapericardial pressures, most commonly in the setting of hypovolemia due to dehydration or blood loss. A more formal definition, based on a single site experience, was described by Sagrista-Sauleda and colleagues[32] as an intrapericardial pressure less than 7 mm Hg, with a post-pericardiocentesis right atrial pressure less than 4 mm Hg and equalization of intrapericardial and right atrial pressures before pericardiocentesis. Importantly, 20% of their patients with cardiac tamponade met these criteria (and 10% of their patients with large pericardial

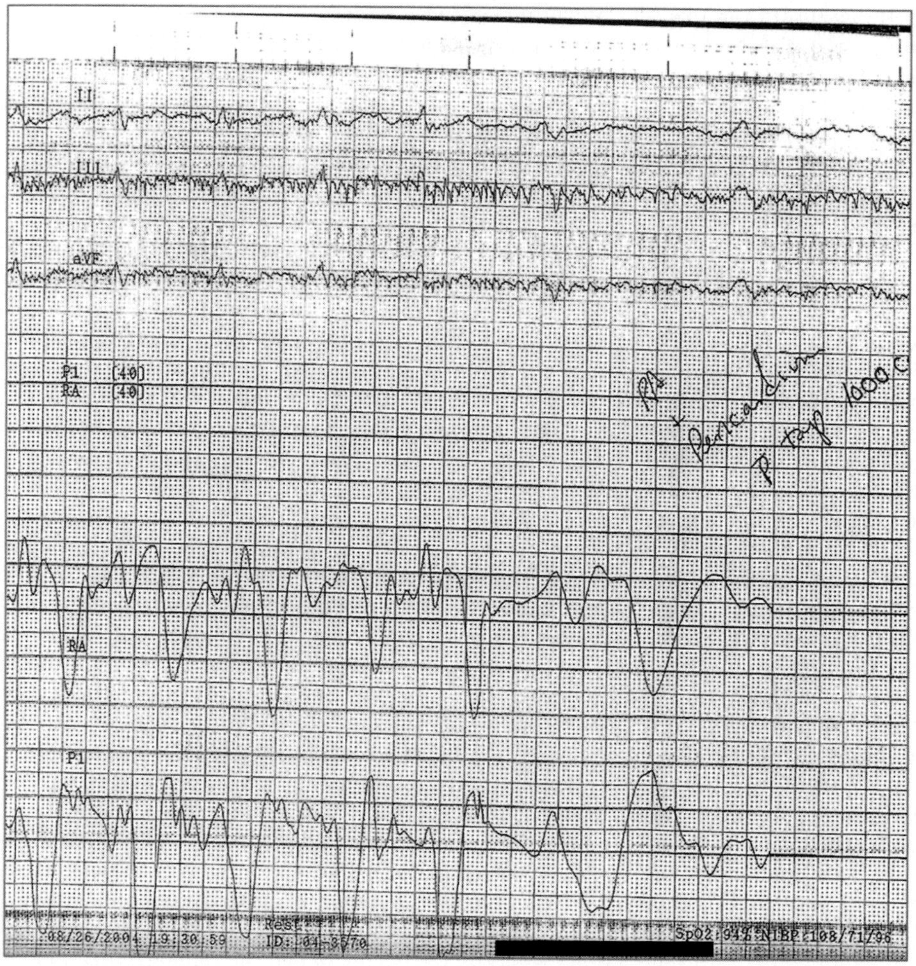

Figure 25-9. Hemodynamic tracings (40 mm Hg scale) obtained one hour after those seen in Figure 25-5. After pericardiocentesis of 1 L of fluid, the pericardial pressure has achieved a mean equivalent to atmospheric pressure (0 mm Hg by convention), while right atrial pressure remains elevated near 22 mm Hg. This is physiology consistent with effusive-constrictive disease. On removal of the effusion, the hemodynamics, including the newly seen steep Y descent, are classic for constriction. This patient had a malignant pericardial effusion. P, intrapericardial pressure; RA, right atrium.

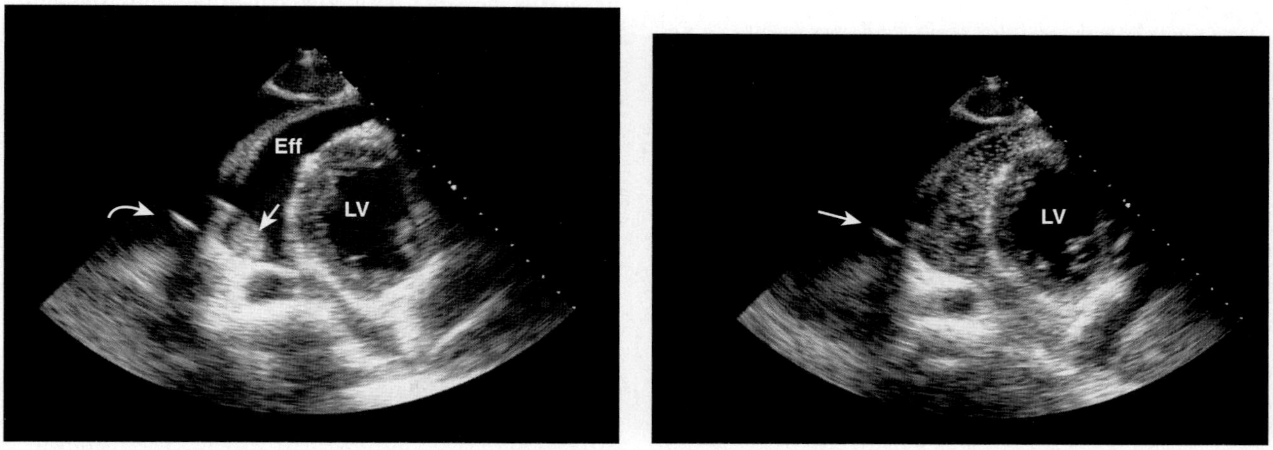

A B

Figure 25-10. Echocardiographic images from a patient with effusive-constrictive disease. **A,** Tamponade. *Curved arrow* points to needle in pericardial space, *straight arrow* points to tumor mass. The pericardium is thickened. **B,** Agitated saline has been injected through the needle *(arrow)* to confirm entry into the pericardial space. Eff, effusion; LV, left ventricle.

effusions), suggesting that low-pressure tamponade, previously the subject primarily of case reports and small series, may be more common than previously appreciated. Because of low pressures, there is a lack of features such as pulsus paradoxus or jugular venous distention, with only 24% demonstrating these classic findings, making the diagnosis significantly more difficult. Fluid challenge may result in more typical findings.

Patients with chronic hypertension in whom tamponade develops occasionally have high blood pressure despite tamponade physiology, presumably because of an exaggerated systemic pressure response to the catecholamine storm associated with tamponade.[33] In this setting, injudicious use of the usual medications to lower blood pressure can result in profound hemodynamic compromise.

SETTINGS IN WHICH TAMPONADE IS SEEN

The Emergency Room

The primary cause of tamponade in the emergency room relates to hemopericardium, although the complete range of medical etiologies can be seen in this setting. Trauma[34] includes gunshot and stab wounds, as well as penetrating and crush wounds to the chest, including those related to automobile accidents. Penetrating wounds are significantly more likely to result in tamponade than crush injuries.[35] Medical presentations with acute hemopericardium include aortic dissection with tamponade, post myocardial infarction rupture, or leaking thoracic aneurysm, situations in which pericardiocentesis may lead to further hemodynamic decompensation,[36,37] as well as hemopericardium secondary to overanticoagulation. In general, acute hemopericardium may be associated with continued hemorrhage as well as clot in the pericardium; the latter makes complete drainage difficult. Clot alone can compress the heart and cause tamponade-like physiology. The clinical presentation of acute intrapericardial hemorrhage is typically shock, and jugular venous distention may or may not be present because of venoconstriction and hypovolemia as previously described. Use of echocardiography in the emergency room in patients with unexplained dyspnea may be an important diagnostic tool.[38]

The Cardiac Catheterization and Electrophysiology Laboratories

Perforation of the heart, including coronary arteries and cardiac chambers, has become an increasingly important cause of pericardial tamponade. Common scenarios include electrophysiology procedures, where relatively stiff catheters are placed in the relatively thin walled structures of the right heart, including the right atrium, right ventricle, and the coronary venous system including the coronary sinus. Anticoagulation, when required for electrophysiology procedures, such as those involving left atrial ablation, raises the risk substantially. Perforation of coronary arteries occurs in particular with atheroablation devices such as those used for rotational atherectomy, directional atherectomy and lasers, with guidewires used in chronic total occlusions or injudiciously manipulated distal to the target lesion, and with oversized balloons and stents.[39] Even with normal sizing, settings such as myocardial bridges or ruptured balloons are associated with vessel perforation or rupture. A third setting is transseptal puncture, a resurgent technique because of burgeoning technologies requiring left atrial access[40] but associated with a significant risk of tamponade.[41] Besides left sided ablations, mitral valvuloplasties, and percutaneous circulatory bypass (with its intake source in the left atrium), transseptal puncture is required for a number of techniques under development, including left atrial appendage occlusion and percutaneous mitral valve repair. Other endovascular procedures associated with tamponade include myocardial biopsy and central venous line placement, as well as erosion of devices implanted across the atrial septum or in the left atrial appendage.[42]

The potentially catastrophic setting of free perforation during coronary interventions is usually readily diagnosable during the procedure, with free flow in the pericardium seen during coronary injection, sometimes before the patient shows any signs of hemodynamic deterioration. This is readily treatable with balloon occlusion of the coronary artery at the perforation site, pericardiocentesis if necessary, and excluding the fenestration with a covered stent. However, lower grade perforations that result in pooling of contrast or small adventitial craters can be more subtle. It is essential to discontinue anticoagulation on such patients and consider heparin reversal, and to ensure that personnel responsible for postprocedure management monitor the patient closely for hypotension and tachycardia. With transseptal punctures, hypotension at any time during the case, but especially after anticoagulation is administered should raise the possibility of tamponade. A quick and relatively specific finding in the catheterization laboratory is straightening and lack of motion of the left heart border on anteroposterior fluoroscopy associated with hypotension (and sometimes reflex bradycardia); rapid intervention is essential in these patients. Hypotension after the procedure should raise the possibility that left atrial access involved a “stitch perforation” whereby the needle exited the right atrium and then entered the left atrium through the pericardial space; this mishap is possible with low punctures and frequently manifests only when catheters are removed from the fenestration at the end of the procedure. In patients who have had pacemaker placement, tamponade can develop acutely or after considerable delay as in the case of lead erosion.[43]

Critical Care Units and Medical Wards

Tamponade in the critical care unit typically is due to complications of myocardial infarction, concomitant sepsis with purulent pericarditis, or hemorrhage into the pericardium because of anticoagulation (either iatrogenic or endogenous) or, most commonly, is secondary to neoplasms. In myocardial infarction, tamponade can be acute, secondary to massive or limited rupture, or somewhat more insidious in onset as part of Dressler’s syndrome, with hemodynamic compromise sometimes exacerbated by anticoagulation. Tamponade also can be iatrogenic, in particular, secondary to placement of various lines through the venous or arterial circulation. Uncommon causes of tamponade, even with pericardial effusions of sometimes significant size, are viral pericarditis, congestive heart failure, uremia, myxedema (Fig. 25-11), and connective tissue disorders.

In patients with malignancy, several possible causes of tamponade are seen, including tumor involvement in the

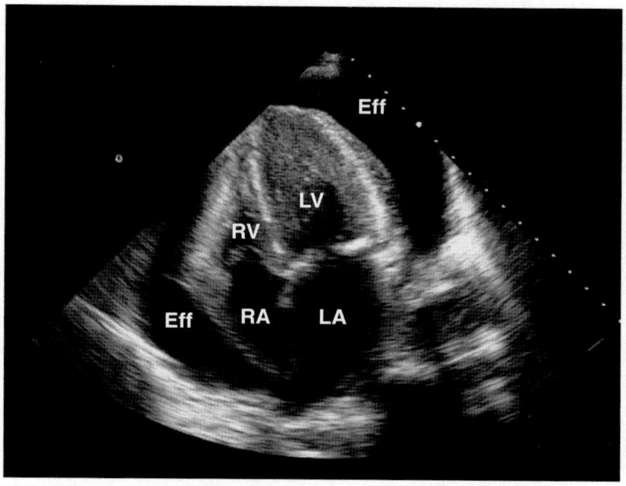

Figure 25-11. Echocardiogram showing large circumferential pericardial effusion in myxedema. Severe tamponade is rare. Eff, effusion; LA, left atrium; LV, left ventricle; RA, right atrium; RV, right ventricle.

pericardium, postradiation pericarditis, graft-versus-host disease, and direct or indirect complications of therapy.[44] Patients with malignancies also are at increased risk for infectious pericarditis, coagulopathies or thrombocytopenia with secondary hemorrhage, and hypothyroid- and hypoalbuminemia-related effusions. AIDS and other immunosuppressed patients similarly are predisposed to infectious tamponade, as well as pericardial tumor involvement, including that from lymphoma. The mechanisms of pericardial effusion in cancer are varied but include direct spread to the pericardium from primary tumors such as lung, mediastinal, and esophageal cancer; hematogenous spread such as with lymphomas; and obstruction of the lymphatic drainage of the heart by tumors in the mediastinum.

Tamponade after cardiac surgery is an important phenomenon, usually occurring as a result of hemorrhagic effusion. Early postoperative tamponade is not uncommon and is important to recognize as a cause of hypotension because it has been reported to occur with a frequency of 5% to 10%, although this generally is thought to be in the 1% range in the modern era.[45] Moderate to large pericardial effusions that do not cause hemodynamic compromise have been much more common.[46] Delayed tamponade after heart surgery, with onset on average at 2 to 3 weeks postoperatively but as late as 6 months or more, occurs in less than 1% of patients but is disproportionately more common in patients undergoing valve surgery, probably related to postoperative anticoagulation in this cohort.[47,48] Delayed tamponade probably is a variant of the more common postcardiotomy syndrome.

Late tamponade typically is due to loculated effusion resulting from formation of adhesions (see Figs. 25-6 and 25-8) during recovery from surgery. Such adhesions can cause decreased cardiac output if they compress the left side of the heart, and in some cases pulmonary edema occurs if obstruction to inflow results. A variety of clinical problems related to increased right-sided heart pressure occur when tamponade involves the right side, including a clinical picture that resembles superior vena cava syndrome; several case reports have described right to left shunting across a patent foramen ovale as well.[49] Pericardiectomy to prevent postoperative tamponade has an uncertain risk-benefit ratio but does appear to decrease the incidence of hemodynamic compromise.[50]

Patients on dialysis present a special diagnostic and management problem. With underdialysis, volume overload can exacerbate chronic fluid accumulation in the pericardial space. Hypotension during or after dialysis may be secondary to inadequate intravascular volume and diminished venous pressure and needs to be avoided as well.

MANAGEMENT

Pericardial tamponade is life-threatening, requiring difficult diagnostic and, in particular, management decisions. When hemodynamics do not suggest significant compromise and effusion is small to moderate in volume, intervention frequently is not necessary and may involve increased risk to the patient, whereas late intervention may be fatal. Typically, the risk associated with pericardiocentesis is inversely related to the volume of accumulated fluid and also is related to the location of the effusion. Thus, relatively small effusions, early in the course of tamponade, usually are located primarily posteriorly because of gravity-dependent accumulation. Waiting until the effusion is large and occupies significant volume anteriorly decreases the risk of percutaneous drainage but increases the possibility of decompensation and death before intervention. Frequent monitoring of hemodynamics and application of sound clinical judgment are essential, but an optimal algorithm does not exist. Comorbid conditions such as endogenous or extrinsic anticoagulation may substantially confound the situation.[51] The clinical decision to drain the effusion percutaneously or to send the patient for thoracotomy will be a function of the clinician's assessment of risk of the former versus the potential advantages of surgery in obtaining pericardial tissue and providing a pericardial window as well. If the percutaneous approach is chosen, performing pericardiocentesis in the cardiac catheterization laboratory has significant advantages. However, the benefit of positioning the pericardial effusion anteriorly, for increased safety during needle entry into the pericardial space, requires that the patient's chest be elevated during the procedure, which typically can be accomplished only to a 20- or 30-degree angle on most catheterization tables because of the image intensifier. A moribund patient frequently needs pericardiocentesis performed at the bedside without fluoroscopic guidance, sometimes without adequate hemodynamic monitoring, and at times without echocardiographic monitoring—all of which are associated with increased risk of failed pericardiocentesis and adverse cardiac events. Detailed discussion of interventions for tamponade can be found in Chapter 6.

Little in the way of medical treatment is clearly therapeutic for tamponade. Hydration in relatively acute tamponade will support right-sided filling in patients with low circulatory volumes, such as are seen in trauma. Patients with chronic tamponade typically have considerable fluid retention, and additional hydration is unlikely to be of benefit. Pressors may be modestly helpful, but for patients with preserved cardiac function, catecholaminergic drugs provide only modest augmentation of cardiac output. Vasodilator therapy is less clearly beneficial, and drugs that decrease preload, such as nitrates and nitroprusside, should be avoided if the patient is hypotensive. Reversal of anticoagulation is essential, both to stop bleeding into the pericardial space and to decrease the risk of trauma to the heart or major blood vessels during pericardiocentesis (e.g., coronary arteries, hepatic vessels). Antibiotic therapy in the setting of purulent pericarditis and tamponade is not expected to acutely relieve hemodynamic decompensation in most settings; postdrainage treatment, including local infusion of drugs, is discussed in Chapter 6. Patients with severe tamponade often are anxious and hypoxic; sedation is hazardous, as is intubation, although the latter is at times necessary. Because of associated positive intrathoracic pressure, ventilation may cause abrupt hemodynamic deterioration. Cardiopulmonary resuscitation using chest compression is unlikely to be effective; immediate pericardiocentesis or thoracotomy will be the only possibility for survival in such cases.

Acknowledgment

The author wishes to acknowledge Priscilla Peters for kindly providing Figures 25-6, 25-8, 25-10, and 25-11.

KEY POINTS

- Pericardial tamponade represents a continuum, ranging from effusions associated with little or no hemodynamic compromise to hemodynamic collapse.
- The primary physiologic feature of tamponade is impairment of cardiac chamber filling due to high intrapericardial pressure, with resultant decrease in cardiac output.
- Acute tamponade occurs after relatively limited accumulation of fluid in the setting of a nondistensible pericardium.
- Chronic tamponade may involve a pericardial effusion of 1 L or more; because hemodynamic decompensation occurs in the steep part of the pressure-volume curve, accumulation of a small amount of additional fluid can result in substantial hemodynamic deterioration.
- Pulsus paradoxus is seen in a variety of conditions besides cardiac tamponade and is absent despite tamponade in a number of settings. A large pericardial effusion and right ventricular collapse, a 10 to 20 mm Hg or larger decrease in systolic pressure with inspiration, and a significant decline in pulse pressure combined are specific for tamponade.
- Right atrial pressure, except in settings such as hypovolemia, usually is significantly elevated, but jugular venous distention may not be seen with acute tamponade.
- Despite markedly elevated right and left atrial pressures, pulmonary vascular congestion usually is not seen.
- Persistent high right atrial pressure after fluid drainage suggests effusive-constrictive disease, most commonly associated with malignancy but also seen with infection and acute pericarditis.
- Management of pericardial tamponade involves determining the optimal timing and method of intervention. Fluid and drug therapy constitute modest adjunctive care only.

REFERENCES

1. Hancock EW: Cardiac tamponade. Med Clin North Am 1979;63:223-237.
2. Little WC, Freeman GL: Pericardial disease. Circulation 2006;113: 1622-1632.
3. Spodick DH: Macrophysiology, microphysiology, and anatomy of the pericardium: A synopsis. Am Heart J 1992;124:1046-1051.
4. Brown KT, Getrajdman GI: Balloon dilation of the superior vena cava (SVC) resulting in SVC rupture and pericardial tamponade: A case report and brief review. Cardiovasc Intervent Radiol 2005;28:372-376.
5. Wynne J, Markis JE, Grossman W: Extrinsic compression of the heart by tumor masquerading as cardiac tamponade. Cathet Cardiovasc Diagn 1978;4:81-85.
6. Watkins MW, LeWinter MM: Physiologic role of the normal pericardium. Annu Rev Med 1993;44:171-180.
7. Hancock EW: Pericardial tamponade. In Parrillo JE, Dellinger RP (eds): Critical Care Medicine: Principles of Diagnosis and Management in the Adult. C.V. Mosby, Philadelphia, 2001, pp 453-463.
8. Ruskin J, Bache RJ, Rembert JC, et al: Pressure-flow studies in man: Effect of respiration on left ventricular stroke volume. Circulation 1973;48: 79-85.
9. Spodick DH: Acute cardiac tamponade. N Engl J Med 2003;349:684-690.
10. Gladych E, Goland S, Attali M, et al: Cardiac tamponade as a manifestation of tuberculosis. South Med J 2001;94:525-528.
11. Keefe DL: Cardiovascular emergencies in the cancer patient. Semin Oncol 2000;27:244-255.
12. Krantz MJ, Lee JK, Spodick DH: Repetitive yawning associated with cardiac tamponade. Am J Cardiol 2004;94:701-702.
13. Beck CS: Two cardiac compression triads. JAMA 1935;104:714-716.
14. Meltser H, Kalaria VG: Cardiac tamponade. Cathet Cardiovasc Interv 2005;64:245-255.
15. Goldstein JA: Cardiac tamponade, constrictive pericarditis, and restrictive cardiomyopathy. Curr Probl Cardiol 2004;29:503-567.
16. Klein LW: Diagnosis of cardiac tamponade in the presence of complex medical illness. Crit Care Med 2002;30:721-723.
17. Akinci SB, Gaine SP, Post W, et al: Cardiac tamponade in an orthotopic liver recipient with pulmonary hypertension. Crit Care Med 2002;30:699-701.
18. Gollapudi RR, Yeager M, Johnson AD: Left ventricular cardiac tamponade in the setting of cor pulmonale and circumferential pericardial effusion. Case report and review of the literature. Cardiol Rev 2005;13:214-217.
19. Jairath UC, Benotti JR, Spodick DH: Cardiac tamponade masking pulmonary embolism. Clin Cardiol 2001;24:485-486.
20. Shabetai R: Pericardial effusion: haemodynamic spectrum. Heart 2004;90:255-256.
21. Levine MJ, Lorell BH, Diver DJ, et al: Implications of echocardiographically assisted diagnosis of pericardial

tamponade in contemporary medical patients: Detection before hemodynamic embarrassment. J Am Coll Cardiol 1991;17:59-65.
22. Shaver JA, Reddy PS, Curtiss EI, et al: Noninvasive/invasive correlates of exaggerated ventricular interdependence in cardiac tamponade. J Cardiol 2001;37(Suppl 1):71-76.
23. Asher CR, Klein AL: Diastolic heart failure: Restrictive cardiomyopathy, constrictive pericarditis, and cardiac tamponade: Clinical and echocardiographic evaluation. Cardiol Rev 2002;10:218-229.
24. Price AS, Leech SJ, Sierzenski PR: Impending cardiac tamponade: A case report highlighting the value of bedside echocardiography. J Emerg Med 2006;30:415-419.
25. Blaivas M, DeBehnke D, Phelan MB: Potential errors in the diagnosis of pericardial effusion on trauma ultrasound for penetrating injuries. Acad Emerg Med 2000;7:1261-1266.
26. Come PC, Riley MF, Fortuin NJ: Echocardiographic mimicry of pericardial effusion. Am J Cardiol 1981;47:365-370.
27. Harries SR, Fox BM, Roobottom CA: Azygos reflux: A CT sign of cardiac tamponade. Clin Radiol 1998;53:702-704.
28. Fowler NO: Cardiac tamponade. A clinical or an echocardiographic diagnosis? Circulation 1993;87:1738-1741.
29. Reddy PS, Curtiss EI, Uretsky BF: Spectrum of hemodynamic changes in cardiac tamponade. Am J Cardiol 1990;66:1487-1491.
30. Sagrista-Sauleda J, Angel J, Sanchez A, et al: Effusive-constrictive pericarditis. N Engl J Med 2004;350:469-475.
31. Sagrista-Sauleda J, Permanyer-Miralda G, Candell-Riera J, et al: Transient cardiac constriction: An unrecognized pattern of evolution in effusive acute idiopathic pericarditis. Am J Cardiol 1987;59:961-966.
32. Sagrista-Sauleda J, Angel J, Sambola A, et al: Low-pressure cardiac tamponade: Clinical and hemodynamic profile. Circulation 2006;114:945-952.
33. Ramsaran EK, Benotti JR, Spodick DH: Exacerbated tamponade: Deterioration of cardiac function by lowering excessive arterial pressure in hypertensive cardiac tamponade. Cardiology 1995;86:77-79.
34. Tyburski JG, Astra L, Wilson RF, et al: Factors affecting prognosis with penetrating wounds of the heart. J Trauma 2000;48:587-590.
35. Grove CA, Lemmon G, Anderson G, et al: Emergency thoracotomy: Appropriate use in the resuscitation of trauma patients. Am Surg 2002;68:313-316.
36. Huang CH, Chang Y, Chan WS, et al: Acute cardiovascular collapse after pericardial drainage in a patient with aortic dissection. Acta Anaesthesiol Taiwan 2005;43:39-42.
37. Isselbacher EM, Cigarroa JE, Eagle KA: Cardiac tamponade complicating proximal aortic dissection. Is pericardiocentesis harmful? Circulation 1994;90:2375-2378.
38. Blaivas M: Incidence of pericardial effusion in patients presenting to the emergency department with unexplained dyspnea. Acad Emerg Med 2001;8:1143-1146.
39. Ellis SG, Ajluni S, Arnold AZ, et al: Increased coronary perforation in the new device era. Incidence, classification, management, and outcome. Circulation 1994;90:2725-2730.
40. Solomon SB: The future of interventional cardiology lies in the left atrium. Int J Cardiovasc Intervent 2004;6:101-106.
41. Turi ZG: Puncturing the septum: Resurgent technique with inherent risk. J Invasive Cardiol 2004;16:3-4.
42. Amin Z, Hijazi ZM, Bass JL, et al: Erosion of Amplatzer septal occluder device after closure of secundum atrial septal defects: review of registry of complications and recommendations to minimize future risk. Cathet Cardiovasc Interv 2004;63:496-502.
43. Eberhardt F, Bode F, Bonnemeier H, et al: Long term complications in single and dual chamber pacing are influenced by surgical experience and patient morbidity. Heart 2005;91:500-506.
44. Retter AS: Pericardial disease in the oncology patient. Heart Dis 2002;4:387-391.
45. Kuvin JT, Harati NA, Pandian NG, et al: Postoperative cardiac tamponade in the modern surgical era. Ann Thorac Surg 2002;74:1148-1153.
46. Stevenson LW, Child JS, Laks H, et al: Incidence and significance of early pericardial effusions after cardiac surgery. Am J Cardiol 1984;54:848-851.
47. Meurin P, Weber H, Renaud N, et al: Evolution of the postoperative pericardial effusion after day 15: The problem of the late tamponade. Chest 2004;125:2182-2187.
48. Mangi AA, Palacios IF, Torchiana DF: Catheter pericardiocentesis for delayed tamponade after cardiac valve operation. Ann Thorac Surg 2002;73:1479-1483.
49. Sandifer DP, Gonzalez JL: Refractory postoperative hypoxemia associated with regional cardiac tamponade and patent foramen ovale. Crit Care Med 1997;25:1608-1611.
50. Asimakopoulos G, Della SR, Taggart DP: Effects of posterior pericardiotomy on the incidence of atrial fibrillation and chest drainage after coronary revascularization: A prospective randomized trial. J Thorac Cardiovasc Surg 1997;113:797-799.
51. Maisch B, Ristic AD: Practical aspects of the management of pericardial disease. Heart 2003;89:1096-1103.

Chapter 26

Severe Sepsis and Multiple Organ Dysfunction

Sergio L. Zanotti-Cavazzoni, R. Phillip Dellinger, and Joseph E. Parrillo

The term sepsis is derived from the Greek word *sepsin*, which means "to make putrid." The relationship between infection and sepsis has been recognized for many years. However, the precise mechanisms by which infection results in sepsis, severe sepsis, septic shock, or multiple organ dysfunction remain to be fully elucidated. Improvements in our understanding of this syndrome have led to the development of novel therapeutic strategies and have increased our appreciation for the complex interactions that exist in sepsis between pathogens and the host response to infection. Despite these advances, severe sepsis remains one of the most significant causes of morbidity and mortality in patients admitted to the intensive care unit (ICU).[1] In this chapter we discuss the current definitions, epidemiology, and pathogenesis of severe sepsis and multiple organ dysfunction. In addition, we review current management options and discuss an approach to treatment based on pathophysiology.

DEFINITIONS

For many years sepsis was loosely applied in clinical practice and was applied to a very heterogeneous patient population. With recognition of this problem, a consensus conference was convened to create standardized definitions and formulate a blueprint to guide future research in sepsis.[2] The term *systemic inflammatory response syndrome* (SIRS) was introduced. SIRS can occur in response to a variety of severe clinical insults and is defined by the presence of two or more of the following conditions: (1) temperature higher than 38°C or lower than 36°C, (2) heart rate greater than 90 beats per minute, (3) respiratory rate higher than 20 breaths per minute or a $Pa{CO_2}$ lower than 32 mm Hg, and (4) white blood cell count more than 12,000 or less than 4000 cells/mm^3. *Sepsis* occurs when SIRS is caused by infection. *Severe sepsis* is sepsis with associated organ dysfunction, hypoperfusion, or hypotension. Hypoperfusion and perfusion abnormalities may include, but are not limited to, lactic acidosis, oliguria, or an acute alteration in mental status. *Septic shock* is defined by the presence of sepsis-induced hypotension (systolic blood pressure less than 90 mm Hg or a reduction of more than 40 mm Hg from baseline in the absence of other causes for hypotension), despite adequate fluid resuscitation along with the presence of perfusion abnormalities.[2]

The introduction of these definitions created a common language that was especially helpful in designing and defining populations for clinical trials.[3] On the other hand, criticism of these definitions pointed out that they were too sensitive and were not useful when applied clinically to individual patients.[4] In 2001, a second consensus conference with a broader representation was convened to revisit the definitions.[5] The conference recommended keeping the 1992 definitions unchanged secondary to lack of new evidence to support new definitions. However, the conference also recommended expanding the diagnostic criteria for sepsis in an effort to enhance recognition at the bedside (Table 26-1). In addition, the PIRO system—consisting of the domains predisposition, insult infection, response, and organ dysfunction—for staging sepsis was proposed. This staging system is in its initial phases, and further development and research are needed before its implementation in clinical practice. Examples and possible measures for the future in each domain are shown (Table 26-2).

EPIDEMIOLOGY

Severe sepsis constitutes a major health care problem. Recent studies have expanded our understanding of the epidemiology and impact of this disease.[6-8] Current estimates of the incidence of severe sepsis in the United States report that approximately 750,000 cases occur per year (3.0 cases per 1000 population).[6] Almost 70% of these cases receive care in a high-dependency unit (ICU, intermediate care unit, or coronary care unit).[6] The inci-

Table 26-1. Diagnostic Criteria for Sepsis in Addition to Infection*	
Clinical findings	Temperature: >38.3°C *or* <36°C Heart rate: >90 beats/min *or* >2 SD above normal value for age Arterial hypotension: Systolic blood pressure (SBP) <90 mm Hg *or* Mean arterial pressure <70 mm Hg *or* Decrease in SBP of >40 mm Hg in adults *or* 1 SD below normal for age Tachypnea Decreased capillary refill or mottling Altered mental status Significant edema or positive fluid balances
Hemodynamic or laboratory findings	Mixed venous oxygen saturation (SvO_2) >70% Cardiac index >3.5 L/min/M² Hyperglycemia in the absence of diabetes White blood cell count: >12,000 cells/μL *or* <4000 cells/μL *or* Normal white with >10% immature forms Plasma C-reactive protein >2 SD above the normal value Plasma procalcitonin 2 SD above the normal value Hyperlactatemia (serum lactate >1 mmol/L)
Evidence of organ dysfunction	Arterial hypoxemia (PaO_2/FIO_2<300) Acute oliguria Serum creatinine increase >0.5 mg/dL Coagulation abnormalities: International Normalized Ratio >1.5 *or* Partial thromboplastin time >60 s Ileus Thrombocytopenia Hyperbilirubinemia

*Criteria include presence of documented or suspected infection plus at least two of the features listed in the table.

dence of severe sepsis and septic shock has risen over time both in North America and in Europe.[6-8] The incidence of severe sepsis is projected to increase by 1.5% every year.[6] These rises in incidence are attributed to an aging population containing a growing number of patients who have compromised immune systems (due to increases in organ transplantation and cancer chemotherapy), are infected with resistant pathogens, and are undergoing prolonged, high-risk surgical interventions.[8] Severe sepsis is more common with age, in males, and in nonwhite patients.[6,8] Before the mid-1980s, gram-negative bacteria were the most common pathogens responsible for severe sepsis. Over the years an increase in proportion of cases from gram-positive bacteria has been reported, and currently, gram-positive bacteria are the predominant pathogens in severe sepsis.[8] The incidence of sepsis due to fungal organisms has increased substantially over the last 20 years.[8] The most common sites of infection are the respiratory system, the bloodstream, and the genitourinary tract.[6,7,9]

Although mortality rates for severe sepsis and septic shock have slightly decreased over time, they still remain elevated (approximately 28% and 55% respectively).[6,7,10] Mortality is higher with age and with larger number of failing organs in black men.[8] Over time the hospital length of stay for patients with sepsis has shortened, and the number of discharges to nonacute medical care facilities has risen.[8] In addition to causing high morbidity and mortality, severe sepsis has a significant economic impact. Estimates report an average cost per patient of $22,000, representing an annual impact to the health care system in excess of $16.5 billion in the United States alone.[6]

PATHOPHYSIOLOGY

Severe sepsis is the end result of complex interactions between infecting organisms and the host response. Important components of this host response in the early phases of sepsis are the immune system, activation of the inflammatory cascade, and alterations in hemostasis. In later stages, organ failure, immunosuppression, and apoptosis play important pathophysiologic roles. Char-

Table 26-2. The PIRO System for Staging Sepsis

Domain	Present	Future
Predisposition	Premorbid conditions, age, and sex	Genetic polymorphism in components of the inflammatory response (e.g., tumor necrosis factor)
Insult infection	Culture and sensitivity testing of pathogens Identification of possible target for source control	Assays of specific microbial products and gene transcript profiles
Response	Systemic inflammatory response syndrome Other signs of sepsis Septic shock Presence of C-reactive protein	Markers of activated inflammation or impaired host responsiveness
Organ dysfunction	Organ dysfunction as number of failing organs or composite scores	Measure of cellular response to insult-apoptosis, cytopathic hypoxia, cell stress

Adapted from Levy M, Fink MP, Marshall JC, et al: 2001 SCCM/ESICM/ACCP/ATS/SIS International Sepsis Definitions Conference. Crit Care Med 2003;31:1250-1256.

acteristics of both the infecting organism and the host response influence the outcome of sepsis. Virulence factors, high burden of infection, and resistance to antibiotics are all organism characteristics associated with higher risk of severe sepsis. A growing body of literature suggests that host responses are influenced by genetic polymorphisms.[11-16] Such influence might offer an explanation as to why some patients have severe sepsis in reaction to a particular pathogen and others do not. We further discuss some of the relevant components of the host response in severe sepsis.

Role of the Immune System in the Early Phases of Sepsis

The immune response to infection takes place through the actions of two pathways, the innate immune system and the adaptive immune system. The goal of the innate immune system is to provide protection in the first minutes to hours after an infectious challenge. Although it was initially thought to be a nonspecific response, research has demonstrated that the innate immune system recognizes pathogens by means of pattern-recognition receptors called *Toll-like receptors* (TLRs; Table 26-3). These receptors bind to highly conserved structures on microorganisms, which are not easily altered by microbes to evade detection and are present on broad groups of organisms.[17] Our current understanding of TLRs suggests that the immune cells use different TLRs to detect several features of an organism, and generate a tailored response to the invading pathogen on the basis of the composite information gained.[17] Activation of TLRs by microorganisms stimulates signaling pathways that increase production of proinflammatory cytokines, such as tumor necrosis factor-alpha (TNF-α), interleukin-1β (IL-1β), and nuclear factor-κB (NF-κB), as well as anti-inflammatory cytokines, such as IL-10.[17,18] TLR activation also results in upregulation of microbial killing mechanisms, such as the production of reactive nitrogen species.[19] TLRs play a pivotal role in initiating the innate immune response and are important regulators of the adaptive immune response to infection. Recognition of these proteins and their functions expanded our understanding of the pathophysiology of sepsis and has provided a new target for therapeutic interventions.[20]

The adaptive immune system amplifies the response initiated by the innate immune system with a higher degree of specificity. In addition to their interactions with the innate immune system, microorganisms stimulate specific cell-mediated and humoral adaptive immune responses. Two types of lymphocytes, B cells and T cells, play an important role in the adaptive immune response. Adaptive immune responses (humoral and cellular) require days to develop. However, they are amnestic through the generation of memory T and B lymphocytes, and in case of reexposure to the same pathogen, they can elicit a faster response. CD4+ T cells are divided into two types, type 1 helper T (Th1) cells and type 2 helper T (Th2) cells. Factors such as type of organism, site of infection, and burden of infection influence the response elicited by T cells. In general, Th1 cells secrete proinflammatory cytokines (TNF-α and interleukin-1β), and Th2 cells anti-inflammatory cytokines (IL-4 and IL-10).[21] B lymphocytes are responsible for releasing immunoglobulins in response to microorganisms. These immunoglobulins bind to organism-specific antigens and enhance their recognition and destruction by other immune cells (natural killer cells and neutrophils). Several other cell types are also involved in the adaptive immune response to infection (Fig. 26-1).

Table 26-3. Role of Toll-Like Receptors (TLRs) in Pathogen Recognition and Pathophysiology of Human Disease

Toll-Like Receptor	Pathogen or Disease State
TLR1	Lyme disease *Neisseria meningitidis*
TLR2	*Myobacterium tuberculosis* Chagas disease Leptospirosis Fungal sepsis Cytomegalovirus viremia
TLR3	Many
TLR4	Gram-negative bacteria Septic shock *Chlamydia trachomatis* *Chlamydia pneumoniae* Certain viruses *M. tuberculosis*
TLR5	Flagellated bacteria, e.g., *Salmonella*
TLR7	Viral infections
TLR8	Viral infections
TLR9	Bacterial and viral infections
TLR10	Unknown

Role of Inflammation

For many years, the prevailing theory has been that sepsis is the result of an uncontrolled inflammatory response.[1,2] This paradigm was based on extensive animal experimentation with models of inflammation that may not necessarily reflect human disease. Animal models of sepsis that used large doses of endotoxin or bacteria created a "cytokine storm." Early blockage of this cytokine storm resulted in improvements in mortality. Most human patients with sepsis, however, have a complex host response that involves activation of both proinflammatory and anti-inflammatory cascades. Early death from overwhelming inflammation is not the norm, and most patients who eventually die have complications related to immunosuppression, apoptosis, and multiple organ failure later in the course of the disease. These differences may partially explain why so many anti-inflammatory compounds worked in animal models yet failed to improve mortality in human clinical trials.

The interplay among proinflammatory cytokines, anti-inflammatory cytokines, and cytokine inhibitors is a dynamic process that influences the host response to sepsis. Proinflammatory cytokines such as TNF-α and IL-1β increase early in sepsis and have overlapping and synergistic effects in further stimulating the inflammatory

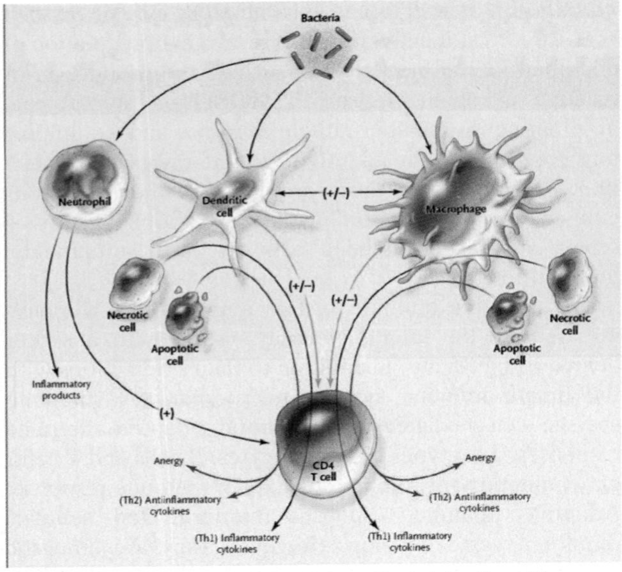

Figure 26-1. Response of immune cells to infection. The immune response to pathogens involves various types of cells. Crosstalk exists between the different cell lines of the immune system (dendritic cells, macrophages, lymphocytes, and neutrophils). The + sign represents upregulation, and the – sign downregulation. Many interactions on the figure have both + and – signs, representing the possibility of either upregulation or downregulation, depending on a variety of factors. (Adapted from Hotchkiss RS: The pathophysiology and treatment of sepsis. N Engl J Med 2003;348:138-150, figure 1, p. 140.)

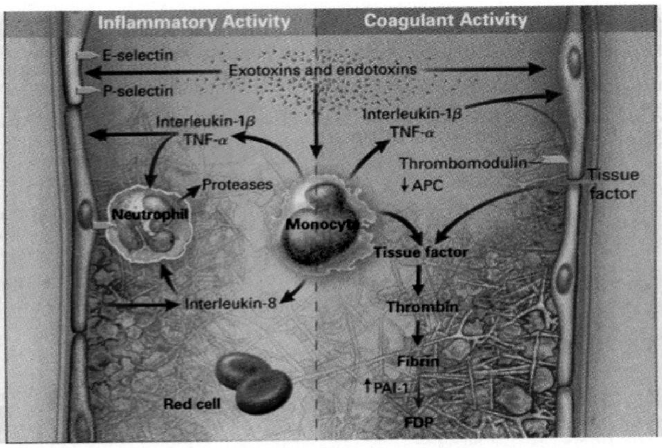

Figure 26-2. Relationship between inflammatory and coagulation systems in sepsis. Monocytes are activated by endotoxins and exotoxins from bacteria and release tumor necrosis factor-alpha (TNF-α) and interleukin-1β (IL-1β). TNF-α and IL-1β activate the inflammatory cascade via neutrophils and the production of other proinflammatory cytokines, and, in combination with tissue factor, also activate the coagulation cascade, with production of fibrin and fibrin degradation products (FDP). APC, activated protein C. (Adapted from Matthay MA: Severe sepsis: A new treatment with both anticoagulant and anti-inflammatory properties. N Engl J Med 2001;344:759-762, figure 1A, p. 761.)

cascade.[22] Later studies using in vitro preparations of myocardial cells and serum from human patients with sepsis have demonstrated that both TNF-α and IL-1β directly depress myocyte contractility.[23] This effect is synergistically larger when myocardial cells are exposed to both TNF-α and IL-1β. Proinflammatory cytokines activate monocytes, macrophages, and neutrophils, stimulate neutrophil margination, and increase gluconeogenesis. In addition, proinflammatory cytokines have an important role in the development of clinical abnormalities such as fever, hypotension, capillary leakage with decreased intravascular volume, and myocardial depression.[22] Proinflammatory cytokines such as macrophage migration inhibitory factor (MIF) and high mobility group 1 (HMG-1) protein have received attention as downstream mediators of inflammation and potential therapeutic targets.[24-27]

The role of anti-inflammatory cytokines in sepsis is still not fully understood. Current understanding suggests that sepsis-induced multiple organ failure and death may be caused, in part, by a shift to an anti-inflammatory phenotype and by apoptosis of key immune cells.[28] This shift is driven partially by increased levels of anti-inflammatory cytokines and results from a shift in helper T-cell populations (from Th1 to Th2).[29] Inflammation plays an important role in the host response to sepsis. It is now apparent that simple therapeutic strategies that block specific proinflammatory cytokines are insufficient to modulate this response. As our understanding of the intricate relationship between proinflammatory and anti-inflammatory responses improves, we might become more successful in modulating these responses to improve patient outcomes.

Alterations of Hemostasis

Another important factor in the pathophysiology of sepsis is the alteration of the hemostatic balance. In sepsis this balance is altered by a rise in procoagulant factors paired with a drop in anticoagulant factors (Fig. 26-2). Under normal conditions the intraluminal vascular surface has anticoagulant properties. During sepsis, stimulation from cytokines promotes expression of tissue factor on endothelial cells, monocytes, and neutrophils.[30] Tissue factor triggers the extrinsic coagulation pathway by activating factor VII. Activation of the extrinsic pathway leads to the formation of thrombin. The intrinsic pathway is triggered by activation of factor XI and leads to amplification of the coagulation cascade with further formation of thrombin. Excessive coagulation is normally counterbalanced by several anticoagulant factors. Anticoagulant factors such as antithrombin III, activated protein C, protein S, and tissue factor pathway inhibitor are decreased in sepsis.[31] These circumstances push the hemostatic balance toward the procoagulant state. Activation of the coagulation cascade leads to a consumption of coagulation factors.

The clinical expression of this phenomenon is disseminated intravascular coagulation (DIC). DIC is characterized by a consumptive coagulopathy, which can raise the risk of bleeding but more commonly in sepsis causes damage by raising the risk of thrombosis. In sepsis the excessive formation of fibrin from thrombin, compounded by the suppression of fibrinolysis and the impairment of anticoagulant pathways, leads to widespread formation of microthrombi. It has been proposed that these microthrombi cause microcirculatory alterations and play an integral role in the pathogenesis of organ failure.[32,33]

MANAGEMENT

Severe sepsis is a medical emergency. When one considers its morbidity and the relationship between number of organ failures and mortality (Fig. 26-3), it makes sense to treat patients on an emergency basis and to institute therapies that can prevent the progression of organ failure and improve outcomes in a time-sensitive fashion. Several therapies for severe sepsis have a potential time-sensitive effect on outcome—that is, they have a higher likelihood of improving outcomes when instituted early than when instituted with time delays (Box 26-1). Although severe sepsis is associated with a higher mortality than other diseases considered medical emergencies, such as trauma, acute ischemic stroke, and acute myocardial infarction, it is still not regarded with the same degree of urgency. This difference may be secondary to difficulties in recognizing severe sepsis early and to a lack of understanding of its consequences and their therapeutic implications on the part of physicians outside the ICU.

In recognition of these problems, the Society of Critical Care Medicine (SCCM), the European Society of Intensive Care Medicine (ESICM), and the International Sepsis Forum (ISF) created the Surviving Sepsis Campaign (SSC). The SSC brings together experts in the field of sepsis from around the world and is endorsed by more than ten international medical societies and the Institute for Healthcare Improvement (www.ihi.gov). The goals of the campaign are to improve standards of patient care, secure funding for research, and ultimately reduce the mortality of severe sepsis by 25% worldwide. In order to achieve these goals, the campaign first published evidence-based practice guidelines and consensus recommendations for the management of patients with severe sepsis.[34] In order to increase the impact of these clinical guidelines at the bedside, the SCC created the concept of "sepsis bundles."[35] The *sepsis resuscitation bundle* should be implemented over the first 6 hours after recognition of a patient with severe sepsis, and the *sepsis management bundle,* over the first 24 hours of admission to the hospital. Small nonrandomized studies have shown that compliance with the bundles and application of their clinical recommendations in the form of protocols can improve patient outcomes.[36,37] The practice guidelines and the sepsis bundles are summarized in Figure 26-4 and Box 26-2.

One of the constructive criticisms of the first SSC guidelines publication was the use of the adapted Sackett evidence-based medicine (EBM) grading system. At the time of the first guidelines process, this system was being used for EBM by both the SCCM and the ACCP. A limitation of this system was that it used quality of evidence as the sole criterion for grading recommendations. Many considered this principle problematic because recommendations that are not amenable to clinical trials will, by definition, have low levels of quality of evidence. For example, in the first guidelines process, early administration of antibiotics received a grade E (expert opinion) rating, whereas interventions such as early goal-directed therapy received a grade B rating on the basis of one large randomized clinical trial. This problem has been remedied in the revision by the addition of a strength of recommendation grading of either 1 (strong) or 2 (weak). Variables used for determining the strength of recommendation include not only quality of evidence but also risk of intervention, cost of intervention, consistency of literature support, and ability to perform clinical trials in the presence of general acceptance of the intervention being graded. Therefore, for example, early use of antibiotics becomes a 1C recommendation in the revision; the 1 (strong) designation is bestowed because (1) clinical trials will never be performed in which subjects with severe sepsis are randomly assigned to receive either immediate or delayed antibiotic therapy and (2) the intervention is known to be both safe and relatively inexpensive. The C grade is related to the change in the level of evidence grades for the revision from five grades (A to E) to four (A to D) as well as to the 2006 retrospective database study supporting the beneficial effect of early antibiotic administration in patients with septic shock.[38]

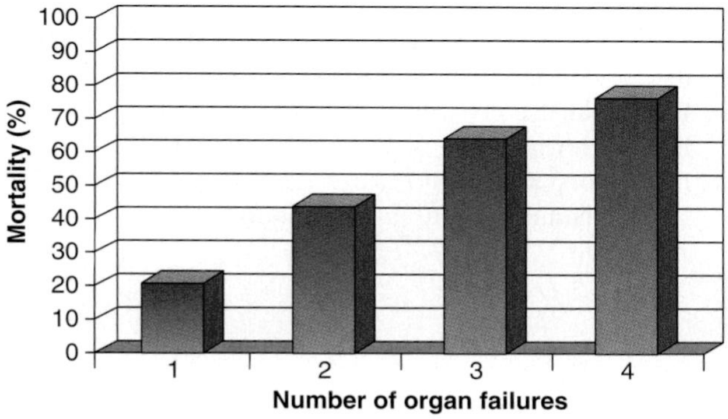

Figure 26-3. Relationship between number of organ failures and mortality. As the number of organ failures rises, mortality from severe sepsis progressively increases. With four organ failures, for example, mortality approaches 80%. (Data from Angus D, Linde-Zwirble WT, Clermont G, et al: Epidemiology of neonatal respiratory failure in the United States: Projections from California and New York. Crit Care Med 2001;29:1303-1310.)

Box 26-1

Therapeutic Interventions for Sepsis That Are Probably Time Sensitive

Antimicrobial treatment
Goal-directed resuscitation
Drotrecogin alfa (activated)
Corticosteroids in shock
Mechanical ventilation
Blood glucose control

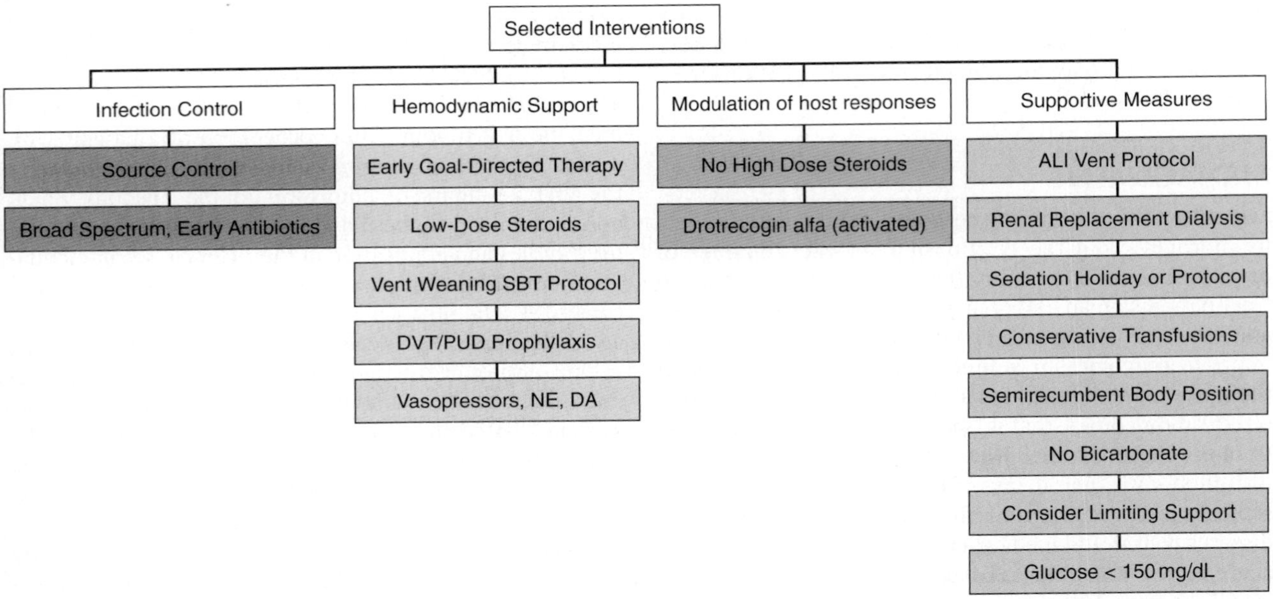

Figure 26-4. Surviving Sepsis Campaign guidelines. Treatment guideline recommendations are grouped according to type of intervention (infection management, hemodynamic support, modulation of the host response, and supportive therapies). ALI, acute lung injury; DA, dopamine; DVT, deep vein thrombosis; NE, norepinephrine; PUD, peptic ulcer disease. (Data from Dellinger RP, Carlet JM, Masur H, et al: Surviving Sepsis Campaign guidelines for management of severe sepsis and septic shock. Crit Care Med 2004;32:858-873.)

Box 26-2

Sepsis Bundles

Sepsis Resuscitation Bundle

To be started immediately and completed within 6 hours:

- Serum lactate measured.
- Blood culture specimens obtained prior to antibiotic administration.
- From the time of presentation, broad-spectrum antibiotics administered within 3 hours for ED admissions and 1 hour for non-ED intensive care unit (ICU) admissions.
- In the event of hypotension and/or lactate >4 mmol/L (36 mg/dL):
  - Deliver an initial minimum of 20 mL/kg of crystalloid (or colloid equivalent).
  - Apply vasopressors for hypotension not responding to initial fluid resuscitation to maintain mean arterial pressure ≥65 mm Hg.
- In the event of persistent hypotension despite fluid resuscitation (septic shock) and/or lactate >4 mmol/L (36 mg/dL):
  - Achieve central venous pressure of ≥8 mm Hg.
  - Achieve central venous oxygen saturation (Scv_{O_2}) of ≥70; achieving a mixed venous oxygen saturation (Sv_{O_2}) of 65% is an acceptable alternative.

Sepsis Management Bundle

To be started immediately and completed within 24 hours:

- Low-dose corticosteroids administered for septic shock in accordance with a standardized hospital policy.
- Drotrecogin alfa (activated) administered in accordance with a standardized hospital policy.
- Blood glucose control maintained at or above lower limit of normal, but >150 mg/dL (8.3 mmol/L).
- Inspiratory plateau pressures kept below 30 cm H_2O for mechanically ventilated patients.

As in other medical emergencies, the first priority in treating patients with severe sepsis should be assessing and optimizing the ABCs of respiration (airway, breathing, and circulation). In conjunction with initial stabilization of physiologic abnormalities, one should initiate appropriate diagnostic interventions to assess potential sources of infection and severity of organ dysfunction. Therapeutic interventions for severe sepsis should be implemented quickly and concomitantly. For the sake of discussion, our approach to treatment of severe sepsis is based on the pathophysiologic abnormalities produced by the syndrome (Fig. 26-5). We discuss in further detail management of the infectious insult, hemodynamic optimization, modulation of the host response, and supportive therapies.

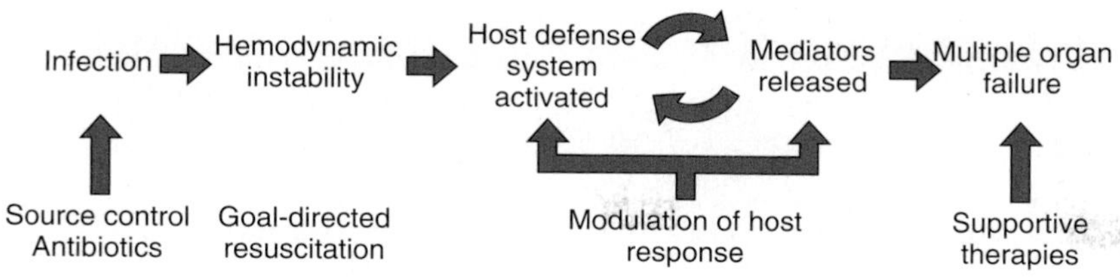

Figure 26-5. Approach to treatment of severe sepsis.

INFECTION MANAGEMENT

Severe sepsis is initiated by an infectious insult. Therefore, infection management constitutes one of the cornerstones of treatment in affected patients. Infection management consists of source control and the administration of appropriate, empirically selected antimicrobial agents that are effective against presumed causative pathogens. Administration of appropriate antibiotics is a time-sensitive intervention. Administration of antibiotics is often delayed, and the delay can result in worse outcomes.[39] Delays in appropriate antibiotic administration are much more likely to result from system failures (e.g., order not written by physician, delay in transport of agent from pharmacy) than from bacteriologic resistance.[40] Current guidelines recommend that appropriate antibiotics be administered to patients with severe sepsis within 1 hour of diagnosis.[34] The 2006 retrospective database study already mentioned was performed in a large group of septic shock patients; its results suggest that every hour that appropriate antibiotic therapy is delayed after onset of hypotension, the odds ratio for death increases in a stepwise manner.[38] The goal should be to administer appropriate antibiotics as soon as possible in patients with severe sepsis. In order to accomplish it, hospitals must examine their individual dynamics and devise systems to optimize antibiotic administration.

Studies in patients with sepsis have reported an incidence of positive blood culture results in the range of 20% to 50%.[8,41-43] Considering the growing need for regimens using broad-spectrum, empirically chosen agents and the need to narrow antimicrobial regimens in order to decrease resistance, obtaining blood culture specimens prior to administration of antibiotics is essential. In most cases one must start antibiotic therapy without bacteriologic confirmation of the causative pathogen. Studies have demonstrated that the appropriateness of initial antibiotic therapy has a significant effect on patient outcomes.[44,45] In one prospective cohort study of critically ill patients, inadequacy of initial antibiotic therapy was associated with statistically significant increase in all-cause and infection-related hospital mortality.[46] Factors associated with administration of inadequate antibiotics included prior administration of antibiotics, bloodstream infections, rising Acute Physiology And Chronic Health Evaluation (APACHE) II scores, and decreasing age.[46] If one considers the detrimental effect on mortality, it is apparent that in patients with severe sepsis, one cannot afford to miss potential causative organisms when empirically selecting an antimicrobial regimen. Choice of antibiotics should be based on the following factors:

- Probable pathogens, based on clinical diagnosis and source of infection (e.g., pneumonia, bloodstream infection, abdominal source)
- Site where infection was acquired (community vs. hospital)
- Results obtained from diagnostic tests such as Gram staining
- Resistance patterns of local and hospital bacterial flora
- Patient comorbidities, drug allergies, and previous antibiotic exposure

Initial antibiotic therapy for severe sepsis should be broad in spectrum and then progressively narrowed as microbiologic data become available. In culture-negative patients, de-escalation of antibiotics may become challenging. In such cases clinical evolution can be used to guide decisions. A detailed discussion of specific antibiotic regimens is beyond the scope of this chapter; for this, the reader is referred to other chapters and to a synopsis offered in Table 26-4.

The term *source control* refers to measures implemented to control the source of infection. Source control interventions can be divided into the three broad categories (1) drainage of an abscess, (2) débridement/drainage/incision of infected tissue, and (3) removal of an infected foreign body.[47] Attention to identifying potential sources amenable to source control measures should be part of the initial evaluation of patients with sepsis. The timing of intervention depends on several factors. When source interventions are simple, such as removal of an infected central venous catheter, they should be implemented immediately. In cases of unstable patients in whom surgery might be required, delaying source control while optimizing hemodynamic status may be appropriate. Finally, for problems such as necrotizing fasciitis, in which delays carry a significant risk of raising mortality, one must proceed to surgery as early as possible. Examples of specific source control measures in patients with sepsis are given in Table 26-5.

Hemodynamic Optimization

Severe sepsis is associated with a host of hemodynamic abnormalities. These abnormalities can ultimately lead to sepsis-induced tissue hypoperfusion if not addressed early and aggressively. The hemodynamic profile of severe sepsis and septic shock is initially characterized by components of hypovolemic, cardiogenic, and distributive shock.[48] In the initial phases of resuscitation, addressing the hypovolemic component is most important. Early in sepsis, increased capillary leak and greater venous capacitance will result in effective hypovolemia with reduced venous return to the heart. Low intravascular volume paired with

Table 26-4. Antibiotic Selection for Sepsis Based on Site of Infection

Site	Bacteria	First-Line Agent(s)	Second-Line Agent(s)
Abdominal			
Primary peritonitis	Enterobacteriaceae *Streptococcus pneumoniae* *Enterococcus faecalis*	Third-generation cephalosporins: Cefotaxime	Quinolones Imipenem-cilastatin Piperacillin-tazobactam
Secondary peritonitis	Aerobic gram-negatives *Bacteroides fragilis* *Enterococcus* species *Pseudomonas aeruginosa* *Candida* species	Ceftriaxone Imipenem-cilastatin Imipenem-cilastatin ± aminoglycoside Imipenem-cilastatin ± aminoglycoside ± amphotericin B	Antipseudomonal β-lactam Third-generation cephalosporin ± metronidazole Quinolone ± metronidazole Third-generation cephalosporin ± aminoglycoside ± amphotericin B
Tertiary peritonitis	*Enterococcus* species *Candida* species *Staphylococcus epidermidis*		Antipseudomonal β-lactam Third-generation cephalosporin ± aminoglycoside ± amphotericin B
Genitourinary	Gram-negatives	Quinolones Third-generation cephalosporins	
Intravascular			
Catheter-related	*Staphylococcus aureus* *S. epidermidis* Gram-negatives	Vancomycin ± extended-spectrum cephalosporin ± aminoglycoside	
Lung			
Early (community-acquired)	*S. pneumoniae* *Legionella* species *Mycoplasma pneumoniae* *Chlamydia* species *S. aureus* *Haemophilus* species *Klebsiella* species	Third-generation cephalosporins plus macrolide ± vancomycin Ceftriaxone Cefotaxime Ceftizoxime	Quinolones Antipseudomonal β-lactam ± quinolone Imipenem-cilastatin ± aminoglycoside
Late (nosocomial)	*P. aeruginosa* *S. aureus* (methicillin-resistant) *Enterobacter* species *Klebsiella* species *Escherichia coli* *Acinetobacter* species	Antipseudomonal β-lactam + vancomycin ± aminoglycoside	Fourth-generation cephalosporin

Table 26-5. Source Control Techniques

Drainage	Intra-abdominal abscess Thoracic empyema Septic arthritis Pyelonephritis, cholangitis
Débridement	Necrotizing fasciitis Infected pancreatic necrosis Intestinal infarction Mediastinitis
Device removal	Infected vascular catheter Urinary catheter Colonized endotracheal tube Infected intrauterine contraceptive device
Definitive control	Sigmoid resection for diverticulitis Cholecystectomy for gangrenous cholecystitis Amputation for clostridial myonecrosis

sepsis-induced myocardial depression will lead to a decrease in stroke volume. Administration of intravascular fluids can alter this early phase of sepsis characterized by hypovolemia, tachycardia, and depressed cardiac output. Initial steps in hemodynamic optimization for patients with severe sepsis should include evaluation for signs of sepsis-induced tissue hypoperfusion. Signs of global hypoperfusion, such as hypotension, tachycardia, oliguria, delayed capillary refill, altered mentation, increased blood lactate level, and low mixed venous oxygen saturation, are helpful, when present, to establish tissue hypoperfusion. However, these signs are not always sensitive, and they must be complemented with assessment of indices of regional hypoperfusion. Patients with severe sepsis should have good venous access. Central venous access is preferred because it can also be used for hemodynamic monitoring.

The importance of early intervention in patients with sepsis-induced tissue hypoperfusion has been highlighted by the results of an early goal-directed therapy (EGDT) clinical trial conducted by Rivers and colleagues.[49] In this study, patients with sepsis-induced hypoperfusion (lactate value >4 mmol/L and/or hypotension after fluid administration) were randomly assigned to receive either standard resuscitation or an EGDT protocol during the first 6 hours after admission to the emergency department. In both groups, end points of resuscitation were as follows: central venous pressure (CVP) = 8-12 mm Hg, mean arterial pressure (MAP) greater than or equal to 65 mm Hg, and urine output greater than or equal to 0.5 mL/kg/hr. In order to achieve these goals, patients were treated with intravenous crystalloids and vasopressors. In the EGDT group, an additional end point was central venous oxygen saturation ($Scvo_2$) greater than or equal to 70%, which was continuously measured from a subclavian or jugular central venous catheter. $ScvO_2$ was used as an index for oxygen delivery. If $ScvO_2$ was less than 70% after targets for CVP and MAP were reached, patients received either packed red blood cells to achieve a hematocrit less than or equal to 30% or dobutamine infusion if the hematocrit value was greater than or equal to 30%. Patients in the EGDT group received more fluids, dobutamine, and transfusions in the first 24 hours. In-hospital mortality was significantly lower in the EGDT group than in the standard therapy group (30.5% vs. 46.5%, respectively; $P = 0.009$). Although the specific merits of each treatment within the EGDT protocol can be debated, the results of this study strongly support early intervention with predefined hemodynamic settings and protocolized care.

As stated before, the initial step in optimizing hemodynamics in patients with severe sepsis is aggressive fluid resuscitation. Although experts agree on the value of early and aggressive volume replacement, controversy persists over the optimal type of fluid. This debate revolves around the use of crystalloids (saline, lactated Ringer's solution) versus colloids (albumin, hydroxyethyl starches). There are no prospective randomized studies in patients with severe sepsis and septic shock that clearly address this issue. Meta-analyses of clinical studies performed in general critical care populations have demonstrated no difference in outcomes between patients treated with crystalloids and those treated with colloids.[50-52] The recently published SAFE (Saline versus Albumin Fluid Evaluation) study involved prospectively randomized assignment of 7000 critically ill patients to receive 4% albumin or 0.9% saline for fluid resuscitation.[53] There were no significant differences between groups in mortality and other secondary outcomes. A subgroup analysis conducted in patients with sepsis revealed a trend toward better outcomes in patients treated with albumin, although this difference did not achieve statistical significance. We believe that achieving end points of resuscitation is more important than the type of fluid used. In North America, consideration for cost differences has made crystalloids the fluid of choice for resuscitating patients with severe sepsis.

Patients with severe sepsis may present with significant intravascular volume depletion. Aggressive fluid boluses are usually required to restore tissue perfusion. It is recommended that patients receive at least 20 mL/kg of crystalloid initially.[34] This may be supplemented with more fluids on the basis of markers of perfusion in repeated boluses of 300 to 500 mL.[54] Current guidelines recommend achieving the following hemodynamic end points of resuscitation during the first 6 hours of treatment: CVP greater than or equal to 8 to 12 mm Hg, MAP greater than or equal to 65 mm Hg, urine output greater than or equal to 0.5 mL/kg/h, and $Scvo_2$ greater than or equal to 70%.[34,55] For further discussion on the pathophysiology and treatment of hemodynamic abnormalities in sepsis, see Chapter 24.

Modulation of the Host Response

Over the years research efforts in severe sepsis have been heavily involved with therapies targeted at modulating the host response. Several pathways and mechanisms have been studied in clinical trials (Table 26-6). Unfortunately, very little success has been found in these endeavors. Initial attempts were aimed at blunting the inflammatory response with nonspecific agents such as high-dose glucocorticoids and ibuprofen.[56-58] Another unsuccessful strategy involved the use of antibodies directed against the lipid A component of endotoxin in patients with gram-negative sepsis.[59-64] However, the area that received the

Table 26-6. Pathways and Mediators of Sepsis, Potential Treatments, and Results of Randomized, Controlled Trials

Pathway	Mediators	Treatment(s)	Results
	Lipopolysaccharide (endotoxin)	Anti lipopolysaccharide	Negative
Inflammatory pathway	Tumor necrosis factor-alpha (TNF-α)	Anti–TNF-α	Negative
	Interleukin-1β	Interleukin-1 receptor antagonist	Negative
	Prostaglandins, leukotrienes	Ibuprofen, high-dose corticosteroids	Negative
	TNF-α receptors	TNF-α receptors	Negative
	Bradykinin	Bradykinin antagonist	Negative
	Platelet-activating factor	Platelet-activating factor acetyl hydrolase	Negative
	Proteases (e.g., elastase)	Elastase inhibitor	Negative
	Nitric oxide	Nitric oxide synthase inhibitor	Negative
Procoagulant pathway	Decreased protein C	Activated protein C	Positive
	Decreased antithrombin III	Antithrombin III	Negative
	Decreased tissue factor-pathway inhibitor	Tissue factor-pathway inhibitor	Negative

Adapted from Russell JA: Management of sepsis. N Engl J Med 2006;355:1699-1713.

greatest attention was modulation of the inflammatory cascade by targeting of specific proinflammatory cytokines such as TNF-α and IL-1β. Multiple clinical trials enrolling thousands of patients tested compounds directed at specific proinflammatory cytokines, among them TNF-α monoclonal antibody, interleukin-1 receptor antagonist, and soluble TNF receptor.[65-72] Unfortunately, none of these compounds improved survival of patients with severe sepsis in randomized studies. The failure of these therapies led to a reappraisal of the pathophysiology, potential therapeutic targets, and clinical trial design in severe sepsis. As the role of the coagulation cascade and its crosstalk with inflammation in sepsis was recognized, a series of new clinical trials took place. Three large trials studied the effects of anticoagulants in severe sepsis (Table 26-7).

Antithrombin III (AT III) is a progressive inhibitor of thrombin and coagulation factor Xa.[73] Studies showed that AT III supplementation attenuated the systemic inflammatory response in patients with severe sepsis.[74] A large (n=2314) multicenter, double-blinded, placebo-controlled trial evaluated the safety and efficacy of AT III in adult patients with severe sepsis.[75] At 28 days there was no difference in mortality between the treatment group and the placebo group (38.9% vs. 38.7%, respectively). Patients who received AT III had a higher risk of bleeding (relative risk >1.7). A subgroup analysis of patients not receiving concomitant heparin therapy showed a trend (statistically nonsignificant) toward reduced mortality at 28 and 90 days with AT III. This specific subgroup of patients with severe sepsis may warrant further investigations. Tissue factor pathway inhibitor (TFPI) has been shown to modulate the extrinsic pathway in preclinical models of severe sepsis. Recombinant human TFPI (tifacogin) was evaluated in clinical trials of patients with severe sepsis. Although the results of a phase II trial suggested a trend toward improved mortality, a large phase III trial, the OPTIMIST (Optimized Phase III Tifacogin in Multicenter International Sepsis Trial) study did not show a mortality benefit in patients treated with this compound.[76,77] Patients treated with tifacogin had a higher risk of bleeding complications irrespective of their baseline International Normalized Ratio values.[76] Studies evaluating different dosing regimens and the application of this drug in patients with pneumonia are still being conducted. Finally, recombinant human activated protein C (rhAPC) was evaluated in clinical trials. A landmark study, PROWESS (Recombinant human protein C Worldwide Evaluation in Severe Sepsis), demonstrated improved 28-day survival in patients with severe sepsis who were treated with rhAPC.[78] We now further discuss the application of rhAPC in modulating the host response in severe sepsis and its effects on outcomes.

Activated Protein C

Protein C is a protein that circulates in the blood in its inactive form. Protein C is converted to activated protein C (APC) by a process that requires thrombin and thrombomodulin. APC plays an important role in modulating endothelia cell function. It has antithrombotic, anti-inflammatory, and profibrinolytic effects.[79] Antithrombotic effects of APC are mediated through inactivation of coagulation factors Va and VIIIa. Profibrinolytic activity is enhanced by APC through increased release of plasminogen activator inhibitor 1. Anti-inflammatory effects of APC result mostly from downregulation of inflammation by inhibiting activity of nuclear factor κB and production of inflammatory cytokines.[80,81] Low levels of protein C are present in a great majority of patients with severe sepsis.[82] Levels of endogenous protein C decrease early in the course of sepsis, before clinical signs and symptoms of organ dysfunction appear. In addition, it has been proposed that lower levels of protein C in patients with sepsis occur in the absence of measurable conversion to APC.[79]

PROWESS, a phase III randomized, double-blind, placebo-controlled, multicenter international study, evaluated the efficacy of drotrecogin alfa (activated) in patients with severe sepsis.[78] This study enrolled 1690 patients and was terminated early after an interim safety analysis found a significantly lower mortality rate in the treatment group than in the placebo group (24.7% vs. 30.8%, respectively; P=.005) and relative and absolute risk reductions (19.4% and 6.1%, respectively). Patients treated with drotrecogin alfa (activated) showed a trend toward higher incidence of bleeding (3.5% vs. 2%, respectively; P=.06). Subgroup analysis demonstrated that patients at higher risk of death, as measured by APACHE II scores (APACHE II ≥25) and number of organ failures (two or more organ failures) received greater benefit from the drug. Angus and colleagues[83] reported, after long-term follow-up, that patients who were treated with drotrecogin alfa (activated) had a longer median survival (9 months) than patients treated with placebo. Once again, beneficial effects of the drug seemed to be greatest in patients with a higher severity of disease. More recently, two further phase IV studies have been published. The ENHANCE trial was a single-arm, open-label

Table 26-7. Trials Using Anticoagulants in Severe Sepsis*

Trial	Compound	N	Mortality for Placebo (%)	Mortality for Treatment (%)	*P*
KyberSept	Antithrombin III	2314	38.7	38.9	NS
OPTIMIST	Tifacogin (recombinant tissue factor pathway inhibitor)	1956	33.9	34.2	NS
PROWESS	Drotrecogin-alfa (recombinant human activated protein C)	1690	30.8	24.7	.005

*Studies referenced in text.

study that enrolled 2375 patients with severe sepsis.[84] This trial evaluated the use of drotrecogin alfa (activated) in a more routine clinical setting beyond the restrictions of a controlled randomized study. The effect of the drug on mortality was similar to that in PROWESS (25.3% in ENHANCE vs. 24.7% in PROWESS). The risk of bleeding during infusion was higher than in PROWESS (3.6% vs. 2.4%, respectively). However, higher rate of postinfusion bleeding observed in the ENHANCE population (3.2% vs. 1.2%) suggests a higher incidence of background bleeding. This could be explained by higher use of the drug in patients with other risk factors for bleeding. One other important observation derived from the ENHANCE trial was the fact that patients who received the drug early (first 24 hours of the enrollment window) seemed to have a greater benefit than those who received it in the second 24 hours of the 48-hour enrollment window. On the basis of this finding, it seems reasonable to treat patients with severe sepsis earlier rather than later once the decision to use drotrecogin alfa (activated) is made. A second phase IV trial, the ADDRESS study, was a randomized, blinded, placebo-controlled trial that evaluated the efficacy of the drug in severe sepsis in patients judged prospectively by the enrolling clinician to have a low risk of death (APACHE II score <25 or single organ failure based on regulation requirements in countries of study entry).[85] This study enrolled 2646 patients and found that treatment with the drug offered no mortality benefit compared with placebo in a population with low risk of death. Serious bleeding events were similar to those reported in PROWESS.

Drotrecogin alfa (activated) is the first approved therapy targeted at modulating the host response in patients with severe sepsis. It has been subject to intensive clinical evaluations to better determine ideal patients and further assess its risk benefit ratio. Currently, the drug is indicated for patients with severe sepsis at high risk of death who are believed to be candidates for aggressive care and have no contraindications related to bleeding or relative contraindications that might outweigh the benefits of the drug (Table 26-8). The drug is administered as a continuous infusion at a dose of 24 μg/kg/h for a total infusion time of 96 hours. The dose is based on the patient's actual body weight. The major complication associated with drotrecogin alpha (activated) is increased risk of serious bleeding. Bleeding associated with this drug seems to be mostly related to procedures and tends to occur during drug infusion. In order to decrease the risk of bleeding, the drug should be suspended 2 hours prior to invasive procedures (establishment of central venous access, thoracentesis) and restarted 2 hours after the procedure is completed.[86] For major surgical procedures, a holding time of 12 hours before and after the surgical procedure are recommended.[86] Because thrombocytopenia can increase the risk of bleeding, it is recommended that therapy with drotrecogin alfa (activated) not be initiated if platelet count is less than 30,000 per μL. Some experts recommend that if the platelet count drops below this value during infusion, that patient should receive platelet transfusion to keep the count above 30,000 per μL.[86]

Table 26-8. Use of Drotrecogin alfa (activated) in Severe Sepsis

Indication	Adult patients with severe sepsis (sepsis associated with acute organ dysfunction) who have a high risk of death (e.g., as determined by APACHE II score or need for vasopressors)
Contraindications	Active internal bleeding Recent (within 3 months) hemorrhagic stroke Recent (within 2 months) intracranial or intraspinal surgery, or severe head trauma Trauma with increased risk of life-threatening bleeding Presence of epidural catheter Intracranial neoplasm, mass lesion, or evidence of cerebral herniation
Warnings	Coagulopathy (platelet count <30,000 cells/μL or International Normalized Ratio >3.0) Concurrent use of heparin Recent use of thrombolytics, acetylsalicylic acid, IIb/IIIa platelet inhibitors, or other anticoagulants Recent (within 6 weeks) gastrointestinal bleed Recent (within 3 months) ischemic stroke Chronic severe hepatic disease Known bleeding diathesis Any condition in which bleeding poses a significant hazard

Even though drotrecogin alfa (activated) is the first drug approved by the U.S. Food and Drug Administration (FDA) for sepsis, its integration into clinical practice has not been without controversy. Beginning with a publication questioning PROWESS trial administration as well as interpretation of results by some writers, including those who had been unsuccessful in their advice to the FDA against approval (as members of the FDA advisory panel) and continuing with a series of publications by these writers and others questioning the validation of the drug's beneficial effect, the use of drotrecogin alfa (activated) has become a controversial and emotional subject within academic critical care.[87-90] Critics of a mandate to use it in severe sepsis cite data that they interpret as supporting (1) bleeding rate with general use higher than that observed in the PROWESS study and (2) failure to substantiate benefit in the APACHE II score of 25 or greater subgroup (whose results drove the beneficial effect analysis of PROWESS) when these subjects were enrolled in a trial that required clinician assessment of low risk of death as a criterion for study inclusion. At the time of publication, this remains a hotly debated issue, and a second confirmatory trial of drotrecogin alfa (activated) is planned.

Supportive Therapies

As in other critical illnesses, patients with severe sepsis require various supportive therapies (Box 26-3). These

Box 26-3

Supportive Care for Patients with Sepsis and Septic Shock

Mechanical ventilation
Prophylaxis against deep vein thrombosis
Prophylaxis against gastrointestinal ulcer
Nutrition
Blood glucose control
Sedation

therapies are general supportive measures that prevent complications associated with critical illness. Improvement in these therapies over the years probably plays a role in the historical decrease in mortality observed in patients with several disease processes, such as severe sepsis and acute respiratory distress syndrome (ARDS). Patients with severe sepsis often present with tachypnea and hypoxemia. Mechanical ventilation is often used for support. Recent studies in patients with ARDS have demonstrated that ventilation strategies using low tidal volume (6 mL/kg) are associated with significantly lower mortality than ventilation with more traditional tidal volumes (12 mL/kg).[91] This is most likely due to a decrease in ventilator-induced lung injury. Current guidelines recommend the use of a protective lung strategy (low tidal volume; inspiratory plateau pressure <30 cm H_2O) in mechanically ventilated patients with severe sepsis.[34] Goals for oxygen saturation should be a SaO_2 greater than or equal to 90%; this can be achieved by increasing the fraction of inspired oxygen (FIO_2), application of positive end-expiratory pressure (PEEP), or both. Patients receiving mechanical ventilation who are clinically improving should be evaluated on a daily basis for weaning from mechanical ventilation. Patients who have severe sepsis and are being mechanically ventilated should be managed with appropriate sedatives and analgesics. For a detailed discussion, see Chapter 20.

Patients with severe sepsis should receive prophylaxis for the development of deep vein thrombosis (DVT). In the absence of contraindications patients should receive pharmacologic DVT prophylaxis. Treatment with low-dose unfractionated heparin (UFH), adjusted-dose UFH, or low-molecular-weight heparin (LMWH) is recommended.[92] Treatment for DVT prophylaxis with UFH or LMWH is not contraindicated during infusion of drotrecogin alfa (activated). Stress ulcer prophylaxis is recommended for all patients with severe sepsis. Histamine H_2 receptor antagonists are more effective than sucralfate in decreasing bleeding risk and transfusion requirements.[93] Proton pump inhibitors have not been assessed in a direct comparison with histamine H_2 receptor antagonists but do demonstrate equivalency and ability to reduce gastric pH.[92]

Severe sepsis is a catabolic state. Metabolic alterations in patients with severe sepsis include breakdown of proteins, carbohydrates, and lipids, negative nitrogen balance, and hyperglycemia with insulin resistance. As with other critically ill patients, those with severe sepsis require adequate nutritional support. Compared with parenteral nutrition, enteral nutrition offers several advantages, including lower cost, preservation of gastric mucosa integrity, lower incidence of infections, and avoidance of parenteral nutritional catheters and their potential complications.[94] In patients who cannot tolerate enteral nutrition, however, parenteral nutrition should be used.[95] Immunomodulation through nutritional supplements has been proposed in patients with severe sepsis but remains experimental at this point.

Hyperglycemia with insulin resistance is common in patients with severe sepsis. This phenomenon is a common feature of the metabolic response to critical illness and stress and has been described after major surgery and in patients with trauma, acute myocardial infarction, and several other disease states. Furthermore, a growing body of literature suggests that hyperglycemia related to critical illness is associated with poor outcomes.[96-100] Proposed mechanisms for this deleterious effect include impaired neutrophil function, increased risk of infection, poor wound healing, and procoagulant state as a consequence of hyperglycemia.[101]

Treatment of critical illness–related hyperglycemia with insulin has been proposed to modulate these effects and improve patient outcomes. Van den Berghe and coworkers[102] studied the effects of tight glycemic control on outcomes in a population of mechanically ventilated patients receiving surgical critical care. In this study patients were randomly assigned to receive either intensive insulin therapy (target serum glucose 80 to 110 mg/dL) or standard therapy (target serum glucose 180 to 200 mg/dL). Patients treated with the intensive insulin regimen had significant improvements in overall ICU mortality rates (4.6% vs. 8.0%). This benefit in mortality was more pronounced among patients who stayed in the ICU longer than 5 days (10.6% vs. 20.2%; $P = .005$). In addition, intensive insulin therapy was associated with reductions of 46% in rate of bloodstream infections, 44% in the incidence of critical illness polyneuropathy, 41% in the need for renal replacement therapy, and 50% in number of transfused units of packed red blood cells. The same group reported the results of a similar study in patients treated in a medical ICU.[103] In this clinical trial, intensive insulin therapy was not associated with better mortality than standard therapy. Intensive insulin therapy was associated with lower mortality in patients who remained in the ICU more than 3 days but with higher mortality in those that remained in the ICU less than 3 days. Prospective identification of these patient groups was difficult.

Although the results of the second trial pose important questions with respect to why the benefit seen in the surgical population were not reproduced in the medical group, there seems to be growing evidence that controlling the hyperglycemia of critical illness is beneficial for patient outcomes. Two questions arise: First, what is the disadvantage of tight glycemic control? Second, what level of glucose should we target? The biggest disadvantage probably relates to the risk of hypoglycemia. In both studies by Van den Berghe and coworkers, hypoglycemia was more common in the intensive insulin therapy group than in the standard group (surgical study, 5.2% vs. 0.7%, respectively, and medical study, 18.7% vs. 3.1%, respectively).[102,103] Concerns about the effects of hypoglycemia on patients in the ICU are well founded. However, it does not appear that short-term hypoglycemia—that is, hypoglycemia that was quickly recognized and treated—carries deleterious consequences.[104] There is no clear answer with respect to what glucose level we should target in patients with severe sepsis. Considering the current available evidence, it is recommended that the serum glucose value be kept below 150 mg/dL in patients with severe sepsis.[34,105] In order to minimize the risk of hypoglycemia, blood glucose monitoring should be performed frequently in patients receiving intensive insulin therapy.

MULTIPLE ORGAN DYSFUNCTION

Multiple organ dysfunction is a common complication of sepsis. Multiple organ dysfunction syndrome (MODS) occurs when two or more organ systems fail sequentially or at the same time in a patient with sepsis. Various organs, such as the brain, heart, lung, kidney, and liver, can be affected in patients with severe sepsis. Often these organs are distant from the site of primary insult, and development of organ failure occurs as a response to complicated interactions and pathophysiologic events. Metabolic and hematologic dysfunctions are also common with severe sepsis and MODS. MODS significantly contributes to higher mortality. Studies have shown that mortality in patients with severe sepsis increases in parallel with increases in number and severity of organ failures.[106,107] Russell and associates[108] evaluated the pattern of organ dysfunction in early sepsis and its relationship with mortality. In this study, clinically significant pulmonary dysfunction, although common early in sepsis, was not associated with 30-day mortality. Early dysfunction of other organs and particularly worsening neurologic, coagulation, and renal dysfunction over the first 3 days were associated with significantly higher 30-day mortality.

Recognition of early organ dysfunction is important because it is likely that early intervention can affect outcomes. The clinical manifestations of MODS for individual organs are summarized in Figure 26-6. The cornerstones of treatment for MODS are based on appropriate treatment for the underlying cause (sepsis) and on early organ-specific support interventions. As discussed previously, early implementation of therapies directed at control of infection, hemodynamic support, and modulation of the host response are key to improving organ dysfunction and patient outcomes. Perhaps, the single most important aspect relates to early and aggressive hemodynamic support. As demonstrated in the study by Rivers and colleagues,[49] goal-directed interventions instituted in the first 6 hours of presentation to the hospital have a tremendous impact on long-term organ function and survival. Modulation of the host response with the use of drotrecogin alfa (activated) has also been shown to improve organ dysfunction.[109] We further discuss some salient features of the pathophysiology of MODS and the use of scoring systems. For a more detailed discussion on organ-specific supportive therapies, the reader is referred to other chapters in this textbook.

Pathophysiology of Multiple Organ Dysfunction Syndrome in Sepsis

The mechanisms that result in the development of MODS in patients with sepsis are still not fully understood. Addi-

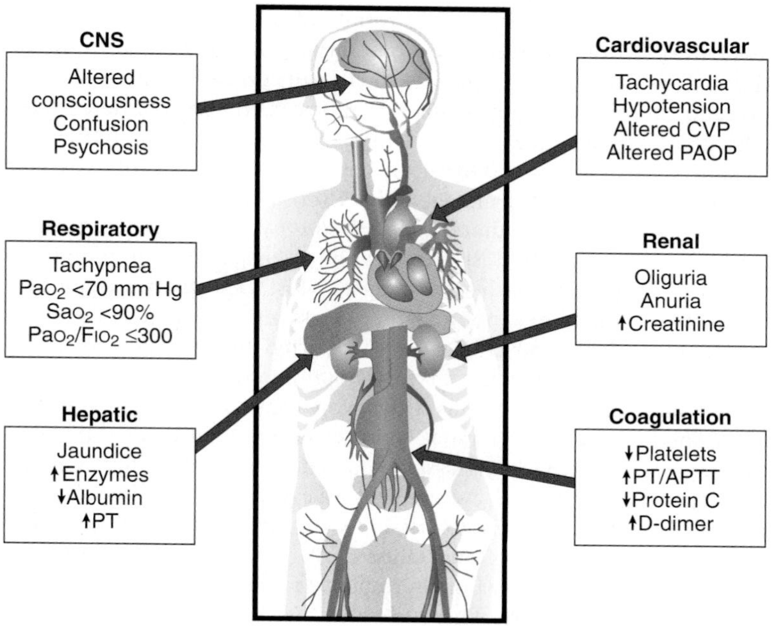

Figure 26-6. Identification of organ failure in severe sepsis. Clinical and laboratory criteria to identify organ failure are shown for each organ system. APTT, activated partial thromboplastin time; CNS, central nervous system; CVP, central venous pressure; PAOP, pulmonary artery occlusion pressure; PT, prothrombin time. (Adapted from Balk RA: Pathogenesis and management of multiple organ dysfunction or failure in severe sepsis and septic shock. Crit Care Clin 2000;16: 337-352.)

tionally, the reason that some patients develop MODS and others do not remains unknown. However, new insights into the pathophysiology of severe sepsis have led to a better understanding of potential mechanisms leading to MODS. In patients in whom MODS develops, the host response to infection becomes sustained and uncontrolled, leading to a complex interaction of inflammatory, anti-inflammatory and procoagulant cascades culminating in the development of organ failure. A key determinant of organ failure seems to be tissue hypoperfusion. Our current knowledge seems to point out two important mechanisms in the development of sepsis-induced tissue hypoperfusion, microvascular dysfunction and cytopathic hypoxia.

In early unresuscitated sepsis, tissue hypoperfusion is to a great extent driven by decreased intravascular volume and the resulting drop in cardiac output (hypovolemic shock).[54] Despite aggressive volume resuscitation, however, many patients still show evidence of tissue hypoperfusion, probably secondary to vasodilation and maldistribution of blood flow (distributive shock).[54] Furthermore, a subset of patients with normalized macrovascular hemodynamic parameters (e.g., blood pressure, CVP, and cardiac output) can still show evidence of sepsis-induced tissue hypoperfusion.[110] New technology has allowed investigators to evaluate the microcirculatory flow in patients with severe sepsis.[111] Redistribution of capillary blood flow has been demonstrated in both animal models and clinical sepsis.[32,33] The importance of this finding has been highlighted by studies demonstrating that functional (impaired blood flow) and structural (shunting, redistribution) abnormalities in microcirculation are associated with death and organ failure in patients with severe sepsis and septic shock.[33,112]

In the early phases of sepsis, decreased oxygen delivery (DO_2) can result in tissue hypoperfusion. However, in late sepsis there is evidence of impaired tissue oxygen utilization even after optimization of DO_2.[113] The inability of cells to use oxygen in the face of adequate DO_2 in sepsis has been termed *cytopathic hypoxia*.[114] Development of cytopathic hypoxia is closely linked to mitochondrial dysfunction. Inability of the mitochondria to use oxygen to produce energy in the form of adenosine triphosphate leads to impaired cellular function. Proposed mechanisms that result in cytopathic hypoxia in sepsis include diminished delivery of pyruvate into the mitochondria, inhibition of mitochondrial enzymes, and activation of poly-(adenosine phosphate-ribosyl) polymerase (PARP).[115] The exact mechanisms leading to organ failure ion sepsis remain unidentified. Organ failure in sepsis is reversible in patients who survive. Furthermore, in patients who do not survive, there is no histopathologic evidence of tissue damage.[28] Hotchkiss and associates[116,117] have described extensive lymphocyte apoptosis in sepsis and have proposed this mechanism as an important driver of the impaired immune response seen in late sepsis and MODS. Finally, multiple organ failure has been hypothesized to be an adaptive metabolic response to overwhelming inflammation in sepsis.[118] The hypothesis holds that multiple organ failure induced by sepsis is primarily a functional abnormality that serves as a protective reactive mechanism and that the decline of organ function is triggered by a decrease in mitochondrial activity. This decrease in mitochondrial activity leads to a reduction in cell metabolism and occurs as a consequence of humoral and mediator-induced changes.[118]

Organ Dysfunction Scoring Systems

Severity of illness scoring systems have been developed and applied in the ICU to describe patient populations. These scoring systems have been useful in predicting expected mortality and comparing different patient populations. The use of general outcome prediction models, such as the APACHE, the Mortality Probability Model (MPM), and the second Simplified Acute Physiologic Score (SAPS), is discussed in detail in Chapter 74. Therefore, this discussion is limited to scoring systems used to specifically assess organ dysfunction.

It is recognized that the risk of death for patients with severe sepsis is directly related to the number of dysfunctional organs. Organ dysfunction scoring systems have been developed as a tool for the clinician to characterize the severity of illness and follow the clinical evolution of patients with sepsis. The more commonly used systems are the Sequential Organ Failure Assessment (SOFA), the Logistic Organ Dysfunction System, and the Multiple Organ Dysfunction Score. Perhaps the most commonly used today is the SOFA score (Table 26-9). It was initially described by Vincent and colleagues[107] to assess the incidence of organ dysfunction in critically ill patients.[107] Using the SOFA scores in patients with severe sepsis, these researchers found that mortality rates were lowest in patients without organ dysfunction (9%) and rose progressively with the number of organ dysfunctions (1 organ, 22%; 2 organs, 38%; 3 organs, 69%; ≥4 organs, 83%).[107] The type of organ dysfunction also affects mortality. Hebert and coworkers[106] used logistic aggression analysis of the results of a simple multiple system organ failure score to determine the odds ratio for death for specific organ system dysfunctions. This study showed that the adjusted odds ratios (OR) for covariates most predictive of mortality were hematologic (OR=6.2), neurologic (OR=4.4), hepatic (OR=3.4), cardiovascular (OR=2.6), and age (OR=1.05). It is important to remember that there are caveats when employing organ dysfunction scores for the management of individual patients with severe sepsis. Most importantly, organ dysfunction is not a static process and it changes over time. Levy and colleagues[119] reported that changes in SOFA score over the first 24 hours were associated with outcomes in patients with severe sepsis. Improvement in cardiovascular, renal, or respiratory failure over the first 24 hours was associated with lower mortality. On the other hand, worsening SOFA scores for these organ systems were associated with higher mortality (approximately 60% mortality rate). Finally, how these scores change over time in response to therapeutic interventions is probably of greater value than an initial organ dysfunction score.

Table 26-9. The Sequential Organ Failure Assessment (SOFA) Score*

Organ System*	Example(s)	Score†				
		0	1	2	3	4
Respiratory	PaO_2/FIO_2 ratio	>400	≤400	≤300	≤200[c]	≤100[c]
Coagulation	Platelet count ($\times10^3$ cells/μL^{-1})	>150	≤150	≤100	≤50	≤20
Liver	Serum bilirubin (mg/dL^{-1})	<1.2	1.2-1.9	2.0-5.9	6.0-11.9	>12.0
Cardiovascular	Hypotension	No hypotension	Mean arterial pressure <70 mm Hg	Dopamine ≤5 μg/kg/min *or* Dobutamine any dose	Dopamine >5 μg/kg/min *or* Epinephrine ≤0.1 μg/kg/min *or* Norepinephrine ≤0.1 μg/kg/min	Dopamine ≥50 μg/kg/min *or* Epinephrine >0.1 μg/kg/min *or* Norepinephrine >0.1 μg/kg/min
Central nervous system	Glasgow Coma Scale score	15	13-14	10-12	6-9	<6
Renal	Serum creatinine (mg/dL^{-1}) *or* Daily urine output (mL)	<1.2	1.2-1.9	2.0-3.4	3.5-4.9 <500	>5 <200

*SOFA scores for each organ system are given with examples.
†Individual scores range from 0 to 4, 0 being normal organ function and 4 representing the most severe organ dysfunction.
Adapted from Vincent JL, de Mendonca A, Cantraine F, et al: Use of the SOFA score to assess the incidence of organ dysfunction/failure in intensive care units: Results of a multicenter, prospective study. Working group on "sepsis-related problems" of the European Society of Intensive Care Medicine. Crit Care Med 1998;26:1793-1800.

KEY POINTS

- Sepsis is the result of a systemic inflammatory response to infection. *Severe sepsis* is defined as sepsis with organ failure.
- The pathophysiology of severe sepsis is complex and involves alterations in the immune system, the inflammatory response, and the coagulation cascade.
- Severe sepsis is common and is associated with high morbidity and mortality.
- Severe sepsis is a medical emergency. Institution of time-sensitive therapeutic interventions is a key factor in modulating and improving outcomes.
- The cornerstones for treatment of sepsis are management of the infection, hemodynamic support, modulation of the host response, and general supportive care.
- Infection management includes the early administration of appropriate antibiotics and institution of source control measures.
- Hemodynamic support consists of early and aggressive fluid resuscitation and maintenance of predefined hemodynamic end points. Studies have shown that early goal-directed therapy for hemodynamic support can improve mortality in patients with severe sepsis.
- Specific antisepsis interventions that modulate the host response have been introduced. Therapies such as recombinant human activated protein C (rhAPC) target multiple pathophysiologic aspects of the sepsis cascade and can improve outcomes.
- To maximize patient outcomes, appropriate supportive therapy must be provided in the ICU: protective lung ventilation, proper nutrition, and prophylaxis against DVT, and glucose control.
- Multiple organ dysfunction syndrome (MODS) occurs when failure of two or more organs develops in a patient with severe sepsis.
- Treatment of MODS is based on treatment of the underlying insult and organ-specific supportive measures.

REFERENCES

1. Stone R: Search for sepsis drugs goes on despite past failures. Science 1994;264:365-367.
2. Bone RC, Balk RA, Cerra FB, et al: Definitions for sepsis and organ failure and guidelines for the use of innovative therapies in sepsis. The ACCP/SCCM Consensus Conference Committee. American College of Chest Physicians/Society of Critical Care Medicine. Chest 1992;101:1644-1655.
3. Trzeciak S, Zanotti-Cavazzoni S, Parrillo JE, Dellinger RP: Inclusion criteria for clinical trials in sepsis: Did the American College of Chest Physicians/Society of Critical Care Medicine consensus conference definitions of sepsis have an impact? Chest 2005;127:242-245.
4. Vincent JL: Dear SIRS, I'm sorry to say that I don't like you. Crit Care Med 1997;25:372-374.

5. Levy MM, Fink MP, Marshall JC, et al: 2001 SCCM/ESICM/ACCP/ATS/SIS International Sepsis Definitions Conference. Crit Care Med 2003;31: 1250-1256.
6. Angus DC, Linde-Zwirble WT, Lidicker J, et al: Epidemiology of severe sepsis in the United States: Analysis of incidence, outcome, and associated costs of care. Crit Care Med 2001; 29:1303-1310.
7. Annane D, Aegerter P, Jars-Guincestre MC, Guidet B: Current epidemiology of septic shock: The CUB-Rea Network. Am J Respir Crit Care Med 2003;168: 165-172.
8. Martin GS, Mannino DM, Eaton S, Moss M: The epidemiology of sepsis in the United States from 1979 through 2000. N Engl J Med 2003;348:1546-1554.
9. Sands KE, Bates DW, Lanken PN, et al: Epidemiology of sepsis syndrome in 8 academic medical centers. JAMA 1997;278:234-240.
10. Friedman G, Silva E, Vincent JL: Has the mortality of septic shock changed with time. Crit Care Med 1998;26: 2078-2086.
11. Arcaroli J, Fessler MB, Abraham E: Genetic polymorphisms and sepsis. Shock 2005;24:300-312.
12. Arcaroli J, Silva E, Maloney JP, et al: Variant IRAK-1 haplotype is associated with increased nuclear factor-kappaB activation and worse outcomes in sepsis. Am J Respir Crit Care Med 2006;173:1335-1341.
13. Barber RC, Aragaki CC, Rivera-Chavez FA, et al: TLR4 and TNF-alpha polymorphisms are associated with an increased risk for severe sepsis following burn injury. J Med Genet 2004;41:808-813.
14. Freeman BD, Buchman TG: Gene in a haystack: Tumor necrosis factor polymorphisms and outcome in sepsis. Crit Care Med 2000;28:3090-3091.
15. Gordon AC, Lagan AL, Aganna E, et al: TNF and TNFR polymorphisms in severe sepsis and septic shock: A prospective multicentre study. Genes Immun 2004;5:631-640.
16. Lin MT, Albertson TE: Genomic polymorphisms in sepsis. Crit Care Med 2004;32:569-579.
17. Underhill DM, Ozinsky A: Toll-like receptors: Key mediators of microbe detection. Curr Opin Immunol 2002;14:103-110.
18. Brower RG, Lanken PN, MacIntyre N, et al: Higher versus lower positive end-expiratory pressures in patients with the acute respiratory distress syndrome. N Engl J Med 2004;351: 327-336.
19. Brightbill HD, Libraty DH, Krutzik SR, et al: Host defense mechanisms triggered by microbial lipoproteins through toll-like receptors. Science 1999;285:732-736.
20. Modlin RL, Brightbill HD, Godowski PJ: The toll of innate immunity on microbial pathogens. N Engl J Med 1999;340:1834-1835.
21. Abbas AK, Murphy KM, Sher A: Functional diversity of helper T lymphocytes. Nature 1996;383: 787-793.
22. Zanotti S, Kumar A, Kumar A: Cytokine modulation in sepsis and septic shock. Expert Opin Investig Drugs 2002;11:1061-1075.
23. Kumar A, Thota V, Dee L, et al: Tumor necrosis factor alpha and interleukin 1beta are responsible for in vitro myocardial cell depression induced by human septic shock serum. J Exp Med 1996;183:949-958.
24. Wang H, Yang H, Tracey KJ: Extracellular role of HMGB1 in inflammation and sepsis. J Intern Med 2004;255:320-231.
25. Czura CJ, Tracey KJ: Targeting high mobility group box 1 as a late-acting mediator of inflammation. Crit Care Med 2003;31(Suppl):S46-S50.
26. Yang H, Ochani M, Li J, et al: Reversing established sepsis with antagonists of endogenous high-mobility group box 1. Proc Natl Acad Sci U S A 2004;101:296-301.
27. Calandra T, Echtenacher B, Roy DL, et al: Protection from septic shock by neutralization of macrophage migration inhibitory factor. Nat Med 2000;6:164-170.
28. Hotchkiss RS, Karl IE: The pathophysiology and treatment of sepsis. N Engl J Med 2003;348: 138-150.
29. Gogos CA, Drosou E, Bassaris HP, Skoutelis A: Pro- versus anti-inflammatory cytokine profile in patients with severe sepsis: A marker for prognosis and future therapeutic options. J Infect Dis 2000;181:176-180.
30. Esmon CT, Taylor FB Jr, Snow TR: Inflammation and coagulation: Linked processes potentially regulated through a common pathway mediated by protein C. Thromb Haemost 1991;66:160-165.
31. Fourrier F, Chopin C, Goudemand J, et al: Septic shock, multiple organ failure, and disseminated intravascular coagulation. Compared patterns of antithrombin III, protein C, and protein S deficiencies. Chest 1992; 101:816-823.
32. Lam C, Tyml K, Martin C, Sibbald W: Microvascular perfusion is impaired in a rat model of normotensive sepsis. J Clin Invest 1994;94:2077-2083.
33. Sakr Y, Dubois MJ, De Backer D, et al: Persistent microcirculatory alterations are associated with organ failure and death in patients with septic shock. Crit Care Med 2004;32:1825-1831.
34. Dellinger RP, Carlet JM, Masur H, et al: Surviving Sepsis Campaign guidelines for management of severe sepsis and septic shock. Crit Care Med 2004; 32:858-873.
35. Levy MM, Pronovost PJ, Dellinger RP, et al: Sepsis change bundles: Converting guidelines into meaningful change in behavior and clinical outcome. Crit Care Med 2004;32(Suppl):S595-S597.
36. Gao F, Melody T, Daniels DF, et al: The impact of compliance with 6-hour and 24-hour sepsis bundles on hospital mortality in patients with severe sepsis: a prospective observational study. Crit Care 2005;9:R764-R770.
37. Micek ST, Roubinian N, Heuring T, et al: Before-after study of a standardized hospital order set for the management of septic shock. Crit Care Med 2006;34:2707-2713.
38. Kumar A, Roberts D, Wood KE, et al: Duration of hypotension before initiation of effective antimicrobial therapy is the critical determinant of survival in human septic shock. Crit Care Med 2006;34:1589-1596.
39. Pittet D, Thievent B, Wenzel RP, et al: Bedside prediction of mortality from bacteremic sepsis: A dynamic analysis of ICU patients. Am J Respir Crit Care Med 1996;153:684-693.
40. Iregui M, Ward S, Sherman G, et al: Clinical importance of delays in the initiation of appropriate antibiotic treatment for ventilator-associated pneumonia. Chest 2002;122:262-268.
41. Blot F, Schmidt E, Nitenberg G, et al: Earlier positivity of central-venous-versus peripheral-blood cultures is highly predictive of catheter-related sepsis. J Clin Microbiol 1998;36:105-109.
42. Leibovici L, Greenshtain S, Cohen O, et al: Bacteremia in febrile patients: A clinical model for diagnosis. Arch Intern Med 1991;151:1801-1806.
43. Weinstein MP, Reller LB, Murphy JR, Lichtenstein KA: The clinical significance of positive blood cultures: A comprehensive analysis of 500 episodes of bacteremia and fungemia in adults. I: Laboratory and epidemiologic observations. Rev Infect Dis 1983;5:35-53.
44. Ibrahim EH, Sherman G, Ward S, et al: The influence of inadequate antimicrobial treatment of bloodstream infections on patient outcomes in the ICU setting. Chest 2000;118:146-155.
45. Leibovici L, Shraga I, Drucker M, et al: The benefit of appropriate empirical antibiotic treatment in patients with bloodstream infection. J Intern Med 1998;244:379-386.
46. Kollef MH, Sherman G, Ward S, Fraser VJ: Inadequate antimicrobial treatment of infections: A risk factor for hospital mortality among critically ill patients. Chest 1999;115:462-474.
47. Jimenez MF, Marshall JC: Source control in the management of sepsis. Intensive Care Med 2001;27(Suppl): S49-S62.
48. Parrillo JE, Parker MM, Natanson C, et al: Septic shock in humans: Advances in the understanding of pathogenesis, cardiovascular dysfunction, and therapy. Ann Intern Med 1990;113:227-242.
49. Rivers E, Nguyen B, Havstad S, et al: Early goal-directed therapy in the treatment of severe sepsis and septic shock. N Engl J Med 2001;345:1368-1377.
50. Choi PT, Yip G, Quinonez LG, Cook DJ: Crystalloids vs. colloids in fluid resuscitation: A systematic review. Crit Care Med 1999;27:200-210.
51. Cook D, Guyatt G: Colloid use for fluid resuscitation: Evidence and spin. Ann Intern Med 2001;135:205-208.
52. Schierhout G, Roberts I: Fluid resuscitation with colloid or crystalloid solutions in critically ill patients: A systematic review of randomised trials. BMJ 1998;316:961-964.
53. Finfer S, Bellomo R, Boyce N, et al; SAFE Study Investigators: A comparison of albumin and saline for fluid resuscitation in the intensive care

unit. N Engl J Med 2004;350:2247-2256.
54. Dellinger RP: Cardiovascular management of septic shock. Crit Care Med 2003;31:946-955.
55. Hollenberg SM, Ahrens TS, Annane D, et al: Practice parameters for hemodynamic support of sepsis in adult patients: 2004 update. Crit Care Med 2004;32:1928-1948.
56. Bernard GR, Wheeler AP, Russell JA, et al: The effects of ibuprofen on the physiology and survival of patients with sepsis. The Ibuprofen in Sepsis Study Group. N Engl J Med 1997;336:912-918.
57. Bone RC, Fisher CJ Jr, Clemmer TP, et al: A controlled clinical trial of high-dose methylprednisolone in the treatment of severe sepsis and septic shock. N Engl J Med 1987;317:653-658.
58. Sprung CL, Caralis PV, Marcial EH, et al: The effects of high-dose corticosteroids in patients with septic shock: A prospective, controlled study. N Engl J Med 1984;311:1137-1143.
59. Bigatello LM, Greene RE, Sprung CL, et al: HA-1A in septic patients with ARDS: Results from the pivotal trial. Intensive Care Med 1994;20:328-334.
60. Derkx B, Wittes J, McCloskey R: Randomized, placebo-controlled trial of HA-1A, a human monoclonal antibody to endotoxin, in children with meningococcal septic shock. European Pediatric Meningococcal Septic Shock Trial Study Group. Clin Infect Dis 1999;28:770-777.
61. McCloskey RV, Straube RC, Sanders C, et al: Treatment of septic shock with human monoclonal antibody HA-1A: A randomized, double-blind, placebo-controlled trial. CHESS Trial Study Group. Ann Intern Med 1994;121:1-5.
62. Smith CR, Straube RC, Ziegler EJ: HA-1A: A human monoclonal antibody for the treatment of gram-negative sepsis. Infect Dis Clin North Am 1992;6:253-266.
63. Wortel CH, von der Mohlen MA, van Deventer SJ, et al: Effectiveness of a human monoclonal anti-endotoxin antibody (HA-1A) in gram-negative sepsis: Relationship to endotoxin and cytokine levels. J Infect Dis 1992;166:1367-1374.
64. Ziegler EJ, Fisher CJ Jr, Sprung CL, et al: Treatment of gram-negative bacteremia and septic shock with HA-1A human monoclonal antibody against endotoxin: A randomized, double-blind, placebo-controlled trial. The HA-1A Sepsis Study Group. N Engl J Med 1991;324:429-436.
65. Abraham E, Anzueto A, Gutierrez G, et al: Double-blind randomised controlled trial of monoclonal antibody to human tumour necrosis factor in treatment of septic shock. NORASEPT II Study Group. Lancet 1998;351:929-933.
66. Abraham E, Laterre PF, Garbino J, et al: Lenercept (p55 tumor necrosis factor receptor fusion protein) in severe sepsis and early septic shock: A randomized, double-blind, placebo-controlled, multicenter phase III trial with 1,342 patients. Crit Care Med 2001;29:503-510.
67. Abraham E, Wunderink R, Silverman H, et al: Efficacy and safety of monoclonal antibody to human tumor necrosis factor alpha in patients with sepsis syndrome: A randomized, controlled, double-blind, multicenter clinical trial. TNF-alpha MAb Sepsis Study Group. JAMA 1995;273:934-941.
68. Dhainaut JF, Yan SB, Margolis BD, et al: Drotrecogin alfa (activated) (recombinant human activated protein C) reduces host coagulopathy response in patients with severe sepsis. Thromb Haemost 2003;90:642-653.
69. Fein AM, Bernard GR, Criner GJ, et al: Treatment of severe systemic inflammatory response syndrome and sepsis with a novel bradykinin antagonist, deltibant (CP-0127): Results of a randomized, double-blind, placebo-controlled trial. CP-0127 SIRS and Sepsis Study Group. JAMA 1997;277:482-487.
70. Fisher CJ Jr, Agosti JM, Opal SM, et al: Treatment of septic shock with the tumor necrosis factor receptor: Fc fusion protein. The Soluble TNF Receptor Sepsis Study Group. N Engl J Med 1996;334:1697-1702.
71. Fisher CJ Jr, Dhainaut JF, Opal SM, et al: Recombinant human interleukin 1 receptor antagonist in the treatment of patients with sepsis syndrome: Results from a randomized, double-blind, placebo-controlled trial. Phase III rhIL-1ra Sepsis Syndrome Study Group. JAMA 1994;271:1836-1843.
72. Opal S, Laterre PF, Abraham E, et al: Recombinant human platelet-activating factor acetylhydrolase for treatment of severe sepsis: results of a phase III, multicenter, randomized, double-blind, placebo-controlled, clinical trial. Crit Care Med 2004;32:332-341.
73. Inthorn D, Hoffmann JN, Hartl WH, et al: Antithrombin III supplementation in severe sepsis: Beneficial effects on organ dysfunction. Shock 1997;8:328-334.
74. Inthorn D, Hoffmann JN, Hartl WH, et al: Effect of antithrombin III supplementation on inflammatory response in patients with severe sepsis. Shock 1998;1:90-96.
75. Warren BL, Eid A, Singer P, et al; KyperSept Trial Study Group: Caring for the critically ill patient: High-dose antithrombin III in severe sepsis. A randomized controlled trial. JAMA 2001;286:1869-1878.
76. Abraham E, Reinhart K, Opal S, et al: Efficacy and safety of tifacogin (recombinant tissue factor pathway inhibitor) in severe sepsis: A randomized controlled trial. JAMA 2003;290:238-247.
77. Abraham E, Reinhart K, Svoboda P, et al: Assessment of the safety of recombinant tissue factor pathway inhibitor in patients with severe sepsis: A multicenter, randomized, placebo-controlled, single-blind, dose escalation study. Crit Care Med 2001;29:2081-2089.
78. Bernard GR, Vincent JL, Laterre PF, et al; Recombinant human protein C Worldwide Evaluation in Severe Sepsis (PROWESS) study group: Efficacy and safety of recombinant human activated protein C for severe sepsis. N Engl J Med 2001;344:699-709.
79. Yan SB, Dhainaut JF: Activated protein C versus protein C in severe sepsis. Crit Care Med 2001;29(Suppl):S69-S74.
80. Joyce DE, Grinnell BW: Recombinant human activated protein C attenuates the inflammatory response in endothelium and monocytes by modulating nuclear factor-kappaB. Crit Care Med 2002;30(Suppl):S288-S293.
81. Schmidt-Supprian M, Murphy C, While B, et al: Activated protein C inhibits tumor necrosis factor and macrophage migration inhibitory factor production in monocytes. Eur Cytokine Netw 2000;11:407-413.
82. Yan SB, Helterbrand JD, Hartman DL, et al: Low levels of protein C are associated with poor outcome in severe sepsis. Chest 2001;120:915-922.
83. Angus DC, Laterre PF, Elterbrand J: The effects of drotrecogin alfa (activated) on long term survival after severe sepsis. Chest 2002;122:51S.
84. Bernard GR, Margolis BD, Shanies HM, et al: Extended evaluation of recombinant human activated protein C United States Trial (ENHANCE US): A single-arm, phase 3B, multicenter study of drotrecogin alfa (activated) in severe sepsis. Chest 2004;125:2206-2216.
85. Abraham E, Laterre PF, Garg R, et al: Drotrecogin alfa (activated) for adults with severe sepsis and a low risk of death. N Engl J Med 2005;353:1332-1341.
86. Fourrier F: Recombinant human activated protein C in the treatment of severe sepsis: An evidence-based review. Crit Care Med 2004;32(Suppl):S534-S541.
87. Eichacker PQ, Natanson C: Increasing evidence that the risks of rhAPC may outweigh its benefits. Intensive Care Med 2007;33:396-399.
88. Minneci PC, Deans KJ, Cui X, et al: Antithrombotic therapies for sepsis: A need for more studies. Crit Care Med 2006;34:538-541.
89. Carlet J: Prescribing indications based on successful clinical trials in sepsis: A difficult exercise. Crit Care Med 2006;34:525-529.
90. Carlet J: Drotrecogin alfa (activated) administration: Too many subgroups. Crit Care Med 2003;31:2564; author reply 2564-2565.
91. Ventilation with lower tidal volumes as compared with traditional tidal volumes for acute lung injury and the acute respiratory distress syndrome. The Acute Respiratory Distress Syndrome Network. N Engl J Med 2000;342:1301-1308.
92. Trzeciak S, Dellinger RP: Other supportive therapies in sepsis: An evidence-based review. Crit Care Med 2004;32(Suppl):S571-S577.
93. Cook D, Guyatt G, Marshall J, et al: A comparison of sucralfate and ranitidine for the prevention of upper gastrointestinal bleeding in patients requiring mechanical ventilation. Canadian Critical Care Trials Group. N Engl J Med 1998;338:791-797.
94. Heyland DK: Nutritional support in the critically ill patients: A critical review of

the evidence. Crit Care Clin 1998;14: 423-440.
95. Heyland DK, MacDonald S, Keefe L, Drover JW: Total parenteral nutrition in the critically ill patient: A meta-analysis. JAMA 1998;280:2013-2019.
96. Finney SJ, Zekveld C, Elia A, Evans TW: Glucose control and mortality in critically ill patients. JAMA 2003;290: 2041-2047.
97. Malmberg K, Norhammar A, Wedel H, Ryden L: Glycometabolic state at admission: Important risk marker of mortality in conventionally treated patients with diabetes mellitus and acute myocardial infarction: long-term results from the Diabetes and Insulin-Glucose Infusion in Acute Myocardial Infarction (DIGAMI) study. Circulation 1999;99:2626-2632.
98. Michaud LJ, Rivara FP, Longstreth WT Jr, Grady MS: Elevated initial blood glucose levels and poor outcome following severe brain injuries in children. J Trauma 1991;31: 1356-1362.
99. Norhammar AM, Ryden L, Malmberg K: Admission plasma glucose: Independent risk factor for long-term prognosis after myocardial infarction even in nondiabetic patients. Diabetes Care 1999;22:1827-1831.
100. Zindrou D, Taylor KM, Bagger JP: Admission plasma glucose: An independent risk factor in nondiabetic women after coronary artery bypass grafting. Diabetes Care 2001;24: 1634-1639.
101. Nylen ES, Muller B: Endocrine changes in critical illness. J Intensive Care Med 2004;19:67-82.
102. van den Berghe G, Wouters P, Weekers F, et al: Intensive insulin therapy in the critically ill patients. N Engl J Med 2001;345:1359-1367.
103. van den Berghe G, Wilmer A, Hermans G, et al: Intensive insulin therapy in the medical ICU. N Engl J Med 2006;354:449-461.
104. Vriesendorp TM, DeVries JH, van Santen S, et al: Evaluation of short-term consequences of hypoglycemia in an intensive care unit. Crit Care Med 2006;34:2714-2718.
105. Cariou A, Vinsonneau C, Dhainaut JF: Adjunctive therapies in sepsis: An evidence-based review. Crit Care Med 2004;32(Suppl):S562-S570.
106. Hebert PC, Drummond AJ, Singer J, et al: A simple multiple system organ failure scoring system predicts mortality of patients who have sepsis syndrome. Chest 1993;10:230-235.
107. Vincent JL, de Mendonca A, Cantraine F, et al: Use of the SOFA score to assess the incidence of organ dysfunction/failure in intensive care units: Results of a multicenter, prospective study. Working group on "sepsis-related problems" of the European Society of Intensive Care Medicine. Crit Care Med 1998;26: 1793-1800.
108. Russell JA, Singer J, Bernard GR, et al: Changing pattern of organ dysfunction in early human sepsis is related to mortality. Crit Care Med 2000;28:3405-3411.
109. Vincent JL, Angus DC, Artigas A, et al: Effects of drotrecogin alfa (activated) on organ dysfunction in the PROWESS trial. Crit Care Med 2003;31:834-840.
110. Zanotti Cavazzoni SL, Dellinger RP: Hemodynamic optimization of sepsis-induced tissue hypoperfusion. Crit Care 2006;10(Suppl 3):S2.
111. Ince C: The microcirculation is the motor of sepsis. Crit Care 2005;9(Suppl 4):S13-S19.
112. Trzeciak S, Dellinger RP, Parrillo JE, et al: Early microcirculatory perfusion derangements in patients with severe sepsis and septic shock: Relationship to hemodynamics, oxygen transport, and survival. Ann Emerg Med 2007;49:88-98;e1-e2.
113. Fink MP: Bench-to-bedside review: Cytopathic hypoxia. Crit Care 2002;6:491-499.
114. Fink M: Cytopathic hypoxia in sepsis. Acta Anaesthesiol Scand Suppl 1997;110:87-95.
115. Fink MP: Cytopathic hypoxia: Is oxygen use impaired in sepsis as a result of an acquired intrinsic derangement in cellular respiration? Crit Care Clin 2002;18:165-175.
116. Hotchkiss RS, Swanson PE, Freeman BD, et al: Apoptotic cell death in patients with sepsis, shock, and multiple organ dysfunction. Crit Care Med 1999;27:1230-1251.
117. Hotchkiss RS, Tinsley KW, Swanson PE, et al: Sepsis-induced apoptosis causes progressive profound depletion of B and CD4+ T lymphocytes in humans. J Immunol 2001;166:6952-6963.
118. Singer M, De Santis V, Vitale D, Jeffcoate W: Multiorgan failure is an adaptive, endocrine-mediated, metabolic response to overwhelming systemic inflammation. Lancet 2004;364:545-548.
119. Levy MM, Macias WL, Vincent JL, et al: Early changes in organ function predict eventual survival in severe sepsis. Crit Care Med 2005;33: 2194-2201.

Chapter 27

Hypovolemic Shock

A. B. J. Groeneveld

Hypovolemic shock can be defined as an acute disturbance in the circulation leading to an imbalance between oxygen supply and demand in the tissues, caused by a decrease in circulating blood volume. An oxygen deficit develops when uptake no longer matches the demand for oxygen and leads to cellular ischemia and ultimately cell death. The condition is life-threatening and, if left untreated, becomes irreversible after a certain period. Rapid and adequate resuscitation is mandatory to save lives. Conversely, hypovolemic shock carries a relatively favorable prognosis, if rapidly and adequately recognized and treated. In this chapter, some aspects of the syndrome are discussed, mainly by reviewing the literature on hemorrhagic shock.

HISTORY AND INCIDENCE

Although hypovolemic shock has been recognized for more than 100 years, Wiggers[1] in 1940 first offered a definition of hypovolemic shock that has remained significant until now: "Shock is a syndrome resulting from depression of many functions, but in which the reduction of the effective circulating blood volume is of basic importance, and in which impairment of the circulation steadily progresses until it eventuates in a state of irreversible circulatory failure." Today, circulatory shock is more precisely defined as an acute decline in global blood flow that compromises the oxygen supply-to-demand ratio in the tissues. Hypovolemic shock can be defined as shock caused by a severe decline in circulating blood volume, mostly caused by trauma and hemorrhage.[2] Hypovolemic shock can occur outside and inside the hospital, in trauma or surgery complicated by excessive loss of blood, but also in the course of burns, gastrointestinal hemorrhage, diarrhea, uncontrolled diabetes mellitus, addisonian crisis, and other conditions (Box 27-1). Some other types of shock, including septic, anaphylactoid, cardiogenic, and burn shock, may be accompanied by hypovolemia. The types of shock not primarily caused by hypovolemia are beyond the scope of this chapter.

PATHOGENESIS AND PATHOPHYSIOLOGY

During hypovolemic shock, the loss of circulating blood volume amounts to 15% to 80%. Hypotension ensues when this loss exceeds about 40%. The prior hydration status, severity and type of injury, coagulation, and resuscitation efforts determine the amount of blood lost after trauma. The severity of shock is determined mainly by the duration and severity of the loss of circulating volume. The pathophysiology of hypovolemic shock concerns primary events, directly relating to the loss of circulating blood volume, and secondary mechanisms, evoked to compensate for this decline, and concerns all components of the circulation. The factors are dealt with together in a general discussion and in a more focused discussion on tissue and organ perfusion and function during hypovolemic shock.

Circulatory Changes

General

Because hypovolemia results in a decrease in preload of the heart and low filling pressures, the cardiac output decreases.[3-9] After unloading of the baroreceptor and activation of the sympathetic nervous system, tachycardia

Box 27-1

Causes of Hypovolemic Shock

Loss of Blood
Internally—rupture of vessels, spleen, liver; extrauterine pregnancy
Externally—trauma; gastrointestinal, pulmonary, renal blood loss

Loss of Plasma
Burn wounds; gastrointestinal losses (diarrhea, ileus, pancreatitis)

Loss of Fluids and Electrolytes
Gastrointestinal and renal losses (uncontrolled diabetes mellitus, adrenocortical insufficiency)

ensues, although some patients may respond with transient sympathetic inhibition and vagal nerve–mediated bradycardia during a sudden, severe loss of circulating blood volume.[3,10-16] Tachycardia partially compensates for the decrease in stroke volume. A moderate decrease in cardiac output can be recognized from a decline in pulse pressure and orthostatic hypotension.[8,17,18] Hypovolemia results in wider than usual swings in central venous pressure (CVP) and systolic arterial blood pressure during the respiratory cycle of spontaneous and mechanical ventilation because of increased sensitivity of the underfilled heart to fluctuations in venous return associated with varying intrathoracic pressure.[19,20] Although activation of the sympathetic nervous system and resulting arterial vasoconstriction during a moderate decrease in cardiac output prevent a severe reduction in arterial blood pressure, a further decrease in cardiac output leads to hypotension and shock.[8,10] Systemic vascular resistance increases early after development of hypovolemic shock, but may decrease in the later stages of shock, and this may herald irreversibility and death, although the increase in resistance (and heart rate) may be transiently attenuated after an imbalance between sympathetic and vagal activity, possibly associated with release of opioids within the central nervous system and into the systemic circulation.[3,6,10,11,13,16,21-23]

Shock is characterized by an oxygen deficit in the tissues.[9,24-26] In the presence of sufficient oxygen, aerobic combustion of 1 mol of glucose yields 38 mol of energy-rich adenosine triphosphate (ATP), which can be hydrolyzed to provide energy for the vital and metabolic functions of the cell.[27] In the absence of oxygen, glucose taken up by cells cannot be combusted because of insufficient uptake of pyruvate into the mitochondrial tricarboxylic acid cycle having a reduced turnover rate. Partly inactivated pyruvate dehydrogenase may play a role in the latter reductions. Pyruvate is converted into lactate, and the lactate-to-pyruvate ratio increases, concomitantly with a reduction in mitochondrial redox potential.[24,27-29] Anaerobic glycolysis in the cytosol ultimately yields, per mol of glucose, 2 mol of ATP.[27] Hydrolysis of ATP yields hydrogen (H^+) ions that lead, when buffers are exhausted, to intracellular and ultimately to extracellular metabolic acidosis.[30] These mechanisms form the basis of the so-called lactic acidosis during hypovolemic shock, whereby the lactate level in arterial blood is elevated above the normal 2 mmol/L associated with acidosis, and constitutes a useful measure of the severity and duration of the oxygen debt in the tissues.[26,27,31-35] Nevertheless, the energy deficit and lactate production in the cells in response to a lack of oxygen can be limited and organ function can be improved by supplying pyruvate and pyruvate dehydrogenase activators, such as dichloroacetate.[27,29,36-38]

The specificity of elevated lactate to pyruvate levels for an oxygen debt in the tissues has been doubted.[27,39] Aerobic glycolysis is probably linked to the membrane Na^+,K^+-ATPase and stimulation of β_2-receptors during sympathetic activation. Catecholamine (epinephrine) secretion may temporarily increase rather than decrease ATPase activity and glycolysis and circulating lactate levels in tissues such as skeletal muscle, without a lack of oxygen and reduced ATP resources, during development and resuscitation from hypovolemic shock.[39,40] Conversely, adrenergic antagonists may reduce lactic acidosis during hypovolemic shock.[39] Epinephrine may increase glycogenolysis. Together, increased glycolytic fluxes independently of oxygen uptake may lead to equal elevations of pyruvate and lactate in the tissues, without the acidosis resulting from ATP hydrolysis after an oxygen deficit.[27] This situation may partly explain why the extent to which changes in the lactate level parallel changes in the anion gap or bicarbonate/base excess concentration during shock and resuscitation is controversial, and why elevated lactate levels sometimes may fail to predict an increase in oxygen uptake during an increase in oxygen delivery.[41-43] This also may explain in part the discrepancies in the course of oxygen-related variables and lactate levels during catecholamine treatment of shock when attempting to boost oxygen delivery.[43]

The lactate level in blood is determined by production, distribution, and elimination.[27] Produced lactic acid in the presence of oxygen may be converted via pyruvate to glucose or oxidized. Bicarbonate is then released. The liver plays a central role in this process, so that the elimination of lactate and clearance from plasma is impaired in case of liver ischemia or prior hepatic disease, even though renal uptake may increase.[27,44,45] Nevertheless, changes in the lactate level in blood, rather than absolute values, mainly reflect changes in production and are a fair measure for the course of shock and the response to therapy, even in the presence of liver disease.[27,46] Although not beyond doubt, the origin of lactate in hypovolemic shock can be skeletal muscle, lung, and gut, particularly if severe liver ischemia, hypoxia, and acidosis in shock attenuates the hepatic uptake of lactate delivered by the gut through the portal vein to the liver.[27,31,44,45,47-49] The respiratory muscles also may contribute to lactic acidosis in a spontaneously breathing patient because, first, the respiratory muscles may demand a share of the cardiac output at the cost of other tissues, and, second, this share may be insufficient to meet oxygen demands of the diaphragm, which may be increased in view of hyperventilation.[34,50-53]

Notwithstanding the aforementioned limitations, an increase in the lactate level in blood and a decrease in the bicarbonate content/base excess or pH and an increase in the anion gap may be fair predictors of morbidity (multiple organ failure [MOF]) and mortality, whereas clearance of lactic acidosis usually indicates a better outcome. A decrease in the blood lactate level during resuscitation from hypovolemic shock is usually a favorable sign and associated with survival, whereas an increase in the lactate level and progressive acidosis usually are associated with morbidity and mortality, even though successful resuscitation may transiently increase the lactate level because of washout of lactate from ischemic tissues.[27,32,33,41,46,54-58] The mentioned variables may serve as guides for resuscitation.

Oxygen Balance

Because insufficient uptake of oxygen relative to demand in the tissues during shock is central, insight into the factors that determine oxygen uptake in shock is important.[25,27] Oxygen delivery is determined by the cardiac output and the content of oxygen in arterial blood, that is, the arterial blood hemoglobin concentration and the saturation of hemoglobin with oxygen. The oxyhemoglobin dissociation curve determines the saturation of hemoglobin with oxygen for a given partial pressure of oxygen (PO_2) in blood. During hypovolemic shock, a decrease in hemoglobin concentration, oxygen saturation, or both aggravates the effect of a decrease in cardiac output in compromising oxygen delivery to the tissues. Cardiac output is determined by preload, afterload, contractility, and heart rate.[7]

During a decrease in oxygen delivery with hypovolemic shock, the body maintains sufficient uptake of oxygen only if the extraction of oxygen increases, and the arteriovenous oxygen content gradient widens, resulting in a decrease in oxygen saturation of venous blood.[6,9,21,22,27,34,40,45,59-68] Associated with the decrease in oxygen delivery, tissue PO_2 declines, and its heterogeneity increases, possibly indicating focal ischemia.[30,45,49,60,69,70] The decline in tissue PO_2 may be even greater than the decrease in draining venous blood because of some increase in microvascular oxygen shunting at low blood flows.[69,70] In animals, it has been shown that the increase in oxygen extraction to compensate for a decrease in oxygen delivery is maximal (but not 100%) if oxygen delivery decreases to less than 8 to 15 mL/kg/min, that is, the critical oxygen delivery (Fig. 27-1).[6,22,27,40,61-63,66,67] Although the critical oxygen delivery may vary widely among studies, following differences in species, basal oxygen needs, and methods to decrease oxygen delivery, data obtained in patients suggest that the critical oxygen delivery in humans also may amount to approximately 8 mL/kg/min.[59,65] During a decrease in oxygen delivery below this critical value in hypovolemic shock, oxygen uptake decreases to less than tissue demand, cellular ischemia ensues, and the body must rely on anaerobic metabolism to meet energy requirements.[9,25,34,40,59,60,62,65-67,71] Blood lactic acidosis results. Conversely, oxygen uptake is supply-dependent if oxygen delivery is lower than the critical value and blood lactate levels are elevated, whereas oxygen uptake may not be supply-dependent if the lactate level in blood is normal.[27,33,43,59,65,71] Treatment of hypovolemic shock, by infusing fluids and blood, is aimed at an increase in cardiac output and the oxygen content of blood and in oxygen delivery above the critical value so that oxygen uptake increases to meet body requirements, the lactate level in blood decreases, and acidosis is ameliorated.[9,27,32-34,43,72-74]

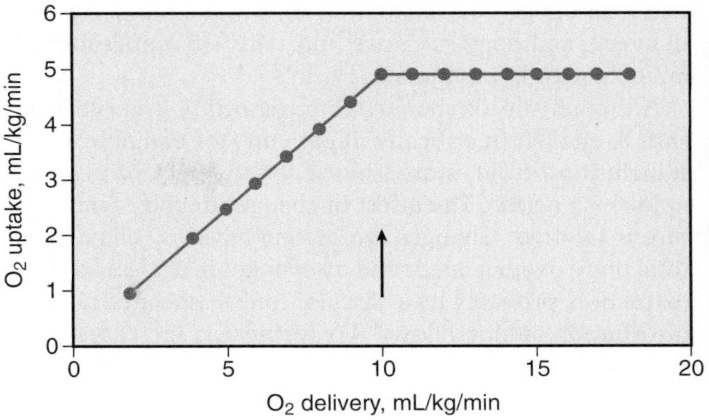

Figure 27-1. Relationship between oxygen uptake and oxygen delivery during progressive hypovolemia. *Arrow* indicates the critical oxygen delivery.

The critical oxygen delivery is a function of the body needs for oxygen and the capability of the body to extract oxygen during a decline in delivery. The body oxygen needs may increase during hypovolemic shock, as a consequence of increased respiratory muscle activity and increased levels of catecholamines in the blood after activation of the sympathetic nervous system, but "downregulation" of the metabolic stimulant effect of catecholamines has been described as well.[13,14,34,40,51,75] The extraction of oxygen is a function of the adaptation of regional blood flow to tissue needs, the number of perfused capillaries and of diffusion distances, and the exchange surface area for oxygen.[64,76] Finally, the position of the oxyhemoglobin dissociation curve could influence critical oxygen extraction. During a reduction in oxygen delivery, however, oxygen uptake is limited by convective transport of oxygen to the tissues, rather than by diffusion of oxygen to respirating mitochondria.[77]

In experimental animals, a change in hemoglobin affinity for oxygen, by altering the storage duration of reinfused blood, hardly changes the critical oxygen extraction, but changes in acid-base status that affect the position of the oxyhemoglobin dissociation curve may have some effect on the oxygen extraction capabilities of the body.[61,77] Acid infusion may increase slightly, and base infusion may reduce oxygen extraction during supply-limited oxygen uptake.[77] Nevertheless, hypercapnia may decrease critical oxygen extraction and increase critical oxygen delivery because of blood flow redistribution.[78] A leftward shift of the oxyhemoglobin dissociation curve may impair maximal oxygen extraction during a reduction in oxygen delivery and may increase mortality in experimental animals with hypovolemic shock.[61]

Although the oxyhemoglobin dissociation curve may shift to the left in critically ill patients, for example, after transfusion of old, stored blood,[79] the effect on oxygen uptake is unclear. The effect of changes in body temperature is twofold: Changes are accompanied by changes in total body oxygen needs and by changes in critical oxygen extraction, probably by a vascular tone–associated altered distribution of blood flow.[62] Hyperthermia increases critical oxygen delivery in hemorrhaged dogs, primarily through an increase in body oxygen needs and despite an increase in critical oxygen extraction, whereas hypothermia, which may be more common in traumatized or hemorrhaged patients, may decrease the critical oxygen delivery.[62] Finally, blood viscosity may influence the extent to which a decrease in circulating blood volume affects oxygen uptake by the tissues. Experimental data suggest, however, that prior anemia does not ameliorate the decrease in oxygen uptake during a decrease in oxygen delivery with hypovolemic shock, indicating that the convective transport of oxygen is the major determinant of oxygen uptake when delivery is impaired, even though prior hemodilution may increase oxygen extraction capabilities and decrease critical oxygen delivery.[6,71]

Taken together, these factors may influence the extent to which oxygen uptake decreases during reduced delivery and how far oxygen delivery should be enhanced during resuscitation from hypovolemic shock. The critical oxygen delivery varies among tissues. The oxygen needs of the kidney may decline during a decrease in renal oxygen delivery because a decrease in renal perfusion may lead to a reduction in glomerular filtration and to a reduction in energy-consuming tubular resorption.[64] In contrast, during progressive hypovolemia, the gut may experience supply dependency of oxygen uptake earlier than nongut tissue, partly because of a higher critical oxygen delivery (higher needs and less extraction of oxygen) and partly because of redistribution of blood flow away from the gut mucosa after more intense vasoconstriction in gut than in nongut tissue.[4,22,64,75,80,81] Respiratory muscle also may have a higher critical oxygen delivery than the body as a whole during progressive hemorrhage.

Concomitantly with an increased arteriovenous oxygen extraction during a decrease in oxygen delivery, the arteriovenous gradient of the carbon dioxide (CO_2) content widens.[8,53,82] The latter is associated with an increase in tissue and venous partial pressure of carbon dioxide (Pco_2) relative to arterial Pco_2 and a decrease in venous pH exceeding the decrease in pH in arterial blood.[45,53,69] This widening of gradient is caused by the Fick principle and a greater decline in cardiac output than in oxygen uptake and CO_2 production in the tissues because of inhibited oxidative metabolism. Nevertheless, the oxygen uptake usually decreases more than CO_2 production, leading to an increase in respiratory quotient.[50,66] This is likely to be caused by buffering of lactic acid by bicarbonate in the tissues and effluent blood, a shift toward glucose instead of fat use for residual oxidation in ischemic tissues, or combinations. The end-tidal expiratory CO_2 fraction decreases in association with a reduction in oxygen uptake and CO_2 production for a given ventilation.[66] Conversely, a decrease in arterial Pco_2 during a decline in CO_2 production versus ventilation may be prevented in part by an increase in deadspace ventilation resulting from a decrease in pulmonary blood flow-to-ventilation ratio.[50] An increase in deadspace ventilation leads to widening of the arterial to expiratory Pco_2.[50]

It has been suggested that the severity and duration of the lack of oxygen—the oxygen debt—accumulated during hypovolemic shock is a major determinant of survival in animals[3,6] and in patients with trauma/hemorrhage and after major surgery.[26,43,83] After trauma and hemorrhage, the defect in circulating blood volume and tissue oxygenation may be greater in patients who develop acute respiratory distress syndrome (ARDS) and MOF than in patients without these complications.[2,41,43,46,84,85] In patients undergoing major surgery, the oxygen deficit during and after surgery may relate directly to the development of postoperative organ damage (i.e., MOF) and demise.[74,83] Conversely, a high oxygen delivery and uptake during resuscitation may be associated with survival, whereas values that may be too low for elevated tissue demands are believed to contribute to ultimate demise, at least in animals with hypovolemic shock and critically ill patients after trauma or major surgery.[9,25,26,43,46,56,68,74,83,84] An increase of oxygen delivery and oxygen uptake to supranormal values has been suggested to improve survival further, although the latter debate has not been settled yet.[9,25,41,43,68,84] Extensive ischemic mitochondrial damage may limit an increase in oxygen consumption during resuscitation and reperfusion.

Macrocirculation

During loss of blood volume, various mechanisms come into play that may counteract the resultant decrease in cardiac output and oxygen delivery and uptake. First, a decrease in cardiac output during hypovolemic shock results in a redistribution of peripheral blood flow.[3,64,75,80,81,86] This redistribution is partly the result of regional autoregulation to maintain blood flow, in which endothelial cells and production of endogenous vasodilators, including endothelial nitric oxide synthase–derived nitric oxide (NO), heme oxygenase–derived carbon monoxide, and metabolic by-products in the tissues including CO_2, potassium, and adenosine, may play a central role.[87-94] Endothelium-derived NO relaxes underlying smooth muscle in the vessel wall, via stimulation of guanylate cyclase and cyclic guanosine monophosphate (cGMP), which can be inhibited by methylene blue.[88,89,95,96] Carbon monoxide also acts via cGMP.[92] Some authors describe that inhibition of endothelial nitric oxide synthase ameliorates early hypotension and even mortality during bleeding.[93] When NO is released, the reactivity to endogenous and exogenous vasoconstrictors may be diminished, even early in hypovolemic shock.[93,97]

Other authors describe endothelial dysfunction in various organs with diminished endothelium-dependent vasorelaxation via NO, which could be overcome by L-arginine, ATP-$MgCl_2$, pentoxifylline, or heparin, so that blockade of endothelial nitric oxide synthase–derived NO may be detrimental.[88-90,97] The opposing vasoconstricting factors include catecholamines, liberated by the activated sympathetic nervous system and the adrenal medulla; direct sympathetic stimulation of the vessel wall; angiotensin II, liberated through an activated renin-angiotensin-aldosterone system; and vasopressin, released by the pituitary in hypovolemic shock.[3,10-14,75,82,98,99] Endothelin is an endothelium-derived potent vasoconstrictor, released on catecholamine stimulation or hypoxia, and its release may contribute to vasoconstriction, particularly in hepatic and renal vascular beds.[100,101] Finally, a decrease in cardiac filling may reduce cardiac secretion of atrial natriuretic peptide A, reducing the vasodilating and diuretic effect of this factor.[102] Levels also may increase as a consequence of diminished renal clearance.[103,104]

Depending on the degree that the mechanisms are operative, the general result of the interplay is that blood flow to intestines, skeletal muscle, and skin is diverted toward vitally more important organs, such as heart and brain, so that the increase of overall peripheral resistance during hypovolemic shock is distributed differently among various organs, with greater increases in gut, skeletal muscle, and skin than in heart and brain.* The kidney also is a target for hypovolemic shock; renal perfusion may be maintained during mild hypotension after hypovolemia, but rapidly decreases if severe hypotension supervenes, and the decrease may exceed that in other organs.[3,14,64,75,87,106] In hypovolemic human volunteers, this redistribution of blood flow accords with the patterns described.[75]

The redistribution of blood flow results in a greater share of oxygen delivery going to organs with high metabolic demand, such as heart and brain, than tissues with less metabolic demands, including skin, skeletal muscle, kidney, gut, and pancreas.[6,14,22,64,81,105,107] The redistribution is probably necessary to optimize the uptake of delivered oxygen to the tissues and partly accounts for the increase in oxygen extraction during a decrease in oxygen delivery.[64,76] In dogs, the ability of the body to extract oxygen diminishes with α-receptor blockade of sympathetic activity, suggesting that redistribution of blood flow aided by the sympathetic nervous system is a major determinant of critical oxygen extraction.[64]

Microcirculation

Vasoconstriction after activation of the sympathetic nervous system during hypovolemia (hemorrhage) occurs in the arteries and medium-sized arterioles, but not in terminal arterioles, which may even dilate, as judged from vital microscopy studies in animals.[4,48,70,80,108] Relatively spared terminal arteriolar blood flow is presumably caused by vasodilating metabolic responses to a decline in nutrient blood flow. Nevertheless, capillary flow usually diminishes, and heterogeneity, both in space and time, may increase, particularly in irreversible shock, and independent of cardiac output.[48,70,76,80,95,109] Increased heterogeneity may serve to augment the ability of tissue to extract oxygen.[76] Traumatic/hypovolemic shock may induce expression of adhesion molecules on primed neutrophils and vascular endothelium and this, together with a reduced flow rate, may promote adherence of neutrophils to endothelium.[95,110-119] This adherence may impair red blood cell flow, particularly in capillaries and postcapillary venules.[48,80,95,111-113,120] Other authors suggest that capillary leukostasis is pressure-dependent and not receptor-dependent and reversible when perfusion pressure has been restored.[121] Finally, endothelial cells may swell and may hamper capillary red and white blood cell flow.[95,109,122] The microcirculation can be visualized, even in humans, by buccal or sublingual orthogonal polarization spectroscopy.[123]

Vasoconstriction is not confined to arteries, but also occurs in the venous vasculature, more in large than in small venules and particularly in the splanchnic area, and this is largely mediated by increased activity of the sympathetic nervous system and vasopressin release.[5,12,69,99,108] Because most of the circulating blood volume is located in small venules, splanchnic venoconstriction results in a decrease in compliance and less volume for a given intravascular pressure in the venous system, increasing return of blood to the heart.[5,7] During hypovolemic shock, the precapillary to postcapillary resistance increases, resulting in a decrease in capillary hydrostatic pressure and in fluid resorption from the interstitial space as opposed to normal filtration from capillary to interstitium, even though interstitial hydrostatic pressure decreases.[4,5,124] This is accompanied by diminished transport of protein from blood to interstitium.[125] Cellular water also is mobilized, unless, at a later stage, the sodium/potassium (Na^+/K^+) pump fails, and the cell swells.[21,126-130] Studies on fluid volumes in hypovolemic shock are not equivocal, but generally suggest that the interstitial and cellular compartments are depleted in favor of the circulating blood volume.[5,126,127]

Mobilization of fluid from the interstitial and cellular compartment can be promoted by plasma hyperosmolarity, through an increase in the glucose concentration.[131,132] This is of primary importance during uncontrolled diabetes mellitus, but also occurs to some extent during hemorrhage.[131] Chronically starved rats with depleted glycogen stores more rapidly die of hypovolemic shock than fed ones, and this can be prevented by prior glucose infusion.[131] In addition, the lymphatics may show increased pumping ability, increasing return of fluid into the systemic circulation independently of the reduced capillary fluid filtration rate.[133] Lymphatic return of interstitial protein and fluid may contribute to repletion of circulating protein and fluid volume.[133] Hemorrhage and hypovolemic shock lead to a decrease in hematocrit and a decrease in plasma proteins through transfer of fluid (and protein) from the interstitial to the intravascular space.[4,5,125] Refilling of the intravascular space diminishes in time after a sudden decrease in circulating volume, when a decline in colloid osmotic pressure, associated with hypoproteinemia, and an increase in hydrostatic pressure accomplish a new steady state in capillary exchange through readjustment of the pericapillary hydrostatic and

*References 3, 10, 12, 14, 15, 21, 22, 29, 64, 75, 86, and 105.

colloid osmotic pressures, which determine fluid and protein transport.[5] Conversely, hypoproteinemia can promote transcapillary fluid transport and expansion of the interstitial space, if hydrostatic pressure returns toward normal (e.g., during crystalloid fluid resuscitation).[127,134-137] During a sudden decrease in circulating blood volume by hemorrhage, some time is needed before the decrease in hematocrit and of proteins in blood is completed, and this decrease is aggravated by nonsanguineous fluid resuscitation.[127,135,138] Finally, increased sympathetic discharge results in contraction of the spleen, releasing red blood cells into the circulation.[14]

Taken together, the mechanisms mentioned partially compensate for a decrease in circulating blood volume and a decrease in cardiac output by promoting venous return to the heart.[7] There are some forms of hypovolemic shock, including traumatic shock, in which local capillary leakage of plasma instead of fluid resorption predominates. Mobilization of intracellular fluid does not play a role during hypotonic hypovolemic shock, with greater losses of sodium than of fluids, as occurs during an addisonian crisis.

Cells

During hypovolemic shock, the oxygen lack in the tissues causes a decline in the mitochondrial production and concentration of high-energy phosphates in the tissues because of greater breakdown than production of these compounds.[24,29,48,139,140] This decline is a function of the severity and duration of regional hypoperfusion relative to oxygen demand. The decrease in the redox status and high-energy phosphates during experimental hypovolemic shock is more pronounced in some tissues (diaphragm, liver, kidney, and gut) than in others (heart and skeletal muscle).[24,39,48,106,140,141]

A decrease in high-energy phosphates heralds irreversible cell injury during ischemia, whereas a less severe decline may result only in prolonged programmed cell death—apoptosis. In animals with hypovolemic shock and in critically ill patients, the circulating levels of ATP can be diminished, and ATP degradation products, including adenosine, inosine, hypoxanthine, and xanthine, can be elevated, suggesting breakdown of ATP following a lack of oxygen in the tissues.[28,29,57,142,143] Conversely, reperfusion is associated with restoration of energy charge, depending on the effect of ischemia, the oxygen demand, and the level of reperfusion. The intravenous administration of energy in the form of ATP-$MgCl_2$ may help tissues (kidney, liver, heart, gut) to recover from ischemia and resume function, independently of the vasodilating effects of the compound.[24,129,144-146] Also, pretreatment with coenzyme Q_{10}, involved in the respiratory chain reactions in mitochondria, has a beneficial effect during hypovolemic shock and resuscitation, at least in dogs.[82,145] Nevertheless, part of the mitochondrial dysfunction after trauma and hypovolemic shock has been suggested to be independent of a lack of oxygen.[54] Near-infrared spectroscopy, which can be applied in animals and patients, may reveal normal absorption spectra for tissue oxyhemoglobin and low mitochondrial cytochrome aa_3 redox status.[54,123,147]

About 60% of the energy produced by respirating cellular mitochondria is needed to fuel the Na^+/K^+ pump of the cell, through which the gradient in electrolyte concentrations and electrical potential over the cell membrane are controlled.[24] In the absence of sufficient ATP because of a decline in production associated with lack of oxygen, the Na^+/K^+ pump is inhibited, and this results, together with a possibly selective increase in cell membrane permeability for ions independently of an energy deficit, in an influx of sodium into and efflux of potassium out of the cell, leading to cellular uptake of fluid.[24,48,110,126,128,148] Measurement of membrane potentials of skeletal muscle and liver in experimental animals has shown that hypovolemic shock rapidly decreases the transmembrane potential (a less negative inner membrane potential), associated with electrolyte and fluid shifts across the cell membrane.[24,48,110,126,128,148] A circulating shock protein also may contribute to these changes, independently of an energy deficit.[126,148] A decrease in activity of the Na^+/K^+ pump may contribute to hyperkalemia because of potassium exchange between cells, interstitial fluid, and vascular space.[39,48,110,126] Finally, calcium (Ca^{++}) influx into cells and their mitochondria inhibits cellular respiration and ultimately contributes to cellular damage and swelling, particularly during resuscitation, and this can be prevented by administration of Ca^{++} antagonists.[24,126,128,130,149,150] Because of cellular influx, the plasma-free Ca^{++} levels may decrease in experimental and human hypovolemic shock.[128,150,151] Intracellular lysosomes lose their integrity so that proteolytic enzymes are released and contribute to cell death.[4,24,107,152] These enzymes eventually may reach the systemic circulation and may damage remote organs.[4,24,107,152]

As has become apparent in past years, the cellular response to stress, such as heat and tissue hypoxia, involves the expression of certain genes, coding for synthesis of the so-called heat-shock proteins, which play an important role in protecting the cells against stress.[153-156] The clinical significance of these molecular cellular changes is unknown. The response may be partially responsible, however, for the decreased susceptibility to hypovolemic shock after hemorrhage in animals with a prior challenge by endotoxin.[111]

Organ Perfusion and Function in Shock

Heart

According to Starling's law of the heart, a change in preload, approximated by the end diastolic volume and determined by the venous return of blood to the heart, directly results in a change in stroke volume, defining myocardial function.[7] The relationship between end diastolic filling pressure and volume reflects compliance. Apart from preload, cardiac output also depends on afterload, which is approximated by the end systolic volume of the heart, and contractility, reflected by the peak systolic pressure-to-volume relationship (maximal elastance).[7,56,157] A diminished response of the stroke work by the heart, that is, the product of stroke volume and arterial blood pressure, to an increase in preload during resuscitation from hypovolemic shock may indicate diminished cardiac contractility (e.g., caused by pre-existent cardiac disease, hypovolemic shock itself, myocardial contusion, or combinations).[4,56,158] The effect of hypovolemic shock on myocardial function in animal models is controversial. Depending on models, methods, and definitions of cardiac dysfunction, some authors describe a decrease, but others describe an unchanged function of the left heart.[4,128,157-161] The latter can be explained if a decrease in contractility of the heart is masked by the inotropic effect of catecholamines and other positive inotropic substances, such as endothelin, liberated during hypovolemic shock, even though receptor-mediated catecholamine responses may decline.[4,23,100,159] Hearts from shocked animals also may show depressed function ex vivo, even at adequate coronary blood flow and oxygen consumption.[161]

Although coronary blood flow may be defended, and the oxygen demands of the heart may decrease associated with a decrease in filling (preload) and arterial blood pressure (afterload) during initial hypovolemic shock, hypotension may become so severe that coronary vasodilation to compensate for a decline in perfusion pressure becomes exhausted, so that myocardial oxygen delivery decreases to less than the oxygen needs of the heart, and ischemia ensues, particularly if tachycardia is present.[3,21,141,161,162] This may occur primarily in endocardium because of more rapidly exhausted vasodilation in endocardium than epicardium and redistribution of blood flow from the inner to the outer layer of the heart.[141] The subendocardium may become ischemic, and patchy necrosis may ensue.[141] Because of regional transmural and intramural differences in vasodilator reserve, myocardial ischemia may be heterogeneously distributed and associated with a diminished redox state, lactate production, and creatine phosphate breakdown.[141,160] Ischemia ultimately may contribute to a decrease in myocardial contractility during hypovolemic shock. Smooth muscle–dependent and, particularly, endothelium-dependent coronary vasomotion may be impaired after hypovolemic shock.[90,163]

Pentoxifylline may improve endothelial and myocardial function.[164] Myocardial edema and compression of capillaries with resultant impairment of diffusion and extraction of oxygen also may contribute to a decrease in regional coronary blood flow, regional myocardial ischemia, and decreased myocardial function in hemorrhaged animals.[128,132,141,161] Hypovolemic shock may induce a decrease in left ventricular compliance.[159] The myocardial dysfunction following a decrease in compliance (diastolic dysfunction) may be particularly pronounced during resuscitation from hypovolemic shock.[157,159] Postischemic failure ("stunning") also may play a role during resuscitation, at least temporarily. Ischemia-reperfusion of the heart results in accumulation of intracellular Ca^{++}.[128] This may impair mitochondrial and sarcoplasmic reticulum function and contribute to impaired cardiac function after hypovolemic shock.[128,159] In dogs, the administration of Ca^{++} blockers may prevent such deterioration during resuscitation from hypovolemic shock.[128] Finally, systemic release or intramyocardial production of negative inotropic substances ("myocardial depressant factors" and endogenous opioids) and inflammatory mediators such as tumor necrosis factor (TNF)-α, interleukin (IL)-6 and platelet activating factor; oxidant damage; metabolic acidosis; diminished adrenoreceptor density; and resultant diminished sensitivity of the heart to circulating catecholamines may contribute to myocardial dysfunction during hypovolemic shock.[11,23,27,37,107,150,160,161,165-168]

The clinical evidence for myocardial dysfunction during hypovolemic shock is scarce.[46,56,162] Nevertheless, it is conceivable that severe hypotension reduces the balance between oxygen delivery and demand of the heart because many patients with hypovolemic shock may be elderly and may have coronary artery disease, compromising coronary vasodilation. For a patient with hypovolemic shock, a decrease in left ventricular compliance, contractility, or both may imply that a relatively high filling pressure would be needed to restore cardiac output during fluid resuscitation.[56,73,161,162,169] The averaged optimal pulmonary capillary wedge pressure, that is, the pressure above which cardiac output does not increase further, may not be elevated in patients with hypovolemic shock (i.e., 12 to 15 mm Hg), although in some patients, abnormally elevated filling pressures may be needed to increase cardiac output, or cardiac output does not increase at all during fluid resuscitation.[56,73,169,170] A diminished function of the heart may hamper restoration of oxygen delivery to the tissues during resuscitation.[9,46,159] Myocardial dysfunction may be greater in nonsurvivors than in survivors.[56] There may be some electrocardiographic or enzymatic evidence for myocardial ischemia and injury, and some patients may experience a myocardial infarction as a complication of severe hypovolemic shock after hemorrhage.[162,171]

Lung

Hypovolemic shock often induces an increase in ventilatory minute volume, resulting in tachypnea or hyperventilation and a decrease in arterial P_{CO_2}.[34,50,51,53,172] Unless complicated by pulmonary abnormalities, these changes are, at least initially, not the result of hypoxemia, but an increase in deadspace ventilation after a decrease in pulmonary perfusion, so that a higher minute ventilation is necessary, for a given CO_2 production, to eliminate CO_2 from the blood and to maintain a normal P_{CO_2} in arterial blood.[34,50,51] Minute ventilatory volume may increase further if a decrease in P_{CO_2} is necessary to compensate for metabolic acidosis after accumulation of lactate in the blood.[27,33,34,50,51,53,172] The imbalance between increased demands of the diaphragm and reduced blood flow in shock finally may lead to respiratory muscle fatigue and a subsequent decline in ventilatory minute volume.[51]

Hypovolemic shock caused by trauma and hemorrhage and followed by extensive transfusion therapy of red blood cell concentrates can be complicated by pulmonary edema and impaired gas exchange.[52,173-178] In some patients, overtransfusion and an elevated filtration pressure (pulmonary artery occlusion pressure [PAOP]) may be responsible. In others, pulmonary edema may be due to a pulmonary vascular injury, however, and increased vascular permeability, at a relatively low PAOP, indicating

ARDS.[52,172,175,176] The reaction to diuretics may help to differentiate between hydrostatic and permeability edema of the lungs. The latter seems relatively rare in polytransfused, polytraumatized patients, unless associated with complications, but other studies suggest that about 30% of patients with severe trauma/hemorrhage may develop ARDS.[175,176,178,179] As measured by the transvascular albumin flux in the lungs, almost 80% of patients with multiple trauma may show increased pulmonary vascular permeability in the disease course.[52] This leak ultimately may contribute to impaired pulmonary mechanics and gas exchange.[52]

Experimental studies are at variance concerning alterations in capillary permeability of the lungs during pure hypovolemic shock and resuscitation.[4,134,172,180,181] According to some investigators, hypovolemic shock following bleeding and transfusion mildly increases transvascular filtration of fluid and proteins and results in accumulation of interstitial fluid, as a consequence of increased permeability,[180] but other authors do not observe such changes.[132,134,180,182] In other animal studies, however, traumatic/hypovolemic shock resulted in extensive morphologic changes of the lung, with endothelial and interstitial edema, accumulation of degranulated neutrophils, and scattered fat emboli, which may resemble the pulmonary changes after traumatic/hypovolemic shock in humans.[172,183-185] As suggested by animal experiments, among others, several factors may play a role, including release of proinflammatory mediators (TNF-α) and priming and activation of blood neutrophils after ischemia-reperfusion, contusion or ischemia-reperfusion of the lungs themselves, pulmonary microemboli of neutrophils, platelets and fat particles from the medulla of fractured long bones, and neutrophilic antibodies or humoral or cellular breakdown products and released cytokines in transfused blood products ("transfusion-related acute lung injury" [TRALI]).[52,117,172,173,178,181,183,185-188] Translocated endotoxin (see the following discussion) also may play a role.[183] Finally, aspiration of foreign material or gastric contents and post-traumatic pneumonia and sepsis may contribute to the development of ARDS in trauma patients. When pulmonary edema has developed, active resorption by alveolar cells becomes necessary for clearance. This process is cylic AMP–dependent and can be disturbed by iNOS-derived NO and peroxynitrite and enhanced by expression of heme oxygenase, at least in animal models. How this translates clinically is unclear.

Brain

Classically, brain perfusion is considered to be relatively spared during progressive hypovolemia because of the extensive autoregulatory capacity of cerebral arteries.[15,187] Regional cerebral blood flow may even increase.[187] In case of autoregulation impairment after neurotrauma, however, brain perfusion may decrease, and subsequent reperfusion may contribute to secondary cerebral damage during hypovolemic shock and resuscitation. Hemorrhagic shock and resuscitation per se also may impair autoregulatory capacity of brain vessels, however, because of endothelial dysfunction and diminished NO-dependent vasodilator reactivity, so that the brain may experience an oxygen deficit and metabolic and functional deterioration.[29,89]

Kidney

Hypovolemic hypotension is an important risk factor for acute renal failure after trauma.[153] During a decrease in cardiac output following progressive hemorrhage, renal blood flow can be maintained because of renal vasodilation, so that the kidneys may not participate in the systemic vasoconstriction that characterizes hypovolemic shock.[3] When blood pressure decreases, however, the renal vessels also constrict, impairing blood flow to the kidneys more than to other organs.[3,14,86,87,106,140] This is partly caused by a baroreflex-mediated increase in sympathetic activity; activation of the renin-angiotensin-aldosterone system; and release of catecholamines, angiotensin II, endothelin, and vasopressin or antidiuretic hormone.[13,14,75]

During prolonged hypovolemic shock, sympathetic inhibition may protect against renal ischemia.[14] Superimposed on a direct effect of renal sympathetic nerve activity, elevated circulating levels of the aforementioned compounds result in renal vasoconstriction. This propensity for vasoconstriction is partly offset if NO and prostaglandins with vasodilatory actions are released intrarenally.[4,87] Inhibition of NO synthesis increases blood pressure, however, and increases renal perfusion and glomerular filtration during hypovolemic shock.[87]

In another study, endothelium-dependent renal vasodilation was impaired after hypovolemic shock.[88] Vasodilating prostaglandins are released through the cyclooxygenase pathway of arachidonic acid metabolism, in response to ischemia, increased sympathetic activity, and angiotensin II, so that renal vasodilation during the early phase of hemorrhage can be blocked by prostaglandin synthesis inhibition, resulting in a profound decrease in blood flow, even if accompanied by an increase in arterial blood pressure.[3] In hypovolemic shock, the balance of these substances favors renal perfusion during a moderate decline in cardiac output and arterial blood pressure, but is unfavorable during a severe decrease in blood pressure so that renal perfusion declines.[3,75,87]

Renal ischemia results in a decrease in glomerular filtration ("prerenal" renal failure) that is less than the decline in blood flow so that the filtration fraction often increases.[139] The latter is caused by greater constriction of efferent than of afferent arterioles in glomeruli, in which high levels of circulating angiotensin II are probably involved. The decrease in glomerular filtration together with an increase in tubular resorption of electrolytes and fluids, mediated by increased levels of antidiuretic hormone released by the pituitary and decreased levels of atrial natriuretic peptide through low atrial filling, results in oliguria or anuria (<0.3 mL/kg/h) and a low sodium content of urine[139] except in cases of uncontrolled diabetes mellitus and adrenocortical insufficiency.

The decrease in renal perfusion during hypovolemic shock is often accompanied by redistribution of blood flow from outer to inner cortex and medulla, which is already borderline hypoxic even in the normal state.[128] If long-lasting and severe, the cortical kidney becomes ischemic, despite a decrease in oxygen needs associated with fewer energy needs for tubular resorption in the presence of less filtration, so that the levels of high-energy phosphates decline.[139,140] Severe and prolonged renal ischemia and metabolic deterioration finally result in acute renal failure with morphologic changes, particularly in proximal tubules and medullary segments (acute tubular necrosis), when an increase in renal perfusion does not immediately restore filtration and diuresis, but rather injures renal structures (reperfusion injury), limiting a return of blood flow and glomerular filtration during resuscitation.[130,139,183,184] This is often recognized by a persistent oliguria and a gradual increase in creatinine and urea levels in blood. In addition, the urinary excretion of tubular cell–derived biomarkers of injury may increase.[104]

Gut

During hypovolemic shock, blood flow from stomach to colon is redistributed to other organs, and this may be primarily mediated by elevated sympathetic activity and increased levels of vasopressin and angiotensin II, even though vascular reactivity to the latter may diminish.* Vasoconstriction may overwhelm NO and other vasodilating mechanisms, and endothelium-dependent vasodilation may be impaired after oxidant endothelial injury.[191] Gut ischemia is aggravated further by the countercurrent mechanism in mucosal (villous) blood flow, promoting diffusional shunting of oxygen from arteries to veins, bypassing tissues. Other studies reported that gut mucosal blood flow may be relatively spared during hypovolemia, however.[76,105] Portal blood flow decreases, and portal blood levels of lactate increase after gut ischemia.[27,49,192]

Gastric mucosal ischemia may result in diminished energy-consuming acid production and may predispose to mucosal stress ulceration.[189,193] Microscopic studies in experimental animals show damage of gastric mucosa, villous epithelium in small bowel, and mucosa of the large bowel after hypovolemic shock.[113,189,194-196] Gastric mucosal ischemia-reperfusion injury after bleeding may be aggravated by gastric acid itself, neutrophils, inflammatory mediators, endothelin, reactive oxygen species (ROS), and proteases.[195,197] Bowel ischemia and mucosal damage during hypovolemic shock in the dog ultimately may lead to leakage of fluid from the bloodstream to the bowel lumen, instead of normal resorption of luminal fluids.[114,194] Diarrhea may contribute to intravascular volume depletion during severe and prolonged hypovolemic shock, at least in animals.

Gut mucosal ischemia, energy depletion, injury, and inflammation may compromise the barrier function of the mucosa, enhancing the likelihood that bacteria and endotoxins in intestinal lumen (large bowel) translocate through the damaged gut wall to lymph nodes, portal venous blood, or both.[143,183,184,196,198-202] The gut epithelial (lumen to plasma) permeability for small molecules also is increased. Indigenous flora, generated toxic ROS, Ca^{++} overload, iNOS, peroxynitrite, phospholipase A_2 activation, cytokines, and activated and adhering neutrophils during ischemia and reperfusion probably all play a role in the injury, promoting hyperpermeability and translocation.[196,202] Mucosal injury and translocation can be inhibited by compounds targeted against these factors.[196] Impaired detoxifying capacity of the Kupffer cells of the liver because of ischemia or pre-existent liver disease may contribute further to bacteria and endotoxins reaching the systemic circulation and contributing to progression of shock, by triggering an inflammation cascade, ultimately resulting in release of vasoactive substances.[4,200,201] This translocation has been shown to contribute to the lethality of hypovolemic shock in experimental animals because clearance or blockade of translocated bacteria and endotoxins is associated with survival, and germ-free animals survive an episode of bleeding more often and longer than ones with a normal intestinal flora.[4,144,201,202] Finally, it has been shown that the absorptive capacity of the gut for carbohydrates, amino acids, and lipids decreases during hypovolemic shock.[149,192] Although enteral feeding during hypovolemic shock and after resuscitation may increase metabolic demands of the gut, there is experimental evidence that luminal application of nutrients, particularly of enterocyte-fueling glutamine, induces an increase in small vessel blood flow, ameliorates damage, and diminishes the likelihood for translocation of endotoxins and bacteria during resuscitation from hemorrhage.[203]

In humans, hypovolemia leads to a decline in hepatosplanchnic perfusion.[75] Stomach mucosal lesions may be common after prolonged hypovolemic shock, but overt bleeding is a relatively rare event, particularly in a rapidly adequately resuscitated patient.[204] Agents that decrease energy-demanding gastric acid production may protect against stress ulcers during mucosal ischemia.[193] The gut is usually quiescent during hypovolemic shock in humans. Ileus is often present, and the patient is managed expectantly until bowel sounds return. Occasionally, a bowel infarction and perforation may complicate hypovolemic shock.[149] As in animals, gut absorptive capacity may decrease.[149] It is likely that these changes are caused in part by gut ischemia. The adequacy of gastrointestinal blood flow can be monitored in humans with the help of a balloon catheter in the stomach (or gut), in which fluid or air is installed, or sublingually or buccally with help of a sensor (tonometry).* The mucosal P_{CO_2} thus measured decreases, and the mucosal-to-blood P_{CO_2} gradient increases, during a decrease in mucosal blood flow relative to demand. An increase of this gradient may occur at an earlier stage than an increase in heart rate or decrease in arterial blood pressure during progressive hypovolemia, constituting a sensitive sign of shock.[205] Gastrointestinal tonometry can be used as a guide for resuscitation.† The clinical occurrence and significance of translocation of intestinal bacteria and endotoxins to mesenteric lymph

*References 3, 13, 14, 22, 80, 81, 97, 105, 140, 189, and 190.

*References 41, 55, 69, 93, 106, 123, 140, 164, 193, and 205-208.

†References 41, 55, 93, 106, 123, 140, 164, 193, and 205-208.

nodes and the bloodstream are unclear, although the capacity of the human gut wall to resorb orally administered small molecules, including lactulose relative to mannitol, may increase, indicating epithelial barrier dysfunction.[55,200,201,207,209-211]

Liver

Liver (microvascular sinusoidal) perfusion declines during hypovolemic shock because of diminished portal and hepatic arterial blood flow, roughly in proportion to the decrease in cardiac output so that in contrast to the gut, there is no angiotensin II–mediated selective vasoconstriction in the hepatic arterial bed.[95,106,140,146,150,164,212-214] Endogenous mechanisms, including release of carbon monoxide and NO, may counteract a decrease in perfusion, which is promoted by thromboxane A_2 and endothelin, unless attenuated by endothelial dysfunction.[92,156] A decrease in blood flow may result in liver ischemia, a decrease in high-energy phosphate contents and clearance function as evidenced by insufficient capacity to clear indocyanine green from blood, and a decrease in the bile excretion rate.[28,45,92,95,143,146,150,212-215] The capacity to clear gut-derived endotoxin and lactate also may decrease, and the ischemic liver produces lactate.[44] Hepatic ischemia may result in a diminished capacity for metabolism of drugs such as lignocaine[216] and for gluconeogenesis from lactate and amino acids, contributing to hypoglycemia in the late stage of hypovolemic shock.[12,140] Hepatic sinuses may become filled with adherent cellular (neutrophilic) aggregates, lining cells may swell, and centrilobular necrosis/apoptosis may finally ensue, with leakage of enzymes into the circulation.[95,164,183,184,213,217] Clinically, there also may be transient elevations of bilirubin and transaminases in blood, and severe abnormalities have been attributed to "ischemic hepatitis," denoting ischemic injury.[218,219] A clinically useful measure of hepatic oxygen deficit is an increase in the plasma ratio of β-hydroxybutyrate to acetoacetate ("keto body ratio"), which occurs concurrently with a decrease in the hepatic mitochondrial redox state.[28,92,95,219]

Spleen

The spleen contracts during hypovolemic shock, probably caused by increased sympathetic activity, and this results in release of red blood cells into the circulation.[3,14] The changes in hematocrit during the early phase of bleeding probably underestimate the severity of plasma losses. The spleen also releases stored platelets.

Pancreas

The pancreas is severely ischemic during hypovolemic shock.[107] This may lead to autodigestion of acinar cells and liberation of pancreatic lysosomal enzymes into the systemic circulation, including proteases and factors with negative inotropic properties on the heart, such as the "myocardial depressant factor," although the latter factor also may come from ischemic gut.[4,107,164] Ligation of the pancreatic duct may be beneficial in experiments, by preventing gut injury and barrier failure, among others.[220]

Inflammatory and Immunologic Changes

During and after hemorrhage, hypovolemic shock, and resuscitation, macrophages, including lung macrophages and Kupffer cells in the liver, may release cytokines, including TNF-α, IL-1, IL-6, and IL-8. This can be ameliorated by blockade of nuclear factor-κB (NF-κB), administration of the macrophage-inhibitor pentoxifylline, or ATP-$MgCl_2$ increasing hepatic blood flow.[145,164,184,185,190,213,221-223] Ischemia per se and the immune consequences of gut barrier injury may play a role in Kupffer cell responses. The reperfused gut, together with the liver, may be a source of systemically released cytokines, as suggested by animal experiments and observations in humans after trauma, and translocated endotoxin may play a role.[55,190,200,201,224-227] During reperfusion after resuscitation, cytokines may induce and amplify the inflammatory response to ischemia and may induce further local and remote organ damage with circulatory changes.[164,185,222,226,227]

Spillover of mediators into the mesenteric lymph or portal and systemic circulations during reperfusion of prior ischemic gut may have deleterious effects on remote organs, by inducing neutrophil activation and adherence, which may contribute to a lung vascular injury with increased permeability.[183,184,186,224,226,227] Circulating levels of proinflammatory cytokines may be of predictive value for remote organ damage, including ARDS, after trauma in patients.[223,224] Endotoxin binding or antibodies and cytokine antibodies may ameliorate remote tissue damage after bleeding, hypovolemic shock, and resuscitation.[183,184] Finally and as mentioned earlier, proinflammatory mediators may be expressed locally in a variety of organs in response to hemorrhagic shock, including heart and lungs, and this is partly under control of α-sympathoadrenergic stimuli, neuroimmune activation, NF-κB, hypoxia-inducible factor, and other factors involved in cell signaling.[228]

Trauma and shock/resuscitation also have been shown to activate the complement and the arachidonic acid systems.[152,229-232] Complement activation may yield potent vasodilating and leukoattractant substances and contribute to remote inflammatory organ damage (ARDS). Ischemia may generate phospholipase A_2, catalyzing arachidonic acid metabolism into prostaglandins via the cyclooxygenase pathway, releasing thromboxane A_2 and prostacyclin, and into leukotrienes via the lipoxygenase pathway.[10,152,231] Thromboxane A_2, released from platelets, neutrophils, and cell membranes, has potent vasoconstricting properties and promotes aggregation of platelets and neutrophils, whereas prostacyclin has vasodilating properties and inhibits platelet and neutrophil aggregation.[231] Leukotrienes have vasoconstricting properties, increase capillary permeability, and attract neutrophils.[152] Vasoconstricting prostaglandins may be involved in tissue damage during ischemia-reperfusion, and vasodilating prostaglandins may be involved in the vasodilated state of terminal hypovolemic shock.[10,230] Another lipid mediator that may be released is platelet-activating factor, but the precise action of this mediator is unclear.[150,168]

Probably of primary importance is the release of xanthine oxidase–generated ROS during ischemia-reperfusion, which may activate macrophages and attract neutrophils, partly mediated by ROS-induced release of cytokines via NF-κB.[191,233] After long-lasting ischemia, activation of the xanthine-oxidase system and formation of uric acid from the ATP breakdown products hypoxanthine and xanthine during reperfusion could liberate ROS, which damage vascular endothelium and parenchymal cell membranes through peroxidation of lipids.[117,186,195,196,233,234] Experimental models indicate that pretreatment with xanthine oxidase inhibitors (allopurinol) or scavengers of ROS including lazaroids may ameliorate microvascular hemodynamics and membrane injury of organs such as the heart and gut and improve survival after resuscitation from hypovolemic shock, although some of these compounds may have more effects than others.[145,191,195,196,233,234]

A study in trauma patients with elevated lipid peroxidation products in plasma showed that superoxide dismutase ameliorated the inflammatory response and MOF.[225] ROS scavengers may inhibit formation of toxic peroxynitrite via NO and ROS and may inhibit breakage of DNA single strands and activation of poly(ADP-ribose) synthetase, which contributes to cellular injury.[91,93,235] The interaction of ROS fueled by oxygen and NO may play a central role in inflammation and vascular tone after perfusion.[91] Similarly, administration of oxygen may bind NO and increase vascular resistance and ROS formation.[91] Some time after hypovolemic shock and resuscitation, iNOS may become active particularly in the gut and liver; circulating NO breakdown products may increase; and inhibition of the excessive NO release may ameliorate hemodynamic changes, organ inflammation, and neutrophil accumulation and function, partly via less peroxynitrite formation, unless too strong or a selective inhibition leads to a decrease in cardiac output.[91,93,156,217] Increased iNOS-derived NO also may be prevented and treated by corticosteroids or adrenocorticotropic hormone (ACTH) fragments.[94,236]

The interplay of these factors may result in endothelial activation throughout the body and an inflammatory reaction, ultimately involving attraction, activation, and endothelial adherence of neutrophils, as shown in animal models of hypovolemic shock after bleeding and ischemia-reperfusion.* Neutrophils release vasoconstricting, platelet-aggregating, and damaging thromboxane A_2 and may inhibit vasodilating prostacyclin, via secreted ROS and proteases such as elastase.[117,224,232,233,237] Neutrophil aggregation and secreted activation products also may also play a role in the reperfusion injury by impairing resumption of small vessel blood flow, even in the presence of a seemingly adequate cardiac output and arterial blood pressure.[48,80,95,112,113,203,231] In humans, the activation of neutrophils after trauma, with increased adhesion molecule expression and propensity for degranulation, is associated with morbidity after trauma, such as development of MOF and predisposition to sepsis.[114,116,117,223,238] After initial leukopenia (neutropenia) following trapping of leukocytes in the microcirculation, activation of the pituitary-adrenal axis and release of corticosteroids and catecholamines during hypovolemic shock result in an increase of circulating neutrophils, following demargination and release from bone marrow, together with eosinopenia and lymphocytopenia.[48,111-114,213] A tertiary decrease of circulating neutrophils in patients with a downhill course may be explained by microcirculatory sequestration.[114] The hemodynamics, organ function, and survival of rats with hypovolemic shock/resuscitation are improved if rats are made neutropenic before the challenge, and this may relate to improved regional and capillary blood flow.[112,231] A monoclonal antibody against or antagonists of neutrophil-endothelial adhesion molecules decrease reperfusion injury in lungs, liver, stomach, and intestines after hypovolemic shock or ruptured aortic aneurysm and may improve survival, at least in animal m odels.[113,117,119,185,233] This does not impair host defense against subsequent bacterial infections.[113]

Hypovolemic shock depresses the immune system, by suppressing the function of lymphocytes, macrophages, and neutrophils, depressing humoral and cellular immune responses, decreasing antigen presentation and delayed hypersensitivity to skin test antigens, and increasing susceptibility to sepsis.[2,110,221,222,238-245] Part of this may be mediated via neuroimmune modulation and resulting efferent sympathetic, adrenergic, and vagal stimulation.[38,94] In patients, the immune defect correlates with the extent and severity of trauma and the degree of blood resuscitation required, but animal experiments document that hemorrhage/resuscitation per se depresses immune function, even though trauma, hypovolemic shock, and blood transfusions may be synergistic in this respect.[222,239,240,245,246] The depression may not depend on the type of trauma and resuscitation fluid. Hemorrhage in experimental animals and patients decreases the capability of lymphocytes to proliferate and to produce lymphokines (IL-2) in response to mitogens, an effect that seems dependent on an energy or NO deficit or on Ca^{++} influx in these cells after ischemia because the defect can be overcome by administration of Ca^{++} influx blockers.[222,239,240,245,246]

The immune consequences of hemorrhage and resuscitation differ among cell populations, however, with some cells expressing enhanced and others diminished inflammatory responses. Increased macrophage production of cytokines during hypovolemic shock and resuscitation may be followed by decreased ability of the cells to release mediators such as TNF-α and to express HLA-DR and to process and present antigens to lymphocytes. This may relate to a cellular energy deficit, accumulation of Ca^{++}, and enhanced prostaglandin E_2 synthesis.[164,221,222,238,241,245] Priming of immune cells may explain in part the increased sensitivity to endotoxin and sepsis after hypovolemic shock, although other authors have described that prior hypovolemic shock and priming decreased the immune response and increased the tolerance to endotoxin or sepsis.[113,182,185,247] The immunodepression after hypovolemic shock and predisposition to sepsis finally may include the release by Kupffer cells, among others, of anti-inflammatory following proinflammatory cytokines, such

*References 10, 111, 113, 116, 152, 164, 186, 195, 213, 226, 230, 232, and 233.

as IL-10, and soluble receptors (receptor antagonists) for proinflammatory cytokines, and this may relate to sepsis-induced MOF, morbidity, and mortality in trauma patients.[245,248]

Hypovolemic shock and gut-derived factors may blunt the increase in bone marrow cytopoiesis after soft tissue trauma and endotoxin and contribute to susceptibility to sepsis.[244,249] Neutrophils may become "downregulated" after initial stimulation by circulating proinflammatory and anti-inflammatory mediators.[110,236,243] Neutrophil dysfunction is evidenced by a diminished potential to migrate and to digest and kill bacteria, perhaps in the presence of an inhibited respiratory burst.[110,186,238,243] In hemorrhaged mice, the infusion of granulocyte colony-stimulating factor or IL-6 after hemorrhage may partly prevent neutrophil defects and protect against mortality from subsequent pulmonary sepsis.[243] Also, the opsonization function of macrophages, that is, the reticuloendothelial system, is depressed so that removal from the circulation of fibrin, cell aggregates, and bacteria by the liver is, at least transiently, impaired.[4,24,165,222,245,250] This may relate to the appearance after hypovolemic/traumatic shock of substances in blood that depress reticuloendothelial system function or to consumption and a decrease of the α_2-glycoprotein fibronectin in plasma, a substance that aids the reticuloendothelial system in opsonization.[4,165,222,250,251] This deficiency may contribute to development of organ failure and might be reversed by infusion of plasma cryoprecipitate.[251]

Otherwise, the immunologic consequences of trauma, hemorrhage, and hypovolemic shock depend on numerous additional factors, including gender and other genetic influences.[238,245] Men may exhibit more immunodepression after trauma/hemorrhage than women. The clinical implication may be that men are more susceptible than women to microbial infections after trauma.[252]

Circulating coagulation factors and platelet counts may decrease after hypovolemic shock and resuscitation, whereas fibrin products may increase. This is the consequence of coagulation activation and fibrinolysis inhibition by endothelial activation, tissue injury, and inflammatory responses, even though dilution after fluid resuscitation may heavily contribute.[179,223,253] Disseminated intravascular coagulation (DIC) and fibrin deposits, if insufficiently removed by the fibrinolytic system, may contribute to a decrease in plasma coagulation factors and to widespread microvascular organ dysfunction.[179,223,254] Proinflammatory responses, some resuscitation fluids, hypothermia, and acidosis may contribute to DIC and the coagulation defect of severe hemorrhagic/traumatic shock.[223] It is still unclear, however, what the gold standard for diagnosing DIC is, what the contribution to organ injury is, and what constitutes the best therapeutic approach.

Hormones and Metabolism

As mentioned before, a severe decrease in cardiac output resulting in a decrease in arterial blood pressure during hypovolemic shock results in activation of the sympathetic nervous system through the baroreceptor reflex and liberation of norepinephrine from nerve endings and epinephrine from adrenal medulla so that circulating levels of these catecholamines increase.[11-13,75,82,98] The insulin secretion by the pancreas is inhibited, and glucagon secretion is enhanced by high circulating norepinephrine levels.[98] The renin-angiotensin-aldosterone system is activated, and the pituitary secretion of antidiuretic hormone (vasopressin) and opioids increases.[11-13,23,98-99] The pituitary response to stress further includes an increase in ACTH with resultant corticosteroid release by the adrenal cortex, unless limited by the so-called relative adrenal insufficiency.[12,98,153] These factors may be essential for survival because prior adrenalectomy decreases survival of animals subjected to hypovolemic shock, and steroid repletion is protective in this respect.[12] This protective effect can be attributed to, among others, less overactivation of the sympathetic nervous system and increased sensitivity of the heart and vasculature to circulating levels of catecholamines.[12]

Finally, the secretion of atrial natriuretic peptide A by the myocardium declines, in response to hypovolemia and diminished wall stress of the atria. These factors result, among others, in tachycardia and a diminished renal excretion of water and salt, to restore circulating blood volume. Endogenous opioids could play a role in maintaining shock by their vasodilating and myocardial depressant properties, however.[11,13,23] Administration of the opioid antagonist naloxone and its derivatives augments arterial blood pressure in hypovolemic shock.[13,23,144,255] Similarly, thyrotropin-releasing hormone depresses the opioid system and increases arterial blood pressure, cardiac function, and survival during hypovolemic shock in animals.[23] Thyroid hormone may have a similar effect.[256]

During hypovolemic shock and cellular ischemia, intermediary metabolism undergoes profound changes, partly caused by an altered hormonal milieu.[98] This situation has been particularly studied after trauma. The early hyperglycemic response to traumatic/hypovolemic shock is the combined result of enhanced glycogenolysis, caused by the hormonal response to stress and elevated epinephrine, cortisol, and glucagon levels; increased gluconeogenesis in the liver, partly mediated by glucagon; and peripheral resistance to the action of insulin, the secretion of which may be diminished shortly after onset of shock, but may be enhanced later after shock.[24,47,98,130] This resistance is most likely the result of an altered hormonal milieu—the increase in circulating epinephrine and cortisol levels. During the late, irreversible stage of hypovolemic shock, however, hypoglycemia supervenes, at least in animal models, because glycogen stores may be depleted and the capacity for gluconeogenesis by the liver may decrease because of ischemia.[12,24,47,110,131]

Increased gluconeogenesis in the liver, and to a lesser extent in the kidneys, follows increased efflux of amino acids such as alanine and glutamine from the muscle to the liver because of breakdown of muscle protein.[98,218] The latter is evidenced by increased urinary losses of nitrogen and a negative nitrogen balance.[98,218] Lactate produced in muscle also can be converted to glucose in the liver.[98]

Finally, fatty acid metabolism undergoes profound changes, with depressed lipolysis, ketogenesis, and combustion of fatty acids during shock and an increase in the resuscitation phase.[98,218] Some investigators regard a deranged intermediary metabolism of primary importance for the eventual outcome of shock, whereas others merely consider these changes as a result of the shock process itself.[218]

Reperfusion and Irreversible Shock

Reperfusion of various organs, including the heart, gut, skeletal muscle, brain, kidneys, and liver, after a transient episode of ischemia, as occurs during hypovolemic shock, results in the so-called reperfusion injury, which limits the possibility for resumption of microvascular tissue blood flow and function of organs, particularly of the liver, even if cardiac output and arterial blood pressure have been restored to normal values.* Redistribution of blood flow during hypovolemia may be only partly attenuated by reperfusion.

Reperfusion after a certain period of shock and diminished oxygen uptake results in an increase in oxygen uptake above baseline levels, provided that oxygen delivery and cellular function are adequate.[43,63,74,98] This repayment of the oxygen debt is largely determined by the increased demands for oxygen to resynthesize ATP from adenosine and phosphates and to rebuild the lost energy stores. This repayment is determined by the extent to which mitochondria are damaged during ischemia and the availability of substrates to resynthesize high-energy phosphates and restore cellular contents of these compounds because the substrates needed for ATP synthesis may have been washed out, necessitating de novo synthesis.[24,143,144] Resuscitation may not completely restore energy levels, the activity of the Na^+/K^+ pump, and the membrane potential of skeletal muscle and liver, necessary to remove accumulated fluid and sodium from the cell.[126,128,143] The relationship between the overshoot in oxygen uptake during reperfusion and the accumulated deficit of oxygen accumulated during ischemia may be poor.[63]

Conversely, the intravenous administration of energy in the form of ATP-$MgCl_2$ or adenosine-regulating compounds such as acadesine may help tissues (kidney, liver, heart, gut) to recover from ischemia and resume function, independently of the vasodilating effects of the compounds, by providing energy, improving the microcirculation, and reducing cell swelling, promoting survival.[24,129,144-146,158] Nevertheless, the ability of organs or the whole body to increase oxygen uptake during reperfusion above normal may be associated with survival in experimental animals with hypovolemic shock and in hypovolemic patients after trauma or major surgery, whereas inability may be associated with ultimate demise.[9,74,83]

Reperfusion not only results in resumption of oxygen delivery, but also of Ca^{++} to the tissues. This Ca^{++} may be taken up by cells and may contribute to the reperfusion injury by damaging cell organelles, inhibiting respiration, and activating proteases and prostaglandin synthesis.[128,130,149,150] Reperfusion injury of heart, gut, kidneys, and liver after resuscitation from hypovolemic shock in animals may be prevented in part by administration of Ca^{++} influx blockers independently of their vasodilating effects, suggesting that Ca^{++} overload is partly responsible for the reperfusion injury.[128,130,149,150] Finally, endothelial damage and swelling and red blood cell aggregation may hamper the regional regulation of blood flow during resuscitation from hypovolemic shock.[80,95,109,122] Neutrophil-mediated endothelial injury may increase capillary permeability and contribute to fluid losses during resuscitation.[112,176,177,259]

If shock syndrome, with hypotension and subnormal oxygen uptake, persists after optimal fluid repletion and attempts at reperfusion with inotropic and vasoactive drugs, the condition can be regarded as irreversible and terminal.[4,9] The term *irreversible shock* has been mainly used in animal experiments, however, in which reinfusion of the shed blood after a certain period is unable to reverse the shock syndrome.[4,260] Various factors may play a role.[4] First, vascular decompensation may contribute to a further decrease in blood pressures and may include diminished constrictive reactivity, dilation of arterioles, and insensitivity to circulating or exogenous catecholamines.[97,108] The decline in vascular resistance may be partly caused by metabolic vasodilation in ischemic and acidotic tissues, overcoming vasoconstrictive influences.[4,10,108] Other factors that may be involved include dysfunction of vascular smooth muscle after induction of iNOS and resultant increased production of vasodilating NO in the vessel wall, activation of low ATP-activated K^+ channels, histamine release, and prostaglandin-induced neurotransmission failure.[10,29,93,94,96,97,140,230,236] Circulating levels of NO breakdown products, nitrate and nitrite, may be elevated already early after hemorrhage in animals and trauma in humans, although other authors described low levels in humans.[261] iNOS upregulation and NO production may be prevented by NO blockers, corticosteroids, or ACTH fragments.[93,94,236] Finally, central cerebral or humoral mechanisms may contribute to the irreversible hemorrhagic shock, and this may relate to endogenous opioids, thyrotropin-releasing hormone, or macrophage-derived anandamide, an endogenous cannabinoid.[13,23,262] Intravenously administered ACTH fragments may have an adrenal-independent central opioid-inhibiting effect, which may help to prevent vascular decompensation and treat hypotension, even clinically.[94]

The decrease in arterial vascular resistance may be particularly pronounced in the tissues, showing most intense vasoconstriction during hypovolemic shock, including gut and skeletal muscle, offsetting the redistribution of blood flow during hypovolemic shock and increasing blood flow to these organs at the expense of blood flow to vital tissues.[10,22] In contrast, venous compliance and resistance increase, leading to peripheral pooling of blood and a decrease in venous return to the heart.[4,164] The latter changes may be particularly pronounced in the

*References 80, 113, 146, 150, 164, 196, 203, 212, 233, 257, and 258.

splanchnic region.[164] During prolonged or irreversible hypovolemic shock, capillary hydrostatic pressure may increase after arteriolar vasodilation and venular constriction (a decrease in the precapillary-to-postcapillary resistance ratio), promoting fluid filtration into the interstitium.[4,5] Capillary permeability also may increase, resulting in a high capillary hydraulic conductance and a decrease in the reflection coefficient for plasma proteins. Increased permeability for proteins increases capillary filtration for a given intravascular hydrostatic pressure and promotes the formation of edema.[176,259] The increase in permeability may be the consequence of endothelial damage by ischemia-reperfusion, possibly involving activated neutrophils and ROS as final mediators. It may contribute further to a decline in circulating blood volume.[5,259] Cells may swell, and this may diminish circulating blood volume further.[4,126,128-130] Expansion of the cellular and interstitial fluid volume at the expense of the intravascular volume is manifested by a preterminal increase of the hematocrit.[4,5,127] Finally, an inflammatory response to ischemic tissue may elicit organ damage and contribute to irreversibility of hypovolemic shock.

Dysfunction of vital organs after prolonged ischemia or patchy necrosis/apoptosis or both may contribute to the irreversibility of hypovolemic shock.[4,113] Reperfusion injury may aggravate organ damage and contribute to irreversible shock.[113,258] The pump function of the heart may diminish after a decrease in systolic contractility and compliance, and this may contribute to irreversibility of shock during resuscitation.[158] Myocardial dysfunction may contribute to the development of pulmonary alveolar edema, if aggressive fluid infusion in attempts to increase cardiac output results in an elevated PAOP.[4] Diminished function of the heart may hamper restoration of oxygen delivery and uptake to the tissues during resuscitation.[9,46,157,158] Damage of the gut mucosa may cause translocation of luminal bacteria and endotoxins from gut lumen to systemic circulation, at least in experimental animals, and the resultant sepsis may contribute to the irreversibility of hypovolemic shock.[4,183,194,196,199-202,211] Taken together, irreversible hypovolemic shock may contribute to MOF and death.[2,204]

CLINICAL FEATURES

Causes

One of the most frequent causes of hypovolemic shock is blood loss after trauma (see Box 27-1), including blood loss during or after major surgery.[2] Ruptured aortic aneurysm and gastrointestinal hemorrhage are other frequent causes of hypovolemic shock. Upper gastrointestinal bleeding can be caused by peptic ulcer disease, reflux esophagitis, variceal bleeding, erosive gastritis (stress ulcer), or aortoduodenal fistula after vascular surgery. Lower gastrointestinal bleeding can result from diverticular disease, carcinomas, or polyps in the colon. Sometimes, massive hemoptysis resulting from a tumor, tuberculosis, fungal infection, or bronchiectasis can be the cause of hypovolemic shock. Hematuria as a result of a tumor or trauma is a rare cause of hypovolemic shock. During multiple trauma, blood loss is essential in causing hypovolemic shock, but trauma itself can activate various mediator systems, with resultant release of vasoactive substances that contribute to the development of shock. In contrast to pure hypovolemic shock, cardiac output can be elevated, and peripheral vascular resistance is often decreased in cases of multiple trauma.[25]

In trauma patients, external blood loss can be accompanied by internal, invisible blood loss after renovascular trauma or major fractures (e.g., of the pelvis or femur). After blunt abdominal trauma, splenic or hepatic ruptures and perforations of hollow viscera are possible. Blunt chest trauma can be accompanied by an aortic rupture, tension pneumothorax, hemothorax or hemopericardium, and tamponade. Nonmechanical causes of hypovolemic shock include uncontrolled diabetes mellitus and acute adrenocortical insufficiency, causing severe renal fluid losses. Acute and severe vomiting (obstruction of the gastric outlet or gut), diarrhea, and burn wounds result in loss of plasma water.

Signs and Symptoms

Hypovolemic shock warrants an early diagnosis, avoiding delay in initial treatment. As soon as possible after admission of the patient, fluid resuscitation should begin via a large-bore catheter in a peripheral vein or a percutaneously inserted central venous catheter. At the same time of initial fluid resuscitation, a history is taken, and a brief but thorough physical examination is performed. The latter serves to establish rapidly the cause and severity of shock. Extensive manipulation of a fractured spine or extremity should be avoided. The history of a patient in hypovolemic shock is mainly determined by its cause. The patient may complain of thirst, diaphoresis, and shortness of breath. The patient's mental state is usually normal, unless shock is severe and the patient becomes apathetic or confused. With less severe cases, the patient is anxious, and with more severe cases, the patient is apathetic.

For a clinical diagnosis of shock, hypotension and clinical signs of organ ischemia should be present. Clinical signs are relatively insensitive for small blood losses (Table 27-1).[205] This sensitivity can be improved by using the shock index, calculated from heart rate divided by systolic blood pressure.[18] The clinician can recognize shock from a decrease in systolic blood pressure to less than 90 mm Hg or a decrease of more than 40 mm Hg below preshock levels, with a reduction in pulse pressure. Hypotension may be so severe that blood pressure is unrecordable noninvasively. There can be a large gradient between invasively and noninvasively measured arterial blood pressure and between central and radial artery pressure during shock and drug-induced vasoconstriction.[263] Hypotension may become particularly marked when the patient sits or stands versus when the patient is supine (orthostatic hypotension).[8,17,18] Postural dizziness, tachycardia, and hypotension are reliable and early signs of hypovolemia, whereas dryness of mucous membranes and axillae, decreased turgor, supine hypotension, and tachycardia and other signs have less diagnostic value.[17,18]

Table 27-1. Clinical Classes of Severity of Hypovolemic Shock after Hemorrhage

	Class I	Class II	Class III	Class IV
Blood loss				
mL	<750	750-1500	>1500-200	>2000
%	<15	15-30	>30-40	>40
Heart rate (beat/min)	<100	>100	>120	>140
Systolic blood pressure	Normal	Normal	Decreased	Decreased
Pulse pressure	Normal	Decreased	Decreased	Decreased
Capillary refill normal	Delayed	Delayed	Delayed	Delayed
Respiratory rate (min)	14-20	20-30	30-40	>35
Urine output (mL/h)	>30	20-30	5-15	Minimal
Mental status	Slightly anxious	Anxious	Confused	Confused and lethargic

Tachycardia may be absent in case of prior use of β-blockers. Elderly patients may have atrial fibrillation and a high ventricular response. Occasionally, bradycardia is present, particularly when vagally mediated fainting supervenes.[16] The peripheral veins are collapsed, and the jugular venous pressure is low. Conversely, an elevated jugular venous pressure should warn the clinician of associated obstruction of the circulation, following pneumothorax, pericardial tamponade, and others, or of pump failure following myocardial contusion or infarction. The respiratory cycle–induced changes in stroke volume and in systolic arterial blood pressure and CVP are exaggerated.[20] Although dependent on tidal volume and respiratory compliance, these variations in a mechanically ventilated patient may constitute fair indices of hypovolemia, so that high variations may predict an increase in cardiac output on fluid loading.[19] Noninvasive, pulse contour–based techniques are suitable for these purposes. Fluid responsiveness also can be predicted by an increase in blood pressure and decrease in stroke volume and pressure variations during leg raising or similar maneuvers. The body temperature may decrease, particularly in elderly patients. The gradient between the ambient and toe temperature may be a fair index of peripheral blood flow and a measure for the severity of hypovolemic shock because a reduction in skin blood flow (cold, clammy skin) is an early and ominous sign of shock in view of selective cutaneous vasoconstriction.[123] Other signs of hypovolemic shock include tachypnea, oliguria/anuria, diaphoresis, cold and clammy skin with diminished capillary refill, and peripheral cyanosis.

The clinical diagnosis of hypovolemic shock is not difficult in the presence of hypotension and visible loss of blood volume, as occurs during trauma (e.g., fractures), gastrointestinal or pulmonary hemorrhage, burn wounds, and diarrhea. Internal hemorrhage after a ruptured aortic aneurysm, blunt abdominal trauma, or hemothorax is difficult to diagnose except when the history of the patient and obvious physical signs, including dullness on thoracic percussion and abdominal distention and tenderness, point to potential internal bleeding. In the case of upper gastrointestinal blood loss, one should look for signs of chronic liver disease, including palmar erythema, spider nevi, and portal hypertension (ascites), because they could predict variceal bleeding as a cause of hypovolemic shock. Brown discoloration of the palms of the hand and mucosal membranes may point to adrenocortical insufficiency, and a smell of acetone in expiratory breath may point to uncontrolled (ketoacidotic) diabetes mellitus.

DIAGNOSTIC APPROACH

General

The diagnostic work-up of a patient with hypovolemic shock should not hamper initial resuscitation. After the history and physical examination, the necessity for further diagnostic procedures depends on the underlying cause of shock.

If trauma and external blood loss are the cause of shock, control of external bleeding, crossmatching of blood, and infusion of fluids and blood components have a higher priority than further diagnostic procedures. Blunt chest trauma can be complicated by aortic rupture, tension pneumothorax, hemothorax or hemopericardium, and tamponade. A chest radiograph can be useful to diagnose these conditions. After blunt abdominal trauma, splenic or hepatic ruptures are possible, and an abdominal tap and analysis of the fluid should be performed to exclude or establish intra-abdominal bleeding or hollow-organ perforation.[264,265] Adjunctive diagnostics, if time permits, may include computed tomography or ultrasonography of the abdomen, to select patients for explorative laparotomy and to avoid negative surgery.[264,265] A ruptured abdominal aortic aneurysm can be diagnosed via ultrasonography or angiography, if the patient's condition allows for the use of such an invasive, time-consuming procedure. Conversely, intra-abdominal pressure may increase considerably, particularly during fluid resuscitation; may impair gut and renal perfusion; and may warrant decompression.[266] The usefulness of emergency aortic clamping or balloon tamponade for massive abdominal hemorrhage is controversial.[267] In the case of gastrointestinal hemorrhage, diagnostic procedures also are performed after initial resuscitation, including gastroscopy for upper gastrointestinal bleeding and sigmoidoscopy for lower gastrointestinal bleeding and angiography. Introduction of a nasogastric tube can be useful to aspirate blood, diagnose bleeding, prevent aspiration during vomiting, and follow the course of bleeding.

Laboratory Investigations

At admission of a patient with suspected hypovolemic shock, blood samples should be taken to determine the hemoglobin/hematocrit and leukocyte and platelet counts; electrolyte, creatinine, and lactate concentrations; arterial blood gases and pH; and blood typing (crossmatching). Immediately after hemorrhage, the hemoglobin content and hematocrit of blood are normal, but they decrease in time with refilling of the plasma compartment, as does the protein content.[127,133,134,138,180,181,268] A high hemoglobin content and hematocrit can be encountered during pure loss of plasma (water), as occurs during burn wounds or severe diarrhea. Acute hypovolemic shock may be accompanied by slight leukopenia followed by leukocytosis.[48,110,112,243,244] If coagulation disorders are suspected (therapy with anticoagulants, liver disease, bleeding tendency), platelet counts and coagulation tests should be performed. Transient thrombocytopenia may ensue if shock is severe, and massive amounts of whole blood are lost and rapidly replaced by erythrocyte concentrates or nonsanguineous fluids (i.e., through dilution). Isolated thrombocytopenia without DIC may occur.

The concentrations of electrolytes (sodium, potassium, chloride) in blood are essentially normal, unless the concentrations in the fluid lost deviate from those in plasma (hypertonic and hypotonic dehydration) and shock is accompanied by severe metabolic acidosis. In the latter example, potassium leaves the cell, potentially leading to hyperkalemia.[110,126] More often, however, less severe forms of shock are accompanied by hypokalemia because of adrenergic receptor–stimulated Na^+,K^+-ATPase. Saline fluid loading or overloading can result in hyperchloremia. Adrenocortical insufficiency may result in hyponatremia, hyperkalemia, and hyperchloremic acidosis, caused by changes in urinary excretion induced by mineralocorticoid deficiency. In a patient with liver disease, the corresponding abnormalities can be found in laboratory studies. In the case of uncontrolled diabetes mellitus, hyperglycemia and glucosuria are observed. As previously mentioned, the glucose concentrations in blood can be elevated in early shock and, occasionally, depressed in late shock. Finally, the concentration of unbound Ca^{++} in blood may diminish during hypovolemic shock after cellular uptake and polytransfusion of red blood cell concentrates, if containing calcium-binding citrate as an anticoagulant.[128,151]

During hypovolemic shock, metabolic acidosis, often associated with an elevated lactate level in blood, is common and of prognostic significance, although the decrease in bicarbonate and base excess may not parallel the increase in lactate.[27,32-34,39,42] The pH can be subnormal after lactic acidosis and a decrease in the bicarbonate content, even if ameliorated by hyperventilation and a decrease in P_{CO_2}.[27,33,34,50,51] The lactate level in blood can be determined rapidly and followed frequently (every 2 hours). The lactate level and its course during treatment also is of prognostic significance during shock because during successful treatment, the lactate level decreases, and the bicarbonate concentration and pH increase, whereas an unchanged or even increased lactate level during resuscitation is usually associated with morbidity, including sepsis and MOF, and mortality.[27,32,33,57] An elevated anion gap, the difference between the sodium on the one hand and the sum of the bicarbonate and chloride concentrations in blood on the other hand, can be a first sign of lactic acidosis, although, as previously mentioned, elevated lactate levels may not be associated with acidosis in the absence of an oxygen deficit.[27] The serum creatinine concentration is initially normal. The urea content increases following "prerenal" renal insufficiency, catabolism, or breakdown of blood in the gut during gastrointestinal hemorrhage. In the urine, the osmolarity is increased.

The sodium content is low, together with a low fractional excretion of sodium,[139] calculated as the quotient of urinary (U) and plasma (P) sodium (Na) and creatinine (creat) concentrations: $FE_{Na} = (U_{na}/P_{na})/(U_{creat}/P_{creat})$. In case of acute renal insufficiency (acute tubular necrosis), the urinary sodium content and fractional excretion are increased.[139] This increased sodium also occurs during adrenocortical insufficiency. Prior diuretic therapy may invalidate this diagnostic tool, however, whereas the fractional excretion of urea may not be affected by diuretics.[104] Tubular injury may be tracked from increased urinary excretion of biomarkers, which may predict the need for renal replacement therapy.[104]

Miscellaneous abnormalities may include elevated levels of nitrate and nitrite, the stable breakdown products of NO.[261] Transient elevations of bilirubin, alkaline phosphatase, γ-glutamyltransferase, and transaminases in blood may be severe and denote ischemic liver damage.[218,219] Elevations of creatinine kinase may be caused by skeletal muscle, cardiac, or, less likely, brain damage. Elevated troponin concentrations specifically may indicate cardiac injury.[162,171]

Monitoring

Noninvasive monitoring of arterial blood pressure to judge the course of shock and its response to treatment suffices for some patients with hypovolemic shock. Nevertheless, there may be substantial differences between the invasive and noninvasive readings of arterial blood pressure, favoring arterial catheterization and invasive monitoring. The gradient between toe and body temperature can be used as a noninvasive index of peripheral perfusion.[123] Urinary output should be measured hourly in patients with shock to judge the adequacy of treatment because transition of oliguria to a diuresis exceeding 40 mL/h is an indicator of adequate renal perfusion.

Unless hypovolemic shock is rapidly reversed by initial infusion of fluids, there is often a need for hemodynamic and respiratory monitoring in the intensive care unit for a patient with hypovolemic shock. The goal of monitoring is to document the course of shock and its reaction to treatment. Complications can be diagnosed in an early phase so that action can be rapidly undertaken, if necessary. Respiratory monitoring is meant to detect, at an early stage, respiratory insufficiency and muscle fatigue, which are caused by an imbalance in oxygen supply to demand and which may necessitate intubation and mechanical ventilatory support.[51]

Arterial blood pressure can be monitored via a catheter in the radial, axillary, or femoral artery, introduced percutaneously using the Seldinger technique, under aseptic conditions. Percutaneous insertion (Seldinger technique) of a double-lumen or triple-lumen central venous catheter may be useful, allowing for more rapid fluid infusion than through a single peripheral cannula. The internal jugular, subclavian, or femoral vein may be used for that purpose. This also permits monitoring of CVP and oxygen saturation. Pressures in the lesser circulation (pulmonary arterial pressure and PAOP) can be measured with the help of a balloon-tipped pulmonary artery catheter inserted percutaneously and advanced under pressure monitoring until the inflated balloon wedges in a pulmonary artery side branch. This catheter also allows for thermodilution measurement of cardiac output and obtaining mixed venous blood for blood gas analysis.[74,269] Together with arterial blood measurement of oxygen variables, this allows the calculation of oxygen delivery, extraction, and uptake.[9,25,74] These calculations may contribute to judging the severity of shock and its response to treatment.[6,9,25,74]

The CVP reflects the filling pressure of the right ventricle, and the PAOP reflects the left atrial pressure and, in the absence of mitral valve disease, the filling pressure of the left ventricle. Under certain circumstances, however, including positive-pressure ventilation or measurement above the level of the left atrium, when the measured pressure is more influenced by alveolar than by venous pressure, the CVP and PAOP may overestimate true (i.e., transmural) right and left atrial pressures. The response of filling pressure and cardiac output to fluid loading, as measured with the central venous or pulmonary artery catheter, is an index of myocardial function and can be useful, particularly in patients with pre-existent cardiac disease.[56,73,169] Measurement of PAOP is important if function or compliance of the left ventricle is altered (e.g., in case of pre-existent heart disease), when the CVP may underestimate PAOP.[56,73] Conversely, the CVP may overestimate PAOP, in case of severe pulmonary hypertension and right ventricular failure. It has been suggested that changes in CVP during fluid loading do not predict changes in PAOP.[73] The intensity and speed of therapy can be guided by the response of filling pressures and cardiac output, as measured with the use of the central venous or pulmonary artery catheter.[9,32,43,56]

These measurements also can help to time, choose, and dose concomitant therapy with inotropic or vasopressor agents. Together with the plasma colloid osmotic pressure, the PAOP determines filtration of fluid across pulmonary capillaries, according to the Starling equation. Monitoring of the PAOP during infusion of fluids may prevent pulmonary edema because infusion can be guided by the filling pressures of the heart. Taken together, data obtained with the pulmonary artery catheter are useful if the hypovolemic origin of shock is not immediately apparent in complicated cases, and if initial therapy is not immediately successful.[9,25,74] The indications for insertion may include a high risk for shock in patients undergoing major surgery and shock of unknown origin when clinical judgment fails to recognize severe hypovolemia. Data obtained with the catheter are of diagnostic value in complicated forms of shock because hypovolemic shock is characterized by low filling pressures and cardiac output and a high peripheral vascular resistance. These characteristics may serve to differentiate from other types of shock.

Difficulties during treatment also may constitute indications for pulmonary artery catheterization, including hypovolemic shock unresponsive to liberal fluid repletion, in the absence of a low jugular venous pressure or CVP, and hypovolemic shock together with pre-existent cardiac disease unresponsive to fluid repletion, if a large discrepancy between CVP and PAOP is suspected and if vasoactive drugs are considered. Monitoring the PAOP may help to lessen the risk for pulmonary edema during fluid loading. Contraindications for pulmonary artery catheterization include those for central venous catheterization. The complications of the technique are discussed elsewhere. Although the use of pulmonary artery catheters is hotly debated, because of lack of direct evidence that they help to increase survival, there are some indications that therapy guided by variables collected with the catheter improves the outcome of selected critically ill patients after trauma or surgery.[9,25,74,270] Nevertheless, the exact hemodynamic and metabolic resuscitation goals are difficult to define, so the usefulness of the pulmonary artery catheter is difficult to prove.[9,43,68,270,271]

As an alternative to the pulmonary artery catheter, various less invasive or even noninvasive (pulse contour–based) systems have been developed that circumvent some of the problems associated with filling pressures as preload indicators and predictors of responsiveness of cardiac output on fluid loading. Among others, the transpulmonary thermodilution technique with detection of thermal changes, after central venous injection of cold dextrose 5% in water in the iliac artery, allows for calculation of cardiac output, global end diastolic volume, and extravascular lung water—measures of cardiac preload, pulmonary fluid filtration, and pulmonary edema.[272] Assessment of cardiac volumes and the ratio of peak systolic pressure to end systolic volume, as done by echocardiography, can be helpful in evaluating heart function further.[157] This technique also evaluates filling of heart and large vessels, when transmural filling pressures are doubted, and suspected cardiac contusion and pericardial tamponade.[273]

Future developments in monitoring the circulation of a patient in hypovolemic shock include continuous monitoring of central venous or mixed venous oxygen saturation, with the help of the fiberoptic technique introduced via catheters, allowing for the continuous evaluation of the oxygen supply-to-demand ratio; right ventricular end diastolic volume monitoring as an index of filling status; and measurement of tissue blood flow, P_{O_2}, P_{CO_2}, and oxygenation by electrodes and optic techniques.* Tissue Po_2 decreases and Pco_2 increases during regional perfusion failure, and these events (in skin, conjunctiva, muscle, or bladder) are probably early signs of hypovolemia following redistribution of blood flow.[8,45,49,60,69,123] The adequacy of gastrointestinal blood flow can be judged noninvasively with the help of a tonometer balloon catheter in the stomach (or gut) or with help of a sensor sublingually or buccally, in which fluid or air is instilled, and the Pco_2 is measured to calculate the mucosal-to-blood Pco_2 gradient, as explained previously.† Fluid treatment guided by the adequacy of gastrointestinal mucosal perfusion, as judged by tonometry, could improve the outcome of hemorrhaged trauma patients compared with resuscitation based on standard hemodynamic variables alone.[41,123,206,208]

Monitoring the end-tidal CO_2 fraction, determined by and directly related to the blood flow–dependent tissue CO_2 production, and the gradient to arterial Pco_2, determined by blood flow–dependent deadspace ventilation, can help to judge the response to resuscitation.[50,66] The use of a balloon-tipped catheter, retrogradely inserted into a peripheral vein to monitor peripheral postcapillary venous pressure, a technique analogous to measurement of PAOP, has not yet gained wide-scale clinical applicability.[124] Hydrostatic pressure measurements in the urinary bladder may reflect the measurements in the abdominal compartment and may help to identify intra-abdominal hypertension and abdominal compartment syndrome.[266] Regional Doppler flow measurements could supplement clinical judgment.[15]

APPROACH TO MANAGEMENT

General

Treatment of shock cannot be delayed, so in practice diagnosis and treatment are done simultaneously. Treatment of hypovolemic shock is aimed at the restoration of the circulation and treatment of the underlying cause. Box 27-2 describes some general guidelines. The main therapeutic goal in hypovolemic shock is to restore circulating blood volume and to optimize oxygen delivery so that oxygen uptake "plateaus" (see Fig. 27-1) and meets tissue needs.[72,271] Optimization of cardiac output, stroke work, and tissue oxygenation and maintenance of arterial blood pressure are physiologically reasonable goals for patients.[43]

Optimization does not imply maximization above levels adequate for tissue needs.[68] Studies by some investigators have suggested that supranormal rather than normal oxygen delivery and consumption may be associated with survival from severe trauma or hemorrhage, including a ruptured aortic aneurysm, and that therapeutic targeting at these values (with oxygen delivery >600 mL/min/m^2 and oxygen consumption >170 mL/min/m^2) improves the outcome of severe trauma in humans.[9,25,41,43,84] These concepts are controversial, however.[271] In any case, resuscitation based on blood pressure alone probably does not fully restore tissue oxygenation, particularly in the case of myocardial dysfunction after shock and resuscitation.[43,56]

Adequate resuscitation from hypovolemic shock should result in a preferably documented or clinically evident increas in oxygen delivery and uptake, a decrease in lactate levels, and amelioration of metabolic acidosis.[9,32-34,43,68,72-74,84,170,271] Concomitantly with the increase in cardiac output, arterial blood pressure increases.[72,73,170] Successful resuscitation in terms of a restored cardiac output and arterial blood pressure may poorly reflect effective recovery of tissue perfusion, however, even though reversal of oliguria is considered as a favorable return of renal perfusion.[30,80,110,130,146,150,164,212] Animal experiments have suggested that early circulatory optimization also ameliorates inflammatory changes after trauma/hemorrhage. In attempts to restore oxygen delivery, hypoxemia should be prevented or corrected. The arterial oxygen saturation, important for the oxygen content of delivered blood, usually exceeds 90% if the Po_2 is greater than 60 mm Hg. If arterial Po_2 is less than 60 mm Hg, supplemental oxygen can be given through a nasal cannula or mask. The patient should be intubated and artificially ventilated, in case of impending respiratory insufficiency. Prophylactic positive end-expiratory pressure in attempts to prevent the development of ARDS in at-risk patients, including patients with traumatic/hemorrhagic shock, is useless.

For the initial stabilization of trauma patients in shock, with severe abdominal trauma or bleeding from lower

Box 27-2

Guidelines for Treatment of Hypovolemic Shock

1. Insert large-bore intravenous catheter; perform laboratory investigations (crossmatching, hemoglobin/hematocrit, thrombocyte count, electrolytes, creatinine, arterial blood gas analysis and pH, lactate, coagulation parameters, transaminases, albumin). Watch for need to supply oxygen, intubation, or artificial ventilation (so that arterial Po_2 >60 mm Hg and oxygen saturation >90%).
2. Resuscitation with fluids is done at a ratio of two thirds crystalloid, one third colloid fluid. At >25% loss of blood volume, give erythrocyte concentrates; at >60% loss, also give fresh frozen plasma (e.g., after about four erythrocyte concentrates and earlier if liver function is disturbed). In case of polytransfusions (>80% loss) and platelet counts <50 × 10^9/L, platelet suspensions should be given. Massive red blood cell transfusion is preferably performed via microfilter.
3. Diagnose and treat underlying cause, concomitantly with guideline no. 2.

*References 30, 45, 49, 54, 60, 69, 123, 124, 147, 206, 271, 274, and 275.

†References 41, 55, 69, 93, 106, 140, 164, 193, 205, 207, and 208.

extremities, passive leg raising has been used, but its beneficial effect on preload-augmented tissue oxygen delivery is controversial.[8,276] The pneumatic antishock garment can be applied as a temporary, immediately lifesaving procedure to (1) stop the hemorrhage and splint pelvic and lower extremity fractures for transportation of the patient after inflation, (2) mobilize blood volume by exerting external pressure on the leg and abdomen, and (3) redirect flow toward vital organs such as the heart and brain.[277-279] Use of the garment and hypertonic saline may act synergistically.[277] The disadvantages of the procedure include aggravation of pressure-dependent and uncontrolled bleeding and ischemia of intra-abdominal organs. Deflation should be gradual, to prevent lethal hypotension after return into the circulation of vasoactive substances and lactic acid from ischemic tissue.[277,278] The use of the pneumatic antishock garment has greatly declined in recent decades. Measures to establish a way to the bloodstream for infusing fluids include insertion of a large-bore catheter in a peripheral vein or, if cannulation of peripheral veins seems impossible because of collapse, a catheter in a central (i.e., jugular/subclavian) vein. The latter catheter also allows monitoring of CVP. The intraosseous route for administration of hypertonic fluids is particularly useful in traumatized children with hypovolemic shock.[280] To this end, a marrow screw is inserted in the sternum or tibia. Fluids can be given by gravity or pressure.

Further treatment of hypovolemic shock depends on the underlying cause. Immediate surgery is warranted in case of extensive trauma and ongoing internal or external blood loss. Massive intra-abdominal bleeding after blunt or penetrating injury may warrant drug therapy with vasopressin or aortic clamping. Gastrointestinal hemorrhage can be stopped by conservative treatment, including histamine$_2$ receptor blockade and endoscopic electrocoagulation or laser coagulation of bleeding peptic ulcers. Bleeding varices can be treated by continuous infusion of vasopressin or somatostatin, a Sengstaken-Blakemore balloon tube, and endoscopic injection sclerotherapy. Surgery is indicated when conservative measures fail (e.g., in the case of peptic ulcer rebleeding) within 48 hours after admission. Apart from fluids, uncontrolled diabetes mellitus necessitates continuous intravenous infusion of insulin (±6 U/h). Acute adrenocortical insufficiency warrants administration of steroids (hydrocortisone 100 mg two to four times daily).

Resuscitation Strategies

The speed with which shock can be reversed depends on the delay from onset to treatment and the severity of shock, as estimated from the clinical condition and hemodynamic status. The speed of fluid infusion can be guided by the clinical condition of the patient, heart rate and blood pressure, diuresis, and determinations every 2 hours of the arterial blood lactate level and acid-base balance.[32] Repeated assessment of jugular venous pressure and auscultation of the lungs are indicated to prevent overhydration and pulmonary edema. If a central venous or pulmonary artery catheter is in place, a fluid challenge protocol can be used (Table 27-2).[32] Monitoring of central venous or pulmonary arterial wedge pressure or preload volumes allows for rapid infusion of solutions and evaluation of the response of oxygen delivery and uptake to resuscitation.[9,25,32,74]

Table 27-2. Fluid Therapy

Guided by	CVP ($cm H_2O$)	PAOP (mm Hg)	Infusion
Start	<8	<10	200 mL/10 min
	<12	<14	100 mL/10 min
	= 12	= 14	50 mL/10 min
During infusion	↑ >5	↑ >7	Stop
After 10 min	= 2	= 3	Continue
	2 > ↑ = 5	3 > ↑ = 7	Wait 10 min
	↑ >5	↑ >7	Stop
After waiting 10 min	Still ↑ >2	Still ↑ >3	Stop
	↑ = 2	↑ = 3	Repeat

10 cm H_2O = 7.3 mm Hg.
CVP, central venous pressure; PAOP, pulmonary artery occlusion pressure.
Adapted from Weil MH, Henning RJ: New concepts in the diagnosis and fluid treatment of circulatory shock. Anesth Analg 1979;58:124.

The usefulness of immediate and vigorous resuscitation in the course of uncontrolled bleeding (e.g., after penetrating vascular trauma) has been challenged in recent years.[269,281-283] Studies have shown that infusion of substantial amounts of nonsanguineous fluids and increasing pressure-dependent bleeding lead to dilution of blood components, coagulation disturbances, and increased mortality, unless the bleeding is controlled before resuscitation.[269,279,282,283] The clinical implication is that resuscitation perhaps should not take place, at least not vigorously, at the scene of the accident when bleeding cannot be controlled and transport to the hospital where the bleeding can be controlled is practicable. This not only may apply to trauma patients, but also perhaps to patients with a ruptured abdominal aneurysm. Authors have proposed slow rather than rapid (but early) infusion rates and "controlled hypotensive" resuscitation (e.g., with help of vasodilators) as long as bleeding is uncontrolled.[279,281,282,284,285] The value of this type of resuscitation with hyperoncotic/hypertonic solutions, including acetate with vasodilating and buffering properties, is debatable.[207,269]

Fluids

The mainstay of treatment of hypovolemic shock is the repletion of circulating blood volume.* During hypovolemic shock, the repletion of intravascular volume is of primary importance to restore cardiac output and oxygen transport to the tissues before repletion of the interstitial and intracellular fluids.[25] Available fluids are described in Tables 27-3 to 27-5. Electrolyte solutions (the crystalloid fluids) are shown in Table 27-3, and high-molecular-weight solutions (the colloid fluids) are shown in Tables 27-4 and

*References 9, 25, 32, 34, 70, 72-74, 170, 206, 271, 282, 286, and 287.

Table 27-3. Crystalloid Fluids

	Na (mmol/L)	K (mmol/L)	Cl (mmol/L)	Ca (mmol/L)	Glucose (mmol/L)	Lactate (mmol/L)	HCO_3^- (mmol/L)	Osmolarity (mOsm/L)
Glucose 5%					278			278
NaCl 0.65%	111		111					222
NaCl 0.9%	154		154					308
NaCl 3%	513		513					1025
NaCl 7.5%	1283		1283					2567
NaCl 30%	5000		5000					10,000
Ringer's lactate	130	4	110	3		27		275
$NaHCO_3$ 1.4%	167						167	334
$NaHCO_3$ 4.2%	500						500	1000
$NaHCO_3$ 8.4%	1000						1000	2000

Table 27-4. Pharmacology of Colloid Fluids

Name	Substance (g/L)	Na (mmol/L)	K (mmol/L)	Cl (mmol/L)	Ca (mmol/L)	Glucose (mmol/L)	Lactate (mmol/L)	Osmolarity (mOsm/L)
Natural Colloids								
Albumin 5%	50	130-160		130-160				308
Albumin 25%	240 g with globulins 10 g	130-160		130-160				1500
Plasma protein fraction 5%	Albumin 44 g with globulins 6 g	130-160	<2			167		290
Gelatin								
Urea-gelatin + electrolytes	35	145	5.1	145	6.25			391
Modified gelatin + electrolytes	30	152	5	100			30	320
Dextran								
Dextran 40 + glucose 5% + NaCl 0.9%	50	154		154		278		278 310
Dextran 40 + glucose 5% + NaCl 0.9%	100	154		154		278		278 310
Dextran 70 + glucose 5% + NaCl 0.9%	60	154		154		278		278 310
Starch (MW)								
Hydroxyethyl starch (130) + NaCl 0.9%	60	154		154				310
Hydroxyethyl starch (200) + NaCl 0.9%	60/100 g	154		154				310
Hydroxyethyl starch (450) + NaCl 0.9%	60	154		154				310
Pentastarch (264) + NaCl 0.9%	100 g	154		154				354

MW, molecular weight.

Table 27-5. Biology of Colloid Fluids

Type	Molecular Weight (D)	Colloid Osmotic Pressure (mm Hg)	Maximal Dose (mL/kg/24 h)	Anaphylactoid Reactions	Coagulation	Diuresis
Albumin	69,000					
5 g/L		20	—	Rare	—	(↓)
25 g/L		100	—	Rare	—	(↓)
Dextran						
40	40,000					
50 g/L		27	40	Rare	↓	↓
100 g/L		170	20	Rare	↓	↓
70	70,000					
60 g/L		59	20	Rare	↓	↓
Gelatin	35,000					
35-40 g/L		26-30	20	Rare	—	—
Starch						
Hydroxyethylstarch, 60 g/L	130,000	36	33	Very rare	(↓)	(↓)
Hydroxyethylstarch, 60 g/L	200,000	25	20	Very rare	(↓)	(↓)
Hydroxyethylstarch, 60 g/L	450,000	30	20	Very rare	(↓)	(↓)
Pentastarch, 100 g/L	264,000	55		Very rare	(↓)	(↓)

↓, decrease; (↓), risk for decrease.

Table 27-6. Changes in Volume of Body Compartments During Infusion of Fluids

Compartment	Glucose 5%	NaCl 0.9%	Hypertonic NaCl	Normal COP Colloids	High COP Colloids
Intravascular	↑	↑	↑↑	↑↑	↑↑↑
Interstitial	↑↑	↑↑	↓	—	↓
Intracellular	↑↑↑	—	↓	—	↓

COP, colloid osmotic pressure.

27-5. In the first group, the hypertonic fluids (i.e., fluids with a higher osmolarity than plasma) are presented. Among the colloid solutions are solutions with a higher colloid osmotic pressure than plasma—the hyperoncotic solutions. Hypertonic and hyperoncotic solutions are plasma expanders because they are able to mobilize cellular and interstitial fluid during resuscitation and to expand plasma volume rapidly.

Table 27-6 shows how the volume of the various compartments is replenished during fluid resuscitation. Because infusion of glucose 5% hardly increases intravascular volume, this solution has no place in resuscitation from hypovolemic shock. Lactated Ringer's solution containing K^+ should not be used during renal insufficiency because of the danger of inducing hyperkalemia. Infusion of lactate-containing solutions during lactic acidosis may be controversial because the capacity of the liver to regenerate bicarbonate from lactate may be impaired.[34] Nevertheless, infusion of lactate-containing solutions such as lactated Ringer's for resuscitation from hypovolemic shock generally does not increase lactate levels (unless in liver failure), worsen acidosis, or adversely affect outcome.[288] In contrast to lactated Ringer's solution,[289] Ringer's ethyl pyruvate solution has anti-inflammatory and cell-protecting actions, which may contribute to less tissue injury and increased survival in animals.[29,38]

The natural colloids consist of albumin and plasma solutions. Albumin is an effective colloidal solution for intravascular volume repletion, and its intravascular half-life is approximately 16 hours.[9,25,136,138,170,287,290-292] For the artificial colloids, the volume-expanding effect and the duration of action generally increase with increasing in vivo molecular weight (Table 27-7). About one third of the hyperoncotic fluids with high molecular weight (dextran 70 and hydroxyethylstarch) may still be in the circulation after 24 hours, whereas dextran 40 is retained for approximately 3 hours. Dextrans and gelatins are, perhaps equally, effective in restoring circulating volume.[293,294] The latter substances might increase tissue blood flow in the microcirculation.

The starch compounds have gained wide interest for the resuscitation of hypovolemic shock.[63,137,168,287,292,295] These

Table 27-7. Distribution of Artificial Colloids 24 Hours after Intravenous Infusion in Normal Volunteers

Colloid	Half-life (h) Concentration in Blood	Plasma (%)*	Urine (%)*	Extravascular (%)*	Overall Survival
Dextran 40	2.5	18	60	22	144 h
Dextran 70	25.5	29	38	33	4-6 wk
Gelatins	3.5	13	65	21	168 h
Hydroxyethylstarch 200	2.5	7	60	33	96 h
Hydroxyethylstarch 450	25.5	38	39	23	17-26 wk

*Of total dose administered.
Adapted from Mishler JM: Systemic plasma volume expanders: Their pharmacology, safety, and clinical efficacy. Clin Haematol 1984;13:75.

colloids are at least as effective as albumin, but less expensive.[136,137,170,292,296] Because the molecular range of the starch compounds varies enormously, the pharmacokinetics are complex.[295] Nevertheless, about 40% of the infused hetastarch (molecular weight >200) still remains in the circulation after 24 hours because 30% of the infused substance may have a half-life of 67 hours. Ninety percent of smaller starch is cleared in 24 hours. The duration of the volume-expanding effect of the starches not only depends on molecular range and concentration, but also on the so-called substitution grade, which is the number of hydroxyethyl groups per glucose unit, and the substitution type, the ratio of C2 to C6 hydroxyethylation.[295] A high molecular weight, high substitution grade, and C2/C6 ratio retard breakdown by plasma amylase and prolong intravascular retention. The residual starch compounds are partly excreted by urine and partly taken up by the reticuloendothelial system. Starch compounds may increase the amylase level in blood and may confound the diagnosis of acute pancreatitis. Experimental evidence shows that some starch compounds, particularly in the 100,000 to 300,000 D molecular weight range, have the advantage over other colloid solutions in "sealing" the capillary endothelium in case of increased permeability after ischemia or trauma, diminishing fluid and protein filtration and preventing edema.[137,177,295,296]

In the resuscitation of hypovolemic shock (e.g., after trauma or burns), the use of hypertonic solutions, with sodium concentrations greater than 0.9%, also has gained wide interest.* The solutions essentially consist of hypertonic sodium chloride, to which often colloids have been added. The combinations include NaCl 7.5% with dextran 70 (6%/10%), NaCl 7.2% with dextran 60 (10%), and NaCl 7.5% with hydroxyethylstarch 6%.[34,63,122,298-301] Hypertonic solutions usually result, at a much lower infusion volume than isotonic solutions (small volume resuscitation), in a rapid hemodynamic improvement, that is, an increase in cardiac output and in oxygen delivery and uptake and arterial blood pressure, in experimental animals and patients with traumatic/hypovolemic shock.[34,63,132,207,280,297-301]

The fluids primarily act through resorption of interstitial and cellular fluid volume and expansion of the plasma volume.[7,132,298] It has been calculated that only 4 mL/kg 7.5% saline solution can increase circulating plasma volume by 8 to 12 mL/kg body weight. A hyperosmolarity-induced increase in cardiac contractility also may contribute to the increase in cardiac output, although this has been doubted.[302] Other potential mechanisms include activation of pituitary and pulmonary osmoreceptors, leading to release of vasopressin and vagal afferent-mediated venoconstriction, and hyperosmolarity-induced arterial vasodilation.[7,63,297,298] Infusion of hypertonic sodium combined with hyperoncotic colloid solutions more rapidly and completely increases cardiac output and arterial blood pressure, and the effects last longer than with infusion of hypertonic or colloid solutions alone.[297-301] During infusion of hypertonic saline, particularly if combined with hyperoncotic colloid solutions, the distribution of peripheral oxygen delivery is reversed to a more favorable pattern with preferential perfusion of vital organs, including gut and kidney.[63,297] The increase in oxygen uptake in bled dogs was less rapid and complete during resuscitation with hypertonic saline plus hydroxyethylstarch, however, than during infusion of relatively large volumes of the latter.[34,63]

The solutions also may ameliorate immunodepression, the translocation of bacteria, and susceptibility to sepsis after hypovolemic shock in rodents.[198,303] Hypertonic solutions (plus dextrans) better restore capillary (hepatic sinusoidal) blood flow and organ function during resuscitation than iso-osmotic fluids because of their ability, among others, to reduce endothelial cell swelling, adhesion molecule expression, and neutrophil activation and adherence compared with normotonic crystalloids such as Ringer's lactate. Hypertonic solutions may prevent lung injury after hemorrhage/resuscitation, probably via these mechanisms.[95,118,122,289,303] Infusion of rapidly acting hypertonic saline, particularly if combined with hyperoncotic colloids, increases survival in bleeding animals compared with infusion of either component or of other isotonic or hypertonic (nonelectrolyte) solutions.[300] Clinical trials also have shown the value of hypertonic solutions in the initial treatment of hypovolemic shock after burns and trauma with uncontrolled bleeding.[118,271,298,300,301] In the resuscitation from shock, hypertonic saline/dextran

*References 34, 63, 118, 122, 198, 207, 271, 280, 287, and 297-301.

favorably compared with isotonic solutions in terms of hemodynamics and survival.[300,301] The use of hypertonic saline solutions warrants close monitoring of plasma sodium levels to prevent excessive hypernatremia and hyperosmolarity.[297-300] Adverse effects of overzealous fluid administration include promotion of pulmonary edema and ascites formation with subsequent aggravation of abdominal compartment syndrome, which may contribute to gut ischemia, abdominal complications, translocation, and renal failure.[266,271]

Fluid Controversies

The choice between available fluids should be guided by the estimated extent and type of fluid losses; their composition and localization; and the properties of infusion fluids, their distribution over body compartments, and, perhaps, the associated costs, which are high for albumin, intermediate for artificial colloids, and relatively low for crystalloid solutions.[132,286,287] Nevertheless, the use of various solutions for resuscitation from hypovolemic shock is hotly debated, partly because the importance of the colloid osmotic pressure for resuscitation and prevention of pulmonary edema is uncertain.[286] Also, the relative merits and detriments of natural and various artificial colloids remain unclear.[286]

Capillary filtration depends on the pericapillary hydrostatic and the colloid osmotic pressure gradient, according to the Starling equation. If, at a given permeability, an imbalance in pressures augments capillary filtration of fluids, a decrease in interstitial colloid osmotic pressure, an increase in interstitial hydrostatic pressure (which also depends on the compliance of the interstitium), and increased lymph flow can, either alone or in combination, partially prevent gross accumulation of interstitial fluid (edema). The colloid osmotic pressure of plasma is primarily determined by the plasma albumin content and normally measures about 24 mm Hg.[32,127,138,304] The pressure can be estimated from albumin and protein concentrations in plasma, but infusion of artificial colloid solutions invalidates this calculation, so proper assessment of plasma colloid osmotic pressure necessitates direct measurement.[138,305] Because of a decrease in circulating plasma protein levels, hypovolemic shock results in a decrease in plasma colloid osmotic pressure.[32,127,134,135,138,180,181] During hypoproteinemia and a reduced plasma colloid osmotic pressure, fluid filtration for a given hydrostatic pressure increases until the pericapillary colloid osmotic pressure gradient decreases, and a new steady state, often at increased lymph flow, has been achieved.[134,136,137] Evoking safety mechanisms, such as a reduced interstitial colloid osmotic pressure and increased lymph flow, may keep the interstitium relatively "dry," and these mechanisms may be more effective in the lung than in the systemic circulation.[134] During hypoproteinemia, the hydrostatic pressure needed to invoke pulmonary edema decreases, however, because of more rapid exhaustion of safety mechanisms.[136,306] Conversely, increased lung water caused by an elevated hydrostatic pressure can be ameliorated by colloid infusion.[306]

For a given increase in hydrostatic pressure, the infusion of crystalloids decreases the plasma colloid osmotic pressure and tends to enhance, if insufficiently compensated by a decrease in the pericapillary colloid osmotic pressure gradient, pulmonary and systemic fluid filtration and interstitial fluid expansion more than infusion of albumin/colloids, which maintain plasma colloid osmotic pressure.[32,127,134-138,170,181,287,291,306] Crystalloid solutions replenish not only the intravascular, but also the interstitial space by increased filtration, whereas colloid fluids tend to primarily fill the former compartment, at least initially.[132,268] Widening of the intravascular-to-interstitial colloid osmotic pressure gradient may prevent increased fluid filtration, but the effect may be transient when some colloids have been filtered along with fluids into the interstitium, and a new steady state of perimicrovascular pressure and draining lymph flow has been established.[137] The mechanism may form the basis for the well-known observation that albumin/colloid solutions yield a twofold to threefold greater expansion of the intravascular space than crystalloids, for a given amount of fluid infused, so that for a given hemodynamic end point, less colloid than crystalloid solution is needed for resuscitation from hypovolemic shock.[25,136,138,170,291-293] In some clinical trials, colloids proved to be superior to crystalloids in resuscitation from hypovolemic shock,[138,170,293] in terms of both the speed and the extent of correction of the hemodynamic abnormalities. Conversely, this may also explain the observations of some investigators that, during resuscitation from hypovolemic shock, pulmonary edema can be prevented in part if the intravascular filtration pressure (i.e., the gradient between plasma colloid osmotic and PAOP) is kept greater than approximately 6 mm Hg, with an elevated risk for pulmonary edema, particularly in case of increased permeability, if the gradient is less than approximately 3 mm Hg, and that resuscitation with colloids less often induces evidence for pulmonary edema than infusion of crystalloids during hypovolemic shock.[32,135,138,170,287,292,293,304,305]

If the permeability for proteins increases, and the reflection coefficient decreases, the hydraulic conductance of the capillary membrane also increases.[134] Increased permeability for proteins increases capillary fluid filtration for a given intravascular hydrostatic pressure and promotes the formation of edema.[292] During increased permeability, the filtration of fluids and expansion of the interstitial fluid space depend more than normally on hydrostatic pressures and less on colloid osmotic pressures because the colloid osmotic pressure gradient is decreased.[134] The differences between the types of solutions in fluid filtration and formation of edema in the lung and peripheral tissues diminish.[307] This may explain in part why some clinical studies did not find a predictive value of the colloid osmotic–pulmonary capillary wedge pressure gradient for pulmonary edema and lack of a difference between fluid types for formation of pulmonary edema and impaired gas exchange during resuscitation from hypovolemic shock.[286,291] Careful animal studies on hypovolemic shock combined with a lung vascular injury showed, however, that colloids are more effective than crystalloids in restoring the circulation, and that the former increased lung water less than the latter, unless permeability was severely increased.[292,307] This can be explained by the fact that, even in case of increased permeability, the reflection coefficient is not zero, and that the pericapillary colloid pressure gradient still exerts some influence on the transcapillary movement of fluids.

Clinical studies on the colloid/crystalloid controversy may be difficult to interpret because of differences in patient populations and end points between fluid types.[286] Lack of similar end points used for resuscitation may partly explain why infusion of colloid solutions increased the risk for pulmonary failure compared with infusion of crystalloids because colloids, owing to their greater intravascular volume-repleting effect, tend to increase hydrostatic filtration pressure in the lung more rapidly than crystalloid fluids, even though colloid osmotic pressure is maintained or increases during infusion of the former and decreases with the latter.[290] The importance of a difference in hydrostatic pressure for the risk of pulmonary edema would be accentuated in case of increased permeability.[290] Finally, pulmonary mechanics, gas exchange, and radiographic changes, used to evaluate the effects of fluid infusions in many studies, may not accurately reflect changes in lung water.[53,170,290-292]

Potential disadvantages of colloid over crystalloid solutions include inhibition of the coagulation system; the risk for anaphylactoid reactions; inhibition of renal salt and water excretion; and perhaps, at least for albumin, depression of myocardial function, possibly owing to binding of Ca^{++}, although this has not been seen in all studies.[169,170] Of all artificial colloids, dextrans affect coagulation most adversely, independently of hemodilution, by interfering with coagulation factors and diminishing thrombocyte and red blood cell aggregation.[308] The gelatins may have some intrinsic effects on the coagulation, whereas the anticoagulant effects of hydroxyethyl starches probably relate to less endothelial release of von Willebrand factor.[279,295,308] Anaphylactoid reactions to artificial colloids are extremely rare and vary from slight fever and skin reactions to life-threatening anaphylactic shock. Starch compounds elicit these reactions less often than dextrans.[295] Large-molecular-weight starches may accumulate in subcutaneous tissues and may cause pruritus, even for weeks after administration.[295] Resuscitation of trauma patients with hydroxyxethyl starch results in less endothelial damage, urinary albumin excretion, and impaired pulmonary gas exchange than resuscitation with gelatins.[177]

Colloids may contribute to the development of acute renal failure, particularly in the case of overadministration, which may be more frequent otherwise with artificial colloids than with albumin/plasma solutions, which can be monitored by measurements of plasma albumin concentrations. As opposed to albumin/plasma, infusion of colloid solutions is often bound to a maximum (see Table 27-5). Side effects may be more frequent with artificial colloid than with albumin/plasma infusion even though the latter carries a very low risk of anaphylactoid reactions and disease transmission. Crystalloid and artificial colloid solutions may activate neutrophil-endothelial interactions and depress macrophage functions much more than albumin does.[289,309] Fresh frozen plasma should not be used solely for the treatment of hypovolemia.[253] In the initial resuscitation from hypovolemic shock, artificial colloids may nevertheless be preferred over natural colloids because the latter are more expensive and less available, even though albumin and plasma solutions are effective volume expanders.

Finally, there is some evidence that the type of fluids infused during hypovolemia may influence the extent and speed with which oxygen uptake is restored: Infusion of colloid (plasma/albumin) solutions in hypovolemic postoperative patients may increase uptake of oxygen, for a given increment in plasma volume and oxygen delivery, more rapidly than infusion of crystalloids.[9,25] This is thought to result in part from increased diffusion distances for oxygen in the tissues subsequent to tissue edema, evoked by massive crystalloid infusion.[9,25,291] Administration of nonbuffered crystalloid solutions such as normal saline carries the risk of hyperchloremic acidosis, which can be avoided by infusion of balanced buffered solutions.[310] Meta-analyses suggest, at least in some groups, a slightly increased mortality risk after resuscitation with natural or artificial colloids versus crystalloids, but the validity of the conclusions has been questioned by more recent meta-analyses.[286,311,312] In the SAFE study comparing albumin and saline for resuscitation in the intensive care unit, a slight but nonsignificant increase in mortality was observed in the trauma subgroup treated by albumin infusions, although animal studies suggest some beneficial, anti-inflammatory effects of albumin resuscitation of hemorrhagic shock.[313]

Acidosis and Optimal Hematocrit

The underlying idea for partial correction of metabolic acidosis is that acidosis is detrimental for, among others, myocardial function, by increasing pulmonary artery pressure and right ventricular afterload and by impairing catecholamine sensitivity, diminishing adrenergic receptors and intracellular Ca^{++} transport necessary for contraction, even if masked by increased sympathetic activity.[37,166] Metabolic acidosis may increase the tendency for life-threatening ventricular arrhythmias and may lessen defibrillation thresholds and vascular tone.[27] The detrimental effects of acidosis are controversial, however. Intracellular acidosis may protect ischemic cells from dying.[37] The need for treatment of metabolic (lactic) acidosis (e.g., by intravenous administration of buffer solutions) remains unclear.[27,36,37,45,53,314,315]

Administration of sodium bicarbonate may carry the risk for aggravation of intracellular acidosis in the tissues because bicarbonate releases CO_2 during buffering, and CO_2 more rapidly traverses the cell membrane than the bicarbonate ion.[27,36,37,53,314,315] Alkali therapy with sodium bicarbonate carries the risks of shifting the oxyhemoglobin curve to the left and impairing tissue oxygenation, a decrease in ionized Ca^{++}, and hypernatremia and osmolarity, although the consequences of these theoretical drawbacks are unclear.[27,37,45] Albeit not beyond doubt, experimental and clinical studies suggest that the administration of buffers such as sodium bicarbonate is not harmful, even though the hemodynamic and metabolic effects of the solution may not surpass those obtained by saline infusion.[27,36,37,45,314,315] In many institutions, small doses of alkali buffers such as sodium bicarbonate (50 to 100 mL of a 4.2%, 0.5 mmol/mL solution) are still given to treat metabolic (lactic) acidosis, if arterial pH is less than 7.2 and acidosis persists despite optimal cardiovascular resuscitation.[27,37]

During sodium bicarbonate infusion, the patient should be hyperventilated to prevent hypercapnia in arterial blood, and bicarbonate doses should be guided by the arterial blood acid-base status, to prevent alkalosis and diminished oxygen release after overadministration.[27,45,314] Prevention of hypercapnia may obviate increased CO_2 diffusion and aggravation of intracellular acidosis.[27,37] The value of buffers, including bicarbonate/carbonate ("carbicarb"), that do not generate CO_2 and prevent aggravation of intracellular acidosis is still controversial.[27,36,314,315] Dichloroacetate is a stimulator of pyruvate dehydrogenase, and the drug may ameliorate lactate accumulation and postresuscitation organ dysfunction, but there is probably no benefit for patient outcome.[27,36,37]

The hematocrit is the main determinant of blood viscosity, and the latter determines, together with the geometric features of the vascular bed, the blood flow through organs.[120] Experimental studies suggest that, during normovolemic hemodilution, normal oxygen delivery is achieved at a range of hematocrit values from 12% to 65% for the heart; 30% to 65% for the brain; 30% to 55% for liver, intestine, and kidney; and 30% to 60% for the whole body because adaptations in vessel diameter and changes in blood flow in this hematocrit range are able to compensate for changes in oxygen content, maintaining a normal oxygen delivery.[86,120,257,316] The "optimal" hematocrit for the whole body may not conform to the regional "optimal" hematocrit.

Because blood is a non-newtonian fluid, so that blood viscosity not only depends on hematocrit, but also on blood flow velocity (shear stress), there may be differences along the vascular profile in blood viscosity, with propensity for red blood cell aggregation in postcapillary venules, where flow velocity is lower than in arterioles, particularly during hypovolemic shock.[4,120] Increased blood viscosity in postcapillary venules may contribute to impaired tissue perfusion during hypovolemic shock.[4] Conversely, the volume status, myocardial function, and vascular tone contribute to blood viscosity so that, for example, the "optimal" hematocrit for oxygen delivery is lower during hypovolemia than hypervolemia.[21,120,316] Finally, red blood cell deformability is decreased in hemorrhagic shock, contributing to increased viscosity.[220]

Taken together, it is hard to define the "optimal" hematocrit for oxygen delivery to the body during hypovolemic shock, even though hematocrit-induced changes in the rheologic properties of blood may contribute to hemodynamic changes in critically ill patients.[21,120,316,317] Most, but not all, authors believe, however, that mild hemodilution (hematocrit approximately 0.30) may benefit delivery and uptake of oxygen in the tissues and promote survival of critically ill patients with hypovolemia, whereas severe hemodilution or hemoconcentration may be detrimental.[9,21,74,120,174,257,317,318] A low hematocrit in the course of hypovolemic shock after major surgery may warrant red blood cell replacement, whereas a high hematocrit may necessitate infusion of nonsanguineous fluids.[9,318] Mild hemodilution may benefit resumption of red blood cell flow and oxygen uptake after prior ischemia.

Blood Products and Substitutes

Regardless of "optimal" hematocrit, resuscitation with blood components may restore tissue oxygen delivery and energy metabolism more rapidly, completely, and persistently than resuscitation with saline during hemorrhage and hypovolemic shock, although this is controversial.[288,310] Nevertheless, it has been suggested that infusion of sodium salts may be essential, and that addition of saline to blood improves survival from hypovolemic shock after hemorrhage because of restoration of the intravascular and the interstitial volume deficits.[297]

In the treatment of hypovolemic shock following hemorrhage, infusion of red blood cells, in the form of erythrocyte concentrates, is crucial.[271,319] This is achieved by autotransfusion from uncontaminated areas during surgery, if possible; by infusion of blood group O Rh-negative donor blood in emergency situations; or by infusion of typed and stored/anticoagulated donor blood. The position of the oxyhemoglobin dissociation curve of old, stored blood is shifted to the left.[61,79] Although this theoretically may impair the delivery and uptake of oxygen in the tissues, the effects of these changes in animal experiments are usually limited.[61,77] The clinical importance of red blood cell oxygen affinity changes in limiting oxygen uptake during anemia, low cardiac output, or fixed organ vessel diameters remains to be established.

Transfusion of substantial amounts of erythrocyte concentrates is preferentially accomplished through a microfilter, to avoid alloimmunization and infusion of neutrophils and other cellular aggregates, which develop in time during storage of blood and which may lodge in the lung, promote pulmonary injury, and impair gas exchange, leading to TRALI.[173,174,178] Today, prior leukocyte-reduced red blood cell concentrates are often used, but it is controversial whether this is associated with less risk. Humoral mediators released in stored blood or during infusion might be responsible in part for pulmonary vascular injury after massive transfusion of blood.[178,188] Nevertheless, massive transfusion, even of leukocyte-reduced red blood cell concentrates, may remain a risk factor for bacterial sepsis, ARDS (TRALI), and MOF, independently from bleeding and indicators of the severity of hypovolemic shock itself.[85,173-175,178,179,188,320,321] Finally, transfusion of donor blood and plasma carries a small risk of transmitting viral infectious diseases and depresses immune function.[288,322]

Because loss of blood also leads to loss of coagulation factors and platelets, and blood concentrations are diluted further during nonsanguineous fluid resuscitation, replenishing plasma levels by infusion of fresh frozen plasma and platelets is usually required.[253,319] The value of prophylactic administration of coagulation factors in a polytransfused patient to prevent bleeding is unclear, however.[151,253] Supplementation of Ca^{++} may be necessary only if more than 12 to 20 U of packed red cells, anticoagulated with Ca^{++}-binding citrate, have been given if rapidly transfused and particularly if liver function is impaired.[151] In our institution, 1 U of fresh frozen plasma is given after every 4 U of packed red cells. If, during resuscitation, the clotting times are prolonged by a factor of 1.5 or more, more fresh frozen plasma is given, and if thrombocyte counts decrease to less 50×10^9/L, platelets are transfused prophylactically. Persistent bleeding warrants a more aggressive approach. The exact place of recombinant factor VIIa, a potent procoagulant, in the treatment of refractory bleeding, has not been settled yet; antifibrinolytic drugs are probably useless.[271,323] The factor stops bleeding and saves blood transfusion, but cost-effectiveness is unclear. Adverse effects include a tendency for thromboembolic events.[323]

To overcome some of the problems associated with donor or autologous red blood cell transfusions, investigators have intensively searched for safe and effective hemoglobin substitutes applicable in humans.[271,324-326] These include chemical oxygen carriers, hemoglobin modifications, and liposome/vesicle-encapsulated hemoglobin.[327] The chemical hemoglobin modifications have been designed to prevent or limit the renal toxicity of free hemoglobin. They include polymerized, modified, cross-linked, and recombinant hemoglobins.[35,328] The use of hemoglobin substitutes has been under clinical investigation. Some nonrecombinant substitutes seemed to increase arterial and, particularly, pulmonary arterial blood pressure more than accounted for by fluid loading, but some compounds have more adverse effects than others.[329] Pulmonary hypertension may relate to the property of hemoglobin to scavenge NO or release endothelin and platelet-activating factor, or combinations, and the use of these solutions is still not without hazard.[329] Diaspirin cross-linked hemoglobin may beneficially influence intracranial hemodynamics during resuscitation from hypovolemic shock.[284] A clinical trial on diaspirin-cross-linked hemoglobin in trauma failed to improve survival over resuscitation with saline, however.[324] The use of hemoglobin substitutes such as perfluorocarbons has not yet reached the stage of widespread, routine clinical practice, although they may effectively carry oxygen in humans and may improve resuscitability from hypovolemic shock following bleeding in animals compared with non–hemoglobin-based solutions.[324-326,330] Further research is ongoing.

Brain Injury and Fluid Resuscitation

Hypovolemia and a decreased mean arterial blood pressure are considered as a major threat for cerebral perfusion in brain injury. The latter creates intracranial hypertension following edema, bleeding, and contusion, so that perfusion is more dependent on pressure than normal. Small volume resuscitation from hypovolemia with hypertonic (and hyperoncotic) solutions could increase mean arterial blood pressure at a small increase in plasma volume and could, by virtue of hypertonicity, decrease cerebral edema and intracranial pressure. The solutions are highly suitable for treatment of multiple trauma that includes the brain.[298,299] Conversely, too much normotonic fluid may aggravate cerebral edema, but too little fluids and under-resuscitation with resulting hypotension and hypoperfusion may do the same. Vasopressor drugs may be useful adjuncts in the initial treatment of hemorrhagic hypotension plus brain injury.

Vasoactive Drugs

Generally, catecholamines do not have a place in the treatment of hypovolemic shock, unless they are used to bridge a period in which infusion fluids are not yet available, or if adequate fluid resuscitation has proved insufficient to reverse hypotension ("irreversible shock") and to increase oxygen delivery to the point that tissue needs are met.[9,43,46,206,275,331] Persistent hypotension despite normovolemia can be caused by a low cardiac output following myocardial dysfunction or by peripheral vasodilation. Data obtained with a pulmonary artery catheter may help to identify these abnormalities, which can be important for choosing among the available vasopressor and inotropic drugs, having widely differing receptor affinities and hemodynamic effects.[9,46]

Treatment with the drugs is best guided by the prevailing hemodynamic profile and aims at optimization of the circulation toward values associated with survival.[9,43,46] Drugs are given as a continuous intravenous infusion, preferably via a central vein. The initial dose is low, and often combinations of drugs are used. The use of catecholamines should be judicious and carefully guided by hemodynamic parameters, to reach predefined hemodynamic goals.[9] β-adrenergic drugs increase cardiac output by inotropic (β_1) or vasodilating (β_2) properties.[9,331] Dopaminergic compounds may preferentially increase splanchnic and renal perfusion, glomerular filtration, and diuresis.[67,275] Dobutamine, having vasodilating β_2 properties, may exert greater effects on delivery and uptake of oxygen than dopamine, at a lower PAOP.[9,331] A decrease in the arterial blood pressure concomitantly with a decreased wedge pressure after dobutamine infusion may warrant additional fluid repletion.[9] Drugs with α-adrenergic activity, such as norepinephrine, increase arterial blood pressure, but this may not lead to a decrease in cardiac output because they may increase venous return to the heart by decreasing venous compliance.[7] The vascular reactivity to vasoconstrictors may diminish in the late phase of shock. Finally, vasopressin and methylene blue, a guanylyl cyclase inhibitor, have been tried to overcome intractable hypotension in this phase.[96,99]

The use of adrenergic drugs is not without hazards. They may enhance the metabolic demands of the body so that the oxygen supply-to-demand ratio is not favorably influenced, even if oxygen delivery is enhanced.[332] Particularly, epinephrine may increase lactic acid levels, independently of oxygen balance.[39] Low-dose dopamine has been shown, at least in bled dogs, to impede oxygen extraction by the gut during a decrease in oxygen supply, probably associated with transmural distribution of blood flow.[67]

In Practice

In practice, the different types of fluids, including isotonic and hypertonic crystalloid and iso-oncotic or hyperoncotic colloid solutions, are often combined in the resuscitation from hypovolemic shock (see Box 27-2). For resuscitation of hypovolemic shock following hemorrhage, typed blood is often not immediately available, even though a blood sample for crossmatching has been sent to the blood bank as soon as possible after admission. If shock is severe and warrants immediate infusion of blood, type O Rh-negative erythrocyte concentrates can be safely used. In the absence of blood, resuscitation should begin with nonsanguineous fluids. During hypovolemic shock, initial resuscitation is often begun with hypertonic and isotonic crystalloids, later supplemented with colloid solutions, and finally accomplished through infusion of erythrocyte concentrates and plasma (Fig. 27-2).

Resuscitation from burn wound shock with loss of plasma also is done with infusion of various combinations of crystalloid and colloid solutions. In the case of uncontrolled diabetes mellitus, profound diarrhea, and acute adrenocortical insufficiency, with loss of plasma water and electrolytes, the infusion of crystalloid solutions usually suffices. These solutions restore intravascular, interstitial, and intracellular (in case of diabetes mellitus) fluids. Changes in the electrolyte concentrations in blood have to be corrected through adaptation of the type and composition of the infusion fluid; in the case of hypokalemia (and in the presence of diuresis), potassium should be supplemented.

Supportive Care

A vomiting patient in hypovolemic shock should be protected against aspiration of gastric contents. The value of

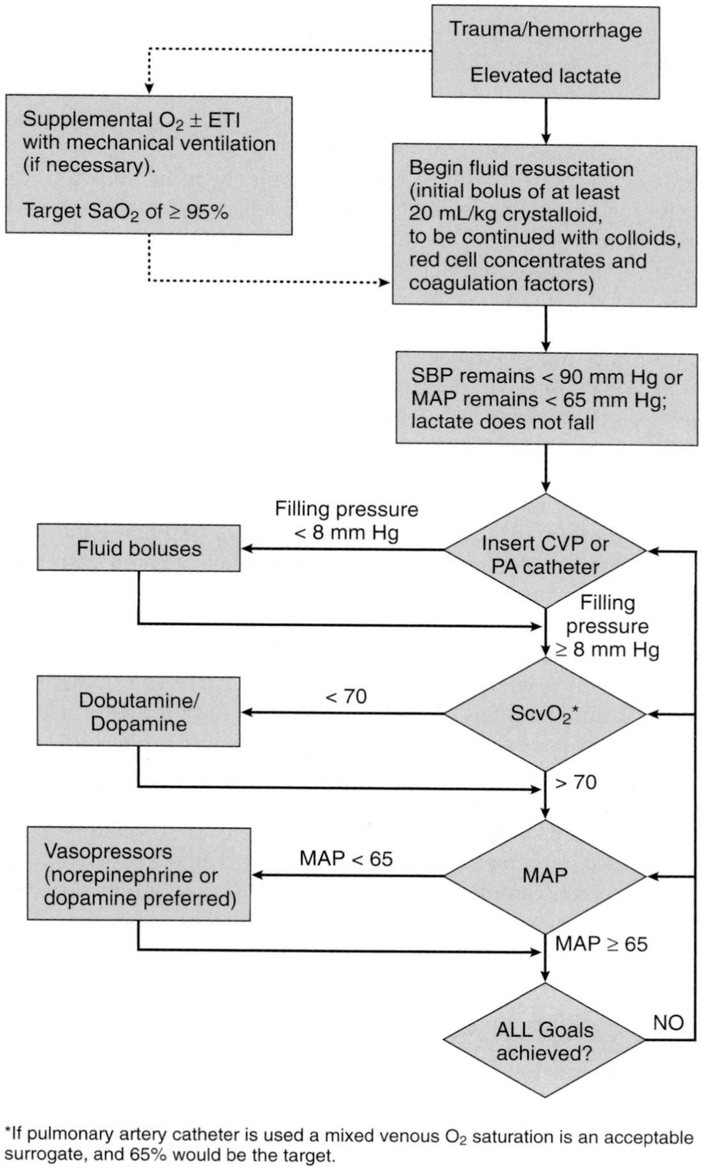

Figure 27-2. Hypovolemic shock management protocol. CVP, central venous pressure; ETI, endotracheal intubation; MAP, mean arterial pressure; PA, pulmonary artery; SaO_2, oxygen saturation; SBP, systolic blood pressure; $ScvO_2$, central venous oxygen saturation.

specific measures for prevention of hemorrhagic gastric mucosal stress ulceration remains controversial.[204] After resuscitation from shock, attention also should be paid to the nutritional status of the patient.[218] It should be judged whether enteral or parenteral nutrition is necessary to improve nitrogen balance and energy intake.[333] Although enteral feeding during hypovolemic shock and after resuscitation may increase metabolic demands of the gut, luminal application of nutrients such as glutamine may induce an increase in mucosal blood flow, ameliorate damage, and diminish the likelihood for translocation of endotoxins and bacteria and of septic complications.[149,203] In addition, there is some evidence that early enteral feeding favorably influences organ function after hemorrhage and reperfusion, in contrast to parenteral feeding, which may have adverse effects.[149] The value of selective decontamination of the digestive tract or luminal absorption of endotoxin to prevent sepsis and its harmful sequelae originating from the gut is still controversial in multiple trauma, although such measures may inhibit the cytokine response to hypovolemic shock in animals.[334]

When treating pain in a patient with extensive trauma, morphinomimetics are cautiously applied even though the drugs may have adverse circulatory effects during hypovolemic shock, which otherwise may be less than in the absence of shock.[11] Because many resuscitated patients after trauma or hemorrhage exhibit hypothermia, partly caused by exhausted energy reserves and infusion of substantial amounts of room temperature infusion fluids, and because hypothermia may denote more severe illness, rewarming infusion fluids may be necessary during resuscitation, and this may prevent some organ dysfunction and perhaps promote survival, despite the increase in oxygen demand with an elevation in body temperature.[57,214,335] In contrast, there also may exist some protective effect of mild hypothermia during bleeding and resuscitation, at least in experiments.

Miscellaneous Therapies

A wide array of experimental drugs has been tried in animal experiments to improve the hemodynamics and survival rate from hypovolemic shock and resuscitation, and some of them have been already mentioned.[145] Blockers of NO synthesis (L-arginine analogues), K^+ channels (oral antidiabetic, sulfonylurea drugs), and poly(ADP-ribose) synthetase have been tried in animal experiments to overcome vascular unresponsiveness early or late after development of hypovolemic shock.[93,94,140,235] ATP-$MgCl_2$ may provide energy to cells, improve the microcirculation, reduce cell swelling, protect tissues from injury, and promote organ function and survival during hypovolemic shock and resuscitation.[24,129,144-146] Ca^{++}-entry blockers have been used to prevent intracellular accumulation of Ca^{++} and further damage of ischemic cells during resuscitation from hypovolemic shock.[50,128,130,145,221,233,242] Opiate antagonists or inhibitors such as naloxone, ACTH, and thyrotropin-releasing hormone been shown to increase arterial blood pressure, decrease inflammation, and improve survival.[11,13,23,24,145,233] Other vasoactive agents, including thyroid hormone, glucagon, and angiotensin inhibitors, with a preferential effect on splanchnic blood flow, also may have beneficial effects in hypovolemic shock.[105,255,256]

Anti-inflammatory drugs include allopurinol, an inhibitor of xanthine oxidase and ROS production, and ROS scavengers, including lazaroids, superoxide dismutase, and adenosine, to prevent ROS injury of cell membranes; some of these agents have been evaluated in clinical trials.[145,191,195,196,225,233,234] It has been suggested that corticosteroids prevent lysosomal disruption and release of toxic proteases (including "myocardial depressant factor"), prevent NO synthesis, and ameliorate the hemodynamic changes and promote survival during hypovolemic shock in animals.[93,165,236,260] Drugs such as pentoxifylline and complement inhibitors may prevent neutrophil-mediated endothelial injury, dysfunction, and downregulation of NO synthesis after bleeding and resuscitation, diminishing endothelium-dependent vasodilation.[119,212] Pentoxifylline may ameliorate not only macrophage cytokine generation, but also adhesion molecule expression and neutrophil activation and aggregation and may improve red blood cell deformability. Administration of pentoxifylline or other methylxanthines may ameliorate reperfusion injury, at least in the rat gut and liver, and survival may be enhanced.[80,115,145,164,203,303]

Heparin and nonanticoagulant heparin sulphate or other analogues may have anti-inflammatory effects and may improve the microcirculation, and administration may partly protect various tissues, including the liver and gut, against reperfusion injury after hypovolemic shock by bleeding.[245,336] Protease inhibitors, such as aprotinin, also may have beneficial effects. Administration of female hormones or inducers such as dehydroepiandrosterone or blockade of testosterone receptors after trauma/hemorrhage and resuscitation partly protects animals from microcirculatory organ dysfunction and immunosuppression, and a wide variety of mechanisms has been implicated.[215] The potential of other immunologic and hormonal agents to treat immunosuppression also has been shown.[215,245] Further drug developments include anticytokine strategies and tissue protective agents interfering with cell stress, apoptosis, or necrosis.[213] Although many experimental drugs have shown some benefit in animal models of hypovolemic shock, in terms of hemodynamics during shock and after resuscitation and ultimate survival, there are no clinical trials substantiating a sustained hemodynamic and survival benefit in humans, even if some have been performed.[24,94,115,119] Finally, cortisol treatment may increase the vascular sensitivity for catecholamines, particularly in patients in whom adrenal cortisol secretion is low relative to severity of disease, the so-called relative adrenal insufficiency.

COMPLICATIONS AND PROGNOSIS

As previously indicated, hypovolemic shock may adversely affect the function of various organs. Even after successful resuscitation from hypovolemic shock, some patients may develop dysfunction of various organ systems (MOF), as evidenced by ARDS, acute renal failure, hyperbilirubinemia, diminished motility and resorptive capacity of the bowel, ischemic colitis, anoxic brain damage, and severe muscle loss, and complications such as acalculous cholecystitis, ischemic perforation of the bowel, and DIC with a bleeding tendency.[2,41,83,201,225,254,321,337] The pathogenesis of the syndrome in humans is still unclear and probably multifactorial, so polytransfusions, ischemia, reperfusion injury, inflammatory reactions, and metabolic changes all may play a role, as previously mentioned.[178,188]

Therapy of the MOF syndrome is supportive and aimed at the replacement of organ function, prevention and treatment of infections, adequate nutrition, and circulatory support.[218] During development of ARDS, the disturbed gas exchange does not respond to liberal oxygen therapy, so intubation and mechanical ventilation are often required for oxygen delivery to the tissues. Further treatment is aimed at diminishing pulmonary edema by judicious manipulation of the hydrostatic pressure in the lungs and the colloid osmotic pressure of plasma (e.g., with help of diuretics), avoiding a decrease in oxygen transport to the tissue. In the case of impending acute renal failure, attempts can be made to promote diuresis by the judicious use of diuretics, if intravascular filling and arterial blood pressure are adequate. If unsuccessful, renal replacement therapy (e.g., by continuous, arteriovenous or venovenous hemofiltration)[338] may be necessary to combat overhydration in the course of resuscitation from hypovolemic shock. There also is some suggestion that the technique, particularly when large ultrafiltration fluid volumes are used, allows for some removal of harmful proinflammatory mediators from the circulation and contributes to hemodynamic stabilization and organ function, independently of renal replacement therapy.[338] It is unclear whether treatment of hypothermia or acidosis ameliorates coagulation disturbances.[179,335] Treatment of the syndrome is controversial and may consist of infusion of heparin, antithrombin III concentrates, fresh frozen plasma, and platelets.[179] If complicated by severe bleeding, the administration of the latter two factors seems nevertheless appropriate to avoid blood loss, even though potentially fueling microvascular thrombosis.

As mentioned, hemorrhage, shock, and resuscitation after trauma may transiently alter immune responses. Together with wounds, this may predispose to susceptibility for bacterial infection and sepsis. Sepsis is a common complication of trauma and is believed to contribute to the development of MOF, including ARDS, in patients ultimately dying in the course of disease.[2,201] Because trauma itself may result in fever and leukocytosis, the recognition of bacterial infection and sepsis in trauma patients is difficult; recognition is aided by infection markers such as circulating C-reactive protein and procalcitonin. Suspected or proven infection should be treated by appropriate antibiotics and drainage, if needed. Despite cardiovascular supportive measures, MOF carries a mortality rate approaching 100% if more than three to four systems fail.[83,201,262]

CONCLUSION

Hypovolemic shock is a life-threatening condition, necessitating prompt diagnosis and therapy to prevent MOF and death. Despite new insights into pathophysiology and new horizons for treatment, the main principles of management remain the rapid and complete repletion of circulating blood volume and treatment of the underlying cause.

KEY POINTS

- Hypovolemic shock is an acute disturbance in the circulation leading to an imbalance between oxygen supply and demand in the tissues, caused by a decline in circulating blood volume.
- Changes in the blood lactate or bicarbonate level reflect the severity and course of shock and roughly predict outcome.
- Compensatory mechanisms evoked during hypovolemic shock attempt to defend vital organ perfusion and function.
- Hypovolemic shock leading to ischemia-reperfusion triggers an inflammatory response, particularly in the gut. The syndrome also is characterized by a diminished immunologic defense.
- The most frequent cause of hypovolemic shock is trauma.
- The main principles for treatment of hypovolemic shock are rapid and complete repletion of circulating blood volume and treatment of the underlying cause. In principle, vasoactive drugs have no place in the treatment of hypovolemic shock.
- Insertion of a pulmonary artery catheter is indicated in case of difficulties in diagnosis, treatment of hypovolemic shock, or both.
- During treatment of hypovolemic shock, repletion of circulating blood volume and oxygen delivery to the tissues is more rapid with infusion of colloid than of crystalloid fluids, unless the latter are hypertonic. Infusion of concentrates of red blood cells is indicated in the case of blood loss.
- The pathogenesis of MOF after hypovolemic shock is multifactorial. The main preventive measure is a rapid restoration of tissue oxygen balance.

REFERENCES

1. Wiggers CJ: Present status of shock problem. Physiol Rev 1942;22:74.
2. Heckbert SR, et al: Outcome after hemorrhagic shock in trauma patients. J Trauma 1998;45:545.
3. Vatner S: Effects of hemorrhage on regional blood flow distribution in dogs and primates. J Clin Invest 1974;54:225.
•4. Zweifach BW, Fronek A: The interplay of central and peripheral factors in irreversible hemorrhagic shock. Prog Cardiovasc Dis 1975;28:147.
5. Rothe CF, Drees JA: Vascular capacitance and fluid shifts in dogs during prolonged hemorrhagic hypotension. Circ Res 1976;38:347.
6. Schwartz S, Frantz RA, Shoemaker WC: Sequential hemodynamic and oxygen transport responses in hypovolemia, anemia and hypoxia. Am J Physiol 1981;241:H864.
7. Bressack MA, Raffin TA: Importance of venous return, venous resistance, and mean circulatory pressure in the physiology and management of shock. Chest 1987;92:906.
8. Wong DH, et al: Changes in cardiac output after acute blood loss and position changes in man. Crit Care Med 1989;17:979.
9. Shoemaker WC, Appel PL, Kram HB: Measurement of tissue perfusion by oxygen transport patterns in experimental shock and in high-risk surgical patients. Intensive Care Med 1990;16:S135.
10. Bond RF, Johnson G III: Vascular adrenergic interactions during hemorrhagic shock. Fed Proc 1985;44:281.
11. Feuerstein G, et al: Effect of morphine on the hemodynamic and neuroendocrine responses to hemorrhage in conscious rats. Circ Shock 1989;27:219.
12. Darlington DN, et al: Corticosterone, but not glucose, treatment enables fasted adrenalectomized rats to survive moderate hemorrhage. Endocrinology 1990;127:766.
13. Schadt JC, Ludbrook J: Hemodynamic and neurohumoral responses to acute hypovolemia in conscious mammals. Am J Physiol 1991;260:H305.
14. Koyama S, et al: Spatial and temporal differing control of sympathetic activities during hemorrhage. Am J Physiol 1992;262:R579.
15. Jørgensen LG, et al: Middle cerebral artery velocity during head-up tilt induced hypovolaemic shock in humans. Clin Physiol 1993;13:323.
16. Victorino GP, Battistella FD, Wisner DH: Does tachycardia correlate with hypotension after trauma? J Am Coll Surg 2003;196:679.
•17. McGee S, Abernethy WB, Simel DL: Is this patient hypovolemic? JAMA 1999;281:1022.
18. Birkhahn RH, et al: Shock index in diagnosing early acute hypovolemia. Am J Emerg Med 2003;23:323.
19. Magder S, Georgiadis G, Cheong T: Respiratory variations in right atrial pressure predict the response to fluid challenge. J Crit Care 1992;7:76.
20. Rooke GA: Systolic pressure variation as an indicator of hypovolemia. Curr Opin Anesthesiol 1995;8:511.
21. Jan K-M, Heldman J, Chien S: Coronary hemodynamics and oxygen utilization after hematocrit variations in hemorrhage. Am J Physiol 1980;239:H326.
22. Nelson DP, et al: Systemic and intestinal limits of O_2 extraction in the dog. J Appl Physiol 1987;63:387.
23. Liu L-M, et al: Effects of thyrotropin-releasing hormone on myocardial adrenoceptors and dopaminergic receptors following hemorrhagic shock in the rat. Shock 1995;3:430.
•24. Chaudry IH: Cellular mechanisms in shock and ischemia and their correction. Am J Physiol 1983;245: R117.
25. Shoemaker WC: Relation of oxygen transport patterns to the pathophysiology and therapy of shock states. Intensive Care Med 1987;13:230.
26. Rixen D, Siegel JH: Bench-to-bedside review: Oxygen debt and its metabolic correlates as quantifiers of the severity of hemorrhagic and post-traumatic shock. Crit Care 2005;9:441.
•27. Mizock BA, Falk JL: Lactic acidosis in critical illness. Crit Care Med 1992;20:80.
28. Nakatani T, et al: Bile and bilirubin excretion in relation to hepatic energy status during hemorrhagic shock and hypoxemia in rabbits. J Trauma 1995;39:665.
29. Mongan PD, et al: Intravenous pyruvate prolongs survival during hemorrhagic shock in swine. Am J Physiol 1999;277:H2253.
30. Sjöberg F, Gustafsson U, Lewis DH: Extracellular muscle surface Po_2 and pH heterogeneity during hypovolemia and after reperfusion. Circ Shock 1991;34:319.
31. Daniel AM, Shizgal HM, MacLean LD: The anatomic and metabolic source of lactate in shock. Surg Gynecol Obstet 1978;147:697.
32. Weil MH, Henning RJ: New concepts in the diagnosis and fluid treatment of circulatory shock. Anesth Analg 1979;58:124.
33. Groeneveld ABJ, et al: Relation of arterial blood lactate to oxygen delivery and hemodynamic variables in human shock states. Circ Shock 1987;22:35.
34. Hannon JP, et al: Oxygen delivery and demand in conscious pigs subjected to fixed-volume hemorrhage and resuscitated with 7.5% NaCl in 6% dextran. Circ Shock 1989;29:205.
35. Siegel JH, et al: Use of recombinant hemoglobin solution in reversing lethal hemorrhagic hypovolemic oxygen debt shock. J Trauma 1997;42:199.
36. Mazer CD, Naser B, Kamel KS: Effect of alkali therapy with $NaHCO_3$ or THAM on cardiac contractility. Am J Physiol 1996;270:R955.
•37. Forsythe SM, Schmidt GA: Sodium bicarbonate for the treatment of lactic acidosis. Chest 2000;117:260.
38. Fink MP: Ethyl pyruvate: A novel anti-inflammatory agent. Crit Care Med 2003;31:S51
39. Luchette FA, et al: Hypoxia is not the sole cause of lactate production during shock. J Trauma 2002;52:415.
40. Revelly J-P, et al: Effect of epinephrine on oxygen consumption and delivery during progressive hemorrhage. Crit Care Med 1995;23:1272.
41. Kirton OC, et al: Failure of splanchnic resuscitation in the acutely injured trauma patient correlates with multiple organ system failure and length of stay in the ICU. Chest 1998;113:1064.
42. Moomey CB, et al: Prognostic value of lactate, base deficit, and oxygen-derived variables in an LD_{50} model of penetrating trauma. Crit Care Med 1999;27:154.
43. Girbes ARJ, Groeneveld ABJ: Circulatory optimisation in patients with or at risk for shock. Clin Intensive Care 2000;11:77.
44. Tashkin DP, Goldstein PJ, Simmons DH: Hepatic lactate uptake during decreased liver perfusion and hypoxemia. Am J Physiol 1972;223:968.
45. Mäkisalo HJ, et al: Effects of bicarbonate therapy on tissue oxygenation during resuscitation of hemorrhagic shock. Crit Care Med 1989;17:1170.
46. Abou-Khalil B, et al: Hemodynamic responses to shock in young trauma patients: Need for invasive monitoring. Crit Care Med 1994;22:633.
47. Pearce FJ, Connett RJ, Drucker WR: Extracellular-intracellular lactate gradients in skeletal muscle during hemorrhagic shock in the rat. Surgery 1985;98:625.
48. Amundson B, Jennische E, Haljamäe H: Correlative analysis of microcirculatory and cellular metabolic events in skeletal muscle during hemorrhagic shock. Acta Physiol Scand 1980;108:147.
49. Soini HO, et al: Peripheral and liver tissue oxygen tension in hemorrhagic shock. Crit Care Med 1992;20:1330.
50. Steenblock U, Mannhart H, Wolff G: Effect of hemorrhagic shock on intrapulmonary right-to-left shunt (Q_s/Q_t) and dead-space (V_D/V_T). Respiration 1976;33:133.
51. Aubier M, et al: Respiratory muscle contribution to lactic acidosis in low cardiac output. Am Rev Respir Dis 1982;126:648.
52. Sturm JA, et al: Increased lung capillary permeability after trauma: a prospective clinical study. J Trauma 1986;26:409.
•53. Adrogué HJ, et al: Arteriovenous acid-base disparity in circulatory failure: Studies on mechanisms. Am J Physiol 1989;257:F1087.
54. Cairns CB, et al: Evidence for early supply independent mitochondrial dysfunction in patients developing multiple organ failure after trauma. J Trauma 1997;42:532.
55. Charpentier C, et al: Is endotoxin and cytokine release related to a decrease in gastric intramucosal pH

after hemorrhagic shock? Intensive Care Med 1997;23:1040.
56. Chang MC, et al: Redefining cardiovascular performance during resuscitation: Ventricular stroke work, power, and the pressure-volume diagram. J Trauma 1998;45:470.
57. Seekamp A, et al: Adenosine-triphosphate in trauma-related and elective hypothermia. J Trauma 1999;47:673.
58. Eberhard LW, et al: Initial severity of metabolic acidosis predicts the development of acute lung injury in severely traumatized patients. Crit Care Med 2000;28:125.
59. Shibutani K, et al: Critical level of oxygen delivery in anesthetized man. Crit Care Med 1983;11:640.
60. Kram HB, et al: Conjunctival and mixed-venous oximeters as early warning devices of cardiopulmonary compromise. Circ Shock 1986;19:211.
61. Schumacker PT, Long GR, Wood LDH: Tissue oxygen extraction during hypovolemia: Role of hemoglobin P50. J Appl Physiol 1987;62:1801.
62. Schumacker PT, et al: Effects of hyperthermia and hypothermia on oxygen extraction by tissues during hypovolemia. J Appl Physiol 1987;63:1246.
63. Reinhart K, et al: O_2 uptake in bled dogs after resuscitation with hypertonic saline or hydroxyethylstarch. Am J Physiol 1989;257:H238.
64. Schlichtig R, Kramer DJ, Pinsky MR: Flow redistribution during progressive hemorrhage is a determinant of critical O_2 delivery. J Appl Physiol 1991;70:169.
•65. Ronco JJ, et al: Identification of the critical oxygen delivery for anaerobic metabolism in critically ill septic and nonseptic patients. JAMA 1993;270:1724.
66. Guzman JA, Rosado AE, Kruse JA: End-tidal partial pressure of carbon dioxide as a noninvasive indicator of systemic oxygen supply dependency during hemorrhagic shock and resuscitation. Shock 1997;8:427.
67. Guzman JA, et al: Dopamine-1 receptor stimulation imparis intestinal oxygen utilization during critical hypoperfusion. Am J Physiol 2002;284:H668.
•68. Bilkovski RN, Rivers EP, Horst HM: Targeted resuscitation strategies after injury. Curr Opin Crit Care 2004;10:529.
69. McKinley BA, Butler BD: Comparison of skeletal muscle P_{O_2}, P_{CO_2}, and pH with gastric tonometric P_{CO_2} and pH hemorrhagic shock. Crit Care Med 1999;27:1869.
70. Sakai H, et al: Changes in resistance vessels during hemorrhagic shock and resuscitation in conscious hamster model. Am J Physiol 1999;276:H563.
71. Van der Linden P, et al: Influence of hematocrit on tissue O_2 extraction capabilities during acute hemorrhage. Am J Physiol 1993;264:H1942.
72. Kaufman BS, Rackow EC, Falk JL: The relationship between oxygen delivery and consumption during fluid resuscitation of hypovolemic and septic shock. Chest 1984;85:336.
73. Packman MI, Rackow EC: Optimum left heart filling pressure during fluid resuscitation of patients with hypovolemic and septic shock. Crit Care Med 1983;11:165.
•74. Shoemaker WC, et al: Prospective trial of supranormal values of survivors as therapeutic goals in high-risk surgical patients. Chest 1988;94:1176.
75. Cooke WH, Ryan KL, Convertino VA: Lower body negative pressure as a model to study progression to acute hemorrhagic shock in humans. J Appl Physiol 2004;96:1249.
76. Connolly HV, Maginniss LA, Schumacker PT: Transit time heterogeneity in canine small intestine: Significance for oxygen transport. J Clin Invest 1997;99:228.
77. Cain SM, Adams RP: O_2 transport during two forms of stagnant hypoxia following acid and base infusions. J Appl Physiol 1983;54:1518.
78. Ward ME: Effect of acute respiratory acidosis on the limits of oxygen extraction during hemorrhage. Anesthesiology 1996;85:817.
79. Myburgh JA, Webb RK, Worthley LIG: The P50 is reduced in critically ill patients. Intensive Care Med 1991;17:355.
80. Flynn WJ, Cryer HG, Garrison RN: Pentoxifylline restores intestinal microvascular blood flow during resuscitated hemorrhagic shock. Surgery 1991;110:350.
81. Reilly PM, et al: The mesenteric hemodynamic response to circulatory shock: An overview. Shock 2001;15:329.
82. Yamada M: Effects of coenzyme Q_{10} in hemorrhagic shock. Crit Care Med 1990;18:509.
•83. Shoemaker WC, Appel PL, Kram HB: Role of oxygen debt in the development of organ failure sepsis, and death in high-risk surgical patients. Chest 1992;102:208.
84. Bishop MH, et al: Prospective, randomized trial of survivor values of cardiac index, oxygen delivery, and oxygen consumption as resuscitation endpoints in severe trauma. J Trauma 1995;38:780.
85. Ciesla DJ, et al: A 12-year prospective study of postinjury multiple organ failure: Has anything changed? Arch Surg 2005;140:432
86. Fan F-C, et al: Effects of hematocrit variations on regional hemodynamics and oxygen transport in the dog. Am J Physiol 1980;238:H545.
87. Lieberthal W, et al: Nitric oxide inhibition in rats improves blood pressure and renal function during hypovolemic shock. Am J Physiol 1991;261:F868.
88. Szabó C, et al: Hemorrhagic hypotension impairs endothelium-dependent relaxations in the renal artery of the cat. Circ Shock 1992;36:238.
89. Szabó C, et al: Role of the L-arginine-nitric oxide pathway in the changes in cerebrovascular reactivity following hemorrhagic hypotension and transfusion. Circ Shock 1992;37:307.
90. Dignan RJ, Wechseler AS, DeMaria EJ: Coronary vasomotor dysfunction following hemorrhagic shock. J Surg Res 1992;52:382.
91. Bitterman H, et al: Effects of oxygen on regional hemodynamics in hemorrhagic shock. Am J Physiol 1996;271:H203.
92. Pannen BHJ, et al: Protective role of endogenous carbon monoxide in hepatic microcirculatory dysfunction after hemorrhagic shock in rats. J Clin Invest 1998;102:1220.
93. Szabó C, Billiar TR: Novel roles of nitric oxide in hemorrhagic shock. Shock 1999;12:1.
94. Guarini S, et al: Adrenocorticotropin reverses hemorrhagic shock in anesthetized rats through the rapid activation of a vagal anti-inflammatory pathway. Cardiovasc Res 2004;63:357-365.
95. Corso CO, et al: Hypertonic saline dextran attenuates leukocyte accumulation in the liver after hemorrhagic shock and resuscitation. J Trauma 1999;46:417.
96. Ghiassi S, et al: Methylene blue enhancement of resuscitation after refractory hemorrhagic shock. J Trauma 2004;57:515.
97. Pieber D, et al: Pressor and mesenteric arterial hyporesponsiveness to angiotensin II is an early event in haemorrhagic hypotension in anaesthetised rats. Cardiovasc Res 1999;44:166.
98. Douglas RG, Shaw JHF: Metabolic response to sepsis and trauma. Br J Surg 1989;76:115.
•99. Morales D, et al: Reversal by vasopressin of intractable hypotension in the late phase of hemorrhagic shock. Circulation 1999;100:226.
100. Chang H, et al: Plasma endothelin level changes during hemorrhagic shock. J Trauma 1993;35:825.
101. Zimmerman RS, Maymind M, Barbee RW: Endothelin blockade lowers total peripheral resistance in hemorrhagic shock recovery. Hypertension 1994;23:205.
102. Perko G, et al: Thoracic impedance and pulmonary atrial natriuretic peptide during head-up tilt induced hypovolaemic shock in humans. Acta Physiol Scand 1994;150:449.
103. Putensen C, et al: Atrial natriuretic factor release during hypovolemia and after volume replacement. Crit Care Med 1992;20:984.
104. Trof RJ, et al: Review: Biomarkers of acute renal injury and renal failure. Shock 2006;26:245.
105. Bond JH, Levitt MD: Effect of glucagon on gastrointestinal blood flow of dogs in hypovolemic shock. Am J Physiol 1980;238:G434.
106. Pellis T, et al: Increases in both buccal and sublingual partial pressure of carbon dioxide reflect decreases of tissue blood flow in a porcine model during hemorrhagic shock. J Trauma 2005;58:817.
107. Lefer AM, Spath JA: Pancreatic hypoperfusion and the production of a myocardial depressant factor in hemorrhagic shock. Ann Surg 1974;179:868.

108. Baker CH, et al: Microvascular responses of intact and adrenal medullectomized rats to hemorrhagic shock. Circ Shock 1988;26:203.
109. Mazzoni MC, et al: Amiloride-sensitive Na^+ pathways in capillary endothelial cell swelling during hemorrhagic shock. J Appl Physiol 1992;73:1467.
110. Davis JM, et al: Neutrophil migratory activity in severe hemorrhagic shock. Circ Shock 1983;10:199.
111. Barroso-Aranda J, et al: Circulating neutrophil kinetics during tolerance in hemorrhagic shock using bacterial lipopolysaccharide. Am J Physiol 1994;266:H415.
•112. Barroso-Aranda J, et al: Granulocytes and no-reflow phenomenon in irreversible hemorrhagic shock. Circ Res 1988;63:437.
113. Sasaki SS, et al: Mild hemorrhagic shock does not enhance the risk of CD 18 blockade to *S. aureus* skin inoculations. J Appl Physiol 1994;76:86.
114. Botha AJ, et al: Early neutrophil sequestration after injury: A pathogenic mechanism for multiple organ failure. J Trauma 1995;39:411.
115. Boldt J, et al: The influence of volume therapy and pentoxifylline infusion on circulating adhesion molecules in trauma patients. Anaesthesia 1996;51:529.
116. Maekawa K, et al: Effects of trauma and sepsis on soluble L-selectin and cell surface expression of L-selectin and CD11b. J Trauma 1998;44:460.
•117. Boyd AJ, et al: A CD18 monoclonal antibody reduces multiple organ injury in a model of ruptured abdominal aortic aneurysm. Am J Physiol 1999;277:H172.
118. Rizoli SB, et al: The immunomodulatory effects of hypertonic saline resuscitation in patients sustaining traumatic hemorrhagic shock: A randomized, controlled, double-blinded trial. Ann Surg 2006;243:47.
119. Harlan JM, Winn RKL: Leukocyte-endothelial interactions: Clinical trials of anti-adhesion therapy. Crit Care Med 2002;30:S214.
120. Voerman HJ, Groeneveld ABJ: Blood viscosity and circulatory shock. Intensive Care Med 1989;15:72.
121. Hansell P, Borgström P, Arfors K-E: Pressure-related capillary leukostasis following ischemia reperfusion and hemorrhagic shock. Am J Physiol 1993;165:H381.
122. Mazzoni MC, et al: Capillary hemodynamics in hemorrhagic shock and reperfusion: In vivo and model analysis. Am J Physiol 1994;267:H1928.
123. De Lima A, Bakker J: Noninvasive monitoring of peripheral circulation. Intensive Care Med 2005;31:1316.
124. Sheldon CA, et al: Peripheral postcapillary venous pressure: A new, more sensitive monitor of effective blood volume during hemorrhagic shock and resuscitation. Surgery 1983;94:399.
125. Tucker VL, et al: Blood to tissue transport in rats subjected to acute hemorrhage and resuscitation. Shock 1995;3:189.
•126. Sayeed MM: Ion transport in circulatory and/or septic shock. Am J Physiol 1987;252:R809.
127. Böck JC, et al: Post-traumatic changes in and effect of colloid osmotic pressure on the distribution of body water. Ann Surg 1989;210:395.
128. Horton JW: Calcium-channel blockade in canine hemorrhagic shock. Am J Physiol 1989;257:R1012.
129. Wang P, Ba ZF, Chaudry IH: ATP-$MgCl_2$ restores the depressed cardiac output following trauma and severe hemorrhage even in the absence of blood resuscitation. Circ Shock 1992;36:277.
130. Wang P, et al: Diltiazem restores cardiac output and improves renal function after hemorrhagic shock and crystalloid resuscitation. Am J Physiol 1992;262:H1435.
131. Alibegovic A, Ljungqvist O: Pretreatment with glucose infusion prevents fatal outcome after hemorrhage in food-deprived rats. Circ Shock 1993;39:1.
132. Moon PF, et al: Fluid compartment in hemorrhaged rats after hyperosmotic crystalloid and hyperoncotic colloid resuscitation. Am J Physiol 1996;270:F1.
133. Boulanger BR, et al: Intrinsic pumping of mesenteric lymphatics is increased after hemorrhage in awake sheep. Circ Shock 1994;43:95.
134. Demling RH, et al: Comparison between lung fluid filtration rate and measured Starling forces after hemorrhagic and endotoxic shock. J Trauma 1980;2:856.
135. McKeen CR, et al: Saline compared to plasma volume replacement after volume depletion in sheep: Lung fluid balance. J Crit Care 1986;1:133.
136. Rackow EC, et al: Effects of crystalloid and colloid fluids on extravascular lung water in hypoproteinemic dogs. J Appl Physiol 1987;62:2421.
137. Myers GA, et al: Effects of pentafraction and hetastarch plasma expansion on lung and soft tissue transvascular fluid filtration. Surgery 1995;117:340.
138. Shippy CR, Shoemaker WC: Hemodynamic and colloid osmotic pressure alterations in the surgical patient. Crit Care Med 1983;11:191.
139. Ratcliffe PJ, et al: Acute renal failure in hemorrhagic hypotension: Cellular energetics and renal function. Kidney Int 1986;30:355.
140. Musser JB, et al: Hemorrhagic shock in swine: Nitric oxide and potassium sensitive adenosine triphosphate channel activation. Anesthesiology 2004;101:399.
141. Miyazaki K, et al: Characterization of energy metabolism and blood flow distribution in myocardial ischemia in hemorrhagic shock. Am J Physiol 1997;273:H600.
142. Grum CM, et al: Evidence for adenosine triphosphate degradation in critically ill patients. Chest 1985;88:763.
143. Van Way CW, et al: Changes in adenine nucleotides during hemorrhagic shock and reperfusion. J Surg Res 1996;66:159.
144. Harkema JM, Chaudry IH: Magnesium-adenosine triphosphate in the treatment of shock, ischemia and sepsis. Crit Care Med 1992;20:263.
145. Harkema JM, et al: Pharmacologic agents in the treatment of ischemia, hemorrhagic shock, and sepsis. J Crit Care 1992;7:189.
146. Wang P, et al: Mechanism of the beneficial effects of ATP-$MgCl_2$ following trauma-hemorrhage and resuscitation: downregulation of inflammatory cytokine (TNF, IL-6) release. J Surg Res 1992;52:364.
147. Crookes BA, et al: Can near-infrared spectroscopy identify the severity of shock in trauma patients? J Trauma 2005;58:806.
148. Eastridge BJ, et al: A circulating shock protein depolarizes cells in hemorrhage and sepsis. Ann Surg 1994;219:298.
149. Singh G, et al: Severe depression of gut absorptive capacity in patients following trauma or sepsis. J Trauma 1994;36:803.
150. Silomon M, et al: Role of platelet-activating factor in hepatocellular Ca^{2+} alterations during hemorrhagic shock. J Surg Res 1997;72:101.
151. Lucas CE, et al: Parathyroid response to hypocalcemia after treatment of hemorrhagic shock. Surgery 1994;96:711.
152. Patel UP, et al: Beneficial effects of combined thromboxane and leukotriene receptor antagonism in hemorrhagic shock. Crit Care Med 1995;23:316.
153. Cabin DE, Buchman RG: Molecular biology of circulatory shock, part III: Human hepatoblastoma (HepG2) cells demonstrate two patterns of shock-induced gene expression that are independent, exclusive and prioritized. Surgery 1990;108:902.
154. Udelsman R, Blake MJ, Holbrook NJ: Molecular response to surgical stress: Specific and simultaneous heat shock protein induction in the adrenal cortex, aorta and vena cava. Surgery 1991;110:1125.
155. Kelly E, et al: Metallothionein and HSP-72 are induced in the liver by hemorrhagic shock and resuscitation but not by shock alone. Surgery 1996;120:403.
•156. Rensing H, et al: Differential expression pattern of heme oxygenase-1/heat shock protein and nitric oxide synthase-II and their impact on liver injury in a rat model of hemorrhage and resuscitation. Crit Care Med 1999;27:2766.
157. Chendrasekhar A, et al: Utility of a bedside Doppler in tracking left ventricular dysfunction related to hemorrhagic shock. Am Surg 1997;63:747.
158. Melton SM, et al: Acadesine during fluid resuscitation from shock and abdominal sepsis. Crit Care Med 1999;27:565.
159. Walley KR, Cooper DJ: Diastolic stiffness impairs left ventricular function during hypovolemic shock in pigs. Am J Physiol 1991;260:H702.
160. Kapoor R, Kalra J, Prasad K: Cardiac depression and cellular injury in hemorrhagic shock and reinfusion:

Role of free radicals. Mol Cell Biochem 1997;176:291.
161. Kline JA, et al: Heart function after severe hemorrhagic shock. Shock 1999;12:454.
162. Karpati PCJ, et al: High incidence of myocardial ischemia during postpartum hemorrhage. Anesthesiology 2004;100:30.
163. Parker JL, et al: Coronary vascular function after hemorrhagic hypotension in dogs. Circ Shock 1993;41:119.
164. Nordin A, et al: Hepatosplanchnic and peripheral tissue oxygenation during treatment of hemorrhagic shock: The effects of pentoxifylline administration. Ann Surg 1998;228:741.
165. Lefer AM: Properties of cardioinhibitory factors produced in shock. Fed Proc 1978;37:2734.
166. Teplinsky K, et al: Effect of lactic acidosis on canine hemodynamics and left ventricular function. Am J Physiol 1990;258:H1193.
167. Meldrum DR, et al: Hemorrhage activates myocardial NFκB and increases TNF-α in the heart. J Mol Cell Cardiol 1997;29:2849.
168. Schurr MJ, et al: Unexpected action of platelet activating factor antagonism after fluid resuscitation from traumatic shock. Surgery 1997;121:493.
169. Dahn MS, et al: Negative inotropic effect of albumin resuscitation for shock. Surgery 1979;86:235.
•170. Rackow EC, et al: Fluid resuscitation in circulatory shock: A comparison of the cardiorespiratory effects of albumin, hetastarch, and saline solutions in patients with hypovolemic and septic shock. Crit Care Med 1983;11:839.
171. Arlati S, et al: Myocardial necrosis in ICU patients with acute non-cardiac disease: A prospective study. Intensive Care Med 2000;26:31.
172. Pretorius JP, et al: The "lung in shock" as a result of hypovolemic-traumatic shock in baboons. J Trauma 1987;27:1344.
173. Reul GJ, et al: Prevention of post-traumatic pulmonary insufficiency. Arch Surg 1973;106:386.
174. Fortune JB, et al: Influence of hematocrit on cardiopulmonary function after acute hemorrhage. J Trauma 1987;27:243.
175. Garber BG, et al: Adult respiratory distress syndrome: A systematic overview of incidence and risk factors. Crit Care Med 1996; 24:687.
176. Pallister I, et al: Prediction of posttraumatic adult respiratory distress syndrome by albumin excretion rate eight hours after admission. J Trauma 1997;42:1056.
177. Allison KP, et al: Randomized trial of hydroxyethyl starch versus gelatin for trauma resuscitation. J Trauma 1999;47:1114.
•178. Silliman CC, McLaughlin NJD: Transfusion-related acute lung injury. Blood Rev 2006;20:139.
179. Spahn DR, Rossaint R: Coagulopathy and blood component transfusion in trauma. Br J Anaesthesia 2005;95:130.
180. Kinnebrew PS, et al: Pulmonary microvascular permeability following *E. coli* endotoxin and hemorrhage. J Appl Physiol 1982;52:403.
181. Gorin AB, Mendiondo G: Permeability of barriers to albumin flux in lungs of sheep resuscitated from hemorrhagic shock. J Appl Physiol 1986;61:2156.
182. Mileski WJ, et al: Sensitivity to endotoxin in rabbits is increased after hemorrhagic shock. J Appl Physiol 1992;73:1146.
183. Bahrami S, et al: Monoclonal antibody to endotoxin attenuates hemorrhage-induced lung injury and mortality in rats. Crit Care Med 1997;25:1030.
184. Bahrami S, et al: Significance of TNF in hemorrhage-related hemodynamic alterations, organ injury, and mortality in rats. Am J Physiol 1997;272:H2219.
185. Ramos-Kelly JR, et al: Upregulation of lung chemokines associated with hemorrhage is reversed with a small molecule multiple selectin inhibitor. J Am Coll Surg 1999;189:546.
186. Fabian TC, et al: Neutrophil CD18 expression and blockade after traumatic shock and endotoxin challenge. Ann Surg 1994;220:552.
187. Waschke KF, et al: Regional heterogeneity of cerebral blood flow response to graded volume-controlled hemorrhage. Intensive Care Med 1996;22:1026.
188. Zallen G, et al: Age of transfused blood is an independent risk factor for postinjury multiple organ failure. Am J Surg 1999;178:570.
189. Cullen JJ, et al: Captopril decreases stress ulceration without affecting gastric perfusion during canine hemorrhagic shock. J Trauma 1994;37:43.
190. Tamion F, et al: Gut ischemia and mesenteric synthesis of inflammatory cytokines after hemorrhagic or endotoxic shock. Am J Physiol 1997;273:G314.
191. Flynn WJ, Pilati D, Hoover EL: Xanthine oxidase inhibition prevents mesenteric blood flow deficits after resuscitated hemorrhagic shock by preserving endothelial function. J Surg Res 1997;68:175.
192. Sodeyama M, et al: The effect of hemorrhagic shock on intestinal amino acid absorption in vivo. Circ Shock 1992;38:153.
•193. Kolkman JJ, Otte JA, Groeneveld ABJ: Gastrointestinal luminal PCO_2 tonometry: An update on physiology, methodology and clinical applications. Br J Anaesth 2000;84:74.
194. Cook BH, Wilson ER, Taylor AE: Intestinal fluid loss in hemorrhagic shock. Am J Physiol 1971;221:1494.
195. Stein HJ, Hinder RA, Oosthuizen MMJ: Gastric mucosal injury by hemorrhagic shock and reperfusion: Protective role of the antioxidant glutathione. Surgery 1990;108:467.
196. Xu D, Lu Q, Deitch EA: Calcium and phospholipase A_2 appear to be involved in the pathogenesis of hemorrhagic shock-induced mucosal injury and bacterial translocation. Crit Care Med 1995;23:125.
197. Kushimoto S, et al: Role of granulocyte elastase in the formation of hemorrhagic shock-induced gastric mucosal lesions in the rat. Crit Care Med 1996;24:1041.
198. Reed LL, et al: The effect of hypertonic saline resuscitation on bacterial translocation after hemorrhagic shock in rats. Surgery 1991;110:685.
199. Arden WA, et al: Scintigraphic evaluation of bacterial translocation during hemorrhagic shock. J Surg Res 1993;54:102.
200. Lemaire LCJM, et al: Bacterial translocation in multiple organ failure: Cause or epiphenomenon still unproven. Br J Surg 1997;84:1340.
201. Moore FA: The role of the gastrointestinal tract in postinjury multiple organ failure. Am J Surg 1999;178:449.
•202. Wells CL, Hess DJ, Erlandsen SL: Impact of the indigenous flora in animal models of shock and sepsis. Shock 2004;22:562.
203. Flynn WJ, Gosche JR, Garrison RN: Intestinal blood flow is restored with glutamine or glucose suffusion after hemorrhage. J Surg Res 1992;52:499.
204. Zeltsman D, et al: Is the incidence of hemorrhagic stress ulceration in surgical critically ill patients affected by modern antacid prophylaxis? Am Surg 1996;62:1010.
205. Hamilton-Davies C, et al: Comparison of commonly used clinical indicators of hypovolaemia with gastrointestinal tonometry. Intensive Care Med 1997;23:276.
•206. Miller PR, Meredith JW, Chang MC: Randomized, prospective comparison of increased preload versus inotropes in the resuscitation of trauma patients: Effects on cardiopulmonary function and visceral perfusion. J Trauma 1998;44:107.
207. Doucet JJ, Hall RI: Limited resuscitation with hypertonic saline, hypertonic sodium acetate, and lactated Ringer's solutions in a model of uncontrolled hemorrhage from a vascular injury. J Trauma 1999;47:956.
208. Hameed SM, Cohn CM: Gastric tonometry: The role of mucosal pH measurement in the management of trauma. Chest 2003;123:465.
209. Gaussorgues P, et al: Bacteremia following cardiac arrest and cardiopulmonary resuscitation. Intensive Care Med 1988;14:575.
210. Harris CE, et al: Intestinal permeability in the critically ill. Intensive Care Med 1992;18:38.
211. Reed LL, et al: Bacterial translocation following abdominal trauma in humans. Circ Shock 1994;42:1.
212. Wang P, et al: Measurement of hepatic blood flow after severe hemorrhage: Lack of restoration despite adequate resuscitation. Am J Physiol 1992;262:G92.
213. Bauer C, et al: Interleukin-1 receptor antagonist attenuates leukocyte-endothelial interactions in the liver after hemorrhagic shock in the rat. Crit Care Med 1995;23:1099.
214. Mizushima Y, et al: Restoration of body temperature to normothermia during resuscitation following

trauma-hemorrhage improves the depressed cardiovascular and hepatocellular functions. Arch Surg 2000;135:175.
215. Szalay L, et al: Estradiol improves cardiac and hepatic function after trauma-hemorrhage: Role of enhanced heat shock protein expression. Am J Physiol Regul Integr Comp Physiol 2006;290:R812.
216. Chandel B, et al: MEGX (monoethylglycinexylidide): A novel in vivo test to measure early hepatic dysfunction after hypovolemic shock. Shock 1995;3:51.
217. Menezes J, et al: A novel nitric oxide scavenger decreases liver injury and improves survival after hemorrhagic shock. Am J Physiol 1999;277:G144.
218. Barton R, Cerra FB: The hypermetabolism multiple organ failure syndrome. Chest 1989;96:1153.
219. Nakatani T, Spolter L, Kobayashi K: Arterial ketone body ratio as a parameter of hepatic mitochondrial redox state during and after hemorrhagic shock. World J Surg 1995;19:592.
220. Cohen DB, et al: Pancreatic duct ligation reduces lung injury following trauma and hemorrhagic shock. Ann Surg 2004;240:885.
221. Ertel W, et al: Immunoprotective effect of a calcium channel blocker on macrophage antigen presentation function, major histocompatibility class II antigen expression, and interleukin-1 synthesis after hemorrhage. Surgery 1990;108:154.
•222. Chaudry IH, et al: Hemorrhage and resuscitation: Immunological aspects. Am J Physiol 1990;259:R663.
223. Nast-Kolb D, et al: Indicators of the posttraumatic inflammatory response correlate with organ failure in patients with multiple injuries. J Trauma 1997;42:446.
•224. Roumen RMH, et al: Cytokine patterns in patients after major vascular surgery, hemorrhagic shock and severe blunt trauma: Relation with subsequent adult respiratory distress syndrome and multiple organ failure. Ann Surg 1993;218:769.
225. Marzi I, et al: Value of superoxide dismutase for prevention of multiple organ failure after multiple trauma. J Trauma 1993;35:110.
226. Upperman JS, et al: Post-hemorrhagic lymph is cytotoxic to endothelial cells and activates neutrophils. Shock 1998;10:407.
227. Hierholzer C, et al: Interleukin-6 production in hemorrhagic shock is accompanied by neutrophil recruitment and lung injury. Am J Physiol 1998;275:L611.
•228. Molina PE: Neurobiology of the stress response: contribution of the sympathetic nervous system to the neuroimmune axis in traumatic injury. Shock 2005;24:3.
229. Spain DA, et al: Complement activation mediates intestinal injury after resuscitation from hemorrhagic shock. J Trauma 1999;46:224.
230. Beamer KC, Daly T, Vargish T: Hemodynamic evaluation of ibuprofen in canine hypovolemic shock. Circ Shock 1987;23:51.
231. Turnage RH, et al: Neutrophil regulation of splanchnic blood flow after hemorrhagic shock. Ann Surg 1995;222:66.
232. Hecke F, et al: Circulating complement proteins in multiple trauma patients: Correlation with injury severity, development of sepsis, and outcome. Crit Care Med 1997;25:2015.
233. Carden DL, et al: Reperfusion injury following circulatory collapse: The role of reactive oxygen metabolites. J Crit Care 1989;4:294.
234. Fleckenstein AE, et al: Comparison of the efficacy of mechanistically different antioxidants in the rat hemorrhagic shock model. Circ Shock 1991;35:223.
•235. Cuzzocrea S: Shock, inflammation and PARP. Pharm Res 2002;52:72.
236. Zingarelli B, Caputi AP, Di Rosa M: Dexamethasone prevents vascular failure mediated by nitric oxide in hemorrhagic shock. Shock 1994;2:210.
237. Tanaka H, et al: Acceleration of superoxide production from leukocytes in trauma patients. Ann Surg 1991;214:187.
238. Guillou PJ: Biological variation in the development of sepsis after surgery or trauma. Lancet 1993;342:220.
239. O'Mahony JB, et al: Depression of cellular immunity after multiple trauma in the absence of sepsis. J Trauma 1984;24:869.
240. Stephan RN, et al: Hemorrhage without tissue trauma produces immunosuppression and enhances susceptibility to sepsis. Arch Surg 1987;122:62.
241. Ertel W, et al: Insights into the mechanisms of defective antigen presentation after hemorrhage. Surgery 1991;110:440.
242. Meldrum DR, et al: Diltiazem restores Il-1, Il-3, Il-6, and IFN-γ synthesis and decreases host susceptibility to sepsis following hemorrhage. J Surg Res 1991;51:158.
243. Abraham E, Stevens P: Effects of granulocyte colony-stimulating factor in modifying mortality from *Pseudomonas aeruginosa* pneumonia after hemorrhage. Crit Care Med 1992;20:1127.
244. Raff G, et al: Hemorrhagic shock abolishes myelopoietic response to turpentine-induced soft tissue injury. J Surg Res 1995;59:75.
245. Angele MK, Faist E: Clinical review: Immunodepression in the surgical patient and increased susceptibility to infection. Crit Care 2002;6:298.
246. Wichmann MW, Ayala A, Chaudry IH: Severe depression of host immune functions following closed-bone fracture, soft-tissue trauma, and hemorrhagic shock. Crit Care Med 1998;26:1372.
247. Zervos EE, et al: Cytokine activation through sublethal hemorrhage is protective against early lethal endotoxic challenge. Arch Surg 1997;132:1216.
248. Lyons A, et al: Major injury induces increased production of interleukin-10 by cells of the immune system with a negative impact on resistance to infection. Ann Surg 1997;226:450.
249. Moore FA, et al: Inadequate granulopoiesis after major torso trauma: A hematopoietic regulatory paradox. Surgery 1990;108:667.
250. Kondo S, et al: Effect of hemorrhagic shock and resuscitation upon hepatic phagocytic clearance and killing of circulating microorganisms. Shock 1996;5:106.
251. Saba TM, et al: Reversal of fibronectin and opsonic deficiency in patients: A controlled study. Ann Surg 1984;199:87.
252. Offner PJ, Moore EE, Biffl WL: Male gender is a risk factor for major infections after surgery. Arch Surg 1999;134:935.
253. Lucas CE, et al: Plasma supplementation is beneficial for coagulation during severe hemorrhagic shock. Am J Surg 1996;171:399.
254. Gando S, Nanzaki S, Kemmotsu O: Disseminated intravascular coagulation and sustained systemic inflammatory response syndrome predict organ dysfunctions after trauma: Application of clinical decision analysis. Ann Surg 1999;229:121.
255. Boeuf B, et al: Naloxone for shock (review). Cochrane Library 2006;1.
256. Dulchavsky SA, et al: Triiodothyronine (T3) improves cardiovascular function during hemorrhagic shock. Circ Shock 1993;39:68.
257. Mesh CL, Gewertz BL: The effect of hemodilution on blood flow regulation in normal and postischemic intestine. J Surg Res 1990;48:183.
258. Ba ZF, et al: Alterations in tissue oxygen consumption and extraction after trauma and hemorrhagic shock. Crit Care Med 2000;28:2837.
259. Abel FL, Wolf MB: Increased capillary permeability to ^{125}I-labeled albumin during experimental hemorrhagic shock. Trans N Y Acad Sci 1973;35:243.
260. Vargish T, et al: Dose-response relationships in steroid therapy for hemorrhagic shock. Am Surg 1977;43:30.
261. Gebhard F, et al: Early posttraumatic increase in production of nitric oxide in humans. Shock 1998;10:237.
262. Wagner JA, et al: Activation of peripheral CB_1 cannabinoid receptors in haemorrhagic shock. Nature 1997;390:518.
263. Dorman T, et al: Radial artery pressure monitoring underestimates central arterial pressure during vasopressor therapy in critically ill surgical patients. Crit Care Med 1998;26:1646.
264. Fang J-F, Chen R-J, Lin B-C: Cell count ratio: New criterion of diagnostic peritoneal lavage for detection of hollow organ perforation. J Trauma 1998;45:540.
265. Elton C, et al: Accuracy of computed tomography in the detection of blunt bowel and mesenteric injuries. Br J Surg 2005,92:1024.
266. Balogh Z, et al: Abdominal compartment syndrome: The cause or effect of postinjury multiple organ failure. Shock 2003;20:483-492.

267. Mitteldorf C, et al: Is aortic occlusion advisable in the management of massive hemorrhage? Experimental study in dogs. Shock 1998;10:141.
268. Drobin D, Hahn RG: Volume kinetics of Ringer's solution in hypovolemic volunteers. Anesthesiology 1999;90:81.
269. Solomonov E, et al: The effect of vigorous fluid resuscitation in uncontrolled hemorrhagic shock after massive splenic injury. J Trauma 2000;28:749.
270. Sandham JD, et al: A randomized, controlled clinical trial of the use of pulmonary artery catheters in high-risk surgical patients. N Engl J Med 2003;348:5.
•271. Moore FA, McKinley BA, Moore EE: The next generation in shock resuscitation. Lancet 2004;363:1988.
272. Groeneveld ABJ, Breukers RMBGE, Verheij J: Clinical value of intrathoracic volumes from transpulmonary indicator dilution. In Pinsky MR, Payen D (eds): Functional Hemodynamic Monitoring. Vincent JL (series editor): Update in Intensive Care Medicine. New York, Springer Verlag, 2005, p 153.
273. Burns JM, et al: The role of transesophageal echocardiography in optimizing resuscitation in acutely injured patients. J Trauma 2005;59:36.
274. Nelson LD: Continuous venous oximetry in surgical patients. Ann Surg 1986;203:329.
275. Nordin A, Mäkisalo H, Häckerstedt K: Dopamine infusion during resuscitation of experimental hemorrhagic shock. Crit Care Med 1994;22:151.
276. Sing RF, et al: Trendelenburg position and oxygen transport in hypovolemic adults. Ann Emerg Med 1995;23:564.
277. Landau EH, et al: Hypertonic saline infusion in hemorrhagic shock treated by military antishock trousers (MAST) in awake sheep. Crit Care Med 1993;21:1554.
278. Chang AK, et al: MAST 96. J Emerg Med 1996;14:419.
279. Roberts I, et al: Is the normalisation of blood pressure in bleeding trauma patients harmful? Lancet 2001;457:385.
280. Sheikh AA, et al: Intraosseous resuscitation of hemorrhagic shock in a pediatric model using a low sodium hypertonic fluid. Crit Care Med 1996;24:1054.
281. Leppäniemi A, et al: Fluid resuscitation in a model of uncontrolled hemorrhage: Too much too early, or too little too late? J Surg Res 1996;63:413.
282. Mapstone J, Roberst I, Evans P: Fluid resuscitation strategies: A systematic review of animal trials. J Trauma 2003;55:571.
•283. Kwan I, et al: Timing and volume of fluid administration for patients with bleeding (review). Cochrane Library 2005;1-11.
284. Novak L, et al: Comparison of standard and alternative prehospital resuscitation in uncontrolled hemorrhagic shock and head injury. J Trauma 1999;47:834.
285. McKinely DA, et al: Nitroprusside in resuscitation of major torso trauma. J Trauma 2000;49:1089.
•286. Choi PTL, et al: Crystalloids vs colloids in fluid resuscitation: A systematic review. Crit Care Med 1999;27:200.
•287. Nolan J: Fluid resuscitation for the trauma patient. Resuscitation 2001;48:57.
288. Singh G, Chaudry KI, Chaudry IH: Crystalloid is as effective as blood in the resuscitation of hemorrhagic shock. Ann Surg 1992;215:377.
289. Rhee P, et al: Human neutrophil activation and increased adhesion by various resuscitation fluids. Crit Care Med 2000;28:74.
290. Weaver DW, et al: Pulmonary effects of albumin resuscitation for severe hypovolemic shock. Arch Surg 1978;113:387.
291. Virgilio RW, et al: Crystalloid vs colloid resuscitation: Is one better? A randomized clinical study. Surgery 1979;85:129.
292. Finch JS, et al: Compared effects of selected colloids on extravascular lung water in dogs after oleic acid-induced lung injury and severe hemorrhage. Crit Care Med 1983;11:267.
293. Modig J: Effectiveness of dextran 70 versus Ringer's acetate in traumatic shock and adult respiratory distress syndrome. Crit Care Med 1986;14:454.
294. Beards SC, et al: Comparison of the hemodynamic and oxygen transport responses to modified fluid gelatin and hetastarch in critically ill patients: A prospective, randomized trial. Crit Care Med 1994;22:600.
295. Treib J, et al: An international view of hydroxyethyl starches. Intensive Care Med 1999;25:258.
296. Zikria BA, et al: A biophysical approach to capillary permeability. Surgery 1989;105:625.
297. Rocha e Silva M, et al: Hyperosmotic sodium salts reverse severe hemorrhagic shock: Other solutes do not. Am J Physiol 1987;253:H751.
298. Younes RN, et al: Hypertonic solutions in the treatment of hypovolemic shock: A prospective, randomized study in patients admitted to the emergency room. Surgery 1992;111:380.
299. Anderson JT, et al: Initial small-volume hypertonic resuscitation of shock and brain injury: Short- and long-term effects. J Trauma 1997;42:592.
300. Wade CE, et al: Efficacy of hypertonic 7.5% saline and 6% dextran-70 in treating trauma: A meta-analysis of controlled clinical studies. Surgery 1997;122:609.
301. Wade CE, et al: Efficacy of hypertonic saline dextran fluid resuscitation for patients with hypotension from penetrating trauma. J Trauma 2003;54:S144.
302. Ogino R, et al: Effects of hypertonic saline and dextran 70 on cardiac contractility after hemorrhagic shock. J Trauma 1998;44:59.
303. Coimbra R, et al: HSPTX protects against hemorrhagic shock resuscitation-induced tissue injury: An attractive alternative to Ringer's lactate. J Trauma 2006;60:41.
304. Rackow EC, Fein IA, Siegel J: The relationship of the colloid osmotic-pulmonary artery wedge pressure gradient to pulmonary edema and mortality in critically ill patients. Chest 1982;82:433.
305. Barclay SA, Bennett D: The direct measurement of plasma colloid osmotic pressure is superior to colloid osmotic pressure derived from albumin or total protein. Intensive Care Med 1987;13:114.
306. Wareing TH, et al: Increased plasma oncotic pressure inhibits pulmonary fluid transport when pulmonary pressures are elevated. J Surg Res 1989;46:29.
307. Pearl RG, et al: Pulmonary effects of crystalloid and colloid resuscitation from hemorrhagic shock in the presence of oleic acid-induced pulmonary capillary injury in the dog. Anesthesiology 1988;68:12.
•308. De Jonge E, Levi M: Effects of different plasma substitutes on blood coagulation: A comparative review. Crit Care Med 2001; 29:1261.
309. Oelschlager BK, et al: Effect of resuscitation with hydroxyethyl starch and lactated Ringers on macrophage activity after hemorrhagic shock and sepsis. Shock 1994;2:141.
310. Mann DV, et al: Superiority of blood over saline resuscitation from hemorrhagic shock: A ^{31}P magnetic resonance spectroscopic study. Ann Surg 1997;226:653.
•311. Cochrane Injuries Group Albumin Reviewers: Human albumin administration in critically ill patients: Systemic review of randomised controlled trials. BMJ 1998;17:235.
312. Roberts I, et al: Colloids versus crystalloids for fluid resuscitation in critically ill patients. Cochrane Database Syst Rev 2004;4:CD000567.
313. Finfer S, et al: A comparison of albumin and saline for fluid resuscitation in the intensive care unit. N Engl J Med 2004;350:2247.
314. Benjamin E, et al: Effects of acid-base correction on hemodynamics, oxygen dynamics, and resuscitability in severe canine hemorrhagic shock. Crit Care Med 1994;22:1616.
315. Beech JS, et al: The effects of sodium bicarbonate and a mixture of sodium bicarbonate and carbonate ("carbicarb") on skeletal muscle pH and hemodynamic status in rats with hypovolemic shock. Metabolism 1994;43:518.
316. Shepherd AP, Riedel GL: Optimal hematocrit for oxygenation of canine intestine. Circ Res 1982;51:233.
317. Scholz PM, et al: Correlation of blood rheology with vascular resistance in critically ill patients. J Appl Physiol 1975;39:1008.
318. Czer LSC, Shoemaker WC: Optimal hematocrit value in critically ill postoperative patients. Surg Gynecol Obstet 1978;147:363.
319. Mortelmans YJ, Vermaut GA, Van Aken H: A simple method for calculating component dilution during fluid resuscitation: The Leuven approach. J Clin Anesth 1994;6:279.

320. Agarwal N, et al: Blood transfusion increases the risk of infection after trauma. Arch Surg 1993;128:171.
321. Moore FA, Moore EE, Sauaia A: Blood transfusion: an independent risk factor for postinjury multiple organ failure. Arch Surg 1997;132:620.
322. Brown E, et al: Effect of resuscitation solutions on the immune status of dogs in hemorrhagic shock. Am Surg 1995;61:669.
•323. Levi M, Peters M, Büller HR: Efficacy and safety of recombinant factor VIIa for treatment of severe bleeding: A systematic review. Crit Care Med 2005;33:883.
324. Sloan EP, et al: Diaspirin cross-linked hemoglobin (DCLHb) in the treatment of severe traumatic hemorrhagic shock: A randomized controlled efficacy trial. JAMA 1999;282:1857.
325. Paxian M, et al: Perfluobron emulsion in prolonged hemorrhagic shock. Anesthesiology 2003;98:1391.
326. Créteur J, Vincent JL: Hemoglobin solutions. Crit Care Med 2003;31:S698.
327. Goins B, et al: Physiological responses, organ distribution, and circulation kinetics in anesthetized rats after hypovolemic exchange transfusion with technetium-99m-labeled liposome-encapsulated hemoglobin. Shock 1995;4:121.
328. Eldridge J, et al: Liver function and morphology after resuscitation from severe hemorrhagic shock with hemoglobin solutions or autologous blood. Crit Care Med 1996;24:663.
329. Johnson JL, et al: Resuscitation of the injured patient with polymerized stroma-free hemoglobin does not produce systemic or pulmonary hypertension. Am J Surg 1998;176:612.
330. Stern SA, et al: Effect of supplemental perfluorocarbon administration on hypotensive resuscitation of severe uncontrolled hemorrhage. Am J Emerg Med 1995;13:269.
331. Shoemaker WC, et al: Comparison of hemodynamic and oxygen transport effects of dopamine and dobutamine in critically ill surgical patients. Chest 1989;96:120.
332. Chioléro R, et al: Effects of catecholamines on oxygen consumption and oxygen delivery in critically ill patients. Chest 1991;100:1676.
333. Bengmark S, Gianotti L: Nutritional support to prevent and treat multiple organ failure. World J Surg 1996;20:474.
334. Lingnau W, et al: Selective intestinal decontamination in multiple trauma patients: Prospective, controlled trial. J Trauma 1997;42:687.
335. Cosgriff N, et al: Predicting lifethreatening coagulopathy in the massively transfused trauma patient: hypothermia and acidoses revisited. J Trauma 1997;42:857.
336. Wang P, et al: Effects of nonanticoagulant heparin on cardiovascular and hepatocellular function after hemorrhagic shock. Am J Physiol 1996;270:H1294.
337. Vivivo G, et al: Risk factors for acute renal failure in trauma patients. Intensive Care Med 1998;24:808.
338. S-Izquierdo Rierra JA, et al: Influence of continuous hemofiltration on the hemodynamics of trauma patients. Surgery 1997;122:902.

Chapter 28

Traumatic Shock and Tissue Hypoperfusion: Nonsurgical Management

David J. Dries

In 1934, Blalock suggested four categories of shock: hypovolemic, vasogenic, neurogenic, and cardiogenic.[1,2] In more recent clinical practice, additional categories of shock have been proposed.[3] Hypovolemic shock, the most common, results from reduction in circulating blood volume. Volume loss may be loss of whole blood, plasma, or extracellular fluid or a combination of all three. Vasogenic shock occurs as a result of changes in the resistance of vessels so that a normal blood volume fails to occupy the available space. Neurogenic shock (spinal shock) is a form of vasogenic shock in which spinal anesthesia or spinal cord injury leads to vasodilation. Septic shock is another form of vasogenic shock in which there is increased capacitance. A decrease in peripheral arterial resistance, a decrease in venous capacitance, and a peripheral arteriovenous maldistribution occur. Cardiogenic shock results from failure of the heart as a pump. Obstructive shock results from mechanical obstruction to cardiac function, as seen with tamponade, tension pneumothorax, or massive pulmonary embolism.[4] Traumatic shock includes several components of the conditions mentioned previously.[5] Hypovolemia caused by blood loss is compounded by neurogenic, cardiogenic, or obstructive shock plus the vasogenic component of maladaptive mediator cascades initiated by tissue injury. Traumatic shock involves hemorrhage in combination with soft tissue trauma and fractures. As a result, study of pure hemorrhagic shock may have limited relevance to the pathophysiologic condition of traumatic shock. Most studies have shown significant differences in the biologic condition of traumatic shock compared with that of pure hemorrhagic shock based on the activation of mediator cascades.[2]

Conflicting observations in literature are due at least in part to the assumption that hemorrhagic shock and traumatic shock are identical insults.[2,3] Pulmonary complications after simple hemorrhage are uncommon in clinical practice, but pulmonary dysfunction is a common comorbid condition after major trauma with attendant soft tissue or long bone injury.[2,6] Activation of mediator systems is far more intense with traumatic shock than with pure hemorrhage.[7] Conflicting data regarding changes in cytokine levels after a traumatic insult are likely due to the fact that systemic cytokine levels do not reflect local production of these mediators. Measurement of tissue levels of mediator production may be necessary to determine accurately whether there is upregulation of various mediator systems after trauma or hemorrhage.

Soft tissue injury alone upregulates mediator systems.[2,8] A small animal study with closed femur fractures showed Kupffer cell activation 30 minutes after injury.[9] Another study assessed the effects of skeletal muscle injury in combination with hemorrhage in a porcine model of hemorrhagic shock. To reach a given physiologic end point (reduction in cardiac index and oxygen delivery), hemorrhage of 40% of the blood volume was required in a pure hemorrhagic shock model. If skeletal muscle injury was added, hemorrhage of only 29% of blood volume was necessary to reach the same end point.[2,10] The ability to maintain cardiac function after hemorrhage was impaired in this study by superimposition of a soft tissue injury, emphasizing the difference between hemorrhagic shock and traumatic shock. A synergy in activation of neuroendocrine and inflammatory mediator systems is likely when traumatic injury and hemorrhagic shock are present.

CLASSIC NEUROENDOCRINE RESPONSE

The essential homeostatic response to acute blood loss is preservation of cerebral and cardiac perfusion with maintenance of normal blood pressure as sensed by carotid body and aortic arch receptors. Peripheral vasoconstriction and curtailment of fluid excretion are seen. Cardiac contractility and peripheral vascular tone also are altered. Pain, hypoxemia, acidosis, infection, changes in temperature, and availability of substrates such as glucose affect this response. A decrease in blood volume alone without hypotension may activate the hypothalamic-pituitary axis. The magnitude of neuroendocrine response depends not only on the volume of blood loss, but also the rate at which blood loss occurs. This response may be modified by patient age, prescribed medications, pre-existing illness, and the use of ethanol or other drugs. With spinal cord transection, operative intervention below the level of injury does not produce typical activation of the hypothalamic-pituitary axis. Similarly, consciousness is unnecessary for activation of this response because it may occur under anesthesia.[2,11-15]

The initial effect seen with hemorrhage is sympathetic vasoconstriction. Capacitance of the circulatory system is reduced, and aortic arch or carotid sinus baroreceptors respond to changes in blood pressure by modulation of sympathetic tone.[2,16] Atrial receptors respond to changes in vascular wall stretch and pressure. Afferent vagal fibers carry signals leading to loss of tonic inhibition of heart rate and immediate activation of thoracolumbar sympathetic outflow with norepinephrine release from postganglionic sympathetic fibers. As blood loss increases, so does the role played by arterial baroreceptors. Another part of this hormonal response is corticotropin-releasing factor production by the hypothalamus, vasopressin release, and growth hormone–releasing factor release.[11]

The clinician sees cool extremities in response to these changes associated with hypovolemia. Venous capacitance also decreases, resulting in accelerated venous return to the heart. Selective arterial vasoconstriction maintains blood flow to the heart and brain until compensation fails. Intense triggering of sympathetic signals is activated when arterial blood pressure decreases to less than 50 mm Hg and is maximally stimulated when systolic blood pressure is less than 15 mm Hg.[2] Although metabolic vasoregulation in the heart and brain helps avoid local vasoconstriction, blood flow to other tissues decreases dramatically. Renal blood flow may be reduced to 5% to 10% of normal with acute hypovolemia. Flow to the splanchnic circulation, skin, and skeletal muscle also decreases. These vasoconstrictor responses are mediated by epinephrine and norepinephrine from the adrenal medulla and local sympathetic activity at the vasculature. With increases in acidosis and hydrogen ion concentration, coronary vasodilation occurs as opposed to constriction of arteries in skeletal muscle and the splanchnic circulation.[3,17,18]

Multiple endocrine responses are seen with trauma and associated hypovolemia. Plasma levels of glucagon, growth hormone, cortisol, and corticotropin (adrenocorticotropic hormone) increase.[2,3,5] The renin-angiotensin-aldosterone axis is stimulated with release of vasoconstrictive angiotensin II. Vasopressin release also occurs after hemorrhage, resulting in water absorption in the distal tubule of the kidney. Vasopressin induces splanchnic vasoconstriction. Research suggests that with prolonged hemorrhage, vasopressin depletion may occur, and supplements of this hormone by clinicians may be warranted. Growth hormone and glucagon promote gluconeogenesis, lipolysis, and glycogenolysis. Catecholamines that inhibit insulin release and hyperglycemia and increase blood osmolarity are thought to shift fluid from cells and the interstitium into the intravascular space. More recent data associate hyperglycemia in the setting of injury with adverse outcome, however. The cellular mechanism for this response remains unclear. Loss of fluid or salt through the kidneys also is limited by these hormonal effects, which serve to conserve the circulating blood volume.[17,19-21]

Compensated acute hypovolemia occurs when the aforementioned mechanisms are sufficient to avoid widespread cellular injury and organ decompensation.[2] If volume loss continues, or resuscitation is inadequate, a cycle of decline occurs with regional perfusion defects leading to tissue and microcirculatory changes. Progression from compensated to decompensated and irreversible shock is often defined in retrospect. Frequently, a patient with acute irreversible hemorrhage has been hypotensive for an extended period and cannot be resuscitated despite fluid administration and use of vasoactive drugs.[22] Presumed mechanisms in this situation include microcirculatory failure with loss of vasomotor response and integrity of the vascular bed. Patients with subacute but ultimately irreversible shock can be resuscitated initially, but progressive organ injury and end-organ dysfunction follow.

INFLAMMATION IN SHOCK AFTER INJURY

In addition to blood loss, extensive research suggests that trauma may be considered an inflammatory disease.[23-26] It has been shown that a variety of mediators and indicators of inflammatory response are elevated in severely injured patients. For many of these factors, it could be shown that they were significantly more elevated in patients eventually dying compared with survivors, and that prediction of outcome is possible with a significant degree of accuracy. Peak inflammatory activity as measured by plasma values has been noted within hours of injury. Although it cannot at present be decided which of these parameters may play a direct pathophysiologic role in development and promotion of inflammatory response and consecutive organ dysfunction, and which is an indicator of this reaction, inflammatory mediators may reflect pathophysiologically relevant disturbances set off by tissue injury and blood loss with consecutive ischemia and reperfusion incidents.[27]

Shock after trauma differs from pure hypovolemic shock in that effects of release of mediators by tissue injury are superimposed on hypovolemia. It also is clear that not all damage after shock is the result of tissue hypoxia, and that much of cellular damage follows reperfusion and subsequent inflammation. Loci of this inflammatory response are the wound, with activation of macrophages and production of proinflammatory mediators, and the microcirculation, with activation of blood elements and the endothelium.[27,28]

CELLULAR ENERGETICS

With blood loss, classic circulatory variables, such as systolic blood pressure, remain normal or supranormal until 30% of blood loss occurs.[2,29] With progressive cellular hypoxia, mitochondria still may be able to metabolize oxygen.[2] Nonetheless, with significant hypovolemia, total oxygen available to tissue is severely reduced, causing anaerobic metabolism, which is energy inefficient because one molecule of glucose is no longer able to contribute to resynthesis of 32 mol of adenosine triphosphate but only to 2 mol. Glucose must reach cells through the circulation, which is critically reduced. In addition, the end product is no longer carbon dioxide, which can be eliminated by ventilation, but lactic acid and hydrogen ions leading to metabolic acidosis. Acidosis drives cellular swelling with loss of extracellular fluid volume into the cells. Lactate finally is metabolized by the liver, which also is hypoxic. Transcapillary refill and lymph flow direct interstitial fluid to increase the circulating blood volume, but ultimately capillaries are damaged by hypoxia and the action of activated neutrophils, which increases interstitial edema. Finally, autoregulation of microcirculation is destroyed, leading to fluid sequestration and sludging in the microvasculature. These factors are responsible for increased diffusion distance for oxygen from capillaries to the mitochondria, which further impairs oxygen extraction. Tissue hypoxia also is the most potent stimulus for proinflammatory activation of macrophages and release of vasoactive or arachidonic acid metabolites, such as prostaglandins and thromboxane. Hypovolemia, shock, and any other cause of brain hypoxia also are detrimental to recovery, particularly in patients with head injury because these conditions induce secondary brain damage.

IMMUNE MEDIATOR CASCADES

Although a variety of initiating events may occur, the subsequent inflammatory response is qualitatively similar.[2] Local activation of the complement cascade produces anaphylatoxins, which are strong attractants and stimulants of neutrophils. Local endothelium expresses endothelial leukocyte adhesion molecules, which attract the neutrophil population. Activated neutrophils also express adhesion molecules, leading to aggregation, margination in the vascular endothelium, and migration through vessel walls at the area of injury. This inflammatory response produces a respiratory burst with formation of oxygen radicals and synthesis of proteolytic enzymes (elastase). Local release of bradykinin, histamine, and prostaglandin induces local vasodilation and increased capillary permeability from macromolecules, resulting in a protein-rich exudate. Local phagocytes release messenger molecules, such as granulocyte-macrophage colony-stimulating factor and macrophage colony-stimulating factor, which activate the bone marrow to produce more inflammatory cells. Neutrophils injure otherwise healthy tissues.[2,30-33]

In a slower response, the monocyte population is attracted to the site of injury, where it differentiates to macrophages and contributes to the inflammatory process by phagocytosing and killing bacteria or disposing of necrotic tissue or both. Macrophages are activated further by triggers such as hypoxia or C5a, macrophage-activating factor, and interleukin (IL)-1-like activity from neutrophils. On stimulation, macrophages release a variety of classes of secretory products, which may be proinflammatory (proteolytic enzymes, oxygen radicals, IL-1, IL-6, tumor necrosis factor) or anti-inflammatory (IL-10, prostaglandin E_2). Macrophage mediators such as prostaglandin E_2, tumor necrosis factor, IL-1, IL-2, and IL-6 provide systemic signals adapting metabolic and defense mechanisms. Macrophages take several days after activation to develop full inflammatory capacity. They also may release nitric oxide and cytotoxic radicals. In the setting of injury, this local inflammatory process spills over to cause an exaggerated systemic response with inflammatory damage to otherwise healthy cells and organs distant to the site of injury. Secondary infection may occur in the compromised host leading to generalized inflammation and multiorgan dysfunction (Table 28-1).[2,34,35]

A wide body of biochemical evidence exists to suggest that shock in trauma is accompanied by systemic inflammation. In the acute phase, activation of complement and neutrophils is important, whereas phase activation of macrophages is seen later.

NEUROIMMUNE RESPONSE TO TRAUMA

More recent work examines the link between the autonomic nervous system and modulation of immune response during traumatic injury. Anatomic interactions with immune-competent cells have been identified, and functional consequences of this interaction in the host are now being examined. Integrated hemodynamic, metabolic, behavioral, and immune responses allowing host adaptation are the stress response.[36-40]

Catecholamines are neurotransmitters that affect immune response humorally through circulating adrenal-derived epinephrine and locally through neuronal release of norepinephrine. There is anatomic evidence of central nervous system (CNS)–lymphoid organ connection through autonomic and sensory fibers and immune tissues, including bone marrow, thymus, spleen, and lymph nodes.[36] This sympathetic innervation of lymphoid organs is found across species and has been confirmed by immunohistochemistry. In bone marrow, myelinated and nonmyelinated fibers are distributed with vascular plexuses

Table 28-1. Inflammatory Mediators Associated with Development of Multiple Organ Dysfunction Syndrome in Injured Patients*

First 24 Hours	Thromboxane B_2 C3a Terminal cytolytic complement complex C-reactive protein Elastase Tumor necrosis factor-α Interleukin-6 Lipofuscin Lactate Antithrombin III
Days 2-5	Elastase Interleukin-6 Lipofuscin Soluble intercellular adhesion molecule 1
Day >8	Elastase Interleukin-1 Interleukin-6 Neopterin Lipofuscin Tumor necrosis factor-α if sepsis

*A variety of inflammatory mediators are associated with soft tissue injury, bony injury, and blood loss associated with various forms of trauma. The time course of mediator appearance in limited studies done to date is suggested in this table. In experimental models and limited clinical data, the presence of soft tissue or bony injury in addition to hemorrhage accelerates and magnifies the production of these mediators over clinical and experimental models where hemorrhage alone is seen.
From Goris RJ: Pathophysiology of shock in trauma. Eur J Surg 2000;166:100-111.

where they influence hematopoiesis and cell migration. In the lungs, noradrenergic nerve fibers supply tracheobronchial smooth muscle and glands. In addition, nerve fibers have been shown throughout the different compartments of the bronchus-associated lymphoid tissue forming close contact with mast cells, cells of the macrophage/monocyte lineage, or other lymph node cells. In the thymus, noradrenergic nerve fibers have been localized in the subcapsular, cortical, and corticomedullary regions associated with blood vessels and intralobular septa branching into cortical parenchyma where they reach to thymocytes.[36,41]

The functional effects of catecholamines on cells of the immune system have been confirmed in human volunteers. In addition, relevance of this control mechanism and the implications for dysregulation have been shown by rapid systemic release of IL-10 and the high incidence of infection in patients with sympathetic storm from accidental or iatrogenic brain trauma.[36] Although detrimental effects of sustained and exaggerated sympathetic nervous system activation on cardiovascular and metabolic homeostasis have long been recognized, attention is now directed to the likelihood of immune dysregulation as well.

The neuroimmune axis is a bidirectional network composed of descending pathways linking the CNS to peripheral immune tissues and a parallel afferent arm linking the immune system with the CNS. The integrity of this loop allows for communication between the CNS and peripheral immune system integrating neuronal and immune signals in the periphery and in the CNS. Cells from the immune system express functional receptors and signal transduction pathway components for several neuroendocrine mediators allowing functional cellular responses to agonist stimulation. Similarly, cells in the CNS are capable of synthesizing, secreting, and responding to inflammatory and immune molecules. There is considerable evidence that the peripheral immune system can signal the brain to elicit a sickness response during infection, inflammation, and injury. Peripheral immune molecules such as cytokines influence CNS action through mechanisms including entry into the brain through a saturable transport mechanism or through areas that lack the blood-brain barrier. Afferent neurons of the vagus nerve also are activated (Fig. 28-1).[42-44]

Severe trauma is characterized by the classic activation of the sympathetic nervous system and, more recently, the important contribution of the inflammatory and neuroimmune response to injury.[36] The sympathetic nervous system has significant anatomic and functional interaction with cells of the immune system and plays an important role in control of the magnitude of early inflammatory response to injury by ensuring expression of adequate cytokine balance.[36] Sympathetic neural pathways exert direct effects on cells of the immune system, affecting cytokine expression, lymphocyte function, and cytotoxic activity. In return, the inflammatory mediators released communicate with the CNS through stimulation of sensory and vagal afferents or by crossing the blood-brain barrier through active transport mechanisms and pathways allowing access to hypothalamic-pituitary structures. Immune-derived mediators, such as cytokines and chemokines, can modulate neurotransmission affecting activation of descending autonomic and neuroendocrine pathways.[36]

FLUID THERAPY

Warmed isotonic electrolyte solutions are recommended for initial resuscitation of traumatic shock by the Committee on Trauma of the American College of Surgeons. This type of fluid provides transient intravascular expansion and stabilizes the intravascular volume by replacing accompanying fluid losses into the interstitial and intracellular spaces. Lactated Ringer's solution is the initial fluid of choice. Normal saline is the currently recommended second choice. Normal saline has the potential to cause hyperchloremic acidosis. This complication is more likely if renal function is compromised (Table 28-2).[45]

An initial warm fluid bolus is given rapidly—usually 1 to 2 L for an adult and 20 mL/kg for a child.[45] Patient response is observed during this initial fluid resuscitation, and subsequent therapeutic decisions are based on this response. The required amount of fluid and blood is difficult to predict on initial evaluation of the patient. A rough guideline promulgated by the American College of Surgeons for the total amount of crystalloid volume acutely required is 3 mL of crystalloid fluid to replace each 1 mL of blood loss, allowing for restitution of plasma volume lost into interstitial and intracellular spaces. It is most important, however, to assess patient response to fluid

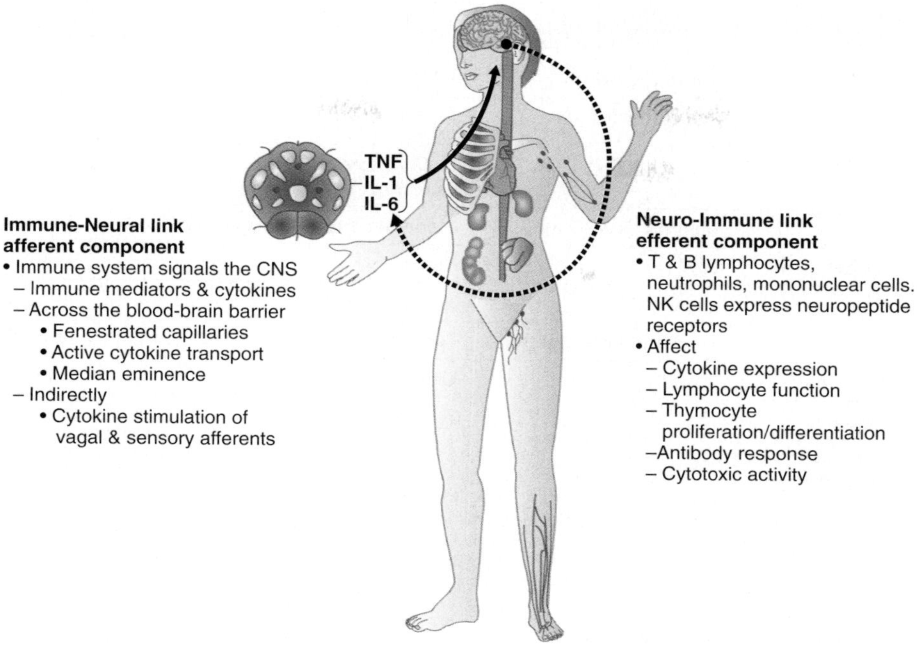

TNF
IL-1
IL-6
Immune-Neural link
afferent component
• Immune system signals the CNS
– Immune mediators & cytokines
– Across the blood-brain barrier
• Fenestrated capillaries
• Active cytokine transport
• Median eminence
– Indirectly
• Cytokine stimulation of vagal & sensory afferents
Neuro-Immune link
efferent component
• T & B lymphocytes, neutrophils, mononuclear cells. NK cells express neuropeptide receptors
• Affect
– Cytokine expression
– Lymphocyte function
– Thymocyte proliferation/differentiation
–Antibody response
– Cytotoxic activity

Figure 28-1. Endocrine, neurologic, and immunologic response to injury is linked through afferent and efferent arcs as described in the text and drawn in this figure. Patients sustaining blunt injury or soft tissue loss in addition to hemorrhage show clinical evidence of increased cytokine and inflammatory mediator production with acceleration of the process described here. The best clinical data in support of this pair of arcs come from patients with traumatic brain injury. CNS, central nervous system; IL-1, interleukin-1; IL-6, interleukin-6; NK, natural killer; TNF, tumor necrosis factor. (From Molina PE: Neurobiology of the stress response: Contribution of the sympathetic nervous system to the neuroimmune axis in traumatic injury. Shock 2005;24:3-10.)

Table 28-2. Estimated Fluid and Blood Losses Based on Patient's Initial Presentation*

	Class I	Class II	Class III	Class IV
Blood loss (mL)	≤750	750-1500	1500-2000	>2000
Blood loss (% blood volume)	≤15%	15-30%	30-40%	>40%
Pulse rate (beats per minute)	<100	>100	>120	>140
Blood pressure	Normal	Normal	Decreased	Decreased
Pulse pressure	Normal or increased	Decreased	Decreased	Decreased
Respiratory rate	14-20	20-30	30-40	>35
Urine output (mL/h)	>30	20-30	5-15	Negligible
Central nervous system/mental status	Slightly anxious	Mildly anxious	Anxious, confused	Confused, lethargic
Fluid replacement (3:1 rule)	Crystalloid	Crystalloid	Crystalloid and blood	Crystalloid and blood

*This is the standard approach to resuscitation of shock after injury as described in the Advanced Trauma Life Support course promulgated by the Committee of Trauma of the American College of Surgeons. The crystalloid of choice used in resuscitation is lactated Ringer's solution. Clinical parameters are used to estimate the degree of blood loss, and fluid resuscitation begins with 1-2 L of lactated Ringer's solution given through large-bore peripheral intravenous lines. Where the response to resuscitation is limited or transient, O-negative or type-specific blood is added to resuscitation as the etiology of shock is sought and additional treatment is employed.
From American College of Surgeons Committee on Trauma: Advanced Trauma Life Support for Doctors, 7th ed., Chicago, American College of Surgeons, 2004, pp 69-85.

resuscitation and evidence of adequate end-organ perfusion as measured by urine output and level of consciousness, rather than provide fluid based on a specific formula. If the amount of fluid required to restore or maintain adequate end-organ function exceeds the above-mentioned estimates, careful reassessment of the situation and exploration for unrecognized injuries or other causes of shock are necessary (Table 28-3).

Crystalloids and Colloids

Plasma and blood were the fluid replacements of choice in traumatic shock until the early 1960s, when a variety of investigators showed the need to replace the extracellular fluid deficit with crystalloid solutions. These observations were followed by a variety of clinical studies comparing colloid, typically albumin, solutions with crystalloids, typically lactated Ringer's solution. Consistent

Table 28-3. Responses to Initial Fluid Resuscitation*

	Rapid Response	Transient Response	No Response
Vital signs	Return to normal	Transient improvement, recurrence of decreased blood pressure and increased heart rate	Remain abnormal
Estimated blood loss	Minimal (10-20%)	Moderate and ongoing (20-40%)	Severe (>40%)
Need for more crystalloid	Low	High	High
Need for blood	Low	Moderate to high	Immediate
Blood preparation	Type and crossmatch	Type specific	Emergency blood release
Need for operative intervention	Possibly	Likely	Highly likely
Early presence of surgeon	Yes	Yes	Yes

*The Advanced Trauma Life Support course advocates ongoing evaluation of patient response to initial fluid administration. Patients with no response frequently require emergent blood transfusion and transfer to the operating room. Patients with transient response also frequently require operative intervention. Most patients, particularly in centers seeing blunt injury, respond rapidly to an initial 1-2 L of crystalloid and are cleared to proceed to more detailed imaging to determine internal injuries after normalization of clinical parameters.
From American College of Surgeons Committee on Trauma: Advanced Trauma Life Support for Doctors, 7th ed., Chicago, American College of Surgeons, 2004, pp 69-85.

with early studies, colloids, when given on an equal volume basis, more effectively increase cardiac output and oxygen transport. Another finding of this early work was the need to give crystalloids in far greater quantities than colloids to achieve consistent hemodynamic objectives.[46,47]

Later studies from the Vietnam era compared resuscitation of patients who were given whole blood and crystalloids with patients given whole blood plus 5% albumin. Fluid infusion volumes were far higher in the patients given crystalloid solutions. There was no evidence of pulmonary edema, and patients treated with crystalloids seemed to fare better than patients treated with resuscitation containing albumin. Albumin seemed to have less effect on restoration of renal function with suggestion of detrimental effects in pulmonary response, myocardial contractility, and coagulation. Large animal models suggested that pulmonary compromise could relate to increased capillary permeability to albumin. Increased losses of albumin to the heart, kidneys, liver, and brain also were reported.[46,48] More extensive studies in injured patients supported reservations regarding the use of albumin. Evaluation of patients randomly selected to receive 150 g of albumin per day intraoperatively and postoperatively noted poorer outcomes than in patients receiving lactated Ringer's solution. Both groups received whole blood and fresh frozen plasma. Patients treated with albumin required greater ventilator support and had poorer oxygenation.[46,49,50] In another carefully conducted trial of patients with multiple trauma, no differences in cardiopulmonary function between patients resuscitated with lactated Ringer's solution and patients given 5% albumin and lactated Ringer's solution were identified.[51] Normal cardiac index was used as a therapeutic end point. To maintain adequate cardiac output, patients who received crystalloids required far more resuscitation volume than patients treated with albumin. These authors concluded that cardiac output was an appropriate end point for resuscitation, and that no advantage was accrued based on the type of fluid employed. A clear cost advantage of crystalloids was identified.[46]

Guyton and Lindsey[52] examined the effect of colloid oncotic pressure on pulmonary edema. They observed that reducing the serum protein level lowered the threshold of left atrial pressure at which pulmonary edema could occur. Zarins and colleagues[53] subsequently showed that a low colloid oncotic pressure alone did not cause an elevation in extravascular lung water. Because of the remarkable efficiency of pulmonary lymphatics, arterial blood gases, shunt fraction, and lung compliance were unchanged despite a 14% increase in body weight caused by infusion of lactated Ringer's solution to keep high pulmonary artery occlusion pressures. No pulmonary edema was created despite the presence of ascites and marked peripheral edema. Demling and coworkers[54] confirmed these findings with a chronic lung lymph fistula in sheep. Holcroft and coworkers[55] produced pulmonary edema in baboons during resuscitation from hemorrhage by continuously administering large volumes of lactated Ringer's solution sufficient to elevate pulmonary artery occlusion pressures 15 mm Hg above baseline levels. With cessation of infusion, filling pressure rapidly returned to normal.

Recent Concerns and Observations

Lactated Ringer's solution has been used as a resuscitation standard for treatment of hypovolemia and hemorrhagic shock. Controversies continue about the use of this solution in resuscitation. One of these controversies involves the hazard of exacerbating lactic acidosis of shock by administration of a lactate-containing solution. In addition, studies suggest that lactated Ringer's solution may have significant effects on immune response by modulating leukocyte function.[56]

A racemic (combination of dextro "D" [right rotary] and levo "L" [left rotary] stereoisomers) lactated Ringer's solution is used as a resuscitation fluid in hemorrhagic shock and has been shown to be superior to normal saline in massive hemorrhage with resuscitation. As lactated

Ringer's solution was introduced, clinical differences between the D-isomers and L-isomers were not appreciated. Intravenous infusion of lactated Ringer's solution at rates used in resuscitation does not seem to increase circulating lactate concentrations in normal hemodynamically stable adults.[57] In animal models of hemorrhagic shock, the "D" stereoisomer of lactated Ringer's solution shows the lowest blood pH and highest plasma lactate concentration compared with Ringer's solutions containing acetate and bicarbonate.[58] Hemorrhage alone did not alter circulating levels of either L-lactate or D-lactate, whereas resuscitation with a lactated Ringer's solution containing a mixture of L-lactate and D-lactate produced a 13-fold elevation in blood D-lactate concentration with no significant elevation in L-lactate levels.[59] Blood lactate in shock, in this respect, reflects not only anoxic tissue production, but also hepatic capacity to clear lactate. The turnover rate of L-lactate, which is more rapidly metabolized by the liver, is 30 minutes. The time to metabolism increases to more than 4 hours in animals with diseased kidneys or liver.[56]

When lactated Ringer's solution containing a mixture of D-lactate and L-lactate is infused, an increase in blood lactate concentration occurs with accumulation of the normally low D-isomer level. Considering the slower elimination of D-lactate from the blood compared with L-lactate even under normal conditions, and a higher toxic potential of D-lactate, its influence on leukocytes may be considerable. Resuscitation with lactated Ringer's solutions containing "D" and "L" stereoisomers, but not with shed blood or 7.5% hypertonic saline, has been shown to increase neutrophil activation in pigs.[56,60] Because of neutrophil activation, which seems to be excessive, the presence of a poorly metabolized D-isomer in clinical racemic Ringer's lactate solutions is a source of laboratory and theoretical concern.

More recent reviews also suggest important differences in safety among colloids. Examination of data comparing colloids with crystalloids must take into account materials employed. When albumin was used as a reference, the incidence ratio for anaphylactoid reactions was 4.51 after administration of hydroxyethyl starch, 2.32 after dextran, and 12.4 after gelatin. Artificial colloid administration was consistently associated with coagulopathy and clinical bleeding, most frequently in cardiac surgery patients receiving starches. Albumin had the lowest rate of total adverse events and serious adverse events.[61] Although albumin is isolated from human plasma, no evidence of viral disease transmission has been consistently identified. Life-threatening anaphylactoid reactions were infrequent for all colloids. Hydroxyethyl starch, as compared with albumin, more than quadrupled the incidence of anaphylactic reactions, whereas dextran more than doubled them. The incidence of these reactions in recipients of gelatin was greater by an order of magnitude than after albumin infusion. Because artificial colloids are derived from nonhuman source materials, they may be recognized as foreign and are more likely to provoke this immune-mediated response. The foreign nature of artificial colloids also may hinder metabolic clearance and promote tissue deposition. On the basis of extensive evidence, albumin is the safest colloid for consideration in resuscitation of traumatic shock.[61] Although factors such as desirability of anticoagulant activity may favor other artificial colloids, this is not true in the setting of injury.

More recent data evaluating administration of albumin in trauma continues to show no benefit over crystalloid solutions. A large meta-analysis of randomized control trials showed no demonstrable benefit in available studies involving surgery or trauma patients.[62] Mechanisms suggested to reduce morbidity in patients receiving albumin do not seem appropriate in the setting of injury. The protective effect of albumin administration in maintaining colloid oncolic pressure and preventing fluid imbalance and pulmonary edema seems unlikely in the setting of injury given work that is already done.[63,64] Conclusions based on experience in trauma may not be relevant in other patient groups, however.

Multicenter data comparing albumin and saline for fluid resuscitation were obtained in Australia and published in 2004.[65] Nearly 7000 patients were randomly assigned to administration of 4% albumin or normal saline for intravascular fluid resuscitation procedures. Mortality and the incidence of single and multiple organ dysfunction were comparable in the two groups. Subset analysis suggests, however, poorer outcomes in the setting of injury. In the subgroup of 140 patients included with principal diagnoses of trauma, a treatment effect seemed to favor administration of saline. In this trial, the increased relative risk of death among patients with trauma compared with patients without trauma resulted from a small excess number of deaths among patients who had trauma with brain injury. The difference in mortality between albumin and saline groups among patients with trauma involving brain injury must be viewed cautiously because the number of involved subjects is small. In the Australian trial, patients with traumatic brain injury constituted only 7% of the study population, and the excess number of deaths in the albumin group was 21. Other parameters that could be helpful in evaluation of the impact of albumin in the setting of brain injury, such as functional neurologic status, were not provided. In contrast with the experience in trauma, the Australian trial suggests some evidence of treatment benefit favoring administration of albumin in patients with severe sepsis. Given contemporary resuscitation technology, factors influencing the choice of resuscitation for critically ill patients include specific clinician concerns, treatment tolerance, safety, and cost.

Hypertonic Plasma Substitutes

Contemporary investigators continue to evaluate alternatives and supplements to lactated Ringer's solution therapy.[66] Although lactated Ringer's solution remains the standard for treatment of hypovolemia because of cost and limited side effects, delayed restoration of intravascular circulating volume with crystalloids has been shown to worsen microvascular flow, endothelial integrity, and tissue oxygenation. Substance-specific benefit with crystalloids on the immune system and endothelium has not been shown by available clinical literature. Experimental, animal, and human studies document negative effects of crystalloids including inappropriate inflammation, endothelial activation, and capillary leakage. A report from the Institute of Medicine raised concern with the Ringer's lactate–based volume replacement strategy because of aggravation of inflammation with resuscitation.[67]

Human albumin is the most expensive plasma substitute and has the best side-effect profile. Beneficial effects in the intensive care unit (ICU) or in resuscitation are absent, however, in the setting of trauma. Other studies using dextrans, gelatins, and starches fail to show an improved benefit-risk profile.[61,62]

Enthusiasm has been generated for hypertonic saline solutions (sodium and chloride concentrations >154 mEq/L) or combination solutions including hypertonic saline and colloids. Hypertonic saline may improve cardiovascular function on a variety of levels, including displacement of tissue fluid into the vascular space, direct vasodilation in the systemic and pulmonary circulation, reduction in venous capacitance, and positive inotropic effects through direct actions on the myocardium. Shock-associated microvascular failure seems to respond better to hypertonic solutions in the laboratory with restoration of vital nutritional blood flow. Hypertonic saline tends to blunt upregulation of leukocyte and endothelial adhesion molecules occurring with isotonic resuscitation of shock. Preclinical studies provide impressive data for improved microcirculation and organ perfusion with decreased inflammation and improved endothelial integrity.[66]

What about the impact of hypertonic saline and associated hypernatremia on head injury?[68] Studies in experimental animals and humans suggest that hypertonic saline may be highly effective in treating head injury, either alone or associated with hemorrhagic hypertension. Tissue swelling in a closed cranium threatens to cause major pressure-induced brain damage or death, and concomitant hemorrhage hypotension reduces cerebral oxygen delivery, resulting in a secondary ischemic insult. Historical data suggest a twofold higher incidence of adverse outcomes in patients with brain injury combined with hypotension. Early data suggest that patients treated with hypertonic saline with dextran are more likely to survive to discharge than individuals treated with standard resuscitation care.[69,70]

Mechanisms by which hypertonic/hyperoncotic resuscitation may be effective in models of head injury and hemorrhage show reduction in water content in noninjured portions of the brain with reduction in intracranial pressure and cerebral edema. In a large animal model, when hypertonic saline was compared with a synthetic colloid, colloid alone had no effect on brain water content.[71,72]

The optimal resuscitation fluid or regimen has yet to be defined. Hypertonic solutions remain on the horizon of opportunity owing to rapid expansion of plasma volume and improvement of hemodynamics, expanding the therapeutic window until patients may be transported to definitive treatment. Optimally, resuscitation as applied clinically and studied in the preclinical setting must be titrated to desired physiologic and metabolic performance objectives.

END POINTS

The Problem

Severely injured trauma patients are at high risk of developing multiple organ failure or death. Initial treatment priorities include appropriate fluid administration and rapid hemostasis.[73,74] Inadequate tissue oxygenation leads to anaerobic metabolism and tissue acidosis. Depth and duration of shock is associated with cumulative oxygen and metabolic debt. Resuscitation is incomplete until the metabolic debt is paid, and tissue acidosis is eliminated with restoration of aerobic metabolism. Many patients seem to be adequately resuscitated based on normalization of vital signs, but have occult hypoperfusion and ongoing tissue acidosis (compensated shock). These individuals are at risk for later organ dysfunction and death.[45]

As stated in the Advanced Trauma Life Support course, the standard of care remains restoration of normal blood pressure, heart rate, and urine output.[45] When these parameters remain abnormal (uncompensated shock), the need for additional resuscitation is obvious. After normalization of these parameters, however, many trauma patients still have evidence of inadequate tissue oxygenation or gastric mucosal ischemia. Recognition of this state and its reversal are crucial to reduce the risk of organ dysfunction or death. The optimal marker of adequate resuscitation in injury remains unclear.[75]

Not all patients can be managed in the same way. More recent literature describing management of neurologic trauma suggests poor outcome with any degree of hypotension during prehospital care, resuscitation, or subsequent in-hospital course. Episodes of hypotension and hypoxia were associated with poor neurologic outcome in a review of more than 700 patients from the Traumatic Coma Data Bank with a Glasgow Coma Scale score less than 9. In this large study, patients without hypotension or hypoxia had a 27% risk of death and a 51% chance of favorable recovery. In the presence of hypotension, with or without hypoxia, the risk of death increased to 65% to 75%. Contrary to the needs of patients with penetrating trauma in whom early aggressive resuscitation may lead to increased bleeding, hypotension should be avoided in head-injured patients. Resuscitation parameters specific to various types of injury have not been reported.[76-78]

Oxygen Delivery Parameters

Shoemaker and various coworkers provided early stimulus to optimization of hemodynamic management in high-risk surgical patients by examining hemodynamic profiles of survivors of surgical shock states versus patients who died.[79] Survivors had significantly higher oxygen delivery and cardiac index values than nonsurvivors. Values correlating with survival included cardiac index greater than 4.5 L/min/m^2, oxygen delivery greater than

600 mL/min/m^2, and oxygen consumption equal to or greater than 170 mL/min/m^2. These initial observations led to a series of articles from Shoemaker's group suggesting reduction in resource consumption and improvement in morbidity and mortality with resuscitation to supranormal oxygen delivery parameters. Initial augmentation of oxygen delivery came with volume loading followed by dobutamine and blood transfusions as needed to a hemoglobin level of 14 g/dL.[80-83]

Attempts by other investigators to replicate these findings met limited success. Moore and coworkers used a resuscitation protocol aimed at maximizing oxygen delivery and found no benefit with resuscitation to achieve supranormal oxygen delivery.[75,84] A variety of studies suggested that patients failing to reach resuscitation goals were at increased risk for multiple organ failure. Other workers noted that patients who did not obtain supranormal oxygen delivery values were at high risk of developing organ failure regardless of treatment strategy.[85,86] Obtaining hemodynamic and oxygen transport parameters seems to be more predictive of survival than useful as a goal for resuscitation, particularly if fluid administration is adequate.

In addition to conflicting outcomes in oxygen transport trials, technical concerns have been raised.[75] These studies cannot be totally blinded. Patients in control groups often obtain similar physiologic end points to those in treatment groups. Other aspects of care were sometimes inconsistent, and entrance criteria varied among investigators. There also is potential mathematical coupling of oxygen delivery and consumption because both are calculated values that share many of the same measured variables.[76] Some clinicians argue that the pathologic relationship between oxygen delivery and consumption trials cannot be accepted with confidence, unless oxygen consumption is measured directly. Finally, use of traditional oxygen delivery and consumption as resuscitative end points requires a pulmonary artery catheter and special expertise for operation and insertion. Routine use of pulmonary artery catheterization or central venous catheters has not been a part of acute trauma resuscitation or emergency medical management.[45,75,76]

Lactate

As an indicator of shock, blood lactate has proved accurate at assessing severity, predicting mortality, and assessing response to resuscitation in the hands of various workers.[75,76] At the cellular level, the explanation is based on oxygen transport principles. With shock and inadequate oxygen delivery, mitochondrial respiration is impaired. The primary cellular fuel, pyruvate, is shunted from its normal aerobic path (conversion by pyruvate dehydrogenase to acetyl coenzyme A and subsequent entry into the tricarboxylic acid cycle) to the anaerobic pathway (conversion to lactate by lactate dehydrogenase). Anaerobic metabolism makes inefficient use of cellular substrate, and high-energy phosphate stores are rapidly depleted. During cellular ischemia, lactate is released into the bloodstream and ultimately converted to glucose in the liver and kidney via the Cori cycle. Because it directly reflects anaerobic metabolism, lactate is thought to serve as a mirror of global hyperperfusion because increasing lactate levels indicate increasing oxygen debt.[76,87]

Initial and peak lactate levels and duration of increased lactate concentration correlate with development of multiorgan dysfunction after trauma.[75] In a study of trauma patient resuscitation, patients normalizing lactate levels at 24 hours survived, whereas patients who normalized lactate levels between 24 and 48 hours had a 25% mortality rate; patients who did not normalize by 48 hours had an 86% mortality rate.[88] Theoretically, severity of metabolic acidosis secondary to tissue hyperperfusion should be reflected in lactate levels, anion gap, and base deficit. This is not a consistent finding among investigators studying trauma resuscitation.[89,90] In addition, although lactate levels are rapidly available, conclusive data tying specific lactate levels and targets to improved resuscitation outcomes are unavailable.

Base Deficit

Inadequate oxygen delivery to tissues leads to anaerobic metabolism. The degree of anaerobiosis is proportional to the depth and severity of hemorrhagic shock, which should be reflected in lactate and base deficit. Arterial pH is not as useful as compensatory mechanisms attempt to normalize this parameter. Serum bicarbonate levels offer better correlation with base deficit (removal of base or addition of the blood).[75,91,92]

Similar to lactate, base deficit has been carefully studied.[75] A greater base deficit has been associated with blood pressure reduction, increased blood loss, and transfusion requirements. A series of studies by Davis and coworkers links base deficit to resuscitation requirements and end-organ dysfunction, such as acute respiratory distress syndrome, renal failure, and coagulopathy. Cytokine and adhesion molecule changes also have been found to parallel changes in base deficit.[93-99]

Base deficit may vary with patient populations. Concern remains in older patients that base deficit is nonspecific and may reflect metabolic acidosis of a variety of etiologies, including renal dysfunction and diabetes.[75,76] Similar to temporal changes in lactate, base deficit variation over time may add to value of this parameter.[91] Patients with elevated base deficit also showed impaired oxygen use reflected in lower oxygen consumption. The timing of base deficit measurement also is important. One study suggested that the worst base deficit in the initial 24 hours was predictive of mortality along with blood pressure and estimated blood loss.[97] Some workers debate whether alcohol intoxication may worsen base deficit for similar levels of injury severity and hemodynamics after trauma. In a large database survey, use of alcohol did not change significant predictive value of admission lactate and base deficit.[100,101] Resuscitation with normal saline (hyperchloremic metabolic acidosis) or lactated Ringer's solution (accumulation of D-lactate) may increase base deficit independent of injury severity. Acidosis associated with hyperchloremia is associated with lower mortality than that from other causes, particularly anaerobic metabolism.[75,102] Base deficit levels and time to normalization of base deficit are similar to those in lactate in that correlation has been established with the need for resuscitation and risk of organ dysfunction and death after injury. Specific thresholds for outcome have not been determined, however, and there are no multicenter data that conclusively show that using base deficit as an end point for resuscitation improves survival.[75]

Gastric Mucosal pH

As systemic perfusion decreases, blood flow to vulnerable organs (brain and heart) is maintained at the expense of other organs (skin, muscle, kidneys, and intestines). Detection of subclinical ischemia to these organs may allow identification of patients requiring additional resuscitation despite normalized vital signs.[75,103] Gastric tonometry is based on the finding that tissue ischemia leads to an increase in tissue partial pressure of carbon dioxide (P_{CO_2}) and subsequent decrease in tissue pH. Because CO_2 diffuses readily across tissues and fluids, the P_{CO_2} of gastric secretions rapidly equilibrates with that in gastric mucosa. For elevation in gastric pH values to be accurate, it is important to withhold gastric feedings and suppress gastric acid secretion. To perform gastric tonometry, a semipermeable balloon is attached to a special nasogastric tube and placed in the stomach. The balloon is filled with saline, and CO_2 is allowed to diffuse into the balloon for a specific time. P_{CO_2} in the saline is then measured. Continuous CO_2 measuring electrodes are sometimes employed. Intramucosal pH is calculated from the Henderson-Hasselbalch equation. The difference between intragastric P_{CO_2} and arterial P_{CO_2}, or the intramucosal pH, correlates with the degree of gastric ischemia.[104]

In studies of a small number of trauma patients, patients with low intramucosal pH (≤ 7.32) were more likely to develop complications or die.[105-107] Patients with normal intramucosal pH fared well. Correlation to other parameters has not been rigorously studied. A larger trial examined the value of intramucosal pH and the gastric mucosal-arterial CO_2 gap (difference between intragastric P_{CO_2} and arterial P_{CO_2}). Ability to predict multiple organ dysfunction and death was maximized with intramucosal pH less than 7.25 and CO_2 gap greater than 18 mm Hg. Similar to studies using blood lactate and base deficit, time course for changes in CO_2 gap or intramucosal pH may be important. Ivatury and associates[108,109] compared changes in intramucosal pH with oxygen transport values. Although intramucosal pH changes paralleled improvement in oxygen transport, delay in achieving intramucosal pH was more predictive of organ system failure than oxygen transport parameters. The gap between gastric mucosal and arterial P_{CO_2} was similarly predictive. After resuscitation, changes in mucosal pH were an early predictor of complications.

Newer fiberoptic technologies increase the ease of gastric mucosal pH assessment.[110] Although this parameter may be predictive of early resuscitation failure, accepted thresholds for failure and outcome data do not support widespread use to guide initial resuscitation after injury (Fig. 28-2).

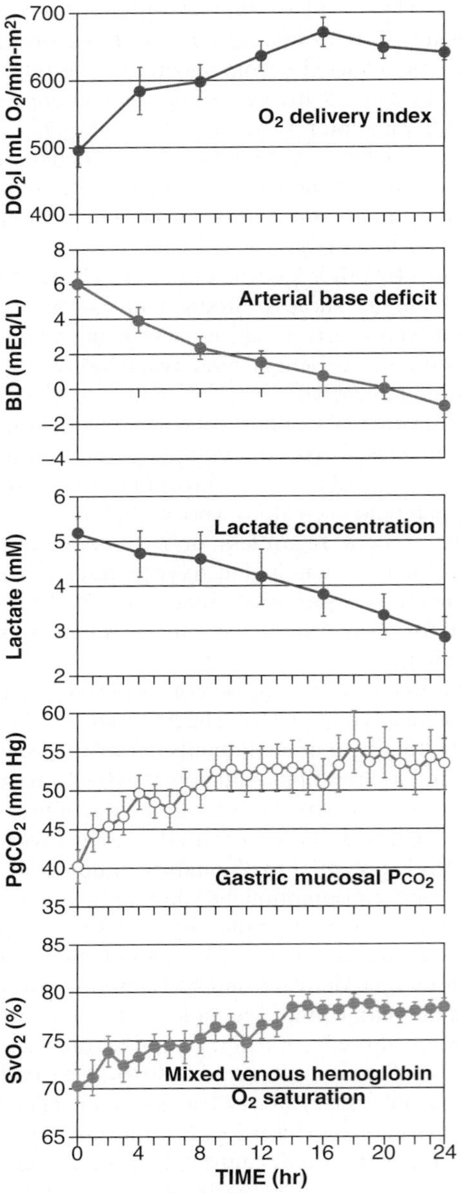

Figure 28-2. Changes in oxygen transport parameters, biochemical indicators of resuscitation success, and local acid-base changes as reflected in gastric mucosal P_{CO_2} are described here. These collected data from McKinley and coworkers suggest the correlation between these common resuscitation parameters. Not all investigators or specific patient groups have complete correspondence among all resuscitation indices, however. (From McKinley BA, Valdivia A, Moore FA: Goal-oriented shock resuscitation for major torso trauma: What are we learning? Curr Opin Crit Care 2003;9:292-299.)

Near-Infrared Spectroscopy

Measurement of skeletal muscle oxyhemoglobin levels by near-infrared spectroscopy offers a noninvasive measurement for monitoring adequacy of resuscitation from normalization of tissue oxygenation.[75,76,104,111] This technology allows simultaneous measurement of tissue partial pressure of oxygen (P_{O_2}), P_{CO_2}, and pH. In human volunteers, cerebral cortex and calf oxygen saturation as measured by near-infrared spectroscopy decreased in proportion to blood loss. Oxygenation index (oxygenated hemoglobin–deoxygenated hemoglobin) also decreased. Studies in injury suggest correlation of tissue oxygen saturation with systemic oxygen delivery, base deficit, lactate, and gastric mucosal P_{CO_2}.[112]

This technology provides information regarding mitochondrial function. Normally, tissue oxyhemoglobin levels reflecting local oxygenation are tightly coupled to cytochrome function, reflecting mitochondrial oxygen consumption. In preliminary studies, where patients showed change in mitochondrial function, even in the absence of abnormality in systemic oxygen transport, multiple organ failure was more likely.[113] Nonetheless, at this time, work in this area is preliminary, and a role for this technology in management of traumatic shock has not been defined.

Adrenal Insufficiency

Adrenal insufficiency is reviewed in Box 28-1.

CLINICAL STRATEGIES

Clinical observations of shock in injury have been made for hundreds of years, but the optimal treatment continues to be debated.[74] Early observations are attributed to Paré, Le Dran, Latta, and Gross.[114,115] Crile and Henderson were among the first to attribute the hemodynamic instability of shock to decreased intravascular volume and to propose therapy based on restoration of intravascular volume with administration of intravenous fluid.[74,115] During the First World War, physiologists Cannon and Bayliss observed patients in clinical shock.[6] These observers noted further that patients with crush injuries despite absence of obvious blood loss also developed signs and symptoms of shock.[116,117] Cannon later suggested the concept of deliberate hypotension in the treatment of wounds to the torso during war with the intent of minimizing internal bleeding until the time at which operative intervention could control the hemorrhage.[118,119] In later studies, other authors reported laboratory models of ongoing arterial hemorrhage and concluded that regardless of the means used to increase blood pressure, either fluid resuscitation or vasopressor, bleeding would increase, with subsequent mortality.[120,121]

Current guidelines for the treatment of hypotension secondary to hemorrhage after trauma recommend rapid infusion of crystalloid solutions to restore blood pressure.[45,119] This premise is based in part on clinical studies and laboratory data showing that hemorrhagic shock in animals produced with controlled blood loss was reversible when blood loss was replaced with two to three times that volume of a crystalloid solution.[122-124] Although controlled hemorrhage is a well-defined laboratory model, resuscitation of a patient with multiple injuries and active or uncontrolled bleeding may represent very different pathophysiology.[74]

In 1950, Wiggers[125] developed a standard hemorrhagic shock model in dogs. He and others showed that severe hypotension over several hours produced a condition in which infusion of withdrawn blood restored arterial pressure only temporarily.[74] After intervals ranging from 30 minutes to 3 hours, arterial pressure declined again. Additional infusions of blood were followed by progressively poorer recovery and more rapid development of circulatory failure, ultimately resulting in the demise of the animal. This decompensatory phase of shock, defining a point at which reinfusion of shed blood could not resuscitate the animal, led to the concept of irreversible

Box 28-1

Adrenal Insufficiency

Check adrenal function in patients who fail to respond to resuscitation.[a-c] Adrenal insufficiency, a rare occurrence in the general population (<0.01%), is seen in 28% of seriously ill patients and 60% of severely injured trauma patients in contemporary series.[d] Severe illness and stress activate the hypothalamic-pituitary-adrenal axis and stimulate the release of corticotropiin (adrenocorticotropic hormone) from the pituitary, which stimulates release of cortisol from the adrenal cortex. This action is an essential component of general adaptation to illness and contributes to maintenance of cellular and organ homeostasis.[a,c]

Although a growing body of literature reviews adrenal insufficiency in critical illness with an emphasis on sepsis, we have seen a significant incidence of adrenal insufficiency, reflected by low serum cortisol levels, in severe injury with or without direct trauma to the brain.[e,f] We suspect adrenal insufficiency in patients who are young and otherwise healthy and require vasoactive drugs in addition to large amounts of resuscitation fluid. Our approach to making the diagnosis of acute adrenal insufficiency is a spot cortisol level. Although a variety of treatment protocols for hormonal replacement exist, we provide 50 mg of hydrocortisone every 6 hours or 100 mg of hydrocortisone every 8 hours for 5 days. Consistent with the treatment threshold reported by Marik and Zaloga,[b,f] we treat if a random cortisol concentration is less than 25 µg/dL. Severely injured patients have been reported to have random cortisol levels greater than 30 µg/dL.[d] Although outcome data are unavailable to suggest the value of adrenal replacement in critically stressed young trauma patients, we have seen the effectiveness of this intervention repeatedly in our own practice.

[a]Cooper MS, Stewart PM: Corticosteroid insufficiency in acutely ill patients. N Engl J Med 2003;348:727-734.
[b]Marik PE, Zaloga GP: Adrenal insufficiency in the critically ill: A new look at an old problem. Chest 2002;122:1784-1796.
[c]Burchard K: A review of the adrenal cortex and severe inflammation: Quest of the "eucorticoid" state. J Trauma 2001;51:800-814.
[d]Offner PJ, Moore EE, Ciesia D: The adrenal response after severe trauma. Am J Surg 2002;184:649-654.
[e]Rivers EP, Gaspari M, Saad GA, et al: Adrenal insufficiency in high-risk surgical ICU patients. Chest 2001;119:889-896.
[f]Marik PE, Zaloga GP: Adrenal insufficiency during septic shock. Crit Care Med 2003;31:141-145.

shock.[126] The approach to resuscitation of cellular, organ, and organism changes after hemorrhagic shock using the Wiggers model has been applied to all types of injury based in part on the elegant experiments of Shires and colleagues[122] and a series of other investigators.[45,46]

Early Limited Resuscitation

Animal Studies

Several large animal studies explored the use of varying degrees of fluid resuscitation in animals receiving injuries leading to uncontrolled hemorrhagic shock. Bickell and coworkers[127] created infrarenal aortotomy using a stainless steel wire in 16 anesthetized Yorkshire swine weighing 23 to 40 kg, which had been instrumented with pulmonary artery and carotid artery catheters. When the wire was pulled, a 5-mm aortotomy with subsequent intraperitoneal hemorrhage followed. Animals were alternately assigned to an untreated control group or a treatment group receiving 80 mL/kg of lactated Ringer's solution as an intravenous bolus. The volume of blood loss and mortality rate were significantly increased in animals treated with lactated Ringer's solution relative to untreated controls. All control animals survived, whereas animals treated with lactated Ringer's solution died in less than 2 hours. Volume of hemorrhage identified in treated animals exceeded 2 L, whereas control animals lost on average less than 800 mL of blood.

Several observations may be made in relation to this widely cited report. First, mortality in the control group was low, leading one to question the severity of injury in the animal model. Second, fluid resuscitation administered, although consistent with replacement of two to three times the volume loss in blood with crystalloid, far exceeds standard resuscitation for a human patient of comparable weight. In addition, the rapidity of fluid administration may have served to diminish further any potential positive impact of fluid administration in this model of injury. The effect seen was reproduced, however, with other types of fluid administration in a comparable injury model. Other large animal studies of hypotensive resuscitation used graded resuscitation protocols.[128,129]

Stern and coworkers[128] examined a swine model combining femoral artery hemorrhage via a catheter to a mean arterial pressure of 30 mm Hg with subsequent intra-abdominal aortic laceration producing a 4-mm tear and uncontrolled intraperitoneal hemorrhage. Three groups of animals were resuscitated to mean arterial pressures of 40 mm Hg, 60 mm Hg, and 80 mm Hg. No untreated control group was employed. Resuscitation was begun when the pulse pressure of each animal reached 5 mm Hg. Animals were resuscitated with saline at 6 mL/kg/min to a maximum of 90 mL/kg, after which resuscitation fluid was changed to shed blood at 2 mL/kg/min to a maximal volume of 24 mL/kg. Animals were observed for 60 minutes or until death. As noted previously, mortality was significantly higher in animals receiving the most aggressive resuscitation compared with less aggressively treated groups. Animals resuscitated most aggressively had higher volumes of intraperitoneal hemorrhage than the two other experimental groups. In addition, oxygen delivery, which was monitored in these animals, was significantly greater in the group resuscitated to a mean arterial pressure of 60 mm Hg than in the two other experimental groups. Similar observations were made in a second report from this same group in a study by Kowalenko and colleagues.[129]

Clinical and preclinical studies focused on early limitation of crystalloid resuscitation and hemorrhagic shock focus on penetrating torso trauma, but do not address initial care of patients with head injury, the leading cause of traumatic death in the United States. Historically, when shock accompanies head injury, the incidence of adverse outcome doubles. Because of the vulnerability of the injured brain to even brief periods of reduced perfusion, guidelines for the management of head injury state that delayed resuscitation cannot be considered applicable in head trauma.[77] Nonetheless, in a large animal model using a standard cerebral injury along with uncontrolled hemorrhage secondary to aortotomy, there was no evidence of increased secondary cerebral ischemia with delayed resuscitation. Conventional resuscitation with lactated Ringer's solution resulted in signs of increased secondary brain injury.[130]

Clinical Studies

Martin and coworkers[131] provided preliminary data in patients on the effect of aggressive versus delayed prehospital resuscitation of uncontrolled hemorrhagic shock after penetrating injury. These workers evaluated the effect of delaying fluid resuscitation until surgical intervention could control the source of hemorrhage on outcome of hypotensive trauma victims. Injury severity was similar in standard resuscitation and delayed resuscitation groups. The rate of survival to hospital discharge was 69% in the delayed resuscitation group and 56% in the standard resuscitation group. The difference between these groups did not reach statistical significance owing to small sample size.

Much attention has been directed to resuscitation of patients after injury owing to a report from Bickell and associates[132] that appeared in the *New England Journal of Medicine*. The authors reported a prospective clinical trial of adults with penetrating truncal trauma who were hypotensive in the field as indicated by a systolic blood pressure less than 90 mm Hg. Patients were randomly assigned to placement of intravascular catheters with standard prehospital and trauma center fluid resuscitation using lactated Ringer's solution or an experimental group in which vascular catheters were placed, but intravenous fluids were not administered until patients reached the operating room. Patients were excluded from this trial if they were noted to have a field revised trauma score of zero consistent with cardiopulmonary arrest or had sustained fatal gunshot wounds to the head with neurologic injury that precluded long-term survival.[27] In addition, patients with penetrating truncal injury who did not require operation were excluded. After 1069 patients were screened during the 37 months of this study, 598 patients were enrolled—309 in an immediate resuscitation group receiving standard fluids according to Advanced Trauma Life Support protocols and 289 in a delayed resuscitation group, which did not receive intravenous fluids until reaching the operating room.[133]

The immediate and delayed resuscitation groups were well matched with respect to age, gender, and anatomic injury as measured by the Injury Severity Score (ISS), Revised Trauma Score (physiologic response to injury) and systolic blood pressure.[134,135] Field response times for prehospital providers in this trial were short, averaging 30 minutes or less. The trauma center interval (i.e., the interval in the hospital before operation) was surprisingly long—44 minutes in the immediate resuscitation group and 52 minutes on average in the group receiving delayed resuscitation. Prehospital fluid administration averaged less than 900 mL in the immediate resuscitation group versus less than 100 mL in the delayed resuscitation cohort. Fluid administration in the trauma center before operation averaged greater than 1600 mL of fluid in the immediate resuscitation group, whereas the delayed resuscitation patients averaged 283 mL of fluid received. Operative blood loss between the study groups was not different. Among the 289 patients who received delayed fluid resuscitation, 203 (70%) survived and were discharged from the hospital. Of the 309 patients who received immediate fluid resuscitation, 193 (62%) survived ($P=.04$). Patients in the delayed resuscitation group displayed a trend toward reduced postoperative complications, including acute respiratory distress syndrome, sepsis syndrome, acute renal failure, coagulopathy, wound infection, and pneumonia, compared with patients in the immediate resuscitation group ($P=.08$).

A subgroup analysis from this study was reported at a subsequent meeting of the American Association for the Surgery of Trauma. When Wall and coworkers[136] examined major subgroups in the patient population reported by Bickell and colleagues, a statistical difference in hospital survival could be shown only in patients who had sustained penetrating cardiac injury.[74] Patients with major vascular injury, solid organ injury requiring operation, or noncardiac thoracic injury had comparable survival in the immediate and delayed resuscitation groups.

Although these early clinical studies represent a remarkable accomplishment in design, organization, and data analysis, many questions remain unanswered. None of the studies reported was blinded, and a randomization scheme was not employed. In the trial of Bickell and colleagues, in which the difference in mortality rested in a difference in survival of a small number of patients in the experimental groups, 22 patients in the delayed resuscitation group were given intravenous fluids in violation of study design.[132] Although these individuals were appropriately included in an intent-to-treat analysis, the impact of selected fluid administration on study outcome is unclear. The authors also have been criticized for excluding patients *after* randomization because of injuries considered too minor (no operative therapy) or too severe (revised trauma score of zero). Exclusion of these patients may invalidate the statistical approach employed and increase the difficulty of the clinician seeking guidance from this work. Finally, time spent in the trauma center by these hypotensive patients with injuries requiring operation was surprisingly long. Although the resuscitation groups described differed statistically in vital signs and hematologic parameters, it is unclear that the differences observed had clinical significance.

Clinical Pathway—Early Resuscitation

In all of the preclinical and clinical work described, the mechanism of injury and survival remains unclear. Among considerations are the impact of fluid resuscitation on early clot formation in the setting of uncontrolled hemorrhage.[74,128] Other workers suggest that rapidity in resuscitation of pulse pressure may relate to mechanical disruption of initial thrombus.[128] Fluid resuscitation may contribute to dilution of clotting factors in the setting of exaggerated bleeding in uncontrolled hemorrhage.[74,119] The data to support these observations are limited. Where clinical data are available, differences in platelet count and prothrombin time favored individuals receiving reduced preoperative fluid administration.[132] None of the deleterious changes observed was sufficient, however, to represent overt coagulopathy. Perhaps the most impressive observation in animals receiving aggressive resuscitation and followed to their demise is progressive hemodilution and associated cardiovascular collapse.[127-129] This observation corresponds to previous work done by Wilkerson, Levy, and various others examining the effect of hemodilution in animals during the development of blood substitutes.[137,138] This negative consequence of aggressive crystalloid resuscitation in uncontrolled hemorrhage seems best supported by available experimental evidence, although clinical data are unavailable.

Despite provocative preclinical and clinical data, there is insufficient evidence to propose practice guidelines or make recommendations. "Uncontrolled" hemorrhage itself remains undefined. This problem is best seen as injury with blood loss occurring in the absence of surgical or mechanical hemostasis or the "control" provided by regulated blood removal through a vascular cannula. It is unclear whether a vascular injury after a torso gunshot wound and a shattered spleen after an automobile crash are different in this regard. The bottom-line message from all of the studies is that elevation of the blood pressure to normal or supranormal levels results in resumption of bleeding from the uncontrolled site, and rebleeding leads to recurrent shock and death of the experimental animal. Other work shows that animals subjected to shock could be successfully resuscitated at lower than "normal" mean arterial pressures if the bleeding site was controlled as part of the resuscitation program. Shock victims resuscitated with electrolyte solutions are subject to progressive hemodilution, and this may lead to death. The lessons that clinicians should learn from this body of data are as follows[45,74,104]:

1. Operation to control bleeding is part of resuscitation.
2. Blood pressure levels are convenient, but possibly misleading end points for shock resuscitation in that resuscitation to normal or supranormal pressures may be

harmful if the effort delays operation to control bleeding or the pressure elevation causes rebleeding. Better end points (e.g., tissue oxygenation or other metabolic parameters) are needed.

3. Extreme hemodilution is possible and dangerous in shock, and the diagnosis of hemorrhagic shock dictates the immediate addition of blood transfusion to the management plan in patients requiring ongoing administration of electrolyte solutions.
4. Resuscitation of traumatic shock, similar to fluid management of a burned patient, requires repeated observation, judgment, and skill and cannot be accomplished by recipe or formula.

The clinical trials that have sought to extend the previously described experimental concepts into the realm of patient care have dealt primarily with blood loss secondary to penetrating injury because this clinical condition is as close a simulation to a pure hemorrhage model as is available in clinical medicine. It is useful to emphasize that multiple blunt injury, multiple wounds, and extensive soft tissue trauma are not similar to pure hemorrhage models in that occult blood and fluid losses and other inflammatory factors exist that make the quantitation of injury severity difficult.

MANAGEMENT OF TRAUMATIC SHOCK IN THE INTENSIVE CARE UNIT

Before admission to the ICU, resuscitation is directed at maintaining blood pressure and reducing heart rate through volume loading with crystalloid and blood products. Relatively simple clinical end points are employed.[45] *This approach should be adequate for 95% of injured patients.* On admission to the ICU, severely injured patients may receive a pulmonary artery catheter to monitor hemodynamics and refine further the direction of resuscitation.[139] A series of early reports by Shoemaker and coworkers proposed that supranormal oxygen delivery (600 mL/min/m^2) and resuscitation to a plateau oxygen consumption were appropriate clinical end points. Although observations of improved hemodynamic response in survivors of injury make intuitive sense, driving injured patients to supranormal hemodynamic performance was not associated with improvement in clinical outcome.[75,81-84] Reduced goals for oxygen delivery (500 mL/min/m^2) are proposed among end points for support of patients receiving pulmonary artery catheter monitoring.[140-142]

Criteria identifying patients warranting consideration of placement of a pulmonary artery catheter and need for ICU resuscitation include major injury (two or more abdominal organs, two or more long bone fractures, complex pelvic fractures, flail chest, or major vascular injury), blood loss (anticipated need >6 U packed red blood cells [PRBC] during the first 12 hours after hospitalization), and metabolic stress (arterial base deficit >6 mEq/L during the first 12 hours after hospital admission). A trauma victim older than 65 years with any two of the previous criteria also warrants consideration of a pulmonary artery catheter and ICU resuscitation. Patients with these criteria who also incurred severe brain injury, defined as Glasgow Coma Scale score less than or equal to 8 in the trauma ICU and abnormality on brain computed tomography scan, were not resuscitated by protocol during development of this approach, unless assessed by the attending neurosurgeon to be at low risk of secondary brain injury with these procedures.[141,142] In my practice, I find that the brain, similar to other organs, benefits from effective resuscitation (Table 28-4).

Table 28-4. Summary of Protocol for Resuscitation of Shock Resulting from Major Torso Trauma*

Intervention	Threshold	Method
Transfuse (PRBC)	DO_2I < 500 mL/min/m^2; hemoglobin <10 g/dL (≥65 years old, <12 g/dL)	1 g hemoglobin/dl/unit PRBC; bolus transfusion, then hemoglobin analysis (bedside), then calculate DO_2I
Volume load (LR)	DO_2I < 500 mL/min/m^2; hemoglobin ≥10 g/dL (≥65 years old, ≥12 g/dL); PCWP < 15 mm Hg (≥65 years old, <12 mm Hg)	1-L LR bolus infusion (≥65 years old, 0.5 L), then measure PCWP, then calculate DO_2I
Starling curve (NS)	DO_2I < 500 mL/min/m^2; hemoglobin ≥10 g/dL (≥65 years old, ≥12 g/dL); PCWP ≥ 15 mm Hg (≥65 years old, ≥12 mm Hg)	0.5- or 0.25-L NS bolus infusion, then measure PCWP and CI: CI-PCWP optimal if ΔCI ≤ −0.3; ΔPCWP ≤ +4 with two consecutive boluses; then calculate DO_2I
Inotrope	DO_2I < 500 mL/min/m^2; hemoglobin 10 g/dL (≥65 years old, ≥12 g/dL); CI and PCWP optimized	Milrinone, 0.1-μg increments to 0.8 μg/kg/min, or dobutamine, 2.5-μg increments to 20 μg/kg/min; calculate DO_2I
Vasopressor	DO_2I < 500 mL/min/m^2; MAP < 65 mm Hg	Norepinephrine, 0.05-μg increments to 0.2 μg/kg/min; measure MAP; calculate DO_2I

*Details of the resuscitation protocol employed by McKinley and coworkers are given. Selected drugs for inotropic and vasopressor support are listed. Patients also are treated to age-appropriate hemoglobin levels and given fluid infusion based on a volume loading protocol until filling pressures and DO_2I are optimized.

CI, cardiac index; CWP, capillary wedge pressure; DO_2I, oxygen delivery index; LR, lactated Ringer's solution; MAP, mean arterial pressure; NS, normal saline; PCWP, pulmonary capillary wedge pressure; PRBC, packed red blood cells.

Modified from McKinley BA, Kozar RA, Cocanour CS, et al: Normal versus supranormal oxygen delivery goals in shock resuscitation: The response is the same. J Trauma 2002;53:825-832.

A sequential approach to shock resuscitation using a pulmonary artery catheter is advocated by McKinley, Moore, and their coworkers.[139,140] Their approach includes a series of interventions including administration of PRBC and lactated Ringer's solution to optimize cardiac index and pulmonary capillary wedge pressure as described in a classic Starling curve. Milrinone, dobutamine, and norepinephrine are used as vasoactive agents as necessary to provide mean arterial pressure greater than 65 mm Hg and oxygen delivery index greater than 500 mL/min/m^2. These patients require large volumes of protocol-directed shock resuscitation (approximately 15 L for oxygen delivery index >500 mL/min/m^2). Significant output volumes also should be expected. This large net positive balance suggests unrecognized ongoing blood loss or extreme fluid shifts between intravascular, interstitial, and intracellular compartments, or both, for severely injured patients (Fig. 28-3).

The protocol-driven approach described has provided a variety of observations.[143] First, even elderly patients respond to ICU resuscitation after injury.[141] In general, the maximal oxygen delivery response is less than that of younger patients, and elderly patients have a greater requirement for inotropic support.[144] Second, a Starling curve generation approach is feasible and reliably improves hemodynamic resuscitation from major trauma. Supranormal resuscitation is neither necessary nor desirable in the management of patients with trauma associated with shock.[139] Third, aggressive resuscitation, particularly in the setting of ongoing bleeding, increases the risk of elevated intra-abdominal pressure and abdominal compartment syndrome.[145] Preload-driven resuscitation may cause bowel edema with subsequent venous obstruction, declining cardiac output, decreased urinary output, and compromise of systemic oxygenation. Finally, although many end points for interventions for goal-directed resuscitation in critical injury exist, systemic oxygen transport is the current state of the art in the most severely injured patients and is the basis for future development of clinical processes for resuscitation of shock caused by major trauma (Fig. 28-4).[143]

The utility of the pulmonary artery catheter in the management of patients with severe injury is suggested by a study using data obtained in the National Trauma Data Bank.[146] From more than 450,000 records, 53,000 patients were reviewed. These patients were admitted between January 1994 and December 2001. Patients survived more than 48 hours and underwent at least one diagnostic or therapeutic procedure. The patients were 60 to 90 years old and distinguished by ISS and initial base deficit. Approximately 2000 patients who had insertion of a pulmonary artery catheter during hospitalization were compared with 51,000 patients who did not. Logistic regression analysis was used to develop a model that examined mortality after injury. Factors included in the model were use of a pulmonary artery catheter, age, emergency department base deficit, ISS, comorbid conditions, mechanism of injury, and specific injury patterns as identi-

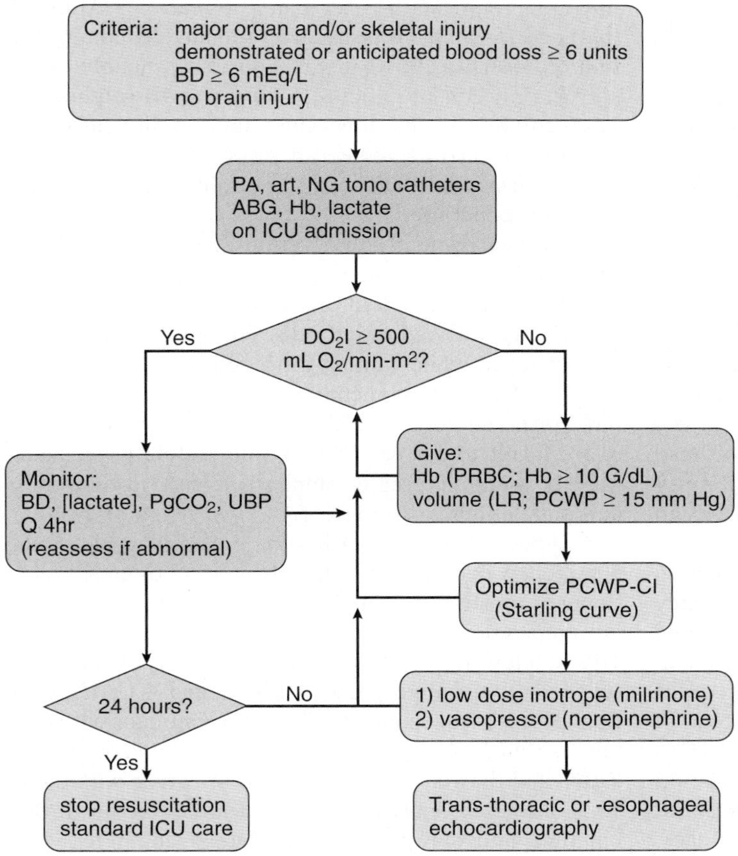

Figure 28-3. A few patients require additional aggressive resuscitation in the ICU. Frequently, these patients require insertion of a pulmonary artery catheter. This protocol is the most widely reported strategy for crystalloid and blood administration in stabilization of these patients coming from a series of articles published by McKinley, Moore, and associates. ABG, arterial blood gas; BD, base deficit; CI, cardiac index; $D0_2I$, oxygen delivery index; Hb, hemoglobin; ICU, intensive care unit; LR, lactated Ringer's; NG, nasogastric; PA, pulmonary artery; PCWP, pulmonary capillary wedge pressure; $PgCO_2$, transgastric oxygen; UBP, urinary bladder pressure. (From Marr AB, Moore FA, Sailors RM, et al: Preload optimization using "Starling curve" generation during shock resuscitation: Can it be done? Shock 2004;21:300-305.)

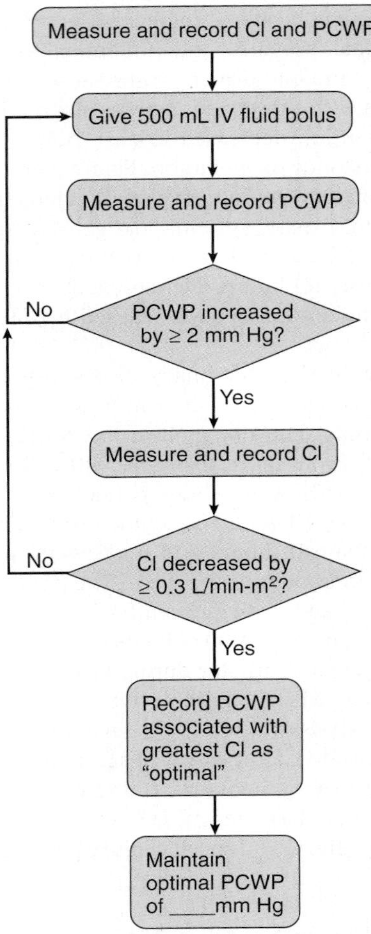

Figure 28-4. This simple algorithm describes a Starling curve protocol for optimization of filling pressures as a part of resuscitation of severely injured patients in the critical care unit where a pulmonary artery catheter is employed. CI, cardiac index; PCWP, pulmonary capillary wedge pressure. (From Marr AB, Moore FA, Sailors RM, et al: Preload optimization using "Starling curve" generation during shock resuscitation: Can it be done? Shock 2004;21:300-305.)

fied by the Abbreviated Injury Scale. Overall, patients managed with a pulmonary artery catheter were older and had a higher ISS, greater emergency department base deficit, and higher mortality (29.7% with pulmonary artery catheter versus 9.8% without pulmonary artery catheter). Patients with spine, abdominal, chest, or head injury and patients with at least one Abbreviated Injury Scale score equal to or greater than 3 were more likely to be managed with a pulmonary artery catheter.

Pulmonary artery catheter use was associated with increased mortality in all subgroups of ISS, emergency department base deficit, and age. As age, base deficit, and ISS increased, however, the risk of death associated with pulmonary artery catheter use decreased, and an apparent benefit of pulmonary artery catheter use emerged. In contrast, less severely injured trauma patients (ISS 16 to 24) and severely injured patients without high admission base deficit (>–5) had increased mortality associated with pulmonary artery catheter placement regardless of age.

Although these observations come from a large database, retrospective study design and subgroup analysis are not optimal for definitive hypothesis testing. Finally, neither timing of placement for pulmonary artery catheters nor cause of death and specific relationship to placement of the pulmonary artery catheter could be conclusively examined by analysis of the National Trauma Data Bank. Nonetheless, these data suggest that injured patients may derive benefit from pulmonary artery catheter–guided resuscitation to avert complications related to persistent perfusion deficits. Further focused examination of patients with risk factors for poor outcome is warranted.[146]

Massive Transfusion

Independent of mechanism of injury, hemorrhagic shock consistently is the second leading cause of early death among injured patients, with only CNS injury consistently more lethal.[147] Severe CNS injury is devastating and has a high rate of prehospital mortality; prevention is the best strategy.[148] Hemorrhagic shock accounts for 30% to 40% of trauma deaths and is more amenable to interventions to reduce mortality and morbidity.[147] In addition, approximately 25% of CNS injuries are complicated by hemorrhagic shock.[149,150] Hemorrhage contributes to death during the prehospital period in 33% to 56% of cases, and exsanguination is the most common cause of death among individuals found dead on arrival of emergency medical services personnel.[151] Hemorrhage accounts for the largest proportion of mortality occurring within the first hour of trauma center care and greater than 80% of operating room deaths after major trauma.[147,152] Although the need for massive transfusion (defined as administration of ≥10 U of PRBC in <24 hours) is probably necessary in only 3% of patients in busy trauma centers, this intervention can be lifesaving, and preliminary data suggest that early aggressive administration of blood products reduces morbidity and mortality and decreases overall product use.[153]

Numerous general observations can be made.[153-155] Most patients receiving massive transfusion are treated initially with crystalloid fluids followed by noncross-matched type O red blood cells. Plasma therapy is typically delayed while waiting for blood typing and plasma thawing. Platelets frequently are not given until patients have received 20 U of PRBC. Coagulopathy is common and difficult to correct. Plasma and platelets are inadequately used and greater emphasis is needed on plasma and platelet administration.

A typical massive transfusion protocol begins in the emergency department when the senior trauma practitioner orders transfusion of O-negative PRBC and invokes an organization-specific massive transfusion protocol.[155,156] This is followed by administration of 4 to 6 U of additional typed or O-negative units of PRBC and 4 U of newly thawed fresh frozen plasma. Therapy continues with containers sent from the blood bank each containing 6 U of PRBC and thawed plasma. Platelets are given with every 12 U of PRBC. Goals are normalization of the prothrombin time and elevation of the platelet count to 50 to

100×10^9/L. The fibrinogen level is checked after 18 U of PRBC, and cryoprecipitate is given if the fibrinogen level is less than 1 g/L. This triggers administration of 10 U of cryoprecipitate.

Recombinant Activated Factor VII

Recombinant activated factor VIIa holds promise for reversing acquired coagulopathy associated with trauma and massive hemorrhage.[157] When bound to exposed tissue factor, normally expressed factor VIIa activates the extrinsic clotting system at the site of injury without causing systemic hypercoagulability. Recombinant activated factor VIIa is an attractive therapeutic candidate for coagulopathy because it bypasses much of the intrinsic coagulation system, is active in the presence of exposed tissue factor, and has a rapid onset and short half-life. Tissue factor exists in high concentrations in the media and is exposed with vessel injury.[158,159]

Large animal and clinical studies have evaluated the role of recombinant activated factor VIIa as a hemostatic agent.[157] Improved clot formation and bleeding control is suggested, and laboratory searches for microthrombi, particularly in animal work, have been negative. The largest clinical database includes more than 200 patients with blunt and penetrating injury. Patients received recombinant activated factor VIIa after 8 units of PRBC with additional doses 1 and 3 hours later. Other treatment was provided according to local standard. In blunt trauma patients, PRBC transfusions were reduced by 2.6 U, and the need for massive transfusion was reduced to a statistically significant degree.[157] No safety issues, including thromboembolic events, were identified. Although laboratory data suggest reduced efficacy with acidosis, recombinant activated factor VIIa seems to be safe in severely injured trauma patients and may be associated with decreased blood product use.[160] Additional multicenter prospective data are required to develop consistent treatment strategies and a role for this expensive agent in patients receiving massive transfusion.

Risks of Early Red Blood Cell Transfusion

Blood transfusion in trauma has been identified as an independent predictor of multiple organ failure, systemic inflammatory response syndrome, increased postinjury infection, and increased mortality in multiple studies.[161] Cumulative risks have been related to the number of units of PRBC transfused, increased storage time of transfused blood, and possibly the presence of leukocytes in donor blood. Many authors have concluded that blood transfusion in an injured patient should be minimized whenever possible.[162]

Large single-institution data sets examined the impact of blood transfusion in postinjury multiple organ failure.[163-165] Variables identified as early independent predictors of multiple organ failure included age older than 55 years, ISS equal to or greater than 25, and greater than 6 U of PRBC in the first 12 hours after admission. Base deficit greater than 8 mEq/L in the first 12 hours and lactate greater than 2.5 mol/L also were independent predictors of multiple organ failure. Subsequent prospective work confirmed the importance of blood transfusion as an independent risk factor for postinjury multiple organ failure after controlling for other indices of shock, including base deficit and lactate. Additional studies of blood product use after injury associate blood transfusion with increased mortality. Potential confounding shock variables, including base deficit, serum lactate, age, gender, race, Glasgow Coma Scale score, and ISS, were controlled in this analysis.

Factors contributing to complications associated with red blood cell transfusion include storage time, increased endothelial adherence of stored red blood cells, nitric oxide binding by free hemoglobin in stored blood, donor leukocytes, host inflammatory response, and reduced red blood cell deformability.[161,166] Nonetheless, transfusion of an injured patient with stored PRBC is the only option for treatment of severe hemorrhagic shock. Although other hemoglobin-based oxygen carriers hold great promise and ultimately may provide better outcomes for injured patients, these materials have not come to be used. In an effort to minimize adverse events, attempts to minimize the use of blood transfusion in injury are appropriate outside major hemorrhage.

SPECIAL PROBLEMS

Abdominal Compartment Syndrome

A compartment syndrome is a condition in which increased pressure within a confined anatomic space adversely affects function and viability of tissues contained within. Confined anatomic spaces associated with compartment syndromes are fascial spaces of the extremities, the globe as in glaucoma, and the cranial cavity as in epidural or subdural hematoma. Abdominal compartment syndrome is a condition in which sustained pressure within the abdominal wall, pelvis, diaphragm, and retroperitoneum adversely affects the function of the gastrointestinal tract and related extraperitoneal organs. Abdominal compartment syndrome is receiving increasing recognition as a complication of massive resuscitation after trauma, burns, or other surgical procedures (Box 28-2). Operative decompression is frequently required. Pressures around 5 to 7 mm Hg in the peritoneal cavity are normal. Short-duration pressure increases frequently occur with coughing, Valsalva maneuvers, defecation, and weightlifting. Intra-abdominal pressure can be nonpathologically increased in obese individuals. Elevated intra-abdominal pressure is a common finding among critically ill medical and surgical patients.[167-169]

The more recent consensus conference on abdominal compartment syndrome has created improved definitions in relation to abdominal compartment syndrome (Table 28-5). For standardization, intra-abdominal pressure should be expressed in mm Hg and measured at end expiration with the patient supine after ensuring that abdominal muscle contractions are absent. The transducer is zeroed at the midaxillary line. The current reference standard for intra-abdominal pressure measurement is pressure measured via an indwelling urinary drainage catheter

Box 28-2

Risk Factors for Intra-abdominal Hypertension and Abdominal Compartment Syndrome

Acidosis (pH<7.2)
Hypothermia (core temperature <33° C)
Polytransfusion (>10 U packed red blood cells/24 h)
Coagulopathy (platelets <55,000/mm³ *or* activated partial thromboplastin time 2× normal or higher *or* prothrombin time <50% *or* international standardized ratio >1.5)
Sepsis (American-European Consensus Conference definitions)
Bacteremia
Intra-abdominal infection or abscess
Peritonitis
Liver dysfunction or cirrhosis with ascites
Mechanical ventilation
Use of positive end-expiratory pressure (PEEP) or the presence of auto-PEEP
Pneumonia
Abdominal surgery, especially with tight fascial closures
Massive fluid resuscitation (>5L colloid or crystalloid/24 h)
Gastroparesis, gastric distention, or ileus
Volvulus
Hemoperitoneum or pneumoperitoneum
Major burns
Major trauma
High body mass index (>30)
Intra-abdominal or retroperitoneal tumors
Prone positioning
Massive incisional hernia repair
Acute pancreatitis
Distended abdomen
Damage control laparotomy
Laparoscopy with excessive inflation pressures
Peritoneal dialysis

From Malbrain ML, Cheatham ML, Kirkpatrick A, et al: Results from the International Conference of Experts on Intra-abdominal Hypertension and Abdominal Compartment Syndrome, I: Definitions. Intensive Care Med 2006;32: 1722-1732.

within the bladder. The recommended technique for measuring intra-abdominal pressure is to clamp the urinary catheter and instill a maximal volume of 25 mL of sterile, room-temperature saline into the bladder with the patient in the supine position. After zeroing a transducer and a stabilization period of at least 30 to 60 seconds, the mean intra-abdominal pressure can be read on a bedside monitor or as the height of the fluid column in urinary drainage tubing.

Intra-abdominal hypertension is defined by a sustained or repeated intra-abdominal pressure greater than 12 mm Hg or an abdominal perfusion pressure less than 60 mm Hg, where abdominal perfusion pressure = mean arterial pressure − intra-abdominal pressure. Abdominal compartment syndrome is present when organ dysfunction occurs as a result of intra-abdominal hypertension. Abdominal compartment syndrome is defined by sustained or repeated intra-abdominal pressure greater than 20 mm Hg or abdominal perfusion pressure less than 60 mm Hg in association with new-onset single or multiple organ system failure. In contrast to intra-abdominal hypertension, abdominal compartment syndrome is not graded, but rather considered as an "all or none" phenomenon.[169,170]

Intra-abdominal hypertension has a variety of physiologic effects. In experimental preparations, animals die as a result of congestive heart failure as abdominal pressure passes a critical threshold. Increased intra-abdominal pressure decreases cardiac output and left and right ventricular stroke work, while increasing central venous pressure, pulmonary artery wedge pressure, and systemic and pulmonary vascular resistance. Abdominal decompression reverses these changes. As both hemidiaphragms are displaced upward with increased intra-abdominal pressure, decreased thoracic volume and compliance are seen. Decreased volume within the pleural cavity causes atelectasis and decreases alveolar clearance. Pulmonary infections also may result. Ventilated patients with abdominal hypertension require increased airway pressure to deliver a fixed tidal volume. As the diaphragm protrudes into the pleural cavity, intrathoracic pressure increases with reduction in cardiac output and increased pulmonary vascular resistance. Ventilation and perfusion abnormalities result, and blood gas measurements show hypoxemia, hypercarbia, and acidosis.[171]

Elevation in intra-abdominal pressure also causes renal dysfunction. Inadequate renal perfusion pressure and renal filtration gradient have been proposed as critical factors in the development of renal insufficiency associated with elevated intra-abdominal pressure. The filtration gradient is the mechanical force across the glomerulus and equals the difference between glomerular filtration pressure and proximal tubular pressure. In the presence of intra-abdominal hypertension, proximal tubular pressure may be assumed to equal intra-abdominal pressure. Glomerular filtration pressure may be estimated as mean arterial pressure minus intra-abdominal pressure. Changes in intra-abdominal pressure may have a greater impact on renal function and urine production than changes in mean arterial pressure. Oliguria is thought to be one of the first signs of intra-abdominal hypertension. Control of intra-abdominal pressure leads to reversal of renal impairment. Oliguria may be seen with intra-abdominal pressure of 15 to 20 mm Hg. Deterioration in cardiac output plays a role in diminished renal perfusion, but even with maintenance of cardiac output, impairment of renal function persists in intra-abdominal hypertension.[167,172-174]

Other organs affected by increased intra-abdominal pressure include the liver, where hepatic blood flow has been shown to decrease with abdominal hypertension.[175,176] It may be assumed that hepatic synthesis of acute-phase proteins, immunoglobulins, and other factors of host defense may be impaired by reduced hepatic blood flow. Other gastrointestinal functions may be compro-

Table 28-5. Consensus Definitions List

Definition 1	IAP is the steady-state pressure concealed within the abdominal cavity
Definition 2	APP=MAP−IAP
Definition 3	FG=GFP−PTP=MAP−2×IAP
Definition 4	IAP should be expressed in mm Hg and measured at end expiration in the complete supine position after ensuring that abdominal muscle contractions are absent and with the transducer zeroed at the level of the midaxillary line
Definition 5	The reference standard for intermittent IAP measurement is via the bladder with a maximal instillation volume of 25 mL sterile saline
Definition 6	Normal IAP is approximately 5-7 mm Hg in critically ill adults
Definition 7	IAH is defined by a sustained or repeated pathologic elevation in IAP≥12 mm Hg
Definition 8	IAH is graded as follows: grade I, IAH 12-15 mm Hg; grade II, IAP 16-20 mm Hg; grade III, IAP 21-25 mm Hg; grade IV, IAP>25 mm Hg
Definition 9	ACS is defined as a sustained IAP>20 mm Hg (with or without an APP<60 mm Hg) that is associated with new organ dysfunction/failure
Definition 10	Primary ACS is a condition associated with injury or disease in the abdominopelvic region that frequently requires early surgical or interventional radiologic intervention
Definition 11	Secondary ACS refers to conditions that do not originate from the abdominopelvic region
Definition 12	Recurrent ACS refers to the condition in which ACS redevelops after previous surgical or medical treatment of primary or secondary ACS

ACS, abdominal compartment syndrome; APP, abdominal perfusion pressure; FG, filtration gradient; GFP, glomerular filtration pressure; IAH, intra-abdominal hypertension; IAP, intra-abdominal pressure; MAP, mean arterial pressure; PTP, proximal tubular pressure.
From Malbrain ML, Cheatham ML, Kirkpatrick A, et al: Results from the International Conference of Experts on Intra-abdominal Hypertension and Abdominal Compartment Syndrome, I: Definitions. Intensive Care Med 2006;32:1722-1732.

mised by increased intra-abdominal pressure. Splanchnic hypoperfusion may begin with an intra-abdominal pressure of 15 mm Hg. Reduced perfusion of intra-abdominal arteries, veins, and lymphatics may create changes in mucosal pH, translocation, bowel motility, and production of gastrointestinal hormones. Finally, intracranial hypertension is seen with chronically increased intra-abdominal pressure. Intracranial hypertension has been shown to decrease when intra-abdominal pressure is reduced in morbidly obese patients and in intracranial injury.

Operative decompression is the method of choice for treatment of patients with intra-abdominal hypertension and associated evidence of organ dysfunction. After decompression, improvements in hemodynamics, pulmonary function, tissue perfusion, and renal function have been shown in a variety of clinical settings. To prevent hemodynamic decompensation during decompression, intravascular volume should be restored, oxygen delivery should be normalized, and hypothermia and coagulation defects should be corrected. The abdomen should be opened in patients with adequate venous access and controlled ventilation. Adjunctive measures to combat reperfusion washout from by-products of anaerobic metabolism include acute use of vasoconstrictor agents to avoid sudden changes in blood pressure. After decompression of the abdomen, the fascial gap is left open using one of a variety of temporary abdominal closure methods.

Extremity Compartment Syndrome

The numerous causes of extremity compartment syndrome include complications of open and closed fractures, arterial injury, temporary vascular occlusion, snakebite, drug abuse, burns, physical exertion, and gunshot wounds. The most common cause of compartment syndrome is muscle injury leading to edema, which is correlated to the amount of tissue damage. Pressure is increased within the closed fascial space first by intracellular swelling followed by hematoma formation if a fracture is present. Because extremities, particularly at the calf, are composed of relatively unyielding fascial compartments, circulatory compromise occurs as tissue pressure increases with resulting ischemia and tissue damage. Leakage of intracellular fluid follows, and a further increase in intracompartmental pressure is seen.[177]

When extremity injuries produce complete ischemia, skeletal muscle that is deprived of oxygen may survive for 4 hours without irreversible damage. Total ischemia of 8 hours' duration produces irreversible change. Peripheral nerves conduct for 1 hour after onset of total ischemia and can survive for 4 hours with only neurapraxic damage. After 8 hours, axonotmesis and irreversible damage occur. Ischemia caused by reduction or cessation of blood flow occurs when the perfusion gradient to a muscle compartment falls below a critical level. Perfusion is related to the compartment pressure. When intracompartmental blood pressure is 25 mm Hg, tissue perfusion in injured tissues is substantially decreased.[177-179]

Fasciotomy should be performed when intracompartmental pressure approaches 25 mm Hg, or if an extremity has been completely ischemic for 6 hours, the patient's clinical condition is worsening, substantial tissue injury is present, or tissue pressure is increasing.[179] Prophylactic treatment is valuable because fasciotomy does not reverse changes caused by initial extremity injury, but can prevent changes resulting from secondary ischemic insults.

Pain, pallor, paralysis, paresthesias, and pulselessness are the classic hallmarks of extremity compartment syndrome. If treatment is not initiated until all of these signs are present, poor results are obtained. Pain and aggravation of pain by passive stretching of the muscles in the involved compartment is the most sensitive clinical finding. Assessment of pain is useful when patients are conscious and can respond cognitively to examination. In unconscious patients at risk for compartment syndrome, tissue pressure measurements may be the only objective criteria for diagnosis. Measurement of compartment pressures is obtained in all extremity compartments at risk and proximal and distal to any fractures. The highest pressure noted should serve as the basis for determining the need for fasciotomy.

Pelvic Fractures

Substantial blunt force is required to disrupt the pelvic ring. The extent of injury is related to the direction and magnitude of force applied. Associated abdominal, thoracic, and head injuries are common. Force applied to the pelvis can cause rotational displacement with opening or compression of the pelvic ring. Other types of displacement seen with pelvic fractures are vertical with complete disruption of the ring and the posterior sacroiliac complex.[180]

Patients with pelvic ring injuries are easily divided into two groups on the basis of clinical presentation—patients who are hemodynamically stable and patients who are hemodynamically unstable.[180] There is a dramatic difference in mortality rates between pelvic fracture patients who are hypotensive and patients who are hemodynamically stable. Hemodynamic stability and biomechanical pelvic instability are separate though related issues, which tend to confuse the clinical picture. The source of bleeding may be multifactorial and not directly related to the pelvic fracture itself. Blood loss secondary to pelvic fracture that contributes to hemodynamic instability is a significant risk factor, however. Early fracture diagnosis and stabilization using external skeletal fixation are crucial in the acute phase of patient management.[181] Treatment of the patient also is directed by response to initial fluid resuscitation. Retroperitoneal bleeding in a pelvic fracture usually arises from a low-pressure source—the cancellous bone at the fracture site or adjacent venous injury. Significant retroperitoneal arterial bleeding occurs in approximately 10% of patients. Clinical evidence has suggested that provisional fracture stabilization using external fixation devices or even wrapping the fractured pelvis in a bed sheet can control low-pressure venous bleeding. Continued, unexplained bleeding after provisional fracture stabilization suggests an arterial source. Angiography with embolization of the involved vessel is indicated. Therapeutic angiography also may be required after abdominal exploration if a rapidly expanding or pulsatile retroperitoneal hematoma is encountered.[182]

KEY POINTS

- Shock after trauma is not the same as simple hemorrhage. Blood loss is combined with an inflammatory component.
- Because of inflammation associated with hemorrhage, the rate and amount of resuscitation are increased after injury compared with hemorrhage outside the setting of trauma.
- The classic neuroendocrine response leading to conservation of salt and water in traumatic shock can be linked to neuroimmune feedback loops, which modulate inflammatory response.
- Although flaws in present crystalloid resuscitation preparations exist, a clear benefit of routinely available colloids has not been shown.
- A variety of metabolic and oxygen transport end points for resuscitation have been identified. In general, these end points change in a consistent fashion after injury. None of the available resuscitation end points is sufficient to limit or guide therapy after injury at this time.
- Resuscitation to supranormal oxygen transport parameters does not improve outcome after injury. A staged approach using a pulmonary artery catheter may be helpful, which should be necessary in less than 5% of injured patients.
- Although massive transfusion may reduce overall blood product requirements in patients with rapid blood loss, limited resuscitation and blood product conservation are seen as appropriate in many injured patients.

REFERENCES

1. Blalock A: Principles of Surgical Care, Shock, and Other Problems. St. Louis, Mosby, 1940.
2. Peitzman AB, Billiar TR, Harbrecht BG, et al: Hemorrhagic shock. Curr Probl Surg 1995;32:925-1002.
3. Spodick DH: Acute cardiac tamponade. N Engl J Med 2003;349:684-690.
4. Moore FA, Moore EE: Initial management of life-threatening trauma. In Souba WW, Fink MP, Jurkovich GJ, et al (eds): ACS Surgery: Principles and Practices 2006. New York, WebMD Professional Publishing, 2006, pp 1125-1144.
5. Goris RJ: Pathophysiology of shock in trauma. Eur J Surg 2000;166:100-111.
6. Horovitz JH, Carrico CJ, Shires GT: Pulmonary response to major injury. Arch Surg 1974;108:349-355.
7. Ayala A, Wang P, Ba ZF, et al: Differential alterations in plasma IL-6 and TNF levels after trauma and hemorrhage. Am J Physiol 1991;260: R167-R171.
8. Bitterman H, Kinarty A, Lazarovich H, et al: Acute release of cytokines is proportional to tissue injury induced by surgical trauma and shock in rats. J Clin Immunol 1991;11:184-192.

9. Huynh T, Currin RT, Tanaka Y, et al: Activation of Kupffer cells in vivo following femur fracture. Arch Surg 1994;129:1324-1329.
10. Rady MY, Kirkman E, Cranley J, et al: A comparison of the effects of skeletal muscle injury and somatic afferent nerve stimulation on the response to hemorrhage in anesthetized pigs. J Trauma 1993;35:756-761.
11. Gann DS, Cross JS: The neuroendocrine response to critical illness. In Barrie PS, Shires GT (eds): Surgical Intensive Care. Boston, Little, Brown, 1993, pp 93-134.
12. Jones MT, Gillman B: Factors involved in the regulation of adrenocorticotropic hormone/beta-lipotropic hormone. Physiol Rev 1988;68:743-818.
13. Bereiter DA, Zaid AM, Gann DS: Effect of rate of hemorrhage on sympathoadrenal catecholamine release in cats. Am J Physiol 1986;250: E69-E75.
14. Bereiter DA, Zaid AM, Gann DS: Effect of rate of hemorrhage on release of ACTH in cats. Am J Physiol 1986;250: E76-E81.
15. Hume DM, Bell CC, Bartter F: Direct measurement of adrenal secretion during operative trauma and convalescence. Surgery 1962;52:174-187.
16. Chernow B, Lake CR, Barton M, et al: Sympathetic nervous system sensitivity to hemorrhagic hypotension in the subhuman primate. J Trauma 1984;24:229-232.
17. Berne RM, Levy MN, Koeppen BM, et al: Physiology, 5th ed. St. Louis, Mosby, 2004.
18. O'Regan RG, Majcherczyk S: Role of peripheral chemoreceptors and central chemosensitivity in the regulation of respiration and circulation. J Exp Biol 1982;100:23-40.
19. Holmes CL, Patel BM, Russell JA, et al: Physiology of vasopressin relevant to management of septic shock. Chest 2001;120:989-1002.
20. Cryer PE: Physiology and pathophysiology of the human sympathoadrenal neuroendocrine system. N Engl J Med 1980;303:436-444.
21. Jeremitsky E, Omert LA, Dunham M, et al: The impact of hyperglycemia on patients with severe brain injury. J Trauma 2005;58:47-50.
22. Wiggers CJ: Experimental hemorrhagic shock. In Wiggers C (ed): Physiology of Shock. New York, Commonwealth, 1950, pp 121-146.
23. Bone RC: Toward a theory regarding the pathogenesis of the systemic inflammatory response syndrome: What we do and do not know about cytokine regulation. Crit Care Med 1996;24:163-172.
24. Rivkind AI, Siegel JH, Guadalupi P, et al: Sequential patterns of eicosanoid, platelet and neutrophil interactions in the evolution of the fulminant post-traumatic adult respiratory distress syndrome. Ann Surg 1989;210:355-373.
25. Waydhas C, Nast-Kolb D, Jochum M, et al: Inflammatory mediators, infection, sepsis, and multiple organ failure after severe trauma. Arch Surg 1992;127:460-467.
26. Deitch EA: Multiple organ failure: Pathophysiology and potential future therapy. Ann Surg 1992;216:117-134.
27. Nast-Kolb D, Waydhas C, Gippner-Steppert C, et al: Indicators of the posttraumatic inflammatory response correlate with organ failure in patients with multiple injuries. J Trauma 1997;42:446-455.
28. Roumen RM, Hendriks T, van der Ven-Jongekrijg J, et al: Cytokine patterns in patients after major vascular surgery, hemorrhagic shock, and severe blunt trauma: Relation with subsequent adult respiratory distress syndrome and multiple organ failure. Ann Surg 1993;218:769-776.
29. van der Kleij AJ, de Koning J, Beerthuizen G, et al: Early detection of hemorrhagic hypovolemia by muscle oxygen pressure assessment: Preliminary report. Surgery 1983;93:518-524.
30. Redl H, Dinges HP, Buurman WA, et al: Expression of endothelial leukocyte adhesion molecule-1 in septic but not traumatic hypovolemic shock in the baboon. Am J Pathol 1991;139:461-466.
31. Anderson BO, Brown JM, Harken AH: Mechanisms of neutrophil-mediated tissue injury. J Surg Res 1991;51:170-179.
32. Henson PM, Johnston RB Jr: Tissue injury in inflammation: Oxidants, proteinases, and cationic proteins. J Clin Invest 1987;79:669-674.
33. Smedly LA, Tonnesen MG, Sandhaus RA, et al: Neutrophil-mediated injury to endothelial cells: Enhancement by endotoxin and essential role of neutrophil elastase. J Clin Invest 1986;77:1233-1243.
34. Nathan CF: Secretory products of macrophages. J Clin Invest 1987;79:319-326.
35. Gordon S: Alternative activation of macrophages. Nat Rev Immunol 2003;3:23-35.
36. Molina PE: Neurobiology of the stress response: Contribution of the sympathetic nervous system to the neuroimmune axis in traumatic injury. Shock 2005;24:3-10.
37. Selye H: A syndrome produced by diverse nocuous agents—1936. J Neuropsychiatry Clin Neurosci 1998;10:230-231.
38. Chrousos GP: The role of stress and the hypothalamic-pituitary-adrenal axis in the pathogenesis of the metabolic syndrome: Neuro-endocrine and target tissue-related causes. Int J Obes Relat Metab Disord 2000;24(Suppl 2): S50-S55.
39. Rozlog LA, Kiecolt-Glaser JK, Marucha PT, et al: Stress and immunity: Implications for viral disease and wound healing. J Periodontol 1999;70:786-792.
40. Bjontorp P: Stress and cardiovascular disease. Acta Physiol Scand Suppl 1997;640:144-148.
41. Felten DL, Felten SY, Carlson SL, et al: Noradrenergic and peptidergic innervation of lymphoid tissue. J Immunol 1985;135(Suppl 2):755S-765S.
42. Rivest S: How circulating cytokines trigger the neural circuits that control the hypothalamic-pituitary-adrenal axis. Psychoneurology 2001;26:761-788.
43. Banks WA, Kastin AJ, Broadwell RD: Passage of cytokines across the blood-brain barrier. Neuroimmunology 1995;2:241-248.
44. Goehler LE, Gaykema RP, Hansen MK, et al: Vagal immune-to-brain communication: A visceral chemosensory pathway. Auton Neurosci 2000;85:49-59.
45. American College of Surgeons Committee on Trauma: Advanced Trauma Life Support for Doctors, 7th ed., Chicago, American College of Surgeons, 2004.
46. Poole GV, Meredith JW, Pennell T, et al: Comparison of colloids and crystalloids in resuscitation from hemorrhagic shock. Surg Gynecol Obstet 1982;154:577-586.
47. Hauser CJ, Shoemaker WC, Turpin I, et al: Oxygen transport responses to colloids and crystalloids in critically ill surgical patients. Surg Gynecol Obstet 1980;150:811-816.
48. Carey LC, Lowery BD, Cloutier CT: Hemorrhagic shock. Curr Probl Surg 1971;8:1-48.
49. Weaver DW, Ledgerwood AM, Lucas CE, et al: Pulmonary effects of albumin resuscitation for severe hypovolemic shock. Arch Surg 1978;113:387-392.
50. Lowe RJ, Moss GS, Jilek J, et al: Crystalloid vs colloid in the etiology of pulmonary failure after trauma: A randomized trial in man. Surgery 1977;81:676-683.
51. Shah DM, Browner BD, Dutton RE, et al: Cardiac output and pulmonary wedge pressure: Use for evaluation of fluid replacement in trauma patients. Arch Surg 1977;112:1161-1168.
52. Guyton AC, Lindsey AW: Effect of elevated left atrial pressure and decreased plasma protein concentration on the development of pulmonary edema. Circ Res 1959;7:649-657.
53. Zarins CK, Rice CL, Smith DE, et al: Role of lymphatics in preventing hypooncotic pulmonary edema. Surg Forum 1976;27:257-259.
54. Demling RH, Manohar M, Will JA, et al: The effect of plasma oncotic pressure on the pulmonary microcirculation after hemorrhagic shock. Surgery 1979;86:323-328.
55. Holcroft JW, Trunkey DD, Carpenter MA: Excessive fluid administration in resuscitating baboons from hemorrhagic shock, and an assessment of the thermodye technic for measuring extravascular lung water. Am J Surg 1978;135:412-416.
56. Koustova E, Stanton K, Gushchin V, et al: Effects of lactated Ringer's solutions on human leukocytes. J Trauma 2002;52:872-878.
57. Didwania A, Miller J, Kassel D, et al: Effect of intravenous lactated Ringer's solution infusion on the circulating lactate concentration: Part 3. Results of a prospective, randomized, double-blind placebo-controlled trial. Crit Care Med 1997;25:1851-1854.
58. Fukuta Y, Kumamoto T, Matsuda A, et al: Effects of various Ringer's

solutions on acid-base balance in rats in hemorrhagic shock and with hepatic dysfunction. Masui 1998;47:22-28.
59. Delman K, Malek SK, Bundz S, et al: Resuscitation with lactated Ringer's solution after hemorrhage: Lack of cardiac toxicity. Shock 1996;5:298-303.
60. Rhee P, Burris D, Kaufmann C, et al: Lactated Ringer's solution resuscitation causes neutrophil activation after hemorrhagic shock. J Trauma 1998;44:313-319.
61. Barron ME, Wilkes MM, Navickis RJ: A systemic review of the comparative safety of colloids. Arch Surg 2004;139:552-563.
62. Vincent JL, Navickis RJ, Wilkes MM: Morbidity in hospitalized patients receiving human albumin: A meta-analysis of randomized, controlled trials. Crit Care Med 2004;32: 2029-2038.
63. Wilkes MM, Navickis RJ: Does albumin infusion affect survival? Review of meta-analytic findings. In Vincent JL (ed): 2002 Yearbook of Intensive Care and Emergency Medicine. Berlin, Springer-Verlag, 2002, pp 454-464.
64. Blunt MC, Nicholson JP, Park GR: Serum albumin and colloid osmotic pressure in survivors and nonsurvivors of prolonged critical illness. Anaesthesia 1998;53:755-761.
65. SAFE Study Investigators: A comparison of albumin and saline for fluid resuscitation in the intensive care unit. N Engl J Med 2004;350:2247-2256.
66. Boldt J: Do plasma substitutes have additional properties beyond correcting volume deficits? Shock 2006;25:103-116.
67. Pope French G, Longenecker DE: Fluid Resuscitation, State of the Science of Treating Combat Casualties and Civilian Injuries. Washington, DC, National Academic Press, 1999.
68. Dubick MA, Bruttig SP, Wade CE: Issues of concern regarding the use of hypertonic/hyperoncotic fluid resuscitation of hemorrhagic hypotension. Shock 2006;25:321-328.
69. Shackford SR, Schmoker JD, Zhuang J: The effect of hypertonic resuscitation on pial arteriolar tone after brain injury and shock. J Trauma 1994;37:899-908.
70. Wade CE, Grady JJ, Kramer GC, et al: Individual patient cohort analysis of the efficacy of hypertonic saline/ dextran in patients with traumatic brain injury and hypotension. J Trauma 1997;42(Suppl):S61-S65.
71. Kempski O, Obert C, Mainka T, et al: "Small volume resuscitation" as treatment of cerebral blood flow disturbances and increased ICP in trauma and ischemia. Acta Neurochir Suppl 1996;66:114-117.
72. Goulin GD, Duthie SE, Zornow MH, et al: Global cerebral ischemia: Effects of pentastarch after reperfusion. Anesth Analg 1994;79:1036-1042.
73. Hirshberg A, Hoyt DB, Mattox KL: Timing of fluid resuscitation shapes the hemodynamic response to uncontrolled hemorrhage: Analysis using dynamic modeling. J Trauma 2006;60:1221-1227.
74. Dries DJ: Hypotensive resuscitation. Shock 1996;6:311-316.
75. Tisherman SA, Barie P, Bokhari F, et al: Clinical practice guideline: Endpoints of resuscitation. J Trauma 2004;57: 898-912.
76. Elliott DC: An evaluation of the end points of resuscitation. J Am Coll Surg 1998;187:536-547.
77. Brain Trauma Foundation: Management and prognosis of severe traumatic brain injury. J Neurotrauma 2000;17:449-627.
78. Chesnut RM, Marshall LF, Klauber MR, et al: The role of secondary brain injury in determining outcome from severe head injury. J Trauma 1993;34:216-222.
79. Shoemaker WC, Appel P, Bland R: Use of physiologic monitoring to predict outcome and to assist in clinical decisions in critically ill postoperative patients. Am J Surg 1983;146:43-50.
80. Shoemaker WC, Appel PL, Kram HB, et al: Prospective trial of supranormal values of survivors as therapeutic goals in high-risk surgical patients. Chest 1988;94:1176-1186.
81. Bishop MH, Shoemaker WC, Appel PL, et al: Relationship between supranormal circulatory values, time delays, and outcome in severely traumatized patients. Crit Care Med 1993;21:56-63.
82. Fleming A, Bishop M, Shoemaker W, et al: Prospective trial of supranormal values as goals of resuscitation in severe trauma. Arch Surg 1992;127: 1175-1181.
83. Bishop MH, Shoemaker WC, Appel PL, et al: Prospective, randomized trial of survivor values of cardiac index, oxygen delivery, and oxygen consumption as resuscitation endpoints in severe trauma. J Trauma 1995;38:780-787.
84. Moore FA, Haenel JB, Moore EE, et al: Incommensurate oxygen consumption in response to maximal oxygen availability predicts postinjury multisystem organ failure. J Trauma 1992;33:58-67.
85. Durham RM, Neunaber K, Mazuski JE, et al: The use of oxygen consumption and delivery as endpoints for resuscitation in critically ill patients. J Trauma 1996;41:32-40.
86. Velmahos GC, Demetriades D, Shoemaker WC, et al: Endpoints of resuscitation of critically injured patients: Normal or supranormal? A prospective randomized trial. Ann Surg 2000;232:409-418.
87. Mizock BA, Falk JL: Lactic acidosis in critical illness. Crit Care Med 1992;20:80-93.
88. Abramson D, Scalea TM, Hitchcock R, et al: Lactate clearance and survival following injury. J Trauma 1993;35:584-589.
89. McNelis J, Marini CP, Jurkiewicz A, et al: Prolonged lactate clearance is associated with increased mortality in the surgical intensive care unit. Am J Surg 2001;182:481-485.
90. Mikulaschek A, Henry SM, Donovan R, et al: Serum lactate is not predicted by anion gap or base excess after trauma resuscitation. J Trauma 1996;40: 218-224.
91. Davis JW, Kaups KL, Parks SN: Base deficit is superior to pH in evaluating clearance of acidosis after traumatic shock. J Trauma 1998;44:114-118.
92. Eachempati SR, Reed RL 2nd, Barie PS: Serum bicarbonate as an endpoint of resuscitation in critically ill patients. Surg Infect (Larchmt) 2003;4:193-197.
93. Davis JW, Shackford SR, Mackersie RC, et al: Base deficit as a guide to volume resuscitation. J Trauma 1988;28: 1464-1467.
94. Falcone RE, Santanello SA, Schulz MA, et al: Correlation of metabolic acidosis with outcome following injury and its value as a scoring tool. World J Surg 1993;17:575-579.
95. Sauaia A, Moore FA, Moore EE, et al: Early predictors of postinjury multiple organ failure. Arch Surg 1994;129:39-45.
96. Kincaid EH, Miller PR, Meredith JW, et al: Elevated arterial base deficit in trauma patients: A marker of impaired oxygen utilization. J Am Coll Surg 1998;187:384-392.
97. Rixen D, Raum M, Bouillon B, et al: Base deficit development and its prognostic significance in posttrauma critical illness: An analysis by the trauma registry of the Deutsche Gesellschaft fur unfallchirurgie. Shock 2001;15:83-89.
98. Davis JW, Parks SN, Kaups KL, et al: Admission base deficit predicts transfusion requirements and risk of complications. J Trauma 1996;41: 769-774.
99. Rixen D, Siegel JH: Metabolic correlates of oxygen debt predict posttrauma early acute respiratory distress syndrome and the related cytokine response. J Trauma 2000;49:392-403.
100. Dunham CM, Watson LA, Cooper C: Base deficit level indicating major injury is increased with ethanol. J Emerg Med 2000;18:165-171.
101. Davis JW, Kaups KL, Parks SN: Effect of alcohol on the utility of base deficit in trauma. J Trauma 1997;43:507-510.
102. Brill SA, Stewart TR, Brundage SI, et al: Base deficit does not predict mortality when secondary to hyperchloremic acidosis. Shock 2002;17:459-462.
103. Dantzker DR: The gastrointestinal tract: The canary of the body? JAMA 1993;270:1247-1248.
104. Harbrecht BG, Alarcon LH, Peitzman AB: Management of shock. In Moore EE, Feliciano DV, Mattox KL (eds): Trauma, 5th ed. New York, McGraw-Hill, 2004, pp 201-226.
105. Roumen RM, Vreugde JP, Goris RJ: Gastric tonometry in multiple trauma patients. J Trauma 1994;36:313-316.
106. Chang MC, Cheatham ML, Nelson LD, et al: Gastric tonometry supplements information provided by systemic indicators of oxygen transport. J Trauma 1994;37:488-494.
107. Miller PR, Kincaid EH, Meredith JW, et al: Threshold values of intramucosal pH and mucosal-arterial CO_2 gap during shock resuscitation. J Trauma 1998;45:868-872.
108. Ivatury RR, Simon RJ, Havriliak D, et al: Gastric mucosal pH and oxygen delivery and oxygen consumption indices in the assessment of adequacy of resuscitation after trauma: A prospective, randomized study. J Trauma 1995;39:128-136.

109. Ivatury RR, Simon RJ, Islam S, et al: A prospective randomized study of end points of resuscitation after major trauma: Global oxygen transport indices versus organ-specific gastric mucosal pH. J Am Coll Surg 1996;183:145-154.
110. Wall P, Henderson L, Buising C, et al: Monitoring gastrointestinal intraluminal PCO_2: Problems with airflow methods. Shock 2001;15:360-365.
111. Soller BR, Cingo N, Puyana JC, et al: Simultaneous measurement of hepatic tissue pH, venous oxygen saturation and hemoglobin by near infrared spectroscopy. Shock 2001;15:106-111.
112. McKinley BA, Marvin RG, Cocanour CS, et al: Tissue hemoglobin O2 saturation during resuscitation of traumatic shock monitored using near infrared spectrometry. J Trauma 2000;48:637-642.
113. Cairns CB, Moore FA, Haenel JB, et al: Evidence for early supply independent mitochondrial dysfunction in patients developing multiple organ failure after trauma. J Trauma 1997;42:532-536.
114. Keynes G: The Apology and Treatise of Ambroise Paré Containing the Voyages Made into Divers Places with Many of His Writings upon Surgery. Chicago, University of Chicago Press, 1952.
115. Simeone FA: Shock, trauma and the surgeon. Ann Surg 1963;158:759-774.
116. Cannon WB: Traumatic Shock. New York, Appleton, 1923.
117. Mapstone J, Roberts I, Evans P: Fluid resuscitation strategies: A systemic review of animal trials. J Trauma 2003;55:571-589.
118. Cannon WB, Fraser J, Cowell EM: The preventive treatment of wound shock. JAMA 1918;70:618-621.
119. Capone AC, Safar P, Stezoski W, et al: Improved outcome with fluid restriction in treatment of uncontrolled hemorrhagic shock. J Am Coll Surg 1995;180:49-56.
120. Shaftan GW, Chiu CJ, Dennis C, et al: Fundamentals of physiologic control of arterial hemorrhage. Surgery 1965;58:851-856.
121. Milles G, Koucky CJ, Zacheis HG: Experimental uncontrolled arterial hemorrhage. Surgery 1966;60:434-442.
122. Shires T, Coln D, Carrico J, et al: Fluid therapy in hemorrhagic shock. Arch Surg 1964;88:688-693.
123. Traverso LW, Lee WP, Langford MJ: Fluid resuscitation after an otherwise fatal hemorrhage, I: Crystalloid solutions. J Trauma 1986;26:168-175.
124. Baue AE, Tragus ET, Wolfson SK Jr, et al: Hemodynamic and metabolic effects of Ringer's lactate solution in hemorrhagic shock. Ann Surg 1967;166:29-38.
125. Wiggers CJ: Physiology of Shock. New York, Commonwealth Publications, 1950.
126. Gann DS, Wright PA: Shock—the final common pathway? In Maull KI (ed): Advances in Trauma Critical Care, Vol 10. St. Louis, Mosby–Year Book, 1995, pp 43-59.
127. Bickell WH, Bruttig SP, Millnamow GA, et al: The detrimental effects of intravenous crystalloid after aortotomy in swine. Surgery 1991;110:529-536.
128. Stern SA, Dronen SC, Birrer P, et al: Effect of blood pressure on hemorrhage volume and survival in a near-fatal hemorrhage model incorporating a vascular injury. Ann Emerg Med 1993;22:155-163.
129. Kowalenko T, Stern S, Dronen S, et al: Improved outcome with hypotensive resuscitation of uncontrolled hemorrhagic shock in a swine model. J Trauma 1992;33:349-353.
130. Novak L, Shackford SR, Bourguignon P, et al: Comparison of standard and alternative prehospital resuscitation in uncontrolled hemorrhagic shock and head injury. J Trauma 1999;47:834-844.
131. Martin RR, Bickell WH, Pepe PE, et al: Prospective evaluation of preoperative fluid resuscitation in hypotensive patients with penetrating truncal injury: A preliminary report. J Trauma 1992;33:354-362.
132. Bickell WH, Wall MJ Jr, Pepe PE, et al: Immediate versus delayed fluid resuscitation for hypotensive patients with penetrating torso injuries. N Engl J Med 1994;331:1105-1109.
133. American College of Surgeons Committee on Trauma: Advanced Trauma Life Support Program for Physicians: Instructor Manual. Chicago, American College of Surgeons, 1993.
134. Champion HR, Sacco WJ, Copes WS, et al: A revision of the trauma score. J Trauma 1989;29:623-629.
135. The Abbreviated Injury Scale, 1990 Revision. Des Plaines, IL, Association for the Advancement of Automotive Medicine, 1990.
136. Wall MJ Jr, Granchi T, Liscum K, et al: Delayed versus immediate resuscitation in patients with penetrating trauma: Subgroup analysis. J Trauma 1995;39:173.
137. Wilkerson DK, Rosen AL, Gould SA, et al: Oxygen extraction ratio: A valid indicator of myocardial metabolism in anemia. J Surg Res 1987;42:629-634.
138. Levy PS, Kim SJ, Eckel PK, et al: Limit to cardiac compensation during acute isovolemic hemodilution: Influence of coronary stenosis. Am J Physiol 1993;265:H340-H349.
139. Marr AB, Moore FA, Sailors RM, et al: Preload optimization using "Starling curve" generation during shock resuscitation: Can it be done? Shock 2004;21:300-305.
140. McKinley BA, Kozar RA, Cocanour CS, et al: Normal versus supranormal oxygen delivery goals in shock resuscitation: The response is the same. J Trauma 2002;53:825-832.
141. McKinley BA, Marvin RG, Cocanour CS, et al: Blunt trauma resuscitation: The old can respond. Arch Surg 2000;135:688-695.
142. McKinley BA, Kozar RA, Cocanour CS, et al: Standardized trauma resuscitation: Female hearts respond better. Arch Surg 2002;137:578-584.
143. McKinley BA, Valdivia A, Moore FA: Goal-oriented shock resuscitation for major torso trauma: What are we learning? Curr Opin Crit Care 2003;9:292-299.
144. Scalea TM, Simon HM, Duncan AO, et al: Geriatric blunt multiple trauma: Improved survival with early invasive monitoring. J Trauma 1990;30:129-136.
145. Balogh Z, McKinley BA, Cocanour CS, et al: Supranormal trauma resuscitation causes more cases of abdominal compartment syndrome. Arch Surg 2003;138:637-643.
146. Friese RS, Shafi S, Gentilello LM: Pulmonary artery catheter use is associated with reduced mortality in severely injured patients: A National Trauma Data Bank analysis of 53,312 patients. Crit Care Med 2006;34:1597-1601.
147. Kauvar DS, Lefering R, Wade CE: Impact of hemorrhage on trauma outcome: An overview of epidemiology, clinical presentations, and therapeutic considerations. J Trauma 2006;60:S3-S11.
148. Bouillon B, Raum M, Fach H, et al: The incidence and outcome of severe brain trauma—design and first results of an epidemiological study in an urban area. Restor Neurol Neurosci 1999;14:85-92.
149. Manley G, Knudson MM, Morabito D, et al: Hypotension, hypoxia, and head injury: Frequency, duration, and consequences. Arch Surg 2001;136:1118-1123.
150. Chesnut RM, Marshall SB, Piek J, et al: Early and late systemic hypotension as a frequent and fundamental source of cerebral ischemia following severe brain injury in the Traumatic Coma Data Bank. Acta Neurochir Suppl (Wien) 1993;59:121-125.
151. Sauaia A, Moore FA, Moore EE, et al: Epidemiology of trauma deaths: A reassessment. J Trauma 1995;38:185-193.
152. Hoyt DB, Bulger EM, Knudson MM, et al: Death in the operating room: An analysis of a multi-center experience. J Trauma 1994;37:426-432.
153. Como JJ, Dutton RP, Scalea TM, et al: Blood transfusion rates in the care of acute trauma. Transfusion 2004;44:809-813.
154. Ketchum L, Hess JR, Hiippala S: Indications for early fresh frozen plasma, cryoprecipitate, and platelet transfusion in trauma. J Trauma 2006;60:S51-S58.
155. Malone DL, Hess JR, Fingerhut A: Massive transfusion practices around the globe and a suggestion for a common massive transfusion protocol. J Trauma 2006;60:S91-S96.
156. Vaslef SN, Knudsen NW, Neligan PJ, et al: Massive transfusion exceeding 50 units of blood products in trauma patients. J Trauma 2002;53:291-296.
157. Holcomb JB: Use of recombinant activated factor VII to treat the acquired coagulopathy of trauma. J Trauma 2005;58:1298-1303.
158. Martinowitz U, Kenet G, Lubetski A, et al: Possible role of recombinant activated factor VII (rFVIIa) in the control of hemorrhage associated with massive trauma. Can J Anaesth 2002;49:S15-S20.
159. Dutton RP, Hess JR, Scalea TM: Recombinant factor VIIa for control of hemorrhage: Early experience in

critically ill trauma patients. J Clin Anesth 2003;15:184-188.
160. Meng ZH, Wolberg AS, Monroe DM 3rd, et al: The effect of temperature and pH on the activity of factor VIIa: Implications for the efficacy of high-dose factor VIIa in hypothermic and acidotic patients. J Trauma 2003;55:886-891.
161. Napolitano L: Cumulative risks of early red blood cell transfusion. J Trauma 2006;60:S26-S34.
162. Silliman CC, Moore EE, Johnson JL, et al: Transfusion of the injured patient: Proceed with caution. Shock 2004;21:291-299.
163. Sauaia A, Moore FA, Moore EE, et al: Early predictors of postinjury multiple organ failure. Arch Surg 1994;129:39-45.
164. Moore FA, Moore EE, Sauaia A: Blood transfusion: An independent risk factor for postinjury multiple organ failure. Arch Surg 1997;132:620-625.
165. Dunne JR, Malone DL, Tracy JK, et al: Allogenic blood transfusion in the first 24 hours after trauma is associated with increased systemic inflammatory response syndrome (SIRS) and death. Surg Infect (Larchmt) 2004;5:395-404.
166. Blajchman MA: The clinical benefits of the leukoreduction of blood products. J Trauma 2006;60:S83-S90.
167. Schein M, Wittmann DH, Aprahamian CC, et al: The abdominal compartment syndrome: The physiological and clinical consequences of elevated intra-abdominal pressure. J Am Coll Surg 1995;180:745-753.
168. Chang MC, Miller PR, D'Agostino R Jr, et al: Effects of abdominal decompression on cardiopulmonary function and visceral perfusion in patients with intra-abdominal hypertension. J Trauma 1998;44:440-445.
169. Cheatham ML, White MW, Sagraves SG, et al: Abdominal perfusion pressure: A superior parameter in the assessment of intra-abdominal hypertension. J Trauma 2000;49:621-627.
170. Malbrain ML, Cheatham ML, Kirkpatrick A, et al: Results from the International Conference of Experts on Intra-abdominal Hypertension and Abdominal Compartment Syndrome, I: Definitions. Intensive Care Med 2006;32:1722-1732.
171. Ivatury RR, Diebel L, Porter JM, et al: Intra-abdominal hypertension and the abdominal compartment syndrome. Surg Clin North Am 1997;77:783-800.
172. Sugrue M, Buist MD, Hourihan F, et al: Prospective study of intra-abdominal hypertension and renal function after laparotomy. Br J Surg 1995;82: 235-238.
173. Sugrue M, Jones F, Janjua KJ, et al: Temporary abdominal closure: A prospective evaluation of its effects on renal and respiratory physiology. J Trauma 1998;45:914-921.
174. Sugrue M, Jones F, Deane SA, et al: Intra-abdominal hypertension is an independent cause of postoperative renal impairment. Arch Surg 1999;134:1082-1085.
175. Diebel LN, Dulchavsky SA, Wilson RF: Effect of increased intra-abdominal pressure on mesenteric arterial and intestinal mucosal blood flow. J Trauma 1992;33:45-49.
176. Diebel LN, Wilson RF, Dulchavsky SA, et al: Effect of increased intra-abdominal pressure on hepatic arterial, portal venous, and hepatic microcirculatory blood flow. J Trauma 1992;33:279-283.
177. Mubarak SJ, Hargens AR: Acute compartment syndromes. Surg Clin North Am 1983;63:539-565.
178. ten Duis HJ, Nijsten MW, Klasen HJ, et al: Fat embolism in patients with an isolated fracture of the femoral shaft. J Trauma 1988;28:383-390.
179. Feliciano DV, Cruse PA, Spjut-Patrinely V, et al: Fasciotomy after trauma to the extremities. Am J Surg 1988;156:533-536.
180. Scalea TM, Burgess AR: Pelvic fractures. In Moore EE, Feliciano DV, Mattox KL (eds): Trauma, 5th ed. New York, McGraw-Hill, 2004, pp 779-807.
181. Gylling SF, Ward RE, Holcroft JW, et al: Immediate external fixation of unstable pelvic fractures. Am J Surg 1985;150:721-724.
182. Ben-Menachem Y, Coldwell DM, Young JW, et al: Hemorrhage associated with pelvic fractures: Causes, diagnosis, and emergent management. AJR Am J Roentgenol 1991;157:1005-1014.

Chapter 29

Anaphylaxis and Anaphylactic Shock

Marilyn T. Haupt

The term *anaphylaxis* refers to a life-threatening event, typically allergic in nature and mediated by immunoglobulin E (IgE). The clinical manifestations are often explosive in onset and may lead to upper airway obstruction, respiratory failure, and circulatory shock. In addition to the classic immune-mediated anaphylactic reaction, other, similar clinical responses without well-defined immune mediation are termed *anaphylactoid reactions, idiopathic anaphylaxis,* and *factitious anaphylaxis.*

The *classic anaphylactic response* is an allergic reaction mediated by IgE.[1] It is classified as a type I reaction according to the Gell and Coombs' classification[2] and has previously been referred to as a *reagin-dependent, immediate hypersensitivity,* or *cytotropic reaction.* The classic anaphylactic reaction has clinical features similar to other, milder type I reactions, such as allergic rhinitis, hives, urticaria, and allergic asthma. Anaphylactic reactions and all type I reactions are characterized by a well-defined immunologic sequence of events that involves antigen-specific and IgE-specific effector cells. When stimulated, these cells release a variety of inflammatory mediators.[3] The effector cells consist of mast cells and basophils, which are based primarily in tissues and in the circulating blood volume. In contrast to other, more limited types of allergic reactions, such as allergic rhinitis and urticaria, anaphylaxis rapidly progresses to a generalized systemic reaction. Agents that produce well-documented IgE-mediated anaphylactic reactions include the penicillins and other antibiotics; latex; venoms from an order of insects known as *Hymenoptera,* which includes bees, wasps, hornets, and fire ants; and many foods (Table 29-1).

Anaphylactoid reactions have clinical features identical to those of classic anaphylactic reactions; however, in an anaphylactoid reaction, IgE and an immune-mediated response cannot be shown. It has been hypothesized that in an anaphylactoid reaction, a nonimmune release of mediators (e.g., from chemical, physical, or osmotic stimuli) from mast cells and basophils is responsible for the clinical syndrome. Agents capable of producing anaphylactoid reactions include radiocontrast dyes, aspirin and other nonsteroidal anti-inflammatory drugs (NSAIDs), and opiates. Exercise-induced anaphylaxis also is considered an anaphylactoid reaction.[4] An association of anaphylactoid reactions with the use of β-blocker drugs has been noted.[5]

Idiopathic anaphylactoid reactions also are clinically identical to classic anaphylactic reactions; however, in these reactions, the specific inciting event and immune mediators are unknown. Idiopathic anaphylactoid reactions typically occur in young adults. These reactions seem to occur more often at night and in the postprandial state. The reactions are rarely fatal and usually result in complete remissions.[6-8]

Factitious anaphylaxis is a type of Munchausen syndrome. Patients with this disorder typically have an acute crisis that resembles anaphylaxis. These reactions may be attributed to a well-defined antigen such as bee venom. Sometimes an inciting agent or event may not be identified.[9-11]

Anaphylaxis may progress to shock, multiple organ failure, and death. Early recognition and rapid implementation of treatment may be lifesaving. It is essential that patients with anaphylaxis be accurately diagnosed so that management can proceed as quickly as possible. Because these severe reactions may continue despite appropriate treatment, and because a recurrence of symptoms after an initial favorable response may occur, patients with anaphylaxis should be admitted to the hospital or intensive care unit for continued monitoring.

HISTORY AND INCIDENCE

Allergic emergencies have been described in humans since ancient times.[12-14] At the turn of the 20th century, a more detailed description of these events was reported by two French physiologists, Portier and Richet.[15] They coined the

Table 29-1. Agents Frequently Associated with Anaphylactic and Anaphylactoid Reactions

Agent	Examples
Antibiotics	Penicillin and penicillin analogues, β-lactam antibiotics, cephalosporins, tetracyclines, erythromycin
Nonsteroidal anti-inflammatory drugs	Salicylates, ibuprofen, indomethacin
Narcotic analgesics	Morphine, codeine, meprobamate
Local anesthetics	Procaine, lidocaine, cocaine
General anesthetics	Thiopental
Muscle relaxants	Suxamethonium, tubocurarine, pancuronium
Blood products and antisera	Red blood cell, white blood cell, and platelet transfusions; gamma globulin; rabies, tetanus, diphtheria antitoxin; snake and spider antivenom
Diagnostic agents	Iodinated radiocontrast agents
Foods	Eggs, milk, nuts, legumes (peanuts, soybeans, kidney beans), fish, shellfish
Venoms	Bees, wasps, hornets, fire ants, scorpions, snakes
Enzymes and other biologic agents	Acetylcysteine, pancreatic enzyme supplements, chymopapain
Extracts of potential allergens used in desensitization	Pollen, food, venom extracts
Chemotherapeutic agents	Cisplatin, cyclophosphamide, daunorubicin, methotrexate
Insulin	Pork, beef, and human insulin
Other drugs	Protamine, chlorpropamide, parenteral iron, iodides, thiazide diuretics

term *anaphylaxis,* which originates from the French word *anaphylactique,* which means "reverse protection." It was believed that these reactions were in contrast to the attenuated or tachyphylactic reactions that commonly protect subjects from reintroduced antigens such as viruses. More recent research defining the role of IgE; the interactions between IgE, antigen, mast cells, basophils, and eosinophils; and the biochemical mediators from these cells has clarified the events leading to clinical anaphylaxis.[1,3,16,17]

The true incidence of the various types of anaphylactic reactions is difficult to determine because these reactions are often spontaneous and unpredictable and are clinically similar to other acute reactions. Estimates of the incidence of the most commonly reported episodes are possible, however. In the United States, penicillin alone probably accounts for several hundred fatalities each year.[18-20] Anaphylaxis to the cephalosporins also is commonly reported.[21] It has been estimated that among patients with an allergic reaction to a penicillin, there is a 3% to 7% rate of allergic reaction to a cephalosporin. Reports of anaphylactic reactions to the newer β-lactam antibiotics are accumulating.[22]

Insects, especially those of the *Hymenoptera* order, account for numerous immediate hypersensitivity reactions. Of the population, 0.5% to 5% has experienced a severe allergic reaction to an insect sting,[23] and 1% of these reactions may lead to life-threatening anaphylaxis.[24] Fire ants are aggressive insects from South America that now reside in the southern United States. In some areas, they have been known to sting 58% of the residents yearly and account for serious allergic reactions.[25]

Snake bites account for probably a dozen or so anaphylactic deaths per year in the United States. Snake bites may be associated with typical anaphylactic symptoms and other problems related to the enzymes, proteins, and peptides in venom. Local tissue necrosis, coagulation problems, hemolysis, and neurologic transmission defects have been described. In the United States, most anaphylactic reactions to snake bites are caused by pit vipers. These include rattlesnakes, water moccasins, and copperheads.[26,27]

The incidence of anaphylactic reactions to food is difficult to determine because acute reactions to food are common. Many reactions to food thought to be anaphylaxis are probably nonallergic reactions, such as food intolerance and food poisoning. Allergic reactions to food have been characterized in 6% of children and 3% to 4% of adults.[28] One emergency department–based study estimated that about 1000 episodes of serious food anaphylaxis occur every year in the United States.[29] Peanuts and tree nuts account for 90% of fatal cases. Common food antigens include peanuts, soybeans, egg whites, and shellfish.[30]

Iodinated contrast agents account for approximately 200 to 800 deaths per year and lead to clinical symptoms similar to anaphylaxis. Although these anaphylactoid reactions are rare, the high mortality rate is attributed to the large number of contrast agents used each year.[31-33]

Latex, used in surgical gloves, balloons, condoms, rubber bands, and many other products, may produce anaphylaxis.[34,35] The use of universal precautions as a result of the acquired immunodeficiency syndrome epidemic has increased the number of reactions to latex in health care workers. Children with spina bifida and genitourinary tract abnormalities are especially susceptible to latex-induced anaphylaxis because of frequent exposure to latex-containing bladder catheters and other products.

Anaphylactic reactions during anesthesia have been described and typically are associated with hypotension and cardiopulmonary arrest. One review suggests that most cases of intraoperative anaphylaxis are from muscle relaxants (e.g., suxamethonium, tubocurarine, pancuronium).[36] Latex, protamine, and blood products also may cause intraoperative anaphylaxis.

Anaphylaxis and other types of IgE-mediated allergic reactions tend to occur in susceptible, genetically predisposed individuals. The reason for the genetic inheritance of sensitivity to the antigens that produce anaphylaxis continues to be speculated. A popular theory is that type I reactions, when confined to an area of parasitic invasion (e.g., intestinal tract), facilitate the killing and removal of parasites and confer a survival advantage to individuals capable of mounting a type I response. Various clinical and laboratory observations support this view.[37-39] The sites of IgE synthesis in laboratory subjects correspond to the sites of entry of many parasites. These sites include the lymphoid tissue of the respiratory tract, the gastrointestinal tract, and the skin. Eosinophils, cells that migrate to the site of antigen introduction in anaphylaxis, elaborate mediators that are toxic to the outer parasitic covering.

When type I reactions to antigen are no longer restricted to local areas because of genetically determined or acquired factors, the release of mediators becomes generalized. Problems typical of a systemic response include increased microvascular permeability, loss of intravascular volume, abnormal vascular reactivity (especially vasodilation), and impaired pulmonary gas exchange. Local IgE-mediated reactions become decompensatory when systemic involvement ensues.

PATHOGENESIS AND PATHOPHYSIOLOGY

Immunologic Events Leading to Mast Cell and Basophil Activation and Mediator Release

When an antigen to which an individual has previously been sensitized is reintroduced, a sequence of events is initiated that lead to mediator release (Fig. 29-1). In classic anaphylaxis, this sequence of events is immunologic in origin. At least several weeks are required between the initial exposure to antigen and a subsequent exposure for clinical manifestations of anaphylaxis to occur. The antigen may be introduced through the skin, respiratory tract, or gastrointestinal tract. Antigen also may be introduced intravenously, usually in association with drug administration. Although most venoms are injected subcutaneously, some may access the circulation through an intravascular route.

Most antigens that produce classic anaphylaxis consist of small bivalent proteins with molecular weights of 10,000 to 70,000 D.[40] In addition, haptens, small chemicals that combine with a host protein, form a complex that functions as an antigen and causes anaphylaxis. Reactive anhydrides or quinones typically found in industrial chemicals function as haptens. The β-lactam groups of penicillins and cephalosporins also may function as haptens. Other drugs, including acetaminophen, isoniazid, and hydralazine, may become haptens after enzymatic conversion in the liver or in other organs. Anaphylactic reactions to polysaccharides, including dextrans and the hydroxyethyl starches (substances often used in synthetic plasma substitutes), are rare, but have been described.[41]

When antigen is reintroduced into the host, it encounters IgE, previously synthesized by plasma cells. IgE, similar to other immunoglobulins, is composed of two heavy chains and two light chains linked by disulfide bonds. Two portions of the molecule have well-defined functions. The Fab portion of the molecule recognizes and binds antigen. The Fc portion of the molecule binds reversibly to receptors on the surface of mast cells and basophils (Fig. 29-2).

The combination of reintroduced antigen with antigen-specific IgE sets the stage for a sequence of biochemical and cellular events that produce the clinical syndrome of anaphylaxis. The bivalent antigen cross-bridges two IgE molecules (see Fig. 29-1). Cross-bridging facilitates the approximation of Fc surface receptors on mast cells and basophils, triggering the release of mediators from

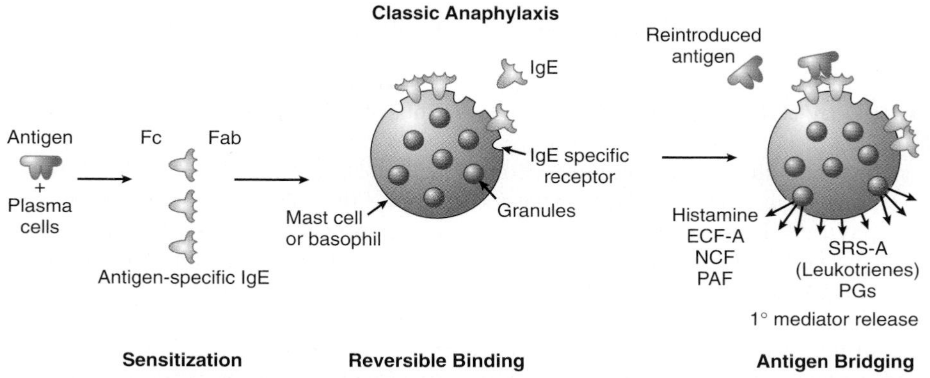

Figure 29-1. The sequence of events leading to mediator release starts with sensitization (initial introduction of a bivalent antigen) and synthesis of antigen-specific IgE. IgE then reversibly binds to mast cells or basophils. When antigen is reintroduced, two cell-bound IgE molecules are linked by the bivalent antigen in a process called *cross-linking.* Cross-linking facilitates the approximation of Fc surface receptors on the mast cell and basophil and initiates a sequence of intracellular biochemical reactions that culminate in mediator release. ECF-A, eosinophil chemotactic factor of anaphylaxis; NCF, neutrophil chemotactic factor; PAF, platelet-activating factor; PGs, prostaglandins; SRS-A, slow-reacting substance of anaphylaxis.

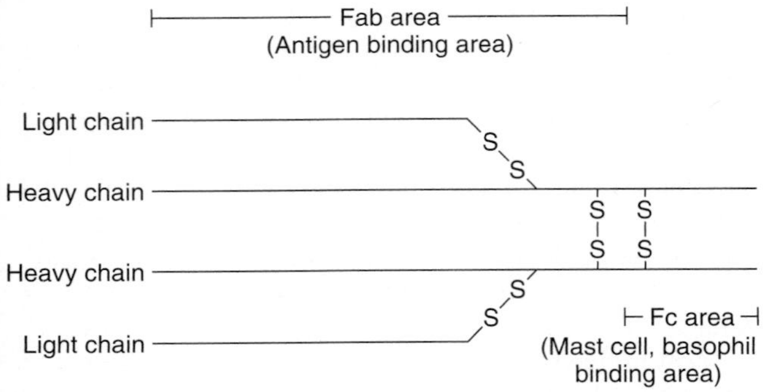

Figure 29-2. The IgE molecule provides immune mediation in classic anaphylactic reactions. Each molecule consists of four polypeptide chains. Two are heavy chains (epsilon [ε]) and are unique to the IgE class of immunoglobulins. Light chains are either kappa (κ) or lambda (λ) chains and may be found in other types of immunoglobulins.

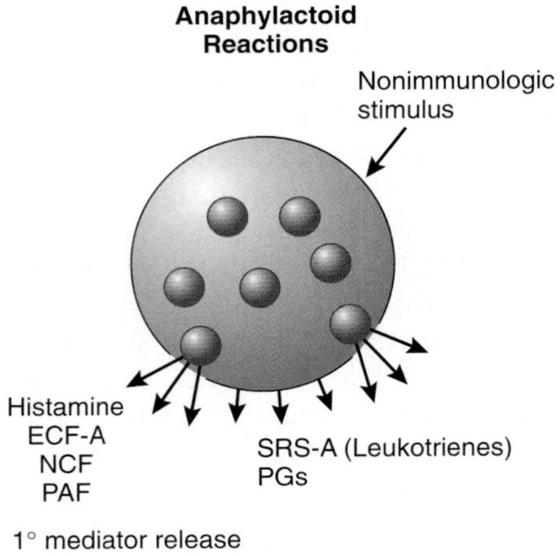

Figure 29-3. In the anaphylactoid reaction, immune mediation cannot be shown. Mediator release is thought to be initiated by stimuli that directly interact with the wall of mast cells or basophils. These may include osmotic, cold, physical, or biochemical stimuli. ECF-A, eosinophil chemotactic factor of anaphylaxis; NCF, neutrophil chemotactic factor; PAF, platelet-activating factor; PGs, prostaglandins; SRS-A, slow-reacting substance of anaphylaxis.

intracellular granules and membrane-based phospholipids. The systemic release of these mediators leads to the pathophysiologic changes that produce the clinical manifestations of anaphylaxis.

Clinical reactions similar to anaphylaxis mediated by immunoglobulins of the IgG class have been described. IgG molecules may combine with antigens, producing an antigen-antibody complex that activates complement. Activation of complement generates C3a and C5a, also known as *anaphylatoxins* because they stimulate mediator release from mast cells and basophils. IgG-mediated reactions are considered type III reactions according to the classification of Gell and Coombs or may be referred to as *Arthus* reactions. These reactions may characterize IgA-deficient individuals who exhibit sudden reactions to blood transfusions. These individuals may develop an antibody of the IgG class to the IgA in the transfused blood product.[41,42] This combination of IgG and IgA antibody activates complement, generates C3a and C5a, and produces a sudden reaction typical of anaphylaxis. Because approximately 1 in 700 individuals is IgA deficient, numerous people are susceptible to this type of blood transfusion reaction.[42] The anaphylactic responses to protamine may be IgG, IgE, or non–immune-mediated.[43-45]

Nonimmunologic Events Leading to Mediator Release

Anaphylactoid reactions are thought to originate from nonimmunologic stimuli (Fig. 29-3). The mediators released during anaphylactoid reactions originate from mast cells and basophils and are identical to the mediators of immune-mediated anaphylaxis. The direct activation of surface receptors on mast cells and basophils by antigen may be responsible for mediator release in anaphylactoid reactions. Iodinated contrast agents, opiates, and highly charged polyionic antibiotics seem to activate surface receptors directly. Physical stimuli, including heat, cold, and hyperosmolar stimuli, also are capable of stimulating mast cells and basophils. Exercise-induced anaphylaxis may be associated with the stimulation of mast cells through cooling of the airways. Anaphylactoid reactions to radiocontrast agents, mannitol, and dextran solutions may be secondary to osmotic stimuli.

Aspirin and other NSAIDs are thought to produce anaphylactoid reactions by facilitating the release of lipoxygenase-derived mediators. The synthesis of these mediators, called *leukotrienes,* is enhanced through NSAID-induced inhibition of the competing cyclooxygenase pathway. Leukotrienes are potent mediators and produce increases in permeability and bronchospasm typical of anaphylaxis. This theory for NSAID-induced anaphylaxis does not account, however, for the observation that most individuals do not experience anaphylactic symptoms after ingesting these drugs. Other theories to account for aspirin and NSAID sensitivity have been postulated and include direct activation of mast cells and basophils and direct activation of the complement cascade.[46] Patients with aspirin sensitivity seem to exhibit sensitivity to a commonly used food coloring called *yellow dye tartrazine.*[47] The mechanism for anaphylactoid reactions to this chemical is unclear, although its structure has similarities to the structure of several NSAIDs.[47]

Cellular Characteristics of Anaphylaxis

Despite the release of similar mediators during anaphylaxis, mast cells and basophils differ in several ways. Mast cells are more abundant than basophils and generally reside in the connective tissue of subcutaneous and submucosal areas. Basophils characteristically circulate in the blood.[48] Despite these differences in location and number, functional differences between the two cell types have not been clearly identified. Both types of cells have receptors for the Fc portion of IgE, and both have granules that bind basic dyes. In addition, the granules of both cells contain histamine and various other mediators that participate in the anaphylactic response.

Eosinophils are commonly identified in the tissues and plasma of patients with anaphylactic and anaphylactoid reactions. These cells typically migrate to the site of antigen introduction. They are attracted by a variety of chemotactic factors, including factors derived from mast cells and basophils, antigen-antibody complexes, histamine, and complement. The granules of eosinophils stain with acidophilic dyes and contain a variety of biochemical mediators that are toxic to helminthic parasites. Substances that inactivate leukotrienes and histamines also are elaborated. Eosinophils function as modulators of the inflammatory response triggered by mast cell and basophil activation.[49,50]

Platelets and polymorphonuclear leukocytes also may be involved in the anaphylactic response. These cells respond to mast cell–derived and basophil-derived chemotactic factors and to tissue injury. They release a variety of mediators that may be responsible for recurrent and late-phase reactions (see the following discussion).

Biochemical Mediators of Anaphylaxis

The biochemical mediators of anaphylaxis are divided into *primary* and *secondary* mediators. Mediators directly released from mast cells and basophils are termed *primary mediators* (Table 29-2). Secondary mediators are released from other cell types in response to primary mediator release (Table 29-3). Primary mediators are subdivided further into *preformed* and *newly synthesized* mediators. Preformed mediators are formed and stored in the intracellular granules of mast cells and basophils. Newly synthesized mediators are derived from the metabolism of arachidonic acid, a phospholipid derived from cell membrane.

Histamine is a well-characterized primary mediator stored and released from the granules of mast cells and basophils. Histamine stimulates H_1 and H_2 receptors located on the surfaces of vascular and bronchial smooth muscle cells. Stimulation of H_1 receptors leads to precapillary arteriolar dilation, contraction of postcapillary

Table 29-2. Physiologic Effects of Primary Mediators of Anaphylaxis Derived from Mast Cells and Basophils

Mediator	Physiologic Effect
Histamine	
H_1-receptor stimulation	Bronchial smooth muscle contraction Increased vascular permeability Cardiac arrhythmias Increased mucus secretion Vasoactive effects (vasodilation, vasoconstriction)
H_2-receptor stimulation	Increased vascular permeability Increased mucus and gastric acid secretion Activation of inhibitory lymphocytes
H_3-receptor stimulation	Inhibition of histamine synthesis and release
Platelet-activating factor	Increased vascular permeability Bronchospasm Aggregation and activation of platelets Attraction of neutrophils and eosinophils
Eosinophil chemotactic factors	Attraction of eosinophils
Neutrophil chemotactic factors	Attraction of neutrophils
Arachidonic acid metabolites	
Prostaglandin D_2	Bronchoconstriction Potentiates leukocyte migration
Prostaglandin E_2	Bronchodilation
Prostaglandin F_2	Bronchoconstriction
Leukotriene C_4, leukotriene D_4, leukotriene E_4	Bronchoconstriction Increased vascular permeability
Leukotriene B_4	Attraction of neutrophils and eosinophils
Enzymes	
Hydrolytic enzymes	Degradation of parasitic and host tissue
Proteases	Degradation of parasitic and host tissue Interaction with complement components, coagulation cascade, and kinin system
Oxidative enzymes	
Superoxide dismutase	Inactivation of oxygen and associated cytotoxic effects
Peroxidase	Inactivation of cytotoxic effects of hydrogen peroxide
Heparin	Anticoagulant activity May assist in the repair of injured tissues
Adenosine	Bronchospasm Regulates mast cell degranulation
Serotonin	Vasoactive effects

Table 29-3. Secondary Mediators of Anaphylaxis and Physiologic Effects

Mediator	Physiologic Effect
Neutrophil, platelet, and eosinophil-derived mediators	Permeability, coagulation changes, proteolysis
Activated complement system	
C3a and C5a	Contract bronchial smooth muscle; increase vascular permeability; attract neutrophils, macrophages, and monocytes
C6-C9	Membrane damage
Activated coagulation cascade	Intravascular coagulation, permeability changes, tissue injury
Activated kinin system (bradykinin)	Increases vascular permeability

venules, and formation of intracellular gaps between capillary endothelial cells. By increasing capillary hydrostatic pressure and permeability, these changes initiate the movement of plasma into the interstitial space. In the lung, H_1 receptor stimulation is associated with bronchial smooth muscle contraction. H_2 receptor stimulation leads to vasodilation, enhanced mucus secretion, increased heart rate and myocardial contractility, increased gastric acid secretion, and inhibition of T cells. The vasoactive and cardiac effects of H_2 receptor stimulation primarily contribute to the clinical manifestations of anaphylaxis.

The family of arachidonic acid metabolites known as *leukotrienes* consists of newly synthesized primary mediators that function as potent vascular permeability agents and bronchoconstrictors. Arachidonic acid metabolism via the cyclooxygenase pathways produces prostaglandins with bronchoconstrictive effects—prostaglandin D_2 and prostaglandin F_2.

The primary mediator release from mast cells and basophils sets the stage for involvement by secondary mediators. Secondary mediators include products of enzyme-dependent cascading biochemical pathways. In addition, secondary mediators may be derived from other involved cells, such as neutrophils, platelets, and eosinophils.

Box 29-1

Intracellular Regulation of Mediator Release by Pharmacologic Agents

Inhibit Release

By increasing cAMP

β-adrenergic drugs (e.g., epinephrine)

Phosphodiesterase inhibitors (e.g., aminophylline, theophylline)

By decreasing cGMP

Anticholinergic drugs (e.g., ipratropium)

Enhance Release

By decreasing cAMP

β-adrenergic blocking agents

α-adrenergic drugs

By increasing cGMP

Cholinergic drugs

cAMP, cyclic adenosine monophosphate; cGMP, cyclic guanosine monophosphate.

Biochemical and Pharmacologic Regulation of Mediator Release

The biochemical regulation of mediator release provides a rationale for the pharmacologic therapy of anaphylaxis. The release of primary mediators is thought to be modified by intracellular levels of cyclic adenosine monophosphate (cAMP) and cyclic guanosine monophosphate (cGMP) and calcium and other bivalent cations. Pharmacologic agents that affect the intracellular levels of these modulators and inhibit mediator release are often used in the treatment of anaphylaxis (Box 29-1).

β_2-adrenergic agonists increase intracellular levels of cAMP by activating adenylate cyclase. This increase in cAMP subsequently inhibits the release of mediators. The methylxanthines aminophylline and theophylline also increase cAMP levels through the inhibition of phosphodiesterase. Because cGMP antagonizes the action of cAMP, agents that decrease cGMP inhibit mediator release. Anticholinergic drugs decrease cGMP levels and may have a role in the treatment of anaphylaxis.

Mediator release from mast cells and basophils is associated with an influx of calcium. Although calcium blocking agents theoretically may be useful in the treatment of anaphylaxis, clinical experience with use of these agents for this condition is lacking. Conversely, calcium administration may be harmful in anaphylaxis because of its association with enhanced mediator release. Other bivalent cations, such as magnesium and manganese, also enhance mediator release.

The complement cascade is activated during anaphylaxis. Classic and alternative pathways of complement activation have been shown. Activated complement leads to the generation of the anaphylatoxins C3a and C5a, which contract smooth muscle; increase vascular permeability; and attract other cells, including neutrophils, macrophages, and monocytes, to the areas involved.[51] Complement components C6 through C9 may cause further membrane damage.

The coagulation cascade and fibrinolytic systems may be activated through Hageman factor (XII). Activation of these pathways can produce intravascular coagulation and tissue injury. The kinin system also is stimulated to produce bradykinin, a mediator of vascular permeability.

Pathophysiologic Effects of Mediators

The numerous mediators released during anaphylactic crisis have many physiologic effects that have been studied extensively in the laboratory. Although it is difficult to determine the specific actions of each mediator in anaphylaxis, the cumulative effects of mediator release have been described in the clinical setting. These effects include abnormalities secondary to increased vascular permeability; vascular resistance changes, primarily vasodilation; and bronchospasm. Autopsies of fatal cases of anaphylaxis reveal edema of the lungs, upper airway (including the larynx and epiglottis), skin, and viscera. Pulmonary congestion is typical in fatal anaphylaxis, and light microscopy often reveals fluid-filled pulmonary alveoli.[52] In another series of fatal cases of anaphylaxis, acute pulmonary emphysema was observed in almost half of cases.[53] This condition is characterized by hyperextended alveoli and thinning of the alveolar septum. Because of the association of acute pulmonary emphysema with laryngeal edema, these fatalities were thought to be caused by upper airway obstruction, with alveolar rupture resulting from forced exhalation against the obstruction.

Cardiac abnormalities, including arrhythmias, reduced contractility, and myocardial ischemia, have been described in anaphylaxis, but seem to be uncommon.[54] These abnormalities may be secondary to the effects of histamine and other mediators on the myocardium. Other contributing factors include circulatory shock, hypotension, increased adrenergic tone, and drugs used to treat anaphylaxis.

Late-Phase or Biphasic Reactions

Anaphylactic and anaphylactoid reactions and other type I allergic reactions may be followed by late-phase reactions (also termed *biphasic reactions*). These reactions typically occur 6 to 12 hours after the initial reaction as a result of the migration of mast cells, basophils, and polymorphonuclear leukocytes into areas of antigen introduction. A secondary wave of mediator release and recurrence of symptoms may be observed.[55-57]

CLINICAL AND HEMODYNAMIC FEATURES

The constellation of clinical signs and symptoms in anaphylaxis may vary widely for individuals; however, severe, rapidly progressive symptoms after exposure to antigen are characteristic. The portal of entry for the antigen, the rate of absorption, and the degree of hypersensitivity to the antigen also influence the clinical presentation. Gastrointestinal symptoms, including nausea, vomiting, abdominal cramps, and diarrhea, may precede more generalized clinical manifestations after ingestion of an antigen. Inhalation of an antigen may be associated with nasal coryza, a sensation of tightness or a lump in the throat, hoarseness, stridor, wheezing, and dyspnea. Introduction of antigen through the skin may produce local pruritus, urticaria, and swelling before progression to systemic symptoms.

The most life-threatening reactions are usually explosive in nature, often occurring within minutes of exposure to the antigen. Victims of these reactions have been noted to describe a feeling of impending doom before more defined symptoms develop. Generalized cutaneous abnormalities include erythema, urticaria, and flushing. Swelling of the periorbital and perioral areas is characteristic. Upper and lower airway abnormalities are common and especially dangerous. Swelling of the posterior pharynx, uvula, tonsils, and vocal cords may develop rapidly. Auscultation of the chest may reveal generalized wheezing and prolongation of expiration. Auscultatory and radiographic signs of pulmonary edema are characteristic of severe episodes. Signs of circulatory shock include hypotension, oliguria, and lactic acidosis from intravascular volume depletion. In some instances, such as the intravenous injection of venom or a drug, circulatory shock may develop without preceding cutaneous and respiratory abnormalities. The clinical features of anaphylaxis may respond quickly to treatment or, in the most severe cases, may last for several hours to several days. An initial favorable response to treatment may be followed by a late-phase reaction—a recurrence of symptoms resulting from a second wave of mediator release approximately 6 to 12 hours after the initial reaction.[55,57]

Hemodynamic descriptions of human anaphylaxis are limited to detailed studies of a few cases. The loss of circulating plasma volume is characteristic and is associated with hemoconcentration, hypotension, tachycardia, decreased cardiac filling pressures, and decreased cardiac output.[58,59] Vasodilation, associated with a decrease in systemic vascular resistance, may contribute to the reduction in venous return and cardiac output. When oxygen delivery decreases to levels below systemic oxygen demands, anaerobic metabolic pathways are activated, and lactic acidosis emerges.[60] Decreases in myocardial contractility seem to be minimal in studies of human anaphylaxis using routine hemodynamic monitoring. This is supported by the observation that most patients with anaphylaxis respond favorably to fluid therapy and do not require inotropic support.[58-62] In a few case reports, reduced myocardial contractility has been observed in association with myocardial ischemia and infarction.[63-68] Some of these adverse cardiac effects have been associated with epinephrine administration, but in some cases, they also have been noted before pharmacologic treatment.[63-68]

Laboratory studies provide more detailed descriptions of the hemodynamic features of anaphylaxis. After antigenic challenge in primates, a transient increase in cardiac output is observed and is followed by decreases in arterial pressure, right and left ventricular filling pressures, and peripheral vascular resistance.[69] The transient increase in cardiac output has been attributed to vasodilation-induced left ventricular unloading or an increase in cardiac contractility or both. Elevated plasma levels of epinephrine, norepinephrine, and histamine have been shown in laboratory animals and humans and may contribute to this increase in contractility.[70,71] Cardiac output eventually decreases when hypotension and shock become established. In human and canine models of anaphylaxis, a reduction in venous return has been observed secondary to vasodilation and pooling of blood in the splanchnic circulation.[72-74] Loss of plasma volume from increased vascular permeability is probably a contributing factor.

When pulmonary edema fluid is sufficiently copious to be sampled from the airway of patients with anaphylaxis, albumin concentrations and oncotic pressures are nearly identical to plasma values. These findings and the association of pulmonary edema with low pulmonary artery wedge pressures suggest that the pulmonary edema in anaphylaxis is noncardiogenic and secondary to increased microvascular permeability.[58] Although transient pulmonary hypertension and increased pulmonary vascular resistance have been observed in primates immediately after antigen challenge,[69] it is unknown whether pulmonary hypertension characterizes human anaphylaxis.

Hemodynamic characteristics of human anaphylaxis are determined by generalized vasodilation and increased vascular permeability, which lead to venous pooling of blood and loss of circulating plasma volume. Permeability edema develops in the lung. Changes in cardiac contractility are not typical of human anaphylaxis; however, reduced contractility may characterize patients who exhibit signs of myocardial ischemia or infarction, especially in association with epinephrine therapy.

MANAGEMENT

Initial Management

The initial assessment of a patient with suspected anaphylaxis should be brief and specific because immediate therapeutic interventions are required. Because a variety of conditions may appear similar to anaphylaxis (Box 29-2), it is important to rule out these events quickly. Vasovagal episodes are among the most common conditions confused with anaphylaxis. Bradycardia, pale skin, and diaphoresis in an acutely ill patient are suggestive of a vasovagal attack, in contrast to the tachycardic, flushed appearance typical of anaphylaxis.

When it is strongly suspected that the patient is experiencing a severe or potentially severe anaphylactic episode, the following steps should proceed rapidly (Fig. 29-4): (1) assurance of a patent airway, (2) removal of toxin at the site of introduction or an attempt to delay the systemic absorption of toxin or both, (3) establishment of intravenous access for fluid therapy, and (4) initiation of pharmacologic support with epinephrine (Box 29-3). A team approach is essential in severe cases of anaphylaxis because the initial assessment and interventions must proceed rapidly and, if possible, simultaneously.

Admission to the hospital is required for all patients experiencing severe anaphylaxis. Hospital personnel should have advanced airway skills and be capable of managing hemodynamic instability. Although symptom recurrence is uncommon in patients who respond favorably to treatment,[74] hospital admission and monitoring is recommended for all patients with severe anaphylaxis because of the potential for late-phase reactions, which may be severe and may occur 12 hours after the initial attack. While in the hospital, the patient should be

Box 29-2

Conditions That Mimic Anaphylaxis

- Vasovagal episodes
- Acute pulmonary events
  - Acute asthmatic attacks
  - Acute pulmonary edema
  - Pulmonary embolus
  - Spontaneous pneumothorax
  - Foreign body aspiration
- Acute cardiac events
  - Supraventricular tachycardias
  - Acute myocardial infarction/ischemia
- Drug overdoses
- Insulin shock
- Carcinoid attacks

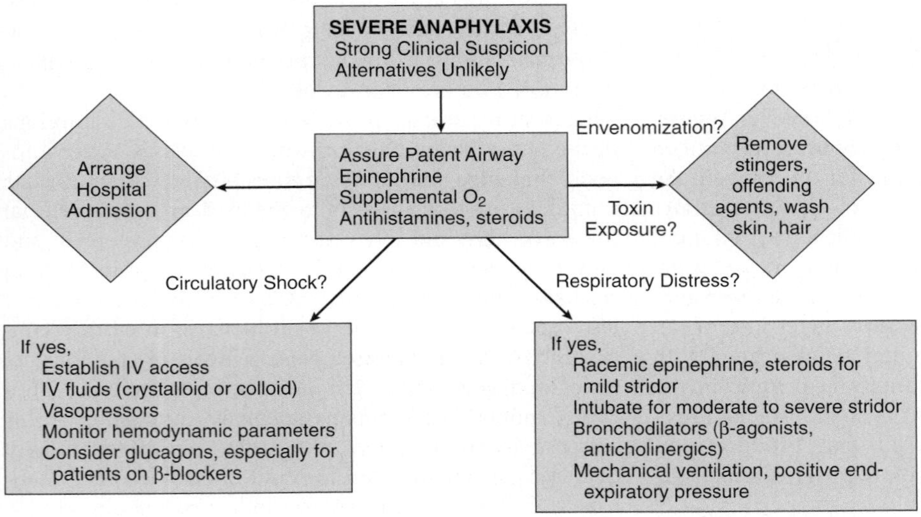

Figure 29-4. Overview of the clinical management of severe anaphylaxis.

Box 29-3

Pharmacologic Approach to the Acute Management of Anaphylaxis

Give epinephrine 0.3-0.5 mL of a 1:1000 solution subcutaneously (for mild cases).
Give epinephrine 3 to 5 mL of a 1:10,000 solution intravenously over 5-10 minutes to be repeated every 15 minutes if needed (for severe cases).
Consider epinephrine 0.3-0.5 mL of a 1:1000 solution injected locally to retard absorption of toxin.
Administer hydrocortisone 100-200 mg intravenously at 4- to 6-hour intervals (for severe cases). Taper rapidly as patient improves.

For Persistent Bronchospasm

Give aminophylline 5-6 mg/kg intravenously loading dose, then 0.4-0.9 mg/kg/min.
Give metaproterenol 0.2-0.3 mL (5% solution) in 2.5 mL normal saline administered by nebulization; repeat every 3-4 hours as needed.
Give ipratropium bromide aerosol (2 puffs) inhaled and repeated at 2-hour intervals.
Provide intravenous fluids according to degree of hemoconcentration or, in more severe cases, hemodynamic factors. Normal saline, Ringer's lactate, 5% human serum albumin, or 6% hydroxyethyl starch may be used.
For continued hypotension and other signs of circulatory shock, one of the following may be tried:
- Epinephrine drip 2-4 mg in 1 L normal saline at 2-4 μg/min
- Norepinephrine drip 4-8 mg in 1 L normal saline at 4-8 μg/min
- Dopamine drip 200 mg in 0.5 L normal saline at 5-16 μg/kg/min

The following may be given if no contraindications:
- Diphenhydramine 25-50 mg orally or intravenously at 4-hour intervals
- Cimetidine 300 mg in 50 mL normal saline given intravenously at 6- to 8-hour intervals

monitored for signs of circulatory shock, respiratory failure, and upper airway obstruction. Blood pressure, urine output, and heart and respiratory rate require frequent evaluation.

The electrocardiogram should be monitored continuously during the acute period because anaphylaxis has been associated with serious arrhythmias and cardiac ischemia. In addition, drugs used to treat anaphylaxis and circulatory shock may precipitate cardiac problems. When signs of circulatory shock and impaired pulmonary gas exchange develop, advanced monitoring with intra-arterial and pulmonary artery catheters is required. As with other types of circulatory shock, fluid therapy, inotropic and vasopressor therapy, and optimization of ventilatory support require titration under hemodynamic guidance to maintain organ perfusion, pulmonary gas exchange, and systemic oxygen delivery.

Close attention to the airway is essential because laryngeal edema is an important cause of morbidity and mortality. Frequent assessment for hoarseness, stridor, and upper airway obstruction is required for patients whose airways are not protected with an endotracheal tube. The head and neck should be positioned to prevent airway obstruction by the tongue. If inspiratory stridor develops, endotracheal intubation should be attempted. Because intubation may be difficult in the presence of laryngeal edema, skilled personnel capable of performing difficult endotracheal intubations and emergency surgical airways should be available.

If intubated patients are unable to breathe spontaneously or have labored respirations, mechanical ventilation should be initiated. Supplemental oxygen should be given to ensure arterial oxygen saturations greater than 90%. Positive end-expiratory pressure and other advanced ventilatory techniques are often necessary when hypoxemia, pulmonary edema, and decreased pulmonary compliance develop.

The site of antigen introduction should be identified. If the patient is unconscious or unaware of the site of antigen introduction, a thorough search of skin surfaces should proceed. Retained stingers from *Hymenoptera* may be found and require complete and immediate removal. If the site of venomization is an extremity, a constricting band should be applied to delay venom absorption. This band should be sufficiently tight to delay venous absorption of venom, but should not interrupt arterial flow to the distal extremity. A solution of epinephrine (see Box 29-3) may be injected locally because local α-adrenergic–mediated vasoconstriction may retard the systemic absorption of venom. The physician should be prepared to reverse α-mediated effects of epinephrine injection with locally injected phentolamine if signs of ischemia or necrosis develop. Sequestered snake venom may be removed by using suction kits or surgical techniques; however, these removal practices are controversial and may enhance the absorption of venom and exacerbate local tissue injury. These practices should be used only by experienced personnel. Thorough washing of the skin should follow exposure to antigen that has contacted the skin surface.

The mainstay of pharmacologic therapy for anaphylaxis is epinephrine. Epinephrine is of proven efficacy in reversing the bronchoconstriction and hypotension associated with anaphylaxis. The β-adrenergic effects of epinephrine inhibit mediator release by increasing intracellular levels of cAMP. In addition, β-adrenergic stimulation reverses bronchospasm, increases myocardial contractility, and increases heart rate. The α-adrenergic vasoconstrictive properties of epinephrine may increase diastolic pressure and enhance coronary flow.

All medical personnel should be aware that two dilutions of epinephrine are commonly available: a 1:1000 and a 1:10,000 dilution. Epinephrine in the 1:10,000 dilution is available in the form of prefilled syringes for rapid intravenous injection and is often used for cardiopulmonary resuscitation.

For mild-to-moderate cases of anaphylaxis, most authorities recommend that 0.3 to 0.5 mL of the 1:1000 solution (0.3 to 0.5 mg) be given subcutaneously. This dose may be repeated at 5- to 10-minute intervals if symptoms do not improve.

For intravenous administration in severe cases, most authors recommend an initial dose of 0.3 to 0.5 mg (i.e., 3 to 5 mL of a 1:10,000 solution). Because several case reports of anaphylaxis have documented cardiac ischemia and acute myocardial infarction after administration of intravenous epinephrine in this dose range,[64,67,71] it is recommended that a starting dose be given slowly and cautiously over 5 to 10 minutes. Repeat administration of epinephrine may be given at intervals of approximately 15 minutes if symptoms do not improve. A retrospective study suggested that more than 35% of anaphylactic reactions require repeat doses of epinephrine.[75] For patients who remain symptomatic after the first dose of epinephrine, an infusion (1 mg in 250 mL of 5% dextrose in water) is an alternative to repeated doses.[67,76] The infusion may be started at 1 μg/min and increased to 4 μg/min if symptoms persist. When possible, cardiac rhythm should be monitored during the administration of epinephrine.

When conventional intravenous access routes are difficult to obtain, alternative routes should be explored, including intravenous administration through the femoral vein or through a vein in the venous plexus under the tongue. A dilute solution of epinephrine also may be injected into the upper airways through an endotracheal tube or through the cricothyroid membrane, where it is reasonably well absorbed through the pulmonary airways.

Fluid therapy is an essential component of anaphylaxis treatment. Fluids reverse the intravascular volume deficits typical of anaphylaxis. Crystalloidal and colloidal fluids are effective. Clinicians should be aware that two to three times as much crystalloid is required compared with colloid to achieve comparable intravascular volume repletion. Reversal of hemoconcentration is a reasonable resuscitative goal for patients who are stable and responding favorably to treatment. In unstable patients with wide fluctuations in vital signs and worsening pulmonary function, fluid therapy should be administered based on hemodynamic measurements. Monitoring with a pulmonary artery catheter may be necessary to achieve this goal.

If hypotension and other signs of circulatory shock persist after the initial administration of epinephrine and fluids, inotropic support is required. Some authorities have recommended a continuous infusion of epinephrine (2 to 4 μg/min) for this purpose. Others suggest that norepinephrine be used (4 to 8 μg/min). Higher dosages of both of these agents may be required if hypotension persists. Dopamine and vasopressin[77] also have been used successfully in anaphylaxis.

Additional Therapeutic Options

When symptoms of anaphylaxis persist after initial treatment with epinephrine and fluids, other pharmacologic agents may be tried. The rationale for use of these agents is based on a basic knowledge of their pharmacologic and cellular actions and on clinical experience in conditions that share clinical features with anaphylaxis (e.g., acute asthma). Because of the unpredictable presentation of anaphylaxis, clinical experience with these drugs is anecdotal and inconclusive. In general, antihistamines, steroids, and inhalational bronchodilators are used routinely.

Antihistamines are logical additions to the pharmacologic management of anaphylaxis because they block mediator release from mast cells and basophils. They block the systemic effects of histamine by competitively inhibiting histamine receptors (H_1 and H_2). They may favorably influence H_1-mediated increases in vascular permeability and contraction of bronchial smooth muscle. Antihistamines also may block H_2 receptors in the myocardium, which mediate increases in heart rate, arrhythmias, atrioventricular conduction delays, and coronary vasoconstriction. Diphenhydramine, an H_1 antagonist, may be given intravenously at 4- to 6-hour intervals in doses of 25 to 50 mg. The H_2 blocker cimetidine (300 mg in 50 mL of normal saline) may be infused intravenously over 5 minutes and repeated at 6- to 8-hour intervals. Other H_2 blockers (e.g., famotidine, ranitidine) are acceptable alternatives.

Corticosteroids should be administered in severe cases of anaphylaxis because they increase tissue responsiveness to β-agonists and inhibit the synthesis of histamine. These agents also may prevent or attenuate late-phase reactions by inhibiting the characteristic secondary wave of mediator release. In severe cases, 100 to 200 mg of hydrocortisone should be given intravenously, repeated at 4- to 6-hour intervals for 24 hours, and rapidly tapered as the patient improves.

Inhalational drugs may be useful in patients with persistent bronchospasm. Inhalational β-agonists include metaproterenol and albuterol. Ipratropium bromide is an inhalational bronchodilator with anticholinergic properties and may have a favorable effect on mediator release by decreasing cGMP levels. This agent may be used in combination with inhalational β-agonists.

Laryngeal edema, if mild, may respond to nebulized racemic epinephrine. Localized vasoconstriction from the α-adrenergic properties of these drugs minimizes edema formation in the larynx and adjacent areas. Racemic epinephrine may be administered by nebulization (0.5 mL of a 2.25% solution diluted in 3.5 mL distilled water). Intravenous corticosteroid therapy also may be useful in this condition. Severe laryngeal edema associated with respiratory distress or stridor should always be treated with intubation of the trachea.

The use of methylxanthines for anaphylaxis is controversial because of poorly documented experience with these agents in humans.[78] In disorders such as asthma, these agents are effective in alleviating bronchospasm, probably secondary to direct effects on smooth muscle. If bronchospasm persists after the use of β-agonists, anticholinergics, and corticosteroids, a loading dose of 5 to 6 mg/kg of aminophylline may be infused over 20 minutes followed by a continuous infusion of 0.2 to 0.9 mg/kg/h. Mild bronchospasm occurring in patients who can take oral medications may be treated with anhydrous theophylline (200 to 400 mg by mouth in divided doses daily).

Several other agents have been used in cases of human anaphylaxis or in laboratory models of anaphylaxis with apparent success. Glucagon, a pancreatic hormone that increases intracellular cAMP levels by activating adenylate cyclase, was effective in a case report of a patient with anaphylaxis who was receiving β-blocker therapy.[79,80] Because calcium enhances mediator release, it has been speculated that calcium blockers might be useful in anaphylaxis. These agents have not been studied in anaphylaxis, however. Their negative inotropic effects may be undesirable in severe anaphylaxis, especially when signs of shock are present. The opiate antagonist naloxone reverses the inhibitory effects of endogenous opiates on the sympathetic nervous system. This agent has been shown to be effective in laboratory models of anaphylaxis.[81] Metaraminol, an α-agonist, has been reported to reverse anaphylaxis in patients under anesthesia.[82] At this time, glucagon, calcium blocking agents, opiate antagonists, and metaraminol have a limited role in the treatment of anaphylaxis. Additional understanding of the physiologic and clinical effects of these drugs in anaphylaxis is required before their routine use can be recommended.

Arrangements must be made for patients who have experienced anaphylaxis to receive follow-up care by a physician experienced in the management of acute allergic events. Skin testing may be required to identify the inciting agent. Instructions in self-treatment after antigen exposure are necessary. Kits are available with injectable epinephrine and oral antihistamines for patients to self-administer.

PROPHYLAXIS AND IMMUNOTHERAPY

If a patient must be treated with a drug that has previously produced severe allergic symptoms or anaphylaxis and no alternative exists, premedication should be implemented. Most authorities recommend premedication with H_1 and H_2 blockers and corticosteroids. Several studies have confirmed that premedication with these agents decreases anaphylactic reactions to radiocontrast media.[83-85] In very-high-risk patients, some authorities believe that epinephrine or isoproterenol should be included as premedication.[86] Because fatal anaphylaxis has been described in patients who received premedication, it is preferable, if clinically possible, to avoid all antigens associated with anaphylaxis.

Methods to desensitize individuals immediately before administration of a drug have been described in detail, especially for penicillin,[87] aspirin,[88] and insulin.[89] These techniques, which involve exposure to antigen in 20- to 30-minute increments, may be unsuccessful, however, and occasional fatalities have been reported.[90-92]

Long-term desensitization may be useful in patients who have experienced anaphylaxis to antigens that are difficult to avoid, especially foods and venoms. This type of immunotherapy involves initial injection of a minute dose of antigen followed by gradual increases in dose at weekly or biweekly intervals according to the patient's tolerance.[93,94] A non-IgE blocking antibody forms and decreases the reactivity of mast cells and basophils to antigen.

Education and acute and long-term desensitization should be the responsibility of physicians experienced in the management of immediate hypersensitivity disorders. The critical care physician is responsible for ensuring the referral of patients who have experienced anaphylaxis to the care of appropriately trained specialists.

KEY POINTS

- Classic anaphylaxis is an IgE-mediated allergic reaction (type I) with acute systemic manifestations.
- Anaphylactoid reactions are clinically identical to classic anaphylaxis and respond similarly to treatment; however, they are not mediated by IgE.
- Mediators derived from mast cells and basophils are responsible for the major pathophysiologic effects of anaphylaxis.
- Eosinophils also release mediators that modulate the inflammatory response of anaphylaxis.
- Mediators from polymorphonuclear leukocytes and platelets are responsible for late-phase reactions after the initial anaphylactic event.
- Histamine, leukotrienes, and prostaglandins are important biochemical mediators of anaphylaxis. Release of these mediators is associated with increased vascular permeability and bronchial smooth muscle constriction.
- Pharmacologic agents that increase cAMP levels inhibit mediator release and may be beneficial in anaphylaxis.
- Agents that decrease cGMP levels (e.g., anticholinergic drugs) also inhibit mediator release.
- Increases in intracellular calcium increase mediator release.
- Fatal anaphylaxis is often associated with upper airway obstruction from laryngeal edema.
- The initial presentation of a patient with anaphylaxis depends on the portal of entry of the antigen and may include a local skin reaction and respiratory, upper airway, and gastrointestinal symptoms.
- Late-phase reactions may occur 6 to 12 hours after the initial anaphylactic event and are associated with a recurrence of symptoms.
- Hemodynamic characteristics of anaphylaxis include tachycardia, hypotension, decreased cardiac distending pressures, and decreased systemic vascular resistance.
- The mainstays of anaphylaxis management are (1) ensure airway patency, (2) remove or delay the absorption of toxins, (3) establish access for fluid

therapy, and (4) initiate pharmacologic support with epinephrine.

- Corticosteroids should be given in severe cases to prevent late-phase reactions.
- Antihistamines (H_1 and H_2 blockers) are routinely given if there are no contraindications. The efficacy of these drugs after anaphylaxis is established is uncertain, however.
- Inhaled β-agonist agents, aminophylline, and inhaled anticholinergic agents may be given for continued bronchospasm.
- All patients who have experienced anaphylaxis should be referred to an appropriately qualified specialist for follow-up. These patients may require allergy testing, desensitization, and premedication strategies.

REFERENCES

•1. Ishizaka T: IgE and mechanisms of IgE mediated hypersensitivity. Ann Allergy 1982;48:313.
2. Gell PGH, Coombs RRA: Classification of allergic reactions responsible for clinical hypersensitivity and disease. In Gell PGH, Coombs RRA, Hachmann PJ (eds): Clinical Aspects of Immunology, 3rd ed. Oxford, Blackwell Scientific, 1975, p 761.
•3. Serafin WE, Austin KF: Mediators of immediate hypersensitivity reactions. N Engl J Med 1987;317:30.
4. Sheffer AL, Austin KF: Exercise-induced anaphylaxis. J Allergy Clin Immunol 1980;6:106.
5. Toogood JH: Risk of anaphylaxis in patients receiving beta-blocker drugs. J Allergy Clin Immunol 1988;81:1.
•6. Lenchner K, Grammer LC: A current review of idiopathic anaphylaxis. Curr Opin Allergy Clin Immunol 2003;3:305:11.
7. Yocum M, Kahn D: Clinical cause of idiopathic anaphylaxis. Ann Allergy 1994;13:370.
8. Grammer L, Shaughnessy M, Harris K, et al: Lymphocyte subsets and activation markers in patients with acute episodes of idiopathic anaphylaxis, Ann Allergy Asthma Immunol 2000;85:368.
9. Hendrix S, Sale S, Zeiss CR, et al: Factitious Hymenoptera allergic emergency: A report of a new variant of Munchausen syndrome. J Allergy Clin Immunol 1981;67:8.
10. McGrath KG, Greenberger PA, Zeiss CR, et al: Factitious allergic disease: Multiple factitious illness and familial Munchausen stridor. Immunol Allergy Pract 1984;6:41.
11. Choy AC, Patterson R, Patterson DR, et al: Undifferentiated somatoform idiopathic anaphylaxis: Nonorganic symptoms mimicking idiopathic anaphylaxis. J Allergy Clin Immunol 1995;96:893.
12. Waddell LA: Egyptian Civilization: Its Sumerian Origin and Real Chronology and Sumerian Origin of Egyptian Hieroglyphs. London, Luzac, 1930.
13. Chafee FH: Insect-sting allergy. J Allergy 1969;43:309.
14. Cohen SG: The pharaoh and the wasp. Allergy Proc 1989;10:149.
15. Portier P, Richet C: De l'action anaphylactique de certains venins. Comput Rend Soc Biol (Paris) 1902;54:170.
16. Murphy RC, Hammarstrom S, Samuelsson B: Leukotriene C: A slow-reacting substance from murine mastocytoma cells. Proc Natl Acad Sci U S A 1979;76:4275.
•17. Lewis RA, Austen KF, Soberman RJ: Leukotrienes and other products of the 5-lipoxygenase pathway: Biochemistry and relation to pathobiology in human diseases. N Engl J Med 1990;323:645.
18. Idsoe O, Guthe T, Willcox RR, et al: Nature and extent of penicillin side-reactions with particular reference to fatalities from anaphylactic shock. Bull World Health Organ 1968;38:159.
19. Park MA, Li JT: Diagnosis and management of penicillin allergy. Mayo Clin Proc 2005;80:405.
20. Weiss ME, Adkinson NF: Immediate hypersensitivity reactions to penicillin and related antibiotics. Clin Allergy 1988;18:515.
21. Kabins SA, Eisenstein B, Cohen S: Anaphylactoid reaction to an initial dose of sodium cephalothin. JAMA 1965;193:165.
•22. Saxon A, Beall GN, Rohr AS, et al: Immediate hypersensitivity reactions to beta-lactam antibiotics. Ann Intern Med 1987;107:204.
•23. Valentine MD: Anaphylaxis and stinging insect hypersensitivity. JAMA 1992;268:2830.
24. Barnard JH: Studies of 400 Hymenoptera sting deaths in the United States. J Allergy Clin Immunol 1973;52:259.
25. DeShazo RD, Butcher BT, Banks WA: Reactions to the stings of the imported fire ant. N Engl J Med 1990;323:462.
26. Russell FE, Carlson RW, Wainschel J, et al: Snake venom poisoning in the United States: Experience with 550 cases. JAMA 1975;233:341.
27. Kunkel DB: Bites of venomous reptiles. Emerg Med Clin North Am 1984;2:563.
•28. Sicherer SH, Sampson HA: Food allergy. J Allergy Clin Immunol 2006;117:S470-S475.
29. Bock SA: The incidence of severe adverse reactions to food in Colorado. J Allergy Clin Immunol 1992;90:683.
30. Bock SA, Munoz-Furlong A, Sampson HA: Fatalities due to anaphylactic reactions to foods. J Allergy Clin Immunol 2001;107:191.
31. Kellerman R: Reactions to radiographic contrast media. Am Fam Physician 1981;23:149.
•32. Cohan RH, Dunnick NR, Bashore TM: Treatment of reactions to radiographic contrast material. AJR Am J Roentgenol 1988;151:263.
33. Lasser EC, Lang J, Sovak M, et al: Steroids: Theoretical and experimental basis for utilization in prevention of contrast media reactions. Radiology 1977;125:1.
34. Sussman GL, Tarlo S, Dolovich J: The spectrum of IgE-mediated responses to latex. JAMA 1991;265:2844.
•35. Slater JE: Latex allergy. J Allergy Clin Immunol 1994;94:139.
36. Galletly DC, Treuren BC: Anaphylactoid reactions during anaesthesia. Anaesthesia 1985;40:329.
37. Johansson SGO, Melvin T, Vahlquist B: Immunoglobulin levels in Ethiopian preschool children with special reference to high concentrations of immunoglobulin E (IgND). Lancet 1968;1:1118.
38. Phils JA, Harrold AJ, Whiteman GV: Pulmonary infiltrates, asthma, and eosinophilia due to *Ascaris suum* infestation in man. N Engl J Med 1972;286:965.
39. Dessein AJ, Parker WL, James SL, et al: IgE antibody and resistance to infection, I: Selective suppression of the IgE antibody response in rats diminishes the resistance and the eosinophil response to *Trichinella spiralis* infection. J Exp Med 1981;153:423.
40. Hernandez-Trujillo VP, Liegerman PL, Chowdhury BA: Drug allergens, haptens, and anaphylatoxins. Clin Allergy Immunol 2004,18:387.
41. Van Arsdel PP: Diagnosing drug allergy. JAMA 1982;247:2576.
42. Vyas GN, Holmdahl L, Perkins A, et al: Serologic specificity of human anti-IgA and its significance in transfusion. Blood 1969;34:573.
43. Best N, Sinosich MJ, Teisner B, et al: Complement activation during cardiopulmonary bypass by heparin-protamine interaction. Br J Anaesth 1984;56:339.
44. Sharath MD, Metzger WJ, Richerson HB, et al: Protamine-induced fatal anaphylaxis. J Thorac Cardiovasc Surg 1985;90:86.
45. Weiss ME, Nyhan D, Zhikang P, et al: Association of protamine IgE and IgG antibodies with life threatening reactions to intravenous protamine. N Engl J Med 1989;320:886.
46. Stevenson DD, Szczeklik A: Clinical and pathological perspectives on aspirin sensitivity and asthma. J Allergy Clin Immunol 2006;118:773.
47. Corder EH, Buckley CE 3rd: Aspirin, salicylate, sulfite, and tartrazine induced bronchoconstriction: Safe doses and case definition in epidemiological studies. J Clin Epidemiol 1995;48:1269-1275.

48. Galli SJ, Wedemeyer J, Tsai M: Analyzing the role of most cells and basophils in host response and other biological responses. Int J Hematol 2002;75:363.
49. Butterworth AE, David JR: Eosinophil function. N Engl J Med 1981;304:154.
50. Weller PF: The immunobiology of eosinophils. N Engl J Med 1991;324:1110.
51. Hugli TE, Muller-Eberhard HJ: Anaphylatoxins: C3a and C5a. Adv Immunol 1978;26:1.
52. Delage C, Irey NS: Anaphylactic deaths: A clinicopathologic study of 43 cases. J Forensic Sci 1972;17:525.
53. James LP, Austen KF: Fatal systemic anaphylaxis in man. N Engl J Med 1964;270:597.
54. Fisher MM: Anaphylaxis. Acute Care 1988-1989;14-15:47.
55. Gleich GJ: The late phase of the immunoglobulin E mediated reaction: A link between anaphylaxis and common allergic disease? J Allergy Clin Immunol 1982;70:160.
56. Naclerio RM, Proud D, Togias AG, et al: Inflammatory mediators in late antigen-induced rhinitis. N Engl J Med 1985;313:65.
57. Lieberman P: Biphasic anaphylactic reactions. Ann Allergy Asthma Immunol 2005;95:217.
•58. Carlson RW, Schaeffer RC, Puri VK, et al: Hypovolemia and permeability pulmonary edema associated with anaphylaxis. Crit Care Med 1981;9:883.
•59. Silverman HJ, Van Hook C, Haponik EF: Hemodynamic changes in human anaphylaxis. Am J Med 1984;77:341.
60. Hanashiro PK, Weil MH: Anaphylactic shock in man: Report of two cases with detailed hemodynamic and metabolic studies. Arch Intern Med 1967;119:129.
61. Fisher M: Blood volume replacement in acute anaphylactic cardiovascular collapse related to anaesthesia. Br J Anaesth 1977;49:1023.
62. Fisher MM, Dicks I: Blood volume replacement in acute anaphylactoid reactions. Anesth Intensive Care 1979;7:375.
63. Booth BH, Patterson R: Electrocardiographic changes in human anaphylaxis. JAMA 1970;211:627.
64. Levine HD: Acute myocardial infarction following a wasp sting. Am Heart J 1976;91:365.
65. Sullivan TJ: Cardiac disorders in penicillin-induced anaphylaxis. JAMA 1982;248:2161.
66. Austin SM, Barooah B, Kim CS: Reversible acute cardiac injury during cefoxitin-induced anaphylaxis in a patient with normal coronary arteries. Am J Med 1984;77:729.
•67. McLean-Tooke AP, Bethune CA, Fay AC, et al: Adrenaline in the treatment of anaphylaxis: what is the evidence? BMJ 2003;327:1332.
68. Raper RF, Fisher MM: Profound reversible myocardial depression after anaphylaxis. Lancet 1988;1:368.
69. Smedegard G, Revenas B, Lundberg C, et al: Anaphylactic shock in monkeys passively sensitized with human reaginic serum, I: Hemodynamics and cardiac performance. Acta Physiol Scand 1981;111:239.
70. Moss J, Fahmy NR, Sunder N, et al: Hormonal and hemodynamic profile of an anaphylactic reaction in man. Circulation 1981;63:210.
71. Hamberger B, Fredholm BB, Farnebo LO: Anaphylaxis and plasma catecholamines. Life Sci 1980;26:1465.
72. Olinger GN, Becker RM, Boncheck LI: Non-cardiogenic pulmonary edema and peripheral vascular collapse following cardiopulmonary bypass: Rare protamine reaction? Ann Thorac Surg 1980;29:20.
73. Enjeti S, Bleeker ER, Smith PL, et al: Hemodynamic mechanisms in anaphylaxis. Circ Shock 1983;11:297.
74. Brady WJ Jr, Luber S, Carter CT, et al: Multiphasic anaphylaxis: An uncommon event in the emergency department. Acad Emerg Med 1997;4:193.
75. Korenblat P, Lundie MJ, Dankner RE: A retrospective study of epinephrine administration for anaphylaxis: How many doses are needed? Allergy Asthma Proc 1999;20:383.
76. ECC Committee, Subcommittees and Task Forces of the American Heart Association: 2005 American Heart Association guidelines for cardiopulmonary resuscitation and emergency cardiovascular care. Circulation 2005;112(24 Suppl):IV-1.
77. Kill C, Wranze E, Wulf H: Successful treatment of severe anaphylactic shock with vasopressin: Two case reports. Int Arch Allergy Immunol 2004;134:260.
78. Ernst ME, Graber MA: Methylxanthine use in anaphylaxis: What does the evidence tell us? Ann Pharmacother 1999;33:1001.
79. Zaloga GP, Delacey W, Holmboe E, et al: Glucagon reversal of hypotension in a case of anaphylactoid shock. Ann Intern Med 1986;105:65.
80. Thomas M, Crawford I: Best evidence report: Glucagon infusion in refractory anaphylactic shock in patients on beta-blockers. Emerg Med J 2005;22:272.
81. Gullo A, Romano E: Naloxone and anaphylactic shock. Lancet 1983;1:819.
82. Heytman M, Rainbird A: Use of alpha-agonists for management of anaphylaxis occurring under anaesthesia: Case studies and a review. Anesthesia 2004;59:1210.
•83. Lasser EC, Berry CC, Talner LB, et al: Pretreatment with corticosteroids to alleviate reactions to intravenous contrast material. N Engl J Med 1987;317:845.
84. Miller WI, Doppman JL, Kaplan AP: Renal arteriography following systemic reaction to contrast material. J Allergy Clin Immunol 1975;56:291.
85. Tramer MR, von Elm E, Loubeyre P, et al: Pharmacologic prevention of serious anaphylactic reactions due to iodinated contrast media: Systemic review. BMJ 2006;333:675.
86. Watkins J: Adverse anaesthetic reactions. Anaesthesia 1985;40:797.
87. Weiss ME, Adkinson NF: Immediate hypersensitivity reactions to penicillin and related antibiotics. Clin Allergy 1988;18:515.
88. Canonica GW: Specific immunotherapy: Still young after one century. Allergy Immunol 2005;37:301.
89. Mattson JR, Patterson R, Roberts M: Insulin therapy in patients with systemic insulin allergy. Arch Intern Med 1975;135:818.
90. Pfaar O, Klimek L: Aspirin desensitization in aspirin intolerance: Update on current standards and recent improvements. Curr Opin Allergy Clin Immunol 2006;6:161.
91. Grieco MH, Dubin MR, Robinson JL, et al: Penicillin hypersensitivity in patients with bacterial endocarditis. Ann Intern Med 1964;60:204.
92. Tuft L: Fatalities following the reinjection of foreign serum: With report of an unusual case. Am J Med Sci 1928;175:325.
93. Graft DF: Venom immunotherapy for stinging insect allergy. Clin Rev Allergy 1987;5:149.
94. Lockey RF: Immunotherapy for allergy to insect stings. N Engl J Med 1990;323:1627.

Chapter 30

Severe Heart Failure

Fredric Ginsberg and Joseph E. Parrillo

Heart failure is a syndrome caused by abnormal cardiac performance that results in signs and symptoms related to salt and fluid retention, increased left ventricular filling pressure, decreased cardiac output, or a combination of these abnormalities. Heart failure is a very common illness, affecting 5 million Americans, women as frequently as men.[1] It is estimated that 1% of the population of Americans older than 65 years are affected by heart failure and that 20% of hospital admissions in patients older than 65 years are due to heart failure.[2] Every year in the United States, 550,000 new cases of heart failure are diagnosed, with a total of nearly 1 million annual hospital discharges and 6.5 million hospital days for patients with a primary diagnosis of heart failure.[1] Nearly 53,000 people in the United States died in 2001 with heart failure as the primary cause. The treatment of heart failure imposes a very large economic burden on the U.S. health care system. Estimated direct and indirect costs of heart failure in 2005 were 25 billion dollars. The majority of these costs was related to the treatment of patients hospitalized with heart failure. Epidemiologic data show significant increases in both the incidence and prevalence of heart failure in the U.S. population over the past decade,[2] likely influenced by both the aging of the population with a higher prevalence of hypertension and improved treatment and survival of patients with ischemic heart disease.[1]

In the American College of Cardiology/American Heart Association (ACC/AHA) Guidelines for the diagnosis and management of chronic heart failure, four stages in the development of heart failure are recognized (Fig. 30-1). This classification emphasizes that there are several medical conditions that put patients at high risk for development of left ventricular dysfunction and the heart failure syndrome. Attention to and appropriate management of these conditions may prevent the development of heart failure. In addition, in patients who have left ventricular dysfunction but who do not yet have heart failure, appropriate therapy can improve prognosis and prevent the development of severe heart failure. Thus, the staging system emphasizes the progressive nature of left ventricular dysfunction and heart failure and identifies evidence-based guidelines for therapy for each stage.[1]

Stage A applies to patients who are at high risk for heart failure but do not have structural heart disease or symptoms of heart failure. These include patients with hypertension, atherosclerotic heart disease, diabetes, obesity, or the metabolic syndrome as well as patients exposed to cardiotoxic medications or with a family history of cardiomyopathy. In Stage B, patients have structural heart disease but no signs or symptoms of heart failure. This group includes those with previous myocardial infarction (MI), those with abnormal left ventricular ejection fraction but no symptoms of heart failure, and those with asymptomatic valvular heart disease. Patients in Stage C have structural heart disease with prior or current symptoms of heart failure. These patients demonstrate shortness of breath, fatigue, and reduced exercise toler-

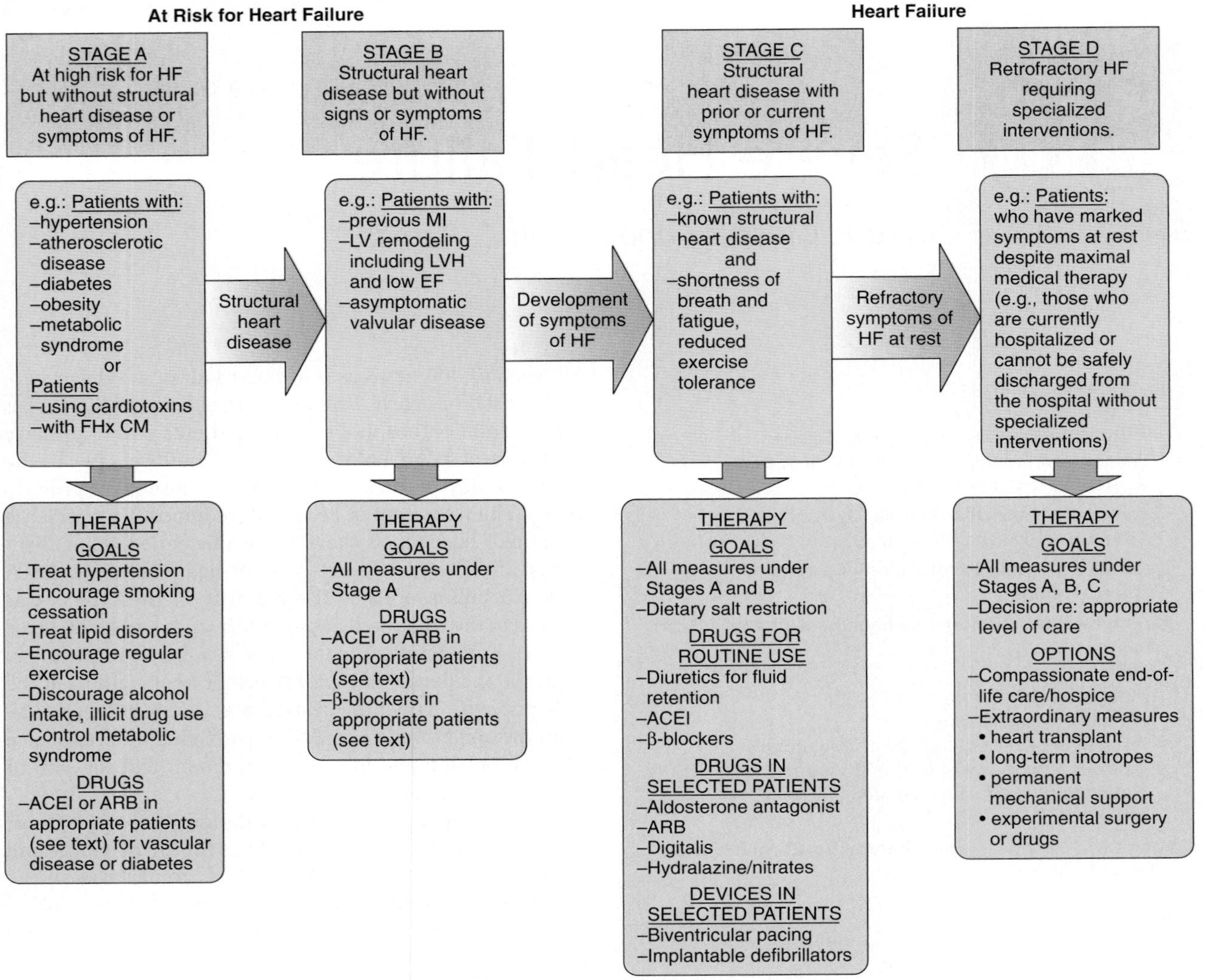

Figure 30-1. Stages in the development of heart failure and recommended therapy by stage. ACEI, angiotensin-converting enzyme inhibitor; ARB, angiotensin receptor blocker; EF, ejection fraction; FHx CM, family history of cardiomyopathy; HF, heart failure; LV, left ventricular; LVH, LV hypertrophy; MI, myocardial infarction. (Redrawn from Hunt S, Abraham WT, Chin M, et al: ACC/AHA 2005 Guideline Update for the Diagnosis and Management of Chronic Heart Failure in the Adult—Summary Article. A report on the American College of Cardiology/American Heart Association Task Force on Practice Guidelines (Writing Committee to Update the 2001 Guidelines for Evaluation and Management of Heart Failure): Developed in collaboration with the American College of Chest Physicians and the International Society for Heart and Lung Transplantation: Endorsed by the Heart Rhythm Society. Circulation 2005;112:1825-1852.)

ance. Stage D applies to patients who have refractory symptoms of heart failure at rest despite maximal medical therapy, who require specialized interventions. Life expectancy is reduced in patients with heart failure, and death can occur either at the end of progressive worsening of the syndrome or suddenly in patients otherwise thought to have been stable.

Manifestations of heart failure can be thought of as due primarily to left ventricular systolic dysfunction or diastolic dysfunction, although clinically many patients experience heart failure with both abnormalities. Systolic heart failure results from the inability of the heart to expel blood normally due to depressed left ventricular contraction. Systolic heart failure can be initiated by a number of conditions that damage left ventricular myocardium. The most common of these conditions are MI and myocardial ischemia due to atherosclerotic coronary artery disease. Other common etiologies of systolic heart failure are hypertension, dilated cardiomyopathy, viral myocarditis, and valvular heart disease (Fig. 30-2A).

Diastolic heart failure is caused by a reduction in left ventricular compliance, which leads to impaired diastolic filling, higher left ventricular diastolic pressures, and increases in pulmonary capillary wedge pressure. Diastolic heart failure is also termed *heart failure in the setting of normal systolic function*. Conditions commonly associated with diastolic heart failure are hypertension, left ventricular hypertrophy, and acute coronary ischemia. Diastolic heart failure is common in elderly populations, especially in women, likely as a result of the progressive diastolic compliance abnormalities seen with aging. Uncommon conditions leading to diastolic heart failure include infiltrative and restrictive cardiomyopathies and chronic constrictive pericarditis (see Fig. 30-2B).

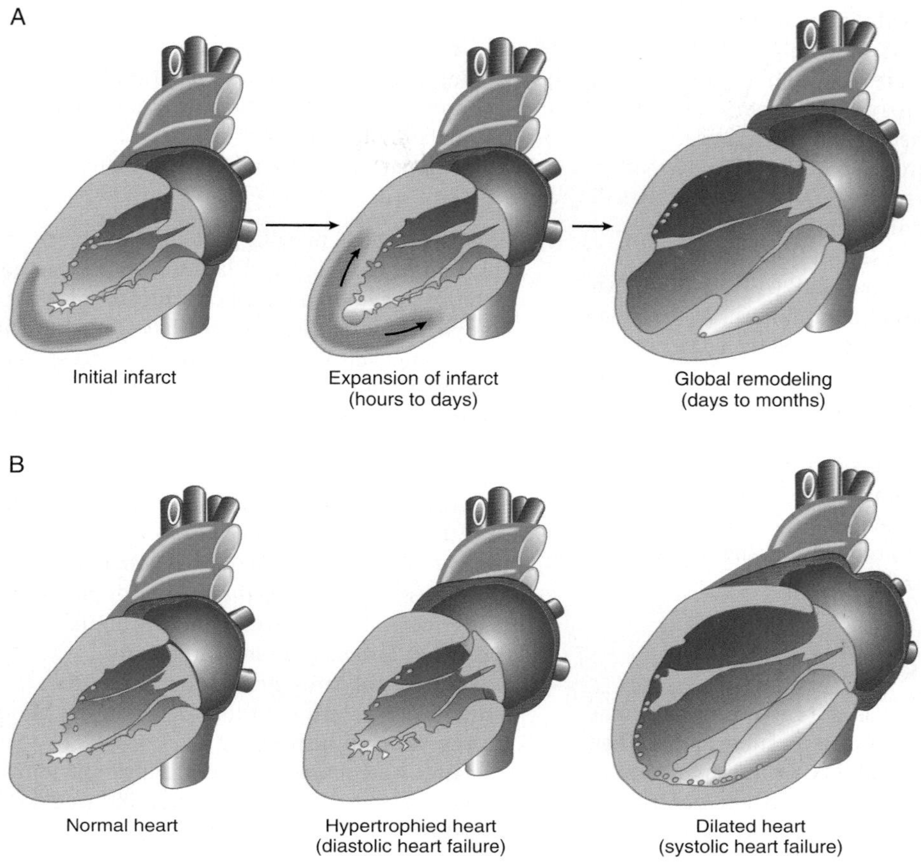

Figure 30-2. A, Left ventricular (LV) remodeling after acute myocardial infarction, resulting in a dilated LV with global systolic dysfunction. **B,** Ventricular remodeling in diastolic and systolic heart failure. Differences in LV morphology in diastolic versus systolic heart failure. (Redrawn from Jessup M, Brozena S: Heart failure. N Engl J Med 2003;348:2007-2018.)

Typical symptoms of heart failure are shortness of breath at rest or with exertion, fatigue, cough, swelling, orthopnea, and paroxysmal nocturnal dyspnea. Physical examination often reveals pulmonary rales, elevated jugular venous pressure, signs of cardiomegaly, third heart sound (S_3) gallop, hepatic enlargement, and edema. Manifestations of more severe heart failure are marked dyspnea at rest possibly leading to respiratory failure, cyanosis, cool extremities, and altered mental state.

The diagnosis of heart failure has traditionally relied on evaluation of symptoms, such as dyspnea and swelling, and of signs detected on physical examination, including pulmonary rales, S_3 gallop, elevated jugular venous pressure, ascites, and edema. Chest radiography and echocardiography, when available, are helpful. However, these signs and symptoms and diagnostic tests are not specific for heart failure, and coexisting conditions such as obesity, chronic lung disease, and deconditioning can add uncertainty to the clinical diagnosis. Thus, heart failure is often both underdiagnosed and overdiagnosed in outpatient and emergency department settings.

Studies have now shown that a serum assay of B-natriuretic peptide (BNP) levels is very helpful in improving the accuracy of diagnosing heart failure. BNP is a 32 amino acid peptide produced by cardiac myocytes in response to pressure-induced wall stretch and tension.[3] The actions of BNP include arterial and venous dilation and natriuresis. A study of 1530 patients presenting to emergency departments with dyspnea showed that knowledge of BNP serum levels leads to greater accuracy of the diagnosis of heart failure than that with clinical judgment alone, from an initial range of 65% to 74% up to the greater accuracy of 81%.[4] BNP levels above 100 pg/mL had a sensitivity of 90% and a specificity of 76% for the diagnosis of heart failure and were very useful for identifying patients with dyspnea due to uncomplicated lung disease, in whom BNP values were less than 100 pg/mL.[5] Patients with BNP values below 100 pg/mL were very unlikely to have heart failure as the cause of dyspnea. Serum BNP measurements should always be used in conjunction with all other clinical data to arrive at the correct diagnosis.

Evaluating BNP levels in heart failure patients in the emergency department also has been shown to decrease the need for hospitalization and decrease the need for intensive care unit (ICU) admissions without affecting 30-day mortality rates.[6] Total hospital stay was shortened by 3 days, cost of treatment was significantly reduced, and time to initiation of definitive therapy in the emergency room was shortened by 30 minutes.

BNP levels correlate with disease severity, because values are higher in patients with more severe heart failure and with worse left ventricular systolic function. Higher levels also have been correlated with a poorer prognosis and can predict a higher risk of functional deterioration and mortality.[7] In a study of 114 patients admitted to the hospital with NYHA class IV heart failure, predischarge BNP level was the most strongly associated of all variables evaluated with death or readmission within 6 months. Values greater than 350 pg/mL had impressive sensitivity and specificity.[8] BNP levels are also high in patients with diastolic heart failure, massive pulmonary embolism, severe pulmonary hypertension, and renal failure as well as in stable patients with chronic dilated cardiomyopathy. BNP levels may initially be low in patients with "flash" pulmonary edema, because they may present to the hospital before significant rises in serum BNP occur.

Serum levels of *N*-terminal pro-BNP (NTpro-BNP) can also be used for the diagnosis of heart failure. *N*-Terminal pro-BNP is the inactive molecule cleaved from the precursor hormone pro-BNP as BNP is produced. NTpro-BNP has a longer half-life than BNP, and is cleared from the serum by the kidneys, so levels are higher in patients with coexisting renal disease. Levels of both NTpro-BNP and BNP are higher in older populations. A cutoff level for NTpro-BNP of 300 pg/mL yielded a positive predictive value of 77% and negative predictive value of 98% for the diagnosis of heart failure.[9,10]

ACUTE, SEVERE HEART FAILURE

Acute heart failure is defined as the rapid onset of signs and symptoms of heart failure due to abnormal cardiac function. It is caused by an inability of the myocardium to maintain cardiac output, at a normal left ventricular diastolic filling pressure, that is sufficient to meet the demands of the peripheral circulation. Left ventricular systolic function may be normal or abnormal in acute heart failure. Acute heart failure is often life-threatening and requires urgent diagnostic and therapeutic interventions, often simultaneously.[11,12]

Several distinct clinical syndromes of acute heart failure can be identified, as follows (Table 30-1)[11]:

1. Patients can present with acute worsening or decompensation of chronic heart failure symptoms, either in the setting of known chronic cardiovascular illness or de novo. These patients do not have shock or pulmonary edema. This is the most common presentation of acute heart failure requiring admission to hospital, occurring in approximately 70% of patients with acute heart failure.[12]
2. Patients may present with acute pulmonary edema with normal blood pressure, often caused by acute MI or acute coronary ischemia.
3. Patients may have pulmonary edema with elevated blood pressure, often in the setting of chronic severe hypertension. Pulmonary edema accounts for roughly 25% of acute heart failure admissions.
4. The presence of cardiogenic shock with heart failure is another distinct presentation, occurring in about 5% of cases of acute heart failure.
5. A smaller percentage of patients present with "high cardiac output heart failure," often induced by sepsis, thyroid disease, or cardiac arrhythmia.

Table 30-1. Acute Heart Failure Syndromes

Syndrome	Onset	Signs and Symptoms	Hemodynamics
Acute decompensated heart failure	Days/weeks	Weakness Dyspnea Rales Third heart sound (S_3) gallop Edema	↑ PCWP ↓ CI Normal or ↑ RAP ↑ SVR
Acute pulmonary edema, normal BP	Abrupt-days	Severe dyspnea Diffuse rales Cyanosis S_3 gallop	↑↑ PCWP Normal or ↓ CI Normal RA Normal or ↑ SVR
Acute pulmonary edema with hypertension	Acute	Severe dyspnea Diffuse rales	↑↑ PCWP Normal CI Normal RAP ↑↑ SVR
Cardiogenic shock	Acute	Hypotension Cyanosis Lethargy Cool, clammy	↑↑ PCWP ↑ RAP ↓↓ CI ↑ SVR
High-output heart failure	Days-weeks	Dyspnea Rales	↑ PCWP ↑ CI ↓ SVR
RV failure	Days-weeks	Hypotension Edema Ascites	Normal or ↑PCWP ↑↑RAP ↓↓ CI

CI, cardiac index; PCWP, pulmonary capillary wedge pressure; RAP, right atrial pressure; SVR, systemic vascular resistance; ↑, increased; ↑↑, markedly increased; ↓, reduced; ↓↓, markedly reduced.

Adapted from Nieminen MS, Bohm M, Cowie MR, et al: Executive Summary of the guidelines on the diagnosis and treatment of acute heart failure. The Task Force on Acute Heart Failure of the European Society of Cardiology. European Heart J 2005;26:384-416; and Gheorghiade M, Zannad F, Sopko G: Acute heart failure syndromes. Circulation 2005;112:3958-3968.

6. Patients may have signs and symptoms of acute right ventricular failure, such as with acute right ventricular MI, massive pulmonary embolism, or cardiac tamponade.

The epidemiology of acute heart failure shows an elderly population with a mean age in the early 70s. In the United States, roughly 80% of patients with acute heart failure have a previous history of heart failure,[12] and in European studies, in one third of patients the diagnosis of heart failure was new.[13] Approximately 40% to 55% of patients have normal or relatively normal left ventricular systolic function; this finding is more common in women than in men. Coronary heart disease is present in 50% to 60% of patients, and hypertension in 72%. Comorbidities are common, including renal disease in 30% of patients, diabetes mellitus in 43%, and chronic obstructive pulmonary disease in roughly 30%.[12-14]

Initial steps in the assessment of patients with acute heart failure from any cause include a history and physical examination. The symptoms of acute heart failure are similar to those of chronic heart failure but are more severe. Patients may present with symptoms of increased lung congestion, such as severe shortness of breath, cough, and orthopnea. Symptoms of tissue hypoperfusion and congestion include fatigue, weakness, confusion, edema, nausea, abdominal pain, and anorexia. Chest pain may indicate acute coronary ischemia.

Physical examination shows pulmonary rales, wheezes, and an S_3 gallop, and may show cardiac murmurs and elevation of jugular venous pressure. The peripheral pulses are weak and thready with diminished cardiac output states. The skin may be cool and clammy, and there may be evidence of cyanosis. Peripheral edema and ascites may indicate concomitant right ventricular failure of longer duration. The presence of pulsus paradoxus should be evaluated if signs of right ventricular failure suggest the presence of cardiac tamponade.

Chest radiography is done urgently. An electrocardiogram (ECG) is needed to assess for signs of ischemia and infarction and to evaluate for arrhythmia. Cardiac rhythm must be monitored continuously. Laboratory examination consists of evaluation of hemoglobin and hematocrit, electrolyte values, renal and liver function, thyroid profile, and cardiac biomarkers (MB portion of creatine kinase [CK-MB] and troponin) to look for evidence of myocardial necrosis. BNP measurements assist in the diagnosis of heart failure in patients presenting with dyspnea and can be followed serially to assess effectiveness of therapy. Pulse oximetry helps assess oxygenation and pulmonary function. Establishment of an arterial line is helpful in managing patients with hypotension or cardiogenic shock. Urgent two-dimensional echocardiography is essential to evaluate left ventricular size and function as well as valvular function. Doppler echocardiographic assessment of hemodynamics is also valuable.

Placement of a pulmonary artery catheter enables the clinician to accurately measure pulmonary capillary wedge pressure, cardiac output, and mixed venous oxygen saturation. It can also help assess the effectiveness of therapy. Whether to *routinely* use pulmonary artery (PA) catheters to assess and manage patients with acute heart failure has been long debated. The ESCAPE trial evaluated the routine use of PA catheterization in patients hospitalized with acute exacerbation of chronic heart failure and left ventricular systolic dysfunction.[15] There was no difference in the primary end point—days alive out of the hospital during 6 months after discharge—between groups managed with and groups managed without a PA catheter. No subgroups were identified in which use of the PA catheter was beneficial. However, a trend toward improvement of initial diuresis, with less deterioration of renal function, was noted in the PA catheter group.[16] The researchers in this study concluded that there was no indication for the routine use of PA catheters in the setting of acute heart failure.

Nevertheless, the PA catheter is often essential for the management of patients with acute severe heart failure or cardiogenic shock. Other indications for PA catheter use are to differentiate pulmonary from cardiac causes of dyspnea, for hemodynamic assessment in patients in whom diagnosis from clinical signs and symptoms is uncertain, and in cases that are not responding to initially prescribed therapies. Pulmonary catheter placement is also necessary as part of the evaluation for cardiac transplantation or the implantation of a ventricular assist device. When a PA catheter is used, hemodynamic targets of therapy include lowering pulmonary capillary wedge pressure to less than 18 mm Hg, lowering mean right atrial pressure to less than 8 mm Hg, and optimization of cardiac output.[16]

Unlike in chronic systolic heart failure, there is a paucity of controlled data to support evidence-based guidelines for the treatment of acute heart failure. Treatment strategies are based on small studies, experience, observation, and a general consensus of opinion. Initial therapies include supplemental oxygen and assessment of the need for ventilatory assistance with external positive airway pressure (PAP; continuous [CPAP] or bilevel [BiPAP]) or endotracheal intubation. Noninvasive positive-pressure ventilation improves oxygenation and pulmonary compliance and decreases work of breathing. It may help avoid endotracheal intubation, which may be required in patients with severe hypercapnia, acidosis, and respiratory muscle fatigue.[11]

Initial medical therapy includes intravenous morphine, which acts as a vasodilator and often reduces heart rate. Intravenous loop diuretics, such as furosemide, offer rapid and effective symptom relief. Intravenous vasodilators are very useful, and intravenous nitroglycerin and intravenous nitroprusside are used most commonly. Beta-blockers should be given early to patients with heart failure and ischemic chest pain, hypertension, or tachyarrhythmias. They should be used with caution in patients with severe heart failure and hypotension. Generally, β-blockers should be continued in patients who were taking these drugs prior to their hospitalization. The use of digoxin and calcium channel blocking agents is generally contraindicated in the acute setting.[12]

The goals of acute therapy are to improve symptoms, optimize blood pressure, lower pulmonary capillary wedge pressure, and improve cardiac output. Treatments to reverse or prevent myocardial injury are instituted, and a search for reversible causes of heart failure must occur. Treatment of arrhythmias is essential. Rapid atrial fibrillation is a common problem in patients with acute heart failure. In the Euroheart Failure Study, 9% of patients hospitalized with acute heart failure had atrial fibrillation during the hospitalization, and 42% had a history of paroxysmal atrial fibrillation.[17] Control of the ventricular response to atrial fibrillation is vital, especially in patients with diastolic heart failure. Such control can rapidly be achieved with the use of intravenous β-blockers such as metoprolol and esmolol, or parenteral digoxin; amiodarone can also be useful. Intravenous diltiazem or verapamil can also be used in patients whose left ventricular systolic function is known to be normal or near normal.

Optimization of other comorbidities, including renal function and pulmonary function, is also important. Finally, initiation of guidelines-based therapy for ischemic heart disease and chronic heart failure must be carried out.

Box 30-1

Factors Indicating a Poor Prognosis in Acute Heart Failure

- Hypotension (systolic blood pressure <115 mm Hg on admission)
- Presence of coronary artery disease
- Elevated blood urea nitrogen and serum creatinine
- Hyponatremia
- Lower left ventricular ejection fraction
- Poorer functional capacity
- Elevated serum biomarkers—B-natriuretic peptide, troponin
- Anemia
- Diabetes mellitus

Adapted from Nieminen MS, Bohm M, Cowie MR, et al: Executive Summary of the guidelines on the diagnosis and treatment of acute heart failure: The Task Force on Acute Heart Failure of the European Society of Cardiology. European Heart J 2005;26:384-416.

Prognosis in Acute Heart Failure

Hospitalization for acute heart failure is associated with a poor prognosis. In-hospital mortality is high, with rates reported at 4% to 8%. The mortality is 9% at 60 to 90 days and 29% at 1 year.[11,12] A 90-day rehospitalization rate of 30% is reported. Several factors have been shown to identify patients with a poorer prognosis. They include reduced left ventricular ejection fraction, low blood pressure on admission with systolic blood pressure less than 115 mm Hg, and higher pulmonary capillary wedge pressure. In the U.S. ADHERE study, a database registry of 62,275 patient admissions for heart failure, the three factors that indicated a poor prognosis for patients admitted with decompensation of chronic heart failure were blood urea nitrogen value higher than 43 mg/dL, systolic blood pressure lower than 115 mm Hg, and creatinine level higher than 2.75 mg/dL.[18] The presence of an elevated blood urea nitrogen value was associated with a four-fold increase in hospital mortality to 8.35%. The presence of all three factors yielded an in-hospital mortality of 19.8%.[18] Other factors that have been associated with increased mortality rates are elevation of serum troponin, hyponatremia, and significant elevations of serum BNP (Box 30-1).[12,17]

Coronary Heart Disease and Heart Failure

Coronary artery disease can lead to acute heart failure via a number of different mechanisms. Acute ischemia can lead to elevation of left ventricular filling pressures and diastolic heart failure. Acute ischemia can also cause "stunning," that is, myocardial dysfunction due to severe and prolonged ischemia, which persists even after normal blood flow is restored. Acute MI can result in necrosis of myocardial tissue and acute left ventricular systolic dysfunction through loss of contractile tissue. Complications of MI such as papillary muscle ischemia, infarction and rupture result in acute, severe mitral regurgitation and acute heart failure. Infarction, necrosis, and rupture of the intraventricular septum results in acute heart failure with cardiogenic shock. Chronic ischemia can cause myocardial dysfunction without infarction, a process termed "hibernation." Often, acute myocardial ischemia is superimposed on a ventricle impaired by chronic ischemia and infarction, so that multiple mechanisms are often operative in patients with chronic coronary disease who present in acute heart failure.[11,19]

In a European observational study of acute heart failure complicating acute coronary syndromes (ACSs) in patients without previous history of heart failure, it was noted that 13% of patients with ACS presented with heart failure on admission.[20] An additional 5.6% experienced heart failure later during hospitalization. The incidence of acute heart failure, 15.6%, was identical in patients with ST segment elevation MI and in those with non–ST segment elevation MI. Eight per cent of patients with unstable angina had heart failure. Prognosis for these patients was poor; in-hospital mortality was 12% for patients who had heart failure on admission and 17.8% of those in whom heart failure developed during hospitalization. This represents a three to four times higher mortality than that in patients with ACS who do not have heart failure.

Several important points regarding acute heart failure and ACS must be stressed. Patients may experience acute heart failure even without echocardiographic evidence of significant left ventricular systolic dysfunction and without myocardial enzyme determinations indicating acute necrosis. The majority of patients with ACS and heart failure do not have left ventricular systolic dysfunction at discharge, and only a minority of these patients have chronic heart failure. These patients have not only a high in-hospital mortality but also high morbidity and mortality after discharge, as well as an 8.5% 6-month mortality; 24% of such patients are rehospitalized within 6 months.[19]

Early aggressive pharmacologic and interventional reperfusion strategies are indicated and must be considered in these patients. Immediate treatment should include the use of intravenous diuretics, intravenous nitroglycerin, and β-blocker therapy. Intra-aortic balloon counterpulsation should be used in patients with signs and symptoms of continued ischemia despite aggressive medical therapies. Coronary angiography is indicated to determine the most appropriate reperfusion strategy.[19]

Acute Heart Failure after Myocardial Infarction

In a large registry of 5573 consecutive patients with acute MI, 42% had heart failure or left ventricular systolic dysfunction during hospitalization.[21] These patients tended to be older, were more commonly female, and were more likely to have had previous MI or coronary bypass surgery. Comorbidities were more commonly present, including peripheral arterial disease, hypertension, diabetes mellitus, and previous stroke. In-hospital mortality rate for these patients was 13%, versus 2.3% for patients with acute MI but without heart failure or left ventricular dysfunction. Mortality rate was 13% to 21% for patients with lung congestion and left ventricular ejection fraction less than 40%. Other complications also occurred more commonly in these patients, including atrial and ventricular arrhythmias, re-infarction, and stroke (Figs. 30-3 and 30-4).

In patients with acute heart failure due to acute MI, rapid reperfusion is the cornerstone of therapy. It may be achieved with thrombolytic therapy, acute coronary angioplasty, or urgent coronary artery bypass surgery. In the GRACE study,[20] revascularization therapies were associated with a lower mortality in patients with ACS and acute heart failure.

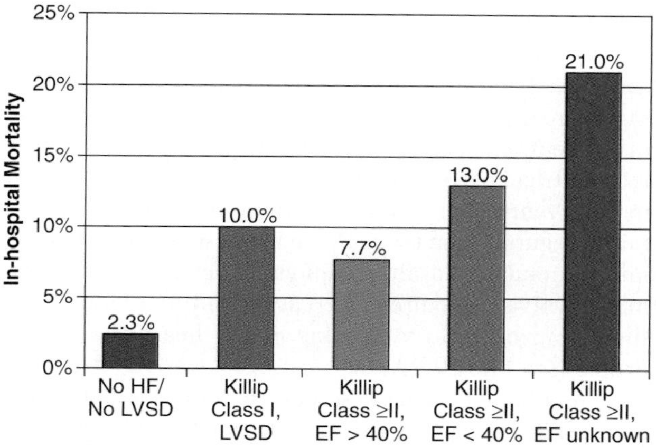

Figure 30-3. In-hospital mortality in patients admitted with acute myocardial infarction, according to presence of heart failure and left ventricular (LV) ejection fraction. EF, ejection fraction; HF, heart failure; Killip class I, patients without evidence of heart failure on physical examination; Killip class II, patients with evidence of heart failure on physical examination; LVSD, LV systolic dysfunction. (Redrawn from Velazquez EJ, Francis GS, Armstrong PW, et al: An international perspective on heart failure and left ventricular systolic dysfunction complicating myocardial infarction: The VALIANT Registry. Eur Heart J 2004;25:1911-1919.)

In patients who have heart failure or significant left ventricular systolic dysfunction (ejection fraction <40%) after MI, a number of pharmacologic therapies have been shown in large placebo-controlled randomized studies to improve mortality and reduce the rate of repeat hospitalization. β-blockers should be part of standard post-MI therapy in these patients. In the CAPRICORN study, a significant 23% relative risk reduction was noted with use of the β-blocker carvedilol.[22] The SAVE study was the first trial to show that the use of an angiotensin-converting enzyme (ACE) inhibitor, captopril, was beneficial in post-MI patients with ejection fractions less than 40%[23]; there was a 5% absolute mortality reduction in 42 months of follow-up. In AIRE, treatment with the ACE inhibitor ramipril, begun 3 to 10 days after MI in patients with post-MI heart failure, resulted in a significant mortality benefit at an average of 15 months of follow-up.[24] Another trial showed that treatment with the ACE inhibitor trandolapril in post-MI patients with ejection fraction less than 35% significantly improved survival at 2 to 4 years of follow-up.[25] Therefore, β-blockers and ACE inhibitors should be started early and continued long term.

The OPTIMAAL study compared the use of the angiotensin receptor blocker losartan with that of captopril in patients with heart failure after MI.[26] There was a nonsignificant reduction in total mortality with the use of captopril. Fewer side effects were associated with the use of losartan. In the VALIANT study, a high dose of the angiotensin receptor blocker valsartan was as effective as an ACE inhibitor in improving survival and reducing cardiovascular morbidity.[27] Thus, angiotensin receptor blockers are recommended in post-MI patients with heart failure who cannot tolerate ACE inhibitors.

Aldosterone blockers have also been shown to be effective in improving prognosis in patients with heart failure or left ventricular dysfunction after MI. These agents are indicated for use in such patients. The EPHESUS study

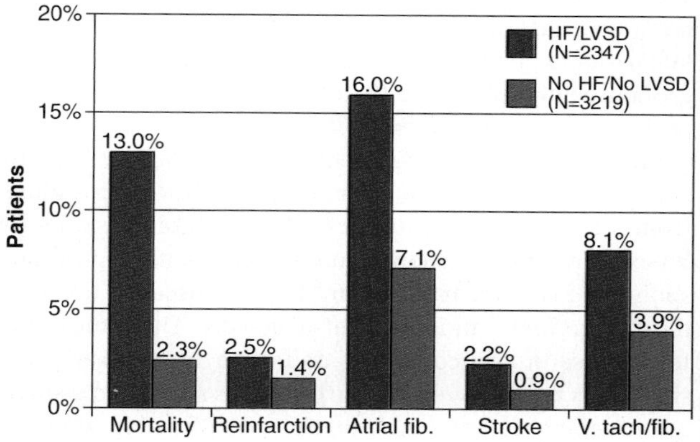

Figure 30-4. In-hospital clinical events among patients with and without heart failure (HF) or left ventricular systolic dysfunction (LVSD) ($P<.001$ for all events except re-infarction). Atrial fib, atrial fibrillation; V. tach/fib, ventricular tachycardia/ventricular fibrillation. (Redrawn from Velazquez EJ, Francis GS, Armstrong PW, et al: An international perspective on heart failure and left ventricular systolic dysfunction complicating myocardial infarction: The VALIANT Registry. Eur Heart J 2004;25:1911-1919.)

showed that eplerenone significantly reduced all cause mortality and repeat hospitalization rates in 16 months of follow-up.[28] Reduction in mortality and sudden cardiac death rates was noted as early as 30 days after initiation of eplerenone therapy.[29]

Acute Myocarditis and Heart Failure

Myocarditis, defined as inflammation of heart muscle, is an uncommon cause of acute heart failure. Severe left ventricular dysfunction and acute heart failure can develop in patients with acute myocarditis. In a minority of cases, myocarditis can manifest as fulminant heart failure and cardiogenic shock, with a high mortality rate.[30,31] A large body of experimental animal data indicates that viral myocarditis leads to activation of immune mechanisms that can also result in chronic dilated cardiomyopathy and chronic heart failure.[30]

An infectious cause of myocarditis is common. Viral agents such as enterovirus and adenovirus have been implicated as causative agents by serologic data and examination of cardiac cell genomes. The protozoa *Trypanosoma cruzi* is the etiologic agent in Chagas' disease, a form of myocarditis endemic in Central and South America that can lead to chronic heart failure. Immune mechanisms are pathogenic in the myocarditis due to giant cell arteritis and the myocarditis associated with progressive systemic sclerosis, systemic lupus erythematosus, and polymyositis.

Myocarditis is a diagnosis made on clinical grounds and should be suspected in patients who present with new-onset heart failure with or without antecedent flulike symptoms. Chest pain may be present. Elevations in leukocyte count, sedimentation rate, and creatinine kinase and troponin levels as well as ECG changes suggestive of myocardial ischemia or infarction may be seen but are not always present. Endomyocardial biopsy may be used to aid diagnosis of myocarditis. However, histologic evidence of both inflammation and myocyte necrosis in biopsy specimens has been very insensitive in making the diagnosis and has a high degree of interobserver variability. For patients in whom myocarditis is suspected on clinical grounds, only 10% to 67% of biopsy results have been positive in reported series.[30,31]

Pharmacologic management of heart failure due to myocarditis is similar to the management of heart failure from other causes. Diuretics, ACE inhibitors, and β-blockers are useful. Many patients experience significant spontaneous improvement in left ventricular function during the first 6 months after diagnosis. The indications for the use of corticosteroids and other immunosuppressive drugs is controversial. Early studies suggested a small improvement in left ventricular ejection fraction with the use of corticosteroids.[32] Other studies suggest targeting immunosuppressive drugs to patients with signs of immune activation.[33] The Myocarditis Treatment Trial showed no significant benefit with immunosuppressive therapy, although there are several problems with the design of this study.[34] On the basis of these studies, we generally recommend a 1- to 3-month trial of corticosteroids and azathioprine in patients with myocarditis and left ventricular dysfunction who do not show spontaneous improvement after 1 to 2 months of conventional heart failure therapies. If the immunosuppressive regimen produces an improvement in ejection fraction, the dosages are tapered over a 6- to 12-month period.[31]

Patients with acute fulminant heart failure and cardiogenic shock may require intravenous vasodilator and inotropic therapy and may be candidates for implantation of a ventricular assist device as a bridge to recovery or transplantation. A number of reported cases of fulminant myocarditis have required mechanical cardiac assistance with ventricular assist devices. When supported aggressively, most patients recover fully to normal ventricular function, and fulminant myocarditis often has a good late prognosis. Therefore, aggressive supportive therapy, including the use of ventricular assist devices, is indicated.[35] Consideration of cardiac transplantation may be necessary for patients who do not show improvement.

CHRONIC LEFT VENTRICULAR SYSTOLIC DYSFUNCTION

Systolic heart failure can be initiated by any one of a number of conditions that damage left ventricular myocardium. This damage leads to a series of systemic maladaptive responses, commonly termed *neurohormonal activation.*[2,36] Two major systems involved in neurohormonal activation are the renin-angiotensin-aldosterone (RAS) system and the sympathetic nervous system.

Activation of the RAS system leads to elevations of renin, angiotensin II, and aldosterone.[36] The effects of these hormones have deleterious consequences for cardiac function. Negative hemodynamic effects include salt and fluid retention, endothelial dysfunction, and vasoconstriction. These agents contribute to a process known as *left ventricular remodeling.*[2,36] In this remodeling, cardiac muscle is affected by myocyte hypertrophy, interstitial fibrosis, and apoptosis (programmed cell death), leading to reduced numbers of myocytes. As a result of remodeling, there is progressive left ventricular dilation, a change in left ventricular geometry, and progressive worsening of left ventricular contractile force. In addition, the change in left ventricular geometry often leads to increasing mitral regurgitation owing to an increase in the size of the mitral annulus and altered physical relationships of the mitral valve structures. Increasing mitral regurgitation then contributes to worsening of the heart failure syndrome (see Fig. 30-2A).

Sympathetic nervous system activation is in part mediated via decreased cardiac output, which results in tachycardia, greater myocardial oxygen consumption, and peripheral vasoconstriction.[37] Renal effects of sympathetic nervous system activation lead to further activation of the RAS system. Higher circulating norepinephrine levels also contribute to myocyte injury and death. Arrhythmias become common. Thus, a detrimental positive feedback loop is established, causing progressive deterioration in left ventricular structure and performance over time. It is clear that these mechanisms are responsible for the progressively worsening nature of chronic heart failure.

The most common causes of chronic systolic heart failure are coronary artery disease, MI, and hypertension. Chronic valvular disease, such as aortic stenosis, aortic insufficiency, and mitral regurgitation, are also common etiologies. Idiopathic dilated cardiomyopathy, familial cardiomyopathy, alcoholic cardiomyopathy, peripartum cardiomyopathy, the chronic phase after acute myocarditis, diabetic cardiomyopathy, and a cardiomyopathy seen in some patients with hyperthyroidism or severe obesity are additional causes.[38-40] Each of these etiologies may demand some specific therapy. However, the medical treatment of chronic systolic heart failure is based on results of many large, randomized, placebo-controlled trials (see later) and is indicated for most causes of this disorder.

When patients are admitted to hospital with acute decompensation of chronic systolic heart failure, the specific reason for a patient's deterioration must be sought and corrected when possible (Box 30-2). Environmental factors such as inadvertent excessive salt and fluid intake or excess alcohol consumption are common. Patient compliance with complicated regimens of multiple medications must be assessed. Emotional and physical stressors should be corrected when feasible.

Box 30-2

Causes of Acutely Decompensated Heart Failure

Environmental Causes
Excess salt and fluid intake
Excess alcohol consumption
Medication noncompliance or misunderstanding
Emotional or physical stress

Adverse Medication Effects
Calcium channel blockers
Antiarrhythmic agents (types 1A, 1C)
Nonsteroidal anti-inflammatory drugs (NSAIDs)
Corticosteroids
Metformin, thiazolidinediones
Cancer chemotherapy

Cardiovascular Conditions
Acute ischemia/infarction
Pulmonary embolism
Uncontrolled hypertension
Arrhythmia
Worsening valvular regurgitation
Endocarditis

Extracardiac Illness
Sepsis, infection, hypoxia
Renal failure, urinary obstruction
Thyroid disease
Anemia, blood loss
Obstructive sleep apnea
Bilateral renal artery stenosis
Worsening of chronic lung disease

Concomitant administration of medications for noncardiac conditions can have detrimental effects. A partial listing includes corticosteroids and nonsteroidal anti-inflammatory drugs (NSAIDs). These can cause fluid retention and can aggravate hypertension. NSAIDs also interfere with the beneficial renal effects of ACE inhibitors and can interfere with the action of loop diuretics.[41] The use of NSAIDs has been reported to raise the risk of hospitalization for heart failure tenfold in patients with a history of heart failure.[14] Metformin and thiazolidinediones can contribute to water retention and aggravate the symptoms and signs of heart failure. Cancer chemotherapies can cause myocardial damage. Cardiac toxicity due to anthracycline chemotherapy is well described. Tyrosine-kinase inhibitors, a newer class of cancer chemotherapy, are also being recognized as agents that can aggravate heart failure and cardiomyopathy.[42] Cardiac medications such as calcium channel blockers and antiarrhythmic drugs can also have direct negative effects on left ventricular contractility. Calcium channel blockers are generally contraindicated in patients admitted with acute decompensated heart failure.[11] Type 1A and type 1C antiarrhythmic drugs are also contraindicated in patients with abnormal left ventricular systolic function.

Acute and chronic extracardiac conditions may also cause heart failure decompensation. Pulmonary embolus, infectious illnesses, and sepsis are common causes. Anemia, blood loss, and thyroid disease must be assessed and corrected. Causes of renal failure are often similar to those of heart failure (e.g., hypertension, vascular disease), and worsening renal function often aggravates heart failure. Obstructive sleep apnea, which can exacerbate heart failure symptoms, can be effectively treated. Influenza and pneumococcal vaccines should be administered to all patients to prevent the cardiac decompensation associated with respiratory infections.

Lastly, coexistent cardiovascular illness can aggravate heart failure. Acute or chronic coronary ischemia should always be suspected, evaluated, and corrected with revascularization strategies when appropriate. Uncontrolled hypertension and cardiac arrhythmias (most commonly, atrial fibrillation and ventricular arrhythmias) frequently accompany left ventricular dysfunction. Worsening valve regurgitation, endocarditis, and bilateral renal artery stenosis are other examples of conditions that can exacerbate heart failure and that are treatable.

Prognosis of Patients Hospitalized with Heart Failure

Despite many advances in heart failure therapy, the prognosis remains poor. Overall, 5-year survival in patients with heart failure is only 50%.[36] In patients for whom heart failure is diagnosed before age 65, men have an 80% 8-year mortality and women a 70% 8-year mortality. Patients hospitalized for treatment of acute decompensated heart failure have a 4% in-hospital mortality,[43] an 11% 30-day mortality, and a 29% 1-year mortality.[13] In a European heart failure database, in-hospital mortality was 6.9%, 12-week readmission rate was 24%, and total mortality at 12 weeks was 13.5%.[44] Recently reported randomized trials of outpatient pharmacologic therapy, reviewed later, show annual mortality rates of approximately 10% in patients with NYHA functional class II to class III heart failure and 20% to 50% annual mortality rates in patients with NYHA class IV disease. Studies of treatment in patients with severe heart failure who are awaiting cardiac transplantation show a 1-year mortality of 75% and 2-year mortality of 92%.[45]

In chronic heart failure, survival relates most closely to severity of left ventricular dysfunction, severity of associated coronary artery disease, and functional class. However, in patients admitted for treatment for decompensated heart failure, short-term prognosis is related most closely to the presence of renal dysfunction, hypotension, myocardial ischemia, and low cardiac output.[43,46]

There is growing recognition that the coexistence of kidney disease significantly worsens the prognosis of patients with heart failure. Kidney disease leads to episodes of volume overload and clinical decompensation. The true prevalence of this "cardio-renal syndrome" is unknown. In up to 50% of patients hospitalized with heart failure, glomerular filtration rate (GFR) drops to less than 60 $mL/min/m^2$, and renal function may worsen in up to 30% of patients admitted with heart failure.[47] Patients with lower left ventricular ejection fractions, lower blood pressure, diabetes mellitus, hypertension, and older age are at higher risk for development of worsening renal function. These patients have longer hospital stays and higher readmission and mortality rates. A meta-analysis of 16 large studies of patients with heart failure showed that 29% of such patients had moderate to severe impairment of renal function. These patients had a more than 100% higher relative mortality risk. Any degree of renal impairment raised the relative mortality risk by approximately 50%.[48] The best treatment strategy for these patients is not clear, because patients with significant renal impairment have generally been excluded from large randomized pharmacologic heart failure trials.

The prognosis for patients who present with heart failure and cardiogenic shock due to acute MI continues to be poor. The in-hospital mortality is 80% to 90% with medical therapy alone, and the rate remains at 40% to 50% even with aggressive supportive therapy and emergency revascularization strategies.[49]

TREATMENT OF ACUTE HEART FAILURE: GENERAL CONSIDERATIONS

Goals for treatment of heart failure can be assessed as either short-term—to reverse acute hemodynamic decompensation in hospitalized patients—or long-term—to prevent rehospitalizations and prolong survival. In patients admitted to the hospital with severe decompensation, short-term goals include improving symptoms by correcting fluid overload and improving hemodynamics, with reduction in pulmonary capillary wedge pressure and an increase in cardiac output. Additional goals are preserving renal function, preventing arrhythmias, and preventing further myocardial necrosis in patients with ischemic and nonischemic disease. Therapies to prevent or attenuate long-term remodeling, which have been shown to improve long-term prognosis, should also be instituted or strengthened while patients are hospitalized.

Long-term goals of therapy include improving symptoms of dyspnea and fatigue and improving exercise tolerance. Treatments shown to reduce mortality must be initiated to decrease the risk of death due to progressive left ventricular failure, reduce the rate of rehospitalization, and lower the risk of sudden arrhythmic death (Box 30-3).

Pharmacologic treatment of heart failure involves combinations of multiple medications. Several drugs have been shown to improve symptoms and functional capacity, decrease the need for repeated hospitalizations, and improve mortality (see later). Therapies are aimed at improving fluid balance as well as reversing the neurohormonal activation responsible for progressive decline in left ventricular function. Pharmacologic agents must be started early in the course of the disease to prevent or attenuate the process of remodeling. Ideally, these therapies are started in the early phase after MI, or when left ventricular dysfunction is first diagnosed, even before the development of clinical symptoms of the heart failure syndrome.

Box 30-3

Goals of Therapy during Hospitalization for Acute Heart Failure

Clinical

- Decreased dyspnea and orthopnea, improved exercise tolerance
- Improved pulmonary function and oxygenation
- Diuresis
- Decreased body fluid weight and edema
- Systolic blood pressure maintained >80 mm Hg

Laboratory

- Normalized serum electrolyte levels
- Optimized renal function
- Decreased serum B-natriuretic peptide levels

Hemodynamics

- Pulmonary capillary wedge pressure <16-18 mm Hg
- Right atrial pressure <8 mm Hg
- Normalized cardiac index

Improve Prognosis

- Treatment of ischemia
- Evidence-based pharmacologic therapy initiated
- Evaluation for use of device therapy (cardiac resynchronization therapy, implantable cardioverter defibrillator)

Adapted from Nieminen MS, Bohm M, Cowie MR, et al: Executive Summary of the guidelines on the diagnosis and treatment of acute heart failure. The Task Force on Acute Heart Failure of the European Society of Cardiology. European Heart J 2005;26:384-416.

The immediate goals of therapy for acute severe heart failure include relieving dyspnea, maximizing improvements in hemodynamic status, and preserving renal function. Therapies should not raise the risk of ischemia, myocyte necrosis, and arrhythmia. Careful serial assessments of patients are mandatory to guide pharmacologic therapy. Signs of heart failure on physical examination are important to monitor, including daily weights, pulmonary rales, the presence of an S_3 gallop, jugular venous pressure, urine output, and pulse oximetry. It is important to note that physical examination findings may be insensitive indicators of hemodynamic status. Tailoring pharmacologic therapy to hemodynamic measurements with use of a pulmonary artery catheter is often helpful and necessary to determine precise baseline measurements of cardiac output and hemodynamic parameters as well as to help guide intensive intravenous drug therapy. Although pulmonary artery pressure monitoring has not been shown to improve prognosis in patients with heart failure, significant adverse effects have also not been demonstrated in such patients.

Aggressive therapy with parenteral vasodilators and diuretics, tailored to an early response in hemodynamic measurements obtained by bedside PA catheter monitoring, has been advocated as an effective method to obtain more rapid and sustained improvement in patients with acute severe heart failure.[50,51] When pulmonary capillary wedge pressure is reduced to less than 16 mm Hg, and right atrial pressure to less than 8 mm Hg, most patients improve both immediately and for the short term during hospitalization. Additional hemodynamic goals include reducing systemic vascular resistance to less than 1200 dynes/sec/cm^{-5}, improving cardiac index to more than 2.6 L/min/m^2, and keeping systolic blood pressure above 80 mm Hg. Pulmonary capillary wedge pressure can be lowered to a normal range of 10 to 12 mm Hg in many patients with significant left ventricular dysfunction, without untoward effects.[50,52]

Improvement in hemodynamics has been obtained with aggressive intravenous vasodilator therapy using intravenous nitroprusside, intravenous nitroglycerin, or nesiritide. The choice of agents depends on matching the specific hemodynamics and clinical picture of the patient's presentation with the predicted effects of each vasodilator.[53-56]

Consecutive patients with severe heart failure were evaluated and classified according to the hemodynamic measurements of PCWP and cardiac index. The patients were described as "dry" when their average pulmonary capillary wedge pressure was less than 17 mm Hg or "wet" when their average pulmonary capillary wedge pressure was 29 mm Hg. The patients were also described as "warm" on the basis of a cardiac index higher than 2.1 L/min/m^2 versus "cold" with a cardiac index less than 1.6 L/min/m^2. The severity of symptoms and physical examination findings did not predict the hemodynamic status as defined by invasive monitoring. In addition, the hemo-dynamic picture did not predict the response to therapy, and survival rates were similar in the four groups. However, the patients with higher cardiac output and lower pulmonary capillary wedge pressures had slightly better outcomes than patients with lower cardiac output and higher pulmonary capillary wedge pressures.[51]

After the initial derangement in hemodynamics has improved with therapy, medical treatments must be instituted and strengthened to try to attain the long-term goals of improvement in cardiac function. Long-term prognosis is directly related to the process of "reverse remodeling," and a lack of a direct relationship between acute hemodynamic status and long-term clinical response has been noted.[17]

PARENTERAL PHARMACOLOGIC MANAGEMENT OF ACUTE HEART FAILURE

Diuretics

Although no randomized clinical trials have been performed, the use of loop diuretics is supported by a long history of clinical success. These agents increase renal excretion of salt and water. The onset of action of intravenous bolus furosemide is 30 minutes, and the action peaks at 1 to 2 hours. The half-life of the medication is 6 hours, so twice-daily dosing is usually required.[41] Other loop diuretics often used are bumetanide and torsemide (Tables 30-2 to 30-4). Patients with chronic heart failure or associated chronic renal insufficiency may exhibit resistance to oral or intravenous bolus loop diuretics. The resistance arises from delayed oral absorption and delivery of a smaller amount of drug to the renal tubule, resulting in lower responsiveness to the drug's diuretic effect. This resistance is associated with a poorer prognosis.[11] Constant delivery of diuretics with intravenous infusions over 8 hours has been shown to result in superior diuresis and natriuresis in comparison with intravenous bolus administration.[57] A low incidence of ototoxicity was seen. Diuretics that act distally in the renal tubule, such as metolazone and the thiazides, or aldosterone blockers

Table 30-2. Loop Diuretics Used for the Treatment of Acute, Severe Heart Failure

Agent	Oral Dose	Initial IV Dose (mg)	Maximum IV Bolus Dose
Bumetanide	0.5-1.0	1.0	4-8
Furosemide	20-40	40	160-200
Torsemide	10-20	10	100-200

IV, intravenous.

Table 30-3. Treatment of Refractory, Diuretic-Resistant Heart Failure

To Loop Diuretic, add:	Dose (mg)
Hydrochlorothiazide	25-50, once or twice daily
or metolazone	2.5-5.0, once or twice daily
or spironolactone	12.5-50, once daily

Table 30-4. Continuous Intravenous (IV) Infusion of Loop Diuretics

Diuretic	Dose
Bumetanide	1 mg IV load then 0.5-2 mg/hour infusion
Furosemide	40 mg IV load then 10-40 mg/hour infusion
Torsemide	20 mg IV load then 5-20 mg/hour infusion

Adapted from Nieminen MS, Bohm M, Cowie MR, et al: Executive Summary of the guidelines on the diagnosis and treatment of acute heart failure. The Task Force on Acute Heart Failure of the European Society of Cardiology. European Heart J 2005;26:384-416.

such as spironolactone, can be added.[1] Hypokalemia, alkalosis, and hypomagnesemia are common side effects of loop diuretics and can potentiate the occurrence of arrhythmias. Electrolyte levels must be carefully monitored during aggressive diuretic therapy.

Diuretics often worsen renal function by altering renal hemodynamics. Some azotemia may need to be accepted to obtain adequate relief of dyspnea and edema. High-dose diuretics may potentiate activation of the RAS system. The dose of loop diuretics should be titrated to the response of patient's symptoms and should be reduced as symptoms improve.

Vasopressin Inhibitors

The use of novel diuretics, the vasopressin inhibitors, is currently being evaluated in clinical trials in the setting of acute heart failure.[58] Vasopressin is a hormone synthesized in the hypothalamus; its major effect is to control free water clearance. It acts through V1a receptors in vascular smooth muscle and myocardium, leading to peripheral and coronary vasoconstriction, myocyte hypertrophy, and positive inotropy. Vasopressin also acts through V2 receptors at the renal tubule collecting ducts to cause free water retention and hyponatremia. Levels of vasopressin are higher in patients with chronic heart failure, and higher vasopressin levels correlate with more severe heart failure. Vasopressin release is stimulated by changes in serum osmolality and cardiac output[59] and leads to vasoconstriction and retention of free water. Inhibition of vasopressin's effects would have theoretical benefits in patients with heart failure.[60] Contrary to the widely used loop diuretics, vasopressin inhibitors theoretically would not cause hypotension or neurohormonal activation and would not aggravate cardiac arrhythmias due to electrolyte depletion.

Three vasopressin antagonists are currently being studied. Conivaptan inhibits V1a and V2 receptors. Tolvaptan and lixivaptan are selective for the V2 receptor. The effects of these medications are increased urine volume and free water excretion, with less sodium loss and therefore a rise in the serum sodium concentration.

The use of conivaptan in patients with NYHA functional class III to class IV heart failure was associated with an increase in urine output and decreases in pulmonary capillary wedge pressure and right atrial pressure without changes in cardiac output.[14] Oral use of tolvaptan was associated with fluid loss and diuresis without change in heart rate, blood pressure, or serum creatinine level. In a small study, tolvaptan had no adverse consequences for renal hemodynamics and resulted in higher renal blood flow than furosemide. There was no depletion of other electrolytes when tolvaptan was used in patients with acute decompensated heart failure.[59] Significant diuresis and weight loss were observed during the first 24 hours. A rise in serum sodium concentration and improvement in hyponatremia were noted within 1 day after treatment with tolvaptan and lixi-vaptan.[60] Long-term results regarding mortality and effects on ventricular remodeling and renal function are pending.

Parenteral Vasodilators

Nitroglycerin

Intravenous nitroglycerin is an effective systemic and coronary vasodilator. It is very useful in heart failure due to acute coronary ischemia, because it improves coronary blood flow. Intravenous nitroglycerin is effective at lowering preload and pulmonary capillary wedge pressure, thereby reducing pulmonary congestion without increasing oxygen demand. It is also an arterial dilator at high doses but is less effective than nitroprusside at reducing afterload. Dosage ranges between 5 and 200 μg/min. A major limitation of the use of intravenous nitroglycerin is the rapid development of tolerance to the drug's effect, which often occurs after only 24 hours of therapy. Thus, having a "nitrate-free" period during the daily dosage regimen is often required to limit the development of tolerance. Oral or topical nitrates are often added to β-blocker and ACE inhibitor therapy in the patient with chronic heart failure if blood pressure allows.

Nitroprusside

Intravenous sodium nitroprusside is a powerful venous and arterial dilator. It is a drug of choice for treating both hypertension-related heart failure with pulmonary edema and severe heart failure due to acute mitral regurgitation. This drug causes a significant reduction of afterload and preload, leading to decreases in right atrial pressure, systemic vascular resistance, mean systemic blood pressure, and pulmonary capillary wedge pressure and a higher cardiac index in patients with heart failure and left ventricular dysfunction. Limitations of nitroprusside include inducing a coronary "steal" syndrome in patients with active coronary ischemia.[41] In addition, toxic metabolites can accumulate with more prolonged administration of nitroprusside; in patients with significant hepatic dysfunction, thiocyanate levels rise, and in patients with renal dysfunction, cyanide is generated. The use of nitroprusside requires hospitalization in the ICU and invasive monitoring with a PA catheter and arterial line. Dosage range is 0.3 to 5.0 μg/kg/min.

Angiotensin-Converting Enzyme Inhibitors

ACE inhibitors are of limited usefulness as parenteral therapy in patients with acute severe heart failure in the urgent setting. Enalaprilat is an intravenous bolus formulation that can be used in patients with chronic heart failure who have been taking oral ACE inhibitors long term and who are now unable to take oral medication. The maximal action occurs in 1 to 4 hours after administration, with a 6-hour duration of action.

Inotropic Drugs, Inodilators, and Vasopressors

Table 30-5 compares the hemodynamics of parenteral vasodilators and inotropic agents.

Dobutamine

Dobutamine is a potent β_1 agonist. It also has β_2- and α-agonist properties. Its major effect is increased myocardial contractility. It also has venodilator properties. At doses of 2.5 to 15 μg/kg/min, dobutamine lowers systemic vascular resistance and pulmonary capillary wedge pressure. This agent also causes a slight rise in heart rate and improves cardiac output. It increases myocardial oxygen demand. Higher doses are associated with vasoconstriction.

A limitation of dobutamine use is that in patients with heart failure, β-adrenergic receptors may be chronically downregulated, limiting its hemodynamic effects. In addition, dobutamine leads to increased myocardial oxygen demand and oxygen consumption, which is detrimental in patients who have active coronary ischemia or have had MI. Higher rates of ventricular arrhythmias have been associated with dobutamine use.[61] In addition, tolerance to dobutamine effects has been demonstrated in patients with infusions lasting more than 24 hours, theoretically as a result of induction of β-adrenergic receptor downregulation.[62]

Milrinone

Milrinone inhibits the action of phosphodiesterase in the myocyte, leading to increased intracellular cyclic adenosine monophosphate (cAMP) and calcium. It is an inotropic agent that acts downstream from the β-adrenergic receptor. Hemodynamic effects include reductions in mean right atrial pressure as well as pulmonary and systemic vascular resistances. When milrinone is given to a patient with heart failure, stroke volume and cardiac output are increased with a slight fall in mean systemic arterial pressure. Milrinone acts as a coronary vasodilator, and there is no net increase in myocardial oxygen consumption. Milrinone tends to lower arterial blood pressure and pulmonary capillary wedge pressure more than dobutamine and has a more prolonged action. There is no tolerance or attenuation of its effect. Milrinone is started as a bolus dose, 50 to 75 μg/kg, with a maintenance infusion of 0.375 to 0.75 μg/kg/min. Doses must be reduced in patients with renal failure. The use of milrinone is limited in patients with hypotension.

Dopamine

The effects of dopamine include increasing renal blood flow at low doses (1-5 μg/kg/min), increasing myocardial contractility and chronotropy through stimulation of β-adrenergic receptors (doses of 3-7 μg/kg/min) and vasoconstriction at higher doses (5-20 μg/kg/min).[61] Dopamine is less useful for treatment of heart failure because its effects result in tachycardia, coronary vasoconstriction, and increases in afterload and oxygen consumption. Dobutamine generally causes a greater rise in cardiac output than dopamine. Dopamine can be used when significant hypotension is part of the hemodynamic picture

Table 30-5. A Comparison of Hemodynamic Effects of Parenteral Vasodilators and Inotropic Agents

	Nitroprusside	Nesiritide	Dobutamine	Milrinone
Mechanism of action	Balanced vasodilator	Vasodilator, natriuretic	β_1-adrenergic receptor stimulator	Phosphodiesterase inhibitor
Heart rate	—	—	Slight ↑	Slight ↑
Arrhythmia	—	—	+	+
Mean right atrial pressure	↓	↓	↓	↓↓
Left ventricular end-diastolic pressure	↓↓	↓↓	↓	↓↓
Mean arterial pressure	↓	↓	—	↓
Systemic vascular resistance	↓↓	↓↓	↓	↓↓
Cardiac index	↑	↑	↑↑	↑↑
dP/dt (inotropy)	—	—	↑↑	↑
Hypotension	+	+	Occasionally	+
Direct Na^+ excretion	—	+	—	—
Other considerations	Increased cyanide and thiocyanate levels with prolonged infusion	Serum B-natriuretic peptide level cannot be followed during infusion	Difficult to use in patients receiving long-term β-blocker therapy	More vasodilator response at higher doses

—, minimal or no effect; +, positive effect; ↑ or ↓, mild increase or decrease, respectively; ↑↑ or ↓↓, moderate increase or decrease, respectively.

and arterial pressure must be restored for adequate end-organ perfusion. Although dopamine at low doses is frequently used as an add-on to inotropic agents in an attempt to increase renal blood flow and augment diuresis, no controlled trials have demonstrated dopamine's usefulness in this setting. No significant benefit of "renal dose dopamine" has been shown in preventing acute renal failure in high-risk patients or in the treatment of established renal failure.[62]

Norepinephrine

Norepinephrine is a sympathomimetic agent with strong α-agonist and weak β-agonist effects. In patients with heart failure, norepinephrine's main effect is to raise blood pressure by increasing systemic vascular resistance with little effect on cardiac output. It also increases myocardial oxygen demand. The use of norepinephrine in the setting of heart failure is restricted to patients with the most severe hypotension that is unresponsive to dopamine and to patients with complicating illnesses such as sepsis.[62] Norepinephrine therapy should be tapered and then discontinued as early as possible. Dosage range is 0.2 to 1 μg/kg/min.

Use of Inotropic Agents

Inotropic drugs are used for patients with persistent hypotension, low cardiac index, and signs of end-organ hypoperfusion. The choice of agent depends on the specific clinical circumstances.[63,64] Dobutamine tends to cause a slight rise in heart rate and has little effect on mean arterial pressure, whereas milrinone often lowers systemic arterial pressure because of its more prominent lowering of systemic vascular resistance.[54,55] Patients who show no response to dobutamine may have a favorable response to milrinone. In the setting of acute heart failure, milrinone, with its more potent vasodilator properties, is used more often than dobutamine. In addition, its effects are not primarily mediated through β-adrenergic receptors, an important consideration in patients receiving concomitant β-blocker therapy.

Several studies have compared vasodilator with inotropic therapy or milrinone with placebo. The use of intravenous inotropic therapy in the form of a 48-hour infusion of milrinone was evaluated as routine therapy in patients admitted with NYHA class III to class IV heart failure when inotropic therapy was judged not to be essential.[65] Compared with standard therapy without milrinone, the addition of milrinone resulted in no improvement in symptom relief, hospital length of stay, or rate of rehospitalization within 60 days. Milrinone was associated with an increased incidence of hypotension and atrial arrhythmias. Thus, milrinone and other inotropic agents are not indicated for routine use in patients with decompensated heart failure.

In the FIRST study of patients with NYHA class III to class IV heart failure, a 14-day average dobutamine infusion was associated with an *increased* risk of morbid events and higher short-term mortality. In patients listed for transplant, with baseline systolic blood pressures less than 100 mm Hg and ejection fractions less than 20%, 12-hour per day infusions of dobutamine and nitroprusside given over an average of 20 days were compared; nitroprusside yielded better relief of symptoms and longer survival.[66] A study of oral milrinone in patients with class IV heart failure was associated with a 53% *increased* risk of mortality compared with placebo.[62] No clinical studies have shown improved short-term or medium-term outcomes with inotropic therapy. The use of inotropic agents has been consistently associated with a *worse* prognosis for survival.[41] These negative outcomes with inotropic agents are believed to be related to their propensity to stimulate sympathetic nervous system activation, thereby raising myocardial oxygen demand, exacerbating serious cardiac arrhythmias, increasing myocardial ischemia, and furthering myocyte loss. Stimulation of chronic hibernating myocardium may also result in myonecrosis.

The use of inotropic agents is not routine and is now restricted to short-term therapy (i.e., less than 72 hours) in patients with severe heart failure and problematic hypotension or critical end-organ hypoperfusion. Clinical examples of situations in which inotropic agents may be useful include cardiogenic shock due to acute MI or right ventricular MI, patients awaiting cardiac transplantation, and patients with end-stage heart failure. According to current ACC/AHA guidelines for the evaluation and management of chronic heart failure, long-term intermittent infusions of a positive inotropic drug as standard therapy for symptomatic systolic dysfunction is *contraindicated.*[1] Continuous intravenous infusion of an inotropic drug can be recommended for palliation of symptoms in patients with refractory end-stage heart failure. In this setting, quality of remaining life takes precedence over prolongation of life. These patients will have been deemed poor candidates for cardiac transplantation or ventricular assist devices. The decision to use inotropic agents in this circumstance is one that should be carefully individualized.

Nesiritide (B-Natriuretic Peptide)

BNP is a hormone produced by ventricular and atrial myocytes in response to stretch from cardiac chamber dilatation. Its effects are counter to those of the RAS system. It causes venous and arterial dilation, coronary vasodilatation, natriuresis, and diuresis. Human BNP can be manufactured by recombinant DNA technology and is available as an intravenous medication, nesiritide, for heart failure therapy. Its hemodynamic effects include rapid reduction in pulmonary capillary wedge pressure and mean right atrial pressure, which were found to exceed the effects of intravenous nitroglycerin in direct comparison.[53] Unlike sympathomimetic drugs, nesiritide is not pro-arrhythmic and does not induce tolerance.[67] It can potentiate the effects of loop diuretics. Some patients show no response to nesiritide, and significant hypotension may limit its use in other patients.[41] Because the hypotensive effects of nesiritide are less marked than nitroprusside, nesiritide can be used without invasive hemodynamic monitoring and can be initiated in emergency department settings. Nesiritide is initiated as an intravenous bolus dose of 2 μg/kg followed by infusion of 0.01 μg/kg/min. When compared with dobutamine in patients with severe heart failure, nesiritide infusion was associated with less tachycardia and ventricular arrhythmia.[61] In another study, there was a trend toward improved survival with nesiritide,[68] and mortality and rehospitalization rates at 6 months have been found to be lower with nesiritide.[67]

A review of multicenter randomized controlled trials of the use of nesiritide in patients with acute decompensated heart failure, however, has raised questions about the drug's safety. A meta-analysis of three randomized trials of nesiritide suggests a slight increase in mortality in patients given nesiritide versus a placebo control group. Eight hundred sixty-two patients were involved, and 30-day mortality with nesiritide was 7.2%, versus 4.0% in control patients (relative risk ratio = 1.74; $P = .056$).[69] There is a concern that this result may be mediated through an adverse effect on renal function, because 21% of patients given nesiritide experienced worsening renal function compared with 15% of the control group.[70] However, a retrospective review of patients receiving intravenous vasoactive medications for acute heart failure indicated mortality rates, adjusted for clinical variables, were equivalent for patients receiving nitroglycerin and those receiving nesiritide. Patients who received intravenous nesiritide or intravenous nitroglycerin had a lower in-hospital mortality rate than those who received dobutamine or milrinone.[71]

A special panel convened to review the safety of nesiritide recommended that the agent be used only in patients admitted to hospital with acute decompensated heart failure and dyspnea at rest. This medication should not be used to replace diuretics, to enhance renal function, or to improve diuresis. It should not be used as an intermittent infusion in an outpatient setting. Additional controlled trials evaluating the use of nesiritide were strongly recommended.[72]

In summary, nesiritide effectively relieves dyspnea and reduces left ventricular filling pressures. It may be safer than the inotropic agents milrinone and dobutamine. Further study is needed to evaluate nesiritide's effect on mortality.

Ultrafiltration

A new approach to the treatment of acute heart failure uses mechanical ultrafiltration. This process removes iso-osmolar extracellular fluid via a convection process.[73] Newer ultrafiltration systems use peripheral arm veins, and central venous access is not required. In a study of 40 patients admitted with heart failure, usual care for heart failure with diuretic therapy was compared with a combination of usual care and ultrafiltration. At 24 hours, average fluid loss with diuretic therapy was 2838 mL, compared with 4650 mL for therapy plus ultrafiltration. Weight loss and improvement in dyspnea were similar in the two therapy groups. Ultrafiltration was not associated with significant changes in heart rate or blood pressure.[74] In another study, 20 patients with acute decompensated heart failure with renal insufficiency and diuretic resistance were treated with an 8-hour course of ultrafiltration. Over 24 hours, an average of 8650 mL of fluid was removed, with an average weight loss of 6 kg during hospitalization. Renal function remained stable, and there was no associated hypotension.[73]

Ultrafiltration offers the potential for rapid and safe removal of fluid and sodium without the negative consequences of electrolyte imbalance, change in renal blood flow, and neurohormonal activation associated with conventional diuretic therapy. Further improvements in the technology as well as further studies will determine whether this therapy has a place in the routine management of acute heart failure.

LONG-TERM PHARMACOLOGIC THERAPY FOR CHRONIC SEVERE HEART FAILURE

Diuretics

Loop diuretics are routinely used in patients with signs or symptoms of fluid retention.[1] Diuretics are continued once patients are euvolemic to prevent reaccumulation of fluid. A flexible dosing schedule, based on daily weights and close telephone contact with a heart failure treatment team member, can be very effective in maintaining a euvolemic state while reducing the frequency of the side effects of diuretics.[50]

Furosemide is the most common loop diuretic used. Bumetanide or torsemide may be helpful in patients with suboptimal responses to furosemide, owing to their more consistent absorption after oral administration.[50,75] Metolazone or a thiazide diuretic can be used in addition to a loop diuretic in patients with more severe heart failure for the synergistic effects. Patients must be periodically monitored for side effects of these agents, including azotemia, hypokalemia, alkalosis, hyponatremia, and hypomagnesemia (Table 30-6).

β-Blockers

Catecholamine levels are higher in heart failure, and higher levels correlate with worse disease severity. Catecholamines have direct negative effects on the myocardium, including induction of myocyte hypertrophy and apoptosis.[37] Clinically, these effects are evident as left ventricular dilation, greater ischemia, higher peripheral vasoconstriction, and cardiac arrhythmia.

β-Blockers interfere with catecholamine-mediated activation of cardiac β-adrenergic receptors, thereby attenuating β-adrenergic receptor–mediated increases in heart rate and oxygen consumption. Effects on remodeling mediated by the sympathetic nervous system can be prevented or attenuated. In addition, the newer agent carvedilol blocks β-adrenergic receptors and also α-adrenergic receptors, which mediate vasoconstriction and increased cardiac contractility.

Several large trials using β-blockers in thousands of patients with chronic heart failure and in post-MI patients with ejection fractions below 40% have demonstrated significant and consistent reductions in the need for rehospitalization for heart failure. Mortality rates are also significantly improved. The BHAT study showed a relative

Table 30-6. Oral Diuretics Recommended for Use in the Treatment of Fluid Retention in Chronic Heart Failure

Drug	Initial Daily Dose(s)	Maximum Total Daily Dose	Duration of Action
Loop Diuretics			
Bumetanide	0.5-1.0 mg once or twice	10 mg	4-6 hours
Furosemide	20-40 mg once or twice	600 mg	6-8 hours
Torsemide	10-20 mg once	200 mg	12-16 hours
Thiazide Diuretics			
Chlorothiazide	250-500 mg once or twice	1000 mg	6-12 hours
Chlorthalidone	12.5-25 mg once	100 mg	24-72 hours
Hydrochlorothiazide	25 mg once or twice	200 mg	6-12 hours
Indapamide	2.5 mg once	5 mg	36 hours
Metolazone	2.5 mg once	20 mg	12-24 hours
Potassium-Sparing Diuretics			
Amiloride	5 mg once	20 mg	24 hours
Spironolactone	12.5-25 mg once	50 mg*	2-3 days
Triamterene	50-75 mg once	200 mg	7-9 hours

*Higher doses may occasionally be used with close monitoring of serum creatinine and potassium levels.
Adapted from Hunt S, Abraham WT, Chin M, et al: ACC/AHA 2005 Guideline Update for the Diagnosis and Management of Chronic Heart Failure in the Adult—Summary Article. A report on the American College of Cardiology/American Heart Association Task Force on Practice Guidelines (Writing Committee to Update the 2001 Guidelines for Evaluation and Management of Heart Failure): Developed in collaboration with the American College of Chest Physicians and the International Society of Heart and Lung Transplantation: Endorsed by the Heart Rhythm Society. Circulation 2005;112:1825-1852.

26% reduction in mortality at 2 years in post-MI patients treated with propranolol.[76,77] The CIBIS II trial, using bisoprolol, showed a 34% relative risk reduction in hospitalizations and mortality at 16 months of therapy.[78] The MERIT-HF study showed a relative reduction of 33% in these end points at 12 months with the use of metoprolol succinate.[79] Patients with more severe heart failure, symptom class III to class IV, with severely reduced ejection fractions (<25%) were studied in the COPERNICUS trial.[80] These patients began therapy with carvedilol in the hospital. At 10.4 months of follow-up, a 35% relative mortality reduction was seen, with improvement in mortality beginning as early as 3 weeks after initiation of therapy (Fig. 30-5). In these trials, β-blockers were not discontinued more frequently than placebo for perceived side effects, and there was no higher risk of heart failure exacerbation with β-blocker therapy than with placebo, even in the early phases of drug administration.[80,81] Several trials with carvedilol have shown an approximate 6% absolute increase in left ventricular ejection fraction after a minimum of 2 years of therapy.[82]

β-Blocker therapy should be instituted for treatment of patients with left ventricular dysfunction, even in the absence of symptoms (ACC/AHA stage B). In patients with heart failure due to systolic dysfunction, β-blockers should be instituted early once patients are deemed euvolemic and the dosage should be titrated up to maximal recommended doses (e.g., metoprolol succinate 200 mg daily or carvedilol 25 mg bid) or maximally tolerated doses. These agents are useful in patients with ischemic and nonischemic cardiomyopathy. β-Blockers should be instituted in "compensated" patients as well, in whom there is a high likelihood of disease progression to symptomatic heart failure within 12 months. This therapy is indicated to be combined with ACE inhibitors in all patients with chronic systolic dysfunction.

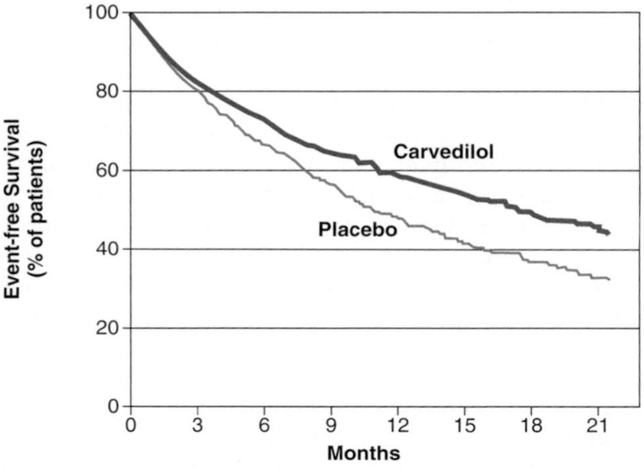

No. of Patients at Risk

Placebo	1133	767	513	377	262	154	88	55
Carvedilol	1156	789	559	431	318	208	122	81

Figure 30-5. All-cause mortality in patients with class III to class IV heart failure, ejection fraction <25%, demonstrating significant survival benefit with carvedilol. (Redrawn from Packer M, Coats A, Fowler M, et al: Effect of carvedilol on survival in severe chronic heart failure. N Engl J Med 2001;344:1651-1658.)

Angiotensin-Converting Enzyme Inhibitors

ACE inhibitors act to decrease the effects of RAS system activation by blocking the conversion of angiotensin I to angiotensin II, thus counteracting the deleterious effects of angiotensin II and aldosterone. Many studies have shown benefits of ACE inhibitor therapy in post-MI patients as well as patients with cardiomyopathy and heart failure. The SOLVD trial, using enalapril in patients with class II to class III heart failure and ejection fractions lower than 35%, showed a 10% relative risk reduction in mortality at 3.5 years.[83] Enalapril given to patients less ill, with asymptomatic left ventricular dysfunction (ejection fractions <35%), in the companion SOLVD trial showed a reduction in the clinical diagnosis of heart failure and a statistically significant reduction in hospitalizations for heart failure at 3 years.[84] A meta-analysis of 32 trials involving 7105 patients and using captopril, enalapril, ramipril, quinapril, or lisinopril found that ACE inhibitors reduce the risk of death and hospitalization due to heart failure.[85] These results indicate that the positive effects of ACE inhibitors are likely to be a class effect rather than specific to a particular agent.

Side effects of these agents include cough, worsening renal function in patients with underlying renal disease or renal artery stenosis, angioneurotic edema, and hyperkalemia. The dose of ACE inhibitors should be increased as renal function and blood pressure allow. Studies have shown that medium doses of ACE inhibitors, compared with low doses, significantly reduce hospitalization rates for heart failure. However, higher doses given routinely do not significantly reduce cardiovascular events further.[86] Additional improvement in symptoms and mortality is thus best achieved by adding β-blocker therapy rather than increasing ACE inhibitor therapy to the highest doses.[87]

In a study of patients older than 65 years who had class II to class III chronic heart failure with an ejection fraction less than 35%, the importance of beginning heart failure therapy with either an ACE inhibitor or a β-blocker was studied. The primary end point was time to death or hospitalization for heart failure. Initiation of the β-blocker bisoprolol was not inferior to the strategy of starting therapy with the ACE inhibitor enalapril. There was also no difference in safety.[88]

Angiotensin Receptor Blockers

Angiotensin receptor blockers (ARBs) work to counter the effects of angiotensin II at the tissue level by blocking angiotensin II receptors. Multiple studies have shown benefits of these medications in patients with heart failure. Large numbers of patients in controlled trials have been studied, and these drugs have been as well studied as the ACE inhibitors. Most often, ARBs were used as a substitute for ACE inhibitors. More recently, they have been evaluated as medications given in combination with ACE inhibitors and β-blockers.

The RESOLVD trial, using candesartan in patients with heart failure and a mean ejection fraction of 27%, showed equivalent mortality rates and similar exercise tolerance and functional class to those of patients treated with enalapril at 3.5 years.[89] ELITE II, a study comparing losartan with captopril in patients with ejection fractions lower than 40%, showed no difference in mortality or congestive heart failure admissions. Losartan was better tolerated because of the lower incidence of problematic cough.[90] The ValHeft 2001 study showed that valsartan as a substitute for ACE inhibitor therapy was associated with a relative 33% risk reduction in mortality in comparison with placebo. A worse mortality was seen for use of valsartan in patients who were already taking both ACE inhibitors and β-blockers, but the small number of patients in this subgroup made conclusions somewhat suspect.[91] In CHARM, candesartan was prescribed for patients with ejection fractions lower than 40%. A 17.5% relative risk reduction in cardiovascular death and congestive heart failure admissions was seen when this ARB was used as a substitute for ACE inhibitors (Fig. 30-6).[92] When candesartan was added to therapy with ACE inhibitors and β-blockers, a 10% relative risk reduction was seen. Significant improvement in outcome and no increase in mortality were demonstrated when this ARB was added to standard therapy,[93] contradicting the findings of ValHeft 2001.

In conclusion, ARBs are an appropriate choice for patients who cannot be maintained on ACE inhibitors because of side effects such as cough. Patients with angioneurotic edema during ACE inhibitor therapy can often be successfully treated with ARBs without experiencing this complication.[94,95] Adding ARBs to ACE inhibitor and β-blocker therapy likely achieves a small additional benefit.

Aldosterone Antagonists

Aldosterone antagonists work to counteract the salt and water retention caused by aldosterone. In addition, this hormone is believed to be involved in the progressive myocardial fibrosis that occurs in the remodeling process. In the RALES trial, the aldosterone antagonist spironolactone was given to patients with class III to class IV heart failure with ejection fraction lower than 35%. A 24% relative risk reduction in mortality was seen in treated patients over 2 years, with reductions in rates of cardiovascular death and need for rehospitalization (Fig. 30-7).[96] Thus the use of these agents is effective in improving outcomes in patients with functional class III to class IV

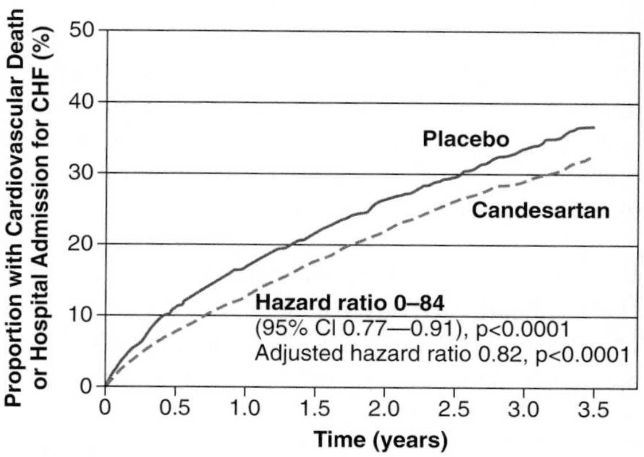

Number at Risk

Candesartan	3803	3563	3271	2215	761
Placebo	3796	3464	3170	2157	743

Figure 30-6. Candesartan was shown to improve outcomes in patients with congestive heart failure (CHF) who were intolerant to angiotensin-converting enzyme inhibitor therapy. CI, confidence interval. (Redrawn from Pfeffer MA, Swedberg K, Granger CB, et al: Effects of candesartan on mortality and morbidity in patients with chronic heart failure: The CHARM-Overall programme. Lancet 2003;362:759-766.)

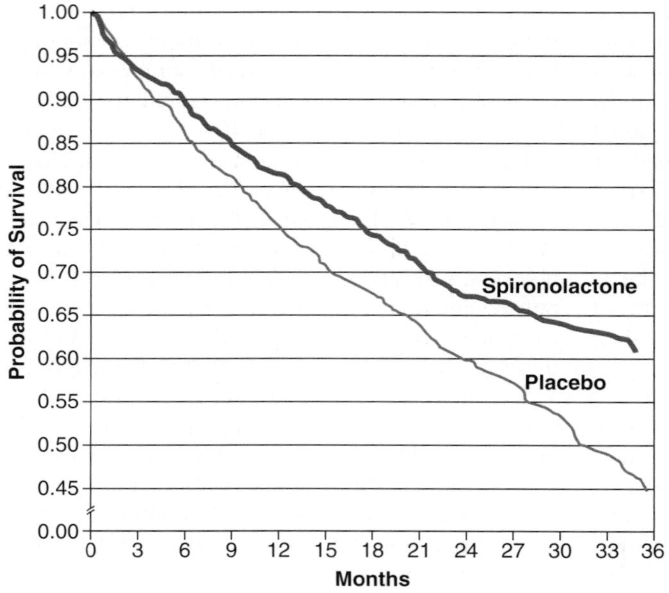

No. at Risk

Placebo	841	775	723	678	628	592	565	483	379	280	179	92	36
Spironolactone	822	766	739	698	669	639	608	526	419	316	193	122	43

Figure 30-7. Kaplan-Meier analysis of the probability of survival among patients in the placebo group and patients in the spironolactone group, treated for class III to class IV heart failure and left ventricular dysfunction. The risk of death was 30% lower among patients in the spironolactone group than among patients in the placebo group (*P*<.001). (Redrawn from Pitt B, Zannad F, Remme W, et al: The effect of spironolactone on morbidity and mortality in patients with severe heart failure. N Engl J Med 1999;341:709-717.)

heart failure. These medications are contraindicated in patients with renal insufficiency and serum creatinine levels higher than 2.5 mg/dL and in patients with baseline serum potassium levels higher than 5.0 mmol/L.

An analysis of a large Canadian health care database showed a substantial rise in the frequency of spironolactone use after the RALES study was published. This greater use was temporally associated with a two to three times higher rate of hospitalization for hyperkalemia.[97] The researchers reporting these findings stressed the need for careful monitoring of serum electrolytes after aldosterone antagonist therapy is initiated. Aldosterone antagonists should be reserved for patients with severe, symptomatic left ventricular systolic dysfunction. They should not be used in patients with preexisting hyperkalemia, which may be present in patients treated with ACE inhibitors. Spironolactone should be initiated at low doses, such as 12.5 mg daily or every other day, especially in elderly patients (Table 30-7).

Combination Hydralazine with Isosorbide Dinitrate

Combination therapy with the vasodilators hydralazine and isosorbide dinitrate (ISDN) was associated with lower mortality than placebo in one study conducted prior to the advent of ACE inhibitors and β-blocker therapy for heart failure.[98] A retrospective analysis of this study suggested that African-American patients may have benefited preferentially. More recently, the A-Heft study enrolled more than 1000 self-described black patients with class II to class IV heart failure and ejection fractions lower than 45%.[99] The use of the combination of hydralazine and ISDN, titrated to a dose of 75 mg hydralazine plus 40 mg ISDN given three times daily, was associated with a 40% relative risk reduction in mortality at 10 months and a

Table 30-7. Inhibitors of the Renin-Aldosterone System and β-Blockers Commonly Used for the Treatment of Patients with Heart Failure and Low Ejection Fraction

Drug	Initial Daily Dose(s)	Maximum Dose(s)
Angiotensin-Converting Enzyme Inhibitors		
Captopril	6.25 mg 3 times	50 mg 3 times
Enalapril	2.5 mg twice	10-20 mg twice
Fosinopril	5-10 mg once	40 mg once
Lisinopril	2.5-5 mg once	20-40 mg once
Perindopril	2 mg once	8-16 mg once
Quinapril	5 mg twice	20 mg twice
Ramipril	1.25-2.5 mg once	10 mg once
Trandolapril	1 mg once	4 mg once
Angiotensin Receptor Blockers		
Candesartan	4-8 mg once	32 mg once
Losartan	25-50 mg once	50-100 mg once
Valsartan	20-40 mg twice	160 mg twice
Aldosterone Antagonists		
Spironolactone	12.5-25 mg once	25 mg once or twice
Eplerenone	25 mg once	50 mg once
β-Blockers		
Bisoprolol	1.25 mg once	10 mg once
Carvedilol	3.125 mg twice	25 mg twice (50 mg twice for patients >85 kg)
Metoprolol succinate extended-release	12.5-25 mg once	200 mg once

Adapted from Hunt S, Abraham WT, Chin M, et al: ACC/AHA 2005 Guideline Update for the Diagnosis and Management of Chronic Heart Failure in the Adult—Summary Article. A report on the American College of Cardiology/American Heart Association Task Force on Practice Guidelines (Writing Committee to Update the 2001 Guidelines for Evaluation and Management of Heart Failure): Developed in collaboration with the American College of Chest Physicians and the International Society of Heart and Lung Transplantation: Endorsed by the Heart Rhythm Society. Circulation 2005;112:1825-1852.

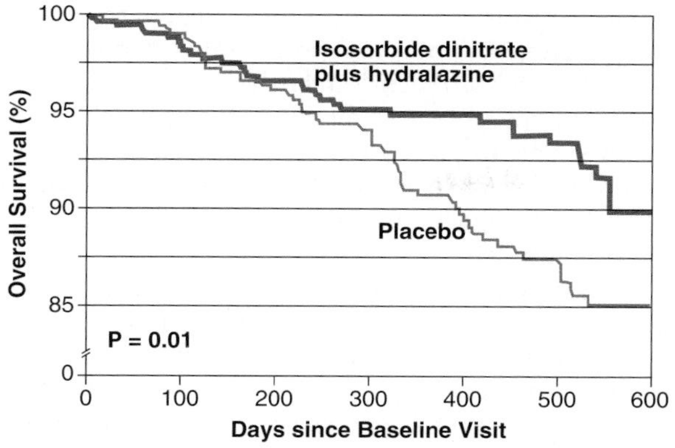

No. at Risk

Placebo	532	466	401	340	285	232	24
Isosorbide dinitrate plus hydralazine	518	463	407	359	313	251	13

Figure 30-8. Significant mortality benefit is seen with the use of a combination of isosorbide dinitrate with hydralazine in black patients with heart failure and left ventricular ejection fraction less than 45%. (Redrawn from Taylor AL, Zieche S, Yancy C, et al: Combination of isosorbide dinitrate and hydralazine in blacks with heart failure. N Engl J Med 2004;351:2049-2057.)

33% relative risk reduction in first hospitalization for heart failure (Fig. 30-8). This therapy was used as add-on treatment with β-blockers, ACE inhibitors, and spironolactone. A hydralazine-ISDN combination tablet is now commercially available and is approved for treatment of heart failure in black patients with heart failure and left ventricular systolic dysfunction.

Digoxin

Digoxin works by inhibiting the myocyte sodium-potassium pump, leading to higher intracellular calcium levels and increased inotropy. However, digoxin is a relatively weak inotropic agent. In addition, it has vagotonic effects. The use of digoxin in heart failure has been studied in large numbers of patients. A lower need for rehospitalization for heart failure was seen with this therapy. However, there was no improvement in overall mortality.[100] Therefore, digoxin is indicated only for patients with symptomatic heart failure, stages C and D.[1] It is also useful in patients with heart failure and atrial fibrillation, to help control the ventricular rate. Digoxin is not useful in the setting of acute heart failure, and it should be avoided in patients with hyopkalemia, bradycardia, or heart block.

Use of Long-Term Pharmacologic Therapy in Patients Hospitalized for Decompensated Heart Failure

In patients hospitalized with acute decompensated heart failure, parenteral therapies are often used to obtain improvement in a patient's symptoms and hemodynamic status. When parenteral medications are tapered off, oral therapy should be resumed, and long-term medications indicated for the treatment of chronic heart failure should be initiated. ACE inhibitors are added in the hospital to therapy for patients who have not been taking them, and doses are maximized in patients already taking them. Low doses of a β-blocker are added when a patient is determined to be stable and euvolemic. Doses of the β-blocker are then titrated up over 6 to 8 weeks to maximal tolerated doses. Aldosterone antagonists should be added at low doses, barring contraindications. Initial improvement in hemodynamics obtained with parenteral therapies can be maintained with this long-term outpatient oral medical therapy. In a study of patients referred for cardiac transplantation, the use of aggressive parenteral therapy, targeted to optimal hemodynamics followed by conversion to appropriate oral therapy, resulted in clinical improvement so that 30% of these patients were able to be removed from transplant lists.[50]

DIASTOLIC HEART FAILURE

Heart failure can occur in patients with normal or relatively normal left ventricular systolic function. It is being increasingly recognized that up to 50% of patients hospitalized with acute heart failure demonstrate primarily diastolic left ventricular dysfunction.[30] There are no uniform definitions to diagnose diastolic heart failure. The European Society of Cardiology has proposed that this diagnosis can be applied to patients who present with clinical signs and symptoms of heart failure, have normal left ventricular systolic function, and have abnormal parameters of diastolic filling as demonstrated on Doppler echocardiography or invasive evaluation of diastolic function. A more practical definition consists of the presence of heart failure and normal systolic function in the absence of primary valve disease.[101]

Diastolic heart failure occurs from impairment of left ventricular filling. This is related to abnormal left ventricular relaxation, which occurs as left ventricular pressure falls during early diastole. There is increased wall stiffness, myocardial hypertrophy, abnormal left ventricular geometry, and impaired compliance.[102] Pathologic findings in patients with primarily diastolic heart failure consist of greater left ventricular wall thickness, increased left ventricular mass-to-volume ratio, myocyte hypertrophy, and larger amounts of collagen in extracellular matrix. Also, myocardial fibrosis and signs of myocardial ischemia are often seen.[103,104] Physiologic findings are impaired left ventricular filling at normal left atrial pressures, thus necessitating an increase in left ventricular filling pressure to maintain cardiac output. This situation leads to chronic pulmonary venous hypertension and pulmonary congestion.[103,105] Patients with diastolic heart failure most often have normal indices of left ventricular systolic performance, function, and contractility.[104]

Diastolic heart failure is a common entity. The reported frequency of diastolic heart failure in the general heart failure population varies according to the definition of the disorder, whether patients with mildly abnormal systolic heart failure (i.e., ejection fraction >40%) are included, and whether systolic function is defined as normal (ejection fraction >50%). Prevalence is also affected by the age range of patients included in studies, by whether solely inpatients or inpatients and outpatients are included, by the proportion of African-American patients studied, and by whether patients studied are treated at an academic referral center or in a community-based setting.[101] The prevalence of diastolic heart failure in population-based studies was 3.1% to 5.5% of patients older than 65 years.[101] The prevalence of diastolic heart failure may be rising.[106] In comparison with patients with systolic heart failure, patients with diastolic heart failure tend to be older, are more commonly women, and have a higher prevalence of hypertension and a lower incidence of coronary artery disease.[105,106] In various studies, up to 40% to 50% of hospital admissions for heart failure are for primarily diastolic heart failure.[103] Up to 72.5% of patients with diastolic heart failure are women, with a 64% to 78% incidence of hypertension or hypertensive heart disease.[107,108] Reported incidences of concomitant diabetes (33% to 46%) and coronary artery disease (26% to 43%) are also high.[107-109] Other common comorbidities are atrial fibrillation, abnormal renal function, and obesity.

In patients who present with heart failure due to diastolic dysfunction, the history and physical findings are indistinguishable from those in patients with systolic heart failure. Presenting blood pressure may be higher, and acute "flash" pulmonary edema may be more common. Common exacerbating factors include severe hypertension, medication noncompliance, myocardial ischemia, and valvular dysfunction. However, in one study, no precipitating factors could be identified in 50% of cases.[106]

The prognosis of patients with diastolic heart failure is serious. Mortality is probably not as poor as in patients with systolic left ventricular dysfunction and heart failure, although one study found similar adjusted and non-adjusted mortality rates at 30 days and 1 year for hospitalized patients with heart failure and left ventricular ejection fraction less than 40% compared with those with ejection fractions over 50%.[111] Morbidity and rehospitalization rates are similar.[102] In-hospital mortality is reported at 4.2%,[107] or four times that for age-matched controls.[112] Annual mortality is variable and likely depends on the cohort of patients being studied; it has been reported in the range of 1.3% to 17.5%.[105] Readmission rates are high, with reported rates of up to 50% at 1 year. Factors that identify patients with a worse prognosis include renal dysfunction, worse functional class, male gender, and advanced age.[112] In the CHARM study of 3025 patients with class II to class IV heart failure and ejection fraction higher than 40%, 18% of patients were rehospitalized over 3.5 years.[113]

Unlike for systolic heart failure, there are few placebo-controlled randomized studies evaluating therapy for diastolic heart failure. However, several basic points are widely agreed upon. Effective treatment of the underlying condition, such as hypertension, diabetes mellitus, or coronary artery disease, is essential. Lowering systolic blood pressure will lower mean left atrial pressure. Control of blood glucose elevations may help retard myocardial fibrosis by lessening cross-linking of myocardial collagen. Control of myocardial ischemia is vital, although there are no convincing controlled data that revascularization will reliably prevent recurrences of diastolic heart failure. Maintenance of sinus rhythm and avoidance of tachycardia are also important.

The CHARM-Preserved Study evaluated the use of the ARB candesartan in comparison with placebo in treating patients with heart failure and preserved systolic function. After an average 3-year follow-up, the combined rates for death from cardiovascular cause or admission for heart failure were similar in the two groups. Candesartan had a moderate impact on preventing hospitalizations due to heart failure.[113]

Medical therapy of diastolic heart failure is focused primarily on alleviating symptoms. Diuretics are effective at improving pulmonary congestion. Lower doses of diuretics are generally used, because higher doses often lead to hypotension in patients with diastolic heart failure, who have small, hypertrophied left ventricles. Long-acting nitrates are also useful to decrease left ventricular filling pressure, pulmonary venous pressure, and dyspnea. Aldosterone antagonists such as spironolactone and eplerenone also have the effect of reducing both hypertension and left ventricular hypertrophy and fibrosis.[114]

β-Blockers can be useful to reduce heart rate and thus improve diastolic filling time. They are also effective medications for hypertension and coronary ischemia. Similarly, calcium channel blockers may improve symptoms of diastolic heart failure by treating hypertension and ischemia and improving diastolic relaxation. The use of ACE inhibitors and ARBs is helpful to lower blood pressure, reduce myocardial fibrosis, and block the adverse effects of the activation of the RAS system. In a retrospective study of patients hospitalized with heart failure and ejection fraction higher than 40%, patients who were prescribed an ACE inhibitor had better quality of life scores, improved functional class, and lower adjusted mortality than those who were not.[109] Therapy with positive inotropic drugs or digoxin is not useful in patients with diastolic heart failure (Table 30-8).[1,114,115]

TREATMENT OF LIFE-THREATENING VENTRICULAR ARRHYTHMIAS

Antiarrhythmic Drugs

Sudden death is a frequent occurrence in patients with heart failure, especially those with cardiomyopathy due to coronary artery disease. Sudden death is presumed to be due to sustained ventricular arrhythmia in the majority of cases. It is estimated that 30% of patients with heart failure and ejection fractions lower than 30% die suddenly. Prophylactic antiarrhythmic drug therapy aimed at reducing this incidence has been evaluated and has been shown to be ineffective. In CAST, patients with coronary artery disease, a history of MI, and frequent PVCs on baseline Holter monitoring had a higher mortality when treated with the class IC antiarrhythmic drugs encainide or flecainide,[116] despite good suppression of the frequency of arrhythmia on follow-up Holter monitoring. This adverse effect on mortality is presumed due to the known potential of these drugs to worsen arrhythmia ("proarrhythmia") in many patients. Therefore, the type IA and type IC antiarrhythmic drugs quinidine, procainamide, disopyramide, flecainide, and propafenone are not useful in prevention of sudden death. They should be used with great caution for treatment of supraventricular arrhyth-

Table 30-8. Recommendations for Treatment of Patients with Heart Failure and Normal Left Ventricular Ejection Fraction

Recommendation	Class*	Level of Evidence†
Physicians should control systolic and diastolic hypertension in accordance with published guidelines.	I	A
Physicians should control ventricular rate in patients with atrial fibrillation.	I	C
Physicians should use diuretics to control pulmonary congestion and peripheral edema.	I	C
Coronary revascularization is reasonable in patients with coronary artery disease in whom symptomatic or demonstrable myocardial ischemia is judged to be having an adverse effect on cardiac function.	IIa	C
Restoration and maintenance of sinus rhythm in patients with atrial fibrillation might be useful to improve symptoms.	IIb	C
The use of β-adrenergic blocking agents, angiotensin-converting enzyme inhibitors, angiotensin II receptor blockers, or calcium antagonists in patients with controlled hypertension might be effective to minimize symptoms of heart failure.	IIb	C
The use of digitalis to minimize symptoms of heart failure is not well established.	IIb	C

*I, There is evidence and/or general agreement that therapy is beneficial, useful and/or effective; IIa, there is conflicting evidence about the usefulness of therapy, but the weight of the evidence is in favor of efficacy; IIb, there is conflicting evidence about the usefulness of therapy, and use is less well established by evidence/opinion.

†A, Data are derived from multiple randomized clinical trials or meta-analysis; C, Only consensus opinion of experts, case studies, or standard of care.

Adapted from Hunt S, Abraham WT, Chin M, et al: ACC/AHA 2005 Guideline Update for the Diagnosis and Management of Chronic Heart Failure in the Adult—Summary Article. A report on the American College of Cardiology/American Heart Association Task Force on Practice Guidelines (Writing Committee to Update the 2001 Guidelines for Evaluation and Management of Heart Failure): Developed in collaboration with the American College of Chest Physicians and the International Society of Heart and Lung Transplantation: Endorsed by the Heart Rhythm Society. Circulation 2005;112: 1825-1852.

mias in patients with heart failure and coronary artery disease, when benefits of therapy outweigh potential risks, and after other agents have failed.

Amiodarone was also studied as primary prevention of sudden death, because the proarrhythmic effect of this medication is much lower than that of type I antiarrhythmics. Six-hundred seventy-five patients with heart failure and ejection fractions lower than 40% were randomly assigned to treatment with either amiodarone or placebo, and there was no survival difference between the two groups at 45 months.[117] There was a trend toward reducing mortality with amiodarone in patients with nonischemic cardiomyopathy. In another study of 1486 post-MI patients with ejection fractions lower than 40% who were randomly assigned to receive amiodarone or placebo, there was no difference in mortality in 21 months, although there was a suggestion of a reduction in deaths due to arrhythmia in the amiodarone group.[118] Unlike in the CAST, a higher risk of death with amiodarone was not observed. Thus, this medication is not helpful in the prevention of sudden cardiac death, but it is considered safe and can be used in patients with heart failure for treatment of supraventricular arrhythmias.

Implanted Cardioverter Defibrillator Therapy

The use of implanted cardioverter defibrillator (ICD) therapy was compared with antiarrhythmic drugs for secondary prevention of sudden cardiac death in patients who had been resuscitated from cardiac arrest or who survived ventricular tachycardia associated with syncope. In the AVID study, 1016 of these patients who also had ejection fractions less than 40% were randomly assigned to receive either ICDs or antiarrhythmic drugs (more than 90% of those patients in the drug group received amiodarone). There was a statistically better survival with ICD therapy at 1, 2, and 3 years of follow-up.[119] In two other studies of similar patients, a nonsignificant reduction in all-cause mortality and arrhythmic death rates was seen with ICDs in comparison with amiodarone,[120,121] and a higher mortality rate was seen with propafenone therapy (a class IC antiarrhythmic).[121] Taken together, these studies have established ICDs as first-line therapy in preference to antiarrhythmic drugs for patients with coronary artery disease and heart failure who have survived cardiac arrest or an episode of sustained ventricular tachycardia.

The effects of ICD therapy on mortality have also been evaluated as primary prevention of arrhythmic death in patients with coronary heart disease, previous MI, and left ventricular dysfunction without symptomatic clinical arrhythmias, and also in patients with nonischemic cardiomyopathy. In MADIT I, patients who had experienced MI, had ejection fractions lower than 35%, and who showed nonsustained ventricular tachycardia on monitoring but did not have symptomatic episodes were studied with electrophysiologic testing and programmed stimulation. Patients were enrolled in this study if they had inducible ventricular tachycardia that was not suppressed by antiarrhythmic therapy. At 2 years of follow-up, total mortality was significantly reduced from 39% in the medically treated group (standard medical therapy with or without amiodarone) to 15% in the ICD group.[122] In the MUSTT study, a similar cohort of patients showed an improvement in mortality, from 55% in patients treated with medication to 24% in patients treated with ICDs, at 5 years.[123] In MADIT II, the patient population was extended to include patients with a history of MI and ejection fractions less than 30%. Importantly in this study, ventricular arrhythmias (either seen on monitoring or induced at electrophysiologic study) were not necessary for inclu-

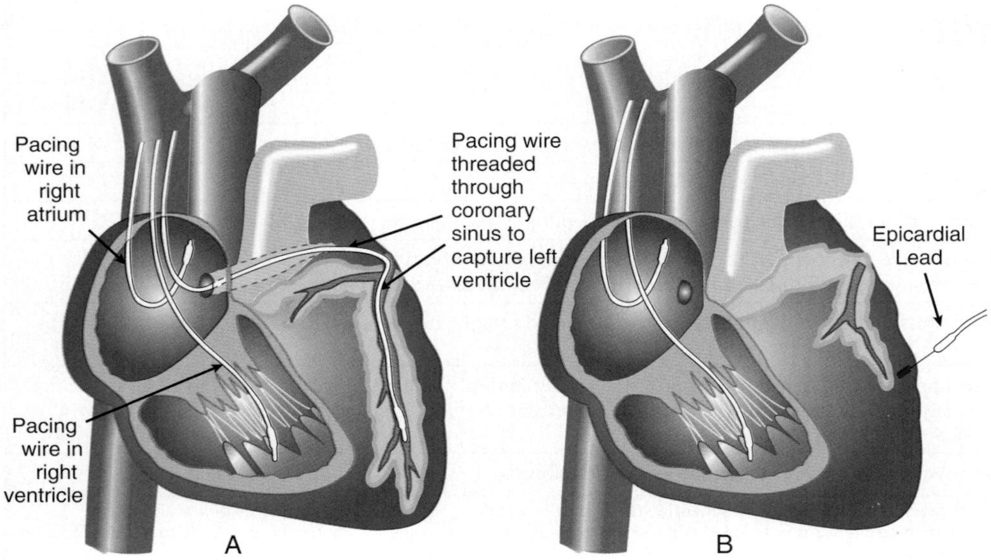

Figure 30-9. A, Placement of pacing wires in biventricular pacing. **B,** Lack of coronary sinus venous branch necessitates epicardial placement of third lead via minimally invasive surgical procedure.

sion. A statistically significant improvement in total mortality was seen in patients treated with ICDs, from 19.8% to 14.2% at 4 years.[124] It should be noted that patients with class IV heart failure were not included in any of these studies.

The SCD-HeFT (Sudden Cardiac-Death-Heart Failure Trial), reported in 2004, enrolled patients with functional class II and III heart failure with left ventricular ejection fractions lower than 35%.[125] Importantly, this study differed from MADIT I and II in that 48% of enrolled patients had nonischemic cardiomyopathy. Primary prevention of sudden cardiac death was compared for standard heart failure pharmacologic therapy, standard therapy combined with amiodarone, and standard therapy plus an ICD. After a mean follow-up of 45.5 months, mortality rates were 29% in the medical group, 28% in the amiodarone group, and 22% in the ICD group, a statistically significant difference. The improvement with ICD therapy was particularly prominent in patients with class II heart failure. Benefits of ICD therapy were seen in patients with both ischemic and nonischemic cardiomyopathy.

In the DEFINITE study, the use of the ICD as primary prevention was evaluated in 458 patients with nonischemic cardiomyopathy in whom ventricular arrhythmia seen on routine monitoring. After a mean follow-up of 29 months, total mortality was not significantly reduced (17.5% with placebo vs. 12% in ICD; $P=.08$), but the rate of sudden death was significantly reduced ($P=.006$).[126] A meta-analysis of all studies in which ICDs were used as primary prevention in patients with nonischemic cardiomyopathy indicated a statistically significant 31% relative risk reduction in favor of ICDs.[127]

Thus, the approved use of ICD therapy for prevention of sudden cardiac death has been extended to prophylactic primary prevention therapy in patients with symptomatic heart failure, class II to IIII, and left ventricular ejection fractions less than 35%, due to both ischemic and nonischemic cardiomyopathy.[128]

DEVICE THERAPY FOR HEART FAILURE

Resynchronization Therapy

In many patients with heart failure, the contraction of the intraventricular septum and left ventricular free wall lacks normal coordination, a condition termed *dyssynchrony*. This problem often coexists with conduction system disease in the His-Purkinje system, marked QRS prolongation being seen on the ECG.[129] In fact, left bundle branch block pattern with long QRS duration is associated with a rise in all-cause mortality in patients with heart failure. Pacemaker therapies have been developed to correct this left ventricular dyssynchrony, involving timed pacing of both left and right ventricles. This approach is called *biventricular pacing* or *resynchronization therapy*. Standard dual-chamber transvenous leads are placed in the right atrium (in the absence of chronic atrial fibrillation) and right ventricle. The left ventricular free wall is also paced via a third electrode passed through the coronary sinus into an epicardial lateral cardiac vein. Alternatively, an epicardial left ventricular lead can be placed via thoracoscopy. The pacemaker is programmed to coordinate timing of atrial stimulation with ventricular stimulation, and septal stimulation via the right ventricle is also synchronized with left ventricular lateral wall stimulation (Fig. 30-9).[129,130]

In the MIRACLE trial, 453 patients with ejection fractions less than 35%, class III to class IV heart failure, and QRS duration greater than 130 msec were treated with resynchronization therapy or standard medical therapy. At 6 months of follow-up, patients receiving biventricular pacing showed a statistically significant improvement in 6-minute walking distance, quality of life score, and functional class, with fewer hospitalizations for recurrent heart failure.[129] No significant mortality improvement was noted during the relatively short follow-up period. An 8% rate of unsuccessful left ventricular lead placement and a 1.2% incidence of serious complications of implantation of the pacemaker device, including coronary sinus dissection or perforation, were found A meta-analysis of three major resynchronization trials in 1634 patients concluded that long-term resynchronization therapy was associated with a statistically significant 51% reduction in rate of death from progressive heart failure.[131]

In the CARE-HF study, resynchronization therapy (without ICD) was evaluated in 813 patients with class III to class IV heart failure due to left ventricular systolic dysfunction, ejection fraction lower than 35%, and either QRS duration longer than 150 msec or QRS duration longer than 120 msec with echocardiographic signs of dyssynchrony.[132] The primary end point, all-cause mortality plus unplanned hospitalization from cardiovascular causes, was reduced from 55% in medically treated patients to 39% in resynchronization patients ($P<.001$) and the rate of all-cause mortality was reduced from 30% to 20% with resynchronization therapy ($P<.002$). Mean follow-up was 29.4 months. Measures of quality of life as well as ejection fractions were improved.

Thus, resynchronization therapy alone, without an ICD, can reduce mortality as well as improve symptoms in patients with chronic heart failure. Currently, resynchronization therapy has been recommended for patients with left ventricular systolic dysfunction, ejection fraction less than or equal to 35%, and QRS duration greater than or equal to 120 msec on ECG, who are in sinus rhythm, and who have persistent class III to class IV heart failure symptoms despite optimal medical therapy.[133]

Combination Devices

Devices combining biventricular pacing and ICD capabilities have been evaluated in patients with systolic heart failure and low ejection fractions, who often have clinical indications for both devices. These devices are used in an attempt to decrease the morbidity and mortality associated with progressive heart failure as well as the mortality associated with sudden life-threatening ventricular arrhythmia. Initial reports indicated that biventricular pacing does not interfere with appropriate ICD detection and termination of ventricular arrhythmias.[134] The COMPANION trial enrolled 1520 patients with advanced heart failure (functional class III to IV), who were in sinus rhythm, and in whom the ECG showed QRS duration longer than 120 msec.[135] Therapies compared were best pharmacologic heart failure therapy, best therapy along with biventricular pacing, and best therapy along with combination biventricular pacing and ICD. Successful implantation was achieved in 87% to 91% of patients in the latter two groups, with a procedural mortality of 0.5% to 0.8%. The primary end points, death from any cause or hospitalization for any cause, with follow-up over 12 months, were 68% in the drug therapy group and 56% in both device groups, a significant difference. One-year rates of death or hospitalization due to cardiovascular cause were 60% in the drug group, with a relative risk reduction of 25% in the biventricular pacing group and 28% in the biventricular pacing–ICD group. The researchers in this study concluded that there was a significant reduction in heart failure hospitalizations with biventricular pacing and an additional significant reduction in mortality when ICD therapy was added. Improvement in both parameters occurred in patients with ischemic and nonischemic cardiomyopathy. Thus, newer combination devices have an important role in providing both symptomatic as well as life-extending benefits to patients with heart failure.

Ventricular Assist Devices

The number of patients in the United States with advanced heart failure due to left ventricular systolic dysfunction, defined as those with symptomatic class III to class IV heart failure, is estimated to be 300,000 to 800,000.[135] Despite appropriate device and pharmacologic therapy, an estimated 60,000 patients have refractory heart failure with high mortality rates. Patients who present with acute heart failure and cardiogenic shock due to acute MI have a very high mortality. In patients with chronic heart failure, factors indicating a very poor prognosis include dependence on parenteral inotropic drugs, class IV symptoms with renal dysfunction precluding the use of ACE inhibitors,[137] refractory congestion, and hypotension preventing β-blocker therapy. Peak oxygen consumption less than 10 mL/kg/min on pulmonary stress testing is also an indicator of poor prognosis. Cardiac transplantation offers an effective therapy for some patients with end-stage heart failure and is currently associated with a 1-year survival exceeding 80%.[136] However, the pool of donor hearts is currently less than 3000 per year and is not growing.[137] Therefore, there is a role for the use of mechanical pumps, called ventricular assist devices (VADs), to replace the function of the failing heart.[138]

VADs are most commonly extracorporeal pumps, used to support the function of the left ventricle. They are inserted via a midline sternotomy (Fig. 30-10). Newer pumps are smaller and can be intracorporeal, implanted in the abdominal wall (Fig. 30-11). Catheter-based pumps, used for short-term hemodynamic support, can provide cardiac output up to 3.5 L/min.[139] Newer VADs can also be used to support both right ventricular and left ventricular function. The power source can be electric or pneumatic and is connected to the device via a percutaneous drive line. Power packs can be small enough to be wearable, so that patients with VADs have greater freedom of movement and can participate in rehabilitation efforts.

VADs can provide normal cardiac output, hemodynamics, and flow to vital organs.[140] VAD technology initially provided pulsatile blood flow, and anticoagulation was required because of a high incidence of embolic complications. Later advances include axial flow pumps, which provide continuous flow,[137] and pumps with textured blood-contacting surfaces, which do not require anticoagulation.[141]

VAD therapy is appropriate for patients with refractory heart failure that is not responding to maximal therapy, with high rates of morbidity and estimated 6-month mortality rates more than 50%. These patients often have the potential for recovery of myocardial function or are candidates for cardiac transplantation. A VAD can also be used as a "bridge" to other interventions (e.g., revascularization) that may lead to recovery of myocardial func-

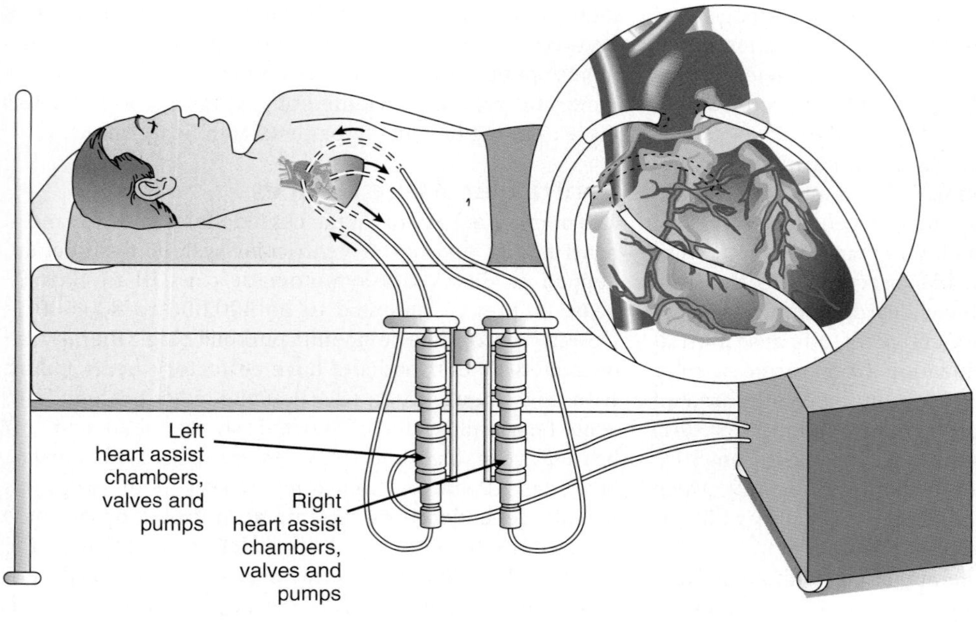

Figure 30-10. Biventricular assist device (BVAD). Blood is removed from the right atrium and injected into the pulmonary artery. Blood is removed from the left atrium and injected into the aorta. This Abiomed BVAD has the ability to completely substitute for left and right heart functions.

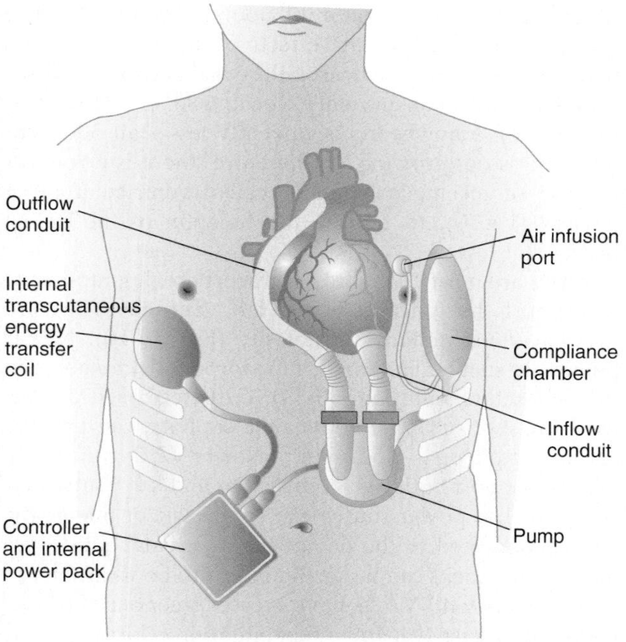

Figure 30-11. A totally implantable left ventricular assist device (LVAD), the LionHeart Left Ventricular Assist System. (Redrawn from Nemeh H, Smedira N: Mechanical treatment of heart failure: The growing role of LVADs and artificial hearts. Cleve Clin J Med 2003;70:223-234.)

tion. Finally, VADs can be used as long-term "destination therapy" (Fig. 30-12).

Clinical conditions in which VAD support can be lifesaving include cardiogenic shock due to acute MI, acute fulminant myocarditis, cardiogenic shock after cardiac surgery, and end-stage dilated cardiomyopathy.[139,140] A 30% mortality has been reported in patients listed for and awaiting heart transplantation, and VADs used in this setting may enable patients to survive until transplantation.[62] Proper patient selection is important. Appropriate hemodynamic indications are persistent hypotension with systolic blood pressure less than 80 mm Hg, with pulmonary capillary wedge pressure greater than 20 mm Hg and cardiac index less than 2 L/min/m^2 despite maximal pharmacologic support with or without the use of intra-aortic balloon counterpulsation. Groups with a worse prognosis with VAD therapy include older patients as well as patients with renal dysfunction (i.e., serum creatinine >3.0 mg/dL), hepatic dysfunction (transaminase and bilirubin levels more than five times normal), neurologic deficits, and abnormal pulmonary function.[142] Contraindications to the use of VADs include severe chronic obstructive pulmonary disease, need for hemodialysis, and uncorrected coagulopathy. Complications of VAD placement are bleeding, air embolism, and right ventricular failure, often due to severe pulmonary hypertension. Complications associated with the longer term use of VADs include sepsis, thromboembolic complications, and device failure.

When VADs are used to support patients awaiting cardiac transplantation, there is a 74% rate of survival to transplantation and a subsequent 91% recovery rate to hospital discharge after transplantation. In recent studies, 50% of VAD recipients have demonstrated enough improvement to be discharged to home to await the transplantation.[136] In patients with fulminant myocarditis, a period of VAD support is often associated with improvement in left ventricular function ("bridge to recovery"), so that the VAD is eventually removed. Aggressive support of critically ill patients with acute fulminant myocarditis, including the temporary use of VADs, has been associated with a 90% long-term survival.[35] In patients with subacute cardiomyopathy and heart failure, there have been case reports of improvement in left ventricular function during VAD therapy lasting 160 to 190 days, such that VADs could be removed, and patients had long-term survival without heart transplantation.[143] During VAD support, which provides maximal left ventricular unloading, neurohormonal and cytokine activation can

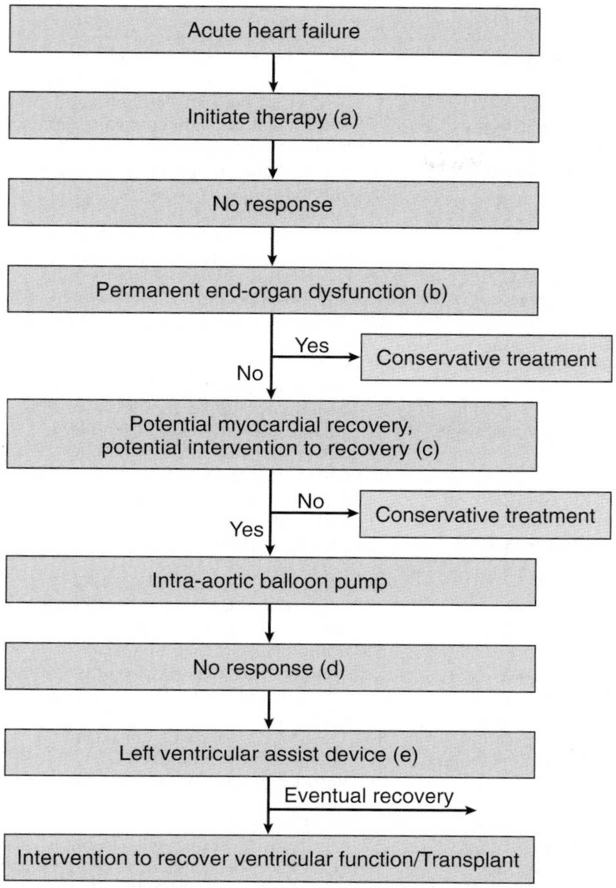

Figure 30-12. Selection of candidates for left ventricular assist devices. (a), No response to conventional treatment of acute heart failure, including appropriate use of diuretics and fluids, intravenous inotropics, and vasodilators. (b), End-organ dysfunction, including severe systemic disease, severe renal failure pulmonary disease or hepatic dysfunction, and permanent central nervous injury. (c), Potential recovery of myocardial function or cardiac function, for example, acute myocardial ischemia, postcardiotomy shock, acute myocarditis, acute valvular heart disease, or candidate for heart transplantation. (d), Absence of clinical improvement after intra-aortic balloon pumping and mechanical ventilation. (e), Final indication may depend on availability of device and experience of cardiovascular team. (Redrawn from Nieminen MS, Bohm M, Cowie MR, et al: Executive summary of the guidelines on the diagnosis and treatment of acute heart failure. The Task Force on Acute Heart Failure of the European Society of Cardiology. Eur Heart J 2005;26:384-416.)

reverse and normalize, and pulmonary hypertension may improve.[138] Intracellular processes indicative of reverse remodeling can be seen, with reversal of cellular phenotypic changes seen in myocytes of the failing heart. Decreased myocyte hypertrophy and left ventricular mass can occur during VAD support.[138,139] It is estimated that less than 10% of patients with chronic heart failure improve enough with VAD therapy for it to be used as a bridge to recovery. However, a period of VAD therapy may improve the overall status of patients with chronic heart failure, enough to enhance their suitability for transplantation.

Lastly, VADs have been evaluated as a long-term treatment, or "destination therapy." The REMATCH trial compared VADs as destination therapy with standard medical therapy in 129 patients with class IV heart failure, ejection fractions less than 25%, and initial dependence on intravenous inotropic therapy.[144] This study showed improved survival and measured quality of life in patients treated with the VAD. Survival at 1 year was 52% for VAD therapy, compared with 25% for medical therapy, and 2-year survival with VAD support was 23% compared with 8% for medical therapy. However, there was a significant 35% complication rate at 2 years with VAD therapy; most common complications were infection, bleeding, and device malfunction. Causes of death in these patients were most often sepsis and device failure, not heart failure.

The use of a total artificial heart as a bridge to cardiac transplantation was reported in 2004. Eighty-one patients at high risk of imminent death due to irreversible biventricular failure, in whom a VAD could not be used, received a biventricular, totally implantable, pulsatile, pneumatic pump.[145] Results compared favorably with those in historical controls: 79% survival to transplant and 70% 1-year survival after transplant. Complications included bleeding, infection, device malfunction, and hepatic dysfunction.

With refinements in design and technologic improvements, long-term mechanical support of the failing left ventricle may be feasible for indefinite periods, especially as the incidence of infectious and thromboembolic complications is reduced. Progress in making these devices smaller and totally implantable will advance treatments toward the goal of a reliable artificial heart.

KEY POINTS

- The ACC/AHA staging of heart failure includes patients at high risk for heart failure, in whom the syndrome has not developed, to emphasize that effective treatment of predisposing conditions can prevent the occurrence of heart failure.
- Serum levels of natriuretic peptides can help in the diagnosis of heart failure in dyspneic patients and can be useful in assessing prognosis.
- In patients with acute heart failure, the presence of myocardial ischemia due to coronary artery disease should be evaluated and treated aggressively.
- β-Blockers and angiotensin-converting enzyme (ACE) inhibitors are the cornerstones of therapy for patients with chronic left ventricular dysfunction who are asymptomatic or have heart failure.
- Successful heart failure therapies lead to "reverse remodeling," with stabilization or improvement in left ventricular size and contractile function.
- Acute or chronic heart failure often develops in the setting of normal left ventricular systolic function, often in elderly patients, especially women, with hypertension and other comorbidities.
- Devices that combine biventricular pacing and automatic defibrillation have been shown to improve exercise tolerance and prolong life in patients with heart failure and severe left ventricular systolic dysfunction.

REFERENCES

1. Hunt S, Abraham WT, Chin M, et al: ACC/AHA 2005 Guideline Update for the Diagnosis and Management of Chronic Heart Failure in the Adult—Summary Article: A report of the American College of Cardiology/ American Heart Association Task Force on Practice Guidelines (Writing Committee to Update the 2001 Guidelines for Evaluation and Management of Heart Failure): Developed in Collaboration with the American College of Chest Physicians and the International Society for Heart and Lung Transplantation: Endorsed by the Heart Rhythm Society. Circulation 2005;112:1825-1852.
2. Jessup M, Brozena S: Heart failure. N Engl J Med 2003;348:2007-2018.
3. Cowie M, Mendez G: B-natriuretic peptide and congestive heart failure. Curr Probl Cardiol 2003;44:264-311.
4. McCullough PA, Nowack PM, McCord J, et al: B-type natriuretic peptide and clinical judgment in emergency diagnosis of heart failure: Analysis from Breathing Not Properly (BNP) Multinational Study Circ 2002;106:416-422.
5. Morrison LK, Harrison A, Krishnaswamy P, et al: Utility of a rapid BNP assay in differentiating congestive heart failure from lung disease in patients presenting with dyspnea. J Am Coll Cardiol 2002;39:202-209.
6. Muller C, Scholer A, Lawle-Kilian K, et al: Use of B-type natriuretic peptide in the evaluation and management of acute dyspnea. N Engl J Med 2004;350:647-654.
7. Maisel A: B-type natriuretic peptide levels: Diagnosis and prognosis in congestive heart failure: What's next? Circulation 2002;105:2328-2331.
8. Logeart D, Thabut G, Jourdian P, et al: Predischarge B-type natriuretic peptide assay for identifying patients at high risk of readmission after decompensated heart failure. J Am Coll Cardiol 2004;43:635-641.
9. Januzzi JL, van Kimmenade R, Lainchbury J, et al: NT-proBNP testing for diagnosis and short-term prognosis in acute destabilized heart failure: In international pooled analysis of 1256 patients. The International Collaborative of NT-proBNP Study. European Heart J 2006;27:330-337.
10. O'Donoghue M, Chen A, Baggish AL, et al: The effects of ejection fraction on *N*-terminal ProBNP and BNP levels in patients with acute CHF: Analysis from the ProBNP Investigation of dyspnea in the Emergency Department (PRIDE) Study. J Cardiac Failure Supplement 2005;11:S9-S14.
11. Nieminen MS, Bohm M, Cowie MR, et al: Executive Summary of the Guidelines on the Diagnosis and Treatment of Acute Heart Failure. The Task Force on Acute Heart Failure of the European Society of Cardiology. European Heart J 2005;26:384-416.
12. Gheorghiade M, Zannad F, Sopko G: Acute heart failure syndromes. Circulation 2005;112:3958-3968.
13. Rudiger T, Harjola V, Muller A, et al: Acute heart failure: Clinical presentation. One year mortality and prognostic factors. Eur J Heart Failure 2005;7:662-670.
14. Sharma M, Teerlink JR: A rational approach for the treatment of acute heart failure: Current strategies and future options. Curr Opin Cardiol 2004;19:254-263.
15. The ESCAPE Investigators and ESCAPE Study Coordinators: Evaluation study of congestive heart failure and pulmonary artery catheterization effectiveness. JAMA 2005;294: 1625-1633.
16. Stevenson LW: Are hemodynamic goals viable in tailoring heart failure therapy? Circulation 2006;113:1020-1027.
17. Jemtel TH, Alt EU: Hemodynamic goals are outdated. Circulation 2006;113:1027-1032.
18. Fonarow GC, Adams KF, Abraham WT: Risk stratification for in-hospital mortality in acutely decompensated heart failure. JAMA 2005;293: 572-580.
19. Velazquez EJ, Pfeffer MA: Acute heart failure complicating acute coronary syndromes. Circulation 2004;109:440-442.
20. Steg PG, Dabbous DH, Feldman LJ, et al: Determinants and prognostic impact of heart failure complicating acute coronary syndromes. Circulation 2004;109:494-499.
21. Velazquez EJ, Francis GS, Armstrong PW, et al: An international perspective on heart failure and left ventricular systolic dysfunction complicating myocardial infarction: The VALIANT registry. European Heart J 2004;25:1911-1919.
22. The CAPRICORN Investigators: Effect of carvedilol on outcome after myocardial infarction in patients with left ventricular dysfunction: The CAPRICORN Randomized Trial. Lancet 2001;357:1385-1390.
23. Pfeffer M, Braunwald E, Moye L, et al: Effect of captopril on mortality and morbidity in patients with left ventricular dysfunction after myocardial infarction. N Engl J Med 1992;327:669-677.
24. The Acute Infarction Ramipril Efficacy (AIRE) Study Investigators: Effect of ramipril on mortality and morbidity of survivors of acute myocardial infarction with clinical evidence of heart failure. Lancet 1993;342:821-828.
25. Kober L, Torp-Pedersen C, Carlsen JE, et al: A clinical trial of the angiotensin-converting-enzyme inhibitor trandolapril in patients with left ventricular dysfunction after myocardial infarction. N Engl J Med 1995;333:670-1676.
26. Dickstein K, Kjekshus J, the OPTIMAAL Steering Committee: Effects of losartan and captopril on mortality and morbidity in high-risk patients after acute myocardial infarction: The OPTIMAAL randomised trial. Lancet 2002;360:752-760.
27. Pfeffer MA, McMurray JJV, Velazquez EJ: Valsartan, captopril, or both in myocardial infarction complicated by heart failure, left ventricular dysfunction, or both. N Engl J Med 2003;349:18931903.
28. Pitt B, Remme W, Zannad F, et al: Eplerenone, a selective aldosterone blocker, in patients with left ventricular dysfunction after myocardial infarction. N Engl J Med 2003;348:1309-1321.
29. Pitt B, White H, Nicolau J: Eplerenone reduces mortality 30 days after randomization following acute myocardial infarction in patients with left ventricular systolic dysfunction and heart failure. J Am Coll Cardiol 2005;46:424-430.
30. Feldman A, McNamara D: Myocarditis. N Engl J Med 2000;19:1388-1398.
31. Parrillo J: Inflammatory cardiomyopathy (myocarditis): Which patients should be treated with anti-inflammatory therapy? Circulation 2001;104:4-6.
32. Parrillo JE, Cunnion R, Epstein S, et al: A prospective randomized controlled trial of prednisone for dilated cardiomyopathy. N Engl J Med 1989;321:1061-1068.
33. Wojnicz R, Nowalany-Kozielska E, Wojciechowska C, et al: Randomized, placebo-controlled study for immunosuppressive treatment of inflammatory dilated cardiomyopathy: Two-year follow-up results. Circulation 2001;104:39-45.
34. Mason J, O'Connell J, Herskowitz A, et al: A clinical trial of immunosuppressive therapy for myocarditis. N Engl J Med 1995;333:269-275.
35. McCarthy R, Boehmer J, Hrubianr F, et al: Long-term outcome of fulminant myocarditis as compared with acute (non-fulminant) myocarditis. N Engl J Med 2002;342:690-695.
36. Wu A, Cody R: Medical and surgical treatment of chronic heart failure. Curr Probl Cardiol 2003;28:225-260.
37. Packer M: Current role of beta-adrenergic blockers in the management of chronic heart failure. Am J Med 2001;110:81S-84S.
38. Asbun J, Villarreal FJ: The pathogenesis of myocardial fibrosis in the setting of diabetic cardiomyopathy. J Am Coll Cardiol 2006;47:693-700.
39. Fadel BM, Ellahham S, Ringel MD: Hyperthyroid heart disease. Clin Cardiol 2000;23:402-408.
40. Alpert MA: Obesity cardiomyopathy: Pathophysiology and evolution of the clinical syndrome. Am J Med Sci 2001;321:225-236.
41. Jain P, Massie B, Gattis W, et al: Current medical treatment for the exacerbation of chronic heart failure resulting in hospitalization. Am Heart J 2003;145:S3-S17.
42. Floyd JD, Nguyen DT, Lobins RL, et al: Cardiotoxicity of cancer therapy. J Clin Oncol 2005;23:7685-7696.
43. Fonarow GC, Adams KF, Abraham WT, et al: Risk stratification for in-hospital mortality in acutely decompensated heart failure. JAMA 2005;293:572-580.
44. Sharma M, Teerlink JR: A rational approach for treatment of acute heart failure: Current strategies and future options. Curr Opin Cardiol 2004;19:254-263.
45. Rose E, Gelijns A, Moskowitz A, et al: Long-term use of a left ventricular

assist device for end-stage heart failure. N Engl J Med 2001;345: 1435-1443.
46. Chin M, Goldman L: Correlates of major complications or death in patients admitted to the hospital with congestive heart failure. Arch Intern Med 1996;156:1814-1820.
47. Geisberg C, Butler J: Addressing the challenges of cardiorenal syndrome. Cleveland Clin J Med 2006;73: 485-491.
48. Smith GL, Lichtman JH, Bracken MB, et al: Renal impairment and outcomes in heart failure: Systematic review and meta-analysis. J Am Coll Cardiol 2006;47:1987-1996.
49. Hochman J, Sleeper L, Webb J, et al: Early revascularization in acute myocardial infarction complicated by cardiogenic shock. SHOCK Investigators. SHould we emergently revascularize OCcluded coronaries for cardiogenic shocK? N Engl J Med 1999;341:625-634.
50. Steimle A, Stevenson L, Chelimsky-Fallick C, et al: Sustained hemodynamic efficacy of therapy tailored to reduce filling pressures in survivors with advanced heart failure. Circulation 1997;96:1165-1172.
51. Stevenson L: Tailored therapy for hemodynamic goals for advanced heart failure. Eur J Heart Fail 1999;1:251-257.
52. Stevenson L, Tillisch J: Maintenance of cardiac output with normal filling pressures in patients with dilated heart failure. Circulation 1986;74: 1303-1308.
53. Publication Committee for the VMAC Investigators: Intravenous nesiritide versus nitroglycerin for treatment of decompensated congestive heart failure: A randomized controlled trial. JAMA 2000;287:1531-1540.
54. Colucci W, Wright R, Jaski B, et al: Milrinone and dobutamine in severe heart failure: Differing hemodynamic effects and individual patient responsiveness. Circulation 1086;73:175-183.
55. Jaski B, Fifer M, Wright R, et al: Positive inotropic and vasodilator actions of milrinone in patients with severe congestive heart failure. J Clin Invest 1985;75:643-649.
56. Colucci W, Elkayam U, Horton D, et al: Intravenous nesiritide, a natriuretic in the treatment of decompensated congestive heart failure. N Engl J Med 2002;343:246-253.
57. Dormans T, Van-Meyel J, Gerlag P, et al: Diuretic efficacy of high dose furosemide in severe heart failure: Bolus injection versus continuous infusion. J Am Coll Cardiol 1996;28:376-382.
58. Gheorghiade M, Gattis W, O'Connor CM, et al: Effects of tolvaptan, a vasopressin antagonist, in patients hospitalized with worsening heart failure. JAMA 2004;291:1963-1971.
59. Goldsmith SR, Gheorghiade M: Vasopressin antagonism in heart failure. J Am Coll Cardiol 2005;46:1785-1791.
60. Orlandi C, Zimmer CA, Cheroghiade M: Role of vasopressin antagonists in the management of acute decompensated heart failure. Curr Heart Fail Rep 2005;2:131-139.
61. Burger A, Horton D, LeGemtel T, et al: Effect of nesiritide (B-type natriuretic peptide) and dobutamine on ventricular arrhythmias in the treatment of patients with acutely decompensated congestive heart failure: The PRECEDENT Study. Am Heart J 2002;144:1102-1108.
62. Chatterjee K, DeMarco T: Role of nonglycosidic inotropic agents: Indications, ethics, and limitations. Med Clin North Am 2003;87:391-418.
63. Leier C, Binkley P: Parenteral inotropic support for advanced congestive heart failure. Prog Cardiovasc Dis 1998;41:207-224.
64. Shah M, Hasselblad V, Stinnett S, et al: Hemodynamic profiles of advanced heart failure: Association with clinical characteristics and long-term outcomes. J Card Fail 2001;7:105-113.
65. Cuffe M, Califf R, Adams K, et al: Short-term intravenous milrinone for acute exacerbation of chronic heart failure: A randomized control trial. JAMA 2002;287:1541-1547.
66. O'Connor C, Gattis W, Uretsky B, et al: Continuous intravenous dobutamine is associated with an increased risk of death in patients with advanced heart failure: Insights from the Flolan International Randomized Survival Trial (FIRST). Am Heart J 1999;138:78-86.
67. Silver M, Horton D, Ghali J, et al: Effect of nesiritide versus dobutamine on short-term outcomes in the treatment of patients with acute decompensated heart failure. J Am Coll Cardiol 2002;39:798-803.
68. Abraham W, Adams K, Fonarow G, et al: Comparison of in-hospital mortality in patients treated with nesiritide versus other parenteral vasoactive medications for acutely decompensated heart failure: An analysis from a large prospective registry database. J Card Fail 2003;9: S81.
69. Sackner-Bernstein JD, Kowalski M, Fox M, Aaronson K: Short-term risk of death after treatment with nesiritide for decompensated heart failure. JAMA 2005;293:1900-1905.
70. Sackner-Bernstein JD, Skopicki HA, Aarronson KD: Risk of worsening renal function with nesiritide in patients with acutely decompensated heart failure. Circulation 2005;111: 1487-1491.
71. Abraham WT, Adams KF, Fonarow GC, et al: In-hospital mortality in patients with acute decompensated heart failure requiring intravenous vasoactive medications. J Am Coll Cardiol 2005;4:57-64.
72. Scios Inc. Dear Health Care Provider Letter (Recommendations of Nesiritide Advisory Panel), July 13, 2005. Available at: http://www.fda.gov/medwatch safety/2005/natrecor2_hcp.pdf
73. Jaski BE, Ha J, Denys BG, et al: Peripherally inserted veno-venous ultrafiltration for rapid treatment of volume overloaded patients. J Card Failure 2003;9:227-231.
74. Bart BA, Boyle A, Bank AJ, et al: Ultrafiltration versus usual care for hospitalized patients with heart failure. J Am Coll Cardiol 2005;46:2043-2053.
75. Philbin EF, Rocco TA Jr, Lindenmuth NW, et al: Systolic versus diastolic heart failure in community practice: Clinical features, outcomes, and the use of angiotensin-converting enzyme inhibitors. Am J Med 2000;109: 605-613.
76. BHAT Trial Research Group: A randomized trial of propranolol in patients with acute myocardial infarction. I: Mortality results. JAMA 1982;747:1707-1714.
77. BHAT Trial Research Group: A randomized trial of propranolol in patients with acute myocardial infarction. II: Morbidity results. JAMA 1983;250:2814-2819.
78. CIBIS II Investigators: The Cardiac Insufficiency Bisoprolol Study II: A randomized trial. Lancet 1999; 353:9-13.
79. The MERIT-HF Study Group: Effects of controlled release metoprolol on total mortality, hospitalizations and well-being in patients with heart failure. JAMA 2000;283:1295-1302.
80. Packer M, Coats A, Fowler M, et al: Effect of carvedilol on survival in severe chronic heart failure. N Engl J Med 2001;344:1651-1658.
81. Krum H, Roecker E, Mohacsi P, et al: Effects on initiating carvedilol in patients with severe chronic heart failure. Results from the COPERNICUS Study. JAMA 2003;289:712-718.
82. Bristow M, Gilbert E, Abraham W, et al: Carvedilol produces dose related improvements in left ventricular function and survival in subjects with chronic heart failure. Circulation 1996;94:2807-2816.
83. The SOLVD Investigators: Effect of enalapril on survival in patients with reduced left ventricular ejection fractions and congestive heart failure. N Engl J Med 1991;325:293-302.
84. The SOLVD Investigators: Effect of enalapril on mortality and the development of heart failure in asymptomatic patients with reduced left ventricular ejection fractions. N Engl J Med 1992;327:685-691.
85. Garg R, Yusuf S: Overview of randomized trials of angiotensin converting enzyme inhibitors on mortality and morbidity in patients with heart failure. JAMA 1995;273:1450-1456.
86. Packer M, Poole-Wilson PA, Armstrong PW, et al: Comparative effects of low and high doses of the angiotensin-converting enzyme inhibitor, lisinopril, on morbidity and mortality in chronic heart failure. Atlas Study Group. Circulation 1999;100:2312-2318.
87. Aronow WS: Epidemiology, pathophysiology, prognosis, and treatment of systolic and diastolic heart failure. Card in Review 2006;14:108-124.
88. Willenheimer R, van Veldhuisen DJ, Silke B, et al: Effect on survival and hospitalization of initiating treatment for chronic heart failure with bisoprolol followed by enalapril, as compared with the opposite sequence. Circulation 2005;112:2426-2435.
89. The RESOLVD Pilot Study Investigators: Comparison of candesartan, enalapril,

and their combination in congestive heart failure. Circulation 1999;100:1056-1064.
90. Pitt B, Poole-Wilson P, Segal R, et al: Effect of losartan compared with captopril on mortality in patients with symptomatic heart failure: Randomized trial—The Losartan Heart Failure Survival Study (ELITE II). Lancet 2000;355:1582-1587.
91. Cohn J, Tognoni G: A randomized trial of the angiotensin receptor blocker valsartan in chronic heart failure. N Engl J Med 2001;345:1667-1675.
92. Granger C, McMurray J, Yusuf S, et al: Effects of candesartan in patients with chronic heart failure and reduced left ventricular systolic function intolerant to angiotensin-converting enzyme inhibitors. The CHARM Alternative Trial. Lancet 2003;362:772-776.
93. Pfeffer MA, Swedberg K, Granger CB, et al: Effects of candesartan on mortality and morbidity in patients with chronic heart failure: The CHARM–Overall programme. Lancet 2003;362:759-766.
94. Manohair P, Pina I: Therapeutic role of angiotensin II receptor blockers in the treatment of heart failure. Mayo Clinic Proc 2003;78:334-338.
95. Sharma D, Buyse M, Pitt B, et al: Meta-analysis of observed mortality data from all controlled double-blind multiple dose studies of losartan in heart failure. Am J Cardiol 2000;85:187-192.
96. Pitt B, Zannad F, Remme W, et al: The effect of spironolactone on morbidity and mortality in patients with severe heart failure. N Engl J Med 1999;341:709-717.
97. Juurlink DN, Mamdani NM, Lee DS, et al: Rates of hyperkalemia after publication of the randomized Aldactone Study. N Engl J Med 2004;351:543-551.
98. Cohn J, Archibald D, Ziesche S, et al: Effect of vasodilator therapy on mortality in chronic congestive heart failure. Results of a Veterans Administration Cooperative Study. N Engl J Med 1986;314:1547-1552.
99. Taylor AL, Zieche S, Yancy C, et al: Combination of isosorbide dinitrate and hydralazine in blacks with heart failure. N Engl J Med 2004;351: 2049-2057.
100. The Digitalis Investigation Group: The effect of digoxin on mortality and morbidity in patients with heart failure. N Engl J Med 1997;336: 525-533.
101. Owan TE, Redfield MM: Epidemiology of diastolic heart failure. Prog Cardiovasc Dis 2005;47:320-332.
102. Leite-Moreira AF: Current perspectives in diastolic dysfunction and diastolic heart failure. Heart 2006;92:712-718.
103. Gaasch WH: Diagnosis and treatment of heart failure based on left ventricular systolic or diastolic dysfunction. JAMA 1994;271: 1276-1280.
104. Aurigemma GP, Zile MR, Gaasch WH: Contractile behavior of the left ventricle in diastolic heart failure. Circulation 2006;113:296-304.
105. Vasan RS, Benjamin EJ, Levy D: Prevalence, clinical features and prognosis of diastolic heart failure: An epidemiologic perspective. J Am Coll Cardiol 1995;26:1565-1574.
106. Owan TE, Hodge DO, Herges RM, et al: Trends in prevalence and outcome of heart failure with preserved ejection fraction. N Engl J Med 2006;355:251-259.
107. Klapholz M, Maurer M, Lowe AM, et al: Hospitalization for heart failure in the presence of a normal left ventricular ejection fraction. J Am Coll Cardiol 2004;43:1432-1438.
108. Devereux RB, Roman MJ, Liu JE, et al: Congestive heart failure despite normal left ventricular systolic function in a population-based sample: The strong heart study. Am J Cardiol 2000;86:1090-1096.
109. Philbin EF, Rocco TA Jr, Lindenmuth NW: Systolic versus diastolic heart failure in community practice: Clinical features, outcomes, and the use of angiotensin-converting enzyme inhibitors. Am J Med 2000;1009: 605-613.
110. Yancy CW, Lopatin M, Stevenson LW, et al: Clinical presentation, management, and in-hospital outcomes of patients admitted with acute decompensated heart failure with preserved systolic function. J Am Coll Cardiol 2006;47:76-84.
111. Bhatia RS, Tu JV, Lee DL, et al: Outcome of heart failure with preserved ejection fraction in a population-based study. N Engl J Med 2006;355:260-269.
112. Franklin KM, Aurigemma GP: Prognosis in diastolic heart failure. Prog Cardiovasc Dis 2005;47:333-339.
113. Yusuf S, Pfeffer MA, Swedberg K, et al: Effects of candesartan in patients with chronic heart failure and preserved left-ventricular ejection fraction: The CHARM-Preserved Trial. Lancet 2003;362(9386):777-781.
114. Little WC, Brucks S: Therapy for diastolic heart failure. Prog Cardiovasc Dis 2005;47:380-388.
115. Zile MR, Baica CF: Alterations in ventricular function: Diastolic heart failure. In Mann DL: Heart Failure: A Companion to Braunwald's Heart Disease. Philadelphia, Saunders, 2004, pp 222-227.
116. The Cardiac Arrhythmia Suppression Trial Investigators Preliminary Report: Effect of encainide and flecainide on mortality in a randomized trial of arrhythmia suppression after myocardial infarction. N Engl J Med 1989;3211:406-412.
117. Singh S, Fletcher R, Fisher S, et al: Amiodarone in patients with congestive heart failure and asymptomatic ventricular arrhythmia. N Engl J Med 1995;333:77-82.
118. Julian D, Camm A, Frangin G, et al: Randomized trial of effect of amiodarone on mortality in patients with left ventricular dysfunction after recent myocardial infarction: EMIAT. Lancet 1997;349:667-674.
119. The AVID Investigators: A comparison of antiarrhythmic drug therapy with implantable defibrillators in patients resuscitated from near-fatal ventricular arrhythmias. N Engl J Med 1997;337:1576-1583.
120. Connolly S, Gent M, Roberts R, et al: Canadian Implantable Defibrillator Study (CIDS): A randomized trial of the implantable cardioverter defibrillator against amiodarone. Circulation 2000;101:1297-1302.
121. Kuck K, Cappato R, Siebels J, et al: Randomized comparison of antiarrhythmic drug therapy with implantable defibrillators in patients resuscitated from cardiac arrest: The Cardiac Arrest Study Hamburg (CASH). Circulation 2000;102:748-754.
122. MADIT Investigators: Improved survival with an implanted defibrillator in patients with coronary disease at high risk for ventricular arrhythmia. N Engl J Med 1995;335:1933-1940.
123. Buxton A, Lee, K, Fisher J, et al: A randomized study of the prevention of sudden death in patients with coronary artery disease. N Engl J Med 1999;341:1882-1890.
124. MADIT II Investigators: Prophylactic implantation of a defibrillator in patients with myocardial infarction and reduced ejection fraction. N Engl J Med 2001;346:877-883.
125. Bardy GH, Lee KL, Mark DB, et al: Amiodarone or an implantable cardioverter defibrillator for congestive heart failure (SCD-HEFT.) N Engl J Med 2005;352:225-237.
126. Kadish A, Dyer A, Daubert JP, et al: Prophylactic defibrillator implantation in patients with non-ischemic dilated cardiomyopathy. N Engl J Med 2004;350:2151-2158.
127. Desai AS, Farg JC, Maisel WH, Baughman KL: Implantable defibrillators for the prevention of mortality in patients with non-ischemic cardiomyopathy: A meta-analysis of randomized controlled trials. JAMA 2004;292:2874-2879.
128. Zipes DP, Camm AJ, Borggrefe M, et al: ACC/AHA/ESC 2006 Guidelines for Management of patients with ventricular arrhythmias and the prevention of Sudden Cardiac Death—Executive Summary; a report of the American College of Cardiology/American Heart Association Task Force and the European Society of Cardiology Committee for Practice Guidelines (Writing Committee to Develop Guidelines for Management of Patients with Ventricular Arrhythmias and the Prevention of Sudden Cardiac Death). J Am Coll Cardiol 2006;48:1064-1108.
129. Abraham W, Fisher W, Smith A, et al: Cardiac resynchronization in chronic heart failure. N Engl J Med 2002;346:1845-1853.
130. Jarcho JA: Biventricular pacing. N Engl J Med 2006;355:288-294.
131. Bradley D, Bradley E, Baughman K, et al: Cardiac resynchronization and death from progressive heart failure: A meta-analysis of randomized control trials. JAMA 2003;289:730-740.
132. Cleland JAF, Danbert J, Erdmann E, et al: The effect of cardiac resynchronization on morbidity and mortality in heart failure. N Engl J Med 352:1539-1549, 2005.
133. Strickberger SA, Conti J, Daoud EG, et al: Patient selection for cardiac resynchronization therapy: From the

Council on Clinical Cardiology Subcommittee on Electrocardiography and Arrhythmias and the Quality of Care and Outcomes Research Interdisciplinary Working Group, in collaboration with the Heart Rhythm Society. Circulation 2005;111: 2146-2150.
134. Young J, Abraham W, Smith A, et al: Combined cardiac resynchronization and implantable cardioversion defibrillation in advanced chronic heart failure. The MIRACLE ICD Trial. JAMA 2003;289:2685-2694.
135. Bristow MR, Saxon LA, Boehmer J, et al: Comparison of medical therapy, pacing and defibrillation in heart failure (COMPANION). N Engl J Med 2004;350:2140-2150.
136. Stevenson LW, Rose EA: Left ventricular assist devices bridges to transplantation, recovery, and destination for whom? Circulation 2003;108:3059-3063.
137. Kittleson M, Hurwitz S, Shah M, et al: Development of circulatory-renal limitations to angiotensin-converting enzyme inhibitors identify patients with severe heart failure and early mortality. J Am Coll Cardiol 2003;41:2029-2035.
138. Felker GM, Rogers JG: Same bridge, new destinations. J Am Coll Cardiol 2006;47:930-932.
139. Mancini D, Burkoff D: Mechanical device-based methods of managing and treating heart failure. Circulation 2005;12:438-448.
140. Goldstein G, Oz M, Rose E: Medical progress: Implantable left ventricular assist devices. N Engl J Med 1998;339:1522-1533.
141. Nemeh H, Smedira N: Mechanical treatment of heart failure. The growing role of LVADs and artificial hearts. Cleve Clin J Med 2003;70:223-234.
142. Aaronson KD, Patel H, Pagani FD: Patient selection for left ventricular assist device therapy. Ann Thorac Surg 2003;75:S29-S35.
143. Muller J, Wallukat G, Weng Y, et al: Weaning from mechanical cardiac support in patients with idiopathic dilated cardiomyopathy. Circulation 1997;96:542-549.
144. Rose E, Gelijas A, Moskowitz A, et al: Long-term use of a left ventricular assist device for end-stage heart failure. N Engl J Med 2001;345: 1435-1443.
145. Copeland JG, Smith RG, Arabia FA, et al: Cardiac replacement with a total artificial heart as a bridge to transplantation. N Engl J Med 2004;351:859-867.

Chapter 31

Acute Coronary Syndromes and Acute Myocardial Infarction

Steven Werns

EPIDEMIOLOGY

The Global Burden of Disease Study identified ischemic heart disease as the leading cause of death in the world in 1990.[1] According to the INTERHEART study, a case-control study of acute myocardial infarction (MI) that enrolled 15,152 cases and 14,820 controls from 52 countries, nine risk factors accounted for greater than 90% of the population-attributable risk of acute MI.[2] Cigarette smoking and abnormal lipids accounted for approximately two thirds of the population-attributable risk of acute MI. Psychosocial factors, abdominal obesity, diabetes, and hypertension were the next most important risk factors. The findings of the study were consistent across all geographic regions and ethnic groups of the world.

The American Heart Association Statistics Committee published a 2007 update of Heart Disease and Stroke Statistics online.[3] Coronary heart disease (CHD), which includes acute MI and other forms of coronary artery disease manifesting acutely, as well as chronic coronary artery disease (CAD), is the single greatest cause of death among American men and women. CHD accounted for 20% of all deaths in the United States in 2004. It is estimated that the number of hospitalizations for acute coronary artery syndromes in the United States in 2004 was 1,565,000. The estimated annual incidence of MI in the United States is 565,000 new attacks and 30,000 recurrent attacks. The economic costs of CHD are staggering and are estimated to include direct costs of $83.6 billion for hospital charges, physician fees, and medications and indirect costs of $68 billion due to lost productivity.[3]

DEFINITIONS

The nomenclature of the acute coronary artery syndromes has undergone significant change in recent years. *Acute coronary syndrome* (ACS) refers to ". . . any constellation of clinical symptoms that are compatible with acute myocardial ischemia."[4] Therefore, the ACS spectrum encompasses unstable angina, non–ST segment elevation myocardial infarction (NSTEMI), and ST segment elevation myocardial infarction (STEMI). The presence or absence in the blood of either troponin or the MB fraction of creatine kinase (CK-MB) determines the distinction between a diagnosis of either unstable angina or myocardial infarction (MI). (For convenience, these and other relevant abbreviations are listed in Table 31-1.) A joint committee of the European Society of Cardiology (ESC) and the American College of Cardiology (ACC) published a revised definition of MI in 2000.[5] The clinical diagnosis of an acute, evolving, or recent MI was defined as a typical rise and gradual fall (for troponin) or more rapid rise and fall (for CK-MB) of biochemical markers of myocardial necrosis, with at least one of the following: ischemic symptoms, development of pathologic Q waves on the electrocardiogram (ECG), ECG changes indicative of ischemia (ST segment elevation or depression), or coronary artery intervention.[5]

The increased sensitivity of troponin compared with CK-MB and the new criteria for the diagnosis of acute MI dictate that many patients who were classified as having unstable angina by the old criteria are now given a diagnosis of acute MI. Among 1851 patients who were enrolled in a prospective study, 538 patients received a diagnosis of acute MI based on dynamic changes in troponin T, compared with only 427 patients when CK-MB was used to diagnose acute MI, representing a 41% increase.[6] A retrospective analysis of 2181 patients with suspected ACS and no ST segment elevation found that the prevalence of acute MI ranged from 9.7% to 22% based on differing troponin-based definitions, compared with 7.8% based on CK-MB alone.[7] Meier and colleagues[8] studied 493 consecutive patients with suspected ACS. 224 patients had elevated CK-MB, and an additional 51 patients had normal CK-MB but elevated troponin I. The latter group was characterized by greater incidence of comorbid conditions and higher 6-month mortality. Among 29,357 patients with non–ST segment elevation ACS who were enrolled in a registry called "Can Rapid Risk Stratification

Table 31-1. Cardiac Critical Care Abbreviations

ACC	American College of Cardiology
ACE	angiotensin-converting enzyme
ACS	acute coronary syndrome
AF	atrial fibrillation
AHA	American Heart Association
APSAC	anisolylated plasminogen–streptokinase activator complex
aPTT	activated partial thromboplastin time
ARB	angiotensin receptor blocker
AVB	atrioventricular block
BNP	brain natriuretic peptide
CABG	coronary artery bypass grafting
CAD	coronary artery disease
CHF	congestive heart failure
CI	confidence interval
CK-MB	MB* fraction of creatine kinase
CT	computed tomography
ECG	electrocardiogram
EF	ejection fraction
ESC	European Society of Cardiology
GP	glycoprotein
IABP	intra-aortic balloon pump
ICH	intracranial hemorrhage
ICU	intensive care unit
ICD	implantable cardioverter-defibrillator
INR	international normalized ratio
IRA	infarct-related artery
LAD	left anterior descending (artery)
LBBB	left bundle branch block
LDL	low-density lipoprotein
LMWH	low-molecular-weight heparin
MI	myocardial infarction
MR	mitral regurgitation
MRI	magnetic resonance imaging
NNT	number needed to treat
NO	nitric oxide
NSTEMI	non–ST segment elevation myocardial infarction
NTG	nitroglycerin
PA	pulmonary artery
PCI	percutaneous coronary intervention
PCWP	pulmonary capillary wedge pressure
RCA	right coronary artery
rPA	reteplase
RVMI	right ventricular myocardial infarction
SK	streptokinase
STEMI	ST segment elevation myocardial infarction
tPA	tissue plasminogen activator
UA	unstable angina
UFH	unfractionated heparin
VF	ventricular fibrillation
VSR	ventricular septal rupture
VT	ventricular tachycardia

*Muscle-brain.

of Unstable Angina Patients Suppress Adverse Outcomes with Early Implementation of the ACC/AHA Guidelines?" (CRUSADE), 18% of patients were CK-MB negative and troponin positive.[9] The risk of in-hospital death was significantly increased among troponin-positive patients regardless of CK-MB status.

The Global Registry of Acute Coronary Events (GRACE) is a prospective observational registry of 26,267 patients with ACS who were admitted to 106 hospitals in 14 countries.[10] (A list of eponyms in use for various cardiac registries and drug trials is provided in Table 31-2.) Among the 10,719 patients (10.4%) with both CK-MB and troponin data, 1110 patients without elevation of CK-MB were diagnosed with acute MI by virtue of elevated troponin. Patients who were troponin negative had similar 6-month mortality regardless of CK-MB status, but patients who were CK-MB negative and troponin positive had a twofold greater hospital case-fatality rate.

PATHOGENESIS

The pathophysiology of the ACSs has been discussed in several excellent reviews.[11,12] James Herrick published an autopsy study in 1912 that attributed acute MI to coronary artery thrombosis.[13] Nevertheless, for many decades investigators debated whether coronary artery thrombi formed in vivo or were merely postmortem artifacts. In the 1970s coronary artery spasm was hypothesized to be an important mechanism in the pathogenesis of acute myocardial ischemia and infarction.[14,15] Although coronary spasm has been well documented as the cause of variant angina,[16] and increased vasoreactivity of the culprit lesion has been demonstrated in patients with unstable angina,[17] a number of studies in the 1980s provided evidence that the usual cause of an ACS is coronary artery thrombosis precipitated by ulceration or rupture of an atherosclerotic plaque, rather than coronary vasospasm.[11]

The coronary angiographic findings published by DeWood and coworkers[18,19] were instrumental in advancing our understanding of the pathogenesis of ACS. Among 192 patients with non–Q wave MI who underwent coronary angiography within 24 hours of peak symptoms, 49 patients (26%) had total occlusion of the infarct-related artery (IRA).[19] The frequency of total occlusion of the IRA was greater among patients who underwent angiography between 72 hours and 7 days after peak symptoms (23/55; 42%). Among 126 patients with Q wave MI who underwent coronary angiography within 4 hours of the onset of symptoms, total occlusion of the IRA was found in 110 patients (87%).[18] Seventy-nine patients underwent emergency coronary artery bypass graft (CABG) surgery, and thrombi were recovered from the coronary arteries in 57 patients. These observations supported the notion that coronary thrombosis is a key event in the pathogenesis of MI and not merely a postmortem event as had been suggested previously.

Angioscopy of coronary arteries in 31 patients with unstable angina or acute MI demonstrated the presence of coronary thrombi in 14 of 15 patients with unstable angina and 15 of 16 patients with acute MI.[20] Grayish white thrombi were observed in 10 of the 14 patients with unstable angina, whereas red thrombi were observed in all 15 patients with acute MI, compared with only 4 of the patients with unstable angina. The different appearances may reflect differences in the age or composition of the thrombi, such as whether the thrombi were platelet-rich or fibrin-rich. A postmortem study of acute coronary lesions in patients with fatal ACS demonstrated that coronary thrombi consisted almost entirely of fibrin in patients with acute MI, whereas patients with unstable angina had

Table 31-2. Cardiac Drug Trial and Registry Eponyms

4S	Scandinavian Simvastatin Survival Study
ACUITY	Acute Catheterization and Urgent Intervention Triage Strategy
AIMI	AngioJet Rheolytic Thrombectomy in Patients Undergoing Primary Angioplasty for Acute Myocardial Infarction
AIRE	Acute Infarction Ramipril Efficacy
APRICOT	Antithrombotics in the Prevention of Reocclusion in Coronary Thrombolysis
ASPECT-2	Antithrombotics in the Secondary Prevention of Events in Coronary Thrombosis-2
ASSENT	Assessment of Safety and Efficacy of a New Thrombolytic
BHAT	Beta-Blocker Heart Attack Trial
CADILLAC	Controlled Abciximab and Device Investigation to Lower Angioplasty Complications
CAPRICORN	Carvedilol Post-Infarct Survival Control in LV Dysfunction
CARE	Cholesterol and Recurrent Events Trial
CAST	Cardiac Arrhythmia Suppression Trial
CLARITY	Clopidogrel as Adjunctive Reperfusion Therapy
COMMIT	Clopidogrel and Metoprolol in Myocardial Infarction Trial
CREATE	Clinical Trial of Reviparin and Metabolic Modulation in Acute Myocardial Infarction Treatment Evaluation
CRUSADE	Can Rapid Risk Stratification of Unstable Angina Patients Suppress Adverse Outcomes with Early Implementation of the ACC/AHA Guidelines
CURE	Clopidogrel in Unstable Angina to Prevent Recurrent Events
DANAMI	Danish Multicenter Randomized Study on Fibrinolytic Therapy versus Acute Coronary Angioplasty for Acute Myocardial Infarction
DAVIT-II	Danish Verapamil Infarction Trial
EPHESUS	Eplerenone Post-Acute Myocardial Infarction Heart Failure Efficacy and Survival Study
EXTRACT	Enoxaparin and Thrombolysis Reperfusion for Acute Myocardial Infarction Treatment
FRISC	Fast Revascularization during Instability in Coronary Artery Disease
GISSI	Gruppo Italiano per lo Studio della Sopravvivenza nell'Infarto Miocardico
GRACE	Global Registry of Acute Coronary Events
GUSTO	Global Utilization of Streptokinase and t-PA for Occluded Coronary Arteries
HINT	Holland Interuniversity Nifedipine/Metoprolol Trial
ICTUS	Invasive versus Conservative Treatment in Unstable Coronary Syndromes
ISIS	International Study of Infarct Survival
LATE	Late Assessment of Thrombolytic Efficacy
LIPID	Long-Term Intervention with Pravastatin in Ischemic Disease Trial
MDPIT	Multicenter Diltiazem Postinfarction Trial
MERLIN	Middlesbrough Early Revascularization to Limit Infarction
MILIS	Multicenter Investigation of the Limitation of Infarct Size
MITI	Myocardial Infarction Triage and Intervention
NRMI	National Registry of MI
OASIS	Organization for the Assessment of Strategies for Ischemic Syndromes
OAT	Occluded Artery Trial
OPTIMAAL	Optimal Trial in Myocardial Infarction with the Angiotensin II Antagonist Losartan
PAMI	Primary Angioplasty in Myocardial Infarction
PROVE IT	Pravastatin or Atorvastatin Evaluation and Infection Therapy
PURSUIT	Platelet Glycoprotein IIb/IIIa in Unstable Angina: Receptor Suppression Using Integrilin Therapy
REACT	Rescue Angioplasty versus Conservative Treatment or Repeat Thrombolysis
RITA-3	Randomized Intervention Trial of Unstable Angina
SAVE	Survival and Ventricular Enlargement
SHOCK	Should We Emergently Revascularize Occluded Coronaries for Cardiogenic Shock?
SMILE	Survival of Myocardial Infarction Long-Term Evaluation
SWORD	Survival With Oral *d*-Sotalol
TACTICS	Treat Angina with Aggrastat and Determine Cost of Therapy with an Invasive or Conservative Strategy
TIMI	Thrombolysis in Myocardial Infarction
TRACE	Trandolapril Cardiac Evaluation
VALIANT	Valsartan in Acute Myocardial Infarction
VANQWISH	Veterans Affairs Non–Q Wave Infarction Strategies in Hospital
WARIS II	Warfarin, Aspirin, Reinfarction Study

coronary thrombi that were composed almost entirely of platelets.[21]

Several groups of investigators performed comparisons of coronary angiograms obtained before and after the onset of ACS.[22-26] Only a small fraction of the culprit arteries had severe (greater than 70% occlusion) stenosis on the initial angiogram, and a majority of the culprit arteries had mild (less than 50% occlusion) stenosis on the initial angiogram. These observations are consistent with the Framingham Heart Study report that among 5144 patients in whom CAD developed, sudden death or acute MI was the initial presentation in 62% of men and 46% of women.[27]

Postmortem pathologic studies and antemortem intravascular ultrasound studies supported the concept that either erosion or rupture of an atherosclerotic plaque is responsible for coronary thrombosis and the ensuing ACS[12,28,29] (Figs. 31-1 and 31-2). Patients with fatal MIs were found to have ruptured plaques with abundant macrophages and T-lymphocytes.[30] Matrix metalloproteinases

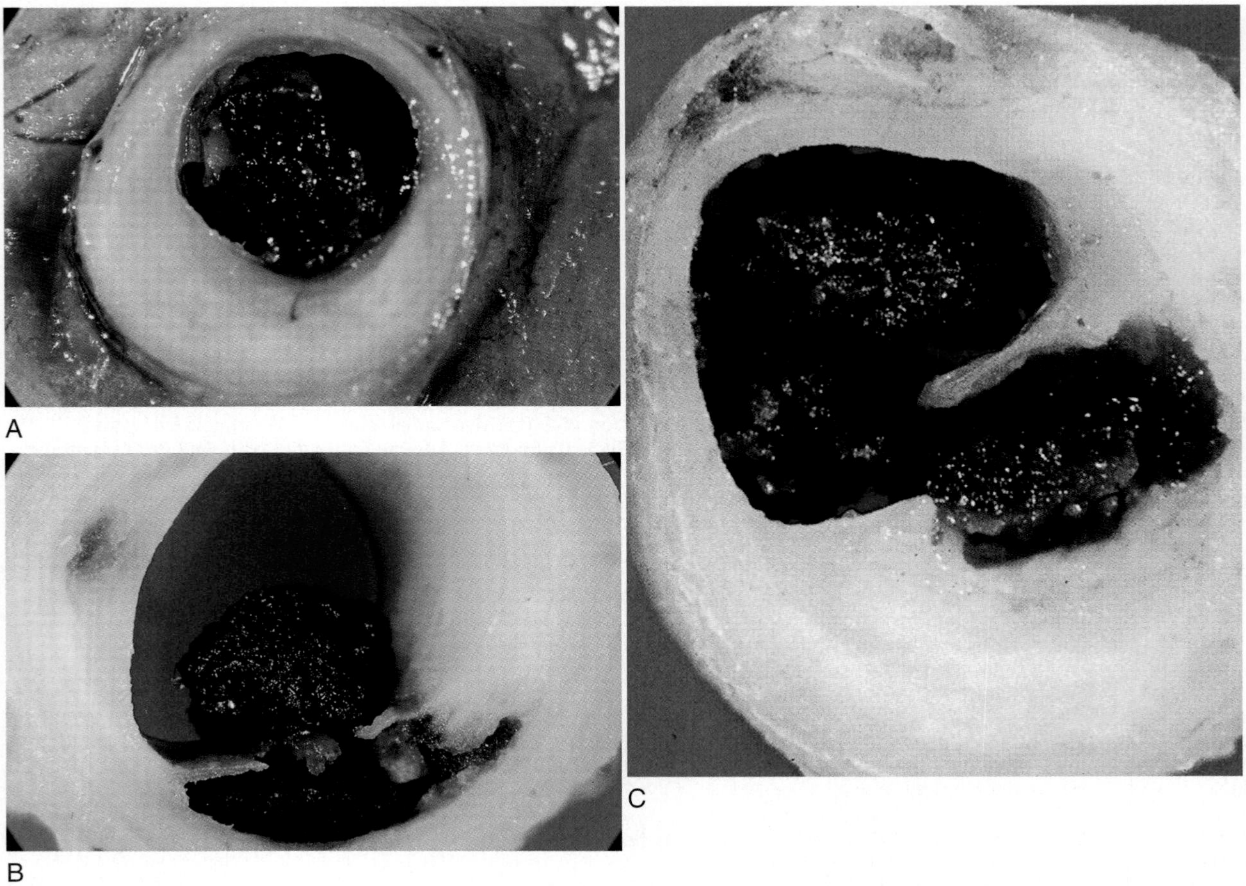

Figure 31-1. Postmortem cross sections of human coronary arteries from patients with acute coronary syndromes. **A,** An acute coronary syndrome may ensue from a thrombus adherent to an erosion on the surface of a plaque that occupies less than 50% of the coronary artery lumen. **B,** Unstable angina or non–ST segment elevation myocardial infarction may result from a nonocclusive thrombus at the site of a ruptured cap. **C,** A thrombus extending from the lipid core through the ruptured cap occludes the coronary artery lumen, the usual cause of ST segment elevation myocardial infarction. (From Davies MJ: The pathophysiology of acute coronary syndromes. Heart 2000;83:361-366.)

derived from human macrophages are able to induce breakdown of the collagen in fibrous caps obtained from human atherosclerotic plaques.[31] Histologic examination of plaque obtained via coronary atherectomy of lesions in patients with either stable angina or ACS revealed that the plaques of ACS patients are characterized by increased infiltration by macrophages and expression of tissue factor and matrix metalloproteinases (e.g., gelatinase), suggesting that macrophage-derived mediators play a role in both erosion or rupture of the fibrous cap and formation of a thrombus at the site of the plaque.[32-34] A thin fibrous cap overlying a lipid-rich core is believed to be a factor that predisposes an atherosclerotic plaque to rupture.[29]

Both angiographic and intravascular ultrasound investigations of patients with ACS have shown that multiple complex or ruptured plaques exist simultaneously, implicating a systemic process in the pathogenesis of plaque rupture.[35,36] Additional evidence of a systemic inflammatory state include activated monocytes in the systemic circulation and elevated serum levels of CD40, a ligand that is released by activated platelets.[37,38] The role of inflammatory mediators in the pathogenesis of ACS may explain the association of acute infection with an increased short-term risk of acute MI.[39,40]

Another common triggering event for an acute MI is heavy physical exertion.[41-43] One report cited evidence that physical exertion, such as shoveling snow, may provoke plaque rupture.[44] The exercised-induced physiologic changes that may trigger an acute MI include increased heart rate, blood pressure, coronary vasoconstriction, plasma catecholamines, and platelet activation.[45] Platelet activation that occurs during exercise may not be

Figure 31-2. Rupture of a vulnerable plaque leads to the activation, adhesion, and aggregation of platelets and the activation of the clotting cascade, resulting in the formation of a thrombus. Acute ST segment elevation myocardial infarction may occur if this process results in complete occlusion of the artery. Alternatively, incomplete coronary artery occlusion may result in non–ST segment elevation myocardial infarction or unstable angina. (From Yeghiazarians Y, Braunstein JB, Askari A, Stone PH: Unstable angina pectoris. N Engl J Med 2000;342:101-114.)

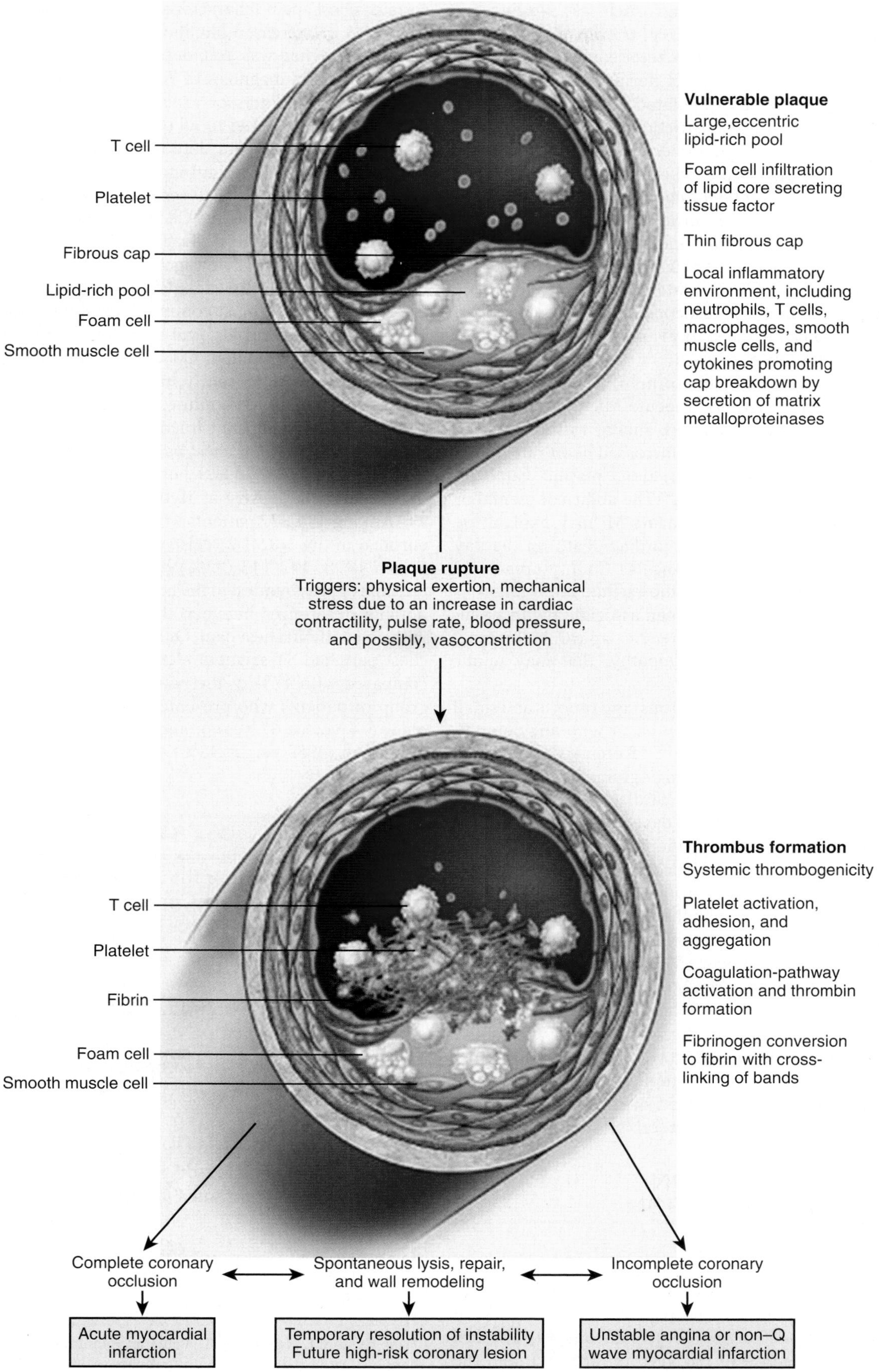
T cell
Platelet
Fibrous cap
Lipid-rich pool
Foam cell
Smooth muscle cell
Vulnerable plaque
Large,eccentric lipid-rich pool
Foam cell infiltration of lipid core secreting tissue factor
Thin fibrous cap
Local inflammatory environment, including neutrophils, T cells, macrophages, smooth muscle cells, and cytokines promoting cap breakdown by secretion of matrix metalloproteinases
Plaque rupture
Triggers: physical exertion, mechanical stress due to an increase in cardiac contractility, pulse rate, blood pressure, and possibly, vasoconstriction
T cell
Platelet
Fibrin
Foam cell
Smooth muscle cell
Thrombus formation
Systemic thrombogenicity
Platelet activation, adhesion, and aggregation
Coagulation-pathway activation and thrombin formation
Fibrinogen conversion to fibrin with cross-linking of bands
Complete coronary occlusion
Spontaneous lysis, repair, and wall remodeling
Incomplete coronary occlusion
Acute myocardial infarction
Temporary resolution of instability Future high-risk coronary lesion
Unstable angina or non–Q wave myocardial infarction

inhibited by antiplatelet drugs such as aspirin and clopidogrel.[46,47] Normal coronary arteries exhibit flow-dependent vasodilation during exercise, while atherosclerotic coronary arteries constrict during exercise because of defective nitric oxide–mediated endothelium-dependent vasodilation.[48] Vasoconstriction would increase shear stress at the site of an atherosclerotic plaque.[49] Increased shear stress may play a role in both activation of platelets and plaque rupture. Angiographic studies have shown that the culprit stenosis is eccentric in a majority of ACS patients.[22] It is believed that increased shear stress may stimulate rupture of an eccentric plaque where the plaque and vessel wall meet.[50] Thus, platelet activation and plaque rupture precipitated by vasoconstriction and increased shear stress may be the critical links between physical exertion and the onset of ACS.

Episodes of anger and other forms of mental stress have been implicated as triggers of acute MI.[51,52] The physiologic effects of mental stress are similar to those caused by physical exertion, including increased heart rate, blood pressure, coronary vasoconstriction, plasma catecholamines, and platelet activation.[45] The ability of mental or emotional stress to trigger an acute MI may explain the increased incidence of sudden cardiac death on the day of an earthquake in the Los Angeles County area[53] and acute MI during the week after the earthquake.[54] Episodes of emotional stress also have been associated with a syndrome of transient left ventricular apical ballooning, known as takotsubo cardiomyopathy, that may mimic evolving acute MI or ACS.[55,56]

Finally, as described in numerous case reports and small series of patients, acute MI may occur with angiographically normal coronary arteries.[57,58] Kereiakes and associates[59] analyzed the coronary angiograms of 810 patients with acute MI who underwent cardiac catheterization at 90 minutes and again 7 to 10 days after receiving fibrinolytic therapy. Eighty-five patients (10.9%) were found to have less than 50% stenotic occlusion of the infarct artery. Thus, spontaneous thrombolysis in a patient with a ruptured plaque and minimal atherosclerosis is one possible cause of a normal coronary angiogram after an acute MI. Frequent causes of acute MI with truly normal coronary arteries are coronary embolism (e.g., in patients with atrial fibrillation or those who have prosthetic heart valves)[60]; coronary spasm (e.g., in patients who abuse cocaine)[61]; and spontaneous coronary artery dissection (e.g., in pregnant or postpartum women).[62] Coronary spasm also has been implicated in the pathogenesis of acute MI after induction of general anesthesia.[58]

ST SEGMENT ELEVATION MYOCARDIAL INFARCTION

Clinical Manifestations

Clinical History

The initial differentiation of ACS from other causes of chest pain is based on the chest pain history, physical examination, presence of risk factors for CAD, and the ECG. A recent review of the literature concluded that certain chest pain characteristics are associated with decreased or increased likelihoods of ACS[63] (Box 31-1). The feature that was found to be associated with the highest risk of a diagnosis of ACS is radiation of pain to one or both shoulders or arms. A prospective study of patients who presented to an emergency department for evaluation of chest pain determined that pain relief by nitroglycerin is not a useful indicator of the presence or absence of ACS.[64] Nitroglycerin relieved chest pain in 35% of patients with active CAD, compared with 41% of patients without active CAD ($P>.2$).[64]

Another literature review included 15 studies published from 1989 to 2002 that identified symptoms of ACS.[65] Chest pain was the most common symptom among both men and women, but atypical symptoms were common, especially among women. Compared with men, women with ACS were significantly more likely to report back and jaw pain, nausea, vomiting, dyspnea, indigestion, and palpitations. A significant fraction of patients with acute MI do not complain of chest pain at the time of presentation.[66,67] A total of 1674 U.S. hospitals contributed patients to the National Registry of Myocardial Infarction (NRMI) 2.[66] Among 434,877 patients with confirmed MI who were enrolled in the NRMI-2 registry between June 1994 and March 1998, 142,445 (33%) did not have chest pain at the time of presentation to the hospital. There were several notable differences between the groups who presented with and without chest pain. Only 23% of patients without chest pain had ST-segment elevation on the initial ECG, compared with 47% of the patients with chest pain. The group of patients who presented without chest pain was older (74 versus 67 years), and had a higher proportion of women (49% versus 38%).

Box 31-1

Risk Stratification for Acute Myocardial Infarction and Acute Coronary Syndrome by Chest Pain History

Low Risk
Pain that is pleuritic, positional, or reproducible with palpation or is described as stabbing

Probable Low Risk
Pain not related to exertion or that occurs in a small inframammary area of the chest wall

Probable High Risk
Pain described as pressure, is similar to that of prior myocardial infarction or worse than prior anginal pain, or is accompanied by nausea, vomiting, or diaphoresis

High Risk
Pain that radiates to one or both shoulders or arms or is related to exertion

From Swap CJ, Nagurney JT: Value and limitations of chest pain history in the evaluation of patients with suspected acute coronary syndromes. JAMA 2005;294:2623-2639.

The absence of chest pain has a major impact on hospital management and outcomes, even among patients who present with ST segment elevation.[66,67] A report from the GRACE registry compared 6385 patients with STEMI and typical symptoms with 541 patients whose presenting symptoms did not include chest pain.[67] Patients without chest pain were significantly less likely to receive in-reperfusion therapy, i.e. fibrinolysis or primary percutaneous coronary intervention (PCI), β-blockers, and aspirin. Perhaps as a consequence of under-treatment, hospital mortality was significantly greater among patients with STEMI and no chest pain than among patients with chest pain (18.7% versus 6.3%; $P>.001$) (Fig. 31-3).

There is a long-standing belief that diabetes is associated with silent myocardial ischemia and painless MI due to autonomic neuropathy. Nevertheless, in the NRMI 2 registry, only 33% of the patients with painless MI had diabetes mellitus, and in the GRACE registry, only 32% of patients with painless ACS had diabetes.[66,67]

Physical Examination

The initial physical examination provides important prognostic information in patients with acute MI. Killip and Kimball published their classic study in 1967.[68] Among 250 patients with acute MI, 81 patients (33%) had no heart failure (Killip class I), 96 (38%) had mild heart failure (Killip class II), 26 (10%) had pulmonary edema (Killip class III), and 47 (19%) had cardiogenic shock (Killip class IV). Respective mortality rates were 6%, 17%, 38%, and 81%. Although the overall mortality for acute MI has decreased since 1967, the Killip class on admission remains a powerful predictor of outcome among patients treated with reperfusion therapy.[69,70] DeGeare and coworkers[70] performed an analysis of 2654 patients with acute MI who were enrolled in three primary angioplasty trials. Patients in Killip class IV were excluded. Increasing Killip class was associated with an increased need for intra-aortic balloon counterpulsation and a greater incidence of renal failure, major arrhythmias, and major bleeding. After controlling for confounding variables, the Killip class on admission remained a multivariate predictor of both in-hospital and 6-month mortality.

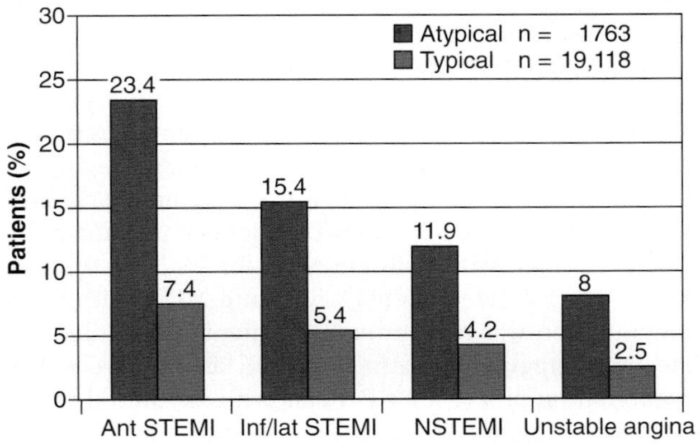

Figure 31-3. In-hospital mortality rate in subgroups with acute coronary syndrome (ACS) according to presenting symptoms. Ant, anterior; Inf/lat, inferior or lateral; NSTEMI, non–ST segment elevation myocardial infarction; STEMI, ST segment elevation myocardial infarction. (From Brieger D, Eagle KA, Goodman SG, et al: Acute coronary syndromes without chest pain, an underdiagnosed and undertreated high-risk group: Insights from the Global Registry of Acute Coronary Events. Chest 2004;126:461-469.)

The physical examination also may provide clues to the diagnosis of causes of chest pain other than ACS. A pericardial friction rub may be audible in patients with pericarditis. Aortic dissection may be associated with diminished or absent pulses. Both diagnoses are important to exclude because they are contraindications to fibrinolytic therapy.

Diagnostic Approach

The ACC/AHA Task Force on Practice Guidelines has published detailed recommendations for the diagnosis and management of patients with ACS.[4,71] Conditions for which there is evidence or general agreement, or both, that a given procedure or treatment is useful and effective are categorized as Class I[71] (not to be confused with Killip class I). Conditions for which there is conflicting evidence or divergence of opinion are categorized as Class II. The weight of evidence or opinion is in favor of usefulness or efficacy for Class IIa conditions, while usefulness or efficacy is less well established for Class IIb conditions. Class III conditions are conditions for which there is evidence and/or general agreement that a procedure/treatment is not useful or effective and may be harmful in some cases.

Electrocardiogram

The ACC/AHA Guidelines for the Management of Patients with ST-Elevation Myocardial Infarction include three Class I indications for an ECG.[71] The first is that all patients with chest discomfort or other symptoms suggestive of STEMI should have a 12-lead ECG within 10 minutes of arrival in the emergency department (and it should be interpreted by an experienced physician). The second is that serial ECGs should be performed at intervals of 5 to 10 minutes in patients with a nondiagnostic initial ECG if the patient remains symptomatic and there is a high clinical suspicion of STEMI. The third is that right-sided ECG leads should be obtained to screen for right ventricular MI in patients with inferior STEMI.

There are two Class I indications for fibrinolytic therapy in patients with STEMI: (1) symptom onset within the prior 12 hours and ST elevation greater than 0.1 mV in at least two contiguous precordial leads or at least two adjacent limb leads; and (2) symptom onset within the prior 12 hours and new or presumably new left bundle branch block (LBBB).[71] The electrocardiographic diagnosis of acute MI in the presence of LBBB is problematic. Although electrocardiographic criteria for diagnosis have been proposed, one study that applied the criteria to 83 patients with LBBB and symptoms suggestive of acute MI found that the ECG algorithm had a sensitivity of only 10%.[72,73]

The ECG provides additional important information in patients with acute MI. Patients with acute inferior STEMI who have ST segment depression in the precordial leads have larger infarctions, more complications post-MI, and a higher mortality rate than patients without precordial ST segment depression.[74] The presence of Q waves in the infarct territory on the initial ECG is an independent predictor of greater 30-day mortality irrespective of the infarct location or time between symptom onset and administration of fibrinolytic therapy.[75] Nevertheless, substantial myocardial salvage is possible despite Q waves on the initial ECG.[76]

The electrocardiographic leads with ST segment elevation have been correlated with occlusions of the left anterior descending (LAD), left circumflex, or right coronary arteries.[77,78] The number of leads with ST segment elevation before reperfusion therapy and the degree of resolution of ST segment elevation after either fibrinolytic therapy or primary angioplasty confer useful prognostic information. The Gruppo Italiano per lo Studio della Sopravvivenza nell'Infarto Miocardico (GISSI) trial investigators reported that in-hospital mortality was directly related to the number of leads with ST segment elevation for both the patients treated with streptokinase and the control group.[79] Treatment with streptokinase significantly reduced in-hospital mortality among patients with ST segment elevation in four or more leads, but not among patients with ST segment elevation that was confined to two or three leads[79] (Fig. 31-4). Early ST segment recovery is associated with improved infarct zone wall motion[80] and greater myocardial salvage as assessed by technetium-99m sestamibi scintigraphy.[81] Also, resolution of ST segment elevation within 90 minutes after either primary angioplasty or fibrinolytic therapy identifies patients with lower mortality at 30 days and 1 year after STEMI.[82-84] Continuous ECG monitoring is customary for detection of arrhythmias and conduction abnormalities.

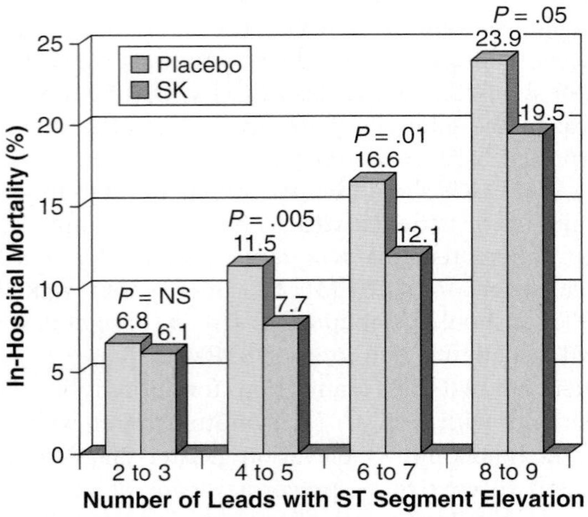

Figure 31-4. In-hospital mortality among patients randomized to the streptokinase (SK) and control groups in the Gruppo Italiano per lo Studio della Sopravvivenza nell'Infarto Miocardico (GISSI-1) trial. Treatment with streptokinase significantly reduced in-hospital mortality among patients with ST segment elevation in 4 or more leads, but not among patients with ST segment elevation that was confined to 2 or 3 leads. NS, not significant. (Data from Mauri F, Gasparini M, Barbonaglia L, et al: Prognostic significance of the extent of myocardial injury in acute myocardial infarction treated by streptokinase (the GISSI trial). Am J Cardiol 1989;63:1291-1295.)

It is important to recognize that ST segment elevation occurs in numerous conditions other than acute MI.[85] The list includes: left ventricular hypertrophy, LBBB, acute pericarditis, hyperkalemia, Brugada syndrome, pulmonary embolism, and left ventricular apical ballooning syndrome (takotsubo cardiomyopathy) [55,85] (Fig. 31-5).

Cardiac Enzymes

Myocardial necrosis is accompanied by the release of several biochemical markers in circulating blood, including creatine kinase, myoglobin, troponins T and I, and lactate dehydrogenase. As noted above, a typical rise and gradual fall of troponin or more rapid rise and fall of CK-MB are required to diagnose an acute, evolving, or recent MI.[5] The ACC/AHA guidelines, however, stress that decisions such as initiation of reperfusion therapy for patients with ST segment elevation and symptoms of STEMI should not be delayed until the results of serum cardiac biomarkers are available.[86]

Although troponin has become the preferred biomarker for myocardial necrosis, numerous other causes of an elevated troponin have been recognized, and several may be associated with chest pain and/or ST segment elevation.[87] An elevated troponin in patients with pulmonary embolism is associated with right ventricular dysfunction and an increased risk of hypotension and death.[88-90] Elevated cardiac troponin also has been reported in patients with acute pericarditis, and patients with ST segment elevation were more likely to have an elevated troponin.[91]

Echocardiography

Echocardiography may be a useful diagnostic tool under a variety of circumstances. A transesophageal echocardiogram may be useful to differentiate STEMI from aortic dissection. Both transthoracic and transesophageal echocardiography are useful in patients with congestive heart failure (CHF) or hypotension to evaluate left and right ventricular function, to rule out cardiac tamponade, and to diagnose ventricular septal rupture or mitral regurgitation (MR). Mitral regurgitation is frequent among patients with uncomplicated MI. Color Doppler echocardiography was performed within 48 hours of admission in a series of 417 consecutive patients with acute MI.[92] Mild mitral regurgitation was present in 121 patients (29%), moderate mitral regurgitation in 21 (5%), and severe mitral regurgitation in 4 (1%).[92] Patients with any mitral regurgitation had higher 30-day and 1-year mortality rates, and mitral regurgitation was independently associated with increased 1-year mortality.[92] Echocardiography performed within 30 days after acute MI revealed mitral regurgitation in 50% of a cohort of 773 patients.[93] A murmur was not detected by cardiac auscultation in 54% of patients with mild and 31% of patients with moderate or severe mitral regurgitation.[93] Among 30-day survivors of an MI, during a mean follow-up period of 4.7 years moderate or

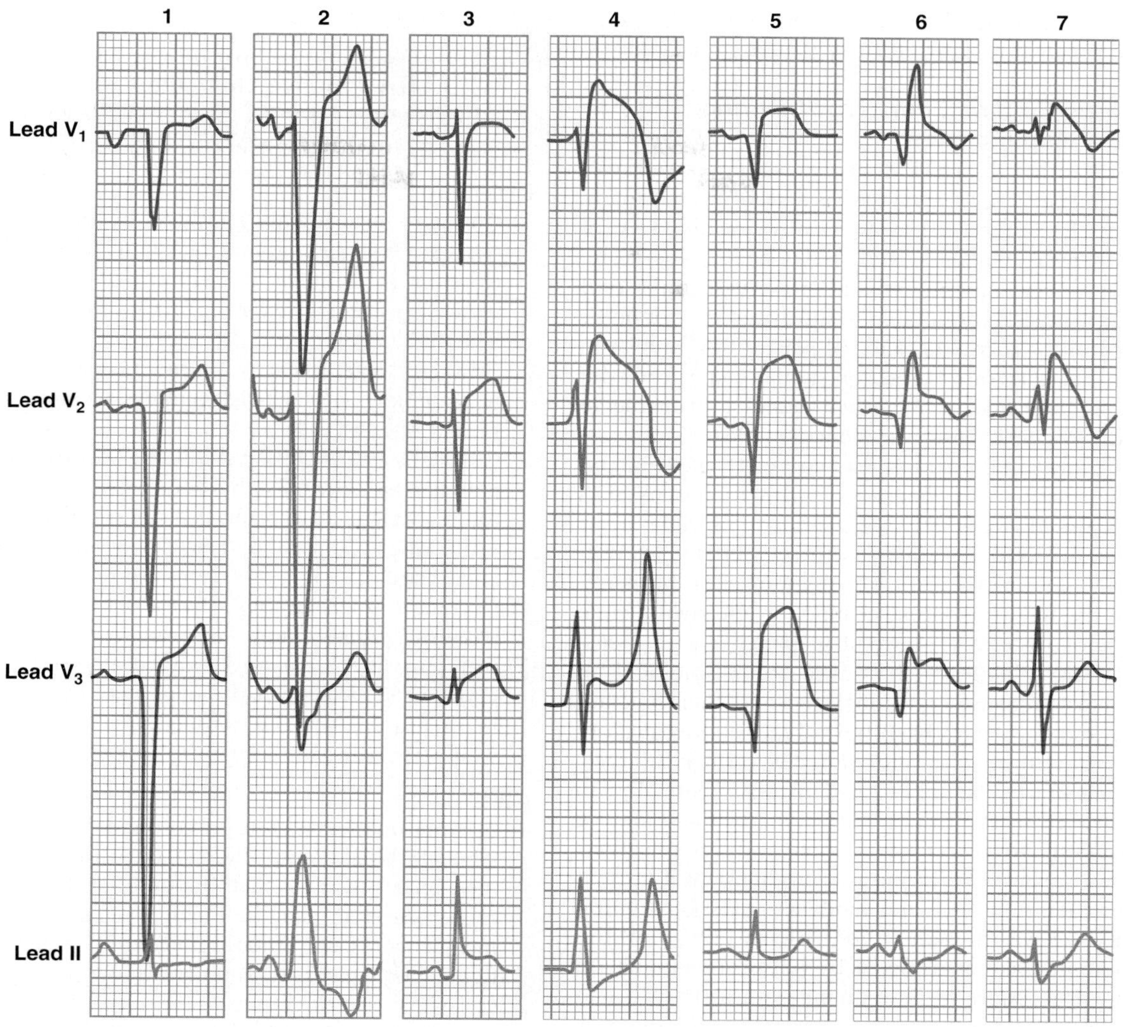

Figure 31-5. ST segment elevation in various conditions. *Tracing 1,* Left ventricular hypertrophy. *Tracing 2,* Left bundle branch block. *Tracing 3,* Acute pericarditis. *Tracing 4,* Hyperkalemia. *Tracing 5,* Acute anteroseptal infarction. *Tracing 6,* Acute anteroseptal infarction and right bundle branch block. *Tracing 7,* Brugada syndrome. (From Wang K, Asinger RW, Marriott HJ: ST-segment elevation in conditions other than acute myocardial infarction. N Engl J Med 2003;349:2128-2135.)

severe mitral regurgitation detected by echocardiography within 30 days of MI was associated with a 55% increase in the relative risk (RR) of death independent of age, gender, left ventricular ejection fraction (EF), and Killip class.[93]

Hemodynamic Monitoring

The value of pulmonary artery catheterization in critically ill patients has been questioned.[94] The evidence base regarding the impact of pulmonary artery catheters on outcome in patients with acute MI is limited to retrospective studies because pulmonary artery catheterization in patients with acute MI has not been evaluated in a prospective, randomized, controlled trial.[95-97] Cohen and associates[97] performed a retrospective analysis of pulmonary artery catheterization in patients with ACS who were enrolled in two large international randomized clinical trials, Global Utilization of Streptokinase and t-PA for Occluded Coronary Arteries (GUSTO) IIb and GUSTO III. The study compared the outcomes in 735 patients who received PA catheters with those in 25,702 patients who did not. Except for patients with cardiogenic shock, mortality at 30 days was significantly greater among patients who received pulmonary artery catheters, both before and after adjustment for baseline differences and subsequent events that may have prompted insertion of a pulmonary artery catheter.

According to the ACC/AHA Guidelines, the Class I indications for pulmonary artery catheter monitoring are (1) progressive hypotension that either is unresponsive to fluid administration or is developing in a patient in whom fluid administration is contraindicated and (2) a suspected mechanical complication, such as a VSD or papillary muscle rupture, if an echocardiogram has not been performed.[71] Intra-arterial pressure monitoring is recommended for patients with systolic blood pressure less than 80 mm Hg, patients with cardiogenic shock, and patients receiving vasopressor and inotropic drugs.[71]

Access site bleeding is a major risk of central line insertion in patients who have received fibrinolytic drugs. The femoral route is preferred, and noncompressible sites, such as the subclavian vein, are relatively contraindicated.

Diagnostic Cardiac Catheterization and Coronary Angiography

Conditions other than STEMI can cause ST segment elevation. Pericarditis, for example, is a relative contraindication to fibrinolytic therapy because of the risk of intrapericardial bleeding and tamponade. Therefore, urgent coronary angiography and primary angioplasty if indicated would be preferable to intravenous fibrinolytic therapy if there is any suspicion of pericarditis. Similarly, diagnostic cardiac catheterization should be performed if clinical findings and noninvasive studies are unable to differentiate aortic dissection from acute MI.

Right heart catheterization and contrast ventriculography can provide useful diagnostic information in patients with suspected acute MI. Measurement of right heart pressures is useful in patients with suspected right ventricular MI and in patients with hypotension. Measurement of the oxygen content of blood in the right atrium and pulmonary artery is useful in patients with a suspected VSD. A contrast left ventriculogram provides an assessment of regional and global left ventricular function and the competence of the mitral valve. Left ventriculography was performed during the index cardiac catheterization in 1976 (95%) of 2082 patients with acute MI who were enrolled in the Controlled Abciximab and Device Investigation to Lower Angioplasty Complications (CADILLAC) trial.[98] Mild mitral regurgitation was present in 192 patients (9.7%), and moderate or severe mitral regurgitation was present in 58 patients (2.9%). Mitral regurgitation was not detected by physical examination in 50% of a cohort of 50 patients with acute MI, and moderately severe or severe mitral regurgitation that was demonstrated by left ventriculography.[99]

Cardiac catheterization is often performed after successful fibrinolysis despite the absence of high-risk indicators but the evidence base for the practice is somewhat limited. A prospective cohort study of 21,912 patients with a first acute MI concluded that revascularization within 14 days of the acute MI was associated with a significant reduction in 1-year mortality (RR 0.47; 95% CI 0.37 to 0.60; $P < .001$).[100] Most of the relevant randomized trials are outdated because they preceded the contemporary practice of coronary stenting and antiplatelet therapy.[101] Several contemporary randomized trials have shown beneficial effects of a routine invasive strategy immediately after fibrinolysis,[102] within 24 hours after fibrinolysis,[103] and 1 to 6 weeks after acute MI.[104]

The 2004 ACC/AHA Practice Guidelines include five Class I recommendations, two Class IIa recommendations, and one Class IIb recommendation for coronary angiography in patients with acute MI[71] (Box 31-2). Coronary angiography is recommended in survivors of STEMI who are candidates for revascularization therapy with spontaneous ischemia, intermediate-risk or high-risk findings on noninvasive testing, hemodynamic or electrical instability, mechanical defects, prior revascularization, or high-risk clinical features.

Box 31-2

ACC/AHA Practice Guidelines for Invasive Evaluation after ST Segment Elevation Myocardial Infarction (STEMI)

Class I

1. Coronary arteriography should be performed in patients with spontaneous episodes of myocardial ischemia or episodes of myocardial ischemia provoked by minimal exertion during recovery from STEMI.
2. Coronary arteriography should be performed for intermediate- or high-risk findings on noninvasive testing after STEMI.
3. Coronary arteriography should be performed if the patient is sufficiently stable before definitive therapy for a mechanical complication of STEMI, such as acute MR, VSR, pseudoaneurysm, or left ventricular aneurysm.
4. Coronary arteriography should be performed in patients with persistent hemodynamic instability.
5. Coronary arteriography should be performed in survivors of STEMI who had clinical heart failure during the acute episode but subsequently demonstrated well-preserved left ventricular function.

Class IIa

1. It is reasonable to perform coronary arteriography when STEMI is suspected to have occurred by a mechanism other than thrombotic occlusion of an atherosclerotic plaque. Such mechanisms would include coronary embolism, certain metabolic or hematologic diseases, and coronary artery spasm.
2. Coronary arteriography is reasonable in STEMI patients with any of the following: diabetes mellitus, left ventricular EF less than 0.40, CHF, prior revascularization, or life-threatening ventricular arrhythmias.

Class IIb

Catheterization and revascularization may be considered as part of a strategy of routine coronary arteriography for risk assessment after fibrinolytic therapy.

Class III

Coronary arteriography should not be performed in survivors of STEMI who are thought not to be candidates for coronary revascularization.

CHF, congestive heart failure; EF, ejection fraction; MR, mitral regurgitation; VSR, ventricular septal rupture.

Modified slightly from Antman EM, Anbe DT, Armstrong PW, et al: ACC/AHA guidelines for the management of patients with ST-elevation myocardial infarction: A report of the American College of Cardiology/American Heart Association Task Force on Practice Guidelines (Committee to Revise the 1999 Guidelines for the Management of Patients with Acute Myocardial Infarction). Circulation 2004;110:e82-e292.

Approach to Management

Figure 31-6 presents an algorithm for the treatment of acute STEMI.

General Considerations

Patients who present to the emergency department with an acute MI will usually be diagnosed and treated before admission to the intensive care unit (ICU). It is not unusual, however, for STEMI to occur in patients receiving ICU treatment for other conditions, such as gastrointestinal bleeding or respiratory failure, or undergoing surgical procedures. As in the patients who present to an ED, prompt performance and interpretation of an ECG constitute a critical initial step in management. Continuous ECG monitoring for arrhythmias is routinely practiced. Patients usually are advanced from nothing-by-mouth (NPO [*nil per os*]) status to clear liquids to a low-fat, low-cholesterol diet as tolerated. Stool softeners should be employed to prevent the hemodynamic effects of constipation.

Oxygen

The effects of supplemental oxygen on ischemic injury was studied by Madias and colleagues.[105] Seventeen patients with acute anterior MI who were not in cardiogenic shock underwent precordial ST segment mapping before and after inhalation of 100% oxygen for 1 hour. The mean arterial partial pressure of oxygen increased from 70 mm Hg on room air to 278 mm Hg during oxygen inhalation. During oxygen inhalation there was a 16% reduction in the sum of all ST segment elevation, with reversion to baseline after oxygen was discontinued. Two hundred patients with suspected acute MI were enrolled in a double-blind, randomized trial of supplemental oxygen versus compressed air.[106] No apparent benefit was observed for oxygen therapy, and the mortality rate was higher in the oxygen group than in the control group (9/80 versus 3/77; P=NS). Although supplemental oxygen is routinely administered to patients with STEMI, according to the ACC/AHA guidelines the only Class I indication for this intervention is an arterial oxygen saturation less than 90%.[71] The guidelines also state that supplemental oxygen can be discontinued after 6 hours in uncomplicated cases.

Analgesia and Sedation

Relief of pain is an important goal in patients with acute MI. According to the most recent ACC/AHA Practice

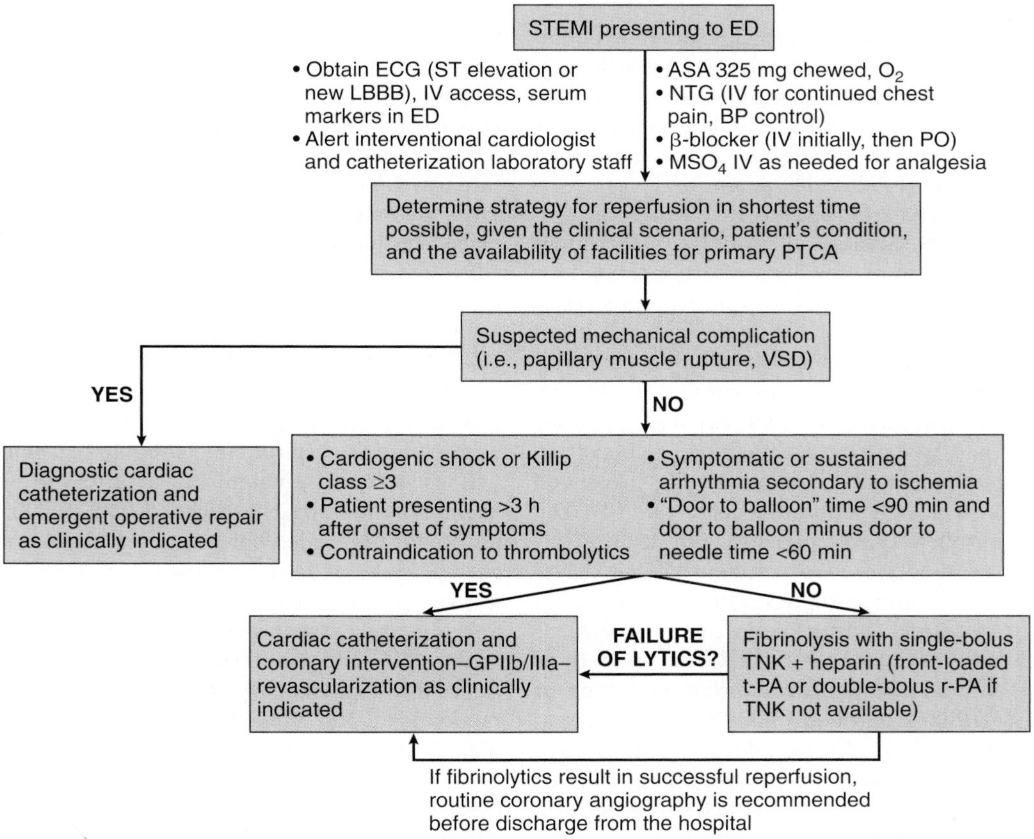

Figure 31-6. Algorithm for the treatment of acute ST segment elevation myocardial infarction (STEMI). *Note:* Nitroglycerin should be used with caution in patients with inferior wall myocardial infarction with possible right ventricular involvement. Nitroglycerin should be avoided altogether in hypotensive patients. ASA, acetylsalicylic acid (aspirin); BP, blood pressure; ECG, electrocardiogram; ED, emergency department; IV, intravenous; LBBB, left bundle branch block; MSO_4, morphine sulfate; NTG, nitroglycerin; PTCA, percutaneous transluminal coronary angioplasty; rPA, recombinant plasminogen activator (replectase); TNK, teneplectase; tPA, tissue plasminogen activator; VSD, ventricular septal defect.

Guidelines, pain associated with STEMI is a Class I indication for intravenous morphine sulfate.[71] There are no published randomized trials of morphine therapy in patients with acute MI. A recent analysis of the CRUSADE registry, however, revealed that use of morphine was associated with a 50% higher mortality in patients with NSTEMI even after risk adjustment.[107] One proposed mechanism of morphine's adverse effect is opioid-induced cortisol deficiency.[108] Until additional data become available, it may be prudent to limit the use of morphine to patients with persistent pain despite treatment with nitrates and a β-adrenergic antagonist.

Nitrates

The ability of sublingual or intravenous nitroglycerin to relieve chest pain in patients with acute MI is well documented.[109] The beneficial physiologic effects of nitrates include vasodilation of peripheral arteries and veins, causing reductions in pulmonary capillary wedge pressure (PCWP), mean arterial pressure and peripheral vascular resistance, thereby decreasing left ventricular preload and afterload and myocardial oxygen demand.[110] Also, vasodilation of the coronary arteries may improve myocardial oxygen supply, especially in patients with a component of coronary spasm.[111] Severe hypotension and bradycardia have been observed after administration of either sublingual or intravenous nitroglycerin in patients with acute MI.[112] Patients with right ventricular MI may experience severe hypotension during administration of nitroglycerin because adequate right ventricular preload is required to maintain cardiac output. Nitroglycerin is contraindicated in patients who have taken phosphodiesterase inhibitors because they potentiate nitroglycerin-induced hypotension.[113]

There are two Class I indications for nitroglycerin in patients with STEMI. Sublingual nitroglycerin (0.4 mg) every 5 minutes for a total of 3 doses is recommended for relief of ischemic discomfort.[71] Intravenous nitroglycerin is indicated for relief of ongoing ischemic discomfort, control of hypertension, or management of pulmonary congestion.[71] It has been proposed that intravenous nitroglycerin may limit myocardial infarct size and expansion.[114] Two large clinical trials, however, were unable to demonstrate significant improvements in mortality by the prolonged administration of nitroglycerin after acute MI.[115,116] The GISSI-3 trial enrolled 19,394 patients with acute MI.[115] Patients who were randomized to treatment with nitroglycerin received intravenous nitroglycerin for 24 hours, followed by transdermal nitroglycerin for 6 weeks.[115] Nitroglycerin did not reduce the 6-week rate of death or clinical heart failure. The Fourth International Study of Infarct Survival (ISIS-4) enrolled 58,050 patients with suspected acute MI in a 2×2×2 factorial study that included randomization to isosorbide mononitrate 60 mg daily or placebo for 28 days.[116] No significant effect of nitroglycerin on mortality was found after 5 weeks or 1 year.

Several studies have investigated the effect of another nitrate, nitroprusside, on hemodynamics and outcome in patients with acute MI.[117-120] Intravenous nitroprusside reduced PCWP and increased cardiac index in patients with acute MI.[117,118] A comparison of intravenous nitroprusside with intravenous nitroglycerin in 10 patients with acute anterior MI demonstrated that ST segment elevation increased during infusion of nitroprusside, whereas it decreased during infusion of nitroglycerin.[117] Experimental data indicate that nitroprusside may exacerbate myocardial ischemia or injury by redistribution of myocardial blood flow from ischemic to nonischemic zones.[117] A Veterans Administration Cooperative Study enrolled 812 patients with acute MI and a PCWP greater than 12 mm Hg in a double-blind, randomized trial of nitroprusside infused for 48 hours.[120] Compared with the placebo group, mortality at 13 weeks was increased by nitroprusside in patients whose infusions started within 9 hours of the onset of pain. A smaller European trial randomized 328 patients with acute MI to infusion of nitroprusside or 5% glucose.[119] The trial was terminated when one-week mortality in the control group was significantly greater than in the nitroprusside group (10.9% versus 3.1%; $P<.05$). The use of nitroprusside in patients with acute MI should probably be reserved for patients with severe hypertension that is unresponsive to treatment with intravenous nitroglycerin.

Aspirin and Other Oral Antiplatelet Agents

The Second International Study of Infarct Survival (ISIS-2) provided definitive evidence that aspirin reduces mortality in patients with acute MI[121] (Fig. 31-7). The study used a 2×2 factorial design to randomize 17,187 patients to four treatment groups: streptokinase, aspirin 160 mg daily for 1 month, both, or neither. Aspirin reduced the rate of in-hospital reinfarction both in the patients who received streptokinase and in the patients who did not receive fibrinolytic therapy. At 35 days, the vascular-cause mortality rate was 9.4% among the patients in the aspirin treatment group patients, compared with 11.8% among those in the placebo group, representing a 23% reduction ($P<.00001$). All-cause mortality also was significantly reduced by aspirin. Also, the combination of aspirin and streptokinase reduced mortality more than did either agent alone. The ACC/AHA Practice Guidelines recommend that patients who present with acute STEMI who have not taken aspirin should receive 162 to 325 mg of non–enteric-coated aspirin, and the aspirin tablets should be chewed.[71]

Reocclusion of a patent infarct artery after successful fibrinolytic therapy is associated with higher in-hospital mortality, reduced event-free survival after hospital discharge, and long-term impairment of regional and global left ventricular function.[122-125] There are conflicting opinions regarding aspirin's effect on reocclusion of an infarct artery.[126,127] The Antithrombotics in the Prevention of Reocclusion in Coronary Thrombolysis (APRICOT) study randomized 300 patients with an open infarct artery within 48 hours after fibrinolysis to three treatment groups: aspirin 325 mg daily, warfarin, or placebo.[128] Cardiac catheterization was performed 3 months later in 248 patients. The reocclusion rates were not significantly different: 32% (24/74) with placebo, 30% (24/81) with warfarin, and 25% (23/93) with aspirin. A pooled analysis of published studies estimated that the incidence of reocclusion after streptokinase or tissue plasminogen activator (tPA) is approximately 11% with aspirin, compared with 25% without aspirin.[126]

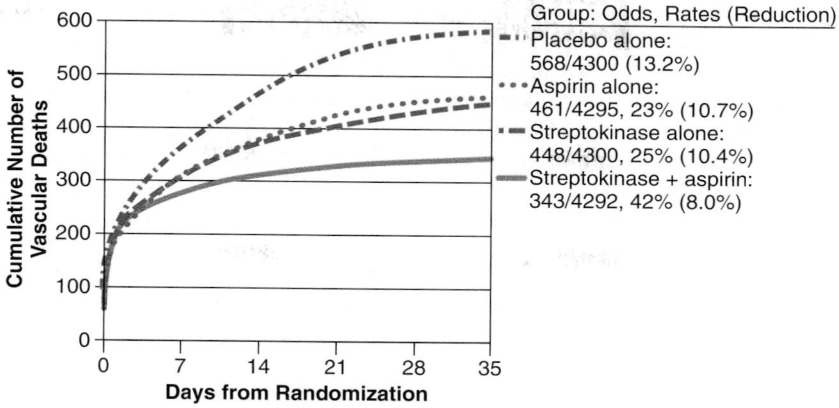

Figure 31-7. Cumulative vascular deaths in the Second International Study of Infarct Survival (ISIS-2). A total of 17,187 patients were enrolled in the study within 24 hours of suspected acute MI. Patients were randomized to receive one of four treatments: aspirin alone, streptokinase alone, both aspirin and streptokinase, or placebo (neither agent). The 35-day vascular death rates and odds reductions (in parentheses) are given for each group. (From Randomised trial of intravenous streptokinase, oral aspirin, both, or neither among 17,187 cases of suspected acute myocardial infarction: ISIS-2. ISIS-2 [Second International Study of Infarct Survival] Collaborative Group. Lancet 1988;2:349-360.)

Recent studies suggest that patients with acute MI should be treated with a combination of aspirin and clopidogrel, an inhibitor of adenosine diphosphate (ADP)-mediated platelet aggregation.[129,130] The Clopidogrel as Adjunctive Reperfusion Therapy (CLARITY) study enrolled 3491 patients who received fibrinolytic therapy for STEMI and randomized them to receive clopidogrel 75 mg daily or placebo in a double-blind fashion.[129] Coronary angiography performed at a median of 84 hours after randomization in each group demonstrated an occluded IRA in 18.4% of the placebo group patients, compared with 11.7% of the clopidogrel group patients ($P<.001$). PCI was performed during the index hospitalization in 1863 (53.4%) of the patients who were enrolled in the CLARITY trial.[131] The combined incidence of cardiovascular death, recurrent MI, or stroke from PCI to 30 days after randomization was significantly lower among patients who were treated with clopidogrel and aspirin compared with the patients who received aspirin alone (3.6% versus 6.2%; adjusted odds ratio 0.54; 95% CI 0.35 to 0.85; $P=.008$).[131] The Clopidogrel and Metoprolol in Myocardial Infarction Trial (COMMIT) randomized 45,852 patients with suspected acute MI to receive treatment with aspirin 162 mg daily plus clopidogrel 75 mg daily or placebo.[130] The in-hospital mortality rate was significantly lower for the clopidogrel group than for the placebo group (7.5% versus 8.1%; $P=.03$). The CLARITY study used a clopidogrel loading dose of 300 mg; the COMMIT study did not employ a loading dose.

Antithrombin Therapy

The rationale for antithrombin therapy in patients with STEMI includes promotion of infarct artery patency, and prevention of deep vein thrombosis, pulmonary embolism, left ventricular mural thrombus, and cerebral embolism. Clinical trials have evaluated both subcutaneous and intravenous unfractionated heparin (UFH) in patients with acute MI who were treated with various fibrinolytic agents. Randomized, controlled clinical trials have shown that adjunctive therapy with intravenous UFH increases the patency of the IRA after administration of tPA.[132,133] A meta-analysis that included 68,000 patients who were enrolled in randomized trials that compared UFH plus aspirin with aspirin alone showed that only 5 lives were saved per 1000 patients who received UFH in addition to streptokinase.[134] The meta-analysis was heavily influenced by two studies, GISSI-2[135] and ISIS-3,[136,137] that enrolled 62,067 patients who were randomly assigned to receive fibrinolytic therapy plus either aspirin alone or aspirin plus subcutaneous UFH. Another meta-analysis was limited to six randomized controlled trials that enrolled 1735 patients who received either intravenous UFH or no heparin after fibrinolytic therapy.[138] The analysis found that addition of intravenous UFH to tPA or streptokinase had insignificant effects on mortality and reinfarction, but the risk of bleeding was significantly increased.[138]

The most recent ACC/AHA guidelines include the following Class IIb recommendation: "It may be reasonable to administer UFH intravenously to patients undergoing reperfusion therapy with streptokinase."[71] Despite evidence that was considered equivocal, the guidelines include the following Class I indications for UFH: "UFH should be given intravenously to patients undergoing reperfusion therapy with alteplase, reteplase, or tenecteplase. . . ."[71] The guidelines recommend treatment for 48 hours and adjustment of the dose of UFH to maintain an activated partial thromboplastin time (aPTT) of 50 to 70 seconds. The recommendation is supported by an analysis of the GUSTO-1 trial that showed that aPTT's greater than 70 seconds were associated with higher risk of death, stroke, and bleeding.[139] The platelet count should be monitored daily during UFH therapy because there is a 3% incidence of heparin-induced thrombocytopenia.[140]

Left ventricular mural thrombus formation after acute MI occurs more commonly after anterior than non–anterior wall MI and is associated with an increased risk of systemic embolization.[141,142] Data are conflicting regarding the incidence of left ventricular thrombus in patients who receive reperfusion therapy. The GISSI-2 study, in which all patients received fibrinolytic therapy, observed left ventricular thrombi in 51 of 180 consecutive patients with a first anterior acute MI who underwent serial echocardiography within 48 hours after the onset of symptoms and before hospital discharge.[143] Another study, however, detected left ventricular thrombi in only 6.4% of patients with acute anterior MI who underwent echocardiography on days 1, 14, and 90 after MI.[144] A double-blind, randomized trial compared a ten-day course of high dose subcutaneous UFH (12,500 units every 12 hours) with low-dose subcutaneous UFH (5000 units every 12 hours) in the prevention of left ventricular thrombus in 221 patients with acute anterior MI who did not receive fibrinolytic therapy.[145] Echocardiography 10 days after MI demonstrated left ventricular thrombi in 10 of 95 patients (11%) in the high-dose group and in 28 of 88 patients (32%) in the low-dose group (P=.0004). A meta-analysis of 7 studies that enrolled 270 patients suggests that systemic anticoagulation in patients with mural thrombi reduces embolic complications.[141]

Several randomized clinical trials[146-148] and meta-analyses[149,150] have been performed to compare low molecular weight heparin (LMWH) with placebo or UFH as adjuncts to fibrinolytic therapy in patients with STEMI. A meta-analysis of 16,943 patients who were enrolled in 4 randomized trials revealed that the end points of death or reinfarction at 7 days and at 30 days were significantly reduced by LMWH compared with placebo.[150] A meta-analysis of 7098 patients who were enrolled in 6 randomized trials revealed that LMWH, compared with UFH, reduced the rates of reinfarction during hospitalization and at 30 days, but the rates of death were not significantly different.[150] The current ACC/AHA guidelines classify LMWH as ". . . an acceptable alternative to UFH as ancillary therapy for patients aged <75 years who are receiving fibrinolytic therapy, provided that significant renal dysfunction is not present."[71]

Based on the results of two large international clinical trials that have been published since the guidelines were written,[148,151] it is possible that the next draft of the guidelines will state that LMWH is the preferred alternative to UFH. Reviparin, a LMWH, was compared with placebo in a trial called the Clinical Trial of Reviparin and Metabolic Modulation in Acute Myocardial Infarction Treatment Evaluation (CREATE).[151] The trial randomized 15,570 patients with STEMI, 73% of whom received fibrinolytic therapy, to treatment with placebo or subcutaneous reviparin twice daily for 7 days. The composite end point of death, myocardial reinfarction, or stroke was significantly lower in the reviparin group both at 7 days (11.0% versus 9.6%; hazard ratio 0.87; 95% CI 0.79 to 0.96; P=.005) and at 30 days (13.6% versus 11.8%; hazard ratio 0.87; 95% CI 0.79 to 0.95; P=.001). Reviparin was associated with a small increase in life-threatening bleeding, but overall, there were 17 fewer major events (death, reinfarction, stroke, or life-threatening bleeding) per 1000 patients who received reviparin.

Enoxaparin, another LMWH, was compared with UFH in a trial called Enoxaparin and Thrombolysis Reperfusion for Acute Myocardial Infarction Treatment (ExTRACT)–TIMI 25.[148] The study was a double-blind, randomized comparison of enoxaparin given subcutaneously twice daily until hospital discharge versus intravenous UFH for 48 hours in 20,506 patients with STEMI. A fibrinolytic agent was received by 99.7% of the patients: 55% received alteplase, 20% received streptokinase, 19% received tenecteplase, and 5.5% received reteplase. The primary end point, death or nonfatal recurrent MI through 30 days, occurred in 12.0% of patients in the UFH group and in 9.9% of patients in the enoxaparin group (P<.001). The rates of major bleeding at 30 days were 1.4% in the UFH group and 2.1% in the enoxaparin group (P<.001), but the rates of intracranial hemorrhage were not significantly different (UFH 0.7%, enoxaparin 0.8%; P=.14).

Fondaparinux, a synthetic pentasaccharide, is a factor Xa inhibitor that binds antithrombin and inhibits factor Xa. The Organization for the Assessment of Strategies for Ischemic Syndromes (OASIS) conducted two trials to evaluate fondaparinux in patients with acute coronary syndromes[152] and STEMI.[153] The OASIS-6 trial was a randomized, double-blind comparison of fondaparinux 2.5 mg daily or control from days 3 through 9 in 12,092 patients with STEMI.[153] Forty-five percent of the patients received fibrinolytic therapy (streptokinase in 73%), 28.9% underwent primary PCI, and 23.7% did not receive any reperfusion therapy. The primary efficacy outcome, death or reinfarction at 30 days, was significantly lower in the fondaparinux group than in the control group (9.7% versus 11.2%; hazard ratio 0.86; 95% CI 0.77 to 0.96; P=.008). Also, fondaparinux significantly reduced the rates of death at day 9, day 30, and the end of the study (3 to 6 months). Significant heterogeneity in the effect of fondaparinux was observed in relation to the reperfusion strategy, with benefit observed in patients who received no reperfusion therapy or a fibrinolytic agent, but not in patients who underwent primary PCI. The rate of severe bleeding was not increased by fondaparinux.

The dose of fondaparinux must be adjusted in patients with renal insufficiency, but adjustment for body weight is not necessary. The anticoagulant effect of the drug cannot be monitored by conventional clotting tests, such as the activated clotting time or partial thromboplastin time. Also, the relatively long half-life of fondaparinux, 17 to 21 hours, conceivably may be viewed as an impediment to early sheath removal and ambulation after cardiac catheterization. Therefore, despite the favorable clinical trial data, it seems unlikely that interventional cardiologists will be quick to adopt fondaparinux as a first-line drug for anticoagulation of patients with acute MI or ACS.

Fibrinolytic Therapy

The dependence of myocardial necrosis on the duration of coronary occlusion was demonstrated using a canine model of MI.[154] The landmark angiographic study performed by DeWood and coworkers[18] confirmed the presence of coronary artery thrombi in patients with STEMI. Although these experimental and clinical observations provided a rationale for fibrinolytic therapy, the initial studies of fibrinolytic agents for acute MI preceded both findings. According to one review of the literature, the first reported use of fibrinolytic therapy for acute MI was in 1958.[155] By 1979 several multicenter studies of intravenous streptokinase had been performed, but the benefit of reperfusion therapy remained unproven, in part because the trial designs were flawed.[156,157]

Effect of Fibrinolysis on Survival

Four well-designed, multicenter randomized trials established that three fibrinolytic agents—streptokinase,[121,158] anisolylated plasminogen–streptokinase activator complex (APSAC) (i.e., anistreplase),[159] and tPA[160]—each reduced short-term and long-term mortality in patients with acute MI. The Fibrinolytic Therapy Trialists' Collaborative Group analyzed nine trials that randomized a total of 58,600 patients with suspected acute MI to a fibrinolytic therapy group or a control group.[161] The absolute risk of death increased with age, but absolute reductions in mortality were comparable among younger and older patients up to 75 years of age. Several trials had upper age limits for enrollment. The remaining trials enrolled 5788 patients 75 years or older and found no significant effect of fibrinolytic therapy on mortality at 35 days (25.3% for the control patients versus 24.3% for patients who received fibrinolytic therapy).[161]

The baseline ECG findings and the elapsed time between the onset of symptoms and the initiation of treatment were significant determinants of the impact of fibrinolytic therapy on mortality at 35 days[161] (Fig. 31-8). The greatest reduction in mortality was observed in patients who presented with either bundle branch block (BBB) (control 23.6% versus fibrinolytic 18.7%) or ST segment elevation in the anterior leads (control 16.9% versus fibrinolytic 13.2%).[161] Fibrinolytic therapy increased mortality among patients with ST segment depression on the baseline ECG.

A linear relationship between the absolute reduction in mortality and the delay from symptom onset to randomization was found among the 45,000 patients who presented with ST elevation or BBB on the ECG.[161] Fibrinolytic therapy produced a significant mortality reduction even among patients who received treatment 7 to 12 hours after the onset of symptoms, but patients who received treatment within the first hour after the onset of their symptoms received the greatest benefit. Patients who receive fibrinolytic therapy within the first hour after symptom onset have the greatest proportional mortality reduction,[162] as well as the highest incidence of so-called aborted MI, defined as maximal creatine kinase level up to twice the upper limit of normal and typical evolution of ECG changes.[163,164] A multicenter trial of fibrinolytic therapy reported that the baseline-adjusted mortality was significantly lower among the 13.3% of patients who had an aborted MI than among those who did not.[163]

Persistent occlusion of the IRA after acute MI is associated with left ventricular remodeling, resulting in increased left ventricular end-systolic volume, a major predictor of survival after acute MI.[165,166] Some evidence suggests that reperfusion later than 6 hours after the onset of symptoms has a favorable effect on ventricular remodeling, with less ventricular dilation observed after successful reperfusion than after no reperfusion therapy.[167,168] Several clinical trials have investigated the effects of fibrinolytic therapy on clinical events in patients who received treatment more than 6 hours after the onset of symptoms. A South American multicenter tial randomized 2080 patients within 7 to 12 hours after the onset of symptoms to receive streptokinase or placebo and found no significant difference in mortality rates in-hospital, after 35 days, and after 1 year.[169] The Late Assessment of Thrombolytic Efficacy (LATE) study randomized 5711 patients who presented with suspected acute MI between 6 and 24 hours after the onset of symptoms to receive tPA or placebo.[170] Treatment with tPA significantly reduced mortality among patients who received treatment within 12 hours of symptom onset: The 35-day mortality rate was 8.9% for the tPA group versus 11.97% for placebo, representing a relative reduction of 25.6% (95% CI 6.3% to 45.0%;

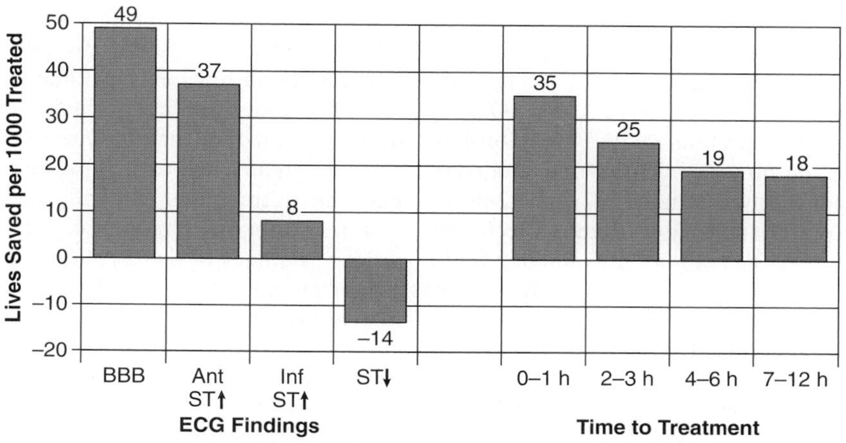

Figure 31-8. The impact of the presenting electrocardiogram (ECG) and the time to treatment on the 35-day mortality of 58,600 patients enrolled in nine randomized trials comparing streptokinase, APSAC (anistreplase), urokinase, or tissue plasminogen activator with placebo or control, expressed as the number of lives saved per 1000 patients who received fibrinolytic therapy. Ant ST, anterior ST segment elevation; APSAC, anisolylated plasminogen–streptokinase activator complex; BBB, bundle branch block; Inf ST, inferior ST segment elevation. (From Indications for fibrinolytic therapy in suspected acute myocardial infarction: Collaborative overview of early mortality and major morbidity results from all randomised trials of more than 1000 patients. Fibrinolytic Therapy Trialists' [FTT] Collaborative Group. Lancet 1994;343:311-322.)

$P=.0229$). Mortality at 35 days was not significantly reduced by administration of tPA to patients who received treatment 12 to 24 hours after symptom onset.

The major causes of delayed fibrinolytic therapy for acute MI are failure of patients to seek medical care[171,172] and delays in administration of fibrinolytic therapy.[173,174] A retrospective review of data for 2409 patients hospitalized with acute MI in Minnesota in 1992 and 1993 reported that 40% of the patients delayed presentation to the hospital more than 6 hours after the onset of symptoms.[171] The ACC/AHA Practice Guidelines set a goal of initiating fibrinolytic therapy within 30 minutes of contact with the medical system.[71] Among 68,430 patients with STEMI who received fibrinolytic therapy and were enrolled in the NRMI-3 and NRMI-4 registries, only 46% of patients received a fibrinolytic drug within 30 minutes of arrival.[174] There was no significant improvement in the so-called door-to-needle time in the 1015 participating hospitals from 1999 to 2002.[174] Pre-hospital administration of fibrinolytic therapy has been investigated as one approach to reducing the delay between symptom onset and reperfusion.[175-177] A meta-analysis of six randomized trials that compared pre-hospital with in-hospital fibrinolytic therapy for acute MI found that the time to fibrinolytic therapy and all-cause in-hospital mortality were significantly reduced by pre-hospital administration of fibrinolytic drugs.[175]

Box 31-3

Definitions of Perfusion in the TIMI Trial

Grade 0 (no perfusion): There is no antegrade flow beyond the point of occlusion.

Grade 1 (penetration without perfusion): The contrast material passes beyond the area of obstruction but "hangs up" and fails to opacify the entire coronary bed distal to the obstruction for the duration of the cineangiographic filming sequence.

Grade 2 (partial perfusion): The contrast material passes across the obstruction and opacifies the coronary bed distal to the obstruction. However, the rate of entry of contrast material into the vessel distal to the obstruction or its rate of clearance from the distal bed (or both) is perceptibly slower than the rate of entry into or clearance from comparable areas not perfused by the previously occluded vessel—e.g., the opposite coronary artery or the coronary bed proximal to the obstruction.

Grade 3 (complete perfusion): Antegrade flow into the bed distal to the obstruction occurs as promptly as antegrade flow into the bed proximal to the obstruction, and clearance of contrast material from the involved bed is as rapid as clearance from an uninvolved bed in the same vessel or the opposite artery.

From Thrombolysis in Myocardial Infarction (TIMI) trial. Phase I findings. TIMI Study Group. N Engl J Med 1985;312:932-936.

Coronary Artery Patency after Fibrinolytic Therapy

Early angiographic studies investigated the rates of coronary reperfusion after intracoronary[178-180] or intravenous administration of fibrinolytic agents.[181] The Thrombolysis in Myocardial Infarction (TIMI) Study Group devised a grading system of coronary patency that has been adopted widely[181] (Box 31-3). Fibrinolysis was judged to be successful if an IRA that was occluded (TIMI grade 0 or 1) before treatment improved to either partial perfusion (TIMI grade 2) or complete perfusion (TIMI grade 3) 90 minutes after the fibrinolytic therapy began.[181] The first TIMI trial revealed that only 31% of occluded arteries were patent (TIMI grade 2 or 3) 90 minutes after intravenous streptokinase, compared with a 62% patency rate after a 3-hour intravenous infusion of tPA ($P<.001$).[182] Subsequent studies that examined the relationship between the TIMI grade flow and clinical outcome concluded that TIMI grade 3 flow, but not TIMI grade 2 flow, improves both in-hospital and long-term mortality after acute MI.[183,184] Therefore, the criteria for evaluating fibrinolytic therapy were revised, and TIMI grade 2 flow is no longer considered a successful outcome.[185]

The GUSTO-I trial randomized 41,021 patients to four fibrinolytic strategies: streptokinase plus subcutaneous UFH, streptokinase plus intravenous UFH, accelerated tPA plus intravenous UFH, or a combination of streptokinase and tPA plus intravenous UFH.[186] Thirty-day mortality was lowest for the accelerated tPA-UFH regimen, 6.3%. A substudy of GUSTO-I included 2431 patients who underwent coronary angiography to assess patency of the IRA.[187,188] TIMI grade 3 flow was achieved 90 minutes after initiation of fibrinolytic therapy in 54% (157/292) of patients in the accelerated tPA-UFH group, compared with 31% of patients who received streptokinase plus UFH (176/576). Analysis of the relationship between patency at 90 minutes and mortality at 30 days regardless of treatment assignment revealed a significant difference between the mortality rate associated with grade 3 flow and the mortality associated with grade 0 or 1 flow (4.4% versus 8.9%; $P=.009$).

The relationship between time to treatment and the mortality reduction by fibrinolytic therapy may be a reflection of several factors. One is that earlier reperfusion achieves greater myocardial salvage.[189] Another factor is that time to treatment may influence the patency rate 90 minutes after administration of certain fibrinolytic drugs.[190] Patency of the IRA 90 minutes after administration of a nonfibrin-specific fibrinolytic drug, such as streptokinase, anistreplase, or urokinase, is lower when patients are first treated beyond 3 hours after the onset of symptoms than when the drugs are administered within 3 hours after onset.[182,190-192] After treatment with tPA or reteplase (rPA), fibrin-specific fibrinolytic agents, the rates of TIMI grade 3 flow are similar for patients who received treatment within 3 hours or at 3 hours or later after the onset of symptoms.[182,191,192] The time-dependent reperfusion efficacy is reflected by the rates of in-hospital mortality. A retrospective analysis of 6 angiographic trials that included 1174 patients found that in-hospital mortality among patients who received nonfibrin-specific drugs was twofold greater for patients treated more than 3 hours after symptom onset compared with patients treated within 3 hours.[192] Among patients who received tPA or rPA, in-hospital mortality did not differ for patients treated within 3 hours of symptom onset or later than 3 hours after symptom onset.

More sophisticated methodologies for assessing myocardial reperfusion have been devised, such as the TIMI Frame Count and TIMI Myocardial Perfusion Grade.[193-195] Application of these methods demonstrated that even among patients with TIMI grade 3 flow after fibrinolytic therapy, clinical outcomes and survival are related to the speed of epicardial flow and the state of myocardial perfusion.[193,194] Therefore, a major goal of recent research has been to determine whether combinations of fibrinolytic and antiplatelet drugs might enhance myocardial reperfusion and achieve further reductions in mortality. Compared with full-dose tPA or rPA, a combination of a reduced dose of either tPA or rPA plus abciximab, a platelet glycoprotein IIb/IIIa (GP IIb/IIIa) inhibitor, was found to increase the rates of TIMI 3 flow at 60 and 90 minutes after administration.[196,197] Unfortunately, a difference in 30-day mortality between standard-dose rPA and half-dose rPA plus full-dose abciximab was not demonstrated by a large clinical trial, GUSTO-V, that enrolled 16,588 patients with evolving STEMI.[198]

Complications of Fibrinolytic Therapy

Intracranial hemorrhage and other hemorrhagic complications are the major risks associated with administration of fibrinolytic therapy.[199,200] The NRMI-2 database accrued 71,073 patients who received tPA for acute MI from June 1, 1994, to September 30, 1996. Intracranial hemorrhage was confirmed by computed tomography (CT) or magnetic resonance imaging (MRI) in 625 patients (0.88%).[200] In-hospital mortality was 53%, and 25.3% of patients with intracranial hemorrhage who survived to hospital discharge had neurologic deficits. A multivariate analysis identified several risk factors that were significantly associated with an increased risk of intracranial hemorrhage: older age, female gender, systolic blood pressure greater than 140 mm Hg, diastolic blood pressure greater than 100 mm Hg, and history of stroke. An aPTT longer than 70 seconds was associated with an increased risk of hemorrhagic stroke in the GUSTO-I trial.[139] Bolus administration of fibrinolytic agents may be associated with an increased risk of intracranial hemorrhage compared with infusion.[201,202] Although phase II trials indicated a statistically nonsignificant reduction in the risk of intracranial hemorrhage, meta-analysis of phase III trials revealed a statistically significant 25% increase in the risk of intracranial hemorrhage with bolus fibrinolytic therapy.[202]

According to the ACC/AHA Guidelines, "The occurrence of a change in neurological status during or after reperfusion therapy, particularly within the first 24 hours after initiation of treatment, is considered to be due to [intracranial hemorrhage] until proven otherwise."[71] When intracranial hemorrhage is suspected, an emergency CT scan should be performed, and fibrinolytic, antiplatelet, and anticoagulant therapies should be discontinued until the diagnosis is ruled out. Cryoprecipitate or fresh frozen plasma should be given to replenish coagulation factors.[71] Protamine should be administered to patients who are receiving UFH. Neurosurgery to evacuate parenchymal hemorrhages or subdural hematomas may improve outcome.[203]

Among 40,903 patients enrolled in the GUSTO-I trial, 1.2% suffered severe bleeding, defined as bleeding that caused hemodynamic compromise that required treatment, and 11.4% experienced moderate hemorrhage, defined as bleeding that required transfusion but did not lead to hemodynamic compromise requiring intervention.[199] The most common sources of moderate and severe bleeding were procedure-related. The rate of moderate or severe bleeding was 6% among patients who underwent no procedures, compared with 17% among patients who underwent coronary angiography, 43% among patients who received a PA catheter, and 50% among patients who received an intra-aortic balloon pump (IABP) or underwent coronary artery bypass surgery. Older age, lower body weight, and female sex were the three strongest independent predictors of hemorrhage. The risk of noncerebral bleeding was greater after streptokinase than after tPA, but the risk of intracranial hemorrhage was greater after tPA.

Patient Selection

The ACC/AHA Guidelines list two Class I indications for fibrinolytic therapy: (1) STEMI with symptom onset within the prior 12 hours and ST elevation greater than 0.1 mV in at least two contiguous precordial leads or at least two adjacent limb leads; and (2) STEMI with symptom onset within the prior 12 hours and new or presumably new LBBB.[71] There is a long list of absolute and relative contraindications to fibrinolytic therapy (Box 31-4). Special attention should be paid to factors that may increase the risk of intracranial hemorrhage, such as a history of such hemorrhage, recent closed head or facial trauma, uncontrolled hypertension, or ischemic stroke within the previous 3 months. PCI is preferable to fibrinolytic therapy in patients with an increased risk of intracranial hemorrhage. Active menstrual bleeding should not be considered a contraindication to fibrinolytic therapy.[204,205] The GUSTO-I trial included 12 menstruating women who received fibrinolytic therapy, 2 of whom required a transfusion for moderate vaginal bleeding.[205] Nontraumatic cardiopulmonary resuscitation also should not be considered a contraindication to fibrinolytic therapy.[204,206]

According to the ACC/AHA guidelines, age greater than 75 years is not a contraindication to fibrinolytic therapy, but the guidelines include a Class IIa indication for primary PCI in patients with STEMI who are 75 years of age or older.[71] Increasing age is a risk factor for death and other adverse events after either primary PCI or fibrinolytic therapy for STEMI.[207] The risk of intracranial hemorrhage after fibrinolytic therapy also increases with advancing age.[200,208] Data are conflicting regarding the

Box 31-4

Contraindications and Cautions for Fibrinolysis in ST Segment Elevation Myocardial Infarction

Absolute Contraindications

Any prior intracranial hemorrhage
Known structural cerebral vascular lesion (e.g., arteriovenous malformation)
Known malignant intracranial neoplasm (primary or metastatic)
Ischemic stroke within 3 months; *exception:* acute ischemic stroke within 3 hours
Suspected aortic dissection
Active bleeding or bleeding diathesis (excluding menses)
Significant closed head or facial trauma within 3 months

Relative Contraindications

History of chronic, severe, poorly controlled hypertension
Severe uncontrolled hypertension on presentation (systolic blood pressure greater than 180 mm Hg or diastolic blood pressure greater than 110 mm Hg)
History of prior ischemic stroke more than 3 months earlier, dementia, or known intracranial pathology not covered in contraindications
Traumatic or prolonged (beyond 10 minutes) CPR or major surgery (within 3 weeks)
Recent (within 2 to 4 weeks) internal bleeding
Noncompressible vascular punctures
For streptokinase/anistreplase: prior exposure (more than 5 days earlier) or prior allergic reaction to these agents
Pregnancy
Active peptic ulcer
Current use of anticoagulants: the higher the INR, the higher the risk of bleeding

CPR, cardiopulmonary resuscitation; INR, international normalized ratio.
From Antman EM, Anbe DT, Armstrong PW, et al: ACC/AHA guidelines for the management of patients with ST-elevation myocardial infarction: A report of the American College of Cardiology/American Heart Association Task Force on Practice Guidelines (Committee to Revise the 1999 Guidelines for the Management of Patients with Acute Myocardial Infarction). Circulation 2004;110:e82-e292.

benefit or lack of benefit of fibrinolytic therapy in patients with STEMI who are older than 75. One analysis of a Medicare database that included 2673 patients aged 76 to 86 found that fibrinolytic therapy conferred a survival disadvantage, with a hazard ratio of 1.38 for 30-day mortality.[209] Fibrinolytic therapy was associated with a 13% reduction in the composite of 1-year mortality and cerebral bleeding in a cohort of 6891 patients 75 years and older with a first STEMI who were enrolled in a Swedish registry.[210] A study performed in the Netherlands randomized 87 patients with acute MI who were older than 75 to primary PCI or streptokinase.[211] The primary composite end point of death, reinfarction, or stroke at 30 days occurred in 4 (9%) patients in the PCI group, compared with 12 (29%) in the streptokinase group (RR 4.3, 95% CI 1.2 to 20.0; *P*=.01). After 1 year, mortality was significantly greater for the streptokinase group than the PCI group (29% versus 11%; RR 3.4, 95% CI 1.0 to 13.5; *P*=.03). One caveat regarding the study is that the mean time from hospital admission to first balloon inflation was 59±19 minutes (range 33 to 120 minutes)—considerably shorter than door-to-balloon times in the United States.

Many patients with acute MI have contraindications to fibrinolytic therapy or do not meet eligibility criteria for fibrinolytic therapy.[212,213] Contraindications such as recent surgery, trauma, or gastrointestinal bleeding would be relatively frequent in patients who develop an acute MI while already hospitalized for another illness. Analysis of patients with STEMI who were enrolled in the NRMI-2, -3 and -4 databases suggested that immediate mechanical reperfusion using either PCI or coronary artery bypass surgery reduced the risk of in-hospital death among patients with contraindications to fibrinolytic therapy.[214]

Percutaneous Coronary Intervention

Dr. Andreas Gruntzig performed the first balloon angioplasty of a coronary artery in 1977.[215] Dr. Peter Rentrop reported his initial experience with PCI for acute MI in 1979.[216,217] O'Neill and colleagues[218] published a randomized trial of PCI compared with intracoronary streptokinase for acute MI in 1986. The most recent meta-analysis identified 23 trials that randomly assigned a total of 7739 patients with STEMI to receive intravenous fibrinolytic therapy or undergo primary PCI, defined as PCI without previous or concomitant fibrinolytic therapy.[219] Numerous other randomized trials have been performed to investigate several other applications of PCI in patients with acute MI. Rescue PCI refers to PCI that is performed after unsuccessful fibrinolytic therpy. After successful fibrinolysis, PCI may be performed immediately, on a routine, deferred basis, or in a selective fashion (e.g., to treat inducible ischemia).

Primary Percutaneous Intervention

Myocardial salvage and long-term mortality are correlated with both the TIMI grade flow and the myocardial blush grade achieved after primary PCI for STEMI.[220-223] TIMI grade 3 flow is achieved in a high percentage of patients who undergo primary PCI for STEMI. The largest clinical trial of PCI compared with fibrinolytic therapy for acute MI was the Danish Multicenter Randomized Study on Fibrinolytic Therapy versus Acute Coronary Angioplasty in Acute Myocardial Infarction (DANAMI-2) study.[224] Immediate angiography was performed in 777 of the 790 (98%) patients who were randomized to undergo PCI. The initial angiogram showed TIMI grade 0 or 1 flow in 68% of patients, and grade 3 flow in 18%. PCI was attempted in 706 patients, resulting in postprocedural flow of TIMI grade 3 in 82%, grade 2 in 16%, and grade 0 or 1 in 2%. The Zwolle Myocardial Infarction Study Group reported the outcome of 1702 patients who underwent PCI for STEMI.[225] Successful PCI, defined as TIMI grade 3 flow and a residual lumen diameter less than 50%, was achieved more often during routine hours (8 AM to 6 PM) than during off-hours (6 PM to 8 AM) (96.2% versus 93.1%; *P*<.01).

Despite the presence of TIMI grade 3 flow, the myocardial blush grade, an indicator of myocardial perfusion, is abnormal in a majority of patients who undergo primary PCI for STEMI.[221,222] Among a cohort of 777 patients who underwent primary PCI for STEMI, normal myocardial blush (grade 3) was achieved in only 148 patients (19%), whereas 236 patients (30%) had blush grade 0 or 1.[221] Multivariate analysis showed that myocardial blush grade was an independent predictor of long-term mortality, with mortality after follow-up for 1.9±1.7 years of 3% for grade 3, 6% for grade 2, and 23% for grade 0 or 1 myocardial blush (*P*<.0001).[221]

Distal embolization of thrombus[226] and microvascular "no reflow"[227] are two of the mechanisms of impaired myocardial perfusion after primary PCI. Distal embolization was observed in 27 of 178 patients (15%) who underwent primary PCI for STEMI.[226] Patients with distal embolization had lower left ventricular EFs at discharge from the hospital and higher long-term mortality. Microvascular obstruction detected by MRI is a prognostic marker for cardiovascular events after acute MI, even after controlling for infarct size.[227] Several randomized trials have been performed to investigate mechanical methods of protecting the coronary microcirculation during PCI for ACS or acute STEMI.[228-234] Use of the X-SIZER thrombectomy catheter (ev3, Inc., Plymouth, Minn.) before coronary angioplasty or stenting appears to reduce distal embolization and improve epicardial flow, myocardial blush, and resolution of ST segment elevation, especially in patients with angiographic evidence of intraluminal thrombus.[228,229,231] The AngioJet Rheolytic Thrombectomy catheter (Possis Medical, Inc., Minneapolis, Minn.) was evaluated in a multicenter, randomized study called the AngioJet Rheolytic Thrombectomy in Patients Undergoing Primary Angioplasty for Acute Myocardial Infarction (AIMI) study.[234] The AIMI trial randomized 480 patients within 12 hours of symptom onset of STEMI to PCI alone or PCI with adjunctive rheolytic thrombectomy. No significant differences were observed in myocardial perfusion blush or resolution of ST segment elevation. Infarct size measured by myocardial perfusion imaging was greater in the thrombectomy group, and major adverse cardiac events were more frequent in the thrombectomy group (6.7% versus 1.7%; *P*=.01). Two different distal embolic protection devices, one that consists of a distal balloon occlusion and aspiration system and another that employs a filter, failed to improve myocardial reperfusion or to reduce infarct size in patients with acute MI.[232,233]

Abciximab, a GP IIb/IIIa inhibitor, has been reported to improve recovery of microvascular perfusion after PCI for acute MI.[235] On the basis of observations from small studies, intracoronary vasodilators, such as adenosine, frequently are employed to treat "no reflow" after PCI.[236-238]

Proponents of primary PCI and fibrinolytic therapy for acute MI have written excellent reviews of the advantages and disadvantages of both reperfusion therapies.[239,240] The evidence base supporting primary PCI for STEMI includes single-center series, multicenter randomized trials, large registries, and several meta-analyses. The Myocardial Infarction Triage and Intervention (MITI) Project Registry described a cohort of patients with acute MI who either underwent primary angioplasty (1050 patients) or received fibrinolytic therapy (2095 patients) at 19 hospitals in Seattle, Washington, between 1988 and 1994.[241] No significant difference in mortality was observed during hospitalization or long-term follow-up between the two groups. The MITI Registry included patients who received streptokinase, while a subsequent NRMI-2 report that was limited to patients who received tPA also found that in-hospital outcomes were similar for both methods of reperfusion.[242] Another cohort study of 20,683 Medicare beneficiaries with acute MI concluded that 30-day and 1-year mortality rates were lower among patients who underwent primary angioplasty than among patients who received fibrinolytic therapy.[243]

The DANAMI-2 trial did not show a significant difference between PCI and fibrinolytic therapy in the rates of death or stroke at 30 days, but the rate of reinfarction at 30 days was significantly lower: 1.6% for the PCI group compared with 6.3% for the fibrinolysis group (*P*<.001).[224] The most recent meta-analysis of PCI versus fibrinolytic therapy included DANAMI-2 and 22 other randomized trials.[219] The trials were rather heterogeneous in design: Stents were used in 12 trials, GP IIb/IIIa inhibitors were used in 8 trials, and 5 trials compared fibrinolytic therapy with PCI performed after transfer from a referral hospital to a hospital that provides invasive cardiac services. The rates of short-term death, nonfatal reinfarction, stroke, and the combined end point of death, nonfatal reinfarction, and stroke were lower for PCI than fibrinolytic therapy (Fig. 31-9). Another analysis pooled the individual patient 6-month follow-up data from 11 randomized trials of PCI versus fibrinolytic therapy for acute MI.[244] At 6 months, the mortality rates were 6.2% for PCI and 8.2% for fibrinolysis (RR 0.73; CI 0.55 to 0.98; *P*=.04).

Analysis of patients enrolled in NRMI-2 showed that in-hospital mortality was 28% lower among patients who underwent primary PCI at hospitals with the highest volume than among those who had PCI at hospitals with the lowest volume (adjusted RR 0.72; CI 0.60 to 0.87; *P*<.001).[245] Among 463 hospitals that performed primary PCI for STEMI and participated in NRMI-4, the hospitals with the greatest relative utilization of primary PCI, versus fibrinolytic therapy, for reperfusion, had shorter door-to-balloon times and lower in-hospital mortality rates.[246] These data may have provided some of the rationale for the ACC/AHA Practice Guidelines regarding the performance of PCI for STEMI.[71] PCI should be performed in a cardiac catheterization laboratory that performs more than 200 PCI procedures per year, including at least 36 cases of primary PCI for STEMI. The operator should perform more than 75 PCI procedures per year.

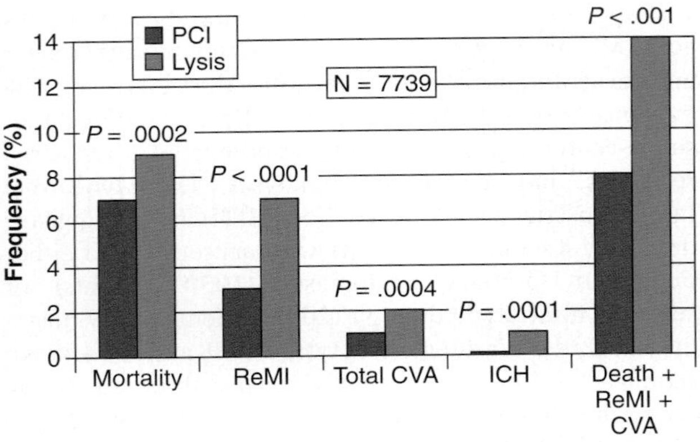

Figure 31-9. Short-term (4 to 6 weeks) clinical outcomes for 7739 patients enrolled in 23 randomized trials comparing fibrinolytic therapy with primary coronary intervention for acute ST segment elevation myocardial infarction. CVA, cerebrovascular accident (stroke); ICH, intracranial hemorrhage; PCI, percutaneous coronary intervention; ReMI, reinfarction. (From Keeley EC, Boura JA, Grines CL: Primary angioplasty versus intravenous thrombolytic therapy for acute myocardial infarction: A quantitative review of 23 randomised trials. Lancet 2003;361:13-20.)

Both the extent of myocardial salvage[189,247] and the mortality benefit[161,248,249] of fibrinolytic therapy and primary PCI are inversely related to the time elapsed between symptom onset and treatment. Among a cohort of 1791 patients with STEMI treated with primary PCI, the relative risk (RR) of death at 1 year increased by 7.5% for each 30-minute delay.[250] Several studies have analyzed the relationship between mortality and the so-called door-to-balloon time, defined as the duration of time between arrival at the hospital and the first balloon inflation.[249,251-253] Although some studies found that in-hospital mortality was not related to the door-to-balloon time,[251] most studies have shown that both in-hospital and late mortality are higher when door-to-balloon time is longer.[249,252,253] Among 2082 patients with acute MI who were enrolled in the CADILLAC trial, door-to-balloon time was an independent predictor of 1-year mortality in patients who presented within 2 hours after the onset of symptoms (n=965; hazard ratio 1.24; 95% CI 1.05 to 1.46; P=.013), but not in patients who presented later than 2 hours (n=944; hazard ratio 0.88; 95% CI 0.67 to 1.15; P=.33).[254]

The ACC/AHA Practice Guidelines set a goal of balloon inflation within 90 minutes of presentation, but observational studies indicate that this goal is seldom achieved.[174,255] Among 33,647 patients with STEMI who underwent primary PCI and were enrolled in the NRMI-3 and NRMI-4 registries, only 35% of patients received treatment within 90 minutes of arrival.[174] No significant improvement in the door-to-balloon time was obtained in the 421 participating hospitals from 1999 to 2002.[174] The time of day and day of week had significant effects on door-to-balloon times.[256] Fifty-four percent of patients who underwent primary PCI were treated during off-hours (weekdays, 5 PM to 7 AM and weekends). Door-to-balloon times exceeded 90 minutes in 74% of patients who underwent PCI during off-hours, compared with 53% of patients treated during regular hours (weekdays, 7 AM to 5 PM) (P<.001). Treatment delays are far greater among patients who are transferred to another hospital to undergo primary PCI.[255] Among 4278 patients who underwent interhospital transfer for primary PCI during the period 1999 to 2002, the median total door-to-balloon time was 180 minutes.[255] Only 4.2% of patients underwent PCI within the benchmark of 90 minutes.[255] Analysis of 23 randomized trials that compared primary PCI with fibrinolytic therapy for STEMI indicated that PCI affords a mortality advantage only if the door-to-balloon time exceeds the door-to-needle time by less than 1 hour.[257]

Several approaches have been suggested to reduce the delay between symptom onset and reperfusion in patients treated by primary PCI. One approach that has been tested is performance of primary PCI at hospitals that have cardiac catheterization laboratories but lack on-site cardiac surgery.[258,259] One trial randomized patients with STEMI to undergo primary PCI (n=225) or receive accelerated tPA (n=226) at 11 community hospitals without on-site cardiac surgery.[259] The composite end point of death, recurrent MI, and stroke was significantly lower among patients treated with primary PCI than among those who received tPA, both 6 weeks after MI (10.7% versus 17.7%; P=.03) and 6 months after MI (12.4% versus 19.9%; P=.03). Another proposed strategy is the diversion of patients with acute MI to a primary PCI hospital, instead of the current practice of transporting patients to the nearest emergency department.[239] A recent survey of 365 hospitals identified six strategies that were significantly associated with a faster door-to-balloon time.[260]

Late reocclusion after successful primary angioplasty is associated with decreased long-term survival.[261] The CADILLAC trial randomized 2082 patients with acute MI to undergo percutaneous transluminal coronary angioplasty (PTCA) or stenting.[262] Although stenting did not improve the myocardial blush score,[263] the angiographic rates of reocclusion of the IRA at 7 months was 5.7% after coronary stenting, compared with 11.3% after PTCA.[262]

Two recent randomized trials compared drug-eluting stents with bare-metal stents for primary PCI of acute STEMI.[264,265] Target-vessel failure at 1 year occurred in 7.3% of patients who received sirolimus-coated stents, compared with 14.3% of patients who received bare-metal stents (P=.004).[264] No differences, however, were observed in the rates of death or recurrent MI between the bare-metal stents and drug-eluting stents.[264,265]

Rescue Percutaneous Coronary Intervention

Compared with TIMI grade 3 flow, TIMI grade 0 or 1 flow at 90 minutes after fibrinolytic therapy is associated with worse left ventricular function and increased mortality rates.[187,188] Compared with complete resolution of ST segment elevation, incomplete resolution of ST segment elevation after fibrinolytic therapy is associated with larger infarct size and greater short-term and long-term mortality.[81,83,266] Therefore, various angiographic or electrocardiographic criteria have been employed to define unsuccessful fibrinolysis and rescue PCI. A report from the TIMI 10B and TIMI 14 trials of fibrinolytic therapy defined rescue PCI as PCI performed between 90 and 150 minutes after the start of therapy for patients with TIMI 0 or 1 flow 90 minutes after the start of therapy.[267] The Middlesbrough Early Revascularization to Limit Infarction (MERLIN) trial defined failed fibrinolytic therapy as failure of the ST segment elevation in the worst lead to have resolved by 50% 60 minutes after the onset of fibrinolytic therapy.[268] The Rescue Angioplasty versus Conservative Treatment or Repeat Thrombolysis (REACT) trial's definition of rescue PCI was PCI performed within 12 hours after failed fibrinolytic therapy, defined as an ECG obtained 90 minutes after the start of fibrinolytic therapy that showed <50% resolution of the ST segment in the lead showing the greatest ST segment elevation.[269] Thus, many of the patients who underwent PCI in the REACT trial would meet the TIMI group's definition of either adjunctive PCI, defined as PCI for patients with TIMI grade 2 or 3 flow, or delayed PCI, defined as PCI longer than 150 minutes after fibrinolytic therapy, rather than rescue PCI as defined by the TIMI group and other investigators.[267] Among patients enrolled in the TIMI 10B and 14 trials, the rate of TIMI grade 3 flow was significantly greater after adjunctive PCI than after rescue PCI (89% versus 78%, $P=.001$),[267] which might account for the REACT trial's 98% (106 of 108 patients) success rate for rescue PCI.[269]

There is conflicting information regarding the impact of rescue PCI on mortality. Among 150 patients who were enrolled in the TIMI 10B trial and had TIMI 0 or 1 flow 90 minutes after fibrinolytic therapy, 2-year mortality was significantly less among the patients who underwent rescue PCI ($n=120$) than among those who did not ($n=30$) ($P=.03$).[270] The randomized trials that compared rescue PCI with conservative therapy were insufficiently powered to detect an effect on mortality. Although differences in trial design and the definition of rescue PCI make it somewhat difficult to compare the results of various trials, at least two meta-analyses of the randomized trials have been published.[271,272] A pooled analysis of the short-term mortality (in-hospital or 30-day) among 942 patients who were enrolled in 5 randomized trials revealed that the risk of death was 36% lower among patients who were randomized to PCI (RR 0.64, 95% CI 0.41 to 1.00, $P=.048$).[271] Another meta-analysis included 6 trials that randomized 908 patients to rescue PCI or conservative therapy.[272] Rescue PCI was not associated with a reduction in all-cause mortality at 6 months (RR 0.69; 95% CI 0.46 to 01.05), but it was associated with significant reductions in the risk of heart failure and reinfarction, and an increased risk of stroke and minor bleeding[272] (Figs. 31-10 and 31-11).

Mortality

Study	PCI	Control	RR (95% CI)
Belenkie et al.	1/16	4/12	0.19 (0.02–1.47)
RESCUE	4/78	7/73	0.53 (0.16–1.75)
TAMI	3/49	1/59	3.61 (0.39–33.64)
RESCUE II	1/14	0/15	3.20 (0.14–72.62)
MERLIN	15/153	17/154	0.89 (0.46–1.71)
REACT	9/144	18/141	0.49 (0.23–1.05)
Total	**33/454 (7.3%)**	**47/454 (10.4%)**	**0.69 (0.46–1.05) *P* = .09**

Absolute risk reduction 3% (95% CI 0%–7%)
NNT 33
Test heterogeneity: χ^2 6.1 df 5 (p 0.30) I^2 18%

Heart Failure

Study	PCI	Control	RR (95% CI)
RESCUE	1/78	5/73	0.19 (0.02–1.56)
TAMI	9/49	14/59	0.77 (0.37–1.63)
MERLIN	37/153	46/154	0.81 (0.56–1.17)
REACT	7/144	11/141	0.62 (0.25–1.56)
Total	**54/424 (12.7%)**	**76/427 (17.8%)**	**0.73 (0.54–1.00) *P* = .05**

Absolute risk reduction 5% (95% CI 0%–9%)
NNT 20
Test heterogeneity: χ^2 2.0 df 3 (p 0.57) I^2 0%

Reinfarction

Study	PCI	Control	RR (95% CI)
TAMI	7/49	10/59	0.84 (0.35–2.05)
MERLIN	11/153	16/154	0.69 (0.33–1.44)
REACT	3/144	12/141	0.24 (0.07–0.85)
Total	**21/346 (6.1%)**	**38/354 (10.7%)**	**0.58 (0.35–0.97) *P* = .04**

Absolute risk reduction 4% (95% CI 0%–9%)
NNT 25
Test heterogeneity: χ^2 2.7 df 2 (p 0.25) I^2 27%

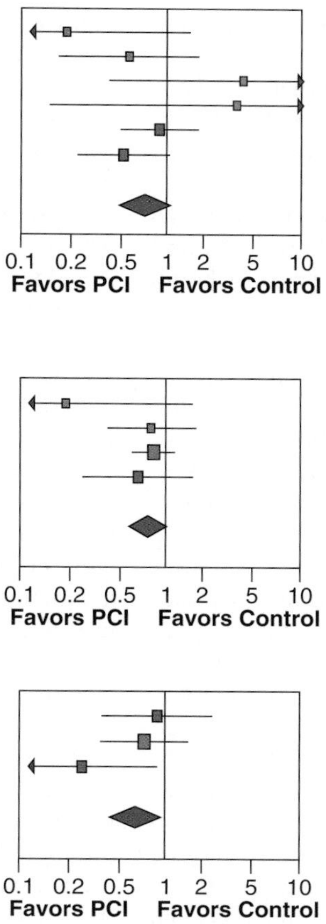

Figure 31-10. Efficacy end points for rescue percutaneous coronary intervention (PCI) versus conservative therapy. CI, confidence interval; MERLIN, Middlesbrough Early Revascularization to Limit Infarction trial; NNT, number needed to treat; REACT, Rescue Angioplasty versus Conservative Treatment or Repeat Thrombolysis trial; RESCUE, Randomized Comparison of Rescue Angioplasty with Conservative Management of Patients with Early Failure of Thrombolysis for Acute Anterior Myocardial Infarction trial; RR, relative risk; TAMI, Thrombolysis and Angioplasty in Myocardial Infarction study. (From Wijeysundera HC, Vijayaraghavan R, Nallamothu BK, et al: Rescue angioplasty or repeat fibrinolysis after failed fibrinolytic therapy for ST-segment myocardial infarction: A meta-analysis of randomized trials. J Am Coll Cardiol 2007;49:422-430.)

Stroke

Study	PCI	Control	RR (95% CI)
MERLIN	7/153	1/154	7.05 (0.88–56.58)
REACT	3/144	1/141	2.94 (0.31–27.90)
Total	**10/297 (3.4%)**	**2/295 (0.7%)**	**4.98 (1.10–22.48) *P* = .04**

Absolute risk reduction 3% (95% CI 0%–5%)
NNH 33
Test heterogeneity: χ^2 0.32 df 1 (p 0.57) I^2 0%

Minor Bleeding

Study	PCI	Control	RR (95% CI)
Belenkie et al.	2/16	1/12	1.50 (0.15–14.68)
MERLIN	17/153	2/154	8.56 (2.01–36.40)
REACT	33/144	8/141	4.04 (1.93–8.44)
Total	**52/313 (16.6%)**	**11/307 (3.6%)**	**4.58 (2.46–8.55) *P* < .001**

Absolute risk reduction 13% (95% CI 8%–18%)
NNH 8
Test heterogeneity: χ^2 1.8 df 2 (p 0.42) I^2 0%

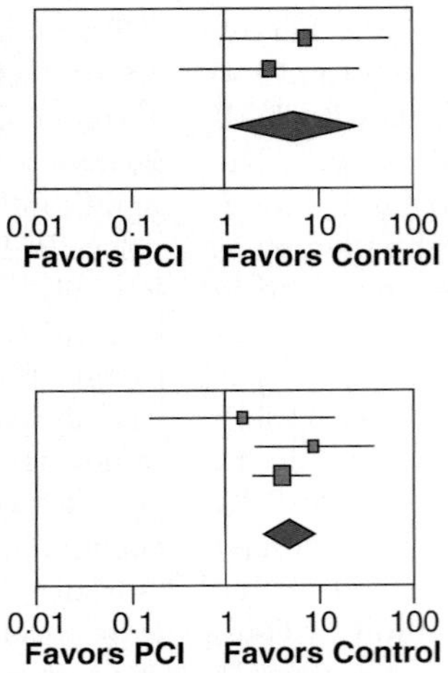

Figure 31-11. Safety end points for rescue percutaneous coronary intervention (PCI) versus conservative therapy. NNH, number needed to harm; other abbreviations as in Figure 31-10. (From Wijeysundera HC, Vijayaraghavan R, Nallamothu BK, et al: Rescue angioplasty or repeat fibrinolysis after failed fibrinolytic therapy for ST-segment myocardial infarction: A meta-analysis of randomized trials. J Am Coll Cardiol 2007;49:422-430.)

Selection of Reperfusion Strategy

There is evidence that reperfusion therapy is underutilized in the United States.[273] The NRMI-2 registry included 84,663 patients with STEMI who presented to the hospital with diagnostic ECG changes on the initial ECG within 6 hours after symptom onset, and without contraindications to fibrinolytic therapy.[273] Despite their eligibility to receive reperfusion therapy, 24% received none (i.e., neither fibrinolytic therapy nor PCI). Age older than 75 years, female gender, lack of chest pain at presentation, and LBBB were independent predictors of failure to receive reperfusion therapy. Among patients enrolled in the NRMI-2 registry, patients in Killip class II or III were less likely to receive reperfusion therapy than patients in Killip class I.[274]

According to the ACC/AHA Practice Guidelines, there are multiple Class I indications for primary PCI but only two Class I indications for fibrinolytic therapy: (1) STEMI with symptom onset within the prior 12 hours and ST elevation greater than 0.1 mV in at least two contiguous precordial leads or at least two adjacent limb leads and (2) STEMI with symptom onset within the prior 12 hours and new or presumably new LBBB.[71] There is no preference for either fibrinolysis or an invasive strategy if the patient presentation is within 3 hours from the onset of symptoms and there is no delay to implementation of the invasive strategy. The guidelines favor fibrinolysis over PCI under the following circumstances: when the duration of symptoms is less than or equal to 3 hours and the door-to-balloon time exceeds the door-to-needle time by more than 1 hour because of transportation delays or other factors; or when PCI is not an option because of either difficult vascular access or lack of access to a skilled cardiac catheterization laboratory.[71] An invasive strategy is preferred under the following circumstances: the diagnosis of STEMI is uncertain; fibrinolysis is contraindicated; the onset of symptoms is more than 3 hours before presentation; the door-to-balloon time is less than 90 minutes and the difference between the door-to-balloon and door-to-needle times is less than 60 minutes; and the patient is in Killip class III or IV (cardiogenic shock).[71]

The ACC/AHA Practice Guidelines provide additional recommendations regarding primary PCI for STEMI. Analysis of the NRMI-2 registry suggested that the risk of in-hospital death was reduced more by primary PCI than by fibrinolytic therapy in patients with CHF.[274] Thus, the ACC/AHA Practice Guidelines recommend primary PCI for patients with severe CHF or pulmonary edema (Killip class III) when the onset of symptoms is within 12 hours.[71] Primary PCI is considered reasonable (a Class IIa recommendation) for patients who present with severe CHF, persistent ischemic symptoms, or hemodynamic or electrical instability 12 to 24 hours after symptom onset.[71] As discussed subsequently, cardiogenic shock within 36 hours of acute MI is considered an indication for primary PCI.

PCI may be preferable to fibrinolytic therapy in patients with acute MI who are classified as high risk by virtue of a TIMI risk score of 5 or higher.[275] Among 1527 patients who were enrolled in the DANAMI-2 trial, no difference in mortality was observed between low-risk patients (TIMI score 0 to 4) who underwent primary PCI and those who received fibrinolytic therapy (8.0% versus 5.6%; P=.11) (Fig. 31-12). The 3-year mortality rate was significantly lower in high-risk patients who underwent PCI than in patients who received fibrinolytic therapy (25.3% versus 36.2%; P=.02) (see Fig. 31-12).

Acute MI in patients who have undergone previous CABG surgery frequently is due to thrombotic occlusion of saphenous vein bypass grafts, rather than occlusion of native coronary arteries.[276,277] Data are limited regarding the efficacy of intravenous fibrinolytic therapy in patients with previous CABG surgery, but in one small study, angiography revealed extensive residual thrombus in the presumed culprit vein grafts.[276] The Second Primary Angioplasty in Myocardial Infarction Trial (PAMI-2) included 58 patients with previous surgery who had either STEMI or NSTEMI.[277] The infarct-related vessel was a native coronary artery in 26 patients (45%) and a bypass graft in 32 patients (55%), including 31 saphenous vein grafts and 1 internal mammary artery graft. PCI was attempted in 72% of the bypass grafts, resulting in TIMI grade 3 flow in only 70.2% of the grafts, compared with 94.3% of native coronary arteries in patients without previous CABG surgery.

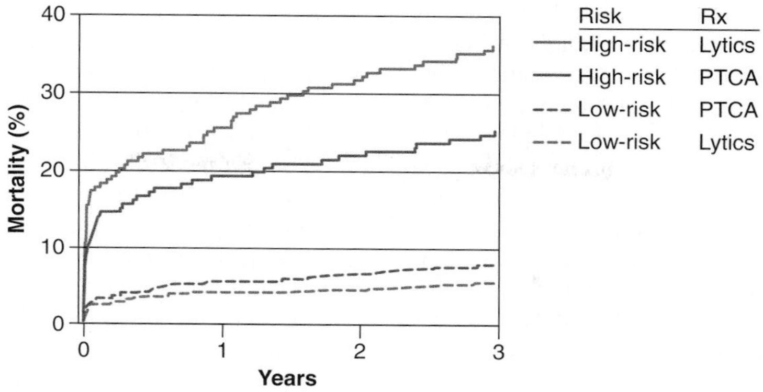

Number at risk

TIMI 0–4	Fx 556	533	531
	PA 578	546	540
TIMI ≥ 5	Fx 207	154	141
	PA 186	150	145

Figure 31-12. Mortality rates for low-risk patients *(dashed lines)* and high-risk patients *(solid lines)* who were randomized to receive fibrinolysis (Fx) *(blue lines)* or primary angioplasty (PA) *(red lines)* in the DANAMI-2 trial. Among 1134 patients who were classified as low risk by virtue of a TIMI risk score of 0 to 4, mortality after fibrinolysis and primary angioplasty was not significantly different. Among 393 patients with a TIMI risk score of 5 or higher, mortality was significantly lower after primary angioplasty compared with fibrinolysis. DANAMI, Danish Multicenter Randomized Study on Fibrinolytic Therapy versus Acute Coronary Angioplasty for Acute Myocardial Infarction; Fx, fibrinolytic therapy; PA, primary angioplasty; PTCA, percutaneous transluminal coronary angioplasty; TIMI, Thrombolysis in Myocardial Infarction study. (From Thune JJ, Hoefsten DE, Lindholm MG, et al: Simple risk stratification at admission to identify patients with reduced mortality from primary angioplasty. Circulation 2005;112:2017-2021.)

Patients presenting more than 12 hours after symptom onset are not considered candidates for fibrinolytic therapy but may benefit from primary PCI.[278] A trial that compared primary PCI with conservative therapy included 365 patients with acute STEMI between 12 and 48 hours after symptom onset.[278] Left ventricular infarct size measured by technetium Tc 99m sestamibi imaging 5 to 10 days after randomization was significantly smaller in patients managed using invasive strategies than in patients managed conservatively (8% versus 13%; $P<.001$). The Occluded Artery Trial (OAT) randomized 2166 patients with total occlusion of the IRA 3 to 28 days after MI to medical therapy or PCI with stenting.[279] PCI did not reduce the occurrence of death, reinfarction, or CHF.

Platelet Glycoprotein IIb/IIIa Receptor Antagonists

Numerous clinical trials have investigated the role of platelet GP IIb/IIIa inhibitors in patients with acute STEMI, either in conjunction with fibrinolytic agents or primary PCI.[280] One rationale of including a GP IIb/IIIa inhibitor in either pharmacologic or mechanical reperfusion strategies is that platelet inhibition may improve myocardial perfusion and enhance salvage of ischemic muscle by reducing distal embolization of platelet aggregates. Another proposed rationale is to achieve coronary artery patency using lower doses of fibrinolytic drugs. In the TIMI 14 trial, 32% of patients had TIMI grade 3 flow 90 minutes after treatment with abciximab alone, whereas TIMI grade 3 flow was achieved in 62% of patients treated with full-dose tPA and in 77% of patients who received half-dose tPA plus abciximab.[196] Also, in patients with TIMI 3 flow 90 minutes after treatment, complete resolution of ST segment elevation, an indirect marker of myocardial perfusion, was more common in patients who received abciximab plus reduced-dose tPA than in those who received tPA alone (69% versus 44%, $P=.0004$).[281] Although the addition of abciximab to either tPA[281] or rPA[197] has been shown to improve angiographic indices of myocardial reperfusion, combination therapy with abciximab and a fibrinolytic drug has not been shown to reduce mortality compared with fibrinolytic therapy alone. A trial that randomized 16,588 patients with acute STEMI to treatment with either standard-dose rPA or half-dose rPA plus full-dose abciximab showed no differences in either 30-day or 1-year mortality.[282] A meta-analysis of 3 fibrinolytic trials that included 23,166 patients who were randomized to receive either abciximab plus half-dose rPA or tenecteplase (TNK) versus full-dose rPA or TNK found that abciximab was associated with a significant reduction in the 30-day rate of reinfarction (2.3% versus 3.6%; $P<.001$) but 30-day mortality was 5.8% for both groups.[280] Therefore, there is no Class I indication for a combination of fibrinolytic agents with GP IIb/IIIa inhibitors in the ACC/AHA Practice Guidelines.[71]

De Luca and associates[280] performed a meta-analysis of eight trials that enrolled a total of 3949 patients who underwent primary PCI and then were randomly assigned to an adjunctive abciximab treatment group or to a control group. Abciximab was associated with a reduction in the rate of reinfarction at 30 days (1.0% versus 1.9%; odds ratio 0.56; 95% CI 0.33 to 0.94; $P=.03$). Long-term (6- to 12-month) mortality was significantly lower among patients treated with abciximab than among control patients (4.4% versus 6.2%; odds ratio 0.69; 95% CI 0.52 to 0.92; $P=.01$). Another meta-analysis pooled trials that compared early versus late administration of abciximab (3 trials) or tirofiban (3 trials) as adjunctive therapy for primary PCI.[283] The trials enrolled 931 patients with STEMI who were randomized to administration of abciximab or tirofiban in the cardiac catheterization laboratory (late administration) or in the ambulance or emergency department (early administration). Early administration of a GP IIb/IIIa inhibitor significantly increased the proportion of patients with TIMI grade 3 flow on the initial angiogram, a possible mechanism for the improved survival associated with adjunctive abciximab in patients undergoing primary PCI for acute MI. A pilot study randomized 100 patients with acute STEMI to administration of tirofiban, another GP IIb/IIIa inhibitor, in the emergency department or in the cardiac catheterization laboratory before undergoing primary PCI.[284] Compared with later administration, early administration of tirofiban was associated with TIMI grade 3 flow in a greater percentage of patients (32% versus 10% [$P<.007$]).[284] Among 2507 patients who were enrolled in four clinical trials and underwent primary PCI, TIMI grade 3 flow before PCI was an independent determinant of survival (odds ratio 2.1, $P=.04$) even when corrected for TIMI grade 3 flow after PCI.[285] Because of the limited number of patients enrolled in the published clinical trials, the ACC/AHA Practice Guidelines Writing Committee assigned a Class IIa recommendation for abciximab as adjunctive therapy for primary PCI for acute STEMI, whereas the other GP IIb/IIIa inhibitors, tirofiban and eptifibatide, received a Class IIb recommendation.[71]

β-Blockers

β-Adrenergic blockers exert both antiarrhythmic and anti-ischemic effects. Experimental studies have shown that β-blockers increase the ventricular fibrillation threshold in ischemic myocardium,[286] and randomized clinical trials have demonstrated that early administration of intravenous followed by oral metoprolol reduces the incidence of ventricular fibrillation in patients with acute STEMI.[287,288]

Experimental studies have shown that β-blockers can limit the extent of myocardial infarction during coronary occlusion because they reduce heart rate, systemic arterial pressure, and myocardial contractility, thereby decreasing myocardial oxygen demand. Clinical data are conflicting, however, regarding the effects of β-blockers on infarct size in patients, with several studies showing reduced infarct size[289,290] and at least one showing no reduction.[291]

Numerous clinical trials have been performed to examine the effects of early or delayed β-blockade on short-term and long-term clinical outcomes in patients with acute MI. Both atenolol[292] and metoprolol[293] administered by intravenous infusion followed by oral administration reduced mortality in patients who did not receive fibrinolytic therapy. A pooled analysis of 27 randomized trials indicated that early β-blockade reduced mortality by 13% in the first week, and the mortality reduction benefit was greatest in the first 2 days.[294]

Subsequent trials have examined the impact of early intravenous β-blockade on the outcome of patients treated with fibrinolytic agents for acute STEMI.[295,296] In the TIMI II-B study 1434 patients who received intravenous tPA for acute STEMI were randomized to immediate or deferred β-blockade.[295] The deferred blockade group received oral metoprolol beginning on day 6, whereas the immediate blockade group received intravenous metoprolol within 2 hours of initiation of tPA, followed by oral metoprolol. The incidence of reinfarction (2.7% versus 5.1%, $P=.02$) and recurrent chest pain (18.8% versus 24.1%, $P<.02$) at 6 days was lower in the immediate group. The GUSTO-I trial protocol recommended that patients without hypotension, bradycardia, or heart failure receive intravenous atenolol as soon as possible after enrollment, followed by oral atenolol daily.[296] Although adjusted 30-day mortality was significantly lower in patients who received atenolol, intravenous atenolol was associated with greater mortality compared with oral treatment alone (odds ratio 1.3; 95% CI 1.0 to 1.5; $P=.02$). Also, administration of intravenous atenolol was associated with increased risks of heart failure, shock, recurrent ischemia, and need for a pacemaker. The Clopidogrel and Metoprolol in Myocardial Infarction Trial (COMMIT) randomized patients with suspected acute MI to treatment with metoprolol (up to 15 mg intravenously, followed by 200 mg/day orally; $n=22{,}929$) or placebo ($n=22{,}923$).[288] Treatment was discontinued either at discharge from the hospital or on day 28 of the hospital stay. 93% of the patients had STEMI, and approximately 54% of the patients received a fibrinolytic agent. The risk of reinfarction during treatment was 18% lower among patients who received metoprolol (2.0% versus 2.5%; $P=.001$). The overall in-hospital mortality rates were 7.7% in the metoprolol treatment group and 7.8% in the placebo group (odds ratio 0.99; 95% CI 0.92 to 1.05; $P=.69$). Allocation to metoprolol was associated with a significant 22% reduction in death attributed to arrhythmia (1.7% versus 2.2%; $P=.0002$), but there was a 29% increase in death attributed to cardiogenic shock among the metoprolol treatment group (2.2% versus 1.7%; $P=.0002$). Although the safety of intravenous β-blockade in patients with acute MI remains uncertain, the ACC/AHA Practice Guidelines Writing Committee assigned a Class I recommendation for prompt oral β-blocker therapy in patients without a contraindication.[71]

At least 32 randomized trials including nearly 27,000 patients have been conducted to determine the effect of β-blockade on long-term survival after acute MI, and several meta-analyses have been published.[294,297,298] The Norwegian Multicenter Study Group randomized 1884 patients to receive double-blind treatment with either oral timolol or placebo beginning 7 to 28 days after acute MI.[299] The cumulative mortality rate at 33 months was 39% lower in the timolol group than in the placebo group (10.6% versus 17.5%; $P=.0005$), and the sudden-death rate at 33 months was reduced by 45% (7.7% versus 13.9%; $P=.0001$). After continued follow-up for up to six years a significant difference in mortality was maintained.[300] The Beta-Blocker Heart Attack Trial (BHAT) demonstrated that treatment with propranolol beginning 5 to 21 days after acute MI also reduced mortality during an average follow-up period of 25 months.[301] Pooled analysis of 31 long-term trials found that β-blocker therapy was associated with a 23% reduction in the odds of death (95% CI 15% to 31%).[298] According to that analysis, the calculated number of patients needed to treat (NNT) for 2 years with a β-blocker to avoid one death is 42, which is less than the calculated NNT for antiplatelet therapy, 153.[298]

The Carvedilol Post-Infarct Survival Control in LV Dysfunction (CAPRICORN) study is an important trial that was not available for inclusion in the pooled analyses discussed earlier.[302] The CAPRICORN study randomized 1959 patients with a left ventricular EF 40% or lower to carvedilol or placebo beginning 3 to 21 days after acute MI. Forty-six percent of the patients had received reperfusion therapy, and 97% had received an angiotensin-converting enzyme (ACE) inhibitor for at least 48 hours before randomization. After an average follow-up period of 1.3 years, a 23% reduction was found for all-cause mortality (12% versus 15%; hazard ratio 0.77; 95% CI 0.60 to 0.98; *P*=.031), identical to that reported in a meta-analysis of previous randomized trials[298] (Fig. 31-13). The CAPRICORN trial supports the conclusion that β-blockade reduces mortality after acute MI even among patients who receive reperfusion therapy and ACE inhibitors for left ventricular dysfunction. Relative contraindications to β-blockade are: PR interval longer than 0.24 second, second-degree or third-degree atrioventricular block, heart rate less than 60, systolic arterial pressure less than 100 mm Hg, moderate or severe left ventricular failure, signs of peripheral hypoperfusion or shock, and active asthma or reactive airway disease.[71] The ACC/AHA Practice Guidelines recommend that patients with moderate or severe left ventricular failure should receive β-blocker therapy with gradual titration of the dose.[71]

Angiotensin-Converting Enzyme Inhibitors and Angiotensin Receptor Blockers

Acute MI triggers neurohormonal activation that is characterized by elevated plasma renin activity and aldosterone, and plasma renin activity was found to be an independent predictor of cardiovascular mortality among patients who were enrolled in the Survival and Ventricular Enlargement (SAVE) trial.[303] ACE inhibitors have been shown to attenuate left ventricular enlargement after acute MI.[304] Multiple clinical trials have demonstrated that ACE inhibitors reduce mortality after acute MI. The GISSI-3 trial randomized 19,394 patients with acute MI, with or without ST segment elevation, to an oral lisinopril treatment group or an open control group within 24 hours of symptom onset.[115] Seventy-one percent of the patients received fibrinolytic therapy. Six-week mortality was 11% lower among patients in the lisinopril treament group than in the control group (6.3% versus 7.1%; odds ratio 0.88; 95% CI 0.79 to 0.99). The ISIS-4 trial randomized 58,050 patients with acute MI to receive oral captopril or placebo within 24 hours of symptom onset.[116] Seventy-nine percent of the patients had ST segment elevation on the initial ECG, and 70% of eligible patients received fibrinolytic therapy, predominantly with streptokinase. Five-week mortality was 7% lower among patients who received captopril than among those in the control group (7.19% versus 7.69%; 95% CI 1% to 13%; *P*=.02). The individual patient data from ISIS-4 and GISSI-3 were combined with the data from two other large trials, creating a database of 98,496 patients, who were randomized to ACE inhibitor treatment or control groups during the acute phase (0 to 36 hours) of acute MI.[305] Thirty-day mortality was 7% lower among patients who received an ACE inhibitor (7.1% versus 7.6%; 95% CI 2% to 11%; *P*=.004). The absolute benefit of ACE inhibitor therapy was greater in patients with anterior MI.

Three additional trials have investigated the efficacy of ACE inhibitors in patients with left ventricular dysfunction or CHF: the SAVE study,[306] the Acute Infarction Ramipril Efficacy (AIRE) study,[307] and the Trandolapril Cardiac Evaluation (TRACE) study.[308] The SAVE study enrolled 2231 patients with an acute MI, no overt CHF, and a left ventricular EF 40% or lower as measured by radionuclide ventriculography.[306] The patients were randomized to double-blind treatment with captopril or placebo 3 to 16 days after acute MI. After an average follow-up period of 42 months, all-cause mortality was reduced by 19% (20% versus 25%; 95% CI 3% to 32%; *P*=.019). The risk reduction was 22% among patients

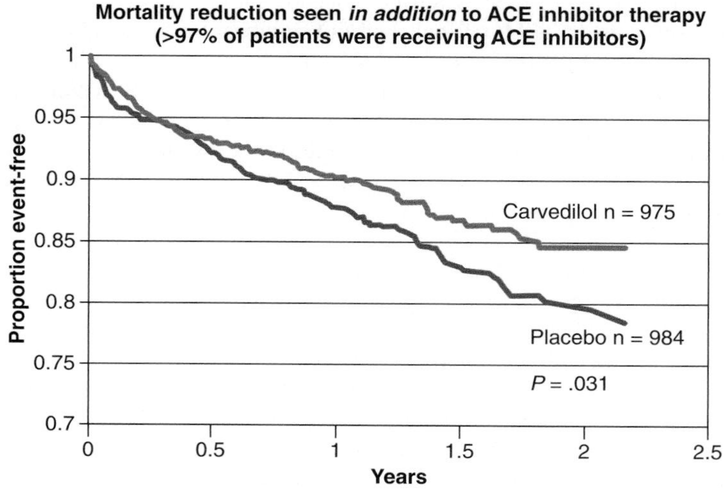

Figure 31-13. Kaplan-Meier estimates of all-cause mortality in the CAPRICORN trial. After an average follow-up period of 1.3 years, there was a 23% reduction in all-cause mortality (carvedilol 12% versus placebo 15%) (hazard ratio 0.77; 95% CI 0.60 to 0.98; *P*=.031). ACE, angiotensin-converting enzyme; CAPRICORN, Carvedilol Post-Infarct Survival Control in LV Dysfunction. (From Dargie HJ: Effect of carvedilol on outcome after myocardial infarction in patients with left-ventricular dysfunction: The CAPRICORN randomised trial. Lancet 2001;357:1385-1390.)

treated with fibrinolytic therapy (33% of the patients) compared with 17% among patients who were not. Captopril reduced the risk of recurrent MI by 25% (95% CI 5% to 40%; P=.015).[309] The AIRE study enrolled 2006 patients with an acute MI and clinical or radiologic evidence of CHF.[307] The patients were randomized to double-blind treatment with ramipril or placebo beginning 3 to 10 days after acute MI. After average follow-ups of 15 months, all-cause mortality was reduced by 27% (17% versus 23%; 95% CI 11% to 40%; P=.002). The TRACE study enrolled 1749 patients with an acute MI and an echocardiographic left ventricular EF 35% or lower.[308] The patients were randomized to double-blind treatment with trandolapril or placebo beginning 3 to 7 days after acute MI. The relative risk (RR) of death from any cause in the trandolapril group, as compared with the control group, was 0.78 (95% CI 0.67 to 0.91; P=.001). After follow-up for a minimum of 6 years, the life expectancy of patients was 4.6 years for patients who received placebo versus 6.2 years for those who were treated with trandolapril, a median increase of 15.3 months.[310] A pooled analysis of the data from individual patients who were enrolled in the SAVE, AIRE, and TRACE trials concluded that the mortality rate after a median treatment duration of 31 months was reduced from 29.1% in control patients to 23.4% in the ACE-inhibitor group (odds ratio 0.74; 95% CI 0.66 to 0.83; P<.0001).[311]

Two randomized clinical trials compared captopril with an angiotensin receptor blocker (ARB) in high-risk acute MI patients: the Optimal Trial in Myocardial Infarction with the Angiotensin II Antagonist Losartan (OPTIMAAL)[312] and the Valsartan in Acute Myocardial Infarction Trial (VALIANT).[313] The OPTIMAAL trial enrolled 5477 patients with acute STEMI who met any of the following entry criteria: symptoms or signs of CHF, left ventricular EF less than 35%, or new anterior Q waves. Fifty-four percent of the patients received fibrinolytic agents. The patients were randomized to double-blind treatment with either losartan, titrated to a target dose of 50 mg daily, or captopril, titrated to a target dose of 50 mg three times daily, within 10 days of symptom onset. After an average follow-up period of 2.7 years, no significant difference in all-cause mortality was found between the losartan and the captopril treatment groups (18% versus 16%; RR 1.13; 95% CI 0.99 to 1.28; P=.07). The prespecified criterion for noninferiority was not satisfied. The VALIANT trial enrolled 14,703 patients with acute MI complicated by clinical or radiographic signs of CHF or reduced left ventricular EF 35% or less by echocardiography or contrast ventriculography 40% or less by radionuclide ventriculography), or both. Approximately 50% of the patients underwent reperfusion therapy; 35%, fibrinolytic therapy; and 15%, primary PCI. Within 10 days after the acute MI, the patients were randomly assigned to three treatment groups: valsartan monotherapy, captopril monotherapy, or the combination of valsartan and captopril. After an average follow-up period of 24.7 months, all-cause mortality was not significantly different for the three groups: valsartan 19.9%, captopril 19.5%, and the combination 19.3%. The investigators concluded that valsartan is at least as effective as captopril, because the criterion for noninferiority of valsartan relative to captopril was met.

Both aldosterone and angiotensin II, a potent stimulus of adrenal aldosterone production, are increased in patients with CHF despite chronic treatment with an ACE inhibitor. Aldosterone exerts numerous adverse cardiovascular effects, including increased myocardial collagen deposition and fibrosis and cardiomyocyte apoptosis.[314] Eplerenone, a selective aldosterone blocker, was studied in a multicenter, international, randomized, double-blind, placebo-controlled trial called The Eplerenone Post-Acute Myocardial Infarction Heart Failure Efficacy and Survival Study (EPHESUS).[315] The EPHESUS investigators enrolled 6632 patients with acute MI complicated by left ventricular dysfunction (EF less than 40%) plus either CHF or diabetes.[315] The patients were randomized to double-blind treatment with eplerenone or placebo beginning 3 to 14 days after acute MI. At the time of enrollment, 86% of the patients were taking an ACE inhibitor or ARB, and 75% were taking a β-blocker. During a mean follow-up period of 16 months, significantly fewer deaths occurred in the eplerenone group (478 of 3319 patients) than in the placebo group (554 of 3313 patients) (14.4% versus 16.7%; RR 0.85; 95% CI 0.75 to 0.96; P=.008). A reduction in the rate of sudden death from cardiac causes (RR .79; 95% CI 0.64 to 0.97; P=.03) also was observed. Serious hyperkalemia, defined as a serum potassium 6.0 mmol/L or more occurred in 5.5% of patients in the eplerenone group versus 3.9% of those in the placebo group (P=.002).

The ACC/AHA Practice Guidelines include the following Class I recommendations regarding inhibitors of the renin-angiotensin-aldosterone system: (1) An ACE inhibitor should be administered orally within the first 24 hours of STEMI to patients with anterior infarction, pulmonary congestion, or left ventricular EF less than 40%, in the absence of hypotension. (2) An ARB should be administered to STEMI patients who are intolerant of ACE inhibitors and who have either clinical or radiological signs of CHF or left ventricular EF less than 40%. (3) An ACE inhibitor should be administered orally during convalescence from STEMI in patients who tolerate them. (4) Long-term aldosterone blockade should be prescribed for post-STEMI patients without significant renal dysfunction or hyperkalemia who are already receiving therapeutic doses of an ACE inhibitor, have a left ventricular EF 40% or less, and have either symptomatic CHF or diabetes.[71] Intravenous ACE inhibitors should not be given within 24 hours of an acute MI because of the risk of hypotension.

Antiarrhythmic Drugs

Both atrial and ventricular arrhythmias are common in patients with acute MI. The incidence of atrial fibrillation was 10.4% among 40,891 patients who were enrolled in the GUSTO-I trial.[316] Patients in whom atrial fibrillation developed after admission were more likely to have a stroke or die within 30 days after acute MI. Among patients enrolled in the TRACE study, which enrolled patients with an acute MI and a left ventricular EF less than 35%, atrial fibrillation occurred in 21% of patients and was associated with a 50% increase in adjusted mortality.[317] Intravenous β-adrenergic blockade is the preferred therapy for patients with sustained atrial fibrillation or atrial flutter that is not associated with hemodynamic compromise, whereas sustained atrial fibrillation or flutter that is associated with hemodynamic compromise is an indication for synchronized cardioversion. Intravenous amiodarone is indicated for treatment of atrial fibrillation that does not respond to electrical cardioversion or recurs after cardioversion. Sustained atrial fibrillation should be treated with anticoagulants.

The incidence of primary ventricular fibrillation, defined as that occurring within 48 hours of acute MI and in the absence of cardiogenic shock or severe CHF, was 4.7% among a cohort of 5020 patients hospitalized for an uncomplicated acute MI in Worcester, Massachusetts, during 11 1-year periods between 1975 and 1997.[318] The incidence of primary ventricular fibrillation in the GISSI-1 trial was not significantly different in the streptokinase and control groups (2.73% versus 2.93%; RR 0.93; 95% CI 0.75 to 1.15).[319] A meta-analysis of 15 randomized trials of fibrinolytic therapy for acute MI confirmed that the likelihood of this arrhythmia is not altered by fibrinolytic therapy, with an incidence of ventricular fibrillation during the first hospital day of 2.99% for both the fibrinolytic treatment and placebo groups.[320] There is evidence, however, that fibrinolytic therapy exerts a protective effect against secondary ventricular fibrillation, defined as ventricular fibrillation in patients with acute MI complicated by CHF or shock.[320,321] Thus, the meta-analysis of 15 fibrinolytic trials found that the odds ratio for the development of ventricular fibrillation at any time during hospitalization in the fibrinolytic treatment group was 0.83 (95% CI 0.76 to 0.90; $P<.0001$).[320]

Primary ventricular fibrillation is an independent predictor of in-hospital mortality whether it occurs early (up to 4 hours) or late (after 4 to 48 hours) after the onset of acute MI.[322] Among 9720 patients with a first STEMI who were enrolled in the GISSI-2 fibrinolytic trial, 356 of the 7755 patients who were in Killip class I at entry developed primary ventricular fibrillation.[322] Early primary ventricular fibrillation occurred in 302 patients (3.7%) and late primary ventricular fibrillation occurred in 54 patients (0.6%); 226 patients had ventricular fibrillation within 1 hour of the onset of acute MI symptoms. In-hospital mortality rates were 13% among patients with late primary ventricular fibrillation (RR 3.80; 95% CI 1.80 to 8.02) and 7% among patients with early primary ventricular fibrillation (RR 2.00; 95% CI 1.29 to 3.12), compared with 4% among patients in Killip class I on admission in whom ventricular fibrillation did not develop. The in-hospital mortality rate associated with primary ventricular fibrillation was much higher in the Worcester Heart Attack Study, with an overall case-fatality rate of 44%, although improved survival was observed in patients who had primary ventricular fibrillation in the 1990s.[318]

Among 11,712 patients enrolled in the GISSI-1 study, secondary ventricular fibrillation occurred in 311 patients (2.7%).[321] The incidence of secondary ventricular fibrillation within 24 hours of acute MI was similar among the patients treated with streptokinase and the control group, while streptokinase halved the frequency of secondary ventricular fibrillation later than 24 hours after admission (27/5860 versus 60/5852; RR 0.45; 95% CI 0.29 to 0.70). The protective effect of streptokinase was even greater among patients who were treated within 3 hours of symptom onset (9/3016 versus 39/3078; RR 0.23; 95% CI 0.12 to 0.45). In-hospital mortality was higher among patients with secondary ventricular fibrillation: 27.1% versus 17.3% for patients in Killip class II (RR 1.77; 95% CI 1.28 to 2.45), and 48.1% versus 35.3% for patients in Killip class III (RR 1.70; 95% CI 0.95 to 3.02). Secondary ventricular fibrillation did not affect in-hospital mortality among the patients in Killip class IV (67.9% with secondary ventricular fibrillation versus 71.9% without secondary ventricular fibrillation; RR 0.83; 95% CI 0.44 to 1.55).

Although primary and secondary ventricular fibrillation both are associated with an increased risk of in-hospital death, patients who survive to be discharged from the hospital after experiencing either type have a good prognosis. Among the patients who were enrolled in the GISSI-1 and GISSI-2 trials and had nonfatal primary ventricular fibrillation, 6-month mortality after hospital discharge among patients with the primary type was not significantly different from that in patients who did not have this arrhythmia.[322,323] In GISSI-2, patients who survived the hospital phase of an acute MI complicated by secondary ventricular fibrillation had a 1-year mortality of 10.4%, compared with 13.9% among patients who did not have secondary ventricular fibrillation (20/193 versus 322/2319; RR 0.72; 95% CI 0.44 to 1.15).[321]

Partly on the basis of the results of one double-blind, randomized study,[324] an editorial published in 1978 concluded that there was justification for routine prophylactic administration of lidocaine to all patients with acute MI to prevent primary ventricular fibrillation.[325] Subsequent studies of prophylactic lidocaine in acute MI, including more than 20 randomized trials and at least 4 meta-analyses, concluded that lidocaine reduces the incidence of ventricular fibrillation but increases mortality.[326] Therefore, according to the ACC/AHA Practice Guidelines that were published in 2004, prophylactic antiarrhythmic therapy is not recommended with use of fibrinolytic agents.[71] Also, the routine use of lidocaine is not indicated for suppression of isolated ventricular premature beats, couplets, runs of accelerated idioventricular rhythm, and nonsustained ventricular tachycardia. The Guidelines favor intravenous amiodarone for treatment of sustained monomorphic ventricular tachycardia.

Although ventricular ectopy is a marker of an increased risk of sudden death in survivors of acute MI, trials of chronic, oral antiarrhythmic drugs have not shown beneficial effects. The Cardiac Arrhythmia Suppression Trial (CAST) I and CAST II found that treatment with the class IC drugs encainide and flecainide, or the class IA drug moricizine, increased mortality in survivors of acute

MI.[327,328] *d*-Sotalol, a potassium channel blocker, also increased mortality among survivors of MI in the Survival with Oral *d*-Sotalol (SWORD) randomized trial.[329] Clinical trials of amiodarone, a class III antiarrhythmic drug, suggested that it may reduce the incidence of ventricular fibrillation or arrhythmic death among survivors of acute MI.[330,331]

The implantable cardioverter-defibrillator (ICD) has become the standard of care for prevention of sudden death in survivors of acute MI.[332] There are two Class I indications for an ICD after STEMI: (1) An ICD is indicated for patients with ventricular fibrillation or hemodynamically significant sustained ventricular tachycardia later than 2 days after STEMI, provided that the arrhythmia is not judged to be due to transient or reversible ischemia or reinfarction. (2) An ICD is indicated for patients without spontaneous ventricular fibrillation or sustained ventricular tachycardia more than 48 hours after STEMI whose STEMI occurred at least 1 month previously, who have a left ventricular EF between 31% and 40%, demonstrated additional evidence of electrical instability (e.g., nonsustained ventricular tachycardia), and have inducible ventricular fibrillation or sustained ventricular tachycardia on electrophysiology testing.[71]

Calcium Antagonists

No Class I indications are provided for calcium channel blockers in patients with acute MI because neither individual clinical trials nor analyses of the pooled results of multiple trials showed a reduction in mortality after acute MI.[297,333,334] A randomized study that compared diltiazem with placebo starting 3 to 15 days after acute MI found that diltiazem therapy was associated with an increased risk of cardiac events in patients with radiographic evidence of pulmonary congestion.[335] The same trial concluded that diltiazem increases the risk of late-onset CHF in patients with a left ventricular EF less than 40%.[336] Thus, there are two Class III recommendations for calcium channel blockers in acute MI: (1) Diltiazem and verapamil are contraindicated in patients with STEMI and associated systolic left ventricular dysfunction and CHF. (2) Nifedipine (immediate-release form) is contraindicated in the treatment of STEMI because of the reflex sympathetic activation, tachycardia, and hypotension associated with its use.[71]

Lipid-Lowering Agents

Numerous trials have evaluated the effects of statins on coronary events in patients with acute and chronic CAD, but none of the trials restricted enrollment to patients with STEMI or provided subgroup analyses of the outcomes among patients with STEMI before enrollment. The Scandinavian Simvastatin Survival Study (4S) was the first clinical trial to demonstrate significant reductions in total mortality and coronary heart disease mortality by treatment with lipid-lowering therapy.[337] Seventy-nine percent of the patients had a history of MI. After a median follow-up period of 5.4 years, total mortality was 12% in the placebo group versus 8% in the patients who were randomly assigned to receive simvastatin (RR 0.70; 95% CI 0.58 to 0.85; $P = .0003$). Also, there was a 37% reduction in the risk of undergoing a myocardial revascularization procedure. The beneficial effects of statin therapy in patients with a history of MI were confirmed by two studies that randomized patients to receive pravastatin 40 mg daily or placebo: the Cholesterol and Recurrent Events (CARE) trial[338] and the Long-Term Intervention with Pravastatin in Ischemic Disease (LIPID) trial.[339] All patients who were enrolled in the CARE trial had a history of MI between 3 and 20 months before enrollment, and 64% of the patients enrolled in the LIPID trial had a history of MI between 3 and 36 months before enrollment.

A diagnosis of hyperlipidemia cannot be excluded during the first week after an acute MI because both total cholesterol and low-density lipoprotein (LDL) cholesterol decrease significantly during the first week after an acute MI.[340] Although the current guidelines recommend a target LDL cholesterol level less than 100 mg per dL, recent data support more aggressive treatment to achieve a goal of LDL cholesterol level less than 70 mg per dL.[341-343] The current ACC/AHA Practice Guidelines include a Class I recommendation for lipid-lowering therapy on hospital discharge of all patients with STEMI regardless of the baseline LDL cholesterol level, with a preference for statins.[71]

Coronary Artery Bypass Graft Surgery

Randomized trials have not been performed to compare surgical reperfusion for acute MI with either conservative medical therapy or reperfusion by means of fibrinolytic therapy or PCI. A nonrandomized study compared the outcomes in 200 patients managed conservatively with those in 187 patients who underwent surgical reperfusion between 1972 and 1976.[344] In-hospital mortality was 5.8% among patients who underwent CABG surgery, compared with 11.5% among patients who did not undergo myocardial reperfusion ($P < .08$). Among the patients who underwent coronary bypass grafting within 6 hours from the onset of symptoms of acute MI, in-hospital mortality was only 2.0% (2/100), compared with 10.3% (9/87) among the patients who underwent surgery more than 6 hours after the onset of symptoms.

Although registry data indicate that CABG surgery within 24 hours of an acute STEMI is associated with a marked increase of in-hospital mortality,[345] emergency surgical revascularization should be considered in certain subsets of patients. Emergency CABG surgery is a reasonable option in patients with cardiogenic shock and coronary anatomy poorly suited for PCI (e.g., severe stenosis of the left main coronary artery). Among patients enrolled in the Should We Emergently Revascularize Occluded Coronaries for Cardiogenic Shock? (SHOCK) trial, survival rates were similar for CABG surgery and for PCI.[346]

Mortality after CABG surgery remains elevated during the first week after an acute MI.[345] Therefore, the guidelines recommend a period of delay before CABG surgery in patients who have incurred a significant decrease in left ventricular function after STEMI. Also, perioperative bleeding is increased in patients who undergo CABG surgery after recent administration of fibrinolytic drugs or antiplatelet agents. The Guidelines recommend that aspirin should not be withheld before elective or nonelective CABG surgery, but that clopidogrel should be withheld for 5 to 7 days before elective surgery.[71]

Management of Complications

Pericarditis and Pericardial Tamponade

Pericarditis, defined as the detection of a pericardial friction rub, was diagnosed in 20% (141/703) of patients who were enrolled in the Multicenter Investigation of the Limitation of Infarct Size (MILIS).[347] The frequency of pericarditis was higher in patients with Q wave MI than in those with non–Q wave MI (25% versus 9%; *P*<.001). Pericarditis was associated with a lower admission left ventricular EF (42% versus 48%; *P*<.001) and a higher incidence of CHF (47% versus 26%; *P*<.001). Pericarditis was accompanied by pleuritic or positional chest pain in 70% of patients. Diagnostic electrocardiographic changes usually are absent in patients with infarction-associated pericarditis.[348] A prospective study of 423 patients with acute MI found that only 1 of the 31 patients with pericardial friction rubs had diagnostic ST segment changes.[348]

The GISSI investigators reported the frequency of pericardial involvement in patients who were enrolled in the GISSI-1 (n=11,806) and GISSI-2 (n=12,381) trials.[349] The incidence of pericardial involvement was lower among patients who received fibrinolytic therapy than among patients in the control groups (6.7% versus 12.0%). Earlier treatment with fibrinolytic therapy was associated with a lower risk of pericardial involvement. Although pericardial involvement was associated with a higher long-term mortality, it was not an independent prognostic factor because it was strongly associated with the extent of infarction as determined by ECG, peak creatine kinase, and echocardiography.

The ACC/AHA Practice Guidelines recommend aspirin for treatment of pericarditis after STEMI.[71] Colchicine or acetaminophen is recommended for patients who do not respond to aspirin. Corticosteroids and nonsteroidal anti-inflammatory drugs are discouraged because of an increased risk of scar thinning and infarct expansion. Finally, anticoagulation should be discontinued if a pericardial effusion is detected.

Hemorrhagic pericarditis and free wall rupture are two potential mechanisms of cardiac tamponade after acute MI. Among 102,060 patients with STEMI who were enrolled in seven randomized clinical trials and received fibrinolytic therapy, cardiac tamponade developed in 1018 patients (1%).[350] Among the patients with tamponade, 153 also had a ventricular septal rupture or acute mitral regurgitation, and 865 had isolated cardiac tamponade. The adjusted 30-day mortality among 7-day survivors with tamponade was significantly increased (hazard ratio 7.9; 95% CI 4.7 to 13.5; *P*<.0001). Pericardial tamponade accounted for 1.4% of patients with cardiogenic shock among 1422 patients with acute MI who were enrolled in either the SHOCK registry or the randomized trial.[351]

Recurrent Ischemia or Infarction

Recurrent infarction (reinfarction) after an initial STEMI is relatively uncommon, but it often is an end point for clinical trials, because reinfarction is associated with increased morbidity and mortality.[352,353] Symptomatic recurrent MI during the index hospitalization occurred in 4.2% (836/20,101) of patients who were enrolled in four clinical trials of various fibrinolytic agents.[353] Recurrent MI occurred a median of 2.2 days after the initial MI and was associated with increased mortality rates at both 30 days (16.4% versus 6.2%; *P*<.001) and 2 years (hazard ratio 2.11, *P*<.001). In-hospital reinfarction occurred in 4.3% of patients (2258/55,911) a median of 3.8 days after fibrinolytic therapy in the GUSTO I and GUSTO III trials.[352] The rates of reinfarction were 4.3% for alteplase, 4.5% for reteplase, and 4.1% for streptokinase (*P*=0.55). Patients with in-hospital reinfarction had higher mortality at 30 days (11.3% versus 3.5%; odds ratio 3.5; *P*<.001) and from 30 days to 1 year (4.7% versus 3.2%; hazard ratio 1.5; *P*<.001).[352] Compared with patients who did not have reinfarction, patients with reinfarction had higher rates of CHF (31.9% versus 13.9%) and cardiogenic shock (15.9% versus 2.4%).

The frequency of recurrent ischemia or reinfarction after an initial STEMI depends on the modality of reperfusion and the adjunctive therapy employed. One of the purported advantages of primary PCI over fibrinolytic therapy is a decreased rate of reinfarction. The 30-day rates of reinfarction in the DANAMI-2 trial were 6.3% (49/782) among patients who were randomized to fibrinolytic therapy compared with 1.6% (13/790) among patients who were assigned to the angioplasty group (*P*<.001).[224] In a meta-analysis of 13 randomized trials of primary angioplasty versus fibrin-specific agents, the frequency of nonfatal reinfarction was 3% (74/2753) among patients randomized to angioplasty, compared with 6% (172/2757) among patients assigned to fibrinolytic therapy (odds ratio 0.42; 95% CI 0.31 to 0.55).[219]

There is evidence that coronary revascularization reduces the risk of reinfarction after fibrinolytic therapy. Among patients who were enrolled in four clinical trials of various fibrinolytic drugs, PCI or CABG surgery was performed during the index hospitalization in 26.1% (5238/20,039) of the patients and was associated with lower rates of both in-hospital recurrent MI (1.4% versus 4.7%, *P*<.001) and 2-year mortality.[353]

A variety of antithrombotic and antiplatelet therapies have been shown to reduce the risk of reinfarction after STEMI. In a trial that randomized 20,506 patients with STEMI to either enoxaparin or UFH as adjunctive treatment after fibrinolytic therapy, the rates of reinfarction at 30 days were 3.0% for the enoxaparin group (309/10,256) compared with 4.5% for the UFH group (458/10,223) (RR 0.67; 95% CI 0.58 to 0.77; *P*<.001).[148] A meta-analysis of 11 clinical trials found that administration of abciximab was associated with a reduction in the 30-day reinfarction rates among patients who underwent primary angioplasty (1.0% versus 1.9%; odds ratio 0.56; 95% CI 0.33 to 0.94; *P*=.03) and among patients who received fibrinolytic therapy (2.3% versus 3.6%; odds ratio 0.64; 95% CI 0.54 to 0.75; *P*<.001).[280]

Numerous clinical trials have investigated the effect of warfarin alone or in combination with aspirin on the risk of reinfarction and other events in patients with ACS, but most of the studies were not restricted to patients with STEMI, the target international normalized ratio (INR) has varied, and conflicting results have emerged.[354,355] The Warfarin Re-Infarction Study randomized 1214 patients to receive placebo or warfarin (target INR 2.8 to 4.8) after an average interval between the index MI and enrollment of 27 days.[356] Approximately 70% of patients had Q waves on the baseline ECG, most patients did not receive reperfusion therapy, and all patients were advised not to take aspirin or other antiplatelet drugs. During an average treatment period of 37 months, the rate of reinfarction was significantly reduced by warfarin compared with placebo (82/607 versus 124/607; RR 34%; 95% CI 19% to 54%; *P*=.0007).

The Antithrombotics in the Secondary Prevention of Events in Coronary Thrombosis-2 (ASPECT-2) study randomized 999 patients to receive one of three antithrombotic regimens: aspirin 80 mg daily, warfarin (target INR 3.0 to 4.0), or the combination of aspirin 80 mg daily and warfarin (target INR 2.0 to 2.5).[357] Patients were enrolled within 8 weeks of hospitalization for either unstable angina (13%) or either Q wave or non–Q wave MI. During a median follow-up period of 12 months the primary composite end point of MI, stroke, or death was significantly less frequent for the two groups that received warfarin, but warfarin did not reduce the risk of MI, and it increased the risk of both major and minor bleeding.

The APRICOT-2 trial randomized 308 patients with a patent IRA within 48 hours after fibrinolytic therapy to receive either aspirin alone (80 mg daily) or aspirin plus warfarin for 3 months (target INR 2.0 to 3.0).[358] The rate of reinfarction during 3 months of follow-up was 2% (3/135) for combination therapy, compared with 8% (11/139) for aspirin alone (*P*<.05). The Warfarin, Aspirin, Reinfarction Study (WARIS II) randomly assigned 3630 patients who were hospitalized for an acute MI to one of three treatment groups: warfarin alone (with a target INR of 2.8 to 4.2), aspirin alone (160 mg daily), or the combination of aspirin 75 mg daily and warfarin (target INR 2.0 to 2.5).[359] Fibrinolytic drugs were administered to 53% to 55% of the patients in each group. During a mean observation period of 4 years, the rates of reinfarction were significantly less in both groups of patients who received warfarin: 9.7% (117/1206) for aspirin alone, 7.4% (90/1216) for warfarin alone (RR 0.74; 95% CI 0.55 to 0.998; *P*=.03), and 5.7% (69/1208) for aspirin plus warfarin (RR 0.56; 95% CI 0.41 to 0.78; *P*<.001). Another study that used a target INR of 1.5 to 2.5 found that the addition of warfarin to aspirin 81 mg daily did not reduce the rate of reinfarction compared with aspirin monotherapy (162 mg daily).[360] The combination of aspirin 80 mg daily with low, fixed-dose warfarin (1 mg or 3 mg) was not superior to aspirin 160 mg daily in patients with a recent STEMI or NSTEMI.[361] Thus, the clinical trials suggest that warfarin is superior to placebo, that the combination of aspirin and warfarin is superior to aspirin alone if the target INR is sufficiently high, and that the risk of major bleeding is increased by adding warfarin to aspirin. Also, the published data should not be extrapolated to patients who receive dual antiplatelet therapy (aspirin plus a thienopyridine) after either fibrinolytic therapy or coronary artery stenting, because most of the patients who were enrolled in the warfarin trials did not receive reperfusion therapy or a thienopyridine.

In the ISIS-2 trial, aspirin reduced the rate of in-hospital reinfarction both in the patients who received streptokinase and in those who did not receive fibrinolytic therapy. Higher platelet counts were associated with an increased risk of reinfarction among patients with STEMI for whom treatment consisted of aspirin plus a fibrinolytic drug.[362] The addition of clopidogrel to aspirin abolishes the increased risk of reinfarction as the platelet count increases.[362] In the CLARITY study, the rate of recurrent MI after fibrinolytic therapy was 4.1% among patients treated with clopidogrel and aspirin, compared with 5.9% among patients who received placebo and aspirin (representing a 31% reduction in odds).[129]

Clinical trials have demonstrated that β-blockers, ACE inhibitors, and statins also reduce the risk of reinfarction after acute MI, although most of the trials enrolled patients with both STEMI and NSTEMI, and subgroup analyses of outcomes in patients with STEMI were not published. Compared with metoprolol started 6 days after tPA for acute STEMI, metoprolol started within 2 hours of tPA was associated with lower rates of reinfarction (5.1% versus 2.7%; *P*=.02) and recurrent chest pain (24.1% versus 18.8%; *P*<.02) at 6 days.[295] The Norwegian Multicenter Study Group randomly assigned 1884 patients to double-blind treatment groups, to receive either oral timolol or placebo, beginning 7 to 28 days after acute MI.[299] The cumulative reinfarction rate at 33 months was 28% lower in the timolol group than in the placebo group (14.4% versus 20.1%; *P*=.0006). The CAPRICORN study randomized 1959 patients with a left ventricular EF of 40% or less to receive carvedilol or placebo beginning 3 to 21 days after acute MI. Forty-six percent of the patients had received reperfusion therapy and 97% had received an ACE inhibitor for at least 48 hours before beginning the study treatment. After an average follow-up period of 1.3 years, the rate of nonfatal MI was significantly lower in the carvedilol group than in the placebo group (3% versus 6%; hazard ratio 0.59; 95% CI 0.39 to 0.90; *P*=.014).

The GISSI 3 trial did not show an effect of lisinopril on the rate of reinfarction after 6 weeks.[115] Although the AIRE[307] and TRACE[308] trials failed to show a significant effect of ramipril or trandolapril on the long-term risk of reinfarction, the SAVE study[306,309] did observe a significant decrease in the reinfarction rate among patients who were randomly selected to receive captopril 3 to 16 days after acute MI. After an average follow-up period of 42 months, captopril reduced the risk of recurrent MI by 25% (95% CI 5% to 40%; *P*=.015).[309] Thus, ACE inhibitors may not reduce the short-term risk of reinfarction after acute MI, but they may decrease the long-term risk of reinfarction.

Numerous trials have evaluated the effects of statins on coronary events in patients with acute and chronic CAD, but none of the trials restricted enrollment to patients with STEMI and many of the trials pooled the data of patients with unstable angina, NSTEMI, and STEMI. All patients who were enrolled in the CARE trial had a history of MI between 3 and 20 months before randomization; 61% were enrolled after a Q wave MI.[338] Although the mean interval from MI to enrollment was 10 months, during a median follow-up period of 5 years there was a significantly lower rate of nonfatal MI among patients who received pravastatin compared with patients who received placebo (6.5% versus 8.3%; RR 23%; 95% CI 4% to 39%; P=.02).[338]

Data are conflicting regarding the benefit of initiating statin therapy within 14 days of the onset of ACS. At least two meta-analyses of relevant randomized controlled trials have been published.[363,364] One analysis of 12 randomized trials concluded that statin therapy initiated within 14 days of hospital admission does not reduce the risk of death, MI, or stroke during the first 4 months after ACS.[363] Another meta-analysis of 13 randomized trials concluded that early statin therapy reduces death and cardiovascular events after 4 months of treatment.[364] A prospective cohort study using data from the Swedish Registry of Cardiac Intensive Care concluded that initiation of statin therapy before discharge was associated with a 25% reduction in 1-year mortality in hospital survivors of acute MI.[365] The current ACC/AHA Practice Guidelines include a Class I recommendation for lipid-lowering therapy on hospital discharge of all patients with STEMI regardless of the baseline LDL cholesterol, with a preference for statins.[71]

Among a cohort of 2301 patients who suffered reinfarction after administration of fibrinolytic therapy in the GUSTO I and Assessment of Safety and Efficacy of a New Thrombolytic 2 (ASSENT 2) clinical trials, reinfarction was treated with repeat fibrinolysis (n=864), with revascularization (n=525), or conservatively (n=835).[366] After adjustment for baseline characteristics, the 30-day mortality was significantly greater in the conservative group, 28%, compared with the repeat fibrinolysis group, 11%, (odds ratio 2.2; 95% CI 1.5 to 3.1; P<.001) or the revascularization group, 11% (odds ratio 2.2; 95% CI 1.4 to 3.3; P<.0001). No significant difference was observed between the revascularization and repeat fibrinolysis groups.

The ACC/AHA Practice Guidelines provide several recommendations regarding the management of recurrent ischemia and reinfarction.[71] They recommend escalation of medical therapy with nitrates, β-blockers, and intravenous anticoagulation. Insertion of an IABP should be considered in patients with hemodynamic instability, poor left ventricular function, or a large area of myocardium at risk. Recurrent ischemic-type chest discomfort is a Class I indication for coronary angiography and PCI or CABG surgery in patients who are considered candidates for revascularization. There is a Class IIa recommendation for readministration of fibrinolytic therapy to patients with ischemic-type chest discomfort and recurrent ST segment elevation who are not considered candidates for revascularization or for whom coronary angiography and PCI cannot be implemented within 60 minutes of the onset of recurrent ischemia. A Class III recommendation regarding streptokinase states that it should not be readministered to patients who received a non–fibrin-specific fibrinolytic agent more than 5 days previously.

Congestive Heart Failure

Wu and colleagues[274] described the outcomes for patients with STEMI who were enrolled in the NRMI-2 database and had CHF on admission (Killip class II or III). A total of 36,303 of 190,518 patients with AMI (19.1%) had CHF on admission; 70.6% were in Killip class II and 29.4% were in Killip class III. Patients who presented with CHF were less likely to receive fibrinolytic therapy or undergo primary PTCA. CHF on admission was a strong independent predictor of in-hospital death (adjusted odds ratio 1.68; 95% CI 1.62 to 1.75).

Hasdai and associates[367] combined the data from four large randomized trials of fibrinolytic therapy for STEMI to describe the incidence, timing, and consequences of mild to moderate CHF in patients with STEMI. Excluding patients with cardiogenic shock, 17,949 of 61,041 (29.4%) patients had mild to moderate CHF. Among the cohort with mild to moderate CHF, 8.7% had CHF only at baseline, 57.6% had CHF only after admission, and 33.7% had CHF at baseline and after admission. The incidence of death was similar for patients without CHF and patients with CHF at baseline that resolved after admission. Patients with CHF that persisted from baseline or developed after admission had a four times greater risk of death at 30 days (8% versus 2%).

There is evidence that patients with STEMI complicated by CHF benefit from early revascularization. Analysis of an Israeli database compared the outcomes of 629 patients with STEMI who presented in Killip class II or III CHF.[368] Mortality at 6 months was lower among patients who underwent PTCA or CABG surgery within 30 days compared with patients who were managed noninvasively (11.6% versus 27.4%; odds ratio 0.40; 95% CI 0.24 to 0.64; P<.0001). Analysis of the NRMI-2 registry suggested that the risk of in-hospital death was reduced more by primary PCI than by fibrinolytic therapy in patients with CHF.[274] Thus, the ACC/AHA Practice Guidelines recommend primary PCI for patients with severe CHF or pulmonary edema (Killip class III) when the onset of symptoms is within 12 hours.[71] Primary PCI is considered reasonable (a Class IIa recommendation) for patients who present with severe CHF, persistent ischemic symptoms, or hemodynamic or electrical instability 12 to 24 hours after symptom onset.[71]

It is important to recognize that CHF also is an important prognostic factor in patients with unstable angina or NSTEMI.[369] Among a cohort of 13,707 patients with a confirmed diagnosis of ACS without prior CHF or cardiogenic shock at the time of presentation to the hospital,

CHF (Killip class II or III) was present at hospital admission in 1778 patients (13%), and CHF developed later during hospitalization in an additional 869 patients (6.3%).[369] The incidence of CHF was similar in patients with STEMI (15.6%) or NSTEMI (15.7%), but less frequent in patients with unstable angina (8.2%). CHF at the time of admission was associated with a four-fold increase in crude in-hospital mortality rates across all three ACS subsets. The cumulative 6-month mortality rate was greater among patients in whom CHF developed during hospitalization (25.3%) than among patients who had CHF at admission (20.7%) or patients who did not have CHF (5.9%).

ACE inhibitors, eplerenone, and β-adrenergic antagonists are believed to improve the long-term survival of patients with MI complicated by CHF.[370] The AIRE study showed that ramipril, initiated 3 to 10 days after acute MI, reduced all-cause mortality by 27% in patients with either STEMI or NSTEMI and clinical or radiologic evidence of CHF.[307] The EPHESUS study randomized patients with either STEMI or NSTEMI and left ventricular EF less than 40%, to eplerenone or placebo beginning 3 to 14 days after the acute MI.[315] Ninety percent of the patients had CHF, documented by the presence of pulmonary rales, a third heart sound, or evidence of pulmonary venous congestion on the chest radiograph. Concomitant medications included β-blockers in 75% of patients and an ACE inhibitor or angiotensin receptor blocker in 86%. At 30 days after randomization, eplerenone reduced the risk of all-cause mortality by 31% (3.2% versus 4.6%; RR 0.69; 95% CI 0.54 to 0.89; P=.004).[371] During a mean follow-up period of 16 months, the all-cause mortality rate was 14.4% in the eplerenone group and 16.7% in the placebo group (RR 0.85; 95% CI 0.75 to 0.96; P=.008).[315]

BHAT, a study that randomized patients to receive propranolol or placebo 5 to 21 days after acute MI, included 710 patients who had a history of CHF before enrollment.[372] After an average follow-up period of 25 months, propranolol reduced total mortality by 27% and sudden death by 47%. A retrospective analysis of the AIRE study was performed to determine the effects of β-blockade on the outcomes for patients with acute MI complicated by CHF.[373] β-Blocker treatment was an independent predictor of reduced risk of total mortality (hazard ratio 0.66; 95% CI 0.48 to 0.90). The CAPRICORN study showed that carvedilol, started 3 to 21 days after MI, reduced all-cause mortality by 33% in patients with a left ventricular EF of 40% or less.[302] Unfortunately, patients with acute MI complicated by CHF are less likely to receive a β-blocker than are patients without CHF.[374]

On the basis of the foregoing evidence, the ACC/AHA Practice Guidelines include eight Class I recommendations for patients with STEMI complicated by pulmonary congestion[71]: (1) An arterial oxygen saturation greater than 90% should be maintained using supplemental oxygen. (2) Morphine sulfate should be given. (3) Patients with a systolic blood pressure 100 mm Hg or higher should receive an ACE inhibitor, beginning with titration of a low dose of a short-acting drug such as captopril. (4) Patients with a systolic blood pressure of 100 mm Hg or higher should receive nitrates. (5) A loop diuretic should be administered to patients with volume overload. (6) Although β-blockade should be initiated before hospital discharge, β-blockers should not be administered acutely to patients with "frank cardiac failure evidenced by pulmonary congestion or signs of a low-output state." (7) Patients already receiving an ACE inhibitor who have a left ventricular EF less than 40% and either symptomatic CHF or diabetes should receive long-term aldosterone blockade unless hyperkalemia (serum potassium greater than 5.0 mEq/L) or significant renal dysfunction (serum creatinine greater than 2.5 mg/dL in men or greater than 2.0 mg/dL in women) is present. (8) Echocardiography should be performed urgently to evaluate left and right ventricular function and to exclude a mechanical complication.

In view of the fact that the relevant clinical trials included patients with both STEMI and NSTEMI, it is logical that treatment of NSTEMI patients with CHF should conform with the practice guidelines as discussed for STEMI patients with CHF. Figure 31-14 presents an algorithm for the emergency management of MI complicated by CHF or hypotension.

Cardiogenic Shock

Cardiogenic shock is defined as decreased cardiac output and evidence of tissue hypoxia in the presence of adequate intravascular volume (see Chapter 23).[375] Cardiogenic shock is the most common cause of death among patients hospitalized with acute MI and accounted for 58% of all deaths within 30 days among 41,021 patients with STEMI who were enrolled in the GUSTO-I trial.[376] The onset of shock usually occurs after admission to the hospital. In a series of 2972 patients in whom cardiogenic shock developed, shock appeared after admission in 2657 (89%), whereas it was present at initial assessment in only 315 patients (11%).[376]

Hochman and colleagues[351] reported the causes of cardiogenic shock among 1422 patients with acute MI who were enrolled in either the registry or the randomized trial known as the Should We Emergently Revascularize Occluded Coronaries for Cardiogenic Shock? (SHOCK) trial. Left ventricular failure was the most common cause of cardiogenic shock, accounting for 78.5% of patients. Additional causes of shock were acute-onset severe mitral regurgitation in 6.9% of patients, ventricular septal rupture in 3.9%, isolated right ventricular shock in 2.8%, and pericardial tamponade in 1.4%.

Both STEMI and NSTEMI are associated with cardiogenic shock. Among 12,084 patients in the GUSTO-IIb trial who did not present with shock, cardiogenic shock developed in 2.5% of patients without ST segment elevation, compared with 4.2% of patients with ST segment elevation (odds ratio 0.58; 95% CI 0.47 to 0.72; $P<.001$).[377] The onset of shock was earlier among patients with ST segment elevation than among patients without ST segment elevation (median 9.6 hours after study entry versus 76.2 hours [$P<.001$]). Thirty-day mortality was 63.0% among shock patients with ST segment elevation on the initial ECG, compared with 72.5% among shock patients without ST segment elevation (P=0.50).

The treatment of patients with cardiogenic shock is multifactorial. Inotropic or vasopressor drugs and an IABP

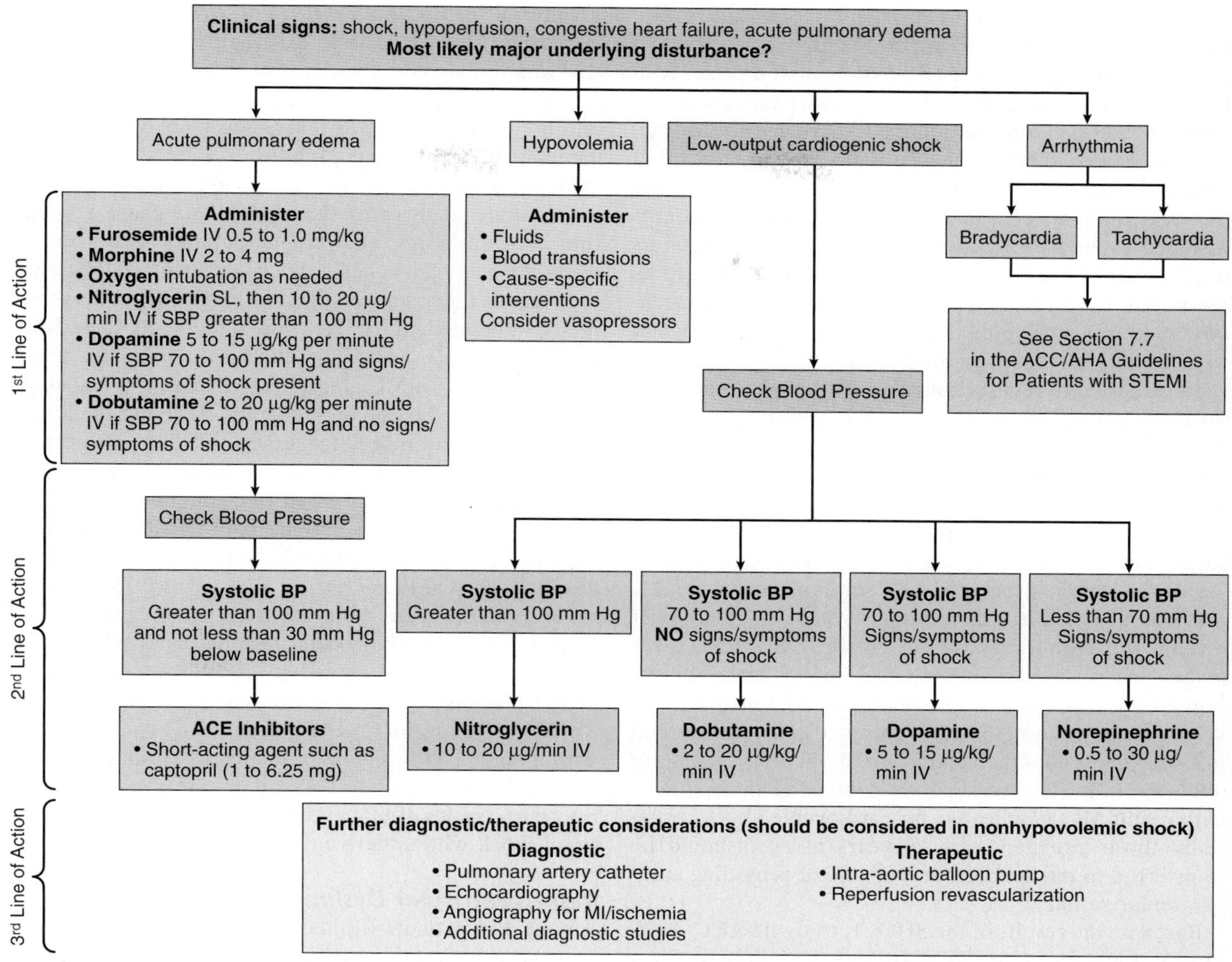

Figure 31-14. Algorithm for emergency management of complicated myocardial infarction (MI). ACE, angiotensin-converting enzyme; BP, blood pressure; IV, intravenous; SBP, systolic BP; SL, sublingual; STEMI, ST segment elevation myocardial infarction. (Data from Guidelines 2000 for cardiopulmonary resuscitation and emergency cardiovascular care: Part 7, the era of reperfusion: Section 1, acute coronary syndromes (acute myocardial infarction). Circulation 2000;102[suppl I]:I-172–I-203.)

are used for hemodynamic support. Mechanical ventilation frequently is required to maintain oxygenation. As discussed later on, revascularization has a major impact on the outcome of patients with cardiogenic shock. A systemic inflammatory response characterized by increased production of nitric oxide (NO) may play a role in the vasodilation and myocardial dysfunction that occur in patients with cardiogenic shock.[378,379] Based on experimental and pilot clinical data that suggested that inhibition of NO synthesis may have favorable hemodynamic and clinical effects in cardiogenic shock,[380] an international, multicenter, randomized, double-blind, placebo-controlled trial was conducted to test tilarginine (L-N^G-monomethyl-arginine), a NO synthase inhibitor, in patients with MI, and open IRA, and refractory cardiogenic shock.[381] The planned enrollment was 658 patients, but after enrollment of 398 patients the 30-day and 6-month mortality rates were not reduced by tilarginine, so the study was terminated based on a prespecified futility analysis.[381]

Patients with cardiogenic shock have been excluded from most of the fibrinolytic trials. The GISSI trial enrolled 280 patients with shock, and the 30-day mortality rates were similar for patients who received streptokinase (69.9%; $n=146$) and those who received placebo (70.1%; $n=134$).[158] Both retrospective observational reports and prospective randomized trials, however, have provided evidence that revascularization accomplished using either PCI or CABG surgery improves outcome in patients with acute MI complicated by cardiogenic shock. Berger and coworkers[382,383] analyzed the impact of early revascularization on the survival of patients with acute MI complicated by cardiogenic shock who were enrolled in the GUSTO-I trial. After adjustment for baseline differences, an aggressive strategy of angiography within 24 hours followed by revascularization if appropriate was associated with reduced mortality at 30 days (odds ratio 0.43; 95% CI 0.34 to 0.54; $P=.0001$)[382] and 1 year (odds ratio 0.6; 95% CI 0.4 to 0.9; $P=.007$).[383]

The SHOCK trial was a landmark randomized study to evaluate early revascularization in patients with cardiogenic shock.[384-386] Patients with cardiogenic shock caused by left ventricular failure complicating acute MI were randomly assigned to either emergency revascularization (n=152 patients) or initial medical stabilization (n=150 patients). An IABP was used in 86% of the patients in both groups. Thrombolytic therapy was administered to 49% of the patients randomized to revascularization, compared with 63% of the patients assigned to initial medical therapy. The median time from randomization to revascularization was 1.4 hours among the patients assigned to revascularization, with 64% of the patients undergoing PCI and 36% undergoing CABG surgery as the initial revascularization procedure. Delayed revascularization was attempted in 21% of the patients assigned to medical therapy, with a median time of 103 hours from randomization to revascularization. Although 30-day survival was not significantly different, 6-month, 1-year, and 6-year survival rates were greater among the patients randomized to early revascularization. The survival rate at 1 year was improved by early revascularization only for patients younger than 75 years of age.[385] The study also found an 18% absolute difference favoring the early revascularization group (51.6% survival versus 33.3% survival; 95% CI, for the difference, 6.1% to 30.4%). At 6 years, the overall survival rates were 32.8% and 19.6% in the early revascularization and initial medical stabilization groups, respectively.[386] Among the 143 hospital survivors, there was a significant difference in 6-year survival (62.4% versus 44.4%; hazard ratio 0.59; 95% CI 0.36 to 0.95; P=.03). The investigators concluded that patients with acute MI complicated by cardiogenic shock, especially those younger than 75 years of age, should be transferred to medical centers capable of providing early revascularization.[385]

Based on the results of the SHOCK trial, the ACC/AHA Practice Guidelines for STEMI include the following Class I recommendation regarding cardiogenic shock: "Early revascularization, either PCI or CABG, is recommended for patients <75 years old with ST elevation or LBBB who develop shock within 36 hours of MI and who are suitable for revascularization that can be performed within 18 hours of shock."[71] The guidelines recommend administration of fibrinolytic therapy to STEMI patients with cardiogenic shock who are unsuitable candidates for invasive strategies. Revascularization, using either PCI or CABG surgery, in patients older than 75 years of age received a Class IIa recommendation.

The IABP also received a Class I recommendation for treatment of cardiogenic shock that is not quickly reversed with pharmacologic therapy.[71] Intra-aortic balloon counterpulsation often improves blood pressure, cardiac output, and coronary blood flow in patients with cardiogenic shock.[387] Experimental studies suggest that an IABP may improve the efficacy of thrombolytic therapy.[388] Recent registry data, however, indicate that only 30% to 50% of patients with cardiogenic shock receive an IABP.[389] The NRMI-2 database included 23,180 patients with acute MI in whom cardiogenic shock developed during hospitalization between 1994 and 1996.[390] An IABP was used in only 31% of patients with cardiogenic shock.

One possible explanation for the underutilization of the IABP in cardiogenic shock is that most patients with acute MI present to hospitals that do not offer PCI or CABG surgery. A second possible explanation for underutilization of ballooon counterpulsation is that the effect of this modality on long-term outcome is uncertain, partly because no randomized trials of use of IABPs in cardiogenic shock have been completed.[389] Several nonrandomized, observational series have been reported.[390-393] A multivariate analysis of the NRMI-2 database revealed that in-hospital mortality among patients with acute MI complicated by cardiogenic shock was significantly greater at hospitals that were classified as low-IABP-volume hospitals, independent of baseline patient characteristics, hospital factors, medications, and revascularization procedures.[394] In the NRMI-2 registry, IABP use was associated with an 18% reduction of in-hospital mortality of patients who received thrombolytic therapy.[390] Of 46 patients with cardiogenic shock who received thrombolytic therapy within 12 hours of acute MI at two community hospitals, 27 received an IABP and 19 did not.[393] Patients managed with an IABP had a significantly higher rate of community hospital survival (93% versus 37%, P=.0002). Twenty-seven patients were transferred to other hospitals and underwent revascularization; hospital survival rate was 74%. Patients who received an IABP had a significantly higher overall 1-year survival rate (67% versus 32%, P=.019). The use of an IABP before PCI was associated with a significantly lower incidence of cardiac arrest or ventricular fibrillation in the cardiac catheterization laboratory in a series of 89 patients with acute MI and cardiogenic shock who underwent primary PTCA.[392]

Right Ventricular Dysfunction and Infarction

Among 416 patients with acute MI who were enrolled in an echocardiographic substudy of the SAVE trial, right ventricular function was an independent predictor of mortality and the development of CHF.[395] The odds of cardiovascular mortality increased 16% for each 5% decrease in the percent change in right ventricular cavity area from end diastole to end systole.

Occlusion of the right coronary artery (RCA) proximal to the acute marginal branches is the most frequent cause of right ventricular infarction, but occlusion of the LAD or a dominant left circumflex coronary artery also may result in right ventricular MI. Although autopsy studies have shown that anterior MI may be associated with a right ventricular infarction, right ventricular MI that is associated with hemodynamic compromise most commonly occurs in patients with an inferior MI because perfusion of the right ventricle occurs predominantly via the right ventricular branches of the RCA.[396,397] In a series of 125 patients with acute inferior MI who underwent emergency coronary angiography, echocardiography performed before coronary reperfusion demonstrated ischemic dysfunction of the right ventricle in 53 (42%) patients.[398] The RCA was the IRA in all patients with right ventricular MI, and depressed flow in the right ventricular branches was evident in each case. Right ventricular branch flow was preserved in patients without right ventricular MI.

Patients with inferior MI complicated by right ventricular infarction have an increased risk of major complications, including death, cardiogenic shock, and ventricular arrhythmias.[399] Cardiogenic shock during hospitalization occurred in 6.9% of a series of 491 patients with inferior MI complicated by right ventricular MI.[399] Patients with right ventricular infarction complicated by cardiogenic shock do not have a better prognosis than patients with cardiogenic shock associated with left ventricular failure.[400] Among a cohort of 1129 patients with acute inferior MI, there was no difference in left ventricular infarct size or function between patients with (n=491) and patients without (n=638) right ventricular MI, indicating that the increased risk of right ventricular MI is due to right ventricular dysfunction, rather than greater left ventricular injury.[399] The impact of right ventricular MI on prognosis may depend on the patient's age.[401] Among a series of 798 consecutive patients with acute inferior MI, 296 (37%) satisfied electrocardiographic and/or echocardiographic criteria for right ventricular infarction.[401] Major complications (45% versus 19%, P<.0001) and in-hospital death (22% versus 6%, P<.0001) occurred more often in patients with than in those without right ventricular MI. The diagnosis of right ventricular MI increased the mortality risk in patients aged 65 or greater, but not among younger patients.

Although numerous electrocardiographic signs of right ventricular MI have been described, ST segment elevation in lead V_4R is the most reliable electrocardiographic indicator of this form of MI.[402] Zehender and associates[403] studied the diagnostic and prognostic value of ST segment elevation in V_4R in a series of 200 consecutive patients with acute inferior MI. ST segment elevation in lead V_4R was present on the initial ECG in 107 patients (54%). Based on the results of autopsy, coronary angiography, right ventriculography, or nuclear scan, or invasive hemodynamic data, ST segment elevation in V_4R had 88% sensitivity, 78% specificity, and 83% diagnostic accuracy for right ventricular MI. ST segment elevation in V_4R was associated with an in-hospital mortality of 31%, compared with 6% among patients without ST segment elevation in V_4R (P<.001). Multivariate analysis of clinical data confirmed that 0.1 mV or greater of ST segment elevation in V_4R was a strong independent predictor of in-hospital death (RR 7.7; 95% CI 2.6 to 23) and major complications (RR 4.7; 95% CI 2.4 to 9).

The triad of hypotension, clear lung fields, and elevated jugular venous pressure should raise a suspicion of right ventricular MI in patients with inferior STEMI, but the triad has a sensitivity of less than 25%.[404] The hemodynamic criteria that have been used to diagnose right ventricular MI are right atrial pressure greater than 10 mm Hg and equal or nearly equal to the pulmonary capillary wedge pressure, or a noncompliant pattern in the right atrium.[405] According to the ACC/AHA Practice Guidelines for STEMI, inferior STEMI with hemodynamic compromise is a Class I indication for recording lead V_4R and an echocardiogram to screen for right ventricular MI.[71] Echocardiographic signs of this disorder include right ventricular dilation, right ventricular asynergy, and abnormal interventricular septal motion.[405] Echocardiography also is valuable to exclude pericardial tamponade because both right ventricular MI and pericardial tamponade may manifest with hypotension and elevated jugular venous pressure.[406]

The ACC/AHA Guidelines emphasize the importance of maintenance of right ventricular preload, reduction of right ventricular afterload, inotropic support of the right ventricle, maintenance of atrioventricular synchrony, and early reperfusion of the IRA.[71] Volume loading plus dobutamine, but not volume loading alone, has been shown to improve cardiac index in patients with acute right ventricular infarction.[407] Systemic vasodilators are poorly tolerated, and hypotension after administration of sublingual nitroglycerin is a common event in patients with right ventricular MI. Short-term inhalation of nitric oxide, a selective vasodilator of the pulmonary circulation, improved cardiac index by 24% in a series of 13 patients with right ventricular infarction and cardiogenic shock.[408]

The status of right atrial function is an important determinant of the hemodynamic consequences of right ventricular MI.[409] Hemodynamic compromise may result if the atrial contribution to ventricular filling is lost in patients with right ventricular MI. Therefore, high-grade atrioventricular block, other bradyarrhythmias, and atrial fibrillation are common causes of hypotension in patients with right ventricular MI. Ventricular pacing may not increase cardiac output in such patients, although atrial pacing and atrioventricular sequential pacing have been shown to improve cardiac output.[410,411] Atrial fibrillation associated with hemodynamic compromise is an indication for electrical cardioversion.

The elevated right atrial pressure in patients with right ventricular MI may cause refractory hypoxemia as a result of increased right-to-left shunting in patients with an atrial septal defect or patent foramen ovale.[408,412] Inhalation of NO reduced right-to-left shunting by 56% in a series of three patients with right ventricular MI.[408] Right-to-left shunting in patients with right ventricular MI also can be treated by percutaneous closure of the patent foramen ovale.[412]

Some evidence indicates that reperfusion of the IRA improves right ventricular function and clinical outcome in patients with MI. Successful PCI of an occluded RCA in patients with right ventricular infarction has been associated with improved right ventricular wall motion within 1 hour[413] and a reduction in right atrial pressure within 8 hours.[414] Three to 5 days after successful PCI, right ventricular function was normal in 95% of patients.[413] In a study of the data for 49 patients with shock and right ventricular MI who were enrolled in the SHOCK trial registry, the in-hospital mortality rate was found to be 65.2% among patients who did not undergo revascularization, compared with 42.3% among patients who underwent PCI or CABG surgery.[400]

Mechanical Causes of Congestive Heart Failure or Low Cardiac Output

Mitral Regurgitation

Among 1976 patients with acute MI who were not in cardiogenic shock and underwent cardiac catheterization within 12 hours of symptom onset, left ventriculography demonstrated mild mitral regurgitation in 192 patients (9.7%) and moderate or severe mitral regurgitation in 58 patients (2.9%).[98] By multivariate analysis, mild mitral regurgitation and moderate or severe mitral regurgitation were the two strongest independent predictors of 1-year mortality. The hazard ratios were 2.40 (95% CI 1.31 to 4.42; P=.005) for mild and 2.82 (95% CI 1.34 to 5.92; P=.006) for moderate or severe mitral regurgitation. The 1-year mortality rates were 2.9% for patients with no mitral regurgitation (n=1726), 8.5% for patients with mild mitral regurgitation (n=192), and 20.8% for patients with moderate or severe mitral regurgitation (n=58).

Acute severe mitral regurgitation accounted for 6.9% of patients with cardiogenic shock among 1422 patients with acute MI who were enrolled in either the SHOCK registry or the randomized trial.[351] The median time from the onset of MI to shock was 12.8 hours.[415] In a postmortem series of 20 cases of papillary muscle rupture, the posteromedial papillary muscle was ruptured in 16 patients and the anterolateral papillary muscle was ruptured in four patients.[416] The greater tendency of the posteromedial papillary muscle to rupture is reflected by the distribution of the IRA in a series of 98 patients with acute mitral regurgitation and cardiogenic shock who were enrolled in the SHOCK studies. The location of the index MI was anterior in 34% of patients and nonanterior in 66%.[415]

The diagnosis of acute severe mitral regurgitation should be suspected in patients with acute onset of pulmonary edema or hypotension. The absence of a loud murmur does not exclude severe mitral regurgitation. The diagnosis can be confirmed by transthoracic or transesophageal echocardiography. The treatment of acute severe mitral regurgitation should include inotropic support, afterload reduction, an IABP, and emergency mitral valve surgery, but mortality is high despite surgical treatment. Among the patients with acute severe mitral regurgitation and cardiogenic shock who were enrolled in the SHOCK registry or the randomized trial, the in-hospital mortality rate was 40% among 43 patients who underwent valve surgery, compared with 71% among 51 patients who did not.[415]

Ventricular Septal Rupture

Among 41,021 patients with STEMI who were enrolled in the GUSTO-I trial, the incidence of ventricular septal rupture was only 0.2% (84/41,021 patients).[417] Acute ventricular septal rupture accounted for 3.9% of patients with cardiogenic shock among 1422 patients with acute MI who were enrolled in either the SHOCK registry or randomized trial.[351]

The clinical manifestations of ventricular septal rupture may include chest pain, dypsnea, and hypotension. A harsh holosystolic murmur may be audible. Cardiogenic shock occurred in 67% of patients in the GUSTO-I trial in whom ventricular septal rupture developed.[417] The diagnosis of ventricular septal rupture can be confirmed by Doppler echocardiography and/or right heart catheterization to measure the oxygen saturation in the right atrium, right ventricle, and pulmonary artery. The median time from MI to diagnosis of ventricular septal rupture was 16 hours among a series of patients with ventricular septal rupture and cardiogenic shock.[418] The electrocardiographic location of the MI was inferior in 26 patients, anterior in 22, both anterior and inferior in 3, and apicolateral in 1 patient.[418] Only 35 of 55 patients underwent coronary angiography, and the IRA was identified in only 26 patients: the RCA in 12, the LAD in 11, and the left circumflex coronary artery in 3 cases.

The location of the IRA may be an important determinant of survival in patients with ventricular septal rupture.[417,419] Among a series of 25 patients with this diagnosis, mortality was greater among patients with inferior MI than among patients with anterior MI.[419] At least two factors may explain the differential outcome of patients with inferior and anterior MI complicated by ventricular septal rupture. First, the right ventricular volume overload caused by the left-to-right shunt may be less tolerated in the presence of ischemia or infarction of the right ventricle, both of which are more common with an inferior MI than an anterior MI. Second, histopathologic studies have shown that complex septal defects that are more difficult to repair surgically are more common in patients with an inferior MI.[420]

An IABP has been shown to decrease the shunt and increase systemic cardiac output in patients with ventricular septal rupture.[421] Therefore, vasodilator therapy and an IABP often are used to stabilize patients before surgical repair of the rupture. The overall in-hospital survival rate among patients with ventricular septal rupture in the SHOCK registry was only 13% (7/55).[418] Although six of the seven survivors underwent surgical repair, mortality was 81% (25/31) in the group of patients who underwent surgery. In the GUSTO-I trial, patients whose rupture was repaired surgically had better 30-day mortality (47%) than patients who received medical treatment (94%).[417] Percutaneous closure of acute ventricular septal rupture may be an option in the future.

Left Ventricular Free Wall Rupture

Rupture of the left ventricular free wall may manifest in any of several ways: pericardial tamponade with acute hemodynamic collapse and immediate death, gradual onset of tamponade and hypotension, or subacute formation of a pseudoaneurysm.[422] Although a 6% rate of cardiac rupture among patients with acute MI often is quoted, recent reports suggest that the rate probably is lower, at least among patients who receive reperfusion therapy. A total of 65 (1.7%) cases of cardiac rupture occurred among 3759 patients with STEMI who received fibrinolytic therapy and were randomized to receive either adjunctive heparin or hirudin.[423] The prevalence of cardiac rupture or pericardial tamponade was 2.3% (28/1190) among patients with cardiogenic shock in the SHOCK registry; 13 patients had both rupture and pericardial tamponade, 9 had tamponade alone, and 6 had rupture alone.[424]

It has been suggested that the incidence of cardiac rupture may be lower after primary PCI than after fibrinolytic therapy. The overall incidence of left ventricular free wall rupture was 2.5% (n=34) among 1375 patients with STEMI who underwent primary PCI (55.4%) or fibrinolytic therapy (44.6%).[425] In a multivariate analysis, primary PCI was independently associated with a lower incidence of rupture, but no significant difference was observed in the incidence of rupture after primary PCI or fibrinolytic therapy (1.8% versus 3.3%; $P=0.686$).

The timing of reperfusion therapy may affect both the risk and the timing of free wall rupture. Death from cardiac rupture appears to occur earlier in patients given fibrinolytic therapy than among patients who do not undergo reperfusion therapy.[426] Honan and associates[427] analyzed the relationship between the risk of cardiac rupture and the timing of fibrinolytic therapy for 58 cases of cardiac rupture among 1638 patients who were enrolled in four randomized trials that compared intravenous streptokinase with no fibrinolytic therapy (in the control group). The odds ratio of cardiac rupture increased significantly with increasing delay in the time to treatment. Regression analysis suggested that treatment within 7 hours after symptom onset reduces the risk of cardiac rupture, whereas treatment later than 17 hours after symptom onset increases the risk of cardiac rupture.[427] Thus, it was hypothesized that early fibrinolytic therapy reduces the risk of rupture by reducing the extent of myocardial necrosis, while late fibrinolytic therapy increases the risk of rupture by promoting hemorrhagic infarction.

The antemortem diagnosis of free wall rupture, pericardial tamponade, and left ventricular pseudoaneurysm usually is confirmed by an echocardiogram. An echocardiogram was obtained in 20 of the 28 patients in the SHOCK registry who had rupture or pericardial tamponade. A pericardial effusion was observed in 15 (75%) and a myocardial tear was detected in 39%.[424] Six patients underwent pericardiocentesis alone, and 21 had surgical repair of the rupture. The in-hospital survival rate was 39.3%.

Cardiac Arrhythmias and Heart Block

Both atrial and ventricular arrhythmias are common in patients with acute MI. The incidence of atrial fibrillation was 10.4% among 40,891 patients who were enrolled in the GUSTO-I trial.[316] Among patients enrolled in the TRACE study, which enrolled patients with an acute MI and a left ventricular EF less than 35%, atrial fibrillation occurred in 21% of patients and was associated with a 50% increase in the adjusted mortality.[317] Management of atrial arrhythmias is discussed in another chapter.

The likelihood of primary ventricular fibrillation (occurring within 48 hours of acute MI and in the absence of cardiogenic shock or severe CHF) is not altered by fibrinolytic therapy, with an incidence of ventricular fibrillation during the first hospital day of 2.99% for both the fibrinolytic and placebo groups.[320] Some evidence, however, suggests that fibrinolytic therapy exerts a protective effect against secondary ventricular fibrillation (occurring in patients with acute MI complicated by CHF or shock).[320,321] Management of ventricular arrhythmias is discussed in Chapter 32.

The incidence of second-degree or third-degree AV block was 6.9% among 75,993 patients with STEMI who received fibrinolytic therapy and were enrolled in a database that combined four randomized clinical trials.[428] Inferior MI was the strongest independent predictor of AV block (odds ratio 3.3; 95% CI 3.1 to 3.5). In comparison with patients without AV block, adjusted mortality was greater at 30 days, 6 months, and 1 year among patients with AV block. The adjusted mortality odds ratios at 1 year were 2.4 (95% CI 2.2 to 2.6) for patients with AV block and inferior MI and 3.3 (95% CI 3.0 to 3.7) for patients with AV block and anterior MI.

UNSTABLE ANGINA AND NON–ST SEGMENT ELEVATION MYOCARDIAL INFARCTION

Clinical Manifestations

Definition

The ACC/AHA Practice Guidelines define *unstable angina* as "an acute process of myocardial ischemia that is not of sufficient severity and duration to result in myocardial necrosis."[4] *NSTEMI* is defined as "an acute process of myocardial ischemia with sufficient severity and duration to result in myocardial necrosis."[4] Thus, NSTEMI is distinguished from unstable angina by the detection of cardiac markers indicative of myocardial necrosis, such as troponin I or T, in patients with NSTEMI.

Clinical History

Criteria for the diagnosis of unstable angina are based on the Canadian Cardiovascular Society (CCS) grading system[429] (Table 31-3). The three principal presentations of unstable angina are angina that occurs at rest, new-onset CCS class III or IV angina, and angina that has increased from class I or II to class III or IV.[430]

Table 31-3. Grading of Angina Pectoris According to Canadian Cardiovascular Society Classification

Class	Description of Stage
I	"Ordinary physical activity does not cause . . . angina," such as walking or climbing stairs. Angina occurs with strenuous, rapid or prolonged exertion at work or recreation.
II	"Slight limitation of ordinary activity." Angina occurs on walking or climbing stairs rapidly; walking uphill; walking or stair climbing after meals; in cold, in wind, or under emotional stress; or only during the few hours after awakening. Angina occurs on walking more than 2 blocks on the level and climbing more than 1 flight of ordinary stairs at a normal pace and under normal conditions.
III	"Marked limitations of ordinary physical activity." Angina occurs on walking 1 to 2 blocks on the level and climbing 1 flight of stairs under normal conditions and at a normal pace.
IV	"Inability to carry on any physical activity without discomfort—anginal symptoms may be present at rest."

Modified from Campeau L: Grading of angina pectoris. Circulation 1976;54:522-523 (Letter).

The GRACE registry analyzed the presenting symptoms of 20,881 patients with STEMI, NSTEMI, or unstable angina.[67] Among the patients with unstable angina and NSTEMI, 5.7% and 12.3%, respectively, presented with symptoms other than chest pain. Patients with unstable angina or NSTEMI who presented with atypical symptoms were less likely to undergo coronary angiography, PCI, or CABG surgery and were less likely to receive heparin, aspirin, or β-blockers. The absence of chest pain among patients with ACS was predictive of an increased risk of in-hospital death.

The risk of death and ischemic events in patients with unstable angina can be predicted by seven variables that are used to calculate a TIMI risk score. Four of the seven variables are derived from the clinical history: age 65 years or older, at least three risk factors for CAD (family history of CAD, hypertension, hypercholesterolemia, diabetes, cigarette smoking), two or more anginal events within the previous 24 hours, and use of aspirin within the previous 7 days.[431]

Physical Examination

As in patients with STEMI, evidence of heart failure at the time of initial presentation has prognostic importance in patients with non–ST elevation ACS. In a database accrued from studies in 26,090 patients with unstable angina or NSTEMI, heart rate, systolic blood pressure, and Killip class were independent predictors of mortality at 30 days and 6 months.[432] Patients in Killip class II, III, or IV constituted only 11% of the population but accounted for 30% of the deaths.

Diagnostic Approach

Electrocardiogram

The admission ECG has prognostic value in patients with ACS.[433,434] Although normal or nonspecific findings on the initial ECG confer a better prognosis than ST segment depression or elevation seen on the ECG, such findings are not predictive of a benign outcome in patients with suspected ACS.[434] The risk of death or reinfarction at 30 days or 6 months is similar in patients with ST segment elevation and in those with ST segment depression; the risk is lower among patients with isolated T wave inversion.[433] The GUSTO-IIb clinical trial enrolled 12,142 patients with symptoms of cardiac ischemia at rest and electrocardiographic signs of myocardial ischemia.[433] After adjustment for factors associated with an increased risk of death or reinfarction, the odds of death or reinfarction at 30 days were 1.68 (95% CI 1.36 to 2.08) in those with ST segment elevation and 1.62 (95% CI 1.32 to 1.98) in those with ST segment depression compared with those who had T wave inversion only on the admission ECG.[433]

The impact of invasive management on outcome in patients with ACS is predicted by the presence or absence of ST segment depression on the admission ECG. Among patients with ACS who were enrolled in the Fast Revascularization during InStability in Coronary Artery Disease (FRISC II) randomized trial comparing early invasive management and a noninvasive strategy, ST segment depression was present at enrollment in 45.5% of patients.[435] Among the patients who presented with ST segment depression, the invasive strategy reduced the risk of death or MI at 12 months from 18.2% to 12.0% (RR 0.66; 95% CI 0.50 to 0.88; $P=.004$). Mortality was reduced from 5.8% to 3.3% (RR 0.58; 95% CI 0.33 to 1.01; $P=.050$). Among the patients without ST segment depression, the corresponding rates of death or MI were 10.4% and 8.9% ($P=0.36$), and the mortality rates were 2.0% and 1.2% ($P=0.26$). A similar dichotomy was found in the Treat Angina with Aggrastat and Determine Cost of Therapy with an Invasive or Conservative Strategy (TACTICS)–TIMI 18 randomized trial of early invasive versus conservative strategies in patients with ACS.[436] Thus, according to the ACA/AHA Practice Guidelines for the management of patients with unstable angina and NSTEMI, new or presumably new ST segment depression is a Class I indication for use of an invasive strategy.[4]

The magnitude[437,438] and the location[439] of ST segment depression also provide independent prognostic information in patients with unstable angina and NSTEMI. Among 1846 patients who were enrolled in the TACTICS—TIMI 18 trial, the magnitude of ST segment depression was a predictor of unsuccessful medical therapy in patients who were randomized to the conservative strategy.[438] The magnitude of ST segment depression was an independent predictor of the extent of CAD among patients who were randomized to the early invasive strategy. After adjustment for baseline characteristics and the degree of troponin elevation, the benefit of an early invasive strategy was greater among patients with ST segment depression of 0.10 mV or greater, compared with patients with 0.05 to 0.09 mV of ST segment depression.

Among a cohort of 432 patients with a first NSTEMI, patients with ST segment depression in two or more lateral leads (I, aVL, V_5, or V_6) had lower left ventricular EFs, more frequent left main coronary artery or three-vessel CAD, and greater in-hospital mortality.[439] Although isolated T wave inversion on the admission ECG is associated with a better prognosis than ST segment depression or elevation, negative T waves in leads V_2 and V_3 are associated with critical stenosis of the proximal LAD and stunning of the myocardium supplied by the LAD.[440,441]

Biochemical Markers

Biochemical markers such as troponin or CK-MB provide both diagnostic and prognostic information. As discussed, the distinction between NSTEMI and unstable angina is based on the blood assays for biochemical markers of myocardial necrosis. Among 1404 patients with unstable angina or NSTEMI who were enrolled in the TIMI IIIB trial, the mortality rate at 42 days was 3.7% (21/573) for patients with a baseline troponin I 0.4 ng per mL or greater, compared with 1.0% (8/831) for patients with a troponin I less than 0.4 ng per ml ($P<.001$).[442] There were significant increases in mortality with increasing levels of troponin I. An elevated troponin in patients with suspected ACS confers a greater risk of death or reinfarction even among patients without significant angiographic

CAD.[443] Patients with ACS who have an elevated troponin, even if the elevation is minor, derive greater benefit from platelet GP IIb/IIIa inhibitors[444,445] or invasive management[446] than do patients without an elevated troponin.

Another biochemical marker that provides prognostic information is brain natriuretic peptide (BNP). An elevated BNP at the time of presentation or after hospital discharge in patients with ACS is an independent predictor of death or new-onset CHF during follow-up.[447,448]

Approach to Management

Figure 31-15 presents an algorithm for the treatment of unstable angina and non–ST segment elevation myocardial infarction. Specific components of management are discussed next.

Anti-ischemic Therapy

Nitrates

The Class I recommendations for anti-ischemic therapy in patients with unstable angina or NSTEMI include nitroglycerin administered initially as a sublingual tablet or spray, followed by intravenous infusion. Although nitroglycerin often relieves chest pain in patients with ACS, nitrates have not been shown to reduce clinical events in patients with unstable angina or NSTEMI. Abrupt cessation of intravenous nitroglycerin may be associated with rebound myocardial ischemia in patients with ACS.[449] After intravenous infusion of nitroglycerin for longer than 24 hours the development of tolerance may require an increase in the dose to maintain efficacy, but 200 μg/min usually is considered the maximum dose.

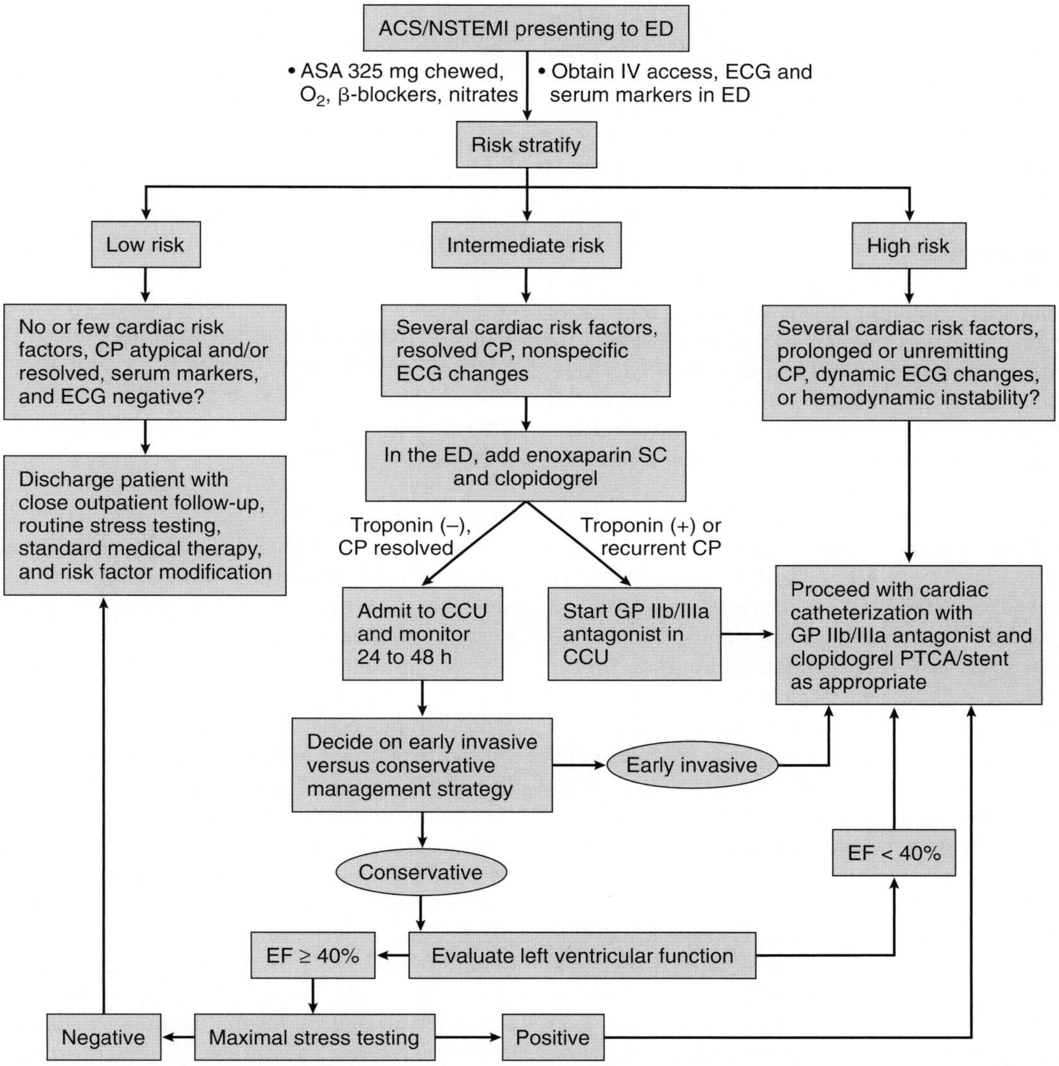

Figure 31-15. Algorithm for the treatment of unstable angina or non–ST segment elevation myocardial infarction. *Note:* Enoxaparin is not recommended for use in patients with known bleeding disorders or significant renal insufficiency (serum creatinine of 2 to 2.5 mg/dL or greater). ACS, acute coronary syndrome; ASA, acetylsalicylic acid (aspirin); CCU, critical care unit; CP, chest pain; ECG, electrocardiogram; ED, emergency department; EF, ejection fraction; IV, intravenous; NSTEMI, non–ST segment elevation myocardial infarction; PTCA, percutaneous transluminal coronary angioplasty; SC, subcutaneous. (From Antman EM, Anbe DT, Armstrong PW, et al: ACC/AHA guidelines for the management of patients with ST-elevation myocardial infarction: A report of the American College of Cardiology/American Heart Association Task Force on Practice Guidelines [Committee to Revise the 1999 Guidelines for the Management of Patients with Acute Myocardial Infarction]. Circulation 2004;110:e82-e292.)

β-Blockers

The Class I recommendations for anti-ischemic therapy in patients with unstable angina or NSTEMI include administration of a β-blocker, beginning with an intravenous dose if there is ongoing chest pain, followed by oral administration. Nevertheless, many patients who are eligible for β-blocker therapy do not receive it, possibly because there are limited data regarding the efficacy of β-blockers in patients with unstable angina or NSTEMI.[450] Clinical trials that evaluated β-blockers in patients with unstable angina were not adequately powered to demonstrate reductions in mortality. A pooled analysis of randomized trials in patients with threatened or evolving MI concluded that β-blockers reduce the risk of MI by 13%.[451] A report from the GRACE registry analyzed the outcomes of 7106 patients with NSTEMI.[450] β-Blocker therapy was initiated within 24 hours of admission in 76% of patients without contraindications. After multivariable logistic regression analysis to adjust for presence of comorbidity, both in-hospital mortality (odds ratio 0.58; 95% CI 0.42 to 0.81) and 6-month mortality (odds ratio 0.75; 95% CI 0.56 to 0.997) were lower among patients who received β-blockers than among patients who did not.

Calcium Antagonists

The Holland Interuniversity Nifedipine/Metoprolol Trial (HINT) found that nifedipine alone increased the risk of MI or recurrent angina, relative to placebo, by 24% in patients with unstable angina.[452] Therefore, the ACC/AHA Practice Guidelines for unstable angina and NSTEMI include a Class III recommendation for immediate-release dihydropyridine calcium antagonists in the absence of a β-blocker.

The Multicenter Diltiazem Postinfarction Trial (MDPIT) randomized 2466 patients to receive diltiazem or placebo 3 to 15 days after acute MI.[335] Approximately 70% of patients met ECG criteria for a Q wave MI and 25% had non–Q wave MI. The percentage of patients with STEMI or NSTEMI was not reported. Total mortality rates for the two treatment groups were nearly identical, but treatment with diltiazem was associated with increased mortality in patients with either radiographic evidence of pulmonary congestion or a left ventricular EF less than 40%. Also, diltiazem was associated with an increased risk of late-onset CHF in patients with a left ventricular EF less than 40%.[336]

Gibson and colleagues[453] performed a post hoc subset analysis of the 817 patients with non–Q wave MI and no pulmonary congestion who were enrolled in two clinical trials: MDPIT and the second Danish Verapamil Infarction Trial (DAVIT-II).[453] The adjusted all-cause mortality was lower among patients who were given diltiazem or verapamil than among those who received placebo (RR 0.65; 95% CI 0.40 to 1.05). Nevertheless, calcium antagonists are not considered first-line therapeutic agents in patients with ACS and are reserved for patients with recurrent ischemia, but no severe left ventricular dysfunction, who have a contraindication to β-blockers.

Intra-aortic Balloon Counterpulsation

Intra-aortic balloon counterpulsation is believed to increase myocardial oxygen supply by increasing diastolic pressure, and to reduce myocardial oxygen demand by afterload reduction of the left ventricle. The indications for an IABP in patients with ACS include refractory ischemia, hypotension, and cardiogenic shock, although this modality should be considered an adjunct to definitive therapies such as percutaneous or surgical myocardial revascularization.

Antiplatelet Therapy

Aspirin

Unstable angina and NSTEMI are Class I indications for aspirin, which should be started as soon as possible and continued indefinitely. The recommendation is based on the results of four small randomized trials. A pooled analysis of the results concluded that aspirin reduces the risk of death or MI by 50% in patients with unstable angina. The optimal dose of aspirin in patients with ACS is uncertain.[454] An aspirin dose of 75 mg/day reduced the risk of MI or death after 1 year in patients with unstable angina or non–Q wave MI who were enrolled in a prospective, randomized, double-blind, placebo-controlled multicenter trial (RR 0.52; 95% CI 0.37 to 0.72).[455] Among 20,521 patients with ACS who were enrolled in the GUSTO IIb and Platelet Glycoprotein IIb/IIIa in Unstable Angina: Receptor Suppression Using Integrilin Therapy (PURSUIT) trials, an aspirin dose 150 mg or greater was associated with a lower risk of MI at 6 months, compared with an aspirin dose less than 150 mg (hazard ratio 0.79; 95% CI 0.64 to 0.98; *P*=.03).[456]

Thienopyridines

Thienopyridines, such as ticlopidine, clopidogrel, and prasugrel, inhibit adenosine diphosphate-induced platelet activation. An open study that randomized patients with unstable angina to ticlopidine or conventional therapy (excluding aspirin) demonstrated a 46% reduction in the risk of vascular death and nonfatal MI.[457] Clopidogrel has a more rapid onset of action and a better safety profile than ticlopidine. The Clopidogrel in Unstable Angina to Prevent Recurrent Events (CURE) trial demonstrated that the combination of clopidogrel and aspirin, compared with aspirin alone, improved outcomes among patients with ACS without ST segment elevation.[458] The ACC/AHA Practice Guidelines recommend that patients with unstable angina or NSTEMI should receive clopidogrel plus aspirin for at least 1 month and for up to 9 months. Also, patients who are unable to take aspirin because of hypersensitivity or gastrointestinal intolerance should be treated with clopidogrel. The optimal loading dose of clopidogrel has not been established.

Clopidogrel should be discontinued at least 5 days before CABG surgery because it is associated with increased perioperative bleeding. Therefore, some practitioners prefer to withhold clopidogrel until the results of diagnostic cardiac catheterization are known. This practice, however, ignores the proven benefit of clopidogrel pretreatment in patients with ACS who undergo PCI[459] or CABG.[460] Also, CABG surgery can usually be deferred for 5 days, and percutaneous revascularization is more frequent than surgical revascularization in patients with ACS.[460] The CURE investigators concluded that the increased bleeding risk in patients who may require CABG surgery is outweighed by the overall reduction in ischemic events among all patients.[460] Thus, a policy of withholding clopidogrel until after coronary angiography may harm more patients than a policy of starting clopidogrel on admission to the hospital.

Platelet Glycoprotein IIb/IIIa Receptor Antagonists

Discontinuation of either UFH or LMWH in patients with unstable angina is associated with a rebound increase in thrombin generation,[461] which may underlie the increase in death and MI that has been observed during the 12 hours after heparin is stopped in patients with ACS.[462,463] Compared with patients who were randomized to a placebo group, patients who were randomized to treatment with a GP IIb/IIIa antagonist, eptifibatide, experienced significantly fewer deaths and MIs during the 12 hours after heparin was terminated.[463]

A retrospective analysis of the PURSUIT trial found that treatment with eptifibatide was associated with improved outcome among patients in whom cardiogenic shock developed during hospitalization for ACS without persistent ST segment elevation.[464] Although randomization to eptifibatide treatment did not affect the occurrence of shock, patients with shock who received eptifibatide had significantly reduced adjusted odds of death at 30 days (odds ratio 0.51; 95% CI 0.28 to 0.94; P=.03). It is unlikely that improved outcome after PCI was responsible for the beneficial effect of eptifibatide because only 25% of the patients with shock in PURSUIT underwent PCI.

Boersma and colleagues[465] performed a meta-analysis of the individual patient data from six trials that randomized 31,402 patients with ACS without persistent ST segment elevation to a GP IIb/IIIa inhibitor treatment group (abciximab, eptifibatide, lamifiban, or tirofiban) or to a control group. Overall, there was a 9% reduction in the odds of death or MI at 30 days (10.8% versus 11.8%; odds ratio 0.91; 95% CI 0.84 to 0.98; P=.015).[465] The baseline troponin value was available in a subset of 11,059 patients (35% of the entire cohort). Among the 45% of patients with a troponin T or I level 0.1 ng/mL or greater there was a 15% reduction in the odds of death or MI at 30 days compared with that for the control group (10.3% versus 12.0%; odds ratio 0.85; 95% CI 0.71 to 1.03). No risk reduction was observed among patients with negative troponins (GP IIb/IIIa inhibitor 7.0% versus control 6.2%; odds ratio 1.17; 95% CI 0.94 to 1.44). Another meta-analysis of the same six trials found that the impact of GP IIb/IIIa antagonists on outcome varied with the revascularization strategy.[466] The reduction of ischemic events was greater among patients who underwent PCI during the index hospitalization (odds ratio 0.82; P=.01) than among patients who were managed medically (odds ratio 0.95; P=0.27).[466] The corresponding number of events prevented per 1000 patients treated was 20 for patients who underwent PCI compared with 4 for patients treated medically.

According to the ACC/AHA Practice Guidelines, patients with unstable angina or NSTEMI in whom cardiac catheterization and PCI are planned should receive one of the three FDA-approved platelet GP IIb/IIIa antagonists, abciximab, eptifibatide, and tirofiban. Patients in whom PCI is not planned should receive eptifibatide or tirofiban, but not abciximab because the GUSTO IV ACS trial failed to show a benefit of abciximab among patients with ACS who did not undergo early coronary revascularization.[467]

GP IIb/IIIa antagonists increase the risk of bleeding, frequently involving the access site used for cardiac catheterization, but the risk of intracranial hemorrhage is not increased.[465] The meta-analysis discussed earlier found that the risk of major bleeding was 2.4% among patients who were randomized to a GP IIb/IIIa antagonist compared with 1.4% among control patients (odds ratio 1.62; 95% CI 1.36 to 1.94; P<.0001).[465] One preventable cause of bleeding is excess dosing of a GP IIb/IIIa antagonist, which occurred in 26.8% of patients with non–ST segment elevation ACS who were enrolled in the CRUSADE registry by 387 hospitals in 2004.[468]

A complete blood count including platelet count should be included in monitoring during administration of GP IIb/IIIa antagonists. A review of eight large placebo-controlled randomized trials, however, concluded that abciximab, but not eptifibatide or tirofiban, increases the incidence of thrombocytopenia.[469]

Antithrombin Therapy

Unfractionated Heparin

At least seven randomized, placebo-controlled trials have compared UFH plus aspirin with aspirin alone in patients with unstable angina, but none of them was adequately powered to detect a reduction in the rate of death or MI during hospitalization. A meta-analysis of six of the trials concluded that the addition of UFH to aspirin reduced the risk of death or MI during treatment by 33% (RR 0.67; 95% CI 0.44 to 1.02; P=.06).[470] Therefore, the ACC/AHA Practice Guidelines include intravenous UFH in the list of Class I recommendations for patients with unstable angina or NSTEMI.[4] The guidelines also recommend daily measurement of hemoglobin or hematocrit and platelet count during treatment with UFH because of the increased risks of bleeding and thrombocytopenia. An analysis of patients who were enrolled in the CRUSADE registry in 2004 found that bleeding was related to excess dosing of UFH, which occurred in 32.8% of patients who received UFH.[468]

As discussed earlier, a rebound increase in thrombin generation with reactivation of unstable angina has been observed after discontinuation of UFH. One clinical trial observed an eight-fold increase in death and a two-fold increase in MI during the 12 hours after heparin was discontinued.[463] The rate of events during the 12 hours after heparin was terminated was significantly lower among patients who were randomized to treatment with eptifibatide than among patients in the placebo group.[463]

Low-Molecular-Weight Heparin

The FRISC study randomized 1506 patients with unstable angina or non–Q wave MI to receive placebo or dalteparin, an LMWH, twice daily for 6 days, followed by once daily for 35 to 45 days.[471] A 63% reduction in the risk of death or MI occurred during the first 6 days (4.8% versus 1.8%; *P*=.001). Subsequently, 21,946 patients with non–ST segment elevation ACS have been enrolled in six randomized trials that compared enoxaparin, another LMWH, with UFH. A meta-analysis of the trials found no significant difference in death at 30 days for enoxaparin versus UFH (3.0% versus 3.0%; odds ratio 1.00; 95% CI 0.85 to 1.17).[472] A statistically significant reduction was observed in the combined end points of death and nonfatal MI at 30 days for enoxaparin versus UFH (10.1% versus 11.0%; odds ratio 0.91; 95% CI 0.83 to 0.99).

Although it had been hypothesized that the risk of bleeding would be less during treatment with LMWH than with UFH, the meta-analysis performed by Petersen and colleagues[472] found no significant difference between enoxaparin and UFH in the rates of blood transfusion or major bleeding at 7 days after initiation of the study treatment. The risk of bleeding during treatment with LWMH may be increased by excess dosing, which occurred in 13.8% of patients who were enrolled in the CRUSADE registry in 2004 and received LMWH.[468]

The most recent ACC/AHA Practice Guidelines, which were written before publication of the meta-analysis just discussed, include a Class IIa recommendation that enoxaparin is preferable to UFH as an anticoagulant in patients with unstable angina or NSTEMI unless CABG surgery is planned within 24 hours.[4] The Guidelines recommend that LMWH be discontinued and UFH used in patients who are going to undergo CABG surgery.

Direct Thrombin Inhibitors

Direct thrombin inhibitors, such as hirudin and bivalirudin, have been evaluated in patients with ACS. The Acute Catheterization and Urgent Intervention Triage Strategy (ACUITY) trial was an open-label, randomized, multicenter trial that compared heparin plus a GP IIb/IIIa antagonist, bivalirudin plus a GP IIb/IIIa antagonist, and bivalirudin alone in patients with moderate-risk or high-risk non–ST segment elevation ACS who were undergoing an early invasive strategy.[473] NSTEMI was present in 59% of patients, and 41% had unstable angina. Compared with patients who received a GP IIb/IIIa antagonist plus UFH or enoxaparin, patients who received bivalirudin alone experienced significantly less non–CABG-related major bleeding (3.0% versus 5.7%; RR 0.53; 95% CI 0.43 to 0.65). Compared with heparin plus a GP IIb/IIIa antagonist, bivalirudin alone resulted in a noninferior rate of the composite ischemia end point (7.3% versus 7.8% respectively; RR 1.08; 95% CI 0.93 to 1.24; *P*=.32). Administration of bivalirudin plus a GP IIb/IIIa antagonist, as compared with heparin plus a GP IIb/IIIa antagonist, resulted in noninferior 30-day rates of the composite ischemia end point (7.7% versus 7.3% respectively; RR 1.07; 95% CI 0.92 to 1.23; *P*=.39) and major bleeding (5.3% versus 5.7% respectively; RR 0.93; 95% CI 0.78 to 1.10; *P*=.38).

Angiotensin-Converting Enzyme Inhibitors

Little information is available regarding the administration of ACE inhibitors to patients with NSTEMI because most of the ACE inhibitor trials did not report subgroup analyses of patients with STEMI or NSTEMI. The Survival of Myocardial Infarction Long-Term Evaluation (SMILE) study enrolled 1556 patients with acute anterior MI who were not eligible for fibrinolytic therapy.[474] The patients were randomized to receive 6-week courses of placebo or zofenopril, an ACE inhibitor. Among the 526 patients with ECG criteria for NSTEMI, death or severe CHF occurred in 10.3% (28/273) of placebo patients and 3.6% (9/253) of zofenopril patients (RR reduction 65%; 95% CI 20% to 80%; *P*=.003).[475] The 1-year mortality rate also was significantly reduced by zofenopril (7.9% versus 15.8%; RR reduction 43%; 95% CI 14% to 57%; *P*=.036).

Lipid-Lowering Therapy

As discussed earlier, the 4S,[337] CARE,[338] and LIPID[339] trials have established the long-term benefits of starting statin therapy 3 months or later after hospitalization for an MI or unstable angina. Analysis of the LIPID trial showed that initiation of pravastatin 40 mg daily 3 to 36 months after hospitalization for unstable angina significantly reduced the risk of several end points, including death (RR 0.74; 95% CI 0.50 to 0.91; *P*=.004) and nonfatal MI (RR 0.67; 95% CI 0.51 to 0.88; *P*=.004).[476]

Data are conflicting regarding the benefit of early initiation of lipid-lowering therapy in patients with ACS. A retrospective analysis of the outcomes in 1616 patients with ACS concluded that statin pretreatment is associated with improved clinical outcome while discontinuation of statins after symptom onset is associated with an increased risk of death and nonfatal MI within 30 days.[477] An observational study that combined data from the GUSTO IIb and PURSUIT trials concluded that prescription of a lipid-lowering drug at hospital discharge was independently associated with a reduced risk of death at 6 months (hazard ratio 0.67; 95% CI 0.48 to 0.95; *P*=.023).[478] Another study of 12,365 patients with ACS concluded that there was no impact of early initiation of statin therapy on death, MI, or severe recurrent ischemia at 90 days.[479]

Numerous randomized trials have investigated the effects of statins on outcomes in patients with ACS. Compared with placebo, treatment with atorvastatin 80 mg daily beginning 24 to 96 hours after hospital admission reduced the rate of recurrent ischemic events at 16 weeks.[480] The Pravastatin or Atorvastatin Evaluation and Infection Therapy–Thrombolysis in Myocardial Infarction 22 (PROVE IT–TIMI 22) study compared atorvastatin

80 mg daily with pravastatin 40 mg daily started within 10 days of hospitalization for an ACS.[341] The primary end point was a composite of death, MI, unstable angina, revascularization, and stroke. The rates for the primary end point at 2 years were 22.4% in the atorvastatin group and 26.3% in the pravastatin group, representing a 16% reduction in the hazard ratio in favor of atorvastatin (95% CI 5% to 26%; P=.005).

At least two meta-analyses of relevant randomized controlled trials have been performed to estimate the effects of early treatment with statins on short-term outcomes in patients with ACS.[363,364] One analysis of 12 randomized trials concluded that statin therapy initiated within 14 days of hospital admission does not reduce the risk of death, MI, or stroke during the first 4 months after ACS.[363] Another meta-analysis of 13 randomized trials concluded that early statin therapy reduces the rates of death and cardiovascular events after 4 months of treatment.[364]

Invasive versus Conservative Management

At least eight randomized trials have compared early invasive and early conservative management strategies for patients with ACS. Patients who are managed by an early conservative strategy undergo coronary angiography if evidence points to spontaneous recurrent ischemia or if results of stress testing are strongly positive despite medical therapy. Patients who are managed using an early invasive strategy undergo routine coronary angiography and coronary revascularization as indicated. Three relatively large trials demonstrated better short-term and long-term outcomes among patients randomized to the early invasive strategy compared with the early conservative strategy: FRISC II,[481-483] TACTICS–TIMI 18,[436] and the Randomized Intervention Trial of Unstable Angina-3 (RITA-3).[484,485] The FRISC II[481-483] and TACTICS–TIMI 18 trials randomized 2457 and 2220 patients, respectively, with unstable angina or NSTEMI to either an early conservative or an early invasive strategy. Both trials found that the early invasive strategy was associated with a lower risk of death or MI at 6 months compared with the early conservative strategy: 9.4% versus 12.1% (RR 0.78; 95% CI 0.62 to 0.98; P=.031) for FRISC II and 7.3% versus 9.5% (odds ratio 0.74; 95% CI 0.54 to 1.00; P<.05) for TIMI 18. The early invasive strategy also was associated with a reduced rate of rehospitalization for ACS in both trials. After follow-up for 2 years in the FRISC II trial, patients who were randomized to the early invasive arm experienced lower rates of MI (9.2% versus 12.7%; RR 0.72; 95% CI 0.57 to 0.91; P=.005) and overall mortality (3.7% versus 5.4%; RR 0.68; 95% CI 0.47 to 0.98; P=.038).[483] The RITA-3 study randomized 1810 patients with non–ST elevation acute coronary syndromes to early invasive or early conservative treatment.[484,485] After a median follow-up period of 5 years, 142 (16.6%) patients randomized to the early intervention group and 178 (20.0%) patients assigned to the early conservative group died or had a nonfatal MI (odds ratio 0.78; 95% CI 0.61 to 0.99; P=.044). The death rates were 12% for the interventional group versus 15% for the conservative group (odds ratio 0.76; 95% CI 0.58 to 1.00; P=.054).

The early invasive strategy confers the greatest benefit in patients who are characterized by high-risk indicators such as ST segment depression[435,436] or elevated troponin.[446] Therefore, according to the ACC/AHA 2002 Guideline Update for the Management of Patients with Unstable Angina and NSTEMI, elevated troponin T or I and new or presumably new ST segment depression are included in a list of 10 high-risk indicators that warrant an early invasive strategy in patients with unstable angina or NSTEMI[4] (Box 31-5). In the absence of high-risk indicators, both the early conservative and the early invasive strategies received Class I recommendations for patients with no contraindications to revascularization.[4]

Although it seems unlikely that the next revision of the guidelines would downgrade the early invasive strategy, one randomized trial[486] and one meta-analysis[487] that were published in 2005 after the most recent guidelines were written suggest that the early invasive strategy may not be superior to the early conservative strategy. The Invasive versus Conservative Treatment in Unstable Coronary Syndromes (ICTUS) trial randomized 1200 patients with non–ST segment elevation ACS and an elevated troponin T (0.03 ng/mL or greater) to early invasive or selective invasive strategies.[486] Revascularization was performed during the initial hospitalization in 76% of patients assigned to the early invasive strategy, compared with 40% of patients assigned to the selective invasive strat-

Box 31-5

ACC/AHA Practice Guidelines: High-Risk Indicators in Patients with Unstable Angina/Non–ST Segment Elevation Myocardial Infarction

1. Recurrent angina/ischemia at rest or with low-level activities despite intensive anti-ischemic therapy
2. Elevated troponin T or troponin I
3. New or presumably new ST segment depression
4. Recurrent angina/ischemia with CHF symptoms, an S_3 gallop, pulmonary edema, worsening rales, or new or worsening MR
5. High-risk findings on noninvasive stress testing
6. Depressed left ventricular systolic function (e.g., EF less than 0.40 on noninvasive study)
7. Hemodynamic instability
8. Sustained ventricular tachycardia
9. PCI within 6 months
10. Prior CABG surgery

CABG, coronary artery bypass graft; CHF, congestive heart failure; EF, ejection fraction; MR, mitral regurgitation; PCI, percutaneous coronary intervention.

From Anderson JL, Adams CD, Antman EM, et al: ACC/AHA 2007 guidelines for the management of patients with unstable angina/non–ST-elevation myocardial infarction: Executive summary: A report of the American College of Cardiology/ American Heart Association Task Force on Practice Guidelines (Writing Committee to Revise the 2002 Guidelines for the Management of Patients with Unstable Angina/Non–ST-Elevation Myocardial Infarction). Circulation 2007;116:803-877.

egy; 79% and 54%, respectively, underwent revascularization within 1 year. The 1-year mortality rate was the same for both groups (2.5%). A diagnosis of MI, defined as an elevation in CK-MB level above the upper limit of normal, within 1 year after randomization was more frequent among patients assigned to the early invasive group than among those in the selective invasive group (15.0% versus 10.0%; RR 1.50; 95% CI 1.10 to 2.04; P=.005). The increased frequency of MI, however, was driven by a greater rate of periprocedural MI (PCI or CABG surgery) among patients who underwent early revascularization, whereas the rate of spontaneous MI was lower among patients who underwent early revascularization. Rehospitalization for angina was less frequent among patients randomized to the early invasive strategy (7.4% versus 10.9%; RR 0.68; 95% CI 0.47 to 0.98; P=.04). The meta-analysis, which did not include the ICTUS trial because it had not been published yet, concluded that a routine invasive strategy was superior to a selective invasive strategy in reducing the risk of MI, severe angina, and rehospitalization.[487] The routine invasive strategy, however, was associated with an increased mortality during the initial hospitalization, which was counterbalanced by a decreased mortality from hospital discharge to the end of follow-up, yielding no significant difference in overall mortality between the two treatment strategies.

The ACC/AHA Practice Guidelines provide recommendations regarding the mode of coronary revascularization in patients with unstable angina or NSTEMI[4] (Table 31-4). Coronary anatomy and left ventricular EF are two of the key factors that determine whether percutaneous or surgical revascularization is preferable in a patient with unstable angina or NSTEMI. Although the guidelines do not specify a preference for PCI or CABG surgery in patients with a non–Q wave MI, periprocedural mortality was greater after CABG surgery than after PCI in The Veterans Affairs Non–Q-Wave Infarction Strategies in Hospital (VANQWISH) trial.[488] Thirty-day mortality was 11.6% after CABG surgery (11/95 patients), compared with 0% after PCI (0/98 patients).[488]

Table 31-4. ACC/AHA Practice Guidelines: Mode of Coronary Revascularization for Unstable Angina/Non–ST Segment Elevation Myocardial Infarction

Extent of Disease	Treatment	Class
Left main disease,* candidate for CABG	CABG PCI	I III
Left main disease, not candidate for CABG	PCI	IIb
Three-vessel disease with EF <0.50	CABG	I
Multivessel disease including proximal LAD with EF <0.50 or treated diabetes	CABG PCI	I IIb
Multivessel disease with EF>0.50 and without diabetes	PCI	I
One- or two-vessel disease without proximal LAD but with large areas of myocardial ischemia or high-risk criteria on noninvasive testing	CABG or PCI	I
One-vessel disease with proximal LAD	CABG or PCI	IIa†
One- or two-vessel disease without proximal LAD with small area of ischemia or no ischemia on noninvasive testing	CABG or PCI	III†
Insignificant coronary stenosis	CABG or PCI	III

*≥50% diameter stenosis.
†Class/level of evidence I/A if severe angina persists despite medical therapy.
ACC, American College of Cardiology; AHA, American Heart Association; CABG, coronary artery bypass grafting; EF, ejection fraction; LAD, left anterior descending (artery); PCI, percutaneous intervention.
From Braunwald E, Antman EM, Beasley JW, et al: ACC/AHA 2002 guideline update for the management of patients with unstable angina and non–ST-segment elevation myocardial infarction: A report of the American College of Cardiology/American Heart Association Task Force on Practice Guidelines (Committee on the Management of Patients with Unstable Angina). Available at: http://www.acc.org/qualityandscience/clinical/guidelines/unstable/incorporated/table20.htm

Long-Term Medical Therapy

Prescription of evidence-based medical therapy at the time of hospital discharge has a major impact on outcome

Box 31-6

ACC/AHA Practice Guidelines: Long-Term Medical Therapy for Patients with Unstable Angina/Non–ST Segment Elevation Myocardial Infarction (NSTEMI)

1. Aspirin 75 to 325 mg per day in the absence of contraindications
2. Clopidogrel 75 mg daily (in the absence of contraindications) when ASA is not tolerated because of hypersensitivity or gastrointestinal intolerance
3. The combination of ASA and clopidogrel for 9 months after unstable angina/NSTEMI
4. β-Blockers in the absence of contraindications
5. Lipid-lowering agents and diet in post-ACS patients, including post-revascularization patients, with LDL cholesterol level greater than 130 mg per dL
6. Lipid-lowering agents if LDL cholesterol level after dietary manipulation is greater than 100 mg per dL
7. ACE inhibitors for patients with CHF, left ventricular dysfunction (EF less than 0.40), hypertension, or diabetes

ACE, angiotensin-converting enzyme; ACS, acute coronary syndrome; ASA, acetylsalicylic acid; CHF, congestive heart failure; EF, ejection fraction; LDL, low-density lipoprotein. Modified slightly from Anderson JL, Adams CD, Antman EM, et al: ACC/AHA 2007 guidelines for the management of patients with unstable angina/non–ST-elevation myocardial infarction: Executive summary: A report of the American College of Cardiology/American Heart Association Task Force on Practice Guidelines (Writing Committee to Revise the 2002 Guidelines for the Management of Patients with Unstable Angina/Non–ST-Elevation Myocardial Infarction). Circulation 2007;116:803-877.

in patients with ACS. Mukherjee and coworkers[489] calculated an appropriateness score based on the use of antiplatelet agents, β-blockers, ACE inhibitors, and lipid-lowering agents in patients with an indication for each class of drugs. The use of combination evidence-based medical therapies was independently associated with lower 6-month mortality among a cohort of 1358 patients with ACS (55% NSTEMI, 30% unstable angina, and 15% STEMI). The odds ratio for death for prescription of all indicated medications versus none of the indicated medications was 0.10 (95% CI 0.03 to 0.42; $P<.0001$).

The ACC/AHA Practice Guidelines for unstable angina and NSTEMI include seven Class I recommendations for long-term medical therapy (Box 31-6).[4] Aspirin 75 to 325 mg daily plus clopidogrel 75 mg daily is recommended for 9 months, and aspirin should be continued indefinitely. β-Blockers are recommended for all patients without contraindications. ACE inhibitors are recommended for patients with CHF, left ventricular EF less than 40%, hypertension, or diabetes. Lipid-lowering agents are recommended in patients with an LDL cholesterol level greater than 100 mg per dL after dietary manipulation.

KEY POINTS

- The ACSs—unstable angina, NSTEMI, and STEMI—all share a common pathophysiology: erosion or rupture of an atherosclerotic plaque that precipitates either nonocclusive or occlusive coronary artery thrombosis.
- Patients with suspected STEMI should have an ECG performed and interpreted within 10 minutes of presentation, and serial ECGs should be performed at intervals of 5 to 10 minutes in patients with a nondiagnostic initial ECG and clinical findings strongly suggestive of STEMI. Right-sided lead tracings should be obtained to screen for right ventricular MI in patients with inferior STEMI.
- The two Class I indications for fibrinolytic therapy in patients with STEMI are (1) symptom onset within the prior 12 hours and ST elevation greater than 0.1 mV in at least two contiguous precordial leads or at least two adjacent limb leads and (2) symptom onset within the prior 12 hours and new or presumably new left bundle branch block.
- Fibrinolytic therapy should be initiated within 30 minutes of presentation.
- Intracranial hemorrhage should be ruled out in any patient with a change in neurologic status during or after fibrinolytic therapy.
- Nitrates are indicated for relief of ischemic discomfort in patients with STEMI, but large clinical trials did not demonstrate a reduction in mortality among patients who received nitroglycerin over prolonged periods after acute MI.
- Aspirin has been shown to reduce mortality in patients with acute MI or unstable angina. Patients with STEMI should receive 162 to 325 mg of non–enteric-coated aspirin, and the aspirin tablets should be chewed.
- The addition of clopidogrel to aspirin has been shown to improve angiographic and clinical outcomes in patients with STEMI or ACS without ST segment elevation.
- A meta-analysis of 23 randomized trials concluded that the rates of short-term death, nonfatal reinfarction, stroke, and the combined end point of all three were lower for primary coronary intervention than for fibrinolytic therapy in patients with STEMI.
- Balloon inflation should occur within 90 minutes of presentation in patients with STEMI who undergo primary coronary intervention.
- Primary coronary intervention is preferable to fibrinolytic therapy in patients with STEMI under the following circumstances: the diagnosis of STEMI is uncertain; fibrinolysis is contraindicated; the door-to-balloon time is less than 90 minutes and the difference between the door-to-balloon and door-to-needle times is less than 60 minutes; and the patient is in Killip class III or IV (pulmonary edema or cardiogenic shock).
- In patients with acute MI early administration of β-blockers reduces the rate of reinfarction and chronic administration improves long-term survival.
- An ACE inhibitor should be administered orally within the first 24 hours of STEMI to patients with anterior infarction, pulmonary congestion, or left ventricular EF less than 40% in the absence of hypotension.
- An angiotensin receptor blocker should be administered to patients with STEMI who are intolerant of ACE inhibitors and have either CHF or a left ventricular EF less than 40%.
- Long-term aldosterone blockade should be prescribed for post-STEMI patients without significant renal dysfunction or hyperkalemia who are already receiving therapeutic doses of an ACE inhibitor, have a left ventricular EF of 40% or less, and have either diabetes or symptomatic CHF.
- Diltiazem and verapamil are contraindicated in patients with STEMI and associated systolic left ventricular dysfunction and CHF.
- Lipid-lowering therapy is indicated at the time of hospital discharge in all patients with STEMI.
- Patients with unstable angina or NSTEMI should receive a GP IIb/IIIa inhibitor and either UH or LMWH.
- An early invasive strategy is favored in patients with unstable angina or NSTEMI who have any of the following high-risk indicators: recurrent angina or ischemia despite intensive anti-ischemic therapy; elevated troponin; new or presumably new ST segment depression; recurrent angina or ischemia with CHF or new or worsening mitral regurgitation; a high-risk noninvasive stress test; left ventricular EF less than 40%; hemodynamic instability; sustained ventricular tachycardia; PCI within the past 6 months; and prior CABG surgery.

REFERENCES

1. Murray CJ, Lopez AD: Mortality by cause for eight regions of the world: Global Burden of Disease Study. Lancet 1997;349:1269-1276.
2. Yusuf S, Hawken S, Ounpuu S, et al: Effect of potentially modifiable risk factors associated with myocardial infarction in 52 countries (the INTERHEART study): Case-control study. Lancet 2004;364:937-952.
3. Rosamond W, Flegal K, Friday G, et al: Heart disease and stroke statistics—2007 update: A report from the American Heart Association Statistics Committee and Stroke Statistics Subcommittee. Circulation 2007;115:e69-e171.
4. Braunwald E, Antman EM, Beasley JW, et al: ACC/AHA 2002 guideline update for the management of patients with unstable angina and non–ST-segment elevation myocardial infarction: A report of the American College of Cardiology/American Heart Association Task Force on Practice Guidelines (Committee on the Management of Patients with Unstable Angina). Available at: http://www.acc.org/clinical/guidelines/unstable/unstable.pdf
5. Alpert JS, Thygesen K, Antman E, et al: Myocardial infarction redefined—a consensus document of The Joint European Society of Cardiology/American College of Cardiology Committee for the redefinition of myocardial infarction. J Am Coll Cardiol 2000;36:959-969.
6. Roger VL, Killian JM, Weston SA, et al: Redefinition of myocardial infarction: Prospective evaluation in the community. Circulation 2006;114:790-797.
7. Kontos MC, Fritz LM, Anderson FP, et al: Impact of the troponin standard on the prevalence of acute myocardial infarction. Am Heart J 2003;146:446-452.
8. Meier MA, Al-Badr WH, Cooper JV, et al: The new definition of myocardial infarction: Diagnostic and prognostic implications in patients with acute coronary syndromes. Arch Intern Med 2002;162:1585-1589.
9. Newby LK, Roe MT, Chen AY, et al: Frequency and clinical implications of discordant creatine kinase-MB and troponin measurements in acute coronary syndromes. J Am Coll Cardiol 2006;47:312-318.
10. Goodman SG, Steg PG, Eagle KA, et al: The diagnostic and prognostic impact of the redefinition of acute myocardial infarction: Lessons from the Global Registry of Acute Coronary Events (GRACE). Am Heart J 2006;151:654-660.
11. Davies MJ: The pathophysiology of acute coronary syndromes. Heart 2000;83:361-366.
12. Fuster V, Moreno PR, Fayad ZA, et al: Atherothrombosis and high-risk plaque: Part I: Evolving concepts. J Am Coll Cardiol 2005;46:937-954.
13. Herrick J: Clinical features of sudden obstruction of the coronary arteries. JAMA 1912;59:2015-2020.
14. Oliva PB, Breckinridge JC: Arteriographic evidence of coronary arterial spasm in acute myocardial infarction. Circulation 1977;56:366-374.
15. Maseri A, L'Abbate A, Baroldi G, et al: Coronary vasospasm as a possible cause of myocardial infarction. A conclusion derived from the study of "preinfarction" angina. N Engl J Med 1978;299:1271-1277.
16. Kaski JC, Tousoulis D, McFadden E, et al: Variant angina pectoris. Role of coronary spasm in the development of fixed coronary obstructions. Circulation 1992;85:619-626.
17. Bogaty P, Hackett D, Davies G, et al: Vasoreactivity of the culprit lesion in unstable angina. Circulation 1994;90:5-11.
18. DeWood MA, Spores J, Notske R, et al: Prevalence of total coronary occlusion during the early hours of transmural myocardial infarction. N Engl J Med 1980;303:897-902.
19. DeWood MA, Stifter WF, Simpson CS, et al: Coronary arteriographic findings soon after non–Q-wave myocardial infarction. N Engl J Med 1986;15:417-423.
20. Mizuno K, Satomura K, Miyamoto A, et al: Angioscopic evaluation of coronary-artery thrombi in acute coronary syndromes. N Engl J Med 1992;326:287-291.
21. Kragel AH, Gertz SD, Roberts WC: Morphologic comparison of frequency and types of acute lesions in the major epicardial coronary arteries in unstable angina pectoris, sudden coronary death and acute myocardial infarction. J Am Coll Cardiol 1991;18:801-808.
22. Ambrose JA, Winters SL, Arora RR, et al: Angiographic evolution of coronary artery morphology in unstable angina. J Am Coll Cardiol 1986;7:472-478.
23. Ambrose JA, Tannenbaum MA, Alexopoulos D, et al: Angiographic progression of coronary artery disease and the development of myocardial infarction. J Am Coll Cardiol 1988;12:56-62.
24. Little WC, Constantinescu M, Applegate RJ, et al: Can coronary angiography predict the site of a subsequent myocardial infarction in patients with mild-to-moderate coronary artery disease? Circulation 1988;78:1157-1166.
25. Nobuyoshi M, Tanaka M, Nosaka H, et al: Progression of coronary atherosclerosis: Is coronary spasm related to progression? J Am Coll Cardiol 1991;18:904-910.
26. Giroud D, Li JM, Urban P, et al: Relation of the site of acute myocardial infarction to the most severe coronary arterial stenosis at prior angiography. Am J Cardiol 1992;69:729-732.
27. Murabito JM, Evans JC, Larson MG, et al: Prognosis after the onset of coronary heart disease. An investigation of differences in outcome between the sexes according to initial coronary disease presentation. Circulation 1993;88:2548-2555.
28. Falk E: Unstable angina with fatal outcome: Dynamic coronary thrombosis leading to infarction and/or sudden death. Circulation 1985;71:699-708.
29. Richardson PD, Davies MJ, Born GV: Influence of plaque configuration and stress distribution on fissuring of coronary atherosclerotic plaques. Lancet 1989;2:941-944.
30. van der Wal AC, Becker AE, van der Loos CM, et al: Site of intimal rupture or erosion of thrombosed coronary atherosclerotic plaques is characterized by an inflammatory process irrespective of the dominant plaque morphology. Circulation 1994;89:36-44.
31. Shah PK, Falk E, Badimon JJ, et al: Human monocyte-derived macrophages induce collagen breakdown in fibrous caps of atherosclerotic plaques. Potential role of matrix-degrading metalloproteinases and implications for plaque rupture. Circulation 1995;92:1565-1569.
32. Moreno PR, Falk E, Palacios IF, et al: Macrophage infiltration in acute coronary syndromes. Implications for plaque rupture. Circulation 1994;90:775-778.
33. Brown DL, Hibbs MS, Kearney M, et al: Identification of 92-kD gelatinase in human coronary atherosclerotic lesions. Association of active enzyme synthesis with unstable angina. Circulation 1995;91:2125-2131.
34. Moreno PR, Bernardi VH, Lopez-Cuellar J, et al: Macrophages, smooth muscle cells, and tissue factor in unstable angina. Implications for cell-mediated thrombogenicity in acute coronary syndromes. Circulation 1996;94:3090-3097.
35. Goldstein JA, Demetriou D, Grines CL, et al: Multiple complex coronary plaques in patients with acute myocardial infarction. N Engl J Med 2000;343:915-922.
36. Rioufol G, Finet G, Ginon I, et al: Multiple atherosclerotic plaque rupture in acute coronary syndrome: A three-vessel intravascular ultrasound study. Circulation 2002;106:804-808.
37. Jude B, Agraou B, McFadden EP, et al: Evidence for time-dependent activation of monocytes in the systemic circulation in unstable angina but not in acute myocardial infarction or in stable angina. Circulation 1994;90:1662-1668.
38. Heeschen C, Dimmeler S, Hamm CW, et al: Soluble CD40 ligand in acute coronary syndromes. N Engl J Med 2003;348:1104-1111.
39. Meier CR, Jick SS, Derby LE, et al: Acute respiratory-tract infections and risk of first-time acute myocardial infarction. Lancet 1998;351:1467-1471.
40. Smeeth L, Thomas SL, Hall AJ, et al: Risk of myocardial infarction and stroke after acute infection or vaccination. N Engl J Med 2004;351:2611-2618.
41. Mittleman MA, Maclure M, Tofler GH, et al: Triggering of acute myocardial infarction by heavy physical exertion. Protection against triggering by regular exertion. Determinants of Myocardial Infarction Onset Study Investigators. N Engl J Med 1993;329:1677-1683.

42. Willich SN, Lewis M, Lowel H, et al: Physical exertion as a trigger of acute myocardial infarction. Triggers and Mechanisms of Myocardial Infarction Study Group. N Engl J Med 1993;329: 1684-1690.
43. Giri S, Thompson PD, Kiernan FJ, et al: Clinical and angiographic characteristics of exertion-related acute myocardial infarction. JAMA 1999;282:1731-1736.
44. Hammoudeh AJ, Haft JI: Coronary-plaque rupture in acute coronary syndromes triggered by snow shoveling. N Engl J Med 1996; 335:2001.
45. Muller JE, Tofler GH, Stone PH: Circadian variation and triggers of onset of acute cardiovascular disease. Circulation 1989;79:733-743.
46. Pamukcu B, Oflaz H, Acar RD, et al: The role of exercise on platelet aggregation in patients with stable coronary artery disease: Exercise induces aspirin resistant platelet activation. J Thromb Thrombolysis 2005;20:17-22.
47. Perneby C, Wallen NH, Hu H, et al: Prothrombotic responses to exercise are little influenced by clopidogrel treatment. Thromb Res 2004;114: 235-243.
48. Gordon JB, Ganz P, Nabel EG, et al: Atherosclerosis influences the vasomotor response of epicardial coronary arteries to exercise. J Clin Invest 1989;83:1946-1952.
49. Vita JA, Treasure CB, Ganz P, et al: Control of shear stress in the epicardial coronary arteries of humans: Impairment by atherosclerosis. J Am Coll Cardiol 1989;14:1193-1199.
50. Davies MJ, Richardson PD, Woolf N, et al: Risk of thrombosis in human atherosclerotic plaques: Role of extracellular lipid, macrophage, and smooth muscle cell content. Br Heart J 1993;69:377-381.
51. Mittleman MA, Maclure M, Sherwood JB, et al: Triggering of acute myocardial infarction onset by episodes of anger. Determinants of Myocardial Infarction Onset Study Investigators. Circulation 1995;92: 1720-1725.
52. Tofler GH, Muller JE: Triggering of acute cardiovascular disease and potential preventive strategies. Circulation 2006;114:1863-1872.
53. Leor J, Poole WK, Kloner RA: Sudden cardiac death triggered by an earthquake. N Engl J Med 1996;334: 413-419.
54. Leor J, Kloner RA: The Northridge earthquake as a trigger for acute myocardial infarction. Am J Cardiol 1996;77:1230-1232.
55. Bybee KA, Kara T, Prasad A, et al: Systematic review: Transient left ventricular apical ballooning: A syndrome that mimics ST-segment elevation myocardial infarction. Ann Intern Med 2004;141:858-865.
56. Wittstein IS, Thiemann DR, Lima JA, et al: Neurohumoral features of myocardial stunning due to sudden emotional stress. N Engl J Med 2005;352:539-548.
57. Raymond R, Lynch J, Underwood D, et al: Myocardial infarction and normal coronary arteriography: A 10 year clinical and risk analysis of 74 patients. J Am Coll Cardiol 1988;11:471-477.
58. Zainea M, Duvernoy WF, Chauhan A, et al: Acute myocardial infarction in angiographically normal coronary arteries following induction of general anesthesia. Arch Intern Med 1994; 154:2495-2498.
59. Kereiakes DJ, Topol EJ, George BS, et al: Myocardial infarction with minimal coronary atherosclerosis in the era of thrombolytic reperfusion. The Thrombolysis and Angioplasty in Myocardial Infarction (TAMI) Study Group. J Am Coll Cardiol 1991;17: 304-312.
60. Prizel KR, Hutchins GM, Bulkley BH: Coronary artery embolism and myocardial infarction. Ann Intern Med 1978;88:155-161.
61. Minor RL, Jr., Scott BD, Brown DD, et al: Cocaine-induced myocardial infarction in patients with normal coronary arteries. Ann Intern Med 1991;115:797-806.
62. Borczuk AC, van Hoeven KH, Factor SM: Review and hypothesis: The eosinophil and peripartum heart disease (myocarditis and coronary artery dissection)—coincidence or pathogenetic significance? Cardiovasc Res 1997;33:527-532.
63. Swap CJ, Nagurney JT: Value and limitations of chest pain history in the evaluation of patients with suspected acute coronary syndromes. JAMA 2005;294:2623-2639.
64. Henrikson CA, Howell EE, Bush DE, et al: Chest pain relief by nitroglycerin does not predict active coronary artery disease. Ann Intern Med 2003;139: 979-986.
65. Patel H, Rosengren A, Ekman I: Symptoms in acute coronary syndromes: Does sex make a difference? Am Heart J 2004;148: 27-33.
66. Canto JG, Shlipak MG, Rogers WJ, et al: Prevalence, clinical characteristics, and mortality among patients with myocardial infarction presenting without chest pain. JAMA 2000;283:3223-3322.
67. Brieger D, Eagle KA, Goodman SG, et al: Acute coronary syndromes without chest pain, an underdiagnosed and undertreated high-risk group: Insights from the Global Registry of Acute Coronary Events. Chest 2004;126:461-499.
68. Killip T 3rd, Kimball JT: Treatment of myocardial infarction in a coronary care unit. A two year experience with 250 patients. Am J Cardiol 1967;20: 457-464.
69. Werns SW, Bates ER: The enduring value of Killip classification. Am Heart J 1999;137:213-215.
70. DeGeare VS, Boura JA, Grines LL, et al: Predictive value of the Killip classification in patients undergoing primary percutaneous coronary intervention for acute myocardial infarction. Am J Cardiol 2001;87: 1035-1038.
71. Antman EM, Anbe DT, Armstrong PW, et al: ACC/AHA guidelines for the management of patients with ST-elevation myocardial infarction: A report of the American College of Cardiology/American Heart Association Task Force on Practice Guidelines (Committee to Revise the 1999 Guidelines for the Management of Patients with Acute Myocardial Infarction). Circulation 2004;110: e82-e292.
72. Sgarbossa EB, Pinski SL, Barbagelata A, et al: Electrocardiographic diagnosis of evolving acute myocardial infarction in the presence of left bundle-branch block. GUSTO-1 (Global Utilization of Streptokinase and Tissue Plasminogen Activator for Occluded Coronary Arteries) Investigators. N Engl J Med 1996;334:481-487.
73. Shlipak MG, Lyons WL, Go AS, et al: Should the electrocardiogram be used to guide therapy for patients with left bundle-branch block and suspected myocardial infarction? JAMA 1999;281:714-719.
74. Peterson ED, Hathaway WR, Zabel KM, et al: Prognostic significance of precordial ST segment depression during inferior myocardial infarction in the thrombolytic era: results in 16,521 patients. J Am Coll Cardiol 1996;128:305-3012.
75. Wong CK, Gao W, Raffel OC, et al: Initial Q waves accompanying ST-segment elevation at presentation of acute myocardial infarction and 30-day mortality in patients given streptokinase therapy: An analysis from HERO-2. Lancet 2006;367:2061-2067.
76. Raitt MH, Maynard C, Wagner GS, et al: Appearance of abnormal Q waves early in the course of acute myocardial infarction: Implications for efficacy of thrombolytic therapy. J Am Coll Cardiol 25:1084-1088.
77. Sgarbossa EB, Birnbaum Y, Parrillo JE: Electrocardiographic diagnosis of acute myocardial infarction: Current concepts for the clinician. Am Heart J 2001;141:507-517.
78. Zimetbaum PJ, Josephson ME: Use of the electrocardiogram in acute myocardial infarction. N Engl J Med 2003;348:933-940.
79. Mauri F, Gasparini M, Barbonaglia L, et al: Prognostic significance of the extent of myocardial injury in acute myocardial infarction treated by streptokinase (the GISSI trial). Am J Cardiol 1989;63:1291-1295.
80. Andrews J, Straznicky IT, French JK, et al: ST-segment recovery adds to the assessment of TIMI 2 and 3 flow in predicting infarct wall motion after thrombolytic therapy. Circulation 2000;101:2138-2143.
81. Dong J, Ndrepepa G, Schmitt C, et al: Early resolution of ST-segment elevation correlates with myocardial salvage assessed by Tc-99m sestamibi scintigraphy in patients with acute myocardial infarction after mechanical or thrombolytic reperfusion therapy. Circulation 2002;105:2946-2949.
82. van't Hof AW, Liem A, de Boer MJ, et al: Clinical value of 12-lead electrocardiogram after successful reperfusion therapy for acute myocardial infarction. Zwolle Myocardial Infarction Study Group. Lancet 1997;350:615-619.
83. Anderson RD, White HD, Ohman EM, et al: Predicting outcome after thrombolysis in acute myocardial infarction according to ST-segment

resolution at 90 minutes: A substudy of the GUSTO-III trial. Global Use of Strategies to Open occluded coronary arteries. Am Heart J 2002;144:81-88.
84. Zeymer U, Schroder K, Wegscheider K, et al: ST resolution in a single electrocardiographic lead: A simple and accurate predictor of cardiac mortality in patients with fibrinolytic therapy for acute ST-elevation myocardial infarction. Am Heart J 2005;149:91-97.
85. Wang K, Asinger RW, Marriott HJ: ST-segment elevation in conditions other than acute myocardial infarction. N Engl J Med 2003;349:2128-2135.
86. Antman EM, Anbe DT, Armstrong PW, et al: ACC/AHA guidelines for the management of patients with ST-elevation myocardial infarction—executive summary: A report of the American College of Cardiology/American Heart Association Task Force on Practice Guidelines (Writing Committee to Revise the 1999 Guidelines for the Management of Patients With Acute Myocardial Infarction). Circulation 2004;110: 588-636.
87. Jeremias A, Gibson CM: Narrative review: Alternative causes for elevated cardiac troponin levels when acute coronary syndromes are excluded. Ann Intern Med 2005;142:786-7891.
88. Meyer T, Binder L, Hruska N, et al: Cardiac troponin I elevation in acute pulmonary embolism is associated with right ventricular dysfunction. J Am Coll Cardiol 2000;36:1632-1636.
89. Konstantinides S, Geibel A, Olschewski M, et al: Importance of cardiac troponins I and T in risk stratification of patients with acute pulmonary embolism. Circulation 2002;106: 1263-1268.
90. Mehta NJ, Jani K, Khan IA: Clinical usefulness and prognostic value of elevated cardiac troponin I levels in acute pulmonary embolism. Am Heart J 2002;145:821-825.
91. Imazio M, Demichelis B, Cecchi E, et al: Cardiac troponin I in acute pericarditis. J Am Coll Cardiol 2003;42:2144-2148.
92. Feinberg MS, Schwammenthal E, Shlizerman L, et al: Prognostic significance of mild mitral regurgitation by color Doppler echocardiography in acute myocardial infarction. Am J Cardiol 2000;86: 903-907.
93. Bursi F, Enriquez-Sarano M, Nkomo VT, et al: Heart failure and death after myocardial infarction in the community: The emerging role of mitral regurgitation. Circulation 2005;111:295-301.
94. Dalen JE: PA catheter-guided therapy does not benefit critically ill patients. Am J Med 2005;118:449-451.
95. Gore JM, Goldberg RJ, Spodick DH, et al: A community-wide assessment of the use of pulmonary artery catheters in patients with acute myocardial infarction. Chest 1987;92:721-727.
96. Zion MM, Balkin J, Rosenmann D, et al: Use of pulmonary artery catheters in patients with acute myocardial infarction. Analysis of experience in 5,841 patients in the SPRINT Registry. SPRINT Study Group. Chest 1990;98:1331-1335.
97. Cohen MG, Kelly RV, Kong DF, et al: Pulmonary artery catheterization in acute coronary syndromes: Insights from the GUSTO IIb and GUSTO III trials. Am J Med 2005;118:482-488.
98. Pellizzon GG, Grines CL, Cox DA, et al: Importance of mitral regurgitation inpatients undergoing percutaneous coronary intervention for acute myocardial infarction: The Controlled Abciximab and Device Investigation to Lower Late Angioplasty Complications (CADILLAC) trial. J Am Coll Cardiol 2004;43:1368-1374.
99. Tcheng JE, Jackman JD, Jr., Nelson CL, et al: Outcome of patients sustaining acute ischemic mitral regurgitation during myocardial infarction. Ann Intern Med 1992;117:18-24.
100. Stenestrand U, Wallentin L: Early revascularisation and 1-year survival in 14-day survivors of acute myocardial infarction: A prospective cohort study. Lancet 2002;359:1805-1811.
101. Beck CA, Eisenberg MJ, Pilote L: Invasive versus noninvasive management of ST-elevation acute myocardial infarction: A review of clinical trials and observational studies. Am Heart J 2005;149:194-199.
102. Scheller B, Hennen B, Hammer B, et al: Beneficial effects of immediate stenting after thrombolysis in acute myocardial infarction. J Am Coll Cardiol 2003;42:634-641.
103. Fernandez-Aviles F, Alonso JJ, Castro-Beiras A, et al: Routine invasive strategy within 24 hours of thrombolysis versus ischaemia-guided conservative approach for acute myocardial infarction with ST-segment elevation (GRACIA-1): A randomised controlled trial. Lancet 2004;364: 1045-1053.
104. Zeymer U, Uebis R, Vogt A, et al: Randomized comparison of percutaneous transluminal coronary angioplasty and medical therapy in stable survivors of acute myocardial infarction with single vessel disease: A study of the Arbeitsgemeinschaft Leitende Kardiologische Krankenhausarzte. Circulation 2003;108:1324-1328.
105. Madias JE, Madias NE, Hood WB Jr: Precordial ST-segment mapping. 2. Effects of oxygen inhalation on ischemic injury in patients with acute myocardial infarction. Circulation 1976;53:411-417.
106. Rawles JM, Kenmure AC: Controlled trial of oxygen in uncomplicated myocardial infarction. BMJ 1976;1:1121-1123.
107. Meine TJ, Roe MT, Chen AY, et al: Association of intravenous morphine use and outcomes in acute coronary syndromes: Results from the CRUSADE Quality Improvement Initiative. Am Heart J 2005;149:1043-1049.
108. Daniell HW: Opioid-induced cortisol deficiency may explain much of the increased mortality after the use of morphine during treatment of acute myocardial infarction. Am Heart J 2005;150:e1.
109. Mikolich JR, Nicoloff NB, Robinson PH, et al: Relief of refractory angina with continuous intravenous infusion of nitroglycerin. Chest 1980;77: 375-379.
110. Armstrong PW, Walker DC, Burton JR, et al: Vasodilator therapy in acute myocardial infarction. A comparison of sodium nitroprusside and nitroglycerin. Circulation 1975;52: 1118-1122.
111. Feldman RL, Pepine CJ, Conti CR: Magnitude of dilatation of large and small coronary arteries of nitroglycerin. Circulation 1981;64:324-333.
112. Come PC, Pitt B: Nitroglycerin-induced severe hypotension and bradycardia in patients with acute myocardial infarction. Circulation 1976;54:624-628.
113. Cheitlin MD, Hutter AM Jr, Brindis RG, et al: ACC/AHA expert consensus document. Use of sildenafil (Viagra) in patients with cardiovascular disease. American College of Cardiology/American Heart Association. J Am Coll Cardiol 1999;33:273-282.
114. Jugdutt BI, Warnica JW: Intravenous nitroglycerin therapy to limit myocardial infarct size, expansion, and complications. Effect of timing, dosage, and infarct location. Circulation 1988;78:906-919.
115. GISSI-3: Effects of lisinopril and transdermal glyceryl trinitrate singly and together on 6-week mortality and ventricular function after acute myocardial infarction. Gruppo Italiano per lo Studio della Sopravvivenza nell'infarto Miocardico. Lancet 1994;343:1115-1122.
116. ISIS-4: A randomised factorial trial assessing early oral captopril, oral mononitrate, and intravenous magnesium sulphate in 58,050 patients with suspected acute myocardial infarction. ISIS-4 (Fourth International Study of Infarct Survival) Collaborative Group. Lancet 1995;345:669-685.
117. Chiariello M, Gold HK, Leinbach RC, et al: Comparison between the effects of nitroprusside and nitroglycerin on ischemic injury during acute myocardial infarction. Circulation 1976;54:766-773.
118. Hockings BE, Cope GD, Clarke GM, et al: Randomized controlled trial of vasodilator therapy after myocardial infarction. Am J Cardiol 1981;48: 345-352.
119. Durrer JD, Lie KI, van Capelle FJ, et al: Effect of sodium nitroprusside on mortality in acute myocardial infarction. N Engl J Med 1982;306: 1121-1128.
120. Cohn JN, Franciosa JA, Francis GS, et al: Effect of short-term infusion of sodium nitroprusside on mortality rate in acute myocardial infarction complicated by left ventricular failure: Results of a Veterans Administration cooperative study. N Engl J Med 1982;306:1129-1135.
121. Randomised trial of intravenous streptokinase, oral aspirin, both, or neither among 17,187 cases of suspected acute myocardial infarction: ISIS-2. ISIS-2 (Second International Study of Infarct Survival) Collaborative Group. Lancet 1988;2:349-360.
122. Ohman EM, Califf RM, Topol EJ, et al: Consequences of reocclusion after successful reperfusion therapy in acute

myocardial infarction. TAMI Study Group. Circulation 1990;82:781-791.
123. Meijer A, Verheugt FW, van Eenige MJ, et al: Left ventricular function at 3 months after successful thrombolysis. Impact of reocclusion without reinfarction on ejection fraction, regional function, and remodeling. Circulation 1994;90:1706-1714.
124. Brouwer MA, Bohncke JR, Veen G, et al: Adverse long-term effects of reocclusion after coronary thrombolysis. J Am Coll Cardiol 1995;26:1440-1444.
125. Nijland F, Kamp O, Verheugt FW, et al: Long-term implications of reocclusion on left ventricular size and function after successful thrombolysis for first anterior myocardial infarction. Circulation 1997;95:111-117.
126. Roux S, Christeller S, Ludin E: Effects of aspirin on coronary reocclusion and recurrent ischemia after thrombolysis: A meta-analysis. J Am Coll Cardiol 1992;19:671-677.
127. Verheugt FW, Meijer A, Lagrand WK, et al: Reocclusion: The flip side of coronary thrombolysis. J Am Coll Cardiol 1996;27:766-773.
128. Meijer A, Verheugt FW, Werter CJ, et al: Aspirin versus coumadin in the prevention of reocclusion and recurrent ischemia after successful thrombolysis: A prospective placebo-controlled angiographic study. Results of the APRICOT Study. Circulation 1993;87:1524-1530.
129. Sabatine MS, Cannon CP, Gibson CM, et al: Addition of clopidogrel to aspirin and fibrinolytic therapy for myocardial infarction with ST-segment elevation. N Engl J Med 2005;352:1179-1189.
130. Chen ZM, Jiang LX, Chen YP, et al: Addition of clopidogrel to aspirin in 45,852 patients with acute myocardial infarction: Randomised placebo-controlled trial. Lancet 2005;366: 1607-1621.
131. Sabatine MS, Cannon CP, Gibson CM, et al: Effect of clopidogrel pretreatment before percutaneous coronary intervention in patients with ST-elevation myocardial infarction treated with fibrinolytics: The PCI-CLARITY study. JAMA 2005;294: 1224-1232.
132. Hsia J, Hamilton WP, Kleiman N, et al: A comparison between heparin and low-dose aspirin as adjunctive therapy with tissue plasminogen activator for acute myocardial infarction. Heparin-Aspirin Reperfusion Trial (HART) Investigators. N Engl J Med 1990;323:1433-1437.
133. Arnout J, Simoons M, de Bono D, et al: Correlation between level of heparinization and patency of the infarct-related coronary artery after treatment of acute myocardial infarction with alteplase (rt-PA). J Am Coll Cardiol 1992;20:513-519.
134. Collins R, Peto R, Baigent C, et al: Aspirin, heparin, and fibrinolytic therapy in suspected acute myocardial infarction. N Engl J Med 1997;336: 847-860.
135. GISSI-2: a factorial randomised trial of alteplase versus streptokinase and heparin versus no heparin among 12,490 patients with acute myocardial infarction. Gruppo Italiano per lo Studio della Sopravvivenza nell'Infarto Miocardico. Lancet 1990;336:65-71.
136. In-hospital mortality and clinical course of 20,891 patients with suspected acute myocardial infarction randomised between alteplase and streptokinase with or without heparin. The International Study Group. Lancet 1990;336:71-75.
137. ISIS-3: A randomised comparison of streptokinase vs tissue plasminogen activator vs anistreplase and of aspirin plus heparin vs aspirin alone among 41,299 cases of suspected acute myocardial infarction. ISIS-3 (Third International Study of Infarct Survival) Collaborative Group. Lancet 1992;339:753-770.
138. Mahaffey KW, Granger CB, Collins R, et al: Overview of randomized trials of intravenous heparin in patients with acute myocardial infarction treated with thrombolytic therapy. Am J Cardiol 1996;77:551-556.
139. Granger CB, Hirsch J, Califf RM, et al: Activated partial thromboplastin time and outcome after thrombolytic therapy for acute myocardial infarction: Results from the GUSTO-I trial. Circulation 1996;93:870-878.
140. Warkentin TE, Levine MN, Hirsh J, et al: Heparin-induced thrombocytopenia in patients treated with low-molecular-weight heparin or unfractionated heparin. N Engl J Med 1995;332: 1330-1335.
141. Vaitkus PT, Barnathan ES: Embolic potential, prevention and management of mural thrombus complicating anterior myocardial infarction: A meta-analysis. J Am Coll Cardiol 1993;22:1004-1009.
142. Nayak D, Aronow WS, Sukhija R, et al: Comparison of frequency of left ventricular thrombi in patients with anterior wall versus non–anterior wall acute myocardial infarction treated with antithrombotic and antiplatelet therapy with or without coronary revascularization. Am J Cardiol 2004;93:1529-1530.
143. Vecchio C, Chiarella F, Lupi G, et al: Left ventricular thrombus in anterior acute myocardial infarction after thrombolysis. A GISSI-2 connected study. Circulation 1991;84:512-519.
144. Greaves SC, Zhi G, Lee RT, et al: Incidence and natural history of left ventricular thrombus following anterior wall acute myocardial infarction. Am J Cardiol 1997;80: 442-448.
145. Turpie AG, Robinson JG, Doyle DJ, et al: Comparison of high-dose with low-dose subcutaneous heparin to prevent left ventricular mural thrombosis in patients with acute transmural anterior myocardial infarction. N Engl J Med 1989;320:352-357.
146. Ross AM, Molhoek P, Lundergan C, et al: Randomized comparison of enoxaparin, a low-molecular-weight heparin, with unfractionated heparin adjunctive to recombinant tissue plasminogen activator thrombolysis and aspirin: Second trial of Heparin and Aspirin Reperfusion Therapy (HART II). Circulation 2001;104: 648-652.
147. Antman EM, Louwerenburg HW, Baars HF, et al: Enoxaparin as adjunctive antithrombin therapy for ST-elevation myocardial infarction: Results of the ENTIRE-Thrombolysis in Myocardial Infarction (TIMI) 23 Trial. Circulation 2002;105:1642-1649.
148. Antman EM, Morrow DA, McCabe CH, et al: Enoxaparin versus unfractionated heparin with fibrinolysis for ST-elevation myocardial infarction. N Engl J Med 2006;354:1477-1488.
149. Theroux P, Welsh RC: Meta-analysis of randomized trials comparing enoxaparin versus unfractionated heparin as adjunctive therapy to fibrinolysis in ST-elevation acute myocardial infarction. Am J Cardiol 2003;91:860-864.
150. Eikelboom JW, Quinlan DJ, Mehta SR, et al: Unfractionated and low-molecular-weight heparin as adjuncts to thrombolysis in aspirin-treated patients with ST-elevation acute myocardial infarction: A meta-analysis of the randomized trials. Circulation 2005;112:3855-3867.
151. Yusuf S, Mehta SR, Xie C, et al: Effects of reviparin, a low-molecular-weight heparin, on mortality, reinfarction, and strokes in patients with acute myocardial infarction presenting with ST-segment elevation. JAMA 2005;293:427-435.
152. Yusuf S, Mehta SR, Chrolavicius S, et al: Comparison of fondaparinux and enoxaparin in acute coronary syndromes. N Engl J Med 2006; 354:1464-1476.
153. Yusuf S, Mehta SR, Chrolavicius S, et al: Effects of fondaparinux on mortality and reinfarction in patients with acute ST-segment elevation myocardial infarction: The OASIS-6 randomized trial. JAMA 2006;295: 1519-1530.
154. Reimer KA, Lowe JE, Rasmussen MM, et al: The wavefront phenomenon of ischemic cell death. 1. Myocardial infarct size vs duration of coronary occlusion in dogs. Circulation 1977;56:786-794.
155. Fletcher A, Alkjaersig N, Smyrniotis F, et al: The treatment of patients suffering from early myocardial infarction with massive and prolonged streptokinase therapy. Trans Assoc Am Physicians 1958;71:287-296.
156. Streptokinase in acute myocardial infarction. European Cooperative Study Group for Streptokinase Treatment in Acute Myocardial Infarction. N Engl J Med 1979;301: 797-802.
157. Sullivan JM: Streptokinase and myocardial infarction. N Engl J Med 1979;301:836-837.
158. Effectiveness of intravenous thrombolytic treatment in acute myocardial infarction. Gruppo Italiano per lo Studio della Streptochinasi nell'Infarto Miocardico (GISSI). Lancet 1086;1:397-402.
159. Long-term effects of intravenous anistreplase in acute myocardial infarction: Final report of the AIMS study. AIMS Trial Study Group. Lancet 1990;335:427-431.
160. Wilcox RG, von der Lippe G, Olsson CG, et al: Trial of tissue plasminogen activator for mortality reduction in acute myocardial infarction. Anglo-Scandinavian Study of Early

Thrombolysis (ASSET). Lancet 1988;2:525-530.
161. Indications for fibrinolytic therapy in suspected acute myocardial infarction: Collaborative overview of early mortality and major morbidity results from all randomised trials of more than 1000 patients. Fibrinolytic Therapy Trialists' (FTT) Collaborative Group. Lancet 1994;343:311-322.
162. Boersma E, Maas AC, Deckers JW, et al: Early thrombolytic treatment in acute myocardial infarction: Reappraisal of the golden hour. Lancet 1996;348:771-775.
163. Taher T, Fu Y, Wagner GS, et al: Aborted myocardial infarction in patients with ST-segment elevation: Insights from the Assessment of the Safety and Efficacy of a New Thrombolytic Regimen-3 Trial Electrocardiographic Substudy. J Am Coll Cardiol 2004;44:38-43.
164. Verheugt FW, Gersh BJ, Armstrong PW: Aborted myocardial infarction: A new target for reperfusion therapy. Eur Heart J 2006;27:901-904.
165. White HD, Norris RM, Brown MA, et al: Left ventricular end-systolic volume as the major determinant of survival after recovery from myocardial infarction. Circulation 1987;76:44-51.
166. Sutton MG, Sharpe N: Left ventricular remodeling after myocardial infarction: Pathophysiology and therapy. Circulation 2000;101:2981-2988.
167. Topol EJ, Califf RM, Vandormael M, et al: A randomized trial of late reperfusion therapy for acute myocardial infarction. Thrombolysis and Angioplasty in Myocardial Infarction-6 Study Group. Circulation 1992;85:2090-2099.
168. Hirayama A, Adachi T, Asada S, et al: Late reperfusion for acute myocardial infarction limits the dilatation of left ventricle without the reduction of infarct size. Circulation 1993;88: 2565-2574.
169. Randomised trial of late thrombolysis in patients with suspected acute myocardial infarction. EMERAS (Estudio Multicentrico Estreptoquinasa Republicas de America del Sur) Collaborative Group. Lancet 1993;342:767-772.
170. Late Assessment of Thrombolytic Efficacy (LATE) study with alteplase 6-24 hours after onset of acute myocardial infarction. Lancet 1993;342:759-766.
171. Gurwitz JH, McLaughlin TJ, Willison DJ, et al: Delayed hospital presentation in patients who have had acute myocardial infarction. Ann Intern Med 1997;126:593-599.
172. Goldberg RJ, Steg PG, Sadiq I, et al: Extent of, and factors associated with, delay to hospital presentation in patients with acute coronary disease (the GRACE registry). Am J Cardiol 2002;89:791-796.
173. Berger AK, Radford MJ, Krumholz HM: Factors associated with delay in reperfusion therapy in elderly patients with acute myocardial infarction: Analysis of the cooperative cardiovascular project. Am Heart J 2000;139:985-992.
174. McNamara RL, Herrin J, Bradley EH, et al: Hospital improvement in time to reperfusion in patients with acute myocardial infarction, 1999 to 2002. J Am Coll Cardiol 2006;47:45-51.
175. Morrison LJ, Verbeek PR, McDonald AC, et al: Mortality and prehospital thrombolysis for acute myocardial infarction: A meta-analysis. JAMA 2000;283:2686-2692.
176. Welsh RC, Ornato J, Armstrong PW: Prehospital management of acute ST-elevation myocardial infarction: A time for reappraisal in North America. Am Heart J 2003;145:1-8.
177. Bonnefoy E, Lapostolle F, Leizorovicz A, et al: Primary angioplasty versus prehospital fibrinolysis in acute myocardial infarction: A randomised study. Lancet 2002;360:825-829.
178. Khaja F, Walton JA Jr, Brymer JF, et al: Intracoronary fibrinolytic therapy in acute myocardial infarction. Report of a prospective randomized trial. N Engl J Med 1983;308:1305-1311.
179. Anderson JL, Marshall HW, Bray BE, et al: A randomized trial of intracoronary streptokinase in the treatment of acute myocardial infarction. N Engl J Med 1983; 308:1312-1318.
180. Kennedy JW, Ritchie JL, Davis KB, et al: Western Washington randomized trial of intracoronary streptokinase in acute myocardial infarction. N Engl J Med 1983;309:1477-1482.
181. The Thrombolysis in Myocardial Infarction (TIMI) trial. Phase I findings. TIMI Study Group. N Engl J Med 1985;312:932-936.
182. Chesebro JH, Knatterud G, Roberts R, et al: Thrombolysis in Myocardial Infarction (TIMI) Trial, Phase I: A comparison between intravenous tissue plasminogen activator and intravenous streptokinase. Clinical findings through hospital discharge. Circulation 1987;76:142-154.
183. Vogt A, von Essen R, Tebbe U, et al: Impact of early perfusion status of the infarct-related artery on short-term mortality after thrombolysis for acute myocardial infarction: Retrospective analysis of four German multicenter studies. J Am Coll Cardiol 1993;21: 1391-1395.
184. Lenderink T, Simoons ML, Van Es GA, et al: Benefit of thrombolytic therapy is sustained throughout five years and is related to TIMI perfusion grade 3 but not grade 2 flow at discharge. The European Cooperative Study Group. Circulation 1995;92:1110-1116.
185. Lincoff AM, Topol EJ: Trickle down thrombolysis. J Am Coll Cardiol 1993;21:1396-1398.
186. An international randomized trial comparing four thrombolytic strategies for acute myocardial infarction. The GUSTO investigators. N Engl J Med 1993;329:673-682.
187. The effects of tissue plasminogen activator, streptokinase, or both on coronary-artery patency, ventricular function, and survival after acute myocardial infarction. The GUSTO Angiographic Investigators. N Engl J Med 1993;329:1615-1622.
188. Simes RJ, Topol EJ, Holmes DR, Jr., et al: Link between the angiographic substudy and mortality outcomes in a large randomized trial of myocardial reperfusion. Importance of early and complete infarct artery reperfusion. GUSTO-I Investigators. Circulation 1995;91:1923-1928.
189. Schomig A, Ndrepepa G, Mehilli J, et al: Therapy-dependent influence of time-to-treatment interval on myocardial salvage in patients with acute myocardial infarction treated with coronary artery stenting or thrombolysis. Circulation 2003;108: 1084-1088.
190. Cannon CP: Timely thrombolysis: Synergism to open arteries and reduce mortality rates. Am Heart J 1999;137:1-3.
191. Steg PG, Laperche T, Golmard JL, et al: Efficacy of streptokinase, but not tissue-type plasminogen activator, in achieving 90-minute patency after thrombolysis for acute myocardial infarction decreases with time to treatment. PERM Study Group. Prospective Evaluation of Reperfusion Markers. J Am Coll Cardiol 1998;31: 776-779.
192. Zeymer U, Tebbe U, Essen R, et al: Influence of time to treatment on early infarct-related artery patency after different thrombolytic regimens. ALKK-Study Group. Am Heart J 1999;137: 34-38.
193. Gibson CM, Murphy SA, Rizzo MJ, et al: Relationship between TIMI frame count and clinical outcomes after thrombolytic administration. Thrombolysis in Myocardial Infarction (TIMI) Study Group. Circulation 1999;99:1945-1950.
194. Gibson CM, Cannon CP, Murphy SA, et al: Relationship of TIMI myocardial perfusion grade to mortality after administration of thrombolytic drugs. Circulation 2000;101:125-130.
195. Gibson CM, Schomig A: Coronary and myocardial angiography: Angiographic assessment of both epicardial and myocardial perfusion. Circulation 2004;109:3096-3105.
196. Antman EM, Giugliano RP, Gibson CM, et al: Abciximab facilitates the rate and extent of thrombolysis: Results of the Thrombolysis in Myocardial Infarction (TIMI) 14 trial. The TIMI 14 Investigators. Circulation 1999;99:2720-2732.
197. Trial of abciximab with and without low-dose reteplase for acute myocardial infarction. Strategies for Patency Enhancement in the Emergency Department (SPEED) Group. Circulation 2000;101:2788-2794.
198. Topol EJ: Reperfusion therapy for acute myocardial infarction with fibrinolytic therapy or combination reduced fibrinolytic therapy and platelet glycoprotein IIb/IIIa inhibition: The GUSTO V randomised trial. Lancet 2001;357:1905-1914.
199. Berkowitz SD, Granger CB, Pieper KS, et al: Incidence and predictors of bleeding after contemporary thrombolytic therapy for myocardial infarction. The Global Utilization of Streptokinase and Tissue Plasminogen Activator for Occluded Coronary Arteries (GUSTO) I Investigators. Circulation 1997;95:2508-2516.
200. Gurwitz JH, Gore JM, Goldberg RJ, et al: Risk for intracranial hemorrhage after tissue plasminogen activator

treatment for acute myocardial infarction. Participants in the National Registry of Myocardial Infarction 2. Ann Intern Med 1998;129:597-604.
201. Mehta SR, Eikelboom JW, Yusuf S: Risk of intracranial haemorrhage with bolus versus infusion thrombolytic therapy: A meta-analysis. Lancet 2000;356: 449-454.
202. Eikelboom JW, Mehta SR, Pogue J, et al: Safety outcomes in meta-analyses of phase 2 vs phase 3 randomized trials: Intracranial hemorrhage in trials of bolus thrombolytic therapy. JAMA 2001;285:444-450.
203. Mahaffey KW, Granger CB, Sloan MA, et al: Neurosurgical evacuation of intracranial hemorrhage after thrombolytic therapy for acute myocardial infarction: Experience from the GUSTO-I trial. Global Utilization of Streptokinase and Tissue-Plasminogen Activator (tPA) for Occluded Coronary Arteries. Am Heart J 1999;138: 493-499.
204. White HD, Van de Werf FJ: Thrombolysis for acute myocardial infarction. Circulation 1998;97: 1632-1646.
205. Karnash SL, Granger CB, White HD, et al: Treating menstruating women with thrombolytic therapy: Insights from the global utilization of streptokinase and tissue plasminogen activator for occluded coronary arteries (GUSTO-I) trial. J Am Coll Cardiol 1995;26:1651-1656.
206. Bottiger BW, Bode C, Kern S, et al: Efficacy and safety of thrombolytic therapy after initially unsuccessful cardiopulmonary resuscitation: A prospective clinical trial. Lancet 2001;357:1583-1585.
207. Holmes DR Jr, White HD, Pieper KS, et al: Effect of age on outcome with primary angioplasty versus thrombolysis. J Am Coll Cardiol 1999;33:412-419.
208. Gore JM, Granger CB, Simoons ML, et al: Stroke after thrombolysis. Mortality and functional outcomes in the GUSTO-I trial. Global Use of Strategies to Open Occluded Coronary Arteries. Circulation 1995;92: 2811-2818.
209. Thiemann DR, Coresh J, Schulman SP, et al: Lack of benefit for intravenous thrombolysis in patients with myocardial infarction who are older than 75 years. Circulation 2000;101:2239-2246.
210. Stenestrand U, Wallentin L: Fibrinolytic therapy in patients 75 years and older with ST-segment-elevation myocardial infarction: One-year follow-up of a large prospective cohort. Arch Intern Med 2003;163:965-971.
211. de Boer MJ, Ottervanger JP, van't Hof AW, et al: Reperfusion therapy in elderly patients with acute myocardial infarction: A randomized comparison of primary angioplasty and thrombolytic therapy. J Am Coll Cardiol 2002;39:1723-1728.
212. Cragg DR, Friedman HZ, Bonema JD, et al: Outcome of patients with acute myocardial infarction who are ineligible for thrombolytic therapy. Ann Intern Med 1991;115:173-177.
213. McCullough PA, O'Neill WW, Graham M, et al: A prospective randomized trial of triage angiography in acute coronary syndromes ineligible for thrombolytic therapy. Results of the medicine versus angiography in thrombolytic exclusion (MATE) trial. J Am Coll Cardiol 1998;32:596-605.
214. Grzybowski M, Clements EA, Parsons L, et al: Mortality benefit of immediate revascularization of acute ST-segment elevation myocardial infarction in patients with contraindications to thrombolytic therapy: A propensity analysis. JAMA 2003;290:1891-1898.
215. Gruntzig A: Transluminal dilatation of coronary-artery stenosis. Lancet 1978;1:263.
216. Rentrop KP, Blanke H, Karsch KR, et al: Initial experience with transluminal recanalization of the recently occluded infarct-related coronary artery in acute myocardial infarction—comparison with conventionally treated patients. Clin Cardiol 1979;2:92-105.
217. Rentrop P, Blanke H, Wiegand V, et al: [Recanalization by catheter of the occluded artery after acute myocardial infarction (transluminal recanalization)]. Dtsch Med Wochenschr 1979;104:1401-1405 [Author's translation].
218. O'Neill W, Timmis GC, Bourdillon PD, et al: A prospective randomized clinical trial of intracoronary streptokinase versus coronary angioplasty for acute myocardial infarction. N Engl J Med 1986; 314:812-818.
219. Keeley EC, Boura JA, Grines CL: Primary angioplasty versus intravenous thrombolytic therapy for acute myocardial infarction: A quantitative review of 23 randomised trials. Lancet 2003;361:13-20.
220. Laster SB, O'Keefe JH Jr, Gibbons RJ: Incidence and importance of thrombolysis in myocardial infarction grade 3 flow after primary percutaneous transluminal coronary angioplasty for acute myocardial infarction. Am J Cardiol 1996;78: 623-626.
221. van't Hof AW, Liem A, Suryapranata H, et al: Angiographic assessment of myocardial reperfusion in patients treated with primary angioplasty for acute myocardial infarction: Myocardial blush grade. Zwolle Myocardial Infarction Study Group. Circulation 1998;97:2302-2306.
222. Stone GW, Peterson MA, Lansky AJ, et al: Impact of normalized myocardial perfusion after successful angioplasty in acute myocardial infarction. J Am Coll Cardiol 2002;39:591-597.
223. Dibra A, Mehilli J, Dirschinger J, et al: Thrombolysis in myocardial infarction myocardial perfusion grade in angiography correlates with myocardial salvage in patients with acute myocardial infarction treated with stenting or thrombolysis. J Am Coll Cardiol 2003;41:925-929.
224. Andersen HR, Nielsen TT, Rasmussen K, et al: A comparison of coronary angioplasty with fibrinolytic therapy in acute myocardial infarction. N Engl J Med 2003;349:733-742.
225. Henriques JP, Haasdijk AP, Zijlstra F: Outcome of primary angioplasty for acute myocardial infarction during routine duty hours versus during off-hours. J Am Coll Cardiol 2003;41:2138-2142.
226. Henriques JP, Zijlstra F, Ottervanger JP, et al: Incidence and clinical significance of distal embolization during primary angioplasty for acute myocardial infarction. Eur Heart J 2002;23:1112-1117.
227. Wu KC, Zerhouni EA, Judd RM, et al: Prognostic significance of microvascular obstruction by magnetic resonance imaging in patients with acute myocardial infarction. Circulation 1998;97:765-772.
228. Beran G, Lang I, Schreiber W, et al: Intracoronary thrombectomy with the X-Sizer catheter system improves epicardial flow and accelerates ST-segment resolution in patients with acute coronary syndrome: A prospective, randomized, controlled study. Circulation 2002;105: 2355-2360.
229. Napodano M, Pasquetto G, Sacca S, et al: Intracoronary thrombectomy improves myocardial reperfusion in patients undergoing direct angioplasty for acute myocardial infarction. J Am Coll Cardiol 2003;42:1395-1402.
230. Antoniucci D, Valenti R, Migliorini A, et al: Comparison of rheolytic thrombectomy before direct infarct artery stenting versus direct stenting alone in patients undergoing percutaneous coronary intervention for acute myocardial infarction. Am J Cardiol 2004;93:1033-1035.
231. Lefevre T, Garcia E, Reimers B, et al: X-sizer for thrombectomy in acute myocardial infarction improves ST-segment resolution: Results of the X-Sizer in AMI for negligible embolization and optimal ST resolution (X AMINE ST) trial. J Am Coll Cardiol 2005;46:246-252.
232. Stone GW, Webb J, Cox DA, et al: Distal microcirculatory protection during percutaneous coronary intervention in acute ST-segment elevation myocardial infarction: A randomized controlled trial. JAMA 2005;293:1063-1072.
233. Gick M, Jander N, Bestehorn HP, et al: Randomized evaluation of the effects of filter-based distal protection on myocardial perfusion and infarct size after primary percutaneous catheter intervention in myocardial infarction with and without ST-segment elevation. Circulation 2006;112: 1462-1469.
234. Ali A, Cox D, Dib N, et al: Rheolytic thrombectomy with percutaneous coronary intervention for infarct size reduction in acute myocardial infarction: 30-day results from a multicenter randomized study. J Am Coll Cardiol 2006;48:244-252.
235. Neumann FJ, Blasini R, Schmitt C, et al: Effect of glycoprotein IIb/IIIa receptor blockade on recovery of coronary flow and left ventricular function after the placement of coronary-artery stents in acute myocardial infarction. Circulation 1998;98:2695-2701.
236. Marzilli M, Orsini E, Marraccini P, et al: Beneficial effects of intracoronary adenosine as an adjunct to primary angioplasty in acute myocardial

infarction. Circulation 2000;101: 2154-2159.
237. Assali AR, Sdringola S, Ghani M, et al: Intracoronary adenosine administered during percutaneous intervention in acute myocardial infarction and reduction in the incidence of "no reflow" phenomenon. Catheter Cardiovasc Interv 2000;51:27-31; discussion 32.
238. Claeys MJ, Bosmans J, De Ceuninck M, et al: Effect of intracoronary adenosine infusion during coronary intervention on myocardial reperfusion injury in patients with acute myocardial infarction. Am J Cardiol 2004;94:9-13.
239. Keeley EC, Grines CL: Primary percutaneous coronary intervention for every patient with ST-segment elevation myocardial infarction: What stands in the way? Ann Intern Med 2004;141:298-304.
240. Brophy JM, Bogaty P: Primary angioplasty and thrombolysis are both reasonable options in acute myocardial infarction. Ann Intern Med 2004;141: 292-297.
241. Every NR, Parsons LS, Hlatky M, et al: A comparison of thrombolytic therapy with primary coronary angioplasty for acute myocardial infarction. Myocardial Infarction Triage and Intervention Investigators. N Engl J Med 1996;335:1253-1260.
242. Tiefenbrunn AJ, Chandra NC, French WJ, et al: Clinical experience with primary percutaneous transluminal coronary angioplasty compared with alteplase (recombinant tissue-type plasminogen activator) in patients with acute myocardial infarction: A report from the Second National Registry of Myocardial Infarction (NRMI-2). J Am Coll Cardiol 1998;31:1240-1245.
243. Berger AK, Schulman KA, Gersh BJ, et al: Primary coronary angioplasty vs thrombolysis for the management of acute myocardial infarction in elderly patients. JAMA 1999;282:341-348.
244. Grines C, Patel A, Zijlstra F, et al: Primary coronary angioplasty compared with intravenous thrombolytic therapy for acute myocardial infarction: Six-month follow up and analysis of individual patient data from randomized trials. Am Heart J 2003;145:47-57.
245. Canto JG, Every NR, Magid DJ, et al: The volume of primary angioplasty procedures and survival after acute myocardial infarction. National Registry of Myocardial Infarction 2 Investigators. N Engl J Med 2000;342:1573-1580.
246. Nallamothu BK, Wang Y, Magid DJ, et al: Relation between hospital specialization with primary percutaneous coronary intervention and clinical outcomes in ST-segment elevation myocardial infarction: National Registry of Myocardial Infarction-4 analysis. Circulation 2006;113:222-229.
247. Liem AL, van't Hof AW, Hoorntje JC, et al: Influence of treatment delay on infarct size and clinical outcome in patients with acute myocardial infarction treated with primary angioplasty. J Am Coll Cardiol 1998;32:629-633.
248. Berger PB, Ellis SG, Holmes DR Jr, et al: Relationship between delay in performing direct coronary angioplasty and early clinical outcome in patients with acute myocardial infarction: Results from the global use of strategies to open occluded arteries in Acute Coronary Syndromes (GUSTO-IIb) trial. Circulation 1999;100:14-20.
249. Cannon CP, Gibson CM, Lambrew CT, et al: Relationship of symptom-onset-to-balloon time and door-to-balloon time with mortality in patients undergoing angioplasty for acute myocardial infarction. JAMA 2000;283:2941-2947.
250. De Luca G, Suryapranata H, Ottervanger JP, et al: Time delay to treatment and mortality in primary angioplasty for acute myocardial infarction: Every minute of delay counts. Circulation 2004;109: 1223-1235.
251. Juliard JM, Feldman LJ, Golmard JL, et al: Relation of mortality of primary angioplasty during acute myocardial infarction to door-to-Thrombolysis in Myocardial Infarction (TIMI) time. Am J Cardiol 91:1401-1405.
252. Brodie BR, Hansen C, Stuckey TD, et al: Door-to-balloon time with primary percutaneous coronary intervention for acute myocardial infarction impacts late cardiac mortality in high-risk patients and patients presenting early after the onset of symptoms. J Am Coll Cardiol 2006;47:289-295.
253. McNamara RL, Wang Y, Herrin J, et al: Effect of door-to-balloon time on mortality in patients with ST-segment elevation myocardial infarction. J Am Coll Cardiol 2006;47:2180-2186.
254. Brodie BR, Stone GW, Cox DA, et al: Impact of treatment delays on outcomes of primary percutaneous coronary intervention for acute myocardial infarction: Analysis from the CADILLAC trial. Am Heart J 2006;151:1231-1238.
255. Nallamothu BK, Bates ER, Herrin J, et al: Times to treatment in transfer patients undergoing primary percutaneous coronary intervention in the United States: National Registry of Myocardial Infarction (NRMI)-3/4 analysis. Circulation 2005;111: 761-767.
256. Magid DJ, Wang Y, Herrin J, et al: Relationship between time of day, day of week, timeliness of reperfusion, and in-hospital mortality for patients with acute ST-segment elevation myocardial infarction. JAMA 2005;294:803-812.
257. Nallamothu BK, Bates ER: Percutaneous coronary intervention versus fibrinolytic therapy in acute myocardial infarction: Is timing (almost) everything? Am J Cardiol 2003;92:824-826.
258. Weaver WD, Litwin PE, Martin JS: Use of direct angioplasty for treatment of patients with acute myocardial infarction in hospitals with and without on-site cardiac surgery. The Myocardial Infarction, Triage, and Intervention Project Investigators. Circulation 1993;88:2067-2075.
259. Aversano T, Aversano LT, Passamani E, et al: Thrombolytic therapy vs primary percutaneous coronary intervention for myocardial infarction in patients presenting to hospitals without on-site cardiac surgery: A randomized controlled trial. JAMA 2002;287: 1943-1951.
260. Bradley EH, Herrin J, Wang Y, et al: Strategies for reducing the door-to-balloon time in acute myocardial infarction. N Engl J Med 2006;355: 2308-2320.
261. Bauters C, Delomez M, Van Belle E, et al: Angiographically documented late reocclusion after successful coronary angioplasty of an infarct-related lesion is a powerful predictor of long-term mortality. Circulation 1999;99:2243-2250.
262. Stone GW, Grines CL, Cox DA, et al: Comparison of angioplasty with stenting, with or without abciximab, in acute myocardial infarction. N Engl J Med 2002;346:957-966.
263. Costantini CO, Stone GW, Mehran R, et al: Frequency, correlates, and clinical implications of myocardial perfusion after primary angioplasty and stenting, with and without glycoprotein IIb/IIIa inhibition, in acute myocardial infarction. J Am Coll Cardiol 2004;44:305-312.
264. Spaulding C, Henry P, Teiger E, et al: Sirolimus-eluting versus uncoated stents in acute myocardial infarction. N Engl J Med 2006;355:1093-1104.
265. Laarman GJ, Suttorp MJ, Dirksen MT, et al: Paclitaxel-eluting versus uncoated stents in primary percutaneous coronary intervention. N Engl J Med 2006;355:1105-1113.
266. de Lemos JA, Antman EM, Giugliano RP, et al: ST-segment resolution and infarct-related artery patency and flow after thrombolytic therapy. Thrombolysis in Myocardial Infarction (TIMI) 14 investigators. Am J Cardiol 2000;85:299-304.
267. Schweiger MJ, Cannon CP, Murphy SA, et al: Early coronary intervention following pharmacologic therapy for acute myocardial infarction (the combined TIMI 10B–TIMI 14 experience). Am J Cardiol 2001;88:831-836.
268. Sutton AG, Campbell PG, Graham R, et al: A randomized trial of rescue angioplasty versus a conservative approach for failed fibrinolysis in ST-segment elevation myocardial infarction: the Middlesbrough Early Revascularization to Limit Infarction (MERLIN) trial. J Am Coll Cardiol 2004;44:287-296.
269. Gershlick AH, Stephens-Lloyd A, Hughes S, et al: Rescue angioplasty after failed thrombolytic therapy for acute myocardial infarction. N Engl J Med 2005;353:2758-2768.
270. Gibson CM, Cannon CP, Murphy SA, et al: Relationship of the TIMI myocardial perfusion grades, flow grades, frame count, and percutaneous coronary intervention to long-term outcomes after thrombolytic administration in acute myocardial infarction. Circulation 2002;105: 1909-1913.
271. Patel TN, Bavry AA, Kumbhani DJ, et al: A meta-analysis of randomized trials of rescue percutaneous coronary intervention after failed fibrinolysis. Am J Cardiol 2006;97:1685-1690.

272. Wijeysundera HC, Vijayaraghavan R, Nallamothu BK, et al: Rescue angioplasty or repeat fibrinolysis after failed fibrinolytic therapy for ST-segment myocardial infarction: A meta-analysis of randomized trials. J Am Coll Cardiol 2007;49:422-430.
273. Barron HV, Bowlby LJ, Breen T, et al: Use of reperfusion therapy for acute myocardial infarction in the United States: Data from the National Registry of Myocardial Infarction 2. Circulation 1998;97:1150-1156.
274. Wu AH, Parsons L, Every NR, et al: Hospital outcomes in patients presenting with congestive heart failure complicating acute myocardial infarction: A report from the Second National Registry of Myocardial Infarction (NRMI-2). J Am Coll Cardiol 2002;40:1389-1394.
275. Thune JJ, Hoefsten DE, Lindholm MG, et al: Simple risk stratification at admission to identify patients with reduced mortality from primary angioplasty. Circulation 2005;112: 2017-2021.
276. Grines CL, Booth DC, Nissen SE, et al: Mechanism of acute myocardial infarction in patients with prior coronary artery bypass grafting and therapeutic implications. Am J Cardiol 1990;65:1292-1296.
277. Stone GW, Brodie BR, Griffin JJ, et al: Clinical and angiographic outcomes in patients with previous coronary artery bypass graft surgery treated with primary balloon angioplasty for acute myocardial infarction. Second Primary Angioplasty in Myocardial Infarction Trial (PAMI-2) Investigators. J Am Coll Cardiol 2000;35:605-611.
278. Schomig A, Mehilli J, Antoniucci D, et al: Mechanical reperfusion in patients with acute myocardial infarction presenting more than 12 hours from symptom onset: A randomized controlled trial. JAMA 2005;293:2865-2872.
279. Hochman JS, Lamas GA, Buller CE, et al: Coronary intervention for persistent occlusion after myocardial infarction. N Engl J Med 2006;355: 2395-2407.
280. De Luca G, Suryapranata H, Stone GW, et al: Abciximab as adjunctive therapy to reperfusion in acute ST-segment elevation myocardial infarction: A meta-analysis of randomized trials. JAMA 2005;293: 1759-1765.
281. de Lemos JA, Antman EM, Gibson CM, et al: Abciximab improves both epicardial flow and myocardial reperfusion in ST-elevation myocardial infarction. Observations from the TIMI 14 trial. Circulation 2000;101: 239-243.
282. Lincoff AM, Califf RM, Van de Werf F, et al: Mortality at 1 year with combination platelet glycoprotein IIb/IIIa inhibition and reduced-dose fibrinolytic therapy vs conventional fibrinolytic therapy for acute myocardial infarction: GUSTO V randomized trial. JAMA 2002;288: 2130-2135.
283. Montalescot G, Borentain M, Payot L, et al: Early vs late administration of glycoprotein IIb/IIIa inhibitors in primary percutaneous coronary intervention of acute ST-segment elevation myocardial infarction: A meta-analysis. JAMA 2004;292: 362-366.
284. Lee DP, Herity NA, Hiatt BL, et al: Adjunctive platelet glycoprotein IIb/IIIa receptor inhibition with tirofiban before primary angioplasty improves angiographic outcomes: Results of the TIrofiban Given in the Emergency Room before Primary Angioplasty (TIGER-PA) pilot trial. Circulation 2003;107:1497-1501.
285. Stone GW, Cox D, Garcia E, et al: Normal flow (TIMI-3) before mechanical reperfusion therapy is an independent determinant of survival in acute myocardial infarction: Analysis from the primary angioplasty in myocardial infarction trials. Circulation 2001;104:636-641.
286. Anderson JL, Rodier HE, Green LS: Comparative effects of beta-adrenergic blocking drugs on experimental ventricular fibrillation threshold. Am J Cardiol 1983;51:1196-1202.
287. Ryden L, Ariniego R, Arnman K, et al: A double-blind trial of metoprolol in acute myocardial infarction. Effects on ventricular tachyarrhythmias. N Engl J Med 1983;308:614-618.
288. Chen ZM, Pan HC, Chen YP, et al: Early intravenous then oral metoprolol in 45,852 patients with acute myocardial infarction: Randomised placebo-controlled trial. Lancet 2005;366:1622-1632.
289. Reduction of infarct size with the early use of timolol in acute myocardial infarction. N Engl J Med 1984;310: 9-15.
290. Roque F, Amuchastegui LM, Lopez Morillos MA, et al: Beneficial effects of timolol on infarct size and late ventricular tachycardia in patients with acute myocardial infarction. Circulation 1987;76:610-617.
291. Roberts R, Croft C, Gold HK, et al: Effect of propranolol on myocardial-infarct size in a randomized blinded multicenter trial. N Engl J Med 1984;311:218-225.
292. Randomised trial of intravenous atenolol among 16 027 cases of suspected acute myocardial infarction: ISIS-1. First International Study of Infarct Survival Collaborative Group. Lancet 1986;2:57-66.
293. Hjalmarson A, Elmfeldt D, Herlitz J, et al: Effect on mortality of metoprolol in acute myocardial infarction. A double-blind randomised trial. Lancet 1981;2:823-827.
294. Yusuf S, Wittes J, Friedman L: Overview of results of randomized clinical trials in heart disease. I. Treatments following myocardial infarction. JAMA 1988;260: 2088-2093.
295. Roberts R, Rogers WJ, Mueller HS, et al: Immediate versus deferred beta-blockade following thrombolytic therapy in patients with acute myocardial infarction. Results of the Thrombolysis in Myocardial Infarction (TIMI) II-B Study. Circulation 1991;83:422-437.
296. Pfisterer M, Cox JL, Granger CB, et al: Atenolol use and clinical outcomes after thrombolysis for acute myocardial infarction: The GUSTO-I experience. Global Utilization of Streptokinase and tPA (Alteplase) for Occluded Coronary Arteries. J Am Coll Cardiol 1998;32: 634-640.
297. Hennekens CH, Albert CM, Godfried SL, et al: Adjunctive drug therapy of acute myocardial infarction—evidence from clinical trials. N Engl J Med 1996;335:1660-1667.
298. Freemantle N, Cleland J, Young P, et al: Beta blockade after myocardial infarction: Systematic review and meta regression analysis. BMJ 1999;318: 1730-1737.
299. Timolol-induced reduction in mortality and reinfarction in patients surviving acute myocardial infarction. N Engl J Med 1981;304:801-807.
300. Pedersen TR: Six-year follow-up of the Norwegian Multicenter Study on Timolol after Acute Myocardial Infarction. N Engl J Med 1985; 313:1055-1058.
301. A randomized trial of propranolol in patients with acute myocardial infarction. I. Mortality results. JAMA 1982;247:1707-1714.
302. Dargie HJ: Effect of carvedilol on outcome after myocardial infarction in patients with left-ventricular dysfunction: The CAPRICORN randomised trial. Lancet 2001;357: 1385-1390.
303. Rouleau JL, Packer M, Moye L, et al: Prognostic value of neurohumoral activation in patients with an acute myocardial infarction: Effect of captopril. J Am Coll Cardiol 1994;24:583-591.
304. St John Sutton M, Pfeffer MA, Plappert T, et al: Quantitative two-dimensional echocardiographic measurements are major predictors of adverse cardiovascular events after acute myocardial infarction. The protective effects of captopril. Circulation 1994;89:68-75, 1994.
305. Indications for ACE inhibitors in the early treatment of acute myocardial infarction: Systematic overview of individual data from 100,000 patients in randomized trials. ACE Inhibitor Myocardial Infarction Collaborative Group. Circulation 1998;97: 2202-2212.
306. Pfeffer MA, Braunwald E, Moye LA, et al: Effect of captopril on mortality and morbidity in patients with left ventricular dysfunction after myocardial infarction. Results of the survival and ventricular enlargement trial. The SAVE Investigators. N Engl J Med 1992;327:669-677.
307. Effect of ramipril on mortality and morbidity of survivors of acute myocardial infarction with clinical evidence of heart failure. The Acute Infarction Ramipril Efficacy (AIRE) Study Investigators. Lancet 1993;342: 821-828.
308. Kober L, Torp-Pedersen C, Carlsen JE, et al: A clinical trial of the angiotensin-converting-enzyme inhibitor trandolapril in patients with left ventricular dysfunction after myocardial infarction. Trandolapril Cardiac Evaluation (TRACE) Study Group. N Engl J Med 1995;333: 1670-1676.
309. Rutherford JD, Pfeffer MA, Moye LA, et al: Effects of captopril on ischemic

events after myocardial infarction. Results of the Survival and Ventricular Enlargement trial. SAVE Investigators. Circulation 1994;90: 1731-1738.
310. Torp-Pedersen C, Kober L: Effect of ACE inhibitor trandolapril on life expectancy of patients with reduced left-ventricular function after acute myocardial infarction. TRACE Study Group. Trandolapril Cardiac Evaluation. Lancet 1999;354:9-12.
311. Flather MD, Yusuf S, Kober L, et al: Long-term ACE-inhibitor therapy in patients with heart failure or left-ventricular dysfunction: A systematic overview of data from individual patients. ACE-Inhibitor Myocardial Infarction Collaborative Group. Lancet 2000;355:1575-1581.
312. Dickstein K, Kjekshus J: Effects of losartan and captopril on mortality and morbidity in high-risk patients after acute myocardial infarction: The OPTIMAAL randomised trial. Optimal Trial in Myocardial Infarction with Angiotensin II Antagonist Losartan. Lancet 2002;360:752-760.
313. Pfeffer MA, McMurray JJ, Velazquez EJ, et al: Valsartan, captopril, or both in myocardial infarction complicated by heart failure, left ventricular dysfunction, or both. N Engl J Med 2003;349:1893-1906.
314. Cohn JN, Colucci W: Cardiovascular effects of aldosterone and post-acute myocardial infarction pathophysiology. Am J Cardiol 2006;97:4F-12F.
315. Pitt B, Remme W, Zannad F, et al: Eplerenone, a selective aldosterone blocker, in patients with left ventricular dysfunction after myocardial infarction. N Engl J Med 2003;348:1309-1321.
316. Crenshaw BS, Ward SR, Granger CB, et al: Atrial fibrillation in the setting of acute myocardial infarction: The GUSTO-I experience. Global Utilization of Streptokinase and TPA for Occluded Coronary Arteries. J Am Coll Cardiol 1997;30:406-413.
317. Pedersen OD, Bagger H, Kober L, et al: The occurrence and prognostic significance of atrial fibrillation/flutter following acute myocardial infarction. TRACE Study Group. Trandolapril Cardiac Evalution. Eur Heart J 1999;20:748-754.
318. Thompson CA, Yarzebski J, Goldberg RJ, et al: Changes over time in the incidence and case-fatality rates of primary ventricular fibrillation complicating acute myocardial infarction: Perspectives from the Worcester Heart Attack Study. Am Heart J 2000;139:1014-1021.
319. Volpi A, Maggioni A, Franzosi MG, et al: In-hospital prognosis of patients with acute myocardial infarction complicated by primary ventricular fibrillation. N Engl J Med 1987;317:257-261.
320. Solomon SD, Ridker PM, Antman EM: Ventricular arrhythmias in trials of thrombolytic therapy for acute myocardial infarction. A meta-analysis. Circulation 1993;88:2575-2581.
321. Volpi A, Cavalli A, Santoro E, et al: Incidence and prognosis of secondary ventricular fibrillation in acute myocardial infarction. Evidence for a protective effect of thrombolytic therapy. Circulation 1990;82: 1279-1288.
322. Volpi A, Cavalli A, Santoro L, et al: Incidence and prognosis of early primary ventricular fibrillation in acute myocardial infarction—results of the Gruppo Italiano per lo Studio della Sopravvivenza nell'Infarto Miocardico (GISSI-2) database. Am J Cardiol 1998;82:265-271.
323. Volpi A, Cavalli A, Franzosi MG, et al: One-year prognosis of primary ventricular fibrillation complicating acute myocardial infarction. The GISSI (Gruppo Italiano per lo Studio della Streptochinasi nell'Infarto Miocardico) investigators. Am J Cardiol 1989;63: 1174-1178.
324. Lie KI, Wellens HJ, van Capelle FJ, et al: Lidocaine in the prevention of primary ventricular fibrillation. A double-blind, randomized study of 212 consecutive patients. N Engl J Med 1974;291: 1324-1326.
325. Harrison DC: Should lidocaine be administered routinely to all patients after acute myocardial infarction? Circulation 1978;58:581-584.
326. Sadowski ZP, Alexander JH, Skrabucha B, et al: Multicenter randomized trial and a systematic overview of lidocaine in acute myocardial infarction. Am Heart J 1999;137:792-798.
327. Echt DS, Liebson PR, Mitchell LB, et al: Mortality and morbidity in patients receiving encainide, flecainide, or placebo. The Cardiac Arrhythmia Suppression Trial. N Engl J Med 1991;324:781-788.
328. Effect of the antiarrhythmic agent moricizine on survival after myocardial infarction. The Cardiac Arrhythmia Suppression Trial II Investigators. N Engl J Med 1992;327:227-233.
329. Waldo AL, Camm AJ, deRuyter H, et al: Effect of *d*-sotalol on mortality in patients with left ventricular dysfunction after recent and remote myocardial infarction. The SWORD Investigators. Survival with Oral *d*-Sotalol. Lancet 1996;348:7-12.
330. Julian DG, Camm AJ, Frangin G, et al: Randomised trial of effect of amiodarone on mortality in patients with left-ventricular dysfunction after recent myocardial infarction: EMIAT. European Myocardial Infarct Amiodarone Trial Investigators. Lancet 1997;349:667-674.
331. Cairns JA, Connolly SJ, Roberts R, et al: Randomised trial of outcome after myocardial infarction in patients with frequent or repetitive ventricular premature depolarisations: CAMIAT. Canadian Amiodarone Myocardial Infarction Arrhythmia Trial Investigators. Lancet 1997;349: 675-682.
332. Moss AJ, Zareba W, Hall WJ, et al: Prophylactic implantation of a defibrillator in patients with myocardial infarction and reduced ejection fraction. N Engl J Med 2002;346:877-883.
333. Held P, Yusuf S, Furberg C: Calcium channel blockers in acute myocardial infarction and unstable angina: An overview. BMJ 1989;299:1187-1192.
334. Teo KK, Yusuf S, Furberg CD: Effects of prophylactic antiarrhythmic drug therapy in acute myocardial infarction. An overview of results from randomized controlled trials. JAMA 1993;270:1589-1595.
335. The effect of diltiazem on mortality and reinfarction after myocardial infarction. The Multicenter Diltiazem Postinfarction Trial Research Group. N Engl J Med 1988;319:385-392.
336. Goldstein RE, Boccuzzi SJ, Cruess D, et al: Diltiazem increases late-onset congestive heart failure in postinfarction patients with early reduction in ejection fraction. The Adverse Experience Committee; and the Multicenter Diltiazem Postinfarction Research Group. Circulation 1991;83:52-60.
337. Randomised trial of cholesterol lowering in 4444 patients with coronary heart disease: The Scandinavian Simvastatin Survival Study (4S). Lancet 1994;344: 1383-1389.
338. Sacks FM, Pfeffer MA, Moye LA, et al: The effect of pravastatin on coronary events after myocardial infarction in patients with average cholesterol levels. Cholesterol and Recurrent Events Trial investigators. N Engl J Med 1996;335:1001-1009.
339. Prevention of cardiovascular events and death with pravastatin in patients with coronary heart disease and a broad range of initial cholesterol levels. The Long-Term Intervention with Pravastatin in Ischaemic Disease (LIPID) Study Group. N Engl J Med 1998;339:1349-1357.
340. Rosenson RS: Myocardial injury: The acute phase response and lipoprotein metabolism. J Am Coll Cardiol 1993;22:933-940.
341. Cannon CP, Braunwald E, McCabe CH, et al: Intensive versus moderate lipid lowering with statins after acute coronary syndromes. N Engl J Med 2004;350:1495-1504.
342. O'Keefe JH, Jr., Cordain L, Harris WH, et al: Optimal low-density lipoprotein is 50 to 70 mg/dL: Lower is better and physiologically normal. J Am Coll Cardiol 2004;43:2142-2146.
343. Cannon CP, Steinberg BA, Murphy SA, et al: Meta-analysis of cardiovascular outcomes trials comparing intensive versus moderate statin therapy. J Am Coll Cardiol 2006;48:438-445.
344. DeWood MA, Spores J, Notske RN, et al: Medical and surgical management of myocardial infarction. Am J Cardiol 1979;44:1356-1364.
345. Lee DC, Oz MC, Weinberg AD, et al: Optimal timing of revascularization: Transmural versus nontransmural acute myocardial infarction. Ann Thorac Surg 2001;71:1197-1202; discussion 1202-1204.
346. White HD, Assmann SF, Sanborn TA, et al: Comparison of percutaneous coronary intervention and coronary artery bypass grafting after acute myocardial infarction complicated by cardiogenic shock: Results from the Should We Emergently Revascularize Occluded Coronaries for Cardiogenic Shock (SHOCK) trial. Circulation 2005;112:1992-2001.

347. Tofler GH, Muller JE, Stone PH, et al: Pericarditis in acute myocardial infarction: Characterization and clinical significance. Am Heart J 1989;117:86-92, 1989.
348. Krainin FM, Flessas AP, Spodick DH: Infarction-associated pericarditis. Rarity of diagnostic electrocardiogram. N Engl J Med 1984;311:1211-1214.
349. Correale E, Maggioni AP, Romano S, et al: Comparison of frequency, diagnostic and prognostic significance of pericardial involvement in acute myocardial infarction treated with and without thrombolytics. Gruppo Italiano per lo Studio della Sopravvivenza nell'Infarto Miocardico (GISSI). Am J Cardiol 1993;71:1377-1381.
350. Patel MR, Meine TJ, Lindblad L, et al: Cardiac tamponade in the fibrinolytic era: Analysis of >100,000 patients with ST-segment elevation myocardial infarction. Am Heart J 2006;151:316-322.
351. Hochman JS, Buller CE, Sleeper LA, et al: Cardiogenic shock complicating acute myocardial infarction—etiologies, management and outcome: A report from the SHOCK Trial Registry. Should We Emergently Revascularize Occluded Coronaries for Cardiogenic Shock? J Am Coll Cardiol 2000;36:1063-1070.
352. Hudson MP, Granger CB, Topol EJ, et al: Early reinfarction after fibrinolysis: Experience from the Global Utilization of Streptokinase and Tissue Plasminogen Activator (Alteplase) for Occluded Coronary Arteries (GUSTO I) and Global Use of Strategies to Open Occluded Coronary Arteries (GUSTO III) trials. Circulation 2001;104:1229-1235.
353. Gibson CM, Karha J, Murphy SA, et al: Early and long-term clinical outcomes associated with reinfarction following fibrinolytic administration in the Thrombolysis in Myocardial Infarction trials. J Am Coll Cardiol 2003;42:7-16.
354. Andreotti F, Testa L, Biondi-Zoccai GG, et al: Aspirin plus warfarin compared to aspirin alone after acute coronary syndromes: An updated and comprehensive meta-analysis of 25,307 patients. Eur Heart J 2006;27:519-526.
355. Rothberg MB, Celestin C, Fiore LD, et al: Warfarin plus aspirin after myocardial infarction or the acute coronary syndrome: Meta-analysis with estimates of risk and benefit. Ann Intern Med 2005;143:241-250.
356. Smith P, Arnesen H, Holme I: The effect of warfarin on mortality and reinfarction after myocardial infarction. N Engl J Med 1990;323:147-152.
357. van Es RF, Jonker JJ, Verheugt FW, et al: Aspirin and coumadin after acute coronary syndromes (the ASPECT-2 study): A randomised controlled trial. Lancet 2002;360:109-113.
358. Brouwer MA, van den Bergh PJ, Aengevaeren WR, et al: Aspirin plus coumarin versus aspirin alone in the prevention of reocclusion after fibrinolysis for acute myocardial infarction: Results of the Antithrombotics in the Prevention of Reocclusion in Coronary Thrombolysis (APRICOT)-2 Trial. Circulation 2002;106:659-665.
359. Hurlen M, Abdelnoor M, Smith P, et al: Warfarin, aspirin, or both after myocardial infarction. N Engl J Med 2002;347:969-974.
360. Fiore LD, Ezekowitz MD, Brophy MT, et al: Department of Veterans Affairs Cooperative Studies Program Clinical Trial comparing combined warfarin and aspirin with aspirin alone in survivors of acute myocardial infarction: Primary results of the CHAMP study. Circulation 2002;105:557-563.
361. Randomised double-blind trial of fixed low-dose warfarin with aspirin after myocardial infarction. Coumadin Aspirin Reinfarction Study (CARS) Investigators. Lancet 1997;350:389-396.
362. Gibson CM, Ly HQ, Murphy SA, et al: Usefulness of clopidogrel in abolishing the increased risk of reinfarction associated with higher platelet counts in patients with ST-elevation myocardial infarction (results from CLARITY–TIMI 28). Am J Cardiol 2006;98:761-763.
363. Briel M, Schwartz GG, Thompson PL, et al: Effects of early treatment with statins on short-term clinical outcomes in acute coronary syndromes: A meta-analysis of randomized controlled trials. JAMA 2006;295:2046-2056.
364. Hulten E, Jackson JL, Douglas K, et al: The effect of early, intensive statin therapy on acute coronary syndrome: A meta-analysis of randomized controlled trials. Arch Intern Med 2006;166:1814-1821.
365. Stenestrand U, Wallentin L: Early statin treatment following acute myocardial infarction and 1-year survival. JAMA 2001;285:430-436.
366. Barbash GI, Birnbaum Y, Bogaerts K, et al: Treatment of reinfarction after thrombolytic therapy for acute myocardial infarction: An analysis of outcome and treatment choices in the Global Utilization of Streptokinase and Tissue Plasminogen Activator for Occluded Coronary Arteries (GUSTO I) and Assessment of the Safety of a New Thrombolytic (ASSENT 2) studies. Circulation 2001;103:954-960.
367. Hasdai D, Topol EJ, Kilaru R, et al: Frequency, patient characteristics, and outcomes of mild-to-moderate heart failure complicating ST-segment elevation acute myocardial infarction: Lessons from 4 international fibrinolytic therapy trials. Am Heart J 2003;145:73-79.
368. Rott D, Behar S, Leor J, et al: Effect on survival of acute myocardial infarction in Killip classes II or III patients undergoing invasive coronary procedures. Am J Cardiol 2001;88:618-623.
369. Steg PG, Dabbous OH, Feldman LJ, et al: Determinants and prognostic impact of heart failure complicating acute coronary syndromes: Observations from the Global Registry of Acute Coronary Events (GRACE). Circulation 2004;109:494-499.
370. Thattassery E, Gheorghiade M: Beta blocker therapy after acute myocardial infarction in patients with heart failure and systolic dysfunction. Heart Fail Rev 2004;9:107-113.
371. Pitt B, White H, Nicolau J, et al: Eplerenone reduces mortality 30 days after randomization following acute myocardial infarction in patients with left ventricular systolic dysfunction and heart failure. J Am Coll Cardiol 2005;46:425-431.
372. Chadda K, Goldstein S, Byington R, et al: Effect of propranolol after acute myocardial infarction in patients with congestive heart failure. Circulation 1986;73:503-510.
373. Spargias KS, Hall AS, Greenwood DC, et al: Beta blocker treatment and other prognostic variables in patients with clinical evidence of heart failure after acute myocardial infarction: Evidence from the AIRE study. Heart 1999;81:25-32.
374. Spencer FA, Meyer TE, Gore JM, et al: Heterogeneity in the management and outcomes of patients with acute myocardial infarction complicated by heart failure: The National Registry of Myocardial Infarction. Circulation 2002;105:2605-2610.
375. Hollenberg SM, Kavinsky CJ, Parrillo JE: Cardiogenic shock. Ann Intern Med 1999;131:47-59.
376. Holmes DR Jr, Bates ER, Kleiman NS, et al: Contemporary reperfusion therapy for cardiogenic shock: The GUSTO-I trial experience. The GUSTO-I Investigators. Global Utilization of Streptokinase and Tissue Plasminogen Activator for Occluded Coronary Arteries. J Am Coll Cardiol 1995;26:668-674, 1995.
377. Holmes DR Jr, Berger PB, Hochman JS, et al: Cardiogenic shock in patients with acute ischemic syndromes with and without ST-segment elevation. Circulation 1999;100:2067-2073.
378. Hochman JS: Cardiogenic shock complicating acute myocardial infarction: Expanding the paradigm. Circulation 2003;107:2998-3002.
379. Kaluski E, Hendler A, Blatt A, et al: Nitric oxide synthase inhibitors in post-myocardial infarction cardiogenic shock—an update. Clin Cardiol 2006;29:482-448.
380. Cotter G, Kaluski E, Milo O, et al: LINCS: L-NAME (a NO synthase inhibitor) in the treatment of refractory cardiogenic shock: A prospective randomized study. Eur Heart J 2003;24:1287-1295.
381. Alexander JH, Reynolds HR, Stebbins AL, et al: Effect of tilarginine acetate in patients with acute myocardial infarction and cardiogenic shock: The TRIUMPH randomized controlled trial. JAMA 2007;297:1657-1666.
382. Berger PB, Holmes DR, Jr., Stebbins AL, et al: Impact of an aggressive invasive catheterization and revascularization strategy on mortality in patients with cardiogenic shock in the Global Utilization of Streptokinase and Tissue Plasminogen Activator for Occluded Coronary Arteries (GUSTO-I) trial. An observational study. Circulation 1997;96:122-127, 1997.
383. Berger PB, Tuttle RH, Holmes DR Jr, et al: One-year survival among patients with acute myocardial infarction complicated by cardiogenic shock, and its relation to early

revascularization: Results from the GUSTO-I trial. Circulation 1999;99:873-878, 1999.
384. Hochman JS, Sleeper LA, Webb JG, et al: Early revascularization in acute myocardial infarction complicated by cardiogenic shock. SHOCK Investigators. Should We Emergently Revascularize Occluded Coronaries for Cardiogenic Shock? N Engl J Med 1999;341:625-634.
385. Hochman JS, Sleeper LA, White HD, et al: One-year survival following early revascularization for cardiogenic shock. JAMA 2001;285:190-192.
386. Hochman JS, Sleeper LA, Webb JG, et al: Early revascularization and long-term survival in cardiogenic shock complicating acute myocardial infarction. JAMA 2006;295:2511-2515.
387. Kern MJ, Aguirre FV, Tatineni S, et al: Enhanced coronary blood flow velocity during intraaortic balloon counterpulsation in critically ill patients. J Am Coll Cardiol 1993;21:359-368.
388. Gurbel PA, Anderson RD, MacCord CS, et al: Arterial diastolic pressure augmentation by intra-aortic balloon counterpulsation enhances the onset of coronary artery reperfusion by thrombolytic therapy. Circulation 1994;89:361-365.
389. Ohman EM, Hochman JS: Aortic counterpulsation in acute myocardial infarction: Physiologically important but does the patient benefit? Am Heart J 2001;141:889-892.
390. Barron HV, Every NR, Parsons LS, et al: The use of intra-aortic balloon counterpulsation in patients with cardiogenic shock complicating acute myocardial infarction: Data from the National Registry of Myocardial Infarction 2. Am Heart J 2001;141: 933-939.
391. Sanborn TA, Sleeper LA, Bates ER, et al: Impact of thrombolysis, intra-aortic balloon pump counterpulsation, and their combination in cardiogenic shock complicating acute myocardial infarction: A report from the SHOCK Trial Registry. SHould we emergently revascularize Occluded Coronaries for cardiogenic shocK? J Am Coll Cardiol 2000;36:1123-1129.
392. Brodie BR, Stuckey TD, Hansen C, et al: Intra-aortic balloon counterpulsation before primary percutaneous transluminal coronary angioplasty reduces catheterization laboratory events in high-risk patients with acute myocardial infarction. Am J Cardiol 1999;84:18-23.
393. Kovack PJ, Rasak MA, Bates ER, et al: Thrombolysis plus aortic counterpulsation: Improved survival in patients who present to community hospitals with cardiogenic shock. J Am Coll Cardiol 1997;29:1454-1458.
394. Chen EW, Canto JG, Parsons LS, et al: Relation between hospital intra-aortic balloon counterpulsation volume and mortality in acute myocardial infarction complicated by cardiogenic shock. Circulation 2003;108:951-957.
395. Zornoff LA, Skali H, Pfeffer MA, et al: Right ventricular dysfunction and risk of heart failure and mortality after myocardial infarction. J Am Coll Cardiol 2002;39:1450-1455.
396. Cabin HS, Clubb KS, Wackers FJ, et al: Right ventricular myocardial infarction with anterior wall left ventricular infarction: An autopsy study. Am Heart J 1987;113:16-23.
397. Andersen HR, Falk E, Nielsen D: Right ventricular infarction: Frequency, size and topography in coronary heart disease: A prospective study comprising 107 consecutive autopsies from a coronary care unit. J Am Coll Cardiol 1987;10:1223-1232.
398. Bowers TR, O'Neill WW, Pica M, et al: Patterns of coronary compromise resulting in acute right ventricular ischemic dysfunction. Circulation 106:1104-1109.
399. Mehta SR, Eikelboom JW, Natarajan MK, et al: Impact of right ventricular involvement on mortality and morbidity in patients with inferior myocardial infarction. J Am Coll Cardiol 2001;37:37-43.
400. Jacobs AK, Leopold JA, Bates E, et al: Cardiogenic shock caused by right ventricular infarction: A report from the SHOCK registry. J Am Coll Cardiol 2003;41:1273-1279.
401. Bueno H, Lopez-Palop R, Perez-David E, et al: Combined effect of age and right ventricular involvement on acute inferior myocardial infarction prognosis. Circulation 1998;98: 1714-1720.
402. Robalino BD, Whitlow PL, Underwood DA, et al: Electrocardiographic manifestations of right ventricular infarction. Am Heart J 1989;118: 138-144.
403. Zehender M, Kasper W, Kauder E, et al: Right ventricular infarction as an independent predictor of prognosis after acute inferior myocardial infarction. N Engl J Med 1993;328: 981-988.
404. Dell'Italia LJ, Starling MR, O'Rourke RA: Physical examination for exclusion of hemodynamically important right ventricular infarction. Ann Intern Med 1983;99:608-611.
405. Kinch JW, Ryan TJ: Right ventricular infarction. N Engl J Med 1994;330: 1211-1217.
406. Lorell B, Leinbach RC, Pohost GM, et al: Right ventricular infarction. Clinical diagnosis and differentiation from cardiac tamponade and pericardial constriction. Am J Cardiol 1979;43:465-471.
407. Dell'Italia LJ, Starling MR, Blumhardt R, et al: Comparative effects of volume loading, dobutamine, and nitroprusside in patients with predominant right ventricular infarction. Circulation 1985;72: 1327-1335.
408. Inglessis I, Shin JT, Lepore JJ, et al: Hemodynamic effects of inhaled nitric oxide in right ventricular myocardial infarction and cardiogenic shock. J Am Coll Cardiol 2004;44:793-798.
409. Goldstein JA, Barzilai B, Rosamond TL, et al: Determinants of hemodynamic compromise with severe right ventricular infarction. Circulation 1990;82:359-368.
410. Topol EJ, Goldschlager N, Ports TA, et al: Hemodynamic benefit of atrial pacing in right ventricular myocardial infarction. Ann Intern Med 1982;96:594-597.
411. Love JC, Haffajee CI, Gore JM, et al: Reversibility of hypotension and shock by atrial or atrioventricular sequential pacing in patients with right ventricular infarction. Am Heart J 108:5-13.
412. Laham RJ, Ho KK, Douglas PS, et al: Right ventricular infarction complicated by acute right-to-left shunting. Am J Cardiol 1994;74: 824-826.
413. Bowers TR, O'Neill WW, Grines C, et al: Effect of reperfusion on biventricular function and survival after right ventricular infarction. N Engl J Med 1998;338:933-940.
414. Kinn JW, Ajluni SC, Samyn JG, et al: Rapid hemodynamic improvement after reperfusion during right ventricular infarction. J Am Coll Cardiol 1995;26:1230-1234.
415. Thompson CR, Buller CE, Sleeper LA, et al: Cardiogenic shock due to acute severe mitral regurgitation complicating acute myocardial infarction: A report from the SHOCK Trial Registry. SHould we emergently revascularize Occluded Coronaries in cardiogenic shocK? J Am Coll Cardiol 2000;36:1104-1109.
416. Vlodaver Z, Edwards JE: Rupture of ventricular septum or papillary muscle complicating myocardial infarction. Circulation 1977;55:815-822.
417. Crenshaw BS, Granger CB, Birnbaum Y, et al: Risk factors, angiographic patterns, and outcomes in patients with ventricular septal defect complicating acute myocardial infarction. GUSTO-I (Global Utilization of Streptokinase and TPA for Occluded Coronary Arteries) Trial Investigators. Circulation 2000;101:27-32.
418. Menon V, Webb JG, Hillis LD, et al: Outcome and profile of ventricular septal rupture with cardiogenic shock after myocardial infarction: A report from the SHOCK Trial Registry. SHould we emergently revascularize Occluded Coronaries in cardiogenic shocK? J Am Coll Cardiol 2000;36:1110-1116.
419. Moore CA, Nygaard TW, Kaiser DL, et al: Postinfarction ventricular septal rupture: The importance of location of infarction and right ventricular function in determining survival. Circulation 1986;74:45-55.
420. Edwards BS, Edwards WD, Edwards JE: Ventricular septal rupture complicating acute myocardial infarction: Identification of simple and complex types in 53 autopsied hearts. Am J Cardiol 1984;54:1201-1205.
421. Gold HK, Leinbach RC, Sanders CA, et al: Intraaortic balloon pumping for ventricular septal defect or mitral regurgitation complicating acute myocardial infarction. Circulation 1973;47:1191-1196.
422. Raitt MH, Kraft CD, Gardner CJ, et al: Subacute ventricular free wall rupture complicating myocardial infarction. Am Heart J 1993;126:946-955.
423. Becker RC, Hochman JS, Cannon CP, et al: Fatal cardiac rupture among patients treated with thrombolytic agents and adjunctive thrombin antagonists: Observations from the Thrombolysis and Thrombin Inhibition in Myocardial Infarction 9 Study. J Am Coll Cardiol 1999;33:479-487.

424. Slater J, Brown RJ, Antonelli TA, et al: Cardiogenic shock due to cardiac free-wall rupture or tamponade after acute myocardial infarction: A report from the SHOCK Trial Registry. Should We Emergently Revascularize Occluded Coronaries for Cardiogenic Shock? J Am Coll Cardiol 2000;36:1117-1122.
425. Moreno R, Lopez-Sendon J, Garcia E, et al: Primary angioplasty reduces the risk of left ventricular free wall rupture compared with thrombolysis in patients with acute myocardial infarction. J Am Coll Cardiol 2002;39:598-603.
426. Becker RC, Gore JM, Lambrew C, et al: A composite view of cardiac rupture in the United States National Registry of Myocardial Infarction. J Am Coll Cardiol 1996;27:1321-1326.
427. Honan MB, Harrell FE Jr, Reimer KA, et al: Cardiac rupture, mortality and the timing of thrombolytic therapy: A meta-analysis. J Am Coll Cardiol 1990;16:359-367.
428. Meine TJ, Al-Khatib SM, Alexander JH, et al: Incidence, predictors, and outcomes of high-degree atrioventricular block complicating acute myocardial infarction treated with thrombolytic therapy. Am Heart J 2005;149:670-674.
429. Campeau L: Grading of angina pectoris. Circulation 1976;54:522-523 (Letter).
430. Braunwald E: Unstable angina. A classification. Circulation 1989;80:410-414.
431. Antman EM, Cohen M, Bernink PJ, et al: The TIMI risk score for unstable angina/non–ST elevation MI: A method for prognostication and therapeutic decision making. JAMA 2000;284:835-842.
432. Khot UN, Jia G, Moliterno DJ, et al: Prognostic importance of physical examination for heart failure in non–ST-elevation acute coronary syndromes: The enduring value of Killip classification. JAMA 2003;290: 2174-2181.
433. Savonitto S, Ardissino D, Granger CB, et al: Prognostic value of the admission electrocardiogram in acute coronary syndromes. JAMA 1999;281: 707-713.
434. Welch RD, Zalenski RJ, Frederick PD, et al: Prognostic value of a normal or nonspecific initial electrocardiogram in acute myocardial infarction. JAMA 22001;86:1977-1984.
435. Diderholm E, Andren B, Frostfeldt G, et al: ST depression in ECG at entry indicates severe coronary lesions and large benefits of an early invasive treatment strategy in unstable coronary artery disease; the FRISC II ECG substudy. The Fast Revascularisation during Instability in Coronary Artery Disease. Eur Heart J 2002;23:41-49.
436. Cannon CP, Weintraub WS, Demopoulos LA, et al: Comparison of early invasive and conservative strategies in patients with unstable coronary syndromes treated with the glycoprotein IIb/IIIa inhibitor tirofiban. N Engl J Med 2001;344:1879-1887.
437. Holmvang L, Clemmensen P, Lindahl B, et al: Quantitative analysis of the admission electrocardiogram identifies patients with unstable coronary artery disease who benefit the most from early invasive treatment. J Am Coll Cardiol 2003;41:905-915.
438. Sabatine MS, Morrow DA, McCabe CH, et al: Combination of quantitative ST deviation and troponin elevation provides independent prognostic and therapeutic information in unstable angina and non–ST-elevation myocardial infarction. Am Heart J 2006;151:25-31.
439. Barrabes JA, Figueras J, Moure C, et al: Prognostic significance of ST segment depression in lateral leads I, aVL, V5 and V6 on the admission electrocardiogram in patients with a first acute myocardial infarction without ST segment elevation. J Am Coll Cardiol 2000;35:1813-1819.
440. de Zwaan C, Bar FW, Janssen JH, et al: Angiographic and clinical characteristics of patients with unstable angina showing an ECG pattern indicating critical narrowing of the proximal LAD coronary artery. Am Heart J 1989;117:657-665.
441. Renkin J, Wijns W, Ladha Z, et al: Reversal of segmental hypokinesis by coronary angioplasty in patients with unstable angina, persistent T wave inversion, and left anterior descending coronary artery stenosis. Additional evidence for myocardial stunning in humans. Circulation 1990;82:913-921.
442. Antman EM, Tanasijevic MJ, Thompson B, et al: Cardiac-specific troponin I levels to predict the risk of mortality in patients with acute coronary syndromes. N Engl J Med 1996;335: 1342-1349.
443. Dokainish H, Pillai M, Murphy SA, et al: Prognostic implications of elevated troponin in patients with suspected acute coronary syndrome but no critical epicardial coronary disease: A TACTICS-TIMI-18 substudy. J Am Coll Cardiol 2005;45:19-24.
444. Heeschen C, Hamm CW, Goldmann B, et al: Troponin concentrations for stratification of patients with acute coronary syndromes in relation to therapeutic efficacy of tirofiban. PRISM Study Investigators. Platelet Receptor Inhibition in Ischemic Syndrome Management. Lancet 1999;354: 1757-1762.
445. Hamm CW, Heeschen C, Goldmann B, et al: Benefit of abciximab in patients with refractory unstable angina in relation to serum troponin T levels. c7E3 Fab Antiplatelet Therapy in Unstable Refractory Angina (CAPTURE) Study Investigators. N Engl J Med 1999;340:1623-1629.
446. Morrow DA, Cannon CP, Rifai N, et al: Ability of minor elevations of troponins I and T to predict benefit from an early invasive strategy in patients with unstable angina and non–ST elevation myocardial infarction: Results from a randomized trial. JAMA 2001;286: 2405-2412.
447. Morrow DA, de Lemos JA, Sabatine MS, et al: Evaluation of B-type natriuretic peptide for risk assessment in unstable angina/non–ST-elevation myocardial infarction: B-type natriuretic peptide and prognosis in TACTICS-TIMI 18. J Am Coll Cardiol 2003;41:1264-1272.
448. Morrow DA, de Lemos JA, Blazing MA, et al: Prognostic value of serial B-type natriuretic peptide testing during follow-up of patients with unstable coronary artery disease. JAMA 2005;294:2866-2871.
449. Figueras J, Lidon R, Cortadellas J: Rebound myocardial ischaemia following abrupt interruption of intravenous nitroglycerin infusion in patients with unstable angina at rest. Eur Heart J 1991;12:405-411.
450. Emery M, Lopez-Sendon J, Steg PG, et al: Patterns of use and potential impact of early beta-blocker therapy in non–ST-elevation myocardial infarction with and without heart failure: The Global Registry of Acute Coronary Events. Am Heart J 2006;152:1015-1021.
451. Yusuf S, Wittes J, Friedman L: Overview of results of randomized clinical trials in heart disease. II. Unstable angina, heart failure, primary prevention with aspirin, and risk factor modification. JAMA 1988;260: 2259-2263.
452. Early treatment of unstable angina in the coronary care unit: A randomised, double blind, placebo controlled comparison of recurrent ischaemia in patients treated with nifedipine or metoprolol or both. Report of The Holland Interuniversity Nifedipine/ Metoprolol Trial (HINT) Research Group. Br Heart J 1986;56:400-413.
453. Gibson RS, Hansen JF, Messerli F, et al: Long-term effects of diltiazem and verapamil on mortality and cardiac events in non–Q-wave acute myocardial infarction without pulmonary congestion: post hoc subset analysis of the multicenter diltiazem postinfarction trial and the second danish verapamil infarction trial studies. Am J Cardiol 2000;86: 275-279.
454. Kong DF, Hasselblad V, Kandzari DE, et al: Seeking the optimal aspirin dose in acute coronary syndromes. Am J Cardiol 2002;90:622-625.
455. Wallentin LC: Aspirin (75 mg/day) after an episode of unstable coronary artery disease: long-term effects on the risk for myocardial infarction, occurrence of severe angina and the need for revascularization. Research Group on Instability in Coronary Artery Disease in Southeast Sweden. J Am Coll Cardiol 1991;18:1587-1593.
456. Quinn MJ, Aronow HD, Califf RM, et al: Aspirin dose and six-month outcome after an acute coronary syndrome. J Am Coll Cardiol 2004;43:972-978.
457. Balsano F, Rizzon P, Violi F, et al: Antiplatelet treatment with ticlopidine in unstable angina. A controlled multicenter clinical trial. The Studio della Ticlopidina nell'Angina Instabile Group. Circulation 1990;82:17-26.
458. Yusuf S, Zhao F, Mehta SR, et al: Effects of clopidogrel in addition to aspirin in patients with acute coronary syndromes without ST-segment elevation. N Engl J Med 2001;345: 494-502.
459. Mehta SR, Yusuf S, Peters RJ, et al: Effects of pretreatment with clopidogrel and aspirin followed by long-term therapy in patients

undergoing percutaneous coronary intervention: The PCI-CURE study. Lancet 2001;358:527-533.
460. Fox KA, Mehta SR, Peters R, et al: Benefits and risks of the combination of clopidogrel and aspirin in patients undergoing surgical revascularization for non–ST-elevation acute coronary syndrome: The Clopidogrel in Unstable Angina to Prevent Recurrent Ischemic Events (CURE) Trial. Circulation 2004;110:1202-1208.
461. Bijsterveld NR, Moons AH, Meijers JC, et al: Rebound thrombin generation after heparin therapy in unstable angina. A randomized comparison between unfractionated and low-molecular-weight heparin. J Am Coll Cardiol 2002;39:811-817.
462. Theroux P, Waters D, Lam J, et al: Reactivation of unstable angina after the discontinuation of heparin. N Engl J Med 1992;327:141-145.
463. Lauer MA, Houghtaling PL, Peterson JG, et al: Attenuation of rebound ischemia after discontinuation of heparin therapy by glycoprotein IIb/IIIa inhibition with eptifibatide in patients with acute coronary syndromes: Observations from the platelet IIb/IIIa in unstable angina: receptor suppression using integrilin therapy (PURSUIT) trial. Circulation 2001;104:2772-2777.
464. Hasdai D, Harrington RA, Hochman JS, et al: Platelet glycoprotein IIb/IIIa blockade and outcome of cardiogenic shock complicating acute coronary syndromes without persistent ST-segment elevation. J Am Coll Cardiol 2000;36:685-692.
465. Boersma E, Harrington RA, Moliterno DJ, et al: Platelet glycoprotein IIb/IIIa inhibitors in acute coronary syndromes: A meta-analysis of all major randomised clinical trials. Lancet 2002;359:189-198.
466. Roffi M, Chew DP, Mukherjee D, et al: Platelet glycoprotein IIb/IIIa inhibition in acute coronary syndromes. Gradient of benefit related to the revascularization strategy. Eur Heart J 2002;23:1441-1448.
467. Simoons ML: Effect of glycoprotein IIb/IIIa receptor blocker abciximab on outcome in patients with acute coronary syndromes without early coronary revascularisation: The GUSTO IV-ACS randomised trial. Lancet 2001;357:1915-1924.
468. Alexander KP, Chen AY, Roe MT, et al: Excess dosing of antiplatelet and antithrombin agents in the treatment of non–ST-segment elevation acute coronary syndromes. JAMA 2005;294:3108-3116.
469. Dasgupta H, Blankenship JC, Wood GC, et al: Thrombocytopenia complicating treatment with intravenous glycoprotein IIb/IIIa receptor inhibitors: A pooled analysis. Am Heart J 2000;140:206-211.
470. Oler A, Whooley MA, Oler J, et al: Adding heparin to aspirin reduces the incidence of myocardial infarction and death in patients with unstable angina. A meta-analysis. JAMA 1996;276:811-815.
471. Low-molecular-weight heparin during instability in coronary artery disease. Fragmin during Instability in Coronary Artery Disease (FRISC) study group. Lancet 1996;347:561-568.
472. Petersen JL, Mahaffey KW, Hasselblad V, et al: Efficacy and bleeding complications among patients randomized to enoxaparin or unfractionated heparin for antithrombin therapy in non–ST-segment elevation acute coronary syndromes: A systematic overview. JAMA 2004;292:89-96.
473. Stone GW, McLaurin BT, Cox DA, et al: Bivalirudin for patients with acute coronary syndromes. N Engl J Med 2006;355:2203-2216.
474. Ambrosioni E, Borghi C, Magnani B: The effect of the angiotensin-converting-enzyme inhibitor zofenopril on mortality and morbidity after anterior myocardial infarction. The Survival of Myocardial Infarction Long-Term Evaluation (SMILE) Study Investigators. N Engl J Med 1995;332:80-85.
475. Borghi C, Bacchelli S, Degli Esposti D, et al: Effects of early angiotensin-converting enzyme inhibition in patients with non–ST-elevation acute anterior myocardial infarction. Am Heart J 2006;152:470-477.
476. Tonkin AM, Colquhoun D, Emberson J, et al: Effects of pravastatin in 3260 patients with unstable angina: Results from the LIPID study. Lancet 2000;356:1871-1875.
477. Heeschen C, Hamm CW, Laufs U, et al: Withdrawal of statins increases event rates in patients with acute coronary syndromes. Circulation 2002;105:1446-1452.
478. Aronow HD, Topol EJ, Roe MT, et al: Effect of lipid-lowering therapy on early mortality after acute coronary syndromes: An observational study. Lancet 2001;357:1063-1068.
479. Newby LK, Kristinsson A, Bhapkar MV, et al: Early statin initiation and outcomes in patients with acute coronary syndromes. JAMA 2002;287:3087-3095.
480. Schwartz GG, Olsson AG, Ezekowitz MD, et al: Effects of atorvastatin on early recurrent ischemic events in acute coronary syndromes: The MIRACL study: A randomized controlled trial. JAMA 2001;285:1711-1718.
481. Invasive compared with non-invasive treatment in unstable coronary-artery disease: FRISC II prospective randomised multicentre study. Fragmin and Fast Revascularisation during Instability in Coronary Artery Disease Investigators. Lancet 1999;354:708-7015.
482. Wallentin L, Lagerqvist B, Husted S, et al: Outcome at 1 year after an invasive compared with a non-invasive strategy in unstable coronary-artery disease: The FRISC II invasive randomised trial. Lancet 200;356:9-16.
483. Lagerqvist B, Husted S, Kontny F, et al: A long-term perspective on the protective effects of an early invasive strategy in unstable coronary artery disease: Two-year follow-up of the FRISC-II invasive study. J Am Coll Cardiol 2002;40:1902-1914.
484. Fox KA, Poole-Wilson PA, Henderson RA, et al: Interventional versus conservative treatment for patients with unstable angina or non–ST-elevation myocardial infarction: The British Heart Foundation RITA 3 randomised trial. Randomized Intervention Trial of Unstable Angina. Lancet 2002;360:743-751.
485. Fox KA, Poole-Wilson P, Clayton TC, et al: 5-year outcome of an interventional strategy in non–ST-elevation acute coronary syndrome: The British Heart Foundation RITA 3 randomised trial. Lancet 2005;366:914-9120.
486. de Winter RJ, Windhausen F, Cornel JH, et al: Early invasive versus selectively invasive management for acute coronary syndromes. N Engl J Med 2005;353:1095-1104.
487. Mehta SR, Cannon CP, Fox KA, et al: Routine vs selective invasive strategies in patients with acute coronary syndromes: A collaborative meta-analysis of randomized trials. JAMA 2005;293:2908-2917.
488. Boden WE, O'Rourke RA, Crawford MH, et al: Outcomes in patients with acute non–Q-wave myocardial infarction randomly assigned to an invasive as compared with a conservative management strategy. Veterans Affairs Non–Q-Wave Infarction Strategies in Hospital (VANQWISH) Trial Investigators. N Engl J Med 1998;338:1785-1792.
489. Mukherjee D, Fang J, Chetcuti S, et al: Impact of combination evidence-based medical therapy on mortality in patients with acute coronary syndromes. Circulation 2004;109:745-749.

Chapter 32

Cardiac Arrhythmias

Lawrence J. Gessman and Richard Trohman

Management of serious cardiac arrhythmias is the shared responsibility of emergency specialists: critical care physicians, cardiologists, and electrophysiologists. The past 10 years have produced only modest changes in acute and subacute therapy of tachyarrhythmias. Antiarrhythmic drugs remain the mainstay of therapy for supraventricular arrhythmias and hemodynamically stable ventricular tachycardia. Temporary pacing remains the "gold standard" of therapy for symptomatic bradyarrhythmias. Permanent pacing is still the only option for treatment of chronic bradycardias. By contrast, dramatic improvement and change have occurred in the chronic therapy of tachyarrhythmias. Most supraventricular tachycardias can now be cured by catheter ablation. Patients with structural heart disease at risk for sudden cardiac death and those resuscitated from hemodynamically unstable ventricular tachyarrhythmias now are managed with implantable defibrillators, with antiarrhythmic drugs used primarily as an adjunct only for patients receiving frequent shocks.

Critical care physicians deal with a plethora of medical and surgical problems in their patients. Arrhythmias may be the primary abnormality or may be secondary to myocardial ischemia, electrolyte imbalance, or toxic or metabolic disturbances due to multisystem organ failure. Optimal management of arrhythmias requires expertise in electrocardiography and clinical pharmacology and a knowledge of arrhythmia precipitants, including proarrhythmia caused by antiarrhythmic drugs.[1] The responsibility of the critical care physician is to facilitate transition from acute to chronic care by referring the patient with an arrhythmia to a cardiologist or an electrophysiologist. Therefore, the major emphasis of this chapter is on acute and chronic care of the patient with an arrhythmia.

BRADYCARDIAS

Bradyarrhythmias and indications and techniques for temporary cardiac pacing are reviewed extensively in Chapter 5. A brief overview is included here to highlight important issues for the intensivist.

Sinus Bradycardia and Sinus Node Dysfunction

Sinus bradycardia is generally defined as periods of sinus rhythm with rates less than 60 beats per minute. In the absence of symptoms, it usually is benign and requires no treatment. Sinus bradycardia is common in young adults (particularly the physically fit). Nocturnal rates of 35 to 40 beats per minute and pauses during sleep of 2 seconds or longer are not uncommon. Sinus arrhythmia, characterized by phasic (respiratory) variation, also is common in young patients with low resting heart rates and enhanced vagal tone. Wandering pacemaker, a variant of sinus arrhythmia characterized by shifting P wave morphologies and periods of junctional rhythm, is likewise found predominantly in young athletic persons.

Pathologic conditions producing sinus bradycardia include increased intracranial pressure, ophthalmologic surgery, cervical and mediastinal tumors, hypothyroidism, hypothermia, gram-negative sepsis, Chagas' disease, depression, and anorexia nervosa. This arrhythmia also is common after cardiac transplantation. β-Blockers, parasympathomimetic agents, calcium antagonists, amiodarone, and lithium commonly produce sinus bradycardia. Digoxin, in therapeutic doses, usually does not markedly affect the sinus node and is relatively safe to use in patients with sinus node dysfunction.[2] Sinus bradycardia complicates 10% to 15% of acute myocardial infarctions and is most common with inferior infarcts. It also may be seen after successful thrombolysis. In the absence of hemodynamic compromise, it is associated with a more favorable prognosis than that for sinus tachycardia.[3]

Short-term pharmacologic enhancement of the sinus rate may be accomplished using atropine, catecholamines, or theophylline. Isoproterenol should be avoided in patients with ischemic heart disease and hypertrophic cardiomyopathy. No safe, reliable drug is available for long-term management of sinus bradycardia. Permanent pacing should be employed to alleviate persistent symptoms.

Sinus bradycardia (with or without atrioventricular block) may occur during periods of autonomic instability. Examples are carotid hypersensitivity and neurocardiogenic syncope. These syndromes have cardioinhibitory (bradycardic), vasodepressor (vasodilatory), and mixed forms. Permanent pacing (which must include the ability to pace the right ventricle for heart block) is well-established therapy for cardioinhibitory carotid sinus hypersensitivity. Its role in neurocardiogenic syncope is more controversial. We believe that neurocardiogenic syncope generally is a benign condition that usually can be managed medically without permanent pacemaker therapy. However, treatment for patients with frequent and severe cardioinhibitory spells, especially for those whose condition is drug refractory or who demonstrate intolerance or in whom asystolic periods exceeding 5 seconds can be demonstrated clinically or during head-up tilt table testing, may include pacemaker therapy.[4]

Sinus node dysfunction may manifest in a variety of ways. These include persistent sinus bradycardia, sinus pause or arrest, sinoatrial exit block, and the bradycardia-tachycardia syndrome.

Type I sinoatrial (SA) exit block is characterized by progressive P-P interval shortening before pauses that are less than two P-P cycles in duration. In type II second-degree SA exit block, the pauses are mathematical multiples of the basic P-P interval. SA exit block usually is transient and often is reversible. Its presence should prompt a search for underlying causes such as enhanced vagal tone, acute myocarditis or infarction, or drug effect (as from digitalis, quinidine, or procainamide).

Symptomatic sinus node dysfunction virtually always requires permanent pacing. Patients with concomitant supraventricular tachycardias may require supplemental antiarrhythmic therapy. Drug therapy may aggravate the bradycardia and probably should be initiated after device placement. Catheter ablation may cure the tachyarrhythmia.

Atrioventricular Block

The various forms of heart block are disturbances of impulse conduction. Heart block may be transient or permanent. The following paragraphs focus on disturbances of atrioventricular (AV) conduction.

First-degree AV block in reality involves no AV block at all. Every atrial impulse is conducted to the ventricles in a delayed fashion such that the PR interval is greater than 200 ms. If the QRS complex on the surface echocardiogram (ECG) is narrow, the delay nearly always is in the AV node. In the presence of a wide QRS, the delay may be in either the AV node or the His-Purkinje system.

Second-degree AV block involves some failure of atrial impulse conduction at times when *physiologic* refractoriness is not operative. The conducted P waves relate to the QRS complexes with recurring PR intervals (they are "associated").

Clinical classification of second-degree AV block as Mobitz type I or II is useful. In Mobitz I (Wenckebach) block, P-P intervals are constant, with gradual PR prolongation before failure of impulse conduction (nonconducted P wave). Although classic Wenckebach block involves simultaneous shortening of successive R-R intervals before AV block, atypical R-R intervals actually are more common. In younger people, Mobitz I AV block with normal QRS complexes generally is benign and does not progress to more advanced AV conduction disturbances. In older patients, the prognosis may be similar to that with Mobitz II block. Mobitz I second-degree AV block may accompany inferior myocardial infarction. The condition is benign, with favorable prognosis, in the absence of hemodynamic compromise. The conduction disturbance usually is transient, and permanent pacing is not required.

Mobitz II AV block is characterized by sudden failure of atrial impulse conduction without prior PR prolongation. This form of AV block frequently heralds development of complete AV block and Adams-Stokes syncope. Mobitz II second-degree AV block in the setting of anterior infarction is associated with pump failure and high mortality rates. Survivors should receive permanent pacemakers.

In general, the surface ECG allows the clinician to localize the site of AV block without the use of invasive electrophysiologic testing, Mobitz type I AV block with a narrow QRS almost always occurs at the AV node. Rarely, Mobitz I second-degree AV block may have an intra-His location. Mobitz I AV block with wide QRS complexes may occur in either the AV node or the His-Purkinje system. Mobitz II second-degree AV block (particularly in the presence of wide QRS complexes) localizes to the His-Purkinje system.

It is important to remember a few general rules to avoid common ECG misinterpretations of second-degree AV block. The 2:1 form of AV block may be nodal or infranodal 2:1 block associated with narrow QRS complexes generally result from AV nodal block. Wide QRS complexes are compatible with block in either the AV node or His-Purkinje system.

In general, atropine improves AV nodal conduction and carotid massage worsens it. These interventions typically have the opposite effect when AV block occurs in the His-Purkinje system. Atropine increases both atrial and ventricular rates in AV nodal block. Likewise, exercise (increased endogenous catecholamines) may reduce the extent of block. Precipitation of second-degree, high-grade or complete AV block during exercise strongly suggests an infranodal site of block.Complete AV block is diagnosed by the presence of independent atrial and ventricular activity on the ECG. When the atrial rhythm is sinus, atrioventricular dissociation is present, with the sinus rate exceeding the ventricular rate. The P-P interval is constant. The R-R interval is constant. The PR interval is variable in a random, non-recurring pattern. Complete AV block also may be present during all varieties of atrial tachycardia.

Complete AV block proximal to the His bundle results in a narrow QRS complex escape rhythm with rates of 50 to 60 beats per minute. Complete infra-His also may result in a narrow QRS escape rhythm with ventricular rates less than 45 beats per minute.

Acquired complete AV block most commonly occurs distal to the His bundle, usually is secondary to a trifascicular conduction disturbance, is potentially life-threatening, and generally is irreversible. A wide QRS escape rhythm with ventricular rates less than 40 beats per minute is the rule. An exception is seen in the setting of inferior infarction, in which recovery of complete (narrow QRS) AV nodal block occurs in greater than 90% of patients (time to recovery, 30 minutes to 16 days).[5]

Drug toxicity, coronary artery disease, and degenerative disease of the conduction system are the most common causes of AV block in adults. Surgery, electrolyte disturbances (such as hyperkalemia), endocarditis, myocarditis (Lyme carditis), tumors, myxedema, rheumatoid nodules, Chagas' disease, calcific aortic stenosis, polymyositis, amyloidosis, sarcoidosis, scleroderma, and vagotonic reflexes all may result in AV block. In truth, the number of factors and conditions that may result in AV block is nearly endless. "Hypervagal" responses (carotid hypersensitivity, neurocardiogenic syncope) may produce transient AV block (see later on).[3]

Congenital complete AV block results from separation of the atrial musculature from the conduction system, or from nodoventricular disconnection. Mortality is highest in neonates, diminishes during childhood and adolescence, and then increases later in life. Patients may be asymptomatic for many years. It is difficult to predict prognosis in individual patients. Persistent ventricular rates less than 50 beats per minute correlate with the development of symptoms and syncope. Symptomatic patients and those patients with left ventricular dilatation should receive permanent pacemakers.

No reliable long-term pharmacotherapy exists for AV block. Transient AV nodal block may be managed with atropine. Infranodal block may be managed with (carefully titrated) isoproterenol until temporary or permanent pacing is established.

Vagally Mediated Sinus Arrest, Bradycardia, and Heart Block

The most common cause of nonconducted P waves during telemetry or Holter recordings is bradycardia-associated AV block. This manifests as sudden (usually nocturnal) block of one or more P waves with or without antecedent PR prolongation. This phenomenon is characterized by P-P prolongation before AV block and is the result of transient increases in vagal tone. Vagally mediated sinus arrest, bradycardia, and heart block often occur in the intensive care unit (ICU) setting as a result of suctioning, gagging, femoral vessel compression (for hemostasis), and a variety of other triggers (listed in Box 32-1). Vagal stimulation may lower blood pressure with or without significant bradycardia. Bradyarrhythmias and hypotension usually resolve when vagal stimulation ceases. Persistent bradycardia or hypotension mediated by vagal tone may require placing the patient in the Trendelenburg position, temporary saline infusion, or intravenous administrationof atropine 0.6 to 1.2 mg to fully resolve the episode.

Box 32-1

Types of Vagally Mediated Heart Block

- Gagging reflexes such as with intubation or placement of a nasogastric tube
- Endotracheal suctioning and irrigation of the carina
- Distention of a visceral organ such as during colonoscopy or bladder irrigation
- Increased intrathoracic pressure as may occur with coughing or excessive tidal volumes on the ventilator
- Direct stimulation of the carotid body, which may occur with vascular surgery in this area
- Increased intracranial pressure and certain neurologic procedures
- Manual compression after femoral artery line removal
- Seizure related
- Neurocardiogenic syncope or simple fainting in patients undergoing painful procedures or possibly in visitors to the intensive care unit

SUPRAVENTRICULAR TACHYCARDIA

Overview

Advances in catheter ablation have placed long-term management of supraventricular tachycardias in the hands of the electrophysiologist. Paroxysmal supraventricular tachycardias and typical atrial flutter are curable in more than 90% of patients who suffer from these maladies. Ablation of atypical atrial flutter also is possible[6,7] and increasingly reliable techniques for catheter-based cure of atrial fibrillation are now available.[8-11]

The substrate for most supraventricular tachycardias is present before admission to an ICU. Notable exceptions include atrial fibrillation (and flutter) after open heart surgery, and multifocal atrial tachycardia (MAT) (which may be transient, requiring no chronic therapy). Conditions such as hypoxemia, electrolyte imbalance, catecholamine excess (endogenous and exogenous), and other metabolic disturbances predispose patients (with or without pre-existing arrhythmic substrates) to tachyarrhythmias (see "Arrhythmogenesis," later on). Intensivists must be prepared for acute management of supraventricular tachycardia. Knowledge of arrhythmia mechanisms, appropriate choices for acute pharmacotherapy, and indications for urgent or emergent direct current cardioversion are requisite.[12]

Premature Atrial Contractions

Premature atrial, junctional, or ventricular beats are common in patients with or without structural heart disease and rarely result in significant alteration of cardiac output. They may occur as a result of enhanced sympathetic tone, metabolic stress, pericarditis, or direct mechanical irritation (as occurs with intracardiac catheters) and may result from the stimulant effects of caffeine, alcohol, intravenous inotropic support, or illicit drugs (such as cocaine). Atrial premature beats may be associated with aberrant conduction and confused with premature ventricular beats, or they may block in the AV node, creating a pause that may be confused with sinus arrest or SA exit block. Atrial premature beats may initiate reentrant supraventricular tachycardias or atrial fibrillation. Premature atrial contractions rarely require treatment, unless they trigger sustained supraventricular tachyarrhythmias.

Paroxysmal Supraventricular Tachycardia

Five types of paroxysmal supraventricular tachycardia (PSVT) are recognized. Atrioventricular nodal reentry tachycardia (AVNRT) is by far the most common and in the past accounted for 50% to 60% of PSVTs evaluated at referral centers.[13] The precise reentrant circuit is not well defined; however, it is clear that the anterior and posterior AV nodal approaches and the perinodal atrial tissue are involved.

AVNRT usually manifests after the age of 20 years[14] and is more common in women than in men. The typical heart rate in AVNRT ranges from 150 to 250 beats per minute. Palpitations, light-headedness, and near-syncope may accompany an episode. True syncope is unusual. Neck pounding (see the following discussion) is virtually pathognomonic.[15] Its absence does not exclude AVNRT.

In 76% to 90% of cases, antegrade conduction proceeds along the posterior (slow) AV nodal approach (pathway), and retrograde conduction along the anterior (fast) AV nodal pathway.[13,14] This is slow-fast AVNRT. Because retrograde conduction is so rapid, atrial and ventricular activation are virtually simultaneous. P waves may not be visible on the surface ECG or may appear in the terminal portion of the QRS complex. Atrial contraction on a closed AV valve may produce neck pounding.[15] Less common (so-called "unusual") variants (fast-slow, slow-slow, and slow–sort of slow) of AV nodal reentry also exist.[14]

Before catheter-based cures became routine, AV reentry (AVRT) was the next most common (accounting for 30%) PSVT.[13] AVRT (also commonly referred to as orthodromic tachycardia) manifests (on average) at a somewhat earlier age than that typical for AVNRT. The antegrade limb of the circuit proceeds down the normal AV nodal His-Purkinje system. The retrograde limb uses an accessory pathway that usually is located along the mitral or tricuspid valve annulus. Because the accessory pathway conducts in only retrograde fashion, it is not seen on surface ECG and therefore is said to be concealed.

Because AVRT proceeds normally antegrade, the QRS complex is generally narrow. The AVRT reentry circuit is to first travel antegrade through the AV node and then through the ventricles before retrograde activation of the atria via the bypass tract. The extra time taken to travel by way of the ventricule creates a longer RP interval during supraventricular tachycardia compared with that seen in AVNRT. Because AVNRT and AVRT activate peri-annular atrial tissue first, P waves (if visible on surface ECG) will be negative in the inferior leads. Upright P waves in these leads indicate atrial (or sinus) tachycardia. AVRT tends to go faster than AVNRT and is more prone to manifest with QRS alternans or left bundle branch block aberrancy.[16,17] A decrease in tachycardia rate on development of bundle branch block ipsilateral to the pathway is characteristic of AVRT. AV block is unusual during AVNRT and *excludes* the diagnosis of AVRT (which requires both atrial and ventricular participation). The presence of AV block strongly suggests the diagnosis of atrial tachycardia.

In the past, intra-atrial reentry, automatic atrial tachycardia, and sinus nodal reentry accounted for the remaining 8% to 10% of PSVTs.[13] Sinus node reentry rarely occurs as an isolated phenomenon.[18]

Approximately 50% of patients with intra-atrial reentry have evidence of structural heart disease.[19] This tachycardia is particularly prone to develop after surgery for congenital cardiac anomalies. Reentry occurs around structural barriers, such as suture lines. In patients without clear-cut structural disease, subtle changes such as scarring and fibrosis provide the substrate for reentry. Automatic atrial tachycardias occur along the crista terminalis, near the ostium of the coronary sinus, along the tricuspid and mitral annuli, in both atrial appendages, and within and in close proximity to the pulmonary veins. They are exquisitely sensitive to catecholamines. Although these tachycardias may manifest in the absence of structural heart disease or obvious precipitants, they also are commonly associated with chronic lung disease, pneumonia, myocardial (atrial) infarction, and acute alcoholic binges. Amphetamine or cocaine abuse also may precipitate automatic atrial tachyarrhythmias.

Reentrant atrial tachycardia tends to be paroxysmal, whereas automatic forms are more likely to be incessant. In both, atrial rates less than 200 beats per minute are characteristic. When the ventricular rate exceeds 120 beats per minute more than 75% of the time, tachycardia-mediated cardiomyopathy may ensue.

As noted, the presence of AV block during tachycardia provides strong evidence that the rhythm disturbance is atrial in origin. Negative P waves are not helpful in differentiating atrial tachycardia from AVNRT or AVRT. An inferior P wave axis with a negative P in lead I is diagnostic of left atrial tachycardia. An inferior P axis, a positive P in lead I, and a P wave morphology different from sinus rhythm can result only from atrial tachycardia.

Sinus node reentry may occur within the sinus node, the perinodal atrial tissue, or both. Although the mechanism may be difficult to prove clinically, most investigators agree that the P wave may be *nearly* identical to sinus rhythm, suggesting that the reentrant exit point may differ slightly from sinus pacemaker beats. Average rates generally are 130 to 140 beats per minute (range 80 to 200).

Approach to Paroxysmal Supraventricular Tachycardia Therapy

Acute management of PSVT should begin with attempts to slow or (transiently) interrupt AV nodal conduction. Vagal maneuvers (such as carotid sinus massage or Valsalva) may be tried first. Adenosine is the initial drug of choice for acute management of PSVT. An initial intravenous dose of 6 mg may be followed (2 minutes) later by 6 mg (if necessary), and 12 mg may be given (2 minutes) later if 6 mg is unsuccessful.

Adenosine should terminate more than 90% of AVNRT and AVRT. This agent also is effective in sinus node reentry. Adenosine also may terminate automatic atrial tachycardias, particularly those originating near the crista terminalis, where vagal innervation is rich. Termination may be transient because of adenosine's short half-life (10 seconds).

Intravenous verapamil (5 to 10 mg is injected over a period of 30 seconds, followed by an additional 5 mg, if necessary, after a 5- to 10-minute interval) or diltiazem (0.25 mg/kg, followed by an additional dose of 0.35 mg per kg, if necessary, after a 15-minute interval) usually is effective for PSVT termination when adenosine fails. AV block without arrhythmia termination (again) suggests the diagnosis of atrial tachycardia. Because of their longer half-lives, intravenous calcium channel blockers also may be effective for treatment of prompt tachycardia recurrence after initial success with adenosine. First-line chronic therapy for supraventricular tachycardia may be pharmacologic, with oral antiarrhythmic drugs (see section on antiarrhythmic drugs), or primary ablation for cure of supraventricular tachycardia (see section on ablation of arrhythmias).

Automatic atrial tachycardia is difficult to manage with pharmacotherapy. Precipitants should be treated or eliminated whenever possible. β-Bblockers may slow atrial rate but rarely restore sinus rhythm. Adenosine may produce sinus rhythm; however, tachycardia generally resumes as soon as the drug is metabolized.[20] Vagal maneuvers may produce AV block but do not terminate these arrhythmias. Clinical successes have been obtained with class IC agents and amiodarone. Flecainide should be avoided in patients with coronary artery disease or significant left ventricular dysfunction. Intravenous flecainide is not available in the United States (see the following discussion). Amiodarone is available for intravenous administration. Intravenous amiodarone may result in hypotension (vasodilation) and but usually does not exacerbate heart failure or cause proarrhythmia in the setting of pre-existing left ventricular dysfunction. Radiofrequency ablation therapy can be effective at curing some automatic atrial tachycardias (see section on ablation of cardiac arrhythmias).

Sinus node reentry may respond to vagal maneuvers, adenosine, verapamil, and digitalis (relatively slow onset of action limits acute application). Acute management of intra-atrial reentry is similar to that for atrial fibrillation in the absence of antegrade accessory pathway conduction (see the following discussion). Emergent or urgent direct current cardioversion is indicated when PSVT results in angina pectoris, congestive heart failure, or hypotension. Techniques for and limitations of direct current cardioversion are discussed later in the chapter. Automatic tachycardias do not respond to direct current cardioversion.

Wolff-Parkinson-White Syndrome and Its Variants

The ECG pattern of Wolff-Parkinson-White syndrome, short PR interval with pre-excitation (delta wave), has a reported prevalence of 0.1% to 0.3% in the general population. It is twice as common in males as in females.

Classic Wolff-Parkinson-White syndrome occurs when the accessory atrioventricular pathway is capable of bidirectional conduction (atrioventricular and ventriculoatrial). Symptomatic presentation usually is during the teenage years or early adulthood. Pregnancy may exacerbate symptoms. The most common tachycardia is atrioventricular reentry (down the AV node and His-Purkinje system, up the bypass tract), identical to AVRT involving a concealed bypass tract. Approximately 25% of patients with a Wolff-Parkinson-White ECG pattern are incapable of retrograde conduction (and therefore do not have orthodromic AVRT). Asymptomatic patients generally have a benign prognosis; however, the initial presentation may be ventricular fibrillation (see the following discussion).[21]

Accessory pathways generally have conduction properties similar to those of myocardium. Decremental conduction (characteristic of the AV node) is uncommon. Pathways may therefore be capable of very rapid antegrade (AV) conduction. In these instances, atrial fibrillation may be associated with irregular wide QRS tachycardia and ventricular rates in excess of 300 beats per minute (Fig. 32-1). Syncope or sudden cardiac death (degeneration to ventricular fibrillation) may ensue.

Regular wide QRS tachycardia in patients with Wolff-Parkinson-White syndrome may have any of several mechanisms. Aberrancy resulting from right or left bundle branch block (fixed or functional) may occur during orthodromic AVRT. As noted, bundle branch block ipsilateral to the accessory pathway may slow tachycardia rate.

Antidromic tachycardia occurs when antegrade conduction proceeds via a free-wall accessory pathway, and retrograde conduction occurs over the normal His-Purkinje–AV nodal route. The ventricles are activated eccentrically beginning at the annular insertion of the accessory pathway. The resulting maximally pre-excited wide QRS rhythm may be difficult to distinguish from ventricular tachycardia. Although accessory pathways

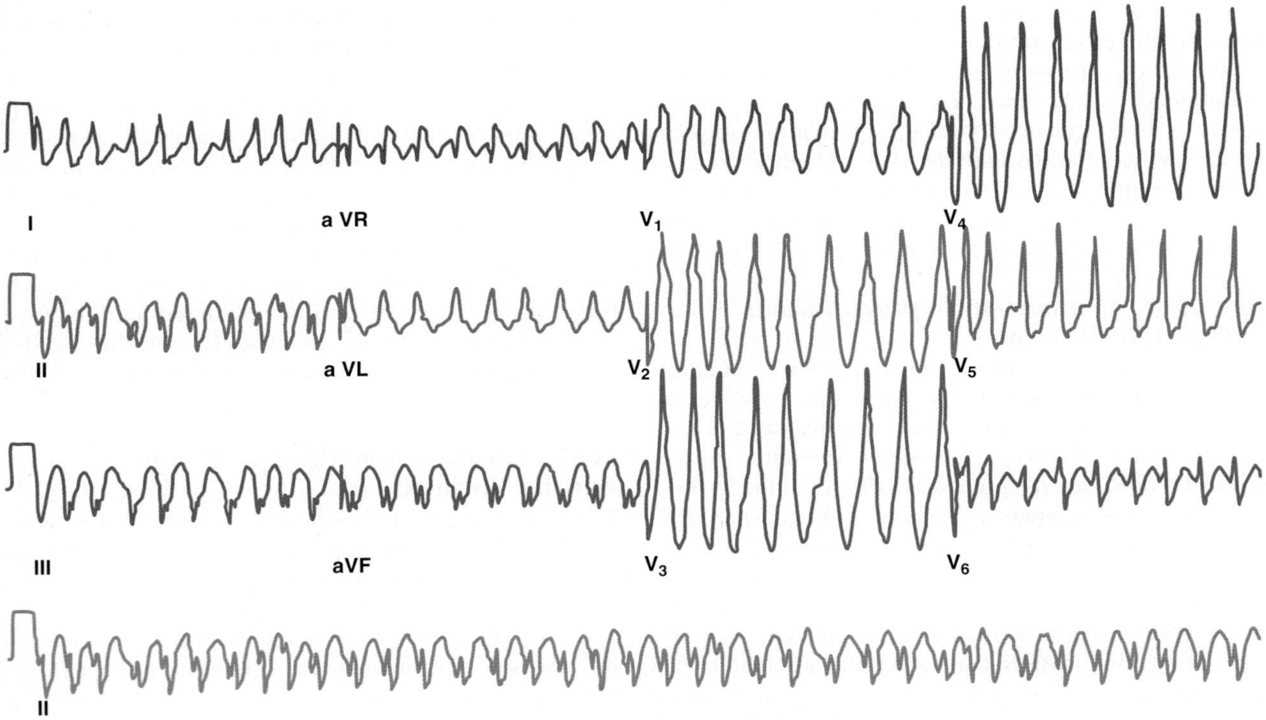

Figure 32-1. A 12-lead electrocardiogram (ECG) tracing from a patient with Wolff-Parkinson-White syndrome showing pre-excited atrial fibrillation with rapid ventricular response. A rapid, "irregularly irregular" wide QRS tachycardia is present. Pre-excited atrial fibrillation, as seen here, may degenerate to ventricular fibrillation. This ECG pattern should be promptly recognized by all practicing clinicians. I, II, III aVR, aVL, aVF, and V_1 to V_6 designate surface ECG leads. (From Trohman RG: Supraventricular tachycardia: Implications for the intensivist. Crit Care Med 2000;28(Suppl 10):N129-N135.)

may be located anywhere along the atrioventricular groove, two variants with characteristic locations deserve mention. Paroxysmal junctional reciprocating tachycardia (PJRT) is a form of AV reentry that may be nearly incessant. The antegrade limb of the circuit is the normal AV conduction system. The retrograde limb is a concealed, decrementally conducting accessory pathway usually located posteroseptally. Incessant tachycardia may result in a tachycardia-mediated cardiomyopathy.

Atriofascicular pathways (Mahaim fibers) connect the right atrium and the right bundle branch. During sinus rhythm, pre-excitation is minimal or absent. Typical Mahaim reentry goes antegrade down the bypass tract and retrograde through the normal conduction system (usually beginning with the right bundle branch). A regular wide QRS pattern results, and a typical left bundle branch block pattern is seen. These pathways conduct antegrade in a decremental fashion (retrograde accessory pathway conduction is absent) and occur much less frequently than typical atrioventricular accessory pathways. Patients with atriofascicular fibers frequently have multiple accessory pathways or AVNRT.[21,22]

Acute Management of Tachycardia Associated with Wolff-Parkinson-White Syndrome

Acute tachycardia treatment depends on characteristics of its QRS complexes. A 12-lead ECG should be obtained whenever possible.

Orthodromic AVRT usually manifests with a narrow QRS complex (functional or fixed bundle branch block can widen the QRS). Treatment should begin with vagal maneuvers. If these do not terminate the tachycardia, intravenous adenosine is the initial drug of choice. These therapeutic interventions interrupt AVRT by creating transient AV nodal conduction block.

Treatment of wide QRS tachycardia should be directed at blocking conduction via the accessory pathway. Although adenosine may terminate antidromic tachycardia (at the AV node), it will not affect atrial tachyarrhythmias conducting rapidly across the accessory pathway. Because of its short half-life adenosine administration poses little risk, unless it precipitates atrial fibrillation.

Intravenous verapamil is contraindicated in the presence of wide QRS tachycardia. Its hypotensive effects may make patients hemodynamically unstable and contribute to the onset of ventricular fibrillation. Intravenous digoxin is not given to patients with Wolff-Parkinson-White syndrome and atrial fibrillation because it may (in approximately one third of patients) enhance antegrade accessory pathway conduction and likewise result in degeneration to ventricular fibrillation.

Patients whose supine systolic blood pressure is greater than 90 mm Hg can be given intravenous procainamide. It is administered in a loading dose of 10 mg per kg infused at a rate not to exceed 50 mg per minute. Blood pressure should be monitored every minute and the infusion rate decreased if hypotension develops. Procainamide will depress conduction across the accessory pathway, decrease ventricular rate, and stabilize the patient. It may also terminate the wide QRS tachycardia. Intravenous ibutilide (1 mg infused over 10 minutes; a second 1-mg dose may be given by infusion after a 10-minute wait, if necessary) also blocks antegrade accessory pathway conduction and is more likely to terminate acute episodes of atrial fibrillation or flutter (see below).[23]

Direct current cardioversion should be available, preferably at the bedside, whenever treatment of a wide QRS tachycardia is undertaken. If, at baseline, the patient exhibits signs of hemodynamic compromise (angina, heart failure, or hypotension), drug therapy should be eschewed and direct current cardioversion employed to promptly restore sinus rhythm. If hemodynamic instability develops during drug therapy, direct current cardioversion should be performed immediately. Direct current cardioversion also should be the next elective therapy when pharmacotherapy is unsuccessful.

Radiofrequency ablation often is primary first-line chronic and curative therapy for patients with Wolff-Parkinson-White syndrome and supraventricular tachycardia (see section on ablation of arrhythmias). Medical therapy for control of supraventricular tachycardia with antiarrhythmic drugs (especially class IC and β-blocker therapy) is usually effective if the patient declines ablation therapy.

Nonparoxysmal Atrioventricular Junctional Tachycardia, Paroxysmal Atrial Tachycardia with Block, and Automatic Atrioventricular Junctional Tachycardia

Nonparoxysmal AV junctional tachycardia occurs primarily in the setting of digitalis toxicity. It also is associated with cardiac surgery, myocardial infarction, and rheumatic fever. Hypokalemia may cause or exacerbate this arrhythmia. Sympathetic stimulation increases the tachycardia rate.

Digitalis toxicity also may precipitate atrial tachycardia (so-called paroxysmal atrial tachycardia with block). This tachycardia usually is managed by withholding digoxin and administering potassium. Lidocaine, phenytoin, and digoxin-specific antigen-binding fragments also may be used.

Automatic AV junctional tachycardia, also known (particularly in pediatrics) as junctional ectopic tachycardia, primarily affects chldren and infants. It often is incessant. In patients without congenital heart disease, it may manifest as a tachycardia-mediated cardiomyopathy.

This tachyarrhythmia results in marked hemodynamic deterioration after corrective surgery for congenital heart disease. It generally appears within 12 hours postoperatively and terminates within a few days if the patient survives. Digitalis, β-blockers, and class IA antiarrhythmics are ineffective in children. Amiodarone (which may suppress tachycardia or control its rate) should be administered when rates less than 150 beats per minute cannot be achieved by other means.[24] In adults, β-blockade may successfully control the rate. Adult automatic AV junctional tachycardia may be difficult to manage medically. Recent reports suggest that catheter ablation can eliminate tachycardia while preserving AV conduction.[25-27]

Multifocal Atrial Tachycardia

MAT generally is regarded to be an automatic arrhythmia. It is characterized by multiple (three or more) morphologically distinct (nonsinus) P waves, atrial rates of 100 to 130 beats per minute, and variable AV block.

MAT commonly is associated with respiratory disease and congestive heart failure. It has been reported in patients with cancer, lactic acidosis, pulmonary emboli, renal disease, and infection. Hypoxemia frequently is present. MAT may be exacerbated by digitalis or theophylline toxicity, hypokalemia, hypomagnesemia, and hyponatremia. These precipitants usually do not result in MAT if respiratory decompensation is absent. Although MAT is (in general) an uncommon arrhythmia, it is relatively common in the critical care setting. Treatment of MAT usually is directed at elimination of the underlying precipitants. Metoprolol (used cautiously when bronchospasm is present) or verapamil may provide (atrial and ventricular) rate control and occasionally restore sinus rhythm.[28,29] Potassium and magnesium supplements may help suppress MAT. Amiodarone also has been useful in restoring sinus rhythm. MAT may, superficially, resemble atrial fibrillation. Careful examination of a 12-lead ECG may be required to distinguish between these two entities. Differentiation is important for proper patient management. MAT does not respond to direct current cardioversion and is not amenable to catheter ablation.

Sinus Tachycardia

Sinus tachycardia usually is a normal reflex response to changes in physiologic, pharmacologic, or pathophysiologic stimuli such as exercise, emotional upset, fever, hemodynamic or respiratory compromise, anemia, thyrotoxicosis, poor physical conditioning, sympathomimetic or vagolytic agents, and abnormal hemoglobins.[30] The resulting increase in cardiac output usually is beneficial. Heart rate generally does not exceed 180 beats per minute, except in young patients, who may achieve rates higher than 200 beats per minute during vigorous exercise.[3] Tachycardia resolves when conditions return to baseline. The differential diagnosis for sinus tachycardia is presented in Table 32-1.

Sinus tachycardia often is present in ICU patients and sometimes is difficult to distinguish from other supraventricular tachycardias. When observed over time, sinus tachycardia will change its rate, with gradual acceleration and gradual deceleration. The P wave morphology of sinus tachycardia should be upright in leads I, II, aVF, and V_4 to V_6. Sinus tachycardia may slow transiently with vagal maneuvers or intravenous adenosine. If adenosine administration produces AV block, the P wave morphology can be clearly seen if a 12-lead ECG is run in rhythm strip mode. A negative P wave in (any of) leads I, II, aVF, and V_4 to V_6 excludes sinus tachycardia. P waves that are negative in lead I suggest a left atrial origin. Differentiation of "high" right atrial tachycardia (positive P waves in II and aVF) waves from sinus tachycardia is more difficult. P

Table 32-1. Differential Diagnosis of Sinus Tachycardia

Etiologic Category	Specific Disorders
Hemodynamic	■ Heart failure—systolic and diastolic heart failure caused by ischemic, valvular, or nonischemic myopathy ■ Loss of circulating blood volume—gastrointestinal bleeding, anemia, shifts of intravascular fluid due to changes in colloidal osmotic pressure or inflammation ■ Septic shock—dehydration ■ Vascular shunts—intracardiac as well as aortovenous malformations, fistulas ■ Pulmonary embolism
Metabolic and neurohumoral	■ Sepsis—infections and inflammatory conditions ■ Hyperthyroidism ■ Paget's disease ■ Pheochromocytoma ■ Carcinoid syndrome ■ Beriberi heart disease ■ Carcinoma ■ Hyperpyrexia ■ Acidosis ■ Exercise
Pharmacologic	■ Sympathomimetic agents—isoproterenol, epinephrine, or dopamine ■ Vagolytic agents, atropine, acopolamine ■ Vasoldilators—nitrates, angiotensin-converting enzyme inhibitors, angiotensin receptor blockers, hydrazine, as well as centrally acting vasodilators ■ Thyroid preparations, caffeine and nicotine ■ Bronchodilators, including theophylline and terbutaline ■ Anesthetic agents, including spinal anesthetics, causing peripheral vasodilation ■ Abused drugs—amphetamines, cocaine, "ecstasy," cannabis
Neurologic/psychological	■ Pain ■ Fear, anxiety, and hysteria ■ Hyper-beta phase of neurocardiogenic syncope ■ Autonomic dysfunction such as with diabetes

wave amplitude in the inferior leads may increase (normally) during sinus tachycardia. Comparison of the 12-lead P wave morphology with that on an older 12-lead ECG tracing (if obtainable) when the patient was clearly in normal sinus rhythm may not result in an exact match.

Atrial Flutter

Although the precise reentrant circuit is unknown, typical atrial flutter traverses (with either counterclockwise or clockwise rotation) through an isthmus formed by the inferior vena cava, tricuspid valve, eustachian ridge, and coronary sinus ostia. Counterclockwise rotation is more common and results in negative "flutter" waves in ECG leads II, III, aVF, and V_6. Atrial activity in lead V_1 is positively directed. Clockwise atrial flutter produces oppositely directed flutter waves in these leads. Atrial rates generally range between 250 and 350 beats per minute; however, slower rates may be seen in the presence of specific pharmacotherapy (which slows conduction within the circuit) or marked right atrial enlargement (presumably caused by a larger circuit). Atrial flutter usually manifests with 2:1 atrioventricular block and ventricular rates of approximately 150 beats per minute.

Pharmacotherapy for (typical and atypical) atrial flutter is similar to that outlined for atrial fibrillation. Special care must be taken to avoid inadvertent precipitation of 1:1 AV conduction and subsequent hemodynamic deterioration. Radiofrequency ablation also can be used as chronic, curative primary therapy for typical atrial flutter (see later section on ablation of arrhythmias).

Atrial Fibrillation

Atrial fibrillation is the most important sustained supraventricular arrhythmia both in frequency and in potential for long-term sequelae. Atrial fibrillation and atrial flutter frequently coexist. More than 2 million people in the United States suffer from atrial fibrillation. The frequency of this arrhythmia increases dramatically after the age of 60.

Atrial fibrillation most often is associated with structural cardiac (diffuse atrial) disease. Unlike in typical atrial flutter, left atrial enlargement is more important than right atrial enlargement in the pathogenesis of atrial fibrillation.[31] The chaotic ECG appearance of this arrhythmia usually is the result of shifting reentrant circuits (multiple wavelet hypotheses). Atrial fibrillation may have focal triggers (usually in one or more pulmonary veins).[8] Causes of atrial fibriilation are listed in Box 32-2.

Acute Management of Atrial Fibrillation

Treatment of atrial fibrillation has three important components: (1) ventricular control; (2) restoration (and maintenance) of sinus rhythm; and (3) prevention of embolic phenomena.

Box 32-2

Causes of Atrial Fibrillation

Increased atrial pressure evaluation, atrium, secondary to:
- Mitral or tricuspid valve disease
- Myocardial disease (primary or secondary, leading to systolic or diastolic dysfunction)
- Semilunar valve abnormalities (causing ventricular hypertrophy)
- Intracardiac tumors or thrombi

Atrial ischemia
- Coronary artery disease

Inflammatory or infiltrative atrial disease
- Pericarditis
- Amyloidosis
- Myocarditis

Age-induced atrial fibrotic changes

Intoxicants
- Alcohol
- Carbon monoxide
- Poison gas

Increased sympathetic activity
- Hyperthyroidism
- Pheochromocytoma
- Anxiety
- Alcohol
- Caffeine
- Drugs

Increased parasympathetic activity

Primary or metastatic disease in or adjacent to the atrial wall

Postoperative
- Cardiac and pulmonary surgery
- Overhydration
- Pericarditis
- Cardiac trauma
- Hypoxia
- Pneumonia

Congenital heart disease
- Particularly atrial septal defect

Neurogenic
- Subarachnoid hemorrhage
- ?Nonhemorrhagic, major stroke

Idiopathic

From Falk RH, Podrid PJ (eds): Atrial Fibrillation: Mechanisms and Management. New York, Raven Press, 1992.

Control of the ventricular rate (Table 32-2) most frequently is achieved using digoxin, β-blockers, calcium channel blockers (verapamil or diltiazem), or combinations of these agents. Verapamil should be administered cautiously to patients with significant left ventricular dysfunction. The time-honored use of digitalis preparations has recently come under considerable scrutiny. Although digoxin is effective in controlling rates at rest, exercise rate control is not often achieved. Digoxin remains appropriate therapy for patients with concomitant left ventricular dysfunction and congestive heart failure. Intravenous diltiazem is effective and well tolerated. Diltiazem may be administered by continuous intravenous infusion. The combination of efficacy, ease of parenteral delivery, and tolerance makes this agent an attractive option in the critical care setting.

A variety of agents may be used to restore sinus rhythm. Patients with adrenergically mediated atrial fibrillation should be managed initially with β-blockers. Sotalol and amiodarone are options in patients with atrial fibrillation refractory to β-blockade alone.

It has become customary to manage acute episodes with intravenous procainamide. This mode of management is appropriate when relatively rapid conversion is desired or if the patient is unable to take medications orally. Dosing and management of associated hypotension have already been discussed. Intravenous procainamide has been reported to restore sinus rhythm in approximately 43% to 65% of patients with atrial fibrillation or flutter.[32]

Ibutilide, a unique class III agent, prolongs action potential, thereby blocking the rapid component of the delayed flow.[33,34] This increase results in QT interval prolongation. Patients receiving intravenous ibutilide should be carefully monitored[33] (on telemetry for 4 to 8 hours) for development of torsades de pointes. Ibutilide is suitable for acute cardioversion; however, prolonged intravenous (or oral) dosing is not available to prevent arrhythmia recurrence. Ibutilide restores sinus rhythm in approximately 30% to 50% of patients with atrial fibrillation and up to 76% of patients with atrial flutter.[32] Ibutilide may be administered safely to patients on concomitant antiarrhythmic agents.[35]

At first glance, the efficacy of intravenous procainamide and that of ibutilide appear to be similar. Newer, direct comparisons of these agents have demonstrated clear superiority of ibutilide in conversion of atrial fibrillation and atrial flutter. Restoration of sinus rhythm with ibutilide occurred in 32% to 51% (atrial fibrillation) of patients and 64% to 76% (atrial flutter), compared with 0% to 5% (atrial fibrillation) and 0% to 14% (atrial flutter) after intravenous procainamide.[33,36,37]

Intravenous amiodarone is (initially) primarily a calcium channel and β-blocker. It may be effective for rate control when other agents fail. The temptation to use intravenous amiodarone to restore sinus rhythm should be tempered by knowledge of its acute electrophysiologic effects. Its class I and, particularly, class III effects take time to occur, making this a poor choice for rapid conversion. Bolus treatment with intravenous amiodarone has been very disappointing (4% conversion) for acute conversion of atrial fibrillation.[32] By contrast, in approximately 20% to 50% of patients with persistent atrial fibrillation (lasting longer than 24 to 48 hours), reversion to sinus rhythm is achieved with sustained administration (loading periods of up to 4 weeks) of oral amiodarone.[38] Intravenous amiodarone may result in less hypotension when used for rate control in the ICU than diltiazem.[39]

Intravenous class IC agents (such as flecainide and propafenone) are the most effective drugs for converting

Table 32-2. Intravenous Drugs for Atrial Fibrillation

Drug	Acute Dose	Maintenance Dose	Comments
Drugs for Rate Control*			
Digoxin	1 mg over 24 h in increments of 0.25-0.5 mg	0.125-0.25 mg	Not very effective in high-catecholamine states; caution with renal disease
Esmolol†	0.5 mg/kg/min for 1 min	0.05-0.2 mg/kg/min	Short half-life; hypotension common
Verapamil	5-20 mg in 5-mg increments	5 to 10-mg boluses every 30 min *or* 0.005 mg/kg/min	Caution with left ventricular dysfunction
Diltiazem	20-25 mg or 0.25-0.35 mg/kg	10-15 mg/hr	Well tolerated; may cause hypotension
Drugs for Cardioversion			
Procainamide	10-15 mg/kg at ≤50 mg/min	2-6 mg/min	May cause hypotension
Amiodarone‡	150 mg over 10 min, then 1 mg/min for 6 h	0.5 mg/min	May cause hypotension; many long-term side effects
Ibutilide	1 mg over 10 min A second dose may be given 10 min after the first	None	Prolongs QT, may cause torsades de pointes May lower energy requirement for direct current cardioversion

Adapted from Falk RH: Control of the ventricular rate in atrial fibrillation. In Falk RH, Podrid PJ (eds): *Atrial fibrillation: Mechanisms and management*, Raven Press, New York, 1992.
*Assumes no pre-excitation.
†Metoprolol and propranolol also may be used.
‡Amiodarone also is effective for rate control.

atrial fibrillation of recent onset. Unfortunately, they are not available in the United States. Ibutilide is more effective than intravenous class IC agents for restoration of sinus rhythm in atrial flutter.[38] Electrical cardioversion remains the most effective way of restoring sinus rhythm in patients with atrial fibrillation. Urgent electrical cardioversion should be contemplated for sustained tachycardias that precipitate angina, heart failure, or hypotension.

Episodes of atrial fibrillation may be precipitated and perpetuated by metabolic disturbances or a hyperadrenergic state. Serial direct current shocks are not appropriate for recurrent (within hours or days) paroxysms (self-terminating episodes) of atrial fibrillation. This scenario is relatively common in ICUs or after cardiac surgery. Appropriate management should include treatment (or removal) of potential precipitants, β-blockade (if tolerated), and institution of specific antiarrhythmic therapy (intravenous procainamide, intravenous or oral amiodarone, oral dofetilide or sotalol) to prevent additional episodes. Restoration of sinus rhythm may be difficult and impractical when a *severe* metabolic derangement or multisystem organ failure is present.[40]

A recent meta-analysis of perioperative prophylactic amiodarone demonstrated decreased incidence of atrial fibrillation and flutter, ventricular tachyarrhythmias, stroke, and reduced length of stay after cardiac surgery.[41] Not all studies included used β-blockade, and the course of therapy was inconsistent among trials. The Prophylactic Oral Amiodarone for the Prevention of Arrhythmias That Begin Early after Revascularization, Valve Replacement, or Repair (PAPABEAR), a large randomized controlled trial, compared perioperative amiodarone with placebo and showed significant reduction in postoperative atrial tachyarrhythmias.[42] Toxicity risks were reduced because amiodarone was used for a short duration. Neither study demonstrated reduction in mortality. The data for perioperative amiodarone in cardiac surgery are compelling; however, incremental benefit beyond β-blockade alone remains unclear. It may still be reasonable to reserve amiodarone for postoperative atrial fibrillation in patients on β-blockers and to limit use of amiodarone to 6 to 12 weeks postoperatively to prevent side effects.

Special Considerations for the Intensivist

Patients in an intensive care setting frequently have active precipitants for reinitiation of atrial or ventricular arrhythmias. Such factors include hypoxemia, excess circulating (endogenous and exogenous) catecholamines, congestive heart failure, fever (sepsis), and pulmonary emboli, to name a few. Many of these conditions have overlapping features as well.

Digoxin, procainamide, dofetilide, and sotalol are excreted renally and must be carefully managed (or avoided) to prevent complications in patients with renal failure or insufficiency. Amiodarone is hepatically excreted and can be used safely in patients with renal insufficiency or renal failure on dialysis.

Drugs administered orally may not be well absorbed, and intravenous agents (procainamide and amiodarone) may cause hypotension. These factors conspire to make prophylaxis against recurrence difficult.

Most digitalis toxicity–related supraventricular arrhythmias show relatively slow heart rates and are reasonably well tolerated hemodynamically. Accelerated junctional rhythm and paroxysmal atrial tachycardia with block tend to terminate spontaneously after digoxin is stopped. Digitalis toxic ventricular tachycardia (classically bidirectional tachycardia) is more serious, but often slow and hemodynamically well tolerated. Dilantin and lidocaine may be effective for control of digitalis-induced ventricular tachycardia. Digoxin antibodies can be used in cases in which watchful waiting or lidocaine is ineffective or poorly tolerated owing to hemodynamic unstability. Electrical cardioversion is contraindicated in the presence of digitalis toxicity. Refractory ventricular fibrillation may ensue.

The intensivist must balance complicated issues before undertaking direct current cardioversion. Strong effort should be focused on avoidance of low-yield attempts. Repeated doses of anesthesia and multiple shocks will ultimately result in further deterioration of critically ill patients. Optimal management of precipitants, careful choices, and monitoring of antiarrhythmic therapy, as well as a solid understanding of cardioversion and defibrillation techniques (see later section on defibrillation), will maximize success. In some cases, atrial fibrillation can be "cured" by radiofrequency ablation, or ventricular rate can be controlled by radiofrequency ablate and pace techniques when medical therapy is ineffective. (See later section on ablation of arrhythmias.)

Anticoagulation

Anticoagulation plays a pivotal role in minimizing the risk of emboli (and strokes) during elective cardioversion of atrial fibrillation.[43] Classic recommendations for management of atrial fibrillation of longer than 48 hours' duration include 3 weeks of therapeutic warfarin (to achieve a prothrombin time [PT]/international normalized ratio [INR] of 2.0-3.0) before direct current shock and (at least) 4 more weeks of warfarin after the procedure. Although emboli may be less frequent with atrial flutter,[43] it is clear that they occur,[44] and the recommendations are the same as for atrial fibrillation.

Special Considerations for the Intensivist

The intensivist rarely sees ideal candidates for classic anticoagulation. Outpatient preparation for an elective cardioversion would be an exception, rather than the rule. Likewise, the intensivist sees many patients with recent or active bleeding (gastrointestinal, intracerebral) and a variety of coagulopathies that make anticoagulation absolutely or relatively contraindicated.

Short-term therapeutic anticoagulation with heparin before cardioversion (followed by warfarin in the usual manner) combined with transesophageal echocardiography (TEE) has gained acceptance as an alternative approach.[45] Data from the ACUTE trial suggested similar embolic rates (0.5% versus 0.8%) comparing conventional and TEE-guided approaches.[46]

TEE is useful for detecting left atrial thrombi. It provides an excellent, minimally invasive view of the left atrial appendage. Patients with obvious thrombi should be anticoagulated for 3 to 6 weeks and have demonstrable resolution of clot before cardioversion is attempted.[45]

The intensivist must carefully weigh the risks and benefits of anticoagulation for each individual patient. Difficult decisions about the safety of both short- and long-term anticoagulation may be compounded by concomitant disease processes. At times, TEE may be the only possible (partial) insurance against emboli. Negative results on TEE, however, do not constitute a guarantee against emboli, and the temptation to routinely substitute TEE for adequate anticoagulation must be avoided.

Direct Current Cardioversion

Deep Sedation for Cardioversion

Direct current shocks should never be administered to a conscious patient. A high-energy shock delivered to an awake patient may result in lifelong emotional trauma and has been appropriately termed a calamity.[47]

Our preferred drug for deep sedation before cardioversion is propofol.[48] Dosing must be individualized. A bolus of 0.5 to 0.6 mg/kg, usually is effective for routine elective cardioversion, but may be excessive in a critically ill patient. Propofol's adverse effects include apnea, bradycardia, hypotension, nausea, and pain and burning at the intravenous injection site that can be minimized by giving local lidocaine at the site. Overdose is treated with ventilation and oxygen, elevation of the legs, increasing flow rates of intravenous fluids, and administration of pressor agents and/or anticholinergic agents.

Regardless of who administers sedation, expert ability to manage the patient's airway must be immediately available. We recommend that an anesthesiologist be present for very-high-risk patients. We use midazolam and fentanyl, in place of propofol, when an anesthesiologist cannot be present.

Technical Aspects

When the capacitors of a defibrillator charge, the device becomes capable of energy delivery (measured in watt-seconds or joules [J]). The energy is composed of voltage and current. Transthoracic current flow is partially determined by electrode placement. A variety of configurations have been employed. We have favored an anteroposterior (parasternal and left infrascapular) pathway for cardioverting atrial fibrillation and flutter and other atrial arrhythmias. This configuration provides the best vectors for energy delivery to the atria[49] (Fig. 32-2). We also have found it to be optimal for patients with an implantable cardioverter-defibrillator (ICD) and epicardial patches.[50]

Most problems with energy delivery have been eliminated with modern external defibrillators that deliver biphasic shocks. Devices with two different biphasic waveforms are available: rectilinear (Zoll Medical, Chelmsford, Mass.) and truncated exponential (Physiocontrol, Redmond, Wash.). Head-to-head comparisons have not found significant differences between these biphasic waveforms. Success rates for conversion of atrial fibrillation range from 87% to 100%.

Self-adhesive pads commonly are used in high-risk patients. They are easy to position precisely. Transthoracic impedance may be higher (70 to 100 ohms) with these

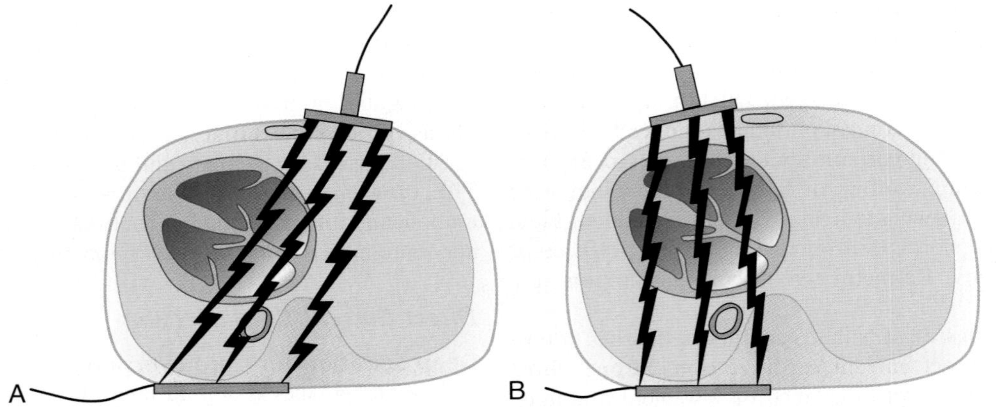

Figure 32-2. Anterior-posterior electrode placement for cardioversion of atrial fibrillation and flutter. **A,** Right parasternal anterior-posterior electrode placement. **B,** Left parasternal anterior-posterior electrode placement. In each instance, the current vector transverses a critical mass of atrial myocardium. The right parasternal position has more of the right atrium between the electrodes and may be advantageous in patients with biatrial pathology. The left parasternal position has a smaller interelectrode distance and less lung between electrodes. It has been advocated for patients with left atrial enlargement. (Adapted from Ewy GA: The optimal technique for electrical cardioversion of atrial fibrillation. Clin Cardiol 1994;17:79-84.)

pads than with metal electrodes (50 ohms). A switch from self-adhesive pads to paddles with pressure is a simple method to increase current delivered per maximum shock and gain additional procedural success.[49] Double patching (Fig. 32-3) is another simple method of lowering the impedance to gain additional procedural success (personal observation, LG).

Although it has been common to recommend an initial monophasic energy of 100 J for atrial fibrillation (with initial success rates of 50%), we agree with Ewy and begin with 200 J.[51] An initial monophasic energy of 360 J for atrial fibrillation lasting longer than 48 hours also has been suggested.[51,52] A similar recommendation of 200 J also applies to biphasic waveforms, particularly for cardioversion in patients with atrial fibrillation of long duration.[45] Optimal monophasic energy delivery for cardioversion of atrial flutter is 100 J.[53] We generally use 100 J for biphasic cardioversion of atrial flutter as well.

R wave synchronization should be ensured during cardioversion of arrhythmias with well-defined QRS complexes. Failure to do so may lead to shock delivery within the "vulnerable period" of the T wave and induction of ventricular fibrillation.

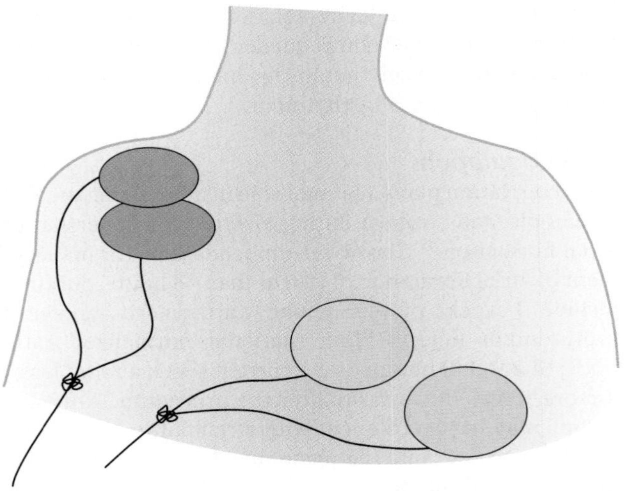

Figure 32-3. Double patching positioned as shown increases electrode surface area, current delivered, and cardioversion-defibrillation shock efficacy.

Determinants of Short- and Long-Term Success of Cardioversion

Electrode size and placement, as well as transthoracic impedance, influence current flow (and procedural outcome). Impedance is in turn influenced by a variety of factors (in addition to those previously described). These include the phase of ventilation (impedance is lower with expiration than with inspiration), distance between electrodes, pressure on electrodes (air does not conduct well), effect of previous discharges (decreased impedance), time between discharges (waiting as long as 3 minutes may provide continued decreases in impedance), and patient body habitus (heavier weight or increased body mass index will decrease success).[49,54]

Poor long-term success in cardioversion of atrial fibrillation relates to arrhythmia duration (longer than 1 year) and large left atrial diameter (greater than 5 cm). Untreated hyperthyroidism, mitral stenosis, or congestive heart failure increases the likelihood of recurrence. Use of concomitant antiarrhythmic drugs (especially amiodarone) may help maintain sinus rhythm. Atrial flutter recurrences are hard to prevent, even with pharmacotherapy. Recurrence of typical atrial flutter should be eliminated with radiofrequency catheter ablation.

Options for Refractory Patients

As noted, the intensivist must weigh the risks and benefits of repeated attempts at direct current cardioversion. Care should be taken to avoid serial futile shocks. Nevertheless, an awareness of available options is essential. Most hospitals have defibrillators that deliver up to 360 J. Standard waveforms have been monophasic (damped sinusoidal or truncated exponential). Newer defibrillators have a biphasic truncated exponential waveform that is more effective per joule output than monophasic waveform defibrillators. Electrode size is an important determinant of transthoracic impedance. Current flow is inversely related to impedance. Optimal paddle size ranges from 8 to 12 cm. A conductive gel or paste must be used between the metal electrodes and the chest skin.[49] Smearing of gel between paddles may deflect energy away from the heart.[55] A switch from monophasic to biphasic defibrillator, or a switch from self-adhesive pads (higher impedance, typically 70 to 100 ohms) to paddles with pressure is a simple method (lower impedance, typically 50 ohms) to increase current delivered per maximum shock, and to promote procedural success. Use of higher-energy transthoracic shocks (720 J) in large patients with atrial fibrillation refractory to 360 J has been reported. Other techniques for increasing success of cardioversion are simultaneous use of two cardioverters, both synchronized via four paddles,[56] and double patching (as shown in Fig. 32-3) using a single defibrillator.

Self-adhesive pads commonly are used in high-risk patients. They are easy to position precisely. Transthoracic impedance may be higher (70 to 100 ohms) with these pads compared with metal electrodes (50 ohms).[49] Double patching can lower electrode impedance by increasing surface area, thereby allowing more current (see Fig. 32-3). Double patching lowers impedance by approximately 20 to 40 ohms and increases current delivery per maximum output shock. In an unpublished series of patients, double patching increased elective cardioversion of atrial fibrillation success rates from 80% (single patch) to 88% (double patch). (personal observation [LG]). On two occasions, double patching was lifesaving when used to defibrillate ventricular fibrillation in two patients, after several 360-J shocks using single patches failed (personal observation [LG]). Double patching is accomplished by splicing the extra electrodes together using conventional electrical wire nuts. Figure 32-3 shows double patch configuration for ventricular defibrillation. A double-patched anterior posterior placement (as in Fig. 32-2) is best for refractory cardioversion of atrial fibrillation.

Internal cardioversion has been used for refractory atrial fibrillation. Internal cardioversion for atrial fibrillation is effective in approximately 70% to 80% of patients refractory to 360 J. Transvenous placement of (both) right atrial coronary sinus multipolar catheters and biphasic shock waveforms markedly reduced energy required for successful cardioversion. Unfortunately, catheter placement may require reduction or discontinuation of anticoagulation, increasing the risk of emboli. Despite very low energy requirements (as low as 2 to 3 J with biphasic waveforms), the procedure remains painful and requires sedation or anesthesia.[57]

Oral Antiarrhythmic Drugs for Treatment of Paroxysmal Atrial Fibrillation, Flutter, and Other Supraventricular Tachycardias

Initiaition of chronic oral antiarrhythmic drug therapy for supraventricular arrhythmias usually is in the realm of practice of general cardiologists and electrophysiologists. Nevertheless, intensivists should be familiar with these agents, as well as current philosophies for their use. The older class IA drugs, including quinidine, procainamide, and disopyramide, now are rarely used because of the risk of QT prolongation and torsades de pointes ventricular tachycardia, low efficacy rates, and poor noncardiac side effect profiles resulting in high drug discontinuation rates.[46,58] The antiarrythmic drugs in common use are described next.

Flecainide (class 1C) is an excellent drug for treatment of all supraventricular tachycardias including atrial fibrillation. It is contraindicated in patients with coronary artery disease or significant left ventricular dysfunction <40%). The typical starting dose is 100 mg given orally twice daily (titrated up to 150 mg twice daily, as needed). Potential adverse effects include proarrhythmia (incessant monomophic ventricular tachycardia), exacerbation of congestive heart failure, and "organization" of atrial fibrillation to atrial flutter with a rapid ventricular response (1:1 conduction). Ventricular proarrhythmia is unlikely in the absence of significant structural heart disease (incidence approximately 2%). Flecainide has very few noncardiac side effects.

Propafenone (class IC) is an equally effective drug for control of supraventricular tachycardia and atrial fibrillation. Newly formulated sustained-release propafenone has more convenient twice-daily dosing, starting at 225 mg orally twice daily, titrated up to 425 mg twice daily if necessary. Sustained-release propafenone was safe and effective in a large outpatient trial (RAFT)[59] and is the only rhythm control drug for atrial fibrillation that is FDA approved for outpatient use. Side effects are similar to those of flecainide, with the addition of a "metallic taste in the mouth" as an unusual noncardiac side effect, which does not require drug discontinuation. Propafenone has mild β-blocking properties but usually not enough to rely on for AV blockade in atrial fibrillation or atrial flutter. Like flecainide, propafenone should not be used in patients with significant structural heart disease.

Sotalol (class III) generally is chosen for patients with coronary artery disease (or other structural heart disease), but can also be a first-line drug for atrial fibrillation in patients with no structural heart disease. It has β-blocking effects and blocks the rapid component of the delayed rectifier potassium current. Sotalol is renally excreted, and doses must be adjusted downward in patients with renal insufficiency. A 3% to 7% risk of torsades de pointes exists with sotalol, with this disturbance usually occurring in the first week of therapy. Other side effects include congestive heart failure, exacerbation of bronchospasm, bradycardia, and fatigue. The starting dose is 80 mg given orally twice daily, titrated up to 160 mg twice daily if necessary and as tolerated. Controversy exists over whether sotalol can be initiated as an outpatient therapy. We recommend hospitalization with telemetry monitoring and daily 12-lead ECGs for safe initiation of sotalol.

Dofetilide (a class III agent) blocks the rapid component of the delayed rectifier potassium current. Similar to other class III drugs, it prolongs the QT interval and can cause torsades de pointes. In the United States, physicians must take a course to permit and certify them to use dofetilide. The drug is dispensed by a national registry system to ensure the physician writing the prescription is certified. Its main advantage is that it has a low proarrhythmia profile (with proper dosing) when used in patients with low ejection fractions. A second virtue is that it does not precipitate or aggravate congestive heart failure (CHF), even if used in patients with low ejection fraction. The dosage range is 125 to 500 μg given twice daily, which is adjusted according to renal function and QT interval prolongation. Inpatient monitoring on a telemetry ward and frequent ECGs (obtained 2 hours after each dose) to monitor the QT are requirements for initiation of dofetilide therapy. The drug is therefore rather inconvenient to use. However, it is the only alternative to amiodarone for treatment of atrial fibrillation in patients with poor left ventricular function. Dofetilide usually is well tolerated, with few noncardiac side effects.

Amiodarone is a class III antiarrhythmic with potassium, sodium, and calcium channel blocking properties. In addition, it is a noncompetitive β-blocker and inhibits peripheral conversion of thyroxine (T_4) to triiodothyronine (T_3). It is considered the best atrial fibrillation rhythm control drug. It is an excellent AV node–blocking drug. Even when the drug fails to achieve rhythm control of atrial fibrillation, it usually will provide good rate control. Amiodarone has an extremely long half-life (a virtue for compliance, but a liability if side effects occur). Like dofetilide, it can be used in patients with low ejection fraction with risk of heart failure exacerbation. Amiodarone does not adversely affect survival and in some studies offered some protection against arrhythmia-related sudden death[60-62] It can cause significant bradycardia but is associated with a very low incidence of ventricular proarrhythmia (less than 1%), despite the fact that it prolongs the QT interval. The drug requires an initial loading dose (regimens vary). A maintenance dose in the range of 200 mg (or less) per day usually can be achieved and is helpful in minimizing side effects. Occasionally, maintenance doses of 400 mg per day are required for supraventricular tachycardia control. Amiodarone's long-term noncardiac side effects are significant and should limit its use in younger patients. Nevertheless, amiodarone is the most frequently prescribed specific antiarrhythmic drug in the United States. Side effects include pulmonary toxicity, polyneuropathy, photosensitivity, bradycardia, hepatic dysfunction, thyroid dysfunction, and ophthalmologic complications. Side effects are correlated with maintenance dose and duration of therapy. Baseline pulmonary function studies with diffusing capacity, chest radiograph, liver and thyroid function studies, and eye examination should be performed before or shortly after the drug is started. We recommend thyroid function tests, liver function tests, and a chest radiograph every 6 months to look for signs of toxicity. It is particularly disturbing that pulmonary toxicity (which may be fatal) may be missed even with careful surveillance.

The AFFIRM trial randomized over 4000 patients to receive rate or rhythm control treatment strategies (plus warfarin sodium in both treatment groups). Because AFFIRM demonstrated no significant stroke, quality of life, or mortality differences with rhythm versus rate control, physicians must consider the risk-benefit ratio of antiarrhythmics to maintain sinus rhythm.[63-65] Patients with brief or minimally symptomatic recurrences of paroxysmal atrial fibrillation, often do not require antiarrhythmic drugs. Patients with troublesome symptoms generally require suppressive antiarrhythmic therapy. Rate control and prevention of thromboembolism are appropriate for both situations.[46]

The 2006 ACC/AHA/ESC guidelines for the management of patients with atrial fibrillation recommend that antiarrhythmic drugs for rhythm control of paroxysmal atrial fibrillation be chosen using an algorithm (Fig. 32-4). This algorithm takes into account whether or not the patient has structural heart disease hypertension with or without "significant" left ventricular hypertrophy (cardiography determined echo wall thickness of 1.4 cm or greater), coronary artery disease.[46] If there is no structural heart disease, or minimal left ventricular hypertrophy only, the therapeutic agents of first choice are, flecainide, propafenone, or sotalol. Second-line therapeutic options include amiodarone, dofetilide, and catheter ablation. If significant left ventricular hypertrophy is present, the treatment of first choice is amiodarone therapy, with catheter ablation considered second-line therapy. If coronary artery disease is present, the treatment of choice is administration of sotalol (because of its β-blocking properties), with second-line therapies including dofetilide, amiodarone, and catheter ablation. If clinical heart failure is present, first-line agents are amiodarone and dofetilide, and second-line therapy is catheter ablation. These guidelines consistently recommend radiofrequency ablation as a second-line therapy, and specify that at least one antiarrhythmic rhythm control drug should be tried before radiofrequency ablative cure of atrial fibrillation is attempted. See the section on radiofrequency ablation of cardiac arrythmias for a discussion of the various methods of ablating atrial fibrillation.

Stroke Prevention

The risk of stroke increases in patients older than 75 years of age. Additional risk factors include history of hypertension, heart failure, left ventricular ejection fraction less than 35%, diabetes mellitus, previous stroke, history of transient ischemic attacks or embolism, mitral stenosis, and the presence of prosthetic heart valve. Patients who are younger than 75 years with normal hearts and "lone" atrial fibrillation (i.e., with none of the aforementioned risk factors) can be anticoagulated with aspirin (81 to 325 mg daily) instead of warfarin sodium.[46]

VENTRICULAR ARRHYTHMIAS

The intensivist must be prepared to recognize and participate in the management of ventricular arrhythmias. However, the long-term management usually is prescribed by cardiologists and electrophysiologists. Therefore, this section concentrates on the intensive care and emergency

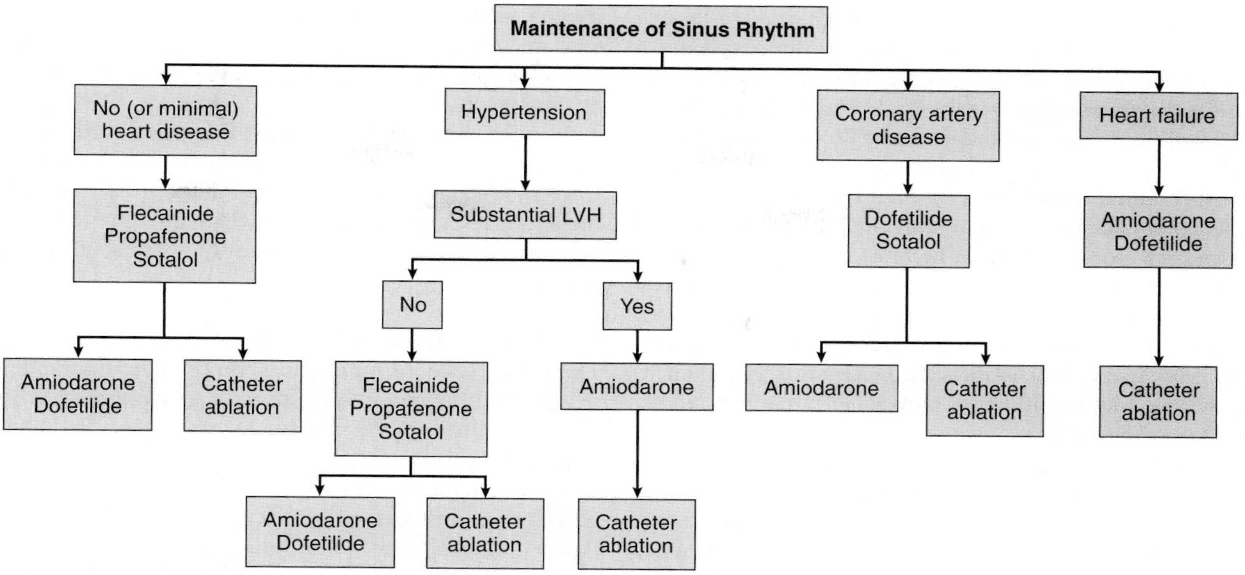

Figure 32-4. 2006 ACC/AHA/ESC guideline algorithm for oral antiarrhythmic drug therapy for maintenance of sinus rhythm in patients with atrial fibrillation. Although the figure suggests that dofetilide is a first-line agent for treatment of coronary artery disease, the text of the guidelines describes it as a second-line agent. LVH, left ventricular hypertension.

treatment of ventricular arrhythmias and briefly addresses chronic therapy. The emergency treatment of cardiac arrest is covered in Chapter 1.

Arrhythmogenesis

Reentry is the most common mechanism for sustained ventricular arrhythmias. Three conditions are required for reentry. The first is the presence of two anatomically contiguous pathways separated by a central region of inexcitable tissue. Second, there must be unidirectional block in one of the pathways. Third, a zone of slow conduction also must be present to allow recovery and excitation of the region of block. Such conditions may be anatomically defined (as in the border zone of an old myocardial infarction scar) or result from functional disturbances in conduction and refractoriness. Gessman and associates[66-68] mapped macro ventricular tachycardia reentry loops in an animal model of ventricular tachycardia, and subsequently in patients. In addition, "cutting" the loop with ice mapping caused ventricular tachycardia termination, providing proof that reentry was the arrhythmia mechanism.

Abnormal automaticity results in spontaneous impulse formation in cells that otherwise do not exhibit pacemaker activity. Diseased cardiac tissue is particularly susceptible to development of abnormal automaticity. This may result in rates faster than the normal pacemaker activity of the sinus node. Automatic cells (in the AV node or the His-Purkinje system) may usurp the sinus node by means of enhanced automaticity in which their depolarization is accelerated by drugs, sympathetic activity, or metabolic disturbances.

Triggered activity occurs when oscillations in membrane potential (called afterdepolarizations) reach the threshold for action potential formation, resulting in abnormal impulse formation. Early afterdepolarizations (EADs) result from delayed inactivation of inward ion currents during the plateau phase of the action potential. EADs appear to be important in the genesis of torsades de pointes (see later). Delayed afterdepolarizations (DADs) result from increased intracellular calcium. Digitalis toxicity is the classic example of DAD-induced triggered activity. Digitalis inhibits the Na^+-K^+ pump, thereby increasing intracellular Na^+, which in turn increases intracellular Ca^{++} via the Na^+-Ca^{++} exchange current.[69]

Metabolic Disturbances and Ischemia

Metabolic disturbances and ischemia are common in the critically ill. Patients may suffer from (synergistic or opposing) effects of multiple abnormalities. In the presence of partial predispositions, arrhythmias may not develop until patients are exposed to factors resulting in abnormal automaticity, conduction, or refractoriness.

Hypokalemia delays repolarization and prolongs action potential duration. This may lead to EADs and triggered arrhythmias. Hypomagnesemia and hypokalemia often coexist. Each is associated with QT prolongation and torsades de pointes. Repletion of Mg^{++} is an important adjunct to the management of hypokalemia. Hypermagnesemia usually is not associated with arrhythmogenesis.

Hyperkalemia suppresses automaticity and slows conduction. The earliest ECG sign is peaked T waves. At high levels (usually 7.0 mEq per L or greater), marked QRS widening (sine wave morphology) may be seen, followed by cardiac arrest. Patients with renal insufficiency may be particularly susceptible. Cardiac effects of severe hyperkalemia may be lethal and require prompt intervention. The most rapid means of countering cardiac toxicity is intravenous administration of 10% calcium chloride. The ECG should be monitored to ensure that signs of hyperkalemia have been reversed. Calcium chloride, although effective emergently, does not lower serum potassium.

Sodium bicarbonate (usual dose 44 to 88 mEq) reduces serum potassium. Regular insulin (10 units) will result in redistribution of K^+ from the extracellular to the intracellular space but does not lower total body potassium stores. Insulin should be followed by 50 mL of 50% glucose.

Further treatment of hyperkalemia involves removal of potassium from the body. The most common is administration of the cation-exchange resin sodium polystyrene sulfonate (Kayexalate). The usual dose is 50 g given two or three times daily. The most effective means of reducing body potassium is dialysis. Care must be taken to avoid precipitous reduction, especially in patients taking digitalis glycosides.[70]

Myocardial ischemia, from coronary artery disease, hemodynamic deterioration, or hypoxemia, can produce a variety of electrophysiologic effects. Acid-base disturbances and exogenous or endogenous catecholamines also can predispose affected patients to ventricular arrhythmias. The role of the sympathetic nervous system in arrhythmogenesis and electrical storm cannot be overemphasized.[69,71,72] Reentry, abnormal automaticity, and triggered activity all may be provoked.

Differential Diagnosis of Wide QRS Tachycardia

Wide QRS tachycardia may be supraventricular or ventricular in origin. The presence of atrial-ventricular dissociation is diagnostic of ventricular tachycardia. In general, supraventricular tachycardia with aberrancy will manifest with a typical bundle branch block pattern, whereas ventricular tachycardia will have more "bizarre" QRS complexes. Pre-excited supraventricular tachycardias may be impossible to distinguish from ventricular tachycardia using ECG criteria alone. A number of algorithms (with good sensitivity and specificity) to help distinguish supraventricular tachycardia from ventricular tachycardia have been proposed.[72]

Algorithms, however, may be difficult to memorize and awkward to carry around (even in miniaturized forms). For tachycardias with a right bundle branch block configuration, a triphasic RSR pattern in lead V_1 favors aberrancy, whereas an R/S size ratio of less than 1 in lead V_6 favors ventricular tachycardia. For tachycardias with a left bundle branch block configuration, each of the following favors the diagnosis of ventricular tachycardia: an initial R wave duration less than 30 ms in V_1, greater than 60 ms from the onset of the R wave to the nadir of the S wave in V_1, any notching in the S wave of V_1 or V_2, or any Q wave in V_6.[73,74]

Approach to Ventricular Arrhythmias in the Critically Ill

New ventricular arrhythmias warrant an assessment of electrolytes, oxygenation, and acid-base status. Routine measurement of cardiac enzymes is not mandatory with the onset of each arrhythmia. The QT interval should be checked via 12-lead ECG. The 12-lead ECG also is useful in distinguishing monomorphic from polymorphic ventricular tachycardia. Dislodgment of intravascular catheters may result in mechanically induced arrhythmias. Catheter position may be confirmed by x-ray examination or fluoroscopy.

A comprehensive discussion of advanced cardiovascular life support (ACLS) is beyond the scope of this chapter. Current recommendations for management of adult cardiac arrest are discussed in Chapter 1 of this book and are summarized in recently published ACLS guidelines.[75,76]

Specific Ventricular Arrhythmias

The occurrence of premature ventricular contractions (PVCs) and nonsustained ventricular arrhythmias in the ICU generally has little immediate importance. Reduction or withdrawal of vasopressors and elimination of metabolic disturbances often will decrease the frequency and severity of nonsustained ventricular tachycardia (NSVT). Acute antiarrhythmic drug therapy is rarely required unless symptoms of hemodynamic compromise occur.

The approach to NSVT that persists after recovery from acute illness depends on the underlying cardiac substrate. Asymptomatic persons without structural disease require no therapy. Patients with coronary artery disease and reduced left ventricular function (to less than 30% to 35%) should be evaluated for ICD therapy (see later on).[62,77,78] If the patient has nonsustained ventricular tachycardia and an ischemic myopathy with an ejection fraction between 35% and 40%, the therapeutic approach is guided by the results of the Multicenter Unsustained Tachycardia Trial (MUSTT).[79,80] If sustained monomorphic ventricular tachycardia is induced during electrophysiologic testing, an ICD is recommended. Most electrophysiologists do not treat asymptomatic NSVT in patients with nonischemic myopathy and ejection fraction greater than 35%. Patients with a nonischemic cardiomyopathy, New York Heart Association (NHYA) class II or III heart failure on "optimal medical therapy" (including a β-blocker, ACE inhibitor, spironolactone, and others), and an ejection fraction of less than 35% also are candidates for a prophylactic ICD.[62] Amiodarone, which has a neutral effect on mortality,[62] may be used to suppress symptomatic NSVT in patients with significant structural heart disease.

Acute management of sustained monomorphic ventricular tachycardia depends primarily on its hemodynamic stability. Unstable tachycardia should be treated promptly with direct current cardioversion. Stable arrhythmias may be treated with intravenous procainamide, amiodarone, or β-blockers. Although lidocaine remains an option, the 2000 International Cardiopulmonary Resuscitation (CPR) guidelines no longer recommend lidocaine as a first-line agent. Antitachycardia pacing may be considered in patients with transvenous or epicardial pacing leads. If these modalities are unsuccessful (or arrhythmia acceleration occurs), direct current cardioversion can be used to restore sinus rhythm. Electrical storm is defined as ventricular tachycardia or ventricular fibrillation occurring more than twice in 24 hours, usually requiring electrical cardioversion or defibrillation.[81]

Although data are limited, β-blockade in conjunction with amiodarone appears to be the most effective therapy for electrical storm.[71,81]

Because the arrhythmic substrate usually is fixed (most commonly, coronary artery disease and prior myocardial infarction), recurrence rates may remain high even after elimination of "reversible" causes.[82,83] Although no definite guidelines exist in the presence of reversible causes, an ICD should be strongly considered in patients with left ventricular dysfunction (if co-morbidity is not prohibitive). Electrophysiologic testing may be useful in patients with coronary artery disease but is much less reliable in patients with nonischemic cardiomyopathy.

Bundle branch reentry accounts for approximately 6% of the cases of monomorphic ventricular tachycardia.[84] This percentage may rise to 40% to 50% in patients with idiopathic dilated cardiomyopathy.[85] Bundle branch reentry should be suspected in patients with marked left ventricular dysfunction (especially nonischemic), intraventricular conduction defects, and wide QRS tachycardia. It may appear after valve replacement surgery. The tachycardia circuit typically uses the right bundle branch as its antegrade limb and the left bundle as its retrograde limb. Tachycardia therefore manifests with classic left bundle branch block morphology. Diagnosis and treatment may be accomplished during a single invasive electrophysiology session. The right bundle branch is easily ablated during sinus rhythm, permitting tachycardia cure without detailed mapping during hemodynamically unstable arrhythmias.[86,87] Although the postablation prognosis has been said to be favorable for patients with isolated bundle branch reentry, patients with residual inducible or spontaneous ventricular tachycardia should be offered ICD therapy. Patients with significant residual infranodal conduction delay (His-ventricular rates longer than 90 ms) after ablation should be considered for permanent pacing (usually with an ICD). It would be reasonable to implant an ICD after ablation in patients with heart failure and ejection fractions less than 35%.

Optimal long-term management of patients with structural heart disease and sustained monomorphic ventricular tachycardia (see later on) is to implant an ICD.[88,89] Hemodynamic stability does not predict a better long-term outcome.[88] Ablation generally is regarded as palliative and is used primarily to reduce the necessary shock frequency in patients with recurrent ventricular tachycardias.[90]

In the absence of QT prolongation, ischemia is the most common cause of polymorphic ventricular tachycardia. Polymorphic ventricular tachycardia/ventricular fibrillation in the early phase (less than 48 hours) of an acute myocardial infarction does not require additional evaluation or treatment. Late polymorphic ventricular tachycardia/ventricular fibrillation complicating myocardial infarction usually occurs when severe heart failure or cardiogenic shock also has been problematic. The initial prognosis usually is determined by hemodynamic recovery rather than arrhythmias.

Ischemia also is a common cause of polymorphic ventricular tachycardia/ventricular fibrillation in the absence of acute infarction. A reduction in or withdrawal of catecholamines should be tried. β-Blockers should be titrated to tolerance. Intra-aortic balloon counterpulsation and acute revascularization should be considered. Pharmacologic therapy with amiodarone may be useful.

The risk of recurrent polymorphic ventricular tachycardia/ventricular fibrillation is high, and the long-term prognosis is poor. Most patients, particularly those with left ventricular dysfunction, should have an ICD implanted if no contraindications exist. Idiopathic ventricular fibrillation may respond to catheter ablation if a single PVC focus (usually from the Purkinje system or the right ventricular outflow tract) is the consistent trigger.[91,92] Coronary artery spasm may result in ventricular fibrillation caused by myocardial ischemia. Recognition of this uncommon cause of cardiac arrest is critical. Medical management of spasm-induced ischemia (primarily with calcium channel blockers) appears to be the treatment of choice. Titration of calcium channel blocker dose to prevent ergonovine-induced spasm eliminated arrhythmia in one small series.[93]

Primary and Secondary Prevention of Ventricular Tachycardia/Ventricular Fibrillation

Although the subject is beyond the realm of acute care, intensivists should have familiarity with primary and secondary prevention of sudden cardiac death. Patients with frequent complex ventricular ectopy, abnormal left ventricular function, or heart failure are at increased risk of sudden death. In 1989, the Cardiac Arrhythmia Suppression Trial (CAST)[94] studied whether suppression of PVCs after myocardial infarction would reduce arrhythmic death. The study was terminated unexpectedly (and stunned the cardiology community) with the unexpected results of increased arrhythmic and total mortality in patients receiving encainide or flecainide for PVC suppression. Since the CAST results were published, a number of trials—MADIT (Multicenter Automatic Defibrillator Trial),[77] MADIT II,[78] MUSST,[79,80] and SCD-HeFT[62]—have demonstrated benefit from ICD prophylaxis in ischemic cardiomyopathy. Amiodarone (widely regarded as the most effective ventricular antiarrhythmic) has a neutral effect on total mortality in ischemic patients. SCD-HeFT provided additional clarification by revealing benefit from ICDs and a neutral effect from amiodarone in nonischemic cardiomyopathy patients with NYHA class II or III heart failure. β-Blockers provide the most effective pharmacologic prophylaxis against sudden death after myocardial infarction and are beneficial in the management of heart failure regardless of its etiology. Because of its neutral effect on mortality, amiodarone may be employed for symptomatic relief as an adjunct to ICD therapy.

Several trials have compared ICDs and amiodarone or other antiarrhythmics in secondary prevention of sudden death.[89,95] The Canadian Implantable Defibrillator Study (CIDS) and the Cardiac Arrest Study Hamburg (CASH) trial demonstrated reduced all-cause mortality with ICDs compared with amiodarone, but neither study reached statistical significance. Amiodarone was comparable to metoprolol in CASH. The Antiarrhythmics versus Implantable Defibrillators (AVID) study demonstrated significant reduction in overall mortality with ICDs compared with antiarrhythmic drug therapy in patients resuscitated from near-fatal ventricular arrhythmias. Amiodarone was used in most patients (90%) in the drug therapy group; a limited number (10%) received sotalol. A meta-analysis of these three trials demonstrated significant relative reduction in total (27%) and arrhythmic (53%) mortality rates with ICDs.[96] ICDs are the therapeutic option of choice for secondary prevention of sudden cardiac death. Because sustained ventricular tachyarrhythmias are not reliably induced during programmed stimulation in nonischemic cardiomyopathy, many electrophysiologists treat unexplained syncope (i.e., with negative results on electrophysiologic testing) in these patients (as secondary prevention) with an ICD.

Less Common Substrates

Serious ventricular arrhythmias are uncommon in the absence of significant left ventricular dysfunction. A few specific entities should be readily recognized by the intensivist.

Idiopathic Ventricular Tachycardia

Idiopathic ventricular tachycardias tend to originate in a "line of fire" from the right ventricular outflow tract (90%), left ventricular outflow tract, aortic cusps, and mitral annulus.[97] They often are facilitated by catecholamine infusion. The most common forms (right ventricular outflow tract tachycardia) have a typical, easily recognizable ECG pattern of left bundle branch block with an inferior frontal lead axis (tall R waves in leads II, III, and aVF). The arrhythmias occur in the absence of apparent structural heart disease. Abnormalities may be detected using magnetic resonance imaging; however they do not definitely correlate with sites of arrhythmogenesis.[98,99]

More than 90% of idiopathic ventricular tachycardias can be cured by catheter ablation.[96] The most reliable method for localizing the site of origin is pace mapping. The 12-lead ECG will exactly match the spontaneous ventricular tachycardia QRS morphology at the site of origin of the ventricular tachycardia. If a perfect 12/12-lead ECG pace map match can be obtained, the site is ablated. These tachycardias are adenosine-sensitive and thought to be the result of cyclic AMP–mediated DADs.[99] These arrhythmias may respond to treatment with β-blockers or calcium channel blockers, which normally are ineffective in other ventricular tachycardias.

Another "idiopathic" left ventricular tachycardia manifests as a relatively narrow right bundle branch block, left axis deviation tachycardia. The ECG and rhythm strip should be examined carefully for P waves. If the P-P is slower and the P waves are dissociated, the diagnosis of ventricular tachycardia, rather than supraventricular tachycardia with aberrancy, is confirmed. This arrhythmia is verapamil-sensitive and can easily be ablated if necessary. The arrhythmia is due to macro-entry in the terminal Purkinje fibers in the left distal third of the apical septum. To ablate it, the lower third of the septum is mapped, looking for the sharpest, earliest Purkinje potential during ventricular tachycardia.[91] A second technique (also using Purkinje potentials) is equally effective.[92] This tachycardia is referred to by several different names, including fascicular ventricular tachycardia, verapamil-sensitive ventricular tachycardia, and Belhassen's ventricular tachycardia.

In patients with ventricular arrhythmias and obvious significant right ventricular disease, the diagnosis of arrhythmogenic right ventricular dysplasia (ARVD)/cardiomyopathy can be made. The left ventricle generally has milder abnormalities. ARVD typically occurs in young patients (80% of patients are diagnosed before the age of 40 years) and is an important cause of sudden cardiac death in this population. It should, however, be emphasized that the overall risk of sudden cardiac death is low (2% to 2.5% per year).[100]

Males are predominantly affected. ARVD is transmitted in an autosomal dominant pattern with variable penetrance (abnormal loci have been mapped to chromosomal regions 14q23, 1q42, 14q12, 2q32, 17q21, and 3p23).[100]

Ventricular arrhythmias in ARVD may be catecholamine dependent and are exacerbated during exercise tolerance testing in 50% of patients. Sotalol and amiodarone seem to be effective in ARVD. Catheter ablation has a palliative, complementary role. Arrhythmia recurrences at new foci may occur after apparent ablative success. Experience with ICDs in ARVD is limited. Patients resuscitated from cardiac arrest or those poorly responsive to (or intolerant of) antiarrhythmic drugs appear to be good candidates.[101]

The congenital long QT syndrome is a manifestation of a variety of ion channel mutations that result in prolonged ventricular repolarization. The three main features of congenital long QT syndrome are (1) prolongation of the rate corrected QT interval (QTc); (2) cardiac arrest secondary to torsades de pointes (Fig. 32-5); and (3) QT prolongation, syncope, or sudden death in family members. Syncope often occurs in association with physical activity, emotional reactions, or acute arousal with auditory stimuli (the specific trigger in a variant of long QT syndrome, LQT2).[102,103] β-Blockers are the mainstay of treatment in patients with long QT syndrome. Permanent pacing is beneficial for patients in whom β-blockade is not effective or in whom excessive bradycardia develops. Limited experience has been reported with left cervicothoracic sympathetic ganglionectomy in patients with drug-refractory long QT syndrome. ICDs are recommended for high-risk patients, including those with recurrent syncope on β-blockers, aborted sudden cardiac death, a strong family history of sudden death, and the Jervell and Lange Nielson syndrome (homozygotes or compound heterozygotes with mutations in KCNQ1 and KCNE1, resulting in abnormal I_{ks} ion current long QT syndrome and hereditary deafness).[104]

Although the short-term effects of gene-specific therapy (e.g., mexiletine or flecainide in patients with sodium channel abnormalities, potassium plus spironolactone in potassium channel defects) on the QT interval are encouraging,[105] long-term data are lacking regarding their ability

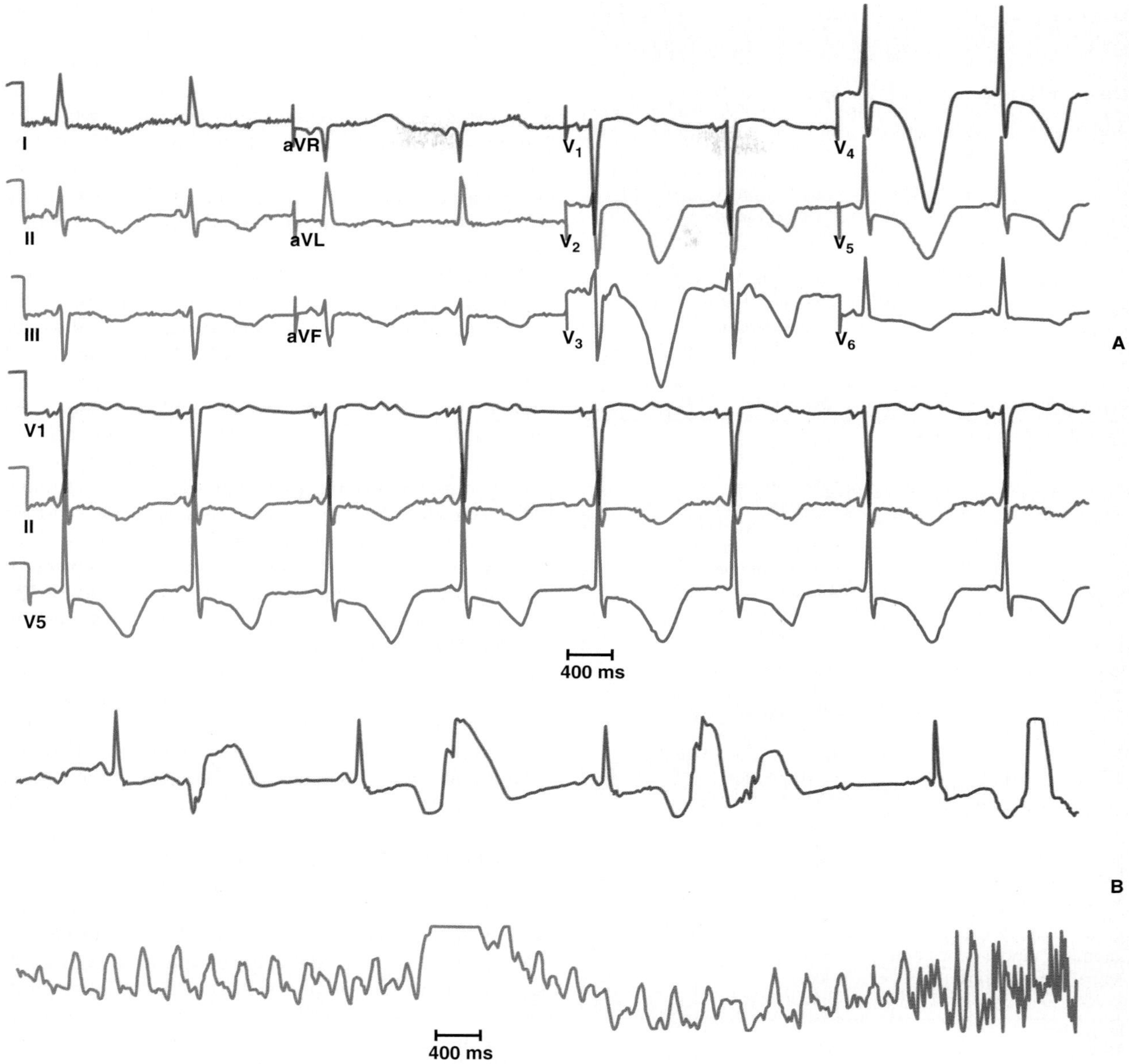

Figure 32-5. A, Marked QT prologation and T wave alternative is a harbinger of electrical instability. **B,** Increasing ventricular ectopy is followed by ventricular fibrillation. (Adapted from Trohman RG, Sahu J: Drug-induced torsades de pointes. Circulation 1999;99:E7.)

to prevent arrhythmias in long QT syndrome. A trial of flecainide for another variant of the syndrome, LQT3, is ongoing.

QT prolongation may be acquired (most commonly caused by drug effects or toxic substances, electrolyte abnormalities, hypothermia, and central nervous system injury). Drug-induced QT prolongation usually is the result of I_{kr} ion current blockade.[34] Intensivists need to be particularly aware of the pharmacologic causes of QT prolongation (Table 32-3). Drug-induced torsades de pointes is managed initially with intravenous magnesium sulfate. Isoproterenol and temporary pacing increase ventricular rates, shorten QT intervals, and help prevent recurrent arrhythmias until the effects of the offending agent diminish.

The Brugada syndrome (first described in 1992) is characterized by right bundle branch block (with ST segment elevation in leads V_1 to V_3), polymorphic ventricular tachycardia, and ventricular fibrillation.[106] Intensivists need to be particularly aware that febrile illnesses may trigger arrhythmic events.[107] Brugada syndrome has been linked to mutation in the sodium channel gene *SCN5A*. This mutation decreases sodium channel activity. It is inherited in an autosomal dominant pattern with variable penetrance. Males are more likely to be affected and have an increased risk of sudden death, probably related to a more prominent transient outward potassium current in men (see later).The ECG abnormality originally was thought to be persistent; however, transient forms (in

Table 32-3. Drugs Reported to Cause Prolongation of the QT Interval or Torsades de Pointes/Ventricular Tachycardia

Drug Category	Specific Agent(s)*
Antiarrhythmic medications	*Class IA* Quinidine Procainamide (metabolized to *N*-acetylprocainamide) Disopyramide *Class III* Dofetilide Ibutilide Sotalol Amiodarone *Class IV* Bepridil†
Promotility medications	Cisapride†
Antimicrobial medications	*Macrolides* Erythromycin Clarithromycin *Fluoroquinolones* Sparfloxacin† *Antiprotozoals* Pentamidine *Antimalarials* Halofantrine Chloroquine
Antipsychotic medications	*Phenothiazine neuroleptics* Thioridazine Chlorpromazine Mesoridazine *Butyrophenone neuroleptics* Droperidol Haloperidol *Diphenylpiperidine neuroleptics* Pimozide
Miscellaneous agents	Arsenic trioxide Methadone
Vitamins, supplements, and herbal preparations	Cesium Licorice Zhigancao

*Partial listing.
†Unavailable or severely limited availability in the United States.
From Gupta A, Lawrence AT, Krishnan K, et al: Current concepts in the mechanisms and management of drug-induced QT prolongation and torsades de pointes. Am Heart J 2007;153:891-899.

which the ECG may be normal for periods of time) have been described.[108] The electrocardiographic abnormalities may be unmasked by procainamide, flecainide, or ajmaline.

The cellular mechanism responsible for the ST segment elevation is early repolarization of the ventricular epicardium as a result of rebalancing of currents at the end of phase I of the action potential. The transient outward potassium current (I_{to}) overwhelms inward currents. The action potential "dome" is abolished at some sites but not others. Propagation of the dome to sites where it is absent may result in so-called *phase II reentry*, the mechanism of arrhythmogenesis.[109] In this instance, diminished sodium channel activity facilitates loss of the action potential dome as a result of a negative shift in the voltage at which phase I begins. Different mutations in SCN5A appear to account for LQT3; however, a recent report suggests a genetic (and perhaps clinical) link between the Brugada syndrome and LQT3.[110] As with long QT syndrome, it appears that genetic heterogenicity exists in the Brugada syndrome.[111] In Japan and Southeast Asia, the Brugada syndrome may account for 40% to 60% of cases of idiopathic ventricular fibrillation. The ICD is the only effective therapeutic intervention against sudden cardiac death.

Catecholaminergic polymorphic ventricular tachycardia (CMPVT) is an inherited disorder with autosomal dominant and autosomal recessant variants. This disorder is characterized by a direct relationship between increased adrenergic activity and arrhythmia onset, progressively complex ventricular ectopy (PVCs to NSVT to sustained polymorphic ventricular tachycardia) with increase in workload, and a structurally normal heart. The polymorphic ventricular tachycardia typically is bidirectional (QRS axis alternates by 180 degrees on a beat-to-beat basis) but also may be irregular without a distinct pattern of QRS vector change.[112] Ventricular tachycardia is reproducibity induced by exercise (usually at sinus rates of 120 to 130 beats per minute). CMPVT typically manifests in childhood as syncope or aborted cardiac arrest. Young boys have the worst prognosis (perhaps they are more sensitive to adrenergic symptoms). β-Blockers are the cornerstone of therapy, and dosing may be titrated according to exercise response. In 40% of patients, arrhythmia control will remain inadequate despite dose optimization during repeat exercise testing. ICDs are the therapeutic option of choice in these patients.[112]

Short-coupled torsades de pointes (SC-TdP) occurs in patients with structurally normal hearts and unremarkable ECG tracings (normal QT intervals). The coupling interval of the initiating beat is invariably less than 300 ms. It is a rare, potentially fatal disorder whose pathophysiology is unknown. The prognosis is poor, and effective pharmacologic therapy (β-blockers, calcium channel blockers) has not been identified. ICDs may be the best option. SC-TdP shares features with idiopathic ventricular tachycardia, and speculation that it may respond to catheter ablation if a single PVC focus (usually from the Purkinje system) is the consistent trigger is not unreasonable.[112]

Short QT syndrome is a heritable primary electrical disease characterized by an abnormally short QT interval (less than 300 ms) and a propensity to atrial fibrillation or sudden cardiac death, or both. As in the long QT syndrome, more than one relevant genetic mutation has been identified. Shortening of effective refractory periods combined with increased dispersion of repolarization is the likely substrate for reentry and life-threatening tachyarrhythmias. The best form of treatment is still unknown, but prevention of atrial fibrillation has been accomplished with propafenone. Implantation of an ICD is recommended for prevention of sudden cardiac death.[113,114]

Patients who experience electrical shock, including being struck by lightning, sustain a wide spectrum of injuries with unique pathophysiologic characteristics that require special management. Patients with serious burns admitted to the ICU are trauma patients and should be treated accordingly. Initial prediction of outcome for patients who have experienced electrical shock is difficult, because the full degree of injury often is not apparent. Sudden cardiac death due to ventricular fibrillation is more common with low-voltage alternating current, whereas asystole is more frequent with electric shocks from direct current or high-voltage alternating current. Potentially fatal arrhythmias are more likely to be caused by horizontal current flow (hand to hand); current passing in a vertical fashion (from head to foot) more commonly causes myocardial tissue damage. Lightning strike is unique because it causes cardiac and respiratory arrest, resulting in a 25% to 30% mortality rate.[115]

Aggressive and prolonged CPR in patients who have experienced electrical shock is indicated for several reasons.[116] First, cardiac arrhythmias and prolonged respiratory arrest may be the only clinical problem, especially in patients struck by lightning. Second, as mentioned, patients who experience electrical shock commonly are young and have few or no comorbid conditions. These young patients may survive prolonged CPR with no or minor sequelae. It is important to remember that keraunoparalysis leading to autonomic dysfunction may masquerade as irreversible neurologic injury in patients who have been electrocuted. For practical purposes, guidelines for CPR as issued by the American Heart Association[75] still apply. The algorithm for asystole acknowledges that "atypical clinical features" need to be considered in deciding whether CPR should be continued after initial unsuccessful attempts.

If more than one person has been electrocuted at a scene of injury, standard triage practices need to be modified, especially in those struck by lightning. Most patients who do not experience cardiac or respiratory arrest will survive.[117] Thus, the usual triage principles should be reversed: First responders should focus initially on patients who appear clinically dead *before* patients who show signs of life are treated.

RADIOFREQUENCY ABLATION OF CARDIAC ARRHYTHMIAS

Because ablation cure rates are so high, radiofrequency ablation has become first-line therapy for supraventricular tachycardia due to AV nodal reentry and bypass tracts, typical atrial flutter (isthmus-dependent, appearing in a "sawtooth" pattern on ECG), some ectopic atrial tachycardias, and both right ventricular outflow tract ventricular tachycardia and fascicular ventricular tachycardia. Radiofrequency ablation is second-line therapy, after at least one or several antiarrhythmic drugs have failed, for atrial fibrillation rate and rhythm control, and for most ventricular tachycardias occurring in patients with ischemic and nonischemic cardiomyopathy. It is important for the intensivist to know when to consider ablation therapy rather than drug therapy. The success and complication rates of a local electrophysiologist for the various radiofrequency ablation procedures also should be known. The success rates for those procedures listed next are typical for the average electrophysiologist. Better success rates are reported in the literature by the "best" high-volume operators. Complication rates are variable, especially for the atrial fibrillation rhythm control procedures, and for ischemic and nonischemic myopathy–palliative ventricular tachycardia ablation procedures. All other radiofrequency procedures are safe in the hands of average electrophysiologists, with serious complication rates in the range of 1% to 2% or less.

Atrial Fibrillation Rate Control

If rate control of atrial fibrillation cannot be achieved with AV node–blocking drugs, such as β-blockers, calcium blockers, digoxin, and amiodarone, then an "ablate and pace" strategy is almost always effective. The technique is to place a cardiac electrode catheter in the area of the fast AV nodal pathway and bundle of His. This is easily accomplished by obtaining a His bundle electrogram and applying radiofrequency energy to the site until complete heart block is created. A temporary right ventricular pacer maintains circulation while a permanent right ventricular or biventricular (BiV) pacemaker is implanted.[118] The rate-responsive feature of the pacemaker will "physiologically" adjust the heart rate in accordance with patient activity level. A vibration sensor in the pacemaker raises heart rate appropriate to exercise level. Wood and colleagues[119] reviewed 21 studies covering 1181 patients and found ablate and pace therapy effective, with fractional shortening evaluated by echocardiography increased from 25% to 32% 90 days after ablate and pace therapy. Treadmill times and patient quality of life scores also improved after ablate and pace therapy. In patients with low or borderline low ejection fraction, a right ventricular pacing-induced cardiomyopathy may develop (as a result of right ventricular apical pacing causing a paced left bundle branch block, leading to septal dyskinesis), further aggravating heart failure. In the PAVE[120] study, an initial ejection fraction of 45% dropped to 40% after 6 months of right ventricular apical pacing in these patients. No drop in borderline or low ejection fraction occurred in patients starting at 45.5% after 6 months of BiV pacing, with ejection fraction remaining at 46%. In patients with borderline or low ejection fractions, and perhaps all patients, AV node ablation should be accompanied by insertion of a biventricular pacemaker.

Atrial Fibrillation Rhythm Control

In paroxysmal atrial fibrillation, the arrhythmia often is triggered by ectopic fast-firing cells located in or near the ostia of pulmonary veins as they insert into the left atrium. The goal of radiofrequency ablation in this disorder is to ablate these cells directly, or encircle and isolate them so they can only depolarize a small portion of the left atrium. Two basic electrophysiologic methods of achieving these goals are available.

The technique of *segmental pulmonary vein ostial ablation*[8,121] is to map and find the trigger cells by placing a halo and radiofrequency ablation mapping catheter from the femoral vein across the atrial septum into each individual pulmonary vein os. The os of each of the four pulmonary veins is mapped to look for pulmonary vein potentials during sinus rhythm, either recorded during sinus rhythm or encouraged to fire using isoproterenol (Isuprel) infusion. The sites of pulmonary vein potentials are then ablated using radiofrequency energy.

The technique of *encircling left atrial ablation*[10,122] is to draw a line of overlapping ablation lesions 1 to 2 cm from the os of each of the four pulmonary veins, essentially encircling all four veins and trapping the pulmonary vein focus. Although the focus still can fire, it can depolarize only local left atrial tissue near the firing site and cannot depolarize the remainder of the atrium.

Morady and colleagues[123] compared both techniques and found the left atrial ablation technique 88% effective at preventing atrial fibrillation reoccurrence at 6 months, compared with the pulmonary vein ostial ablation success rate of 67% at 6 months. Complications can be serious, including cardiac perforation[6,7] with tamponade, hemothorax, perforation of the esophagus with atrioesophageal fistula, pulmonary vein stenosis,[124] creation of new left atrial flutter with rapid ventricular rate, stroke, and death. The only complication among 80 patients reported by Morady and colleagues was left atrial flutter in one patient. In clinical practice, however, higher complication rates (especially causing new rapid left atrial flutter) are much more common.

The two techniques just described target the triggers of atrial fibrillation. A new technique of targeting complex, multicomponent electrograms and continuous electrical activity[10,125] aims at interrupting wavelets of reentry that sustain atrial fibrillation. This technique often is added to the pulmonary vein or left atrial ablation technique.

Atrial Flutter

Isthmus-dependent or typical right atrial flutter is a reentrant arrhythmia that produces a classic ECG pattern of sawtooth P waves in leads II, III, and aVF. Whether traveling clockwise or counterclockwise around the right atrium, the arrhythmia always passes through the right atrial isthmus (tissue between the tricuspid annulus, coronary sinus os, and inferior vena cava). If an ablation line is drawn across the isthmus, it blocks the flutter in both directions. This is accomplished by placing an ablation catheter into the right ventricle through the femoral vein, and pulling the catheter back and across the tricuspid annulus. Ablation energy is turned on as the catheter is moved from tricuspid annulus to the junction of the right atrium and inferior vena cava, essentially blocking any flutter wave from crossing the isthmus. Radiofrequency ablation of typical atrial flutter is over 90% effective.

Atrioventricular Node Reentry Supraventricular Tachycardia

The anatomic AV node (what the pathologist sees on histologic examination) is a compact structure that is located in the anterior tricuspid value annulus contiguous with the bundle of His. Specialized atrial conduction pathways enter this compact node anteriorly (called fast pathways) and posteriorly (called slow pathways). The slow pathways actually are located at the tricuspid annulus near the coronary sinus os, several centimeters away from the compact AV node and His bundle. During sinus rhythm, conduction over the fast pathway beats the slow pathway and forms the PR interval on the ECG. During supraventricular tachycardia, conduction usually is antegrade down the slow pathway and retrograde up the fast pathway. The first beat of supraventricular tachycardia often displays a "jump" or prolongation of the PR interval as conduction antegrade shifts from fast to slow pathway, and then blocks in the fast pathway. The fast pathway has time to recover as conduction proceeds down the slow pathway and then after recovery travels up the fast pathway retrograde to maintain the reentry loop. This reentry loop is more safely ablated by placing the radiofrequency catheter anatomically in the area of the slow pathway. When the slow pathway is heated and damaged by radiofrequency energy, an accelerated junctional tachycardia occurs for several seconds, marking the end point of the ablation. Because the slow pathway is far from the compact AV node, fast pathway, and His bundle, heart block is rarely produced (less than 1% complication rate). The older ablation technique of fast pathway ablation resulted in obligatory first-degree heart block, with a much higher rate of complete heart block, and has been abandoned. The cure rate for slow-pathway radiofrequency ablation of AV node reentry supraventricular tachycardia is greater than 95%.

Supraventricular Tachycardia Due to Concealed or Overt Wolff-Parkinson-White Syndrome

Ablation of accessory pathways requires mapping the atrial side of the mitral and tricuspid annulus to look for bypass tract potentials, or the earliest site of retrograde atrial activation during induced supraventricular tachycardia, or during right ventricular pacing. This corresponds with the location of the atrial insertion of the bypass tract. This site is targeted with a radiofrequency ablation catheter, with radiofrequency energy applied for approximately 1 minute. After delivery of radiofrequency energy, if ablation of the bypass tract was successful, then retrograde VA conduction during ventricular pacing is either absent or present in a central pattern via the AV node. Supraventricular tachycardia is no longer inducible, and the delta wave during sinus rhythm disappears. The success rate for left-sided bypass tracts is 90% to 95%. Right-sided bypass tracts and septal tracts are slightly harder to ablate, with slightly lower success rates.

Ectopic Atrial Tachycardia

An analysis of the surface ECG during induced or spontaneous atrial tachycardia gives an initial indication of the general location of the focus (right atrium with upright P waves in leads I and aVL, versus left atrium with negative P in leads I and aVL). An inferior location would be negative in leads II, III, and aVF. The atrial chamber most likely to harbor the focus is then carefully mapped, usually using an anatomic mapping system. The site of earliest atrial activation relative to the P wave marks the ablation target. The success rate for atrial tachycardia ablation is highly dependent on whether the arrhythmia can be induced and maintained long enough for mapping in the electrophysiology studies laboratory. The reported success rates are quite variable but are lower than for AV nodal or macroreentrant supraventricular tachycardia due to bypass tracts.

Right Ventricular Outflow Tract Ventricular Tachycardia

If the ventricular tachycardia can be induced in the electrophysiology laboratory, a catheter is moved around the right ventricular outflow tract until the local electrogram recorded from the catheter tip precedes the earliest QRS activity on surface ECG by at least 20 to 30 ms. This site is then ablated. If the right ventricular outflow tract ventricular tachycardia can be only transiently induced and will not maintain in a sustained mode, a 12-lead ECG of the ventricular tachycardia is obtained. During sinus rhythm, a pace map of the right ventricular outflow tract is made by making repeated 12-lead ECG recordings from various right ventricular outflow tract pacing sites. The paced 12-lead ECG will exactly match the spontaneous ventricular tachycardia QRS at the site of origin of ventricular tachycardia. If a perfect 12-lead ECG–pace map match can be obtained, the site is ablated. Right ventricular outflow tract ventricular tachycardia can be successfully ablated, if even still partially inducible, in 80% to 90% of cases.

Fascicular Ventricular Tachycardia

A mapping catheter is placed into the left ventricle transseptally or through the aortic valve. The lower third of the septum is mapped to look for a prominent Purkinje spike that looks like a His bundle spike. Ventricular tachycardia is then induced. This site should record a spike potential electrogram occurring before the onset of the right bundle branch block left axis QRS, which this arrhythmia usually displays. The spike may still be seen during induced supraventricular tachycardia. This is the site of radiofrequency ablation.

Bundle Branch Reentry Ventricular Tachycardia

Bundle branch reentry supraventricular tachycardia can be ablated by ablating the right bundle branch. A catheter is placed in the His bundle area and advanced slightly to record a right bundle potential. This is the site of radiofrequency energy delivery, to purposely create a right bundle branch block. These patients typically have other supraventricular tachycardias or risk of sudden death due to very poor ventricular function and still require an ICD.

The primary success rates for ablation of all other ventricular tachycardias caused by ischemic and nonischemic cardiomyopathy are low. Accordingly, the primary therapy for these tachycardias is placement of an ICD. Ablation therapy is attempted only for patients getting frequent shocks from a morphologically definable monomorphic supraventricular tachycardia. The details of supraventricular tachycardia mapping are far beyond the scope of this chapter.

PACEMAKERS AND IMPLANTABLE DEFIBRILLATORS

The intensivist is increasingly likely to encounter patients with pacemakers or implantable defibrillators. Modern devices have sophisticated diagnostic and therapeutic options. A detailed discussion of antiarrhythmia device managment is beyond the scope of this chapter. Some useful tips for the nonelectrophysiologist are presented in this section. Interested readers may refer to several reviews for more detailed information.[4,126-129]

Magnet application may be useful for pacemaker identification, termination of reentrant arrhythmias, and temporary inhibition of ICD tachycardia therapies. Three pacemaker companies make more than 90% of the pacemakers used in the United States. The device manufacturers have no standardized programmers, so the device brand must be known in order to bring the company-specific programmer to the patient. Medtronic pacemakers usually respond to magnet application by pacing at 85 beats per minute; Guidant (recently renamed Boston Scientific) devices, at 100 beats per minute, and St. Jude devices, at 98.6 beats per minute. Pacemakers will return to the programmed lower rate limit when the magnet is removed. Clinicians also can find out if a patient has a Medtronic pacemaker or implantable defibrillator by calling 1-800-MEDTRONIC; a Guidant device, by calling 1-800-CARDIAC; and a St. Jude device, by calling 1-800-PACEICD. Access to technical experts also is available via these telephone numbers.

Magnet application may terminate slow reentrant atrial and ventricular tachycardias by creating a competitive, asynchronous paced rhythm that interrupts the reentrant circuit. If this maneuver is used, a defibrillator should be present in case underdrive pacing accelerates the arrhythmia.

Magnet application inhibits ICD tachyarrhythmia therapies. This feature is useful to avoid shocks from oversensing of electromagnetic interference (as from Bovie use during surgery), or recurrent shocks despite hemodynamically stable tachyarrhythmias. Programmable options that allow the device to be disabled (rather than temporarily inhibited) by magnet applications are potentially dangerous and should be avoided.

Most pacemakers and ICDs provide some or all of the following features: heart rate histograms, date-time stamped arrhythmia diagnostics including storage of electrograms during a tacharrhythmia, and mode switch data. Important questions that device interrogation can answer include the following: (1) Does the rate histogram indicate whether the patient is adequately β-blocked (2) On the date (and time) of syncope or palpitations, was an arrhythmia logged in device memory? (3) What is the diagnosis of the real time or stored arrhythmia? (4) What frequency and duration of atrial tachyarrhythmias will result in mode switches (to a nonatrial tracking mode to avoid rapid P-synchronous ventricular pacing)?

Pacing at rates greater than 70 beats per minute is useful to prevent drug-induced TdP. Rate-smoothing algorithms also may be helpful in preventing drug-induced TdP. Atrial (assuming 1:1 AV conduction) or ventricular pacing at 80 beats per minute may help prevent TdP and TdP "storm"[4,130] in patients with congenital long QT syndrome.

Tiered ICD therapy provides antitachycardia pacing (as well as cardioversion and defibrillation) to terminate reentrant arrhythmias. This feature can be useful to limit shock delivery.[131-133] This feature is complex and may result in arrhythmia acceleration and hemodynamic compromise. Programming of this feature should be performed only by electrophysiologists.

Antiarrhythmic drugs can slow the rate of ventricular tachycardia (particularly sodium channel blockers that decrease conduction velocity) and can raise pacing thresholds and defibrillation thresholds (DFTs). Antiarrhythmics may reduce ventricular tachycardia rates below the programmed ICD detection rate. This leaves the arrhythmia undetected and untreated. Amiodarone (and other drugs) may raise DFTs, rendering ICD therapy ineffective. Sotalol has the potential to lower DFTs and may be a better adjuvant choice in patients with high baseline values. We recommend noninvasive programmed stimulation and DFT testing after antiarrhythmics are initiated or dosing is adjusted.

Cardiac resynchronization therapy (CRT), or biventricular pacing, is an important therapeutic option with drug-refractory NYHA class III or IV congestive heart failure, left ventricular ejection fraction up to 35%, and a major left-sided conduction delay (QRS duration greater than 120 ms). The underlying rhythm should be sinus or atrial fibrillation, with a ventricular response slow enough to allow continuous biventricular stimulation and capture. Biventricular pacing most frequently is used as part of an ICD system (CRT-D). Acute and chronic congestive heart failure contributes to the need for tachyarrhythmia treatment in ICD recipients. Although small trials (93 patients in total) have shown that biventricular pacing diminished ventricular arrhythmias, these results were not confirmed in larger trials.[4]

A typical arrhythmia time/date–stamped electrogram interrogated from a Guidant pacemaker is shown in Figure 32-6. A typical set of histograms from a Medtronic ICD indicating worsening CHF due to paroxysmal atrial fibrillation is shown in Figure 32-7. Pace termination of supraventricular tachycardia by means of the ventricular lead of a St. Jude VVI-ICD is shown in Figure 32-8.

CONCLUSIONS

The intensivist must have a keen awareness of patterns, mechanisms, precipitants, and treatment of cardiac arrhythmias. The intensivist must remember that *all* antiarrhythmic therapies (pharmacologic and nonpharmacologic) have the potential for adverse effects. Reducing and eliminating arrhythmia precipitants may be safer and more effective than dramatic interventions. Antiarrhythmic drugs should be chosen carefully and the patient monitored closely. Direct current cardioversion should be used aggressively when the situation is emergent, cautiously when elective, and eschewed when futile. Ablation is effective therapy for most supraventricular tachycardias, idiopathic ventricular tachycardia, and bundle branch reentry and may be used as adjuvant therapy for patients with frequent appropriate ICD shocks. ICDs are the therapy of choice for primary and secondary prevention in patients with structural heart disease. Consultation with a cardiac electrophysiologist should be considered a routine part of the critical care physician's armamentarium.

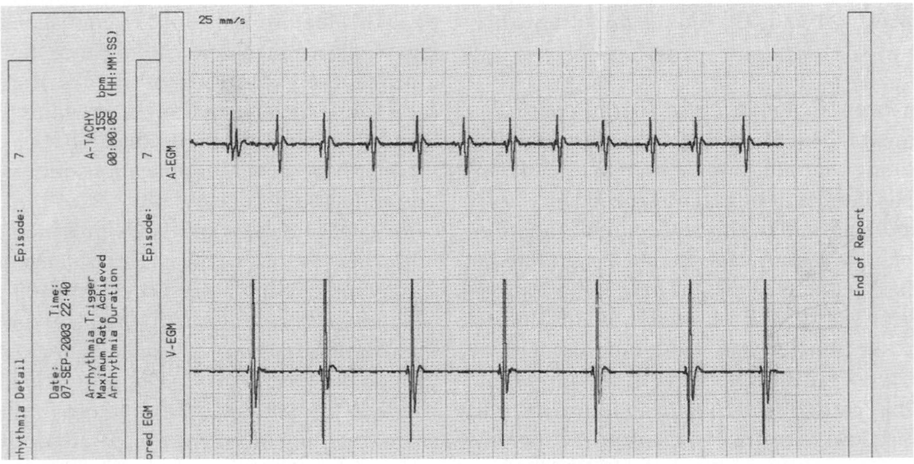

Figure 32-6. Guidant pacemaker interrogation showing the date and time of occurrence for an outpatient episode of atrial tachycardia that was logged in the device memory. The device also saved an atrial and ventricular electrogram of the arrhythmia, clearly showing atrial tachycardia with block to the ventricle as the cause, on that date, of the patient's clinically occurring palpitations. Atrial tachycardia with block is a potential result of digitalis toxicity, which needs to be ruled out.

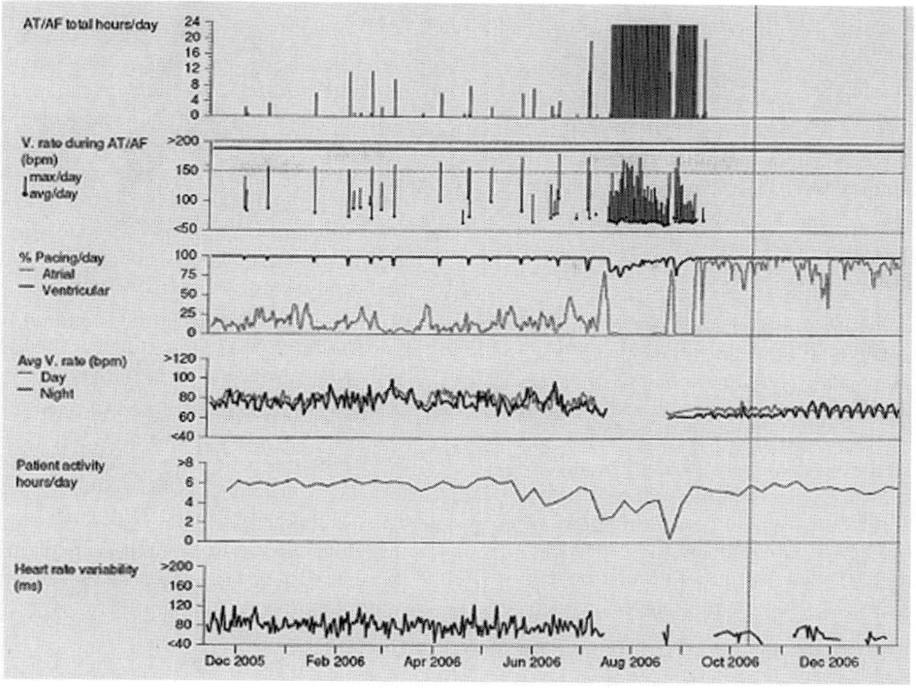

Figure 32-7. Histogram data interrogated from a Medtronic implantable cardioverter-defibrillator (ICD). Atrial fibrillation burden, ventricular rate during atrial fibrillation, percentage time of atrial and ventricular pacing, average atrial and ventricular rates, patient activity, and heart rate variability all are plotted in graphic format for a 1-year period, from December 2005 to December 2006. Note that the patient had infrequent, brief episodes of paroxysmal atrial fibrillation, sometimes with rapid ventricular response between December 2005 and July 2006. The patient went into persistent atrial fibrillation in July and August of 2006 with variable but sometimes rapid (80 to 170 beats per minute) ventricular response, associated with a marked decrease in physical activity. Amiodarone, started in August 2006, seems to have suppressed paroxysmal atrial fibrillation completely from September to December 2006, with return to the patient's previous physical activity level. All of this information was obtained by simply interrogating this ICD.

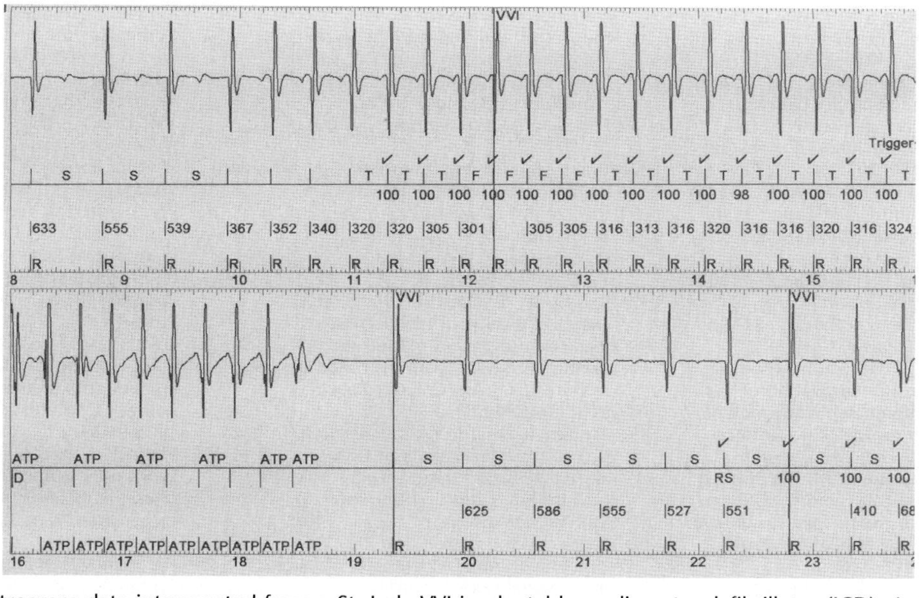

Figure 32-8. Electrogram data interrogated from a St. Jude VVI implantable cardioverter-defibrillator (ICD). A stored annotated electrogram from the ventricular lead of the ICD is shown. After several beats at cycle length of 555 ms, there is sudden onset of a regular tachycardia at cycle length 305 to 316 ms (approximately 190 to 200 beats per minute) that looks exactly like the ventricular electrogram of the patient's basic rhythm before and after termination of the arrhythmia. The device reports that the QRS electrogram is 98% to 100% similar to the patient's natural QRS, suggesting supraventricular tachycardia. The arrhythmia rate, however, exceeds the programmed ventricular tachycardia detection rate, so the device triggers antitachycardia pacing (labeled ATP), which successfully terminates the supraventricular tachycardia.

KEY POINTS

- Intensivists managing arrhythmias must have expertise in electrocardiography, pharmacokinetics, pharmacodynamics, and bedside clinical acumen.
- All antiarrhythmic therapies (pharmacologic and nonpharmacologic) have the potential for adverse effects.
- Patients in an intensive care setting frequently have active arrhythmia precipitants. They include hypoxemia, excess circulating catecholamines, congestive heart failure, fever (sepsis), pulmonary emboli, electrolyte, and other metabolic disturbances. Reducing or eliminating arrhythmia precipitants may be safer and more effective than dramatic antiarrhythmic interventions.
- Direct current cardioversion of tachyarrhythmias should be used aggressively when emergent (angina pectoris, congestive heart failure, hypotension), cautiously when elective, and eschewed when futile. The critical care physician must carefully weigh the risks and benefits of direct current cardioversion for each patient.
- Left ventricular dysfunction is the most important predictor of cardiac mortality in patients with ventricular arrhythmias. Long-term management of sustained ventricular arrhythmias in the setting of structural heart disease is usually best accomplished with an implantable cardioverter-defibrillator.
- Diagnosis and management of complex arrhythmias may be facilitated by consultation with a cardiac electrophysiologist.
- Ablation of cardiac arrhythmias often is now first-line elective therapy for most supraventricular tachycardias and some ventricular tachycardias.
- Data and electrograms stored in permanent pacemakers and ICDs can easily be assessed to help the intensivist determine the patient's past history and the frequency, rate, and duration of arrhythmias.
- Antiarrhythmic drugs can raise pacing and defibrillator thresholds and change supraventricular tachycardia and supraventricular tachycardia rates, necessitating device reprogramming

REFERENCES

1. Trohman RG, Parrillo JE: Arrhythmias: Perspectives for the critical care physician. Crit Care Med 28:N115, 2000.
2. Rubenstein JJ, Schulman CL, Yurchak PM, DeSanctis RW: Clinical spectrum of the sick sinus syndrome. Circulation 1972;46:5-13.
3. Zipes DP: Specific arrhythmias: Diagnosis and treatment. In Zipes DP (ed): Heart Disease. Philadelphia, WB Saunders, 1997.
4. Trohman RG, Kim MH, Pinski SL: Cardiac pacing: The state of the art. Lancet 2004;364:1701-1719.
5. DeGuzman M, Rahimtoola SH: What is the role of pacemakers in patients with coronary artery disease and conduction abnormalities? Cardiovasc Clin 1983;13:191-207.
6. Kall JG, Rubenstein DS, Kopp DE, et al: Atypical atrial flutter originating in the right atrial free wall. Circulation. 2000;101:270-279.
7. Jais P, Hocini M, Weerasoryia R, et al: Atypical left atrial flutters. Card Electrophysiol Rev 2002;6:371-377.
8. Haissaguerre M, Jais P, Shah DC, Garrigue S, et al: Electrophysiological end point for catheter ablation of atrial fibrillation initiated from multiple pulmonary venous foci. Circulation 2000;101:1409-1417.
9. Shah DC, Haissaguerre M, Jais P, et al: Electrophysiologically guided ablation of the pulmonary veins for the curative treatment of atrial fibrillation. Ann Med 2000;32:408-416.
10. Pappone C, Santinelli V: The who, what, why, and how-to guide for circumferential pulmonary vein ablation. J Cardiovasc Electrophysiol 2004;15:1226-1230.
11. Nademanee K, Schwab M, Porath J, Abbo A: How to perform electrogram-guided atrial fibrillation ablation. Heart Rhythm 2006;3:981-984.
12. Trohman RG: Supraventricular tachycardia: Implications for the intensivist. Crit Care Med 2000;28: N129-N135.
13. Tchou PJ, Trohman RG: Supraventricular tachycardias. In Dale DC, Federman DD (eds): Scientific American Medicine. New York, WebMD, 2003.
14. Utomo K, Wang Z, Lazzara R, Jackman WM: Atrioventricular nodal reentrant tachycardia: Electrophysiologic characteristics of four forms and implications for the reentrant circuit. In Zipes DP, Jalife J (eds): Cardiac Electrophysiology: From Cell to Bedside, 3rd ed. Philadelphia, WB Saunders, 2000, pp 504-521.
15. Gursoy S, Steurer G, Brugada J, et al: Brief report: The hemodynamic mechanism of pounding in the neck in atrioventricular nodal reentrant tachycardia. N Engl J Med 1992;327:772-774.
16. Knight BP, Ebinger M, Oral H, et al: Diagnostic value of tachycardia features and pacing maneuvers during paroxysmal supraventricular tachycardia. J Am Coll Cardiol 2000;36:574-582.
17. Morady F, DiCarlo LA Jr, Baerman JM, et al: Determinants of QRS alternans during narrow QRS tachycardia. J Am Coll Cardiol 1987;9:489-499.
18. Sanders WE Jr, Sorrentino RA, Greenfield RA, et al: Catheter ablation of sinoatrial node reentrant tachycardia. J Am Coll Cardiol 1994;23:926-934.
19. Swerdlow CD, Liem LB: Atrial and junctional tachycardias. In Zipes DP, Jalife J (eds): Cardiac Electrophysiology: From Cell to Bedside, 3rd ed. Philadelphia, WB Saunders, 2000, pp 742-755.
20. Engelstein ED, Lippman N, Stein KM, Lerman BB: Mechanism-specific effects of adenosine on atrial tachycardia. Circulation 1994;89:2645-2654.
21. Blomstrom-Lundqvist C, Scheinman MM, Aliot EM, et al: ACC/AHA/ESC guidelines for the management of patients with supraventricular arrhythmias—executive summary. A report of the American College of Cardiology/American Heart Association Task Force on Practice Guidelines and the European Society of Cardiology Committee for Practice Guidelines (writing committee to develop guidelines for the management of patients with supraventricular arrhythmias) developed in collaboration with NASPE-Heart Rhythm Society. J Am Coll Cardiol 2003;42:1493-1531.
22. Prystowsky EN, Yee R, Klein GJ: Wolff-Parkinson-White syndrome. In Zipes DP, Jalife J (eds): Cardiac Electrophysiology: From Cell to Bedside, 4th ed. Philadelphia, WB Saunders, 2004 (Serial).
23. Glatter KA, Dorostkar PC, Yang Y, et al: Electrophysiological effects of ibutilide in patients with accessory pathways. Circulation 2001;104: 1933-1939.
24. Villain E, Vetter VL, Garcia JM, et al: Evolving concepts in the management of congenital junctional ectopic tachycardia. A multicenter study. Circulation 1990;81:1544-1549.
25. Hamdan MH, Badhwar N, Scheinman MM: Role of invasive electrophysiologic testing in the evaluation and management of adult patients with focal junctional tachycardia. Card Electrophysiol Rev 2002;6:431-435.
26. Scheinman MM, Gonzalez RP, Cooper MW, et al: Clinical and electrophysiologic features and role of

catheter ablation techniques in adult patients with automatic atrioventricular junctional tachycardia. Am J Cardiol 1994;74:565-572.
27. Trohman RG, Haery C, Pinski SL: Focal radiofrequency catheter ablation of an irregularly irregular supraventricular tachycardia. Pacing Clin Electrophysiol 1999;22:360-362.
28. Hanau SP, Solar M, Ansura EL: Metoprolol in the treatment of multifocal atrial tachycardia. Cardiovasc Rev Rep 1984;1182.
29. Levine JH, Michael JR, Guarnieri T: Treatment of multifocal atrial tachycardia with verapamil. N Engl J Med 1985;312:21-25.
30. Dougherty AH, Schroth G, Ilkiw RL: Episodic tachycardia in a 12-year-old girl. Circulation 1995;92:268-273.
31. Stevenson JP, Pinski SL, McLaughlin VV, et al: Right atrial enlargement: An innocent bystander in the pathogenesis of atrial fibrillation. Circulation 1999;100:I-212 (Abstract).
32. Murray KT: Ibutilide. Circulation 1998;97:493.
33. Gupta A, Lawrence AT, Krishnan K, et al: Current concepts in the mechanisms and management of drug-induced QT prolongation and torsades de pointes. Am Heart J 2007;153:891-899.
34. Roden DM: Ibutilide and the treatment of atrial arrhythmias. A new drug—almost unheralded—is now available to U.S. physicians. Circulation 1996;94:1499-1502.
35. Sahu J, Volgman AS, Abi-Mansour P, et al: Ibutilide is safe for cardioversion of atrial fibrillation in patients on concomitant antiarrhythmic agents. Pacing Clin Electrophysiol 1999;22: 743 (Abstract).
36. Volgman AS, Carberry PA, Stambler B, et al: Conversion efficacy and safety of intravenous ibutilide compared with intravenous procainamide in patients with atrial flutter or fibrillation. J Am Coll Cardiol 1998;31:1414-1419.
37. Stambler BS, Wood MA, Ellenbogen KA: Antiarrhythmic actions of intravenous ibutilide compared with procainamide during human atrial flutter and fibrillation: Electrophysiological determinants of enhanced conversion efficacy. Circulation 1997;96:4298-4306.
38. Van G, I, Tuinenburg AE, Schoonderwoerd BS, et al: Pharmacologic versus direct-current electrical cardioversion of atrial flutter and fibrillation. Am J Cardiol 1999;84:147R-151R.
39. Delle Karth G, Geppert A, Neunteufl T, et al: Amiodarone versus diltiazem for rate control in critically ill patients with atrial tachyarrhythmias. Crit Care Med 2001;29:1149-1153.
40. Trohman RG, Parrillo JE: Direct current cardioversion: Indications, techniques, and recent advances. Crit Care Med 2000;28:N170-N173.
41. Aasbo JD, Lawrence AT, Krishnan K, et al: Amiodarone prophylaxis reduces major cardiovascular morbidity and length of stay after cardiac surgery: A meta-analysis. Ann Intern Med 2005;143:327-336.
42. Mitchell LB, Exner DV, Wyse DG, et al: Prophylactic Oral Amiodarone for the Prevention of Arrhythmias that Begin Early After Revascularization, Valve Replacement, or Repair: PAPABEAR: A randomized controlled trial. JAMA 2005;294:3093-3100.
43. Arnold AZ, Mick MJ, Mazurek RP, et al: Role of prophylactic anticoagulation for direct current cardioversion in patients with atrial fibrillation or atrial flutter. J Am Coll Cardiol 1992;19:851-855.
44. Lanzarotti CJ, Olshansky B: Thromboembolism in chronic atrial flutter: Is the risk underestimated? J Am Coll Cardiol 1997;30:1506-1511.
45. Fuster V, Ryden LE, Cannom DS, et al: ACC/AHA/ESC 2006 guidelines for the management of patients with atrial fibrillation: Full text: A report of the American College of Cardiology/American Heart Association Task Force on Practice Guidelines and the European Society of Cardiology Committee for Practice Guidelines (writing committee to revise the 2001 guidelines for the management of patients with atrial fibrillation) developed in collaboration with the European Heart Rhythm Association and the Heart Rhythm Society. Europace 2006;8:651-745.
46. Asher CR, Klein AL: Transesophageal echocardiography to guide cardioversion in patients with atrial fibrillation: ACUTE trial update. Card Electrophysiol Rev 2003;7:387-391.
47. Kowey PR: The calamity of cardioversion of conscious patients. Am J Cardiol 1988;61:1106-1107.
48. Bryson HM, Fulton BR, Faulds D: Propofol. An update of its use in anaesthesia and conscious sedation. Drugs 1995;50:513-559.
49. Ewy GA: The optimal technique for electrical cardioversion of atrial fibrillation. Clin Cardiol 1994;17: 79-84.
50. Pinski SL, Arnold AZ, Mick M, et al: Safety of external cardioversion/defibrillation in patients with internal defibrillation patches and no device. Pacing Clin Electrophysiol 1991;14:7-12.
51. Ewy GA: Optimal technique for electrical cardioversion of atrial fibrillation. Circulation 1992;86: 1645-1647.
52. Joglar JA, Hamdan MH, Ramaswamy K, et al: Initial energy for elective external cardioversion of persistent atrial fibrillation. Am J Cardiol 2000;86: 348-350.
53. Pinski SL, Sgarbossa EB, Ching E, Trohman RG: A comparison of 50-J versus 100-J shocks for direct-current cardioversion of atrial flutter. Am Heart J 1999;137:439-442.
54. Saliba W, Juratli N, Chung MK, et al: Higher energy synchronized external direct current cardioversion for refractory atrial fibrillation. J Am Coll Cardiol 1999;34:2031-2034.
55. Caterine MR, Yoerger DM, Spencer KT, et al: Effect of electrode position and gel-application technique on predicted transcardiac current during transthroacic defibrillation. Ann Emerg Med 1997;29:588-595.
56. Kerber R, Spencer K, Kallok M, et al: Overlapping sequential pulses. A new waveform for transthoracic defibrillation. Circulation 1994;89:2369-2379.
57. Murgatroyd FD, Slade AK, Sopher SM, et al: Efficacy and tolerability of transvenous low energy cardioversion of paroxsmal atrial fibrillation in man. J Am Coll Cardiol 1995;35:1347-1353.
58. Coplen SE, Antman EM, Berlin JA, et al: Efficacy and safety of quinidine therapy for maintenance of sinus rhythm after cardioversion. A meta-analysis of randomized control trials. Circulation 1990;82:1106-1116.
59. Pritchett EL, Page RL, Carson M for the Rythmol Atrial Fibrillation Trial (RAFT) Investigators: Efficacy and safety of sustained-release propafenone (propafenone SR) for patients with atrial fibrillation. Am J Cardiol 2003;92:941-946.
60. Cairns JA, Connolly SJ, Roberts R, Gent M: Randomised trial of outcome after myocardial infarction in patients with frequent or repetitive ventricular premature depolarisations: CAMIAT. Canadian Amiodarone Myocardial Infarction Arrhythmia Trial Investigators. Lancet 1997;349: 675-682.
61. Julian DG, Camm AJ, Frangin G, et al: Randomised trial of effect of amiodarone on mortality in patients with left-ventricular dysfunction after recent myocardial infarction: EMIAT. European Myocardial Infarct Amiodarone Trial Investigators. Lancet 1997;349:667-674.
62. Bardy GH, Lee KL, Mark KL, et al: Amiodarone or an implantable cardioverter defibrillator for congestive heart failure (Sed Heft Trial). N Engl J Med 2005;352:225-237.
63. Wyse DG, Waldo AL, DiMarco JP, et al: A comparison of rate control and rhythm control in patients with atrial fibrillation. N Engl J Med 2002;347: 1825-1833.
64. Jenkins LS, Brodsky M, Schron E, et al: Quality of life in atrial fibrillation: The Atrial Fibrillation Follow-up Investigation of Rhythm Management (AFFIRM) study. Am Heart J 2005;149: 112-120.
65. Sherman DG, Kim SG, Boop BS, et al: Occurrence and characteristics of stroke events in the Atrial Fibrillation Follow-up Investigation of Sinus Rhythm Management (AFFIRM) study. Arch Intern Med 2005;165: 1185-1191.
66. Gessman LJ, Agarwal JB, Endo T, Helfant RH: Localization and mechanism of ventricular tachycardia by ice mapping 1 week after the onset of myocardial infarction in dogs. Circulation 1983;68:657-666.
67. Gessman LJ, Endo T, Egan J, et al: Dissociation of the site of origin from the site of cryo-termination of ventricular tachycardia. Pacing Clin Electrophysiol 1983;6:1293-1305.
68. Gallagher JD, Del Rossi AJ, Fernandez J, et al: Cryothermal mapping of recurrent ventricular tachycardia in man. Circulation 1985;71:732-739.
69. Ramaswamy K, Hamdan MH: Ischemia, metabolic disturbances, and arrhythmogenesis: Mechanisms and

management. Crit Care Med 2000;28: N151-N157.
70. Pastay SO, Braunwald E: Renal disorders and heart disease. In Braunwald E (ed): Heart Disease. Philadelphia, WB Saunders, 1988.
71. Nademanee K, Taylor R, Bailey WE, et al: Treating electrical storm: sympathetic blockade versus advanced cardiac life support-guided therapy. Circulation 2000;102: 742-747.
72. Brugada P, Brugada J, Mont L, et al: A new approach to the differential diagnosis of a regular tachycardia with a wide QRS complex. Circulation 1991;83:1649-1659.
73. Kindwall KE, Brown J, Josephson ME: Electrocardiographic criteria for ventricular tachycardia in wide complex left bundle branch block morphology tachycardias. Am J Cardiol 1988;61:1279-1283.
74. Wellens HJ, Bar FW, Lie KI: The value of the electrocardiogram in the differential diagnosis of a tachycardia with a widened QRS complex. Am J Med 1978;64:27-33.
75. Kinsara AJ: Guidelines 2000 for advanced cardiopulmonary resuscitation emergency cardiovascular care. Circulation 2000;104:E45.
76. ECC Committee, Subcommittees and Task Forces of the American Heart Association: 2005 American Heart Association guidelines for cardiopulmonary resuscitation and emergency cardiovascular care. Circulation 2005;112(24 Suppl): IVI-203.
77. Moss AJ, Hall WJ, Cannom DS, et al: Improved survival with an implanted defibrillator in patients with coronary disease at high risk for ventricular arrhythmia. Multicenter Automatic Defibrillator Implantation Trial Investigators. N Engl J Med 1996;335:1933-1940.
78. Moss AJ, Zareba W, Hall WJ, et al: Prophylactic implantation of a defibrillator in patients with myocardial infarction and reduced ejection fraction. N Engl J Med 2002;346:877-883.
79. Buxton AE, Lee KL, Fisher JD, et al: A randomized study of the prevention of sudden death in patients with coronary artery disease. Multicenter Unsustained Tachycardia Trial Investigators. N Engl J Med 1999;341:1882-1890.
80. Buxton AE, Lee KL, DiCarlo L, et al: Electrophysiologic testing to identify patients with coronary artery disease who are at risk for sudden death. Multicenter Unsustained Tachycardia Trial Investigators. N Engl J Med 2000;342:1937-1945.
81. Credner SC, Klingenheben T, Mauss O, et al: Electrical storm in patients with transvenous implantable cardioverter-defibrillators: Incidence, management and prognostic implications. J Am Coll Cardiol 1998;32:1909-1915.
82. Kim SG, Hallstrom A, Love JC, et al: Comparison of clinical characteristics and frequency of implantable defibrillator use between randomized patients in the Antiarrhythmics vs Implantable Defibrillators (AVID) trial and nonrandomized registry patients. Am J Cardiol 1997;80:454-457.
83. Pinski SL, Yao Q, Epstein AE, et al: Determinants of outcome in patients with sustained ventricular tachyarrhythmias: The Antiarrhythmics versus Implantable Defibrillators (AVID) study registry. Am Heart J 2000;139: 804-813.
84. Caceres J, Jazayeri M, McKinnie J, et al: Sustained bundle branch reentry as a mechanism of clinical tachycardia. Circulation 1989;79:256-270.
85. Tchou P, Jazayeri M, Caceres JA: Bundle branch reentrant ventricular tachycardia. Am Heart J 1988;116: 1647-1648.
86. Tchou P, Jazayeri M, Denker S, et al: Transcatheter electrical ablation of right bundle branch. A method of treating macroreentrant ventricular tachycardia attributed to bundle branch reentry. Circulation 1988;78:246-257.
87. Langberg JJ, Desai J, Dullet N, Scheinman MM: Treatment of macroreentrant ventricular tachycardia with radiofrequency ablation of the right bundle branch. Am J Cardiol 1989;63:1010-1013.
88. Raitt MH, Renfroe EG, Epstein AE, et al: "Stable" ventricular tachycardia is not a benign rhythm: Insights from the Antiarrhythmics versus Implantable Defibrillators (AVID) registry. Circulation 2001;103:244-252.
89. A comparison of antiarrhythmic-drug therapy with implantable defibrillators in patients resuscitated from near-fatal ventricular arrhythmias. The Antiarrhythmics versus Implantable Defibrillators (AVID) Investigators. N Engl J Med 1997;337:1576.
90. Strickberger SA, Man KC, Daoud EG, et al: A prospective evaluation of catheter ablation of ventricular tachycardia as adjuvant therapy in patients with coronary artery disease and an implantable cardioverter-defibrillator. Circulation 1997;96: 1525-1531.
91. Haissaguerre M, Shoda M, Jais P, et al: Mapping and ablation of idiopathic ventricular fibrillation. Circulation 2002;106:962-967.
92. Haissaguerre M, Shah DC, Jais P, et al: Role of Purkinje conducting system in triggering of idiopathic ventricular fibrillation. Lancet 2002;359:677-678.
93. Myerburg RJ, Kessler KM, Mallon SM, et al: Life-threatening ventricular arrhythmias in patients with silent myocardial ischemia due to coronary-artery spasm. N Engl J Med 1992; 326:1451-1455.
94. The Cardiac Arrhythmia Suppression Trial (CAST) Investigators: Preliminary report: Effect of encainide and flecainide on mortality in a randomized trial of arrhythmia suppression after myocardial infarction. N Engl J Med 1989;321: 406.
95. Connolly SJ, Hallstrom AP, Cappato R, et al: Meta-analysis of the implantable cardioverter defibrillator secondary prevention trials. AVID, CASH and CIDS studies. Antiarrhythmics vs Implantable Defibrillator study. Cardiac Arrest Study Hamburg. Canadian Implantable Defibrillator Study. Eur Heart J 2000;21:2071-2078.
96. Varma N, Josephson ME: Therapy of "idiopathic" ventricular tachycardia. J Cardiovasc Electrophysiol 1997; 8(1):104-116.
97. Chen Q, Kirsch GE, Zhang D, et al: Genetic basis and molecular mechanism for idiopathic ventricular fibrillation. Nature 1998;392:293.
98. Carlson MD, White RD, Trohman RG, et al: Right ventricular outflow tract ventricular tachycardia: Detection of previously unrecognized anatomical abormalities using cine magnetic imaging. J Am Coll Cardiol 1994;24:720.
99. Markowitz SM, Litvak BL, Ramirez de Arellano EAM, et al: Adenosine-sensitive ventricular tachycardia: Right ventricular abnormalities delineated by magnetic resonance imaging. Circulation 1997;96:1192.
100. Trohman RG, Sahu J: Arrhythmogenic right ventricular dysplasia. Curr Treat Opt Cardiovasc Med 1999;1:259.
101. Marcus FI, Fontaine G: Arrhythmogenic right ventricular dysplasia/cardiomyopathy: A review. Pacing Clin Electrophysiol 1995;18:1298.
102. Wilde AA, Jongbloed RJ, Doevendans PA, et al: Auditory stimuli as a trigger for arrhythmic events differentiate HERG-related (LQTS2) patients from KVLQT1-related patients (LQTS1). J Am Coll Cardiol 1999;33:327-332.
103. Schwartz PJ, Priori SG, Spazzolini C, et al: Genotype-phenotype correlation in the long-QT syndrome: Gene-specific triggers for life-threatening arrhythmias. Circulation 2001;103: 89-95.
104. Zareba W, Moss AJ, Daubert JP, et al: Implantable cardioverter defibrillator in high-risk long QT syndrome patients. J Cardiovasc Electrophysiol 2003;14: 337-341.
105. Windle JR, Geletka RC, Moss AJ, et al: Normalization of ventricular repolarization with flecainide in long QT syndrome patients with SCN5A:DeltaKPQ mutation. Ann Noninvasive Electrocardiol 2001;6: 153-158.
106. Brugada P, Brugada J: Right bundle branch block, persistent ST segment elevation and sudden cardiac death: A distinct clinical and electrocardiographic syndrome. A multicenter report. J Am Coll Cardiol 1992;20:1391-1396.
107. Pasquie JL, Sanders P, Hocini M, et al: Fever as a precipitant of idiopathic ventricular fibrillation in patients with normal hearts. J Cardiovasc Electrophysiol 2004;15:1271-1276.
108. Brugada J, Brugada P: Right bundle branch block, persistent ST segment elevation and sudden cardiac death: A distinct clinical and electrocardiographic syndrome: A multicenter report. J Am Coll Cardiol 1992;20(6):1391-1396.
109. Gussak I, Antzelevitch C, Bjerregaard P, et al: The Brugada syndrome: Clinical, electrophysiologic and genetic aspects. J Am Coll Cardiol 1999;33:5-15.
110. Priori SG, Napolitano C, Schwartz PJ, et al: The elusive link between LQT3

and Brugada syndrome: The role of flecainide challenge. Circulation 2000;102:945-947.
111. Priori SG, Napolitano C, Gasparini M, et al: Clinical and genetic heterogeneity of right bundle branch block and ST-segment elevation syndrome: A prospective evaluation of 52 families. Circulation 2000;102: 2509-2515.
112. Napolitano C, Priori SG: Catecholaminergic polymorphic ventricular tachycardia and short-coupled torsades de pointes. In Zipes D, Jalife J (eds): Cardiac Electrophysiology: From Cell to Bedside, 4th ed. Philadelphia, WB Saunders, 2004.
113. Bjerregaard P, Gussak I: Short QT syndrome. Ann Noninvasive Electrocardiol 2005;10:436-440.
114. Bjerregaard P, Gussak I: Short QT syndrome: Mechanisms, diagnosis and treatment. Nat Clin Pract Cardiovasc Med 2005;2:84-87.
115. Spies C, Trohman RG: Narrative review: Electrocution and life-threatening electrical injuries. Ann Intern Med 2006;145:531-537.
116. Kobernick M: Electrical injuries: Pathophysiology and emergency management. Ann Emerg Med 1982;11:633-638.
117. Cooper MA: Lightning injuries: Prognostic signs for death. Ann Emerg Med 1980;9:134.
118. Trohman RG, Simmons TW, Moore SL, et al: Catheter ablation of the atrioventricular junction using radiofrequency energy and a bilateral cardiac approach. Am J Cardiol 1992;70:1438-1443.
119. Wood MA, Brown-Mahoney C, Kay GN, et al: Clinical outcome after ablation and pace therapy: With analysis. Circulation 2000;101: 1138-1144.
120. Doshi RN, Daoud EG, Fellows C, et al: LV based cardiac stimulation post AV node ablation evaluation (the PAVE Study). J Cardiovasc Electrophysiol 2005;16:1166-1167.
121. Takahashi Y, O'Neill MD, Jonsson A, et al: How to interpret and identify pulmonary vein recordings with the lasso catheter. Heart Rhythm 2006;3:748-750.
122. Oral H, Scharf C, Chugh A, et al: Catheter ablation for paroxysmal atrial fibrillation. Circulation 2003;108:2355-2360.
123. Morady F: Radio-frequency ablation as treatment for cardiac arrhythmias. N Engl J Med 1999;340:534-544.
124. Hsu LF, Jais P, Hocini M, et al: Incidence and prevention of cardiac tamponade complicating ablation for atrial fibrillation. Pacing Clin Electrophysiol 2005;28(Suppl 1): S106-S109.
125. Nademanee K, McKenzie J, Kosar ET, et al: A new approach for catheter ablation of atrial fibrillation: mapping of the electrophysiologic substrate. J Am Coll Cardiol 2004;43:2044-2053.
126. Pinski SL, Trohman RG: Implantable cardioverter-defibrillators: Implications for the nonelectrophysiologist. Ann Intern Med 1995;122:770-777.
127. Pinski SL, Trohman RG: Permanent pacing via implantable defibrillators. Pacing Clin Electrophysiol 2000;23:1667-1682.
128. Pinski SL, Trohman RG: Interference in implanted cardiac devices, Part I. Pacing Clin Electrophysiol 2002;25: 1367-1381.
129. Pinski SL, Trohman RG: Interference in implanted cardiac devices, Part II. Pacing Clin Electrophysiol 2002;25:1496-1509.
130. Pinski SL, Eguia LE, Trohman RG: What is the minimal pacing rate that prevents torsades de pointes? Insights from patients with permanent pacemakers. Pacing Clin Electrophysiol 2002;25:1612-1615.
131. Wathen MS, Sweeney MO, Degroot PJ, et al: Shock reduction using antitachycardia pacing for spontaneous rapid ventricular tachycardia in patients with coronary artery disease. Circulation 2001;104:796-801.
132. Wathen MS, Degroot PJ, Sweeney MO, et al: Prospective randomized multicenter trial of empirical antitachycardia pacing versus shocks for spontaneous rapid ventricular tachycardia in patients with implantable cardioverter-defibrillators: Pacing Fast Ventricular Tachycardia Reduces Shock Therapies (PainFREE Rx II) trial results. Circulation 2004;110: 2591-2596.
133. Wathen M: Implantable cardioverter defibrillator shock reduction using new antitachycardia pacing therapies. Am Heart J 2007;153:44-52.

Chapter 33

Valvular Heart Disease in Critical Care

Zoltan G. Turi

The profile of valvular heart disease in the critical care setting has evolved substantially over the past several decades. Aortic stenosis, mitral insufficiency, and aortic insufficiency are the most common valve diseases seen in the intensive care unit, but hypertrophic obstructive cardiomyopathy and mitral stenosis remain important entities as well. Patients with valvular heart disease in critical care units typically fall into one of two categories: (1) those who are critically ill because of valvular dysfunction or (2) those in whom valvular disease represents an important comorbidity. Many patients present without prior diagnosis of heart valve disease, either because the progression has been insidious and the disease not previously diagnosed or because the onset has been acute. Improvements in technology and the ubiquitous availability of echocardiography have improved diagnosis, while clinician skills at integrating physical examination and other data have generally atrophied during this same time frame.

Rheumatic heart disease accounted for 50% or more of admissions for heart disease in the first half of the 20th century, with congenital heart disease representing the other major indication for valve surgery through the 1960s.[1] With evolving technology and an increase in average life expectancy, heart valve surgery has shifted to valve repair, as well as replacement for a variety of acquired valvulopathies. The therapeutic armamentarium, once limited to minimal supportive medical therapy, then solely to valve replacement, has expanded to a variety of surgical repair techniques; a multitude of tissue and mechanical valve options for replacement; and, most recently, an expanding set of percutaneous interventions including percutaneous valve implantation. In addition, various mechanical devices for temporary hemodynamic support are important adjuncts to the management of patients with valvular heart disease in the critical care setting.

Diagnosis of valvular heart disease in the critical care setting is challenging, with lack of a quiet environment for auscultation; comorbidities that affect physical findings; and stress, infection, or metabolic abnormalities that result in tachycardia and shorter intervals for evaluation of heart sounds. Patients in a low output state have softer heart sounds and murmurs as well. In addition, clinical reliance on physical examination has fallen, as has the ability to make accurate diagnosis of valve disease.[2] A delay in recognizing the presence of significant valve disease continues to occur frequently, and some patients who have had prior routine medical outpatient care nevertheless present with undiagnosed valvular heart disease.[3] The currently accepted thresholds for mild, moderate, and severe valvular heart disease are shown in Table 33-1.

AORTIC STENOSIS

With the aging of the population, aortic stenosis (AS) has moved to the forefront in frequency of valvular heart disease encountered in older populations. The prevalence is surprisingly high; in patients 85 years of age, more than 8% of a random general population survey had Doppler-derived aortic valve area estimates of 1 cm^2 or less (Fig. 33-1),[4] consistent with severe AS by the 2006 ACC/AHA guidelines.[5] Thus AS should be considered in the differential diagnosis of each elderly critical care patient with hemodynamic instability. The possibility of AS should be dismissed only after considering physical examination, electrocardiographic and, where applicable, echocardiographic and invasive findings, all of which have potential limitations in achieving accurate diagnosis as discussed subsequently.[6]

Table 33-1. Classification of Severity of Valvular Heart Disease Based on ACC/AHA Guidelines

A. Left-sided Valve Disease			
	Aortic Stenosis		
Indicator	**Mild**	**Moderate**	**Severe**
Jet velocity (m/sec)	<3.0	3-4	>4
Mean gradient (mm Hg)*	<25	25-40	>40
Valve area (cm^2)	>1.5	1-1.5	<1
Valve area index (cm^2/m^2)			<0.6
	Mitral Stenosis		
	Mild	**Moderate**	**Severe**
Mean gradient (mm Hg)*	<5	5-10	>10
Pulmonary artery systolic pressure (mm Hg)	<30	30-50	>50
Valve area (cm^2)	>1.5	1-1.5	<1.0
	Aortic Regurgitation		
	Mild	**Moderate**	**Severe**
Qualitative			
Angiographic grade	1+	2+	3-4+
Color Doppler jet width	Central jet, width <25% of LVOT	Greater than mild but no signs of severe AR	Central jet, width >65% LVOT
Doppler vena contracta width (cm)	<0.3	0.3-0.6	>0.6
Quantitative (cath or echo)			
Regurgitant volume (mL/beat)	<30	30-59	≥60
Regurgitant fraction (%)	<30	30-49	≥50
Regurgitant orifice area (cm^2)	<0.1	0.1-0.29	≥0.30
Additional essential criteria			
Left ventricular size			Increased
	Mitral Regurgitation		
	Mild	**Moderate**	**Severe**
Qualitative			
Angiographic grade	1+	2+	3-4+
Color Doppler jet area	Small, central jet (<4 cm^2 or <20% LA area)	Signs of MR greater than mild present but no criteria for severe MR	Vena contracta width >0.7 cm with large central MR jet (area >40% of LA area) or with a wall-impinging jet of any size, swirling in LA
Doppler vena contracta width (cm)	<0.3	0.3-0.69	≥0.7
Quantitative (cath or echo)			
Regurgitant volume (mL/beat)	<30	30-59	≥60
Regurgitant fraction (%)	<30	30-49	≥50
Regurgitant orifice area (cm^2)	<0.2	0.2-0.39	≥0.4
Additional essential criteria			
Left atrial size			Enlarged
Left ventricular size			Enlarged
B. Right-sided Valve Disease	**Characteristic**		
Severe tricuspid stenosis:	Valve area <1 cm^2		
Severe tricuspid regurgitation:	Vena contracta width >0.7 cm and systolic flow reversal in hepatic veins		
Severe pulmonic stenosis:	Jet velocity >4 m/sec or maximum gradient >60 mm Hg		
Severe pulmonic regurgitation:	Color jet fills outflow tract; dense continuous wave Doppler signal with a steep deceleration slope		

*Valve gradients are flow dependent and when used as estimates of severity of valve stenosis should be assessed with knowledge of cardiac output or forward flow across the valve.

AR, aortic regurgitation; cath, catheterization; echo, echocardiography; LA, left atrial/atrium; LVOT, left ventricular outflow tract; MR, mitral regurgitation.

From Bonow RO, Carabello BA, Chatterjee K, et al: ACC/AHA 2006 guidelines for the management of patients with valvular heart disease: A report of the American College of Cardiology/American Heart Association Task Force on Practice Guidelines (writing committee to revise the 1998 guidelines for the management of patients with valvular heart disease) developed in collaboration with the Society of Cardiovascular Anesthesiologists and endorsed by the Society for Cardiovascular Angiography and Interventions and the Society of Thoracic Surgeons. J Am Coll Cardiol 2006;48:e1-148.

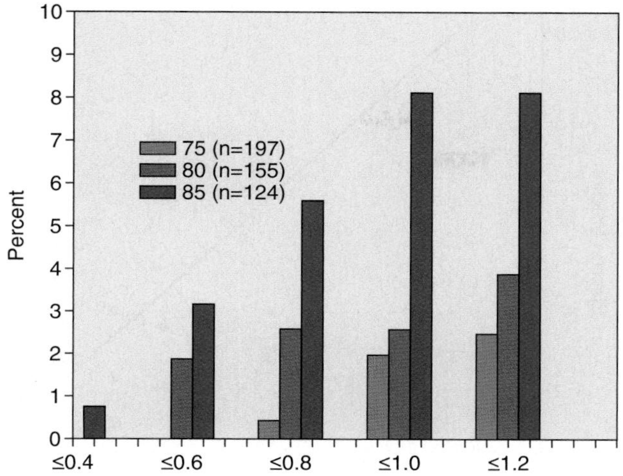

Figure 33-1. Doppler-derived estimates of aortic valve area at ages 75, 80, and 85 years from a randomized sampling of individuals in the general population. Bars represent percent of individuals with valve areas at or below the thresholds on the abscissa (in cm^2). (Data from Lindroos M, Kupari M, Heikkila J, et al: Prevalence of aortic valve abnormalities in the elderly: An echocardiographic study of a random population sample. J Am Coll Cardiol 1993;21:1220-1225.)

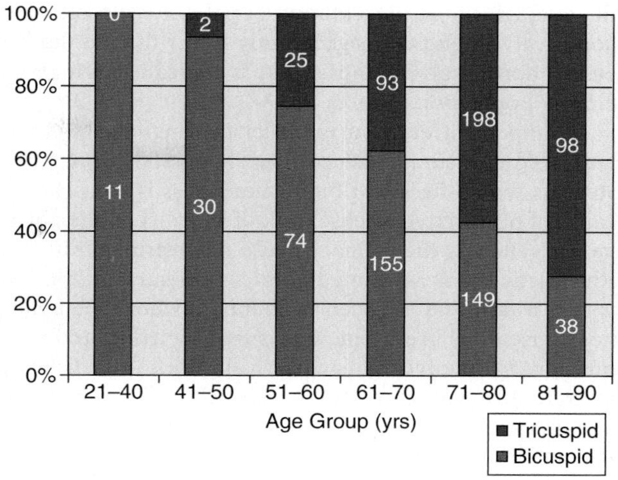

Figure 33-2. Distribution by age group of bicuspid versus tricuspid aortic valves in patients undergoing aortic valve replacement for aortic stenosis. (Modified from Roberts WC, Ko JM: Frequency by decades of unicuspid, bicuspid, and tricuspid aortic valves in adults having isolated aortic valve replacement for aortic stenosis, with or without associated aortic regurgitation. Circulation 2005;111:920-925.)

Pathophysiology

AS represents a continuum, from hemodynamically insignificant congenital and atherosclerotic disease to end-stage decompensation secondary to severe valvular obstruction. The congenital pathway is typically secondary to a bicuspid aortic valve, the most common congenital cardiac anomaly if mitral valve prolapse is excluded, occurring in approximately 1.5% of the population[7] and originally described by DaVinci in 1513.[8] The most common acquired anomaly is typically referred to as *degenerative disease*, an atherosclerotic process that represents a continuum from aortic valve sclerosis, which is not associated with a significant gradient, to a densely calcified aortic valve with severe outflow obstruction. Although the etiology of aortic valve stenosis in patients undergoing aortic valve replacement has shifted to calcific tricuspid aortic valve disease from bicuspid and rheumatic disease, this remains an age-related phenomenon, with a predominance of bicuspid aortic valve disease in patients younger than age 70 (Fig. 33-2).[9]

Aortic Valve Sclerosis

Aortic valve *sclerosis* is an important disease entity, although usually not because of hemodynamic considerations. Defined as calcification and thickening of the aortic valve without significant outflow obstruction (gradient <20 to 25 mm Hg), it is present in nearly 30% of the population older than age 65 and nearly 50% by age 85[10] and is associated with a 50% increase in 5-year cardiovascular mortality.[11] Its incidence is as high as 15-fold greater than aortic valve stenosis; the two diagnoses can be differentiated from one another by hemodynamics and physical examination findings discussed subsequently. In keeping with the primary atherosclerotic nature of aortic sclerosis, it is associated with increasing age, male gender, hypertension, smoking, elevated low-density lipoprotein and lipoprotein(a) levels, and diabetes.[10] The primary importance of aortic valve sclerosis is that it provides a window on the overall presence of vascular disease, in particular coronary artery disease.[12] Thus there should be a high index of suspicion of vascular disease in any patient with aortic valve sclerosis managed in the critical care setting.

Patients with aortic sclerosis do progress to aortic valve stenosis; a study of more than 2000 patients with valve thickening showed progression to severe AS in 2.5% over an average time interval of 7 years.[13] The fact that so-called degenerative disease of the aortic valve is absent in nearly half of octogenarians is also important to consider because it implies that it is not only aging but other factors that result in leaflet thickening, calcification, and stenosis. In the Helsinki Aging Study from which data are reflected in Figure 33-1, additional analysis demonstrated that not only age but also hypertension and low body mass index independently predicted calcification of the aortic valve, and age and serum ionized calcium were independently associated with valvular stenosis.[14] In general the process of sclerosis and then stenosis of the aortic valve appears, like atherosclerosis in general, to be an active inflammatory process, with deposition of lipoproteins, local inflammation with T lymphocyte and macrophage infiltration, fibroblast proliferation, and eventually osteoblast and bone formation.[15] Similar to other vascular disease, endothelial disruption likely leads to the initial lipid deposition in the leaflet tissues. The areas of early focal plaque formation appear at the loci of greatest stress: on the aortic side of the leaflets at the flexion points. Because bicuspid valves have greater mechanical stress, the average age at presentation of patients with bicuspid aortic valve stenosis is significantly lower than in the tricuspid aortic valve stenosis that is typically seen in an elderly population.[16]

An important element in understanding calcific AS is lack of commissural fusion; unlike rheumatic mitral valve stenosis where fusion of the commissures is the primary cause of obstructive disease, lack of mobility of the aortic valve leaflets is the primary cause of obstruction in AS. Rheumatic AS *is* associated with commissural fusion but is now a rare finding, even in countries where rheumatic heart disease is prevalent, and is usually associated with mitral valve involvement and typically aortic insufficiency as well. More obscure etiologies, such as unicuspid and quadricuspid aortic valve disease are uncommon, although presentation can be delayed to adulthood. In the case of unicuspid aortic valves there is a strong association with aortic stenosis,[17] whereas with quadricuspid aortic valves there is a high incidence of significant aortic insufficiency.[18]

Normal aortic valve area ranges from 3 to 4 cm^2. Significant resistance to outflow does not occur until the valve orifice is reduced more than 50%. Based on the simple hydraulic principle of Poiseuille's law, a 50% reduction in valve diameter results in approximately a 16-fold increase in resistance. In practice, as the resistance to outflow rises, the left ventricle is subject to pressure overload, resulting in compensatory hypertrophy. This in turn normalizes wall stress because the latter is proportional to chamber diameter times pressure divided by wall thickness (the LaPlace principle). The degree of wall thickness is variable: In patients with inadequate hypertrophic response, wall stress is inordinately high and there is early dilation and dysfunction.[19] In patients with a profound hypertrophic response disproportionate to valvular resistance, wall stress actually falls below normal and ejection fraction becomes supranormal,[20] a phenomenon that appears to be more common in women with AS. The ejection fraction for any degree of wall stress is predictable,[19] and patients who have disproportionately poor ejection phase indices (afterload mismatch) typically manifest left ventricular (LV) dysfunction beyond the depression that would be associated with high wall stress (Fig. 33-3),[21] a phenomenon described under low-gradient, low-output AS that follows.

LV hypertrophy, although it reduces wall stress, has several features that may be deleterious. With progressive hypertrophy, diastolic pressures may rise as LV compliance decreases, resulting in increased LV filling pressures. In addition, the myocardial supply-demand relationship is deleteriously affected by hypertrophy in this setting. With increased wall stress and increased wall mass, myocardial oxygen demand is increased; at the same time coronary flow reserve is decreased in AS,[22] and in later stages of the disease diastolic perfusion pressure is lowered. Because of abnormal flow reserve, conventional testing for ischemia in the setting of significant aortic valve stenosis has inadequate specificity to identify the presence or absence of hemodynamically significant concomitant coronary artery disease.[23]

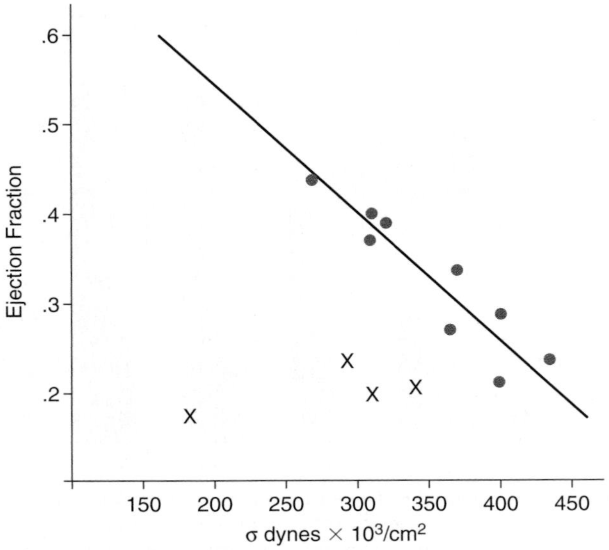

Figure 33-3. The relationship between ejection fraction and wall stress in patients with aortic stenosis. The patients (each represented by an "X") whose ejection fraction was disproportionately lower than the regression line had a poor overall outcome. In these patients ejection phase indices were depressed despite a low transvalvular gradient, a phenomenon suggesting intrinsic contractile dysfunction. (From Carabello BA, Green LH, Grossman W, et al: Hemodynamic determinants of prognosis of aortic valve replacement in critical aortic stenosis and advanced congestive heart failure. Circulation 1980;62:42-48.)

Other features associated with AS that are important in the critical care setting include abnormal platelet function and decreased levels of von Willebrand factor,[24] with associated bleeding risk that improves with aortic valve replacement. Another associated cause of bleeding is gastrointestinal angiodysplasia associated with aortic valve stenosis,[25] possibly exacerbated by the concomitant presence of von Willebrand syndrome.

The progression of AS is highly variable, but with the onset of moderately severe disease, the estimated mean decrease in valve area is on the order of 0.1 cm^2/year.[26] Certain demographics and noninvasive findings appear to predict the rate of progression, including age older than 50 years and moderate to severe valve calcification.[27] The issue of progression is particularly important in patients who are asymptomatic of the disease because aortic valve replacement before it is necessary is undesirable but must be weighed against the risk of sudden death. The latter has been studied in a number of longitudinal studies and is rare if patients are followed prospectively. The patients who are most likely to require early intervention are those with peak Doppler systolic velocities greater than 4 m/sec or who have a rapid increase in serial transvalvular Doppler velocity measurements.[26,27] This threshold has been confirmed by other series.[28] Once patients become symptomatic, with a classic triad of heart failure, angina, or syncope, hemodynamic deterioration can be rapid with significant associated mortality.[29]

Diagnosis

Physical Examination

The hallmarks of the physical examination relate to the contour of the aortic pressure upstroke, with a low volume and delayed carotid upstroke (pulsus parvus et tardus), a late peaking systolic ejection murmur, and a diminished or absent aortic second sound. Figure 33-4 demonstrates the hemodynamics that manifest in an abnormal carotid pulse contour; unlike the brisk upstroke of LV pressure over time (dP/dt), the aortic pressure is slow to rise and of significantly lower volume. An ejection click may be present in young patients with congenital AS, but with increasing calcification of the valve, mobility decreases to a point at which an ejection click becomes unlikely. The aortic component of the second heart sound, reflecting deceleration and closure of the aortic valve, is diminished or absent in severe AS where the thickened aortic valve leaflets are poorly mobile, have little deceleration, and drift rather than snap shut. The murmur of AS is characteristically a crescendo-decrescendo murmur that is late peaking, consistent with the timing of the peak gradient as seen in Figure 33-4, and is typically best heard over the right upper sternum and clavicle. It reflects the high-velocity systolic jet directed into the ascending aorta. A second component, described by Gallavardin as a musical component, is best heard at the left lower sternal border. The latter confounds diagnosis because the murmur is sug-gestive of mitral regurgitation (MR), but in its true form it is purely second to aortic valve stenosis. Because handgrip raises resistance to LV ejection, the murmur should decrease if it is a true Gallavardin phenomenon, whereas when it is secondary to MR, it should increase.[30]

Unfortunately none of these findings has sufficiently high sensitivity or specificity for AS or for differentiating moderate from severe disease.[3] Many patients with AS, particularly the elderly with stiff noncompliant vessels, will have a wide pulse pressure even with declining cardiac output and may have systolic hypertension. Hypotension may not be seen until late stages of the disease. The loudness of the murmur, which correlates to some degree with severity, is also not specific because body habitus and a variety of other factors affect the acoustics transmitted across the chest. Most importantly, in severe AS, as the cardiac output drops, the gradient generated decreases as well. In this setting the murmur may be quite soft, although sometimes still high pitched because of the high velocity across a tight constriction. A useful means of differentiating aortic sclerosis from stenosis is that in the former the systolic ejection murmur heard over the right sternum is typically mid peaking and mild to moderate in intensity, and it features a well-preserved aortic second sound. Although the physical findings described are variable, presence of the aortic second heart sound tends to reliably exclude severe AS.[31]

Noninvasive Evaluation

In contrast to the physical examination, echocardiographic techniques have progressively improved over the past several decades and availability in the critical care setting in industrialized nations is ubiquitous. The characteristic echocardiographic features of AS are decreased valve leaflet mobility, calcification in all except congenital AS in adolescents and young adults, and an augmented Doppler velocity that generally allows accurate estimation of the gradient. In congenital bicuspid AS in young adults, when commissural fusion is dominant, a characteristic doming pattern is seen, but this disappears with progressive valve calcification. The severity of calcification correlates with extent of obstruction by middle age; and typically Doppler signal velocity with peak and mean pressure gradient and valve area by continuity equation provide an accurate overall assessment. However, gradient is highly dependent on flow across the valve, and in low output states the gradient may result in underestimation of severity of disease; in high output states such as in patients with augmented cardiac output caused by inotropic stimulation, endogenous high catecholamine states, and sepsis, the gradient may be disproportionately higher than the severity of stenosis would suggest. The latest ACC/AHA guidelines describe the threshold for severe AS as antegrade jet velocity greater than 4 m/sec, gradient greater than 40 mm Hg, and aortic valve area less than 1 cm^2, with the caveat that the gradient and jet velocity depend

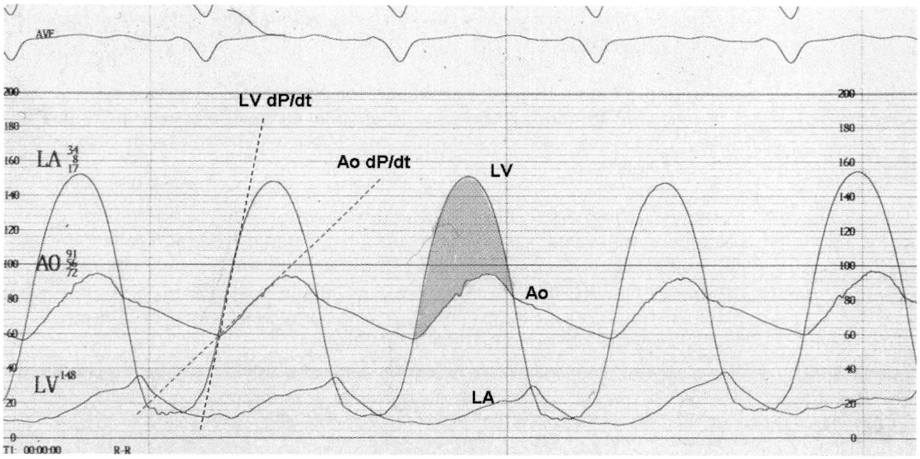

Figure 33-4. Left ventricular (LV), aortic (Ao), and left atrial (LA) pressure on 200 mm Hg scale, 100 mm/sec paper speed. The aortic valve gradient is filled in yellow. The dramatic difference in the slope of left ventricular (LV dP/dt, *dashed blue line*) and aortic pressure upstroke (Ao dP/dt, *dashed red line*) and the low pulse pressure (≈ 30 mm Hg) in this patient with classic severe aortic valve stenosis is demonstrated.

on the overall transvalvular flow[5] (see Table 33-1). Importantly, antegrade flow across the aortic valve does not equal cardiac output in patients with confounding conditions, including aortic insufficiency. Finally, although most practitioners do not index the valve area, it is important to appreciate that in patients with large body surface areas, disease that might be considered moderate in smaller patients may be functionally severe.

Several caveats need to be considered before acceptance of noninvasive data in the critical care setting. Inadequate acoustic windows in some patients and difficulty in positioning patients on respirators and with multiple lines in place do limit echocardiographic imaging. Technical errors in recording and interpretation result in significant misdiagnosis: errors in recording angle, inadvertent imaging of MR jets instead of aortic outflow, assessing proximal velocity instead of the transvalvular signal, and selecting signals in the setting of arrhythmias that are not representative of mean heart beats can all lead to skewed assessment of valve disease severity.[32] Further, a number of other potential confounding variables can lead to overestimation or underestimation of the severity of AS,[6,33] and valve area calculations by the continuity equation in a low-flow setting may be inaccurate.[34] Nevertheless, there is a trend toward a shift in the gold standard from catheter-derived to Doppler-derived determination of AS severity, and cardiac catheterization is no longer indicated for hemodynamic assessment of aortic valve disease severity when noninvasive findings are unequivocal.[5]

The echocardiogram provides important additional information including severity of LV hypertrophy, LV function and size, and concomitant disease of other heart valves. The presence of regional wall motion abnormalities, in the absence of a conduction disturbance, suggests concomitant coronary artery disease. The electrocardiogram (ECG) in AS is typically abnormal and frequently features LV hypertrophy, with ST segment abnormalities in the lateral leads typically described as a strain pattern.[35] Although occasionally mistaken for anterior ischemia or infarction, with loss of R voltage across the precordium and occasionally with narrow QS complexes, the ECG is not specific for severity of AS. With increasing calcification of the perivalvular tissues, heart block is seen, typically late in the course of the disease.

Cardiac Catheterization

Cardiac catheterization *is* indicated in patients in whom the noninvasive data are equivocal, and coronary angiography is indicated in a range of settings identified in Table 33-2. The hemodynamics of AS are best recorded with a catheter or catheters placed simultaneously on either side of the aortic valve.[6,36] Unfortunately most laboratories

Table 33-2. Indications for Cardiac Catheterization in Patients with Valvular Heart Disease

General indications:	1. When noninvasive findings are inconclusive or discordant with clinical findings or inadequate imaging is obtained 2. Right heart catheterization when clinical decision making will be influenced by hemodynamics not otherwise obtainable
Coronary angiography should be performed:*	Class I 1. Before valve surgery or percutaneous balloon commissurotomy in patients with chest pain, other objective evidence of ischemia, decreased LV systolic function, history of CAD, or coronary risk factors 2. In patients with apparently mild to moderate valvular heart disease but progressive angina, objective evidence of ischemia, decreased LV systolic function, or overt congestive heart failure 3. Before valve surgery or percutaneous balloon commissurotomy in men 35 years and older, premenopausal women aged 35 years and older who have coronary risk factors, and postmenopausal women Class II Surgery without coronary angiography is reasonable for patients having emergency valve surgery for acute valve regurgitation, aortic root disease, or infective endocarditis Class IIb Coronary angiography may be considered for patients undergoing catheterization to confirm the severity of valve lesions before valve surgery without preexisting evidence of CAD, multiple coronary risk factors, or advanced age Class III 1. Coronary angiography is not indicated in young patients undergoing nonemergency valve surgery when no further hemodynamic assessment by catheterization is deemed necessary and there are no coronary risk factors, no history of CAD, and no evidence of ischemia 2. Patients should not undergo coronary angiography before valve surgery if they are severely hemodynamically unstable

*From Bonow RO, Carabello BA, Chatterjee K, et al: ACC/AHA guidelines for the management of patients with valvular heart disease: A report of the American College of Cardiology/American Heart Association Task Force on Practice Guidelines (writing committee to revise the 1998 guidelines for the management of patients with valvular heart disease) developed in collaboration with the Society of Cardiovascular Anesthesiologists and endorsed by the Society for Cardiovascular Angiography and Interventions and the Society of Thoracic Surgeons. J Am Coll Cardiol 2006;48:e1-148.
CAD, coronary artery disease; LV, left ventricular.

record femoral artery pressure in lieu of central aortic pressure or do a catheter pullback in lieu of simultaneous pressure tracings; both techniques can result in significant misinterpretation of the severity of aortic valve disease.[37] A variety of other errors in catheterization laboratory pressure measurements makes the catheter-derived valve area generally more variable than desirable in all except a few laboratories, including inherent errors in estimating rather than measuring oxygen consumption and in assuming that the Gorlin constant (originally established for a limited subset of patients[38]) and the valve area itself remain constant under varying loading conditions.[34] In the catheterization laboratory as well, transvalvular flow is underestimated if there is concomitant aortic insufficiency, resulting in overestimation of the severity of aortic valve disease.

Low-Gradient, Low-Output Aortic Stenosis

The critical care unit patient with a low to moderate gradient (typically <30 mm Hg) across the aortic valve in the setting of low cardiac output represents an important conundrum (and should be differentiated from the aortic *sclerosis* patient with low gradient not associated with depressed output). In general the rules of hydraulics demonstrate that valve area is proportional to flow divided by the square root of the gradient.[38] Thus when the valve area is fixed, increased flow is associated with an exponential rise in gradient when valve areas are less than 1 cm^2 (Fig. 33-5). When a patient in the critical care setting has depressed cardiac output and a low gradient across the aortic valve, there are two possible interpretations of these findings: either the patient has mild to moderate AS and poor LV function, or the patient has severe AS with a low ejection fraction appropriate to high wall stress (see Fig. 33-3) and secondary depression of cardiac output. In the case of the former, increasing flow results in better opening of the aortic valve, with only mild to moderate increase in gradient and an increase in the calculated valve area of 0.3 cm^2 or greater.[39] In the latter case, a fixed obstruction to outflow exists and increasing transvalvular flow results in dramatic increase in gradient. In addition to increasing flow across the valve in these patients, typically with dobutamine infusion,[40] the echocardiogram can be useful in several other ways[41]: Calcification is suggestive of fixed outflow obstruction and, if severe, suggests that the underlying pathology is severe AS rather than LV dysfunction. Preserved LV contractile reserve, with significant rise in stroke volume (>20%), peak velocity (>0.6 m/second), or mean transvalvular gradient (>10 mm Hg) at the time of dobutamine infusion is an additional useful marker. Lack of contractile reserve has been associated with lower operative survival[42] (6% vs. 33% in one study), although it should not be the sole parameter for the decision on whether or not to operate because patients who survive may manifest significant recovery in LV function postoperatively[43] and low contractile reserve should not preclude surgery in patients who do have severe fixed obstruction because their prognosis without surgery is abysmal.[44]

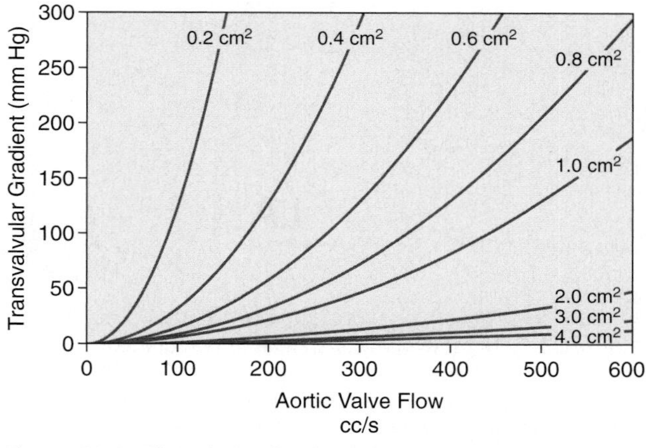

Figure 33-5. The relationship between transvalvular flow and transvalvular gradient for given valve areas. An exponential rise in gradient occurs when flow is increased with valve areas in the severe stenosis range (<1 cm^2). The curve demonstrates that change in gradient is proportional to the square of change in flow; thus doubling the flow rate results in a fourfold increase in gradient. (From Gorlin R, Gorlin SG: Hydraulic formula for calculation of the area of the stenotic mitral valve, other cardiac valves, and central circulatory shunts. Am Heart J 1951;41:1-29.)

Therapy

Medical Management

Medical management is aimed solely at patient stabilization because pharmacologic intervention has never been shown to prolong life and can achieve modest hemodynamic improvement at best. In the critical care setting the approach to the patient with AS normally parallels treatment of corresponding degrees of heart failure, albeit with caution, because the normal therapeutic approach to heart failure can be deleterious or fatal in the setting of severe AS. The traditional heart failure therapies of digitalis glycosides, diuretics, and angiotensin-converting enzyme (ACE) inhibitors need to be used with care because reduction in preload can cause hypotension, decreased cardiac output, and a downward spiral into refractory shock. In patients with small-volume hypertrophic left ventricles, cardiac output is particularly preload dependent.

Atrial arrhythmias, in particular atrial fibrillation (AF), can lead to abrupt and severe decompensation because of loss of the atrial contraction component of LV filling. Cardioversion in the critical care setting is particularly helpful in severely decompensated patients, and maintenance of sinus rhythm in patients who are otherwise suitable (e.g., left atrium <6 cms, recent onset of AF, and absence of clot in the left atrium by transesophageal echocardiography) should be a priority.

Vasodilator therapy, in particular nitroprusside, has been used in the critical care setting in patients with severe LV dysfunction and severe AS.[45] In a select group of patients not dependent on inotropes, cardiac output rose significantly and there was overall hemodynamic improvement. Similarly, intra-aortic balloon pumping has been used, although there are only isolated case reports of efficacy.[46,47] As would be expected, both nitroprusside and intra-aortic balloon pumping result in afterload reduction and some increase in transvalvular flow along with some increase in aortic valve gradient.

Hemodynamic monitoring is essential for the pharmacologic management of decompensated severe AS patients in the critical care setting. Because of the dependence on preload, a fine threshold exists between optimal filling pressures and pulmonary edema. Vasodilator therapy as described earlier results in peripheral vasodilation, but because of the fixed obstruction to outflow it may not provide sufficient increase in stroke volume and cardiac output to maintain systemic blood pressure. Inotropic agents are frequently required, and patients with inadequate contractile reserve may show limited improvement. β-blockers are relatively dangerous, although tachycardia is hemodynamically unfavorable, even in sinus rhythm. β-blockade, if employed, should be used with great caution. β-Blockers decrease contractility and, in addition, an increase in heart rate may be the only remaining compensatory mechanism for low stroke volume because of the fixed resistance to outflow. Patients with severe AS can enter a death spiral in which hemo-dynamic recovery becomes impossible.

Lipid-lowering therapy and converting enzyme inhibitors have been the subject of substantial investigation,[48] although their role is in the chronic setting rather than during critical care. Although design issues may have muddled outcomes, a prospective randomized trial failed to show clear benefits of atorvastatin in slowing disease progression.[49] Some preliminary evidence suggests potential benefits of ACE inhibitors in decreasing progression of aortic valve calcification,[50] but the available clinical data do not show slowing of AS progression.[51] Both lipid-lowering and converting enzyme inhibitors need to be tested in larger populations earlier in the course of aortic valve disease.

Percutaneous Interventions

Balloon aortic valvuloplasty is a temporizing measure for patients who are hemodynamically unstable and are at high risk for aortic valve replacement. Although the procedure is therapeutic and indicated in congenital AS in children and young adults, the risk/benefit ratio in patients beyond their 20s is usually unfavorable. Because calcific AS is associated with open commissures and ossified leaflets, abrupt balloon inflation exerts its effect by improving leaflet compliance through the formation of multiple, usually microscopic, fracture lines in the calcified tissues. Stretching of the commissures is temporary, and any hemodynamic benefit of the latter resolves within hours. The leaflets lose their improved compliance within weeks to months, and the aortic valve area typically returns to baseline.

The acute hemodynamic results (Fig. 33-6) are poor compared with those of aortic valve replacement, with a 50% reduction in gradient and an increase in aortic valve area of only 0.2 to 0.3 cm^2.[52] The in-hospital mortality was close to 10% in the National Heart, Lung and Blood Institute registry[53] and is substantially higher in patients with hemodynamic decompensation and multiorgan failure. Most valves have restenosed within a few months, with a recent series showing an 87% mortality rate after

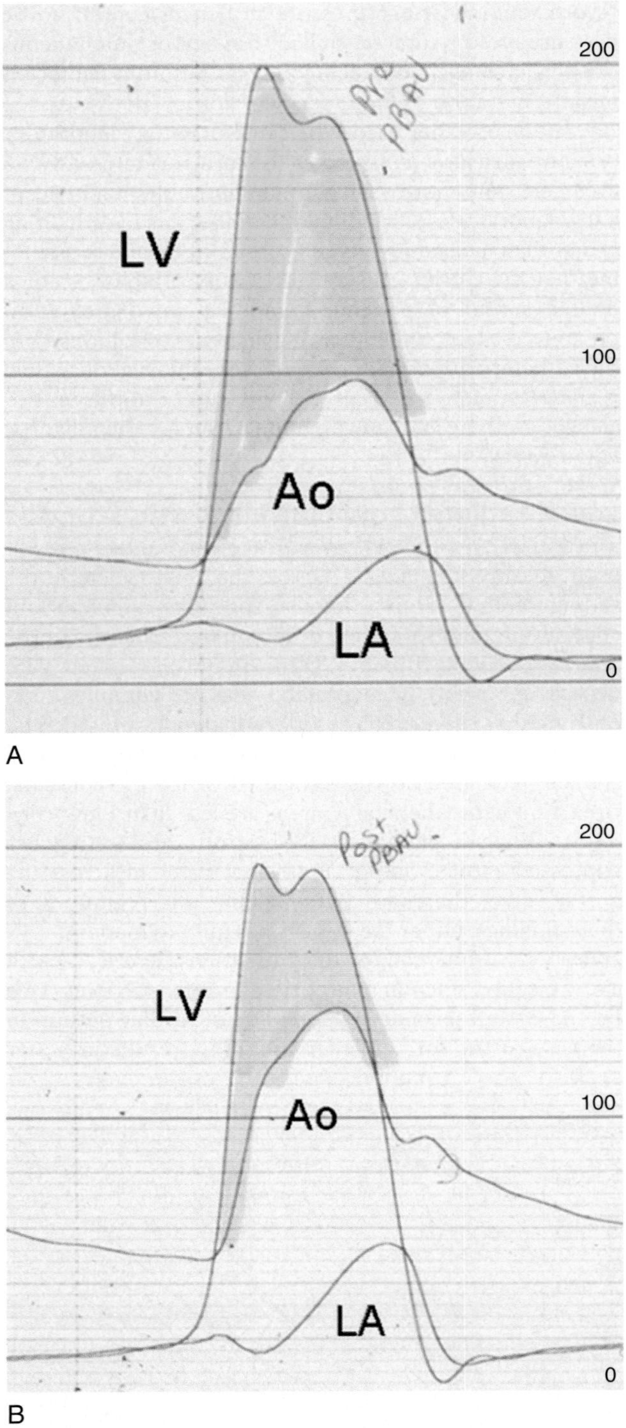

Figure 33-6. Hemodynamic response to percutaneous balloon aortic valvuloplasty. Tracings show before **(A)** and after **(B)** balloon dilation on 200 mm Hg scale. A successful 50% reduction in gradient occurs, but residual gradient remains 50 mm Hg, still in the severe category. The pulse pressure has increased from 60 mm Hg to 90 mm Hg, the peak aortic systolic pressure has increased to 140 mm Hg from 100 mm Hg, and the left ventricular pressure upslope can be seen to have improved dramatically. Ao, aorta; LA, left atrium; LV, left ventricle.

a median of less than 7 months,[54] and no benefit for long-term outcomes has been shown. Indeed, the overall clinical course is not influenced by balloon valvotomy.[55] Nevertheless, it can serve as a bridge to aortic valve replacement in select patients with multiple comorbidities and is an alternative but low efficacy measure for patients who are not candidates for aortic valve replacement. It is not an alternative to surgery for patients who can undergo valve replacement, even for most patients at relatively high risk for the latter.

Several settings in which balloon aortic valvuloplasty was previously considered to have a role are no longer included as indications in the 2006 ACC/AHA guidelines.[5] These include preoperative balloon dilation in patients undergoing noncardiac surgery[56]; in general all but decompensated patients can withstand general anesthesia as long as careful hemodynamic monitoring and anesthesia management are performed.[57] Patients who require urgent noncardiac surgery in the setting of severe symptomatic AS do have a significant perioperative risk,[58] and preoperative aortic valve replacement should be considered if at all possible. Balloon aortic valvuloplasty has also been proposed as a tool to differentiate myocardial dysfunction from severe AS with secondary LV dysfunction in low-gradient, low-output AS.[59] The latter patients typically demonstrated substantial improvement in stroke volume and ejection fraction after balloon dilation, but dobutamine stress testing is a far safer, less morbid screening tool.

A percutaneous intervention of increasing likelihood to be important in the critical care setting is percutaneous aortic valve replacement. Several technologies are undergoing pilot or pivotal trials, initially using an antegrade transseptal approach[60] but now limited to transfemoral or open chest apical approaches.[61] The early results, while incorporating learning curves, device development, and a significant number of complications, are promising overall.[62] Most of the experience to date has been with patients with severe AS and severe comorbidities, which likely contribute to the high early morbidity and mortality rates.

Aortic Valve Replacement

Aortic valve replacement remains the treatment of choice for severe AS. Class I indications are severe AS (valve area less than 1 cm^2) with symptoms or, regardless of symptoms, if patients have severe AS and are undergoing coronary artery bypass, are undergoing surgery of the aorta or other heart valves, or have LV dysfunction. A long list of class II indications generally focuses on patients who do not meet class I criteria but are thought to be at increased risk of rapid disease progression or hemodynamic compromise. In addition, patients with moderate AS who undergo other cardiac surgery generally have simultaneous aortic valve replacement. Survival after aortic valve replacement is excellent if LV function is preserved, with operative mortality in ideal candidates as low as 1%. In these patients, age-matched survival is not significantly different from patients without AS.[63] In the setting of LV dysfunction, however, postoperative life expectancy is relatively poor.[64] Nevertheless, conservative therapy for severe aortic stenosis remains an undesirable alternative: A recent review of 453 patients treated without surgery despite severe AS had 1-year, 5-year, and 10-year survival rates of only 62%, 32%, and 18%, respectively[65] with the worst survival in patients with renal failure, pulmonary hypertension, age older than 75 years, diminished ejection fraction, and congestive heart failure.

AORTIC INSUFFICIENCY

The overall prevalence of moderate or severe aortic insufficiency (AI) in the United States, as shown in the Framingham Offspring Study, ranged from 0.3% in the fifth decade of life to 2.2% for patients aged 70 to 83.[66] The frequency is age and male gender related. The diagnosis of AI is more difficult and the treatment issues in many ways more complex than for AS, with less of a clear dichotomy in the decision tree for valve replacement. AI needs to be considered in light of its acuity: Acute AI is usually associated with life-threatening comorbidities and the resultant acute regurgitation places great stress on the left ventricle and may itself be fatal. In contrast, chronic AI may evolve from clinically insignificant to requiring surgery over decades. Unlike AS, it is not primarily a disease of the aging process (although it does occur more frequently with increasing age) and is typically secondary to one of an extensive list of systemic or structural pathologies that result in insufficiency of the aortic valve. Acute AI frequently requires urgent surgery, whereas chronic AI may be managed by watchful waiting and some limited options for medical therapy.

Pathophysiology

Acute AI is generally associated with leaflet involvement by endocarditis or disruption of the aortic valve's annular structure by dissection or trauma. Chronic AI, by contrast, is caused by congenital valve abnormalities, most importantly bicuspid aortic valve disease, or by the degenerative process described earlier associated with aortic stenosis. Conditions that distort the annulus and aortic root including systemic hypertension have been considered to be important causes of secondary AI, although the association between chronic AI and systemic hypertension remains to be confirmed.[66,67] Rheumatic AI, almost invariably associated with mitral valve involvement as well, remains prevalent in developing countries but is an uncommon cause of AI in industrialized nations.

In general, etiologies of AI (Table 33-3) have been divided into those that affect the leaflets primarily and those that affect the root and annulus. The former includes bicuspid and other aortic valve abnormalities, endocarditis, rheumatic aortic valve disease, the atherosclerotic process described earlier, connective tissue disorders, antiphospholipid syndrome (Libman-Sacks endocarditis), and toxicity from anorectic drugs.[68] The aortic root and annulus are affected by a variety of comorbidities that dilate the aortic root; Marfan and Ehlers-Danlos syndromes; osteogenesis imperfecta; chronic aortic dissection; syphilitic aortitis; connective tissue disorders; and, along with the valve leaflets, ankylosing spondylitis.

In isolated acute AI, the sudden onset of regurgitation imposes a large-volume load on the left ventricle in diastole prior to an adaptive process being in place. The abrupt rise in pressure is reflected by parallel development of left atrial and pulmonary vascular hypertension, frequently resulting in pulmonary edema. Because the compliance of a previously unaffected left ventricle is not sufficient to allow adequate dilation to absorb the regurgitant volume, the ventricle operates on the steep portion of its pressure-volume curve, with inadequate stroke volume to accommodate the high regurgitant flow. The effective (net) forward stroke volume (antegrade flow minus retrograde filling) is therefore low, compensated to some degree by tachycardia, but frequently insufficient to maintain normal cardiac output. This phenomenon is exaggerated in patients with preexistent LV hypertrophy in whom the ventricle is already operating on the steep portion of its pressure-volume curve, and particularly severe decompensation is seen when the left ventricle is small and hypertrophic. Critical care settings for the latter unfortunately include many of the common scenarios for acute AI including endocarditis in the setting of aortic stenosis and aortic dissection in patients with hypertension and a dilated aortic root.[5]

Table 33-3. Etiologies of Acute and Chronic Aortic Insufficiency

Acute	Infective endocarditis Aortic dissection Trauma
Chronic	Dilation of the aorta Systemic hypertension Bicuspid aortic valve Calcific degenerated aortic valve disease Rheumatic aortic valve disease Infective endocarditis Myxomatous degeneration Aortic dissection Marfan syndrome Trauma Ankylosing spondylitis Syphilis Rheumatoid arthritis Osteogenesis imperfecta Giant cell aortitis Ehlers-Danlos syndrome Subaortic stenosis Ventricular septal defect with cusp prolapse Anorectic drug reaction

Acute severe AI results in near approximation of aortic and LV pressures at end diastole, with consequent deleterious effects on coronary perfusion of the subendocardium (Fig. 33-7). Because coronary perfusion pressure is the difference between diastolic pressure in the aortic root and subendocardial pressure in the LV cavity, the decrease in aortic diastolic pressure and rise in subendocardial pressure that are hallmarks of acute AI can result in profound subendocardial ischemia, especially in patients with preexistent hypertrophy or patients with underlying coronary artery disease. In addition, because afterload and wall stress in this setting are increased, there is a rise in myocardial oxygen demand simultaneous with a fall in supply, occasionally leading to cardiogenic shock and death. Acute AI also results in early closure of the mitral valve as LV diastolic pressure rises above left atrial pressure, a phenomenon that has potential protective benefits for the pulmonary circulation.

In contrast, chronic AI features a host of adaptive processes by the left ventricle including progressive dilation, increased compliance, and hypertrophy. As with AS, hypertrophy results in lower wall stress but AI features an increase in afterload combined with progressive LV dilation and somewhat less hypertrophy, resulting in significantly higher wall stress than seen in compensated AS.[69] End diastolic dilation of the left ventricle allows for larger stroke volumes to compensate for regurgitant fractions,

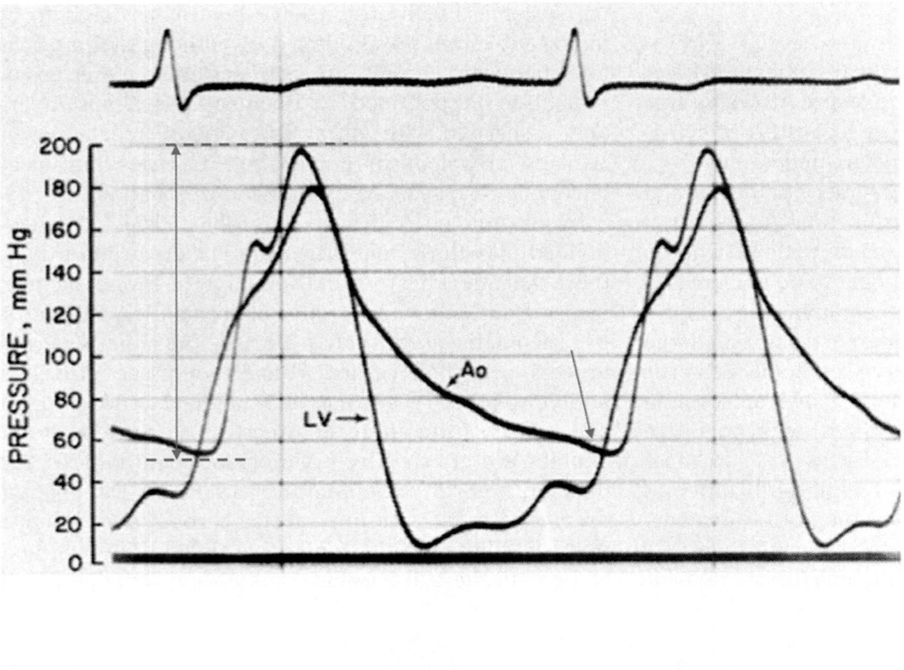

Figure 33-7. The hemodynamics of acute aortic insufficiency. The wide pulse pressure (150 mm Hg difference between peak and minimum aortic pressure *[blue arrow]*) and near diastasis of left ventricular and aortic pressure late in diastole *(red arrow)* are demonstrated. Ao, aorta; LV, left ventricle. (Modified from Grossman W: Profiles in valvular heart disease. In Baim D [ed]: Grossman's Cardiac Catheterization, Angiography and Intervention. Philadelphia, Lippincott Williams & Wilkins, 2006, p 654.)

which may be in the range of 50% or greater. With combined pressure and volume overload, unique among the valve disorders discussed in this chapter, LV adaptations allow for maintenance of normal overall function until ventricular remodeling and hypertrophy are no longer sufficient to maintain forward stroke volume and ejection fraction. With increasing wall stress and LV dilation, LV contractility is eventually impaired, at which point filling pressures begin to rise (or rise further) and patients become symptomatic. Coronary flow reserve in AI, as with AS, is impaired,[70] and, combined with increased demand and the need for additional perfusion for a hypertrophic myocardium, may result in significant ischemia. The onset of symptoms may be abrupt, especially with new onset of atrial tachyarrhythmias or sudden increase in cardiac output demand such as with exertion or infection.

Although acute aortic insufficiency represents a relative or absolute medical emergency, chronic AI may have an insidious course over decades. Some insight into the rate of progression of chronic AI is provided by a meta-analysis incorporated into the most recent ACC/AHA guidelines.[5] In a review of nine admittedly heterogeneous studies incorporating nearly 600 primarily asymptomatic or mildly symptomatic patients with AI, average progression to symptoms with or without LV systolic dysfunction was 4.3% annually, and sudden death occurred in 0.2% annually.[5] Although this rate of progression is modest, patients do not necessarily develop symptoms before developing LV dysfunction or sudden death.[71] Age, end systolic dimensions,[72] and rate of deterioration of end systolic dimension and ejection fraction[73] are more sensitive tools for predicting outcome in chronic AI.

In contrast, in the setting of *symptomatic* AI that does not fall in the acute severe category, annual mortality of 6% to 25% has been described, depending on severity of symptoms. By the 10-year follow-up, 75% had undergone aortic valve replacement or died.[74]

Diagnosis

Physical Examination

The hallmarks of *acute* severe AI include features consistent with congestive heart failure and low cardiac output including tachycardia, dyspnea, and signs of impaired cardiac output such as peripheral vasoconstriction. The wide pulse pressure that is a hallmark of AI may or may not be seen, in part because it is dependent on LV compliance. The classic aortic insufficiency murmur may not be heard because of the limited gradient between the aorta and LV during diastole when LV diastolic pressures in some cases approach systemic diastolic. Tachycardia and diminished effective forward flow in acute AI may offset the augmented systolic and wide pulse pressure seen in later stages of the disease, and these patients may have normal or occasionally diminished pulses, although more moderate acute AI may feature the more classic findings. Early closure of the mitral valve may result in a soft first heart sound, and distortions of leaflet anatomy may result in lack of a distinct aortic second sound. In some cases absence of a second heart sound in a patient presenting with cardiogenic shock may be the most prominent physical finding.[68]

The dramatic physical findings in *chronic* AI are among the most familiar to physicians and trainees. A wide pulse pressure results primarily because of increased stroke volume, which augments systolic pressure,[75] and low aortic diastolic pressures because of volume runoff into the left ventricle. This in turn results in a large variety of associated eponymous physical findings including bounding carotid and peripheral pulses (Corrigan's and water hammer pulses, respectively); Hill's sign (dramatically higher systolic pressure in the legs than the arms because of the exaggerated effect of harmonics on systolic pressure waveforms, variously described as having a 20 or 40 mm Hg threshold); Duroziez's sign (to and fro murmur over the femoral arteries); and Traube's sign ("pistol shot" sound over the femoral artery during simultaneous compression). With LV dilation, the apical impulse is displaced laterally.

The intensity of the classic diastolic decrescendo murmur heard over the left midsternal border generally correlates well with the severity of AI,[76] although in later stages of decompensation (or in acute AI), when the gradient between the aorta and the left ventricle disappears in later stages of diastole, the murmur typically shortens. When the murmur is better heard over the right (rather than left) sternal border, the etiology of the AI may be secondary to a dilated aortic root rather than a primary leaflet abnormality.[77] Two other murmurs are frequently heard with moderate to severe AI: a systolic ejection murmur consistent with increased transvalvular flow and on occasion an Austin-Flint murmur. The latter is the apical diastolic rumble occasionally confused with mitral stenosis and thought to originate from vibration of the anterior mitral leaflet caused by the diastolic regurgitant jet originating at the aortic valve; it has been described only in the setting of severe AI.[77] In rheumatic AI, if a diastolic rumble is heard, mitral stenosis should be excluded. An S3 gallop is most likely to be present when severe AI occurs in a setting of depressed LV function[78] but may merely reflect substantial volume loading; the finding is not specific.

Noninvasive Evaluation

As with aortic stenosis, noninvasive assessment has replaced cardiac catheterization for determining severity of AI. It provides both structural and physiologic information including visualization of the leaflets, annulus, and aortic root; semiquantitative assessment of the severity of AI; and characterization of LV size, hypertrophy, and function, as well as other structural heart disease. Transesophageal echocardiography has superior diagnostic sensitivity to transthoracic echo for certain parameters, in particular for detection of valvular vegetations.[79] A wide range of techniques for measurement of AI severity including width of the color Doppler jet compared with size of the LV outflow tract, width of the vena contracta, regurgitant volume, regurgitant fraction, and regurgitant orifice area are described in Chapter 8. The correlation of these parameters with severity of AI is listed in Table 33-1. Additional findings of importance are rate of jet velocity deceleration as diastasis is achieved between aortic and LV diastolic pressures and duration of diastolic flow reversal in the aorta.[80] In addition to echocardiography, cine MRI can assess severity of aortic insufficiency, size of chamber volumes, LV mass, wall thickness, and systolic function.[81] LV size and function have also been followed serially by radionuclide ventriculography.[82]

The size and function of the LV have been used to set thresholds at which aortic valve replacement should be considered. The ACC/AHA guidelines[5] and the European Society of Cardiology guidelines[83] have set slightly different values for classes I and II recommendations. The echocardiogram-based recommendations, which vary with clinical settings, use thresholds that include LV end diastolic dimension greater than 70 to 75 mm and end systolic dimension greater than 50 to 55 mm, aortic root dimension greater than 50 to 55 mm (the lower threshold is for patients with bicuspid valves or Marfan syndrome),[83] and ejection fraction less than 50%. As the observational data have grown, these numbers have shifted slightly from the familiar "rule of 55's," which recommended surgery for asymptomatic patients with ejection fraction less than 55% or LV end systolic dimension greater than 55 mm. An important consideration is that the end systolic and end diastolic dimensions should be adjusted downward for patients with small body surface area. Keeping in mind that these threshold values can be confounded by comorbidities that affect chamber size and function including ischemic and other forms of cardiomyopathy, as well as multivalvular disease, is important.

The ECG was once an important tool in the serial assessment of patients with AI. Similar to AS, features of LV hypertrophy may be present. Progression of LV dilation and dysfunction were thought to correlate with development of an LV strain pattern, a phenomenon that has been confirmed recently.[84] As a result, the use of digitalis glycosides, which can cause a similar strain pattern, was discouraged in order to maintain relative specificity of the finding. Conduction disturbances remain an important feature, particularly heart block in the setting of endocarditis, discussed subsequently.

Cardiac Catheterization

As with the other valvular diseases discussed in this chapter, cardiac catheterization is indicated only for patients with inconclusive noninvasive findings or when noninvasive findings are discordant with the rest of the clinical picture. Typical findings include a wide aortic pulse pressure and an exaggerated rise in LV diastolic pressure, reflecting continuous retrograde filling during diastole (see Fig. 33-7). Cardiac catheterization in this setting normally includes aortic root angiography; although the latter requires a significant dye load (typically 30 mL/second for 2 seconds) to be diagnostically accurate. The hallmark of severe aortic insufficiency is greater opacification of the left ventricle than the aorta. The indications for coronary angiography in this setting are listed in Table 33-2.

Therapy

Medical Management

In acute AI, medical therapy is targeted to stabilization pending aortic valve replacement. Nitroprusside has been the standard for reducing peripheral vascular resistance and improving net forward flow across the aortic valve since the 1970s.[85] The use of arterial vasodilators is more complex when the patient is already hypotensive, and a combination of inotropes and afterload reduction should be considered. Although afterload reduction in this setting is highly beneficial, the otherwise optimal combination of afterload reduction and augmented pressure normally provided by intra-aortic balloon pumping in cardiogenic shock (see Chapters 7 and 33) is not a viable choice in AI. Counterpulsation during diastole increases the severity of AI with potentially catastrophic consequences; it represents an absolute contraindication to the intra-aortic balloon pump.

Besides vasodilator therapy, maneuvers to raise the heart rate may be helpful, especially in patients who are bradycardic or have a normal heart rate. Tachycardia disproportionately decreases the diastolic filling period, thereby decreasing the duration of regurgitation across the aortic valve. Both isoproterenol or electrical pacing to raise the heart rate have been used with therapeutic benefit.

In *chronic* AI, the evidence base is incomplete and somewhat controversial. The general consensus is that asymptomatic patients with mild to at most moderate AI with normal LV function who are not hypertensive do not require or benefit from vasodilator therapy.[71,73] Only when patients are not surgical candidates is vasodilator use in chronic AI a class I indication.[5] Class II indications are short-term treatment to optimize the patient's hemodynamic status prior to aortic valve replacement and, more controversially, long-term therapy for asymptomatic patients with severe AI but preserved LV function. Two important studies with divergent results have been performed: One, using nifedipine, appeared to demonstrate some slowing of progression to need for aortic valve replacement compared with patients on digoxin.[86] The second, a placebo-controlled study, failed to demonstrate clear benefits of vasodilator therapy with either nifedipine or an ACE inhibitor,[87] but there are concerns regarding the size of the study, dose of drug used, and modest severity of disease at baseline. Oral vasodilators that have been described as having potential therapeutic benefit include several dihydropyridine calcium channel blockers (nifedipine and felodipine), as well as hydralazine. The appropriateness of vasodilator therapy regardless of severity of disease is clearer in patients with systemic hypertension, in whom reduction of afterload has dual benefits. The dose of drug should be sufficient to show at least some reduction in systolic pressure. There is no evidence base to recommend other forms of medical therapy, such as nitrates or drugs commonly used to treat congestive heart failure to prevent progression of disease in chronic asymptomatic AI. In the critical care setting, however, inotropes and vasodilators are appropriate if patients have congestive heart failure or a low output state, or both.

Aortic Valve Replacement

Two factors primarily determine when a patient should be referred for valve replacement: the presence of symptoms, and findings of LV systolic dysfunction.[5] Surgery results in superior long-term survival than medical therapy alone for symptomatic patients.[74,88] Similarly, patients with LV dysfunction have an inverse correlation between ejection fraction and mortality.[89] Three ACC/AHA class I indications for surgery, all for patients with *severe* AI, exist: (1) patients who have symptoms regardless of LV function; (2) patients with LV systolic dysfunction (EF less than or equal to 50%) regardless of symptoms; and (3) patients undergoing coronary bypass surgery or surgery on other heart valves or the aorta.

ACC/AHA Class II indications use the thresholds defined by LV dimensions, again for patients with *severe* AI, using 55 mm as the end systolic threshold and 75 mm as the end diastolic threshold, but lowering those values by 5 mm when the rate of LV dilation is progressive or when patients have deteriorating exercise tolerance or an abnormal hemodynamic response to exercise. Patients with only moderate AI who are undergoing surgery on the aorta or coronary bypass are also considered to have class II indications.

The question of whether it is ever too late to perform aortic valve replacement in patients with AI has been raised.[75] Because the disease involves high afterload and wall stress, there is postoperative improvement in ejection fraction[90] even in patients with severe baseline LV dysfunction. In general there is substantial reversal of the physiologic adaptations required by chronic severe AI in the postoperative state.[91] Nevertheless, delay in referring patients for surgery is deleterious, with significant negative impact on outcomes[92]; the prognosis is adversely affected both by the severity and duration of LV dysfunction.[93] This includes a fourfold increase in operative mortality for patients with EF less than 35% (14%) compared with those with EF greater than 50% (3.7%). Thus the trend has been for earlier referral of symptomatic patients and more aggressive noninvasive monitoring for early detection of deterioration in LV function or dimensions.

Special consideration should be given to patients with acute aortic valve endocarditis. Deteriorating hemodynamics, as well as extension of infection as manifest by progressive heart block and ring abscess formation on echo (Fig. 33-8), are among several factors that mandate early surgery[94]; despite the semielective nature of the operation (with an operative mortality of close to 10%) and the theoretical risk of an infected prosthesis, the long-term outcomes have been satisfactory, with 75% 10-year survival after hospital discharge.[95]

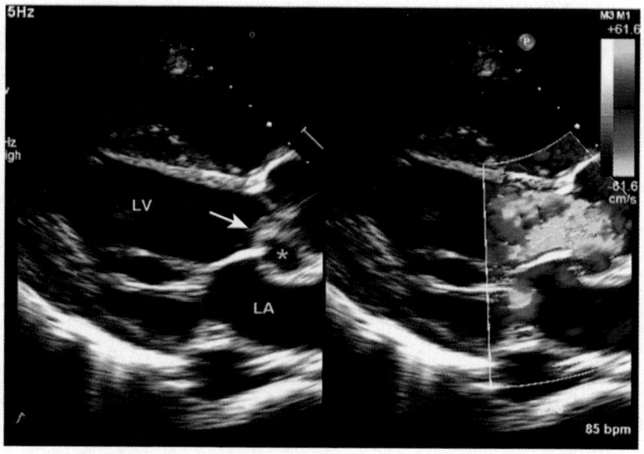

Figure 33-8. Vegetation *(arrow)*. On right is wide-open aortic insufficiency—the jet fills the outflow tract. Asterisk on left refers to walled-off echolucent abscess cavity. LA, left atrium; LV, left ventricle.

MITRAL REGURGITATION

Anatomically and physiologically, the mitral valve is the most complex of the heart valves, dependent for function on a complex interaction between leaflets, annulus, commissures, and the supporting apparatus consisting of chordae tendineae tethered to the papillary muscles (Fig. 33-9). Distortion or dysfunction of any of the elements and changes in function and geometry of the left ventricle and left atrium can all have a significant impact on flow across the mitral valve. In addition, unlike other valvulopathies, the mitral valve is highly dependent on the myocardial circulation. In contrast with the relatively passive nature of opening and closing of the aortic valve, mitral valve motion is an active process reflecting not just cyclical pressure variations but tethering and dynamic interaction with the supporting apparatus. As with AI, mitral insufficiency (MR) has acute and chronic manifestations and chronic (rather than acute) insufficiency is more common. However, acute MR has a much larger variety of etiologies than acute AI and the overall incidence is higher. Data from the Framingham Offspring Study revealed a prevalence of moderate or greater MR from 0.9% of women in the fifth decade of life, to 11.2% of men between ages 70 and 83, and correlated with age, low body mass, and systemic hypertension.[66] As with aortic insufficiency, ventricular function predicts overall outcomes. Chronic MR can both cause and be the result of LV remodeling and heart failure and, when secondary to LV dysfunction, is associated with a significantly poorer overall prognosis than LV dysfunction without secondary MR.[96]

Pathophysiology

Fundamental understanding of the pathophysiology of MR has expanded substantially in the past 2 decades. In particular, awareness of the role of the subvalvular apparatus in preserving LV function and data demonstrating the need for earlier referral to surgery have resulted in significant changes in clinical and surgical practice, leading to substantial improvement in outcomes.[97]

As with AI, MR results in volume overloading of the LV. Unlike AI, the afterload is not increased and overall LV ejection is enhanced rather than impaired by loading

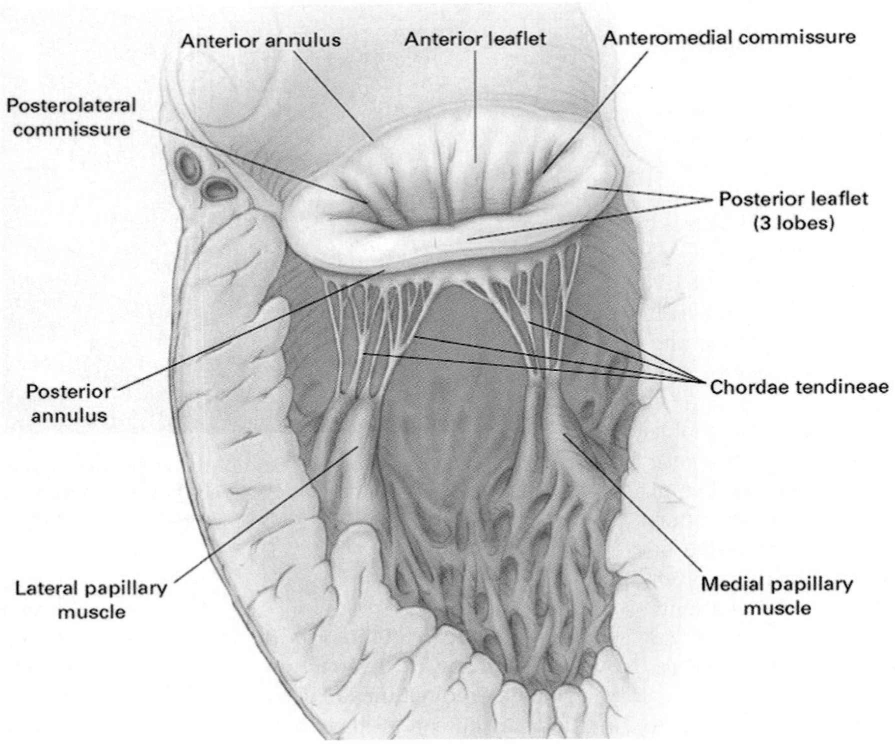

Figure 33-9. Structure of the mitral valve, its surrounding apparatus, and relationship to the left ventricle. Each component can contribute to the presence and extent of mitral regurgitation. (From Otto CM: Evaluation and management of chronic mitral regurgitation. N Engl J Med 2001;345:740-746.)

conditions, although in significant MR half or more of the ejection is retrograde into the left atrium. The incompetent mitral valve acts as a second pathway for blood ejection, which reduces afterload in a setting in which preload is increased, thus potentiating ejection via the Frank-Starling mechanism. The combination ultimately may raise ejection fraction to supranormal early in the course of the disease. As a result, patients with "normal" ejection fraction may already have significant impairment in LV function.[98] Adaptations to the volume loading include lengthening of the myocytes, which increases LV volume. Progressive MR eventually results in contractile dysfunction. Relatively early in the course of the disease, the sympathetic nervous system is activated as a compensatory mechanism to volume loading and decreased forward ejection.[99] Chronic high sympathetic tone results in secondary myocardial damage[100] and has been postulated as the rationale for potential benefit from beta blockade in chronic MR.[101] Over time, although some hypertrophy develops, the predominant response to volume overload without pressure overload is enlargement of chamber size. Extrapolating the LaPlace relationship, which is manifestly protective of wall stress in AS, the progressive expansion of LV dimensions in MR without similar compensatory hypertrophy results in increasing wall stress, which in turn results in increasing MR. In a similar manner, a second vicious cycle is caused by the effect of MR on LV chamber size, which, as it enlarges, results in stretching of the annulus, further exacerbating MR.[102] Thus chronic MR can both cause and be the result of LV remodeling and heart failure.

The etiologies of MR vary by geography, with mitral valve prolapse being the most common in industrialized nations. Rheumatic MR remains common in developing countries. The etiologies of acute MR include ischemic MR, endocarditis, chordal rupture, papillary muscle dysfunction, and a variety of pathologies affecting prosthetic valves (Table 33-4). The most likely causes of acute MR in the critical care setting are ischemia, including acute myocardial infarction, and infectious endocarditis, and should be considered in any patient who develops sudden hemodynamic decompensation in the peri-infarction period or who has known endocarditis. Chronic MR is secondary to a variety of structural, degenerative, connective tissue, inflammatory, and ischemic disorders, as well as congenital abnormalities outlined in Table 33-4.

The classic teaching has been that acute MR secondary to ischemia was caused by papillary muscle dysfunction, most likely secondary to ischemia of the posteromedial papillary muscle, which is dependent on a single blood supply from the right coronary artery. The anterolateral papillary muscle typically has dual circulation from the left anterior descending and circumflex coronary arteries, specifically from a diagonal branch and a circumflex marginal branch. The source of papillary muscle circulation is in fact variable, and on occasion the anterior papillary muscle also has a single blood supply.[103] The role of impaired circulation to the papillary muscle as the cause of ischemic MR has been revisited,[104] and evidence to date suggests that ischemic MR is secondary to alterations in ventricular geometry and leaflet tethering rather than dysfunction caused solely by impaired circulation to the papillary muscle during ischemia,[105] although alterations in papillary muscle geometry can be seen in chronic ischemic MR.[106] The hemodynamics of dynamic, ischemic MR are shown in Figure 33-10.

Table 33-4. Etiologies of Acute and Chronic Mitral Insufficiency

Acute	*Mitral annular disorders* Infective endocarditis (with abscess) Trauma (e.g., valve surgery) Paravalvular leak Surgical—suture interruption Infection *Mitral leaflet disorders* Infective endocarditis (with perforation or vegetation interfering with coaptation) Trauma Atrial myxoma Myxomatous degeneration Systemic lupus erythematosus (Libman-Sacks lesions) *Chordal rupture* Spontaneous Myxomatous degeneration Mitral valve prolapse Marfan syndrome Ehlers-Danlos syndrome Infective endocarditis Acute rheumatic fever Trauma *Papillary muscle disorders* Coronary artery disease Acute global left ventricular dysfunction Infiltrative diseases (amyloidosis, sarcoidosis) Trauma *Primary mitral valve prosthetic disorders* Bioprosthetic cusp perforation Bioprosthetic cusp degeneration Mechanical failure (e.g., strut fracture) Immobilized disc or ball
Chronic	*Inflammatory* Rheumatic heart disease Systemic lupus erythematosus Scleroderma *Degenerative* Myxomatous degeneration (mitral valve prolapse) Marfan syndrome Ehlers-Danlos syndrome Pseudoxanthoma elasticum Calcification of mitral valve annulus *Infective* Endocarditis *Structural* Ruptured chordae tendineae Spontaneous Secondary to: Myocardial infarction Trauma Mitral valve prolapse Endocarditis Rupture or dysfunction of papillary muscle (ischemia or infarction) Dilation of mitral valve annulus and left ventricular cavity Congestive cardiomyopathies Aneurysmal dilation of the left ventricle Hypertrophic cardiomyopathy Paravalvular prosthetic leak *Congenital* Mitral valve clefts or fenestrations Parachute mitral valve abnormality in association with other congenital disorders

From Otto C, Bonow RO: Valvular heart disease. In Libby P, Bonow RO, Mann DL, Zipes DP (eds): Braunwald's Heart Disease. A Textbook of Cardiovascular Medicine. Philadelphia, Saunders, 2008, p 1657.

Analysis of thrombolysis in myocardial infarction data showed a 27% incidence of MR most commonly in the setting of anterior rather than inferior myocardial infarction, although these values vary widely by criteria and techniques used for screening, with incidence ranging from 11% to 59%.[107] A Mayo Clinic review of more than 1300 acute myocardial infarction patients found moderate to severe MR in 12% and found it to be an independent predictor of both heart failure and survival.[108] It is associated with multivessel coronary artery disease, as well as prior infarction.[109]

Papillary muscle rupture is a rare but potentially catastrophic cause of flail leaflets and represents a surgical emergency.[110] In addition to the typical acute myocardial infarction setting, it may be secondary to trauma and isolated other etiologies such as postpartum Ehlers-Danlos syndrome.[111] Other etiologies of acute MR to consider (see Table 33-4) include spontaneous chordal rupture, infectious endocarditis with distortion of the valve leaflets or chordal rupture, and prosthetic valve dysfunction including paravalvular prosthetic valve leak. In patients with sudden onset of acute MR, retrograde flow is typically into a normal-sized and relatively noncompliant left atrium unless preexisting atrial hypertension has been present. The sudden volume loading immediately places the left atrium on the steep portion of its pressure-volume curve, which commonly causes acute pulmonary edema. As is the case with acute AI, the left ventricle is unable to adapt acutely and effective forward stroke volume is decreased. In the setting of myocardial infarction in particular, patients with acute MR may develop cardiogenic shock.

The classic hemodynamic response, a giant V wave, is shown in Figure 33-11. Differentiating a giant V wave from a prominent pulmonary artery pressure wave form can be difficult in the critical care setting, and repeated attempts to obtain a wedge pressure when the catheter is already in wedge position may result in iatrogenic pulmonary artery hemorrhage.

Diagnosis

Physical Examination

In acute MR the abrupt rise of left atrial pressure results from torrential retrograde flow, although the gradient between the left atrium and LV may narrow substantially near the end of systole because of the substantial rise in left atrial pressure as shown in Figure 33-11. Thus the systolic murmur may decrease in intensity prior to the onset of the aortic second sound. A systolic thrill may be noted. The sudden and severe left atrial hypertension typically results in pulmonary edema with accompanying physical findings, as well as an increase in the pulmonic second sound and paradoxical splitting of the second heart sound. Because the adaptive mechanisms are not yet in place, features of LV volume overload are not seen, although a prominent precordial impulse, reflecting increased (albeit retrograde) ejection, may be noted. Unlike AI, the pulse pressure is not increased and may be reduced to reflect the lower forward stroke volume.

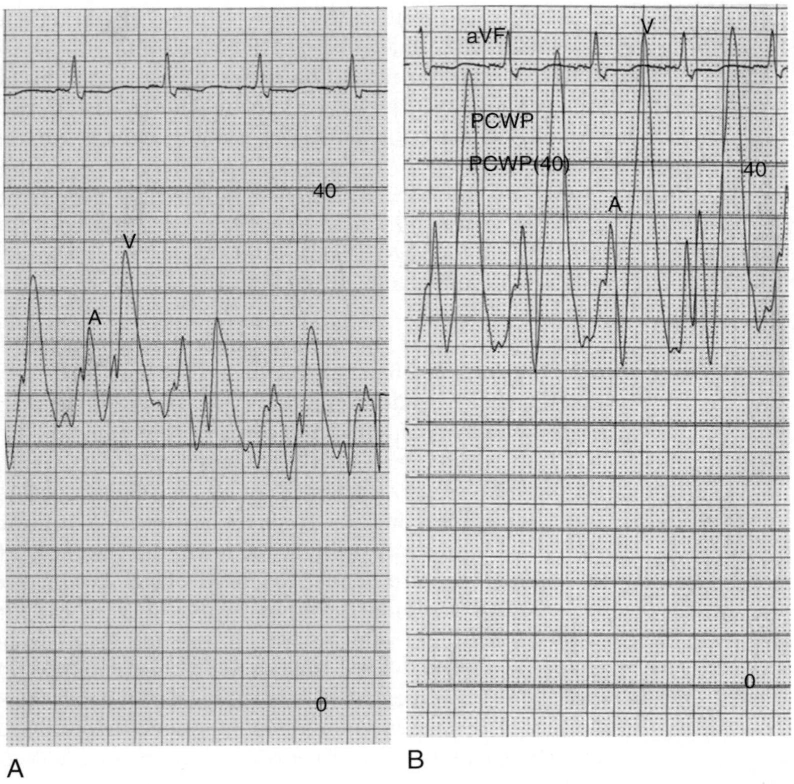

Figure 33-10. Dynamic mitral insufficiency in a patient with transient left ventricular dysfunction after recent acute myocardial infarction. The panel on the left demonstrates hemodynamics on 40 mm Hg scale at baseline **(A).** Note elevated filling pressures at a mean of 24 mm Hg with V waves at average height of 32 mm Hg. The panel on the right **(B)** shows tracings recorded a few minutes later. Mean pulmonary capillary wedge pressure rose to 33 mm Hg with V waves to 48 mm Hg. A, A wave; PCWP, pulmonary capillary wedge pressure; V, V wave.

In chronic MR, precordial features of volume overload include a displaced point of maximal impulse and prominent precordial pulsation. An S3 gallop is heard, especially with marked dilation of the LV,[78] and a diastolic flow murmur representing increased transvalvular flow (rather than mitral stenosis) may be present. The first heart sound may be soft, reflecting lack of brisk apposition of the mitral valve leaflets. The murmur of MR commences immediately following the first heart sound, reflecting the observation that a significant amount of regurgitation takes place during what would otherwise be isovolumic systole (which normally commences immediately following mitral valve closure). The murmur of chronic MR is characteristically blowing; may be medium or high pitched; is best heard at the apex; radiates to the axilla and left scapula (when severe); and extends throughout systole, reflecting the presence of a relatively high gradient throughout LV ejection.

The location of radiation can provide a clue to the affected leaflet: anteriorly directed jets result from posterior leaflet dysfunction, and conversely anterior leaflet prolapse results in a murmur best heard toward the patient's back. Because the Gallavardin phenomenon in AS mimics an MR murmur, it is important to differentiate these two when possible (AS and MR frequently occur concurrently, given the high LV systolic pressure with the former). The murmur of MR differs because it is holosystolic and increases rather than decreases with handgrip.

The intensity of the MR murmur reflects a number of phenomena relating to size of the gradient, compliance of the LV and left atrium, and contractility of the LV but does not correlate well with extent of MR; thus the murmur may be difficult to hear or inaudible, especially in the critical care setting.[112]

Noninvasive Evaluation

Echocardiography provides visualization of the multiple structures responsible for causing MR including the valve leaflets, annulus, chordae tendineae papillary muscles, and left ventricle (see Fig. 33-9). Transesophageal echo provides superior imaging of the valve including assessment for vegetations in case endocarditis is suspected and better visualization of flail leaflets; it is particularly useful when the transthoracic views are incomplete or inadequate. In general, transesophageal echo is superior for fully assessing characteristics of the mitral regurgitant jet[113] and provides additional information in evaluating mitral valve morphology and motion. As with AI, Doppler methods allow assessment of the width of the regurgitant jet and size of the vena contracta, and semiquantitative measures of the regurgitant volume, regurgitant jet, and effective orifice area (see Table 33-1) are discussed in detail in Chapter 8. In patients presenting with acute heart failure and a hyperdynamic LV, acute MR should always be considered.

Cardiac Catheterization

Although the indications for cardiac catheterization (see Table 33-2) are similar as for AS and AI, an additional consideration is included as a class I indication: to assess pulmonary artery pressures at rest and if necessary with exercise to evaluate appropriateness for surgery (see valve

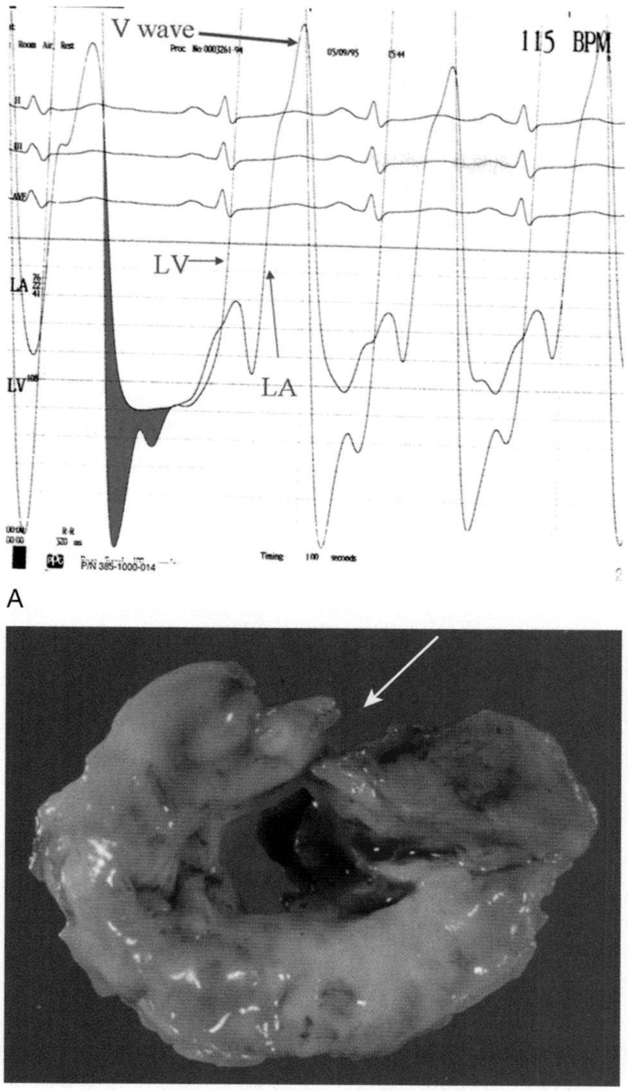

Figure 33-11. Hemodynamics **(A)** of severe MR (40 mm Hg scale) with giant V wave (to ≈ 70 mm Hg) late in systole. As LA pressure rises in acute severe MR, the gradient between the LV and LA pressure tracing is reduced and may result in a decrease in intensity of the murmur in late systole. The markedly thickened mitral valve **(B)** was excised from this patient after being torn *(arrow)* during balloon mitral commissurotomy. Elimination of mitral stenosis gradient *(area in A, filled in red)* is demonstrated. LA, left atrium; LV, left ventricle; MR, mitral valve insufficiency.

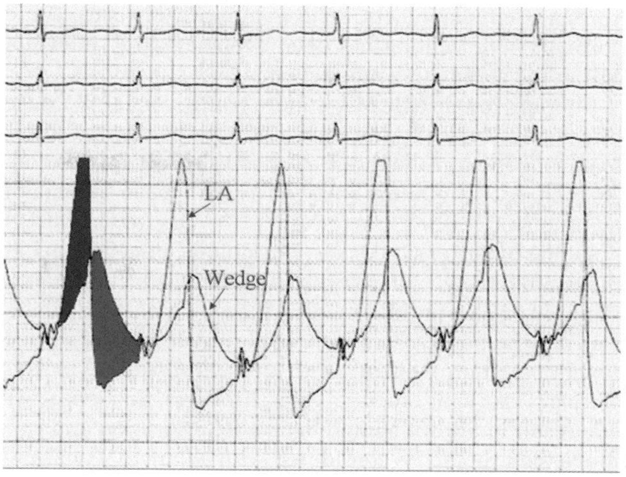

Figure 33-12. Underestimation of the left atrial V wave by pulmonary wedge pressure recording in the setting of severe mitral insufficiency (MR). The tracings show simultaneous left atrial and pulmonary artery wedge pressures in a patient with chronic severe MR because of paravalvular leak (40 mm Hg scale). The V wave on the wedge tracings is approximately 28 mm Hg, but on direct left atrial pressure measurement obtained by transseptal puncture is 44 mm Hg. The gradients between wedge pressure and left atrial pressure during systole *(area filled in blue)* and during diastole *(area filled in red)* represent artifact because of damping and phase delay of pressure waveforms reflected across the pulmonary vascular bed. The effect of this damping is gross underestimation of the severity of the V wave and overestimation of any gradient between the left atrium (LA) and left ventricle; these in turn result in underestimation of severity of MR and overestimation of the severity of mitral stenosis when pulmonary wedge pressures are used. The mean of the two pressures is exactly the same.

replacement indications later). The size of the V wave is not an accurate indicator of MR severity and is not used as a decision-making criterion for surgery because it may be unremarkable even in severe MR when there is high left atrial compliance. In addition, the size of the V wave is typically recorded by wedge rather than direct left atrial pressure, which can result in significant underestimation of the severity of MR (Fig. 33-12). Right heart catheterization and oxygen saturation sampling allow differentiation between the two most common causes of abrupt mechanical deterioration in acute MI: severe MR and ventricular septal defect. Both conditions can feature a large V wave because of sudden volume loading of a noncompliant left atrium: secondary to retrograde flow across the mitral valve in the case of acute MR and antegrade flow of shunted blood from the LV across the pulmonary circulation in the case of a ventricular septal defect.

Medical Management Therapy

For acute, severe, symptomatic MR, the primary medical therapy consists of aggressive vasodilation with nitroprusside. It provides improved aortic flow, diminishes MR, and decreases left-sided filling pressures. In the setting of acute MR with shock, nitroprusside alone is usually considered undesirable because of poor end organ perfusion if further hypotension is caused by the drug. Intra-aortic balloon pumping is highly effective in this setting[114] (see Chapter 7) because it lowers aortic impedance, improves cardiac output, and decreases regurgitant fraction at the same time as it restores blood pressure. A combination of an inotrope (typically dobutamine; a vasoconstrictor should be avoided) and nitroprusside can have similar salutary effects. When the acute MR is dynamic (i.e., occurs and resolves abruptly), the etiology is frequently acute ischemia, and consideration should be given to evaluating the coronary circulation. In a small number of cases, acute coronary intervention has been documented to alleviate MR in the setting of acute ischemia.[115]

Therapy for chronic MR is more controversial. Because afterload is typically not increased, the benefits of afterload reduction are without clear physiologic foundation. As such, ACE inhibitors have consistently been shown not to be effective for chronic MR.[116-118] When concomitant systemic hypertension exists, physiologic benefits appear more convincing.[119] If patients have LV dysfunction superimposed on chronic MR, medical therapy with ACE inhibitors may be beneficial, and several studies have observed functional improvement with resychronization in this setting.[120] As with other valvular disorders, new-onset AF can result in abrupt hemodynamic deterioration and cardioversion should be considered with adjunctive pharmacotherapy to maintain sinus rhythm and rate control. Because of the sympathetic activation previously discussed, β-blockers appear to be beneficial[121,122] and may have additive benefit when used in combination with ACE inhibitors.[123] Both classes of drugs appear to be therapeutic when used after mitral valve repair.[124]

Mitral Valve Surgery

Three types of surgery are performed on the mitral valve: repair, replacement with preservation of the subvalvular apparatus and attachments, and replacement with transection of the chordae. Mitral valve repair has been consistently shown to improve outcomes compared with mitral valve replacement, both acutely and long term, with a fourfold lower operative mortality and a 30% improvement in 10-year survival.[125] With mitral valve replacement, patients who nevertheless have the chordal apparatus preserved have superior long-term outcomes compared with those who have the chords transected.[126] An additional benefit of repair is the avoidance of anticoagulation if patients are in sinus rhythm compared with replacement with a mechanical valve where anticoagulation is required.

In general, the timing of surgery for chronic MR should be prior to the onset of LV dysfunction. The most commonly used markers are symptoms and echocardiographic parameters including LV ejection fraction less than 60%.[5] Patients who develop class III or IV symptoms, even transiently, have a nearly 10-fold increase in annual mortality,[127] with evidence that early surgery in the setting of severe MR improves overall survival. The 60% threshold for surgery has been shown to correlate with postoperative LV function[128] as well as survival.[129] More recently the effective regurgitant orifice has been shown to be strongly predictive of 5-year mortality, with patients having an orifice of greater than or equal to 40 mm^2 having an odds ratio of death greater than 5 : 1 compared with patients with orifice size of less than or equal to 20 mm^2.[130] Preoperative end systolic diameter of 40 mm or less has also been associated with superior outcomes. Patients with AF in general have a worse prognosis,[131] although in large part because of embolic events rather than LV dysfunction, as do patients with pulmonary hypertension or right heart failure, or both.[132] Mitral valve surgery, even in the setting of depressed ejection fraction, may result in postoperative return to normal function.[133] Comparison of long-term outcomes between operated and medically treated patients with asymptomatic MR has invariably favored the former,[130] although much of the data depend on nonrandomized registry data. In general, the key to improved function and outcomes is preserving the integrity of the submitral apparatus,[134] and comparison of successful repair versus replacement has indicated that high-volume institutions (>140 mitral operations/ year) have the best results with nearly twice the rate of successful repair as low-volume institutions.[135]

A common teaching has been that repair or replacement of the mitral valve eliminates the "pop-off valve" represented by incompetent leaflets, resulting in dramatically increased afterload postoperatively. In turn, if significant preoperative LV dysfunction were present, the LV would fail, with hemodynamic deterioration and subsequent mortality. In fact, careful investigation has demonstrated that postoperative deterioration of LV function was secondary to disruption of chordal integrity[136] and elimination of the favorable effects of the submitral apparatus on valvular-ventricular interaction rather than the elimination of a low-pressure decompression pathway. Afterload following mitral valve surgery with chordal transection does in fact increase, whereas patients subjected to mitral valve surgery with preservation of the chordal apparatus had decreased LV chamber volume and, in keeping with the LaPlace equation, *reduced* afterload.[137] Thus the recommendations regarding LV ejection fraction for surgery have changed dramatically, and successful repair of mitral valves in series of patients with EF less than 25% has been reported with operative risk of less than or equal to 5%.[138] The operative risk is in the 1% to 2% range for symptomatic patients with LV dysfunction but higher ejection fraction.[139] Similarly, the Society of Thoracic Surgeons database has reported mortality of approximately 5% with EF less than or equal to 30% but 3% with EF greater than 30%.[140] Propensity analysis of patients eligible for mitral valve repair who did or did not undergo the procedure has not shown a survival advantage in patients with mean ejection fraction less than 25%,[124] although a randomized trial has not been reported. Similarly, concomitant mitral valve surgery in patients undergoing CABG with moderate or greater MR did not clearly improve short-term survival.[141] Combining mitral valve surgery with a mesh placed around the heart to help prevent dilation and thus lower wall stress may have additional benefit for patients with MR and LV dysfunction.[139] Only in the setting of an ejection fraction of less than 30% or end systolic dimension greater than 55 mm, as well as anatomy or surgical experience that suggests chordal preservation is unlikely, do the current guidelines recommend medical therapy alone.

In symptomatic acute severe MR, mitral valve surgery is a class I indication regardless of level of LV function. Both with infective endocarditis;[94] as well as with papillary muscle rupture, surgery is mandated to be performed with as little delay as possible.[142] However, the overall risk

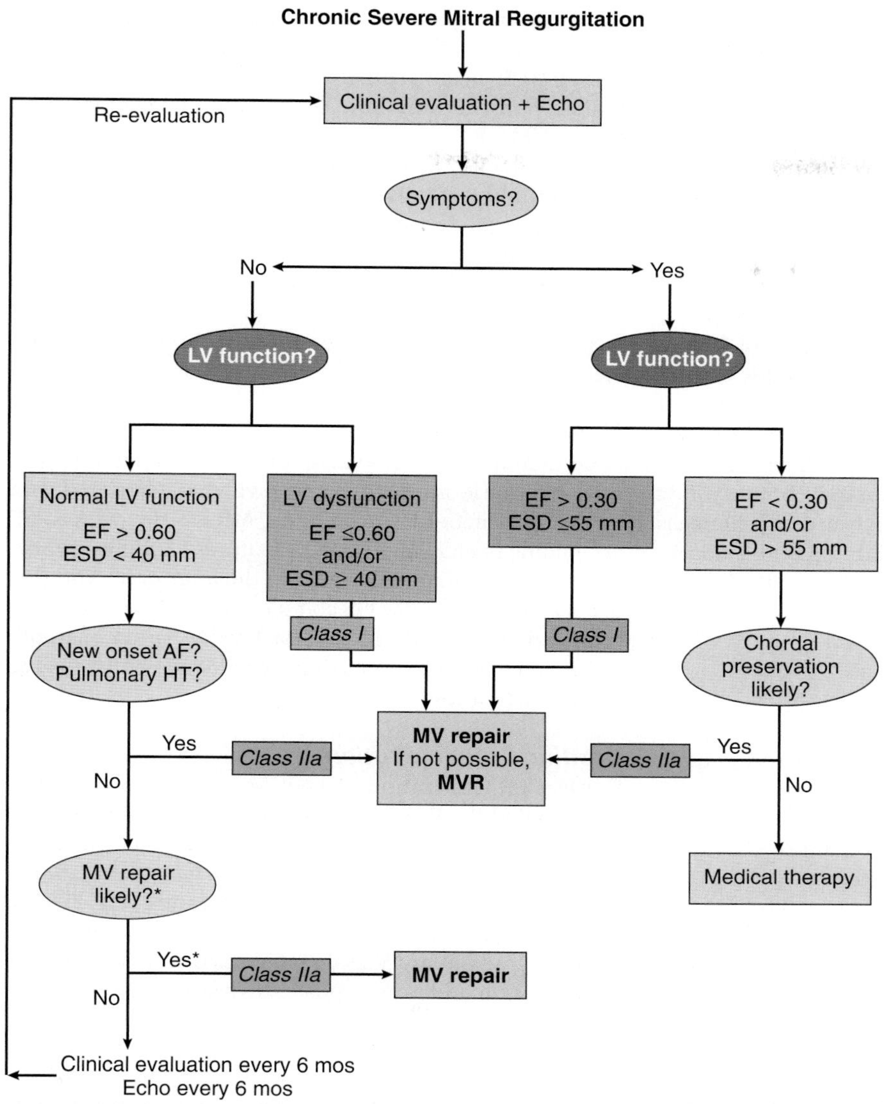

Figure 33-13. Algorithm for management of patients with chronic severe mitral regurgitation. *Mitral valve repair may be performed in asymptomatic patients with normal left ventricular (LV) function if performed by an experienced surgical team and if the likelihood of successful mitral valve (MV) repair is greater than 90%. AF, atrial fibrillation; EF, ejection fraction; ESD, end-systolic dimension; HT, hypertension; MVR, mitral valve replacement. (From Bonow RO, Carabello BA, Chatterjee K, et al: ACC/AHA 2006 guidelines for the management of patients with valvular heart disease: A report of the American College of Cardiology/American Heart Association Task Force on Practice Guidelines [writing committee to revise the 1998 guidelines for the management of patients with valvular heart disease] developed in collaboration with the Society of Cardiovascular Anesthesiologists and endorsed by the Society for Cardiovascular Angiography and Interventions and the Society of Thoracic Surgeons. J Am Coll Cardiol 2006;48:e1-148.)

of mortality when MR accompanies acute myocardial infarction is substantially enhanced,[143] a phenomenon noted in patients undergoing emergent percutaneous intervention as well.[144] Chronic severe MR is much more complex, and the management algorithm is outlined in Figure 33-13. Percutaneous alternatives to mitral valve repair are in earlier stages of development and testing than percutaneous aortic valve replacement; the techniques including edge-to-edge approximation and annuloplasty, are less comprehensive than the standard surgical approaches being mimicked.[145]

SELECTED OTHER VALVULAR HEART DISORDERS

HYPERTROPHIC OBSTRUCTIVE CARDIOMYOPATHY

Although a disease of the heart muscle rather than a primary valvular disorder, hypertrophic obstructive cardiomyopathy (HOCM) has important features of LV outflow obstruction and concomitant MR. The clinical presentation, physical examination, noninvasive and invasive findings, and overall management differ in general from AS or MR, and HOCM represents an important consideration for patients in critical care units.

Pathophysiology

The hallmark of HOCM is dynamic obstruction of the LV outflow tract with eccentric hypertrophy; many variations exist, and obstruction is not always at the subvalvular level. Only approximately one fourth to one third of patients with hypertrophic cardiomyopathy (HCM) have a resting gradient of 30 mm Hg or greater.[146] HCM is found in approximately 0.2% of the population[147] and is defined as hypertrophy of the LV that is not secondary to hypertrophic stimuli such as systemic hypertension or AS. Contrary to conventional wisdom, the majority of patients with HCM were found to have provokable gradients with exercise in a single large-volume center[148] (likely with some skewing from the nature of its referral population). The genetics of HCM have been studied extensively and, although complex, there is a familial association in a majority of patients. Although the clinical course may be generally benign in patients without risk factors for adverse events,[149] it is the most common cardiac cause of sudden death in young adults[150] and leads to heart failure, rhythm disturbances, and occasional sudden death in older patients. The patients at high risk for sudden death, comprising only about 10% to 20% of those within the HCM population, include those with prior cardiac arrest or sustained ventricular tachycardia, those with a family history of HCM and sudden death, hypotensive response to exercise, and severe LVH with wall thickness of 30 mm or greater.[151] A resting gradient across the outflow tract of more than 30 mm Hg alone predicts an increased risk of sudden death or development of moderate to severe congestive heart failure,[146] and there may be higher risk with very high gradients.[152] Because of impaired coronary flow reserve[153] and severe hypertrophy, myocardial ischemia is a potentially important factor in acute patient management; there is also an association between HOCM and myocardial coronary bridging.[154]

Diagnosis

Physical Examination

The physical examination in HOCM features abrupt early rise in systolic pressure followed by obstruction to LV outflow, resulting in a blunted pressure rise later in systole. This translates to the spike and dome pattern characteristic of HOCM on palpation of the carotid pulse. The typically hypertrophic septum (1.3 to 1.5 times the thickness of the posterior wall and typically 18 mm or greater in clinically significant HOCM) obstructs the outflow tract after initial ejection as LV volume decreases. Physiologic maneuvers or clinical states that lower LV volume abruptly such as standing, dehydration, or use of diuretics can substantially exacerbate the gradient and increase the intensity of the systolic ejection murmur characteristic of HOCM. Because the obstruction begins after the initial brisk ejection of blood from the ventricle, the onset of murmur is late after the first heart sound. It is best heard over the left base of the heart. In contrast to AS, the murmur typically does not radiate to the carotids, does not extend throughout systole, and decreases with squatting. The blunting of the carotid upstroke, so characteristic of AS, is not seen because of the vigorous early ejection.

Noninvasive Evaluation

Abnormalities of mitral valve function are common. Systolic anterior motion of the mitral valve is associated with further obstruction[155]; in addition, MR is a typical secondary finding in HOCM. The ECG features LV hypertrophy, strain, and prominent Q waves in the inferior and precordial leads, with narrow QS complexes being common. The echocardiogram is diagnostic for HOCM, providing both an anatomic basis and physiologic evidence of the degree of obstruction (Fig. 33-14).

Cardiac Catheterization

Cardiac catheterization in HOCM may reveal the standard triad of the Brockenbrough-Braunwald-Morrow sign in the postextrasystolic heart beat: increase in the gradient between LV and aorta, decrease in systemic blood pressure, and narrowing of the pulse pressure (Fig. 33-15). Other stimuli that increase outflow obstruction and increase gradient are Valsalva maneuver and amyl nitrite inhalation, in addition to postextrasystolic potentiation.

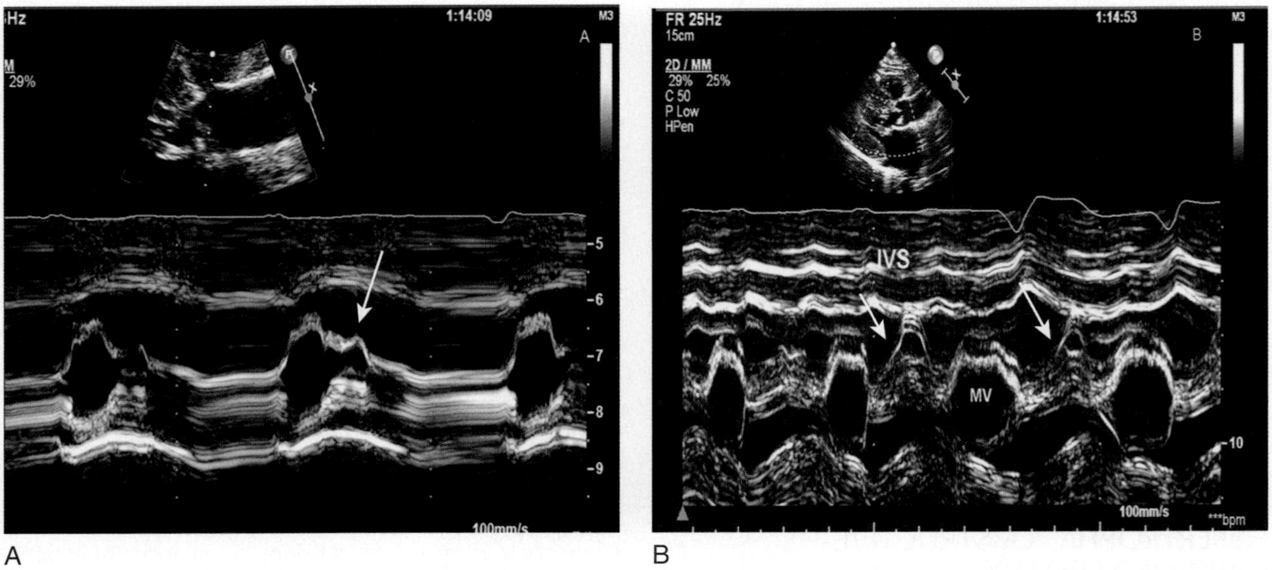

Figure 33-14. A, M-mode of hypertrophic obstructive cardiomyopathy with aortic valve opening showing the effect of midsystolic outflow obstruction; after initial normal opening, the aortic valve leaflets remain only partially separated because of diminished transvalvular flow *(arrow)*. **B,** Systolic anterior motion of the anterior mitral leaflet with apposition against outflow tract *(arrows)*. The severely hypertrophied septum on two-dimensional view is shown at the top of each panel.

Therapy

Medical Management

The management of critically ill patients with HOCM focuses on several core principles: optimizing LV volumes, specifically increasing preload while *not* decreasing afterload, decreasing contractility, and maintaining the patient in sinus rhythm. Thus the typical regimen of diuretics, vasodilators, and inotropes used in most patients presenting with congestive heart failure who do not have HOCM can severely exacerbate the outflow gradient and lead to further decompensation or death[156] (as can intra-aortic balloon pumping); somewhat counterintuitively in this setting, negative inotropes, in particular β-blockers, combined with volume loading can stabilize patients.[157,158] Other negative inotropes including verapamil and disopyramide appear to have favorable hemodynamic effects and may represent an alternative to β-blockade.[159] In the patient in shock, if vasopressors are required, agents such as phenylephrine, which are primarily peripheral vasoconstrictors, should be used rather than inotropic agents. Verapamil has negative inotropic benefits and some utility as an antiarrhythmic agent, as well as diastolic relaxation properties, and has been used successfully in both chronic therapy, as well as the acutely decompensated patients with HOCM.[160] Verapamil does have some potentially undesirable vasodilator properties and can cause synergistic depression of conduction and contractility in combination with β-blockade; the effects of combined therapy, if used, should be monitored closely.[161]

Patients with hypertrophic heart disease are highly dependent on the atrial contribution to cardiac output,[162] and patients with obstruction in particular depend on the additional LV filling from atrial contraction. AF is a cause of acute decompensation in HOCM patients, and cardioversion should be considered acutely. AF occurred in approximately one fourth of patients with HCM followed for 9 years and is predictive of heart failure–related death and stroke.[163] In terms of the latter, patients with HCM and AF appear particularly predisposed to thromboembolic events;[164] anticoagulation has been shown to reduce the incidence significantly.[165] Left atrial size and function predict the onset of AF.[166] The Maze procedure and catheter ablation of left atrial pathways have been used successfully in small series to prevent recurrent AF.[167,168] Amiodarone has been particularly effective for the maintenance of sinus rhythm in the population with AF and HCM[169] and may also have additional efficacy in preventing sudden death in patients with episodes of nonsustained ventricular tachycardia.[170,171] Ventricular fibrillation appears to be the primary cause of sudden death and can be prevented with implantable defibrillators for either primary or secondary prevention, with activation of the devices in 5% to 11% of patients annually depending on indications for placement[172]; episodes of sustained ventricular tachycardia and a history of prior sudden death place patients in the highest risk category.

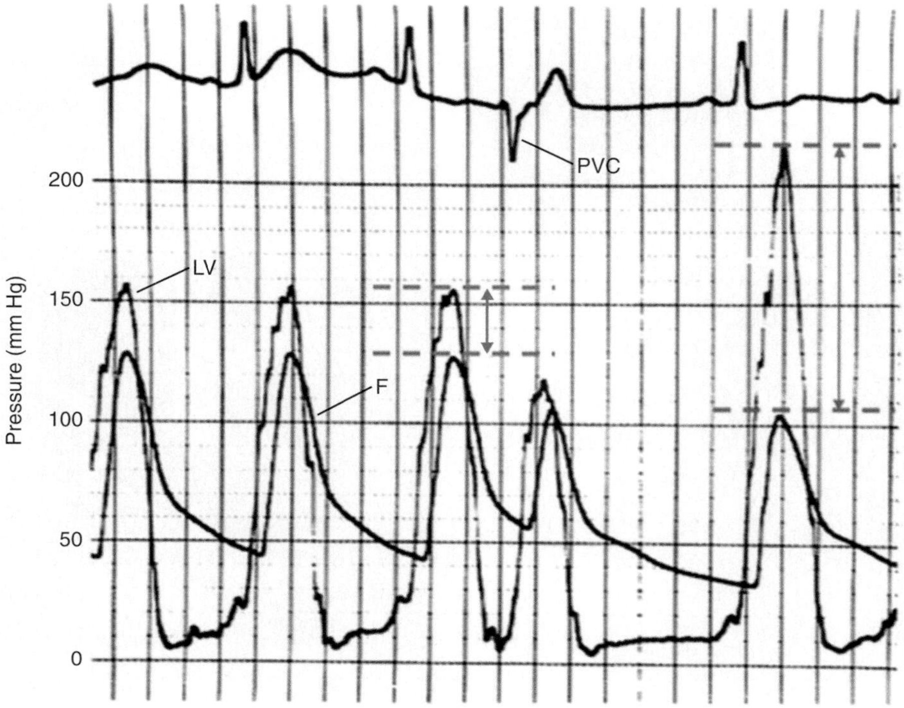

Figure 33-15. The Brockenbrough-Braunwald-Morrow sign. Dramatic exaggeration of the resting gradient in the postextrasystolic beat, with lower systemic pressure, and narrowed pulse pressure (difference between femoral systolic and diastolic pressure) are demonstrated—all hallmarks of dynamic outflow obstruction. *Dashed lines* represent left ventricle (LV) and aortic systolic pressures at rest *(green)* and after a premature ventricular contraction (PVC) *(red);* the gradient rises from a basal 30 mm Hg *(double-sided green arrow)* to approximately 130 mm Hg *(double-sided red arrow).* (Modified from Pollock SG: Pressure tracings in obstructive cardiomyopathy. N Engl J Med 1994;331:238.)

Percutaneous Intervention or Surgery

Once patients develop refractory symptoms despite pharmacologic management and have significant obstruction to LV outflow, surgical myomectomy or alcohol septal ablation must be considered. The choice is controversial and depends on LV and coronary anatomy, comorbidities, severity of coexistent mitral valve or other potentially surgical heart disease, and a variety of other clinical issues; equivalence of outcomes with the less invasive percutaneous approach has not been demonstrated.[173] Typical thresholds for intervention are a resting peak instantaneous gradient of 50 mm Hg or more, although depending on degree of symptoms and provokability, a variety of other thresholds have been applied.[151] Mitral valve replacement can frequently be avoided, especially in patients without intrinsic mitral disease, in whom MR is largely abolished by myomectomy and relief of the outflow gradient.[174] In patients with intrinsic mitral valve disease, or for a variety of other anatomic considerations, mitral valve surgery including use of low-profile prostheses is used.[151] Dual chamber pacing, once considered therapeutically effective,[175] with theoretical benefit from asynchronous septal contraction and secondary reduction in outflow tract gradient, has not been shown to have clear therapeutic benefit in randomized clinical trials, with the most likely functional benefits occurring in a limited subset of elderly patients.[176]

MITRAL VALVE STENOSIS

Mitral valve stenosis (MS) is primarily a rheumatic disorder and, as such, has become increasingly uncommon in industrialized nations. Nevertheless, the disease remains prevalent in developing countries and a small but significant number of patients continue to present in the critical care setting throughout the world. Rheumatic MS involves disease of both the valve leaflets and submitral apparatus and may involve the valve ring as well (Fig. 33-16). Although MS is primarily caused by rheumatic deformity and scarring of the valve leaflets and subvalve with fusion of the commissures, a variety of disorders result in leaflet and annular calcification that also create obstruction between the left atrium and left ventricle. Most notably, mitral annular calcification, present in 6% of patients undergoing routine echocardiography,[177] is more prevalent in the elderly, women, smokers, and patients on dialysis (who have high parathyroid hormone levels). It may present with severe nonrheumatic mitral stenosis, although MR is a more common association.[177,178] A variety of uncommon other etiologies account for less than 1% of cases of MS.[179]

Pathophysiology

The physiologic hallmark of mitral stenosis is obstruction to left atrial outflow resulting in rising left atrial and pul-

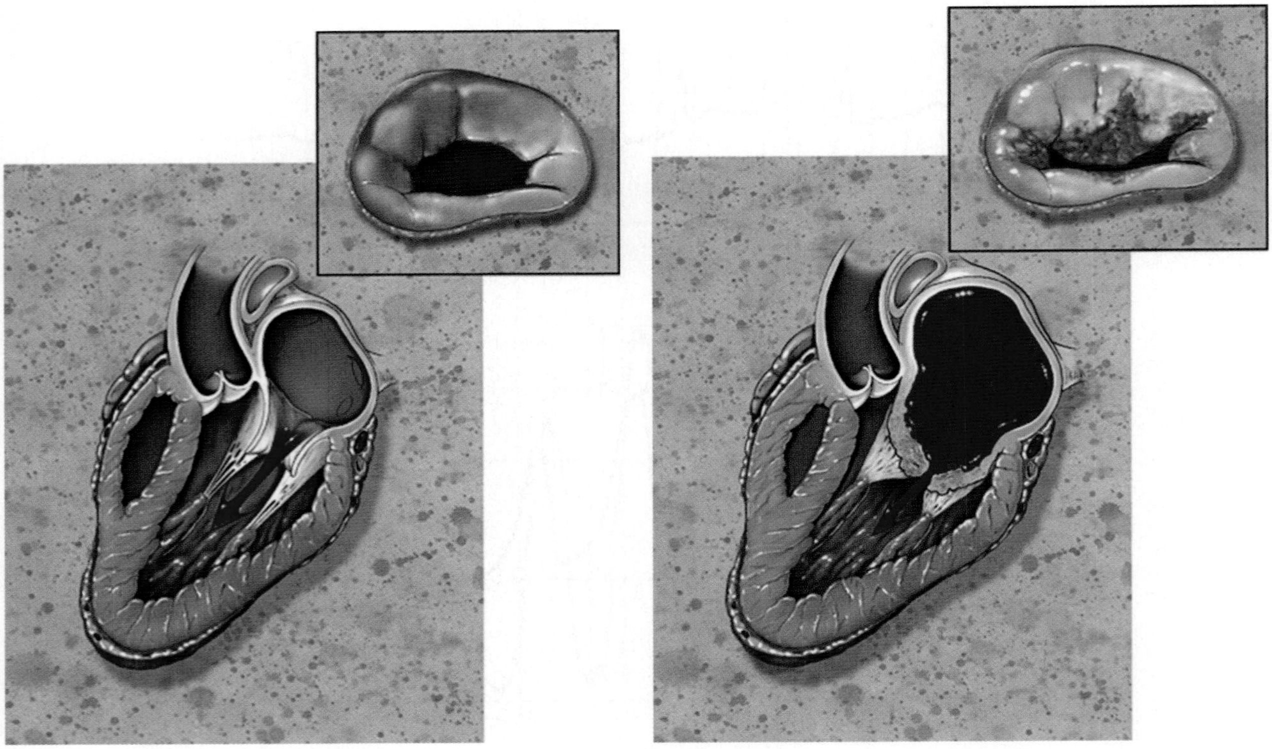

A B

Figure 33-16. Long axis view during diastole of the mitral apparatus, left atrium, and left ventricle in a normal patient **(A)** and with mitral stenosis **(B).** Cross-sectional views of the left atrial surface of the valve are shown in the inset. With mitral stenosis, the valve opening is restricted with a characteristic doming appearance, the commissures are fused, the leaflets are thickened, the subvalvular apparatus is deformed, and some calcification is noted. The left atrium is enlarged. (From Turi ZG: Cardiology patient page. Mitral valve disease. Circulation 2004;109:e38-e41.)

monary pressures (the extent of the latter depends to a significant degree on left atrial compliance). The normal mitral valve is in the range of 4 to 6 cm^2, and patients typically do not become symptomatic until valve areas decrease significantly below 2 cm^2 (see Table 33-1). As valve area decreases, an additional pressure gradient is required to maintain transvalvular flow (see Fig. 33-5). Because antegrade flow is entirely during diastole, and the diastolic filling period shortens or lengthens disproportionately with increase or decrease in heart rate respectively, the gradient is highly flow dependent. In MS, as with virtually all valvulopathies, cardiac output is potentially highly dependent on maintenance of sinus rhythm; because the influence on cardiac output is exaggerated by the need for active left atrial pumping across a stenotic orifice, atrial contraction is particularly important in MS. A frequent mode of presentation is acute congestive heart failure in a patient with MS who suddenly develops AF; the concomitant loss of atrial contraction and high ventricular rate with short diastolic filling period frequently results in pulmonary edema.

Diagnosis

Physical Examination

The diagnosis of MS on physical examination is frequently missed, in part because it is uncommonly seen by most practitioners outside of developing countries. Besides findings suggestive of congestive heart failure with a low output in the critical care setting, several findings correlate strongly with mitral stenosis. A right ventricular lift may occur in patients with advanced and chronic pulmonary hypertension, and occasionally a palpable pulmonic second sound is felt. Both S_1 and P_2 are increased early in the course of the disease; with progressive deformity of the subvalvular apparatus, S_1 may become quite soft as mitral valve closure velocity decreases. The opening snap is preserved until the end stages of mitral stenosis, and the severity of the disease correlates inversely with the length of time between S_2 and the opening snap. The diastolic rumble may not be heard if the patient is not placed in the lateral decubitus position and is difficult to hear in the critical care setting. Presystolic accentuation is the result of increased flow in late diastole caused by atrial contraction in patients in sinus rhythm. The diagnosis is often missed in both the outpatient and critical care settings,[180] and patients are sometimes treated for years for bronchitis, pneumonia, or asthma, when in fact the presentation is congestive heart failure with the underlying disease process being MS.

Noninvasive Evaluation

The echocardiogram is the primary tool for diagnosis of MS. The typical hockey stick appearance of the rheumatic anterior mitral leaflet is caused by partial restriction of mobility (Fig. 33-17). Other important characteristics of the mitral leaflets are degree of thickening, mobility, and calcification, all of which, along with extent of subvalvular disease, help to address suitability for balloon dilation or commissurotomy rather than valve replacement.[181] It is important to differentiate rheumatic MS from severe nonrheumatic MS, as shown in Figure 33-17. Transesophageal echo provides the requisite sensitivity to detect left atrial thrombus prior to balloon commissurotomy or cardioversion. Severity of mitral stenosis is graded by physiologic and anatomic criteria: The former depend on Doppler interrogation of transvalvular flow, with peak velocity used to estimate the gradient; rate of decompression of the left atrial pressure, or pressure half time, correlates inversely with valve area. The valve area is frequently directly measured using planimetry of a cross-sectional view. Because these methods have potential for error, a number of alternative methodologies have been proposed,[182-184] although there is no agreement on a gold standard.[185] As with aortic stenosis, dramatic increase in gradient accompanies increased flow related to exercise or dobutamine infusion[186] (Figs. 33-18 and 33-19). Cardiac catheterization may be required if the noninvasive data are inconclusive; there is a tendency for the pulmonary wedge pressure/LV gradient to overestimate the severity of mitral stenosis

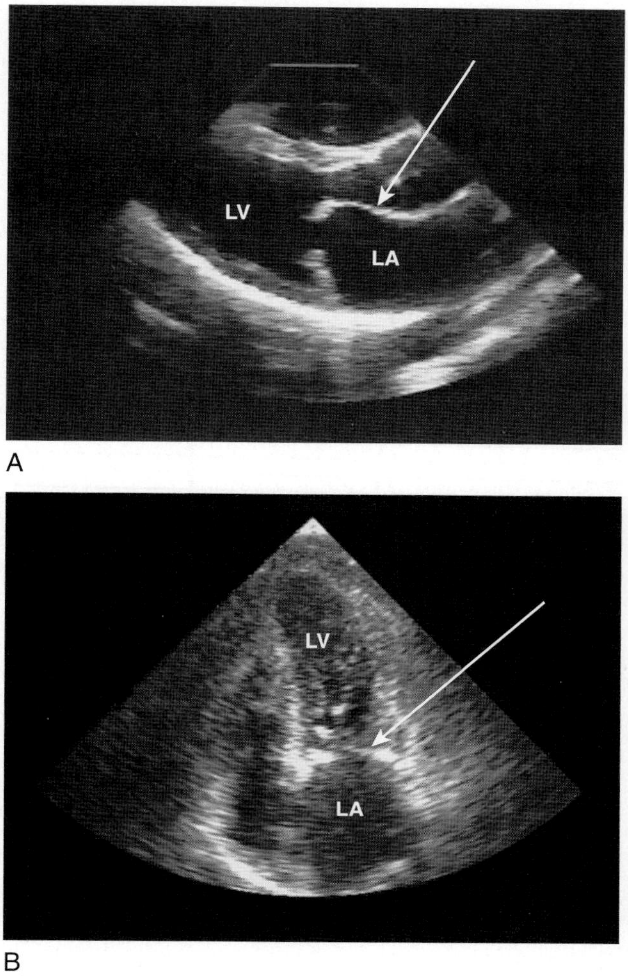

Figure 33-17. Two appearances of stenotic mitral valves. **A,** The parasternal long axis view shows typical rheumatic deformity with a hockey stick appearance of the anterior mitral leaflet *(arrow).* **B,** The four-chamber view is from a patient with a significant gradient across the mitral orifice; this patient was on dialysis, did not have rheumatic heart disease, and demonstrated significant calcification of the mitral leaflets and annulus *(arrow).* LA, left atrium; LV, left ventricle.

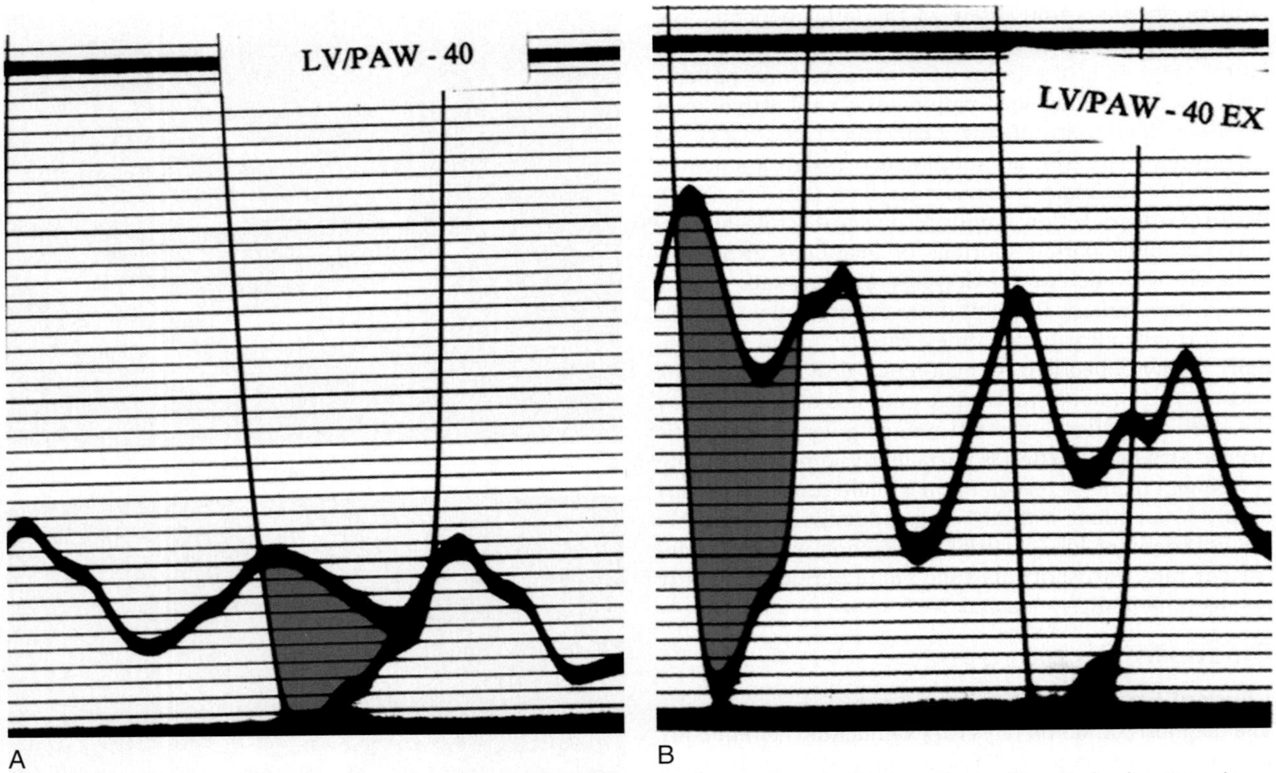

Figure 33-18. Effect of exercise and increased heart rate on mitral valve gradient *(red)* in a patient with mitral valve stenosis (40 mm Hg scale). The tracing at left **(A)** shows a mean gradient of approximately 5 mm Hg with diastasis late in diastole; with increased heart rate and cardiac output **(B),** the gradient rose to a mean of approximately 20 mm Hg, a fourfold increase. LV, left ventricle; PAW, pulmonary artery wedge.

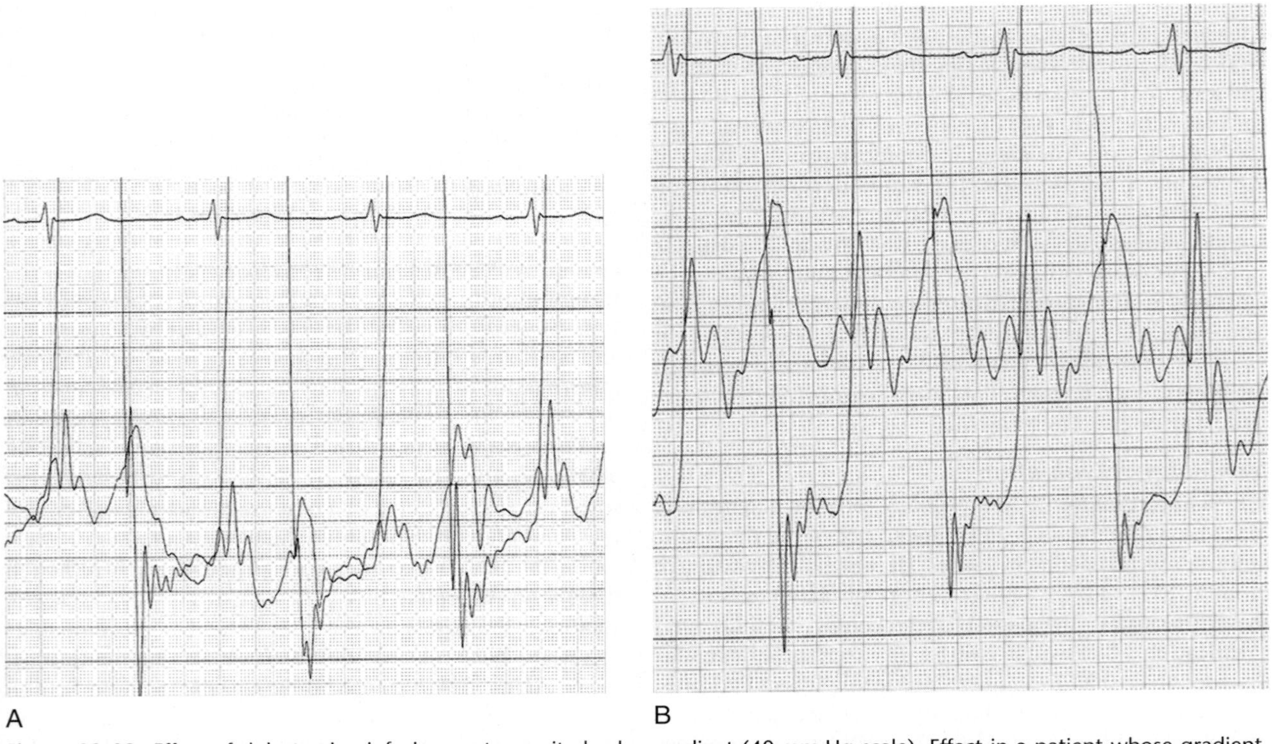

Figure 33-19. Effect of dobutamine infusion on transmitral valve gradient (40 mm Hg scale). Effect in a patient whose gradient was nearly abolished at rest **(A)** and was augmented dramatically with infusion of dobutamine **(B).**

compared with left atrial/LV gradient measurement[187] (Fig. 33-20). Cardiac catheterization can also be used to assess pulmonary artery pressures and response to exercise if the clinical and noninvasive pictures are discordant.[5]

Therapy

Medical Therapy

Medical therapy specifically aimed at improving hemodynamics in mitral stenosis is basically twofold: slowing the heart rate and anticoagulation. In sinus rhythm, β-blockade is the preferred therapy; patients with significant bronchospasm or with coexistent, usually secondary severe pulmonary hypertension with or without right heart failure may not tolerate β-blockers. Diltiazem or low doses of β-blocker combined with diltiazem or verapamil are sometimes used in this setting. With combined therapy, care should be exercised that severe heart rate slowing or atrioventricular block does not occur, and verapamil may not be tolerated in right heart failure. For the acutely decompensated patient with MS, diuretics; nitrates; inotropes (preferably agents that do not raise heart rate); and, to a lesser degree, arterial vasodilator therapy may all be beneficial.

Approximately 30% of patients with MS are thought to develop AF, with the risk increased by progressive increase in left atrial size. The risk of embolic events, especially stroke, is substantially higher than in AF patients without MS[188] (up to 15% in unanticoagulated patients), possibly in part because of a hypercoagulopathy and increased platelet activation associated with MS,[189] making the use of anticoagulation essential. It is not uncommon for the presenting finding to be an embolic event in a previously undiagnosed MS patient. Even in the setting of sinus rhythm,[5] if spontaneous echo contrast is seen in the MS patient or left atrial size is greater than 55 mm, anticoagulation may decrease stroke risk[189] and it should also be used in the sinus rhythm patient with prior embolic event or with left atrial thrombus detected by transesophageal echocardiography.

In the setting of new-onset AF and acute decompensation, cardioversion should be considered. Regardless of chronicity, heart rate slowing is essential; digoxin, β-blockers, diltiazem, or verapamil alone or in combination may be beneficial. Rate control only at rest is inadequate; many patients with low resting heart rates become tachycardic with minimal exercise. This is a vicious cycle because the tachycardia may be a response to inadequate stroke volume; the tachycardia then lowers diastolic

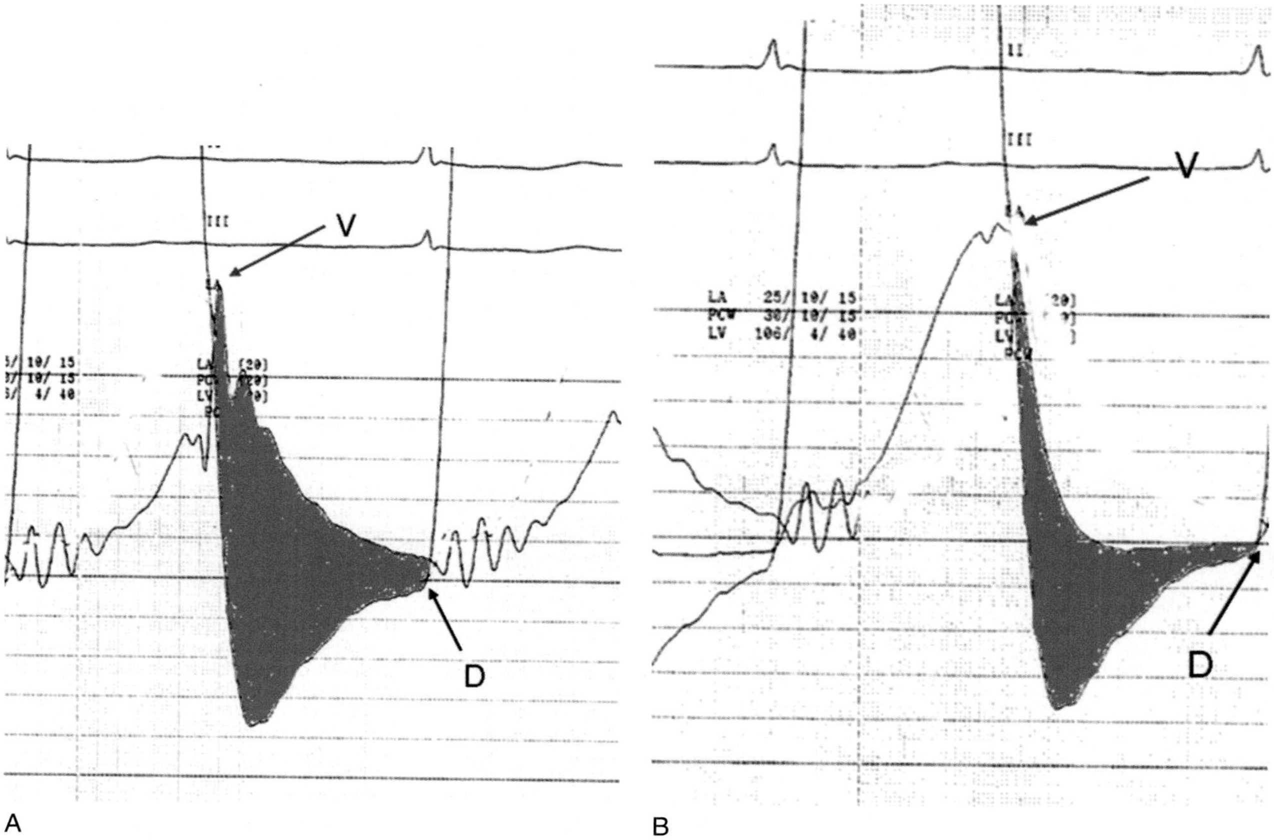

Figure 33-20. Effect of using pulmonary wedge pressure **(A)** or direct left atrial pressure **(B)** to assess gradient *(in red)* between the left atrium and left ventricle in mitral stenosis (40 mm Hg scale). Using the wedge pressure, the gradient appears to be approximately twice as great as when left atrial pressure is used. Rapid decompression of left atrial pressure is shown in the tracing on the right. The findings are consistent with mixed mitral stenosis and regurgitation, with the dominant physiology being secondary to mitral insufficiency. In both tracings, diastasis (D) is noted by end diastole, a feature not consistent with severe mitral stenosis except in marked bradycardia. The V wave height is similar in both tracings, unlike in Figure 33-12. The two tracings above were recorded a few seconds apart.

filling period and further exacerbates the gradient. Control of tachycardia is important beyond its hemodynamic benefit; it also helps avoid tachycardia-induced cardiomyopathy.[190]

Percutaneous Intervention or Surgery

Percutaneous balloon mitral valvuloplasty is equivalent or superior to surgery in patients with favorable valve anatomy,[191,192] characterized by mild to moderate impairment of leaflet mobility, valve thickness, valve calcification, and subvalvular disease, the components of the Wilkins-Weyman echo score.[193] The scoring system has been shown to correlate with long-term outcomes.[194] Surgery should be reserved for patients with unfavorable anatomy, more than mild MR, or persistent thrombus in the left atrium despite anticoagulation.[5] The threshold for percutaneous or surgical intervention is a mitral valve area of 1.5 cm^2 or less. If patients are symptomatic and have favorable anatomy or if they are asymptomatic but have pulmonary hypertension (>50 mm Hg systolic at rest or >60 mm Hg with exercise), they have class I indications. Patients who have unfavorable anatomy and are functional class III or IV are considered to have a class II indication, especially if they are poor candidates for surgery. Asymptomatic patients with new-onset AF and favorable anatomy and symptomatic patients with mild MS (valve area >1.5 cm^2) who have pulmonary artery pressure greater than 60 mm Hg, wedge pressure 25 mm Hg or greater, or gradient 15 mm Hg or greater during exercise are also considered class II candidates.[5]

Acknowledgment

The author wishes to acknowledge Priscilla Peters for kindly providing Figures 33-8, 33-14, and 33-17.

KEY POINTS

- Valvular heart disease in the critical care setting ranges from the primary cause of acute decompensation to a comorbidity of varying degrees of clinical significance.
- Valvulopathy affects not only valve anatomy but also cardiac structure and function and overall hemodynamics; it is essential to consider all four elements in diagnosis and management.
- AS in the critical care setting requires careful titration of need to maintain cardiac output, avoid hypotension, and replace the aortic valve early if AS is the primary cause of symptoms.
- Low-gradient, low-output AS requires increasing cardiac contractility or transvalvular flow, or both, to differentiate severe AS from primary myocardial dysfunction.
- Acute aortic and mitral insufficiency in the decompensated patient benefits from vasodilator therapy; vasodilator treatment of chronic aortic and mitral insufficiency in asymptomatic patients does not have the benefit of a compelling evidence base.
- Intra-aortic balloon counterpulsation is useful in hemodynamically decompensated MR patients, of some benefit in severely ill AS patients but contraindicated with HOCM and particularly in patients with AI.
- AF exacerbates hemodynamic deterioration in valvulopathies; if left atrial size is less than 6 cm and thrombus is not present, cardioversion and maintenance of sinus rhythm are highly beneficial.
- There are now only limited indications for prophylactic therapy with antibiotics for endocarditis prevention for the valvulopathies described in this chapter,[195] primarily the presence of prosthetic cardiac valves and history of previous infectious endocarditis.

REFERENCES

1. Passik CS, Ackermann DM, Pluth JR, et al: Temporal changes in the causes of aortic stenosis: A surgical pathologic study of 646 cases. Mayo Clin Proc 1987;62:119-123.
2. Mangione S, Nieman LZ, Gracely E, et al: The teaching and practice of cardiac auscultation during internal medicine and cardiology training. A nationwide survey. Ann Intern Med 1993;119:47-54.
3. Das P, Pocock C, Chambers J: The patient with a systolic murmur: Severe aortic stenosis may be missed during cardiovascular examination. QJM 2000;93:685-688.
4. Lindroos M, Kupari M, Heikkila J, et al: Prevalence of aortic valve abnormalities in the elderly: An echocardiographic study of a random population sample. J Am Coll Cardiol 1993;21:1220-1225.
5. Bonow RO, Carabello BA, Chatterjee K, et al: ACC/AHA 2006 guidelines for the management of patients with valvular heart disease: A report of the American College of Cardiology/American Heart Association Task Force on Practice Guidelines (writing Committee to Revise the 1998 guidelines for the management of patients with valvular heart disease) developed in collaboration with the Society of Cardiovascular Anesthesiologists endorsed by the Society for Cardiovascular Angiography and Interventions and the Society of Thoracic Surgeons. J Am Coll Cardiol 2006;48:e1-148.
6. Turi ZG: Whom do you trust? Misguided faith in the catheter- or Doppler-derived aortic valve gradient. Catheter Cardiovasc Interv 2005;65:180-182.
7. Braverman AC, Guven H, Beardslee MA, et al: The bicuspid aortic valve. Curr Probl Cardiol 2005;30:470-522.
8. daVinci L: Notes on the valves of the heart and flow of blood within it, with illustrative drawings. 1513.
9. Roberts WC, Ko JM: Frequency by decades of unicuspid, bicuspid, and tricuspid aortic valves in adults having isolated aortic valve replacement for aortic stenosis, with or without associated aortic regurgitation. Circulation 2005;111:920-925.
10. Stewart BF, Siscovick D, Lind BK, et al: Clinical factors associated with calcific aortic valve disease. Cardiovascular Health Study. J Am Coll Cardiol 1997;29:630-634.
11. Otto CM, Lind BK, Kitzman DW, et al: Association of aortic-valve sclerosis with cardiovascular mortality and morbidity in the elderly. N Engl J Med 1999;341:142-147.
12. Carabello BA: Aortic sclerosis—a window to the coronary arteries? N Engl J Med 1999;341:193-195.
13. Cosmi JE, Kort S, Tunick PA, et al: The risk of the development of aortic stenosis in patients with "benign" aortic valve thickening. Arch Intern Med 2002;162:2345-2347.
14. Lindroos M, Kupari M, Valvanne J, et al: Factors associated with calcific aortic valve degeneration in the elderly. Eur Heart J 1994;15:865-870.
15. Freeman RV, Otto CM: Spectrum of calcific aortic valve disease:

Pathogenesis, disease progression, and treatment strategies. Circulation 2005;111:3316-3326.
16. Beppu S, Suzuki S, Matsuda H, et al: Rapidity of progression of aortic stenosis in patients with congenital bicuspid aortic valves. Am J Cardiol 1993;71:322-327.
17. Novaro GM, Mishra M, Griffin BP: Incidence and echocardiographic features of congenital unicuspid aortic valve in an adult population. J Heart Valve Dis 2003;12:674-678.
18. Tutarel O: The quadricuspid aortic valve: A comprehensive review. J Heart Valve Dis 2004;13:534-537.
19. Gunther S, Grossman W: Determinants of ventricular function in pressure-overload hypertrophy in man. Circulation 1979;59:679-688.
20. Carroll JD, Carroll EP, Feldman T, et al: Sex-associated differences in left ventricular function in aortic stenosis of the elderly (see comments). Circulation 1992;86:1099-1107.
21. Carabello BA, Green LH, Grossman W, et al: Hemodynamic determinants of prognosis of aortic valve replacement in critical aortic stenosis and advanced congestive heart failure. Circulation 1980;62:42-48.
22. Nemes A, Forster T, Varga A, et al: How can coronary flow reserve be altered by severe aortic stenosis? Echocardiography 2002;19:655-659.
23. Nemes A, Forster T, Thury A, et al: The comparative value of the aortic atherosclerosis and the coronary flow velocity reserve evaluated by stress transesophageal echocardiography in the prediction of patients with aortic stenosis with coronary artery disease. Int J Cardiovasc Imaging 2003;19:371-376.
24. Vincentelli A, Susen S, Le Tourneau T, et al: Acquired von Willebrand syndrome in aortic stenosis. N Engl J Med 2003;349:343-349.
25. Pate GE, Mulligan A: An epidemiological study of Heyde's syndrome: An association between aortic stenosis and gastrointestinal bleeding. J Heart Valve Dis 2004;13:713-716.
26. Otto CM, Burwash IG, Legget ME, et al: Prospective study of asymptomatic valvular aortic stenosis. Clinical, echocardiographic, and exercise predictors of outcome (see comments). Circulation 1997;95:2262-2270.
27. Rosenhek R, Binder T, Porenta G, et al: Predictors of outcome in severe, asymptomatic aortic stenosis. N Engl J Med 2000;343:611-617.
28. Pellikka PA, Sarano ME, Nishimura RA, et al: Outcome of 622 adults with asymptomatic, hemodynamically significant aortic stenosis during prolonged follow-up. Circulation 2005;111:3290-3295.
29. Iivanainen AM, Lindroos M, Tilvis R, et al: Natural history of aortic valve stenosis of varying severity in the elderly. Am J Cardiol 1996;78:97-101.
30. Giles TD, Martinez EC, Burch GE: Gallavardin phenomenon in aortic stenosis. A possible mechanism. Arch Intern Med 1974;34:747-749.
31. Munt B, Legget ME, Kraft CD, et al: Physical examination in valvular aortic stenosis: Correlation with stenosis severity and prediction of clinical outcome. Am Heart J 1999;137:298-306.
32. Baumgartner H: Hemodynamic assessment of aortic stenosis: Are there still lessons to learn? J Am Coll Cardiol 2006;47:138-140.
33. Baumgartner H, Stefenelli T, Niederberger J, et al: "Overestimation" of catheter gradients by Doppler ultrasound in patients with aortic stenosis: A predictable manifestation of pressure recovery. J Am Coll Cardiol 1999;33:1655-1661.
34. Burwash IG, Thomas DD, Sadahiro M, et al: Dependence of Gorlin formula and continuity equation valve areas on transvalvular volume flow rate in valvular aortic stenosis. Circulation 1994;89:827-835.
35. Yankopoulos NA, Haisty WK, Pipberger HV: Computer analysis of the orthogonal electrocardiogram and vectorcardiogram in 257 patients with aortic valve disease. Am J Cardiol 1977;40:707-715.
36. Bae JH, Lerman A, Yang E, et al: Feasibility of a pressure wire and single arterial puncture for assessing aortic valve area in patients with aortic stenosis. J Invasive Cardiol 2006;18:359-362.
37. Assey ME, Zile MR, Usher BW, et al: Effect of catheter positioning on the variability of measured gradient in aortic stenosis. Cathet Cardiovasc Diagn 1993;30:287-292.
38. Gorlin R, Gorlin SG: Hydraulic formula for calculation of the area of the stenotic mitral valve, other cardiac valves, and central circulatory shunts. Am Heart J 1951;41:1-29.
39. deFilippi CR, Willett DL, Brickner ME, et al: Usefulness of dobutamine echocardiography in distinguishing severe from nonsevere valvular aortic stenosis in patients with depressed left ventricular function and low transvalvular gradients. Am J Cardiol 1995;75:191-194.
40. Burwash IG: Low-flow, low-gradient aortic stenosis: From evaluation to treatment. Curr Opin Cardiol 2007;22:84-91.
41. Grayburn PA: Assessment of low-gradient aortic stenosis with dobutamine. Circulation 2006;113:604-606.
42. Monin JL, Quere JP, Monchi M, et al: Low-gradient aortic stenosis: Operative risk stratification and predictors for long-term outcome: A multicenter study using dobutamine stress hemodynamics. Circulation 2003;108:319-324.
43. Quere JP, Monin JL, Levy F, et al: Influence of preoperative left ventricular contractile reserve on postoperative ejection fraction in low-gradient aortic stenosis. Circulation 2006;113:1738-1744.
44. Lange RA, Hillis LD: Dobutamine stress echocardiography in patients with low-gradient aortic stenosis. Circulation 2006;113:1718-1720.
45. Khot UN, Novaro GM, Popovic ZB, et al: Nitroprusside in critically ill patients with left ventricular dysfunction and aortic stenosis. N Engl J Med 2003;348:1756-1763.
46. Theleman KP, Grayburn PA, Roberts WC: Mitral "annular" calcium forming a complete circle "O" causing mitral stenosis in association with a stenotic congenitally bicuspid aortic valve and severe coronary artery disease. Am J Geriatr Cardiol 2006;15:58-61.
47. Folland ED, Kemper AJ, Khuri SF, et al: Intraaortic balloon counterpulsation as a temporary support measure in decompensated critical aortic stenosis. J Am Coll Cardiol 1985;5:711-716.
48. Baumgartner H: Aortic stenosis: medical and surgical management. Heart 2005;91:1483-1488.
49. Cowell SJ, Newby DE, Prescott RJ, et al: A randomized trial of intensive lipid-lowering therapy in calcific aortic stenosis. N Engl J Med 2005;352:2389-2397.
50. O'Brien KD, Probstfield JL, Caulfield MT, et al: Angiotensin-converting enzyme inhibitors and change in aortic valve calcium. Arch Intern Med 2005;165:858-862.
51. Rosenhek R, Rader F, Loho N, et al: Statins but not angiotensin-converting enzyme inhibitors delay progression of aortic stenosis. Circulation 2004;110:1291-1295.
52. Kuntz RE, Tosteson AN, Berman AD, et al: Predictors of event-free survival after balloon aortic valvuloplasty. N Engl J Med 1991;325:17-23.
53. NHLBI Balloon Valvuloplasty Registry: Percutaneous balloon aortic valvuloplasty. Acute and 30-day follow-up results in 674 patients from the NHLBI Balloon Valvuloplasty Registry. Circulation 1991;84:2383-2397.
54. Klein A, Lee K, Gera A, et al: Long-term mortality, cause of death, and temporal trends in complications after percutaneous aortic balloon valvuloplasty for calcific aortic stenosis. J Interv Cardiol 2006;19:269-275.
55. Lieberman EB, Bashore TM, Hermiller JB, et al: Balloon aortic valvuloplasty in adults: Failure of procedure to improve long-term survival. J Am Coll Cardiol 1995;26:1522-1528.
56. Roth RB, Palacios IF, Block PC: Percutaneous aortic balloon valvuloplasty: Its role in the management of patients with aortic stenosis requiring major noncardiac surgery. J Am Coll Cardiol 1989;13:1039-1041.
57. Torsher LC, Shub C, Rettke SR, et al: Risk of patients with severe aortic stenosis undergoing noncardiac surgery. Am J Cardiol 1998;81:448-452.
58. Christ M, Sharkova Y, Geldner G, et al: Preoperative and perioperative care for patients with suspected or established aortic stenosis facing noncardiac surgery. Chest 2005;128:2944-2953.
59. Safian RD, Warren SE, Berman AD, et al: Improvement in symptoms and left ventricular performance after balloon aortic valvuloplasty in patients with aortic stenosis and depressed left ventricular ejection fraction. Circulation 1988;78:1181-1191.
60. Cribier A, Eltchaninoff H, Bash A, et al: Percutaneous transcatheter implantation of an aortic valve prosthesis for calcific aortic stenosis:

First human case description. Circulation 2002;106:3006-3008.
61. Lichtenstein SV, Cheung A, Ye J, et al: Transapical transcatheter aortic valve implantation in humans: Initial clinical experience. Circulation 2006;114: 591-596.
62. Cribier A, Eltchaninoff H, Tron C, et al: Treatment of calcific aortic stenosis with the percutaneous heart valve: Mid-term follow-up from the initial feasibility studies: The French experience. J Am Coll Cardiol 2006;47:1214-1223.
63. Lindblom D, Lindblom U, Qvist J, et al: Long-term relative survival rates after heart valve replacement. J Am Coll Cardiol 1990;15:566-573.
64. Connolly HM, Oh JK, Schaff HV, et al: Severe aortic stenosis with low transvalvular gradient and severe left ventricular dysfunction: Result of aortic valve replacement in 52 patients. Circulation 2000;101:1940-1946.
65. Varadarajan P, Kapoor N, Bansal RC, et al: Clinical profile and natural history of 453 nonsurgically managed patients with severe aortic stenosis. Ann Thorac Surg 2006;82:2111-2115.
66. Singh JP, Evans JC, Levy D, et al: Prevalence and clinical determinants of mitral, tricuspid, and aortic regurgitation (the Framingham Heart Study). Am J Cardiol 1999;83:897-902.
67. Kim M, Roman MJ, Cavallini MC, et al: Effect of hypertension on aortic root size and prevalence of aortic regurgitation. Hypertension 1996;28:47-52.
68. Bekeredjian R, Grayburn PA: Valvular heart disease: Aortic regurgitation. Circulation 2005;112:125-134.
69. Grossman W, Jones D, McLaurin LP: Wall stress and patterns of hypertrophy in the human left ventricle. J Clin Invest 1975;56:56-64.
70. Ardehali A, Segal J, Cheitlin MD: Coronary blood flow reserve in acute aortic regurgitation. J Am Coll Cardiol 1995;25:1387-1392.
71. Borer JS, Hochreiter C, Herrold EM, et al: Prediction of indications for valve replacement among asymptomatic or minimally symptomatic patients with chronic aortic regurgitation and normal left ventricular performance. Circulation 1998;97:525-534.
72. Tarasoutchi F, Grinberg M, Spina GS, et al: Ten-year clinical laboratory follow-up after application of a symptom-based therapeutic strategy to patients with severe chronic aortic regurgitation of predominant rheumatic etiology. J Am Coll Cardiol 2003;41:1316-1324.
73. Bonow RO, Lakatos E, Maron BJ, et al: Serial long-term assessment of the natural history of asymptomatic patients with chronic aortic regurgitation and normal left ventricular systolic function. Circulation 1991;84:1625-1635.
74. Dujardin KS, Enriquez-Sarano M, Schaff HV, et al: Mortality and morbidity of aortic regurgitation in clinical practice. A long-term follow-up study. Circulation 1999;99:1851-1857.
75. Carabello BA: Is it ever too late to operate on the patient with valvular heart disease? J Am Coll Cardiol 2004;44:376-383.
76. Desjardins VA, Enriquez-Sarano M, Tajik AJ, et al: Intensity of murmurs correlates with severity of valvular regurgitation. Am J Med 1996;100:149-156.
77. Harvey WP: Cardiac pearls. Dis Mon 1994;40:41-113.
78. Tribouilloy CM, Enriquez-Sarano M, Mohty D, et al: Pathophysiologic determinants of third heart sounds: A prospective clinical and Doppler echocardiographic study. Am J Med 2001;111:96-102.
79. Baddour LM, Wilson WR, Bayer AS, et al: Infective endocarditis: diagnosis, antimicrobial therapy, and management of complications: A statement for healthcare professionals from the Committee on Rheumatic Fever, Endocarditis, and Kawasaki Disease, Council on Cardiovascular Disease in the Young, and the Councils on Clinical Cardiology, Stroke, and Cardiovascular Surgery and Anesthesia, American Heart Association: Endorsed by the Infectious Diseases Society of America. Circulation 2005;111:e394-e434.
80. Zoghbi WA, Enriquez-Sarano M, Foster E, et al: Recommendations for evaluation of the severity of native valvular regurgitation with two-dimensional and Doppler echocardiography. J Am Soc Echocardiogr 2003;16:777-802.
81. Kozerke S, Schwitter J, Pedersen EM, et al: Aortic and mitral regurgitation: quantification using moving slice velocity mapping. J Magn Reson Imaging 2001;14:106-112.
82. Bonow RO: Radionuclide angiography in the management of asymptomatic aortic regurgitation. Circulation 1991;84:I296-I302.
83. Vahanian A, Baumgartner H, Bax J, et al: Guidelines on the management of valvular heart disease: The Task Force on the Management of Valvular Heart Disease of the European Society of Cardiology. Eur Heart J 2007;28:230-268.
84. Badano L, Rubartelli P, Giunta L, et al: Relation between ECG strain pattern and left ventricular morphology, left ventricular function, and DPTI/SPTI ratio in patients with aortic regurgitation. J Electrocardiol 1994;27:189-197.
85. Miller RR, Vismara LA, DeMaria AN, et al: Afterload reduction therapy with nitroprusside in severe aortic regurgitation: Improved cardiac performance and reduced regurgitant volume. Am J Cardiol 1976;38:564-567.
86. Scognamiglio R, Rahimtoola SH, Fasoli G, et al: Nifedipine in asymptomatic patients with severe aortic regurgitation and normal left ventricular function. N Engl J Med 1994;331:689-694.
87. Evangelista A, Tornos P, Sambola A, et al: Long-term vasodilator therapy in patients with severe aortic regurgitation. N Engl J Med 2005;353:1342-1349.
88. Klodas E, Enriquez-Sarano M, Tajik AJ, et al: Optimizing timing of surgical correction in patients with severe aortic regurgitation: Role of symptoms. J Am Coll Cardiol 1997;30:746-752.
89. Chaliki HP, Mohty D, Avierinos JF, et al: Outcomes after aortic valve replacement in patients with severe aortic regurgitation and markedly reduced left ventricular function. Circulation 2002;106:2687-2693.
90. Taniguchi K, Nakano S, Kawashima Y, et al: Left ventricular ejection performance, wall stress, and contractile state in aortic regurgitation before and after aortic valve replacement. Circulation 1990;82:798-807.
91. Roman MJ, Klein L, Devereux RB, et al: Reversal of left ventricular dilatation, hypertrophy, and dysfunction by valve replacement in aortic regurgitation. Am Heart J 1989;118:553-563.
92. Tornos P, Sambola A, Permanyer-Miralda G, et al: Long-term outcome of surgically treated aortic regurgitation: Influence of guideline adherence toward early surgery. J Am Coll Cardiol 2006;47:1012-1017.
93. Bonow RO, Picone AL, McIntosh CL, et al: Survival and functional results after valve replacement for aortic regurgitation from 1976 to 1983: Impact of preoperative left ventricular function. Circulation 1985;72:1244-1256.
94. Middlemost S, Wisenbaugh T, Meyerowitz C, et al: A case for early surgery in native left-sided endocarditis complicated by heart failure: Results in 203 patients. J Am Coll Cardiol 1991;18:663-667.
95. Pompilio G, Brockmann C, Bruneau M, et al: Long-term survival after aortic valve replacement for native active infective endocarditis. Cardiovasc Surg 1998;6:126-132.
96. Trichon BH, Felker GM, Shaw LK, et al: Relation of frequency and severity of mitral regurgitation to survival among patients with left ventricular systolic dysfunction and heart failure. Am J Cardiol 2003;91:538-543.
97. Carabello BA: The pathophysiology of mitral regurgitation. J Heart Valve Dis 2000;9:600-608.
98. Starling MR, Kirsh MM, Montgomery DG, et al: Impaired left ventricular contractile function in patients with long-term mitral regurgitation and normal ejection fraction. J Am Coll Cardiol 1993;22:239-250.
99. Mehta RH, Supiano MA, Oral H, et al: Compared with control subjects, the systemic sympathetic nervous system is activated in patients with mitral regurgitation. Am Heart J 2003;145:1078-1085.
100. Nagatsu M, Zile MR, Tsutsui H, et al: Native beta-adrenergic support for left ventricular dysfunction in experimental mitral regurgitation normalizes indexes of pump and contractile function. Circulation 1994;89:818-826.
101. Tsutsui H, Spinale FG, Nagatsu M, et al: Effects of chronic beta-adrenergic blockade on the left ventricular and cardiocyte abnormalities of chronic canine mitral regurgitation. J Clin Invest 1994;93:2639-2648.
102. Carabello BA: Ischemic mitral regurgitation and ventricular

remodeling. J Am Coll Cardiol 2004;43:384-385.
103. Kim TH, Seung KB, Kim PJ, et al: Images in cardiovascular medicine. Anterolateral papillary muscle rupture complicated by the obstruction of a single diagonal branch. Circulation 2005;112:e269-e270.
104. Kaul S, Spotnitz WD, Glasheen WP, et al: Mechanism of ischemic mitral regurgitation. An experimental evaluation. Circulation 1991;84: 2167-2180.
105. Levine RA, Schwammenthal E: Ischemic mitral regurgitation on the threshold of a solution: from paradoxes to unifying concepts. Circulation 2005;112:745-758.
106. Jouan J, Tapia M, Cook C, et al: Ischemic mitral valve prolapse: Mechanisms and implications for valve repair. Eur J Cardiothorac Surg 2004;26:1112-1117.
107. Bursi F, Enriquez-Sarano M, Jacobsen SJ, et al: Mitral regurgitation after myocardial infarction: A review. Am J Med 2006;119:103-112.
108. Bursi F, Enriquez-Sarano M, Nkomo VT, et al: Heart failure and death after myocardial infarction in the community: The emerging role of mitral regurgitation. Circulation 2005;111:295-301.
109. Birnbaum Y, Chamoun AJ, Conti VR, et al: Mitral regurgitation following acute myocardial infarction. Coron Artery Dis 2002;13:337-344.
110. Nishimura RA, Gersh BJ, Schaff HV: The case for an aggressive surgical approach to papillary muscle rupture following myocardial infarction: From paradise lost to paradise regained. Heart 2000;83:611-613.
111. Seve P, Dubreuil O, Farhat F, et al: Acute mitral regurgitation caused by papillary muscle rupture in the immediate postpartum period revealing Ehlers-Danlos syndrome type IV. J Thorac Cardiovasc Surg 2005;129:680-681.
112. Schreiber TL, Fisher J, Mangla A, et al: Severe "silent" mitral regurgitation. A potentially reversible cause of refractory heart failure. Chest 1989;96:242-246.
113. Castello R, Fagan L Jr, Lenzen P, et al: Comparison of transthoracic and transesophageal echocardiography for assessment of left-sided valvular regurgitation. Am J Cardiol 1991;68:1677-1680.
114. Dekker AL, Reesink KD, van der Veen FH, et al: Intra-aortic balloon pumping in acute mitral regurgitation reduces aortic impedance and regurgitant fraction. Shock 2003;19:334-338.
115. Le Feuvre C, Metzger JP, Lachurie ML, et al: Treatment of severe mitral regurgitation caused by ischemic papillary muscle dysfunction: Indications for coronary angioplasty. Am Heart J 1992;123:860-865.
116. Wisenbaugh T, Sinovich V, Dullabh A, et al: Six month pilot study of captopril for mildly symptomatic, severe isolated mitral and isolated aortic regurgitation. J Heart Valve Dis 1994;3:197-204.
117. Levine HJ, Gaasch WH: Vasoactive drugs in chronic regurgitant lesions of the mitral and aortic valves. J Am Coll Cardiol 1996;28:1083-1091.
118. Host U, Kelbaek H, Hildebrandt P, et al: Effect of ramipril on mitral regurgitation secondary to mitral valve prolapse. Am J Cardiol 1997;80:655-658.
119. Tischler MD, Rowan M, LeWinter MM: Effect of enalapril therapy on left ventricular mass and volumes in asymptomatic chronic, severe mitral regurgitation secondary to mitral valve prolapse. Am J Cardiol 1998;82:242-245.
120. Breithardt OA, Sinha AM, Schwammenthal E, et al: Acute effects of cardiac resynchronization therapy on functional mitral regurgitation in advanced systolic heart failure. J Am Coll Cardiol 2003;41:765-770.
121. Starling MR: Is prophylactic beta-adrenergic blockade appropriate in mitral regurgitation: Impact of cellular pathophysiology. Adv Cardiol 2004;41:25-35.
122. Capomolla S, Febo O, Gnemmi M, et al: Beta-blockade therapy in chronic heart failure: Diastolic function and mitral regurgitation improvement by carvedilol. Am Heart J 2000;139:596-608.
123. Nemoto S, Hamawaki M, De Freitas G, et al: Differential effects of the angiotensin-converting enzyme inhibitor lisinopril versus the beta-adrenergic receptor blocker atenolol on hemodynamics and left ventricular contractile function in experimental mitral regurgitation. J Am Coll Cardiol 2002;40:149-154.
124. Wu AH, Aaronson KD, Bolling SF, et al: Impact of mitral valve annuloplasty on mortality risk in patients with mitral regurgitation and left ventricular systolic dysfunction. J Am Coll Cardiol 2005;45:381-387.
125. Enriquez-Sarano M, Schaff HV, Orszulak TA, et al: Valve repair improves the outcome of surgery for mitral regurgitation. A multivariate analysis. Circulation 1995;91: 1022-1028.
126. Horskotte D, Schulte HD, Bircks W, et al: The effect of chordal preservation on late outcome after mitral valve replacement: A randomized study. J Heart Valve Dis 1993;2:150-158.
127. Ling LH, Enriquez-Sarano M, Seward JB, et al: Clinical outcome of mitral regurgitation due to flail leaflet. N Engl J Med 1996;335:1417-23.
128. Matsumura T, Ohtaki E, Tanaka K, et al: Echocardiographic prediction of left ventricular dysfunction after mitral valve repair for mitral regurgitation as an indicator to decide the optimal timing of repair. J Am Coll Cardiol 2003;42:458-463.
129. Enriquez-Sarano M, Tajik AJ, Schaff HV, et al: Echocardiographic prediction of survival after surgical correction of organic mitral regurgitation. Circulation 1994;90:830-837.
130. Enriquez-Sarano M, Avierinos JF, Messika-Zeitoun D, et al: Quantitative determinants of the outcome of asymptomatic mitral regurgitation. N Engl J Med 2005;352:875-883.
131. Eguchi K, Ohtaki E, Matsumura T, et al: Pre-operative atrial fibrillation as the key determinant of outcome of mitral valve repair for degenerative mitral regurgitation. Eur Heart J 2005;26:1866-1872.
132. Borer JS, Hochreiter CA, Supino PG, et al: Importance of right ventricular performance measurement in selecting asymptomatic patients with mitral regurgitation for valve surgery. Adv Cardiol 2002;39:144-152.
133. Starling MR: Effects of valve surgery on left ventricular contractile function in patients with long-term mitral regurgitation. Circulation 1995;92: 811-818.
134. Wisenbaugh T: Unexpected, dismal left ventricular function after surgery for mitral regurgitation: There is just no excuse for it anymore. J Am Coll Cardiol 2003;42:464-465.
135. Gammie JS, O'Brien SM, Griffith BP, et al: Influence of hospital procedural volume on care process and mortality for patients undergoing elective surgery for mitral regurgitation. Circulation 2007;115:881-887.
136. Sarris GE, Miller DC: Valvular-ventricular interaction: The importance of the mitral chordae tendineae in terms of global left ventricular systolic function. J Card Surg 1988;3:215-234.
137. Rozich JD, Carabello BA, Usher BW, et al: Mitral valve replacement with and without chordal preservation in patients with chronic mitral regurgitation. Mechanisms for differences in postoperative ejection performance. Circulation 1992;86:1718-1726.
138. Bolling SF: Mitral reconstruction in cardiomyopathy. J Heart Valve Dis 2002;11(Suppl 1):S26-S31.
139. Acker MA, Bolling S, Shemin R, et al: Mitral valve surgery in heart failure: Insights from the Acorn Clinical Trial. J Thorac Cardiovasc Surg 2006;132: 568-77.
140. Haan CK, Cabral CI, Conetta DA, et al: Selecting patients with mitral regurgitation and left ventricular dysfunction for isolated mitral valve surgery. Ann Thorac Surg 2004;78:820-825.
141. Trichon BH, Glower DD, Shaw LK, et al: Survival after coronary revascularization, with and without mitral valve surgery, in patients with ischemic mitral regurgitation. Circulation 2003;108(Suppl 1): II103-II110.
142. Minami H, Mukohara N, Obo H, et al: Papillary muscle rupture following acute myocardial infarction. Jpn J Thorac Cardiovasc Surg 2004;52:367-371.
143. Lamas GA, Mitchell GF, Flaker GC, et al: Clinical significance of mitral regurgitation after acute myocardial infarction. Survival and Ventricular Enlargement Investigators. Circulation 1997;96:827-833.
144. Pellizzon GG, Grines CL, Cox DA, et al: Importance of mitral regurgitation inpatients undergoing percutaneous coronary intervention for acute myocardial infarction: The Controlled Abciximab and Device Investigation to Lower Late Angioplasty Complications (CADILLAC) trial. J Am Coll Cardiol 2004;43:1368-1374.
145. Davidson MJ, White JK, Baim DS: Percutaneous therapies for valvular

heart disease. Cardiovasc Pathol 2006;15:123-129.
146. Maron MS, Olivotto I, Betocchi S, et al: Effect of left ventricular outflow tract obstruction on clinical outcome in hypertrophic cardiomyopathy. N Engl J Med 2003;348:295-303.
147. Maron BJ, Gardin JM, Flack JM, et al: Prevalence of hypertrophic cardiomyopathy in a general population of young adults. Echocardiographic analysis of 4111 subjects in the CARDIA Study. Coronary Artery Risk Development in (Young) Adults. Circulation 1995;92:785-789.
148. Maron MS, Olivotto I, Zenovich AG, et al: Hypertrophic cardiomyopathy is predominantly a disease of left ventricular outflow tract obstruction. Circulation 2006;114:2232-2239.
149. Spirito P, Chiarella F, Carratino L, et al: Clinical course and prognosis of hypertrophic cardiomyopathy in an outpatient population. N Engl J Med 1989;320:749-755.
150. Epstein SE, Maron BJ: Sudden death and the competitive athlete: Perspectives on preparticipation screening studies. J Am Coll Cardiol 1986;7:220-230.
151. Maron BJ: Hypertrophic cardiomyopathy: A systematic review. JAMA 2002;287:1308-1320.
152. Maki S, Ikeda H, Muro A, et al: Predictors of sudden cardiac death in hypertrophic cardiomyopathy. Am J Cardiol 1998;82:774-778.
153. Krams R, Ten Cate FJ, Carlier SG, et al: Diastolic coronary vascular reserve: A new index to detect changes in the coronary microcirculation in hypertrophic cardiomyopathy. J Am Coll Cardiol 2004;43:670-677.
154. Sorajja P, Ommen SR, Nishimura RA, et al: Myocardial bridging in adult patients with hypertrophic cardiomyopathy. J Am Coll Cardiol 2003;42:889-894.
155. Sherrid MV, Gunsburg DZ, Moldenhauer S, et al: Systolic anterior motion begins at low left ventricular outflow tract velocity in obstructive hypertrophic cardiomyopathy. J Am Coll Cardiol 2000;36:1344-1354.
156. Ghani MF, Parker BM: Hypotension, heart block and reversed pulsus alternans in a patient with hypertrophic subaortic stenosis following digitalis and diuretic therapy. Chest 1974;65:695-698.
157. Hamid MS, Gimeno JR, Valdes M, et al: Reversal of acute pulmonary oedema with beta-blockers in hypertrophic cardiomyopathy. Eur J Echocardiogr 2003;4:71-72.
158. Sherrid MV, Pearle G, Gunsburg DZ: Mechanism of benefit of negative inotropes in obstructive hypertrophic cardiomyopathy. Circulation 1998;97:41-47.
159. Sherrid MV, Barac I, McKenna WJ, et al: Multicenter study of the efficacy and safety of disopyramide in obstructive hypertrophic cardiomyopathy. J Am Coll Cardiol 2005;45:1251-1258.
160. Cohen IL, Fein IA, Nabi A: Reversal of cardiogenic shock and asystole in a septic patient with hypertrophic cardiomyopathy on verapamil. Crit Care Med 1990;18:775-776.
161. Borja J, Izquierdo I, Guindo J: Hypertrophic cardiomyopathy. Combination of beta blockers and verapamil may be risky. BMJ 2006;333:97.
162. Yamaji K, Fujimoto S, Yutani C, et al: Does the progression of myocardial fibrosis lead to atrial fibrillation in patients with hypertrophic cardiomyopathy? Cardiovasc Pathol 2001;10:297-303.
163. Olivotto I, Cecchi F, Casey SA, et al: Impact of atrial fibrillation on the clinical course of hypertrophic cardiomyopathy. Circulation 2001;104:2517-2524.
164. Shigematsu Y, Hamada M, Mukai M, et al: Mechanism of atrial fibrillation and increased incidence of thromboembolism in patients with hypertrophic cardiomyopathy. Jpn Circ J 1995;59:329-336.
165. Maron BJ, Olivotto I, Bellone P, et al: Clinical profile of stroke in 900 patients with hypertrophic cardiomyopathy. J Am Coll Cardiol 2002;39:301-307.
166. Losi MA, Betocchi S, Aversa M, et al: Determinants of atrial fibrillation development in patients with hypertrophic cardiomyopathy. Am J Cardiol 2004;94:895-900.
167. Chen MS, McCarthy PM, Lever HM, et al: Effectiveness of atrial fibrillation surgery in patients with hypertrophic cardiomyopathy. Am J Cardiol 2004;93:373-375.
168. Duytschaever M, Vijgen J, Tavernier R: Atrial fibrillation in hypertrophic cardiomyopathy: another indication for circumferential pulmonary vein ablation? Acta Cardiol 2006;61: 193-196.
169. Robinson K, Frenneaux MP, Stockins B, et al: Atrial fibrillation in hypertrophic cardiomyopathy: A longitudinal study. J Am Coll Cardiol 1990;15:1279-1285.
170. Cecchi F, Olivotto I, Montereggi A, et al: Prognostic value of non-sustained ventricular tachycardia and the potential role of amiodarone treatment in hypertrophic cardiomyopathy: Assessment in an unselected non-referral based patient population. Heart 1998;79:331-336.
171. Spirito P, Seidman CE, McKenna WJ, et al: The management of hypertrophic cardiomyopathy. N Engl J Med 1997;336:775-785.
172. Maron BJ, Shen WK, Link MS, et al: Efficacy of implantable cardioverter-defibrillators for the prevention of sudden death in patients with hypertrophic cardiomyopathy. N Engl J Med 2000;342:365-373.
173. Ralph-Edwards A, Woo A, McCrindle BW, et al: Hypertrophic obstructive cardiomyopathy: Comparison of outcomes after myectomy or alcohol ablation adjusted by propensity score. J Thorac Cardiovasc Surg 2005;129: 351-358.
174. Yu EH, Omran AS, Wigle ED, et al: Mitral regurgitation in hypertrophic obstructive cardiomyopathy: Relationship to obstruction and relief with myectomy. J Am Coll Cardiol 2000;36:2219-2225.
175. Fananapazir L, Epstein ND, Curiel RV, et al: Long-term results of dual-chamber (DDD) pacing in obstructive hypertrophic cardiomyopathy. Evidence for progressive symptomatic and hemodynamic improvement and reduction of left ventricular hypertrophy. Circulation 1994;90:2731-2742.
176. Maron BJ, Nishimura RA, McKenna WJ, et al: Assessment of permanent dual-chamber pacing as a treatment for drug-refractory symptomatic patients with obstructive hypertrophic cardiomyopathy. A randomized, double-blind, crossover study (M-PATHY). Circulation 1999;99:2927-2933.
177. Movahed MR, Saito Y, Ahmadi-Kashani M, et al: Mitral annulus calcification is associated with valvular and cardiac structural abnormalities. Cardiovasc Ultrasound 2007;5:14.
178. Willens HJ, Chirinos JA, Hennekens CH: Prevalence and clinical correlates of mitral annulus calcification in Hispanics and non-Hispanic whites. J Am Soc Echocardiogr 2007;20:191-196.
179. Bonow RO, Braunwald E: Valvular heart disease. In Zipes DP, Libby P, Bonow RO, Braunwald E (eds): Braunwald's Heart Disease; A Textbook of Cardiovascular Medicine. Philadelphia, Elsevier, 2005, pp 1553-1632.
180. Thibault GE: Clinical problem-solving. Studying the classics. N Engl J Med 1995;333:648-652.
181. Wilkins GT, Weyman AE, Abascal VM, et al: Percutaneous balloon dilatation of the mitral valve: An analysis of echocardiographic variables related to outcome and the mechanism of dilatation. Br Heart J 1988;60:299-308.
182. Messika-Zeitoun D, Brochet E, Holmin C, et al: Three-dimensional evaluation of the mitral valve area and commissural opening before and after percutaneous mitral commissurotomy in patients with mitral stenosis. Eur Heart J 2007;28:72-79.
183. Uzun M, Baysan O, Erinc K, et al: A simple different method to use proximal isovelocity surface area (PISA) for measuring mitral valve area. Int J Cardiovasc Imaging 2005;21: 633-640.
184. Abaci A, Oguzhan A, Unal S, et al: Application of the vena contracta method for the calculation of the mitral valve area in mitral stenosis. Cardiology 2002;98:50-59.
185. Palacios IF: What is the gold standard to measure mitral valve area postmitral balloon valvuloplasty? [editorial; comment]. Cathet Cardiovasc Diagn 1994;33:315-316.
186. Mohan JC, Patel AR, Passey R, et al: Is the mitral valve area flow-dependent in mitral stenosis? A dobutamine stress echocardiographic study. J Am Coll Cardiol 2002;40:1809-1815.
187. Schoenfeld MH, Palacios IF, Hutter AM Jr, et al: Underestimation of prosthetic mitral valve areas: Role of transseptal catheterization in avoiding unnecessary repeat mitral valve surgery. J Am Coll Cardiol 1985;5:1387-1392.

188. Carabello BA: Modern management of mitral stenosis. Circulation 2005;112:432-437.
189. Topaloglu S, Boyaci A, Ayaz S, et al: Coagulation, fibrinolytic system activation and endothelial dysfunction in patients with mitral stenosis and sinus rhythm. Angiology 2007;58: 85-91.
190. Schumacher B, Luderitz B: Rate issues in atrial fibrillation: Consequences of tachycardia and therapy for rate control. Am J Cardiol 1998;82: 29N-36N.
191. Reyes VP, Raju BS, Wynne J, et al: Percutaneous balloon valvuloplasty compared with open surgical commissurotomy for mitral stenosis. N Engl J Med 1994;331:961-967.
192. Turi ZG, Reyes VP, Raju BS, et al: Percutaneous balloon versus surgical closed commissurotomy for mitral stenosis. A prospective, randomized trial. Circulation 1991;83:1179-1185.
193. Heger JJ, Wann LS, Weyman AE, et al: Long-term changes in mitral valve area after successful mitral commissurotomy. Circulation 1979;59:443-448.
194. Palacios IF, Sanchez PL, Harrell LC, et al: Which patients benefit from percutaneous mitral balloon valvuloplasty? Prevalvuloplasty and postvalvuloplasty variables that predict long-term outcome. Circulation 2002;105:1465-1471.
195. Wilson W, Taubert KA, Gewitz M, et al: Prevention of infective endocarditis. Guidelines from the American Heart Association. A guideline from the American Heart Association Rheumatic Fever, Endocarditis, and Kawasaki Disease Committee, Council on Cardiovascular Disease in the Young, and the Council on Clinical Cardiology, Council on Cardiovascular Surgery and Anesthesia, and the Quality of Care and Outcomes Research Interdisciplinary Working Group. Circulation 2007; Apr 19 (Epub ahead of print).

Chapter 34

Acute Aortic Dissection

Jonathan H. Cilley, Jr., and Robert J. March

HISTORICAL BACKGROUND

In 1819, Laennec[1] introduced the term *aortic dissection* to describe an intimal tear distal to the aortic valve and a longitudinal space within the aortic wall in a 67-year-old man who had died suddenly. The first reference to this problem was by Sennertus[2] in 1650. Nicholls[3] in 1728 stated, "An aneurysm may rupture or rupture of the inner layers only may occur allowing for expansion of the outer lumen." Years later, his autopsy report described the aortic dissection and pericardial tamponade causing the death of King George II[4] in 1760. Peacock,[5] in 1863, reported findings in 80 patients in which he described the three stages of the disease as (1) intimal tear, (2) propagation of the dissecting hematoma with possible rupture, and (3) recanalization of the lumen. It is still not entirely clear whether the precipitating event is the intimal tear or an intramural hematoma with subsequent intimal rupture.

Although he did not recognize the associated cardiovascular complications, in 1896 Marfan described the connective tissue anomaly that bears his name.[6] In 1910, Osler[7] described aortic dissection as causing angina pectoris. Additional understanding came from Erdheim[8] in 1929, when he compared the characteristic morphologic features of dissection to those of syphilitic and atherosclerotic disorders of the aorta. The dire outcome of acute dissection was further documented by Shennan[9] in 1934.

In the first operation deemed "successful" for an acute dissection or its complications, as reported by Gurin and colleagues[10] in 1935, a fenestration procedure to correct vascular compromise of the right leg in a 43-year-old man was performed. Although dividing the septum separating the true and false channels restored blood flow to the leg, the patient succumbed to renal failure. In 1955 Shaw[11] provided additional description of reentry or internal fenestration procedures, which permit decompression of the false lumen into the distal vasculature. Also in 1955, DeBakey[12] treated a dissection of the descending thoracic aorta by resecting the aneurysmal segment, reapproximating the dissected layers, and graft interposition. Morris, Henly, and DeBakey[13] used a similar approach in 1963 to repair an ascending aortic dissection complicated by aortic valvular insufficiency. Wheat and colleagues[14] in 1965 described the use of β-adrenergic blockade and antihypertensives in the aggressive treatment of descending aortic dissections and in preparing anterior dissections for operative intervention. They established the importance of controlling blood pressure as the initial therapy.

INCIDENCE AND CLASSIFICATION

The most common catastrophe affecting the aorta is dissection, which occurs in approximately 5 to 10 patients per 1 million population between the ages of 50 and 70 years, with males affected by a 3:1 margin over females. This incidence is two to three times that of rupture of an abdominal aortic aneurysm. At least 2000 cases are diagnosed in the United States each year.[15] Dissection is rare in patients younger than 40 years, with the exception of pregnant women, persons with bicuspid aortic valves,[16] and patients with a familial predisposition such as in Marfan syndrome, Ehler-Danlos syndrome, or other connective tissue disorders.

Several classifications for aortic dissection have been proposed. The following criteria are applied to acute dissections, which by definition are less than 2 weeks old.

1. DeBakey and associates proposed the first classification scheme in 1965.[17] Based on the origin of the dissection and its distal progression, the *DeBakey classification* identified three types of dissection. In types I and II (Figs. 34-1 and 34-2), the intimal tear is in the ascending aorta. In type II, the dissection is confined to the ascending aorta but in type I extends distal to the arch. In type III, it originates in the proximal descending aorta. Rarely (5%), retrograde dissection occurs from the descending aortic tear back into the arch or even the ascending aorta. If that happens, the dissection is still considered type III based on the

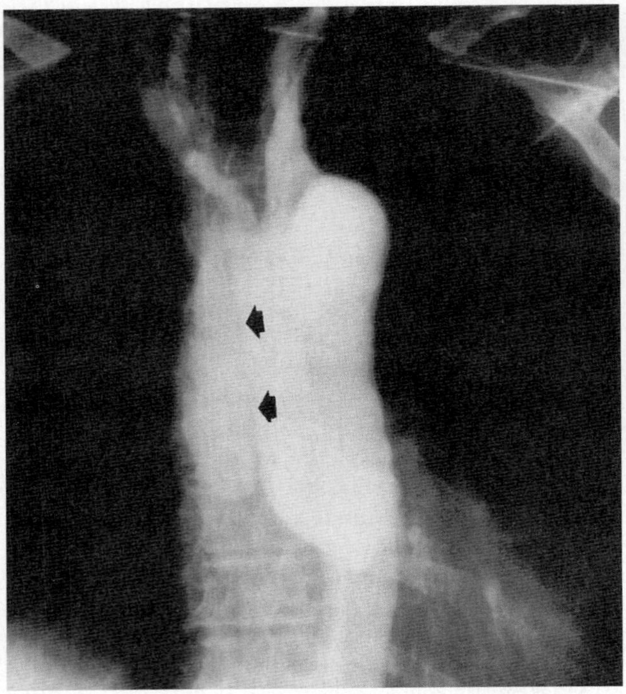

Figure 34-1. Stanford type A (DeBakey type II, anterior) dissection. The aortogram demonstrates the intimal septum *(arrows)* between the true and false lumens. The dissection begins just above the aortic valve and extends into the innominate artery.

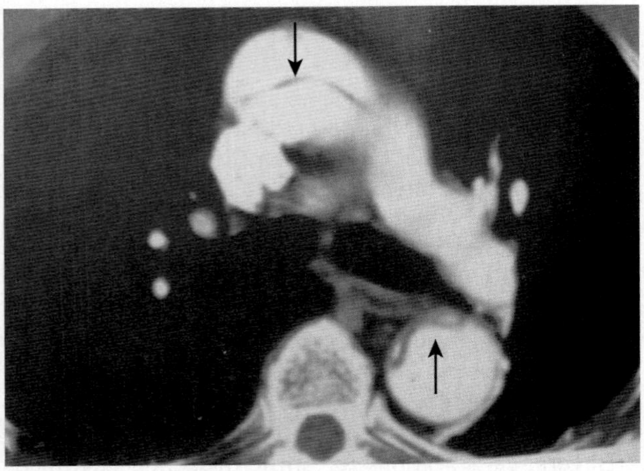

Figure 34-2. Contrast-enhanced CT scan demonstrates a type A (DeBakey type I) dissection with an intimal flap in the ascending aorta *(top arrow)*. The dissection extends into the descending aorta, where there is compression of the true lumen by the false *(bottom arrow)*. (From Gilkeson RC, Kolodny S: Computed tomography and magnetic resonance imaging of the thoracic aorta. In Haaga JR, Lanzieri CF, Gilkeson RC [eds]: CT and MR Imaging of the Whole Body, 4th ed. Mosby, St. Louis, 2003, p 1044.)

origin of the tear, although the treatment would be as for type II or I.

2. In 1970, Daily and associates[18] proposed the original *Stanford classification* based on the extent of aortic involvement, regardless of the site of intimal tear. All dissections involving the ascending aorta were classified as type A and those involving only the descending thoracic aorta as type B (Fig. 34-3).
3. In an attempt to simplify the classifications (because both DeBakey type I and type II dissections are approached via sternotomy), Najafi and colleagues[19] grouped them together as anterior dissections. The type III dissections they called posterior. Anterior dissections also are referred to as ascending or proximal, as opposed to posterior, which are descending or distal—all relative to the left subclavian artery.

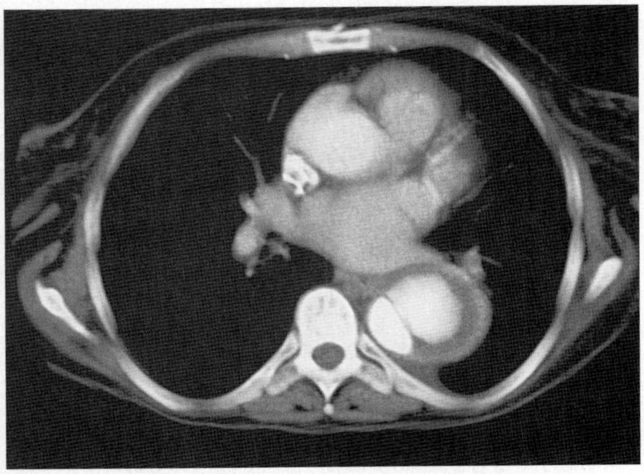

Figure 34-3. Stanford type B (DeBakey type III, posterior) dissection. The contrast-enhanced CT scan shows a chronically enlarged descending aorta with partial thrombosis of the false lumen. The true lumen is compressed medially.

ETIOLOGIC AND PATHOPHYSIOLOGIC CONSIDERATIONS

With relatively consistent histopathologic findings, aortic dissection generally is thought to result from deterioration of the fibrous structure of the media, specifically elastin and collagen breakdown.[20] This end result is cystic medial degeneration, a feature shared by hereditary disorders such as Marfan syndrome and Ehler-Danlos syndrome (arterial type IV)[21-23] that may be seen in the arterial wall before development of an aneurysm or dissection. Even in dissections not associated with a particular syndrome, cystic medial degeneration is found. Atherosclerotic changes may be observed, especially in the older patient.

A variety of commonalities become apparent when large series are evaluated. More than 70% of patients with aortic dissection have had or have systemic hypertension at the time of diagnosis.[24,25] It has been suggested that the higher the blood pressure, the greater the probability of aortic dissection. For example, coarctation of the aorta is associated with an increased risk of dissection. In patients with coarctation, acute dissection usually occurs proximal rather than distal to the coarctation.[26] Propensity for dissection is increased by uncontrolled hypertension, whereas reduction of blood pressure clearly lowers its incidence. Despite the increased risk of acute dissection associated with elevated blood pressure, hypertension cannot be viewed as the sole cause of aortic dissection.

Although pregnancy has been invoked as a risk factor for aortic dissection, the number of patients affected is small, and coexistent predisposing factors such as hypertension have not been well documented. Rarely, dissection is the consequence of blunt thoracic trauma, usually a severe deceleration injury from a motor vehicle accident or fall. Most commonly, with that mode of injury, an intimal tear occurs at the aortic isthmus, and a localized hematoma results without propagation of a dissection. Bicuspid aortic valve[16] and coarctation of the aorta are associated with an increased risk of aortic dissection.

Along with the introduction of arterially invasive technology comes iatrogenic aortic dissection. It may result from antegrade or retrograde arterial perfusion during cardiopulmonary bypass (CPB)[27] or intra-aortic balloon counterpulsation.[28] The switch from femoral arterial to direct aortic cannulation for CPB was prompted to some extent by the number of dissections encountered related to groin cannulation. A dissection may originate at any site of clamp application or at any aortotomy, whether for cannulation or for anastomosis.[29,30] The risk of type A dissection is increased after aortic valve replacement, especially with aortic diameters greater than 5 cm.[31,32] Diagnostic angiography and cardiac catheterization have also been complicated by aortic dissection.

With spontaneous dissection it is unclear whether rupture of the intima is caused by hemorrhage within a diseased media or whether a defect in the intima itself is the initial event leading to dissection. Typically, clinical aortic dissection begins with a transverse defect in the intima and evolves by longitudinal disruption of the media for approximately two thirds of the aortic circumference. The hematoma advances within the media of the artery and may extend to the aortic bifurcation or beyond. When all types of dissection are considered, the primary tear is found in the ascending aorta in two thirds of patients. In approximately one fourth, it occurs in the proximal portion of the descending aorta, and in nearly one tenth, the defect occurs in the aortic arch. A second tear (reentry) will be found distally in 15% of patients and is in the abdominal aorta or iliac arteries. Rarely, no tear can be identified, suggesting that defective vasa vasorum or medial necrosis may be the inciting event. Intramural hematoma can precede aortic dissection and when present within the ascending aorta ought to be treated with operative intervention because of the increased risk of dissection or rupture.[33,34]

A number of factors come into play when the dissection is propagated. These include blood pressure, left ventricular contractility, turbulence, and steepness of the pulse wave (dP/dt)—that is, change in pressure over time. In an experimental model, the pulse pressure is the most critical force in propagating the dissection.[35] Once blood under pressure enters the media, dissection of the entire aorta takes only a few seconds.[27] The outer wall, encompassing the false lumen and usually consisting of little more than adventitia, is exceedingly thin and therefore vulnerable to rupture. This explains the near-instantaneous death of many patients who suffer aortic dissection. A few days after the onset of the process, aortic wall necrosis may develop, further increasing the risk of rupture. In one series of 34 necropsies, 62% of the specimens revealed aortic wall necrosis.[36]

Although identical histopathologic features are not found in all aortic dissections, the gross pathologic findings usually are similar. A tear in the ascending aorta commonly involves the right lateral wall, and the dissection follows along the greater curvature of the aortic arch. This explains the frequency with which the brachiocephalic arteries are involved in type A dissection.

Despite the intimal tear occurring most frequently in the ascending aorta, the descending aorta is the most commonly involved segment because in the great majority of patients, dissection of the ascending aorta extends into the descending thoracic aorta. It is uncommon for a descending aortic dissection (DeBakey type III) to exhibit retrograde extension back into the ascending aorta. Dissections limited to the ascending aorta (DeBakey type II) are quite uncommon.[20]

Branches of the aorta along the course of dissection may shear off and become occluded or can remain in continuity with either the true or the false lumen. Moreover, a branch itself could dissect—a more likely consequence with a large artery. These several anatomic variations help to explain the diverse signs and symptoms associated with acute aortic dissection.

In the acute phase (the first 2 weeks), aortic enlargement is diffuse but generally does not reach aneurysmal proportions. Blood almost always extravasates through the thinned-out adventitia, forming a hematoma, which may be localized or quite extensive. Significant anemia can result. Rupture is the most common cause of death in the acute phase; the most frequent site of rupture is into the pericardial cavity, causing tamponade. Central neurologic injury can result from compromise of the arch vessels. Other causes of death with involvement of the aortic root include myocardial infarction from coronary ostial compromise and acute left-sided heart failure from severe aortic regurgitation. Rare complications include aortic-arterial or aortic–right ventricular fistula or high-degree heart block resulting from retrograde dissection into the aortic root and septum. Over time, the thin wall of the residual pseudoaneurysm tends to enlarge and become weaker and can eventually rupture—hence the need for routine follow-up evaluation. Spontaneous thrombosis of the false lumen rarely occurs, but a distal reentry site may help decompress that false lumen and increase chances of survival. Long-term survival has been postulated to be related to the distance of the proximal tear from the aortic valve; once healing has occurred, the longer the false channel, the longer the survival.[20]

The mortality rate from acute type A dissection has been variously reported in early series as high as 1% to 2% per hour in the first 48 hours after the onset of symptoms.[9,25] More recent data from Hagan and associates, collected in the International Registry of Acute Aortic Dissection (IRAD), reported a 58% in-hospital mortality rate in medically treated patients[37]—a marked improvement attributable to better medical therapy, but still indicative of the devastating nature of the disease.

Any dissected descending thoracic aorta may rupture freely into the left pleural space. The dissected abdominal aorta is at risk for contained rupture into the retroperitoneal space or free rupture into the peritoneal cavity. Significant compression of the true lumen by the false lumen can cause obstruction and distal malperfusion. Occlusion may rarely occur from circumferential loss of intima such that intussusception of the intima and the media occurs. Spinal cord ischemia, renal failure, intestinal ischemia, and lower limb malperfusion may be consequences of dissection in the descending aorta regardless of the site of origin. Although the incidence of serious malperfusion-related complications from descending aortic dissection is relatively low, the associated mortality rate is very high.[33] The prognosis is more favorable if the origin of any dissection involving the descending aorta is beyond the left subclavian artery, sparing the brachiocephalic branches, and if a reentry site is present.

SYMPTOMS AND PHYSICAL FINDINGS

The great majority (more than 85%) of patients with aortic dissection have chest pain as the presenting symptom (Box 34-1).[25] The pain often is described as ripping or tearing, and its onset, location, and pattern of radiation may give valuable clues to its cause. Sudden-onset, excruciating anterior chest pain that radiated or traveled to the interscapular region, neck, back, or epigastrium is a classic presentation for dissection originating in the ascending aorta. Interscapular pain with radiation to the lower back and abdomen may point to a descending aortic problem. There may have been associated syncope or temporary weakness of the lower limbs. If the brachiocephalic vessels are affected, hemiplegia may result, or paraplegia if spinal cord ischemia has occurred. The patient often is in severe distress, with tachycardia (from pain or heart failure, or both) and tachypnea. Hypertension is likely to be present. Hypotension is an ominous finding because it often correlates with a life-threatening complication such as hemopericardium with tamponade, aortic rupture, myocardial ischemia from coronary artery compromise, or left ventricular failure from acute aortic valvular insufficiency.[25] Loss of pulse in an arm or one or both legs may be falsely interpreted as an embolic phenomenon. Acute renal failure can occur, although one kidney usually is perfused through either the true or the false lumen. Acute abdominal findings, resulting from intestinal ischemia or infarction, are a sign of mesenteric arterial obstruction. Ecchymosis is very rarely seen acutely but may be observed later on the lower back, chest, or abdomen with significant leakage of blood from the involved aorta. A new murmur of aortic regurgitation is an excellent diagnostic clue but is found in only 50% of patients with ascending aortic dissection. No such murmur may be associated with acute aortic valve insufficiency if ventricular failure has developed from the acute volume overload.

Box 34-1

Acute Aortic Dissection: Symptoms, Signs, and Complications

Most Common Symptoms

Sudden-onset excruciating chest pain, often ripping or tearing in quality
Substernal if dissection originates in ascending aorta
Interscapular if process originates in descending aorta
Near-syncope or syncope

Signs

Hypertension usually present
Decrease or absence of one or more peripheral pulses after onset of chest pain
Inconsistent pulse volume often revealed on successive examinations of peripheral pulses
Murmur of aortic valve regurgitation possibly present.
Without ischemic ECG changes, aortic dissection must be ruled out
With ischemic ECG changes, aortic dissection must still be excluded

Complications

Rupture of false lumen causing pericardial tamponade, hemothorax, intraperitoneal or retroperitoneal hemorrhage
Involvement of one or more aortic branches in the dissection (partial or total obstruction or disruption) resulting in organ malperfusion; possible related clinical presentations: myocardial infarction, cerebrovascular accident (hemiplegia, coma), and/or intestinal, renal, spinal cord (paraplegia), and/or extremity ischemia; symptoms often transient
Distended false lumen or invagination of circumferentially torn intima/media may cause partial or complete aortic obstruction, leading to malperfusion distally
Acute aortic valve incompetence leading to left ventricular failure and pulmonary edema; diastolic murmur of aortic regurgitation highly suggestive of aortic dissection, but present only 50% of the time

Confusion with myocardial infarction can be resolved in many situations by performing a electrocardiogram (ECG). Left ventricular hypertrophy is quite commonly seen. A nonischemic ECG tracing favors a diagnosis other than infarction. An ECG tracing that indicates myocardial ischemia or infarction, however, does not rule out aortic dissection.

Patients who experience dissection originating in the ascending aorta generally are younger than those with more distal dissections (nearly 10 years' difference in mean age).[38] Sudden death can occur from rupture within the pericardium or chest or from shearing off of one or both coronary arteries at their ostia. Careful monitoring of peripheral pulses is necessary because changes in presence and quality can constitute important clues as to the diagnosis. Unfortunately, few patients will remain hemodynamically stable over the long term without treatment, but in an occasional case the acute dissection goes undiagnosed.

DIAGNOSIS AND IMAGING MODALITIES

Physician awareness and a high index of suspicion are critical to the timely diagnosis of aortic dissection. Occasionally treatment is delayed for days while a variety of conditions are searched for and not found; then an evaluation specifically for aortic dissection is undertaken almost as an afterthought. This delay in diagnosis can be detrimental and sometimes fatal because the dissection may extend and the aorta may become necrotic.[36]

When a patient seen in the emergency department for chest pain has a normal ECG tracing, acute aortic dissection should be suspected and the patient should be evaluated and managed accordingly. Pain control and treatment of blood pressure should be initiated as rapidly as possible. The principal diagnostic goal is confirmation of the dissection with localization of its origin and extent, visualization of major arterial branches and their relationship to the true or false lumen, and detection of associated complications. A variety of imaging modalities have been used successfully, each with specific strengths and weaknesses (Table 34-1). Appropriate use of any imaging techniques must take into account the patient-specific circumstances, the availability of a particular test, and the clinician's experience in performing and interpreting it.

Table 34-1. Comparison of Diagnostic Imaging Modalities for Evaluation of Aortic Dissection

	CT/CTA	TEE	MRI/MRA
Accuracy with classic dissection	+++	+++	+++
Accuracy with dissection variants	+++	+	+++
Visualization of entire aorta	+++	−	+++
Branch artery involvement	+++	+	+++
Coronary artery involvement	++	++	++
Aortic valve involvement	+	+++	+
Entry/reentry tear localization	+++	+	+++
Rupture	+++	++	+++
Objectivity/reproducibility	+++	+	+++
Portability	−	+++	−
Availability	+++	++	+
Speed	+++	++	+
Ease of monitoring patients	+++	+++	−
Patient comfort/lack of invasiveness	+++	−	+

CT, computed tomography; CTA, computed tomographic angiography; MRI, magnetic resonance imaging; MRA, magnetic resonance angiography; TEE, transesophageal echocardiography.
From Kapustin AJ, Litt HI: Diagnostic imaging for aortic dissection. Semin Thorac Cardiovasc Surg 2005;17:221.

The chest film is almost never diagnostic by itself but may increase clinical suspicion, especially if comparison with previous films can be made. A normal appearance on the chest film in no way excludes the diagnosis, but a variety of abnormalities seen on a plain film should allow the next study performed to confirm the diagnosis. Findings that may be seen with aortic dissection include a widened superior mediastinum, significant discrepancy between the diameters of the ascending and descending segments of the aorta, aortic outline irregularity, a localized density on the aortic arch distal to the left subclavian artery, and the presence of intimal calcification more than 1 cm from the outer shadow of the aorta. Other, even less specific findings may include deviation of the trachea to the right due to enlargement of the aortic knob, left pleural effusion, and increased cardiothoracic ratio.

Before the general availability of computed tomography (CT) and computed tomographic angiography (CTA), the aortogram including images enhanced by digital subtraction was considered the "gold standard" for evaluation and diagnosis of aortic dissection. Aortography has since fallen into disfavor as the diagnostic study of choice owing in part to its invasive nature and a relatively high false-negative rate.[39] Although it can be used even in critically ill patients, its sensitivity is lower than for CT and its specificity is no better. Reliance on contrast does not ensure direct visualization of a thrombosed lumen or intramural hematoma, or occasionally even comfirm the presence of a second, false lumen.[40] Nevertheless, endovascular intervention in the management of dissections with stenting across intimal tears, fenestration of intimal flaps, and opening occluded branch vessels has brought a resurgence in the use of catheter aortography,[41,42] but for therapy rather than for diagnosis.

Early-generation CT was hampered by technical factors resulting in false-positive and false-negative results often requiring catheter aortography for confirmation.[43] The advent of the spiral (helical) CT, followed by the introduction of multidetector CT in the late 1990s, has changed the way in which the diagnosis of aortic dissection is made[44,45] (see Fig. 34-3). Data collected from 1996 to 1998 by the International Registry of Acute Aortic Dissection showed that CT was used as the primary diagnostic modality in 61% of the cases. Transthoracic echocardiography (TTE) or transesophageal echocardiography (TEE), or a combination of both, was used in 33%. Catheter aortography at 4.4% and magnetic resonance imaging (MRI) at 1.8% were rarely used.[37]

The technological limitations of the early generation of CT equipment have been overcome by the use of helical (spiral) multidetector scanners with ECG-triggering or ECG-gating that can eliminate both motion and streak artifact.[46,47] Furthermore, currently available spiral multidetector scanner technology allows volume-rendered three-dimensional reconstruction of CT angiograms (Fig. 34-4) that are superior to MR images.[44,48]

Like aortography, CT requires the administration of iodinated contrast medium and does expose the patient

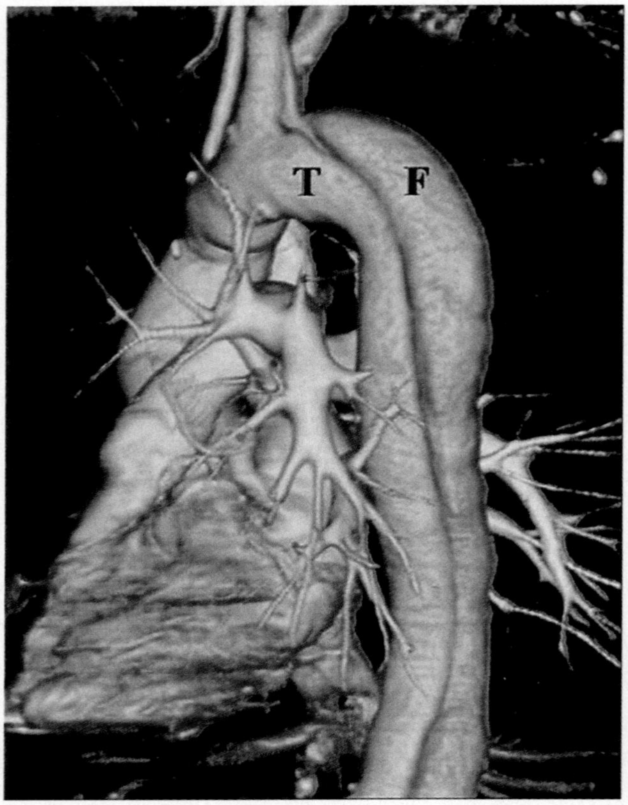

Figure 34-4. Volume-rendered enhanced image from computed tomographic angiography study showing true (T) and false (F) lumens in the descending thoracic aorta. (From Kapustin AJ, Litt HI: Diagnostic imaging for aortic dissection. Semin Thorac Cardiovasc Surg 2005;17:219.)

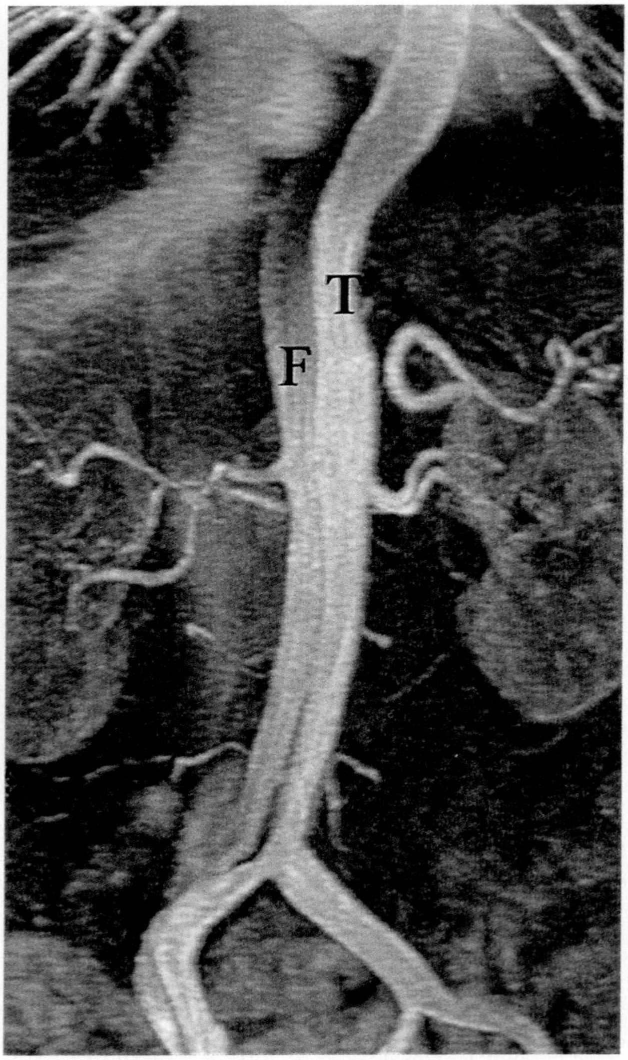

Figure 34-5. Image from gadolinium-enhanced magnetic resonance angiographic study demonstrating both true (T) and false (F) lumens in the abdominal aorta. Each lumen supplies a different renal artery. (From Kapustin AJ, Litt HI: Diagnostic imaging for aortic dissection. Semin Thorac Cardiovasc Surg 2005;17:221.)

to ionizing radiation, either of which could be contraindicated.

MRI also has proved to be an excellent method for evaluating the thoracic aorta. Its findings are similar to those of CT, the most reliable diagnostic finding being demonstration of two lumens separated by an intimal flap. Gadolinium-enhanced magnetic resonance angiography (MRA) allows the visualization of blood flow, which can be used to detect the presence and magnitude of aortic regurgitation or to demonstrate communication between the true and false lumens at the site of an intimal tear. An intimal flap can be identified in most cases (Fig. 34-5), except when the false lumen is completely thrombosed. With expert interpretation, the diagnostic accuracy of MRI for aortic dissection approaches 100%.[49] Disadvantages are that it should not be performed in patients with pacemakers or defibrillators, aneurysm clips, or ferrous metal implants and that it cannot be easily performed in patients with claustrophobia or on life support equipment (ventilators, monitors, intravenous infusion pumps). Image acquisition, despite advances in the technology, is more time consuming than with CT, and availability still remains an issue. Because it entails no radiation exposure, MRI has been recommended as the appropriate initial study for stable patients[50] and is the modality of choice for long-term follow-up evaluation.[45]

Because two-dimensional echocardiography is readily available and noninvasive and can be performed rapidly in the emergency department or intensive care unit (ICU), TTE should be performed early in the evaluation of any patient in whom the diagnosis of ascending aortic dissection is seriously entertained. Pericardial fluid can be seen; if an effusion is present, signs of tamponade can be identified. TTE can help identify aortic dissection if multiple views are obtained—specifically, suprasternal, subcostal, and right parasternal.[51] The intimal flap floats within the lumen, with motion that is "out of sync" with the movement of surrounding structures. To minimize the chance of a false-positive result, the flap should be visualized in more than one view. The addition of color Doppler helps to identify flow artifacts (as opposed to an intimal flap) within the ascending aorta by demonstrating flow between the true and false channels at the site of an intimal tear and by showing a difference in the timing or direction of flow within the two lumens.[52] In acute aortic regurgitation, the typical diastolic murmur often is absent: color Doppler permits detection and quantification of aortic regurgitation. TTE is especially useful for diagnosing dissections involving the ascending aorta but is much less sensitive for descending dissections.[39] If a dissection is not visualized, finding regional wall motion abnormalities may suggest an alternative diagnosis such as coronary ischemia.

TEE (Fig. 34-6) can be performed safely on most critically ill patients in a monitored setting.[53,54] To avoid precipitating hypertension, tachycardia, or gagging and straining in a patient with suspected dissection, conscious sedation should be administered. By using a multiplane transducer (omniprobe), nearly all of the thoracic aorta can be visualized, including most of the arch. The area from the distal ascending aorta to the midarch, however, is difficult to evaluate with TEE because of interposition of the airway between the esophagus and the aorta.[55] The sensitivity of TEE for thoracic aortic dissection is close to 100%, but specificity is lower, owing primarily to linear (reverberation) artifacts sometimes visualized within the ascending aorta, which may simulate an intimal flap.[50] Color flow Doppler should be used during TEE to identify flow through or on either side of any suspected intimal flap (Fig. 34-7). TEE also is helpful in evaluating involvement of the coronary ostia and aortic valve. As with TTE, regional and overall ventricular wall motion can be evaluated and the presence of pericardial effusion can be determined. TEE has been used successfully as the only diagnostic procedure before emergency operative repair.[56]

Evaluation of a patient for suspected aortic dissection may employ CT, TTE or TEE (or both), or MRI as the initial modality (after a plane chest film). (Figure 34-8 presents a decision tree for diagnosis of suspected aortic dissection.) Which study to perform depends on what other major diagnosis is most important to exclude. Patient stability also plays an important role. In the presence of hypotension or myocardial ischemia, a screening TTE can be rapidly performed. Because the equipment is portable, a TTE or TEE examination can be easily accomplished without transporting the patient from the monitored setting. A CT is the appropriate initial study if pulmonary embolism or pneumonia is under consideration. In a stable patient with blood pressure differential between the arms, either CT or MRI is suitable.[43] As part of the evaluation phase of acute aortic dissection, contrast aortography has little role.[45] It probably will play an ever-

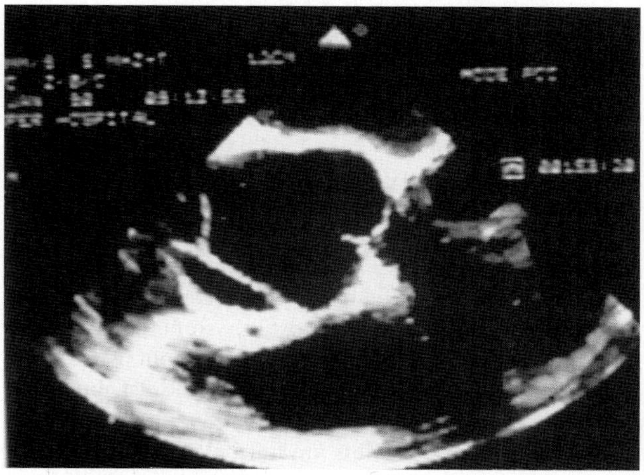

Figure 34-6. Transesophageal echocardiogram image showing intimal flap in ascending aorta extending to the aortic annulus. (Courtesy of Priscilla Peters, Cooper University Hospital, Camden, NJ.)

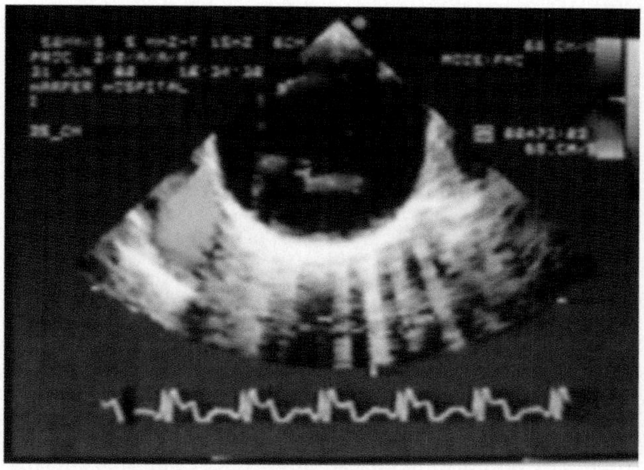

Figure 34-7. Image from transesophageal echocardiogram revealing an intimal flap in the descending aorta. Color Doppler shows flow through two fenestrations in the flap. (Courtesy of Priscilla Peters, Cooper University Hospital, Camden, NJ.)

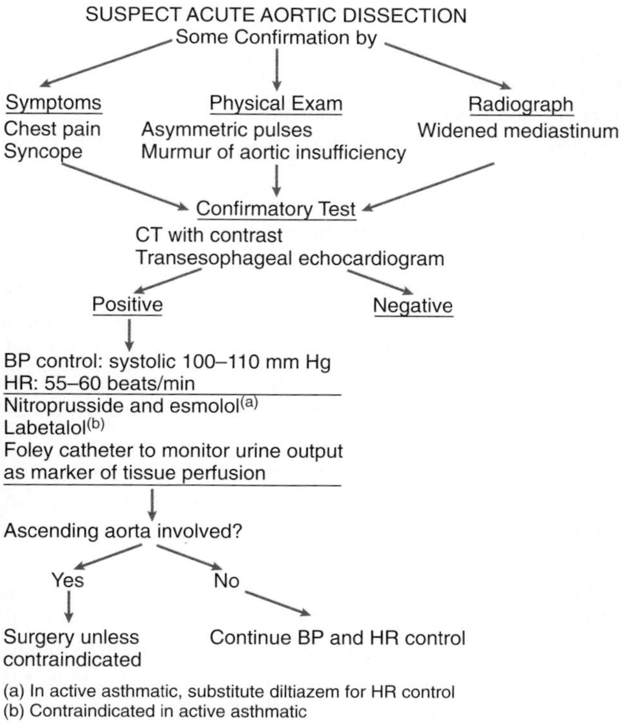

Figure 34-8. Algorithm for confirming a suspected case of acute aortic dissection. BP, blood pressure; CT, computed tomography; HR, heart rate.

increasing role in therapy as percutaneous catheter-based intervention to treat the dissection or its complications becomes more prevalent.[40,41] If operative therapy is indicated, and time and patient stability permit, TEE may be performed before the patient is moved to the operating room in order to help surgeons, anesthesiologists, and perfusionists plan for the conduct of the operation. In any case, unless a known contraindication such as esophageal disease would make passage of the probe hazardous, intraoperative TEE should be undertaken to evaluate both the aortic valve and ventricular function before and after CPB.

Often a patient arrives in the ICU from a referring institution having already had a CT scan as the initial screening test. If adequate information is gained from evaluating the CT findings, therapy can start immediately. Should the diagnosis be in question, however, further studies to elucidate the type of dissection and its extent are warranted.

THERAPEUTIC CONSIDERATIONS

Operative Approach

With few exceptions, surgeons agree that acute dissections involving the ascending aorta or proximal arch are best treated by operation. Such surgery relieves or prevents the life-threatening complications of aortic regurgitation, coronary artery disruption, neurologic compromise, and rupture into the pulmonary artery, the interventricular septum, or most commonly the pericardial sac.[17,57-60] Contraindications to surgical treatment are few and include coma, massive stroke, extensive bowel infarction, and bilateral renal infarctions—all evidence of severe malperfusion. These preoperative malperfusion syndromes may be associated with excessive mortality (89%) when surgery is immediately undertaken. Deeb and coworkers reported improved outcome in those patients with an average delay of 21 days, during which a mortality rate of 5%, from aortic rupture, was observed.[58,61]

Acute dissection arising in the descending aorta that is complicated by rupture, persistent or recurrent pain (a symptom of progression), vascular compromise not amenable to catheter-based fenestration or stenting, or dilatation greater than 6.5 cm is best treated surgically.[33,62] Dissection associated with Marfan syndrome should be treated surgically in most cases because of the high probability of rupture or recurrent dissection.

The goal of surgical therapy is to resect the most dangerously involved segment of aorta, reapproximate the dissected layers both proximally and distally, and reestablish aortic continuity.

Immediate operation yields the best results for acute dissection complicated by aortic regurgitation. The method used to restore aortic valve competence is controversial. Some surgeons consider valve replacement mandatory; others have reported excellent results with reconstructive surgery.[58,63,64] Current practice favors graft replacement of only the affected segment of the ascending aorta, unless the patient has Marfan syndrome or annuloaortic ectasia, in which case insertion of a valved conduit with coronary reimplantation is advisable.[65-67] In a Stanford series of 32 patients managed by graft replacement of the ascending aorta, only two (13%) subsequently required valve replacement. Occasionally, malperfusion of vital arteries may occur; for example, disruption of both renal arteries may cause anuria. Restoration of blood flow to the kidneys should precede management of the thoracic aortic dissection. The same is true for intestinal ischemia caused by interruption of blood flow into the celiac and superior mesenteric arteries.

Anterior or type A dissections are approached through a median sternotomy. CPB is initiated using the femoral artery[68] or right axillary artery[69] and a double-stage right atrial venous cannula. Intraoperative TEE, along with cerebral oximetry, is used to detect malperfusion that may occur with the use of femoral artery perfusion. A short period of hypothermic circulatory arrest without, or a longer period with, retrograde cerebral perfusion (via the superior vena cava), or a still longer period with antegrade cerebral perfusion (via balloon-tipped catheters in the innominate and left carotid arteries), can be used during an open distal anastomosis,[70] depending on the extent of aorta that requires replacement. A tear extending into the arch, or occurring primarily in the arch and extending into the descending aorta will require ascending aorta and either hemiarch or full arch replacement. If the brachiocephalic vessels can be included together as a Carrell (island) patch, that should be done. Extensive dissection involving those vessels may require a multibranched arch graft with individual artery anastomosis. If total arch replacement is necessary, leaving an "elephant trunk" segment of prosthetic graft in the descending aorta can facilitate endovascular stent-graft deployment, either antegrade through the open aorta at the same time or retrograde later.[71,72] Once the distal anastomosis is complete, the aorta and brachiocephalic vessels are "de-aired" and the graft is clamped. CPB is restarted and if the false lumen is pressurized or the graft is not, the perfusion cannula is changed from wherever it was placed to the newly inserted graft. The aortic root is then addressed as the patient is rewarmed.

As the intimal tear will be found in the ascending aorta in two thirds of the patients, it can be resected with only ascending graft replacement. With involvement of a coronary artery, or if the intimal defect extends down into the sinus of Valsalva, aortic root replacement with a valved conduit most often is needed. Any condition that would compromise a good long-term result, such as Marfan syndrome, a connective tissue disorder, or annuloaortic ectasia, should be treated by root replacement. Dissection involving a coronary artery ostium sometimes can be repaired with reconstruction of the ostium but usually will require coronary artery bypass grafting to the distribution(s) of the affected vessel.

If the aortic valve leaflets are normal and regurgitation is caused by prolapse of the commissures, resuspension of the commissures should restore valvular competence. The layers of the aorta are reapproximated using polytetrafluoroethylene (Teflon) felt or "biologic glue."[70,73,74] and a graft is placed. Valve-sparing aortic root replacement may be performed in those patients who have a long life expectancy. This complex procedure requires resection of all aorta distal to the annulus, creation of neo-sinuses, and coronary artery reimplantation, with reconstitution of aortic lumen continuity.[75]

When surgery is required because of aortic size or complications, dissection involving the descending thoracic aorta (posterior or type B) is approached through a left posterolateral thoracotomy. Resection of the proximal descending aorta including the site of the intimal tear, along with any significantly dilated distal segments, is sufficient. Although this can be performed by means of a simple cross-clamp technique, it is no longer recommended; rather, use of some type of "left heart bypass" (LHB) to provide proximal decompression and distal perfusion is preferable. Coselli[76] and coworkers reported a series of 1250 patients in which LHB was clearly superior to no LHB at prevention of neurologic injury associated with thoracoabdominal aortic surgery. There are various ways in which this can be accomplished: femoral-femoral bypass, use of a pump oxygenator, or left atrial–femoral bypass using only a pump.

Perioperative Therapy

DeBakey and associates[12] introduced surgical therapy for acute dissection in 1955. Medical therapy before surgical intervention for patients with anterior dissections and as the definitive therapy for patients with uncomplicated posterior dissections was first advocated by Wheat and coworkers[14] 10 years later. Current treatment of aortic dissection depends on the site of origin and the extent of the dissecting process. As initially described by Wheat and colleagues, medical therapy has two important objectives: rapidly lowering arterial blood pressure in hypertensive patients and reducing the force of left ventricular contraction in all patients. The basis for β-blocker therapy in normotensive patients is an experimental model of aortic dissection in which cardiac ejection velocity constituted the major shearing force that tended to initiate and propagate dissection.[35]

Immediate initiation of medical therapy is imperative. The patient is admitted to the ICU, where vital signs are continuously monitored. Blood pressure should be determined in both upper extremities. Carotid pulses should be palpated for equality. Intra-arterial pressure monitoring permits precise control of blood pressure during administration of potent hypotensive agents. For type A dissection, a radial artery (chosen by whichever side has the higher blood pressure) or left femoral arterial line should be used and care taken that the patient's highest blood pressure is being monitored. If possible, the right femoral artery and vein should remain unviolated in order to facilitate cannulation for CPB during operative intervention. For type B dissection, invasive blood pressure monitoring is best done via the right radial artery. In any patient who will require operative intervention, use of a Swan-Ganz pulmonary artery catheter that allows cardiac filling pressures, cardiac output, and mixed venous oxygen saturation ($S\bar{v}O_2$) all to be determined continuously is helpful. Drugs should be administered intravenously, rather than orally, to achieve rapid onset of action and to keep the stomach as empty as possible.

Therapy designed to reduce dP/dt is part of initial management for all patients including those who have become pain free and are normotensive. The heart rate is lowered to 60 to 75 beats per minute. The systolic pressure is rapidly reduced to the lowest level tolerated while adequate end organ function is maintained, usually 100 to 120 mm Hg, with a mean blood pressure of 60 to 75 mm Hg. Observation of mental status, ECG and blood pressure monitoring, and insertion of a bladder catheter are helpful in ascertaining adequacy of perfusion to the brain, heart, and kidneys, respectively.

A traditional approach has been to administer esmolol, given intravenously first as a loading dose and then as a continuous infusion, to achieve a heart rate of approximately 60 to 75 beats per minute, followed by intravenous nitroprusside to lower the blood pressure further if necessary to achieve the target (Table 34-2). Alternatively, metoprolol, with a longer duration of action than for esmolol, may be given by intravenous bolus. β-Blockade should be accomplished first because nitroprusside (a potent vasodilator) administered alone increases the shearing force by increasing dP/dt. Labetalol, which is a selective α_1-blocker with nonselective β-blockading action (the α/β effect ratio for intravenous therapy is 7:1), can reduce blood pressure without reflex tachycardia. It does cause vasodilatation and therefore must be used with caution. In patients with a contraindication to β-blockade (severe bronchospasm, symptomatic bradycardia, severe congestive heart failure), an alternative is the calcium channel blocker diltiazem given as an intravenous infusion after a loading dose. Intravenous administration of morphine sulfate is useful for pain control and also to help control blood pressure. Before a definitive diagnostic procedure is performed, the patient's blood pressure should be stabilized.

The pain of aortic dissection usually subsides once progression of the disease is halted and can be used as a therapeutic marker.

Most clinicians consider medical therapy the treatment of choice for uncomplicated posterior or type B dissection.[77] Some also use it for uncomplicated and stable anterior or type A dissection in patients who are poor surgical candidates. Medical management may be considered for dissections originating in the aortic arch and for patients with ascending aortic dissection who have exceedingly high risk of death, such as the very elderly.[78]

Prevention of postoperative hypertension is crucial. Successful repair of an ascending dissection effectively eliminates the acute risks, and because most dissections originating in the ascending aorta extend into the descending aorta, intensive medical therapy will still be required. Lifelong control of hypertension is mandatory because good control of blood pressure significantly reduces the incidence of late false channel aneurysm development to 10% to 20% from 50%[17,79,80] and minimizes the incidence of redissection or rupture. Periodic evaluation of the aorta using noninvasive testing modalities such as CT

Table 34-2. Drugs Used in Medical Therapy for Acute Aortic Dissection

Drug	Dosage	Effects	Contraindications	Comments
Esmolol	Load 500 μg/kg IV, titrate from 150-350 μg/kg/min	↓dP/dt ↓Heart rate ↓MAP	Hypotension Bronchospasm Severe heart failure Heart block	β_1-Selectivity lost at doses >350 μg/kg/min If needed, add vasodilator to lower MAP
Metoprolol	5 mg IV q5 min×3, then 5 mg IV q4-6h	As for esmolol	As for esmolol	Inject over 3-5 min
Labetalol	20 mg IV q10 min, then 20-80 mg IV q4-6h *or* IV infusion 1-3 mg/min	Vasodilatation (α-blockade)	As for esmolol	Inject over 2 min Labetalol α/β 7:1 200 mg/160 mL D_5W (1 mg/mL)
Nitroprusside	IV infusion 0.3-10 μg/kg/min	Vasodilatation ↑dP/dt ↓MAP Reflex ↑heart rate	Hypotension Caution in renal failure	Use with β-blockade to avoid ↑dP/dt Cyanide toxicity
Nicardipine	IV infusion 5-15 mg/min IV	Vasodilatation Slight ↑dP/dt	Caution in severe liver disease	↓Clearance in severe liver disease
Diltiazem	Load 10-20 mg IV Titrate 5-15 mg/h	↓Heart rate ↓MAP Slight ↓dP/dt	Hypotension Heart block	Inject over 2 min Use if β-blocker is contraindicated

dP/dt, rate of rise in blood pressure; IV, intravenous; MAP, mean arterial pressure.

or MRI is essential for timely discovery of potentially life-threatening complications such as ongoing aneurysmal dilatation.

The usual spectrum of postoperative complications are encountered, including hemorrhage, renal and pulmonary insufficiency, perioperative myocardial infarction, low-cardiac output syndrome, bowel necrosis, cerebrovascular accident, paraplegia, deep venous thrombosis, and pulmonary embolism. Regrettably, most patients subjected to surgery for any type of dissection are not cured because of the persistence of the false lumen and its propensity to enlarge over time—hence the need for permanent antihypertensive treatment.

Options to Open Surgery

Recent advances in catheter-based technology, including endovascular stent-grafting, have been applied, with various degrees of success, to descending aortic disease including dissection. In theory, coverage of the site of intimal disruption with a covered stent would seem the ideal treatment. A practical advantage to endovascular therapy is its less invasive nature. Endoluminal stent-grafts delivered by a femoral approach have been used to treat complicated descending dissections.[81,82] A covered stent is deployed to treat the primary intimal tear, and bare metal stents are placed to obliterate the false channel and restore renal and mesenteric flow if compromised.

In an acute setting, restoring visceral blood flow by balloon fenestration of the septum between a true and a false lumen may obviate the need for a major transabdominal or retroperitoneal surgical revascularization procedure in a desperately ill patient.[83,84]

Although technical success as reported in the European Collaborators on Stent Graft Techniques for Thoracic Aortic Aneurysm and Dissection Repair (EUROSTAR) and the United Kingdom Thoracic Endograft Registry[85] was very high, and mortality was lower than for open treatment, the appropriate timing of the endovascular therapy remains unclear. Stent-graft deployment in a newly dissected descending aorta was complicated by retrograde dissection causing a type A dissection in just under 7%, with an associated mortality rate of 40%.[86] Bortone and associates found that because of false lumen progression and the presence of multiple reentry points, nearly two thirds of patients did not get technically satisfactory results when the stent-graft placement was delayed.[87] Some devices may serve better in acute situations and others in chronic ones. Proper patient selection will remain the most significant predictor of success. As with any emerging technology, improvements in endovascular stent-grafts and their delivery and fixation systems will continue.

OUTCOMES AND PROGNOSIS

The rationale for surgical treatment of acute type A dissection is universally recognized. Patients with acute ascending aortic dissection treated medically fare far worse than those with dissection involving the descending aorta. The current 6-month and 10-year survival rates reported for type A dissection managed medically are 43% and 27%, respectively; for type B dissection they are 90% and 50%.[37,66]

Operative mortality rates for patients undergoing surgery for acute dissection involving the ascending aorta range from 8.6% to 25%.[33,70,75,88,89] Long-term survival has improved and can be expected to be approximately 90% at 1 year,[33,90] from 71% to 89% at 5 years, and from 54% to 66% at 10 years.[75,88,89] A significant decline in postoperative mortality related to ascending dissections has been observed during the last 25 years, particularly in those centers in which dissections are frequently treated. This may be due in part to survival of some patients after the initial dissection for long enough to be referred to a tertiary center.[33] Alternately, recognizing that some patients suffering serious visceral, renal, or extremity malperfusion represented an excessive surgical risk caused the surgery to be delayed until their condition improved.[61] Intimal tear extension requiring reconstruction that includes hemiarch replacement has been reported variously as being associated with increased operative risk[57,88] and also as risk neutral.[90,91] The use of biologic glue to strengthen the dissected aortic wall and obliterate the false lumen at the anastomotic sites, although not universally accepted, decreases acute suture line bleeding. Neurologic injury, low cardiac output, and bleeding are the principal causes of death.

Little controversy exists over the treatment of choice for the acute type B variety. For most patients, unless life- or limb-threatening complications occur, medical therapy is considered superior to surgical treatment, although neither confers a significant advantage in long-term survival benefit.[92,93] If a complication such as rupture necessitating emergency surgery arises, however, the mortality rate can approach 50%. Fortunately, this situation occurs less than 10% of the time. Mortality is still high if operation is required within the acute (first 2 weeks) time frame.[33] Analysis of all early postoperative complications shows a much lower stroke rate than with repair of ascending dissections, although the incidence of pulmonary complications and spinal cord injury is higher.

Percutaneous interventions have been applied successfully to restore visceral and extremity perfusion, limiting the need for open revascularization. Patients treated primarily with endovascular stent-grafts for descending aortic dissection were considered to be high-risk candidates for open repair. The optimal timing for stent-grafting in type B dissections has not been established. Midterm results at 1 year were very favorable when compared with surgery.[85,94]

Immediate and intensive medical stabilization with administration of a β-blocker to control blood pressure and shearing force, expeditious operative intervention when indicated, use of endovascular technology when appropriate, and careful long-term follow-up evaluation have improved outcomes for patients with aortic dissection. Because the technology of the most recently introduced therapeutic modality (endovascular stent-graft) is still undergoing change, the optimal approach to aortic dissection remains in evolution.

KEY POINTS

- Dissection is the most common aortic catastrophe.
- An abnormal ECG tracing does not exclude aortic dissection.
- Immediate initiation of medical therapy for aortic dissection is imperative; start as soon as the diagnosis is suspected.
- Aortography should no longer be considered the "gold standard" for the diagnosis of aortic dissection. CT and CTA are more sensitive and more specific and generally are more readily available.
- The goals of imaging are to confirm the diagnosis of dissection, define its origin, ascertain its extent and the involvement of major arterial branches, and identify complications.
- It is important to look at the full CT scan, not just the report.
- TEE is extremely valuable in the ICU and operating suite to help plan operative strategy.
- MRI and MRA have excellent diagnostic accuracy and provide the best imaging for long-term follow-up evaluation.
- Acute dissection complicated by aortic regurgitation is best treated by immediate operation.
- Contraindications to early surgical therapy for type A aortic dissection include conditions representing evidence of severe malperfusion: coma, massive stroke, extensive bowel infarction, and bilateral renal infarctions.
- Medical therapy is the treatment of choice for uncomplicated type B dissection.
- Acute type B dissection complicated by rupture, persistent or recurrent pain, malperfusion not amenable to catheter-based intervention, or dilatation greater than 6.5 cm should be treated surgically.
- Dissection complicating Marfan syndrome should be treated surgically because of the high incidence of recurrent dissection or rupture.

REFERENCES

1. Laennec RTH: De l'ascultations médiate, ou traité du diagnostic des maladies des poumons et du coeur, fondé principalemente sur ce nouveau moyen d'exploration. JA Brosson & JD Chaudé, Paris, 1819.
2. Sennertus D: Cap. 42. Op Omn Lib 1650;5:306.
3. Nicholls F: Some observations on aneurysms in general and in particular on the foregoing. Proc Soc Lond 1728;35:440.
4. Nicholls F: Observations concerning the body of His Late Majesty. Philos Trans London 1762;52:265.
5. Peacock TB: Report of cases of dissecting aneurysm. Trans London Pathol Soc 1863;14:87.
6. Marfan A: Un cas de deformation congenitale des quatre membres, plus prononcée aux extremités, caracterisée par l'allongement des os avec un certain degré d'amincissement. Soc Hop Paris Bull Mem 1896;13:220-226.
7. Osler W: The Lumlian lectures on angina pectoris (lecture II). Lancet 1910;1:810.
8. Erdheim J: Medionecrosis aortae idiopathica. Virchows Arch Pathol 1929;273:454.
9. Shennan T: Dissecting aneurysms. Medical Research Clinical Special Report Series No. 193. His Majesty's Stationery Office, London, 1934.
10. Gurin D, Bulmer JW, Derby R: Dissecting aneurysm of the aorta: Diagnosis and operative relief of acute arterial obstruction due to this cause. N Y State J Med 1935;35:1200.
11. Shaw RS: Acute dissecting aortic aneurysms: Treatment by fenestration of the internal wall of the aneurysm. N Engl J Med 1995;253:331.
12. DeBakey ME, Cooley DA, Creech O Jr: Surgical considerations of dissecting

aneurysm of the aorta. Ann Surg 1955;142:586.
13. Morris GC Jr, Henly WS, DeBakey ME: Correction of acute dissecting aneurysm of aorta with valvular insufficiency. JAMA 1963;184:63.
14. Wheat MW, Palmer RF, Bartley TD, et al: Treatment of dissecting aneurysms of the aorta without surgery. J Thorac Cardiovasc Surg 1965;50:364.
15. Isselbacher EM, Eagle KA, Desanctis RW: Diseases of the aorta. In Braunwald E (ed): Heart Disease: A Textbook of Cardiovascular Medicine. WB Saunders, Philadelphia, 1997.
16. Braverman AC, Guven H, Beardslee MA, et al: The bicuspid valve. Curr Prob Cardiol 2005;30(9):470-522.
17. DeBakey ME, Henly WS, Cooley DA, et al: Surgical management of dissecting aneurysms of the aorta. J Thorac Cardiovasc Surg 1965;49:130.
18. Daily PO, Trueblood HW, Stinson EB, et al: Management of acute aortic dissections. Ann Thorac Surg 1970;10:237.
19. Najafi H, Dye WS, Javid H, et al: Acute aortic regurgitation secondary to aortic dissection: Surgical management without valve replacement. Ann Thorac Surg 1972;14:474.
20. Roberts WC: Aortic dissection: Anatomy, consequences, and causes. Am Heart J 1981;101:195.
21. Svensson LG, Crawford ES: Aortic dissection and aortic aneurysm surgery: Clinical observations, experimental investigations, and statistical analysis. Curr Probl Surg 1992;29:915.
22. Spittell PC, Spittell JA, Joyce JW, et al: Clinical features and differential diagnosis of aortic dissection: Experience with 236 cases. Mayo Clinic Proc 1993;68:642.
23. Larson EW, Edwards WD: Risk factors for aortic dissection: A necropsy study of 161 cases. Am J Cardiol 1984;53:849.
24. Edwards JE: Aneurysms of the thoracic aorta complicating coarctation. Circulation 1973;48:195.
25. Hirst AE Jr, Johns VJ Jr, Kime SW Jr: Dissecting aneurysm of the aorta: A review of 505 cases. Medicine (Baltimore) 1958;37:217.
26. Abbott ME: Congenital cardiac disease. In McCrae T (ed): Osler's Modern Medicine, 3rd ed, vol 4. Lea & Febiger, Philadelphia, 1927.
27. Najafi H: Vascular complications of extracorporeal circulation. In Cordell AR, Ellison RG (eds): Complications of Intrathoracic Surgery. Little, Brown, Boston, 1979.
28. Isner JM, Cohen SR, Virmani R, et al: Complications of the transaortic balloon counterpulsation device: Clinical and morphologic observations in 45 necropsy patients. Am J Cardiol 1980;45:260.
29. Muna WF, Spray TL, Morrow AG, Roberts WC: Aortic dissection after aortic valve replacement in patients with valvular stenosis. J Thorac Cardiovasc Surg 1977;74:65.
30. Nicholson WJ, Crawley IS, Logue RB, et al: Aortic root dissection complicating coronary bypass surgery. Am J Cardiol 1978;41:103.
31. Pieters F, Widdershoven J, Gerardy A, et al: Risk of aortic dissection after aortic valve replacement. Am J Cardiol 1993;72:1043.
32. Borger MA, Preston M, Ivanov J, et al: Should the ascending aorta be replaced more frequently in patients with bicuspid aortic valve disease? J Thorac Cardiovasc Surg 2004;128(5):677-683.
33. Gallo A, Davies RR, Coe MP, et al: Indications, timing, and prognosis of operative repair of aortic dissections. Semin Thorac Cardivasc Surg 2005;17:224-235.
34. Coady MA, Rizzo JA, Elefteriades JA: Pathologic variants of aortic dissections. Penetrating atherosclerotic ulcers and intramural hematomas. Cardiol Clin 1999;17(4):637-657.
35. Prokop EK, Wheat MR, Palmer RF: Hydrodynamic forces in dissecting aneurysm: In vitro studies in a Tygon model and in dog aortas. Circ Res 1970;27:121.
36. Barsky SH, Rosen S: Aortic infarction following dissecting aortic aneurysm. Circulation 1978;58:876.
37. Hagan PG, Nienaber CA, Isselbacher EM, et al: The International Registry of Acute Aortic Dissection (IRAD): New insights into an old disease. JAMA 2000;283:897-903.
38. Miller DC, Stinson EB, Oyer PE, et al: Operative treatment of aortic dissections: Experience with 125 patients over a sixteen-year period. J Thorac Cardiovasc Surg 1979;78:365.
39. Cigarroa JE, Isselbacher EM, DeSanctis RW, Eagle KA: Diagnostic imaging in the evaluation of suspected aortic dissection: Old standards and new directions N Engl J Med 1993;328:35.
40. Shuford WH, Sybers RG, Weens HS: Problems in the aortographic diagnosis of dissecting aneurysm of the aorta. N Engl J Med 1969;280:225-231.
41. Prendergast BD, Boon NA, Buckenham T: Aortic dissection: Advances in imaging and endoluminal repair. Cardiovasc Intervent Radiol 2002;25:95-97.
42. Hartnell GG, Gates J: Aortic fenestration: A why, when, how-to guide. Radiographics 2005;25:175-189.
43. Vasile N, Mathieu D, Keita K, et al: Computed tomography of thoracic aortic dissection: accuracy and pitfalls. J Comp Assist Tomogr 1986;10:211.
44. Hamada S, Takamiya M, Kimura K, et al: Type A aortic dissection: Evaluation with ultrafast CT. Radiology 1992;183:155.
45. Kapustin AJ, Litt HI: Diagnostic imaging for aortic dissection. Semin Thorac Cardiovasc Surg 2005;17:214-223.
46. Rubin GD, Shiau MC, Leung AN, et al: Aorta and iliac arteries: Single versus multiple detector-row helical CT angiography. Radiology 2000;215:670-676.
47. Roos JE, Willmann JK, Weishaupt D, et al: Thoracic aorta: Motion artifact reduction with retrospective and prospective electrocardiography-assisted multi-detector row CT. Radiology 2002;222:271-277.
48. Rubin GD: CT angiography of the thoracic aorta. Semin Roentgenol 2003;38:115-134.
49. Nienaber CA, Spielmann RP, Kodolitsch Y, et al: Diagnosis of thoracic aortic dissection. Circulation 1992;85:434.
50. Nienaber CA, Von Kodolitsch Y, Volkmar N, et al: The diagnosis of thoracic aortic dissection by noninvasive imaging procedures. N Engl J Med 1993;328:1-9.
51. Granato JE, Dee P, Gibson RS: Utility of two-dimensional echocardiography in suspected ascending aortic dissection. Am J Cardiol 1985;56:123.
52. Iliceto S, Nanda NC, Rizzon P, et al: Color Doppler evaluation of aortic dissection. Circulation 1987;75:748.
53. Adachi H, Omoto R, Kyo S, et al: Emergency surgical intervention of acute aortic dissection with the rapid diagnosis by transesophageal echocardiography. Circulation 1991;84:III-14.
54. Pearson AC, Castello R, Labovitz AJ, et al: Safety and utility of transesophageal echocardiography in the critically ill patient. Am Heart J 1990;119:1083.
55. Blanchard DG, Kimura BJ, Dittrich HC, DeMaria AN: Transesophageal echocardiography of the aorta. JAMA 1994;272:546.
56. Chan KL: Impact of transesophageal echocardiography on the treatment of patients with aortic dissection. Chest 1992;101:406.
57. Crawford ES, Kirklin JW, Naftel DC, et al: Surgery for acute ascending aortic dissection: Should the arch be included? J Thorac Cardiovasc Surg 1992;103:46-59.
58. Kouchoukos NT, Marshal WG Jr: Treatment of ascending aortic dissection in Marfan's syndrome. J Cardiac Surg 1986;1:333.
59. Miller DC: Surgical management of aortic dissections: Indications, perioperative management, and long-term results. In Doroghazi RM, Slater EE (eds): Aortic Dissection. McGraw-Hill, New York, 1983.
60. Najafi H: Aortic dissection. In Sabiston DC Jr, Spencer FC (eds): Gibbon's Surgery of the Chest. WB Saunders, Philadelphia, 1983.
61. Deeb GM, Williams DM, Bolling SF, et al: Surgical delay for acute type A dissection with malperfusion. Ann Thorac Surg 2002;64:1669-1677.
62. Borst HG, Heinemann MK, Stone CD: Surgical Treatment of Aortic Dissection. Churchill Livingstone, New York, 1996.
63. Bentall H, DeBono A: A technique for complete replacement of the ascending aorta. Thorax 1968;23:338.
64. Najafi H, Dye WS, Javid H, et al: Aortic insufficiency secondary to aortic root aneurysm and/or dissection. Arch Surg 1975;110:1401.
65. Masuda Y, Yamada Z, Morooka N, et al: Prognosis of patients with medically treated aortic dissections. Circulation 1991;84(suppl III):III-7.
66. Najafi H: Descending aortic aneurysm: Update of surgical management. Ann Thorac Surg 1993;55(4):1042.
67. Cachera JP, Vouhe PR, Loisance DY, et al: Surgical management of acute dissections involving the ascending aorta: Early and late results in 38 patients. J Thorac Cardiovasc Surg 1981;82:576.
68. Fusco DS, Shaw RK, Tranquilli M, et al: Femoral cannulation is safe for type A dissection repair. Ann Thorac Surg 2004;78:1285-1289.

69. Svensson LG, Blackstone EH, Rajeswaran J, et al: Does the arterial cannulation site for circulatory arrest influence stroke risk? Ann Thorac Surg 2004;78:1274-1284; discussion 1274-1284.
70. Bavaria JE, Brinster DR, Gorman RC, et al: Advances in the treatment of acute type A dissection: An integrated approach. Ann Thorac Surg 2002;74: S1848-S1852; discussion S1857-S1863.
71. Szeto WY, Gleason TG: Operative management of ascending aortic dissections. Semin Thorac Cardiovasc Surg 2005;17:247-255.
72. Kato M, Kuratani E, Kaneko M, et al: The results of total arch graft implantation with open stent-graft placement for type A aortic dissection. J Thorac Cardiovasc Surg 2002;134:531-540.
73. Chao HH, Torchiana DF: BioGlue: Albumin/glutaraldehyde sealant in cardiac surgery. J Card Surg 2003;18:500-503.
74. Raanani E, Georghiou GP, Kogan A, et al: "BioGlue" for the repair of aortic insufficiency in acute aortic dissection. J Heart Valve Disease 2004;13:734-737.
75. Kallenbach K, Oelze T, Salcher R, et al: Evolving strategies for treatment of acute aortic dissection type A. Circulation 2004;110:II243-II249.
76. Coselli JS: The use of left heart bypass in the repair of thoracoabdominal aortic aneurysms: Current techniques and results. Semin Thorac Cardiovasc Surg 2003;15:326-332.
77. Glower DD, Fann JI, Speier RH, et al: Comparison of medical and surgical therapy for uncomplicated descending aortic dissection. Circulation 1990;82(5 Suppl):iv39-iv46.
78. Centofanti P, Flocco R, Ceresa F, et al: Is surgery always mandatory for type A aortic dissection? Ann Thorac Surg 2006;82:1658-1664.
79. DeBakey ME, McCollum CH, Crawford ES, et al: Dissection and dissecting aneurysms of the aorta: Twenty-year follow-up of 527 patients treated surgically. Surgery 1982;92:1118.
80. Lemole GM, Strong MD, Spagna PM, Karmilowicz NP: Improved results for dissecting aneurysms: Intraluminal sutureless prosthesis. J Thorac Cardiovasc Surg 1982;83:249.
81. Mitchell RS: Endovascular solutions for diseases of the thoracic aorta. Cardiol Clin 1999;17(4):822.
82. Mitchell RS, Ishimaru S, Criado FJ, et al: Third International Summit on Thoracic Aortic Endografting: Lessons from long-term results of thoracic stent-graft repairs. J Endovasc Ther 2005;12:89-97.
83. Williams DM, Lee YD, Hamilton BH, et al: The dissected aorta: Percutaneous treatment of ischemic complications-principles and results. J Vasc Interv Radiol 1997;8(4):605-625.
84. Panneton JM, Teh SH, Cherry KJ, et al: Aortic fenestration for acute or chronic aortic dissection: An uncommon but effective procedure. J Vasc Surg 2000;32:711-720.
85. Leurs LJ, Bell R, Degrieck Y, et al: Endovascular treatment of thoracic aortic diseases: Combined experience from the EUROSTAR and United Kingdom Thoracic Endograft Registries. J Vasc Surg 2004;40:670-679.
86. Neuhauser B, Czermak BV, Fish J, et al: Type A dissection following endovascular thoracic aortic stent-graft repair. J Endovasc Ther 2005;12:74-81.
87. Bortone AS, Schena S, D'Agostino D, et al: Immediate versus delayed endovascular treatment of post-traumatic aortic pseudoaneurysms and type B dissections: Retrospective analysis and premises to the upcoming European trial. Circulation 2002;106:1234-1240.
88. Ehrlich MP, Ergin MA, McCullough JN, et al: Results of immediate surgical treatment of all acute type A dissections. Circulation 2000;102: III248-III252.
89. Driever R, Botsios S, Schmitz E, et al: Long-term effectiveness of operative procedures for Stanford type A aortic dissections. Cardiovasc Surg 2003;11:265-272.
90. Shiono M, Mitsumasa H, Akira S, et al: Validity of a limited ascending and hemiarch replacement for acute type A aortic dissection. Ann Thorac Surg 2006;82:1665-1669.
91. Moon MR, Sundt TM III, Pasque MK, et al: Does the extent of proximal or distal resection influence outcome for type A dissections? Ann Thorac Surg 2001;71:1244-1249; discussion 1249-1250.
92. Umana JP, Lai DT, Mitchell RS, et al: Is medical therapy still the optimal treatment strategy for patients with acute type B aortic dissections? J Thorac Cardiovasc Surg 2002;194:896-910.
93. Roseborough G, Burke J, Sperry J, et al: Twenty year experience with acute distal thoracic aortic dissections. J Vasc Surg 2004;40(2):235-246.
94. Peterson BG, Eskandari MK: Endovascular repair of descending aortic dissections. Semin Thorac Cardiovasc Surg 2005;17:268-273.

Chapter

35 Hypertensive Crises

Sergio L. Zanotti-Cavazzoni

Hypertension is a common clinical disorder. Estimates indicate that almost 30% of the United States adult population suffers from elevated blood pressure.[1] Furthermore, one third of these patients are unaware of their diagnosis, and of those who are diagnosed and treated, only 34% have adequate control of their blood pressure.[2] Severe elevations in blood pressure—hypertensive crises—will occur in approximately 1% of patients with chronic hypertension.[1,3] Hypertensive crises constitute a clinical problem that intensivists (i.e., intensive care physicians) will encounter in the hospital setting. Unfortunately, a paucity of clinical studies evaluating optimal therapeutic strategies and a lack of consideration for key pathophysiologic aspects have led to common misunderstandings and pitfalls in the management of patients with hypertensive crises.

DEFINITIONS

According to the seventh report of the Joint National Committee (JNC) on Detection, Evaluation, and Treatment of High Blood Pressure, hypertension is classified into three stages: *Prehypertension, Stage 1,* and *Stage 2*[3] (Table 35-1). The terms "malignant hypertension" and "accelerated hypertension" have been abandoned. These terms were used to describe severe elevations in blood pressure associated with advanced retinopathy, the equivalent of Keith-Wagener-Barker stages III and IV. Prognosis for these clinical entities has improved dramatically with the advent of effective drugs for hypertension. In addition, studies have demonstrated that retinopathy as measured by the Keith-Wagener-Barker classification does not correlate with severity of hypertension or outcomes.[4]

Hypertensive crises are defined as severe elevations in blood pressure. Although some authors have suggested a threshold value for diastolic blood pressure of 120 mm Hg, it is preferable to evaluate acute elevations of blood pressure within the context of each case and with consideration of the effects of a given blood pressure on organ function in the individual patient. For example, an acute rise in diastolic blood pressure to 100 mm Hg can cause significant damage in a previously normotensive person, whereas a diastolic pressure of 130 mm Hg may be tolerated in a patient with a history of uncontrolled hypertension. As discussed later on, these patients will require different therapeutic approaches. A traditional and useful clinical approach has been to classify hypertensive crises as either hypertensive emergencies or hypertensive urgencies.

A *hypertensive emergency* is characterized by severe elevation in blood pressure associated with the presence of acute end-organ damage. Hypertensive emergencies require immediate control of blood pressure, within 1 to 2 hours, to prevent further organ damage. This will usually require the use of intravenous medications and invasive monitoring (using an arterial line) in a high-dependency unit such as the intensive care unit (ICU). The principal systems susceptible to acute end-organ damage from severe elevations in blood pressure are the central nervous, cardiovascular, and renal systems (Fig. 35-1). Several clinical situations are associated with hypertensive emergencies (Box 35-1). The absolute level of blood pressure and the time course of this elevation will determine the development of a hypertensive emergency. However, acute end-organ damage can occur at different blood pressure values in different patients. Therefore, it is more useful to define hypertensive emergencies by the presence of acute end-organ damage than by specific values for systolic or diastolic blood pressure. In addition to immediate therapeutic interventions, patients with hypertensive emergency may require further diagnostic evaluation to determine the cause of their elevated blood pressure. Depending on the population studied, from 20% to 50% of patients presenting with a hypertensive emergency will have a secondary cause of hypertension identified.[5]

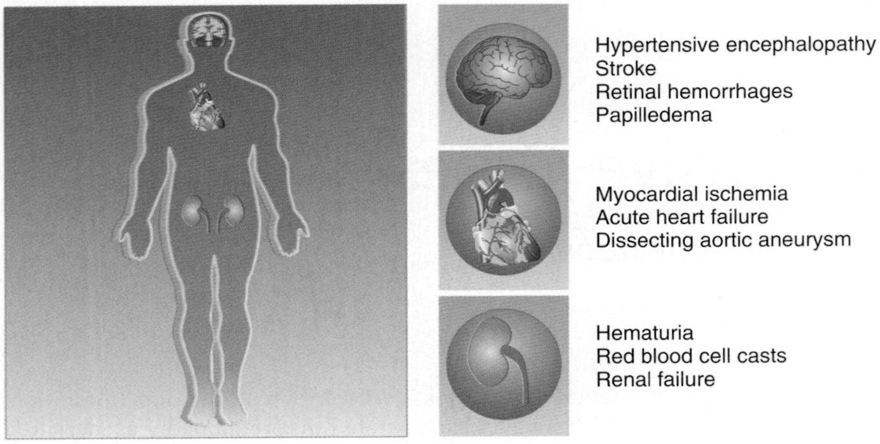

Figure 35-1. End-organ failure in hypertensive emergency.

Table 35-1. Classification of Hypertension (JNC VII)

BP Classification	SBP (mm Hg)		DBP (mm Hg)
Normal	<120	*and*	<80
Prehypertension	120-139	*or*	80-89
Stage 1 hypertension	140-159	*or*	90-99
Stage 2 hypertension	≥160	*or*	≥100

BP, blood pressure; DPB, diastolic blood pressure; JNC VII, Seventh report of the Joint National Committee on Prevention, Detection, Evalulation, and Treatment of High Blood Pressure; SBP, systolic blood pressure.

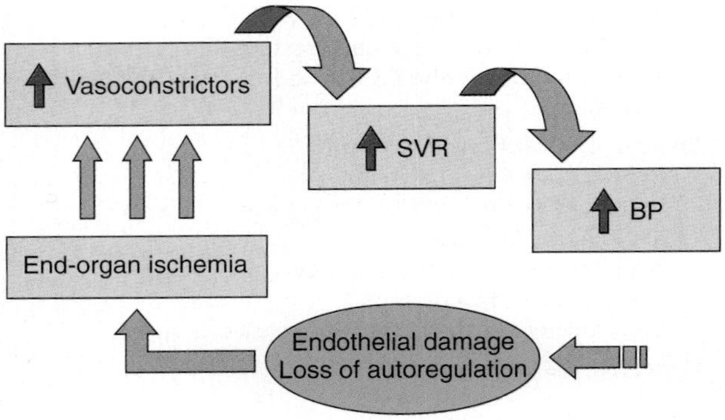

Figure 35-2. Pathophysiology of hypertensive emergency. Increase in humoral vasoconstrictors leads to increased systemic vascular resistance (SVR), which raises blood pressure. As blood pressure increases, endothelial damage results in loss of autoregulation and organ ischemia. Organ ischemia increases release of vasoconstrictors, and a vicious circle is initiated. BP, blood pressure.

Box 35-1

Hypertensive Emergencies

- Hypertensive encephalopathy
- Cerebrovascular accident
- Acute aortic dissection
- Acute left ventricular failure
- Acute myocardial infarction
- Acute renal failure
- Preeclampsia/eclampsia
- Catecholamine excess states
- Postoperative hypertension

A *hypertensive urgency* is characterized by marked elevations of blood pressure without evidence of acute end-organ damage. In hypertensive urgencies the blood pressure can be lowered more gradually, over 24 to 48 hours. This usually can be accomplished with oral medications and does not require invasive hemodynamic monitoring in an ICU. Hypertensive urgencies can be associated with chronic stable organ dysfunction, such as in stable angina, chronic renal insufficiency, or previous cerebrovascular accident, without evidence of acute end-organ damage.

PATHOPHYSIOLOGY

The underlying pathophysiology of hypertensive crises still is not fully understood. The transition from mild hypertension or normotension to a hypertensive crisis usually is precipitated by an event that leads to an abrupt increase in blood pressure. Situations associated with this event may include cessation of hypertensive medications with potential rebound effects, consumption of illicit drugs, and severe pain, as well as several clinical syndromes. Blood pressure is determined by the product of cardiac output and systemic vascular resistance ($BP = CO \times SVR$). In most hypertensive crises, the initial rise in blood pressure is secondary to increased systemic vascular resistance. The rise in systemic vascular resistance is believed to be caused by humoral vasoconstrictors.[6] With the increase in blood pressure, mechanical stress on the arteriolar wall leads to endothelial damage and fibrinoid necrosis of the arterioles.[6,7] Vascular damage leads to loss of autoregulatory mechanisms, ischemia, and acute end-organ damage, which prompts further release of vasoconstrictors, thereby initiating a vicious circle[6,7] (Fig. 35-2).

APPROACH TO MANAGEMENT

The management of patients with hypertensive crises often is associated with pitfalls resulting from poor understanding of the underlying process and lack of clear end points for treatment. Common pitfalls include treating "numbers" without evaluating the individual patient for acute end-organ damage and misuse of intravenous drugs leading to a precipitous drop in blood pressure. A methodical approach to patients with severe elevations in blood pressure can help establish safe and effective treatment. The following three questions should be used to guide treatment for patients in hypertensive crisis: (1) Should the blood pressure be lowered acutely? (2) How much should the blood pressure be lowered? (3) Which medication should be used to lower the blood pressure? These considerations, discussed next, provide a framework for the management of patients with hypertensive crises.

Should the Blood Pressure Be Lowered Acutely?

The key consideration in whether blood pressure should be lowered immediately is the presence or absence of acute end-organ damage. As previously discussed, patients with a hypertensive emergency will have evidence of acute end-organ damage and require immediate reduction of blood pressure. By contrast, patients with hypertensive urgency and no evidence of acute end-organ damage do not require immediate reduction of blood pressure regardless of absolute values for blood pressure. A systematic clinical evaluation can determine the presence of acute end-organ failure.

A focused history should determine previous diagnosis of hypertension, medication history, use of illicit drugs or over-the-counter agents with potential hypertensive effects, and presence of signs or symptoms consistent with neurologic, visual, cardiac, or renal dysfunction. Physical examination should confirm vital signs; it is very important to measure blood pressure adequately and in both upper extremities. Pulses also should be checked in all extremities because inequalities in blood pressure or pulses can exist with aortic dissection. In addition, a thorough neurologic and cardiopulmonary examination should evaluate for possible signs of end-organ failure such as altered mentation, new focal neurologic deficits, or cardiogenic pulmonary edema. Funduscopic examination of the eyes should complement the physical examination. Signs such as acute papillary edema and new retinal hemorrhages support the presence of acute end-organ damage. A set of simple diagnostic tests can complete the evaluation for acute end-organ damage. Abnormalities in levels of blood urea nitrogen (BUN) or serum creatinine and on urinalysis (red blood cell casts) suggest renal involvement. An electrocardiogram to rule out active ischemia and a chest film to assess for pulmonary edema or signs of aortic pathology are helpful to evaluate the cardiopulmonary system. Other tests such as computed tomography scans of the head may be indicated in patients with neurologic deficits. An algorithm to estabish the presence of acute end-organ damage is presented in Figure 35-3.

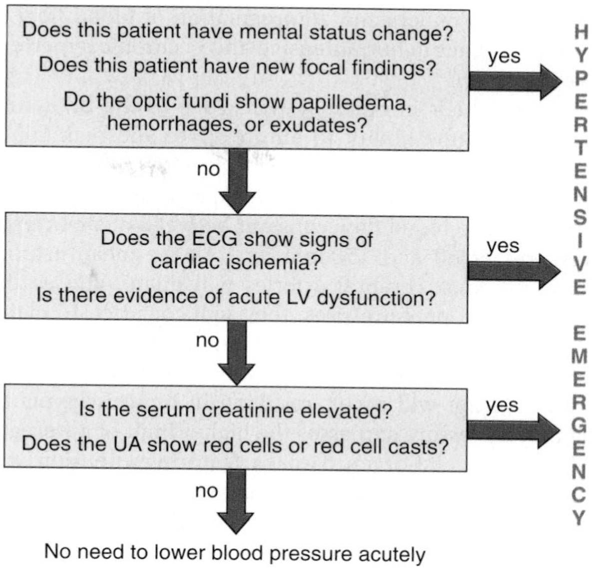

Figure 35-3. Evaluation algorithm for hypertensive emergency. Systematic evaluation for possible acute end-organ damage can proceed according to this scheme. If the answer to any of the questions is "yes," the patient has a hypertensive emergency and blood pressure should be lowered acutely. If the answer to all questions is "no," the patient does not have a hypertensive emergency and the blood pressure can be lowered gradually. ECG, electrocardiogram; LV, left ventricular; UA, urinalysis.

If the clinical evaluation reveals evidence of acute end-organ damage, the patient's blood pressure should be lowered acutely. If a systematic evaluation of the patient fails to uncover such evidence, however, the blood pressure does not require immediate reduction. In these patients with hypertensive urgency, a gradual reduction of blood pressure over 24 to 48 hours with oral agents is indicated. In some instances it may be difficult to establish whether end-organ damage is acute or chronic. A common clinical presentation in this respect is that of a patient with severe elevations of blood pressure and an abnormal creatinine concentration. In such patients, old records may help define the acuity of organ dysfunction. If this is not possible, however, the clinical decision regarding treatment must be based on specific findings for the individual patient. In equivocal cases, it probably is better to treat as if acute end-organ damage is present.

How Much Should the Blood Pressure Be Lowered?

Once the decision to lower a patient's blood pressure acutely is made, the next step should be to establish a therapeutic target for the blood pressure. The goals for treating hypertensive emergencies are to lower the blood pressure to a point at which acute end-organ damage is prevented and, at the same time, to avoid iatrogenic damage caused by abrupt falls in blood pressure leading to hypoperfusion. To accomplish these goals, it is important to understand autoregulation of blood flow in different organs in normotensive and in chronic hypertensive states.

Vascular beds in organ systems such as the brain and kidney have the ability to autoregulate and maintain a constant blood flow through a range of mean arterial pressures. Under normal conditions, cerebral autoregulation will keep blood flow constant between mean arterial pressures of 60 and 150 mm Hg.[8] As the mean arterial pressure drops, cerebral arteries will dilate, and as the mean arterial pressure rises, they will constrict, to maintain constant blood flow to the brain. When the blood pressure falls below the lower limit of autoregulation, hypoperfusion will occur, resulting in brain ischemia. If the blood pressure surpasses the higher limit of autoregulation, acute end-organ damage from hypertension will occur. In the case of the brain, this may result in hypertensive encephalopathy. Studies in animal models and in humans have shown that chronic hypertension will lead to compensatory functional and structural changes in the arterial circulation.[9,10] These changes will result in a shift to the right of the autoregulatory curve for a given vascular bed.[11] Autoregulatory curves for cerebral blood flow in healthy persons and in patients with chronic hypertension are shown in Figure 35-4.

This pathophysiologic paradigm has important therapeutic implications. Patients with chronic hypertension will have a higher tolerance to elevations in blood pressure, because their autoregulatory curve is shifted to the right. This explains why many patients present with severely elevated blood pressure and no evidence of acute end-organ damage. With rapid reductions in blood pressure to "normal" levels, however, the lower autoregulatory capacity of the circulation may be exceeded in a chronically hypertensive patient. This phenomenon explains the hypoperfusion of vital organs and the development of renal failure or cerebral ischemia (or both) often seen when blood pressure is lowered too far or too fast.[12] In view of these issues, a reasonable goal for most hypertensive emergencies is to lower the mean arterial pressure by 15% to 25% over periods of several minutes to hours, depending on the clinical situation.[13] Reduction of blood pressure to normal levels may be warranted in special situations such as the presence of aortic dissection or a postoperative hypertensive emergency in a previously normotensive patient. Special considerations also may apply in patients with severe elevations of blood pressure within the context of an acute stroke. For patients with hypertensive urgency, acute lowering of blood pressure is not recommended; instead, a gradual reduction of blood pressure levels over 24 to 48 hours should be achieved.

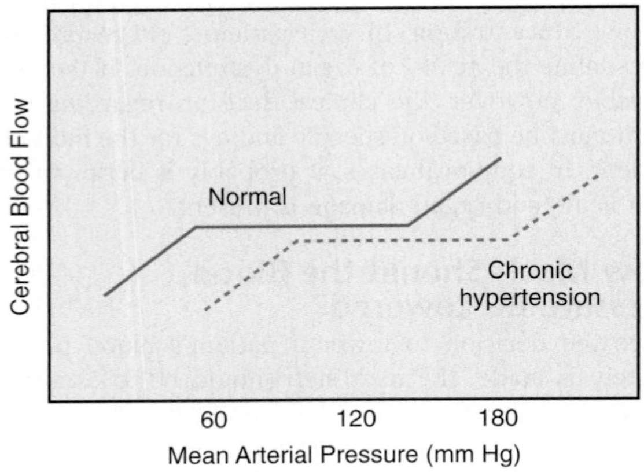

Figure 35-4. Autoregulation of cerebral blood flow. Cerebral blood flow autoregulation curves are depicted for normotensive *(solid purple line)* and chronic hypertensive *(dashed blue line)* states.

Which Medication Should Be Used to Lower the Blood Pressure?

The ideal medication to treat a hypertensive emergency should have a rapid onset of action, high potency, immediate reversibility, no risk of tachyphylaxis, and minimal or no adverse effects. Although no perfect medication exists, several agents with some of these characteristics are summarized in Table 35-2. A limited number of studies have compared agents in terms of clinical outcome. With no clear outcome data, the selection of a particular agent is based on the clinical scenario, pharmacologic characteristics of the drug, and availability. Parenteral agents that are useful in treating hypertensive emergencies are discusssed next (in alphabetical order).

Esmolol

Esmolol is an ultra-short-acting cardioselective, β-adrenergic agent that can be administered intravenously for the treatment of hypertensive emergencies.[14] Esmolol has a rapid onset of action (within 2 minutes), a short elimination half-life (approximately 9 minutes), and a rapid duration of effect (within 15 to 30 minutes after stopping infusion).[15] Esmolol is rapidly metabolized by red blood cells and is not dependent on renal or hepatic function.[15] Such properties enable easy titration of the drug and make it attractive for use in situations of hypertensive emergency associated with intense adrenergic responses or tachycardia.

This agent is available for intravenous use, both as a bolus and as a continuous infusion. The usual dose is 0.5 mg per kg as a loading dose, followed by a maintenance infusion of 25 to 300 μg per kg per minute titrated to the individual patient's response.[15]

Esmolol has been found to be effective in controlling postoperative hypertension and tachycardia in several clinical studies.[16-18] The drug also has been used successfully for treating hypertensive emergencies in various other clinical situations.[19,20] Esmolol seems to be more effective in patients with both high blood pressure and tachycardia in whom problematic issues with β-blockade (such as in severe systolic cardiac dysfunction or asthma) are absent. It often is used in conjunction with other agents to achieve a better response.

Fenoldopam

Fenoldopam is a selective dopamine agonist that causes systemic and renal vasodilation by stimulating dopamine D_1 receptors.[21,22] Fenoldopam is administered intrave-

Table 35-2. Pharmacologic Agents Used in Treating Hypertensive Emergencies

Drug	Dosing	Elimination Half life	Onset of Action	Duration of Effect	Advantages	Disadvantages
Enalaprilat	1.25 mg IV q6h, increment by 1.25 mg q12-24h to max dose of 5 mg q6h	—	15 min	12-24 h	No significant adverse effects	Requires shorter dosing interval or a large dose for efficacy
Esmolol	50 μg/kg/min bolus, then infuse 50-300 μg/kg/min	9 min	2 min	18-30 min	Easily titratable; cardioselectivity	Use with caution in patients with heart failure or asthma
Fenoldopam	Initial dose, 0.1 μg/kg/min with titration every 15 min, no bolus	5-10 min	5 min	30-60 min	Induces both a diuresis and natriuresis	Use with caution in patients with glaucoma
Labetalol	Bolus 20 mg, then 20-80 mg every 10 min for maximum dose of 300 mg; infuse at 0.52-2 mg/min	5 h	2-5 min	2-4 h	No reflex tachycardia	Use with caution in patients with asthma, heart failure, or bradycardia
Nicardipine	Initial dose 5 mg/h, to maximum of 15 mg/h	40-60 min	10-20 min	1-4 h	Minimal cardiodepressant effects; minimal dose adjustments required	Possible adverse effects: hypotension, headache, and flushing
Nitroprusside	Initial dose 0.25 μg/kg/min; maximum dose 8-10 μg/kg/min	14 min	Within seconds	3-4 min	Immediate onset of effect	Hypotension; coronary steal; cyanide toxicity; light sensitivity; frequent monitoring required

nously and has a rapid onset of action (5 minutes) and a short duration of action (30 to 60 minutes).[22] It is rapidly metabolized by conjugation in the liver to inactive metabolites that are excreted by the kidney. The plasma elimination half-life is approximately 5 to 10 minutes.[22]

Fenoldopam is administered as a continuous infusion (without a bolus dose), at an initial dose of 0.1 μg per kg of body weight per minute; this dose is titrated by 0.05 to 0.1 μg per kg per minute to achieve the desired effect, up to a maximum dose of 1.6 μg per kg per minute.[21]

The most common adverse effects of the drug are related to its vasodilator properties and include hypotension, headache, reflex tachycardia, and flushing.[21] Fenoldopam also increases intraocular pressure and should be used with caution in patients with glaucoma.[23] Fenoldopam has been demonstrated to be safe and effective in postoperative hypertension.[24] Two clinical studies in severely hypertensive patients found fenoldopam to be comparable in efficacy to sodium nitroprusside.[25,26]

Because of its effects on the renal vasculature and its ability to increase urine output, fenoldopam has been proposed as a renal-protective drug. A number of small clinical studies report conflicting results in this respect. A recent meta-analysis, however, found improved renal function and decreased mortality in critically ill patients with acute kidney injury treated with fenoldopam.[27] In the setting of a hypertensive emergency, protective effects of fenoldopam on renal function have not been confirmed. Because it does not affect renal function adversely and is not associated with increased toxicity in the setting of renal failure, however, it may be a useful alternative to sodium nitroprusside in patients with hypertensive emergency and renal failure.

Labetalol

Labetalol is a combined α- and β-adrenergic receptor blocker that currently is approved for both oral and intravenous use in the treatment of hypertension. Labetalol lowers blood pressure by decreasing systemic vascular resistance by α_1-blockade and at the same time counteracts the reflex tachycardia from vasodilation through its β-blocker effect.[28,29] Labetalol reduces peripheral vascular resistance while maintaining cerebral, renal, and coronary blood flow. Unlike other β-blockers, labetalol does not reduce cardiac output. When administered intravenously it has a rapid onset of action (2 to 5 minutes), with peak hypotensive effect occurring within 5 to 10 minutes and the effect lasting 2 to 4 hours.[30] The drug is metabolized primarily by the liver and has a plasma elimination half-life of approximately 5 hours.[28]

Labetalol usually is administered intravenously in a loading dose of 20 mg, followed by incremental doses of 20 to 80 mg every 10 minutes until the target blood pressure is achieved or a maximal dose of 300 mg. An alternative regimen is a continuous infusion starting at a rate of 1 to 2 mg per minute and titrated upwards to achieve a desired blood pressure end point.

Adverse effects of labetalol include orthostatic hypotension, bronchospasm (the drug should be avoided in asthma patients), heart failure, and significant bradycardia (it should be avoided in the presence of sinus bradycardia or heart block greater than first degree). Labetalol has been shown to be effective in a wide range of clinical situations associated with hypertensive emergencies.[28,29,31-34]

Nicardipine

Nicardipine is a short-acting calcium channel antagonist that produces selective arteriolar dilation. Nicardipine decreases systemic vascular resistance without producing reflex tachycardia, while maintaining or increasing cardiac output.[35] Intravenous nicardipine has a rapid onset of action (the major effect lasts 10 to 15 minutes, and the plasma elimination half-life is 40 to 60 minutes), making it easily titratable in treating hypertensive emergencies.[36,37]

An initial dose of 5 mg per hour is recommended, with increases in the infusion rate by 2.5 mg per hour every 5 to 15 minutes (to a maximum rate of 15 mg per hour) until the desired hemodynamic response is achieved. Once the target blood pressure is achieved, the infusion rate can be reduced to 3 mg per hour and adjusted to maintain the desired end point. The drug is rapidly distributed throughout the body and is metabolized by the liver into inactive metabolites.

Nicardipine should be avoided or used cautiously in patients with aortic stenosis, patients with cardiomyopathy receiving β-blockers, and patients with impaired hepatic function. Several studies have documented the utility and safety of nicardipine in patients with hypertensive emergencies. Randomized studies have demonstrated that nicardipine is similar in efficacy to nitroprusside for the management of postoperative hypertension.[36,38]

Nitroprusside

For many years, sodium nitroprusside was the standard intravenous drug administered for hypertensive emergencies and remains a viable alternative today. Nitroprusside is a potent balanced arterial and venous vasodilator that decreases both cardiac afterload and preload. Nitroprusside has a rapid onset of action (2 to 3 minutes) and a short serum half-life (1 to 2 minutes) and can be easily titrated.[39] Because of its potent effects on blood pressure, use of nitroprusside requires invasive hemodynamic monitoring (using an arterial line for continuous blood pressure monitoring). Nitroprusside infusion typically is begun at 0.3 μg per kg of body weight per minute and increased by 0.2 to 1.0 μg per kg per minute every 3 to 5 minutes as needed until a maximum rate of 2 μg per kg per minute is attained.

Cyanide and thiocyanate are metabolites of nitroprusside with potential toxic effects. Cyanide is released nonezymatically from nitroprusside. Cyanide is converted to thiocyanate by the liver. Finally, the kidney excretes thiocyanate. The total dose of nitroprusside and the presence of liver or renal dysfunction increase the risk of toxicity. Cyanide toxicity can be associated with lactic acidosis, mental status changes, and hypotension. Signs of thiocyanate toxicity include delirium, headaches, nausea, abdominal pain, and muscular spasms.[40] To reduce possible toxicity, the duration of treatment with nitroprusside should be limited and the maintenance rate of infusion should not exceed 2 μg per kg per minute. In patients requiring higher doses of nitroprusside, an infusion of thiosulfate is recommended to decrease risk of toxicity.[41] Hydroxocobalamin also has been demonstrated to prevent and treat possible cyanide toxicity associated with the use of nitroprusside. Despite these concerns, nitroprusside has been used successfully in the treatment of hypertensive emergencies for many years, and with proper precautions, toxicity is seldom encountered.

Other Agents

Several other agents have been used for treating severely elevated blood pressure. Many of them have been abandoned secondary to the emergence of safer and more efficacious alternatives. Nevertheless, despite some limitations compared with the drugs previously discussed, a few additional agents may be useful in particular situations.

Nitroglycerin directly interacts with nitrate receptors to produce predominantly venous dilation. Because of its favorable effects on coronary perfusion and its ability to reduce preload, it is a drug well suited for treating hypertensive emergency associated with myocardial ischemia or acute left ventricular failure.[42] Several clinical studies have shown the safety and efficacy of nitroglycerin for the treatment of hypertension after cardiac surgery.[43-45] Nitroglycerin is administered as a continuous infusion. The starting infusion rate is 5 μg per minute, which can be titrated up to a maximum of 200 μg per minute.

Phentolamine is an α-adrenergic blocking agent that may be used for the management of catecholamine-induced hypertensive emergencies, such as with pheochromocytoma.[46] Phentolamine is administered intravenously in 1- to 5-mg boluses. The effects are immediate and may last up to 15 minutes. This drug may cause arrhythmias and angina. Once the blood pressure is controlled, a long-acting α-adrenergic–blocking agent such as oral phenoxybenzamine can be started.

Enalaprilat is an angiotensin-converting enzyme (ACE) inhibitor that can be administered intravenously. It has an onset of action within 15 minutes, and its duration of action is 12 to 24 hours.[47,48] The usual dose is 1.25 mg given intraveously every 6 hours, titrated by increments of 1.25 mg at 12- to 24-hour intervals to a maximum dose of 5 mg every 6 hours.[49] The degree of blood pressure reduction with enalaprilat is correlated directly with the pretreatment levels of angiotensin II and plasma renin activity.[50] Enalaprilat is especially useful in hypertensive emergency associated with scleroderma crises.[51]

Hydralazine is a vasodilator that has been used in pregnancy-related hypertensive crises for many years. It has unpredictable effects on blood pressure, however, and a long half-life. Nicardipine and labetalol are better choices for treating hypertensive emergencies in pregnant patients in the ICU.

SPECIFIC CLINICAL CONSIDERATIONS

Hypertensive Encephalopathy

When rises in mean arterial pressure exceed the upper limits of the cerebral blood flow autoregulatory curve, endothelial damage with extravasation of plasma proteins can lead to cerebral edema.[52] Hypertensive encephalopathy, the clinical manifestation of this phenomenon, is characterized by headache, visual disturbances, confusion, and focal or generalized weakness. If untreated, it can lead to coma and death.[53] Magnetic resonance imaging has demonstrated that a majority of the cases involve the cortical regions of the brain.[54] Recently, however, hypertensive encephalopathy with brainstem involvement also has been described.[55,56]

The differential diagnosis of hypertensive encephalopathy includes several neurologic syndromes (Box 35-2). These should be quickly ruled out with the use of imaging of the brain and other pertinent diagnostic tests. Treatment should be instituted immediately. The goal is to reduce the mean arterial pressure by 15% to 20% within the first 1 to 2 hours.[57] The hallmark of hypertensive encephalopathy is clinical improvement with resolution of symptoms once the blood pressure is controlled. Caution should be taken not to worsen neurologic function as a result of hypoperfusion caused by lowering the mean arterial pressure (MAP) excessively. Drugs suitable for treating hypertensive encephalopathy include nitroprusside, nicardipine, labetalol, and fenoldopam.

Box 35-2

Differential Diagnosis of Hypertensive Encephalopathy

Ischemic stroke
Intracerebral hemorrhage
Subarachnoid hemorrhage
Subdural hematoma
Epidural hematoma
Central nervous system vasculitis
Brain mass
Seizure disorder
Central nervous system infection
Drug toxicity
Withdrawal syndrome

Hypertensive Crisis in Cerebrovascular Accidents

The optimal management of hypertension after cerebrovascular accidents is controversial. Hypertension is common after both ischemic and hemorrhagic strokes. Extreme elevations in blood pressure have been associated with poor outcomes after ischemic and hemorrhagic cerebrovascular accidents.[58,59] Significant elevations in blood pressure after stroke raise concerns for potential reinfarction, development of cerebral edema, increase in hemorrhage size, or hemorrhagic transformation of ischemic lesions. A well-described finding after an acute stroke is impairment of the ability of the cerebrovasculature to autoregulate blood flow.[60] During this period, flow to the brain is highly pressure dependent. Further neurologic deterioration from aggressive pharmacologic lowering has been reported.[61] Current guidelines recommend withholding therapy for hypertension in the acute phase of ischemic strokes unless the patient will receive thrombolysis or evidence of concomitant acute end-organ damage or excessive elevation in blood pressure (arbitrarily selected as systolic blood pressure higher than 220 mm Hg or diastolic blood pressure higher than 120 mm Hg) is present.[62] For hemorrhagic strokes, current recommendations are to maintain a MAP of 130 mm Hg or less in patients with history of hypertension and a MAP of 100 mm Hg or less in patients who underwent craniotomy.[63] Current guidelines are summarized in Tables 35-3 and 35-4.

Acute Aortic Dissection

Aortic dissection is one of the most feared complications of hypertension. It is caused by a tear in the intima of the aorta that is then propagated by the aortic pulse wave. The aortic pulse wave (dP/dt) is dependent on myocardial

Table 35-3. Guidelines for Treatment of Hypertension in Ischemic Cerebrovascular Accidents

Clinical Parameter	Treatment
Patients* Not *Eligible for Thrombolysis	
SBP<220 *or* DBP<120 mm Hg	No treatment
SBP>220 *or* DBP 121-140 mm Hg	Labetalol or nicardipine to 10-15% reduction
DBP>140 mm Hg	Nitroprusside to 10-15% reduction More labetalol or nicardipine
Patients Eligible for Thrombolysis	
Before Thrombolytic Therapy	
SBP>185 *or* DBP>110 mm Hg	Labetalol or nitropaste
During or after Thrombolytic Therapy	
SBP 180-230 *or* DBP 105-120 mm Hg	Labetalol
SPB>230 *or* DBP 121-140 mm Hg	Labetalol or nicardipine
DBP>140 mm Hg	Nitroprusside

DPB, diastolic blood pressure; MAP, mean arterial pressure; SBP, systolic blood pressure.

Table 35-4. Guidelines for Treatment of Hypertension in Hemorrhagic Cerebrovascular Accidents

Clinical Parameter	Treatment
SBP<180 and DBP<105 mm Hg MAP<130 mm Hg	No treatment
SBP 180-230 *or* DBP 105-140 mm Hg MAP 130-160 mm Hg	Labetalol, esmolol, nicardipine, enalaprilat
SBP>230 *or* DBP>140 mm Hg MAP>160 mm Hg	Nitroprusside Nicardipine±labetalol

DPB, diastolic blood pressure; MAP, mean arterial pressure; SBP, systolic blood pressure.

contractility, heart rate, and blood pressure. Additional risk factors for aortic dissection include advanced atherosclerosis, connective tissue diseases, and aortic coarctation.[64]

Aortic dissections are classified as type A (proximal to the left subclavian artery, involving the ascending aorta) or type B (distal to the left subclavian artery, involving the descending aorta).[64] The presenting symptom usually is severe, sharp chest pain of abrupt onset. The chest radiograph may reveal a widened mediastinum. The diagnosis is best made with contrast-enhanced computed tomography or transesophageal echocardiography.[65] Type A dissections usually require surgery to prevent serious complications such as acute aortic insufficiency, hemopericardium, and cardiac tamponade.[66] Type B dissection often is managed medically. The goal of treatment is rapid reduction of dP/dt. Mean arterial pressure and heart rate must be controlled in order to achieve this goal. In patients with aortic dissection, the mean arterial pressure should be reduced to normal values as quickly as possible. Combination of a vasodilator (nitroprusside) with a β-blocker to prevent reflex tachycardia commonly is recommended. Labetalol is an alternative to the combination of nitroprusside and a beta-blocker[67] (see Chapter 34).

Hypertensive Crises in Pregnancy

Hypertension is a common complication of pregnancy and is responsible for 18% of maternal deaths in the United States.[68] The spectrum of disease ranges from mild increases in blood pressure to severe pregnancy-related syndromes with hypertensive emergencies such as preeclampsia and eclampsia.[69] Hypertension in pregnancy is defined as a systolic blood pressure of 140 mm Hg or greater or a diastolic pressure of 90 mm Hg or greater. *Preeclampsia* is a pregnancy-specific condition defined by new-onset hypertension, proteinuria (excretion of greater than 300 mg of protein per 24 hours), and development of pathologic edema. *Eclampsia* is defined by the development of seizures or coma in a pregnant patient with preeclampsia. The challenge in pregnant patients with hypertensive crises is to lower the blood pressure enough to prevent maternal end-organ damage while minimizing acute changes in placental perfusion that could have a negative impact on the well-being of the fetus. Treatment of severe preeclampsia and eclampsia includes delivery of the fetus, magnesium sulfate for prevention and treatment of seizures, and appropriate blood pressure control. The goal is to reduce the diastolic blood pressure to 100 mm Hg or the mean arterial pressure by 20%.

Historically, hydralazine has been preferred in pregnant patients for its safety profile with respect to the fetus. As suggested by recent data, however, it may not be the most effective or safe agent for this patient population.[70] For pregnant patients who require acute lowering of blood pressure in the ICU, drugs such as labetalol and nicardipine probably are better options.[71,72] Nitroprusside is reserved for refractory cases because of concerns with potential fetal cyanide toxicity. Finally, ACE inhibitors such as enalaprilat are contraindicated in the second and third trimesters because of the associated increase in fetal and neonatal morbidity and mortality.

Postoperative Hypertension

Postoperative hypertension warranting consideration of immediate parenteral treatment has been arbitrarily defined as a systolic blood pressure greater than 190 mm Hg or a diastolic blood pressure less than 100 mm Hg, or both, on two consecutive readings after surgery. Previous history of hypertension, high body mass index, age, and the grade of surgical stress are recognized risk factors for the development of postoperative hypertension.[73] Marked increases in arterial blood pressure in the immediate postoperative period can result in serious complications such as heart failure, arrhythmia, myocardial ischemia, wound hemorrhage, and cerebral hemorrhage.[74] In view of the deleterious effects of prolonged postoperative hypertension, many authors have recommended aggressive treatment.[74] The goal of treatment is similar to that with other hypertensive emergencies: to decrease blood pressure to safe levels and at the same time avoid complications related to hypotension. Although some clinicians believe that postoperative hypertension should be treated aggressively because of the potential for acute end-organ damage, others recommend evaluating for possible causes of hypertension such as pain, hypercarbia, hypoxemia, and urinary retention before initiation of antihypertensive drugs. Because most patients in the postoperative period are unable to take oral medications, even patients with no clear evidence of acute end-organ damage will receive intravenous medications. In patients with a previous history of hypertension, a reasonable goal is to reduce mean arterial pressure by 20%. In patients with no previous history of hypertension, the goal is to reduce blood pressure to normal levels.

Nitroprusside, labetalol, and nicardipine all have been extensively studied in cardiac, vascular, and neurosurgical settings. Nitroglycerin commonly is used in post–coronary artery bypass surgery, and fenoldopam has been proposed for use in clinical settings with increased risk of renal ischemia.

Catecholamine-Associated Hypertensive Crisis

Hypertensive crisis related to excess catecholamines can result from several causes. Ingestion of sympathomimetic agents (amphetamines, cocaine, phencyclidine, and certain diet pills), decongestants (ephedrine, pseudoephedrine), and other agents (atropine, alkaloids) can result in excessive catecholamine release and hypertension. Withdrawal from β-blocking or α-blocking agents can lead to a rapid surge in catecholamines with resultant hypertension. In such cases, reinstituting the particular drug may be sufficient to treat the elevated blood pressure. Additional causes include pheochromocytoma, autonomic dysfunction (e.g., Guillain-Barré syndrome), and ingestion of tyramine in conjunction with monoamine oxidase inhibitor therapy. As a general rule, in catecholamine-related hypertension the use of β-blockers for initial therapy should be avoided. Loss of β-adrenergic–mediated vasodilation leaves α-mediated vasoconstriction unopposed, potentially leading to further elevation in blood pressure.

Pheochromocytoma is a rare tumor that produces excess catecholamine and can cause severe hypertension. Symptoms and signs commonly associated with pheochromocytoma include headache, palpitations, diaphoresis, abdominal pain, anxiety, and hypertension. Some patients may present with orthostatic symptoms. For hypertensive emergencies associated with pheochromocytoma, the drug of choice is phentolamine. Once blood pressure is controlled, a β-blocker can be added to manage the tachycardia. For less critical situations or after acute hypertension is controlled, the oral agent phenoxybenzamine can be used.

HYPERTENSIVE URGENCY

Hypertensive urgency refers to a clinical situation characterized by severe elevation of blood pressure without evidence of acute end-organ damage. This is a common clinical situation that often is mismanaged. Too often clinicians have the impulse to treat numbers, which risks causing more harm to the patient from precipitous drops in blood pressure. Despite markedly elevated blood pressure, patients with hypertensive urgency are at low risk of immediate complications. Morbidity from elevated blood pressure occurs over months to years. Therefore, it is more important to start patients with hypertensive urgency on a good long-term oral regimen and reduce the blood pressure gradually over 24 to 48 hours. It is important to avoid the use of medications that have the potential to produce abrupt drops in blood pressure, with the potential for significant damage from resultant hypoperfusion.[12,75] In this respect, practices such as the use of sublingual nifedipine in hypertensive urgency have been abandoned because of the potential hazard to the patient.[76,77] Often, restarting a previously effective drug regimen is all that is needed to manage the hypertensive urgency. Physicians often feel compelled to treat elevated blood pressures immediately and feel a false sense of security if they see the numbers improve quickly. In the absence of acute end-organ damage, however, this therapeutic strategy has higher potential for causing damage and is not based on a clear scientific rationale.

KEY POINTS

- Hypertension is a common clinical disorder, with an estimated 30% of the U.S. adult population suffering from elevated blood pressure.
- A *hypertensive emergency* is a severe elevation in blood pressure associated with the presence of acute end-organ damage.
- The treatment of a hypertensive crisis is guided by (1) whether the blood pressure should be lowered acutely; (2) how much it should be lowered; and (3) what medication should be used.
- The ideal medication to treat a hypertensive emergency would have a rapid onset of action, high potency, immediate reversibility, no risk of tachyphylaxis, and minimal or no adverse effects.
- Parenteral agents with specific indications in the treatment of hypertensive crises include esmolol, fenoldopam, labetalol, nicardipine, and nitroprusside.

REFERENCES

1. Burt VL, Whelton P, Roccella EJ, et al: Prevalence of hypertension in the U.S. adult population. Results from the Third National Health and Nutrition Examination Survey, 1988-1991. Hypertension 1995;25(3):305-313.
2. Hajjar I, Kotchen TA: Trends in prevalence, awareness, treatment, and control of hypertension in the United States, 1988-2000. JAMA 2003;290(2):199-206.
3. National Heart, Lung and Blood Institute: Seventh report of the Joint National Committee on Prevention, Detection, Evalulation, and Treatment of High Blood Pressure (JNC VII). National Institutes of Health, Bethesda, Md, 2003 (NIH 03-5233).
4. Fuchs FD, Maestri MK, Bredemeier M, et al: Study of the usefulness of optic fundi examination of patients with hypertension in a clinical setting. J Hum Hypertens 1995;9(7):547-551.
5. Houston MC: Pathophysiology, clinical aspects, and treatment of hypertensive crises. Prog Cardiovasc Dis 1989;32(2):99-148.
6. Ault MJ, Ellrodt AG: Pathophysiological events leading to the end-organ effects of acute hypertension. Am J Emerg Med 1985;3(6 Suppl):10-15.
7. Wallach R, Karp RB, Reves JG, et al: Pathogenesis of paroxysmal hypertension developing during and after coronary bypass surgery: A study of hemodynamic and humoral factors. Am J Cardiol 1980;46(4):559-565.
8. Strandgaard S, Paulson OB: Cerebral autoregulation. Stroke 1984;15(3):413-416.
9. Johansson B: Regional cerebral blood flow in acute experimental hypertension. Acta Neurol Scand 1974;50(3):366-372.
10. Johansson BB, Nilsson B: Cerebral vasomotor reactivity in normotensive and spontaneously hypertensive rats. Stroke 1979;10(5):572-576.
11. Strandgaard S: Autoregulation of cerebral blood flow in hypertensive patients. The modifying influence of prolonged antihypertensive treatment on the tolerance to acute, drug-induced hypotension. Circulation 1976;53(4):720-727.
12. Yanturali S, Akay S, Ayrik C, Cevik AA: Adverse events associated with aggressive treatment of increased blood pressure. Int J Clin Pract 2004;58(5):517-519.

13. Calhoun DA, Oparil S: Treatment of hypertensive crisis. N Engl J Med 1990;323(17):1177-1183.
14. Barbier GH, Shettigar UR, Appunn DO: Clinical rationale for the use of an ultra-short acting beta-blocker: Esmolol. Int J Clin Pharmacol Therapeut 1995;33(4):212-218.
15. Wiest D: Esmolol. A review of its therapeutic efficacy and pharmacokinetic characteristics. Clin Pharmacokinet 1995;28(3):190-202.
16. Girard D, Shulman BJ, Thys DM, et al: The safety and efficacy of esmolol during myocardial revascularization. Anesthesiology 1986;65(2):157-164.
17. Gold MI, Sacks DJ, Grosnoff DB, et al: Use of esmolol during anesthesia to treat tachycardia and hypertension. Anesth Analg 1989;68(2):101-104.
18. Gray RJ, Bateman TM, Czer LS, et al: Comparison of esmolol and nitroprusside for acute post-cardiac surgical hypertension. Am J Cardiol 1987;59(8):887-891.
19. Mooss AN, Hilleman DE, Mohiuddin SM, Hunter CB: Safety of esmolol in patients with acute myocardial infarction treated with thrombolytic therapy who had relative contraindications to beta-blocker therapy. Ann Pharmacother 1994;28(6):701-703.
20. Stumpf JL: Drug therapy of hypertensive crises. Clin Pharm 1988;7(8):582-591.
21. Oparil S, Aronson S, Deeb GM, et al: Fenoldopam: a new parenteral antihypertensive: Consensus roundtable on the management of perioperative hypertension and hypertensive crises. Am J Hypertens 1999;12(7):653-664.
22. Post JBT, Frishman WH: Fenoldopam: A new dopamine agonist for the treatment of hypertensive urgencies and emergencies. J Clin Pharmacol 1998;38(1):2-13.
23. Elliott WJ, Karnezis TA, Silverman RA, et al: Intraocular pressure increases with fenoldopam, but not nitroprusside, in hypertensive humans. Clin Pharmacol Ther 1991;49(3):285-293.
24. Goldberg ME, Cantillo J, Nemiroff MS, et al: Fenoldopam infusion for the treatment of postoperative hypertension. J Clin Anesthes 1993;5(5):386-391.
25. Panacek EA, Bednarczyk EM, Dunbar LM, et al: Randomized, prospective trial of fenoldopam vs sodium nitroprusside in the treatment of acute severe hypertension. Fenoldopam Study Group. Acad Emerg Med 1995;2(11):959-965.
26. Pilmer BL, Green JA, Panacek EA, et al: Fenoldopam mesylate versus sodium nitroprusside in the acute management of severe systemic hypertension. J Clin Pharmacol 1993;33(6):549-553.
27. Landoni G, Biondi-Zoccai GG, Tumlin JA, et al: Beneficial impact of fenoldopam in critically ill patients with or at risk for acute renal failure: A meta-analysis of randomized clinical trials. Am J Kidney Dis 2007;49(1):56-68.
28. Dimich I, Lingham R, Gabrielson G, et al: Comparative hemodynamic effects of labetalol and hydralazine in the treatment of postoperative hypertension. J Clin Anesthes 1989;1(3):201-206.
29. Leslie JB, Kalayjian RW, Sirgo MA, et al: Intravenous labetalol for treatment of postoperative hypertension. Anesthesiology 1987;67(3):413-416.
30. Donnelly R, Macphee GJ: Clinical pharmacokinetics and kinetic-dynamic relationships of dilevalol and labetalol. Clin Pharmacokinet 1991;21(2):95-109.
31. Mabie WC, Gonzalez AR, Sibai BM, Amon E: A comparative trial of labetalol and hydralazine in the acute management of severe hypertension complicating pregnancy. Obstet Gynecol 1987;70(3 Pt 1):328-333.
32. Michael CA: Intravenous labetalol and intravenous diazoxide in severe hypertension complicating pregnancy. Aust N Z J Obstet Gynaecol 1986;26(1):26-29.
33. Morel DR, Forster A, Suter PM: I.V. labetalol in the treatment of hypertension following coronary-artery surgery. Br J Anaesth 1982;54(11):1191-1196.
34. Orlowski JP, Shiesley D, Vidt DG, et al: Labetalol to control blood pressure after cerebrovascular surgery. Crit Care Med 1988;16(8):765-768.
35. Lambert CR, Hill JA, Nichols WW, et al: Coronary and systemic hemodynamic effects of nicardipine. Am J Cardiol 1985;55(6):652-656.
36. Efficacy and safety of intravenous nicardipine in the control of postoperative hypertension. IV Nicardipine Study Group. Chest 1991;99(2):393-398.
37. Wallin JD, Fletcher E, Ram CV, et al: Intravenous nicardipine for the treatment of severe hypertension. A double-blind, placebo-controlled multicenter trial. Arch Intern Med 1989;149(12):2662-2669.
38. David D, Dubois C, Loria Y: Comparison of nicardipine and sodium nitroprusside in the treatment of paroxysmal hypertension following aortocoronary bypass surgery. J Cardiothorac Vasc Anesth 1991;5(4):357-361.
39. Cohn JN, Burke LP: Nitroprusside. Ann Intern Med 1979;91(5):752-757.
40. Robin ED, McCauley R: Nitroprusside-related cyanide poisoning. Time (long past due) for urgent, effective interventions. Chest 1992;102(6):1842-1845.
41. Hall VA, Guest JM: Sodium nitroprusside–induced cyanide intoxication and prevention with sodium thiosulfate prophylaxis. Am J Crit Care 1992;1(2):19-25; quiz 6-7.
42. Yusuf S, Collins R, MacMahon S, Peto R: Effect of intravenous nitrates on mortality in acute myocardial infarction: An overview of the randomised trials. Lancet 1988;1(8594):1088-1092.
43. Flaherty JT, Magee PA, Gardner TL, et al: Comparison of intravenous nitroglycerin and sodium nitroprusside for treatment of acute hypertension developing after coronary artery bypass surgery. Circulation 1982;65(6):1072-1077.
44. Kaplan JA, Dunbar RW, Jones EL: Nitroglycerin infusion during coronary-artery surgery. Anesthesiology 1976;45(1):14-21.
45. Tobias MA: Comparison of nitroprusside and nitroglycerine for controlling hypertension during coronary artery surgery. Br J Anaesth 1981;53(8):891-897.
46. Vaughan CJ, Delanty N: Hypertensive emergencies. Lancet 2000;356(9227):411-417.
47. De Marco T, Daly PA, Liu M, et al: Enalaprilat, a new parenteral angiotensin-converting enzyme inhibitor: Rapid changes in systemic and coronary hemodynamics and humoral profile in chronic heart failure. J Am Coll Cardiol 1987;9(5):1131-1138.
48. DiPette DJ, Ferraro JC, Evans RR, Martin M: Enalaprilat, an intravenous angiotensin-converting enzyme inhibitor, in hypertensive crises. Clin Pharmacol Ther 1985;38(2):199-204.
49. Rutledge J, Ayers C, Davidson R, et al: Effect of intravenous enalaprilat in moderate and severe systemic hypertension. Am J Cardiol 1988;62(16):1062-1067.
50. Hirschl MM, Binder M, Bur A, et al: Impact of the renin-angiotensin-aldosterone system on blood pressure response to intravenous enalaprilat in patients with hypertensive crises. J Hum Hypertens 1997;11(3):177-183.
51. Strauss R, Gavras I, Vlahakos D, Gavras H: Enalaprilat in hypertensive emergencies. J Clin Pharmacol 1986;26(1):39-43.
52. Gifford RW Jr, Westbrook E: Hypertensive encephalopathy: Mechanisms, clinical features, and treatment. Prog Cardiovasc Dis 1974;17(2):115-124.
53. Chester EM, Agamanolis DP, Banker BQ, Victor M: Hypertensive encephalopathy: A clinicopathologic study of 20 cases. Neurology 1978;28(9 Pt 1):928-939.
54. Schilling S, Hartel C, Gehl HB, Sperner J: MRI findings in acute hypertensive encephalopathy. Eur J Neurol 2003;10(3):329-330.
55. Uchino M, Haga D, Nomoto J, et al: Brainstem involvement in hypertensive encephalopathy: A report of two cases and literature review. Eur Neurol 2007;57(4):223-226.
56. Biousse V, Newman NJ, Chang GY: Brainstem involvement in hypertensive encephalopathy: Clinical and radiological findings. Neurology 2004;63(9):1759-1760; author reply 1760.
57. Williams O, Brust JC: Hypertensive encephalopathy. Curr Treat Options Cardiovasc Med 2004;6(3):209-216.
58. Aslanyan S, Weir CJ, Lees KR: Elevated pulse pressure during the acute period of ischemic stroke is associated with poor stroke outcome. Stroke 2004;35(6):e153-e155.
59. Dandapani BK, Suzuki S, Kelley RE, et al: Relation between blood pressure and outcome in intracerebral hemorrhage. Stroke 1995;26(1):21-24.
60. Powers WJ: Acute hypertension after stroke: The scientific basis for treatment decisions. Neurology 1993;43(3 Pt 1):461-467.
61. Ahmed N, Nasman P, Wahlgren NG: Effect of intravenous nimodipine on blood pressure and outcome after acute stroke. Stroke 2000;31(6):1250-1255.
62. Adams HP Jr, Adams RJ, Brott T, et al: Guidelines for the early management of patients with ischemic stroke: A scientific statement from the Stroke Council of the American Stroke

Association. Stroke 2003;34(4): 1056-1083.
63. Broderick JP, Adams HP Jr, Barsan W, et al: Guidelines for the management of spontaneous intracerebral hemorrhage: A statement for healthcare professionals from a special writing group of the Stroke Council, American Heart Association. Stroke 1999;30(4):905-915.
64. Prisant LM, Nalamolu VR: Aortic dissection. J Clin Hypertens 2005;7(6):367-371.
65. Sommer T, Fehske W, Holzknecht N, et al: Aortic dissection: A comparative study of diagnosis with spiral CT, multiplanar transesophageal echocardiography, and MR imaging. Radiology 1996;199(2):347-352.
66. DeBakey ME, McCollum CH, Crawford ES, et al: Dissection and dissecting aneurysms of the aorta: twenty-year follow-up of five hundred twenty-seven patients treated surgically. Surgery 1982;92(6):1118-1134.
67. Grubb BP, Sirio C, Zelis R: Intravenous labetalol in acute aortic dissection. JAMA 1987;258(1): 78-79.
68. Koonin LM, MacKay AP, Berg CJ, et al: Pregnancy-related mortality surveillance—United States, 1987-1990. MMWR CDC Surveill Summ 1997;46(4):17-36.
69. Vidaeff AC, Carroll MA, Ramin SM: Acute hypertensive emergencies in pregnancy. Crit Care Med 2005;33(10 Suppl):S307-S312.
70. Magee LA, Cham C, Waterman EJ, et al: Hydralazine for treatment of severe hypertension in pregnancy: Meta-analysis. BMJ (Clin Res Ed) 2003;327(7421):955-960.
71. Awad K, Ali P, Frishman WH, Tejani N: Pharmacologic approaches for the management of systemic hypertension in pregnancy. Heart Dis 2000;2(2):124-132.
72. Jannet D, Carbonne B, Sebban E, Milliez J: Nicardipine versus metoprolol in the treatment of hypertension during pregnancy: A randomized comparative trial. Obstet Gynecol 1994;84(3): 354-359.
73. Nishigaki R, Ito A, Kamei J, et al: Risk factors for development of postoperative hypertension. Meth Find Exp Clin Pharmacol 2001;23(4): 203-207.
74. Gal TJ, Cooperman LH: Hypertension in the immediate postoperative period. Br J Anaesth 1975;47(1): 70-74.
75. Zeller KR, Von Kuhnert L, Matthews C: Rapid reduction of severe asymptomatic hypertension. A prospective, controlled trial. Arch Intern Med 1989;149(10):2186-2189.
76. Grossman E, Messerli FH, Grodzicki T, Kowey P: Should a moratorium be placed on sublingual nifedipine capsules given for hypertensive emergencies and pseudoemergencies? JAMA 1996;276(16):1328-1331.
77. Rehman F, Mansoor GA, White WB: "Inappropriate" physician habits in prescribing oral nifedipine capsules in hospitalized patients. Am J Hypertens 1996;9(10 Pt 1): 1035-1039.

Chapter 36

General Principles of Postoperative Intensive Care Unit Care

Michael J. Hockstein and Philip S. Barie

Regionalization within a health care structure allows for more efficient control and use of limited resources. The intensive care unit (ICU) contains specially trained staff and a variety of support devices, such as mechanical ventilators, intra-aortic balloon pumps, ventricular assist devices, and dialysis machines, which in most cases cannot be used elsewhere. Optimally, the location of a patient is determined by matching the patient's needs with a location's resources and expertise.

Generally, the surgical ICU is where experience, manpower, skills, and technology converge to provide services that cannot be provided anywhere else within the hospital. Highly skilled nurses, often greater in number than the patients themselves, work intimately with intensivists and ancillary staff in an environment designed to stabilize, diagnose, and treat simultaneously the most acutely ill patients. ICU management by intensivists allows for an economic and a morbidity and mortality advantage.[1] The surgical ICU combines experienced personnel with critically ill postoperative patients to facilitate this special care and allows for safe and efficient patient throughput. Such efficiency allows for greater institutional procedural volume, which, when paired with surgeon procedural volume, has been shown to be associated with reduced mortality.[2]

Classic postoperative indications for ICU admission include advanced age or prolonged duration of the operation, both criteria without specifically defined thresholds. Other factors, such as the need for mechanical ventilation, volume resuscitation, or administration of vasoactive medications, make ICU care unavoidable. Monitoring of level of consciousness, airway, bleeding, pulses, rhythm, acidosis, urine output, and global perfusion also is facilitated by ICU admission. Identifying patients who *may need* postoperative ICU care can be difficult. Although there are quantitative ways to assess risk and mortality (APACHE, SAPS, MPM, Possum), most physicians do not use these tools to determine postoperative ICU admission. Many of these prediction models are applied to patients already in the ICU and have not been validated as preadmission screening tools. Scoring systems may have good general mortality prediction, but lack calibration for all patient populations.[3] Although extremely useful to describe severity of illness of populations, the accuracy for single patients is significantly less, and physicians may predict mortality better than scoring systems.[4] Admission criteria based on priority, diagnosis, and objective parameter models have been published by the Task Force of the American College of Critical Care Medicine and the Society of Critical Care Medicine.[5]

POSTOPERATIVE EVALUATION

Obtaining a comprehensive medical and surgical history is a fundamental step in understanding a patient in the surgical ICU. The written medical record should contain all of the elements necessary to assemble the story up until the time of ICU admission, although deciphering a chart, particularly when it is long, requires time, detective skills, and patience. Data gathering usually begins by word of mouth from the providers delivering the patient. Certain questions are common to virtually all admissions, as follows:

1. How old is the patient?
2. What are the highlights of the medical/surgical history?
3. Was the operation elective or emergent?
4. What operation was performed, and what are the details of the surgery?
5. Are there any drains?

6. What are the current ventilator settings if the patient is intubated?
7. What medications is the patient receiving currently?
8. Where are the vascular access points? Were they placed under sterile conditions?
9. What was the intubation and anesthetic course like?
10. What were the complications, if any?

Age, comorbidities, and emergency operations all affect mortality. The details of the operation are key, often aided by diagrams in the chart. Resections, diversions, anastomoses, transplantations, use of prosthetic materials and other surgical findings are some of the details that should be obtained. In addition, the type and location of each drain must be accounted for. Only by knowing where a drain is placed can a care provider know how to interpret the quantity and quality of the effluent. Each drain or wire must be labeled correctly. Also, the completion of wound closure must be ascertained (skin and fascia closed?). Finally, if the operation was incomplete, the health care provider needs to inquire about intentions to return to the operating room for staged or incomplete procedures.

The significance of the anesthesia record should not be minimized. The details about trends in gas exchange, blood pressure, urine output, medications, and summary fluid balance should be reviewed. Always identify if the intubation was easy or difficult. Reviewing the ventilator settings that were used in the operating room sheds some light on any possible gas exchange difficulties and provides a first opportunity to make corrections. Tidal volumes in the operating room are often much larger than those used in the ICU. Identification of current medications and the purpose of each help to formulate short-term therapeutic strategies. Elements such as the duration of the case and the volumes of resuscitation fluids, blood products, urine output, and other fluid losses all factor into assessing the adequacy of intraoperative resuscitation. Patients are virtually always in positive fluid balance at the end of the case. Typical postoperative maintenance intravenous fluid rates are 80 to 125 mL/h, but can be substantially higher in the presence of ongoing intravascular volume loss. Isotonic fluids are the most appropriate maintenance fluids. It is useful to inquire the last time the patient received narcotics, benzodiazepines, or paralytics. If paralytics were used, were reversal agents given? Finally, any intraoperative laboratory values, particularly ones that require immediate attention, should be ascertained.

When time permits, attention should be directed back to the medical record. The clinician should scan the history and physical examination, progress notes, and consultations and develop a cohesive story line of events that led up to the operation. Did the illness have an impact on nutrition or functional state? How are other comorbidities or past operations related to the current presentation? The past medical history and the medication list should be scrutinized; the two are complementary. Inclusion of a disease in the past medical history and absence of an expected medication warrants further investigation (and vice versa). The medication list should be scanned in particular for antiseizure medications, bronchodilators, antihypertensives, antiarrhythmics, anticoagulants, diuretics, steroids, and insulin. It must be decided which medications must be continued in the immediate postoperative period and which can be temporarily delayed. If antibiotics were administered preoperatively, the clinician should identify what they were and how long had they been given and for what indication. In general, if administered preoperatively, bronchodilators, steroids, and insulin are resumed postoperatively. Long-acting antihypertensives should be avoided in the early postoperative period, and short-acting intravenous agents should be used to control hypertension. Diuretics should be avoided in the immediate postoperative period unless directed by invasive monitoring or required because of some other medical necessity. The use of early postoperative β-blockade in patients with coronary artery disease is encouraged if the overall hemodynamic performance allows. Most other medications can be safely delayed until the postoperative patient has shown satisfactory cardiopulmonary performance and stability.

Postoperative laboratory, imaging, and electrocardiogram studies should be selected on a case-by-case basis. Patients who have been moved from operating room table to bed and then transported for any distance are at risk for displacement of tubes and catheters. The admission chest radiograph allows for the evaluation of intravascular catheter and endotracheal, nasogastric, and thoracostomy tube positions in addition to visualization of the pleural, mediastinal, and parenchymal structures. Measurements of blood counts and chemistries are usually routine, but may be deemed unnecessary if preoperative or intra-operative values were unremarkable, and the operation was uneventful. Laboratory abnormalities should be followed closely until a favorable trend is established. Patients at risk for perioperative myocardial injury or with new intraoperative arrhythmias should have an electrocardiogram and possibly cardiac enzyme determination.

The physical examination of the patient completes the initial postoperative evaluation. It starts as a cursory survey and concludes as a detailed examination. *The examination should expose all parts of the patient that can be accessed, and the examiner should inspect and palpate the patient.* Areas that are not under examination should be kept covered to preserve body temperature. If the bed sheets are being changed, it presents an opportunity to examine the back of the patient. An initial assessment of the vital signs, skin, pulses, and urine output provides preliminary insight into clinical perfusion (Table 36-1).

The endotracheal tube, if present, needs to be secured adequately. The health care provider should listen for obvious air leaks around the cuff. The presence of nasal or oral gastric tubes should be noted. All drainage tubes should be identified, and the quality and quantity of output should be scrutinized: Is it serous? Sanguineous? Bilious? Drainage from raw, inflamed surfaces is often serosanguineous. Frankly bloody drainage in quantities of more than 100 mL/h may suggest surgical bleeding or coagulopathy. All intravascular catheters should be identi-

Table 36-1. Support for Adequate Clinical Perfusion
Mean arterial blood pressure >70 mm Hg
Heart rate <100 beats per minute
Warm, pink skin without cyanosis or mottling over the digits, thighs, or knees
Palpable pulses
Good capillary refill
Clear yellow urine >0.5-1 mL/kg/h

fied with the goal of determining which should be retained for use and which should be removed. Diagnostic catheters often remain unnoticed—and unused—particularly when in femoral vessels. Intravenous catheters not placed under sterile conditions should be removed immediately.

The neurologic examination may be suboptimal if the patient is still under the effects of anesthesia. Reducing or temporarily withholding narcotics and sedation can provide a window to complete a neurologic assessment. If further analgesia or sedation is still required, it may be resumed after the neurologic assessment.

Intubation, general anesthesia, and mechanical ventilation can result in a variety of airway or parenchymal injuries. Breath sounds should be equal bilaterally. Asymmetry can be caused by atelectasis (possibly endotracheal tube malposition), pleural effusions, or pneumothorax and can be excluded by careful review of the chest x-ray. Examination of the respiratory system should include evaluation of thoracostomy tubes and the mechanical ventilator if present. Except in the case of pneumonectomy, thoracostomy tubes should be placed to suction pending demonstration of sustained lung inflation or resolution of significant drainage. The mechanical ventilator settings and airway pressures should be noted. The clinician should ensure satisfactory initial oxygen saturation and avoid excessive tidal volumes. End-tidal carbon dioxide monitoring facilitates adjustment in ventilation and progress in weaning. Routine blood gas analysis is unnecessary.

The cardiovascular examination is primarily directed at assessment of adequate clinical perfusion. Impressions from the initial survey of clinical perfusion plus any available data from invasive monitoring can be used to assess appropriate hourly maintenance fluid rate and the need for further volume resuscitation. Cardiac surgery patients may have mediastinal drains and pacing wires. The former should be connected to suction, and the quantity and quality of drainage should be scrutinized. Pacing wires should be tested for function on admission and can be capped if pacing is not needed. If a postoperative patient comes to the ICU with a permanent pacemaker or an implantable cardiac defibrillator, the device should be interrogated for mode and function at the earliest convenience.

In contrast to the lungs and heart, which can be imaged easily and whose function can be monitored objectively, the abdomen and its contents cannot be evaluated handily. The persistence of anesthesia or administration of narcotics can remove many of the signs and symptoms typically relied on to signal problems. Examination should focus on baseline location and quantity of pain, presence of abdominal distention, firmness to palpation, and quality and quantity of effluent from drains. Bleeding and progressive visceral edema can cause a rapid distention and loss of compliance of the abdomen, often before other findings occur, such as reduction in hemoglobin concentration, urine output, and blood pressure. Frequent follow-up examinations compared with baseline data may be the earliest way of recognizing an intra-abdominal catastrophe. Knowing where the tip of each abdominal drain lies is necessary to evaluate the effluent. A drain lying outside the bowel or biliary system should not drain succus or bile. A drain that suddenly shows these fluids may herald loss of integrity of a surgical repair or de novo perforation. Unexplained or unexpected changes in the quantity of effluent from a drain also are notable. Abdominal wounds are not always closed at the end of an operation. The clinician needs to determine if the skin or fascia has been left open and, if so, what kind of temporary closure is employed. Surgical or traumatic wounds, regardless of location on the body, should be examined for closure integrity, erythema, and induration.

Examination of pulses is important after vascular surgical procedures. Scheduled reassessments should document the presence and strength of pulses. Sudden reduction or loss or pulse signal can represent proximal vascular occlusion. Baseline cyanosis and mottling of extremities should be noted for subsequent comparison.

Evaluation of a postoperative trauma patient in the ICU can be restricted by the presence of dressings and immobilizing casts and neck collars. Sometimes only toes or fingers are visible for examination. Should the mechanism of injury increase the risk of muscle swelling and compartment syndromes, the practitioner should perform fasciotomy, measure intravesical pressure, or reopen the abdominal incision to facilitate examination of muscle compartments, depending on location. Postoperative admission to the ICU is a good opportunity to look for injuries missed during the initial evaluation and management period.

RECOVERY FROM ANESTHESIA

Postoperative Resuscitation

Assessment

"Adequate resuscitation" is a state, often temporary, which allows for good clinical perfusion and physiologic stability. Patients with good clinical perfusion (expected heart rates, blood pressures, and urine outputs: absence of acidosis) may require no further resuscitation other than maintenance intravenous fluids. Subtle abnormalities in any of these parameters may suggest a more serious physiologic derangement warranting further investigation and intervention. Resuscitation is the process of optimizing macroscopic and microscopic metabolic substrate delivery with the goal of avoiding an imbalance between supply and demand. The most fundamental concept is to ensure adequate oxygen delivery (Do_2) and meet the oxygen consumption ($\dot{V}o_2$) needs of tissues and organelles. Because the moment when $\dot{V}o_2$ exceeds Do_2 is difficult to determine, resuscitation "targets" serve as proxy markers of adequate Do_2. Resuscitation targets are reproducible, quantifiable values, such as pressures, outputs, metabolites, inflammatory mediators, or oxygen saturations, which represent therapeutic goals. Resuscitation targets provide an important opportunity for study and outcome validation. Despite the seemingly simple logic of employing resuscitation targets, few of these therapeutic goals have been shown to improve clinical outcome. Even routine data derived from a pulmonary artery catheter have not been shown to improve outcome in patients undergoing surgery with decompensated cardiogenic shock or acute lung injury.[6,7]

Management Theory

Restoration of "normal" blood pressure, heart rate, and urine output do not ensure adequate Do_2, particularly at the level of the microvasculature.[8] Evaluation and optimization of blood pressure, filling pressures, heart rate, and rhythm often occur simultaneously, particularly in unstable patients (Fig. 36-1). Overzealous resuscitation and supranormal Do_2 not only do not improve outcome, but also may be detrimental.[9] Not all patients require the same type of resuscitation. Although the fundamental

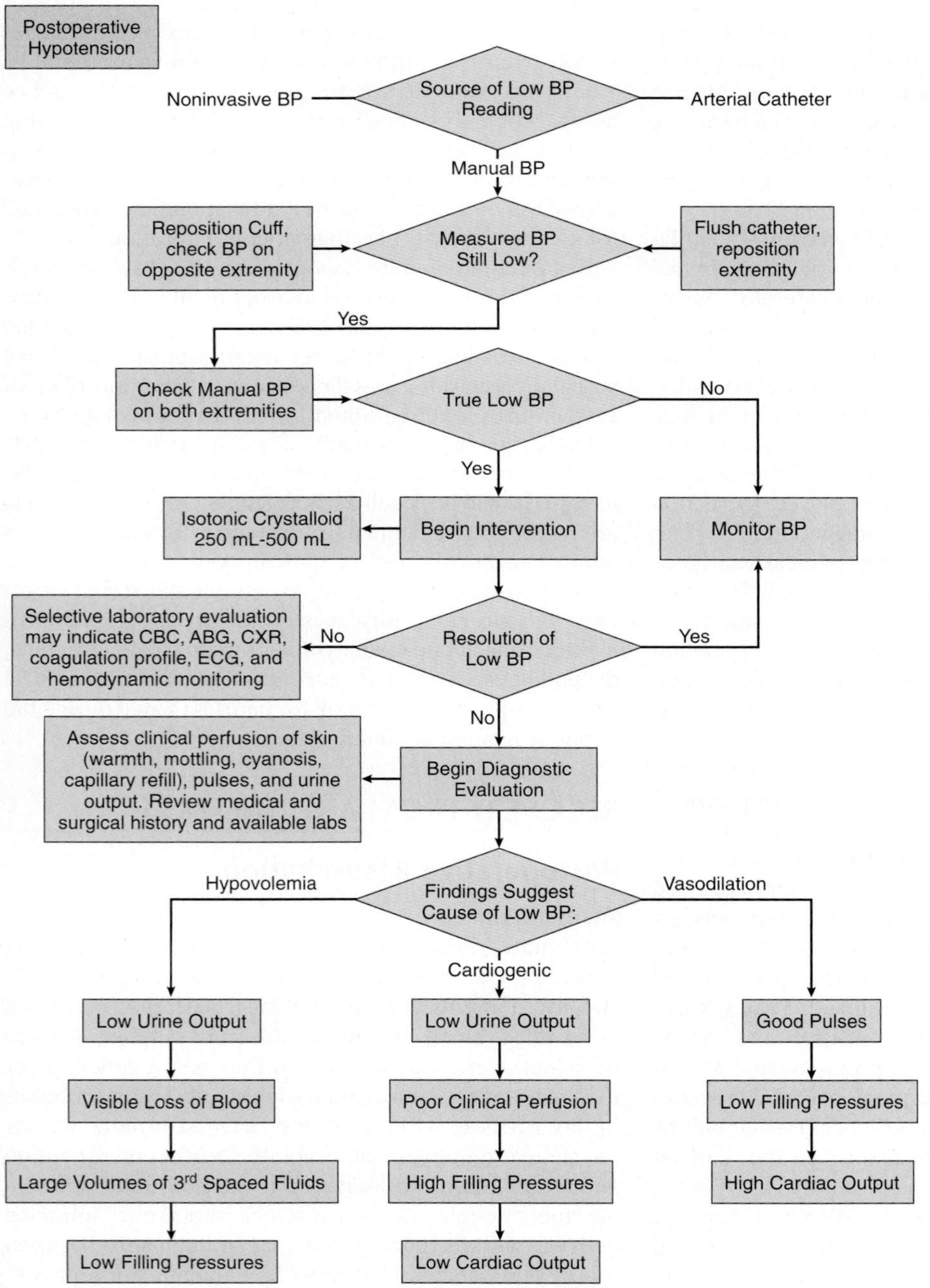

Figure 36-1. Approach to managing postoperative hypotension. ABG, arterial blood gases; BP, blood pressure; CBC, complete blood count; CXR, chest x-ray; ECG, electrocardiogram.

principles are the same, the particular resuscitation end points may differ among the different types of shock.[10,11] For example:

- Early goal-directed therapy in patients with septic shock, as described by Rivers and colleagues,[12] has been shown to reduce morbidity, mortality, and resource consumption. In early goal-directed therapy for sepsis, volume resuscitation targets central venous pressures of 8 to 12 mm Hg followed by the addition of vasoactive agents to keep the mean arterial pressure at 65 to 90 mm Hg.
- In patients with penetrating trauma, attaining "normal" filling and systemic pressures before hemostasis may result in undesirable hemodilution, coagulopathy, bleeding, and less favorable outcomes.[10]

Although these two examples illustrate possible differences in initial blood pressure goals, the therapeutic principles of ensuring adequate D_{O_2} can be applied to all forms of shock. Targeted resuscitation strategies provide an orderly approach to resuscitation, monitoring, and outcome validation. In general, such strategies optimize cardiovascular performance and concurrently measure markers of adequate global D_{O_2} and tissue use. Increased serum lactate concentration, decreased mixed venous oxygen saturation, and decreased central venous oxygen saturation are the proxy markers for inadequate global D_{O_2}. Noninvasive techniques have reduced the need to obtain physiologic data by the use of a pulmonary artery catheter.[13] Normal values of mixed venous oxygen saturation and central venous oxygen saturation do not guarantee normal use of oxygen in the tissues, however, particularly at the regional level. Appropriate targets for microcirculatory resuscitation remain elusive. Gastric tonometry, sublingual capnography, near-infrared spectroscopy, and orthogonal polarization spectral imaging are some of the current unvalidated technologies available to assess the effectiveness of resuscitation at the regional level.[14]

Resuscitation products should target the intravascular components that are inadequate, including red blood cell concentrates, platelets, coagulation factors, and acellular resuscitation fluids. Fluid type, bolus volume, and maintenance rate must be individualized. The optimal resuscitation fluid effectively should expand the intravascular space and minimize the inflammatory response (particularly in hemorrhagic shock[15,16]). All resuscitation fluids leak to some degree out of the intravascular space into the interstitium of the extracellular space. Hypotonic resuscitation fluids are inappropriate for volume resuscitation because of their inability to remain exclusively in the extracellular space. Volume per volume, hypertonic fluids cause more intravascular expansion than isotonic fluids. Hypertonic fluids yield no better outcomes than isotonic crystalloids, however, in the resuscitation of trauma patients. Similarly, isotonic crystalloids are at least as efficacious or may be better than colloids to reach the same end points.[14]

Metabolic consequences are associated with virtually all resuscitation fluids. Ringer's lactate can activate neutrophils and cause a potent inflammatory response.[17] Hypertonic saline and dextran combinations cause less of an inflammatory response but any mortality benefit is unproved.[18,19] Greater than 1 L of hypertonic saline typically results in the development of hypernatremia. Resuscitation exclusively with isotonic NaCl results in a hyperchloremic acidosis. Hetastarch can cause coagulopathy if greater than 1.5 L is given. All acellular resuscitation fluids, if given in sufficient quantities, cause dilutional anemia. Despite this confusing and contradictory collection of recommendations, no single resuscitation fluid is satisfactory on its own.

Temperature Control

Postoperative patients can come to the ICU with moderate-to-severe hypothermia. Heat is lost in the operating room as a result of vasodilation from volatile anesthetics, cool intravenous fluids and air temperature, large open surfaces, and evaporation. Excluding patients with potentially anoxic central nervous system injuries,[20] hypothermia complicates initial postoperative care by creating an in vivo coagulopathy, even when in vitro coagulation studies (normalized to 37°C) are normal. In trauma patients, reduction in enzyme activity and platelet function, leading to abnormal fibrin polymerization, occurs at temperatures less than 34° C.[21] Care must be taken when administering large volumes of cold blood products or even room temperature crystalloids. Fluid warming devices are available not only to prevent, but also to treat hypothermia. All patients with postoperative hypothermia less than 36° C should be actively warmed with forced air blankets, and when normothermia has been achieved, patients should be kept covered to prevent heat loss. Active warming does not cause peripheral vasodilation and subsequent hypotension, and it does not paradoxically cause core cooling owing to heat exchange in cold extremities.

Awakening from Anesthesia

Before successful resuscitation, sedation, analgesia, and anxiolysis should be maintained to facilitate patient comfort and to prevent interference with medical care (e.g., mechanical ventilation or motor activity jeopardizing airway, drains, and intravenous catheters). Selected agents should have minimal hemodynamic sequelae and relatively short duration of action so that frequent neurologic assessment can be performed. Daily interruption of continuous sedation has been shown to reduce ICU length of stay, duration of mechanical ventilation, and incidence of post-traumatic stress disorder.[22,23] The use of standardized sedation scales may obviate the need for daily interruption of sedation, while maintaining the benefits of continuous sedation.

Narcotics such as fentanyl, morphine, and hydromorphone make ideal first-line analgesics. Delivered by continuous infusion and supplemented as needed, successful analgesia reduces pain-driven tachycardia and hypertension and facilitates cough and deep breathing. The sensation of anxiety is a potent dysphoric stimulus that can result in restlessness and interfere with care. Anxiety can be treated with short-acting intravenous benzodiazepines, such as lorazepam. Very short-acting benzodiazepines, such as midazolam, are less useful because of the dosing frequency necessary to prevent symptoms from returning. Narcotics and benzodiazepines, when given in sufficient dose, can reduce greatly the level of consciousness. This may be a desired effect in a patient who has persistent restlessness that competes with mechanical ventilation or provision of care. If further reduction of level of consciousness is necessary, propofol or dexmedetomidine can be added and titrated to desired effect. Dexmedetomidine, a weak analgesic, can reduce narcotic requirements.[24] Propofol has no intrinsic analgesic properties, however. In a patient who has serious pain, neither propofol nor dexmedetomidine should be used without the concurrent administration of a narcotic. The use of most agents mentioned can be limited by their tendency to reduce blood pressure.

When patients are resuscitated adequately, consideration can be given to awakening from residual sedation. On arrival to the surgical ICU or recovery room, unconsciousness, if present, is due to the residual effects of volatile anesthetics, narcotics, benzodiazepines, and paralytics. The effects of volatile anesthetics can persist for 20 to 60 minutes after their discontinuation, particularly if the agent is fat-soluble, the patient is obese, and the case was long. Paralytics can have longer than expected duration of action, and this should be suspected when a postoperative patient remains very weak (cannot perform a 10-second head lift) or does not move. A train-of-four twitch monitor can address this issue. Persistent chemical paralysis can be reversed with neostigmine and glycopyrrolate.

Re-entry into consciousness may be accompanied by disorientation, anxiety, pain, and varying degrees of restlessness. In the absence of underlying encephalopathy, it is usually possible to get patients to follow commands, answer questions, and participate in the extubation process. The discomfort of an endotracheal tube can lead to unplanned self-extubation. It is important for the bedside care provider to maintain control of the recovery process by ensuring analgesia and anxiolysis. Small doses of narcotic or benzodiazepine or both can usually correct these problems without inducing further sedation and delay of extubation.[25] Patients with encephalopathy resulting from sepsis or shock may not recover a level of consciousness that allows participation in the weaning process. It is controversial whether such a patient should be extubated (avoiding the complications of prolonged extubation) or remain intubated until the ability to protect the airway is more certain. Dexmedetomidine can reduce restlessness without respiratory suppression and may be useful to facilitate extubation of a restless patient. Patients who require sedation for an extended time should receive doses of medication no higher than necessary to achieve the therapeutic target. Sedation scales, such as the Ramsay and Richmond Agitation Sedation Scale,[26] are useful to avoid oversedation and ultimately promote earlier liberation from mechanical ventilation. See Chapter 20 for a comprehensive discussion of sedation and analgesia.

Postoperative Extubation

Liberation from mechanical ventilation requires clinical readiness to begin weaning and demonstration of adequate physiologic reserve before extubation. Clinical readiness assesses completion of perioperative tasks at hand and questions any need for early return to the operating room. Resuscitation should be complete, hemostasis should be achieved, metabolic acidosis should be resolving, vasoactive support and gas exchange abnormalities should be minimized, anesthetic agents should be cleared, the ability to protect the airway should be present, and the patient should be awake and reasonably cooperative. These criteria have not been validated clinically, but similar consensus guidelines have been published.[27] Daily, if not more frequent, reassessment of clinical readiness is necessary to determine if it is reasonable to consider weaning.[28]

Patients who are ready clinically to progress to extubation should have an assessment of physiologic reserve. Having the patient breathe without mechanical assistance allows observation of respiratory rate, mechanical coordination of chest and abdomen, vital signs, end-tidal carbon dioxide concentration, and subjective comfort. If the patient was not mechanically ventilated preoperatively, the perioperative course has been uneventful after 60 to 90 minutes, the patient is comfortable with stable vital signs, and no tachypnea or respiratory muscle dyssynchrony is present, extubation can usually proceed.

Patients who do not achieve these basic criteria may require continued mechanical ventilation that maximizes patient comfort and unloads the respiratory muscles. These patients require a structured, evidence-based approach to ventilator weaning and assessment of adequate physiologic reserve. For more detailed information on weaning, refer to Chapter 44.

BEST PRACTICES

Achieving optimal outcomes should be pursued by providing optimal care. This is especially true for patients with longer length of stay. Effort should be expended pursuing interventions that have been shown to reduce complications, cost, morbidity, and mortality. Because a postoperative ICU patient is different in many ways from other ICU patients, some of these fundamental practices are applied with slight nuance and warrant additional mention.

Prevention of Venous Thromboembolism and Deep Venous Thrombosis

All postoperative ICU patients should be considered for venous thromboembolism (VTE) or deep venous thrombosis (DVT) prophylaxis. For *general surgery* patients with moderate to high risk[29] of VTE or DVT, prevention is anticoagulant based. Low-dose unfractionated heparin twice a day or low-molecular-weight heparin once a day should be continued in the absence of postoperative bleeding or instituted if not started intraoperatively. Patients at higher risk for VTE/DVT should receive low-dose unfractionated heparin three times a day or low-molecular-weight heparin once a day. Very-high-risk patients should receive mechanical prophylaxis via sequential compression devices (SCD), in addition to low-dose unfractionated heparin or low-molecular-weight heparin. In general surgery patients with a high risk of postoperative bleeding, mechanical prophylaxis should be the initial preventive modality until the risk of bleeding has decreased enough to allow for anticoagulant prophylaxis.

Neurosurgical procedures or the use of neuraxial analgesia also require special consideration. Anticoagulant prophylaxis should not be in effect while epidural catheters are placed or removed and should be used with caution while an epidural catheter is in place. Patients undergoing intracranial surgery should receive mechanical prophylaxis with SCD. Anticoagulant prophylaxis should be added in patients at high risk for VTE/DVT beginning 24 hours postoperatively.[29]

Trauma patients constitute an extremely heterogeneous group, making it difficult to study the strategies of VTE/DVT prophylaxis. There is disagreement in the literature about valid independent risk factors for VTE/DVT in trauma patients. Older age, spinal fractures, spinal cord injuries, traumatic brain injuries, prolonged mechanical ventilation, pelvic fractures, venous injuries, and multiple major operative procedures are often cited. In trauma patients, there are few large, prospective, randomized studies validating the efficacy of any method of VTE/DVT prevention.[30] Low-dose unfractionated heparin, which has proven efficacy in the general surgery population, is no better than absence of prophylaxis in a trauma patient.[31] Low-molecular-weight heparin given twice daily does offer a statistical benefit, however, in the prevention VTE/DVT in trauma patients.[32] Trauma patients without significant risks for bleeding should begin anticoagulant prophylaxis or postoperatively. Data are insufficient to make recommendations as to when anticoagulant prophylaxis in trauma patients with brain injury or liver or spleen fracture is safe. Waiting 72 hours in the former and 48 hours in the latter, after bleeding has ceased, are conservative times to delay. In trauma patients at high risk for bleeding, mechanical prophylaxis can be used, although benefit is unproved. In selected trauma patients, expected to have prolonged immobilization or with significant risks for bleeding, inferior vena cava filters may be placed as VTE prophylaxis.[30] Inferior vena cava filters should not be used as a primary prophylactic strategy in trauma patients.[29] If available, removable filters should be considered. SCD cannot be applied to lower extremities with fractures, fasciotomies, or external fixators. Compression devices applied to the feet may be used as a substitute for SCD, but have not been shown to be as efficacious as leg devices. In a trauma patient at high risk for VTE/DVT, the addition of mechanical prophylaxis to anticoagulant prophylaxis may be useful, but synergistic benefit is unproved.

Stress Ulcer Prophylaxis

Stress-related mucosal disease (SRMD) is manifest as diffuse gastric mucosal petechiae, erosions (loss of epithelium, necrosis, and hemorrhage), and discrete ulcers. SRMD can progress to clinically significant bleeding resulting in hemodynamic instability and need for transfusion. It can develop as early as 24 hours after ICU admission. Patients at risk for SRMD include critically ill patients who require mechanical ventilation for greater than 48 hours and patients with coagulopathy (risk associated with the presence of shock only approached statistical significance).[33] Other patients are at low risk for clinically significant bleeding. The risk of clinically significant bleeding increases with the severity of illness, duration of mechanical ventilation, increased length of stay, and low intragastric pH. Hemodynamic compromise secondary to acute blood loss occurs in only a small percentage of patients with SRMD, but it is associated with a significantly increased mortality rate.[34]

Because of the morbidity and mortality associated with the complications of SRMD, it is important to identify patients at risk for SRMD and employ effective prophylaxis before bleeding occurs. Although early enteral nutrition has many benefits, the effects of enteral nutrition on SRMD are controversial and should not be used as a sole prophylactic strategy.[35] Pharmacologic prophylaxis targets mucosal protection or the suppression of acid secretion. Proton-pump inhibitors may be a good first choice for SRMD prophylaxis owing to degree of acid suppression, duration of action, lack of tolerance, and cost, but data are lacking. Parenteral H_2 receptor antagonists may offer a cost advantage over proton-pump inhibitors. Prophylaxis with sucralfate is not preferred because of the efficacy profile of acid-suppression therapies and a higher rate of bleeding with sucralfate prophylaxis.

Preventing Nosocomial Pneumonia

Postoperative patients should be encouraged to take deep breaths, cough, ambulate, and use incentive spirometry. Iatrogenic spread of bacteria can be reduced by the enforcement of hand washing and by the use of appropriate barrier protection when performing procedures.[36] Semirecumbent body positioning, keeping the head of bed elevated more than 30 degrees, has been shown to reduce ventilator-associated pneumonia in mechanically ventilated patients.[37] Placing the bed in reverse Trendelenburg position can simulate this elevation without flexing the back, as could be difficult in trauma patients or patients with large open abdomens. Before deflating the cuff of an endotracheal tube for tube removal or position change, ensure that secretions are suctioned clear from above the cuff.[36] Endotracheal tubes designed to provide drainage to the subglottic area above the tube's cuff have been shown to reduce the risk of ventilator-associated pneumonia.[38] The use of 0.12% chlorhexidine oral rinse has been associated with reductions in the rate of ventilator-associated pneumonia in surgical ICU patients and should be part of good oral hygiene.[39] Although there is evidence that selective digestive decontamination beyond the oropharynx also can reduce the risk of ventilator-associated pneumonia, it is unclear how the routine use of this technique would affect antimicrobial resistance.[40] The use of noninvasive ventilation in patients with exacerbations of chronic obstructive pulmonary disorder and congestive heart failure is associated with reductions in rates of nosocomial pneumonia, but there are few studies evaluating application of this technique in the management of postoperative respiratory failure. Use of noninvasive ventilation may be associated with a higher mortality rate when used to manage failed extubation (see Chapter 44).[41]

Management of Agitation and Delirium

Delirium is a major problem in postoperative ICU patients.[42] Previously believed to be an expected and unavoidable result of critical illness that resolves with clinical improvement, it is now known to be a significant marker of increased morbidity,[43] resource use, and long-term cognitive deficit. Delirium is an acute, variable change in mental status with inattention and either altered level of consciousness or disorganized thinking. Occurring in about 70% to 80% of ICU patients, delirium had been underdiagnosed until validated assessment tools such as the Confusion Assessment Method for the ICU (CAM-ICU) became available.[44] Delirium is believed to be due to imbalances between the stimulatory and inhibitory neurotransmitters, particularly an increase in dopaminergic and decrease in γ-aminobutyric acid and cholinergic activity. Risk factors include age, pre-existing dementia, sepsis, metabolic abnormalities, and medications. The use of benzodiazepines, narcotics, anticholinergics, and antipsychotics is associated with a substantial increase in risk. It is currently unclear whether prevention or treatment of delirium changes clinical outcomes such as mortality and long-term cognitive deficits.

Preventive strategies include avoidance of hypoxemia (Fig. 36-2), correction of metabolic disturbances, restoration of sleep/wake cycles, adequate pain control, minimization of unnecessary physical and auditory stimulation, frequent reorientation (particularly with family involvement), and early mobilization.[42] Pharmacologic treatment of delirium is suboptimal because the same medications intended to reduce disorganized thought may simultaneously increase sedation, prolonging the undesired state. Benzodiazepines may aggravate disorganized thought and should not be used to treat delirium. Haloperidol is the most commonly prescribed neuroleptic to treat delirium,[45] although its efficacy is yet to be validated. Until efficacy of any pharmacologic intervention is shown, medications should be used in the lowest doses possible for as brief a time as possible.

Management of Hyperglycemia

Hyperglycemia in a critically ill patient can be due to diabetes mellitus (established or new) or stress-induced release of counter-regulatory mediators. It is associated with increased mortality after acute myocardial infarction, stroke, and severe traumatic brain injury. Hyperglycemia also is associated with reduced functional outcome after neurologic injury, the development of polyneuropathy in critically ill patients, increased rates of infectious complications in the postoperative period, and defective collagen formation in wound healing.

More recent literature has shown that outcomes can be improved with more intensive monitoring and treatment of hyperglycemia in postoperative patients requiring continued ICU stay. Animal studies have shown improvement in survival and neurologic outcome in models of cerebral ischemia and head trauma.[46] In a large prospective study of cardiac surgery patients, tight glycemic control with intravenous insulin was associated with a significant reduction in deep sternal surgical site infections compared with glycemic control with subcutaneous insulin.[47] Tight glycemic control with insulin also has been shown to improve mortality attributable to infection, reduce polyneuropathy, and reduce the need for mechanical ventilation.[48]

It is increasingly clear that correction of hyperglycemia, rather than supplementation of insulin, is responsible for the beneficial effects. A vigilant approach to monitoring and an urgent and efficacious treatment of hyperglycemia needs to be implemented. Unreliable subcutaneous absorption, extreme or labile hyperglycemia, and inconsistent caloric intake are reasons to use short-acting, continuous intravenous insulin rather than slower-onset, longer-acting subcutaneous insulin. Insulin therapy should target a blood glucose range of 80 to 110 mg/dL.

POSTOPERATIVE NUTRITION

Postoperative surgical patients are exposed to unique nutritional challenges as a result of the enhanced metabolic demands of wound healing and the abnormalities of bowel motility, anastomotic function, and swallowing. Nutritional support provides calories for metabolic processes, reduces catabolism of protein stores as an energy source, supplies substrate for anabolic processes, and provides an opportunity to reduce net protein losses in the face of ongoing protein catabolism. In an otherwise well-nourished postoperative patient, beginning nutritional support may be unnecessary, unless it is anticipated that oral nutrition would be delayed for 7 days.[49] There are considerably fewer studies showing nutritional support strategies that work in the postoperative patient than ones that do not work.[50]

Timing and Route

There are three routes of nutritional support—enteral nutrition, parenteral nutrition, and oral feedings. With respect to outcomes, it is important to consider not only the route of administration, but also the timing. Neither enteral nutrition nor parenteral nutrition seems to have an effect on *mortality* whether given preoperatively or postoperatively.[51] *Preoperative* nutritional support seems to benefit only severely malnourished patients by reducing complication rates.[52,53] Parenteral nutrition, which requires vascular access, is associated with complications related to non–catheter-related infection and catheter-related bloodstream infection.[51] In addition to avoiding the complications associated with parenteral nutrition, enteral nutrition possibly reduces gut mucosal atrophy and bacterial translocation. In perioperative patients, sufficient evidence is lacking, however, to suggest that the effect of enteral nutri-

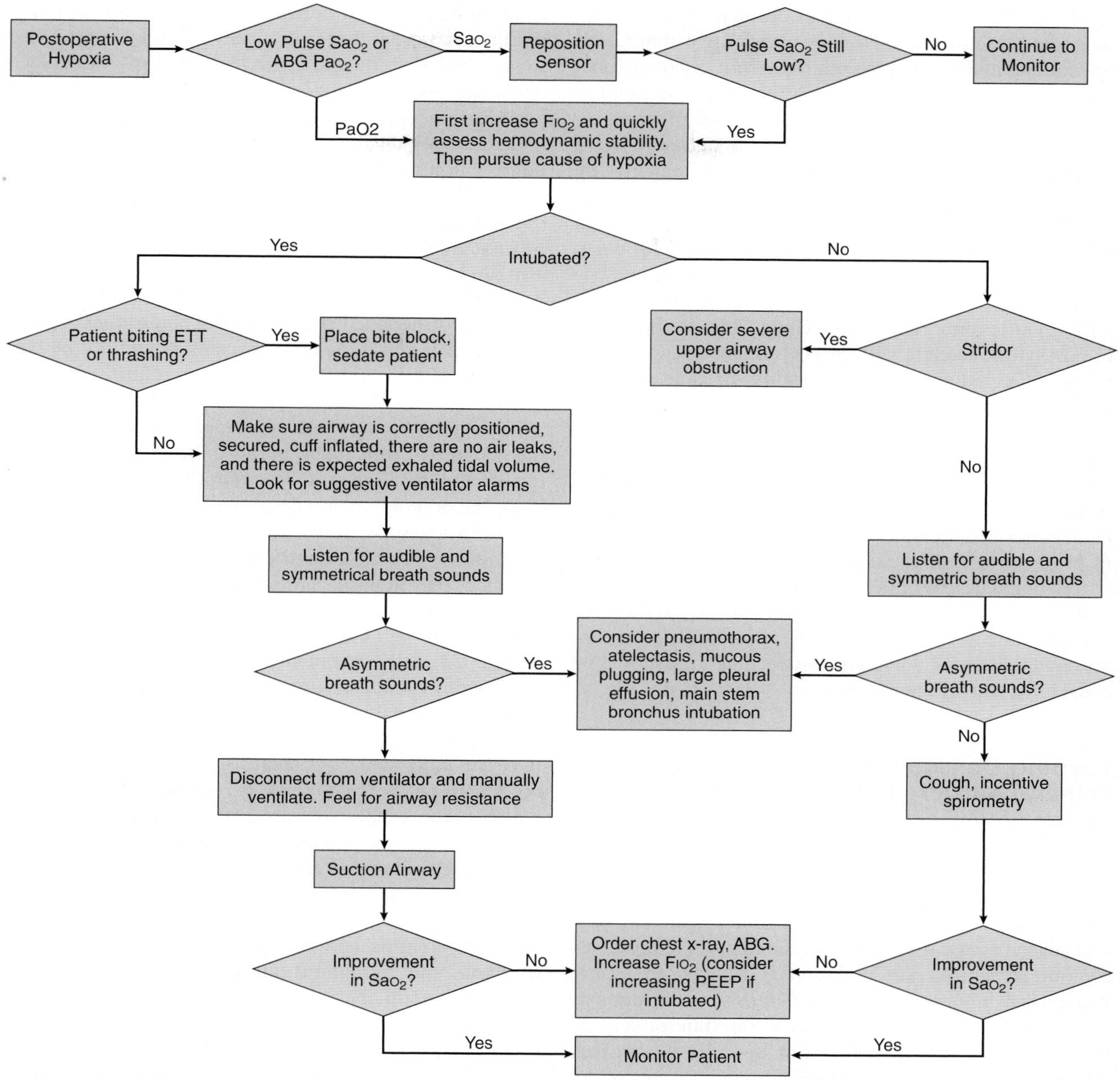

Figure 36-2. Approach to managing postoperative hypoxemia. ABG, arterial blood gas; ETT, endotracheal tube; Fio_2, fraction of inspired oxygen; Pao_2; arterial oxygen tension; PEEP, positive end-expiratory pressure; Sao_2; arterial oxygen saturation.

tion on the gut barrier has any outcome advantage over parenteral nutrition.[54,55] Enteral nutrition has been shown to be associated with a lower risk of infection compared with parenteral nutrition.[56] Early enteral nutrition also has been shown to be associated with a shorter length of stay and lower incidence of infections compared with delayed enteral nutrition.[57] Enteral nutrition is the preferred route over parenteral nutrition because of the reduction in complications and cost. Early postoperative parenteral nutrition does not improve clinical outcomes and should be reserved only for patients who are unable to receive timely enteral nutrition.[58]

The combination of parenteral nutrition and early enteral nutrition has no advantage over early enteral nutrition alone in patients who are not malnourished.[59] Patients who are malnourished or are not expected to be tolerating oral feedings at nutritional goal by about postoperative day 7 should begin enteral nutrition as soon as bowel function permits. If otherwise adequately nourished postoperative ICU patients are expected to be tolerating oral feedings at nutritional goal by postoperative day 7, early enteral nutrition may not provide substantial benefit. Finally, patients who are able to take oral feedings but are unable to consume an amount equal to the nutritional goal require supplemental nutrition, typically enteral nutrition.

When the decision is made to deliver enteral nutrition, tube feedings should be increased quickly in volume to reach nutritional goal. The initial destination for enteral nutrition is the stomach. Nothing about laparotomy itself precludes enteral nutrition with the return of bowel function (e.g., bowel sounds, flatus). Although bowel motility continues through surgery or returns shortly thereafter, gastroparesis is common postoperatively and may result in delayed gastric emptying. It may be recognized by abdominal distention, high daily nasogastric output (>500 mL/d), or high residual volume in the stomach (>300 mL). Gastroparesis has the potential to delay achieving delivery of adequate enteral nutrition and has resulted in a trend toward delivering enteral nutrition via a postpyloric route. There is no clinical benefit, however, to postpyloric feeding with respect to incidence of pneumonia, ICU length of stay, mortality, or time to reach nutritional goal compared with the prepyloric route.[60] Gastroparesis often can be improved with prokinetic agents, such as metoclopramide or erythromycin.[61] It is reasonable to continue gastric enteral nutrition in the presence of gastric residual volumes of 150 to 300 mL as long as the patient is not experiencing nausea, vomiting, or progressive abdominal distention or has any evidence of functional gastric outlet obstruction or ileus. The nasogastric route of feeding is preferred, but if establishing stomach function is anticipated to be problematic, implantation placement of a jejunostomy feeding tube should be considered during laparotomy.

Feeding Considerations in General Surgery Patients

Patients requiring esophageal resection may present with some degree of malnutrition. It is important to resume nutritional support as soon as technically possible after the operation. These patients have fragile anastomoses in their chests, however, which usually have a suction catheter placed across the repair to decompress the postanastomotic structures. An oral diet is delayed to ensure mechanical integrity of the anastomosis. Some patients have a distal feeding tube placed at the time of surgery so that enteral nutrition does not need to be delayed. Patients who cannot receive oral or enteral nutrition by postoperative day 7 should be considered for early institution of parenteral nutrition.

Gastric surgery may result in delayed gastric emptying. Vagal denervation can cause some degree of gastroparesis, and functional outlet obstruction may occur owing to edema at the site of anastomosis. Gastric enteral nutrition cannot be started until gastric emptying improves. If it seems that gastric enteral nutrition would be unacceptably delayed, a more distal enteral route should be secured, or parenteral nutrition should be started. Patients with new gastrostomies, whether placed percutaneously or via an open procedure, rarely have postoperative motility disturbances. It is common, however, to wait for 24 hours before use of gastronomy feeding tubes.

Postoperative ICU patients with manipulation, resection, or diversion of the bowel may have a transient ileus. Small bowel hypomotility, if present, resolves 6 to 8 hours after surgery, and some absorptive capacity is present even without normal peristalsis.[62,63] Large bowel hypomotility, if present, begins to resolve 24 hours postoperatively, heralded by the passage of flatus. Recognized postoperatively as abdominal distention on physical examination or a nonobstructed gas pattern on abdominal x-ray, ileus usually resolves over 24 to 72 hours with conservative therapy including nasogastric suctioning. Refractory ileus in the absence of mechanical obstruction should suggest some unresolved inflammatory process. In the absence of such unresolved problems, ileus also can be improved with prokinetic agents. Neostigmine has been successful in decompressing acute colonic pseudo-obstruction.[64] The presence of enterotomy repairs, bowel anastomoses, or new ostomies should not be barriers to enteral nutrition with the return of bowel function.[65]

Nutritional support in the presence of an enterocutaneous fistula is problematic because enteral nutrition can exacerbate fistula output. This output, particularly when high, can perpetuate or worsen malnutrition owing to the loss of nitrogen. With the exception of some colocutaneous fistulas, conservative therapy consists of bowel rest (nothing per mouth), parenteral nutrition, control of infection, correction of electrolyte disturbances, and local wound care. High-output fistulas may require a daily nonprotein calorie complement based on 1.5 to 2 times the basal energy expenditure plus 1.5 to 2.5 g/protein to satisfy nutritional needs.[66]

Acute pancreatitis is treated commonly in the surgical ICU. In mild acute pancreatitis, enteral nutrition has no effect on outcome and is recommended only in patients who cannot tolerate oral nutrition after 5 to 7 days.[67] In severe acute pancreatitis, the therapeutic pendulum has swung from bowel rest and parenteral nutrition back toward early enteral nutrition. Although no differences in mortality have been shown in severe acute pancreatitis between groups treated with enteral nutrition and parenteral nutrition, the early enteral nutrition group has significant reductions in stress response, infections, surgical interventions, and length of stay.[68,69] Early enteral nutrition can be given equally effectively via gastric or postpyloric destinations when started at low volumes and incremented slowly toward nutritional goal.[70]

WOUND HEALING AND CARE

Physiology and Biology of Wound Healing

Many tissues in the body respond to injury by undergoing a reparative process, which can be described histologically, biochemically, chronologically, or functionally. There are many ways to label these processes, but a simple and useful paradigm includes inflammatory, proliferative, and remodeling phases.[71,72] The process begins with hemostasis, inflammation, and generation of an extracellular matrix on which proliferating cells can attach. Wound healing is locally coordinated by cytokines and facilitated by systemically mobilized cellular elements and noncellular substrate. Ultimately, the normal healing process ends with collagen maturation. Collagen develops its tensile strength through intermolecular cross-linking of fibrils into larger and longer bundles. By 1 week's time, in the absence of extraordinary tension, the wound has developed enough mechanical integrity to allow for suture removal. The collagen mass undergoes continual synthesis and degradation as weaker, randomly oriented collagen fibers are reorganized into stronger, linear, highly cross-linked bundles aligned toward mechanical stress placed on the wound. This remodeling process may last 6 to 12 months. In normal circumstances, these phases tend to be sequential with generous overlap between the end of one phase and the beginning of the next.

Surgical site infection, the presence of necrotic tissue, ischemia, and poor surgical closure technique all can contribute to failed wound healing and possibly wound dehiscence. Whether a surgical wound purposely closed by *primary intention* or an open wound left to close slowly by granulation and wound contraction *(secondary intention)*, the healing processes are similar. Successful healing of a closed surgical wound yields mechanical integrity by virtue of high tensile strength. Successful healing in an open wound may be measured by epithelialization with the promise of satisfactory mechanical integrity (scarring) over time. Understanding these interrelated processes facilitates logical wound care and helps to avoid diversions from normal wound healing.

Epithelialization and Wound Care

Development of an epithelial barrier begins within hours of injury. In partial-thickness wounds, the source of epithelial repopulation is remaining dermal structures, sweat glands, and hair follicles. Epithelial cells from the basal layers of the wound migrate across the underlying extracellular matrix, reforming the characteristic basal to apical differentiation, until migration halts in the center of the wound because of contact inhibition. Wound coverage can be complete 24 to 48 hours after a clean surgical incision is closed by primary intention. At this time, no further wound protection is necessary, and skin cleansing with water is permitted. Bacteria, necrotic tissue, wound exudates, inflammatory cells, inflammatory mediators, and desiccation all retard re-epithelialization. Deeper or open wounds also show delayed epithelialization. Open wounds first must fill in with proliferating fibroblasts, capillaries, and a loose extracellular matrix made of collagen and proteoglycans (granulation tissue) before epithelialization can occur. Such tissue is of poor mechanical integrity.

The ability of epithelialization to occur from the margin of the wounds over the granulation tissue depends on the presence of adequate angiogenesis, absence of bacterial burden, the provision of a moist environment, and the removal of excess necrosis and proteinaceous exudates (which contain proteases and inflammatory mediators and support bacterial growth). With optimal circumstances, the maximal rate of epithelialization from the margins occurs at 1 to 2 mm/d. As the epithelial cells mature and stratification progresses, keratinization occurs.

Without moist, occlusive dressings over superficial wounds, a scab forms, delaying epithelialization. Only with clot proteolysis can the wound be resurfaced successfully. If the wound is kept moist with an occlusive dressing,[73] however, and accumulated exudates and necrotic tissue are removed frequently, epithelialization can occur. Small amounts of wound exudates and necrotic tissue can be removed with frequent, moist dressing changes and water irrigation; larger amounts may require surgical débridement. The optimal wound dressing provides a moist environment, has absorptive reserve to trap wound exudates, possesses bacteriostatic properties, and does not adhere to the wound. Large, open wounds may be dressed with moist gauze at the surface and reinforced with dry gauze packing (wet-to-dry dressing). Absorptive capacity is limited, however, and frequent dressing changes are required. Dressings made of hydrocolloids, materials that incorporate high-capacity absorptive materials into a self-adhering occlusive backing, are useful for open wounds of moderate size and allow for less frequent dressing changes. More recently, the vacuum-assisted closure has gained popularity for the management of large open wounds. Vacuum-assisted closure therapy is the combination of moderate suction applied above an absorptive surface, such as a towel or sponge, which is covered by an occlusive plastic drape. This application provides for continual removal of wound exudates and edema and may improve local perfusion and promote wound contraction.[74]

Optimizing Wound Healing

Management of Hyperglycemia

Hyperglycemia is common in postoperative critically ill patients and is associated with poor outcome in a variety of conditions. In the current context, hyperglycemia is associated with impaired immune response, infection, and impaired wound healing.[46] Although the optimal glucose range has not been validated, a target of 80 to 110 mg/dL is reasonable. Hypoglycemia and hyperglycemia are to be avoided.

Antibiotics

The routine use of systemic antibiotics to aid wound healing, in the absence of actual surgical site infection, should be avoided. Wound surfaces are typically colonized by bacteria, and this colonization is not detrimental to wound healing. An increased bacterial load, more than the typical colonization, may impede wound healing, however. Distinguishing between common colonization and an increased bacterial burden requires microbiologic confirmation. Simple swab cultures lack specificity, and quantitative tissue cultures revealing greater than 10^5 organisms/g may be necessary to identify true bacterial burden. Topical antibiotics are commonly applied to wound surfaces, but the benefits of topical antibiotics are not well documented.[72] The incorporation of silver into dressing materials adds bacteriostatic properties and may be useful to limit bacterial overgrowth in the wound.

Nutrition in Wound Healing

Nutritional deficiencies can impede wound healing. Large, open wounds are metabolically demanding and may be a source of substantial protein loss. Daily dietary goals of calorie and protein need to be increased accordingly. Deficiencies of vitamins and minerals (micronutrients) are infrequent, but should be suspected in malnourished (including unusual dietary habits) patients, elderly patients, and patients who have been receiving parenteral nutrition. Vitamin and mineral supplementation should accompany dietary calorie and protein in patients with deficiencies, but the benefit of pharmacologic doses of these micronutrients in the absence of deficiency is unproved. Vitamin A is required for proper fibroblast proliferation, collagen cross-linking, and epithelialization. Vitamin A may reverse the inhibitory effects of steroids on the inflammatory phase of wound healing and may be useful in steroid-dependent patients with poorly healing wounds.[75] Vitamin C is needed for hydroxylation of lysine and proline in collagen formation (see earlier). The benefit of vitamin C supplementation in patients receiving a normal diet is not validated. Zinc is an essential trace mineral for protein synthesis, cell division, and protein synthesis; however, its supplementation has not been shown to be beneficial in patients who are not zinc deficient.[75] Glucosamine is required for the synthesis of hyaluronic acid, an abundant component of the extracellular matrix, but also lacks clinical validation of benefit.

Surgical Site Infections

Infections of surgical incisions are referred to as surgical site infections (SSIs).[76,77] SSIs are *superficial* incisional SSIs when limited to skin and subcutaneous tissues above the fascia or *deep* incisional SSIs if extending below. Intracavitary SSIs are referred to as organ-space SSIs. The surgical site becomes inoculated either inward from the skin or outward from the structures beneath the incision. Most SSIs are caused by the gram-positive cocci found on the skin, such as *Staphylococcus aureus, Staphylococcus epidermidis,* and *Enterococcus* species. The type of the operation also can influence the causative organisms of the SSI such that enteric aerobic gram-negative rods (*Escherichia, Enterobacter*) and anaerobic organisms (*Bacteroides*) are more likely after intestinal or head and neck surgery.[76]

Skin and bowel preparations are used preoperatively to reduce bacterial numbers. These techniques, in addition to the use of narrow-spectrum "prophylactic" systemic antibiotics, have reduced the incidence of SSIs. Administration of prophylactic antibiotics beyond 24 hours, even in the presence of colonic perforation or shock, does not contribute further to reducing the rate of SSIs, however.[78] In addition, prolonged use of prophylactic antibiotics may result in the emergence of multiple drug–resistant strains of organisms, *Clostridium difficile* colitis, nosocomial pneumonia, and catheter-related infections.[79] It is important to discontinue prophylactic antibiotics before the benefits of such therapy are overshadowed by the risks that their continuation brings with them.

The first rule of wound evaluation is "Take off the dressing and look at the wound." Wounds should be evaluated at least daily for progression of healing and for development of infection. Normally healing surgical incisions should be dry with a minimal dry scab at the point of closure. The edges should have at most a 3- to 4-mm border of erythema and induration when fresh, which should resolve over about 1 week. Nonpurulent drainage is not likely to be infected. Clear drainage from the wound may simply be escaping subcutaneous edema fluid. Wounds with an enlarging border of erythema and induration, without fluctuance or drainage, particularly when painful to palpation, suggest cellulitis or infection of deeper structures. Fluctuance and drainage may be from an abscess beneath the wound. Drainage that is turbid or frankly purulent should suggest true SST. SSIs require opening of the incision for irrigation and drainage. Antibiotics may not be needed for uncomplicated SSIs, which respond to this intervention and local care.[76]

More complicated SSIs require systemic antibiotics directed at the likely pathogens. Culture of pus collected aseptically is useful to guide therapy, but simple swab cultures of the wound surface are of low specificity because of the presence of wound colonizers. Necrotizing SSIs can spread rapidly through soft tissues and involve the fascia (necrotizing fasciitis). Necrotizing soft tissue infections can have subtle findings at the skin surface (e.g., an advancing border of erythema), while forging a destructive path just below. Wounds that dehisce superficially or at the fascia should suggest infection or technically inadequate closure. Dehiscence almost always requires surgical evaluation. When an abdominal wound has open skin, evaluation for status of the fascial closure is needed. The mechanical integrity can be evaluated by gently probing the closure with sterile cotton-tipped swabs. The edges of these wounds should show yellow fat or pink granulation. Dark gray, nonviable tissue should be obvious on inspection and should be débrided.

Drains

Few things in the postoperative patient are more puzzling and sometimes intimidating than drains. Seemingly simple in construction and intuitive in purpose, the efficacy of these devices and their application are quite limited. A study of the history of drainage is a study in the evolution of medicine and surgery itself. The earliest description of drains shows their application for the removal of fluid from large cavities, such as the pleural space, abdomen, and bladder, and for the treatment of wounds.

Drains can be classified on many levels.[80] Drains with one end open to the atmosphere are known as "open" systems and constitute most early devices. Before the recognition of germ theory, it was not appreciated that open systems provided a free route for entrance of etiologic agents into the body. Some open systems employed a filter at the open end to limit the ability of microorganisms to enter the system. "Closed" systems of drainage have no opening to the atmosphere directly; fluid collection terminates in a bag or canister.

Structurally, drains can be classified as "hollow" or "capillary." Hollow drains take on many shapes, but all have one or multiple internal lumens and have fenestrations throughout a portion of their length, sometimes including their ends. Fenestrations must be large enough to allow fluid and debris to enter, but not so large as to allow significant portions of tissue, such as omentum or intestine, to enter. Such migration into the drain has been the cause of drain failure, tissue adhesion, and organ injury. Capillary-type drains leverage the physical interaction, which occurs between liquids and the walls of thin tubes and fibers. Structurally, capillary-type devices are made from tufts of thin fibers, fabrics (e.g., gauze), or thin tubes.

Drains can be classified as "passive" or "active." Passive drains provide a route of low resistance to the body's exterior and are driven by capillary action and pressure gradients. Capillary-type drains are classified as passive drains. Active drains use an external source of negative pressure to establish a pressure gradient. Active drainage of deep recesses is classified as sump drainage. Sump drains were ultimately modified so that an additional lumen running alongside the primary lumen supplied atmospheric gas into the drainage site to prevent the intestine and omentum from occluding the fenestra.[81] Sump drains are used to drain the gastrointestinal tract and abscess cavities. Active drainage employing a closed system is used to obliterate potential spaces, particularly under skin/muscle flaps or other wounds.

Drains should be soft and flexible, but not so much that the lumen collapses with suction. Irritating materials, such as latex rubber, should be avoided (except in cases where development of a fibrous tract is desired, such as in T-tube biliary drainage). Siliconized materials (Silastic) and polyvinyl chloride are commonly used in contemporary drainage systems.

Drains also are classified as therapeutic or prophylactic.[82] Therapeutic drainage is intended to remove necrotic debris, pus, or fistula drainage or to prevent premature closure of wounds. Prophylactic drainage is intended to prevent the accumulation of blood, pus, bile, pancreatic secretions, intestinal contents, and fluids. In the historical literature of medicine and surgery, it was noted that patients with ovariotomy developed accumulations of blood and fluid in the pelvis. It was believed that this fluid, in stagnation, would decompose and release toxins whose absorption resulted in fatal outcomes. In 1882, drains were used to "remove from cavities fluids liable to undergo putrefactive changes if retained and to cleanse such cavities by injection of disinfectants."[80]

The popularity of drainage in certain applications waxed and waned owing to its controversial effect on outcome, particularly mortality. When surgeons abandoned the use of abdominal drains during World War II, mortality decreased by 50% compared with World War I.[83] The use of prophylactic drains, particularly in abdominal surgery, was equally controversial. Capillary-based systems, which did more to prevent drainage of necrotic or purulent material than facilitate its removal, ultimately fell out of favor. Complications increased from use of multiple or unnecessary drains and included ventral hernias, pain on removal, omental penetration of the drain's fenestrations, intestinal obstruction, adhesions (occasionally pulling omentum or bowel into the abdominal wall), fecal fistulas, and persistent sinus tracts. The pioneering surgeon Halsted believed that good surgical technique and obliteration of dead-space obviated the need for drainage in nonseptic instances. He believed that drains "invariably produce some necrosis of tissue with which it comes in contact and enfeebles the power of resistance of tissues towards organisms. But, given necrotic tissue plus infections, drains become almost indispensable."[80] Prophylactic drainage ultimately gave way to therapeutic drainage. In the 1920s, indications for drains included the "presence of free purulent material in considerable quantity . . . and the presence of an abscess sac."[80]

Currently, the indications for drainage include the following:

- Removal of cerebrospinal fluid (CSF) from the brain's ventricles or spinal cord for the purpose of reducing pressure in a closed space and improving perfusion pressure
- Removal of blood or fluid from the subdural space to prevent compression or shift of intracranial contents
- Closure of certain soft tissue wounds to minimize dead space and remove excess fluid and debris; often seen in neck surgery, breast surgery, and certain reconstructive procedures
- Drainage of the pleural space in the event of pneumothorax, hemothorax, or large pleural effusions
- Drainage of the pericardium to treat large pericardial effusions
- Drainage of abscess cavities; drains can be placed directly in the operating room or percutaneously with the guidance of imaging technologies
- Drainage of existing fistulas to create a controlled route of elimination; includes drainage of bile or pancreatic secretions, succus, or stool
- Surveillance drainage over the sites of complicated procedures involving the stomach, duodenum, pancreas, and rerouting anastomoses

Placement of surveillance drains is controversial because of the risk of creating a fistula by the drains themselves. In the event of a catastrophic breach in enteral integrity, such as the highly morbid duodenal stump "blow-out," early identification and controlled drainage may be facilitated.

In general, the following questions must be answered for all drains:

1. What is the intended anatomic location of the drain?
2. How can location be confirmed?
3. What is the expected quantity and quality of the drain's output?
4. Is the drain functioning normally?
5. When should a drain be removed and by what criteria?

Only by knowing the intended anatomic location of a given drain can a clinician determine the best way to confirm location and assess function. The visual location of a drain on physical examination does not ensure proper placement; a thoracostomy tube seen to penetrate the chest wall may not be in the pleural space, and a gastrostomy tube seen to penetrate the abdominal wall does not guarantee that the tip lies in the stomach. Sometimes the location of a drain cannot be confirmed, such as drains left in the peritoneum. This leaves only assessment of quantity and quality of drain output as a guide to the drain's proper function. For these reasons, it is useful to know certain characteristics of specific drains.

The most common drains seen after neurosurgical procedures are the subdural drain and the ventriculostomy. The former drain is usually a Silastic drain left in the subdural space to drain blood or fluid after craniotomy. There is no way to confirm its location. These drains typically drain about 20 to 30 mL of serosanguineous fluid per hour until tapering off to minimal drainage after about 6 hours. Frankly bloody drainage, particularly when in higher volumes or persisting longer than a few hours, suggests active bleeding that requires correction of coagulopathy or neurosurgical intervention. The ventriculostomy tube, also made of Silastic, has its tip located in a lateral ventricle. The proper tip location can be confirmed by seeing a pulsatile waveform when the catheter has continuous pressure monitoring and by seeing CSF output. About 450 mL of CSF is produced a day; the volume of CSF drained depends on the height of the drainage system's external port relative to the height of the catheter's tip in the ventricle and the ability of the arachnoid granulations to reabsorb CSF. The fluid may be clear or sanguineous depending on the intracranial pathology. CSF that changes from clear or serosanguineous to frankly bloody suggests a serious problem, particularly in subarachnoid hemorrhage. Declining or absent CSF drainage or loss of a pulsatile waveform suggests tube occlusion by clot or malposition and requires neurosurgical attention.

Thoracostomy tubes are placed to drain pleural effusions and treat pneumothorax. Thoracostomy tubes can be inadvertently placed subcutaneously. Proper location is confirmed by chest radiograph. The tube may be intentionally positioned in many orientations; however, the most proximal "sentinel" hole should always lie within the pleural space, and the tube should not be kinked. A properly functioning, correctly located thoracostomy tube should show a cycling of intrapleural pressure with respiration when the drainage system is on "water seal." Absence of cycling may suggest tube occlusion or inappropriate location. Bubbling across the water seal suggests an air leak, but does not indicate the source of the leak. Persistence of the bubbles across the water seal when the thoracostomy tube is clamped close to the chest wall indicates a leak in the drainage system, not in the lung. Variable amounts of suction can be applied to the thoracostomy tube, particularly when draining an effusion or reinflating a lung after pneumothorax. Initial suction of –20 cm H_2O is applied. Persistence of sanguineous drainage greater than 100 to 200 mL/h for 2 to 3 hours after the correction of hypothermia and coagulopathy suggests surgical bleeding and requires attention. When fluid drainage has diminished to about 100 to 200 mL/d or air leaks have ceased, external suction can be removed, and the water seal alone can be used to prevent lung collapse. If effusions or pneumothorax do not return, as assessed on chest radiograph, the thoracostomy tube can be removed.

Nasogastric or orogastric tubes are used to decompress the stomach or provide a route for nutrition. Double-lumen sump tubes should never have the secondary port clamped to prevent mucosal injury in the presence of suction. Inadvertent placement in the airways can be disastrous if enteral feedings are administered. Confirmation of gastric placement cannot be guaranteed by listening over the epigastrium during insufflation. Correct placement on radiograph is recognized by identifying the distal tip well below the diaphragm. Salivary and gastric output can be 0.75 to 1.5 L/d each. Continuous gastric suction can result in significant volume loss, leading to metabolic alkalosis. Gastric suction should be maintained until resolution of enteral obstructions or ileus. When the daily volume of gastric aspirate is less than 200 to 300 mL, gastric suction can be discontinued as long as nausea, vomiting, or abdominal distention does not result.

The color of gastric aspirate should be clear or yellow-green. Large volumes of bilious aspirate suggest the distal port of the drain is positioned beyond the pylorus. "Coffee grounds" or frank blood in the aspirate suggests bleeding in the stomach or duodenum. The stomach also can be accessed by placement of a surgical or percutaneous endoscopically assisted gastrostomy. These tubes infrequently migrate out of the stomach to lie in the peritoneum. Should acute abdominal pain or absence of typical gastric drainage occur in a patient with a recently placed gastrostomy, a radiographic contrast study of the gastrostomy should be done to exclude tube migration. The liver produces 500 to 1500 mL of bile daily. Drainage of the common bile duct via a T-tube is used after complicated biliary surgery, often for obstruction. The drainage tube itself causes a modest inflammatory reaction resulting in the formation of a fibrous tract. The drainage system is closed, without suction, and terminates in a collection bag. Significant reduction or cessation of biliary output may suggest either obstruction or malposition of the T-tube or resolution of the obstruction.

With the exception of drains placed in abscess cavities and to control the direction of pancreatic and enteral fistula output, drains left in the abdominal cavity are seen less frequently than in the past. Drains left in the peritoneum should have relatively little output. Confirmation of their location is usually unnecessary. A change in the quality or quantity of drainage is important to note. New bile, succus entericus, or stool in a drain suggests a breach in the integrity of some part of the viscera and requires investigation or surgical attention.

Drains placed in subcutaneous spaces or areas of reconstruction are placed to gentle suction to obliterate potential spaces and remove excessive fluid and blood collection. Confirmation of absolute location is generally unnecessary. The quality of the fluid should be serous to serosanguineous in volumes less than 100 mL hourly for the first 3 to 6 hours postoperatively before tapering off. Frankly bloody drainage in higher volumes or of longer durations suggests surgical bleeding in the absence of coagulopathy.

KEY POINTS

- Optimally, the location of a patient in the ICU is determined by matching the patient's needs with a location's resources and expertise. Such efficiency allows for greater institutional procedural volume, which, when paired with surgeon procedural volume, has been shown to be associated with reduced mortality.
- The postoperative evaluation should include a thorough evaluation of the patient's medical and surgical history and a physical examination, which should encompass all parts of the patient that can be accessed by sight and touch.
- "Adequate resuscitation" is a state, often temporary, which allows for good clinical perfusion and physiologic stability. The most fundamental concept is to ensure adequate DO_2 and meet $\dot{V}O_2$ needs of tissues and organelles.
- Resuscitation targets are reproducible, quantifiable values, such as pressures, outputs, metabolites, inflammatory mediators, or oxygen saturations, that represent therapeutic goals. Targeted resuscitation strategies optimize cardiovascular performance and concurrently measure markers of adequate global DO_2 and tissue use.
- Analgesics should be administered as the patient is resuscitated from anesthesia to facilitate comfort and avoid interference with medical care.
- Resuscitation should be complete, with hemostasis achieved, metabolic acidosis resolving, vasoactive support and gas exchange abnormalities minimized, anesthetic agents cleared, the ability to protect the airway present, and the patient awake and reasonably cooperative.
- Nutritional support provides calories for metabolic processes, reduces cannibalism of protein stores as an energy source, supplies substrate for anabolic processes, and provides an opportunity to reduce net protein losses in the face of ongoing protein catabolism.
- Successful healing of a closed surgical wound yields mechanical integrity by virtue of high tensile strength. Successful healing in an open wound may be measured by epithelialization with the promise of satisfactory mechanical integrity (scarring) over time.
- The ability of epithelialization to occur from the margin of the wounds over the granulation tissue depends on the presence of adequate angiogenesis, the absence of bacterial burden, the provision of a moist environment, and the removal of excess necrosis and proteinaceous exudates (which contain proteases and inflammatory mediators and harbor bacterial growth).
- The first rule of wound evaluation is: "Take off the dressing and look at the wound." Wounds should be evaluated at least daily for progression of healing and for development of infection.
- Only by knowing the intended anatomic location of a given drain can a clinician determine the best way to confirm location and assess its function.

REFERENCES

1. Pronovost PJ, Needham DM, Waters H, et al: Intensive care unit physician staffing: Financial modeling of the Leapfrog standard. Crit Care Med 2004;32:1247-1253.
2. Peterson ED, Coombs LP, DeLong ER, et al: Procedural volume as a marker of quality for CABG surgery. JAMA 2004;291:195-201.
3. Arabi Y, Al Shirawi N, Memish Z, et al: Assessment of six mortality prediction models in patients admitted with severe sepsis and septic shock to the intensive care unit: A prospective cohort study. Crit Care 2003;7:R116-R122.
4. Sinuff T, Adhikari NK, Cook DJ, et al: Mortality predictions in the intensive care unit: Comparing physicians with scoring systems. Crit Care Med 2006;34:878-885.
5. Guidelines for intensive care unit admission, discharge, and triage. Task Force of the American College of Critical Care Medicine, Society of Critical Care Medicine. Crit Care Med 1999;27:633-638.
6. Shah MR, Hasselblad V, Stevenson LW, et al: Impact of the pulmonary artery catheter in critically ill patients: Meta-analysis of randomized clinical trials. JAMA 2005;294:1664-1670.
7. National Heart, Lung, and Blood Institute Acute Respiratory Distress Syndrome (ARDS) Clinical Trials Network, Wheeler AP, Bernard GR, Thompson BT et al: Pulmonary-artery versus central venous catheter to guide treatment of acute lung injury. N Engl J Med 2006;354:2213-2224.
8. Vincent JL, De Backer D: Microvascular dysfunction as a cause of organ dysfunction in severe sepsis. Crit Care 2005;9(Suppl 4):S9-S12.
9. Gattinoni L, Brazzi L, Pelosi P, et al: A trial of goal-oriented hemodynamic therapy in critically ill patients. SvO_2 Collaborative Group. N Engl J Med 1995;333:1025-1032.
10. Bickell WH, Wall MJ, Pepe P, et al: Immediate versus delayed fluid resuscitation for hypotensive patients with penetrating torso injuries. N Engl J Med 1994;331:1105-1109.
11. Kowalenko T, Stern S, Dronen S, et al: Improved outcome with hypotensive resuscitation of uncontrolled hemorrhagic shock in a swine model. J Trauma 1992;33:349-353, discussion 361-362.
12. Rivers E, Nguyen B, Havstad S, et al: Early goal-directed therapy in the treatment of severe sepsis and septic shock. N Engl J Med 2001;345: 1368-1377.
13. Pinsky MR, Vincent JL: Let us use the pulmonary artery catheter correctly and only when we need it. Crit Care Med 2005;33:1119-1122.
14. Bilkovski RN, Rivers EP, Horst HM: Targeted resuscitation strategies after injury. Curr Opin Crit Care 2004;10:529-538.
15. Kristiansson M, Soop M, Shanwell A, et al: Prestorage versus bedside white blood cell filtration of red blood cell concentrates: Effects on the content of cytokines and soluble tumor necrosis factor receptors. J Trauma 1996;40: 379-383.
16. Alam HB, Stanton K, Koustova E, et al: Effect of different resuscitation strategies on neutrophil activation in a swine model of hemorrhagic shock. Resuscitation 2004;60:91-99.
17. Rhee P, Burris D, Kaufmann C, et al: Lactated Ringer's solution resuscitation causes neutrophil activation after hemorrhagic shock. J Trauma 1998;44:313-319.
18. Wade CE, Kramer GC, Grady JJ, et al: Efficacy of hypertonic 7.5% saline and 6% dextran-70 in treating trauma: A meta-analysis of controlled clinical studies. Surgery 1997;122: 609-616.
19. Choi SH, Lee SW, Hong YS, et al: Selective inhibition of polymorphonuclear neutrophils by resuscitative concentration of hypertonic saline. Emerg Med J 2006;23:119-122.
20. Sanders AB: Therapeutic hypothermia after cardiac arrest. Curr Opin Crit Care 2006;12:213-217.
21. Watts DD, Trask A, Soeken K, et al: Hypothermic coagulopathy in trauma: Effect of varying levels of hypothermia on enzyme speed, platelet function,

and fibrinolytic activity. J Trauma 1998;44:846-854.
22. Kress JP, Gehlbach B, Lacy M, et al: The long-term psychological effects of daily sedative interruption on critically ill patients. Am J Respir Crit Care Med 2003;168:1457-1461.
23. Schweickert WD, Gehlbach BK, Pohlman AS, et al: Daily interruption of sedative infusions and complications of critical illness in mechanically ventilated patients. Crit Care Med 2004;32: 1272-1276.
24. Coursin DB, Coursin DB, Maccioli GA: Dexmedetomidine. Curr Opin Crit Care 2001;7:221-226.
25. Guler T, Unlugenc H, Gundogan Z, et al: A background infusion of morphine enhances patient-controlled analgesia after cardiac surgery. Can J Anaesth 2004;51:718-722.
26. Ely EW, Truman B, Shintani A, et al: Monitoring sedation status over time in ICU patients: Reliability and validity of the Richmond Agitation-Sedation Scale (RASS). JAMA 2003;289: 2983-2991.
27. MacIntyre NR, Cook DJ, Ely EW, et al; American College of Chest Physicians; American Association for Respiratory Care; American College of Critical Care Medicine: Evidence-based guidelines for weaning and discontinuing ventilatory support: A collective task force facilitated by the American College of Chest Physicians; the American Association for Respiratory Care; and the American College of Critical Care Medicine. Chest 2001;120(6 Suppl):375S-395S.
28. MacIntyre NR: Evidence-based ventilator weaning and discontinuation. Respir Care 2004;49:830-836.
29. Geerts WH, Pineo GF, Heit JA, et al: Prevention of venous thromboembolism. The Seventh ACCP Conference on Antithrombotic and Thrombolytic Therapy. Chest 2004;126(3 Suppl):338S-400S.
30. Knudson MM, Ikossi DG, Khaw L, et al: Thromboembolism after trauma: An analysis of 1602 episodes from the American College of Surgeons National Trauma Data Bank. Ann Surg 2004;240: 490-496, discussion 496-498.
31. Rogers FB, Cipolle MD, Velmahos G, et al: Practice management guidelines for the prevention of venous thromboembolism in trauma patients: The EAST practice management guidelines work group. J Trauma 2002;53:142-164.
32. Geerts WH, Jay RM, Code KI, et al: A comparison of low-dose heparin with low-molecular-weight heparin as prophylaxis against venous thromboembolism after major trauma. N Engl J Med 1996;335:701-707.
33. Cook DJ, Fuller HD, Guyatt GH, et al: Risk factors for gastrointestinal bleeding in critically ill patients. Canadian Critical Care Trials Group. N Engl J Med 1994;330:377-381.
34. Steinberg KP: Stress-related mucosal disease in the critically ill patient: Risk factors and strategies to prevent stress-related bleeding in the intensive care unit. Crit Care Med 2002;30(6 Suppl): S362-S364.
35. Stollman N, Metz DC: Pathophysiology and prophylaxis of stress ulcer in intensive care unit patients. J Crit Care 2005;20:35-45.
36. Tablan OC, Anderson LJ, Besser R, et al: Guidelines for preventing health-care-associated pneumonia, 2003: Recommendations of CDC and the Healthcare Infection Control Practices Advisory Committee. MMWR Recomm Rep 2004;53(RR-3):1-36.
37. Drakulovic MB, Torres A, Bauer TT, et al: Supine body position as a risk factor for nosocomial pneumonia in mechanically ventilated patients: A randomised trial. Lancet 1999;354: 1851-1858.
38. Dezfulian C, Shojania K, Collard HR, et al: Subglottic secretion drainage for preventing ventilator-associated pneumonia: A meta-analysis. Am J Med 2005;118:11-18.
39. Genuit T, Bochicchio G, Napolitano LM, et al: Prophylactic chlorhexidine oral rinse decreases ventilator-associated pneumonia in surgical ICU patients. Surg Infect (Larchmt) 2001;2:5-18.
40. Flanders SA, Collard HR, Saint S: Nosocomial pneumonia: State of the science. Am J Infect Control 2006;34: 84-93.
41. Esteban A, Frutos-Vivar F, Ferguson ND, et al: Noninvasive positive-pressure ventilation for respiratory failure after extubation. N Engl J Med 2004;350: 2452-2460.
42. Pandharipande P, Jackson J, Ely EW: Delirium: Acute cognitive dysfunction in the critically ill. Curr Opin Crit Care 2005;11:360-368.
43. Ely EW, Shintani A, Truman B, et al: Delirium as a predictor of mortality in mechanically ventilated patients in the intensive care unit. JAMA 2004;291: 1753-1762.
44. Ely EW, Inouye SK, Bernard GR, et al: Delirium in mechanically ventilated patients: Validity and reliability of the confusion assessment method for the intensive care unit (CAM-ICU). JAMA 2001;286:2703-2710.
45. Ely EW, Stephens RK, Jackson JC, et al: Current opinions regarding the importance, diagnosis, and management of delirium in the intensive care unit: A survey of 912 healthcare professionals. Crit Care Med 2004;32:106-112.
46. Khoury W, Klausner JM, Ben-Abraham R, et al: Glucose control by insulin for critically ill surgical patients. J Trauma 2004;57:1132-1138.
47. Furnary AP, Zerr KJ, Grunkemeier GL, et al: Continuous intravenous insulin infusion reduces the incidence of deep sternal wound infection in diabetic patients after cardiac surgical procedures. Ann Thorac Surg 1999;67: 352-360, discussion 360-362.
48. van den Berghe G, Wouters P, Weekers F, et al: Intensive insulin therapy in the critically ill patients. N Engl J Med 2001;345:1359-1367.
49. Guidelines for the use of parenteral and enteral nutrition in adult and pediatric patients. J Parenter Enteral Nutr 2002;26(1 Suppl):1SA-138SA.
50. Huckleberry Y: Nutritional support and the surgical patient. Am J Health Syst Pharm 2004;61:671-682, quiz 683-684.
51. Peter JV, Moran JL, Phillips-Hughes J: A metaanalysis of treatment outcomes of early enteral versus early parenteral nutrition in hospitalized patients. Crit Care Med 2005;33:213-220, discussion 260-261.
52. Perioperative total parenteral nutrition in surgical patients. The Veterans Affairs Total Parenteral Nutrition Cooperative Study Group. N Engl J Med 1991;325: 525-532.
53. Heyland DK, MacDonald S, Keefe L, et al: Total parenteral nutrition in the critically ill patient: A meta-analysis. JAMA 1998;280:2013-2019.
54. MacFie J: Enteral versus parenteral nutrition: The significance of bacterial translocation and gut-barrier function. Nutrition 2000;16:606-611.
55. Lipman TO: Grains or veins: Is enteral nutrition really better than parenteral nutrition? A look at the evidence. J Parenter Enteral Nutr 1998;22:167-182.
56. Braunschweig CL, Levy P, Sheean PM, et al: Enteral compared with parenteral nutrition: A meta-analysis. Am J Clin Nutr 2001;74:534-542.
57. Marik PE, Zaloga GP: Early enteral nutrition in acutely ill patients: A systematic review. Crit Care Med 2001;29:2264-2270.
58. Silk DB, Green CJ: Perioperative nutrition: Parenteral versus enteral. Curr Opin Clin Nutr Metab Care 1998;1:21-27.
59. Dhaliwal R, Jurewitsch B, Harrietha D, Heyland DK: Combination enteral and parenteral nutrition in critically ill patients: Harmful or beneficial? A systematic review of the evidence. Intensive Care Med 2004;30: 1666-1671.
60. Marik PE, Zaloga GP: Gastric versus post-pyloric feeding: A systematic review. Crit Care 2003;7:R46-R51.
61. Lacy BE, Weiser K: Gastric motility, gastroparesis, and gastric stimulation. Surg Clin North Am 2005;85:967-987, vi-vii.
62. Woods JH, Erickson LW, Condon RE, et al: Postoperative ileus: A colonic problem? Surgery 1978;84:527-533.
63. Ward N: Nutrition support to patients undergoing gastrointestinal surgery. Nutr J 2003;2:18.
64. Ponec RJ, Saunders MD, Kimmey MB: Neostigmine for the treatment of acute colonic pseudo-obstruction. N Engl J Med 1999;341:137-141.
65. Malhotra A, Mathur AK, Gupta S: Early enteral nutrition after surgical treatment of gut perforations: A prospective randomised study. J Postgrad Med 2004;50:102-106.
66. Gonzalez-Pinto I, Gonzalez EM: Optimising the treatment of upper gastrointestinal fistulae. Gut 2001; 49(Suppl 4):iv-22-iv-31.
67. Meier R, Ockenga J, Pertkiewicz M, et al: ESPEN guidelines on enteral nutrition: Pancreas. Clin Nutr 2006;25:275-284.
68. Marik PE, Zaloga GP: Meta-analysis of parenteral nutrition versus enteral nutrition in patients with acute pancreatitis. BMJ 2004;328: 1407.
69. McClave SA, Chang WK, Dhaliwal R, Heyland DK, et al: Nutrition support in acute pancreatitis: A systematic review

of the literature. J Parenter Enteral Nutr 2006;30:143-156.
70. Kumar A, Singh N, Prakash S, et al: Early enteral nutrition in severe acute pancreatitis: A prospective randomized controlled trial comparing nasojejunal and nasogastric routes. J Clin Gastroenterol 2006;40:431-434.
71. Deodhar AK, Rana RE: Surgical physiology of wound healing: A review. J Postgrad Med 1997;43:52-56.
72. Cohen IK, Diegelman RF: Wound healing. In Mulholland MW, Lillemoe KD, Doherty GM, et al: Greenfield's Surgery: Scientific Principles and Practice, 4th ed. Philadelphia, Lippincott Williams & Wilkins, 2006.
73. Winter GD, Scales JT: Effect of air drying and dressings on the surface of a wound. Nature 1963;197:91-92.
74. Moues CM, Vos MC, van den Bemd GJ, et al: Bacterial load in relation to vacuum-assisted closure wound therapy: A prospective randomized trial. Wound Repair Regen 2004;12:11-17.
75. MacKay D, Miller AL: Nutritional support for wound healing. Altern Med Rev 2003;8:359-377.
76. Barie PS, Eachempati SR: Surgical site infections. Surg Clin North Am 2005;85:1115-1135, viii-ix.
77. Horan TC, Gaynes RP, Martone WJ, et al: CDC definitions of nosocomial surgical site infections, 1992: A modification of CDC definitions of surgical wound infections. Infect Control Hosp Epidemiol 1992;13: 606-608.
78. Velmahos GC, Toutouzas KG, Sarkisyan G, et al: Severe trauma is not an excuse for prolonged antibiotic prophylaxis. Arch Surg 2002;137:537-541.
79. Namias N, Harvill S, Ball S, et al: Cost and morbidity associated with antibiotic prophylaxis in the ICU. J Am Coll Surg 1999;188:225-230.
80. Moss JP: Historical and current perspectives on surgical drainage. Surg Gynecol Obstet 1981;152: 517-527.
81. Robinson JO: Surgical drainage: An historical perspective. Br J Surg 1986;73:422-426.
82. Memon MA, Memon MI, Donohue JH: Abdominal drains: A brief historical review. Isr Med J 2001;94: 164-166.
83. Smith SR, Gilmore OJ: Surgical drainage. Br J Hosp Med 1985;33:308, 311, 314-315.

Chapter 37

Management of the Patient after Cardiac Surgery

Robert G. Johnson and C. Allen Bashour

A postoperative cardiac surgery patient may be admitted to the cardiovascular intensive care unit (ICU) with any combination of conditions including hypotension, low cardiac output, atrial and ventricular arrhythmias, cardiac irritability, hypothermia, pulmonary dysfunction, low urine output, coagulopathy, and postoperative bleeding. Laboratory abnormalities including lactic acidemia, hypoxemia, hypokalemia, anemia, thrombocytopenia, leukocytosis, and poor glycemic control are encountered frequently in the early postoperative period. These findings are superimposed on preoperative cardiac pathology that has been partially or completely corrected (e.g., incomplete myocardial revascularization or poor left ventricular function). Cardiac surgery patients also may have one or more comorbidities, including seizure disorder, cerebrovascular or peripheral vascular disease, chronic atrial fibrillation (AF), systemic or pulmonary hypertension, chronic obstructive pulmonary disease/asthma, renal insufficiency, and diabetes. Despite these challenges, management of these patients under a protocol-driven system produces successful results in most cases.

The first part of this chapter outlines the sequential steps involved in the care of routine cardiac surgical patients. The second part provides additional details about managing complications. Although there are no universally accepted criteria that separate routine post–cardiac surgery patients from complicated ones, the criteria listed in Box 37-1 may help distinguish the two. Many of the postoperative complications that occur in patients undergoing cardiac surgery are the same as those seen in other critically ill postoperative surgical patients. As such, other chapters provide information that pertains to these shared complications. This chapter focuses primarily on the postoperative care that distinguishes cardiac patients from other surgical patients.

INITIAL POSTOPERATIVE EVALUATION

After cardiac surgery, patients are transferred to the next care setting, which is usually an ICU. After successful transfer to the ICU, the operating room (OR) and ICU personnel converge with assigned tasks to ensure patient stability. This involves confirmation of a secure airway and proper connection to the ventilator (if the patient was not extubated in the OR). Attention is given to initial peak inspiratory pressures and tidal volumes, adequate ventilation, and normal range pulse oximetry. In the absence of specific contraindications (see Box 37-1), ventilator weaning begins shortly after arrival in the ICU. Most patients with truly difficult tracheal intubations are allowed to awaken briefly for neurologic assessment and are then sedated. Elective extubation may be planned for the morning of the first postoperative day.

Active rewarming is initiated to decrease the risk of dysrhythmias and postoperative bleeding and to permit

Box 37-1

Early Postoperative Conditions or Criteria That Mitigate Against the Initiation of Ventilator Weaning on Arrival in the ICU after Cardiac Surgery*

Primary Adverse Criteria
- Hemodynamic instability (due to)
  - Atrial or ventricular arrhythmias
  - Low cardiac index (<2 L/m^2)
  - Hypotension, unexplained or uncontrolled
  - High level of inotropic or pressor support
- Ventilatory dysfunction
  - Low PaO_2/FIO_2 ratio
  - Difficult airway-intubation
- Excessive postoperative bleeding (>200-300 mL/h)
- Hypothermia
- Mechanical ventricular assist
- Open sternum

Secondary Adverse Criteria
- Intra-aortic balloon pump counterpulsation support
- Long-standing pulmonary hypertension
- Operation type
  - Acute myocardial infarction
  - Acute ventricular septal defect
  - Acute mitral regurgitation (papillary muscle rupture)
  - Descending aortic aneurysm

*Notably few of these are absolute contraindications to ventilator weaning, but they warrant consideration in the aggregate (see text).
FIO_2, fraction of inspired oxygen; PaO_2, partial pressure of oxygen in arterial blood.

ventilator weaning if the patient's initial temperature is less than 36° C.[1] Shivering (micro or gross) secondary to a cytokine-mediated inflammatory response (not hypothermia) may occur during the early postoperative period. Shivering should be controlled promptly to prevent increased arterial carbon dioxide tension ($PaCO_2$) and acidemia, the latter of which increases the risk of dysrhythmias and diminishes the effectiveness of pressors and inotropes. The treatment of postoperative shivering begins with adequate sedation (fentanyl or propofol drips or both) followed by an ongoing assessment to determine the need for a muscle-relaxing agent. Steroid administration also may be considered to counter the inflammatory response that produces postoperative shivering. Meperidine (Demerol) does not effectively control shivering in this patient group.[2]

The patient's cardiac output on admission to the ICU is usually measured by pulmonary artery catheter thermodilution. To assess hemodynamic stability, the initial results are compared with the last values obtained from the OR. Whether or not the patient has a pulmonary artery catheter, he or she should be assessed first clinically for adequate tissue perfusion by evaluating and measuring core body temperature, extremity temperature and appearance (warmth and pulses), neurologic recovery (time to return of consciousness), and hourly volume of urine output. Cardiac rate and rhythm are compared with preoperative values. Frequent premature ventricular contractions usually can be suppressed by correcting hypo-kalemia (usually from postoperative diuresis) and administering magnesium (it is unnecessary to check magnesium levels routinely). Premature ventricular contractions also may indicate an underlying problem, however, as simple as a coiled pulmonary artery catheter in the right ventricle, ischemia owing to incomplete revascularization, or a technical problem that involves the coronary artery graft (kinking or thrombosis). Frequent premature atrial contractions may indicate that AF is imminent. Atrial and ventricular epicardial pacing wires are usually present, and if the patient is being paced, the setting should be in demand mode (AAI, VVI, or DDD) and mean amplitude output thresholds should be noted along with the underlying rhythm. If an implantable cardioverter defibrillator is present, it usually should be reactivated. Mediastinal or pleural chest tubes, or both, if present, are connected to 10 to 20 cm H_2O suction empirically, and the presence of air leaks is documented as chest tube output is monitored.

This initial assessment should occur in the context of a prior exchange of information from the OR surgeon and anesthesiologist to the ICU staff (see later section on transfer from the operating room to the ICU). The purpose of the initial evaluation is to determine if the patient's condition has changed since leaving the OR and is intended to provide a baseline for the ensuing early postoperative hours in the ICU when return to consciousness, hemodynamic stability, pulmonary and renal function, postoperative bleeding, and extubation parameters are continuously assessed. The initial evaluation is analogous to that outlined in the advanced trauma life support curriculum because it includes a rapid evaluation of the patient's airway and ventilatory and circulatory status followed by a more comprehensive patient evaluation. The same patient parameters first communicated (Box 37-2; see also section on transfer from the operating room to the ICU) from the OR are re-evaluated during the secondary evaluation. Neurologic function and peripheral pulses are assessed. A baseline 12-lead electrocardiogram (ECG), chest radiograph, and blood tests (arterial blood gas, electrolytes, hemogram, and prothrombin time/partial thromboplastin time) are obtained. The postoperative chest radiograph is reviewed to confirm proper endotracheal tube position (exclude right main stem intubation or an endotracheal tube placement that is too high), pulmonary artery catheter position (the most common improper position is too distal, which increases the risk of pulmonary artery rupture and ventricular arrhythmias), hemothorax, pneumothorax, or subcutaneous emphysema. Oxygen saturation and hemodynamic parameters are assessed to provide a baseline.

OUTCOME RISK PREDICTION AND ASSESSMENT

The goal for each cardiac surgery patient is an uncomplicated recovery, and it is important to evaluate continuously whether optimal care is being provided. There are

Box 37-2

Communication between the Operating Room and the ICU

Communication between the operating room and the ICU must occur before or at the time of transfer of a critically ill patient. This communication may be standardized, including the following intraoperative elements:

- Pulmonary
  - Tracheal intubation experience
  - Oxygenation or ventilation difficulties
- Cardiac
  - What was accomplished compared with what was planned
  - Current, postwean condition of the patient
  - Hemodynamics
  - Pacemaker setting and underlying rhythm
- Temperature
- Urine output
- Current bleeding
- Current pharmacologic management
- Laboratory tests
  - Trends through the operation
  - Pending

well-established outcome prediction models for patients undergoing cardiac surgery—Northern New England Cardiovascular Disease Study Group,[3] Veterans Administration,[4] Society of Thoracic Surgeons,[5] Health Data Research,[6] revised application of the Parsonnet score,[7] EuroScore[8], and Cleveland Clinic Severity Score.[9] These outcome models have been tested and validated in patient populations that are different from the populations used to derive them. Baseline patient variables common to many of these models and associated with outcome include age, gender, body mass index, reoperation, emergency operation, left ventricular function, creatinine, chronic pulmonary disease, peripheral vascular disease, diabetes, and albumin.[2-7,10] These risk prediction models may be used to help inform individual patients and their families about the operative risk, although they offer little certainty in an individual case. Although it might be attractive to think that an individual patient's risk could be reduced by modifying his or her preoperative variables, this approach is not evidence-based for each and every risk variable. Statistically significant risk factors may be markers for poorer outcomes without being an actual cause of a poorer outcome.

Other, subclinical, baseline patient parameters have been associated with an adverse outcome, such as low serum antiendotoxin[11] core antibody. The presence of antibodies directed against platelet factor 4–heparin complexes[12] is associated with increased morbidity and mortality after cardiac operations. A genetic predisposition to increased cytokine release in response to cardiopulmonary bypass (CPB) and the ensuing inflammatory response is another subclinical correlate of poorer outcomes after cardiac surgery.[13,14] An array of specific genotype polymorphisms also have been linked to postcardiac surgical

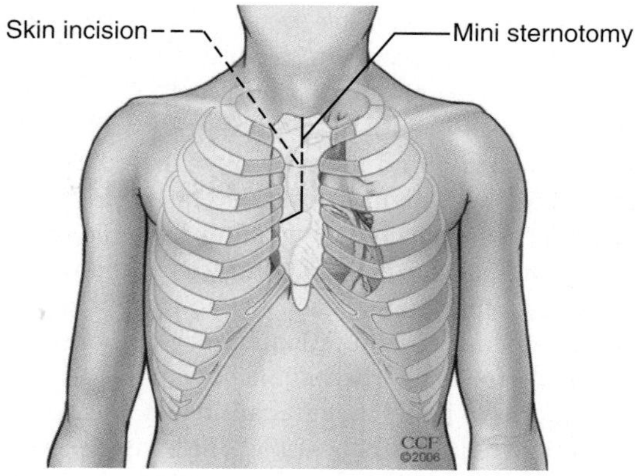

Figure 37-1. Mini sternotomy incision. (Reprinted with permission of the Cleveland Clinic.)

bleeding and myocardial infarction.[15,16] None of these subclinical correlates of outcome is routinely assessed, and the influence they might have on patient outcome has not yet been well established.

INTRAOPERATIVE EVENTS

Some understanding of cardiac surgical care in the OR is important for optimal postoperative care. Cardiac surgical operative and anesthesia management varies across the spectrum of procedures (coronary revascularization, valve repair and replacement, great vessel surgery, and cardiac remodeling procedures), surgeons, anesthesiologists, and institutions. Detailed discussions about intraoperative management can be found in specialized cardiothoracic surgical and anesthesia textbooks, but there are a few specific and broadly applicable concepts that have an impact on the postoperative care of cardiac surgical patients. This section highlights selected aspects of intraoperative cardiac surgical care and attempts to establish their relevance to postoperative care.

Operative Approach

Access to the operative field may vary from less invasive to full sternotomy or thoracotomy. Although a full sternotomy was long the standard for all cardiac procedures, smaller incisions (ministernotomy and mini–anterior thoracotomy) have been used since the 1990s, especially in valve procedures (Fig. 37-1). Although there is less tissue trauma, the only improved outcome consistently reported in these patients has been a decreased need for transfusions.[17] A decrease in initial intubation time, ICU length of stay, and major morbidity and mortality has not been firmly established.

Use of Cardiopulmonary Bypass

Use of extracorporeal circulation with an oxygenator is still essential for most cardiac operations. CPB induces an inflammatory response that does not occur in operations without CPB.[18,19] CPB requires arterial cannulation (distal ascending aorta or femoral, subclavian, or axillary arteries) for "inflow" to the patient and venous cannulation for "outflow" (right atrium or inferior and superior vena cavae) to the pump itself (Fig. 37-2).

Blood from the venous system drains by gravity (or assisted by vacuum suction) from the right heart and the lungs. The lungs are deprived of pulmonary arterial flow and mechanical ventilation during CPB. The patient's drained venous blood must be oxygenated before being returned to the patient (most centers employ membrane or hollow fiber exchange oxygenator technology). Contact between blood and artificial surfaces (cannulae, tubing, connectors, and membranes or hollow fibers) induces cytokine release and an inflammatory response. Heparin anticoagulation is nearly universally employed to prevent the initiation of platelet aggregation and activation of the coagulation cascade that would otherwise be associated with such blood–artificial surface contact. Activated clotting times are used to regulate the adequacy of the heparinization. Heparin-coated CPB circuits decrease the heparin dose required to achieve effective anticoagulation and may have other beneficial effects as well.[20,21] Alternative anticoagulant protocols are used in patients when heparin is contraindicated (e.g., in patients with heparin-induced thrombocytopenia[22]).

The extracorporeal CPB circuit requires a variable volume of fluid (pump prime) that dilutes the patient's circulating volume. This can be minimized by using lower volume circuits. Heat is lost extracorporeally, so a warming/cooling bath is required to regulate body temperature. Certain operations are conducted at low temperatures to protect the central nervous system[23] and spinal cord.

CPB induces a cytokine-mediated and genetically variable inflammatory response in patients undergoing cardiac surgery.[18] This inflammatory response can lead to coagulation abnormalities on top of those that are already present (pharmacologic, dilutional, consumptive, and hypothermic). Inflammation associated with CPB or cytokine-mediated inflammation also is associated with variable degrees of acute lung injury (nonventilated, possibly ischemic lungs),[24-26] embolic events (cannulation of an atherosclerotic aorta, incomplete anticoagulation), and end-organ dysfunction (nonpulsatile low mean arterial pressure [MAP] perfusion).

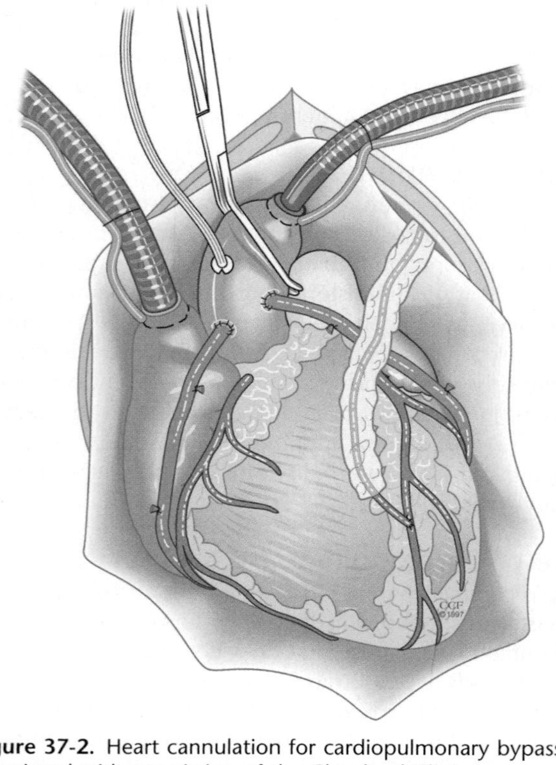

Figure 37-2. Heart cannulation for cardiopulmonary bypass. (Reprinted with permission of the Cleveland Clinic.)

Decreased systemic vascular resistance (vasoplegia) related to CPB-induced inflammation or hypothermia commonly occurs.[27] Whether it is a result of dilution (colloid, oncotic changes), inflammation (increased capillary permeability), ischemia-reperfusion, or some combination thereof, CPB patients routinely experience capillary leak and mild to severe extravascular "third-space" fluid sequestration. The associated weight gain seen after CPB is well documented, but most significant is the correlation between the lowest hematocrit on CPB and outcome.[28,29] Technological evolution has improved medical equipment and operative techniques (anticoagulation methods, centripetal pumps, heparin-coated tubing, membrane/fiber as opposed to bubble oxygenators), but despite these improvements, derangements associated with CPB (e.g., hemodilution, coagulopathy, and inflammation) still affect the postoperative course.

Comparing outcomes between on-pump and off-pump cardiac operations is informative. Revascularization procedures do not require an "open heart" and can be performed without CPB use.[30] Off-pump coronary artery surgery is performed on the beating heart with the aid of stabilization devices used to steady the segment of the coronary artery selected for bypass grafting (Fig. 37-3).

Off-pump coronary artery bypass (OPCAB) is employed in 13.8% to 70.8% of coronary artery revascularization procedures in centers that report its use.[30] As with less invasive procedures, and despite avoiding CPB and cardiac ischemia (no cross-clamping), there is no consensus that overall outcome is improved with OPCAB despite a reported decrease in proinflammatory cytokine release.[31] A decrease in coagulopathy and postoperative chest tube output with OPCAB has reduced preoperative transfusion requirements. Several investigations have reported that OPCAB is associated with better early neurologic outcomes (improved cognitive test performance; fewer central nervous system ischemic events),[32] shorter initial intubation time, decreased ICU length of stay, decreased need for inotrope and pressor therapy, and a lower incidence of postoperative AF.[31] Other investigations have reported no difference, however, in same outcomes between OPCAB and coronary artery bypass grafting (CABG) with CPB.[31,33-35] Selection of patients for one technique or the other varies widely across centers, and uniform selection criteria have not been established.[36,37]

Hypothermic Circulatory Arrest

In patients undergoing complex procedures, such as complete correction in infants or great vessel operations in adults, hypothermic circulatory arrest is made possible by CPB. Postoperative neurologic complications correlate

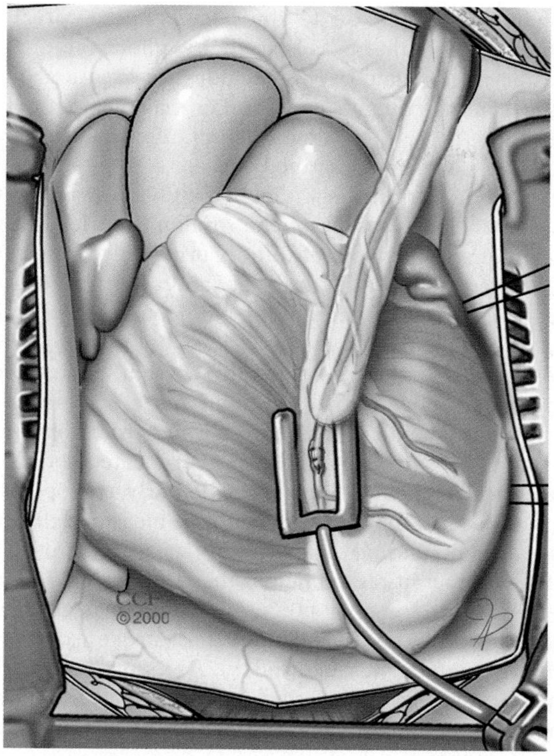

Figure 37-3. Heart stabilizing device for off-pump coronary artery bypass surgery. (Reprinted with permission of the Cleveland Clinic.)

directly with the duration of hypothermic circulatory arrest; most patients tolerate 30 minutes or less well, although up to 60 minutes may be tolerated without obvious adverse outcomes. Details of hypothermic circulatory arrest management (central nervous system monitoring, pharmacologic adjuncts, and pH management) can be found elsewhere.[38]

Procedure Performed

The type of procedure performed affects the postoperative care of cardiac surgical patients. Of particular relevance is the condition of the patient before the operation, as discussed in the previous risk assessment section. The preoperative state of the myocardium (e.g., acutely ischemic or acutely failing) influences the outcome. It is widely recognized that the operative time is associated with outcome. Although CPB and aortic cross-clamp time are associated with morbidity and mortality, the exact relationship between time and outcome is not well elucidated.[39-41] Completing the surgical objective and minimizing total CPB time are important because prolonged or multiple CPB runs may have as harmful an effect on outcome as incomplete correction of cardiac pathology. When cross-clamp, or myocardial ischemic, time is greatly prolonged to complete the surgical objective, adequate myocardial protection is even more critical.

In some centers, when multiple arterial grafts—particularly radial arterial conduits—are used, a calcium channel blocker infusion is started in the OR and continued for 12 to 24 hours to prevent vasospasm. Other centers have not experienced significant problems with postoperative myocardial ischemia owing to arterial conduit vasospasm and have discontinued this practice because of calcium channel blocker–induced systemic hypotension.

As stated before (see Box 37-2), the surgeon's and anesthesiologist's assessment of the operation and details of any problems that were encountered during the operation must be communicated to the ICU staff. This information includes the completeness of revascularization, perioperative echocardiographic findings, and knowledge of any details of the operation that could affect the perioperative course, such as a fragile aorta or a tenuous suture line. These and other intraoperative events that potentially could have an impact on the postoperative course should be communicated to the individuals involved in postoperative care directly by those with first-hand information, when possible.

Weaning from Cardiopulmonary Bypass

After CPB, the empty heart is filled by decreasing venous drainage to the extracorporeal pump. Blood previously draining into the pump fills the right ventricle and is ejected into the pulmonary circulation through the lungs that are being ventilated and then into the left atrium and left ventricle. This usually uneventful process of allowing the heart to refill and begin ejecting can be problematic if a patient was not completely revascularized (owing to poor distal coronary artery targets) or if a patient has inadequate myocardial protection (because of cardioplegia not being well delivered or distributed through the coronary circulation). Air embolism to the coronary circulation (right coronary artery is the most common) may occur as the heart begins to eject. This usually manifests as ischemic ECG changes, ventricular arrhythmias, and hemodynamic instability that may necessitate a rapid return to CPB. Uneventful separation from CPB requires a coordinated effort between the surgeon, anesthesiologist, and perfusionist.

Transesophageal echocardiography has become invaluable in assessing left and right ventricular function, regional wall motion abnormalities, cardiac chamber air, and valvular function before the initial CPB separation attempt. The determinants of cardiac function—rate, rhythm, contractility, preload, and afterload—should be optimized before the initial weaning attempt. This can be accomplished with pacing to increase heart rate if indicated (usually 80-90 beats per minute), volume administration (colloid or crystalloid), antiarrhythmic agents, inotropes, or vasopressors (based on echocardiography findings). The postoperative ICU staff should be informed of any difficulties encountered during weaning from CPB and what was required to wean successfully.

Use of mechanical cardiac support is considered when separation from CPB is difficult. If required, the most commonly employed device is the intra-aortic balloon pump (IABP), which reduces afterload and augments coronary blood flow during diastole. Overall, use of the IABP has decreased significantly since the 1990s. The frequency of intraoperative and postoperative placement has decreased as *preoperative* placement, in the coronary care unit or catheterization laboratory, has increased.[42] Preoperative insertion now exceeds postoperative insertion (a change since the 1990s).[42] A decrease in the number of balloons placed for unstable angina because of aggressive percutaneous catheter–based interventions might explain the decrease in preoperative use, but the shift in proportion of preoperative compared with intraoperative and postoperative IABP insertions must be accounted for by greater preoperative recognition of a population of patients that might need placement intraoperatively (preoperative heart failure) or improved OR management of patients who previously had IABP insertion after CPB or both. It is recognized that the placement of an IABP after CPB, whether in the operating room or postoperatively, is associated with a higher mortality than when employed preoperatively (28% versus 9% mortality[43]). Patients with intraoperative insertion have a better survival at 1 year than do patients with postoperative IABP insertion.[44] The evidence suggests that improved survival is favored by the institution of an IABP at the earliest appropriate point in a patient's course.

In addition to a rationale for earlier (preoperative) IABP use, there are other reasons for decreased post-CPB IABP placement. Although a causal relationship has not been firmly established, intraoperative evaluation and management techniques such as an increased use of intraoperative transesophageal echocardiography and the phosphodiesterase inhibitor, milrinone, have likely contributed to the decreased need for IABP use intraoperatively. Transesophageal echocardiography identifies underlying pathophysiology that can be corrected or treated with modalities other than IABP, and phosphodiesterase inhibitor use augments catecholamine support and acts to provide afterload reduction (the pharmacologic equivalent of the IABP). Ineffective prolonged weaning attempts may delay the decision to insert a mechanical support device and result in hypothermia, acidemia, coagulopathy, and an increased inflammatory response. In such situations, the actual placement of a mechanical device may occur at a time when benefit from the device has passed.

TRANSFER FROM THE OPERATING ROOM TO THE INTENSIVE CARE UNIT

The period from chest closure through transport and admission to the ICU is a critical time in the postoperative management of a cardiac surgery patient. The increased potential for hemodynamic instability coincides with patient transport. Communication is essential to convey the important details of the operative procedure: what was accomplished compared with what was planned, tracheal intubation experience, oxygenation or ventilation difficulties, the condition of the patient (hemodynamics, pacemaker setting and underlying rhythm, temperature, bleeding), and the current pharmacologic management (see Box 37-2). In many institutions, intraoperative parameters can be visualized in real time on the monitor in the patient's ICU bed space. This can give ICU personnel some insight into events that may affect the patient's early postoperative course. Transportation of the patient requires appropriate monitors, infusion pumps, and ventilator support. On admission to the postoperative care unit, communication that was started by phone before the transfer is completed. This includes information about changes in the patient's condition or management during transport. At the same time, the initial evaluation of the patient is started as described earlier.

Patient monitoring begins immediately on arrival to the ICU and includes heart rate and rhythm (four-lead ECG), transcutaneous oxygen saturation, urine output by catheter drainage, chest tube drainage, and a central pressure line (central venous catheter or pulmonary artery catheter). The initial hemodynamic assessment takes into consideration the patient's heart rate, rhythm, contractility, and preload and afterload and compares those parameters with values obtained preoperatively and just before transfer from the OR. This assessment is repeated serially to detect hemodynamic changes in the early postoperative period. Cardiac contractility cannot be measured directly, but is estimated using cardiac output measurements. Clinically, contractility is defined as the relationship between preload (central venous pressure or pulmonary capillary wedge pressure) and systolic function (stroke work index or more commonly cardiac index). Assessing contractility requires invasive monitoring (transesophageal echocardiography, pulmonary artery catheter) and serial preload measurements.

The decision to use a pulmonary artery catheter in patients undergoing cardiac surgery is made by the anesthesiologist and surgeon, usually preoperatively. Routine pulmonary artery catheter use is unnecessary.[45] Patients with a pulmonary artery catheter often need larger amounts of fluid than similar patients managed without a pulmonary artery catheter.[46] Selection criteria for pulmonary artery catheter use in cardiac surgery patients are not well established, but the data support selective, rather than universal, use. Many surgeons and anesthesiologists agree that off-pump cases require the intraoperative use of a pulmonary artery catheter or transesophageal echocardiography or both.

EARLY POSTOPERATIVE MANAGEMENT

Although cardiac surgery patients as a group today have higher patient acuity and undergo more complex primary and reoperative surgical procedures than the patients of only a decade ago, their hospital morbidity and mortality are decreasing. This is primarily due to advances in surgery and anesthesia and improved perioperative care. Recognition of subtle abnormalities in the early postoperative period is required to keep these patients on course to an uneventful recovery. This section is a discussion of routine early postoperative patient management. More complex patients are discussed in subsequent sections of this chapter.

Ventilator Weaning

Patients who are not weaned and extubated in the OR as part of an accelerated recovery or "fast-track" protocol are usually candidates for weaning and extubation within a few hours after coming to the ICU. A protocol-driven and respiratory therapist–managed reduction in initial postoperative intubation time has been achieved in many ICUs.[47] Some institutions use inclusion/exclusion criteria for selecting patients to be weaned under a fast-track or accelerated recovery protocol.[1,48] Other units employ a protocol wherein all patients are initially included, and a patient is excluded only when he or she does not meet the parameters for advancement. Patients who are not candidates for early (within 4 hours) extubation are usually sedated after a normal neurologic examination is confirmed and may remain intubated during the first post-operative night (see Box 37-1).

Intensive Care Unit Length of Stay

Initial intubation time is associated with ICU length of stay.[1] Most cardiac surgery patients can be extubated early and transferred out of the ICU within 24 hours. Rapid patient turnover is achieved in ICUs that use care pathways based on patient parameters and not the length of stay.[49] Patient-based parameters for a diuresis protocol would be based on a patient's weight relative to the preoperative weight, their blood urea nitrogen/creatinine and their cardiac index/preload, not based on time ("postoperative day 1"). When time-based parameters are used, they should be based on hours rather than days. Pacing wires might be routinely removed after any 12-hour period with no need for pacing or antidysrhythmic therapy, rather than "on postoperative day 2." Timing of chest tube removal may be based on volume and character of the drainage, rather than on an experientially derived time or postoperative day.

Pain Management

It is well recognized that adequate postoperative pain management can reduce pulmonary complications and ICU stay after cardiac surgery. A standard sternotomy is generally less painful than a thoracotomy or an alternative approach that may require more chest wall retraction. It is common for patients to experience more pain related to the chest tube entry sites than from the sternotomy.

Coughing can cause mechanical stress on the wound. External support can be provided by having the patient hug a pillow or blanket roll. This also can serve as an effective pain-reducing adjunct to pharmacologic therapy. The goal is to keep the patient as pain-free as possible without depressing the respiratory drive or cough reflex. ICU staff should ensure that efforts to avoid oversedation do not lead to inadequate pain management, which limits chest excursion and often results in atelectasis and prolonged ICU stays owing to pulmonary complications.

Opioid analgesia (intravenous morphine sulfate or fentanyl) is the most common early treatment. Intravenous patient-controlled analgesia has been an effective pain control method if intermittent dosing is inadequate. The addition of nonsteroidal anti-inflammatory drugs (ketorolac tromethamine, 15 to 30 mg intravenously in adults every 6 hours) if there are no contraindications[50] (e.g., renal insufficiency in elderly patients and diabetics, history of gastrointestinal ulcers, bleeding, or reflux disease) is a helpful adjunct in selected patients. Most patients can be transitioned to oral narcotics (oxycodone) with or without acetaminophen within 24 hours after their operation. Dexmedetomidine, an α_2-adrenoceptor agonist, is a useful sedative agent with analgesic properties that can reduce the analgesic requirement of the postoperative patient for a 24-hour period without suppressing respiratory drive.

Hemodynamic Support

Volume administration in the early postoperative period is guided by hemodynamic findings, such as sinus tachycardia, low central venous pressure, low pulmonary artery diastolic pressure, low pulmonary artery occlusion pressure (wedge pressure) when associated with hypotension, and a low cardiac index. Transthoracic echocardiography can be used to assess cardiac chamber size and adequacy of atrial and ventricular filling and to exclude other causes of hypotension, such as cardiac tamponade. A variety of intravenous fluids are used in post–cardiac surgery patients. Colloids and crystalloids are equally effective, and hypertonic salt solutions[51] or hetastarch (1500 mL) may be used to reduce the volume administered.[52]

These stressed patients are typically in a sodium-avid, potassium-excreting state. Fluid requirements vary in the early postoperative period (lower requirements are seen in off-pump cases), with some patients requiring 2 to 3 L of fluid in the first 12 hours. Elevation of central venous or pulmonary artery diastolic pressure to an arbitrary target in the face of other evidence of satisfactory cardiac output (e.g., adequate urine output) is undesirable. These patients can have an increased requirement for fluid owing to the inflammatory response, fluid sequestration, increased chest tube output, and diuresis, but it also is important to recognize that an excessive fluid requirement is often a sign of a significant problem, such as cardiac tamponade or postoperative hemorrhage.

Impaired preoperative ventricular function predicts the need for postoperative inotropic support usually for 36 hours or more, as does a prolonged and complex operation or one that incompletely achieves the therapeutic objectives. Before considering inotropic support, it is important that normal filling pressures are achieved. The preoperative and intraoperative ventricular compliance (change in volume per change in pressure) is important if one is to assess compliance or contractility changes postoperatively. Decreased compliance may mirror decreased systolic function or reflect diastolic dysfunction alone (without systolic impairment as measured by end-systolic volume). Inotrope preferences vary from center to center. Short-term (<12 hours) contractility support with a single agent may be necessary. Low-dose epinephrine (0.02 μg/kg/min) or dobutamine (2-10 μg/kg/min) can be used in patients with a low cardiac index. Milrinone (0.375 to 0.75 μg/kg/min) can be used in patients with a low index and right ventricular dysfunction or elevated pulmonary or systemic vascular resistance.

Inotropic support is especially important for patients with moderate to severe preoperative ventricular function. Each inotropic drug has its advantages and disadvantages related to the drug's chronotropic and vasoconstrictor or dilatory effects.[53] Recognizing the need to initiate or maintain inotropic support during the early postoperative period should be based on an understanding of preoperative ventricular function, intraoperative events, and perioperative transesophageal echocardiography findings. Mild cardiac dysfunction, even after uneventful operations, may occur and continue for 48 hours or more after the operation. Severe cardiac dysfunction is addressed further in the section on low cardiac output.

Low MAP in the presence of adequate cardiac filling and cardiac output (normal contractility) is the usual indication for vasopressor support in the early postoperative period. In this setting, systemic vascular resistance (arithmetic calculation using mean aortic pressure and cardiac output) is low. Administration of vasopressors that increase afterload should be considered only after cardiac contractility is optimized and the patient has an adequate circulating volume. More profound low resistance states are addressed subsequently.

Atrial and ventricular epicardial pacing wires are routinely placed at the end of the procedure in most centers, although they may be used selectively.[54] In the setting of bradycardia without atrial arrhythmias, atrial pacing, if atrioventricular conduction is preserved, or sequential atrioventricular pacing, when it is not, increases cardiac output more than ventricular pacing alone by increasing the frequency of ejection of an atrially augmented stroke volume. As many patients today take β-blockers and are bradycardic, atrial pacing is a useful means of improving cardiac output in the early postoperative period. Just as one may use intravenous fluids and filling pressures or cardiac index to create a compliance (Frank-Starling) curve for a given patient at a given time, the determination of the optimal heart rate and pacing mode at a given moment in a given patient also is appropriate. A patient may have improved cardiac output with a lower intrinsic rate, possibly as a result of greater atrioventricular synchrony and time for more complete ventricular filling, than at a higher atrial or atrioventricular sequential rate. Given the benefits of atrioventricular synchrony and the contribution of atrial contraction, few patients benefit from pure ventricular pacing, unless their intrinsic rate is less than 70 beats per minute, and atrial pacing is not possible because of loss of atrial capture.

Renal Function

Subclinical renal dysfunction (e.g., measurable by creatinine clearance change from preoperative levels) occurs universally after CPB operations, and clinically apparent renal insufficiency is associated with a significant increase in mortality.[55] It is important to recognize impaired renal function and identify the cause. After cardiac operations with CPB, diuresis is expected because total body water (and sodium) is increased, even though most of the excess fluid is not in the vascular space. Urine output of 0.5 to 1 mL/kg/h generally indicates normal renal function and perfusion. Abnormal renal function can be classified as prerenal (inadequate preload), postrenal (obstruction), renal (usually ischemia-induced or toxin-induced acute tubular necrosis), and pseudorenal (increase in creatinine or blood urea nitrogen in the absence of renal dysfunction—drug-induced gastrointestinal bleeding). Optimization of preload is the best first option to improve renal function because low urine output in the early postoperative period is commonly due to inadequate effective circulating blood volume. The urinary drainage catheter should be evaluated to ensure it is working properly and is not obstructed. After prerenal and postrenal causes have been ruled out, investigations directed at identifying renal causes should be started (see the following section on renal failure).

Along with optimizing the cardiac output with volume, attention should be paid to inadequate perfusion pressures, especially after CPB in the setting of chronic renal insufficiency. Patients with long-standing hypertension generally continue to require higher renal perfusion pressures to prevent acute tubular necrosis. Matching preoperative MAP must be tempered by the recognition that a higher than normal (but appropriate for the patient) MAP also may increase the risk of postoperative bleeding, especially at aorta suture line and arterial cannulation sites. As noted previously, these patients retain significant fluid volume, and that volume, much of it extravascular, is mobilized and diuresed over hours and days postoperatively. Some institutions use routine pharmacologic diuresis with loop diuretics, continuously or as intermittent boluses, to achieve a target hourly volume output.

Pharmacologic diuresis speeds the return to a patient's preoperative weight, but its use needs to be tempered with careful attention to intravascular volume assessment (central pressure monitoring, blood urea nitrogen elevation) to avoid inducing or exacerbating renal dysfunction.[56] Diuretics are useful when a fluid-overloaded patient (increased weight to preoperative weight) has adequate filling pressures, as determined by central venous pressure or pulmonary artery diastolic pressure (PAD) and satisfactory cardiac function, and in patients in whom there is no longer an ongoing fluid requirement (to maintain filling pressures, output, or MAP). Their routine use in low-risk patients has not been shown, however, to improve clinical outcome beyond an earlier return to baseline weight.[56]

Electrolyte Abnormalities

Hypokalemia is common after cardiac surgery because these patients retain sodium and excrete urinary potassium. Serum potassium should be monitored frequently, especially in high urine output in the early postoperative period because hypokalemia increases the risk of ventricular arrhythmias. The risk for postoperative ventricular arrhythmia can be reduced by maintaining serum potassium within a normal range.[57] Potassium replacement should be based on frequent serum values, with modification in renal insufficiency or acid-base abnormalities or both. Hypomagnesemia also is common, and because the therapeutic window for magnesium is so broad in patients with normal renal function, its repletion usually can be readily accomplished without the need to check levels repeatedly. The administration of magnesium (also a predominantly intracellular cation) has been shown, in at least one study, to decrease the incidence of ventricular dysrhythmias.[58] Hypocalcemia (seen with the use of cardioplegia solutions) is common, but associated with the dilution of serum proteins; it should be managed using the serum ionized calcium concentration. Calcium repletion has an often transient, inotropic and pressor benefit.

Glycemic Control

Hyperglycemia in postoperative cardiac patients is common and usually accompanies the increased endogenous and exogenous catecholamine levels induced by surgical stress. Depending on the classification of diabetes (diet, oral, or insulin therapy), 40% of patients having cardiac operations have a diagnosis of diabetes. It has been shown that excellent glycemic control that begins in the OR reduces morbidity (infectious) and mortality after cardiac operations.[59] Independent of a diagnosis of diabetes, tight glucose control in one institution's experience (serum glucose <130 mg/dL on 50% of samples) necessitated insulin drip therapy in 90% of post-CABG patients (57% of whom had no diagnosis of diabetes preoperatively). Associated with this tight control was a decreased incidence of mediastinitis.[60]

Antiplatelet Therapy

After CABG, most institutions begin antiplatelet therapy (aspirin 81 mg) 6 hours after ICU admission if the chest tube output is minimal (<50 mL/h) and the patient has been extubated. Otherwise, it is started on the morning of postoperative day 1. This antiplatelet regimen is continued in-definitely because of its benefits on conduit patency and amelioration of intimal hyperplasia. Patients who have undergone OPCAB do not experience the routine coagulopathy seen with CPB, and there is concern about early thrombosis,[61,62] leading some authors to reverse heparin incompletely with protamine in the OR, or to initiate more postoperative anticoagulation earlier[63] using heparin or clopidogrel (Plavix), or both. With these protocols, the patient must be stable and have minimal chest tube drainage.

Blood Transfusion

Many patients have low hematocrits (<28%) after cardiac surgery. The degree of anemia that is tolerated should not be dictated by protocol or a number, but individualized based on oxygen delivery reserve. This requires assessing the patient's cardiopulmonary function; if a patient's cardiac output and oxygenation are barely satisfactory, and, even more importantly, if significant support is required to maintain that level of function, the patient's oxygen delivery reserve is limited. Other factors that should be considered in the early transfusion decision are the completeness of operative repair or revascularization and the ongoing rate of red blood cell loss from the chest tubes. The disadvantages of permissive, dilutional anemia have been well documented,[64] as have the risks and adverse outcomes associated with blood transfusion.[65-67] There is no universal transfusion trigger, and otherwise healthy patients undergoing primary operations usually can tolerate a very low hematocrit (20% to 22%). The decision to transfuse red blood cells should be based on the need to improve oxygen delivery, remembering that older cells take up and release oxygen less effectively. If the cardiac index is optimal, increasing oxygen-carrying capacity may be the only way to improve oxygen delivery, but it should not be the first-line therapy.

Atrial Fibrillation (AF) Prevention

Despite preventive efforts, the incidence of postoperative AF remains high (25% to 40%) after cardiac operations. Postoperative AF increases morbidity and mortality and ICU and hospital length of stay.[68] Some centers start AF prophylaxis regimens 24 to 48 hours (or 6 days) before surgery to prevent new-onset postoperative AF. These regimens use amiodarone (400 mg orally two to three times a day) with or without a β-blocker.[69] Although numerous studies show some benefit (lower incidence of postoperative AF) with such protocols, most of the available evidence shows that β-blockers alone decrease the incidence of AF[70,71] (e.g., metoprolol, 12.5 mg to 100 mg two to four times a day, or sotalol, 80 mg twice a day, adjusted for renal dysfunction.) with few side effects when started on the first postoperative day.[72]

Antibiotic Prophylaxis

The role of antistaphylococcal prophylaxis just before and after cardiac surgery is well established. Termination of this regimen varies from center to center. No published data show the benefit of more than three doses,[73] or 24 hours of postoperative coverage. It is common practice, however, for antibiotics to be given until the mediastinal and pleural chest tubes are removed.

Intra-aortic Balloon Pump Weaning

As noted elsewhere in this chapter, most patients with an IABP on arrival in the post–cardiac surgery unit have had the device percutaneously placed preoperatively in the catheterization laboratory. Appropriate management requires knowing the indication for its placement. In patients with unstable angina or left critical anatomy (usually a left main, with or without proximal right coronary artery obstruction), the balloon often can be weaned as soon as the bleeding risks associated with removal are considered back to baseline. This may occur before extubation while the patient is still sedated. These are patients whose indication for IABP insertion has been corrected by the operation, and who do not require significant inotropic support, so the device is withdrawn in the early postoperative hours.

Less common and more challenging are the patients who had an IABP inserted for hemodynamic instability or cardiogenic shock preoperatively. In these patients, weaning from mechanical support may occur only after pharmacologic support (inotropes and vasopressors) has been weaned to a level that would allow them to be reinstituted or increased to support the patient after IABP removal. These are patients in whom a trial of ventilator weaning on IABP may be appropriate because the balloon unloads the afterload increases seen by a poor ventricle during awakening and ventilator weaning. In such patients, the IABP may be removed after extubation, but often ventilatory failure predominates, and the balloon weaning end points (minimal or no pharmacologic support) are reached well before extubation is an option. In these patients, mechanical support is weaned (decreasing the balloon augmentation ratio from

1:1 to 1:2 to 1:3, or by decreasing the balloon inflation volume). A normal response is to see the native (unloaded) systolic pressure increase as the MAP remains steady over 30 to 60 minutes. If these criteria are met, the balloon usually can be safely removed.

Patients who have an IABP placed intraoperatively may have had "prophylactic" mechanical support initiated, and, if on minimal pressor and inotrope support, with an anatomically corrective procedure, the device may be removed before extubation as noted earlier. IABPs placed after CPB as an adjunct to weaning (see earlier) are frequently needed for days before successful weaning.

Routine Order Sets

The post–cardiac surgery setting routinely makes good use of preprinted orders that, ideally, reflect a system-wide patient care pathway for the "typical" patient. It is important to review and revise these orders regularly to ensure that they remain appropriate in light of changes in accepted treatment principles and the institution's patient population. The review and revision of these order sets should include a review of patient care pathways or protocols. Protocol modifications should be part of a process involving surgeons, anesthesiologists, intensivists, nurses, respiratory therapists, pharmacists, infectious disease specialists, and nephrologists.

EARLY POSTOPERATIVE COMPLICATIONS

After complex cardiac operations, given the general illness of these patients, it may be unclear what constitutes a "complicated" versus "routine" postoperative course. After most *noncardiac* operations, bleeding more than 500 mL in 2 hours, a hematocrit of 23%, and the need for vasopressor therapy would be considered to be a complication. As noted previously, however, these findings are not inconsistent with an "uncomplicated" course after cardiac surgery. "Complications" in complicated patients after complex operations might be best defined as conditions that occur in less than 20% of post–cardiac surgery patients and, in most instances, depending on the criteria applied, in less than 10% of patients. Such complications also might be defined as complications that increase the risk of mortality or are associated with an increased use of resources or length of hospital stay compared with the "usual" post–cardiac surgery patient.

Low Cardiac Output

As noted previously, a patient's preoperative cardiac function and intraoperative events largely determine the early cardiac performance and the need for preload increases and inotropic support (Fig. 37-4). In patients with preexisting heart failure or profound postoperative failure, combination therapy is commonly used. Dopamine or epinephrine plus a phosphodiesterase inhibitor (milrinone) may complement each other (working on either side of the cyclic adenosine monophosphate pathway to improve contractility). This combination reduces afterload (milrinone as a peripheral phosphodiesterase inhibitor), whereas higher doses of epinephrine or dopamine cause vasoconstriction. Although vasopressors are not ideal in left heart failure, they are necessary at times to support adequate perfusion pressure, inclusive of the need for coronary perfusion with high end-diastolic pressures (coronary blood flow is directly related to the MAP or diastolic aortic pressure, minus the end diastolic pressure).

Norepinephrine bitartrate (Levophed) or phenylephrine (Neo-Synephrine) may be used initially, but in all cases, the first step should be to optimize preload.

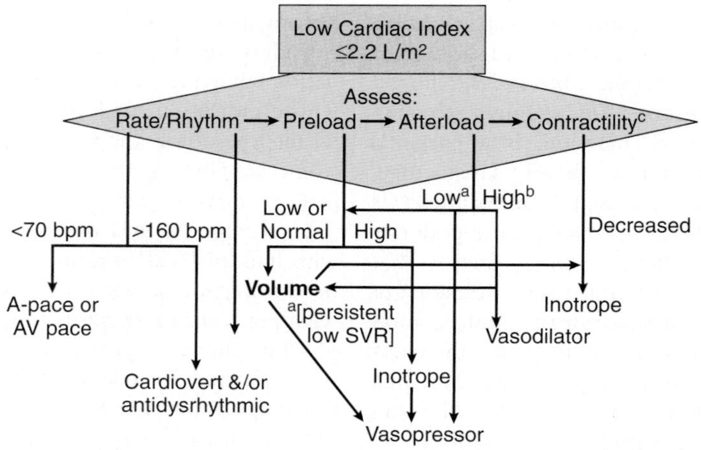

Figure 37-4. Simplified algorithm for assessment and management of decreased cardiac index postoperatively. Beginning with the assessment and management of the rate and rhythm, the evaluation continues through to contractility by virtue of assessing and managing preload and afterload. The underlying cause of decreased cardiac index must be considered as well, as discussed in the text. [a]Low afterload or SVR requires reassessment of the preload and correction to optimize volume and cardiac index before instituting vasopressor agent. [b]High afterload or pulmonary vascular resistance may be a sign of mild hypovolemia and requires a reassessment of preload before employing a vasodilator that may decrease preload further. [c]Contractility is the final link in evaluating a decreased cardiac index and usually is evaluated as preload is treated or assessed with a volume challenge to assess the ventricular compliance or the dynamics of the Frank-Starling relationship or both. A-pace, atrial pacing; AV, atrioventricular; SVR, systemic vascular resistance.

Inotropes can be administered before vasoconstrictors. At least one study reported improved coronary flow with norepinephrine[74] compared with phenylephrine. Both are effective, however, in working through different mechanisms to increase systemic vascular resistance. Calcium also can be an effective, albeit temporary, vasoconstrictor when ionized levels are low-normal. Arginine vasopressin has been used, especially after other pressors are ineffective, and particularly in patients who have chronic heart failure (reduced levels of antidiuretic hormone[75]). Vasopressin, similar to phenylephrine, is a pure vasoconstrictor, and when used at higher doses (>0.04 U/min), it may reduce splanchnic, coronary artery, renal cortical, and skin blood flow, negating the benefit of the increased MAP in an individual patient.[76] The subsequent section on vasodilatory shock discusses the appropriate use of vasopressin at higher doses.

Acidemia is common in post-CPB patients and is usually metabolic (lactate) and self-limited in patients whose ongoing oxygen demands are being met. There may be a component of respiratory acidemia present, which usually can be corrected over time in an adequately ventilated patient who has normal or near-normal pulmonary compliance. Modification (rather than complete correction) of metabolic acidemia with sodium bicarbonate (slowly administered) can be considered if the arterial pH is less than the range of 7.20 to 7.25, and the ventilatory function is satisfactory (to allow exhalation of the carbon dioxide load). Otherwise, there is no role for bicarbonate use in this setting. Acidemia is the result of lactate accumulation from low perfusion pressures during CPB, and it gradually corrects itself with adequate postoperative cardiac output. More important than the absolute increase in the serum lactate or base deficit postoperatively is its persistence. This implies ongoing inadequate oxygen delivery, and the cause must be identified and corrected because of the increased risk of arrhythmias and reduced effectiveness of inotropes and pressors in this setting.

Few drugs augment cardiac output as efficiently as IABP counterpulsation, which decreases myocardial oxygen demand by reducing myocardial wall tension during systole by afterload reduction (balloon deflation). It also increases oxygen supply by increasing coronary blood flow during diastole (balloon inflation). Device insertion is often delayed as other measures are tried and fail, and some early benefit of reducing heart work and increasing oxygen delivery is lost (see earlier section on intraoperative events). Complications can occur during IABP insertion and removal (bleeding, emboli, thrombosis, vessel or plaque disruption) and if it is malpositioned within the aorta (too high—interferes with circulation to the head; too low—can impair renal blood flow). The IABP also can interfere with distal lower extremity perfusion and lead to compartment syndrome. Other options for postoperative mechanical assistance of the failing heart include left ventricular assist devices. Left or right ventricular assistance may be provided by insertion of an Abiomed (Danvers, MA) or other ventricular assist device.

Solitary right heart assistance with extracorporeal membrane oxygenation is more commonly and successfully used after congenital heart operations than after adult operations. With any of these devices, but particularly extracorporeal membrane oxygenation, it is common to leave the sternum open and covered by a sterile dam or dressing to avoid cardiac and pulmonary compression. A detailed description of the use of these and other mechanical devices is beyond the scope of this chapter, but three important points should be made. First, some degree of anticoagulation is needed given the artificial surface contact. The risk of bleeding in these patients is very high. Second, these devices are very "preload" dependent, and volume or cannula position is commonly the cause of low pump outputs. Third, and perhaps the most challenging issue regarding these devices, is the timing of their insertion. If a mechanical device is to be used, it would be of greatest benefit if used before end-organ dysfunction or coagulopathy or both develop. There is a relatively high usage threshold because of the increased resources and risks associated with insertion and maintenance.

Most important is the careful evaluation of the underlying etiology of low cardiac output after an operation. In revascularized patients, ischemia secondary to early graft failure must be considered and may require emergent left heart catheterization to establish graft patency. Graft thrombosis in the early postoperative period is most often a technical issue ranging from inadequate distal outflow to graft kinking or entrapment during chest closure or anastomotic narrowing at the proximal or distal sites. Prosthetic valve dysfunction (entrapment), valve repair disruption, and pericardial tamponade are among the possible complications that manifest as a deterioration in cardiac function, and these are discussed next.

Vasodilatory Shock

Occasionally, a patient presents (generally within the first 6 hours of operation) with profound hypotension and a normal to slightly above-normal cardiac index. This is not a common occurrence because more commonly hypotension is associated with lower than normal cardiac indices, and it is the cardiac function that must be addressed first. In a retrospective examination of post-CABG patients with cardiac indices equal to or greater than 2.5 L/m^2 and persistent hypotension (MAP < 70 mm Hg), the incidence was seen to be only 2.5%.[27] Preoperative use of angiotensin-converting enzyme inhibitors was identified as an independent predictor for this vasodilatory state. Prolonged CPB times and the inflammatory state also have been associated with its occurrence. Managing this condition requires attention to ventricular filling pressures because they are often low and the use, often in high doses, of vasopressors, such as phenylephrine, 40 to 180 μg/min, or vasopressin, greater than 0.04 U/min, titrated to achieve an appropriate increase in the MAP.

Myocardial Ischemia or Infarction

Acute ECG changes localized to a grafted or ungraftable myocardial territory indicate ongoing ischemia and possibly graft failure (Fig. 37-5). If the global function is normal (filling pressures and cardiac index), the patient should have serial evaluation of that function and the

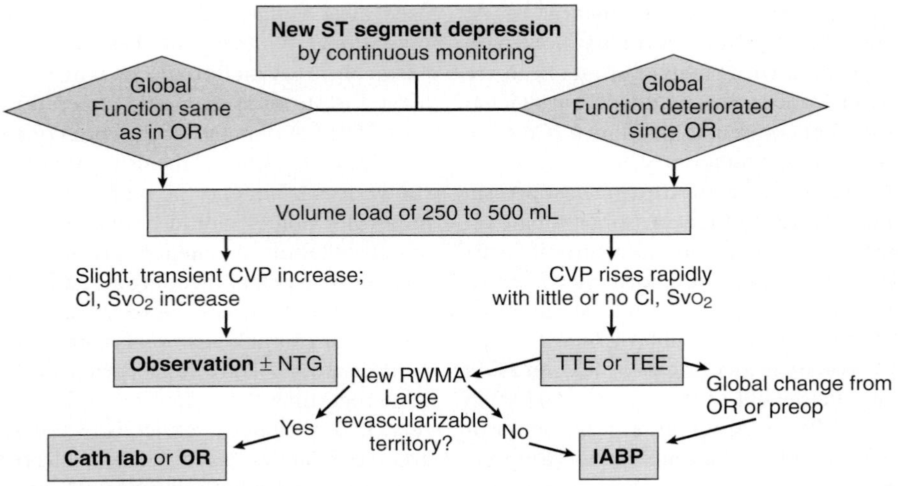

Figure 37-5. Postoperative ST segment depression in a patient may occur early after cardiac surgery, particularly in a post–coronary artery bypass graft patient with difficult distal or arterial conduits. Spasm or occlusion must be considered, as should the potential myocardial territory involved—its size and its potential revascularizability. A poor distal vessel or conduit limitations may not be amenable to further revascularization attempts, whereas a large, intraoperatively satisfactory graft to a large territory may be an obvious candidate for prompt revision. Because percutaneous techniques also may salvage a territory, knowledge of the preoperative angiogram and the location of any new regional wall motion abnormality (RWMA) should guide the choice of catheterization laboratory or operating room (OR). CI, cardiac index; CVP, central venous pressure; IABP, intra-aortic balloon pulsation; NTG, nitroglycerin; Svo_2, venous oxygen saturation; TEE, transesophageal echocardiography; TTE, transthoracic echocardiography.

evolution of the ECG changes. If filling pressure is elevated (with or without decreased cardiac output), echocardiography should be performed to look for new wall motion abnormalities (compared with the previous intraoperative study). A surgeon may then decide, depending on the area's size and the graft and native vessel anatomy, whether left heart catheterization is indicated, and whether operative revision or a catheter-based intervention is appropriate. Nitroglycerin may be used during this time, but it is unlikely to increase coronary flow to the threatened myocardium sufficiently. Modest ECG changes in the form of ST-T segment elevation that span the precordium and the limb leads in a hemodynamically stable patient are common and presumably represent pericardial changes (inflammation) associated with the operation itself. Although postoperative cardiac enzyme (troponin T) levels are still measured routinely on the first postoperative day in some centers, this seems to do little in terms of improving the outcome or management. There may be some prognostic value, however, if there is a high index of suspicion that ischemia is present or infarction has occurred.

Cardiac Tamponade

Appropriately called the "great masquerader," cardiac tamponade can manifest with sudden drama (often, clues were missed) or insidiously, even under close scrutiny. Classically, patients who have been draining a significant amount of mediastinal blood develop clots in the chest tubes or drains (blood slowly accumulating should be defibrinated in the pericardium and does not clot) and slowly develop increased filling pressures. Mean aortic pressure, cardiac output, and urine output decrease. In some cases, when the bleeding is acute, or the chest tubes are simply not draining loculated blood, tamponade physiology can occur in the absence of *apparent* mediastinal "chest tube" hemorrhage. Cardiac tamponade is best diagnosed by echocardiography. If the study is unremarkable and clinical suspicion remains high, however, the best course of action is to re-explore the mediastinum in the OR. Transthoracic echocardiography may not be able to detect cardiac tamponade caused by a small accumulation of blood that is compressing the right atrium and impairing venous return.

Cardiac tamponade is best managed by reopening the sternum in the OR and evacuating the clot and blood. Identification of the hemorrhagic source or any underlying coagulopathy or both is fundamental. Many patients have no clearly identifiable bleeding site. Some units are prepared to provide an appropriate environment for sternal exploration without a return to the OR. Rarely, in any postoperative unit, in the face of desperate and acute decompensation, it may be necessary to open the chest and evacuate a clot immediately without transfer to the OR despite a lack of good lighting and a sterile environment. In such situations, suction and instruments still are needed. It is important to be aware of the operation details if possible in advance because bypass conduits can be easily disrupted, and exploration for a source of bleeding is more efficient if one is familiar with the operative field. Initially, just opening the chest usually can relieve tamponade. Manipulating the heart should be avoided until good lighting and exposure are obtained, unless it is obvious that hemostasis is required (most of these patients are not exsanguinating). Complete reopening of the sternotomy with lighting, retraction, and suction not only relieves the tamponade, but also it may permit direct control of the bleeding site. Adequate perfusion, despite tamponade physiology, allows a patient to be returned to the OR for evacuation of blood or clot, complete re-exploration, and chest closure. Emergent re-exploration in the ICU may be associated with an increased risk of wound infection.[77,78]

Postoperative Hemorrhage

"Mechanical" or "surgical" bleeding (defined here as site-specific, not purely coagulopathic) from a leaking or disrupted suture line or an uncoagulated, unligated branch can develop slowly or suddenly. A brief period of hypertension occasionally occurs just before an increase in mediastinal tube blood output, and in other cases the output increases steadily from that observed in the OR or during transfer. Institutional protocols vary, but the absence of clear evidence of coagulopathy (acidemia, hypothermia) and postoperative chest tube bleeding greater than 500 mL in the first hour, greater than 300 mL in the second, and greater than 200 mL in the third or any hour thereafter should lead one to consider the need for a return to the OR for mediastinal exploration. Lower thresholds are used for minimally invasive approaches. Every effort is made in the OR during the initial operation to correct diffuse bleeding. Although nearly all patients who have undergone cardiac operations with CPB have some degree of coagulopathy, increased chest tube output *with clot formation* in the chest tubes is usually not entirely due to coagulopathy.

Specific therapy should be directed at causes of postoperative bleeding, such as hypothermia, acidemia, thrombocytopenia, platelet dysfunction, hemodilution, and consumption of coagulation factors. Empiric therapy based on patient-specific and operation-specific factors (preoperative antiplatelet or warfarin [Coumadin] therapy) may be initiated while awaiting the results of coagulation studies. Re-exploration is associated with identification of one or more bleeding sites that benefit from surgical therapy in most instances,[79] but in 30% to 40% of cases, continued coagulopathy or no specific bleeding site is found.[80] At least one retrospective study confirms a widely observed phenomenon that re-exploration and evacuation of clots (associated with blood product administration) are associated with resolution of excessive hemorrhage, even in the absence of an identified site of bleeding.[81] The use of activated factor VII as a means of rescuing a patient with unresponsive coagulopathy has been shown to be of marginal to significant benefit without major thrombotic complications.[82,83]

Pulmonary Complications

The treatment of pulmonary dysfunction is described elsewhere in this textbook. As with postoperative cardiac dysfunction, patients with compromised preoperative pulmonary function can be expected to have it exacerbated postoperatively. There are patients with preoperative cardiogenic pulmonary dysfunction who improve, often quite promptly, after their operation (e.g., especially patients with mitral stenosis, acute mitral regurgitation, or severe aortic stenosis). Unanticipated, new-onset pulmonary dysfunction is usually due to acute lung injury and is associated with inflammation and hemodilution of CPB, particularly after long operations. After CPB, the lung may be the target of remote organ injury. Systemic reperfusion-inflammation may occur or the lung itself may be injured by its own ischemia-reperfusion (no ventilation or pulmonary blood flow during CPB, sustained only by bronchial, nonpulsatile flow). Regardless of the mechanism, some pulmonary dysfunction is universal.[24,26] Manifestations include decreased pulmonary compliance, large alveolar-arterial gradients, and bronchoconstriction.

The management of these patients is similar to patients with acute lung injury (PaO_2/FIO_2 ratio <300 mm Hg) or its more severe form, acute respiratory distress syndrome (PaO_2/FIO_2 ratio <200 mm Hg). This always requires adequate sedation and often necessitates muscle relaxation (paralytics) to coordinate patient breathing better with the ventilator and to increase chest wall compliance. A cerebral monitor (e.g., BIS; Aspect Medical Systems, Norwood, MA) may be used to indicate the level of sedation if long-term sedation is required. Muscle relaxation also makes equal or inversed inspiratory-to-expiratory cycle time ratios, often required in these patients, better tolerated. Postinjury lung protective strategies, such as low stretch tidal volume (6 mL/kg) are administered by pressure control ventilation. Early in the patient's course, high positive end-expiratory pressure may be required to allow FIO_2 levels to decrease to less than 60%, which minimizes the risk of secondary lung injury owing to free radical production. The reduced tidal volumes minimize the risk of volutrama, but also decrease minute ventilation, which results in hypercapnia. This is allowed as long as the pH remains greater than 7.25 (permissive hypercapnia). In most patients, acute lung injury may occur as part of the systemic inflammatory response and does not progress into more severe forms such as acute respiratory distress syndrome. With these lung-protective measures, inverse ratio ventilation and muscle relaxation are not typically required. Most lung dysfunction in the initial postoperative period is due to atelectasis, which usually responds well to higher positive end-expiratory pressure levels. Other causes include copious thick secretions, especially a mucus plug with partial lung collapse (which may require bronchoscopy), volume overload, and occasionally right main stem intubation. The latter should be corrected as soon as the initial postoperative chest radiograph is reviewed to avoid atelectasis or lung collapse, which is usually seen on the left side.

Other pulmonary complications include pneumothorax, hemothorax (bleeding not adequately drained by pleural or mediastinal chest tubes), and bronchial obstruction with lobar collapse. The chest x-ray can lead to the correct diagnosis and treatment (chest tube thoracostomy, bronchoscopy). Rarely, abdominal compartment syndrome from massive interstitial edema or acute bleeding may occur after a long CPB run. In such cases, the peak inspiratory pressures are quite high, and the abdomen is quite turgid. Laparotomy and temporary expanded closure may be lifesaving in rare patients. The diagnosis of a paralyzed or palsied diaphragm generally awaits the first x-ray after weaning from positive-pressure ventilation, but diaphragmatic dysfunction secondary to phrenic nerve injury (hypothermal, retractor stretch, or direct injury with mammary dissection) may delay or make impossible weaning from ventilatory support.

Atrial Fibrillation

The incidence of postoperative AF increases with age and occurs in up to 40% of the patient population (and 80% of octogenarians).[33] If AF is acute and associated with hemodynamic instability, it requires direct current cardioversion. This should be done either immediately or after the administration of an antiarrhythmic agent, such as amiodarone or procainamide. The requirement to monitor serum procainamide and *N*-acetyl procainamide levels with procainamide and its associated side effects (hypotension, lupus-like syndrome, gastrointestinal upset, and arrhythmias) have markedly reduced its use in favor of amiodarone. If direct current cardioversion is required, the patient's airway function should be ensured, and the need for tracheal intubation should be assessed to protect the airway (e.g., full stomach or obtunded patient). Reliable central or peripheral venous access should be obtained. In AF that has lasted longer than 48 hours, echocardiography should be performed to rule out thrombus. Sedation with etomidate (0.2 mg/kg) with or without fentanyl allows energy to be delivered (starting at 50 J [biphasic] for flutter and 75 to 100 J for fibrillation, up to 200 J and a maximum of three attempts) in a ventricular sensing, synchronized mode. External wires (or pads, if applied) may be used if sinus bradycardia or asystole transiently occurs.

Most patients tolerate the AF well enough to be treated solely with pharmacologic agents. There is no clear evidence that favors either rate or rhythm control.[84] With either therapy, an equal number of patients have been shown to be in a sinus rhythm weeks after their operation. During rate-controlled AF or atrial flutter, anticoagulation must be maintained, first with heparin and then with warfarin. Rate control or control of the ventricular response may be obtained with calcium channel blockers or β-blockers. Digoxin, previously commonly employed to control the rate, has fallen out of favor owing to newer, more effective agents and its own pro–ventricular arrhythmia effect. Pharmacologic conversion with amiodarone[85] (150 to 300 mg intravenous loading dose over 10 minutes followed by a continuous infusion of 0.5 to 1 mg/min) is commonly employed for hemodynamically stable AF that occurs in the ICU. After conversion, the drug can be administered orally and ultimately discontinued and reinstituted long-term if the AF recurs. The risk of AF diminishes over time, and patients discharged on amiodarone typically remain on it for 6 weeks postoperatively. There is no clear evidence, however, to support a specific duration of treatment or prophylaxis.[85] Thyroid and pulmonary toxicity of amiodarone are risks that must be considered, but the drug is usually well tolerated short-term.

Neurologic Complications

Neurologic complications can be classified as generalized (global) or focal. Focal deficits may be transient or permanent. Except in their most severe form, neurologic complications cannot be completely assessed until the patient returns to consciousness and is weaned from the ventilator. A new focal abnormality is usually evaluated by a computed tomography scan. Computed tomography for nonfocal, cognitive dysfunction rarely yields new information that is helpful to the patient's management (other than showing no evidence of an acute, new injury, such studies most often show old, chronic changes, such as atrophy or lacunar infarcts), and in all cases, the patient must be stable enough to be transported if the institution does not have a portable scanner. The risk factors for neurologic injury post–cardiac surgery have been well studied,[86,87] but reliable prevention is impossible. The cause of stroke may be embolic or low flow ("watershed" events). Patients with descending thoracic aortic operations are at significant risk for spinal cord ischemia intraoperatively, and, rarely, delayed injury (days postoperatively) may occur.

Renal Dysfunction and Failure

Some mild degree of renal dysfunction occurs after CPB in virtually all patients.[88] Acute renal failure occurs in 30% of patients, and 1% to 2% require dialysis.[89] Preexisting renal dysfunction is a predictor of postoperative acute renal failure. Although a variety of strategies have been tried, including furosemide, low or "renal" dose dopamine, mannitol,[90] fenoldopam,[91] and *N*-acetylcysteine,[92] none has proved uniformly successful in reducing the incidence or improving the outcome of this complication. Acute renal failure after cardiac surgery has been shown to be an *independent* predictor (adjusted for a host of comorbidities predictive of renal failure and death) of early mortality.[93]

Other Early Complications

Hypertension may occur postoperatively. It is often considered a "favorite" problem because it has many favorable, pharmacologic remedies. Hypertensive patients generally have a long history of hypertension, and sodium nitroprusside infusions (starting dose, 0.1 to 0.5 μg/kg/min maintenance dose, 0.75 to 3 μg/kg/min, maximum dose, 10 μg/kg/min) offer a means of vasodilation that can be finely titrated. Attention to the cumulative dose (time and drug volume), particularly in patients with renal dysfunction, is necessary to avoid cyanide toxicity. Thiocyanate levels can be drawn to avoid this complication. β-blockade with short-acting esmolol infusions may be appropriate in some patients with satisfactory cardiac function, but should be used cautiously in patients with sinus tachycardia who might be manifesting compensation for low stroke volume secondary to hypovolemia. In patients with preoperative inadequately treated, long-standing hypertension, excessive control of the mean arterial blood pressure (even in the normal range) postoperatively may be associated with low urine output (<0.5 mL/kg/h), azotemia, and acute renal injury.

As noted earlier, lactic acidemia—manifested by low pH, bicarbonate, and base deficits often up to 10—is not unusual after CPB. If the patient's cardiac and urine output are deemed adequate, and the patient is warming and waking up, such deficits should not be treated with bicarbonate. Increasing recurrent or worsening levels of acidemia or even sustained moderate acidemia should trigger evaluation of cardiac function, renal function, and the less likely but more insidious possibility of gastrointestinal or extremity ischemia. In most cases, the acidemia that occurs in the first 6 hours after operation is deemed to be reflective of a prior oxygen supply/demand imbalance during CPB, which usually corrects itself within 12 hours as long as normal cardiac output is maintained.

Gastrointestinal complications include ulcer/upper gastrointestinal hemorrhage (gastritis or peptic), bowel ischemia, pseudomembranous colitis, and pancreatitis. These complications, although rare, are serious because they often are diagnosed late or in association with other major complications. Predictive factors include a longer CPB time, peripheral vascular disease, long-term steroid use, and low left ventricular ejection fraction.[94,95] A gastritis and stress ulcer prophylaxis regimen for patients in critical care should include H_2 blockers.

INTERMEDIATE-TERM POSTOPERATIVE COMPLICATIONS

Patients whose length of stay in the ICU lasts 48 hours or more have generally manifested one or more major complications. These include asystole or bradycardia (<30 beats per minute), atrial arrhythmias, ventricular dysrhythmias (ventricular tachycardia/ventricular fibrillation), low cardiac output, prolonged need for an IABP, an open chest, heart block, focal or global neurologic event, seizures, encephalopathy, alcohol withdrawal, pulmonary dysfunction (acute lung injury or acute respiratory distress syndrome), inability to wean from ventilator support, diaphragm dysfunction, pulmonary embolism, renal failure requiring dialysis, sepsis syndrome, and gastrointestinal bleeding. Each of these conditions is covered elsewhere in this chapter or other chapters. Intermediate-term management specific to cardiac surgery patients includes the following points.

Tracheostomy to assist in weaning from the ventilator should be considered in appropriate patients.[96] In years past, a patient with a median sternotomy was considered to require weeks of healing before a tracheostomy (potentially communicating with the middle mediastinum) could be performed. At present, percutaneous tracheostomy performed at the bedside seems to have at least similar clinical outcomes at a significantly reduced cost compared with the open procedure.[97] Tracheostomy timing is based on the determination at some time interval (e.g., 1 to 2 weeks) of a patient's likelihood of successful weaning over the next week. If at that time, successful weaning is unlikely, a tracheostomy should be considered. It also should be considered at the end of the second week of mechanical ventilation if weaning has not occurred. A tracheostomy is more comfortable for the patient, facilitates easier oral care, and allows for easier continued weaning (continuous positive airway pressure/tracheostomy collar trials and nocturnal rest periods). Suctioning a tracheostomy is easier and more effective than through an endotracheal tube. Finally, with a tracheostomy a patient can more readily be transferred out of the ICU to a step-down unit or a unit specialized in ventilator weaning (when nutrition and weaning are primary management issues).

Bradycardia and Complete Heart Block

In the early postoperative period, bradycardia is managed with epicardial wires and an external pacemaker. If low heart rate remains a problem, a permanent pacemaker may be required. Older patients are given the lowest dose of a β-blocker because AF prophylaxis may manifest profound sinus bradycardia and then tachycardia when the β-blocker is discontinued. This may be viewed as the serendipitous diagnosis of tachycardia-bradycardia syndrome, and, especially if β-blockers are indicated to treat tachycardia, a permanent pacemaker may be required. Other patients may manifest some degree of atrioventricular block that precludes appropriate response to exercise or, worse, is present at rest. These patients often had valve procedures or myomyectomy for asymmetric septal hypertrophy, and although some have atrioventricular block from the OR forward in time, others develop the condition after hours of apparent atrioventricular conduction. Experiences vary regarding the time one must wait to allow atrioventricular node recovery, as may occur after conduction tissue edema subsides. Drugs that decrease atrioventricular node conduction should be stopped if possible to allow appropriate assessment of atrioventricular nodal function. With the temporary pacing wires in place, if high (increasing) mean amplitude output levels are required to pace the heart, temporary pacemaker backup may be considered. A permanent dual-lead pacemaker lead system works well in this situation and should begin to be considered at days 3 to 5, depending on mean amplitude output levels, in a stable patient without atrioventricular node recovery.

Sternal Infection and Mediastinitis

Sternal wound infections may be classified as superficial or deep (mediastinitis). Most patients are discharged from the ICU before this diagnosis is made. The condition usually manifests as sternal instability (sternal click), purulent drainage, or a low-grade fever. The risk factors for such infections are well established,[77] and their prevention includes the use of prophylactic antibiotics initiated before the operation and readministered (every 4 hours in some centers and "as directed" in others) during CPB. As noted, there is no solid evidence that continued prophylactic dosing after three doses increases effectiveness, but many institutional protocols continue prophylaxis until the chest tubes are removed.

TRANSFER FROM THE INTENSIVE CARE UNIT

Most patients are ready to be transferred to a less intensive postoperative care environment within 24 hours. Early discharge generally is not associated with increased readmission rates because patients with longer ICU stays are more likely to be readmitted.[98] As with transfer to the ICU from the OR, transfer out of the ICU to the regular nursing floor requires effective coordination with the staff in the next care setting. Clear communication with the nursing staff from one unit to the next based on a protocol-driven patient care pathway is important. Telemetry is essential for these patients for at least the first 48 hours. Some centers use an intermediate care (step-down) unit before a predischarge care setting. In this age of shorter hospital stays, most patients can be discharged to home or rehabilitation from the post-ICU telemetry unit within 5 days.

CONCLUSION

Post–cardiac surgery patients are routinely complex patients because of the gravity of their preoperative condition and the magnitude of their intraoperative treatment. Most of the complexities that these patients present are seen in other patients in the postsurgical ICU, but these patients are unique by virtue of the routine combination of these conditions. These patients are best cared for in a multidisciplinary, well-functioning (communicating) system that appreciates their complexity and makes use of thoughtfully designed, well-followed care pathways applicable to the usual patient. In this way, most of these complex patients become "routine," and patients whose condition deviates from the usual are readily identified, and the appropriate treatment is instituted.

KEY POINTS

- Patient transfer from the OR to the ICU is optimized by *standardized communication* regarding intraoperative factors such as (1) the operation performed versus the operation planned, (2) ease of weaning from bypass or support used currently or both, and (3) current assessment of hemodynamics and oxygen delivery.
- A post–cardiac surgical unit and its patients benefit from *standardization of protocols* managing a variety of common issues that include (1) ventilatory weaning that is not routinely physician dependent; (2) pain and sedation pharmacologic regimens; (3) AF management with pharmacologic regimens; (4) glycemic control with insulin drips (<150 to 170 mg/dL) for all patients, with or without known diabetes; (5) pacing wire removal or cutting indications and technique; and (6) chest tube removal indications and technique.
- Individualization of patient management is dictated not only by intraoperative events, but also by *preoperative conditions,* such as the following: (1) Hypertension poorly controlled preoperatively should not be overcontrolled postoperatively. (2) Poor preoperative ventricular compliance persists, or becomes worse, early after operation, often requiring an upward adjustment in the desired filling pressure. (3) Decreased oxygenation generally is worse early postoperatively, and strategies that protect from volutrauma must be implemented to avoid a short-term problem becoming a long-term one. (4) Similar to the exacerbation of lung dysfunction, preoperative renal insufficiency often, at least transiently, is worsened, requiring a primary focus first on maintaining renal perfusion and second on avoiding overaggressive early diuresis.
- *Mediastinal bleeding* more than a threshold rate, such as 500 mL in the first hour, 300 mL in the second hour, and 200 mL in any hour thereafter, when associated with chest tube clotting, strongly suggests the need to re-explore the patient's mediastinum.
- *Blood transfusion triggers* are not specific for hematocrit and hemoglobin above a baseline value of 20% to 21% in the healthiest patients, but all others require an assessment of their symptoms, signs, oxygen delivery capacity, and bleeding risks.
- *Cardiac tamponade* manifests dramatically or suddenly, and diagnosis requires a high index of suspicion in unanticipated states of decreasing urine output and elevated filling pressures.
- *Length of stay* in the ICU is best optimized when specific criteria are defined as the trigger for discharge to the next unit.

REFERENCES

1. van Mastrigt GA, Maessen JG, Heijmans J, et al: Does fast-track treatment lead to a decrease of intensive care unit and hospital length of stay in coronary artery bypass patients? A meta-regression of randomized clinical trials. Crit Care Med 2006;34:1624-1634.
2. Yared JP, Starr NJ, Hoffmann-Hogg L, et al: Dexamethasone decreases the incidence of shivering after cardiac surgery: A randomized, double-blind, placebo-controlled study. Anesth Analg 1998;87:795-799.
3. O'Connor GT, Plume SK, Olmstead EM, et al: Multivariate prediction of in-hospital mortality associated with coronary artery bypass graft surgery. Northern New England Cardiovascular Disease Study. Circulation 1992;85:2110-2118.
4. Grover FL, Shroyer AL, Hammermeister K, et al: A decade's experience with quality improvement in cardiac surgery using the Veterans Affairs and Society of Thoracic Surgeons national databases. Ann Surg 2001;234:464-472.
5. Shroyer ALW, Coombs LP, Peterson ED, et al: The Society of Thoracic Surgeons: 30-day operative mortality and morbidity risk models. Ann Thorac Surg 2003;75:1856-1865.
6. Health Data Research: Merged cardiac registry. http://www.healthdataresearch.com/mcr_file.htm (accessed July 15, 2007).
7. Bernstein AD, Parsonnet V: Bedside estimation of risk as an aid for decision-making in cardiac surgery. Ann Thorac Surg 2000;69:823-828.
8. Roques F, Nashef SAM, Michel P, et al: Risk factors and outcome in European cardiac surgery: analysis of the EuroSCORE multinational database of 19030 patients. Eur J Cardiothorac Surg 1999;15:816-823.
9. Higgins TL, Estafanous FD, Loop GJ, et al, Cleveland Clinic Foundation: Stratification of morbidity and mortality outcome by preoperative risk factors in coronary artery bypass patients: A clinical severity score. JAMA 1992;267:2344-2348.
10. Higgins TL, Estafanous FG, Loop FD, et al: Stratification of morbidity and mortality outcome by preoperative risk factors in coronary artery bypass patients: a clinical severity score. JAMA 1992;267:2344-2348.
11. Bennett-Guerrero E, Ayuso L, Hamilton-Davies C, et al: Relationship of preoperative antiendotoxin core antibodies and adverse outcomes following cardiac surgery. JAMA 1997;277:646-650.
12. Bennett-Guerrero E, Slaughter TF, White WD, et al: Preoperative anti-PF4/heparin antibody level predicts adverse outcome after cardiac surgery. J Thorac Cardiovasc Surg 2005;130:1567-1572.
13. Yende S, Quasney MW, Tolley E, et al: Association of tumor necrosis factor

gene polymorphisms and prolonged mechanical ventilation after coronary artery bypass surgery. Crit Care Med 2003;31:133-140.
14. Waterer GW, Wunderink RG: Science review: genetic variability in the systemic inflammatory response. Crit Care 2003;7:308-314.
15. Welsby IJ, Podgoreanu MV, Phillips-Bute B, et al: Perioperative Genetics and Safety Outcomes Study (PEGASUS) Investigative Team. Genetic factors contribute to bleeding after cardiac surgery. J Thromb Haemost 2005;3:1206-1212.
16. Liet JM, Kuster A, Denizot S, et al: Effects of hydroxyethyl starch on cardiac output in hypotensive neonates: a comparison with isotonic saline and 5% albumin. Acta Paediatr 2006;95:555-560
17. Khan NE, De Souza A, Mister R, et al: A randomized comparison of off-pump and on-pump multivessel coronary-artery bypass surgery. N Engl J Med 2004;350:21-28.
18. Franke A, Lante W, Fackeldey V, et al: Pro-inflammatory cytokines after different kinds of cardio-thoracic surgical procedures: Is what we see what we know? Eur J Cardiothorac Surg 2005;28:569-575.
19. Royston D: The inflammatory response and extracorporeal circulation. J Cardiothorac Vasc Anesth 1997;11:341-354.
20. Øvrum E, Tangen G, Tølløfsrud S, et al: Heparin-coated circuits and reduced systemic anticoagulation applied to 2500 consecutive first-time coronary artery bypass grafting procedures. Ann Thorac Surg 2003;76:1144-1148.
21. Lappegård KT, Fung M, Bergseth G, et al: Effect of complement inhibition and heparin coating on artificial surface-induced leukocyte and platelet activation. Ann Thorac Surg 2004;77:932-941.
22. Edwards JT, Hamby JK, Worrall NK: Successful use of argatroban as a heparin substitute during cardiopulmonary bypass: Heparin-induced thrombocytopenia in a high-risk cardiac surgical patient. Ann Thorac Surg 2003;75:1622-1624.
23. Murkin JM: The role of CPB management in neurobehavioral outcomes after cardiac surgery. Ann Thorac Surg 1995;59:1308-1311.
24. Taggart DP, el-Fiky M, Carter R, et al: Respiratory dysfunction after uncomplicated cardiopulmonary bypass. Ann Thorac Surg 1993;56:1123-1128.
25. DeFoe GR, Ross CS, Olmstead EM, et al: Lowest hematocrit on bypass and adverse outcomes associated with coronary artery bypass grafting. Northern New England Cardiovascular Disease Study Group. Ann Thorac Surg 2001;71:769-776.
26. Clark SC: Lung injury after cardiopulmonary bypass. Perfusion 2006;21:225-228.
27. Mekontso-Dessap A, Houël R, Soustelle C, et al: Risk factors for post-cardiopulmonary bypass vasoplegia in patients with preserved left ventricular function. Ann Thorac Surg 2001;71:1428-1432.
28. DeFoe GR, Ross CS, Olmstead ES, et al: Lowest hematocrit on bypass and adverse outcomes associated with coronary artery bypass grafting. Ann Thorac Surg 2001;71:769-776.
29. Ranucci M, Biagioli B, Scolletta S, et al: Lowest hematocrit on cardiopulmonary bypass impairs the outcome in coronary surgery: An Italian Multicenter Study from the National Cardioanesthesia Database. Tex Heart Inst J 2006;33: 300-305.
30. Mack MJ, Pfister A, Bachand D, et al: Comparison of coronary bypass surgery with and without cardiopulmonary bypass in patients with multivessel disease. J Thorac Cardiovasc Surg 2004;127:167-173.
31. Sellke FW, DiMaio JM, Caplan LR, et al: Comparing on-pump and off-pump coronary artery bypass grafting: Numerous studies but few conclusions: A scientific statement from the American Heart Association Council on Cardiovascular Surgery and Anesthesia in Collaboration With the Interdisciplinary Working Group on Quality of Care and Outcomes Research. Circulation 2005;111: 2858-2864.
32. Lee JD, Lee SJ, Tsushima WT, et al: Benefits of off-pump bypass on neurologic and clinical morbidity: A prospective randomized trial. Ann Thorac Surg 2003;76:18-26.
33. Cohn WE, Sirois CA, Johnson RG: Atrial fibrillation after minimally invasive coronary artery bypass grafting: A retrospective, matched study. J Thorac Cardiovasc Surg 1999;117:298-301.
34. Lund C, Sundet K, Tennoe B, et al: Cerebral ischemic injury and cognitive impairment after off-pump and on-pump coronary artery bypass grafting surgery. Ann Thorac Surg 2005;80: 2126-2131.
35. Tomic V, Russwurm S, Moller E, et al: Transcriptomic and proteomic patterns of systemic inflammation in on-pump and off-pump coronary artery bypass grafting. Circulation 2005;112:2912-2920.
36. Kshettry VR, Flavin TF, Emery RW, et al: Does multivessel, off-pump coronary artery bypass reduce postoperative morbidity? Ann Thorac Surg 2000;69:1725-1731.
37. Brown JM, Poston RS, Gammie JS, et al: Off-pump versus on-pump coronary artery bypass grafting in consecutive patients: decision-making algorithm and outcomes. Ann Thorac Surg 2006;81:555-561.
38. Kouchoukos NT, Daily BB, Rokkas CK, et al: Hypothermic bypass and circulatory arrest for operations on the descending thoracic and thoracoabdominal aorta. Ann Thorac Surg 1995;60:67-76.
39. Boldt J, Brenner T, Lehmann A, et al: Is kidney function altered by the duration of cardiopulmonary bypass? Ann Thorac Surg 2003;75:906-912.
40. Bitkover CY, Gardlund B: Mediastinitis after cardiovascular operations: A case-control study of risk factors. Ann Thorac Surg 1998;65:36-40.
41. Duke T, Butt W, South M, et al: Early markers of major adverse events in children after cardiac operations. J Thorac Cardiovasc Surg 1997;114:1042-1052.
42. Baskett RJF, O'Connor GT, Hirsch GM, et al: A multicenter comparison of intraaortic balloon pump utilization in isolated coronary artery bypass graft surgery. Ann Thorac Surg 2003;76: 1988-1992.
43. Christenson JT, Cohen M, Ferguson JJ, et al: Trends in intraaortic balloon counterpulsation complications and outcomes in cardiac surgery. Ann Thorac Surg 2002;74:1086-1091.
44. Ramnarine IR, Grayson AD, Dihmis WC, et al: Timing of intra-aortic balloon pump support and 1-year survival. Eur J Cardiothorac Surg 2005;27:887-892.
45. Schwann TA, Zacharias A, Riordan CJ, et al: Safe, highly selective use of pulmonary artery catheters in coronary artery bypass grafting: An objective patient selection method. Ann Thorac Surg 2002;73:1394-1401.
46. Stewart RD, Psyhojos T, Lahey SJ, et al: Central venous catheter use in low-risk coronary artery bypass grafting. Ann Thorac Surg 1998;66:1306-1311.
47. Konstantakos AK, Lee JH: Optimizing timing of early extubation in coronary artery bypass surgery patients. Ann Thorac Surg 2000;69:1842-1845.
48. Ely EW, Meade MO, Haponik EF, et al: Mechanical ventilator weaning protocols driven by nonphysician health-care professionals: Evidence-based clinical practice guidelines. Chest 2001;120:454S-463S.
49. van Mastrigt GA, Heijmans J, Severens J, et al: Short-stay intensive care after coronary artery bypass surgery: randomized clinical trial on safety and cost-effectiveness. Crit Care Med 2006;34:65-75.
50. Roediger L, Larbuisson R, Lamy M: New approaches and old controversies to postoperative pain control following cardiac surgery. Eur J Anaesthesiol 2006;23:539-550.
51. Sirieix D, Hongnat JM, Delayance S, et al: Comparison of the acute hemodynamic effects of hypertonic or colloid infusions immediately after mitral valve repair. Crit Care Med 1999;27:2159-2165.
52. Liet J, Kuster A, Denizot S, et al: Effects of hydroxyethyl starch on cardiac output in hypotensive neonates: A comparison with isotonic saline and 5% albumin. Acta Paediatr 2006;95: 555-560.
53. St Andre AC, DelRossi A: Hemodynamic management of patients in the first 24 hours after cardiac surgery. Crit Care Med 2005;33:2082-2093.
54. Bethea BT, Salazar JD, Grega MA, et al: Determining the utility of temporary pacing wires after coronary artery bypass surgery. Ann Thorac Surg 2005;79:104-107.
55. Abu-Omar Y, Ratnatunga C: Cardiopulmonary bypass and renal injury. Perfusion 2006;21:209-213.
56. Lim E, Ali ZA, Attaran R, et al: Evaluating routine diuretics after coronary surgery: A prospective randomized controlled trial. Ann Thorac Surg 2002;73:153-155.
57. Johnson RG, Shafique T, Sirois C, et al: Potassium concentrations and ventricular ectopy: A prospective, observational study in post-cardiac

surgery patients. Crit Care Med 1999;27:2430-2434.
58. England MR, Gordon G, Salem M, et al: Magnesium administration and dysrhythmias after cardiac surgery: A placebo-controlled, double-blind, randomized trial. JAMA 1992;268:2395-2402.
59. Furnary AP, Gao G, Grunkemeier GL, et al: Continuous insulin infusion reduces mortality in patients with diabetes undergoing coronary artery bypass grafting. J Thorac Cardiovasc Surg 2003;125:1007-1021.
60. Carr JM, Sellke FW, Fey M, et al: Implementing tight glucose control after coronary artery bypass surgery. Ann Thorac Surg 2005;80:902-909.
61. Mariani MA, Gu YJ, Boonstra PW, et al: Procoagulant activity after off-pump coronary operation: Is the current anticoagulation adequate? Ann Thorac Surg 1999;67:1370-1375.
62. Kim K-B, Lim C, Lee C, et al: Off-pump coronary artery bypass may decrease the patency of saphenous vein grafts. Ann Thorac Surg 2001;72: S1033-S1037.
63. Onorati F, Olivito S, Mastroroberto P, et al: Perioperative patency of coronary artery bypass grafting is not influenced by off-pump technique. Ann Thorac Surg 2005;80:2132-2140.
64. Weisel RD, Charlesworth DC, Mickleborough LL, et al: Limitations of blood conservation. J Thorac Cardiovasc Surg 1984;88:26-38.
65. Thurer RL: Blood transfusion in cardiac surgery. Can J Anaesth 2001;48 (4 Suppl):S6-S12.
66. Spiess BD: Transfusion of blood products affects outcome in cardiac surgery. Semin Cardiothorac Vasc Anesth 2004;8:267-281.
67. Koch CG, Li L, Duncan AI, et al: Transfusion in coronary artery bypass grafting is associated with reduced long-term survival. Ann Thorac Surg 2006;81:1650-1657.
68. Gillespie EL, Coleman CI, Sander S, et al: Effect of prophylactic amiodarone on clinical and economic outcomes after cardiothoracic surgery: A meta-analysis. Ann Pharmacother 2005;39:1409-1415.
69. Auer J, Weber T, Berent R, et al: A comparison between oral antiarrhythmic drugs in the prevention of atrial fibrillation after cardiac surgery: The pilot Study of Prevention of Postoperative Atrial Fibrillation (SPPAF), a randomized, placebo-controlled trial. Am Heart J 2004;147:636-643.
70. Kailasam R, Palin CA, Hogue CW Jr: Atrial fibrillation after cardiac surgery: An evidence-based approach to prevention. Semin Cardiothorac Vasc Anesth 2005;9:77-85.
71. Mooss AN, Wurdeman RL, Sugimoto JT, et al: Amiodarone versus sotalol for the treatment of atrial fibrillation after open heart surgery: The Reduction in Postoperative Cardiovascular Arrhythmic Events (REDUCE) trial. Am Heart J 2004;148:641-648.
72. Gillespie EL, Coleman CI, Sander S, et al: Effect of prophylactic amiodarone on clinical and economic outcomes after cardiothoracic surgery: A meta-analysis. Ann Pharmacother 2005;39:1409-1415.
73. Edwards FH, Engelman RM, Houck P, et al: The Society of Thoracic Surgeons Practice Guideline Series: Antibiotic prophylaxis in cardiac surgery, Part I: Duration. Ann Thorac Surg 2006;81:397-404.
74. DiNardo JA, Bert A, Schwartz MJ, et al: Effects of vasoactive drugs on flows through left internal mammary artery and saphenous vein grafts in man. J Thorac Cardiovasc Surg 1991;102:730-735.
75. Argenziano M, Chen JM, Choudhri AF, et al: Management of vasodilatory shock after cardiac surgery: Identification of predisposing factors and use of a novel pressor agent. J Thorac Cardiovasc Surg 1998;116:973-980.
76. Dunser MW, Mayr AJ, Ulmer H, et al: The effects of vasopressin on systemic hemodynamics in catecholamine-resistant septic and postcardiotomy shock: A retrospective analysis. Anesth Analg 2001;93:7-13.
77. Gummert JF, Barten MJ, Hans C, et al: Mediastinitis and cardiac surgery—an updated risk factor analysis in 10,373 consecutive adult patients. Thorac Cardiovasc Surg 2002;50:87-91.
78. Borger MA, Rao V, Weisel RD, et al: Deep sternal wound infection: Risk factors and outcomes. Ann Thorac Surg 1998;65:1050-1056.
79. Hall TS, Brevetti GR, Skoultchi AJ, et al: Re-exploration for hemorrhage following open heart surgery differentiation on the causes of bleeding and the impact on patient outcomes. Ann Thorac Cardiovasc Surg 2001;7:352-357.
80. Hall TS, Sines JC, Spotnitz AJ, et al: Hemorrhage related reexploration following open heart surgery: The impact of pre-operative and post-operative coagulation testing. Cardiovasc Surg 2002;10:146-153.
81. Pelletier MP, Solymoss S, Lee A, et al: Negative reexploration for cardiac postoperative bleeding: Can it be therapeutic? Ann Thorac Surg 1998;65:999-1002.
82. Karkouti K, Beattie WS, Wijeysundera DN, et al: Recombinant factor VIIa for intractable blood loss after cardiac surgery: A propensity score-matched case-control analysis. Transfusion 2005;45:26-34.
83. von Heymann C, Redlich U, Jain U, et al: Recombinant activated factor VII for refractory bleeding after cardiac surgery—a retrospective analysis of safety and efficacy. Crit Care Med 2005;33:2241-2246.
84. Lee JK, Klein GJ, Krahn AD, et al: Rate-control versus conversion strategy in postoperative atrial fibrillation: Trial design and pilot study results. Card Electrophysiol Rev 2003;7:178-184.
85. Martinez EA, Bass EB, Zimetbaum P: Pharmacologic control of rhythm: American College of Chest Physicians guidelines for the prevention and management of postoperative atrial fibrillation after cardiac surgery. Chest 2005;128:48S-55S.
86. D'Agostino RS, Svensson LG, Neumann DJ, et al: Screening carotid ultrasonography and risk factors for stroke in coronary artery surgery patients. Ann Thorac Surg 1996;62:1714-1723.
87. Bucerius J, Gummert JF, Borger MA, et al: Stroke after cardiac surgery: A risk factor analysis of 16,184 consecutive adult patients. Ann Thorac Surg 2003;75:472-478.
88. Lombardi R, Ferreiro A, Servetto C: Renal function after cardiac surgery: Adverse effect of furosemide. Ren Fail 2003;25:775-786.
89. Rosner MH, Okusa MD: Acute kidney injury associated with cardiac surgery. Clin J Am Soc Nephrol 2006;1:19-32.
90. Sirivella S, Gielchinsky I, Parsonnet V: Mannitol, furosemide, and dopamine infusion in postoperative renal failure complicating cardiac surgery. Ann Thorac Surg 2000;69:501-506.
91. Ranucci M, Soro G, Barzaghi N, et al: Fenoldopam prophylaxis of postoperative acute renal failure in high-risk cardiac surgery patients. Ann Thorac Surg 2004;78:1332-1338.
92. Burns KEA, Chu MWA, Novick RJ, et al: Perioperative N-acetylcysteine to prevent renal dysfunction in high-risk patients undergoing CABG surgery: A randomized controlled trial. JAMA 2005;294:342-350.
93. Chertow GM, Levy EM, Hammermeister KE, et al: Independent association between acute renal failure and mortality following cardiac surgery. Am J Med 1998;104:343-348.
94. Mercado PD, Farid H, O'Connell TX, et al: Gastrointestinal complications associated with cardiopulmonary bypass procedures. Am Surg 1994;60:789-792.
95. Khan JH, Lambert AM, Habib JH, et al: Abdominal complications after heart surgery. Ann Thorac Surg 2006;82:1796-1801.
96. Byhahn C, Rinne T, Halbig S, et al: Early percutaneous tracheostomy after median sternotomy. J Thorac Cardiovasc Surg 2000;120:329-334.
97. Bacchetta MD, Girardi LN, Southard EJ, et al: Comparison of open versus bedside percutaneous dilatational tracheostomy in the cardiothoracic surgical patient: Outcomes and financial analysis. Ann Thorac Surg 2005;79:1879-1885.
98. Cohn WE, Sirois C, Lisbon A, et al: Surgical intensive care unit recidivism after cardiac operations. Chest 1999;116:688-692.

PART

III

CRITICAL CARE PULMONARY DISEASE

Chapter 38

Acute Respiratory Failure

David P. Gurka and Robert A. Balk

Acute respiratory failure is commonly encountered in the intensive care unit setting and may be the primary diagnosis necessitating the admission or a complication of the patient's medical condition(s) or their treatment. Remembering that the respiratory failure may be the result of a variety of causes and may not directly involve the lungs or the respiratory muscles is important.[2] It has been said the body is like a chain composed of links that represent the brain, peripheral nervous system, upper airway, lower airway, respiratory muscles, cardiovascular system, and lungs (Fig. 38-1).[2] Respiratory failure may result when any of the links become sufficiently dysfunctional or weak. Like a chain, the body is only as strong as its weakest link and respiratory failure may result when a component of the chain becomes sufficiently compromised. Common causes of hypoxemic and hypercapnic respiratory failure are listed in Box 38-2. This chapter reviews the basic mechanisms and clinical manifestations of types 1 and 2 respiratory failure and concludes with a more in-depth discussion of acute lung injury and ARDS, which are clinical disorders in the type 1 category.

ACUTE RESPIRATORY FAILURE—TYPES 1 AND 2

Acute respiratory failure is defined as the inability of the respiratory system to meet the oxygenation, ventilation, or metabolic requirements of the patient.[1] Although the main function of the lungs appears to be related to gas exchange (i.e., oxygenation and ventilation), it should be remembered that the lung is a metabolically active organ as well.[1,2] Respiratory failure has been divided into two main types. Type 1 is hypoxemic respiratory failure, and type 2 is hypercapnic with or without hypoxemic respiratory failure.[2] More simply stated, type 1 respiratory failure is oxygenation failure and type 2 is ventilatory failure. Operationally, type 1 respiratory failure is defined by a partial pressure of oxygen in arterial blood ($Pa{O_2}$) less than 60 mm Hg and type 2 respiratory failure is defined by a partial pressure of carbon dioxide in arterial blood ($Pa{CO_2}$) of greater than 50 mm Hg (Box 38-1). The respiratory failure can be acute or chronic in nature, related to the onset and duration of the failure.[2,3] Some patients may present with an acute deterioration or worsening of their chronic respiratory dysfunction.[4] This is termed *acute-on-chronic respiratory failure.*

HYPOXEMIC RESPIRATORY FAILURE

Basic Mechanisms

Hypoxemic respiratory failure refers to the inability of the respiratory system to maintain satisfactory levels of oxygen in the arterial blood.[3] The five basic mechanisms of hypoxemia are listed in Box 38-3. Ventilation-perfusion abnormality is the most commonly encountered abnormality.[2,3] Multiple mechanisms may even be instrumental in the respiratory failure in an individual patient. Most of the abnormalities will improve with the administration of supplemental oxygen, except for a shunt abnormality where the $Pa{O_2}$ continues to be low despite the administration of high levels of supplemental oxygen. The shunt may be either intracardiac (such as a right-to-left shunt through a probe-patent foramen ovale) or intrapulmonary (as seen with pneumonia or the acute respiratory distress syndrome [ARDS]).[5,6] A diffusion abnormality is infrequently the cause of hypoxemia in clinical practice and typically is only significant in the setting of tachycardia, high cardiac outputs, and when the diffusion capacity is below 25% of predicted.[3]

Box 38-1

Definition of Respiratory Failure

Type 1
PaO_2 <60 mm Hg
Type 2
$PaCO_2$ >50 mm Hg

Assessment of Oxygenation

The hallmark of type 1 respiratory failure is hypoxemia, which is primarily determined by assessing the PaO_2 through an arterial blood gas. An estimate of the oxygenation status of a patient can be obtained using the noninvasive pulse oximeter and assessing the oxygen saturation of the patient. An appreciation of the sigmoid shape of the oxyhemoglobin dissociation curve allows for a rough estimation of the PaO_2 (Fig. 38-2). The curve will shift rightward or leftward related to changes in the pH, $PaCO_2$, temperature, and PO_4^{-2} concentration.[7] As mentioned

Box 38-2

Common Causes of Hypoxemic and Hypercapnic Respiratory Failure

Brain
Bulbar poliomyelitis
Central alveolar hypoventilation
Cerebrovascular accident
Cerebral malignancy
Drug overdose (e.g., narcotic, sedative/hypnotic)
Encephalitis and meningitis
Pontine herniation
Postoperative anesthetic depression

Spinal Cord
Amyotrophic lateral sclerosis
Cervical cordotomy
Guillain-Barré syndrome
Poliomyelitis
Spinal cord trauma

Neuromuscular System
Acute intermittent porphyria
Botulism
Cholinergic crisis
Curariform drugs
Electrolyte disorders (e.g., hypophosphatemia, hypomagnesemia)
Hypokalemic periodic paralysis
Multiple sclerosis
Myasthenia gravis
Myxedema
Neuromuscular blocking antibiotics (e.g., polymyxin, streptomycin)
Organophosphate insecticides
Peripheral neuritis
Polymyositis
Respiratory muscle fatigue—critical illness poly-neuropathy/polymyopathy
Tetanus

Upper Airway
Epiglottitis and laryngotracheitis
Large tonsils and adenoids
Obstructive sleep apnea
Postintubation laryngeal edema
Tracheal obstruction
Vocal cord paralysis

Thorax and Pleura
Chest wall burn with eschar formation
Chest wall trauma—flail chest
Kyphoscoliosis
Massive abdominal distention
Massive obesity
Muscular dystrophy
Large pleural effusion/pleural fibrosis
Pneumothorax
Rheumatoid spondylitis
Thoracoplasty

Cardiovascular System
Cardiogenic pulmonary edema
Left ventricular failure
Mitral stenosis
Biventricular failure
Fat embolism
Snake bite
Uremia
Volume overload
Pulmonary veno-occlusive disease

Lower Airway and Alveoli
Acute respiratory distress syndrome (ARDS)
Aspiration
Asthma
Atelectasis
Bronchiectasis
Bronchiolitis
Chronic obstructive pulmonary disease
Cystic fibrosis
Interstitial lung disease
Massive bilateral pneumonia
Near-drowning
Pancreatitis
Pulmonary contusion
Radiation lung injury
Sepsis
Smoke inhalation
Surgical resection of lung parenchyma

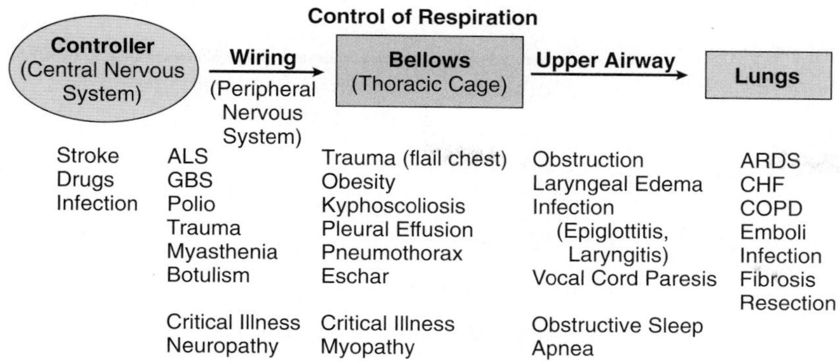

Figure 38-1. Control of respiration. ALS, amyotrophic lateral sclerosis; ARDS, acute respiratory distress syndrome; CHF, congestive heart failure; COPD, chronic obstructive pulmonary disease; GBS, Guillain-Barré syndrome; Myasthenia, myasthenia gravis or the Eaton-Lambert myasthenic syndrome.

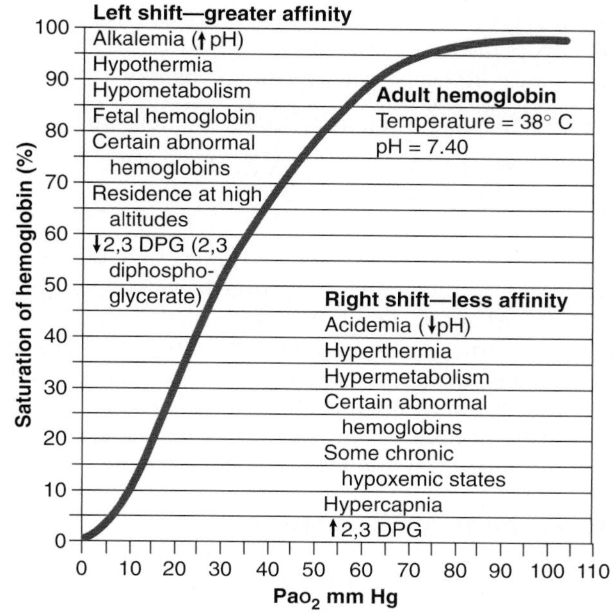

Figure 38-2. Oxyhemoglobin dissociation curve.

Box 38-3

Mechanisms of Hypoxemia

- Inadequate P_{AO_2}
  - Alveolar hypoventilation
  - Decreased F_{IO_2}
- $\dot{V}/\dot{Q}$ mismatch
- Shunt
  - Intrapulmonary
  - Intracardiac
- Diffusion abnormality
- Low $M\bar{v}O_2$

earlier, Box 38-3 lists the five basic causes of hypoxemia. Determination of the arterial blood gas and knowledge of the exact F_IO_2 allows for the calculation of the alveolar-arterial oxygen gradient (A-a gradient) using the formula $P_{AO_2} - Pa_{O_2}$ = A-a gradient, where the $P_{AO_2} = F_{IO_2}(P_B - P_{H_2O}) - Pa_{CO_2}/R$.[3]

P_{AO_2}	Partial pressure of oxygen in the alveolus
Pa_{O_2}	Partial pressure of oxygen in the arterial blood
F_IO_2	Fraction of inspired oxygen
P_B	Barometric pressure
PH_2O	Water vapor pressure at standard temperature and pressure
Pa_{CO_2}	Partial pressure of carbon dioxide in the arterial blood
R	Respiratory quotient (R = 0.8)

The A-a gradient is not F_IO_2 independent and will increase as the F_IO_2 increases. Because of this F_IO_2 dependency, some have preferred to evaluate oxygenation abnormalities by calculating the Pa_{O_2}/P_{AO_2} ratio, which is independent of the F_{IO_2}.[3] For simplicity's sake, many individuals use the Pa_{O_2}/F_{IO_2} ratio as a measure of oxygenation abnormality because this entails a simple calculation using easily obtained variables. Because this formula is used in the definition of acute lung injury and the acute respiratory distress syndrome, it has gained wide-scale acceptance.[8] The shunt fraction or venous admixture can also be calculated after a patient is given 100% oxygen to breathe and has reached steady-state oxygenation.

HYPERCAPNIC RESPIRATORY FAILURE

Hypercapnic respiratory failure can be the result of a variety of disorders as listed in Box 38-2.[9] Acute hypercapnic respiratory failure, also termed *acute ventilatory failure,* occurs when a patient's arterial blood gas reveals acute respiratory acidemia with a Pa_{CO_2} of greater than 50 mm Hg. This definition is not generally applicable to patients with severe chronic obstructive lung disease or neuromuscular disorders, who have developed a compensatory metabolic alkalemia in response to their chronic hypercapnia. However, these patients may have acute exacerbations or comorbid conditions that cause them to decompensate into acute-on-chronic respiratory failure.

In steady-state conditions the rate of CO_2 production ($\dot{V}CO_2$) equals the rate of CO_2 elimination.[9] Carbon dioxide elimination ($\dot{V}CO_2$) is equal to the alveolar ventilation (V_A) multiplied by the partial pressure of carbon dioxide in the alveolar gas (P_{ACO_2}). Thus the equation for carbon dioxide production is $\dot{V}CO_2 = V_A \times P_{ACO_2}$. In the pulmonary capillary, carbon dioxide is readily diffusible through the endothelial and epithelial cell membranes down a substantial concentration gradient of approximately 45 to 50 mm Hg (normal pulmonary arterial CO_2

[Pa_{CO_2}] versus essentially zero for the partial pressure of carbon dioxide in room air [Pi_{CO_2}]) so that the alveolar and capillary blood partial pressures of CO_2 are equal ($P_{ACO_2} = Pa_{CO_2}$).

Not all respired air is effective alveolar ventilation because some of the total tidal ventilation (V_T) ventilates nonperfused areas or dead space (V_D) (both anatomic and pathologic). This relationship between tidal volume, dead-space volume, and alveolar volume can be expressed as[3]:

$$V_T = V_A + V_D \quad \text{or} \quad V_A = V_T - V_D$$

The minute ventilation (V_E) is equal to the sum of the dead space ventilation (V_D) and the alveolar ventilation (V_A) or $V_E = V_D + V_A$. Combining and rearranging terms from these various equations yields the following relationship of carbon dioxide production and alveolar ventilation with the Pa_{CO_2}.[3]

$$Pa_{CO_2} \approx \frac{\dot{V}_{CO_2}}{V_T - V_D}$$

Therefore elevated Pa_{CO_2} can result from a combination of any of three clinical alterations; increased CO_2 production, decreased tidal ventilation, or increased dead space ventilation.[9] Increased CO_2 production arises from hypermetabolic states such as exercise, fever, sepsis, burns, trauma, excessive carbohydrate intake, and hyperthyroidism.[9] In isolation, these relatively common conditions rarely induce hypercapnic respiratory failure because the normal physiologic response to an elevated arterial blood CO_2 (P_aCO_2) concentration is to increase minute (and therefore alveolar) ventilation to maintain eucapnia and a normal pH. Only those patients who are unable to increase their effective alveolar ventilation as a result of neuromuscular disorders affecting the muscles of respiration, the presence of excessive ventilation/perfusion ($\dot{V}/\dot{Q}$) mismatching, or increased deadspace ventilation develop hypercapnic respiratory failure caused by elevated CO_2 production.

Ventilatory deficiencies, either decreased tidal ventilation and/or increased dead space ventilation, that result in hypercapnic respiratory failure can be differentiated by using the alveolar-to-arterial oxygen gradient equation. The P_{AO_2}–Pa_{O_2} difference breathing room air is normally less than 10 to 15 mm Hg when simple alveolar hypoventilation is responsible for the hypoxemia noted on blood gas analysis. An increased P_{AO_2}–Pa_{O_2} difference suggests a parenchymal lung process, usually associated with $\dot{V}/\dot{Q}$ abnormalities, to account for the additional hypoxemia in these patients with hypercapnic respiratory failure.

Decreased tidal volume hypoventilation can be caused by disorders affecting any component of the "neuromuscular sequence" starting in the central nervous system (CNS) and ending at the muscles of respiration (see Fig. 38-1). Among the more common causes are CNS depressants such as narcotics and sedatives, which diminish respiratory drive; cerebral vascular disorders, especially those that involve the brainstem, which impair the efferent signals to breathe; and disorders of neuromuscular

Box 38-4

Decreased Respiratory Muscle Strength and/or Endurance

Disorders of the phrenic nerve

- Guillain-Barré syndrome
- Poliomyelitis

Respiratory muscle atrophy

Disorders of neuromuscular transmission

- Myasthenia gravis
- Ventilator dependence
- Malnutrition
- Myopathy
- Critical illness polyneuropathy/myopathy

Altered diaphragmatic force-length relationship

- Dynamic hyperinflation and diaphragmatic flattening

transmission such as myasthenia gravis and the paraneoplastic Eaton-Lambert myasthenic syndrome (Box 38-4).[10,11] Abnormal respiratory mechanics can result from airflow obstruction, chest wall deformities, and loss of lung volume. Disorders that increase the respiratory load, such as a circumferential chest burn eschar or flail chest, or impair function of the respiratory muscles, such as kyphoscoliosis, will also lead to hypoventilation.

Assessment of Ventilation

The hallmark feature of inadequate ventilation is the presence of an elevated Pa_{CO_2} with or without the presence of hypoxemia.[3,9] In the adult population the best method to detect an elevated Pa_{CO_2} is with an arterial blood gas measurement. Noninvasive evaluation of ventilation in the critically ill adult, using end-tidal CO_2 (Pet_{CO_2}) measurements or transcutaneous CO_2 (Ptc_{CO_2}) determinations, is not as reliable as it is in the healthy adult or the neonate, respectively.[7]

CLINICAL MANIFESTATIONS

The risk factors for developing acute respiratory failure include the postoperative state, pre-existing chronic illness, malnutrition, advanced age, morbid obesity, chronic bronchitis, and cigarette smoking. The clinical manifestations of respiratory distress may be subtle and nonspecific or may be obvious to even the untrained observer. The patient with respiratory distress may have an abnormal respiratory rate (too high or low) or display an irregular pattern of breathing. The patient with respiratory distress may evidence gasping ventilation, nasal flaring, or use of the accessory muscles of respiration. Intercostal retractions may be seen, and the patient may exhibit paradoxical respiratory movement. Typically, patients with acute respiratory failure, whether type 1 or type 2, will have altered heart rate and blood pressure. The majority will evidence a sympathetic response with tachycardia and hypertension, but patients may be hypotensive and bradycardic. Cardiac arrhythmias may be seen in both type 1 and type 2 respiratory failure. Patients with acute respiratory failure will usually be in distress and often appear apprehensive.[2,9] Many will be diaphoretic and have altered mental status or level of consciousness. Hypercapnic patients may demonstrate signs of a respiratory encephalopathy including somnolence, coma, asterixis, seizures, tremors, or myoclonic jerks. Papilledema and congested conjunctiva may be present. Type 1 respiratory failure patients may appear cyanotic.[9]

ACUTE LUNG INJURY AND ACUTE RESPIRATORY DISTRESS SYNDROME

Since the initial 1967 description of acute catastrophic respiratory failure in 12 patients, who were subsequently declared to have the adult respiratory distress syndrome (ARDS), there has been a great deal of research and clinical study attempting to understand the mechanism of injury and improve the outcome of these critically ill patients.[12-15] The hallmark of this disorder was the rapid onset of acute hypoxemic respiratory failure that was characterized by refractory hypoxemia despite the administration of high concentrations of supplemental oxygen, decreased pulmonary compliance, diffuse, bilateral radiographic infiltrates, the absence of left heart failure, and histologic evidence of alveolar damage with hyaline membrane formation, which was followed by fibrosis of the lung.[8,12,13] The subsequent 10 to 20 years of ARDS management were associated with extremely high mortality rates, at times approaching 90%, despite the provision of extremely aggressive supportive care.[16-21] Some of the initial clinical and basic investigations that attempted to improve the outcome of patients with ARDS were hampered by the lack of uniformly accepted definitions and management strategies employed in the care of these patients.[22-25] An American-European Consensus Conference defined acute lung injury (ALI) and ARDS in an attempt to eliminate confusion related to terminology for these conditions.[22,23] The definitions are clinically based and regard ALI as a continuum with the more severe oxygenation abnormalities reflective of ARDS. Among the main benefits of the uniform definition would be improved communication and enhanced clinical trial design (Box 38-5).

Box 38-5

American-European Consensus Conference Definition of Acute Lung Injury and ARDS

Acute Lung Injury

Acute onset of respiratory failure
Bilateral chest infiltrates on frontal radiograph
Absence of elevated left heart filling pressure (PAOP <18 mm Hg)
PAO_2/FIO_2 <300 mm Hg

Acute Respiratory Distress Syndrome

Acute onset of respiratory failure
Bilateral chest infiltrates on frontal radiograph
Absence of elevated left heart filling pressure (PAOP <18 mm Hg)
PAO_2/FIO_2 <200 mm Hg

PAOP, pulmonary artery occlusion pressure.

The American-European Consensus Conference definition of ALI and ARDS has recently come under attack related to a reported discrepancy between the clinical and pathologic findings in individuals felt to have died with ARDS.[26] In a Spanish study conducted by Esteban and colleagues,[26] one third of the people who died with a clinical diagnosis of ARDS did not have histologic evidence of diffuse alveolar damage on postmortem examination. In addition, diffuse alveolar damage, the hallmark pathologic finding of ARDS, was evident in 10% of patients who died without a clinical diagnosis of ARDS. A subsequent study evaluated the sensitivity and specificity of the three clinical definitions of ARDS.[27] The study evaluated the Murray Lung Injury Score, the American-European Consensus Conference Definition of ARDS, and a Delphi Definition that incorporated oxygenation abnormality, x-ray findings, clinical onset, compatible clinical scenario, and absence of left heart failure.[27] The combination of Lung Injury Score greater than 2.5 with either the American European Consensus Conference Definition or the Delphi definition of ARDS resulted in the best combination of sensitivity and specificity. At this time, the majority of clinical trials and clinicians continue to use the American-European Consensus Conference Definition, but it is likely that further refinements in the definition will occur in the future.[28]

Remembering that ALI and ARDS are part of a syndrome and that no specific laboratory test is pathognomonic for the diagnosis is important.[8,22,28] As evident from the three definitions of ARDS discussed earlier, the abnormalities on a chest radiograph are a key component to the clinical diagnosis.[27] The American-European Consensus Conference Definition requires the presence of bilateral pulmonary infiltrates for the diagnosis of both ALI and ARDS.[22] When 21 experts were given 28 chest radiographs to evaluate for the presence of bilateral pulmonary infiltrates, they only agreed 43% of the time and one third of the time five or more individuals differed in their interpretation.[29] The range of ALI/ARDS diagnoses was from 36% to 71%.[29]

Risk Factors for ALI and ARDS

It has been recognized that ALI and ARDS may arise in association with a number of clinical conditions (Box 38-6).[8,18,22,28,30-34] The most common clinical risk factor for the development of ARDS is sepsis.[8,22,34] Various studies report that approximately 5% to 40% of septic patients will develop this complication.[8,19,33] Shock (prolonged hypotension) and the systemic inflammatory response syndrome (SIRS) are also common risk factors. Other frequently encountered clinical risk factors include multiple emergency transfusions; aspiration injury; near-drowning; pancreatitis; trauma (particularly lung contusion,

Box 38-6

Common Clinical Risk Factors for ARDS

Sepsis and the systemic inflammatory response syndrome (SIRS)
Prolonged hypotension/shock
Trauma (long bone fractures, lung contusion, fat embolism)
Acid aspiration
Near-drowning
Multiple emergency blood product transfusions
Pancreatitis
Disseminated intravascular coagulation (DIC)
Post–cardiopulmonary bypass
Burn injury

Box 38-7

Common Pulmonary and Extrapulmonary Causes of ALI and ARDS

Direct Pulmonary Causes
Pneumonia
Acid aspiration
Inhalational lung injury
Lung contusion
Chest trauma
Near-drowning

Extrapulmonary Causes
Sepsis—systemic inflammatory response syndrome
Shock—hypotension
Pancreatitis
Trauma (fat embolism)
Post–cardiopulmonary bypass
Massive transfusion therapy
Burns

fat emboli from long bone fractures); burns; cardiopulmonary bypass; and disseminated intravascular coagulation (DIC). These clinical risk factors are synergistic, and when more than one of the clinical risk factors is present, the likelihood of ARDS is greater than just the sum of the collective risk factors.[8,18] The clinical risk factor associated with the development of ARDS appears to greatly influence the expected outcome. Whether ALI and ARDS arise from a direct pulmonary insult or from an extra-pulmonary cause impacts the subsequent response to positive end-expiratory pressure (PEEP) and ventilatory support (Box 38-7).[20] Age also has an impact on the likelihood for ALI and ARDS development.[35] Older individuals have a greater likelihood of developing ARDS from most of the risk factors noted earlier. In the setting of trauma the risk for ARDS seems to peak in the sixth and seventh decades and then decline.[35]

Negative pressure (postobstructive) pulmonary edema (NPPE or POPE) is a type of noncardiogenic pulmonary edema that can manifest as ALI or ARDS.[36] It is rare (five cases reported from a large tertiary medical intensive care unit in 4 years),[37] can range in severity from mild hypoxemia treated with low-flow supplemental oxygen to profound hypoxemia requiring mechanical ventilation, and may even present as alveolar hemorrhage.[38-42] It is believed to be caused by increased vascular permeability caused by alveolar and capillary damage caused by the rapid resolution of large levels of negative intrathoracic pressure (generated by attempting to inspire against an occluded airway) by removal of the airway obstruction.[43,44] This leads to a protein-rich alveolar exudate impairing gas exchange in mild-to-moderate cases and leaking of capillary blood into the alveoli in more severe circumstances. Most of the reported cases are related to surgical procedures: thyroidectomy,[45,46] septorhinoplasty,[47] tonsillectomy/adenoidectomy,[48] mandibular open reduction and internal fixation,[49] or cryosurgery for a tracheal obstruction.[50] Nonoperative conditions leading to NPPE have included laryngospasm,[51,52] occlusion of an endotracheal tube,[53,54] excessive tube thoracostomy suction pressure,[55] nonlethal hanging,[56] and even hiccups.[57,58] The common element is the rapid relief of a large airway occlusion. Patients often have no underlying cardiopulmonary disorders. NPPE may account for a small percentage of immediate postoperative extubation failures, particularly if an unrecognized mainstem intubation is present in an awakening and spontaneously breathing patient. Clinical manifestations of hypoxemia and respiratory distress may be delayed up to 6 hours.[44] Therapy is supportive with supplemental oxygen and, if needed, positive pressure ventilation (invasive or noninvasive).

Incidence and Prevalence of ALI and ARDS

The exact incidence and prevalence of ALI and ARDS are unknown at the present time.[8,35] Early reports suggested that there were 150,000 patients with ARDS each year in the United States.[8,30,33,59] This led to an estimated incidence of 75 cases per 100,000 population. Proposed estimates have suggested that the incidence of ARDS ranges from 1.5 to 64 cases per 100,000 population.[35,59,60] The proposed incidence appears to be dependent on the country reporting the data and the definition used (Box 38-8).[8,33,35] A recent study evaluated the incidence and outcome of ALI in mechanically ventilated patients aged 15 or older cared for at 21 hospitals in and around King County, Washington over a 15-month observation period.[35] The crude incidence of ALI was 78.9 per 100,000 person-years, and the incidence of ARDS was 58.7 per 100,00 person-years. On the basis of their results, the authors estimated the annual number of U.S. episodes was 190,600 cases of ALI and 141,500 cases of ARDS. The authors also observed a relationship between increasing age and increased incidence and mortality related to ALI and ARDS.

Clinical Manifestations

A variable initial clinical presentation, primarily reflecting the underlying disease process and the overall condition of the patient, may exist. However, when the ALI/ARDS become clinically apparent, the patient is noted to be in significant distress associated with dyspnea, tachypnea,

Box 38-8

Incidence of ARDS

1985 Canary Island Conference	1.5/100,000 person-years
1990 Utah	4.8-8.3/100,000 person-years
1991 Berlin	3/100,000 person-years
1995 Maryland	10.5-14.2/100,000 person-years
1997 Sweden/ Denmark	13.5/100,000 person-years
2002 Australia	28/100,000 person-years
2005 Seattle	58.7-64/100,000 person-years

Adapted from Bersten AD, Edibam C, Hunt T, et al: Incidence and mortality of acute lung injury and the acute respiratory distress syndrome in three Australian States. Am J Respir Crit Care Med 2002;165:443-448; Rubenfeld GD, Neff MJ: Epidemiology of acute lung injury: A public health perspective. In Matthay MA (ed): Acute Respiratory Distress Syndrome. New York, Marcel Dekker, 2003, p 40, and Rubenfeld GD, Caldwell E, Peabody E, et al: Incidence and outcomes of acute lung injury. N Engl J Med 2005;353:1685-1693.

visible signs of respiratory distress, and an increased work of breathing.[8,22,30,33] The typical presentation is manifest as an acute catastrophic complication in a patient who has one or more of the clinical risk factors for the development of this form of ALI. As previously stated, the precipitating injury need not directly involve the pulmonary system.[8,33,61] Past definitions have emphasized the need to exclude patients with previous or known chronic pulmonary or cardiovascular diseases.[20-22,28] Recent definitions exclude patients with elevated left heart filling pressures and chronic infiltrative lung disease as the cause of the radiographic or physiologic alterations.[22]

The hallmark of ARDS is the presence of hypoxemia despite the administration of high concentrations of inspired oxygen, evidence of an increase in the shunt fraction, a decrease in pulmonary compliance, and an increase in the deadspace ventilation.[8,25] The chest radiographic manifestation of both ALI and ARDS is the presence of diffuse, bilateral pulmonary infiltrates with a normal cardiac silhouette. Recent reports have cautioned that even among trained experts there is often disagreement concerning the interpretation of the chest radiograph.[29,59,62] Chest computed tomography has also demonstrated that the radiographic injury is not homogeneous and has a predominance in the dependent portions of the lung.[8,40] The presence of left heart failure and elevated left ventricular filling pressures should be eliminated either clinically or through the placement of a pulmonary artery catheter and measurement of the pulmonary capillary wedge pressure to ensure that it is less than 18 mm Hg.[22] Importantly, ARDS is a clinical syndrome and the diagnosis is made clinically, not on the basis of a single radiograph, ABG, or laboratory test.

Pathologic Manifestations

Typically, type 1 alveolar cells comprise the major gas exchange surface of the alveolus and are integral to the maintenance of the permeability barrier function of the alveolar membrane.[8] Type 2 pneumocytes are the progenitors of type 1 cells and are responsible for surfactant production and homeostasis.[8] During ALI there is damage to the capillary endothelial and the alveolar epithelial cells.[8] Cellular injury and alteration of the normal barrier function results in a permeability defect that gives way to flooding of the alveoli with protein-rich fluid and inflammatory cells.[8,30,63] This results in the alteration of pulmonary mechanics, physiology, and gas exchange.[8,63-65] In addition, there is the alteration of alveolar surfactant that results directly from damage to the type 2 pneumocyte and from the inactivation and dilution of alveolar surfactant from the protein and fluid that have entered into the alveolar space, respectively.[66,67] Surfactant dysfunction can lead to atelectasis and a further reduction in pulmonary compliance.[8,66,67] In addition, dysfunction of the alveolar epithelial cells can impair the resorption of fluid from the alveolar space, which augments the parenchymal injury process and gas exchange abnormalities.[8,68]

The observed pathological findings in ALI and ARDS depend on the timing of the tissue sampling. During the initial stages of clinically evident lung injury there is histologic evidence of diffuse alveolar damage.[8] Histologic features of the injury include microthrombi composed of platelets and white blood cells within the capillary lumen, denudation of the alveolar epithelial lining cells, swelling of the capillary endothelial cells, interstitial and alveolar infiltration by polymorphonuclear leukocytes (PMNLs), and hyaline membrane formation within the alveoli.[8] Grossly, the lungs appear heavy and wet. Later, areas of type 3 collagen deposition with fibrosis will be present.[68] An intense inflammatory reaction involving PMNLs, activated monocytes, macrophages, and endothelial cells is present in the fibroproliferative phase of lung injury.[67-70] Pro- and anti-inflammatory molecules produced by these activated cells may be found in the circulating blood and/or bronchoalveolar lavage (BAL) fluid.[70-72] This phase may be followed by fibrosis, but this fibrosis does not appear to have the same permanence as typical fibrosis would have and may actually resolve over time in survivors of the injury.[73]

Pathophysiology of ALI and ARDS

Controversy exists over whether ALI/ARDS develops as a result of epithelial or endothelial cell injury.[8,13,74,75] Both sites of injury and cells are important for maintenance of normal barrier function and are capable of initiating an inflammatory response. In the majority of clinical settings the initial site of the ALI involves the capillary endothelial cell, which may be the initial manifestation of a "pan-endothelial cell injury" resulting from SIRS.[72] Endothelial cell injury compromises the integrity of the vascular barrier and results in transudation of fluid and inflammatory mediators into the interstitial tissues and ultimately into the alveoli.[8,13] The frequent occurrence and early involvement of lung dysfunction as a component of multiple organ dysfunction/failure lends support to the hypothesis of a panendothelial cell injury as one of the target injuries in the setting of SIRS.[76]

The complex pathophysiologic processes that culminate in the production of ALI and ARDS involves a delicate balance between the body's proinflammatory and anti-inflammatory responses to the inciting clinical event.[72,76] The balance that exists between the various inflammatory molecules or mediators and the endogenous compensatory responses evoked by the inflammatory response will dictate whether or not lung injury and other forms of organ dysfunction will develop.[70] The ensuing interaction between SIRS and the compensatory antiinflammatory response syndrome (CARS) will thus determine whether a patient successfully deals with an injury or is predisposed to develop organ dysfunction (excessive SIRS response) or immunosuppression and infectious complications (excessive CARS response).[72,76] This mixed antagonistic response syndrome (MARS) is actually the prevailing condition that may have tremendous impact on the eventual fate of the critically ill patient.[76]It is likely that some or all of the potential mediators listed in Box 38-9 are instrumental in the initiation, augmentation, propagation and/or maintenance of ALI/ARDS.

Management Strategies

Until now, management of patients with ALI and ARDS has been predominantly one of support (Box 38-10).[8,19,22,24,30,33,77] The high mortality rates seen in patients with ALI and ARDS have prompted a search for improved understanding of the pathophysiologic processes involved in the production and propagation of the injury, as well as evaluation of innovative adjuvant therapies that may prove to be the specific cure for improving the outcome of these patients.[8,19,22-24,30,33] Initial attention must be directed to the identification of the predisposing underlying clinical condition(s), and there should be specific treatment directed at the underlying or predisposing disorder.[8,22-24] The recognition of sepsis and infection as frequent causes of ALI and ARDS should prompt an aggressive search for undiagnosed foci of infection and the administration of appropriate antimicrobial treatment and use of surgical drainage procedures as indicated.[16,18,78] Successful management strategies mandate this thorough investigation for occult sources of infection or an exaggerated proinflammatory response.[32] This is particularly true in the patient who fails to improve and manifests a persistent SIRS response.[32]

The cornerstone of supportive management is the provision of mechanical ventilatory support.[8,22-24] Recent experimental and clinical data report significant survival benefit from the use of lung protective ventilatory support strategies.[79,80] The primary goal of this support is to improve oxygenation and ensure that the lung is allowed to heal and avoid augmentation of the existing injury. Use of nonprotective ventilatory support strategies may have a role in the persistent proinflammatory response and the development of multiple organ dysfunction syndrome (MODS) and/or multiple organ failure (MOF).[79-81]

Box 38-9

Potential Mediators of Acute Lung Injury

Proinflammatory Molecules and Cells
Polymorphonuclear leukocytes (PMNLs)
Tissue macrophages and monocytes
Platelets
Arachidonic acid metabolites

- Prostaglandins, prostacyclin, thromboxane
- Leukotrienes

Cytokines (interleukins 1,2,6,8,15, TNF, G-CSF)
Soluble adhesion molecules
Platelet-activating factor (PAF)
Complement and activation of the complement cascade
Various kinins (e.g., bradykinin)
Endorphins
Histamine and serotonin
Proteolytic enzymes

- Elastase and lysosomal enzymes

Protein kinase, tyrosine kinase
Toxic oxygen metabolites

- Superoxide, hydroxyl radical, hydrogen peroxide, peroxynitrite, etc.

Endotoxin and other bacterial and microbial toxins
Activation of the coagulation cascade
Neopterin
Plasminogen activator inhibitor-1 (PAI-1)
CD-14
Vasoactive neuropeptides
Monocyte chemoattractant protein (MCP)-1 and 2

Potential Anti-inflammatory Molecules
Interleukin 1 receptor antagonist (IL-1ra)
Type 2 interleukin 1 receptor
IL-4
IL-10
IL-13
Transforming growth factor β (TGF-β)
Epinephrine
Soluble TNF receptor (sTNFr)
Leukotriene B_4 receptor antagonist
Soluble CD-14
Lipopolysaccharide (LPS) binding protein

Mechanical Ventilation of ALI/ARDS

See Chapter 11 for a more detailed discussion of mechanical ventilation of ALI/ARDS. Over the past decade there has been increasing recognition that the ventilatory support strategy used in the management of patients with ALI and ARDS may produce or augment lung injury and/or impair the healing process (Box 38-11).[82-87] These fears initially arose from the results of experimental animal studies that demonstrated clinical, physiological, and histological evidence of ALI, similar to that observed in

Box 38-10

Basic Management Strategies for Patients with ALI and ARDS

Identify and treat underlying/predisposing cause of ALI/ARDS
Ventilatory support

- Lung protective ventilatory support strategy
- Application of PEEP (per ARDSnet protocol)

Restore and maintain hemodynamic function

- Conservative fluid replacement strategy using goal-oriented approach
- Vasopressor and inotropic support as needed to meet goals

Prevent complications of critical illness

- Stress ulcer (stress-related mucosal disease) prophylaxis
- Preventive strategies for PE and DVT
- Prevent infections such as ventilator-associated pneumonia (VAP)
- Control glucose and metabolic function
- Prevent development of multiple organ dysfunction/failure

Ensure adequate nutrition
Avoid oversedation and medication errors
Using weaning protocol with spontaneous breathing trials when ready to wean
Cautious use of steroids for fibroproliferative phase (avoid if patient has received neuromuscular blocking drugs)

Box 38-11

Ventilator-Associated Lung Injury

Volutrauma
Atelectotrauma
Biotrauma
Barotrauma
Air embolism/translocation

patients with ARDS, when the animals were ventilated with large tidal volumes or were given high inflation pressures.[84-87] The alveolar overdistention produced by these ventilatory modes was felt to be the critical element in production of the lung injury.[84-87] Lung injury could result from the administration of large tidal volumes or the administration of positive pressure or negative pressure breaths that were sufficient to produce alveolar overdistention (termed *volutrauma*).[86-88] Other mechanisms that could potentially result in lung injury were the repetitive recruitment-derecruitment of distal airways (termed *atelectotrauma*) and alveoli or the disruption of alveoli resulting in translocation of organisms or air emboli.[86,87] Alveolar overdistention can also give rise to systemic inflammatory molecules that may contribute to the SIRS response and drive the development of MODS/MOF.[81,87] This has been termed *biotrauma*.[87] Interestingly, the lung injury produced by high inflation pressures or large tidal volumes in these experimental models could be ameliorated by the addition of therapeutic amounts of PEEP.[86,87] Subsequent human studies have evaluated the distribution of the radiographic lung injury in ARDS patients as determined by the use of computed tomography (CT) scans of the chest and have noted the dependent nature of the injury.[63,89] The injury to the lungs was not diffuse and homogeneous as once believed. These dependent areas of injury comprised regions of alveolar flooding from the gravitational accumulation of lung water, areas of lung injury, and normal lung regions. The relatively normal ventral (nondependent) lung has been referred to as the "baby lung," and the injured (dependent) lung has been called the "sponge lung."[29,89] With the use of higher tidal volumes, PEEP, or high distending pressures, there was evidence of alveolar overdistention, particularly in the areas of normal lung. A multicenter trial of low versus traditional tidal volume ventilation in patients with ALI/ARDS demonstrated increased proinflammatory cytokines in the serum and bronchoalveolar lavage fluid (BALF) of patients ventilated with the larger traditional tidal volumes, supporting the concept of biotrauma from alveolar overdistention.[81]

Pulmonary barotrauma (pneumomediastinum, pneumopericardium, pneumoperitoneum, pneumothorax, subcutaneous emphysema, pulmonary interstitial emphysema, and air embolism) is a well-recognized complication of ventilatory support and is found in 7% to 15% of patients with ALI/ARDS.[90] Some studies have reported an association of pulmonary barotrauma with increased mortality or increased length of stay.[85,90] A retrospective review of a large septic ARDS database failed to detect an adverse effect of pneumothoraces or air leaks on outcome in this patient population.[91] In actuality, the ventilator-induced lung disease from alveolar overdistention is also a form of barotrauma, or what should more appropriately be termed *volutrauma*.[87]

For the past 2 decades there has been a great deal of controversy concerning the "best" ventilatory support strategy to use for patients with ALI/ARDS.[79,80,82-84,87,92-106] Some authors advocated high-frequency ventilation, whereas others favored low-frequency ventilation with or without extracorporeal CO_2 removal.[98,104,106] Some centers used pressure control instead of volume control, and some experts felt that inverse ratio ventilation was required to improve gas exchange in patients with ARDS.[96,98] Others used high PEEP, whereas some claimed benefit from airway-pressure release ventilation.[107-111]

In an attempt to determine the importance of the ventilatory support strategy on the outcome of patients with ALI/ARDS and the potential for ventilator-induced lung injury (VILI) to develop in critically ill adults, a number of controlled clinical trials were conducted.[82,83,93-95] Trials were designed to evaluate low versus more traditional tidal volumes in the management of patients with lung injury. Prospective, randomized, controlled trials of low tidal volume ventilatory strategies revealed conflicting results.[93-95,112] In an attempt to answer the question concerning the value of using smaller tidal volumes, the NHLBI ARDS Network, a 10-center network supported by the NIH to evaluate treatment protocols for ARDS, has published the results from a trial designed to test the low versus high stretch management of patients with ALI and ARDS.[83] This study compared low tidal volumes (6 mL/kg of ideal body weight) against conventional tidal volumes (12 mL/kg of ideal body weight). A protocol governed the use of PEEP according to the F_{IO_2} required to meet the oxygenation goals. A weaning protocol was used once the patient was on a reduced amount of ventilatory support. The study design called for the enrollment of 1000 patients and included interim analyses after every 200 patients to determine if there was a need to stop the study early for either efficacy or safety concerns. The trial was terminated after 861 patients were enrolled, following the determination of a significant (22% relative reduction) decrease in mortality associated with the use of low tidal volumes (39.8% vs. 31%; P = .007). A significant difference occurred between the low and high tidal volume groups in length of stay, ventilator days, and development of MODS.[83] No difference occurred in the development of barotrauma between the two ventilator support strategies. On further analysis, this survival benefit was present irrespective of the patient's BMI.[113]

The use of lower tidal volumes typically results in a controlled hypoventilation or permissive hypercapnia and can lead to hypercapnic acidosis.[97] Some experimental animal models of lung injury suggest that hypercapnic acidosis may be beneficial to the lung and produce less lung injury as measured by extravascular lung water (Box 38-12).[113]

PEEP is also a major component of the ventilatory support strategy for the patient with ALI/ARDS.[8] In fact, PEEP may actually have a direct therapeutic role in the prevention of ventilator-induced lung injury, as noted in some of the experimental models of VILI.[85,101,107,108,110,114-119] The use of PEEP has assisted the recruitment of atelectatic lung units, prevented recruitment-derecruitment, increased the functional residual capacity (FRC), decreased the shunt fraction, and allowed for a reduction to a less toxic F_{IO_2} while still maintaining adequate oxygen saturation and tissue oxygen delivery.[108,109,116-118] The application of the "right amount" of PEEP has recently taken on a more sophisticated approach. The ability to construct a pressure-volume curve to reflect the compliance of the patient's lung has allowed for the identification of both the lower and upper inflection points (Fig. 38-3).[119] Maintaining a PEEP level above the lower inflection point should potentially avoid the repetitive opening and closing of alveoli and the development of shear forces from the recruitment-derecruitment process, which may participate in the production or propagation of lung injury. If too much PEEP is applied, there may be overdistention of alveoli, which can potentiate volutrauma or barotrauma and have adverse consequences on pulmonary mechanics, hemodynamic function, and lung healing. Constructing pressure volume curves to determine the "best PEEP" is a difficult undertaking and requires the patient to be heavily sedated or paralyzed and the use of a calibrated super-syringe. Determining the precise lower inflection point on the inspiratory inflation curve is difficult, and the compliance curves may change (along with the inflection points) over time as the patient's lung compliance changes. To simplify the determination of adequate PEEP, the ARDS Network ventilatory support protocol used a monogram for PEEP levels on the basis of the F_{IO_2} requirements and the goal of maintaining a P_{AO_2} between 55 and 80 mm Hg.[83] For the protocol, end-inspiratory plateau pressure was kept lower than or equal to 30 cm H_2O and the pH was maintained in the 7.30 to 7.45 range. Despite the demonstrated significant improvement in mortality associated with this protocol, some felt that additional benefit could be seen with the use of higher levels of PEEP. A subsequent large, prospective, randomized controlled trial conducted by the ARDS network evaluated the PEEP protocol from the initial trial (PEEP levels from 5 to 24 cm H_2O) versus higher levels of PEEP.[120] During the study there was a change to a higher PEEP strategy to ensure a difference in the amount of applied PEEP between the two treatment arms. No significant difference in deaths before discharge home, breathing without assistance by day 28, ventilator-free days, intensive care unit–free days, organ failure–free days, or barotrauma was found.[120]

Box 38-12

Potential Benefits of Hypercapnia in Patients with ALI and ARDS

↓ TNF-α release by alveolar macrophages
↓ PMNL-endothelial cell adhesion
↓ Xanthine oxidase activity
↓ NFκB
↓ NOS activity
↓ Production of IL-8 and TOR from PMNLs

From Kregenow DA, Rubenfeld GD, Hudson LD, Swenson ER: Hypercapnic acidosis and mortality in acute lung injury. Crit Care Med 2006;34:1-7.

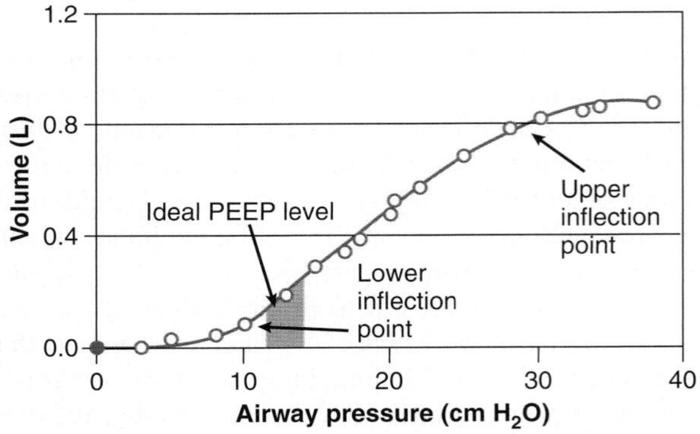

Figure 38-3. Pulmonary volume-pressure curve. PEEP, positive end-expiratory pressure. (Modified from Hospital Pulmonary Disease Board Review Manual 2000;7:7.)

PEEP has the potential to have profound hemodynamic consequences in selected patients and clinical circumstances, and it is important to closely monitor patients with hemodynamic, echocardiographic, or other sophisticated monitors if there is a question of the adequacy of cardiac function when PEEP is applied.[6,107,108,110] The effect of PEEP may not be the same in the supine and prone positions. Apparently there is an enhanced ability to recruit alveoli when the patient is in the prone position as compared with the supine position when the patient is on the same amount of PEEP.[121] There may be a different responsiveness to the use of PEEP depending on whether the ARDS results from a direct pulmonary injury or a nonpulmonary process that gives rise to ALI.[29]

Despite the survival benefits demonstrated by the use of lung protective ventilatory support strategy, there has not been universal adoption of this technique of ventilatory support for all patients with ALI and ARDS. Reasons for this slower than expected incorporation into daily practice are many and varied and certainly go beyond lack of awareness. Young and coworkers[122] reported on the tidal volume used to ventilate ARDS patients at three large New England university hospitals. Prior to the publication and subsequent education of the 2000 ARDS Network results, the tidal volume averaged 12.3 mL/kg predicted body weight (9.8 mL/kg measured body weight). After the publication of the study results, the tidal volume dropped to 10.6 mL/kg predicted body weight (8 mL/kg measured body weight).

Fluid Management and Vasoactive Support

Controversy also surrounds the approach to fluid management and oxygen delivery in the critically ill patient with ALI.[123-134] Patients with ALI often require aggressive management to restore and maintain appropriate hemodynamic function.[135-136] The SAFE trial demonstrated that resuscitation with saline is as beneficial as resuscitation with albumin in critically ill patients with shock.[137] Correcting shock and hemodynamic derangements in patients with ALI and ARDS is important because these are potential causes for the lung injury and may result in organ dysfunction/failure.[136] Several studies have reported increased survival associated with low pulmonary capillary occlusion pressure in the setting of ARDS/ALI.[123,125] Concern for the potential to compromise organ perfusion and predispose to the development of organ system dysfunction and the subsequent development of MODS/MOF led to additional studies from the ARDS Network to evaluate a liberal versus conservative fluid replacement strategy (FACTT trial).[138] In addition, this trial was designed to evaluate the utility and safety of using a pulmonary artery (PA) catheter to guide volume replacement as opposed to a central venous catheter.[139] The safety and potential benefits of using PA catheters in the critically ill has been an area of controversy for the past 20 years.[140] Ten years ago, Connors and coworkers reported a lack of benefit and possible harm associated with the use of PA catheters in critically ill patients in the SUPPORT database.[141]

In a prospective, randomized, controlled trial of PA catheters versus no PA catheters in the management of 676 adult patients with shock and/or ARDS, there was no difference in organ failure–free days, ventilator-free days, vasopressor-free days, or days in the ICU or hospital.[142] This trial did not have an algorithm to direct management based on the hemodynamic data obtained from the use of the PA catheter. The ARDS Network trial evaluated liberal versus conservative fluid management on the basis of the central venous catheter (central venous pressure [CVP]) data versus PA catheter (PA occlusion pressure [PAOP]) data in 1000 patients with established ALI.[139] The use of a PA catheter did not significantly change 60-day survival or days of unassisted breathing in comparison with the use of a central venous catheter.[139] There was no difference between the groups in lung or renal function, use of vasopressors, renal replacement therapy, or hypotension. The PA catheter group did have twice as many catheter-related complications, predominantly in the form of arrhythmias, compared with the central venous catheter group.

The liberal fluid management arm of the FACTT trial had an average net gain of almost 7 L over the first 7 days, whereas the conservative fluid management group averaged a loss of 136 mL over 7 days of cumulative fluid balance.[138] The use of the conservative fluid management strategy was associated with a significant improvement in oxygenation index and lung injury score and increased the number of ventilator-free days compared with the more liberal strategy. There was no difference in the development of shock or the need for renal replacement therapy between the two fluid management strategies.[138]

In the past, some have advocated treatment strategies designed to increase tissue oxygen delivery to "supernormal" levels by hypertransfusing the patient or by using inotropes to increase the cardiac output.[127,129,131] The theoretical benefit of these maneuvers had primarily been demonstrated in surgical patients or as a mathematical end point when the oxygen delivery and oxygen consumption were both derived from calculated variables.[126] Clinical trials have yielded conflicting results and have often been complicated by an inability to drive up the tissue oxygen delivery in a sizeable number of the study population.[126-128] In addition, some trials have demonstrated the potential for some harm to be associated with this practice.[128] A large prospective, randomized clinical trial did not demonstrate a survival benefit associated with "supranormal" oxygen delivery, and this management strategy is no longer being pursued.[143]

Basic Management of ALI/ARDS

ALI/ARDS patients are also at risk for the complications that commonly complicate the course of the critically ill. Most of these complications are preventable, and prophylactic strategies should be employed whenever possible. Common complications include deep venous thrombosis and pulmonary embolism, stress-related gastrointestinal hemorrhage, ventilator-associated pneumonia and nosocomial infections, metabolic abnormalities, critical illness polyneuropathy, and malnutrition.[144-148] Anticipation and prevention of these complications is vitally important. Prophylactic strategies to prevent stress-related mucosal disease and gastrointestinal bleeding using H_2 blockers, proton pump inhibitors, or possibly early enteral nutrition should occur in all patients unless otherwise contraindicated.[148-149] Deep vein thrombosis and pulmonary embolism prophylaxis should also be administered unless there are contraindications.[149] The use of enteral nutrition is also important to prevent stress-related gastrointestinal bleeding and to maintain the normal barrier function of the gastrointestinal mucosa.[148,150-152] Loss of the gastrointestinal barrier function has been associated with the translocation of bacteria and/or toxins into the mesenteric lymph nodes and portal circulation, which may be the fuel that leads to or perpetuates the injury process.[153] Nutritional support is also important to maintain the proper level of immune function and potentially to prevent the development of malnutrition in the catabolic critically ill patient. The use of enteral formulas designed to enhance the immune response with increased amounts of arginine, glutamine, or selected fatty acids remains controversial. The use of enteral formulas with increased amounts of eicosapentaenoic acid and γ-linolenic acid has been shown to improve organ dysfunction and improve oxygenation in clinical trials but has not been demonstrated to improve survival in patients with ALI and ARDS.[154,155]

Recent studies have stressed the importance of glycemic control to prevent hyperglycemia using infusions of insulin and frequent monitoring of blood sugar.[156,157] In a study of predominantly postoperative patients managed with intensive insulin to maintain the blood sugar between 80 and 110 mg/dL, there was a significant improvement in ICU and hospital survival.[156] One of the main reasons for this improved survival was a fourfold reduction in the development of MOF with a proven sepsis focus in the intensive insulin management group.[156] A recently published study from the same group of investigators conducted in a medical intensive care unit (MICU) population did not show a similar survival advantage with intensive insulin management in the overall study population.[157] The significant improvement in survival was demonstrable in the subgroup of patients who remained in the MICU for 3 or more days.[157]

A major goal of management should be the prevention of nosocomial or secondary infections/sepsis and multiple organ dysfunction/failure because these two conditions are currently responsible for the high mortality rate seen in patients with ALI and ARDS.[19,78,144-146] Ventilator-associated pneumonia (VAP) is a frequent complication in critically ill ventilated patients. As previously mentioned, prevention of VAP should be a primary management goal for patients with ALI and ARDS. Detection of a complicating VAP can be difficult in the setting of the pulmonary radiographic infiltrates seen in patients with ALI and ARDS. Diagnosis of VAP and identification of the offending pathogen often requires the use on bronchoscopy with BAL or protected specimen brushes coupled with semi-quantitative culture results.[144,146] Recent data suggest that identifying the soluble triggering receptor expressed on myeloid cells (sTREM) may be beneficial in the detection of VAP but does not identify the specific etiologic organism.[158] European investigators have been enthusiastic about the technique of selective digestive decontamination (SDD) as a method to decrease nosocomial lung infections in the critically ill patient.[159] Keeping the head of the bed elevated above 30 degrees is also effective at preventing VAP.[149] Additional measures designed to decrease the development of VAP include continuous subglottic suction, coated endotracheal tubes, closed suction systems, and kinetic therapy.[149] Development of complications has been associated with increased morbidity, length of stay, cost of care, and possibly mortality.[148,149]

Encountering ventilatory support–related complications in the management of patients with ALI and ARDS is common. These complications include pulmonary barotrauma and VAP, which may be associated with increased morbidity and mortality.[7,148] Pulmonary barotrauma has been reported to develop in approximately 7% to 15% of patients with ALI.[90] When a pneumothorax is detected in a mechanically ventilated patient, prompt recognition and chest tube insertion are required to prevent the development of tension physiology.[90]

Having abnormalities in oxygenation and/or requiring high concentrations of supplemental oxygen and/or PEEP during the management of patients with ALI and ARDS is common. Various strategies have been developed in an attempt to improve oxygenation and lessen FIO_2 requirements in these patients. Included in these strategies are recruitment maneuvers, prone positioning, sighs, surfactant replacement therapy, partial liquid ventilation, inhaled nitric oxide, and enhanced edema clearance.[121,160-180] These techniques remain investigational at this time and should be subjected to rigorous evaluation to adequately determine their ability to improve outcome for patients with ALI and ARDS. Importantly, the use of higher tidal volumes (12 mL/kg ideal body weight) in the ARDS Network trial was associated with an improvement in oxygenation but a significantly decreased survival in patients with ALI and ARDS.[83]

Recruitment maneuvers represent an attempt to open the atelectatic distal airways and alveoli on the border of the collapsed flooded alveoli that comprise the dependent area of radiographic lung injury.[87] Some experts believe that this maneuver should precede the provision of PEEP and ventilator support in the early phases of ALI.[181] The maneuver is accomplished by increasing the PEEP to 35 to 50 cm H_2O and holding that level of pressure for 30 seconds. The ARDS network attempted to define the value of a recruitment maneuver in 43 patients with ARDS by randomly assigning them to a recruitment maneuver with 35 to 40 cm H_2O for 30 seconds versus a sham recruitment maneuver.[170] The recruitment maneuver was assessed on the basis of a sustained improvement in oxygenation as judged by the ability to titrate PEEP/FIO_2 on the basis of the network algorithm and changes in lung compliance. There was no significant difference in the magnitude or duration of the oxygenation effect, compliance, or change in PEEP/FIO_2 titration. The group that received a recruitment maneuver did have a greater decrease in blood pressure during the maneuver.

Patients with ARDS may improve their oxygenation abnormalities when they are placed in the prone position.[160-165] This position may be more physiologic for most mammals and result in improved secretion removal, ventilation perfusion matching, and better aeration of the dorsal lung units.[164] The prone position may also prevent the heart from collapsing the left lower lobe and enhance the recruitment effects of PEEP by stabilizing the more flexible ventral chest wall.[164] A number of trials have demonstrated an improvement in oxygenation during and after being placed in a prone position.[162-165] One prospective randomized trial designed to demonstrate survival advantage failed to do so.[166] A number of potential complications can result from the process of changing the patient from a supine to a prone position.[173,174] Included in the list of potential complications are tube/catheter malposition/problems, pressure sores, blindness, and difficulty with patient assessment and resuscitation.[173,174] Prone positioning should be considered in patients with low risk for such a position change who require high FIO_2 despite optimization of ventilator strategy.

Inhaled Nitric Oxide

Inhaled nitric oxide is a bronchial and vascular smooth muscle dilator that also decreases platelet adherence and aggregation.[182] It has been shown to improve oxygenation by improving ventilation/perfusion relationships in the lung.[175,182,183] A reduction in pulmonary artery pressure and pulmonary vascular resistance also occurs. These beneficial pulmonary effects are associated with minimal systemic effect from the inhaled nitric oxide because it is rapidly inactivated when the nitric oxide enters the circulation and is taken up by red blood cells. Two prospective, randomized, placebo-controlled clinical trials failed to demonstrate an improvement in survival despite the early improvement in oxygenation associated with the administration of inhaled nitric oxide.[179,180]

Surfactant Replacement Therapy

Surfactant abnormalities are present in patients with ALI and ARDS related to decreased production, inactivation by alveolar proteins and proteolytic enzymes, and dilution by the alveolar fluid.[169] Theoretically, surfactant replacement should produce a survival benefit, just as it does in the infant respiratory distress syndrome.[168,169] Anzueto and colleagues[167] reported no difference in hemodynamic function, oxygenation, length of stay, duration of mechanical ventilation, and survival in 725 sepsis-induced ARDS patients who were prospectively randomized into a placebo-controlled trial of Exosurf (artificial surfactant) versus placebo. The researchers believe that the lack of associated surfactant proteins might account for the lack of efficacy. Trials are continuing to evaluate recombinant forms of surfactant replacement that include surfactant proteins.[168] A meta-analysis from a group of small trials evaluating recombinant surfactant protein C replacement in patients with ARDS noted an improvement in oxygenation but no survival benefit.[168] Further investigation is continuing at this time.

Enhanced Edema Clearance

Accumulated fluid in the alveolus could potentially worsen the gas exchange, as well as produce adverse pulmonary mechanics with an increased work of breathing. Recent strategies designed to improve edema clearance either using aquaporins or increasing the activity of the Na/K pump could potentially provide a benefit to patients with ALI and ARDS. The BALTI trial evaluated the use of intravenous β-agonist (Salbutamol) in patients with ALI and demonstrated a significant decrease in extravascular lung water at day 7.[176] The salbutamol-treated group also had lower end-inspiratory plateau pressures, and there was a trend toward a lower Murray Lung Injury Score. This group also had more supraventricular arrhythmias. The amount of edema in the lung can also be increased when there is a low oncotic pressure. To evaluate the potential benefit of infusing albumin and furosemide as opposed to furosemide alone to patients with ALI, Martin and colleagues[178] conducted a randomized control trial in 40 hypoproteinemic patients with ALI. The albumin-infused group had an improvement in oxygenation, total protein, net fluid loss, increased number of shock-free days, and less hypotension. Although this is a small study, it does suggest a potential benefit of this maneuver in the hypoproteinemic ALI/ARDS patients. Further investigation is necessary to determine the benefit of edema clearance strategies in the management of ALI patients.

Experimental/Innovative Therapies

In an attempt to reduce the high mortality rate associated with ALI and ARDS, a number of experimental and innovative therapeutic approaches have been evaluated. A majority of these approaches target abnormalities that either produce or result from the systemic inflammatory response that is felt to be central to the pathogenesis of the injury. To date, none of these approaches has been demonstrated to offer significant benefit in well-conducted, prospective, randomized, controlled, multicentered clinical trials. These approaches have included the early administration of high-dose corticosteroids, prostaglandin E_1, nonsteroidal antiinflammatory drugs, antiendotoxin and anticytokine therapy, inhaled nitric oxide, surfactant therapy, antioxidant therapy, positional changes, and partial liquid ventilation.[161-165,168,175,179,180,184-220]

Many investigations in experimental animal models of ALI have demonstrated benefit from pretreatment and early treatment with high-dose corticosteroids.[184-187] Similar benefit has been observed with a number of nonsteroidal antiinflammatory agents in experimental animal models of lung injury.[188,196,197,221] Unfortunately, the use of antiinflammatory strategies in humans with sepsis and/or ARDS has repeatedly failed to demonstrate significant benefit.[181,189,191,192,222,223] In fact, in subgroup analysis there was evidence of potential harm in patients with renal dysfunction who were administered high-dose methylprednisolone for treatment of severe sepsis and septic shock.[192] To further complicate this clinical situation, it has been demonstrated that a significant proportion of patients with septic shock and other critical illnesses have relative adrenal insufficiency as defined by the inability to elevate the plasma cortisol level more than 9 μg/dL after ACTH stimulation.[223] This relative adrenocortical deficiency has been implicated as a potential cause of the persistent shock state and impaired perfusion. However, these patients have not always been responsive to the administration of steroids, and the adrenergic hyporesponsiveness may be related to sepsis-induced nitric oxide production, desensitization, and/or down-regulation of α and β adrenergic receptors.[223] Lower-dose, more physiologic steroid replacement may restore the α and β adrenergic responsiveness and potentially turn off the inflammatory reaction to allow for better healing and less injury.[223-225] Attempts to prevent the development of ALI/ARDS in high-risk patients with severe sepsis and septic shock with high-dose corticosteroids have not been shown to prevent the development of ARDS, improve the reversal of ARDS, or improve the outcome from ARDS.[192]

Steroid therapy has been shown to be beneficial in patients with severe *Pneumocystis jiroveci (carinii)* pneumonia and ALI and possibly in patients with fat embolism.[184] In the patient with adrenal insufficiency, stress dose steroids should be administered. The use of corticosteroids to treat patients with established ALI/ARDS is controversial and is discussed later. Ibuprofen, a nonsteroidal anti-inflammatory drug, failed to significantly improve the outcome of patients with severe sepsis or septic shock and failed to prevent the development of ARDS in a prospective, randomized, placebo-controlled, multicentered clinical trial.[122]

A plethora of clinical trials have evaluated "antimediators" that have targeted the potential proinflammatory compounds that can be identified in the blood or BAL of patients at risk for or diagnosed with ALI and ARDS.[8,79,198,226,227] Despite encouraging results from preclinical experimental animal and early clinical studies, these innovative strategies have failed to demonstrate a significant survival benefit.[8,192,199,202-204,207-215] Attempts to change the inflammatory response by changing the ratio of omega 3:6 fatty acids have evaluated the potential benefit of an enteral nutritional formula rich in eicosapentaenoic acid and γ-linoleic acid.[154] A large, multicentered, prospective, randomized trial demonstrated an improvement in lung injury score, oxygenation, and organ dysfunction as compared with an isocaloric, isonitrogenous enteral formulation.[154] Unfortunately, there was not a survival benefit seen.

Pentoxifylline and lisophylline are xanthine derivatives that were felt to have utility in the management of sepsis and ALI. Pentoxifylline is a rheologic agent that has the ability to inhibit toxic oxygen radical release, decrease platelet aggregation, decrease phagocytosis, diminish the response to PAF stimulation, and inhibit the release of TNF into the systemic circulation. Clinical evaluation of this treatment strategy by the NIH ARDS Network found no significant benefit.[226]

A number of clinical trials evaluated the potential benefit of anticoagulant agents such as antithrombin III, activated protein C, and tissue factor pathway inhibitor (TFPI) to prevent or treat the microthrombosis of the microcirculatory bed that occurs in sepsis and could result in ALI/ARDS as an early manifestation of MODS/MOF.[227-230] To date, none of these strategies has been found to decrease the development of or improve the outcome of ALI/ARDS.

ALI/ARDS may be produced or worsened by the elaboration of toxic oxygen radicals from the activated inflammatory cells.[8] The abundant production of toxic oxygen radicals may overwhelm the ability of the endogenous oxygen radical scavengers, superoxide dismutase (SOD), catalase, and the glutathione redux cycle. The administration of antioxidants such as N-acetylcysteine, procysteine, vitamin E, β-carotene, and vitamin C have been evaluated in the prevention and/or management of patients with ALI/ARDS.[135,219,231,232] No survival benefit was seen associated with the administration of N-acetylcysteine or procysteine versus control in patients with ALI/ARDS.[219]

Prevention of ALI and ARDS

Two published trials have demonstrated a significant reduction in the development of ARDS in surgical patients when ketoconazole, an imidazole thromboxane A_2 synthetase inhibitor, was administered to an at-risk population of patients.[233-234] When ketoconazole was used in the treatment of patients with established ARDS as part of the ARDS Network clinical trials, there was no reported benefit on survival.[235] We must wait for further evaluation of this agent as a prevention in a group of patients at high risk for the development of ALI and ARDS before we make our final judgment concerning the ability of ketoconazole to prevent ALI. At present no other agents appear to be promising in the prevention of ARDS.

Fibroproliferative Phase of Acute Lung Injury

An improved understanding of the injury and repair phase of ARDS has resulted in the recognition of the late fibroproliferative phase of the ALI.[8,70-73,236] This stage of the injury/repair process is characterized by replacement of damaged epithelial cells and accumulation of mesenchymal cells and connective tissue products in the airspaces and the intra-acinar microvessels.[68-70] Clinical manifestations include fever, leukocytosis, diffuse alveolar infiltrates on the chest radiograph, and persistent inflammatory mediators in the serum.[68-70] Gallium scans demonstrate an increase in pulmonary uptake, and BAL typically contains markers of inflammation and type 3 procollagen peptide.[68] Physiologic manifestations include the worsening of static pulmonary compliance, abnormal gas exchange, increased dead space ventilation, pulmonary hypertension, and lack of PEEP response.[236] This picture of persistent inflammation requires a dedicated approach to ensure that there is not an ongoing uncontrolled infectious process that has not been adequately addressed.[236] Once it is determined that this state is not the result of inadequately treated infection, therapy with corticosteroids is used by some experts.[236] Several anecdotal reports have suggested that this therapy may have potential efficacy in patients with a persistent inflammatory response.[184,236] A small, single-center, prospective, randomized, placebo-controlled, double-blind clinical trial in 24 patients with the fibroproliferative phase of ARDS demonstrated an improvement in survival, lung function, and organ system dysfunction.[237] This study has been criticized because it included the crossover of patients at day 10 and had a smaller study population than a previously reported uncontrolled trial from the same center.[237]

The use of steroid rescue for the patient with persistent ARDS or the fibroproliferative phase of ARDS was evaluated by the NIH-sponsored ARDS Network.[238] The study prospectively randomized 180 patients with ARDS for greater than or equal to 7 days into a placebo-controlled trial of methylprednisolone versus placebo. The primary efficacy outcome was alive at home at 60 days. Patients with septic shock, a defined need for corticosteroid therapy, disseminated fungal infection, or undrained abscess were excluded. The trial was conducted over 6 years and included a modification of the study protocol that included a reduction in the number of subjects from 400 to 180 and an increase in the inclusion PaO_2/FiO_2 ratio. The use of methylprednisolone was associated with an early improvement in mortality, PaO_2/FiO_2 ratio, blood pressure, ventilator, and ICU-free days. An increase in the white blood cell count and glucose level related to steroid administration occurred, along with a decrease in body temperature. No difference was measured in the primary efficacy end point and 60-day mortality, and no significant difference in 180-day outcome occurred between the two groups. The steroid treatment was not associated with an increase in serious infections. In fact, there was more pneumonia and septic shock seen in the placebo group than the steroid-treated group. Unfortunately, the use of steroids was associated with more neuropathy and myopathy, but it is important to note that 30% of the steroid-treated patients were receiving neuromuscular blocking drugs.[238] For now, the use of rescue steroids remains controversial on the basis of the disparate results of these published studies.

Multiple Organ Dysfunction/Failure

A frequent complication of an exaggerated proinflammatory state in the setting of sepsis, SIRS, and ARDS is the development of organ system dysfunction.[8,19,33,78,239] This dysfunction may involve single or multiple organs.[153,239] A recent consensus conference has suggested that the dysfunction of two or more organs such that normal homeostasis cannot be maintained in the setting of a systemic inflammatory response to a variety of insults is considered MODS.[240] This dysfunction may be partial or complete, reversible or irreversible.[153] A continuum of abnormalities ranging from dysfunction to failure for each organ is probable.[153] Unfortunately, as of this time there has been no consensus on the threshold that separates these two phenomena or the threshold between reversible and irreversible organ system dysfunction.[153]

MODS and MOF are the most common causes of death in the noncoronary intensive care unit.[8,19,239,241,242] Many authorities consider ALI and ARDS as the earliest manifestation of an uncompensated systemic inflammatory process with excessive proinflammatory component.[76,162] One hypothesis for this injury suggests that in the absence of a direct injury to a specific organ, there must be multiple inflammatory insults to produce the clinically apparent MODS/MOF.[153] This has been called the "two-hit hypothesis."[153] This hypothesis suggests that an initial sensitizing insult is followed within a specific period of time by a second insult that is capable of initiating a more profound proinflammatory response because the target cells have been upregulated or primed by the initial insult.[153] Multiple combinations of direct injury, ischemic injury, circulating humoral or inflammatory mediators, translocation of endotoxin and/or colonic bacteria, altered rheologic properties of the blood cells, or iatrogenic effects of the therapy administered may interact in the eventual production of MODS/MOF.[153]

Prognosis in Acute Lung Injury

Recent studies report a significant reduction in the mortality rate from ARDS using lung protective ventilatory support and proper levels of PEEP.[8,83,241,243] Current trials report mortality rates in the range of 30% to 60% in comparison with the 60% to 90% of the past.[8,83,244,245] The 30-day mortality rate seen in patients enrolled in the NIH-sponsored ECMO trial of the 1970s was 91% with both conventional and ECMO treatment.[244] Older reports from large tertiary referral centers documented mortality rates of 90% for patients with gram-negative septic shock and ARDS.[245] A large multicenter trial of inhaled surfactant in 725 patients with septic-induced ARDS demonstrated survival rates of 60% at 28 days in both the treatment and the control groups.[167] Today the mortality rate from ARDS appears to depend on the cause of the injury, the patient's underlying disease status, patient age, and institutional factors.[35,243] This improvement in mortality mandates the use of a concomitant control group as opposed to using historical controls in the assessment of new innovative therapeutic strategies.

The most common causes of death in patients with ARDS continues to be from MOF and recurrent sepsis.[3,8,17,33,241,242] Less than 20% of patients die because of the inability to adequately oxygenate or ventilate them.[241] The complexities of the balance between the proinflammatory and anti-inflammatory processes that encompass the pathophysiologic response of this injury direct the response from organ dysfunction secondary to an overzealous proinflammatory reaction to infectious complications. These complications result from the immune suppression of a predominant antiinflammatory response.[72,246] When infection is present, the lung is a frequent site for the process and may be extremely difficult to diagnose.[32,78,144,145] Patients with pulmonary infections were found to typically have a septic clinical picture without definitive positive culture results.[32] On the other hand, in patients who were found to have positive blood cultures without antemortem identification of a specific site, the site of occult infection was commonly found to be in the abdomen at postmortem examination.[32] The detection of elevated levels of soluble triggering receptor expressed on myeloid cells in the serum or BAL may be a marker for the presence of an infection.[158] This assay may improve the diagnosis of a complicating pulmonary infection in the setting of ARDS and other critical illnesses.[158] Predictors of high mortality rates from ARDS include the development of multiple organ dysfunction/failure, development of secondary sepsis, concomitant cancer, and the presence of cirrhosis or hepatic dysfunction.[17]

After recovery from ALI, the prognosis appears to be reasonably good. A recent report found that 85% of ARDS survivors discharged from the ICU were still alive 2 years later.[247] Although most ARDS survivors have initial abnormalities in pulmonary function quality of life, the majority return to near their baseline pulmonary function status within 3 to 6 months.[248,249] The major residual abnormality in pulmonary function is a restrictive pulmonary defect and a reduction in the carbon monoxide diffusion capacity.[248,249] These alterations may result in exercise desaturation in some patients or, more commonly, a decrease in timed walked distance.[248,249] When observed over the next 1 to 2 years, their pulmonary function did not improve a great deal after this initial improvement.[247,250] However, most patients continue to experience exercise limitation at 2 years, despite the fact that 65% have returned to work.[247]

Survivors of ARDS have been found to have a decreased health-related quality of life, increased respiratory symptoms, insomnia, depression, anxiety, and post-traumatic stress disorder.[251-253] ARDS survivors have been found to have a clinically significant reduction in their physical function and increased pulmonary symptoms in comparison with the matched survivors of critical illness.[251-255] Elderly patients, older than 70 years of age, seem to have worse outcomes with an increase in mortality rate compared with ARDS patients who are younger than 70 years of age.[253] Continued evaluation is necessary to determine the long-term impact of the injury on the survivors of ALI and ARDS.

FUTURE CONSIDERATIONS

The growing knowledge of molecular biology and the elaborate mechanisms that govern a person's response to injury, repair, and cell death will likely have a major role in the management of patients with ALI and ARDS. Individuals with increased risk for ALI and ARDS development will no doubt be identified on the basis of their genetic profile. This knowledge will likely affect future management. In years to come, scientists may potentially modify the genetic makeup or the biologic response of a susceptible individual by inserting selected genes or modifying the transcription or function of various regulatory proteins.

SUMMARY

Acute respiratory failure is the inability of the respiratory system to meet the oxygenation (type 1 or hypoxemic failure) or ventilation (type 2 or hypercapneic failure) requirements of the patient. Hypoxemic respiratory failure is defined as a P_{AO_2} of less than 60 mm Hg and is the result of one of six potential mechanisms: low inspired F_{IO_2}, hypoventilation, ventilation-perfusion mismatching, shunt, low $M_{\bar{v}}O_2$ (pulmonary arterial oxygenation), or diffusion impairment. The exact etiology may be elucidated by analysis of the alveolar-arterial oxygen gradient, response to the administration of supplemental oxygen, and the clinical context. Hypercapneic or ventilatory failure is defined as a P_{ACO_2} of greater than 50 mm Hg, generally with acidemia; it can be acute, chronic, or acute-on-chronic and is the result of one of three potential mechanisms: hypoventilation, increased dead space ventilation, or increased CO_2 production. Clinical manifestations can range from adrenergic sympathetic hyperactivity (tachycardia and hypertension) to tachypnea and respiratory distress to encephalopathy with somnolence. Therapy is with supplemental oxygen, assisted ventilation with or without high levels of PEEP, or both.

ALI/ARDS continues to have a significant morbidity and mortality rate despite the advances in understanding and management that have occurred over the past decades. Major advances have occurred in our understanding of the pathogenesis and in our ability to adequately provide the required support while the injury is allowed to heal. Attention has been directed on improved ventilatory support, the use of local and systemic therapies, and attempts at prevention of injury in high-risk patient populations. Despite recent improvements in management and knowledge of the pathophysiologic alterations likely involved, the mortality rate continues to be unacceptably high. Recent improvements in prognosis have occurred, primarily in those patients younger than age 60. Remembering the systemic nature of the injury and developing effective preventive and reparative strategies is important as we look to the future of ALI and ARDS management. Repair of the acutely injured lung, whether from the initial event, the ventilator, or complicating infection is an important target and may be more achievable than attempting to prevent the initial injury or intervene early enough to prevent the development of ARDS.

KEY POINTS

- Both type 1 and type 2 acute respiratory failure are common problems in the ICU and may represent the primary reason for ICU admission or be a complication arising in the critically ill patient.
- The arterial blood gas (ABG) is the cornerstone for the diagnosis and management of the patient with acute respiratory failure.
- The American-European Consensus Conference has operationally defined the acute respiratory distress syndrome (ARDS) and suggested that there is a continuum of injury from ALI to the more severe form, ARDS. The degree of oxygenation abnormality distinguishes the two.
- The most common clinical risk factors for the development of ARDS include sepsis, SIRS, hypotension, shock, trauma, near-drowning, and aspiration injury.
- The pathophysiology of ALI and ARDS represents a complex mixture of anti-inflammatory and proinflammatory responses, activation of the coagulation system, abnormal function of the microcirculation,

and altered surfactant function. Alterations affect both the capillary endothelium and the epithelial lining cells.

- At this time the management of patients with ALI and ARDS is primarily supportive, but it is important to provide specific treatment directed at the underlying predisposing cause of the injury along with the provision of adequate ventilatory, circulatory, and nutritional support. Complications of critical illness should be anticipated, and prophylactic strategies should be adopted when possible.
- The concept of ventilator-induced lung injury has now been supported by the results of recent clinical trials demonstrating a survival benefit associated with the use of lower tidal volumes to avoid alveolar overdistention.
- The proper amount of PEEP therapy is important in the management of patients with ALI and ARDS to avoid alveolar overdistention and the repetitive collapse and recruitment-derecruitment of alveoli and small airspaces.
- The use of steroids to treat the fibroproliferative phase of ARDS remains a controversial area. If there is no active untreated infectious process and there is a persistent inflammatory process in the lung, there may be a benefit associated with corticosteroid therapy; however, a recent multicenter trial conducted by the ARDS network did not find a survival benefit at 60 days.
- Although the overall prognosis in ARDS has been improving, there is still a mortality rate that ranges from 30% to 60%.

REFERENCES

1. Greene KE, Peters JI: Pathophysiology of acute respiratory failure. Clin Chest Med 1994;15:1-12.
2. Balk RA, Bone RC: Acute respiratory failure. Med Clin North Am 1983;67:351-356.
3. Tisi GM: Pulmonary Physiology in Clinical Medicine, 2nd ed. Baltimore, Williams & Wilkins, 1983, pp 3-41.
4. Derenne JP, Fleury B, Pariente R: Acute respiratory failure of chronic obstructive pulmonary disease. Am Rev Respir Dis 1988;138:1006-1033.
5. Chen WJ, Kuan P, Lien WP, Lin FY: Detection of patent foramen ovale by contrast transesophageal echocardiography. Chest 1992;101:1515-1520.
6. Cujec B, Polasek P, Mayers I, Johnson D: Positive end-expiratory pressure increases the right-to-left shunt in mechanically ventilated patients with patent foramen ovale. Ann Intern Med 1993;119:887-894.
7. Tobin MJ: Respiratory monitoring in the intensive care unit. Am Rev Respir Dis 1988;138:1625-1642.
8. Ware LB, Matthay MA: The acute respiratory distress syndrome. N Engl J Med 2000;342:1334-1349.
9. Weinberger SE, Schwartzstein RM, Weiss JW: Hypercapnia. N Engl J Med 1989;321:1223-1231.
10. Parsons PE: Respiratory failure as a result of drugs, overdoses, and poisonings. Clin Chest Med 1994;15:93-101.
11. Anzueto A, Peters JI, Tobin MJ, et al: Effects of prolonged controlled mechanical ventilation on diaphragmatic function in healthy adult baboons. Crit Care Med 1997;25:1187-1190.
12. Ashbaugh DG, Bigelow DB, Petty TL, Levine BE: Acute respiratory distress in adults. Lancet 1967;2:319-323.
13. Matthay MA, Zimmerman GA: Acute lung injury and the acute respiratory distress syndrome: Four decades of inquiry into pathogenesis and rational management. Am J Respir Crit Cell Mol Biol 2005;33:319-327.
14. Jain R, DalNogare A: Pharmacological therapy for acute respiratory distress syndrome. Mayo Clin Proc 2006;81:205-212.
15. Manthous CA: ARDS redux. Clin Pulm Med 2006;13:121-127.
16. Petty T: Indicators of risk, course, and prognosis in adult respiratory distress syndrome (ARDS). Am Rev Respir Dis 1985;132:471.
17. Doyle RL, Szaflarski N, Modin GW, et al: Identification of patients with acute lung injury: Predictors of mortality. Am J Resp Crit Care Med 1995;152:1818-1824.
18. Fowler AA, Hamman RF, Good JT, et al: Adult respiratory distress syndrome: Risk with common predispositions. Ann Intern Med 1983;98:593-597.
19. Balk, RA, Bone RC: Adult respiratory distress syndrome. Med Clin North Am 1983;67:685-700.
20. Gattinoni L, Pelosi P, Suter PM, et al: Acute respiratory distress syndrome caused by pulmonary and extrapulmonary disease. Different syndromes? Am J Respir Crit Care Med 1998;158:3-11.
21. Pepe P, Potkin R, Holtman Reus D, et al: Clinical predictors of the adult respiratory distress syndrome. Am J Surg 1982;144:124-130.
22. Bernard GR, Artigas A, Brigham KL, et al: The American-European Consensus Conference on ARDS: Definitions, mechanisms, relevant outcomes, and clinical trial coordination. Am J Respir Crit Care Med 1994;149:818-824.
23. Artigas A, Bernard GR, Carlet J, et al: The American-European Consensus Conference on ARDS, Part 2. Am J Respir Crit Care Med 1998;157:1332-1347.
24. American Thoracic Society: Round table conference: Acute lung injury. Am J Respir Crit Care Med 1998;158:675-679.
25. Abraham E: Toward new definitions of acute respiratory distress syndrome. Crit Care Med 1999;27:237-238.
26. Esteban A, Fernancez-Segoviano P, Frutos-Villar F, et al: Comparison of clinical criteria for the acute respiratory distress syndrome with autopsy findings. Ann Intern Med 2004;131:440-445.
27. Ferguson ND, Frutos-Vivar F, Esteban A, et al: Acute respiratory distress syndrome: Underrecognition by clinician and diagnostic accuracy of three clinical definitions. Crit Care Med 2005;33:2228-2234.
28. Luce JL: The imperfect diagnosis of acute respiratory distress syndrome. Crit Care Med 2005;33:2419-2420.
29. Rubenfeld GD, Caldwell E, Granton J, et al: Interobserver variability in applying a radiographic definition for ARDS. Chest 1999;116:1347-1353.
30. Fulkerson WJ, MacIntyre N, Stamler J, Crapo JD: Pathogenesis and treatment of the adult respiratory distress syndrome. Arch Intern Med 1996;156:29-38.
31. Zilberberg MD, Epstein SK: Acute lung injury in the medical ICU. Am J Respir Crit Care Med 1998;157:1159-1164.
32. Seidenfeld JJ, Pohl DF, Bell RC, et al: Incidence, site, and outcome of infections in patients with the adult respiratory distress syndrome. Am Rev Respir Dis 1986;134:12-16.
33. Kollef MH, Schuster DP: The acute respiratory distress syndrome. N Engl J Med 1995;332:27-37.
34. Brun-Buisson C, for the ALIVE Study Group: Epidemiology and outcome of acute lung injury in European intensive care units: Results from the Alive Study. Intensive Care Med 2004;30:51-61.
35. Rubenfeld GD, Caldwell E, Peabody E, et al: Incidence and outcomes of acute lung injury. N Engl J Med 2005;353:1685-1693.
36. Ackland GL, Mythen MG: Negative pressure pulmonary edema as an unsuspected imitator of acute lung injury/ARDS. Chest 2005;127:1867-1868.
37. Koh MS, Hsu AA, Eng P: Negative pressure pulmonary edema in the medical intensive care unit. Intensive Care Med 2003;29:1601-1604.
38. Patel AR, Bersten AD: Pulmonary haemorrhage associated with negative-pressure pulmonary oedema: A case report. Crit Care Resusc 2006;8:115-116.
39. Sow Nam Y, Garewal D: Pulmonary hemorrhage in association with negative pressure edema in an intubated patient. Acta Anaesthesiol Scand 2001;45:911-913.
40. Broccard AF, Liaudet L, Aubert JD, et al: Negative pressure post-tracheal

extubation alveolar hemorrhage. Anesth Analg 2001;92:273-275.
41. Dolinski SY, MacGregor DA, Scuderi PE: Pulmonary hemorrhage associated with negative-pressure pulmonary edema. Anesthesiology 2000;93:888-890.
42. Schwartz DR, Maroo A, Malhotra A, Kesselman H: Negative pressure pulmonary hemorrhage. Chest 1999;115:1194-1197.
43. Oswalt CE, Gates GA, Holmstrom MG: Pulmonary edema as a complication of acute airway obstruction. JAMA 1977;238:1833-1835.
44. Tarrac SE: Negative pressure pulmonary edema—a postanesthesia emergency. J Perianesth Nurs 2003;18:317-323.
45. Ikeda H, Asato R, Chin K, et al: Negative-pressure pulmonary edema after resection of mediastinum thyroid goiter. Acta Otolaryngol 2006;126:886-888.
46. Sharma ML, Beckett N, Gormley P: Negative pressure pulmonary edema following thyroidectomy. Can J Anaesth 2002;49:215.
47. Westreich R, Sampson I, Shaari CM, Lawson W: Negative-pressure pulmonary edema after routine septorhinoplasty: Discussion of pathophysiology, treatment, and prevention. Arch Facial Plast Surg 2006;8:8-15.
48. Thomas CL, Palmer TJ, Shipley P: Negative pressure pulmonary edema after a tonsillectomy and adenoidectomy in a pediatric patient: Case report and review. AANA J 1999;67:425-430.
49. Lloyd C, Kamisetty A: Negative pressure pulmonary edema following open reduction and internal fixation of a fractured mandible. Oral Surg Oral Med Oral Pathol Oral Radiol Endod 2003;95:2.
50. Gupta S, Richardson J, Pugh M: Negative pressure pulmonary oedema after cryotherapy for tracheal obstruction. Eur J Anaesthesiol 2001;18:189-191.
51. Jouan ZT, Jawan B, Lee JH: Pulmonary edema complicated by post-extubation laryngospasm: A case report. Changgeng Yi Xue Za Zhi 1997;20:309-312.
52. Murray-Calderon P, Connolly MA: Laryngospasm and noncardiogenic pulmonary edema. J Perianesth Nurs 1997;12:89-94.
53. Dicpinigaitis PV, Mehta DC: Postobstructive pulmonary edema induced by endotracheal tube occlusion. Intensive Care Med 1995;21:1048-1050.
54. Liu EH, Yih PS: Negative pressure pulmonary oedema caused by biting and endotracheal tube occlusion—a case for oropharyngeal airways. Singapore Med J 1999;40:174-175.
55. Memtsoudis SG, Rosenberger P, Sadovnikoff N: Chest tube suction-associated unilateral negative pressure pulmonary edema in a lung transplant patient. Anesth Analg 2005;101:38-40.
56. Kaki A, Crosby ET, Lui AC: Airway and respiratory management following non-lethal hanging. Can J Anaesth 1997;44:445-450.
57. Stuth EA, Stucke AG, Berens RJ: Negative-pressure pulmonary edema in a child with hiccups during induction. Anesthesiology 2000;93:282-284.
58. Mandal NG: Negative-pressure pulmonary edema in a child with hiccups during induction. Anesthesiology 2001;94:378-379.
59. Moss M, Goodman PL, Heinig M, et al: Establishing the relative accuracy of three new definitions of the adult respiratory distress syndrome. Crit Care Med 1995;23:1629-1637.
60. Goss CH for the ARDS Network: Incidence of acute lung injury in the United States. Crit Care Med 2003;31:1607-1611.
61. Hudson L: New therapies for ARDS. Chest 1995;108:79S-91S.
62. Gattinoni L, D'Andrea L, Pelosi P, et al: Regional effects and mechanism of positive-end expiratory pressure in early adult respiratory distress syndrome. JAMA 1993;269: 2122-2127.
63. Weiland JE, Davis WB, Holter JF, et al: Lung neutrophils in the adult respiratory distress syndrome. Am Rev Respir Dis 1986;133:218-225.
64. Puybasset L, Cluzel P, Chao N, et al: CT Scan ARDS Group: A computed tomography scan assessment of regional lung volume in acute lung injury. Am J Respir Crit Care Med 1998;158:1644-1655.
65. Hechtam, HB, Valeri R, Shepro D: Role of humoral mediators in adult respiratory distress syndrome. Chest 1984;86:623-627.
66. Shirley Jr HH, Wolfram CG Waserman K, Mayerson HS: Capillary permeability to macromolecules: Stretched pore phenomenon. Am J Physiol 1957;190:189-193.
67. Enhorning G: Surfactant replacement in adult respiratory distress syndrome. Am Rev Respir Dis 1989;140:281-283.
68. Clark JG, Milberg JA, Steinberg KP, Hudson LD: Type III procollagen peptide in the adult respiratory distress syndrome. Ann Intern Med 1994;122:17-23.
69. Fowler AA, Hamman RF, Zerbe GO, et al: Adult respiratory distress syndrome. Am Rev Respir Dis 1985;132:472-478.
70. Meduri GU, Kohler G, Headley S, et al: Inflammatory cytokines in the BAL of patients with ARDS: Persistent elevation over time predicts poor outcome. Chest 1995;108:1303-1314.
71. Meduri GU, Headley S, Tolley E, et al: Plasma and BAL cytokine response to corticosteroid rescue treatment in late ARDS. Chest 1995;108:1315-1325.
72. Meduri GU, Headley S, Kohler G, et al: Persistent elevation of inflammatory cytokines predicts a poor outcome in ARDS: Plasma IL-1β and IL-6 levels are consistent and efficient predictors of outcome over time. Chest 1995;107:1062-1073.
73. Martin C, Papazian L, Payan MJ, et al: Pulmonary fibrosis correlates with outcome in adult respiratory distress syndrome. Chest 1995;107:196-200.
74. Matthay MA, Robriquet L, Fang X: Alveolar epithelium: Role in lung fluid balance and acute lung injury. Proc Am Thorac Soc 2005;2:206-213.
75. Martin TR, Hagimoto N, Nakamura M, Matute-Bello G: Apoptosis and epithelial injury in the lungs. Proc Am Thorac Soc 2005;2:214-220.
76. Bone RC, Grodzin CJ, Balk RA: Sepsis: A new hypothesis for pathogenesis of the disease process. Chest 1997;117:235-243.
77. Fan E, Needham DM, Stewart TE: Ventilatory management of acute lung injury and acute respiratory distress syndrome. JAMA 2005;294:2889-2896.
78. Bell RC, Coalson JJ, Smith JD, Johanson WG Jr: Multiple organ system failure and infection in adult respiratory distress syndrome. Ann Intern Med 1983;99:293-298.
79. Suter PM: Lung inflammation in ARDS—friend or foe? N Engl J Med. 2006;354:1739-1742.
80. Marini JJ, Kelsen SG: Retargeting ventilatory objectives in adult respiratory distress syndrome. Am Rev Respir Dis 1992;146:2-3.
81. Ranieri VM, Suter PM, Tortorella C, et al: Effect of mechanical ventilation on inflammatory mediators in patients with acute respiratory distress syndrome. JAMA 1999;282:54-61.
82. Amato MBP, Barbas CSV, Medeiros DM, et al: Effect of a protective ventilation strategy on mortality in the acute respiratory distress syndrome. N Engl J Med 1998;338:347-354.
83. The Acute Respiratory Distress Syndrome Network: Ventilation with lower tidal volumes as compared with traditional tidal volumes for acute lung injury and the acute respiratory distress syndrome. N Engl J Med 2000;342:1301-1308.
84. Slutsky AS, Tremblay LN: Multiple system organ failure: Is mechanical ventilation a contributing factor? Am J Respir Crit Care Med 1998;157:1721-1725.
85. Dreyfuss D, Saumon G: Ventilator induced lung injury: Lessons from experimental studies. Am J Respir Crit Care Med 1998;157:294-323.
86. Parker JC, Hernandez LA, Peevy KJ: Mechanisms of ventilator induced lung injury. Crit Care Med 1993;21:131-143.
87. Pinhu L, Whitehead T, Evans T, Griffiths M: Ventilator-associated lung injury. Lancet 2003;361:332-340.
88. Meade MO, Cook DJ, Kernerman P, Bernard G: How to use articles about harm: The relationship between high tidal volumes, ventilating pressures, and ventilator-induced lung injury. Crit Care Med 1997;25:1915-1922.
89. Vieira ARR, Puybasset L, Richecoeur J, et al: A lung computed tomographic assessment of positive end-expiratory pressure-induced lung overdistention. Am J Respir Crit Care Med 1998;158:1571-1577.
90. Marini JJ: Lung mechanics in the adult respiratory distress syndrome. Clin. Chest Med 1990;11:673-690.
91. Weg JG, Anzueto A, Balk RA, et al: The relation of pneumothorax and other air leaks to mortality in the acute respiratory distress syndrome. N Engl J Med 1998;338:341-346.
92. Hickling KG, Henderson SJ, Jackson R: Low mortality associated with low volume, pressure limited ventilation

with permissive hypercapnia in severe adult respiratory distress syndrome. Intensive Care Med 1990;16:372-377.
93. Stewart TE, Meade MO, Cook DJ, et al: Evaluation of a ventilatory strategy to prevent barotrauma in patients at high risk for acute respiratory distress syndrome. N.Engl J Med 1998;338:355-361.
94. Brochard L, Roudot-Thoraval F, Roupie E, et al: Tidal volume reduction for prevention of ventilator-induced lung injury in acute respiratory distress syndrome. Am J Respir Crit Care Med 1998;158:1831-1838.
95. Brower RG, Shanholtz CB, Fessler HE, et al: Prospective, randomized, controlled clinical trial comparing traditional versus reduced tidal volume ventilation in acute respiratory distress syndrome patients. Crit Care Med 1999;27:1492-1498.
96. East TD, Bohm SH, Wallace CJ, et al: A successful computerized protocol for clinical management of pressure control inverse ratio ventilation in ARDS patients. Chest 1992;101: 697-710.
97. Kacmarek RM, Hickling KG: Permissive hypercapnia. Respir Care 1993;38: 373-387.
98. Morris AH, Wallace CJ, Menlove RL, et al: Randomized clinical trial of pressure-controlled inverse ratio ventilation and extracorporeal CO_2 removal for adult respiratory distress syndrome. Am J Respir Crit Care Med 1994;149:295-305.
99. Kiiski R, Takala J, Kari A, Milic-Emili J: Effect of tidal volume on gas exchange and oxygen transport in the adult respiratory distress syndrome. Am Rev Respir Dis 1992;146:1131-1135.
100. East TD: The magic bullets in the war on ARDS: Aggressive therapy for oxygenation failure. Respiratory Care 1993;38:690-704.
101. Hall JB: Respiratory system mechanics in adult respiratory distress syndrome: Stretching our understanding. Am J Respir Crit Care Med 1998;158:1-2.
102. Mergoni M, Martelli A, Volpi A, et al: Impact of positive end-expiratory pressure on chest wall and lung pressure-volume curve in acute respiratory failure. Am J Respir Crit Care Med 1997;156:846-854.
103. Hickling KG, Wright T, Laubscher K, et al: Extreme hypoventilation reduces ventilator-induced lung injury during ventilation with low positive end-expiratory pressure in saline-lavaged rabbits. Crit Care Med 1998;26: 1690-1697.
104. Peek GJ, Moore HM, Moore N, et al: Extracorporeal membrane oxygenation for adult respiratory failure. Chest 1997;112:759-764.
105. Marik PE, Krikorian J: Pressure-controlled ventilation in ARDS: A practical approach. Chest 1997;112:1102-1106.
106. Gluck E, Heard S, Patel C, et al: Use of ultrahigh frequency ventilation in patients with ARDS. Chest 1993;103:1413-1420.
107. Pesenti A: PEEP: Blood gas cosmetics or a therapy for ARDS? Crit Care Med 1999;27:253-254.
108. Myers J, Reilley T, Cloutier CT: Effect of positive end-expiratory pressure on extravascular lung water in porcine acute respiratory failure. Crit Care Med 1988;16:52.
109. Carvalho CRR, Barbas CSV, Medeiros DM, et al: Temporal hemodynamic effects of permissive hypercapnia associated with ideal PEEP in ARDS. Am J Respir Crit Care Med 1997;156:1458-1466.
110. Zwissler B, Schosser R, Schwickert C, et al: Perfusion of the interventricular septum during ventilation with positive end-expiratory pressure. Crit Care Med 1999;19:1414.
111. Pepe PE, Hudson LD, Carrico CJ: Early application of positive end-expiratory pressure in patients at risk for the adult respiratory distress syndrome. N Engl J Med 1984;311;261-266.
112. Amato MB, Barbos CS, Medeiros DM, et al: Beneficial effects of the "open lung approach" with low distending pressures in acute respiratory distress syndrome. Am J Respir Crit Care Med 1995;152:1835-1846.
113. O'Brien JM Jr, Welsh CH, Fish RH, et al: Excess body weight is not independently associated with outcome in mechanically ventilated patients with acute lung injury. Ann Intern Med 2004;140:338-345.
114. Laffey JG, Engelberts D, Kavanagh BP: Buffering hypercapnic acidosis worsens acute lung injury. Am J Resp Crit Care Med 2000;161:141-146.
115. Kregenow DA, Rubenfeld GD, Hudson LD, Swenson ER: Hypercapnic acidosis and mortality in acute lung injury. Crit Care Med 2006;34:1-7.
116. Walther SM, Domino KB, Glenny RW, Hiastala MP: Positive end-expiratory pressure redistributes perfusion to dependent lung regions in supine but not in prone lambs. Crit Care Med 1999;27:37-45.
117. Neumann P, Berglund JE, Mondejar EF, et al: Effect of different pressure levels on the dynamics of lung collapse and recruitment of oleic-acid-induced lung injury. Am J Respir Crit Care Med 1998;158:1636-1643.
118. Ruiz-Bailen M, Fernandez-Mondejar E, Hurtado-Ruiz B, et al: Immediate application of positive-end expiratory pressure is more effective than delayed positive-end expiratory pressure to reduce extravascular lung water. Crit Care Med 1999;27:380-384.
119. Jonson B, Richard JC, Straus C, et al: Pressure-volume curves and compliance in acute lung injury. Am J Respir Crit Care Med 1999;159: 1172-1178.
120. The National Heart, Lung, and Blood Institute Acute Respiratory Distress Syndrome (ARDS) Clinical Trials Network: Higher versus lower positive end-expiratory pressures in patients with the acute respiratory distress syndrome. N Engl J Med 2004;351: 327-336.
121. Mure M, Glenny RW, Domino KB, Hlastala MP: Pulmonary gas exchange improves in the prone position with abdominal distention. Am J Respir Crit Care Med 1998;157:1785-1790.
122. Young MP, Manning HL, Wilson DL, et al: Ventilation of patients with acute lung injury and acute respiratory distress syndrome: Has new evidence changed clinical practice? Crit Care Med 2004;32:1260-1265.
123. Humphrey H, Hall J, Sznajder I, et al: Improved survival in ARDS patients associated with a reduction in pulmonary capillary wedge pressure. Chest 1990;97:1176-1180.
124. Hudson LD: Fluid management strategy in acute lung injury. Am Rev Resp Dis 1992;145:988-989.
125. Mitchell JP, Schuller D, Calandrino FS, Schuster DP: Improved outcome based on fluid management in critically ill patients requiring pulmonary artery catheterization. Am Rev Respir Dis 1992;145:990-998.
126. Russell JA, Phang PT: The oxygen delivery/consumption controversy: Approaches to management of the critically ill. Am J Respir Crit Care Med 1994;149:533-537.
127. Tuchschmidt J, Fried J, Aziz M, Rackow E: Elevation of cardiac output and oxygen delivery improves outcome in septic shock. Chest 1992;102: 216-220.
128. Hayes MA, Timmins AC, Yau EHS, et al: Elevation of systemic oxygen delivery in the treatment of critically ill patients. N Engl J Med 1994;330: 1717-1722.
129. Ronco JJ, Fenwick JC, Tweeddale MG, et al: Identification of the critical oxygen delivery for anaerobic metabolism in critically ill septic and nonseptic humans. JAMA 1993;270: 1724-1730.
130. Yu M, Takanishi D, Myers SA, et al: Frequency of mortality and myocardial infarction during maximizing oxygen delivery: A prospective, randomized trial. Crit Care Med 1995;23: 1025-1032.
131. Shoemaker WC, Appel PL, Kram HB, et al: Prospective trial of supranormal values of survivors as therapeutic goals in high-risk surgical patients. Chest 1988;94:1176-1186.
132. Bishop MH, Shoemaker WC, Appel WC, et al: Prospective, randomized trial of survivor values of cardiac index, oxygen delivery, and oxygen consumption as resuscitation endpoints in severe trauma. J Trauma Inj Infect Crit Care 1995;38:780-787.
133. Yu M, Levy MM, Smith P, et al: Effect of maximizing oxygen delivery on morbidity and mortality rates in critically ill patients: A prospective, randomized, controlled study. Crit Care Med 1993;21:830-837.
134. Hayes MA, Yau EHS, Timmins AC, et al: Response of critically ill patients to treatment aimed at achieving supranormal oxygen delivery and consumption. Chest 1993;103:886-895.
135. Goldstein G, Luce JM: Pharmacologic treatment of the adult respiratory distress syndrome. Clin Chest Med 1990;11:773-787.
136. Rivers EP: Fluid-management strategies in acute lung injury-liberal, conservative, or both? N Engl J Med 2006;354:2598-2600.
137. The SAFE Study Investigators: A comparison of albumin and saline for fluid resuscitation in the intensive care unit. N Engl J Med 2004;350:2247-2256.

138. The National Heart, Lung, and Blood Institute Acute Respiratory Distress Syndrome (ARDS) Clinical Trials Network: Comparison of two fluid management strategies in acute lung injury. N Engl J Med 2006;354:2564-2575.
139. The National Heart, Lung, and Blood Institute Acute Respiratory Distress Syndrome (ARDS) Clinical Trials Network. Pulmonary-artery versus central venous catheter to guide treatment of acute lung injury. N Engl J Med 2006;354:2213-2224.
140. Shure D: Pulmonary-artery catheters—peace at last? N Engl J Med 2006;354:2273-2274.
141. Connors AF Jr, Speroff T, Dawson N, et al: The effectiveness of right heart catheterization in the initial care of critically ill patients. JAMA 1996;276:889-897.
142. Richard C, Warszawski J, Anguel N, et al: Early use of the pulmonary artery catheter and outcomes in patients with shock and acute respiratory distress syndrome: A randomized controlled trial. JAMA 2003;290:2713-2720.
143. Gattinoni L, Brazzi L, Pelosi P, et al: A trial of goal-oriented hemodynamic therapy in critically ill patients. N Engl J Med 1995;333:1025-1032.
144. Chastre J, Trouillet JL, Vaugnat A, et al: Nosocomial pneumonia in patients with acute respiratory distress syndrome. Am J Respir Crit Care Med 1998;157:1165-1172.
145. Winer-Muram HT, Steiner RM, Gurney JW, et al: Ventilator-associated pneumonia in patients with adult respiratory distress syndrome: CT evaluation. Radiology 1998;208:193-199.
146. Meduri GU, Reddy RC, Stanley T, El-Zeky F: Pneumonia in acute respiratory distress syndrome. Am J Respir Crit Care Med 1998;158:870-875.
147. Delclaux C, Roupie E, Blot F, et al: Lower respiratory tract colonization and infection during severe acute respiratory distress syndrome. Am J Respir Crit Care Med 1997;156:1092-1098.
148. Pingleton SK: Complications of acute respiratory failure. Am Rev Respir Dis 1988:137:1463-1493.
149. Patel G, Liberman J, Gurka D, et al: Complications of critical illness: Rationale for prophylactic strategies. Clin Pulm Med 2005;12:258-268.
150. Noseworthy TW, Cook DJ: Nosocomial pneumonia, prophylaxis against gastric erosive disease, and the clinically important gastrointestinal bleeding: Where do we stand? Crit Care Med 1993;21:1814-1816.
151. Bonten MJM Gaillard CA, Van Der Gest S, et al: The role of intragastric acidity and stress ulcer prophylaxis on colonization and infection in mechanically ventilated ICU patients. Am J Respir Crit Care Med 1995;152:1825-1834.
152. Prodhom G, Leuenberger P, Koerfer J, et al: Nosocomial pneumonia in mechanically ventilated patients receiving antacid, ranitidine, or sucralfate as prophylaxis for stress ulcer. Ann Intern Med 1994;120:653-662.
153. Balk RA: Pathogenesis and management of multiple organ dysfunction or failure in severe sepsis and septic shock. Crit Care Clin 2000;16:337-352.
154. Gadek JE, DeMichele SJ, Karlstad MD, et al: Effect of enteral feeding with eicosapentaenoic acid, γ-linolenic acid, and antioxidants in patients with acute respiratory distress syndrome. Crit Care Med 1999;27:1409-1420.
155. Singer P, Theilla M, Fisher H, et al: Benefit of an enteral diet enriched with eicosapentaenoic acid and gamma-linolenic acid in ventilated patients with acute lung injury. Crit Care Med 2006;34:1033-1036.
156. Van den Berghe G, Wouters P, Weekers F, et al: Intensive insulin therapy in critically ill patients. N Engl J Med 2001;345:1359-1367.
157. Van den Berghe G, Wilmer A, Hermans G, et al: Intensive insulin therapy in the medical ICU. N Engl J Med 2006;354:449-461.
158. Gibot S, Cravoisy A, Levy B, et al: Soluble triggering receptor expressed on myeloid cells and the diagnosis of pneumonia. N Engl J Med 2004;350:451-458.
159. Jacobs S, Foweraker JE, Roberts SE: Effectiveness of selective decontamination of digestive tract (SDD) in an ICU with a policy encouraging a low gastric pH. Clin Intensive Care 1992;3:52-58.
160. Chatte G, Sab JM, Dubois JM, et al: Prone position in mechanically ventilated patients with severe acute respiratory failure. Am J Respir Crit Care Med 1997;155:473-478.
161. Broccard AF, Shapiro RS, Schmitz LL, et al: Influence of prone position on the extent and distribution of lung injury in a high tidal volume oleic acid model of acute respiratory distress syndrome. Crit Care Med 1997;25:16-27.
162. Vollman KM, Bander JJ: Improved oxygenation utilizing a prone positioner in patients with acute respiratory distress syndrome. Intensive Care Med 1996;22: 1105-1111.
163. Lamm WJE, Graham MM, Albert RK: Mechanism by which the prone position improves oxygenation in acute lung injury. Am J Respir Crit Care Med 1994;150:184-193.
164. Pelosi P, Tubiolo D, Mascheroni D, et al: Effects of the prone position on respiratory mechanics and gas exchange during acute lung injury. Am J Respir Crit Care Med 1998;157:387-393.
165. Mure M, Martling C, Lindahl S: Dramatic effect on oxygenation in patients with severe acute lung insufficiency treated in the prone position. Crit Care Med 1997;25: 1539-1544.
166. Mancebo J, Fernandez R, Blanch L, et al: A multicenter trial of prolonged prone ventilation in severe acute respiratory distress syndrome. Am J Respir Crit Care Med 2006;173: 1233-1239.
167. Anzueto A, Baughman RP, Guntupalli KK, et al: Aerosolized surfactant in adults with sepsis induced ARDS. N Engl J Med 1996;22:1417-1421.
168. Spragg RG, Lewis JF, Walmrath HD, et al: Effect of recombinant surfactant protein C-based surfactant on the acute respiratory distress syndrome. N Engl J Med 2004;351:884-892.
169. Haas CF, Weg JG: Exogenous surfactant therapy: An update. Resp Care 1996;41:397-414.
170. The National Heart, Lung, and Blood Institute Acute Respiratory Distress Syndrome (ARDS) Clinical Trials Network. Effects of recruitment maneuvers in patients with acute lung injury and acute respiratory distress syndrome ventilated with high positive end-expiratory pressure. Crit Care Med 2003;31:2592-2597.
171. Lim C-M, Jung H, Koh Y, et al: Effect of alveolar recruitment maneuver in early acute respiratory distress syndrome according to antiderecruitment strategy, etiological category of diffuse lung injury, and body position of the patient. Crit Care Med 2003;31:411-418.
172. Pelosi P, Bottino N, Chiumello D, et al: Sigh in supine and prone position during acute respiratory distress syndrome. Am J Respir Crit Care Med 2003;167:521-527.
173. Gattinoni L, Vagginelli F, Carlesso E, et al: Decrease in P_{ACO_2} with prone position is predictive of improved outcome in acute respiratory distress syndrome. Crit Care Med 2003;31:2727-2733.
174. Guerin C, Gaillard S, Lemasson S, et al: Effect of systematic prone positioning in hypoxemic acute respiratory failure: A randomized controlled trial. JAMA 2004;292:2379-2387.
175. Griffiths MJD, Evans TW: Inhaled nitric oxide therapy in adults. N Engl J Med 2005;353:2683-2695.
176. Perkins GD, McAuley DF, Thickett DR, Gao F: The β-agonist lung injury trial (BALTI). Am J Respir Crit Care Med. 2006;173:281-287.
177. Kacmarek RM, Wiedemann HP, Lavin PT, et al: Partial liquid ventilation in adult patients with acute respiratory distress syndrome. Am J Respir Crit Care Med 2006;173:882-889.
178. Martin GS, Moss M, Wheeler AP, et al: A randomized, controlled trial of furosemide with or without albumin in hypoproteinemic patients with acute lung injury. Crit Care Med 2005;33:1681-1687.
179. Dellinger RP, Zimmerman JL, Taylor RW, et al: Effects of inhaled nitric oxide in patients with acute respiratory distress syndrome: Results of a randomized phase II trial. Crit Care Med 1998;26:15-23.
180. Taylor RW, Zimmerman JL, Dellinger RP, et al: Low-dose inhaled nitric oxide in patients with acute lung injury: A randomized controlled trial. JAMA 2004;291:1603-1609.
181. Marini JJ: Are recruiting maneuvers necessary when ventilating acute respiratory distress syndrome? Crit Care Med 2003;31:2701-2703.
182. Rossaint R, Falke KJ, Lopez F, et al: Inhaled nitric oxide for the adult respiratory distress syndrome. N Engl J Med 1993;328:399-405.
183. Luhr O, Nathorst-Westfelt U, Lundin S, et al: A retrospective analysis of nitric

oxide inhalation in patients with severe acute lung injury in Sweden and Norway. Acta Anaesthesiol Scand 1997;41:1238-1246.
184. Jantz MA, Sahn SA: Corticosteroids in acute respiratory failure. Am J Respir Crit Care Med 1999;160:1079-1100.
185. Hinshaw LB, Archer LT, Beller-Todd BK, et al: Survival of primates in lethal septic shock following delayed treatment with steroid. Circ Shock 1981;8:291-300.
186. Brigham KL, Bowers RE, McKeen CR: Methylprednisolone prevention of increased lung vascular permeability following endotoxemia in sheep. J Clin Invest 1981;67:1103-1110.
187. Hollenbach SJ, DeGuzman LR, Bellamy RF: Early administration of methylprednisolone promotes survival in rats with intra-abdominal sepsis. Circ Shock 1986;20:161-168.
188. Rinaldo JE, Dauber JH: Effect of methylprednisolone and ibuprofen, an nonsteroidal antiinflammatory agent, on bronchoalveolar inflammation following endotoxemia. Circ Shock 1985;16:195-203.
189. Metz CR, Sibbald WK: Anti-inflammatory therapy for acute lung injury. A review of animal and clinical studies. Chest 1991;100:1110-1119.
190. Bernard GR, Luce JM, Sprung CL, et al: High dose corticosteroids in patients with the adult respiratory distress syndrome. N Engl J Med 1987;317:1565-1570.
191. Luce JM, Montgomery AB, Marks JD, et al: Ineffectiveness of high-dose methylprednisolone in preventing parenchymal lung injury and improving mortality in patients with septic shock. Am Rev Respir Dis 1988;138:62-68.
192. Bone RC, Fisher Jr. CJ, Clemmer TP, et al: A controlled clinical trial of high-dose methylprednisolone in the treatment of severe sepsis and septic shock. N Engl J Med 1987;317:653-658.
193. Silverman HJ, Slotman G, Bone RC, et al: Effects of prostaglandin E_1 on oxygen delivery and consumption in patients with the adult respiratory distress syndrome. Chest 1990;98:405-410.
194. Holcroft JW, Vassar MJ, Weber CJ: Prostaglandin E_1 and survival in patients with the adult respiratory distress syndrome: A prospective trial. Ann Surg 1986;203:371-378.
195. Bone RC, Slotman G, Maunder R, et al: Randomized, double-blind, multicenter study of prostaglandin E_1 in patients with adult respiratory distress syndrome. Chest 1989;96:114-119.
196. Rinaldo JE, Pennock B: Effects of ibuprofen on endotoxin-induced alveolitis: Biphasic dose response and dissociation between inflammation and hypoxemia. Am J Med Sci 1986;291:29-38.
197. Balk RA, Jacobs RF, Tryka AF, et al: Ibuprofen effects on neutrophil function and acute lung injury. Crit Care Med 1988;16:1121-1127.
198. Parsons PE, Worthen GS, Moore EE, et al: The association of circulating endotoxin with the development of the adult respiratory distress syndrome. Am Rev Respir Dis 1989;140:294-301.
199. Fisher CJ, Dhainaut FA, Opal SM, et al: Recombinant human interleukin 1 receptor antagonist in the treatment of patients with sepsis syndrome. JAMA 1994;271:1836-1848.
200. Fink MP, O'Sullivan BP, Menconi MJ, et al: A novel leukotriene B_4-receptor antagonist in endotoxin shock: A prospective, controlled trial in a porcine model. Crit Care Med 1993;21:1825-1837.
201. Marra MN, Thornton MB, Snable JL, et al: Endotoxin-binding and neutralizing properties of recombinant bactericidal/permeability-increasing protein and monoclonal antibodies HA-1A and E5. Crit Care Med 1994;22:559-565.
202. Abraham E, Wunderink R, Silverman H, et al: Efficacy and safety of monoclonal antibody to human tumor necrosis factor α in patients with sepsis syndrome. JAMA 1995;273:934-941.
203. Abraham E, Baughman R, Fletcher E, et al: Liposomal prostaglandin E_1 (TLC C-53) in acute respiratory distress syndrome: A controlled, randomized, double-blind, multicenter clinical trial. Crit Care Med 1999;27:1478-1485.
204. Opal SM, Fisher CJ, Dhainaut J-FA, et al: Confirmatory interleukin-1 receptor antagonist trial in severe sepsis: A phase III, randomized, double-blind, placebo-controlled, multicenter trial. Crit Care Med 1997;25:1115-1124.
205. Reinhart K, Wiegand-Lohnert C, Grimminger F, et al: Assessment of the safety and efficacy of the monoclonal anti-tumor necrosis factor antibody-fragment, MAK 195F, in patients with sepsis and septic shock: A multicenter, randomized, placebo-controlled, dose-ranging study. Crit Care Med 1996;24:733-742.
206. McCloskey RV, Straube RC, Sanders C; the CHESS Trial Study Group: Treatment of septic shock with human monoclonal antibody HA-1A. Ann Intern Med 1994;121:1-5.
207. Abraham E, Anzueto A, Gutierrez G, et al: Double-blind randomized controlled trial of monoclonal antibody to human tumour necrosis factor in treatment of septic shock. Lancet 1998;351:929-933.
208. Abraham E, Glauser MP, Butler T, et al: p55 tumor necrosis factor receptor fusion protein in the treatment of patients with severe sepsis and septic shock. JAMA 1997;277:1531-1538.
209. Sörensen J, Kald B, Tagesson C, Lindahl M. Platelet-activating factor and phospholipase A_2 in patients with septic shock and trauma. Intensive Care Med 1994;20:555-561.
210. Bone RC, Balk RA, Fein AM; the E5 Sepsis Study Group: A second large controlled clinical study of E5, A monoclonal antibody to endotoxin: Results of a prospective, multicenter, randomized, controlled trial. Crit Care Med 1995;23:994-1005.
211. Greenman RL, Schein RM, Martin MA, et al: A controlled clinical trial of E-5 murine monoclonal IgM antibody to endotoxin in the treatment of gram-negative sepsis. JAMA 1991;266:1097-1102.
212. Angus DC, Birmingham MC, Balk RA, et al: E-5 murine monoclonal antiendotoxin antibody in gram-negative sepsis: A randomized controlled trial. JAMA 2000;283:1723-1730.
213. Ziegler EJ, Fisher CJ Jr, Sprung CL, et al: Treatment of gram negative bacteremia and septic shock with HA-1A human monoclonal antibody against endotoxin. A randomized, double-blind, placebo-controlled trial. N Engl J Med 1991;324:429-436.
214. Goldie AS, Fearon KCH, Ross JA, et al: Natural cytokine antagonists and endogenous antiendotoxin core antibodies in sepsis syndrome. JAMA 1995;274:172-177.
215. Zwissler B, Kemming G, Habler O, et al: Inhaled prostacyclin (PGI_2) versus inhaled nitric oxide in adult respiratory distress syndrome. Am J Respir Crit Care Med 1996;154:1671-1677.
216. Dhainaut JF, Tenaillon A, Hemmer M, et al: Confirmatory platelet-activating factor receptor antagonist trial in patients with severe gram negative bacterial sepsis: A phase III, randomized, double-blind, placebo-controlled, multicenter trial. Crit Care Med 1998;26:1963-1971.
217. Metzler M, Balk R, Schuster D, et al: An evaluation of recombinant human platelet activating factor acetylhydrolase (rPAF-AH) in patients at risk for developing acute respiratory distress syndrome (ARDS). Crit Care Med 1999;27:A85.
218. Zeni F, Freeman B, Natanson C: Anti-inflammatory therapies to treat sepsis and septic shock: A reassessment. Crit Care Med 1997;25;1095-1100.
219. Bernard GR, Wheeler AP, Arons MM, et al: A trial of antioxidants N-acetylcysteine and procysteine in ARDS. Chest 1997;112:164-172.
220. Hirschl RB, Pranikoff T, Wise C, et al: Initial experience with partial liquid ventilation in adult patients with the acute respiratory distress syndrome. JAMA 1996;275:383-389.
221. Bernard GR, Reines HD, Halushka PV, et al: Prostacyclin and thromboxane A2 formation is increased in human sepsis syndrome. Effects of cyclooxygenase inhibition. Am Rev Respir Dis 1991;144:1095-1101.
222. Bernard GR, Wheeler AP, Russell JA, et al: The effects of ibuprofen on the physiology and survival of patients with sepsis. N Engl J Med 1997;336:912-918.
223. Sprung CL, Caralis PV, Marcial EH, et al: The effects of high-dose corticosteroids in patients with septic shock: A prospective, controlled study. N Engl J Med 1984;311:1137-1143.
224. Annane D, Sebille V, Troche G, et al: A 3-level prognostic classification in septic shock based on cortisol levels and cortisol response to corticotropin. JAMA 2000;283:1038-1045.
225. Annane D, Sebille V, Bellissant E, et al: Effect of low doses of corticosteroids in septic shock patients with or without early acute respiratory distress syndrome. Crit Care Med 2006;34:22-30.
226. The ARDS clinical trials network: Randomized, placebo-controlled trial of lisofylline for early treatment of

acute lung injury and acute respiratory distress syndrome. Crit Care Med 2002;30:1-6.
227. Fourrier F, Chopin C, Huart JJ, et al: Double-blind, placebo-controlled trial of antithrombin III concentrates in septic shock with disseminated intravascular coagulation. Chest 1993;104:882-888.
228. Fourrier F, Chopin C, Goudemand J, et al: Septic shock, multiple organ failure, and disseminated intravascular coagulation. Compared patterns of antithrombin III, protein C, and protein S deficiencies. Chest 1992;101:816-823.
229. Goldfarb RD, Glock D, Johnson K, et al: Randomized, blinded, placebo-controlled trial of tissue factor pathway inhibitor in porcine septic shock. Shock 1998;10:258-264.
230. Bernard GR, Vincent JL, Laterre PF, et al: Efficacy and safety of recombinant human activated protein C for severe sepsis. N Engl J Med 2001;344:699-709.
231. Brochard L: Clinical trials in acute respiratory distress syndrome: What is ARDS? Crit Care Med 1999;27:1657-1658.
232. Jepsen S, Herlevson P, Knudsen P, et al: Antioxidant treatment with N-acetylcysteine during adult respiratory distress syndrome: A prospective, randomized, placebo-controlled study. Crit Care Med 1992;20:918-924.
233. Slotman GJ, Burchard KW, D'Arezzo A, et al:. Ketoconazole prevents acute respiratory failure in critically ill surgical patients. J Trauma 1988;28:648-654.
234. Yu M, Thomas G: A double-blind, prospective, randomized trial of ketoconazole, a thromboxane synthetase inhibitor, in the prophylaxis of the adult respiratory distress syndrome. Crit Care Med. 1993;21:1635-1642.
235. Wiedemann HP, Fisher CH, Kormara J, et al: Ketoconazole for early treatment of acute lung injury and acute respiratory distress syndrome. JAMA 2000;183:1995-2002.
236. Meduri GU, Headley AS, Golden E, et al: Effect of prolonged methylprednisolone therapy in unresolving acute respiratory distress syndrome: A randomized controlled trial. JAMA 1998;280:159-165.
237. Meduri GU, Chinn AJ, Leeper KV, et al: Corticosteroid rescue treatment of progressive fibroproliferation in late ARDS. Chest 1994;105:1516-1527.
238. The National Heart, Lung, and Blood Institute Acute Respiratory Distress Syndrome (ARDS) Clinical Trials Network. Efficacy and safety of corticosteroids for persistent acute respiratory distress syndrome. N Engl J Med 2006;354:1671-1684.
239. Bone RC, Balk R, Slotman G, et al: Adult respiratory distress syndrome: Sequence and importance of development of multiple organ failure. Chest 1992;101:320-326.
240. Bone RC, Balk RA, Cerra FB, et al: American College of Chest Physicians/Society of Critical Care Medicine Consensus Conference: Definitions for sepsis and organ failure and guidelines for the use of innovative therapies in sepsis. Chest 1992;101:1644-1655.
241. Suchyta MR, Clemmer TP, Orne JF Jr, et al: Increased survival of ARDS patients with severe hypoxemia (ECMO criteria). Chest 1991;99:951-955.
242. Montgomery AB, Stager MA, Carrico CJ, Hudson LD: Causes of mortality in patients with the adult respiratory distress syndrome. Am Rev Respir Dis 1985;132:485-489.
243. Milberg JA, Davis DR, Steinberg KP, Hudson LD: Improved survival of patients with acute respiratory distress syndrome (ARDS): 1983-1993. JAMA 1995;273:306-309.
244. Zapol WM, Snider MT, Hill JD, et al: Extracorporeal membrane oxygenation in severe acute respiratory failure. A randomized prospective study. JAMA 1979;242:2193-2196.
245. Fein AM, Lippman M, Holtzman H, et al: The risk factors, incidence, and prognosis or ARDS following septicemia. Chest 1983;83:40-42.
246. Faist E, Wichmann M, Kim C: Immunosuppression and immunomodulation in surgical patients. Curr Opin Crit Care 1997;3:293-298.
247. Cheung AM, Tansey CM, Tomlinson G, et al: Two-year outcomes, health care use, and costs of survivors of acute respiratory distress syndrome. Am J Respir Crit Care Med 2006;174:538-544.
248. Elliott CG: Pulmonary sequelae in survivors of the adult respiratory distress syndrome. Clin Chest Med 1990;11:789-800.
249. Peters JI, Bell RC, Prihoda TJ, et al: Clinical determinants of abnormalities in pulmonary functions in survivors of the adult respiratory distress syndrome. Am Rev Respir Dis 1989;139:1163-1168.
250. Herridge MS, Cheung Am, Tansey CM, et al: One year outcomes in survivors of the acute respiratory distress syndrome. N Engl J Med 2003;348:683-693.
251. Heyland DK, Groll D, Caeser M: Survivors of acute respiratory distress syndrome: Relationship between pulmonary dysfunction and long-term health-related quality of life. Crit Care Med 2005;33:1549-1556.
252. Angus DC, Musthafa AA, Clermont G, et al: Quality-adjusted survival in the first year after acute respiratory distress syndrome. Am J Respir Crit Care Med 2001;163:1389-1394.
253. Ely EW, Wheeler AP, Thompson BT, et al: Recovery rate and prognosis in older persons who develop acute lung injury and the acute respiratory distress syndrome. Ann Intern Med 2002;136:25-36.
254. Davidson TA, Caldwell ES, Curtis JR, et al: Reduced quality of life in survivors of acute respiratory distress syndrome compared with critically ill control patients. JAMA 1999;281:354-360.
255. Weinert CR, Gross CR, Kangas JR, et al: Health related quality of life after acute lung injury. Am J Respir Crit Care Med 1997;156:1120-1128.

Chapter 39

Life-Threatening Asthma

S. Sujanthy Rajaram and R. Phillip Dellinger

EPIDEMIOLOGY OF LIFE-THREATENING ASTHMA

In 2003, approximately 20 million Americans were diagnosed with asthma. Asthma ranks within the top 10 prevalent conditions causing limitation of activity, and an estimated annual health care cost of $16.1 billion was reported in 2004.[1,2] Prevalence of asthma in the United States is about 5%, and worldwide it is estimated to be 7.2% (10% children, 6% adults). In children, prevalence of asthma is higher in boys than in girls (3 : 2, 6 to 11 years old; 8 : 5, 12 to 17 years old), but in adults asthma is more prevalent in women.[2,3] Populations at risk for asthma and asthma-related deaths include racial and ethnic minorities. Patients in urban settings (lower socioeconomic status) have high risk for asthma and often have poorly controlled asthma.[4-6] A bimodal distribution of development of asthma places the risk greatest between 15 and 24 years old and older than 55 years.[7] African Americans have been reported to have a greater prevalence of asthma and greater likelihood of mortality from asthma compared with whites.[8,9]

TRIGGERS OF ACUTE ASTHMA

Common triggers for acute asthmatic attacks include air pollutants, respiratory tract infection, and allergen exposure. An association of panic-type anxiety and life-threatening asthma has been suggested. Box 39-1 contains a comprehensive list of precipitating factors.

MORTALITY FROM ASTHMA

In the 1960s, a global alarm was sounded when sharp epidemic increases in asthma death rates were reported.[10] Deaths approximately doubled in the United States from 1980 to 1995.[3] After a long period of steady increase, asthma mortality and morbidity rates have continued to decline for the past 4 years.[2]

Seasonal variations in asthma mortality have been reported.[11-13] In patients 5 to 44 years old, death from asthma peaks in the summer months, although hospitalizations peak during the winter months. In older asthmatic patients, a different distribution of mortality is seen, with hospitalizations and mortality peaking in the winter months. Older patients with asthma also have been shown to have fewer symptoms of dyspnea with methacholine-induced obstruction.[14]

Polynesians, African Americans, and black South Africans all have been reported to have higher asthma mortality rates. Likely reasons include genetic predisposition or poor management of severe asthma attacks because of reduced or delayed use of health care services and lower level of understanding. Self-medication also may play a role. Pendergraft and colleagues[15] reported among 29,430 admissions in the United States with a primary diagnosis of asthma, 10.1% were admitted to intensive care units (ICUs), and 2.1% were intubated. The risk of in-hospital death was significantly higher in patients who were intubated and with comorbidities.

Box 39-1

Precipitating Factors for Severe Asthma

Atopy: Genetic factors (inherited predisposition to allergic diseases)[16,140]
Environmental factors: Allergens—9% (e.g., dust mites, dog, cats, cockroaches)
Upper respiratory tract infection—23%
Allergic rhinitis[16]
Pneumonia—9%
Medications: Aspirin, nonsteroidal anti-inflammatory drugs; β-receptor blockers, angiotensin-converting enzyme inhibitors[16]
Premenstrual worsening; postmenopausal hormone replacement therapy[10,16]
Occupational asthma[16]
Inhaled irritants (e.g., heroin,[18,136] cocaine, smoking)
Reflux esophagitis
Sinusitis
Cold: viral infections[25,137]
Exercise
Emotional stress; strong association with panic disorder[138]
Tapering of steroids—3%
Noncompliance—32%

Data from references 4 and 8.

CLASSIFICATION

About 5% of asthma patients have "difficult asthma" (asthma difficult to control with maximal recommended doses of inhaled medications, in particular inhaled corticosteroids). Most of these patients meet the criteria for severe asthma or may have chronic mild or moderate disease with acute exacerbations.[16] Two clinical patterns of life-threatening asthma have been reported.[17] A more serious type is the slow onset of life-threatening asthma characterized by onset over days to weeks, copious amounts of mucoid secretions with intense eosinophilic infiltration, and resistance to bronchodilator therapy. This is described as "slow onset–late arrival," or type 1, pattern and accounts for 80% to 85% of fatal asthma.[18,19] Sudden-type asthma is characterized by onset over hours with acute deterioration, absence of large quantities of airway secretions with no mucous plugs but neutrophil infiltration of the submucosa, typically a marked response to bronchodilators, and quick recovery in most circumstances. This is described as "sudden asphyxic asthma," or type 2, scenario of asthma death. Sudden-type asthma accounts for about 15% to 20% of fatal asthma.[18,19]

PATHOPHYSIOLOGY AND IMMUNOLOGY

The pathophysiologic processes leading to pulmonary function abnormalities in severe life-threatening asthma are bronchial smooth muscle contraction, bronchial inflammation–associated mucosal edema, and mucous plugging. Obstruction of air flow leads to low ventilation-perfusion areas and hypoxemia.[20] Expiratory obstruction decreases forced expiratory volume in the first second (FEV_1). The hallmark of asthma is a decreased FEV_1/forced vital capacity (FVC) ratio. A severely asthmatic individual is unable to complete expiration because of expiratory airway resistance and tachypnea-induced limited expiratory time leading to air trapping and an increasing functional residual capacity and a decreased FVC. The hyperinflation produces increased work of breathing. Edema and increased airway secretions also compromise inspiratory flow and, when combined with hyperinflation, often lead to high peak inspiratory pressures in a patient whose lungs are being mechanically ventilated. The cause of respiratory arrest in asthmatics is usually failure of the inspiratory muscles with ventilatory arrest.

Manthous and Goulding[21] studied the effect of intravascular volume status on deadspace fraction in mechanically ventilated patients with severe asthma. They noted a mean increase in deadspace ventilation of 4.2% in response to intravascular volume expansion with 250 to 500 mL of normal saline solution.

Characteristic findings of fatal asthma are airways showing infiltration with neutrophils and eosinophils, degranulated mast cells, sub–basement membrane thickening, loss of epithelial cell integrity, occlusion of bronchial lumen by mucus, hyperplasia and hypertrophy of bronchial smooth muscle, and hyperplasia of goblet cells. Asthma is an inflammatory response evidenced by the presence of cytokines that mediate inflammation and chemotactic chemokines in bronchoalveolar lavage fluid and pulmonary secretions. Some cytokines initiate inflammatory response by activating transcription factors, which act on genes that encode inflammatory cytokines, chemokines, adhesion molecules, and other proteins that induce and perpetuate inflammation. Adhesion molecules provide a mechanism for the adhesion of inflammatory cells to the endothelium and migration of these cells from the circulation into the lamina propria, epithelium, and the airway lumen itself.[22]

Busse and colleagues[23] described the immunology of allergic inflammation in asthma. IgE antibodies are linked to the severity of asthma. The release of cytokines depends on cross-linking of IgE by allergen. IgE antibodies are synthesized and released by B cells; briefly circulate in the blood; and bind to high-affinity IgE receptors on the surface of mast cells in tissues and peripheral blood basophils and low-affinity IgE receptors on lymphocytes, eosinophils, platelets, and macrophages.

The early phase of asthma (usually resolves within 1 hour) is characterized by inhaled allergen precipitating acute constriction of smooth muscles by release of histamines and leukotrienes from mast cells. A prolonged late phase (4 to 6 hours later) occurs as a result of cytokines and chemokines generated by resident inflammatory cells (mast cells, macrophages, epithelial cells) and recruited inflammatory cells (lymphocytes, eosinophils) and causes further obstruction of airflow. Numerous cytokines regulate the function of eosinophils and other cells in asthma. Interferon-γ is elevated in severe asthma during the acute phase. Data also suggest that interferon-γ contributes to the activation of eosinophils and likely augments inflammation. There are two types of helper $CD4^+$ T lymphocyte cells. Type 1 helper (Th1) T cells produce interleukin (IL)-2 and interferon-γ, which are essential for cellular defense mechanisms. Type 2 helper (Th2) T cells produce cytokines (IL-4, IL-5, IL-6, IL-9, and IL-13) that mediate allergic inflammation.[24] Balance between the Th1-type and Th2-type cytokine response contributes to the cause and evolution of atopic diseases, including asthma. The increasing prevalence of asthma in Western countries has led to the "hygiene hypothesis."[25,26] The immune system in newborns is primarily Th2 cells, and a timely and appropriate environmental stimulus is needed to create a balanced immune response. Alteration in the number of infections in early life, widespread use of antibiotics, adoption of the Western lifestyle, and repeated exposure to allergens may affect the balance between Th1-type and Th2-type cytokine responses and increase the likelihood of immune response by Th2 cells and lead to asthma.[22] Evidence continues to underscore the importance of immune factors in the development of asthma and resulting inflammatory process. This particular strategy and insight into the mechanisms of these processes would be important for future treatment of acute severe asthma.[27]

Asthma Genetics

Asthma and atopy are complex phenotypes that are influenced by genetic and environmental factors. About 79 genes have been associated with asthma or atopy phenotype. ADAM-33 gene has been associated with asthma. A locus on the short arm of chromosome 20 has been linked to asthma and bronchial hyperresponsiveness. If further investigations confirm that ADAM-33 is an asthma gene, future studies should enhance understanding of asthma and lead to new therapeutic targets.[28] As Ober and Hoffjan[29] described, such "molecular phenotyping" of patients with asthma and atopic diseases may generate informed decisions regarding treatment, laying the foundation for genomic medicine in the next decade.

SYMPTOMS AND SIGNS

Wheezing may be expiratory and inspiratory and correlates with the degree of obstruction if adequate air movement is present.[21] Absence of wheezing is an ominous finding in a severely distressed asthmatic patient because it implies minimal air movement and is a harbinger of respiratory arrest. Contraction of the sternocleidomastoid muscles and other accessory muscles indicates severe obstruction ($FEV_1 < 1$).[30] Intense inspiratory effort leads to large swings in intrathoracic pressure and to an accentuated pulsus paradoxus (representing a decreased stroke volume during inspiration). Pulsus paradoxus is often appreciated during routine blood pressure measurement in acute severe bronchospasm because systolic blood pressure decreases dramatically during inspiration (this decrease is <10 mm Hg in normal individuals).[31] A decrease of more than 15 mm Hg in a patient in an acute asthma episode is associated with severe reduction in FEV_1.

Ominous signs and findings during an acute severe asthma episode include diaphoresis, inability to recline or talk, peak expiratory flow rate (PEFR) less than 60 L/min, and use of accessory muscles. In acute severe asthma, lung hyperinflation occurs secondary to increased expiratory airflow resistance, short expiratory time, high ventilatory demands, and increased postinspiratory activity of the inspiratory muscles. The presence of these factors in variable degrees does not allow the respiratory cycle to reach a static equilibrium volume at the end of expiration. Inspiration begins at a volume in which the respiratory system exhibits a positive elastic recoil pressure called intrinsic positive-end expiratory pressure (PEEP), or auto-PEEP. This phenomenon is described as dynamic hyperinflation. Dynamic hyperinflation produces a significant decrease in systemic venous return to the heart, leading to a decrease in left ventricular diastolic filling. Also problematic is the increase in left ventricular afterload as a result of large negative intrathoracic pressure swings during inspiration. Pulmonary artery pressure also may be increased secondary to lung hyperinflation resulting in increased right ventricular afterload. These events combine to produce pulsus paradoxus.[18]

All that wheezes is not asthma. Other entities to consider are upper airway obstruction and "cardiac asthma." Upper airway obstruction should be considered in patients at risk (e.g., tracheal stenosis in patients who were previously intubated) and when there is no response to therapy in a patient with no history of asthma. If the patient's status would tolerate it, flow volume loops may be diagnostic. Likewise, wheezing that dissipates with intubation should make one suspect upper airway obstruction. Paradoxical vocal cord movement can stimulate asthma.[32] Patients with acute left ventricular failure may wheeze as a result of interstitial fluid compression of bronchioles and edema-associated bronchiolar smooth muscle contraction.[33]

OBJECTIVE MEASUREMENT OF OBSTRUCTION

During an asthmatic attack, all indices of expiratory flow are significantly reduced, including FEV_1; FEV_1/FVC; PEFR; maximal expiratory flows at 75% (MEF_{75}), 50% (MEF_{50}), and 25% of vital capacity (MEF_{25}); and maximal expiratory flow between 25% and 75% of the FVC ($MEF_{25\text{-}75}$). With acute asthmatic crisis, high functional residual capacity, total lung capacity, and residual volume are observed.[18]

Although spirometry is the best objective measure of airway obstruction, a severely ill asthmatic patient is rarely able to perform the necessary full FVC maneuver. Objective assessment of airway obstruction in a severe asthmatic usually can be made by measuring the PEFR because this measurement requires patient cooperation only in the early part of the FVC maneuver. Because the greatest expiratory flow rates exist in early expiration, most patients are able to produce a reliable PEFR value. Normal expiratory flow rates vary considerably with age, sex, and height. In adults, a PEFR less than 100 to 125 L/min implies severe obstruction to air flow. Failure to improve PEFR significantly with initial aggressive bronchodilator therapy is the best predictor of morbidity in a patient with acute severe asthma.

LABORATORY AND RADIOGRAPHIC DATA

Asymmetric breath sounds or chest pain should alert the physician to the possibility of pneumothorax and mandates an early chest radiograph. An increased white blood cell count may be produced by asthma alone in the absence of infection; β-receptor agonists and theophylline shift potassium intracellularly. Hypokalemia-induced dysrhythmias could occur after intensive bronchodilator therapy in elderly patients or in patients receiving other therapies that predispose to hypokalemia, such as steroidal and diuretic medications. Creatine phosphokinase (non-MB fraction) may be increased as a result of the strenuous activity of ventilatory muscles.[34] Severe asthma may cause right-sided heart strain as shown on electrocardiogram; this resolves with clinical improvement. Arterial blood gas assessment adds little to the early management of acute asthma. The early stage of asthma usually reveals mild hypoxemia, hypocapnia, and respiratory alkalosis. A non–anion gap acidosis also may be observed in patients with severe asthma if several days of hyperventilation have led to renal compensation with bicarbonate wasting to compensate for the respiratory alkalosis. As the severity of obstruction increases, arterial carbon dioxide ($Pa{CO_2}$) normalizes and then increases as a sign of impending respiratory collapse. After initial therapy, arterial blood gases may be useful for decisions regarding hospital admission or tracheal intubation. Most asthma patients respond dramatically to initial therapy; arterial blood gases obtained when the patient is first seen are rarely predictive of outcome or useful clinically.

Early attention should be directed toward aggressive therapeutic intervention. A normal $Pa{CO_2}$ level in a distressed asthmatic patient despite aggressive in-hospital therapy should alert the physician to respiratory fatigue and the danger of respiratory arrest. Respiratory acidosis may be preceded by a lactate-induced anion gap metabolic acidosis.[35] This lactic acidosis is likely caused by a combination of failing inspiratory muscles, aggressive use of β-agonist therapy, and decreased liver perfusion resulting from increased intrathoracic pressure and blood flow diverted to the muscles of respiration. Lactic acidosis occurs more commonly in men and with administration of parenteral β-agonists.[36,37]

INPATIENT ADMISSION DECISIONS

Conditions typically requiring hospitalization for a patient with severe asthma are listed in Box 39-2.

Box 39-2

Conditions Typically Requiring Hospitalization for a Patient with Severe Asthma

Acute respiratory acidosis despite aggressive bronchodilator therapy
Pneumonia
Pneumothorax
Initial PEFR<60 L/min (assumes full cooperation)
Inability to raise PEFR to 200 L/min despite aggressive therapy
Inability to boost baseline bronchodilator regimen
Multiple visits to emergency department for severe asthma attack
History of tracheal intubation or ICU admission because of asthma[37,73,140]

PEFR, peak expiratory flow rate.

DRUG THERAPY

Oxygen

If pulse oximetry confirms the presence of hypoxemia, oxygen should be given to maintain oxygen saturation at greater than 92%.[10] A transient decrease in arterial oxygen tension has been shown in some patients after initiation of β-adrenergic agonist therapy in severe asthma.[38] Mechanisms of this decrease relate to some combination of β_2-induced vasodilation in areas of decreased ventilation and increase in pulmonary blood flow resulting from a β_1 inotropic and chronotropic effect. Saturation may decrease initially during bronchodilator therapy with β-agonists, which produce vasodilation and may increase intrapulmonary shunting.[39] Studies in children suggest that aerosolized salbutamol administration may cause hypoxemia during acute episodes of asthma if the drug is administered without oxygen. Most published data show that salbutamol does not have a clinically important effect on oxygenation in asthmatic adults. This seems to be true for stable and acute asthma; however, these studies in adults exclude the most severe exacerbations more likely to be associated with marked hypoxemia.[40] Because inhaled β-agonist should be given in this circumstance, the only clinical response is to treat any worsening of oxygenation that occurs with additional oxygen.

Moloney and colleagues[41] showed that bronchoconstriction induced by dry air challenge can be prevented by humidifying inspired air. Humidification of inspired air should be achieved with a heated cascade humidifier. The use of heat and moisture exchangers is discouraged because they increase the deadspace and add to the expiratory airway resistance.[41]

β-Adrenergic Therapy

Inhaled β_2-Selective Agonist (Albuterol or Salbutamol)

Albuterol is the cornerstone of treatment for acute exacerbation in patients with acute asthma. Initial therapy in an acutely ill asthma patient, as recommended by the National Asthma Education and Prevention Program Update,[27] is 2.5 to 5 mg of albuterol (0.5 to 1 mL of 0.5% solution in 5 mL of normal saline solution) by nebulization every 20 minutes for three doses (for optimal delivery, dilute aerosols to a minimum of 3 mL at gas flow of 6 to 8 L/min), followed by 2.5 to 10 mg every 1 to 4 hours as needed, or 10-15 mg/h continuously, and the titration is based on response and severity of symptoms. Continuous nebulization should be considered in the most severe patients.[33,38,39] Tachycardia and hypokalemia may occur with continuously nebulized albuterol.[43] β_2-selective agents delivered parenterally or orally lose much of the β_2 selectivity, which provides the rationale for inhalation treatment as the cornerstone of therapy.

Adequate delivery of β-agonists can be accomplished by a metered-dose inhaler (MDI) with spacer during acute bronchospasm if proper technique is used and doses are increased. Four puffs of albuterol (0.36 mg) delivered with a spacer should be expected to be equipotent to 2.5 mg of albuterol by nebulization in patients with severe disease. It is advisable to deliver the β-agonist by nebulization in most acutely ill asthma patients because nebulization requires minimal coordination and cooperation of the patient and less bedside instruction and supervision by health care professionals. Many randomized controlled clinical studies over the last several decades have compared β-agonists delivered by MDIs or by nebulizer. Most studies show similar responses.[44-48] Protocols typically include methods that ensure proper use of the MDI, however. Greater amounts of drug delivery are required with nebulized therapy to produce the same effect as that seen with an MDI with a spacer. To initiate therapy with nebulized albuterol and then switch to an MDI with spacer after the patient has improved and stabilized may be cost-effective.[49,50] When aerosol β-agonists are delivered in intubated patients and patients receiving mechanical ventilatory support, much of the physiologic effect is lost as a result of deposition onto the endotracheal tube.[50] Doubling the dose that would be used in a nonintubated patient is recommended.

Aggressive inhaled β-agonist therapy is preferred to intravenous albuterol because the same end point usually can be achieved with less risk for toxicity.[51] Intravenous albuterol (if available) may be considered as an alternative when patients with life-threatening asthma have failed to respond to inhaled therapy. Oral β_2-selective agents should not be used as primary treatment for patients with acute asthma because the therapeutic-to-toxicity ratio is less than with inhaled agents. Effects of corticosteroids and β_2-agonists on airflow obstruction may be additive.

Levalbuterol, 0.63 mg, is equivalent to racemic albuterol, 1.25 mg, for efficacy and side effects. Levalbuterol is available as 0.63 mg/3 mL and 1.25 mg/3 mL nebulizer solutions. The recommended adult dose of levalbuterol is 1.25 to 2.5 mg every 20 minutes for three doses, then 1.25 to 5 mg every 1 to 4 hours as needed, or 5 to 7.5 mg/h continuous nebulization.[27]

Subcutaneous β-Agonist Therapy (Epinephrine or Terbutaline)

Subcutaneous β-agonist therapy has a disadvantageous therapeutic-to-toxicity ratio compared with inhaled β_2-selective agonists. Although there is no proven value of systemic therapy over aerosol therapy, rapid delivery of β-agonists to the airway may be beneficial in seriously ill asthmatic patients who are at imminent risk for respiratory arrest or in need of intubation and at low risk for β-agonist cardiac toxicity (young asthmatics). In this circumstance, a combination of inhaled and subcutaneously administered β-agonists may be useful.[52] The subcutaneous epinephrine dose for adults is 0.3 to 0.5 mL of a 1:1000 dilution(1 mg/mL), depending on age and weight; it may be repeated in the initial management every 20 minutes for three times. An alternative subcutaneous β-agonist agent is subcutaneous terbutaline, 0.25 mg, which can be repeated every 20 minutes for three doses.[27,39] When subcutaneous terbutaline is compared with subcutaneous epinephrine, equal cardiac side effects are seen.[53] No clinical studies document benefit of subcutaneous terbutaline over subcutaneous epinephrine. Terbutaline is, however, the parenteral agent of choice in pregnancy. β_1-adrenergic stimulators are given subcutaneously with caution to the elderly and to patients with documented or suspected coronary artery disease.

Anecdotal reports have suggested the success of epinephrine administration through the endotracheal tube after respiratory arrest from asthma.[54] Prospective trials are needed in this area. Despite the lack of confirmatory studies, in an asthma patient with respiratory arrest, it may be considered.

Corticosteroids

Corticosteroids are an essential part of in-hospital asthma therapy. The National Institutes of Health expert panel recommendation is intravenous methylprednisolone, 120 to 180 mg/d in three or four divided doses for 48 hours, for patients admitted to the hospital, with tapering as clinically tolerated, typically 60 to 80 mg/day until peak expiratory flow reaches 70% of predicted or personal best.[55] Numerous clinical studies have shown benefit of corticosteroids in treating patients admitted to the hospital with acute severe asthma.[56-58] The typical initial adult dose of methylprednisolone is 125 mg (dose range 40-250 mg).[39,59] No differences in clinical effects between oral and intravenous forms of corticosteroid therapy have been proved.[60]

Some trials show improvement following initiation of steroids after a patient's condition was refractory to initial therapy. Others show benefit when corticosteroid therapy is initiated early in the course of an acute asthma episode. Most corticosteroid benefit is thought to be delayed for approximately 6 hours, although a potential for earlier beneficial effect has been postulated. The delay in effect may reflect the time necessary for steroids to induce upregulation of new β_2-receptors and reversal of β_2-receptor desensitization and downregulation. Some patients show corticosteroid resistance. Numerous studies have evaluated corticosteroid dose in treatment of acute severe asthma.

In a hospitalized asthma patient, intravenous dose selection should be between 40 and 125 mg given intravenously every 6 hours for the first day. We typically initiate a dose of 60 mg of methylprednisolone every 6 hours in hospitalized asthmatic patients. Dose reduction should be targeted to clinical response, with conversion to oral steroids as the patient improves. Potential benefits of corticosteroids are listed in Box 39-3.

Inhaled Anticholinergic Therapy with Ipratropium

Although ipratropium achieves less bronchodilation at peak effect than β-agonist and less predictable clinical response, the effect is likely to be additive to albuterol. Most published evidence supports the addition of ipratropium to inhaled β-agonist therapy for admitted acute asthma patients. It produces clinically modest improvement in lung function compared with albuterol alone.[61] Although some studies have failed to show benefit from the addition of ipratropium, most single studies and a meta-analysis support combined therapy.[62-73]

The National Institutes of Health expert panel's recommended dose of ipratropium is 0.5 mg by nebulizer every 30 minutes for three doses, then every 2 to 4 hours as needed.[74] Onset of action is slow (20 minutes), with peak effectiveness at 60 to 90 minutes and no systemic side effects.[39] A hand-held mouthpiece nebulizer system should be used for nebulization because contamination of the ocular area with precipitation of narrow-angle glaucoma may occur in susceptible individuals if a facemask is used for delivery of an anticholinergic agent. Ipratropium may be combined with the nebulized albuterol dose. The deposition of ipratropium may be enhanced, however, when it follows albuterol-induced bronchodilation. In a patient with severe asthma, ipratropium may produce a clinically significant response within minutes of administration, as opposed to the longer delay to response in chronic obstructive pulmonary disease patients with chronic stable disease. If ipratropium is delivered by MDI (0.018 mg/puff), 4 to 8 puffs per treatment is recommended.

Theophylline

Theophylline is an effective bronchodilator compared with placebo in patients with acute bronchospasm. Inhaled β-agonists are accepted to be superior to theophylline as single agents for acute bronchospasm. Consensus opinion and meta-analysis support no significant additive clinical benefit with the addition of theophylline to a full course of inhaled β-agonists.[75] Although a few studies have shown physiologic benefits evident at 24 or 48 hours,[76,77] the addition of theophylline to high-dose inhaled β-agonist and corticosteroid therapy in patients with acute severe asthma seems to offer no clear-cut or substantial clinical benefit.[78,79] Because theophylline toxicity is a potential problem, the use of theophylline should be limited to patients who are already on theophylline at the time of admission or patients with life-threatening asthma who fail to respond to other therapy after admission. If the decision is made to use theophylline, the guidelines in Box 39-4 may be useful. Methylxanthines are infrequently used for acute asthma because of unpredictable pharmacokinetics and known side effects.[39]

Magnesium Sulfate

Magnesium has multifactorial actions relative to potential reversal of bronchoconstriction, which is based on characteristics of inhibition of the calcium channel and decreased acetylcholine release. Hashimoto and colleagues[80] showed that 40% of asthmatic patients exhibited magnesium deficiency, and that low magnesium erythrocyte concentrations reflected decreased magnesium stores in patients with bronchial asthma.

A Cochrane meta-analysis concluded that use of intravenous magnesium sulfate improves pulmonary function and decreases hospital admissions in acute severe asthma,

Box 39-3

Potential Benefits of Corticosteroids in the Treatment of Asthma

- Enhancement of β_2-receptor responsiveness by upregulating β_2-receptors on airway smooth muscle
- Decrease in capillary basement membrane permeability; decrease vascular leak from endothelial cells
- Decreased leukocyte attachment; decreased number of eosinophils, mast cells, and dendritic cells
- Modulation of calcium migration intracellularly
- Reduction in airway mucus production
- Suppression of IgE receptor binding
- Interruption of arachidonic acid inflammatory pathways
- Decreased airway smooth muscle contraction, mucosal edema, and airway inflammation
- Airway remodeling
- Decreased cytokine and mediator production from epithelial cells

Box 39-4

Guidelines for Theophylline Use

- If the patient has not been receiving a theophylline preparation, a loading dose of aminophylline 5 mg/kg over 15 to 30 minutes is recommended.
- After the loading dose is given, administer aminophylline by continuous infusion with an infusion pump at a rate of 0.6 mg/kg/h.
- Factors that decrease aminophylline clearance and necessitate a reduction of continuous infusion rates include cimetidine use, macrolide use, congestive heart failure, and liver disease.
- Do not use theophylline in the presence of tachyarrhythmia.
- All patients who have been receiving a theophylline preparation should have a theophylline level determined before the loading dose is administered.
- Target a therapeutic range of serum theophylline of 6 to 12 μg/mL to minimize risk for toxicity. A 1 mg/kg intravenous aminophylline dose increases the serum concentration by approximately 2 μg/mL, with considerable scatter.

particularly in patients with severe exacerbations.[81] Inhaled magnesium sulfate improves pulmonary function during acute exacerbations of asthma, although it fails to show alterations in clinically important outcomes, such as hospital admissions.[34] Magnesium sulfate can improve pulmonary function modestly[82] and when dosed appropriately has no significant side effect profile.

Traditionally, 2 g of magnesium sulfate is administered over 20 minutes. Repeat doses, if used, require careful monitoring of magnesium levels and assessment for clinical manifestations of toxicity. Magnesium therapy should be avoided in the presence of renal insufficiency.

Heliox

Heliox (mixture of helium and oxygen optimally effective at a 70:30 mix) has been shown to improve the delivery and deposition of nebulized albuterol. If a patient requires more than 30% oxygen, it cannot be used. Heliox may be useful in acute severe asthma refractory to conventional treatment. There are no data to support the use of heliox as the initial treatment for acute severe asthma.[83,84] Heliox is available in mixtures of 60:40, 70:30, and 80:20. Helium is less dense than air and can be delivered through a tight-fitting nonrebreathing mask or, in an intubated patient, through the ventilatory circuit. Heliox results in decreased large airway resistance. One might anticipate that the role of heliox would be limited by the fact that heliox improves flow in large turbulent airways, and most of the obstruction in asthma is in the peripheral airways. Studies have nonetheless shown the ability of heliox to decrease inspiratory and expiratory resistance in severe asthma. Its potential to decrease PEEP not set on the ventilator (auto-PEEP) might be particularly useful. Heliox may augment carbon dioxide removal by facilitating carbon dioxide movement across the endothelial-epithelial barrier compared with the presence of a mixture of oxygen and nitrogen as the carrier gas. Heliox also has been shown to improve oxygenation, which may allow higher helium concentrations to be delivered.[85]

Other

Antibiotics

Antibiotic therapy in an asthma patient is indicated only if bacterial infection is present. The Telithromycin, Chlamydophilia, and Asthma (TELECAST) study[86] reported that, in patients presenting for unscheduled care because of an acute asthma exacerbation, treatment with telithromycin showed a significant improvement in FEV_1 over placebo at the end of a 10-day treatment period. One of the primary efficacy end points, improvement in asthma symptom scores, was significantly greater in the telithromycin group than placebo.[86] An editorial by Little[87] points to the possible anti-inflammatory effects of macrolides in the treatment of asthma, but stops short of recommending this as standard therapy at this time.

Fluids

If the patient is volume depleted, normal saline or lactated Ringer's solution is used to re-establish adequate intravenous volume. There is no evidence that excess volume replacement liquefies or facilitates loosening of secretions. Chest physiotherapy and other maneuvers to mobilize secretions physically also are not recommended.[88] Nebulization of acetylcysteine is not indicated and may irritate the airways. Saline solution and acetylcysteine have been successfully used as part of bronchial lavage with fiberoptic bronchoscopy in patients with severe asthma.

Ketamine

Ketamine is an intravenous analgesic agent that has bronchodilator properties, but may stimulate bronchial secretions and may cause tachycardia, hypertension, delirium, and lowering of seizure threshold.[89] So far no trials have been published to prove its effectiveness.[39] When intubation of a severe acute asthmatic is required, and in the absence of hypertension and known seizure disorder, however, it seems an optimal induction agent. It also may be used in life-threatening situations where conventional therapy has failed.

Leukotriene Antagonists

Leukotriene antagonists improve lung function and are often used in the management of chronic asthma, but their role in acute asthma is unclear.

Omalizumab (Anti-IgE Antibody)

Recombinant anti-IgE antibody (omalizumab) improves asthma control in severely allergic asthmatics, reducing inhaled steroids and rescue medication requirement and improving asthma-related quality of life.[90] Its role in acute severe asthma is unstudied. The delay in onset of effect likely makes its impact less likely.

Strunk and Bloomberg[91] reported patients likely to benefit from omalizumab are patients with evidence of sensitization to perennial aeroallergens who require high doses of inhaled corticosteroids that have a potential for adverse effects, patients with frequent exacerbations of asthma, and patients with severe disease-related noncompliance. Total IgE levels should be measured in all patients, and the recommended dose, 0.016 mg/kg body weight per international unit of IgE every 4 weeks, should be administered subcutaneously at 2- or 4-week intervals.[91] Strunk and Bloomberg[91] recommended adding omalizumab in a compliant patient with severe asthma, after a trial of leukotriene modifiers or extended-release theophylline proved ineffective.

NONTRADITIONAL THERAPY OF SEVERE BRONCHOSPASM

Asthmatic patients who fail to respond to conventional therapy should be considered for nontraditional therapy. Nontraditional treatment alternatives include intensification of β-agonist therapy beyond routinely recognized standards, general anesthetic agents, and bronchial lavage. Continuous intravenous albuterol has been used in Europe, but is unavailable in the United States. It is unlikely that it adds any additional benefit over increasing the aggressiveness of treatment with inhaled bronchodilators. Intravenous isoproterenol and terbutaline have been used in children, but are not recommended in adults.

In a patient with refractory severe asthma who is receiving mechanical ventilatory support, anecdotal success with isoflurane or halothane anesthesia, intravenous thiopental, and rectally administered ether has been reported.[92-95] Intravenous ketamine has the potential for administration in the ICU and is likely the best alternative for anesthetic therapy.[96] Que and Lusaya[97] anecdotally showed significant improvement when using sevoflurane induction for emergency cesarean section in a woman with severe life-threatening asthma. Maternal and neonatal outcome were good. Propofol has been reported to relax smooth muscle in arteries and veins, and bronchodilator effect has been suggested.[98,99] A case series report showed temporally related improvement in severe asthmatic bronchospasm after propofol infusion.[100]

Although anecdotal success has been reported, critically ill mechanically ventilated asthmatic patients are poor candidates for bronchial lavage because the procedure itself would exacerbate auto-PEEP and decrease oxygenation.[101-103] The procedure is likely to produce a significant increase in auto-PEEP and worsening of hypoxemia. Anecdotal success has been shown with the use of plasma exchange in refractory life-threatening status asthmaticus in pregnancy.[103] The measurement of preplasma and postplasma exchange complement factors and immunoglobulin revealed 50% elimination. Glucagon, a rapid-acting smooth muscle relaxant with a short half-life, also has been studied for potential benefit in acute severe asthma.[105] In a small study of 21 glucagon-treated (0.03 mg/kg) patients and 25 placebo-treated patients, no differences were found. Successful bronchodilation was defined as a PEFR increase of 60 L/ min at 10 minutes. Standard bronchodilator therapy also was administered. Finally, rapid improvement in a mechanically ventilated asthma patient refractory to medical therapy was temporally related to addition of 15 ppm of inhaled nitric oxide to the inspiratory circuit.[106]

ACUTE SEVERE ASTHMA IN PREGNANCY

Asthma complicates 3% to 12% of pregnancies and is perhaps the most common serious medical problem to complicate pregnancy.[107,108] Exacerbations occur in approximately 20% of all pregnant women with asthma and can occur any time during gestation, but tend to occur late in the second trimester. Acute attacks of asthma during labor are rare.[108] Simultaneous management of the mother and the fetus is a challenge. The goal in approaching a pregnant patient with severe asthma is to prevent maternal hypoxemia.[19]

Studies of pregnancy-associated asthma reveal an increased incidence of maternal and fetal complications, which include preeclampsia, perinatal mortality, low birth weight, and preterm infants.[109] The risk of uncontrolled asthma is considered to outweigh any risk associated with the use of recommended medications for asthma. It is important that a physician skilled in the management of asthma be involved in the patient's care. Uterine contractions are common during asthma exacerbation and usually do not progress to preterm labor. When more than one β-adrenergic tocolytic agent is being administered simultaneously (systemically and inhaled), the possibility of excessive systemic effects should be considered. This is particularly true as it pertains to maternal and fetal tachycardia. One study compared perinatal outcomes in 259 pregnant women treated with inhaled β_2-adrenergic agonists with 101 pregnant women with asthma not treated with inhaled β_2-agonists and with 295 pregnant women without asthma and found no difference in rates of perinatal mortality, congenital malformations, preterm delivery, or delivery of low-birth-weight infants.[110] There also were no differences in Apgar scores, rates of complications of labor or delivery, or postpartum bleeding.

Cydulka and colleagues[111] found that pregnant women with asthma exacerbation were less likely to receive oral steroid treatment in the emergency department on discharge than nonpregnant women with asthma. In addition, at 2-week follow-up, pregnant women were almost three times more likely to report ongoing exacerbation. More recent studies show oral steroid use associated with an increased risk of preterm delivery, although it is difficult to separate the effect of the medication from the effect of exacerbation.[112]

Asthma exacerbations have the potential to lead to severe problems for the fetus. During pregnancy, asthma exacerbations should be managed aggressively. During pregnancy, acute severe asthma is treated initially with inhaled short-acting β-agonist by MDI or nebulizer, one to three doses in the first hour; oxygen; and if no response, oral systemic corticosteroids. If there is severe exacerbation of asthma (PEFR<50%), β-agonist could be given continuously or every 20 minutes, combined with inhaled ipratropium bromide. Fetal assessment and monitoring should be done until the patient is stabilized. To control asthma, there are limited data using leukotriene receptor antagonists in humans during pregnancy, although reassuring animal data are available. Studies and clinical evidence confirm safety of theophylline at recommended doses (to serum concentrations of 5 to 12 μg/mL) during pregnancy. There were higher levels of reported side effects and discontinuation of the medication, however. The experimental animal studies confirm the association of high-dose theophylline and adverse pregnancy outcomes in animals.[113]

MECHANICAL VENTILATION IN ASTHMA PATIENTS

Indications

Kearney and coworkers[114] examined the requirement for mechanical ventilation in severely asthmatic patients in a single hospital that used standardized guidelines for deciding on institution of mechanical ventilation. They concluded that over time there was an increased percentage of severe asthma cases requiring mechanical ventilation, but morbidity and mortality had decreased in this group.

Endotracheal intubation should be strongly considered at the time of presentation if the patient has central cyanosis, mental status changes, or a depressed level of consciousness. Inability to oxygenate or ventilate the lungs of an asthmatic patient adequately mandates tracheal intubation. A sustained respiratory rate greater than 40 breaths per minute may imply impending respiratory fatigue and mandates consideration of tracheal intubation. Zimmerman and associates[115] evaluated 69 consecutive patients admitted to the hospital who received tracheal intubation for severe asthma. Clinical respiratory distress was the primary reason for intubation (based on chart review), followed by acute hypercapnia, hypoxemia, respiratory arrest, and altered mental status. The decision to intubate patients is most frequently made based on clinical deterioration. Patients other than those intubated in association with cardiac arrest had an excellent prognosis.

An increasing arterial $Paco_2$ despite aggressive therapy is an ominous sign. Although an elevated $Paco_2$ is not an indication for intubation, an increasing $Paco_2$ despite aggressive therapy typically calls for intubation and mechanical ventilation. Nowak and colleagues[116] showed that an elevated $Paco_2$ correlates with FEV_1 less than 25% of age-predicted values. Another sign of imminent respiratory failure is paradoxical breathing. Normally, as the diaphragm contracts, it moves caudad, and the abdomen moves out. When the diaphragm fails, it moves cephalad to fix the ribcage and assist the intercostal muscles of inspiration, and in that circumstance the abdomen moves in with inspiration. The intubation technique should be the one in which the operator feels most proficient. The largest endotracheal tube practical should be selected to decrease the degree of auto-PEEP.

Aerosol Delivery

Aerosol delivery in an intubated patient receiving mechanical ventilatory support poses a significant problem because the nebulized agent reaching the lung parenchyma is markedly reduced, with most of the agent deposited in the endotracheal tube, probably because of its 90-degree curve.[50] It is important to connect the ventilator circuit nebulizer system as close to the patient as possible and to consider increasing the amount of active agent in each treatment, usually double the dose used in a nonintubated patient. An MDI with a spacer is generally accepted as being as effective in delivering bronchodilator medication in patients receiving mechanical ventilation as nebulized therapy, and it costs less. Either method may give varying delivery based on technique and ventilator and patient variables.

Sedation and Analgesia

Sedation and analgesia are almost always required in preparation for intubation in a patient with a severe asthma episode. Sedation and analgesia generally should be avoided in nonintubated patients with asthma, unless they are used as part of premedication for intubation. After the patient is intubated successfully and mechanical ventilation has been instituted, a combination of benzodiazepines or propofol and opioids should be administered during initial mechanical ventilator therapy.

Neuromuscular Blockade

Some patients require neuromuscular blocking agents (NMBAs), especially early in their ventilatory course to control respiratory rate in the presence of life-threatening auto-PEEP. Neuromuscular blockade also may be required in some patients to facilitate intubation. Neuromuscular blockade, when combined with steroid therapy, increases the risk for prolonged blockade after discontinuation of the NMBA and should be discontinued as soon as possible in this population. Status asthmaticus patients receiving mechanical ventilation who are given corticosteroids and NMBAs are at risk for developing prolonged weakness after discontinuation of NMBAs. Prolonged neuromuscular blockade is ideally avoided. If NMBAs are used, attempts to withdraw neuromuscular blockade over 24 to 48 hours after intubation are advised.

If the patient is to be continuously paralyzed, a peripheral nerve stimulator should be used to limit paralysis to no less than a recording of one or two twitches in response to a train-of-four stimulus, as opposed to higher degrees of paralysis. The rationale for neuromuscular blockade is to control the rate, and patient attempts to trigger ideally can be controlled with a three-twitch or four-twitch response. Prolonged neuromuscular blockade may lead to persistent neuromuscular weakness after withdrawal of neuromuscular blockade therapy. This situation is particularly likely to occur in patients with renal impairment, in female patients, in patients with hypophosphatemia, in patients with higher degrees of paralysis, and in patients in whom corticosteroids are given concomitantly. Patients with persistent neuromuscular blockade associated with the combined use of NMBAs and systemic steroids typically exhibit proximal and distal muscle weakness. Creatine kinase may be elevated, and myoglobinuria may be present. Steroid myopathy, by contrast, primarily involves proximal muscles, and the creatine kinase level is normal.[117]

Griffin and associates[118] described acute myopathy associated with prolonged neuromuscular blockade after discontinuation of nondepolarizing muscle blockade in three asthma patients. These patients had received pancuronium or vecuronium for 10 to 14 days in addition to methylprednisolone, 320 to 750 mg/d. The weaning process was more prolonged because of muscle weakness. Muscle biopsy specimens show muscle necrosis and degeneration of type 1 and type 2 muscle fibers.

David and colleagues[119] described electromyography findings in acute myopathy after combined use of steroids and paralytic agents in the treatment of status asthmaticus. Electromyography findings are consistent with a myopathic process without evidence of neuromuscular transmission disorder or generalized neuropathy. Not all of the patients reported by these authors showed significant myonecrosis or elevated creatine kinase. Some patients improved rapidly after the diagnosis, whereas others improved more slowly.

If NMBAs are needed for longer than 24 hours, they should be discontinued daily to ensure patient arousal. More recent evidence indicates that properly administered, continuously infused NMBA is associated with a decreased incidence of prolonged blockade compared with intermittent bolus therapy.[120] Prolonged muscle paralysis may lead to a denervated state with an increased number of steroid receptors.[121,122] The additive effect of NMBAs and steroids may be related to this finding. In patients with asthma, cisatracurium is the first-choice NMBA because it is eliminated by esterase degradation and spontaneous breakdown in the serum.[19]

Initiating Mechanical Ventilation

The strategy of mechanical ventilation is to avoid excessive airway pressures and reduce dynamic hyperinflation.[42] To achieve this goal, it may be necessary to allow "controlled hypoventilation" or "permissive hypercapnia."[123] Recommended initial ventilator settings are tidal volume of 8 mL/kg ideal body weight and a frequency of 10 to 14 breaths per minute, minute ventilation less than 10 L/min, and expiratory time increased and targeted to avoid auto-PEEP and to achieve arterial oxygen saturation greater than 90%. If volume ventilation is used, peak inspiratory flow rates should be set at 60 to 80 L/min with a decelerating waveform.[42] The use of noncompressible tubing facilitates lowering of inspiratory time and adds to expiration time. Total volume is reduced to 6 mL/kg ideal body weight or less to achieve inspiratory plateau pressure (IPP) of less than 30 cm H_2O. The way to minimize hyperinflation is to minimize inspiratory time, while providing adequate oxygenation and ventilation, considering permissive hypercapnia in the latter case. Controlled mechanical ventilation may be required during initial ICU stay and requires heavy sedation and analgesia, or more typically sedation, analgesia, and muscle paralysis. Assisted controlled ventilation without heavy sedation or sedation/paralysis predisposes the patient to hyperinflation if the patient's breathing rate is high. Heavy sedation or sedation/paralysis reduces carbon dioxide production, facilitates measurement of end inspiratory and end expiratory pressures, and facilitates mechanical ventilation of severely asthmatic patients. Pressure-control ventilation is discouraged because of fluctuating high airway resistance and intrinsic PEEP. Keeping the peak alveolar pressures low (IPP of <30 cm H_2O) prevents overdistention of alveoli distal to the least obstructed airway.[42]

Auto–Positive End-Expiratory Pressure

Definition and Predisposing Factors

Auto-PEEP occurs when ventilator settings result in an inspiratory-to-expiratory ratio that does not allow adequate expiratory time for total exhalation of the delivered ventilator breath. Because airways obstruction increases expiratory time, mechanically ventilated asthma patients are at increased risk for auto-PEEP.[124] After the first breath delivered in a setting conducive to auto-PEEP, the next breath is delivered before complete emptying of the first breath. With each subsequent breath that fails to empty completely, end-inspiratory and end-expiratory lung volumes increase, as do flow and pressure at end expiration. The increase in lung volume predisposes to the risk of barotraumas, and elevations of intrathoracic pressure decrease cardiac output.

With volume ventilation, end-inspiratory lung volume and peak alveolar pressure increase until barotrauma occurs, the peak pressure limit alarm setting is exceeded and total volume decreases, or equilibrium is reached. Equilibrium is established as a result of the distention-induced larger caliber of airways (reduced resistance to expiratory flow), and the increased lung recoil (caused by increased end-inspiratory lung volume), eventually allowing complete emptying of the delivered tidal volume. Equilibrium is reached, however, with significant end-expiratory flow still occurring when the next ventilator breath is delivered.

With pressure-control ventilation, the onset and worsening of acute PEEP decreases delivered tidal volume at the set applied pressure because tidal volume is determined by the ventilator system pressure that is constant and the intrathoracic pressure in the patient, which is increasing. The continued expiratory flow at end expiration represents positive pressure relative to atmospheric pressure. PEEP exists, even though it is not set on the ventilator (auto-PEEP). Auto-PEEP may be associated with significant increases in mean intrathoracic pressure. This condition may be accompanied by associated hypotension (decreased venous return to heart) and barotrauma (pneumothorax).

Diagnosis and Treatment

When there is no other obvious cause (e.g., tension pneumothorax), auto-PEEP should be suspected clinically in an intubated asthmatic patient who is hypotensive after institution of mechanical ventilation. A higher minute ventilation, likely to occur in assist control mode ventilation in an awake asthma patient, predisposes to auto-PEEP. Auto-PEEP is treated by decreasing total inspiratory time and is best accomplished by decreasing the rate; controlling and minimizing ventilator rate is the most important target of treatment of auto-PEEP. This requires heavy sedation in most cases and NMBAs in some, at least for a short time. Decreasing tidal volume also is effective but less efficient. If hypotension resolves, increasing expiratory time is a diagnostic and a therapeutic maneuver. Unless inspiratory flow rate was set inappropriately low (<80 L/min), shortening the total inspiratory time by increasing flow rate is a less effective way of decreasing auto-PEEP and may hyperinflate areas of lung with short time constants for filling. The inspiratory-to-expiratory ratio is not a good barometer for risk for auto-PEEP. Absolute time of expiration for each breath and size of tidal volume are direct correlates of risk for and treatment of auto-PEEP. Auto-PEEP can be detected easily with graphic flow displays showing expiratory gas flow still present at the onset of the next inspiration.

Auto-PEEP can be measured with the occlusion technique or esophageal balloon technique. Occlusion of the expiratory and inspiratory circuit of the ventilator just before the onset of the next breath causes the pressure in the lungs and ventilator circuit to equilibrate. The displayed pressure represents the level of auto-PEEP. With the esophageal balloon technique, the negative deflection in esophageal pressure (representing pleural pressure) from the onset of inspiratory effort to the onset of inspiratory flow represents the inspiratory muscle pressure necessary to counterbalance the end-expiratory elastic recoil of the respiratory system and represents the amount of auto-PEEP.

In the absence of an esophageal balloon device, the ability to reflect accurately the auto-PEEP–related pressure at the alveolar level in an intubated patient depends on a prolonged end-expiratory hold (3 to 4 seconds) and the absence of patient inspiratory or expiratory effort during measurement. This measurement is unlikely to be accurate, unless the patient is heavily sedated or sedated/paralyzed. Unless full equilibration to a no-flow state is allowed at end inspiration with the system closed to the ventilator, the auto-PEEP level exerted at the alveolar level is typically underestimated. The typical end-expiratory hold used in clinical practice of 0.4 to 1 second is less likely to provide a reliable measurement.

Increased Work of Breathing with Auto–Positive End-Expiratory Pressure

Auto-PEEP in the presence of assisted ventilation modes (assist control and synchronized intermittent mandatory ventilation) implies that the patient must initiate gas flow by producing an inspiratory effort equal to not only the sensitivity setting of inspiratory triggering, but also the level of auto-PEEP. Extrinsic PEEP normally has no indication, however, in acute severe asthma during controlled mechanical ventilation. If it is not advantageous or possible to eliminate auto-PEEP in the patient with assisted ventilation modes, applying or increasing ventilator-set PEEP to a level slightly below total PEEP would decrease patient effort necessary to trigger the ventilator breath.[42] Inappropriately set ventilator PEEP offers additional risks to the patient, and this approach is recommended only by health care professionals well schooled in the intricacies of mechanical ventilation.

Barotrauma

The risk for barotrauma in an intubated asthma patient correlates best with peak alveolar pressure as estimated by IPP. The amounts of measured auto-PEEP and peak inspiratory pressures are less reliable predictors. Peak inspiratory pressure, although correlating to some degree with IPP and end-inspiratory lung volume, also reflects resistance in the endotracheal tube and tracheobronchial tree, which may be considerable in the presence of a small endotracheal tube, airway secretions, mucosal thickening, and bronchoconstriction.

In a heavily sedated or sedated/paralyzed patient, IPP measurement is the best means for estimating peak alveolar pressure and the best indicator of hyperinflation and risk for barotraumas because closure of airways toward the end of expiration may lead to underestimation of hyperinflation.[125] In the presence of normal chest wall and abdominal compliance factors, an IPP equal to or greater than 30 cm H_2O puts the patient at risk for exceeding maximal alveolar size (total lung capacity). Decreases in IPP are usually accomplished by using low tidal volumes and minimizing auto-PEEP. In a paralyzed patient, the collection of the total exhaled volume of gas obtainable with 20 to 60 seconds of apnea allows the measurement of end inspired volume above apnea functional residual capacity. This volume may be 3 L despite the use of small tidal volumes.[126]

Because high IPP is reduced by lowering tidal volume, a reduction in the tidal volume directly decreases the risk for barotrauma as does any maneuver that decreases auto-PEEP. If, after heavy sedation or sedation/paralysis, the IPP remains 30 cm H_2O or greater despite decreases in tidal volume to the lowest value that allows an acceptable pH, typically greater than or equal to 7.20, the use of bicarbonate infusion to allow acceptable pH with further reduction of tidal volume may be considered.[127]

The concept of reducing the tidal volume and accepting a higher Pa_{CO_2} and lower pH is called *permissive hypercapnia.*[128,129] Permissive hypercapnia is relatively safe in asthma and well tolerated in the absence of contraindications, such as increased intracranial hypertension and pregnancy.[10,89,130] Physicians are uncomfortable to allow Pa_{CO_2} to become greater than 80 100 mm Hg, but several case reports described short durations of hypercapnia (>150 mm Hg) as well tolerated, and one report described Pa_{CO_2} of 200 mm Hg for 10 hours with no consequences reported.[37,74,131] Permissive hypercapnia limits volutrauma and hemodynamic consequences of increased intrathoracic pressures. In normoxic states, acute hypercapnia has limited potential for inducing severe intracellular acidosis. If permissive hypercapnia results in pH less than 7.2, increased sedation and paralysis and methods of decreasing carbon dioxide production, such as reducing fever, overfeeding, and patient effort, should be considered. In the absence of tissue hypoperfusion or volume overload, iatrogenic compensation for acute respiratory acidosis with intravenous bicarbonate administration is appropriate. In severe acidosis, large amounts of bicarbonate may be necessary to elevate the pH substantially, potentially leading to volume overload.[42]

Permissive hypercapnia should be considered in the mechanically ventilated asthmatics with life-threatening asthma, severe hyperinflation, and inability to achieve a satisfactory IPP without producing an unacceptable acidemia. Permissive hypercapnia is well tolerated in most patients, even when Pa_{CO_2} is 90 mm Hg (12 kPa), as long as pH remains greater than or equal to 7.20. It should be avoided, however, in the presence of increased intracranial pressure and clinically significant myocardial dysfunction and during pregnancy to avoid fetal distress.

Noninvasive Positive-Pressure Ventilation

Noninvasive positive-pressure ventilation (NPPV) is a safe treatment and can reduce the need for intubation in a selected group of patients with severe asthma and hypercapnia, who fail to improve with initial medical management.[132] Fernandez and colleagues[132] further describe the rationale for NPPV in severe asthma is its potential for improving alveolar ventilation, decreasing the risk of respiratory muscle fatigue. Mask continuous positive airway pressure (CPAP) produces bronchodilation and decreases the airway resistance, reverses atelectasis, and promotes removal of secretions.[133] The work of the diaphragm and the inspiratory muscles is reduced, and intrinsic PEEP may be offset. In addition, CPAP decreases the adverse hemodynamic effects of large negative inspiratory swings in pleural pressure,[133] which compromise right and left ventricular performance.[132] NPPV potentially may enhance delivery of inhaled β-agonists. One study showed a small but statistically significant greater improvement in PEFR when NPPV was used for initial β-agonist delivery.[134] A nonrandomized study by Meduri and associates[135] reported a reduction in Pa_{CO_2} and improvement in dyspnea with the use of NPPV in 17 episodes of asthma with acute respiratory failure.

CPAP, as opposed to NPPV, has been studied in asthmatic patients after induction of bronchospasm with aerosolized histamine.[133] CPAP of 12 cm H_2O increased the minimal pleural pressure and decreased swings in transdiaphragmatic pressure. Although ventilation increased, the inspiratory work per liter decreased significantly, as did the pressure time product for the inspiratory muscles. Functional residual capacity increased slightly. The authors concluded that CPAP produced a load on the inspiratory muscles, improving their efficiency and decreasing the energy cost of inspiration. Despite the potential for benefit of NPPV or CPAP in selected patients in severe acute asthma, it should be used with caution pending controlled clinical trials. Ram and colleagues[136] also concluded in a Cochrane analysis that application of NPPV in status asthmaticus, despite some promising preliminary results, remains controversial. If NPPV is used, initial setting should be an expiratory positive airway pressure (CPAP or PEEP) of about 5 cm H_2O and inspiratory pressure (or pressure support) of approximately 8 cm H_2O. If tidal volumes are shallow (<7 mL/kg), inspiratory pressure can be increased gradually by 2 cm H_2O every 15 minutes, to a goal to reduce the respiratory rate to less than 25 breaths per minute.[42] Peak pressures greater than 15 to 20 cm H_2O rarely can be tolerated without mask leaks or discomfort or claustrophobia.[19] See Box 39-5 for contraindications for NPPV.[1]

See Box 39-6 for complications of asthma. Figure 39-1 is an algorithm that shows the approach to acute life-threatening asthma.

Box 39-5

Contraindications for Noninvasive Positive-Pressure Ventilation

Uncooperative or obtunded patients
Hemodynamic instability
Cardiac or respiratory arrest
Encephalopathy
Facial surgery or deformity
High risk for aspiration
Nonrespiratory organ failure
Severe upper gastrointestinal bleeding
Unstable arrhythmia
Upper airway obstruction

From Stather DR, Stewart TE: Clinical review: Mechanical ventilation in severe asthma. Crit Care 2005;9:581-587.

Box 39-6

Complications of Acute Severe Asthma

Pneumothorax
Pneumomediastinum
Subcutaneous emphysema
Pneumopericardium
Tracheoesophageal fistula (mechanically ventilated patients)
Myocardial ischemia (coronary artery disease patients)
Mucous plugging and atelectasis
Theophylline toxicity
Lactic acidosis
Electrolyte disturbances—hypokalemia, hypophosphatemia, hypomagnesemia
Myopathy
Anoxic brain injury

From Papiris S, Kotanidou A, Malagari K, et al: Clinical review: Severe asthma. Crit Care 2002;6:30-44.

KEY POINTS

- The cause of respiratory arrest in asthmatic patients is usually failure of the inspiratory muscles with ventilatory arrest.
- Ominous signs and findings in a patient with acute severe asthma, if not quickly reversed, include diaphoresis, inability to recline, inability to talk, increased Pa_{CO_2}, PEFR less than 60 L/min, and use of accessory muscles.
- Pathophysiology of asthma consists of three key abnormalities: bronchoconstriction, airway inflammation, and mucous impaction.
- The ADAM-33 gene is significantly associated with asthma.
- Inhaled β-agonists are the cornerstone of medical therapy for hospitalized severe asthmatics. The addition of steroids and ipratropium is recommended.

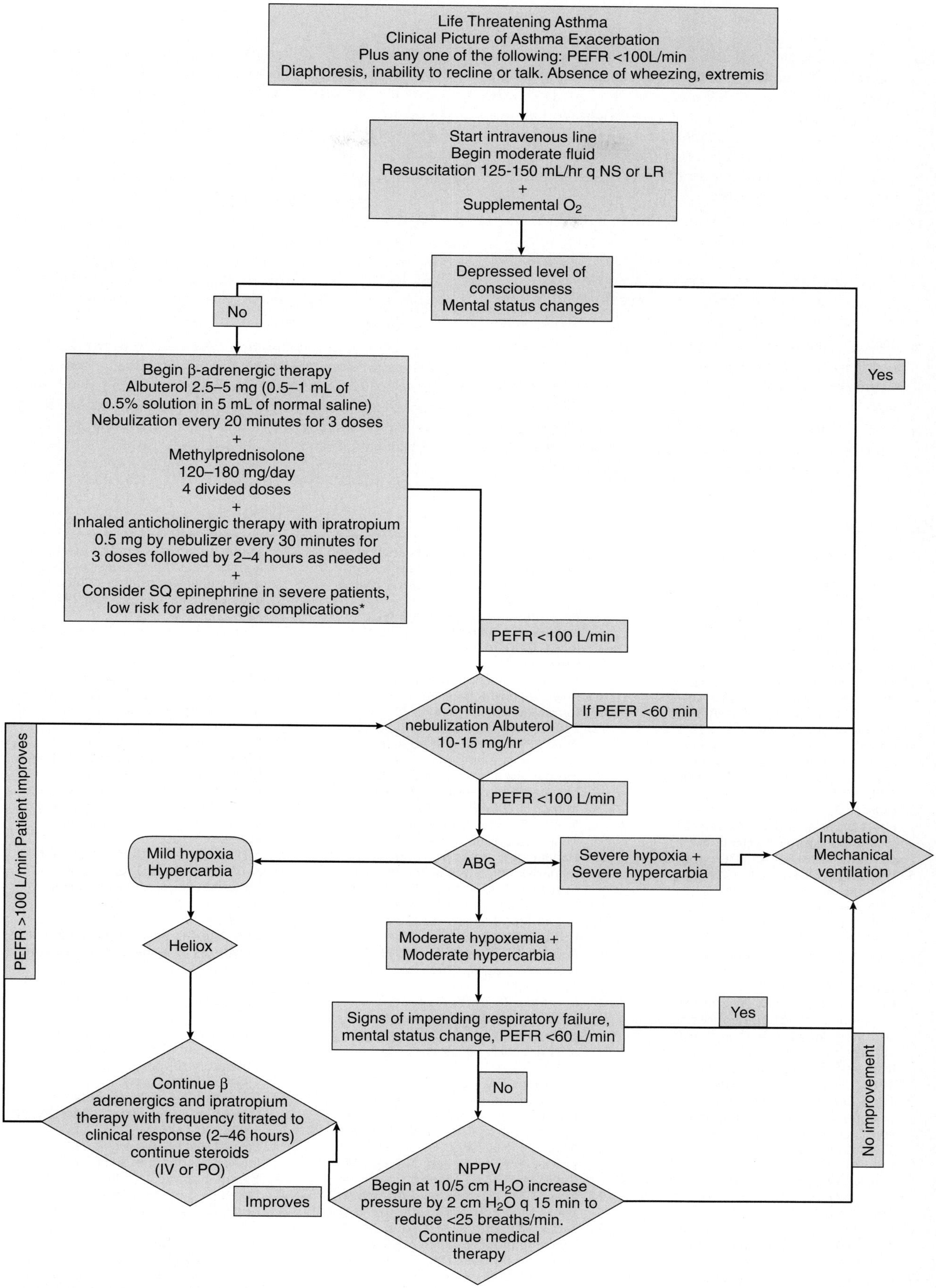

Figure 39-1. Approach to acute life-threatening asthma. *Check for hypokalemia and treat. ABG, arterial blood gas; LR, lactated Ringer's; NPPV, noninvasive positive pressure ventilation; NS, normal saline; PEFR, peak expiratory flow rate.

- Adequate delivery of β-agonists can be accomplished by use of an MDI with a spacer during acute bronchospasm if proper technique is used and doses are increased. It is advisable to deliver the β-agonist by nebulization in most acutely ill asthma patients because nebulization requires minimal coordination and cooperation of the patient and less bedside instruction and supervision by health care professionals.
- Larger doses and more frequent dosing intervals for inhaled β-agonist therapy are needed in acute severe asthma because of decreased deposition at the site of action (low tidal volumes and narrowed airways), alteration in dose-response curve, and altered duration of activity. Continuous nebulization is an option.
- Theophylline is not recommended for general use in hospitalized patients with acute asthma. Intravenous magnesium is recommended for the most severe asthma attacks.
- Although there is no proven value of systemic therapy over aerosol therapy, rapid delivery of β-agonists to the airway may be beneficial in seriously ill asthmatic patients who are at imminent risk for respiratory arrest or need intubation and who are at low risk for β-agonist cardiac toxicity (young asthmatics). In these patients, a combination of inhaled and subcutaneously administered β-agonists in this circumstance may be useful.
- If NMBAs are used, attempts to withdraw these agents over the first 24 to 48 hours after intubation are advised.
- Auto-PEEP is treated by decreasing total inspiratory time. Increasing expiratory time is best accomplished by decreasing rate. Decreasing tidal volume also is effective. Prolonging expiratory time is a diagnostic and a therapeutic maneuver.
- The concept of reducing the tidal volume to decrease alveolar inflation and accepting a higher $PaCO_2$ and lower pH is called permissive hypercapnia and should be considered in asthma patients undergoing mechanical ventilation therapy with life-threatening asthma, severe hyperinflation, and high IPP.

REFERENCES

1. Stather DR, Stewart TE: Clinical review: Mechanical ventilation in severe asthma. Crit Care 2005;9:581-587.
2. Trends in Asthma Morbidity and Mortality. New York, American Lung Association Epidemiology and Statistics Unit Research and Program Services, May 2005.
3. Forecasted state-specific estimates of self-reported asthma prevalence—United States, 1998. MMWR Morb Mortal Wkly Rep 1998;47:1022-1102.
4. Carr W, Zeitel L, Weiss K: Variations in asthma hospitalizations and deaths in New York City, Am J Public Health 1992;82:59.
5. Marder D, Targonski P, Orris P, et al: Effect of racial and socioeconomic factors on asthma mortality in Chicago. Chest 1992;101(Suppl):426.
6. Weiss KB, Wagener DK: Changing patterns of asthma mortality: Identifying target populations at high risk (comments). JAMA 1990;264:1683.
7. Serafini U: Can fatal asthma be prevented? A personal view. Clin Exp Allergy 1992;22:576.
8. Evans RD, Mullally DI, Wilson RW, et al: National trends in the morbidity and mortality of asthma in the US: Prevalence, hospitalization and death from asthma over two decades: 1965-1984. Chest 1987;91(6 Suppl):65.
9. Turkeltaub PC, Gergen PJ: Prevalence of upper and lower respiratory conditions in the US population by social and environmental factors: Data from the second National Health and Nutrition Examination Survey, 1976 to 1980 (NHANES II), Ann Allergy 1991;67(2 Pt 1):147.
10. Rodrigo GJ, Rodrigo C, Hall JB: Acute asthma in adults: A review. Chest 2004;125:1081-1102.
11. Nicholas T, Hansell A, Strachan D: The contribution of "holiday deaths" to seasonal variations in asthma mortality in England and Wales. Clin Exp Allergy 1999;29:1415.
12. Khot A, Burn R: Seasonal variation and time trends in childhood asthma in England and Wales: 1975-81. BMJ 1984;289:233.
13. Weiss KB: Seasonal trends in U.S. asthma hospitalizations and mortality. JAMA 1990;263:2323.
14. Killian KJ, Watson R, Otis J, et al: Symptom perception during acute bronchoconstriction. Am J Respir Crit Care Med 2000;162:490.
15. Pendergraft TB, Stanford RN, Beasley R, et al: Rates and characteristics of intensive care unit admissions and intubations among asthma-related hospitalizations. Ann Allergy Asthma Immunol 2004;93:29-35.
16. Strek ME: Difficult asthma. Proc Am Thorac Soc 2006;3:116-123.
17. Hananel JI, Barbers RG: Critical care management of the asthmatic patient. Curr Opin Pulm Med 1998;4:4.
18. Papiris S, Kotanidou A, Malagari K, et al: Clinical review: Severe asthma. Crit Care 2002;6:30-44.
19. Rodrigo GJ, Rodrigo C, Hall JB: Acute asthma in adults. Chest 2004;125:1081-1102.
20. Rodriguez-Roisin R: Acute severe asthma: Pathophysiology and pathobiology of gas exchange abnormalities. Eur Respir J 1997;10:1359.
21. Manthous CA, Goulding P: The effect of volume infusion on dead space in mechanically ventilated patients with severe asthma. Chest 1997;112:843.
22. Rosen FS, MacKay I: The immunology series comes to an end. N Engl J Med 2001;345:1343-1344.
23. Busse WW, Lemanske RF: Asthma. N Engl J Med 2001;344:350-362.
24. Sad S, Marcotte R, Mosmann TR: Cytokine induced differentiation of precursor mouse CD8+ T cells into cytotoxic CD8+ T cells Eth 1 or The 2 cytokines. Immunity 1995;2:27-29.
25. Strachan DP: Hay fever, hygiene, and household size. BMJ 1989;299:1259-1260.
26. Mattes J, Karmaus W: The use of antibiotics in the first year of life and development of asthma: Which comes first? Clin Exp Allergy 1999;29:729-732.
27. National Asthma Education and Prevention Program: Expert Panel Report: Guidelines for the Diagnosis and Management of Asthma: Update on Selected Topics 2002. NIH publication no. 02-5074. Bethesda, MD, National Institutes of Health, 2003, p 122.
28. Shapiro SD, Owen CA: ADAM-33 surfaces as an asthma gene. N Engl J Med 2002;347:936-938.
29. Ober C, Hoffjan S: Asthma genetics 2006: The long and winding road to gene discovery. Genes Immun 2006;7:95-100.
30. McFadden ER Jr, Kiser R, DeGroot WJ: Acute bronchial asthma: Relations between clinical and physiologic manifestations. N Engl J Med 1973;288:221.
31. Gerschke GL, Baker FJ, Rosen P: Pulsus paradoxus as a parameter in treatment of the asthmatic. J Am Coll Emerg Physicians 1977;6:191.
32. Murray DM, Lawler PG: All that wheezes is not asthma: Paradoxical vocal cord movement presenting as severe acute asthma requiring ventilatory support. Anesthesia 1998;53:1006.
33. Fishman AP: Cardiac asthma—a fresh look at an old wheeze. N Engl J Med 1989;320:1346.
34. Blitz M, Blitz S, Beasely R, et al: Inhaled magnesium sulfate in the treatment of acute asthma. Cochrane Database Syst Rev 2005;CD 003898.
35. Appel D, Rubenstein R, Schrager K, et al: Lactic acidosis in severe asthma. Am J Med 1983;75:580.
36. O'Connell MB, Iber C: Continuous intravenous terbutaline infusions for adult patients with status asthmaticus. Ann Allergy 1990;64:213.
37. Yanos J, Wood LD, Davis K, et al: The effect of respiratory and lactic acidosis

on diaphragm function. Am Rev Respir Dis 1993;147:616.
38. Harris L: Comparison of the effect on blood gases, ventilation, and perfusion of isoproterenol-phenylephrine and salbutamol aerosols in chronic bronchitis with asthma. J Allergy Clin Immunol 1972;49:63.
39. 2005 American Heart Association Guidelines for Cardiopulmonary Resuscitation and Emergency Cardiovascular Care. Part 10.5: Near fatal asthma. Circulation 2005;112: IV-142.
40. Inwald D, Roland M, Kuitert L, et al: Oxygen treatment for acute severe asthma. BMJ 2001;323:98-100.
41. Moloney E, O'Sullivan S, Hogan T, et al: Airway dehydration: A therapeutic target in asthma? Chest 2002;121:1806-1811.
42. Oddo M, Feihl F, Schaller MD, et al: Management of mechanical ventilation in acute severe asthma: Practical aspects. Intensive Care Med 2006;32:501-510.
43. Lin RY, Smith AJ, Hergenroeder P: High serum albuterol levels and tachycardia in adult asthmatics treated with high-dose continuously aerosolized albuterol. Chest 1993;103:221.
44. Idris AH, McDermott MF, Raucci JC, et al: Emergency department treatment of severe asthma: Metered-dose inhaler plus holding chamber is equivalent in effectiveness to nebulizer. Chest 1993;103:655.
45. Rodrigo G, Rodrigo C: Comparison of salbutamol delivered by nebulizer or metered-dose inhaler with a pear-shaped spacer in acute asthma. Curr Ther Res Clin Exp 1993;54:797.
46. Rodrigo C, Rodrigo G: Salbutamol treatment of acute severe asthma in the ED: MDI versus hand-held nebulizer. Am J Emerg Med 1998;16:637.
47. Robertson D: Dose-response study of albuterol by inhaler or nebulizer for acute asthma. Drug Therap 1994;24:40.
48. Mandelberg A, Chen E, Noviski N, et al: Nebulized wet aerosol treatment in emergency department—is it essential? Chest 1997;112:1501.
49. Jasper AC, Mohsenifar Z, Kahan S, et al: Cost-benefit comparison of aerosol bronchodilator delivery methods in hospitalized patients. Chest 1987;91:614.
50. MacIntyre NR, Silver RM, Miller CW, et al: Aerosol delivery in intubated, mechanically ventilated patients. Crit Care Med 1985;13:81.
51. Salmeron S, Brochard L, Mal H, et al: Nebulized versus intravenous albuterol in hypercapnic acute asthma: A multicenter, double-blind, randomized study. Am J Respir Crit Care Med 1994;149:1466.
52. Appel D, Karpel P, Sherman M: Epinephrine improves expiratory airflow rates in patients with asthma who do not respond to inhaled metaproterenol sulfate. J Allergy Clin Immunol 1989;84:90.
53. Amory DW, Burnham SC, Cheney FW: Comparison of the cardiopulmonary effects of subcutaneously administered epinephrine and terbutaline in patients with reversible airway obstruction. Chest 1975;67:279.
54. Liebman JB: Should epinephrine be administered exclusively by the endotracheal route in respiratory arrest secondary to asthma? Am J Emerg Med 1997;15:106.
55. National Asthma Education and Prevention Program: Expert Panel Report: Guidelines for the Diagnosis and Management of Asthma: Update on Selected Topics 2002. NIH publication no. 02-5074. Bethesda, MD, National Institutes of Health, 2003.
56. Kelly HW, Murphy S: Corticosteroids for acute, severe asthma. DICP 1991;25:72-79.
57. Jantz MA, Shan SA: Corticosteroids in acute respiratory failure. Am J Respir Crit Care Med 1999;160:1079.
58. Haskell RJ, Wong BM, Hansen JE: A double-blind, randomized clinical trial of methylprednisolone in status asthmaticus. Arch Intern Med 1983;143:1324.
59. Lin RY, Pesola GR, BakalchuckL, et al: Rapid improvement of peak flow in asthmatic patients treated with parenteral methylprednisolone in the emergency department: A randomized controlled study. Ann Emerg Med 1999;33:487.
60. Ratto D, Alfaro C, Sipsey J, et al: Are intravenous corticosteroids required in status asthmaticus? JAMA 1988;260:527.
61. Aaron SD: The use of ipratropium bromide for the management of acute severe asthma exacerbation in adults and children: A systematic review. J Asthma 2001;38:521-530.
62. Summers QA, Tarala RA: Nebulized ipratropium in the treatment of asthma. Chest 1990;97:430.
63. O'Driscoll BR, Taylor RJ, Horsley MG, et al: Nebulized salbutamol with and without ipratropium bromide in acute airflow obstruction. Lancet 1989;24:1418.
64. Higgins RM, Stradling JR, Lane DJ: Should ipratropium bromide be added to beta-agonists in treatment of acute severe asthma? Chest 1988;94:718.
65. Rebuck AS, Chapman KB, Abboud P: Nebulized anticholinergic and sympathomimetic treatment of asthma and chronic airways disease in the emergency room. Am J Med 1987;82:59.
66. Bryant DH: Nebulized ipratropium bromide in the treatment of acute asthma. Chest 1987;88:24.
67. Ward MJ, Macfarlane JT, Davies D: A place for ipratropium bromide in the treatment of severe acute asthma. Br J Dis Chest 1985;79:374.
68. Roesler J, Reynaert MS: A comparison of fenoterol and fenoterol-ipratropium nebulisation treatment in acute asthma. Acta Therap 1987;13:571.
69. Karpel JP, Schacter EN, Fanta C, et al: A comparison of ipratropium and albuterol vs albuterol alone for the treatment of acute asthma. Chest 1996;110:611.
70. Garrett JE, Town GI, Rodwell P, et al: Nebulized salbutamol with and without ipratropium bromide in the treatment of acute asthma. J Allergy Clin Immunol 1997;100:165.
71. Fitzgerald JM, Grunfeld A, Pare PD, et al: The clinical efficacy of combination nebulized anticholinergic and adrenergic bronchodilators vs nebulized adrenergic bronchodilator alone in acute asthma. Chest 1997;111:311.
72. Lanes SF, Garrett JE, Wentworth CE, et al: The effect of adding ipratropium bromide to salbutamol in the treatment of acute asthma. Chest 1998;114:365.
73. Stoodley RG, Aaron SD, Dales RE: The role of ipratropium bromide in the emergency management of acute asthma exacerbation: A meta-analysis of randomized clinical trials. Ann Emerg Med 1999;34:8.
74. U.S. Department of Health and Human Services, National Institutes of Health, National Heart, Lung, and Blood Institute: Practical Guide for the Diagnosis and Management of Asthma. NIH publication no. 97-4053. Bethesda, MD, National Institutes of Health, 1997.
75. Littenberg B: Aminophylline in severe, acute asthma: A metaanalaysis. JAMA 1988;259:1678.
76. Huang D, O'Brien RG, Harman E, et al: Does aminophylline benefit adults admitted to the hospital for an acute exacerbation of asthma? Ann Intern Med 1993;119:1155.
77. Kelly HW, Murphy S: Should we stop using theophylline for the treatment of the hospitalized patient with status asthmaticus. DICP 1989;23:995-998.
78. Coleridge J, Cameron P, Epstein J, et al: Intravenous aminophylline confers no additional benefit in acute asthma treated with intravenous steroids and inhaled bronchodilators. N Z Med J 1993;23:348.
79. Rodrigo C, Rodrigo G: Treatment of acute asthma: Lack of therapeutic benefit and increase of the toxicity from aminophylline given in addition to high doses of salbutamol delivered by metered-dose inhaler. Chest 1994;106:1071.
80. Hashimoto Y, Nishimura Y, Maeda H, et al: Assessment of magnesium status in patients with bronchial asthma. J Asthma 2000;37:489.
81. Rowe BH, Bretzlaff JA, Bourdon C, et al: Magnesium sulfate for treating exacerbations of acute severe asthma in the emergency department. Cochrane Database Syst Rev 2000; CD001490.
82. Silverman RA, Osborn H, Runge J, et al: IV magnesium in the treatment of severe asthma: A multicenter randomized controlled trial. Chest 2002;122:489-497.
83. Rodrigo GA, Rodrigo C, Pollack CV, et al: Use of helium-oxygen mixture in the treatment of acute asthma: A systematic review. Chest 2003;123:891-896.
84. Reuben AD, Harris AR: Heliox for asthma in the emergency department: A review of the literature. Emerg Med J 2004;21:131-135.
85. Schaeffer EM, Pohlman A, Morgan S, et al: Oxygenation in status asthmaticus improves during ventilation with helium-oxygen. Crit Care Med 1999;27:2666.
86. Johnston SL, Blasi F, Black PN, et al: The effect of telithromycin in acute exacerbations of asthma. N Engl J Med 2006;354:1589-1600.
87. Little FF: Treating acute asthma with antibiotics—not quite yet. N Engl J Med 2006;354:1632-1634.

88. Corbridge T, Hall JB: State of the art: The assessment and management of adults with status asthmaticus. Am J Respir Crit Care Med 1995;151:1296.
89. Stather DR, Stewart TE: Clinical review: Mechanical ventilation in severe asthma. Crit Care 2005;9:581-587.
90. Holgate ST, Chuchalin AG, Hebert J, et al: Efficacy and safety of a recombinant anti-immunoglobulin E antibody in severe allergic asthma. Clin Exp Allergy 2004;34:632-638.
91. Strunk RC, Bloomberg GD: Omalizumab for asthma. N Engl J Med 2006;354:2689-2695.
92. Rosseel P, Lauwers LF, Baute L: Halathane treatment in life-threatening asthma. Intensive Care Med 1985;11:241.
93. Schwartz SH: Treatment of status asthmaticus with halothane. JAMA 1984;251:2688.
94. Robertson CE, Sinclair CJ, Steedman D, et al: Use of ether in life-threatening acute severe asthma. Lancet 1985;1:187.
95. Grunberg G, Cohen JD, Keslin J, et al: Facilitation of mechanical ventilation in status asthmaticus with continuous intravenous thiopental. Chest 1991;99:1216.
96. Corssen G, Gutierrez J, Reves JG, et al: Ketamine in the anaesthetic management of asthmatic patients. Anesth Analg 1972;51:588.
97. Que JC, Lusaya VO: Sevoflurane induction for emergency cesarean section in a parturient in status asthmaticus. Anesthesiology 1999;90:1475.
98. Bentley GN, Gent JP, Goodchild CS: Vascular effects of propofol: Smooth muscle relaxation in isolated veins and arteries. Pharm Pharmacol 1989;41:797.
99. Gigarini I, Bonnet F, Lorino AM, et al: Comparison of the effects of fentanyl on respiratory mechanics under propofol or thiopental anaesthesia. Acta Anaesth Scand 1990;34:253.
100. Pedersen CM: The effect of sedation with propofol on postoperative bronchoconstriction in patients with hyperreactive airway disease. Intensive Care Med 1992;18:45.
101. Lang DM, Simon RA, Mathison DA, et al: Safety and possible efficacy of fiberoptic bronchoscopy with lavage in the management of refractory asthma with mucous impaction. Ann Allergy 1991;67:324.
102. Henke CA, Hertz M, Gustafson P: Combined bronchoscopy and mucolytic therapy for patients with severe refractory status asthmaticus on mechanical ventilation: A case report and review of the literature. Crit Care Med 1994;22:1880.
103. Millman M, Goodman AH, Goldstein IM, et al: Status asthmaticus: Use of acetylcysteine during bronchoscopy and lavage to remove mucous plugs. Ann Allergy 1983;50:85.
104. Franzen D, Günther H, Borberg H, et al: Plasma exchange: An option for the treatment of life-threatening status asthmaticus in pregnancy. Eur Respir J 1999;13:938.
105. Wilber ST, Wilson JE, Blanda M, et al: The bronchodilator effect of intravenous glucagon in asthma exacerbation: A randomized, controlled trial. Ann Emerg Med 2000;36:427.
106. Rishani R, El-Khatib M, Mroueh S: Treatment of severe status asthmaticus with nitric oxide. Pediatr Pulmonol 1999;28:451.
107. Venkataraman MT, Shanies HM: Pregnancy and asthma. J Asthma 1997;34:265.
108. Murphy VE, Clifton VL Gibson PG: Asthma exacerbations during pregnancy: Incidence and association with adverse pregnancy outcomes. Thorax 2006;61:169-176.
109. Schatz M, Zeiger RS, Hoffman CP: Intrauterine growth is related to gestational pulmonary function in pregnant asthmatic women. Chest 1990;98:389.
110. Schatz M, Zeiger RS, Harden KM, et al: The safety of inhaled beta-agonist bronchodilators during pregnancy. J Allergy Clin Immunol 1988;82:686.
111. Cydulka RK, Emerman CL, Schreiber D, et al: Acute asthma among pregnant women presenting to the emergency department. Am J Respir Crit Care Med 1999;160:887.
112. Murphy VE, Gibson P, Talbot PI, et al: Severe asthma exacerbations during pregnancy. Obstet Gynecol 2005;106(5 Pt 1):1046-1054.
113. Quick Reference from the Working Group Report on Managing Asthma during Pregnancy: Recommendations for Pharmacologic Treatment Update 2004. NIH publication no. 05-3279. Bethesda, MD, National Institutes of Health, 2004.
114. Kearney SE, Graham DR, Atherton ST: Acute severe asthma treated by mechanical ventilation: A comparison of the changing characteristics over a 17 year period. Respir Med 1998;92:716.
115. Zimmerman JL, Dellinger RP, Shah AN, et al: End tracheal intubation and mechanical ventilation in severe asthma. Crit Care Med 1993;21:1727.
116. Nowak RM, Tomlanovich MC, Sarker DD, et al: Arterial blood gases and pulmonary function testing in acute bronchial asthma: Predicting patient outcomes. JAMA 1983;249:2043.
117. Layzer R: Neuromuscular Manifestations of Systemic Disease. Philadelphia, Davis, 1985.
118. Griffin D, Fairman N, Coursin D, et al: Acute myopathy during treatment of status asthmaticus with corticosteroids and steroidal muscle relaxants. Chest 1992;102:510.
119. David WS, Roehr CL, Leatherman JW: EMG findings in acute myopathy with status asthmaticus, steroids and paralytics: Clinical and electrophysiologic correlation. Electromyogr Clin Neurophysiol 1998;38:371.
120. De Lemos JM, Carr RR, Shalansky KF: Paralysis in the critically ill: Intermittent bolus pancuronium compared with continuous infusion. Crit Care Med 1999;27:2648.
121. Drachman D, Stanley E, Pestronik A: Neural regulation of muscle properties. In Serrantrice G, et al (eds): Neuromuscular Diseases. New York, Raven Press, 1984.
122. DuBois DC, Almon RR: A possible role for glucocorticoids in denervation atrophy. Muscle Nerve 1981;4:370.
123. Feihl F, Perret C: Permissive hypercapnea: How permissive should we be? Am J Respir Crit Care Med 1994;150:1722-1737.
124. Smyth RJ: Ventilatory care in status asthmaticus. Can Respir J 1998;5:485.
125. Leatherman JW, Ravenscraft SA, Iber C, et al: Does measured auto-PEEP accurately reflect the degree of dynamic hyperinflation during mechanical ventilation of status asthma? Am Rev Respir Dis 1993;147:877A.
126. Tuxen DV, Williams TJ, Scheinkestel CD, et al: Use of a measurement of pulmonary hyperinflation to control the level of mechanical ventilation in patients with acute severe asthma. Am Rev Respir Dis 1992;146:1136.
127. Menitove SM, Goldring RM: Combined ventilator and bicarbonate strategy in the management of status asthmaticus. Am J Med 1983;74:898.
128. Bidani A, Tzouanakis AE, Cardenas VJ, et al: Permissive hypercapnia in acute respiratory failure. JAMA 1994;272:957.
129. Tuxen DV: Permissive hypercapnic ventilation. Am J Respir Crit Care Med 1994;150:870.
130. Mutlu GM, Factor P, Schwartz DE, et al: Severe status asthmaticus: Management with permissive hypercapnea and inhalation anesthesia. Crit Care Med 2002;30:477-480.
131. Adnet E, Plaisance P, Borron SW, et al: Prolonged severe hypercapnia complicating near fatal asthma in a 35-year-old woman. Intensive Care Med 1998;24:1335.
132. Fernandez MM, Villagra A, Blanch L, et al: Non-invasive mechanical ventilation in status asthmaticus. Intensive Care Med 2001;27:486-492.
133. Martin JG, Shore S, Engel LA: Effect of continuous positive airway pressure on respiratory mechanics and pattern of breathing in induced asthma. Am Rev Respir Dis 1982;126:817.
134. Pollack CV, Fleisch KB, Dowsey K: Treatment of acute bronchospasm with β-adrenergic agonist aerosols delivered by a nasal bilevel positive airway pressure circuit. Ann Emerg Med 1995;26:552.
135. Meduri G, Cook TR, Turner RE, et al: Noninvasive positive pressure ventilation in status asthmaticus. Chest 1996;110:767.
136. Ram FS, Wellington S, Rowe B, et al: Non-invasive positive pressure ventilation for treatment of respiratory failure due to severe acute exacerbations of asthma. Cochrane Database Syst Rev 2005;3:CD004360.
137. Cygan J, Trunsky M, Corbridge T: Inhaled heroin-induced status asthmaticus: Five cases and a review of the literature. Chest 2000;117:272.
138. Tan WC: Viruses in asthma exacerbations. Curr Opin Intern Med 2005;4:178-183.
139. Hasler G, Gergen PJ, Kleinbaum DG, et al: Asthma and panic in young adults. Am J Respir Crit Care Med 2005;171:1224-1230.
140. Turner MO, Noertjojok K, Vedal S, et al: Risk factors for near-fatal asthma. Am J Respir Crit Care Med 1998;157(6 Pt 1):1804-1809.

Chapter 40

Chronic Obstructive Pulmonary Disease

Guillermo Domínguez-Cherit, Juan Gabriel Posadas-Calleja, and Delia Borunda

The American Thoracic Society recommends that the term *chronic obstructive pulmonary disease* (COPD) be applied to patients who have chronic bronchitis or emphysema or both with significant airflow limitation that does not change significantly over several months of observation, differentiating these patients from patients with asthma.[1] This chapter focuses on the management of patients who have COPD with acute respiratory failure (ARF).

DEFINITIONS

ARF is defined by arterial blood gas analysis. In a patient without underlying lung disease, ARF is defined by a arterial oxygen tension (PaO_2) of less than 50 mm Hg (breathing fraction of inspired oxygen [FIO_2] 0.21 at sea level).[2] In a patient with COPD, it is difficult to define ARF by arterial blood gas analysis without knowledge of baseline arterial blood gas levels. Clinical data, such as worsening of daily baseline symptoms, cough, tachypnea, and deterioration of mental status, also must be considered. A decrease in PaO_2 from baseline and an increase in arterial carbon dioxide tension ($PaCO_2$) with acidemia is a common presentation of ARF in COPD.

BACKGROUND

COPD is a common, costly, and preventable disease that has implications for worldwide health. In the United States, COPD is the fourth leading cause of death,[3] exceeded only by heart attacks, cancer, and stroke.[4] Among 28 industrialized countries, the United States ranks 12th in COPD mortality for men and 7th for women.[3] It has been estimated that 16 million Americans have symptomatic COPD. During 1993, COPD cost roughly $15 billion distributed among physician consultations, hospitalizations, and other health care resources.[5]

COPD has had a similar effect on health and mortality throughout the developed and underdeveloped world, and many of the important issues surrounding COPD in the United States apply elsewhere.[6] Worldwide, COPD is the only leading cause of death that still has an increasing mortality, and it has been estimated that by 2020, COPD will be fifth among the most burdensome conditions to society.[3] COPD is a disease that is essentially totally preventable by avoiding smoking tobacco.

PATHOPHYSIOLOGY

The main pathophysiologic feature in COPD is the limitation to expiratory flow.[7] Chronic expiratory flow limitation and hyperinflation are the mechanical hallmarks of COPD.[8] Expiratory airflow limitation results from many factors; among them narrowing of the peripheral airways,[9] mucous hypersecretion,[10] and impaired ciliary clearance[11] are the most important. COPD consists of a combination of chronic bronchitis and emphysema. In patients with chronic bronchitis, bronchial mucosal edema[9] and hyperplasia[10] contribute to the obstruction. In emphysematous patients, there is a destruction of the elastic supporting structure with decreased elastic recoil.[12]

Although carbon dioxide (CO_2) retention depends on the severity of airflow limitation, there is considerable variability in the relationship of Pa_{CO_2} to forced expiratory volume in 1 second (FEV_1) and total lung resistance,[13] best explained by contribution of deadspace and minute ventilation. In stable COPD patients with severe airflow obstruction, shallow breathing is the main factor associated with CO_2 retention.[14] In stable COPD patients, the diaphragm is less effective than in normal subjects, and with increasing airflow obstruction and hyperinflation, the contribution of the ribcage muscle to the generation of ventilatory pressure increases.[15] Abdominal muscles are recruited during expiration in patients with severe COPD, and the expiratory increase in gastric pressure is directly related to intrinsic positive end-expiratory pressure (PEEP). During acute bronchoconstriction, COPD patients with severe airflow obstruction increase the inspiratory recruitment of the ribcage muscles relative to the diaphragm. This recruitment is associated with abdominal muscle contraction and a reduction in abdominal volume at end expiration, which contributes to intrinsic PEEP. Dynamic hyperinflation can be overestimated during chronic and acute airway obstruction if abdominal muscle function is not evaluated.[13,14]

During a COPD exacerbation, all of the aforementioned factors contribute to the increase in airflow limitation, often resulting in air trapping, increased work of breathing,[16] reduction in chest wall and lung compliance,[8,17] and development of intrinsic PEEP, which requires the patient to generate increased negative pleural pressure to initiate inspiratory flow.[18] The consequence is the ominous combination of an increase in the work of breathing[19] and a reduction in the mechanical capabilities of the respiratory muscles. As the muscles of inspiration lengthen in response to severe air trapping, the optimal length-tension relationship is exceeded.[20]

The worsening gas exchange and the deterioration of the arterial blood gas values during acute exacerbations in patients with severe COPD can be explained by several factors: respiratory muscle fatigue,[21] increases in deadspace ventilation, alveolar hypoventilation, and worsening of ventilation-perfusion matching.[22] Minute ventilation may be normal early in an exacerbation, but the respiratory rate is generally increased.[23] There is an associated increase in physiologic deadspace that impairs CO_2 elimination and may result in acidemia.[24] The hypoxemia seen during exacerbations results from the combination of two factors—alveolar hypoventilation[25] and worsening of ventilation-perfusion matching.[26,27] Increases in ventilation-perfusion heterogeneity are attributed to (1) a reduction in the effectiveness of hypoxic vasoconstriction as a protective mechanism as pulmonary artery pressure increases and vasodilating inflammatory mediators are released[27] and (2) the failure to redirect perfusion away from inadequately ventilated regions because of the reduction in cross-sectional area of the pulmonary vascular bed.

CLINICAL MANIFESTATIONS

Most COPD patients with acute exacerbations initially show some combination of increasing cough, worsening of dyspnea, increased sputum production, purulent sputum, or increase in viscosity of the sputum, rather than a deterioration noted by laboratory or respiratory function parameters. Symptoms may come on slowly over several days or acutely, depending on the severity of the underlying disease. Often, patients have a history of upper respiratory tract infection. Patients generally appear in acute distress. Vital signs typically show tachycardia and tachypnea, and blood pressure can be reduced in response to the effect of intrinsic PEEP. Use of accessory inspiratory muscles may be seen with increasing severity of exacerbations. With inspiration, the diaphragm normally moves down as it contracts, forcing the abdominal contents out. With diaphragmatic fatigue, the diaphragm no longer functions as a primary muscle of inspiration, but instead assists the intercostal muscles' inspiratory effort by fixing the ribcage. This action is associated with a rise in the diaphragm, and the abdomen moves in instead of out as it does with normal inspiration. This is called *paradoxical breathing*.[28] This sign implies respiratory muscle fatigue and often imminent ventilatory failure and respiratory arrest.[29] Wheezing and other auscultatory findings of obstruction also are present. Cyanosis is an insensitive manifestation, but when seen denotes severe hypoxemia. Patients with severe acute CO_2 retention may present in coma.

PRECIPITATING FACTORS

Although the precise cause of acute exacerbation is poorly understood, it has been associated with numerous precipitating factors, as follows:

- Bacterial or viral infection[30,31]
- Environmental factors[32,33]
- Pulmonary embolism[34]
- Medication failure or patient noncompliance[35]
- Other

Exacerbation occurs more commonly with increasing baseline severity of COPD. At present, there is a clear understanding in regard to deterioration as measured by physiologic parameters; however, there is little knowledge regarding histopathologic features during a COPD exacerbation.[36] The importance of this information relates to the presence or absence of invading pathogens and the degree of lung and airway structure alterations.[37] Histologic findings, as defined in the literature, include vascular congestion of the airway mucosa[38] and plasma exudation,[39] perhaps triggered by inflammation.[40] These findings could contribute to the airway narrowing, which, along with goblet cell hyperplasia[9] and mucus hypersecretion,[10] can quickly narrow the already compromised small airway geometry. All of these factors produce nonbronchospastic flow limitation.

Infections

Infectious agents are the major cause of acute exacerbation of COPD. Respiratory viruses are associated with 30% of exacerbations with or without a superimposed bacterial infection.[41]

Several studies have been conducted to investigate airway bacterial infections as etiologic factors involved in COPD exacerbations.[42-44] At present, there seems to be an agreement that the major pathogens isolated from sputum during acute exacerbation are *Haemophilus influenzae, Streptococcus pneumoniae,* and *Moraxella catarrhalis*[45]; however, all of these bacteria can be isolated in patients during the stable phases of COPD.[46,47] Atypical bacteria, mostly *Chlamydia pneumoniae,* have been implicated in approximately 10% of acute exacerbations.[48,49] Other potential microorganisms that should be considered include other *Streptococcus* species, enteric gram-negative bacilli, and *Legionella*.[50] The role of bacterial pathogens isolated from the respiratory tract during an acute exacerbation has become better defined by application of bronchoscopic protected brush sampling with quantitative or semiquantitative cultures. When properly defined, 80% of acute exacerbations are likely to be infectious in origin.[31,51-53]

Environmental Factors

Environmental factors are among the noninfectious causes of COPD exacerbation that should be investigated as precipitating causes.[33,54-57] Air pollution is implicated as a trigger of exacerbations[58]; however, a direct cause-and-effect relationship has been difficult to establish over the last 50 years.[59] From an epidemiologic viewpoint, definitive evidence exists regarding a role of air pollutants in the increased death rates seen in cities during periods of heavy pollution.[60] The dramatic increase in motor vehicle traffic has produced a relative increase in the levels of newer pollutants, such as ozone and fine-particulate air pollution. Elucidation of the mechanisms of the harmful effects of these pollutants should allow improved risk assessment for patients with airway diseases who are susceptible to the effects of these air pollutants.

Pulmonary Thromboembolism

Pulmonary thromboembolism (PTE) can precipitate acute COPD exacerbations through impairment of gas exchange or increases in pulmonary vascular pressures.[61,62] Some evidence suggests that deep venous thrombosis occurs in more than 5 million people each year. More than 500,000 people eventually develop PTE, which is the primary cause of death in more than 100,000 patients annually in the United States.[63] The precise incidence of PTE in COPD is unknown. Studies in COPD patients have found pulmonary embolus in 50% of autopsies. PTE risk factors inherent to COPD are sedentary lifestyle, right ventricular failure, right ventricular mural thrombi, and secondary polycythemia.[64] Patients with COPD also have been shown to have increased platelet aggregation and increased plasma β-thromboglobulin.[64]

Thirty percent of untreated thromboembolic patients die.[63] Diagnosing PTE as the precipitating factor in acute COPD exacerbation is crucial (Fig. 40-1). The diagnosis of PTE is extremely difficult in COPD exacerbation, however. Nonetheless, the approach to diagnosis is similar to that used with other patients.[34,65] Most patients with COPD have an indeterminate ventilation-perfusion scan, usually making this scan unhelpful in evaluation for PTE.[66] For patients with such indeterminate results (low or intermediate probability), noninvasive testing of the lower extremity should be conducted.[69,70] If positive results for deep venous thrombosis are obtained, anticoagulation therapy must be initiated. It has been proposed that use of newer D-dimer assays also may have a role as a diagnostic tool; however, even with a sensitivity of 98%, specificity is

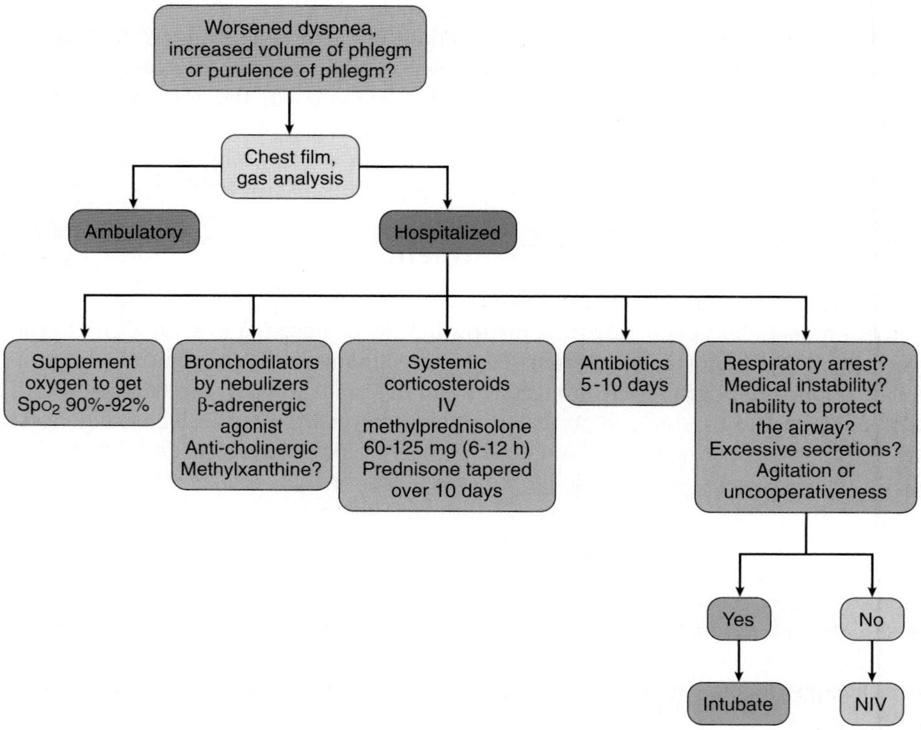

Figure 40-1. Diagnosis and management of chronic obstructive pulmonary disease. NIV, noninvasive ventilation.

problematic, with a value of 39%.[71] When the diagnosis is still in doubt (intermediate-probability scan and negative leg study or low-probability scan and negative leg study with intermediate clinical probability of PTE), helical computed tomography (CT) or conventional pulmonary angiography may be required. Although the safety of pulmonary angiography in patients with cor pulmonale has been questioned, data from the PIOPED (Prospective Investigation of Pulmonary Embolism Diagnosis) study support safety and accuracy in patients with COPD.[66] Helical CT has become an increasingly accepted technique and is the method of choice for direct visualization of pulmonary emboli. The quantitative assessment of tissue perfusion may yield more important information for patient management than the direct visualization of emboli by CT alone.[67] Enhanced multislice helical CT with thin collimation can be used to analyze precisely the subsegmental pulmonary arteries and may identify even more distal pulmonary arteries.[68] More recent data suggest that helical CT may be an alternative to angiography, particularly when results are not discordant with pretest clinical probability of pulmonary emboli, and when combined with other tests that support CT findings (D-dimer, leg ultrasound, lung scanning). Helical CT may have adequate sensitivity and specificity in the COPD population (see Chapter 45).

Medication Failure or Noncompliance

Many acute COPD exacerbations can be explained by inadequate pharmacologic therapy or noncompliance with pharmacologic therapy. These are likely underestimated causes of exacerbation in COPD patients. It also is possible that patients overmedicate, leading to toxic drug effects of cardiac, gastrointestinal, or metabolic nature. Certain pharmacologic interactions can precipitate toxicity or loss of effect of one drug, and the physician must ascertain whether newer medications for other conditions have recently been added to the patient's therapeutic regimen.[35,72,73]

Other Causes

Clinical decompensation in patients with stable COPD also may occur as a result of acute congestive heart failure or cardiac arrhythmia. One study found that 27% of COPD patients die as a result of coronary disease.[74] This is likely because of the shared risk factor of cigarette smoking. Other causes of exacerbation include sleep-disordered breathing,[75-78] vocal cord paralysis, tumor or scarring from prior intubations, and development of spontaneous pneumothorax.[79,80] Finally, pleural effusion can produce respiratory deterioration, especially in patients with poor respiratory reserve.[81]

INITIAL MANAGEMENT

Because chronic airflow obstruction cannot be reversed, acute management of COPD is directed at reversible pathogenetic mechanisms, including pulmonary infection, airway tissue inflammation, bronchoconstriction, and support of failing muscular function.

Oxygen

Oxygen remains the mainstay of initial therapy in most COPD exacerbations. Relief of hypoxemia, and consequently of hypoxemic pulmonary vasoconstriction, decreases pulmonary vascular resistance, with variable effects on the ventilation-perfusion ratio.[82,83] Oxygen delivery may increase as a result of increases in oxygen arterial content and anticipated improved right-sided heart function. One study showed, however, that relief of hypoxemia did not increase cardiac output.[84]

Hypercapnia is well tolerated when it is chronic.[85-87] Oxygen should be administered cautiously in patients who have chronic hypercapnia, however, because it is known to lead to clinically significant increases in $Pa{CO_2}$ in certain COPD patients as a result of changes in the physiologic deadspace and perhaps suppression of the respiratory drive.[88,89] Acute increases in $Pa{CO_2}$ are more likely to occur in patients with elevated baseline $Pa{CO_2}$. A randomized study showed that although oxygen administration worsened hypercarbia and respiratory acidosis, these changes were well tolerated in most patients.[90] Oxygen therapy should not be withheld in acutely ill hypoxemic patients because tissular hypoxia can lead to acute organ dysfunction.

Oxygen should be initiated at a low $F{IO_2}$ and slowly titrated up as necessary with vigilant monitoring to document improvement and stabilization in $Pa{O_2}$, with special attention paid to maintaining the oxyhemoglobin at 90% or greater without producing dangerous decreases in pH as a result of increases in CO_2. These dangerous increases in $Pa{CO_2}$ typically are associated with worsening mental status. In some circumstances, acceptance of oxyhemoglobin saturation levels less than 90% may be a better option than intubation and mechanical ventilation. Nasal cannulas or Venturi masks can be used to initiate a low $F{IO_2}$. Either a nasal cannula at a flow rate of 1 L/min or a Venturi mask initially at the lowest setting (25%) is appropriate for initiating oxygen in patients known or suspected to be chronic CO_2 retainers. In the presence of acute severe hypoxemia in patients with impending respiratory failure, high-flow oxygen therapy may be in the patient's best interest, regardless of the risk for CO_2 retention.[91]

Drug Treatment

Bronchodilators

Bronchodilator therapy is indicated in acute COPD exacerbations, even in patients without clinical wheezing. Although intravenous bronchodilators are available (methylxanthines or in some countries β_2-selective agonists), inhaled delivery of β_2-selective agonists and ipratropium is the therapy of choice for acute exacerbations of COPD because of the advantageous benefit-to-toxicity ratio. Bronchodilator treatment in acutely ill COPD patients has been shown to decrease inspiratory muscle loading, with an increase in FEV_1 and a decrease in functional residual capacity and dynamic hyperinflation.[92] In mechanically ventilated patients, a reduction in expiratory resistance and dynamic hyperinflation (measured as a decrease in intrinsic PEEP) has been described.[93]

There is no strong evidence supporting use of one inhaled β_2-selective agonist over another. The widespread use of inhaled β-agonists has been accompanied by clinical concern of cardiac complications in elderly patients and patients with coronary artery disease. In a study on clinically stable COPD or asthma patients with a history of myocardial ischemia, no ischemic events, arrhythmias, or tachycardias were observed, however, when commonly used doses of salbutamol were administered.[94] In high-risk cardiac patients, ipratropium may be preferred over β-agonists because of the decreased chance of cardiac side effects. Although ipratropium bromide is widely used in stable COPD patients with improvement of pulmonary mechanics and essentially no toxicity, its use as the sole therapy in acute exacerbations is not recommended[95-97] because it has a less predictable clinical response compared with β-agonists in this population.[98]

Tiotropium bromide is a cholinolytic bronchodilator that antagonizes muscarinic receptors and dissociates more slowly from M_1 and M_3 than from M_2 and subsequently has a long duration of action. Tiotropium reduces the number of exacerbations, increases time to first exacerbation, and improves lung function significantly compared with ipratropium. Tiotropium produces superior bronchodilation and improvements in dyspnea and health-related quality of life compared with ipratropium and salmeterol in patients with COPD. The use of tiotropium is associated with sustained reduction of lung hyperinflation at rest and during exercise.[99] Its benefits in acute exacerbation have not been fully shown, however.[100] Superiority of combination β-agonist and ipratropium bromide also is controversial, with some reports showing clinical improvement with combined use,[101,102] and others showing no difference from the improvement achieved with inhaled β-agonist therapy alone.[103-106] In acute severe exacerbations of COPD, we recommend combination therapy.

Although parenteral use of theophylline compounds is not recommended as part of initial therapy of COPD exacerbation, it may be considered in admitted patients who are unresponsive to β-agonist, ipratropium, and steroid therapy. Magnesium sulfate therapy, although reported in a few case reports to be temporarily associated with improvement,[107] is not recommended as therapy in COPD exacerbation.

Aerosol Delivery

Classically, aerosolized drugs in acutely ill, nonintubated patients have been administered with pressure-driven jet nebulizers. More recent investigations have shown, however, that with proper technique and attachments, inhaled therapy can be delivered effectively with commercial metered-dose inhalers (MDIs) or dry-powder inhalers, without a decrease in pharmacologic effects. There is no clinical difference whether aerosol therapy is administered via nebulized wet aerosols, MDIs, or dry-powder inhalers, as long as appropriate dosing and techniques are used.[108-111] Of these three alternatives, an MDI is the most often used. A spacing device, which enhances lower airway drug deposition, is indicated when used for acute exacerbations to ensure adequate drug delivery.[112] Some reports have shown, however, that patients with extremely impaired airway function receive a suboptimal dose when an MDI with spacer is used; a twofold to fourfold increase in drug dosage is recommended.[113-115] In the most severely tachypneic and dyspneic patients, nebulizers are still the best option to ensure optimal drug delivery.

Most modern commercial mechanical ventilators have a built-in nebulization system, which allows easily achievable synchronized administration during mechanical inspirations and avoids manipulation of the ventilator circuitry. An MDI also is an option for use in mechanically ventilated patients.[116] In these patients, a review of published reports found no differences when comparing drug delivery using an MDI or a nebulizer.[117]

Corticosteroids

Systemic parenteral corticosteroids were routinely used over the years in the medical therapy of hospitalized COPD patients, despite no conclusive evidence supporting their efficacy.[106,118,119] Until more recently, reports advocating corticosteroid use were primarily based on chronic stable patients and outpatient acute exacerbations.[120,121] Although some studies showed clinical improvement in FEV_1 in patients with acute exacerbations,[122,123] one report found no differences when comparing methylprednisolone with placebo.[124] Systemic corticosteroids have been shown to improve respiratory mechanics in mechanically ventilated patients, with a decrease in airway resistance and dynamic air trapping.[125] In a report that described corticosteroid responders and nonresponders among hospital patients with acute exacerbations of COPD, failure to respond correlated with a 100-mL increase in FEV_1 during the first two post-treatment measures.[121]

In a study by Niewoehner and colleagues,[126] COPD patients with exacerbations were randomly assigned within the first 12 hours of admission to receive 125 mg of methylprednisolone intravenously every 6 hours for 72 hours, followed by a 4-day oral steroid taper (group 1) or a 2-week taper (group 2). Group 3 received placebo only (no steroids). FEV_1 improved faster in groups 1 and 2 compared with the placebo group, and hospital stay was shorter in groups 1 and 2 compared with the placebo group. No difference was noted between groups 1 and 2. This study supports the use of steroids with a short (4-day) taper in COPD patients admitted with exacerbation.

Antibiotics

Because bacteria are often found in the lower respiratory tract of COPD patients,[31,51-53] and infection is a common precipitating factor of COPD exacerbations, antibiotic therapy seems a reasonable consideration. This is a controversial area, however, with some authors recommending antibiotic therapy and others not.[132,133] We believe that antibiotic therapy benefits select groups of patients with COPD exacerbations. A randomized, double-blind study by Anthonisen and coworkers[134] and a meta-analysis of randomized trials between 1957 and 1992 by Saint and colleagues[135] support a small but clinically significant antibiotic benefit in COPD patients (defined as more rapid improvement in peak flow and fewer hospital days). Patients who are most likely to benefit have increasing shortness of breath associated with a change in sputum character or increased sputum production. Destache and associates[136] classified antibiotics for treatment of COPD exacerbation as first-line (amoxicillin, trimethoprim/sulfamethoxazole, tetracycline, erythromycin), second-line (cephradine, cefuroxime, cefaclor, cefprozil), and third-line antibiotics (amoxicillin/clavulanate, azithromycin, ciprofloxacin); greater efficacy was shown with the third-line antibiotics. In a retrospective study, Adams and associates[137] reported similar results.

Although routine sputum cultures are advisable in all patients with COPD exacerbations, invasive techniques (transtracheal aspirates,[138,139] bronchoscopic aspirates, or protected specimen brushing[51,52,140,141]) are not indicated. Exceptions include culture-negative, community-acquired pneumonia not responding to therapy and ventilator-associated pneumonia.[142-145] Because many COPD patients have airway colonization by bacteria, without clinical signs of infection and exacerbation, there is no clear significance of a positive culture in a COPD patient; however, in the presence of exacerbation associated with an alteration in sputum character or quantity, potentially pathogenic organisms grown from sputum should be covered with an appropriate antibiotic.[146]

A more recent review shows that in COPD exacerbations with increased cough and sputum purulence, antibiotics reduce the relative risk of short-term mortality by 77%, the relative risk of treatment failure by 53%, and the relative risk of sputum purulence by 44%. This review supports antibiotics for patients with COPD exacerbations with increased cough and sputum purulence who are moderately or severely ill.[147]

Other Drugs

Although central respiratory stimulants (analeptics) have been used in COPD patients with acute respiratory acidosis with the rationale that stimulation of central respiratory centers would increase respiratory drive and avoid respiratory acidosis, this group of drugs has a very narrow therapeutic threshold and the potential to produce seizures. Analeptics are not recommended for routine therapy of COPD-associated hypocarbia.[148] Other central respiratory stimulants (e.g., doxapram, almitrine mesylate) are potential options; however, they are not approved by the U.S. Food and Drug Administration for use in COPD patients[149,150] and have not been shown in clinical studies to decrease the incidence or duration of mechanical ventilation.[151]

Hemodynamic Support

Fluid Management

COPD patients often have chronic pulmonary hypertension, which may worsen with COPD exacerbation because of hypoxic vasoconstriction, dynamic lung hyperinflation, and, in mechanically ventilated patients, intrinsic PEEP. This may lead to acute or worsening right ventricular failure. In one study, the prevalence of right ventricular failure in terminal COPD patients was 66%, and the prevalence of left ventricular failure was only 6%.[152] As in other patients with right ventricular failure, hemodynamic stability is related to maintenance of mean arterial pressure. Mean systemic pressure potentially can be increased in these patients by increasing intravascular volume or by selectively improving compliance of the pulmonary vascular bed.[153] Intravenous fluid challenge is the initial step in hemodynamic support in the presence of hemodynamic compromise. These patients often have peripheral edema, and fluids are often restricted to treat this cosmetic effect. Diuretics also may have been administered, leading to loss of intravascular volume, decreased venous return, decreased cardiac output, and hypotension.

Likewise, because pulmonary hypertension produces chronically elevated right ventricular pressures, fluid challenge potentially could worsen the hemodynamic status of patients with cor pulmonale. Overzealous fluid administration may increase right ventricular pressure to the point that it produces a shift in the interventricular septum and a reduction in left ventricular compliance and filling. Currently, no consensus or guidelines exist concerning invasive pulmonary artery catheterization in this group of patients; however, in patients remaining hypotensive after initial volume challenge or in patients with organ perfusion abnormalities and biventricular failure, invasive monitoring may be clinically useful.

Inotropics and Vasodilators

In patients who remain hemodynamically unstable despite fluid therapy, adrenergic therapy is advised. Although some literature recommends adrenergic therapy of right ventricular failure using norepinephrine[154,155] or dobutamine,[156] we could find no controlled trials of adrenergic drug therapy in hemodynamically unstable COPD patients. Because pulmonary embolism patients have a hemodynamic derangement similar to that of COPD patients with right ventricular failure, however, dobutamine seems a reasonable choice in attempts to increase right ventricular function and to increase cardiac output in a normotensive patient with decreased tissue perfusion. In the presence of hypotension, dobutamine would be used in combination with a inotrope vasopressor such as norepinephrine or dopamine. Nitroglycerin has been shown in one study to enhance right ventricular performance when added to dobutamine.[157] Nitroglycerin should be administered cautiously in patients who may have suboptimal right ventricle filling. Digoxin has no anticipated clinical utility in right ventricular failure, unless it is associated with left ventricular failure or arrhythmias that respond to digoxin.[158-160]

Although vasodilators have been used in clinical trials of COPD with right ventricular failure,[161-168] there is no consistent evidence of clinical outcome benefit. Inhaled nitric oxide, a selective pulmonary vasodilator with a short half-life and no systemic vasodilator properties, has shown variable results in patients with exacerbation of COPD.[169-173]

Secretion Management

Although mucous hypersecretion has not been linked with mortality,[174] enhancing clearance of secretions improves respiratory mechanics, accelerates recovery from acute exacerbations, and adds to patient comfort. Chest physical therapy has no role in the management of exacerbation of COPD. One report found no differences in sputum volume or arterial blood gases when chest physiotherapy (expansion exercises, postural drainage, and vibrations) was compared with conventional therapy.[175] This result was substantiated in an additional study.[176] Some studies have shown that postural drainage, percussion, directed cough, and vibrations produce a significant decline in FEV_1, which is not observed with postural drainage and directed cough alone.[177,178] Bronchoscopy also has no role in the routine management of central airway secretions. It rarely may be used in patients with large-volume atelectasis associated with significant symptoms, who are not responding to conventional therapy.

Although more recent reports describe a decreased rate of COPD exacerbations with orally administered *N*-acetylcysteine in ambulatory patients,[179-181] its use in acutely ill COPD patients remains to be established. It is not recommended for aerosol delivery in COPD exacerbation. Novel pharmacotherapeutic targets are being investigated, including inhibitors of nerve activity (e.g., large conductance calcium-activated potassium, BKCa, channel activators), tachykinin receptor antagonists, epoxygenase inducers (e.g., benzafibrate), inhibitors of mucin exocytosis (e.g., anti-myristoylated alanine-rich C kinase substrate [MARCKS], peptide, and Munc-18B blockers), inhibitors of mucin synthesis and goblet cell hyperplasia (e.g., epidermal growth factor, receptor tyrosine kinase inhibitors, p38 mitogen-activated protein [MAP], kinase inhibitors, MAP kinase/extracellular signal-regulated kinase [MEK/ERK] inhibitors, human calcium-activated chloride [hCACL2] channel blockers, and retinoic acid receptor-a antagonists), inducers of goblet cell apoptosis (e.g., Bax inducers or Bcl-2 inhibitors), and purinoceptor P(2Y2) antagonists to inhibit mucin secretion or P(2Y2) agonists to hydrate secretions.[182]

Nutritional Support

Chapter 83 discusses overall nutritional support of critically ill patients; highlights of some issues directly related to COPD patients follow. Malnutrition has been recognized as a factor that increases mortality[183,184] in COPD. Weight gain has been associated with decreased mortality.[185] Nutritional status tends to decline markedly during acute illness in COPD patients,[186-188] and patients may not recover to their previous nutritional state during convalescence, with recurrent exacerbations leading to a stepwise decline in nutritional status over time.[189] Studies have shown that skeletal muscle mass is directly related to muscle dysfunction in COPD patients.[185] Nutritional status has been correlated with weaning outcome.[190] Short-term studies of oral supplemental feeding or enteral feeding have shown increases in body weight and improvement in immunologic markers and respiratory muscle function.[191-193] Nutritional support has been shown to produce improvement in lung function in hospitalized patients with acute exacerbation of COPD.[194]

Special care must be taken to avoid overfeeding patients with COPD exacerbation because excess calories, particularly if carbohydrate-rich, elevate total oxygen consumption and CO_2 production, which may complicate management in patients with hypercapnia.[195-199] In one study of mechanically ventilated patients, enteral nutrition was administered with a fixed carbohydrate content, and an association between total caloric intake and CO_2 production when providing nutritional support to COPD patients with ARF was noted. It has been recommended that enteral alimentation provide total calories 1.25 to 1.3 times the resting energy expenditure of the patient with a respiratory quotient target of 0.7 to 0.8 and limiting carbohydrate calories to 40% of total calories.[200]

NONINVASIVE MECHANICAL VENTILATION

Despite adequate and aggressive treatment, patients with exacerbation of COPD may require mechanical ventilatory support. The frequency of this support varies among series, reaching 74%.[201] This respiratory support may be of two types—invasive or noninvasive ventilation. Noninvasive positive-pressure ventilation (NPPV) using a nasal mask or facemask has proved efficacious in ARF caused by COPD in several clinical studies, with success rates of 65% in some series.[202-204] One randomized trial studied the use of NPPV in COPD exacerbation associated with manifestations of respiratory failure and showed decreases in the need for endotracheal intubation, length of hospital stay, and in-hospital mortality rate.[205] A case-control study was performed in patients with acute exacerbation of COPD who received at least 2 hours of NPPV as the central ventilation therapy and patients who had the same risk predictive characteristics but did not receive NPPV.[206] The investigators concluded that the use of NPPV was associated with a lower risk of nosocomial infections, less antibiotic use, shorter length of stay in the intensive care unit (ICU), and lower mortality. In a prospective study with 122 patients affected by COPD complicated by ARF and treated with noninvasive ventilation, the schedule of noninvasive ventilation provided sessions of 2 to 6 hours twice daily; the authors concluded that noninvasive ventilation may be useful to avoid intubation in approximately 80% of patients with COPD complicated by moderate to severe hypercapnic respiratory failure.[207]

Physiologic Effects

The mechanism of action of NPPV is the same as that for invasive ventilation. Supra-atmospheric pressures are applied intermittently through the airways, increasing transpulmonary pressure and insufflating the lungs. Exhalation is a passive process related to the elastic recoil properties of the lung. The major salutary effects of NPPV are its ability to decrease the work of breathing and improve alveolar ventilation, while resting respiratory musculature. Improvement in gas exchange results from an increase in alveolar ventilation without observable changes in ventilation-perfusion matching.[208] Transdiaphragmatic pressure, diaphragmatic pressure-time product, and diaphragmatic electromyographic amplitude all are decreased by the application of NPPV-delivered pressure support ventilation (PSV) to patients with exacerbations of COPD.[209] NPPV may prevent the development of muscle fatigue by providing support during respiratory crisis, decreasing the need for tracheal intubation and its related complications. In mechanically ventilated patients with auto-PEEP, the addition of externally applied PEEP produced decreases in the work of breathing by allowing triggering of the ventilator with less negative inspiratory effort.

Potential physiologic benefits of NPPV in COPD patients include improvement in tidal volume, gas exchange, respiratory rate, heart rate, oxygenation, and diaphragm activity and a reduction in arterial CO_2 with a concomitant improvement in pH. When these beneficial responses occur, they are typically seen in the first several hours after beginning NPPV.

Indications

According to the consensus statement of the American Association of Respiratory Care,[210] initiation of noninvasive ventilation in COPD patients is recommended when two or more of the following criteria are present:

- Respiratory distress with moderate to severe dyspnea
- pH less than 7.35 with a Pa_{CO_2} greater than 45 mm Hg
- Respiratory rate of 25 breaths per minute or more

Implementation of Noninvasive Positive-Pressure Ventilation

One critical item in this respiratory modality is the interface for the application of NPPV; this can be accomplished with a facemask, nasal mask, or oronasal mask and the recently introduced helmet. The nasal mask has less deadspace, causes less claustrophobia, minimizes potential complications in case of vomiting, and allows expectoration and oral intake of fluids without the need to remove the mask. Facemasks are preferable in severely dyspneic patients, however, because the nasal resistance to breathing is decreased with combined nose and mouth air entry. Also, opening of the mouth during nasal NPPV produces loss of tidal volume, which decreases effectiveness. No study has made a direct comparison of the efficacy of one or the other type of masks. In our opinion, the facemask is optimal for initial use in most patients with severe respiratory distress.

As for the ventilatory mode, several choices are available, including assist control (either volume ventilation or pressure-control ventilation) and PSV. Randomized, controlled trials of NPPV in COPD exacerbations have shown efficacy using a wide variety of modes.[201-204]

PSV was shown in one study to be better tolerated than assist-control mask ventilation, with greater patient-ventilator synchrony, presumably related to the patient's ability to regulate independently the depth and pattern of breathing.[210] Another study found, however, that assist-control volume-cycled ventilation delivered by mask reduced the work of breathing to a greater extent than PSV, but was no more effective than mask PSV in preventing intubation among COPD patients.[211] Bilevel positive airway pressure has become the preferred mode of NPPV administration in COPD patients because it is generally as comfortable as PSV, but produces greater improvements in gas exchange and reduces the work of breathing more effectively than PSV alone.[212,214] With NPPV PSV, tidal volume may vary with changes in airway resistance and lung compliance.

Selection of the Ventilator

Several types of ventilators specifically designed for NPPV, with pressure-limited and volume-cycled modes, are available. Advantages of specific ventilators made for NPPV include smaller size, portability, and less expense. Standard microprocessor-controlled ventilators used for invasive ventilation also can be used. These ventilators offer numerous advantages over portable units made for NPPV, including the following:[215,216]

- Precisely measured and high concentrations of oxygen can be delivered.
- Separate inspiratory and expiratory tubing minimizes CO_2 rebreathing.
- Large mask leaks or patient disconnection can be more readily detected.
- Monitoring and alarm features are more sophisticated.

Initial Approach and Maintenance

Explaining the procedure in depth to the patient facilitates cooperation, acceptance, and success. The facemask is recommended for initial use in most patients. Close surveillance and monitoring by health care personnel, ideally in a step-down or ICU bed, are advised. The patient should be made NPO (nothing by mouth) during initial ventilation until success of NPPV is clear.

For PSV ventilation, the initial inspiratory support pressure is set at 5 to 8 cm H_2O above the end-expiratory pressure setting and raised slowly over time as tolerated to achieve the target Pa_{CO_2}. With the assist-control volume-cycled mode, the starting tidal volume is 10 mL/kg ideal body weight and adjusted up or down for tolerance and effect on Pa_{CO_2}. The patient-triggered PSV mode is usually tolerated better in most patients. PSV is set at 5 to 8 cm H_2O above end-expiratory pressure and then titrated up to the desired tidal volume. There is evidence supporting an efficient breathing pattern as the primary goal during NPPV.[216] When using ventilators made for NPPV, we recommend the use of an oxygen cannula plugged directly into the entry port located at the mask, titrating oxygen flow to desired pulse oximetry values. Tidal volume is increased gradually according to patient tolerance, targeting a reduction in Pa_{CO_2} of 5 to 10 mm Hg and focusing on the pH target over a specific Pa_{CO_2} level. With ventilators made for NPPV, the end-expiratory pressure (synonymous with PEEP) is typically set at 4 to 5 cm H_2O to facilitate ventilator function. With standard ventilators, this is unnecessary, although an initial end-expiratory pressure of 4 to 5 cm H_2O may minimize the effects of auto-PEEP.

Patients who respond to NPPV typically have rapid synchronization with the ventilator and a decrease in respiratory rate, heart rate, and $Pa{CO_2}$ during the first several hours of ventilation.[218] In the absence of these improvements over the first several hours, intubation and invasive mechanical ventilation are advisable. One report found an additional clinical response when heliox was added to NPPV.[219,220]

Weaning

Weaning from NPPV may be accomplished by progressively decreasing the levels of inspiratory positive pressure support, by permitting the patient to be intermittently off NPPV for increasing lengths of time, or by a combination of both strategies. In general, it is useful to wean patients by progressively lengthening the period of spontaneous breathing without NPPV. When the crisis is over, many patients can be weaned relatively quickly. In contrast to invasive ventilation, NPPV can be reinstituted easily and quickly if the patient shows signs of fatigue or intolerance to spontaneous breathing. The use of nocturnal NPPV may be needed during the early weaning period and may be continued at home in some patients.[221]

Studies have analyzed weaning outcome in intubated COPD patients, comparing NPPV with conventional weaning methods. Results showed that NPPV reduced weaning time, shortened ICU length of stay, decreased the incidence of nosocomial pneumonia, and improved 60-day survival rates.[222,223] NPPV also has been used successfully in another study of postextubation hypercarbia patients.[224] A meta-analysis concluded that the use of NPPV to facilitate weaning in mechanically ventilated patients with predominantly COPD is associated with promising, but insufficient, evidence of net clinical benefit at present.[225]

Complications

Adverse hemodynamic effects resulting from NPPV are unusual. One study failed to find hypotension, acute arrhythmias, or significant changes in cardiac output assessed by Doppler echocardiography.[226] Many studies suggest that the risk of nosocomial pneumonia in patients treated by NPPV is decreased compared with that of intubated patients.[221,224]

INVASIVE MECHANICAL VENTILATION

Invasive ventilation is indicated for patients who are not suited for NPPV or who fail NPPV (see following discussion). The need for invasive mechanical ventilation may be an ominous sign. Patients with acute exacerbation of COPD requiring invasive mechanical ventilation have a higher ICU mortality and in-hospital mortality compared with nonventilated patients.[227]

Initial Approach and Maintenance

Ventilation Modes

Mechanical ventilation of COPD should lead to a significant decrease in excessive respiratory work. Patient-triggered ventilation modes, either assist-control or synchronized intermittent mandatory ventilation, typically accomplish this goal. Special care must be taken, however, because if these modes are not adequately adjusted to fit the characteristics of the patient, an increase in respiratory work results.[228]

PSV has been extensively used and reviewed in the literature.[229,230] In COPD patients, PSV has been shown to decrease inspiratory effort as the applied pressure is increased; however, the response among patients varied significantly.[231] At higher levels of support pressure, many patients show an activation of the respiratory muscles during the late phase of inflation, with the potential to produce ventilation dyssynchrony. This may be more common in patients with longer time constants and patients who require higher inspiratory flows delivered for longer periods.[228] We recommend that ventilation be provided as total support during the initial phase of respiratory management (assist-control volume ventilation or high-level PSV).

Inspired Oxygen

The goal of oxygenation should be to maintain an oxyhemoglobin saturation of at least 90% to 92%. In dark-skinned patients, pulse oximetry may overestimate oxyhemoglobin saturation, and in these patients, we recommend targeting pulse oximetry values of 95% to ensure adequate oxygenation.[232] Although there is no clear-cut clinical evidence that allows determination of the $F{IO_2}$ threshold of concern for oxygen toxicity, based on animal studies of oxygen toxicity in normal lungs, attempts to lower $F{IO_2}$ to 0.6 or less by the end of the first 24 hours of mechanical ventilation is a reasonable goal.[233]

Intrinsic Positive End-Expiratory Pressure

Before discussing ventilation settings in COPD complicated with ARF, a discussion of intrinsic PEEP (auto-PEEP, dynamic hyperinflation) is in order. Intrinsic PEEP occurs in the presence of insufficient exhalation times. The respiratory system is prevented from returning to its resting state at the end of the expiration. *Auto-PEEP,* or intrinsic PEEP, is the positive difference between alveolar pressure and airway pressure at the end of expiration minus extrinsic positive pressures (PEEP or continuous positive airway pressure). When mechanical ventilation induces hyperinflation, alveolar pressure remains continually positive during both phases of the respiratory cycle. If the next inspiration is held at the end of expiration, expiratory flow continues.

Intrinsic PEEP is typically not detected on the pressure gauge of the ventilator because it is open to the atmosphere except for a very brief moment at the end of expiration. If the expiration port of the circuit is occluded at end expiration in a relaxed patient with a delay of next inspiration, the pressure inside the lungs and in the circuit begins to equilibrate; if occlusion is sufficiently prolonged, intrinsic PEEP may be recorded.[234]

Auto-PEEP has numerous hemodynamic and mechanical consequences. When auto-PEEP is profound, barotrauma may occur. Hemodynamic consequences of auto-PEEP effect are more common with decreased venous return, decreased stroke volume, and hypotension. Auto-PEEP also increases respiratory work. This is represented by an increase of workload during spontaneous inspiration and by a depression in the sensitivity of ventilator triggering. Auto-PEEP is treated by decreasing inspiration time and increasing expiratory time. This is best done by decreasing rate and tidal volume.

Sensitivity

The setting of the optimal triggering threshold is more difficult in COPD patients, especially if dynamic lung hyperinflation (intrinsic PEEP, auto-PEEP) exists. This is because the patient needs to generate a negative pressure equal to intrinsic PEEP before interfacing with the preset sensitivity on the ventilator. When auto-PEEP is high, the patient may exert significant inspiratory effort before the triggering threshold is reached, another cause of dyssynchrony. If the sensitivity of the ventilator has been placed at a very sensitive level, the ventilator may cycle inappropriately and can cause serious respiratory alkalosis, especially in the absence of significant auto-PEEP. Many ventilators have flow-triggered options, and although theoretically flow triggering may reduce patient effort, more recent reports fail to show differences when flow triggering is compared with newer pressure-triggering devices, even in COPD patients, although it is known that flow-triggered ventilators work better when the patient has elevated requirements of inspiratory flow.[235,236]

Inspiratory Flow Rate

High inspiratory flow rates help satisfy the demands of most dyspneic or tachypneic COPD patients; it decreases the likelihood of dynamic hyperinflation and intrinsic PEEP. This decreases inspiratory time and increases expiratory time, minimizing auto-PEEP. An improvement in gas exchange has been found when inspiratory flows were increased from 40 to 60 L/min in COPD patients.[237]

Tidal Volume

In patients with known or suspected auto-PEEP, smaller tidal volumes (6 to 8 mL/kg) may be necessary to prevent alveolar overdistention, dynamic hyperinflation, and barotrauma.

Respiratory Rate

In the presence of auto-PEEP or a strong predisposition for auto-PEEP, elevations in respiratory rate must be avoided because expiratory time would be significantly decreased. Although synchronized intermittent mandatory ventilation with low spontaneous tidal volume may control minute ventilation, it has variable effects on auto-PEEP and may increase respiratory workload significantly. For these reasons, controlled mechanical ventilation with heavy sedation or sedation/paralysis may be the optimal approach.

Positive End-Expiratory Pressure

In the past, PEEP was avoided in patients with COPD because of the concern of worsening dynamic hyperinflation. Now it is known that application of extrinsic PEEP slightly lower than intrinsic PEEP may facilitate ventilator triggering because alveolar pressure now needs to be decreased to only below the level of the external PEEP, instead of below the level of atmospheric pressure, decreasing the work required to trigger the inspiration.[238,239]

Weaning

In general, restoration of respiratory muscle function requires approximately 24 to 48 hours of mechanical ventilation.[240-242] Before weaning COPD patients from mechanical ventilation, the premorbid condition that triggered ARF should be corrected, and an adequate neuromuscular competency-to-workload ratio should be achieved. The strategy for facilitating weaning from the ventilator should include an increase in inspiratory force and a decrease in the load on the respiratory system. See Chapter 44 for a comparison of various weaning techniques.

Extubation with Noninvasive Ventilation

In certain patient populations, the use of NPPV as a bridge to successful weaning is advocated. Extubation is immediately followed with institution of NPPV, and NPPV is subsequently weaned. There is evidence that in selected patients, however, the use of NPPV could delay reintubation, and this delay was associated with increased mortality.[243]

PROGNOSIS

The outcome for a COPD patient with ARF depends on the severity of the COPD, the trigger for ARF, and avoidance of ICU complications. In patients who require mechanical ventilation for acute exacerbation, overall in-hospital mortality is greater than 20%.[244] For elderly patients, the mortality is greater than 50%.[245] In a multicenter study of patients 65 years old or older, mortality was 30% at hospital discharge, 41% at 90 days, 47% at 180 days, and 59% at 1 year.[225] The time course and recovery after COPD exacerbation in a cohort of 101 patients with a mean FEV_1 of 41.9% has been reported.[246] Patients recorded daily morning peak expiratory flow rate after the onset of the exacerbation. Median recovery time for peak expiratory flow rate was 6 days. Recovery of peak expiratory flow rate to baseline values was complete in only 75.2% of exacerbations at 35 days, and 7.1% of exacerbations had still not returned to baseline at 91 days.[246]

TERMINAL CARE FOR END-STAGE PATIENTS

All patients with severe end-stage COPD should be well educated about their prognosis and limitations of therapy.

Some patients may elect not to be mechanically ventilated when COPD is in the late stage, and the likelihood of extubation is extremely low. Others may choose short-term ventilation only in hopes of a reversible cause. Others may choose long-term ventilation with tracheostomy and home or special facility mechanical ventilation. Emotional and psychological support should be given for end-stage patients and their families.

KEY POINTS

- Worldwide, COPD is the only leading cause of death that still has an increasing mortality, and it has been estimated that by 2020, COPD will be fifth among the most burdensome conditions to society.
- Abdominal muscles are recruited during expiration in patients with severe COPD, and the expiratory increase in gastric pressure is directly related to intrinsic PEEP. Dynamic hyperinflation can be overestimated during chronic and acute airway obstruction if abdominal muscle function is not evaluated.
- Although the precise cause of acute exacerbation is poorly understood, it has been associated with numerous precipitating factors, including bacterial or viral infection, environmental factors, pulmonary embolism, medication failure, and patient noncompliance.
- Acute increases in $Pa{CO_2}$ with administration of supplemental oxygen are more likely to occur in patients with elevated baseline $Pa{CO_2}$.
- In high-risk cardiac patients, tiotropium may be preferred over β-agonists because of the decreased chance of cardiac side effects.
- When an MDI is used for acute exacerbations, the addition of a spacing device, which enhances lower airway drug deposition, is indicated to ensure adequate drug delivery. In the most severely tachypneic and dyspneic patients, nebulizers are still the best option to ensure optimal drug delivery.
- More recent literature supports the use of steroids with a short (4-day) taper in COPD patients admitted with exacerbation.
- Amoxicillin/clavulanate, azithromycin, and ciprofloxacin have shown superiority over amoxicillin, trimethoprim/sulfamethoxazole, tetracycline, erythromycin, cephradine, cefuroxime, cefaclor, and cefprozil in the treatment of COPD exacerbation.
- *N*-acetylcysteine in ambulatory patients is not recommended for aerosol delivery in COPD exacerbation.
- Nutritional support has been shown to produce improvements in lung function in hospitalized patients with acute exacerbation of COPD.
- Potential physiologic benefits of NPPV in COPD include improvement in tidal volume, gas exchange, respiratory rate, heart rate, oxygenation, and diaphragm activity and a reduction in $Pa{CO_2}$ with a concomitant improvement in pH. When these beneficial responses occur, they are typically seen in the first several hours after beginning NPPV.
- If the expiration port of the circuit is occluded at end expiration in a relaxed patient with a delay of next inspiration, the pressure inside the lungs and in the circuit begins to equilibrate; if occlusion is sufficiently prolonged, intrinsic PEEP may be recorded.
- Auto-PEEP has numerous hemodynamic and mechanical consequences.
- Auto-PEEP is treated by decreasing inspiration time and increasing expiratory time. This is best done by decreasing rate and tidal volume.

REFERENCES

1. Dantzker DR, Pingleton SK, Pierce JA, et al: Standards for the diagnosis and care of patients with chronic obstructive pulmonary disease (COPD) and asthma: Official statement of the American Thoracic Society. Am Rev Respir Dis 1987;136:225.
2. Seriff NS, Khan F, Lazo BJ: Acute respiratory failure. Med Clin North Am 1973;57:1539.
3. National Center of Health Statistics: Vital Health Stat Series No. 10, 1998, p 193.
4. National Heart, Lung, and Blood Institute: NHLBI Morbidity and Mortality Chartbook. Washington, DC, Department of Health and Human Services, National Institutes of Health, 1998.
5. National Lung Health Education Program (NLHEP): Strategies in preserving lung health and preventing COPD and associated diseases. Chest 1998;113:123S.
6. Murray CJL, Lopez AD: Evidence-based health policy: Lessons from the Global Burden of Disease Study. Science 1996;274:740.
7. Hyatt RE: The interrelationship of pressure, flow and volume during various respiratory maneuvers in normal and emphysematous patients. Am Rev Respir Dis 1961;83:676.
8. Gottfried SB: The role of PEEP in mechanically ventilated patients. In Roussos C, Marini JJ (eds): Ventilatory Failure. Berlin, Springer-Verlag, 1991.
9. Hogg JC, Macklem PT, Thurlbeck WM, et al: Site and nature of airway obstruction in chronic obstructive lung disease. N Engl J Med 1968;278:1355.
10. Reid LM: Pathology of chronic bronchitis. Lancet 1954;1:275.
11. Wanner A: The role of mucus in chronic obstructive pulmonary disease. Chest 1990;97(Suppl):11S.
12. Thurlbeck WM: Pathophysiology of chronic obstructive pulmonary disease. Clin Chest Med 1990;11:389.
13. Scano G, Gorini M, Duranti R, et al: Physiological changes during severe airflow obstruction in chronic obstructive pulmonary disease. Heart Lung 2000;29:124.
14. Gorini M, Misuri G, Corrado A, et al: Breathing patterns and carbon dioxide retention in severe chronic obstructive pulmonary disease. Thorax 1996;51:677.
15. American Thoracic Society: Skeletal muscle function in chronic obstructive pulmonary disease: A statement of the American Thoracic Society and European Respiratory Society. Am J Respir Crit Care Med 1999;159:S1.
16. Tantucci C, Grassi V: Flow limitation: An overview. Chest 1999;116:488.
17. Stubbing DG, Penegelly LD, Morse JLC: Pulmonary mechanics during exercise in subjects with chronic air-flow obstruction. J Appl Physiol 1980;49:511.
18. Marini JJ: Monitoring during mechanical ventilation. Clin Chest Med 1988;9:73.
19. Smith TC, Marini JJ: Impact of PEEP on lung mechanics and work of

breathing in severe airflow obstruction. J Appl Physiol 1988;65:1488.
20. Tobin MJ, Perez W, Guenther SM, et al: The pattern of breathing during successful and unsuccessful trial of waning during mechanical ventilation. Am Rev Respir Dis 1986;134:111.
21. Cohen CA, Zagelbaum G, Gross D, et al: Clinical manifestation of inspiratory muscles fatigue. Am J Med 1982;73:308.
22. Jeffrey AA, Warren PM, Flenley DC: Acute hypercarbic respiratory failure in patients with chronic obstructive lung disease: Risk factors and of guidelines for management. Thorax 1992;47:34.
23. Aubier M, Murciano D, Milic-Emili J: Effects of administration of O2 on ventilation and blood gases in patients with chronic obstructive pulmonary disease during acute respiratory failure. Am Rev Respir Dis 1980;122:747.
24. Juan G, Calverley P, Talamo C: Effect of carbon dioxide on diaphragmatic function in human beings. N Engl J Med 1984;310:874.
25. Garay SM, Turini GM, Goldring RM: Sustained reversal of chronic hypercapnia in patients with alveolar hypoventilation syndromes: Long term maintenance with noninvasive nocturnal mechanical ventilation. Am J Med 1981;70:269.
26. Derenne JP, Fleury B, Pariente R: Acute respiratory failure of chronic obstructive disease. Am Rev Respir Dis 1988;138:1006.
•27. Barbera JA, Roca J, Ferrer A, et al: Mechanisms of worsening gas exchange during acute exacerbations of chronic obstructive pulmonary disease. Eur Respir J 1997;10:1285.
28. Tobin MJ, Perez W, Guenther SM, et al: Does rib cage-abdominal paradox signify respiratory muscle fatigue? J Appl Physiol 1987;63:851.
29. Yanos J, Keamy MF, Leisk L: The mechanisms of respiratory arrest in inspiratory loading and hypoxemia. Am Rev Respir Dis 1990;141:933.
30. Mc Hardy VU, Inglis JM, Calder MA, et al: A study of infective and other factors in exacerbations of chronic bronchitis. Br J Dis Chest 1980;74:228.
•31. Soler N, Torres A, Ewig S, et al: Bronchial microbial patterns in severe exacerbations of chronic obstructive pulmonary disease. Am J Respir Crit Care Med 1998;157:1498.
32. Dockery DW, Pope AC, Xu X, et al: An association between air pollution and mortality in six U.S. cities. N Engl J Med 1993;329:1753.
33. Cifuentes LA, Vega J, Köpfer K, Lave L: Effect of the fine fraction of particulate matter versus the coarse mass and other pollutants on daily mortality in Santiago, Chile. J Air Waste Manag Assoc, 2000;50: 1287-1298.
34. Lippmann M, Fein A: Pulmonary embolism in the patients with chronic obstructive disease. Chest 1981;79:39.
35. Ziment I: Pharmacologic therapy in obstructive airway disease. Clin Chest Med 1990;11:461.
36. Pare PD, Hegele RG, Hogg JC: The lung pathology of acute exacerbation of chronic obstructive pulmonary disease. In Derenne JP, Whitelaw WA, Similowski T (eds): Lung Biology in Health and Disease, vol 92. New York, Marcel Dekker, 1996.
37. Voelkel NF, Tuder R: COPD exacerbation. Chest 2000;117:376S.
38. Persson CGA: Airway epithelium and microcirculation. Eur Respir Rev 1994;4:352.
39. Persson CGA, Erjefalt JS, Andersson M, et al: Extravasation, lamina propria flooding and lumenal entry of bulk plasma exudates in mucosal defense, inflammation and repair. Pulm Pharmacol 1996;9:129.
•40. Di Stefano A, Capelli A, Lusuardi M, et al: Severity of airway limitation is associated with airway inflammation in smokers. Am J Respir Crit Care Med 1998;158:1277.
41. Sethi S: Infectious etiology of acute exacerbations of chronic bronchitis. Chest 2000;117:380S.
42. Gump DW, Phillips CA, Forsyth BR, et al: Role of infection in chronic bronchitis. Am Rev Respir Dis 1976;113:465.
43. Buscho RO, Saxta D, Shultz PS, et al: Infections with viruses and *Mycoplasma pneumoniae* during exacerbation of chronic bronchitis. J Infect Dis 1978;137:377.
44. Smith CB, Golden C, Kanner R, et al: Association of viral and *Mycoplasma pneumoniae* infections with acute respiratory illness in patients with chronic obstructive pulmonary disease. Am Rev Respir Dis 1980;121:225.
45. Murphy TS, Sethi S: Bacterial infection in chronic obstructive pulmonary disease. Am Rev Respir Dis 1992;146:1067.
46. Tager I, Speizer FE: Role of infection in chronic bronchitis. N Engl J Med 1975;292:563.
47. Schreiner A, Bjerkestrand G, Digranes A, et al: Bacteriological findings in the transtracheal aspirate from patients with acute exacerbation of chronic bronchitis. Infection 1978;6:54.
48. Blasi F, Legnani D, Lombardo VM, et al: *Chlamydia pneumoniae* infection in acute exacerbations COPD. Eur Respir J 1993;6:19.
49. Miyashita N, Niki Y, Nakajima M, et al: *Chlamydia pneumoniae* infections in patients with diffuse panbronchiolitis and COPD. Chest 1998;114:969.
50. Eller J, Ede A, Schaberg T, et al: Infective exacerbation of chronic bronchitis: Relation between bacteriologic etiology and lung function. Chest 1998;113:1542.
•51. Monso E, Ruiz J, Rosell A, et al: Bacterial infection in chronic obstructive pulmonary disease: A study of stable and exacerbated outpatients using the protected specimen brush. Am J Respir Crit Care Med 1995;152:1316.
52. Fagon JY, Chastre J, Trouillet JL, et al: Characterization of bronchial microflora during acute exacerbation of chronic bronchitis. Am Rev Respir Dis 1990;142:1004.
53. Pela R, Marchesani FF, Agostinelli C, et al: Airways microbial flora in COPD patients in stable clinical conditions and during exacerbation: A bronchoscopic investigation. Monaldi Arch Chest Dis 1998;53:262.
54. California Department of Public Health: Clean Air for California: Initial Report of the Air Pollution Study Project. San Francisco, State of California Department of Public Health, 1955.
55. Dockery DW, Pope AC, Xu X, et al: An association between air pollution and mortality in six U.S. cities. N Engl J Med 1993;329:1753.
56. Delfino RJ, Becklake MR, Hanley JA: The relationship of urgent hospital admission for respiratory illness to photochemical air pollution levels in Montreal. Environ Res 1994;67:1.
57. Higgins IT, D'Arcy JB, Gibbon DI, et al: Effects of exposures to ambient ozone on ventilatory lung function in children. Am Rev Respir Dis 1990;141:1136.
58. Thurston GD, Ito K: Epidemiological studies of ozone exposure effects. In Holgate ST, Samet JM, Koren HS, et al (eds): Air Pollution and Health. London, Academic Press, 1999.
59. Schwartz J: PM10, ozone and hospital admissions for the elderly in Minneapolis-St. Paul, Minnesota. Arch Environ Health 1994;49:366.
60. Bates DV: Setting the stage: Critical risks. In: Environmental Health Risks and Public Policy: Decision Making in Free Societies. Seattle, University of Washington Press, 1994.
61. Baum GL, Fisher FD: The relationship of fatal pulmonary insufficiency with cor pulmonale, right-sided mural thrombi and pulmonary emboli: A preliminary report. Am J Med Sci 1960;240:609.
62. Moser K, Lemoine J, Natchtwey R, et al: Deep venous thrombosis a pulmonary embolism: Frequency in a respiratory intensive unit. JAMA 1981;246:1422.
63. Dalen JE, Alpert JS: Natural history of pulmonary embolism. In Sasahara AA, Sonnenblick EH, Lesch M (eds): Pulmonary Embolism. New York, Grune & Stratton, 1975.
64. Cordova C, Musca A, Violi F, et al: Platelet hyperfunction in patients with chronic airway obstruction. Eur J Respir Dis 1985;66:9.
65. Fanta CH, Wright TC, McFaden ER Jr: Differentiation of recurrent pulmonary emboli from chronic obstructive pulmonary disease as a cause of cor pulmonale. Chest 1981;79:92.
66. PIOPED Investigators: Value of ventilation/perfusion scan in acute pulmonary embolism: Results of the PIOPED. JAMA 1990;263:2753.
67. Wildberger JE, Schoepf UJ, Mahnken AH, et al: Approaches to CT perfusion imaging in pulmonary embolism. Semin Roentgenol 2005;40:64-73.
68. Coche E, Pawlak S, Dechambre S, et al: Peripheral pulmonary arteries: Identification at multi-slice spiral CT with 3D reconstruction. Eur Radiol 2003;13:815-822.
69. Lensing AW, Pradoni P, Brandjes D, et al: Detection of deep venous

thrombosis by real time B-mode ultrasonography. N Engl J Med 1989;320:342.
70. Wheeler HB, O'Donnell JA, Anderson FA, et al: Occlusive impedance phlebography: A diagnostic procedure for venous thrombosis and pulmonary embolism. Prog Cardiovasc Dis 1974;17:199.
71. Bounameaux H, Cirafici D, DeMoerloose P, et al: Measurement of the D-dimer in patients as a diagnostic aid in suspected pulmonary embolism. Lancet 1991;37:196.
72. Barnes PB: Strategies for novel COPD therapies. Pulm Pharmacol Ther 1999;12:67.
73. Siafakas NM, Bouros D: Management of acute exacerbation of chronic obstructive pulmonary disease. In Postma DS, Siafakas NM (eds): Management of Chronic Obstructive Pulmonary Disease, vol 3. European Respiratory Monograph. Sheffield, UK, European Respiratory Society Journals, 1998.
74. Kuller L, Ockene J, Townsend M, et al: The epidemiology of pulmonary function and COPD mortality in the multiple risk factor intervention trial. Am Rev Respir Dis 1989;140:76S.
75. Douglas NJ, White DP, Pickett CK, et al: Respiration during sleep in normal man. Thorax 1982;37:840.
76. Douglas NJ, White DP, Weil JV, et al: Hypercapnic ventilatory response in sleeping adults. Am Rev Respir Dis 1982;126:758.
77. Gould GA, Gugger M, Molloy J, et al: Breathing pattern and eye movement density during REM sleep in man. Am Rev Respir Dis 1988;138:874.
78. Catterall JR, Calverley PMA, MacNee W, et al: Mechanism of transient nocturnal hypoxemia in hypoxic chronic bronchitis and emphysema. J Appl Physiol 1985;59:1698.
79. Videm V, Pillgram-Larsen J, Ellingsen O, et al: Spontaneous pneumothorax in chronic obstructive pulmonary disease: Complications, treatment and recurrences. Eur J Respir Dis 1987;71:365.
80. Chistensen EE, Dietz GW: Subpulmonic pneumothorax in patients with chronic obstructive pulmonary disease. Radiology 1976;121:33.
81. Estenne M, Yernault JC, DeTrayer A: Mechanism of relief of dyspnea after thoracentesis in patients with large pleural effusions. Am J Med 1983;74:813.
•82. Hunt JM, Copland J, McDonald CF, et al: Cardiopulmonary response to oxygen therapy in hypoxaemic chronic airflow obstruction. Thorax 1989;44:930.
83. MacNee W, Wathen CG, Flenley DC, et al: The effects of controlled oxygen therapy on ventricular function in patients with stable and decompensated cor pulmonale. Am Rev Respir Dis 1988;137:1289.
84. Esteban A, Cerda E, De La Cal MA, et al: Hemodynamic effects of oxygen therapy in patients with acute exacerbations of chronic obstructive pulmonary disease. Chest 1993;104:471.
85. Meissner HH, Franklin C: Extreme hypercapnia in a fully alert patient. Chest 1992;102:1298.
86. Potkin RT, Swenson ER: Resuscitation from severe acute hypercapnia. Chest 1992;102:1742.
87. Carroll GC, Rothenberg DM: Carbon dioxide narcosis. Chest 1992;102: 986.
88. Robinson TD, Freiberg DB, Regnis JA, et al: The role of hypoventilation and ventilation-perfusion redistribution in oxygen-induced hypercapnia during acute exacerbations of chronic obstructive pulmonary disease. Am J Respir Crit Care Med 2000;161:1524.
•89. Hanson CW III, Marshall BE, Frasch HF, et al: Causes of hypercarbia with oxygen therapy in patients with chronic obstructive pulmonary disease. Crit Care Med 1996;24:23.
90. Agusti AG, Carrera M, Barbe F, et al: Oxygen therapy during exacerbations of chronic obstructive pulmonary disease. Eur Respir J 1999;14:934.
91. Wasserman K: Uses of oxygen in the treatment of acute respiratory failure secondary to obstructive lung disease. Monaldi Arch Chest Dis 1993;48:509.
92. Duranti R, Misuri G, Gorini M, et al: Mechanical loading and control of breathing in patients with severe chronic obstructive pulmonary disease. Thorax 1995;50:127.
93. Bernasconi M, Brandolese R, Poggi R, et al: Dose-response effects and time course of effects of inhaled fenoterol on respiratory mechanics and arterial oxygen tension in mechanically ventilated patients with chronic airflow obstruction. Intensive Care Med 1990;16:108.
94. Rossinen J, Partanen J, Stenius-Aarniala B, et al: Salbutamol inhalation has no effect on myocardial ischaemia, arrhythmias and heart-rate variability in patients with coronary artery disease plus asthma or chronic obstructive pulmonary disease. J Intern Med 1998;243:361.
95. American Thoracic Society: Standards for the diagnosis and care of patients with chronic obstructive pulmonary disease. Am J Respir Crit Care Med 1995;152:S77.
96. Rennard SI, Serby CW, Ghafouri M, et al: Extended therapy with ipratropium is associated with improved lung function in patients with COPD: A retrospective analysis of data from seven clinical trials. Chest 1996;110:62.
97. Demirkan K, Kuhl D, Headley AS, et al: Can we justify ipratropium therapy as initial management of acute exacerbations of COPD? Pharmacotherapy 1999;19:838.
•98. Karpel JP: Bronchodilator responses to anticholinergic and beta-adrenergic agents in acute and stable COPD. Chest 1991;99:871.
99. Niewoehner DE, Rice K, Cote C, et al: Prevention of exacerbations of chronic obstructive pulmonary disease with tiotropium, a once-daily inhaled anticholinergic bronchodilator: A randomized trial. Ann Intern Med 2005;143:317-326.
100. Gross NJ: Tiotropium bromide. Chest 2004;126:1946-1953.
101. The COMBIVENT Inhalation Solution Study Group: Routine nebulized ipratropium and albuterol together are better than either alone in COPD. Chest 1997;112:1514.
102. Shrestha M, O'Brien T, Haddox R, et al: Decreased duration of emergency department treatment of chronic obstructive pulmonary disease exacerbations with the addition of ipratropium bromide to beta-agonist therapy. Ann Emerg Med 1991;20:1206.
103. Koutsogiannis Z, Kelly AM: Does high dose ipratropium bromide added to salbutamol improve pulmonary function for patients with chronic obstructive airways disease in the emergency department? Aust N Z J Med 2000;30:38.
104. Moayyedi P, Congleton J, Page RL, et al: Comparison of nebulised salbutamol and ipratropium bromide with salbutamol alone in the treatment of chronic obstructive pulmonary disease. Thorax 1995;50:834.
•105. Kuhl DA, Agiri OA, Mauro LS: Beta-agonists in the treatment of acute exacerbation of chronic obstructive pulmonary disease. Ann Pharmacother 1994;28:1379.
106. Fernández A, Muñoz J, de la Calle B, et al: Comparison of one versus two bronchodilators in ventilated COPD patients. Intensive Care Med 1994;20:199.
107. Skorodin MS, Tenholder MF, Yetter B, et al: Magnesium sulfate in exacerbations of chronic obstructive pulmonary disease. Arch Intern Med 1995;155:496.
108. Mandelberg A, Chen E, Noviski N, et al: Nebulized wet aerosol treatment in emergency department: Is it essential? Comparison with large spacer device for metered-dose inhaler, Chest 1997;112:1501.
109. Laursen LC: Clinical efficacy and safety of Turbuhaler as compared to pressurized MDIs—beta 2-agonists. J Aerosol Med 1994;7:S59.
•110. Appleton S, Jones T, Poole P, et al: Ipratropium bromide versus short acting beta-2 agonists for stable chronic obstructive pulmonary disease. Cochrane Database Syst Rev 2006;19:CD001387.
111. Berry RB, Shinto RA, Wong FH, et al: Nebulizer vs spacer for bronchodilator delivery in patients hospitalized for acute exacerbations of COPD. Chest 1989;96:1241.
112. Tobin MJ, Jenouri G, Danta I, et al: Response to bronchodilator drug administration by a new reservoir aerosol delivery system and a review of other auxiliary delivery systems. Am Rev Respir Dis 1982;126:670.
113. Nilsestuen J, Fink J, Witek T Jr, et al: AARC clinical practice guidelines: Selection of aerosol delivery device. Respir Care 1992;37:891.
114. Newhouse MT, Dolovich M: Aerosol therapy of reversible airflow obstruction. Chest 1987;91:58S.
115. Newhouse MT, Dolovich MB: Control of asthma by aerosols. N Engl J Med 1986;315:870.

116. Fernández A, Lázaro A, Garc'a A, et al: Bronchodilators in patients with chronic obstructive pulmonary disease on mechanical ventilation: Utilization of metered-dose inhalers. Am Rev Respir Dis 1990;141:164.
117. Coleman DM, Kelly HW, McWilliams BC: Therapeutic aerosol delivery during mechanical ventilation. Ann Pharmacother 1996;30:644.
118. Wood-Baker R, Walters EH: Corticosteroids for acute exacerbations of chronic obstructive pulmonary disease. Cochrane Database Syst Rev 2000;2:CD001288.
119. Jantz MA, Sahn SA: Corticosteroids in acute respiratory failure. Am J Respir Crit Care Med 1999;160:1079.
120. Thompson WH, Nielson CP, Carvalho P, et al: Controlled trial of oral prednisone in outpatients with acute COPD exacerbation. Am J Respir Crit Care Med 1996;154:407.
•121. Koyama H, Nishimura K, Mio T, et al: Response to oral corticosteroid in patients with chronic obstructive pulmonary disease. Intern Med 1992;31:1179.
122. Niewoehner DE, Collins D, Erbland ML: Relation of FEV_1 to clinical outcomes during exacerbations of chronic obstructive pulmonary disease. Department of Veterans Affairs Cooperative Study Group. Am J Respir Crit Care Med 2000;161:1201.
123. Albert RK, Martin TR, Lewis SW: Controlled clinical trial of methylprednisolone in patients with chronic bronchitis and acute respiratory insufficiency. Ann Intern Med 1980;92:753.
124. Emerman CL, Connors AF, Lukens TW, et al: A randomized controlled trial of methylprednisolone in the emergency treatment of acute exacerbations of COPD. Chest 1989;95:563.
125. Rubini F, Rampulla C, Nava S: Acute effect of corticosteroids on respiratory mechanics in mechanically ventilated patients with chronic airflow obstruction and acute respiratory failure. Am J Respir Crit Care Med 1994;149:306.
126. Niewoehner DE, Erbland ML, Deupree RH, et al: Effect of systemic glucocorticoids on exacerbations of chronic obstructive pulmonary disease. N Engl J Med 1999;340:1941.
127. Balbi B, Majori M, Bertacco S, et al: Inhaled corticosteroids in stable COPD patients: Do they have effects on cells and molecular mediators of airway inflammation? Chest 2000;117:1633.
128. Yildiz F, Kaur AC, Ilgazli A, et al: Inhaled corticosteroids may reduce neutrophilic inflammation in patients with stable chronic obstructive pulmonary disease. Respiration 2000;67:71.
129. Burge PS, Calverley PM, Jones PW, et al: Randomised, double blind, placebo controlled study of fluticasone propionate in patients with moderate to severe chronic obstructive pulmonary disease: The ISOLDE trial. BMJ 2000;320:1297.
130. Senderovitz T, Vestbo J, Frandsen J, et al: Steroid reversibility test followed by inhaled budesonide or placebo in outpatients with stable chronic obstructive pulmonary disease. The Danish Society of Respiratory Medicine. Respir Med 1999;93:715.
131. Calverley PM: The role of corticosteroids in chronic obstructive pulmonary disease. Semin Respir Crit Care Med 2005;26:235.
132. Hirschmann JV: Do bacteria cause exacerbations of COPD? Chest 2000;118:193.
133. Murphy TF, Sethi S, Niederman MS: The role of bacteria in exacerbations of COPD: A constructive view. Chest 2000;118:204.
134. Anthonisen NR, Manfreda J, Warren CPW, et al: Antibiotic therapy in exacerbations of chronic obstructive pulmonary disease. Ann Intern Med 1987;106:196.
•135. Saint S, Bent S, Vittinghoff E, et al: Antibiotics in chronic obstructive pulmonary disease exacerbations: A meta-analysis. JAMA 1995;273:957.
136. Destache CJ, Dewan N, O'Donohue WJ, et al: Clinical and economic considerations in the treatment of acute exacerbations on chronic bronchitis. J Antimicrob Chemother 1999;43:107.
137. Adams S, Melo J, Anzueto A: Effect of antibiotics on the recurrence rates of chronic obstructive pulmonary disease. Chest 1997;112:22S.
138. Irwin RS, Erickson AD, Pratter ME, et al: Prediction of tracheobronchial colonization in current cigarette smokers with chronic obstructive bronchitis. J Infect Dis 1982;145:234.
139. Bjerkestrand G, Digranes A, Schreiner A: Bacteriologic findings in transtracheal aspirates from patients with chronic bronchitis and bronchiectasis. Scand J Respir Dis 1975;56:201.
140. Monso E, Rosell A, Bonet G, et al: Risk factors for lower airway bacterial colonization in chronic bronchitis. Eur Respir J 1999;13:338.
141. Martínez JA, Rodríguez E, Bastida T, et al: Quantitative study of the bronchial bacterial flora in acute exacerbations of chronic bronchitis. Chest 1994;105:976.
142. Baughman RP, Pina E: Infections in acute exacerbation of chronic bronchitis: What are they and how do we know? Semin Respir Crit Care Med 2000;21:87.
143. Sánchez Nieto JM, Torres A, García Córdoba F, et al: Impact of invasive and noninvasive quantitative culture sampling on outcome of ventilator-associated pneumonia: A pilot study. Am J Respir Crit Care Med 1998;157:371.
144. Jourdain B, Novara A, Jolly Guillou ML, et al: Role of quantitative cultures of endotracheal aspirates in the diagnosis of nosocomial pneumonia. Am J Respir Crit Care Med 1995;152:241.
145. Meduri GU, Chastre J: The standardization of bronchoscopic techniques for ventilator-associated pneumonia. Chest 1992;102:557S.
146. Gay P: Pharmacologie des stimulans respiratoires. Bull Eur Physiopathol Respir 1979;14:775.
147. Ram F, Rodriguez-Roisin R, Granados-Navarrete A, et al: Antibiotics for exacerbations of chronic obstructive pulmonary disease. Cochrane Database Syst Rev 2006;19: CD004403.
148. Powles ACP, Tuxen DU, Mahood CB: The effect of intravenously administrated almitrine, a peripheral chemorreceptor agonist on patient with chronic airflow obstruction. Am Rev Respir Dis 1983;127:284.
149. Melot C, Naeije R, Rothschild T, et al: Improvement in ventilation:perfusion matching by almitrine in COPD. Chest 1983;83:528.
150. Naeije R, Melot C, Mols P, et al: Effects of almitrine in decompensated chronic respiratory insufficiency. Bull Eur Physiopathol Respir 1981;17:153.
•151. Moser KM, Luchsinger PC, Adamson JS, et al: Respiratory stimulation with intravenous doxapram in respiratory failure. N Engl J Med 1973;288:427.
152. Vizza CD, Lynch JP, Ochoa LL, et al: Right and left ventricular dysfunction in patients with severe pulmonary disease. Chest 1998;113:576.
153. Goldberg HS, Rabson J: Control of cardiac output by systemic vessels. Am J Cardiol 1981;47:696.
154. Martin C, Perrin G, Saux P, et al: Effects of norepinephrine on right ventricular function in septic shock patients. Intensive Care Med 1994;20:444.
155. Hirsch LJ, Rooney MW, Wat SS, et al: Norepinephrine and phenylephrine effects on right ventricular function in experimental canine pulmonary embolism. Chest 1991;100:796.
156. Angle MR, Molloy DW, Penner B, et al: The cardiopulmonary and renal hemodynamic effects of norepinephrine in canine pulmonary embolism. Chest 1989;95:1333.
157. Juilliere Y, Feldmann L, Perrin O, et al: Beneficial cumulative role of both nitroglycerin and dobutamine on right ventricular systolic function in congestive heart failure patients awaiting heart transplantation. Int J Cardiol 1995;52:17.
158. Mathur PN, Powles ACP, Pugsley SO, et al: Effect of long-term administration of digoxin on exercise performance in chronic airflow obstruction. Eur J Respir Dis 1985;66:273.
159. Brown SE, Pakron FJ, Milne N, et al: Effects of digoxin on exercise capacity and right ventricular function during exercise in chronic airflow obstruction. Chest 1984;85:187.
160. Mathur PN, Powles ACP, Pugsley SO, et al: Effect of digoxin on right ventricular function in severe chronic airflow obstruction. Ann Intern Med 1981;95:283.
161. Mols P, Huynh CH, Dechamps P, et al: Acute effects of nifedipine on systolic and diastolic ventricular function in patients with chronic obstructive pulmonary disease. Chest 1993;103:1381.
162. Kalra L, Bone MF: Effect of nifedipine on physiologic shunting and oxygenation in chronic obstructive

pulmonary disease. Am J Med 1993;94:419.
163. Gassner A, Sommer G, Fridrich L, et al: Differential therapy with calcium antagonists in pulmonary hypertension secondary to COPD: Hemodynamic effects of nifedipine, diltiazem, and verapamil. Chest 1990;98:829.
164. Agostoni P, Doria E, Galli C, et al: Nifedipine reduces pulmonary pressure and vascular tone during short- but not long-term treatment of pulmonary hypertension in patients with chronic obstructive pulmonary disease. Am Rev Respir Dis 1989;139:120.
165. Corriveau ML, Rosen BJ, Keller CA, et al: Effect of posture, hydralazine, and nifedipine on hemodynamics, ventilation, and gas exchange in patients with chronic obstructive pulmonary disease. Am Rev Respir Dis 1988;138:1494.
166. Corriveau ML, Vu-Dinh Minh, Dolan GF: Long-term effects of hydralazine on ventilation and blood gas values in patients with chronic obstructive pulmonary disease and pulmonary hypertension. Am J Med 1987;83:886.
167. Keller CA, Shepard JW Jr, Chun DS, et al: Effects of hydralazine on hemodynamics, ventilation, and gas exchange in patients with chronic obstructive pulmonary disease and pulmonary hypertension. Am Rev Respir Dis 1984;130:606.
168. Brent BN, Matthay RA, Mahler DA, et al: Relationship between oxygen uptake and oxygen transport in stable patients with chronic obstructive pulmonary disease: Physiologic effects of nitroprusside and hydralazine. Am Rev Respir Dis 1984;129:682.
169. Brent BN, Berger HJ, Matthay RA, et al: Contrasting acute effects of vasodilators (nitroglycerin, nitroprusside, and hydralazine) on right ventricular performance in patients with chronic obstructive pulmonary disease and pulmonary hypertension: A combined radionuclide-hemodynamic study. Am J Cardiol 1983;51:1682.
170. Baigorri F, Joseph D, Artigas A, et al: Inhaled nitric oxide does not improve cardiac or pulmonary function in patients with an exacerbation of chronic obstructive pulmonary disease, Crit Care Med 1999;27:2153.
171. Germann P, Ziesche R, Leitner C, et al: Addition of nitric oxide to oxygen improves cardiopulmonary function in patients with severe COPD. Chest 1998;114:29.
172. Yoshida M, Taguchi O, Gabazza EC, et al: Combined inhalation of nitric oxide and oxygen in chronic obstructive pulmonary disease. Am J Respir Crit Care Med 1997;155:526.
173. Blanch L, Joseph D, Fernandez R, et al: Hemodynamic and gas exchange responses to inhalation of nitric oxide in patients with the acute respiratory distress syndrome and in hypoxemic patients with chronic obstructive pulmonary disease. Intensive Care Med 1997;23:51.
174. Peto R, Speizer FE, Cochrane AL, et al: The relevance in adults of air-flow obstruction, but not of mucus hypersecretion, to mortality from chronic lung disease. Am Rev Respir Dis 1983;128:491.
175. Anthonisen P, Riis P, Sogaard-Andersen T: The value of lung physiotherapy in the treatment of acute exacerbations in chronic bronchitis. Acta Med Scand 1964;175:715.
176. Oldenburg FA, Dolovich MB, Montgomery JM, et al: Effects of postural drainage, exercise and cough on mucus clearance in chronic bronchitis. Am Rev Respir Dis 1979;120:739.
177. Wollmer P, Ursing K, Midgren B, et al: Inefficiency of chest percussion in the physical therapy of chronic bronchitis. Eur J Respir Dis 1985;66:233.
178. Campbell AH, O'Conell JM, Wilson F: The effect of chest physiotherapy upon the FEV_1 in chronic bronchitis. Med J Aust 1975;1:33.
179. Grandjean EM, Berthet P, Ruffmann R, et al: Efficacy of oral long-term N-acetylcysteine in chronic bronchopulmonary disease: A meta-analysis of published double-blind, placebo-controlled clinical trials. Clin Ther 2000;22:209.
180. Pela R, Calcagni AM, Subiaco S, et al: N-acetylcysteine reduces the exacerbation rate in patients with moderate to severe COPD. Respiration 1999;66:495.
181. Hansen NC, Skriver A, Brorsen-Riis L, et al: Orally administered N-acetylcysteine may improve general well-being in patients with mild chronic bronchitis. Respir Med 1994;88:531.
182. Rogers DF, Barnes PJ: Treatment of airway mucus hypersecretion. Ann Med 2006;38:116.
183. Gray DK, Gibbons L, Shapiro SH, et al: Nutritional status and mortality in chronic obstructive pulmonary diseases. Am J Respir Crit Care Med 1996;153:961.
184. Donahoe M, Rogers RM: Nutritional assessment and support in chronic obstructive pulmonary disease. Clin Chest Med 1990;11:487.
185. Wilson DO, Rogers RM, Wright EC, et al: Body weight in chronic obstructive pulmonary disease. The National Institutes of Health Intermittent Positive-Pressure Breathing Trial. Am Rev Respir Dis 1989;139:1435.
186. Rochester DF: Body weight and respiratory muscle function in chronic obstructive pulmonary disease. Am Rev Respir Dis 1986;134:446.
187. Vandenbergh E, Woestijne vdKP, Gyselen A: Weight changes in the terminal stages of chronic obstructive pulmonary disease. Am Rev Respir Dis 1967;95:556.
188. Schols A, Slangen J, Volovics L, et al: Weight loss is a reversible factor in the prognosis of chronic obstructive pulmonary disease. Am J Respir Crit Care Med 1998;157:1791.
189. Driver AG, McAlevy MT, Smith JL: Nutritional assessment of patients with chronic obstructive pulmonary disease and acute respiratory failure. Chest 1982;82:568.
•190. Hunter AMB, Carey MA, Larsh HW: The nutritional status of patients with chronic obstructive pulmonary disease. Am Rev Respir Dis 1981;124:376.
191. Bernard S, LeBlanc P, Whittom F, et al: Peripheral muscle weakness in patients with chronic obstructive pulmonary disease. Am J Respir Crit Care Med 1998;158:629.
192. Bassili HR, Deitel M: Effect of nutritional support on weaning patients off mechanical ventilators. J Parenter Enteral Nutr 1981;5:161.
193. Whittaker JS, Ryan CF, Buckley PA, et al: The effects of refeeding on peripheral and respiratory muscle function in malnourished chronic pulmonary disease patients. Am Rev Respir Dis 1990;142:283.
194. Fuenzalida CE, Petty TL, Jones ML, et al: The immune response to short-term nutritional intervention in advanced chronic obstructive pulmonary disease. Am Rev Respir Dis 1990;142:49.
195. Wilson DO, Rogers RM, Sanders MH, et al: Nutritional intervention in malnourished patients with emphysema. Am Rev Respir Dis 1986;134:672.
196. Saudny Unterberger H, Martin JG, Gray DK: Impact of nutritional support on functional status during an acute exacerbation of chronic obstructive pulmonary disease. Am J Respir Crit Care Med 1997;156:794.
197. Rose W: Total parenteral nutrition and the patient with chronic obstructive pulmonary disease. J Intrav Nurs 1992;15:18.
198. Dark DS, Pingleton SK, Kerby GR: Hypercapnia during weaning. Chest 1985;88:141.
199. Covelli HD, Black JW, Olsen MS, et al: Respiratory failure precipitated by high carbohydrate loads. Ann Intern Med 1981;95:579.
200. Talpers SS, Romberger DJ, Bunce SB, et al: Nutritionally associated increased carbon dioxide production. Chest 1992;102:551.
201. Brochard L, Mancebo J, Wysocki M, et al: Noninvasive ventilation for acute exacerbations of chronic obstructive pulmonary disease. N Engl J Med 1995;333:817.
202. Bott J, Carroll MP, Conway JH, et al: Randomized controlled trial of nasal ventilation in acute respiratory failure due to chronic obstructive airways disease. Lancet 1993;341:1555.
203. Collaborative Research Group of Noninvasive Mechanical Ventilation for Chronic Obstructive Pulmonary Disease: Early use of non-invasive positive pressure ventilation for acute exacerbations of chronic pulmonary disease: A multicentre randomized controlled trial. Chin Med J 2005;118:2034.
•204. Kramer N, Meyer TJ, Meharg J, et al: Randomized, prospective trial of noninvasive positive pressure ventilation in acute respiratory failure. Am J Respir Crit Care Med 1995;151:1799.
205. Brochard L, Mancebo J, Wysocki M, et al: Noninvasive ventilation for

acute exacerbations of chronic obstructive pulmonary disease. N Engl J Med 1995;333:817.
206. Girou E, Schortgen F, Delclaux C, et al: Association of noninvasive ventilation with nosocomial infections and survival in critically ill patients. JAMA 2000;284:2361.
•207. Carratu P, Bonfitto P, Dragonieri S, et al: Early and late failure of noninvasive ventilation in chronic obstructive pulmonary disease with acute exacerbation. Eur J Clin Invest 2005;35:404.
208. Diaz O, Iglesia R, Ferrer M, et al: Effects of noninvasive ventilation on pulmonary gas exchange and hemodynamics during acute hypercapnic exacerbations of chronic obstructive pulmonary disease. Am J Respir Crit Care Med 1997;156:1840.
•209. Brochard L, Isabey D, Piquet J, et al: Reversal of acute exacerbations of chronic obstructive lung disease by inspiratory assistance with a face mask. N Engl J Med 1990;323:1523.
210. Bach JR, Brougher P, Hess DR, et al: Consensus, statement: Noninvasive positive pressure ventilation. Respir Care 1997;42:365.
211. Vitacca M, Rubini F, Foglio K, et al: Non-invasive modalities of positive pressure ventilation improve the outcome of acute exacerbations in COLD patients. Intensive Care Med 1993;19:450.
212. Girault C, Richard J-C, Chevron V, et al: Comparative physiologic effects of noninvasive assist-control and pressure support ventilation in acute hypercapnic respiratory failure. Chest 1997;111:1639.
213. Appendini L, Patessio A, Zanaboni S, et al: Physiologic effects of positive end expiratory pressure and mask pressure support during exacerbations of chronic obstructive pulmonary disease. Am J Respir Crit Care Med 1994;149:1069.
214. Kacmarek RM: Characteristics of pressure-targeted ventilators used for noninvasive positive pressure ventilation. Respir Care 1997;42:380.
215. Ferguson GT, Gilmartin M: CO2 rebreathing during BiPAP respiratory assistance. Am J Respir Crit Care Med 1995;151:1126.
216. Diaz O, Iglesia R, Ferrer M, et al: Effects of noninvasive ventilation on pulmonary gas exchange and hemodynamics during acute hypercapnic exacerbations of chronic obstructive pulmonary disease. Am J Respir Crit Care Med 1997;156:1840.
217. Anton A, Guell R, Gomez J, et al: Predicting the result of noninvasive ventilation in severe acute exacerbations of patients with chronic airflow limitation. Chest 2000;117:828.
218. Jaber S, Fodil R, Carlucci A, et al: Noninvasive ventilation with helium-oxygen in acute exacerbations of chronic obstructive pulmonary disease. Am J Respir Crit Care Med 2000;161:1191.
219. Jolliet P, Tassaux D, Thouret JM, et al: Beneficial effects of helium : oxygen versus air : oxygen noninvasive pressure support in patients with decompensated chronic obstructive pulmonary disease. Crit Care Med 1999;27:2422.
•220. Garrod R, Mikelsons C, Paul EA, et al: Randomized controlled trial of domiciliary noninvasive positive pressure ventilation and physical training in severe chronic obstructive pulmonary disease. Am J Respir Crit Care Med 2000;162:1335.
221. Girault C, Daudenthun I, Chevron V, et al: Noninvasive ventilation as a systematic extubation and weaning technique in acute-on-chronic respiratory failure: A prospective, randomized controlled study. Am J Respir Crit Care Med 1999;160:86.
222. Nava S, Ambrosino N, Clini E, et al: Noninvasive mechanical ventilation in the weaning of patients with respiratory failure due to chronic obstructive pulmonary disease: A randomized, controlled trial. Ann Intern Med 1998;128:721.
223. Hilbert G, Gruson D, Portel L, et al: Noninvasive pressure support ventilation in COPD patients with postextubation hypercapnic respiratory insufficiency. Eur Respir J 1998;11:1349.
224. Confalonieri M, Gazzaniga P, Gandola L, et al: Haemodynamic response during initiation of non-invasive positive pressure ventilation in COPD patients with acute respiratory failure. Respir Med 1998;92:331.
225. Burns KE, Adhikari NK, Meade MO: A meta-analysis of non invasive weaning to facilitate liberation from mechanical ventilation. Can J Anaesth 2006;53:305-315.
•226. Antonelli M, Conti G, Rocco M, et al: A comparison of noninvasive positive pressure ventilation and conventional mechanical ventilation in patients with acute respiratory failure. N Engl J Med 1998;339:429.
227. Seneff MG, Wagner DP, Wagner RP, et al: Hospital and 1-year survival of patients admitted to intensive care units with acute exacerbation of chronic obstructive pulmonary disease. JAMA 1995;274:1852.
228. Braschi A, Iotti G, Rodi G, et al: Dynamic pulmonary hyperinflation (DPH) during intermittent mandatory ventilation (IMV). Intensive Care Med 1988;14:589.
229. Brochard L: Pressure support ventilation. In Tobin MJ (ed): Principles and Practice of Mechanical Ventilation. New York, McGraw-Hill, 1994.
230. MacIntyre NR: Respiratory function during pressure support ventilation. Chest 1986;89:117.
231. Jubran A, Van de Graaff WB, Tobin MJ: Variability of patient-ventilator interaction with pressure support ventilation in patients with COPD. Am J Respir Crit Care Med 1995;152:129.
232. Jubran A, Tobin MJ: Reliability of pulse oximetry in titrating supplemental oxygen therapy in ventilator-dependent patients. Chest 1990;97:1420.
233. Slutsky AS: Mechanical ventilation. American College of Chest Physicians' Consensus Conference. Chest 1993;104:1833.
234. Pepe PE, Marini JJ: Occult positive end expiratory pressure in mechanically ventilated patients with airflow obstruction. Am Rev Respir Dis 1982;126:166.
235. Sydow M, Golisch W, Buscher H, et al: Effect of low-level PEEP on inspiratory work of breathing in intubated patients, both with healthy lungs and with COPD. Intensive Care Med 1995;21:887.
•236. Sassoon C, Del Rosario N, Fei R, et al: Influence of pressure- and flow-triggered synchronous intermittent mandatory ventilation on inspiratory muscle work. Crit Care Med 1994;22:1933.
237. Connors AF, McCaffree DR, Gray BA: Effect of inspiratory flow rate on gas exchange during mechanical ventilation. Am Rev Respir Dis 1981;124:537.
•238. Petrof BJ, Legaré M, Goldberg P, et al: Continuous positive airway pressure reduces work of breathing and dyspnea during weaning from mechanical ventilation in severe chronic obstructive pulmonary disease. Am Rev Respir Dis 1990;141:281.
239. Smith TC, Marini JJ: Impact of PEEP on lung mechanics and work of breathing in severe airflow obstruction. J Appl Physiol 1988;65:1488.
240. Grassino A, Macklem PT: Respiratory muscle fatigue and ventilator failure. Ann Rev Med 1984;35:625.
241. Braun NMT, Faulkner J, Hughes RL, et al: When should respiratory muscles be exercised? Chest 1983;84:76.
242. Kaelin RM, Assimacopoulos A, Chevrolet JC: Failure to predict six-month survival of patients with COPD requiring mechanical ventilation by analysis of simple indices. Chest 1987;92:971.
243. Caples SM, Gay PC: Noninvasive positive pressure ventilation in the intensive care unit. Crit Care Med 2005;33:2651.
244. Petty TL: Acute respiratory failure in COPD. In Petty TL (ed): Chronic Obstructive Pulmonary Disease, 2nd ed. New York, Marcel Dekker, 1985.
244. Swinburne AJ, Fedullo AJ, Bixby K, et al: Respiratory failure in the elderly: Analysis of outcome after treatment with mechanical ventilation. Arch Intern Med 1993;153:1657.
246. Seemungal TA, Donaldson GC, Bhowmik A, et al: Time course and recovery of exacerbations in patients with chronic obstructive disease. Am J Respir Crit Care Med 2000;161:1608.

Chapter 41

Hypoventilation and Respiratory Muscle Dysfunction

Franco Laghi

Hypercapnic respiratory failure is a state in which ventilation is insufficient to maintain a normal arterial tension of carbon dioxide ($Paco_2$) for the level of metabolic activity (measured by CO_2 production, $\dot{V}co_2$).[1] Under steady-state conditions, the relationship between $Paco_2$, alveolar ventilation ($\dot{V}_A$), and $\dot{V}co_2$ is given by the following equation:

$$Paco_2 = (\dot{V}co_2/\dot{V}_A) \times K$$

where K is usually stated as 0.863 using standard units (mL/min for $\dot{V}co_2$, L/min for $\dot{V}_A$, and mm Hg for pressure). The term $\dot{V}_A$ represents the portion of minute ventilation ($\dot{V}_E$) that reaches the terminal gas exchange units; it is calculated as follows:

$$\dot{V}_A = \dot{V}_E - \dot{V}_D$$

where $\dot{V}_D$ equals deadspace ventilation. A reduction in $\dot{V}_A$ may result from an inadequate $\dot{V}_E$ or an increase in $\dot{V}_D$ (resulting from an increase in true $\dot{V}_D$ or a functional increase in $\dot{V}_D$ secondary to lung regions with high ventilation-perfusion ($\dot{V}_A/\dot{Q}$) relationships).*

Hypercapnia is synonymous with alveolar hypoventilation (for the patient's level of carbon dioxide production). Alveolar hypoventilation can result from diminished neuromuscular capacity and higher respiratory load (Fig. 41-1).[2] Isolated impairments in gas exchange—i.e., conditions in which the alveolar-arterial O_2 gradient† is increased—usually do not cause hypercapnia.[3] When gas exchange is impaired, however, the magnitude of neuromuscular derangements or increased respiratory load, which may cause hypercapnia are less than the corresponding derangements when gas exchange is normal. Conditions in which gas exchange contributes to hypercapnia are usually characterized by ventilation-perfusion inequality. When gas exchange is impaired, total minute ventilation may actually be increased despite a concurrent decrease in alveolar ventilation.

DECREASED NEUROMUSCULAR CAPACITY

Disease states that may result in decreased neuromuscular capacity and thus in alveolar hypoventilation consist of those characterized by decreased respiratory center output and those characterized by respiratory muscle weakness and respiratory muscle fatigue.

Decreased Respiratory Center Output

Isolated decreases in respiratory drive can produce ventilatory failure without distress. Potential causes include sedative overdose,[1] hypothyroidism,[4] metabolic alkalosis,[5] semistarvation,[6] and central alveolar hypoventilation syndrome. Central alveolar hypoventilation syndrome can be either idiopathic (i.e., primary alveolar hypoventilation, or Ondine's curse) or secondary to a neurologic lesion

*Terminology of dead space is confusing. Anatomic dead space is made up of the conducting airways (nose, mouth, pharynx, larynx, trachea, bronchi, and bronchioles). Alveolar dead space is made up of alveoli that receive some or no blood flow, which does not match ventilation (units with very high $\dot{V}_A/\dot{Q}$ ratio). Physiologic dead space is the sum of anatomic dead space and alveolar dead space.[1]

†The alveolar-arterial O_2 gradient (A-aDo_2) is calculated as $PAo_2 - Pao_2$, where PAo_2 (alveolar O_2 tension) can be estimated according to the following simplified alveolar gas equation:

$$PAo_2 = FIo_2 \times (PB - PH_2O) - Paco_2/R$$

where FIo_2 is fractional concentration of inspired O_2 (about 0.21 when breathing room air), PB is barometric pressure (about 760 mm Hg at sea level), PH_2O is water vapor pressure (usually taken as 47 mm Hg at 37° C), and R is respiratory exchange ratio of the whole lung. The R is calculated as CO_2 production ÷ O_2 consumption ($\dot{V}co_2/\dot{V}o_2$). R is normally about 0.8. In steady state, R is determined by the relative proportions of free fatty acids, protein, and carbohydrate consumed by the tissues. In this equation, it is assumed that alveolar Pco_2 and $Paco_2$ are the same (usually they nearly are). In healthy young subjects (≤30 years old) breathing air at sea level, A-aDo_2 is usually <10 mm Hg, but it rises to as much as 28 mm Hg in healthy 60-year-old subjects.[1]

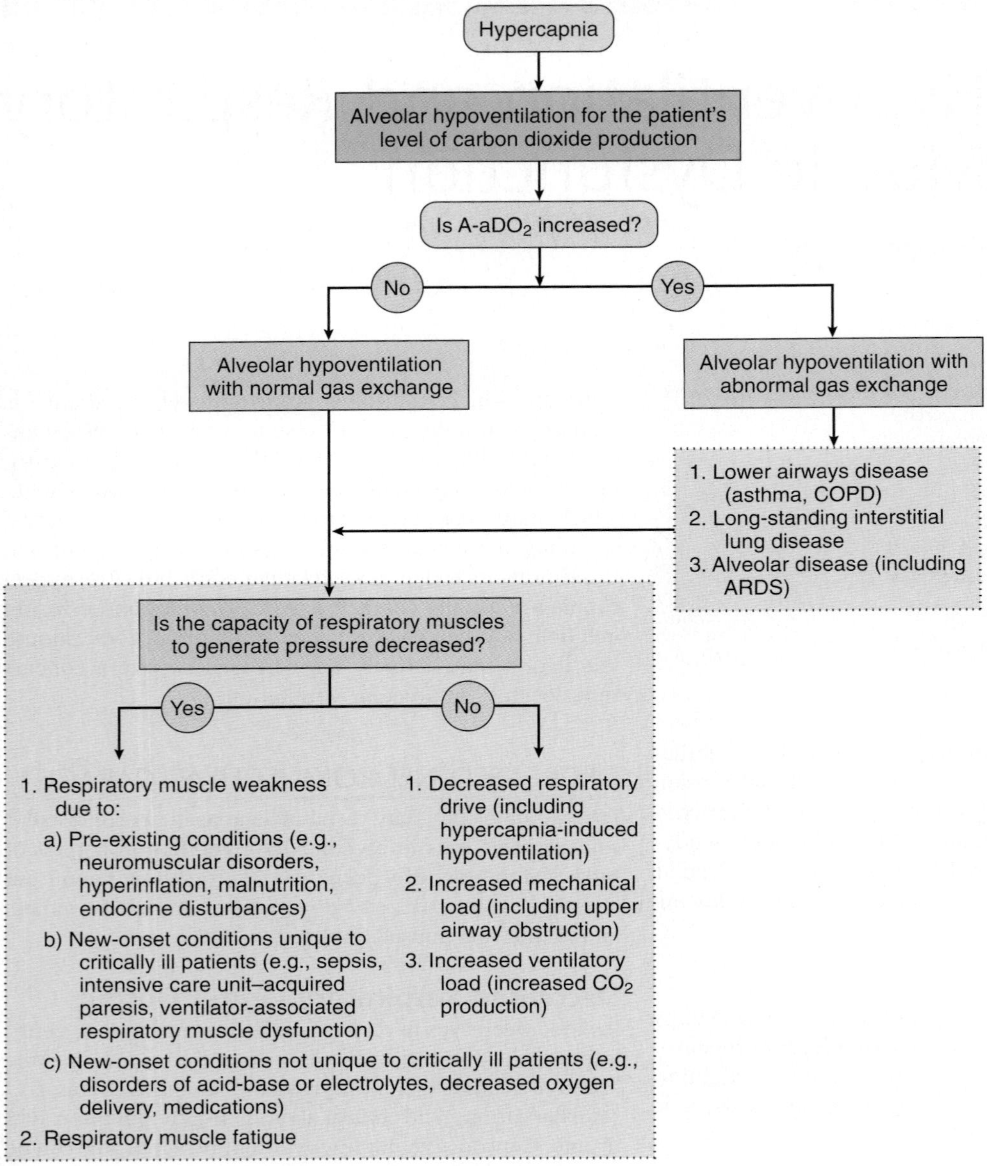

Figure 41-1. Diagnostic approach to critically ill patient with hypercapnia. A-aDO_2, alveolar-arterial difference in partial pressure of oxygen; ARDS, acute respiratory distress syndrome; COPD, chronic obstructive pulmonary disease.

such as trauma, infection (e.g., poliomyelitis), infarction, Shy-Drager syndrome, demyelination and obesity hypoventilation syndrome.[4] An elevated drive in patients with respiratory distress and ventilatory failure, however, does not necessarily translate into full respiratory muscle recruitment (Fig. 41-2).[7-9] It follows that, in some patients, a decrease in drive relative to the partial pressure of carbon dioxide may be contributing to CO_2 retention. Whether sleep deprivation decreases respiratory drive remains controversial.[10,11]

Respiratory Muscle Weakness

Detection of Respiratory Muscle Weakness in Critically Ill Patients

Measurements of airway pressure during maximal voluntary inspiratory efforts are used to evaluate global inspiratory muscle strength.[12] In healthy subjects, maximum inspiratory airway pressure is usually more negative than −80 cm H_2O.[12] In mechanically ventilated patients recovering from an episode of acute respiratory failure, maximum inspiratory airway pressure can range from less negative than −20 cm H_2O to about −100 cm H_2O.[9,13,14] Values of maximal airway pressure during voluntary maneuvers depend greatly on a level of motivation and comprehension of the maneuver (often not obtainable in critically ill patients). Thus, in patients requiring short-term mechanical ventilation, measurements of maximum inspiratory airway pressure commonly do not differentiate between patients in whom a trial of weaning will be successful and those in whom the trial will fail.[14-16]

In contrast to the voluntary nature of maximal voluntary inspiratory efforts, transdiaphragmatic pressures elicited by single stimulations of the phrenic nerves—or twitch pressure—are independent of patients' motivation and eliminate the influence of the central nervous system.[12] Activation can be achieved with either an electrical stimulator[17] or a magnetic stimulator,[17] although the latter is

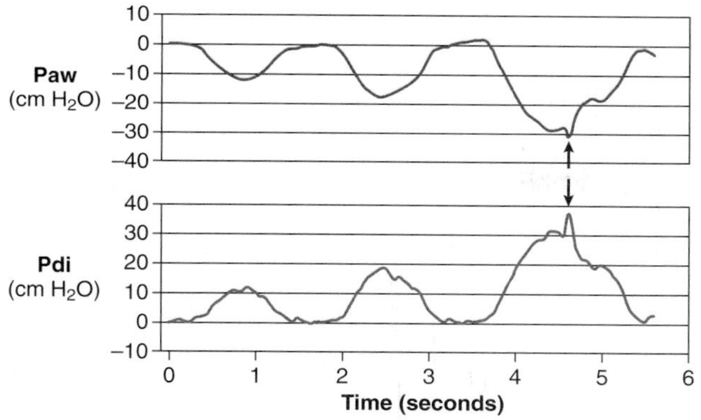

Figure 41-2. Continuous recordings of airway pressure (Paw) and transdiaphragmatic pressure (Pdi) during airway occlusion in a patient with chronic obstructive pulmonary disease (COPD) after an unsuccessful trial of spontaneous breathing. Phrenic nerve stimulation (*arrows*) during the maximal inspiratory effort resulted in a detectable superimposed twitch. That a twitch could be superimposed during the maximal effort indicates that diaphragmatic activation was incomplete.

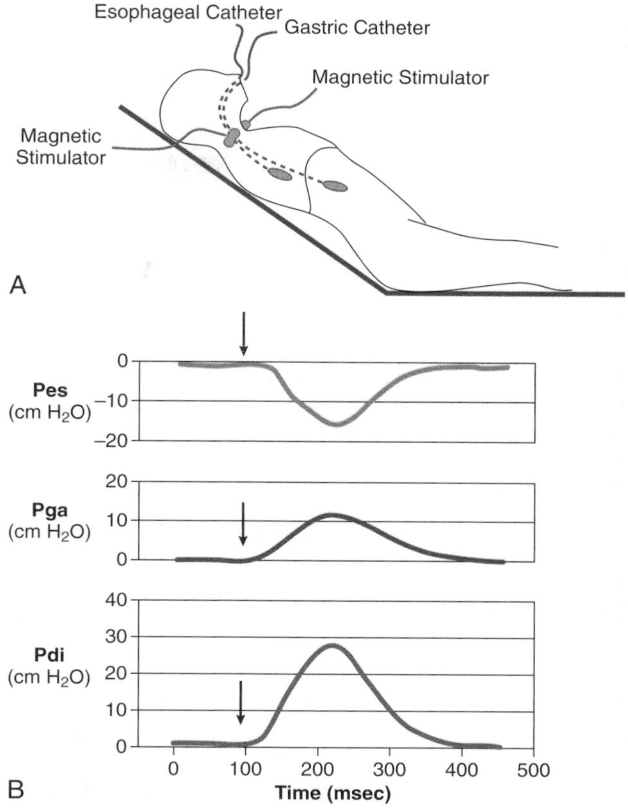

Figure 41-3. Recording of transdiaphragmatic twitch pressure. **A,** An esophageal balloon and a gastric balloon are passed through the nares. Magnetic stimulation of the phrenic nerves elicits diaphragmatic contraction. **B,** Continuous recordings of esophageal (Pes) and gastric (Pga) pressures and transdiaphragmatic pressure (Pdi)—calculated by subtracting Pes from Pga. Phrenic nerve stimulation (*arrows*) results in contraction of the diaphragm with consequent drop in intrathoracic pressure (negative defection of Pes) and rise in intra-abdominal pressure (positive deflection of Pga). These swings in pressure are responsible for the transdiaphragmatic twitch pressure. The smaller the transdiaphragmatic twitch pressure, the smaller the force generation capacity of the diaphragm.

easier to use in mechanically ventilated patients (Fig. 41-3).[15,18,19]

In healthy volunteers, magnetic stimulation elicits twitch pressures averaging 31 to 39 cm H_2O.[12] In patients with severe chronic obstructive pulmonary disease (COPD), twitch pressures average 19 to 20 cm H_2O.[20,21] The transdiaphragmatic twitch pressure value in patients recovering from an episode of acute respiratory failure is about half that recorded in ambulatory patients with severe COPD (Fig. 41-4).[15,18,19] This marked reduction in twitch pressure[18,19] indicates the presence of respiratory muscle weakness in most of these patients. Respiratory muscle weakness in critically ill patients can result from pre-existing or new-onset conditions.

Weakness Due to Pre-existing Conditions

Pre-existing conditions that can cause respiratory muscle weakness in critically ill patients include disorders such as neuromuscular disorders, malnutrition, endocrine disorders, and hyperinflation. The existence of pre-existing conditions can be recognized before or during the development of acute ventilatory failure or after it is already established.[4,22-25]

Neuromuscular Disorders

The capacity of the respiratory muscles to generate tension can be reduced in disorders such as stroke, amyotrophic lateral sclerosis, spinal cord injuries, poliomyelitis, Guillain-Barré syndrome, neuropathies due to massive intoxications of arsenic[26] or thallium,[27] chronic inflammatory demyelinating polyneuropathy, axonopathy of acute intermittent porphyria, myasthenia gravis, acid maltase deficiency, and muscular dystrophies such as myotonic dystrophy (the most common adult form of muscular dystrophy).[4,28,29] In the case of Guillain-Barré syndrome, the condition may precede admission to the intensive care unit (ICU) or may be triggered by a condition such as trauma, major surgery, or an infective illness that was the cause for ICU admission in the first place.[4]

Hypercapnic respiratory failure usually occurs when respiratory muscle strength falls to 39% of the predicted normal value.[30] However, Gibson and colleagues[31] described several patients with neuromuscular disorders in whom the partial pressure of CO_2 was normal despite decreases in respiratory muscle strength to less than 20% of predicted. Conversely, some patients with only moderate respiratory muscle weakness displayed hypercapnia (Fig. 41-5).[31] In other words, reductions in muscle strength do not consistently predict alveolar hypoventilation in this setting.

Hyperinflation

Hyperinflation is a common pre-existing problem in patients with obstructive lung diseases such as COPD,[4] cystic fibrosis,[32] bronchiolitis,[33] and lymphangioleiomyo-

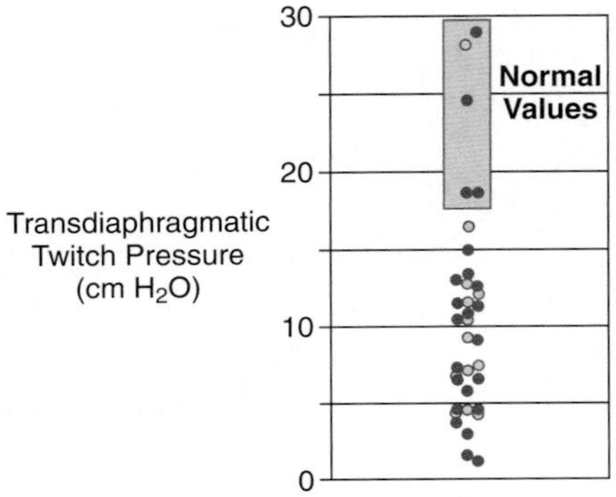

Figure 41-4. Transdiaphragmatic twitch pressure recorded in mechanically ventilated patients recovering from episodes of acute respiratory failure. The *red box* represents the range of transdiaphragmatic twitch pressures recorded in ambulatory patients with severe chronic obstructive pulmonary disease (COPD). Most mechanically ventilated patients had evidence of diaphragmatic weakness. Data from Cattapan et al[18] (*open circles*) and Watson et al[19] (*closed circles*). (From Laghi F: Assessment of respiratory output in mechanically ventilated patients. Respir Care Clin North Am 2005;11:173-199.)

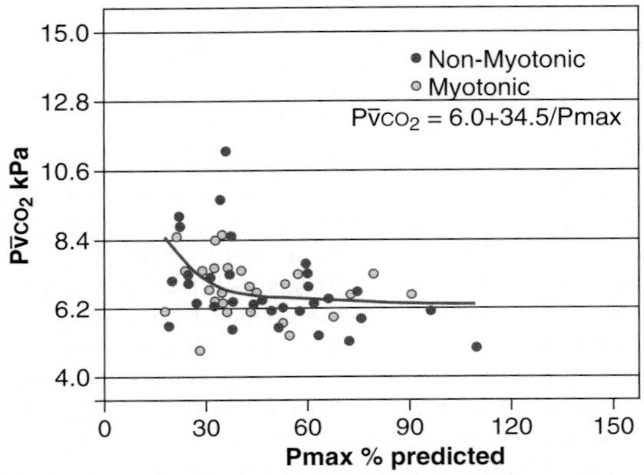

Figure 41-5. Relationship between muscle strength and mixed venous partial pressure of CO_2 ($P\bar{v}CO_2$) in patients with respiratory muscle weakness. Respiratory muscle strength is the arithmetic sum of maximum static inspiratory and expiratory mouth pressures ($Pmax = P_I max + P_E max$). The *open circles* represent data from patients with myotonic dystrophy, and the *closed circles* data from patients with a variety of nonmyotonic muscle diseases. As respiratory muscle weakness became more severe, $P\bar{v}CO_2$ rose, although considerable variability was observed among patients. The regression lines were similar in the myotonic and nonmyotonic patients. (From Gibson GJ, Gilmartin JJ, Veale D, et al: Respiratory muscle function in neuromuscular disease. In Jones NL, Killian KJ [eds]: Breathlessness: The Campbell Symposium. Hamilton, Ont, Boehringer-Ingelheim, 1992.)

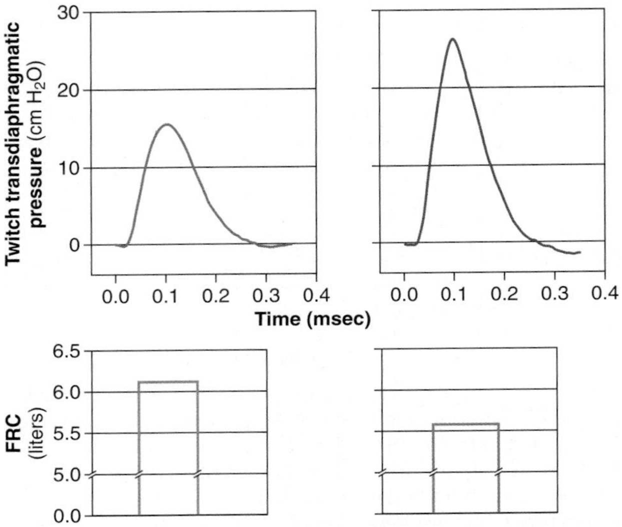

Figure 41-6. Twitch transdiaphragmatic pressure elicited by phrenic nerve stimulation (*upper panels*) and functional residual capacity (FRC) (*lower panels*) in a patient with severe emphysema before (*left*) and after (*right*) lung volume reduction surgery. The increase in transdiaphragmatic pressure after surgery was in part due to a decrease in the operating lung volume as demonstrated by the decrease in functional residual capacity. (Data from Laghi F, Jubran A, Topeli A, et al: Effect of lung volume reduction surgery on neuromechanical coupling of the diaphragm. Am J Respir Crit Care Med 1998;157:475-483.)

matosis.[4] The severity of pre-existing hyperinflation commonly worsens in patients experiencing an exacerbation of COPD.[34] Hyperinflation can also occur de novo in patients with pneumonia, acute respiratory distress syndrome, and chest trauma.[34,35] Hyperinflation has a number of adverse effects on inspiratory muscle function: The inspiratory muscles operate at an unfavorable position of the length-tension relationship (Fig. 41-6)[36]; flattening of the diaphragm reduces the size of the zone of apposition, so that diaphragmatic contraction causes less effective rib cage expansion.[4] Hyperinflation has also an adverse effect on the elastic recoil of the thoracic cage.[4] This means that the inspiratory muscles must work not only against the elastic recoil of the lungs but also against that of the thoracic cage. The functional consequences of dynamic hyperinflation are probably the main causes of ventilatory failure in patients with COPD.[37] Impairment of inspiratory muscle function, however, is less likely in patients with acute respiratory distress syndrome, because they breathe at a low lung volume despite dynamic hyperinflation.[35,38]

Malnutrition

Malnutrition is highly prevalent among critically ill patients requiring mechanical ventilation[39,40] and is associated with poor prognosis.[40] Malnutrition decreases muscle mass and respiratory muscle strength both in humans[41,42] and in laboratory animals.[43-45]

Short-term malnutrition in adolescent rats and long-term malnutrition in adult rats causes atrophy of all fiber types: fatigue-resistant (type I, type IIa) and fatigue-sensitive (type IIb, type IIx) (Table 41-1).[44,46] In old rats, long-term malnutrition causes a decrease in type IIb fibers and a relative increase in type I and IIa fibers of the diaphragm.[43] The decrease in muscle mass and the shift in the type of myosin heavy chain are responsible for a decrease in total muscle force output[43] and for greater

Table 41-1. Characteristics of Types of Muscle Fibers*

Characteristic	Type I	Type IIa	Type IIx	Type IIb
Contractile properties:				
Velocity of shortening	+	++	+++	++++
Tetanic force	+	+	++	++
Endurance	++++	+++	++	+
Work efficiency†	+++	++	++	+
Histochemistry:				
Mitochondrial volume density	+++	+++	++	+
Adenosine triphosphate (ATP) consumption rate	+	++	+++	++++
Oxidative enzymes	+++	+++	++	+
Glycolytic enzymes	+	++	+++	++++
Glycogen	+	++	++	+++
Capillary supply	+++	+++	++	+
Diameter	+	++	++	+++

*A single myosin heavy-chain isoform (MHCI) is typically expressed within an adult skeletal muscle fiber. Fibers classified as type I, IIa, IIx, and IIb express I (or slow), IIa, IIx, and IIb, respectively. Type IIx fibers have been reported in peripheral muscles of humans and animals and in the diaphragm of animals. Type IIx fibers have not been reported in the human diaphragm. More than one MHCI is expressed in a few fibers (about 14% of adult rat diaphragm coexpresses MHCIs IIb and IIx, and less than 1% coexpresses MHCIs I and IIa).[258] Although the velocity of muscle contraction depends primarily on the MHCI, the velocity of muscle relaxation is mainly determined by troponin C calcium binding and release and by calcium reuptake by the sarcoendoplasmic reticulum calcium–adenosine triphosphatase (SERCA). Several SERCA isoenzymes have been identified: SERCA 1 is expressed in type II fibers (fast calcium reuptake); and SERCA 2a is expressed in type I (slow calcium reuptake).[211] The density of pumping sites largely accounts for different rates of calcium uptake in fast- and slow-twitch muscle fibers.[211] Despite this separation of tasks, velocity of contraction and velocity of relaxation tend to parallel each other; type II fibers contract and relax with a greater velocity than type I fibers. Slower velocity of relaxation allows fusion of repetitive twitches at lower frequencies of stimulation than with fast relaxations. Impairment of SERCA activity has been implicated in the development of fatigue and in disease states, including heart failure and corticosteroid myopathy.
†Amount of work performed per unit of ATP consumed.
From Laghi F, Tobin MJ: Disorders of the respiratory muscles. Am J Respir Crit Care Med 2003;168:10-48.

resistance to fatigue.[43,45] Likely mechanisms contributing to respiratory muscle atrophy in malnutrition include proteolysis of myofibrillar proteins by the ubiquitin-proteasome proteolytic system (Fig. 41-7) and apoptosis.[4,47] Apoptosis can be triggered by local and circulating tumor necrosis factor-α and by release of cytochrome *c* from the mitochondria.[48,49]

Long-term malnutrition superimposed on emphysema produces a decrease in total force production, atrophy (more so of type II fibers), and improved capillarity of the diaphragm in hamsters.[50] Diaphragmatic endurance is increased in hamsters with emphysema, but the combination of long-term malnutrition and emphysema reduces endurance to the level of normal animals.[50] The studies in animals are confounded by the use of semistarvation[43,45,46,50] (which also decreases energy expenditure) to achieve weight loss. In previously healthy humans, starvation reduces oxygen consumption by 30% to 40%.[51,52] In patients with anorexia nervosa, in whom weight loss is due to voluntary caloric restriction, energy expenditure is usually not different from that in controls.[53] In patients with COPD, involuntary weight loss occurs without caloric restriction, and energy expenditure is usually increased.[54]

In patients with COPD, inspiratory muscle strength is about 30% less in poorly nourished patients than in well-nourished patients with equivalent airway obstruction.[54] Similarly, malnourished patients with anorexia nervosa can present with inspiratory muscle strength reduced to 35% to 50% of that predicted,[42] impairment of respiratory muscle endurance[55] and hypercapnic ventilatory response,[55] and, occasionally, hypercapnia at rest.[42] In malnourished patients, inspiratory weakness,[42,54,55] fatigability,[54] and dyspnea[54] are partially reversible with nutritional support. The process is slow, and in laboratory animals, it can take months of refeeding for muscle mass to return to normal values.[56] To date, it remains unclear whether malnutrition by itself can cause sufficient respiratory muscle weakness to produce hypoventilation. It is more likely for malnutrition to be a contributory factor and not a sole cause of hypercapnic respiratory failure.

Endocrine Disturbances

Endocrine disturbances, such as hypothyroidism,[57] hyperthyroidism,[49,58-60] and acromegaly,[61] can adversely affect respiratory muscle function. Proteolysis of myofibrillar proteins by the ubiquitin-proteasome proteolytic system[47] (see Fig. 41-7) is probably responsible for respiratory muscle catabolism and weakness of hyperthyroidism.[49] This mechanism is implicated in the muscle wasting associated with acidosis, renal failure, denervation, cancer, diabetes, acquired immunodeficiency syndrome (AIDS), trauma, and burns.[47] In contrast to other endocrine disturbances, respiratory muscle weakness is unusual in patients with Cushing's syndrome.[62]

Weakness Due to New-Onset Conditions

New-onset respiratory muscle weakness in critically ill patients may result from conditions unique to these patients, which include ventilator-associated respiratory muscle dysfunction, sepsis-associated myopathy, and ICU-acquired paresis. New-onset respiratory muscle weakness may also result from conditions or factors that are not unique to critically ill patients, such as acid-base

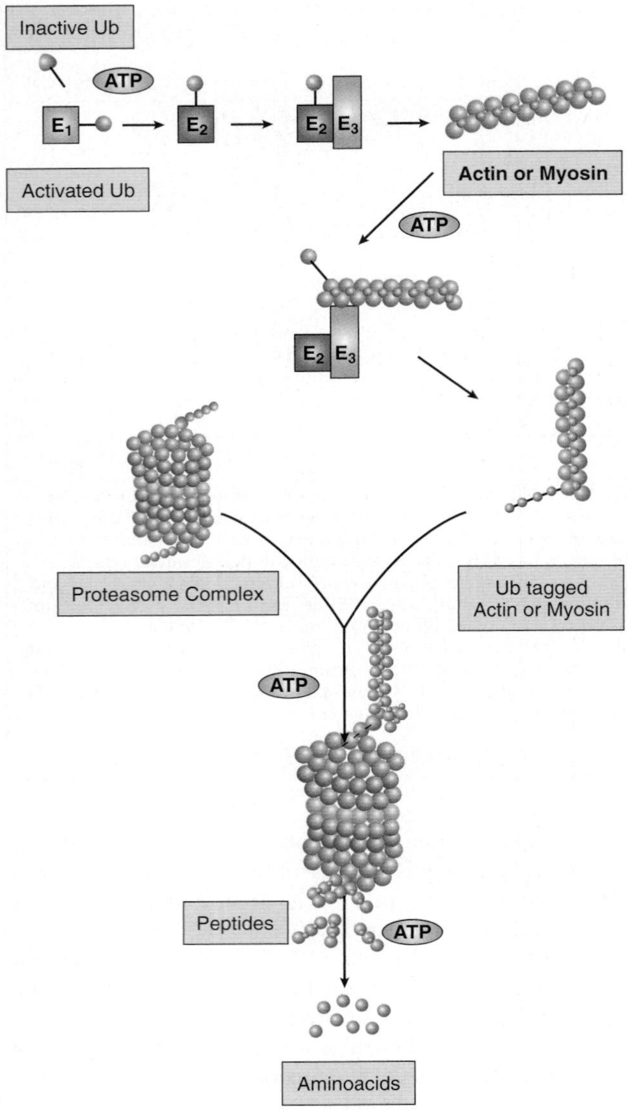

Figure 41-7. Ubiquitin-proteasome degradation of contractile proteins. The first step in degradation of actin and myosin is activation of ubiquitin (Ub) by a first enzyme, E_1—a process requiring adenosine triphosphate (ATP). Activated ubiquitin interacts with a second enzyme, E_2, a carrier protein. Ub and E_2 join a third enzyme, E_3. E_3 transfers activated Ub to actin and myosin. The cycle is repeated until a chain of Ub is bound to the contractile proteins. The chain of Ub binds to one end of a proteasome complex in a process requiring ATP. The Ub chain is subsequently removed (allowing reuse of Ub), and actin and myosin are unfolded and pushed into the core of the proteasome. Multiple enzymes within the core degrade actin and myosin into small peptides. The peptides are extruded from the proteasome and degraded to amino acids by peptidases in the cytoplasm. The ubiquitin-proteasome system degrades myofibrillar proteins only after they have been cleaved and released by other proteolytic pathways—i.e., the ubiquitin-proteasome pathway cannot degrade intact myofibrillar proteins. (From Laghi F, Tobin MJ: Disorders of the respiratory muscles. Am J Respir Crit Care Med 2003;168:10-48.)

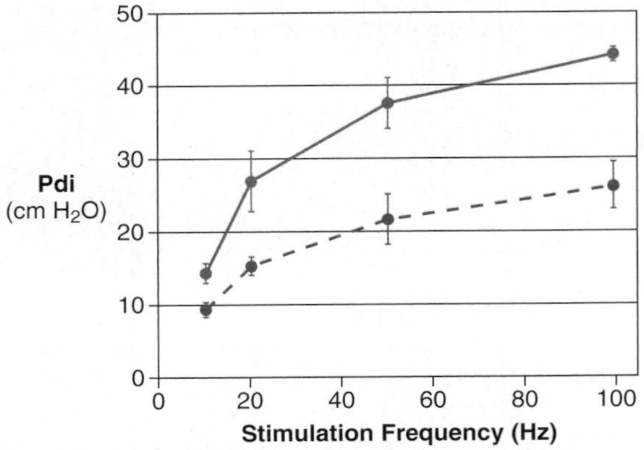

Figure 41-8. Transdiaphragmatic pressure (Pdi) response to phrenic nerve stimulation before (*blue line*) and after (*red line*) 11 days of mechanical ventilation. That the transdiaphragmatic pressure recorded after 11 days of mechanical ventilation shows a decrease in response to all stimulation frequencies suggests ventilator-associated diaphragmatic dysfunction. (Modified from Anzueto A, Peters JI, Tobin MJ, et al: Effects of prolonged controlled mechanical ventilation on diaphragmatic function in healthy adult baboons. Crit Care Med 1997;25:1187-1190.)

disorders, electrolyte disturbances, decreased oxygen delivery, and medications. Respiratory muscle weakness due to conditions that are unique to critically ill patients are often associated with alterations in respiratory muscle structure, whereas that due to nonunique conditions is not necessarily associated with such alterations. Recovery from respiratory muscle weakness (if it occurs at all) is slow when the weakness is caused by alterations in muscle structure. In contrast, recovery of respiratory muscle weakness due to a condition that is not necessarily associated with alteration in muscle structure is usually quick once the underlying triggering factor has been corrected.

Ventilator-Associated Respiratory Muscle Dysfunction

In laboratory animals, controlled mechanical ventilation delivered for 1 to 11 days can decrease diaphragmatic force generation by 20% to more than 50% (Fig. 41-8)[63-69] and can cause similar decreases in diaphragmatic endurance.[68] The reduction in force is out of proportion to both the decrease in diaphragmatic mass[64,69] and the decrease in cross-sectional area of muscle fibers.[64] The reduction in force has been related to the extent of myofibril damage and mitochondrial swelling (rabbits) (Fig. 41-9)[65] and with a decrease in muscle fibers expressing type I myosin isoforms (rats).[64] The reduction in force has been also related to increases in both muscle fibers expressing type IIa myosin heavy chains (rabbits)[65] and hybrid muscle fibers coexpressing type I and type II myosin isoforms (rats).[64] Impairment of membrane depolarization or excitation/contraction coupling may contribute to the decrease in respiratory muscle strength.[67]

Several mechanisms, including structural injury,[65,70,71] oxidative stress,[72-75] muscle fiber remodeling,[64,74,76] myofiber proteolysis,[74,77] and muscle atrophy[64,69,74,77,78] appear

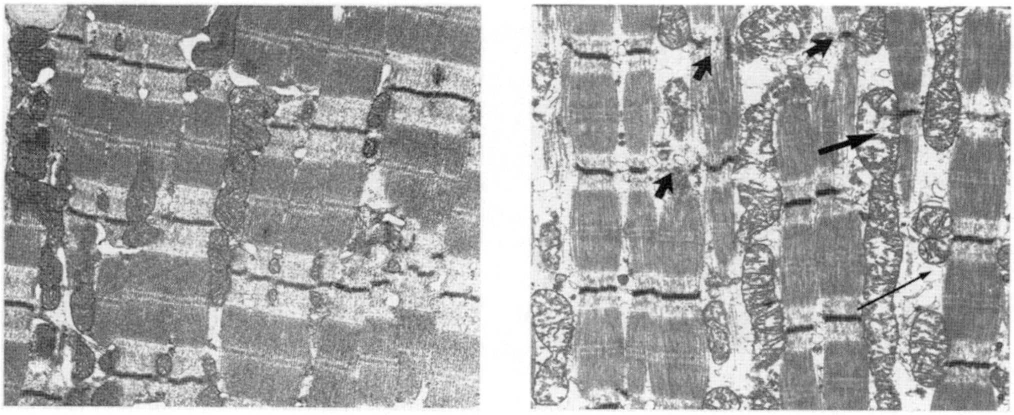

Figure 41-9. Electron microscopy of the diaphragm (longitudinal section) of a rabbit under control conditions (**A,** specimen processed with 1100-mOsm fixative) and of a rabbit after 3 days of controlled mechanical ventilation (**B,** specimen processed with 500-mOsm fixative). The control rabbit has an intact ultrastructure. The mechanically ventilated rabbit shows several areas of disrupted myofibrils (*short thick arrows*), the mitochondria are swollen (*long thick arrow*) and have abnormal cristae, and the intermyofibril space contains lipid droplets (*long thin arrow*), indicating decreased lipid uptake by the mitochondria. (From Laghi F, Tobin MJ: Disorders of the respiratory muscles. Am J Respir Crit Care Med 2003;168:10-48. Electron micrographs provided by Dr. Catherine S. H. Sassoon, Long Beach VA Hospital and University of California, Irvine, California.)

to be responsible for ventilator-associated respiratory muscle dysfunction. Myofiber proteolysis could result from ubiquitin-proteasome proteolysis[74,77]—which can be triggered by activation of E_3-ubiquitin ligases such as MuRF1 and MAFbx (see Fig. 41-7)[79]—and by proteolysis by the lysosomal proteolytic system and the calcium-dependent calpain system.[74,80,81] It has been speculated that use of dantrolene to avert an increase in intracellular calcium (which is necessary for calpain-mediated proteolysis) or use of antioxidants might prevent the muscle damage resulting from mechanical ventilation.[72] Of interest, antioxidant supplementation (vitamin E and vitamin C) in critically ill surgical patients was associated with a decrease in the duration of mechanical ventilation.[82] Whether the decrease in duration of mechanical ventilation was, at least in part, due to the potential positive effects of antioxidants on the respiratory muscles remains to be demonstrated.

In animal models, ventilator settings can affect the extent of ventilator-associated respiratory muscle dysfunction.[66] In rabbits, assist-control mechanical ventilation causes a nonsignificant decrease in diaphragm muscle contractility, which contrasts with the 48% decrease recorded with controlled mechanical ventilation.[66] This observation raises the important question whether maintenance of partial diaphragmatic activity or intermittent loading of the diaphragm could prevent the harm done to diaphragmatic function by mechanical ventilation.[83]

In limb muscles, structural abnormalities associated with disuse are worse when the length of the muscle is kept short.[84] Loss of stretch-induced stimulation of protein synthesis may be responsible for the worse structural abnormalities observed when a muscle's length is kept short.[85] On these grounds, investigators have hypothesized that ventilator-associated respiratory muscle dysfunction could be amplified by the use of positive end-expiratory pressure.[83]

Whether ventilator-associated respiratory muscle dysfunction occurs in humans is unclear. In a retrospective study of 13 infants who received uninterrupted ventilator assistance for at least 12 days before death, most diaphragmatic fibers appeared atrophic (Fig. 41-10).[86] The development of atrophy was suggested by a smaller diaphragmatic muscle mass in these infants than in 26 infants who died after receiving mechanical ventilation for 7 days or less.[86] These data are supported by a preliminary report by Levine and associates,[87] who compared costal diaphragm biopsies of six brain-dead organ donors maintained on controlled mechanical ventilation for 18 to 72 hours with those of nine patients ventilated for less than 2 hours during surgery (to remove solitary pulmonary nodules). In this preliminary report, prolonged controlled mechanical ventilation was associated with 40% atrophy of slow fibers and 36% atrophy of fast fibers.[87] Atrophy was coupled with greater ubiquitin-proteasome proteolysis.[77]

Considering that decreases in protein synthesis seem to contribute to ventilator-associated respiratory muscle dysfunction,[77,88] it would seem biologically plausible that administration of anabolic factors—such as growth hormone—might be of benefit in ventilated patients. Unfortunately, when growth hormone has been administered to patients requiring prolonged mechanical ventilation, duration of mechanical ventilation was not decreased nor was muscle strength increased.[89] Of concern is the report that recombinant growth hormone can raise mortality in critically ill patients.[90]

Sepsis-Associated Myopathy

Sepsis, a common occurrence in critically ill patients, can produce ventilatory failure by causing respiratory muscle dysfunction and raising metabolic demands.[91] Septic animals demonstrate failure of both neuromuscular transmission (due to increased sarcolemmal electric

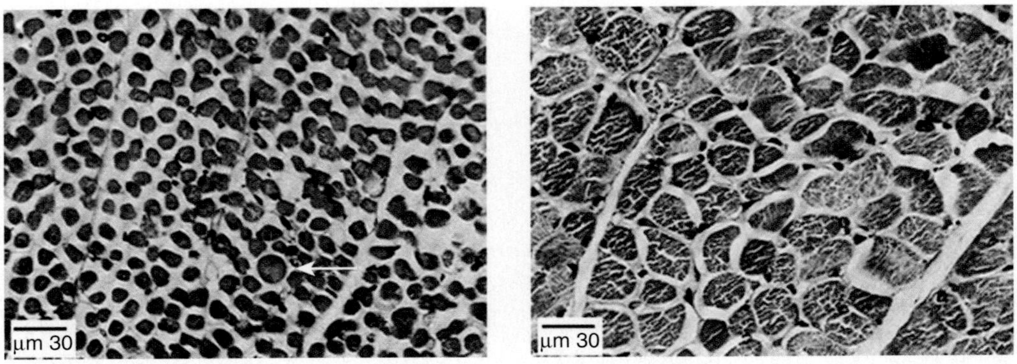

A B

Figure 41-10. Photomicrographs of transverse sections of diaphragm from an infant ventilated from birth until death at day 47 **(A)** and from an infant ventilated from birth until accidental death at day 3. (The *white arrow* indicates a developing myofiber also known as Wohlfart myofiber.) **(B)** Prolonged mechanical ventilation was associated with reduction in myofiber cross-sectional area. (Modified from Knisely AS, Leal SM, Singer DB: Abnormalities of diaphragmatic muscle in neonates with ventilated lungs. J Pediatr 1988;113:1074-1077.)

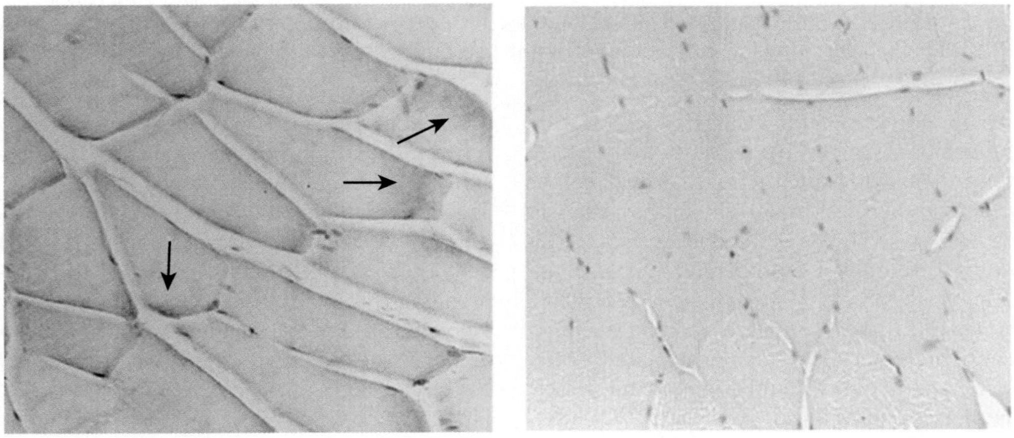

A B

Figure 41-11. A, A sample of gastrocnemius muscle obtained from an adult Sprague-Dawley rat injected 12 hours earlier with *Escherichia coli* endotoxin (20 mg/kg). The section was stained with an antibody to inducible nitric oxide synthase. Positive staining (*brown coloration, arrows*) is evident inside the fibers. **B,** A sample of gastrocnemius muscle obtained from a rat injected 12 hours earlier with normal saline. No positive staining response is evident. (From Laghi F, Tobin MJ: Disorders of the respiratory muscles. Am J Respir Crit Care Med 2003;168:10-48. Photomicrographs provided by Dr. Sabah N. Hussain, Royal Victoria Hospital, Montreal.)

potential)[92-94] and excitation-contraction coupling.[91,95] Mechanisms responsible for failure of excitation-contraction coupling include the cytotoxic effect of nitric oxide and its metabolites,[96,97] free radicals,[98-101] ubiquitin-proteasome proteolysis,[47,49,91,102,103] and, possibly, decrease in nicotinic acetylcholine receptors.[104] Local dysregulation of the circulation and Krebs cycle may also contribute.[91]

Nitric oxide, a free radical that has a negative inotropic effect on the heart and skeletal muscle, is produced in large amounts during sepsis by a nitric oxide synthase inducible by lipopolysaccharide and several cytokines (Fig. 41-11).[105] Greater expression of inducible nitric oxide synthase in the diaphragm during sepsis is associated with morphologic evidence of widespread damage to the myofiber membrane, or sarcolemma (Fig. 41-12).[93] Although diaphragmatic contractions enhance this sepsis-induced sarcolemmal injury,[106] early mechanical ventilation reduces sarcolemmal injury and the associated diaphragmatic dysfunction.[107] The beneficial effects of resting the diaphragm with the use of mechanical ventilation are not coupled with a decrease in either oxidative stress or the expression of inducible nitric oxide synthase in the muscle.[107] These observations suggest the existence of a detrimental interaction of two independent stressors (oxidative and biomechanical stresses) on the sarcolemma during sepsis.[107]

To determine whether the inducible nitric oxide synthase pathway contributes to impaired skeletal muscle contractility in humans, Lanone and coworkers[108] obtained samples of the rectus abdominis muscle in 16 septic patients and 21 control subjects. The muscles of the patients had lower contractile force and increased inducible nitric oxide synthase expression (mRNA and protein) and activity. Immunohistochemical studies showed the generation of peroxynitrite (a highly reactive oxidant formed by the reaction of nitric oxide with superoxide

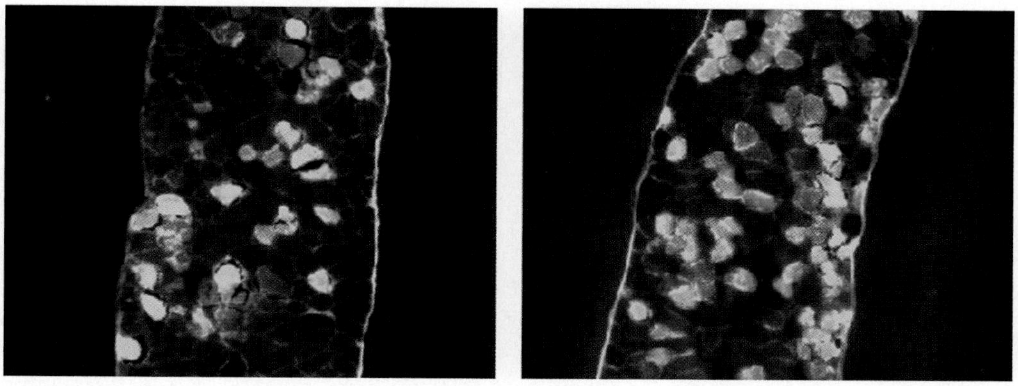

Figure 41-12. **A,** A strip of diaphragm obtained from a C57BL/6 mouse injected 12 hours earlier with normal saline. The strip was stimulated for 3 minutes (50 Hz, 300-ms duration) and then immersed for 90 minutes in Krebs solution containing a fluorescent probe, Procion orange 14 (0.15, wt/vol). **B,** A strip of diaphragm obtained from a C57BL/6 mouse injected 12 hours earlier with *Escherichia coli* endotoxin (20 mg/kg). Stimulation and staining were conducted as described for **A.** Sarcolemmal damage, indicated by yellow staining, was increased by endotoxin. (From Laghi F, Tobin MJ: Disorders of the respiratory muscles. Am J Respir Crit Care Med 2003;168:10-48. Photomicrographs provided by Dr. Sabah N. Hussain, Royal Victoria Hospital, Montreal.)

anion). Exposure of control muscles to the amount of peroxynitrite found in patients caused an irreversible decrease in force generation. These data suggest that sepsis reduces muscle force through the production of nitric oxide and its toxic by-products.

Production of nitric oxide in sepsis may be protective and not solely deleterious.[100,106,109,110] In mice deficient in inducible[109] or constitutive (neuronal) nitric oxide synthase,[106] endotoxin caused a greater decline in diaphragmatic contractility than in nondeficient mice. This finding contrasts with the observation that nitric oxide synthase inhibitors prevent muscle dysfunction in septic rats.[93,97,105] Although the results may be species-dependent,[106] the data underscore that nitric oxide has both antioxidant and prooxidant actions.[111]

In addition to nitric oxide and its derivatives, several other oxygen-derived free radicals (superoxide anion, hydroxyl radicals, hydrogen peroxide) contribute to the reduced contractility of the diaphragm in sepsis.[98-101] This greater expression of oxygen-derived free radicals in sepsis is accompanied by enhanced activity of the antioxidant enzyme superoxide dismutase[101] and increased expression of the heme oxygenase-1 pathway.[99] The heme oxygenase-1 pathway is a powerful cellular system that protects against oxidative stress and contractile fatigue during sepsis.[99] Administration of an inhibitor (zinc protoporphyrin IX) or an inducer (hemin) of heme oxygenase activity respectively enhances or reduces the oxidative stress and contractile failure of the diaphragm in a rat model of sepsis.[99] In septic rats, lower diaphragmatic contractility can also be improved by the administration of specific scavengers of superoxide ions, hydrogen peroxide, and hydroxyl radicals.[101]

Intensive Care Unit–Acquired Paresis

While cared for in the ICU, critically ill patients can experience muscle weakness and, occasionally, paralysis. Some of these patients have evidence of axonal degeneration and denervation atrophy (Fig. 41-13).[4] This constellation of findings is known as *critical illness polyneuropathy* (Table 41-2).[112] Cytokines[113] and low-molecular-weight neurotoxins,[114] released during episodes of sepsis or when multiple organ failure develops, are thought to be responsible for this axonal degeneration. Critical illness polyneuropathy has been considered one of the manifestations of multiple organ failure syndrome. Sepsis and multiple organ failure, however, are not essential prerequisites for the development of critical illness polyneuropathy.[115,116] Tight control of hyperglycemia may reduce both the risk of polyneuropathy and the duration of mechanical ventilation.[117]

In other patients, rather than axonopathy, there is evidence of isolated myopathy (i.e., critical illness myopathy).[4] Patients in whom isolated myopathy develops often have been treated with corticosteroids and neuromuscular blocking agents (e.g., patients with status asthmaticus).[4] Muscle biopsies demonstrate a general decrease in myofibrillar protein content and a selective loss of thick filaments (myosin) within type I and type II fibers (Fig. 41-14). Animal models of critical illness myopathy suggest that medical denervation with paralytic agents causes an upregulation of glucocorticoid receptors in the muscle.[118] If the animal subsequently receives high-dose corticosteroids, depletion of thick myosin filaments occurs.[118] Although a decrease in thick-filament proteins may be important for prolonged weakness,[119] this decrease is probably not the cause of the acute paralysis,[120] particularly in patients with compound motor action potentials of low amplitude.[121] Impaired muscle membrane excitability is probably more important during the acute stage.[120,122]

In the last few years it has become increasingly apparent that critical illness neuropathy and myopathy often coexist.[113,116,122-125] It has become common to refer to

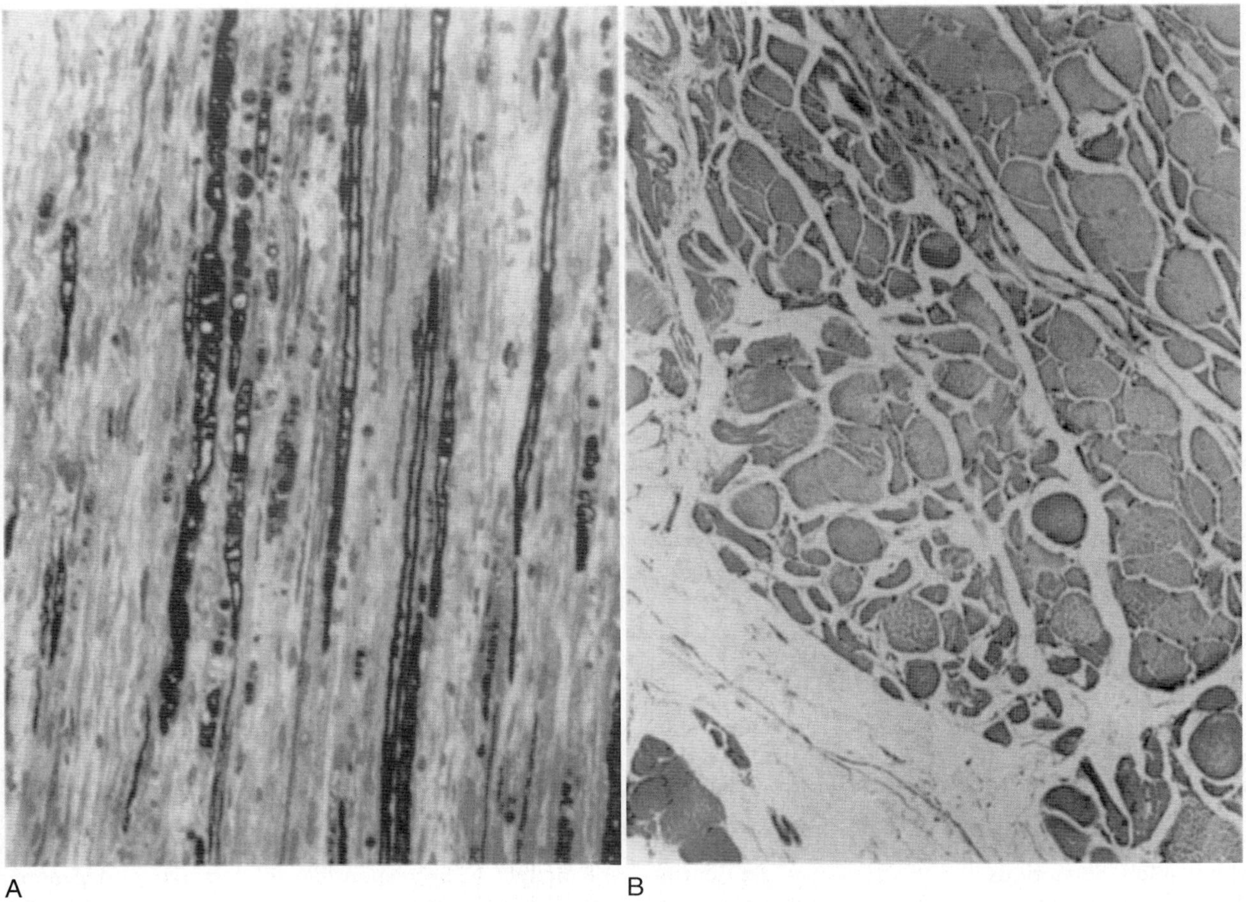

Figure 41-13. Transverse sections of a peripheral motor nerve (deep peroneal nerve, **A**) and of a skeletal muscle (intercostal, **B**) in patients in whom profound weakness developed after a prolonged hospital course characterized by sepsis, multiple organ failure syndrome, and inability to be weaned from mechanical ventilation. **A,** The long thin dark structures are myelin sheaths that contain axons. The axons are degenerating and dying. After death, they disintegrate. The myelin surrounding the disintegrating axons collapses around the axonal debris to form *ovoids of myelin*—seen better on the lateral portions of the *left* micrograph. **B,** Amid muscle fibers that are normal in size and shape are atrophic fibers that appear small and have developed contours with acute angles. These findings are consistent with denervation atrophy secondary to axonal degeneration, so-called critical illness polyneuropathy. (From Zochodne DW, Bolton CF, Wells GA, et al: Critical illness polyneuropathy: A complication of sepsis and multiple organ failure. Brain 1987;110:819-841.)

patients who become weak while in the ICU as a result of acquired neuropathy and/or myopathy (not associated with a known disorder) as simply having ICU-acquired paresis.[122,123,125] ICU-acquired paresis has been reported to be an independent risk factor of prolonged weaning.[125]

The functional outcome of ICU-acquired paresis is not uniform. Approximately 50% to 60% of patients experience complete recovery (ability to breathe spontaneously and to walk independently) over a period of 2 weeks to 6 months or longer.[119,126,127] About 30% experience severe persistent disability with tetraparesis, tetraplegia, or paraplegia.[126] Other investigators report even worse outcome: Only 2 of 10 patients in one study left the hospital.[124] Whether it is possible to prevent ICU-acquired paresis in patients recovering from severe acute illness and whether the prevention would result in shorter duration of mechanical ventilation remains unknown.

Acid-Base Disorders

Alkalosis, either metabolic or respiratory, does not affect skeletal muscle strength[128-30] and might improve endurance.[128] Whether acidosis, either metabolic or respiratory, impairs respiratory muscle function remains controversial. Because the contractile response to metabolic acidosis and respiratory acidosis are not necessarily the same,[131,132] they are discussed separately.

Metabolic Acidosis Until recently, there was little doubt that metabolic acidosis could decrease muscle contractility.[133,134] Purported mechanisms included reduction of actin-myosin cross-bridge activation by H^+ competitive inhibition of Ca^{2+} binding to troponin C, reduced transition of actin-myosin cross-bridges from low-force to high-force state, and inhibition of myofibrillar adenosine triphosphatase (ATPase), glycolytic rate, and maximal shortening velocity, and inhibition of sarcoplasmic

Table 41-2. Electromyographic Findings*

Finding	Axonal Injury	Myelin Injury	Neuromuscular Conduction Defect	Myopathy
Compound muscle action potential (amplitude)†	Reduced	Normal to slightly reduced	Normal‡	Normal
Sensory nerve action potential (amplitude)§	Reduced	Normal to reduced	Normal	Normal
Conduction velocity	Normal to slightly reduced	Reduced	Normal	Normal
Spontaneous muscle depolarization¶	Present	Absent	Absent	None to present
Amplitude of compound muscle action potential with stimulation at 3 Hz‖	Unchanged	Unchanged	Decreased	Unchanged
Motor unit activation	Decreased	Decreased	Normal	Increased

*Examples of injuries and deficits: axonal injury, critical illness myopathy; myelin injury, Guillain-Barré syndrome; neuromuscular conduction defect, myasthenia, prolonged neuromuscular blockade; myopathy, critical illness myopathy. Although features of myopathy can be recorded by electromyographic studies, electromyography cannot always distinguish critical illness myopathy from critical illness polyneuropathy, and muscle biopsies may be needed.
†Elicited by motor nerve stimulation.
‡Decreased in the Lambert-Eaton syndrome.
§Elicited by sensory nerve stimulation.
¶Spontaneous muscle depolarization (caused by denervation) is detected as presence of fibrillation potentials and positive sharp waves.
‖Repetitive nerve stimulation is performed to exclude neuromuscular transmission defects such as prolonged neuromuscular paralysis.
From Laghi F, Tobin MJ: Disorders of the respiratory muscles. Am J Respir Crit Care Med 2003;168:10-48.

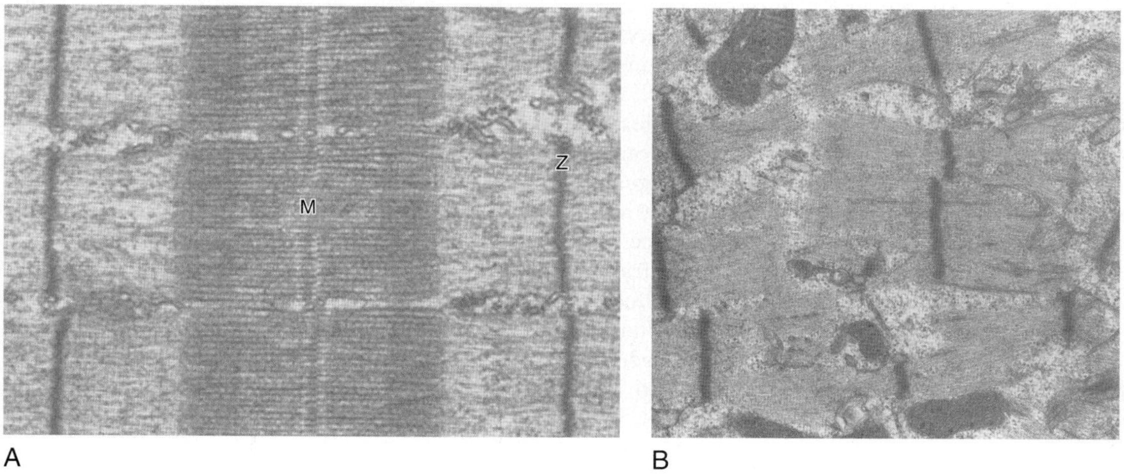

Figure 41-14. Electron micrographs of normal skeletal muscle **(A)** and skeletal muscle from a patient who received steroids and the neuromuscular blocking agent vecuronium during a hospitalization with status asthmaticus followed by flaccid quadriplegia **(B).** Compared with the normal structure, the patient specimen shows extensive loss of thick (myosin) myofilaments and relative preservation of thin (actin) filaments. Muscle strength returned to normal 2 months after discontinuation of vecuronium. M, M-line formed by myosin filaments and M-line proteins; Z, Z-disk formed by a lattice of filaments that join the actin filaments of one sarcomere with the actin filaments of the adjacent sarcomere. (**A,** from Eisenberg BR. In Bradley WG, Gardner-Medwin D, Walton JN [eds:] Recent Advances in Myology. Amsterdam, Excerpta Medica, 1975; and **B,** from Danon MJ, Carpenter S: Myopathy with thick filament [myosin] loss following prolonged paralysis with vecuronium during steroid treatment. Muscle Nerve 1991;14:1131-1139.)

ATPase with reduction of sarcoplasmic Ca^{2+} reuptake leading to reduced release of Ca^{2+} from the sarcoplasmic reticulum.[135]

Despite the biologic plausibility, investigators have reported no effect[132,136] or marginal effect[137] of metabolic acidosis on respiratory muscle function. Yanos and colleagues[132] assessed maximal transdiaphragmatic pressure elicited by tetanic stimulation of the phrenic nerves in seven anesthetized dogs during respiratory acidosis (pH 7.1) and during lactic acidosis (pH 7.1). They observed a fall in maximal diaphragm strength with respiratory acidosis (−18%, $P<.05$), but not with lactic acidosis (+3%). Similarly, when Coast and associates[137] exposed isolated strips of rat diaphragm to different concentrations of lactic acid, they recorded decreases in force when the pH was lowered to 6.8—but only after the muscle strips were stressed with 75 contractions (25 Hz, 250-ms train duration, one train per second). Contractility was not affected when the pH was decreased to 6.8 to 7.2 at rest or after the set of 75 contractions delivered at a pH of 7.1 to 7.2.[137]

These negative results are in line with reports of some—but not all[138,139]—recent investigations questioning the inhibitory role of metabolic acidosis on limb muscle contractility at physiologic temperatures.[140-143] For instance, Nielsen and coworkers[143] reported that metabolic acidosis (pH 6.80) counteracts the detrimental effects of increased extracellular K^+ concentration (which occurs with forceful contractions) on the excitability and force generation of the rat soleus muscle. In humans, Degroot and colleagues[141] measured intracellular H^+ concentration during sustained isometric foot plantar flexion. In contrast to what would be expected if acidosis caused decrease in contractility, Degroot and colleagues[141] reported a decrease in intracellular H^+ concentration during the first 10 seconds of exercise when force was declining, and a rise in intracellular H^+ concentration immediately after exercise when force partially recovered.[141] Whether severe metabolic acidosis in humans might impair skeletal function by causing a reduced central nervous system drive remains to be demonstrated.[133]

Acute Respiratory Acidosis There are contrasting reports on the effect of acute respiratory acidosis on respiratory muscle contractility.[129,130,132,144] In anesthetized dogs, diaphragmatic contractility decreases at an equal pace with the severity of acute respiratory acidosis[129] (but has no effect on gastrocnemius muscle contractility[132]). Similarly, in healthy volunteers, acute increases of arterial carbon dioxide to 54 mm Hg (corresponding to a pH of about 7.29) reduces the capacity of the unfatigued diaphragm to generate pressure by 10% to 30% (Fig. 41-15).[130] Such reduction in pressure generation is even greater when arterial carbon dioxide is increased to 63 mm Hg (corresponding to a pH of about 7.22).[130] Acute respiratory acidosis decreases respiratory muscle endurance[130,145] and can increase the extent of diaphragmatic fatigue at the conclusion of 2 minutes of maximal voluntary ventilation.[146] Despite greater voluntary activation of the diaphragm,[147] hypercapnic patients with COPD generate lower maxi-mal static inspiratory pressures than patients with normocapnia.[148,149]

A direct inhibitory effect of acute respiratory acidosis[129,130,132,145,146] on respiratory muscle contractility and respiratory muscle endurance could provide a potential mechanism for the rapid clinical deterioration that can occur with severe asthma and during COPD exacerbations.[130] Yet the human data suggesting a direct deleterious effect of acute respiratory acidosis on respiratory muscle function[130,145,146,148] are not uniform. Some investigators report no change in diaphragmatic contractility[144,146] (but decrease in force of the adductor pollicis[144]) when acute respiratory acidosis causes a decrease in pH to about 7.16 to 7.27,[144,150] no change in the maximum relaxation rate of the diaphragm,[150] and no effect in the extent of diaphragmatic fatigue 20 to 90 minutes after loading.[146]

For several reasons it is difficult to reconcile the conflicting data reported in the literature on the effects of acute respiratory acidosis on respiratory muscle contractility. First, the nonsignificant 12% decrease in diaphragmatic contractility (twitch pressure) recorded during acute hypercapnia in 12 healthy subjects in one study[144] raises the possibility of type II error. Second, it is impossible to state that more severe acidosis was responsible for the different results in human investigations if one considers the comparable pH values of the studies with negative[144] and positive[130] results. Third, it is unlikely that the different frequencies of stimulation used to assess the respiratory muscles[130,144,146] are responsible for the contrasting results, because when present, acidosis-associated decrease in contractility is frequency inependent.[129] Moreover, the following three additional considerations further cloud our understanding of any interaction (if present) between acute respiratory acidosis and respiratory muscle contractility:

1. Respiratory acidosis (pH 6.50-6.88) may actually enhance, and not depress, skeletal muscle contractility.[143,151]

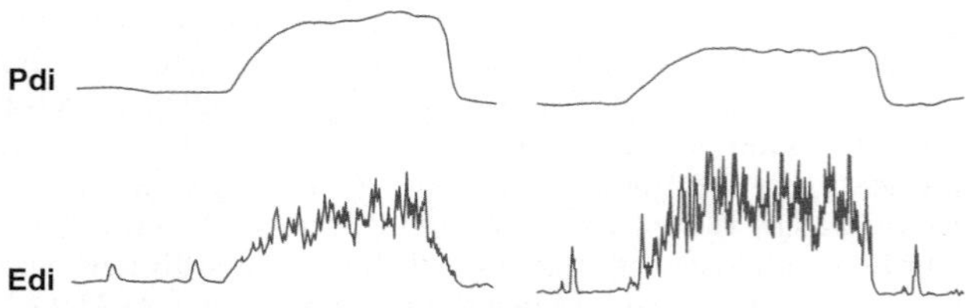

Figure 41-15. Transdiaphragmatic pressure (Pdi) and electrical activity of the diaphragm (Edi) during a voluntary isometric contraction in a healthy subject during normocapnia (*left panels*) and during acute hypercapnia (end-tidal CO_2, 7.5%; *right panels*). For a given Edi during hypercapnia, the pressure output of the diaphragm was decreased. (From Juan G, Calverley P, Talamo C, et al: Effect of carbon dioxide on diaphragmatic function in human beings. N Engl J Med 1984;10:874-879.)

2. Whether comorbidities that often affect hypercapnic patients such as sepsis, decreased cardiac function, and impaired respiratory mechanics could act synergistically with acute hypercapnia in worsening respiratory muscle function is unknown.
3. Whether equivalent levels of pH occurring as a result of acute or acute-on-chronic respiratory acidosis may or may not have the same effect on respiratory muscle function is also unknown.

Electrolyte Disturbances

Respiratory muscle function may be impaired by decreased levels of phosphate,[152] calcium,[153] magnesium,[154] and potassium.[155]

Aubier and coworkers[152] studied the effects of severe hypophosphatemia (0.55±0.18 mmol/L) on diaphragmatic function in eight patients with acute respiratory failure who were being mechanically ventilated. Diaphragmatic function was quantified before and after phosphorus replacement therapy through recording of the transdiaphragmatic twitch pressure elicited by phrenic nerve stimulation. Correction of hypophosphatemia was accompanied by a significant increase in transdiaphragmatic twitch pressure—that is, from 9.8±3.8 cm H_2O before phosphate infusion to 17.3±6.5 cm H_2O after phosphate infusion ($P<.001$). Changes in the serum phosphorus level and transdiaphragmatic pressure were well correlated ($r=0.73$). These results strongly suggest that hypophosphatemia can impair the contractile properties of the diaphragm during acute respiratory failure.

The same investigators assessed the effects of hypocalcemia on diaphragmatic function in 12 anesthetized dogs.[153] A continuous infusion of the chelating agent ethylene glycol-bis (B aminoethylether)-*N,N'*-tetraacetic acid (EGTA) was used to produce hypocalcemia. Over the two hours of observation, a progressive reduction in diaphragmatic force production paralleled the progressive reduction in ionized serum calcium.

Hypomagnesemia, a common occurrence in the ICU, can also cause respiratory muscle weakness. Dhingra and associates[154] reported improvements in maximal inspiratory and expiratory pressures in 17 hypomagnesemic patients after magnesium replacement therapy but not after placebo therapy.

Disorders or conditions such as post-hypercapnic alkalosis, renal tubular acidosis, primary hyperaldosteronism, gastrointestinal potassium losses, use of diuretics, thyrotoxic periodic paralysis, familial hypokalemic paralysis, use of β_2-adrenergic agonists, and licorice ingestion can cause severe hypokalemia. When the serum potassium concentration decreases below 2.0 to 2.5 mEq/L, patients may have muscular weakness (including respiratory muscle weakness) and arrhythmias. Hypokalemia-associated respiratory muscle weakness can lead to respiratory failure and death.[155]

Decreased Oxygen Delivery

Laboratory animals with cardiogenic shock[156] or with septic shock[91,157] die of respiratory failure. Death is not caused by pulmonary disease per se but by an inability of the respiratory muscles to maintain adequate ventilation. This inability to maintain adequate ventilation is caused by insufficient oxygen delivery to the respiratory muscles.[4]

Whether the decrease in oxygen delivery to the respiratory muscles—or the respiratory centers—during shock is sufficient to reduce respiratory muscle performance and cause hypoventilation in patients, although likely,[158] remains to be determined. A nonrandomized study by Kontoyannis and associates[159] in 28 patients with cardiogenic shock provides support for the view that hemodynamic instability could reduce respiratory muscle performance in patients with shock. Compared with nonventilated patients, ventilated patients were weaned from an intra-aortic balloon pump more often, and their survival was greater.[159] These results are in line with the observation of Viires and colleagues,[160] who reported lower metabolic requirements by the diaphragm after institution of mechanical ventilation in dogs with cardiogenic shock.

Hemodynamic situations less extreme than shock that could still affect respiratory muscle performance are failed attempts at spontaneous respiration during weaning from mechanical ventilation. Jubran and coworkers[161] investigated the importance of hemodynamic performance in determining weaning outcome in 8 ventilator-supported patients in whom a trial of spontaneous breathing failed and 11 patients who tolerated a trial and were successfully extubated. Immediately before the trial, mixed oxygen venous saturation values were not different in the two groups. Mixed venous oxygen saturation progressively decreased over the course of the trial in the failure group, whereas it remained unchanged in the success group (Fig. 41-16A). Although the calculated oxygen demand values were similar in the two groups, the manner in which the demands were met differed in the groups. In the success group, oxygen transport increased, resulting mainly from an increase in cardiac index; in the failure group, the rise in demand was met by an increase in oxygen extraction, resulting in a decrease in mixed venous oxygen saturation (Fig. 41-16B). Although increased, the oxygen extraction ratio at the end of the trial in the failure group was close to the ratio reported to signify the onset of anaerobic metabolism (0.60)[162] in only two patients, who had ratios of 0.50 and 0.56. The ability of the failure group to deal with respiratory muscle energy demands through aerobic pathways is probably related to the capacity of the diaphragm to achieve higher blood flow than most other skeletal muscles.[163] During loading, the diaphragm rapidly increases oxygen extraction to a plateau of about 55% to 65%; further rises in oxygen demand are achieved by increases in blood flow.[164,165] The diaphragmatic musculature appears to be extremely resistant to hypoxic stress, and animals can maintain a ventilation that is sufficient to avoid hypercapnia until phrenic vein P_{O_2} falls to 12 mm Hg.[163] Likewise, investigators have found that an oxygen tension of about 10 mm Hg in the phrenic vein is

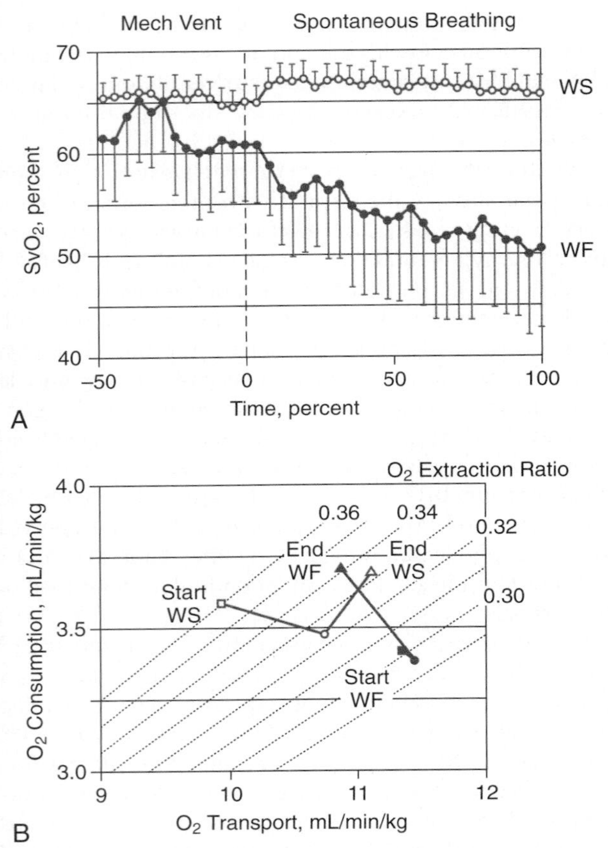

Figure 41-16. A, Mixed venous oxygen saturation (Svo_2) during mechanical ventilation and a trial of spontaneous breathing in 11 patients in whom ventilator weaning was successful (WS, *open symbols*) and in 8 patients in whom it failed (WF, *closed symbols*). During mechanical ventilation, Svo_2 values were similar in the two groups (P=.28). Between the onset (*dashed line*) and the end of the trial, Svo_2 decreased in the failure group (P<0.01), whereas it remained unchanged in the success group (P=.48). Over the course of the trial, Svo_2 was lower in the failure group than in the success group (P<0.02). *Bars* indicate SE. **B,** Oxygen transport, oxygen consumption, and isopleths of oxygen extraction ratio in the success (WS, *open symbols*) and failure (WF, *closed symbols*) groups during mechanical ventilation (*squares*) and at the onset (*circles*) and end (*triangles*) of a spontaneous breathing trial. See text for details. (Modified from Jubran A, Marthu M, Dries E, et al: Continuous recordings of mixed venous oxygen saturation during weaning from mechanical ventilation and the ramifications thereof. Am J Respir Crit Care Med 1998;158:1763-1769.)

the threshold associated with the onset of diaphragmatic lactate production[166] and the development of fatigue.[167] The lowest mixed venous oxygen tension recorded by Jubran and coworkers[161] was 26 mm Hg, which is above the threshold for onset of diaphragmatic lactate production. This association must be interpreted with caution, however, because mixed venous blood contains effluents from many tissue beds other than the diaphragm. The investigation by Jubran and coworkers[161] is the first documentation that when challenged by an increase in mechanical load,[13] the respiratory muscles of critically ill patients do not appear to switch from aerobic to anaerobic metabolism.

High variability in hemodynamic response during failure to wean has been reported by Zakynthinos and associates[16] In a study similar to the Jubran investigation,[161] Zakynthinos and associates[16] recorded a drop in mixed venous oxygen saturation and a rise in oxygen consumption (met mainly by an increase in oxygen extraction) in 9 of 18 patients in whom a trial of weaning had failed. In the other 9 patients, however, mixed venous oxygen saturation and oxygen consumption were not affected by the weaning trial. It is unclear whether the lack of interaction between weaning failure and oxygen consumption was due to depression of the respiratory centers, limited capacity to extract oxygen, or limited cardiac reserve.[168]

Medications

Weakness can result from direct myotoxic effects of some medications; examples are blockade of myocyte glycoprotein synthesis and electron transport caused by inhibitors of the hydroxy-methylglutaryl coenzyme A reductase or nucleoside analogues used in patients with human immunodeficiency virus.[169-172] Weakness can also result with use of neuromuscular blocking agents and aminoglycosides, which interfere with neuromuscular transmission.[173,174]

Paralysis, including of the respiratory muscles, can persist after discontinuation of neuromuscular blocking agents.[174-176] Prolonged neuromuscular blockade has been defined as 2,[174] 4,[176] or 6 hours[175] of paralysis after discontinuation of neuromuscular blocking agents. Prolonged blockade is estimated to occur in 12% to 44% of patients receiving pancuronium or vecuronium for 1 day or longer.[174-176] The risk with use of vecuronium is higher in patients with renal failure.[174,176] Accumulation of metabolites of the neuromuscular blocking agents is responsible for the prolonged blockade.[174] Recovery from prolonged neuromuscular blockade begins within 2 days of the last dose,[174,175] a process contrasting with the prolonged course of critical illness myopathy or neuropathy.[119,127,177,178] Train-of-four monitoring of the dose of a neuromuscular blocking agent with a peripheral nerve stimulator may hasten recovery.[176]

Limitations in the Current Classification of Respiratory Muscle Weakness

When one is studying respiratory muscle weakness leading to hypoventilation in critically ill patients it is necessary to bear in mind the current limited understanding of these conditions, as follows:

1. The distinction between pre-existing conditions and new-onset conditions can be arbitrary.
2. Conditions that are pre-existing (malnutrition and hyperinflation) can worsen during the course of an unrelated critical illness.
3. The nosology is often unsatisfactory. Consider the nebulous distinction between ICU-acquired paresis and sepsis-associated myopathy or between ICU-acquired paresis and ventilator-associated respiratory muscle dysfunction.

4. Conditions in which respiratory muscle weakness is associated with muscle damage can display also some degree of muscle atrophy—for example, the diaphragmatic atrophy in cases of ventilator-associated respiratory muscle dysfunction.
5. Laboratory specificity to differentiate the various conditions causing weakness in the ICU is limited.
6. In any given patient, more than one mechanism may be responsible for respiratory muscle weakness.
7. Respiratory muscle weakness can be combined with depressed drive—for example, in the setting of hypercapnia-induced hypoventilation.

Respiratory Muscle Fatigue

Contractile fatigue occurs when a sufficiently large respiratory load is applied over a sufficiently long period.[17,179-187] Contractile fatigue can be brief or prolonged. Short-lasting fatigue results from accumulation of inorganic phosphate,[142,188,189] failure of the membrane electrical potential to propagate beyond T tubules,[190] and to a much lesser extent intramuscular acidosis.[191-193] Short-lasting fatigue appears to have a protective function, because it can prevent injury to the sarcolemma caused by forceful muscle contractions.[194] Long-lasting fatigue[180] is consistent with the development of, and recovery from, muscle injury.[194,195] Load-induced injury occurs in two phases: an acute injury immediately after muscle contraction[194] and a delayed or secondary injury.[196-198]

Immediately after intense loading, muscles display apoptosis,[199] vacuolization of the sarcoplasmic reticulum, sarcoplasmic damage,[194] loss of the normal alignment between adjacent myofibrils,[197] sarcomeric disruption,[200] and Z-band streaming (Fig. 41-17).[201] Z-band streaming is attributed to a loss of protein elements in the Z-band, such as α-actinin and vimentin.[201] Several mechanisms may contribute to the acute injury. The first is shear forces resulting from high intramuscular tension[194] and eccentric contractions.[202,203] Eccentric contractions (contraction of muscle while it is stretched by external forces) occur in the diaphragm during the postinspiratory activity that occurs with acute bronchoconstriction[202] or in morbidly obese patients.[204] Eccentric contractions also occur within regions of the costal diaphragm during external inspiratory resistive loading.[205] Second, activation of calpain (by contraction-associated influx of calcium in the myocyte) causes lysis of myofibrillar proteins.[198] Calpain is a calcium-dependent nonlysosomal protease that degrades myofibrillar proteins, such as desmin, vimentin, tropomyosin, α-actinin and C-protein, but not actin or myosin heavy chains.[201] Oxidation during forceful contraction makes myofibrillar proteins more susceptible to calpain degradation.[201] Third, muscle contractions increase muscle temperature, which degrades muscle proteins.[196] Fourth, damage can result from excessive production of reactive oxygen species (superoxide anions, hydrogen peroxide, and hydroxyl radicals).[182,201,206-210] Reactive oxygen species are, however, essential for normal force production,[210] probably because they maintain an adequate redox state of sarcoplasmic reticulum proteins, such as the ryanodine receptors (calcium release channels)[211,212] and sarcoendoplasmic reticulum calcium–adenosine triphosphatase (SERCA) (an enzymatic pump responsible for reuptake of calcium from the cytosol).[210,211] In human (in vivo, skeletal[207] and diaphragm[182] muscles) and in animal experiments (in vivo, dog's diaphragm),[208] oxidative stress may account for up to 50% of the loss in sustainable force resulting from fatigue during loading.[213] Hypercapnia and reduction in diaphragmatic length (hyperinflation)—common in patients with acute

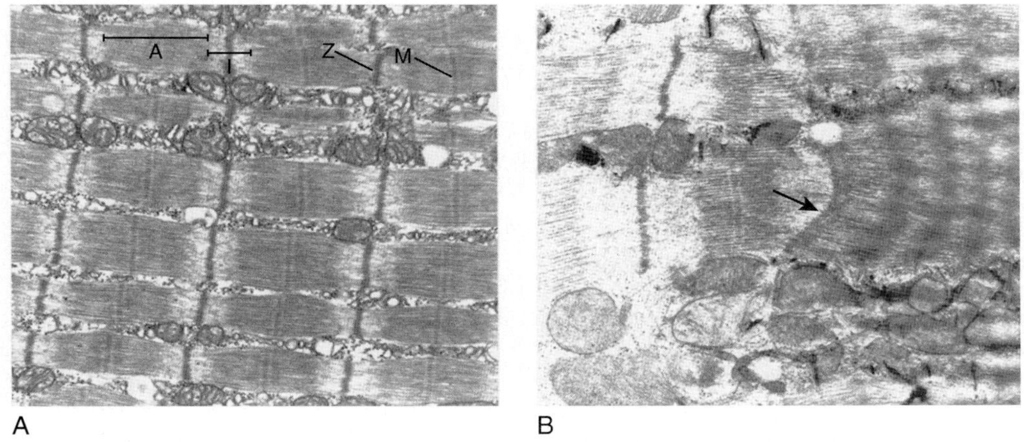

Figure 41-17. Electron micrographs of longitudinal sections from the costal diaphragm of a healthy control hamster **(A)** and a hamster exposed to 6 days of resistive loading **(B)**. **A,** Normal sarcomeres with distinct A-bands, I-bands, Z-bands, and M-lines that are aligned between adjacent myofibrils. **B,** Load-induced damage, recognizable from the Z-band streaming (*arrow*) and disruption of sarcomeric structure (right section of **B**) with loss of distinct A-bands and I-bands. Z-band streaming is attributed to a loss of cytoskeletal protein elements such as desmin, α-actinin, and vimentin. Magnification for both micrographs: ×16,500. (From Laghi F, Tobin MJ: Disorders of the respiratory muscles. Am J Respir Crit Care Med 2003;168:10-48. Electron micrographs provided by Drs. David C. Walker and Darlene W. Reid, University of British Columbia, Vancouver.)

respiratory failure—and a decrease in inspiratory muscle force generation (secondary to central or peripheral fatigue) can reduce superoxide release and thus protect the diaphragm from excessive damage and fatigue.[209] Strenuous muscle contractions also activate heme oxygenase (a microsomal enzyme of the inducible heat-stress protein family),[214] which has a defensive role against oxidative stress.[99] The role of nitric oxide derivatives in oxidative stress and fatigue is controversial.[210]

Delayed or secondary injury involves 7% to 9% of the diaphragm[195,201,215] and is characterized by focal necrosis, flocculent degeneration of the sarcoplasm, influx of inflammatory cells (in vivo inspiratory resistive loading in rabbits),[195,215] and disruption of the sarcolemma and sarcomeres.[201,216] The injury occurs days after exposure to high-intensity loads that have been sustained over a couple of hours[195,215] or moderate-intensity loading applied intermittently over several days.[216] Delayed diaphragmatic injury is proportional to the load[195] and peaks 3 days after application of the load (in vivo inspiratory threshold loading in rats).[198] Delayed injury decreases diaphragmatic force production at rest and increases fatigability both in vivo[195] and in vitro.[215] The decrease in force production depends on the intensity of the preceding load in healthy subjects[179,195] and in rabbits.[195] Free radicals, already present during acute injury, are still being produced 3 days after loading.[215] Free radical scavengers, however, do not completely prevent the loss of diaphragmatic force associated with delayed injury,[215] indicating that other mechanisms are involved.

The loss of force is disproportionate to the amount of muscle injured (as observed under light microscopy) [195,213]; susceptibility to calpain-mediated injury is increased in damaged muscle[201]; free radicals are produced long after loading[215]; and the respiratory muscles contract constantly to sustain life. These four facts carry two important clinical implications. First, muscle injury may cause a substantial decrease in force production.[217] Second, additional injury may occur because of persistent loading, coexisting malnutrition, abnormal arterial blood gases, or medications (e.g., glucocorticoids).[217]

In limb muscles, a repair process begins within 12 hours of the muscle injury resulting from excessive load (rat model).[218] Satellite cells (small mononucleated stem cells located between the basal lamina and sarcolemma of a muscle fiber) proliferate, differentiate, and fuse with existing myofibers.[218-220] Insulin-like growth factor 1, hepatocyte growth factor, and fibroblast growth factor appear to modulate this response.[218] Repair may explain the lessening of diaphragmatic injury between the third and fourth days after loading (threshold loading in rats).[198] Whether this repair process occurs in critically ill patients is unknown.

Modest intermittent resistive loading (2 hours a day over 4 days), equivalent to that in patients with lung disease, can disrupt sarcomeres and the sarcolemma of diaphragmatic fibers in dogs.[216] The sarcolemma disruption involves more type I than type II fibers.[216] This mechanism may occur in patients. The proportion of abnormal fibers in the diaphragm was correlated with airflow obstruction in 21 patients with forced expiratory volume in the first second (FEV_1) values ranging from 16% to 122% of predicted.[217] Abnormalities consisted of myofibers with internally located nuclei (Fig. 41-18), lipofuscin pigmentation (sign of oxidative stress), small angulated fibers, inflammation, and necrosis; these abnormalities occupied 4% to 34% of the diaphragm.[217] At a subcellular level, sarcomere disruption has also been reported.[200] The density of sarcomere disruption (i.e., number of areas containing disrupted sarcomeres expressed as $n/100\ \mu m^2$) in 18 patients with COPD was twice that seen in 11 control subjects, and it was correlated with FEV_1 ($r = -0.59$) and with the ratio of residual volume to total lung capacity ($r = 0.80$).[200] In the same investigation, a subset of 7 patients with COPD and 5 control subjects breathed through a threshold resistor until task failure (inspiratory load).[200] Compared with the unloaded state, the density of sarcomere disruptions increased by 89% in the loaded healthy subjects and by 38% in the loaded patients. The density of disruptions, however, was about two times greater in the patients with COPD after loading as compared with the unloaded healthy subjects[200]—39.0 versus 19.5 sarcomere disruptions per $100\ \mu m^2$. Diaphragmatic damage has been reported in patients dying of asphyxia, sudden infant death syndrome, and status asthmaticus.[221-223]

Whether or not either short-lasting or long-lasting contractile fatigue of the respiratory muscles develops in critically ill patients is not clear. Patients in whom a trial of weaning from mechanical ventilation fails are at particular risk for development of fatigue because they experience marked increases in respiratory load.[9,13,34] The addition of a new injury to the respiratory muscles (secondary to the development of contractile fatigue) might be the ultimate

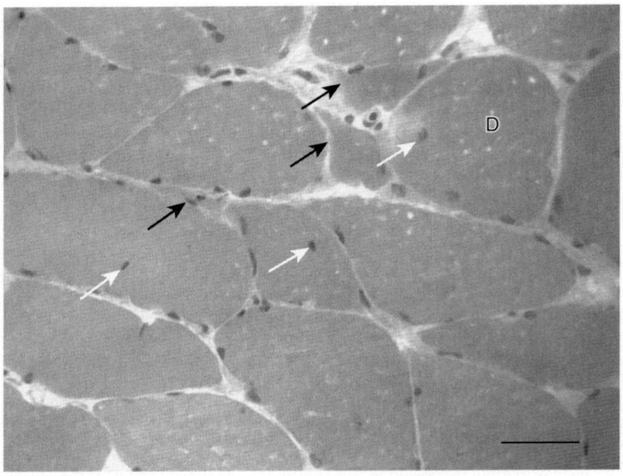

Figure 41-18. Microscopy of diaphragm from a patient with chronic obstructive pulmonary disease (COPD) (FEV_1 27% of predicted) stained with hematoxylin and eosin. Note internal nuclei (*white arrows*), small atrophic fibers (*black arrows*), and degeneration (D). Scale bar=50 microns. (From Laghi F, Tobin MJ: Disorders of the respiratory muscles. Am J Respir Crit Care Med 2003;168:10-48. Photomicrograph provided by Dr. Darlene W. Reid, University of British Columbia, Vancouver.)

determinant of whether or not some patients are ever successfully weaned from ventilation. Circumstantial evidence of contractile fatigue in patients experiencing respiratory distress has been reported.[13,224-226] Because of technical limitations,[224-226] these early data did not provide proof of contractile fatigue.[12,227]

Laghi and associates[15] measured the contractile response of the diaphragm to phrenic nerve stimulation in nine patients in whom a weaning trial failed; seven patients who were successfully weaned served as control subjects. The weaning failure patients experienced a greater respiratory load. Moreover, the *tension-time index* of the diaphragm—an index of the diaphragmatic effort of inspiration normalized by its maximal pressure output,[228] which is calculated by multiplying two ratios, the respiratory duty cycle (inspiratory time divided by the time of a total respiratory cycle) and the mean inspiratory pressure per breath divided by maximum inspiratory pressure—was greater in the failure group than in the success group ($P = .01$). Nevertheless, not a single patient demonstrated a decrease in transdiaphragmatic twitch pressure elicited by phrenic nerve stimulation (Fig. 41-19). The failure of fatigue to develop is surprising because in seven of the nine weaning failure patients the tension-time index exceeded 0.15 (the putative threshold for task failure and fatigue).

The most likely reason fatigue did not develop in these patients is that physicians re-instituted mechanical ventilation before it could develop. The relationship between tension-time index and the length of time that a load can be sustained until task failure follows an inverse-power function. Bellemare and Grassino[228] expressed the relationship as time to task failure = 0.1 (tension-time index)$^{-3.6}$. The increase in tension-time index over the course of the weaning trial[15] and predicted time to task failure[228] are shown in Figure 41-20. At the point that the physicians reinstituted mechanical ventilation, patients were predicted to be an average of 13 minutes away from task failure. Moreover, the time to task failure was underestimated because diaphragmatic recruitment during maximal voluntary contractions was incomplete.[15] In other words, patients show clinical manifestations of severe respiratory distress for a substantial time before fatigue develops. In an intensive care setting, these clinical

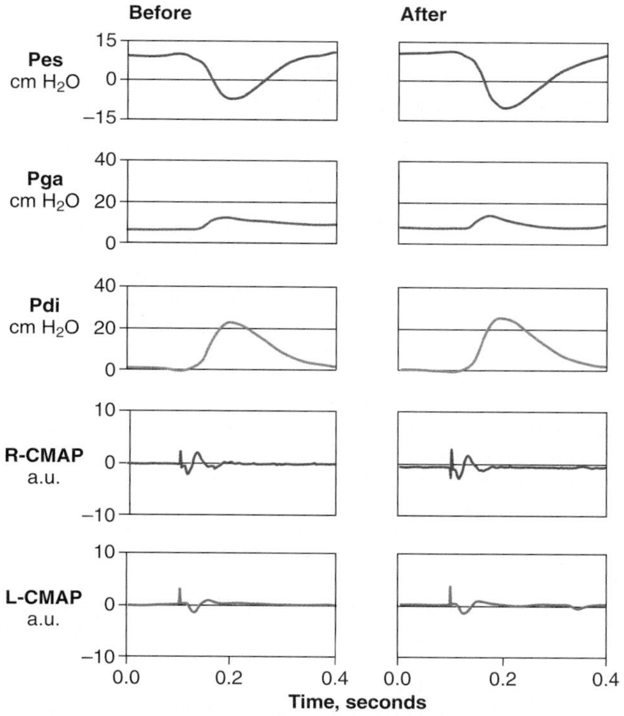

Figure 41-19. Esophageal pressure (Pes), gastric pressure (Pga), transdiaphragmatic pressure (Pdi), and compound motor action potentials of the right (R-CMAP) and left (L-CMAP) hemidiaphragms after phrenic nerve stimulation before and after a failed trial of weaning. The end-expiratory value of Pes and the amplitude of the right and left CMAPs were the same before and after the trial, indicating that the stimulations were delivered at the same lung volume and that the stimulations achieved the same extent of diaphragmatic recruitment. The amplitude of twitch Pdi elicited by phrenic nerve stimulation was the same before and after weaning. (From Laghi F, Cattapan SE, Jubran A, et al: Is weaning failure caused by low-frequency fatigue of the diaphragm? Am J Respir Crit Care Med 2003;167:120-127.)

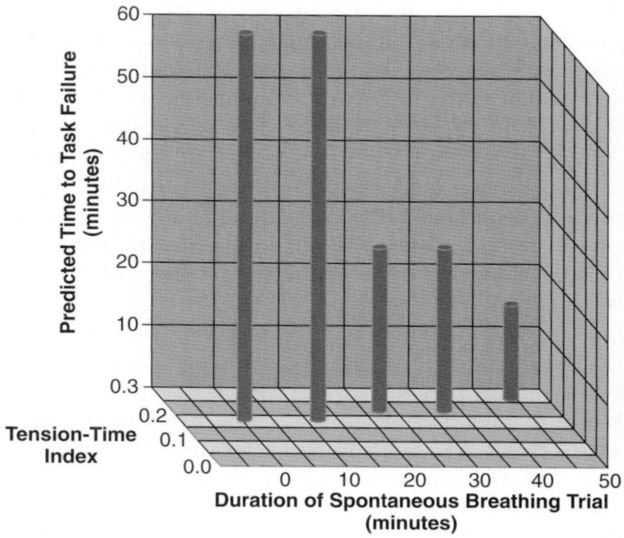

Figure 41-20. The interrelationship between the duration of a spontaneous breathing trial, tension-time index of the diaphragm, and predicted time to task failure in 9 patients in whom a trial of weaning from mechanical ventilation failed. The patients breathed spontaneously for an average of 44 minutes before a physician terminated the trial. At the start of the trial, tension-time index was 0.17, and the formula of Bellemare and Grassino[28] (see text for details) predicted that patients could sustain spontaneous breathing for another 59 minutes before task failure developed. As the trial progressed, tension-time index rose and predicted time to the development of task failure decreased. At the end of the trial, the tension-time index reached 0.26; that patients were predicted to sustain spontaneous breathing for another 13 minutes before development of task failure clarifies why patients did not show a decrease in diaphragmatic twitch pressure. In other words, physicians interrupted the trial on the basis of clinical manifestations of respiratory distress before sufficient time elapsed for development of contractile fatigue. (From Laghi F, Tobin MJ: Disorders of the respiratory muscles. Am J Respir Crit Care Med 2003;168:10-48.)

signs lead attendants to re-institute mechanical ventilation before fatigue has time to develop.

Studies in animals[191,229-231] support the finding that patients do not develop long-lasting contractile fatigue of the respiratory muscles. Inspiratory loading in animals causes respiratory failure and acidosis before force output decreases or substrate is depleted in the diaphragm,[191,229-231] suggesting that central[228,229,232] and reflex mechanisms[233,234] affect the breathing pattern[192] and α-motoneuron firing rates[235] in response to loading. Two neural pathways may convey information from the respiratory muscles to the central nervous system.[228,233,234,236,237] One pathway transmits information from mechanoreceptors (Golgi tendon organs and muscle spindles)[233,238] in the dorsal column, relaying it to the brainstem and thalamus before reaching the sensomotor cortex.[239] This pathway may participate in proprioceptive control of the respiratory muscles, integrating movements originating in the motor cortex.[232] The second pathway consists of vagal[227,228,231] and possibly phrenic nerve afferents (group IV phrenic afferent fibers)[233] that reach the amygdala after relaying in the brainstem and then projecting to the mesocortex (cingulated gyrus).[228] This pathway may deal with respiratory nociception,[232,240] such as dyspnea (through the relay in the amygdala),[241] and with the ventilatory response to carbon dioxide (through the relay in the brainstem, ventral cerebellum, and limbic system).[232,240,242] In addition to these two pathways projecting to the central nervous system, there is evidence for the existence of a spinal pathway responsible for phrenic-to-phrenic reflex inhibition.[234] An increase in carbon dioxide concentration during loading may also protect the respiratory muscles by decreasing production of reactive oxygen species.[209]

Resistive breathing causes hypercapnia without affecting diaphragmatic force output or aerobic metabolism (assessed by ^{31}P nuclear magnetic resonance spectroscopy) in spontaneously breathing piglets.[13,192,243] The hypoxia combined with resistive breathing caused a decrease in diaphragmatic force and inadequate oxidative metabolism, as reflected by accumulation of inorganic phosphorus and reduced phosphocreatine.[192] Force output and oxidative metabolism returned to baseline values with normoxia despite persistent loading.[192] The investigators speculated that loading produces a decrease in central activation (to the point of ventilatory failure), which decreases metabolic demands and prevents peripheral fatigue; additional stress of hypoxia may overwhelm this defense mechanism and cause peripheral fatigue.[192] Hypoxemia can also induce degradation of myofibrillar proteins.[244]

In hypoxia, the respiratory centers are impaired at a higher oxygen tension than the respiratory muscles,[167,245] making it difficult to decipher the effects of hypoxemia on the respiratory muscles. Animals demonstrate severe alveolar hypoventilation and respiratory arrest before the tension-generating ability of the diaphragm has begun to decrease.[167,245] As previously stated, it is unknown whether, in patients with shock,[158] decreases in oxygen delivery to the respiratory muscles[161,246] or respiratory centers can be sufficient to cause hypoventilation.

INCREASED RESPIRATORY LOAD

Increased respiratory load can result from greater mechanical load and/or larger ventilatory requirements.

Increased Mechanical Load

Patients in acute respiratory failure usually experience an increased mechanical load.[9,13,15,34,243,247-249] These patients typically have a 30% to 50% greater inspiratory resistance,[13,15,34] 100% greater dynamic elastance,[9,13] and 100% to 200% greater intrinsic positive end-expiratory pressure (PEEP)[9,13,15] than similar patients who are not in acute respiratory failure. The pressure output of the inspiratory muscles—quantified by calculation of the *pressure-time product* of inspiration—is almost equally divided in offsetting intrinsic PEEP, elastic recoil, and inspiratory resistance (Fig. 41-21).[13,243] Abnormal mechanics arise from bronchoconstriction, bronchial edema, pulmonary edema,[13] and lung inflammation.[247,248] Rapid shallow

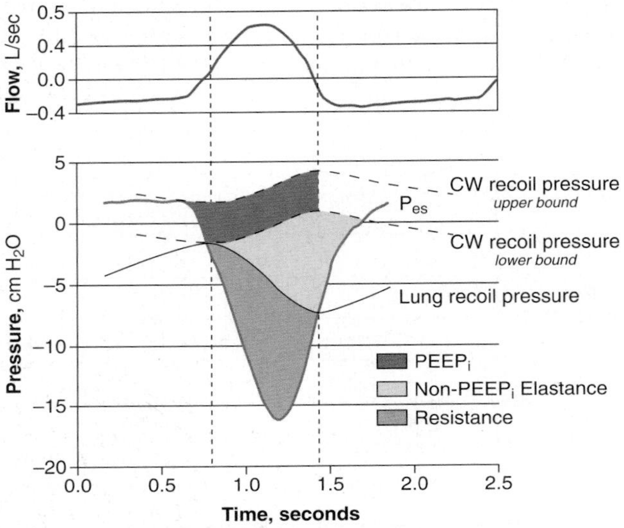

Figure 41-21. Quantification of the pressure output of the inspiratory muscles with the pressure-time product of inspiration. Flow (inspiration upward) and pressure tracings during spontaneous breathing. Recoil pressures of the chest wall (CW) and lung are calculated from dynamic elastances of the chest wall and lung, respectively, and lung volume. Upper-bound inspiratory pressure-time product (PTP) is calculated with use of the integral of the difference between esophageal pressure (Pes) and upper-bound CW recoil pressure from the onset of the rapid decrease in Pes to the transition from inspiratory to expiratory flow. The component of PTP due to intrinsic positive end-expiratory pressure ($PEEP_i$) is computed with use of the integral of the difference between the upper and lower bounds of CW recoil pressure from the onset of rapid decrease in Pes to the transition from inspiratory to expiratory flow. The component of PTP due to non-$PEEP_i$ elastance is computed with use of the integral of the difference between lung recoil pressure and lower-bound CW recoil pressure from the onset of inspiratory flow to the moment of transition from inspiratory to expiratory flow. The resistive fraction of PTP is computed with use of the integral of the difference between Pes and lung recoil pressure. The *vertical interrupted lines* represent points for zero flow. (From Jubran A, Tobin MJ: Pathophysiologic basis of acute respiratory distress in patients who fail a trial of weaning from mechanical ventilation. Am J Respir Crit Care Med 1997;155:906-915.)

breathing can aggravate the abnormalities in lung elastance, intrinsic PEEP, and carbon dioxide clearance.[13,34] Expiratory muscle recruitment can also increase intrinsic PEEP and breathing effort.[250] In some patients, greater mechanical load results from upper airway obstruction, one of the most urgent and potentially lethal medical emergencies.[1] Complete airway obstruction lasting for as little as 4 to 6 minutes can cause irreversible brain damage.[1] The upper airway, which encompasses the passage between the nares and carina, can be obstructed from functional or anatomic causes. Among the first are vocal cord paralysis and laryngospasm. Among the second are trauma, burn, infections, foreign bodies, and tumors. Functional and anatomic obstruction can occur postoperatively in patients with redundant pharyngeal soft tissue (sleep apnea) and loss of muscle tone related to the postanesthetic state.[1]

Increased Ventilatory Requirements

Increased ventilatory requirements can result from increases in carbon dioxide production, deadspace ventilation, and respiratory drive. Carbon dioxide production can rise as a result of sepsis,[91] fever, shivering, drugs (salicylates), lipogenesis,[251,252] or a shift in utilization of fuels from lipids (respiratory quotient [RQ]=0.7) to carbohydrates (RQ=1.0).[253] A rise in carbon dioxide production can be only a contributory factor to, not a sole cause of, hypercapnic respiratory failure.[3]

The ratio of deadspace volume to tidal volume is normally 0.30. The ratio increases up to 0.65 in patients with severe COPD,[254] acute respiratory distress syndrome,[255] and other severe lung diseases.[3] Patients can compensate for such an increase in deadspace volume by doubling minute ventilation.[3] Such a rise in minute ventilation poses a minor challenge when respiratory mechanics and respiratory muscles are normal; for example, hypercapnia is uncommon with pulmonary vascular disease.[3] Accordingly, an increase in deadspace ventilation should never be considered the primary mechanism responsible for hypercapnic respiratory failure unless there is a concurrent abnormality in the control of breathing or in the mechanical load of the respiratory muscles or in their contractile performance.[3]

Stimulation of pulmonary irritant or J receptors, neurologic lesions, sepsis, and toxins can inappropriately increase respiratory drive. Whether or not an inappropriately heightened drive places sufficient stress on the respiratory muscle to cause respiratory muscle fatigue and, consequently, hypoventilation remains to be determined.

HYPERCAPNIA-INDUCED HYPOVENTILATION

Severe hypercapnia depresses the central nervous system and decreases respiratory motor output.[252] A vicious circle can arise, whereby hypercapnia causes depressed drive, leading to more hypercapnia.[256,257] The possibility of hypercapnia-induced hypoventilation is supported by reports of successful resolution of hypercapnic respiratory failure in some patients after short-term infusion of the respiratory stimulant doxapram.[256,257]

SUMMARY

A relative or absolute decrease in respiratory muscle output is responsible for alveolar hypoventilation and hypercapnic respiratory failure. The number of distinct clinical entities that result in hypercapnia is vast, and often there is more than one disease process in the same patient—for example, hyperinflation-associated respiratory muscle weakness and ventilation-perfusion inequality in patients with COPD. The relative or absolute decrease in respiratory muscle output in patients with hypercapnia may stem from a reduction in respiratory drive, excess mechanical load on the respiratory muscles, and respiratory muscle weakness (see Fig. 41-1). Whether respiratory muscle fatigue is responsible for hypercapnic respiratory failure is an important issue that has yet to be resolved.

KEY POINTS

- *Hypercapnia* is synonymous with *alveolar hypoventilation* (for the patient's level of carbon dioxide production).
- A relative or absolute drop in respiratory muscle output is responsible for alveolar hypoventilation.
- Isolated impairments in gas exchange usually do not cause hypercapnia.
- When gas exchange is impaired, the magnitude of neuromuscular impairment or increased respiratory load conducive to hypercapnia can be less than the corresponding derangements when gas exchange is intact.
- Respiratory drive is elevated in many patients with acute ventilatory failure. This finding does not necessarily exclude the possibility that during episodes of ventilatory failure, the central nervous system is not fully recruiting the respiratory muscles and may be contributing to CO_2 retention.
- In critically ill patients, respiratory muscle weakness is probably responsible for a large number of cases of alveolar hypoventilation.
- Metabolic disturbances such as hypophosphatemia, hypomagnesemia, hypokalemia, and hypocalcemia can cause respiratory muscle weakness.
- Hyperinflation places the respiratory muscles in a mechanical disadvantage to generate the driving pressure of the respiratory system.
- Hyperinflation can occur during episodes of respiratory distress even in patients without history of airway disease (e.g., asthma or COPD).
- The role of respiratory muscle fatigue in causing hypercapnic respiratory failure remains to be determined.
- Severe hypercapnia can in itself be conducive to alveolar hypoventilation through depression of respiratory drive.
- It is still unclear whether respiratory or metabolic acidosis has a clinically relevant direct effect on respiratory muscle contractility.

REFERENCES

1. Laghi F, Tobin MJ: Indications for mechanical ventilation. In Tobin MJ (ed): Principles and Practice of Mechanical Ventilation. New York, McGraw-Hill, 2006, pp 129-162.
2. West JB: Pulmonary Pathophysiology: The Essentials, 6th ed. Philadelphia, Lippincott Williams & Wilkins, 2003.
3. Younes M: Mechanisms of ventilatory failure. Curr Pulmonol 1993;14: 243-292.
4. Laghi F, Tobin MJ: Disorders of the respiratory muscles. Am J Respir Crit Care Med 2003;168:10-48.
5. Webster NR, Kulkarni V: Metabolic alkalosis in the critically ill. Crit Rev Clin Lab Sci 1999;36:497-510.
6. Baier H, Somani P: Ventilatory drive in normal man during semistarvation. Chest 1984;85:222-225.
7. Tobin MJ, Perez W, Guenther SM, et al: The pattern of breathing during successful and unsuccessful trials of weaning from mechanical ventilation. Am Rev Respir Dis 1986;134: 1111-1118.
8. Sassoon CS, Mahutte CK: Airway occlusion pressure and breathing pattern as predictors of weaning outcome. Am Rev Respir Dis 1993;148:860-866.
9. Purro A, Appendini L, De Gaetano A, et al: Physiologic determinants of ventilator dependence in long-term mechanically ventilated patients. Am J Respir Crit Care Med 2000;161: 1115-1123.
10. Cooper KR, Phillips BA: Effect of short-term sleep loss on breathing. J Appl Physiol 1982;53:855-858.
11. Spengler CM, Shea SA: Sleep deprivation per se does not decrease the hypercapnic ventilatory response in humans. Am J Respir Crit Care Med 2000;161:1124-1128.
12. Tobin MJ, Laghi F: Monitoring respiratory muscle function. In Tobin MJ (ed): Principles and Practice of Intensive Care Monitoring. New York, McGraw-Hill, 1998, pp 497-544.
13. Jubran A, Tobin MJ: Pathophysiologic basis of acute respiratory distress in patients who fail a trial of weaning from mechanical ventilation. Am J Respir Crit Care Med 1997;155: 906-915.
14. Yang KL, Tobin MJ: A prospective study of indexes predicting the outcome of trials of weaning from mechanical ventilation. N Engl J Med 1991;324:1445-1450.
15. Laghi F, Cattapan SE, Jubran A, et al: Is weaning failure caused by low-frequency fatigue of the diaphragm? Am J Respir Crit Care Med 2003;167:120-127.
16. Zakynthinos S, Routsi C, Vassilakopoulos T, et al: Differential cardiovascular responses during weaning failure: Effects on tissue oxygenation and lactate. Intensive Care Med 2005;31:1634-1642.
17. Laghi F, Harrison MJ, Tobin MJ: Comparison of magnetic and electrical phrenic nerve stimulation in assessment of diaphragmatic contractility. J Appl Physiol 1996;80:1731-1742.
18. Cattapan SE, Laghi F, Tobin MJ: Can diaphragmatic contractility be assessed by airway twitch pressure in mechanically ventilated patients? Thorax 2003;58:58-62.
19. Watson AC, Hughes PD, Louise HM, et al: Measurement of twitch transdiaphragmatic, esophageal, and endotracheal tube pressure with bilateral anterolateral magnetic phrenic nerve stimulation in patients in the intensive care unit. Crit Care Med 2001;29:1325-1331.
20. Polkey MI, Kyroussis D, Hamnegard CH, et al: Diaphragm strength in chronic obstructive pulmonary disease. Am J Respir Crit Care Med 1996;154:1310-1317.
21. Laghi F, Jubran A, Topeli A, et al: Effect of lung volume reduction surgery on diaphragmatic neuromechanical coupling at 2 years. Chest 2004;125:2188-2195.
22. Oomman A, Gurtoo A: Acute intermittent porphyria as a cause of acute respiratory failure. J Indian Med Assoc 2002;100:44, 46.
23. Tyagi A, Chawla R, Sethi AK, et al: Respiratory failure in acute intermittent porphyria. J Assoc Physicians India 2002;50:443-445.
24. Vodoff MV, Cremer R, Martinot A, et al: [Acute respiratory insufficiency revealing myasthenia gravis: Apropos of 3 cases]. Arch Pediatr 1997;4:845-848.
25. Vaidya H: Case of the month: Unusual presentation of myasthenia gravis with acute respiratory failure in the emergency room. Emerg Med J 2006;23:410-413.
26. Greenberg C, Davies S, McGowan T, et al: Acute respiratory failure following severe arsenic poisoning. Chest 1979;76:596-598.
27. Vergauwe PL, Knockaert DC, Van Tittelboom TJ: Near fatal subacute thallium poisoning necessitating prolonged mechanical ventilation. Am J Emerg Med 1990;8:548-550.
28. Henderson RD, Sandroni P, Wijdicks EF: Chronic inflammatory demyelinating polyneuropathy and respiratory failure. J Neurol 2005;252:1235-1237.
29. Trend PS, Wiles CM, Spencer GT, et al: Acid maltase deficiency in adults: Diagnosis and management in five cases. Brain 1985;108:845-860.
30. Braun NM, Arora NS, Rochester DF: Respiratory muscle and pulmonary function in polymyositis and other proximal myopathies. Thorax 1983;38:616-623.
31. Gibson GJ, Gilmartin JJ, Veale D, et al: Respiratory muscle function in neuromuscular disease. In Jones NL, Killian KJ (eds): Breathlessness. The Campbell Symposium. Hamilton, Ontario, Boehringer-Ingelheim, 1992, pp 66-73.
32. Alison JA, Regnis JA, Donnelly PM, et al: End-expiratory lung volume during arm and leg exercise in normal subjects and patients with cystic fibrosis. Am J Respir Crit Care Med 1998;158:1450-1458.
33. Bloch KE, Weder W, Boehler A, et al: Successful lung volume reduction surgery in a child with severe airflow obstruction and hyperinflation due to constrictive bronchiolitis. Chest 2002;122:747-750.
34. Vassilakopoulos T, Zakynthinos S, Roussos C: The tension-time index and the frequency/tidal volume ratio are the major pathophysiologic determinants of weaning failure and success. Am J Respir Crit Care Med 1998;158:378-385.
35. Koutsoukou A, Armaganidis A, Stavrakaki-Kallergi C, et al: Expiratory flow limitation and intrinsic positive end-expiratory pressure at zero positive end-expiratory pressure in patients with adult respiratory distress syndrome. Am J Respir Crit Care Med 2000;161:1590-1596.
36. Laghi F, Jubran A, Topeli A, et al: Effect of lung volume reduction surgery on neuromechanical coupling of the diaphragm. Am J Respir Crit Care Med 1998;157:475-483.
37. Coussa ML, Guerin C, Eissa NT, et al: Partitioning of work of breathing in mechanically ventilated COPD patients. J Appl Physiol 1993;75:1711-1719.
38. Pelosi P, Cereda M, Foti G, et al: Alterations of lung and chest wall mechanics in patients with acute lung injury: Effects of positive end-expiratory pressure. Am J Respir Crit Care Med 1995;152:531-537.
39. Laaban JP, Kouchakji B, Dore MF, et al: Nutritional status of patients with chronic obstructive pulmonary disease and acute respiratory failure. Chest 1993;103:1362-1368.
40. Faisy C, Rabbat A, Kouchakji B, et al: Bioelectrical impedance analysis in estimating nutritional status and outcome of patients with chronic obstructive pulmonary disease and acute respiratory failure. Intensive Care Med 2000;26:518-525.
41. Kim J, Heshka S, Gallagher D, et al: Intermuscular adipose tissue-free skeletal muscle mass: Estimation by dual-energy X-ray absorptiometry in adults. J Appl Physiol 2004;97: 655-660.
42. Murciano D, Rigaud D, Pingleton S, et al: Diaphragmatic function in severely malnourished patients with anorexia nervosa: Effects of renutrition. Am J Respir Crit Care Med 1994;150:1569-1574.
43. Ameredes BT, Watchko JF, Daood MJ, et al: Growth hormone restores aged diaphragm myosin composition and performance after chronic undernutrition. J Appl Physiol 1999;87:1253-1259.
44. Lewis MI, Li H, Huang ZS, et al: Influence of varying degrees of malnutrition on IGF-I expression in the rat diaphragm. J Appl Physiol 2003;95:555-562.
45. Lewis MI, Lorusso TJ, Zhan WZ, et al: Interactive effects of denervation and malnutrition on diaphragm structure and function. J Appl Physiol 1996;81:2165-2172.
46. Lewis MI, Feinberg AT, Fournier M: IGF-I and/or growth hormone preserve diaphragm fiber size with moderate

malnutrition. J Appl Physiol 1998;85:189-197.
47. Mitch WE, Goldberg AL: Mechanisms of muscle wasting: The role of the ubiquitin-proteasome pathway. N Engl J Med 1996;335:1897-1905.
48. Lewis MI: Apoptosis as a potential mechanism of muscle cachexia in chronic obstructive pulmonary disease. Am J Respir Crit Care Med 2002;166:434-436.
49. Tawa NE Jr, Odessey R, Goldberg AL: Inhibitors of the proteasome reduce the accelerated proteolysis in atrophying rat skeletal muscles. J Clin Invest 1997;100:197-203.
50. Lewis MI, Monn SA, Zhan WZ, et al: Interactive effects of emphysema and malnutrition on diaphragm structure and function. J Appl Physiol 1994;77:947-955.
51. Winick M: Preface. In Winick M (ed): Hunger Disease: Studies by the Jewish Physicians in the Warsaw Ghetto. New York, John Wiley & Sons, 1979, p ii.
52. Fliederbaum J: Clinical aspects of hunger disease in adults. In Winick M (ed): Hunger Disease: Studies by the Jewish Physicians in the Warsaw Ghetto. New York, John Wiley & Sons, 1979, pp 11-36.
53. Bossu C, Galusca B, Normand S, et al: Energy expenditure adjusted for body composition differentiates constitutional thinness from both normal subjects and anorexia nervosa. Am J Physiol Endocrinol Metab 2007;292:E132-E137.
54. Schols AM, Soeters PB, Mostert R, et al: Physiologic effects of nutritional support and anabolic steroids in patients with chronic obstructive pulmonary disease: A placebo-controlled randomized trial. Am J Respir Crit Care Med 1995;152:1268-1274.
55. Ryan CF, Whittaker JS, Road JD: Ventilatory dysfunction in severe anorexia nervosa. Chest 1992;102:1286-1288.
56. Lanz JK Jr, Donahoe M, Rogers RM, et al: Effects of growth hormone on diaphragmatic recovery from malnutrition. J Appl Physiol 1992;73:801-805.
57. Martinez FJ, Bermudez-Gomez M, Celli BR: Hypothyroidism: A reversible cause of diaphragmatic dysfunction. Chest 1989;96:1059-1063.
58. Norrelund H, Hove KY, Brems-Dalgaard E, et al: Muscle mass and function in thyrotoxic patients before and during medical treatment. Clin Endocrinol (Oxf) 1999;51:693-699.
59. Goswami R, Guleria R, Gupta AK, et al: Prevalence of diaphragmatic muscle weakness and dyspnoea in Graves' disease and their reversibility with carbimazole therapy. Eur J Endocrinol 2002;147:299-303.
60. Siafakas NM, Milona I, Salesiotou V, et al: Respiratory muscle strength in hyperthyroidism before and after treatment. Am Rev Respir Dis 1992;146:1025-1029.
61. Iandelli I, Gorini M, Duranti R, et al: Respiratory muscle function and control of breathing in patients with acromegaly. Eur Respir J 1997;10:977-982.
62. Mills GH, Kyroussis D, Jenkins P, et al: Respiratory muscle strength in Cushing's syndrome. Am J Respir Crit Care Med 1999;160:1762-1765.
63. Powers SK, Shanely RA, Coombes JS, et al: Mechanical ventilation results in progressive contractile dysfunction in the diaphragm. J Appl Physiol 2002;92:1851-1858.
64. Yang L, Luo J, Bourdon J, et al: Controlled mechanical ventilation leads to remodeling of the rat diaphragm. Am J Respir Crit Care Med 2002;166:1135-1140.
65. Sassoon CS, Ciaozzo VJ, Manka A, et al: Altered diaphragm contractile properties with controlled mechanical ventilation. J Appl Physiol 2002;92:2585-2595.
66. Sassoon CS, Zhu E, Caiozzo VJ: Assist-control mechanical ventilation attenuates ventilator-induced diaphragmatic dysfunction. Am J Respir Crit Care Med 2004;170:626-632.
67. Radell PJ, Remahl S, Nichols DG, et al: Effects of prolonged mechanical ventilation and inactivity on piglet diaphragm function. Intensive Care Med 2002;28:358-364.
68. Anzueto A, Peters JI, Tobin MJ, et al: Effects of prolonged controlled mechanical ventilation on diaphragmatic function in healthy adult baboons. Crit Care Med 1997;25:1187-1190.
69. Le Bourdelles G, Viires N, Boczkowski J, et al: Effects of mechanical ventilation on diaphragmatic contractile properties in rats. Am J Respir Crit Care Med 1994;149:1539-1544.
70. Radell P, Edstrom L, Stibler H, et al: Changes in diaphragm structure following prolonged mechanical ventilation in piglets. Acta Anaesthesiol Scand 2004;48:430-437.
71. Capdevila X, Lopez S, Bernard N, et al: Effects of controlled mechanical ventilation on respiratory muscle contractile properties in rabbits. Intensive Care Med 2003;29:103-110.
72. Hussain SN, Vassilakopoulos T: Ventilator-induced cachexia. Am J Respir Crit Care Med 2002;166:1307-1308.
73. Shanely RA, Coombes JS, Zergeroglu AM, et al: Short-duration mechanical ventilation enhances diaphragmatic fatigue resistance but impairs force production. Chest 2003;123:195-201.
74. Shanely RA, Zergeroglu MA, Lennon SL, et al: Mechanical ventilation-induced diaphragmatic atrophy is associated with oxidative injury and increased proteolytic activity. Am J Respir Crit Care Med 2002;166:1369-1374.
75. Zergeroglu MA, McKenzie MJ, Shanely RA, et al: Mechanical ventilation-induced oxidative stress in the diaphragm. J Appl Physiol 2003;95:1116-1124.
76. Radell P, Edstrom L, Stibler H, et al: Changes in diaphragm structure following prolonged mechanical ventilation in piglets. Acta Anaesthesiol Scand 2004;48:430-437.
77. Nguyen T, Friscia M, Kaiser LR, et al: Ventilator-induced proteolysis in human diaphragm myofibers [abstract]. Proc Am Thorac Soc 2006;3:A259.
78. Capdevila X, Lopez S, Bernard N, et al: Effects of controlled mechanical ventilation on respiratory muscle contractile properties in rabbits. Intensive Care Med 2003;29:103-110.
79. Bodine SC, Latres E, Baumhueter S, et al: Identification of ubiquitin ligases required for skeletal muscle atrophy. Science 2001;294:1704-1708.
80. DeRuisseau KC, Shanely RA, Akunuri N, et al: Diaphragm unloading via controlled mechanical ventilation alters the gene expression profile. Am J Respir Crit Care Med 2005;172:1267-1275.
81. DeRuisseau KC, Kavazis AN, Deering MA, et al: Mechanical ventilation induces alterations of the ubiquitin-proteasome pathway in the diaphragm. J Appl Physiol 2005;98:1314-1321.
82. Nathens AB, Neff MJ, Jurkovich GJ, et al: Randomized, prospective trial of antioxidant supplementation in critically ill surgical patients. Ann Surg 2002;236:814-822.
83. Sassoon CS: Ventilator-associated diaphragmatic dysfunction. Am J Respir Crit Care Med 2002;166:1017-1018.
84. Goldspink DF, Morton AJ, Loughna P, et al: The effect of hypokinesia and hypodynamia on protein turnover and the growth of four skeletal muscles of the rat. Pfluger's Arch 1986;407:333-340.
85. Goldspink DF, Morton AJ, Loughna P, et al: The effect of hypokinesia and hypodynamia on protein turnover and the growth of four skeletal muscles of the rat. Pfluger's Arch 1986;407:333-340.
86. Knisely AS, Leal SM, Singer DB: Abnormalities of diaphragmatic muscle in neonates with ventilated lungs. J Pediatr 1988;113:1074-1077.
87. Levine S, Nguyen T, Friscia M, et al: Ventilator-induced atrophy in human diaphragm myofibers [abstract]. Proc Am Thorac Soc 2006;3:A27.
88. Shanely RA, Van Gammeren D, DeRuisseau KC, et al: Mechanical ventilation depresses protein synthesis in the rat diaphragm. Am J Respir Crit Care Med 2004;170:994-999.
89. Pichard C, Kyle U, Chevrolet JC, et al: Lack of effects of recombinant growth hormone on muscle function in patients requiring prolonged mechanical ventilation: A prospective, randomized, controlled study. Crit Care Med 1996;24:403-413.
90. Takala J, Ruokonen E, Webster NR, et al: Increased mortality associated with growth hormone treatment in critically ill adults. N Engl J Med 1999;341:785-792.
91. Hussain SN: Respiratory muscle dysfunction in sepsis. Mol Cell Biochem 1998;179:125-134.
92. Leon A, Boczkowski J, Dureuil B, et al: Effects of endotoxic shock on diaphragmatic function in mechanically ventilated rats. J Appl Physiol 1992;72:1466-1472.
93. Lin MC, Ebihara S, El Dwairi Q, et al: Diaphragm sarcolemmal injury is induced by sepsis and alleviated by nitric oxide synthase inhibition. Am J

Respir Crit Care Med 1998;158: 1656-1663.
94. Aarli JA, Skeie GO, Mygland A, et al: Muscle striation antibodies in myasthenia gravis. Diagnostic and functional significance. Ann N Y Acad Sci 1998;841:505-515.
95. Callahan LA, Nethery D, Stofan D, et al: Free radical-induced contractile protein dysfunction in endotoxin-induced sepsis. Am J Respir Cell Mol Biol 2001;24:210-217.
96. Boczkowski J, Lisdero CL, Lanone S, et al: Endogenous peroxynitrite mediates mitochondrial dysfunction in rat diaphragm during endotoxemia. FASEB J 1999;13:1637-1646.
97. El Dwairi Q, Comtois A, Guo Y, et al: Endotoxin-induced skeletal muscle contractile dysfunction: Contribution of nitric oxide synthases. Am J Physiol 1998;274:C770-C779.
98. Supinski G, Nethery D, DiMarco A: Effect of free radical scavengers on endotoxin-induced respiratory muscle dysfunction. Am Rev Respir Dis 1993;148:1318-1324.
99. Taille C, Foresti R, Lanone S, et al: Protective role of heme oxygenases against endotoxin-induced diaphragmatic dysfunction in rats. Am J Respir Crit Care Med 2001;163:753-761.
100. Javesghani D, Magder SA, Barreiro E, et al: Molecular characterization of a superoxide-generating NAD(P)H oxidase in the ventilatory muscles. Am J Respir Crit Care Med 2002;165:412-418.
101. Fujimura N, Sumita S, Aimono M, et al: Effect of free radical scavengers on diaphragmatic contractility in septic peritonitis. Am J Respir Crit Care Med 2000;162:2159-2165.
102. Tiao G, Fagan J, Roegner V, et al: Energy-ubiquitin-dependent muscle proteolysis during sepsis in rats is regulated by glucocorticoids. J Clin Invest 1996;97:339-348.
103. Laghi F: Curing the septic diaphragm with the ventilator. Am J Respir Crit Care Med 2002;165:145-146.
104. Tsukagoshi H, Morita T, Takahashi K, et al: Cecal ligation and puncture peritonitis model shows decreased nicotinic acetylcholine receptor numbers in rat muscle: Immunopathologic mechanisms? Anesthesiology 1999;91:448-460.
105. Boczkowski J, Lanone S, Ungureanu-Longrois D, et al: Induction of diaphragmatic nitric oxide synthase after endotoxin administration in rats: Role on diaphragmatic contractile dysfunction. J Clin Invest 1996;98:1550-1559.
106. Comtois AS, Barreiro E, Huang PL, et al: Lipopolysaccharide-induced diaphragmatic contractile dysfunction and sarcolemmal injury in mice lacking the neuronal nitric oxide synthase. Am J Respir Crit Care Med 2001;163:977-982.
107. Ebihara S, Hussain SN, Danialou G, et al: Mechanical ventilation protects against diaphragm injury in sepsis: Interaction of oxidative and mechanical stresses. Am J Respir Crit Care Med 2002;165:221-228.
108. Lanone S, Mebazaa A, Heymes C, et al: Muscular contractile failure in septic patients: Role of the inducible nitric oxide synthase pathway. Am J Respir Crit Care Med 2000;162:2308-2315.
109. Comtois AS, El Dwairi Q, Laubach VE, et al: Lipopolysaccharide-induced diaphragmatic contractile dysfunction in mice lacking the inducible nitric oxide synthase. Am J Respir Crit Care Med 1999;159:1975-1980.
110. Afulukwe IF, Cohen RI, Zeballos GA, et al: Selective NOS inhibition restores myocardial contractility in endotoxemic rats; however, myocardial NO content does not correlate with myocardial dysfunction. Am J Respir Crit Care Med 2000;162:21-26.
111. Wink DA, Mitchell JB: Chemical biology of nitric oxide: Insights into regulatory, cytotoxic, and cytoprotective mechanisms of nitric oxide. Free Radic Biol Med 1998;25:434-456.
112. Bolton CF, Laverty DA, Brown JD, et al: Critically ill polyneuropathy: Electrophysiological studies and differentiation from Guillain-Barré syndrome. J Neurol Neurosurg Psychiatry 1986;49:563-573.
113. Faragher MW, Day BJ: A practical approach to weakness in the intensive care unit. In Cros D (ed): Peripheral Neuropathy: A Practical Approach to Diagnosis And Management. Philadelphia, Lippincott Williams & Wilkins, 2001, pp 370-386.
114. Druschky A, Herkert M, Radespiel-Troger M, et al: Critical illness polyneuropathy: Clinical findings and cell culture assay of neurotoxicity assessed by a prospective study. Intensive Care Med 2001;27:686-693.
115. Hund EF, Fogel W, Krieger D, et al: Critical illness polyneuropathy: Clinical findings and outcomes of a frequent cause of neuromuscular weaning failure. Crit Care Med 1996;24:1328-1333.
116. Latronico N, Fenzi F, Recupero D, et al: Critical illness myopathy and neuropathy. Lancet 1996;347:1579-1582.
117. Van den Berghe G, Wouters P, Weekers F, et al: Intensive insulin therapy in the critically ill patients. N Engl J Med 2001;345:1359-1367.
118. Rouleau G, Karpati G, Carpenter S, et al: Glucocorticoid excess induces preferential depletion of myosin in denervated skeletal muscle fibers. Muscle Nerve 1987;10:428-438.
119. Larsson L, Li X, Edstrom L, et al: Acute quadriplegia and loss of muscle myosin in patients treated with nondepolarizing neuromuscular blocking agents and corticosteroids: Mechanisms at the cellular and molecular levels. Crit Care Med 2000;28:34-45.
120. Rich MM, Teener JW, Raps EC, et al: Muscle is electrically inexcitable in acute quadriplegic myopathy. Neurology 1996;46:731-736.
121. Rich MM, Bird SJ, Raps EC, et al: Direct muscle stimulation in acute quadriplegic myopathy. Muscle Nerve 1997;20:665-673.
122. Lefaucheur JP, Nordine T, Rodriguez P, et al: Origin of ICU acquired paresis determined by direct muscle stimulation. J Neurol Neurosurg Psychiatry 2006;77:500-506.
123. De Jonghe B, Sharshar T, Lefaucheur JP, et al: Paresis acquired in the intensive care unit: A prospective multicenter study. JAMA 2002;288:2859-2867.
124. Faragher MW, Day BJ, Dennett X: Critical care myopathy: An electrophysiological and histological study. Muscle Nerve 1996;19:516-518.
125. De Jonghe B, Bastuji-Garin S, Sharshar T, et al: Does ICU-acquired paresis lengthen weaning from mechanical ventilation? Intensive Care Med 2004;30:1117-1121.
126. Latronico N, Shehu I, Seghelini E: Neuromuscular sequelae of critical illness. Curr Opin Crit Care 2005;11:381-390.
127. Leatherman JW, Fluegel WL, David WS, et al: Muscle weakness in mechanically ventilated patients with severe asthma. Am J Respir Crit Care Med 1996;153:1686-1690.
128. Roberts PA, Loxham SJ, Poucher SM, et al: Bicarbonate-induced alkalosis augments cellular acetyl group availability and isometric force during the rest-to-work transition in canine skeletal muscle. Exp Physiol 2002;87:489-498.
129. Schnader JY, Juan G, Howell S, et al: Arterial CO_2 partial pressure affects diaphragmatic function. J Appl Physiol 1985;58:823-829.
130. Juan G, Calverley P, Talamo C, et al: Effect of carbon dioxide on diaphragmatic function in human beings. N Engl J Med 1984;310:874-879.
131. Jackson DC, Arendt EA, Inman KC, et al: 31P-NMR study of normoxic and anoxic perfused turtle heart during graded CO2 and lactic acidosis. Am J Physiol 1991;260:R1130-R1136.
132. Yanos J, Wood LD, Davis K, et al: The effect of respiratory and lactic acidosis on diaphragm function. Am Rev Respir Dis 1993;147:616-619.
133. Cairns SP: Lactic acid and exercise performance: Culprit or friend? Sports Med 2006;36:279-291.
134. Keeton RB, Binder-Macleod SA: Low-frequency fatigue. Phys Ther 2006;86:1146-1150.
135. Gladden LB: Lactate metabolism: A new paradigm for the third millennium. J Physiol 2004;558:5-30.
136. Vogiatzis I, Georgiadou O, Giannopoulou I, et al: Effects of exercise-induced arterial hypoxaemia and work rate on diaphragmatic fatigue in highly trained endurance athletes. J Physiol 2006;572:539-549.
137. Coast JR, Shanely RA, Lawler JM, et al: Lactic acidosis and diaphragmatic function in vitro. Am J Respir Crit Care Med 1995;152:1648-1652.
138. Knuth ST, Dave H, Peters JR, et al: Low cell pH depresses peak power in rat skeletal muscle fibres at both 30 degrees C and 15 degrees C: Implications for muscle fatigue. J Physiol 2006;575:887-899.
139. Kristensen M, Albertsen J, Rentsch M, et al: Lactate and force production in skeletal muscle. J Physiol 2005;562:521-526.
140. Posterino GS, Dutka TL, Lamb GD: L(+)-lactate does not affect twitch and

tetanic responses in mechanically skinned mammalian muscle fibres. Pfluger's Arch 2001;442:197-203.
141. Degroot M, Massie BM, Boska M, et al: Dissociation of [H+] from fatigue in human muscle detected by high time resolution 31P-NMR. Muscle Nerve 1993;16:91-98.
142. Westerblad H, Allen DG, Lannergren J: Muscle fatigue: Lactic acid or inorganic phosphate the major cause? News Physiol Sci 2002;17:17-21.
143. Nielsen OB, de Paoli F, Overgaard K: Protective effects of lactic acid on force production in rat skeletal muscle. J Physiol 2001;536:161-166.
144. Mador MJ, Wendel T, Kufel TJ: Effect of acute hypercapnia on diaphragmatic and limb muscle contractility. Am J Respir Crit Care Med 1997;155:1590-1595.
145. Schnader J, Howell S, Fitzgerald RS, et al: Interaction of fatigue and hypercapnia in the canine diaphragm. J Appl Physiol 1988;64:1636-1643.
146. Rafferty GF, Lou HM, Polkey MI, et al: Effect of hypercapnia on maximal voluntary ventilation and diaphragm fatigue in normal humans. Am J Respir Crit Care Med 1999;160:1567-1571.
147. Topeli A, Laghi F, Tobin MJ: The voluntary drive to breathe is not decreased in hypercapnic patients with severe COPD. Eur Respir J 2001;18:53-60.
148. Begin P, Grassino A: Inspiratory muscle dysfunction and chronic hypercapnia in chronic obstructive pulmonary disease. Am Rev Respir Dis 1991;143:905-912.
149. Braun NMT, Rochester DF: Respiratory muscle function in chronic obstructive pulmonary disease (COPD) [abstract]. Am Rev Respir Dis 1977;115:A91.
150. Vianna LG, Koulouris N, Moxham J: Lack of effect of acute hypoxia and hypercapnia on muscle relaxation rate in man. Rev Esp Fisiol 1993;49:7-15.
151. Ranatunga KW: Effects of acidosis on tension development in mammalian skeletal muscle. Muscle Nerve 1987;10:439-445.
152. Aubier M, Murciano D, Lecocguic Y, et al: Effect of hypophosphatemia on diaphragmatic contractility in patients with acute respiratory failure. N Engl J Med 1985;313:420-424.
153. Aubier M, Viires N, Piquet J, et al: Effects of hypocalcemia on diaphragmatic strength generation. J Appl Physiol 1985;58:2054-2061.
154. Dhingra S, Solven F, Wilson A, et al: Hypomagnesemia and respiratory muscle power. Am Rev Respir Dis 1984;129:497-498.
155. Stedwell RE, Allen KM, Binder LS: Hypokalemic paralyses: A review of the etiologies, pathophysiology, presentation, and therapy. Am J Emerg Med 1992;10:143-148.
156. Aubier M, Trippenbach T, Roussos C: Respiratory muscle fatigue during cardiogenic shock. J Appl Physiol 1981;51:499-508.
157. Hussain SN, Simkus G, Roussos C: Respiratory muscle fatigue: A cause of ventilatory failure in septic shock. J Appl Physiol 1985;58:2033-2040.
158. Ronco JJ, Fenwick JC, Tweeddale MG, et al: Identification of the critical oxygen delivery for anaerobic metabolism in critically ill septic and nonseptic humans. JAMA 1993;270:1724-1730.
159. Kontoyannis DA, Nanas JN, Kontoyannis SA, et al: Mechanical ventilation in conjunction with the intra-aortic balloon pump improves the outcome of patients in profound cardiogenic shock. Intensive Care Med 1999;25:835-838.
160. Viires N, Sillye G, Aubier M, et al: Regional blood flow distribution in dog during induced hypotension and low cardiac output: Spontaneous breathing versus artificial ventilation. J Clin Invest 1983;72:935-947.
161. Jubran A, Mathru M, Dries D, et al: Continuous recordings of mixed venous oxygen saturation during weaning from mechanical ventilation and the ramifications thereof. Am J Respir Crit Care Med 1998;158:1763-1769.
162. Weber KT, Kinasewitz GT, Janicki JS, et al: Oxygen utilization and ventilation during exercise in patients with chronic cardiac failure. Circulation 1982;65:1213-1223.
163. Reid MB, Johnson RL Jr: Efficiency, maximal blood flow, and aerobic work capacity of canine diaphragm. J Appl Physiol 1983;54:763-772.
164. Robertson CH Jr, Foster GH, Johnson RL Jr: The relationship of respiratory failure to the oxygen consumption of, lactate production by, and distribution of blood flow among respiratory muscles during increasing inspiratory resistance. J Clin Invest 1977;59:31-42.
165. Rochester DF, Bettini G: Diaphragmatic blood flow and energy expenditure in the dog: Effects of inspiratory airflow resistance and hypercapnia. J Clin Invest 1976;57:661-672.
166. Rochester DF, Briscoe AM: Metabolism of the working diaphragm. Am Rev Respir Dis 1979;119:101-106.
167. Bark H, Supinski G, Bundy R, et al: Effect of hypoxia on diaphragm blood flow, oxygen uptake, and contractility. Am Rev Respir Dis 1988;138:1535-1541.
168. Richard C, Teboul JL: Weaning failure from cardiovascular origin. Intensive Care Med 2005;31:1605-1607.
169. Rodriguez JA, Crespo-Leiro MG, Paniagua MJ, et al: Rhabdomyolysis in heart transplant patients on HMG-CoA reductase inhibitors and cyclosporine. Transplant Proc 1999;31:2522-2523.
170. Masters BA, Palmoski MJ, Flint OP, et al: In vitro myotoxicity of the 3-hydroxy-3-methylglutaryl coenzyme A reductase inhibitors, pravastatin, lovastatin, and simvastatin, using neonatal rat skeletal myocytes. Toxicol Appl Pharmacol 1995;131:163-174.
171. Sugiyama S: HMG CoA reductase inhibitor accelerates aging effect on diaphragm mitochondrial respiratory function in rats. Biochem Mol Biol Int 1998;46:923-931.
172. Cote HC, Brumme ZL, Craib KJ, et al: Changes in mitochondrial DNA as a marker of nucleoside toxicity in HIV-infected patients. N Engl J Med 2002;346:811-820.
173. Hasfurther DL, Bailey PL: Failure of neuromuscular blockade reversal after rocuronium in a patient who received oral neomycin. Can J Anaesth 1996;43:617-620.
174. Segredo V, Caldwell JE, Matthay MA, et al: Persistent paralysis in critically ill patients after long-term administration of vecuronium. N Engl J Med 1992;327:524-528.
175. de Lemos JM, Carr RR, Shalansky KF, et al: Paralysis in the critically ill: Intermittent bolus pancuronium compared with continuous infusion. Crit Care Med 1999;27:2648-2655.
176. Rudis MI, Sikora CA, Angus E, et al: A prospective, randomized, controlled evaluation of peripheral nerve stimulation versus standard clinical dosing of neuromuscular blocking agents in critically ill patients. Crit Care Med 1997;25:575-583.
177. de Seze M, Petit H, Wiart L, et al: Critical illness polyneuropathy: A 2-year follow-up study in 19 severe cases. Eur Neurol 2000;43:61-69.
178. Hirano M, Ott BR, Raps EC, et al: Acute quadriplegic myopathy: A complication of treatment with steroids, nondepolarizing blocking agents, or both. Neurology 1992;42:2082-2087.
179. Laghi F, Topeli A, Tobin MJ: Does resistive loading decrease diaphragmatic contractility before task failure? J Appl Physiol 1998;85:1103-1112.
180. Laghi F, D'Alfonso N, Tobin MJ: Pattern of recovery from diaphragmatic fatigue over 24 hours. J Appl Physiol 1995;79:539-546.
181. Mador JM, Rodis A, Diaz J: Diaphragmatic fatigue following voluntary hyperpnea. Am J Respir Crit Care Med 1996;154:63-67.
182. Travaline JM, Sudarshan S, Roy BG, et al: Effect of *N*-acetylcysteine on human diaphragm strength and fatigability. Am J Respir Crit Care Med 1997;156:1567-1571.
183. McKenzie DK, Bigland-Ritchie B, Gorman RB, et al: Central and peripheral fatigue of human diaphragm and limb muscles assessed by twitch interpolation. J Physiol 1992;454:643-656.
184. Moxham J, Morris AJ, Spiro SG, et al: Contractile properties and fatigue of the diaphragm in man. Thorax 1981;36:164-168.
185. Bellemare F, Bigland-Ritchie B: Central components of diaphragmatic fatigue assessed by phrenic nerve stimulation. J Appl Physiol 1987;62:1307-1316.
186. Similowski T, Straus C, Attali V, et al: Cervical magnetic stimulation as a method to discriminate between diaphragm and rib cage muscle fatigue. J Appl Physiol 1998;84:1692-1700.
187. Yan S, Lichros I, Zakynthinos S, et al: Effect of diaphragmatic fatigue on control of respiratory muscles and ventilation during CO_2 rebreathing. J Appl Physiol 1993;75:1364-1370.
188. Dahlstedt AJ, Katz A, Westerblad H: Role of myoplasmic phosphate in contractile function of skeletal muscle: Studies on creatine kinase-deficient mice. J Physiol 2001;533:379-388.
189. Dahlstedt AJ, Katz A, Wieringa B, et al: Is creatine kinase responsible for fatigue? Studies of isolated skeletal

muscle deficient in creatine kinase. FASEB J 2000;14:982-990.
190. Westerblad H, Lee JA, Lannergren J, et al: Cellular mechanisms of fatigue in skeletal muscle. Am J Physiol 1991;261:C195-C209.
191. Nichols DG, Buck JR, Eleff SM, et al: Diaphragmatic fatigue assessed by 31P-magnetic resonance spectroscopy in vivo. Am J Physiol 1993;264: C1111-C1118.
192. Radell PJ, Eleff SM, Nichols DG: Effects of loaded breathing and hypoxia on diaphragm metabolism as measured by ^{31}P-NMR spectroscopy. J Appl Physiol 2000;88:933-938.
193. Westerblad H, Bruton JD, Lannergren J: The effect of intracellular pH on contractile function of intact, single fibres of mouse muscle declines with increasing temperature. J Physiol 1997;500:193-204.
194. Zhu E, Comtois AS, Fang L, et al: Influence of tension time on muscle fiber sarcolemmal injury in rat diaphragm. J Appl Physiol 2000;88:135-141.
195. Jiang TX, Reid WD, Road JD: Delayed diaphragm injury and diaphragm force production. Am J Respir Crit Care Med 1998;157:736-742.
196. Armstrong RB: Initial events in exercise-induced muscular injury. Med Sci Sports Exerc 1990;22:429-435.
197. Armstrong RB, Ogilvie RW, Schwane JA: Eccentric exercise-induced injury to rat skeletal muscle. J Appl Physiol 1983;54:80-93.
198. Reid WD, Belcastro AN: Time course of diaphragm injury and calpain activity during resistive loading. Am J Respir Crit Care Med 2000;162:1801-1806.
199. Podhorska-Okolow M, Sandri M, Zampieri S, et al: Apoptosis of myofibres and satellite cells: Exercise-induced damage in skeletal muscle of the mouse. Neuropathol Appl Neurobiol 1998;24:518-531.
200. Orozco-Levi M, Lloreta J, Minguella J, et al: Injury of the human diaphragm associated with exertion and chronic obstructive pulmonary disease. Am J Respir Crit Care Med 2001;164:1734-1739.
201. Reid WD, Huang J, Bryson S, et al: Diaphragm injury and myofibrillar structure induced by resistive loading. J Appl Physiol 1994;76:176-184.
202. Martin J, Powell E, Shore S, et al: The role of respiratory muscles in the hyperinflation of bronchial asthma. Am Rev Respir Dis 1980;121:441-447.
203. Wilcox PG, Wakai Y, Walley KR, et al: Tumor necrosis factor alpha decreases in vivo diaphragm contractility in dogs. Am J Respir Crit Care Med 1994;150:1368-1373.
204. Sampson MG, Grassino AE: Load compensation in obese patients during quiet tidal breathing. J Appl Physiol 1983;55:1269-1276.
205. Wakai Y, Leevers AM, Road JD: Regional diaphragm shortening measured by sonomicrometry. J Appl Physiol 1994;77:2791-2796.
206. Vassilakopoulos T, Katsaounou P, Karatza MH, et al: Strenuous resistive breathing induces plasma cytokines: Role of antioxidants and monocytes. Am J Respir Crit Care Med 2002;166:1572-1578.
207. Reid MB, Stokic DS, Koch SM, et al: *N*-Acetylcysteine inhibits muscle fatigue in humans. J Clin Invest 1994;94:2468-2474.
208. Supinski G, Nethery D, Stofan D, et al: Effect of free radical scavengers on diaphragmatic fatigue. Am J Respir Crit Care Med 1997;155:622-629.
209. Stofan DA, Callahan LA, DiMarco AF, et al: Modulation of release of reactive oxygen species by the contracting diaphragm. Am J Respir Crit Care Med 2000;161:891-898.
210. Reid MB: Invited Review: Redox modulation of skeletal muscle contraction: What we know and what we don't. J Appl Physiol 2001;90:724-731.
211. Aubier M, Viires N: Calcium ATPase and respiratory muscle function. Eur Respir J 1998;11:758-766.
212. Bers DM: Cardiac excitation-contraction coupling. Nature 2002;415:198-205.
213. Reid MB: Redox modulation of skeletal muscle contraction by reactive oxygen and nitric oxide. In Hargreaves M (ed): Biochemistry of Exercise X. Champaign, Ill, Human Kinetics, 1999, pp 155-166.
214. Essig DA, Borger DR, Jackson DA: Induction of heme oxygenase-1 (HSP32) mRNA in skeletal muscle following contractions. Am J Physiol 1997;272:C59-C67.
215. Jiang TX, Reid WD, Road JD: Free radical scavengers and diaphragm injury following inspiratory resistive loading. Am J Respir Crit Care Med 2001;164:1288-1294.
216. Zhu E, Petrof BJ, Gea J, et al: Diaphragm muscle fiber injury after inspiratory resistive breathing. Am J Respir Crit Care Med 1997;155: 1110-1116.
217. Macgowan NA, Evans KG, Road JD, et al: Diaphragm injury in individuals with airflow obstruction. Am J Respir Crit Care Med 2001;163:1654-1659.
218. Adams GR, Haddad F, Baldwin KM: Time course of changes in markers of myogenesis in overloaded rat skeletal muscles. J Appl Physiol 1999;87:1705-1712.
219. Corfield DR, Roberts CA, Guz A, et al: Modulation of the corticospinal control of ventilation by changes in reflex respiratory drive. J Appl Physiol 1999;87:1923-1930.
220. Robertson TA, Papadimitriou JM, Grounds MD: Fusion of myogenic cells to the newly sealed region of damaged myofibres in skeletal muscle regeneration. Neuropathol Appl Neurobiol 1993;19:350-358.
221. Silver MM, Smith CR: Diaphragmatic contraction band necrosis in a perinatal and infantile autopsy population. Hum Pathol 1992;23:817-827.
222. Douglass JA, Tuxen DV, Horne M, et al: Myopathy in severe asthma. Am Rev Respir Dis 1992;146:517-519.
223. Deshmukh S, Rao R, Harke A: Clinicopathological correlation of diaphragmatic contraction band necrosis in a neonatal and infantile population—an autopsy study. Indian J Pathol Microbiol 1999;42:345-353.
224. Efthimiou J, Fleming J, Spiro SG: Sternomastoid muscle function and fatigue in breathless patients with severe respiratory disease. Am Rev Respir Dis 1987;136:1099-1105.
225. Cohen CA, Zagelbaum G, Gross D, et al: Clinical manifestations of inspiratory muscle fatigue. Am J Med 1982;73:308-316.
226. Goldstone JC, Green M, Moxham J: Maximum relaxation rate of the diaphragm during weaning from mechanical ventilation. Thorax 1994;49:54-60.
227. Tobin MJ, Walsh JM, Laghi F: Monitoring of respiratory neuromuscular function. In Tobin MJ (ed): Principles and Practice of Mechanical Ventilation. New York:, McGraw-Hill, 1994, pp 945-966.
228. Bellemare F, Grassino A: Effect of pressure and timing of contraction on human diaphragm fatigue. J Appl Physiol 1982;53:1190-1195.
229. Radell PJ, Eleff SM, Traystman RJ, et al: In vivo diaphragm metabolism: Comparison of paced and inspiratory resistive loaded breathing in piglets. Crit Care Med 1997;25:339-345.
230. Sassoon CS, Gruer SE, Sieck GC: Temporal relationships of ventilatory failure, pump failure, and diaphragm fatigue. J Appl Physiol 1996;81:238-245.
231. Adams JM, Farkas GA, Rochester DF: Vagal afferents, diaphragm fatigue, and inspiratory resistance in anesthetized dogs. J Appl Physiol 1988;64:2279-2286.
232. Straus C, Zelter M, Derenne JP, et al: Putative projection of phrenic afferents to the limbic cortex in humans studied with cerebral evoked potentials. J Appl Physiol 1997;82:480-490.
233. Hill JM: Increase in the discharge of muscle spindles during diaphragm fatigue. Brain Res 2001;918:166-170.
234. Speck DF, Revelette WR: Attenuation of phrenic motor discharge by phrenic nerve afferents. J Appl Physiol 1987;62:941-945.
235. Marsden CD, Meadows JC, Merton PA: Isolated single motor units in human muscle and their rate of discharge during maximal voluntary effort. J Physiol 1971;217:12P-13P.
236. Attali V, Mehiri S, Straus C, et al: Influence of neck muscles on mouth pressure response to cervical magnetic stimulation. Am J Respir Crit Care Med 1997;156:509-514.
237. Peiffer C, Poline JB, Thivard L, et al: Neural substrates for the perception of acutely induced dyspnea. Am J Respir Crit Care Med 2001;163:951-957.
238. Macefield G, Hagbarth KE, Gorman R, et al: Decline in spindle support to alpha-motoneurons during sustained voluntary contractions. J Physiol 1991;440:497-512.
239. Zifko UA, Young BG, Remtulla H, et al: Somatosensory evoked potentials of the phrenic nerve. Muscle Nerve 1995;18:1487-1489.
240. Corfield DR, Fink GR, Ramsay SC, et al: Evidence for limbic system activation during CO_2 breathing in man. J Physiol 1995;488:77-84.
241. Bernard JF, Huang GF, Besson JM: The parabrachial area: Electrophysiological evidence for an involvement in visceral nociceptive processes. J Neurophysiol 1994;71:1646-1660.

242. Gozal D, Hathout GM, Kirlew KA, et al: Localization of putative neural respiratory regions in the human by functional magnetic resonance imaging. J Appl Physiol 1994;76:2076-2083.
243. Appendini L, Purro A, Patessio A, et al: Partitioning of inspiratory muscle workload and pressure assistance in ventilator-dependent COPD patients. Am J Respir Crit Care Med 1996;154:1301-1309.
244. Simpson JA, van Eyk JE, Iscoe S: Hypoxemia-induced modification of troponin I and T in canine diaphragm. J Appl Physiol 2000;88:753-760.
245. Nava S, Bellemare F: Cardiovascular failure and apnea in shock. J Appl Physiol 1989;66:184-189.
246. Maldonado A, Bauer TT, Ferrer M, et al: Capnometric recirculation gas tonometry and weaning from mechanical ventilation. Am J Respir Crit Care Med 2000;161:171-176.
247. Zakynthinos SG, Vassilakopoulos T, Roussos C: The load of inspiratory muscles in patients needing mechanical ventilation. Am J Respir Crit Care Med 1995;152:1248-1255.
248. D'Angelo E, Calderini E, Robatto FM, et al: Lung and chest wall mechanics in patients with acquired immunodeficiency syndrome and severe *Pneumocystis carinii* pneumonia. Eur Respir J 1997;10:2343-2350.
249. Gattinoni L, Pelosi P, Suter PM, et al: Acute respiratory distress syndrome caused by pulmonary and extrapulmonary disease: Different syndromes? Am J Respir Crit Care Med 1998;158:3-11.
250. Parthasarathy S, Jubran A, Tobin MJ: Cycling of inspiratory and expiratory muscle groups with the ventilator in airflow limitation. Am J Respir Crit Care Med 1998;158:1471-1478.
251. Covelli HD, Black JW, Olsen MS, et al: Respiratory failure precipitated by high carbohydrate loads. Ann Intern Med 1981;95:579-581.
252. Kellog RH: Central chemical regulation of respiration. In Fenn WO, Rahn H (eds): Handbook of Physiology. Washington, DC, American Physiological Society, 1964, p 513.
253. Efthimiou J, Mounsey PJ, Benson DN, et al: Effect of carbohydrate rich versus fat rich loads on gas exchange and walking performance in patients with chronic obstructive lung disease. Thorax 1992;47:451-456.
254. Pitcher WD, Cunningham HS: Oxygen cost of increasing tidal volume and diaphragm flattening in obstructive pulmonary disease. J Appl Physiol 1993;74:2750-2756.
255. Nuckton TJ, Alonso JA, Kallet RH, et al: Pulmonary dead-space fraction as a risk factor for death in the acute respiratory distress syndrome. N Engl J Med 2002;346:1281-1286.
256. Costello R, Deegan P, Fitzpatrick M, et al: Reversible hypercapnia in chronic obstructive pulmonary disease: A distinct pattern of respiratory failure with a favorable prognosis. Am J Med 1997;102:239-244.
257. Moser KM, Luchsinger PC, Adamson JS, et al: Respiratory stimulation with intravenous doxapram in respiratory failure: A double-blind co-operative study. N Engl J Med 1973;288:427-431.
258. Sieck GC, Prakash YS: Cross-bridge kinetics in respiratory muscles. Eur Respir J 1997;10:2147-2158.

Chapter 42

Nonpulmonary Causes of Respiratory Failure

Ramya Lotano

An estimated 20% of respiratory failure is a result of nonpulmonary causes such as disorders that affect the upper airway, chest wall, muscles of respiration, and nervous system. Hypoventilation is the primary pathophysiological etiology of all of these disorders.[1]

HYPOVENTILATION

Pathophysiology (Fig. 42-1)

Hypoventilation is defined as alveolar ventilation that is inappropriately low for metabolic demands. Alveolar (A) and arterial (a) $Pa{CO_2}$ are elevated. Arterial pressure is decreased. Alveolar hypoventilation exists when arterial $P{CO_2}$ increases above the normal range of 37 to 43 mm Hg.[2-7]

Hypoventilation is associated with arterial hypoxemia (when breathing room air oxygen) and a raised arterial $P{CO_2}$. The rise in $Pa{CO_2}$ as a result of hypoventilation can be calculated using the *alveolar ventilation equation*.[8] In a single-compartment lung model, alveolar $P{CO_2}$ and $P{O_2}$ are inversely related according to the alveolar air equation. An increase in alveolar $P{CO_2}$ is associated with an obligatory fall in alveolar $P{O_2}$. During hypercapnia, the alveolar minus arterial $P(A - a){O_2}$ difference predicted by this model (while breathing room air) is "normal." Regarding the combination of hypercapnia and a normal $P(A - a){O_2}$ difference as a requirement to diagnose nonpulmonary disorders associated with hypoventilation is common clinical practice. However, these disorders are also commonly complicated by microatelectasis, retention of secretions, and bronchopneumonia, which cause abnormal ventilation/perfusion inequality and increase the $P(A - a){O_2}$ difference. Conversely, the $P(A - a){O_2}$ difference has been shown to be an unreliable index of abnormal gas exchange in the presence of substantial hypercapnia. For these reasons, a normal $P(A - a){O_2}$ difference is not helpful in differentiating pulmonary from nonpulmonary causes of respiratory failure. The alveolar partial pressure of oxygen is calculated with the formula:

$$P_{A}{O_2} = P_{I}{O_2} - Pa{CO_2}\left(F_{I}{O_2} + \frac{1 - F_{I}{O_2}}{R}\right)$$

where $F_{I}{O_2}$ is the inspired oxygen fraction (0.21 in all calculations) in the dry gas, $P_{I}{O_2}$ is the inspired $P{O_2}$, and R is the respiratory exchange ratio (assumed to be 0.8). In other words, the flow of CO_2 molecules across the alveolar membrane per minute is divided by the flow of O_2 molecules across the membrane per minute. $Pa{CO_2}$ is the ideal alveolar carbon dioxide tension.

This important equation indicates that the level of $P{CO_2}$ in alveolar gas and in arterial blood is inversely related to the alveolar ventilation.

This is true only if a steady state of alveolar ventilation and carbon dioxide production rate exist. In clinical practice it is common to consider the combination of hypercapnia and a normal $P(A - a){O_2}$ difference as a requirement to diagnose nonpulmonary disorders associated with hypoventilation.[9] However, hypoventilation-induced atelectasis causing abnormal gas exchange will result in an increase in $P(A - a){O_2}$ difference.[10] In the presence of substantial hypercapnia, an abnormal alveolar-to-arterial oxygen difference may not rule out a nonpulmonary cause of hypoventilation.

MECHANISMS UNDERLYING CHRONIC ALVEOLAR HYPOVENTILATION (see Fig. 42-1)

Defects in the metabolic control system result in hypoventilation when abnormalities in blood gases and cerebral acid base status are not sensed or if sensed do not produce an appropriate change in motor output of the medullary respiratory neurons. Patients with such defects fail to breathe normally in response to metabolic respiratory stimuli, but because the behavioral control system,

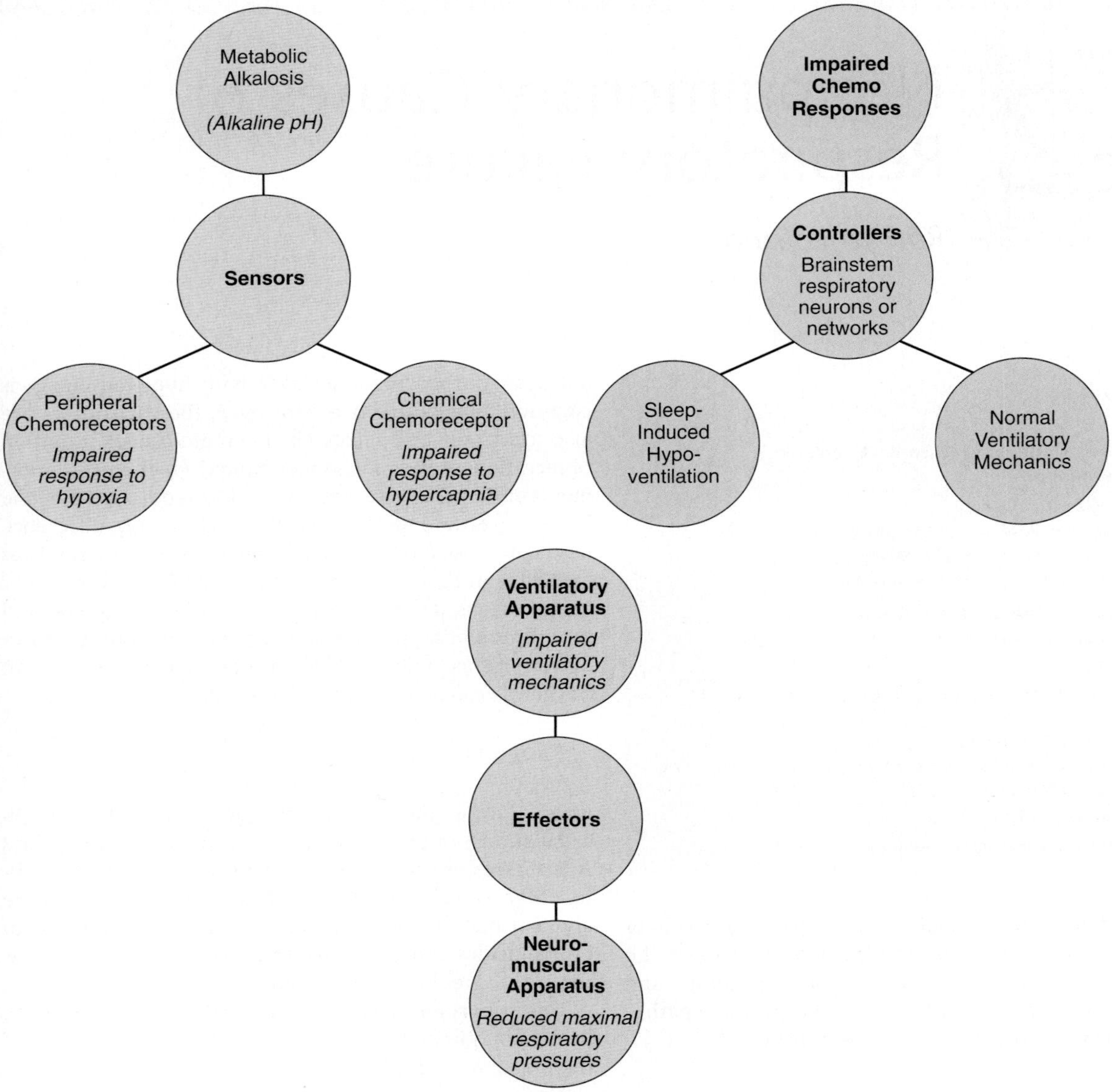

Figure 42-1. Mechanisms underlying chronic alveolar hypoventilation.

respiratory motor pathways, and ventilatory apparatus are intact, they are capable of voluntarily driving respiration. As a result, patients with defects in the metabolic control system typically demonstrate normal ventilatory mechanics, but they have impaired responses to metabolic respiratory stimuli and often hypoventilate severely during sleep, when ventilation is critically dependent on the metabolic control system.[1,3,11-17] As a result of chronic hypoventilation, these patients have a primary respiratory acidosis leading to a secondary increase in extracellular bicarbonate ion concentration.[18,19]

In contrast, patients with a primary metabolic alkalosis may develop secondary hypoventilation as a compensatory response. This type of hypoventilation represents not a defect in respiratory control but rather an appropriate response of the metabolic control system to a disturbance in acid-base status. It is said that patients with metabolic alkalosis "shouldn't" breathe, in contrast to those with control defects, who "won't" breathe, and those with mechanical defects, who "can't" breathe. However, the degree of hypoventilation that develops in response to metabolic alkalosis depends on several factors, including associated electrolyte disturbances and the sensitivity of the peripheral chemoreceptors to the accompanying hypoxemia.[19,20] Therefore patients with weak hypoxic responsiveness tend to hypoventilate more than do patients with brisk hypoxic responsiveness.

Chronic hypoventilation resulting from defects in effector elements of the respiratory system represents disturbances of ventilatory motor and mechanical function, and these defects do not in themselves mean that the metabolic control system is defective. Because the same effector elements also serve the behavioral control system, these patients are usually unable to breathe normally even when consciously attempting to do so. Hence such defects are characterized either by reductions in the maximum inspiratory pressures that can be generated voluntarily or by impairment of lung volumes and flow rates.[21] In the presence of such neural or mechanical defects, coexisting disturbances in respiratory control are often difficult to identify because the neuromuscular or mechanical defect may preclude normal responses to chemical respiratory stimuli even when the control system is intact.[1]

ETIOLOGIC CLASSIFICATION

Plum and Leigh[22,23] described nonrespiratory causes of respiratory failure. Causes of hypoventilation include depression of the respiratory center by drugs such as morphine derivatives and barbiturates; diseases of the brainstem such as encephalitis; abnormalities of the spinal cord conducting pathways such as high cervical dislocation; anterior horn cell diseases including poliomyelitis that affect the phoenix nerves or supplying intercostal muscles; diseases of nerves to respiratory muscles (e.g., Guillain-Barré syndrome); diseases of the myoneural junction such as myasthenia gravis; diseases of the respiratory muscles themselves such as progressive muscular dystrophy; thoracic cage abnormalities (e.g., crushed chest); upper airway obstruction (e.g., thymoma); hypoventilation associated with extreme obesity (Pickwickian syndrome); and other miscellaneous causes such as metabolic alkalosis and idiopathic states.[2] In all these conditions the lungs are normal.

Respiratory Failure from Neuromuscular Disease

Neuromuscular diseases are accompanied by variable degrees of involvement of the muscles of inspiration and expiration. The clinical manifestations reflect the compromise of both muscle groups.[24] Disorders of respiratory control and those of peripheral neuromuscular disease are shown in Tables 42-1 and 42-2, respectively.

Tests of Respiratory Muscle Strength

Respiratory muscle weakness is the hallmark of most neuromuscular disease. Simple tests measure maximal inspiratory and expiratory pressures (PI_{max} and PE_{max}). These tests are conducted by measuring airway pressures while requiring the patient to make maximal inspiratory and expiratory efforts against a closed airway at low or high volumes, respectively.[25] Respiratory muscle force is dependent on age, sex, and lung volume. PI_{max} and PE_{max} of greater than 60 to 80 cm H_2O excludes significant neuromuscular weakness. Abnormally low values are not diagnostic but indicate a need for further assessment.

The classic example of chronic alveolar hypoventilation secondary to brainstem disease is that seen in bulbar poliomyelitis or encephalitis. Secondary causes of alveolar hypoventilation are usually signified by features of the underlying disease.

Tests of Respiratory Control and Drive

If the tests of pulmonary function testing are unremarkable, indicating no parenchymal, neuromuscular, or chest wall disease accounting for the patient's hypercapnia or abnormal ventilation, tests of respiratory control are indicated.

These tests include measurement of hypoxic and hypercapnic ventilatory responses (because ventilatory response to hypoxia and hypercarbia can be potentially hazardous, O_2 saturation and end tidal CO_2 tension should be monitored); analysis of breathing pattern; mouth occlusive pressure (measurement of maximal pressure generated during the first 0.1 second of normal inspiratory effort when the airway is occluded); and elastic and resistive load testing (by breathing through progressively narrower tubes while sensation of dyspnea is measured by the Borg scale).

Electromyography permits more direct measurements of respiratory muscle strength. Respiratory muscle fatigue is indicated by paradoxical respirations or *respiratory alternans.* The mechanism consists of intermittent decreases or cessation of the contribution of the diaphragm to the inspiratory effort. It has been assumed that this pattern of muscle recruitment indicates diaphragmatic fatigue.[26]

CLINICAL RECOGNITION AND MANIFESTATIONS

Alveolar hypoventilation exists when arterial P_{CO_2} increases above the normal range. In clinically important hypercarbia, P_{CO_2} typically ranges from 50 to 70 mm Hg. Lethargy, confusion, and a depressed level of consciousness are seen as a result of hypercapnia. An increase in intracranial pressure and cerebral blood flow, as well as a decrease in myocardial contractility, occur.[2] The oxyhemoglobin dissociation curve shifts to the right, which leads to an increase in the release of oxygen to the tissues.

In the acute form, progressive weakness of respiratory muscles leads to rapid reduction in vital capacity followed by respiratory failure with hypoxemia and hypercarbia. Symptoms are those of acute respiratory failure including dyspnea, tachypnea, and tachycardia. In the chronic form, impairment of the respiratory muscles affects mechanical properties of the lungs and chest wall, decreases the ability to clear secretions, and eventually may alter the function of the central respiratory centers. Symptoms include orthopnea, fatigue, disturbed sleep, and hypersomnolence.[27]

Significant hypoxemia may coexist with chronic hypercapnia or occur with the onset of additional acute pulmonary disorders. Administration of supplemental oxygen is expected to worsen hypercapnia. Major processes that contribute are worsening of ventilation perfusion mismatching caused by an attenuation of hypoxic pulmonary vasoconstriction, decrease in the binding affinity of hemoglobin for CO_2 (Haldane effect), and a decrease in minute ventilation. Importantly, the clinician must be aware that it is imperative to provide supplemental oxygen to maintain adequate tissue oxygenation. This precaution will avoid potentially life-threatening consequences; however, in the spontaneously breathing patient, the lowest F_{IO_2} that produces acceptable oxygenation should be chosen. The major adverse effect seen in patients with

Table 42-1. Disorders of Ventilatory Control

Disorder	Associations	Mechanism
Metabolic alkalosis[54]	Maintenance of metabolic alkalosis for any length of time means that renal homeostatic mechanisms for HCO_3^- excretion have been disrupted.	Impaired autonomic control of ventilation. Voluntary control remains intact.
Ondine's curse[55,56] (congenital or acquired central alveolar hypoventilation)	Usually caused by congenital hypoventilation syndrome but can be from surgical incisions into the second cervical segment to relieve intractable pain.[57] Can also be seen in medullary infarction in an intermittent form.[58-60]	Impaired automatic control of ventilation. Voluntary ventilation remains intact. Classically the patient "forgets to breathe" when asleep. Patient maintains relatively normal blood gas while awake.[3,61]
Carotid body resection[62]	Introduced in Japan in 1940s as a treatment for asthma.[63,64] Also seen after bilateral endarterectomy for carotid vascular disease.	Depressed hypoxic ventilatory drive during exercise. Generally eucapnic at rest. Destruction of peripheral chemoreceptors.[65,66]
Cheyne-Stokes respiration[67,68]	Commonly associated with cardiac disease; can also be seen in neurologic disease sedation, sleep, altitude acclimatization.[69]	Delay between changes in ventilation and detection of the resulting arterial P_{CO_2} by the central chemoreceptors maintains a cyclic pattern of respiration.
Myxedema	In critically ill patients, laboratory differentiation between severe hypothyroidism and the euthyroid-sick syndromes is difficult and may require measurement of free hormone levels.	Respiratory muscle weakness. Depression of ventilatory drive.[70-72]
Starvation	Nutritional intervention can return muscle ventilatory function to normal levels. Furthermore, it seems likely that the ventilatory drive can be influenced by dietary intake of amino acids and glucose.	Decreased ventilatory drive, decreased respiratory muscle function, alterations of lung parenchyma and depressed lung defense mechanisms.
Drug effects	Opiates, barbiturates, benzodiazepines	Should be used judiciously in patients with preexisting hypoventilation.
	Medroxyprogesterone*	Increases ventilatory drive in normal males leading to about 5 mm fall in Pa_{CO_2}. Used in obesity hypoventilation syndrome.[73-75]
	Theophylline*	Increases hypoxic ventilatory response and prevents the fall in hypoxic ventilatory response.
	Acetazolamide*	Efficacy and side effects of long-term use are unknown. Small, crossover study reduced central apnea in patients with congestive heart failure.[76]

*Effects used for treatment.

hypercapnia with use of supplemental oxygen is an abrupt discontinuation of oxygen leading to hypoxemia.[28-30]

When hypoventilation is not caused by decreased central nervous system drive, neuromuscular weakness, or bellows dysfunction, tachypnea is a relatively early manifestation that can be seen in association with near-normal maximum respiratory pressures.[31] Orthopnea that develops within seconds of lying down is a classic symptom of patients with diaphragmatic paralysis. The pathophysiology of dyspnea resulting from gravitational influences and the mechanical function of the diaphragm during water immersion, another manifestation of diaphragmatic paralysis, are discussed by McCool and Mead.[32] Normal diaphragm contraction is associated with a downward movement of the diaphragm and outward movement of the abdomen. When subjects with diaphragmatic paralysis are observed in a supine posture, a paradoxical inward motion of the abdomen can be observed during inspiration. Because these patients are unable to develop transdiaphragmatic pressure gradients, the abdominal contents are drawn toward the chest by the inspiratory fall in pleural pressure generated by the accessory muscles of respiration.[33]

PATIENT MANAGEMENT

Respiratory Failure

Respiratory failure is defined as a failure to maintain adequate gas exchange and is characterized by abnormalities of arterial blood gas tensions. *Type 1 failure* is defined

Table 42-2. Disorders of Peripheral Neuromuscular System

Site of Disease	Disease	Type of Respiratory Failure
Spinal Cord		
Space-occupying lesions	Syringomyelia Multiple sclerosis[77] Mass	Chronic respiratory failure Chronic respiratory failure Chronic respiratory failure
Anterior horn cell lesions	Poliomyelitis[5,16,78] Amyotrophic lateral sclerosis	Chronic respiratory failure Chronic respiratory failure
Inhibiting neuronal blockade	Tetanus	Acute respiratory failure
Any level	Traumatic injury	Acute respiratory failure
Motor Nerves		
Peripheral neuropathy	Phrenic nerve injury[54] Beriberi[79] Guillain-Barré[80] Critical illness polyneuropathy[81,82] Lyme disease[83] Diphtheria[84]	Acute/chronic respiratory failure Chronic respiratory failure Chronic respiratory failure Chronic respiratory failure Chronic respiratory failure Acute respiratory Failure
Neuromuscular junction	Tick paralysis[85] Organophosphate poisoning Botulism[86] Eaton-Lambert syndrome Myasthenia gravis[5,31]	 Acute respiratory failure Acute respiratory failure Acute respiratory failure Acute/chronic respiratory failure
Muscle Involvement		
Dystrophies	Muscular dystrophy[5,31,87-89] Myotonic dystrophy[90,91]	Chronic respiratory failure Chronic respiratory failure
Myopathy	Polymyositis, dermatomyositis, and other collagen vascular diseases[92] Malnutrition[93] Thyroid, adrenal, pituitary glands Metabolic-acid-base, electrolyte[4,18-20]	Chronic respiratory failure Chronic respiratory failure Chronic respiratory failure Acute respiratory failure
Disorders of the Chest Wall	Obesity hypoventilation[4,94-96] Asphyxiating thoracic dystrophy[97] Fibrothorax[98] Thoracoplasty[98] Ankylosing spondylitis[98] Flail chest	Acute/chronic respiratory failure Acute/chronic respiratory failure Acute/chronic respiratory failure Acute/chronic respiratory failure Acute/chronic respiratory failure Acute/chronic respiratory failure

by a PaO_2 of less than 60 mm Hg with a normal or low $PaCO_2$. *Type 2 failure* is defined by a PaO_2 of less than 60 mm Hg and a $PaCO_2$ of greater than 50 mm Hg. Respiratory failure can be acute, acute on chronic, or chronic. Although not always clear cut, this distinction is important in deciding on the location of patient treatment and the most appropriate treatment strategy, particularly in type 2 respiratory failure:

- *Acute* hypercapnic respiratory failure: the patient will have no, or minor, evidence of preexisting respiratory disease, and arterial blood gas tensions will show a high $PaCO_2$, low pH, and normal bicarbonate.
- *Chronic* hypercapnic respiratory failure: evidence of chronic respiratory disease, high $PaCO_2$, near normal pH, high bicarbonate.
- *Acute-on-chronic* hypercapnic respiratory failure: an acute deterioration in an individual with significant preexisting hypercapnic respiratory failure, high $PaCO_2$, low pH, high bicarbonate.[34]

Acute Respiratory Failure Caused by Neuromuscular Disease

Involvement of the inspiratory and expiratory muscle groups in neuromuscular disease occurs to variable degrees.[24,35] Inspiratory muscle fatigue occurs as muscle weakness progresses or because of excessive ventilatory demands, as in systemic infection. Respiratory rate increases as a usual response to preserve minute ventilation. Work of breathing is increased in tachypnea due to *increased dead-space ventilation* and by *decreased relative time spent in expiration.* Blood flow to respiratory muscles is compromised because this occurs primarily during expiration.[35] Weakness of inspiratory muscles predisposes to atelectasis because of reduced tidal volume and vital capacity. The elastic recoil of the stretched thoracic and lung tissue provides driving pressure for airflow. Therefore expiratory muscle weakness has less impact on respiratory ventilation and mechanics. Essential function of the expiratory muscle is that of generation of an effective cough and clearance of secretions.

Respiratory clinical manifestations include tachypnea, abdominal paradox, respiratory alternans, and small tidal volume.

The risk of respiratory failure increases significantly when the vital capacity (VC) falls below 15 mL/kg, particularly if there is a clear downward trend. Serial measurements of vital capacity at the bedside are helpful in this situation.[36,37] Careful assessments of ability to protect airway, oxygenation, ability to ventilate, and chest radiographs are essential in determining need for assistance with ventilation.[38] Ideally, ventilatory support should be initiated in the setting of impending respiratory failure, when there has been a clear downward trend, rather than having to initiate after the development of cardiovascular instability. Noninvasive ventilation or endotracheal intubation with initiation of positive pressure ventilation is indicated at this time. An anticipatory approach avoids risks associated with emergent intubation and minimizes complications.[39-41]

Supportive care is an important factor. Nutritional support, psychological and emotional support, physical therapy, range of motion exercises to prevent joint malalignment, tendon shortening and skin care to prevent pressure sores, and prevention of thromboembolic disease should be initiated as soon as possible.

Noninvasive Positive Pressure Ventilation

In a patient with intact bulbar function, noninvasive ventilation should be the ventilatory support of choice because of its efficacy, convenience, and portability. Progression of underlying disease will ultimately require invasive ventilation.

Noninvasive ventilation (NIV) is widely used for acute and chronic respiratory failure. If arterial blood gas tensions do not improve, the level of support can be increased. If the aim is to abolish muscle effort completely, there is little to be gained by increasing the level of inspiratory pressure above 20 cm H_sO (chest wall deformity) or 25 cm H_sO (chronic obstructive pulmonary disease).[42,43] NIV is widely considered to be an effective treatment in patients with chronic ventilatory failure caused by chest wall deformity and neuromuscular disease.[44]

When to Use Noninvasive Ventilation in Nonpulmonary Causes of Respiratory Failure[45]

Patients

- Chest wall deformity
- Neuromuscular disorder
- Decompensated OSA

Blood Gases

- Respiratory acidosis ($Pa\text{CO}_2 > 50$ mm Hg, pH < 7.35 or $H^+ > 45$ nmol/L) that persists despite maximal medical treatment and appropriate controlled oxygen therapy (patients with pH < 7.25 or $H^+ > 56$ nmol/L respond less well and should be managed in an intensive care unit).
- Low A-a oxygen gradient (patients with severe life-threatening hypoxemia are more appropriately managed by tracheal intubation).

Clinical State

- Sick but not moribund
- Able to protect airway
- Conscious and cooperative
- Hemodynamically stable
- No excessive respiratory secretions
- Few comorbidities

Contraindications Excluded

- Facial burns/trauma/recent facial or upper airway surgery
- Vomiting
- Fixed upper airway obstruction
- Undrained pneumothorax

Premorbid State

- Potential for recovery to quality of life acceptable to the patient
- Patient's wishes considered

Contraindications to Noninvasive Ventilation[34]

- Facial trauma/burns
- Recent facial, upper airway, or upper gastrointestinal tract* surgery
- Fixed obstruction of the upper airway
- Inability to protect airway*
- Life-threatening hypoxemia*
- Hemodynamic instability*
- Severe comorbidity*
- Impaired consciousness*
- Confusion/agitation*
- Vomiting
- Bowel obstruction*
- Copious respiratory secretions*
- Focal consolidation on chest radiograph*
- Undrained pneumothorax*

Chronic Respiratory Failure

Prolonged mechanical ventilation is defined by the Centers for Medicare and Medicaid Services in the United States as greater than 21 days of mechanical ventilation for at least 6 hours per day.[46] Most patients requiring prolonged

*NIV may be used despite the presence of these contraindications if it is to be the "ceiling" of treatment.

mechanical ventilation will have a tracheostomy placed to facilitate comfort, communication, and chronic ventilator facility or home ventilation placement. Common problems among patients undergoing prolonged mechanical ventilation are similar to those on short-term ventilation including the following[47-50]:

- Infections (e.g., pneumonia, line sepsis, *Clostridium difficile* colitis)
- Ileus
- Renal failure
- Pneumothorax
- Seizures
- Tracheal bleeding
- Laryngeal edema
- Development of tracheal granulation tissue
- Tracheoesophageal fistula formation
- Loss of airway patency because of unplanned extubation or decannulation

CHRONIC VENTILATORY-ASSIST DEVICES

Methods of chronic mechanical ventilation include noninvasive and invasive techniques (Tables 42-3 and 42-4). Ventilatory-assist devices have been used for chronic respiratory failure for decades. Initially, negative-pressure ventilators were used, but this approach was soon replaced by the use of volume-cycled ventilation delivered by a tracheostomy. Because this patient population was in a terminal stage without other treatment options, tracheostomy and chronic ventilation became the standard of therapy if the patient wanted to continue aggressive care.

Major ethical considerations surround the institution of chronic ventilatory support.[51] This issue is evolving rapidly because of the widespread availability of relatively inexpensive technology. Guidelines have been published recently regarding clinical indications and management strategies for the use of noninvasive positive pressure ventilation, although they are based on inadequate data.[52,53] The discussion about ventilatory assistance should occur before an emergent setting. Adequate and unbiased information should be given to patients so that they can make an informed decision. Different ventilatory methods and modes of delivery should be discussed with patients, including the possibility of foregoing any type of mechanical ventilation. Patient and caregiver quality of life and satisfaction have only recently been investigated in this population, and many unanswered questions remain.[124] Management of the terminal phase can also be difficult.

KEY POINTS

- A normal $P(A - a)O_2$ difference should not be required as a diagnostic criterion for nonpulmonary causes of respiratory failure.
- The etiologic classification of nonpulmonary disorders causing respiratory failure consists of the following broad categories: disorders of ventilatory control, neuromuscular disorders, disorders of the chest wall, and upper airway obstruction.
- Clinical recognition of these disorders depends on familiarity with the physiologic consequences of chronic hypoxia and hypercapnia, the signs and symptoms of respiratory muscle weakness, and their effects on pulmonary function tests.
- The approach to the management of acute respiratory failure does not differ in principle from the approach used in lung diseases.
- Noninvasive nocturnal ventilatory support has gained acceptance as a means of controlling diurnal hypercapnia and providing respiratory muscle rest.

Table 42-3. Ventilatory-Assist Devices

Mode of Ventilation	Example	Advantages	Disadvantages	Applications
Abdominal displacement	Pneumobelt (Fig. 42-2A through C)	Noninvasive	Requires sitting. Skin abrasions at points of contact.	Diaphragm paralysis or weakness, high cord lesions, mainly for daytime use. Typical settings rate 16-24; pressure 35-50 cm H_2O.
		Portable	Upper airway obstruction.	
	Rocking bed (Fig. 42-3)	Simplicity	Not portable.	Diaphragm paralysis or weakness, mainly for nocturnal use. Typical settings 12-16/min.

Continued

Table 42-3. Ventilatory-Assist Devices—cont'd

Mode of Ventilation	Example	Advantages	Disadvantages	Applications
Diaphragmatic pacing (Fig. 42-4)			Motion sickness.	Intact phrenic nerve and diaphragm muscle; high cord lesion and central hypoventilation.
Expiratory aids.[99] Manually assisted coughing ("quad" coughing), cough in-exsufflator percussionator, Hayek oscillator (Fig. 42-5)				Peak cough flow augmentation in patients with expiratory muscle weakness.
Glossopharyngeal breathing				Postpolio and muscular dystrophy patients. Respiratory muscle weakness, but upper airway function is intact.
Negative-pressure ventilation	Pneumosuit (Fig. 42-6)	Portable	Difficulty applying suit. Cumbersome. Upper airway obstruction.	Typical settings: Pressure −20 to −40 cm H_2O.[101] Rate 14-18.
	Chest cuirass	Allows speech and feeding Portable.	Fitting difficulties. Upper airway obstruction.	Typical settings: Pressure −20 to −40 cm H_2O.[101] Rate 14-18.
	Iron lung (Fig. 42-7)	Reliable	Confining. Not portable.	Second line for patients if nasal ventilation fails. Typical settings: Rate 12-14. Pressure −12 to −25 cm H_2O.
Positive-pressure ventilation			Upper airway obstruction	Mode of first choice. Nasal route preferred, oronasal or mouthpiece if nasal unsuccessful. Typical settings Rate 12-24; Inspiratory pressure 10-20 cm H_2O Expiratory pressure 12-15 cm H_2O.
Volume-cycled	PLV-100 and 102 (Respironics, Inc)	Allows tidal volume adjustment		
	Companion 2801 (Mallinckrodt, Inc)			
	LP 6 Plus	High/low airway pressure alarms		
	LP 10	Apnea alarms		
Pressure-cycled	Quantum PSV	Usually used noninvasively		
	BI-PAP S/T	Mandatory rate available		
	KnightStar 335			
	VPAP Adapt SV ResMed Inc.			Adaptive-servo ventilator is designed specifically to treat central sleep apnea (CSA) in all its forms. Adapts to the patient's ventilatory needs on a breath-by-breath basis and automatically calculates a target ventilation. Adjusts the pressure support to achieve it.

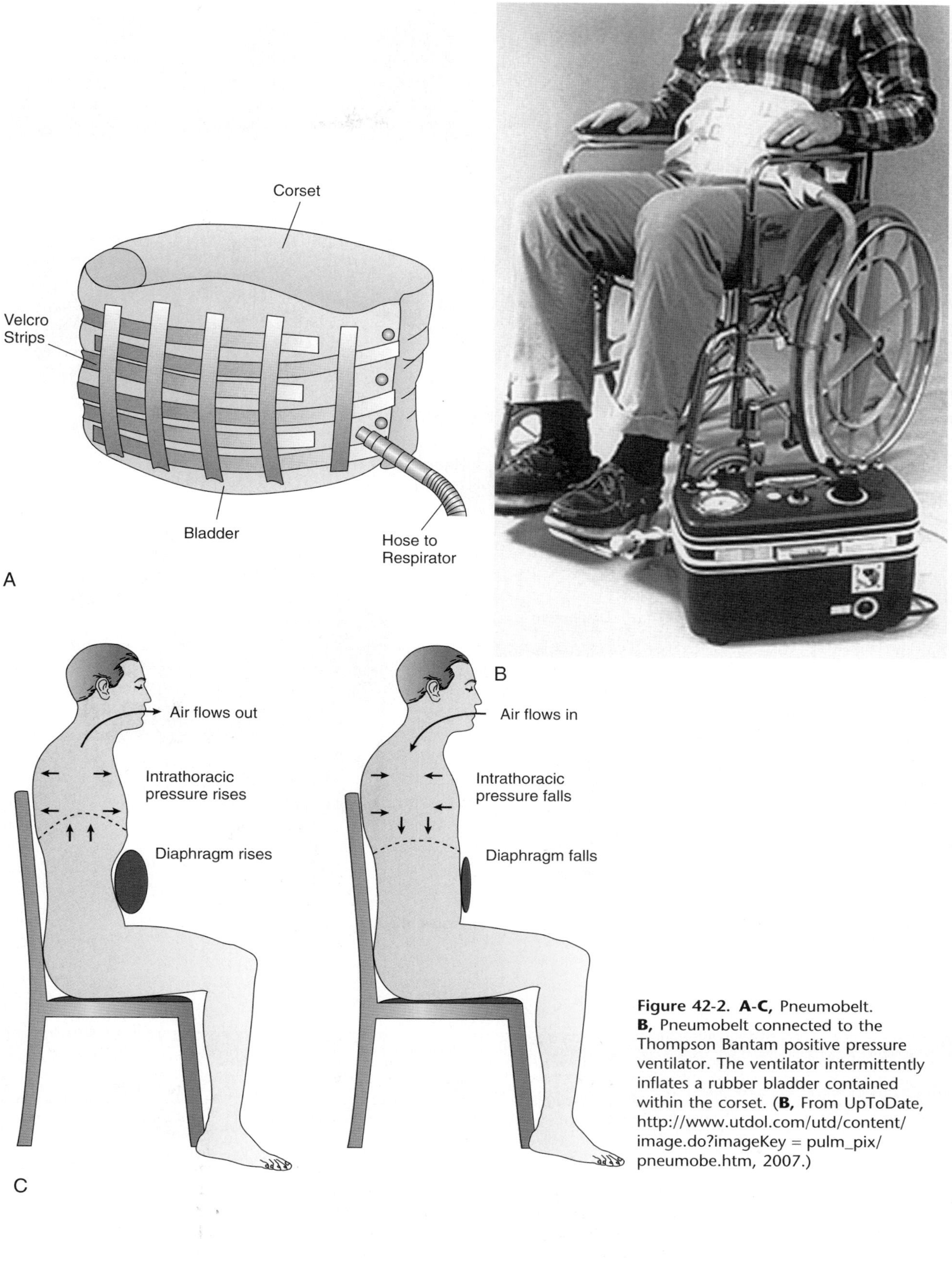

Figure 42-2. A-C, Pneumobelt. **B,** Pneumobelt connected to the Thompson Bantam positive pressure ventilator. The ventilator intermittently inflates a rubber bladder contained within the corset. (**B,** From UpToDate, http://www.utdol.com/utd/content/image.do?imageKey = pulm_pix/pneumobe.htm, 2007.)

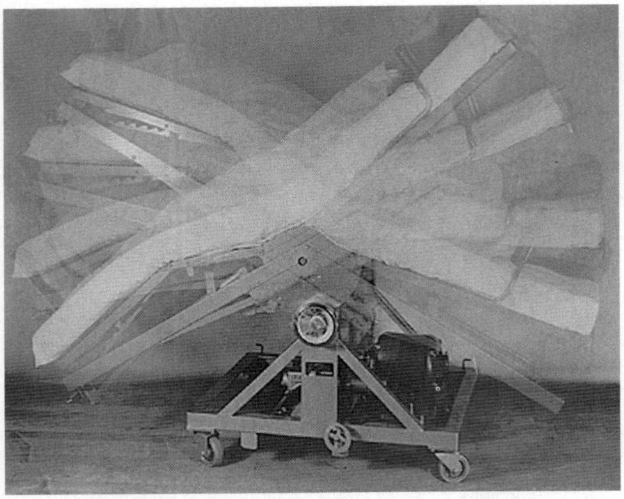

Figure 42-3. Rocking bed.

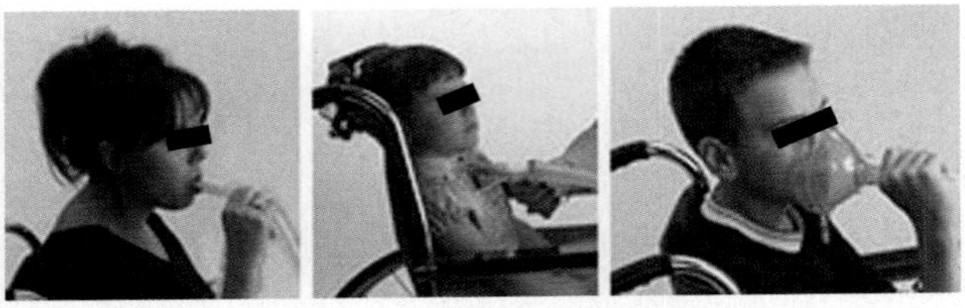

Figure 42-5. Patients using cough assist devices.

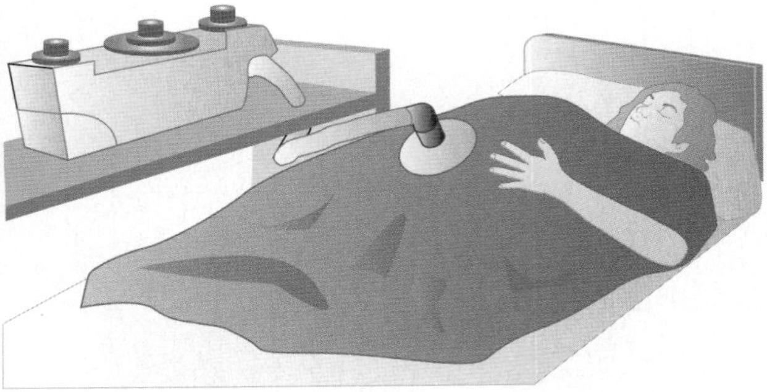

Figure 42-6. Pneumosuit.

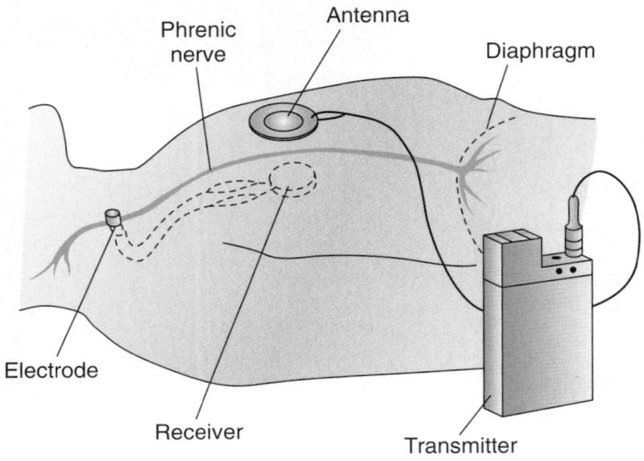

Figure 42-4. Diaphragmatic pacer.

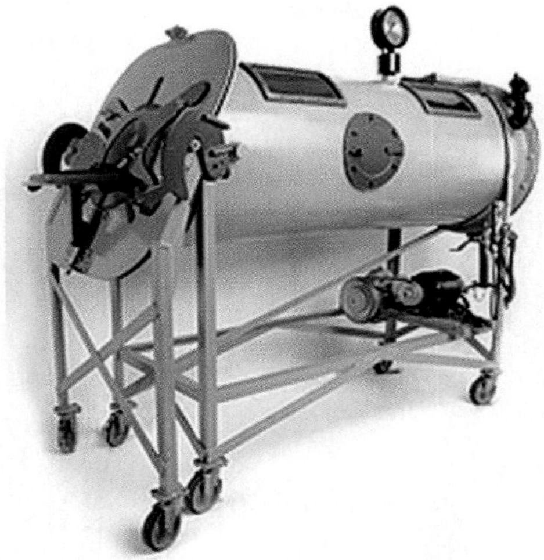

Figure 42-7. Iron lung.

Table 42-4. Interfaces for Ventilatory-Assist Devices

Mode of Delivery	Example	Advantages	Disadvantages
Noninvasive	Nasal mask (Fig. 42-8)	Avoids tracheostomy complications Less claustrophobia	Mouth leak Patent nares required Nasal bridge ulceration Patient cooperation required
	Nasal pillows (Fig. 42-9)	Avoids tracheostomy complications	Mouth leak
	Oronasal mask (Fig. 42-10)	Avoids tracheostomy complications	Poor seal Aspiration risk Cannot speak
	Mouthpiece (Fig. 42-11)	Avoids tracheostomy complications	Increased secretions Cannot speak
Invasive	Tracheostomy (Fig. 42-12)	Allows suctioning	Surgical procedure required

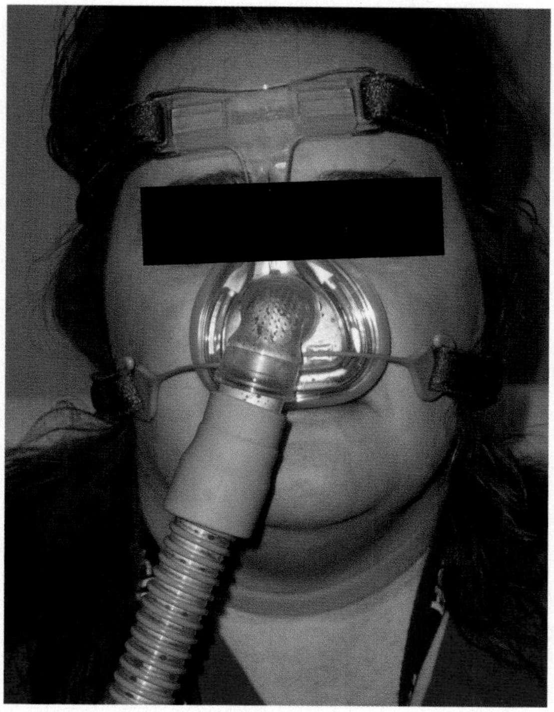

Figure 42-8. Nasal mask.

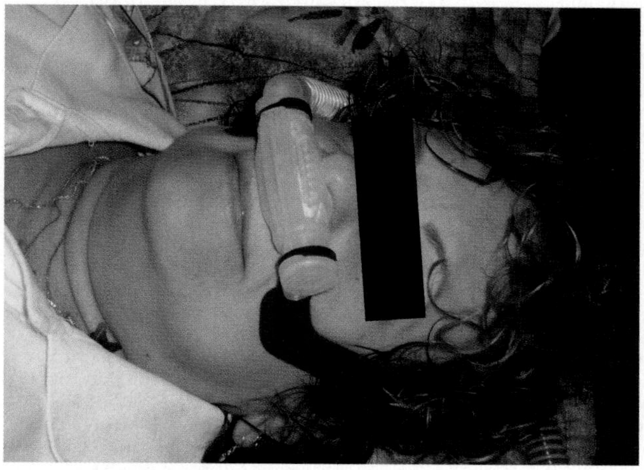

Figure 42-9. Nasal pillows.

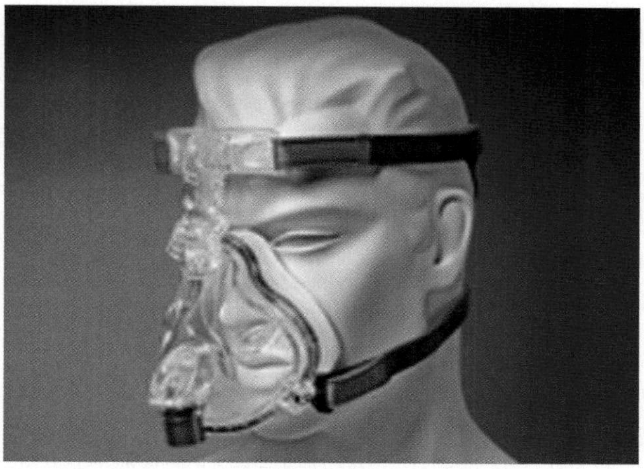

Figure 42-10. Oronasal mask. (Courtesy of Respironics, Murrysville, PA.)

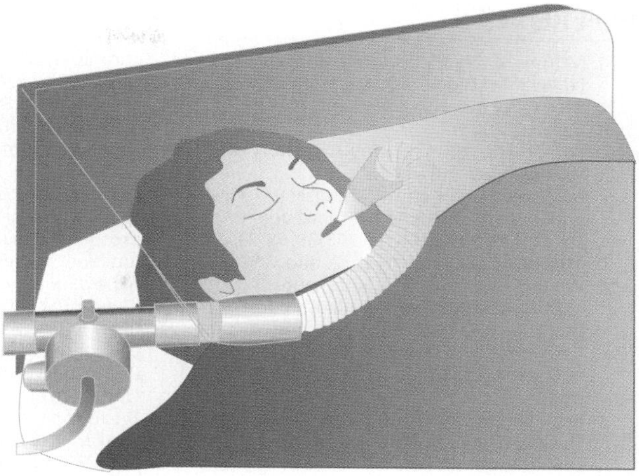

Figure 42-11. Mouthpiece.

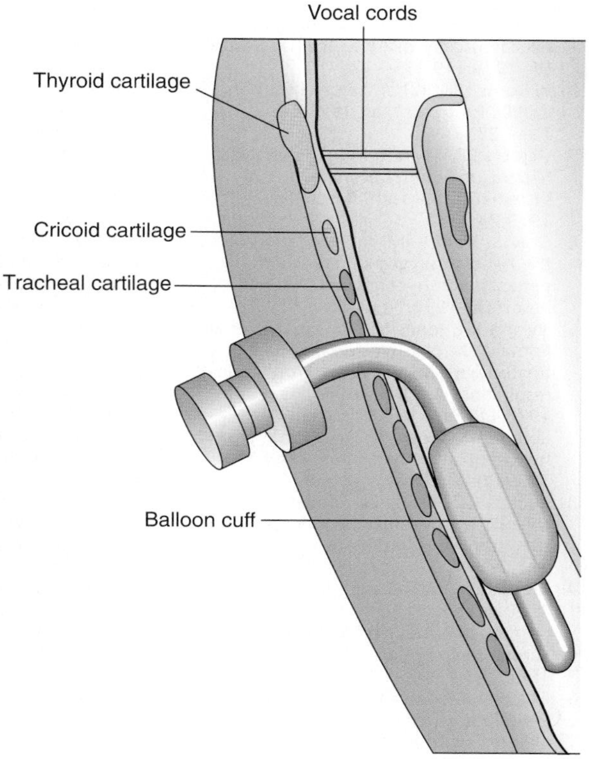

Figure 42-12. Completed tracheostomy.

REFERENCES

1. Murray M, Nadel J: Murray and Nadel's Textbook of Respiratory Medicine, 4th ed., Philadelphia, Elsevier, 2005.
2. Karnad DR, Apte SJ, Supe AN: Effect of venous hypercarbia and hyperventilation on myocardial contractility in canine haemorrhagic shock. J Postgrad Med 1993;39:68-71.
3. Mellins RB, Balfour HH Jr, Turino GM, Winters RW: Failure of automatic control of ventilation (Ondine's curse). Medicine 1970;49:487-504.
4. Rochester DF, Enson Y: Current concepts in the pathogenesis of the obesity-hypoventilation syndrome. Am J Med 1974;57:402-420.
5. Davis J, Goldman M, Loh L, et al: Diaphragm function and alveolar hypoventilation. Q J Med 1976;45:87-100.
6. Goldstein R: Hypoventilation: Neuromuscular and chest wall disorders. Clin Chest Med 1992;13:507-521.
7. Newsom-Davis J: The diaphragm and neuromuscular disease. Am Rev Respir Dis 1979;119:115-117.
8. Williams MH Jr: Ventilatory failure in COPD. Postgrad Med 1973;54:124-128.
9. Demers RR, Irwin R: Management of hypercapneic respiratory failure: A systematic approach. Respir Care 1979;24:328.
10. Gray B, Blalock JM: Interpretation of the alveolar oxygen difference in patients with hypercapnia. Am Rev Respir Dis 1991;143:4-8.
11. Hyland RH, Jones NL, Powles AC, et al: Primary alveolar hypoventilation treated with nocturnal electrophrenic respiration. Am Rev Respir Dis 1978;117:165-172.
12. Rodman T, Close HP: The primary hypoventilation syndrome. Am J Med 1959;26:808-817.
13. Rhoads GG, Brody JS: Idiopathic alveolar hypoventilation: Clinical spectrum. Ann Intern Med 1969;71:271-278.
14. McNicholas WT, Carter JL, Rutherford R, et al: Beneficial effect of oxygen in primary alveolar hypoventilation with central sleep apnea. Am Rev Respir Dis 1982;125:773-775.
15. Gozal D, Marcus CL, Shoseyof D, et al: Peripheral chemoreceptor function in children with the congenital hypoventilation syndrome. J Appl Physiol 1993;74:379-387.
16. Hsu AA, Staats BA: "Postpolio" sequelae and sleep-related disordered breathing. Mayo Clin Proc 1998;73:216-224.
17. Spengler CM, Gozal D, Shea SA: Chemoreceptive mechanisms elucidated by studies of congenital central hypoventilation syndrome. Respir Physiol 2001;129:247-255.
18. Schwartz WB, Brackett NC Jr, Cohen JJ: The response of extracellular hydrogen ion concentration to graded degrees of chronic hypercapnia: The physiologic limits of the defense of pH. J Clin Invest 1965;44:291-301.
19. Goldring RM, Turino GM, Heinemann HO: Respiratory-renal adjustments in chronic hypercapnia in man. Am J Med 1971;51:772-784.
20. Heinemann HO, Goldring RM: Bicarbonate and the regulation of ventilation. Am J Med 1974;57:361-370.
21. Jackson CE, Rosenfeld J, Moore DH, et al: A preliminary evaluation of a prospective study of pulmonary function studies and symptoms of hypoventilation in ALS/MND patients. J Neurol Sci 2001;191:75-78.
22. Plum F, Leigh RJ: Abnormalities of central mechanisms. In Horbein TF (Ed.), Lung Biology in Health and Disease (Vol. 17), Regulation of Breathing (Part 2). New York, Marcel Dekker, 1981, pp 989-1057.
23. Plum F: Neurological integration of behavioral and metabolic control of breathing. In Porter R (Ed.), Breathing. Hering-Breuer Centenary Symposium. London, Churchill, 1970.
24. Roussos C, Macklem PT: The respiratory muscles. N Engl J Med 1982;307:786-797.
25. ATS/ERS statement on respiratory muscle testing. Am J Respir Crit Care Med 2002;166:518-624.
26. Zagelbaum G, Gross DA: Clinical manifestations of inspiratory muscle fatigue. Am J Med 1982;73:308-316.
27. Sivak ED, Shefner JM, Sexton J: Neuromuscular disease and hypoventilation. Curr Opin Pulm Med 1999;5:355-362.
28. Dick CR, Liu Z, Sassoon CS, et al: O_2-induced change in ventilation and ventilatory drive in COPD. Am J Respir Crit Care Med 1997;155:609-614.
29. Sassoon CS, Hassell KT, Mahutte CK: Hyperoxic-induced hypercapnia in stable chronic obstructive pulmonary disease. Am Rev Respir Dis 1987;135:907-911.
30. Kelsen SG, Fleegler B, Altose MD: The respiratory neuromuscular response to hypoxia, hypercapnia, and obstruction to airflow in asthma. Am Rev Respir Dis 1979;120:517-527.
31. Gibson GJ, Pride NB, Davis JN, Loh LC: Pulmonary mechanics in patients with respiratory muscle weakness. Am Rev Respir Dis 1977;115:389-395.
32. McCool FD, Mead J: Dyspnea on immersion: Mechanisms in patients with bilateral diaphragm paralysis. Am Rev Respir Dis 1989;139:275-276.
33. Davis J, Goldman M, Loh L, Casson M: Diaphragm function and alveolar hypoventilation. Q J Med 1976;45:87-100.
34. Wyatt J, Bellis F: British Thoracic Society guidelines on non-invasive ventilation. Emerg Med J 2002;19:435.
35. Roussos C, Koutsoukou A: Respiratory failure. Eur Respir J Suppl 2003;47:3s-14s.
36. Rabinstein AA, Wijdicks EF: Warning signs of imminent respiratory failure in neurological patients. Semin Neurol 2003;23:97-104.
37. Ropper AH: The Guillain-Barré syndrome. N Engl J Med 1992;326:1130-1136.
38. MacDuff A, Grant IS: Critical care management of neuromuscular disease, including long-term ventilation. Curr Opin Crit Care 2003;9:106-112.
39. Newton-John H: Prevention of pulmonary complications in severe Guillain-Barré syndrome by early assisted ventilation. Med J Aust 1985;142:444-445.
40. Ropper AH, Kehne SM: Guillain-Barré syndrome: Management of respiratory failure. Neurology 1985;35:1662-1665.
41. Loh L: Neurological and neuromuscular disease. Br J Anaesth 1986;58:190-200.
42. Tuggey JM, Elliott MW: Titration of non-invasive positive pressure ventilation in chronic respiratory failure. Respir Med 2006;100:1262-1269.
43. International Consensus Conferences in Intensive Care Medicine: Noninvasive positive pressure ventilation in acute respiratory failure. Am J Respir Crit Care Med 2001;163:283-291.
44. Turkington PM, Elliott MW: Rationale for the use of non-invasive ventilation in chronic ventilatory failure. Thorax 2000;55:417-423.
45. Wyatt J, Bellis F: British Thoracic Society guidelines on non-invasive ventilation. Emerg Med J 2002;192:192-211.
46. MacIntyre NR, Epstein SK, Carson S, et al: Management of patients requiring prolonged mechanical ventilation: Report of a NAMDRC consensus conference. Chest 2005;128:3937-3954.
47. Ding LW, Wang HC, Wu HD, et al: Laryngeal ultrasound: A useful method in predicting post-extubation stridor. A pilot study. Eur Respir J 2006;27:384-389.
48. Chatila WM, Criner GJ: Complications of long-term mechanical ventilation. Respir Care Clin N Am 2002;8:631-647.
49. Kalb TH, Lorin S: Infection in the chronically critically ill: Unique risk profile in a newly defined population. Crit Care Clin 2002;18:529-552.
50. Chung YH, Chao TY, Chiu CT, Lin MC: The cuff-leak test is a simple tool to verify severe laryngeal edema in patients undergoing long-term mechanical ventilation. Crit Care Med 2006;34:409-414.
51. Polkey MI, Lyall RA, Davidson AC, et al: Ethical and clinical issues in the use of home non-invasive mechanical ventilation for the palliation of breathlessness in motor neurone disease. Thorax 1999;54:367-371.
52. Robert D, Willig TN, Leger P, Paulus J: Long-term nasal ventilation in neuromuscular disorders: Report of a consensus conference. Eur Respir J 1993;6:599-606.
53. Clinical indications for noninvasive positive pressure ventilation in chronic respiratory failure due to restrictive lung disease, COPD, and nocturnal hypoventilation—a consensus conference report. Chest 1999;116:521-534.
54. Tuller MA, Mehdi F: Compensatory hypoventilation and hypercapnia in primary metabolic alkalosis. Report of

three cases. Am J Med 1971;50: 281-290.
55. Weese-Meyer: Idiopathic congenital central hypoventilation syndrome: Diagnosis and management. American Thoracic Society. Am J Respir Crit Care Med 1999;160:368-373.
56. Fishman AP: The syndrome of chronic alveolar hypoventilation. Bull Physiopathol Respir 1972;8:971-980.
57. Mullan S, Hosobuchi Y: Respiratory hazards in high cervical percutaneous cordotomy. J Neurosurg 1968;28: 291-297.
58. Lassman A, Mayer SA: Paroxysmal apnea and vasomotor instability following medullary infarction. Arch Neurol 2005;62:1286-1288.
59. Bogousslavsky J, Khurana R, Deruaz JP, et al: Respiratory failure and unilateral caudal brainstem infarction. Ann Neurol 1990;28:668-673.
60. Severinghaus JW: Pathophysiologic aspects of the regulation of respiration. Bull Mem Acad R Med Belg 1979;134:261-271.
61. Severinghaus JW: Respiration. Ann Rev Physiol 1962;24:421-470.
62. Wade JG, Larson CP Jr, Hickey RF, et al: Effect of carotid endarterectomy on carotid chemoreceptor and baroreceptor function in man. N Engl J Med 1970;282:823-829.
63. Winter B: Bilateral carotid body resection for asthma and emphysema. A new surgical approach without hypoventilation or baroreceptor dysfunction. Int Surg 1972;57: 458-466.
64. Winter B: Carotid body resection. Controversy—confusion—conflict. Ann Thorac Surg 1973;16:648-659.
65. Lugliani R, Whipp BJ, Seard C, Wasserman K: Effect of bilateral carotid body resection on ventilatory control at rest and during exercise in man. N Engl J Med 1971;285: 1105-1111.
66. Winter B: Bilateral carotid body resection for asthma and emphysema. Respir Ther 1972;57:458-466.
67. Cherniack NS, Longobardo GS: Cheyne-Stokes breathing. An instability in physiologic control. N Engl J Med 1973;288:952-957.
68. Kasai T, Narui K, Dohi T, et al: Efficacy of nasal bi-level positive airway pressure in congestive heart failure patients with Cheyne-Stokes respiration and central sleep apnea. Circ J 2005;69:913-921.
69. Cherniack NS, Longobardo G, Evangelista CJ: Causes of Cheyne-Stokes respiration. Neurocrit Care 2005;3:271-279.
70. Zwillich C, Peirson DJ, Hofeldt FD, et al: Ventilatory control in myxedema and hypothyroidism. N Engl J Med 1975;292:662-665.
71. Nordqvist P, Dhuner KG, Stenberg K, et al: Myxoedema coma and carbon dioxide-retention. Acta Med Scand 1960;166:189-194.
72. Massumi R, Winnacker JL: Severe depression of the respiratory center in myxedema. Am J Med 1964;36: 876.
73. Sutton FD Jr, Zwillich CW, Creagh CE, et al: Progesterone for outpatient treatment of Pickwickian syndrome. Ann Intern Med 1975;83:476-479.
74. Skatrud JB, Dempsey JA, Kaiser DG: Ventilatory response to medroxyprogesterone acetate in normal subjects: Time course and mechanism. J Appl Physiol 1978;44: 393-344.
75. Kryger M, McCullough RE, Collins D, et al: Treatment of excessive polycythemia of high altitude with respiratory stimulant drugs. Am Rev Respir Dis 1978;117:455-464.
76. Javaheri S: Acetazolamide improves central sleep apnea in heart failure: A double-blind, prospective study. Am J Respir Crit Care Med 2006;173: 234-237.
77. Berlin L, Kurtzke JF, Guthrie TC: Acute respiratory failure in multiple sclerosis and its management. AMA Arch Neurol Psychiatry 1953;69:394-395.
78. Lane DJ, Hazleman B, Nichol PJ: Late onset respiratory failure in patients with previous poliomyelitis. Q J Med 1974;43:551-568.
79. Fujita I, Sata T, Gondo K, et al: Cardiac beriberi (shoshin beriberi) caused by excessive intake of isotonic drink. Acta Paediatr Jpn 1992;34:466-468.
80. Zifko U, Chen R: The respiratory system. Baillieres Clin Neurol 1996;5:477-495.
81. Dhand UK: Clinical approach to the weak patient in the intensive care unit. Respir Care 2006;51:1024-1040; discussion 1040-1041.
82. Latronico N, Peli E, Botteri M: Critical illness myopathy and neuropathy. Curr Opin Crit Care 2005;11:126-132.
83. Abbott RA, Hammans S, Margarson M, Aji BM: Diaphragmatic paralysis and respiratory failure as a complication of Lyme disease. J Neurol Neurosurg Psychiatry 2005;76:1306-1307.
84. Popova LM, Avdiunina IA, Alferova VP, et al: Respiratory insufficiency in adults with diphtheric polyneuropathy. Anesteziol Reanimatol 1996;Mar-April: 9-13.
85. Grattan-Smith PJ, Morris JG, Johnston HM, et al: Clinical and neurophysiological features of tick paralysis. Brain 1997;120:1975-1987.
86. FitzGerald S, Lyons R, Ryan J, et al: Botulism as a cause of respiratory failure in injecting drug users. Ir J Med Sci 2003;172:143-144.
87. Coccagna G, Mantovani M, Parchi C, et al: Alveolar hypoventilation and hypersomnia in myotonic dystrophy. J Neurol Neurosurg Psychiatry 1975;38:977-984.
88. Inkley SR, Oldenburg FC, Vignos Jr PJ: Pulmonary function in Duchenne muscular dystrophy related to stage of disease. Am J Med 1974;56:297-306.
89. Hukins CA, Hillman DR: Daytime predictors of sleep hypoventilation in Duchenne muscular dystrophy. Am J Respir Crit Care Med 2000;161: 166-170.
90. Denis J, Cornu P, Laffay J, et al: Myotonic dystrophy and acute respiratory insufficiency. Sem Hop 1977;53:1683-1688.
91. Rimmer KP, Golar SD, Lee MA, Whitelaw WA: Myotonia of the respiratory muscles in myotonic dystrophy. Am Rev Respir Dis 1993;148:1018-1022.
92. Martyn JB, Wong MJ, Huang SH: Pulmonary and neuromuscular complications of mixed connective tissue disease: A report and review of the literature. J Rheumatol 1988;15:703-705.
93. Saka M, Balkan A, Demirci N, Sarikayalar U: Pulmonary function and nutrition. Tuberk Toraks 2003;51: 461-466.
94. Berger KI, Ayappa I, Chatr-Amontri B, et al: Obesity hypoventilation syndrome as a spectrum of respiratory disturbances during sleep. Chest 2001;120:1231-1238.
95. Lopata M, Onal E: Mass loading, sleep apnea, and the pathogenesis of obesity hypoventilation. Am Rev Respir Dis 1982;126:640-645.
96. Phipps PR, Starritt E, Caterson I, Grunstein RR: Association of serum leptin with hypoventilation in human obesity. Thorax 2002;57: 75-76.
97. Zizka J, Rehulova E, Juttnerova V, Balicek P: Asphyxiating thoracic dystrophy. Cesk Pediatr 1979;34:98-99.
98. Bergofsky E: Respiratory failure in disorders of the thoracic cage. Am Rev Respir Dis 1979;119:643-669.
99. Bach JR, Ishikawa Y, Kim H: Prevention of pulmonary morbidity for patients with Duchenne muscular dystrophy. Chest 1997;112:1024-1028.
100. Kasai T, Narui K, Dohi T, et al: First experience of using new adaptive servo-ventilation device for Cheyne-Stokes respiration with central sleep apnea among Japanese patients with congestive heart failure: Report of four clinical cases. Circ J 2006;70:1148-1154.
101. Linton DM: Cuirass ventilation: A review and update. Crit Care Resusc 2005;7:22-28.

Chapter 43

Pneumonia: Considerations for the Critically Ill Patient

Michael S. Niederman

Pneumonia is the sixth leading cause of death in the United States and the number one cause of death from infectious diseases. The patient with pneumonia is managed in the intensive care unit (ICU) when severe forms of community-acquired pneumonia (CAP) are present or when a hospitalized patient develops a life-threatening nosocomial pneumonia (NP). A newly defined entity, health care–associated pneumonia (HCAP), is a form of NP that arises in patients who have been in contact with environments such as nursing homes and hemodialysis centers that expose them to the multidrug-resistant bacteria present in the hospital; these patients frequently develop severe pneumonia.[1,2] In the ICU almost 90% of episodes of NP occur in patients who are being mechanically ventilated for other reasons, and this is termed *ventilator-associated pneumonia* (VAP). The elderly account for a disproportionate number of critically ill patients with all forms of pneumonia, often because they commonly have comorbid illness that predisposes them to more severe forms of infection, and their short- and long-term mortality is higher than that of younger patients.[3] In all forms of severe pneumonia, antibiotic resistance is an increasing problem, especially among pneumococci in CAP, and with *Pseudomonas aeruginosa*, *Acinetobacter* spp., extended-spectrum β-lactamase–producing gram-negatives, and methicillin-resistant *Staphylococcus aureus* (MRSA) in VAP and HCAP.[1,2] Although patients with HIV infection and those with other immunocompromising diseases commonly develop pneumonia, the approach to managing these patients is very specific and different from that used in immunocompetent patients. Therefore these populations are not discussed here.

Pneumonia is unusual among medical illnesses because its pathogenesis, therapy, and prevention can be discussed, but there is tremendous controversy about how to best diagnose its presence. Although the clinical definition requires the presence of a new radiographic infiltrate and supporting clinical information for the presence of infection, the diagnosis of ventilator-associated pneumonia is imprecise, and most physicians are relegated to managing patients from this imperfect perspective. Considerable controversy exists about whether a more precise and accurate bacteriologic definition of pneumonia would lead to improved patient outcome, with some recent studies focusing on this issue.[2,4,5] Numerous other controversies related to pneumonia therapy and prevention are also debated among critical care physicians and are discussed in this chapter.

DEFINITIONS OF SEVERE PNEUMONIA, RISK FACTORS, AND PROGNOSIS

Among patients with CAP admitted to the hospital, 10% to 20% require care in the ICU and the rates are higher in elderly patients.[6,7] No uniform definition of severe pneumonia exists, but patients who need ICU care are often those with either respiratory failure (hypoxemic or hypercarbic) requiring mechanical ventilation or noninvasive ventilation; septic shock; or other clinical features of serious illness such as respiratory rate greater than 30 breaths per minute, systolic blood pressure (BP) less than 90 mm Hg or diastolic BP less than 60 mm Hg, multilobar infiltrates, PaO_2/FIO_2 ratio less than 250, confusion, or destabilization of another serious medical problem.[1,8] In patients with severe CAP, the expected mortality rate for those admitted to the ICU is 35% to 40%, but higher rates have been observed if the majority of ICU-admitted patients are mechanically ventilated, implying that the prognosis is worse if ICU care is first provided late in the course of illness.[9] One recent study found that CAP accounted for 5.9% of all ICU admissions in the United Kingdom and that 59% were admitted within the first 2 days of hospital stay. In this group, 55% were mechanically ventilated on ICU entry and the mortality rate was lowest (46%) in those admitted within the first 2 days, compared with those admitted later in the course of hospital illness.[9] On the basis of a number of studies, a reasonable benchmark is that approximately 60% of all ICU CAP patients will be mechanically ventilated at the time of admission.[6,7,10]

Among those with VAP, mortality rates can be as high as 50% to 70%, and case-control studies have documented mortality directly attributable to the presence of pneumonia.[11] Antibiotic-resistant organisms may add to the mortality rate of VAP, not because of increased virulence but rather because these organisms are often not anticipated and, when present, are often initially treated with ineffective antibiotic regimens.[12] HCAP is a form of NP that includes patients with pneumonia developing any time during their hospital stay (including on admission) who have been exposed to the drug-resistant bacteria present in the health care environment. This includes any patient with a history of hospitalization in the past 3 months, admission from a long-term care facility, need for dialysis or home infusion therapy, home wound care, or antibiotic therapy in the past 3 months.[2,13]

A number of studies have defined the risk factors for severe forms of CAP and VAP, as well as the clinical parameters associated with an increased risk for patient mortality.

Risk Factors for Severe Forms of Community-Acquired Pneumonia

Most patients with severe CAP (45% to 65%) have coexisting illnesses, and patients who are chronically ill have an increased likelihood of developing a complicated pneumonic illness (Box 43-1).[1,14] The most common chronic illnesses in these patients are respiratory diseases such as chronic obstructive lung disease (COPD), cardiovascular disease, and diabetes mellitus. In addition, certain habits such as cigarette smoking and alcohol abuse are also quite common in those with severe CAP, and cigarette smoking has been identified as a risk factor for bacteremic pneumococcal infection.[15] Other common illnesses in those with CAP include malignancy and neurologic illness (including seizures). Milder forms of pneumonia may be more severe on presentation if patients have not received antibiotic therapy prior to hospital admission. In addition, genetic differences in the immune response may predispose certain individuals to more severe forms of infection and adverse outcomes and may be reflected by a family history of severe pneumonia or adverse outcomes from infection.[16]

Box 43-1

Risk Factors for Developing Severe Community-Acquired Pneumonia

Advanced age (older than 65)
Comorbid illness
Chronic respiratory illness (including COPD), cardiovascular disease, diabetes mellitus, neurologic illness, renal insufficiency, malignancy
Cigarette smoking (risk for pneumococcal bacteremia)
Alcohol abuse
Absence of antibiotic therapy prior to hospitalization
Failure to contain infection to its initial site of entry
Immune suppression
Genetic polymorphisms in the immune response

Risk Factors for Mortality from Community-Acquired Pneumonia

In a meta-analysis of 33,148 patients with CAP, the overall mortality rate was 13.7%, but those admitted to the ICU had a mortality rate of 36.5%.[17] Eleven prognostic factors were significantly associated with different odds ratios (ORs) for mortality: male sex (OR = 1.3), pleuritic chest pain (OR = 0.5), hypothermia (OR = 5.0), systolic hypotension (OR = 4.8), tachypnea (OR = 2.9), diabetes mellitus (OR = 1.3), neoplastic disease (OR = 2.8), neurologic disease (OR = 4.6), bacteremia (OR = 2.8), leukopenia (OR = 2.5), and multilobar infiltrates (OR = 3.1). In other studies the clinical features that predict a poor outcome (Box 43-2) include advanced age (older than 65 years), preexisting chronic illness of any type, the absence of fever on admission, respiratory rate greater than 30 breaths per minute, diastolic or systolic hypotension, elevated blood urea nitrogen (BUN) (>19.6 mg/dL), profound leukopenia or leukocytosis, inadequate antibiotic therapy, need for mechanical ventilation, hypoalbuminemia, and the presence of certain "high-risk" organisms (type III pneumococcus, *S. aureus*, gram-negative bacilli, aspiration organisms, or postobstructive pneumonia). Other studies have found that when CAP patients have a delay in the initiation of appropriate antibiotic therapy of more than 4 hours, mortality is increased.[18-20]

Prognostic scoring approaches have been applied to predict mortality in CAP patients, and two prominent systems are the pneumonia severity index (PSI) and a modification of the British Thoracic Society rule, referred to as *CURB-65*.[8,21-23] The PSI is a complex scoring system that places patients into one of five risk groups for death on the basis of age, presence of male sex, comorbid illness, and certain laboratory and physical findings. This tool is good for predicting mortality, but it heavily weights age and comorbidity and does not account for the social needs of patients, so it may not help to define the optimal site of care for a given patient. The CURB-65 approach assesses the presence of confusion, elevated

Box 43-2

Risk Factors for a Poor Outcome from Community-Acquired Pneumonia

Patient-Related Factors
Male sex
Absence of pleuritic chest pain
Nonclassic clinical presentation (nonrespiratory presentation)
Neoplastic illness
Neurologic illness
Age older than 65 years
Family history of severe pneumonia or death from sepsis

Abnormal Physical Findings
Respiratory rate greater than 30 breaths per minute on admission
Systolic (<90 mm Hg) or diastolic (<60 mm Hg) hypotension
Tachycardia (>125 beats/min)
High fever (>40°C) or afebrile
Confusion

Laboratory Abnormalities
BUN >19.6 mg/dL
Leukocytosis or leukopenia
Multilobar radiographic abnormalities
Rapidly progressive radiographic abnormalities during therapy
Bacteremia
Hyponatremia (<130 mmol/L)
Multiple organ failure
Respiratory failure
Hypoalbuminemia
Arterial pH <7.35
Pleural effusion

Pathogen-Related Factors
High-risk organisms
Type III pneumococcus, *Staphylococcus aureus*, gram-negative bacilli (including *Pseudomonas aeruginosa*), aspiration organisms, severe acute respiratory syndrome
Possibly high levels of penicillin resistance (minimum inhibitory concentration of at least 4 mg/L) in pneumococcus

Therapy-Related Factors
Delay in initial antibiotic therapy (more than 4 to 6 hours)
Initial therapy with inappropriate antibiotic therapy
Failure to have a clinical response to empiric therapy within 72 hours

BUN, respiratory rate greater than 30 breaths per minute, low blood pressure (either systolic <90 mm Hg or diastolic <60 mm Hg), and whether the patient is at least 65 years old. If 3 of these 5 criteria are present, the predicted mortality rate is greater than 20%.[22,23]

Prognostic scoring systems have been used to define the need for ICU admission, with the suggestion that ICU care be considered for those in PSI classes IV and V or those with a CURB-65 score of 3 or higher.[8,23] This may not always be effective because up to 37% of those admitted to the ICU are in PSI classes I to III, and risk for death (which PSI can measure) is not always the same as need for intensive care.[8] Conversely, patients in higher PSI classes do not always need ICU care if they fall into these high-mortality-risk groups because of advanced age and comorbid illness, in the absence of physiologic findings of severe pneumonia. Neither of the current prognostic scoring systems is ideal by itself for defining the need for ICU care, and both can be regarded only as providing decision support information that must be supplemented by clinical assessment and judgment. In addition, the two scoring approaches should be viewed as being complementary to one another.[24] For example, in one recent study that compared the PSI with the CURB-65, both were good for predicting mortality and in identifying low-mortality-risk patients. However, the CURB-65 appeared to be more discriminating in defining mortality risk in the severely ill.[23] In another study, Ewig and colleagues[25] examined the 10 criteria in the 1993 American Thoracic Society guidelines to define severe CAP. They found that need for ICU was defined by the presence of two of three minor criteria (systolic BP <90, multilobar disease, $Pa{O_2}/F{IO_2}$ ratio <250) or one of two major criteria (need for mechanical ventilation or septic shock).[25] On the basis of these observations, the 2001 ATS guidelines for CAP recommend that severe CAP could be defined on the basis of the presence of these features.[1]

Other investigators have shown that the use of early and effective empiric therapy can improve survival in the setting of severe CAP. Retrospective data have shown a reduced mortality for admitted CAP patients who are treated within 4 hours of arrival to the hospital, compared with those who are treated later.[18] Ineffective initial empiric therapy was a potent predictor of death, being associated with a 60% mortality rate, compared with an 11% mortality rate for those who received initial effective therapy.[10] Similarly, in other studies of CAP, the combined use of a β-lactam and a macrolide antibiotic was associated with a lower mortality than if other therapies were given.[26,27]

Among patients with severe CAP, another important prognostic finding is clinical evolution, as reflected by radiographic progression during therapy.[6] The elderly with CAP often have a higher risk of dying than other populations, in part because adverse prognostic features are particularly common in this population.[3] In one series the mortality rate of nursing home–acquired pneumonia was 32%, compared with a mortality rate of 14% in other patients with CAP.[28] One factor that may explain this finding is that older patients often have atypical clinical presentations of pneumonia, which may lead to their being diagnosed at a later, more advanced stage of illness, resulting in an increased risk of death.[29] In part, as a consequence of these unusual clinical presentations, when these patients come to the hospital for evaluation, there are often delays in establishing the correct diagnosis. This leads to delays in initiating timely therapy and further increases the risk of dying.[20] Older patients from nursing homes who present with pneumonia are now included in a separate category, HCAP (discussed earlier).

Risk Factors for Ventilator-Associated Pneumonia

Mechanical ventilation for more than 2 days is the most important risk factor for NP, but other identified risks include being older than 60 years of age, malnutrition (serum albumin <2.2 g/dL), acute lung injury (acute respiratory distress syndrome [ARDS]), coma, burns, recent abdominal or thoracic surgery, multiple organ failure, transfusion of greater than 4 units of blood, transport from the ICU, prior antibiotic therapy, elevation of gastric pH (by antacids or histamine–type 2 blocking agents), large-volume aspiration, use of a nasogastric tube (rather than a tube placed in the jejunum or a tube inserted through the mouth), use of inadequate endotracheal tube cuff pressure, prolonged sedation and paralysis, maintaining patients in the supine position in bed, use of total parenteral nutrition feeding rather than enteral feeding, and repeated reintubation.[2] When a patient is mechanically ventilated, the risk of pneumonia is greatest in the first 5 days (3% per day). It declines thereafter to a risk of 2% per day for days 6 to 10 and to a rate of 1% per day or lower after this.[30] Noninvasive ventilation for respiratory failure is associated with a much lower risk of pneumonia than endotracheal intubation.

The relation between pneumonia and ARDS is particularly interesting. As many as one third of all cases of ARDS may be the result of pneumonia, and in some series pneumonia is the most common cause of acute lung injury. Not only can a variety of CAPs serve as a cause of ARDS, but secondary NP is the most common infection acquired by patients with established ARDS.[31-33] However, it has been shown that when patients with ARDS develop pneumonia, it is generally a late event, occurring after at least 7 days of mechanical ventilation.[32]

Pneumonia also presents a particular problem in the postoperative patient, particularly after elective thoracic, cardiac, or abdominal surgery. Other surgical groups that are at high risk for pneumonia include the victims of major trauma, particularly those suffering head injury and blunt chest trauma. When a patient has a pulmonary contusion, it may be difficult to distinguish this process from secondary lung infection on the basis of clinical and radiographic findings.

Risk Factors for Mortality from Ventilator-Associated Pneumonia

The factors associated with the greatest impact on attributable mortality are the accuracy and timeliness of initial antibiotic therapy. Use of the wrong therapy or delays in the initiation of therapy are the most important predictors of VAP mortality.[11,12,34] Initial appropriate therapy (using an agent to which the etiologic pathogen is sensitive) can reduce mortality, but administration of correct therapy at a later date, after initially incorrect therapy, may not effectively reduce mortality.[34] The benefit of accurate empiric therapy may not apply to all patients, but may be greatest for those infected with *P. aeruginosa* or *S. aureus*[35] and for those without the most severe degree of multiple organ dysfunction at the time of therapy.[36] For some patients, even using the correct therapy does not reduce mortality if it is not given in adequate doses and if the therapy does not reach the site of infection.

Closely related to appropriateness of initial therapy is the ability to decrease the number and/or spectrum of antimicrobial therapy once culture data become available, referred to as "de-escalation." Several recent studies have demonstrated that the use of de-escalation is associated with lower mortality compared with escalation or compared with a strategy of making no effort to reduce antibiotic therapy.[37,38] The choice of how to administer a specific agent can also affect outcome, and one study of MRSA VAP found that the mortality with intermittent infusion of vancomycin was twice as high as when this agent was administered by continuous infusion.[39] Other risk factors for mortality include prolonged duration of ventilation, coma on admission, creatinine greater than 1.5, transfer from another ward to the ICU, the presence of certain "high-risk" pathogens (particularly an antibiotic-resistant organism such as *P. aeruginosa*, *Acinetobacter* spp., or *S. aureus*), bilateral radiographic abnormalities, age older than 60 years, an ultimately fatal underlying condition, shock, prior antibiotic therapy, multiple-system organ failure, nonsurgical primary diagnosis, or a rising APACHE score during pneumonia therapy (Box 43-3).[2,40]

Box 43-3

Risk Factors for Mortality from Nosocomial Pneumonia

Physiologic Findings
Respiratory failure
Coma on admission
Multiple system organ failure
Acute physiology and chronic health evaluation II score rising to greater than 20 at 72 hours after diagnosis

Laboratory Findings
Creatinine >1.5 mg/dL
Gram-negative pneumonia, especially *Pseudomonas aeruginosa.* or *Acinetobacter* infection
Infection with any drug-resistant pathogen
Bilateral radiographic abnormalities
Fungal pneumonia
Polymicrobial infection

Historical Data
Prior antibiotic therapy
Age older than 60 years
Underlying fatal illness
Prolonged mechanical ventilation
Inappropriate antimicrobial therapy
Transfer to the intensive care unit from another ward

Although a number of host and bacteriologic factors enhance the mortality risk of NP, developing a superinfection, as opposed to a primary NP, is a particularly ominous finding. Rello observed that pulmonary superinfection had a 67% mortality, whereas primary NP had a 38% mortality rate.[41] In earlier studies, Graybill[42] observed a 62% mortality rate with superinfection pneumonia, compared with a 40% mortality rate for primary nosocomial lung infection. These data, as well as information from Fagon and colleagues[43] and Trouillet and colleagues,[44] emphasize the important role of prior antibiotics in enhancing mortality, an outcome that is likely the result of secondary infection by more virulent pathogens. As a result, antibiotic use has two pivotal roles in prognosticating outcome from NP: outcome is improved if the correct therapy is chosen, but if this therapy is followed by superinfection, then mortality is much more likely, generally because these infections involve difficult-to-treat, drug-resistant organisms.

PATHOGENESIS

General Overview

Pneumonia results when host defenses are overwhelmed by an infectious pathogen. This may occur because the patient has an inadequate immune response, often as the result of underlying comorbid illness; because of anatomic abnormalities (endobronchial obstruction, bronchiectasis); or because of therapy-induced dysfunction of the immune system (corticosteroids, endotracheal intubation).[2,45,46] In addition, genetic variations in the immune response make some patients prone to overwhelming infection because of an inadequate response and others prone to acute lung injury because of an excessive immune response.[16] In fact, the failure to localize the immune response to the respiratory site of initial infection may explain why some patients develop acute lung injury and sepsis because the inflammatory response extends to the entire lung and systemic circulation.[47] Pneumonia can even occur in patients who have an adequate immune system, if the host defense system is overwhelmed by a large inoculum of bacteria (massive aspiration) or by a particularly virulent organism to which the patient has no preexisting immunity or to which the patient has an inability to form an adequate immune response. With this paradigm in mind, it is easy to understand why previously healthy individuals develop infection with virulent pathogens such as viruses (influenza), *Legionella pneumophila*, *Mycoplasma pneumoniae*, *Chlamydophila pneumoniae*, and *Streptococcus pneumoniae*. However, for chronically ill patients, it is possible for them to be infected not by these virulent organisms but also by organisms that are not highly virulent. Because of host defense impairments, organisms that commonly colonize these patients can cause infection as a result of immune responses that are inadequate. These organisms include enteric gram-negative bacteria (*Escherichia coli*, *Klebsiella pneumoniae*, *P. aeruginosa*, *Acinetobacter* spp.) and fungi (*Aspergillus* and *Candida* spp.).

Bacteria can enter the lung via several routes, but aspiration from a previously colonized oropharynx is the most common way that patients develop pneumonia. Although most pneumonias result from micro-aspiration, patients can also aspirate large volumes of bacteria if they have impaired neurologic protection of the upper airway (stroke, seizure) or gastrointestinal illnesses that predispose to vomiting. Other routes of entry include inhalation, which applies primarily to viruses, *Legionella pneumophila* and *Mycobacterium tuberculosis*; hematogenous dissemination from extra-pulmonary sites of infection (right-sided endocarditis); and direct extension from contiguous sites of infection. In critically ill hospitalized patients, bacteria can also enter the lung from a colonized stomach (spreading retrograde to the oropharynx, followed by aspiration), a colonized or infected maxillary sinus, and colonization of dental plaque, or they can enter the lung directly via the endotracheal tube (from the hands of staff members). Recent studies have shown that the use of nasal tubes (into the stomach or trachea) can predispose to sinusitis and pneumonia, but that a gastric source of pneumonia pathogens in ventilated patients is not common.[48,49]

Role of Respiratory Therapy Equipment and Endotracheal Tubes

The endotracheal tube bypasses the filtration and host defense functions of the upper airway and can act as a conduit for direct inoculation of bacteria into the lung. This route may be particularly important if bacteria colonize the inside of the endotracheal tube itself.[50,51] This can occur if tracheobronchial organisms reach the endotracheal tube, a site where they are able to proliferate free from any impediment by the host defense system. Bacteria commonly grow at this location in a biofilm, which promotes the growth of multidrug-resistant organisms.[51] The biofilm represents a "sequestered nidus" of infection on the inside of the endotracheal tube, and particles can be dislodged every time the patient is suctioned. This is one of the mechanisms explaining the strong association between endotracheal intubation and pneumonia. Given the presence of biofilm in endotracheal tubes, it may be tempting to regularly reintubate patients and use a fresh tube, but this approach is not recommended because reintubation is itself a risk factor for VAP.[52]

Just as a patient's own tracheobronchial flora can spread to the endotracheal tube and amplify to large numbers, a similar phenomenon can occur in respiratory therapy equipment and in ventilator circuits.[53,54] Ventilator circuit colonization studies indicate that the greatest numbers are found at sites closest to the patient, not the ventilator, suggesting that circuit contamination originates from the patient.[53] One highly contaminated site is the condensation in the tubing, and this material can inadvertently be inoculated into patients if the tubing is not handled carefully. Because condensate colonization occurs in 80% of tubings within 24 hours, it does not appear that frequent ventilator circuit changes are useful or even able to reduce the risk of pneumonia; in one study, tubing changes every 24 hours (rather than every 48 hours) served as a risk factor for pneumonia.[55] Although most patients have ventilator tubing changed every 48 hours, several studies have shown no increased risk of infection if tubing is never changed or changed infrequently.[56,57] The use of heat moisture exchangers may be one way to avoid this problem, but they have had an inconsistent effect on preventing VAP. In addition, frequent changes of heat moisture exchangers (i.e., every 24 hours) have not been shown to have an impact on the incidence of VAP, and heat moisture exchangers should be changed no more frequently than every 48 hours.[58]

CLINICAL FEATURES OF PNEUMONIA

Historical Information

Pneumonia is generally characterized by symptoms of fever, cough, purulent sputum production, and dyspnea in a patient with a new or progressive lung infiltrate, with or without an associated pleural effusion. In nonventilated patients, cough is the most common finding. Cough is present in up to 80% of all CAP patients but is less common in those who are elderly, those with serious comorbidity, or individuals coming from nursing homes. Patients with CAP and an intact immune system generally have classic pneumonia symptoms, but the elderly patient can have a nonrespiratory presentation with symptoms of confusion, falling, failure to thrive, altered functional capacity, or deterioration in a preexisting medical illness such as congestive heart failure.[59] The absence of clear-cut respiratory symptoms and an afebrile status have themselves been predictors of an increased risk of death. Pleuritic chest pain is also commonly seen in patients with CAP, and in one study its absence was also identified as a poor prognostic finding.[60]

Certain clinical conditions are associated with specific pathogens in patients with CAP, and these associations should be evaluated when obtaining a history (Table 43-1).[1] For example, if the presentation is subacute, following contact with birds, rats, or rabbits, then the possibility of psittacosis, leptospirosis, tularemia, or plague should be considered. *Coxiella burnetii* (Q fever) is a concern with exposure to parturient cats, cattle, sheep, or goats; *Francisella tularensis* with rabbit exposure; hantavirus with exposure to mice droppings in endemic areas; *C. psittaci* with exposure to turkeys or infected birds; and Legionella with exposure to contaminated water sources (saunas). Following influenza, superinfection with pneumococcus, *S. aureus* including MRSA, and *Hemophilus influenzae* should be considered. With travel to endemic areas in Asia, the onset of respiratory failure after a preceding viral illness should lead to suspicion of a viral

Table 43-1. Likely Microbiologic Etiology and Host Epidemiology of CAP and NP/VAP

Epidemiology	Suspected Pathogen
Community-Acquired	
Alcoholism	Pneumococcus (including drug-resistant organisms), anaerobes, *H. influenzae, K. pneumoniae,* tuberculosis
Splenic dysfunction (sickle cell disease)	Pneumococcus, *H. influenzae*
COPD	Pneumococcus, *H. influenzae, M. catarrhalis*
Recent influenza infection	Pneumococcus, *S. aureus* (including MRSA), *H. influenzae,* enteric gram-negatives
High-risk aspiration	Anaerobes, enteric gram-negative bacilli
Neutropenia (including chronic corticosteroid therapy)	Gram-negative bacilli (esp. *P. aeruginosa*); *Aspergillus*
HIV infection (risk groups: intravenous drug abuser, tuberculosis, hemophilia, homosexual)	Pneumococcus, *H. influenzae, Pneumocystis jerovicii*
Rabbit exposure	*Francisella tularensis*
Exposure to farm animals, parturient cats	*Coxiella burnetii* (Q fever)
Exposure to mouse droppings	Hantavirus
Nursing Home–Acquired (no prior antibiotics and good functional status)	Pneumococcus (including drug-resistant organisms) and other organisms of CAP
Nursing Home–Acquired (prior antibiotics or poor functional status)	Gram-negative bacilli (including *P. aeruginosa, Acinetobacter* spp., ESBL-producing *Enterobacteriaceae*), *S. aureus* (including MRSA)
Hospital-Acquired and VAP	Gram-negative bacilli (including *P. aeruginosa, Acinetobacter* spp., ESBL-producing *Enterobacteriaceae*), *S. aureus* (including MRSA) Consider local microbiology

CAP, community-acquired pneumonia; COPD, chronic obstructive pulmonary disease; ESBL, extended-spectrum β-lactamase; MRSA, methicillin-resistant *Staphylococcus aureus;* NP/VAP, nosocomial pneumonia/ventilator-associated pneumonia.

pneumonia, which could be severe acute respiratory syndrome (SARS) or avian influenza.[61] Endemic fungi (coccidioidomycosis, histoplasmosis, and blastomycosis) occur in well-defined geographic areas and may present acutely with symptoms that overlap with acute bacterial pneumonia.

NP patients often present with less definitive clinical findings, particularly in those who are mechanically ventilated, and the clinical diagnosis is made in patients with a new or progressive radiographic infiltrate, along with some indication that infection is present (fever, purulent sputum, or leukocytosis). Recently, the Clinical Pulmonary Infection Score (CPIS) has been applied to patients with VAP. Six criteria are scored on a scale from 0 to 2 for each, and pneumonia is diagnosed with a total score of at least 6 (out of a maximum of 12).[62] The criteria are (1) fever, (2) purulence of sputum, (3) white blood cell count, (4) oxygenation, (5) degree of radiographic abnormality, and (6) the presence of pathogens in the sputum. Many studies have documented that VAP is diagnosed more often clinically than can be confirmed microbiologically, and the diagnosis is further obscured by the fact that most mechanically ventilated patients are colonized by *enteric gram-negative bacteria*. Thus the finding of potential pathogens in the sputum has no diagnostic value. In addition, some patients can have purulent sputum and fever, without a new infiltrate, and be diagnosed with purulent tracheobronchitis, an infectious complication of mechanical ventilation that may also require antibiotic therapy but is not pneumonia.[2]

In taking a history from a patient with NP, it is important to identify any risk factors for drug-resistant organisms. For ventilated patients, these include prolonged ICU stay (>5 days), recent antibiotic therapy, and the presence of health care–associated pneumonia.[2,44] In CAP patients, risk factors for drug-resistant pneumococcus include recent β-lactam therapy, exposure to a child in daycare, alcoholism, immune suppression, and multiple medical comorbidities.[1,63]

Physical Examination

Physical findings of pneumonia include tachypnea, crackles, rhonchi, and signs of consolidation (egophony, bronchial breath sounds, dullness to percussion). Patients should also be evaluated for signs of pleural effusion. In addition, extrapulmonary findings should be sought to rule out metastatic infection (arthritis, endocarditis, meningitis) or to add to the suspicion of an "atypical" pathogen such as *M. pneumoniae* or *C. pneumoniae*, which can lead to such complications as bullous myringitis, skin rash, pericarditis, hepatitis, hemolytic anemia, or meningoencephalitis. One of the most important ways to recognize severe CAP early in the course of illness is to carefully count the respiratory rate.[64,65] In the elderly, an elevation of respiratory rate can be the initial presenting sign of pneumonia, preceding other clinical findings by as much as 1 to 2 days. Tachypnea is present in more than 60% of all patients, more often in the elderly than in younger patients with pneumonia.[65] In addition, the counting of respiratory rate can identify the patient with severe illness, who commonly has a rate greater than 30 breaths per minute.

ETIOLOGIC PATHOGENS

Community-Acquired Pneumonia

Even with extensive diagnostic testing, an etiologic agent is defined in only about half of all patients with CAP, pointing out the limited value of diagnostic testing and the possibility that we do not know all the organisms that can cause CAP. The most common cause of CAP is pneumococcus *(S. pneumoniae)*, an organism which is frequently (at least 40% of the time) resistant to penicillin or other antibiotics, leading to the term *drug-resistant S. pneumoniae* (DRSP). Fortunately, most penicillin resistance in the United States is still more commonly of the "intermediate" type (penicillin minimum inhibitory concentration, or MIC, of 0.1 to 1.0 mg/L) and not of the high-level type (penicillin MIC of 2.0 or more).[66] Pneumococcal resistance to other antibiotics is also common, including macrolides and trimethoprim-sulfamethoxazole, but the clinical relevance and impact on outcome of these in vitro findings is uncertain, and most experts believe that only organisms with a penicillin MIC of greater than 4 mg/L lead to an increased risk of death.[67]

All patients with severe CAP should be considered to be at risk for DRSP and, in addition, those admitted to the ICU can have infection with atypical pathogens, which accounts for up to 20% of infections, either as primary infection or as co-pathogens. The identity of these organisms varies over time and geography. In some areas, *Legionella* is a common cause of severe CAP, whereas in others *Chlamydophila pneumoniae* or *M. pneumoniae* predominate.[68] Other important causes of severe CAP include *H. influenzae; S. aureus*, which includes MRSA (especially after influenza); and enteric gram-negatives (including *P. aeruginosa*) in patients with appropriate risk factors (particularly bronchiectasis and steroid-treated COPD). Recently, a toxin-producing strain of MRSA has been described to cause CAP in patients after influenza and other viral infections. This community-acquired MRSA is biologically and genetically distinct from the MRSA that causes NP, being more virulent and necrotizing and associated with the production of the Panton-Valentine Leukocidin (PVL).[69,70] Viruses can be a cause of severe CAP including influenza virus, as well as parainfluenza virus and epidemic viruses such as coronavirus (which caused SARS) and avian influenza.[61] Viral pneumonia (SARS and influenza) can lead to respiratory failure, and occasionally tuberculosis or endemic fungi can result in severe pneumonia.

Unusual etiologies should be considered, especially in patients who have epidemiologic risk factors for specific pathogens, as discussed earlier. In addition, certain "modifying factors" may be present that increase the likelihood of CAP caused by certain pathogens.[1] Thus the risk factors for DRSP include β-lactam therapy in the past 3 months, alcoholism, age older than 65 years, immune suppression, multiple medical comorbidities, and contact with a child in day care.[1,63] Risk factors for gram-negatives include residence in a nursing home, underlying cardiopulmonary disease, multiple medical comorbidities, probable aspiration, recent hospitalization, and recent antibiotic therapy. Many of these patients who are at risk for gram-negatives would now be reclassified as having health care–associated pneumonia (HCAP).[2,13] Some ICU patients are at risk for pseudomonal infection, whereas others are not, and the risk factors for *P. aeruginosa* infection are structural lung disease (bronchiectasis), corticosteroid therapy (>10 mg prednisone/day), broad-spectrum antibiotic therapy for more than 7 days in the past month, previous hospitalization, and malnutrition.[2] Although aspiration has often been considered a risk factor for anaerobic infection, a study of severe CAP in elderly patients with aspiration risk factors found that this population is likely to have gram-negative infection and, using sensitive microbiologic methods, anaerobes were uncommon.[71]

Nosocomial Pneumonia

All patients with this illness are at risk for infection with a group of bacteria referred to as "core organisms," which include pneumococcus, *H. influenzae*, methicillin-sensitive *S. aureus*, and nonresistant gram-negatives (*E. coli*, *Klebsiella* spp., *Enterobacter* spp., *Proteus* spp., and *Serratia marcescens*). In addition, some patients are also at risk for infection with other organisms, depending on the presence of risk factors such as prolonged hospitalization (>5 days), prior antibiotic therapy, recent hospitalization (within 90 days), recent antibiotic therapy, residence in a nursing home, or need for chronic care outside the hospital.[2,44] Patients with these risk factors can possibly be infected with multidrug-resistant (MDR) gram-positive and gram-negative organisms including MRSA, *P. aeruginosa*, and *Acinetobacter* spp. Recognition of the multiple risk factors associated with these resistant pathogens has made it clear that there are patients with "early-onset" NP (within the first 4 days of hospitalization) who can be infected with MDR organisms. In addition, up to 40% of patients with VAP have polymicrobial infection, involving multiple pathogens.[72]

Most data on NP bacteriology come from patients with VAP, and the etiology in nonventilated patients is presumed to be similar on the basis of the presence of risk factors for drug-resistant pathogens. In patients with VAP, infection with enteric gram-negatives is more common than infection with gram-positives, although the frequency of MRSA infection is increasing in this population, as is infection with *Acinetobacter* spp.[73] HCAP patients have been included in the NP guidelines as being a group at risk for infection with MDR gram-positive and gram-negatives.[2] Although most ICU-admitted patients with this illness are infected with these organisms, one study of nursing home patients requiring mechanical ventilation for severe pneumonia showed that these organisms were not present if the patient with severe pneumonia had not received antibiotics in the preceding 6 months and was also of a good functional status (as defined by activities of daily living).[74]

In approaching the bacteriology of NP, it is important to recognize that each hospital, as well as each ICU within a given hospital, can have its own unique flora and antibiotic susceptibility patterns, and thus therapy needs to be adapted to the organisms in a given institution, which can change over time.[75] In addition, it is especially important to know this information because antibiotic resistance is a common factor contributing to initially inappropriate empiric antibiotic therapy. Choosing the wrong empiric therapy has been a particular problem for organisms such as *P. aeruginosa*, *Acinetobacter* spp., and MRSA.[12] These highly resistant organisms can be present in up to 60% of patients who develop VAP after at least 7 days of ventilation and who have also received prior antibiotic therapy.[2,44]

Need for Respiratory Isolation

Patients with certain suspected pathogens should be placed in respiratory isolation to protect both the staff and other patients from infection with these organisms. This includes primarily airborne pathogens that spread via the aerosol route and includes any patient who is suspected of having tuberculosis, influenza, respiratory syncytial virus, or any other epidemic viral infection. Tuberculosis should be considered in any patient with a history of a preceding indolent pneumonia and in those with severe pneumonia and a history of HIV infection or recent immigration from endemic areas of infection. Patients with MRSA and highly resistant gram-negatives may need gown, glove, and mask precautions to avoid spread of these difficult-to-treat bacteria.

DIAGNOSTIC ISSUES

Diagnostic testing is performed for two purposes: (1) to define the presence of pneumonia and (2) to identify the responsible pathogen. In all forms of pneumonia, a chest radiograph is used to identify the presence of a lung infiltrate, but in some clinical settings, especially in suspected VAP, there can be noninfectious causes for the radiographic abnormality. Chest radiographic patterns are generally not useful for identifying the etiology of CAP, although findings such as pleural effusion (pneumococcus, *H. influenzae*, *M. pneumoniae*, pyogenic streptococci) and cavitation (*P. aeruginosa*, *S. aureus*, anaerobes, MRSA, tuberculosis) can suggest certain groups of organisms. Defining the etiologic pathogens in patients with CAP is often difficult because up to half of all such patients have no identified etiology, even with extensive diagnostic testing including cultures of blood and sputum. On the other hand, those with VAP commonly have bacteria present in samples of lower respiratory tract secretions, but the presence of a positive culture cannot reliably distinguish infection from colonization.

Community-Acquired Pneumonia

For patients with CAP, a chest radiograph not only confirms the presence of pneumonia but can be used to identify complicated and severe illness, if the patient has findings such as multilobar infiltrates, cavitation, or a loculated pleural effusion (suggesting an empyema). Although diagnostic testing is valuable in patients with CAP, therapy should never be delayed for the sole purpose of facilitating testing because delays in therapy have been associated with increased mortality. All CAP patients admitted to the ICU should have a chest radiograph, blood and lower respiratory tract (sputum, endotracheal aspirate, bronchoalveolar lavage, or bronchoscopic specimen) cultures, an arterial blood gas, and routine hematologic and blood chemistry testing. If the patient has a moderate-sized pleural effusion, this should be tapped and the fluid sent for culture and biochemical analysis. Patients with severe CAP should have two sets of blood cultures, and these are more likely to be positive if the patient has not received antibiotics at the time of sampling or if there are signs of systolic hypotension, tachycardia, dehydration, or an elevated white blood cell count.[76] The presence of bacteremia may not worsen prognosis but does allow identification of drug-resistant organisms, and most positive blood cultures in CAP reveal *Pneumococcus*.

Sputum culture should be accompanied by a Gram stain to guide interpretation of the culture results, but not to focus initial antibiotic therapy. In some situations, Gram stain can be used to broaden initial empiric therapy by enhancing the suspicion for organisms that are not covered in routine empiric therapy (such as *S. aureus* being suggested by the presence of clusters of gram-positive cocci, especially during a time of epidemic influenza). Routine serologic testing is not recommended. However, in patients with severe illness, the diagnosis of *Legionella pneumophila* can be made by urinary antigen testing, which is the test that is most likely to be positive at the time of admission, but a test that is specific only for serogroup I infection.[1,77] Examination of concentrated urine for pneumococcal antigen may also be valuable. Bronchoscopy is not indicated as a routine diagnostic test but may be necessary in some patients with severe forms of CAP to establish an etiologic diagnosis. In these patients the results of diagnostic testing can often be used to focus the initially broad-spectrum empiric therapy to a simpler regimen.[78]

Nosocomial Pneumonia

NP is diagnosed when a patient has been in the hospital for at least 48 to 72 hours and then develops a new or progressive infiltrate on chest radiograph, accompanied by at least 2 of the following 3: fever, leukocytosis, and purulent sputum. As mentioned, these clinical findings may be sensitive but not specific for infection, and efforts to improve the clinical diagnosis of pneumonia have involved the previously mentioned CPIS.[79] Many patients with suspected NP can have other diagnoses that can be suggested by the rapidity of the clinical response and by the nature of the clinical findings. These diagnoses include atelectasis and congestive heart failure (rapid clinical resolution) or, in the case of a lack of response to therapy, inflammatory lung diseases, extrapulmonary infection (sinusitis, central line infection, intraabdominal infection), or the presence of an unusual or drug-resistant pathogen. In addition, the presence of pathogenic organisms in sputum culture is not diagnostic because this finding cannot separate oropharyngeal and tracheobronchial colonization from parenchymal lung infection. The situation is further complicated because some ventilated patients can have nosocomial infectious tracheobronchitis, an illness with all the clinical features of pneumonia but with no new lung infiltrate, and this illness may also require antibiotic therapy and involve the same pathogens as VAP.[2]

In an effort to make the diagnosis more secure, and to avoid the overuse of antibiotics, some investigators have used quantitative sampling of lower respiratory secretions collected either bronchoscopically (bronchoalveolar lavage, protected specimen brush) or nonbronchoscopically (endotracheal aspirate, nonbronchoscopic catheter lavage), particularly in patients with suspected VAP. When quantitative cultures are collected, some investigators have defined the presence of pneumonia by the growth of bacteria at a concentration above a predefined threshold concentration.[4,5] Although the results can guide therapy decisions, most clinicians use antibiotic therapy, regardless of quantitative culture data, in patients who have clinical signs of sepsis and suspected pneumonia. Regardless of whether quantitative cultures are used, all patients with suspected NP should have a lower respiratory tract culture collected prior to the start of antibiotic therapy. If this is not a quantitative culture, then a sputum or tracheal aspirate should be obtained and the findings reported "semiquantitatively" as light, moderate, or heavy growth of bacteria.[2,5] Unfortunately, a negative culture is difficult to interpret if the patient has had initiation or change in antibiotic therapy in the preceding 72 hours. If, however, either a quantitative or semiquantitative culture is negative or does not show a highly resistant pathogen, and antibiotics have not been changed in the past 72 hours, the therapy can often be stopped or focused to a narrower spectrum.[2,80]

THERAPY

For all patients with severe pneumonia, algorithms for initial empiric therapy have been developed on the basis of the most likely etiologic pathogens in a given patient and clinical setting. If diagnostic testing reveals a specific etiologic pathogen, therapy can be focused on the results. In addition, as mentioned earlier, if an anticipated pathogen is not present in a diagnostic sample, it may be possible to stop empiric coverage of that organism (Fig. 43-1).

General Considerations

Until recently, combination empiric antibiotic therapy for severe pneumonia was universally given by physicians working in ICUs. The rationale for this approach was to provide broad antimicrobial coverage, prevent the emergence of resistance during therapy, and potentially provide synergistic activity if a β-lactam antibiotic was combined with an aminoglycoside (for *P. aeruginosa* pneumonia). However, only with bacteremic *P. aeruginosa* pneumonia has combination therapy (generally with an aminoglycoside and a β-lactam) been shown to be

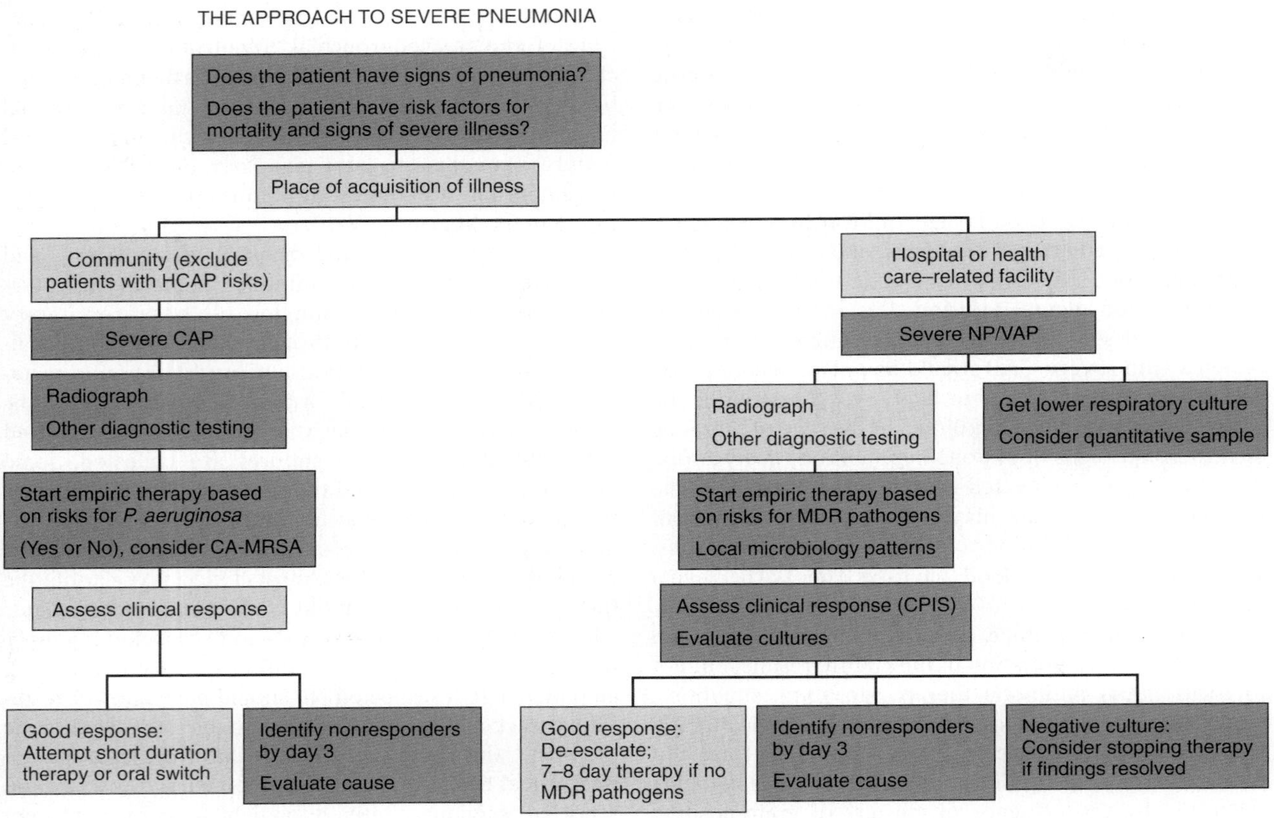

Figure 43-1. Algorithmic approach to managing severe pneumonia. Patients are categorized into community-acquired pneumonia and nosocomial pneumonia/ventilator-associated pneumonia. Each group undergoes diagnostic testing, followed by empiric therapy based on the most likely etiologic pathogens. The resulting clinical response is used to guide the duration of therapy or to decide whether to broaden the differential diagnosis to other processes. CA-MRSA = community-acquired MRSA; CAP = community-acquired pneumonia; MDR = multidrug resistant; NP = nosocomial pneumonia; VAP = ventilator-associated pneumonia.

superior to monotherapy.[81,82] One practical problem to this approach is the aminoglycosides themselves, a class of antibiotics with a narrow therapeutic-to-toxic ratio, and a high incidence of nephrotoxicity, particularly in elderly patients. When these drugs are used, it is important to use enough antibiotic to achieve high peak serum levels to optimize efficacy but to also avoid elevated trough levels, which correlate with toxicity. When peak serum levels have been monitored, levels of more than 7 μg/mL for gentamicin and tobramycin and more than 28 μg/mL for amikacin have been associated with more favorable outcomes.[83]

One other limitation of aminoglycosides is their relatively poor penetration into bronchial secretions, achieving only 40% of the serum concentrations at this site. In addition, antimicrobial activity is reduced at the low pH levels that are common in the bronchial secretions of patients with pneumonia. These concerns may explain the finding in one study that the addition of an aminoglycoside to imipenem had no added efficacy for severe NP and only added renal toxicity.[84] In addition, a meta-analysis of the value of adding an aminoglycoside to a β-lactam in critically ill patients, including many with pneumonia, found no therapeutic benefit.[82] It has now become standard to administer aminoglycosides by combining the total 24-hour dose into a single dose, rather than in divided doses.

This approach is theoretically possible because of the prolonged postantibiotic effect of aminoglycosides, and it is hoped that once-daily dosing can improve efficacy, reduce (or at least not increase) toxicity, and reduce the need for monitoring of serum levels. In one meta-analysis, this approach proved to have little advantage with regard to efficacy or safety.[85] Despite these findings, if aminoglycosides are used, once-daily dosing is recommended because it is simpler and requires less intensive monitoring (measuring only trough levels).

Recently, the development of newer cephalosporins, carbapenems, other β-lactams, and quinolones with high potency and broad antibacterial activity, as well as resistance to degradation by bacterial β-lactamases, has permitted the introduction of monotherapy, even in the patient with severe NP, provided that certain high-risk organisms are absent (*P. aeruginosa, Acinetobacter* spp., and MRSA). In the absence of these highly resistant pathogens, antibiotics that have been effective as monotherapy for severe VAP include imipenem, meropenem, cefepime, ciprofloxacin, high-dose levofloxacin (750 mg daily), and piperacillin/tazobactam.[2,86-90] In the patient with severe pneumonia, it is usually necessary to start therapy with multiple agents, but after tracheal aspirate or other lower respiratory tract cultures become available, it is usually possible to "de-escalate" to monotherapy, particularly if a highly resistant organism is absent.[80]

In some circumstances monotherapy should not be used: (1) in any patient with severe CAP because the efficacy of this approach has not been demonstrated; (2) in suspected bacteremic infection with *P. aeruginosa;* (3) in the empiric therapy of VAP, if the patient has risk factors for infection with MDR pathogens; and (4) if the patient has NP and both *S. aureus* and *P. aeruginosa* are identified in culture as the etiologic pathogens. Monotherapy should never be attempted with a third-generation cephalosporin because of the possibility of emergence of resistance during therapy as a result of production of chromosomal β-lactamases by the *Enterobacteriaceae* group of organisms.[2]

If *P. aeruginosa* is a target organism of therapy, antibiotics with efficacy against this pathogen are necessary. Anti-pseudomonal β-lactam antibiotics include the penicillins piperacillin, azlocillin, mezlocillin, ticarcillin, and carbenicillin; the third-generation cephalosporins ceftazidime and cefoperazone; the fourth-generation cephalosporin cefepime; the carbapenems imipenem and meropenem; the monobactam aztreonam (which can be used in the penicillin-allergic patient); and the β-lactam/β-lactamase inhibitor combinations ticarcillin/clavulanate and piperacillin/tazobactam. Other antipseudomonal agents include the quinolone ciprofloxacin; high-dose levofloxacin; and the aminoglycosides (amikacin, gentamicin, tobramycin).

Community-Acquired Pneumonia

For ICU-admitted CAP, initial therapy should be directed at DRSP, *Legionella* and other atypical pathogens, enteric gram-negatives, and other selected organisms on the basis of epidemiologic risk assessment. Therapy is chosen, depending on whether or not the patient is at risk for *P. aeruginosa* ("modifying" risk factors listed earlier). In all the treatment algorithms, no ICU-admitted CAP patient should receive empiric monotherapy, even with one of the new quinolones.[1] This recommendation is based on the fact that the efficacy (especially for meningitis complicating pneumonia), effective dosing and safety of quinolone monotherapy has not been established for ICU-admitted CAP patients. In one recent study comparing levofloxacin with a β-lactam/quinolone combination, the single-agent regimen was not shown to be effective for patients in septic shock and for those treated with mechanical ventilation.[91]

Recommended therapy for severe CAP, in the absence of pseudomonal risk factors, should be with a selected intravenous β-lactam (e.g., cefotaxime, ceftriaxone, ertapenem, a β-lactam/β-lactamase inhibitor combination) combined with either an intravenous macrolide or an intravenous antipneumococcal quinolone (levofloxacin or moxifloxacin). For patients with pseudomonal risk factors, therapy can be with a two-drug regimen using an anti-pseudomonal β-lactam (imipenem, meropenem, piperacillin/tazobactam, cefepime) plus ciprofloxacin (the most active anti-pseudomonal quinolone) or levofloxacin (750 mg daily). An alternative is a three-drug regimen using an anti-pseudomonal β-lactam plus an aminoglycoside plus either an intravenous antipneumococcal quinolone (levofloxacin or moxifloxacin) or a macrolide.[1,92]

In addition to the antibiotic approach to therapy outlined earlier, there are several other considerations in the management of CAP. These include providing the first dose of therapy as soon as possible (within 4 hours of arrival in the hospital) and providing coverage in all patients for atypical pathogens using either a macrolide or a quinolone in the regimen on the basis of the data that such an approach reduces mortality.[26,27,93] Even in patients with pneumococcal bacteremia, the use of combination therapy (generally with the addition of atypical pathogen coverage to pneumococcal coverage) has been associated with reduced mortality compared with monotherapy.[93] In addition, certain adjunctive therapies should be considered including oxygen, chest physiotherapy (if at least 30 mL of sputum daily and a poor cough response), aerosolized bronchodilators, and corticosteroids (if hypotension and possible relative adrenal insufficiency are present). An analysis of the use of activated protein C for patients with septic shock demonstrated that 35% of the patients in the pivotal clinical trial had underlying CAP and that activated protein C was most effective for those CAP patients with an APACHE II score of greater than 25, a PSI class of IV or V, and a CURB-65 score of at least 2. Patients with pneumococcal infection and inadequate therapy also benefited, although the benefit was minimal in those treated with adequate therapy.[94] In addition to their value in patients with relative adrenal insufficiency, corticosteroids may be helpful in severe CAP because of their immunomodulating effect. One randomized controlled trial of 48 patients compared hydrocortisone infusion (240 mg/day) with placebo and found that steroid therapy reduced mortality, length of stay, and duration of mechanical ventilation.[95] These findings require other studies to confirm the benefit of this adjunctive therapy.

Information on the proper duration of therapy in patients with CAP, especially those with severe illness, is scarce. Even in the presence of pneumococcal bacteremia, short durations of therapy may be possible, with a rapid switch from intravenous to oral therapy in responding patients. Generally, *S. pneumoniae* can be treated for 5 to 7 days if the patient is responding rapidly and has received accurate empiric therapy at the correct dose. The presence of extrapulmonary infection (such as meningitis) and the identification of certain pathogens (e.g., bacteremic *S. aureus*, *P. aeruginosa*) may require longer durations of therapy. Identification of *L. pneumophila* pneumonia may require at least 14 days of therapy, depending on severity of illness and host defense impairments, although recent data have shown that quinolone therapy may be the best approach to management and that durations as short as 5 days with levofloxacin 750 mg may be effective.[96] The switch to oral therapy, even in severely ill patients, may be facilitated by the use of quinolones, which are highly bioavailable and achieve the same serum levels with oral therapy as with intravenous therapy.

Currently, there is controversy about the need for empiric therapy directed against community-acquired MRSA. Most experts recommend that this organism be targeted in patients with severe, necrotizing CAP following a viral illness, particularly influenza. Optimal therapy has not been defined. Vancomycin alone may not be sufficient and has led to clinical failure, presumably because it is not active against the PVL toxin that accompanies community-acquired MRSA. For this reason, it may be necessary to add clindamycin to vancomycin or to use linezolid because both of these latter agents can inhibit toxin production.[70]

Nosocomial Pneumonia

Antibiotic therapy should be given promptly at the first clinical suspicion of pneumonia, and empiric therapy should be dictated by considering whether the patient is at risk for infection with MDR pathogens, primarily because of the presence of recent antibiotic therapy, a prolonged hospital stay, or the development of infection after residing in a nursing home or other chronic care setting (such as a dialysis center) or if there are other risk factors for HCAP. Patients without risks for MDR pathogens can be treated for the "core pathogens" listed earlier, generally with a monotherapy regimen of a second-generation or non-pseudomonal third-generation cephalosporin, a β-lactam/β-lactamase inhibitor combination, ertapenem, or a quinolone (levofloxacin or moxifloxacin).[2] If the patient is allergic to penicillin, therapy can be with a quinolone or the combination of clindamycin and aztreonam. Probably not all HCAP patients need therapy directed against MDR pathogens, and monotherapy has been successful in the absence of MDR pathogens. MDR pathogens are not likely in HCAP patients who do not have at least two of the following: severe infection, recent antibiotic therapy in the past 6 months, poor functional status.[71]

In the selection of an empiric therapy regimen, it is necessary to know which antibiotic the patient has recently received (within the past 14 days) and to choose an agent that is in a different class because repeated use of the same class of antibiotic may drive resistance to that class, especially if the pathogen is *P. aeruginosa*.[97] Similar findings have been made for patients with bacteremic pneumococcal pneumonia and CAP, and repeat use of an agent within 3 months may mean that the patient is being treated with an agent to which pneumococcus is more likely to be resistant.[98] In addition, the recent use of quinolones may present a particular problem because, in the ICU, recent quinolone therapy may predispose to not only quinolone-resistant organisms but also to infection with MDR pathogens, extended-spectrum β-lactamase producing gram-negatives, and MRSA.[99] For all patients with VAP, it is important to use the correct dose of antibiotic (see Box 43-4 for recommended doses for patients with normal renal function).[2]

Although it is possible to identify, on the basis of risk factors, the patient who is likely to be infected with MDR pathogens, it is important to realize that each hospital and each ICU has its own unique organisms and patterns of antimicrobial resistance and that these patterns change over time. Therefore it is necessary to monitor local patterns of resistance and to choose empiric therapy that is likely to be effective in a given clinical setting.[75] One other concept that has been incorporated into some studies of empiric therapy is that of "antibiotic rotation," which means the standard empiric regimens are intentionally varied over time to expose bacteria to different antibiotics and thus minimize the selection pressure for resistance. In some studies this approach has been effective in reducing the incidence of infection with resistant organisms.[100] One limitation of antibiotic rotation is that it may mean the use of the same regimen repeatedly in the same patient, and this may itself be a risk factor for selecting for resistance. In addition, there are unanswered questions about how long each cycle of therapy should last, what agents should be cycled, how effective the approach is for medical versus surgical patients, and whether cycling should focus on gram-positive and gram-negative organisms.[101]

Patients at risk for MDR pathogens generally require combination therapy rather than monotherapy. Combination therapy is most valuable because it provides broad-spectrum coverage, thereby minimizing the chance of initially inappropriate therapy. Recent data have shown that combination therapy using an aminoglycoside with a β-lactam is no more effective than monotherapy with a β-lactam for severe infections including those caused by *P. aeruginosa*, but dual-pseudomonal therapy is still recommended for patients at risk for this pathogen in order to minimize the chance of initially ineffective therapy.[2,82] The empiric therapy for patients at risk for MDR pathogens should include an aminoglycoside or quinolone (ciprofloxacin or high-dose levofloxacin) plus an anti-pseudomonal β-lactam (imipenem, meropenem, piperacillin/tazobactam, aztreonam, or cefepime). If the patient is at risk for a second ICU-acquired infection (and most are), it may be prudent to use an aminoglycoside for the first episode of infection, reserving the quinolone for

Box 43-4

Doses of Selected Antibiotics for Ventilator-Associated Pneumonia (Normal Renal Function)

Ciprofloxacin: 400 mg every 8 hours; Levofloxacin 750 mg every day
Imipenem 1 gm every 8 hours or 500 mg every 6 hours; meropenem 1 gm every 6 to 8 hours
Piperacillin/tazobactam 4.5 gm every 6 hours
Cefepime 1 to 2 gm every 8 to 12 hours
Ceftazidime 2 gm every 8 hours
Gentamicin or tobramycin 7 mg/kg/d or amikacin 20 mg/kg/d
Linezolid 600 mg every 12 hours
Vancomycin 15 mg/kg every 12 hours

any subsequent infection, because of concern about quinolone induction of MDR, which could limit subsequent therapy options.[102] If the patient is suspected of having MRSA because of a tracheal aspirate Gram stain showing gram-positive organisms or because of other risk factors, a third drug should be added. This could be either linezolid or vancomycin, and recent data have suggested the superiority of linezolid for both survival and clinical cure in patients who have been documented to have MRSA VAP.[103]

Many patients with NP will get an initial empiric therapy that is broad-spectrum, and thus it is important to consider "de-escalation" of the initial regimen as serial clinical and microbiologic data become available (see Fig. 43-1).[80] If the patient has received a broad-spectrum regimen and the cultures do not show MDR organisms, then the patient can finish therapy with any of six monotherapy regimens that have been documented to be effective for severe VAP, in the absence of MDR organisms: ciprofloxacin, imipenem, meropenem, piperacillin/tazobactam, cefepime, and high-dose levofloxacin. If *P. aeruginosa* is present, combination therapy with a β-lactam and aminoglycoside should continue for 5 days, after which the patient can be switched to monotherapy with an agent to which the organism is sensitive.[2] When de-escalation has been used, meaning either the switch to a more narrow spectrum regimen, the use of fewer drugs, or both, mortality in VAP has been reduced, compared with when patients do not have de-escalation.[37,38,80] Many unrealized opportunities exist for using this approach in patients with *P. aeruginosa* infection and sensitive pathogens and in those with a good clinical response and negative respiratory tract cultures.[80]

If the lower respiratory tract cultures are negative, it may be possible to stop therapy (especially if an alternative diagnosis is suspected) or to shorten the duration of therapy. In addition, if cultures show that the initial empiric regimen was appropriate and if the patient has a good clinical response (reflected by a drop in the CPIS), then it may be possible to reduce the duration of therapy to as little as 7 to 8 days, although this may not be pos-sible if the etiologic pathogen is *P. aeruginosa* or MRSA.[104]

Adjunctive therapeutic measures are necessary in some patients including chest physiotherapy, aerosolized bronchodilators, and mucolytic agents. For selected patients who are infected with highly resistant organisms and are not responding to systemic antibiotics, it may be valuable to add aerosolized antibiotics (e.g., gentamicin, tobramycin, colistin, ceftazidime). Aerosolized administration of antibiotics offers the advantage of achieving high concentrations of antibiotics at the site of infection. As a result, it may be possible to overcome the problems of poor lung penetration of certain agents (aminoglycosides) and provide the high levels of antibiotics that are necessary to kill certain resistant organisms. Locally administered antibiotics are rarely absorbed, and systemic toxicity is minimized. Despite these theoretical advantages, many efficacy questions remain to be answered by clinical trials. Pending more information, locally instilled or aerosolized antibiotics are not usually recommended for routine treatment of pneumonia but may have a role as adjunctive therapy in patients with MDR organisms not responding to systemic therapy.[105]

EVALUATION OF NONRESPONDING PATIENTS

Because pneumonia is a clinical syndrome, not all patients with this diagnosis actually have lung infection and some may be infected with an unusual or nonsuspected pathogen. In addition, some patients can develop complications of the illness or its therapy, and all of these situations may lead to an apparent nonresponse to therapy.

With effective therapy, most patients with CAP become afebrile by days 3 to 5, and most have a clinical response by day 3. Similarly, even with VAP, most patients have some improvement, particularly in oxygenation, by day 3.[2,62] Nonresponding patients with either CAP or VAP should be evaluated for alternative diagnoses (inflammatory lung disease, atelectasis, heart failure, malignancy, pulmonary hemorrhage, pulmonary embolus, a nonpneumonic infection); a resistant or unusual pathogen (including tuberculosis and fungal infection); a pneumonia complication (empyema, lung abscess, drug fever, antibiotic-induced colitis); or a secondary site of infection (central line infection, intra-abdominal infection) (Box 43-5). The evaluation of a nonresponding patient should be individualized but may include CT scanning of the

Box 43-5

Mimics of Infectious Pneumonia in the Mechanically Ventilated Patient: Consider in the Nonresponding Patient

Nonpneumonia Diagnoses
- Primary pulmonary malignancy: lung cancer, lymphoma
- Metastatic cancer: including tumor emboli, lymphangitic spread of cancer
- Pulmonary vasculitis: including Wegener's granulomatosis, Goodpasture's syndrome
- Alveolar hemorrhage
- Pulmonary emboli and/or infarction
- Atelectasis
- Pleural effusion
- Acute respiratory distress syndrome
- Heart failure
- Extrapulmonary infection: central line, intra-abdominal
- Lung contusion after thoracic trauma

Iatrogenic Processes
- Drug-induced pneumonitis
- Aspiration of enteral feeding
- Pulmonary artery catheter complications
- Hemorrhage
- Infarction
- Pneumothorax

chest, pulmonary angiography, bronchoscopy, and occasionally open lung biopsy.

PREVENTION

Prevention of CAP is important for all groups of patients, especially the elderly patient, who is at risk for both a higher frequency of infection and a more severe course of illness. Appropriate patients should be vaccinated with both pneumococcal and influenza vaccines, and cigarette smoking should be stopped in all at-risk patients. Even for the patient who is recovering from CAP, immunization while in the hospital is appropriate to prevent future episodes of infection. The evaluation of all patients for vaccination need and the provision of information about smoking cessation are now performance standards used to evaluate the hospital care of CAP patients. If there is uncertainty about whether the patient has recently been vaccinated, it is probably best to give a pneumococcal vaccination because repeat administration, even more often than recommended, is not generally associated with an adverse reaction.[106] Hospital-based immunization is recommended. One study found that among 1633 patients with pneumonia treated in the hospital, 62% had been hospitalized in the preceding 4 years.[107] In addition, 80% of these patients had a high-risk condition that would have qualified them to receive pneumococcal vaccine. On the basis of these observations, it seems likely that many cases of CAP could be prevented if pneumococcal vaccine were given to all hospitalized patients who qualify for the vaccine, regardless of why they are hospitalized.

Although no single method can reliably prevent NP, multiple small interventions may have benefit, especially those focused on modifiable risk factors for infection. Recently, these interventions have been combined into "ventilator bundles," which have been demonstrated to reduce the incidence of VAP if applied carefully.[108,109] Most of these bundles include multiple interventions, so it is difficult to know which individual manipulations are most valuable. Successful bundles have included interventions such as elevation of the head of the bed to 30 degrees (to avoid the risk of aspiration present with the supine position), daily interruption of sedation to attempt weaning, peptic ulcer disease prophylaxis, endotracheal tube suctioning (possibly with a closed suction system), hand washing, careful oral care, and tight control of blood glucose.[110] Despite the success of this approach, one recent randomized study has demonstrated a lack of benefit and feasibility of routine head-of-the-bed elevation.[111]

Other widely used measures in mechanically ventilated patients are avoidance of large inocula of bacteria into the lung (careful handling of ventilator circuit tubing); mobilization of respiratory secretions (frequent suctioning, use of rotational bed therapy in selected individuals); nutritional support (enteral preferred over parenteral); placing of feeding tubes into the small bowel (to avoid aspiration, which is more likely with stomach tubes); and avoidance of large gastric residuals when giving enteral feeding. In addition, any tube inserted into the stomach or trachea should be inserted through the mouth and not the nose, whenever possible, to avoid obstructing the nasal sinuses and prevent nosocomial sinusitis, which can lead to NP.[110] A specially adapted endotracheal tube that allows for continuous aspiration of subglottic secretions may interrupt the oropharyngeal to tracheal transfer of bacteria and reduce the incidence of pneumonia.[112] Because endotracheal intubation is a risk for pneumonia, noninvasive positive pressure ventilation should be used whenever possible. This approach is associated with a lower pneumonia risk than traditional mechanical ventilation. Prophylactic systemic or topical antibiotics have no specific role, but some data suggest that patients with coma caused by stroke or head trauma and those who may have aspirated during an emergent intubation may benefit from a 24-hour course of systemic antibiotics.[113] "Selective digestive decontamination," which includes systemic and topical intestinal antibiotics, remains controversial as a method to reduce the incidence of pneumonia. Literature support exists in some selected populations. This approach carries the risk of promoting antibiotic resistance.[2]

KEY POINTS

- NP is the hospital-acquired infection most likely to lead to the death of patients. Typically the crude mortality rate of this infection is 50%, with even higher rates seen in patients who are mechanically ventilated. Of all patients who die with NP, from one third to one half of these deaths are the direct result of infection termed "attributable mortality."
- A good, simple predictor of a poor outcome from CAP is the presence of at least 3 of the CURB-65 indicators: confusion, admission blood urea nitrogen greater than 19.6 mg/dL, low blood pressure (systolic blood pressure <90 mm Hg, or diastolic blood pressure lower than 60 mm Hg), a respiratory rate higher than 30 breaths per minute, and age of at least 65.
- The most important risk factor for mortality in patients with VAP is inappropriate antibiotic therapy. Other risk factors for mortality include respiratory failure, coma on admission, bilateral radiographic abnormalities, and infection with resistant organisms.
- A number of common therapeutic interventions increase the risk of hospital-acquired pneumonia and should be chosen carefully. These include endotracheal intubation, corticosteroids, antibiotics, immunosuppressives, total parenteral nutrition, and certain strategies for feeding enterally and providing prophylaxis for intestinal bleeding.
- The most common pathogen for CAP is pneumococcus, with *Legionella pneumophila* and other atypical pathogens being a major concern in patients with severe CAP.
- Enteric gram-negative bacteria are the most common pathogens causing NP, but MDR pathogens including gram-negatives and *Staphylococcus aureus* (including MRSA) can also occur, particularly when the patient has been in the hospital for at least 5 days and has received antibiotic therapy before the onset of pneumonia.

- NP is often treated after making a clinical diagnosis, but this clinical approach is overly sensitive, and some patients who satisfy a clinical definition of pneumonia will have other disease processes.
- Invasive diagnostic methods can be used to quantify the bacteriology of NP patients but may not always identify all patients with pneumonia, particularly in the presence of prior antibiotic therapy. Methodologic questions make these tools controversial in patient management, and it is uncertain if they favorably alter patient outcome.
- Each ICU has its own unique bacteriology, and this information should be considered when choosing empiric therapy of NP.
- In choosing an antibiotic for a patient with severe pneumonia, take a history of recent antibiotic use and avoid using any agent prescribed in the past 3 months for a patient with CAP and any agent prescribed in the past 2 weeks for a patient with VAP.
- Although initial empiric antibiotic therapy of severe pneumonia is necessarily broad-spectrum, efforts should be made to re-evaluate clinical response and microbiologic data to narrow the spectrum of therapy and the number of drugs. This can usually be done after 3 days, and patients with a good clinical response can have the duration of therapy reduced to 7 to 10 days.
- If the patient has not improved after 3 days of therapy, it is necessary to determine if there is another disease process other than pneumonia or if the infection is caused by a drug-resistant or unsuspected pathogen.
- In treating patients with severe pneumonia it is important to use the correct dose of the correct antibiotic. Using too low a dose can be a factor leading to poor outcome.
- CAP can be prevented by the use of vaccines, particularly in hospital-based programs. The most widely used strategy for NP prevention is the use of "ventilator bundles," which may be valuable if carefully applied, but the impact of each individual component is unknown.

REFERENCES

1. Niederman MS, Mandell LA, Anzueto A, et al: Guidelines for the management of adults with community-acquired lower respiratory tract infections: Diagnosis, assessment of severity, antimicrobial therapy and prevention. Am J Respir Crit Care Med 2001;163:1730-1754.
2. Niederman MS, Craven DE, Bonten MJ, et al: Guidelines for the management of adults with hospital-acquired, ventilator-associated, and healthcare-associated pneumonia. Am J Respir Crit Care Med 2005;171:388-416.
3. Kaplan V, Clermont G, Griffin MF, et al: Pneumonia: Still the old man's friend? Arch Intern Med 2003; 163:317-323.
4. Fagon JY, Chastre J, Wolff M, et al: Invasive and noninvasive strategies for management of suspected ventilator-associated pneumonia: A randomized trial. Ann Intern Med 2000;132: 621-630.
5. The Canadian Critical Care Trials Group. A randomized trial of diagnostic techniques for ventilator-associated pneumonia. N Engl J Med 2006;355:2619-2630.
6. Torres A, Serra-Batlles J, Ferrer A, et al: Severe community-acquired pneumonia. Epidemiology and prognostic factors. Am Rev Respir Dis 1991;144:312.
7. Pachon J, Prados MD, Capote F, et al: Severe community-acquired pneumonia: Etiology, prognosis, and treatment. Am Rev Respir Dis 1990;142:369.
8. Ewig S, de Roux A, Bauer T, et al: Validation of predictive rules and indices of severity for community acquired pneumonia. Thorax 2004;59:421-427.
9. Woodhead M, Welch CA, Harrison DA, et al: Community-acquired pneumonia on the intensive care unit: Secondary analysis of 17,869 cases in the ICNARC case mix programme database. Crit Care 2006;10(Suppl 2): S1.
10. Leroy O, Santre C, Beuscart C: A 5-year study of severe community-acquired pneumonia with emphasis on prognosis in patients admitted to an ICU. Intensive Care Med 1995;21:24.
11. Heyland DK, Cook DJ, Griffith L, et al: The attributable morbidity and mortality of ventilator-associated pneumonia in the critically ill patient. The Canadian Critical trials group. Am J Respir Crit Care Med 1999;159:1249-1256.
12. Kollef MH: Inadequate antimicrobial treatment: an important determinant of outcome for hospitalized patients. Clin Infect Dis 2000;31(Suppl 4):131-138.
13. Kollef MH, Shorr A, Tabak YP, et al: Epidemiology and outcomes of health-care-associated pneumonia: Results from a large US database of culture positive patients. Chest 2005;128: 3854-3862.
14. Ruiz M, Ewig S, Torres A, et al: Severe community-acquired pneumonia: Risk factors and follow-up epidemiology. Am J Respir Crit Care Med 1999; 160:923-929.
15. Nuorti JP, Butler JC, Farley MM, et al: Cigarette smoking and invasive pneumococcal disease. N Engl J Med 2000;342:681-689.
16. Waterer GW, Quasney MW, Cantor RM, et al: Septic shock and respiratory failure in community-acquired pneumonia have different TNF polymorphism associations. Am J Respir Crit Care Med. 2001;163: 1599-1604.
17. Fine MJ, Smith MA, Carson CA, et al: Prognosis and outcomes of patients with community-acquired pneumonia. A meta-analysis. JAMA 1996;275: 134-141.
18. Houck PM, Bratzler DW, Nsa W, et al: Timing of antibiotic administration and outcomes for Medicare patients hospitalized with community-acquired pneumonia. Arch Intern Med 2004; 164:637-644.
19. Waterer GW, Kessler LA, Wunderink RG: Delayed administration of antibiotics and atypical presentation in community-acquired pneumonia. Chest 2006;130:11-15.
20. Meteresky ML, Sweeney TA, Getzow MB, et al: Antibiotic timing and diagnostic uncertainty in Medicare patients with pneumonia: Is it reasonable to expect all patients to receive antibiotics within 4 hours? Chest 2006;130:16-21.
21. Fine MJ, Auble TE, Yealy DM, et al: A prediction rule to identify low-risk patients with community-acquired pneumonia. N Engl J Med 1997;336:243-250.
22. Lim WS, van der Erden MM, Laing R, et al: Defining community acquired pneumonia severity on presentation to hospital: An international derivation and validation study. Thorax 2003; 58:377-382.
23. Aujesky D, Auble TE, Yealy DM, et al: Prospective comparison of three validated prediction rules for prognosis in community-acquired pneumonia. Am J Med 2005;118:384-392.
24. Niederman MS, Feldman C, Richards GA: Combining information from prognostic scoring tools for CAP: An American view on how to get the best of all worlds. Eur Resp J 2006;27:9-11.
25. Ewig S, Ruiz M, Mensa J, et al: Severe community-acquired pneumonia: Assessment of severity criteria. Am J Respir Crit Care Med 1998;158: 1102-1108.
26. Gleason PP, Meehan TP, Fine JM, et al: Associations between initial antimicrobial therapy and medical outcomes for hospitalized elderly patients with pneumonia. Arch Intern Med 1999;159:2562-2572.

27. Houck PM, MacLehose RF, Niederman MS, et al: Empiric antibiotic therapy and mortality among Medicare pneumonia inpatients in 10 Western atates: 1993, 1995, and 1997. Chest 2001;119:1420-1426.
28. Marrie TJ, Blanchard W: A comparison of nursing home-acquired pneumonia patients with patients with community-acquired pneumonia and nursing home patients without pneumonia. J Am Geriatr 1997;45:50.
29. Starczewski AR, Allen SC, Vargas E, et al: Clinical prognostic indices of fatality in elderly patients admitted to hospital with acute pneumonia. Age Ageing 1988;17:181.
30. Cook DJ, Walter SD, Cook RJ: Incidence of and risk factors for ventilator-associated pneumonia in critically ill patients. Ann Intern Med 1998;129:433-440.
31. Sutherland KR, Steinberg KP, Maunder RJ, et al: Pulmonary infection during the acute respiratory distress syndrome. Am J Respir Crit Care Med 1995; 152:550-556.
32. Chastre J, Trouillet JL, Vuagnet A, et al. Nosocomial pneumonia in patients with acute respiratory distress syndrome. Am J Respir Crit Care Med 1998;157:1165-1172.
33. Seidenfeld JJ, Pohl DF, Bell RD, et al: Incidence, site, and outcome of infections in patients with the adult respiratory distress syndrome. Am Rev Respir Dis 1986;134:12.
34. Luna CM, Vujacich P, Niederman MS, et al: Impact of BAL data on the therapy and outcome of ventilator associated pneumonia. Chest 1997;111:676-685.
35. Dupont H, Mentec H, Sollet JP, Bleichner G: Impact of appropriateness of initial antibiotic therapy on the outcome of ventilator-associated pneumonia. Intensive Care Med 2001;27:355-362.
36. Clec'h C, Timsit JF, De Lassence A, et al: Efficacy of adequate antibiotic therapy in ventilator-associated pneumonia: Influence of disease severity. Intensive Care Med 2004;30:1327-1333.
37. Kollef MH, Morrow LE, Niederman MS, et al: Clinical characteristics and treatment patterns among patients with ventilator-associated pneumonia. Chest 2006;129:1210-1218.
38. Soo Hoo GW, Wen E, Nguyen TV, Goetz MD: Impact of clinical guidelines in management of severe hospital-acquired pneumonia. Chest 2005;128:2778-2787.
39. Rello J, Sole-Violan J, Sa-borges M, et al: Pneumonia caused by oxacillin-resistant Staphylococcus aureus treated with glycopeptides. Crit Care Med 2005;33:1983-1987.
40. Chastre J, Fagon JY: Ventilator-associated pneumonia. Am J Respir Crit Care Med 2002;165:867-903.
41. Rello J, Quintana E, Ausina V, et al: Incidence, etiology, and outcome of nosocomial pneumonia in mechanically ventilated patients. Chest 1991;100:439.
42. Graybill JR, Marshall LW, Charache P, et al: Nosocomial pneumonia: A continuing major problem. Am Rev Respir Dis 1973;108:1130.
43. Fagon JY, Chastre J, Hance A, et al: Nosocomial pneumonia in ventilated patients: A cohort study evaluation attributable mortality and hospital stay. Am J Med 1993;94:281.
44. Trouillet J-L, Chastre J, Vuagnat A, et al: Ventilator-associated pneumonia caused by potentially drug-resistant bacteria. Am J Respir Crit Care Med 1998;157:531.
45. Skerrett SJ, Niederman MS, Fein AM: Respiratory infections and acute lung injury in systemic illness. Clin Chest Med 1989;10:469.
46. Campbell GD, Niederman MS, Broughton WA, et al: Hospital-acquired pneumonia in adults: Diagnosis, assessment of severity, initial antimicrobial therapy, and preventative strategies: A consensus statement. Am J Respir Crit Care Med 1996;153:1711.
47. Niederman MS, Ahmed QA: Inflammation in severe pneumonia: Act locally, not globally. Crit Care Med 1999;27:2030.
48. Niederman MS, Craven DE: Devising strategies for preventing nosocomial pneumonia: Should we ignore the stomach? Clin Infect Dis 1997;24:320.
49. Holzapfel L, Chastang C, Demingeon G, et al: A randomized study assessing the systematic search for maxillary sinusitis in nasotracheally mechanically ventilated patients: Influence of nosocomial maxillary sinusitis on the occurrence of ventilator-associated pneumonia. Am J Respir Crit Care Med 1999;159:695.
50. Sottile FD, Marrie TJ, Prough DS, et al: Nosocomial pulmonary infection: Possible etiologic significance of bacterial adhesion to endotracheal tubes. Crit Care Med 1986;14:265.
51. Prince AS: Biofilms, antimicrobial resistance, and airway infection. N Engl J Med 2002;347:1110-1111.
52. Torres A, Gatell JM, Aznar E, et al: Re-intubation increases the risk for nosocomial pneumonia in patients needing mechanical ventilation. Am J Respir Crit Care Med 1995;152:137.
53. Craven DE, Goularte TA, Make BJ: Contaminated condensate in mechanical ventilator circuits: A risk factor for nosocomial pneumonia. Am Rev Respir Dis 1984;129:625.
54. Craven DE, Lichtenberg DA, Goularte TA, et al: Contaminated medication nebulizers in mechanical ventilator circuits. Source of bacterial aerosols. Am J Med 1984;77:834.
55. Craven DE, Connolly MG, Jr., Lichtenberg DA, et al. Contamination of mechanical ventilators with tubing changes every 24 or 48 hours. N Engl J Med 1982;306:1505.
56. Dreyfuss D, Djedaini K, Weber P, et al: Prospective study of nosocomial pneumonia and of patient and circuit colonization during mechanical ventilation with circuit changes every 48 hours versus no change. Am Rev Respir Dis 1991;143:738.
57. Hess D, Burns E, Romagnoli D, et al: Weekly ventilator circuit changes: A strategy to reduce costs without affecting pneumonia rates. Anesthesiology 1995;82:902.
58. Djedaini K, Billiard M, Mier L, et al: Changing heat and moisture exchangers every 48 hours rather than 24 hours does not affect their efficacy and the incidence of nosocomial pneumonia. Am J Respir Crit Care Med 1995;152:1562.
59. Metaly JP, Schulz R, Li Y-H, et al: Influence of age on symptoms at presentation in patients with community-acquired pneumonia. Arch Intern Med 1997;157:1453-1459.
60. Fine MJ, Orloff JJ, Arisumi D, et al: Prognosis of patients hospitalized with community-acquired pneumonia. Am J Med 1990;88:1N-8N.
61. Lapinsky SE, Hawryluck L: ICU management of severe acute respiratory syndrome. Intensive Care Med 2003;29:870-875.
62. Luna CM, Blanzaco D, Niederman MS, et al: Resolution of ventilator-associated pneumonia: Prospective evaluation of the clinical pulmonary infection score as an early clinical predictor of outcome. Crit Care Med 2003;31:676-682.
63. Clavo-Sánchez AJ, Girón-González JA, López-Prieto D, et al: Multivariate analysis of risk factors for infection due to penicillin-resistant and multidrug-resistant Streptococcus pneumoniae: A multicenter study. Clin Infect Dis 1997;24:1052.
64. Van Eeden SF, Coetzee AR, Joubert JR: Community-acquired pneumonia-factors influencing intensive care admission. S Afr Med J 1988;73:77.
65. McFadden JP, Price RC, Eastwood HD, Briggs RS: Raised respiratory rate in elderly patients: A valuable physical sign. Br Med J 1982;284:626-627.
66. Doern GV, Richter SS, Miller A, et al: Antimicrobial resistance among Streptococcus pneumoniae in the United States: Have we begun to turn the corner on resistance to certain antimicrobial classes? Clin Infect Dis 41:139-148, 2005.
67. Feikin DR, Schuchat A, Kolczak M, et al: Mortality from invasive pneumococcal pneumonia in the era of antibiotic resistance, 1995-1997. Am J Public Health 2000;90:223-229.
68. Ruiz M, Ewig S, Torres A, et al: Severe community-acquired pneumonia: Risk factors and follow-up epidemiology. Am J Respir Crit Care Med 1999;160:923-929.
69. Francis JS, Doherty MC, Lopatin U, et al: Severe community-onset pneumonia in healthy adults caused by methicillin-resistant Staphylococcus aureus carrying the Panton-Valentine leukocidin genes. Clin Infect Dis 2005;40:100-107.
70. Micek ST, Dunne M, Kollef MH: Pleuropulmonary complications of Panton-Valentine leukocidin-positive community-acquired methicillin-resistant Staphylococcus aureus: Importance of treatment with antimicrobials inhibiting exotoxin production. Chest 2005;128:2732-2738.
71. El-Solh AA, Pietrantoni C, Bhat A, et al: Microbiology of severe aspiration pneumonia in institutionalized elderly. Am J Respir Crit Care Med 2003;167: 1650-1654.
72. Fagon JY, Chastre J, Domart Y, et al: Nosocomial pneumonia in patients receiving continuous mechanical

ventilation: prospective analysis of 52 episodes with use of a protected specimen brush and quantitative culture techniques. Am Rev Respir Dis 1989;139:877.
73. Gaynes R, Edwards JR, and the National Nosocomial Infections Surveillance System: Overview of infections caused by Gram-negative bacilli. Clin Infect Dis 2005;41:848-854.
74. El Solh AA, Pietrantoni C, Bhat A, et al: Indicators of potentially drug-resistant bacteria in severe nursing home-acquired pneumonia. Clin Infect Dis 2004;39:474-480.
75. Rello J, Sa-Borges M, Correa H, et al: Variations in etiology of ventilator-associated pneumonia across four treatment sites. Implications for antimicrobial prescribing practices. Am J Respir Crit Care Med 1999;160: 608-613.
76. Metersky ML, Ma A, Bratzler DW, Houck PM: Predicting bacteremia in patients with community-acquired pneumonia. Am J Respir Crit Care Med 2004;169:342-347.
77. Plouffe JF, File TM, Breiman RF, et al: Reevaluation of the definition of Legionnaires' disease: Use of the urinary antigen assay. Clin Infect Dis 1995;20:1286.
78. Rello J, Bodi M, Mariscal D, et al: Microbiological testing and outcome of patients with severe community-acquired pneumonia. Chest 2003;123:174-180.
79. Pugin J, Auckenthaler R, Mili N, et al: Diagnosis of ventilator-associated pneumonia by bacteriology analysis of bronchoscopic and nonbronchoscopic "blind" bronchoalveolar lavage fluid. Am Rev Respir Dis 1991;143:1121.
80. Niederman MS: The importance of de-escalating antimicrobial therapy in patients with ventilator-associated pneumonia. Semin Respir Crit Care Med 2006;27:45-50.
81. Hilf M, Yu VL, Sharp J, et al: Antibiotic therapy for Pseudomonas aeruginosa bacteremia: Outcome correlations in a prospective study of 200 patients. Am J Med 1989;87:540.
82. Paul M, Benuri-Silbiger I, Soares-Weiser K, Liebovici L: β-lactam monotherapy versus β-lactam-aminoglycoside combination therapy for sepsis in immunocompetent patients: Systematic review and meta-analysis of randomized trials. BMJ 2004;328: 668.
83. Moore RD, Smith CR, Lietman PS: Association of aminoglycoside plasma levels with therapeutic outcome in gram-negative pneumonia. Am J Med 1984;77:657.
84. Cometta A, Baumgartner JD, Lew D, et al: Prospective randomized comparison of imipenem monotherapy with imipenem plus netilmicin for treatment of severe infections in nonneutropenic patients. Antimicrob Agents Chemother 1994;38:1309.
85. Hatala R, Dinh T, Cook DJ: Once-daily aminoglycoside dosing in immunocompetent adults: A meta analysis. Ann Intern Med 1996;124: 717.
86. Fink MP, Snydman DR, Niederman MS, et al: Treatment of severe pneumonia in hospitalized patients: Results of a multicenter, randomized, double-blind trial comparing intravenous ciprofloxacin with imipenem-cilastatin. Antimicrob Agents Chemother 1994;38:547.
87. Jaccard C, Troillet N, Harbarth S, et al: Prospective randomized comparison of imipenem-cilastatin and piperacillin-tazobactam in nosocomial pneumonia or peritonitis. Antimicrob Agents Chemother 1998;42:2966-2972.
88. West M, Boulanger BR, Fogarty C, et al: Levofloxacin compared with imipenem/cilastatin followed by ciprofloxacin in adult patients with nosocomial pneumonia: A multicenter, prospective, randomized, open-label study. Clin Ther 2003;25: 485-506.
89. Chapman TM, Perry CM: Cefepime: A review of its use in the management of hospitalized patients with pneumonia. Am J Respir Med 2003;2:75-107.
90. Sieger B, Berman SJ, Geckler RW, et al: Meropenem Lower Respiratory Infection Group. Empiric treatment of hospital-acquired lower respiratory tract infections with meropenem or ceftazidime with tobramycin: A randomized study. Crit Care Med 1997;25:1663-1670.
91. Leroy O, Saux P, Bedos JP, Caulin E: Comparison of levofloxacin and cefotaxime combined with ofloxacin for ICU patients with community-acquired pneumonia who do not require vasopressors. Chest 2005;128:172-83.
92. File TM, Niederman MS: Antimicrobial therapy of community-acquired pneumonia. Infect Dis Clin N Am 2004;18:993-1016.
93. Waterer GW, Somes GW, Wunderink RG: Monotherapy may be suboptimal for severe bacteremic pneumococcal pneumonia. Arch Intern Med 2001;161:1837-1842.
94. Laterre PF, Garber G, Levy H, et al: Severe community-acquired pneumonia as a cause of severe sepsis: Data from the PROWESS study. Crit Care Med 33:952-961, 2005.
95. Confalonieri M, Urbino R, Potena A, et al: Hydrocortisone infusion for severe community-acquired pneumonia: A preliminary randomized study. Am J Respir Crit Care Med 2005;171:242-248.
96. Yu VL, Greenberg RN, Zadeikis N, et al: Levofloxacin efficacy in the treatment of community-acquired legionellosis. Chest 2004;125: 2135-2139.
97. Trouillet JL, Vuagnat A, Combes A, et al: Pseudomonas aeruginosa ventilator-associated pneumonia: Comparison of episodes due to piperacillin-resistant versus piperacillin-susceptible organisms. Clin Infect Dis 2002;34:1047-1054.
98. Vanderkooi OG, Low DE, Green K, et al: Predicting antimicrobial resistance in invasive pneumococcal infections. Clin Infect Dis 2005;40: 1288-1297.
99. Nseir S, Di Pompeo C, Soubrier S, et al: First-generation fluoroquinolone use and subsequent emergence of multiple drug-resistant bacteria in the intensive care unit. Crit Care Med 2005;33:283-289.
100. Kollef MH, Vlasnik J, Sharpless L, et al: Scheduled change of antibiotic classes: A strategy to decrease the incidence of ventilator-associated pneumonia. Am J Respir Crit Care Med 1997;156: 1040-1048.
101. Niederman MS: Is crop rotation of antibiotics the solution to a resistant problem in the ICU? Am J Respir Crit Care Med 1997;156:1029-1031.
102. Niederman MS: Reexamining quinolone use in the intensive care unit: Use them right or lose the fight against resistant bacteria. Crit Care Med 2005;33:443-444.
103. Wunderink RG, Rello J, Cammarata SK, et al: Linezolid vs. vancomycin: Analysis of two double-blind studies of patients with methicillin-resistant Staphylococcus aureus nosocomial pneumonia. Chest 2003;124: 1789-1797.
104. Chastre J, Wolff M, Fagon JY, et al: Comparison of 8 vs. 15 days of antibiotic therapy for ventilator-associated pneumonia in adults: A randomized trial. JAMA 2003;290: 2588-2598.
105. Michalopoulos A, Kasiakou SK, Mastora Z, et al: Aerosolized colistin for the treatment of nosocomial pneumonia due to multidrug-resistant gram-negative bacteria in patients without cystic fibrosis. Crit Care 2005;9:R53-59.
106. Walker FJ, Singleton RJ, Bulkow LR, et al: Reactions after 3 or more doses of pneumococcal polysaccharide vaccine in adults in Alaska. Clin Infect Dis 2005;40:1730-1735.
107. Fedson DS, Harward MP, Reid RA, et al: Hospital-based pneumococcal immunization: Epidemiologic rationale from the Shenandoah study. JAMA 1990;264:1117.
108. Zack JE, Garrison T, Trovillion E, et al: Effect of an educational program aimed at reducing the occurrence of ventilator associated pneumonia. Crit Care Med 2002;30:2407-2412.
109. Concanour CS, Peninger M, Domonoske BD, et al: Decreasing ventilator-associated pneumonia in a trauma ICU. J Trauma 2006;61: 122-130.
110. Tablan OC, Anderson LJ, Besser R, et al: Guidelines for preventing health-care-associated pneumonia, 2003. MMWR 2004;53(RR-3):1-36.
111. Van Nieuwenhoven CA, Vandenbroucke-Grauls C, van Tiel FH, et al: Feasibility and effects of the semirecumbent position to prevent ventilator-associated pneumonia: A randomized study. Crit Care Med 2006;34:396-402.
112. Vallés J, Artigas A, Rello J, et al: Continuous aspiration of subglottic secretions in preventing ventilator-associated pneumonia. Ann Intern Med 1995;122:179.
113. Sirvent JM, Torres A, El-Ebiary M, et al: Protective effect of intravenously administered cefuroxime against nosocomial pneumonia in patients with structural coma. Am J Respir Crit Care Med 1997;155:1729-1734.

Chapter 44

Weaning from Mechanical Ventilation

Martin J. Tobin

Mechanical ventilation is often lifesaving, but it is associated with numerous complications.[1,2] Accordingly, it is imperative to disconnect patients from the ventilator at the earliest feasible time. Deciding the right time to initiate this disconnection process, usually referred to as *weaning,* is one of the greatest challenges in critical care medicine.[3] If a physician is too conservative and postpones the initiation of weaning, the patient is placed at an increased risk of life-threatening, ventilator-associated complications. Conversely, if weaning is begun prematurely, the patient may suffer cardiopulmonary or psychological decompensation of sufficient severity to set back a patient's clinical course.[4]

This chapter reviews the pathophysiology of weaning failure, weaning-predictor testing, different weaning techniques, and extubation.

PATHOPHYSIOLOGY OF WEANING FAILURE

After patients have been disconnected from the ventilator, up to 25% experience respiratory distress severe enough to necessitate the reinstitution of mechanical ventilation.[5,6] Our understanding of why ventilator discontinuation fails in some patients has advanced considerably in recent years. The pathophysiologic mechanisms of weaning failure can be divided into those occurring at the level of the respiratory control system, mechanics of the lung and chest wall, the respiratory muscles, the cardiovascular system, and gas-exchange properties of the lung.[4]

Control of Breathing

Many weaning-failure patients develop hypercapnia. Accordingly, it had been thought that these patients were experiencing an acute decrease in minute ventilation consequent to a decrease in respiratory center output.[3] Measurements of respiratory center drive, using mean inspiratory flow (V_T/T_I) or airway occlusion pressure ($P_{0.1}$), have consistently revealed an increase, not a decrease, in respiratory drive in weaning-failure patients.[4,7,8]

Weaning-failure patients, however, exhibit marked abnormalities in respiratory timing, specifically marked shortening of inspiratory time (T_I), which is coupled with shortening of expiratory time (T_E). The decrease in both T_I and T_E means that respiratory frequency (f) is markedly elevated. The shortening of T_I combined with a normal mean inspiratory flow (V_T/T_I) results in a marked decrease of tidal volume (V_T).[7] This combination (elevated f and decreased V_T) is referred to as *rapid shallow breathing*—now recognized as the physiological hallmark of weaning failure (Fig. 44-1).[3]

Respiratory Mechanics

The most detailed study of respiratory mechanics during weaning trials was carried out by Jubran and Tobin.[9,10] Immediately before commencement of a trial of spontaneous breathing, patients who went on to tolerate or fail the trial showed little or no difference in detailed measurements of passive respiratory mechanics.[10] Resistance, elastance, and intrinsic positive end-expiratory pressure ($PEEP_i$) were equivalent in the two groups.

During the course of the trial, all of these variables became more abnormal in the weaning-failure patients than in the weaning-success patients (Fig. 44-2).[9] Respiratory resistance increased progressively, reaching about seven times the normal value at the end of the trial. Pulmonary elastance increased, reaching five times the normal value. Intrinsic PEEP more than doubled over the course of the trial. A similar pattern has been observed by other investigators.[11] The observation that respiratory mechanics were equivalent in weaning-success and weaning-failure patients immediately before a weaning trial but deteriorated immediately in the weaning-failure patients indicates that some mechanism associated with

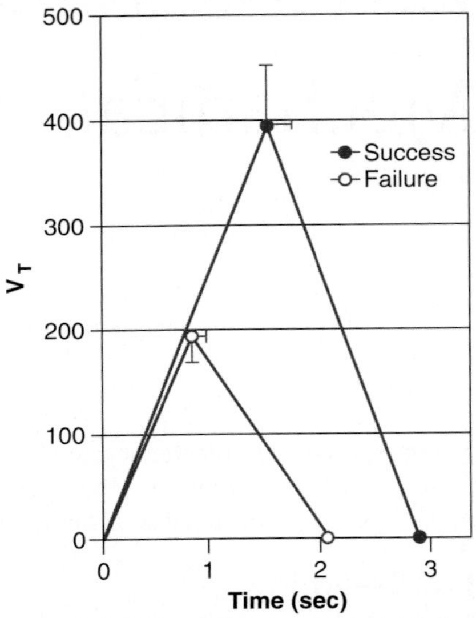

Figure 44-1. The mean respiratory cycle during spontaneous breathing in 7 weaning-failure and 10 weaning-success patients. The early termination of inspiratory time in the weaning-failure patients leads to a decrease in tidal volume (V_T). The decrease in inspiratory time, coupled with a decrease in expiratory time, results in a faster respiratory frequency. Bars represent 1 SE. (Redrawn from Tobin MJ, Perez W, Guenther SM, et al: The pattern of breathing during successful and unsuccessful trials of weaning from mechanical ventilation. Am Rev Respir Dis 1986;134:1111-1118.)

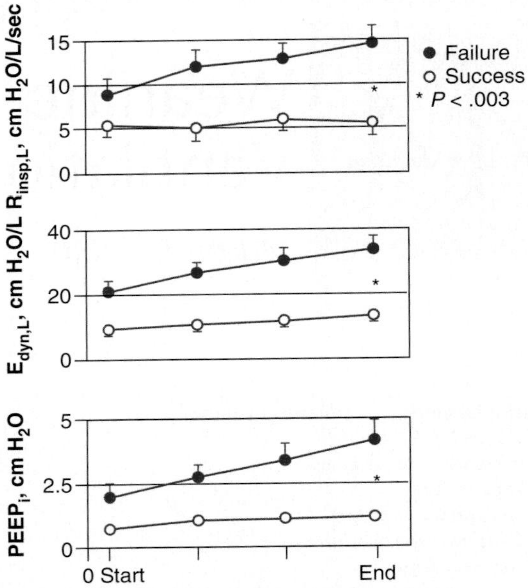

Figure 44-2. Inspiratory resistance of the lung ($R_{insp,L}$), dynamic lung elastance ($E_{dyn,L}$), and intrinsic positive end-expiratory pressure (PEEP$_i$) in 17 weaning-failure patients and 14 weaning-success patients. Data displayed were obtained during the second and last minute of a T-tube trial, and at one third and two thirds of the trial duration. Between the onset and end of the trial, the failure group developed increases in $R_{insp,L}$ ($P < .009$), $E_{dyn,L}$ ($P < .0001$), and PEEP$_i$ ($P < .0001$) and the success group developed increases in $E_{dyn,L}$ ($P < .006$) and PEEP$_i$ ($P < .02$). Over the course of the trial, the failure group had higher values of $R_{insp,L}$ ($P < .003$), $E_{dyn,L}$ ($P < .006$) and PEEP$_i$ ($P < .009$) than the success group. (Redrawn from Jubran A, Tobin MJ: Pathophysiologic basis of acute respiratory distress in patients who fail a trial of weaning from mechanical ventilation. Am J Respir Crit Care Med 1997;155:906-915.)

the act of spontaneous breathing causes the worsening of respiratory mechanics that leads to weaning failure.

Patient Effort

To compensate for the marked worsening of respiratory mechanics, patients need to make a greater inspiratory effort. It had been thought that inability to make sufficient inspiratory effort might be responsible for weaning failure.[3] Investigators have quantified inspiratory effort through measurements of work of breathing and pressure-time product.[12,13] These studies consistently show that weaning-failure patients make a greater inspiratory effort than do weaning-success patients (Fig. 44-3).[9,14]

Respiratory Muscles

In reviewing research on the respiratory muscles, it is useful to distinguish between respiratory muscle strength and endurance (the inverse of fatigue). Overall strength of the inspiratory muscles is usually assessed by measuring maximal inspiratory pressure (P_{Imax}).[12] Most investigators have found that values of P_{Imax} are largely similar in weaning-success and weaning-failure patients.[4,9,14] A fundamental limitation of the P_{Imax} technique is its total dependence on patient motivation and cooperation.[15] Employing phrenic nerve stimulation (twitch-interpolation technique), Laghi and colleagues[14] found that P_{Imax} values in weaning-failure patients underestimated inspiratory muscle strength. Moreover, these investigators observed that 6 of 10 weaning-failure patients had twitch transdiaphragmatic pressure (P_{di}) values below 10 cm H_2O. (Healthy subjects have values of 35 to 39 cm H_2O.) Thus, contrary to current thinking, respiratory muscle weakness may be quite common in weaning-failure patients.

For several years, investigators had suspected that many weaning-failure patients develop respiratory muscle fatigue.[3] The question went untested because of the difficulty of obtaining reliable measurements of fatigue in critically ill patients. The most direct measure of diaphragmatic fatigue is to stimulate the phrenic nerves and record the resulting transdiaphragmatic pressure.[12] Laghi and colleagues[14] employed this technique in 11 weaning-failure and 8 weaning-success patients before and after a T-tube trial. No patient in either group exhibited a fall in twitch pressure. This result was surprising. Related analyses disclosed why. Failure patients became progressively distressed during the trial, leading clinicians to reinstate ventilator support before patients had breathed long enough to develop fatigue (Fig. 44-4).[15,16] In other words, monitoring clinical signs of distress provides sufficient warning to avoid respiratory muscle fatigue.

Cardiovascular Performance

During a weaning trial, patients can experience substantial increases in right- and left-ventricular afterload.[17,18]

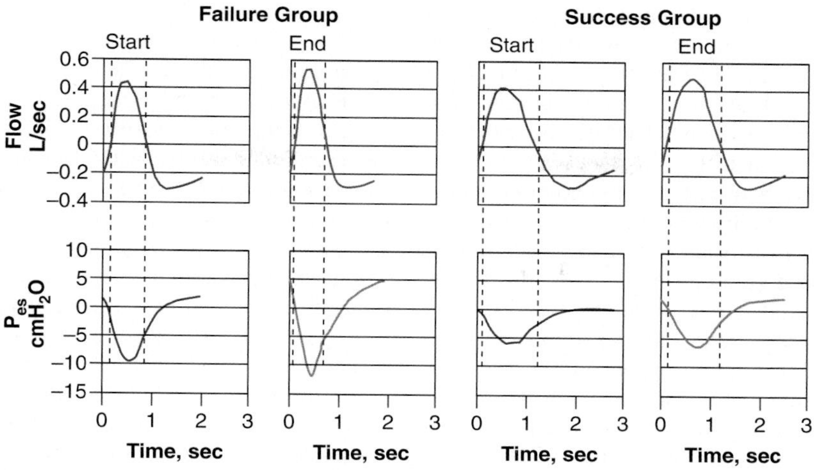

Figure 44-3. Ensemble average plots of flow and esophageal pressure (P_{es}) at the start and end of a T-tube trial in 17 weaning-failure patients and 14 weaning-success patients. At the start of the trial, the inspiratory excursion in P_{es} was greater in the failure patients, and it increased further by the end of the trial. To generate these plots, flow and P_{es} tracings were divided into 25 equal time intervals over a single respiratory cycle for each of the 5 breaths for each patient in the 2 groups. For a given patient, the five breaths from the start of the trial were then superimposed and aligned with respect to time, and the average at each time point was calculated. The group mean tracings were then generated by ensemble averaging of the individual mean from each patient. The same procedure was performed for breaths at the end of the trial. (Redrawn from Jubran A, Tobin MJ: Pathophysiologic basis of acute respiratory distress in patients who fail a trial of weaning from mechanical ventilation. Am J Respir Crit Care Med 1997;155:906-915.)

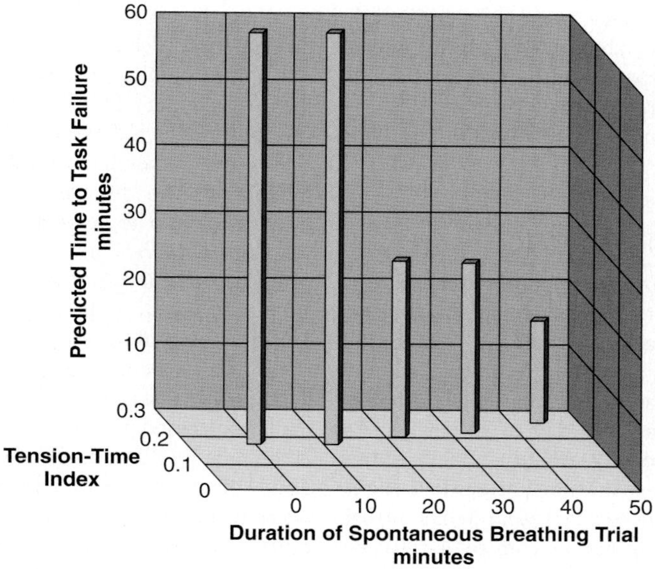

Figure 44-4. Interrelationship between the duration of a spontaneous breathing trial, tension-time index of the diaphragm, and predicted time to task failure in nine patients who failed a trial of weaning from mechanical ventilation. The patients breathed spontaneously for an average of 44 minutes before a physician terminated the trial. At the start of the trial, the tension-time index was 0.17, and the formula of Bellemare and Grassino[16] (see text for details) predicted that patients could sustain spontaneous breathing for another 59 minutes before developing task failure. As the trial progressed, the tension-time index increased and the predicted time to development of task failure decreased. At the end of the trial, the tension-time index reached 0.26. That patients were predicted to sustain spontaneous breathing for another 13 minutes before developing task failure clarifies why patients did not develop a decrease in diaphragmatic twitch pressure. In other words, physicians interrupted the trial on the basis of clinical manifestations of respiratory distress, before patients had sufficient time to develop contractile fatigue. (Redrawn from Laghi F, Tobin MJ: Disorders of the respiratory muscles. Am J Respir Crit Care Med 2003;168:10-48.)

These afterload increases most likely result from associated increases in negative swings of intrathoracic pressure. At the completion of a weaning trial, the level of oxygen consumption is equivalent in weaning-success and weaning-failure patients. How the cardiovascular system meets the oxygen demand differs in the two groups of patients. In weaning-success patients, oxygen demand is met through an increase in oxygen delivery, mediated by the expected increase in cardiac output on discontinuation of positive-pressure ventilation.[18] In weaning-failure patients, oxygen demand is met through an increase in oxygen extraction; these patients have a relative decrease in oxygen delivery.[18] The greater oxygen extraction causes a substantial decrease in mixed venous oxygen saturation, contributing to the arterial hypoxemia that occurs in some patients.[18]

Gas Exchange

Because a primary goal of mechanical ventilation is to improve gas exchange, one expects some deterioration in gas exchange with the resumption of spontaneous breathing. Studies employing the multiple inert-gas technique have revealed that the ventilation-perfusion maldistribution and acute hypercapnia observed in weaning-failure patients is produced primarily by shallow breathing (low V_T).[3] About half of weaning-failure patients experience an increase in Pa_{CO_2} of 10 mm Hg or more over the course of a spontaneous breathing trial.[9] The hypercapnia is not usually a consequence of a decrease in minute ventilation. Instead, it results from rapid, shallow breathing, which causes an increase in dead-space ventilation. In a small proportion of weaning-failure patients, primary depression of respiratory drive may be responsible for the hypercapnia.[7]

WEANING PREDICTOR TESTING

In randomized trials of different weaning techniques, most patients who had received mechanical ventilation for a week or longer were able to tolerate ventilator discontinuation on the first day that weaning-predictor tests were measured.[5,6] Many of these patients probably would have tolerated extubation a day or so earlier. As such, one of the main sources of weaning delay is the failure of the physician to *think* that the patient just *might* come off the ventilator. Psychological research has shown that delays in decision making result from over-reliance on algorithms and rules and insufficient attention to the pretest probability of a condition.[4] By undertaking diagnostic testing (via weaning predictor tests) early in the patient's clinical course, it is possible to speed up the weaning process.

Pitfalls in Use of Weaning-Predictor Tests

Physicians commonly view diagnostic testing in monolithic terms: a test is a test is a test. In reality, diagnostic testing has to satisfy two very different tasks: One is screening, the other is confirmation.[19] The characteristics of these test types differ, and a single diagnostic test rarely fulfills both functions.[19]

The fundamental job of a weaning-predictor test is screening.[4] Because the goal is to not miss anybody with the condition under consideration, a good screening test has a low rate of false-negative results; to achieve this goal, a higher false-positive rate is acceptable. Thus an ideal screening test has a high sensitivity.[4,19] Some authors have used likelihood ratio as a method for assessing the reliability of a weaning-predictor test for screening.[20,21] Likelihood ratio is not precisely suited to screening-test evaluation because it includes test components not directly focused on screening (true-negative and false-positive rates), as well as components vital for screening (true-positive and false-negative rates); the former clouds the contribution of the vital components.[19]

Weaning involves the use of three diagnostic tests in sequence: measurement of predictors, a weaning trial, and a trial of extubation. The sequential nature of the testing gives rise to particular problems in studies undertaken to investigate the reliability of a (preexisting) predictor test. One is spectrum bias. This occurs when a new study population contains fewer (or more) sick patients than the population in which a diagnostic test was originally developed.[19,22] A second is test-referral bias. This occurs when the results of a test under evaluation are used to select patients for a reference-standard test, such as use of a weaning-predictor test to select patients for a reference-standard test (passing a weaning trial that leads to extubation).[19,22]

A third factor that affects studies of the reliability of a predictor test is base-rate fallacy.[22,23] Consider a diagnostic test for a disease that has a false-positive rate of 5% and false-negative rate of 0%, and the incidence of the disorder (under consideration) is 1 per 1000 persons. A randomly selected person undergoes diagnostic testing. The result comes back positive. What is the chance this person has the disease? More than 80% of physicians answer 95%. The correct answer is 1.96%.[23] Physicians who answer 95% are failing to take into account the pretest probability of the disorder. Thus they fall into the trap of base-rate fallacy.

Pretest probability is a physician's estimate of the likelihood of a particular condition (weaning outcome) before a diagnostic test is undertaken.[4] Post-test probability (typically expressed as positive- or negative-predictive value) is the new likelihood after the test results are obtained. A good diagnostic test achieves a marked increase (or decrease) in the post-test probability (over pretest probability). For every test in every medical subspecialty, the magnitude of change between pretest probability and post-test probability is determined by Bayes' theorem.[22] Three factors (alone) determine the magnitude of the pretest to post-test change: sensitivity, specificity, and pretest probability. Sensitivity and specificity are commonly assumed to remain constant for a test. In truth, test-referral bias, a common occurrence in studies of weaning tests, leads to major changes in sensitivity and specificity.[19] Likewise, major changes in pretest probability arise as a consequence of spectrum bias.[19] All of these factors need to be carefully considered when reading a study that evaluates the reliability of a weaning-predictor test.

Respiratory Frequency-to-Tidal Volume Ratio (f/V_T)

The ratio of respiratory frequency to tidal volume (f/V_T) is measured during 1 minute of spontaneous breathing (Fig. 44-5).[24] Measurements of f/V_T in the presence of pressure support or CPAP will result in inaccurate predictions of weaning outcome.[4] The higher the f/V_T ratio, the more severe the rapid, shallow breathing and the greater the likelihood of unsuccessful weaning. An f/V_T ratio of 100 best discriminates between successful and unsuccessful attempts at weaning.[24]

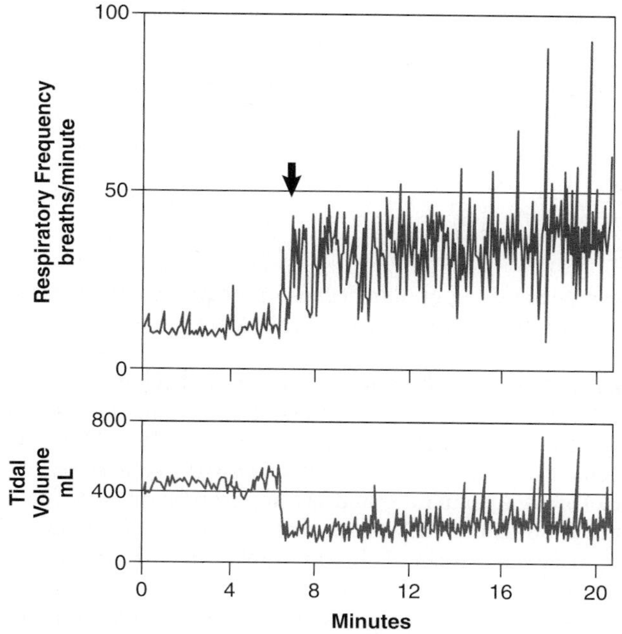

Figure 44-5. A time-series, breath-by-breath plot of respiratory frequency and tidal volume in a patient who failed a weaning trial. The arrow indicates the point of resuming spontaneous breathing. Rapid, shallow breathing developed almost immediately after discontinuation of the ventilator. (Redrawn from Tobin MJ, Perez W, Guenther SM, et al: The pattern of breathing during successful and unsuccessful trials of weaning from mechanical ventilation. Am Rev Respir Dis 1986;134:1111-1118.)

The initial evaluation of f/V_T was reported in 1991.[24] Since then, this test has been evaluated in more than 25 studies. Reported sensitivity ranges from 0.35 to 1.[22] Specificity ranges from 0 to 0.89.[22] At first glance, this wide scatter suggests that f/V_T is an unreliable predictor of weaning outcome. Many of the investigators, however, ignored the possibility of test-referral bias and spectrum bias.[4] The Evidence-Based Medicine Task Force of the American College of Chest Physicians (ACCP) undertook a meta-analysis of the studies.[21] The task force calculated pooled likelihood ratios for f/V_T and judged the summated values to signify that f/V_T was not as reliable a predictor of weaning success as some believed, although concluding that both an RR greater than 38 breaths/minute and an f/V_T ratio of greater than 100 breaths/L/minute did decrease the probability of successful extubation.[20,21] The studies included in the meta-analysis, however, exhibited significant heterogeneity in pretest probability of successful outcome.[22] Such marked heterogeneity prohibits the undertaking of a reliable meta-analysis.[25,26] When data from the studies (included in the meta-analysis) were entered into a Bayesian model with pretest probability as the operating point, the reported positive-predictive values were significantly correlated with the values predicted by the original report on f/V_T,[24] $r = 0.86$ ($P < .0001$); likewise, reported negative-predictive values were correlated with the values predicted, $r = .82$ ($P < .0001$) (Figs. 44-6 and 44-7).[22]

The primary job of a weaning-predictor test is screening, which requires a high sensitivity.[4,19] The average sensitivity in all of the studies on f/V_T was 0.89, and 85% of the studies reveal sensitivities higher than 0.90.[22] This sensitivity compares well with commonly used diagnostic tests: creatine phosphokinase (CPK) for the diagnosis of acute myocardial infarction, sensitivity of 0.94; chest radiograph for lung cancer, 0.60; stress echocardiography for myocardial ischemia, 0.60; and echocardiography for

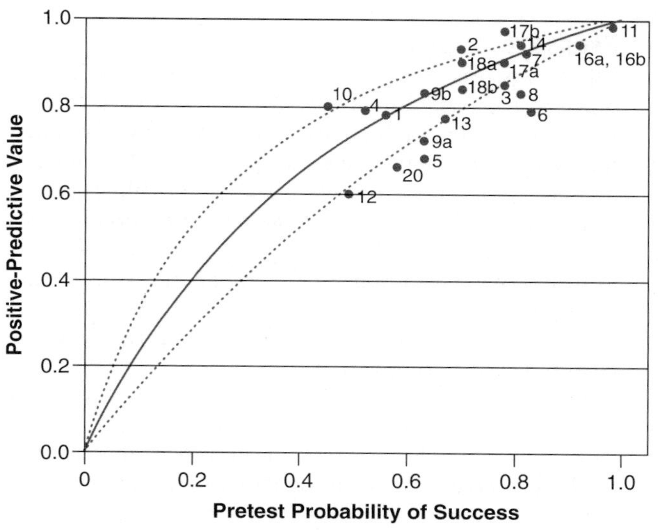

Figure 44-6. Positive-predictive value (post-test probability of successful outcome) for f/V_T plotted against pretest probability of successful outcome. The curve is based on the sensitivity and specificity originally reported by Yang and Tobin[24] and Bayes' formula for 0.01-unit increments in pretest probability between 0.00 and 1.00.[22] The lines represent the upper and lower 95% confidence intervals for the predicted relationship of the positive predictive values against pretest probability. The observed positive-predictive value in a study is plotted against the pretest probability of weaning success (prevalence of successful outcome). (Redrawn from Tobin MJ, Jubran A: Variable performance of weaning-predictor tests: Role of Bayes' theorem and spectrum and test-referral bias. Intensive Care Med 2006;32:2002-2012.)

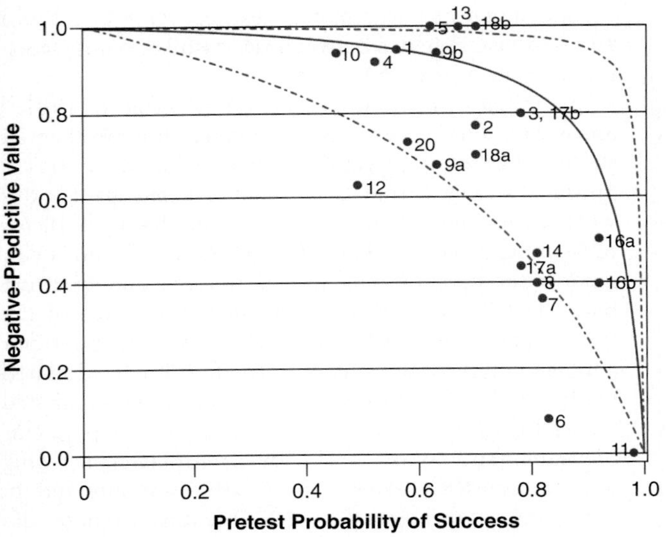

Figure 44-7. Negative-predictive value (post-test probability of unsuccessful outcome) for f/V_T. The curve, its 95% confidence intervals, and placement of a study on the plot are described in the legend of Figure 44-6. The observed negative-predictive value in a study is plotted against the pretest probability of weaning success (prevalence of successful outcome). Of note is that study #11 has a negative-predictive value of 0.00 and specificity of 0.00. These values suggest that f/V_T is an unreliable test (and this will also be the natural conclusion reached by a meta-analysis of likelihood ratio). Instead, a negative-predictive value of 0.00 and specificity of 0.00 are predicted for the pretest probability of weaning success of 98.2% reported in study #11. (Redrawn from Tobin MJ, Jubran A: Variable performance of weaning-predictor tests: Role of Bayes' theorem and spectrum and test-referral bias. Intensive Care Med 2006;32:2002-2012.)

diagnosis of endocarditis, 0.37.[4] The sensitivity of a spontaneous breathing trial is unknown.

Because screening is the primary purpose of a weaning-predictor test, it is important that the test be performed early in a patient's ventilator course. Figures 44-6 and 44-7, however, reveal that pretest probability of weaning success was 75% or higher in more than half the studies of weaning-predictor tests. In other words, most physicians are postponing (inappropriately) the undertaking of weaning-predictor tests. A simple way for a physician to assess his or her own timeliness in initiating weaning is to estimate the number of times he or she obtained positive results on weaning-predictor tests over the preceding 6 months. If a physician working in a typical medical intensive care unit estimates that he (or she) obtained positive results 70% or more of the time, he should consider that he is being too slow in initiating weaning.

WEANING TRIALS

When a screening test is positive, the clinician proceeds to a confirmatory test.[19] The goal of a positive result on a confirmatory test is to rule in a condition:[19] The likelihood of a patient tolerating a trial of extubation is high. An ideal confirmatory test has a low rate of false-positive results (i.e., a high specificity).[19] Unfortunately, the specificity of a spontaneous breathing trial is not known. Indeed, its specificity will never be known because its determination would require an unethical experiment: extubating all patients who fail a weaning trial and counting how many require reintubation.[4]

Multiple T-Tube Trials

Of the four methods available for conducting a weaning trial, the use of repeated T-tube trials, several times a day, is the oldest method.[3] The patient receives an enriched supply of oxygen through a T-tube circuit. Initially 5 to 10 minutes in duration, T-tube trials are extended and repeated several times a day until the patient can sustain spontaneous ventilation for several hours. This approach has become unpopular because it requires considerable time on the part of intensive care staff.

Intermittent Mandatory Ventilation

For many years, intermittent mandatory ventilation (IMV) was the most popular method of weaning.[3] With IMV, the mandatory rate from the ventilator is reduced in steps of 1 to 3 breaths per minute, and an arterial blood gas is obtained about 30 minutes after each rate change.[27] Unfortunately, titrating the number of breaths from the ventilator in accordance with the results of arterial blood gases can produce a false sense of security. As few as two to three positive-pressure breaths per minute can achieve acceptable blood gases, but these values provide no information regarding the patient's work of breathing (which may be excessive).[4] At IMV rates of 14 breaths per minute or fewer, patient inspiratory efforts are increased to a level likely to cause respiratory muscle fatigue.[28,29] Moreover, this occurs not only with the intervening spontaneous breaths but also with ventilator-assisted breaths. Consequently, use of IMV may actually contribute to the development of respiratory muscle fatigue or prevent its recovery.

Pressure Support

When pressure support is used for weaning, the level of pressure is reduced gradually (decrements of 3 to 6 cm H_2O) and titrated on the basis of the patient's respiratory frequency.[30] When the patient tolerates a minimal level of pressure support, he or she is extubated. What exactly constitutes a "minimal level of pressure support" has never been defined.[31] For example, pressure support of 5 to 8 cm H_2O is widely used to compensate for the resistance imposed by the endotracheal tube and ventilator circuit.[32] A patient who can breathe comfortably at this level of pressure support can reasonably tolerate extubation. But if the upper airways are swollen because an endotracheal tube has been in place for several days, the work engendered by breathing through the swollen airways is about the same as that caused by breathing through an endotracheal tube.[32] Accordingly, any amount of pressure support overcompensates and may give misleading information about the likelihood that a patient can tolerate extubation.

Once-Daily T-Tube Trials

The fourth method of weaning is to perform a single daily T-tube trial, lasting for 30 to 120 minutes. If this trial is successful, the patient is extubated. If the trial is unsuccessful, the patient is given at least 24 hours of respiratory muscle rest with full ventilator support before another trial is performed.[4]

Comparison of Weaning Methods

Until the early 1990s, it was widely believed that all weaning methods were equally effective, and the physician's judgment was regarded as the critical determinant.[3] But the results of randomized, controlled trials clearly indicate that the period of weaning is as much as three times as long with IMV as with trials of spontaneous breathing.[5,6] In a study involving patients with respiratory difficulties on weaning, trials of spontaneous breathing halved the weaning time as compared with pressure support[6]; in another study, the weaning time was similar with the two methods.[5] Performing trials of spontaneous breathing once a day is as effective as performing such trials several times a day but much simpler.[6] In patients not expecting to pose any particular difficulty with weaning, a half-hour trial of spontaneous breathing is as effective as a 2-hour trial.[33]

Weaning by Protocol versus Usual Care

Six randomized controlled trials have compared the use of protocols for weaning versus usual care. The reports of Kollef and colleagues,[34] Marelich and colleagues,[35] and Ely and colleagues[36] are viewed as evidence for the superiority of a protocol approach to weaning with all three trials concluding benefit.

In the trial by Kollef and colleagues, patients assigned to usual care were significantly sicker than the patients assigned to protocol management in that ICU; this confounding factor weakens the assertion that protocol weaning was superior. Furthermore, no advantage for weaning by protocol was observed in three of the four ICUs in this study.[34]

Marelich and colleagues[35] studied weaning by protocol in two ICUs and found significant advantage in only one of the two units. The study of Ely and colleagues[36] is not a straightforward comparison of protocol versus nonprotocol care. All of the patients in the intervention arm were weaned by T-tube or flow-by trials, whereas 76% of the patients in the nonintervention arm were managed by IMV alone or in combination with pressure support. Physiological studies and randomized trials have repeatedly shown that IMV is the least effective weaning modality.[5,6,28,29] The fundamental difference in techniques between the two groups makes it difficult to form a conclusion about the efficacy of a protocol per se. The report of Ely and colleagues[36] may instead support the conclusion, as previously found in the reports of Brochard and colleagues[5] and Esteban and colleagues,[6] that IMV slows weaning.

The report of Namen and colleagues[37] showed that in neurosurgical patients a protocol based on traditional respiratory physiology variables was not useful; however, the combination of respiration physiology plus neurologic measures did assist weaning. Randolph and colleagues found that use of a protocol had no beneficial effect on weaning failure or weaning duration.[38]

On reflection, it is not surprising that the use of a protocol may not improve weaning outcome. One needs to make a distinction between the use of algorithms in research protocols and their subsequent application in everyday practice. The algorithm in a research protocol is specified with exacting precision.[39] For example, if f/V_T less than 100 is the nodal point for advancement to a T-tube trial, then patients with an f/V_T of 100 will undergo the trial, whereas patients with a f/V_T of 101 will return to mechanical ventilation for another 24 hours. An experienced clinician, however, would think it unwise to blindly comply with a protocol that decided an entire day of ventilator management on a one-unit difference in a single measurement of f/V_T (or any other weaning predictor).[40] Instead, an intelligent physician customizes the knowledge generated by research to the particulars of each patient. The intelligent application of physiological principles is likely to outperform an inflexible application of a protocol. This is supported by a study demonstrating no benefit of protocolized weaning in a closed-ICU with generous physician staffing and structured rounds.[41]

EXTUBATION

Decisions about weaning and decisions about extubation are commonly combined.[42] When a patient tolerates a weaning trial without distress, a clinician feels reasonably confident that the patient will be able to sustain spontaneous ventilation after extubation. Before removing the endotracheal tube, however, the clinician must also judge whether or not the patient will be able to maintain a patent upper airway after extubation.

Of patients who are expected to tolerate extubation without difficulty, approximately 10% to 20% fail and require reintubation.[5,6] Mortality among patients who require reintubation is more than six times as high as mortality among patients who can tolerate extubation.[33] The reason for the higher mortality is unknown. It might be related to the development of new problems after extubation or to complications associated with reinsertion of a new tube. A more likely explanation is that the need for reintubation reflects greater severity of the underlying illness.[42]

Because of the high mortality associated with reintubation, clinicians are eager to avoid this problem. The major diagnostic test used to predict the success of an extubation attempt is a weaning trial. In contrast to the many studies that have evaluated the reliability of diagnostic tests that predict the outcome of a trial of weaning, the diagnostic accuracy of weaning trials in predicting the outcome of a trial of extubation is unknown.[42] Moreover, the accuracy is impossible to determine because the experiments necessary to measure the sensitivity and specificity of a weaning trial (for predicting extubation outcome) are unethical.

CONCLUSION

In conclusion, to minimize the likelihood of either delayed weaning or premature extubation, a two-step diagnostic strategy is recommended: measurement of weaning predictors followed by a weaning trial. Because each step constitutes a diagnostic test, clinicians must be mindful of the scientific principles of diagnostic testing when interpreting the information generated by each step. The critical step is for the physician to contemplate the possibility that a patient *just might* be able to tolerate weaning. Such diagnostic triggering is assisted through use of a screening test, which is the rationale for measurement of weaning-predictor tests. Importantly, one should not postpone this first step by waiting for a more complex diagnostic test, such as a T-tube trial. Many complex facets of pulmonary pathophysiology impinge on weaning management. Thus weaning requires individualized care at a high level of sophistication.

KEY POINTS

- Most patients who fail a trial of weaning from mechanical ventilation do so because of a markedly increased respiratory load, which, in turn, is secondary to severe worsening of respiratory mechanics over the course of the weaning trial.
- Less common reasons for weaning failure include weakened respiratory muscles or impaired cardiovascular performance; primary abnormalities of the respiratory centers or intra-pulmonary shunt are uncommon mechanisms of weaning failure.
- Several studies suggest that most patients weaned successfully could have tolerated the weaning attempts had they been initiated a day or more earlier. Such data emphasize the need for the early use of screening tests.
- The primary goal of a screening test is to not miss anybody with the condition; thus the test should have a high sensitivity. The ratio of respiratory frequency to tidal volume (f/V_T) has been evaluated in more than 25 studies; its average sensitivity is 0.89.
- Weaning involves the undertaking of three diagnostic tests in sequence. The sequential nature of the testing predisposes to the occurrence of test-referral bias and spectrum bias.
- Of the techniques used for a weaning trial, intermittent mandatory ventilation (IMV) has been repeatedly shown to be inferior to the use of T-tube trials or pressure support.
- Six randomized trials have evaluated the usefulness of protocols in the management of weaning. Three studies observed no benefit with the use of protocols. Two of the remaining three studies had major methodological problems, leaving only one study supporting the use of protocols.

REFERENCES

1. Tobin MJ: Advances in mechanical ventilation. N Engl J Med 2001;344:1986-1996.
2. Tobin MJ (ed): Principles and Practice of Mechanical Ventilation, 2nd ed. New York, McGraw-Hill, 2006.
3. Tobin MJ: Remembrance of weaning past: The seminal papers. Intensive Care Med 2006;32:1485-1493.
4. Tobin MJ, Jubran A: Weaning from mechanical ventilation. In Tobin MJ (ed): Principles and Practice of Mechanical Ventilation, 2nd ed. New York, McGraw-Hill, 2006, pp 1185-1220.
5. Brochard L, Rauss A, Benito S, et al: Comparison of three methods of gradual withdrawal from ventilatory support during weaning from mechanical ventilation. Am J Respir Crit Care Med 1994;150: 896-903.
6. Esteban A, Frutos F, Tobin MJ, et al: A comparison of four methods of weaning patients from mechanical ventilation. Spanish Lung Failure Collaborative Group. N Engl J Med 1995;332: 345-350.
7. Tobin MJ, Perez W, Guenther SM, et al: The pattern of breathing during successful and unsuccessful trials of weaning from mechanical ventilation. Am Rev Respir Dis 1986;134: 1111-1118.
8. Sassoon CS, Te TT, Mahutte CK, et al: Airway occlusion pressure. An important indicator for successful weaning in patients with chronic obstructive pulmonary disease. Am Rev Respir Dis 1987;135:107-113.
9. Jubran A, Tobin MJ: Pathophysiologic basis of acute respiratory distress in patients who fail a trial of weaning from mechanical ventilation. Am J Respir Crit Care Med 1997;155:906-915.
10. Jubran A, Tobin MJ: Passive mechanics of lung and chest wall in patients who failed or succeeded in trials of weaning. Am J Respir Crit Care Med 1997;155: 916-921.
11. Vassilakopoulos T, Zakynthinos S, Roussos C: The tension-time index and the frequency/tidal volume ratio are the major pathophysiologic determinants of weaning failure and success. Am J Respir Crit Care Med 1998;158: 378-385.
12. Tobin MJ, Laghi F: Monitoring of respiratory muscle function. In Tobin MJ (ed): Principles and Practice of Intensive Care Monitoring. New York, McGraw-Hill, 1998, pp 497-544.
13. Tobin MJ: Monitoring respiratory mechanics in spontaneously breathing patients. In Tobin MJ (ed): Principles and Practice of Intensive Care Monitoring. New York, McGraw-Hill, 1998, pp 617-654.
14. Laghi F, Cattapan SE, Jubran A, et al: Is weaning failure caused by low-frequency fatigue of the diaphragm? Am J Respir Crit Care Med 2003;167:120-127.
15. Laghi F, Tobin MJ: Disorders of the respiratory muscles. Am J Respir Crit Care Med 2003;168:10-48.
16. Bellemare F, Grassino A: Effect of pressure and timing of contraction on human diaphragm fatigue. J Appl Physiol 1982;53:1190-1195.
17. Lemaire F, Teboul JL, Cinotti L, et al: Acute left ventricular dysfunction during unsuccessful weaning from mechanical ventilation. Anesthesiology 1988;69:171-179.
18. Jubran A, Mathru M, Dries D, et al: Continuous recordings of mixed venous oxygen saturation during weaning from mechanical ventilation and the ramifications thereof. Am J Respir Crit Care Med 1998;158: 1763-1769.
19. Feinstein AR: Clinical Epidemiology: The Architecture of Clinical Research. Philadelphia, Saunders, 1985.
20. MacIntyre NR, Cook DJ, Ely EW Jr, et al: Evidence-based guidelines for weaning and discontinuing ventilatory support: A collective task force facilitated by the American College of Chest Physicians; the American Association for Respiratory

Care; and the American College of Critical Care Medicine. Chest 2001;120(Suppl 6):375S-395S.
21. Meade M, Guyatt G, Cook D, et al. Predicting success in weaning from mechanical ventilation. Chest 2001;120:400S-424S.
22. Tobin MJ, Jubran A: Variable performance of weaning-predictor tests: Role of Bayes' theorem and spectrum and test-referral bias. Intensive Care Med 2006;32:2002-2012.
23. Casscells W, Schoenberger A, Graboys TB: Interpretation by physicians of clinical laboratory results. N Engl J Med 1978;299:999-1001.
24. Yang KL, Tobin MJ: A prospective study of indexes predicting the outcome of trials of weaning from mechanical ventilation. N Engl J Med 1991;324: 1445-1450.
25. Brand R, Kragt H: Importance of trends in the interpretation of an overall odds ratio in the meta-analysis of clinical trials. Stat Med 1992;11:2077-2082.
26. Schmid CH, Lau J, McIntosh MW, et al: An empirical study of the effect of the control rate as a predictor of treatment efficacy in meta-analysis of clinical trials. Stat Med 1998;17:1923-1942.
27. Sassoon CS: Intermittent mechanical ventilation. In Tobin MJ (ed): Principles and Practice of Mechanical Ventilation, 2nd ed. New York, McGraw-Hill, 2006, pp 201-220.
28. Marini JJ, Smith TC, Lamb VJ: External work output and force generation during synchronized intermittent mechanical ventilation. Effect of machine assistance on breathing effort. Am Rev Respir Dis 1988;138:1169-1179.
29. Imsand C, Feihl F, Perret C, et al: Regulation of inspiratory neuromuscular output during synchronized intermittent mechanical ventilation. Anesthesiology 1994;80:13-22.
30. Brochard L: Pressure-support ventilation. In Tobin MJ (ed): Principles and Practice of Mechanical Ventilation, 2nd ed. New York, McGraw-Hill, 2006, pp 221-250.
31. Jubran A, Van de Graaff WB, Tobin MJ: Variability of patient-ventilator interaction with pressure support ventilation in patients with chronic obstructive pulmonary disease. Am J Respir Crit Care Med 1995;152: 129-136.
32. Straus C, Louis B, Isabey D, et al: Contribution of the endotracheal tube and the upper airway to breathing workload. Am J Respir Crit Care Med 1998;157:23-30.
33. Esteban A, Alia I, Tobin MJ, et al: Effect of spontaneous breathing trial duration on outcome of attempts to discontinue mechanical ventilation. Spanish Lung Failure Collaborative Group. Am J Respir Crit Care Med 1999;159:512-518.
34. Kollef MH, Shapiro SD, Silver P, et al: A randomized, controlled trial of protocol-directed versus physician-directed weaning from mechanical ventilation. Crit Care Med 1997;25:567-574.
35. Marelich GP, Murin S, Battistella F, et al. Protocol weaning of mechanical ventilation in medical and surgical patients by respiratory care practitioners and nurses: Effect on weaning time and incidence of ventilator-associated pneumonia. Chest 2000;118:459-467.
36. Ely EW, Baker AM, Evans GW, et al: The prognostic significance of passing a daily screen of weaning parameters. Intensive Care Med 1999;25:581-587.
37. Namen AM, Ely EW, Tatter SB, et al: Predictors of successful extubation in neurosurgical patients. Am J Respir Crit Care Med 2001;163:658-664.
38. Randolph AG, Wypij D, Venkataraman ST, et al: Effect of mechanical ventilator weaning protocols on respiratory outcomes in infants and children: A randomized controlled trial. JAMA 2002;288:2561-2568.
39. Morris AH: Algorithm-based decision making. In Tobin MJ (ed): Principles and Practice of Intensive Care Monitoring, 1st ed. New York, McGraw-Hill, 1998, pp 1355-1381.
40. Tobin MJ: Of principles and protocols and weaning. Am J Respir Crit Care Med 2004;169:661-662.
41. Krishnan JA, Moore D, Robeson C, et al: A prospective, controlled trial of a protocol-based strategy to discontinue mechanical ventilation. Am J Respir Crit Care Med 2004;169:673-678.
42. Tobin MJ, Laghi F: Extubation. In Tobin MJ (ed): Principles and Practice of Mechanical Ventilation, 2nd ed. New York, McGraw-Hill, 2006, pp 221-1238.

Chapter 45

Pulmonary Embolism

John D. Buckley, Daniel R. Ouellette, and John Popovich, Jr.

The anatomic structure of the pulmonary vasculature is associated with functional attributes. One function of the pulmonary vasculature dictated by structure is filtration of the circulatory system. Diverse materials entering into the systemic venous circulation may lodge in the pulmonary vasculature. Clinical syndromes may occur depending on the quantity and nature of the filtered material and on the physiologic reserves of the individual.[1] The most common and clinically important of these syndromes is pulmonary thromboembolism, a complication of deep venous thrombosis (DVT). Pulmonary thromboembolism and DVT are different manifestations of the same disease, namely venous thromboembolism (VTE). Other similar clinical syndromes of importance to the critical care practitioner are the sequelae produced by the embolization of air, fat, infected clots, amniotic fluid, tumor, inorganic substances, and fecal matter.

Pulmonary thromboembolism is the focus of this chapter because of the relative clinical importance of this problem to the critical care practitioner. More than 600,000 patients suffer pulmonary embolism (PE) in the United States every year. Pulmonary thromboembolism may cause or contribute to death in up to 200,000 individuals annually.[2-5] When patients present to medical attention with hemodynamic instability, the in-hospital mortality rate may be as high as 31%.[6] Pulmonary thromboembolism thus represents a common critical illness.

In this chapter we discuss the clinical implications, diagnostic strategies, and management of pulmonary thromboembolism. Our discussion is then extended to other types of embolic phenomena encountered in critically ill patients.

PATHOPHYSIOLOGIC EFFECTS OF PULMONARY EMBOLI

Life-threatening pulmonary thromboemboli may be caused by a massive embolus in a physiologically normal person or may be caused by a submassive embolus in a person with impaired physiologic reserves. This is understood when one learns that not only will two thirds of patients who die from pulmonary thromboembolism die within 1 hour of presentation, but that anatomically massive pulmonary emboli will account for only half of the deaths.[7] Figure 45-1 depicts the conceptual relationship between the size of the pulmonary embolus, the cardiopulmonary reserves of the patient, and the outcomes from pulmonary thromboembolism. The term *major pulmonary thromboembolism* has been coined to describe any pulmonary thromboembolus that results in a hemodynamically significant event.[8] This definition provides a useful perspective for the critical care practitioner.

In patients with pulmonary thromboembolism, hemodynamic instability is an important predictor of survival (Table 45-1).[7] The Urokinase Pulmonary Embolism Trial (UPET)[9] demonstrated that the presence of hemodynamic decompensation was associated with a sevenfold increase in mortality. The International Cooperative Pulmonary Embolism Registry (ICOPER)[10] confirmed these results by demonstrating a fourfold increase in mortality for those patients with hemodynamic instability. Because of the associations between outcome from pulmonary thromboembolism and shock or hypotension, aggressive intervention in patients thought to have pulmonary thromboembolism who are in shock may have important therapeutic consequences. Wood speaks of the "golden hour" of major PE in which timely diagnosis and treatment are crucial.[7]

The principal pathophysiologic effects of pulmonary thromboembolism result from the acute impaction of material into pulmonary circulation and the resulting vascular obstruction and humoral mediator release.[1] In nonhematogenous obstruction of the pulmonary vasculature, obliteration of 60% to 70% of the vascular tree is required to cause an elevation of the pulmonary artery pressure.[11-15] However, only 25% to 30% of the vascular tree must be obstructed in pulmonary thromboembolism for elevation of the pulmonary artery pressure to be realized.[1,15,16] Therefore factors other than simple mechanical obstruction of the pulmonary vascular system must play a role in the elevation of the pressures in the pulmonary circuit during pulmonary thromboembolism (Fig. 45-2). Neural and humoral mediators play an important role in the hemodynamic consequences of PE. Medium-sized pulmonary arteries, pulmonary arterioles, and pulmonary veins are constricted by pathways mediated by neural and humoral stimuli.[15] Constriction of small pulmonary arteries and pulmonary arterioles decreases pulmonary artery compliance.[17] Constriction of pulmonary veins causes movement of blood away from the pulmonary venous compartment.[1]

Cardiac failure in major PE results from increased vascular resistance to right ventricular output (see Fig. 45-2). The pressure load increases in the right ventricle in response to the increased resistance resulting from the embolic phenomenon. This leads to increased ventricular wall stress and cardiac ischemia.[7] The mathematical

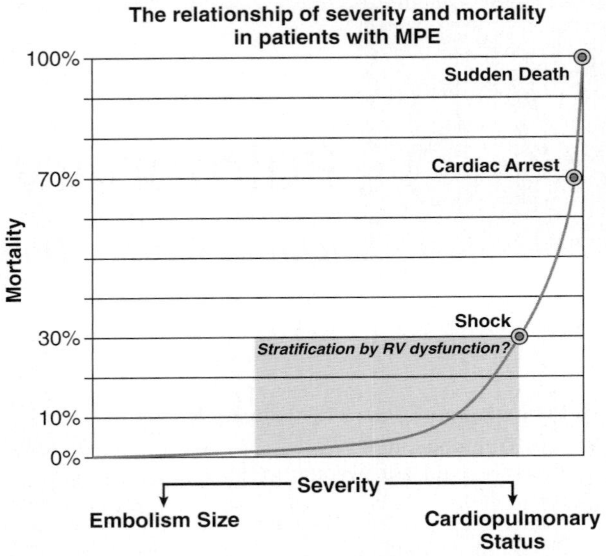

Figure 45-1. Outcomes in pulmonary embolism. (Adapted with permission from Wood KE: Major pulmonary embolism: Review of a pathophysiological approach to the golden hour of hemodynamically significant pulmonary embolism. Chest 2002;121:877-905.)

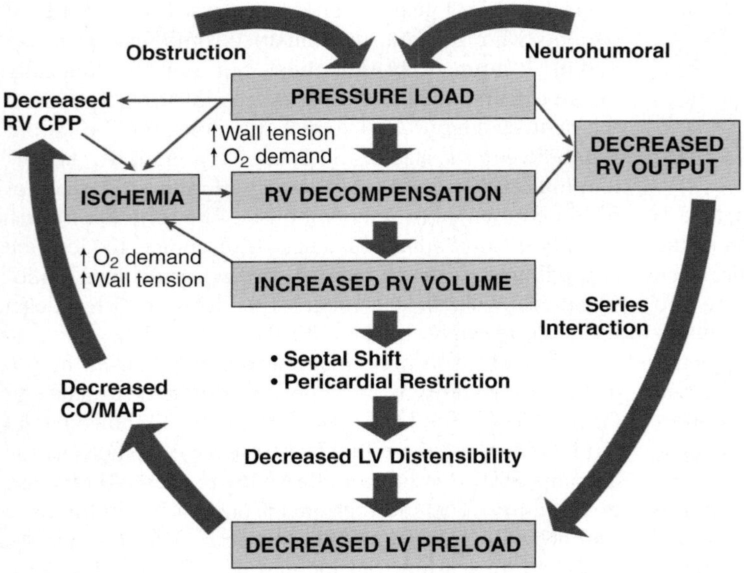

Figure 45-2. Pathophysiologic cycle of massive pulmonary embolism. CO, cardiac output; CPP, coronary perfusion pressure; LV, left ventricle; MAP, mean arterial pressure; RV, right ventricle. (Adapted with permission from Wood KE: Major pulmonary embolism: Review of a pathophysiologic approach to the golden hour of hemodynamically significant pulmonary embolism. Chest 2002;121:877-905.)

Table 45-1. Relationships among Shock, Embolism Size, and Outcome*

Study	Shock Patients	Nonshock Patients	Patients with Massive PEs in Shock	Patients with Nonmassive PEs in Shock	Patients with Massive PEs Not in Shock	Patients with Nonmassive PEs Not in Shock
UPET[9] (*n* = 160)[†]	9/36	91/6	12/18	4/100	88/5	96/6
Alpert et al[192] (*n* = 136)[‡]	21/25	79/5	38/32	11/11	62/7	90/4

*Values given as patients, %/mortality, %.
[†]Treatment with heparin or urokinase.
[‡]Treatment with heparin or ligation.
UPET, Urokinase Pulmonary Embolism Trial.

relationships between flow (Q), pressure (P), and resistance (R) are seen in Equation 1.

$$Q = \Delta P/R$$

During the early phase of pulmonary embolization, compensation allows flow to be maintained. Compensation occurs as a result of sympathetic-mediated tachycardia and right ventricular dilation based on the Frank-Starling concept.[7] Ultimately, right ventricular output falls in response to increased right ventricular wall stress and ischemia. When this happens, left ventricular preload is diminished. Left ventricular compliance may also diminish as a result of several factors.[18-20] Because the right ventricle is dilated as a result of the pressure load of a PE, the interventricular septum undergoes a leftward shift, which results in diminished left ventricular compliance. Additionally, the dilation of the right ventricle leads to increased constrictive forces by the pericardium, which causes diminished left ventricular compliance. The decrease in left ventricular preload and the decrease in left ventricular compliance have important effects on left ventricular function. Left ventricular output falls, and hypotension ensues.

The increased vascular resistance in the pulmonary circuit during venous thromboembolism is related not only to anatomic obstruction by thrombus but also to increased pulmonary vascular resistance caused by neural reflexes, release of humoral factors from platelets or endothelium, activation of humoral factors in serum, and hypoxia.

The von Bezold-Jarisch reflex, which includes the clinical signs of apnea, bradycardia, and hypotension, may be evoked by pulmonary emboli.[1] The afferent portion of this loop is believed to be constituted by J-receptors and pulmonary C-fibers located in the lung.[21-24]

The efferent loop of the von Bezold-Jarisch reflex is mediated by the vagus nerve.[25] It has been observed that blockade of the vagus nerve eliminates the von Bezold-Jarisch reflex but does not prevent the increase in pulmonary artery or right ventricular pressures seen with pulmonary embolus.[26] One reason that pulmonary embolus may cause increased pressures in the pulmonary circuit in the presence of cholinergic blockade is that increased sympathetic tone may also lead to neurogenic pulmonary vasoconstriction in pulmonary embolus.[27,28] Although sympathetic vasoconstriction is not an important phenomenon in normal pulmonary vasculature, it may be important when an elevated pulmonary artery pressure is present, as occurs during pulmonary embolus. Sympathetic vasoconstrictive innervation extends through the entire pulmonary vascular system, whereas vasodilating innervation exists only in arteries that have a diameter greater than 700 μm.[29] At rest in the normal pulmonary vasculature, vascular tone is either absent or low.[1] Interestingly, the effects of sympathomimetics and acetylcholine on pulmonary vascular resistance and tone are different depending on whether the pulmonary artery pressure is normal or elevated (Table 45-2).[1] These differential effects have important implications regarding sympathetic stimulation during the course of a pulmonary embolus.

Table 45-2. Effects of Some Sympathomimetics and of Acetylcholine on Pulmonary Artery Pressure (PAP) as a Function of Resting PAP

	Normal Baseline PAP	Increased Baseline PAP
Epinephrine	Constricts	Dilates
Norepinephrine	Constricts	Constricts, dilates
Phenylephrine	Constricts	Constricts, dilates
Acetylcholine	Constricts, dilates	Dilates

Following pulmonary thromboembolism, a complex series of events occurs in part resulting from the release and activation of a variety of humoral factors. Platelet activation and aggregation are important events that occur with thrombus formation. Evidence indicates that platelet activity is an ongoing process during pulmonary venous thromboembolism, even if the thrombus was formed at a remote location.[30] A number of mediators are released or activated as a consequence of platelet activation that affects the pulmonary vasculature (Table 45-3).[27,31] Although the normal, intact pulmonary endothelium has inherent anticoagulant and vasodilating effects, the disrupted pulmonary vascular endothelium may promote vasoconstrictive and procoagulant activities.[32] Factors promoting endothelial disruption during pulmonary thromboembolism include increased pulmonary arterial pressure, high shear stress, hypoxia and ischemia, neutrophil activation, and the toxic effect of fibrin and its degradation products.[1] Factors produced by endothelial cells that affect thrombosis and vasomotor tone are presented in Figure 45-3.[33]

Abnormalities of gas exchange and pulmonary function result from pulmonary emboli. Hypoxemia is a common sequela of pulmonary thromboembolism. Hypoxemia may occur from a variety of mechanisms. These include the development of ventilation/perfusion mismatching in underventilated regions of lung parenchyma, intracardiac shunting through a patent foramen ovale in the setting of high right-sided pressures, intrapulmonary shunting through areas of atelectasis, and a decrease in cardiac output leading to a decrease in the mixed venous oxygen saturation. Hypoxemia itself may promote endothelial damage, as noted earlier, and thus lead to pulmonary vasoconstriction. Hypoxemia may also promote a prothrombotic and antifibrinolytic state.[1]

Pulmonary thromboembolism also may lead to underperfused but ventilated areas of lung parenchyma. This creates a *deadspace effect*.[34] Eugene Robin proposed in 1959 that areas of the lung that are well ventilated but poorly perfused following pulmonary thromboembolism should contribute a volume of gas to an end-tidal gas collection relatively bereft of carbon dioxide compared with the arterial carbon dioxide partial pressure.[34] The partial pressure of CO_2 in an end-tidal gas collection has been shown to fall in pulmonary thromboembolism; it has been suggested that the fall in end-tidal CO_2 occurs when more than 25% of the pulmonary vasculature is occluded.[1]

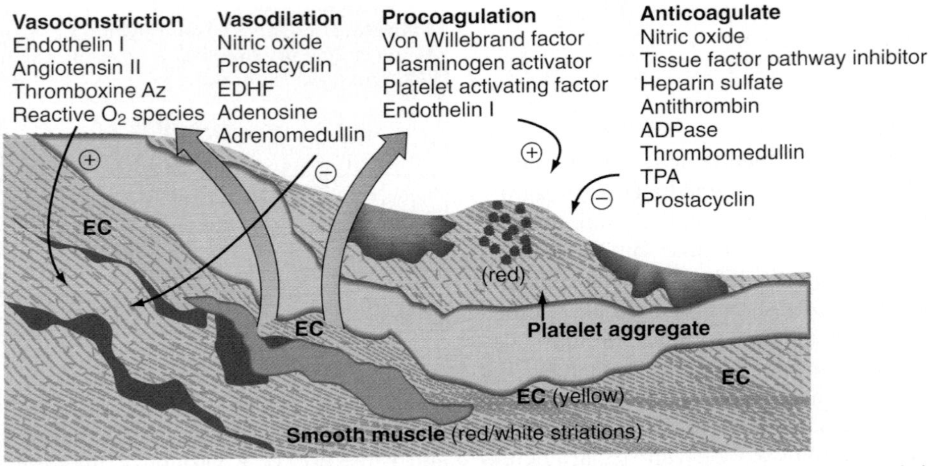

Figure 45-3. Factors produced by endothelial cells that affect thrombosis and vasomotor tone. EC, endothelial cell.

Table 45-3. Examples of Mediators Affecting the Aggregatory-Pulmonary Vasomotor Balance after Pulmonary Embolism

	Prothrombotic/Vasoconstrictive Effect	Antithrombotic/Vasodilative Effect
Serotonin	Vasoconstriction	Production of NO
ADP	Vasoconstriction, platelet recruitment	Production of NO
Thrombin	Vasoconstriction activates platelets	Production of NO and PG-I_2
ACh	Vasoconstriction	NO production
Catecholamines	Vasoconstriction at normal PAP	NO production, vasodilation at ↓ PAP
Leukotrienes	Vasoconstriction	Production of NO
Bacterial toxins, cytokines	Tissue factor expression	NO production
Shear stress	Endothelial cell damage	Production of NO
ROS	Inhibition of NO production	Vasodilation, production of PG-I_2
NO	Inhibition of NO production	Vasodilation, inhibition of platelet and leukocyte activation, ↓ ROS, inhibition of GPIIb/IIIa and several integrins, ↓ tissue factor
AT-II	Inhibition of NO production (via ↑ ROS), ↑ ET-1, ↑ catecholamines	Production of NO
ET-1	Vasoconstriction, ↑ coagulability (↑ FVIII, ↓ AT, ↓ tPA)	Release of NO and EDHF
PDGF	Vasoconstriction, ↑ platelets	Production of PG-I_2
PAF	Vasoconstriction, ↑ platelet and leukocyte adhesion to endothelium	Production of NO

Many humoral mediators and physical factors have opposing effects on hemostasis, as well as vasomotor control. The information contained in this table is not comprehensive.
ACh, acetylcholine; ADP, adenosine diphosphate; AT, antithrombin; AT-II, angiotensin II; EDHF, endothelium-derived hyperpolarizing factor; ET-1, endothelin-1; FVIII, coagulation factor VIII; GPIIb/IIIa, glycoprotein IIb/IIIa; NO, nitric oxide; PAF, platelet activating factor; PAP, pulmonary artery pressure; PDGF, platelet-derived growth factor; PG-I_2, prostacyclin; ROS, reactive oxygen species; tPA, tissue plasminogen activator.
Data from references 27 and 31.

However, a variety of cardiopulmonary conditions lead to abnormalities in the end-tidal CO_2 levels, so this measurement is unreliable as a specific diagnostic test.

VENOUS THROMBOEMBOLI

Venous thromboembolism (VTE) is particularly important to the critical care practitioner in that, similar to sepsis, it can be a primary reason for admission to the critical care unit or a complication of other critical illness. As a primary critical illness, VTE usually presents with either respiratory distress and/or hemodynamic collapse (major pulmonary embolus). As a complication of other critical illness, VTE must be considered in the differential diagnosis of a myriad of frequent clinical occurrences complicating the critically ill, such as worsening hypoxemia, cardiac dysrhythmias, hemodynamic alterations, chest pain, and fever.

Incidence and Epidemiology

The true incidence of pulmonary thromboembolism is difficult to accurately determine because of inaccuracies in ascertaining the correct clinical diagnosis. Much of the previous literature contains figures both underestimating and overestimating the incidence of PE. Various autopsy data provide wide ranges in estimates of major pulmonary emboli associated with death. Likewise, death certificates, discharge summary data, and other data sources have significant errors in the accuracy of diagnosis. Estimates of the annual incidence of VTE range from 23 to 100 per 100,000 population.[2,4,35] Advanced age is a significant risk factor, as demonstrated in a longitudinal study of 855 men followed from the ages of 50 to 80 years, in which the cumulative incidence of a venous thromboembolic event was 0.5% by the age of 50 years and increased to 10.7% by the age of 80 years.[36] Even more disturbing are estimates that only 10% to 30% of all cases are accurately diagnosed antemortem.[37] The incidence of VTE as a cause of critical illness and requiring admission to an intensive care unit is unknown. Most studies suggest approximately 15% to 20% of patients with diagnosed PE have either significant hemodynamic compromise, manifested by shock or syncope, or significant respiratory compromise manifested by hypoxemia or respiratory distress.[38,39] In a cross-sectional study of 100 medical ICU patients, one third had evidence of DVT on serial ultrasounds of lower and upper extremities.[40] Approximately 10% of patients referred to the PIOPED-I study were hospitalized in a medical or surgical critical care unit.[39]

Table 45-4. Risk Factors for Venous Thromboembolism (VTE)

Strong Risk Factors	Fracture of hip, pelvis, leg Hip or knee replacement surgery Major trauma Major general surgery Spinal cord injury
Moderate Risk Factors	Arthroscopic knee surgery Indwelling central venous catheters Malignancy Congestive heart failure Respiratory failure Estrogen therapy Paralytic stroke Postpartum period Previous VTE Thrombophilia
Weak Risk Factors	Bed rest for more than 3 days Immobility caused by sitting Advanced age Laparoscopic surgery Obesity Antepartum period Varicose veins

From Blann AD, Lip GY: Venous thromboembolism. BMJ 2006;332:215-219.

Risk Factors

Most clinically significant pulmonary emboli, estimated as high as 95%, emanate from the deep veins of the lower extremity.[41-43] The proximal deep veins of the leg are the most common sites of origin of clots that embolize to the pulmonary circulation. Pulmonary thromboembolism and deep vein thrombosis should be viewed as different clinical presentations of the same disease process.

Virchow first described general risk factors for the development of deep venous thrombosis in the nineteenth century.[44] Stasis, vascular wall abnormalities, and hypercoagulability predispose patients to the development of venous thrombosis. Patients with a variety of critical illnesses are at an increased risk of developing VTE.[45,46] Unfortunately, accurate data on critically ill patients in intensive care units are not available. Additional information about this heterogenous patient population is provided in a later section.

Many risk factors for VTE have been identified and are outlined in Table 45-4.[47] Several acquired and inherited hypercoagulable states have been shown to increase the risk of PE. Several of these conditions, collectively known as thrombophilia, are presented in Box 45-1.

Box 45-1

Conditions Associated with Thrombophilia

Malignancy
Activated protein C resistance
Antiphospholipid antibody syndrome
Prothrombin gene mutation 2021A
Protein C or S deficiency
Factor V Leiden mutation
Antithrombin deficiency
Estrogen therapy

Role of Deep Venous Thrombosis

Deep venous thrombosis probably forms from a platelet aggregate nidus to form a fibrin clot, usually in the inferior aspect of a venous valve or a site of specific vascular disruption, such as an indwelling catheter site.[48] A general consensus suggests that clinically significant deep venous thromboses and pulmonary emboli originate by proximal extension of calf DVT. Under the proper coagulation conditions, a clot may propagate quickly to form a red fibrin and platelet aggregation. Clots that continue to propagate have a greater risk to break apart and lead to embolization. This generally occurs more frequently in the first few days after clot formation. Clots that do not continue to propagate resolve by either fibrinolysis or organization.[49,50] These processes generally occur within 7 days of clot formation.

Clinical Manifestations

Clinical manifestations of pulmonary emboli vary significantly and are nonspecific. Classic symptoms such as acute dyspnea, pleuritic chest pain, hemoptysis, and syncope may not be present in some cases of substantial embolization. Physical findings also may be nonspecific. More than 65% of patients initially suspected of having a pulmonary embolus on the basis of clinical suspicion prove not to have this disease.[39,42,85] These data underscore the difficulty in establishing the diagnosis of PE clinically, emphasizing the importance of heightened awareness and reliance on further testing to diagnose this disorder.

Patients with PE admitted to critical care units usually have either massive pulmonary emboli, symptomatic PE in the setting of other cardiopulmonary disease, or secondary complications of pulmonary emboli or its treatment such as arrhythmias or gastrointestinal hemorrhage. Massive PE presents with acute cardiorespiratory symptoms and signs generally attributed to right ventricular output failure or ischemia.[52] Sudden cardiopulmonary arrest, often with bradyarrhythmias and pulseless electrical activity, may be the reason for admission to the critical care unit. Efforts to resuscitate such patients are often futile because of the failure to overcome right ventricular outflow obstruction and develop life-sustaining peripheral perfusion pressures. The absence of a pressure pulse developing during closed chest massage should suggest the diagnosis of massive PE. Closed chest percussion has been reported to fragment experimental clots and restore some perfusion; this has also been anecdotally reported from angiography studies of PE.

Other manifestations of extensive pulmonary emboli include significant anxiety with a sense of impending doom, substernal chest discomfort, syncope, shock, and acute cor pulmonale. The chest discomfort is usually described as sudden in onset, oppressive, unrelenting, and nonradiating. This pain is often difficult to distinguish from severe angina pectoris or dissecting thoracic aortic aneurysm. In fact, a component of the chest pain may be truly anginal, related to right ventricular ischemia. Syncope may be the result of either low cardiac output or vagally mediated bradyarrhythmias.[53] Manifestations of acute cor pulmonale include distended neck veins, a prominent and often palpable pulmonic component of the second heart sound, right ventricular S_3 or S_4 gallops, and pulsus paradoxus. Sepsis, right ventricular infarction, tension pneumothorax, pericardial tamponade, superior vena caval obstruction, restrictive or hypertrophic cardiomyopathies, and pre-existing chronic cor pulmonale with superimposed acute illness must be considered in this differential.

Less dramatic presentations of PE often occur in patients with preexisting cardiopulmonary disease. Nonmassive pulmonary emboli may present as an exacerbation of congestive heart failure or chronic obstructive lung disease, leading to gas exchange abnormalities severe enough to require expectant monitoring or active treatment in a critical care setting. Often the presenting clinical manifestations are dictated by the principal underlying disease. Tachypnea and/or hypoxemia out of proportion to the estimated severity of the exacerbation should raise clinical suspicion, as should prior embolic disease, significant risk factors, signs of right-sided cardiac ischemia, or unusual radiographic findings (such as pleura-based infiltrates with effusion or focal oligemia).

Occult PE may occur in critically ill patients who often have risk factors. Immobilization, sepsis, and invasive venous catheters are often present in intensive care patients, leading to a potentially increased risk of venothrombotic complications. Clinical suspicion must remain high, in that many of the manifestations of pulmonary emboli in this population are easily attributed to other processes. Supraventricular tachycardia, episodic hypoxemia or hypocapnia, unexplained fever, pleuritic chest discomfort, and pulmonary infiltrates may be some of the subtle manifestations of PE in this population. Hemodynamic alterations, such as abrupt cardiac output reductions with increases in pulmonary arterial pressure (if these parameters are being monitored), may suggest the diagnosis. Unfortunately, all of these findings are nonspecific, and patients often require invasive testing or CT scan to diagnosis PE in this setting. Underdiagnosis of pulmonary embolus in the critically ill patient may occur because patients may not be stable to transfer to the radiology suite for invasive radiologic studies, as well as because these patients have multiple comorbidities, which can confound the diagnosis.

Electrocardiograms are generally nonspecific in pulmonary embolic disease, although manifestations of right-sided heart strain (new right axis deviation or a new right bundle branch block) may signal the presence of massive embolization. Chest radiographs are also nonspecific in assessing PE but may point to another disease process such as pneumothorax or mucous plugging to explain the acute syndrome of concern.[54] Patients with PE in the PIOPED-I study were more likely to have findings of an elevated hemidiaphragm, hypovascularity, pleural-based opacities, and focal oligemia (Westermark's sign) and be less likely to have diffuse pulmonary edema.[51] Arterial blood gases often show hypoxemia or an increase in alveolar-arterial oxygen gradient, but the magnitude of the oxygenation deficit does not differentiate between at-risk individuals with or without documented PE. Because arterial blood gases may be completely normal in pulmonary embolus, such testing is not helpful in differentiating pulmonary embolus from other diagnostic possibilities.

Diagnostic Tests

Chest Radiography

Chest radiography, as noted earlier, is used in the general clinical evaluation of patients with possible PE to both exclude other causes of the acute clinical syndrome and to identify radiographic patterns attributed to PE. The PIOPED-I investigators studied radiographs of patients with the proven diagnosis of PE compared with a group of patients in whom the diagnosis was excluded, noting that certain radiographic patterns were more common in PE. Pleural-based infiltrates, focal oligemia, and hypovascularity were more common in the PE–positive group. Unfortunately, these findings did not have high sensitivity or specificity for the disorder.[39]

Ventilation-Perfusion Nuclear Scans

With the improving performance of spiral CT at detecting pulmonary thromboembolism, ventilation-perfusion lung scanning is being performed less often yet remains a valuable diagnostic test. The sensitivity and specificity of this technique was established in a general representative American population by the PIOPED-I study.[39] In a sophisticated analysis of well-performed, multiple ventilation and perfusion images compared with a gold standard of selective pulmonary angiography, ventilation-perfusion lung scans were interpreted using consensus criteria. Scans were interpreted as near normal–normal, low probability, intermediate probability, and high probability for PE. The sensitivity of all abnormal scans in aggregate was high (>98%), but the specificity for all scans is approximately 10%.

In a smaller study of 104 patients, revised PIOPED-I criteria for interpreting ventilation-perfusion scans and a "gestalt" interpretation by experienced nuclear radiologists demonstrated improved accuracy over the original PIOPED-I criteria for assessing the likelihood of PE.[53] High probability scans provide useful information, especially when combined with a high pretest clinical suspicion for PE (positive predictive value of 96%).[39] When a high probability scan is associated with an intermediate- or low-likelihood clinical assessment, the positive predictive values fall to 88% and 56%, respectively. However, the majority of angiographically proven pulmonary emboli in the PIOPED-I study had ventilation-perfusion scans that were not high probability. Normal or near-normal scans are also useful studies. When these scan results are paired with a low-likelihood clinical assessment, the negative predictive value is 98%.[39] Unfortunately, normal and high probability scans account for less than 30% of all ventilation-perfusion scans. Of the low probability scans in the PIOPED study, 16% had evidence of PE on pulmonary angiography, and other studies suggest that low-probability scans may miss up to 40% of pulmonary emboli.[39,54] The disappointing results of these studies have led many authors to combine low-probability and indeterminate scans, referring to them as *nondiagnostic ventilation-perfusion scans*.[54-57]

Other cardiopulmonary diseases diminish the clinical utility of ventilation-perfusion scans by increasing the prevalence of nondiagnostic scans.[58] High probability scans may occur in patients because of chronic obstructive pulmonary disease (COPD). In general, nondiagnostic scans are more likely to occur in COPD patients than in patients without pre-existing cardiopulmonary disease.[59] Lung scans are not useful to either establish or rule out the diagnosis of PE in more than 80% of cases. A similar disadvantage of ventilation-perfusion lung scans is noted in critically ill patients with prior cardiopulmonary disease. Nevertheless, ventilation-perfusion lung scans can be performed in the critically ill, even if patients are receiving mechanical ventilation. Despite the limited ventilation component under positive pressure respiration, the perfusion component is not significantly affected by mechanical ventilation. Ventilation-perfusion scans remain a useful tool in patients with contraindications to pulmonary angiography or CT angiography.

Echocardiography

Recent advancements in echocardiography may result in this technology playing a useful role in the diagnosis of PE. Compared with several other diagnostic tests for PE, echocardiography is noninvasive, fast, and can be performed at the bedside in the intensive care unit. In a cohort of 132 patients suspected of having pulmonary emboli, transthoracic echocardiographic parameters in patients proven to have pulmonary emboli differed from patients with normal perfusion scans or angiograms in that they had greater right ventricular and lesser left ventricular diameters.[60] In another study of 49 patients with suspected pulmonary emboli and evidence of right ventricular overload on transthoracic echocardiography, transesophageal echocardiography correctly identified 80% of the documented pulmonary emboli in the proximal and lobar pulmonary arteries with 100% specificity.[61] Echocardiography has been proposed as a useful tool to identify PE patients at high risk of death and possible candidates for thrombolytic therapy (see following discussion).[62] In a recent review of 3468 patients with pulmonary emboli and normal vital signs, 30% to 40% had evidence of right ventricular strain or failure on echocardiography.[63] A negative echocardiogram does not rule out the presence of a PE. Another use of ultrasound technology is the transthoracic imaging of the lung parenchyma.

Lower Extremity Studies

Documenting acute deep vein thrombosis with lower extremity studies is useful in evaluating critically ill patients suspected of having pulmonary emboli. Venography has largely been replaced by duplex ultrasonography because it is noninvasive, safe, and can be performed at the bedside. Duplex ultrasonography combines determination of vein compression and Doppler blood flow, and has demonstrated greater than 90% sensitivity and nearly 99% specificity for proximal deep vein thrombosis in patients suspected of having concomitant deep venous thrombosis. However, this falls significantly for below-the-knee thrombosis.[65,66] This high degree of accuracy requires sophisticated equipment and skilled technicians.

Computed Tomography

Technical advancements in computed tomography (CT) with intravenous contrast media now provide markedly improved resolution of pulmonary arteries. These spiral (or helical) CT angiograms (CTAs) play a growing role in evaluating patients suspected of having pulmonary emboli. First-generation spiral CT scanners had a single detector that "spiraled" around a patient to obtained data for images. Newer generations have multiple detectors that collect data simultaneously and permit faster imaging. Faster imaging minimizes respiratory motion artifact and obtains more images during peak concentrations of IV contrast in the pulmonary arteries. Clinical trials assessing the test performance characteristics of CT angiography have consistently shown good specificity (81% to 100%), with sensitivity varying as low as 53% with early single-detector spiral CTAs to more than 80% with multiple detectors.[67] The recent PIOPED-II study examined four-detector CT angiography in 824 patients suspected of having PE. Of 773 patients with interpretable CT angiograms, the overall sensitivity and specificity were 83% and 96%, respectively. When CT venography (CTV) of the pelvis and thighs was included (no additional contrast material), the overall CTA/CTV sensitivity and specificity were 90% and 95%, respectively.[68]

After considering the pretest clinical probability of pulmonary thromboembolism, the post-test positive and negative predictive values for spiral CT are included in Table 45-5.

Newer multidetector row spiral CT systems (16 to 64 detectors) provide even better resolution, especially when data are synchronized with the patient's ECG (Fig. 45-4).[69] These CT scans likely have better test performance characteristics than those reported in PIOPED-II.

The wide range of test performance characteristics throughout the literature results from different patient populations, generation of technology, and a variety of reference standards. Clinical outcome studies have suggested that the negative likelihood ratio of a negative CT angiogram is comparable with directed catheter pulmonary angiography.[70] As CT technology continues to improve, even the traditional gold standard of catheter-directed pulmonary angiography is being questioned.[69] However, interpreting CT angiography results in critically ill patients must be done with some caution because most of the published studies on CT angiography including PIOPED-II did not include critically ill patients. Additional clinical studies in critically ill patients will be necessary to clearly define the role of spiral CT. CT angiography adds another advantage over other diagnostic tests by providing extensive information related to other cardiopulmonary diseases. This added utility will likely enhance its role in the evaluation of patients presenting with a variety of cardiopulmonary diseases.

Table 45-5. Negative and Positive Predictive Values (NPV and PPV) of CT Angiography (CTA) Alone and CT Angiography Combined with CT Venography (CTA/CTV)

	CTA NPV	CTA/CTV NPV	CTA PPV	CTA/CTV PPV
Low pretest probability	96%	97%	58%	57%
Moderate pretest probability	89%	92%	92%	90%
High pretest probability	60%	82%	96%	96%

From Stein PD, for the PIOPED-II Investigators: Multidetector computer tomography for acute pulmonary embolism. N Engl J Med 2006;354:2317-2327.

Magnetic Resonance Imaging

Magnetic resonance angiography (MRA) is evolving as an alternative diagnostic test for PE. Like CT angiography, gadolinium-enhanced MRA technology has advanced in recent years. In a review of three clinical trials investigating MRA involving 184 subjects, the sensitivity ranged from 77% to 100% with specificity ranging from 95% to 98%.[71] The advantages of MRA include the avoidance of pulmonary artery catheterization, ionizing radiation, and nephrotoxic contrast material. The current prolonged scanning times and limited availability compared to CT angiography may limit the use of MRA. As this technology undergoes more testing, and becomes more feasible, it

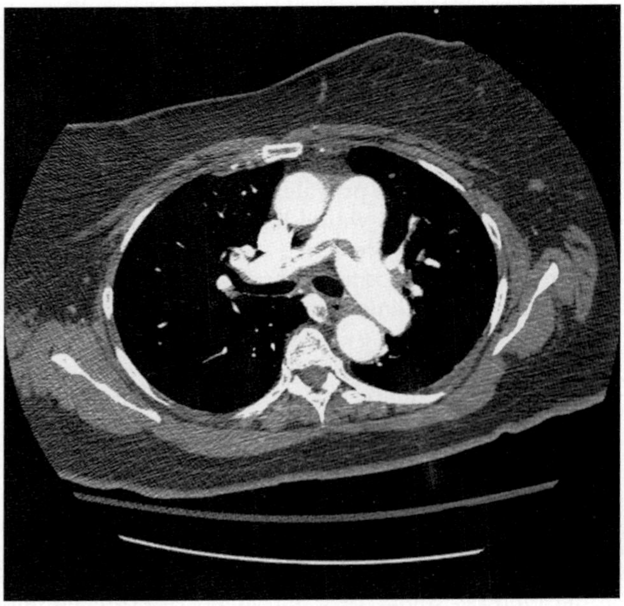

A

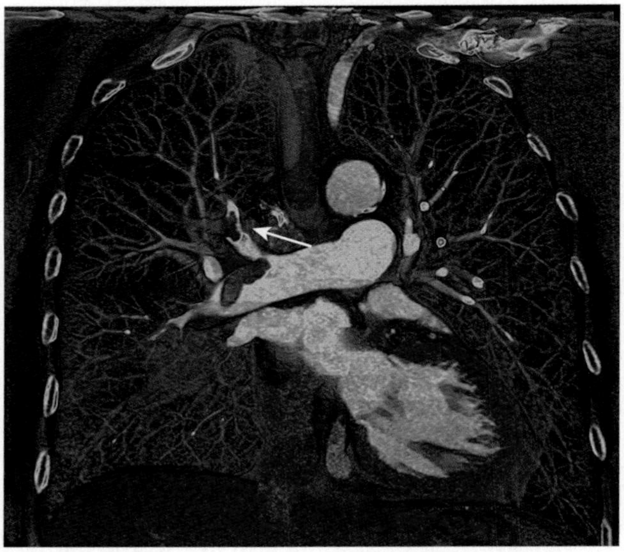

B

Figure 45-4. Single-detector **(A)** and 64-detector **(B)** CT angiogram images. (From Schoepf UJ, Savino G, Lake DR, et al: The age of CT pulmonary angiography. J Thorac Imaging 2005;20:273-279.)

may emerge as another valuable tool in diagnosing PE. The potential value of this technology is emphasized by the 40% of eligible patients for PIOPED-II who could not be enrolled because of contraindication to dye infusion, 30%.[68]

D-Dimer

D-dimers are specific degradation products of cross-linked fibrin. Elevated whole blood levels greater than 500 ng/mL are seen in nearly all patients with PE.[72-74] However, D-dimer levels are also elevated in many other clinical conditions such as recent surgery, malignancy, trauma, severe infection, pregnancy, disseminated intravascular coagulation, and liver disease.[75,76] This lack of specificity of elevated D-dimer levels does not help identify PE, but low levels may help exclude PE from a differential diagnosis. A review of published literature demonstrated a negative predictive value (NPV) of 94.2% for D-dimer levels less than 500 ng/mL when detected by ELISA. Newer rapid ELISA determination permits practical use in critically ill patients suspected of having PE. Clinical outcome studies have demonstrated that combining a low pretest probability with a negative D-dimer makes VTE unlikely.[77-79] However, clinicians should use caution in patients other than low-risk outpatients because the role of D-dimers has not been clearly established.

Directed-Catheter Pulmonary Angiography

Historically, the gold standard for the diagnosis of PE has been the directed-catheter pulmonary angiogram, but this may be replaced by ever-improving CT angiography. However, when CTA is nondiagnostic, directed-catheter pulmonary angiography may remain an important diagnostic test. The well-performed pulmonary angiogram has a sensitivity and specificity for acute PE of more than 95%.[39] In other words, a negative pulmonary angiogram essentially rules out clinically important pulmonary emboli. Proper technique is essential to prevent injection artifacts, which would make subsequent interpretation of angiograms difficult. Complications from pulmonary angiography are rare in experienced hands.[80,81] Of the 1111 angiograms performed in the PIOPED-I study, major complications occurred in only 14 (1.2%) patients including death in 5 (0.45%), respiratory arrest or failure in 4, renal failure in 3, and hemorrhage requiring transfusion in 2.[80] Minor complications and transient complications occurred in 60 (5.4%) patients. Of the 210 pulmonary angiograms performed in PIOPED-II, the only reported complication was transient acute renal insufficiency in one patient. No other complications were identified.[68]

The role of directed catheter pulmonary angiography is diminishing because of the improving characteristics, ease, safety, and availability of CT angiography. When diagnostic certainty is unequivocally mandatory, such as critical illness with hemodynamic or respiratory compromise, when thrombolytic agents, vena caval interruption, or surgical embolectomy are contemplated, or when therapy with anticoagulants carries substantial risk, pulmonary angiography still has a role, albeit a shrinking one. Large clinical trials comparing CT angiography with directed catheter pulmonary angiography do not exist and are unlikely to be conducted. As fewer invasive studies are performed, the technical expertise will likely decrease, contributing to a lower utility as a diagnostic test.

Diagnostic Strategies

Perhaps the most critical step in the diagnosis of PE is the development of a clinical suspicion of the diagnosis. This clinical suspicion is based on a compiled assessment of risk factors, symptoms, signs, electrocardiogram, chest radiograph, and laboratory blood studies. Synthesizing a pretest probability for pulmonary thromboembolism can be done by both subjective and objective means. At least two investigations have suggested that experienced clinicians can, with reasonable accuracy, differentiate high (>80%) and low (<20%) probability for PE in patient populations.[39,42] Less experienced clinicians can rely on several objective clinical assessments such as the Wells, Geneva, and revised Geneva criteria.[82-86] Unfortunately, the false-negative and false-positive values of clinical assessment alone make further studies necessary for diagnosis. Nevertheless, clinicians can make appropriate prior probability estimates to enhance the clinical usefulness of further diagnostic studies. These further studies can be separated into predominantly radiologic techniques aimed at making or excluding the diagnosis of pulmonary thromboembolism and studies used to ascertain the diagnosis of deep venous thrombosis of the legs.

Evaluating patients for the presence or absence of pulmonary thromboembolism in the intensive care unit presents several unique challenges. These patients have more risk factors for the development of thromboembolic diseases, yet the diagnostic tests are often difficult to interpret in these patients. Transporting hemodynamically unstable patients for diagnostic imaging studies can be risky, but the need for diagnostic certainty is often critical.

The link between deep vein thrombosis and pulmonary thromboembolism provides an additional diagnostic approach to patients suspected of having pulmonary thromboemboli. Many patients with proximal deep venous thrombosis have lung scans suggestive of PE.[87,88] Autopsy series suggest that proximal deep vein thrombosis is the most common source of pulmonary emboli found at this time. Therefore an alternative to the definitive pursuit of a diagnosis of PE is an attempt to establish the diagnosis of deep venous thrombosis. If the diagnosis of DVT is confirmed, additional testing for PE can usually be deferred. The documentation of venous thrombosis of the popliteal vein or higher commits one to treat with anticoagulants for a similar duration and intensity, as in the treatment of established PE. However, obtaining a duplex ultrasound or impedance plethysmography (IPG) in an ICU patient suspected of having a PE may not be a useful screening test. In several series of patients suspected of having a PE, duplex ultrasonography as an initial test revealed positive results in only 8% to 15% of patients, yet prevalence of concomitant PE was not rigorously determined.[89-92] Bedside testing with either duplex ultrasonography or IPG may be useful when immediately available.[95] However, when pursuing a diagnosis of pulmonary thromboembolism in patients without concomitant signs and symptoms of DVT, consider bypassing these tests and proceed directly to ventilation-perfusion scan or CT angiography.

A general diagnostic algorithm for the diagnosis of PE centers on the initial performance of a clinical assessment. For low-risk outpatients, the clinician should obtain a D-dimer with a validated assay and, if negative, pursue other diagnoses. If there are concomitant signs and symptoms of DVT, duplex ultrasonography or IPG, if readily available, should be obtained. Otherwise, the clinician should pursue CT angiography. If the patient has a history of contrast allergy or renal insufficiency, one should pursue a ventilation-perfusion scan. If the pretest probability of PE differs from the test results, the diagnosis remains uncertain and additional testing is usually necessary. Nondiagnostic CT angiograms are often the result of poor intravenous contrast, and repeat studies may be more definitive.

Patients in extremis are often too ill to travel out of an intensive care unit for diagnostic testing. Bedside transesophageal echocardiography with or without duplex ultrasonography may be useful in these patients, depending on availability and technical expertise. However, negative echocardiograms (no RV dysfunction) do not rule out PE, only PE as a cause of hypotension. An algorithm for the evaluation of critically ill patients suspected of having a pulmonary thromboembolism is presented in Figure 45-5.

Approach to Management

The major difference in the management of critically ill patients with PE versus non–critically ill patients is in the requirement for general monitoring, respiratory support, and hemodynamic augmentation. Most patients with PE do not need to be admitted to a critical care unit unless they are experiencing some cardiopulmonary aberration requiring anticipatory monitoring or active treatment. Exceptions might include settings where adequate infusion of heparin and monitoring of its effects cannot be performed on general nursing units, as well as the antici-

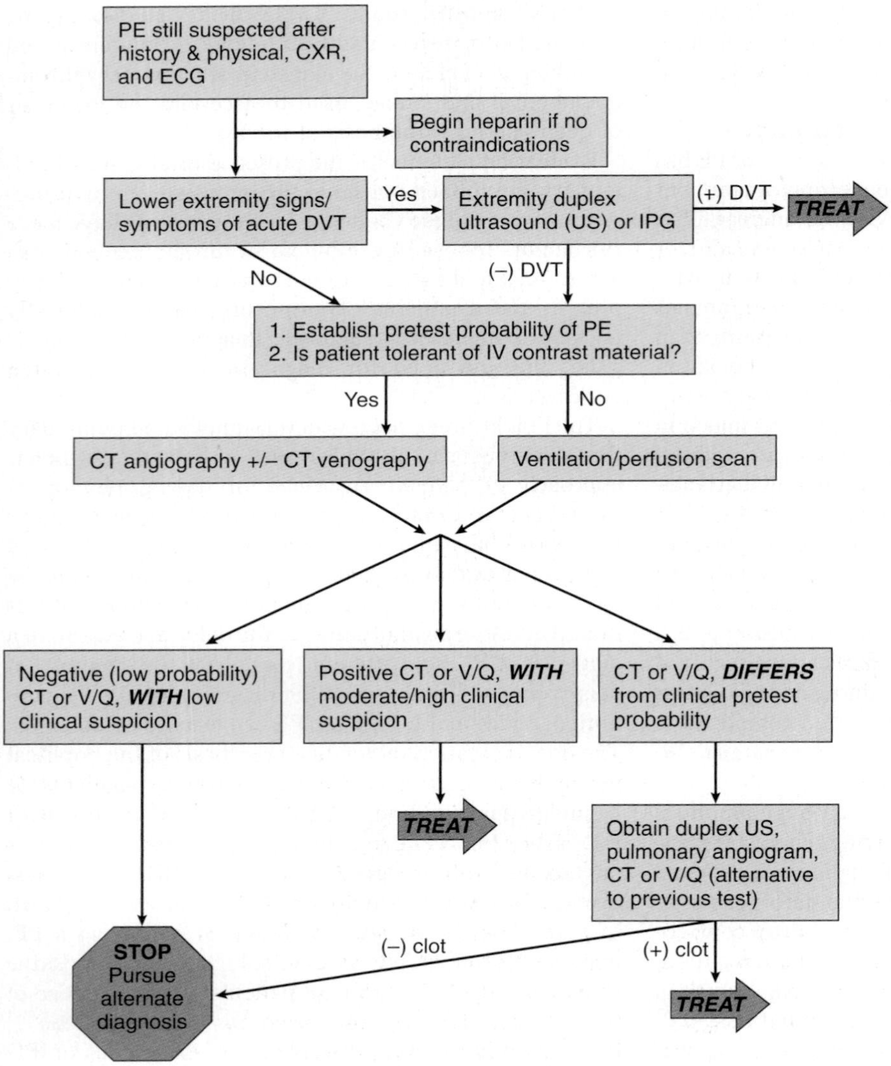

Figure 45-5. Diagnostic algorithm for pulmonary thromboembolism in critically ill patients. Consider transesophageal echocardiography (if available) for hemodynamically unstable patients. CT, computed tomography; CXR, chest x-ray; DVT, deep venous thrombosis; ECG, electrocardiogram; IPG, impedance plethysmography; PE, pulmonary embolism; US, ultrasonography; V/Q, ventilation-perfusion.

pated need for possible escalation of therapy (marked RV dysfunction on echocardiography, large clot burden, or severe underlying cardiopulmonary disease).

Critically ill patients with pulmonary emboli should be monitored with continuous electrocardiogram, noninvasive measurement of blood pressure, and pulse oximetry. Bedrest is often necessary for other reasons, although there is no significant evidence suggesting ambulation increases the risk of embolization of deep vein thromboses. Pain and anxiety should be treated with narcotic analgesics such as morphine sulfate and low-dose anxiolytic agents. Neurologic status, neck vein distention, cardiac rhythm, peripheral perfusion, and urine output should be monitored. Arterial catheterization should be instituted in patients with significant hemodynamic compromise. At least two large-bore (larger than 20 gauge) intravenous catheters should be placed peripherally. More invasive procedures, such as central venous catheterization, repetitive intravenous or intra-arterial blood draws, or needle diagnostic procedures, should be carefully considered if thrombolytic therapy is anticipated. A complete blood count, prothrombin time, activated partial thromboplastin time (or thrombin clotting time), platelet count, and stool for hemoglobin should be obtained.

All patients with PE should be assessed for adequacy of oxygenation with pulse oximetry or radial arterial blood gas analysis. Supplemental oxygen should be delivered to achieve an arterial oxygen saturation of at least 90% (arterial PO_2 >60 mm Hg). Higher arterial oxygen tension may be of some benefit in the alleviation of hypoxic-induced pulmonary vasoconstriction. Endotracheal intubation and mechanical ventilation is indicated for conventional reasons, such as oxygenation refractory to high levels of inspired oxygen by nonrebreather mask delivery, respiratory acidosis, or shock. The role of positive end-expiratory pressure (PEEP) is somewhat debated in PE with refractory hypoxemia despite mechanical ventilation, although anecdotal reports suggest some patients may be significantly responsive to this modality.[96] The potential impairment of RV preload from PEEP may be outweighed by the improvements in alveoli recruitment and decreased transmural pressure gradients in some patients. Noninvasive mechanical ventilation has not been extensively studied in these patients and is generally not recommended at this time.

Patients with shock and PE pose a particularly difficult challenge to the critical care practitioner. Cardiac dysrhythmia should be corrected, in that restoration of sinus rhythm may significantly improve right ventricular performance. Hypotensive patients with pulmonary emboli should receive a challenge of volume expansion in the absence of clinical evidence of cardiogenic pulmonary edema. Volume challenges of 100 to 200 mL crystalloid every 10 minutes with repetitive hemodynamic assessment are warranted. Some patients' shock states from PE may improve with fluid resuscitation despite high right ventricular filling pressures, on the basis of the possibility of expanding blood volume to aerated lungs previously underperfused from pulmonary arterial vasoconstriction.[97] Rising right atrial or central venous pressures with unimproved or deteriorating hemodynamic status should indicate that volume expansion is not improving and may be deteriorating right ventricular function.[98,99] In the hypotensive patient, increases in right ventricular filling pressure, estimated by right atrial mean or central venous pressures, without corresponding increases in systemic blood pressure, may cause a critical decrease in this RV perfusing pressure (aortic mean pressure minus right ventriculare mean pressure). The onset of right ventricular ischemia and acute deterioration in right ventricular pump function corresponds with the reduction of this critical pressure. The role of specific inotropes and vasopressors is less clear in hemodynamically compromised patients with pulmonary thromboembolism. Although published data in humans are lacking, animal studies suggest that norepinephrine (hypotensive patient), dobutamine (normotensive patient), or a combination of the two (hypotensive patient) may have advantages over other agents in the PE patient with tissue hypoperfusion.[100]

Heparin

The principal acute therapy for pulmonary thromboembolism is anticoagulation with unfractionated intravenous heparin (UFH) or low-molecular-weight heparin (LMWH).[101] With a strong clinical suspicion for pulmonary thromboembolism and/or deep venous thrombosis, heparin therapy should be initiated unless there is a contraindication, such as active or recent hemorrhage. Early treatment and adequacy of anticoagulation is critical.[102] Unfractionated heparin is usually delivered in a continuous infusion and monitored by determinations of the activated partial thromboplastin time (aPTT). Assays for aPTT vary among laboratories, and therapeutic ranges for aPTT should be established locally on the basis of corresponding anti-Xa activity by the amidolytic assay. For patients requiring large daily doses of UFH, consider directly measuring the anti-Xa level for dosing guidance.[101]

For unfractionated heparin, a weight-based dosing nomogram appears to be the most effective dosing regimen.[103] In a randomized clinical trial, patients receiving a weight-based heparin regimen reached the targeted prolongation of the aPTT sooner than conventional dosing that consisted of a 5000-unit bolus with 1000 units per hour infusion.[104] In addition, fewer recurrent thromboembolic events occurred in the weight-based dosing group and comparable bleeding complications. Heparin requirements are usually largest in these first few days. After 48 to 72 hours, aPTT can be measured on a daily basis for the duration of therapy. Experts generally concur that subtherapeutic levels of anticoagulation in the first few days after initial embolization are associated with an increased risk of recurrence of pulmonary embolization.[105]

Multiple clinical trials have shown LMWHs to be at least as effective and just as safe as UFH in the initial management of pulmonary thromboembolism.[101,106-108]

LMWHs vary in size from 4 to 7 kD. When compared with UFH, the various LMWHs have greater bioavailability, longer half-lives, and more predictable anticoagulant responses when administered subcutaneously in fixed doses.[107,109,110] Inhibition of Factor Xa is predictable and usually does not require monitoring.[101,111-113] Deciding between administering LMWH versus UFH requires consideration of a number of variables including cost, ease of administration, need for rapid reversibility, and need for monitoring. The Seventh ACCP Conference on Antithrombotic Therapy recommends LMWH for acute, submassive pulmonary thromboembolism and UFH in patients with severe renal failure and life-threatening pulmonary thromboembolism.[101]

With any heparin therapy, platelet counts should be monitored at least every other day for signs of heparin-induced thrombocytopenia (HIT).[114,115] HIT is an immune-mediated process that usually begins after 5 days of therapy and resolves only after discontinuation of heparin. Previous heparin exposure may prompt HIT to occur within the first few days of heparin therapy. HIT is associated with low platelet counts and evidence of arterial and venous thrombosis, and it develops in approximately 2% of patients receiving unfractionated heparin.[115] The incidence is lower in patients receiving LMWHs.[116] However, should HIT develop with unfractionated heparin, switching to a low-molecular-weight form is contraindicated because of nearly 100% cross-reactivity.[114] If platelet counts drop below 100,000/μL, or more than 50% from baseline after day 5 of heparin, heparin should be discontinued. Therapy for HIT with other anticoagulants such as hirudin, other direct thrombin inhibitors (e.g., argatroban, lepirudin, bivalirudin), or factor Xa inhibitors (e.g., fondiparinux or danaparoid) should be considered with any evidence of thrombosis.[115] Vitamin K antagonists (e.g., warfarin) are ineffective in HIT and may cause harm, so its use should be delayed until resolution of the HIT.[117]

Thrombolytic Therapy

Despite years of investigation, the specific role of thrombolytic agents in the treatment of PE is still debated and requires individualization. Thrombolytic therapy rapidly clears clots from the deep venous and pulmonary arterial vasculature. Thrombolytic agents are superior to heparin in the resolution of pulmonary emboli, as assessed by improvements in pulmonary angiography, lung scan, or hemodynamic derangements.[38,118] Nevertheless, mortality improvement and other meaningful outcome parameters have not been clearly demonstrated in randomized clinical trials.[118-125] Although careful selection of patients has diminished hemorrhagic complications of thrombolytics, the risk of significant hemorrhage with this therapy is significantly greater than in patients treated with conventional anticoagulant therapy of heparin and warfarin.[125] This is especially so in the critical care unit, where patients may be harboring clinically unrecognized bleeding sites such as upper gastrointestinal abnormalities that have previously clotted. These "good" clots will be indiscriminately lysed through systemic thrombolysis, potentially leading to hemorrhagic complications. Furthermore, critically ill patients often have contraindications to thrombolytics, and multiple invasive lines in critical care patients serve as additional bleeding sites for complications. The clinical advantage of thrombolytic agents in the critical care unit is in patients with persistent hypotension (requiring vasopressor) or refractory hypoxemia despite aggressive interventions, where rapid reduction in clot occluding the pulmonary vasculature may be hemodynamically beneficial.[123,126] Patients with hemodynamic instability and PE should be considered for thrombolytic therapy if there are no bleeding tendencies or absolute contraindications. Intrapulmonary arterial infusion of thrombolytic agents has not been shown to improve clot lysis or reduce hemorrhagic complications.[126] Given the current evidence, thrombolytic agents should be used only for massive pulmonary thromboembolism with significant hemodynamic compromise or refractory hypoxemia. The optimal agent and infusion strategy remains uncertain.[101,127]

Inferior Vena Cava Filters

Patients with PE and a contraindication to anticoagulation or a major complication of anticoagulation therapy should be considered for placement of an inferior vena cava (IVC) filter.[101,128] In selected patients receiving anticoagulation therapy, the additional use of an IVC filter should also be considered in the following situations: (1) recurrent thromboembolism despite adequate anticoagulation, (2) the presence of a large free-floating caval thrombus, (3) chronic recurrent PE with pulmonary hypertension, and (4) patients who have had surgical embolectomy or pulmonary endarterectomy. Retrievable filters are gaining increasing attention in patients with high risks for bleeding (e.g., trauma victims and neurosurgical patients) or current contraindications for anticoagulation that will abate early during periods of desired anticoagulation because of their temporary benefit while waiting for recovery and safe use of anticoagulants. Several case series have reported success, but at the time of this writing, no randomized clinical trials have been performed.[129] The procedure of choice is the intravenous percutaneous insertion under fluoroscopic guidance of an IVC filter. Several different filters have been studied, and long-term complications using these devices are low, with patency rates of 95% to 98%.[130,131]

Prophylaxing against pulmonary emboli with IVC filters in patients with known deep vein thrombosis who will receive anticoagulation therapy remains controversial. In a randomized clinical trial of IVC filter placement in 400 patients with deep vein thrombosis and high risk of PE, two patients with IVC filters developed PE over a 2-year period compared with 9 patients without IVC filters (odds ratio [OR] 0.22; 95% CI, 0.05 to 0.90). However, this group experienced a higher deep vein thrombosis recurrence rate over 2 years (OR 1.87; 95% CI, 1.10 to 3.20).[132] In a subsequent report of the same patients 8 years later, the trends continued with fewer PEs in the IVC filter group (cumulative rate of 6% vs. 15%) and more recurrent DVTs (36% vs. 27%).[133] Multiple trauma patients have been identified as having a high risk of developing PE, yet the reported prevalence of DVT varies tremendously and it is unclear whether this group is more likely to benefit from prophylactic placement of an IVC filter.[134] Insertion of IVC filters can be performed at the bedside in the intensive care unit, and it has been shown to be safe and more cost effective than traditional locations such as the operating room and interventional radiology suite.[135]

Embolectomy

Pulmonary embolectomy should be considered only in patients who have massive PE, preferably documented by pulmonary angiography, persistence of shock despite medical management, and failure or contraindication of thrombolytic therapy.[101] The aggressive therapy of open-chest pulmonary embolectomy requires an experienced cardiac surgical team to be immediately available.[136] Survival rates vary from 25% to 89% among several case series likely reflecting different surgical techniques and patient selection.[101,137] Recently, ablative, angioplastic, and suction catheter techniques have been used in limited series.[138-141] The eventual role of such techniques awaits further study.

Long-Term Therapy and Newer Agents

Long-term therapy for pulmonary thromboembolism is similar to that for DVT. Warfarin therapy is generally started on the first day of heparin therapy in uncomplicated PE, although it may be prudent to delay this for several days in critically ill patients because of the uncertainty of their clinical course.[142] Overlap of warfarin and heparin should be continued for at least 2 days once the INR is therapeutic, with longer duration of therapy considered in patients with larger clot burdens seen with massive PE and/or iliofemoral venous thrombosis. The optimal long-term duration of warfarin is patient-specific, depending on ease of administration and monitoring in a therapeutic range, bleeding risks and complications, and drug interactions. Decisions on duration are best left to the outpatient setting. In general, 3 months of therapy may be appropriate for patients with identifiable and reversible risk factors. A minimum of 6 or 12 months may be best for patients with idiopathic PE or underlying malignancy.[101]

Newer anticoagulants are gaining attention in the long-term treatment of PE. These new agents act in more predictable ways on factors VII, Xa, and thrombin, obviating the general need for pharmacologic monitoring. Although most studies focus on DVT prophylaxis, many agents could play a growing role in the treatment of acute PE. Three months of fondaparinux was comparable with heparin plus warfarin in safety and efficacy in an open-label study of 2213 patients with pulmonary thromboembolism.[143] Ximelagatran appears just as effective in treating DVT as LMWH and warfarin with comparable bleeding risks but may have some hepatic toxicity when used long term.[144] These agents and others will require further investigation of efficacy and safety before widely replacing warfarin therapy.

Prognosis

PE is a potentially lethal disorder in which anticoagulation significantly improves survival. Patients with PE have 1-year mortality rates from recurrent VTE more than 3 times greater than patients with DVT alone (1.5% vs. 0.4%).[145] Mortality without anticoagulation is approximately 30%, whereas mortality with anticoagulation is 8%. In the PIOPED-I study, 399 patients with PE were analyzed for clinical outcome.[146] Treatment for PE was given to 94% of these patients, with 73% receiving conventional anticoagulation with heparin and warfarin, 10% receiving an IVC filter, and 6% receiving thrombolytic therapy. Death from PE occurred in 10 patients (2.5%). One half of the deaths occurred in the 24 hours after clinical onset, and 90% of the deaths occurred within 2 weeks of initial onset. The death rate at 1 year for PIOPED-I patients diagnosed with PE was 23.8%, which was not significantly different from the 18.9% in patients found to be negative for PE at the time of study entry. On multivariate factor analysis, the conditions associated with death and their corresponding relative risk were cancer, 3.8; left-sided congestive heart failure, 2.7; and chronic lung disease, 2.2. Of the 399 patients with documented PE, 33 (8.3%) demonstrated diagnosed recurrence of PE within the 1-year follow-up period. Sixteen (48%) of these recurrences were noted in the first week after diagnosis, and 15 (45%) patients with recurrences died in the year after diagnosis. Most importantly, of the 10 patients who died of PE, 9 demonstrated recurrence of the disease. The important conclusions regarding clinical outcome of PE from this study are (1) when properly diagnosed and treated, clinically apparent PE was an uncommon cause of death; (2) PE recurs in a minority of properly treated cases but is frequently associated with those patients dying acutely of PE; (3) most deaths in the year after diagnosis of PE are caused by other underlying disease; and (4) patients with PE who had cancer, congestive heart failure, or chronic lung disease had a higher risk of dying in 1 year than did other patients with PE.

The anatomic size of emboli does not correlate well with mortality. This underscores the importance of underlying cardiopulmonary disease, chronic lung disease, or prior pulmonary vascular disease such as previous pulmonary emboli in reducing the pulmonary vascular cross-sectional area, upon which even a small embolus would be poorly tolerated hemodynamically and possibly result in death. Patients with pulmonary emboli who do not have shock generally have a low mortality, even if the embolus is anatomically massive. Mortality in patients with pulmonary emboli and shock is significantly higher, with estimates as high as 33%.[9]

Pulmonary emboli resolve by fibrinolysis or organization mechanisms. With proper therapy, most pulmonary emboli clear within 2 weeks of occurrence, which is an important consideration for diagnostic purposes in evaluating persistent perfusion scan abnormalities and clinical manifestations attributable to pulmonary hypertension.[50]

Prophylaxis

Deep venous thrombosis prophylaxis is effective at reducing death. In several meta-analyses of surgical patients, prophylactic measures reduced the development of thromboembolic events by more than 50% and also the VTE-attributable mortality.[147,148] Almost all critically ill patients have significant risk factors for venous thromboembolism.[149] The advent of safe and effective prophylaxis strategies makes all critical care patients candidates for some form of preventive therapy on the basis of risk factors present in this population of patients. Several studies suggest that more than 85% of hospitalized patients are receiving some sort of DVT prophylaxis.[150-152] VTE prophylactic measures are growing in intensive care units with quality care initiatives targeting this intervention via bundled care pathways.[153]

Although many interventions have been shown to decrease the incidence of venous thromboembolism, the ideal intervention in critically ill patients depends on numerous factors and is complex.[154] General recommendations from the American College of Chest Physicians are summarized in Table 45-6.[154]

VENOUS AIR EMBOLI

Venous air embolism occurs whenever air at a pressure higher than venous blood pressure comes into communication with the venous circulation.[155] The most common procedure in which venous air embolism may occur is intravenous catheterization, especially with large-bore catheters. Surgical procedures such as neurosurgical cases performed with patients in the sitting position and obstetrical procedures that expose large veins have also been commonly associated with venous air embolism. Thoracic procedures, traumatic injuries, mechanical ventilation with barotrauma, and decompression sickness are less common causes of the syndrome.[156,157]

The pathophysiology of venous air embolism has predominantly been studied in laboratory animal experi-

Table 45-6. Venous Thromboembolism Prophylaxis

Patient Group	Intervention	Grade of Evidence
Surgical patients		
General, vascular, gynecologic, and urologic surgery		
Low risk (minor procedure and age younger than 40 y)	Early mobilization	1C+
Moderate risk	LDUH 5000 U twice a day or LMWH <3400 U daily	1A
High risk (age older than 60 y, major procedure, comorbidities)	LDUH 5000 U tid or LMWH >3400 U daily	1A
Patients at high risk of bleeding complications	Mechanical prophylaxis with GCS and/or IPC	1A
Trauma	LMWH when considered safe IPC or GCS when high risk of bleeding complications	1A 1B
Orthopedic surgery		
THR, TKA, HFS	Higher dose LMWH, fondaparinux, or adjusted-dose warfarin	Grade 1C+ to 1A
Knee arthroscopy	Early mobilization	2B
Neurosurgery		
Spinal cord Injury Intracranial procedures Burns	LMWH once primary hemostasis is evident IPC with or without GCS IPC and/or GCS *plus* heparin (LDUH or LMWH) LMWH or LDUH	1B 1A 2B 1C+
Acutely ill medical patients		
Bed confined with one or more additional risk factors	LDUH or LMWH	1A
Medical patients with contraindications to anticoagulation	GCS or IPC	1C+

GCS, graduated compression stockings; HFS, hip fracture surgery; IPC, intermittent pneumatic compression; LDUH, low-dose unfractionated heparin; LMWH, low-molecular-weight heparin; THR, total hip replacement; TKA, total knee arthroplasty; VFP, venous foot pump.
Adapted from Geerts WH, Pineo GF, Heit JA, et al: Prevention of venous thromboembolism: The Seventh ACCP Conference on Antithrombotic and Thrombolytic Therapy. Chest 2004;126:338S-400S.

ments. In addition to the mechanical obstruction of the pulmonary arterial circuit, air emboli rapidly become a nidus for platelet aggregation, fibrin deposition, and lipid accumulation. Endothelial cell injury directly from air and indirectly from vasoactive platelet products may lead to arteriolar and capillary leakage of pulmonary edema.[158] The amount of air necessary to cause the syndrome in man has not clearly been determined. Extrapolation from animal experiments suggests that air infused at 20 mL per second probably will cause symptoms, whereas 75 to 100 mL per second is likely to be fatal. Nevertheless, through a medium-bore catheter, such as a 14-gauge device, 5 cm H_2O gradient pressure will produce an airflow rate of more than 60 mL per second, sufficiently large enough to cause symptoms and, possibly, death.[159]

The clinical syndrome of air embolism is an abrupt onset of agitation, dyspnea, tachypnea, and tachycardia.[160] Wheezing may occur, although initially the chest is often silent. The so-called "mill-wheel" murmur is a loud, continuous slapping noise heard best at the left sternal border. This is probably attributable to right ventricular beating against subpulmonic air. Airway pressures may rise as a result of bronchoconstriction produced by the air embolism.[161] Pulmonary arterial pressures generally rise abruptly without a rise in pulmonary capillary wedge pressure. Laboratory studies are nonspecific, although chest radiography may demonstrate air in the right heart, pulmonary artery, or hepatic circulation.[162] Diagnosis can occasionally be demonstrated with echocardiography.[163]

Therapy for venous air embolism begins by placing the patient on 100% oxygen and positioning the patient in the left lateral decubitus or Trendelenburg position to divert air from the pulmonary outflow tract. Closed-chest cardiac message may restore circulation in cardiac arrest because the air may be dissipated.[164] Placement of a pulmonary arterial catheter into the RV outflow tract may allow aspiration of air from the circulation. Vigorous early treatment of this syndrome and resulting complications, such as the adult respiratory distress syndrome, probably has resulted in an improved prognosis from this disorder in the past several years. In a series of 113 patients with venous air embolism, 69% recovered without sequelae, 26% developed sequelae, and 5% died.[165] During high-risk surgical procedures, monitoring devices such as pulmonary artery catheterization, end-tidal CO_2 assessment, Doppler analysis of right heart flow, and transesophageal ultrasonography have all been used in early detection of air embolism.[166] Nevertheless, awareness of preventive measures such as the use of Trendelenburg positioning during central venous catheterization (to increase central venous pressure) and the use of positive pressure ventilation during neurosurgical procedures performed in the upright position are key elements in preventing this syndrome.

FAT EMBOLI

The fat embolism syndrome is characterized by the development of pulmonary and cerebral dysfunction, fever, and hypoxemia in association with long bone fractures.[167] Other commonly associated findings are petechiae over the chest, neck and axillae, retinal fat, fat in clotted blood, lipiduria, and diffuse pulmonary infiltrates. Although the essential aspects of the syndrome have been debated, the major criteria for the diagnosis include only cerebral dysfunction, fever, and hypoxemia in the appropriate clinical setting. Multiple lower-extremity long bone fractures are the most common risk factor for the development of fat embolism syndrome. Singular fractures, especially of the upper extremity, are far less likely to cause this syndrome. The incidence of the syndrome is at least 10% after long bone or pelvic fracture when prospectively evaluated.[168]

Although simple fat embolism may be a pathologic finding of variable clinical significance, patients with the fat embolism syndrome have fat emboli in multiple organs, which show extensive damage from this embolization. The pulmonary vasculature contains fat globules with associated platelet and fibrin accumulation. Intrapulmonary hemorrhage with diffuse sterile pneumonitis and pulmonary edema are usually demonstrated. Fat, platelet, and fibrin conglomerations also plug cerebral arterioles. Ischemia and distal hemorrhage are typical of cerebral lesions, as well as lesions in other vascular beds such as the liver, kidney, and heart. The fat embolism syndrome is likely to occur in stages, with the initial mechanical obstruction phase leading to a secondary endothelial injury phase initiated by the intravascular fat.[169] The role of coagulation system activation in the secondary injury phase is probable; disseminated intravascular coagulation is not infrequently associated with severe fat embolism syndrome.[170]

The pathophysiologic debate regarding fat embolism syndrome is largely related to questions of the origin of fat emboli. The two basic theories are a physicochemical theory, proposing fat emboli arise from circulating lipoproteins, and a mechanical theory, proposing that the fat originates from bone marrow.[171,172]

The clinical syndrome of fat embolism is distinctive from other embolic disorders in onset and associated findings. The vast majority of cases occur within 48 hours of injury, with approximately 20% of cases occurring within several hours. The syndrome generally presents as an acute, but not abrupt, onset of dyspnea, tachypnea, and mental status change. The mental status change may range from restlessness and confusion to coma. The mental status changes often occur prior to significant respiratory abnormalities and are initially out of proportion to the degree of hypoxemia demonstrated. Almost all patients are febrile. Most demonstrate petechiae, usually best noticed in the buccal mucosa or axillary folds. Funduscopic examination may be fruitful in the demonstration of hemorrhage and new fluffy exudates. Chest radiograph demonstrates diffuse bilateral infiltrates compatible with the adult respiratory distress syndrome.

Bronchoalveolar lavage has been reported to be a useful technique in identifying patients with the fat embolism syndrome.[169,173] The staining of cells with oil red O after recovery by a standard 150- to 200-mL lavage can identify intracellular fat droplets. In patients with definite fat embolism syndrome, 63% (range of 31% to 82%) of macrophages recovered by bronchoalveolar lavage demonstrated fat droplets by this technique, whereas fat staining was positive in less than 2% of cells recovered by lavage from trauma patients with no clinical evidence of the syndrome, patients with ARDS, or normal volunteers.[169]

Therapy for fat embolism syndrome is largely prophylactic and supportive. Early fixation of long bone fractures appears to decrease the incidence of fat embolism syndrome and other adverse respiratory outcomes. Altering the surgical technique during orthopedic procedures has been demonstrated to reduce the incidence of echocardiographic evidence of fat and bone marrow embolism.[174] High-dose corticosteroids, although advocated by some, have not been validated and would not likely benefit only if given prophylactically.[175] Other speculated therapies such as glucose and insulin, alcohol infusion, and heparin therapy have theoretical benefit but have not been shown to be effective in conclusive scientific studies.

AMNIOTIC FLUID EMBOLI

The embolization of vernix caseosa (the "waxy" or "cheesy" white substance found coating the skin of newborn humans) and meconium mucin into the venous circulation produces an abrupt syndrome of tachypnea, pulmonary edema, and respiratory failure in women during labor.[176,177] The overall frequency of amniotic fluid embolism is probably less than 1 in 8000, but the frequency of this disorder in women who die during delivery is high. Conditions that promote tearing or leaking of the fetal membrane, such as especially forceful uterine contractions during "strong" labor, predispose to amniotic fluid embolism. Cesarean section, multiparity, advanced maternal age, dead fetus syndrome, placenta previa, and abruptio placentae may also be risk factors.[178]

Amniotic fluid embolism syndrome should be differentiated from embolization of trophoblasts during molar pregnancies. Placental trophoblasts embolize to the lung during normal pregnancies, although large numbers embolize and produce an embolic syndrome, with rare exceptions, only with molar pregnancies.

The pathophysiology of amniotic fluid embolism consists of three phases.[156,179] As in most cases of PE, the first phase involves mechanical obstruction of the pulmonary vasculature. The second phase is the production of a systemic response similar to anaphylaxis. During this phase, systemic vasodilation, endothelial injury, and pulmonary vasoconstriction produce the clinical findings of pulmonary edema and shock. The third phase is the development of disseminated intravascular coagulation, initiated by the release of thromboplastin-like amniotic products.[177] This phase leads to the potentiated hemorrhage, which complicates nearly all cases of amniotic fluid embolism that survive greater than 1 hour. The clinical syndrome consists of dyspnea, shock, chills, and hemorrhage occurring either during labor or within 24 hours after delivery. Shock is often the initial finding and may be especially profound if complicated by hemorrhage. Physical findings are consistent with acute noncardiogenic pulmonary edema. Right heart catheterization generally demonstrates significant elevations of pulmonary artery pressures with normal or low pulmonary capillary wedge pressures. Laboratory studies show an elevated white blood cell count and often a disseminated intravascular coagulation profile, especially in patients demonstrating hemorrhage. Chest radiography demonstrates alveolar infiltrates.

The diagnosis of amniotic fluid embolism is contingent on the demonstration of fetal squamous cells in the lung.[180] Clusters of fetal squamous cells may be demonstrated in lung biopsy, sputum, or blood drawn from the pulmonary vasculature through a pulmonary artery catheter.[181] The cells are easily identified using Wright's stain and by polarized microscopy, the latter because of their birefringent characteristic. The accuracy of diagnosis using these techniques is unknown.

Therapy for amniotic fluid embolism is generally supportive with the use of conventional therapy for shock, the adult respiratory distress syndrome, and disseminated intravascular coagulation. Despite modern support for these complications, amniotic fluid embolism carries a grave prognosis; studies from before 1960 demonstrated an 80% fatality rate.[177] No indications that modern supportive techniques have reduced this number exist.

SEPTIC PULMONARY EMBOLI

Hussey first described septic pulmonary emboli in 1945.[182] Septic pulmonary emboli are dislodged infected clots from either peripheral vein septic thrombophlebitis or right-sided endocarditis.[183,184] Tricuspid endocarditis in intravenous drug abusers was the cause of at least one half of cases reported. The remaining cases generally are equally split in frequency from endogenously and exogenously produced sites. The most common causes of endogenous peripheral thrombi are pelvic thrombophlebitis from delivery or abortion; deep vein thrombophlebitis related to cellulitis, osteomyelitis, or subcutaneous abscesses; and jugular venous thrombophlebitis from infections of the head and neck. Infected intravascular devices such as central venous catheters, dialysis shunts, and pacemaker wires commonly cause septic thrombophlebitis and resultant emboli. Foreign infected material that may be injected during illicit drug use can also produce the syndrome. With the more frequent use of monitoring catheters in the intensive care unit, the syndrome has been recognized more frequently as a complication of critical care. Infected pulmonary artery catheters have been associated with a high rate of right-sided endocarditis. Of importance in these cases is that the pulmonary valve may either be infected alone or in association with the tricuspid valve to cause a nidus of septic emboli. Isolated pulmonary valvular endocarditis is almost always caused by a prior infected pulmonary artery catheter.[185]

Septic PE are generally associated with pulmonary infarction. Whereas infarction is often not produced by bland pulmonary emboli caused by the adequacy of collateral circulation, associated inflammation occurring with septic pulmonary emboli causes a reduction of collateral blood flow, leading to infarction and abscess production. Much of the resultant clinical syndrome is caused by this distinctive process of vascular occlusion and associated inflammation.[183]

The clinical syndrome of septic PE is distinct from bland PE, with findings dominated by fever, shaking chills, and pleuritic chest pain in a patient from the population predisposed to septic thrombophlebitis. As opposed to bland embolism, the symptoms are rarely transient or evanescent, and dyspnea is not a major clinical manifestation. Hemoptysis is not infrequent, although massive hemoptysis is rare. Physical examination often discloses the primary site of the septic thrombophlebitis. Laboratory studies support an underlying septic process, although sputum and blood cultures are variably positive. Common organisms include *Staphylococcus aureus*, alpha hemolytic streptococcal, enterococcal, gram-negative, and anaerobic species. Fungal septic thrombophlebitis and embolism should be considered in neutropenic patients with chronic indwelling intravenous catheters.

The chest radiograph is essential to the diagnosis of septic pulmonary emboli, and in many critically ill patients is the reason for clinical suspicion of the diagnosis.[186,187] Multiple bilateral nodular densities often with a lower lobe predisposition ranging in size from a few millimeters to several centimeters are usually apparent. Crops of new nodular densities appear sequentially over days. The mature nodular densities have a tendency to expand in size, cavitate, or become pleural-based wedge-like densities. Over the course of time, hilar and mediastinal adenopathy and pleural effusions, often complicated, are apparent.

Therapy for septic pulmonary emboli consists of both medical and surgical management depending upon the site of the septic thrombophlebitis and the response of the process to medical therapy alone. General medical support with oxygen and pain control is necessary, but critical care is necessary only for patients with significant cardiopulmonary embarrassment. Appropriate antibiotics and removal of indwelling intravenous catheters is essential for almost all cases. Patients with non-cardiac foci should probably be treated with heparin.[188,189] The optimal duration of anticoagulation required in these cases is unknown. Many patients with erratic fever from septic thrombophlebitis, such as within the pelvic veins, may not show defervescence until heparinization is used. Patients with persistent fever, positive blood culture, and persistent septic pulmonary emboli should be considered medical failures and considered for drainage of potential abscesses, vascular resection, and vein ligation. Femoral vein septic thrombophlebitis from illicit intravenous "groin" injections are often associated with deep fascial abscesses, which should be identified by ultrasonography or computerized axial tomographic scanning for anticipated surgical drainage. Pleural effusions should be diagnostically sampled and drained by tube thoracostomy if complicated by empyema. Right-sided endocarditis often requires surgery if the patient does not respond to antibiotic treatment. Heparin is not indicated in right-sided endocarditis.

Prognosis is dependent on the general medical condition of the patient and the underlying septic process. Most patients do not have either long-term venous or pulmonary effects of this type of PE.

TUMOR EMBOLI

The embolization of tumor into the pulmonary arterial vasculature has been reported with multiple types of carcinoma and sarcoma.[156] Tumor that invades the systemic capillary and venous circuit or reaches the thoracic duct and central venous circulation by lymphatic invasion may gain access to the pulmonary circulation. Tumor emboli are generally fragments of tumor with associated thrombus that simply mechanically obstruct the pulmonary arterial vasculature. These emboli usually do not evoke a major nonmechanical response, which differentiates tumor emboli from other forms of pulmonary emboli. Tumor emboli may progress to pulmonary parenchymal metastases, but this does not always occur. Although tumor emboli may be seen in up to 25% of patients dying of neoplasia, less than one fourth of these patients have respiratory symptoms attributed significantly to these emboli.[190] The frequency of pulmonary tumor emboli is related to the type of primary tumor. Autopsy data suggest the overall frequency of significant tumor emboli causing a distinct respiratory syndrome is less than 3%. The more common neoplasms to cause tumor embolism to the lungs are cancers from the breast, prostate, and stomach, along with hepatoma, hypernephroma, and choriocarcinoma.[191]

The clinical presentation of pulmonary tumor emboli may be precipitous, suggesting thrombotic PE. More frequently the presentation is more insidious, with the development of pulmonary hypertension, cor pulmonale, and progressive severe hypoxemia. Cancer patients with advanced tumor stage are more likely to develop this syndrome. In these cases, usual diagnostic evaluation for deep venous thrombosis and/or thrombotic PE should be performed to rule out these more common complications of advanced malignancy. The performance of cytologic evaluation of blood aspirated from the pulmonary artery through a pulmonary artery catheter has been proposed as a diagnostic maneuver in critically ill patients in whom the diagnosis is considered.[181]

No specific therapy exists for pulmonary tumor embolism. Heparin is not indicated in this group of patients. Pulmonary embolectomy has been performed in massive tumor pulmonary emboli with satisfying results; such aggressive therapy should only be considered in patients with otherwise reasonable tumor containment and preexistent functional status. Prognosis for most patients with pulmonary tumor emboli is grim, with most patients dying within 3 months of diagnosis.

MISCELLANEOUS PULMONARY EMBOLI

An assortment of other inorganic and organic material may cause pulmonary emboli.[156] Intravenous drug abusers may inject a number of insoluble materials such as talc crystals and cotton fiber, which may lodge within the pulmonary vasculature and produce a fibrogenic and thrombogenic response. Parasites, mechanical devices, and endogenous material such as feces, bile, bone marrow, and cerebral tissue have also been reported to cause or be confused with acute PE syndromes in the proper clinical setting.

KEY POINTS

The most common and clinically important PE syndrome is thromboembolism, although many other diverse materials may embolize to the pulmonary circulation, causing similar but unique syndromes.

- Impaction of material into the pulmonary circulation causes acute cardiovascular and pulmonary effects; the degree of pathophysiologic derangement relates both to the magnitude of mechanical obstruction produced by the embolism and the secondary and unique effects of the embolic material.
- Most clinical risk factors center on Virchow's triad of stasis, vascular wall abnormalities, and hypercoagulability. Inherited and acquired forms of hypercoagulability include malignancy, Factor V Leiden mutation, antiphospholipid antibody syndrome, antithrombin-III deficiency, and protein C and protein S deficiency.
- The clinical manifestations of PE are nonspecific and require specific testing to establish the diagnosis.
- The link between deep vein thrombosis and pulmonary embolism allows one to establish the clinically equivalent diagnosis of proximal deep vein thrombosis, through contrast venography or noninvasive studies such as Doppler duplex ultrasonography.
- Determining a pretest probability for VTE is essential when interpreting the results of diagnostic tests.
- A nonelevated whole blood D-dimer level performed by an ELISA can usually safely exclude VTE in low-risk outpatients.
- Spiral CT angiography has emerged as the leading test in the evaluation of patients suspected of having a pulmonary thromboembolism, with image quality improving yearly.
- The management of PE in the acutely ill requires careful attention to cardiopulmonary support and early initiation of adequate anticoagulation with heparin.
- Thrombolytic agents should be reserved for patients with PE who demonstrate persistent hypotension or refractory hypoxemia despite medical optimization and/ or where rapid reduction in clot occluding the pulmonary vasculature may be hemodynamically beneficial.
- Venous thromboembolism prophylaxis strategies are necessary for nearly all critical care patients.
- The most common and important nonthrombotic PE syndromes are venous air, fat, amniotic fluid, septic PE, and tumor embolism.

REFERENCES

1. Stratmann G, Gregory GA: Neurogenic and humoral vasoconstriction in acute pulmonary thromboembolism. Anesth Analg 2003;97:341-354.
2. Anderson FA Jr, Wheeler HB, Goldberg RJ, et al: A population-based perspective of the hospital incidence and case-fatality rates of deep vein thrombosis and pulmonary embolism. The Worcester DVT Study. Arch Intern Med 1991;151:933-938.
3. Lilienfeld DE, Chan E, Ehland J, et al: Mortality from pulmonary embolism in the United States: 1962 to 1984. Chest 1990;98:1067-1072.
4. Dalen JE, Albert JS: Natural history of pulmonary embolism. In AA Sasahara, EH Sonnenblick, M Lesch (ed): Pulmonary Embolism. New York, Grune & Stratton, 1975.
5. Clagett GP, Anderson FA Jr, Heit J, et al: Prevention of venous thromboembolism. Chest 1995;108(4 Suppl):312S-334S.
6. Kasper W, Konstantinides S, Geibel A, et al: Management strategies and determinants of outcome in acute major pulmonary embolism: Results of a multicenter registry. J Am Coll Cardiol 1997;30:1165-1171.
7. Wood KE: Major pulmonary embolism: review of a pathophysiologic approach to the golden hour of hemodynamically significant pulmonary embolism. Chest 2002;121:877-905.
8. Hoagland PM: Massive pulmonary embolism. In SZ Goldhaber (ed): Pulmonary Embolism and Deep Venous Thrombosis. Philadelphia, WB Saunders, 1985.
9. Urokinase pulmonary embolism trial: Phase 1 results: A cooperative study. JAMA 1970;214:2163-2172.
10. Goldhaber SZ, Visani L, De Rosa M: Acute pulmonary embolism: Clinical outcomes in the International Cooperative Pulmonary Embolism Registry (ICOPER). Lancet 1999;353:1386-1389.
11. Smith G, Smith AN: The role of serotonin in experimental pulmonary embolism. Surg Gynecol Obstet 1955;101:691-700.
12. Malik A, Johnson A: Role of humoral mediators in the pulmonary vascular response to pulmonary embolism. In Weir E, Reeves J (eds): Pulmonary Vascular Physiology and Pathophysiology. New York, Marcel Dekker, 1989, pp 445-468.
13. Alpert JS, Godtfredsen J, Ockene IS, et al: Pulmonary hypertension secondary to minor pulmonary embolism. Chest 1978;73:795-797.
14. Moser K, Guisan M, Bartimmo E: Resolution rates of experimental venous thromboemboli. In Moser K, Stein M (eds): Pulmonary Thromboembolism. Chicago, Year Book Medical Publishers, 1971, pp 104-113.
15. Nelson JR, Smith JR: The pathologic physiology of pulmonary embolism. A physiologic discussion of the vascular reactions following pulmonary arterial obstruction by emboli of varying size. Am Heart J 1959;58: 916-932.
16. Lewis JW Jr, Bastanfar M, Gabriel F, Mascha E: Right heart function and prediction of respiratory morbidity in patients undergoing pneumonectomy with moderately severe cardiopulmonary dysfunction. J Thorac Cardiovasc Surg 1994;108: 169-175.
17. Elliott CG: Pulmonary physiology during pulmonary embolism. Chest 1992;101(4 Suppl):163S-171S.
18. Taylor RR, Covell JW, Sonnenblick EH, Ross J Jr: Dependence of ventricular distensibility on filling of the opposite ventricle. Am J Physiol 1967;213: 711-718.
19. Jardin F, Dubourg O, Gueret P, et al: Quantitative two-dimensional echocardiography in massive pulmonary embolism: Emphasis on ventricular interdependence and leftward septal displacement. J Am Coll Cardiol 1987;10:1201-1206.
20. Belenkie I, Dani R, Smith ER, Tyberg JV: Ventricular interaction during experimental acute pulmonary embolism. Circulation 1988;78: 761-768.
21. Widdicombe J: Reflex mechanisms in pulmonary thromboembolism. In Moser K, Stein M (eds): Pulmonary Thromboembolism. Chicago, Year Book Medical Publishers, 1971, pp 178-186.
22. Stein M, Levy SE: Reflex and humoral responses to pulmonary embolism. Prog Cardiovasc Dis 1974;17:167-174.
23. Chen HF, Lee BP, Kou YR: Mechanisms of stimulation of vagal pulmonary C fibers by pulmonary air embolism in dogs. J Appl Physiol 1997;82:765-771.
24. Chen HF, Kou YR: Vagal and mediator mechanisms underlying the tachypnea caused by pulmonary air embolism in dogs. J Appl Physiol 2000;88: 1247-1253.
25. Katz S, Horres AD: Medullary respiratory neuron response to pulmonary emboli and pneumothorax. J Appl Physiol 1972;33:390-396.

26. Comroe JH Jr, Van Lingen B, Stroud RC, Roncoroni A: Reflex and direct cardiopulmonary effects of 5-OH-tryptamine (serotonin); their possible role in pulmonary embolism and coronary thrombosis. Am J Physiol 1953;173:379-386.
27. Hyman A: Autonomic control of the pulmonary circulation. In Weir E, Reeves J (eds): Pulmonary Vascular Physiology and Pathophysiology. New York, Marcel Dekker, 1989, pp 291-319.
28. Aviado DM, Guevara Aviado D: The Bezold-Jarisch reflex. A historical perspective of cardiopulmonary reflexes. Ann N Y Acad Sci 2001;940:48-58.
29. Haberberger R, Schemann M, Sann H, Kummer W: Innervation pattern of guinea pig pulmonary vasculature depends on vascular diameter. J Appl Physiol 1997;82:426-34.
30. Thomas DP, Gurewich V, Ashford TP: Platelet adherence to thromboemboli in relation to the pathogenesis and treatment of pulmonary embolism. N Engl J Med 1966;274:953-956.
31. Blaise G: Endothelium at rest. In Spiess B (ed): The Relationship Between Coagulation, Inflammation and Endothelium: A Pyramid Towards Outcome. Philadelphia, Lippincott Williams & Wilkins, 2000, pp 31-78.
32. Boyle E, Morgan E, Verrier E: The endothelium disturbed: The procoagulant response. In Spiess B (ed): The Relationship Between Coagulation, Inflammation, and Endothelium: A Pyramid Towards Outcome. Philadelphia, Lippincott Williams & Wilkins, 2000, pp 79-89.
33. Schmeck J, Heller A, Groschler A, et al: Impact of endothelin-1 in endotoxin-induced pulmonary vascular reactions. Crit Care Med 2000;28:2851-2857.
34. Robin ED, Julian DG, Travis DM, Crump CH: A physiologic approach to the diagnosis of acute pulmonary embolism. N Engl J Med 1959;260:586-591.
35. White RH: The epidemiology of venous thromboembolism. Circulation 2003;107(23 Suppl 1):I4-8.
36. Hansson PO, Welin L, Tibblin G, Ericsson H: Deep vein thrombosis and pulmonary embolism in the general population. "The Study of Men Born in 1913." Arch Intern Med 1997;157: 1665-1670.
37. Goldhaber SZ, Hennekens CH, Evans DA, et al: Factors associated with correct antemortem diagnosis of major pulmonary embolism. Am J Med 1982;73:822-826.
38. Urokinase pulmonary embolism trial: A cooperative study. Circulation 1973;47(Suppl)II1-108.
39. Value of the ventilation/perfusion scan in acute pulmonary embolism. Results of the prospective investigation of pulmonary embolism diagnosis (PIOPED). The PIOPED Investigators [see comments]. JAMA 1990;263: 2753-2759.
40. Hirsch DR, Ingenito EP, Goldhaber SZ: Prevalence of deep venous thrombosis among patients in medical intensive care. JAMA 1995;271:335-337.
41. Havig O: Deep vein thrombosis and pulmonary emboli. Acta Chir Scand 1977;Suppl 1:478.
42. Hull RD, Hirsh J, Carter CJ, et al: Pulmonary angiography, ventilation lung scanning and venography for clinically suspected pulmonary emboli with abnormal perfusion scans. Ann Intern Med 1983;98:891–899.
43. Sevitt S, Gallagher NG: Venous thrombosis and pulmonary embolism: A clinicopathologic study in injured and burned patients. Br J Surg 1961;48:475.
44. Virchow RLK: Gesammelte Abhandlungen zur Wissenschaftlichen. In Buchhandlung GH-G (ed): Thrombose and Emboli. Berlin, 1862.
45. Ibarra-Perez C, Lau-Cortes E, Comenero-Zubiate S, et al: Prevalence and prevention of deep venous thrombosis of the lower extremities in high-risk pulmonary patients. Angiology 1988;39:505.
46. Kierkegaard A, Norgren L, Olsson C, et al: Incidence of deep vein thrombosis in bed-ridden non-surgical patients. Acta Med Scand 1987;222:409.
47. Blann AD, Lip GY: Venous thromboembolism. BMJ 2006;332:215-219.
48. Dalen JE, Bauds JS, Brooke HL, et al: Resolution rate of acute pulmonary embolism in man. N Engl J Med 1969;280:1194.
49. McIntyre KM, Sasahara AA: Determinants of right ventricular function and hemodynamics after pulmonary embolism. Chest 1974;65:534.
50. Sharma GVRK, McIntyre KM, Sharma S, et al: Clinical and hemodynamic correlates in pulmonary embolism. Clin Chest Med 1984;5:421.
51. Thames MD, Albert J, Dalen JE: Syncope in patients with pulmonary embolism. JAMA 1977;238:2509.
52. Kelly, Elliot LP: The radiographic evaluation of the patient with suspected pulmonary thromboembolic disease. Med Clin North Am 1974;59:3.
53. Sostman DH, Coleman RE, DeLong DM, et al: Evaluation of revised criteria for ventilation-perfusion scintigraphy in patients with suspected pulmonary embolism. Radiology 1994;193:103-107.
54. American Thoracic Society Clinical Practice Guideline. The Diagnostic Approach to Acute Venous Thromboembolism. Am J Respir Crit Care Med 1999;160:1043-1066.
55. Legere BM, Dweik RA, Arroliga AC: Venous thromboembolism in the intensive care unit. Clin Chest Med 1999;20:367-384.
56. Goodman LR, Lipchik RJ: Diagnosis of acute pulmonary embolism: Time for a new approach. Radiology 1996;199:25-27.
57. Perrier A, Buswell L, Bounameaux H, et al: Cost-effectiveness of noninvasive diagnostic aids in suspected pulmonary embolism. Arch Intern Med 1997;157:2309-2316.
58. Stein PD, Coleman RE, Gottschalk A, et al: Diagnostic utility of ventilation/perfusion lung scans in acute pulmonary embolism is not diminished by pre-existing cardiac or pulmonary disease. Chest 1991;100:604.
59. Lesser BA, Leeper KV Jr, Stein PD, et al: The diagnosis of acute pulmonary embolism in patients with chronic obstructive pulmonary disease. Chest 1992;102:17.
60. Nazeyrollas P, Metz D, Jolly D, et al: Use of transthoracic Doppler echocardiography combined with clinical and electrocardiographic data to predict acute pulmonary embolism. Eur Heart J 1996;17:779-786.
61. Pruszczyk P, Torbicki A, Pacho R, et al: Noninvasive diagnosis of suspected severe pulmonary embolism: Transesophageal echocardiography vs spiral CT [see comments]. Chest 1997;112:722-728.
62. Kreit JW: The impact of right ventricular dysfunction on the prognosis and therapy of normotensive patients with pulmonary embolism. Chest 2004;125:1539-1545.
63. Gibson NS, Sohne M, Buller HR: Prognostic value of echocardiography and spiral computed tomography in patients with pulmonary embolism. Curr Opin Pulm Med 2005;11: 380-384.
64. Mathis G, Blank W, Reissig A, et al: Thoracic ultrasound for diagnosing pulmonary embolism: A prospective multicenter study of 352 patients. Chest 2005;128:1531-1538.
65. Lensing AW, Prandoni P, Brandjes D, et al: Detection of deep-vein thrombosis by real-time B-mode ultrasonography. N Engl J Med 1989;320:342-345.
66. Cronon JJ, Dorman GS: Deep venous thrombosis: Ultrasound assessment using vein compression. Radiology 1987;162:191.
67. Remy-Jardin M, Tillie-Leblond I, Szapiro D, et al: CT angiography of pulmonary embolism in patients with underlying respiratory disease: Impact of multislice CT on image quality and negative predictive value. Eur Radiol 2002;12:1971-1978.
68. Stein PD for the PIOPED-II Investigators: Multidetector Computer Tomography for Acute Pulmonary Embolism. N Engl J Med 2006;354: 2317-2327.
69. Schoepf UJ, Savino G, Lake DR, et al: The age of CT pulmonary angiography. J Thorac Imaging 2005;20:273-279.
70. Quiroz R, Kucher N, Zou KH, et al: Clinical validity of a negative computed tomography scan in patients with suspected pulmonary embolism: A systematic review. JAMA 2005;293:2012-2017.
71. Stein PD, Woodard PK, Hull RD, et al: Gadolinium-enhanced magnetic resonance angiography for detection of acute pulmonary embolism: An in-depth review. Chest 2003;124: 2324-2328.
72. Ginsberg JS, Brill-Edwards PA, Demers C, et al: D-dimer in patients with clinically suspected pulmonary embolism. Chest 1993;104: 1679-1684.
73. Bounameaux H, Cirafici P, de Moerloose P, et al: Measurement of D-dimer in plasma as diagnostic aid in suspected pulmonary embolism. Lancet 1991;337:196-200.

74. Ginsberg JS, Kearon C, Douketis J, et al: The use of D-dimer testing and impedance plethysmographic examination in patients with clinical indications of deep venous thrombosis. Arch Intern Med 1997;157:1077-81.
75. Foti M, Gurwich V: Fibrin degradation products and impedance plethysmography. Arch Intern Med 1980;140:903-906.
76. Whitake A, Rowe E, Pasci P, et al: Identification of D-dimer E complex in disseminated intravascular coagulation. Thromb Res 1980;18:453-459.
77. Rodger MA, Bredeson CN, Jones G, et al: The bedside investigation of pulmonary embolism diagnosis study: A double-blind randomized controlled trial comparing combinations of 3 bedside tests vs ventilation-perfusion scan for the initial investigation of suspected pulmonary embolism. Arch Intern Med 2006;166:181-187.
78. Le Gal G, Righini M, Roy PM, et al: Value of D-dimer testing for the exclusion of pulmonary embolism in patients with previous venous thromboembolism. Arch Intern Med 2006;166:176-180.
79. Stein PD, Hull RD, Patel KC, et al: D-dimer for the exclusion of acute venous thrombosis and pulmonary embolism: A systematic review. Ann Intern Med 2004;140:589-602.
80. Stein PD, Athanasoulis C, Alavi A, et al: Complications and validity of pulmonary angiography in acute pulmonary embolism. Circulation 1992;85:462.
81. Perlmutt LM, Braun SD, Neuman GE, et al: Pulmonary arteriography in the high risk patient. Radiology 1987;162:187.
82. Wicki J, Perneger TV, Junod AF, et al: Assessing clinical probability of pulmonary embolism in the emergency ward: a simple score. Arch Intern Med 2001;161:92-97.
83. Sanson BJ, Lijmer JG, Mac Gillavry MR, et al: Comparison of a clinical probability estimate and two clinical models in patients with suspected pulmonary embolism. ANTELOPE-Study Group. Thromb Haemost 2000;83:199-203.
84. Wells PS, Anderson DR, Rodger M, et al: Excluding pulmonary embolism at the bedside without diagnostic imaging: Management of patients with suspected pulmonary embolism presenting to the emergency department by using a simple clinical model and D-dimer. Ann Intern Med 2001;135:98-107.
85. Wells PS, Ginsberg JS, Anderson DR, et al: Use of a clinical model for safe management of patients with suspected pulmonary embolism. Ann Intern Med 1998;129:997-1005.
86. Chagnon I, Bounameaux H, Aujesky D, et al: Comparison of two clinical prediction rules and implicit assessment among patients with suspected pulmonary embolism. Am J Med 2002;113:269-275.
87. Huisman MV, Buller HR, Cate JW, et al: Unexpected high prevalence of silent pulmonary embolism in patients with deep venous thrombosis. Chest 1989;95:498.
88. Moser KM, LeMoine JR: Is embolic risk conditioned by location of deep venous thrombosis? Ann Intern Med 1981;94:439.
89. Fowl RJ, Strothman GB, Bleba J, et al: Inappropriate use of venous duplex scans: An analysis of indications and results. J Vasc Surg 1996;23:881-886.
90. Lipsky DA, Shepard AD, McCarthy BD, et al: Noninvasive venous testing in the diagnosis of pulmonary embolism: The impact on decision making. J Vasc Surg 1997;26:757-763.
91. Matteson B, Langsfeld M, Schermer C, et al: Role of venous duplex scanning in patients with suspected pulmonary embolism. J Vasc Surg 1996;24:768-773.
92. Bendick PJ, Catto S, Cornelius P, et al: Outcome of duplex ultrasound testing for DVT relative to referral source. J Vasc Technol 1994;18:5-8.
93. Davidson BL, Elliot CG, Lensing AW: Low accuracy of color Doppler ultrasound in the detection of proximal leg vein thrombosis in asymptomatic high-risk patients. Ann Intern Med 1992;117:735-738.
94. Harris LM, Curl GR, Booth FV, et al: Screening for asymptomatic deep vein thrombosis in surgical intensive care patients. J Vasc Surg 1997;26:765-769.
95. Perrier A, Roy PM, Aujesky D, et al: Diagnosing pulmonary embolism in outpatients with clinical assessment, D-dimer measurement, venous ultrasound, and helical computed tomography: A multicenter management study. Am J Med 2004;116:291-299.
96. Orta Da, Tucker NH, Green LE, et al: Severe hypoxemia secondary to pulmonary embolization treated successfully with the use of a CPAP (continuous positive airway pressure) mask. Chest 1978;74:588.
97. Hauser CJ, Shoemaker WC: Volume loading in massive acute pulmonary embolus. Crit Care Med 1979;7:304.
98. Laver MB, Strauss WH, Pohost GM: Right and left ventricular geometry: adjustments during acute respiratory failure. Herbert Shubin Memorial Lecture. Crit Care Med 1975;7:509.
99. Ghignone M, Girling L, Prewitt RM: Volume expansion vs noradrenaline in treatment of a low cardiac output complicating an acute increase in right ventricular afterload in dogs. Anesthesiology 1984;60:48.
100. Layish DT, Tapson VF: Pharmacologic hemodynamic support in massive pulmonary embolism. Chest 1997;111:218-224.
101. Buller HR, Agnelli G, Hull RD, et al: Antithrombotic therapy for venous thromboembolic disease: The Seventh ACCP Conference on Antithrombotic and Thrombolytic Therapy. Chest 2004;126(3 Suppl):401S-428S.
102. Basu D, Gallus A, Hirsh J, et al: A prospective study of the value of monitoring heparin treatment with the activated partial thromboplastin time. N Engl J Med 1975;292:1046.
103. Hyers TM, Hull RD, Weg JG: Antithrombotic therapy for venous thromboembolic disease. Chest 1995;108:335S-351S.
104. Raschke RA, Reilly BM, Guidry JR, et al: The weight-based heparin dosing nomogram compared with "standard care" nomogram. Ann Intern Med 1993;119:874-881.
105. Hull RD, Raskob GE, Rosenbloom D, et al: Optimal therapeutic level of heparin therapy in patients with venous thrombosis. Arch Intern Med 1992;152:1589.
106. Low-molecular-weight heparin in the treatment of patients with venous thromboembolism. The Columbus Investigators. N Engl J Med 1997;337:657-662.
107. Simonneau G, Sors H, Chargonnier B: A comparison of low-molecular-weight heparin with unfractionated heparin for acute pulmonary embolism. N Engl J Med 1997;337:663-669.
108. de Valk HW, Banga JD, Wester JW, et al: Comparing subcutaneous danaparoid with intravenous unfractionated heparin for the treatment of venous thromboembolism. A randomized controlled trial. Ann Intern Med 1995;123:1-9.
109. Hirsh J, Levine MN: Low molecular weight heparin. Blood 1992;79:1-17.
110. Ginsberg JS: Management of venous thromboembolism. N Engl J Med 1996;337:663-669.
111. Siragusa S, Cosmi B, Piovella F, et al: Low-molecular-weight heparins and unfractionated heparin in the treatment of patients with acute venous thromboembolism: Results of a meta-analysis [see comments]. Am J Med 1996;100:269-277.
112. Walenga JM, Hoppensteadt D, Fareed J: Laboratory monitoring of the clinical effects of low molecular weight heparins. Thromb Res Suppl 1991;14:49-62.
113. Harenberg J, Wurzner B, Zimmermann, et al: Bioavailability and antagonization of the low molecular weight heparin CY 216 in man. Thromb Res 1986;44:549-554.
114. Warkentin TE, Kelton JG: Heparin induced thrombocytopenia. Prog Hemost Thromb 1991;10:1.
115. Warkentin TE, Greinacher A: Heparin-induced thrombocytopenia: Recognition, treatment, and prevention: The Seventh ACCP Conference on Antithrombotic and Thrombolytic Therapy. Chest 2004;126(3 Suppl):311S-337S.
116. Fabris F, Luzzatto G, Stefani PM, et al. Heparin-induced thrombocytopenia [In Process Citation]. Haematologica 2000;85(1):72-81.
117. Warkentin TE, Chong BH, Greinacher A: Heparin-induced thrombocytopenia: Towards consensus. Thromb Haemost 1998;79:1-7.
118. Urokinase-streptokinase pulmonary embolism trial: Phase 2 results, a cooperative study. JAMA 1974;229:1606.
119. Arcasoy SM, Kreit JW: Thrombolytic therapy of pulmonary embolism: A comprehensive review of current evidence. Chest 1999;115:1695-1707.
120. Goldhaber SZ, Kessler CM, Heit J, et al: Randomized controlled trial of recombinant tissue plasminogen activator versus urokinase in the treatment of acute pulmonary embolism. Lancet 1988;2:293-298.

121. Goldhaber SZ, Kessler CM, Heit JA, et al: Recombinant tissue-type plasminogen activator versus a novel dosing regimen of urokinase in acute pulmonary embolism: A randomized controlled multicenter trial. J Am Coll Cardiol 1992;20:24-30.
122. Meneveau N, Schiele F, Vuillemenot A, et al: Streptokinase vs alteplase in massive pulmonary embolism: A randomized trial assessing right heart hemodynamics and pulmonary vascular obstruction. Eur Heart J 1997;18:1141-1148.
123. Meneveau N, Schiele F, Metz D, et al: Comparative efficacy of two-hour regimen of streptokinase versus alteplase in acute massive pulmonary embolism: Immediate clinical and hemodynamic outcome and one-year follow-up. J Am Coll Cardiol 1998;31:1057-1063.
124. Meyer G, Sors H, Charbonnier B, et al: Effects of intravenous urokinase versus alteplase on total pulmonary resistance in acute massive pulmonary embolism: A European multicenter double-blind trial. J Am Coll Cardiol 1992;19: 239-245.
125. Thabut G, Thabut D, Myers RP, et al: Thrombolytic therapy of pulmonary embolism: A meta-analysis. J Am Coll Cardiol 2002;40:1660-1667.
126. Leeper KV, Popovich J, Lesser BA, et al: Treatment of massive acute pulmonary embolism: The use of low doses of intra-pulmonary arterial streptokinase combined with full doses of systemic heparin. Chest 1988;93:234.
127. Capstick T, Henry MT: Efficacy of thrombolytic agents in the treatment of pulmonary embolism. Eur Respir J 2005;26:864-874.
128. Kanter B, Moser KM: The Greenfield vena cava filter. Chest 1988;93:170.
129. Millward SF: Temporary and retrievable inferior vena cava filters: Current status. J Vasc Interv Radiol 1998;9:381-387.
130. Nicholson AA, Ettles DF, Paddon AJ, et al: Long-term follow-up of the Bird's Nest IVC Filter. Clin Radiol 1999;54: 759-764.
131. Wittenberg G, Kueppers V, Tschammler A, et al: Long-term results of vena cava filters: Experiences with the LGM and the Titanium Greenfield devices. Cardiovasc Intervent Radiol 1998;21:225-229.
132. Decousus H, Leizorovicz A, Parent F, et al: A clinical trial of vena caval filters in the prevention of pulmonary embolism in patients with proximal deep-vein thrombosis. Prevention du Risque d'Embolie Pulmonaire par Interruption Cave Study Group [see comments]. N Engl J Med 1998;338:409-415.
133. Eight-year follow-up of patients with permanent vena cava filters in the prevention of pulmonary embolism: The PREPIC (Prevention du Risque d'Embolie Pulmonaire par Interruption Cave) randomized study. Circulation 2005;112:416-422.
134. Venet C, Berger C, Tardy B, et al: [Prevention of venous thromboembolism in polytraumatized patients. Epidemiology and importance]. Presse Med 2000;29:68-75.
135. Tola JC, Holtzman R, Lottenberg L: Bedside placement of inferior vena cava filters in the intensive care unit. Am Surg 1999;65:833-837.
136. Mattox KL, Feldman RW, Beall AC Jr, et al: Pulmonary embolectomy for acute massive pulmonary embolism. Ann Surg 1982;195:726.
137. Aklog L, Williams CS, Byrne JG, Goldhaber SZ: Acute pulmonary embolectomy: A contemporary approach. Circulation 2002;105: 1416-1419.
138. Koning R, Cribier A, Gerber L, et al: A new treatment for severe pulmonary embolism: Percutaneous rheolytic thrombectomy. Circulation 1997;96: 2498-2500.
139. Schmitz-Rode T, Janssens U, Schild HH, et al: Fragmentation of massive pulmonary embolism using a pigtail rotation catheter [see comments]. Chest 1998;114:1427-1436.
140. Stahr P, Rupprecht HJ, Voigtlander T, et al: A new thrombectomy catheter device (AngioJet) for the disruption of thrombi: An in vitro study. Catheter Cardiovasc Interv 1999;47:381-389.
141. Uflacker R, Strange C, Vujic I: Massive pulmonary embolism: Preliminary results of treatment with the Amplatz thrombectomy device. J Vasc Interv Radiol 1996;7:519-528.
142. Hull RD, Raskob GE, Rosenbloom D, et al: Heparin for 5 days as compared with 10 days in the initial treatment of proximal venous thrombosis. N Engl J Med 1990;322:1260.
143. Buller HR, Davidson BL, Decousus H, et al: Subcutaneous fondaparinux versus intravenous unfractionated heparin in the initial treatment of pulmonary embolism. N Engl J Med 2003;349:1695-1702.
144. Fiessinger JN, Huisman MV, Davidson BL, et al: Ximelagatran vs low-molecular-weight heparin and warfarin for the treatment of deep vein thrombosis: A randomized trial. JAMA 2005;293:681-689.
145. Douketis JD, Kearon C, Bates S, et al: Risk of fatal pulmonary embolism in patients with treated venous thromboembolism. JAMA 1998;279:458-462.
146. Carson JL, Kelley MA, Duff A, et al: Clinical course of pulmonary embolism. N Engl J Med 1992;326: 1240.
147. Clagett GP, Reisch JS: Prevention of venous thromboembolism in general surgical patients. Results of a meta-analysis. Ann Surg 1988;208:227-240.
148. Collins R, Scrimgeour A, Yusuf S, et al: Reduction on fatal pulmonary embolism and venous thrombosis by perioperative administration of subcutaneous heparin. Overview of results of randomized trials in general, orthopedic, and urologic surgery. N Engl J Med 1988;337:657-662.
149. Neuhaus A, Bentz RR, Weg JG: Pulmonary embolism in respiratory failure. Chest 1978;73:460.
150. Pingleton SK, Bone RC, Pingleton WW, et al: Prevention of pulmonary emboli in a respiratory intensive care unit: efficacy of low-dose heparin. Chest 1981;79:647-650.
151. Ryskamp RP, Trottier SJ: Utilization of venous thromboembolism prophylaxis in a medical-surgical ICU. Chest 1998;113:162-164.
152. Samama MM, Cohen AT, Darmon JY, et al: A comparison of enoxaparin with placebo for the prevention of venous thromboembolism in acutely ill medical patients. Prophylaxis in Medical Patients with Enoxaparin Study Group. N Engl J Med 1999;341:793-800.
153. Crunden E, Boyce C, Woodman H, Bray B: An evaluation of the impact of the ventilator care bundle. Nurs Crit Care 2005;10:242-246.
154. Geerts WH, Pineo GF, Heit JA, et al: Prevention of venous thromboembolism: The Seventh ACCP Conference on Antithrombotic and Thrombolytic Therapy. Chest 2004;126(3 Suppl):338S-400S.
155. O'Quin RJ, Lakshminarayan S: Venous air embolism. Arch Intern Med 1982;142:2173.
156. Adler DS: Nonthrombotic pulmonary embolism. In SZ Goldhaber (ed): Pulmonary embolism and deep venous thrombosis. Philadelphia, WB Saunders, 1985.
157. Marini JJ, Culver BH: Systemic gas embolism complicating mechanical ventilation in the adult respiratory distress syndrome. Ann Intern Med 1989;110:699.
158. Albertine KH: Lung injury and neutrophil density during air embolization in sheep after leukocyte depletion with nitrogen mustard. Am Rev Respir Dis 1988;138:1444.
159. Butler BD, Hills BA: Transpulmonary passage of venous air emboli. J Appl Physiol 1985;59:543.
160. Campkin TV, Perks JS: Venous air embolism. Lancet 1973;1:235.
161. Sloan TB, Kimovec MA: Detection of venous air embolism by airway pressure monitoring. Anesthesiology 1986;64:645.
162. Kizer KW, Goodman PC: Radiographic manifestations of venous air embolism. Radiology 1982;144:35.
163. Marcus RH, Weinert L, Neumann A, et al: Venous air embolism. Diagnosis by spontaneous right-sided contrast echocardiography. Chest 1991;99:784-785.
164. Ericsson JA, Gottlieb JD, Sweet RB: Closed-chest cardiac massage in the treatment of venous air embolism. N Engl J Med 1964;270:1353.
165. Boussuges A, Blanc P, Molenat F, et al: [Prognosis in iatrogenic gas embolism]. Minerva Med 1995;86:453-457.
166. Furuya H, Suzuki T, Okumua F, et al: Detection of air embolism by transesophageal echocardiography. Anesthesiology 1983;58:124.
167. Dines DE, Linscheld RL, Didier DE: The fat-embolism syndrome. Mayo Clin Proc 1972;47:237.
168. Fabian TC, Hoots AV, Stanford DS, et al: Fat embolism syndrome: Prospective evaluations in fracture patients. Crit Care Med 1990;18:42.
169. Chastre J, Fagon JY, Soler P, et al: Bronchoalveolar lavage for rapid diagnosis of the fat embolism syndrome in trauma patients. Ann Intern Med 1990;113:583.
170. Guenther CA, Braun TE: Fat embolism syndrome. Chest 1981;79:143.

171. Gossling HR, Pelligrini VD: Fat embolism syndrome. A review of the pathophysiological basis of treatment. Clin Orthop 1982;165:68.
172. Hulman G: Pathogenesis of non-traumatic fat embolism. Lancet 1988;1:1366.
173. Osakabe Y, Takahashi Y: Utility of bronchoalveolar lavage for the diagnosis of fat emboli syndrome. Nihon Kokyuki Gakkai Zasshi 1998;36:953-958.
174. Pitto RP, Hamer H, Fabiani R, et al: Prophylaxis against fat and bone-marrow embolism during total hip arthroplasty reduces the incidence of postoperative deep-vein thrombosis: A controlled, randomized clinical trial. J Bone Joint Surg Am 2002;84-A: 39-48.
175. Kallenbach J, Lewis M, Zaltman M, et al: Low dose corticosteroid prophylaxis against fat embolism. J Trauma 1987;27:1173.
176. Steiner PE, Lushbaugh CC: Maternal pulmonary embolism by amniotic fluid. JAMA 1941;117:1245.
177. Aguillon A, Andjus T, Grayson A , et al: Amniotic fluid embolism: A review. Ostet Gynecol Surv 1962;17:619.
178. Moore J, Baldisseri MR: Amniotic fluid embolism. Crit Care Med 2005;33(10 Suppl):S279-285.
179. Courtney LD: Amniotic fluid embolism. Obstet Gynecol Surv 1974;29:169.
180. Dolyniuk M, Orfei E, Vania H, et al: Rapid diagnosis of amniotic fluid embolism. 1983;61:28S.
181. Masson RG, Ruggieri J: Pulmonary microvascular cytology: A new diagnostic application of the pulmonary artery catheter. Chest 1985;88:908.
182. Hussey HH, Katz S: Septic pulmonary infarction. Ann Intern Med 1945;22:526.
183. MacMillan JC, Milstein SH, Samson PC: Clinical spectrum of septic pulmonary embolism and infarction. J Thorac Cardiovasc Surg 1978;75:670.
184. Fred HL, Harle TS: Septic pulmonary embolism. Chest 1969;55:483.
185. Rowley KM, Clubb KS, Smith GJW, et al: Right-sided endocarditis as a consequence of flow directed pulmonary artery catheterization: A clinicopathological study of 55 autopsied patients. N Engl J Med 1984;311:1152.
186. Jaffe RB, Koschmann EB: Septic pulmonary emboli. Radiology 1970;96:527.
187. Osei C, Berger HW, Nicholas P: Septic pulmonary infarction: Clinical and radiographic manifestations in 11 patients. Mt Sinai J Med 1979;45:145.
188. Dunn LJ, Van Voorhis LW: Enigmatic fever and pelvic thrombophlebitis. N Engl J Med 1967;276:275.
189. Ledger WJ, Peterson EP: The use of heparin in the management of pelvic thrombophlebitis. Surg Cynecol Obstet 1970;113:1115.
190. Winterbauer RH, Elfenbein IB, Ball WC: Incidence and clinical significance of tumor embolization to the lungs. Am J Med 1968;45:271.
191. Bassiri AG, Haghighi B, Ramona LD, et al: Pulmonary tumor embolism. Am J Respir Crit Care Med 1997;155: 2089-2095.
192. Alpert JS, Smith R, Carlson J, et al: Mortality in patients treated for pulmonary embolism. JAMA 1976;236:1477-1480.

Chapter 46 Pulmonary Hypertension

Lewis J. Rubin

The pulmonary circulation is normally a low-resistance circuit capable of accommodating the entire right ventricular output at a pressure and resistance that are a fraction of those in the systemic circulation, even when pulmonary blood flow increases markedly with physical activity. Elevations in pulmonary artery pressure give rise to an increased impedance to right ventricular ejection; sustained increases in afterload eventually result in right heart dysfunction, producing symptoms predominantly attributable to a reduced cardiac output. When pulmonary hypertension is severe or long-standing, overt right heart failure ensues and is frequently the prominent clinical manifestation of pulmonary vascular disease. Although the term *cor pulmonale* is often equated with right heart failure, it is best defined as pulmonary hypertension in the setting of acute or chronic respiratory disease. Right heart failure is a late manifestation of pulmonary hypertension, and its presence is not required to entertain a diagnosis of cor pulmonale. Indeed, patients with acute cor pulmonale may manifest little evidence of overt right heart failure.

PATHOGENESIS AND PATHOPHYSIOLOGY

Pulmonary vascular disease can be classified on the basis of the site in the pulmonary vasculature where the vascular insult originates. Processes such as left ventricular failure and mitral valve disease cause pulmonary artery hypertension (PAH) primarily by raising postcapillary (venous) pressure, necessitating an increased pulmonary arterial pressure to maintain flow through the lung circuit. In this setting the gradient between the pulmonary artery diastolic and pulmonary capillary wedge or left atrial pressure is relatively small (3 to 5 mm Hg), and the histopathologic changes in the arterial tree are relatively mild, consisting of medial hypertrophy and intimal changes that are potentially reversible. In contrast, conditions that primarily affect the pulmonary arteries and arterioles produce an increased pulmonary arteriovenous pressure gradient; pathologically, these vascular abnormalities range from mild intimal proliferation to obliteration of the vessels and may be highly reversible or irreversible, depending on the etiology and severity.

The differentiation between precapillary and postcapillary pulmonary hypertension has important therapeutic and prognostic implications. This can be accomplished clinically by using measurements of pressure and flow obtained by catheterization of the right heart to calculate vascular resistances.

The total resistance across the pulmonary circuit (total pulmonary resistance [TPR]) is defined as follows:

$$\frac{\text{Mean pulmonary artery pressure (mm Hg)}}{\text{cardiac output (L/min)}}$$

The resistance across the pulmonary arterial circuit (pulmonary vascular resistance [PVR]) is defined as follows:

$$\frac{\text{Mean pulmonary artery pressure} - \text{pulmonary capillary wedge pressure (mm Hg)}}{\text{cardiac output (L/min)}}$$

Thus, patients with postcapillary pulmonary hypertension tend to have a TPR elevated out of proportion to the increase in PVR, whereas precapillary pulmonary hypertension is usually characterized by a PVR that approximates the TPR.

This hemodynamic disparity in vascular resistances is helpful in differentiating the primary site of disease in most cases, but there are two exceptions. First is pulmonary veno-occlusive disease, which is characterized pathologically by obliteration of the small- and medium-sized pulmonary veins, yet the pulmonary capillary wedge pressure measured with a pulmonary artery flotation catheter may be normal. This occurs because the wedge pressure reflects downstream pressure in the large pulmonary veins that drain blood largely from those capillary-venule networks, which are unaffected and do not readily communicate with diseased capillary-venule circuits. Thus, the PVR approximates the TPR in the setting of postcapillary hypertension. Second, most patients with mitral valve disease undergoing valve replacement manifest a prompt fall in pulmonary artery pressure postoperatively, resulting from the alleviation of the downstream obstruction to flow. However, long-standing mitral valve disease can result in persistent precapillary hypertension, characterized pathologically by extensive arterial remodeling, despite correcting the cause of increased venous pressure.

A classification of pulmonary hypertension based on causative disease is shown in Box 46-1. *Secondary pulmonary hypertension* is the term used to describe pulmonary vascular disease that is the result of disorders that primarily alter the structure or function of the lung or diseases that affect the lung circulation as part of a systemic illness. Primary, or idiopathic, pulmonary artery hypertension (IPAH) is a disorder in which pulmonary artery pressure is increased in the absence of a clinically demonstrable cause.

Figure 46-1 depicts the factors contributing to the development of pulmonary hypertension in the setting of respiratory disease. Alveolar hypoxia, which is a common feature of many forms of acute or chronic respiratory disease, produces constriction of pulmonary arteries.[1] Although the precise mechanism responsible for hypoxic pulmonary vasoconstriction remains unknown, it appears to be an intrinsic property of pulmonary smooth muscle cells and is dependent on the availability of extracellular calcium and the state of the cellular membrane voltage-activated potassium channels. Hypercapnia or acidosis, which frequently accompanies obstructive lung disease and may be particularly conspicuous in the setting of acute respiratory failure, potentiates the pulmonary vascular hypoxic pressor response. Although acute hypoxic pulmonary vasoconstriction is readily reversible upon restoration of a normal gas exchange milieu, chronic hypoxia results in vascular remodeling, which is both slowly and incompletely responsive to correction of the derangements in ventilation and gas exchange. Mechanical obstruction of the vasculature by hyperinflated bullae may also play a role in developing pulmonary hypertension in the setting of severe emphysema and may contribute to worsening pulmonary vascular dynamics during acute decompensations. Chronic hypoxia often leads to compensatory polycythemia, which can produce hyperviscosity, further impeding blood flow through the lung circulation. A loss of the cross-sectional surface area of the vasculature as a result of widespread destruction of normal lung parenchyma may serve as an additional factor, causing pulmonary arterial pressure to be elevated in conditions such as advanced bullous emphysema or fibrotic diseases of the lung. Finally, thromboembolism can result in an acute decompensation in the setting of chronic cardiopulmonary disease by raising pulmonary artery pressure directly as a result of vascular obstruction by thrombus, by release of vasoactive substances at

Box 46-1

Nomenclature and Classification of Pulmonary Hypertension*

- Pulmonary arterial hypertension (PAH)
  - Sporadic (IPAH)
  - Familial (FPAH)
  - Related to:
    - Collagen vascular disease
    - Congenital systemic to pulmonary shunts (large, small, repaired or non-repaired)
    - Portal hypertension
    - Human immunodeficiency virus infection
    - Drugs and toxins
    - Other (glycogen storage disease, Gaucher's disease, hereditary hemorrhagic telangiectasia, hemoglobinopathies, myeloproliferative disorders, splenectomy)
  - Associated with significant venous or capillary involvement
    - Pulmonary veno-occlusive disease
    - Pulmonary capillary hemangiomatosis
- Pulmonary venous hypertension
  - Left-sided atrial or ventricular heart disease
  - Left-sided valvular heart disease
- Pulmonary hypertension associated with hypoxemia
  - Chronic obstructive pulmonary disease
  - Interstitial lung disease
  - Sleep disordered breathing
  - Alveolar hypoventilation disorders
  - Chronic exposure to high altitude
- Pulmonary hypertension caused by chronic thrombotic and/or embolic disease
  - Thromboembolic obstruction of proximal pulmonary arteries
  - Thromboembolic obstruction of distal pulmonary arteries
  - Pulmonary embolism (tumor, parasites, foreign material)
- Miscellaneous
  - Sarcoidosis, histiocytosis X, lymphangiomatosis, compression of pulmonary vessels (adenopathy, tumor, fibrosing mediastinitis)

*Modified from Rubin LJ: Diagnosis and management of pulmonary arterial hypertension: ACCP evidence-based clinical practice guidelines. Chest 2004;126(Suppl):1S-92S.

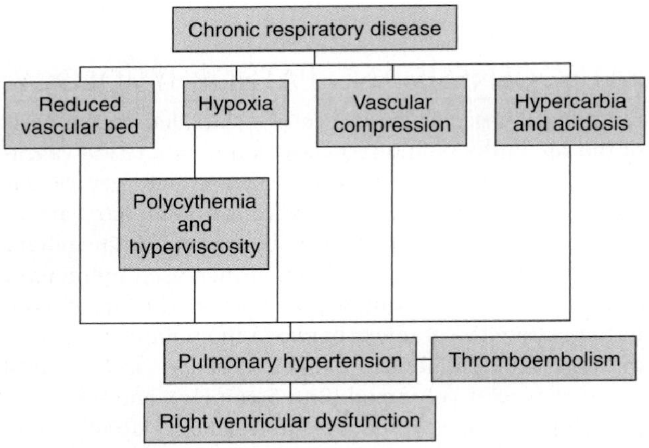

Figure 46-1. Factors responsible for the pathogenesis of pulmonary hypertension in the setting of chronic respiratory disease (cor pulmonale).

the site of thrombosis, or by worsening intrapulmonary gas exchange and potentiating hypoxic pulmonary vasoconstriction.

Elevations in pulmonary artery pressure occur frequently in patients with adult respiratory distress syndrome (ARDS). In addition to the factors listed previously, release of vasoactive mediators as a result of the underlying inflammatory process contributes to the pulmonary vascular process.[2]

Patients with connective tissue diseases may develop pulmonary hypertension either as part of a systemic vasculopathy or as the primary manifestation of their illness. The vasculature may also be secondarily affected as a result of parenchymal lung disease, such as pulmonary fibrosis in systemic sclerosis. Finally, pulmonary vasospasm (pulmonary Raynaud's phenomenon) has been observed in some patients with connective tissue diseases, particularly those who experience typical Raynaud's phenomenon.

IPAH is a condition of unknown cause in which the pulmonary vasculature is the exclusive target of the disease process.[3,4] The mechanism responsible for developing pulmonary vascular disease is unclear, but a number of conditions have been associated with this disorder.[5] Pulmonary hypertension has resulted from ingesting diet suppressants chemically similar to amphetamines, which suggests that these agents may either induce vasoconstriction directly or alter the metabolism or intracellular transport of circulating vasoactive substances such as serotonin. It has also been suggested that this potential mechanism causes the pulmonary vascular disease that has occurred in patients ingesting rapeseed oil (toxic oil syndrome) and contaminated L-tryptophan. Pulmonary hypertension may also complicate portal hypertension, possibly because of an undefined vasotoxin that may bypass hepatic metabolism and injure the lung circulation. Extracts from the plant species *Crotalaria,* which are used in parts of Africa and the Caribbean to make herbal tea, have also been implicated in IPAH pathogenesis in several patients. Furthermore, administering the monocrotaline derivative of this plant to laboratory animals results in severe necrotizing pulmonary arteritis and subsequent development of chronic pulmonary vascular disease. Pulmonary vascular disease that is pathologically identical to IPAH has also been observed in patients who test positive for antibodies to the human immunodeficiency virus.

IPAH occurs twice as often in women as in men. Individuals at any age may be affected, but the disease is most common between the ages of 20 and 50 years. On occasion, there is a family history of IPAH, and a mutation in the Bone Morphogenetic Protein Receptor-2 (*BMPR2*) gene, a member of the transforming growth factor beta (TGFβ) superfamily, has been identified as the genetic basis for the familial inheritance in many cases.

CLINICAL MANIFESTATIONS

Patients with pulmonary hypertension often present with subtle and nonspecific symptoms. The most common symptoms accompanying pulmonary hypertension include exertional dyspnea, fatigue, chest pain that is often described by patients as a substernal pressure suggestive of angina pectoris, and syncope. Syncope is particularly noteworthy because it implies a markedly impaired cardiac output and is a poor prognostic sign. Similarly, the presence of edema or anasarca implies right heart failure and portends an ominous prognosis. Raynaud's phenomenon is reported to occur in up to 25% to 30% of patients with IPAH, although it is far more common in pulmonary hypertension secondary to connective tissue diseases. Hoarseness and a nonproductive cough may result from compression of the recurrent laryngeal nerve by massively dilated proximal pulmonary arteries.

A meticulous physical examination may not only suggest the presence of pulmonary vascular disease but also provide clues to its cause. Examination of the jugular venous pulse may demonstrate elevated venous pressure, suggesting right heart volume overload, as well as prominent *a* or *cv* waves, indicating altered right ventricular compliance and tricuspid regurgitation, respectively. Examination of the chest may disclose abnormalities that point to an underlying specific cause of pulmonary vascular disease, such as obstructive lung disease or restriction from chest cage deformities. The findings on cardiac examination may vary, depending on the cause and severity of the process. Patients with severe, chronic pulmonary hypertension usually manifest a prominent right ventricular impulse along the parasternal region; a right-sided fourth heart sound and pulmonic component to the second heart sound (P_2) may also be palpable. In contrast, the point of maximal cardiac impulse is frequently in the subxiphoid region in patients with cor pulmonale resulting from severe obstructive lung disease. Auscultation of the heart may disclose an accentuated P_2, right-sided S_4 gallop, or a pulmonic ejection click. An S_3 gallop, indicating right heart failure, is a serious prognostic finding. The murmur of tricuspid insufficiency, audible along the lower right sternal border and increasing with inspiration, is a common finding in advanced pulmonary hypertension. On occasion, a murmur of pulmonic insufficiency may be heard at the left second intercostal space and the parasternal area. Fixed splitting of the second heart sound should raise the suspicion of an unsuspected atrial septal defect. Short systolic bruits heard during auscultation of the lungs may indicate a partially occlusive thrombus in the larger pulmonary arteries.

Because a normal right ventricle can acutely increase systolic pressure only to a level of approximately 40 to 45 mm Hg in response to an acute pulmonary vascular insult without resulting in overt right heart failure and cardiogenic shock, the physical findings in acute pulmonary hypertension are usually less dramatic than those in established, long-standing hypertensive pulmonary vascular disease.

Hepatomegaly, ascites, or edema suggests right heart failure, and peripheral cyanosis implies a markedly reduced cardiac output. In contrast, central cyanosis may indicate a right-to-left shunt, which may result from congenital heart disease with Eisenmenger's syndrome, pulmonary arteriovenous malformations, or the opening of the foramen ovale as a result of right atrial pressure and volume overload. Digital clubbing does not occur in IPAH, and its presence suggests that pulmonary hypertension is from parenchymal lung disease, congenital heart disease, or hepatic cirrhosis.

DIAGNOSTIC APPROACH

A variety of laboratory tests are useful in both establishing a diagnosis of pulmonary hypertension and determining its cause. Chest radiography may disclose evidence of parenchymal lung disease or demonstrate right ventricular and pulmonary vascular prominence (Fig. 46-2). The finding of Kerley's B lines on the chest radiograph of a patient with pulmonary hypertension but a normal left heart shown by cardiac catheterization or echocardiography suggests pulmonary veno-occlusive disease. Electrocardiography may show the characteristic signs of right ventricular hypertrophy including a QRS axis greater than 110 degrees, RSR^1 complex in V_1 and V_2, and an incomplete right bundle branch block.

The findings are generally much less prominent in patients with underlying lung disease, owing both to the displacement of the heart in the thorax in patients with hyperinflation and to the tendency for cor pulmonale to be a milder form of pulmonary hypertension than other causes. The presence of an $S_1Q_3T_3$ pattern on the electrocardiogram (ECG) is strongly suggestive of an acute right ventricular pressure overload state, such as massive acute pulmonary thromboembolism. Prominent, peaked *p* waves in the inferior and right precordial leads (p pulmonale) is a nonspecific finding on ECG and may appear and disappear in patients with acute, reversible airflow obstruction in the absence of pulmonary hypertension. Echocardiography may demonstrate right-sided chamber enlargement, flattening of the interventricular septum during systole, or coexistent left ventricular or mitral valve disease (Fig. 46-3). A pericardial effusion may also be present and is suggestive of either a connective tissue disease or right atrial pressure overload. Doppler studies can determine the presence and magnitude of tricuspid regurgitation, which may be a useful means of noninvasively estimating pulmonary artery systolic pressure. Intravenous injection of agitated saline or hydrogen peroxide during echocardiographic study may disclose an intracardiac shunt.

The presence and severity of pulmonary hypertension correlate closely with the degree of impairment in lung

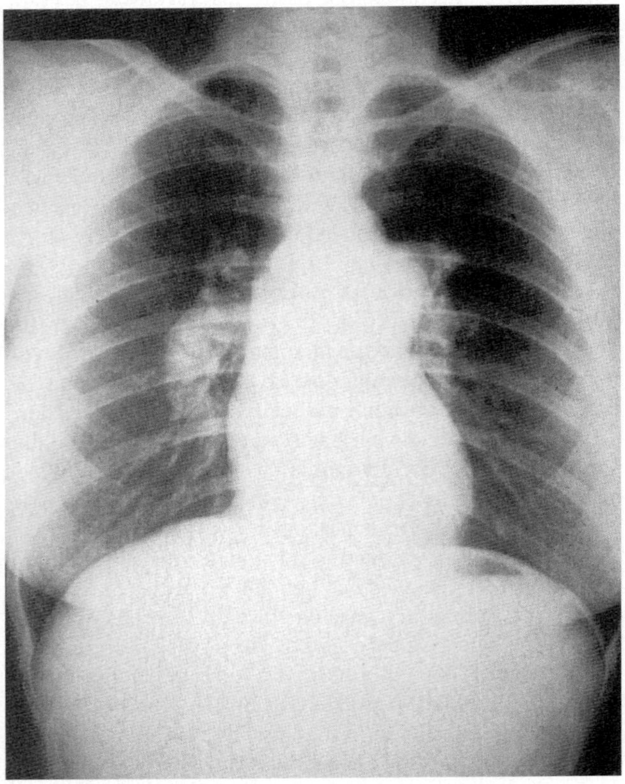

Figure 46-2. Posteroanterior chest radiograph in a patient with pulmonary hypertension. The proximal pulmonary arteries are enlarged, and the right ventricular configuration is prominent.

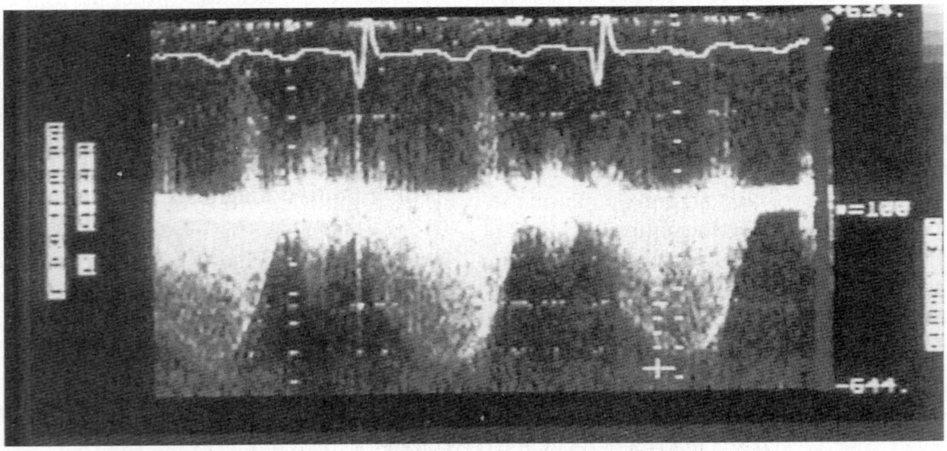

Figure 46-3. Doppler examination of the tricuspid valve showing a regurgitant jet, which can be used to estimate pulmonary artery systolic pressure.

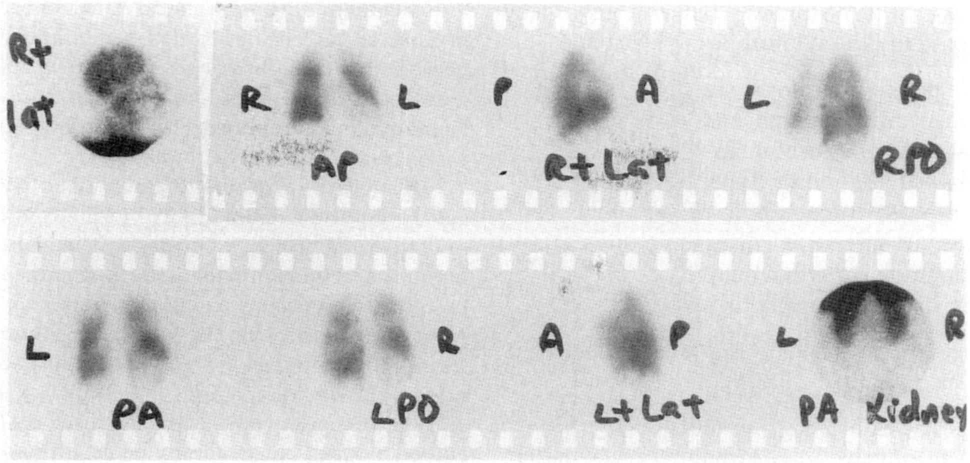

Figure 46-4. Perfusion lung scan in a patient with primary pulmonary hypertension. The distribution of perfusion is homogeneous.

function in patients with chronic parenchymal lung disease. In general, patients with chronic airflow obstruction are likely to have pulmonary hypertension when the 1-second forced expiratory volume (FEV_1) falls below 1 L.[6,7] In chronic restrictive lung disease, pulmonary hypertension is usually present when the vital capacity or the diffusing capacity is below 50% of predicted levels. Additionally, arterial blood gas measurements while the patient breathes ambient air may suggest chronic hypoxemia, which may be important not only in establishing an etiology but also in guiding the initial approach to therapy. Worsening pulmonary hypertension during acute exacerbations is likely in individuals with severe chronic parenchymal disease.

Chronic thrombotic occlusion of the pulmonary vasculature should be considered in any patient with unexplained pulmonary hypertension because it is potentially curable by thromboendarterectomy.[8] Radioisotope lung scanning is a safe and reliable method of assessing the distribution of ventilation and perfusion in the lungs. Patients with IPAH usually manifest a homogeneous pattern of perfusion, whereas scans from patients with chronic thromboembolism exhibit multiple perfusion defects of varying sizes (see Fig. 46-6). Scanning over the head or kidneys may demonstrate an unsuspected right-to-left shunt (Fig. 46-4). Patients with veno-occlusive disease may have a mottled appearance on perfusion scan,[9] although this is not always the case. Patients in whom a distinction between IPAH and chronic thromboembolic disease cannot be made noninvasively should undergo pulmonary arteriography (Figs. 46-5, 46-6, and 46-7). Similarly, consideration should be given to acute pulmonary thromboembolism in a patient with chronic cor pulmonale who experiences a sudden clinical deterioration in the absence of clear signs of progression of the underlying parenchymal lung disease.

In patients with pulmonary vascular disease secondary to connective tissue diseases, serologic studies are usually abnormal and at high titers. Some patients with IPAH also

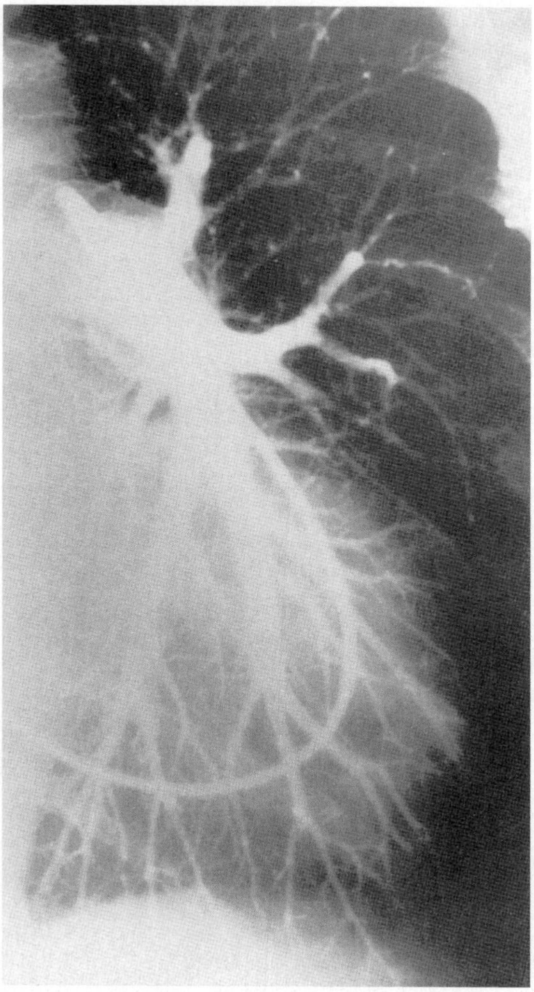

Figure 46-5. Pulmonary angiogram in a patient with idiopathic pulmonary artery hypertension. The proximal vessels are dilated, with peripheral pruning and a loss of the normal arborization pattern in the absence of intraluminal filling defects.

may have positive serologic studies,[10] but these are usually in nonspecific patterns and at low titers. Other studies that may be useful in the diagnostic workup of unexplained pulmonary hypertension include the following:

- High-resolution computed tomography scanning of the chest to exclude occult interstitial disease, particularly when the chest radiograph is normal but pulmonary function is substantially impaired
- Magnetic resonance imaging to exclude fibrosing mediastinitis and proximal thrombosis of the pulmonary vasculature
- Polysomnography to evaluate the presence of sleep-disordered breathing

Complete cardiac catheterization should be performed in patients with unexplained, severe pulmonary hypertension to exclude congenital heart disease, proximal or peripheral pulmonic stenosis, and valvular heart disease.

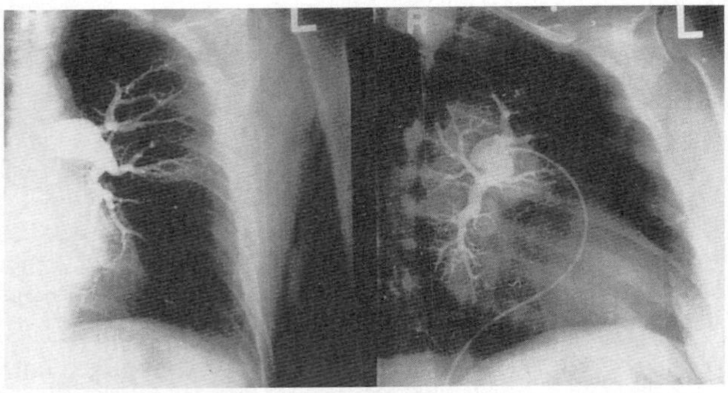

Figure 46-6. Pulmonary angiogram in a patient with chronic thromboembolic pulmonary hypertension. Large areas of the lung are avascular, and there is abrupt cutoff of several pulmonary arteries.

The pulmonary artery pressure often approaches systemic levels in IPAH, chronic thromboembolic disease, and connective tissue diseases and tends to be more modestly elevated in most forms of acute or chronic cor pulmonale. Hemodynamic monitoring may also help guide the management of acute cor pulmonale.

In most cases a cause of the pulmonary vascular disease can be ascertained on clinical grounds. However, for a definitive diagnosis to be made, it may be necessary to obtain a specimen of lung tissue from patients with severe pulmonary hypertension who have confusing evidence on physical examination or ancillary laboratory testing. Open lung biopsy is the preferred approach, although it carries an increased risk of complications in patients with severe pulmonary vascular disease. Thoracoscope-guided biopsies can generally be performed safely in such patients and involve considerably lower risks and complications than traditional approaches. Because the small specimen sizes preclude establishing a pathologic diagnosis, transbronchial biopsy via the fiberoptic bronchoscope is not a suitable alternative to open lung biopsy in the setting of unexplained pulmonary vascular disease (Fig. 46-8).

APPROACH TO MANAGEMENT

Initially the management of pulmonary hypertension should be directed toward treating the underlying cause, if one exists. Improving gas exchange and airflow in patients with cor pulmonale resulting from chronic obstructive airway disease usually ameliorates the pulmonary hypertension to some degree. Patients with interstitial lung disease and pulmonary hypertension may show marked hemodynamic improvement when lung function is improved with corticosteroid or immunosuppressive

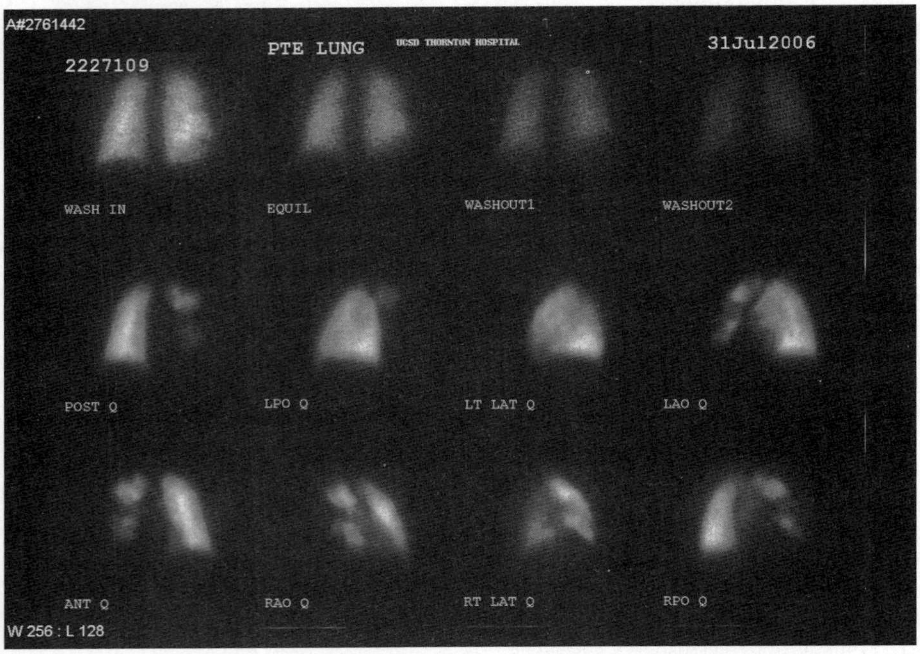

Figure 46-7. Ventilation-perfusion lung scan in a patient with chronic thromboembolic pulmonary hypertension showing normal ventilation and multiple large perfusion defects.

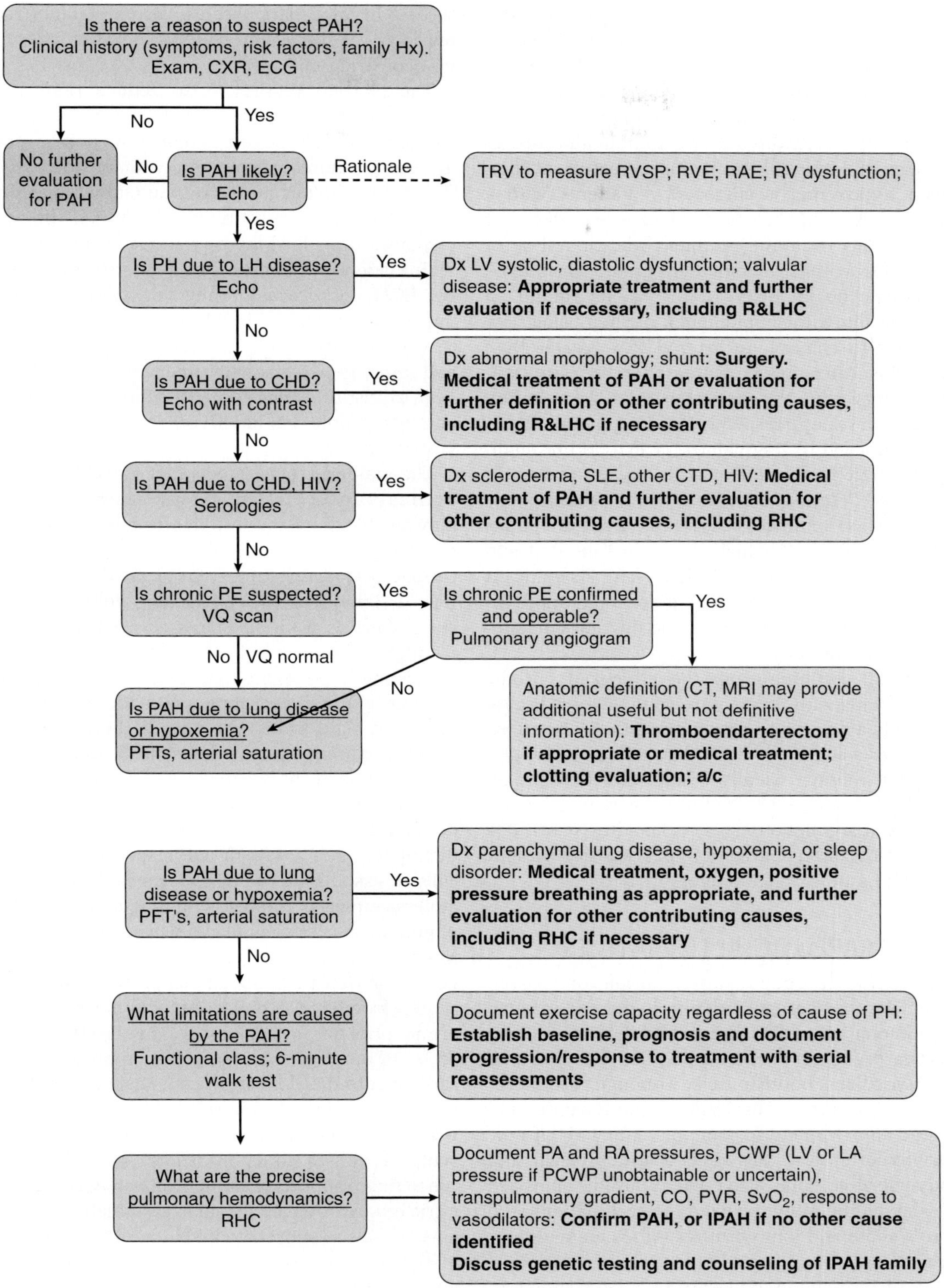

Figure 46-8. Diagnostic algorithm for suspected pulmonary artery hypertension. a/c, anticoagulation; CHD, congenital heart disease; CO, cardiac output; CTD, connective tissue disease; Dx, diagnosis; echo, echocardiography; Hx, history; IPAH, idiopathic pulmonary artery hypertension; LA, left atrial; LH, left heart; LV, left ventricular; PAH, pulmonary artery hypertension; PCWP, pulmonary capillary wedge pressure; PE, pulmonary embolism; PFT, pulmonary function test; PVR, pulmonary vascular resistance; RAE, right atrial enlargement; RHC, right heart catheterization; R&LHC, right and left heart catheterization; RV, right ventricular; RVE, right ventricular enlargement; SvO_2, mixed venous oxygen saturation; TRV, peak velocity of TR jet. (From Rubin LJ: Diagnosis and management of pulmonary arterial hypertension: ACCP evidence-based clinical practice guidelines. Chest 2004;126(Suppl):1S-92S.)

therapy. Because hypoxia is a major contributor to both acute and chronic cor pulmonale, correction of hypoxemia is an important component of the therapeutic approach to affected patients. Although the hemodynamic effects of low-flow supplemental oxygen in patients with chronic obstructive lung disease are variable and slow in achieving maximal effect,[11] survival is increased substantially when hypoxemia is corrected.[12] Patients with a stable arterial partial pressure of oxygen (PO_2) of 55 mm Hg or less breathing ambient air, or a PO_2 of 59 mm Hg or less with (1) a hematocrit greater than 55%, (2) p pulmonale on an ECG, or (3) edema should be treated chronically with supplemental oxygen using flow rates sufficient to achieve an arterial PO_2 greater than 60 mm Hg. Flow rates may be increased for activity or at night in patients who experience arterial desaturation with exercise or sleep, respectively. In general, IPAH patients with normal resting values for PO_2 do not manifest hemodynamic improvement with oxygen therapy.[13] However, acute deteriorations from further compromise of cardiac function or lower respiratory tract infections can result in hypoxemia, which is poorly tolerated and should be treated aggressively. Patients with a significant right-to-left shunt do not usually experience an improvement in oxygenation to an appreciable degree with supplemental oxygen therapy.

Polycythemia, resulting from the effects of chronic hypoxia in patients with severe parenchymal lung disease or congenital heart disease, may contribute to elevations in PVR by increasing blood viscosity. Although supplemental oxygen therapy usually results in a decrease in hematocrit in these patients, this response may be incomplete.[12] Isovolemic phlebotomy to a hematocrit of 50% to 55% may reduce the degree of hyperviscosity without compromising tissue oxygen delivery.[14]

OTHER THERAPEUTIC ALTERNATIVES

Vasodilator therapy for pulmonary hypertension is based on the premises that vasoconstriction is present in some forms of pulmonary vascular disease and these drugs may exert their vasorelaxant properties in pulmonary, as well as systemic vascular, smooth muscle. Although vasodilator therapy may produce substantial hemodynamic and symptomatic improvement in some patients with chronic pulmonary hypertension,[5] this effect is not universal, and serious adverse effects may also result. Thus this approach to therapy should be individualized for each patient, and the patient's acute and long-term responses meticulously monitored.

A variety of systemic vasodilators have been shown to reduce pulmonary artery pressure in experimentally induced pulmonary hypertension including hydralazine, calcium channel blockers (nifedipine, diltiazem, and verapamil), prostaglandins E_1 and I_2 (epoprostenol, PGI_2, prostacyclin), adenosine, nitrates (nitroglycerin and nitroprusside), and inhaled nitric oxide. These agents have also been used to treat selected patients with either idiopathic or secondary pulmonary hypertension, but with little success in large part because chronic pulmonary hypertension is a disease of vasoproliferation more so than vasoconstriction.[15]

The goal of therapy is to reduce right ventricular afterload and increase cardiac output and systemic oxygen delivery. A substantial reduction in pulmonary arterial pressure concomitant with an increased stroke volume and an unchanged or minimally reduced systemic arterial pressure constitutes the optimal hemodynamic response to medical therapy and is frequently associated with evidence of regression of right heart abnormalities by ECG, echocardiography, or catheterization[16] and improved survival.[17] This ideal response is seen in response to vasodilators in less than 20% of patients with IPAH and rarely in patients with other forms of PAH. The decision to institute long-term vasodilator therapy in these patients should be based on individual assessment of vasoreactivity.

The major adverse effects that vasodilator administration may produce include (1) systemic hypotension, which may result either from systemic vasodilation in the absence of any pulmonary vascular effect or from a reduced cardiac output resulting from negative inotropic properties of some drugs; (2) worsening pulmonary hypertension, which is from an increased cardiac output flowing through a vascular bed with a fixed resistance; and (3) worsening hypoxemia, due either to increased perfusion to poorly ventilated lung units (decreased ratio)[18] or increased right-to-left shunting if the systemic vascular effect predominates. Patients with right heart failure appear to be at the greatest risk for adverse effects from vasodilator administration.[15] However, no other reliable demographic or clinical parameters are available for predicting whether a patient will respond acutely or chronically to vasodilator therapy. Because the risk of sustained adverse effects is greatest with long-acting agents, the use of potent, short-acting, titratable vasodilators to test vasoreactivity has been advocated. Adenosine, epoprostenol, and nitric oxide are the agents most commonly used for acute vasodilator testing. A reduction in mean pulmonary artery pressure by at least 10 mm Hg to a level below 35 to 40 mm Hg, accompanied by a normal or increased cardiac output and no significant change in systemic blood pressure, is generally considered a positive response that warrants a trial of chronic oral vasodilator therapy. The acute responses to epoprostenol have been useful in predicting responsiveness to orally active drugs.[19] Inhaled nitric oxide produces a similar vasodilation of the pulmonary vessels as epoprostenol but has the added advantage of pulmonary vascular selectivity with little or no systemic effect.

In the few IPAH patients who demonstrate pulmonary vasoreactivity with acute vasodilator testing, long-term calcium channel blocker therapy is the standard of care. For the nonresponders, oral endothelin receptor antagonists, phosphodiesterase inhibitors, and subcutaneously or inhaled delivery of prostacyclin analogues are now approved therapies for PAH and have revolutionized the care of patients with this condition. Continuous infusion of intravenous epoprostenol therapy, which has been shown to improve quality of life, exercise capacity, hemodynamics, and survival in IPAH patients, is now reserved for the most severely ill patients with PAH.[20,21] Epoprostenol may also benefit other selected patients with secondary small vessel pulmonary hypertension.[22,23] Patients with severe pulmonary hypertension are at risk for fatal pulmonary thromboembolic events because of their sedentary lifestyle, venous insufficiency, and dilated right heart chambers with sluggish pulmonary blood flow. Even a small vascular thrombotic occlusion may be lethal in a patient with a compromised pulmonary vascular bed that possesses the capability neither to recruit unused vessels nor to dilate functional vasculature in response to an acute insult. Accordingly, prophylactic anticoagulation has been advocated for patients with severe nonthrombotic pulmonary hypertension, and survival may be improved in those receiving anticoagulants.[17,24] However, anticoagulant therapy is not without risk in this setting, and life-threatening side effects including hemoptysis from spontaneously ruptured pulmonary vessels may occur. If warfarin therapy is contemplated, the international normalized ratio should be monitored frequently and maintained between 2 and 2.5. Adjusted-dose subcutaneous heparin may be a suitable alternative to warfarin, although it is more cumbersome to administer and its use should be reserved for patients who have a greater risk of complications with warfarin. Acutely ill patients with nonthrombotic pulmonary hypertension should receive low-dose heparin subcutaneously during the acute illness.

Diuretics can help treat right heart failure by reducing the degree of hepatic congestion and peripheral edema. In addition, patients with right heart failure and hypoxemia because of a right-to-left shunt may experience improved oxygenation with diuresis, owing to the reduced transatrial pressure gradient. However, diuretics should be used cautiously in this setting because decreasing right ventricular preload may result in a reduction in cardiac output. Also, diuretic-induced hypokalemia and alkalosis may be poorly tolerated.

Cardiac glycosides have little use in the acute or chronic management of pulmonary vascular disease, with the exception of supraventricular tachyarrhythmias or biventricular failure.[25] Furthermore, patients with chronic respiratory disease are at an increased risk of developing toxicity with these agents.[26]

Atrial septostomy may temporarily improve right heart function and symptoms (ascites, edema, syncope) in selected patients who are refractory to standard therapy. An atrial septal defect is created using progressively larger catheter balloons. By creating a right-to-left shunt, the right atrial pressure is reduced and left heart filling is increased. Some degree of hypoxemia is inevitable but may be offset by improvements in systemic oxygen delivery. This procedure may serve as a bridge to transplantation, but it is a high-risk procedure that should only be performed in specialized centers.[27,28]

Combined heart-lung transplantation has been considered the surgical treatment of choice for severe pulmonary hypertension that is refractory to medical management.[29] However, the dearth of suitable organ donors and the limited number of centers with the expertise to perform this procedure have limited its availability. Both single-lung or bilateral-lung transplantation result in marked improvement in right heart function in patients with isolated pulmonary vascular disease without the need to transplant the heart.[30]

Because the course of pulmonary vascular disease is variable, it is difficult to determine the ideal time to consider transplantation in an individual patient. However, patients with symptoms that substantially limit their lifestyle and are unresponsive to medical therapy may be suitable candidates for lung transplantation. Patients with evidence of severe and irreversible right heart dysfunction, significant disease affecting the left side of the heart or coronary circulation, or complex congenital cardiac defects should be considered only for combined heart-lung transplantation. Organ rejection and opportunistic infections constitute the major causes of morbidity and mortality after transplantation. Whether idiopathic diseases such as IPAH will recur in transplanted lungs is unknown.

Despite the continued increase in the number of candidates awaiting transplantation, the availability of donor lungs has remained relatively fixed at a level insufficient to meet demand. This has led to an increase in the average wait to receive an organ (approximately 24 months) and an increase in the number of candidates who die while awaiting a transplant.[31] Fortunately, continuous epoprostenol has resulted in such significant improvement in selected patients that they are able to survive the wait to transplantation and, in others, medical therapy has obviated the need for transplant.

The treatment of choice for chronic thrombotic pulmonary hypertension is pulmonary thromboendarterectomy.[8] However, only an organized thrombus in the proximal vessels is approachable by this technique. Preoperative evaluation should include complete pulmonary angiography to determine the site and extent of thrombosis. Marked hemodynamic improvement frequently results from successful removal of organized thrombus. Patients with acute cor pulmonale resulting from massive pulmonary embolism should be evaluated for emergent embolectomy if death is imminent and there is insufficient time for thrombolytic therapy to affect enough clot lysis to restore the integrity of the pulmonary vascular bed.

PROGNOSIS

In the settings of both chronic obstructive pulmonary disease and ARDS, the presence of cor pulmonale contributes significantly to shortened survival.[2,6] The 3-year survival in patients with severe airflow obstruction and a PVR 3 to 4 times normal is less than 10% to 15%.[6,32] Survival is similarly influenced by the presence of pulmonary hypertension in chronic restrictive lung diseases and connective tissue diseases.

Death from IPAH depends mainly on the state of the right ventricle. Patients with symptoms of severe right heart dysfunction, such as syncope, and hemodynamic evidence of impaired right ventricular function, such as reduced cardiac output or mixed venous saturation and elevated right atrial pressure, usually succumb to the disease within 1 to 2 years.[33] Patients with milder symptoms and relatively well-preserved right heart function survive longer, although the course is highly variable. Medical therapy appears to have had a significant impact on survival.

KEY POINTS

- The term *cor pulmonale* should be used to connote pulmonary hypertension in the setting of parenchymal lung disease or primary pulmonary vascular disease rather than right heart failure; the latter is a late manifestation of cor pulmonale.
- Precapillary forms of pulmonary hypertension are characterized by comparable elevations in the total pulmonary and pulmonary vascular resistances, respectively, and by an elevated pulmonary arterial-venous pressure gradient; they can thus be differentiated from postcapillary causes. These hemodynamic features are useful for approaching the differential diagnosis of pulmonary vascular disease.
- Patients with pulmonary vascular disease often present with nonspecific complaints including exertional dyspnea and chest pain. Syncope, indicative of an inability to increase cardiac output during physical activity, is a particularly ominous prognostic sign.
- A meticulous and thorough approach to elucidate the cause of pulmonary vascular disease is important for clarifying the prognosis and guiding therapy.
- Therapy should be directed toward improving lung function and gas exchange in patients with underlying parenchymal lung disease or ventilatory dysfunction, although the maximal hemodynamic responses to therapy in this setting are often delayed.
- Vasodilator therapy may be considered in patients with persistent pulmonary hypertension in whom vasoconstriction is thought to be a significant contributor and should be initiated cautiously and under careful monitoring of pulmonary and systemic hemodynamics and gas exchange.
- Treatment of PPH with intravenous epoprostenol has been shown to improve hemodynamics and quality of life and prolong survival in patients who do not respond to calcium channel blockers.
- Patients with severe pulmonary hypertension resulting from chronic thromboembolic disease should be evaluated for their candidacy for thromboendarterectomy, which offers the potential of surgically restoring the integrity of the pulmonary vasculature.
- Heart-lung or lung transplantation should be considered in patients with severe pulmonary hypertension in the absence of a systemic disease. Because the waiting time on a transplant list may exceed 1 year, patients should be evaluated and listed at the earliest suggestion that right heart function is compromised and unresponsive to medical therapy.

REFERENCES

1. Yuan JXJ (ed): Hypoxic Pulmonary Vasoconstriction: Cellular and Molecular Mechanisms. Boston, Kluwer Academic Publishers, 2004.
2. Cranshaw JH, Evans TW: Effects of lung injury on the pulmonary circulation. In Peacock A, Rubin LJ (eds): Pulmonary Circulation—Diseases and Their Management, 2nd ed. London, Arnold Publishers, 2004, pp 518-531.
3. Bjornsson J, Edwards WD: Primary pulmonary hypertension: A histopathologic study of 80 cases. Mayo Clin Proc 1985;60:16.
4. Rich S, Dantzker DR, Ayres SM, et al: Primary pulmonary hypertension: A national prospective study. Ann Intern Med 1987;107:216.
•5. Rubin LJ: Diagnosis and management of pulmonary arterial hypertension: ACCP evidence-based clinical practice guidelines. Chest 2004;126(Suppl):1S-92S.
6. Burrows B, Kettle LJ, Niden AH, et al: Patterns of cardiovascular dysfunction in chronic obstructive lung disease. N Engl J Med 1972;286:912.
•7. Salvaterra CG, Rubin LJ: Investigation and management of pulmonary hypertension in chronic obstructive pulmonary disease. Am Rev Respir Dis 1993;148:1414.
8. Hoeper M, Meyer E, Simonneau G, Rubin LJ: Chronic thromboembolic pulmonary hypertension. Circulation 2006;113:2011-2020.
9. Bailey CL, Channick RN, Auger WR, et al: High probability perfusion lung scans in pulmonary veno-occlusive disease. Am J Resp Crit Care Med 2000;162:1974-1978.
10. Rich S, Kieras K, Hart K, et al: Antinuclear antibodies in primary pulmonary hypertension. J Am Coll Cardiol 1986;8:1307.
11. Timms RM, Khaja FU, Williams GW, et al: Hemodynamic response to oxygen therapy in chronic obstructive pulmonary disease. Ann Intern Med 1985;102:29.
12. Nocturnal Oxygen Therapy Trial Group: Continuous or nocturnal oxygen therapy in hypoxemic chronic obstructive airways disease: A clinical trial. Ann Intern Med 1980;93:391.
13. Morgan JM, Griffiths M, du Bois RM, et al: Hypoxic pulmonary vasoconstriction in systemic sclerosis and primary pulmonary hypertension. Chest 1991;99:551.
14. Weisse AB, Moschos CB, Frank MJ, et al: Hemodynamic effects of staged hematocrit reduction in patients with stable cor pulmonale and severely elevated hematocrit levels. Am J Med 1975;58:92.
15. Rubin LJ: Therapy of pulmonary hypertension: The evolution from vasodilators to antiproliferative agents. Am J Resp Crit Care Med 2002;166:1308-1309.
16. Rich S, Brundage BH: High-dose calcium channel blocking therapy for primary pulmonary hypertension; evidence for long-term reduction in pulmonary arterial pressure and regression of right ventricular hypertrophy. Circulation 1987;76:135.
17. Sitbon O, Humbert M, Jais X, et al: Long-term response to calcium channel blockers in idiopathic pulmonary arterial hypertension. Circulation 2005;111:3105-3111.

18. Melot C, Naeije R, Mols P, et al: Effects of nifedipine on ventilation/perfusion matching in primary pulmonary hypertension. Chest 1983;89:497.
19. Barst RJ: Pharmacologically induced pulmonary vasodilation in children and young adults with primary pulmonary hypertension. Chest 1986;89:497.
20. Sitban O, Brenot F, Denjean A, et al: Inhaled nitric oxide as a screening vasodilator agent in primary pulmonary hypertension. Am J Respir Crit Care Med 1995;151:384.
•21. Barst RJ, Rubin LJ, Long WA, et al: A comparison of continuous intravenous epoprostenol (prostacyclin) with conventional therapy for primary pulmonary hypertension. N Engl J Med 1996;334:296.
•22. Rubin LJ, Badesch DB: Evaluation and management of the patient with pulmonary arterial hypertension. Ann Intern Med 2005;143:282-292.
23. Badesch DB, Tapson VF, McGoon MD, et al: Continuous intravenous epoprostenol for pulmonary hypertension due to the scleroderma spectrum of disease. Ann Intern Med 1999;132:425.
24. Fuster V, Steele PM, Edwards WD, et al: Primary pulmonary hypertension: Natural history and the importance of thrombosis. Circulation 1984;70:580.
25. Mathur PN, Powles P, Pugsley SO, et al: Effect of digoxin on right ventricular function in severe chronic airflow obstruction: A controlled clinical trial. Ann Intern Med 1981;95:283.
26. Green LH, Smith TW: The use of digitalis in patients with pulmonary disease. Ann Intern Med 1977;87:459.
27. Rothman A, Sklansky MS, Lucas VW, et al: Atrial septostomy as a bridge to lung transplantation in patients with severe pulmonary hypertension. Am J Cardiol 1999;84:682.
28. Sandoval J, Gaspar J, Pulido T, et al: Graded balloon dilation atrial septostomy in severe primary pulmonary hypertension. A therapeutic alternative for patients nonresponsive to vasodilator treatment. J Am Coll Cardiol 1998;32:297.
29. Reitz BA, Wallwork JL, Hunt SA, et al: Heart-lung transplantation. Successful therapy for patients with pulmonary vascular disease. N Engl J Med 1982;306:557.
30. Pasque MK, Trulock EP, Kaiser LD, et al: Single lung transplantation for pulmonary hypertension. Three month hemodynamic follow-up. Circulation 1991;84:2275.
31. United Network for Organ Sharing (UNOS) Scientific Registry Data (http://www.unos. org).
32. Traver GA, Cline MG, Burrows B: Predictors of mortality in chronic obstructive pulmonary disease. Am Rev Respir Dis 1979;119:895.
•33. D'Alonzo GG, Barst RJ, Ayres SM, et al: Survival in patients with primary pulmonary hypertension: Results from a national prospective registry. Ann Intern Med 1991;115: 343.

Chapter 47

Massive Hemoptysis

Susan Garwood, Charlie Strange, and Steven A. Sahn

Massive hemoptysis is defined as the expectoration of blood in quantities sufficient to be life threatening. Hemoptysis comes from the Greek words *haima*, meaning blood, and *ptysis*, meaning spitting. Clinical definitions of massive hemoptysis have arbitrarily selected between 200 to 1000 mL of coughed blood over 24 hours, with the majority choosing 600 mL. Fortunately, massive hemoptysis is rare, occurring in 1% to 4% of patients with hemoptysis.[1,2] However, mortality rates as high as 80%[3,4] suggest that all hemoptysis, regardless of amount, should be taken seriously. This chapter focuses on the pathogenesis of vascular injury and clinical manifestations of hemoptysis within the framework of common diagnoses.

HISTORY

The history of hemoptysis is closely linked to tuberculosis with few alternative etiologies for bleeding considered until the advent of rigid bronchoscopy in the 1900s. The placement of many hemoptysis patients with a variety of diseases in tuberculosis sanitariums likely added to the concordance of tuberculosis and hemoptysis.

The increased use of flexible bronchoscopy, high-resolution computed tomography, and vascular embolization has changed the scope of massive hemoptysis in the past 3 decades. A broadened differential diagnosis and new treatment options have altered morbidity and mortality in this patient subset.

INCIDENCE

Hemoptysis varies in amount from intermittent blood-streaked sputum to massive arterial bleeding with asphyxiation or exsanguination. Incidence studies have been problematic because of the vagaries of definition. However, in a series of 4331 admissions to a pulmonary and thoracic surgery service over 32 months, 67 patients (1.5%) with 600 mL or more hemoptysis in a 48-hour period were seen.[5] In 46 of 67 patients, 600 mL of hemoptysis occurred over 16 hours or less. The incidence of blood-streaked sputum is obviously much higher with estimates of 10% to 15% of patients admitted to a pulmonary service.

PATHOGENESIS

Anatomic Considerations

The lung is unique among the visceral organs in that it receives a dual blood supply from different circulations. Because hemoptysis can occur from either the pulmonary or bronchial circulation, an anatomic understanding of each of these systems is important.

Pulmonary Circulation

The pulmonary artery bifurcates into left and right main pulmonary arteries after it leaves the right heart through the pulmonic valve. Normal pulmonary artery blood pressures are approximately 25/8 mm Hg in an adult man yet may rise to approach systemic pressures in both pulmonary parenchymal and pulmonary vascular diseases. Nevertheless, pulmonary hypertension alone rarely produces hemoptysis.

Prospective arteriographic series for hemoptysis in which both pulmonary and bronchial circulations have been studied do not exist. Pulmonary arterial bleeding, although significantly less frequent than bronchial artery bleeding, has been noted in a wide variety of destructive pulmonary lesions including tuberculosis, lung abscess, and aspergilloma.[6] Aneurysms of the pulmonary artery, arteriovenous malformations, and pulmonary artery rupture have also been reported but are nonetheless rare.

Bronchial Circulation

Bleeding from the bronchial circulation has been estimated to cause 88% of the cases of massive and submassive hemoptysis.[7] Although the bronchial circulation was described in association with inflammatory lesions of the lung in the 1500s by Leonardo da Vinci, more recent descriptions of bronchial artery anatomy provide insight into the smaller communications that exist. The bronchial arteries arise from the descending aorta with considerable anatomic variation. The one or two bronchial arteries that supply each lung in the majority of individuals[8,9] arise from the area near the first and second intercostal arteries. Particularly on the right side, the bronchial arteries may arise directly from the proximal first intercostal artery. The arteries course along the trachea, major bronchi, and bronchioles and have terminal communications with the pulmonary capillaries or pulmonary venules. The small-vessel bronchial supply to the trachea and major bronchi drains into the azygos vein with direct communication to the superior vena cava. Aneurysmal dilation of bronchial arteries (Dieulafoy's vascular malformation) has been noted in some patients with hemoptysis, and it can occasionally be visualized endobronchially and noted on bronchial arteriography.[10]

A direct anastomotic communication between the bronchial and pulmonary arterioles has been sought to explain the preservation of lung parenchyma after injuries to the pulmonary vascular supply. Series of anatomic studies in normal humans have found that intermeshing of pulmonary and bronchial capillary networks is the most common anastomotic arrangement that prevents pressurization of the pulmonary arterioles with systemic pressures.[11] However, in chronic inflammatory diseases of the airways, anatomic anastomoses have been found that allow direct pressurization of the pulmonary artery with systemic pressures.[12] The extent to which these vascular communications are related to hemoptysis remains unknown.

Bronchial arteries vasodilate in the presence of cholinergic; β_2-adrenergic; and some nonadrenergic, noncholinergic agonists. Although the effect of β_2 agonists on the course of hemoptysis remains unstudied, the balance between improved mucociliary clearance of blood affected by β_2 agonists and detrimental bronchial artery dilation should be considered.[13] Alternatively, anticholinergics vasoconstrict and provide therapeutic alternatives for bronchodilation.

Other physiochemical maneuvers can influence bronchial blood flow—cold air causes blanching of the human airway,[14] humidified air decreases bronchial blood flow compared with dry gas,[15] and increased alveolar pressure decreases bronchial blood flow by applied pressure at the capillaries.[11]

Nonbronchial Systemic Collateral Circulation

In diseases of the lung associated with inflammation, neovascularization of the lung parenchyma occurs from many sources. Although proliferation of the bronchial circulation is the most common mechanism to extend the vascular supply, an extensive network of systemic arteries may neovascularize the lung after crossing the pleural space. This most commonly occurs in diseases that produce pleural scarring, such as in aspergillomas and cystic fibrosis. Anatomically these collaterals commonly arise from the intercostal, subclavian, axillary, and phrenic arteries. However, nonbronchial collaterals have also been described from the internal mammary, thyrocervical, carotid, and even the coronary arteries. Suspicion that these vessels may be involved in a patient is heightened by previous bronchial artery embolizations, the presence of pleural disease, and the absence of bronchial arteries supplying an area of lung parenchyma on initial bronchial arteriography.

Pulmonary Venous Abnormalities

Bleeding from the pulmonary veins is best characterized in cardiac disease such as mitral stenosis or mitral regurgitation. Focal varices of the pulmonary veins that are occasionally visualized on chest radiography, but are best characterized on the venous phase of pulmonary arteriography, have been described.[16,17]

COMMON CAUSES OF HEMOPTYSIS

Six common medical disorders account for 90% of the cases of massive hemoptysis. Infection or malignancy comprises 70%. However, almost any of the many causes of hemoptysis (Box 47-1) can become massive on rare occasions. Because the etiology of the hemoptysis is often unknown at the time of presentation, evaluation and

Box 47-1

Causes of Focal Pulmonary Hemorrhage

Iatrogenic
Bronchoscopy
Lung biopsy
Swan-Ganz catheterization
Transtracheal aspirate

Infectious
Lung abscess
Mycetoma
Necrotizing pneumonia (*Staphylococcus aureus,* gram-negative aerobes, *Legionella,* actinomycosis, *Stenotrophomonas, Kytococcus sedentarius,* leptospirosis)
Parasitic infection (paragonimiasis, amebiasis, ascariasis, clonorchiasis, echinococciasis, hookworm infestation, strongyloidiasis, trichinosis, schistosomiasis)
Parenchymal fungal infection (aspergillosis, mucormycosis, coccidioidomycosis, maduromycosis, botryomycosis)
Tuberculosis (active or inactive)
Viral tracheitis
Herpetic tracheobronchitis

Interstitial Lung Diseases
Lymphangioleiomyomatosis (LAM)
Sarcoidosis
Tuberous sclerosis
Pneumoconiosis
Langerhans cell granulomatosis

Miscellaneous
Amyloidosis
Bronchogenic cyst
Broncholithiasis
Bronchopleural fistula
Endometriosis
Foreign body
Tracheopathia osteoplastica
Lipoid pneumonia
Organophosphate aspiration
Chronic pancreatitis

Neoplastic
Bronchial adenoma
Lung cancer
Tracheal tumors (mucoepidermoid, squamous cell, adenoid cystic, glomus)
Pulmonary blastoma
Pleuropulmonary angiosarcoma
Sarcoma (synovial, myofibroblastic)
Clear cell tumor
Metastatic disease (prostate, renal, breast, ovarian)
Tracheobronchial schwannoma

Pulmonary Airway Diseases
Bronchiectasis
Bronchitis
Granulomatous tracheobronchitis (ulcerative colitis, Crohn's disease, Wegener's granulomatosis)
Cystic fibrosis
Bullous emphysema

Pulmonary Embolism
Systemic cholesterol embolism

Traumatic
Blunt chest trauma
Penetrating injury
Ruptured bronchus
Lightning injury
Thoracic splenosis

Vascular
Intralobar sequestration
Pulmonary artery aneurysms
Behçet's disease, Hughes-Stovin syndrome, traumatic pseudoaneurysms
Acquired arteriovenous malformation
Osler-Weber-Rendu syndrome (hereditary hemorrhagic telangiectasia)
Takayasu's arteritis
Aortic aneurysms
Tracheal-innominate artery fistulas
Scimitar syndrome
Cava-bronchial fistulas
Dieulafoy's disease of bronchus
Ventriculopulmonary fistula
Hemangioma (sclerosing, cavernous, tracheal)

stabilization are often carried out empirically. Hints at specific diagnoses are obtained by history, physical examination, chest radiography, and chest computed tomography.

Table 47-1 lists the underlying causes of hemoptysis in representative series from the past 3 decades. Major differences in the incidence of respective diseases are found between clinical centers that likely depend on patient demographics and disease frequency in the community. The other variable that influences disease frequency is the rate of bleeding. In a single series, chronic bronchitis accounted for 47% of cases when hemoptysis was less than 20 mL in 24 hours. When hemoptysis of greater than 200 mL in 24 hours was considered, chronic bronchitis dropped in frequency to 27% of cases.[1]

Chronic Bronchitis

Chronic bronchitis is rarely the cause of massive hemoptysis. Yet when all cases of hemoptysis are evaluated, chronic bronchitis emerges as a diagnosis made commonly with a history of chronic sputum production or the bronchoscopic finding of reddened airways during diagnostic studies. However, caution should be exercised in ascribing hemoptysis to bronchitis alone in that many of these

Table 47-1. Causes of Hemoptysis from Recent Series of More Than 50 Patients

Investigators	*N*	Demographics	Cancer* (%)	Bronchitis (%)	Other Infections (%)	Active TB (%)	Lung Abscess (%)	Bronchiectasis (%)	Cause Unknown (%)	Miscellaneous (%)
Conlan et al,[184] 1983	123	(South Africa)	5	0	12	38	5	30	1	9
Corey and Hla,[22] 1987	59	(Veterans Hospital)	34	25	7	5	0	3	7	19
Johnston et al,[1] 1989	148	All bronchoscopy (Kansas)	19	37	8	7	2	3	4	20
Santiago et al,[185] 1991	264	All bronchoscopy (Veterans Hospital)	29	23	10	6	2	<1	22	8
Knott-Craig et al,[186] 1993	120	(South Africa)	5	0	6	23	2	51†	8	5
McGuinness et al,[187] 1994	57	All bronchoscopy (Bellevue Hospital)	12	5	12	16	0	25	19	5
DiLeo et al,[142] 1995	424	Inpatients (Louisiana)	24	32	11	1	0	4	20	8
Coss-Bu et al,[188] 1997	246	Pediatric inpatients (Texas)	3	0	7	1	0	65‡	4	20
Hirshberg,[189] 1997	208	Inpatients and outpatients (Israel)	19	18	15	1	1	20	8	18
Abal et al,[190] 2001	52	Inpatients (Kuwait)	0	5.8	0	15.4	0	38.5	25	1.9
Fidan et al,[191] 2002	108	Inpatients (Turkey)	34.2	1.9	10.2	17.6	0	25	0	11.1
Revel et al,[145] 2002	80	ICU with massive/large hemoptysis (France)	11	0	10	19	0	31	10	19
Reechairpichitkul et al,[192] 2005	101	Inpatients (Thailand); massive hemoptysis	10.9	0	16.9	20.8	6.9	33.7	0	10.8

*Bronchogenic cancer, metastatic cancer, or leukemia.
†All post-tuberculous.
‡All except a single case from cystic fibrosis.

patients are cigarette smokers and are at risk for bronchogenic carcinoma.

The pathologic lesions responsible for bleeding are likely dilated bronchial arteries that can be eroded during active inflammation of the airways.[18] Because many of these patients have normal chest radiographs and a normal or nonfocal bronchoscopy, the extent of the evaluation in such patients remains controversial. In a study of 196 bronchoscopy patients with hemoptysis and a nonlocalizing or normal chest radiograph, the best predictors of bronchogenic carcinoma were age older than 50, male sex, and smoking more than 40 pack-years. When 2 of the 3 variables were combined with hemoptysis greater than 30 mL per day, 100% of bronchogenic carcinoma patients were identified.[19]

Lung Cancer

Lung cancer is associated with hemoptysis in 20% to 30% of cases and may be the presenting manifestation.[20,21] Although the clinical course of hemoptysis is often that of chronic blood-streaked sputum, the frequency with which massive hemoptysis occurs as a terminal event remains unappreciated.[22] Massive hemoptysis is most commonly associated with squamous cell type[23]; cavitation within the carcinoma[24]; and central endobronchial position, occasionally with invasion into the pulmonary arteries. The blood supply to most lung carcinomas is derived from diffuse neovascularization from the bronchial circulation, making bronchial artery embolization effective in some cases.

Other less common cancers can bleed when found in the lung. Kaposi's sarcoma has a high incidence of bloody pleural effusions and hemoptysis. Angiosarcomas are vascular tumors that may bleed continuously from small tumor sites.[25] Choriocarcinomas may bleed profusely, particularly after initiation of chemotherapy. Metastatic disease including renal, ovarian, and breast cancer have rarely been associated with hemoptysis.

Bronchiectasis

Bronchiectasis is characterized by abnormal dilation of the bronchi with altered mucociliary clearance, persistent bacterial colonization, chronic inflammation in the bronchial mucosa, and submucosal neovascularization that makes hemoptysis common. A variable prevalence of hemoptysis (25% to 91%) has been recorded in a series of bronchiectasis patients.[26,27]

Hemoptysis in bronchiectasis can present as a single life-threatening episode but is more commonly heralded by intermittent blood streaking intermixed with purulent sputum. In patients without a previous diagnosis, the evaluation can be difficult because chest radiography can be normal or the alveolarized blood can obscure abnormalities. Suspicion of the diagnosis warrants broad-spectrum antibiotics to cover the usually multiple organisms causing infection. Although bronchography has demonstrated abnormalities in 27% of one series of patients with hemoptysis,[28] it has been supplanted by high-resolution chest computed tomography (CT).

Massive hemoptysis occurs in 5% to 70% of patients with cystic fibrosis (CF) with significant morbidity and mortality.[29,30] Origin of the bleeding is most often upper lobe bronchial or systemic arteries. This subset of patients is difficult to treat because of minimal pulmonary reserve in the majority of patients at the time of their hemoptysis. Pulmonary resections are reserved for patients with mild disease and recurrent focal bleeding when all other measures have failed.[30] Prevalence is increased in older patients with reduced lung function (forced expiratory volume in 1 second [FEV_1] <40%) and strongly associated with *Staphylococcus aureus* and diabetes.[31] While *Pseudomonas aeruginosa* remains the predominant pathogen associated with decline in lung function, its presence has not translated into an increased incidence of hemoptysis. Treatment should be aimed at aggressive empiric antibiotic coverage to include *S. aureus* until cultures return. Inhaled tobramycin and dornase alpha use were associated with a lower hemoptysis incidence and should be considered in long-term management.[31] Endobronchial occlusion and bronchial artery embolization,[32,33] however, remain the mainstays of therapy for control of massive hemoptysis in cystic fibrosis. Serious consideration for lung transplantation should be given to patients with an FEV_1 less than 30% and massive hemoptysis because their 2-year mortality approaches 60%.[31]

Tuberculosis

The resurgence of tuberculosis with unabated growth in many parts of the world mandates consideration of the disease whenever hemoptysis occurs. Hemoptysis complicates the course of approximately 25% of tuberculosis cases[34,35] and is more commonly found with cavitary disease. The pathologic lesion that causes hemoptysis in tuberculosis is often Rasmussen's aneurysm, a small aneurysm of the pulmonary circulation positioned within a cavity wall. Bleeding from the bronchial circulation can also complicate bronchial erosions in active tuberculosis, and study of both circulations is occasionally necessary in cases in which resection for local disease is not possible.

Although all patients suspected of having hemoptysis secondary to tuberculosis should be placed in respiratory isolation, active pulmonary tuberculosis is found in only a third of such cases. However, hemoptysis can occur through a variety of mechanisms related to previous lung destruction. Posttuberculous bronchiectasis remains a common cause of hemoptysis[36] that requires antibacterial therapy. Hemoptysis has also been reported in miliary tuberculosis, although the mechanism is unknown.

Because tuberculosis is often focal with normal lung parenchyma in the remainder of the lung, serious consideration should be given to resection in cases of massive hemoptysis. Unfortunately, there is no reliable mechanism to predict which patients are at risk for recurrent massive hemoptysis during the long course of antituberculous therapy.

Lung Abscess

Anaerobic lung abscesses are commonly found in areas prone to aspiration. The indolent course of these infections allows time for hypertrophy of the bronchial circulation within the walls of the abscess cavity. Additionally, these cavities may enlarge and erode into major pulmonary arteries and other thoracic vessels, including the aorta.[37] With either of these abnormalities, bleeding can be massive and recurrent. Although the abscesses are focal and amenable to surgery, the patient who chronically aspirates because of alcoholism or dementia may have other contraindications for surgery.

Other Pulmonary Infections

Although hemoptysis can complicate any bacterial or fungal pneumonia, massive hemoptysis remains rare unless tissue necrosis is present. Tissue necrosis is a hallmark of anaerobic, staphylococcal, and actinomycotic[38] pneumonias but can occur with many different bacterial causes. Septic pulmonary emboli, particularly from staphylococcal species, have a high incidence of concomitant lung cavitation.[39] Mycotic pulmonary artery aneurysms may also be hidden within pneumonias that can be diagnosed and treated at pulmonary arteriography.[40]

Hemoptysis is particularly common in fungal pneumonias that invade the vasculature. Invasive *Aspergillus* can be found in nonimmunosuppressed patients with chronic obstructive pulmonary disease (COPD)[41] but is more commonly found in the persistently neutropenic patient. A characteristic radiographic pattern of cavitation and hemoptysis follows the return of neutrophils and should be anticipated in these patients.[42,43] The use of prophylactic surgery to resect areas of infarcted lung tissue has been advocated[44,45] because of the high mortality associated with medical management of the hemoptysis. Nevertheless, such surgery remains high risk, and controlled trials have not been performed.

Although rarer, invasive pulmonary mucormycosis[46] may produce similar findings. Hemoptysis complicates primary coccidioidal infections in 15% of cases and may approach a 50% incidence in patients with chronic coccidioidal cavities. Histoplasmosis, cryptococcosis, and blastomycosis can also present with hemoptysis.

Frequent hemoptysis is a hallmark of the parasitic diseases paragonimiasis,[47] echinococcosis,[48] strongyloidiasis, and ancylostomiasis.

Pulmonary Embolism

Hemoptysis occurs in approximately 30% of patients with thrombotic pulmonary emboli. Characteristically, hemoptysis is low grade and requires no specific therapy. Because diagnoses of pulmonary emboli are usually made without bronchoscopy, this diagnosis rarely appears in series of hemoptysis, which are usually bronchoscopic series. Hemoptysis usually implies some degree of pulmonary infarction with potential disruption of either vascular supply.

Paradoxically, this cause of bleeding must be treated with anticoagulants to prevent propagation of deep venous thrombi. No clinical series of pulmonary embolism hemoptysis patients has been assembled to determine the incidence of worsening hemoptysis after heparin or thrombolytics. However, in one series of patients who died from pulmonary emboli, hemoptysis was present in only 3% of patients.[49] From these data the risk of death from further emboli appears to be higher than the risk of intensified bleeding.

Pulmonary embolism is considered in the differential diagnosis of hemoptysis, and suspicion should be heightened in the presence of thrombosis risk factors, multicentric bleeding sites, or pleuritic chest pain.

Nonthrombotic emboli have also been associated with hemoptysis. Septic emboli usually respond to antibiotics alone. Ethiodol embolization after lymphangiography may present with hemoptysis up to 10 days after the procedure.[50]

LESS COMMON CAUSES OF HEMOPTYSIS

Aspergillus Fungus Balls

Hemoptysis occurs in more than half of patients with pulmonary *Aspergillus* fungus balls.[51] The cavity walls are richly vascularized by branches of the bronchial circulation, yet enlargement of these cavities may also extend into large branches of the pulmonary artery.[6] The mechanism of hemoptysis is likely multifactorial from secondary bacterial invasion of the *Aspergillus* cavity, microinvasion of the cavity wall by *Aspergillus* (semi-invasive aspergillosis), or less commonly by truly invasive disease. Therapy of hemoptysis depends on the underlying cause for the cavitary lung disease. *Aspergillus* fungus balls complicating tuberculosis or lung abscess cavities may be isolated and amenable to resection considering the recurrent nature of the bleeding. Fungus balls complicating sarcoidosis usually occur in patients with bilateral upper lobe cavitary disease (stage IV), in which underlying lung function prohibits resection.

Therapy of hemoptysis remains supportive in the first few hours. Alveolarized blood or an air-fluid level in the cavity often obscures an adequate evaluation of the surrounding lung parenchyma. Systemic antifungal therapy remains controversial because there is not a well-defined means to diagnose semi-invasive disease.[52,53] Intracavitary amphotericin B, however, instilled via a transthoracic catheter has proved successful at dissolution and sclerosis of the cavity with excellent control of hemoptysis and is a viable option in patients who are poor surgical candidates.[54,55] Alternatively, antifungal therapy with ketoconazole,[56] miconazole,[57] or amphotericin B[58] has been given endobronchially for fungus ball dissolution and hemoptysis control, but these techniques are effective in less than half of patients.[59] External beam radiotherapy of 3.5 Gy given once per week has been used as an adjunctive measure in nonoperable patients.[60]

Surgery remains the therapy of choice in patients with adequate pulmonary reserve. Simple aspergilloma (no abnormality in surrounding lung) has an excellent response to surgical resection, most commonly a lobectomy. Complex aspergilloma with surrounding pleural and parenchymal involvement usually requires pneumonectomy and is associated with variable success.[61]

Cardiovascular Causes

Mitral stenosis is one of the most common cardiac abnormalities that can present with hemoptysis.[62] The risk of hemoptysis is likely related to the elevation of pulmonary venous pressure and the rapidity with which the stenosis has developed. Diagnostically, the opening snap or diastolic murmur can be difficult to elicit in the emergency department in the presence of massive pulmonary hemorrhage and airway rhonchi; however, the chest radiograph may suggest that mitral stenosis is the culprit. Because the bleeding may be focal, this diagnosis should be specifically discounted before an emergent pulmonary resection is entertained.

Other causes of increased pulmonary venous pressure, such as mitral regurgitation or severe congestive cardiomyopathy, may also produce hemoptysis that usually presents with radiographic pulmonary edema and a prodrome of pink frothy sputum. Fibrosing mediastinitis,[63] pulmonary veno-occlusive disease,[64] and congenital pulmonary venous stenosis[65] are less common causes of pulmonary venous congestion.

Rarely, hemoptysis will occur from systemic venous hypertension in severe biventricular heart failure by azygous vein hypertension and dilation. Because the azygous vein drains the trachea and major bronchi, the submucosal dilated venous plexus of the trachea can be friable and produce major hemoptysis.

Catamenial Hemoptysis

Catamenial hemoptysis is suggested by a cyclical history of hemoptysis that occurs with the onset of menses. It is part of the spectrum of thoracic endometriosis syndrome (TES), which also includes catamenial pneumothorax, hemothorax, and pulmonary nodules.[66] Parenchymal endometriosis is characterized by endometrial tissue in the peripheral portions of the lung that changes in size throughout the menstrual cycle. These changes can be noted on serial CT scan,[67] which remains the most useful diagnostic tool because histopathologic confirmation has been documented in only one third of cases.[68] Pathogenesis is unknown but thought to be related to lymphatic or hematogenous embolization from the uterus or pelvis. Patients often have a prior history of obstetric or gynecologic procedures.

Treatment remains controversial and includes hormonal therapy or surgery to remove endometrial implants. Hormone therapy is expensive, carries significant adverse effects, and has a high recurrence rate with cessation of therapy. Surgery results in minimal morbidity with little risk of recurrence but requires exact preoperative localization with CT and bronchoscopy.[69]

Interstitial Lung Disease

Only a few of the interstitial lung diseases are prone to hemoptysis. Lymphangioleiomyomatosis (LAM) is a disease of smooth muscle proliferation around pulmonary lymphatics, airways, and vasculature. Any of the triad of hemoptysis, pneumothorax, or chylothorax should suggest the diagnosis in a female of childbearing age.[70] The airway granulomas of sarcoidosis have also been associated with hemoptysis, although the presence of traction bronchiectasis may be a more common cause. Additionally, the erosion of calcified hilar lymph nodes into the vasculature can produce hemoptysis. The other interstitial lung diseases that have associated hemoptysis usually have diffuse alveolar hemorrhage.

Broncholithiasis

Broncholithiasis is an infrequent but significant cause of hemoptysis. The typical patient has had an established diagnosis of mediastinal calcification from granulomatous disease. Previous histoplasmosis, sarcoidosis, or tuberculosis are most common. Broncholithiasis is diagnosed by bronchoscopy when any degree of lymph node calcification is visualized in the bronchial lumen. Symptoms of cough, chest pain, airway obstruction, and hemoptysis can be seen. Lithoptysis, coughing out a broncholith, can also confirm the diagnosis.

Therapy of hemoptysis involves broncholith removal. Broncholith removal by rigid or flexible bronchoscopy is usually successful when the broncholith is free. When broncholiths are partially embedded in the airway wall, removal is best facilitated by rigid bronchoscopy (successful in 48% of cases in one recent series)[71] or by thoracic surgery. Surgical options include lymph node resection with or without bronchoplasty or lobectomy. A recent surgical series had a 34% complication rate and a 15% rate of recurrent or persistent disease.[72]

DIFFUSE ALVEOLAR HEMORRHAGE

Diffuse alveolar hemorrhage (DAH) most commonly presents abruptly and may or may not be associated with frank hemoptysis. The early manifestations are often confused with other alveolar filling processes such as pulmonary edema, bacterial pneumonia, or the acute respiratory distress syndrome (ARDS). Consideration of DAH is prompted by the rapidly changing chest radiograph, the presence of renal dysfunction, other systemic manifestations of a vasculitis, the association of hemoptysis, and the common finding of anemia. Unfortunately, the many causes of DAH are often differentiated on the basis of laboratory tests that may not be routine in many hospitals. Furthermore, specific therapy is often not begun until a definitive diagnosis has been established by biopsy.

The differential diagnosis of DAH is listed in Box 47-2. Although some of these diseases have no specific therapy, establishing a diagnosis and instituting supportive care avoids unnecessary diagnostic and therapeutic maneuvers. However, many of the vasculitides are only stabilized with aggressive immunosuppressive therapy, which would not be appropriate for many infectious diseases that can also present with the same apparent features in a chest radiograph.

Bronchoscopy with transbronchial biopsy and bronchoalveolar lavage is usually performed in a patient with unknown pulmonary infiltrates in the intensive care unit (ICU). Although often not sufficient to establish a specific diagnosis, finding a bloody lavagate, hemosiderin-laden

Box 47-2

Causes of Diffuse Alveolar Hemorrhage

Immunologic
Antibasement-membrane antibody (ABMA) disease (Goodpasture's syndrome)
Vasculitides associated with circulating or in situ immune complexes
- Systemic lupus erythematosus
- Mixed connective tissue disease
- Henoch-Schönlein syndrome
- Essential mixed cryoglobulinemia
- Tumor-related vasculitis
- Endocarditis-related vasculitis
- Polyarteritis nodosa
- Systemic necrotizing vasculitis

Vasculitides associated with antineutrophil cytoplasmic antibodies (ANCA)
- Wegener's granulomatosis
- Microscopic polyangiitis
- Idiopathic necrotizing-crescentic glomerulonephritis

Rapidly progressive glomerulonephritis (RPGN)
Associated with other connective tissue diseases, patho physiology unknown
- Rheumatoid arthritis
- Progressive systemic sclerosis
- Behçet's disease

Associated with other renal diseases
- IgA nephropathy
- Diabetic nephropathy

Associated with precipitating antibodies to milk (Heiner's syndrome)
Idiopathic pulmonary hemosiderosis
Primary antiphospholipid antibody syndrome

Chemical or Drug Related
Amiodarone
D-penicillamine
Isocyanates
Nitrofurantoin
Retinoic acid
Trimellitic anhydride
"Crack" cocaine
Sirolimus
Propothiouracil-induced vasculitis
Erlotinib
Bevacizumab
Gemcitabine
Infliximab

Transplant Related
Bone marrow transplant
Renal transplant
Lung transplant

Bleeding Diathesis
Thrombocytopenia
Leukemia with diffuse alveolar damage
Viral pneumonia
Bacterial or fungal sepsis
Radiation
Chemotherapy toxic to lung
Blast counts >80,000 mm^3
Extrinsic anticoagulants/thrombolytics
Warfarin overdose
Tissue plasminogen activator
Platelet glycoprotein IIb/IIIa inhibitors
Coagulopathies
Cirrhosis
DIC

Infections
Legionnaires' disease

Pulmonary Venous Hypertension
Mitral stenosis
Mitral regurgitation
Pulmonary capillary hemangiomatosis
Pulmonary veno-occlusive disease
Fibrosing mediastinitis
Congenital heart disease

Diffuse Lung Injury
Negative pressure pulmonary hemorrhage
Breath-hold diving
Postictal neurogenic pulmonary edema

macrophages, and the lack of specific pathogens can presumptively yield a diagnosis of DAH. For a patient who is not severely ill, an enhanced alveolar uptake of carbon monoxide may suggest the diagnosis.[73]

The diagnosis of DAH is best made by quantitation of hemosiderin in alveolar macrophages obtained by BAL. A Prussian blue stain is graded by the cytopathologist by the methods of Kahn and colleagues[74]; hemosiderin scores above 100 are virtually diagnostic of alveolar hemorrhage. Hemosiderin-laden macrophages may not appear in BAL fluid until 48 to 72 hours after acute hemorrhage, resulting in a low sensitivity for hemosiderin scores in this setting.[75]

Immunologic Lung Disease

The differential diagnosis of DAH is narrowed significantly if renal abnormalities are present. Although these pulmonary-renal syndromes can often be stabilized with high-dose corticosteroids alone pending further evaluation, directed therapy depends on the measurement of specific auto-antibodies and evaluation of a renal biopsy.

Alveolar hemorrhage is a hallmark of anti-basement-membrane antibody disease (Goodpasture's disease). This disease is 75% male-predominant and follows a flulike prodrome in 30% of patients. Pulmonary hemorrhage is the initial manifestation in 90%, and an abnormal urinalysis is found in 80%. An iron-deficiency anemia from sequestration of iron within pulmonary alveolar macrophages is commonly associated with the disease. The IgG antibodies reacting to a component of type IV collagen are found in linear deposits on the basement membrane of both alveoli and glomeruli and are circulating in 90% of cases.[76] In the appropriate clinical setting, the presence of circulating anti-GBM antibodies is sufficient to make a diagnosis without tissue and institute plasmapheresis with or without plasma exchange for severe pulmonary or renal disease. After initial stabilization, corticosteroids and immunosuppressive medications will usually prevent further antibody production. Treatment with an anti-CD20 monoclonal antibody (rituximab) is also an option for patients intolerant of or refractory to standard therapy.[77]

Steroids alone are usually sufficient to treat alveolar hemorrhage associated with the immune complex vasculitides. These disorders are usually associated with hypocomplementemia and an elevated titer of antinuclear antibody. Systemic lupus erythematosus (SLE) is the most frequent of the immune complex disorders causing alveolar hemorrhage. SLE rarely presents with alveolar hemorrhage without other manifestations of active disease. Although the alveolar hemorrhage of SLE usually occurs from acute lupus pneumonitis, the high incidence of pneumonia, congestive heart failure, and aspiration in these patients makes a presumptive diagnosis problematic. Lupus pneumonitis usually stabilizes on 1 to 1.5 mg/kg/day methylprednisolone.

Diffuse alveolar hemorrhage also complicates other connective tissue diseases and systemic vasculitides with or without immune complex deposition. Mixed connective tissue disease, cryoglobulinemia, periarteritis nodosa, progressive systemic sclerosis, rheumatoid arthritis, Behçet's disease, endocarditis and tumor-related vasculitis, Henoch-Schönlein syndrome, and systemic necrotizing vasculitis have all been described in association with DAH. Specific diagnosis depends on the nonpulmonary features of disease presentation.

Alveolar hemorrhage is an unusual manifestation of Wegener's granulomatosis.[78] The classic triad of renal dysfunction, upper airway pathology, and pulmonary infiltrates is present in less than 20% of patients at presentation; however, pulmonary infiltrates are present in 45%.[79] The pulmonary findings are characterized by nodules that may cavitate, lobar infiltrates that are often fleeting, upper airway obstruction from the granulomatous inflammation that follows airway ulceration, prominent interstitial markings with or without hilar and mediastinal adenopathy, or alveolar hemorrhage. Antineutrophil antibodies against proteinase 3 in cytoplasmic granules (c-ANCA) are found in the serum of 85% to 90% of patients with active Wegener's granulomatosis and are 97% specific for the diagnosis.[80]

Among the many causes of rapidly progressive crescentic glomerulonephritis (RPGN) are small vessel vasculitides such as microscopic polyangiitis that are associated with pulmonary hemorrhage in a third of patients.[81,82] Therapy of these vasculitides and Wegener's granulomatosis usually includes corticosteroids and immunosuppressive therapy. In patients with life-threatening respiratory failure, extracorporeal membrane oxygenation (ECMO) has proved lifesaving in patients with ANCA positive vasculitides and SLE awaiting onset of systemic therapy.[83,84] Novel use of recombinant factor VIIa has also been reported with lifesaving effects in this setting, but optimal dosage and frequency of this drug remain unstudied.[85]

Idiopathic Pulmonary Hemosiderosis

Significant proportions of cases of DAH remain idiopathic. Idiopathic pulmonary hemosiderosis (IPH) is characterized by repetitive episodes of hemorrhage that occur without obvious precipitating factors. Open lung biopsy fails to demonstrate immune complexes, and no other organ system is affected. Therapy with corticosteroids and occasionally cyclophosphamide has been attempted, although no controlled trials have been done. In the pediatric patient, a syndrome of hemosiderosis in association with precipitating antibodies to cow milk antigens may be responsive to withdrawal of all milk products.[86] Whether similar antigenic mechanisms are operational in adult patients with IPH is unknown.

Immunocompromised Host

Diffuse alveolar hemorrhage complicates both autologous and allogenic bone marrow transplantation in up to 21% of cases.[87,88] Risk factors include age younger than 40 years, the presence of underlying solid tumors, renal insufficiency, and severe mucositis. The typical presentation is characterized by occurrence near the time of leukocyte recovery and is heralded by high fever and diffuse pulmonary infiltrates that prompt bronchoalveolar lavage. Typically the lavagate gets progressively bloody over serial aliquots, and no pathogenic organisms are recovered on bacterial, fungal, or viral culture. Mortality has been reported from 80% to 100% despite aggressive supportive care[87,89] but may be improved with corticosteroid therapy.[90] The optimal dosage and duration of corticosteroid treatment remains controversial, but standard regimens include 1 g/day methylprednisolone administered for 3 days and thereafter tapered over 2 months.[90] The addition of recombinant Factor VIIa to patients with life-threatening DAH refractory to steroids has been reported with positive outcomes. [91] More recent reports[88] reveal a favorable prognosis in patients with early (first 30 days) versus late DAH and autologous versus allogenic transplants with an overall mortality of 48%.

A similar syndrome characterized by fever and pulmonary infiltrates has been noted after renal transplantation and may occur in 5% of patients. Hemoptysis is rare with this presentation. Evaluation should attempt to exclude infectious causes of pulmonary deterioration, particularly invasive *Aspergillus*, as this remains the most common cause of alveolar hemorrhage in the immunocompromised host.

Pulmonary capillaritis following lung transplant also can result in DAH. Hemoptysis is seen in up to 25% of cases with fulminant respiratory failure in 18%.[92] This form of acute allograft rejection appears less responsive to corticosteroid therapy than acute lung rejection but has a more favorable response to plasmapheresis. No long-term adverse effects on allograft function are apparent.

Bleeding Diathesis

Although hemoptysis may occur with intrinsic coagulopathies,[93] extrinsic anticoagulants,[94] thrombocytopenia,[95] or fibrinolytics,[96] patients at risk should undergo bronchoscopy to exclude the possibility of bronchogenic carcinoma[97] in the proper clinical setting. Usually the disorders of hemostasis are not in themselves solely responsible for hemoptysis, and bleeding can usually be ascribed to the combined presence of another cause, often as insignificant as an upper respiratory infection.

Leukemia patients may be particularly susceptible to DAH when chemotherapy-induced thrombocytopenia is combined with diffuse alveolar damage from any of multiple causes. Viral infections, sepsis, radiation, chemotherapy with pulmonary toxicity, and leukostasis from blast counts exceeding 80,000 per mm^3 may all produce diffuse alveolar damage in leukemia.[98] Therapy is directed toward correction of thrombocytopenia and supportive care of lung injury.

Drug-Induced Alveolar Hemorrhage

A unique cause of drug-induced DAH is seen in patients who inhale freebase (crack) cocaine.[99] The clinical presentation includes fever, dyspnea, hypoxemia, and hemoptysis within 2 hours of inhaling crack. The histology reveals diffuse alveolar damage, alveolar hemorrhage, and interstitial and intra-alveolar inflammatory cell infiltration notable for the prominence of eosinophils. High-dose corticosteroids have been used with success, although in many patients the condition resolves spontaneously.

Other drug-induced DAH is rare, but causative drugs include amiodarone,[100] nitrofurantoin,[101] D-penicillamine,[102] retinoic acid,[103] propothiouracil,[104] infliximab,[105] inhaled resins containing trimellitic anhydride,[106] and various chemotherapeutic agents.[107-110]

VASCULAR ABNORMALITIES

Almost all blood vessels that course through the thoracic cavity have been associated with fistula formation to an airway with resultant hemoptysis. Often this occurs concomitant with endovascular infection, congenital or acquired stenoses, or aneurysms of these vessels or following chest surgery.

Some of the rare vascular-to-airway fistulas that have been described include (1) carotid artery to trachea in a patient with occult laryngeal cancer[111]; (2) various abdominal arterial supplies to pulmonary sequestrations[112]; (3) syphilitic aneurysms of the ascending aorta and other thoracic arteries to pulmonary parenchyma[113]; (4) coronary artery bypass grafts to pulmonary parenchyma[114]; (5) splenopulmonary shunt in portal hypertension following splenectomy[115]; (6) left ventricular pseudoaneurysms[116] to pulmonary parenchyma; and (7) vena caval-bronchial fistulas.[117] Two of the more common bronchovascular communications, aortobronchial fistulas and pulmonary artery aneurysms, deserve comment.

Aortobronchial Fistulas

Dissecting aortic aneurysms are often of subacute or chronic duration with variable degrees of inflammation around the dissection. As an aneurysm enlarges it may cause lung compression, pleural adhesions, and dissection of blood into the pulmonary parenchyma. Particularly in situations where an aortic graft has been previously placed, aortic graft infection may also be present. The net result is an often stuttering course of hemoptysis marked by sudden large bleeds. Therapy is surgical, although these operations are difficult in the presence of graft infections and failed prior operations.

Pulmonary Artery Aneurysms

Aneurysms of the pulmonary artery remain rare causes of hemoptysis.[118] Mycotic aneurysms are commonly caused by *Mycobacterium tuberculosis,* syphilis, *S. aureus,* and streptococcal species. Poststenotic dilation may occur in congenital pulmonary artery strictures. Structural vascular abnormalities such as Marfan syndrome can also affect the pulmonary arteries.

Behçet's disease, characterized by oral ulcers, uveitis, arthritis, and cutaneous vasculitis, is the only common systemic vasculitis that affects the pulmonary arteries.[119] These often multiple aneurysms can resolve with high-dose corticosteroid therapy or cyclophosphamide.[120,121]

An idiopathic syndrome, characterized by fatal hemoptysis from pulmonary artery aneurysms, associated with fever and recurrent superficial and deep venous thromboembolism, was originally reported in 1959 by Hughes and Stovin.[122] Cases of the Hughes-Stovin syndrome continue to be reported.[123] Although an infectious cause is suspected, the organism remains elusive.

Arteriovenous Malformations

Pulmonary arteriovenous malformations (PAVMs) present with progressive hypoxemia, paradoxical emboli, or bleeding complications including hemoptysis or hemothorax.[124] Although the majority of these lesions are likely congenital telangiectasias that have enlarged over years,[125] acquired arteriovenous malformations (AVMs) have been noted after chest surgery and trauma and have been associated with actinomycosis, schistosomiasis, cirrhosis, and metastatic carcinoma.[126] The hereditary Osler-Weber-Rendu disease (OWR) is associated with hemorrhagic telangiectasias in many organ systems. Approximately 15% of OWR patients have pulmonary arteriovenous aneurysms,[127] and up to 36% of patients with a single PAVM and 57% of patients with multiple PAVMs have OWR.[128] Bronchial artery telangiectasias with bleeding[129] have also been described, although the pathogenic relationship to pulmonary artery telangiectasias remains speculative. Treatment of PAVMs, particularly if hemoptysis has developed, is to embolically obliterate the lesion.[130] This should be done by an experienced operator because paradoxical emboli to the systemic arterial circulation are more than a theoretical concern.

Trauma

Hemoptysis following major trauma requires emergent thoracic surgical consultation and management. Although some cases will be simple lung contusions that manifest as a focal radiographic abnormality apparent on the first radiograph, with blood-streaked sputum present, approximately 15% of thoracic traumas need early exploration. The majority of cases with hemoptysis need bronchoscopy to localize bleeding and exclude a tracheobronchial rupture, which can be clinically silent for weeks. The most common reason for emergent thoracotomy remains pulmonary hemorrhage. Pneumonorrhaphy (suture repair of the lung) is preferred for minor injuries; lobectomy and pneumonectomy, performed for more severe injuries, carry mortality rates of 55% and 89%, respectively.[131]

Lung laceration is common after penetrating pulmonary injury. However, it can also occur after blunt thoracic trauma in which sheer forces of acceleration or deceleration leave intraparenchymal lacerations involving airways or vasculature. Continued bleeding into the lung can present with rupture into the pleural space (hemothorax), intraparenchymal hematoma formation, or hemoptysis. Monitoring the rate of hemoptysis often helps guide therapy.

Thoracic splenosis is a rare and remote event from the time of trauma. In this condition, splenic tissue is transported across the diaphragm after penetrating injury, where it becomes functional and vascularized within the lung. Hemoptysis may thereafter occur spontaneously.

Vascular Access and Monitoring Catheters

Inflation of Swan-Ganz catheters needs to occur in the proximal pulmonary circulation, with capillary wedge occlusion pressures obtained over 20 seconds or less. More distal and prolonged inflation can cause fatal pulmonary artery dissection, pseudoaneurysm formation,[132] or pulmonary artery rupture.[133,134] Endovascular damage may predispose to thrombus formation and pulmonary infarction. Preventive measures include noting the insertion distance during placement of the catheter such that full inflation is required to obtain an occlusion pressure, slowly inflating balloon and easing inflation when occlusion pressure is obtained (never inflating against resistance), full inflation of the balloon to prevent the Swan-Ganz tip from projecting beyond the balloon, and daily monitoring of catheter position with chest radiography.

Once hemoptysis has occurred with a PA catheter in place, this herald bleed, particularly if associated with a concomitant infiltrate in the appropriate position on the chest radiograph, should be a warning to proceed to angiography for diagnosis. Risk factors for a morbid course include concomitant anticoagulation, advanced age, and presence of pulmonary hypertension.[135] Surgical resection of the involved lobe or angiographic ablation of the involved pulmonary artery has been successful in aborting the 50% to 90% incidence of recurrent and often fatal hemoptysis.[136] These PA injuries probably remain underdiagnosed, imposing a selection bias on fatal courses. Nevertheless, in patients with adequate pulmonary vascular reserve, an arteriographic ablation that will likely recanalize in the future is reasonable therapy to prevent massive hemoptysis.

Other successful interventions for acute conditions have included proximal reinflation of the PA catheter to stop blood flow to the PA segment that is bleeding[137]; high levels (18 mm Hg) of positive end-expiratory pressure to decrease the pulmonary artery to bronchial pressure gradient[138]; resumption of cardiopulmonary bypass for patients in cardiac surgery[139]; and operative banding of the pulmonary artery, which can be unclamped 48 hours later.

Factitious Hemoptysis

Well-publicized cases of factitious hemoptysis have sensitized physicians to this unique form of Munchausen's syndrome.[140] However, red sputum from clofazimine use[141] may be less well known.

DIAGNOSTIC APPROACH

Localization

The most emergent diagnostic issue is localization of the site of bleeding. Regardless of the amount of hemoptysis, localization allows further diagnostic and therapeutic work to continue.

Because blood in the mouth can occur from the gastrointestinal tract or from diverse sites in the sinuses, nasal airway, or upper airway proximal to the larynx, an initial evaluation will necessitate bleeding localization. One recent series of hemoptysis patients found an upper airway source of bleeding in 10%.[142] The characteristics of the expectorated blood and presentation of the patient often help in differentiating hemoptysis from upper airway or gastrointestinal sources (Table 47-2). pH testing (low pH expected in gastric hemorrhage) and observation of expectorated sputum can be done quickly at the bedside.

All patients with hemoptysis need a baseline evaluation that consists of a physical examination and chest radiograph. In a series of 105 patients[2] the physical examination demonstrated unilateral findings in 47 patients, with correct identification of the bleeding lung in 45 patients. However, 58 patients (55%) had nonlocalizing examinations (normal examination or bilateral abnormalities). The high specificity of a focal examination suggests that

Table 47-2. Features of Hemoptysis and Patient Presentation

Hemoptysis	Clinical Presentation
Blood usually bright red	Often dyspneic
Portion of blood usually frothy	Hypoxemia
pH alkaline	Preceding cough common
Blood usually mixed with sputum	Anemia and melena uncommon
Alveolar macrophages may be present	

selective intubation might be guided in emergent situations by focal examination.

The chest radiograph is helpful in patients with hemoptysis. Apart from the ability to suggest specific diagnoses, the radiograph helps in localization of bleeding in approximately 60% of cases.[2] However, blood in the alveoli can obscure an underlying pulmonary pathologic condition; be most intense in areas distant from lung inflammation; and be present bilaterally, making localization of the bleeding site problematic.

Chest Computed Tomography

The role of chest CT continues to evolve in the diagnosis of acute hemoptysis. It is most commonly used for patients with occult hemoptysis to exclude small or peripheral lung carcinomas,[143] broncholithiasis,[144] aspergillomas, or bronchiectasis. Previous reports have noted that routine use of CT in addition to fiberoptic bronchoscopy had little clinical impact.[143] However, in a series of 80 patients with massive hemoptysis, emergency high-resolution computed tomography (HRCT) was not only equivalent to bronchoscopy in localizing bleeding (70% vs. 73%), but it was more efficient than bronchoscopy for identifying the cause of bleeding (77% vs. 8%). Findings on HRCT also directly affected treatment in more than 30% of the patients in this study.[145]

HRCT also allows the adequate prediction of nonbronchial systemic arterial supplies, which can be the cause of bleeding in massive hemoptysis and a significant cause of recurrent bleeding after successful bronchial artery embolization.[146] The addition of contrast can further increase the yield by identifying vascular abnormalities (i.e., thoracic aneurysm or AVMs) that would allow for more timely surgical referral. Additional modalities including CT angiography, multiplanar reconstruction, and endobronchial simulation (i.e., virtual bronchoscopy) have also recently been introduced and will likely increase the diagnostic yield of CT even further as these techniques become more mainstream. CT, except in unstable patients, should therefore be performed in patients prior to bronchoscopy to efficiently guide management.

Bronchoscopy

Although the diagnostic yield of bronchoscopy remains low in cases other than endobronchial carcinoma, it remains a vital tool in the management of acute massive hemoptysis in unstable patients. Localization of bleeding allows for immediate intervention including appropriate patient positioning, endobronchial tamponade, selective intubation, endobronchial infusions, laser photocoagulation, and guidance for referral to bronchial artery embolization or surgical resection. Recent studies, however, have suggested that patients with lateralizing radiography and known causation who are candidates for bronchial arterial embolization do not need prior bronchoscopy unless bronchoscopic airway management is necessary.[147,148] This strategy can avoid delays in definitive therapy, reduce cost, and avoid the risk of airway compromise from sedation associated with bronchoscopy.

During massive hemoptysis the rigid bronchoscope has some advantages over flexible fiberoptic instruments. Ventilation is secured through the bronchoscope lumen, suctioning is not impeded, and visualization is less likely to be permanently impaired. The flexible instrument has advantages of subsegmental localization and visualization of the upper lobes. Because the two bronchoscopes have complementary properties, they are often used together. The rigid bronchoscope is used to secure ventilation and localize the bleeding lung; the flexible scope passed through the rigid scope allows for further diagnostic work.

MANAGEMENT

The major management issues depend on the rate of bleeding. The classic study by Crocco and colleagues[5] demonstrated that in patients with 600 mL of hemoptysis in less than 4 hours the incidence of death was 71%, compared with 22% and 5% mortality if 600 mL of hemoptysis occurred in 4 to 16 hours and 16 to 48 hours, respectively. Optimal care of the bleeding patient depends on the precise quantitation of bleeding. Sputum containers placed hourly at the bedside allow precise measurement to continue through hospitalization.

Therapy to control minor and moderate hemoptysis can usually proceed along diagnostic channels. However, massive hemoptysis must be investigated within a framework of expeditious therapy to stabilize and resuscitate the patient. Figure 47-1 is a suggested algorithm for management. The frustrating inability to determine when and whether an individual patient's hemoptysis will accelerate[149] suggests that all patients with a blood loss of more than 200 mL should be hospitalized in an area in which airway support can be rapidly initiated if necessary.

Endotracheal Intubation

Endotracheal intubation is difficult in the patient with massive hemoptysis. Because airway suctioning, ventilation, and bronchoscopy depend on endotracheal tube diameter, the largest possible tube that will fit through the laryngeal orifice is appropriate. Because endotracheal tubes of larger size can be applied through the mouth, an orotracheal intubation is preferred.[150] A second reason to use the orotracheal route is to have the length available for selective mainstem intubations.

Because the patient's physical examination and chest radiograph will often define the bleeding lung, an effort to protect the airway to the normal lung is often attempted. With a single-lumen endotracheal tube already in place, the two mechanisms to localize ventilation to one lung include selective intubation of one of the mainstem bronchi and selective endobronchial tamponade.[151]

Selective bronchial intubation is easiest in a patient with a bleeding left lung. Because of the leftward displacement of the carina in the majority of humans, an endotracheal tube advanced downward will almost always intubate the right main bronchus. Unfortunately, the right upper lobe bronchus is so close to the carina that the usual right mainstem intubation also causes right upper lobe atelectasis. The ability to ventilate and oxygenate a patient with the right lower and right middle lobes alone depends on the underlying cardiopulmonary reserve.

Intubation of the left main bronchus is facilitated by placing the patient in a right lateral decubitus position to shift the mediastinum rightward. Angulation of the endotracheal tube curvature toward the left and progression of the tube over a coudé catheter may be helpful. Either of these selective intubations is easily facilitated by a bronchoscope.

Double-Lumen Endotracheal Tubes

An alternative airway management technique for trained individuals is placement of a double-lumen endotracheal tube.[152] The independent isolation of each mainstem bronchus allows for single-lung ventilation to be secured. The smaller suction ports of each independent lumen can cause difficulty in suctioning blood.[153] Endobronchial evaluation requires a pediatric bronchoscope or double-lumen tube removal once bleeding has been controlled. Although the double-lumen tube allows rapid airway stabilization in experienced hands, proximal airway carcinomas should be anticipated as likely reasons that a tube cannot be easily passed.

Other endotracheal tubes with movable, built-in blocking balloons have been successful in the patient with massive bleeding.[154] As with all of these specialized techniques, familiarity with endotracheal tubes before the emergency is always appropriate.

Endobronchial Tamponade

An emerging mechanism to control acute bleeding is the use of endobronchial tamponade with balloon-tipped catheters.[155] Briefly, a 100-cm Fogarty catheter or Arndt endobronchial blocker is directed to the bleeding bron-

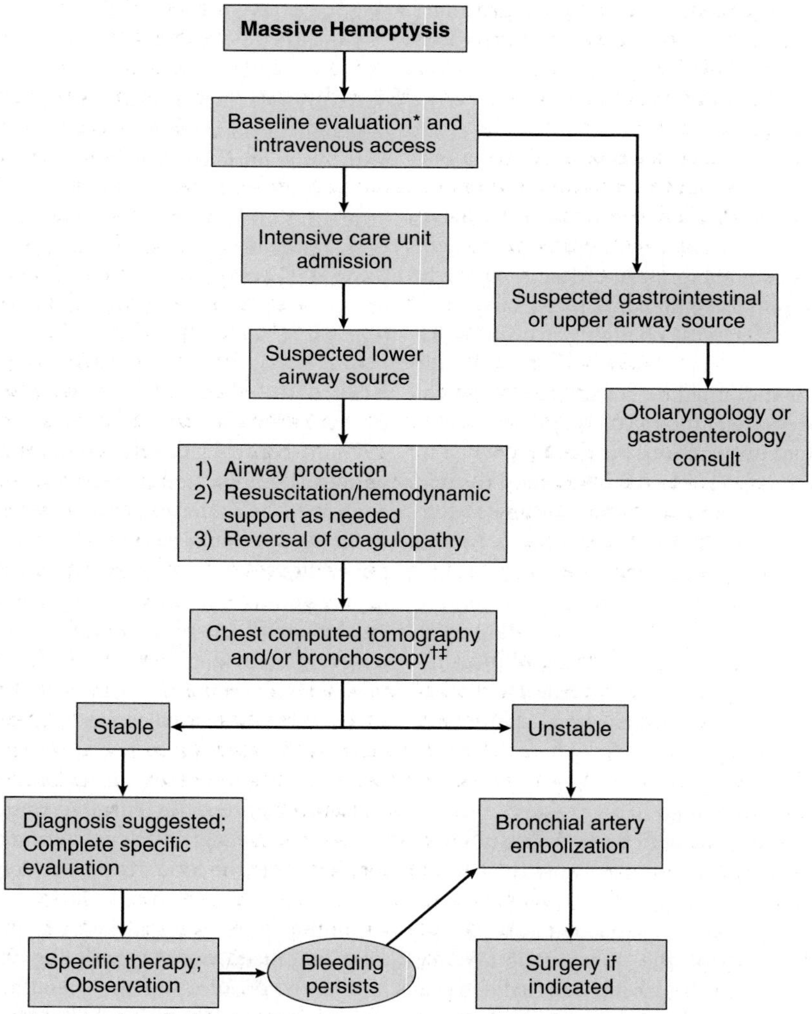

Figure 47-1. Massive hemoptysis.
*History and physical examination, complete blood count, coagulation panel, type and cross match, chest radiograph, arterial blood gas. †Local availability and patient stability should guide choice; computed tomography preferred initial evaluation in stable patient. ‡Local measures including iced saline, vasoconstrictors, balloon catheters, YAG-laser, electrocautery, and/or fibrin glue can be used endobronchially.

chus with the fiberoptic bronchoscope. By advancing the blocker to the smallest subsegment to which bleeding can be visualized, bleeding can be contained and diagnostic workup can continue. Swan-Ganz catheters can also be used for this purpose,[156] although they must be carried to the bleeding site on the outside of the bronchoscope by the *bronchoscopic shuttle technique*.[157] Multiple catheters can be placed if hemoptysis is multifocal and catheters can be left in place for 48 hours or more.[158]

Patient Positioning

A patient with massive bleeding should be positioned with the bleeding lung down to keep bleeding contained to one lung. Once an airway is secured, the optimal patient position becomes more controversial. Clotting of blood in a dependent lung has the potential to tamponade bleeding, yet clotted blood in the proximal airway has attendant problems, with lung collapse and atelectasis. Furthermore, if the pulmonary circulation is bleeding, it can be influenced by gravity by placing the bleeding segment higher than other areas of the chest. By converting that segment to a zone 1 condition in which alveolar pressure is higher than PA pressure, bleeding can be decreased.

Expectant Therapy

Cough suppression has been recommended for the majority of patients with massive hemoptysis. Most commonly, moderate doses of codeine are used; they can be reversed for patient oversedation by narcotic antagonists. Although no prospective study has evaluated the efficacy of cough suppression on patient outcome, the large swings in intrathoracic pressure that occur with coughing are likely to be detrimental.

The additional factor that must be considered in cough suppression is the necessary removal of blood clots that can cause endobronchial obstruction. Particularly when a central airway lesion is responsible for bleeding, the suctioning necessary to remove blood clots may be associated with rebleeding and perpetuation of a vicious cycle. Blood clots left unsuctioned, however, may cause atelectasis detrimental to patient weaning from the ventilator. Although endobronchial streptokinase (1000 IU/mL; total dose 30,000 to 80,000 IU) has been used for dissolution of central blood clots,[159] airway stabilization can usually be obtained with serial bronchoscopies and suctioning alone.

Laser Photocoagulation

The Nd-YAG or argon laser has been used successfully for airway carcinoma with persistent hemoptysis. Recognizing that carcinomatous bleeding is usually progressive and can be life threatening, aggressive photocoagulation of the endobronchial site may provide the only possibility for palliation after chemotherapy and radiation have been exhausted. Success has been reported in approximately 60% of cancer patients with hemoptysis.[160] Appropriate training, however, is imperative to ensure appropriate patient selection and avoid catastrophic complications such as tracheal fire or vessel perforation.[161]

Endobronchial Infusions

Although a variety of materials have been infused into the airway through the bronchoscope in an attempt to control bleeding, no studies have been published comparing the materials with each other or with other modalities of therapy. Nevertheless, the potential advantage of these agents is their administration during the same procedure as endobronchial balloon tamponade. Fibrinogen-thrombin mixtures have been used in Japan and Spain to provide a hemostatic clot in the area of bleeding with good success.[162,163] Although commercial fibrinogen is not available in the United States for patient use, cryoprecipitate-thrombin or thrombin alone remain other theoretically beneficial alternatives. Oxidized regenerated cellulose mesh, a biodegradable cellulose fabric, is an alternative procoagulant used in patients with massive hemoptysis with a 98% success rate in a series of 57 patients.[164] Once deployed in the area of hemorrhage, it absorbs blood, swelling into a gelatinous mass that promotes tamponade and coagulation. Endobronchial sealing with n-butyl cyanoacrylate, a biocompatible glue with prothombotic properties, has also been used with good success in small case series.[165]

Topical vasoconstrictors including iced saline lavage,[166] topical epinephrine,[167] and vasopressin or vasopressin derivatives[168,169] have also been used effectively for airway bleeding in anecdotal reports. The likely mechanism is vasoconstriction of bronchial arteries. Although a survey of chest physicians at the 1998 ACCP meeting revealed little faith in these methods,[170] reports indicate they are a safe, effective alternative in patients without access to bronchial artery embolization (BAE) or surgery, or unstable in need of a temporizing intervention until definitive therapy is available.

Bronchial Artery Embolization

Bronchial artery embolization (BAE) was first described in 1974 to control massive hemoptysis in the nonsurgical patient.[171] Subsequent studies on safety and efficacy have confirmed immediate, safe control of hemoptysis in 77% to 95% of patients, resulting in more frequent and earlier referral to BAE in the majority of centers. [170] It should not be viewed as definitive therapy because there is a high incidence of recurrent bleeding, which warrants inpatient observation in all patients undergoing BAE. The incidence of recurrence is not uniform in all lung diseases, however, with higher recurrence rates in aspergillomas[7] and lung cancers.[172] Nevertheless, the acute cessation of massive hemoptysis allows for a more controlled evaluation of the patient for potentially curative surgery.

The BAE begins with localization of the bronchial arteries supplying the lobe that is bleeding. A formal bronchial arteriogram is performed (1) to ensure that there is no communication to the anterior spinal artery, (2) to determine whether a vascular pathologic condition is present,[173] and (3) to ensure that the bleeding area of lung parenchyma is served by the vessel. Only rarely will a vascular blush indicative of bleeding be observed, usually in massively bleeding patients.[174] More commonly, hypervascularity or an enlarged and tortuous vessel will be found that can be embolized. Arteriographic technique usually

Table 47-3. Mortality According to the Rate of Bleeding

	Surgical Management		Nonsurgical Nonoperable Management			
	Number of Patients	Deaths	Number of Patients	Deaths	Number of Patients	Deaths
600 mL in <4 h	11	4 (36%)	6	6 (100%)	11	10 (91%)
600 mL/4-16 h	10	1 (10%)	3	1 (33%)	5	2 (40%)
600 mL/16-48 h	11	1 (9%)	0	0	10	0

begins with injection of a contrast medium in the descending aorta just below the left subclavian artery. Bronchial arteries supplying the majority of the lung and phrenic arteries supplying the lung bases can usually be identified. Identification of anomalous origins of the bronchial arteries may require a full arch aortogram in some patients.[175] For pathologic conditions of the lower lung, a selective phrenic artery injection is used if the entire lung is not visualized by bronchial injections. Rarely, these lower injections may demonstrate a pulmonary sequestration that has a 5% risk of causing fatal hemoptysis.[176] For pathologic conditions of the upper lung zone, a unilateral subclavian artery injection is done to exclude nonbronchial systemic collateral arteries.

No studies have evaluated the optimal embolization material for hemoptysis control. Gelatin sponge particles, polyvinyl alcohol fragments, or liquid polymers with a predetermined polymerization time have all been used with success. Velour, polyurethane particles of varying size, metal coils, protein macroaggregates, and fibrinogen-thrombin mixtures[177] have also been instilled. Liquid sclerosants, such as absolute alcohol or Gelfoam powder, should be used with caution because they may pass into the smallest vessels at the bronchial surface, producing bronchial necrosis.[178,179]

Significant complications remain rare when proper technique is employed. The most devastating complication is embolization of the anterior spinal artery, which arises from the bronchial artery circulation in approximately 5% of normal patients. However, with proliferation of the bronchial artery circulation, as occurs in cystic fibrosis, communication to the anterior spinal artery may be found in up to 55% of cases.[180] By performing high-quality bronchial arteriograms to define vascular anatomy and avoiding the anterior spinal artery by wedging the arteriography catheter distal to its takeoff (or by avoiding the vessel altogether), a safe procedure can almost always be ensured. The recent introduction of microcatheter technology (i.e., "superselective" catheterization) allows achievement of a more distal, safe catheter position and has greatly reduced the number of aborted procedures and complications arising from anterior spinal artery embolization.

Recurrent hemoptysis in the first few days after bronchial artery embolization occurs in approximately 10% of patients and may occur from several causes. For the patient who continues to bleed during the procedure, the appropriate blood vessel usually has not been embolized. In one series of persistently bleeding patients, 26 of 28 cases (93%) without an initial response to BAE were found to have a pulmonary arterial source for the bleeding.[179] Other common causes include bleeding from nonbronchial systemic vessels, particularly if not evaluated initially, and lysis of the hemostatic plug in the embolized bronchial artery.

Long-term control of hemoptysis is closely related to the underlying lung disease. Because bronchial artery neovascularization or recanalization is related to the degree of bronchial inflammation, diseases particularly likely to rebleed include bronchiectasis, *Aspergillus* fungus balls, and lung carcinoma, with rebleeding rates approaching 50%[7,181] at 2 years. Recent use of "superselective" embolization, which provides less of a stimulus for neovascularization, may improve these recurrence rates.[182]

Surgery

The major controversy in therapy of massive hemoptysis is whether the evolving conservative management techniques including endobronchial tamponade and bronchial artery embolization are better than emergent surgery in improving the high mortality rates associated with massive hemoptysis. Given the high success rates of BAE and low associated morbidity and mortality, attempts at more conservative techniques are now considered the first-line therapy over emergent surgery, which carries mortality rates as high as 15% to 30%.[5] Absolute indications for surgery do not exist, but patients with vascular pathology (e.g., leaking aortic aneurysm, AVMs, pulmonary artery rupture, chest trauma); focal fungal disease or bronchiectasis; or failed bronchial artery embolization should be considered for urgent surgery in the setting of massive hemoptysis.

The surgical experience of Crocco and colleagues[5] (Table 47-3) represents the largest series of massive hemoptysis patients in which the amount and timing of bleeding have been reported for both operable and nonoperable patients. The group with the highest mortality rate was that in which patients expectorated 600 mL of blood in 4 hours or less. All 6 potentially operable patients who did not go to surgery died, compared with 4 of 11 (36%) in the operated group who died. Although patients with 600 mL of expectorated blood in 4 to 16 hours still may have a sudden fatal bleeding episode, there is usually time to pursue the alternative interventions of endobronchial tamponade and bronchial artery embolization.

The issues that become important in assessment of a patient for thoracic surgery include the underlying cardiopulmonary reserve, precise localization of bleeding, and the focality of the patient's disease. Unfortunately, the safety of the large intrathoracic pressure swings involved with bedside spirometry in a massively bleeding patient has not been established. Because alveolarized blood can produce significant chest restriction on spirometry, a functional assessment is often obtained on the basis of premorbid exercise tolerance.

Patients with fibrosis and adhesions between the lung and chest wall, commonly seen in tuberculosis, fungal disease, and bronchiectasis, have significant surgical risks because they often require pneumonectomy. Physiologic lung exclusion, in which the bronchus and pulmonary artery of the involved lobe or lung are surgically interrupted, leaving the pulmonary veins intact, appears to be a viable alternative in such patients. In a series of 20 patients, Dhaliwal and colleagues[183] reported control of bleeding in all patients with no mortality and no significant morbidity.

The decision regarding surgery for massive hemoptysis is a difficult one that often must be made in the emergency department, without all the historical facts present. The availability of bronchial artery embolization and endobronchial tamponade may provide time for a reasoned decision to be made regarding surgery in all but the most rapidly bleeding patients.

KEY POINTS

- A few medical diseases account for 90% of the causes of massive hemoptysis. Massive hemoptysis is more common with lung cancer, bronchiectasis, tuberculosis, and lung abscess than with chronic bronchitis, pneumonia, and pulmonary emboli, which are usually submassive.
- DAH carries an extensive differential diagnosis that is narrowed considerably if renal abnormalities are present.
- Vascular abnormalities of either the bronchial or pulmonary circulation can cause massive hemoptysis. Specific diagnosis often requires angiography.
- Evaluation and stabilization of the massive hemoptysis patient are often carried out empirically because the cause of hemoptysis is often unknown at the time of presentation.
- A physical examination is helpful in localizing an acutely bleeding lung in some patients with massive hemoptysis. Definitive diagnosis and localization require a complementary approach with bronchoscopy and high-resolution computed tomography.
- Airway stabilization, if necessary, should be provided by an orotracheal tube of large caliber to allow for future bronchoscopic intervention.
- Endobronchial tamponade may be performed with a Fogarty catheter or selectively with an Arndt blocker through a fiberoptic bronchoscope to stabilize an asphyxiating patient.
- Bronchial artery embolization, if available, should be used as the initial therapeutic modality in most patients.
- Many issues determine which patients are optimally treated with surgery to stop hemoptysis. The most important factors include the rate of hemoptysis, underlying diagnosis, and extent of cardiopulmonary reserve.

REFERENCES

1. Johnston RN, Lockhart W, Ritchie RT, et al: Hemoptysis. Br Med J 1960;1:592.
2. Pursel SE, Lindeskog GE: Hemoptysis. Am Rev Respir Dis 1961;84:329.
3. Gourin A, Garzon AA: Operative treatment of massive hemoptysis. Ann Thorac Surg 1974;18:52.
4. Adams FV: Respiratory tract hemorrhage: Guide to emergency management. Hosp Med 1978;14:66.
5. Crocco JA, Rooney JJ, Fankushen DS, et al: Massive hemoptysis. Arch Intern Med 1968;121:495.
6. Remy J, Lemaitre L, Lafitte JJ, et al: Massive hemoptysis of pulmonary arterial origin: Diagnosis and treatment. AJR 1984;143:963.
7. Remy J, Remy-Jardin M, Voisin C: Endovascular management of bronchial bleeding. In Butler J (ed): The Bronchial Circulation. New York, Marcel Dekker, 1992.
8. Cauldwell WE, Siekert RG, Lininger RE, et al: The bronchial arteries. Surg Gynecol Obstet 1948;86:395.
9. Liebow AA: Patterns of origin and distribution of the major bronchial arteries in man. Am J Anat 1965;117:19.
10. Katoh O, Yamada H, Hiura K, et al: Bronchoscopic and angiographic comparison of bronchial arterial lesions in patients with hemoptysis. Chest 1987;91:486.
11. Charan NB, Albert RK, Lakshminarayan S, et al: Factors affecting bronchial blood flow through bronchopulmonary anastomoses in dogs. Am Rev Respir Dis 1986;134:85.
12. Liebow AA, Hales MR, Lindskog GF: Enlargement of the bronchial arteries and their anastomoses with the pulmonary arteries in bronchiectasis. Am J Path 1949;25:211.
13. Ullah MI, Fegan O: Potential hazard of nebulised salbutamol in patients with haemoptysis. Br Med J (Clin Res Ed) 1983;286:844.
14. McFadden ER: Respiratory heat and water exchange; physiological and clinical implications, J Appl Physiol 1983;54:331.
15. Agostoni P, Arena V, Doria E, et al: Inspired gas relative humidity affects systemic to pulmonary bronchial blood flow in humans. Chest 1990;97:1377.
16. Ferretti GR, Arbib F, Bertrand B, et al: Haemoptysis associated with pulmonary varices: Demonstration using computed tomographic angiography. Eur Respir J 1998;12:989.
17. Umaya T, Monden Y, Harada K, et al: Pulmonary varices: A case report and review of the literature. Jpn J Surg 1988;18:359.
18. Spark RP, Sobonya RE, Armbruster RJ, et al: Pathologic bronchial vasculature in a case of massive hemoptysis due to chronic bronchitis. Chest 1991;99:504.
19. Poe RH, Israel RH, Marin MG, et al: Utility of fiberoptic bronchoscopy in patients with hemoptysis and a nonlocalizing chest roentgenogram. Chest 1988;93:70-75.
20. Moersch HJ: Clinical significance of hemoptysis. JAMA 1952;148:1461.
21. Hamilton W, Peters TJ, Round A, et al: What are the clinical features of lung

cancer before the diagnosis is made? A population based case-control study. Thorax 2005;60:1059-1065.
22. Corey R, Hla KM: Major and massive hemoptysis: reassessment of conservative management. Am J Med Sci 1987;294:301.
23. Miller RR, McGregor DH: Hemorrhage from carcinoma of the lung, Cancer 1980;46:200.
24. Panos RJ, Barr LF, Walsh TJ, Silberman HJ: Factors associated with fatal hemoptysis in cancer patients. Chest 1988;94:1008.
25. Palvio DH, Paulsen SM: Primary angiosarcoma of the lung presenting as intractable hemoptysis. Thorac Cardiovasc Surg 1987;35:105.
26. Field EC: Bronchiectasis. A long term follow-up of medical and surgical cases from childhood. Arch Dis Child 1969;44:551.
27. Baum GL, Racz I, Bubis JJ, et al: Cystic disease of the lung: Report of eighty-eight cases with an ethnologic relationship. Am J Med 1966;40:578.
28. Jones DK, Cavanagh P, Shneerson JM, et al: Does bronchography have a role in the assessment of patients with haemoptysis? Thorax 1985;40:668.
29. Porter DK, Van Every MJ, Anthracite RF, et al: Massive hemoptysis in cystic fibrosis. Arch Intern Med 1983;143:287.
30. Porter DK, Van Every MJ, Mack JW Jr: Emergency lobectomy for massive hemoptysis in cystic fibrosis. J Thorac Cardiovasc Surg 1983;86:409.
31. Flume PA, Yankaskas JR, Ebeling M, et al: Massive hemoptysis in cystic fibrosis. Chest 2005;128:729-738.
32. Sweezey NB, Fellows KE: Bronchial artery embolization for severe hemoptysis in cystic fibrosis. Chest 1990;97:1322.
33. Brinson GM, Noone PG, Mauro MA, et al: Bronchial artery embolization for the treatment of hemoptysis in patients with cystic fibrosis. Am J Respir Crit Care Med 1998;157:1951.
34. Levitt N: Clinical significance of hemoptysis. J Mich Med Soc 1951;50:606.
35. Minor GR: Haemorrhage in pulmonary tuberculosis. Am Rev Tuberc 1943;48: 109.
36. Stinghe RV, Mangiulea VG: Hemoptysis of bronchial origin occurring in patients with arrested tuberculosis. Am Rev Respir Dis 1970;101:84.
37. Rogol PR: Fatal hemoptysis due to lung abscess and pulmoaortic fistula. Chest 1988;94:441.
38. Hamer DH, Schwab LE, Gray R: Massive hemoptysis from thoracic actinomycosis successfully treated by embolization. Chest 1992;101:1442.
39. Silverman NA, Levitsky S, Spigos DG, et al: Massive hemoptysis and recurrent tricuspid infective endocarditis in a heroin addict. Chest 1982;82:195.
40. Renie WA, Rodeheffer RJ, Mitchell S, et al: Balloon embolization of a mycotic pulmonary artery aneurysm. Am Rev Respir Dis 1982;126:1107.
41. Pittokopitis K, Herriott DT, Shirey JK: Massive fatal hemoptysis secondary to invasive aspergillosis in a patient with COPD. Chest 1983;83:583.
42. Albeda SM, Talbot GH, Gerson SC, et al: Pulmonary cavitation and massive hemoptysis in invasive pulmonary aspergillosis. Am Rev Respir Dis 1985;131:115.
43. Kibbler CC, Milkins SR, Bhamra A, et al: Apparent pulmonary mycetoma following invasive aspergillosis in neutropenic patients. Thorax 1988;43:108.
44. Wong K, Waters CM, Walesby RK: Surgical management of invasive pulmonary aspergillosis in immunocompromised patients. Eur J Cardiothorac Surg 1992;6:18.
45. Pedhorecky I, Urschel J, Anderson T: Resection of invasive pulmonary aspergillosis in immunocompromised patients. Ann Surg Oncol 2000;7:312.
46. Watts WJ: Bronchopleural fistula followed by massive fatal hemoptysis in a patient with pulmonary mucormycosis. A case report. Arch Intern Med 1983;143:1029.
47. Razaque MA, Mutum SS, Singh TS: Recurrent haemoptysis? Think of paragonimiasis. Trop Doct 1991;21:153.
48. Sandberg T, Dernevik L, Gatzinsky P, et al: Pulmonary hydatidosis—an unusual cause of recurrent hemoptysis. Lakartidningen 1991;88:2989.
49. Morgenthaler TI, Ryu JH: Clinical characteristics of fatal pulmonary embolism in a referral hospital. Mayo Clinic Proc 1995;70:417.
50. Marglin SI, Castellino: Severe pulmonary hemorrhage following lymphography. Cancer 1979;43:482.
51. Rafferty P, Biggs BA, Crompton GK, et al: What happens to patients with pulmonary aspergilloma? Analysis of 23 cases. Thorax 1983;38:579.
52. Shale J, Faux JA, Lane DJ: Trial of ketoconazole in non-invasive aspergillosis. Thorax 1987;42:26.
53. Jennings TS, Hardin TC: Treatment of aspergillosis with itraconazole. Ann Pharmacother 1993;27:1206-1211.
54. Cochrane LJ, Morano JU, Norman JR, et al: Use of intracavitary amphotericin B in a patient with aspergilloma and recurrent hemoptysis. Am J Med 1991;90:654.
55. Rumbak M, Kohler G, Eastrige C, et al: Topical treatment of life threatening haemoptysis from aspergillomas. Thorax 1996;51:253-255.
56. Guleria R, Gupta D, Jindal SK: Treatment of pulmonary aspergilloma by endoscopic intracavitary instillation of ketoconazole. Chest 1993;103: 1301.
57. Hamamoto T, Watanabe K, Ikemoto H: Endobronchial miconazole for pulmonary aspergilloma. Ann Intern Med 1983;98:1030.
58. Hargis JL, Bone RC, Stewart J, et al: Intracavitary amphotericin B in the symptomatic pulmonary aspergilloma. Am J Med 1980;68:389.
59. Yamada H, Kohno S, Koga H, et al: Topical treatment of pulmonary aspergilloma by antifungals. Chest 1993;103:1421.
60. Falkson C, Sur R, Pacella J: External beam radiotherapy: a treatment option for massive haemoptysis caused by mycetoma. Clin Oncol (R Coll Radiol) 2002;14:233-235.
61. Shiraishi Y, Katsuragi N, Nakajima Y, et al: Pneumonectomy for complex aspergilloma: Is it still dangerous? Eur J Cardiothorac Surg 2006;29:9-13.
62. Scarlat A, Bodner G, Liron M: Massive haemoptysis as the presenting symptom in mitral stenosis. Thorax 1986;41:413.
63. Hicks, GL Jr: Fibrosing mediastinitis causing pulmonary artery and vein obstruction with hemoptysis. NY State J Med 1983;83:242.
64. Cohn RC, Wong R, Spohn WA, et al: Death due to diffuse alveolar hemorrhage in a child with pulmonary veno-occlusive disease. Chest 1991;100:1456.
65. Reid JM, Jamieson MP, Cowan MD: Unilateral pulmonary vein stenosis. Br Heart J 1986;55:599.
66. Joseph J, Sahn SA: Thoracic endometriosis syndrome: New observations from an analysis of 110 cases. Am J Med 1996;100:164-170.
67. Hertzanu Y, Hernier D, Hirsch M: Computed tomography of pulmonary endometriosis, Comput Radiol 1987;11:81.
68. Wood DJ, Krishnan K, Stocks P, et al: Catamenial haemoptysis: A rare cause. Thorax 1993;48:1048-1049.
69. Alifano M, Trisolini R, Cancellieri A, et al: Thoracic endometriosis: Current knowledge. Ann Thorac Surg 2006;81:761-769.
70. Taylor JR, Ryu J, Colby TV, et al: Lymphangioleiomyomatosis: Clinical course in 32 patients. N Engl J Med 1990;323:1254.
71. Olson EJ, Utz JP, Prakash UB: Therapeutic bronchoscopy in broncholithiasis. Am J Respir Crit Care Med 1999;160:766.
72. Potaris K, Miller DL, Trastek VF, et al: Role of surgical resection in broncholithiasis. Ann Thorac Surg 2000;70:248.
73. Ewan PW, Jones HA, Rhodes CG, et al: Detection of intrapulmonary hemorrhage with carbon monoxide uptake. N Engl J Med 1976;295:1391.
74. Kahn FW, Jones JM, England DM: Diagnosis of pulmonary hemorrhage in the immunocompromised host. Am Rev Respir Dis 1987;136:155.
75. Sherman JM, Winnie G, Thomassen MJ, et al: Time course of hemosiderin production and clearance by human pulmonary macrophages. Chest 1984;86:409-411.
76. Wilson CB, Dixon FJ: Anti-glomerular basement membrane antibody-induced glomerulonephritis. Kidney Int 1973;3:74.
77. Arzoo K, Sadeghi S, Liebman HA: Treatment of refractory antibody mediated autoimmune disorders with an anti-CD20 monoclonal antibody (rituximab). Ann Rheum Dis 2002;61:922-924.
78. Myers JL, Katzenstein AL: Wegener's granulomatosis presenting with massive pulmonary hemorrhage and capillaritis. Am J Surg Pathol 1987;11:895.
79. Hoffman GS, Kerr GS, Leavitt RY, et al: Wegener granulomatosis: An analysis of 158 patients. Ann Intern Med 1992;116:488.
80. Kallenberg CGM, Mulder AHL, Tervaert JWC: Antineutrophil

cytoplasmic antibodies: A still-growing class of autoantibodies in inflammatory disorders. Am J Med 1992;93:675.
81. Cohen Tervaert JW, Goldschmeding R, Elema JD, et al: Autoantibodies against myeloid lysosomal enzymes in crescentic glomerulonephritis. Kidney Int 1990;37:799.
82. Savage COS, Winearls CG, Evans DJ, et al: Microscopic polyarteritis: Presentation, pathology and prognosis. Q J Med 1985;56:467.
83. Ahmed SH, Aziz T, Cochran J, et al: Use of extracorporeal membrane oxygenation in a patient with diffuse alveolar hemorrhage. Chest 2004;126;305-309.
84. Tandon M, Reynolds HN, Borg U, et al: Life-threatening acute systemic lupus erythematosus: survival after multiple extracorporeal modalities: A place for the multipotential extracorporeal service. ASAIO J 2000;46:146-149.
85. Henke D, Falk RJ, Gabriel DA: Successful treatment of diffuse alveolar hemorrhage with activated factor VII. Ann Intern Med 2004;140:493-494.
86. Boat TF, Polmar SH, Whitman V, et al: Hyperreactivity to cow milk in young children with pulmonary hemosiderosis and cor pulmonale secondary to nasopharyngeal obstruction. J Pediatr 1975;87:23.
87. Robbins RA, Linder J, Stahl MG, et al: Diffuse alveolar hemorrhage in autologous bone marrow transplant recipients. Am J Med 1989;87:511.
88. Afessa B, Tefferi A, Litzow MR, et al: Outcome of diffuse alveolar hemorrhage in hematopoietic stem cell transplant recipients. Am J Respir Crit Care Med 2002;166:1364-1368.
89. Jules-Elysee K, Gulati S, Stover DE, et al: Pulmonary complications in autologous bone marrow transplantation. Am Rev Respir Dis 1990;141:A604.
90. Chao NJ, Duncan SR, Long GD, et al: Corticosteroid therapy for diffuse alveolar hemorrhage in autologous bone marrow transplant recipients. Ann Intern Med 1991;114:145.
91. Pastores SM, Papadopoulos E, Voigt L, et al: Diffuse alveolar hemorrhage after allogeneic hematopoietic stem-cell transplantation: Treatment with recombinant factor VIIa. Chest 2003;124:2400-2403.
92. Astor TL, Weill D, Cool C, et al: Pulmonary capillaritis in lung transplant recipients: Treatment and effect on allograft function. J Heart Lung Transplant 2005;24:2091-2097.
93. Kagalwalla AF, Rahman A, Taleb A, et al: Pulmonary hemorrhage in association with auto-immune chronic active hepatitis. Chest 1993;103:634.
94. Finley TN, Aronow A, Cosentino AM, et al: Occult pulmonary hemorrhage in anticoagulated patients. Am Rev Respir Dis 1975;112:23.
95. Fireman Z, Yust I, Abramov AL: Lethal occult pulmonary hemorrhage in drug-induced thrombocytopenia. Chest 1981;78:358.
96. Basher AW, Oduwole A, Bhalodkar NC, et al: Fatal hemoptysis during coronary thrombolysis. J Thromb Thrombolysis 1996;3:87.
97. Small M, Lowe GD, Davidson K, et al: Bronchial carcinoma in von Willebrand's disease: Successful removal after hemostasis with lyophilized cryoprecipitate. Arch Intern Med 1983;143:1604.
98. Smith LJ, Katzenstein AA: Pathogenesis of massive pulmonary hemorrhage in acute leukemia. Arch Intern Med 1982;142:2149.
99. Forrester JW, Steel AW, Waldron JA, et al: Crack lung: An acute pulmonary syndrome with a spectrum of clinical and histopathologic findings. Am Rev Respir Dis 1990;142:462.
100. Ravishankar R, Samuels LE, Kaufman MS, et al: Amiodarone-associated hemoptysis. Am J Med Sci 1998;316:390.
101. Bucknall CE, Adamson MR, Banham SW: Non fatal pulmonary haemorrhage associated with nitrofurantoin. Thorax 1987;42:475.
102. Sternlieb I, Bennet B, Scheinberg IW: D-penicillamine-induced Goodpasture's syndrome in Wilson's disease. Ann Intern Med 1975;83:673.
103. Nicolls MR, Terada LS, Tuder RM, et al: Diffuse alveolar hemmorrhage with underlying pulmonary capillaritis in the retinoic acid syndrome. Am J Respir Crit Care Med 1998;158:1302.
104. Nakamori Y, Tominaga T, Inoue Y, et al: Propylthiouracil (PTU)-induced vasculitis associated with antineutrophil antibody against myeloperoxidase (MPO-ANCA). Intern Med 2003;42:529-533.
105. Panagi S, Palka W, Korelitz BI, et al: Diffuse alveolar hemorrhage after infliximab treatment of Crohn's disease. Inflamm Bowel Dis 2004;10:274-277.
106. Herbert FA, Orford R: Pulmonary hemorrhage and edema due to inhalation of resins containing trimellitic anhydride. Chest 1979;76:546.
107. Carron PL, Cousin L, Caps T, et al: Gemcitabine-associated diffuse alveolar hemorrhage. Intensive Care Med 2001;27:1554.
108. de Gramont A, Van Cutsem E: Investigating the potential of bevacizumab in other indications: Metastatic renal cell, non-small cell lung, pancreatic and breast cancer. Oncology 2005;69(Suppl 3):46-56.
109. Tammaro KA, Baldwin PD, Lundberg AS: Interstitial lung disease following erlotinib (Tarceva) in a patient who previously tolerated gefitinib (Iressa). J Oncol Pharm Pract 2005;11:127-130.
110. Vlahakis NE, Rickman OB, Morgenthaler T: Sirolimus-associated diffuse alveolar hemorrhage. Mayo Clin Proc 2004;79:541-545.
111. Dellinger RP, Savage PJ, Carruth C, et al: Tracheocarotid fistula secondary to laryngeal carcinoma presenting as massive hemoptysis. Chest 1983;84:222.
112. Hayakawa K, Soga T, Hamamoto K, et al: Massive hemoptysis from a pulmonary sequestration controlled by embolization of aberrant pulmonary arteries: Case report. Cardiovasc Intervent Radiol 1991;14:345.
113. Boundy K, Bignold LP: Syphilitic aneurysm of the right subclavian artery presenting with hemoptysis. Aust NZ J Med 1987;17:533.
114. Nielsen JF, Stentoft J, Aunsholt NA: Haemoptysis caused by aneurysm of saphenous bypass graft to a coronary artery. Scand J Thor Cardiovasc Surg 1988;22:189.
115. Escoffier JM, Le Treut YP, Antoni M, et al: Severe hemoptysis due to portal hypertension. Responsibility of acquired splenopulmonary shunt and treatment by proximal splenorenal anastomosis. Gastroenterol Clin Biol 1991;15:974.
116. Adkins MS, Laub GW, Pollock SB, et al: Left ventricular pseudoaneurysm with hemoptysis. Ann Thorac Surg 1991;51:476.
117. Winkler TR, Hanlin RJ, Hinke TD, et al: Unusual cause of hemoptysis: Hickman-induced cava-bronchial fistula. Chest 1992;102:1285.
118. Bartter T, Irwin RS, Nash G: Aneurysms of the pulmonary arteries. Chest 1988;94:1065.
119. Cadman EC, Lundberg WB, Mitchell MS: Pulmonary manifestations in Behçet's syndrome. Arch Intern Med 1976;136:944.
120. Stricker H, Malinverni R: Multiple, large aneurysms of pulmonary arteries in Behçet's disease. Arch Intern Med 1989;149:925.
121. Aktogu S, Erer OF, Urpek G, et al: Multiple pulmonary arterial aneurysms in Behçet's disease: Clinical and radiologic remission after cyclophosphamide and corticosteroid therapy. Respiration 2002;69:178-181.
122. Hughes JP, Stovin PGI: Segmental pulmonary artery aneurysms with peripheral venous thrombosis. Br J Dis Chest 1959;53:19.
123. Riantawan P, Yodtasurodom C, Chotivatanapong T, et al: Hughes-Stovin syndrome: A case report and review of the literature. J Med Assoc Thai 1999;82:312-16.
124. Swanson KL, Prakash UB, Stanson AW: Pulmonary arteriovenous fistulas: Mayo Clinic experience 1982-1997. Mayo Clin Proc 1999;74:671.
125. Teragaki M, Akioka K, Mitsutaka Y, et al: Case report: Hereditary hemorrhagic telangiectasia with growing pulmonary arteriovenous fistulas followed for 24 years. Am J Med Sci 1988;195:545.
126. Prager RL, Laws KH, Bender HW Jr: Arteriovenous fistula of the lung. Ann Thorac Surg 1983;26:231.
127. Hodgson CH, Burchell HB, Good CA, et al: Hereditary hemorrhagic telangiectasia and pulmonary arteriovenous fistula: Study of a large family. N Engl J Med 1959;26:625.
128. Bosher LH Jr, Blake Da, Byrd BR: An analysis of the pathologic anatomy of pulmonary arteriovenous aneurysms with particular reference to the applicability of local excision. Surgery 1959;45:91.
129. Lincoln MJ, Shigeoka JW: Pulmonary telangiectasia without hypoxemia. Chest 1988;93:1097.
130. Terry PB, Barth KH, Kaufman SL, et al: Balloon embolization for treatment of pulmonary arteriovenous fistulas. N Engl J Med 1980;302:1189.
131. Thompson DA, Rowlands BJ, Walker WD, et al: Urgent thoracotomy for

pulmonary or tracheobronchial injury. J Trauma 1988;28:276.
132. Kron IL, Piepgrass W, Carabello B: False aneurysm of the pulmonary artery: A complication of pulmonary artery catheterization. Ann Thorac Surg 1982;33:629.
133. Culpepper JA, Setter M, Rinaldo JE: Massive hemoptysis and tension pneumothorax following pulmonary artery catheterization. Chest 1982;82:380.
134. Brandstetter RD, Alarakhia N, Coli L, et al: Distal kinking of a pulmonary artery catheter as a cause of fatal hemoptysis. N Y State J Med 1984;84:521.
135. Pape LA, Haffajee CI, Markis JE, et al: Fatal pulmonary hemorrhage after use of the flow-directed balloon-tipped catheter. Ann Intern Med 1979;90:344.
136. Dieden JD, Louis FA: Renner JW: Pulmonary artery false aneurysms secondary to Swan-Ganz pulmonary artery catheters. AJR 1987;149:901.
137. Thomas R, Siproudhis L, Laurent JF, et al: Massive hemoptysis from iatrogenic balloon catheter rupture of pulmonary artery: Successful early management by balloon tamponade. Crit Care Med 1987;5:272.
138. Scuderi PE, Prough DS, Price JD, et al: Cessation of pulmonary artery catheter-induced endobronchial hemorrhage associated with the use of PEEP. Anesth Analg 1983;62:236.
139. Rice PL, Pifarre R, El-Etr A, et al: Management of endobronchial hemorrhage during cardiopulmonary bypass. J Thorac Cardiovasc Surg 1981;81:800.
140. Duffy TP: The red baron. N Engl J Med 1992;327:408.
141. Girdhar A, Venkatesan K, Chauhan SL, et al: Red discoloration of the sputum by clofazimine simulating haemoptysis—a case report. Lepr Rev 1992;61:47.
142. DiLeo MD, Amedee RG, Butcher RB: Hemoptysis and pseudohemoptysis: The patient expectorating blood. Ear Nose Throat J 1995;74:822.
143. Haponik EF, Britt J, Smith PL, et al: Computed chest tomography in the evaluation of hemoptysis. Chest 1987;91:80.
144. Shin MS, Ho KJ: Broncholithiasis: Its detection by computed tomography in patients with recurrent hemoptysis of unknown etiology. J Comput Tomogr 1983;7:189.
145. Revel MP, Fournier LS, Hennebicque AS, et al: Can CT replace bronchoscopy in the detection of the site and cause of bleeding in patients with large or massive hemoptysis? AJR 2002;179:1217-1224.
146. Yoon W, Kim YH, Kim JK, et al: Massive hemoptysis: Prediction of nonbronchial systemic arterial supply with chest CT. Radiology 2003;227:232-238.
147. Hsiao EI, Kirsch CM, Kagawa FT, et al: Utility of fiberoptic bronchoscopy before bronchial artery embolization for massive hemoptysis. AJR 2001;177:861-867.
148. Ramakantan R, Bandekar VG, Gandhi MS, et al: Massive hemoptysis due to pulmonary tuberculosis: Control with bronchial artery embolization. Radiology 1996;200:691-694.
149. Bobrowitz ID, Ramakrishna S, Young-Soo S: Comparison of medical vs surgical treatment of major hemoptysis. Arch Intern Med 1983;143:1343.
150. Katakov WN, Ault MJ: Endotracheal intubation in massive hemoptysis: Advantages of the orotracheal route (letter). Crit Care Med 1989;17:968.
151. Gourin A, Garzon AA: Control of hemorrhage in emergency pulmonary resection for massive hemoptysis. Chest 1975;68:120.
152. Strange C: Double lumen endotracheal tubes. Clin Chest Med 1991;12:497.
153. Garzon AA, Cerruti MM, Golding ME: Exsanguinating hemoptysis. J Thorac Cardiovasc Surg 1982;84:829.
154. Inoue H, Shohtsu A, Ogawa J, et al: Endotracheal tube with movable blocker to prevent aspiration of intratracheal bleeding. Ann Thorac Surg 1984;37:497.
155. Saw EC, Gottlieb LS, Yokoyama T, et al: Flexible fiberoptic bronchoscopy and endobronchial tamponade in the management of massive hemoptysis. Chest 1976;70:589.
156. Jolliet P, Soccal P, Chevrolet J: Control of massive hemoptysis by endobronchial tamponade with a pulmonary artery balloon catheter. Crit Care Med 1992;20:1730.
157. Haruno MM, Williams JH: The flexible fiberoptic bronchoscopic shuttle. Chest 1992;102:944.
158. Feloney JP, Balchum OJ: Repeated massive hemoptysis. Chest 1978;74:683.
159. Maxwell SL, Stauffer JL: Endobronchial streptokinase for relief of tracheobronchial obstruction by blood clots. Chest 1992;101:1738.
160. Hetzel MR, Nixon C, Edmondstone WM, et al: Laser therapy in 100 tracheobronchial tumours. Thorax 1985;40:341.
161. Turner JF Jr, Wang KP: Endobronchial laser therapy. Clin Chest Med 1999;20:107-122.
162. Tsukamoto T, Sasaki H, Nakamura H: Treatment of hemoptysis patients by thrombin and fibrinogen-thrombin infusion therapy using a fiberoptic bronchoscope. Chest 1989;96:473.
163. De Gracia J, de la Rosa D, Catalan E, et al: Use of endoscopic fibrinogen-thrombin in the treatment of severe hemoptysis. Respir Med 2003;97:790-795.
164. Valipour A, Kreuzer A, Koller H, et al: Bronchoscopy-guided topical hemostatic tamponade therapy for the management of life-threatening hemoptysis. Chest 2005;127: 2113-2118.
165. Bhattacharyya P, Dutta A Samanta AN, et al: New procedure: Bronchoscopic endobronchial sealing: A new mode of managing hemoptysis. Chest 2002;121:2066-2069.
166. Conlan AA, Hurwitz SS: Management of massive haemoptysis with the rigid bronchoscope and cold saline lavage. Thorax 1980;35:901.
167. Dupree H, Lewejohann J, Gleiss J, et al: Fiberoptic bronchoscopy of intubated patients with life threatening hemoptysis. World J Surg 2001;25:104-107.
168. Tuller C, Tuller D Tamm M, et al: Hemodynamic effects of endobronchial application of orinpressin versus terlipressin. Respiration 2004;71:397-401.
169. Breuer H, Charchut S, Worth C: Endobronchial versus intravenous application of vasopressin derivative Glypressin during diagnostic bronchoscopy. Eur Respir J 1989;2:225-228.
170. Haponik EF, Fein A, Chin Robert: Managing life threatening hemoptysis: Has anything really changed? Chest 2000;118:1431-1435.
171. Remy J, Viosin C, Dupois C, et al: Traitement des hemoptysies par embolisation de circulation systemique. Ann Radiol 1974;17:5.
172. Hayakawa K, Tanaka F, Torizuka T, et al: Bronchial artery embolization for hemoptysis: Immediate and long-term results. Cardiovasc Intervent Radiol 1992;15:154.
173. Servois V, Denys A, Silbert A: Mycotic aneurysm of the bronchial artery: A rare cause of hemoptysis. AJR 1992;159:428.
174. Rabkin JE, Astafjev VI, Gothman LN, et al: Transcatheter embolization in the management of pulmonary hemorrhage. Radiology 1987;163:361.
175. McPherson S, Routh WD, Nath H, et al: Anomalous origin of bronchial arteries: Potential pitfall of embolotherapy for hemoptysis. J Vasc Interv Radiol 1990;1:86.
176. Imgrund SP, Goldberg SK, Walkenstein MD, et al: Clinical diagnosis of massive hemoptysis using the fiberoptic bronchoscope. Crit Care Med 1985;13:438.
177. Bense L: Intrabronchial selective coagulative treatment of hemoptysis. Chest 1990;97:990.
178. Naar CA, Soong J, Clore F, et al: Control of massive hemoptysis by bronchial artery embolization with absolute alcohol. AJR 1983;140:271.
179. Ivanick MJ, Thorwarth W, Donohue, et al: Infarction of the left main-stem bronchus: A complication of bronchial artery embolization. AJR 1983;141:535.
180. Cohen AM, Doershuk CF, Stern RC: Bronchial artery embolization to control hemoptysis in cystic fibrosis. Radiology 1990;175:401.
181. Katoh O, Kishikawa T, Yamada H, et al: Recurrent bleeding after arterial embolization in patients with hemoptysis. Chest 1990;97:541.
182. Tanaka N, Yamakado K, Murashima S, et al: Superselective bronchial artery embolization for hemoptysis with a coaxial microcatheter system. J Vasc Interv Radiol 1997;8:65.
183. Dhaliwal RS, Saxena P, Puri D, et al: Role of physiological lung exclusion in difficult lung resections for massive hemoptysis and other problems. Eur J Cardiothorac Surg 2001;20:25-29.
184. Conlan AA, Hurwitx SS, Krige L, et al: Massive hemoptysis. J Thorac Cardiovasc Surg 1983;85:120.
185. Santiago S, Tobias J, Williams AJ: A reappraisal of the causes of

hemoptysis. Arch Intern Med 1991; 151:2449-2451.
186. Knott-Craig CJ, Oostuizen G, Rossouw G, et al: Management and prognosis of massive hemoptysis: Recent experience with 120 patients. J Thorac Cardiovasc Surg 1993;105:394.
187. McGuinness G, Beacher JR, Harkin T, et al: Hemoptysis:prospective high-resolution CT/bronchoscopic correlation. Chest 1994;105:1155.
188. Coss-Bu JA, Sachdeva RC, Bricker JT: Hemoptysis: A 10-year retrospective study. Pediatrics 1997;100:37.
189. Hirshberg B, Biran I, Glazer M, et al: Hemoptysis: Etiology, evaluation, and outcome in a tertiary referral hospital. Chest 1997;112:440.
190. Abal AT, Nair PC, Cherian J: Haemoptysis: Aetiology, evaluation and outcome—a prospective study in a third world country. Respir Med 2001;95:548-552.
192. Fidan A, Ozdogan S, Oruc O, et al: Hemoptysis: A retrospective analysis of 108 cases. Respir Med 2002;96: 677-680.
192. Reechaipichitkul W, Latong S: Etiology and treatment outcomes of massive hemoptysis. Southeast Asian J Trop Med Public Health 2005;36: 474-480.

Chapter

48 Pneumothorax and Barotrauma

Ankur A. Karnik and Ashok M. Karnik

HISTORY

Pneumothorax (PTX), the accumulation of air in the pleural space, results from a break in the visceral or parietal pleura. Hippocrates was perhaps the first physician to suspect the presence of air in the pleural space in one of his patients, but it was in 1803 that the term *pneumothorax* was used for the first time.[1] Although Laennec[2] gave the first clinical description of pneumothorax in 1819, it was not until 1901 that this entity was demonstrated on a chest radiograph published in the *Lancet*.[3] In the eighteenth and nineteenth centuries, pneumothoraces were believed to be the result of tuberculosis. This belief was laid to rest when Kjaergaard,[4] in 1932, described the occurrence of this condition in otherwise healthy young adults. Definitive therapy for the condition became available with the advent of tube thoracostomy, employed by Hewett in 1876.[5]

INCIDENCE

Weissberg and Refaely[6] reported on 1199 patients with pneumothorax. Of 865 male and 334 female patients, 60.3% of the pneumothoraces were spontaneous, 33.6% were traumatic, and 6.1% were iatrogenic. Chen and colleagues,[7] in their university-based teaching hospital ICU, found that of 60 patients who developed pneumothorax while in the ICU, 58% were related to procedures, most commonly thoracentesis.

The reported recurrence rates of pneumothorax vary widely, depending on the type of pneumothorax and the duration of follow-up. A compilation of 11 studies showed that the recurrence rate in "primary" spontaneous pneumothorax (PSP) ranged from 16% to 52% with a mean recurrence rate of 30% in those without definitive preventive treatment.[8] Table 48-1 categorizes episodes of pneumothorax seen at Nassau University Medical Center, a 530-bed hospital and trauma center in the suburbs of New York City.

PATHOPHYSIOLOGY

Etiology

Conventionally, PSP has been defined as a pneumothorax that occurs spontaneously in a patient who has no underlying lung disease. However, a condition is unlikely to remain "primary" or "idiopathic" as we gain understanding about this disease process. Diagnoses labeled as "primary" then shift into the category of "secondary."

Emphysema-Like Changes

Understanding the development of PTX in a patient who has known blebs and bullae is easy. However, computed tomography (CT) can detect abnormalities predisposing to PSP in patients with normal chest radiograph. CT has demonstrated emphysema-like changes (ELCs) in patients with PSP. Bense and others[9] reported on 27 nonsmoking cases of spontaneous pneumothorax (SP) who were not deficient in alpha-1 antitrypsin. In 22 cases (81%), CT showed ELCs. These changes were found mainly in the upper and peripheral regions. No ELCs were detected in the control group. Other investigators[10,11] have also reported similar findings on CT in their cases of PSP.

Pleural Porosity

Although the previously mentioned studies support the role of ELCs in the pathogenesis of PSP, ELCs are not the sole cause of PSP.[12,13] Air leak is not seen at the site of ruptured ELC in each patient during surgical intervention for PSP. Moreover, an air leak can be present in areas where no ELCs are seen. This has led to the concept of "pleural porosity."[14,15] Noppen and colleagues[14] have

Table 48-1. Episodes of Pneumothorax (PTX) Seen at Nassau University Medical Center

Type of PTX	2001	2002	2003	2004	2005	2006
Spontaneous PTX	20	14	21	15	30	23
Iatrogenic PTX	21	24	27	8	26	20
Traumatic PTX without open wound	44	42	65	68	61	76
Traumatic PTX with open wound	11	10	7	5	6	8
Total	96	90	120	96	123	127

described a patient with recurrent PSP in whom inhalation of aerosolized fluorescein followed by autofluorescence thoracoscopy allowed in vivo localization of various areas of extensive subpleural fluorescein accumulation, which were not visible with normal white thoracoscopy. This has led to the concept of "porous" pleura.[15]

Smoking

In a study on 138 Swedish patients, Bense and colleagues[16] found that smoking increased the risk of developing PSP 9-fold in women and 22-fold in men. Although cessation of smoking appears to reduce the risk of recurrence,[17] continued smoking increases the risk of recurrence.[18] Cottin and colleagues[19] found that in 79 smokers who underwent surgery for recurrence or persistence of PSP, 70 (88.6%) had evidence of respiratory bronchiolitis. Smit and colleagues[20] performed spirometrically controlled high-resolution CT density measurements in 41 patients with SP and found that the mean lung density was lower in patients with pneumothorax. They hypothesized that peripheral airway inflammation leads to airway obstruction with a check valve phenomenon, causing air trapping and development of pneumothorax. No correlation was found between air trapping and smoking habit or ELCs.

Genetics

Although rare, familial inheritance of pneumothorax has been reported.[21,22] The analyses suggest two possible models of inheritance: an autosomal dominant gene with incomplete penetrance and an X-linked recessive gene. The occurrence of recurrent SP in a Finnish brother and his sisters also raises the possibility of autosomal recessive inheritance.[23] As in SP, patients with Marfan syndrome are tall, and pneumothorax is a common pulmonary complication. Marfan syndrome is caused by the mutation in the *FBN1* gene on chromosome 15. This gene is responsible for the formation of 10- to 12-nm microfibrils in the extracellular matrix of connective tissue. Cardy and colleagues[24] hypothesized that familial SP is caused by a connective tissue disorder that exhibits mendelian inheritance and postulated *FBN1* as the causative gene. Another interesting syndrome in which patients develop SP has been described. Brit-Hogg-Dube (BHD) is an autosomal dominant cancer syndrome characterized by benign skin and renal tumors, pleuropulmonary blebs and cysts, and SP. The gene has been mapped to chromosome 17p11.2 and recently identified, expressing a novel protein called folliculin.[25,26]

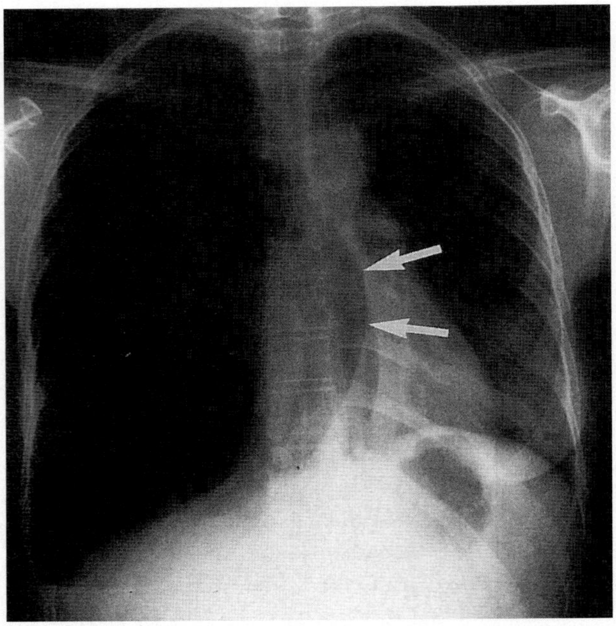

Figure 48-1. Radiograph of a patient with tension pneumothorax showing shift of the mediastinum to the opposite side.

Effect of Pneumothorax on Cardiopulmonary Physiology

As a result of a breach in the visceral or parietal pleura, air enters the pleural space. When the amount of air is large and the increase in intrapleural pressure great, the mediastinum shifts to the opposite side and the diaphragm is depressed (Fig. 48-1). A decrease in vital capacity, functional residual capacity, total lung capacity, and oxygen transfer occurs.[27] In a large pneumothorax, the arterial oxygen pressure (PaO_2) falls and the alveolar-arterial oxygen pressure difference [$P(A\text{-}a)O_2$] increases. The factors that lead to hypoxemia during a large pneumothorax are anatomic shunt,[28] hypoventilation,[29] and relative overperfusion of partially collapsed, underventilated lungs.[30] Anthonisen[31] reported that in patients with pneumothorax, airway closure occurs at low lung volumes and suggested that this was the main cause of ventilation maldistribution in such patients.

Animal studies suggest that the progressive hypoxemia with increasing pneumothorax is primarily the result of increasing degrees of pulmonary vascular shunting associated with increasing parenchymal collapse.[32]

CLASSIFICATION

The classification given in Box 48-1 combines the circumstances of occurrence of pneumothorax, the etiologic factors, and the state of the underlying lung. When pneumothorax occurs without trauma and is not iatrogenically induced, it is called *SP*. SP occurring in an otherwise healthy person is called *PSP*, as mentioned earlier. Secondary SP (SSP) occurs in patients with a variety of underlying lung diseases. Other interesting categories of SP are catamenial pneumothorax, pneumothorax in drug addicts and acquired immunodeficiency syndrome (AIDS) patients, and familial SP.

Box 48-1

Classification of Pneumothorax and Barotrauma

A. Spontaneous pneumothorax
  a. Primary spontaneous pneumothorax (PSP)
    1. In healthy young adults
    2. Familial spontaneous pneumothorax
  b. Secondary spontaneous pneumothorax (SSP)
    1. Secondary to underlying lung disease
    2. In drug abusers
    3. In AIDS patients
    4. Catamenial pneumothorax
B. Nonspontaneous pneumothorax
  a. Traumatic pneumothorax
  b. Iatrogenic pneumothorax
    1. Barotrauma and pneumothorax associated with mechanical ventilation
    2. Accidental
      During diagnostic procedures: Transbronchial lung biopsy and aspiration, subclavian vein catheterization, thoracentesis, electrophysiologic testing
      During therapeutic procedures: CPR, surgical tracheostomy, percutaneous tracheostomy, pulmonary function testing, acupuncture, incorrect position of nasogastric tube, secondary to radiation and chemotherapy, laparoscopic cholecystectomy, hyperbaric oxygen
C. Special situations
  a. Pneumothorax ex vacuo
  b. Sports-related pneumothorax
  c. Barotrauma unrelated to mechanical ventilation
  d. Postoperative air spaces
  e. Barotrauma in airplane passengers, pilots, divers, and other causes of barotrauma
  f. Spontaneous pneumothorax following contralateral pneumonectomy
  g. Spontaneous pneumothorax in pregnancy
  h. SARS, CPR

AIDS, acquired immunodeficiency syndrome; CPR, cardiopulmonary resuscitation; SARS, severe acute respiratory syndrome.

Spontaneous Pneumothorax

Primary Spontaneous Pneumothorax

Investigators have found subpleural blebs or bullae at apices on chest radiographs and at thoracotomy in patients with SP.[33] The pathogenesis of these blebs and the factors that lead to their rupture remain controversial.

PSP is classically seen in previously healthy young men with an asthenic body habitus. Melton and colleagues[34] found that the incidence of PSP rose with increasing height among adults of both sexes, more so in males. It reached a figure of more than 200 per 100,000 person-years for those 76 inches or taller. It has been suggested that the greater prevalence of SP in tall, thin males is the result of a combination of circumstances. In an extremely long and narrow chest, the apical alveoli are underperfused; such alveoli are more readily torn by gravitational stress. Inherited weakness of connective tissue might also contribute to the pathogenesis, as suggested by the numerous reports of SP in families and concurrent occurrence of SP in twins.[35] Morrison and colleagues[36] have reported a family exhibiting spontaneous pneumothorax in a father and three offspring and suggested that isolated autosomal dominant pneumothorax may be a distinct entity.

Most patients with SP are heavy smokers. In one series,[37] 72% of all patients were smokers. An increase in cigarette consumption during a particular year was followed within 1 to 2 years by an increased incidence of SP; the reverse occurred with decreased cigarette consumption.[38] Smoking increases the relative risk of developing SP about 9-fold in women and 22-fold among men, and there is a statistically significant dose-response relationship between smoking and SP.[39]

Secondary Spontaneous Pneumothorax

Pneumothorax Secondary to Underlying Lung Disease

In adults, SP has been reported to occur as a result of a large variety of diseases including asthma, staphylococcal septicemia, pulmonary infarction, sarcoidosis, idiopathic pulmonary hemorrhage, pulmonary alveolar proteinosis, familial fibrocystic pulmonary dysplasia, tuberous sclerosis, cryptogenic fibrosing alveolitis, eosinophilic granuloma, coccidioidomycosis, echinococcal disease, chronic obstructive pulmonary disease (COPD), Shaver's disease (bauxite pneumoconiosis), lymphangioleiomyomatosis, von Recklinghausen's disease, gastropleural and colopleural fistulas through the diaphragm into the left pleural cavity, radiation therapy to the thorax, Wegener's granulomatosis, cystic fibrosis, acute bacterial pneumonia, and as a complication of the chemotherapy used in the treatment of malignancy and pulmonary metastases from a variety of malignancies.[40]

The most common cause of secondary SP, however, is COPD. SP in COPD patients is a serious complication with excessive morbidity and mortality.[8,41] The clinical presentation of pneumothorax in COPD patients is often atypical—pain may be absent, anxiety and breathlessness may predominate and be out of proportion to the collapsed lung, and the classic sign of hyperresonance may not be helpful because of the underlying emphysema. The air leak in these patients is usually large, and the tissues slow to heal, so it is weeks before the tubes can be taken out.[42]

Pneumothorax in Drug Abusers

When the peripheral veins of chronic abusers of drugs become obliterated because of a sclerotic or infectious process, the individual may attempt to use larger veins in the groin or neck. Attempted subclavicular or supraclavicular injection ("pocket shoot") of drugs in the street setting has led to unilateral or bilateral pneumothoraces.[43-47] Douglas and Levison[47] found that the incidence of pneumothoraces is equal in both sexes and that it is less of a problem in teenagers (because they are unwilling to invade the clearly dangerous territory of neck veins or because they have not yet exhausted the peripheral veins) and in addicts older than 40 years of age (probably because either conservation alters their behavior or they do not survive to their fifth decade). It was also noted that although most drug users describe using small (21- or 22-gauge) needles, a large, complete, or tension pneumothorax usually develops. Quite often the pneumothorax is bilateral.[43,45]

Pneumothorax in Acquired Immune Deficiency Syndrome Patients

Since the first report of spontaneous pneumothorax in patients with AIDS in 1984 by Wollschlager and colleagues,[48] numerous other authors[49-60] have reported on the occurrence of pneumothorax in these patients.

SP is an uncommon event (0.06%) in the general population and occurs rarely in association with infectious pneumonia.[61] Spontaneous pneumothorax in patients with AIDS has become the leading cause of nontraumatic pneumothorax in this population.[62] With the diagnosis of AIDS, a patient's risk of sustaining a nontraumatic pneumothorax increases to 450 times that of general population.[63] A high incidence (2% to 9%) has been reported in patients with AIDS and *Pneumocystis carinii* pneumonia (PCP).[58,59,64] *Pneumocystis carinii,* which was thought to be a protozoan, has been renamed as *Pneumocystis jerovici* and is now classified as an Archiascomycetous fungus.[65] Mechanical ventilation and bronchoscopy are quite often required in AIDS patients, and these two factors further increase the chance of pneumothorax occurring in these patients.[53,66] In patients with AIDS, the pneumothorax is frequently bilateral, recurrent, and not responsive to conservative therapy.[67,68] Most often it is related to the infection with *P. jerovici,* but other infections like *Mycobacterium tuberculosis, M. avium intracellulare,* pulmonary cytomegalovirus, *Pneumococcus* organisms,[53] or pulmonary toxoplasmosis[69] may be associated. In a study of 144 patients of AIDS with PCP, the overall mortality was reported to be 21.5%; pneumothorax was found to be one of the seven factors that predicted 90-day mortality.[70]

The exact pathogenesis of the pneumothorax in these patients is not clear. In AIDS patients who have or have had active PCP, large confluent areas of thin-walled blebs, distributed randomly on the surface of each lobe, have been reported.[53] It has been postulated that the cystic changes may result from a check-valve mechanism caused by airway inflammation and resultant partial airway obstruction or may be the result of disordered parenchymal architecture secondary to chronic infection and inflammation.[54,55]

Various investigators[51,55,58] have pointed out that the incidence of spontaneous pneumothorax is especially high in those patients who receive aerosolized pentamidine for PCP prophylaxis. This has been attributed to poor distribution of the aerosolized pentamidine at the periphery of the lung, which allows the development of a peripheral necrotizing pneumonitis, producing a bronchopleural fistula with resultant pneumothorax.[58] Alternately, an ongoing acute infection in inadequately treated areas may eventually result in cystic dilation of distal airway.[55] Martinez and colleagues[51] have suggested that the sulfite in the isethionate component of the aerosol may cause an irritant cough, resulting in a rupture of the cysts. It has been found that low diffusing capacity of lung for carbon monoxide before pentamidine therapy for secondary prophylaxis is associated with an increased risk of bilateral pneumothoraces and increased mortality in these patients.[60]

Catamenial Pneumothorax

A "catamenial pneumothorax" is defined as a spontaneous or recurrent pneumothorax occurring within 72 hours from the onset of menstruation. Alifano and colleagues[71] described 32 women with spontaneous pneumothorax who had been referred for surgical treatment. In eight cases (25%), the catamenial character of the pneumothorax was recognized by clinical history. In all eight cases, the pneumothorax was recurrent (one to four previous episodes) and right sided. A diaphragmatic abnormality was found in all eight cases. Two mechanisms have been described for pneumothorax related to endometriosis. The most common is the movement of endometrial implants to the diaphragm, preferentially to the right side because of the recognized peritoneal circulation up from the pelvis to the right side. These implants then create channels or "holes" through the diaphragm that allow the implants or air to move into the chest. The second and much less frequent cause of endometrial implants in the chest is through the venous implants that lodge in the lung itself.[72] Clinical manifestations of thoracic endometriosis include chest pain, dyspnea, and hemoptysis. Bilateral pneumothoraces and concurrent hemothorax, hemoptysis, chest pain, and pneumothorax have been described.[73]

Nonspontaneous Pneumothorax

Traumatic Pneumothorax

Traumatic pneumothorax most often occurs as a result of penetrating injury but may also occur with closed chest trauma consequent to alveolar rupture from thoracic compression, fracture of a bronchus, esophageal rupture, or rib fractures that lacerate the pleura.[74,75] Traumatic pneumothorax can be subclassified into open, closed, tension, or hemopneumothorax. A tension pneumothorax needs to be managed immediately by letting the air out with a large-bore needle. Open pneumothorax should have a moist sterile gauze pack placed over the open wound, followed by a chest tube. Hemopneumothorax requires insertion of a chest tube.[76]

Increasing use of computed tomography (CT) scan to evaluate blunt abdominal trauma has revealed a new diagnostic entity that has been called *occult pneumothorax*.[77-82] In the series of trauma patients reported by Hill and colleagues,[83] there were 67 patients (71 pneumothoraces) who were seen to have a pneumothorax on CT that was not seen on admission chest radiograph. The management of these pneumothoraces is controversial. Wolfman and colleagues,[84] reporting on 44 occult pneumothoraces, suggested that most small (minuscule) occult pneumothoraces can be managed by close observation. Moderate-sized pneumothoraces can also be managed by observation if the patient is not on a ventilator, but most of the anterolateral pneumothoraces need chest tube placement.

Iatrogenic Pneumothorax

The leading causes of iatrogenic pneumothorax are transthoracic needle aspiration (24% to 36%), subclavian venipuncture (22% to 23%), and thoracentesis (20% to 31%). Positive pressure ventilation has been reported to be the causative factor in only 7% of all iatrogenic pneumothoraces. Most patients require treatment for 4 to 7 days, and hospitalization is prolonged in only a small number of patients because of this complication.[85,86]

Barotrauma and Pneumothorax in Mechanically Ventilated Patients

An important complication of mechanical ventilation is barotrauma. In one of the series,[87] 15 of 430 patients receiving ventilatory support for longer than 12 hours developed pneumothorax. More recently, Lassence and colleagues[88] reported that iatrogenic pneumothorax occurred in 3% of intensive care unit patients. Risk factors were AIDS, acute respiratory distress syndrome (ARDS), or cardiogenic pulmonary edema at admission, body weight less than 80 kg, central vein or pulmonary artery catheter insertion, and use of inotropic agents during the first 24 hours.

When the lungs are exposed to high volumes, tissue disruption may occur. Air passes along bronchovascular bundles to the lung hilum and then to other interstitial spaces and may enter pleural or pericardial cavities.[89]

In a ventilated patient, a rise in peak and plateau pressures should alert the clinician to the possible complication of pneumothorax.[90] Petersen and Baier[91] reported a 43% incidence of barotrauma in patients who required a peak airway pressure above 70 cm H_2O. An early radiologic feature and a harbinger of life-threatening barotrauma is the presence of pulmonary interstitial emphysema. Pulmonary interstitial emphysema manifests radiologically as small parenchymal cysts, circular cuffs around larger pulmonary vessels projected end-on (perivascular halos), small dots representing small peripheral vessels surrounded by areas of radiolucency, linear streaks of air radiating toward the hilum, and large cystic collections of air and subpleural air.[92,93] The air, having entered the interstitium, then dissects proximally along bronchovascular sheaths toward the lung hilum and mediastinum. Once in the mediastinum, the accumulated air takes the path of least resistance and may produce subcutaneous emphysema, pneumopericardium, pneumoperitoneum, or retroperitoneum (Fig. 48-2). If the mediastinal pressure rises abruptly or if decompression via these routes is not sufficient, the mediastinal parietal pleura may rupture, resulting in pneumothorax. Entry of gas into the pulmonary circulation may produce systemic air embolism.[94] Even pneumoscrotum has been described as an unusual complication of barotrauma.[95] Pneumomediastinum can produce several interesting radiographic signs such as pneumopericardium, continuous diaphragm sign, continuous left hemidiaphragm sign, Naclerio's sign, V sign at confluence of brachiocephalic veins, thymic spinnaker-sail sign, ring-round-the-artery sign, and extrapleural sign.[96]

Previous studies had shown that the factors that predispose to barotrauma are high peak and mean airway pressures, positive end-expiratory pressure (PEEP), use of volume-cycled ventilators, intubation of the right

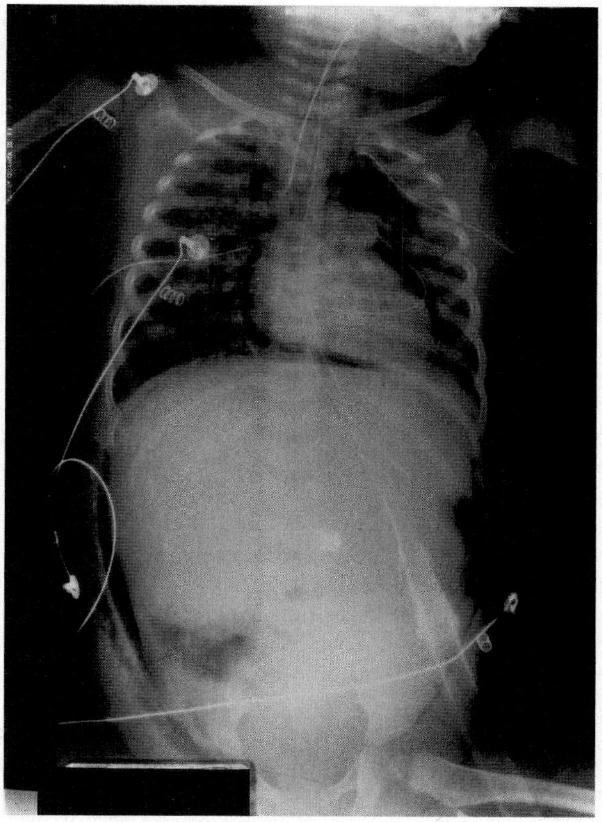

Figure 48-2. Infant with respiratory distress syndrome. The radiograph shows cysts and linear streaks of air, pneumopericardium, pneumoperitoneum, and subcutaneous emphysema. Although the radiograph belongs to an infant, it illustrates well the features of early barotrauma and its late complications.

bronchus, chronic airways obstruction, and aspiration pneumonia.[97-100] However, some studies[101,102] have shown that the incidence of barotrauma is independent of airway pressure. Experts now accept that pulmonary edema and lung injury during mechanical ventilation are the consequence of "volutrauma" rather than "barotrauma."[103] The best treatment for barotrauma is early recognition, and prevention-delayed treatment has a mortality of 31%.[97] The recommended preventive measures are to decrease peak airway pressure by decreasing tidal volume, peak flow, and ventilatory rate; to use the best PEEP; and to employ assist-control mode, independent lung ventilation, and high-frequency positive pressure ventilation.[100] In a study published by the Acute Respiratory Distress Syndrome Network, it was found that treatment with a ventilator strategy designed to protect the lungs from excessive stretch resulted in decreased mortality and increased the number of days without ventilator use in patients with acute lung injury and acute respiratory distress syndrome.[104]

Pneumothorax after Fiberoptic Bronchoscopy and Needle Biopsy of the Lung

After a literature review of more than 9000 procedures of fiberoptic bronchoscopy (FOB) with transbronchial biopsy, Milam and colleagues[105] found that the rate of pneumothorax was 1.9%. After analyzing their series of patients who had undergone FOB with transbronchial biopsy, Milam and colleagues,[105] Frazier and colleagues,[106] and Blasco and colleagues [107] concluded that an immediate postbronchoscopic chest radiograph rarely provides clinically useful information and that in FOB without transbronchial biopsy, an immediate postbronchoscopy radiograph is not necessary. In a study published in June 2006, Izbicki and colleagues[108] also concluded that in asymptomatic patients, routine radiograph after transbronchial biopsy is not necessary. When biopsies are performed, the following groups of patients should be considered for postbronchoscopy radiograph: comatose or mentally retarded patients, patients receiving positive-pressure ventilation, patients with severe respiratory compromise as a result of disease or surgery, patients with bullous disease, patients who complain of chest pain, and outpatients. Pneumothorax after bronchoalveolar lavage without biopsy is extremely rare. Similarly, the complication of pneumothorax after transbronchial needle aspiration is also low (1 of 152 patients).[109]

The incidence of pneumothorax after percutaneous needle biopsy[110-113] is much higher and ranges from 17% to 43%. Although some authors have found that a more central location of the lesion, COPD, and lung hyperinflation increase the risk of pneumothorax,[114-115] others found no correlation between development of pneumothorax and spirometric parameters or the presence of obstructive airways disease.[111,116] However, Kazerooni and others[117] found that in patients with emphysema, there is a high incidence of pneumothorax after transthoracic needle aspiration; there is rapid development of pneumothorax in these cases, requiring chest tube placement. Delayed pneumothorax after percutaneous fine needle aspiration, although extremely unusual, has been reported in two cases and patients should be warned of this possible complication.[118] More recently, Choi and colleagues[119] reported on their series of 458 patients who had undergone transthoracic needle biopsy (TTNB). A follow-up chest radiograph was obtained immediately and 3 hours, 8 hours, and 24 hours after the biopsy procedure. A pneumothorax that developed after 3 hours was defined as delayed pneumothorax. Pneumothorax developed in 100 of the 458 patients (21.8%), and delayed pneumothorax developed in 15 patients (3.3%). Female gender and absence of emphysematous changes correlated with an increased rate of delayed pneumothorax.

Pneumothorax after Thoracentesis

The reported incidence of pneumothorax after thoracentesis ranges from 5.7% to 19.2%.[120-124] Various mechanisms may explain the pneumothoraces that occur after thoracentesis: the lung may be punctured at the time of needle entry or after the fluid has been withdrawn or a small amount of air may be drawn into the chest during aspiration or along the needle track if high negative intrapleural pressures develop.[125] Raptopoulos and colleagues[126] found that ultrasonographically guided thoracentesis, use of the smallest possible needle, and aspiration of the smallest possible amount of fluid are complicated by pneumothorax significantly less often than thoracentesis done with conventional techniques. Age, sex, underlying lung condition, overall clinical condition, size of the effusion, and type of tap (diagnostic or therapeutic) had no significant effect on the occurrence of pneumothorax after thoracentesis. In a recent review article, Feller-Kopman[127] concluded that the use of ultrasound for thoracentesis has been associated with improved yield and reduced complication rate and is quickly becoming the standard of care for procedural guidance.

Colt and colleagues,[128] reporting on 255 thoracenteses performed in 205 adult patients, found that hospitalization status, critical illness, effusion size or type, presence of loculations, operator, needle type, amount of fluid withdrawn, occurrence of dry tap, and type of thoracentesis were not associated with increased frequency of pneumothorax. The only predictor showing significant correlation was repeated thoracentesis. After an analysis of 506 thoracenteses in 370 patients, Aleman and colleagues[129] concluded that, in asymptomatic patients, the risk of developing pneumothorax was so low that the practice of obtaining a routine chest radiograph may not be justified. Chakrabarti and colleagues[130] reported the use of blind percutaneous pleural biopsy by Abrams needle in 75 patients; pneumothorax was seen in eight patients (11%), with only two patients requiring specific intervention.

Pneumothorax Resulting from Nasogastric Feeding Tubes

In 1978 James[131] first reported pneumothorax as a complication of passing a narrow-bore nasogastric tube. Since that time numerous authors[132-139] have reported this complication.

Narrow-bore feeding tubes are particularly likely to give rise to pneumothorax because of the tube's small diameter (2.7 mm), self-lubricating properties, and wire stylet—all of which permit their undetected entry into the tracheobronchial tree, perforation of pulmonary tissue, and lodging in the pleural cavity.[134] Other factors associated with increased risk of a misplaced feeding tube include the presence of an endotracheal or tracheostomy tube (these may increase pulmonary passage of the tube by preventing glottis closure and perhaps by inhibiting swallowing), altered mental status, denervation of airways, esophageal stricture, enlargement of the heart, and neuromuscular weakness.[137] The clinical signs commonly used to ascertain correct placement of the feeding tube may be misleading. Normally, to confirm the correct placement of a feeding tube in the stomach, a small amount of air is injected. This produces a characteristic gurgle in the left upper quadrant of the abdomen, but a "pseudoconfirmatory gurgle" with a feeding tube in the chest has been reported.[133] Aspiration of large amounts of fluid through the tube is also taken to be a test of correct placement into the stomach, but delayed aspiration of a large quantity of undigested enteral feeding solution from the pleural space, mistaken for gastric contents, has been reported.[132]

Pneumothorax after Percutaneous Dilational Tracheostomy

Percutaneous tracheostomy was first described in 1955. In 1985, Ciaglia and colleagues[140] described percutaneous dilational tracheostomy (PDT). Fikkers and colleagues[141] described cases of subcutaneous emphysema and pneumothorax after percutaneous tracheostomy in a series of 326 cases. They described 7 of their own cases which had developed complications to include subcutaneous emphysema, mediastinal emphysema, and pneumothorax. Their review of literature showed that the incidence of subcutaneous emphysema was 1.4% and that of pneumothorax 0.8%. Findings associated with PTX included difficult PDT and the use of a fenestrated cannula.

Special Situations

Pneumothorax Ex Vacuo

Development of air in the pleural space after partial resolution of total bronchial obstruction,[142] as a complication of lobar collapse,[143] and after therapeutic thoracentesis for malignant effusions[144] has been described. Acute lobar collapse results in a sudden increase in negative pleural pressure surrounding the collapsed lobe. Although the parietal and visceral pleural surfaces remain intact, the gas originating from the ambient tissues and blood is drawn into the pleural space, producing a pneumothorax called *pneumothorax ex vacuo*. Recognition of this type of pneumothorax is crucial because managing it requires relieving the bronchial obstruction rather than inserting a chest tube. The diagnosis of trapped lung requires documentation of chronicity and absence of pleural inflammation, pleural malignancy, or endobronchial lesion. The pathognomonic radiographic sign of a trapped lung is the pneumothorax ex vacuo, characterized as a small to moderate-sized air collection after evacuation of effusion.[145]

Sports-Related Pneumothorax

Experts have recognized that sports-related air leaks and pneumothorax occur more frequently than the literature suggests. Levy and colleagues[146] and Patridge and colleagues[147] each described three cases of pneumothorax or pneumomediastinum caused by blunt trauma sustained during a contact sport. Kizer and colleagues[148] identified 20 patients who had sustained a spontaneous or traumatic air leak while engaged in an outdoor sport.

Barotrauma Unrelated to Mechanical Ventilation

Although traditionally the term *barotrauma* has been used to describe development of extra alveolar air in a patient on mechanical ventilation, there are other situations in which, because of increased intraalveolar pressure, air leaks out of alveoli. Pulmonary barotrauma (PBT) of ascent is a well-known complication of compressed air diving. Tetzlaff and colleagues[149] found that preexisting small lung cysts or end-expiratory flow limitation may increase the risk of PBT, although Neuman and colleagues[150] contested these conclusions. Some experts have suggested that even minor forms of PBT should be considered a contraindication to further diving because the divers are prone to recurrences that can occur even at shallow depths.[151] Clinically significant PBT has been reported from self-inflating bag-valve devices,[152] after inflation of party balloons,[153] as a result of blast injury,[154,155] during submarine escape training,[156] after automobile air bag deployment,[157] and in a normal healthy volunteer after repeated measurements of maximal respiratory pressure.[158]

CLINICAL FEATURES

The clinical features of pneumothorax depend on its size, the underlying lung condition, and whether the pneumothorax is tension in type. PSP usually develops in tall, thin males while the patients are at rest. Most often the onset of symptoms is not related to physical exertion. Surprisingly, many patients do not seek medical attention immediately after developing symptoms. In one series,[159] 18% of patients waited for more than 1 week after developing symptoms. Chest pain and dyspnea are the two main symptoms associated with the development of pneumothorax. In one series of 39 patients, all patients had one of the two symptoms and 25 of 39 patients (64%) had both.[160] The chest pain is sudden in onset; pleuritic in nature initially; and then becomes a persistent dull ache, localized to the affected site. The degree of dyspnea depends on the size of the pneumothorax and the condition of the underlying lung. Cough, malaise, orthopnea, or hemoptysis may be the presenting symptoms.

Small pneumothoraces (<25%) may not be detectable clinically, especially in a patient with emphysema. Larger pneumothorax may produce tachycardia and tachypnea. Decreased motion, vocal resonance, and breath sounds on the side of pneumothorax; hyperinflation; and

duced by the redundant skinfold, can be differentiated from the line of pneumothorax by the following three features: (1) the lung markings are present peripheral to the skinfold; (2) the skinfold has a wavy appearance; and (3) in the skinfold, there is a gradual increase in radiodensity as the line is approached from the hilum. However, in the presence of a consolidated lung, a pneumothorax presents as an edge instead of a line.[181]

When pneumothorax is strongly suspected clinically but a pleural line is not clearly seen, possibly because of an overlying rib, gas in the pleural space can be detected by either of two procedures: (1) radiography in the erect posture (potentially more diagnostic with full expiration) or (2) radiography in the lateral decubitus position with a horizontal x-ray beam. Some authors,[182-184] however, have suggested that the expiratory film does not increase diagnostic capability.

The diagnosis of pneumothorax in the critically ill patient is more difficult to establish. The following four variables occur statistically more often in patients with initial failure to diagnose pneumothorax: mechanical ventilation, atypical radiographic location of pneumothorax, altered mental status, and development of pneumothorax after peak physician staffing hours.[185]

In the ICU setting, radiographs are typically obtained in the supine position, making pneumothorax diagnosis more difficult. In the supine position the gas within the pleural space rises to the highest point in the hemithorax, which, in this position, is the anterior costophrenic sulcus. Various authors have described the depression and clear visualization of the diaphragm anteriorly, creating a "double" appearance to the diaphragm, a deep lateral costophrenic angle on the involved side ("the deep sulcus sign") (Fig. 48-4), an unusually distinct cardiac apex and pericardial fat tags, and increased hyperlucency of the upper abdominal quadrants.[186-190] A sharp line outlining the descending aorta may be produced by air trapped behind the inferior pulmonary ligament. Any of these findings should lead to a prompt cross-table lateral or decubitus study or a CT scan to establish the diagnosis of pneumothorax.

Although not done commonly for the diagnosis of pneumothorax, CT of the chest may detect an unsuspected pneumothorax in a critically ill patient (Fig. 48-5).[191] In view of the difficulty of clinically diagnosing pneumothorax in critically ill patients, Hall and colleagues[192] have recommended daily chest radiographs for this group of patients. In those patients who are treated with PEEP, interstitial gas may be seen as an early sign of barotrauma: More than 50% of these go on to develop features of barotrauma.[92] The interstitial gas is manifested radiographically by cystic changes, linear streaks along the bronchi and vessels, halos of gas around vessels, and subpleural gas. CT scan may also be useful to detect pneumothorax in complex cystic lung diseases.[193]

Ultrasound examination is not used in the routine diagnosis of pneumothorax but may be of diagnostic utility. During the ultrasound examination, a kind of back-and-forth movement of lung ("lung sliding"), synchronized with respiration, is normally seen. Lichtenstein and Menu[194] found that absence of lung sliding was suggestive of pneumothorax. In a normal subject, in vertical orientation, the ultrasound screen shows artifacts rising from the pleural line and spreading to the edge of the screen ("comet-tail" artifacts). Lichtenstein and colleagues,[195] in a more recent report, concluded that ultrasound detection of "comet-tail" artifact at the anterior wall allows complete pneumothorax to be excluded.

MANAGEMENT

The goals of management of pneumothorax are (1) to rid the pleural space of air and allow re-expansion of the lung with the least possible morbidity and (2) to decrease the

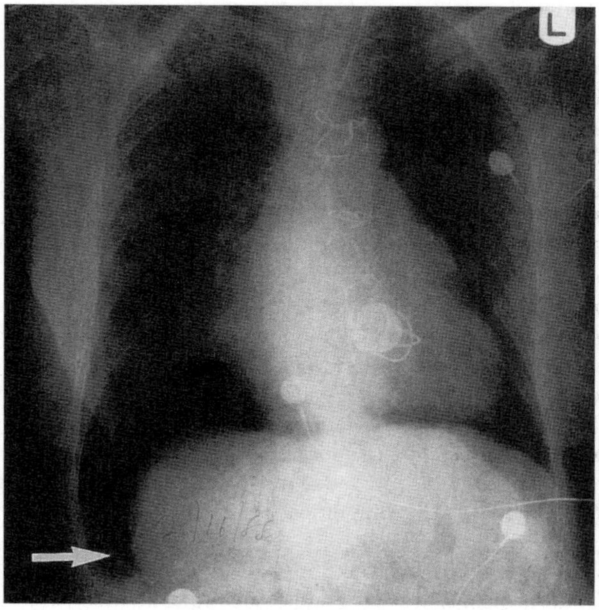

Figure 48-4. The deep sulcus sign in a supine patient.

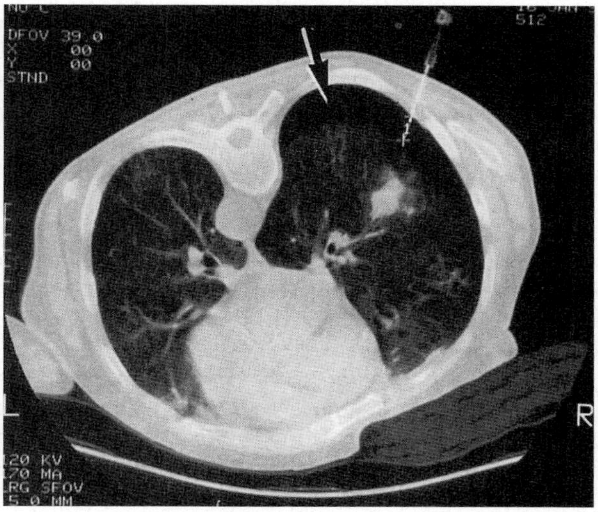

Figure 48-5. Computed tomography scan of chest showing pneumothorax.

likelihood of recurrence. Approaches for the management of the initial episode include observation, supplemental oxygen, simple aspiration of the pneumothorax, or tube thoracostomy. The choice of therapy in a given patient depends on various factors such as the size of pneumothorax, whether the pneumothorax is primary or secondary, the condition of the lungs, the clinical stability of the patient, the occupation of the patient, and whether the pneumothorax has occurred in a special setting. For prevention of recurrence, chest tube placement with pleurodesis or various surgical interventions including thoracotomy or video-assisted thoracic surgery (VATS) may be necessary. However, as a postal survey of 3000 American College of Chest Physicians (ACCP) members showed, there exists marked practice variation in the clinicians' approaches to the management of spontaneous pneumothorax and bronchopleural fistula. This was partially explained by differences between pulmonologists and thoracic surgeons.[196] Many new recommendations that suggest a shift from the previous practices have been made and are discussed later.[197]

Management of the First Episode of Pneumothorax

Estimating Size of Pneumothorax

A number of methods have been described to measure the size of pneumothorax.[198-200] Engdahl and colleagues[201] found that the size of pneumothorax measured from a chest radiograph did not correlate with CT, whereas the size of pneumothorax as estimated by CT correlated well with the amount of air aspirated in 12 of 16 patients treated with drainage. They suggested that the decision to treat should be based on clinical status and, if it is considered important to determine the size, CT should be used.

Various approaches to the management of pneumothorax are discussed in subsequent sections.

Expectant Therapy

An estimated 1.25% of the volume of pneumothorax is absorbed each 24 hours. Therefore if a patient has a 20% pneumothorax, it will take 16 days for the air to be absorbed spontaneously. Different authors have used different sizes of pneumothorax in recommending expectant management: less than 15%,[199] less than 25%,[56,76] or an apical collapse of less than 4 cm and lateral collapse of less than 1 cm.[202]

The absorption of gas from the pleural space depends, besides other factors, on the gradient between the partial pressure in the capillaries and in the pleural space. On room air, the net gradient is only 54 mm Hg, whereas it exceeds 550 mm Hg when the patient is on 100% oxygen.[199] Studies[203,204] have shown that administering 100% oxygen increases absorption of air fourfold to sixfold. Hospitalized patients with any type of pneumothorax, who are not subjected to aspiration of air or tube thoracostomy, should be treated with supplemental oxygen at high concentrations.[199]

Removal of Air from Pleural Space

In those patients whose pneumothorax is large (more than 20% to 25%), progressive, or tension type; who are symptomatic; have an underlying chronic lung disease; are on a ventilator; or who have a recurrent pneumothorax, the pleural space air needs to be removed by various therapeutic means rather than be allowed to be absorbed spontaneously. The following methods have been used for the removal of air.

Simple Aspiration

Inserting an intercostal tube is a traumatic, painful procedure associated with a risk of hemorrhage. If connected to an underwater seal, the tube confines the patient to bed, thereby increasing the risk of thromboembolism and prolonging the duration of hospitalization. In view of these disadvantages, some investigators have treated pneumothorax by simple aspiration.[205-208] Simple aspiration is usually performed in the second intercostal space in the midclavicular line. The catheter is connected to a three-way tap with the exit tube placed under water to ensure correct direction of airflow. Resistance is felt as the reexpanded lung impinges on the cannula. A confirmatory chest radiograph is performed.

A large tension pneumothorax needs to be evacuated immediately. Thoracocentesis using a catheter (e.g., Seldinger technique) that is advanced into the pleural cavity by means of a metal needle, a butterfly needle, or a regular disposable needle is fraught with danger because the lung may be punctured. Wung and colleagues[209] have described the use of a spring-loaded Veress needle (American Cystoscope Makers, Inc., Stamford, Conn.) for emergency thoracentesis. This needle consists of a slender spring-loaded inner tube, which is blunt tipped and has a side aperture, enclosed in a 16-gauge sharp needle. The spring action allows the inner needle to retract while the outer needle is puncturing the chest wall but lets it spring out as soon as the pleural cavity is punctured.

Simple aspiration is a technique with low morbidity that is well tolerated and allows the patient to be mobile and return to work rapidly. It may be used as the initial procedure in the absence of signs of tension.[210] Unfortunately, simple aspiration leaves the patient with a 10% to 50% chance of recurrence.[159,204-206] However, in a recent randomized, prospective, multicenter pilot study involving 60 patients with the first episode of PSP, Noppen and colleagues[211] reported that manual aspiration seemed equally effective as chest tube drainage and was safe, well tolerated, and feasible as an outpatient procedure in the majority of patients. Devanand and colleagues,[212] after a meta-analysis of three randomized controlled trials (RCTs) with a combined total of 194 patients, concluded that simple aspiration is advantageous in the initial management of PSP because of shorter hospitalization. No significant difference in recurrence was reported at 1 year using either modality, but the efficacy data were inconclusive.

Tube Thoracostomy

Modern chest tubes are made of clear plastic with varying internal diameters, multiple holes and distance markers, and radiopaque stripes that outline the proximal drainage hole. They are pliable but not supple enough to kink.

The second intercostal space in the midclavicular line is generally chosen for insertion of the tube because the area is wide and avascular. The tube is inserted using the trocar or blunt dissection method. Most institutions now prefer the latter. After insertion the tube is directed anteroapically and secured to prevent accidental removal. The tube is then connected to a water-seal drainage or a drainage system.[213] To avoid the risk of reexpansion pulmonary edema, it is recommended that negative suction not be applied in the absence of a bronchopleural fistula.[214]

Bell and colleagues,[215] in 102 chest tube removals in 69 trauma patients, found that the post–chest tube removal pneumothoraces rates did not differ whether the chest tube was removed at end-expiration or end-inspiration. In the absence of trauma and with good aseptic technique, prophylactic antibiotics are not recommended.

The complications associated with thoracostomy that have been reported in the literature include laceration of the lung, spleen, liver, and stomach; intercostal artery bleeding; infarction of a peripheral segment of the lung aspirated into the drainage part of the chest tube; and delayed pulmonary perforation and subcutaneous emphysema.[213,216] A blocked tube may result in a residual pleural space with the development of empyema.[217]

Percutaneous Pneumothorax Catheter

A number of authors[218,219] have described the use of small lumen catheters for treating a simple pneumothorax. In view of the ease of insertion, good response, and low incidence of complications, it has been suggested that a small lumen catheter may be a useful alternative to tube thoracotomy. Although catheter failure included kinking, malposition, inadvertent removal by the patient, occlusion of the tube or valve by pleural fluid, and large air leak, no complication attributable to tube placement occurred.[218] Liu and colleagues[220] reported their experience with the use of pigtail catheters in 50 patients versus traditional chest tube in 52 patients and found that the pigtail drainage was no less effective than the traditional chest tube.

The questions pertaining to chest tubes such as small-bore tube versus large-bore tube, whether to apply suction or not, and whether the tube should be taken out at the end of inspiration or expiration have been discussed nicely by Baumann should be[15] in a review article in 2006. These points are summarized in the management algorithms given later.

Thoracic Vent

Samelson and colleagues[221] and Martin and colleagues[222] have described their experiences with the thoracic vent (one-way valve feature) in managing simple pneumothorax. The thoracic vent is inserted in the second intercostal space in the midclavicular line. The authors point out that this device has the advantage of a urethane tube that does not kink, a self-contained one-way valve, and a unique signal diaphragm that reflects pleural pressure; however, the device is not suitable for use in patients who are expected to have large-volume or protracted air leaks.

Prevention of Recurrence

As mentioned earlier, the initial episode of spontaneous pneumothorax may be managed by simple observation or drainage. Once the initial episode of pneumothorax has resolved, the decision as to the need for measures to prevent recurrence must be made. In the following groups of patients, further management needs to be planned after the resolution of pneumothorax: recurrent pneumothorax, patients with chronic air leak, patients with demonstrable large bullae, and patients who live in remote areas or pursue an occupation in which a recurrence could be a hazard (e.g., airline personnel or divers).

Different recurrence rates have been reported by various authors and range from 20% to 52%.[1,202,223,224] The following are *established* risk factors for recurrence: more than one previous episode, COPD, air leak for more than 48 hours during the first episode, and large cysts seen on radiograph. The following are *possible* risk factors for recurrence: nonoperative management of first episode (versus tube drainage) and tube drainage for only 24 hours during first episode (versus 3 to 4 days). Further management in these high-risk groups is aimed at preventing recurrence. The following approaches have been used.

Chemical pleurodesis via chest tube, at thoracotomy, or VATS can be used to institute preventive measures.

Chemical Sclerosis (Pleurodesis)

Pleurodesis (adhesion of visceral and parietal pleura) can be done by introducing the sclerotic agent via a chest tube, or it can be done in the operating room with open thoracotomy or thoracoscopy. However, there is no consensus about the timing or method of pleurodesis.[225] A practical approach is outlined later in the management algorithm.

Because sterile tetracycline is no longer available, intrapleural instillation of doxycycline has been used as an alternative for pleurodesis.[226] Talc, finely powdered magnesium silicate, is another effective pleural irritant, producing fibrosis and adhesions. Numerous complications and side effects such as fever, pain, infection, and respiratory failure have been reported with its use,[227] but Lange and colleagues[228] found that although talc may result in mild restrictive respiratory impairment in long-term follow-up, it was not clinically significant and there were no recorded cases of mesothelioma.

In the past, patients with failed pleurodesis underwent surgical intervention. Thoracic surgery in such patients is complicated by partial pleural symphysis. Also, previous chemical pleurodesis makes lung transplantation more difficult technically. In view of these concerns, Kirby and Ginsberg[76] recommend that chemical pleurodesis be used only in selected patients who are too ill for surgery.

Surgery

The objectives of surgical treatment are to obtain full reexpansion of the affected lung, control complications, tackle the underlying lung problem, and prevent recurrence through pleural sclerosis by mechanical abrasion or pleurectomy.

Indications

Surgical management during the first episode of SP is indicated under the following circumstances: 3% to 4% of patients have a persistent leak resulting from a large fistula that needs to be closed surgically; about 5% of patients have frank hemothorax, and surgical intervention is required in these patients to control the bleeding; a trapped lung may fail to reexpand, and decortication is required in such cases. If the patient is a diver, airline pilot, or lives in a remote area, surgery should be considered after the first episode to prevent a recurrence.

Surgical Approach

Apical bullous disease can be surgically approached by a transaxillary approach[76,229] or through the auscultation triangle.[230] In a young female, a cosmetically acceptable scar is produced by a submammary anterolateral incision.[210] In an older individual with difficult pneumothorax complicated by other problems, a formal posterolateral thoracotomy is recommended.[76,210,229] If bilateral pleurectomy is required, a midline sternotomy is preferred. This permits access to both pleural cavities with minimum interference with respiratory function and causes minimal postoperative pain.[210]

Surgical Techniques

Sites of air leaks and obvious bullae are oversewn.[229] With modern stapling instruments, blebs and bullae can be excised easily with an airtight seal, without sacrificing a great amount of normal underlying lung tissue.[76] If one large cyst is fed by a major bronchial branch, then control of the feeding bronchus and marsupialization or plication of the bulla is performed. Segmentectomy and lobectomy to deal with underlying pathology are rarely necessary.[210]

Obliteration of pleural space can be achieved by abrasion of the pleura with a dry gauze sponge, apical pleurectomy,[210] or an extensive pleurectomy.[231] When bilateral pleurectomy is advisable, it should be done in stages, 10 to 30 days apart. In most of the cases, blebectomy and pleural abrasion are sufficient.

In their study, Murray and colleagues[232] suggested an entirely different approach to the problem of recurrent pneumothorax. They used a limited axillary thoracotomy as primary treatment for recurrent pneumothorax, without a preoperative chest tube.

Thoracoscopic Surgery

Modern thoracoscopy allows minimally invasive access to the chest cavity. It allows full visualization of the lung and pleura and, when combined with resection of blebs and pleurodesis or pleurectomy, results in a low recurrence rate, minimal patient discomfort, and rapid recovery. Identified bullae can be treated with a variety of modalities.[233-235] Chemical or mechanical pleurodesis can be performed during VATS.[236-238] Thoracoscopic identification and treatment of bronchopleural fistulas are also possible in patients with prolonged air leaks despite chest tube drainage.[239] Bilateral VATS has been found to be a safe and efficacious procedure for patients with bilateral bullous disease and patients presenting with simultaneous or nonsimultaneous bilateral SP.[240,241]

Management under Special Circumstances

Pneumothorax in AIDS Patients

Pneumocystis jerovici pneumonia–related pneumothorax is complicated by a virulent form of necrotizing subpleural lesions, which result in diffuse air leaks that are refractory to the standard treatment.[52,57] Asymptomatic patients can be observed. An aggressive stepped-care management with large-bore intercostal tube drainage, chemical pleurodesis, and early video-assisted thoracic talc poudrage has been recommended for symptomatic patients.[242] In patients with an air leak persisting for more than 7 days, thoracotomy with stapling of blebs and mechanical pleurodesis has been recommended. When chemical pleurodesis is unsuccessful and open surgical pleurectomy is not desirable because of the patient's underlying disease, morbidity, and poor prognosis, thoracoscopic pleural ablation offers a therapeutic alternative.[239]

Pneumothorax in Cystic Fibrosis

Pleurodesis as an initial step in the management of pneumothorax in cystic fibrosis is considered contraindicated because it results in extensive pleural adhesions that jeopardize subsequent lung transplantation.[243] Therefore Noyes and Orenstein[244] have recommended a stepwise management of pneumothorax in cystic fibrosis. If initial tube thoracostomy does not bring resolution of air leak within 5 days, blebectomy should be performed. If blebectomy proves unsuccessful, with either continuing air leak or recurrence, a definitive pleural ablative procedure should be undertaken.

Catamenial Pneumothorax and Pneumothorax Complicating Pregnancy

The initial episode of catamenial pneumothorax is managed in the usual manner. Recurrences, which occur 72 hours before or after menstrual flow, are managed by pleurodesis or hormonal treatment.[245] Therapeutic options include oral contraceptive pills, danazol, progestational agents, and gonadotropin-releasing hormone (GnRH) analogues.[72] Thoracotomy should be considered if the patient is unable to take ovulation-suppressing drugs, has a recurrent pneumothorax while on drugs, or wants to become pregnant. At thoracotomy, any diaphragmatic defects should be closed, any subpleural blebs should be oversewn, and pleural abrasion should be performed to effect a pleurodesis.[246,247] A patient who has a previous or current catamenial pneumothorax is at increased risk for barotrauma with positive pressure ventilation and represents a unique challenge to the anesthetist. Postoperative hormonal therapy is often required to prevent recurrences. Hysterectomy or tubal ligation may benefit selected patients.[72] Pneumothorax complicating pregnancy is managed in the usual way, but in view of the high rate of recurrence of pneumothorax during parturition, thoracotomy with resection of apical blebs (if present) should be considered.[248]

Pneumothorax in Air Travelers

Air or gas trapped in body cavities expands in direct proportion to the decrease in atmospheric pressure. At an altitude of 10,000 feet, a pneumothorax will increase 1.5 times in size.[249] If a patient with pneumothorax, especially secondary to COPD, has to be transported, the following precautions should be taken: (a) the ability of the patient to take supplemental oxygen without causing alveolar hypoventilation must be established before the flight and supplemental oxygen administered during the flight; (b) a chest tube with a Heimlich flutter valve should be in place; and (c) the patient should travel with a medically knowledgeable companion.[250]

Management of Pneumothorax in Severe Acute Respiratory Syndrome

The 2002 epidemic of the severe acute respiratory syndrome (SARS) brought several ethical issues associated with new, severe epidemic diseases into sharp focus. Of the six cases described by Sihoe,[251] pneumothoraces were bilateral in three patients, mechanical ventilation was indicated in three patients, and two patients died. Air leaks or recurrences occurred in all four patients who accepted chest tubes. These air leaks took 14 to 31 days to resolve. Peripheral leukocytes and serum lactate dehydrogenase were higher in SARS patients with pneumothorax. These complications reflected severe pathologic changes in lung tissues and the strong pulmonary and systemic inflammatory responses that accompany SARS. During the SARS epidemic, health care providers were at risk, with substantial risk for those who performed bronchoscopy. By the end of the epidemic, approximately 30% of reported cases were in health care workers and some died. Felice[252] concluded that if multiple management options are available and they can be expected to result in equivalent, optimal patient outcomes, options that pose lesser risks to health care providers should be selected.

Management of Pneumothorax in Lymphangioleiomyomatosis

Lymphangioleiomyomatosis (LAM) is a rare and frequently fatal disease that exclusively affects women of childbearing age. Thin-walled cyst formation occurs in the pulmonary parenchyma, and lung function declines progressively. The LAM Pleural Disease Consensus Group reviewed the responses to a questionnaire by 395 patients. Of these, 260 patients (incidence, 66%) reported at least one spontaneous pneumothorax during their lifetime and 200 out of 260 (77%) indicated that they had subsequent pneumothoraces.[253] Because of the morbidity and cost associated with multiple recurrences, the authors recommended early, definitive intervention, preferably at the time of the initial pneumothorax. Although pleurodesis may be associated with an increased risk of perioperative bleeding with lung transplantation, their data suggested that the complications are manageable and do not preclude successful transplantation.

Persistent Pulmonary Air Leak and Bronchopleural Fistula

A persistent pulmonary air leak, which may occur as a result of pneumothorax or after pulmonary resection, is a difficult and frustrating problem to manage. Conventionally, the air leak persisting for more than 7 days is called *bronchopleural fistula* and it is not an uncommon problem. In the series reported by Chee and colleagues,[254] the overall incidence of bronchopleural fistula was 34.6%. In pulmonary resection cases, Cerfolio and colleagues,[255] on univariate analysis, found that the increased age and the following findings on pulmonary function testing predicted air leak on postoperative day one: low forced expiratory volume in 1 second/forced vital capacity ratio (FEV_1/FVC), increased residual volume/total lung capacity ratio (RV/TLC), increased RV, and increased functional residual capacity (FRC). In the patients with air leaks who are managed by tube thoracostomy, Cerfolio and colleagues[255] found that conversion from suction to a water seal is an effective way of sealing an expiratory air leak. If the leak persists beyond 7 days, tube thoracostomy is deemed to have failed and a more definitive treatment is planned. Such cases are usually managed surgically, but patients who are unfit or unwilling for surgery pose a management dilemma. Chemical pleurodesis may be tried but does not succeed if the lung has failed to expand. In such a situation, autologous "blood patch" pleurodesis has been found useful.[256,257] Kinoshita and colleagues[258] have described a technique for such cases. They used a large amount of diluted fibrin glue for pleurodesis in patients with intractable pneumothorax or intrapleural dead space and found it useful. If pleurodesis also fails, the leak is localized during fiber-optic bronchoscopy and the fistula is sealed by using a sealant.[259] Pectoral myoplasty, in which the right pectoralis major muscle was transferred into the thorax and draped over the area of lung with multiple leaks, has been used when other interventions fail.[260] Murata and colleagues[261] have described a closure with intravenous administration of a coagulation factor XIII concentrate. Ferguson and colleagues[262] reported closure of a persistent distal bronchopleural fistula using a one-way endobronchial valve designed for the treatment of emphysema.

COMPLICATIONS RELATED TO MANAGEMENT

Ziskind and colleagues,[263] in 1965, described a case of pneumothorax in which accidental application of high, negative intrapleural pressure led to acute pulmonary edema. Since that time, *unilateral expansion pulmonary edema* has been recognized as a complication that can occur during the management of pneumothorax (Fig. 48-6). Re-expansion pulmonary edema tends to occur with greater frequency in patients 20 to 39 years of age, when there is complete collapse of the lung, when the pneumothorax has remained untreated for more than 72 hours, and when rapid re-expansion occurs secondary to the application of negative pressure; age-related changes in the older patients seem to afford some protection.[214,264] The exact pathogenesis of re-expansion pulmonary edema is not known, but various factors such as bronchial obstruction,[265] decrease in surfactant,[266] and increased capillary permeability[267,268] have been implicated. The development of *bilateral re-expansion pulmonary edema*

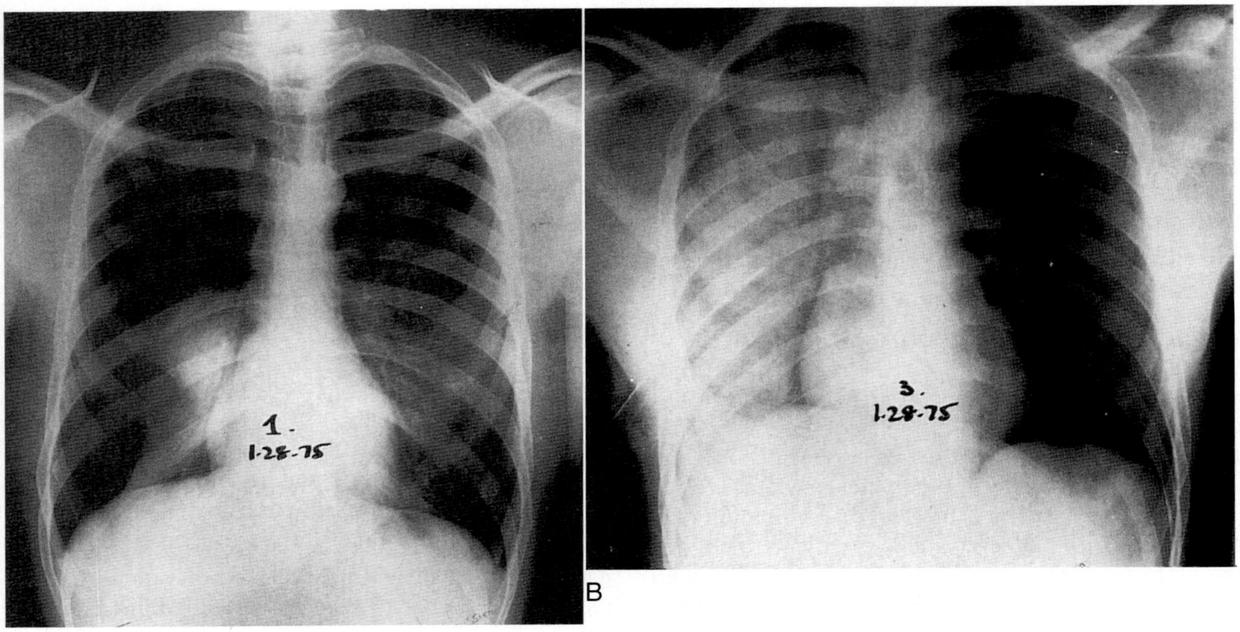

Figure 48-6. **A,** Large pneumothorax. **B,** Re-expansion pulmonary edema.

after unilateral pleurodesis in a young male without heart disease might suggest that forces leading to ipsilateral reexpansion pulmonary edema also affect the contralateral lung.[269]

Pavlin and colleagues[270] have described three cases of *re-expansion hypotension* that followed rapid evacuation of persistent unilateral pneumothorax. Besides the presence of pulmonary collapse for more than 3 days, the other risk factors were significant arterial hypoxemia during pneumothorax, an elevated or rising hemoglobin and hematocrit level, and development of respiratory distress after insertion of a pleural drain. The mechanism of hypotension and shock after pulmonary re-expansion is not clear, but volume depletion and myocardial depression possibly play a role.

Slow expansion by intermittent clamping of the chest tube, especially in high-risk patients, may prevent both reexpansion edema and reexpansion hypotension.[214,270] Paradoxically, vigorous fluid therapy may be advantageous in preserving circulation dynamics despite coexisting pulmonary edema. Myocardial stimulants may be useful if myocardial depression is suspected.[270] Diuretics have been used to manage re-expansion pulmonary edema[214] but may prove dangerous in the presence of hypovolemia and shock.[271] It has been recommended that a more logical approach in patients with shock and hypoxemia may be to use mechanical ventilation with PEEP, which would reduce further fluid shift into the re-expanded lung. Plasma expanders, fluid replacement, and vasopressor therapy can be used as needed.[270,272]

Development of *tension pneumothorax* has been reported after inadvertent, improper attachment of a Heimlich valve.[273,274]

GUIDELINES FOR MANAGING PNEUMOTHORAX

A more aggressive approach to managing pneumothorax has been advocated recently.[275] Guidelines for managing pneumothorax have been published.[276,277]

Pneumothorax size: American College of Chest Physician (ACCP) guidelines define a small pneumothorax as less than 3 cm in apex-to-cupola distance; British Thoracic Society (BTS) guidelines define a small pneumothorax as a visible rim of less than 2 cm between the lung margin and chest wall.

Stable patient: The ACCP defines a stable patient as one who has all of the following: respiratory rate less than 24 breaths per minute; heart rate greater than 60 beats per minute or less than 120 beats per minute; normal blood pressure; room air saturation of greater than 90%; and ability to speak in whole sentences.

Imaging of pneumothorax: Expiratory chest radiographs are not recommended for the routine diagnosis. A lateral view or a lateral decubitus film should be performed if the posteroanterior (PA) view is normal and the suspicion for pneumothorax is high. BTS guidelines recommend CT scan to differentiate a pneumothorax from complex lung disease, when aberrant tube placement is suspected, and when plain radiograph is obscured by surgical emphysema. The ACCP panel did not achieve consensus regarding the role of CT.

Management of chest tubes: Some controversy exists regarding the size of the tube in various situations and the use of suction. According to BTS, there is no evidence that large tubes (20 to 24 French [Fr]) are any better than smaller tubes (10 to 14 Fr) in the management of pneumothorax. However, a small chest tube may need to be replaced by a larger tube if leaking persists and creates management difficulty.

A PRACTICAL APPROACH TO THE MANAGEMENT OF PNEUMOTHORAX

The clinician finds it most practical to use a “roadmap” in different clinical scenarios. The difference between didactic medicine and bedside medicine is that the former is taught in a classroom and begins with a “diagnosis”; the latter starts at the bedside with a clinical scenario as the starting point. Figure 48-7 represents an algorithmic approach to management that is based on the ACCP and BTS guidelines and practical experience. It can be applied to most patients with pneumothoraces.

Acknowledgments

The authors thank Faroque Khan, MB, MACP, for valuable advice and for contributing most of the radiographs; Dvorah Balsam, MD, for Fig. 48-2; and Leonard Octavius Barrett, MD, FACS, Chief of Thoracic Surgery at NUMC, for his comments regarding the surgical therapy.

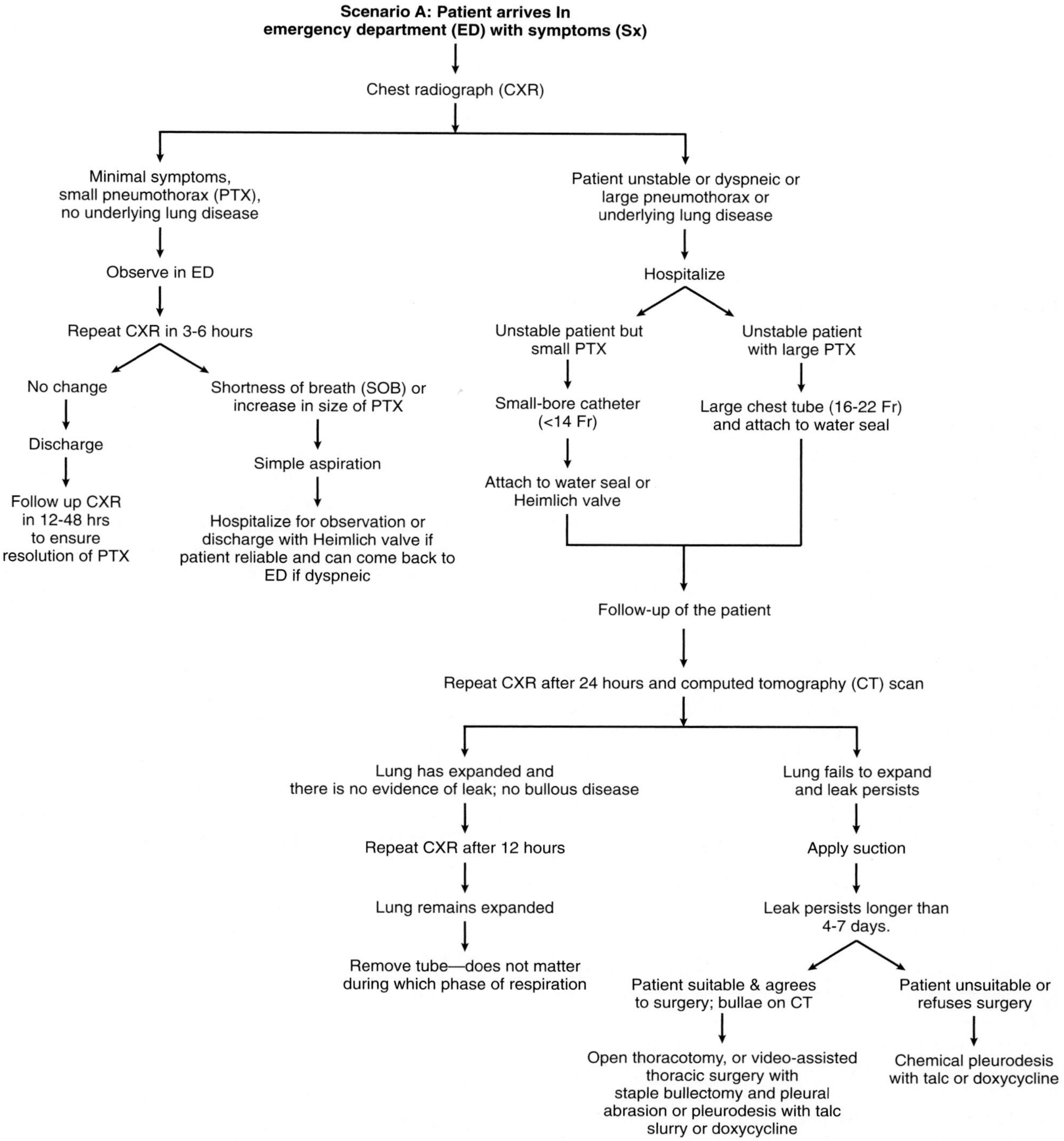

Figure 48-7. Algorithmic approach to the management of pneumothorax.

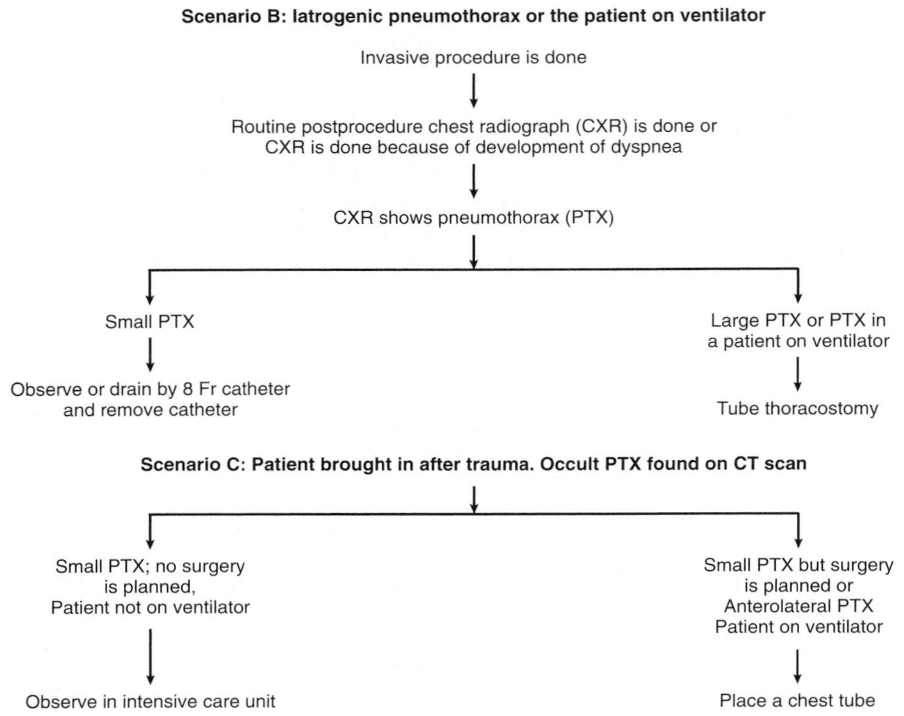

Figure 48-7, cont'd. Algorithmic approach to the management of pneumothorax.

KEY POINTS

- PSP occurs primarily in tall, thin, previously healthy young men, most of whom are smokers. Chest radiograph often shows apical subpleural blebs or bullae. Rupture of these bullae is *not* related to physical activity but may be related to changes in atmospheric pressure. COPD is the most common cause of secondary pneumothorax. Presentation of pneumothorax in COPD is often atypical and causes excessive morbidity and mortality.
- A high incidence of pneumothorax occurs in AIDS patients, related to PCP and the mechanical ventilation and bronchoscopy that are commonly required in these patients. In this group of patients, pneumothorax is frequently bilateral, recurrent, and unresponsive to conservative therapy.
- Traumatic pneumothorax, which occurs as a result of a penetrating injury, may occur with closed chest trauma.
- PTX is a common complication of mechanical ventilation. Interstitial emphysema is a harbinger of this complication. High peak and mean airway pressures, PEEP, use of volume-cycled ventilators, intubation of right mainstem bronchus, chronic airways obstruction, and aspiration pneumonia increase the incidence.
- Pneumothorax ex vacuo, sports-related pneumothorax, and barotrauma unrelated to mechanical ventilation are interesting conditions that are not common, but they are important to be aware of.
- Simultaneous bilateral pneumothoraces and "shifting pneumothoraces" are rare but interesting conditions and may develop because of persistent pleuro-pleural communication called *iatrogenic buffalo chest.*
- An immediate postbronchoscopy chest radiograph is rarely useful but should be done in certain groups of patients (e.g., comatose, mentally retarded, ventilated, or with respiratory compromise).
- PTX induced by a misplaced small-bore feeding tube is not uncommon. Clinical signs may be misleading.
- A visceral pleural line with absence of lung markings peripherally is the classic radiographic sign of PTX. When the chest radiograph is obtained in the supine position, the signs are very different.
- The approach to management of a PTX is dictated by the clinical condition rather than merely the size of the PTX, which is best estimated by CT scan of the chest. Expectant therapy is recommended for a small PSP in a stable patient. Reabsorption of air is hastened by 100% oxygen.
- Air can be removed by simple aspiration, a small lumen catheter, or tube thoracostomy. Unstable patients with large secondary PTXs must be managed with tube thoracostomy.
- A staged approach is recommended for chest tube removal. In PSP cases, the tube can be removed 6 to 12 hours after evidence of air leak was last seen; this waiting period is 12 to 24 hours in secondary PTX.
- Definitive management of recurrent pneumothorax or persistent leak can be done by open thoracotomy or video-assisted thoracoscopy associated with pleurodesis, pleural abrasion, parietal pleurectomy, or bullectomy. In

patients unsuitable or unwilling for surgery, chemical pleurodesis via a chest tube may be done.

- PTX tends to recur in patients with cystic fibrosis. Blebectomy, without stripping the pleura, is recommended in these patients so that they may remain transplant candidates. Pleurodesis should not be done in these cases because adhesion development jeopardizes subsequent lung transplantation.
- PTX in pregnancy is managed in the usual manner initially. In view of the high recurrence rates during parturition, thoracotomy with resection of blebs should be considered.
- Re-expansion pulmonary edema is an important complication and can be prevented by slow expansion in high-risk patients.

REFERENCES

1. Getz SB, Beasley WE: Spontaneous pneumothorax. Am J Surg 1983;145:823.
2. Laennec RT: De l'auscultation mediate: JA Brosson and JS Chaude, Paris 1819. Cited by Ransdell HT, McPherson: Management of spontaneous pneumothorax. Arch Surg 1963;87:1023.
3. Joseph M, Goulston K, Grant AF, et al: Spontaneous pneumothorax. Med J Aust 1964;1:1.
4. Kjaergaard H: Spontaneous pneumothorax in the apparently healthy. Acta Med Scand 1932;43(Suppl)1:159. Cited by Kirby TJ, Ginsberg RJ: Management of the pneumothorax and barotrauma. Clin Chest Med 1992;13:97.
5. Hewett FC: Thoracentesis: The plan of continuous aspiration. BMJ 1876;1: 317.
6. Weissberg D, Refaely Y: Pneumothorax. Experience with 1,199 patients. Chest 2000;117:1279.
7. Chen K, Jerng J, Liao W, et al: Pneumothorax in the ICU. Patient outcomes and prognostic factors. Chest 2002;122:678.
8. Schramel F, Postmus P, Vanderschueren R: Current aspects of spontaneous pneumothorax. Eur Respir J 1997;10: 1372.
9. Bense L, Lewander R, Eklund G, et al: Nonsmoking, non-alpha 1- antitrypsin deficiency-induced emphysema in nonsmokers with healed spontaneous pneumothorax identified by computed tomography of the lungs. Chest 1993;103:433.
10. Lesur O, Delorme N, Fromaget J, et al: Computed tomography in the etiologic assessment of idiopathic spontaneous pneumothorax. Chest 1990;98:341.
11. Mitlehner W, Friedrich M, Dissmann W: Value of computed tomography in the detection of bullae and blebs in patients with primary spontaneous pneumothorax. Respiration 1992;59:221.
12. Smit HJM, Wienk MATP, Schreurs AJM, et al: Do bullae indicate a predisposition to recurrent pneumothorax? Br J Radiol 2000;73:356.
13. Noppen M: Management of primary spontaneous pneumothorax. Curr Opin Pul Med 2003;9:272.
14. Noppen M, Stratakos G, Verbanck S, et al: Fluorescein-enhanced autofluorescence thoracoscopy in primary spontaneous pneumothorax. Am J Respir Crit Care Med 2004;170:680.
15. Baumann MH: Management of spontaneous pneumothorax. Clin Chest Med 2006;27:369.
16. Bense L, Eklund G, Wiman L-G: Smoking and the increased risk of contracting spontaneous pneumothorax. Chest 1987;92:1009.
17. Sadikot RT, Greene T, Meadows K, Arnold EA: Recurrence of pneumothorax. Thorax 1997;52:805.
18. Smit H, Chatrou, Postmus P: The impact of spontaneous pneumothorax, and its treatment, on the smoking behavior of young adult smokers. Respir Med 1998;92:1132.
19. Cottin V, Streichenberger N, Gamondes J-P, et al: Respiratory bronchiolitis in smokers with spontaneous pneumothorax. Eur Respir J 1998;12:702.
20. Smit HJM, Golding RP, Schramel FMNH, et al: Lung density measurements in spontaneous pneumothorax demonstrate air trapping. Chest 2004;125:2083.
21. Morrison P, Lowry R, Nevin N: Familial primary spontaneous pneumothorax consistent with true autosomal dominant inheritance. Thorax 1998;53:151.
22. Morrison P, Lowry R, Nevin N: Familial primary spontaneous pneumothorax consistent with true autosomal dominant inheritance. Thorax 1998;53:151.
23. Koivisto PA, Mustonen A: Primary spontaneous pneumothorax in two siblings suggests autosomal recessive inheritance. Chest 2001;119:1610.
24. Cardy CM, Maskell NA, Handford PA, et al: Familial spontaneous pneumothorax and FBN1 mutations. Am J Respir Crit Care Med 2004;169:1260.
25. Khoo SK, Giraud S, Kahnoski K, et al: Clinical and genetic studies of Brit-Hogg-Dube syndrome. J Med Genetics 2003;40:906.
26. Butnor KJ, Guinee DG Jr: Pleuropulmonary pathology of Birt-Hogg- Dube syndrome. Am J Surg Pathol 2006;30:395.
27. Peters JI, Sako EY: Pneumothorax. In Fishman AP (ed): Fishman's Pulmonary Diseases and Disorders, ed 2, vol 1. New York, McGraw-Hill, 1998.
28. Norris RM, Jones JG, Bishop JM: Respiratory gas exchange in patients with spontaneous pneumothorax. Thorax 1968;23:427.
29. Dines DE, Clagett OT, Payne WS: Spontaneous pneumothorax in emphysema. Mayo Clin Proc 1970;45:481.
30. Moran JF, Jones RH, Wolfe WG: Regional pulmonary function during experimental unilateral pneumothorax in the awake state. J Thorac Cardiovasc Surg 1977;74:396.
31. Anthonisen NR: Regional lung function in spontaneous pneumothorax. Am Rev Respir Dis 1977;115:873.
32. Rutherford RB, Hurt HH Jr, Brickman RD, et al: The pathophysiology of progressive tension pneumothorax. J Trauma 1968;8:212.
33. Ohata M, Suzuki H: Pathogenesis of spontaneous pneumothorax with special reference to the ultrastructure of emphysematous bullae. Chest 1980;77:771.
34. Melton LJ III, Hepper NGG, Offord KP: Influence of height on the risk of spontaneous pneumothorax. Mayo Clin Proc 1981;56:678.
35. Sugiyama Y, Maeda H, Yotsumoto H, et al: Familial spontaneous pneumothorax. Thorax 1986;41:969.
36. Morrison PJ, Lowry RC, Nevin NC: Familial primary spontaneous pneumothorax consistent with true autosomal dominant inheritance. Thorax 1998;53:151.
37. Hart GJ, Stokes TC, Couch AHC: Spontaneous pneumothorax in Norfolk. Br J Dis Chest 1983;77:164.
38. Bense L, Wilman LG: Time relation between sale of cigarettes and the incidence of spontaneous pneumothorax. Eur J Respir Dis 1987;71:362.
39. Bense L, Eklund G, Odont D, et al: Smoking and the increased risk of contracting spontaneous pneumothorax. Chest 1987;92:1009.
40. Fraser RS, Muller NL, Colman N, et al: Pneumothorax. In Fraser RS, Muller NL, Colman N, Paré PD (eds): Fraser and Paré's Diagnosis of Diseases of the Chest, 4th ed, vol IV. Philadelphia, WB Saunders, 1999.
41. Videm V, Pillgram-Larsen J, Ellingsen O, et al: Spontaneous pneumothorax in chronic obstructive pulmonary disease: Complications, treatment and recurrences. Eur J Respir Dis 1987;71:365.
42. Vukich DJ: Diseases of the pleural space. Med Clin North Am 1989;7:309.
43. Lewis JW Jr, Groux N, Elliott JP Jr, et al: Complications of attempted central venous injection performed by drug abusers. Chest 1980;78:613.
44. Moss GS, Young Q: Man's worst enemy—himself. Chest 1980;78:551.
45. Cohen HL, Cohen SW: Spontaneous bilateral pneumothorax in drug addicts. Chest 1984;86:645.

46. Wisdom K, Nowak RM, Richardson HH, et al: Alternate therapy for traumatic pneumothorax in "pocket-shooters." Ann Emerg Med 1986;15:428.
47. Douglas RE, Levison MA: Pneumothorax in drug abusers: An urban epidemic? Am Surg 1986: 52:377.
48. Wollschlager CM, Khan FA, Chitkara RK, et al: Pulmonary manifestations of acquired immunodeficiency syndrome (AIDS). Chest 1984;85:197.
49. Sherman M, Levin D, Breidbart D: Pneumocystis carinii pneumonia with spontaneous pneumothorax: A report of three cases. Chest 1986;90:609.
50. Joe L, Gordin F, Parker RH: Spontaneous pneumothorax with *Pneumocystis carinii* infection: Occurrence in patients with acquired immuno-deficiency syndrome. Arch Intern Med 1986;146:1816.
51. Martinez CM, Romanelli A, Mullen MP, et al: Spontaneous pneumothoraces in AIDS patients receiving aerosolized pentamidine (letter). Chest 1988;94:1317.
52. Afessa B, Green WR, Williams WA, et al: Pneumocystis carinii pneumonia complicated by lymphadenopathy and pneumothorax. Arch Intern Med 1988;148:2651.
53. Byrnes TA, Brevig JK, Yeoh CB: Pneumothorax in patients with immunodeficiency syndrome. J Thorac Cardiovasc Surg 1989;98:546.
54. Pinsk R, Rogers LF: Cystic parenchymal changes associated with spontaneous pneumothorax in an HIV-positive patient. Chest 1990;97:1471.
55. Newsome GS, Ward DJ, Pierce PF: Spontaneous pneumothorax in patients with acquired immunodeficiency syndrome treated with prophylactic aerosolized pentamidine. Arch Intern Med 1990;150:2167.
56. McClellan MD, Miller SB, Parsons PE, et al: Pneumothorax with *Pneumocystis carinii* pneumonia in AIDS: Incidence and clinical characteristics. Chest 1991;100:1224.
57. Shanley DJ, Luyckx BA, Haggerty MF, et al: Spontaneous pneumothorax in AIDS patients with recurrent *Pneumocystis carinii* pneumonia despite aerosolized pentamidine prophylaxis. Chest 1991;99:502.
58. Sepkovitz KA, Telzak EE, Gold JWM, et al: Pneumothorax in AIDS. Ann Intern Med 1991;114:455.
59. Truitt T, Bagheri K, Safirstein BH: Spontaneous pneumothorax in *Pneumocystis carinii* pneumonia: Common or uncommon? AJR Am J Roentgenol 1992;158:916.
60. Renzi PM, Corbeil C, Chasse M, et al: Bilateral pneumothoraces hasten mortality in AIDS patients receiving secondary prophylaxis with aerosolized pentamidine: Association with a lower DCO prior to receiving aerosolized pentamidine. Chest 1992;102:491.
61. Love L, King JC: Spontaneous pneumothorax complicating pneumonia. Ann Intern Med 1954;40:153.
62. Spivak H, Keller S: Spontaneous pneumothorax in the AIDS population. Am Surgeon 1996;62:753.
63. Becker CE, Reynolds M, Roy TM: Treatment of pneumothorax in the patients with AIDS. J Ky Med Assoc 1996;94:59.
64. Fleisher AG, McElvaney G, Lawson L, et al: Surgical management of spontaneous pneumothorax in patients with acquired immunodeficiency syndrome. Ann Thorac Surg 1988;45:21.
65. Sidhu GS, Cassai ND, Pei Z: *Pneumocystis carinii:* An update. Ultrastruct Pathol 2003;27:115.
66. Orenstein M, Webber CA, Cash M, et al: Value of bronchoalveolar lavage in the diagnosis of pulmonary infection in acquired immune-deficiency syndrome. Thorax 1986;41:345.
67. Asboe D, Fisher M, Nelson MR, et al: Pneumothorax in AIDS: Case reviews and proposed clinical management. Genitourin Med 1996;72:258.
68. Alkhuja S, Badhey K, Miller A: Simultaneous bilateral pneumothorax in an HIV-infected patient. Chest 1997;112:1417.
69. Libanore M, Bicocchi R, Sighinolfi L, et al: Pneumothorax during pulmonary toxoplasmosis in an AIDS patient (letter). Chest 1991;100:1184.
70. Azoulay E, Parrot A, Flahault A, et al: AIDS-related *Pneumocystis carinii* pneumonia in the era of adjunctive steroids. Am J Respir Crit Care Med 1999;160:493.
71. Alifano M, Roth T, Broet SC, et al: Catamenial pneumothorax. A prospective study. Chest 2003;124:1004.
72. Hazelrigg SR: Secondary spontaneous pneumothorax. Catamenial pneumothorax. Chest 2003;124:781.
73. Johnson MM: Catamenial pneumothorax and other thoracic manifestations of endometriosis. Clinics in Chest Med 2004;25:311.
74. Guest JL, Anderson JN: Major airway injury in closed chest trauma. Chest 1977;72:63.
75. Amauchi W, Birolini D, Branco PD, et al: Injuries to the tracheobronchial tree in closed trauma. Thorax 1983;38:923.
76. Kirby TJ, Ginsberg RJ: Management of the pneumothorax and barotrauma. Clin Chest Med 1992;13:97.
77. Garramone RR Jr, Jacobs LM, Sahdev P: An objective method to measure and manage occult pneumothorax. Surg Gynecol Obstet 1991;173:257.
78. Collins JC, Levine G, Waxman K: Occult traumatic pneumothorax: Immediate tube thoracostomy versus expectant management. Am Surg 1992;58:743.
79. Wolfman NT, Gilpin JW, Bechtold RE, et al: Occult pneumothorax in patients with abnormal trauma: CT studies. J Comput Assist Tomogr 1993;17:56.
80. Bridges KG, Welch G, Silver M, et al: CT detection of occult pneumothorax in multiple trauma patients. J Emerg Med 1993;11:179.
81. Enderson BL, Abdalla R, Frame SB, et al: Tube thoracostomy for occult pneumothorax: A prospective randomized study of its use. J Trauma Inj Infect Crit Care 1993;35:726.
82. Collins JA, Samra GS: Failure of chest x-rays to diagnose pneumothoraces after blunt trauma. Anaesthesia 1998;53:69.
83. Hill SL, Edmisten T, Holtzman G, et al: The occult pneumothorax: An increasing diagnostic entity in trauma. Am Surg 1999;65:254.
84. Wolfman NT, Myers WS, Glauser SJ, et al: Validity of CT classification on management of occult pneumothorax: A prospective study. AJR 1998;171:1317.
85. Sassoon CS, Light RW, O'Hara VS, et al: Iatrogenic pneumothorax: Etiology and morbidity. Results of a Department of Veterans Affairs cooperative study. Respiration 1992;59:215.
86. Despars JA, Sassoon CSH, Light RW: Significance of iatrogenic pneumothoraces. Chest 1994;105:1147.
87. Zimmerman JE, Dunbar BS, Klingenmaier CH: Management of subcutaneous emphysema, pneumomediastinum, and pneumothorax during respirator therapy. Crit Care Med 1975;3:69.
88. de Lassence A, Timsit J-F, Tafflet M, et al: Pneumothorax in the intensive care unit: Incidence, risk factors and outcome. Anesthesiology 2006;104:5.
89. Leith DE: Barotrauma in human research (editorial). Crit Care Med 1976;4:159.
90. Marino PJ (ed): The ICU Book, 3rd ed. Philadelphia, Lippincott Williams & Wilkins, 2007, p 466.
91. Petersen GW, Baier H: Incidence of pulmonary barotrauma in a medical ICU. Crit Care Med 1983;11:67.
92. Johnson TH, Altman AR: Pulmonary interstitial gas: First sign of barotrauma due to PEEP therapy. Crit Care Med 1979;7:532.
93. Woodring JH: Pulmonary interstitial emphysema in the adult respiratory distress syndrome. Crit Care Med 1985;13:786.
94. Jantz MA, Pierson DJ: Pneumothorax and barotrauma. Clin Chest Med 1994;15:75.
95. Varon J, Busch LE, Sternbach GL: Another complication of barotrauma (letter). Chest 1992;102:1306.
96. Bejvan SM, Godwin JD: Pneumomediastinum: Old signs and new signs. AJR 1996;166:1041.
97. Steir M, Ching N, Roberts EB, et al: Pneumothorax complicating continuous ventilatory support. J Thorac Cardiovasc Surg 1974;67:17.
98. Bone RC, Francis PB, Pierce AK: Pulmonary barotrauma complicating positive end expiratory pressure (abstract). Am Rev Respir Dis 1975;111:921.
99. de Latorre FJ, Tomasa A, Klamburg J: Incidence of pneumothorax and pneumomediastinum in patients with aspiration pneumonia requiring ventilatory support. Chest 1977;72: 141.
100. Haake R, Schlichtig R, Ulstad DR, et al: Barotrauma: Pathophysiology, risk factors and prevention. Chest 1987;91:608.
101. Weg JG, Anzueto A, Balk RA, et al: The relation of pneumothorax and other air leaks to mortality in the acute respiratory distress syndrome. N Engl J Med 1998;338:341.

102. Stewart TE, Meade MO, Cook DJ, et al: Evaluation of a ventilator strategy to prevent barotrauma in patients at high risk for acute respiratory distress syndrome. N Engl J Med 1998;339:355.
103. Dreyfuss D, Saumon G: Ventilator-induced lung injury. Lessons from experimental studies. Am J Respir Crit Care Med 1998;157:294.
104. The Acute Respiratory Distress Syndrome Network: Ventilation with lower tidal volumes as compared with traditional tidal volumes for acute lung injury and the acute respiratory distress syndrome. N Engl J Med 2000;342:1301.
105. Milam MG, Evins AE, Sahn SA: Immediate chest roentgenography following fiberoptic bronchoscopy. Chest 1989;96:477.
106. Frazier WD, Pope TL Jr, Findely LJ: Pneumothorax following transbronchial biopsy: Low diagnostic yield with routine chest roentgenograms. Chest 1990;97:539.
107. Blasco LH, Hernandez IMS, Grarrido UV, et al: Safety of the transbronchial biopsy in outpatients. Chest 1991;99:562.
108. Izbicki G, Shitrit D, Yarmolovsky A, et al: Is routine chest radiography after transbronchial biopsy necessary? A prospective study of 350 cases. Chest 2006;129:1561.
109. Reichenberger F, Weber J, Tamm M, et al: The value of transbronchial needle aspiration in the diagnosis of peripheral pulmonary lesions. Chest 1999;116:704.
110. Poe RH, Kallay MC, Wicks CM, et al: Predicting risk of pneumothorax in needle biopsy of the lung. Chest 1984;85:232.
111. Hill PC, Spagnolo SV, Hockstein MJ: Pneumothorax with fine-needle aspiration of thoracic lesions. Is spirometry a predictor? Chest 1993;104:1017.
112. Falguera M, Nogues A, Ruiz-Gonzalez A, et al: Transthoracic needle aspiration in the study of pulmonary infections in patients with HIV. Chest 1994;106:697.
113. Larscheid RC, Thorpe PE, Scott WJ: Percutaneous transthoracic needle aspiration biopsy: A comprehensive review of its current role in the diagnosis and treatment of lung tumors. Chest 1998;114:704.
114. Miller KS, Fish GB, Stanley JH, et al: Prediction of pneumothorax rate in percutaneous aspiration of the lung. Chest 1988;93:742.
115. Fish GD, Stanley JH, Miller KS, et al: Postbiopsy pneumothorax: Estimating the risk by chest radiography and pulmonary function tests. AJR Am J Roentgenol 1988;150:71.
116. Anderson CL, Crespo JS, Lie TH: Risk of pneumothorax not increased by obstructive lung disease in percutaneous needle biopsy. Chest 1994;105:1705.
117. Kazerooni EA, Hartker FW III, Whyte RI, et al: Transthoracic needle aspiration in patients with severe emphysema. A study of lung transplant candidates. Chest 1996;109:616.
118. Traill ZC, Gleeson FV: Delayed pneumothorax after CT-guided percutaneous fine needle aspiration lung biopsy. Thorax 1997;52:581.
119. Choi C-M, Um S-W, Yoo C-G et al. Incidence and risk factors of delayed pneumothorax after transthoracic needle biopsy of the lung. Chest 2004;126:151,
120. Shepard JW: Thoracentesis: a safer needle, Am Rev Respir Dis 1980; 121(suppl):188.
121. Collins TR, Sahn SA: Thoracentesis: complications, patient experience and diagnostic value, Am Rev Respir Dis 1983;127:A114.
122. Kohan JM, Poe RH, Israel RH, et al: Value of chest ultrasonography versus decubitus roentgenography for thoracentesis. Am Rev Respir Dis 1986;133:1124.
123. Seneff MG, Corwin RW, Gold LH, et al: Complications associated with thoracentesis. Chest 1986;90:97.
124. Grogan DR, Irwin RS, Channick R, et al: Complications associated with thoracentesis: A prospective, randomized study comparing three different methods. Arch Intern Med 1990;150:873.
125. Swinburne AJ, Bixby K, Fedullo AJ, et al: Pneumothorax after thoracentesis (letter). Arch Intern Med 1991;151:2095.
126. Raptopoulos V, Davis LM, Lee G, et al: Factors affecting the development of pneumothorax associated with thoracentesis. AJR Am J Roentgenol 1991;156:917.
127. Feller-Kopman D: Ultrasound-guided thoracentesis. Chest 2006;129:1709.
128. Colt HG, Brewer N, Barbur E: Evaluation of patient-related and procedure-related factors contributing to pneumothorax following thoracentesis. Chest 1999;116:134.
129. Aleman C, Alegre J, Armadans L, et al: The value of chest roentgenography in the diagnosis of pneumothorax after thoracentesis. Am J Med 1999;107:340.
130. Chakrabarti B, Ryland I, Sheard J, et al: The role of Abrams percutaneous pleural biopsy in the investigation of exudative pleural effusion. Chest 2006;129:1549.
131. James RH: An unusual complication of passing a narrow bore nasogastric tube, Anesthesia 1978;33:716.
132. Hollimon PW, McFee AS: Pneumothorax attributable to nasogastric tube. Arch Surg 1981;116:970.
133. Torrington KG, Bowman MA: Fatal hydrothorax and empyema complicating a malpositioned nasogastric tube. Chest 1981;79:240.
134. Hand RW, Kempster M, Levy JH, et al: Inadvertent transbronchial insertion of narrow-bore feeding tubes into the pleural space. JAMA 1984;251:2396.
135. Scholten DJ, Wood TL, Thompson DR: Pneumothorax from nasogastric feeding tube insertion: A report of five cases. Am Surg 1986;52:381.
136. Wendell GD, Lenchner GS, Promisloff RA: Pneumothorax complicating small-bore feeding tube placement. Arch Intern Med 1991;151:599.
137. Dobranowski J, Fitzgerald JM, Baxter F, et al: Incorrect positioning of nasogastric feeding tubes and the development of pneumothorax. Can Assoc Radiol J 1992;43:35.
138. Kiwak MG, McLoud TC, Dedrick CG, et al: Entriflex feeding tube: Need for care in using it. AJR Am J Roentgenol 1984;143:1341.
139. Marderstein EL, Simmons RL, Ochoa JB: Patient safety: Effect of institutional protocols on adverse events related to feeding tube placement in the critically ill. J Am Coll Surg 2004; 199:39.
140. Ciaglia P, Firsching R, Syniec C: Elective percutaneous dilational tracheostomy: A new simple bedside procedure; preliminary report. Chest 1985;87:715 (Abstract).
141. Fikkers BG, van Veen JA, Kooloos JG, et al: Emphysema and pneumothorax after percutaneous tracheostomy. Case reports and an anatomic study. Chest 2004;125:1805.
142. Nishioka M, Fukuoka M, Nakagawa K, et al: Spontaneous pneumothorax following partial resolution of total bronchial obstruction. Chest 1993;104:160.
143. Woodring JH, Baker MD, Stark P: Pneumothorax ex vacuo. Chest 1996;110:1102.
144. Boland GW, Gazelle GS, Girard MJ, et al: Asymptomatic hydropneumothorax after therapeutic thoracentesis for malignant pleural effusion. AJR Am J Roentgenol 1998;170:943.
145. Jantz MA, Antony VB: Pleural fibrosis. Clin Chest Med 2006;27:181.
146. Levy AS, Bassett F, Lintner S, et al: Pulmonary barotrauma: Diagnosis in American football players. Three cases in three years. Am J Sports Med 1996;24:227.
147. Patridge RA, Coley A, Bowie R, et al: Sports-related pneumothorax. Ann Emerg Med 1997;30:539.
148. Kizer KW, MacQuarrie MB: Pulmonary air leaks resulting from outdoor sports. A clinical series and literature review. Am J Sports Med 1999;27:517.
149. Tetzlaff K, Reuter M, Leplow B, et al: Risk factors for pulmonary barotrauma in divers, Chest 1997;112:654.
150. Neuman TS, Clausen JL: Recommend caution in defining risk factors for barotrauma in divers (letter). Chest 1998;114:1791.
151. Raymond LW: Pulmonary barotrauma and related events in divers. Chest 1995;107:1648.
152. Silbergleit R, Lee DC, Blank-Reid C, et al: Sudden severe barotrauma from self-inflating bag-valve devices. J Trauma 1996;40:320.
153. Mumford AD, Ashkan K, Elborn S: Clinically significant pulmonary barotrauma after inflation of party balloons. BMJ 1996;313;1619.
154. Oppenheim A, Pizov R, Pikarsky A, et al: Tension pneumoperitoneum after blast injury: Dramatic improvement in ventilatory and hemodynamic parameters after surgical decompression. J Trauma 1998;44:915.
155. Pizov R, Oppenheim-Eden A, Matot I, et al: Blast lung injury from an explosion on a civilian bus. Chest 1999;115:165.

156. Broome CR, Jarvis LJ, Clark RJ: Pulmonary barotrauma in submarine escape training. Thorax 1994;49:186.
157. Morgenstern K, Talucci R, Kaufman MS, et al: Bilateral pneumothorax following airbag deployment. Chest 1998;114:624.
158. Manco JC, Terra-Filho J, Silva GA: Pneumomediastinum, pneumothorax and subcutaneous emphysema following the measurement of maximal expiratory pressure in a normal subject. Chest 1990;98:1530.
159. Seremetis MG: The management of spontaneous pneumothorax. Chest 1970;57:65.
160. Vail WJ, Alway AE, England NJ: Spontaneous pneumothorax. Chest 1960;38:512.
161. Scadding JG, Wood P: Systolic clicks due to left sided pneumothorax. Lancet 1939;2:1208.
162. Roelandt J, Willems J, van der Hauwaert LG, et al: Clicks and sounds (whoops) in left sided pneumothorax: Clinical and phonocardiographic study. Dis Chest 1969;56:31.
163. Desser KB, Bechimol A: Clicks secondary to pneumothorax confounding the diagnosis of mitral valve prolapse. Chest 1977; 71:523.
164. Sataline LR, Kraus T: Horner's syndrome occurring with spontaneous pneumothorax. N Engl J Med 1965;272:1227.
165. Aston SJ, Rosove M: Horner's syndrome occurring with spontaneous pneumothorax. N Engl J Med 1972;287:1098.
166. Widder D: Ptosis associated with iatrogenic pneumothorax: A false lateralizing sign. Arch Intern Med 1982;142:145.
167. Orriols R: A new physical sign in pneumothorax. Ann Intern Med 1987;107:255.
168. Wiedemann HP, Matthay MA, Matthay RA: Cardiovascular-pulmonary monitoring in the intensive care unit (part 2). Chest 1984;85:656.
169. Glauser FL, Polatty RC, Sessler CN: Worsening oxygenation in the mechanically ventilated patient: causes, mechanisms, and early detection. Am Rev Respir Dis 1988;138:458.
170. Schorlemmer GR, Khouri RK, Murray GF, et al: Bilateral pneumothoraces secondary to iatrogenic buffalo chest; an unusual complication of median sternotomy and subclavian catheterization. Ann Surg 1984;199:372 (Abstract).
171. Paranjpe DV, Wittich GR, Hamid LW, et al: Frequency and management of pneumothoraces in heart-lung transplant recipients. Radiology 1994;190:255 (Abstract).
172. Wittich GR, Kusnick CA, Starness VA, et al: Communication between the two pleural cavities after major cardiothoracic surgery: Relevance to percutaneous intervention. Radiology 1992;184:461 (Abstract).
173. Engler CE, Olson PN, Engler CM, et al: Shifting pneumothorax after heart-lung transplantation. Radiology 1992;185:715 (Abstract).
174. Johri S, Berlin D, Sanders A: Bilateral pneumothoraces after unilateral transthoracic needle biopsy of a lung nodule. Chest 2003;123:1297.
175. Sayar A, Turna A, Metin M, et al: Simultaneous bilateral spontaneous pneumothorax report of 12 cases and review of literature. Acta Chir Belg 2004;104:572 (Abstract).
176. Copeland RB, Omenn GS: Electrocardiogram changes suggestive of coronary artery disease in pneumothorax: Their reversibility with upright posture. Arch Intern Med 1970;125:151.
177. Walston A, Brewer DL, Kitchens CS, et al: The electrocardiographic manifestations of spontaneous left pneumothorax. Ann Intern Med 1974;80:375.
178. Ruo W, Rupani G: Left tension pneumothorax mimicking myocardial ischemia after percutaneous central venous cannulation. Anesthesiology 1992;76:306.
179. Alikhan M, Biddison JH: Electrocardiographic changes with right-sided pneumothorax. South Med J 1998;91:677.
180. Strizik B, Forman R: New ECG changes associated with a tension pneumothorax. Chest 1999;115:1742.
181. Buckner CB, Harmon BH, Pallin JS: The radiology of abnormal intrathoracic air. Curr Probl Diagn Radiol 1988;17:43.
182. Bradley M, Williams C, Walshaw MJ: The value of routine expiratory chest films in the diagnosis of pneumothorax. Arch Emerg Med 1991;8:115.
183. Seow A, Kazerooni EA, Cascade PN, et al: Comparison of upright inspiratory and expiratory chest radiographs for detecting pneumothoraces. AJR 1996;166:313.
184. Schramel FM, Golding RP, Haakman CDE, et al: Expiratory chest radiographs do not improve visibility of small apical pneumothoraces by enhanced contrast. Eur Respir J 1996;9:406.
185. Kollef MH: Risk factors for the misdiagnosis of pneumothorax in the intensive care unit. Crit Care Med 1991;19:906.
186. Rhea JT, van Sonnenberg E, McLoud TC: Basilar pneumothorax in the supine adult. Radiology 1979;133:593.
187. Gordon R: The deep sulcus sign. Radiology 1980;136:25.
188. Ziter FMH, Westcott JL: Supine subpulmonary pneumothorax. AJR Am J Roentgenol 1981;137:699.
189. Chiles C, Ravin CE: Radiographic recognition of pneumothorax in the intensive care unit. Crit Care Med 1986;14:677.
190. Swensen SJ, Peters SG, LeRoy AJ, et al: Radiology in the intensive care unit. Mayo Clin Proc 1991;66:396.
191. Roddy LH, Unger KM, Miller WC: Thoracic computed tomography in the critically ill patient. Crit Care Med 1981;9:515.
192. Hall JB, White SR, Karrison T: Efficacy of daily routine chest radiographs in intubated, mechanically ventilated patients. Crit Care Med 1991;19:689.
193. Phillips GD, Trotman-Dickenson B, Hodson ME, et al: Role of CT in management of pneumothorax in patients with complex cystic lung disease. Chest 1997;112:275.
194. Lichtenstein DA, Menu Y: A bedside ultrasound sign ruling out pneumothorax in the critically ill. Chest 1995;108:1345.
195. Lichtenstein D, Meziere G, Biderman P, et al: A comet-tail artefact: An ultrasound sign ruling out pneumothorax. Intensive Care Med 1999;25:383.
196. Baumann MH, Strange C: The clinician's perspective on pneumothorax management. Chest 1997;112:822.
197. Olsen CM: Spontaneous pneumothorax management guidelines previewed. Pulm Rev 2000;5:1.
198. Rhea JT, DeLuca SA, Greene RE: Determining the size of pneumothorax in the upright patient. Radiology 1982;144:733.
199. Light RW, Broaddus VC: Pneumothorax, chylothorax, hemothorax and fibrothorax. In Murray JF, Nadel JA (eds): Textbook of Respiratory Medicine, 3rd ed. Philadelphia, WB Saunders Company, 2000.
200. Choi BG, Park SH, Yun EH, et al: Pneumothorax size: Correlation of supine anteroposterior with erect posteroanterior chest radiographs. Radiology 1998;209:567.
201. Engdahl O, Toft T, Boe J: Chest radiograph—a poor method for determining the size of a pneumothorax. Chest 1993;103:26.
202. Cannon WB, Mark JBD, Jamplis RW: Pneumothorax: A therapeutic update. Am J Surg 1981;142:26.
203. Chernick V, Avery ME: Spontaneous alveolar rupture at birth. Pediatrics 1963;32:816.
204. Northfield TC: Oxygen therapy for spontaneous pneumothorax. BMJ 1971;4:86.
205. Hamilton AAD, Archer GJ: Treatment of pneumothorax by simple aspiration. Thorax 1983;38:934.
206. Jones JS: A place for aspiration in the treatment of spontaneous pneumothorax. Thorax 1985;40:66.
207. Archer GJ, Hamilton AAD, Upadhya R, et al: Results of simple aspiration of pneumothoraces. Br J Dis Chest 1985;79:177.
208. Brochard L, Dreyfuss D, Andrivet P, et al: Spontaneous pneumothorax (SP): Comparison of simple aspiration and tube thoracostomy. Am Rev Respir Dis 1991;143(Suppl):A659.
209. Wung JT, Raker R, Driscoll JM Jr, et al: A spring-loaded needle for emergency evacuation of pneumothorax. Crit Care Med 1978;6:378.
210. Harvey JE, Jeyasingham K: The difficult pneumothorax. Br J Dis Chest 1987;81:209.
211. Noppen M, Alexander P, Driesen P, et al: Manual aspiration versus chest tube drainage in first episodes of primary spontaneous pneumothorax. A multicenter, prospective, randomized pilot study. Am J Respir Crit Care Med 2002;165:1240.
212. Devanand A, Koh MS, Ong TH, et al: Simple aspiration versus chest-tube insertion in the management of primary spontaneous pneumothorax:

A systematic review. Respir Med 2004;98:579.
213. Miller KS, Sahn SA: Chest tubes: indications, techniques, management and complications. Chest 1987;91:258.
214. Shaw TJ, Caterine JM: Recurrent re-expansion pulmonary edema. Chest 1984;86:784.
215. Bell RL, Ovadia P, Abdullah F, et al: Chest tube removal: End-inspiration or end-expiration? J Trauma 2001;50:674.
216. Resnick DK: Delayed pulmonary perforation: A rare complication of the tube thoracostomy. Chest 1993;103:311.
217. Streitz JM Jr, Karlson KJ: Complications of percutaneous dart therapy in management of pneumothorax. Chest 1991;99:1549.
218. Conces DJ, Tarver RD, Gray WC, et al: Treatment of pneumothoraces utilizing small caliber chest tubes. Chest 1988;94:55.
219. Laub M, Milman N, Muller D, et al: Role of small caliber chest tube drainage for iatrogenic pneumothorax. Thorax 1990;45:748.
220. Liu CM, Hang LW, Chen WK, et al: Pigtail tube drainage in the treatment of spontaneous pneumothorax. Am J Emerg Med 2003;21:241.
221. Samelson SL, Goldberg EM, Ferguson MK: The thoracic vent: Clinical experience with a new device for treating simple pneumothorax. Chest 1991;100:880.
222. Martin T, Fontana G, Olak J, et al: Use of a pleural catheter for the management of simple pneumothorax. Chest 1996;110:1169.
223. Gobbel WG Jr, Rhea WG Jr, Nelson IA, et al: Spontaneous pneumothorax. J Thorac Cardiovasc Surg 1963;46:331.
224. Hart GJ, Stokes TC, Couch AHC: Spontaneous pneumothorax in Norfolk. Br J Dis Chest 1983;77:164.
225. Heffner JE, Huggins JT. Management of secondary spontaneous pneumothorax. There is confusion in the air. Chest 2004;124:1190.
226. Heffner JE, Unruh LC: Tetracycline pleurodesis: adios, farewell, adieu. Chest 1992;101:5.
227. Kennedy L, Sahn SA: Talc pleurodesis for the treatment of pneumothorax and pleural effusion. Chest 1994;106:1215.
228. Lange P, Mortensen J, Groth S: Lung function 22-35 years after treatment of idiopathic spontaneous pneumothorax with talc poudrage or simple drainage. Thorax 1988;43:559.
229. Weeden D, Smith GH: Surgical experience in the management of spontaneous pneumothorax, 1972-82. Thorax 1983;38:737.
230. Lau OJ, Shawkat S: Pleurectomy through the triangle of auscultation. Thorax 1982;37:945.
231. Behl PR, Holden MP: Pleurectomy for recurrent pneumothorax (letter). Chest 1983;84:785.
232. Murray KD, Matheny RG, Howanitz EP, et al: A limited axillary thoracotomy as primary treatment for recurrent spontaneous pneumothorax. Chest 1993;103:137.
233. Wakabayashi A: Thoracoscopic ablation of blebs in the treatment of recurrent or persistent spontaneous pneumothorax. Ann Thorac Surg 1989;48:651.
234. Torre M, Belloni P: Nd:YAG laser pleurodesis through thoracoscopy: New curative therapy in spontaneous pneumothorax. Ann Thorac Surg 1989;47:887.
235. Nathason LK, Shimi SM, Wood RAB, et al: Videothoracoscopic ligation of bulla and pleurectomy for spontaneous pneumothorax. Ann Thorac Surg 1991;52:316.
236. Kimmel RD, Karp MP, Cascone JJ, et al: Talc pleurodesis during videothoracoscopy for *Pneumocystis carinii* pneumonia-related pneumothorax. A new technique. Chest 1994;105:314.
237. Tschopp JM, Brutsche M, Frey JG: Treatment of complicated spontaneous pneumothorax by simple talc pleurodesis under thoracoscopy and local anesthesia. Thorax 1997;52:329.
238. Nkere UU, Griffin SC, Fountain SW: Pleural abrasion: A new method of pleurodesis. Thorax 1991;46:596.
239. Colt HG: Thoracoscopy: New frontiers. Pulm Perspect 1992;9:1.
240. Ayed AK: Bilateral video-assisted thoracoscopic surgery for bilateral spontaneous pneumothorax. Chest 2002;122:223.
241. Watanabe S, Sakasegawa K, Kariatsumari K, et al: Bilateral video-assisted thoracoscopic surgery in the supine position for primary spontaneous pneumothorax. Thorac Cardiovasc Surg 2004;52:42.
242. Wait MA, Dal Nogare AR: Treatment of AIDS-related spontaneous pneumothorax. A decade of experience. Chest 1994;106:693.
243. Griffith BP, Hardesty RL, Trento A, et al: Heart-lung transplantation: Lessons learned and future hopes. Ann Thorac Surg 1987;43:6.
244. Noyes BE, Orenstein DM: Treatment of pneumothorax in cystic fibrosis in the era of lung transplantation (editorial). Chest 1992;101:1187.
245. Slabbynck H, Laureys M, Impens N, et al: Recurring catamenial pneumothorax treated with a Gn-RH analogue. Chest 1991; 100:851.
246. Lillington GH, Mitchell SP, Wood GA: Catamenial pneumothorax. JAMA 1972;219:1328.
247. Stern H, Toole AL, Merino M: Catamenial pneumothorax. Chest 1980;78:480.
248. Terndrup TE, Bosco SF, McLean ER: Spontaneous pneumothorax complicating pregnancy—case report and review of the literature. J Emerg Med 1989;7:245.
249. AMA Commission on Emergency Medical Services: Medical aspects of transportation board commercial aircraft. JAMA 1982;247:1007.
250. Stonehill RB, Fess SW: Commercial air transportation of a patient recovering from pneumothorax. Chest 1973;63:300.
251. Sihoe ADL, Wong RHL, Lee ATH, et al: Severe acute respiratory distress syndrome complicated by spontaneous pneumothorax. Chest 2004;125:2345.
252. Felice GA: SARS, pneumothorax and our response to epidemics. Editorial. Chest 2004;125:1982.
253. Almoosa KF, Ryu JH, Mendez J, et al: Lymphangioleiomyomatosis. Management of pneumothorax in lymphangioleiomyomatosis. Effects on recurrence and lung transplantation complications. Chest 2006;129:1274.
254. Chee CBE, Abisheganaden J, Yeo JKS, et al: Persistent air leak in spontaneous pneumothorax-clinical course and outcome. Resp Med 1998;92:757.
255. Cerfolio RJ, Tummala RP, Holman WL, et al: A prospective algorithm for the management of air leaks after pulmonary resection. Ann Thorac Surg 1998;66:1726.
256. Dumire R, Crabbe MM, Mappin FG, et al: Autologous "blood patch" pleurodesis for persistent pulmonary air leak. Chest 1992;101:64.
257. Ando M, Yamamoto M, Kitagawa C, et al: Autologous blood patch pleurodesis for secondary spontaneous pneumothorax with persistent air leak. Resp Med 1999;93:432.
258. Kinoshita T, Miyoshi S, Katoh M, et al: Intrapleural administration of a large amount of diluted fibrin glue for intractable pneumothorax. Chest 2000;117:790.
259. Baumann MH, Sahn SA: Medical management and therapy of bronchopleural fistulas in the mechanically ventilated patient. Chest 1990;97:721.
260. Gilby EM, McLean NR, Morritt GN: Pectoral myoplasty for recurrent pneumothorax: An extrathoracic solution to an intrathoracic problem. Ann R Coll Surg England 1999;81:154.
261. Murata A, Kouno A, Yamamato K, et al: The treatment of refractory pneumothorax in diffuse panbronchiolitis by intravenous administration of coagulation factor XIII concentrate. J Nippon Med Sch 2006;73:89 (Abstract).
262. Ferguson JS, Sprenger K, Van Natta T: Closure of a bronchopleural fistula using bronchoscopic placement of an endobronchial valve designed for the treatment of emphysema. Chest 2006;129:479.
263. Ziskind MM, Weill H, George RA: Acute pulmonary edema following treatment of spontaneous pneumothorax with excessive negative intrapleural pressure. Am Rev Respir Dis 1965;92:632.
264. Matsuura Y, Nomimura T, Murakami H, et al: Clinical analysis of reexpansion pulmonary edema. Chest 1991;100:1562.
265. Childress ME, Moy G, Mottram M: Unilateral pulmonary edema resulting from treatment of spontaneous pneumothorax. Am Rev Respir Dis 1971;104:119.
266. Miller WC, Toon R, Palat H, et al: Experimental pulmonary edema following re-expansion of pneumothorax. Am Rev Respir Dis 1973;108:664.
267. Sprung CL, Loewenherz JW, Baier H, et al: Evidence for increased permeability in reexpansion pulmonary edema. Am J Med 1981;71:497.

268. Wilkinson PD, Keegan J, Davies SW, et al: Changes in pulmonary microvascular permeability accompanying re-expansion oedema: Evidence from dual isotope scintigraphy. Thorax 1990;45:456.
269. Ragozzino MW, Greene R: Bilateral reexpansion pulmonary edema following unilateral pleurocentesis. Chest 1991;99:506.
270. Pavlin DJ, Raghu G, Rogers TR, et al: Reexpansion hypotension: A complication of rapid evacuation of prolonged pneumothorax. Chest 1986;89:70.
271. Henderson AF, Banham SW, Moran F: Re-expansion pulmonary edema: A potentially serious complication of delayed diagnosis of pneumothorax. BMJ 1985;291:593.
272. Wong CF, Cohen MAH, Chan MS: PEEP ventilation—the treatment for life-threatening re-expansion pulmonary edema. Respir Med 1991;85:69.
273. Mainini SE, Johnson FE: Tension pneumothorax complicating small-caliber chest tube insertion. Chest 1990;97:759.
274. Spouge AR, Thomas HA: Tension pneumothorax after reversal of a Heimlich valve. AJR Am J Roentgenol 1992;158:763.
275. Baumann MH, Strange C: Treatment of spontaneous pneumothorax. A more aggressive approach? Chest 1997;112:789.
276. Baumann MH, Strange C, Heffner JE, et al: Management of spontaneous pneumothorax. An American College of Chest Physicians Delphi Consensus Statement. Chest 2001;119:590.
277. Henry M, Arnold T, Harvey J, on behalf of the BTS Pleural Disease Group, a subgroup of the BTS Standards of Care Committee: BTS guidelines for the management of spontaneous pneumothorax. Thorax 2003;58(Suppl)2:ii, 39.

Chapter 49

Toxic Gas, Fume, and Smoke Inhalation

M. Sean Kincaid, Sam R. Sharar, and Leonard D. Hudson

Inhalation injuries can be divided into two groups—those occurring with acute exposure (e.g., smoke inhalation at the scene of a fire) and those occurring with chronic exposure (e.g., cigarette smoking or occupational exposure to asbestos). The evaluation and treatment of these two types of inhalation injury are quite different. The latter requires the use of long-term surveillance techniques, a high reliance on epidemiologic analyses, and often intervention at a political/societal level to achieve a measurable impact on injury, usually with emphasis on injury prevention. A discussion of these chronic and occupational inhalation injuries is beyond the scope of this chapter; other sources cover them in depth.[1]

Acute exposure to toxic gases, fumes, or smoke can result in a wide spectrum of pulmonary or systemic disease, or both. In extreme cases the inhalation of toxic gases can result in massive casualties, such as the 1984 industrial gas leak of methyl isocyanate in Bhopal, India, which killed an estimated 3800 people,[2] or the intentional exposure to purportedly nonlethal gases in the 2002 Moscow theater incident that killed 127 individuals.[3] More commonly, however, inhalation of toxic substances occurs in small numbers of individuals in structural fires, isolated chemical accidents, or recreational drug use.

Because the mechanism of injury involves direct exposure of the respiratory airway or alveolar epithelium to irritant chemicals, acute or severe pulmonary dysfunction, or both, can often occur, requiring rapid assessment, diagnosis, and critical care intervention. Conversely, certain toxic gases (e.g., carbon monoxide) cause little pulmonary injury but rapidly cross the alveolar-capillary barrier to produce nonpulmonary organ injury from systemic exposure, whereas others simply alter physiology in a deleterious manner (e.g., respiratory depression and bradycardia from an inhaled fentanyl derivative).

The goal of this chapter is to provide the information necessary for the direct assessment and management of individuals with commonly seen inhalation injuries, especially those that cause pulmonary dysfunction. To that end, we emphasize smoke inhalation—occurring as an isolated event or associated with a concomitant cutaneous burn injury—as a paradigm of the approach to managing inhalation injuries.

HISTORY AND INCIDENCE

Civilian Disasters with Smoke Inhalation

Despite earlier reports linking smoke inhalation in patients rescued from fire scenes to their subsequent development of pulmonary dysfunction, the first thoughtful analysis of respiratory tract injury in cutaneous burn and smoke inhalation victims came from the 1942 Cocoanut Grove nightclub fire in Boston.[4] A total of 491 victims died either at the fire scene or during hospitalization. As identified by Cope[5] in his summary of the hospitalized victims, the onset of pulmonary insufficiency was delayed, being measured in hours rather than minutes. Many victims died with no sign of cutaneous burn injury. Cherry-red lips (consistent with carbon monoxide poisoning) were a regular feature on early physical examination. Soot in the oropharynx, combined with crowing respirations, indicated upper airway compromise and pending airway obstruction. Cope observed that the sequence of respiratory compromise in these victims was similar to that seen in World War I victims of phosgene poisoning,[6] an observation further confirmed by pulmonary histopathologic study. Despite the compelling evidence of inhalation injury in these victims, the possibility of an iatrogenic component of the pulmonary edema leading to respiratory failure (e.g., caused by excessive resuscitation) remains controversial because there were somewhat different clinical experiences in patients treated at Boston City Hospital.[7] In addition to furthering our understanding of smoke inhalation injury, this nightclub fire led to significant changes in the fire code. Because of a single revolving door at the main entrance and inadequate emergency exits, many people died simply because of the delay in leaving the building.

The importance of carbon monoxide poisoning in victims of isolated smoke inhalation injury during fires was further demonstrated in the 1980 MGM Grand Hotel fire in Las Vegas. Although only a small number of burn injuries occurred, 84 people died at the scene, primarily from carbon monoxide intoxication. By contrast, the efficacy of prompt assessment and treatment of smoke inhalation was demonstrated: in more than 400 individuals who received hospital evaluation for smoke inhalation injury, mortality was less than 1%, and the rate of significant complications (myocardial infarction, respiratory failure, or pneumonia) was low, only 1% for each.[8] More recent experience with institutional fires has supported this finding that with prompt medical care, the fatalities are predominantly those that occur at the scene from inhalation injury.[9] This fire, which caused numerous deaths because of smoke traveling upward through elevator shafts and stairwells, also resulted in changes to the fire code to improve public safety.

The Stardust Nightclub fire that claimed 48 lives in Dublin in 1981 added a great deal to our understanding of smoke inhalation injury because the disaster site was meticulously reconstructed and the event reenacted for scientific study. A review of these experimental studies[10] details the extreme life-threatening environmental conditions that can be produced in this type of fire. Within minutes, visibility was reduced to less than 1 m and ambient temperatures reached 1160°C (2120°F). Near the fire, dramatic changes in inhaled gas concentrations were noted, with oxygen reduced to less than 2% and carbon monoxide increased to greater than 3%. Hydrogen cyanide was measured at 250 ppm, and hydrogen chloride was measured at 8500 ppm.

Toxic Gas Inhalation

Already experienced with the use of tear gas (chloroacetophenone) in civilian demonstrations, the French first introduced this substance in the context of chemical warfare against the Germans in 1914.[11] The use of phosgene as an agent of chemical warfare was subsequently introduced by the Germans at the Battle of Ypres in 1915 and was called the *Green Cross* by German artillery.[12] In the 1920s the Germans, Soviets, and Japanese all developed active programs for the research and manufacture of toxic gases including mustard gas. It was from workers in these manufacturing plants that the neoplastic hazards of multiple and long-term exposures were first identified. Concurrent with the use of mustard gases by the Chinese and Italians in military encounters in the 1930s, the Germans developed and stockpiled large quantities of a different class of inhaled toxin with anticholinesterase properties: the organophosphates. Despite both sides in the conflict having access to these new "nerve gas" agents, these and other chemical agents were never used in military ventures during World War II, in accordance with the 1925 Chemical Weapons Convention that prohibited first use of such weapons. Despite the subsequent 1972 Biologic Weapons Convention that prohibited production and stockpiling of both chemical and biologic weapons, military use of nitrogen mustards was documented as recently as the 1980 Iran-Iraq War[13] and the 1988 Iraqi-Kurd Civil War.[14] In addition, inhaled chemical and biologic weapons have been used on a small scale as acts of terrorism in incidents such as the 1994 and 1995 sarin gas attacks in Japan[15] and the 2001 spread of anthrax through the U.S. mail.[16]

Incidence of Inhalation Injury

The incidence of inhalation injury caused by exposure to toxic gases or smoke is difficult to quantify. Burn injury ranges between the third and sixth most common cause of unintentional injury-related death across all age ranges,[17] but the incidence of inhalation injury is uncertain because the frequency of smoke inhalation injury in victims of fire varies with diagnostic criteria. The incidence may be as low as 2% to 15% when single or restrictive criteria based on history and physical examination are used, but as high as 20% to 30% when based on objective tests such as fiberoptic bronchoscopy or radionuclide scanning.[18] The overall incidence of smoke inhalation in the United States has fallen, primarily as a result of the legislated use of home smoke detection monitors. As of 2004 approximately 96% of homes in the United States had at least one smoke detector.[19] Further improvements in prevention have been hindered by the difficulty of ensuring that monitors remain functional, however. Although progress has been made with the development of the 10-year lithium battery and with hard-wired smoke detectors, many are intentionally disabled by the home occupants. It has been estimated that 60% to 70% of all deaths from house fires can be attributed to carbon monoxide poisoning, whereas only 25% to 30% are the result of burn injury.[20]

The unintentional death rate in the United States from carbon monoxide generated by motor vehicle exhaust is roughly 1 per 100,000 population for each decade of age group between 15 and 90 years, equivalent to the rate of unintentional death from all other gases and vapors (excluding structural fires).[20] The corresponding suicide rate for carbon monoxide generated by motor vehicle exhaust ranges from 2 to 4 per 100,000 for each decade of age group between 20 and 90 years and is maximal in the fifth decade of life. Unintentional poisoning by natural gas has decreased 10-fold since the 1940s, with the increased reliance in the United States on electric stoves and home heating by electricity and oil.

PATHOGENESIS

Smoke Inhalation Injury

The inhalation of combustion (flaming) or pyrolysis (smoldering) products in smoke from a fire causes direct tissue injury to the respiratory tract by two primary mechanisms: heat and chemical irritation. In addition, inhalation of certain toxic substances (e.g., carbon monoxide, cyanide) found in smoke can result in systemic effects beyond the confines of the lung. Finally, smoke inhalation concomitant with cutaneous burn injury occurs more frequently than either injury alone.[21] Because extensive cutaneous burn injury results in release of a variety of inflammatory mediators from injured skin and circulating leukocytes that can independently cause pulmonary dysfunction, the apparent pulmonary injury in victims with both smoke inhalation and burns is more severe than in individuals with either injury alone.

Respiratory Tract Heat Injury

Injury to the respiratory tract as a consequence of inhaling hot gas is usually immediate and consists of mucosal and submucosal edema, erythema, hemorrhage, and ulceration. Temperatures in excess of 1000° C have been recorded at fire scenes and are quite capable of causing significant airway injury. However, thermal injury is usually limited to the upper airway (above the vocal cords) and trachea for two reasons. First, the nasopharynx and oropharynx together provide an effective mechanism for heat exchange because of their relatively large surface area and associated air turbulence, as well as their mucosal water lining, which acts as a heat reservoir.[22] Second, sudden exposure to hot air may trigger reflex closure of the vocal cords, reducing the potential for lower airway injury.[23] Animal experiments stimulated by the Boston Cocoanut Grove fire demonstrated that significant heat exchange also occurs in the airway segment between the vocal cords and the tracheal bifurcation, further protecting the lower airway. Combustion products delivered by means of transoral cannula in dogs at the level of the larynx decreased in temperature from greater than 300° C to 50° C when measured at the carina.[24] The clinical result of these anatomic and physical characteristics of the upper airway is that the lower airway is rarely exposed to hot, ambient gas at a fire scene. The one exception to these observations is in cases of superheated steam inhalation, in which, because of energy released in the respiratory tract as the steam condenses to water, severe injury has been reported in the lower airways, with measurable injury in the alveoli.[24] In this setting, steam at 100° C at the larynx may still be greater than 90° C at the carina.

Respiratory Tract Chemical Injury

One of the greatest complexities in studying smoke inhalation injuries, as well as a major variable that can determine the extent of injury, is the vast array of toxic products released during combustion or pyrolysis.[25] The type and quantity of smoke constituents produced depend on the type of fuel burned, whether burning occurs in a high- or low-oxygen environment, and the actual heat of combustion. For example, combustion of polyvinyl chloride (PVC) products commonly used as construction materials results in carbon monoxide production of 429 mg/g if the temperature rise is 3° C/minute, but only 269 mg/g if the temperature rise is significantly greater at 50° C/minute.[26] In addition, combustion of even a single fuel source (rarely the case in actual civilian fires) can result in a long list of chemical products.

The mechanisms of direct respiratory tract injury by each of these many smoke constituents are incompletely understood.[27] Inhaled smoke can produce pulmonary injury by direct chemical irritation, by interference with normal physiologic mechanisms (e.g., inhibition of mucociliary clearance or surfactant inactivation), or through oxidative or other tissue injury. The relative contribution of each mechanism in a given patient depends on a number of factors. This section focuses on the injury mechanisms of smoke constituents within the respiratory tract; a discussion of the mechanisms of systemic injury by toxic gases and fumes (including those produced in fires) follows in the next section.

Smoke inhalation can cause direct epithelial damage at all levels of the respiratory tract, from oropharynx to alveolus. The anatomic level at which damage occurs depends on the ventilatory pattern, the smoke constituents (e.g., particulate concentration, particulate size, and chemical components), and the anatomic distribution of particulate deposition. The clinical correlation between smoke type and anatomic level of inhalation injury in the respiratory tract has been reported by Alexeeff and colleagues,[28] who exposed spontaneously breathing rats to smoke from three fuel types—Douglas fir, polyurethane (high cyanide content), and polyvinyl chloride (high hydrogen chloride content). In histopathologic examination, all animals sustained immediate subglottic epithelial disruption and evidence of retained secretions and cellular debris that resolved over 21 days. However, rats exposed to fir smoke had their injury localized to the trachea and mainstem bronchi, whereas those exposed to polyurethane smoke primarily developed injury of the smaller conducting airways; PVC-exposed animals sustained even more distal injury, including alveolar disruption and pulmonary edema. These data suggest that the anatomic level of airway injury after smoke inhalation depends on smoke type; these findings may help explain the spectrum of physiologic abnormalities that can present with smoke inhalation.

Smoke exposure at the alveolar level also causes inactivation of endogenous surfactant. The effect is the immediate development of atelectasis that is slowly reversible with normal ventilation, as shown in open-chest animal studies.[29] In vitro analysis of lung extracts from these animals shows a threefold increase in minimum surface tension after smoke inhalation, indicating the tendency for alveolar collapse (Fig. 49-1). This effect on surfactant is aggravated by regional hypoventilation as a result of small airway obstruction, resulting in significant alveolar atelectasis, intrapulmonary shunt, and subsequent hypoxemia.

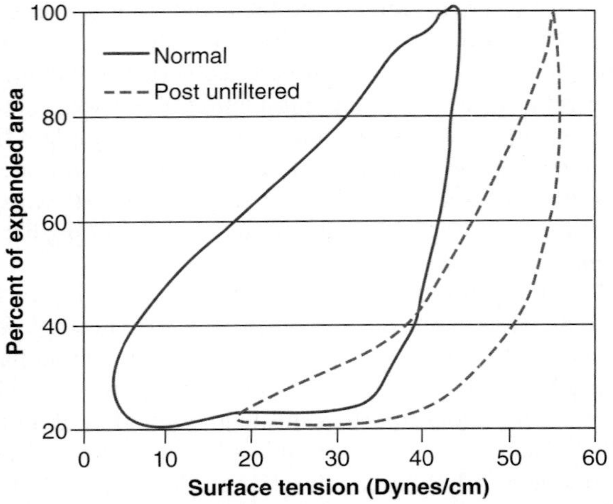

Figure 49-1. Surfactant analysis (determined by in vitro surface balance) of lung extracts taken from normal dogs and from dogs receiving 2 minutes of continuous exposure to smoke generated by combustion of fir plywood and kerosene. After smoke inhalation, there is a rapid and marked increase in the minimum surface tension, indicating either that less surfactant is available or that endogenous surfactant is no longer active. (From Nieman GF, Clark WR, Was SD, Webb WR: The effect of smoke inhalation on pulmonary surfactant. Ann Surg 1980;191:171.)

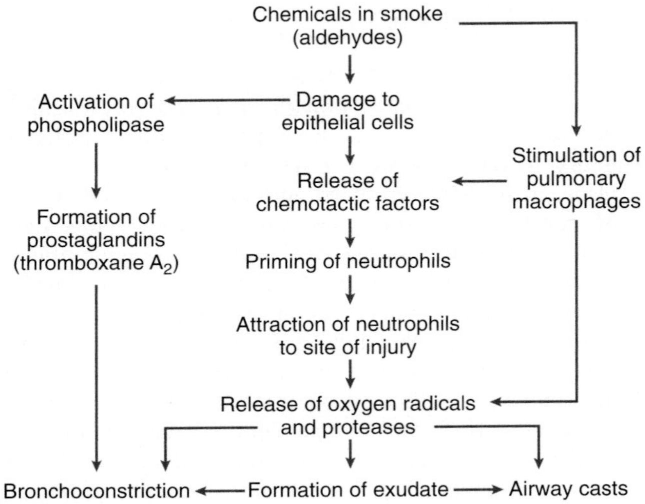

Figure 49-2. Pathophysiology of tracheobronchial damage by smoke inhalation. (From Traber LD, Herndon DN: Pathophysiology of smoke inhalation. In Haponik EF, Munster AM [eds]: Respiratory Injury: Smoke Inhalation and Burns. New York, McGraw-Hill, 1990.)

Chemical irritation of the respiratory tract causes an acute inflammatory response, with an initial approximately 10-fold increase in bronchial blood flow.[30] Concurrent with this is the stimulation of intrapulmonary macrophages, the release of chemotactic factors, the activation of circulating neutrophils that localize to the site of injury,[31] and the release of oxygen radicals and tissue proteases (Fig. 49-2) that results in changes in vascular permeability.[32,33] The result is the development of airway edema that, when combined with sloughing of necrotic epithelial mucosa and impairments of mucociliary clearance of secretions, produces airway obstruction in both small and large airways and a resultant ventilation inhomogeneity. The physiologic consequence is mismatched ventilation and perfusion, which results in hypoxemia.

A few individuals with smoke inhalation present clinically with immediate evidence of severely abnormal gas exchange and injury to the alveoli and have a clinical picture consistent with acute lung injury (ALI). This injury is more likely after inhalation with smoke generated from plastics,[34] after combined smoke inhalation and burn injury,[35] and after the onset of sepsis in patients with smoke inhalation and burn injury.[36,37] Reproducible models of both combined burn and inhalation injury,[38] as well as inhalation injury with sepsis, have been produced in sheep,[39] using cotton smoke insufflation with either concomitant burn or subsequent *Pseudomonas aeruginosa* instillation, respectively. The pulmonary edema observed in these models results from increased permeability of the pulmonary capillary endothelium and increased bronchial blood flow, which, in combination with impaired hypoxic pulmonary vasoconstriction, result in impaired gas exchange.[40] One factor that likely contributes to the pulmonary pathology is the increased nitric oxide (NO) production through upregulation of inducible NO synthase (iNOS).[41] As a vasodilator, NO not only increases blood flow in the lung but also impairs the lung's ability to direct blood away from nonventilated regions, resulting in ventilation-perfusion mismatch. NO may also react with other oxygen species to form peroxynitrite,[42] which causes tissue injury and thus gives rise to the increased capillary permeability and pulmonary edema. Further impairment of pulmonary function likely occurs as a result of airway obstruction by mechanisms described earlier.[43] In the sheep model, therapies that target NO production have been shown to decrease lung injury,[44,45] as have interventions to decrease free radicals[46] and mitigate cellular response to reactive nitrogen species.[47] Neutrophil protease is likely involved in airway injury, as inhaled antiprotease decreased fluid movement into the lung, and minimized smoke-related degradation in gas exchange in this sheep model.[48] Finally, both inhaled heparin and systemic activated protein C improve lung function, presumably via a decrease in airway obstruction.[49,50]

Cutaneous burn injury results in the systemic release of inflammatory mediators including prostaglandins and oxidants that can aggravate pulmonary injury independent of smoke inhalation. Thromboxane-A_2 released from burned tissue causes a variety of changes in the lung including pulmonary hypertension, reduced dynamic compliance, and increased lipid peroxidation.[51] Oxidants are generated as a consequence of neutrophil activation and increased xanthine oxidase[52] and contribute to lung injury. Finally, decreased plasma oncotic pressure caused by the loss of plasma protein through increasingly permeable vessels in both burned and unburned tissue creates an abnormal oncotic pressure gradient in the lung that, when combined with pulmonary hypertension, results in transient hydrostatic pulmonary edema.[53] These changes help explain the observations of comorbidity[21,54,55] in cases of combined inhalation and burn injuries. A recent study by Holm and colleagues[56] evaluating extravascular lung water in burn patients with inhalation injury calls into question the long-held belief that accumulation of fluid in the lung plays a significant role in poor pulmonary function in these patients, however.[56] Holm argues that pulmonary fluid accumulation may occur later in these patients, particularly in combination with sepsis, but not in the early resuscitation stage. This apparent conflict between animal and human studies may be explained by the differences in smoke constituents and other reasons, in particular varying severity of injury: the patients in Holm's study purportedly had combined burn and inhalation injury, yet none of the patients had an elevated carboxyhemoglobin level; in contrast, animal models of combined injury may have carboxyhemoglobin levels as high as 70%,[57] thus suggesting severe inhalation injury.

Toxic Gas Inhalation Injury

Toxic gases and fumes have origins in the combustion of certain fuels or from direct manufacture. The two toxic gases most commonly responsible for injury by inhalation, carbon monoxide and hydrogen cyanide, play major roles in smoke inhalation injury. Although inhalation of these compounds is usually accidental, these compounds are also associated with purposeful injury by attempted suicide or capital punishment. Highly water-soluble gases (e.g., aldehydes, ammonia, sulfur dioxide) and poorly soluble gases (e.g., phosgene, nitrogen dioxide) are also discussed. Of the long list of other industrial and recreational inhalants, little is known of their cellular pathogenesis. The clinical manifestations of their use are described in the subsequent section.

Carbon monoxide is a colorless, odorless, and tasteless gas with an affinity for hemoglobin 230 to 270 times that of oxygen. It is the product of incomplete combustion of carbonaceous fuels. Once inhaled and absorbed, carbon monoxide avidly binds to hemoglobin to form carboxyhemoglobin (COHb). COHb interferes with oxygen delivery to tissues by at least four mechanisms. First, in contrast to its high affinity for hemoglobin, oxygen has low affinity for COHb, resulting in decreased oxygen-carrying capacity in blood. Second, COHb shifts the oxygen-hemoglobin dissociation curve to the left, thereby decreasing oxygen unloading from normal hemoglobin at the tissue level. A further effect of carbon monoxide occurs at the tissue level, where it interferes with aerobic cellular metabolism. It inhibits the cytochrome oxidase a_3 complex, resulting in less effective intracellular respiration. Finally, carbon monoxide may also bind to myoglobin in both cardiac and skeletal muscle to cause direct toxicity. These mechanisms, in combination with the hypoxic environment found in many fires, act in concert to deprive cellular metabolism of essential oxygen.[58] In addition, carbon monoxide acts in the central nervous system (CNS) through multiple mechanisms[59] to cause early neurologic depression and late neuroanatomic abnormalities, with neurocognitive and affective impairment.[60]

Hydrogen cyanide, a common product of polyurethane combustion, also interferes with normal oxygen utilization at the tissue level but is a more effective inhibitor of cellular respiration than carbon monoxide. By inhibiting the final step of oxidative phosphorylation at the cytochrome a_3 level, cyanide halts aerobic metabolism, inducing lactic acidosis and cellular asphyxia. The effects of cyanide are specifically injurious to tissues with little anaerobic reserve, such as that of the CNS. Because of similar cellular injury mechanisms, combined exposure to cyanide and carbon monoxide (as occurs in many cases of smoke inhalation) results in a synergistic decrease in tissue oxygen utilization.[61] Although this effect is a plausible source of harm in humans, critical analysis of deaths from fire data has failed to demonstrate synergism and has yielded conflicting results with respect to the contribution of cyanide to human deaths.[58]

The water solubility of a toxic gas is a major determinant of whether airway or alveolar injury occurs. When inhaled, the highly soluble organic aldehydes produced by combustion/pyrolysis (e.g., formaldehyde, acetaldehyde, acrolein) rapidly dissolve into the water lining the mucosa of the upper and lower airways, causing direct epithelial injury. The result is epithelial necrosis, edema, and submucosal hemorrhage, primarily in the lower airways. Ammonia is also highly soluble and reacts with respiratory tract water to form ammonium hydroxide, a strong alkali. Inhaled sulfur dioxide becomes similarly hydrated and then oxidized to form both sulfurous and sulfuric acid. These caustic acids (including hydrogen chloride) and bases all cause significant mucosal coagulation and liquefaction necrosis, producing a similar injury pattern to that of the aldehydes. By contrast, phosgene, a compound of low water solubility, is deposited more distally in the respiratory tract, where it is hydrolyzed to hydrogen chloride and produces alveolar epithelial injury, pneumonia, and pulmonary edema. The nitrogen mustards, also poorly soluble, are converted to sulfonium ion, which is an alkylating agent causing DNA cross-linking, and produce subsequent injury to rapidly dividing epithelium in the respiratory tract and gut. Nitrogen mustard–induced airway injuries are characterized by hemorrhagic inflammation that can result in severe erosions of the airway wall and subsequent airway stenosis. The organophosphates (e.g., sarin, tabun) are anticholinesterase agents that affect cholinergically controlled glands and the smooth muscle respiratory tract to cause hypersecretion, bronchorrhea, and bronchospasm.

Lacrimatory agents including tear gas (chloroacetophenone) and related compounds are used in riot control. These agents are potent irritators of all mucous membranes, causing severe pain, upper airway edema (usually without stridor), and copious secretion production. At higher doses the distal respiratory tract can also be involved, resulting in pulmonary edema and intra-alveolar hemorrhage. Deaths from tear gas–induced pulmonary injury have been reported.[62,63]

CLINICAL MANIFESTATIONS

Respiratory Tract Injury

As suggested earlier, smoke inhalation can result in injury at three anatomic levels: upper airway, lower airway, and alveolus. Edema develops acutely in the upper airway (oral stoma, oropharynx, and larynx) and can lead to frank airway obstruction within 12 to 24 hours, if not sooner. Airway obstruction at the glottic level is often heralded by hoarse voice or stridor. Severe oropharyngeal edema can interfere with usual airway maintenance maneuvers such as laryngoscopy and endotracheal intubation and may necessitate surgical creation of an airway in the cricothyroid membrane. Acute inflammation and epithelial sloughing in the lower airways causes necrotic tracheobronchitis, retained secretions, and increased airway resistance. Wheezing, coughing, and production of carbonaceous sputum can be observed. The physiologic manifestations of these changes are atelectasis, mismatched ventilation and perfusion, and hypoxemia. In the rare cases of alveolar injury after an isolated instance of smoke inhalation, frothy sputum and cyanosis occur as a consequence of atelectasis, pulmonary edema, and intrapulmonary shunt and are often preceded by more subtle signs of hypoxemia (e.g., tachypnea and labored respirations in the absence of wheezing).

Systemic Responses

The cardinal physiologic manifestation of carbon monoxide poisoning is tissue hypoxia, particularly in the CNS and cardiovascular system. Patients with underlying coronary, cerebrovascular, and pulmonary diseases may be more sensitive to carbon monoxide intoxication, exhibiting signs of coronary ischemia (e.g., angina),[64] neurologic deficits, or respiratory failure, respectively. As COHb levels increase, symptoms progress as shown in Table 49-1, although with considerable variability among victims because of host factors. Consistent with the findings of poor peripheral oxygen delivery because of altered hemoglobin, blood gas analysis demonstrates normal arterial P_{O_2} but dramatically reduced arterial and mixed venous oxygen contents and mixed venous P_{O_2}.

Table 49-1. Signs and Symptoms of Carbon Monoxide Intoxication

Carboxyhemoglobin Level (%)	Clinical Manifestations
5-10	Mild headache, confusion
11-20	Throbbing headache, blurred vision, flushing of skin
21-30	Disorientation, nausea, impaired manual dexterity
31-40	Irritability, dizziness, vomiting, syncope
41-50	Tachypnea, tachycardia
50 and above	Coma, seizures, respiratory failure, death

From Sharar SR, Heimbach DM, Hudson LD: Management of inhalation injury in patients with and without burns. In Haponik EF, Munster AM (eds): Respiratory Injury: Smoke Inhalation and Burns. New York, McGraw-Hill, 1990.

Because cyanide intoxication results in severely impaired tissue oxygen utilization, arterial and mixed venous P_{O_2} and corresponding oxygen contents are normal. However, because anaerobic metabolism is maximal, significant metabolic and lactic acidoses are present. In fact, plasma lactate concentrations have been demonstrated to correlate with blood cyanide concentrations in human victims of smoke inhalation.[65] As with carbon monoxide poisoning, individuals with underlying cardiac or CNS dysfunction are less tolerant of cyanide intoxication than are normal individuals. Neurologic impairments (e.g., altered level of consciousness, dizziness, headache) appear early, usually preceded only by tachypnea and tachycardia. Unfortunately, these latter signs are easily confused with those of carbon monoxide poisoning, hypoxemia, or anxiety and are thus not specific for cyanide poisoning. The tachypnea of cyanide intoxication is transient, however, and is followed by respiratory depression.

Although smoke inhalation may also result in elevated blood levels of lead, no clinically relevant lead toxicity has yet been reported in this setting.[66]

Recreational inhalants (e.g., nitrous oxide, toluene, gasoline and other hydrocarbons, Freon, amyl nitrite) are popular not only because they are easy to obtain but also because their systemic manifestations of euphoria and hallucinations exceed their pulmonary effects. Nonetheless, adverse side effects are possible with these substances. Nitrous oxide inhaled from whipped cream dispensers ("whippets") have been associated with peripheral neuropathy caused by contaminating neurotoxins such as toluene and phenol.[67] Nitrous oxide also inhibits intracellular methionine synthase activity and can produce megaloblastic bone marrow depression.[68] Toluene is an organic solvent of a class similar to carbon tetrachloride and trichloroethylene. Inhalation of these substances causes significant hepatic, renal, and neurologic damage but little pulmonary injury. Chronic gasoline sniffing can lead to irreversible encephalopathy, characterized by dementia, ataxia, chorea, tremor, and myoclonus.[69] Freon is also a neurotoxin, but in addition has been shown to induce fatal cardiac dysrhythmias when inhaled at high concentrations.[70] The manifestations of amyl nitrite inhalation are many including neurologic, cardiovascular, and hematologic effects. The historical use of amyl nitrite for the treatment of angina speaks to its powerful vasodilating properties. Peripheral vasodilation and tachycardia accompany the euphoria produced by larger doses of this substance but can extend to syncope and cardiovascular collapse at high doses.

DIAGNOSTIC APPROACH

Diagnostic Alternatives in Smoke Inhalation

Given the multiple manifestations of smoke inhalation injury described earlier, making a definitive diagnosis can be difficult. If one assumes that each victim of smoke exposure is at risk for injury, then what becomes clinically relevant is making a diagnosis that will specifically affect the treatment of any anatomic and physiologic abnormalities. Although specialized studies can be helpful in certain cases, detailed history taking, comprehensive physical examination, and standard laboratory tests will rapidly and safely confirm most inhalation injuries. The specialized examinations for diagnosis of inhalation injury include direct laryngoscopy, fiberoptic nasopharyngoscopy, chest radiography, nuclear medicine imaging, computed tomography (CT) scanning, fiberoptic bronchoscopy, and laser Doppler endoscopy. These techniques were reviewed and extensively described by Haponik.[71] The indications for these more specialized examinations remain controversial. We contend, as supported later, that clinical assessment and less invasive laboratory tests, together with direct laryngoscopy by a skilled examiner when indicated, provide an adequate basis for determining the need for observation, airway control, and more expensive and invasive supportive therapy, and that the specialized examinations are unnecessary or only rarely indicated because they fail to affect management.

In obtaining a history, one should emphasize data specific to the smoke exposure itself and the type of therapy instituted before the patient was hospitalized. Information that the exposure occurred in a closed space such as a building or an automobile indicates that smoke was less diluted by ambient air, resulting in greater pulmonary exposure to carbon monoxide and smoke constituents than in an open-space exposure. Knowing the duration of exposure is also helpful because it correlates with the severity of lung injury.[72] Information on the probable fuel types burned at the scene can alert the clinician to the possibility of parenchymal lung damage, such as after plastic smoke inhalation.[28] Finally, a knowledge of both transport time from the accident scene and of oxygen therapy administered en route can allow "back-calculation" of the peak COHb reached at the accident scene and give a more accurate estimate of the degree of smoke inhalation.

A screening physical examination should be performed, emphasizing the face (facial burn, singed nasal vibrissae, or a perioral burn, suggesting upper airway smoke exposure); oropharyngeal airway (edema, stridor, or soot impaction suggesting significant smoke inhalation); chest auscultation (wheezing or rhonchi, suggesting injury to lower airways); level of consciousness (decreased with hypoxemia, carbon monoxide, or cyanide poisoning); and the presence of specific neurologic defects that might be associated with carbon monoxide intoxication. Laboratory evaluation should include arterial blood gases, COHb, and cyanide or lactate determinations.

Direct laryngoscopy requires only a laryngoscope, topical anesthesia, and a cooperative, awake patient but is usually performed in the process of securing the upper airway with an endotracheal tube. The examination can be performed at the bedside but is difficult in the presence of significant perioral and oropharyngeal edema. It requires an operator with a knowledge of normal laryngeal anatomy and the procedural skill to obtain a satisfactory examination with minimal patient discomfort. Fiberoptic nasopharyngoscopy is an alternative that does not require laryngoscopic skills or use of extensive topical anesthesia, but it yields a limited examination in inexperienced hands.

Chest radiography, although safely performed at the bedside, is notoriously insensitive in detecting a severely injured lung early after smoke exposure.[73] False-negative rates as high as 92% have been reported,[21] although the use of a semiquantitative grading scale can improve sensitivity and specificity of the examination by 48 hours after injury.[74] Later in the course of the injury, chest radiography is useful, particularly in intubated patients, for assisting in the diagnosis of new pulmonary infection or acute respiratory distress syndrome (ARDS).

Xenon-133 scanning, which defines ventilated regions of the lung, has long been available to demonstrate abnormal ventilation, which occurs in but is not specific to inhalation injury.[75] In addition, technetium-99m hexamethylpropylene amine oxime (99mTc HMPAO) has been demonstrated to accumulate in the lung following smoke inhalation and is therefore a potentially noninvasive method of detecting inhalation injury.[76] The inconvenience of transporting a critically ill patient to the nuclear medicine suite along with the uncertain added value of these tests over history, physical examination, and a few laboratory tests have prevented both Xenon-133 and 99mTc HMPAO scans from becoming commonly used in the setting of smoke inhalation.

A CT scan of the chest has been shown in animal models to be more sensitive in detecting atelectasis after smoke inhalation than either xenon-133 scanning or chest radiography.[77] In a limited number of patients, CT was found to have a 23% false-negative rate, superior to that of chest radiography (92%) but equivalent to xenon-133 scanning (14%). The abnormalities found on CT scan appear to represent atelectasis because they resolve quickly in those victims who recover uneventfully. Like nuclear scans, CT examination requires transport to the radiology suite and is of little value in unstable or critically ill victims. More recently, high-resolution multislice CT scans have been used to perform "virtual bronchoscopies" in patients with presumed inhalation injury.[78] The clinical utility of this technique is not clear at this point, however.

Fiberoptic bronchoscopy has been described by some authors as the gold standard for diagnosis of inhalation injury.[79-81] This technique allows visualization of upper airway, glottis, and tracheobronchial structures to the level of lobar bronchi. Findings of erythema, soot deposition, epithelial ulceration, and edema are all pathognomonic of injury. However, the procedure requires both specialized equipment and skilled personnel and may not influence therapy beyond what is suggested by other more routine examinations. Furthermore, the procedure may be hazardous in some high-risk patients.[82] One potential use of bronchoscopy, however, is in combination with endoscopic laser flowmetry to quantify hyperemia in the tracheobronchial tree associated with lung injury.[83] Laser flowmetry has not entered mainstream clinical use in patients with inhalation injury, however.

To help determine the role of bronchoscopy in patients with smoke inhalation we studied 100 consecutive patients admitted to our regional burn unit who had presented with at least one of the usual clinical warning signs of inhalation injury (closed-space smoke exposure, facial burn, singed nasal vibrissae, perioral burn, pharyngeal edema, hoarseness, carbonaceous sputum, bronchorrhea, or wheezing). We then performed fiberoptic bronchoscopy and tested for correlation with multivariate analysis. A 96% correlation was found between positive bronchoscopic findings and the clinical triad of closed-space fire, COHb levels greater than 10%, and carbonaceous sputum. If only two items of the clinical triad were present, the correlation dropped to 70%; if only one was present, the correlation was less than 30%. No other positive correlations were detected. On the basis of these observations and the limitations of fiberoptic bronchoscopy, as described earlier, we favor the use of history-taking, clinical examination, and laboratory studies in making the diagnosis of inhalation injury and reserve the fiberoptic bronchoscopy for exceptional cases (e.g., expansion of lobar atelectasis, removal of obstructing intrabronchial secretions).

As with other causes of lower airway obstruction, diagnosis is made by physical examination (e.g., wheezing); pulmonary function testing; or, in more severe cases, arterial blood gas analysis. Respiratory failure because of alveolar injury is suggested by tachypnea or dyspnea and confirmed by the usual laboratory procedures (e.g., arterial blood gas and chest radiography).

Diagnostic Alternatives in Toxic Gas Inhalation

The characteristic physical sign of carbon monoxide intoxication—cherry red lips—is subtle and unreliable. The diagnosis of carbon monoxide poisoning, regardless of the mechanism of exposure, is definitively made by measuring the arterial COHb level. To assess the degree of intoxication, COHb levels should be obtained as soon as possible after inhalation. A knowledge of transport time from the accident scene, oxygen therapy administered en route, and the kinetics of carbon monoxide elimination will allow "back-calculation" of an estimated COHb level at the accident scene, most easily accomplished using an appropriate nomogram. Although COHb levels do not correlate with the development of respiratory failure,[23] this estimated peak COHb level will more accurately reflect the degree of carbon monoxide exposure and raise the proper index of suspicion for associated manifestations of severe smoke inhalation and carbon monoxide inhalation (e.g., neuropsychiatric sequelae; see the following). Serial COHb determinations in individuals with severe intoxication (COHb>30%) will help ensure adequate therapy and elimination of carbon monoxide.

As described earlier, arterial Po_2 measurements will usually be normal in cases of carbon monoxide or cyanide exposure; if abnormal, they suggest the presence of other parenchymal lung injury. Specific assessment of hemoglobin (oxyhemoglobin and COHb) by co-oximetry is critical in the diagnostic work-up. Calculated oxygen content determinations based on Po_2 levels alone are invalid. Furthermore, pulse oximetry is unreliable in the presence of carbon monoxide poisoning because COHb is not detected by this device. Because only oxyhemoglobin and deoxyhemoglobin are detected, a falsely elevated oxygen saturation reading will be obtained in the presence of COHb (Fig. 49-3).[84]

Cyanide intoxication results in abnormal neurologic findings including altered level of consciousness, dizziness, and headache, as well as tachycardia and tachypnea, followed by bradypnea. Blood cyanide levels can be measured,[85] although this assay may not be available in many centers. Because aerobic metabolism is severely affected in these individuals, lactic acidosis is a common diagnostic feature. Plasma lactate measurements have been shown to correlate with cyanide levels and provide an alternative diagnostic tool.[65]

Diagnosis of most toxic gas inhalations is made by history and supplemented by associated findings on physical examination. Laboratory methods to confirm diagnosis are in many cases highly technical, expensive, and impractical because of their infrequent use. Of the substances most commonly abused by recreational inhalation (marijuana, cocaine, phenylcyclidine, and heroin), objective evidence of use is generally obtained by identification of the drug or its metabolites in urine, or both. Such testing is qualitative because an individual's intake, absorption, metabolism, and renal excretion of each drug are variable. Radioimmunoassay and gas chromatography or mass spectrometry are the most common techniques used; these are discussed elsewhere.[86]

Bronchoalveolar lavage is a useful tool for sampling the lower respiratory tract, although its use in toxic gas inhalation to detect specific toxins is limited by the high solubil-

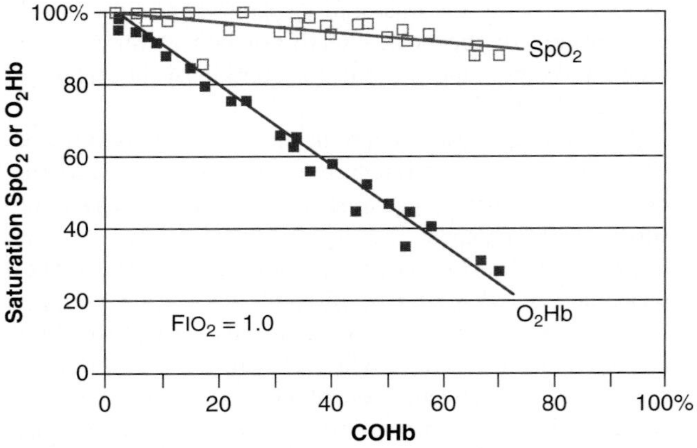

Figure 49-3. Oxyhemoglobin saturation as measured by pulse oximetry (Spo_2) and by co-oximetry (O_2Hb) in the presence of carboxyhemoglobin (COHb) in dogs ventilated with oxygen FIO_2 of 1 and varied concentrations of carbon monoxide. Spo_2 consistently overestimates the true oxyhemoglobin saturation. At FIO_2 1, the overestimation of O_2Hb is approximately 1% for every 1% COHb. (Modified from Barker SJ, Tremper KK: The effect of carbon monoxide inhalation on pulse oximetry and transcutaneous Po_2. Anesthesiology 1987;66:677.)

ity of most inhaled toxins and their transient residence in epithelial lining fluid. However, bronchoalveolar lavage has known utility for sampling cell populations and inflammatory mediators in the airspaces after toxin inhalation[87] and can yield insight into the pathogenesis of generalized inflammatory lung injuries. Although it has been used in the detection of inhalational lung injury resulting from nitrogen mustard exposure[88] and some occupational particle exposures,[89] it is in general not a reliable tool for diagnostic purposes specific to inhaled toxins. In addition, there is at present no apparent role for bronchoalveolar lavage in the treatment of acute or chronic inhalational lung disease. Bronchoscopy, however, has been described for therapeutic laser photoresection and stent placement in large airways of patients with nitrogen mustard-induced strictures.[88]

APPROACH TO MANAGEMENT

Upper Airway Injury

As described previously, hoarseness, stridor, or severe pharyngeal edema suggests an upper airway at risk for obstruction, a lethal complication. In these cases the airway should be aggressively secured with endotracheal intubation early in the hospital course, rather than just observing the patient, because inflammation will result in further edema and reduction in airway caliber for the first 24 to 36 hours after injury. Observation carries the risks of unwitnessed airway obstruction and increasingly difficult laryngoscopy and intubation because of progressive edema. If signs of a more mild upper airway injury are present (facial burn, singed nasal vibrissae, or perioral burn without the upper airway signs noted earlier), a safe alternative is observation in a high-visibility unit where skilled personnel and equipment are immediately available for securing the airway. These management guidelines may be modified according to available resources.

Endotracheal intubation by the oral or nasal route is acceptable, the choice primarily depending on the skill and experience of the operator. Long-term intubation is uncommon because airway compromise in cases of isolated inhalation injury usually resolves within 2 to 5 days. Before extubation, airway patency can be assessed by deflating the tube cuff and listening for ventilation around the tube or by fiberoptic nasopharyngoscopy. The cuff leak test remains controversial, however, because of a significant false-positive rate[90]; an absent cuff leak should not preclude extubation except in unusual circumstances (e.g., obvious airway edema or known difficult intubation). Such assessment is difficult in children because of their smaller anatomy, the use of uncuffed endotracheal tubes, and the increased incidence of postextubation stridor and reintubation. The incidence of postextubation stridor in these victims has been reported as high as 47%, compared with only 4% in elective pediatric surgical patients.[91] The treatment of postextubation stridor includes administration of racemic epinephrine and helium-oxygen mixtures. For these and other high-risk patients, extubation should be performed only in the presence of individuals capable of reintubating the child; in extreme cases this is best done with the patient under general anesthesia in the operating room.

The administration of steroids in the acute period after smoke inhalation is not recommended as a means of protecting against airway obstruction caused by edema. Although their anti-inflammatory effects may reduce the peak edema response, steroids require hours to take effect and do not guarantee airway patency. After isolated inhalation injury in humans, steroidal agents have been shown to be of no benefit,[8,92] and in cases of combined inhalation and burn injuries, their use is associated with higher mortality and infection rates.[93] Steroids may be of use, however, in patients who are dependent on exogenous steroidal therapy for preexisting medical illness or patients who present with severe bronchospasm that is unresponsive to bronchodilators.

In individuals at high risk of developing postextubation stridor or requiring reintubation for partial airway obstruction following inhalation injury (e.g., pediatric victims of smoke inhalation, as noted previously), the use of humidified oxygen and nebulized racemic epinephrine may be of use. Ventilation with 60% helium in oxygen may be of additional benefit by producing a lower density of gas that decreases the work of breathing by up to 30%.[94] This technique has been shown to be useful in pediatric smoke inhalation patients[95,96] and deserves further study in the context of other inhalation injuries.

Lower Airway Injury

Tracheobronchitis, commonly seen in victims of smoke and toxic gas inhalation, produces wheezing, coughing, and retained secretions. The ventilation/perfusion mismatch in these patients can result in mild to moderate hypoxemia, depending on the degree of underlying lung disease. Therefore supplemental oxygen should be routinely administered. The cause of increased airway resistance is more often decreased airway caliber (from mucosal-submucosal edema and retained secretions) than true bronchospasm. The efficacy of bronchodilators in these patients has not been well studied, although a trial of therapy is most often attempted, certainly in those with preexistent bronchospastic disease. Nebulized or metered dose therapy with β_2-agonists or racemic epinephrine are most commonly used. Steroids are only indicated after isolated inhalation injury for patients with underlying severe bronchospastic disease or those with preexisting dependence on exogenous steroids. Anticholinergic agents (atropine or ipratropium bromide) have the theoretical advantage of reducing reflex bronchospasm caused by chemical irritation of the airways but have not been carefully studied in this setting. Finally, aggressive pulmonary toilet and chest physiotherapy are essential for mobilizing retained secretions and preventing worsening atelectasis in a critically ill patient whose physical activity is restricted. In one study of intubated pediatric burn-inhalation injury victims,[97] prophylactic administration of aerosolized heparin and the mucolytic acetylcysteine has been shown to reduce atelectasis, reintubation rates, and mortality, compared with standard pulmonary toilet and may be of particular use in young patients or those with severe lower airway injury and retained secretions. Finally, ventilator strategies should be designed to minimize auto-PEEP (positive end-expiratory pressure) in this setting, much as one would in patients with status asthmaticus.

Alveolar Injury

As mentioned previously, alveolar injury is uncommon, except in certain cases of plastic smoke or poorly soluble toxin inhalation and in cases of combined inhalation and burn injury. When alveolar injury occurs, the presenting sign is usually hypoxemia, as diagnosed by pulse oximetry or, preferably (especially in the presence of COHb), arterial blood gas analysis. Most inhalation victims receive supplemental oxygen, so significant alveolar-arterial oxygen gradients can be missed by pulse oximetry because saturation levels of less than 95% do not occur until arterial PO_2 is less than 80 mm Hg. Arterial blood gas analysis is therefore the monitoring procedure of choice in assessing oxygenation after an inhalation injury. Initial therapy should always include administration of high-flow oxygen to supplement oxygenation and to reduce COHb in cases of carbon monoxide inhalation. Upper airway patency must be ensured and airway resistance minimized with chest physiotherapy or bronchodilators, or both. Central hypoventilation caused by carbon monoxide or cyanide poisoning should be treated immediately with endotracheal intubation and assisted ventilation, and efforts made to reverse intoxication.

The need for mechanical ventilation to supplement oxygenation is determined by repeated blood gas measurements. As a guideline, the PaO_2/FIO_2 (P/F) ratio may be calculated without mixed venous blood sampling and used as an approximation of the shunt fraction. A P/F ratio above 300 indicates mild to moderate injury, usually requiring only supplemental oxygen therapy. A P/F ratio below 300 (and certainly below 200) is evidence of serious parenchymal lung injury and usually indicates a need for intubation and ventilation with high inspired oxygen fractions or the use of PEEP. Because of the frequent presence of acute atelectasis after alveolar exposure to smoke, PEEP can be particularly useful. The National Institutes of Health ARDS Network trial comparing 6 mL/kg with 12 mL/kg tidal volume in patients with acute lung injury showed a reduction in mortality with the lower tidal volume. The trial excluded burn victims and thus included few, if any, patients with smoke inhalation injury.[98] However, there is no strong conceptual reason to expect that lungs exposed to smoke injury would behave in a manner different from that of other widespread lung injury. Therefore we recommend following the ARDS Network protocol limiting tidal volume to avoid alveolar overdistention with propagation of the lung injury (see Chapter 11),[98,99] even though published evidence to support this strategy in this setting is not currently available.

Numerous novel methods of mechanical ventilation are used in some centers in patients with inhalation injury. High-frequency percussive ventilation is one technique that has several potential benefits including improved secretion clearance, lower peak airway pressures, and less hemodynamic impairment. It may also improve oxygenation over conventional ventilation and thus allow use of lower FIO_2, another possible advantage.[100] High-frequency oscillatory ventilation has been used extensively at some burn centers for patients with inhalation injury and ARDS, both in the ICU and in the operating room, with good success in reversal of oxygenation failure.[101] Unfortunately, the limited availability of these types of ventilators and the lack of useful outcome data prevent their widespread use. Another unusual method of managing patients with respiratory failure from inhalation injury is extracorporeal membrane oxygenation (ECMO), which has been used successfully on a limited basis in adults but lacks adequate research demonstrating its effect on outcome.[102]

Prophylactic administration of antibiotics in the acute treatment of inhalation injury is not indicated; their use has not been shown to protect against the development of pulmonary infection.[103] However, specific antibiotics are indicated for clinically apparent pneumonia, which may subsequently develop. Careful surveillance for bacterial pneumonia is required in cases of combined smoke inhalation and cutaneous burn injury because of the increased incidence of this complication (30% to 50% in burn patients with concomitant inhalation injury) and its associated increased mortality.[21,54]

Respiratory Tract Management in Patients with Concomitant Cutaneous Burn Injury

Aside from the changes in upper airway anatomy after smoke inhalation described previously, concomitant burn injury can complicate attempts at endotracheal intubation as a result of associated changes in the response to muscle relaxants commonly used to achieve skeletal muscle paralysis before laryngoscopy is performed. Beginning approximately 2 to 5 days after a burn injury, skeletal muscle acetylcholine receptors undergo a quantitative and functional change. They are upregulated across the muscle membrane as an isoform that may be persistently depolarized by choline, a metabolite of acetylcholine and succinylcholine.[104] The end result is a dramatically increased hyperkalemic response to succinylcholine,[105,106] with the increased potential for transient but severe ventricular dysrhythmias. Thus nondepolarizing muscle relaxants with rapid onset of action (e.g., rocuronium) are indicated for use during tracheal intubation in burn patients beginning at 2 to 5 days after their injuries. In addition, these patients are relatively resistant to nondepolarizing neuromuscular relaxants and may require one and a half to three times the usual intubating dose of atracurium,[107] metocurine,[108] or rocuronium[109] to achieve proper intubating conditions.

The presence of circumferential full-thickness thorax burns can produce a restrictive lung defect that may dramatically interfere with positive-pressure ventilation and require immediate treatment with chest wall escharotomy. Escharotomies through skin to subcutaneous fat are made in the anterior axillary line bilaterally, extending from the clavicle to the costal margin. If the abdomen is involved with the burn, the inferior margins of the escharotomy may be connected transversely.

Formation of a tracheostomy in burn patients is controversial. Clearly, if the upper airway is in danger of imminent obstruction and endotracheal intubation attempts are unsuccessful, emergent cricothyroidotomy is indicated. The timing of conversion from prolonged endotracheal intubation to tracheostomy remains controversial, however, with significant variability between institutions and clinicians. Patients with anterior neck burns who require elective tracheostomy should undergo excision and grafting of the area 5 to 7 days before creation of the tracheostomy. This technique minimizes pulmonary and burn wound infectious complications associated with the procedure.[110,111] One recent trend in airway management has been the percutaneous technique over conventional surgical tracheostomy. The surgical procedure requires transport of a critically ill patient to the operating room, and with that the utilization of resources such as operating room time, anesthesiology, and ancillary staff. Percutaneous tracheostomies, however, can be performed at the bedside in the ICU by the intensivist. This method has become increasingly popular since the introduction of the Ciaglia technique in 1985.[112] In addition to the time and financial savings of the percutaneous tracheostomy, recent evidence has demonstrated that it has a lower rate of infectious and bleeding complications than the open surgical technique.[113] In addition, percutaneous tracheostomy has been favorably evaluated both in burn patients[114] and burn patients with inhalation injury.[115]

Management of Systemic Effects

Carbon monoxide is a major source of morbidity in the setting of smoke inhalation. Successful management of carbon monoxide toxicity requires its rapid diagnosis, via COHb levels, and prompt displacement of carbon monoxide from circulating hemoglobin by administering high inspired oxygen concentrations. The elimination half-life of carbon monoxide in someone breathing room air is as long as 250 minutes, but this number decreases to approximately 50 minutes in someone breathing 100% oxygen and then decreases even further, to under 30 minutes, when one breathes 2.5 atmospheres hyperbaric oxygen.[116]

Hyperbaric oxygen therapy is therefore an attractive intervention for patients with carbon monoxide toxicity. Traditionally its use has been considered in the setting of patients with severe carbon monoxide toxicity, as indicated by loss of consciousness, neurologic deficit, myocardial ischemia, pulmonary edema, or severe metabolic acidosis,[117] but its benefits apart from more rapid clearance of carbon monoxide have remained unclear. A randomized trial published in 2002 by Weaver and colleagues[118] appeared to provide evidence of the benefit of hyperbaric oxygen in the setting of carbon monoxide poisoning. This study demonstrated a reduced incidence of cognitive sequelae in patients who underwent three hyperbaric oxygen treatments within a 24-hour period. Recent criticism of the Weaver study in a Cochrane review again raises doubts as to the utility of hyperbaric oxygen in this setting.[119] It is probably still appropriate to administer hyperbaric oxygen for the treatment of severe carbon monoxide toxicity when practical considerations such as the availability of a hyperbaric oxygen chamber permit its use.

When one does use hyperbaric oxygen therapy for carbon monoxide toxicity, the appropriate frequency and duration of therapy remains unknown. Numerous protocols exist, but none has been demonstrated to be superior. A recent randomized clinical trial has attempted to address this question by treating patients either with three 30-minute periods of 100% oxygen at 2.4 atmospheres or with a protocol of two 23-minute periods at 3 atmospheres and two 25-minute periods at 2 atmospheres.[120] The study was not adequately powered to detect a difference between the protocols, but perhaps a future multicenter trial will provide more guidance on how best to administer hyperbaric oxygen to the patient with carbon monoxide toxicity.

Management of cyanide inhalation is problematic because of the difficulty in definitive diagnosis of intoxication. Treatment is indicated for any patient meeting the previously described clinical criteria (e.g., appropriate history and unexplained metabolic acidosis) or with cyanide levels greater than 0.2 mg/L. Treatment should always include high inspired oxygen concentrations. Cyanide is enzymatically detoxified by hepatic rhodanese, requiring sulfate as a substrate. The resulting thiocyanate product is inactive and is excreted in the urine. Unfortunately, this hepatic conversion of cyanide is slow and often limited by the availability of sulfate. Standard treatment therefore involves the temporary diversion of cyanide into other minor metabolic pathways while supplemental sulfate (thiosulfate) is given to accelerate the detoxification reaction. A three-step cyanide antidote package is commonly available. Amyl nitrite is first administered by inhalation (15 to 30 seconds each minute) while sodium nitrite solution is prepared. This solution is injected (300 mg in 10 mL in an adult) over 2 to 4 minutes, with careful monitoring of blood pressure. These two steps produce methemoglobin, which combines with cyanide to yield nontoxic cyanmethemoglobin. The amount of sodium nitrite injected is limited to keep methemoglobin levels below 40%; above this level, toxic effects from hypoxia begin to appear.[121] Finally, sodium thiosulfate (12.5 g in 50 mL 5% dextrose) is injected over a 10-minute period as a more definitive treatment. Using another diversion pathway, intravenous hydroxycobalamin (vitamin B_{12}) may be given up to 10 grams to produce the inactive cyanocobalamin. Cyanide shunted to these minor pathways must eventually be detoxified by hepatic rhodanese; careful observation of these patients (blood gases and cyanide or lactate levels) is therefore warranted for 24 to 48 hours. In the setting of inhalation injury, in which concurrent carbon monoxide poisoning or significant ventilation-perfusion mismatch may already impair oxygen delivery, the risk of further harm through the production of methemoglobin is a concern that has led some authors to change their approach to the management of cyanide toxicity. One review suggests avoiding amyl nitrite and sodium nitrite altogether; the authors argue for hydroxycobalamin first and then adding sodium thiosulfate for more significant poisoning.[122]

A discussion of the treatment of systemic effects associated with the inhalation of the wide variety of industrial, military, and recreational abuse substances is beyond the scope of this chapter; the reader is referred to other sources.[11,86]

PROGNOSIS

Outcome

A number of studies examining outcome following smoke inhalation have produced similar findings.[21,55,123,124] They support the notion that mortality and morbidity after isolated smoke inhalation are low but not negligible (<10%). The addition of cutaneous burn injury or pul-monary sepsis, or both, to inhalation injury dramatically increases the mortality rate (30% to 70%). Clark and colleagues[21] reported 8% mortality for patients with inhalation injury without burn and 31% mortality for those with concomitant smoke inhalation and burn injury. Elderly persons, the very young, and obese individuals are especially high-risk groups, particularly in the context of concomitant smoke inhalation and burn. This increased risk is likely because of the presence of underlying pulmonary disease (the elderly and obese) or smaller anatomic dimensions that exacerbate lower airway injury (children).

Preliminary efforts to describe an "inhalation injury severity score" and to prognosticate outcome are reported for victims of combined burn and inhalation injuries.[125] The P/F ratio calculated after fluid resuscitation (typically 24 to 48 hours after injury) is a better predictor than the P/F ratio calculated at admission; a postresuscitation P/F ratio of greater than 300 is associated with a significantly greater chance of patient survival than a ratio less than 300. In addition, a composite injury severity score based on P/F ratio, chest radiography, and peak airway pressure measured on days 0, 1, and 7 correlated with survival. Further studies are required, however, to confirm these initial findings and expand them to the adult patient population.

Outcome data for victims of other toxic gas or fume inhalation are sparse because of the relative infrequency of these various presentations. The reader is referred to other sources for brief discussions of these data.[11,86]

PULMONARY COMPLICATIONS

A summary of the frequency of the major acute pulmonary complications seen after smoke inhalation or burn injury, or both, is shown in Tables 49-2 and 49-3. As outlined previously, the primary complications of isolated smoke inhalation are asphyxia, tracheobronchitis, airway obstruction, pulmonary edema, and pneumonia. The incidence and distribution of these complications increase with the presence of concomitant burn injury. A variety of other pulmonary complications commonly seen in the context of generalized pulmonary critical care have also been reported after smoke inhalation including pleural effusion, aspiration, pneumothorax, and pulmonary embolism. (These are discussed in detail elsewhere in this text.)

Long-term complications of smoke inhalation injury include laryngeal, tracheal, and bronchial stenosis, bronchiectasis, reactive airway disease, chronic bronchitis, and restrictive pulmonary defects at the parenchymal level.

Table 49-2. General Impact of Clinical Respiratory Complications in Burn Victims

	Smoke Inhalation Only	Cutaneous Burn Only	Both Smoke Inhalation and Burns Present
Asphyxia	+++	+	++++
Upper airway obstruction	+	0	++++
Tracheobronchitis	++	0	++++
Permeability edema			
Toxic	+	++	++++
Septic	+	+++	++++
Hydrostatic edema	0	+++	++++
Pneumonia	+	+++	++++
Pulmonary embolism	0	+	+
Mortality	+	++	++++
Likelihood of residual respiratory impairment	+	+	+
Need for intubation, mechanical ventilation	+	++	++++
Relative duration, cost of hospitalization	+	++	++++

From Haponik EF, Munster AM: Diagnosis, impact, and classification of inhalation injury. In Haponik EF, Munster AM (eds): Respiratory Injury: Smoke Inhalation and Burns. New York, McGraw-Hill, 1990.

Table 49-3. Incidence of Respiratory Complications after Smoke Inhalation and Burns*

	Pruitt et al 1962-1963 (*n*=308)	Pruitt et al 1967 (*n*=389)	Venus et al 1976-1977 (*n*=998)	Dimick et al 1972-1981 (*n*=1271)
Pulmonary edema	27 (8.8%)	21 (5.4%)	45 (4.5%)	—
Pneumonia	70 (23%)	56 (14.4%)	29 (2.9%)	204 (16%)
Atelectasis	8 (2.6%)	10 (2.6%)	11 (11%)	—
Respiratory burn	—	—	—	160 (12.6%)
Pleural effusion	—	7 (2%)	—	—
Smoke inhalation injury	3 (1%)	1	—	—
Aspiration with asphyxia	—	2	—	—
Analgesia-related respiratory depression	1	1	—	—
Pulmonary embolism	2	3 (1%)	—	28 (2.2%)
Chest wall defects, fractured ribs	1	2	—	—
Tracheostomy complications	47 (15%)	26 (7%)	—	—
Subglottic stenosis	—	—	2 (2%)	—
Pneumothorax	1	0	5 (5%)	17 (1.3%)
Exacerbation of chronic bronchitis	—	1	—	—

*Note the decreasing incidence of pulmonary edema and tracheostomy complications concurrent with changes in clinical practice, whereas the incidence of pneumonia and atelectasis is relatively constant.
From Haponik EF, Munster AM: Diagnosis, impact, and classification of inhalation injury. In Haponik EF, Munster AM (eds): Respiratory Injury: Smoke Inhalation and Burns. New York, McGraw-Hill, 1990.

Although laryngeal and tracheal stenosis can result from inhalation injury itself, these injuries are usually aggravated by translaryngeal intubation or tracheostomy. Bronchiectasis is a nonspecific response seen after various types of airway inflammation. Inhalation injury may cause bronchiectasis by initiating a submucosal inflammatory reaction that weakens supporting elements of the bronchial wall. Bronchiectasis following inhalation injury can be severe and has been reported to lead to hypercapnic respiratory failure and cor pulmonale.[126] The development of reactive airway disease has been documented after exposure to a variety of environmental irritants[127] and sulfur dioxide.[128] Its development following a single episode of smoke or fume inhalation has been thought to be rare and is more likely to occur after multiple exposures (e.g., firefighters). However, recent reports have documented long-term changes in pulmonary function tests after single exposures. They appear to be correlated with either COHb[129] or inhalation of polyvinyl chloride products.[130] Restrictive lung defects and persistent abnormal gas exchange can occur after uncomplicated inhalation injury, although these cases are rare. These abnormalities are more likely to occur when inhalation injury has been complicated by ARDS, but they are usually mild.[131]

KEY POINTS

- Despite ambient atmospheric temperatures that can exceed 1000°C at fire scenes, thermal injury to the respiratory tract is uncommon because of efficient heat exchange in the nasopharynx and oropharynx. The term *pulmonary burn* is a misnomer.
- Respiratory tract injury following smoke inhalation is the result of chemical irritation and an acute inflammatory response, resulting in epithelial disruption, tissue edema, and occasionally inflammatory cell infiltration. In most cases isolated smoke inhalation results in pulmonary dysfunction that is self-limited and resolves within 2 to 4 days.
- Smoke inhalation injury is common in both upper and lower airways but infrequent at the alveolar level in cases of isolated smoke inhalation. The anatomic level of injury is in part determined by the type of smoke inhaled, which in turn is determined by the type of fuel burned.
- Smoke inhalation injury at the upper airway level is manifested by soft tissue edema and carries the risk of life-threatening airway obstruction. Diagnosis is made by history and physical examination, and treatment involves early provision of a secure airway (e.g., endotracheal intubation). Steroid administration is unreliable or ineffective in reducing acute soft tissue edema and is harmful in the patient with concomitant burns.
- Smoke inhalation injury at the lower airway level is manifested by airway edema resulting in wheezing and ventilation/perfusion mismatching. Diagnosis is made by history, physical examination, and blood gas analysis.

Fiberoptic bronchoscopy is one of several alternative techniques that can assist in diagnosis. Treatment is supportive with chest physiotherapy, supplemental oxygen, and perhaps bronchodilators. Mechanical ventilation may be necessary in severe cases.

- Smoke inhalation injury at the alveolar level results in surfactant inactivation and atelectasis. Pulmonary edema is uncommonly seen, unless there is significant concomitant cutaneous burn or systemic sepsis.
- Carbon monoxide inhalation can occur in the context of smoke inhalation or as an isolated event (e.g., suicide attempt). Carbon monoxide combines with circulating hemoglobin and intracellular cytochrome to decrease both oxygen delivery and utilization. Treatment is with supplemental oxygen and, in severe cases, hyperbaric oxygen.
- Pulse oximetry is an unreliable indicator of oxygenation in the context of carbon monoxide poisoning because of mechanical factors of pulse oximeter design. In this instance, only co-oximetry will accurately measure blood hemoglobin saturation.
- Hydrogen cyanide inhalation is a common complication of smoke inhalation, particularly when polyurethane is burned. Cyanide halts aerobic cellular metabolism at the cytochrome level, producing cellular asphyxia. Treatment involves the temporary shunting of cyanide into other metabolic pathways (e.g., methemoglobin by administration of nitrites) until hepatic rhodanese can convert cyanide into inactive thiocyanate.
- Tear gas (chloroacetophenone) is primarily a lacrimatory agent but at high doses can cause upper airway obstruction and pulmonary edema.
- Because of upregulation of nonjunctional acetylcholine receptors, burn victims respond abnormally to muscle relaxants used for pharmacologic paralysis. Depolarizing agents (e.g., succinylcholine) produce acute, life-threatening hyperkalemia. By contrast, burn patients are resistant to nondepolarizing agents (e.g., vecuronium).

REFERENCES

1. Singh N, Davis GS. Review: Occupational and environmental lung disease. Curr Opin Pulm Med 2002;8:117-125.
2. Broughton E: The Bhopal disaster and its aftermath: A review. Environ Health 2005;4:6.
3. Wax PM, Becker CE, Curry SC: Unexpected "gas" casualties in Moscow: A medical toxicology perspective. Ann Emerg Med 2003;41:700-705.
4. Cope O, et al: Symposium on the management of the Cocoanut Grove burns at the Massachusetts General Hospital. Ann Surg 1943;117:801-965.
5. Cope O: Care of the victims of the Cocoanut Grove fire at the Massachusetts General Hospital. N Engl J Med 1943;229:138.
6. Winternitz MC: Pathology of war gas poisoning. Princeton, NJ, Yale University Press, 1920.
7. Finland M, Davidson SC, Levenson SM: Clinical and therapeutic aspects of the conflagration injuries in the respiratory tract sustained by victims of the Cocoanut Grove disaster. Medicine 1946;25:215-283.
8. Robinson NB, Hudson LD, Riem M, et al: Steroid therapy following isolated smoke inhalation injury. J Trauma 1982;22:876.
9. Mahoney EJ, Harrington DT, Biffl WL, et al: Lessons learned from a nightclub fire: Institutional disaster preparedness. J Trauma 2005;58:487-491.
10. Davies JWL: Toxic chemicals versus lung tissue—an aspect of inhalation injury revisited. J Burn Care Rehab 1986;7:213.
11. Urbanetti JS: Battlefield chemical inhalation injury. In Loke J (ed): Pathophysiology and Treatment of Inhalation Injuries. New York, Marcel Dekker, 1988.
12. Zellner PR: The 1990 Everett Idris Evans Memorial lecture: The inhalation injury. J Burn Care Rehab 1990;11:487.
13. Baker DJ: Chemical and biologic warfare. In Grande CM (ed): Textbook of Trauma, Anesthesia, and Critical Care. St. Louis, Mosby, 1993.
14. Hay A, Roberts G: The use of poison gas against the Iraqi Kurds: Analysis of bomb fragments, soil, and wool samples. JAMA 1990;263:1065-1066.
15. Yanagisawa N, Morita H, Nakajima T: Sarin experiences in Japan: Acute toxicity and long-term effects. J Neurol Sci 2006;249:76-85.
16. Hsu VP, Handzel T, Hayslett J, et al: Opening a *Bacillus anthracis*–containing envelope, Capitol Hill, Washington, DC: The public health response. Emerging Infectious Diseases. 2002;8:1039-1043.
17. Centers for Disease Control and Prevention: Web-based Injury Statistics Query and Reporting System (WISQARS). Available at http://www.cdc.gov/ncipc/wisqars Accessed May 17, 2007.
18. Herndon DN, Thompson PB, Brown M, et al: Diagnosis, pathophysiology, and treatment of inhalation injury. In Boswick JA (ed): The Art and Science of Burn Care. Rockville, Md, Aspen Publishers, 1987.
19. Ahrens M: U.S. Experience with Smoke Alarms. NFPA Fire Analysis & Research Division. Quincy, Mass, November, 2004.
20. Baker SP, O'Neill B, Karpf RS: The Injury Fact Book. Lexington, Mass, DC Heath, 1984.
21. Clark WR, Bonaventura M, Myers W: Smoke inhalation and airway management at a regional burn unit: 1974-1983. Part I: Diagnosis and consequences of smoke inhalation. J Burn Care Rehab 1989;10:52.
22. Walker JEC, Wells RE, Merril EW: Heat and water exchange in the respiratory tract. Am J Med 1961;30:259.
23. Achauer BM, Allyn PA, Furnas DW, et al: Pulmonary complications of burns: The major threat to the burn patient. Ann Surg 1973;177:31.
24. Moritz AR, Henriques FC, McLean R: The effects of inhaled heat on the air passages and lungs: An experimental investigation. Am J Pathol 1945;21:311.
25. Lowry WT, Juarez L, Petty CS, Roberts B: Studies of toxic gas production during actual structural fires in the Dallas area. J Forens Sci 1985;30:59.
26. Terrill JB, Montgomery RR, Reinhardt CF: Toxic gases from fires. Science 1978;200:1343.
27. Crapo RO: Causes of respiratory injury. In Haponik EF, Munster AM (eds): Respiratory Injury: Smoke Inhalation and Burns. New York, McGraw-Hill, 1990.
28. Alexeeff GV, Lee YC, Thorning D, et al: Pulmonary tissue reaction in response to smoke. J Fire Sci 1987;4:427.
29. Nieman GF, Clark WR, Was SD, et al: The effect of smoke inhalation on pulmonary surfactant. Ann Surg 1980;191:171.
30. Kramer GC, Herndon DN, Linares HA, et al: Effects of inhalation injury on airway blood flow and edema formation. J Burn Care Rehab 1989;10:45.
31. Demarest GB, Hudson LD, Altman LC: Impaired alveolar macrophage chemotaxis in patients with acute smoke inhalation. Am Rev Respir Dis 1979;119:279.
32. Traber DL, Herndon DN: Pathophysiology of smoke inhalation. In Haponik EF, Munster AM (eds): Respiratory Injury: Smoke Inhalation and Burns. New York, McGraw-Hill, 1990.
33. Riyami BM, Tree R, Kinsella J, et al: Changes in alveolar macrophage, monocyte, and neutrophil cell profiles after smoke inhalation injury. J Clin Pathol 1990;43:43.
34. Dyer RF, Esch VH: Polyvinyl chloride toxicity in fires. JAMA 1976;235:393.
35. Zawacki BE, Jung RC, Joyce J, et al: Smoke, burns and the natural history of inhalation injury in fire victims:

A correlation of experimental and clinical data. Ann Surg 1977;185:100.
36. Tranbaugh RF, Elings VB, Christensen JM, et al: Effect of inhalation injury on lung water accumulation. J Trauma 1983;23:597.
37. Tranbaugh RF, Lewis FR, Christensen JM, et al: Lung water changes after thermal injury: The effect of crystalloid resuscitation and sepsis. Ann Surg 1980;192:479.
38. Soejima K, Schmalstieg FC, Sakurai H, et al: Pathophysiological analysis of combined burn and smoke inhalation injuries in sheep. Am J Physiol Lung Cell Mol Physiol 2001;280:L1233-241.
39. Murakami K, Bjertnaes LJ, Schmalstieg FC, et al: A novel animal model of sepsis after acute lung injury in sheep. Crit Care Med 2002;30:2083-2090.
40. Enkhbaatar P, Traber DL: Pathophysiology of acute lung injury in combined burn and smoke inhalation injury. Clin Sci (Lond) 2004;107:137-143.
41. Soejima K, Traber LD, Schmalstieg FC, et al: Role of nitric oxide in vascular permeability after combined burns and smoke inhalation injury. Am J Respir Crit Care Med 2001;163: 745-752.
42. Hughes MN: Relationships between nitric oxide, nitroxyl ion, nitrosonium cation and peroxynitrite. Biochim Biophys Acta 1999;1411:263-272.
43. Cox RA, Burke AS, Soejima K, et al: Airway obstruction in sheep with burn and smoke inhalation injuries. Am J Respir Cell Mol Biol 2003;29:295-302.
44. Enkhbaatar P, Murakami K, Shimoda K, et al: Ketorolac attenuates cardiopulmonary derangements in sheep with combined burn and smoke inhalation injury. Clin Sci (Lond) 2003;105:621-628.
45. Enkhbaatar P, Murakami K, Shimoda K, et al: The inducible nitric oxide synthase inhibitor BBS-2 prevents acute lung injury in sheep after burn and smoke inhalation injury. Am J Respir Crit Care Med 2003;167: 1021-1026.
46. Morita N, Traber MG, Enkhbaatar P, et al: Aerosolized alpha-tocopherol ameliorates acute lung injury following combined burn and smoke inhalation injury in sheep. Shock 2006;25: 277-282.
47. Shimoda K, Murakami K, Enkhbaatar P, et al: Effect of poly(ADP ribose) synthetase inhibition on burn and smoke inhalation injury in sheep. Am J Physiol Lung Cell Mol Physiol 2003;285:L240-L249.
48. Niehaus GD, Kimura R, Traber LD, et al: Administration of a synthetic antiprotease reduces smoke-induced lung injury. J Appl Physiol 1990;69:694-699.
49. Murakami K, McGuire R, Cox RA, et al: Heparin nebulization attenuates acute lung injury in sepsis following smoke inhalation in sheep. Shock 2002;18:236-241.
50. Maybauer MO, Maybauer DM, Fraser JF, et al: Recombinant human activated protein C improves pulmonary function in ovine acute lung injury resulting from smoke inhalation and sepsis. Crit Care Med 2006;34:2432-2438.
51. Jin L, Lalonde C, Demling RH: Lung dysfunction after thermal injury in relation to prostanoid and oxygen radical release. J Appl Physiol 1986;61:103.
52. Youn YK, Lalonde C, Demling R: Oxidants and the pathophysiology of burn and smoke inhalation injury. Free Radical Biol Med 1992;12:409.
53. Demling RH, Niehaus G, Perea A, et al: Effect of burn-induced hypoproteinemia on pulmonary transvascular fluid filtration rate. Surgery 1979;85:339.
54. Shirani KZ, Pruitt BA, Mason AD: The influence of inhalation injury and pneumonia on burn mortality. Ann Surg 1987;205:82.
55. Tredget EE, Shankowsky HA, Taerum TV, et al: The role of inhalation injury in burn trauma. A Canadian experience. Ann Surg 1990;212:720.
56. Holm C, Tegeler J, Mayr M, et al: Effect of crystalloid resuscitation and inhalation injury on extravascular lung water: Clinical implications. Chest 2002;121:1956-1962.
57. Soejima K, Schmalstieg FC, Sakurai H, et al: Pathophysiological analysis of combined burn and smoke inhalation injuries in sheep. Am J Physiol Lung Cell Mol Physiol 2001;280: L1233-1241.
58. Alarie Y: Toxicity of fire smoke. Crit Rev Toxicol 2002;32:259-289.
59. Coburn RF: Mechanisms of carbon monoxide toxicity. Prev Med 1979;8:310-322.
60. Jasper BW, Hopkins RO, Duker HV, Weaver LK: Affective outcome following carbon monoxide poisoning: A prospective longitudinal study. Cogn Behav Neurol 2005;18: 127-134.
61. Norris JC, Moore SJ, Hume AS: Synergistic lethality induced by the combination of carbon monoxide and cyanide. Toxicology 1986;40:121.
62. Chapman AJ, White C: Death resulting from lacrimatory agents. J Forens Sci 1978;23:527.
63. Stein AA, Kirwan WE: Chloracetophenone (tear gas) poisoning: A clinico-pathologic report. J Forensic Sci 1964;9:374.
64. Williams J, Lewis RW, Kealey GP: Carbon monoxide poisoning and myocardial ischemia in patients with burns. J Burn Care Rehab 1992;13: 210.
65. Baud FJ, Barriot P, Toffis V, et al: Elevated blood cyanide concentrations in victims of smoke inhalation. N Engl J Med 1991;325:1761.
66. Lahn M, Sing W, Nazario S, et al: Increased blood lead levels in severe smoke inhalation. Am J Emerg Med 2003;21:458-460.
67. Sahenk Z, Mendell JR, Couri D, Nachtman J: Polyneuropathy from inhalation of N_2O cartridges through a whipped cream dispenser. Neurology 1978;28:485.
68. Koblin DD, Waskell L, Watson JE, et al: Nitrous oxide inactivates methionine synthetase in human liver. Anesth Analg 1982;61:75.
69. Fortenberry JD: Gasoline sniffing. Am J Med 1985;79:740.
70. Garriot J, Petty CS: Death from inhalant abuse: Toxicological and pathological evaluation of 34 cases. Clin Toxicol 1980;16:305.
71. Haponik EF: Clinical and functional assessment. In Haponik EF, Munster AM (eds): Respiratory Injury: Smoke Inhalation and Burns. New York, McGraw-Hill, 1990.
72. Kimura R, Traber LD, Herndon DN, et al: Increasing duration of smoke exposure induces more severe lung injury in sheep. J Appl Physiol 1988;64:1107.
73. Putnam CL, Loke J, Matthay RA, et al: Radiographic manifestations of acute smoke inhalation. Am J Roentgenol 1977;129:865.
74. Peitzman AB, Shires GT III, Teixidor HS, et al: Smoke inhalation injury: Evaluation of radiographic manifestations and pulmonary dysfunction. J Trauma 1989;29:1232.
75. Schall GL, McDonald HD, Carr LB, Capozzi A: Xenon ventilation-perfusion lung scans. The early diagnosis of inhalation injury. JAMA 1978;240: 2441-2445.
76. Shiau YC, Liu FY, Tsai JJ, et al: Usefulness of technetium-99m hexamethylpropylene amine oxime lung scan to detect inhalation lung injury of patients with pulmonary symptoms/signs but negative chest radiograph and pulmonary function test finding after a fire accident—a preliminary report. Ann Nucl Med 2003;17:435-438.
77. Clark WR, Grossman ZD, Nieman GF, et al: Positive computed tomography of dog lungs following severe smoke inhalation: Diagnosis of inhalation injury. J Burn Care Rehab 1982;3:207.
78. Gore MA, Joshi AR, Nagarajan G, et al: Virtual bronchoscopy for diagnosis of inhalation injury in burn patients. Burns 2004;30:165-168.
79. Hunt JL, Agee RN, Pruitt BA: Fiberoptic bronchoscopy in acute inhalation injury. J Trauma 1975;15:641.
80. Moylan JA, Adib K, Birnbaum M: Fiberoptic bronchoscopy following thermal injury. Surg Gynecol Obstet 1975;140:541.
81. Wanner A, Cutchavree A: Early recognition of upper airway obstruction following smoke inhalation. Am Rev Respir Dis 1973; 180:1421.
82. Pegg SP, Kinckley VM: Adjunct role of scintigraphy and bronchoscopy in the early diagnosis of respiratory burns. Burns 1977;4:86.
83. Loick HM, Traber LD, Hurst C, et al: Endoscopic laser flowmetry: A valid method for detection and quantitative analysis of inhalation injury. J Burn Care Rehab 1991;12:313.
84. Barker SJ, Tremper KK: The effect of carbon monoxide inhalation on pulse oximetry and transcutaneous P_{O_2}. Anesthesiology 1987;66:677.
85. Feldstein M, Klendshoj NJ: The determination of cyanide in biologic fluids by microdiffusion analysis. J Lab Clin Med 1954;44:166.
86. Loke J, Rowley R, Kleber HD, et al: Inhalational drug abuse. In Loke J (ed): Pathophysiology and treatment of inhalation injuries. New York, Marcel Dekker, 1988.
87. Henderson RF, Benson JM, Hahn FF, et al: New approaches for the

evaluation of pulmonary toxicity: Bronchoalveolar lavage fluid analysis. Fund Appl Toxicol 1985;5:451.
88. Freitag L, Firusian N, Stanatis G, Greschuchna D: The role of bronchoscopy in pulmonary complications due to mustard gas inhalation. Chest 1991;100:1436.
89. Young KR, Reynolds HY: Bronchoalveolar lavage in inhalation lung toxicity. In Loke J (ed): Pathophysiology and Treatment of Inhalation Injuries. New York, Marcel Dekker, 1988.
90. De Backer D: The cuff-leak test: What are we measuring? Crit Care 2005; 9:31-33.
91. Kemper KJ, Benson MS, Bishop MJ: Predictors of postextubation stridor in pediatric trauma patients. Crit Care Med 1991;19:352.
92. Levine BA, Petroff PA, Slade CL, et al: Prospective trials of dexamethasone and aerosolized gentamicin in the treatment of inhalation injury in the burned patient. J Trauma 1978;18:188.
93. Moylan JA, Chan CK: Inhalation injury-an increasing problem. Ann Surg 1978;183:34.
94. Skrinskas G, Hyland RH, Hutcheon MA: The use of helium-oxygen mixtures in the management of acute upper airway obstruction. Can Med Assoc J 1983;128:555.
95. Kemper KJ, Ritz RH, Benson MS, et al: Helium-oxygen mixture in the treatment of postextubation stridor in pediatric trauma patients. Crit Care Med 1991;19:356.
96. Rodeberg DA, Easter AJ, Washam MA, et al: Use of a helium-oxygen mixture in the treatment of postextubation stridor in pediatric patients with burns. J Burn Care Rehabil 1995;16:476.
97. Desai MH, Mlcak R, Richardson J, et al: Reduction in mortality in pediatric patients with inhalation injury with aerosolized heparin/N-acetylcystine [correction of acetylcystine] therapy. J Burn Care Rehabil 1998;19:210-212.
98. The Acute Respiratory Distress Syndrome Network: Ventilation with lower tidal volumes as compared with traditional tidal volumes for acute lung injury and the acute respiratory distress syndrome. N Engl J Med 2000;342:1301.
99. Ware LB, Matthay MA: The acute respiratory distress syndrome. N Engl J Med 2000;342:1334.
100. Reper P, Wibaux O, Van Laeke P, et al: High frequency percussive ventilation and conventional ventilation after smoke inhalation: A randomised study. Burns 2002;28:503-508.
101. Cartotto R, Ellis S, Smith T: Use of high-frequency oscillatory ventilation in burn patients. Crit Care Med 2005;33:S175-S181.
102. Thompson JT, Molnar JA, Hines MH, et al: Successful management of adult smoke inhalation with extracorporeal membrane oxygenation. J Burn Care Rehabil 2005;26:62-66.
103. Levine BA, Petroff PA, Slade CL, et al: Prospective trials of dexamethasone and aerosolized gentamicin in the treatment of inhalation injury in the burned patient. J Trauma 1978; 18:188.
104. Martyn JA, Richtsfeld M: Succinylcholine-induced hyperkalemia in acquired pathologic states: Etiologic factors and molecular mechanisms. Anesthesiology 2006;104:158-169.
105. Shaner PJ, Brown RL, Kirksey F, et al: Succinylcholine induced hyperkalemia in burned patients-1. Anesth Analg 1969;48:764.
106. Tolmie JD, Joyce TH, Mitchell GD: Succinylcholine changes in the burned patient. Anesthesiology 1967;28:467.
107. Dwersteg JF, Pavlin EG, Heimbach DM: Patients with burns are resistant to atracurium. Anesthesiology 1986;65: 517.
108. Martyn JA, Goudsouzian RS: Metocurine requirements and plasma concentration in burned paediatric patients. Br J Anaesth 1983;55:263.
109. Han T, Kim H, Bae J, et al: Neuromuscular pharmacodynamics of rocuronium in patients with major burns. Anesth Analg 2004;99:386-392.
110. Wachtel TL, Frank DH, Frank HA: Management of burns of the head and neck. Head Neck Surg 1981; 3:458.
111. Robinson L, Miller RH: Smoke inhalation injuries. Am J Otolaryngol 1986;7:375.
112. Ciaglia P, Firshing R, Syniec C: Elective percutaneous dilatational tracheostomy: A new simple bedside procedure: Preliminary report. Chest 1985;87:715-719.
113. Delaney A, Bagshaw SM, Nalos M: Percutaneous dilatational tracheostomy versus surgical tracheostomy in critically ill patients: A systematic review and meta-analysis. Crit Care 2006;10:R55.
114. Caruso DM, Al-Kasspooles MF, Matthews MR, et al: Rationale for "early" percutaneous dilatational tracheostomy in patients with burn injuries. J Burn Care Rehabil 1997;18:424-428.
115. Gravvanis AI, Tsoutsos D, Iconomou TG, Papadopoulos SG: Percutaneous versus conventional tracheostomy in burned patients with inhalation injury. World J Surg 2005;29:1571-1575.
116. Pace N, Strajman E, Walker EL: Acceleration of carbon monoxide elimination in man by high pressure oxygen. Science 1950; 111:652-654.
117. Tibbles PM, Edelsberg JS: Hyperbaric-oxygen therapy. N Engl J Med 1996;334:1642-1648.
118. Weaver LK, Hopkins RO, Chan KJ, et al: Hyperbaric oxygen for acute carbon monoxide poisoning. N Engl J Med 2002;347:1057-1067.
119. Juurlink DN, Buckley NA, Stanbrook MB, et al: Hyperbaric oxygen for carbon monoxide poisoning. Cochrane Database Syst Rev 2005 Jan 25;(1): CD002041.
120. Hampson NB, Dunford RG, Ross DE, Wreford-Brown CE: A prospective, randomized clinical trial comparing two hyperbaric treatment protocols for carbon monoxide poisoning. Undersea Hyperb Med 2006;33:27-32.
121. Vogel SN, Sultan TR: Cyanide poisoning. Clin Toxicol 1981;18:367.
122. Megarbane B, Delahaye A, Goldgran-Toledano D, Baud FJ: Antidotal treatment of cyanide poisoning. J Chin Med Assoc 2003;66:193-203.
123. Haponik EF, Summer WR: Respiratory complications in burned patients: Pathogenesis and spectrum of inhalation injury. J Crit Care 1987; 2:49.
124. Thompson PB, Herndon DN, Traber DL, Abstron S: Effect on mortality of inhalation injury. J Trauma 1986; 26:163.
125. Brown DL, Archer SB, Greenhalgh DG, et al: Inhalation injury severity scoring system: A quantitative method. J Burn Care Rehabil 1997;17:552.
126. Slutzker AD, Kinn R, Said SI: Bronchiectasis and progressive respiratory failure following smoke inhalation. Chest 1989;95:1349.
127. Hargreave FE, Dolovich J, O'Byrne PM, et al: The origin of airway hyperresponsiveness. J Allergy Clin Immunol 1986;78:825.
128. Rabinovitch S, Greyson ND, Weiser W, Hoffstein V: Clinical and laboratory features of acute sulfur dioxide inhalation poisoning: Two-year follow-up. Am Rev Respir Dis 1989;139:556.
129. Kinsella J, Carter R, Reid WH, et al: Increased airway reactivity after smoke inhalation. Lancet 1991;337:595.
130. Moisan TC: Prolonged asthma after smoke inhalation: A report of three cases and a review of previous reports. J Occup Med 1991;33:458.
131. Elliott CG, Morris AH, Cengiz M: Pulmonary function and exercise gas exchange in survivors of adult respiratory distress syndrome. Am Rev Respir Dis 1981;123:492.

Chapter 50

Immunologic Lung Disease in the Critically Ill

Gregory A. Schmidt and Gary W. Hunninghake

Pulmonary defense mechanisms have evolved to respond to a variety of inhaled agents. Although these defense mechanisms are usually beneficial to the host, they can go astray, leading to inflammatory lung injury. Immunologic lung disease can arise in any anatomic compartment of the lung. Examples include the airways in bronchiolitis obliterans, the parenchyma in idiopathic pulmonary fibrosis (IPF), and blood vessels in vasculitis. In each instance these illnesses may prove severe enough to merit intensive care unit management for diagnosis and treatment. The large variety of immunologic lung diseases tend to share two features during critical illness. First, restrictive lung physiology is generally present, so the risk of lung overdistention and associated ventilator-induced lung injury is real. Secondly, pulmonary hypertension may complicate management of the circulation. Early recognition and treatment of immunologic lung diseases are essential to avoid permanent lung damage or death.

The focus of this chapter is immunologic lung disease. The emphasis is on those disorders that are likely to present to the medical intensivist. Asthma and neuromuscular diseases are covered elsewhere in this book and are not reviewed here.

IDIOPATHIC PULMONARY FIBROSIS

Idiopathic pulmonary fibrosis is a disorder of unknown etiology characterized by inflammation of the lower respiratory tract that usually leads to irreversible scarring. Current and former smokers are at increased risk, and there may be an inherited susceptibility to develop this disease.[1-3] IPF most commonly presents as an outpatient illness with the insidious onset of exertional dyspnea and cough. On examination of the lungs, coarse crackles are found and clubbing of the fingers is characteristic.[3] Chest radiographs may show a spectrum of findings from peripheral reticular densities to end-stage honeycombed lung.[3] Alveolar infiltrates are unusual unless the patient has a concurrent lung cancer, pneumonia, or heart disease. The lung computed tomography (CT) findings most closely associated with a pathologic diagnosis of IPF are lower-lung honeycombing and upper-lung irregular lines.[4] The histology of IPF reveals lesions characterized by inflammation, fibroblastic foci, areas of fibrosis, and remodeling of the lung parenchyma. This type of lesion is also called *usual interstitial pneumonitis*. The pulmonary fibrosis appears to follow collapse of involved alveoli.

The basement membranes of adjacent alveoli join to form what appears to be a single, thickened alveolar septum. For this reason, the lungs of patients with IPF exhibit restrictive physiology with decreased lung volumes, decreased parenchymal compliance, and a loss of functional capillary beds leading to a reduction in the diffusing capacity.[5] In this manner the functionally smaller lungs of the patient with IPF resemble the lungs of patients with the acute respiratory distress syndrome (ARDS). This concept is supported by CT findings of heterogeneous disease involvement in the lungs of patients with both IPF and ARDS. This parallel can be used as a framework for managing tidal volumes during mechanical ventilation of IPF patients with respiratory failure. If large tidal volumes (or excessive inflation pressures) are used, relatively normal areas of lung will be overdistended, potentially exacerbating lung injury. Limiting tidal volumes to 6 mL/kg predicted body weight in patients with acute lung injury (ALI) or ARDS saves lives.[6] Similar data are not available regarding safe parameters for ventilating patients with chronic restrictive lung diseases, but limiting tidal volumes to roughly 6 mL/kg (and raising the rate accordingly) carries little risk. Moreover, retrospective analysis of mechanically ventilated patients without ALI/ARDS suggests that large tidal volumes may produce ALI (odds ratio 1.3 for each mL above 6 mL/kg predicted body weight).[7] Because there is little evidence that intrinsic positive end expiratory pressure (PEEP) plays a physiologically important role in respiratory failure in patients with IPF, more rapid ventilatory rates may be tolerated.[5] This may allow ventilation without resorting to permissive hypercapnia, which may aggravate pulmonary hypertension.[8,9] As in the ARDS lung, it seems likely that nonfunctional, diseased lung units exist alongside those with essentially normal function. However, unlike the acutely injured lung, atelectatic lung units available for recruitment through the use of elevated end expiratory pressure are rare in IPF. There is probably little clinical advantage to using high PEEP in IPF patients; in fact, high levels of PEEP may be detrimental by overdistending the lung, as well as by contributing to cor pulmonale, as described later.

Another clinicopathologic process to consider in the ventilatory management of the patient with IPF is pulmonary hypertension. Pulmonary artery pressures are chronically elevated in advanced IPF, and their pressure increases further with the increased cardiac output that accompanies exercise, fever, and hypercarbia.[9,10] Pulmonary hypertension may eventually lead to cor pulmonale because of increased right ventricular afterload.[11] Mechanical ventilation may interact adversely with pulmonary hypertension in the patient with IPF. Positive pressure ventilation, alone, impairs right heart function, and this effect is exaggerated by PEEP.[12] PEEP increases afterload by increasing pulmonary vascular resistance.[13] The resulting increase in wall tension decreases right ventricular perfusion pressure, which leads to myocardial ischemia.[13,14] Right ventricular ischemia may cause further dysfunction and dilation of the right heart, in addition to diastolic dysfunction of the left ventricle (through ventricular interdependence), producing a cycle of progressively deteriorating circulatory function.[11] Thus it is important to minimize further increases in pulmonary artery pressure and to maintain adequate systemic pressure to preserve perfusion of the right ventricle. Additionally, adequate oxygenation is essential to prevent reflex increases in pulmonary artery pressure and to maintain peripheral oxygen delivery. Finally, hypercapnia, which tends to raise pulmonary artery pressures, should generally be avoided. Because predicting the degree of pulmonary hypertension in IPF is difficult—and the need to avoid increases in pulmonary artery pressures is so important—we advocate liberal use of echocardiography. Other forms of monitoring, such as central venous saturation measurement or pulmonary artery catheterization, might also be useful. When acute-on-chronic cor pulmonale compromises the circulation, dobutamine or norepinephrine is often helpful.[15] Inhaled nitric oxide or inhaled prostacyclin probably plays some role, at least to buy time in the critically impaired patient.[16,17] The role of newer pulmonary vasodilators such as bosentan and sildenafil in patients with acute cor pulmonale is unclear.

Death in patients with IPF is most often directly attributable to progression of the underlying disease, even when the disease is only of moderate severity.[3,18] Nevertheless, the clinician should seek treatable complicating conditions before making the difficult decision to withhold mechanical ventilatory support. Other causes of respiratory failure in IPF include congestive heart failure, bronchogenic carcinoma, pulmonary embolism, and infection. Left ventricular failure is often found in association with IPF. These patients often have many of the risk factors (e.g., smoking, hyperlipidemia) that are associated with the development of atherosclerosis. For this reason, left ventricular failure may result from ischemic heart disease. Two other factors that may contribute to left ventricular failure in these individuals are systemic arterial hypertension and right ventricular failure. Hypoxemia may exacerbate these effects. A search for potentially treatable left ventricular failure should be considered in the deteriorating IPF patient.

Patients with IPF have about a 14-fold excess risk of developing lung cancer.[19] These malignancies are difficult to detect on an already abnormal chest radiograph and often cause rapid deterioration in the IPF patient. Treatment options for malignancy are often limited by poor pulmonary reserve. However, the diagnosis of lung cancer may greatly alter therapeutic planning. Furthermore, relieving airway obstruction and postobstructive infection may significantly palliate dyspnea.

Pulmonary embolism can also cause rapid deterioration and respiratory failure in IPF patients. Ventilation-perfusion scans often reveal nonsegmental perfusion defects and inhomogeneous areas of poor ventilation as a result of the IPF alone, so the utility of these scans in diagnosing pulmonary emboli is limited.[20] Pulmonary angiography or helical CT scanning should be considered if it can be performed safely.[20] We recommend empiric long-term anticoagulation for individuals with advanced IPF and severe pulmonary hypertension who are suspected of having pulmonary embolism but for whom a diagnostic evaluation is unfeasible.[21]

Pulmonary infection is also difficult to document in patients with end-stage IPF and is a frequent cause of rapid decline in these patients. Many end-stage patients who die of respiratory failure have an infection as the inciting event. Only subtle changes on the chest radiograph are present in most of these patients. Computed tomography scanning may show alveolar infiltrates. Strong consideration should be given to the use of antibiotics in all IPF patients who suffer an acute respiratory decline. Bronchoalveolar lavage or protected brush specimens from the distal airway may identify specific bacterial pathogens. Often the organism is not identified, and broad-spectrum antibiotics are used. The end-stage fibrotic lung has grossly distorted airways and multiple cystic airspaces, so this empiric coverage should be designed to also cover anaerobic organisms. In our experience, long courses of antibiotics are frequently required to adequately treat respiratory infections in IPF. We use 10 to 14 days of intravenous antibiotics followed by a prolonged course of oral therapy (6 to 12 weeks) aimed at treating anaerobic organisms.

An important factor to consider in patients with advanced IPF who develop respiratory failure is that this disease is largely irreversible. Although many exciting new therapies are under investigation, current treatments are largely ineffective in reversing the decline in lung function.[22-4] Most patients with IPF who are in respiratory failure do not respond to corticosteroid therapy.[25] Cytotoxic therapy, such as cyclophosphamide 1.5 mg/kg/day, can be tried, but there is little evidence that this alters survival. In a study of 38 IPF patients admitted to an intensive care unit, 61% died in the hospital and, of the survivors, 92% died at a median of 2 months after discharge.[26] If patients are young, have early disease, or may be diagnosed with interstitial lung disease other than IPF, an open lung biopsy should be considered to exclude alternative treatable diseases. Recently, lung transplantation has become a viable option for some patients with end-stage IPF. It is imperative that physicians caring for these patients familiarize themselves with the referral protocols and policies of their respective regional transplant centers.

HAMMAN-RICH SYNDROME

Hamman-Rich syndrome, more recently called *acute interstitial pneumonia* (AIP), is a rapidly progressive interstitial pneumonia first described by Hamman and Rich.[27] The mean age of patients is 50 to 60 with a broad range and perhaps an increased risk for males.[27,28] The patients often describe a prodromal viral-like respiratory illness. This is typically followed by subacute progressive dyspnea, fever, and nonproductive coughing.

AIP usually evolves over 1 to 3 months and, in some instances, within 1 to 2 weeks after the onset of symptoms. Signs of right heart failure may exist, and diffuse or basilar crackles may be found on auscultation of the lung. Diffuse, bilateral interstitial infiltrates are characteristic on chest radiograph. The findings on CT scan include diffuse patchy alveolar ground glass infiltrates. Laboratory studies may show a leukocytosis with neutrophilia. Hypoxemia may be profound. Pulmonary function tests in patients without respiratory failure show a restrictive defect, generally without evidence of airway obstruction.[28]

For many years experts believed that this disease was simply a rapidly progressive form of IPF; now it is felt that this disease is more related to ARDS. The pathology of AIP is characterized by diffuse, active fibrosis, with proliferating fibroblasts and minimal collagen. These findings appear acute and relatively uniform in age and resemble the organizing stage of diffuse alveolar damage as seen in ARDS.[29]

The prognosis of acute interstitial pneumonitis is poor, with only about a 40% short-term survival. Supportive care may involve ventilatory support. Antibiotics to treat possible underlying infection and corticosteroids to treat inflammation have been used in many cases but the efficacy of these treatments is unproved.[28] In one small series, early efforts to exclude infection combined with lung-protective ventilation and high-dose corticosteroid therapy led to success in 8 of 10 patients.[30] We recommend rigorous exclusion of an infectious etiology including open lung biopsy, if necessary, before considering any immunosuppressive therapy.

ALVEOLAR HEMORRHAGE SYNDROMES

Perhaps the most striking immunologically mediated lung diseases are those that present with alveolar hemorrhage. These disorders require prompt diagnosis and management. We limit our comments here to the disorders that most commonly present as alveolar hemorrhage: Goodpasture's syndrome, Wegener's granulomatosis (WG), microscopic polyangiitis, catastrophic antiphospholipid syndrome, systemic lupus erythematosus (SLE), and idiopathic pulmonary hemosiderosis. Box 50-1 provides a

Box 50-1

Causes of Immune/Idiopathic Alveolar Hemorrhage

Goodpasture's Syndrome

Wegener's Granulomatosis

Other Systemic Vasculitides/Collagen Vascular Diseases
Microscopic polyangiitis
Catastrophic antiphospholipid antibody syndrome
Systemic lupus erythematosus
Henoch-Schönlein purpura
Behçet's disease
Essential mixed cryoglobulinemia
Rheumatoid arthritis
Progressive systemic sclerosis
Mixed connective tissue disease

Alveolar Hemorrhage and Glomerulonephritis Unrelated to Goodpasture's Syndrome, Vasculitis, or Collagen Vascular Disease*

Thrombotic Thrombocytopenic Purpura

Membranoproliferative Glomerulonephritis

Immunoglobulin A Nephropathy

Diffuse Endocapillary Proliferative Glomerulonephritis

Focal Proliferative Glomerulonephritis

Alveolar Hemorrhage Resulting from Drugs or Chemicals
D-penicillamine
Trimellitic anhydride
Isocyanates
Nitrofurantoin
Amiodarone
Propylthiouracil
Infliximab

Idiopathic Pulmonary Hemosiderosis

*Idiopathic alveolar hemorrhage with pauci-immune necrotizing or crescentic glomerulonephritis is classified as nonspecific systemic vasculitis (presumptive).

Adapted from Leatherman JW: Diffuse alveolar hemorrhage in immune and idiopathic disorders. In Lynch JP III, De Remee R (eds): Immunologically Mediated Pulmonary Diseases. Philadelphia, JB Lippincott, 1991.

more complete list of disorders that can lead to alveolar hemorrhage.

An essential goal of managing patients with alveolar hemorrhage is prompt diagnosis of the underlying disorder (Fig. 50-1). The first step is to document alveolar hemorrhage. The classic triad of hemoptysis, anemia, and diffuse infiltrates on chest radiograph strongly suggests alveolar hemorrhage, yet many patients with significant alveolar hemorrhage do not have hemoptysis.[31] Consequently, the absence of hemoptysis does not exclude the presence of alveolar hemorrhage. Thus diffuse pulmonary infiltrates, respiratory distress, and anemia associated with clinical evidence of glomerulonephritis or other conditions associated with vasculitis should arouse suspicion for alveolar hemorrhage, even in the absence of hemoptysis.

Before any specific therapy is instituted, it is important to document the presence of alveolar hemorrhage. Other processes that result in diffuse alveolar filling must be excluded, such as inflammatory exudate from infection, cardiogenic pulmonary edema, and ARDS. In addition, one should exclude hemorrhage from cancer, bronchitis, bronchiectasis, excessive anticoagulation, or an endogenous coagulation defect. Perhaps the most valuable test for documenting alveolar hemorrhage is bronchoscopy with bronchoalveolar lavage. Blood-tinged lavage fluid or frank blood in the airways is usually present.[32] Another test that can be used is to stain alveolar macrophages retrieved by lavage for hemosiderin. Normal individuals will have few hemosiderin-laden macrophages in bronchoalveolar lavage (BAL), but the intensity of staining and percentage of cells staining positive have been found to be predictive of alveolar hemorrhage.[33,34] We feel, however, that this test is of questionable clinical value. If patients have sufficient acute bleeding to cause infiltrates on chest radiograph, this should be seen easily in the lavage fluid. If the only evidence for hemorrhage is the presence of hemosiderin-laden macrophages, we would propose that the acute infiltrates are the result of another cause. Similarly, the negative predictive value of this test can be questioned because it may take up to 48 hours for intracellular hemosiderin accumulation after an acute bleed.[35] Documentation of an elevated diffusion capacity for carbon monoxide (DLCO) is also a means of evaluating for alveolar hemorrhage.[36,37] Bowley and coworkers[37] demonstrated the usefulness of this measure as a sensitive index of recurrent alveolar hemorrhage in patients undergoing treatment.

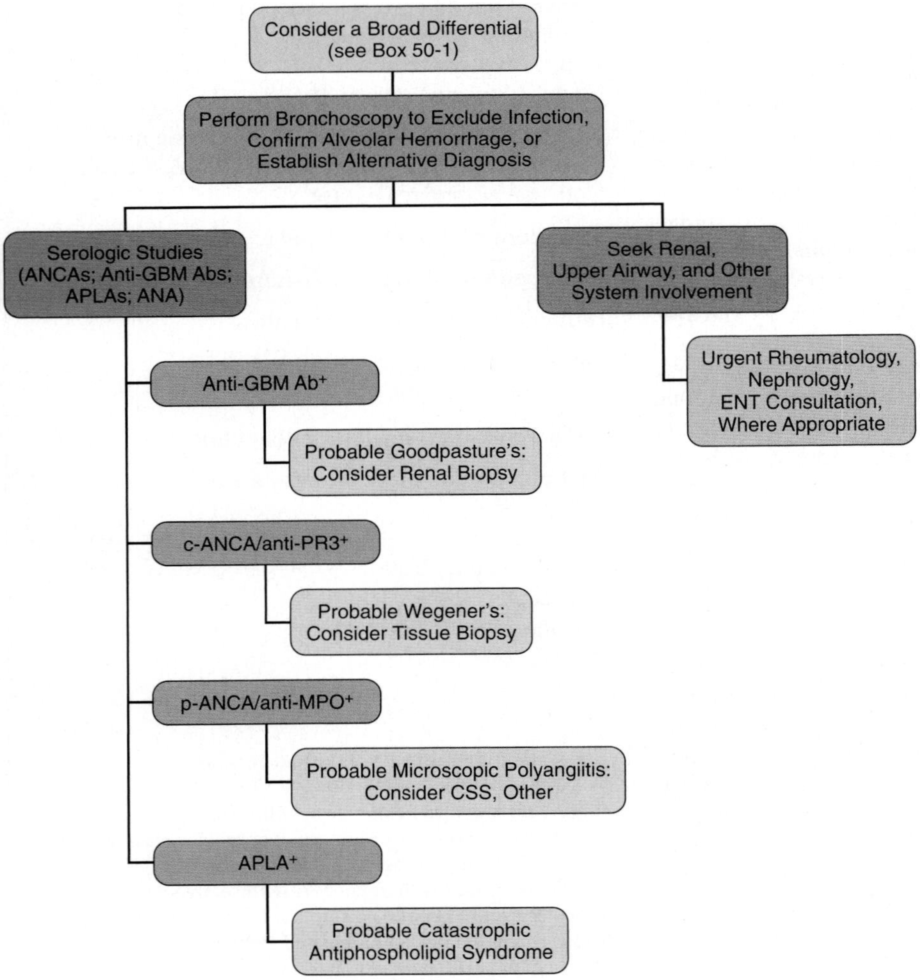

Figure 50-1. Diagnosis and management of alveolar hemorrhage syndromes. ANA, anti-nuclear antibodies; ANCA, anti-neutrophil extoplasmic antibody; Anti-GBM Abs, anti-glomerular basement membrane antibodies; anti-MPO, anti-myeloperoxidase antibodies; anti-PR3, anti-proteinase antibodies; APLAs, anti-phospholipid antibodies; CSS, Churg-Strauss syndrome; ENT, ear, nose, and throat.

Goodpasture's Syndrome

Goodpasture's syndrome accounts for 20% to 30% of the cases of alveolar hemorrhage.[38] This disease is a classic pulmonary-renal syndrome with a high mortality from alveolar hemorrhage or renal failure if untreated. Antibasement membrane antibody is a universal finding in this disease. Antibody deposition along the glomerular basement membrane undoubtedly contributes to the renal pathology of this disease[38]; however, other cofactors, in addition to anti-GBM antibody may be necessary for alveolar hemorrhage to develop. A higher incidence of alveolar hemorrhage has been reported in smokers with anti-GBM antibody disease.[39] Experimental studies also showed that exposure to 100% oxygen in animals with circulating antibasement membrane antibody resulted in alveolar hemorrhage, whereas unexposed animals did not develop lung disease.[40]

A 2:1 ratio of males to females exists with a median age of 21 years in patients with Goodpasture's syndrome.[41,42] Alveolar hemorrhage is the most common presentation of Goodpasture's syndrome. Evidence of renal involvement is usually present; however, some patients may only have microscopic hematuria.[38] Untreated, Goodpasture's syndrome carries a mortality approaching 100%, the cause of death being equally divided between uremia and alveolar hemorrhage.[41] With early dialysis, plasma exchange, and immunosuppression, however, the acute mortality of the disease is about 27%, with the single most common cause of death being infection.[43]

The evaluation of patients suspected of having Goodpasture's syndrome should include confirmation of alveolar hemorrhage, evaluation for renal disease, and testing for antibasement membrane antibody. Circulating antibasement membrane antibody can be demonstrated in more than 95% of patients through radioimmunoassay or enzyme-linked immunosorbent assay (ELISA).[44] Kidney biopsy should also be considered to confirm the diagnosis and to document the extent of glomerular loss. The characteristic glomerular lesion shows strong linear deposition of immunoglobulin G (IgG) along glomerular capillaries.[38] Other histologic features include segmental, necrotizing, crescentic glomerulonephritis indistinguishable from that found in other forms of vasculitis. Walker and colleagues[43] demonstrated that patients with greater than 85% crescents on biopsy were significantly less likely to regain renal function. Lung biopsy is rarely necessary and often nonspecific.

Treatment consists of dialysis, plasma exchange, and immunosuppressive therapy. Immunosuppression usually includes both cyclophosphamide and corticosteroids.[38,45] Dialysis should be performed early to reverse uremic platelet dysfunction and to prevent fluid overload because both factors may perpetuate alveolar hemorrhage. Mechanical ventilation may be necessary to provide respiratory support, as well as to facilitate clearing blood from the airways. When mechanical ventilatory support is used, efforts should be made to select lung-protective tidal volumes and to minimize the fraction of inspired oxygen. We also aggressively treat possible respiratory infection because it may precipitate and perpetuate alveolar hemorrhage. If the patient has received drugs that impair platelet function, such as aspirin, we also administer platelets in cases of life-threatening hemorrhage. Alveolar hemorrhage generally responds within 1 to 3 days to this treatment.[46] In refractory cases, there has been anecdotal response to mycophenolate or to anti-CD20 antibody. Once the patient has recovered, the importance of maintenance cyclophosphamide in preventing recurrent alveolar hemorrhage cannot be overemphasized.[38,46,47]

Wegener's Granulomatosis

Another form of vasculitis that commonly presents as alveolar hemorrhage is WG. This disorder is characterized by a granulomatous vasculitis involving the upper and lower airways and is associated with rapidly progressive renal failure. WG represented 15% of the cases of alveolar hemorrhage in a series reported by Leatherman.[38] The incidence of pulmonary hemorrhage in this disorder is reported to vary between 12% and 30%.[48,49] Clinical findings that may suggest a diagnosis of WG include nodules visible on a chest radiograph and evidence of upper airway involvement including chronic otitis media, sinusitis, nasal septal perforation, or tracheal stenosis.[50] Eye involvement with either proptosis or extraocular muscle entrapment may occur.[50] Skin lesions may include petechiae, palpable purpura, ulcers, vesicles, papules, and subcutaneous nodules.[48] Musculoskeletal findings include myalgias, arthralgias, and pauciarticular or migratory arthritis. Neurologic manifestations include sensoryneural deafness, mononeuritis multiplex, and cranial nerve palsies.[48,50] Subglottic tracheal stenosis or obstruction can occur in these patients and should be considered before endotracheal intubation is undertaken. In up to 10% of patients, tracheostomy may be required to manage the airway sometime during the course of their illness.[50]

Laboratory findings in WG include leukocytosis, anemia, thrombocytosis, and an elevated erythrocyte sedimentation rate. A valuable laboratory test is the antineutrophil cytoplasmic antibody (ANCA), which detects IgG directed at a variety of neutrophil and monocyte antigens. Clinically important ANCAs are of two types: antiproteinase 3 antibodies (anti-PR3) and antimyeloperoxidase antibodies (anti-MPO). When serum containing these antibodies is applied to neutrophils and stained by indirect immunofluorescence, anti-PR3 produces a cytoplasmic pattern of staining (c-ANCA), whereas anti-MPO produces a perinuclear or nuclear pattern (p-ANCA). Both anti-PR3 (seen almost exclusively in WG) and anti-MPO (which may be seen in pauci-immune rapidly progressive glomerulonephritis, Churg-Strauss syndrome, and microscopic polyangiitis) can be measured more directly by ELISA. The sensitivity of ANCA has been reported to be 80% to 96% in patients with active generalized (e.g., having renal involvement) WG, and generally these patients have both c-ANCA and anti-PR3 positivity. In the ANCA-associated systemic vasculitides, which include WG, alveolar hemorrhage has been found in patients who have tested positive for either c-ANCA or p-ANCA (see "Microscopic Polyangiitis" later). More recently, the presence of an immunoglobulin M (IgM) isotype of ANCA has been strongly associated with alveolar hemorrhage; conversely, patients lacking IgM ANCA may have a low risk for alveolar hemorrhage.[51] Frequently, the diagnosis of WG relies on tissue examination. Biopsies of upper airway lesions are probably acceptable in nonemergent situations where diagnosis can be delayed. However, in the case of severe alveolar hemorrhage, there is frequently an emergent need for diagnosis so that effective treatment can be instituted. An open lung biopsy often provides the diagnosis. Potential infectious etiologies, especially mycobacterial and fungal pathogens, can also be excluded. Fauci and coworkers have developed a scheme of major and minor criteria for WG on the basis of histology. Three major pathologic manifestations were identified including parenchymal necrosis, vasculitis, and granulomatous inflammation[52]; however, in 18% of biopsies, less distinctive histologic features were the predominant findings. If definitive tissue biopsy cannot be obtained, a WG with alveolar hemorrhage diagnosis should be based on the histologic finding of a small vessel vasculitis or crescentic glomerulonephritis, together with compelling clinical evidence of WG consisting of cavitary pulmonary nodules or characteristic upper airway involvement.[38] Moreover, the presence of a positive c-ANCA test can help to confirm the diagnosis.

The recommended treatment for alveolar hemorrhage resulting from WG includes high-dose corticosteroids and cyclophosphamide.[38,53] We recommend that patients who are critically ill receive intravenous methylprednisolone at doses up to 1 g daily for the first 3 days in addition to cyclophosphamide at 3 to 5 mg/kg for 3 to 5 days. After this period, the prednisone dosage is reduced to 1 mg/kg/day and cyclophosphamide continued at 1.5 mg/kg/day. Most patients respond favorably to this regimen, but mortality remains substantial, often because of renal failure or sepsis. Plasma exchange or intravenous immunoglobulin may be useful in patients with life-threatening diffuse alveolar hemorrhage or when disease persists despite corticosteroids and cyclophosphamide.[54] Other rescue therapies have included trimethoprim-sulfamethoxazole, rituximab,[55] antitumor necrosis factor antibodies, and antilymphocyte antibodies. The supportive measures described earlier for alveolar hemorrhage in Goodpasture's syndrome also apply to this disease.

Microscopic Polyangiitis

Microscopic polyangiitis (MPA) is a systemic, small-vessel vasculitis. Symptoms may begin subtly with weeks to months of fever, weight loss, malaise, and myalgias. ICU admission is often precipitated by life-threatening diffuse alveolar hemorrhage, and MPA is probably the most common vasculitis to present this way. Renal failure caused by crescentic, rapidly progressive, focal segmental necrotizing glomerulonephritis can predate ICU admission or be recognized concurrently but eventually develops in nearly all cases without treatment. Joint and skin manifestation are occasionally seen, as well as peripheral nerve and gastrointestinal involvement. Most patients will have positive ANCA with specificity for MPO (p-ANCA), although some will be c-ANCA positive. Some patients initially suspected of having MPA will ultimately develop granulomatous upper airway disease, and the diagnosis is changed to WG.

Treatment requires high-dose corticosteroids and cyclophosphamide in the same doses as for WG. Intravenous immunoglobulin may be effective in difficult cases. Factor VIIa has also been tried, and the rescue therapies described earlier for WG may also be effective. For the patient with respiratory failure caused by alveolar hemorrhage, ventilator guidelines for acute lung injury/ARDS should be followed. Once a patient survives the acute alveolar hemorrhage, there are reasonable prospects for long-term survival, although this depends to a large degree on whether renal function recovers.

Catastrophic Antiphospholipid Syndrome

The term *antiphospholipid syndrome* was coined to describe patients with systemic thrombosis or recurrent fetal loss having increased antiphospholipid antibodies in the circulation. A subset presenting with widespread vascular thrombosis and a fulminating clinical course, often involving respiratory failure, was subsequently called the *catastrophic antiphospholipid syndrome* (CAPS).[56] This syndrome can occur in those without a recognized rheumatologic disease but also in those with SLE or other diseases.

CAPS has been generally considered a noninflammatory, thrombotic disease leading to widespread ischemia and necrosis, producing multiorgan failure and death. More recently, however, cases of alveolar hemorrhage have been described in the setting of antiphospholipid syndrome in which thrombosis was not evident clinically or pathologically. These authors proposed that a nonthrombotic mechanism for pulmonary capillaritis and alveolar hemorrhage should be sought.[57]

Infections, trauma, procedures, drugs, and malignancy have been implicated as precipitating factors. Clinically there is often evidence of widespread arterial and venous occlusions. Renal, pulmonary, and central nervous systems are most often affected. Multiple pulmonary manifestations have been reported including pulmonary thromboembolism, pulmonary hypertension, and acute lung injury in addition to diffuse alveolar hemorrhage. Serologic findings include elevated titers of anticardiolipin antibody or the lupus anticoagulant. Increased β_2-glycoprotein I has been linked to CAPS.[58]

Treatment generally involves immunosuppression along the lines of treatment for other immune alveolar hemorrhage syndromes. Plasmapheresis may be effective.[59] The role for anticoagulation in the acute setting of alveolar hemorrhage is uncertain, but we recommend first establishing control of bleeding with immunosuppressive therapy and plasmapheresis, then later instituting antithrombotic treatment.

Systemic Lupus Erythematosus

In patients with SLE, a wide variety of lung lesions are found. Histologic evidence of alveolar hemorrhage can be found in 40% of patients at autopsy [60] Massive alveolar hemorrhage is uncommon, being reported in only 5% of patients in one series of 99 patients with SLE and lung involvement.[61] Although massive alveolar hemorrhage may be the presenting manifestation of SLE, this is uncommon.[62,63] The clinical presentation of alveolar hemorrhage in SLE is similar to other alveolar hemorrhage syndromes; however, fever as high as 39°C to 40°C may be a prominent feature.[61] At the time of alveolar hemorrhage, patients often manifest other typical clinical manifestations of SLE, particularly nephritis, highlighting the systemic nature of this disease.[64]

The etiology of alveolar hemorrhage in SLE is not entirely clear. In some patients, antiphospholipid antibodies, as discussed earlier, may play a role.[65] Pathologic studies of open lung biopsies have not always demonstrated immune complex deposition.[60,63] Patients with SLE often show a microscopic angiitis on biopsy.[62,64] Considerable clinical overlap between the alveolar hemorrhage syndrome and acute lupus pneumonitis exists.[60,64] Because treatment of both lesions is similar, we recommend separating these two pulmonary manifestations on clinical grounds without the need for open lung biopsy, as long as infection has been adequately excluded.

Infection is the most important factor to exclude in diagnosing alveolar hemorrhage in the patient with SLE. At least half of the patients with SLE who present with infiltrates should be expected to have an infectious etiology.[60] Because many of these patients are receiving immunosuppressive therapy and because SLE is associated with impaired cellular immunity, the differential diagnosis for infectious agents is broad and includes bacterial, fungal, mycobacterial, and viral and parasitic pathogens. Bronchoscopy with lavage and transbronchial biopsies are the logical procedures used to search for an infectious cause. Open lung biopsy may be necessary in some cases.

Mortality from SLE-associated alveolar hemorrhage is variable in small series, ranging from about 20% to more than 85%.[38,63,64] Many patients develop respiratory failure, and the need for mechanical ventilation is associated with an increased mortality.[64] This high risk for respiratory failure is multifactorial, with contributions from alveolar hemorrhage, a high prevalence of underlying atelectasis, and diaphragmatic weakness.[66,67] We recommend treating these patients with both high-dose corticosteroids and cyclophosphamide in a regimen similar to that used for WG.

Idiopathic Pulmonary Hemosiderosis

The diagnosis of idiopathic pulmonary hemosiderosis is, by definition, one of exclusion. The syndrome is typically an illness that presents in infancy or childhood.[68] The disease is characterized by recurrent episodes of alveolar hemorrhage, although often these episodes may be subclinical.[69] There have been familial clusters of cases.[70,71] Some cases of unexplained alveolar hemorrhage with onset during adulthood have been reported. The specific treatment of this illness is not clear. Most patients do well during the acute episode with supportive care alone, but there may be a short-term benefit from corticosteroid therapy. Long-term corticosteroid treatment has been described in some cases.

CRYPTOGENIC ORGANIZING PNEUMONIA

Cryptogenic organizing pneumonia (COP), also termed *idiopathic bronchiolitis obliterans with organizing pneumonia* (BOOP) frequently presents as an acute illness with respiratory failure. This disease often responds well to therapy without residual respiratory deficit, if timely diagnosis and treatment are undertaken. COP presents throughout adult life and shows no particular demographic associations.[72] The presenting symptoms include cough, dyspnea, or both in more than two thirds of cases. Flulike symptoms are present in 14%, and patients usually present with subacute symptoms within 3 months.[73,74] Examination of the lung reveals dry crackles in 50% to 75% of cases. Wheezing and finger clubbing are rarely seen. Up to 12% of patients can be expected to present with a normal physical examination.[73,74]

The chest radiograph most often shows patchy alveolar infiltrates scattered throughout all lung fields. Interstitial infiltrates and nodular densities may be seen.[74,75] Some reports suggest that interstitial densities on chest radiograph may be associated with a worse prognosis.[76] High-resolution computed tomography (HRCT) of the chest shows predominantly subpleural or peribronchial areas of air space consolidation, small nodules, or both in almost all cases.[77] These changes are not pathognomonic for COP, but the HRCT images may be useful for directing biopsies to abnormal areas. The results of physiologic testing characteristically reveal a restrictive ventilatory defect with reduced lung volumes.[73,74] Obstructive flow defects are seen only in smokers.[74] The DLCO is frequently abnormal, out of proportion to the other pulmonary function tests.[73] Resting and exercise-induced hypoxemia are almost always present.

Bronchoalveolar lavage usually shows increased cellularity. An increased percentage of lymphocytes, neutrophils, or eosinophils may exist, but this finding does not help distinguish COP from other lung diseases.[74] Transbronchial lung biopsy should be performed in these patients, but the diagnosis may be difficult to make because the tissue samples obtained are often not large enough.[73,78] Transbronchial biopsy is useful to rule out other disorders, especially infections. The gold standard for diagnosis is the open lung biopsy.[73] Findings include patchy areas of intraluminal polyps of granulation tissue and constrictive bronchiolitis, organizing inflammation within the alveolar ducts, interstitial mononuclear cell infiltrate of variable density, alveolar space foam cells, and the absence of honeycombing or extensive interstitial fibrosis.[79]

COP may be associated with systemic diseases, certain inhalational exposures, or a drug reaction. A viral etiology is hypothesized for at least a proportion of the cases of idiopathic COP.[80] An association between COP and connective tissue diseases, especially rheumatoid arthritis, exists.[81-83] COP has been reported in association with human immunodeficiency virus infection.[84] Radiation therapy has been suggested to cause COP.[85] Smoking free-base cocaine may cause COP, in addition to causing other pulmonary problems.[86] Thus it appears that COP may appear secondary to a variety of pulmonary insults and may represent an aberrant healing process in the distal airspace.

The mortality of COP is about 5%.[73] Typically prednisone is used to treat this disease at a dose of 1 mg/kg/day. For the critically ill patient in the intensive care unit, higher doses of parenteral corticosteroids can be used. Additional immunosuppression with cyclophosphamide is usually not required in COP and is associated with a high rate of complications.[87,88] When respiratory failure develops, the ventilatory management of COP is similar to that in patients with IPF, except that chronic pulmonary hypertension and right ventricular failure are less of a problem.

CONNECTIVE TISSUE DISEASES

Rheumatologic disorders affect the lungs in a variety of ways. Alveolar hemorrhage is discussed earlier. Interstitial fibrosis, vasculitis, pulmonary hypertension, and respiratory muscle weakness are mechanisms by which the patient with connective tissue disease may develop respiratory failure. This section focuses on those rheumatologic disorders most likely to be encountered in an intensive care unit.

Lupus Pneumonitis

SLE is a systemic disorder characterized by widespread inflammation of serosal surfaces, skin, connective tissues, kidney, lung, and other organ systems. The characteristic finding of SLE is the presence of circulating autoantibodies, particularly antinuclear antibodies, and immune complexes. Pleuropulmonary involvement is common.[89] For the purposes of this discussion, we define lupus pneumonitis as any acute presentation of respiratory disease and pulmonary infiltrates, associated with SLE, that is neither infection nor frank alveolar hemorrhage (see previous discussion). Matthay found acute presentation of lung disease in 11% of patients hospitalized for SLE.[90] In 50% of these patients, lupus pneumonitis was the presenting manifestation of SLE, which is distinctly unusual in SLE-associated alveolar hemorrhage.[64]

The patients typically have dyspnea, cough, and pleuritic chest pain. Fever and tachypnea are also frequently present. The chest radiograph characteristically shows bilateral basilar or diffuse infiltrates, but unilateral infiltrates may be present and atelectasis may be a prominent feature. An accompanying pleural effusion is often present.[89-91] Cyanosis and basilar rales are often found on physical examination. The arterial blood gas frequently shows severe hypoxemia. Histopathologic findings on open lung biopsy are variable and may include areas of desquamative or usual interstitial pneumonia, cryptogenic organizing pneumonia, and microscopic alveolar hemorrhage. Pulmonary infarction is associated with anticardiolipin antibody, and focal atelectasis from respiratory muscle weakness can be seen.[81,90,92] The rapidity of clinical deterioration can be alarming. The mortality rate for patients who present with the characteristic clinical features of lupus pneumonitis can be up to 50% despite treatment.[90,92] The treatment of these patients usually includes high-dose corticosteroids. Cyclophosphamide and azathioprine have been used in cases of progressive disease.[81,91,92] In patients with acute, severe neurological lupus, cyclophosphamide was more effective than high-dose corticosteroids.[93] We recommend the initial use of both cyclophosphamide and high-dose corticosteroids in a regimen similar to that used to treat vasculitis (see previous discussion). Before initiating immunosuppressive therapy, it is essential to exclude infection with bronchoscopy or open lung biopsy. Maintaining a high suspicion for infection in the patient who is unresponsive to immunosuppression or who shows clinical deterioration despite treatment is also important.

Rheumatoid Arthritis

Rheumatoid arthritis (RA) is a disease of subacute and chronic inflammation characterized by erosive arthritis that is usually symmetric, affecting mainly the peripheral joints. A positive rheumatoid factor is present in at least 75% of cases. RA, like SLE, has a variety of associated pleuropulmonary manifestations that can present during the course of illness.[89] It is important for the intensivist to recognize the spectrum of lung disease associated with RA because many of the findings on chest radiograph can be ascribed to relatively benign disease.[94] Moreover, even moderately severe chronic pulmonary disease may go undetected because it is obscured by musculoskeletal limitations. Two of the more common forms of rheumatoid involvement that present with severe lung disease are interstitial fibrosis and COP.

Interstitial fibrosis is a relatively common finding in patients who have RA. In the overwhelming majority of patients, this is an incidental finding and is asymptomatic.[95] The clinical course of RA-associated interstitial lung disease is typically much more benign than that seen in IPF; however, a subset of patients presents with fulminant interstitial lung disease associated with RA.[96] Like IPF, the physical examination frequently shows Velcro-like rales, and the chest radiograph in the more severe cases typically shows diffuse bilateral reticular or reticulonodular infiltrates.[96]

Patients with RA are generally admitted to the ICU with sepsis rather than complications of the arthritis itself.[97] Most of these patients have been treated previously with corticosteroids or other immunosuppressive regimens. Airway management may be particularly challenging because many RA patients have limited mouth opening, atlanto-axial instability, or cricoarytenoid arthritis. Fiberoptic intubation is a necessary skill for safely managing patients with rheumatoid arthritis and ventilatory failure.

RA is the most common connective tissue disease to present with COP. This illness typically presents with a subacute onset of dyspnea. The presentation and pathology of COP associated with RA are indistinguishable from idiopathic COP.[83,98] Diagnosis usually requires an open lung biopsy to define the histology. In a few patients the diagnosis is made by transbronchial biopsy. Bronchoscopy should be undertaken before immunosuppressive therapy to rule out infection. Treatment of this disorder is identical to the treatment of COP, but the prognosis for RA-associated COP appears to be worse.[99] For this reason, we consider cyclophosphamide earlier to treat this disease when it does not respond rapidly to corticosteroids.

Progressive Systemic Sclerosis

Progressive systemic sclerosis (PSS) and the related disorder, the CREST (calcinosis, Raynaud's phenomena, esophageal dysmotility, sclerodactyly, telangiectasis) syndrome, are disorders characterized by fibrosing inflammation of the skin with variable visceral involvement. Patients with PSS and CREST develop interstitial lung disease that histopathologically resembles the lung fibrosis associated with RA and IPF.[100] The prevalence of pulmonary fibrosis detected by chest radiograph is approximately 36% in PSS and 20% in CREST.[101] The clinical presentation is indistinguishable from other secondary causes of pulmonary fibrosis. Many of these patients also have chronic aspiration resulting from esophageal dysfunction, which can precipitate and exacerbate pulmonary inflammation and fibrosis.[102]

The diagnosis of lung disease in PSS and CREST usually does not require an open lung biopsy. Pulmonary function tests characteristically reveal a restrictive ventilatory defect with low lung volumes.[103] The detection of circulating autoantibodies may be helpful in diagnosing these diseases.[89] Anticentromere antibody presence is associated with a lower incidence of pulmonary fibrosis in CREST.[104,105] Anti-SCL-70 antibody presence is associated with a higher incidence of pulmonary fibrosis.[106] Bronchoscopy can be used to evaluate for an infectious process and to look for vegetable matter or lipid-laden macrophages, which may suggest chronic aspiration. Treatment of interstitial lung disease associated with PSS or CREST with cyclophosphamide has been shown effective in the National Institutes of Health Scleroderma Lung Study by improving physiology, dyspnea, and quality of life. Nevertheless, the prognosis remains poor. The role of steroids is unproved.

Pulmonary hypertension is another common manifestation of lung involvement in PSS and the CREST syndrome. This can occur without evidence of other lung disease, but it is often associated with interstitial disease. When accompanying interstitial lung disease, pulmonary hypertension is often more prominent than one would expect from the degree of interstitial lung disease alone. The prevalence of pulmonary hypertension in PSS has been found to be about 33%. In CREST the prevalence of pulmonary hypertension is at least as high.[107] The etiology of pulmonary hypertension in these disorders is not well understood. Some experts have speculated that early in the course of disease there is a period of vascular reactivity associated with Raynaud's phenomenon.[108] This period is hypothesized to be followed by a period of increased pulmonary pressures associated with local hypoxia.[109] Finally, there is vascular remodeling with intimal thickening and loss of capillary beds.[110]

The patient with pulmonary hypertension may present with exertional dyspnea or impending respiratory failure, but pulmonary hypertension may also be asymptomatic.[107] Physical findings include those features commonly associated with PSS or CREST. Findings suggestive of cor pulmonale may be present including jugular venous distention with prominent A waves, loud or palpable S2, left parasternal lift, and an S4 gallop that increases with inspiration. Although approximately 88% specific, the physical examination is only about 63% sensitive to identifying definite pulmonary hypertension in PSS.[107] The single best marker of underlying pulmonary hypertension is a low DLCO. When the DLCO is below 40% to 55% of predicted normal values, pulmonary hypertension is likely to be present.[107,111] The sensitivity of this finding, irrespective of the presence of interstitial lung disease, is about 87% with a specificity of 88%.[107,111] The electrocardiogram may show right bundle branch block, right ventricular hypertrophy, or right atrial enlargement. Echocardiography is highly specific for pulmonary hypertension if a Doppler gradient analysis of tricuspid regurgitation suggests pulmonary hypertension.[112] The gold standard has been pulmonary artery catheterization with documentation of an elevated pulmonary artery pressure and a normal pulmonary capillary wedge pressure.

Early intervention with vasodilating agents may alter the course of pulmonary hypertension by preventing progression that is dependent on high pulmonary artery pressures or by ameliorating angiogenesis or fibrosis. Bosentan, the dual endothelin receptor inhibitor, has been found effective in clinical trials of subjects with pulmonary hypertension including those with scleroderma.[113] Other treatments such as prostanoids, endothelin receptor blockers, and sildenafil may play a role in chronic management of the patient with pulmonary hypertension. In the acute ICU setting, treatment of acute-on-chronic cor pulmonale generally involves seeking treatable precipitants, infusing rapidly acting vasoactive drugs such as dobutamine, and giving short-acting pulmonary vasodilators such as inhaled nitric oxide or inhaled prostacyclin. In mechanically ventilated patients, tidal volumes should be limited to reduce the potential for superimposing acute lung injury.

HYPERSENSITIVITY PNEUMONITIS

Hypersensitivity pneumonitis, in the majority of cases, does not result in an illness that requires critical care management. The cases that do present acutely are important to identify because these patients respond well to treatment. Furthermore, identifying an inciting exposure can prevent serious relapse or progression to chronic lung disease. Acute and subacute hypersensitivity pneumonitis are the most likely forms of this illness to result in admission to the intensive care unit. The etiology of hypersensitivity pneumonitis involves exposure to an airborne agent (Table 50-1).[114] Associated symptoms include malaise, myalgia, fever, nonproductive cough, and dyspnea.[115] The patient's history may reveal an onset of symptoms within 4 to 6 hours of the exposure to a previously sensitized antigen.[116] The physical examination

Table 50-1. Hypersensitivity Pneumonitis (Extrinsic Allergic Alveolitis) Reported Associations

Disease	Source of Particles
Farmer's lung	"Moldy" hay, grain, silage
Bird fancier's, breeder's, or handler's lung	Avian droppings or feathers
Humidifier or air-conditioner lung	Contaminated water in humidification and air-conditioning systems
Chemical worker's lung	Polyurethane foam, varnishes, lacquer
Bagassosis	"Moldy" bagasse (sugar cane)
Malt worker's lung	Moldy barley
Mushroom worker's lung	Mushroom compost
Sequoiosis	Redwood sawdust
Maple bark disease	Maple bark
Woodworker's lung	Oak, cedar, mahogany dusts; pine and spruce pulp
Cheese washer's lung	Moldy cheese
Suberosis	Cork dust
Sauna taker's lung	Contaminated sauna water
Pituitary snuff taker's lung	Heterologous pituitary snuff
Coffee worker's lung	Coffee beans
Miller's lung	Infested wheat flour
Fish meal worker's lung	Fish meal
Furrier's lung	Animal pelts
Lycoperdonosis	Lycoperdon puffballs
Compost lung	Compost
Wood trimmer's disease	Contaminated wood trimmings
Thatched roof disease	Dried grasses and leaves
Streptomyces albus HSP	Contaminated fertilizer
Cephalosporium HSP	Contaminated basement (sewage)
Detergent worker's disease	Detergent
Japanese summer house HSP	House dust? Bird droppings
Potato riddler's lung	"Moldy" hay around potatoes
Tobacco worker's disease	Mold on tobacco
Hot tub lung	Mold on ceiling
Winegrower's lung	Mold on grapes
Laboratory worker's HSP	Laboratory rat
Tapwater lung	Contaminated tapwater
Pauli's HSP	Laboratory reagent
Woodman's disease	Oak and maple trees

Adapted from Richerson HB, Bernstein IL, Fink JN, et al: Guidelines for the clinical evaluation of hypersensitivity pneumonitis. Report of the Subcommittee on Hypersensitivity Pneumonitis. J Allergy Clin Immunol 1989;84:839.

frequently reveals diffuse basilar lung crackles. The chest radiograph findings vary from normal to nodular or diffuse fluffy infiltrates. A predilection for involvement of the lung bases exists.[117] The HRCT scan in the acute phase shows diffuse airspace consolidation that evolves to a fine nodular or reticulonodular pattern over the course of days to weeks. Laboratory studies generally show a leukocytosis with a leftward shift in neutrophils. Eosinophilia is variably present, usually at low levels.[115] A polyclonal gammopathy may be present. Specific serum precipitins should be interpreted only as evidence of exposure, not as definitive evidence of disease. Rheumatoid factor may be present in as high as 50% of cases.[115,116] Pulmonary function tests usually show restrictive defects with maintenance of expiratory flow rates.[118]

Bronchoalveolar lavage nearly always shows increased cellularity.[119] In the acute phase of illness, within 24 to 48 hours of the onset of symptoms, BAL typically shows a predominance of neutrophils; as the illness progresses, BAL shows a predominance of lymphocytes, up to as high as 80%.[120-122] Most of the lymphocytes are suppressor/cytotoxic (CD_8, supressor cytotoxic; CD_4, helper) T-cells. The presence of many foamy macrophages in the BAL is also highly suggestive of hypersensitivity pneumonitis. Histopathology of transbronchial biopsies or open lung biopsy shows an inflammatory process involving both the airspaces and the interstitium. A mononuclear cell infiltration with many lymphocytes exists. Foamy histiocytes and plasma cells can frequently be seen. Interstitial, often poorly formed, noncaseating granulomas may be present.[114,118,123]

The differential diagnosis of acute hypersensitivity pneumonitis should include other causes of interstitial pneumonitis such as COP or acute interstitial pneumonia (Hamman-Rich syndrome). Organic dust toxic syndrome also occurs under similar environmental exposures as hypersensitivity pneumonitis but represents an acute response to inhaled bacterial and fungal cell wall products.[124] This illness tends to be more acute, resolves spontaneously, and often appears in case clusters because the response is not a specific allergic hypersensitivity. Atypical community-acquired pneumonia should also be considered in the critically ill patient. BAL and transbronchial biopsies are helpful in evaluating for an infectious etiology. After the diagnosis of hypersensitivity pneumonitis is made, treatment usually includes corticosteroids and environmental counseling to avoid repeated exposure.

SUMMARY

Patients with immunologic lung diseases can present with fulminant respiratory failure requiring care in an intensive care unit. These conditions require a high index of suspicion because they may mimic many atypical pneumonia syndromes.[125] An efficient management strategy must include a rapid diagnosis; aggressive supportive care; and, often, therapy with immunosuppressive agents. Patients with an established diagnosis may already have received potent corticosteroids or cytotoxic therapy and are at great risk of opportunistic infection that can mimic a flare of their underlying immunologic lung disease.[88,126] In addition, although in many cases immunomodulatory therapies have greatly altered the course of these diseases, treatment remains nonspecific with considerable toxicity. Indeed, in some series up to half of disease-related deaths can be attributed to treatment toxicity including infections and secondary malignancies.[48] Supportive management generally entails lung-protective ventilation and, in appropriate patients, surveillance for pulmonary hypertension.

KEY POINTS

- Immunologic lung disease may present with fulminant respiratory failure. Appropriate diagnosis requires a high index of suspicion combined with a thorough history and physical examination.
- Pulmonary infection may mimic, exacerbate, or result from the treatment of any immunologic lung disease. Lower airway sampling through bronchoalveolar lavage, parenchymal brushing, or biopsy may be required to exclude infectious etiologies.
- Respiratory failure as a manifestation of end-stage IPF portends a grave prognosis. Looking for other potentially treatable causes of impaired lung function such as infection, myocardial ischemia, heart failure, pulmonary embolic disease, or malignancy is important.
- When respiratory failure complicates IPF or fibrosis associated with connective tissue diseases, lung-protective ventilatory strategies should be used and the potential role of concurrent pulmonary hypertension should be considered.
- Bronchoscopy with lavage sampling of the distal airspace is a valuable tool in the documentation of alveolar hemorrhage and the exclusion of infection.
- Prompt institution of anti-inflammatory therapy after diagnosing COP or hypersensitivity pneumonitis may result in little or no long-term pulmonary dysfunction.

REFERENCES

1. Bitterman PB, Rennard SI, Keogh BA, et al: Familial idiopathic pulmonary fibrosis: Evidence of lung inflammation in unaffected family members. N Engl J Med 1986; 314:1343.
2. Carrington CB, Gaensler EA, Coutu RE, et al: Natural history and treated course of usual and desquamative interstitial pneumonia. N Engl J Med 1978;298:801.
3. Turner-Warwick M, Burrows B, Johnson A: Cryptogenic fibrosing alveolitis: Clinical features and their influence on survival. Thorax 1980;35:171.
4. Hunninghake GW, Lynch DA, Galvin JR, et al: Radiologic findings are strongly associated with a pathological diagnosis of usual interstitial pneumonia. Chest 2003;124:1215.
5. Nava S, Rubini F: Lung and chest wall mechanics in ventilated patients with end stage idiopathic pulmonary fibrosis. Thorax 1999;54:390.
6. The Acute Respiratory Distress Syndrome Network: Ventilation with lower tidal volumes as compared with traditional tidal volumes for acute lung injury and the acute respiratory distress syndrome. N Engl J Med 2000;342:1301.
7. Gajic O, Dara SI, Mendez JL, et al: Ventilator-associated lung injury in patients without acute lung injury at the onset of mechanical ventilation. Crit Care Med 2004;32:1817.
8. Carvalho CR, Barbas CS, Medeiros DM, et al: Temporal hemodynamic effects of permissive hypercapnia associated with ideal PEEP in ARDS. Am J Respir Crit Care 1997;156:1458.
9. Thorens JB, Jolliet P, Ritz M, et al: Effects of rapid permissive hypercapnia during mechanical ventilation for the acute respiratory distress syndrome. Intens Care Med 1996;22:182.
10. Nadrous HF, Pellikka PA, Krowka MJ, et al: Pulmonary hypertension in patients with idiopathic pulmonary fibrosis. Chest 2005;128:2393.
11. Schulman DS, Biondi JW, Matthay RA, et al: Differing responses in right and left ventricular filling, loading and volumes during positive end-expiratory pressure. Am J Cardiol 1989;64:772.
12. Biondi JW, Schulman DS, Matthay RA: Effects of mechanical ventilation on right and left ventricular function. Clin Chest Med 1988;9:55.
13. Schulman DS, Biondi JW, Matthay RA, et al: Effect of positive end-expiratory

pressure on right ventricular performance. Importance of baseline right ventricular function. Am J Med 1988;84:57.
14. Mebazaa A, Karpati P, Renaud E, et al: Acute right ventricular failure-from pathophysiology to new treatments. Intensive Care Med 2004;30:185.
15. Prewitt RM, Ghigone M: Treatment of right ventricular dysfunction in acute respiratory failure. Crit Care Med 1983;11:346.
16. Theodoraki K, Rellia P, Thanopoulos A, et al: Inhaled iloprost controls pulmonary hypertension after cardiopulmonary bypass. Can J Anaesth 2002;49:963.
17. Bhorade S, Christenson J, O'Connor M, et al: Response to inhaled nitric oxide in patients with acute right heart syndrome. Am J Respir Crit Care Med 1999;159:571.
18. Martinez FJ, Safrin S, Weycker D, et al: The clinical course of patients with idiopathic pulmonary fibrosis. Ann Intern Med 2005;142:963.
19. Turner-Warwick M, Lebowitz M, Burrows B, et al: Cryptogenic fibrosing alveolitis and lung cancer. Thorax 1980;35:496.
20. Pochis WT, Krasnow AZ, Collier BD, et al: Idiopathic pulmonary fibrosis. A rare cause of scintigraphic ventilation-perfusion mismatch. Clin Nuc Med 1990;15:321.
21. Kubo H, Nakayama K, Yanai M, et al: Anticoagulant therapy for idiopathic pulmonary fibrosis. Chest 2005;128:1475.
22. Collard HR, Ryu JH, Douglas WW, et al: Combined corticosteroid and cyclophosphamide therapy does not alter survival in idiopathic pulmonary fibrosis. Chest 2004;125:2169.
23. Raghu G, Brown KK, Bradford WZ, et al: A placebo-controlled trial of interferon gamma-1b in patients with idiopathic pulmonary fibrosis. N Engl J Med 2004;350:125.
24. Hunninghake GW: Antioxidant therapy for idiopathic pulmonary fibrosis. N Engl J Med 2005;353:2285.
25. Parambil JG, Myers JL, Ryu JH: Histopathologic features and outcome of patients with acute exacerbation of idiopathic pulmonary fibrosis undergoing surgical lung biopsy. Chest 2005;128:3310.
26. Saydain G, Islam A, Afessa B, et al: Outcome of patients with idiopathic pulmonary fibrosis admitted to the intensive care unit. Am J Respir Crit Care Med 2002;166:839.
27. Hamman L, Rich AR: Acute diffuse interstitial fibrosis of the lungs. Bull Johns Hopkins Hosp 1944;74:177.
28. Olson J, Colby TV, Elliott CG: Hamman-Rich syndrome revisited. Mayo Clin Proc 1990;65:1538.
29. Katzenstein ALA, Myers JL: Idiopathic pulmonary fibrosis. Am J Respir Crit Care Med 1998;157:1301.
30. Suh GY, Kang EH, Chung MP, et al: Early intervention can improve clinical outcome of acute interstitial pneumonia. Chest 2006;129:753.
31. Bradley J: The pulmonary hemorrhage syndromes. Clin Chest Med 1982;3:593.
32. Robbins RA, Linder J, Stahl MG, et al: Diffuse alveolar hemorrhage in autologous bone marrow transplant recipients. Am J Med 1989;87:511.
33. Perez M, Losa GJ, Garcia MM, et al: Hemosiderin-laden macrophages in bronchoalveolar lavage fluid. Acta Cytol 1992;36:26.
34. Kahn FW, Jones JM, England DM: Diagnosis of pulmonary hemorrhage in the immunocompromised host. Am Rev Respir Dis 1987;136:155.
35. Sherman JM, Winnie G, Thomassen MJ, et al: Time course of hemosiderin production and clearance by human pulmonary macrophages. Chest 1984;86:409.
36. Ewan PW, Jones HA, Rhodes CG, et al: Detection of intrapulmonary hemorrhage with carbon monoxide uptake. Application in Goodpasture's syndrome. N Engl J Med 1976;295:1391.
37. Bowley N, Hughes JM, Steiner RE: The chest x-ray in pulmonary capillary haemorrhage: Correlation with carbon monoxide uptake. Clin Radiol 1979;30:413.
38. Leatherman JW: Diffuse alveolar hemorrhage in immune and idiopathic disorders. In Lynch JP III, De Remee R (eds): Immunologically Mediated Pulmonary Diseases. Philadelphia, JB Lippincott, 1991.
39. Donaghy M, Rees M: Cigarette smoking and lung haemorrhage in glomerulonephritis caused by autoantibodies to glomerular basement membrane. Lancet 1983;8364:1390.
40. Jennings I, Rohold JA, Pressman D, et al: Experimental antialveolar basement membrane antibody-mediated pneumonitis. J Immunol 1981;127:129.
41. Benoit FL, Rulon DB, Theil GB: Goodpasture's syndrome. Am J Med 1964;37:424.
42. Young KR: Pulmonary-renal syndromes. Clin Chest Med 1989;10:655.
43. Walker RG, Scheinkestel C, Becker GJ, et al: Clinical and morphological aspects of the management of crescentic anti-glomerular basement membrane antibody (anti-GBM) nephritis/Goodpasture's syndrome. Quart J Med 1985;54:75.
44. Fish AJ, Kieppel M, Jeraj K, et al: Enzyme immunoassay of anti-glomerular basement membrane antibodies. J Lab Clin Med 1985;105:700.
45. Levy JB, Turner AN, Rees AJ, et al: Long-term outcome of anti-glomerular basement membrane antibody disease treated with plasma exchange and immunosuppression. Ann Intern Med 2001;134:1033.
46. Johnson JP, Moore J, Austin HA, et al: Therapy of anti-glomerular basement membrane antibody disease: Analysis of prognostic significance of clinical pathologic and treatment factors. Medicine 1985;64:219.
47. Lockwood CM, Rees M, Pearson TA, et al: Immunosuppression and plasma-exchange in the treatment of Goodpasture's syndrome. Lancet 1976;1:711.
48. Hoffmann GS, Kerr GS, Leavitt MD, et al: Wegener's granulomatosis: An analysis of 158 patients. Ann Intern Med 1992;116:488.
49. Misset B, Glotz D, Escudier B, et al: Wegener's granulomatosis presenting as diffuse pulmonary hemorrhage. Intens Care Med 1991;17:118.
50. McDonald TJ, DeRemee RA: Wegener's granulomatosis. Laryngoscope 1983;93:220.
51. Esnault VL, Soleimani B, Keogan MT, et al: Association of IgM with IgG ANCA in patients presenting with pulmonary hemorrhage. Kidney Int 1992;41:1304.
52. Travis WD, Hoffman GS, Leavitt RY, et al: Surgical pathology of the lung in Wegener's granulomatosis. Review of 87 open lung biopsies from 67 patients. Am J Surg Pathol 1991;15:315.
53. Jantz MA, Sahn SA: Corticosteroids in acute respiratory failure. Am J Respir Crit Care Med 1999;160:1079.
54. Frankel SK, Cosgrove GP, Fischer A, et al: Update in the diagnosis and management of pulmonary vasculitis. Chest 2006;129:452.
55. Stasi R, Stipa E, Poeta GD, et al: Long-term observation of patients with anti-neutrophil cytoplasmic antibody-associated vasculitis treated with rituximab. Rheumatology 2006[Epub ahead of print].
56. Asherson RA: The catastrophic antiphospholipid syndrome. J Rheumatol 1992;19:508.
57. Deane KD, West SG: Antiphospholipid antibodies as a cause of pulmonary capillaritis and diffuse alveolar hemorrhage: A case series and literature review. Semin Arthritis Rheum 2005;35:154.
58. Abinader A, Hanly AJ, Lozada CJ: Catastrophic antiphospholipid syndrome associated with anti-beta-2-glycoprotein I IgA. Rheumatol 1999;38:84.
59. Waterer GW, Latham B, Waring JA, et al: Pulmonary capillaritis associated with the antiphospholipid antibody syndrome and rapid response to plasmapheresis. Respirology 1999;4:405.
60. Miller LR, Greenherg SD, McLarty JW: Lupus lung. Chest 1985;88:265.
61. Onomura K, Nakata H, Tanaka Y, et al: Pulmonary hemorrhage in patients with systemic lupus erythematosus. J Thorac Imag 1991;6:57.
62. Myers JL, Katzenstein AA: Microangiitis in lupus-induced pulmonary hemorrhage. Am J Clin Pathol 1986;85:552.
63. Mintz G, Galindo LF, Fernandez DJ, et al: Acute massive pulmonary hemorrhage in systemic lupus erythematosus. J Rheumatol 1978;5:39.
64. Zamora MR, Warner ML, Tuder R, et al: Diffuse alveolar hemorrhage and systemic lupus erythematosus. Clinical presentation, histology, survival, and outcome. Medicine 1997;76:192.
65. Nguyen VA, Gotwald T, Prior C, et al: Acute pulmonary edema, capillaritis and alveolar hemorrhage: Pulmonary manifestations coexistent in antiphospholipid syndrome and

systemic lupus erythematosus? Lupus 2005;14:557.
66. Thompson PJ, Dhillon DP, Ledingham J, et al: Shrinking lungs, diaphragmatic dysfunction, and systemic lupus erythematosus. Am Rev Respir Dis 1985;132:926.
67. Gibson CJ, Edmonds JP, Hughes GR: Diaphragm function and lung involvement in systemic lupus erythematosus. Am J Med 1977;63:926.
68. Morgan PG, Turner WM: Pulmonary haemosiderosis and pulmonary haemorrhage. Br J Dis Chest 1981;75:225.
69. Cutz E: Idiopathic pulmonary hemosiderosis and related disorders in infancy and childhood. Perspect Pediatr Pathol 1987;11:47.
70. Beckerman R, Taussig L, Pinnas J: Familial idiopathic pulmonary hemosiderosis. Am J Dis Child 1979;133:609.
71. Thaell JF, Greipp PR, Stubbs SE, et al: Idiopathic pulmonary hemosiderosis: Two cases in a family. Mayo Clin Proc 1978;53:113.
72. Epler GR: Bronchiolitis obliterans organizing pneumonia: Definition and clinical features. Chest 1992;102:8.
73. Epler GR, Colby TV, McLoud TC, et al: Bronchiolitis obliterans organizing pneumonia. N Engl J Med 1985;312:152.
74. King TJ, Mortenson RL: Cryptogenic organizing pneumonitis. The North American experience. Chest 1992;102:18.
75. Flowers JR, Clunie G, Burke M, et al: Bronchiolitis obliterans organizing pneumonia: The clinical and radiological features of seven cases and a review of the literature. Clin Radiol 1992;45:371.
76. Cordier JF, Loire R, Brune J: Idiopathic bronchiolitis obliterans organizing pneumonia. Definition of characteristic clinical profiles in a series of 16 patients. Chest 1989;96:999.
77. Muller NL, Staples CA, Miller RR: Bronchiolitis obliterans organizing pneumonia: CT features in 14 patients. Am J Roentgenol 1990;154:983.
78. Kitaichi M: Differential diagnosis of bronchiolitis obliterans organizing pneumonia. Chest 1992;102:44.
79. Colby TV: Pathologic aspects of bronchiolitis obliterans organizing pneumonia. Chest 1992;102:38.
80. Marinopoulos GC, Huddle KR, Wainwright H: Obliterative bronchiolitis: virus induced? Chest 1991;99:243.
81. Gammon RB, Bridges TA, Al NH, et al: Bronchiolitis obliterans organizing pneumonia associated with systemic lupus erythematosus. Chest 1992;102:1171.
82. Yousem SA, Colby TV, Carrington CB: Lung biopsy in rheumatoid arthritis. Am Rev Respir Dis 1985;131:770.
83. Rees JH, Woodhead MA, Sheppard MN, et al: Rheumatoid arthritis and cryptogenic organizing pneumonitis. Resp Med 1991;85:243.
84. Allen J, Wewers M: HIV-associated bronchiolitis obliterans organizing pneumonia. Chest 1989;96:197.
85. Kaufman J, Komorowski R: Bronchiolitis obliterans. A new clinical-pathologic complication of irradiation pneumonitis. Chest 1990;97:1243.
86. Patel RC, Dutta D, Schonfeld SA: Free-base cocaine use associated with bronchiolitis obliterans organizing pneumonia. Ann Intern Med 1987;107:186.
87. McLoud TC, Epler GR, Colby TV, et al: Bronchiolitis obliterans. Radiology 1986;159:1.
88. Sen RP, Walsh TE, Fisher W, et al: Pulmonary complications of combination therapy with cyclophosphamide and prednisone. Chest 1991;99:143.
89. Hunninghake GW, Fauci AS: Pulmonary involvement in the collagen vascular diseases. Am Rev Resp Dis 1979;119:471.
90. Matthay RA, Schwarz MI, Petty TH, et al: Pulmonary manifestations of systemic lupus erythematosus: Review of twelve cases of acute lupus pneumonitis. Medicine 1975;54:397.
91. Pines A, Kaplinsky N, Olchovsky D, et al: Pleuro-pulmonary manifestations of systemic lupus erythematosus: Clinical features of its subgroups. Prognostic and therapeutic implications. Chest 1985;88:129.
92. Pertschuk LP, Moccia LF, Rosen Y, et al: Acute pulmonary complications in systemic lupus erythematosus. Immunofluorescence and light microscopic study. Am J Clin Path 1977;68:553.
93. Barile-Fabris L, Ariza-Andraca R, Olgun-Ortega L, et al: Controlled clinical trial of IV cyclophosphamide versus IV methylprednisolone in severe neurological manifestations in systemic lupus erythematosus. Ann Rheum Dis 2005;64:620.
94. Helmers R, Galvin J, Hunninghake GW: Pulmonary manifestations associated with rheumatoid arthritis. Chest 1991;100:235.
95. Salorinne Y: Single-breath pulmonary diffusing capacity. Reference values and application in connective tissue diseases and in various lung diseases. Scand J Resp Dis Suppl 1976;96:1.
96. Hakala M: Poor prognosis in patients with rheumatoid arthritis hospitalized for lung fibrosis. Chest 1988;93:114.
97. Dedhia HV, DiBartolomeo A: Rheumatoid arthritis. Crit Care Clin 2002;18:841.
98. Van Thiel U, van der Burg S, Groote AD, et al: Bronchiolitis obliterans organizing pneumonia and rheumatoid arthritis. Eur Resp J 1991;4:905.
99. Geddes DM, Corrin B, Brewerton DA, et al: Progressive airway obliteration in adults and its association with rheumatoid disease. Q J Med 1977;46:427.
100. Harrison NK, Myers AR, Corrin B, et al: Structural features of interstitial lung disease in systemic sclerosis. Am Rev Respir Dis 1991;144:706.
101. Alton E, Turner-Warwick M: Lung involvement in scleroderma. In Jayson M, Black CM (eds): Systemic sclerosis. New York, John Wiley, 1988.
102. Johnson DA, Drane WE, Curran J, et al: Pulmonary disease in progressive systemic sclerosis. A complication of gastroesophageal reflux and occult aspiration? Arch Intern Med 1989;149:589.
103. Bagg LR, Hughes DT: Serial pulmonary function tests in progressive systemic sclerosis. Thorax 1979;34:224.
104. Owens GR, Fino GJ, Herbert DL, et al: Pulmonary function in progressive systemic sclerosis. Comparison of CREST syndrome variant with diffuse scleroderma. Chest 1983;84:546.
105. Steen VD, Ziegler GL, Rodnan GP, et al: Clinical and laboratory associations of anticentromere antibody in patients with progressive systemic sclerosis. Arth Rheum 1984;27:125.
106. Manoussakis MN, Constantopoulos SH, Gharavi AE, et al: Pulmonary involvement in systemic sclerosis. Association with anti-Scl 70 antibody and digital pitting. Chest 1987;92:509.
107. Ungerer RG, Tashkin DP, Furst D, et al: Prevalence and clinical correlates of pulmonary arterial hypertension in progressive systemic sclerosis. Am J Med 1983;75:65.
108. Ohar JM, Robichaud AM, Fowler AA, et al: Increased pulmonary artery pressure in association with Raynaud's phenomenon. Am J Med 1986;81:361.
109. Morgan JM, Griffiths M, du Bois RM, et al: Hypoxic pulmonary vasoconstriction in systemic sclerosis and primary pulmonary hypertension. Chest 1991;99:551.
110. Salerni R, Rodnan GP, Leon DF, et al: Pulmonary hypertension in the CREST syndrome variant of progressive systemic sclerosis (scleroderma). Ann Intern Med 1977;86:394.
111. Steen VD, Graham G, Conte C, et al: Isolated diffusing capacity reduction in systemic sclerosis. Arth Rheum 1992;35:765.
112. Murata I, Kihara H, Shinohara S, et al: Echocardiographic evaluation of pulmonary arterial hypertension in patients with progressive systemic sclerosis and related syndromes. Japanese Circ J 1992;56:983.
113. Rubin LJ, Badesch DB, Barst RJ, et al: Bosentan therapy for pulmonary arterial hypertension. N Engl J Med 2002;346:896.
114. Costabel U: The alveolitis of hypersensitivity pneumonitis. Eur Respir J 1988;1:5.
115. Fink JN: Hypersensitivity pneumonitis. In Lynch JP III, DeRemee RA: Immunologically mediated pulmonary diseases. Philadelphia, JB Lippincott, 1991.
116. Salvaggio JE, Robert A: Cooke memorial lecture. Hypersensitivity pneumonitis. J Aller Clin Immunol 1987;79:558.
117. Gurney JW: Hypersensitivity pneumonitis. Radiol Clin N Am 1992;30:1219.
•118. Richerson HB, Bernstein IL, Fink JN, et al: Guidelines for the clinical

evaluation of hypersensitivity pneumonitis. Report of the Subcommittee on Hypersensitivity Pneumonitis. J Aller Clin Immunol 1989;84:839.

119. Semenzato G: Current concepts on bronchoalveolar lavage cells in extrinsic allergic alveolitis. Respiration 1988;1:59.
120. Salmeron S, Brochard L, Rain B, et al: Early neutrophil alveolitis after rechallenge in drug-induced alveolitis. Thorax 1988;43:647.
121. Fournier E, Tonnel AB, Gosset P, et al: Early neutrophil alveolitis after antigen inhalation in hypersensitivity pneumonitis. Chest 1985;88:563.
122. Semenzato G, Chilosi M, Ossi E, et al: Bronchoalveolar lavage and lung histology. Comparative analysis of inflammatory and immunocompetent cells in patients with sarcoidosis and hypersensitivity pneumonitis. Am Rev Respir Dis 1985;132:400.
123. Richerson HB: Hypersensitivity pneumonitis-pathology and pathogenesis. Clin Rev Allergy 1983;1:469.
124. Von Essen S, Robbins RA, Thompson AB, et al: Organic dust toxic syndrome: An acute febrile reaction to organic dust exposure distinct from hypersensitivity pneumonitis. J Toxicol 1990;28:389.
125. Gross TJ, Chavis AD, Lynch JP: Noninfectious pulmonary diseases masquerading as community-acquired pneumonia. Clin Chest Med 1991;12:363.
126. Weiss DJ, Greenfield JW, O'Rourke KS, et al: Systemic cytomegalovirus infection mimicking an exacerbation of Wegener's granulomatosis. J Rheumatol 1993;20:155.

PART

IV

CRITICAL CARE INFECTIOUS DISEASE

Chapter 51

Nosocomial Infection in the Intensive Care Unit

Dennis G. Maki, Christopher J. Crnich, and Nasia Safdar

Intensive care units (ICUs) have contributed greatly to the survival of patients with trauma, shock states, and other life-threatening conditions[1-3] but are associated with a greatly increased risk of nosocomial (hospital-acquired) infection. Rates of nosocomial infection in patients requiring more than 1 week of advanced life support within an ICU are three to five times higher than in hospitalized patients who do not require ICU care.[4-8] Infection, usually nosocomial, is the most common cause of death, directly or indirectly, of patients who survive the early period after major trauma or full-thickness burns and is the most commonly identified cause of multiple-organ dysfunction syndrome.[9-11]

Although most of this book focuses on the diagnosis and management of critically ill patients in the ICU, nosocomial infections are clearly one of the most common and serious complications of ICU care and are usually a consequence of invasive monitoring or life support therapies. Thus they are greatly preventable, and it is appropriate that measures to prevent nosocomial infections be addressed.

Much has been learned over the past decade about the epidemiology of nosocomial infection acquired in the ICU. Published guidelines for prevention are now available, based increasingly on randomized trials that have established the efficacy of specific control measures. Knowledge and technology of asepsis with regard to surgery and high-risk medical devices are now sufficiently advanced that, if applied consistently, the risk of nosocomial infection can be greatly reduced.[12-15]

INCIDENCE AND PROFILE

Definitions

Obtaining meaningful data on rates of nosocomial infection that can form the basis for comparisons within a hospital and, especially, among hospitals and that can also be used to monitor secular trends and document the efficacy or lack of efficacy of control measures must begin with clear, unambiguous definitions. Although there are no standardized definitions for infection at specific sites that are universally accepted by clinicians or investigators, the Centers for Disease Control and Prevention (CDC) has published definitions for the purpose of surveillance of nosocomial infection within hospitals, which most U.S. centers and an increasing number of hospitals around the world have adopted (Box 51-1).[16] For research purposes, more stringent definitions for specific infections will usually be necessary,[17] especially for pneumonia.[18]

Incidence

The incidence of hospital-acquired infection is most commonly expressed as the number of infections per 100 patients hospitalized and is highest in burn units,[7,19] surgical ICUs,[5-7,19-22] and ICUs for low-birth-weight neonates (5% to 30%),[4,23,24] with intermediate risk in medical ICUs[4,5,7,19,22,25] and pediatric ICUs[4] (5% to 7%) and lowest risk in coronary care units (1% to 2%) (Table 51-1).[4,7,8,19]

Recognizing that the risk of nosocomial infection within ICUs is heavily influenced by the length of stay and that the length of stay ranges widely among ICUs in the same hospital and among different hospitals,[26] the CDC has advocated the use of rates expressed per 1000 patient-days to permit more meaningful intrainstitutional and, especially, interhospital comparisons.[26,27] Furthermore, recognizing the powerful influence of exposure to invasive devices on susceptibility to infection[28,29] and the great variation in use of devices among different ICUs in the same hospital and among different hospitals,[26] the CDC has further recommended surveillance of device-associated nosocomial infections expressed as infections per 1000 device-days.[26,27] Representative rates of device-associated nosocomial infection in U.S. hospitals that are members of the CDC's National Nosocomial Infection Surveillance System (NNIS),[30] which can be used for intrahospital and interhospital comparisons are shown in Table 51-2. In the future, device-associated infection rates will be sought in accreditation reviews by the Joint Commission on the Accreditation of Healthcare Organizations (JCAHO)[31] as this influential organization continues to move toward measurement of patient outcomes as the most effective way to improve patient care in the United States.

Profile and Secular Trends

Approximately 40% of endemic nosocomial infections within ICUs are catheter-related urinary tract infections, and 25% are pneumonias—most associated with endotracheal intubation and mechanical ventilatory support. Up to 10% of patients hospitalized in a medical-surgical ICU for more than 72 hours acquire a nosocomial bloodstream infection, most commonly from an intravascular device.[26,32,33] Postoperative surgical site infections and intra-abdominal infections; nosocomial bacteremias; and gastrointestinal infections, especially antibiotic-associated *Clostridium difficile* colitis,[34] account for the remainder.[4-8,26]

Nearly 50% of nosocomial infections in the ICU are caused by aerobic gram-negative bacilli, especially *Pseudomonas aeruginosa, Enterobacter* species, or *Serratia marcescens;* and 35% are caused by gram-positive cocci, most commonly coagulase-negative staphylococci or *Staphylococcus aureus* or, increasingly, resistant enterococci (Fig. 51-1).[35] Almost 15% are caused by *Candida* species,[35] but filamentous fungi such as *Aspergillus* and *Zygomycetes* are being increasingly encountered in patients with hematologic malignancy or those who received solid organ transplants.[36-38] Viruses such as respiratory syncytium virus (RSV)[39] and rotaviruses[40] are important pathogens in pediatric ICUs. *Legionella* species now account for up to 10% of nosocomial pneumonias in centers that make efforts to diagnose *Legionella* infections.[41]

Table 51-1. Reported Rates of Nosocomial Infection in ICUs

		Rate (Per 100 Discharges) by Type of ICU					
Authors	**Study Period**	**Neonatal**	**Pediatric**	**Coronary**	**Medical**	**Surgical**	**Burn**
Hemming et al.[599]	1970-1974	24.3					
Northey et al.[20]	1972-1973					27.3	
Daschner et al.[22]	1976-1979				3.6	35.3	
Caplan and Hoyt[21]	1977-1978					50.9	
Goldmann et al.[23,24]	1977-1979 1980-1981	5.2 0.9					
Donowitz et al.[25]	1979-1980				18		
Wenzel et al.[19]	1980-1982			2	7	8	64
Craven et al.[5]	1980-1983				3.5	61.6	
Brown et al.[4]	1981-1983	5.9	6.2	1.8	11.2		
Nystrom et al.[6]	1983-1984					26	
Chandrasekar et al.[7]	1984-1985			6.6	13.9	35	29.8
Schandorf et al.[8]	1984-1985			4.6			

Box 51-1

Definitions for Nosocomial Infection of the Centers for Disease Control and Prevention

Primary Bloodstream Infection*

1. Recognized pathogen isolated from blood culture AND pathogen is not related to infection from another site (other than site of an intravascular device)

OR

2. One of the following: fever (>38° C), chills, or hypotension AND any of the following:
   a. Common skin contaminant isolated from two blood cultures drawn on separate occasions AND organism is not related to infection at another site
   b. Common skin contaminant isolated from blood culture from patient with intravascular access device AND physician institutes appropriate antimicrobial therapy AND organism is not related to infection at another site
   c. Positive antigen test on blood AND organism is not related to infection at another site

OR

3. Patient ≤12 months of age has one of the following: fever (>38° C), hypothermia (<37° C), apnea, or bradycardia AND one of the following:
   a. Common skin contaminant isolated from two blood cultures drawn on separate occasions AND organism is not related to infection at another site (other than site of an intravascular device)
   b. Common skin contaminant isolated from blood culture from patient with intravascular access device AND physician institutes appropriate antimicrobial therapy AND organism is not related to infection at another site
   c. Positive antigen test on blood AND pathogen is not related to infection at another site

Clinically Defined Pneumonia (PNU1)

1. For any patient, two or more serial chest radiographs with one or more of the following: new or progressive *and* persistent infiltrate, consolidation, cavitation, AND at least *one* of the following:
   - Fever (>38° C or >100.4° F) with no other recognized cause
   - Leukopenia (<4000 WBC/mm^3) or leukocytosis (12,000 WBC/mm^3)
   - For adults >70 years old, altered mental status with no other recognized cause

   AND at least *two* of the following:

   - New onset of purulent sputum or change in character of sputum, increased respiratory secretions, or increased suctioning requirements
   - New onset of worsening cough, dyspnea, or tachypnea
   - Rales or bronchial breath sounds
   - Worsening gas exchange (e.g., O_2 desaturation [e.g., $PaO_2/FIO_2 \leq 240$]), increased oxygen requirements, or increased ventilation demands

OR

2. For infant ≤ 1 year old, two or more serial chest radiographs with one or more of the following: new or progressive *and* persistent infiltrate, consolidation, cavitation, or pneumatocele AND worsening gas exchange (e.g., O_2 desaturation [e.g., $PaO_2/FIO_2 \leq 240$]), increased oxygen requirements, or increased ventilation demands AND at least *three* of the following:
   - Temperature instability with no other recognized cause
   - Leukopenia (<4000 WBC/mm^3) or leukocytosis (≥12,000 WBC/mm^3) and left shift (≥10% band forms)
   - New onset of purulent sputum, change in character of sputum, increased respiratory secretions, or increased suctioning requirements
   - Apnea, tachypnea, nasal flaring with retraction of chest wall, or grunting
   - New onset of worsening cough, dyspnea, or tachypnea
   - Wheezing, rales, or rhonchi
   - Cough
   - Bradycardia (<100 beats/min) or tachycardia (>170 beats/min)

OR

3. Alternate criteria for child >1 OR < 12 years old, two or more serial chest radiographs with one or more of the following: new or progressive *and* persistent infiltrate, consolidation, cavitation, AND at least *three* of the following:
   - Fever (>38° C or >100.4° F) with no other recognized cause
   - Leukopenia (<4000 WBC/mm^3) or leukocytosis (≥12,000 WBC/mm^3)
   - New onset of purulent sputum, change in character of sputum, increased respiratory secretions, or increased suctioning requirements
   - New onset of worsening cough, dyspnea, or tachypnea
   - Rales or bronchial breath sounds
   - Worsening gas exchange (e.g., O_2 desaturation [e.g., $PaO_2/FIO_2 \leq 240$]), increased oxygen requirements, or increased ventilation demands

Laboratory-Defined Pneumonia (PNU2)

1. Two or more serial chest radiographs with one or more of the following: new or progressive *and* persistent infiltrate, consolidation or cavitation, AND at least *one* of the following:

Continued

Box 51-1

Definitions for Nosocomial Infection of the Centers for Disease Control and Prevention—cont'd

- Fever (>38° C or >100.4° F) with no other recognized cause
- Leukopenia (<4000 WBC/mm^3) or leukocytosis (≥12,000 WBC/mm^3)
- For adults ≥ 70 years old, altered mental status with no other recognized cause

AND at least *one* of the following:

- New onset of purulent sputum, change in character of sputum, increased respiratory secretions, or increased suctioning requirements
- New onset of worsening cough, dyspnea, or tachypnea
- Rales or bronchial breath sounds
- Worsening gas exchange (e.g., O_2 desaturation [e.g., $PaO_2/FIO_2 \leq 240$]), increased oxygen requirements, or increased ventilation demands

AND at least one of the following:

- Positive growth in blood culture not related to another source of infection
- Positive growth in culture of pleural fluid
- Positive quantitative culture from minimally contaminated lower respiratory tract specimen (e.g., bronchoalveolar lavage or protected specimen brushing)
- ≥5% bronchoalveolar lavage–obtained cells contain intracellular bacteria on direct microscopic examination (e.g., Gram stain)
- Histopathologic examination shows at least *one* of the following evidences of pneumonia:
  - Abscess formation or foci of consolidation with intense neutrophil accumulation in bronchioles and alveoli
  - Positive quantitative culture of lung parenchyma
  - Evidence of lung parenchyma invasion by fungal hyphae or pseudohyphae

Asymptomatic Urinary Tract Infection

1. An indwelling urinary catheter is present within 7 days before urine is cultured AND patient has no fever (>38° C), urgency, frequency, dysuria, or suprapubic tenderness AND has urine culture of ≥ 10^5 organisms/mL urine with no more than two species or organisms

OR

2. No indwelling urinary catheter is present within 7 days before the first of two urine cultures with > 10^5 organisms/mL urine of the same organism with no more than two species of organisms AND patient has no fever (>38° C), urgency, frequency, dysuria, or suprapubic tenderness

Sinusitis

1. Organism isolated from culture of purulent material obtained from sinus cavity

OR

2. One of the following: fever (>38° C), pain or tenderness over the involved sinus, headache, purulent exudate, or nasal obstruction AND either of the following:
   a. Positive transillumination
   b. Radiographic evidence of infection

Gastroenteritis

1. Acute onset of diarrhea (liquid stools for >12 hours) with or without vomiting or fever (>38° C) AND no likely noninfectious cause (e.g., diagnostic tests, therapeutic regimen, acute exacerbation of a chronic condition, psychologic stress)

OR

2. Two of the following with no other recognized cause: nausea, vomiting, abdominal pain, or headache AND any of the following:
   a. Enteric pathogen isolated from stool culture or rectal swab
   b. Enteric pathogen detected by routine or electron microscopy examination
   c. Enteric pathogen detected by antigen or antibody assay on feces or blood
   d. Evidence of enteric pathogen detected by cytopathic changes in tissue culture (toxin assay)
   e. Diagnostic single antibody titer (IgM) or fourfold increase in paired serum samples (IgG) for pathogen

*All intravascular device-related bloodstream infections are classified with primary bloodstream infections.
From Horan TC, Gaynes RP: Surveillance of nosocomial infections. In Mayhall CG (ed): Hospital Epidemiology and Infection Control, 3rd ed. Philadelphia, Lippincott Williams & Wilkins, 2004, pp 1659-1702.

The microbial profile of infections at individual sites in ICU patients is shown in Table 51-3. There has been an unrelenting increase in nosocomial infections caused by intrinsically resistant organisms during the past decade, especially coagulase-negative staphylococci, *S. aureus,* enterococci, *P. aeruginosa* and other resistant gram-negative bacilli, and *Candida.*[32,35,42,43] Moreover, the incidence of infection caused by organisms with *acquired* resistance, especially methicillin-resistant *S. aureus* (MRSA); enterococci resistant to vancomycin (VRE), ampicillin, or both drugs; and gram-negative bacilli resistant to extended-spectrum beta-lactams and fluoroquinolones, has increased even more sharply (Fig. 51-2).[44]

Nosocomial infections acquired in the ICU clearly differ from infections acquired in non-ICU patient care units within the same institutions. Overall rates

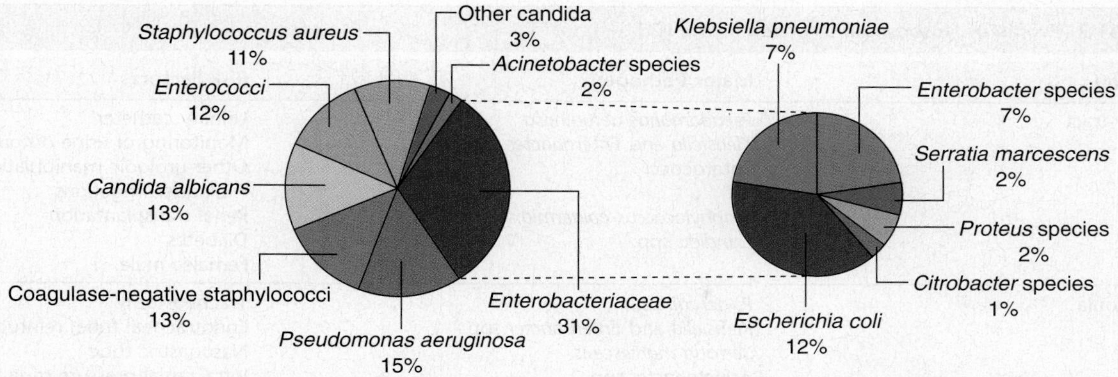

Figure 51-1. Microbiology of nosocomial infection in the intensive care unit (ICU). Based on 13,317 infections occurring in ICU patients in 97 participating U.S. hospitals in the Centers for Disease Control's National Nosocomial Infections Surveillance System (NNIS), January 1992 through July 1997. (Data from Richards MJ, Edwards JR, Culver DH, Gaynes RP: Nosocomial infections in medical intensive care units in the United States. National Nosocomial Infections Surveillance System. Crit Care Med 1999;27:887-892.)

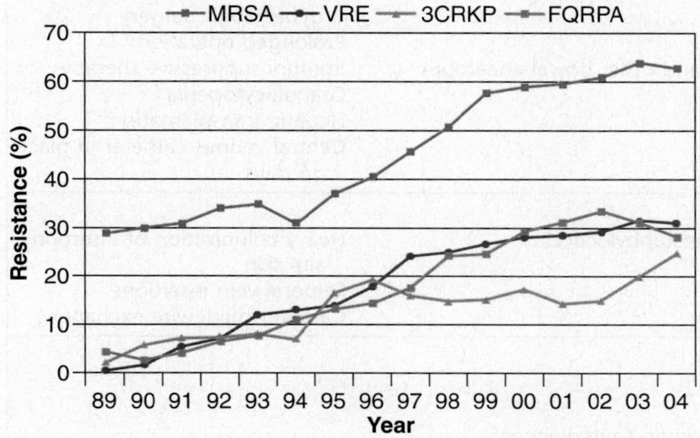

Figure 51-2. Temporal trends in the proportion of isolates resistant to antibiotics among pathogenically important bacteria in U.S. intensive care units (ICUs), National Nosocomial Infections Surveillance System (NNIS) 1989-2004. FQRPA, *Pseudomonas aeruginosa* resistant to fluoroquinolones; MRSA, methicillin-resistant *Staphylococcus aureus;* 3CRKP, *Klebsiella pneumoniae* resistant to third-generation cephalosporins; VRE, vancomycin-resistant enterococcus. (From Centers for Disease Control and Prevention: Trends in antibiotic resistance in National Nosocomial Infections Surveillance (NNIS) system hospitals, 1989-2004. http://www.cdc.gov/ncidod/dhqp/pdf/ar/ICU_RESTrend1995-2004.pdf Accessed January 15, 2007.)

Table 51-2. Rates of Device-Related Nosocomial Infection in U.S. Hospital ICUs, Expressed per 1000 Device-Days*

		Rate (No. of Cases Per 1000 Device-Days)	
Type of Infection	**Type of ICU**	**Median**	**25th to 75th Percentile of Hospitals**
Catheter-associated urinary tract infection	PICUs	3.6	1.6-6.1
	MICUs	4.7	2.5-7.1
	SICUs	3.8	2.3-6.5
Ventilator-associated pneumonia	PICUs	2.3	0.9-4.8
	MICUs	3.7	2.1-6.2
	SICUs	8.3	4.7-12.2
Central line–associated bloodstream infections	PICUs	5.2	3.0-8.1
	MICUs	3.9	2.4-6.4
	SICUs	3.4	2.0-5.9

*From the nearly 300 hospitals in the Centers for Disease Control and Prevention's National Nosocomial Infections Surveillance System (NNIS) study, 1992-2004.
ICU, intensive care unit; MICU, medical ICU; PICU, pediatric ICU; SICU, surgical ICU.
From National Nosocomial Infections Surveillance (NNIS) System Report: Data Summary from January 1992 through June 2004, issued October 2004. Am J Infect Control 2004;32:470-485.

are two to three times higher, and rates of ventilator-associated pneumonia (VAP) and primary bacteremia—most of which originate from intravascular devices—are 10 times higher. A far greater proportion of ICU-acquired infections are caused by antibiotic-resistant bacteria because the intensive antimicrobial therapy characteristic of modern-day ICUs grossly distorts patients' microflora. Moreover, more than half of all nosocomial epidemics now occur among the 10% of hospitalized patients confined to an ICU.[19,32] Finally, the risk of occupationally

Table 51-3. Profile of Nosocomial Infection in the ICU

Infection	Major Pathogen	Risk Factors
Urinary tract	*Pseudomonas aeruginosa* *Klebsiella* and *Enterobacter* spp. Enterococci *Staphylococcus epidermidis* *Candida* spp.	Urinary catheter Monitoring of urine output Other urologic manipulation or bladder irrigations Renal transplantation Diabetes Female>male
Pneumonia	*P. aeruginosa* *Klebsiella* and *Enterobacter* spp. *Serratia marcescens* *Acinetobacter* spp. *Staphylococcus aureus* Oral anaerobes Immunosuppression	Tracheostomy Endotracheal tube, reintubation Nasogastric tube Intracranial pressure monitoring Stress ulcer prophylaxis with H_2 blocker or antacids Immunosuppression Granulocytopenia
Postsurgical wound	*Staphylococcus aureus* *Escherichia coli* and other gram-negative bacilli Enterococci *Bacteroides fragilis* and other bowel anaerobes	Trauma, especially penetrating abdominal injury Gastrointestinal or radical gynecologic surgery Prolonged operation Immunosuppressive therapy Granulocytopenia Hepatic transplantation Central venous catheter in place >5 days
Bacteremia from intravascular devices Catheter related	Coagulase-negative staphylococci *S. aureus* *Candida* spp.	Heavy colonization of insertion site skin Femoral vein insertions Catheter guidewire exchanges
Contaminated infusate	*Enterobacter* spp. *S. marcescens* *Citrobacter* spp. *Pseudomonas cepacia* or *Xanthomonas maltophilia*	
Antibiotic-associated diarrhea or colitis	*Clostridium difficile*	Prolonged antibiotic therapy, especially with clindamycin or broad-spectrum β-lactams Enteral tube feeding
Candidemia	*Candida* spp.	Broad-spectrum, prolonged antimicrobial therapy Mucosal or urinary colonization Central venous catheter Hyperalimentation Renal failure

Modified from Maki DG: Nosocomial infection. In Parrillo JE (ed): Current Therapy in Critical Care Medicine, 2nd ed. Philadelphia, BC Decker, 1991.

acquired infection among health care workers (HCWs), particularly by bloodborne viruses and herpes simplex virus (HSV), is highest among ICU personnel, as contrasted with those who work in non-ICU patient care units (see Protection of Health Care Workers in the Intensive Care Unit later).

MORBIDITY AND ECONOMIC IMPACT

Nosocomial infections have a considerable impact on morbidity and mortality and are estimated to affect more than 2 million patients in U.S. hospitals annually.[45] Table 51-4 summarizes major studies that have examined mortality, length of stay, and costs associated with the major nosocomial infections in U.S. hospitals.[2-18] Nosocomial infections have been ascribed by the National Institute of Medicine to be responsible for more than 80,000 hospital deaths each year and in 1995 resulted in more than $5 billion in excess health care costs.[45] Considering that nosocomial infections acquired by ICU patients account for nearly half of all infections in most hospitals, progress in reducing the incidence of infection acquired within ICUs could produce substantial economic benefits.

Table 51-4. Estimated Extra Days, Extra Charges, and Deaths Associated with Nosocomial Infections in U.S. Hospitals as Reported in Recent Major Studies

Infection	Description	Average Extra Days in Hospital or ICU Per Infection	Average Extra Charges or Costs per Infection ($)	Excess Mortality	
				Unadjusted	Attributable
Postoperative Surgical Wound Infection					
Kirkland et al, 1999[600]	CABG, vascular surgery, abdominal surgery, orthopedic surgery	6.5	3,089	NR	4.3%
Whitehouse et al, 2002[601]	Orthopedic surgery	14	17,708	NR	0.0%
Hollenbeak et al, 2000[602]	Deep chest infection following CABG	20	20,012	NR	19.4%
McGarry et al, 2004[603]	All major surgical procedures; only *S. aureus* infections included	13	53,625	NR	16.8%
Herwaldt et al, 2006[604]	All major surgical procedures	NR	3,021	1.2%	0%
Ventilator-Associated Pneumonia					
Fagon et al, 1993[605]	Medical and surgical patients	13	NR	NR	27.1%
Heyland et al, 1999[606]	Medical and surgical patients	4.3	NR	NR	5.8%
Bercault et al, 2001[607]	Medical and surgical patients	5	NR	NR	27.4%
Rello et al, 2002[608]	Medical and surgical patients	11	40,000	NR	0%
Warren et al, 2003[609]	Medical and surgical patients	25	11,897	16%	NR
Cocanour et al, 2005[610]	Trauma patients	15	57,158	NR	0%
Bloodstream Infection					
Pittet et al, 1994[264]	Surgical ICU	24	40,000	NR	35%
Digiovine et al, 1999[265]	Adult ICU	10	34,508	NR	4%
Slonim et al, 2001[611]	Pediatric ICU	22	35,000	NR	13%
Warren et al, 2006[612]	Adults	7.5	11,971	23%	NR
Catheter-Associated Urinary Tract Infection					
Bryan et al, 1984[469]	Medical and surgical patients	NR	NR	NR	12%
Tambyah et al, 2002[472]	Medical and surgical patients	NR	589	NR	NR

PATHOGENESIS AND EPIDEMIOLOGY

Pathogenesis

The occurrence of nosocomial infection reflects the conjunction in space and time of a pathogenic microbe and a vulnerable patient, catalyzed by events associated with hospitalization and the patient's care. Many patients admitted to an ICU are intrinsically more susceptible to infection because of underlying diseases or conditions associated with impaired immunity such as cancer, trauma,[46] or advanced age[47] or because of immunosuppression associated with malnutrition[48] or therapy with corticosteroids,[49] cancer chemotherapeutic agents,[50] or other immunosuppressive drugs.[51] Moreover, many drugs have indirect effects that increase susceptibility to infection, such as narcotics or sedatives that impair the capacity to protect the airway, or antacids or H_2-histamine receptor antagonists that neutralize gastric acidity, producing gastric overgrowth by gram-negative bacilli,[52] increasing the risk of nosocomial pneumonia.[53] Even transfusion therapy produces immunosuppression and increases the risk of nosocomial infection.[54]

Moreover, most nosocomial pathogens exhibit resistance to antibiotics (see Figs. 51-1 and 51-2),[42,43,55-58] and many are also more virulent because of (1) their capacity to subsist or even multiply in aqueous reservoirs for prolonged periods (e.g., pseudomonads[59] or *Legionella pneumophila*[60]); (2) the elaboration of endotoxins (e.g., all of the gram-negative bacilli) or exotoxins (*P. aeruginosa*,[61] *C. difficile*,[62] or *S. aureus*[63]); or (3) the production of adhesions[64] or exoglycocalyx[65] (e.g., coagulase-negative staphylococci), conferring the capacity to adhere avidly and form biofilms on biologic and prosthetic surfaces resistant to host defenses[66] and even antibiotics.[67] Because most patients in ICUs receive broad-spectrum antibiotics, resistant nosocomial organisms have an enormous ecologic advantage and, in Darwinian fashion, predictably supplant the normal cutaneous, respiratory, and gastrointestinal flora.

In most cases, colonization is the first step in the progression to nosocomial infection,[68] especially if the patient is already vulnerable because of underlying disease, if the organism is more virulent or resistant to antibiotics, or if the patient has invasive medical devices that assist invasion by colonizing organisms, bypassing or further impairing host defenses.

Reservoirs and Transmission

The epidemiology of an infection consists of the reservoirs and mode or modes of transmission of the pathogen or pathogens and those factors associated with an increased (or decreased) risk of infection. *Understanding the epidemiology of an infection is essential to developing effective strategies for its prevention.*

In the ICU the major reservoir of nosocomial organisms is the infected or colonized patient (Fig. 51-3).[28] Whereas *Streptococcus pneumoniae,*[69] *Mycobacterium tuberculosis,*[70-72] *Legionella,*[41] *Aspergillus* and *Zygomycetes,*[36-38] measles,[73] rubella,[74] and influenza A[75] are transmitted by the airborne route, the best evidence suggests that most aerobic bacteria—particularly *S. aureus,*[76] enterococci,[29] and the enteric gram-negative bacilli[77]; many viruses such as hepatitis A, RSV,[78] and rotaviruses[79]; *C. difficile*[80]; and even *Candida*[81]—are spread in the ICU on the hands of medical personnel, who themselves are not infected or even permanently colonized. Surgery and exposure to invasive devices of all types greatly amplify transmission, colonization, and susceptibility to infection.[28,82]

Outbreaks of *S. aureus*[83] or group A streptococcal infection[84] usually indicate a health care provider who is a carrier of the epidemic strain. Airborne spread of gram-negative bacilli is probably rare unless unusual environmental circumstances generate massively contaminated aerosols.[85]

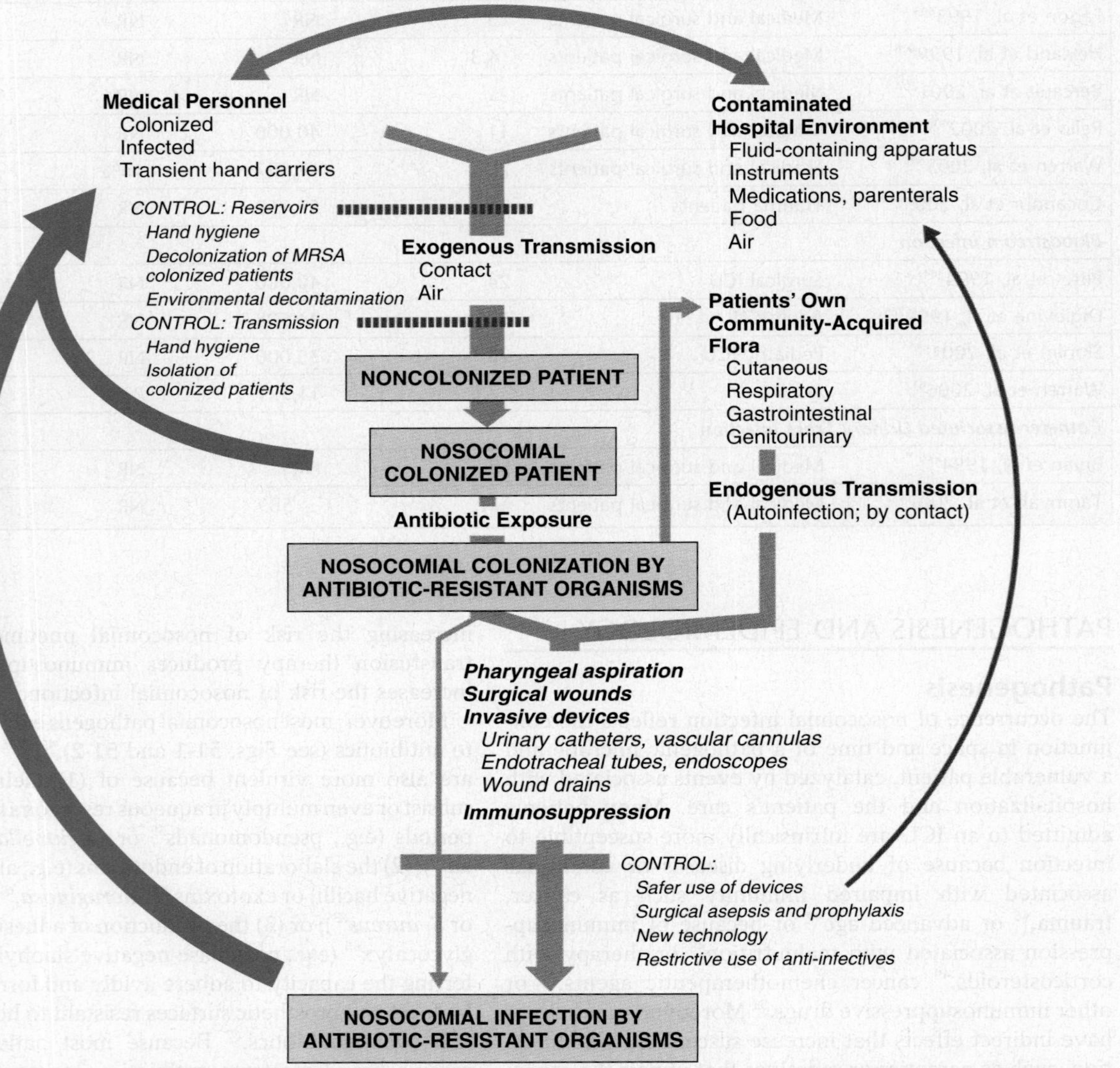

Figure 51-3. The epidemiology of nosocomial infection. Transmission occurs mainly by contact spread and, to a much lesser extent, the airborne route. Aspiration, surgical wounds, and exposure to invasive medical devices enormously amplify transmission, colonization, and susceptibility to infection. (From Maki DG: Control of colonization and transmission of pathogenic bacteria in the hospital. Ann Intern Med 1978;89[Suppl]:777-780.)

Increasing evidence suggests that many nosocomial infections acquired in the ICU derive from resistant organisms of enteric origin[86-89] or present on skin[86,87] or in the lower respiratory tract[88] on admission to the ICU. This explains the failure of conventional infection control practices, based on the use of barriers, to prevent extrinsically acquired infection.[90] Whereas food[91] and even enteral feeding preparations[92] are often heavily contaminated by microorganisms, studies have not conclusively linked such contamination to disease.

Nosocomial organisms originating from colonized or infected patients are readily perpetuated and spread in contaminated medical apparatus or devices[28] such as urine-collection receptacles,[93] respiratory therapy equipment,[94,95] transducers used for hemodynamic monitoring,[96] dialysis machines,[97,98] and fiberoptic bronchoscopes and endoscopes.[95,99-101] Given the implicit close proximity of vulnerable ICU patients and the HCWs who have repeated contact with them each day, it is almost predictable that the ICU is a milieu within the hospital uniquely conducive to the epidemic infection, especially infections caused by antibiotic-resistant pathogens.

Although successful immune enhancement could in theory create a protective final barrier against infection by nosocomial organisms, the unique features of nosocomial infection—enormous microbial heterogeneity, pervasive effects of invasive devices and procedures, and often large infecting inocula—can overwhelm the healthiest patient's immune defenses. *Measures to eradicate reservoirs of nosocomial pathogens and to block transmission, based on a thorough understanding of epidemiology, seem much more likely to be protective at present.*

Risk Factors

Risk factor analysis using powerful statistical techniques of multivariable analysis can identify the circumstances that put a patient at increased risk for nosocomial infection and further guide the development of preventive strategies. Risk factors based on prospectively collected data and, in most cases, the use of multivariable analysis are listed in Table 51-3 for urinary tract infection,[102,103] pneumonia,[104,105] postoperative surgical infection,[106] intravascular device-related bloodstream infection,[107] ventriculostomy-associated meningitis,[108] antibiotic-associated colitis,[34,109] and deep *Candida* infection.[110-112]

Critical care medicine is synonymous with cutting-edge, high-tech medicine; mechanical ventilatory support; hemodynamic monitoring; total parenteral nutrition; hemodialysis; intracranial pressure monitoring; innovative forms of surgery; and a huge arsenal of drugs, especially anti-infectives of every genre. This technology, more than anything else, has forced critical care medicine to accept the necessity for nosocomial infection control. In general, invasive devices of all types are far more important in determining susceptibility to nosocomial infection than underlying diseases (see Tables 51-3 and 51-5). However, this should be viewed as welcome news: There is far more hope for reducing nosocomial infections in the coming decade by innovative improvements in aseptic technique and advances in the technology of invasive devices than by breakthroughs that will reverse the ravages of chronic organ failure or degenerative diseases such as type 1 diabetes mellitus.

Table 51-5. Significant Risk Factors for Nosocomial Infection in the ICU as Determined by Multivariate Analysis of Prospectively Collected Databases

Type of ICU (Investigators)	Risk Factors	Approximate Magnitude of Increased Risk*
Pediatric ICU[23,613]	Patent ductus arteriosus	28.2
	Low birth weight	—†
	Endotracheal tube	7
	Hyperalimentation	5.9
	Surgery	—
	High fraction inspired oxygen	—
	Umbilical catheter	—
	Blood product therapy	—
	Central venous catheter	—
	Mechanical ventilatory support	—
Adult medical and surgical ICUs[5]	Urinary catheter >10 days	3.2
	ICU confinement >3 days	2.5
	Intracranial pressure monitor	2.5
	Arterial line	1.5
	Shock	2.5

*Relative risk or odds ratio: values >1 denote significantly increased risk of infection, and ratios <1, decreased risk, vis-à-vis a protective effect.
†Not reported or indeterminant (e.g., zero denominator).

GENERAL CONTROL MEASURES

Hospital Infection Control Programs

Beginning in the late 1960s, scattered U.S. hospitals began to establish infection control programs to conduct surveillance, to develop infection control policies, and especially to try to implement control measures more consistently.[113] In 1976 JCAHO added to its requirements for hospital accreditation the establishment of a formal infection control program.

In the early 1970s the CDC undertook determining the effectiveness of nosocomial infection surveillance and control programs in the United States through the auspices of the Study of the Efficacy of Nosocomial Infection Control (SENIC). The goals of SENIC were to determine the extent to which infection control programs had been adopted by U.S. hospitals and to ascertain how much these programs had reduced rates of nosocomial infection. SENIC was launched by a survey of all U.S. hospitals to determine the characteristics of infection control programs and was completed in 1975-1976 by a review of more than 339,000 patient medical records in 338 randomly selected hospitals.[114]

The SENIC found that hospitals reduced their nosocomial infection rates by approximately 32% if their surveillance and infection control program included four components: (1) emphasis on both surveillance and an infection control program, (2) at least one full-time infection control practitioner for every 250 beds, (3) a trained hospital epidemiologist, and (4) surveillance of surgical wound infections *with* feedback of wound infection rates to practicing surgeons.[115] However, the relative importance of each component varied for the four major types of nosocomial infections (surgical wound infections, urinary tract infections, bloodstream infections, and pneumonia).[115,116] SENIC suggests that nearly one third of all nosocomial infections are in theory preventable, whereas a 1983 survey of surveillance and control programs in a random sample of U.S. hospitals found that failure to implement all essentials of the program, particularly to have an adequate number of infection control practitioners or a trained hospital epidemiologist or to disseminate wound infection rates to surgeons, was greatly limiting the potential for prevention: U.S. hospitals were estimated to be preventing only 9% of all infections.[117]

It is hoped that surveillance and control programs will continue to evolve. Prevention of nosocomial infections is a major priority of the U.S. Public Health Service,[118] JCAHO,[31] and the Institute of Medicine.[119] With the shift to prospective-payment reimbursement, hospitals now have a powerful financial incentive to reduce their rates of nosocomial infection,[120] and it can be anticipated that efforts to prevent hospital-acquired infections will assume ever greater importance.

JCAHO now mandates that all hospitals have an active program for surveillance, prevention, and control of hospital-acquired infections, which begins with an institutional infection control committee with representation from the major clinical services and hospital departments including the institution's ICUs. The most essential members of the infection control program are the infection control practitioner(s), usually registered nurse(s), and the hospital epidemiologist, usually a physician with training in infectious diseases or microbiology, who implement the policies developed by the committee, educate hospital personnel about nosocomial infection control, and investigate suspected outbreaks (Box 51-2).

Box 51-2

Facets of a Hospital Infection Control Program

- Active infection control committee, with representation from major departments and services including the intensive care units (ICUs)
- Surveillance of nosocomial infections, especially in each ICU
- Comprehensive and regularly updated institutional policies and procedures for prevention of nosocomial infection:
  - Surveillance of nosocomial infections
  - Isolation and universal precautions
  - Sterilization and disinfection
  - Indications for and management of invasive procedures and devices
    - All types of intravascular catheters
    - Hemodynamic monitoring
    - Tracheostomy and endotracheal intubation
    - Mechanical ventilation and other respiratory therapy
    - Bronchoscopy and gastrointestinal endoscopy
    - Anesthesia and the operating room
    - Hemodialysis
    - Intra-aortic balloon pumps
    - Cardiopulmonary bypass
    - Intracranial pressure monitoring
- Antimicrobial stewardship program
- Guideline for investigation of an epidemic
- Strong liaison with clinical microbiology laboratory
  - Representation on the Infection Control Committee
  - Laboratory-based surveillance
  - Monitoring and reporting of trends in antimicrobial susceptibility
  - Retaining important isolates
  - Microbiologic support of all infection control activities
  - Subtyping of isolates for investigations or studies
- Educational programs for new employees, periodic updates dealing with nosocomial infection control
- Active employee health department:
  - Free immunizations (hepatitis B, measles, mumps, rubella, varicella, pertussis, influenza A)
  - Tuberculin screening
  - Postexposure protocols
- Quality assurance review of implementation of infection control policies and practices

Modified from Maki DG: Nosocomial infection. In Parrillo JE (ed): Current Therapy in Critical Care Medicine, 2nd ed. Philadelphia, BC Decker, 1991.

Surveillance of nosocomial infections is the cornerstone of an effective infection control program and offers numerous potential benefits[116,121]: (1) It permits determination of baseline (expected) infection rates, assisting recognition of outbreaks and evaluation of new policies and control measures; (2) it identifies institutional problems that require attention, permitting focused infection control efforts and education; (3) it provides reliable data that can be disseminated to individual departments, increasing awareness and involvement of individual staff members; (4) it increases the visibility of the infection control staff on patient care units, providing an opportunity for consultation and ad hoc education; and (5) it facilitates the earliest discovery of patients with communicable infections, permitting timely institution of isolation precautions to limit spread. Because total surveillance (of all infections) is labor intensive, most hospitals now focus their surveillance efforts on infections that are associated with high morbidity (e.g., nosocomial pneumonia), that greatly increase health care costs (e.g., postcardiac surgery sternotomy infections), that are caused by antibiotic-resistant organisms with potential for spread (e.g., MRSA,

genic bacteria, indirectly, through contact with HCWs' hands and equipment (see Fig. 51-3). This indirect route of infection is of particular importance in the ICU, where all patients are heavily exposed to invasive devices and have a high risk of infection. In the ICU the inanimate environment may become a reservoir for the transmission of resistant nosocomial organisms such as MRSA,[155,156] *C. difficile,*[80,157] VRE[152,158] and gram-negative bacilli such as *Klebsiella* spp., *Acinetobacter* spp., and *Enterobacter* organisms.[159,160] Studies have shown that enhanced surface decontamination with hypochlorite-containing cleaning solutions has been necessary to terminate outbreaks caused by *C. difficile*[161] and *Acinetobacter baumanii.*[153]

Although the ICU environment cannot be made microbe free, certain organizational, architectural, and environmental issues must be addressed with the design or remodeling of an ICU. The capacity to systematically improve the care of critically ill patients and prevent nosocomial infection requires a structural foundation on which the processes of care can be optimized (i.e., make it easy for HCWs to do it right and difficult to do it wrong). Accountability for compliance with critical policies and procedures and ongoing assessment of outcomes needs to be built into the administrative structure of the ICU.

An ICU must be adequately staffed to allow the processes of care to be carried out but also assure a high level of compliance with essential infection control measures such as hand hygiene and barrier isolation. Adequate staffing cannot be overemphasized; numerous studies have found greatly increased rates of nosocomial infection when ICUs are staffed suboptimally or when staffing requirements are met with temporary personnel who are unfamiliar with ICU infection control policies and procedures.[162,163] In a large nosocomial outbreak of *Enterobacter cloacae* infection in a neonatal ICU, Harbarth and colleagues[164] found that infection rates during periods of understaffing were strikingly higher than during periods with adequate levels of staffing (RR=6, 95% CI=2.2 to 16.4). The effects of understaffing are likely multiple; however, erosion of basic hygienic practices with excessive patient-to-staff ratios likely explains much of this phenomenon.[165]

Many of the published recommendations for ICU architectural design[166] are empiric, and evidence that they reduce rates of nosocomial infection is, by and large, lacking. Although more research is necessary before specific features of ICU design achieve a level of evidence sufficient for an evidence-based guideline, certain facets of the ICU layout deserve attention:

- ICUs should be located in areas that limit traffic flow to essential ICU personnel.
- ICU facilities should be designed with ICU professionals in mind, ensuring appropriate space, resources, and environment for day-to-day operations.[166] Recognizing the growing variety and complexity of life support equipment required for the care of many patients, each cubicle or room should provide a minimum of 11 m^2 per bed.[167] The area should be large enough to accommodate the bed and all equipment yet allow immediate access to the patient at all times from both sides of the bed. Adequate space must also be provided for storage of nursing supplies. Facilities for disposal of biohazardous waste (e.g., bedpan flushers); for cleaning, reprocessing, and storage of ICU equipment; and for storage of housekeeping supplies should be separate from patient care areas. Single-patient rooms may increase the likelihood of handwashing being done and improve compliance with isolation practices, reducing the risk of cross-infection. For example, Mulin and colleagues[168] found that converting from an open unit to single rooms in their ICU greatly reduced rates of patient colonization with *A. baumanii,* and Shirani and colleagues[169] found that renovation of their burn unit to include separate bed enclosures reduced rates of nosocomial infection by 48%.[169]
- Materials used for fixtures, furniture, and other surfaces should be smooth and easy to clean; surfaces made of porous materials foster bacterial colonization.[170]
- An adequate number of sinks must be available for convenient handwashing by ICU personnel. Ideally, a sink should be located at the *entrance* of each cubicle or patient room to encourage handwashing by all entering personnel who will have contact with the patient or the immediate environment.[171,172] Separate sinks should be used for cleaning and reprocessing contaminated equipment. Sinks and sink drains are normally contaminated by pseudomonads,[173] although their role in the epidemiology of nosocomial infection is as yet unclear. However, sinks should be designed to minimize aerosol formation and splashback.
- All ICUs should be equipped with one or more class A isolation rooms,[200] which include an anteroom for gowning and handwashing and the necessary modifications (negative pressure, roofline exhaust) to permit it to be used for patients with tuberculosis or other airborne infections such as chickenpox, measles, disseminated HSV infection or a highly contagious emerging pathogen such as the severe acute respiratory syndrome (SARS) human coronavirus. If an ICU treats bone marrow transplant patients or other patients with prolonged severe granulocytopenia, positive-pressure isolation rooms using high-efficiency particle-arrest (HEPA) filters should be available. Isolation rooms for patients with infections transmitted by the respiratory route or to protect profoundly granulocytopenic patients must be kept closed to maintain control over the direction of airflow.
- A centralized, filtered air-handling system that provides at least six room-exchanges per hour is essential.[167,174] Ideally, each patient's room should have the capacity of being set at positive or negative pressure with respect to the rest of the unit; if it cannot be, the room should be maintained permanently at positive pressure.

A variety of microorganisms including bacteria, mycobacteria, fungi, and parasites can be isolated from hospital water and have been implicated in endemic and epidemic nosocomial infections.[175] Many of these outbreaks were caused by bacteria typically thought of as "water" organisms such as *P. aeruginosa,*[173] *Stenotrophomonas maltophilia,*[176] and *A. baumanii*[153,177,178]; however, the most important and epidemiologically linked hospital water pathogen is the *Legionella* group.[179]

Nosocomial legionellosis was first described in 1979,[180] and it is estimated that up to 50% of cases of legionellosis are acquired in the health care setting,[181] with a mortality rate that approaches 30%.[182] Contamination of hospital potable water remains underappreciated despite studies showing that *Legionella* species can be recovered from 12% to 70% of hospital water systems,[183] and a number of studies in which nosocomial cases were identified only when specific diagnostic and surveillance methods were employed.[184,185] Characteristics of hospital water systems that are associated with *Legionella* contamination include piping systems with dead-ends that facilitate stagnation, large-volume water heaters that result in inefficient heating of hospital water, sediment build-up, water heater temperatures <60° C and tap water temperatures <50° C, maintaining water pH>8 and receiving municipal water untreated with monochloramine.[186-188]

Despite the ubiquity of water systems colonized with *Legionella* species and studies demonstrating a correlation between the level of colonization and risk of infection, the CDC does not recommend routine surveillance of hospital water systems,[181] although this stance is controversial.[183] Researchers from Pittsburgh, Pennsylvania, and the Allegheny County Health Department have recommended a more proactive stepwise approach that involves initial surveillance of hospital water for *Legionella* contamination, regardless of the presence or absence of institutional nosocomial legionellosis, followed by continued surveillance based on the level of water contamination found or the presence of institutional legionellosis.[183]

Legionella species are resistant to chlorine and heat, making it challenging to eradicate them from contaminated hospital water systems.[188] Attempts to hyperchlorinate hospital water have been partially successful if chlorine levels are continuously maintained between 2 and 6 parts per million at all times but produce rapidly accelerated corrosion of water pipes and are expensive.[189] Thermal eradication is feasible, using a "heat-and-flush" method to raise water tank temperatures to greater than 70° C and distal water sites to >60° C for short periods of time.[190] Although effective, super-heating is labor intensive and there is the constant fear that patients or health care personnel may sustain scald injuries if they wash or shower with tap water during a flushing period. The use of technologies such as instantaneous steam heat for incoming water[190] and ultraviolet light[191] are technically feasible with newer hospital water systems but may be incompatible with older hospital water systems.

Perhaps the most attractive, effective, safe, and cost-efficient method for *Legionella* eradication may be the use of continuous copper-silver ionization systems to sterilize hospital water systems. These systems have been well studied over the past decade and have proved to be highly effective for reliably eradicating *Legionella* contamination of hospital water and, most importantly, for eliminating nosocomial legionellosis in institutions when other interventions have failed.[192] In our own institution, two clusters of nosocomial legionellosis prompted a retrospective review that identified 10 cases over a 11-year period. Surveillance of the hospital water system found that 75% of all samples contained low levels of *L. pneumophila,* which were shown to be clonally related to the 10 cases of nosocomial legionellosis. Installation of a continuous copper-silver ionization system led to complete eradication of *Legionella* from water samples, and no further cases of nosocomial legionellosis have been identified at our institution since 1995, among 255,000 patients hospitalized.

Reliable Sterilization Procedures, Chemical Disinfectants, and Antiseptics

Reliable sterilization, disinfection, and antisepsis embrace virtually all measures aimed at prevention of nosocomial infection. *Critical* objects, which are introduced directly into the bloodstream or into other normally sterile areas of the body, such as surgical instruments, cardiac catheters, and implanted devices, must be reliably sterile and sterilized with steam, gas, hydrogen peroxide gas, or chemical sterilization. *Semicritical* items, which come into contact with intact mucous membranes, such as fiberoptic endoscopes, endotracheal tubes, or ventilator circuit tubing, can be decontaminated between patients by pasteurization or the use of high-level chemical disinfection with glutaraldehyde, peracetic acid, hydrogen peroxide, ethyl alcohol, or hypochlorite. *Noncritical* items, which normally come into contact only with intact skin, such as blood pressure cuffs or electrocardiograph electrodes, require hygienic cleansing or low-level disinfection with an iodophor, hypochlorite, quaternary ammonium or phenolic disinfectants, or alcohol.[193,194] The lone exception to this classification scheme is devices that pose a risk of transmitting prion-related diseases. Transmissible spongiform encephalopathies such as Creutzfeldt-Jakob disease (CJD) and variant CJD (vCJD) have gained considerable attention over the past decade and have only recently been addressed in published disinfection and sterilization guidelines.[195] Prions are not readily inactivated by conventional disinfection and sterilization procedures.[193] As a result, devices that pose a risk for transmission of prion-related diseases should undergo special sterilization procedures after cleaning that involve sodium hydroxide followed by low-temperature autoclaving (121° C) or high-temperature autoclaving (132° C for 1 hour or 134° C for 18 minutes).[194] Despite concerns that procedures involving semicritical items such as endoscopes and bronchoscopes may pose a risk for transmission of prion-related infections, there has not been a single report of CJD or vCJD associated with these devices. As a result, current guidelines recommend that only critical items and semicritical items that have come in contact with neurologic tissue (e.g., brain, spinal cord, eye tissue) should undergo special prion inactivation sterilization procedures.[194,196]

Numerous epidemics of gram-negative infection have been described in association with respiratory therapy equipment,[94,95] diagnostic equipment such as bronchoscopes and endoscopes,[95,99-101] and solutions used for cutaneous antisepsis.[197,198] Most of these outbreaks were traced to improper procedures or malfunction of automated systems used for the disinfection and sterilization of medical devices, although a number of epidemics in years past arose as a result of extrinsic contamination of solutions used for cutaneous antisepsis.[197,198] For these reasons, the importance of strict adherence to recommended policies and procedures for cleaning and reprocessing medical equipment used in the ICU cannot be overemphasized.

Endoscopes and bronchoscopes are essential diagnostic and therapeutic instruments in the ICU. Although most postendoscopy nosocomial infections are caused by inoculation of colonizing mucosal flora into normally sterile, vulnerable anatomic sites during the procedure, numerous epidemics have been traced to contaminated endoscopes.[95,99-101] Following use for bronchoscopy, endoscopes are typically contaminated with 6×10^4 colony-forming units (CFUs/mL).[199] All endoscopes are considered semicritical medical devices by the Spaulding classification and therefore require high-level disinfection following use.[196] In order to ensure their safe use, flexible endoscopes should be reprocessed with the following procedures: (1) physical cleaning to reduce microbial bioburden and remove organic debris; (2) high-level disinfection—glutaraldehyde and automated chemical sterilizing systems that use peracetic acid are most commonly used in the United States—with adequate contact time between the disinfectant and device surface; (3) following disinfection, rinsing with sterile or filtered tap water to remove dis-infectant residue; (4) flushing of all channels with 70% to 90% ethyl or isopropyl alcohol; and (5) drying with forced air.[196] Devices used with endoscopes that violate mucosal barriers, such as biopsy forceps, need to be reprocessed as critical medical items with full sterilization.[196] Other devices used in the delivery of respiratory care are also considered semicritical under the Spaulding classification and therefore should be reprocessed in a manner similar to endoscopes prior to reuse.[131]

Iodophors (e.g., 10% povidone-iodine), until recently, have been the most common agents used for cutaneous disinfection in North America. However, a large, prospective, randomized trial of cutaneous antiseptics used for drawing blood cultures recently showed that chlorhexidine was superior to 10% povidone-iodine and was associated with a more than twofold reduced rate of contaminated blood cultures (OR=0.40, 95% CI 0.21 to 0.75, P=.004).[200] Moreover, a recent meta-analysis examining the impact of different cutaneous antiseptic agents found that chlorhexidine was superior to povidone-iodine for both the prevention of intravascular catheter colonization and catheter-related bloodstream infection.[201] On the basis of these and other recent studies,[202,203] chlorhexidine-containing solutions are the preferred cutaneous antiseptics for insertion of intravascular devices in the ICU.[129] Whatever agent is used, it is essential that it be applied with vigorous scrubbing for a minimum of 1 minute to allow adequate time for germicidal activity.

Hand Hygiene

The major reservoir of nosocomial infection in the ICU is infected or colonized patients, and the major mode of spread of most nosocomial bacterial pathogens, many viruses, and even *Candida* from patient to patient is by transient carriage on the hands of medical personnel (see Fig. 51-3). Studies in our center of hand carriage of nosocomial pathogens by ICU personnel, using a simple rinse technique to quantify the transient flora,[204] have shown that, on average, approximately 60,000 CFUs (or 4.6 logs) are recovered from the hands of ICU personnel randomly sampled (Table 51-6). Nearly half of persons cultured at any point in time will be found to be carrying gram-negative bacilli, and 10% will be carrying *S. aureus.*[205] Serial culturing has shown that all ICU personnel, at various times, carry gram-negative bacilli and that nearly two thirds carry *S. aureus.* Carriage of both gram-negative bacilli and *S. aureus* is typically transient: sampling persons every other day over a prolonged period has shown *S. aureus* or the same gram-negative species in consecutive cultures only 16% of the time; prolonged carriage of a single gram-negative species seems to be rare—but has been reported.[206]

Hygienic handwashing before undertaking invasive procedures, handling open wounds, or having manual contact with high-risk patients (e.g., newborns or patients in ICUs) or after touching a source or object likely to be contaminated has been recognized since the time of Semmelweis and Lister as one of the most basic and

Table 51-6. Studies of Microorganisms Carried on the Hands of Hospital Personnel Working in a Neurosurgery Unit, University of Wisconsin Hospital

	All Microorganisms	Gram-Negative Bacilli	*Staphylococcus aureus*
Mean $\log_{10}$ CFU±SD, recovered from persons' hands* (range of individuals' means)	4.59±0.69 (3.31-5.76)	1.04±0.44 (0.29-1.93)	0.44±0.44 (0-1.45)
% All cultures positive	100	44.5	11.2
% All individuals positive at least once*	100	100	64

*Based on 6 to 34 cultures obtained at random times from each of 25 employees working in the unit over a 4-month period.
CFU, colony-forming units; SD, standard deviation.
From Maki DG: Control of colonization and transmission of pathogenic bacteria in the hospital. Ann Intern Med 1978;89:777-780.

important infection control measures. Despite universal acknowledgement of handwashing as a cornerstone of nosocomial infection control programs, compliance rates much above 50% have been difficult to achieve and handwashing rates among HCWs have ranged from 9% to 50% in numerous observational studies.[165,207,208] Recent investigations have undertaken to better understand the reasons for poor compliance in the face of the compelling evidence that hand hygiene is essential for prevention of nosocomial infection,[165] identifying cutaneous irritation, inconvenient sink location, time constraints, high workload, and understaffing. Of concern, risk factors for noncompliance with hand hygiene include being a physician (rather than a nurse); working in an ICU; and, paradoxically, engaging in patient-care activities with a high risk of cross-transmission.[165] Interventions to redress these deficiencies have included targeted education; feedback; convenient location of sinks and hand hygiene agents; use of alternative, less irritative hand hygiene agents; hand care lotions or creams[209]; and patient education.[210]

Studies done with working hospital staff have shown that hygienic handwashing with an antiseptic-containing agent reduces the count of microorganisms on the hands of the user far more effectively than handwashing with a nonmedicated soap.[204] Repeated use of some antiseptics such as chlorhexidine has a cumulative suppressive effect on the transient hand flora. Routine use of an antiseptic-containing handwashing agent could, in theory, enhance the effectiveness of the handwashing that is done. Moreover, if an agent that exhibits prolonged antimicrobial activity, such as chlorhexidine, is used, it might also confer protection against contaminants acquired between handwashings.[204] However, antiseptic-containing handwashing agents are more expensive and often more irritating to the skin. Irritation can result in dermatitis and, paradoxically, increased colonization by gram-negative bacilli.[211]

Clearly, antiseptic-containing soaps are more effective in removing microorganisms from the hands of users, but will routine use of these agents for hygienic handwashing reduce the incidence of nosocomial infection in patients? Discontinuation of hexachlorophene for handwashing by personnel and bathing of infants in the United States in 1973 was followed by a marked upsurge in *S. aureus* infections in nurseries,[212] and use of chlorhexidine-containing handwashing agents was considered an essential measure for control of hospital outbreaks caused by multiply resistant *Klebsiella*[213] and MRSA.[214,215] However, since Semmelweis' study, few studies have prospectively evaluated the efficacy of antiseptic-containing handwashing agents for reducing *endemic* nosocomial infections, particularly infections caused by gram-negative bacilli.[211,216]

In 1982 a comparative sequential trial of three handwashing agents—a nonmedicated tissue soap, 10% povidone-iodine (Betadine Scrub), and 4% chlorhexidine (Hibiclens)—was undertaken in the trauma-surgical ICU of the University of Wisconsin Hospital.[211] Each agent was used exclusively for approximately 6 weeks, during which time hand cultures of ICU personnel were done at random and surveillance of infection in patients was carried out. Risk factors for infection in patients hospitalized during the use of each agent were comparable: Nearly two thirds of the patients in each period required ventilatory support and hemodynamic monitoring, and almost all had urinary catheters. The incidence of nosocomial infection in all groups was expectedly high, but it was 30% lower during the use of the two antiseptic-containing handwashing agents than during the use of the nonmedicated soap ($P<.001$). Povidone-iodine was irritating to the hands of most staff, and chlorhexidine had a slightly drying effect but was well tolerated, comparable with the nonmedicated soap.

In a similar study at the University of Iowa Hospital, Massanari and Heirholzer[216] did not find significant differences in the rates of nosocomial infection when nonmedicated soap was used exclusively as compared with alternating cycles during which 4% chlorhexidine (Hibiclens) was used in surgical ICUs; however, the incidence of infection in the medical ICU was 50% lower during use of chlorhexidine ($P<.05$).

In the largest multiple-crossover prospective study—1894 adult patients in three ICUs—of the relative efficacy of antiseptic-containing handwashing agents used by personnel in ICUs, Doebbeling and colleagues[217] found that the use of 4% chlorhexidine (Hibiclens) was associated with a 30% reduction in nosocomial infections (OR=0.73), as contrasted with rates when a 60% alcohol hand-rinsing agent (Cal-Stat) was used. Both regimens were well tolerated.

Recently, alcohol-based, waterless hand rubs have become the agents of choice for hand hygiene and are now universally used in U.S. hospitals because of their convenience and broad-spectrum activity.[210] Alcohols have the most rapid and pronounced bactericidal action and greatly reduce the time needed for hand disinfection. A vigorous 1-minute rubbing with a sufficient volume of alcohol to wet the hands completely has been shown to be highly effective at reducing the density of skin flora.[218] Ethanol, iso- and n-propanol are the constituents of most commercially available alcohol-based hand rubs; at equal concentrations, n-propanol is most effective and ethanol, the least. However, all have limited efficacy with gross soilage so that visibly soiled hands should always be washed with antiseptic soap and water.[171] Moreover, at least 3 mL of an alcohol-based rub is necessary to completely coat the hands and achieve optimal degerming. The use of alcohol hand rubs or gels will be augmented by making conveniently located calibrated dispensers widely available. However, many HCWs prefer individual containers that can be carried in a pocket, which makes it difficult to ensure that an adequate volume is used with each application.

Few trials have been conducted to evaluate the efficacy of alcohol-containing hand rubs for reducing nosocomial infection. Most are quasi-experimental before-after studies, and most have shown a short-term reduction in nosocomial infection rates with use of alcohol-containing hand rubs.[172,219,220]

The major factor limiting acceptance of alcohol products for hand antisepsis in the past was desiccation and irritation of skin. This is now obviated by incorporating emollients into alcohol-based hand rubs, which has enhanced acceptance by HCWs and may augment antibacterial activity by slowing the evaporation of alcohol.[221] A recent randomized clinical trial in 50 ICU HCWs compared a conventional 2% chlorhexidine gluconate wash with water to a waterless alcohol-based hand rub (61% ethanol with emollients) and showed that use of the waterless alcohol-based product produced significantly less skin scaling and irritation[222]; unfortunately, degerming was not assessed.

A recent review describes in detail the various hand hygiene agents available and their spectrum of activity.[210] Recommendations for hand hygiene by the CDC have recently been published (Table 51-7),[171] emphasizing hand antisepsis with an antiseptic-containing soap or detergent or an alcohol-based hand rub: (1) before and after direct contact with patients or the environment and equipment in the immediate vicinity of the patient and (2) before performing invasive procedures such as insertion of an intravascular device or urinary catheter. Use of skin care products—lotions or creams—to minimize irritant contact dermatitis associated with frequent handwashing and improve compliance with hand hygiene practices is highly recommended.

Institutional commitment is essential to improve compliance with recommended hand hygiene practices. The CDC guideline recommends that institutions (1) monitor and record adherence to hand hygiene by ward or service; (2) provide feedback to HCWs about their performance and (3) monitor the volume of alcohol hand rubs used per 1000 patient-days.[171]

Clearly, further studies are necessary, particularly large comparative trials in which rates of nosocomial infection, rather than levels of cutaneous colonization, are used as the index of comparison. In the meantime the available data indicate that routine use of a chlorhexidine-containing product or alcohol-containing product will be more effective than use of a nonmedicated soap for hand hygiene in the high-risk areas of the hospital, such as ICUs, where cross-infection is most likely to occur.

Isolation Precautions for Communicable Infections

Isolation, the use of special precautions in the care of infected patients, is the only means of curtailing the spread of contagious microorganisms and preventing epidemics, especially in ICUs, where the risk of cross-infection is highest. Although requiring all persons entering an infected patient's room to wear gloves and a gown, possibly even a mask, may seem ritualistic and almost archaic, each aspect of the isolation procedure is directed at interrupting a potential mode of spread and is based on the known epidemiology of the infecting organism.[223] To be maximally effective, however, isolation procedures require compliance by each person coming into contact with the patient, including physicians. Isolation is also indicated, usually for the entirety of hospitalization, for all patients infected or known to be colonized by antibiotic-resistant nosocomial pathogens such as MRSA, gram-nega-

Table 51-7. Recommendations for Routine Hand Hygiene from the Centers for Disease Control and Prevention Guideline

Recommendation	Level of Evidence*
■ When hands are visibly dirty or contaminated with proteinaceous material or are visibly soiled with blood or other body fluids, wash hands with either a nonantimicrobial soap and water or an antimicrobial soap and water	IA
■ If hands are not visibly soiled, use an alcohol-based hand rub or, alternatively, wash hands with an antimicrobial soap and water for the following situations: Before direct contact with patients Before putting on sterile gloves when inserting a central vascular catheter Before inserting urinary catheter, peripheral vascular catheter, or other invasive procedure not requiring surgery After contact with patient's intact skin After contact with body fluids, mucous membranes, and wound dressings if hands are not visibly soiled Moving from a contaminated body site to a clean body site during patient care After contact with inanimate objects in the immediate vicinity of the patient After removing gloves	IB
■ Before eating and after using a restroom, wash hands with a nonantimicrobial soap and water or with an antimicrobial soap and water	IB
■ Antimicrobial-impregnated wipes are not a substitute for using an alcohol-based hand rub or antimicrobial soap	IB
■ If exposure to *Bacillus anthracis*, wash hands with nonantimicrobial soap and water or antimicrobial soap and water	II

*Categorization of recommendations: IA: strongly supported for implementation and strongly supported by well-designed experimental, clinical or epidemiologic studies. IB: strongly recommended for implementation and supported by certain clinical or epidemiologic studies and by strong theoretical rationale. IC: required for implementation, as mandated by federal or state regulation or standard. II: suggested for implementation and supported by suggestive clinical or epidemiologic studies or by strong theoretical rationale. No recommendation: unresolved issue: practices for which insufficient evidence or no consensus exists about efficacy.
Modified from Boyce JM, Pittet D: Recommendations of the Healthcare Infection Control Practices Advisory Committee and the HICPAC/SHEA/APIC/IDSA Hand Hygiene Task Force. MMWR Recommend Rep 2002;16:1-45.

tive bacilli resistant to aminoglycosides or third-generation cephalosporins, or VRE; in such cases, isolation has been shown to be effective in reducing endemic infections[224,225] (Figs. 51-5 and 51-6) and in controlling outbreaks.[225]

Isolation Systems

Most U.S. hospitals subscribe to one of two CDC isolation systems developed by panels of experts. The simplest system, *category-specific* isolation precautions, issued by the CDC in 1970,[223] groups diseases in seven categories by infections for which similar precautions are indicated: wound and skin precautions, enteric precautions, discharge precautions, blood precautions, respiration isolation, strict isolation, and protective isolation. Guidelines for *disease-specific* isolation precautions, issued in 1983,[226] consider each infectious disease individually, so only those precautions indicated to interrupt transmission of that specific disease are used. Disease-specific precautions minimize unnecessary isolation procedures; however, they are more complicated and may be implemented most effectively by a computerized system.

An alternative, simpler system, *body substance isolation,* has gained adherents and focuses on the isolation of potentially infectious body substances, such as blood, feces, urine, sputum, wound drainage, and other body fluids, of *all* patients through the use of simple barrier precautions—primarily gloves, gowns, plastic aprons, and masks or goggles. These barriers should be used when potentially infectious secretions are likely to soil or splash the clothing, skin, or face of the HCW.[227] Body substance isolation provides sufficient flexibility to augment the basic precautions taken with each patient, as needed, and adds private rooms with masks for infections transmitted by the airborne route. A criticism of this simpler system

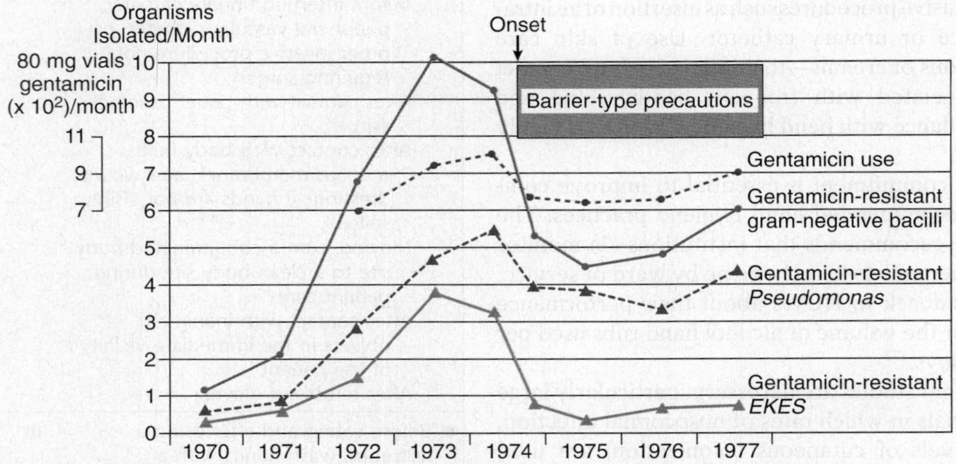

Figure 51-5. Impact of implementing barrier-type precautions (gown and gloves) with patients known to be colonized or infected by gram-negative bacilli resistant to gentamicin. Frequency of infections by gentamicin-resistant gram-negative bacilli and gentamicin use at Michael Reese Medical Center, 1970-1977. Data are plotted as the monthly average, and the averages for the first 7 and last 5 months of 1974 are plotted separately to demonstrate the effect of barrier-type precautions implemented in August 1974. *EKES, Escherichia coli, Klebsiella pneumoniae, Enterobacter* species, and *Serratia* species. (From Weinstein RA, Nathan C, Gruensfelder R, et al: Endemic aminoglycoside resistance in gram-negative bacilli: epidemiology and mechanisms. J Infect Dis 1980;141:338-345.)

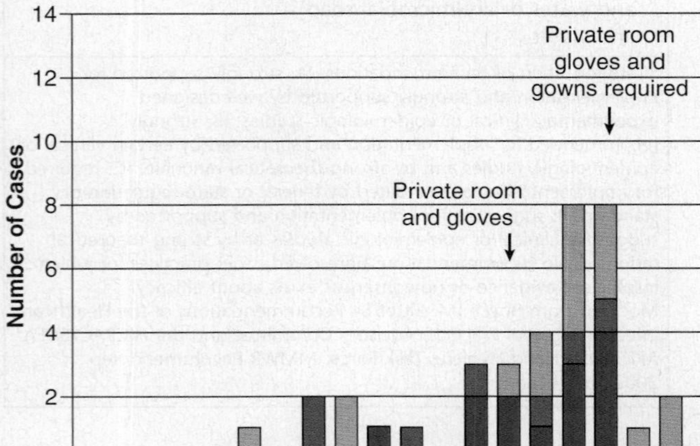

Figure 51-6. Impact of specific control measures on an institutional outbreak of vancomycin-resistant *Escherichia faecium.* Cases, by date of first positive culture for the epidemic strains (from January 1991 to December 1992). Number of cases=case patients in the intensive care unit (ICU) at time of first positive culture for the epidemic strain×other patients with previous exposure to the ICU×case patients never in the ICU. (From Boyce JM, Opal SM, Chow JW, et al: Outbreak of multidrug-resistant *Enterococcus faecium* with transferable vanB class vancomycin resistance. J Clin Microbiol 1994;32:1148-1153.)

has been the reduced emphasis on handwashing when gloves are removed.[228]

The most recent CDC guideline, currently in draft form,[174] separates basic precautions into (1) *standard precautions* designed for the care of all patients in hospitals, regardless of their diagnosis or presumed infection status, and (2) additional *transmission-based precautions* designed for the care of specified patients who are known or suspected to be infected with highly transmissible or epidemiologically important pathogens. Standard precautions synthesize the major features of universal blood and body fluid precautions and are designed to reduce the risk of transmission of microorganisms from patient to patient and from patient to HCW, from both recognized and unrecognized sources of infection in the hospital. Transmission-based precautions are divided into three subgroups on the basis of the mode of transmission: contact precautions, droplet precautions, and airborne precautions. Contact precautions are recommended with multidrug-resistant bacteria that can be acquired by contact with the colonized patient or environmental surfaces or objects. Droplet precautions provide additional measures for transmission by large-particle droplets, such as during suctioning or bronchoscopy. Airborne precautions are added to standard precautions for care of patients with tuberculosis and other microorganisms transmitted by the airborne route. In general, transmission-based precautions usually specify a private room—always for airborne precautions.

Special Issues in the ICU

An environmental issue pertaining to isolation may be most relevant in the ICU, namely, the greater potential for fomites or environmental surfaces to contribute to the spread of nosocomial infection, especially with antibiotic-resistant microorganisms. Although previous studies have not been able to demonstrate that the inanimate hospital environment, particularly surfaces, walls, or floors, contribute materially to the occurrence of nosocomial infection,[154,155] accumulating evidence suggests that this may not necessarily be true for ICUs, where uniform exposure to invasive devices makes patients unduly susceptible. A number of careful studies of the epidemiology of ICU-acquired infection with resistant organisms such as MRSA,[155,156] *C. difficile,*[80,157] and VRE[152,158,229] have shown heavy contamination of the inanimate environment immediately contiguous to the patient by strains implicated in nosocomial infections occurring in patients. Even if gloves are being worn as part of protective isolation or universal precautions, the possibility of transmission of microorganisms from the environment to patients on the gloved hands of HCWs is real. Prolonged wearing of gloves in the ICU, which is common, may increase the risk of nosocomial cross-infection, expanding the epidemiologic role of the inanimate environment with certain pathogens such as MRSA or VRE.[229]

Similarly, the use of common stethoscopes, sphygmomanometers, or electronic thermometers with multiple patients provides further opportunity for organisms to spread. Although stethoscopes are commonly contaminated by nosocomial organisms,[230] their role in cross-infection is less clear.[230] On the other hand, spread of VRE[231] and *C. difficile*[232] has been traced to contamination of electronic thermometers. All surfaces contiguous to the ICU patient should be wiped down with the general hospital disinfectant at least daily, and *each ICU patient should have a dedicated stethoscope and sphygmomanometer.* The use of electronic temperature measuring devices on multiple patients within an ICU bears reevaluation, unless stringent efforts are made to assure reliable decontamination of the device after each use.

As discussed, many nosocomial infections appear to derive from organisms carried on the hands of ICU personnel, who during the working day have contact with multiple patients. To improve nursing care and reduce the risk of cross-infection, ICUs must have an adequate number of staff. Although the optimal nurse/patient ratio for patients in an ICU is not known, increased rates of infection and outbreaks have occurred when nurses have been assigned to multiple critically ill patients who require complicated nursing care.[163] One-to-one nurse/patient ratios may significantly reduce the risk of cross-infection.

To contain the spread of certain resistant organisms in the ICU (e.g., MRSA, VRE), *cohort nursing* is strongly recommended. In cohort nursing, the care of patients known to be infected (or colonized) by the organism is provided by nurses (and respiratory therapists) who will not provide care during that shift for noninfected patients, and the nursing care of noninfected patients is restricted to personnel who will not have contact with infected patients, except in an emergency. Cohorting of patients known to be colonized or infected with MRSA is widely practiced but has not been adequately studied. In one recent prospective study, the authors found that there was no evidence of increased transmission of MRSA when patients were not cohorted.[233]

Tuberculosis

The upsurge in tuberculosis since 1985, particularly the numerous nosocomial outbreaks caused by multidrug-resistant strains,[70-72,234,235] demonstrates the importance of isolation precautions to prevent the spread of tuberculosis within hospitals, especially within ICUs.[126] New guidelines[126] reemphasize the importance of air control by mandating the use of private negative-pressure rooms, combined with the use of ultraviolet lights or ventilatory modifications in which all air exiting the room is either filtered or exhausted directly to the roofline, away from hospital intake vents. Isolation room doors must be kept closed to maintain control over the direction of airflow, and all persons who enter a room in which tuberculosis isolation precautions are in effect must wear a disposable particulate respirator such as a dust-mist mask or a HEPA-filter mask. Gowns and gloves usually are not indicated. All ICUs should have one or more negative-pressure isolation rooms for the care of patients requiring respiratory isolation for tuberculosis and other airborne infections such as chickenpox or disseminated herpes zoster, disseminated HSV infection or emerging, highly contagious airborne infections such as SARS. To reduce the risk of contaminating a ventilator or discharging *M. tuberculosis* into the environment, when mechanically ventilating a patient with suspected or confirmed pulmonary tuberculosis, a bacterial filter capable of filtering particles ≥0.3 μm in size, with a filter efficacy of greater than 95%, should be placed on the patient's endotracheal tube or at the expiratory side of the breathing circuit of a ventilator.[126] ICU patients with tuberculosis not requiring mechanical ventilation should wear a surgical mask if leaving the negative-pressure isolation rooms for radiographic or other procedures.[126]

Standard Precautions

The world epidemic of AIDS and evidence that more than 1 million persons in the United States are silent carriers of the human immunodeficiency virus (HIV) have engendered great concern among HCWs regarding the risk of exposure to HIV in the workplace. In 1987 the CDC and the Department of Labor issued detailed guidelines for *Universal Blood and Body Fluid Precautions*[236,237] to prevent exposure of HCW workers and patients to potentially hazardous blood or body fluids. Universal precautions were based on the concept that all blood and body fluids that might be contaminated with blood should be treated as infectious because patients with bloodborne infections can be asymptomatic or unaware they are infected. The relevance of universal precautions to other aspects of disease transmission was recognized, and in 1996 the CDC expanded the concept and changed the term to *Standard Precautions*.[238] Standard precautions integrate and expand the elements of universal precautions into a standard of care designed to protect health care personnel and patients from pathogens that can be spread by blood or any other body fluid, excretion, or secretion. Standard precautions apply to contact with (1) blood; (2) all body fluids, secretions, and excretions (except sweat), regardless of whether they contain blood; (3) nonintact skin; and (4) mucous membranes.

Gloves are recommended for venipunctures, insertion of intravascular devices, and whenever it can be anticipated that the hands could become contaminated by blood or another high-risk body fluid. If there is potential for splatter or contamination of clothing, a gown is added. When there is potential for aerosolization of body fluids, such as during surgery, intubation, endoscopy, or insertion of an arterial catheter, a mask and eye shielding are included. Because the vast majority of occupationally related HIV infections have involved needle sticks or other sharps injuries, every effort must be made to avert such injuries that could result in percutaneous inoculation of HIV or other bloodborne viruses.[236,239]

Because prophylactic use of barrier precautions appears to be of some benefit for prevention of nosocomial infection[169,240,241] and all U.S. hospitals are currently mandated to follow standard precautions, it has been suggested that the use of gloves for all patient contacts, as is now common in many U.S. hospitals, should implicitly reduce the risk of nosocomial infection in general. However, this has not been demonstrated and there is concern that standard precautions might paradoxically increase the risk of nosocomial cross-infection.[242] In most U.S. hospitals it is still common to observe ICU personnel, many of whom routinely wear gloves for all patient contacts to protect themselves, put on gloves, touch heavily contaminated areas (e.g., an open wound or tracheostomy), and then, without removing the gloves, proceed to write in the patient's chart, answer the telephone, or care for another patient. This occurs because the health care providers have forgotten that although the gloves may protect themselves, the gloves must be immediately discarded after use to prevent cross-contamination of hazardous pathogens to other vulnerable sites on the same patient or transmission to other patients or the ICU environment. Before the era of AIDS and universal precautions, health care professionals were oriented toward protecting the patient and likely to wash their hands when exposed to potential contamination. Now the focus is centripetal, and many HCWs unfortunately view all precautions as measures to protect themselves. Thus prolonged wearing of gloves can result in heavy contamination of the gloves[243] and increase the risk of nosocomial cross-infection among patients.[229,244] It also puts the HCW worker at increased risk of dermatitis and allergic reactions to glove material.[245] *Standard precautions do not obviate the need for designated isolation precautions for patients with communicable infections.* The greatly expanded use of gloves as part of standard precautions in hospitals must now be accompanied by educational programs on how to use gloves effectively and in a manner that will not jeopardize patients. Staff must be strongly encouraged to wash their hands after removing gloves, especially after performing a bloody procedure, because blood often penetrates defects in gloves and can be found on the hands of the wearer.[246] Moreover, if the gloved HCW has had hands-on contact with a patient colonized by MRSA or VRE, the process of removing the gloves will result in contamination of the hands of the HCW by these organisms up to one third of the time.

Antibiotic Stewardship

There is a world crisis in antibiotic resistance (Fig. 51-2),[247,248] which reflects in greatest measure the heavy use of systemic antibiotics worldwide over the past 30 years, especially in hospitals. Antimicrobial therapy has its greatest ecologic impact in the close confines of the ICU. Most nosocomial outbreaks caused by antibiotic-resistant microorganisms[249,250] have occurred in patients hospitalized in an ICU. Antibiotic pressure, which promotes the exchange of genes encoding drug resistance by a variety of transfer mechanisms (Fig. 51-7),[251] has been shown to be the single most important factor predisposing patients to nosocomial infection with resistant organisms. Modern-day ICUs are the breeding grounds for the multiply resistant bacteria that are now being encountered in hospitals throughout the world: methicillin-resistant staphylococci; VRE; *Enterobacter, Serratia, Citrobacter, Proteus-Providencia*, and *P. aeruginosa* resistant to fluoroquinolones, aminoglycosides, or extended-spectrum beta-lactams.[55-58,247] Broad-spectrum antimicrobial therapy

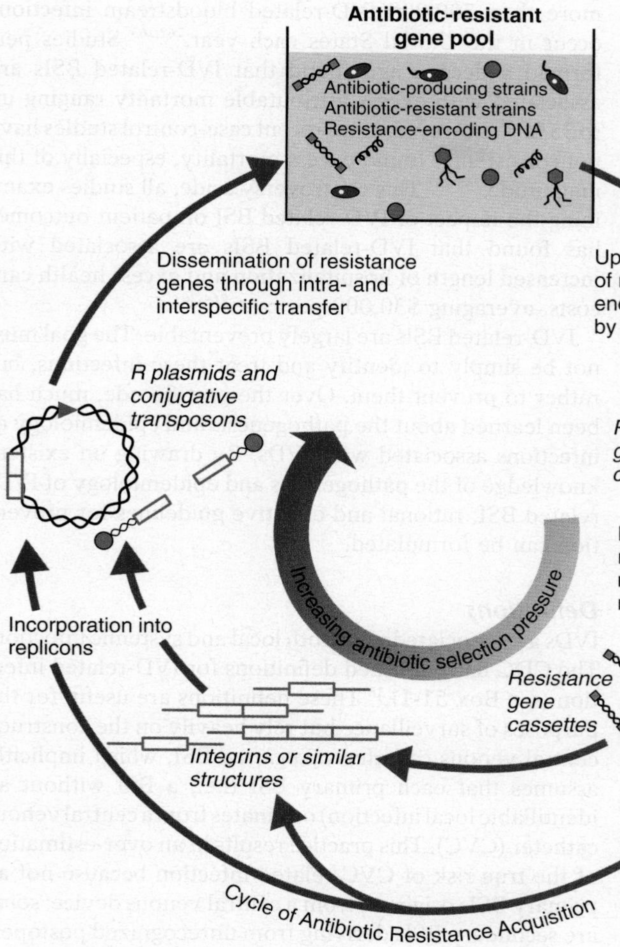

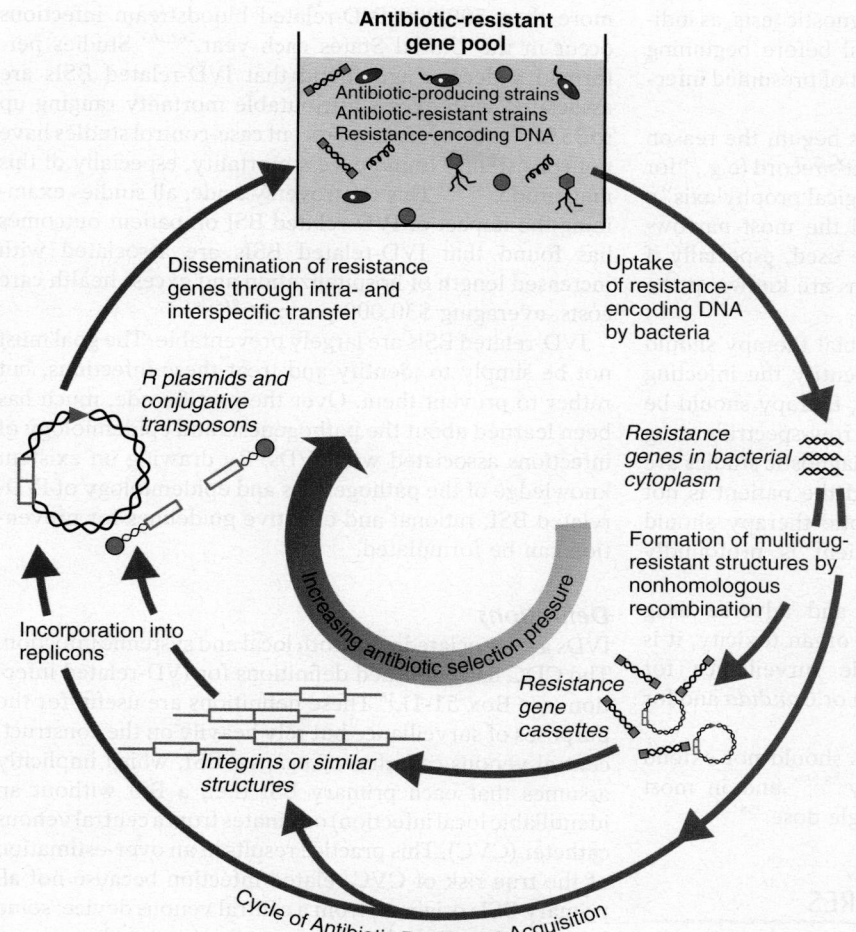

Figure 51-7. Schematic depicting the route by which antibiotic-resistant genes are acquired by bacteria in response to selection pressure of antibiotic use. The resistance gene pool represents all potential sources of DNA encoding antibiotic-resistant determinants in the environment; this includes hospitals, farms, or other microenvironments where antibiotics are used to control bacterial development. After uptake of single- or double-stranded DNA by the bacterial host, the incorporation of the resistance genes into stable replicons (DNA elements capable of autonomous replication) may occur by several different pathways that have not yet been identified. The involvement of integrins, as shown here, has been demonstrated for a large class of transposable elements in the *Enterobacteriaceae.* The resulting resistance plasmids could exist in linear or circular form in bacterial hosts. The final step in the cycle, dissemination, is brought about by one or more gene transfer mechanisms. (From Davies J: Inactivation of antibiotics and the dissemination of resistance genes. Science 1994;264:375-382.)

is the root cause of antibiotic-associated diarrhea and colitis caused by *C. difficile*.[80]

Clearly, antimicrobials are widely overused and misused; more than 75% of patients in U.S. ICUs, other than coronary care units, receive antimicrobial agents, whereas studies indicate that more than half of hospitalized patients receiving antimicrobial therapy have no evidence of infection or clear justification to be receiving antibiotics.[252] Moreover, within ICUs, a high proportion of the antibiotics used are broad-spectrum–extended-spectrum penicillins, third-generation cephalosporins, carbapenems, aminoglycosides, or fluoroquinolones. Greater efforts must be directed to improving the use of systemic antibiotics, especially within ICUs.

JCAHO now mandates that hospitals periodically review their use of antimicrobial agents through the use of antimicrobial audits.[31] Such audits should scrutinize the need for antimicrobial therapy—clear evidence of infection or clear justification for prophylactic use, the appropriateness of the regimen selected, and monitoring for therapeutic efficacy and side effects during therapy.[253] Educational programs and institutional guidelines for antimicrobial use that permit the hospital staff to construct guidelines and policies based on local needs and judgments, aided by published criteria, have been shown to materially improve antimicrobial use within the hospital.[252,254] Other important methods for controlling antimicrobial use include a restricted formulary, the policies of the clinical microbiology laboratory on reporting of susceptibility testing, and automatic stop orders for surgical prophylaxis.[252] Many institutions also place expensive or the most broad-spectrum drugs (e.g., third-generation cephalosporins, carbapenems, amikacin, ciprofloxacin, fluconazole, ganciclovir, lipid-associated amphotericin B) on a restricted list, requiring physicians who wish to use the agents to justify their use to a representative of the institutional antibiotic review committee.[255] Such programs greatly reduce use of restricted antibiotics and are gaining ever-wider acceptance.

Excellent resources,[256,257] including other chapters in this book (Chapters 21, 52), are available to guide the selection and use of anti-infective drugs in critically ill patients. However, several principles can reduce unnecessary antimicrobial therapy and improve the use of the drugs that are given:

1. Fever without other indications of infection should not mandate automatically beginning antimicrobial therapy in an ICU patient.
2. Unless antimicrobial therapy is being given for surgical prophylaxis, it is most likely being given for treatment of suspected or proved infection. Gram-stained smears,

cultures, and other appropriate diagnostic tests, as indicated, should be done without fail before beginning antimicrobial therapy for treatment of presumed infection in an ICU patient.

3. Whenever antimicrobial therapy is begun, the reason should be documented in the patient's record (e.g., "for treatment of pneumonia," "for surgical prophylaxis").
4. When possible, a single drug and the most narrow-spectrum drug or drugs should be used, especially if the infecting organism or organisms are known at the outset.
5. The need for continued antimicrobial therapy should be reassessed daily. If cultures identify the infecting microorganism or microorganisms, therapy should be modified, aiming for the most narrow-spectrum drug or drugs likely to be effective. If diagnostic studies are negative after 48 to 72 hours and the patient is not exhibiting signs of sepsis, antibiotic therapy should be discontinued, unless the patient is profoundly granulocytopenic.
6. Beyond monitoring for efficacy and adverse drug effects such as hypersensitivity or organ toxicity, it is essential that monitoring include surveillance for superinfection by resistant bacteria or *Candida* and for *C. difficile* diarrhea.
7. Surgical antimicrobial prophylaxis should not extend beyond 24 hours postoperatively[258,259] and in most operations can be limited to a single dose.[258]

SPECIFIC CONTROL MEASURES

As noted earlier, most nosocomial infections, especially in immunologically competent patients and in ICUs, are causally related to surgical operations or exposure to invasive devices of various types (see Tables 51-2 and 51-3). Comprehensive guidelines for the prevention of infection with procedures or devices that pose the greatest risk (urinary catheters,[130,260] endotracheal intubation and mechanical ventilatory support,[131] intravascular catheters and infusion therapy,[129] hemodialysis[261] and surgery[258]) have been published and can form the basis for institutional policies and procedures. Health care professionals working in ICUs are obligated to be informed about prevention of infection associated with the procedures they perform and the devices with which they work daily.

Intravascular Device–Related Bloodstream Infection

Impact

Obtaining and maintaining reliable vascular access has become one of the most essential features of modern-day intensive care. Unfortunately, vascular access is associated with substantial and generally underappreciated potential for producing iatrogenic disease, particularly bloodstream infection (BSI) originating from infection of the percutaneous intravascular device (IVD) used for vascular access-IVD-related (IVDR) BSI, often referred to as "line sepsis." Nearly 60% of all nosocomial bacteremias derive from vascular access in some form,[17] and it is estimated that more than 500,000 IVD-related bloodstream infections occur in the United States each year.[262,263] Studies performed a decade ago found that IVD-related BSIs are associated with excess attributable mortality ranging up to 35%[264]; however, more recent case-control studies have not consistently found excess mortality, especially of this magnitude.[265-267] This controversy aside, all studies examining the impact of IVD-related BSI on patient outcomes has found that IVD-related BSIs are associated with increased length of hospitalization and excess health care costs, averaging $30,000 per case.[264-267]

IVD-related BSIs are largely preventable. The goal must not be simply to identify and treat these infections, but rather to prevent them. Over the past decade, much has been learned about the pathogenesis and epidemiology of infections associated with IVDs. By drawing on existent knowledge of the pathogenesis and epidemiology of IVD-related BSI, rational and effective guidelines for prevention can be formulated.

Definitions

IVDs are associated with both local and systemic infection. The CDC has published definitions for IVD-related infection (see Box 51-1).[16] These definitions are useful for the purposes of surveillance but rely heavily on the construct, central venous catheter–*associated* BSI, which implicitly assumes that each primary BSI (i.e., a BSI without an identifiable local infection) originates from a central venous catheter (CVC). This practice results in an over-estimation of the true risk of CVC-related infection because not all primary BSIs originate from a central venous device; some are secondary BSIs deriving from unrecognized postoperative surgical site or intra-abdominal infections or nosocomial pneumonias or originate from other vascular devices such as peripheral venous catheters or arterial catheters used for hemodynamic monitoring.

By applying molecular subtyping techniques[107,268,269] to the results of semiquantitative or quantitative cultures of the removed IVD and blood cultures or the results of cultures of blood drawn through the IVD and a separate concomitant percutaneous peripheral blood culture, it is now possible to reliably determine whether an IVD was the source of a nosocomial BSI. Using these new diagnostic techniques allows formulation of simple but more rigorous definitions for IVD-related infection (Table 51-8), which we believe bear consideration as the standard for randomized trials and epidemiologic studies of IVD-related infection.[17]

Recognition and Diagnosis

Clinical Features

Recent evidence-based guidelines provide the best current information on the evaluation of the ICU patient with fever or other signs of sepsis.[270] Before any decision regarding initiation of antimicrobial therapy or removal of an IVD, the patient must be thoroughly examined to identify *all* plausible sites of infection including VAP, catheter-associated urinary tract infection, surgical site infection, antibiotic-associated colitis, and line sepsis.

Table 51-8. Proposed Definitions for Intravascular Device-Related (IVDR) Colonization, Local Infection, and Bloodstream Infection (BSI) Based on Microbiologic Confirmation of the IVD as the Source

IVD colonization	(i) A positive semiquantitative* (or quantitative†) culture of the implanted portion or portions of the IVD; (ii) absence of signs of local or systemic infection.
Local IVD infection	(i) A positive semiquantitative* (or quantitative†) culture of the removed IVD or a positive microscopic examination or culture of pus or thrombus from the cannulated vessel; (ii) clinical evidence of infection of the insertion site (i.e., erythema, induration or purulence); but (iii) absence of systemic signs of infection and negative blood cultures, if done.
IVDR BSI	*If the IVD is removed:* (i) A positive semiquantitative* (or quantitative†) culture of the IVD or a positive culture of the catheter hub or infusate (or positive microscopic examination or culture of pus or thrombus from the cannulated vessel) *and* one or more positive blood cultures, ideally percutaneously drawn, concordant for the same species, ideally by molecular subtyping methods; (ii) clinical and microbiologic data disclose no other clear-cut source for the BSI. *If the IVD is retained:* (i) If quantitative blood cultures are available, cultures drawn both from the suspect IVD and a peripheral vein (or another IVD) are both positive and show a marked step-up in quantitative positivity (≥fivefold) in the IVD-drawn culture; (ii) clinical and microbiologic data disclose no other clear-cut source for the BSI. or (i) If automated monitoring of incubating blood cultures is available, blood cultures drawn concomitantly from the suspect IVD and a peripheral vein (or another IVD) show both are positive, but the IVD-drawn blood culture turns positive more than 2 hr before the peripherally drawn culture; (ii) clinical and microbiologic data disclose no other clear-cut source for the BSI.

*Roll plate of cannula segment(s) >15 colony-forming units (CFUs).
†Sonication culture of cannula segment(s) ≥10^3 CFUs.
Modified from Crnich CJ, Maki DG: The role of intravascular devices in sepsis. Curr Infect Dis Rep 2001;3:497-506.

Table 51-9. Clinical, Epidemiologic, and Microbiologic Features of Intravascular Device-Related Bloodstream Infection

Nonspecific	Suggestive of Device-Related Etiology
Fever	Patient unlikely candidate for sepsis (e.g., young, no underlying diseases)
Chills, shaking rigors*	Source of sepsis inapparent, no identifiable local infection
Hypotension, shock*	Intravascular device in place, especially central venous catheter
Hyperventilation, respiratory failure	Inflammation or purulence at insertion site
Gastrointestinal*	Abrupt onset, associated with shock
Abdominal pain	Bloodstream infection caused by staphylococci (especially coagulase-negative staphylococci), *Corynebacterium* spp., *Candida, Trichophyton, Fusarium,* or *Malassezia* species†
Vomiting	
Diarrhea	
Neurologic*	Very high-grade (>25 CFU/mL) candidemia
Confusion	Cluster of cryptogenic infusion-associated bloodstream infections caused by *Enterobacter cloacae, Pantoea agglomerans,* or *Serratia marcescens**†
Seizures	
	Sepsis refractory to antimicrobial therapy or dramatic improvement with removal of cannula and infusion*

*Commonly seen in overwhelming gram-negative sepsis originating from contaminated infusate, peripheral suppurative phlebitis, or septic thrombosis of a central vein.
†Conversely, bacteremia caused by streptococci, aerobic gram-negative bacilli, or anaerobes is unlikely to derive from an intravascular device.
Modified from Maki DG, Mermel LA: Infections due to infusion therapy. In Bennett JV, Brachman PS (eds): Hospital Infections, 4th ed. Boston, Lippincott-Raven, 1998.

Despite the challenge of identifying the source of a patient's signs of sepsis,[270] several clinical, epidemiologic, and microbiologic findings point strongly toward an IVD as the source of a septic episode (Table 51-9).[262,271] Patients with an abrupt onset of signs and symptoms of sepsis without any identifiable local infection such as pneumonia or surgical site infection should prompt suspicion of infection of an IVD. The presence of inflammation or purulence at the catheter insertion site is now uncommon in patients with IVD-related BSI.[272] However, if inflammation, especially any purulence, is seen in combination with signs and symptoms of sepsis, it is highly likely the patient has IVD-related BSI and should prompt removal of the device. Finally, recovery of certain microorganisms in multiple blood cultures, such as staphylococci, *Corynebacterium* or *Bacillus* species, or *Candida* or *Malassezia* strongly suggests infection of an IVD.

Blood Cultures

Starting anti-infective drugs for suspected or presumed infection in the critically ill patient without first obtaining blood cultures from two separate sites, *at least one of which is drawn from a peripheral vein by percutaneous venipuncture,* is indefensible. The volume of blood cultured is essential to maximize the sensitivity of blood cultures for diagnosis of bacteremia or candidemia: in adults, obtaining at least 20 mL, ideally 30 mL, per drawing (each specimen containing 10 mL or 15 mL, inoculated into aerobic and anaerobic media) significantly improves the yield as compared with obtaining only 5 mL at each drawing and culturing a smaller total volume.[273,274] In adults, if at least 30 mL of blood is cultured, 99% of detectable bacteremias should be identified.[273,275] Similar operating characteristics are achieved in the pediatric population using a weight-based graduated volume approach to blood cultures.[276] Standard blood cultures drawn through CVCs provide excellent sensitivity for diagnosis of BSI but are less specific than cultures obtained from a peripheral vein.[277,278] If the patient has a long-term multilumen catheter, it may be reasonable to obtain a specimen from each lumen of the catheter because studies have found discordance (≈30%) among cultures obtained from different lumens of the same catheter.[279]

Every effort must be made to prevent introduced contamination when drawing blood cultures because a single contaminated blood culture has been shown to prolong hospitalization by 4 days and increase the costs of hospitalization by $4100 to $4400.[280,281] Tincture of iodine, isopropyl alcohol, chlorhexidine, or povidone-iodine *combined* with alcohol rather than povidone-iodine *alone* should be used for skin antisepsis prior to venipuncture for blood cultures, recognizing that studies have shown significantly reduced rates of contamination with use of these agents.[200,281,282] Up to 30% of blood cultures positive for coagulase-negative staphylococcus (CNS) represent true infection[283,284]; however, the majority of single positive cultures represent contamination,[284] a finding that should reemphasize the need to obtain cultures from *two* separate sites whenever BSI is suspected.

Cultures of Removed Intravascular Devices

Removal and direct culture of the IVD has historically been the gold standard for confirming the presence of IVD-related BSI, particularly with short-term IVDs. Studies have shown that culturing catheter segments semiquantitatively on solid media[285] or quantitatively in liquid media (e.g., removing the adherent organisms by sonication[286]) provides superior sensitivity and specificity for diagnosis of IVD-related BSI, with a strong correlation between high colony counts and line sepsis. Growth of greater than or equal to 15 CFUs from a catheter segment by semiquantitative culture or growth of greater than or equal to 10^3 CFUs from a catheter cultured after sonication with accompanying local inflammation or signs of sepsis indicates local catheter infection. Significant growth in the absence of local or systemic inflammation suggests colonization of the device; if continued vascular access is necessary, a new device should be placed in a *new* location rather than replacing it with a new one in the same location by guidewire exchange.

Although recent studies[287] have suggested that quantitative methods (e.g., sonication) are superior to the semiquantitative methods (e.g., roll plate), other studies have shown them to be equivalent.[288,289] Because hub contamination progressing to intraluminal colonization is the primary route of infection for long-term devices (e.g., devices in place >10 days), quantitative techniques may be superior to semiquantitative techniques in detecting infections from these types of devices because they remove organisms from both the internal and external surface of catheters.[289] In contrast, semiquantitative methods may be preferred over quantitative methods in cases of suspected infection related to a short-term device (e.g., devices in place <10 days) because the primary route of infection in this setting is caused by extraluminal ingress of skin organisms at the catheter insertion site and the semiquantitative method is simple, less expensive, and allows identification of the infecting organisms a day earlier.

Direct and impression Gram stains[290] or acridine orange stains[289] of intravascular segments of removed catheters have shown excellent correlation with quantitative techniques for culturing catheters and can permit rapid diagnosis of catheter-related infection.

To rigorously identify the mechanism of IVD-related BSI in prospective studies, it is necessary to culture *all* potential sources of microorganisms at the time of catheter removal (Fig. 51-8): skin of the insertion site, each catheter hub, infusate from each lumen, as well as implanted catheter segments. If the results of these cultures appear to link a BSI with microorganisms isolated from one or more portions of the device by phenotypic criteria, efforts then need to be made to conclusively establish concordance, *beyond* speciation and antimicrobial susceptibility pattern, using one or more molecular subtyping systems such as multi-locus enzyme electrophoresis, plasmid profile, or restriction-enzyme digestion of genomic DNA analyzed by pulsed-field electrophoresis.[268,269,274,291]

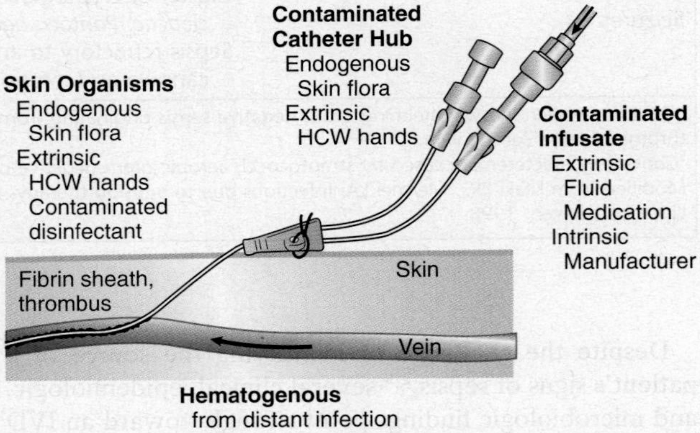

Figure 51-8. Potential sources of infection of a percutaneous IVD: the contiguous skin flora, contamination of the catheter hub and lumen, contamination of infusate, and hematogenous colonization of the IVD from distant, unrelated sites of infection. HCW, health care worker. (From Crnich CJ, Maki DG: The promise of novel technology for the prevention of intravascular device-related bloodstream infection. I. Pathogenesis and short-term devices. Clin Infect Dis 2002;34:1232-1242.)

Diagnosis of Infection with Implanted Long-Term Intravascular Devices

The methods described earlier require removal of the device for confirmation of IVD-related BSI. This can pose formidable challenges to management with long-term, surgically implanted IVDs such as Hickman and Broviac catheters, cuffed and tunneled hemodialysis catheters, and subcutaneous central venous ports. Only 15% to 45% of long-term IVDs that are removed for suspected infection are truly colonized or infected at the time of removal.[292-295] To avoid unnecessary removal of IVDs, methods have been developed to diagnose IVD-related BSI while allowing the device to remain in place: (1) paired quantitative blood cultures drawn from the IVD and percutaneously from a peripheral vein[289] and (2) differential time to positivity (DTP) of paired standard blood cultures, one drawn from the IVD and the other from a peripheral vein.[296]

If a laboratory has available an automated quantitative system for culturing blood (e.g., Isolator lysis-centrifugation system, Wampole Laboratories, Cranbury, NJ), quantitative blood cultures drawn through the IVD *and* concomitantly by venipuncture from a peripheral vein (or another IVD) can permit the diagnosis of IVD-related bacteremia or fungemia to be made with sensitivity and specificity in the range of 80% to 95%,[289] without removal of the catheter, if empiric antimicrobial therapy has not yet been initiated. IVD-drawn cultures demonstrating 5- to 10-fold higher concentrations of microorganisms per milliliter, as compared with counts of the same micro-organism obtained in a culture drawn from a peripheral vein, confirm the presence of IVD-related BSI.

The differential-time-to-positivity (DTP) of paired blood cultures, one drawn through the IVD and the second, concomitantly from a peripheral vein, has also been shown to reliably identify IVD-related BSI of long-term IVDs if the blood culture drawn from the IVD turns positive 2 or more hours before the culture drawn peripherally. In studies of patients with long-term IVDs, the sensitivity and specificity of DTP ranged from 82% to 94% and 88% to 91%, respectively.[289,296] The performance of DTP in short-term IVDs has recently been examined, with disappointing results,[297] a finding that is not entirely unexpected given the predominant extraluminal route of infection with these devices.

Detection of Contaminated Infusate

To diagnose infection caused by contaminated infusate, a sample of IV fluid, aspirated from the line, should be cultured quantitatively and qualitatively[285]; concordance with positive peripheral blood cultures, without another identifiable source for the patient's BSI, definitively implicates infected infusate as the cause of the BSI. Anaerobic culture techniques are not necessary unless blood or another biologic product is involved.

Incidence

Prospective studies, in which every attempt was made to conclusively identify the presence of an IVD-related BSI, show that every type of IVD carries some risk of causing BSI; however, the magnitude of risk varies greatly, depending on the type of device (Table 51-10).[298] The device that poses the greatest risk of IVD-related BSI today is the

Table 51-10. Rates of Intravascular Device–Related Bloodstream Infection Caused by Various Types of Devices Used for Vascular Access in Adults

					Rates of IVD-Related Bloodstream Infection			
					Per 100 Devices		Per 1000 IVD-days	
Device	Studies, *n*	Catheters, *n*	IVD-days, *n*	BSIs, *n*	Pooled mean	95% CI	Pooled mean	95% CI
Peripheral IV catheters	11	10,910	28,720	13	0.1	0.1-0.2	0.5	0.2-0.7
Arterial catheters	14	4366	21,397	37	0.8	0.6-1.1	1.7	1.2-2.3
Short-term, nonmedicated central venous catheters	79	20,226	322,283	883	4.4	4.1-4.6	2.7	2.6-2.9
Pulmonary artery catheters	13	2057	8143	30	1.5	0.9-2.0	3.7	2.4-5
Hemodialysis catheters:								
Temporary, noncuffed	16	3066	51,840	246	8	7-9	4.8	4.2-5.3
Long-term, cuffed, and tunneled	16	2806	373,563	596	21.2	19.7-22.8	1.6	1.5-1.7
Peripherally inserted central catheters (PICCS):	15	3566	105,839	112	3.1	2.6-3.7	1.1	0.9-1.3
Long-term tunneled and cuffed central venous catheters	29	4512	622,535	1013	22.5	21.2-23.7	1.6	1.5-1.7
Subcutaneous venous ports	14	3007	983,480	81	3.6	2.9-4.3	0.1	0-0.1

BSI, bloodstream infection; TPN, total parenteral nutrition.
Modified from Maki DG, Kluger DM, Crnich CJ: The risk of bloodstream infection in adults with different intravascular devices: A systematic review of 200 published prospective studies. Mayo Clin Proc 2006;81:1159-1171.

CVC in its many forms (see Table 51-10): short-term, noncuffed, single-lumen or multilumen catheters inserted percutaneously into the subclavian or internal jugular vein have shown rates of catheter-related BSI in the range of 3% to 5% (2 to 3 per 1000 IVD-days).[298] Far lower rates of infection have been encountered with surgically implanted cuffed Hickman or Broviac catheters and subcutaneous central venous ports (1 and 0.2 per 1000 IVD-days, respectively).[298] Contrary to popular belief, peripherally inserted central catheters (PICCs) used in inpatients and arterial catheters are associated with rates of catheter-related BSI approaching those seen with short-term, noncuffed, and nontunnelled, multilumen CVCs—up to 2.1[299] and 3.4[300] BSIs per 1000 IVD-days, respectively.

Pathogenesis and Risk Factors

Two major sources of IVD-related BSI exist: (1) colonization of the IVD, *catheter-related infection* and (2) contamination of the fluid administered through the device, *infusate-related infection*.[262] Contaminated infusate is the cause of most *epidemic* IVD-related BSIs; in contrast, catheter-related infections are responsible for most *endemic* IVD-related BSIs.[17]

In order for microorganisms to cause catheter-related infection, they must first gain access to the extraluminal or intraluminal surface of the device, where they can adhere and become incorporated into a biofilm that allows sustained infection and hematogenous dissemination.[301] Microorganisms gain access to the bloodstream by one of three mechanisms (see Fig. 51-8): (1) skin organisms invade the percutaneous tract, probably assisted by capillary action, at the time of insertion or in the days following; (2) microorganisms contaminate the catheter hub (and lumen) when the catheter is inserted over a percutaneous guidewire or later manipulated; or (3) organisms are carried hematogenously to the implanted IVD from remote sources of local infection such as pneumonia.

With *short-term* IVDs (e.g., in place <10 days) such as peripheral IV catheters; arterial catheters; and noncuffed, nontunneled CVCs, most device-related BSIs are of cutaneous origin, from the insertion site, and gain access extraluminally, occasionally intraluminally at insertion with the guidewire.[302,303] In contrast, contamination of the catheter hub and luminal fluid is the predominant mode of invasive infection with *long-term* IVDs (e.g., in place >10 days) such as cuffed Hickman- and Broviac-type catheters, subcutaneous central ports, and PICCs.[304,305]

Also important is recognizing that infusate (parenteral fluid, blood products, or IV medications) administered through an IVD can also occasionally become contaminated and produce device-related BSI. Contaminated fluid is fortunately an infrequent cause of endemic infusion-related infection with most short-term IVDs; it is, however, an important cause of BSIs with arterial catheters used for hemodynamic monitoring and long-term IVDs such as Hickman or Broviac catheters, cuffed hemodialysis CVCs, and subcutaneous central venous ports.[303,306,307]

Most nosocomial *epidemics* of infusion-related BSI have been traced to contamination of infusate by gram-negative bacilli, introduced during its manufacture (intrinsic contamination) or during its preparation and administration in the hospital (extrinsic contamination).[143,308] If an epidemic is suspected, the epidemiologic approach must be methodical and thorough yet expeditious, directed toward establishing the bona fide nature of the putative epidemic infections (i.e., ruling out "pseudoinfections")[242] and confirming the existence of an epidemic; defining the reservoirs and modes of transmission of the epidemic pathogens; and, most importantly, controlling the epidemic, quickly and completely. Control measures are predicated on accurate delineation of the epidemiology of the epidemic pathogen. The essential steps in dealing with a suspected nosocomial outbreak have recently been reviewed (and are discussed later).[262]

In recent years the factors associated with an increased risk of IVD-related BSI have become better delineated (Table 51-11). Prolonged hospitalization and severity of illness clearly influence the risk, and clinical states such as granulocytopenia, AIDS, and bone marrow transplanta-

Table 51-11. Risk Factors for Intravascular Device–Related Bloodstream Infection with Short-Term Intravascular Devices

Risk Factors (No. of Studies)	Relative Risk or Odds Ratio
Underlying Disease:	
AIDS (2)	4.8
Neutropenia (2)	1-15.1
GI disease (1)	2.4
Surgical service (1)	4.4
ICU/CCU placement (3)	0.4-6.7
Extended hospitalization (3)	1-6.7
Other intravascular devices (2)	1-3.8
Systemic antibiotics (3)	0.1-0.5
Active infection at another site (2)	8.7-9.2
High APACHE III score (1)	4.2
Mechanical ventilation (1)	2-2.5
Transplant patient (1)	2.6
Features of Insertion:	
Difficult insertion (1)	5.4
Maximal sterile barriers (1)	0.2
Tunneling (2)	0.3-1
Insertion over a guidewire (8)	1-3.3
Insertion Site:	
Internal jugular vein (6)	1-3.3
Subclavian vein (5)	0.4-1
Femoral vein (2)	3.3-4.8
Defatting insertion site (1)	1
Use a multilumen catheter (8)	–6.5
Catheter Management:	
Routine change of IV set (2)	1
Staffing in SICU (nurse-to-patient ratio) (1)	
1 : 2	61.5
1 : 1.5	15.6
1 : 1.28	4
1 : 1	1
Inappropriate catheter usage (1)	5.3
Duration of catheterization >7 days (5)	1-8.7
Colonization of catheter hub (3)	17.9-44.1
Parenteral nutrition (2)	–4.8

Modified from Safdar NS, Kluger DM, Maki DG: A review of risk factors for catheter-related infection caused by percutaneously inserted, noncuffed central venous catheters: Implications for preventive strategies. Medicine 2002;81:466-479.

tion have been associated with fourfold to sixfold increased rates of IVD-related BSI.[309,310] However, the features of the IVD, its insertion, and its maintenance appear to have far greater impact on the overall risk of infection. In 289 patients, Merrer and colleagues[311] found that insertion of an IVD in the femoral versus the subclavian vein was associated with a greatly increased risk of infection (20 versus 3.7 BSIs per 1000 IVD-days, $P<.001$) and thrombotic complications (21.5% versus 1.9%, $P<.001$).[311] Moreover, Robert and colleagues[312] found that patients with primary BSI were more likely to have received care during times when there was a lower nursing-to-patient ratio and a higher proportion of temporary ("float") nurses rather than the fulltime nursing staff.[312]

Microbiology

Figure 51-9 summarizes the microbial profile of IVD-related BSI from 159 published prospective studies.[313] As might be expected from knowledge of the pathogenesis of these infections, skin microorganisms account for the largest proportion of these infections.

Strategies for Prevention

Recommendations for the prevention of IVD-related BSIs were published by the Hospital Infection Control Practices Advisory Committee (HICPAC) several years ago.[129] Table 51-12 summarizes the recommendations of the 2001 HICPAC guideline for the prevention of IVD-related BSI and scores each recommendation on the basis of the quality of the available scientific evidence. It must be reaffirmed that measures for prevention of any nosocomial infection must, wherever possible, be based on the best understanding of pathophysiology and epidemiology and, whenever possible, controlled clinical trials.

At-Device Insertion

1. *Choice of catheter and site of device insertion:* Obviously, the choice of IVD inserted into a patient will be guided primarily by that patient's particular needs (e.g., hemodialysis versus fluid administration). However, the astute clinician can mitigate much of the risk associated with vascular access by choosing the best device for the task at hand and inserting the IVD in a location associated with the least risk of infection. Studies suggest that multilumen IVDs are associated with a higher risk of infection than single-lumen catheters.[314] That said, if a patient has need for multiple infusions, inserting several single lumen catheters will pose greater risks than a single multilumen catheter.

   To date, there have been no randomized studies designed to evaluate the optimal location for placement of short-term CVCs. However, the data accumulated from numerous observational studies suggest that the lowest risk of IVD-related BSI is seen with subclavian vein insertion and the highest risk with femoral vein insertion, with an intermediate level of risk associated with jugular vein insertions.[303,311]

   The femoral vein is often used for central venous access, especially on nonsurgical services, because of the ease of cannulation and the lower risk of mechanical complications from insertion (i.e., bleeding or pneumothorax). Unfortunately, prospective studies evaluating the risk of femoral vein device placement have shown that CVCs placed in the femoral vein are more likely to be colonized at the time of removal than catheters placed in the internal jugular vein (RR=4.7, CI=2 to 8.8, $P=.0001$)[315] and are associated with an increased risk of IVD-related BSI when compared with CVCs placed in the subclavian vein (4.4% versus 1.5%, $P=.07$).[311] Furthermore, recent prospective studies have found higher rates of catheter-related deep vein thrombosis with femoral catheters, in the range of 7% to 25%.[310,311] In general, we believe femoral access should be used only if emergent access is required, the inexperience of the operator limits placement in the upper body, or there is a contraindication to placement in the upper body (no available sites, an extensive burn, or severe coagulopathy). If a short-term CVC must be placed in the femoral vein or artery, we believe it is important that the catheter insertion site be located at least 2 inches (5 cm) below the inguinal crease or an intertriginous area, which is heavily colonized with bowel organisms and yeasts; this also allows a more secure protective dressing to be affixed.

   In contrast to short-term CVCs, observational studies of hemodialysis catheters have not been able to confirm a lower rate of infection with catheters inserted in the subclavian vein as compared with those inserted in the internal jugular vein,[316] although there is still excess risk associated with femoral vein placement.[317] More importantly, prospective studies of catheters used for hemodialysis have demonstrated a significant risk of great vein thrombosis and stenosis in catheters inserted

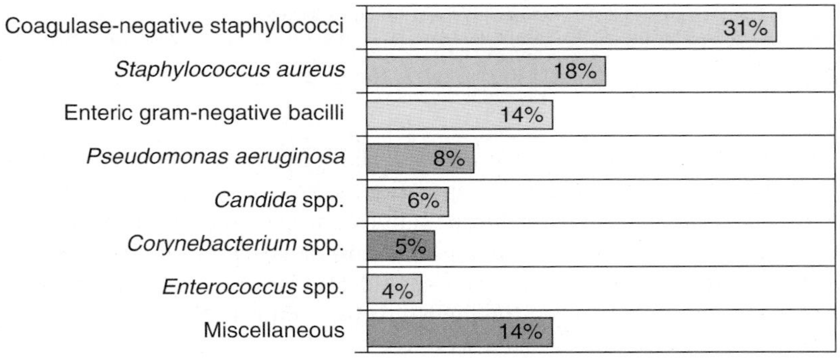

Figure 51-9. Microbial profile of intravascular device–related bloodstream infection based on an analysis of 159 published prospective studies. (Modified from Maki DG, Kluger DM, Crnich CJ: The microbiology of intravascular device-related (IVDR) infection in adults: An analysis of 159 prospective studies and implications for prevention and treatment. In Abstracts and Proceedings from the 40th Annual Meeting of the Infectious Disease Society of America. Chicago, Infectious Disease Society of America, 2002.)

Table 51-12. Summary of CDC/HICPAC Guideline for Prevention of IVD-Related Bloodstream Infection

Recommendation	Strength of Evidence*
General measures	
■ Educate all health care workers involved with IVD care and maintenance	IA
■ Ensure adequate nursing staffing levels in ICUs	IB
Surveillance	
■ Monitor institutional IVD infection rates of IVD-related BSI	IA
■ Express rates of CVC-related BSI per 1000 CVC-days	IB
At-catheter insertion	
■ Aseptic technique:	
Hygienic hand care before insertion or manipulation of any IVD	IA
Clean or sterile gloves during insertion and manipulation of noncentral IVDs	IC
Maximal barrier precautions during insertion of CVCs: mask, cap, sterile gown, gloves, drapes	IA
■ Dedicated IVD team strongly recommended	IA
■ Cutaneous antisepsis: first choice, chlorhexidine; however, tincture of iodine, an iodophor, or 70% alcohol are acceptable (no recommendations for use of chlorhexidine in infants younger than 2 months, unresolved issue)	IA
■ In adults, other than hemodialysis catheters (jugular site preference), use a subclavian site rather than a jugular or femoral site for CVC access (in pediatric patients, no recommendations for preferred site, unresolved issue)	IA
■ Use of sutureless securement device	NR
■ Sterile gauze or a semipermeable polyurethane dressing to cover site	IA
■ No systemic or topical antibiotics at insertion	IA
Maintenance	
■ Remove IVD as soon as no longer required	IA
■ Monitor IVD site daily	IB
■ Change dressing of CVC insertion site at least weekly	II
■ Do not use topical antibiotic ointments	IA
■ Change needless IV systems at least as frequently as the administration set; replace caps no more frequently than every 3 days or per manufacturer's recommendations	II
■ Complete lipid infusions within 12 hr	IB
■ Replace administration sets no more frequently than every 72 hr. When lipid-containing admixtures or blood products are given, sets should be replaced every 24 hr; with propofol, every 6-12 hr	IA
■ Replace peripheral IVs every 72-96 hr	IB
■ Do not routinely replace CVCs or PICCs solely for prevention of infection	IB
■ Do not remove CVCs or PICCs solely because of fever unless IVD infection is suspected, but replace catheter if there is purulence at the exit site, especially if the patient is hemodynamically unstable and IVD-related BSI is suspected	II
Technology	
■ Use antimicrobial-coated or antiseptic-impregnated CVC in adult patients if institutional rate of BSI is high despite consistent application of preventive measures and catheter likely to remain in place >5 days (no data or recommendations for pediatric patients)	IB
■ Use chlorhexidine-impregnated sponge dressing for adolescent or adult patients with uncuffed CVCs or other catheters likely to remain in place >5 days (no recommendation for children, do not use in neonates younger than 7 days old or gestational age younger than 26 wk)	NR
■ Use prophylactic antibiotic lock solution *only* in patients with long-term IVDs who have continued to experience IVD-related BSIs despite consistent application of infection control practices	II

*Taken from CDC/HICPAC system of weighting recommendations based on scientific evidence. **IA**, strongly recommended for implementation and supported by well-designed experimental, clinical, or epidemiological studies. **IB**, strongly recommended for implementation and supported by some experimental, clinical, or epidemiological studies and a strong theoretical rationale. **IC**, required by state or federal regulations, rules, or standards. **II**, suggested for implementation and supported by suggestive clinical or epidemiological trials or a theoretical rationale. **Unresolved issue**, an unresolved issue for which evidence is insufficient or no consensus regarding efficacy exists. **NR**, no recommendation for or against at this time.

BSI, bloodstream infection; CVC, central venous catheter; ICU, intensive care unit; IV, intravenous; IVD, intravascular device.

Modified from O'Grady NP, Alexander M, Dellinger EP, et al: Guidelines for the prevention of intravascular catheter-related infections. Clin Infect Dis 2002;35:1281-1307.

into the subclavian vein that approaches 40% to 50% as compared with rates of 0% to 10% with catheters inserted into the internal jugular vein.[318,319] On the basis of these data, internal jugular vein insertion is preferable to subclavian vein insertion for central access for hemodialysis.

2. *Barrier precautions:* Hand hygiene with an antiseptic-containing preparation, either conventional handwashing with chlorhexidine (2% to 4%) or with a waterless alcohol rub or gel,[171] must always precede the insertion of an IVD and should also precede subsequent handling of the device or its administration set.[129] A new

pair of disposable, nonsterile gloves, using a "no-touch" technique, is adequate for the placement of peripheral IV catheters in most patients; however, *sterile gloves* should be used during insertion in high-risk patients such as those with granulocytopenia. *Sterile* gloves are strongly recommended for placement of all other types of IVDs that are associated with a 1% or higher risk of associated bacteremia, specifically arterial catheters and all types of centrally placed devices including PICCs.[129]

Studies have shown that the use of *maximal barriers* including a long-sleeved, sterile surgical gown, mask, cap and large sterile drape, and sterile gloves significantly reduces the risk of CVC-related BSI (0.08 BSIs with maximal barriers versus 0.5 BSIs per 1000 IVD-days without maximal barriers, $P=.02$).[320] The use of maximal barriers has further been shown to be highly cost effective.[320] Considering that of all IVDs, CVCs are most likely to produce nosocomial BSI, a strong case can be made for *mandating* maximal barrier precautions during the insertion of *all* central IVDs.[129] They are not necessary, however, for arterial catheters used for hemodynamic monitoring, during which sterile gloves and a sterile fenestrated drape will suffice.[321]

3. *IV teams:* Good technique is also essential. Studies have shown that the use of special IV therapy teams, consisting of trained nurses or technicians who can assure a consistent and high level of aseptic technique during catheter insertion and in follow-up care of the catheter, have been associated with substantially lower rates of catheter-related BSI and are cost effective.[322,323] But even if an institution does not have an IV team, it can greatly reduce its rate of IVD-related BSI by formal education of nurses and physicians and stringent adherence to IVD care protocols.[324,325]
4. *Cutaneous antisepsis:* Given the evidence for the importance of cutaneous microorganisms in the pathogenesis of short-term IVD-related infections, measures to reduce colonization of the insertion site would seem of the highest priority, particularly the choice of chemical antiseptics for disinfection of the site. Nine randomized, prospective trials comparing a chlorhexidine-containing antiseptic to either povidone-iodine or alcohol for preparation of the skin prior to insertion of a short-term IVD have been reported.[201-203,326] In the largest study to date, a randomized trial in 1050 CVCs and arterial catheters placed in a university hospital ICU, cutaneous antisepsis with 1% tincture of chlorhexidine showed a highly significant reduction in IVD-related BSIs compared with an iodophor ($RR=0.35$, $P<.01$).[326] More recently, a meta-analysis that examined results from eight of the nine aforementioned studies found that use of chlorhexidine was associated with a nearly 50% reduction in the risk of IVD-related compared with povidone-iodine ($RR=0.49$, 95% $CI=0.28$ to 0.88).[201]

Insertion Site Care and IVD Maintenance

1. *IVD dressings:* IVDs can be dressed with sterile gauze and tape or with a sterile transparent, semipermeable, polyurethane film dressing. The available data suggest that the two types of dressings are equivalent in terms of their impact on IVD-related BSI with peripheral IVs and short-term CVCs.[327-329] In contrast, results from studies of arterial catheters have found that polyurethane dressings greatly increase the risk of IVD-related BSI.[327,330] As a result, polyurethane dressings should probably not be used on arterial catheters until future studies confirm their safety.
2. *Topical antimicrobial ointments:* In theory, application of a topical antimicrobial agent to the catheter insertion site should confer some protection against microbial invasion. Clinical trials of a topical combination antibacterial ointment containing polymyxin, neomycin, and bacitracin with peripheral IVs have shown marginal benefit,[331] but the use of polyantibiotic ointments has been associated with a fivefold increased frequency of *Candida* infection, limiting their utility.[331,332]

The topical antibacterial mupirocin, which is active primarily against gram-positive organisms, was shown in one study to significantly reduce colonization of internal jugular catheters without increasing colonization by *Candida* spp.,[333] and a more recent study by Sesso and colleagues[334] showed significant reductions in hemodialysis catheter colonization (3.17 versus 14.27 per 1000 IVD-days, $P = <.001$) and *S. aureus* IVD-related BSIs (0.71 versus 8.92 BSIs per 1000 IVD-days, $P = <.001$).[334] Unfortunately, resistance of *S. aureus*[335] and coagulase-negative staphylococci[336] rapidly emerges during wide-scale mupirocin use,[337] which contravenes its use as a topical agent for the prevention of IVD-related BSI at this time.[129]

Three prospective studies of topical povidone-iodine ointment applied to central venous catheter sites have failed to show a statistical benefit to its use,[331,338,339] but a single comparative trial in subclavian hemodialysis catheters showed that the use of topical povidone-iodine ointment was associated with a fourfold reduction in the incidence of IVD-related *S. aureus* BSI.[340] Therefore if a topical agent is to be used with hemodialysis catheters, an iodophor may be most desirable.

3. *Replacement of the device:* Studies have shown that peripheral IVs may be safely left in place for up to 96 hours if the patient and the insertion site is monitored closely.[341] Studies have suggested that the duration of peripheral catheterization may be prolonged even further,[342] but, viewing reports of increasing nosocomial *S. aureus* bacteremias linked to prolonged peripheral venous catheterization,[343] more studies are required before this can become considered acceptable routinely.

Scheduled replacement of short-term, noncuffed, nontunneled CVCs has long been practiced in many centers; however, some studies have called this practice into question.[344] Moreover, a meta-analysis found no benefit to routine replacement of short-term CVCs.[345] On the basis of these data, there appears to be no indication for scheduled replacement of short-term CVCs that are functioning well and show no clinical signs of infection.

4. *Guidewire exchanges of CVCs:* The management of CVCs that must be replaced, either because of mechanical malfunction or suspected infection, deserves special attention. Replacement of CVCs by guidewire exchange is associated with a reduced risk of mechanical complications[344,345]; however, it is also associated with an increased risk of the newly placed CVC becoming infected and causing CVC-related BSI.[344] As a result, if circumstances necessitate guidewire exchange for placement of a new catheter (e.g., the patient has limited sites for access, is morbidly obese, or is at high risk of mechanical complications because of underlying coagulopathy), the same strict aseptic technique, which includes full barrier precautions, must be used. However, the tip and/or intracutaneous segment(s) of the removed CVC should routinely be sent for culture to determine whether the insertion tract is colonized. If it is, the newly inserted CVC should be promptly removed and a new CVC placed percutaneously in a new site. If the tract is not colonized, the newly exchanged CVC can remain in the old insertion site.

   Although small studies have found some utility of guidewire exchange in the management of CVCs suspected of being infected,[346,347] we believe that, in the absence of randomized studies demonstrating its safety, guidewire exchange generally should not be performed if there is suspicion of IVD-related BSI, especially if there are signs of local infection such as purulence or erythema at the insertion site or signs of systemic sepsis without a source. In these cases the old catheter should be removed and cultured, and a new catheter should be inserted in a new site.
5. *Replacing the delivery system:* Whereas most infusion-related BSIs are caused by infection of the device used for vascular access, infusate can occasionally become contaminated and cause endemic BSIs.[303,348] If an infusion runs continuously for an extended period, the cumulative risk of contamination increases, and there is further risk that contaminants can grow to concentrations that could produce BSI in the recipient of the fluid. For more than 25 years, most U.S. hospitals have routinely replaced the entire delivery system of patients' IV infusions at 24- or 48-hour intervals[349] to reduce the risk of BSI from extrinsically contaminated fluid. Prospective studies indicate that IV delivery systems need not be replaced more frequently than every 72 to 96 hours, including infusions used for total parenteral nutrition or any infusions in ICU patients[341,350]; extending the duration of use can permit cost savings to hospitals.[350]

   Four clinical settings might be regarded as exceptions to using 72 hours as an interval for routine set change[350]: (1) administration of blood products, (2) administration of lipid emulsion, (3) arterial pressure monitoring, and (4) suspicion of an epidemic of infusion-related BSI. In these circumstances, it may be most prudent for administration sets to be changed routinely at 24- or 48-hour intervals.

   Arterial infusions used for hemodynamic monitoring appear to be more vulnerable to becoming contaminated during use and producing endemic[348] or epidemic septicemia,[96] caused by gram-negative bacilli. If the infusion for hemodynamic monitoring is set up so that the fluid flows continuously through the system, thus eliminating a blind stagnant column of fluid, extrinsic contamination appears to be greatly reduced and may even eliminate the need to replace the administration set, transducer assembly, and other components of the system at frequent intervals.[351,352] If disposable transducers are used, there appears to be no need to replace the transducer assembly and other components of the delivery system more frequently than every 4 days,[351] and it may be safe to replace them even less frequently.[352]
6. *Anticoagulation:* Thrombus formation on an intravascular device is associated with an increased risk of infection.[353,354] Two prospective studies have been performed to examine the efficacy of warfarin anticoagulation for reducing rates of IVD-associated thrombosis with long-term IVDs.[355,356] Both studies found that use of warfarin in a dose of 1 mg/day was associated with significantly reduced rates of thrombosis with long-term IVDs, although no data were provided on rates of IVD-related BSI.

   The use of prophylactic heparin for reducing rates of IVD-related thrombosis and infection has been evaluated in a meta-analysis.[357] Examining a variety of different administration techniques in 14 randomized controlled studies, Randolph and colleagues[357] concluded that systemic heparinization significantly reduced the risk of IVD-associated thrombosis (RR=0.43, CI=0.23-0.78) and device colonization (RR=0.18, CI=0.06 to 0.6) but failed to show a reduction in IVD-related BSIs. Heparin-bonded pulmonary artery catheters may be less prone to IVD-related BSI than nonheparinized catheters.[303,358,359]

   On the basis of these studies, low-level anticoagulation with warfarin is warranted for long-term IVDs as long as there is no contraindication (bleeding diathesis, brain tumor, or predilection to falls) and the INR is maintained below 1.6.[355] For short-term IVDs, the use of low-dose subcutaneous heparin is more appropriate; it is commonly given to patients with CVCs or arterial lines as part of ICU thromboembolism prophylaxis.

Novel Technology

Despite compliance with recommended guidelines, many centers continue to have high rates of IVD-related BSI. Novel technology holds much promise (Table 51-13). Innovative technologies designed to reduce the risk of IVD-related BSI have proved to be not only effective but also to reduce health care costs, both with short-term and long-term IVDs.[301,360]

1. *Novel securement devices:* Recently, a novel sutureless device for securing noncuffed vascular catheters has

Table 51-13. Novel Technology for Prevention of IVD-Related Bloodstream Infection That Has Been Examined in Randomized Clinical Trials

Chlorhexidine For Cutaneous Antisepsis
Securement Devices
Topical anti-infective creams or ointments
Polymyxin, neomycin, bacitracin polyantibiotic ointment
Povidone-iodine ointment
Mupirocin ointment
Dressings
Transparent, polyurethane film dressings
Hyperpermeable polyurethane dressings
Hydrocolloid dressings
Chlorhexidine-impregnated sponge dressings
Innovative IVD Design
Cuffed and tunneled CVCs
Subcutaneous central venous ports
Attachable silver-impregnated cuffs
Peripherally inserted central venous catheters (PICCs)
Anti-Infective–Coated Catheters
Benzalkonium chloride–impregnated catheters
Chlorhexidine–silver sulfadiazine–coated catheters
Cefazolin-coated catheters
Minocycline-rifampin–coated catheters
Silver-impregnated catheters
Anti-Infective Catheter Hubs
Iodinated chamber
External povidone-iodine-saturated sponge cap
Anti-Infective Lock Solutions for Long-Term IVDs
Gentamicin
Vancomycin
Vancomycin/ciprofloxacin
Trisodium citrate/gentamicin
Minocycline/ethylenediaminetetraacetic acid (EDTA)
Ethanol
Taurolidine
Scheduled (Prophylactic) Thrombolysis with Urokinase

CVC, central venous catheter; IVD, intravascular device.
Modified from Crnich CJ, Maki DG: The promise of novel technology for the prevention of intravascular device-related bloodstream infection. I. Pathogenesis and short-term devices. Clin Infect Dis 2002;34:1232-1242 and 1362-1368.

become available (StatLock, Venetec International). In a randomized trial of the device, premature loss of pediatric PICCs caused by accidental extrusion and PICC-associated thrombosis was significantly reduced,[361] and in two additional trials the incidence of catheter-related BSI was significantly reduced with the use of the novel securement device, both in adults and children with PICCs.[361,362]

The promise of this device for reducing infection may derive from elimination of a festering skin suture wound contiguous to the newly inserted catheter and minimizing to-and-fro movement of the catheter, which may promote invasion of the tract by cutaneous microorganisms through capillary action.[363]

2. *Novel dressings:* Studies of polyurethane dressings, which contain antiseptics such as povidone-iodine or ionized silver, have been disappointing. However, on the basis of demonstrated superiority of chlorhexidine for cutaneous disinfection of access sites, a novel chlorhexidine-impregnated sponge dressing has been developed (Biopatch, Johnson and Johnson Medical, Inc.). It maintains a high concentration of the antiseptic on the insertion site under the dressing. The largest study to date found that use of the chlorhexidine-impregnated sponge dressing was associated with a 60% reduction in catheter-related BSI (RR=0.37, P=.01).[364] Although there were no adverse side effects associated with the use of this dressing in this trial in adults, a pediatric trial found that 15% of low-birth-weight neonates developed local dermatotoxicity.[365]
3. *Anti-infective impregnated catheters:* Intravascular devices directly coated or impregnated with antimicrobials or antiseptics have been intensively studied over the past decade. Eighteen randomized trials evaluating the efficacy of chlorhexidine-silver-sulfadiazine– or minocycline-rifampin–impregnated CVCs have been published in full article or abstract form since 1994.[268,269,291,366,367]

Of the 16 published studies that examined the effect of antimicrobial-impregnated CVCs on rates of CVC-related BSI, 12 found either a statistically significant reduction or a strong trend toward a reduction in rates of CVC-related BSI.[366,367] Aggregate analysis of the 15 studies that compared antimicrobial-impregnated CVCs with nonimpregnated CVCs,[366,367] encompassing a total of 4250 CVCs, shows that antimicrobial-impregnated CVCs are associated with a 40% reduction in CVC-related BSI (61 BSIs/2129 devices versus 101 BSIs/2118 devices, OR 0.60, 95% CI=0.44 to 0.82, P=.001), a result remarkably similar to the findings of three published meta-analyses.[301,368,369]

Finally, two rigorous and sophisticated economic analyses have found that antimicrobial-impregnated CVCs are cost effective.[370,371] Veenstra and colleagues showed that antimicrobial-impregnated CVCs remained cost effective even if the cost of a CVC-related BSI was as low as $687 per case; cost savings were $196 per antimicrobial-impregnated CVC when a more realistic cost of a CVC-related BSI of $9738 was used in the analysis.[370] Shorr and colleagues[371] showed that use of antimicrobial-impregnated CVCs was associated with a cost savings of $9600 per CVC-related BSI prevented and that $165 to $280 would be saved for every patient who received an antimicrobial-impregnated CVC.

On the basis of this large body of data, two national advisory panels have recommended the use of antimicrobial-impregnated CVCs *in clinical settings where, despite rigorous application of other preventive interventions, rates of IVD-related BSI remain unacceptably high* (i.e., ≥3.3 BSIs per 1000 IVD-days).[129,372]
4. *Antimicrobial lock solutions:* Given the importance of hub contamination and intraluminal colonization in the genesis of IVD-related BSI with long-term IVDs,

intraluminal instillation of an antibiotic or antiseptic solution has the potential to reduce the risk of BSI associated with these devices. Six randomized, prospective trials have examined a vancomycin-containing antibiotic lock solution for the prevention of IVD-related BSI, the largest of which found that use of a vancomycin or vancomycin/ciprofloxacin lock solution reduced the risk of IVD-related BSI nearly 80% (P=.005), with no evidence that the use of the lock solution promoted colonization or infection by vancomycin-resistant bacteria or fungi.[373,374] Yet concern about the emergence of resistance with prophylactic antibiotic-containing lock solutions has limited their wider acceptance to date. *However, the use of prophylactic antibiotic lock solution is considered acceptable in the 2001 HICPAC Guideline if a patient with an essential long-term IVD has continued to experience recurrent IVD-related BSIs despite consistent application of infection control practices.*[129]

Various other prophylactic lock solutions have been studied as a means of preventing IVD-related BSI including trisodium citrate/gentamicin,[375] minocycline/ethylenediaminetetraacetic acid (EDTA),[376] ethanol,[377] and taurolidine-containing solutions.[378] Concerns about increased IVD complication rates[378] and drug-related toxicity[375] associated with the use of certain types of lock solutions, combined with the limited number of patients who have been studied while receiving these agents, precludes their routine use at this time.

5. *Catheter hubs:* A novel catheter hub that contains a chamber filled with iodinated alcohol has been shown to be effective in preventing colonization of IVDs in an animal model.[379] Use of this same hub model in some clinical studies has demonstrated significantly lower rates of IVD colonization compared with IVDs with control hubs.[380,381] One clinical trial has also demonstrated reduced rates of IVD-related BSIs with use of this hub (4% versus 16%, P <.01). A subsequent study also showed a reduction in hub-related IVD-related BSIs (1.7% versus 7%, P<.049), but overall rates of IVD-related BSIs in both groups were similar.[381] Another study was unable to find any benefit with regards to IVD colonization or IVD-related BSI with use of the novel hub.[382] This device is not yet available in the United States and until further studies more conclusively demonstrate its benefit, its use cannot be recommended at this time.

Ventilator-Associated Pneumonia

Incidence and Impact

Hospital-acquired pneumonia (HAP) is defined as pneumonia that develops more than 48 hours after hospitalization.[383] VAP is a subset of HAP and is defined as pneumonia that occurs more than 48 to 72 hours after initiating mechanical ventilation.[383] Nearly 300,000 episodes of HAP occur in U.S. hospitals each year.[384] More than 90% of HAPs occur in patients undergoing mechanical ventilation, and 10% to 20% of mechanically ventilated patients will develop VAP.[385] VAP is the second most common nosocomial infection in U.S. ICUs participating in the National Nosocomial Infection Surveillance (NNIS) program with median rates of VAP ranging from 2.3 cases per 1000 ventilator-days in pediatric units to 11.4 cases per 1000 ventilator-days in trauma units (Table 51-14).[133] VAP increases length of hospitalization by 6.1 days and health care costs by $10,019 when compared with matched controls who had not developed VAP.[385] More importantly, VAP is associated with more nosocomial deaths than is infection at any other site[386]—at least 50,000 deaths in U.S. centers annually—and increases hospital mortality at least twofold in affected individuals.[385]

Pathogenesis

In the normal nonsmoking host, multiple host defense mechanisms contribute to protection against pneumonia.[387] The respiratory tract above the vocal cords is normally heavily colonized by bacteria, but unless the person has chronic bronchitis or has had respiratory tract instrumentation, the lower respiratory tract is normally sterile; although healthy adults aspirate frequently during sleep, the lower airways and pulmonary parenchyma of healthy, nonsmoking persons without lung disease are remarkably free of microbial colonization.[388] The major defense mechanisms include anatomic airway barriers, the cough reflex, mucus,[389] and mucociliary clearance.[390] Below the terminal bronchioles, the cellular and humoral immune systems are essential components of host defense.[391] Alveolar macrophages and leukocytes remove particulate matter and potential pathogens, elaborate cytokines that activate the systemic cellular immune response and act as antigen-presenting cells to the humoral arm of immunity.[392] Immunoglobulins and complement opsonize bacteria and bacterial products within the respiratory tract, assisting phagocytosis.

In the mechanically ventilated patient, numerous factors conspire to compromise host defenses: Critical illness, comorbidities, and malnutrition impair the immune system.[393,394] Endotracheal intubation thwarts the cough reflex; compromises mucociliary clearance; injures the tracheal epithelial surface; and provides a direct conduit for bacteria from the mouth, hypopharynx, and stomach to gain direct access to the lower respiratory tract.[395] Moreover, the cuff of the endotracheal tube allows pooling of oropharyngeal secretions in the subglottic region, forming an ideal medium for microbial growth, which periodically leaks around the cuff into the trachea. It would probably be more accurate pathogenically to rename VAP as "endotracheal intubation–related pneumonia." This combination of impaired host defenses and continuous exposure of the lower respiratory tract to large numbers of potential pathogens through the endotracheal tube puts the mechanically ventilated patient at great jeopardy of developing VAP.

In order for microorganisms to cause VAP, they must first gain access to the normally sterile lower respiratory

Table 51-14. Ventilator-Associated Pneumonia Rates*

Type of ICU	No. of Units	Ventilator-days	Pooled Mean	Percentile				
				10%	25%	50% (Median)	75%	90%
Coronary	59	76,145	4.4	0	1.9	4	6.8	9.8
Cardiothoracic	47	98,358	7.2	1.2	2.9	6.3	12.6	15.5
Medical	92	268,518	4.9	0.5	2.1	3.7	6.2	8.9
Major teaching	99	320,916	5.4	1.2	2.6	4.6	7.2	9.9
All others	109	351,705	5.1	1.7	2.9	5.1	6.7	8.9
Neurosurgical	29	45,073	11.2	0	2.4	6.2	13.5	16.8
Pediatric	52	133,995	2.9	0	0.9	2.3	4.8	8.1
Surgical	98	253,900	9.3	2.2	4.7	8.3	12.2	17.9
Trauma	22	63,137	15.2	4.3	8	11.4	16.6	25.3
Burn	14	23,117	12	—	—	—	—	—
Respiratory	6	18,838	4.9	—	—	—	—	—

$$\text{*}\frac{\text{Number of ventilator–associated pneumonias}}{\text{Number of ventilator–days}} \times 1000$$

ICU, intensive care unit.

From National Nosocomial Infections Surveillance System Report, Data Summary from January 1992 through June 2004. Available at: www.cdc.gov/ncidod/dhqp/pdf/nnis/2004NNISreport.pdf (Accessed May 10, 2007)

tract, where they can adhere to the mucosa and produce sustained infection. Microorganisms gain access by one of four mechanisms (Fig. 51-10): (1) aspiration of microbe-laden secretions, either from the oropharynx directly or, secondarily, by reflux from the stomach into the oropharynx, then into the lower respiratory tract[396-398]; (2) inhalation of contaminated air or medical aerosols[399]; (3) direct extension of a contiguous infection such as a pleural space infection[400]; or (4) hematogenous carriage of microorganisms to the lung from remote sites of local infection such as an IVD-related BSI.[401]

Although numerous epidemics of VAP have been caused by contaminated aerosols or medical respiratory devices,[94,95,100] the preponderance of evidence suggests that most endemic VAPs derive from aspiration of oropharyngeal organisms[395,402]:

- The oropharynx of critically ill patients is rapidly colonized with the pathogens that cause VAP, especially aerobic gram-negative and *S. aureus*.[393]
- Studies in which multiple anatomic sites are cultured simultaneously over time have shown that the pathogenic microorganisms implicated in VAP are usually first recovered from the oropharynx and later from the tracheobronchial tree and stomach.[396-398,403] Moreover, heavy oropharyngeal colonization is a powerful independent predictor of subsequent tracheobronchial colonization and VAP.[398]
- Reducing oropharyngeal colonization with topical antimicrobials and antiseptics has been shown to significantly reduce the risk of VAP.[404-407]

By this route, aspiration of oropharyngeal contents containing a large microbial inoculum overwhelms host defenses already compromised by critical illness and the presence of an endotracheal tube, readily leading to the development of VAP.

Microbiology

Pathogens causing VAP may be part of the host's endogenous flora at the time of hospitalization or may be acquired exogenously after admission to the health care institution, from the hands, apparel or equipment of HCWs, hospital environment, and use of invasive devices (see Fig. 51-10). The normal flora of the oropharynx in the nonintubated patient without critical illness is composed predominantly of viridans streptococci, *Haemophilus* species, and anaerobes. Salivary flow and proteins (immunoglobulin, fibronectin) are the major host factors maintaining the normal flora of the mouth (and dental plaque). Aerobic gram-negative bacilli are rarely recovered from the oral secretions of healthy patients.[408] During critical illness, especially in ICU patients, the oral flora shifts dramatically to a predominance of aerobic gram-negative bacilli and *S. aureus*.[393] Bacterial adherence to the orotracheal mucosa of the mechanically ventilated patient is assisted by reduced mucosal IgA and increased protease production, exposed and denuded mucous membranes, elevated airway pH, increased numbers of airway receptors for bacteria because of acute illness, and antimicrobial use.

Early-onset VAP, which manifests within the first 4 days of hospitalization, is most often caused by community-acquired pathogens, such as *S. pneumoniae* and *Haemophilus* species (Fig. 51-11).[409] However, the microbial spectrum of VAP shifts to typical nosocomial pathogens with increasing lengths of mechanical ventilation and exposure to broad-spectrum antimicrobials (see Fig. 51-11).[409] That the preponderance of episodes of VAP have a late onset is supported by the fact that the most

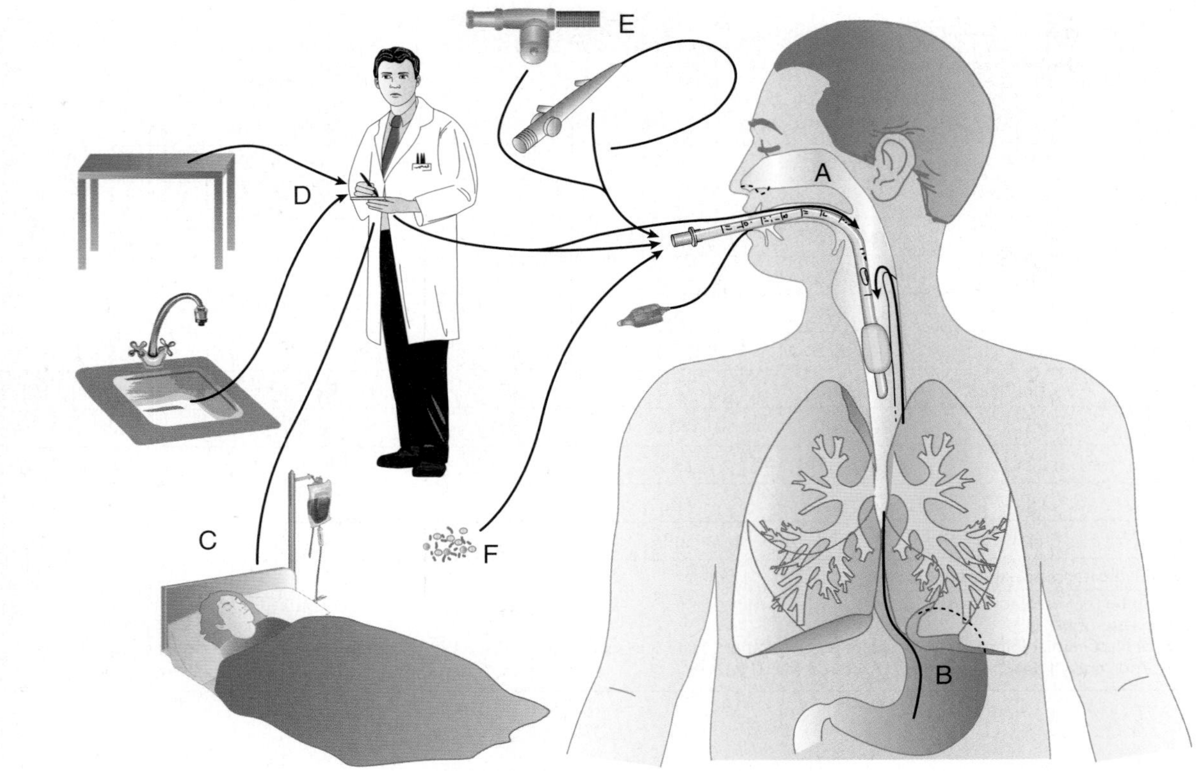

Figure 51-10. Routes of colonization/infection in mechanically ventilated patients. Colonization of the aerodigestive tract may occur endogenously **(A** and **B)** or exogenously **(C** through **F).** Exogenous colonization may result in primary colonization of the oropharynx or may be the result of direct inoculation into the lower respiratory tract during manipulations of respiratory equipment **(D),** during use of respiratory devices **(E),** or from contaminated aerosols **(F).** (From Crnich CJ, Safdar NS, Maki DG: The role of the intensive care environment in the pathogenesis and prevention of ventilator-associated pneumonia. Respir Care 2005;50:813-836.)

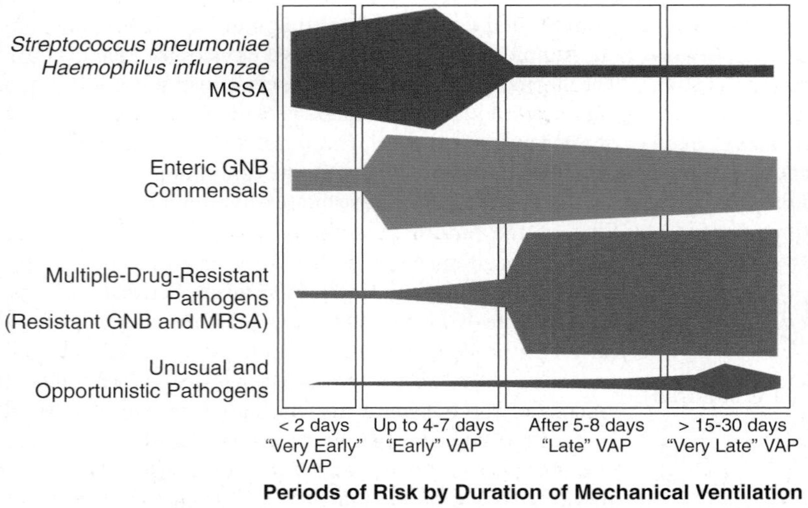

Figure 51-11. Microbial causes of ventilator-associated pneumonia based on increasing length of mechanical ventilation. The relative importance of each microbial category is indicated by the thickness of the bars as they progress through each stage from left to right. GNB, gram-negative bacilli; MRSA, methicillin-resistant *S. aureus;* MSSA, methicillin-susceptible *S. aureus*; VAP, ventilator-associated pneumonia. (From Park DR: The microbiology of ventilator-assisted pneumonia. Respir Care 2005;50:742-765.)

common pathogens recovered from mechanically ventilated patients with pneumonia are *P. aeruginosa, S. aureus,* and the Enterobacteriaceae (Fig. 51-12).[409,410] VAP is polymicrobial in up to 20% to 40% of cases. The role of anaerobic bacteria in VAP is not well defined.

Diagnosis

Hospitals participating in the CDC's National Nosocomial Infection Surveillance system (NNIS) use a standardized definition for HAP[16] (see Box 51-1) on the basis of three clinical criteria developed empirically more than 3 decades ago[411]: (1) systemic signs of infection—fever, tachycardia, and leukocytosis; (2) a new or worsening infiltrate on chest radiograph; and (3) bacteriologic evidence of infection from positive qualitative cultures of endotracheal aspirates. Unfortunately, even when used in combination, the specificity of clinical criteria is poor, with an overall diagnostic accuracy of approximately 60% in published studies.[412,413]

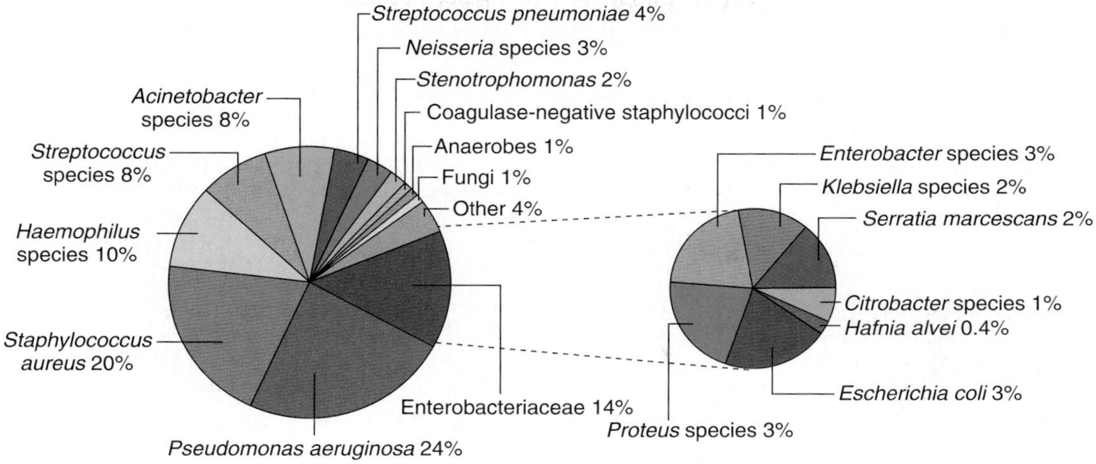

Figure 51-12. Microbial etiology of ventilator-associated pneumonia. The relative proportions of microbial causes of ventilator-associated pneumonia from 1689 bronchoscopically confirmed cases involving 2490 individual isolates reported in 24 published studies. (From Park DR: The microbiology of ventilator-assisted pneumonia. Respir Care 2005;50:742-765.)

For this reason, most experts have advocated routine use of invasive procedures when VAP is suspected—bronchoalveolar lavage (BAL), cultures of protected specimen brush (PSB) samples obtained by bronchoscopy, or blind (mini)-BAL, on the grounds that these diagnostic techniques have comparable sensitivity, greater specificity, and superior accuracy than clinical criteria alone.[410,414-417] Whether more rigorous clinical criteria such as the clinical pneumonia infection score (CPIS),[418] for example, or the use of quantitative cultures of endotracheal aspirates improve diagnostic accuracy without the need for invasive procedures is an unsettled issue.[419]

Although invasive procedures—BAL, PSB, and mini-BAL—are clearly more specific than clinical criteria, their impact on patient outcomes is much less clear.[420,421] Fagon and colleagues[420] found that patients with suspected VAP who were managed using an invasive diagnostic approach—bronchoscopic-guided PSB or BAL—had a significantly reduced 14-day mortality, reduced antibiotic-days, and reduced 28-day mortality on multivariate analysis, compared with patients managed using a clinical diagnostic approach (HR=0.65, 95% CI=0.46 to 0.91, P=.01).[420] Recently, however, Heyland and colleagues[421] found in a large multicenter Canadian trial that 28-day mortality and targeted antimicrobial use was identical among patients randomized to an invasive versus a clinical diagnostic approach. This study has been criticized for its exclusion of subjects at high risk for infection with antimicrobial-resistant pathogens.[422] In the absence of definitive data demonstrating the superiority of either approach, the recent American Thoracic Society–Society of Critical Care Medicine–Infectious Disease Society of America joint guideline acknowledges that both diagnostic approaches are useful and acceptable when evaluating patients with suspected VAP. This puts great weight on an initial Gram stain of a deep tracheal aspirate, however, if no microorganisms are seen, it can be concluded that it is unlikely the patient has bacterial VAP.[383]

Risk Factors

A number of independent risk factors have been shown to increase the likelihood of developing VAP (Table 51-15).[131,410] In general, these risk factors can be categorized as (1) factors that increase the likelihood or duration of mechanical ventilation, (2) factors that increase colonization of the oropharynx and gastric mucosa, (3) factors that increase the likelihood of aspiration, and (4) host factors that increase susceptibility to infection.

Prolonged mechanical ventilation or reintubation, or both, are the most powerful predictors of developing VAP. Cunnion and colleagues[423] found that mechanical ventilation in excess of 24 hours was associated with a 12-fold increased risk of developing VAP, and Trouillet found that ventilation longer than 7 days was associated with a sixfold increased risk.[424] Emergent reintubation also carries a high risk of aspiration and was associated with a sixfold increased risk of VAP in a retrospective study.[425]

Poor dental hygiene increases the bacterial burden in the oropharynx and is an independent risk factor for nosocomial pneumonia.[426] Likewise, a high gastric pH (>5) is associated with greatly increased bacterial colonization of the gastric contents,[427] as well as an increased risk of VAP.[428] A number of studies have found that exposure to antacids or H_2-blockers is associated with an increased risk of VAP,[53] although this has not been a universal finding.[429]

Depressed levels of consciousness, nasogastric tubes, and endotracheal tubes are ubiquitous in the ICU and all increase a patient's risk of aspiration. That an altered level of cognition is associated with an increased risk of aspiration is supported by surveillance data showing increased rates of VAP in trauma and neurosurgical ICUs.[133] Joshi

Table 51-15. Independent Risk Factors for Ventilator-Associated Pneumonia in Multivariate Analysis of Published Studies

Host Factors	Intervention Factors
Serum albumin, <2.2 g/dL	H_2 blockers±antacids
Age, ≥60 yr	Paralytic agents, continuous intravenous sedation
Adult respiratory distress syndrome (ARDS)	Receipt of >4 units of blood
Chronic obstructive pulmonary disease or other chronic pulmonary diseases	Intracranial pressure monitoring
Coma or impaired consciousness	Mechanical ventilation in excess of 48 hr
Burns, trauma	Positive end-expiratory pressure
Organ failure	Frequent ventilator circuit changes
Advanced severity of illness	Reintubation
Large-volume gastric aspiration	Nasogastric tube
Gastric colonization and gastric pH	Supine head position
Upper respiratory tract colonization	Transport out of the intensive care unit
Sinusitis	Prior antibiotic therapy

Modified from Chastre J, Fagon JY: Ventilator-associated pneumonia. Am J Resp Crit Care Med 2002;165:867-903.

and colleagues[430] found that the use of a nasogastric tube was an independent predictor of VAP in a multivariate analysis (OR 6.5, 95% CI 2.1 to 19.8). Finally, as noted, endotracheal tubes allow pooling of hypopharyngeal secretions that can leak around the cuff directly into the trachea, and a supine position appears to increase the risk of aspiration around the cuff.[431]

Host factors also contribute to an increased risk of developing VAP (see Table 51-15). Conditions such as advanced age, increased severity of illness, and the post-surgical state are rarely modifiable. However, poor nutritional status,[397] oversedation,[432] transfusion therapy,[433] and exposure to broad-spectrum antimicrobials[424] are associated with an increased risk of VAP and are under the control of the clinician.

Prevention

With an understanding of pathogenesis and epidemiology in hand, clinicians caring for mechanically ventilated patients can implement preventive strategies that can materially reduce the risk of VAP (Table 51-16). Both the CDC HICPAC and Canadian Critical Care Trials Group offer evidence-based guidelines for the prevention of VAP.[131,434] Their recommendations are very similar, with minor differences. The Canadian guideline focuses exclusively on specific interventions for the prevention of VAP,[434] whereas the HICPAC guideline incorporates additional guidance for the prevention of nosocomial influenza, legionellosis, and invasive filamentous fungal infections in the hospital.[131] Recommendations from both guidelines can be divided into general, nonpharmacologic, and pharmacologic preventive measures (see Table 51-16).[435] The general measures employed to reduce VAP including education, infection control, hand hygiene, and reliable disinfection and sterilization of respiratory care equipment are discussed elsewhere in this chapter.

Nonpharmacologic Preventive Measures

Avoiding prolonged intubation and reintubation—if avoiding intubation altogether is not feasible—offers the greatest promise for reducing an individual patient's risk of developing VAP.[425] The use of noninvasive ventilation in order to avoid endotracheal intubation has been shown to be successful in reducing rates of nosocomial pneumonia in a number of studies[436,437] and may abrogate the need for reintubation in selected patients who prematurely extubate themselves.[131] The implementation of weaning protocols has also been shown to significantly reduce the duration of mechanical ventilation,[438,439] health care costs,[438,439] and institutional rates of VAP.[440,441] Early tracheostomy—within 1 week of intubation—has been advocated as a method for reducing the risk of VAP in patients likely to require prolonged mechanical ventilation. However, randomized trials, admittedly of limited power, have not found significant benefit with this approach[442] and early tracheostomy is not currently recommended by most authorities.[131,434]

As noted earlier, supine positioning of the mechanically ventilated patient's head has been shown to increase the risk of gastro-esophageal-pharyngeal aspiration.[431] A simple solution to this threat is to elevate the head of the patient's bed 35 to 45 degrees. Drakulovic and colleagues[443] found that patients whose torso and head were kept elevated at 45 degrees had much lower rates of microbiologically confirmed pneumonia compared with patients cared for in a 0-degree supine position (5% versus 23%, $P = .018$).[443] In reality, maintaining elevation of the head in excess of 45 degrees on a consistent basis is actually quite difficult and uncommonly achieved in practice. A recent randomized study that sought to maintain head elevation above 45 degrees for 85% of the study period found that head elevation in the intervention arm only averaged 28.1 degrees.[444] Perhaps as a result of failure to successfully achieve adequate elevation, no reductions in the rate of VAP were seen.

Although data on the effect that comprehensive oral care has on risk of infection are limited,[445] maintaining adequate dental hygiene is considered an important component of VAP prevention.[131] Binkley and colleagues[446] found that although a majority of nurses caring for patients undergoing mechanical ventilation appreciated the

Table 51-16. Recommendations for the Prevention of Ventilator-Associated Pneumonia

Preventive Measures	HICPAC Grade*	CCCTG Recommendation
General Measures		
■ Educate all health care workers involved with the care of mechanically ventilated patients on the risks and methods of preventing ventilator-associated pneumonia	IA	—
■ Perform adequate hand hygiene between patient contacts	IA	—
■ Use gloves for handling respiratory secretions or objects contaminated with respiratory secretions	IB	—
■ Conduct surveillance for bacterial pneumonia in ICU patients using NNIS definitions. Include data on causative organisms and their antimicrobial susceptibility patterns. Express data as rates to assist intrahospital comparisons	IB	—
■ Do not routinely perform cultures of patients, equipment, or environment in the absence of an outbreak	II	—
■ Thoroughly clean all devices to be sterilized and disinfected	IA	—
■ Use steam sterilization or wet heat pasteurization for reprocessing of heat-stable semicritical devices and low-temperature sterilization for heat- or moisture-sensitive devices	IA	—
■ Use sterile water for rinsing reusable semicritical devices	IB	—
■ Change ventilator circuit only when they become soiled	IA	Recommended
■ Periodically drain and discard condensate from ventilator circuits	IB	—
■ Clean, disinfect, rinse with sterile water, and dry in-line nebulizers between treatments on the same patient	IB	—
■ When possible, use aerosolized medications in single-use vials	IB	—
Nonpharmacologic Measures to Reduce Pneumonia		
■ Oral (non-nasal) intubation	IB	Recommended
■ Remove nasogastric and endotracheal tubes as soon as clinically feasible	IB	—
■ Avoid unnecessary reintubation	II	—
■ When feasible, use noninvasive ventilation to avoid the need for intubation or reintubation	II	—
■ Early tracheostomy	—	No recommendation
■ Semirecumbent positioning of the patient	II	Recommended
■ Implement a comprehensive oral-hygiene program for mechanically ventilated patients	II	—
■ If feasible, use an endotracheal catheter that allows for continuous or frequent subglottic suctioning	II	Consider
■ Humidification with heat and moisture exchanger (HME)	NR	Recommended†
■ Closed multiuse catheters for airway secretion suctioning	NR	Recommended
■ Kinetic bed therapy	NR	Consider
Pharmacologic Measure to Reduce Pneumonia		
■ Immunize all patients at risk for pneumococcal infection	IA	—
■ Immunize all patients at risk for influenza	IA	—
■ Routine use of chlorhexidine oral rinse	NR	—
■ Targeted use of chlorhexidine oral rinse in postcardiac surgery patients	II	—
■ Oral decontamination with topical antimicrobial agents	NR	—
■ Preferential use of sucralfate for stress bleeding prophylaxis	NR	Not recommended
■ Selective digestive decontamination	NR	Not recommended‡
■ Acidification of gastric feedings	NR	—
■ Systemic antimicrobials to prevent development of pneumonia	NR	Not recommended‡
■ Cycling of antibiotic classes to reduce resistance in the ICU	NR	

*Taken from CDC/HICPAC system of weighting recommendations based on scientific evidence. **IA**, strongly recommended for implementation and supported by well-designed experimental, clinical, or epidemiological studies. **IB**, strongly recommended for implementation and supported by some experimental, clinical, or epidemiological studies and a strong theoretical rationale. **IC**, required by state or federal regulations, rules or standards. **II**, suggested for implementation and supported by suggestive clinical or epidemiological trials or a theoretical rationale. **Unresolved issue**, an unresolved issue for which evidence is insufficient or no consensus regarding efficacy exists. **NR**, no recommendation for or against at this time.

†Recommended in patients without hemoptysis or high minute ventilation. Exchanger should be replaced weekly.

‡Topical or systemic antimicrobial agents alone are not recommended. Insufficient evidence on antibiotic resistance and cost-effectiveness exists to recommend combination topical and systemic therapy.

CCCTG, Canadian Critical Care Trials Group; HICPAC, Healthcare Infection Control Practices Advisory Committee.

Modified from Tablan OC, Anderson LJ, Besser R, et al: Guidelines for preventing health-care-associated pneumonia, 2003: Recommendations of CDC and the Healthcare Infection Control Practices Advisory Committee. MMWR Recomm Rep 2004;53(RR-3):1-36 and Dodek P, Keenan S, Cook D, et al: Evidence-based clinical practice guideline for the prevention of ventilator-associated pneumonia. Ann Intern Med 2004;141:305-313.

importance of dental hygiene, the methods used to provide this varied considerably. Until more data are available on specific dental hygienic practices, it is recommended that mechanically ventilated patients have their teeth brushed daily, undergo oral cleansing every 2 to 4 hours, undergo routine suctioning to reduce accumulation of fluids in the oropharynx, and have a mouth moisturizer applied to their lips to prevent cracking.[447] The periodic instillation of a topical oral antiseptic solution is an additional promising intervention[447] and is discussed under pharmacologic preventive measures later.

The use of a modified endotracheal tube that has a separate ventral drainage tube for continuous or intermittent suctioning of subglottic secretions has been evaluated in a number of studies.[448,449] Subglottic suctioning reduced the rate of VAP significantly in all but one of these studies.[449] However, in this latter study, the time to onset of VAP was delayed significantly (5.9 days versus 2.9 days, $P=.006$),[449] and recent evidence-based guidelines have recommended the use of endotracheal tubes that allow for suctioning of subglottic secretions.[131,434] Nevertheless, the use of an endotracheal tube that allows for subglottic suctioning did not reduce the duration of mechanical ventilation or ICU mortality in the studies done, which, coupled with the increased cost of the tube and propensity of the suction lumen to occlude, has limited wider adoption of this technology in practice.[450]

The evidence that heat and moisture exchangers (HMEs) are associated with a reduced risk of VAP is mixed. Only one of six published trials found a statistically significant reduction in VAP with use of HMEs (RR 0.41, 95% CI 0.20 to 0.86, $P=.02$).[451] However, pooling data from a recent systematic review[452] and a subsequently published randomized trial[453] shows that HMEs reduce the risk of VAP by 38% (RR 0.62, 95% CI 0.43 to 0.89, $P=.012$). The use of HMEs has been recommended by authors of a systematic review[454] and is currently recommended by the Canadian Critical Care Trials Group.[434] However, HICPAC made no recommendation for the use of HMEs because five of six published trials failed to demonstrate a statistically significant reduction in the rate of VAP.[131] Heat exchange moisturizers become readily occluded in patients with airway hemorrhage and can increase airway resistance. As a result, they should not be used in patients with hemoptysis or those requiring a high-minute ventilation.[434] Finally, the membranes of HMEs can become colonized with bacteria and should be replaced weekly, according to current guidelines.[434]

The availability of in-line multiuse suction catheters abrogates the need to open and manipulate the endotracheal circuit, theoretically reducing the risk of exogenous contamination.[455] Despite their theoretical benefit, prospective studies have not consistently showed that in-line suction catheters are associated with a reduced risk of VAP.[456-458] Although in-line suction catheters do not appear to increase the risk of VAP, they are more time efficient for nursing personnel and respiratory therapists, and are more cost effective than open suction catheters.[434] Kollef and colleagues[459] found that rates of VAP were identical in patients randomized to as-needed changes of their in-line suction catheter versus those who had their catheter changed every 24 hours (14.7% versus 14.8%). As a result, there is no compelling evidence that in-line suction catheters should be periodically changed, unless clinically indicated.

Pharmacologic Preventive Measures

Antacids and H_2-blockers have been used extensively in the ICU setting to prevent stress ulcer bleeding but have been associated with an increased risk of developing of VAP because they lead to bacterial overgrowth of the gastric contents.[53] Sucralfate prevents stress ulcer bleeding without reducing gastric pH but is more difficult to administer and is less effective than acid-reducing agents.[429] The results of clinical trials examining these two competing strategies for preventing gastrointestinal hemorrhage in the ICU have been mixed, with earlier trials favoring the use of sucralfate.[53] However, more recently published trials suggest only a small incremental increased risk of VAP with H_2-blockers[429,460,461] and most experts feel that this risk is more than offset by their superior capacity to prevent stress ulcer bleeding.[131,434]

Selective digestive decontamination (SDD) is one of the most extensively studied preventive interventions in critical care medicine, yet the role for SDD continues to generate vigorous debate as to its overall benefit.[462,463] A more detailed discussion on the risks and benefits of this intervention is provided later in this chapter. Most U.S. experts believe that SDD has the potential to increase infection caused by multiresistant bacteria, particularly in settings with high rates of endemic antimicrobial resistance.[464,465] Until well-designed multicenter trials are done, proving that SDD does not adversely effect the ICU ecology, it is likely that North American guidelines will continue to discourage its use.[131,434]

The isolated use of parenteral antimicrobials for prevention of VAP has not met with much success,[464] but selective antimicrobial decontamination of the oropharynx, without the use of enteral or systemic agents, reduced the risk of VAP nearly 70% (RR=0.33, 95% CI 0.16 to 0.67, $P=.001$) in a recent trial.[405] This study reemphasized the primary role of oropharyngeal colonization in the pathogenesis of VAP but engenders the same concerns as SDD over its potential for promoting antimicrobial resistance. However, it has facilitated the idea that topical decolonization of the oropharynx with *nonantimicrobial* agents might be able to materially reduce the risk of VAP without the potential for emergence of antimicrobial resistance. A recent meta-analysis of seven randomized trials that enrolled 914 mechanically ventilated patients found that topical chlorhexidine applied to the oropharynx reduced the risk of VAP by nearly 30% (RR=0.74, 95% CI 0.56 to 0.96, $P=.02$), although there was no significant impact on mortality.[407] The beneficial effects of chlorhexidine appear to be most pronounced in post–cardiac surgery patients,[466,467] prompting HICPAC to recommend its use in this subpopulation.[131]

Catheter-Associated Urinary Tract Infection

Incidence and Impact

Each year, urinary catheters are inserted in more than 5 million patients in acute-care hospitals and extended-care facilities.[468] Catheter-associated urinary tract infection (CAUTI) is the most common nosocomial infection in hospitals and nursing homes, comprising more than 40% of all institutionally acquired infections.[133]

Nosocomial bacteriuria or candiduria develops in up to 25% of patients requiring a urinary catheter for more than 7 days, with a daily risk of 5%.[468] CAUTI is the second most common cause of nosocomial bloodstream infection[469]; some studies have also found increased mortality associated with CAUTI.[470] Although most CAUTIs are asymptomatic,[471] rarely extend hospitalization, and add only $500 to $1000 to the direct costs of acute-care hospitalization,[472] asymptomatic infections commonly precipitate unnecessary antimicrobial-drug therapy.[473] CAUTIs comprise perhaps the largest institutional reservoir of nosocomial antibiotic-resistant pathogens, the most important of which are multidrug-resistant Enterobacteriaceae other than *Escherichia coli* such as *Klebsiella, Enterobacter, Proteus,* and *Citrobacter; Pseudomonas aeruginosa;* enterococci and staphylococci; and *Candida* spp.[474]

Pathogenesis

Excluding rare hematogenously derived pyelonephritis, caused almost exclusively by *S. aureus,* most microorganisms causing endemic CAUTI derive from the patient's own colonic and perineal flora or from the hands of health care personnel and gain access to the patient's urinary tract during catheter insertion or manipulation of the collection system.[260] Organisms gain access in one of two ways. Extraluminal contamination may occur early, by direct inoculation when the catheter is inserted, or later, by organisms ascending from the perineum by capillary action in the thin mucous film between the external catheter surface and the urethral wall. Intraluminal contamination occurs by reflux of microorganisms gaining access to the catheter lumen from failure of closed drainage or contamination of urine in the collection bag. Recent studies suggest that CAUTIs most frequently stem from microorganisms gaining access to the bladder extraluminally,[475] but both routes are important.

Most infected urinary catheters are covered by a thick biofilm containing the infecting microorganisms embedded in a matrix of host proteins and microbial exoglycocalyx.[476] A biofilm forms on the intraluminal or extraluminal surface of the implanted catheter, or both, usually advancing in a retrograde fashion. The role of the biofilm in the pathogenesis of CAUTI has not been established. However, anti-infective–impregnated and silver-hydrogel catheters, which inhibit adherence of microorganisms to the catheter surface, significantly reduce the risk of CAUTI,[477] particularly infections caused by gram-positive organisms or yeasts, which are most likely to be acquired extraluminally from the periurethral flora. These data suggest that microbial adherence to the catheter surface is important in the pathogenesis of many, but not all, CAUTIs. Infections in which the biofilm does not play a pathogenic role are probably caused by mass transport of intraluminal contaminants into the bladder by retrograde reflux of microbe-laden urine when a catheter or collection system is moved or manipulated.

Prevention

Several catheter-care practices are universally recommended to prevent or at least delay the onset of CAUTI[260]: most importantly, avoiding unnecessary catheterizations; considering using a condom catheter in a male or a suprapubic catheter; having trained professionals insert catheters aseptically; removing the catheter as soon as no longer needed; maintaining uncompromising closed drainage; ensuring dependent drainage as much as possible; minimizing manipulations of the system; and separating catheterized patients geographically on the patient care unit.

As noted earlier, technologic innovations to prevent nosocomial infection are most likely to be effective if they are based on a clear understanding of the pathogenesis and epidemiology of the infection. Novel technologies must be designed to block CAUTI by either the extraluminal or intraluminal routes, or both. Medicated catheters, which reduce adherence of microorganisms to the catheter surface, may confer the greatest benefit for preventing CAUTI. Two catheters impregnated with anti-infective solutions have been studied in randomized trials, one impregnated with the urinary antiseptic nitrofurazone[478] and the other with a new broad-spectrum antimicrobial-drug combination, minocycline and rifampin.[479] Both catheters showed a modest reduction in bacterial CAUTIs; however, the studies were small, and the risk of selection of antimicrobial drug–resistant uropathogens was not satisfactorily resolved. Silver compounds have also been studied for coating urinary catheters. A meta-analysis of eight randomized trials comparing silver oxide or silver alloy catheters with standard nonimpregnated catheters found that silver alloy, but not silver oxide, catheters were associated with a reduced risk of CAUTI.[480] Recommendations for the prevention of CAUTI are summarized in Table 51-17.

Control of Antibiotic Resistance

During the past 55 years, more than 14 different classes of parenteral antimicrobials and several hundred antimicrobial compounds have been introduced into clinical use. In the 1960s, public health officials confidently declared that the war against infectious diseases was almost over. Unfortunately, it is not clear which side will be victorious. Although the greatest strides in our struggles with infectious diseases have resulted from improvements in hygiene and social conditions, the growing losses of our antibiotic armamentarium as a result of surging bacterial resistance could ultimately be disastrous for ICU patients if the tide is not stemmed.

Table 51-17. Recommendations for Prevention of Catheter-Associated Urinary Tract Infection

Recommendation	Strength of Recommendation*
■ Educate personnel in correct techniques of catheter insertion and care.	I
■ Catheterize only when necessary.	I
■ Emphasize hand hygiene.	I
■ Insert catheter using aseptic technique and sterile equipment.	I
■ Secure catheter properly.	I
■ Maintain closed sterile drainage.	I
■ Obtain urine samples aseptically.	I
■ Maintain unobstructed urine flow.	I
■ Periodically re-educate personnel in catheter care.	II
■ Use smallest suitable bore catheter.	II
■ Avoid irrigation unless needed to prevent or relieve obstruction.	II
■ Refrain from daily meatal care with either of the regimens discussed in text.	II
■ Do not change catheters at arbitrary fixed intervals.	II
■ Consider alternative techniques of urinary drainage before using an indwelling urethral catheter.	III
■ Replace the collecting system when sterile closed drainage has been violated.	III
■ Spatially separate infected and uninfected patients with indwelling catheters.	III
■ Avoid routine bacteriologic monitoring.	III
■ Consider the use of a nitrofurantoin or silver hydrogel catheter.	NR**

*Novel technology was not addressed in this guideline.
Category I, strongly recommended for adoption; Category II, moderately recommended for adoption; Category III, weakly recommended for adoption.
Modified from Wong ES: Guideline for prevention of catheter-associated urinary tract infections. Am J Infect Control 1983;11:28-36.

Evolution of Antibiotic Resistance in Intensive Care Units

Antimicrobial resistance has evolved through several phases. In the 1970s and 1980s, resistance of aerobic gram-negative bacilli was the major concern, and *P. aeruginosa,* with its broad range of intrinsic and acquired resistances, was the quintessential nosocomial pathogen. By the 1990s, the availability of antibiotics from a variety of distinct classes—aminoglycosides, broad-spectrum penicillins (e.g., piperacillin), monobactams (e.g., aztreonam), carbapenems (e.g., imipenem), β-lactam–beta-lactamase inhibitors (e.g., piperacillin-tazobactam), trimethoprim-sulfamethoxazole, and fluoroquinolones—promised a respite from concerns about resistance in aerobic gram-negative bacilli. During this period, however, gram-positive cocci gained prominence, and MRSA β-lactam–resistant coagulase-negative staphylococci and VRE became the major problem nosocomial pathogens. Antibiotic pressure, deriving first from the widespread use of third-generation cephalosporin antibiotics in hospitals, is often cited as a major factor in the emergence of MRSA. Co-emerging as nosocomial pathogens with MRSA have been methicillin-resistant coagulase-negative staphylococci, which have become the leading cause of IVD-related BSI and prosthesis-related surgical site infections.

In the early 1990s VRE burst onto the hospital and ICU scene in the United States and within a few years became entrenched in most tertiary medical centers. Heavy use of vancomycin, often as empiric treatment in response to concerns about MRSA, was probably the initial factor driving the emergence of VRE. In most settings, however, exposure to cephalosporins and antimicrobials with antianaerobic activity have emerged as the greatest risk factors for nosocomial colonization or infection by VRE. The mid-1990s witnessed growing problems with resistance in fungi and shifts to non–*Candida albicans* species, representing the effects of heavy empirical use of azoles such as fluconazole in hospitals during this period.

The ICU component of the CDC's NNIS system powerfully reaffirms the rapidly rising rates of bacterial resistance in U.S. ICUs during the past 20 years (see Fig. 51-2).[133]

Forces Driving Resistance

To a large extent, emergence of antimicrobial resistance reflects the combined effects of genetic selection, antibiotic pressures, and the frequency of cross-infection in ICUs. For some resistance mechanisms (e.g., extended-spectrum β-lactamases [ESBLs] that confer resistance to third-generation cephalosporins such as ceftazidime), a shift of single amino acid in existing resistance genes can lead to new, inactivating enzymes. For other resistant bacteria, such as penicillin-resistant pneumococci, multiple resistance genes must be cobbled together in a specific, exacting sequence, which may take years to evolve, emerge, and spread.

Antibiotic pressures provide the necessary Darwinian forces that amplify these genetic changes.[481] Usually, resistance emerges to a specific agent that is used most heavily and, hence, provides the greatest pressure. In some instances, genetic linkage of resistance mechanisms to unrelated classes of antimicrobials results in the capacity of heavy use of one drug class to select for resistance to a different class. For example, use of trimethoprim-sulfamethoxazole has been associated statistically with emergence of ceftazidime-resistant *E. coli* and *K. pneumoniae* as a result of linkage on a single plasmid of genes that encode production of ESBLs and trimethoprim-sulfamethoxazole resistance. A large proportion of extended-spectrum β-lactamase producing gramnegative bacilli are also resistant to fluoroquinolones.[482,483]

In epidemiologic and clinical studies of antibiotic resistance, there is always a proportion of patients in whom resistance is found without exposure to the problem antibiotic. These patients usually have other important risk factors, such as increased severity of underlying disease, extremes of age, presence of invasive devices, recent surgery, or proximity to patients who are infected or colonized with antibiotic-resistant bacteria. In these cases the presence of antibiotic-resistant strains is most often the consequence of patient-to-patient spread, usually on the contaminated hands of HCWs; occasionally, spread results from a contaminated common source, such as an inadequately cleaned piece of equipment. Studies of HCW hand hygiene show that rates of handwashing between patient contacts range from 25% to 50%, at best, and are inadequate to control resistance, especially in ICUs, where the staff are extremely busy and less likely to be attentive to hand hygiene.[165]

Controlling Antimicrobial Resistance in the Intensive Care Unit

Stemming the tide of antimicrobial resistance requires a multifaceted approach (see Box 51-3), especially in ICUs, where antibiotic pressures and lapses in hospital hygiene are usually greatest. First, active surveillance for resistant bacteria is essential to provide an understanding of local problems and needs. To support surveillance and treatment, cultures must be obtained from suspected sites of infection before empiric antibiotic therapy is initiated. The benefit of routine surveillance cultures (e.g., periodic cultures of sputum specimens or rectal swabs) for assessing rates of colonization by resistant bacteria in ICUs will depend on how such cultures are used.

Second, when rates of resistance begin to increase, molecular typing, such as by pulsed-field gel electrophoresis, can differentiate spread of a single strain (clonal expansion)—which suggests person-to-person or common source transmission—from spread of multiple strains (polyclonal expansion), which suggests emergence of resistance in individual patients as a result of antibiotic pressures or exogenous introduction of multiple resistant strains. Often, these problems—clonal and polyclonal—coexist.

Third, the importance of hand hygiene must be stressed at all times. Aggressive hand hygiene campaigns, with adherence monitoring and feedback of ward and even individual results, may achieve compliance rates as high as 70%. For some situations (e.g., when there is a large resistance iceberg and extensive patient colonization by antibiotic resistant bacteria), these levels of adherence may not be sufficient to control cross-infection. Response to this problem has been to encourage "universal gloving," in addition to wider use of alcohol-based hand rubs (a "belt-and-suspender" approach) to bridge the gap left by incomplete attention to hand hygiene even in the best of circumstances. Use of universal gloving has been successful in controlling spread of aminoglycoside-resistant gram-negative bacilli in ICUs and *C. difficile*-related diarrhea.[224,241] Because patients' intact skin and the environment in patient rooms may be a source of resistant bacteria, such as VRE, we recommend that disposable examination gloves be worn for all contact with ICU patients or their environment. Because gloves are not a total barrier, they must be removed and hands disinfected by an alcohol hand rub between patient contacts.

Fourth, antimicrobial stewardship is essential (see Table 51-18).[253] The primary goal of antimicrobial stewardship is to optimize clinical outcomes while minimizing unintended consequences of antimicrobial use such as toxicity, emergence of resistance, and *C. difficile*-associated diarrhea. Because antimicrobial use drives antimicrobial resistance, the frequency of inappropriate antimicrobial use can be used as a surrogate marker for antimicrobial resistance. Both antimicrobial stewardship and a comprehensive infection control program are essential to limiting the emergence and transmission of antimicrobial-resistant pathogens. Most studies assessing the utility of antimicrobial stewardship have focused on adults in ICUs, where the burden of antimicrobial resistance is greatest.

A comprehensive evidence-based stewardship program to combat antimicrobial resistance is typically a multifaceted, multidisciplinary program; the size and complexity of the management team and the specific measures applied to optimize prescribing vary on the basis of local antimicrobial use patterns, resistance trends, and available resources. The two core strategies that provide the foundation for a successful antimicrobial stewardship program are (1) prospective audits, with intervention and feedback; and (2) formulary restriction and preauthorization.[253]

Several studies have shown that prospective audits of antimicrobial use with intervention and feedback are an effective means of reducing inappropriate antimicrobial use.[484,485] In a randomized trial conducted at a 600-bed tertiary teaching hospital, inpatients receiving parenteral antimicrobial therapy were randomized to an intervention group that received suggestions for optimal antimicrobial use from an infectious diseases physician or to no interventions. Physicians in the intervention group implemented 85% of the suggestions they received, which resulted in 1.6 fewer days of parenteral therapy and $400 savings per patient. Similar results have been noted in trials undertaken in community hospitals.[484] If daily review of antimicrobial use is not feasible, review of antimicrobial usage 3 days a week may still have a significant impact. Effective audit with intervention and feedback can be undertaken most easily with automated computer surveillance of antimicrobial use, allowing the targeting of specific units where the problems are greatest.

Formulary restriction and preauthorization requirements for specific agents are now common in most hospitals. Antimicrobial restriction is unequivocally the most effective method of controlling antimicrobial use.[486,487] However, it is unclear whether antimicrobial restriction achieves the more important outcome, reducing antimicrobial resistance. Several studies of outbreaks of *C. difficile*-associated diarrhea have shown abrupt cessation of the outbreak following restriction (and greatly reduced use) of one or more key antimicrobials such as clindamy-

Table 51-18. Recommendations for Developing an Institutional Program to Enhance Antimicrobial Stewardship

Recommendation	Level of Evidence
■ Create a multidisciplinary antimicrobial stewardship team, including an infectious disease physician and a clnical pharmacist with infectious disease training	A-II
■ Include, if possible, a clinical microbiologist, an information systems specialist, an infection control professional, and hospital epidemiologist	A-III
■ Foster collaboration between the antimicrobial stewardship team and the hospital infection control committee	A-III
■ Create a climate of support and collaboration between the antimicrobial stewardship team and the hospital administration and medical staff leadership	A-III
■ Develop infrastructure to measure antimicrobial use and track use on ongoing basis	A-II
■ Employ a system of prospective audit of antimicrobial use with direct interaction and feedback to the prescriber by an infectious disease physician or a clinical pharmacist with infectious disease training	A-I
■ Use formulary restrictions and preauthorization requirement to reduce antimicrobial use and cost	A-II
■ Provide education to health care providers regarding stewardship strategies	A-III
■ Education must be combined with active interventions to improve antimicrobial prescribing practices	B-II
■ Develop evidence-based multidisciplinary guidelines incorporating local microbiology and resistance patterns to improve antimicrobial utilization	A-I
■ No recommendation can be made regarding antimicrobial cycling as a means of preventing or reducing antimicrobial resistance	C-II
■ Use antimicrobial order forms as a component of antimicrobial stewardship	B-II
■ No recommendation can be made regarding the routine use of combination therapy to prevent emergence of resistance	C-II
■ Streamline or de-escalate antimicrobial therapy on the basis of culture results	A-II
■ Optimize antimicrobial dosing on the basis of individual patient characteristics, causative organisms, site of infection, and pharmacokinetic and pharmacodynamic characteristics of the drug	A-II
■ Use health care information technology such as electronic medical records, computerized physician order entry and clinical decision support to improve antimicrobial prescribing	B-II
■ Use computer-based surveillance for more efficient targeting of antimicrobial interventions, tracking of resistance patterns, identification of nosocomial infections and adverse drug reactions	B-II
■ Engage the clinical microbiology laboratory to participate in antimicrobial stewardship by providing patient-specific culture and susceptibility data and by assisting infection control efforts in the surveillance of resistant organisms and in the molecular epidemiologic investigation of outbreaks	A-III
■ Determine the impact of antimicrobial stewardship by measuring process and outcomes	B-III

Based on the Infectious Diseases Society of America grading system for ranking recommendations in clinical guidelines. A, good evidence to support a recommendation for use; B, moderate evidence to support a recommendation for use; C, poor evidence to support a recommendation for use; I, evidence from>1 properly randomized, controlled trial; II, evidence from>1 well-designed clinical trial, without randomization; from cohort or case-controlled analytic studies; from multiple time-series; III, evidence from expert opinion.
Modified from Dellit TH, Owens RC, McGowan JE Jr, et al: Infectious Diseases Society of America and the Society for Healthcare Epidemiology of America guidelines for developing an institutional program to enhance antimicrobial stewardship. Clin Infect Dis 2007;44:159-177.

cin or third-generation cephalosporins.[486] However, other studies have documented inexorably rising resistance rates in nosocomial pathogens despite a rigorous program of antimicrobial restriction.[488] One explanation for this increase in resistance may be the compensatory increase in usage of broad-spectrum antimicrobials other than the restricted agent, thus counteracting any benefit of restriction. Furthermore, restricting use of a single drug to reduce antimicrobial resistance may be ineffective because cross-resistance in bacterial species to more than one class of antimicrobials is the rule in nosocomial organisms.

One or both of the core strategies should be adopted and supplemented by close collaboration among a core antimicrobial stewardship team, infection control personnel, health care providers, and hospital administration.

Beyond the two major mechanisms of antimicrobial stewardship mentioned earlier, other elements that should be incorporated into an institutional antimicrobial stewardship program include education of health care pro-viders; however, passive educational efforts such as conference presentations, teaching sessions, and provision of guidelines are only marginally effective in the absence of other active interventions.[489] Clinical practice guidelines are being introduced with increasing frequency; however, the impact of these guidelines on provider behavior and clinical outcomes has been difficult to measure. Guidelines tailored to local antimicrobial resistance patterns and antimicrobial use trends may have more impact than a generic clinical pathway.

Interest has been sparked in ICUs by the reborn concept of antibiotic cycling.[490,491] The most recent experiences have evaluated switch therapy[492] for empiric antibiotic use, rather than actual cycling, and have shown beneficial reductions in resistance among gram-negative bacilli[493] and in the prevalence of VRE. Such approaches, as well as true cycling through different antimicrobial classes, may be effective over limited periods in closed environments such as ICUs, by transiently reducing selection pressure and thus resistance to the restricted agent. Yet studies have thus far not shown a consistent long-term benefit with cycling, and mathematical models do not predict that cycling will be an effective measure to reduce antimicrobial resistance.[494]

Antimicrobial order forms reduce antimicrobial usage through the use of automatic stop orders and the requirement for physician justification.[495] Streamlining or de-escalation of therapy based on culture data is an essential component of appropriate antimicrobial use, with studies showing substantial reductions in days of antimicrobial use and cost savings.[496,497]

Computer order entry provides needed information at the moment in a neutral, nonjudgmental, fact-based format; this system is efficient, well accepted, and holds the promise to change prescribing behaviors materially.[498,499]

Effective antimicrobial stewardship programs can be financially self-supporting and improve patient care. Studies have shown reductions in antimicrobial usage from 22% to 36%, with annual savings of $200,000 to $900,000 in larger teaching hospitals and community hospitals. A recent guideline from the Infectious Diseases Society of America and the Society for Healthcare Epidemiology of America provides detailed recommendations for developing institutional programs of antimicrobial stewardship, which are summarized in Table 51-18.[253]

AVANT GARDE CONTROL MEASURES

Selective Digestive Decontamination

Intense interest has arisen in Europe and the United States[457-459] over the use of "selective digestive decontamination" (SDD) for prevention of bacterial pneumonia and other nosocomial infections in mechanically ventilated ICU patients. This novel therapy is based on the premise that the upper respiratory tract flora exists in a continuum with the gastrointestinal flora and that these mucosal microorganisms make up the major reservoir of pathogens causing pneumonia and many other nosocomial infections, especially in mechanically ventilated patients. Most ventilated ICU patients have a nasogastric tube that provides a direct conduit for reflux of microorganisms from the heavily colonized stomach to the oropharynx, from which organisms gain access to the lower respiratory tract.

SDD consists of four components: (1) a broad-spectrum parenteral antibiotic given for approximately 3 days to treat infections incubating at the time of the admission to the ICU; (2) topical antimicrobials (usually polymyxin E, tobramycin, and amphotericin B) periodically applied to the oropharynx and instilled into the gut for a variable period, usually for the entire duration of ICU stay, to reduce the mucosal burden of gram-negative bacteria and yeasts while preserving the anaerobic flora; (3) a re-emphasized adherence to hand hygiene to prevent nosocomial transmission of bacteria, in some European centers, empiric barrier isolation; and (4) serial surveillance cultures of the oropharynx and rectum to monitor the efficacy of the treatment.[500,501]

Eleven meta-analyses assessing the efficacy of SDD for reducing infection and mortality have been published (Table 51-19).[502-512] All have found a reduction in pneumonia. Some, but not all, have found reduced mortality. However, a recent review showed that the results of the meta-analyses were inversely related to study design,[513] which in the case of SDD may overestimate its efficacy. Most studies and meta-analyses of SDD did not make a distinction between parenteral and topical SDD; the few meta-analyses that undertook subgroup analyses found that topical antibiotics alone reduced infection but not mortality.[507]

The greatest deterrent to widespread acceptance of SDD is the fear that it will promote the emergence and spread of antimicrobial resistant microorganisms. Antibiotic pressure is without question the single most powerful force driving the selection of resistant microorganisms and any strategy for prevention of infection in the ICU that has the potential to increase infections caused by multiresistant organisms must be approached very cautiously. A number of studies underlie the concern of promoting antimicrobial resistance with SDD. Numerous studies have documented major shifts in the microbial ecology of the ICU with the use of SDD.[514-516] In a study by Lingnau and colleagues,[514] 4.5 years of SDD with ciprofloxacin led to a marked increase in MRSA infection from 17% to 81% and of ciprofloxacin-resistant *S. aureus* from 33% to 80%. The number of infections caused by other multiresistant bacteria such as *Acinetobacter* was also increased by SDD.[514]

A distinction must also be made between the risk to an individual receiving SDD of infection caused by a resistant pathogen and the institutional risk of an increased prevalence of antimicrobial-resistant organisms related to the use of SDD. Although both consequences are undesirable, given the skyrocketing rates of endemic nosocomial MRSA and VRE infections worldwide, any—however small—potential for increased antimicrobial resistance must be taken seriously. In order to better address this issue, well-designed, cluster-randomized trials that employ multilevel modeling and specifically address the effects of SDD on antimicrobial resistance across the entire spectrum of microbial pathogens at the institutional level are necessary. Until such data are available, we believe that continued North American concerns about the effects of SDD on antimicrobial resistance are justified, particularly in institutions where MRSA and VRE are endemic, which encompasses virtually all larger hospitals. Given that other effective measures for prevention of nosocomial infection exist, we believe that SDD should be restricted to select patients, such as certain trauma patients, or as a potential adjunctive control measure for a nosocomial outbreak caused by multiply resistant organisms.[517]

Table 51-19. Meta-Analyses of Randomized Controlled Trials of Selective Digestive Decontamination

Study, yr	No. of RCTs included	Description	Pneumonia Point Estimate OR or RR (95% CI)	Mortality Point Estimate OR or RR (95% CI)
Vandenbroucke, 1991[502]	6	Medical and surgical patients	0.12 (0.08-0.19)	0.70 (0.45-1.09)
SDD Trialists Collaborative Group, 1993[503]	22	Medical and surgical patients	0.37 (0.31-0.43)	0.90 (0.79-1.04)
Kollef, 1994[504]	16	Medical and surgical patients	0.28 (0.21-0.38)	0.90 (0.74-1.1)
Heyland et al, 1994[505]	25	Medical and surgical patients	0.46 (0.39-0.56)	0.87 (0.79-0.97)
Hurley et al, 1995[506]	26	Medical and surgical patients	0.35 (0.30-0.42)	0.86 (0.74-0.99)
D'Amico et al, 1998[507]	33	Medical and surgical patients	0.35 (0.29-0.41)	0.88 (0.78-0.98)
Nathens et al, 1999[508]	21	Medical and surgical patients	Medical: 0.45 (0.33-0.62) Surgical: 0.19 (0.15-0.26)	Medical: 0.91 (0.71-1.18) Surgical: 0.70 (0.52-0.93)
Safdar et al, 2004[509]	4	Liver transplant patients	0.88 (0.73-1.09)*	0.82 (0.22-2.45)
Liberati et al, 2004[510]	36	Medical and surgical patients	0.35 (0.29-0.41)	0.78 (0.68-0.89)
Silvestri et al, 2005[511]	42	Medical and surgical patients	0.30 (0.17-0.53)†	NR
Silvestri et al, 2007[512]	51	Medical and surgical patients	0.73 (0.59-0.90)‡	0.80 (0.69-0.94)

*Overall infection.
†Fungal infections.
‡Bloodstream infection.

Recent randomized trials have identified several novel measures for prevention of VAP such as semi-recumbent positioning[443] and subglottic suction endotracheal tubes.[518] We believe that these approaches are ecologically more attractive control measures for ventilated ICU patients than prophylactic topical and systemic antibiotics.

Pre-emptive Barrier Isolation

Having fewer patients in a room, improving the facilities for handwashing, and using cohort nursing (i.e., assigning each nurse to designated patients) have reduced the incidence of endemic nosocomial infection in neonatal and pediatric ICUs.[169,519] Complicated forms of protective isolation have reduced the high rates of nosocomial infection in patients with profound granulocytopenia[520] or full-thickness burns.[169,240] Moreover, the routine use of gowns and gloves on a special pediatric unit was associated with a marked decline in the incidence of nosocomial infection with RSV,[78] and the routine use of gloves for all patient contacts was shown to reduce the incidence of nosocomial *C. difficile* infection nearly fivefold in a large veterans hospital.[241]

Unfortunately, the few studies that have prospectively evaluated protective isolation of ICU patients have been performed in newborns and pediatric patients and have yielded conflicting and generally disappointing results[521-524]; however, most of these studies had major weaknesses in design.[243] More recently, several studies have shown that pre-emptive use of barrier precautions can effectively reduce the spread of multiresistant organisms such as MRSA or VRE in epidemic[525,526] and endemic settings (Table 51-20).[78,241,522,527-535] If colonization by nosocomial organisms could be prevented or at least delayed until invasive devices are removed, the incidence of infection might be significantly reduced.

One major prospective trial that assessed the efficacy of simple protective isolation—which we prefer to call *pre-emptive barrier precautions*—to reduce the incidence of nosocomial infection during pediatric intensive care studied 70 high-risk children over 30 months who were not immunosuppressed but who required prolonged mechanical ventilatory support and exposure to invasive devices in a pediatric ICU and were randomized to receive standard care without any special precautions or pre-emptive barrier isolation, with the use of disposable non-woven polypropylene gowns and nonsterile latex gloves for all patient contacts.[527] Risk factors predisposing patients to infection were comparable in the two groups. Nosocomial colonization occurred later among isolated patients (median 12 versus 7 days) and was associated with subsequent infection in 2 patients, as compared with 12 patients given standard care. Among children who were isolated, the interval before the first infection was significantly longer (median, 20 versus 8 days), the daily infection rate was twofold lower (86 versus 44 infections per 1000 ICU days), and there were 50% fewer days with fever. The benefit of isolation was most notable after 7 days of ICU care. Isolation was well tolerated by patients and their families. Unannounced monitoring showed that children in each group were touched and handled indiscernibly by hospital personnel and families.

The study concluded that the use of disposable high-barrier gowns and gloves for the care of select high-risk children who require prolonged ICU care can substantially reduce the incidence of nosocomial infection, is well tolerated, and does not compromise the delivery of care. Simple forms of protective isolation as a general control measure would also seem preferable to attempts to suppress nosocomial colonization with SDD. Further studies

Table 51-20. Studies of Pre-emptive Barrier Isolation to Contain Spread of Multiresistant Organisms

Pre-emptive Barrier Isolation Precautions for All High-Risk Patients	Control of Epidemic Spread: No. of Outbreaks	Control of Epidemic Spread: No. (%) Totally Controlled	Control of Endemic Infections: Before-After and Nonrandomized Trials: Author	Before-After and Nonrandomized Trials: RR (95% CI)	Randomized Trials: Author	Randomized Trials: RR (95% CI)
Methicillin-resistant *Staphylococcus aureus*	2[525]	2 (100)[525]	Safdar[532]	0.36 (0.13-0.98)*	No studies	
Vancomycin-resistant *Enterococcus*	2[525,526]	2 (100)[525,526]	Montecalvo[534] Slaughter[531] Morris[535] Srinivasan[533] **All studies**	0.22 (0.05-0.92)* 2.66 (1.00-6.77)† 1.18 (NR)† 0.47 (NR)* 0.22-2.66	No studies	
Resistant gram-negative bacilli	none		McManus[614]	0.38 (0.31-0.46)*	No studies	
Clostridium difficile	none		Johnson[241]	0.19 (NR)*	No studies	
Other						
Necrotizing enterocolitis			Agbayani[522]	0.13 (0.02-0.84)*		
Respiratory syncytial virus			Leclair[78]	0.34 (0.17-0.60)*		
All nosocomial infections			Slaughter[531]	1.51 (0.74-3.12)†	Slota[528] Klein [527] Koss[530]	0.48 (NR)* 0.19 (0.05-0.70)* 1.86 (1.10-3.16)*

*$P < 0.05$
†$P > 0.05$

are necessary to determine the cost effectiveness of prophylactic barrier precautions in the ICU and especially the efficacy of protective isolation in adult surgical ICUs, where the incidence of nosocomial infection is as high as 35%. Studies should also determine the relative importance of wearing a gown, as compared with wearing gloves alone.

Patients with prolonged severe granulocytopenia or those who are receiving high dosages of corticosteroids, usually as part of immunosuppressive regimens to prevent transplant rejection, are at risk for invasive pulmonary infection caused by *Aspergillus* species, *Zygomycetes,* and other filamentous airborne fungi, which is associated with high mortality.[36-38,536] The risk of invasive infection appears to be directly related to the counts of airborne fungi, and numerous outbreaks have been linked to building construction or failure of air-control systems. Studies have shown that the isolation of vulnerable patients in positive-pressure rooms with spore-free HEPA-filtered air greatly reduces the risk of invasive infection.[36,38] HEPA-filtered ICU rooms should be available for the care of patients who have received bone marrow or solid organ transplants and who require intensive care, especially in the early post-transplant period or during the treatment of rejection, when dosages of immunosuppressive drugs are high.

Pre-emptive use of barrier isolation precautions (gowns and gloves) and providing dedicated patient care items such as stethoscopes and sphygmomanometers in all high-risk patients from the time of admission is a simple and effective strategy to prevent HCWs from acquiring hand contamination by multiresistant organisms when having contact with patients with unrecognized colonization or infection and to block transmission to other as yet uncolonized patients.

APPROACH TO A NOSOCOMIAL EPIDEMIC

As noted earlier, most nosocomial epidemics now occur in ICUs. If an epidemic is suspected, the epidemiologic approach must be methodical and thorough yet expeditious, directed toward establishing the bona fide nature of the putative epidemic infections (i.e., ruling out "pseudoinfections"[242]); confirming the existence of an epidemic (i.e., ruling out a "pseudoepidemic"[242]); defining the reservoirs and modes of transmission of the epidemic pathogens; and, most importantly, controlling the epidemic quickly and completely. Control measures are predicated on accurate delineation of the epidemiology of the epidemic pathogen.

Each hospital, through its infection control committee, must be prepared administratively to carry out an investigation and implement needed control measures. The essential steps in dealing with a suspected outbreak of nosocomial bloodstream infection have been reviewed previously (Box 51-3).[143] To illustrate the approach to a nosocomial epidemic, the epidemiologic investigation of an unusual and complicated outbreak of infusion-related bacteremia[307] is reviewed:

During a 2-week period in late March 1985, three patients in a university hospital developed primary nosocomial bacteremia with a similar nonfermentative gram-negative bacillus. All three patients had had open-heart surgery between March 11 and March 25 (Fig. 51-13) and became bacteremic 48 to 148 hours after the operation.

The bloodstream pathogen in each case was shown to be *Pseudomonas pickettii* biovariant 1. The organism was also cultured from the intravenous fluid of two of the patients at the time because, serendipitously, during the outbreak most adult patients in the hospital receiving intravenous fluids were participating in a study of intravenous catheter dressings:[537] As part of the study protocol, specimens were routinely obtained from patients' intravenous fluid when the catheter was removed. Review of nearly 1000 cultures of intravenous fluid from the infusions of participants in the study since its outset 3 months earlier showed that three additional surgical patients operated on in March had had intravenous fluid cultures positive for *P. pickettii* biovariant 1 (see Fig. 51-13), even though none had shown clinical signs of bacteremia.

Box 51-3

Evaluation of a Suspected Epidemic of Nosocomial Infections

Administrative preparedness
- Immediately retrieve putative epidemic isolates for confirmation of identity through species and subtyping by one or more methods:
  - Biotyping
  - Antimicrobial susceptibility pattern (antibiogram)
  - Serotyping
  - Phage-typing
  - Bacteriocin typing
  - SDS-PAGE protein electrophoresis
  - Immunoblot pattern
  - Multifocus enzyme electrophoresis
  - Restriction enzyme digestion and restriction fragment polymorphism patterns
  - DNA probes

Preliminary evaluations and control measures
- Identify and characterize individual cases in time, place, risk factors
- Strive to identify source of infections
- Ascertain whether cases represent true infections, rather than "pseudoinfections"
- Ascertain whether cases represent a true epidemic, rather than a "pseudoepidemic"
- Develop and implement provisional control measures
- Intensify surveillance to detect each new case
- Review general infection control policies and procedures
- Determine the need for assistance, especially extramural (local, state, CDC)

Epidemiologic investigations
- Clinicoepidemiologic studies, especially case-control studies
- Microbiologic studies

Develop and implement definitive control measures

Confirm control of epidemic by intensified follow-up surveillance

Report the findings
- Intramurally
- State Health Department, CDC

Publish the report

Modified from Maki DG, Mermel LA: Infections due to infusion therapy. In Bennett JV, Brachman PS (eds): Hospital Infections, 4th ed. Boston, Lippincott-Raven, 1998.

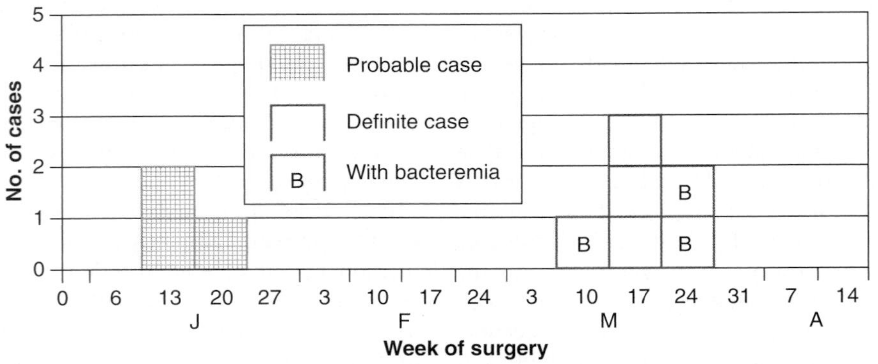

Figure 51-13. Epidemic curve for an outbreak of *Pseudomonas pickettii* bacteremias and contaminated intravenous infusions traced to contaminated fentanyl given intravenously. Isolates from blood or intravenous fluid of six definite cases (March 1985) were available for reconfirmation and subtyping as *P. pickettii* biovariant 1; isolates from intravenous fluid of three probable cases (January 1985) were not available for retesting but were considered likely to have also been *P. pickettii* biovariant 1 on review of the results of 20 biochemical tests common to these three and the six confirmed isolates. (From Maki DG, Klein BS, McCormick RD, et al: Nosocomial *Pseudomonas pickettii* bacteremias traced to narcotic tampering. A case for selective drug screening of health care personnel. JAMA 1991;265:981-986.)

Molecular subtyping by restriction enzyme digestion and pulsed-field electrophoresis to delineate restriction polymorphism patterns showed all six isolates to be the clonal. Three more patients who had been operated on in January had had intravenous fluid that cultured positive for a similar nonfermentative gram-negative bacillus; although the three isolates were no longer available, the results of screening by AP-20E biochemical panel (API Analytab, Inc.) at the time were identical to those of the six patients with *P. pickettii* contamination of intravenous fluid, with or without associated bacteremia.

All three septic patients had had multiple positive blood cultures and were clinically in septic shock. *P. pickettii* had not been isolated from any local site of infection such as the urinary tract, lower respiratory tract, or surgical wound in any of the patients.

Review of nosocomial bacteremias over the past 7 years showed that *P. pickettii* had not previously been identified in any positive blood cultures from the institution, indicating that the cluster of three cases and six instances of contaminated infusate without bacteremia represented a true epidemic and, with the results of the subtyping, a common source epidemic.

The CDC and the manufacturer were contacted: None of more than 70 NNIS hospitals had reported *P. pickettii* bacteremias in the past year, and the manufacturer had never identified contamination with *P. pickettii* in quality control microbiologic sampling of its fentanyl before distribution or received any complaints from users about suspected contamination of their fentanyl. Moreover, a survey of surrounding Wisconsin hospitals that also used the manufacturer's fentanyl revealed none experiencing nosocomial bacteremias with *P. pickettii.*

Table 51-21. Case-Control Analysis of Risk Factors for Bacteremia or Contaminated Intravenous Fluid with *Pseudomonas Pickettii*

	Cases (*n*=9)	Controls* (*n*=19)	*P* Value
Age, Mean	50 yr	46 yr	NS†
Duration of Surgery, Mean	4.0 hr	3.7 hr	NS
Type of Surgery			
Cardiovascular	5 (55)	3 (16)	NS
General	4 (45)	16 (84)	
Intravenous Fluids			
Lactated Ringer's	8 (89)	11 (58)	NS
Dextrose in Ringer's lactate	5 (55)	14 (74)	NS
Saline 0.9%	6 (67)	4 (21)	NS
Blood products	7 (78)	4 (21)	NS
Albumin, fresh frozen plasma	4 (44)	2 (10)	NS
Intraoperative Intravenous Medications			
Pentothal	4 (45)	13 (68)	NS
Lidocaine	5 (55)	5 (26)	NS
Pancuronium	5 (55)	4 (21)	NS
Heparin	5 (55)	0 (0)	<.001
Cefazolin	9 (100)	10 (53)	NS
Fentanyl	9 (100)	9 (47)	.05
Volume of intravenous fentanyl, mean	61.6 mL	16.8 mL‡	<.001

*Patients randomly selected who had had surgery on the same day as cases but who had negative cultures of intravenous fluid from their infusion begun in the operating room.
†Not significant at $P<.05$.
‡For the nine control patients who received fentanyl.
From Maki DG, Klein BS, McCormick RD, et al: Nosocomial *Pseudomonas pickettii* bacteremias traced to narcotic tampering. A case for selective drug screening of health care personnel. JAMA 1991;265:981-986.

A case-control study comparing the 9 cases, all of whom had had recent surgery, with 19 operated patients who had had negative intravenous fluid cultures in the intravenous dressing study (Table 51-21), showed that all 9 cases but only 9 of the 19 operated control cases had received fentanyl intravenously in the operating room ($P=.05$; the mean total dose given to the 9 cases was far greater than that given to control patients who received the drug, 3080 μg versus 840 μg, $P<.001$).

In the hospital at the time, fentanyl was used only in the operating rooms as part of balanced anesthesia. The drug was received in 20-mL ampules from the manufacturer, and each week one of three pharmacy technicians, by rotation, drew into sterile syringes all fentanyl likely to be needed the following week in the operating rooms. Each day, one of the technicians delivered enough predrawn syringes to the operating rooms to meet the needs of the cases being done that day. Cultures of predrawn fentanyl in syringes in the central pharmacy, prompted by the findings of the case-control study, showed that twenty (40%) of fifty 30-mL syringes sampled were contaminated by *P. pickettii*, in a concentration of greater than 10^4 CFU/mL; none of thirty-five 5- or 2-mL syringes showed contamination ($P=.001$).

Extensive culturing within the central pharmacy was negative for evidence of environmental contamination by *P. pickettii* with one exception: *P. pickettii* biovariant 1, with an identical antimicrobial susceptibility pattern and restriction enzyme fragment pattern to the epidemic strain recovered from blood cultures or patients' intravenous infusions, was cultured in a concentration of 28 to 80 CFU/mL from five specimens of distilled water drawn from a tap in the central pharmacy. The epidemic strain was shown to multiply well in the fentanyl solution, attaining concentrations exceeding 10^4 CFU/mL within 48 hours.

A second case-control study suggested strongly that the epidemic was caused by theft of fentanyl from 30-mL syringes by one pharmacy staff member and replacement by distilled water that the individual thought was sterile but which, unfortunately, was contaminated by *P. pickettii.* The pharmacy member resigned early in the investigation and no longer works in the hospital. On April 29, 1985, the hospital's system for providing fentanyl and other narcotics to the operating rooms was changed; narcotics are no longer predrawn into syringes in the central pharmacy but are delivered to the operating rooms in unopened vials or ampules, and anesthesiologists' orders for narcotics are filled by a staff pharmacist assigned to the operating room. No further bacteremias with *P. pickettii* have occurred since March 25, 1985 (see Fig. 51-13), and cultures of more than 6000 samples of hospitalized patients' intravenous fluid in research studies since then have shown no further contamination by *P. pickettii*.

This outbreak illustrates the power of genetic subtyping[147] and case-control analyses to identify the cause of an epidemic. It further illustrates the potential for contamination of parenteral drugs or admixtures and the extraordinary range of epidemiologic mechanisms of nosocomial bloodstream infection deriving from such contamination.[107]

If epidemiologic or microbiologic studies suggest or indicate intrinsic contamination of a widely distributed commercial product or device, the local and state health authorities, U.S. Food and Drug Administration, CDC, and manufacturer should be informed immediately. Remaining products should be quarantined and retained for evaluation by the public health authorities.

PROTECTION OF HEALTH CARE WORKERS IN THE INTENSIVE CARE UNIT

HCWs in general, but especially those working in ICUs who are exposed daily to critically ill patients, many of whom have contagious but undiagnosed infections, are at increased risk of acquiring occupationally related infections including tuberculosis; herpes simplex virus infection; chickenpox; cytomegalovirus infection; hepatitis A, B, or C; HIV infection; influenza; measles; rubella; mumps; pertussis; and viral conjunctivitis.[538-540]

Fortunately, the risk posed by many of these infections can be eliminated by immunization of the HCW.[541] The Advisory Committee on Immunization Practices (ACIP) last made recommendations for the vaccination of HCWs in 1997[542]; however, a number of new developments in vaccine-preventable diseases have emerged since these guidelines were last published, and a considerable number of occupational infections exist for which there are currently no vaccines.

General Precautions against Biohazardous Exposure

All hospitals, as mandated by JCAHO,[31] must have an employee health service and written protocols for the management of biohazardous exposures (Box 51-4).[125,543] Such protocols permit expeditious and comprehensive evaluation and timely administration of postexposure prophylaxis (PEP) with antiretrovirals after HIV exposure, immune serum globulin or hepatitis B immune globulin after exposure to hepatitis A or B, or antimicrobial prophylaxis after exposure to contagious bacterial pathogens such as *Neisseria meningitidis* or *Bordetella pertussis*.

The single greatest measure a hospital can take to reduce the risk of biohazardous exposures is to implement a comprehensive program that actively monitors occupational exposures,[544] educates HCWs about the consequences and ways to prevent exposures,[545] and advocates for and rigorously evaluates new safety technologies as a means of reducing exposures further.[546]

The importance of uncompromising compliance with universal precautions to protect HCWs from unknowing exposure to HIV and other bloodborne viruses has been discussed. *Importantly, the greatest emphasis in training on universal precautions should be placed on measures to prevent needle sticks and other sharps injuries,*[543] *prohibition of recapping used needles, and making impervious needle disposal containers*[547] *available at the bedside of each ICU patient.*[548] The use of engineered controls such as needleless systems holds the greatest promise for effecting a material reduction in hazardous sharps injuries.[546]

Vaccine-Preventable Diseases

Hepatitis B

Percutaneous exposure of an unvaccinated HCW to blood from a patient who is hepatitis B surface antigen (HBsAg) positive carries considerable risk of seroconversion (23% to 37%) and development of clinical disease (1% to 6%).[125] This risk is greatly magnified if the source patient is hepatitis B e antigen (HBeAg) positive: the risk of seroconversion is 37% to 62%, and the risk of developing clinical disease is 22% to 31%.[125] The introduction of the recombinant hepatitis B vaccine in 1986 has greatly reduced the risk of occupationally acquired disease, and it is recommended that all HCWs receive a complete series of immunizations at 0, 1, and 6 months.[542] Furthermore, ACIP recommends that all HCWs have documentation of protective serum titers (hepatitis B surface antibody [HBsAb] serum titer=10 IU/mL) 1 to 2 months after completion of their primary series. Those HCWs who do not mount protective titers should undergo a secondary immunization series.[542] HCWs exposed to hepatitis B who have not developed protective titers after a primary or secondary immunization series or who have not completed a primary immunization series should be given postexposure prophylaxis (PEP) as detailed by the U.S. Public Health Service.[125]

Measles, Mumps, and Rubella

Reported cases of measles, mumps, and rubella have declined steadily in the United States since the introduction of mandatory childhood immunizations.[549-551] However, epidemics of measles and, more recently, mumps, continue to be a problem in many parts of the country.[552,553] Severe measles in susceptible HCWs who themselves exposed additional patients while in the incubation phase of infection have been well described in the literature.[73,554] As a result, it is recommended that all HCWs born after 1956 have documented immunity to measles and rubella by either (1) laboratory evidence of a protective titer; (2) physician documentation of clinical measles and rubella; or (3) documentation of appropriate vaccination against measles and rubella.[542] Although ACIP is less stringent with regards to documentation of immunity to mumps, it is recommended that HCWs receive the trivalent measles, mumps, rubella (MMR) vaccine rather than single vaccines.[542] When nonimmune HCWs are exposed to measles, PEP with MMR vaccination has been shown to reduce the likelihood of developing fulminant disease.[555] Measles immunoglobulin is another PEP option for nonimmune HCWs who have a contraindication to immunization—pregnancy—but only provides temporary protection.[555]

Box 51-4

Guidelines for Prevention and Management of Biohazardous Injuries in the Hospital*

1. Hospital personnel must be made more personally aware of the potential catastrophic sequelae of sharps injuries and other biohazardous exposures and of guidelines for prevention. This must be conveyed in initial orientation programs for all new personnel including physicians and by periodic updates on each patient care unit and presentations at staff conferences. The topic can also be periodically reviewed in the hospital's newsletter for personnel. Prominently placed posters warning of the hazards of sharps injuries and listing simple precautions to avert such injuries, especially in areas where sharps are heavily used, may also be of value.
2. Sharps disposal units should be made widely and conveniently available throughout the hospital, especially in locations that facilitate their immediate use: in individual patient rooms, nursing stations, pharmacy units, and utility rooms; in all clinical laboratories; on anesthesia carts; and in each operating room. Receptacles should be made of impervious material such as plastic or metal and should be emptied according to an established routine by personnel who have been properly instructed. Disposal units should consist of impervious receptacles into which a used needle and syringe or other sharp can be immediately dropped without handling it further. If it is necessary to remove a used needle from a syringe or Vacutainer, an instrument should always be used.
3. Recapping or resheathing of used needles must be strongly discouraged except when rare circumstances do not permit immediate disposal, in which case capping must be done using a "one-handed technique" or special sheath.
4. Medical or nursing personnel must be apprised of the importance of obtaining adequate assistance when administering injections or infusion therapy to patients who may not be able to cooperate.
5. Personnel must be apprised of the need to use extreme care in cleaning up after procedures that involve needles or other sharps such as lumbar punctures, thoracentesis, or central venous catheter placement.
6. A strong institutional commitment to the continuous evaluation and selective adoption of technology-based approaches to prevention of sharps injuries will have the greatest impact.
7. With accidental sharps injuries, unless the injury occurred with a clean sharp not used on a patient, the injury should be immediately reported to the employee health service, where work-related injuries in general can be evaluated and managed most consistently and inexpensively and surveillance of all work-related injuries can be assisted. A mechanism to ensure prompt management of biohazardous injuries 24 hours a day (including during nights and weekends by emergency department personnel who have been trained in the institutional biohazardous injury protocol) must be available.

   All hospital personnel who render care or services to patients including all staff physicians, house officers, and health care students should be covered by this institutional service to ensure consistent reporting and treatment of injuries.

   Employee health service personnel should meet with each employee sustaining a biohazardous injury, ascertain the exact reason for the accident, and review how to prevent a similar injury in the future. Particular attention should be given to those HCWs who have sustained repeated injuries to identify accident-prone activities or individuals or high-risk work situations that should be modified.
8. Institutions should carry out continuous surveillance and reporting of all biohazardous injuries, which can form the basis for preventive programs and determine their effectiveness. Risk management personnel should include sharps injury reduction as a major institutional priority.
9. Management of sharps injuries: It is beyond the scope of this review to provide a comprehensive protocol for management of sharps injuries; however, it is imperative that all hospitals have a protocol that provides unambiguous guidelines for management, specifically the following:
   a. Clear definitions of biohazardous injuries
   b. Procedures for immediate care of the injury at the time of occurrence (e.g., squeezing the puncture wound to induce bleeding, disinfection with a virucidal agent, such as an iodophor)
   c. Procedures to determine expeditiously the magnitude of risk (i.e., screening the source patient for evidence of active infection by hepatitis B virus; hepatitis C virus; and HIV). With regard to HIV screening, the protocol must be in compliance with state statutes governing HIV testing.
   d. The responsibilities of the injured HCW; the worker's supervisor; the employee health service; and, after working hours, the emergency department
   e. Guidelines for postexposure immunoprophylaxis and drug therapy, especially with exposures to the following:
      Hepatitis A, B, and C
      HIV
      Jakob-Creutzfeldt disease
      Syphilis
      Malaria
      Bacteremia
   f. Follow-up of the exposed HCW, especially following exposures to HIV; hepatitis B virus; and hepatitis C virus
   g. Administrative follow-up of all injuries, to minimize recurrences, and institutional surveillance of biohazardous injuries
   h. Periodic review of the protocol, with revision as indicated

*The Biohazardous Exposure Protocol of the University of Wisconsin Hospital and Clinics is available from the authors on request.
Modified and updated from McCormick RD, Meisch MG, Ircink FG, Maki DG: Epidemiology of hospital sharps injuries: A 14-year prospective study in the pre-AIDS and AIDS eras. Am J Med 1991;91:301S-307S.

Varicella

Occupational acquisition of varicella-zoster virus (VZV) is well described, with transmission rates among susceptible HCWs ranging from 2% to 16% in published studies.[541,556] Infected HCWs pose a threat for transmission to other susceptible patients, and HCWs, when compared with persons who acquire varicella during adolescence, often experience more severe disease,[557] particularly if pregnant.[558] All HCWs should be asked about a history of primary varicella. In the absence of a positive history, all HCWs should undergo serologic testing to confirm seropositivity or be immunized with the live, attenuated vaccine.[559] Susceptible HCWs should not care for patients with suspected or confirmed varicella or zoster infections, particularly if pregnant. In the event of an accidental exposure, susceptible HCWs should undergo varicella immunization within 72 hours of exposure on the basis of studies demonstrating a reduced risk of developing clinical infection and attenuated clinical disease.[560] The routine use of varicella-zoster immune globulin (VZIG) for PEP of susceptible HCWs exposed to VZV is not recommended.[559] Rather, the decision to administer VZIG should be guided by the presence of risk factors that increase the risk of severe disease (e.g., pregnancy or other immunodeficient conditions such as advanced AIDS).

Influenza

Influenza is responsible for 114,000 hospitalizations and 36,000 deaths in the United States each year.[561] Nosocomial outbreaks of influenza are common and serve to put HCWs at considerable risk of acquiring and transmitting influenza to others.[562,563] These outbreaks impose considerable economic burden on health care institutions and increase adverse events among HCWs and patients alike.[564] Influenza immunization of HCWs has significantly reduced days of febrile illness and sick leave in randomized controlled trials,[565,566] and surveys suggest that HCWs tend to view influenza immunization as a means of protecting themselves from illness.[567,568] However, accumulating evidence suggests that influenza immunization of HCWs also significantly reduces rates of influenza-related morbidity and mortality among potentially exposed patients in a variety of health care settings.[569-571] Moreover, expanding influenza rates of HCWs has been shown to be cost saving from an institutional perspective.[572] Despite this evidence, voluntary immunization rates among U.S. HCWs remain disappointingly low—in the range of 40%.[573] For these reasons, some experts are beginning to call for mandatory influenza immunization of HCWs (i.e., a condition of employment) in much the same way that hepatitis B and MMR vaccinations are mandatory for HCWs in most hospitals.[574]

Pertussis

HCWs are at increased risk of developing pertussis as a result of waning immunity in adulthood,[575] and numerous pertussis epidemics among HCWs have been reported in recent years.[576,577] Pertussis outbreaks are associated with considerable economic consequences,[577,578] and studies have shown that routinely providing a pertussis booster to HCWs in the form of tetanus toxoid, reduced diphtheria toxoid, and acellular pertussis adsorbed vaccine (Tdap) is cost effective.[577] The National Foundation of Infectious Diseases (NFID) and ACIP have recommended that all HCWs undergo booster immunization with Tdap, although these recommendations have not yet been endorsed by the U.S. Department of Health and Human Services.[579]

Non–Vaccine-Preventable Diseases of Major Interest

Herpetic Whitlow

Primary HSV paronychia has long been an occupational hazard of being an ICU nurse or physician[580,581] and is usually associated with a great deal of pain and discomfort, fever, and lymphadenitis. Leave from work for 2 to 3 weeks is not uncommon. One of the most compelling reasons for ICU HCWs to routinely wash their hands after contact with an ICU patient and to wear gloves during any contact with a patient's airway—including gloves on *both* hands during tracheal suctioning—is to protect themselves from this miserable condition.

Tuberculosis

Numerous reports of tuberculosis (TB) outbreaks in hospitals and other health care settings in the early and mid-1990s reminded the health care community of the risk associated with the care of patients with active pulmonary tuberculosis.[70-72,234] The feature common to most of these outbreaks was failure to recognize patients with active pulmonary tuberculosis. The most important measure for preventing the transmission of tuberculosis is to (1) rapidly identify and isolate patients with suspected tuberculosis and (2) promptly initiate appropriate therapy when tuberculosis is confirmed, to reduce the duration of infectiousness.[582] Updated guidelines for the prevention of nosocomial TB have recently been published that stress the importance of administrative, environmental, and personal respiratory protection controls.[126] Implementation of these recommendations has led to remarkable reductions in nosocomial transmission rates.[235]

Hepatitis C

Nearly 4 million persons in the United States are infected with hepatitis C virus (HCV), which is responsible for 8000 to 10,000 deaths every year.[583] Although the already high and rising prevalence of HCV infection in the population potentially exposes HCWs to occupationally acquired infection, most studies have failed to find a higher seroprevalence to HCV among HCWs than in the general population.[584] However, at least one study found that a previous history of a needle stick injury is associated with an increased risk of HCV infection,[585] and pooled analyses of published studies suggest that the seroconversion rate following a percutaneous injury involving HCV-positive persons is about 0.5%, a risk that is similar to that seen with percutaneous injuries involving needle stick exposures to HIV.[584] Current guidelines for the management of HCWs exposed to HCV only recommend serologic testing and measurement of serum alanine aminotransferase (ALT) levels, with or without HCV PCR testing, at baseline and again 4 to 6 months later, and do not make specific treatment recommendations.[125] However, these recommendations may undergo modification in the near future in light of studies demonstrating sustained virological responses to interferon monotherapy in excess of 90% in patients with acute-onset HCV infection.[586,587]

Human Immunodeficiency Virus

Although the risk of occupationally acquired HIV infection is low, it is not zero. As of 2002, there have been 57 probable and an additional 139 possible cases of occupationally acquired HIV in the United States.[588] The vast majority involved percutaneous injuries from hollow-bore needles contaminated with blood.[584] Other types of sharps injuries are less likely to transmit HIV, and only a single documented case of occupational HIV transmission caused by a body fluid exposure other than blood—bloody pleural fluid—has been reported in the literature.[589] Although no randomized trials exist, there are considerable data from animal[590] and observational studies[591] to suggest that PEP with antiretrovirals can significantly reduce the likelihood of HIV transmission following a high-risk exposure. For this reason, the U.S. Public Health Service has issued detailed recommendations on occupational HIV PEP with the choice and number of drugs driven by characteristics of the HCW, type of exposure, and characteristics of the source patient.[592]

GOALS FOR THE FUTURE

Clearly, nosocomial infection is one of the most important causes of iatrogenic morbidity and mortality in patients who require prolonged life-support care in an ICU. Much has been learned over the past 3 decades about the relative risks and especially the pathogenesis and epidemiology of these infections, information that has provided the scientific underpinnings for preventive strategies that have proved effective. However, there is an urgent need for better research to prevent nosocomial infection in ICU patients (Box 51-5),[593] particularly with respect to strategies to prevent colonization by multiresistant microorganisms, and to prevent infection even if colonization has already occurred.[28]

Most of our understanding of the epidemiology of nosocomial infection, especially in ICUs, is based on studies of epidemics. Well-designed studies are necessary to better define the epidemiology of *endemic* nosocomial infections, especially those caused by resistant staphylococci, enterococci and gram-negative bacilli, and yeasts. The importance of hand carriage of pathogens by hospital personnel, the role of airborne transmission in the ICU, and the relevance of contamination of the inanimate hospital environment by resistant pathogens all need to be better delineated, as well as the factors influencing nosocomial colonization and superinfection by resistant bacteria and yeasts.

In addition, larger and more sophisticated studies, using multivariate techniques of statistical analysis to define risk factors for the major forms of nosocomial infection in the ICU, are necessary to guide allocation of infection control resources and to target future research efforts.

Considering that the period of greatly increased susceptibility to infection of ICU patients is limited—until the invasive devices have been removed—a major commitment must be made to devise and evaluate strategies for blocking transmission of organisms between patients and preventing, or at least delaying, nosocomial colonization.

One of the oldest yet most important infection control measures—hand hygiene—is still done almost indifferently by HCWs in most hospitals including within ICUs. Innovative approaches are necessary to improve the frequency *and the quality* of handwashing after patient contacts likely to result in acquisition of nosocomial organisms. Exactly how should hands be washed for maximal benefit and with what agents? The question can be posed: Could very frequent handwashing, which approaches 40 times per 8-hour shift in neonatal ICUs, increase the potential for transmission of microorganisms, such as methicillin-resistant coagulase-negative staphylococci? Should the frequency of handwashing, as well as the agents used, be critically reexamined? Beyond a certain frequency, more may not necessarily be better. Should handwashing machines, which substantially augment degerming,[594,595] be adopted widely? Could regular application of chlorhexidine-containing evaporative lotions, used without water, replace some of the conventional handwashing or at least compensate for the suboptimal handwashing currently practiced?[221,596,597] Large clinical trials, ideally in multiple centers, are necessary to ascertain the efficacy or lack of efficacy of innovative approaches to hand degerming in reducing *infections* in high-risk patients, particularly in nurseries and ICUs.

Whereas SDD with topical nonabsorbable antibiotics has shown promise for the prevention of nosocomial respiratory infection in ICU patients, as noted, the potential effect on the microbial ecology of the ICU must be viewed with caution, and the cost-benefit and long-term effects of SDD need better clarification. The uses of simple barrier precautions to prevent colonization and infection have shown promise and warrant further study, especially in ICUs.

Studies have shown that the use of dedicated intravenous therapy teams, consisting of trained nurses or technicians to ensure a high level of aseptic technique during catheter insertion and in follow-up care of the catheter, has been associated with greatly reduced rates of catheter-related infection and appears to be cost effective.[322,323,598] The use of teams of trained ICU personnel to insert all urethral catheters and provide follow-up care for these catheters, all intravascular devices, and percutaneous tubes in the ICU deserves study.

Remarkably, there have been few comparative clinical trials of the various chemical antiseptics available for disinfecting skin before inserting intravascular devices or assisting in surgery or studies of antiseptic handwashing agents. Large, randomized clinical trials, ideally in multiple centers, are necessary in which *infection,* rather than

Box 51-5

Directions for Future Research in Nosocomial Infection Control

Studies to better define the epidemiology of endemic nosocomial infections:

- Especially those caused by resistant staphylococci, gram-negative bacilli, and *Candida*
- The relevance of hand carriage of pathogens by hospital personnel
- The role of airborne transmission
- The relative importance of contamination of the inanimate hospital environment, especially with methicillin-resistant *S. aureus, C. difficile,* and other resistant organisms
- The biologic factors influencing colonization by nosocomial organisms
- The factors governing superinfection by resistant bacteria and *Candida*
- Better understanding of risk factors predisposing to infection, especially in the ICU, to guide allocation of resources in infection control and focus research efforts

Innovative strategies to prevent nosocomial colonization and interrupt cross-infection, especially in ICUs:

- New approaches to improving compliance with and improving the effectiveness of handwashing between patients
- Various types of barrier precautions (forms of protective isolation)
- The true efficacy and cost-benefit of selective digestive decontamination; the ecologic effects of long-term use must be assessed carefully
- Dedicated device-care teams
- Large, randomized clinical trials of the various cutaneous antiseptics available, with infection, rather than colonization, as the index of comparison, for handwashing by personnel, site disinfection with invasive devices, patient bathing, and decolonization

Research on devices:

- Innovative designs to implicitly reduce contamination
- Colonization-resistant polymers, possibly incorporating antimicrobials onto the surface or into the polymer itself
- Better techniques of use to enhance safety
- Cost-effective "needleless" systems to protect health care personnel
- Improved laboratory tests to identify infection more accurately and rapidly, especially tracheobronchitis and pneumonia, to reduce unnecessary antibiotic therapy yet permit early therapy to avert progression to life-threatening sepsis
- Measures to restrict and improve the use of antibiotics, especially in ICUs
- Expanded, more effective approaches to education in infection control for health care personnel, especially physicians, with respect to handwashing, use of isolation, invasive devices, and use of antibiotics

Modified from Maki DG: Risk factors for nosocomial infection in intensive care. "Devices vs. nature" and goals for the next decade. Arch Intern Med 1989;149:30-35.

cutaneous colonization or positive cultures, is used as the index of comparison.

Considerable evidence indicates that the material used in construction of an implanted device plays an important role in the pathogenesis of device-related infection, namely, whether the material provides an attractive surface for adherence by pathogenic microorganisms such as coagulase-negative staphylococci. Studies are necessary to delineate fully the molecular mechanisms of microbial adherence to prosthetic surfaces to develop new materials intrinsically resistant to colonization for use with implantable devices and to design devices that intrinsically deny microbial access.

Increased use of diagnostic tests has greatly increased awareness of infectious diseases. Improved laboratory techniques to identify infection more accurately and rapidly, especially methods to reliably distinguish colonization of the lower respiratory tract from early infection that merits antimicrobial therapy, could greatly reduce unnecessary antimicrobial therapy yet detect infections earlier, before they progress to sepsis with multiple-organ failure.

Antimicrobials are not used optimally in most ICUs, and there is much overuse in hospitals, particularly of extended-spectrum penicillins and cephalosporins, imipenem, and quinolones. Antibiotic pressure has had a powerful effect on the hospital microbial ecology and, as noted previously, on the profile of nosocomial infection, especially in ICUs. We must and can do better.

Last, but certainly not least, many physicians remain remarkably oblivious to the most basic precepts of infection control, and nurses are in general far better informed and are a more effective force for ensuring compliance with infection control practices. More effective ways to communicate essential information on nosocomial infection control to hospital personnel, especially with regard to handwashing, aseptic use of devices, and antibiotic therapy, and to apply it more consistently in all hospitals, would have vast immediate benefits.

KEY POINTS

- Patients in modern-day ICUs experience rates of nosocomial infection three to five times higher than non-ICU hospitalized patients. Rates of primary bacteremia and nosocomial pneumonia are up to 10 times higher.
- Patients who are severely immunocompromised or who are critically ill and have high severity of illness scores have a substantially increased risk of nosocomial infection. However, most nosocomial infections in the ICU appear causally to be most directly related to life-saving technology, particularly invasive devices such as endotracheal tubes and mechanical ventilatory support, urethral and intravascular catheters, and intraventricular catheters, which facilitate colonization by nosocomial organisms and greatly increase vulnerability to infection.
- The major reservoir of bacterial nosocomial pathogens, and possibly *Candida* as well, in the ICU is the colonized or infected patient. Most infections begin with nosocomial colonization by organisms acquired from the hands of noncolonized HCWs. Increasing evidence suggests that antibiotic-resistant organisms, particularly MRSA, resistant enterococci, and *C. difficile,* may also be acquired from the inanimate environment immediately surrounding the patient. *Mycobacterium tuberculosis, Legionella, Aspergillus,* influenza A virus, varicella-zoster virus, measles, mumps, and the new highly virulent SARS human coronavirus are transmitted by the airborne route.
- ICUs are uniquely conducive to the epidemic spread of nosocomial organisms of all types, especially antibiotic-resistant bacteria and even *Candida;* more than half of all hospital epidemics occur in ICUs.
- An active, visible institutional infection control program can prevent up to one third of nosocomial infections. Surveillance of infection, whether total or focused, and education of all personnel are the most essential components of the program.
- Use of a chlorhexidine-containing agent for handwashing between patients will reduce endemic nosocomial infections in the ICU by at least 30%. The regular use of waterless alcohol-containing hand rubs or gels may provide comparable benefit in prevention of cross-infection.
- Stringent attention to isolation precautions, especially disposable gloves and a gown for contacts with patients known to be infected or colonized by resistant organisms, is mandatory to minimize cross-infection and prevent outbreaks. Misuse of gloves as part of universal precautions may, paradoxically, increase the risk of nosocomial infection.
- Modern-day ICUs must have adequate numbers of special negative-pressure isolation rooms for the care of patients with suspected or proven pulmonary tuberculosis and other airborne infections, such as varicella-zoster virus.
- Patients who have undergone recent bone marrow transplants or who have received intensive chemotherapy and are experiencing prolonged severe granulocytopenia should receive ICU care in special HEPA-filtered positive-pressure isolation rooms to protect them from devastating deep *Aspergillus* and other filamentous fungal infection.
- Meticulous attention to aseptic technique and the use of *maximal* barrier precautions—long-sleeved sterile surgical gown, mask and head cover, as well as sterile gloves—during the insertion of central venous catheters; the use of 2% chlorhexidine solutions for cutaneous antisepsis; avoiding insertion into the femoral veins; and prompt removal of catheters as soon as they are no longer necessary can reduce the incidence of catheter-related bloodstream infection at least threefold.
- Studies suggest that the prophylactic use of simple barrier precautions, vis-à-vis protective isolation, may provide protection against all types of ICU-acquired infection. Protective isolation is more appealing ecologically than the use of SDD.
- Measures to avert needle sticks and other sharps injuries are the most important aspect of universal precautions; these measures are necessary to protect the HCWs from HIV and other bloodborne viruses.
- A crisis of antibiotic resistance exists in ICUs. The progressive increase in antibiotic resistance of nosocomial staphylococci (methicillin), gram-negative bacilli (aminoglycosides and expanded-spectrum beta-lactams), and enterococci (vancomycin or ampicillin), and the sixfold increase in *Candida* infections during the past 2 decades indicates that it is of highest priority to reduce antimicrobial pressure within ICUs.
- Novel technology holds the greatest promise for prevention of nosocomial infection in general, particularly the development of medical devices that are intrinsically resistant to infection.
- Identifying more effective ways to communicate knowledge of infection control to hospital personnel, especially with regard to handwashing, aseptic use of devices, and antibiotic therapy, and to apply it consistently in all hospitals would have vast immediate benefits.

REFERENCES

1. Knaus WA, Draper EA, Wagner DP, Zimmerman JE: An evaluation of outcome from intensive care in major medical centers. Ann Intern Med 1986;104:410-418.
2. Reynolds HN, Haupt MT, Thill-Baharozian MC, Carlson RW: Impact of critical care physician staffing on patients with septic shock in a university hospital medical intensive care unit. JAMA 1988;260:3446-3450.
3. Ron A, Aronne LJ, Kalb PE, et al: The therapeutic efficacy of critical care units. Identifying subgroups of patients who benefit. Arch Intern Med 1989;149:338-341.
4. Brown RB, Hosmer D, Chen HC, et al: A comparison of infections in different ICUs within the same hospital. Crit Care Med 1985;13:472-476.
5. Craven DE, Kunches LM, Lichtenberg DA, et al: Nosocomial infection and fatality in medical and surgical intensive care unit patients. Arch Intern Med 1988;148:1161-1168.
6. Nystrom B, Frederici H, von Euler C: Bacterial colonization and infection in

an intensive care unit. Intensive Care Med 1988;14:34-38.
7. Chandrasekar PH, Kruse JA, Mathews MF: Nosocomial infection among patients in different types of intensive care units at a city hospital. Crit Care Med 1986;14:508-510.
8. Schandorf WA, Brown RB, Sands M, Hosmer D: Infections in a coronary care unit. Am J Cardiol 1985;56: 757-759.
9. Miller RM, Polakavetz SH, Hornick RB, Cowley RA: Analysis of infections acquired by the severely injured patient. Surg Gynecol Obstet 1973;137:7-10.
10. Marshall WG Jr, Dimick AR: The natural history of major burns with multiple subsystem failure. J Trauma 1983;23:102-105.
11. Pine RW, Wertz MJ, Lennard ES, et al: Determinants of organ malfunction or death in patients with intra-abdominal sepsis. A discriminant analysis. Arch Surg 1983;118:242-249.
12. Centers for Disease Control and Prevention. Monitoring hospital-acquired infections to promote patient safety—United States, 1990-1999. MMWR Morb Mortal Wkly Rep 2000;49:149-153.
13. Berenholtz SM, Pronovost PJ, Lisett PA, et al: Eliminating catheter-related bloodstream infection in the intensive care unit. Crit Care Med 2004;32: 2014-2020.
14. Reduction in central line-associated bloodstream infections among patients in intensive care units—Pennsylvania, April 2001-March 2005. MMWR Morb Mortal Wkly Rep 2005;54:1013-1016.
15. Pronovost P, Needham D, Berenholtz S, et al: An intervention to decrease catheter-related bloodstream infections in the ICU. N Engl J Med 2006;355: 2725-2732.
16. Horan TC, Gaynes RP: Surveillance of nosocomial infections. In Mayhall CG (ed): Hospital Epidemiology and Infection Control, 3rd ed. Philadelphia, Lippincott Williams & Wilkins, 2004, pp 1659-1702.
17. Crnich CJ, Maki DG: The role of intravascular devices in sepsis. Curr Infect Dis Rep 2001;3:497-506.
18. Wunderink RG, Mayhall CG, Gibert C: Methodology for clinical investigation of ventilator-associated pneumonia. Epidemiology and therapeutic intervention. Chest 1992;102(5 Suppl 1):580S-588S.
19. Wenzel RP, Thompson RL, Landry SM, et al: Hospital-acquired infections in intensive care unit patients: An overview with emphasis on epidemics. Infect Control 1983;4:371-375.
20. Northey D, Adess ML, Hartsuck JM, Rhoades ER: Microbial surveillance in a surgical intensive care unit. Surg Gynecol Obstet 1974;139:321-325.
21. Caplan ES, Hoyt N: Infection surveillance and control in the severely traumatized patient. Am J Med 1981;70:638-640.
22. Daschner FD, Frey P, Wolff G, et al: Nosocomial infections in intensive care wards: A multicenter prospective study. Intensive Care Med 1982;8:5-9.
23. Goldmann DA, Durbin WA Jr, Freeman J: Nosocomial infections in a neonatal intensive care unit. J Infect Dis 1981;144:449-459.
24. Goldmann DA, Freeman J, Durbin WA Jr: Nosocomial infection and death in a neonatal intensive care unit. J Infect Dis 1983;147:635-641.
25. Donowitz LG, Wenzel RP, Hoyt JW: High risk of hospital-acquired infection in the ICU patient. Crit Care Med 1982;10:355-357.
26. Jarvis WR, Edwards JR, Culver DH, et al: Nosocomial infection rates in adult and pediatric intensive care units in the United States. National Nosocomial Infections Surveillance System. Am J Med 1991;91: 185S-191S.
27. Nosocomial infection rates for interhospital comparison: Limitations and possible solutions. A Report from the National Nosocomial Infections Surveillance (NNIS) System. Infect Control Hosp Epidemiol 1991;12: 609-621.
28. Maki DG: Control of colonization and transmission of pathogenic bacteria in the hospital. Ann Intern Med 1978;89(5 Pt 2 Suppl):777-780.
29. Wenzel RP, Osterman CA, Donowitz LG, et al: Identification of procedure-related nosocomial infections in high-risk patients. Rev Infect Dis 1981;3:701-707.
30. Emori TG, Culver DH, Horan TC, et al: National nosocomial infections surveillance system (NNIS): Description of surveillance methods. Am J Infect Control 1991;19:19-35.
31. Joint Commission on Accreditation of Healthcare Organizations. Comprehensive Accreditation Manual for Hospitals. Oak Brook, Ill, JCAHO, 2007.
32. Maki DG: Nosocomial bacteremia. An epidemiologic overview. Am J Med 1981;70:719-732.
33. Richards MJ, Edwards JR, Culver DH, Gaynes RP: Nosocomial infections in combined medical-surgical intensive care units in the United States. Infect Control Hosp Epidemiol 2000;21: 510-515.
34. Kelly CP, Pothoulakis C, LaMont JT: *Clostridium difficile* colitis. N Engl J Med 1994;330:257-262.
35. Richards MJ, Edwards JR, Culver DH, Gaynes RP: Nosocomial infections in medical intensive care units in the United States. National Nosocomial Infections Surveillance System. Crit Care Med 1999;27:887-892.
36. Rhame FS, Streifel AJ, Kersey JH Jr, McGlave PB: Extrinsic risk factors for pneumonia in the patient at high risk of infection. Am J Med 1984;76:42-52.
37. Sherertz RJ, Belani A, Kramer BS, et al: Impact of air filtration on nosocomial *Aspergillus* infections. Unique risk of bone marrow transplant recipients. Am J Med 1987;83:709-718.
38. Walsh TJ, Dixon DM: Nosocomial aspergillosis: Environmental microbiology, hospital epidemiology, diagnosis and treatment. Eur J Epidemiol 1989;5:131-142.
39. Sinnott JTt, Gilchrist LS, Ellis L: Respiratory syncytial virus. Infect Control Hosp Epidemiol 1988;9: 465-468.
40. Cone R, Mohan K, Thouless M, Corey L: Nosocomial transmission of rotavirus infection. Pediatr Infect Dis J 1988;7:103-109.
41. Hart CA, Makin T: Legionella in hospitals: A review. J Hosp Infect 1991;18(Suppl A):481-489.
42. Banerjee SN, Emori TG, Culver DH, et al: Secular trends in nosocomial primary bloodstream infections in the United States, 1980-1989. National Nosocomial Infections Surveillance System. Am J Med 1991;91:86S-89S.
43. Schaberg DR, Culver DH, Gaynes RP: Major trends in the microbial etiology of nosocomial infection. Am J Med 1991;91:72S-75S.
44. Centers for Disease Control and Prevention: Trends in antibiotic resistance in National Nosocomial Infections Surveillance (NNIS) system hospitals, 1989-2004. Available at http://www.cdc.gov/ncidod/dhqp/pdf/ar/ICU_RESTrend1995-2004.pdf (Accessed January 15, 2007)
45. Weinstein RA: Nosocomial infection update. Emerg Infect Dis 1998;4: 416-420.
46. Ayala A, Perrin MM, Wagner MA, Chaudry IH: Enhanced susceptibility to sepsis after simple hemorrhage. Depression of Fc and C3b receptor-mediated phagocytosis. Arch Surg 1990;125:70-74; discussion 4-5.
47. Gardner ID: The effect of aging on susceptibility to infection. Rev Infect Dis 1980;2:801-810.
48. Gorse GJ, Messner RL, Stephens ND: Association of malnutrition with nosocomial infection. Infect Control Hosp Epidemiol 1989;10:194-203.
49. Fauci AS, Dale DC, Balow JE: Glucocorticosteroid therapy: Mechanisms of action and clinical considerations. Ann Intern Med 1976;84:304-315.
50. Santos GW, Owens AH Jr, Sensenbrenner LL: Effects of selected cytotoxic agents on antibody production in man; a preliminary report. Ann N Y Acad Sci 1964;114: 404-423.
51. Rubin RH: Infection in the renal and liver transplant patient. In Rubin RH, Young LS (eds): Clinical Approach to Infection in the Compromised Host. New York, Plenum, 1988.
52. Atherton ST, White DJ: Stomach as source of bacteria colonising respiratory tract during artificial ventilation. Lancet 1978;2:968-969.
53. Messori A, Trippoli S, Vaiani M, et al: Bleeding and pneumonia in intensive care patients given ranitidine and sucralfate for prevention of stress ulcer: Meta-analysis of randomised controlled trials. BMJ 2000;321: 1103-1106.
54. Agarwal N, Murphy JG, Cayten CG, Stahl WM: Blood transfusion increases the risk of infection after trauma. Arch Surg 1993;128:171-176; discussion 6-7.
55. Wenzel RP, Nettleman MD, Jones RN, Pfaller MA: Methicillin-resistant *Staphylococcus aureus:* Implications for the 1990s and effective control measures. Am J Med 1991;91:221S-227S.
56. Gray JW, Pedler SJ: Antibiotic-resistant enterococci. J Hosp Infect 1992;21: 1-14.

57. McGowan JE Jr: Antibiotic resistance in hospital bacteria: Current patterns, modes of appearance or spread, and economical impact. Rev Med Microbiol 1991;2:161-169.
58. Sanders CC, Sanders WE Jr: beta-Lactam resistance in gram-negative bacteria: global trends and clinical impact. Clin Infect Dis 1992;15:824-839.
59. Favero MS, Carson LA, Bond WW, Petersen NJ: *Pseudomonas aeruginosa:* Growth in distilled water from hospitals. Science 1971;173:836-838.
60. Wadowsky RM, Wolford R, McNamara AM, Yee RB: Effect of temperature, pH, and oxygen level on the multiplication of naturally occurring *Legionella pneumophila* in potable water. Appl Environ Microbiol 1985;49:1197-1205.
61. Cross AS, Sadoff JC, Iglewski BH, Sokol PA: Evidence for the role of toxin A in the pathogenesis of infection with *Pseudomonas aeruginosa* in humans. J Infect Dis 1980;142:538-546.
62. Tucker KD, Carrig PE, Wilkins TD: Toxin A of *Clostridium difficile* is a potent cytotoxin. J Clin Microbiol 1990;28:869-871.
63. Schlievert PM, Shands KN, Dan BB, et al: Identification and characterization of an exotoxin from *Staphylococcus aureus* associated with toxic-shock syndrome. J Infect Dis 1981;143: 509-516.
64. Tojo M, Yamashita N, Goldmann DA, Pier GB: Isolation and characterization of a capsular polysaccharide adhesin from *Staphylococcus epidermidis.* J Infect Dis 1988;157:713-722.
65. Falcieri E, Vaudaux P, Huggler E, et al: Role of bacterial exopolymers and host factors on adherence and phagocytosis of *Staphylococcus aureus* in foreign body infection. J Infect Dis 1987;155:524-531.
66. Vaudaux P, Lew D, Waldvogel FA: Host-dependent pathogenic factors in foreign body infection: A comparison between *Staphylococcus epidermidis* and *S. aureus*. Zentralbl Bakteriol Suppl 1987;16:189-193.
67. Gristina AG, Jennings RA, Naylor PT, et al: Comparative in vitro antibiotic resistance of surface-colonizing coagulase-negative staphylococci. Antimicrob Agents Chemother 1989;33:813-816.
68. von Eiff C, Becker K, Machka K, et al: Nasal carriage as a source of *Staphylococcus aureus* bacteremia. Study Group. N Engl J Med 2001;344:11-16.
69. Moore EP, Williams EW: Hospital transmission of multiply antibiotic-resistant *Streptococcus pneumoniae.* J Infect 1988;16:199-200.
70. Pearson ML, Jereb JA, Frieden TR, et al: Nosocomial transmission of multidrug-resistant *Mycobacterium tuberculosis.* A risk to patients and health care workers. Ann Intern Med 1992;117: 191-196.
71. Griffith DE, Hardeman JL, Zhang Y, et al: Tuberculosis outbreak among healthcare workers in a community hospital. Am J Resp Crit Care Med 1995;152:808-811.
72. Frieden TR, Sherman LF, Maw KL, et al: A multi-institutional outbreak of highly drug-resistant tuberculosis: Epidemiology and clinical outcomes. JAMA 1996;276:1229-1235.
73. Atkinson WL, Markowitz LE, Adams NC, Seastrom GR: Transmission of measles in medical settings—United States, 1985-1989. Am J Med 1991;91:320S-324S.
74. Poland GA, Nichol KL: Medical students as sources of rubella and measles outbreaks. Arch Intern Med 1990;150:44-46.
75. Oliveira EC, Lee B, Colice GL: Influenza in the intensive care unit. J Intensive Care Med 2003;18:80-91.
76. Hare R, Thomas CG: The transmission of *Staphylococcus aureus.* BMJ 1956;2:840-844.
77. Reybrouck G: Role of the hands in the spread of nosocomial infections. J Hosp Infect 1983;4:103-110.
78. Leclair JM, Freeman J, Sullivan BF, et al: Prevention of nosocomial respiratory syncytial virus infections through compliance with glove and gown isolation precautions. N Engl J Med 1987;317:329-334.
79. Raad, II, Sherertz RJ, Russell BA, Reuman PD: Uncontrolled nosocomial rotavirus transmission during a community outbreak. Am J Infect Control 1990;18:24-28.
80. McFarland LV, Mulligan ME, Kwok RY, Stamm WE: Nosocomial acquisition of *Clostridium difficile* infection. N Engl J Med 1989;320:204-210.
81. Reagan DR, Pfaller MA, Hollis RJ, Wenzel RP: Characterization of the sequence of colonization and nosocomial candidemia using DNA fingerprinting and a DNA probe. J Clin Microbiol 1990;28:2733-2738.
82. Dougherty SH: Pathobiology of infection in prosthetic devices. Rev Infect Dis 1988;10:1102-1117.
83. Nakashima AK, Allen JR, Martone WJ, et al: Epidemic bullous impetigo in a nursery due to a nasal carrier of *Staphylococcus aureus:* Role of epidemiology and control measures. Infect Control 1984;5:326-331.
84. Viglionese A, Nottebart VF, Bodman HA, Platt R: Recurrent group A streptococcal carriage in a health care worker associated with widely separated nosocomial outbreaks. Am J Med 1991;91:329S-333S.
85. Grieble HG, Bird TJ, Nidea HM, Miller CA: Chute-hydropulping waste disposal system: A reservoir of enteric bacilli and pseudomonas in a modern hospital. J Infect Dis 1974;130:602-607.
86. Olson B, Weinstein RA, Nathan C, et al: Epidemiology of endemic *Pseudomonas aeruginosa:* Why infection control efforts have failed. J Infect Dis 1984;150:808-816.
87. Olson B, Weinstein RA, Nathan C, et al: Occult aminoglycoside resistance in *Pseudomonas aeruginosa:* Epidemiology and implications for therapy and control. J Infect Dis 1985;152:769-774.
88. Weinstein RA: Endemic emergence of cephalosporin-resistant *Enterobacter:* Relation to prior therapy. Infect Control 1986;7(2 Suppl):120-123.
89. Flynn DM, Weinstein RA, Nathan C, et al: Patients' endogenous flora as the source of "nosocomial" *Enterobacter* in cardiac surgery. J Infect Dis 1987;156:363-368.
90. Weinstein RA: Epidemiology and control of nosocomial infections in adult intensive care units. Am J Med 1991;91:179S-184S.
91. Shooter RA, Gaya H, Cooke EM, et al: Food and medicaments as possible sources of hospital strains of *Pseudomonas aeruginosa.* Lancet 1969;1:1227-1229.
92. Thurn J, Crossley K, Gerdts A, et al: Enteral hyperalimentation as a source of nosocomial infection. J Hosp Infect 1990;15:203-217.
93. Rutala WA, Kennedy VA, Loflin HB, Sarubbi FA Jr: *Serratia marcescens* nosocomial infections of the urinary tract associated with urine measuring containers and urinometers. Am J Med 1981;70:659-663.
94. Cobben NA, Drent M, Jonkers M, et al: Outbreak of severe *Pseudomonas aeruginosa* respiratory infections due to contaminated nebulizers. J Hosp Infect 1996;33:63-70.
95. Crnich CJ, Safdar N, Maki DG: The role of the intensive care unit environment in the pathogenesis and prevention of ventilator-associated pneumonia. Respir Care 2005;50:813-836; discussion 36-8.
96. Mermel LA, Maki DG: Epidemic bloodstream infections from hemodynamic pressure monitoring: Signs of the times. Infect Control Hosp Epidemiol 1989;10:47-53.
97. Favero MS, Petersen NJ, Boyer KM, et al: Microbial contamination of renal dialysis systems and associated health risks. Trans Am Soc Artif Intern Organs 1974;20A:175-183.
98. Berkelman RL, Godley J, Weber JA, et al: *Pseudomonas cepacia* peritonitis associated with contamination of automatic peritoneal dialysis machines. Ann Intern Med 1982;96:456-458.
99. Alvarado CJ, Stolz SM, Maki DG: Nosocomial infections from contaminated endoscopes: A flawed automated endoscope washer. An investigation using molecular epidemiology. Am J Med 1991;91: 272S-280S.
100. Weber DJ, Rutala WA: Lessons from outbreaks associated with bronchoscopy. Infect Control Hosp Epidemiol 2001;22:403-408.
101. Srinivasan A, Wolfenden LL, Song X, et al: An outbreak of *Pseudomonas aeruginosa* infections associated with flexible bronchoscopes. N Engl J Med 2003;348:221-227.
102. Platt R, Polk BF, Murdock B, Rosner B: Risk factors for nosocomial urinary tract infection. Am J Epidemiol 1986;124:977-985.
103. Garibaldi RA, Burke JP, Dickman ML, Smith CB: Factors predisposing to bacteriuria during indwelling urethral catheterization. N Engl J Med 1974;291:215-219.
104. Celis R, Torres A, Gatell JM, et al: Nosocomial pneumonia. A multivariate analysis of risk and prognosis. Chest 1988;93:318-324.
105. Craven DE, Kunches LM, Kilinsky V, et al: Risk factors for pneumonia and fatality in patients receiving continuous mechanical ventilation. Am Rev Respir Dis 1986;133:792-796.

106. Nichols RL: Surgical wound infection. Am J Med 1991;91:54S-64S.
107. Maki DG: Infections caused by intravascular devices used for infusion therapy: Pathogenesis, prevention and management. In Bisno AL, Waldvogel FA (eds): Infections Associated with Indwelling Medical Devices, 2nd ed. Washington, DC, ASM Press, 1994.
108. Mayhall CG, Archer NH, Lamb VA, et al: Ventriculostomy-related infections. A prospective epidemiologic study. N Engl J Med 1984;310:553-559.
109. Bleichner G, Thomas O, Sollet JP: Diarrhea in intensive care: diagnosis and treatment. Int J Antimicrob Agents 1993;3:33.
110. Wey SB, Mori M, Pfaller MA, et al: Risk factors for hospital-acquired candidemia. A matched case-control study. Arch Intern Med 1989;149:2349-2353.
111. Bross J, Talbot GH, Maislin G, et al: Risk factors for nosocomial candidemia: A case-control study in adults without leukemia. Am J Med 1989;87:614-620.
112. Fraser VJ, Jones M, Dunkel J, et al: Candidemia in a tertiary care hospital: Epidemiology, risk factors, and predictors of mortality. Clin Infect Dis 1992;15:414-421.
113. Infection surveillance and control programs in U.S. hospitals: An assessment. MMWR Morb Mortal Wkly Rep 1978;27.
114. Haley RW, Quade D, Freeman HE, et al: Study on efficacy of nosocomial infection control (SENIC project): Summary of study design. Am J Epidemiol 1980;111:472-485.
115. Haley RW, Culver DH, White JW, et al: The efficacy of infection surveillance and control programs in preventing nosocomial infections in US hospitals. Am J Epidemiol 1985;121:182-205.
116. Haley RW: The development of infection surveillance and control programs. In Bennett JV, Brachman PS (eds): Hospital Infections, 4th ed. Philadelphia, Lippincott-Raven Publishers, 1998, pp 53-64.
117. Haley RW, Morgan WM, Culver DH, et al: Hospital infection control: Recent progress and opportunities under prospective payment. Am J Infect Control 1985;13:97-108.
118. U.S. Department of Health and Human Services. Healthy People 2010. Washington, DC, U.S. Government Printing Office, 2000.
119. Institute of Medicine. To Err is Human: Building a Safer Health System. Washington, DC, National Academy Press, 1999.
120. Haley RW, White JW, Culver DH, Hughes JM: The financial incentive for hospitals to prevent nosocomial infections under the prospective payment system. An empirical determination from a nationally representative sample. JAMA 1987;257:1611-1614.
121. Goldmann DA: Nosocomial infection control in the United States of America. J Hosp Infect 1986;8:116-128.
122. Haley RW: Managing Hospital Infection Control for Cost-Effectiveness. Chicago, American Hospital Association, 1986.
123. Wenzel RP, Pfaller MA: Infection control: the premier quality assessment program in United States hospitals. Am J Med 1991;91:27S-31S.
124. Scheckler WE: Interim report of the Quality Indicator Study Group. Infect Control Hosp Epidemiol 1994;15: 265-268.
125. Updated U.S. Public Health Service Guidelines for the Management of Occupational Exposures to HBV, HCV, and HIV and Recommendations for Postexposure Prophylaxis. MMWR Recomm Rep 2001;50(RR-11):1-52.
126. Jensen PA, Lambert LA, Iademarco MF, Ridzon R: Guidelines for preventing the transmission of *Mycobacterium tuberculosis* in health-care settings, 2005. MMWR Recomm Rep 2005;54:1-141.
127. Rutala WA, Mayhall CG: Medical waste. Infect Control Hosp Epidemiol 1992;13:38-48.
128. Rutala WA, Odette RL, Samsa GP: Management of infectious waste by US hospitals. JAMA 1989;262: 1635-1640.
129. O'Grady NP, Alexander M, Dellinger EP, et al: Guidelines for the prevention of intravascular catheter-related infections. Clin Infect Dis 2002;35: 1281-1307.
130. Wong ES: Guideline for prevention of catheter-associated urinary tract infections. Am J Infect Control 1983;11:28-36.
131. Tablan OC, Anderson LJ, Besser R, et al: Guidelines for preventing health-care-associated pneumonia, 2003: Recommendations of CDC and the Healthcare Infection Control Practices Advisory Committee. MMWR Recomm Rep 2004;53(RR-3):1-36.
132. Jones RN: Global epidemiology of antimicrobial resistance among community-acquired and nosocomial pathogens: A five-year summary from the SENTRY Antimicrobial Surveillance Program (1997-2001). Semin Respir Crit Care Med 2003;24:121-134.
133. National Nosocomial Infections Surveillance (NNIS) System Report, data summary from January 1992 through June 2004, issued October 2004. Am J Infect Control 2004; 32:470-485.
134. McGowan JE, Weinstein RA: The role of the laboratory in control of nosocomial infection. In Bennett JV, Brachman PS (eds): Hospital Infections, 4th ed. Philadelphia, Lippincott-Raven Publishers, 1998, pp 143-164.
135. Bouam S, Girou E, Brun-Buisson C, et al: An intranet-based automated system for the surveillance of nosocomial infections: Prospective validation compared with physicians' self-reports. Infect Control Hosp Epidemiol 2003;24:51-55.
136. Wright MO, Perencevich EN, Novak C, et al: Preliminary assessment of an automated surveillance system for infection control. Infect Control Hosp Epidemiol 2004;25:325-332.
137. Ernst EJ, Diekema DJ, BootsMiller BJ, et al: Are United States hospitals following national guidelines for the analysis and presentation of cumulative antimicrobial susceptibility data? Diagn Microbiol Infect Dis 2004;49:141-145.
138. Lautenbach E, Nachamkin I: Analysis and presentation of cumulative antimicrobial susceptibility data (antibiograms): Substantial variability across medical centers in the United States. Infect Control Hosp Epidemiol 2006;27:409-412.
139. Zapantis A, Lacy MK, Horvat RT, et al: Nationwide antibiogram analysis using NCCLS M39-A guidelines. J Clin Microbiol 2005;43:2629-2634.
140. National Committee for Clinical Laboratory Standards (NCCLS). Analysis and presentation of cumulative antimicrobial susceptibility test data: Approved standard. NCCLS document M39-A. Wayne, Pa, NCCLS, 2002.
141. Pestotnik SL, Classen DC, Evans RS, Burke JP: Implementing antibiotic practice guidelines through computer-assisted decision support: Clinical and financial outcomes. Ann Intern Med 1996;124:884-890.
142. McGregor JC, Weekes E, Forrest GN, et al: Impact of a computerized clinical decision support system on reducing inappropriate antimicrobial use: A randomized controlled trial. J Am Med Inform Assoc 2006;13:378-384.
143. Maki DG: Epidemic nosocomial bacteremias. In Wenzel RP (ed): Handbook of Hospital Infection. Boca Raton, Fla, CRC Press, 1981, pp 371-512.
144. Tenover FC: Rapid detection and identification of bacterial pathogens using novel molecular technologies: Infection control and beyond. Clin Infect Dis 2007;44:418-423.
145. Thorburn K, Kerr S, Taylor N, van Saene HK: RSV outbreak in a paediatric intensive care unit. J Hosp Infect 2004;57:194-201.
146. Quindos G: New microbiological techniques for the diagnosis of invasive mycoses caused by filamentous fungi. Clin Microbiol Infect 2006;12(Suppl 7):40-52.
147. Herwaldt LA, Pfaller MA, Weber S: Microbial molecular techniques. In Thomas JC, Weber DJ (eds): Epidemiologic Methods for the Study of Infectious Diseases. New York, Oxford University Press, 2001, pp 163-191.
148. Poutanen SM, Tompkins LS: Molecular methods in nosocomial epidemiology. In Wenzel RP (ed): Prevention and Control of Nosocomial Infections. Philadelphia, Lippincott Williams & Wilkins, 2003, pp 481-499.
149. Schwartz DH, Laeyendecker OB, Arango-Jaramillo S, et al: Extensive evaluation of a seronegative participant in an HIV-1 vaccine trial as a result of false-positive PCR. Lancet 1997;350:256-259.
150. Lievano FA, Reynolds MA, Waring AL, et al: Issues associated with and recommendations for using PCR to detect outbreaks of pertussis. J Clin Microbiol 2002;40:2801-2805.
151. Boyce JM, Potter-Bynoe G, Chenevert C, King T: Environmental contamination due to methicillin-resistant *Staphylococcus aureus*: Possible infection control implications. Infect Control Hosp Epidemiol 1997;18:622-627.

152. Bonten MJ, Hayden MK, Nathan C, et al: Epidemiology of colonisation of patients and environment with vancomycin-resistant enterococci. Lancet 1996;348:1615-1619.
153. Aygun G, Demirkiran O, Utku T, et al: Environmental contamination during a carbapenem-resistant *Acinetobacter baumannii* outbreak in an intensive care unit. J Hosp Infect 2002;52: 259-262.
154. Maki DG, Alvarado CJ, Hassemer CA, Zilz MA: Relation of the inanimate hospital environment to endemic nosocomial infection. N Engl J Med 1982;307:1562-1566.
155. McGowan JE Jr: Environmental factors in nosocomial infection: A selective focus. Rev Infect Dis 1981;3:760-769.
156. Boyce JM, White RL, Causey WA, Lockwood WR: Burn units as a source of methicillin-resistant *Staphylococcus aureus* infections. JAMA 1983;249: 2803-2807.
157. Samore MH, Venkataraman L, DeGirolami PC, et al: Clinical and molecular epidemiology of sporadic and clustered cases of nosocomial *Clostridium difficile* diarrhea. Am J Med 1996;100:32-40.
158. Duckro AN, Blom DW, Lyle EA, et al: Transfer of vancomycin-resistant enterococci via health care worker hands. Arch Intern Med 2005;165: 302-307.
159. Getchell-White SI, Donowitz LG, Groschel DH: The inanimate environment of an intensive care unit as a potential source of nosocomial bacteria: Evidence for long survival of *Acinetobacter calcoaceticus.* Infect Control Hosp Epidemiol 1989;10: 402-407.
160. Neely AN: A survey of gram-negative bacteria survival on hospital fabrics and plastics. J Burn Care Rehabil 2000;21:523-527.
161. Mayfield JL, Leet T, Miller J, Mundy LM: Environmental control to reduce transmission of Clostridium difficile. Clin Infect Dis 2000;31:995-1000.
162. Needleman J, Buerhaus P, Mattke S, et al: Nurse-staffing levels and the quality of care in hospitals. N Engl J Med 2002;346:1715-1722.
163. Hugonnet S, Harbarth S, Sax H, et al: Nursing resources: A major determinant of nosocomial infection? Curr Opin Infect Dis 2004;17:329-333.
164. Harbarth S, Sudre P, Dharan S, et al: Outbreak of *Enterobacter cloacae* related to understaffing, overcrowding, and poor hygiene practices. Infect Control Hosp Epidemiol 1999;20: 598-603.
165. Pittet D, Mourouga P, Perneger TV: Compliance with handwashing in a teaching hospital. Ann Intern Med 1999;130:126-130.
166. Harvey MA: Critical-care-unit bedside design and furnishing: Impact on nosocomial infections. Infect Control Hosp Epidemiol 1998;19:597-601.
167. du Moulin G: Minimizing the potential for nosocomial pneumonia: Architectural, engineering, and environmental considerations for the intensive care unit. Eur J Clin Microbiol Infect Dis 1989;8:69-74.
168. Mulin B, Rouget C, Clement C, et al: Association of private isolation rooms with ventilator-associated *Acinetobacter baumanii* pneumonia in a surgical intensive-care unit. Infect Control Hosp Epidemiol 1997;18:499-503.
169. Shirani KZ, McManus AT, Vaughan GM, et al: Effects of environment on infection in burn patients. Arch Surg 1986;121:31-36.
170. Carter CD, Barr BA: Infection control issues in construction and renovation. Infect Control Hosp Epidemiol 1997;18:587-596.
171. Boyce JM, Pittet D, Healthcare Infection Control Practices Advisory Committee: Society for Healthcare Epidemiology of America. Association for Professionals in Infection Control. Infectious Diseases Society of America. Hand Hygiene Task Force Guideline for Hand Hygiene in Health-Care Settings: Recommendations of the Healthcare Infection Control Practices Advisory Committee and the HICPAC/SHEA/APIC/IDSA Hand Hygiene Task Force. Infect Control Hosp Epidemiol 2002;23(12 Suppl):S3-40.
172. Pittet D, Hugonnet S, Harbarth S, et al: Effectiveness of a hospital-wide programme to improve compliance with hand hygiene. Lancet 2000;356:1307-1312.
173. Trautmann M, Michalsky T, Wiedeck H, et al: Tap water colonization with *Pseudomonas aeruginosa* in a surgical intensive care unit (ICU) and relation to *Pseudomonas* infections of ICU patients. Infect Control Hosp Epidemiol 2001;22:49-52.
174. Garner JS, Healthcare Infection Control Practices Advisory Committee: Guideline for isolation precautions in hospitals. Am J Infect Control 2007;(in press).
175. Anaissie EJ, Penzak SR, Dignani MC: The hospital water supply as a source of nosocomial infections: A plea for action. Arch Intern Med 2002;162:1483-1492.
176. Weber DJ, Rutala WA, Blanchet CN, et al: Faucet aerators: A source of patient colonization with *Stenotrophomonas maltophilia.* Am J Infect Control 1999;27:59-63.
177. Simor AE, Lee M, Vearncombe M, et al: An outbreak due to multiresistant *Acinetobacter baumannii* in a burn unit: Risk factors for acquisition and management. Infect Control Hosp Epidemiol 2002;23:261-267.
178. Wang SH, Sheng WH, Chang YY, et al: Healthcare-associated outbreak due to pan-drug resistant *Acinetobacter baumannii* in a surgical intensive care unit. J Hosp Infect 2003;53:97-102.
179. Sabria M, Yu VL: Hospital-acquired legionellosis: Solutions for a preventable infection. Lancet Infect Dis 2002;2:368-373.
180. Haley CE, Cohen ML, Halter J, Meyer RD: Nosocomial Legionnaires' disease: A continuing common-source epidemic at Wadsworth Medical Center. Ann Intern Med 1979;90: 583-586.
181. Centers for Disease Control and Prevention: Guidelines for preventing health-care-associated pneumonia, 2003. Recommendations of the CDC and the Healthcare Infection Control Practices Advisory Committee. MMWR Morb Mortal Wkly Rep 2004;53(RR-3).
182. Benin AL, Benson RF, Besser RE: Trends in Legionnaires disease, 1980-1998: Declining mortality and new patterns of diagnosis. Clin Infect Dis 2002;35: 1039-1046.
183. Yu VL: Resolving the controversy on environmental cultures for *Legionella:* A modest proposal. Infect Control Hosp Epidemiol 1998;19:893-897.
184. Kool JL, Fiore AE, Kioski CM, et al: More than 10 years of unrecognized nosocomial transmission of Legionnaires' disease among transplant patients. Infect Control Hosp Epidemiol 1998;19:898-904.
185. Lepine LA, Jernigan DB, Butler JC, et al: A recurrent outbreak of nosocomial Legionnaires' disease detected by urinary antigen testing: Evidence for long-term colonization of a hospital plumbing system. Infect Control Hosp Epidemiol 1998;19:905-910.
186. Alary M, Joly JR: Factors contributing to the contamination of hospital water distribution systems by legionellae. J Infect Dis 1992;165:565-569.
187. Kool JL, Bergmire-Sweat D, Butler JC, et al: Hospital characteristics associated with colonization of water systems by Legionella and risk of nosocomial legionnaires' disease: A cohort study of 15 hospitals. Infect Control Hosp Epidemiol 1999;20:798-805.
188. Fields BS, Benson RF, Besser RE: Legionella and Legionnaires' disease: 25 years of investigation. Clin Microbiol Rev 2002;15:506-526.
189. Helms CM, Massanari RM, Wenzel RP, et al: Legionnaires' disease associated with a hospital water system. A five-year progress report on continuous hyperchlorination. JAMA 1988;259: 2423-2427.
190. Muraca PW, Yu VL, Goetz A: Disinfection of water distribution systems for Legionella: A review of application procedures and methodologies. Infect Control Hosp Epidemiol 1990;11:79-88.
191. Farr BM, Gratz JC, Tartaglino JC, et al: Evaluation of ultraviolet light for disinfection of hospital water contaminated with Legionella. Lancet 1988;2:669-672.
192. Stout JE, Yu VL: Experiences of the first 16 hospitals using copper-silver ionization for Legionella control: Implications for the evaluation of other disinfection modalities. Infect Control Hosp Epidemiol 2003;24:563-568.
193. Rutala WA, Weber DJ: Disinfection and sterilization in health care facilities: What clinicians need to know. Clin Infect Dis 2004;39:702-709.
194. Rutala WA, Weber DJ: Guideline for disinfection and sterilization in healthcare facilities: Recommendations of the CDC Healthcare Infection Control Practices Advisory Committee. MMWR Morb Mortal Wkly Rep 2007;(in press).
195. Knight R: Creutzfeldt-Jakob disease: A rare cause of dementia in elderly persons. Clin Infect Dis 2006;43:340-346.
196. Nelson DB, Jarvis WR, Rutala WA, et al: Multi-society guideline for reprocessing flexible gastrointestinal endoscopes. Society for Healthcare Epidemiology of America. Infect

Control Hosp Epidemiol 2003;24:532-537.
197. Centers for Disease Control and Prevention: Contaminated povidone-iodine solution—Texas. MMWR Morb Mortal Wkly Rep 1989;38:133-134.
198. Panlilio AL, Beck-Sague CM, Siegel JD, et al: Infections and pseudoinfections due to povidone-iodine solution contaminated with Pseudomonas cepacia. Clin Infect Dis 1992;14: 1078-1083.
199. Alfa MJ, Sitter DL: In-hospital evaluation of orthophthalaldehyde as a high level disinfectant for flexible endoscopes. J Hosp Infect 1994;26: 15-26.
200. Mimoz O, Karim A, Mercat A, et al: Chlorhexidine compared with povidone-iodine as skin preparation before blood culture. A randomized, controlled trial. Ann Intern Med 1999;131:834-837.
201. Chaiyakunapruk N, Veenstra DL, Lipsky BA, Saint S: Chlorhexidine compared with povidone-iodine solution for vascular catheter-site care: A meta-analysis. Ann Intern Med 2002;136: 792-801.
202. Maki DG, Ringer M, Alvarado CJ: Prospective randomised trial of povidone-iodine, alcohol, and chlorhexidine for prevention of infection associated with central venous and arterial catheters. Lancet 1991;338:339-343.
203. Humar A, Ostromecki A, Direnfeld J, et al: Prospective randomized trial of 10% povidone-iodine versus 0.5% tincture of chlorhexidine as cutaneous antisepsis for prevention of central venous catheter infection. Clin Infect Dis 2000;31:1001-1007.
204. Maki DG, Zilz MA, Alvarado CJ: Evaluation of the antibacterial efficacy of four agents for handwashing. In Nelson JC, Grassi C (eds): Current chemotherapy and infectious disease: Proceedings of the 11th International Congress on Chemotherapy and the 19th Interscience Conference on Antimicrobial Agents and Chemotherapy; 1980. Washington, DC, American Society for Microbiology, 1980.
205. Horn WA, Larson EL, McGinley KJ, Leyden JJ: Microbial flora on the hands of health care personnel: Differences in composition and antibacterial resistance. Infect Control Hosp Epidemiol 1988;9:189-193.
206. Larson EL: Persistent carriage of gram-negative bacteria on hands. Am J Infect Control 1981;9:112-119.
207. Graham M: Frequency and duration of handwashing in an intensive care unit. Am J Infect Control 1990;18:77-81.
208. Larson E: A causal link between handwashing and risk of infection? Examination of the evidence. Infect Control 1988;9:28-36.
209. McCormick RD, Buchman TL, Maki DG: Double-blind, randomized trial of scheduled use of a novel barrier cream and an oil-containing lotion for protecting the hands of health care workers. Am J Infect Control 2000;28:302-310.
210. Pittet D, Boyce JM: Hand hygiene and patient care: Pursuing the Semmelweiss legacy. Lancet Infect Dis 2001;0:9.
211. Maki DG, Hecht J: Antiseptic-containing handwashing agents reduce nosocomial infections: a prospective study. In Proceedings of the 22nd Interscience Conference on Antimicrobial Agents and Chemotherapy; 1982. Miami Beach, Fla, American Society for Microbiology, 1982.
212. Kaslow RA, Dixon RE, Martin SM, et al: *Staphylococcal* disease related to hospital nursery bathing practices. A nationwide epidemiologic investigation. Pediatrics 1973;51: 418-429.
213. Casewell M, Phillips I: Hands as route of transmission for Klebsiella species. BMJ 1977;2:1315-1317.
214. Bartzokas CA, Paton JH, Gibson MF, et al: Control and eradication of methicillin-resistant *Staphylococcus aureus* on a surgical unit. N Engl J Med 1984;311:1422-1425.
215. Onesko KM, Wienke EC: The analysis of the impact of a mild, low-iodine, lotion soap on the reduction of nosocomial methicillin-resistant *Staphylococcus aureus:* A new opportunity for surveillance by objectives. Infect Control 1987;8: 284-288.
216. Massanari RM: A crossover comparison of antiseptic soaps on nosocomial infection rates in intensive care units. Am J Infect Control 1984;12.
217. Doebbeling BN, Stanley GL, Sheetz CT, et al: Comparative efficacy of alternative hand-washing agents in reducing nosocomial infections in intensive care units. N Engl J Med 1992;327:88-93.
218. Rotter ML: Arguments for alcoholic hand disinfection. J Hosp Infect 2001;48(Suppl A):S4-8.
219. Gordin FM, Schultz ME, Huber RA, Gill JA: Reduction in nosocomial transmission of drug-resistant bacteria after introduction of an alcohol-based handrub. Infect Control Hosp Epidemiol 2005;26:650-653.
220. Lai KK, Fontecchio S, Melvin Z, Baker SP: Impact of alcohol-based, waterless hand antiseptic on the incidence of infection and colonization with methicillin-resistant *Staphylococcus aureus* and vancomycin-resistant enterococci. Infect Control Hosp Epidemiol 2006;27:1018-1024.
221. Larson EL, Eke PI, Laughon BE: Efficacy of alcohol-based hand rinses under frequent-use conditions. Antimicrob Agents Chemother 1986;30:542-544.
222. Larson EL, Aiello AE, Bastyr J, et al: Assessment of two hand hygiene regimens for intensive care unit personnel. Crit Care Med 2001;29: 944-951.
223. Centers for Disease Control and Prevention: Isolation techniques for use in hospitals. Washington, DC, U.S. Government Printing Office, 1975.
224. Weinstein RA, Nathan C, Gruensfelder R, Kabins SA: Endemic aminoglycoside resistance in gram-negative bacilli: Epidemiology and mechanisms. J Infect Dis 1980;141:338-345.
225. Muto CA, Jernigan JA, Ostrowsky BE, et al: SHEA guideline for preventing nosocomial transmission of multidrug-resistant strains of *Staphylococcus aureus* and enterococcus. Infect Control Hosp Epidemiol 2003;24:362-386.
226. Garner JS, Simmons BP: Guideline for isolation precautions in hospitals. Infect Control 1983;4(4 Suppl): 245-325.
227. Lynch P, Cummings MJ, Roberts PL, et al: Implementing and evaluating a system of generic infection precautions: Body substance isolation. Am J Infect Control 1990;18:1-12.
228. Garner JS, Hughes JM: Options for isolation precautions. Ann Intern Med 1987;107:248-250.
229. Karanfil LV, Murphy M, Josephson A, et al: A cluster of vancomycin-resistant *Enterococcus faecium* in an intensive care unit. Infect Control Hosp Epidemiol 1992;13:195-200.
230. Garner TK, Rimland D: Stethoscopes and infections. JAMA 1982;248:310.
231. Livornese LL Jr, Dias S, Samel C, et al: Hospital-acquired infection with vancomycin-resistant *Enterococcus faecium* transmitted by electronic thermometers. Ann Intern Med 1992;117:112-116.
232. Brooks SE, Veal RO, Kramer M, et al: Reduction in the incidence of *Clostridium difficile*–associated diarrhea in an acute care hospital and a skilled nursing facility following replacement of electronic thermometers with single-use disposables. Infect Control Hosp Epidemiol 1992;13:98-103.
233. Cepeda JA, Whitehouse T, Cooper B, et al: Isolation of patients in single rooms or cohorts to reduce spread of MRSA in intensive-care units: prospective two-centre study. Lancet 2005;365:295-304.
234. Agerton T, Valway S, Gore B, et al: Transmission of a highly drug-resistant strain (strain W1) of *Mycobacterium tuberculosis*. Community outbreak and nosocomial transmission via a contaminated bronchoscope. JAMA 1997;278:1073-1077.
235. Maloney SA, Pearson ML, Gordon MT, et al: Efficacy of control measures in preventing nosocomial transmission of multidrug-resistant tuberculosis to patients and health care workers. Ann Intern Med 1995;122:90-95.
236. Recommendations for prevention of HIV transmission in health-care settings. MMWR Morb Mortal Wkly Rep 1987;36(Suppl 2):1S-18S.
237. Update: Universal precautions for prevention of transmission of human immunodeficiency virus, hepatitis B virus, and other bloodborne pathogens in health-care settings. MMWR Morb Mortal Wkly Rep 1988;37:377-382, 87-88.
238. Edmond M: Isolation. Infect Control Hosp Epidemiol 1997;18:58-64.
239. Occupational exposure to bloodborne pathogens—OSHA. Final rule. Fed Regist 1991;56:64004-64182.
240. Burke JF, Quinby WC, Bondoc CC, et al: The contribution of a bacterially isolated environment to the prevention of infection in seriously burned patients. Ann Surg 1977; 186:377-387.
241. Johnson S, Gerding DN, Olson MM, et al: Prospective, controlled study of vinyl glove use to interrupt *Clostridium*

difficile nosocomial transmission. Am J Med 1990;88:137-140.
242. Maki DG: Through a glass darkly. Nosocomial pseudoepidemics and pseudobacteremias. Arch Intern Med 1980;140:26-28.
243. Doebbeling BN, Pfaller MA, Houston AK, Wenzel RP: Removal of nosocomial pathogens from the contaminated glove. Implications for glove reuse and handwashing. Ann Intern Med 1988;109:394-398.
244. Maki DG, McCormick RD, Zilz MA, et al: A MRSA outbreak in an SICU during universal precautions: New epidemiology for nosocomial MRSA: Downside for universal precautions. In Proceedings and Abstracts of the 30th Interscience Conference on Antimicrobial Agents and Chemotherapy; 1990, Atlanta, American Society for Microbiology, 1990.
245. Bubak ME, Reed CE, Fransway AF, et al: Allergic reactions to latex among health-care workers. Mayo Clin Proc 1992;67:1075-1079.
246. Kennedy PB, Gwaltney JMJ: Brief report: The detection of blood on gloved hands of central sterile supply personnel and cleaned instruments used for procedures on patient units. Infect Control Hosp Epidemiol 1988;9:117-118.
247. Neu HC: The crisis in antibiotic resistance. Science 1992;257: 1064-1073.
248. Kunin CM: Resistance to antimicrobial drugs—a worldwide calamity. Ann Intern Med 1993;118:557-561.
249. Jarvis WR: Nosocomial outbreaks: the Centers for Disease Control's Hospital Infections Program experience, 1980-1990. Epidemiology Branch, Hospital Infections Program. Am J Med 1991;91:101S-106S.
250. Martone WJ, Jarvis WR, Culver DH, et al: Incidence and nature of endemic and epidemic nosocomial infections. In Bennett JE, Brachman PS (eds): Hospital Infections, 3rd ed. Boston, Little, Brown, 1992.
251. Davies J: Inactivation of antibiotics and the dissemination of resistance genes. Science 1994;264:375-382.
252. Marr JJ, Moffet HL, Kunin CM: Guidelines for improving the use of antimicrobial agents in hospitals: A statement by the Infectious Diseases Society of America. J Infect Dis 1988;157:869-876.
253. Dellit TH, Owens RC, McGowan JE Jr, et al: Infectious Diseases Society of America and the Society for Healthcare Epidemiology of America guidelines for developing an institutional program to enhance antimicrobial stewardship. Clin Infect Dis 2007;44:159-177.
254. Avorn J, Harvey K, Soumerai SB, et al: Information and education as determinants of antibiotic use: Report of Task Force 5. Rev Infect Dis 1987;9: S286-296.
255. Collier J, Foster J: Management of a restricted drugs policy in hospital: The first five years' experience. Lancet 1986;2:331.
256. Bartlett JC: Pocketbook of Infectious Disease Therapy. Baltimore, Williams & Wilkins, 1993.
257. Sanford JP, Gilbert DN: Guide to Antimicrobial Therapy. Dallas, Antimicrobial Therapy, 1994.
258. Mangram AJ, Horan TC, Pearson ML, et al: Guideline for Prevention of Surgical Site Infection, 1999. Centers for Disease Control and Prevention (CDC) Hospital Infection Control Practices Advisory Committee. Am J Infect Control 1999;27:97-132.
259. DiPiro JT, Cheung RP, Bowden TA Jr, Mansberger JA: Single dose systemic antibiotic prophylaxis of surgical wound infections. Am J Surg 1986;152:552-559.
260. Maki DG, Tambyah PA: Engineering out the risk for infection with urinary catheters. Emerg Infect Dis 2001;7:342-347.
261. National Kidney Foundation: III. NKF-K/DOQI Clinical Practice Guidelines for Vascular Access: Update 2000. Am J Kidney Dis 2001;37(1 Suppl 1): S137-181.
262. Maki D, Mermel L: Infections due to infusion therapy. In Bennett JV, Brachman PS (eds): Hospital Infections, 4th ed. Philadelphia, Lippincott-Raven, 1998, pp 689-724.
263. Mermel LA: Prevention of intravascular catheter-related infections. Ann Intern Med 2000;132:391-402.
264. Pittet D, Tarara D, Wenzel RP: Nosocomial bloodstream infection in critically ill patients. Excess length of stay, extra costs, and attributable mortality. JAMA 1994;271:1598-1601.
265. Digiovine B, Chenoweth C, Watts C, Higgins M: The attributable mortality and costs of primary nosocomial bloodstream infections in the intensive care unit. Am J Respir Crit Care Med 1999;160:976-981.
266. Soufir L, Timsit JF, Mahe C, et al: Attributable morbidity and mortality of catheter-related septicemia in critically ill patients: A matched, risk-adjusted, cohort study. Infect Control Hosp Epidemiol 1999;20:396-401.
267. Rello J, Ochagavia A, Sabanes E, et al: Evaluation of outcome of intravenous catheter-related infections in critically ill patients. Am J Respir Crit Care Med 2000;162:1027-1030.
268. Maki DG, Stolz SM, Wheeler S, Mermel LA: Prevention of central venous catheter-related bloodstream infection by use of an antiseptic-impregnated catheter. A randomized, controlled trial. Ann Intern Med 1997;127:257-266.
269. Raad I, Darouiche R, Dupuis J, et al: Central venous catheters coated with minocycline and rifampin for the prevention of catheter-related colonization and bloodstream infections. A randomized, double-blind trial. Ann Intern Med 1997;127: 267-274.
270. O'Grady NP, Barie PS, Bartlett J, et al: Practice parameters for evaluating new fever in critically ill adult patients. Crit Care Med 1998;26:392-408.
271. Mermel LA, Farr BM, Sherertz RJ, et al: Guidelines for the management of intravascular catheter-related infections. Clin Infect Dis 2001; 32:1249-1272.
272. Safdar N, Maki DG: Inflammation at the insertion site is not predictive of catheter-related bloodstream infection with short-term, noncuffed central venous catheters. Crit Care Med 2002;30:2632-2635.
273. Mermel LA, Maki DG: Detection of bacteremia in adults: Consequences of culturing an inadequate volume of blood. Ann Intern Med 1993;119:270-272.
274. Dobbins BM, Kite P, Wilcox MH: Diagnosis of central venous catheter related sepsis—a critical look inside. J Clin Pathol 1999;52:165-172.
275. Weinstein MP, Murphy JR, Reller LB, Lichtenstein KA: The clinical significance of positive blood cultures: A comprehensive analysis of 500 episodes of bacteremia and fungemia in adults. II. Clinical observations, with special reference to factors influencing prognosis. Rev Infect Dis 1983;5: 54-70.
276. Gaur AH, Giannini MA, Flynn PM, et al: Optimizing blood culture practices in pediatric immunocompromised patients: Evaluation of media types and blood culture volume. Pediatr Infect Dis J 2003;22:545-552.
277. DesJardin J, Falagas M, Ruthazer R, et al: Clinical utility of blood cultures drawn from indwelling central venous catheters in hospitalized patients with cancer. Ann Intern Med 1999;131: 641-647.
278. Norberg A, Christopher NC, Ramundo ML, et al: Contamination rates of blood cultures obtained by dedicated phlebotomy vs intravenous catheter. JAMA 2003;289:726-729.
279. Robinson JL: Sensitivity of a blood culture drawn through a single lumen of a multilumen, long-term, indwelling, central venous catheter in pediatric oncology patients. J Pediatr Hematol Onc 2002;24:72-74.
280. Bates DW, Goldman L, Lee TH: Contaminant blood cultures and resource utilization. The true consequences of false-positive results. JAMA 1991;265:365-369.
281. Little JR, Murray PR, Traynor PS, Spitznagel E: A randomized trial of povidone-iodine compared with iodine tincture for venipuncture site disinfection: Effects on rates of blood culture contamination. Am J Med 1999;107:119-125.
282. Strand CL, Wajsbort RR, Sturmann K: Effect of iodophor vs iodine tincture skin preparation on blood culture contamination rate. JAMA 1993;269: 1004-1006.
283. Herwaldt LA, Geiss M, Kao C, Pfaller MA: The positive predictive value of isolating coagulase-negative staphylococci from blood cultures. Clin Infect Dis 1996;22:14-20.
284. Finkelstein R, Fusman R, Oren I, et al: Clinical and epidemiologic significance of coagulase-negative staphylococci bacteremia in a tertiary care university Israeli hospital. Am J Infect Control 2002;30:21-25.
285. Maki DG, Jarrett F, Sarafin HW: A semiquantitative culture method for identification of catheter-related infection in the burn patient. J Surg Res 1977;22:513-520.
286. Raad, II, Sabbagh MF, Rand KH, Sherertz RJ: Quantitative tip culture methods and the diagnosis of central venous catheter-related infections.

Diagn Microbiol Infect Dis 1992;15:13-20.
287. Siegman-Igra Y, Anglim AM, Shapiro DE, et al: Diagnosis of vascular catheter-related bloodstream infection: A meta-analysis. J Clin Microbiol 1997;35:928-936.
288. Kristinsson KG, Burnett IA, Spencer RC: Evaluation of three methods for culturing long intravascular catheters. J Hosp Infect 1989;14:183-191.
289. Safdar N, Fine JP, Maki DG: Meta-analysis: methods for diagnosing intravascular device-related bloodstream infection. Ann Intern Med 2005;142:451-466.
290. Collignon P, Chan R, Munro R: Rapid diagnosis of intravascular catheter-related sepsis. Arch Intern Med 1987;147:1609-1612.
291. Darouiche RO, Raad II, Heard SO, et al: A comparison of two antimicrobial-impregnated central venous catheters. N Engl J Med 1999;340:1-8.
292. Ryan JJ, Abel R, Abbott W, et al: Catheter complications in total parenteral nutrition. A prospective study of 200 consecutive patients. N Engl J Med 1974;290:757-761.
293. Sitzmann JV, Townsend TR, Siler MC, Bartlett JG: Septic and technical complications of central venous catheterization. A prospective study of 200 consecutive patients. Ann Surg 1985;202:766-770.
294. Tacconelli E, Tumbarello M, Pittiruti M, et al: Central venous catheter-related sepsis in a cohort of 366 hospitalised patients. Eur J Clin Microbiol Infect Dis 1997;16:203-209.
295. Gowardman JR, Montgomery C, Thirlwell S, et al: Central venous catheter-related bloodstream infections: An analysis of incidence and risk factors in a cohort of 400 patients. Intensive Care Med 1998;24:1034-1039.
296. Blot F, Nitenberg G, Chachaty E, et al: Diagnosis of catheter-related bacteraemia: A prospective comparison of the time to positivity of hub-blood versus peripheral-blood cultures. Lancet 1999;354:1071-1077.
297. Rijnders BJ, Verwaest C, Peetermans WE, et al: Difference in time to positivity of hub-blood versus nonhub-blood cultures is not useful for the diagnosis of catheter-related bloodstream infection in critically ill patients. Crit Care Med 2001;29: 1399-1403.
298. Maki DG, Kluger DM, Crnich CJ: The risk of bloodstream infection in adults with different intravascular devices: A systematic review of 200 published prospective studies. Mayo Clin Proc 2006;81:1159-1171.
299. Safdar N, Maki DG: The risk of catheter-related bloodstream infection with peripherally-inserted central venous catheters used in inpatients [abstract #K-1435]. In Abstracts and Proceedings from the 41st International Conference of Antimicrobial Agents and Chemotherapy. [abstract #K-1435]: Washington, DC, American Society of Microbiology, 2001, p 428.
300. Safdar N, Maki DG: The incidence and pathogenesis of catheter-related bloodstream infection with arterial catheters [abstract #K-81]. In Abstracts and Proceedings from the 42nd Interscience Conference on Antimicrobial Agents and Chemotherapy. Washington, DC, American Society of Microbiology, 2002, p 299.
301. Crnich CJ, Maki DG: The promise of novel technology for the prevention of intravascular device-related bloodstream infection. I. Pathogenesis and short-term devices. Clin Infect Dis 2002;34:1232-1242.
302. Maki DG, Cobb L, Garman JK, et al: An attachable silver-impregnated cuff for prevention of infection with central venous catheters: A prospective randomized multicenter trial. Am J Med 1988;85:307-314.
303. Mermel LA, McCormick RD, Springman SR, Maki DG: The pathogenesis and epidemiology of catheter-related infection with pulmonary artery Swan-Ganz catheters: A prospective study utilizing molecular subtyping. Am J Med 1991;91:197S-205S.
304. Linares J, Sitges-Serra A, Garau J, et al: Pathogenesis of catheter sepsis: A prospective study with quantitative and semiquantitative cultures of catheter hub and segments. J Clin Microbiol 1985;21:357-360.
305. Raad I, Costerton W, Sabharwal U, et al: Ultrastructural analysis of indwelling vascular catheters: A quantitative relationship between luminal colonization and duration of placement. J Infect Dis 1993;168: 400-407.
306. Maki D, Ringer M: Prospective study of arterial catheter-related infection: Incidence, sources of infection and risk factors [abstract]. In Abstracts and Proceedings from the 29th Interscience Conference on Antimicrobial Agents and Chemotherapy. Washington, DC, American Society of Microbiology, 1989, p 1075.
307. Maki DG, Klein BS, McCormick RD, et al: Nosocomial *Pseudomonas pickettii* bacteremias traced to narcotic tampering. A case for selective drug screening of health care personnel. JAMA 1991;265:981-986.
308. Maki D: The epidemiology and prevention of nosocomial bloodstream infections [abstract]. In Programs and Abstracts of the Third International Conference on Nosocomial Infections. Washington, DC, American Society of Microbiology, 1990, p 3.
309. Safdar N, Kluger DM, Maki DG: A review of risk factors for catheter-related bloodstream infection caused by percutaneously inserted, noncuffed central venous catheters: Implications for preventive strategies. Medicine 2002;81:466-479.
310. Crnich CJ, Maki DG: Infections caused by intravascular devices: Epidemiology, pathogenesis, diagnosis, prevention, and treatment. In APIC Text of Infection Control and Epidemiology, 2nd ed. Washington, DC, Association for Professionals in Infection Control and Epidemiology, 2005, p 24.1-6.
311. Merrer J, De Jonghe B, Golliot F, et al: Complications of femoral and subclavian venous catheterization in critically ill patients: A randomized controlled trial. JAMA 2001;286: 700-707.
312. Robert J, Fridkin SK, Blumberg HM, et al: The influence of the composition of the nursing staff on primary bloodstream infection rates in a surgical intensive care unit. Infect Control Hosp Epidemiol 2000;21: 12-17.
313. Maki DG, Kluger DM, Crnich CJ: The microbiology of intravascular device-related (IVDR) infection in adults: An analysis of 159 prospective studies and implications for prevention and treatment [abstract]. In Abstracts and Proceedings from the 40th Annual Meeting of the Infectious Disease Society of America. Chicago, Infectious Disease Society of America, 2002.
314. Dezfulian C, Lavelle J, Nallamothu BK, et al: Rates of infection for single-lumen versus multilumen central venous catheters: A meta-analysis. Crit Care Med 2003;31:2385-2390.
315. Goetz AM, Wagener MM, Miller JM, Muder RR: Risk of infection due to central venous catheters: Effect of site of placement and catheter type. Infect Control Hosp Epidemiol 1998;19:842-845.
316. Moss AH, Vasilakis C, Holley JL, et al: Use of a silicone dual-lumen catheter with a Dacron cuff as a long-term vascular access for hemodialysis patients. Am J Kidney Dis 1990;16: 211-215.
317. Oliver MJ, Callery SM, Thorpe KE, et al: Risk of bacteremia from temporary hemodialysis catheters by site of insertion and duration of use: A prospective study. Kidney Int 2000;58:2543-2545.
318. Cimochowski GE, Worley E, Rutherford WE, et al: Superiority of the internal jugular over the subclavian access for temporary dialysis. Nephron 1990;54:154-161.
319. Schillinger F, Schillinger D, Montagnac R, Milcent T: Post catheterisation vein stenosis in haemodialysis: Comparative angiographic study of 50 subclavian and 50 internal jugular accesses. Nephrol Dial Transplant 1991;6: 722-724.
320. Raad, II, Hohn DC, Gilbreath BJ, et al: Prevention of central venous catheter-related infections by using maximal sterile barrier precautions during insertion. Infect Control Hosp Epidemiol 1994;15:231-238.
321. Rijnders BJ, Van Wijngaerden E, Wilmer A, Peetermans WE: Use of full sterile barrier precautions during insertion of arterial catheters: A randomized trial. Clin Infect Dis 2003;36:743-748.
322. Tomford JW, Hershey CO, McLaren CE, et al: Intravenous therapy team and peripheral venous catheter-associated complications. A prospective controlled study. Arch Intern Med 1984;144:1191-1194.
323. Soifer NE, Borzak S, Edlin BR, Weinstein RA: Prevention of peripheral venous catheter complications with an intravenous therapy team: A randomized controlled trial. Arch Intern Med 1998;158:473-477.
324. Sherertz RJ, Ely EW, Westbrook DM, et al: Education of physicians-in-training can decrease the risk for

vascular catheter infection. Ann Intern Med 2000;132:641-648.
325. Eggimann P, Harbarth S, Constantin M, et al: Impact of a prevention strategy targeted at vascular-access care on incidence of infections acquired in intensive care. Lancet 2000;355:1864-1868.
326. Maki DG, Knasinski V, Narans LL, Gordon BJ: A randomized trial of a novel 1% chlorhexidine-75% alcohol tincture versus 10% povidone-iodine for cutaneous disinfection with vascular catheters [abstract #142]. In Abstracts and Proceedings from the 31st Annual Society for Healthcare Epidemiology of America Meeting. Toronto, Society for Healthcare Epidemiology of America, 2001, p 70.
327. Maki D, Will L: Colonization and infection associated with transparent dressings for central venous, arterial, and Hickman catheters: A comparative trial [abstract #1241]. In Abstracts and Proceedings from the 24th Interscience Conference on Antimicrobial Agents and Chemotherapy. Washington, DC, American Society of Microbiology, 1984, p 991.
328. Maki DG, Stolz SS, Wheeler S, Mermel LA: A prospective, randomized trial of gauze and two polyurethane dressings for site care of pulmonary artery catheters: Implications for catheter management. Crit Care Med 1994;22:1729-1737.
329. Maki D, Mermel LA, Martin M, et al: A highly semipermeable polyurethane dressing does not increase the risk of CVC-related BSI: A prospective, multicenter, investigator-blinded trial [abstract J-64]. In Abstracts and Proceedings from the 36th Interscience Conference on Antimicrobial Agents and Chemotherapy. Washington, DC, American Society for Microbiology, 1996, p 230.
330. Ricard P, Martin R, Marcoux JA: Protection on indwelling vascular catheters: Incidence of bacterial contamination and catheter-related sepsis. Crit Care Med 1985;13: 541-543.
331. Maki DG, Band JD: A comparative study of polyantibiotic and iodophor ointments in prevention of vascular catheter-related infection. Am J Med 1981;70:739-744.
332. Flowers RHd, Schwenzer KJ, Kopel RF, et al: Efficacy of an attachable subcutaneous cuff for the prevention of intravascular catheter-related infection. A randomized, controlled trial. JAMA 1989;261:878-883.
333. Hill RL, Fisher AP, Ware RJ, et al: Mupirocin for the reduction of colonization of internal jugular cannulae—a randomized controlled trial. J Hosp Infect 1990;15:311-321.
334. Sesso R, Barbosa D, Leme IL, et al: *Staphylococcus aureus* prophylaxis in hemodialysis patients using central venous catheter: Effect of mupirocin ointment. J Am Soc Nephrol 1998;9:1085-1092.
335. Miller MA, Dascal A, Portnoy J, Mendelson J: Development of mupirocin resistance among methicillin-resistant *Staphylococcus aureus* after widespread use of nasal mupirocin ointment. Infect Control Hosp Epidemiol 1996;17:811-813.
336. Zakrzewska-Bode A, Muytjens HL, Liem KD, Hoogkamp-Korstanje JA: Mupirocin resistance in coagulase-negative staphylococci, after topical prophylaxis for the reduction of colonization of central venous catheters. J Hosp Infect 1995;31: 189-193.
337. Perez-Fontan M, Rosales M, Rodriguez-Carmona A, et al: Mupirocin resistance after long-term use for *Staphylococcus aureus* colonization in patients undergoing chronic peritoneal dialysis. Am J Kidney Dis 2002;39:337-341.
338. Prager RL, Silva J: Colonization of central venous catheters. South Med J 1984;77:458-461.
339. Maki D, Will L: Study of polyantibiotic and povidone-iodine ointments on central venous and arterial catheter sites dressed with gauze or polyurethane dressing [abstract]. In Abstracts and Proceedings from the 26th Interscience Conference on Antimicrobial Agents and Chemotherapy. Washington, DC, American Society of Microbiology, 1986, p 1041.
340. Levin A, Mason AJ, Jindal KK, et al: Prevention of hemodialysis subclavian vein catheter infections by topical povidone-iodine. Kidney Int 1991;40: 934-938.
341. Lai KK: Safety of prolonging peripheral cannula and i.v. tubing use from 72 hours to 96 hours. Am J Infect Control 1998;26:66-70.
342. Bregenzer T, Conen D, Sakmann P, Widmer AF: Is routine replacement of peripheral intravenous catheters necessary? Arch Intern Med 1998;158: 151-156.
343. Pujol M, Hornero A, Saballs M, et al: Clinical epidemiology of bacteremia due to peripheral vascular catheter infections. In 43rd International Conference on Antimicrobial Agents and Chemotherapy [abstract K-2040]; 2003. Washington, DC, American Society of Microbiology, 2003.
344. Cobb DK, High KP, Sawyer RG, et al: A controlled trial of scheduled replacement of central venous and pulmonary-artery catheters. N Engl J Med 1992;327:1062-1068.
345. Cook D, Randolph A, Kernerman P, et al: Central venous catheter replacement strategies: A systematic review of the literature. Crit Care Med 1997;25:1417-1424.
346. Robinson D, Suhocki P, Schwab SJ: Treatment of infected tunneled venous access hemodialysis catheters with guidewire exchange. Kidney Int 1998;53:1792-1794.
347. Beathard GA: Management of bacteremia associated with tunneled-cuffed hemodialysis catheters. J Am Soc Nephrol 1999;10:1045-1049.
348. Maki DG, Hassemer CA: Endemic rate of fluid contamination and related septicemia in arterial pressure monitoring. Am J Med 1981;70:733-738.
349. Maki DG, Goldman DA, Rhame FS: Infection control in intravenous therapy. Ann Intern Med 1973;79:867-887.
350. Maki DG, Botticelli JT, LeRoy ML, Thielke TS: Prospective study of replacing administration sets for intravenous therapy at 48- vs 72-hour intervals. 72 hours is safe and cost-effective. JAMA 1987;258:1777-1781.
351. Luskin RL, Weinstein RA, Nathan C, et al: Extended use of disposable pressure transducers: A bacteriologic evaluation. JAMA 1986;255:916-920.
352. Shinozaki T, Deane RS, Mazuzan JE Jr, et al: Bacterial contamination of arterial lines. A prospective study. JAMA 1983;249:223-225.
353. Raad, II, Luna M, Khalil SA, et al: The relationship between the thrombotic and infectious complications of central venous catheters. JAMA 1994;271:1014-1016.
354. Mehall JR, Saltzman DA, Jackson RJ, Smith SD: Fibrin sheath enhances central venous catheter infection. Crit Care Med 2002;30:908-912.
355. Boraks P, Seale J, Price J, et al: Prevention of central venous catheter associated thrombosis using minidose warfarin in patients with haematological malignancies. Br J Haematol 1998;101:483-486.
356. Bern MM, Lokich JJ, Wallach SR, et al: Very low doses of warfarin can prevent thrombosis in central venous catheters. A randomized prospective trial. Ann Intern Med 1990;112: 423-428.
357. Randolph AG, Cook DJ, Gonzales CA, Andrew M: Benefit of heparin in peripheral venous and arterial catheters: Systematic review and meta-analysis of randomised controlled trials. BMJ 1998;316:969-975.
358. Mermel LA, Maki DG: Infectious complications of Swan-Ganz pulmonary artery catheters. Pathogenesis, epidemiology, prevention, and management. Am J Respir Crit Care Med 1994;149: 1020-1036.
359. Mermel LA, Stolz SM, Maki DG: Surface antimicrobial activity of heparin-bonded and antiseptic-impregnated vascular catheters. J Infect Dis 1993;167:920-924.
360. Crnich CJ, Maki DG: The promise of novel technology for the prevention of intravascular device-related bloodstream infection. II. Long-term devices. Clin Infect Dis 2002;34: 1362-1368.
361. Schears GJ: Summary of product trials for 10,164 patients: Comparing an intravenous stabilizing device to tape. J Infus Nurs 2006;29:225-231.
362. Yamamoto AJ, Solomon JA, Soulen MC, et al: Sutureless securement device reduces complications of peripherally inserted central venous catheters. J Vasc Interv Radiol 2002;13:77-81.
363. Cooper GL, Schiller AL, Hopkins CC: Possible role of capillary action in pathogenesis of experimental catheter-associated dermal tunnel infections. J Clin Microbiol 1988;26:8-12.
364. Maki DG, Mermel LA, Kluger DM, et al: The efficacy of a chlorhexidine-impregnated sponge (biopatch) for the prevention of intravascular catheter-related infection—a prospective, randomized, controlled, multicenter trial [abstract #1430]. In

Abstracts and Proceedings from the 40th Interscience Conference on Antimicrobial Agents and Chemotherapy. Washington, DC, American Society for Microbiology, 2000, p 422.
365. Garland JS, Alex CP, Mueller CD, et al: A randomized trial comparing povidone-iodine to a chlorhexidine gluconate-impregnated dressing for prevention of central venous catheter infections in neonates. Pediatrics 2001;107:1431-1436.
366. Crnich CJ, Maki DG: Are antimicrobial-impregnated catheters effective? When does repetition reach the point of exhaustion? Clin Infect Dis 2005;41: 681-685.
367. Crnich CJ, Maki DG: Are antimicrobial-impregnated catheters effective? Don't throw out the baby with the bathwater. Clin Infect Dis 2004;38: 1287-1292.
368. Veenstra DL, Saint S, Saha S, et al: Efficacy of antiseptic-impregnated central venous catheters in preventing catheter-related bloodstream infection: A meta-analysis. JAMA 1999;281: 261-267.
369. Marin MG, Lee JC, Skurnick JH: Prevention of nosocomial bloodstream infections: Effectiveness of antimicrobial-impregnated and heparin-bonded central venous catheters. Crit Care Med 2000;28: 3332-3338.
370. Veenstra DL, Saint S, Sullivan SD: Cost-effectiveness of antiseptic-impregnated central venous catheters for the prevention of catheter-related bloodstream infection. JAMA 1999;282:554-560.
371. Shorr AF, Humphreys CW, Helman DL: New choices for central venous catheters. Chest 2003;124:275-284.
372. Saint S: Prevention of intravascular catheter-associated infections. In Shojania KG, Duncan BW, McDonald KM, Wachter RM (eds): Making Health Care Safer: A Critical Analysis of Patient Safety Practices. Rockville, Md, Agency for Healthcare Research and Quality, 2001, pp 163-184.
373. Henrickson KJ, Axtell RA, Hoover SM, et al: Prevention of central venous catheter-related infections and thrombotic events in immunocompromised children by the use of vancomycin/ciprofloxacin/heparin flush solution: A randomized, multicenter, double-blind trial. J Clin Oncol 2000;18:1269-1278.
374. Garland JS, Alex CP, Henrickson KJ, et al: A vancomycin-heparin lock solution for prevention of nosocomial bloodstream infection in critically ill neonates with peripherally inserted central venous catheters: A prospective, randomized trial. Pediatrics 2005;116:e198-205.
375. Dogra GK, Herson H, Hutchison B, et al: Prevention of tunneled hemodialysis catheter-related infections using catheter-restricted filling with gentamicin and citrate: A randomized controlled study. J Am Soc Nephrol 2002;13:2133-2139.
376. Raad I, Hachem R, Tcholakian RK, Sherertz R: Efficacy of minocycline and EDTA lock solution in preventing catheter-related bacteremia, septic phlebitis, and endocarditis in rabbits. Antimicrob Agents Chemother 2002;46:327-332.
377. Maki DG, Crnich CJ, Safdar N: Successful use of a 25% alcohol lock solution for prevention of recurrent CVC-related bloodstream infection in a patient on home TNA [abstract #K-671]. In Abstracts and Proceedings from the 42nd Interscience Conference on Antimicrobial Agents and Chemotherapy. Washington, DC, American Society for Microbiology, 2002, p 320.
378. Allon M: Prophylaxis against dialysis catheter-related bacteremia with a novel antimicrobial lock solution. Clin Infect Dis 2003;36: 1539-1544.
379. Segura M, Alia C, Valverde J, et al: Assessment of a new hub design and the semiquantitative catheter culture method using an in vivo experimental model of catheter sepsis. J Clin Microbiol 1990;28:2551-2554.
380. Segura M, Alvarez-Lerma F, Tellado JM, et al: A clinical trial on the prevention of catheter-related sepsis using a new hub model. Ann Surg 1996;223: 363-369.
381. Leon C, Alvarez-Lerma F, Ruiz-Santana S, et al: Antiseptic chamber-containing hub reduces central venous catheter-related infection: A prospective, randomized study. Crit Care Med 2003;31:1318-1324.
382. Luna J, Masdeu G, Perez M, et al: Clinical trial evaluating a new hub device designed to prevent catheter-related sepsis. Eur J Clin Microbiol Infect Dis 2000;19:655-662.
383. Guidelines for the management of adults with hospital-acquired, ventilator-associated, and healthcare-associated pneumonia. Am J Respir Crit Care Med 2005;171:388-416.
384. McEachern R, Campbell GD Jr: Hospital-acquired pneumonia: Epidemiology, etiology, and treatment. Infect Dis Clin North Am 1998;12: 761-779.
385. Safdar N, Dezfulian C, Collard HR, Saint S: Clinical and economic consequences of ventilator-associated pneumonia: A systematic review. Crit Care Med 2005;33:2184-2193.
386. Gross PA, Neu HC, Aswapokee P, et al: Deaths from nosocomial infections: Experience in a university hospital and a community hospital. Am J Med 1980;68:219-223.
387. Zhang P, Summer WR, Bagby GJ, Nelson S: Innate immunity and pulmonary host defense. Immunol Rev 2000;173:39-51.
388. Laurenzi GA, Potter RT, Kass EH: Bacteriologic flora of the lower respiratory tract. N Engl J Med 1961;265:1273-1278.
389. Lillehoj ER, Kim KC: Airway mucus: Its components and function. Arch Pharm Res 2002;25:770-780.
390. Salathe M, Wanner A: Nonspecific host defenses: Mucociliary clearance and cough. In Niederman M (ed): Respiratory Infections. Philadelphia, Saunders, 1994, pp 17-32.
391. Zeiher BG, Hornick DB: Pathogenesis of respiratory infections and host defenses. Curr Opin Pulm Med 1996;2:166-173.
392. Strieter RM, Belperio JA, Keane MP: Host innate defenses in the lung: The role of cytokines. Curr Opin Infect Dis 2003;16:193-198.
393. Johanson WG, Pierce AK, Sanford JP: Changing pharyngeal bacterial flora of hospitalized patients. Emergence of gram-negative bacilli. N Engl J Med 1969;281:1137-1140.
394. Sigalet DL, Mackenzie SL, Hameed SM: Enteral nutrition and mucosal immunity: implications for feeding strategies in surgery and trauma. Can J Surg 2004;47:109-116.
395. Safdar N, Crnich CJ, Maki DG: The pathogenesis of ventilator-associated pneumonia: Its relevance to developing effective strategies for prevention. Respir Care 2005;50:725-739; discussion 39-41.
396. de Latorre FJ, Pont T, Ferrer A, et al: Pattern of tracheal colonization during mechanical ventilation. Am J Respir Crit Care Med 1995;152:1028-1033.
397. George DL, Falk PS, Wunderink RG, et al: Epidemiology of ventilator-acquired pneumonia based on protected bronchoscopic sampling. Am J Respir Crit Care Med 1998;158:1839-1847.
398. Ewig S, Torres A, El-Ebiary M, et al: Bacterial colonization patterns in mechanically ventilated patients with traumatic and medical head injury. Incidence, risk factors, and association with ventilator-associated pneumonia. Am J Respir Crit Care Med 1999;159: 188-198.
399. Hamill RJ, Houston ED, Georghiou PR, et al: An outbreak of Burkholderia (formerly Pseudomonas) cepacia respiratory tract colonization and infection associated with nebulized albuterol therapy. Ann Intern Med 1995;122:762-766.
400. Estes RJ, Meduri GU: The pathogenesis of ventilator-associated pneumonia: I. Mechanisms of bacterial transcolonization and airway inoculation. Intensive Care Med 1995;21:365-383.
401. Alcon A, Fabregas N, Torres A: Hospital-acquired pneumonia: Etiologic considerations. Infect Dis Clin North Am 2003;17:679-695.
402. Bonten MJ, Gaillard CA, de Leeuw PW, Stobberingh EE: Role of colonization of the upper intestinal tract in the pathogenesis of ventilator-associated pneumonia. Clin Infect Dis 1997;24: 309-319.
403. Bonten MJ, Kullberg BJ, van Dalen R, et al: Selective digestive decontamination in patients in intensive care. The Dutch Working Group on Antibiotic Policy. J Antimicrob Chemother 2000;46: 351-362.
404. Pugin J, Auckenthaler R, Lew DP, Suter PM: Oropharyngeal decontamination decreases incidence of ventilator-associated pneumonia. A randomized, placebo-controlled, double-blind clinical trial. JAMA 1991;265: 2704-2710.
405. Bergmans DC, Bonten MJ, Gaillard CA, et al: Prevention of ventilator-associated pneumonia by oral decontamination: A prospective, randomized, double-blind, placebo-controlled study. Am J Resp Crit Care Med 2001;164:382-388.

406. Koeman M, van der Ven AJ, Hak E, et al: Oral decontamination with chlorhexidine reduces the incidence of ventilator-associated pneumonia. Am J Respir Crit Care Med 2006;173:1348-1355.
407. Chlebicki MP, Safdar N: Topical chlorhexidine for prevention of ventilator-associated pneumonia: A meta-analysis. Crit Care Med 2007;35:595-602.
408. Meduri GU, Estes RJ: The pathogenesis of ventilator-associated pneumonia: II. The lower respiratory tract. Intensive Care Med 1995;21:452-461.
409. Park DR: The microbiology of ventilator-associated pneumonia. Respir Care 2005;50:742-763.
410. Chastre J, Fagon JY: Ventilator-associated pneumonia. Am J Resp Crit Care Med 2002;165:867-903.
411. Johanson WG Jr, Pierce AK, Sanford JP, Thomas GD: Nosocomial respiratory infections with gram-negative bacilli. The significance of colonization of the respiratory tract. Ann Intern Med 1972;77:701-706.
412. Fagon JY, Chastre J, Hance AJ, et al: Evaluation of clinical judgment in the identification and treatment of nosocomial pneumonia in ventilated patients. Chest 1993;103:547-553.
413. Montravers P, Fagon JY, Chastre J, et al: Follow-up protected specimen brushes to assess treatment in nosocomial pneumonia. Am Rev Respir Dis 1993;147:38-44.
414. Cook DJ, Fitzgerald JM, Guyatt GH, Walter S: Evaluation of the protected brush catheter and bronchoalveolar lavage in the diagnosis of nosocomial pneumonia. J Intensiv Care Med 1991;6:196-205.
415. Cook DJ, Brun-Buisson C, Guyatt GH, Sibbald WJ: Evaluation of new diagnostic technologies: Bronchoalveolar lavage and the diagnosis of ventilator-associated pneumonia. Crit Care Med 1994;22: 1314-1322.
416. Torres A, El-Ebiary M: Bronchoscopic BAL in the diagnosis of ventilator-associated pneumonia. Chest 2000;117(4 Suppl 2):198S-202S.
417. Shorr AF, Sherner JH, Jackson WL, Kollef MH: Invasive approaches to the diagnosis of ventilator-associated pneumonia: A meta-analysis. Crit Care Med 2005;33:46-53.
418. Pugin J, Auckenthaler R, Mili N, et al: Diagnosis of ventilator-associated pneumonia by bacteriologic analysis of bronchoscopic and nonbronchoscopic "blind" bronchoalveolar lavage fluid. Am Rev Respir Dis 1991;143: 1121-1129.
419. Fabregas N, Ewig S, Torres A, et al: Clinical diagnosis of ventilator associated pneumonia revisited: Comparative validation using immediate post-mortem lung biopsies. Thorax 1999;54:867-873.
420. Fagon JY, Chastre J, Wolff M, et al: Invasive and noninvasive strategies for management of suspected ventilator-associated pneumonia. A randomized trial. Ann Intern Med 2000;132:621-630.
421. Heyland D, Dodek P, Muscedere J, Day A: A randomized trial of diagnostic techniques for ventilator-associated pneumonia. N Engl J Med 2006;355: 2619-2630.
422. Kollef MH: Diagnosis of ventilator-associated pneumonia. N Engl J Med 2006;355:2691-2693.
423. Cunnion KM, Weber DJ, Broadhead WE, et al: Risk factors for nosocomial pneumonia: Comparing adult critical-care populations. Am J Respir Crit Care Med 1996;153:158-162.
424. Trouillet JL, Chastre J, Vuagnat A, et al: Ventilator-associated pneumonia caused by potentially drug-resistant bacteria. Am J Resp Crit Care Med 1998;157:531-539.
425. Torres A, Gatell JM, Aznar E, et al: Re-intubation increases the risk of nosocomial pneumonia in patients needing mechanical ventilation. Am J Resp Crit Care Med 1995;152: 137-141.
426. Fourrier F, Duvivier B, Boutigny H, et al: Colonization of dental plaque: A source of nosocomial infections in intensive care unit patients. Crit Care Med 1998;26:301-308.
427. du Moulin GC, Paterson DG, Hedley-Whyte J, Lisbon A: Aspiration of gastric bacteria in antacid-treated patients: A frequent cause of postoperative colonisation of the airway. Lancet 1982;1:242-245.
428. Daschner F, Reuschenbach K, Pfisterer J, et al: The effect of stress ulcer prevention on the incidence of pneumonia in artificial respiration. Anaesthetist 1987;36:9-18.
429. Cook D, Guyatt G, Marshall J, et al: A comparison of sucralfate and ranitidine for the prevention of upper gastrointestinal bleeding in patients requiring mechanical ventilation. Canadian Critical Care Trials Group. N Engl J Med 1998;338:791-797.
430. Joshi N, Localio AR, Hamory BH: A predictive risk index for nosocomial pneumonia in the intensive care unit. Am J Med 1992;93:135-142.
431. Torres A, Serra-Batlles J, Ros E, et al: Pulmonary aspiration of gastric contents in patients receiving mechanical ventilation: The effect of body position. Ann Intern Med 1992;116:540-543.
432. Schweickert WD, Gehlbach BK, Pohlman AS, et al: Daily interruption of sedative infusions and complications of critical illness in mechanically ventilated patients. Crit Care Med 2004;32:1272-1276.
433. Taylor RW, Manganaro L, O'Brien J, et al: Impact of allogenic packed red blood cell transfusion on nosocomial infection rates in the critically ill patient. Crit Care Med 2002;30: 2249-2254.
434. Dodek P, Keenan S, Cook D, et al: Evidence-based clinical practice guideline for the prevention of ventilator-associated pneumonia. Ann Intern Med 2004;141:305-313.
435. Kollef MH: The prevention of ventilator-associated pneumonia. N Engl J Med 1999;340:627-634.
436. Brochard L, Mancebo J, Wysocki M, et al: Noninvasive ventilation for acute exacerbations of chronic obstructive pulmonary disease. N Engl J Med 1995;333:817-822.
437. Girou E, Schortgen F, Delclaux C, et al: Association of noninvasive ventilation with nosocomial infections and survival in critically ill patients. JAMA 2000;284:2361-2367.
438. Ely EW, Baker AM, Dunagan DP, et al: Effect on the duration of mechanical ventilation of identifying patients capable of breathing spontaneously. N Engl J Med 1996;335:1864-1869.
439. Kollef MH, Shapiro SD, Silver P, et al: A randomized, controlled trial of protocol-directed versus physician-directed weaning from mechanical ventilation. Crit Care Med 1997;25: 567-574.
440. Dries DJ, McGonigal MD, Malian MS, et al: Protocol-driven ventilator weaning reduces use of mechanical ventilation, rate of early reintubation, and ventilator-associated pneumonia. J Trauma 2004;56:943-951.
441. McLean SE, Jensen LA, Schroeder DG, et al: Improving adherence to a mechanical ventilation weaning protocol for critically ill adults: Outcomes after an implementation program. Am J Crit Care 2006;15: 299-309.
442. Rodriguez JL, Steinberg SM, Luchetti FA, et al: Early tracheostomy for primary airway management in the surgical critical care setting. Surgery 1990;108:655-659.
443. Drakulovic MB, Torres A, Bauer TT, et al: Supine body position as a risk factor for nosocomial pneumonia in mechanically ventilated patients: A randomised trial. Lancet 1999;354: 1851-1858.
444. van Nieuwenhoven CA, Vandenbroucke-Grauls C, van Tiel FH, et al: Feasibility and effects of the semirecumbent position to prevent ventilator-associated pneumonia: A randomized study. Crit Care Med 2006;34:396-402.
445. Schleder B, Stott K, Lloyd RC: The effect of a comprehensive oral care protocol on patients at risk for ventilator-associated pneumonia. J Advocate Health Care 2002;4:27-30.
446. Binkley C, Furr LA, Carrico R, McCurren C: Survey of oral care practices in US intensive care units. Am J Infect Control 2004;32:161-169.
447. Cutler CJ, Davis N: Improving oral care in patients receiving mechanical ventilation. Am J Crit Care 2005;14:389-394.
448. Valles J, Artigas A, Rello J, et al: Continuous aspiration of subglottic secretions in preventing ventilator-associated pneumonia. Ann Intern Med 1995;122:179-186.
449. Kollef MH, Skubas NJ, Sundt TM: A randomized clinical trial of continuous aspiration of subglottic secretions in cardiac surgery patients. Chest 1999;116:1339-1346.
450. Cook D, Ricard JD, Reeve B, et al: Ventilator circuit and secretion management strategies: A Franco-Canadian survey. Crit Care Med 2000;28:3547-3554.
451. Kirton OC, DeHaven B, Morgan J, et al: A prospective, randomized comparison of an in-line heat moisture exchange filter and heated wire humidifiers: Rates of ventilator-associated early-onset (community-acquired) or late-onset (hospital-acquired) pneumonia and

incidence of endotracheal tube occlusion. Chest 1997;112:1055-1059.
452. Cook D, De Jonghe B, Brochard L, Brun-Buisson C: Influence of airway management on ventilator-associated pneumonia: Evidence from randomized trials. JAMA 1998;279:781-787.
453. Kollef MH, Shapiro SD, Boyd V, et al: A randomized clinical trial comparing an extended-use hygroscopic condenser humidifier with heated-water humidification in mechanically ventilated patients. Chest 1998;113:759-767.
454. Collard HR, Saint S, Matthay MA: Prevention of ventilator-associated pneumonia: An evidence-based systematic review. Ann Intern Med 2003;138:494-501.
455. Mayhall CG: The Trach Care closed tracheal suction system: A new medical device to permit tracheal suctioning without interruption of ventilatory assistance. Infect Control Hosp Epidemiol 1988;9:125-126.
456. Deppe SA, Kelly JW, Thoi LL, et al: Incidence of colonization, nosocomial pneumonia, and mortality in critically ill patients using a Trach Care closed-suction system versus an open-suction system: Prospective, randomized study. Crit Care Med 1990;18:1389-1393.
457. Johnson KL, Kearney PA, Johnson SB, et al: Closed versus open endotracheal suctioning: costs and physiologic consequences. Crit Care Med 1994;22:658-666.
458. Combes P, Fauvage B, Oleyer C: Nosocomial pneumonia in mechanically ventilated patients, a prospective randomised evaluation of the Stericath closed suctioning system. Intensive Care Med 2000;26:878-882.
459. Kollef MH, Prentice D, Shapiro SD, et al: Mechanical ventilation with or without daily changes of in-line suction catheters. Am J Resp Crit Care Med 1997;156(2 Pt 1):466-472.
460. Bonten MJ, Gaillard CA, van der Geest S, et al: The role of intragastric acidity and stress ulcus prophylaxis on colonization and infection in mechanically ventilated ICU patients. A stratified, randomized, double-blind study of sucralfate versus antacids. Am J Respir Crit Care Med 1995;152:1825-1834.
461. Thomason MH, Payseur ES, Hakenewerth AM, et al: Nosocomial pneumonia in ventilated trauma patients during stress ulcer prophylaxis with sucralfate, antacid, and ranitidine. J Trauma 1996;41:503-508.
462. Silvestri L, Petros AJ, Viviani M, et al: Selective decontamination of the digestive tract and ventilator-associated pneumonia (part 1). Respir Care 2006;51:67-69; author reply 70-72.
463. van Saene HK, Damjanovic V, Silvestri L, et al: Selective decontamination of the digestive tract and ventilator-associated pneumonia (part 2). Respir Care 2006;51:72-75.
464. Bonten MJ: Selective digestive tract decontamination—will it prevent infection with multidrug-resistant gram-negative pathogens but still be applicable in institutions where methicillin-resistant *Staphylococcus aureus* and vancomycin-resistant enterococci are endemic? Clin Infect Dis 2006;43(Suppl 2):S70-74.
465. Bonten MJ, Krueger WA: Selective decontamination of the digestive tract: Cumulating evidence, at last? Semin Respir Crit Care Med 2006;27:18-22.
466. DeRiso AJ II, Ladowski JS, Dillon TA, et al: Chlorhexidine gluconate 0.12% oral rinse reduces the incidence of total nosocomial respiratory infection and nonprophylactic systemic antibiotic use in patients undergoing heart surgery. Chest 1996;109:1556-1561.
467. Houston S, Hougland P, Anderson JJ, et al: Effectiveness of 0.12% chlorhexidine gluconate oral rinse in reducing prevalence of nosocomial pneumonia in patients undergoing heart surgery. Am J Crit Care 2002;11:567-570.
468. Warren JW: The catheter and urinary tract infection. Med Clin North Am 1991;75:481-493.
469. Bryan CS, Reynolds KL: Hospital-acquired bacteremic urinary tract infection: Epidemiology and outcome. J Urol 1984;132:494-498.
470. Platt R, Polk BF, Murdock B, Rosner B: Reduction of mortality associated with nosocomial urinary tract infection. Lancet 1983;1:893-897.
471. Tambyah PA, Maki DG: Catheter-associated urinary tract infection is rarely symptomatic: A prospective study of 1497 catheterized patients. Arch Intern Med 2000;160:678-682.
472. Tambyah PA, Knasinski V, Maki DG: The direct costs of nosocomial catheter-associated urinary tract infection in the era of managed care. Infect Control Hosp Epidemiol 2002;23:27-31.
473. Nicolle LE: Catheter-related urinary tract infection. Drug Aging 2005;22:627-639.
474. Wazait HD, Patel HR, Veer V, et al: Catheter-associated urinary tract infections: Prevalence of uropathogens and pattern of antimicrobial resistance in a UK hospital (1996-2001). BJU Int 2003;91:806-809.
475. Tambyah PA, Halvorson KT, Maki DG: A prospective study of pathogenesis of catheter-associated urinary tract infections. Mayo Clin Proc 1999;74:131-136.
476. Saint S, Chenoweth CE: Biofilms and catheter-associated urinary tract infections. Infect Dis Clin North Am 2003;17:411-432.
477. Johnson JR, Kuskowski MA, Wilt TJ: Systematic review: Antimicrobial urinary catheters to prevent catheter-associated urinary tract infection in hospitalized patients. Ann Intern Med 2006;144:116-126.
478. Maki DG, Knasinski V, Halvorson KT, et al: A prospective, randomized, investigator-blinded trial of a novel nitrofurazone-impregnated urinary catheter [abstract M49]. Infect Control Hosp Epidemiol 1997;18(Suppl):50.
479. Darouiche RO, Smith JA Jr, Hanna H, et al: Efficacy of antimicrobial-impregnated bladder catheters in reducing catheter-associated bacteriuria: A prospective, randomized, multicenter clinical trial. Urology 1999;54:976-981.
480. Saint S, Elmore JG, Sullivan SD, et al: The efficacy of silver alloy-coated urinary catheters in preventing urinary tract infection: A meta-analysis. Am J Med 1998;105:236-241.
481. Wright GD: The antibiotic resistome: The nexus of chemical and genetic diversity. Nat Rev Microbiol 2007;5:175-186.
482. Lautenbach E, Fishman NO, Bilker WB, et al: Risk factors for fluoroquinolone resistance in nosocomial *Escherichia coli* and *Klebsiella pneumoniae* infections. Arch Intern Med 2002;162:2469-2477.
483. Lautenbach E, Strom BL, Bilker WB, et al: Epidemiological investigation of fluoroquinolone resistance in infections due to extended-spectrum beta-lactamase-producing *Escherichia coli* and *Klebsiella pneumoniae.* Clin Infect Dis 2001;33:1288-1294.
484. Fraser GL, Stogsdill P, Dickens JD Jr, et al: Antibiotic optimization. An evaluation of patient safety and economic outcomes. Arch Intern Med 1997;157:1689-1694.
485. Solomon DH, Van Houten L, Glynn RJ, et al: Academic detailing to improve use of broad-spectrum antibiotics at an academic medical center. Arch Intern Med 2001;161:1897-1902.
486. Pear SM, Williamson TH, Bettin KM, et al: Decrease in nosocomial *Clostridium difficile*–associated diarrhea by restricting clindamycin use. Ann Intern Med 1994;120:272-277.
487. Quale J, Landman D, Saurina G, et al: Manipulation of a hospital antimicrobial formulary to control an outbreak of vancomycin-resistant enterococci. Clin Infect Dis 1996;23:1020-1025.
488. Lautenbach E, LaRosa LA, Marr AM, et al: Changes in the prevalence of vancomycin-resistant enterococci in response to antimicrobial formulary interventions: Impact of progressive restrictions on use of vancomycin and third-generation cephalosporins. Clin Infect Dis 2003;36:440-446.
489. Bantar C, Sartori B, Vesco E, et al: A hospitalwide intervention program to optimize the quality of antibiotic use: Impact on prescribing practice, antibiotic consumption, cost savings, and bacterial resistance. Clin Infect Dis 2003;37:180-186.
490. Warren DK, Hill HA, Merz LR, et al: Cycling empirical antimicrobial agents to prevent emergence of antimicrobial-resistant gram-negative bacteria among intensive care unit patients. Crit Care Med 2004;32:2450-2456.
491. Merz LR, Warren DK, Kollef MH, et al: The impact of an antibiotic cycling program on empirical therapy for gram-negative infections. Chest 2006;130:1672-1678.
492. McGowan JE Jr: Minimizing antimicrobial resistance in hospital bacteria: Can switching or cycling drugs help? Infect Control 1986;7:573-576.
493. Gerding DN: Antimicrobial cycling: lessons learned from the aminoglycoside experience. Infect

Control Hosp Epidemiol 2000;21(1 Suppl):S12-17.
494. Bonhoeffer S, Lipsitch M, Levin BR: Evaluating treatment protocols to prevent antibiotic resistance. Proc Natl Acad Sci U S A 1997;94:12106-12111.
495. Durbin WA Jr, Lapidas B, Goldmann DA: Improved antibiotic usage following introduction of a novel prescription system. JAMA 1981;246:1796-1800.
496. Kollef MH: Hospital-acquired pneumonia and de-escalation of antimicrobial treatment. Crit Care Med 2001;29:1473-1475.
497. Kollef MH: Providing appropriate antimicrobial therapy in the intensive care unit: Surveillance vs. de-escalation. Crit Care Med 2006;34:903-905.
498. Burke JP, Pestotnik SL: Antibiotic use and microbial resistance in intensive care units: Impact of computer-assisted decision support. J Chemother 1999;11:530-535.
499. Evans RS, Classen DC, Pestotnik SL, et al: A decision support tool for antibiotic therapy. Proc Annu Symp Comput Appl Med Care 1995:651-655.
500. Stoutenbeek CP, van Saene HK: Prevention of pneumonia by selective decontamination of the digestive tract (SDD). Intensive Care Med 1992;18(Suppl 1):S18-23.
501. van Saene HK, Stoutenbeek CC, Stoller JK: Selective decontamination of the digestive tract in the intensive care unit: Current status and future prospects. Crit Care Med 1992;20:691-703.
502. Vandenbroucke-Grauls CM, Vandenbroucke JP: Effect of selective decontamination of the digestive tract on respiratory tract infections and mortality in the intensive care unit. Lancet 1991;338:859-862.
503. Meta-analysis of randomised controlled trials of selective decontamination of the digestive tract. Selective Decontamination of the Digestive Tract Trialists' Collaborative Group. BMJ 1993;307:525-532.
504. Kollef MH: The role of selective digestive tract decontamination on mortality and respiratory tract infections. A meta-analysis. Chest 1994;105:1101-1108.
505. Heyland DK, Cook DJ, Jaeschke R, et al: Selective decontamination of the digestive tract. An overview. Chest 1994;105:1221-1229.
506. Hurley JC: Prophylaxis with enteral antibiotics in ventilated patients: Selective decontamination or selective cross-infection? Antimicrob Agents Chemother 1995;39:941-947.
507. D'Amico R, Pifferi S, Leonetti C, et al: Effectiveness of antibiotic prophylaxis in critically ill adult patients: Systematic review of randomised controlled trials. BMJ 1998;316: 1275-1285.
508. Nathens AB, Marshall JC: Selective decontamination of the digestive tract in surgical patients: A systematic review of the evidence. Arch Surg 1999;134:170-176.
509. Safdar N, Said A, Lucey MR: The role of selective digestive decontamination for reducing infection in patients undergoing liver transplantation: A systematic review and meta-analysis. Liver Transpl 2004;10:817-827.
510. Liberati A, D'Amico R, Pifferi, et al: Antibiotic prophylaxis to reduce respiratory tract infections and mortality in adults receiving intensive care. Cochrane Database Syst Rev 2004(1):CD000022.
511. Silvestri L, van Saene HK, Milanese M, Gregori D: Impact of selective decontamination of the digestive tract on fungal carriage and infection: Systematic review of randomized controlled trials. Intensive Care Med 2005;31:898-910.
512. Silvestri L, van Saene HK, Milanese M, et al: Selective decontamination of the digestive tract reduces bacterial bloodstream infection and mortality in critically ill patients. Systematic review of randomized, controlled trials. J Hosp Infect 2007;65:187-203.
513. van Nieuwenhoven CA, Buskens E, van Tiel FH, Bonten MJ: Relationship between methodological trial quality and the effects of selective digestive decontamination on pneumonia and mortality in critically ill patients. JAMA 2001;286:335-340.
514. Lingnau W, Berger J, Javorsky F, et al: Changing bacterial ecology during a five-year period of selective intestinal decontamination. J Hosp Infect 1998;39:195-206.
515. Leone M, Albanese J, Antonini F, et al: Long-term (6-year) effect of selective digestive decontamination on antimicrobial resistance in intensive care, multiple-trauma patients. Crit Care Med 2003;31:2090-2095.
516. Saunders GL, Hammond JM, Potgieter PD, et al: Microbiological surveillance during selective decontamination of the digestive tract (SDD). J Antimicrob Chemother 1994;34:529-544.
517. Paterson DL, Singh N, Rihs JD, et al: Control of an outbreak of infection due to extended-spectrum beta-lactamase—producing *Escherichia coli* in a liver transplantation unit. Clin Infect Dis 2001;33:126-128.
518. Dezfulian C, Shojania K, Collard HR, et al: Subglottic secretion drainage for preventing ventilator-associated pneumonia: A meta-analysis. Am J Med 2005;118:11-18.
519. Haley RW, Bregman DA: The role of understaffing and overcrowding in recurrent outbreaks of staphylococcal infection in a neonatal special-care unit. J Infect Dis 1982;145:875-885.
520. Levine AS, Siegel SE, Schreiber AD, et al: Protected environments and prophylactic antibiotics. A prospective controlled study of their utility in the therapy of acute leukemia. N Engl J Med 1973;288:477-483.
521. Evans HE, Akpata SO, Baki A, Behrman RE: Bacteriologic and clinical evaluation of gowning in a premature nursery. J Pediatr 1971;78:883-886.
522. Agbayani M, Rosenfeld W, Evans H, et al: Evaluation of modified gowning procedures in a neonatal intensive care unit. Am J Dis Child 1981;135: 650-652.
523. Donowitz LG: Failure of the overgown to prevent nosocomial infection in a pediatric intensive care unit. Pediatrics 1986;77:35-38.
524. Artru F, Brun Y, Firholz P, Deleuze R: Prevention of hospital-acquired infection. Efficacy of isolation procedures in a neurological intensive care unit (ICU). Nouv Presse Med 1979;8:1065-1069.
525. Maki DG, Zilz MA, McComick R: The effectiveness of using preemptive barrier precautions routinely (protective isolation) in all high-risk patients to prevent nosocomial infection with resistant organisms, especially MRSA, VRE and C. difficile. In Abstracts and Proceedings of the 34th Annual Meeting of the Infectious Disease Society of North America; 1996. New Orleans, Infectious Disease Society of America, 1996.
526. van Voorhis J, Destefano L, Sobek S, et al: Impact of barrier precautions and cohorting on a monoclonal outbreak of vancomycin-resistant enterococcus faecium (VRE). In Abstracts and Proceedings of the 7th Annual Meeting of the Society for Healthcare Epidemiology of America; 1997. St. Louis, Society for Healthcare Epidemiology of America, 1997.
527. Klein BS, Perloff WH, Maki DG: Reduction of nosocomial infection during pediatric intensive care by protective isolation. N Engl J Med 1989;320:1714-1721.
528. Slota M, Green M, Farley A, et al: The role of gown and glove isolation and strict handwashing in the reduction of nosocomial infection in children with solid organ transplantation. Crit Care Med 2001;29:405-412.
529. McManus AT, Goodwin CW, Pruitt BA Jr: Observations on the risk of resistance with the extended use of vancomycin. Arch Surg 1998;133:1207-1211.
530. Koss WG, Khalili TM, Lemus JF, et al: Nosocomial pneumonia is not prevented by protective contact isolation in the surgical intensive care unit. Am Surg 2001;67:1140-1144.
531. Slaughter S, Hayden MK, Nathan C, et al: A comparison of the effect of universal use of gloves and gowns with that of glove use alone on acquisition of vancomycin-resistant enterococci in a medical intensive care unit. Ann Intern Med 1996; 125:448-456.
532. Safdar N, Marx J, Meyer N, Maki DG: The effectiveness of preemptive enhanced barrier precautions for controlling MRSA in a burn unit. In Abstracts and Proceedings of the 43rd InterScience Conference on Antimicrobial Agents and Chemotherapy; 2003. Chicago, American Society of Microbiology, 2003.
533. Srinivasan A, Song X, Ross T, et al: A prospective study to determine whether cover gowns in addition to gloves decrease nosocomial transmission of vancomycin-resistant enterococci in an intensive care unit. Infect Control Hosp Epidemiol 2002;23:424-428.
534. Montecalvo MA, Jarvis WR, Uman J, et al: Infection-control measures reduce transmission of vancomycin-resistant enterococci in an endemic setting. Ann Intern Med 1999;131:269-272.

535. Morris JG Jr, Shay DK, Hebden JN, et al: Enterococci resistant to multiple antimicrobial agents, including vancomycin. Establishment of endemicity in a university medical center. Ann Intern Med 1995;123: 250-259.
536. Castaldo P, Stratta RJ, Wood RP, et al: Clinical spectrum of fungal infections after orthotopic liver transplantation. Arch Surg 1991;126:149-156.
537. Maki DG, Ringer M: Evaluation of dressing regimens for prevention of infection with peripheral intravenous catheters. Gauze, a transparent polyurethane dressing, and an iodophor-transparent dressing. JAMA 1987;258:2396-2403.
538. Patterson WB, Craven DE, Schwartz DA, et al: Occupational hazards to hospital personnel. Ann Intern Med 1985;102:658-680.
539. Gestal JJ: Occupational hazards in hospitals: Risk of infection. Br J Ind Med 1987;44:435-442.
540. Rogers B: Health hazards in nursing and health care: An overview. Am J Infect Control 1997;25:248-261.
541. Nora Jr JJ, Doebbeling BN: New vaccines and vaccination programs for hospital staff members. In Wenzel RP (ed): Prevention and Control of Nosocomial Infections, 4th ed. Philadelphia, Lippincott Williams & Wilkins, 2003, pp 413-429.
542. Immunization of health-care workers: Recommendations of the Advisory Committee on Immunization Practices (ACIP) and the Hospital Infection Control Practices Advisory Committee (HICPAC). MMWR Recomm Rep 1997;46(RR-18):1-42.
543. McCormick RD, Meisch MG, Ircink FG, Maki DG: Epidemiology of hospital sharps injuries: A 14-year prospective study in the pre-AIDS and AIDS eras. Am J Med 1991;91:301S-307S.
544. Lee JM, Botteman MF, Nicklasson L, et al: Needlestick injury in acute care nurses caring for patients with diabetes mellitus: A retrospective study. Curr Med Res Opin 2005;21: 741-747.
545. Haiduven DJ, DeMaio TM, Stevens DA: A five-year study of needlestick injuries: Significant reduction associated with communication, education, and convenient placement of sharps containers. Infect Control Hosp Epidemiol 1992;13:265-271.
546. Tuma S, Sepkowitz KA: Efficacy of safety-engineered device implementation in the prevention of percutaneous injuries: A review of published studies. Clin Infect Dis 2006;42:1159-1170.
547. Goldwater PN, Law R, Nixon AD, et al: Impact of a recapping device on venepuncture-related needlestick injury. Infect Control Hosp Epidemiol 1989;10:21-25.
548. McCormick RD, Maki DG: Epidemiology of needle-stick injuries in hospital personnel. Am J Med 1981;70:928-932.
549. van Loon FP, Holmes SJ, Sirotkin BI, et al: Mumps surveillance—United States, 1988-1993. MMWR CDC Surveill Summ 1995;44:1-14.
550. Centers for Disease Control and Prevention: Epidemiology of measles—United States, 2001-2003. MMWR Morb Mortal Wkly Rep 2004;53: 713-716.
551. Centers for Disease Control and Prevention: Elimination of rubella and congenital rubella syndrome—United States, 1969-2004. MMWR Morb Mortal Wkly Rep 2005;54:279-282.
552. Centers for Disease Control and Prevention: Measles—United States, 2005. MMWR Morb Mortal Wkly Rep 2006;55:1348-1351.
553. Centers for Disease Control and Prevention: Update: Multistate outbreak of mumps—United States, January 1-May 2, 2006. MMWR Morb Mortal Wkly Rep 2006;55:559-563.
554. Davis RM, Orenstein WA, Frank JA Jr, et al: Transmission of measles in medical settings. 1980 through 1984. JAMA 1986;255:1295-1298.
555. Watson JC, Hadler SC, Dykewicz CA, et al: Measles, mumps, and rubella—vaccine use and strategies for elimination of measles, rubella, and congenital rubella syndrome and control of mumps: Recommendations of the Advisory Committee on Immunization Practices (ACIP). MMWR Recomm Rep 1998;47:1-57.
556. Weber DJ, Rutala WA, Hamilton H: Prevention and control of varicella-zoster infections in healthcare facilities. Infect Control Hosp Epidemiol 1996;17:694-705.
557. Choo PW, Donahue JG, Manson JE, Platt R: The epidemiology of varicella and its complications. J Infect Dis 1995;172:706-712.
558. Enders G, Miller E, Cradock-Watson J, et al: Consequences of varicella and herpes zoster in pregnancy: Prospective study of 1739 cases. Lancet 1994;343:1548-1551.
559. Prevention of varicella: Recommendations of the Advisory Committee on Immunization Practices (ACIP). Centers for Disease Control and Prevention. MMWR Recomm Rep 1996;45:1-36.
560. Prevention of varicella. Update recommendations of the Advisory Committee on Immunization Practices (ACIP). MMWR Recomm Rep 1999;48:1-5.
561. Bridges CB, Harper SA, Fukuda K, et al: Prevention and control of influenza. Recommendations of the Advisory Committee on Immunization Practices (ACIP). MMWR Recomm Rep 2003;52:1-34; quiz CE1-4.
562. Salgado CD, Farr BM, Hall KK, Hayden FG: Influenza in the acute hospital setting. Lancet Infect Dis 2002;2: 145-155.
563. Stott DJ, Kerr G, Carman WF: Nosocomial transmission of influenza. Occup Med 2002;52:249-253.
564. Dash GP, Fauerbach L, Pfeiffer J, et al: APIC position paper: Improving health care worker influenza immunization rates. Am J Infect Control 2004;32: 123-125.
565. Nichol KL, Lind A, Margolis KL, et al: The effectiveness of vaccination against influenza in healthy, working adults. N Engl J Med 1995;333:889-893.
566. Wilde JA, McMillan JA, Serwint J, et al: Effectiveness of influenza vaccine in health care professionals: A randomized trial. JAMA 1999;281: 908-913.
567. Nichol KL, Hauge M: Influenza vaccination of healthcare workers. Infect Control Hosp Epidemiol 1997;18:189-194.
568. Canning HS, Phillips J, Allsup S: Health care worker beliefs about influenza vaccine and reasons for non-vaccination—a cross-sectional survey. J Clin Nurs 2005;14:922-925.
569. Carman WF, Elder AG, Wallace LA, et al: Effects of influenza vaccination of health-care workers on mortality of elderly people in long-term care: A randomised controlled trial. Lancet 2000;355:93-97.
570. Salgado CD, Giannetta ET, Hayden FG, Farr BM: Preventing nosocomial influenza by improving the vaccine acceptance rate of clinicians. Infect Control Hosp Epidemiol 2004;25: 923-928.
571. Hayward AC, Harling R, Wetten S, et al: Effectiveness of an influenza vaccine programme for care home staff to prevent death, morbidity, and health service use among residents: Cluster randomised controlled trial. BMJ 2006;333:1241.
572. Burls A, Jordan R, Barton P, et al: Vaccinating healthcare workers against influenza to protect the vulnerable—is it a good use of healthcare resources? A systematic review of the evidence and an economic evaluation. Vaccine 2006;24:4212-4221.
573. Walker FJ, Singleton JA, Lu P, et al: Influenza vaccination of healthcare workers in the United States, 1989-2002. Infect Control Hosp Epidemiol 2006;27:257-265.
574. Hoffmann CJ, Perl TM: The next battleground for patient safety: Influenza immunization of healthcare workers. Infect Control Hosp Epidemiol 2005;26:850-851.
575. Wendelboe AM, Van Rie A, Salmaso S, Englund JA: Duration of immunity against pertussis after natural infection or vaccination. Pediatr Infect Dis J 2005;24(5 Suppl):S58-61.
576. Centers for Disease Control and Prevention: Pertussis outbreak among adults at an oil refinery—Illinois, August-October 2002. MMWR Morb Mortal Wkly Rep 2003;52:1-4.
577. Calugar A, Ortega-Sanchez IR, Tiwari T, et al: Nosocomial pertussis: Costs of an outbreak and benefits of vaccinating health care workers. Clin Infect Dis 2006;42:981-988.
578. Ward A, Caro J, Bassinet L, et al: Health and economic consequences of an outbreak of pertussis among healthcare workers in a hospital in France. Infect Control Hosp Epidemiol 2005;26:288-292.
579. Rusk J: ACIP recommends Tdap vaccine for health care workers. Infectious Disease News 2006. Available at http://www.infectiousdiseasenews.com/200603/frameset.asp?article-tdap.asp (Accessed July 5, 2007)
580. Adams G, Stover BH, Keenlyside RA, et al: Nosocomial herpetic infections in a pediatric intensive care unit. Am J Epidemiol 1981;113:126-132.
581. Klotz RW: Herpetic whitlow: An occupational hazard. AANA J 1990;58:8-13.

582. Glassroth J, Crnich CJ: Pulmonary infections caused by mycobacterial species. In Crapo JD, Glassroth J, Karlinsky JB, King TE (eds): Baum's Textbook of Pulmonary Diseases, 7th ed. Philadelphia, Lippincott Williams & Wilkins, 2003.
583. Butt AA, Singh N: Hepatitis C: Prevention, therapy, and role of transplantation. In Wenzel RP (ed): Prevention and Control of Nosocomial Infections, 4th ed. Philadelphia, Lippincott Williams & Wilkins, 2003, pp 215-228.
584. Jagger J, De Carli G, Perry JL, et al: Occupational exposure to blood-borne pathogens: Epidemiology and prevention. In Wenzel RP (ed): Prevention and Control of Nosocomial Infections, 4th ed. Philadelphia, Lippincott Williams & Wilkins, 2003, pp 430-466.
585. Polish LB, Tong MJ, Co RL, et al: Risk factors for hepatitis C virus infection among health care personnel in a community hospital. Am J Infect Control 1993;21:196-200.
586. Wiegand J, Buggisch P, Boecher W, et al: Early monotherapy with pegylated interferon alpha-2b for acute hepatitis C infection: The HEP-NET acute-HCV-II study. Hepatology 2006;43:250-256.
587. Jaeckel E, Cornberg M, Wedemeyer H, et al: Treatment of acute hepatitis C with interferon alfa-2b. N Engl J Med 2001;345:1452-1457.
588. Centers for Disease Control and Prevention: Surveillance of healthcare personnel with HIV/AIDS, as of December 2002. Available at http://www.cdc.gov/ncidod/dhqp/bp_hiv_hp_with.html Accessed January 15, 2007.
589. Oksenhendler E, Harzic M, Le Roux JM, et al: HIV infection with seroconversion after a superficial needlestick injury to the finger. N Engl J Med 1986;315:582.
590. Black RJ: Animal studies of prophylaxis. Am J Med 1997;102:39-44.
591. Cardo DM, Culver DH, Ciesielski CA, et al: A case-control study of HIV seroconversion in health care workers after percutaneous exposure. Centers for Disease Control and Prevention Needlestick Surveillance Group. N Engl J Med 1997;337:1485-1490.
592. Panlilio AL, Cardo DM, Grohskopf LA, et al: Updated U.S. Public Health Service guidelines for the management of occupational exposures to HIV and recommendations for postexposure prophylaxis. MMWR Recomm Rep 2005;54:1-17.
593. Maki DG: Risk factors for nosocomial infection in intensive care. "Devices vs. nature" and goals for the next decade. Arch Intern Med 1989;149:30-35.
594. Decker LA, Gross A, Miller FC, et al: A rapid method for the presurgical cleansing of hands. Obstet Gynecol 1978;51:115-117.
595. Vesley D, Langholz AC, Timmermann TA: Evaluation of a mechanical handwashing device with germicidal and non-germicidal products. In Program and Abstracts of the 15th Annual Meeting of the Association for the Professionals in Infection Control; 1988. Dallas, Association for the Professionals of Infection Control, 1988.
596. Maki DG, McCormick R, Alvarado CJ, et al: Clinical evaluation of the degerming efficacy of seven agents for handwashing in hospitals. In Program and Abstracts of the 24th Interscience Conference on Antimicrobial Agents and Chemotherapy; 1984. Washington, DC, American Society for Microbiology, 1984.
597. Morrison AJ Jr, Gratz J, Cabezudo I, Wenzel RP: The efficacy of several new handwashing agents for removing non-transient bacterial flora from hands. Infect Control 1986;7:268-272.
598. Soifer N, Edlin B, Weinstein R, Group MIS: A randomized IV team trial [abstract]. In Abstracts and Proceedings from the 29th Interscience Conference on Antimicrobial Agents and Chemotherapy. Washington, DC, American Society of Medicine, 1989, p 1076.
599. Hemming VG, Overall JC Jr, Britt MR: Nosocomial infections in a newborn intensive-care unit. Results of forty-one months of surveillance. N Engl J Med 1976;294:1310-1316.
600. Kirkland KB, Briggs JP, Trivette SL, et al: The impact of surgical-site infections in the 1990s: Attributable mortality, excess length of hospitalization, and extra costs. Infect Control Hosp Epidemiol 1999;20:725-730.
601. Whitehouse JD, Friedman ND, Kirkland KB, et al: The impact of surgical-site infections following orthopedic surgery at a community hospital and a university hospital: Adverse quality of life, excess length of stay, and extra cost. Infect Control Hosp Epidemiol 2002;23:183-189.
602. Hollenbeak CS, Murphy DM, Koenig S, et al: The clinical and economic impact of deep chest surgical site infections following coronary artery bypass graft surgery. Chest 2000;118:397-402.
603. McGarry SA, Engemann JJ, Schmader K, et al: Surgical-site infection due to *Staphylococcus aureus* among elderly patients: Mortality, duration of hospitalization, and cost. Infect Control Hosp Epidemiol 2004;25:461-467.
604. Herwaldt LA, Cullen JJ, Scholz D, et al: A prospective study of outcomes, healthcare resource utilization, and costs associated with postoperative nosocomial infections. Infect Control Hosp Epidemiol 2006;27:1291-1298.
605. Fagon JY, Chastre J, Hance AJ, et al: Nosocomial pneumonia in ventilated patients: A cohort study evaluating attributable mortality and hospital stay. Am J Med 1993;94:281-288.
606. Heyland DK, Cook DJ, Griffith L, et al: The attributable morbidity and mortality of ventilator-associated pneumonia in the critically ill patient. The Canadian Critical Trials Group. Am J Respir Crit Care Med 1999;159:1249-1256.
607. Bercault N, Boulain T: Mortality rate attributable to ventilator-associated nosocomial pneumonia in an adult intensive care unit: A prospective case-control study. Crit Care Med 2001;29:2303-2309.
608. Rello J, Ollendorf DA, Oster G, et al: Epidemiology and outcomes of ventilator-associated pneumonia in a large US database. Chest 2002;122:2115-2121.
609. Warren DK, Shukla SJ, Olsen MA, et al: Outcome and attributable cost of ventilator-associated pneumonia among intensive care unit patients in a suburban medical center. Crit Care Med 2003;31:1312-1317.
610. Cocanour CS, Ostrosky-Zeichner L, Peninger M, et al: Cost of a ventilator-associated pneumonia in a shock trauma intensive care unit. Surg Infect 2005;6:65-72.
611. Slonim AD, Kurtines HC, Sprague BM, Singh N: The costs associated with nosocomial bloodstream infections in the pediatric intensive care unit. Pediatr Crit Care Med 2001;2:170-174.
612. Warren DK, Quadir WW, Hollenbeak CS, et al: Attributable cost of catheter-associated bloodstream infections among intensive care patients in a nonteaching hospital. Crit Care Med 2006;34:2084-2089.
613. Mullett MD, Cook EF, Gallagher R: Nosocomial sepsis in the neonatal intensive care unit. J Perinatol 1998;18:112-115.
614. McManus AT, Mason AD Jr, McManus WF, Pruitt BA Jr: A decade of reduced gram-negative infections and mortality associated with improved isolation of burned patients. Arch Surg 1994;129:1306-1309.

Chapter 52

Principles Governing Antimicrobial Therapy in the Intensive Care Unit

John Godke and George Karam

For many years, classic approaches to infectious diseases centered on recognition of pathogens involved in a disease process and the selection of antibiotic therapy based on the susceptibility of the organism. Recent years have brought increasing awareness of a broader set of concepts that affect clinical outcomes and should therefore influence antibiotic prescribing. Playing a pivotal role in this change has been an evolving worldwide epidemic of antibiotic resistance, at a time when development of new classes of antibiotics, especially those directed at multidrug-resistant gram-negative pathogens, is not occurring to a significant degree.[1] In the era of what the Infectious Diseases Society of America (IDSA) has termed "bad bugs, no drugs,"[2] much attention has been directed toward a process of *antibiotic stewardship,* which is based on adherence to variables in antibiotic use that result in optimal clinical outcomes while simultaneously preserving the efficacy of antimicrobial agents that exist today. In a joint 2007 guideline paper for the development of an institutional program to enhance antimicrobial stewardship, the IDSA and the Society for Healthcare Epidemiology of America (SHEA) wrote on the importance of education as an essential element in any program designed to influence prescribing behavior.[3] This chapter focuses on the elements of antibiotic stewardship that play a clinically relevant role in the use of antibiotics prescribed to patients in intensive care units (ICUs).

In the critical care setting, the selection of optimal antibiotic therapy often entails a two-stage process: empiric therapy, followed by directed therapy once the pathogen and type of infection are clearly identified. Figure 52-1 incorporates this progression in antibiotic therapy and summarizes some principles that contribute to the overall goal of preserving the antibiotic armamentarium while simultaneously attempting to achieve optimal clinical efficacy—the components of antibiotic stewardship. A challenge for the critical care physician is to recognize that antibiotic therapy for critically ill patients has potential ramifications for other patients in that unit over the weeks to follow. If antibiotic-resistant organisms or organisms with certain virulence factors are selected by some pattern of antibiotic use, those pathogens can become part of the ICU's ecology and can then be transmitted to other patients over a period that may span weeks. See Figure 52-2 for clinical examples of the principles of empiric therapy. In recognition of such complications that may be imposed by antibiotic therapy, this chapter discusses those variables that influence both empiric therapy and directed therapy. Knowledge of these variables is essential in clinical practice and can serve as the basis for the insights necessary for an enhanced level of antibiotic prescribing.

ADEQUACY OF INITIAL EMPIRIC ANTIBIOTIC THERAPY

An important question in the management of patients with serious infections is whether any modifiable variables exist that have a positive impact on clinical outcome. For many years, the impression was that antibiotic therapy could be adjusted at day 2 or 3 into a clinical course once either bacterial susceptibility was known or the clinical course of the patient had been defined, with no negative aspects of such changes. Beginning in the 1990s, several reports challenging this tenet were published regarding such infectious disease processes as sepsis and ventilator-associated pneumonia (VAP).[4-9] In these reports, the term *inadequate* was used to describe those situations in which the organism causing an infection was not covered, as indicated by in vitro susceptibility, by the antibiotic regimen initially ordered. The published studies were characterized by variability in sample size, inconclusiveness regarding whether organisms isolated were true

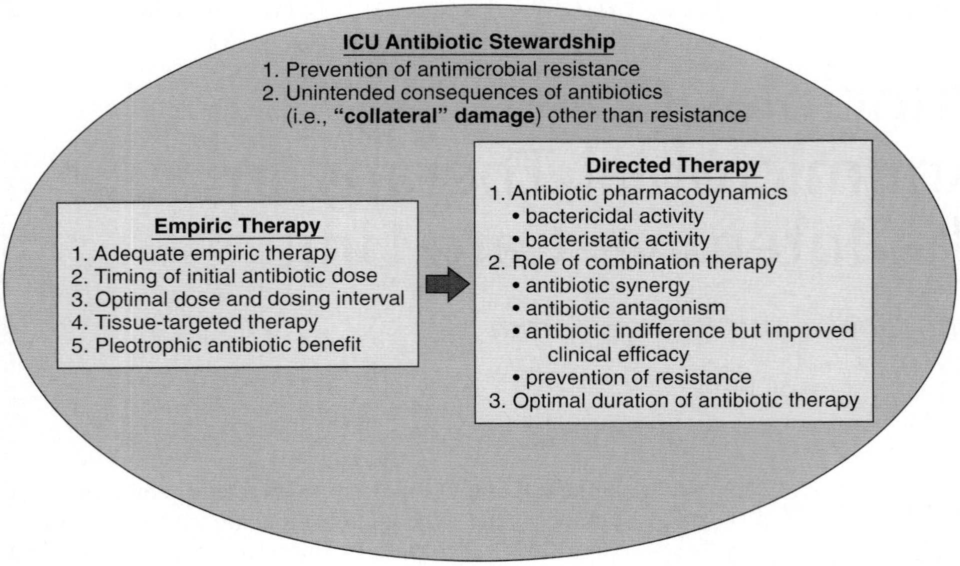
ICU Antibiotic Stewardship
1. Prevention of antimicrobial resistance
2. Unintended consequences of antibiotics
(i.e., "collateral" damage) other than resistance
Empiric Therapy
1. Adequate empiric therapy
2. Timing of initial antibiotic dose
3. Optimal dose and dosing interval
4. Tissue-targeted therapy
5. Pleotrophic antibiotic benefit
Directed Therapy
1. Antibiotic pharmacodynamics
• bactericidal activity
• bacteristatic activity
2. Role of combination therapy
• antibiotic synergy
• antibiotic antagonism
• antibiotic indifference but improved clinical efficacy
• prevention of resistance
3. Optimal duration of antibiotic therapy

Figure 52-1. Principles governing antibiotic therapy in the intensive care unit. This concept map lists principles that influence antibiotic prescription for an individual patient, first in empiric and then in directed therapy. Antibiotic selection at all times occurs within the context of the entire intensive care unit, raising principles relevant to antibiotic stewardship that may conflict or compete with those influencing individual antibiotic prescription.

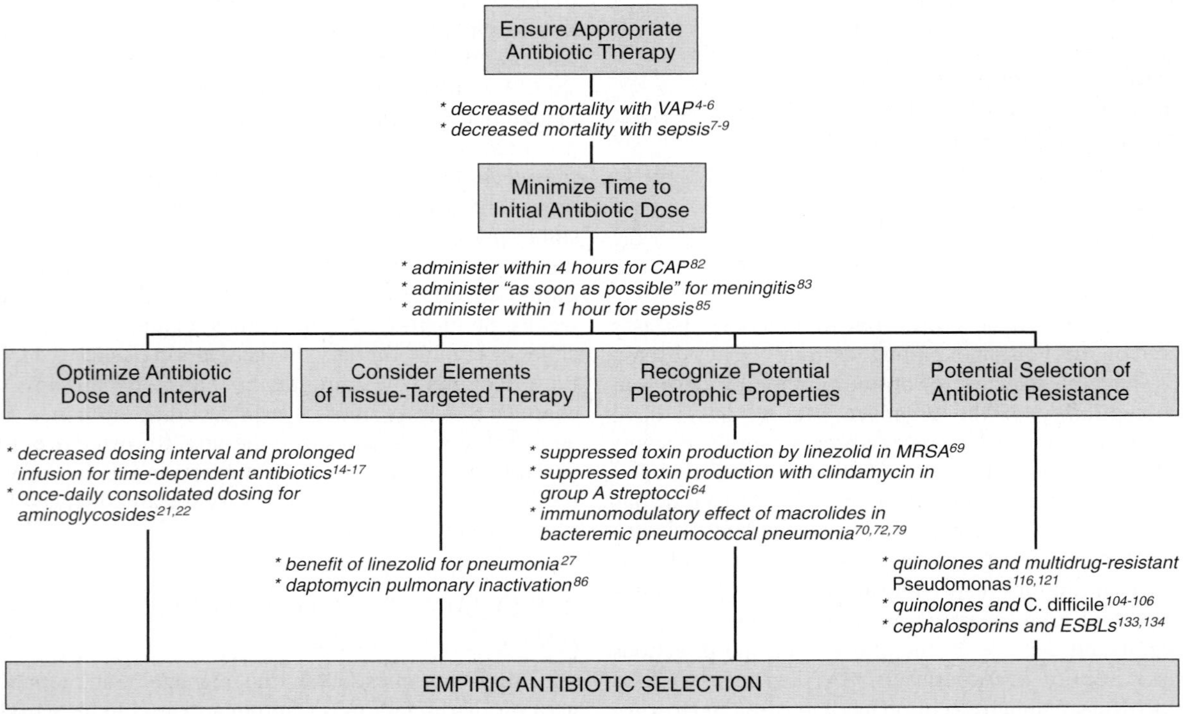
Ensure Appropriate Antibiotic Therapy
* decreased mortality with VAP[4-6]
* decreased mortality with sepsis[7-9]
Minimize Time to Initial Antibiotic Dose
* administer within 4 hours for CAP[82]
* administer "as soon as possible" for meningitis[83]
* administer within 1 hour for sepsis[85]
Optimize Antibiotic Dose and Interval
Consider Elements of Tissue-Targeted Therapy
Recognize Potential Pleotrophic Properties
Potential Selection of Antibiotic Resistance
* decreased dosing interval and prolonged infusion for time-dependent antibiotics[14-17]
* once-daily consolidated dosing for aminoglycosides[21,22]
* suppressed toxin production by linezolid in MRSA[69]
* suppressed toxin production with clindamycin in group A streptococci[64]
* immunomodulatory effect of macrolides in bacteremic pneumococcal pneumonia[70,72,79]
* benefit of linezolid for pneumonia[27]
* daptomycin pulmonary inactivation[86]
* quinolones and multidrug-resistant Pseudomonas[116,121]
* quinolones and C. difficile[104-106]
* cephalosporins and ESBLs[133,134]
EMPIRIC ANTIBIOTIC SELECTION

Figure 52-2. Selection of empiric antibiotic therapy in the intensive care unit. This algorithm incorporates specific examples from the text to illustrate how empiric antibiotic–prescribing principles can sequentially or concurrently influence the ultimate selection of an appropriate empiric agent.

pathogens or only colonizers, and lack of consistent identification of confounding factors that may contribute to mortality, and on the basis of such variables, it is not possible to prove irrefutably that such adequate therapy decreased mortality. Nevertheless, conclusions from multiple studies concerned with adequate versus inadequate initial therapy in seriously ill patients in ICUs have led to the interpretation that initial inadequate therapy contributed to mortality.[10]

Shortly after the reports emphasizing the importance of getting initial antibiotic therapy right, a growing awareness of variables other than the initial choice of antibiotic that influenced clinical outcomes in ICU patients began to emerge. In a 2005 joint guideline for management of patients with hospital-acquired pneumonia (HAP), VAP, and health care–associated pneumonia (HCAP), the American Thoracic Society (ATS) and the IDSA suggested modified definitions for the terms used in the selection of antibiotic therapy.[11] As a replacement for the term *inadequate* used in earlier reports to denote those situations in which the initial antibiotic selected did not match the susceptibility of the organism that subsequently grew,[4-9] *inappropriate* was the term used to define that scenario. *Adequate* was adopted to refer to therapy that included not only the correct antibiotic based on the susceptibility of the organism but also optimal dose, correct route of administration to ensure penetration at the site of infection, and use of combination therapy if necessary.[11]

A review of the literature suggests that other variables also play important roles in the determination of optimal clinical outcomes in patients in the ICU, including timing of antibiotic administration and certain pharmacologic properties of the agents selected. Awareness of such factors is important in the development of the knowledge base regarding adequate antibiotic therapy and its effect on both morbidity and mortality. These factors, in addition to those proposed in the ATS/IDSA guidelines,[11] are discussed next.

Optimal Dose

As the literature regarding the treatment of infections in the ICU has evolved over the years, studies have identified several elements that influence the dose of an antibiotic that is most likely to result in the best clinical efficacy. The manner in which antibiotics kill bacteria varies among different classes of drugs, but the two pharmacodynamic categories of killing that have been best categorized are time-dependent killing and concentration-dependent killing.[12] In time-dependent killing, which also has been referred to as concentration-independent killing, maximum bacterial killing occurs when the drug concentration remains constantly above the minimal inhibitory concentration (MIC). Examples of antibiotics that demonstrate this type of antimicrobial killing property include β-lactam drugs and vancomycin. In concentration-dependent killing, maximum bacterial killing occurs when the peak drug concentration is approximately 10 times the MIC of the drug. Examples of agents with this type of pharmacodynamic property are fluoroquinolones and aminoglycosides. The relevance of such antibiotic properties in the management of patients with serious infections has been well demonstrated in a number of reports.

The pharmacologic properties of vancomycin have been nicely summarized and include emphasis on the fact that vancomycin exhibits time-dependent killing.[13] Accordingly, the length of time that concentrations of vancomycin are maintained above the pathogen's MIC is critical to bacterial eradication, with a key variable for clinical success in pneumonia being the percentage of time that drug levels in the alveolar space exceed the MIC. As drug levels decline, organisms have the potential to begin to regrow, with a detrimental effect being clinical failure. This principle may contribute to an understanding of why certain patients with lung infection caused by a gram-positive organism sensitive to vancomycin do not respond optimally to vancomycin administered every 12 hours. In such a setting, use of a dosing schedule of every 6 hours seems to be a more rational approach.

Because a goal with time-dependent antibiotics is to maintain levels above the MIC of the organism for as long as possible during the dosing cycle, emphasis has recently been placed on use of extended-infusion dosing for this purpose. The efficacy of extended dosing has been examined for both β-lactam antibiotics and vancomycin. In a study of 194 patients with infection caused by *Pseudomonas aeruginosa*, piperacillin-tazobactam was administered intravenously either every 4 to 6 hours over 30 minutes or every 8 hours over 4 hours.[14] The 14-day mortality rate was significantly lower among patients who received extended-infusion therapy than among patients who received intermittent-infusion therapy (12.2% versus 31.6%, respectively; *P*=.04). In a study designed to assess blood levels of antibiotic based on both dose and pattern of administration, meropenem was administered to two study groups, each with 8 healthy volunteers.[15] One group received 500 mg as an intravenous infusion over 30 minutes three times a day versus a 250-mg loading dose followed by a 1500-mg continuous infusion over 24 hours; the second group received 1000 mg as an intravenous infusion over 30 minutes three times a day versus a 500-mg loading dose followed by a 3000-mg continuous infusion over 24 hours. Pharmacokinetic calculations were performed, and the data were extrapolated by Monte Carlo simulations for 10,000 simulated subjects for pharmacodynamic evaluation. The results of the analyses of the probability of MIC attainment with the high dose were 4 mg per liter with continuous infusion and 0.5 mg per liter with intermittent infusion. With the low dose, results were 2 mg per liter with continuous infusion and 0.25 mg per liter with intermittent infusion. Such data emphasize how intermittent infusion of a low dose of a time-dependent drug may result in MICs adequate to treat relatively sensitive organisms such as *Klebsiella pneumoniae* but may result in less-than-optimal killing of organisms that have intrinsically higher MICs (for example, *P. aeruginosa*). The efficacy of continuous-infusion vancomycin also has been reported.[16,17]

It has been shown in animal infection models that dosage regimens providing the same total amount of aminoglycoside given at 12-hour intervals or 24-hour intervals may be at least equally effective as dosage regimens that continuously provide inhibitory concentrations.[18-20] The postantibiotic effect (PAE), in which microbial killing persists despite loss of detectable serum levels, complements the concentration-dependent killing of gram-negative bacilli exhibited by aminoglycosides, and the two may serve as the basis for once-daily aminoglycoside therapy.[21] It has been suggested that giving the same total dose in larger concentration less often will result in better killing, longer PAE period, and reduced aminoglycoside toxicity that has been associated with elevated trough levels. Such pharmacologic and clinical data were the foundation for the move toward once-daily aminoglycoside dosing.

In such a dosing schedule, the single doses of gentamicin or tobramycin that have been used once daily have included 5 mg per kg and 7 mg per kg of body weight. The experience with once-daily therapy using 7 mg per kg in 2184 adult patients has been reported.[22] Excluded from such therapy were patients with ascites, burns involving greater than 20% total body surface area, pregnancy, end-stage renal disease requiring dialysis, and enterococcal endocarditis. The reported review stated that it was unnecessary to draw standard peak and trough samples and that monitoring could be completed by obtaining a single random blood sample between 6 and 14 hours after the start of an aminoglycoside infusion. The dosing interval could be subsequently adjusted in accordance with a nomogram which was provided. Several important observations were made in this large group of patients: (1) Despite the prolonged drug-free period, bacterial regrowth was not clinically evident; (2) no increase in either ototoxicity or nephrotoxicity was found; and (3) efficacy was promoted in a cost-effective manner.[22] A meta-analysis evaluating the safety and efficacy of once-daily aminoglycosides in 1200 patients from 16 trials found no difference concerning efficacy and safety between single-dose and multiple-dose regimens.[23]

To achieve optimal clinical benefits while minimizing the unintended consequences of selecting resistant bacteria, multiple variables should be considered simultaneously when concentration-dependent drugs are used in the treatment of serious infections. In a study of lower respiratory tract infections caused by *P. aeruginosa,* ciprofloxacin was administered intravenously as a dose of 200 to 300 mg every 12 hours.[24] Resistance emerged at a rate greater than 70% during therapy. This was similar to the 75% rate predicted by a pharmacodynamic study.[25] By contrast, a randomized comparison of imipenem and ciprofloxacin for treatment of nosocomial pneumonia used a ciprofloxacin regimen of 400 mg given intravenously every 8 hours and noted emergence of resistance during therapy in 33% of cases in which *Pseudomonas* was the causative pathogen.[26] This rate of emergence of resistance was similar to the 38% predicted by the pharmacodynamic study previously cited.[25] These data emphasize the importance of considering not only the dosing interval but also the dose of antibiotic administered when concentration-dependent drugs are used in serious infections.

Penetration at the Site of Infection: Tissue-Targeted Therapy

The importance of antibiotic pharmacokinetic properties, as a determinant of therapeutic success, has recently received heightened attention for the treatment of pneumonia caused by multidrug-resistant gram-positive cocci. Pulmonary pharmacokinetics have been used as a justification for the greater treatment success of linezolid, when compared with vancomycin in traditional regimens, for pneumonia caused by methicillin-resistant *Staphylococcus aureus* (MRSA).[27-30] Understanding the relevance of pharmacokinetic properties will help the critical care physician navigate through the recent published literature for these infections.

Pulmonary pharmacokinetics specifically addresses the tissue penetration and distribution of antibiotics within the lung.[31] Early studies dealing with the relevance of antibiotic penetration in infections occurring in the ICU were related to aminoglycosides and fluoroquinolones. Although aminoglycoside levels in the interstitium of the lung are good, levels in pulmonary secretions reach a mean of only about 20% of the concomitant serum level.[32] By contrast, the concentrations of quinolones in lung tissue significantly exceed the concomitant serum concentrations, and levels in bronchial secretions also have been reported to exceed those in serum.[33] Despite the fact that quinolones have better penetration into the lung and less potential for nephrotoxicity than has been shown for aminoglycosides, available data show a trend toward improved survival in patients with VAP treated with an aminoglycoside-containing, but not with quinolone-containing, combination.[34] A concern with fluoroquinolones in combination therapy directed against gram-negative organisms is the selection of resistance, particularly in organisms such as *P. aeruginosa,* in which the resistance may be to multiple classes of antibiotics.[35] Because of the coexistent potential for clinical efficacy but nephrotoxicity with aminoglycosides, some investigators have suggested, on the basis of clinical trials, discontinuation of the aminoglycoside after 5 days if the patient is improving.[36]

Existing pharmacokinetic evidence testifies to the extremely poor lung tissue penetration of vancomycin. Cruciani and associates investigated vancomycin pharmacokinetics in 30 human lung tissue sections after administration of a 1-g dose over 1 hour.[37] A comparison of serum-to-tissue concentration over the dosing interval was used to generate a graph allowing determination of a concentration ratio. Overall, the serum-to-lung tissue concentration ratio was determined to be 21%. Not surprisingly, investigation has confirmed even poorer penetration into epithelial lining fluid.[38] These data raise concern that the traditional dosing regimens of vancomycin (1 g given intravenously every 12 hours) and established target serum trough concentrations (5 to 10 μg/mL) will generate lung tissue concentrations below the MIC for *Staphylococcus aureus.* The issues surrounding suboptimal vancomycin dosing are reflected in the 2005 published ATS/IDSA guidelines for treatment for adults with HAP, VAP, and HCAP, in which it was noted that retrospective pharmacokinetic modeling suggested that the vancomycin failures may be related to inadequate dosing and in which the recommendation was made that trough levels for vancomycin should be 15 to 20 μg/mL.[11]

In contrast with the poor pulmonary pharmacokinetic properties of vancomycin, several studies of linezolid confirm excellent lung penetration in healthy volunteer subjects and with in vitro modeling.[39-41] Boselli and coworkers investigated the steady-state plasma pharmacokinetic variables and epithelial lining fluid concentrations of linezolid administered to critically ill patients with VAP.[42] Epithelial lining fluid concentrations of linezolid approximated 100% of corresponding plasma values, with drug concentrations that exceeded the susceptibility breakpoint (4 mg/mL) for *S. aureus* throughout the greater part of the dosing interval. The same 2005 ATS guideline statement that raises concern about poor vancomycin pharmacokinetics recognizes the potential pharmacokinetic advantage of linezolid, which may be due to the higher penetration of linezolid into epithelial lining fluid.[11]

To date, no prospective, randomized, controlled trial has been published to compare dose-intensified vancomycin and linezolid for the treatment of MRSA pneumonia. Even so, the principle of antibiotic pharmacokinetics has supported the conclusion that linezolid is superior to vancomycin in traditional dosing regimens for MRSA pneumonia based on retrospective analysis of the two multinational, double-blind, randomized studies published to date.[27]

Role of Combination Therapy

Synergy

In discussions of combination therapy, one of the most frequently cited justifications is for the achievement of synergy, in which antimicrobial combinations are more effective than single agents. The best-recognized example of the clinical relevance of synergistic antimicrobial therapy is in treatment of enterococcal endocarditis, in which treatment with penicillin or ampicillin alone has been associated with a high rate of relapse when compared with therapy with penicillin or ampicillin in combination with streptomycin or gentamicin.[43,44] Discussions of combination therapy have raised the question of whether the use of multiple drugs in the treatment of an infection may be associated with enhanced clinical outcomes. For example, in the treatment of bacteremia with *S. aureus,* some investigators have used a semisynthetic penicillinase-resistant penicillin (e.g., nafcillin or oxacillin) in combination with a brief course (3 to 5 days) of an aminoglycoside based on data showing more rapid clearing of bacteremia.[45] Data from this trial did not show a decrease in mortality in the study population of nonaddicts with primarily left-sided endocarditis caused by *S. aureus* when compared with those patients who received nafcillin alone. For *P. aeruginosa,* the mechanism of synergy between antipseudomonal penicillins and aminoglycosides is similar to that of enterococci, with enhanced uptake of the aminoglycoside in the presence of the penicillin.[46] Despite this microbiologic observation, the presence or absence of synergy in this setting seemed less important in a trial assessing outcomes in patients with *P. aeruginosa* bacteremia than did the administration of combination therapy given in an attempt to prevent the emergence of resistance.[47]

In contrast with synergy, in which combination therapy is beneficial, a question that sometimes is raised about patients in an ICU is whether the components of a combination regimen may have an antagonistic effect. The classic example of such an effect was with the treatment of pneumococcal meningitis in the 1950s, in which the fatality rate among patients who received penicillin alone was 21%, in contrast with 79% among those who received both penicillin (a bactericidal agent) plus chlortetracycline (a bacteristatic agent).[48] The clinical importance of the concept of antagonism has gained increasing significance in the era of community-associated methicillin-resistant *S. aureus* (CA-MRSA), which may occur in alarmingly high rates within a community, resulting in life-threatening community-acquired infections that require admission to an ICU. The plight of the critical care clinician has been further expanded with data demonstrating the lack of predictability of methicillin resistance versus methicillin susceptibility in community strains of *S. aureus.*[49] Compounding this clinical dilemma is the published evidence supporting the fact that MRSA is an independent predictor of mortality, ICU length of stay, and overall cost of care.[50-53] Because a limited number of therapeutic options exist for the treatment of severe, invasive MRSA infections, effort has been made to identify the in vitro activity of antibiotic combinations that may have clinical applicability.[54-56] This includes the potential for not only a synergistic but also an antagonistic effect.

In a study using 10 different stains of *S. aureus,* an overall pattern of antibiotic indifference was noted when linezolid was combined with fusidic acid, rifampin, and gentamicin. Of special concern was the finding of slight antagonism and reduced bactericidal effect when linezolid was combined with ciprofloxacin and vancomycin against the same strains of staphylococci.[54] A subsequent study using the checkerboard broth microdilution method tested linezolid in combination with 28 different antimicrobial agents, including vancomycin and several fluoroquinolones, and demonstrated no antagonistic effect.[57] Antibiotic indifference was again reproduced with vancomycin by Sahuquillo and colleagues, but antagonism with levofloxacin was noted in two of the five *S. aureus* isolates tested.[55]

The rabbit model of aortic valve endocarditis was used to evaluate 5-day treatment regimens of linezolid alone, vancomycin alone, and linezolid in combination with vancomycin in 40 rabbits infected with an MRSA strain.[57] Vancomycin-treated rabbits demonstrated greater mean reductions in valvular vegetation bacterial counts than those in the other treatment groups ($P = .05$). Vancomycin also sterilized aortic valve vegetations in three of eight rabbits; by contrast, none of the rabbits treated with linezolid had sterile aortic valve vegetations. A noteworthy finding in this study was that the treatment regimen of linezolid plus vancomycin lowered the peak linezolid levels in serum to below those obtained with regimens with linezolid alone. Even though in vitro synergy testing revealed additive or indifferent activity between the two drugs, in vivo antagonism was demonstrated using the rabbit model. A potential explanation offered by the investigators for the observed antagonism between vancomycin and linezolid was the effect of combining a bacteriostatic agent such as linezolid with a bactericidal drug like vancomycin. The observed reduction in peak linezolid levels in serum with the combination of the two drugs was thought to suggest a role for additional mechanisms in the interaction between the two antibiotics. Unfortunately, the clinical significance of these findings is not yet known.

In the absence of definitive data on optimal management of *S. aureus* infections in seriously ill patients, a pattern has emerged in some health care systems to prescribe combination therapy for this pathogen. The overall assessment of the data is that antibiotic indifference, or no combination effect, appears to best characterize the drug interaction profile of linezolid; however, because some data, albeit unsubstantiated in controlled clinical trials, seem to cast doubt on the advisability of its combination with vancomycin[54] and the fluoroquinolones,[55] it is important for the critical care clinician to be aware of such a possibility in the crafting of empiric antibiotic regimens for seriously ill patients.

Enhanced Efficacy against a Pathogen

A common question in clinical medicine is whether combination therapy will result in increased efficacy against a pathogen via a mechanism other than synergy. In an attempt to find a more definitive answer to this clinically relevant question, a meta-analysis of 64 trials with 7586 patients comparing β-lactam monotherapy versus β-lactam plus an aminoglycoside in immunocompetent patients with sepsis was conducted.[58] This report did not identify a statistically significant advantage of combination therapy among the 1835 patients with gram-negative infections for whom the data were analyzed. In contrast with the results in the previously cited study,[47] no improved survival was observed for the 426 patients who had infection caused by *P. aeruginosa*. An additional finding was that the rates of development of resistance did not differ in the two treatment groups. Nephrotoxicity, however, developed significantly more often in those patients who received combination therapy.

Prevention of the Emergence of Resistance

Combination therapy for *P. aeruginosa* commonly has been used in an attempt to prevent the emergence of resistance. Despite the importance of this subject, no definitive data are available to prove that combination therapy will prevent the emergence of *Pseudomonas* resistance[59]; however, results of clinical trials[26] and concern about this possibility based on limited data have been the basis for such recommendations. In a meta-analysis of eight randomized controlled clinical trials, β-lactam monotherapy and β-lactam plus aminoglycoside combination therapy were compared to assess if combination therapy may decrease the risk of emergence of resistance.[60] Among initially antimicrobial-susceptible isolates in this analysis, combination therapy was not associated with a beneficial effect on the development of antimicrobial resistance. In the meta-analysis of 64 trials comparing β-lactam monotherapy and β-lactam plus aminoglycoside combination therapy in immunocompetent patients with sepsis, no difference in the rate of development of resistance was observed.[58]

Increased Opportunity for Achieving Appropriate Therapy

Even though issues of synergy and reduction in the emergence of resistance frequently are invoked in discussions of combination therapy, the relevant data do not prove consistent benefits. In patients in the intensive care setting, an important advantage of combination therapy is that it provides the clinician with broader antibacterial coverage for potentially multidrug-resistant microorganisms.[61] In addition, because inappropriate initial therapy may result in increased mortality, a combination of antibiotics has the potential benefit of providing coverage against a pathogen that may not be the most likely on a statistical basis but is a reasonable consideration in life-threatening clinical settings confronting the critical care physician.

Immunomodulating Effect of Antibiotics

Although antibiotics traditionally are classified according to their chemical structure and spectrum of coverage, additional properties that have important clinical implications are being discovered. The interaction of antibiotics with host immune response, bacterial population kinetics, and bacterial gene expression for exotoxin production are examples of pleotropic properties of antibiotics. For the critical care physician, this is especially relevant in the treatment of life-threatening infection caused by gram-positive cocci and may be the basis for combination therapy in the treatment of infections caused by such pathogens.

Streptococcal toxic shock syndrome is a clinical infection in which bacterial exotoxins are produced and act as host superantigens, precipitating shock, multiple organ failure, and death. Although *Streptococcus pyogenes* demonstrates exquisite in vitro sensitivity to penicillin, experimental studies of infection by this pathogen have demonstrated reduced efficacy against organisms in the stationary phase of bacterial growth. This phenomenon has been termed the Eagle effect, whereby high organism population density and slow organism division make treatment with an antibiotic dependent on cell wall synthesis ineffective.[62] The Eagle effect has been used as a justification for use of clindamycin, which is a bacteristatic antibiotic, in the treatment of toxic shock syndrome. In addition, clindamycin is an antibiotic that inhibits bacterial protein synthesis, and this pharmacodynamic property is independent of the stage of bacterial growth.[63] Clindamycin inhibits bacterial exotoxin production, facilitates phagocytosis of *Streptococcus pyogenes* by inhibiting M protein synthesis, and suppresses the production of penicillin-binding proteins. Evidence exists that clindamycin demonstrates immunomodulatory effects, suppressing monocyte synthesis of tumor necrosis factor-α (TNF-α).[64,65] All of these pleotropic qualities have resulted in the recommendation for clindamycin use in necrotizing skin or soft tissue infections and toxic shock syndrome caused by *S. pyogenes*.[63]

The dramatic increase worldwide of highly virulent, community-acquired infection with CA-MRSA has resulted in increasing reports of necrotizing skin and soft tissue infections and necrotizing pneumonia confronting the critical care physician.[66-68] CA-MRSA virulence has been attributed to expression of several virulence factors: α-hemolysins, toxic shock syndrome toxin-1 (TSST-1), staphylococcal enterotoxin B, and Panton-Valentine leukocidin (PVL). The association of staphylococcal virulence with the current CA-MRSA epidemic prompted Stevens and colleagues to investigate the impact of antibiotics on the expression of virulence-associated exotoxin genes.[69] These investigators were able to demonstrate markedly suppressed in vitro production of staphylococcal toxin genes by clindamycin and linezolid, such that no PVL production was noted up to 12 hours after antibiotic administration. Of interest, subinhibitory concentrations of the cell wall–active agent nafcillin were found to increase toxin production. These findings led the investigators to conclude that protein synthesis inhibition is an important consideration in the selection of antimicrobial agents for treatment of serious infections caused by toxin-producing gram-positive cocci.[69]

A growing body of evidence exists to support the benefit of macrolide therapy for bacteremic pneumonia caused by *Streptococcus pneumoniae*.[70-78] Although multiple explanations have been proposed, efficacy appears to extend beyond the drug's spectrum of activity. The *macrolide* class of antibiotics exerts a broad range of immunomodulatory effects: suppression of harmful interleukin host responses and inhibition of neutrophil oxidant burst and degranulation.[70,72,79] These pleotropic effects have received an increasing focus of attention and further illustrate how immune modulation influences recommendations for therapy in the intensive care setting.

Timing

The impact of the timing of antibiotic therapy has been addressed in several ways with regard to patients in the ICU. In an analysis based on 107 consecutive patients receiving mechanical ventilation and antibiotic treatment for VAP, Iregui and colleagues noted that 30.8% (33 of 107) received antibiotic treatment that was delayed for 24 hours or more after initially meeting diagnostic criteria for VAP and were classified as having initially delayed appropriate antibiotic therapy (IDAAT).[80] Two major variables were identified in these patients with IDAAT: (1) a delay in writing an antibiotic order (in 75.8% of the cases); and (2) the presence of a bacterial species resistant to the initially prescribed antibiotic regimen (in 18.2%). The investigators found that hospital mortality rate was 69.7% for the patients with IDAAT, in contrast with only 28.4% for the patients without IDAAT ($P<.01$). An earlier study noted that even when patients with VAP were changed to a regimen that covered the pathogen based on a susceptibility report, the increase in mortality with inadequate therapy was not eliminated.[4] Acknowledgment of this finding was the basis for the statement that secondary modifications of an initially failing antibiotic regimen do not substantially improve the outcome for critically ill patients.[81] These results challenge the clinician to order antibiotics that cover the involved pathogens even before culture results are obtainable. In the empiric approach to VAP, the more easily modifiable major factor contributing to IDAAT is the prevention of delay in writing the antibiotic order.

The importance of antibiotic timing in patients with community-acquired pneumonia was assessed in a retrospective cohort study of pneumonia in 18,209 Medicare patients.[82] In this trial, conducted in a random sample of inpatients 65 years of age or older with community-acquired pneumonia who had not received antibiotics as out-patients, the influence on clinical outcome was assessed for use of antibiotics prescribed according to standard guidelines published at the time of the analysis and not identification of pathogens isolated from the patients. Of the patients who received antibiotics within 4 hours of hospital arrival, 83.2% were prescribed a guideline-recommended regimen, in contrast with 71.8% of the patients who received antibiotics after 4 hours of arrival. The results of this analysis suggested that administering antibiotics within 4 hours of hospital arrival was associated with decreased mortality and length of stay. Offered by the investigators as a plausible biologic mechanism explaining the results is that antibiotics may interrupt or minimize the effects of the acute lung injury process that occurs as part of the systemic inflammatory response in patients with bacterial pneumonia.

The ISDA practice guidelines for management of adult patients with meningitis note the lack of prospective clinical data on the relationship of the timing of antimicrobial administration of antimicrobial agents to clinical outcome in patients with bacterial meningitis.[83] Data from a retrospective cohort study of 269 adult patients with community-acquired bacterial meningitis provide some insights into the timing of antibiotic therapy in the absence of definitive recommendations.[84] In this trial, the baseline clinical features of hypotension, altered mental status, and seizures were associated with adverse outcome. Using these three factors, the investigators created a prognostic model to predict clinical outcome based on the stratification of patients into three stages of risk: low (defined as none of the clinical features); intermediate (1 clinical feature), or high risk (2 or more clinical features). The results demonstrated that a delay in initiation of antimicrobial therapy after patient arrival in the emergency department was associated with adverse clinical outcome when the patient's condition advanced from a low- or intermediate-risk stage to a high-risk stage of prognostic severity. Using these and other data, the IDSA acknowledged that evidence for definitive recommendations is inadequate and concluded that a reasonable assumption is to administer treatment for bacterial meningitis before the infection advances to a high level of clinical severity.[83] Referring to meningitis as a "neurologic emergency," the guideline recommended that appropriate therapy for meningitis be initiated as soon as possible after the diagnosis is considered to be likely.[83] In support of the importance of prompt timing, this document also noted the potential in certain patients for administration of antibiotics before hospital admission if the patient initially presents outside the hospital.

For the critical care clinician, sepsis is a clinical entity in which adequate antibiotic therapy has been associated with improved clinical outcomes.[7-9] In recognition of the importance of prompt therapy in influencing clinical outcomes in patients with sepsis, the 2004 Surviving Sepsis Campaign guidelines offered a specific recommendation regarding the timing of antimicrobial therapy for the septic patient: "Intravenous antibiotic therapy should be started within the first hour of recognition of severe sepsis, after appropriate cultures have been obtained."[85]

Special Pharmacologic Properties

As the focus of antibiotic research has expanded beyond the characterization of in vitro properties for a particular agent, the importance of antibiotic performance at the in vivo target tissue level is becoming increasingly recognized. It was with the 2003 introduction of a novel antibiotic, daptomycin, for treatment of infections caused by resistant gram-positive cocci that the relevance of "organ-specific deactivation" initially was described.[86] Daptomycin is an intravenous cyclic lipopeptide with rapid, concentration-dependent killing and bactericidal activity against a broad spectrum of gram-positive cocci.[87-89] It demonstrates a unique mechanism of action, with calcium-dependent insertion into the phospholipid bacterial cell membrane. This results in cell depolarization via potassium efflux, causing disruption of DNA, RNA, and protein synthesis.[90]

Two multicenter, randomized, controlled, evaluator-blinded trials, totaling 1092 patients with complicated skin and soft tissue infections, demonstrated improved efficacy of daptomycin treatment when compared with traditional therapy with penicillinase-resistant penicillin or vancomycin.[91] As a result, daptomycin, at a daily dose of 4 mg per kg (for patients with creatinine clearance greater than 30 mL per minute), received U.S. Food and Drug Administration (FDA) approval for the treatment of complicated skin and soft tissue infections. A more recent randomized, open-label trial investigated use of daptomycin in *S. aureus* bacteremia and endocarditis.[92] This trial prompted FDA approval of daptomycin for treatment of *S. aureus* bacteremia, including right-sided endocarditis, at a daily intravenous dose of 6 mg per kg.

Phase 3 clinical trials also were conducted for the treatment of community-acquired pneumonia in hospitalized patients. Despite daptomycin's potent in vitro bactericidal activity against *Streptococcus pneumoniae,* clinical outcomes were disappointing and inferior to those with the comparator, ceftriaxone. Although daptomycin is known to exhibit poor penetration into epithelial lining fluid, the reason for treatment failure was not fully elucidated until Silverman and colleagues described a unique organ-specific inactivation process.[86] Daptomycin's inactivation was linked to its mechanism of bactericidal action: calcium-dependent membrane lipid binding.[86,90,93,94] Using a mouse model, investigators were able to demonstrate drug sequestration and inactivation by binding to phospholipid vesicles that are found in pulmonary surfactant.[86] For this reason, daptomycin is not considered an appropriate therapeutic agent for treatment of pneumonia, largely because of the presence of surfactant at the target tissue. This phenomenon appears to be unique to daptomycin[86] but raises the question of unrecognized organ-specific interaction for other classes of antibiotics and other target organs.

Recent antibiotic developments have introduced the possibility of managing life-threatening infections with antimicrobial agents administered at a prolonged dosing interval. A long drug half-life ($T_{1/2}$) is conducive to completion of treatment courses in the outpatient setting and maximizes patient compliance. In the context of critical care, exploiting an antibiotic's $T_{1/2}$ historically has been used in settings such as hemodialysis with end-stage renal disease. Less frequent antibiotic dosing diminishes the burden of intravenous access and increases the possibility of treatment outside of an intensive care environment.

A novel lipoglycopeptide, dalbavancin, can be administered with weekly intravenous dosing owing to a $T_{1/2}$ of approximately 8 to 9 days. Dalbavancin demonstrates a spectrum of antimicrobial activity against *Staphylococcus, Enterococcus,* and *Streptococcus* (including resistant strains). A phase 2 open-label, randomized, controlled trial has compared dalbavancin with vancomycin for the treatment of catheter-related bloodstream infections.[95] Enrollment in this trial was small, limiting statistical conclusions, but dalbavancin demonstrated overall treatment success. A phase 3 noninferiority trial for the treatment of complicated skin and soft tissue infections demonstrated comparable clinical efficacy for weekly dalbavancin and linezolid (88.9% and 91.2%, respectively).[96] The clinical role and applicability of dalbavancin remain to be determined but may signal a possible trend by the pharmaceutical industry to develop antibiotics that will allow intermittent dosing.

UNINTENDED CONSEQUENCES OF ANTIBIOTIC THERAPY

For many years, traditional teaching about antibiotics focused on three classic parameters: efficacy, safety, and cost-effectiveness. With respect to safety, the major considerations were allergic reactions and adverse effects. In the new era of "bad bugs and no drugs,"[2] an important new safety issue should be added: unintended consequences of antibiotic therapy. An insightful report termed such unintended consequences the "collateral damage" of antibiotics, in which some unwanted event occurs in the process of trying to achieve clinical efficacy through antibiotic killing.[97] In this report, *collateral damage* referred to the ecologic adverse effect of selecting drug-resistant organisms and the unwanted development of colonization or infection with multidrug-resistant organisms. In the worldwide epidemic of antibiotic resistance, this probably is the best-characterized form of collateral damage to date. Some important new considerations recently described in the literature, however, may influence initial antibiotic selection for serious infections in the ICU.

The increasing prevalence of MRSA infections in patients in the critical care setting has required an ongoing evaluation of factors that propagate and sustain such a pattern of resistance. The role of inadequate hand washing in the spread of nosocomial MRSA in hospitals has been well known for many years.[98] As rates of MRSA have increased in infections such as HAP,[99] increased emphasis has been placed on other variables that potentially may contribute to the role that MRSA now plays as the etiologic agent of HAP and VAP. In recognition of the infectious disease concept that colonization by a pathogen often is an antecedent event leading to clinical disease produced by that pathogen, attention has been directed to factors that may increase colonization by MRSA. One piece of preliminary evidence is provided in a report by

Bisognano and colleagues, who evaluated the occurrence and frequency of increased adhesion in clinical isolates of fluoroquinolone-resistant MRSA and methicillin-susceptible *S. aureus* (MSSA) that was mediated by fluoroquinolone-induced increases in fibronectin-binding proteins (FnBPs).[100] In this report, 8 of 10 MRSA isolates and 4 of 6 MSSA isolates with *grlA* and *gyrA* mutations exhibited significant increases in attachment to fibronectin-coated surfaces after growth in the presence of one-fourth the MIC of ciprofloxacin. The response was abolished by pretreatment with rifampin, and an interpretation by the investigators was that this indicated an effect at the level of transcription. Although this report does not prove that suboptimal levels of fluoroquinolones contribute in a clinically significant way to increased production of FnBP(s) and higher levels of bacterial attachment, the data do challenge the clinician to consider possible unintended antibiotic consequences as a possible explanation for increasing rates of infection with MRSA.

A problem that has gained increasing attention in recent years has been infection by strains of *Clostridium difficile* with markedly increased levels of toxin production. The analysis of this problem has occurred on multiple levels, but an intriguing prospect has been raised by the potential for certain classes of antibiotics to create genetic damage, with a resultant increase in the rate of mutations that leads to either antibiotic resistance or other untoward effects. Spontaneous mutations that lead to bacterial resistance occur with a frequency that generally is in the range from 10^{-6} to 10^{-8}.[25] Hypermutation has been used to refer to a situation in which the mutation rate exceeds that recognized for spontaneous mutations.[101] Certain factors may lead to genetic damage in bacteria with a resultant increase in the potential for a mutation that can lead to resistance, and antibiotics that have an effect on DNA have been shown with in vitro experiments to potentially contribute to this predisposition to resistance.[101] The SOS response, which is named after the International Morse Code distress signal and refers to an inducible DNA repair system, has been nicely described by Beaber and colleagues, who propose it as a means for promoting horizontal dissemination of antibiotic resistance genes.[102] Important background information from that report includes the role of integrating conjugative elements (ICEs), which are capable of cell-to-cell transfer with integration into the new cell's chromosome and which can then allow expression of a variety of resistance genes. Normally, repressors are in place to decrease the expression of activators for ICE transfer. The SOS response occurs when DNA damage alleviates the repression induced by a variety of environmental factors as well as by certain antibiotics, including fluoroquinolones. As demonstrated by Beaber and colleagues, ciprofloxacin can cause genetic damage that can induce transfer of certain ICEs; this may represent a mechanism by which therapeutic agents can promote the spread of antibiotic resistance genes.[102] Similar data have been published furthering the contention that altered expression of *SOS* and other stress response genes is among the many global changes that can result from exposure to antibiotics.[103]

The data regarding the role of antibiotics in causing DNA damage that leads to increased resistance via hypermutation become relevant when one considers potential mechanisms for the increasing toxin production in *C. difficile* that has led to such problems as toxic megacolon, bowel perforation, and death. In an attempt to better understand outbreaks of clinical disease caused by toxin-producing strains of *C. difficile,* the genetics of epidemic strains were studied.[104,105] In these studies, an 18-base-pair deletion in the *tcdC* gene, which normally downregulates production of toxins A and B, was noted. An additional finding was the presence of binary toxin genes. These factors were thought to contribute to the hyperproduction of toxin expressed in clinical outbreaks. The epidemiologic analysis of these outbreaks identified fluoroquinolone therapy as a risk factor in recent *C. difficile* outbreaks.[104-106] If the fluoroquinolones are indeed contributors to the outbreaks, what remains unanswered is whether the antibiotic exposure–selected spontaneous mutants led to the DNA damage associated with increased toxin production, or was involved in some other manner. Regardless of the findings, these preliminary observations challenge the critical care clinician to again consider the potential of unintended antibiotic consequences in the selection of empiric antibiotic therapy in seriously ill patients.

The effect of antibiotics on toxin production has been studied in gram-positive organisms. In a study investigating the effects that cell wall–active antibiotics and protein synthesis inhibitors have on transcription and translation of genes for PVL, α-hemolysin (AH), and TSST-1, it was demonstrated that subinhibitory concentrations of nafcillin induced and prolonged messenger RNA (mRNA) expression for PVL, AH, and TSST-1.[69] A clinical interpretation of these data suggested by the investigators is that inadvertent use of β-lactam antibiotics to treat methicillin-resistant *S. aureus* infections may contribute to worse outcomes.

Even though such processes as DNA damage leading to hypermutation and increases in virulence factors are important considerations in discussions about unintended consequences, the most mature knowledge base related to the collateral damage of antibiotics is the risk of these agents to contribute to the expression of bacterial resistance.

CLINICIAN RESPONSES TO MULTIDRUG RESISTANCE

In the studies addressing increased mortality rates associated with inadequate initial antimicrobial therapy for serious infections,[4-9] unanticipated bacterial resistance was a frequent reason for not initially selecting a drug to which the organism was susceptible. An important insight is provided in the study by Trouillet and colleagues, who evaluated the risk factors for resistance in patients with VAP.[107] The conclusions of that study were that use of antibiotics within the past 15 days and mechanical ventilation of at least 7 days' duration were the most important. When these two parameters were used in subcategories to evaluate the predisposition for selecting resistant organisms, antibiotic use was a more influential factor than was mechanical ventilation. This fact highlights the dual role that antibiotics play in the ICU: (1) treatment of infection and (2) potential selection of the resistant organisms that lead to the next episode of infection. The challenge for the clinician is to achieve the appropriate degree of balance between these two opposing effects.

Increasing the sophistication of antibiotic prescribing in the ICU is an understanding of those factors that lead to the expression of antibiotic resistance. Although resistance in gram-negative bacilli may occur by means of several mechanisms, one that provides a foundation for understanding resistance is related to β-lactamase production in gram-negative organisms. To effectively address the issues of how β-lactamases are affected by clinical usage of antibiotics and how these enzymes influence management of critically ill patients, the clinician needs a clinically relevant approach to β-lactamases. One such method is to divide them into the categories of type I enzymes and non–type I enzymes.

Type I β-lactamases are chromosomally mediated, with production controlled by the *ampC* gene (hence the term *ampC β-lactamases*). These enzymes characteristically are produced by *Serratia, P. aeruginosa,* indole-positive *Proteus, Citrobacter,* and *Enterobacter.* (These bacteria may be remembered as the "SPICE bugs," a mnemonic derived from the first letters of their names. Some authors substitute *Acinetobacter* for indole-positive *Proteus* and use the mnemonic SPACE.) According to data from the Centers for Disease Control and Prevention's National Nosocomial Infections Surveillance (NNIS) system, nosocomial infections of urine, lung, skin, or blood are caused about 20% of the time by one of these pathogens.[108] Even though these pathogens do not always produce type I enzymes, this potential does exist and must be taken into consideration if initial antibiotic therapy is to be appropriate. Traditionally, the four classes of antibiotics stated to have the most predictable stability in the presence of type I β-lactamases are aminoglycosides, carbapenems (e.g., imipenem, meropenem, doripenem, ertapenem), fluoroquinolones, and fourth-generation cephalosporins (e.g., cefepime). Because type I β-lactamases have an affinity for cephalosporins (and have therefore been referred to by some authors as cephalosporinases), it is understandable that third-generation cephalosporins are not predictably stable in the presence of type I enzymes.[109] Also lacking stability are the β-lactamase inhibitors—clavulanic acid, sulbactam, and tazobactam—of which tazobactam is the most likely to resist destruction by these enzymes.

Certain antibiotics may contribute to a microorganism's ability to produce type I β-lactamases. Two mechanisms for this have been described in the literature: (1) induction and (2) the selection of spontaneous mutant strains (previously referred to as stable de-repression).[110] As described by Sanders and Sanders,[110] an organism with the potential to produce type I β-lactamases was incubated overnight in the presence of antibiotic. After this incubation, an assay was done for type I β-lactamase, and when it was detectable, the process was described as induction. Strong inducing antibiotics identified in this report were cefoxitin, imipenem, and clavulanic acid. Of note, when the inducing antibiotic was removed, the β-lactamase production ceased before the next dose of drug was due to be given. Of importance is that induction was described as a reversible in vitro phenomenon.[110]

As previously noted, type I β-lactamases are chromosomally mediated, with the control gene for the production of this enzyme being the *ampC* gene. The regulation of *ampC* production is controlled through the regulatory *ampR* gene. These facts are pivotal in understanding the mechanism by which induction occurs in vitro.[111] Because β-lactam antibiotics do not go beyond the bacterial cell wall, they do not have the ability to directly turn on either the *ampR* or the *ampC* gene. What has been proposed is that these antibiotics bind to penicillin-binding proteins (PBPs), forming an antibiotic-PBP complex, which then sends a signal into the cytoplasm of the cell. The result is activation of the *ampR* gene, which then turns on the *ampC* gene, culminating in the production of type I β-lactamase. When the antibiotic is stopped, the antibiotic-PBP complex is eliminated, with cessation of the signal entering the cytoplasm of the cell. The *ampC* gene is turned off, and the type I β-lactamase production ceases. Hence, the induction described in gram-negative organisms is a reversible process without genetic change in the exposed organism. In the years since the description of induction as an in vitro phenomenon, no definitive evidence has been accumulated demonstrating that induction in gram-negative organisms leads to clinically significant resistance in patients.

What has been proved to occur in patients is the second mechanism—selection of spontaneous mutant strains of bacteria.[110] In the organisms that have the ability to produce type I β-lactamases, the enzymes normally are under repressor control, and the organisms initially appear susceptible to a large number of antimicrobial agents. In those gram-negative organisms such as *Enterobacter* that have the ability to produce type I β-lactamase, a certain number (often in the 10^{-6} to 10^{-7} range) will have a spontaneous mutation that allows them to express type I β-lactamase.[110] When certain broad-spectrum antibiotics are given, the sensitive non-mutated organisms are killed; however, the genetic mutant strains proliferate and become the predominant organisms. Because a genetic change has occurred in the spontaneous mutant bacteria that are selected, the type I β-lactamase production continues even when the inciting antibiotic is stopped. Most notable of the antibiotics that have been described in the literature to select these stably de-repressed mutants are the third-generation cephalosporins.[112,113]

A clinically relevant lesson can be learned from the story of how type 1 β-lactamases lead to the expression of resistance. In the overwhelming majority of instances with gram-negative organisms, antibiotics do not lead to induction of resistance, in which a genetic predisposition exists, is nonactive at the moment, but is reversibly turned on after exposure to an antibiotic. What occurs clinically is that resistant strains that already have the turned-on genetics for resistance exist but are present in too small a number to be clinically detected. With antibiotic therapy, sensitive strains of the bacteria are killed, leaving the resistance mutants unencumbered and therefore able to reproduce at a clinically detectable level. This process of selection, not induction, is the basis for most of the resistance that is encountered in the clinical setting.

An understanding of this concept takes on significance with the increasingly common problem in ICUs of the development of resistance to multiple antibiotics. Referred to as multidrug-resistant organisms, these pathogens may be the cause of clinical failure of antibiotic treatment if an inappropriate therapeutic regimen is used. A common mistake in clinical practice is to assume that the major predisposition to a pattern of resistance is the overuse of the broadest category of antibiotic to which a pathogen is resistant. Several examples are important in the understanding of this concept.

A classic example of multi-drug resistance in gram-negative organisms is the resistance in *P. aeruginosa*. Multiple resistance mechanisms regulated by genetic operons on the chromosome of *P. aeruginosa* have been described, including efflux pumps, *ampC* β-lactamases, and outer membrane porin closure.[114]

Efflux pumps are three-component systems, contained within the bacterial cell wall, that allow bacteria to eliminate antibiotics that have entered. Initially described in 1980 as a mechanism of resistance in tetracyclines, efflux was recognized in 1988 as a contributor to fluoroquinolone resistance.[115] In recent years, the contribution of efflux to clinical resistance has broadened, with important implications for treatment of VAP. The composition of this system has been nicely detailed.[116,117] The pump itself (also referred to as the transporter) lies in the cytoplasmic membrane and is designated MexB, MexD, or MexF. It is attached via a linker lipoprotein (MexA, MexC, or MexE) in the periplasm, which lies between the outer and inner membranes of the bacterial cell wall. This second component is linked to the third component, the exit portal (OprM, OprJ, or OprN), which lies in the outer membrane. These three components of the efflux pump normally are under repressor gene control and therefore are not clinically active.

P. aeruginosa has several efflux systems, with MexAB-OprM and MexEF-OprN having particular clinical significance: The MexAB-OprM system contributes to both intrinsic and acquired resistance; and the MexEF-OprN system contributes only to acquired resistance.[118] The MexAB-OprM system is expressed constitutively in cells grown in standard laboratory media, where it contributes to intrinsic resistance to a number of antimicrobials, including fluoroquinolones and β-lactams.[119] The contribution of MexAB-OprM to β-lactam efflux is interesting from two perspectives: (1) reports of efflux of β-lactam antibiotics have been comparatively rare; and (2) β-lactams act on periplasmic rather than cytoplasmic targets, in contrast with all other MexAB-OprM antibiotic substrates. Of the β-lactams, only carbapenems appear to be poor substrates for MexAB-OprM. The different carbapenems vary with regard to their susceptibility to efflux. Meropenem is subject to efflux, and expression of the MexAB-OprM efflux system has been correlated with resistance to meropenem.[120] By contrast, imipenem is not subject to efflux.[118] It has been suggested that this may be due to the need for efflux systems with MexAB-OprM to access their substrates within the cytoplasmic membrane, with meropenem being much more amphiphilic than imipenem, which appears not to be substrates for MexAB-OprM.[120]

The ability of fluoroquinolones to select certain *nfxc* (*mexT*) mutants has been discussed.[116,121] In addition to resistance to fluoroquinolones, these mutants may have decreased susceptibility and even clinical resistance to carbapenems (e.g., imipenem, meropenem) that occurs on the basis of either closure of porin channels in the outer membrane of the bacterial cell wall (with resultant impermeability) or upregulation of an efflux pump (which allows the bacteria to eliminate drug that has penetrated the organism's cell wall). Such newly recognized information may help explain patterns of increasing carbapenem resistance in health care institutions in which carbapenem use has not recently increased. Several antibiotic efflux systems have been characterized in *P. aeruginosa,* with the MexAB-OprM system constitutively expressed in virtually all isolates.[119] Substrates for this pump include fluoroquinolones, tetracyclines, piperacillin, cefepime, aztreonam, and certain carbapenems. It is noteworthy that not all carbapenems are subject to efflux. For example, imipenem does not appear to be a substrate for MexAB-OprM, whereas meropenem may be extruded by this pump because of its hydrophobic side chain.[118,122]

For infections such as HAP and VAP, in which *P. aeruginosa* is a pathogen targeted with empiric therapy and for which fluoroquinolones are offered as an option in the initial regimen,[11,123-125] data on the risk of fluoroquinolones leading to multidrug resistance via efflux mechanisms become especially noteworthy.

The experience with carbapenem-resistant *Acinetobacter baumannii* in Brooklyn, New York, provides an important insight into the problem of selection for resistance by one class of antibiotic to an entirely different class. In a study to evaluate the endemicity of *A. baumannii,* all unique patient isolates of this pathogen were collected from 15 Brooklyn hospitals over a 3-month period.[126] Antibiotic susceptibilities, the genetic relatedness of resistant isolates, using ribotype profiles, and the relationship between antibiotic use and resistance rates were determined. Among the 224 carbapenem-resistant strains of *A. baumannii,* ribotyping demonstrated that one strain accounted for two thirds of the isolates and was present in all of the 15 participating hospitals. The strongest predisposition to selection for this pathogen was cephalosporin use. Known *A. baumannii* resistance mechanisms include chromosomally associated β-lactamases and porin protein mutations,[127] so it can be assumed that this represents selection of carbapenem-resistant mutant strains by the cephalosporins.

A retrospective analysis of critically ill trauma patients with late-onset gram-negative pneumonia showed that the antibiotic most associated with pneumonia due to

Stenotrophomonas maltophilia was cefepime.[128] These data on cephalosporins as a risk factor for *S. maltophilia* infection are similar to those in an earlier report that identified use of ceftazidime and imipenem as associated with similar rates of *S. maltophilia* acquisition in hospitalized patients.[129] The suggestion by these reports is that broad-spectrum agents, more so than one specific agent, may kill sensitive bacteria and allow pathogens such as *Stenotrophomonas* to become clinically expressed.

One of the alarming trends in the worldwide epidemic of antibiotic resistance has been the increasing prevalence of carbapenem-hydrolyzing β-lactamases. These carbapenemases have occurred as both metallo-based enzymes (class B in the Ambler system of β-lactamase classification) as well as serine-based enzymes (classes A and D).[130] Among the class A carbapenemases are enzymes produced by *Klebsiella pneumoniae* and referred to as KPC enzymes. A clinical report described a group of infections caused by *Klebsiella* species in which 45% of *K. pneumoniae* strains produced extended-spectrum β-lactamases (ESBLs), with 3.3% of the strains carrying KPC-2 carbapenem-hydrolyzing enzymes.[131] In an attempt to understand this outbreak, the investigators studied the prior antibiotic exposure in the patients from whom these KPC-2 enzymes were isolated. Most had received a β-lactam or fluoroquinolone, but only 20% had received a carbapenem. The overall 14-day mortality rate in patients who were bacteremic with these pathogens was 47%. Most isolates were from a single ribotype, suggesting inadequate infection control as a mechanism for dispersing the resistant pathogens selected by antibiotic pressure. As in the reports of carbapenem-resistant *Acinetobacter* and *Stenotrophomonas* just described, KPC enzyme–producing bacteria may be the product of selection by antibiotics other than carbapenems.

A more common problem than that of carbapenemases in *Klebsiella* is the production of extended-spectrum β-lactamases (ESBLs), which also are produced by such pathogens as *E. coli, Enterobacter,* and *Proteus*. Described first in the 1980s, these enzymes may occur on the basis of a change of only one amino acid in the β-lactamases normally produced by these pathogens.[132] Despite the minimal structural change, the enzymes have the capacity to inactivate many broad-spectrum β-lactam drugs. Of note, use of any of several classes of antibiotics, notably third-generation cephalosporins and fluoroquinolones, has been identified as a risk factor for selecting ESBLs.[133,134] The standard techniques that have been used around the world for ESBL detection have included disk diffusion, but as nicely reviewed, the breakpoints for susceptibility vary according to regions of the world, with the breakpoints in the United States being higher than those reported from other geographic areas.[132] This difference becomes noteworthy when it is considered that ESBL production has been detected in up to 36% of ceftriaxone-susceptible isolates and 19% of ceftazidime-susceptible isolates.[135] This pattern of hidden resistance can be the basis for inappropriate therapy, because the test used to identify a pattern of resistance may not be sensitive enough to do so. The resistance that occurs in such ESBL producers is of importance for the clinician in initial antibiotic selection in two regards. With β-lactam antibiotic therapy, even antibiotics that generally are stable in the presence of β-lactamases may not have predictable activity. Inferior outcomes associated with extended-spectrum cephalosporins, such as cefepime and β-lactam/β-lactamase inhibitor combinations such as piperacillin-tazobactam, have been described[136]; this finding has been attributed to inoculum effect, with diminished susceptibility as the size of the inoculum is increased from 10^5 to 10^7 organisms.[136,137] An alternative explanation for the lack of activity by certain β-lactam antibiotics has been proposed by Craig and Bhavnani.[138] As the number of bacterial colony-forming units (CFUs) increases from 5×10^5 to 5×10^7, approximately 100 times more β-lactamase is released from bacteria lysed after antibiotic exposure. Variations in antibiotic efficacy may rest on the increased release of enzyme in infections with larger inoculums of organisms (for example, pneumonia and intra-abdominal abscess) and not on the size of the inoculum alone. Thus, in vitro susceptibility may not predict in vivo outcome for treatment of infectious diseases. Because inadequate therapy of infection caused by ESBL-producing organisms has been associated with increased mortality,[136] it is important for clinicians to be aware of such information.

Even though ESBLs are β-lactamases, certain non–β-lactam antibiotics are not efficacious in infections with ESBL-producing gram-negative bacilli. The resistance genes for aminoglycosides are located on the same plasmid carrying genetic elements for ESBL production. As a result, gentamicin and tobramycin resistance may occur in ESBL producers.[137] With fluoroquinolones, multiple mechanisms may contribute to quinolone resistance in ESBL producers. Topoisomerase mutations may be associated with decreased binding. The *qnr* gene codes for a protein that wraps around DNA gyrase, thereby preventing quinolones from attaching to target binding sites.[139] In addition, ESBL-producing organisms may possess efflux pumps, and because fluoroquinolones are subject to extrusion from bacteria by means of these pumps, efflux is a potential mechanism of quinolone resistance in ESBL producers.[140] Complicating the problem with ESBLs is that these pathogens have now been described as the cause of community outbreaks, which usually manifest as urinary tract infections caused by *E. coli.*[141]

The foregoing examples of carbapenem resistance in *Pseudomonas, Acinetobacter, Stenotrophomonas,* and *Klebsiella* underscore an important concept in antimicrobial therapy for the critical care clinician, for whom such patterns of resistance are becoming increasingly prevalent in the ICU. When multidrug resistance occurs, it cannot be predictably assumed that such resistance is on the basis of exposure to the broadest class of antibiotic to which the organism is resistant. To accept such a flawed assessment could result in limited use of that class of antibiotic, which could then shift to increased use of the actual class of antibiotic that led to the pattern of resistance. The other clinically relevant observation in all of these recently described outbreaks is that inadequate infection control contributed to the spread of resistant strains that had been selected by antibiotics.[126,131,136]

DURATION OF THERAPY

Because antibiotics may be a risk factor for resistance,[107] it is important in the process of antibiotic stewardship to identify opportunities to minimize exposure to these therapeutic agents. One possibility is with the duration of therapy. Often the decisions regarding traditional durations of therapy find their basis not in controlled trials or prospective studies, but rather in expert opinion; however, trials in VAP have challenged some of the classic tenets.

Dennesen and coworkers[142] evaluated the response to antimicrobial therapy administered according to ATS guidelines in 27 patients diagnosed with VAP in a study that initially used a bronchoalveolar lavage (BAL) along with clinical parameters to confirm the diagnosis of VAP but subsequently used semiquantitative tracheal aspirates for microbiologic surveillance. All patients in this study received appropriate antibiotic therapy. After initiation of antibiotic therapy, T_{max} (maximal temperature over a 24-hour period), PaO_2/FiO_2 (ratio used to quantify impairment of oxygen gas exchange in the lung), WBC count, and semiquantitative cultures of endotracheal aspirate were monitored. Resolution of clinical parameters occurred primarily within the first 6 days of therapy. Using cultures of endotracheal aspirates, the investigators found that colonization with *P. aeruginosa* persisted throughout the duration of treatment, whereas colonization with *S. aureus, H. influenzae,* and *S. pneumoniae* resolved shortly after initiation of therapy. Acquired colonization, predominantly with resistant pathogens such as *P. aeruginosa* or members of Enterobacteriaceae, usually occurred in week 2 and frequently preceded a recurrent episode of lung infection. On the basis of these data, it was suggested that 7 days may be an appropriate duration of therapy for patients with VAP.

Ibrahim and colleagues[143] evaluated a clinical guideline for the treatment of VAP using 7 days of therapy. A total of 102 patients were prospectively evaluated, 50 before institution of the guidelines and 52 after institution. In addition to more frequent choice of adequate initial antibiotic treatment after implementation of the clinical guideline, patients also had shorter antibiotic courses when treated under the guideline. No mortality difference was noted between the two groups. As was the case with the study by Denneson and coworkers,[142] a second episode of VAP was more likely to occur in the patients receiving the longer, traditional duration of therapy.

Chastre and associates[144] conducted a prospective, multicenter, randomized, double-blind study of 401 patients with VAP confirmed by quantitative cultures obtained by bronchoscopic protected specimen brush (PSB) or BAL, or both. Only patients who had received initial appropriate antibiotic therapy were included. Therapy was divided into two categories: short course, which was given for 8 days in 197 patients, versus long course, which was given for 15 days in 204 patients. Clinical efficacy was similar between the short course and long course groups. Because slightly more patients with nonfermenting gram-negative bacilli assigned to the 8-day regimen had pulmonary infection recurrences, the investigators were unable to demonstrate the noninferiority of the 8-day regimen for infection by such pathogens compared with the 15-day course of therapy. Multiresistant pathogens more frequently caused recurrences in patients who received the 15-day regimen. Even though the findings from this study do not definitively prove that therapy for HAP or VAP can be limited to 7 days, they lend support to the findings by Dennesen[142] and Ibrahim[143] and their colleagues.

MINIMIZING CLINICAL RESISTANCE

In the absence of a significant pipeline of antibiotics for treating multidrug-resistant organisms, it is important for the clinician to use antibiotics judiciously so that currently available agents are active for as long as possible. Several approaches toward achieving this goal have been described.

For many years, the standard approach to antibiotic prescribing occurred in a homogeneous manner in which a single or limited numbers of antibiotics were used as the "workhorse" agents in empiric therapy.[145] Such an approach to antibiotic prescribing often was associated with restricted formularies, the thought being that limiting broad-spectrum agents might prevent the emergence of resistance. Unfortunately, this approach did not take into consideration that the inadequate therapy in seriously ill patients might not be reversible when the initial antibiotics were changed to the correct agents once susceptibilities were known. In addition, it was during this era of restricted formularies that the proliferation of bacterial resistance began to occur. Because an inherent risk with homogeneous antibiotic use is the selective pressure that when applied can lead to resistance, other approaches must be considered.

Heterogeneous antibiotic use, in which antibiotic selection is based not on hospital mandates but rather on issues related both to the patient and the pathogens involved in the infectious process, may decrease selective pressure.[145] Heterogeneity can be achieved in any of several ways. One such approach that has been advocated is cycling of antibiotics, referred to by some authors as "crop rotation." The rationale is that changing the first-line agent for empiric therapy in a hospital or even in a specific unit on a regular predefined basis will, at least to some degree, lead to heterogeneity. A cycling protocol studied initially in four academic centers in the United States but completed in two used cefepime, ciprofloxacin or levofloxacin, imipenem, and piperacillin/tazobactam rotated at 3- to 4-month intervals in two medical ICUs.[146] The defined outcome in the study was acquisition and prevalence of resistance in *P. aeruginosa*. A total of 1942 patients were studied over 31 months; 392 *P. aeruginosa* isolates were collected, with 42% from surveillance swabs. No change in either the incidence of VAP or acquisition of *P. aeruginosa* was noted, with the prevalence increasing in one hospital from 8.3 to 26.9 patients per 1000 admissions during the study period.

It has been acknowledged that the cumulative evidence to date suggests that antibiotic cycling has limited efficacy for preventing antibiotic resistance.[147] In response to the lack of predictable efficacy of cycling in preventing resistance, a strategy by which multiple or all classes of antibiotics are available for use (i.e., antibiotic heterogeneity) has been suggested as part of a broader effort aimed at curtailing antibiotic resistance within ICUs. As a potential alternative to cycling, a mathematical model was developed to compare antibiotic cycling with *mixing,* in which antibiotic variation is random as opposed to the regulation that occurs with cycling.[148] The premise for such a comparison is that mixing imposes greater fluctuation in selective conditions, thereby yielding greater heterogeneity than occurs with cycling. In this study, the results were underlaid by a simple ecologic explanation that led to the conclusion that cycling is unlikely to be effective and may even hinder resistance control and that mixing may yield more favorable results in terms of preserving antibiotic susceptibility.

In contrast with homogeneous antibiotic use, which was developed to control resistance, heterogeneous use is aimed at managing resistance.[145] Because resistance at some level is an inevitable part of medical practice, the latter approach seems more insightful.

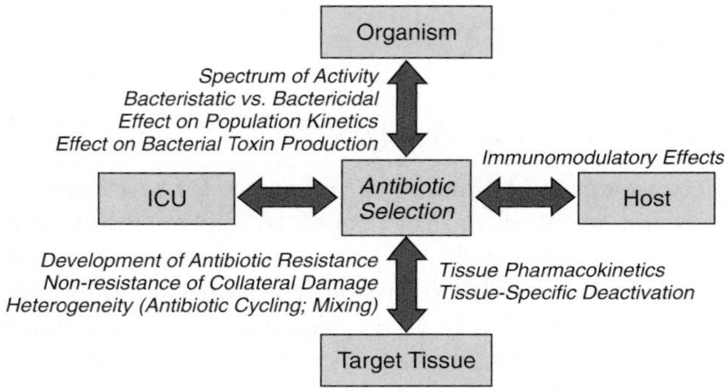

Figure 52-3. The interplay of antibiotic selection with principles relevant to host, organism, intensive care unit, and target tissue. Adequate antibiotic therapy is dictated by more than matching spectrum of antibiotic activity with a pathogen's in vitro susceptibility.

CONCLUSIONS

At a time when bacterial resistance is becoming more prevalent but during which antibiotic development is relatively stagnant, the critical care clinician is faced with the somewhat daunting challenge of achieving clinical efficacy without compromising the antibiotic armamentarium that exists at present. For this to be accomplished, the interplay of several important concepts will drive the decision process. As depicted in Figure 52-3, these considerations include the organism, the host, and the targeted tissue, as well as specific issues related to the ICU itself.

Armed with the knowledge of these variables, health care providers now have the foundation for achieving the first goal of antibiotic stewardship—education.[3] Nevertheless, in the recently developed guideline for antibiotic stewardship, it was acknowledged that education alone, without incorporation of active intervention, is only marginally effective in changing antimicrobial prescribing practices and has not demonstrated a sustained effect.[3] An understanding of the principles governing antimicrobial selection in the ICU should better position critical care clinicians for practicing the art of antibiotic prescribing in a manner that both achieves efficacy for optimal outcome and preserves the integrity of the antibiotics available for this task.

KEY POINTS

- Initial appropriate antibiotic therapy (defined as matching antibiotic to pathogen susceptibility), with early dose administration, reduces mortality in the treatment of serious infections.
- Adequate antibiotic therapy extends beyond appropriate therapy and includes dose optimization, ensuring target tissue penetration, and consideration of combination therapy.
- Empiric and directed antibiotic regimens for the individual patient also are influenced by factors that the critical care physician must recognize: time- versus concentration-dependent killing; synergy versus antagonism; immunomodulatory antibiotic properties; inhibition of bacterial protein synthesis; and organ-specific deactivation.
- In selecting antibiotics for serious infections, the clinician should consider not only the individual therapeutic efficacy but also the potential for unintended antibiotic consequences, such as selection of resistant microorganisms.
- Because antibiotic therapy is a risk factor for selecting resistant microorganisms, antibiotics should not be broader in coverage, or given longer, than necessary. Initial broad and aggressive antibiotic therapy should be rapidly de-escalated to focused therapy as soon as is clinically possible.
- It is important to recognize that resistance to a class of antibiotics may be selected by therapy with an entirely different class of drugs.
- Knowledge of the mechanisms by which antibiotic-resistant bacteria are selected may lead to more judicious patterns of antibiotic use that may help to manage the evolving patterns of resistance that are occurring globally.

REFERENCES

1. Talbot GH, Bradley J, Edwards JE Jr, et al: Bad bugs need drugs: An update on the development pipeline from the Antimicrobial Availability Task Force of the Infectious Diseases Society of America. Clin Infect Dis 2006;42: 657-668.
2. Infectious Diseases Society of America: Bad bugs, no drugs. July 2004. Available at www.idsociety.org/badbugsnodrugs
3. Dellit TH, Owens RC, McGowan JE, et al: Infectious Diseases Society of America and the Society for Healthcare Epidemiology of America guidelines for developing an institutional program to enhance antimicrobial stewardship. Clin Infect Dis 2007;44:159-177.
4. Luna CM, Vujacich P, Niederman MS, et al: Impact of BAL data on therapy and outcome of ventilator-associated pneumonia. Chest 1997;111:676-685.
5. Rello J, Gallego M, Mariscal D, et al: The value of routine microbial investigation in ventilator-associated pneumonia. Am J Respir Crit Care Med 1997;156:196-200.
6. Kollef MH, Ward S: The influence of mini-BAL cultures on patient outcomes: Implications for the antibiotic management of ventilator-associated pneumonia. Chest 1998;113:412-420.
7. Ibrahim EH, Sherman G, Ward S, et al: The influence of inadequate antimicrobial treatment of bloodstream infection on patient outcomes in the ICU setting. Chest 2000;118:146-155.
8. Harbarth S, Garbino J, Pugin J, et al: Inappropriate initial antimicrobial therapy and its effect on survival in a clinical trial of immunomodulating therapy for severe sepsis. Am J Med 2003;115;529-535.
9. Vallés J, Rello J, Ochagavía A, et al: Community-acquired bloodstream infection in critically ill adult patients: Impact of shock and inappropriate antibiotic therapy on survival. Chest 2003;123:1615-1624.
10. Kollef MH: Inadequate antimicrobial treatment: An important determinant of outcome for hospitalized patients. Clin Infect Dis 2000;31(Suppl 4): S131-S138.
11. American Thoracic Society/Infectious Diseases Society of America: Guidelines for the management of adults with hospital-acquired, ventilator-associated, and healthcare-associated pneumonia. Am J Respir Crit Care Med 2005;171:388-416.
12. Ebert SC, Craig WA: Pharmacodynamic properties of antibiotics: Application to drug monitoring and dosage regimen design. Infect Control Hosp Epidemiol 1990;11:319-326.
13. Bodi M, Ardanuy C, Rello J. Impact of gram-positive resistance on outcome of nosocomial pneumonia. Crit Care Med 2001;29 (Suppl):N82-N86.
14. Lodise TP, Lomaestro B, Drusano GL: Piperacillin-tazobactam for *Pseudomonas aeruginosa* infection: Clinical implications of an extended-infusion dosing strategy. Clin Infect Dis 2007;44:357-363.
15. Krueger W, Bulitta J, Kinzig-Schippers M, et al: Evaluation by Monte Carlo simulation of the pharmacokinetics of two doses of meropenem administered intermittently or as a continuous infusion in healthy volunteers. Antimicrob Agents Chemother 2005;49:1881-1889.
16. Wysocki M, Delatour F, Faurisson F, et al: Continuous versus intermittent infusion of vancomycin in severe staphylococcal infections: Prospective multicenter randomized study. Antimicrob Agents Chemother 2001;45:2460-2467.
17. Rello J, Paiva JA, Baraibar J, et al: International conference for the development of consensus on the diagnosis and treatment of ventilator-associated pneumonia. Chest 2001;120:955-970.
18. Gerber AU, Craig WA, Brugger HP, et al: Impact of dosing intervals on activity of gentamicin and ticarcillin against *Pseudomonas aeruginosa* in granulocytopenic mice. J Infect Dis 1983;147:910-917.
19. Kapusnik JE, Hackbarth CJ, Chambers HL, et al: Single, large, daily dosing versus intermittent dosing of tobramycin for treating experimental pseudomonas pneumonia. J Infect Dis 1988;158:7-12.
20. Powell SH, Thompson WL, Luthe MA, et al: Once daily vs. continuous aminoglycoside dosing: Efficacy and toxicity in animal and clinical studies of gentamicin, netilmicin, and tobramycin. J Infect Dis 1983;147: 918-932.
21. Vogelman B, Craig WA: Kinetics of antimicrobial activity. J Pediatr 1986;108:835-840.
22. Nicolau DP, Freman CD, Belliveau PP, et al: Experience with a once-daily aminoglycoside program administered to 2,184 adult patients. Antimicrob Agents Chemother 1995;39:650-655.
23. Galloe AM, Graudal N, Christensen HR, Kampmann JP: Aminoglycosides: Single or multiple daily dosing? A meta-analysis on efficacy and safety. Eur J Clin Pharmacol 1995;48:39-43.
24. Peloquin CA, Cumbo TJ, Nix DE, et al: Evaluation of intravenous ciprofloxacin in patients with nosocomial lower respiratory tract infections: Impact of plasma concentrations, organism, minimum inhibitory concentration, and clinical condition on bacterial eradication. Arch Intern Med 1989;149:2269-2273.
25. Drusano GL, Louis A, Deziel M, Gumbo T: The crisis of resistance: Identifying drug exposures to suppress amplification of resistant mutant subpopulations. Clin Infect Dis 2006;42:525-532.
26. Fink MP, Snydman DR, Niederman MS, et al: Treatment of severe pneumonia in hospitalized patients: Results of a multicenter, randomized, double-blind trial comparing intravenous ciprofloxacin with imipenem-cilastatin. The Severe Pneumonia Study Group. Antimicrob Agents Chemother 1994; 38:547-557.
27. Wunderink RG, Rello J, Cammarata SK, et al: Linezolid vs vancomycin: Analysis of two double-blind studies of patients with methicillin-resistant *Staphylococcus aureus* nosocomial pneumonia. Chest 2003;124: 1789-1797.
28. Kollef MH, Rello J, Cammarata SK, et al: Clinical cure and survival in gram-positive ventilator-associated pneumonia: Retrospective analysis of two double-blind studies comparing linezolid with vancomycin. Intensive Care Med 2004;30:388-394.
29. Rubinstein E, Cammarata S, Oliphant T, et al: Linezolid (PNU-100766) versus vancomycin in the treatment of hospitalized patients with nosocomial pneumonia: A randomized, double-blind, multicenter study. Clin Infect Dis 2001;32:402-412.
30. Wunderink RG, Cammarata SK, Oliphant TH, et al: Continuation of a randomized, double-blind, multicenter study of linezolid versus vancomycin in the treatment of patients with nosocomial pneumonia. Clin Ther 2003;25:980-992.
31. Honeybourne D: Antibiotic penetration into lung tissues. Thorax 1994;49: 104-106.
32. Thys JP, Klastersky J, Mombelli G: Peak or sustained antibiotic levels for optimal tissue penetration. J Antimicrob Chemother 1981;8(Suppl C):29-36.
33. Berre J, Thys JP, Husson M, et al: Penetration of ciprofloxacin in bronchial secretions after intravenous administration. J Antimicrob Chemother 1988;22:499-504.
34. Fowler RA, Flavin KE, Barr J, et al: Variability in antibiotic prescribing patterns and outcomes in patients with clinically suspected ventilator-associated pneumonia. Chest 2003;123:835-844.
35. Niederman M: Reexamining quinolone use in the intensive care unit: Use them right or lose the fight against resistant bacteria. Crit Care Med 2005;33:443-444.
36. Gruson D, Hilbert G, Vargas F, et al: Rotation and restricted use of antibiotics in a medical intensive care unit: Impact on the incidence of ventilator-associated pneumonia caused by antibiotic resistant gram-negative bacteria. Am J Respir Crit Care Med 2000;162:837-843.
37. Cruciani M, Gatti G, Lazzarini L, et al: Penetration of vancomycin into human lung tissue. J Antimicrob Chemother 1996;38:865-869.
38. Lamer C, de Beco V, Soler P, et al: Analysis of vancomycin entry into pulmonary lining fluid by bronchoalveolar lavage in critically ill patients. Antimicrob Agents Chemother 1993;37:281-286.
39. Conte JE Jr, Golden JA, Kipps J, Zurlinden E: Intrapulmonary pharmacokinetics of linezolid. Antimicrob Agents Chemother 2002;46:1475-1480.
40. Honeybourne D, Tobin C, Jevons G, et al: Intrapulmonary penetration of linezolid. J Antimicrob Chemother 2003;51:1431-1434.
41. MacGowan, Alasdair P: Pharmacokinetic and

pharmacodynamic profile of linezolid in healthy volunteers and patients with gram-positive infections. J Antimicrob Chemother 2003;51(Suppl 2):ii17-ii25.
42. Boselli E, Breilh D, Rimmele T, et al: Pharmacokinetics and intrapulmonary concentrations of linezolid administered to critically ill patients with ventilator-associated pneumonia. Crit Care Med 2005;33:1529-1533.
43. Moellering RC Jr, Wennersten C, Weinberg AN: Studies on antibiotic synergism against enterococci. I. Bacteriologic studies. J Lab Clin Med 1971;77:821-828.
44. Rahal JJ Jr: Antibiotic combinations: The clinical relevance of synergy and antagonism. Medicine 1978;57: 179-195.
45. Korzeniowski O, Sande MA: The national collaborative endocarditis study group: Combination antimicrobial therapy for *Staphylococcus aureus* endocarditis in patients addicted to parenteral drugs and in nonaddicts. Ann Intern Med 1982;97:496-503.
46. Moellering RC Jr, Eliopoulos GM: Principles of anti-infective therapy. In Mandell GL, Bennett JE, Dolin R (eds): Mandell, Douglas, and Bennett's Principles and Practice of Infectious Diseases, 6th ed. Philadelphia, Churchill Livingstone, 2005, pp 242-253.
47. Hilf M, Yu VL, Sharp JA, et al: Antibiotic therapy for *Pseudomonas aeruginosa* bacteremia: Outcome correlations in a prospective study of 200 patients. Am J Med 1989;87: 540-546.
48. Lepper MH, Dowling HF: Treatment of pneumococcic meningitis with penicillin compared with penicillin plus aureomycin. Arch Intern Med 1951;88:489-494.
49. Miller LG, Perdreau-Remington F, Bayer AS: Clinical and epidemiologic characteristics cannot distinguish community-associated methicillin-resistant *Staphylococcus aureus* infection from methicillin-susceptible *S. aureus* infection: A prospective investigation. Clin Infect Dis 2007;44:471-482.
50. Blot SI, Vandewoude KH, Hoste EA, Colardyn FA: Outcome and attributable mortality in critically ill patients with bacteremia involving methicillin-susceptible and methicillin-resistant *Staphylococcus aureus.* Arch Intern Med 2002; 162:2229-2235.
51. Cosgrove SE, Sakoulas G, Perencevich EN, et al: Comparison of mortality associated with methicillin-resistant and methicillin-susceptible *Staphylococcus aureus* bacteremia: A meta-analysis. Clin Infect Dis 2003;36:53-59.
52. Shorr SF, Combes A, Kollef MH, Chastre J: Methicillin-resistant *Staphylococcus aureus* prolongs intensive care unit stay in ventilator-associated pneumonia, despite initially appropriate antibiotic therapy. Crit Care Med 2006;34:700-706.
53. Shorr SF, Tabak YP, Gupta V, et al: Morbidity and cost burden of methicillin-resistant *Staphylococcus aureus* in early onset ventilator-associated pneumonia. Crit Care 2006;10:R97.
54. Grohs P, Kitzis MD, Gutmann L: In vitro bactericidal activities of linezolid in combination with vancomycin, gentamicin, ciprofloxacin, fusidic acid, and rifampin against *Staphylococcus aureus.* Antimicrob Agents Chemother 2003;47:418-420.
55. Sahuquillo AJM, Colombo GM, Gil BA, et al: In vitro activity of linezolid in combination with doxycycline, fosfomycin, levofloxacin, rifampicin, and vancomycin against methicillin-susceptible *Staphylococcus aureus.* Rev Esp Quimioter 2006;19:252-257.
56. Sweeney MT, Zurenko GE: In vitro activities of linezolid combined with other antimicrobial agents against staphylococci, enterococci, pneumococci, and selected gram-negative organisms. Antimicrob Agents Chemother 2003;47: 1902-1906.
57. Chiang F-Y, Climo M: Efficacy of linezolid alone or in combination with vancomycin for treatment of experimental endocarditis due to methicillin-resistant *Staphylococcus aureus.* Antimicrob Agents Chemother 2003;47:3002-3004.
58. Paul M, Benuri-Silbiger I, Soares-Weiser K, Leibovici L: β-Lactam monotherapy versus β-lactam-aminoglycoside combination therapy for sepsis in immunocompetent patients: Systematic review and meta-analysis of randomised trials. BMJ 2004;328: 668-681.
59. Allan JD: Antibiotic combinations. Med Clin North Am 1987;71:1074-1091.
60. Bliziotis IA, Samonis G, Vardakas KZ, et al: Effect of aminoglycoside and beta-lactam combination therapy versus beta-lactam monotherapy on the emergence of antimicrobial resistance: A meta-analysis of randomized, controlled trials. Clin Infect Dis 2005;41:149-158.
61. Harbarth S, Nobre V, Pittet D: Does antibiotic selection impact patient outcome? Clin Infect Dis 2007;44: 87-93.
62. Eagle H: Experimental approach to the problem of treatment failure with penicillin. I. Group A streptococcal infection in mice. Am J Med 1952;13:389-399.
63. Bisno AL, Stevens DL: Streptococcal infections of skin and soft tissues. N Engl J Med 1996;334:240-245.
64. Stevens DL, Bryant AE, Hackett SP: Antibiotic effects on bacterial viability, toxin production, and host response. Clin Infect Dis 1995;20(Suppl 2): S154-S157.
65. Gemmell CG, Peterson PK, Schmeling D, et al: Potentiation of opsonization and phagocytosis of *Streptococcus pyogenes* following growth in the presence of clindamycin. J Clin Invest 1981;67:1249-1256.
66. Francis JS, Doherty MC, Lopatin U, et al: Severe community-onset pneumonia in healthy adults caused by methicillin-resistant *Staphylococcus aureus* carrying the Panton-Valentine leukocidin genes. Clin Infect Dis 2005;40:100-107.
67. Miller LG, Perdreau-Remington F, Rieg G, et al: Necrotizing fasciitis caused by community-associated methicillin-resistant *Staphylococcus aureus* in Los Angeles. N Engl J Med 2005; 352: 1445-1453.
68. Fridkin SK, Hageman JC, Morrison M, et al: Methicillin-resistant *Staphylococcus aureus* disease in three communities. N Engl J Med 2005;352:1436-1444.
69. Stevens DL, Ma Y, Salmi DB, et al: Impact of antibiotics on expression of virulence-associated exotoxin genes in methicillin-sensitive and methicillin-resistant *Staphylococcus aureus.* Clin Infect Dis 2007;195:202-211.
70. Baddour LM, Yu VL, Klugman KP, et al: Combination antibiotic therapy lowers mortality in severely ill patients with pneumococcal bacteremia. Am J Respir Crit Care Med 2004;170:440-444.
71. Garcia VE, Mensa J, Martinez JA, et al: Lower mortality among patients with community-acquired pneumonia treated with a macrolide plus a beta-lactam agent versus a beta-lactam agent alone. Eur J Clin Microbiol Infect Dis 2005;24:190-195.
72. Martinez FJ: Monotherapy versus dual therapy for community-acquired pneumonia in hospitalized patients. Clin Infect Dis 2004;38(Suppl 4): S328-S340.
73. Martinez JA, Horcajada JP, Almela M, et al: Addition of a macrolide to a beta-lactam–based empirical antibiotic regimen is associated with lower in-hospital mortality for patients with bacteremic pneumococcal pneumonia. Clin Infect Dis 2003;36:389-395.
74. Mufson MA, Stanek RJ: Bacteremic pneumococcal pneumonia in one American city: A 20-year longitudinal study, 1978-1997. Am J Med 1999;107:34S-43S.
75. Mufson MA, Stanek RJ: Revisiting combination antibiotic therapy for community-acquired invasive *Streptococcus pneumoniae* pneumonia. Clin Infect Dis 2006;42:304-306.
76. Waterer GW: Monotherapy versus combination antimicrobial therapy for pneumococcal pneumonia. Curr Opin Infect Dis 2005;18:157-163.
77. Waterer GW, Somes GW, Wunderink RG: Monotherapy may be suboptimal for severe bacteremic pneumococcal pneumonia. Arch Intern Med 2001;161:1837-1842.
78. Weiss K, Low DE, Cortes L, et al: Clinical characteristics at initial presentation and impact of dual therapy on the outcome of bacteremic *Streptococcus pneumoniae* pneumonia in adults. Can Respir J 2004;11: 589-593.
79. Vázquez EG, Mensa J, Martínez A, et al: Lower mortality among patients with community-acquired pneumonia treated with a macrolide plus a beta-lactam agent versus a beta-lactam agent alone. Eur J Clin Microbiol Infect Dis 2005;24:190-195.
80. Iregui M, Ward S, Sherman G, et al: Clinical importance of delays in the initiation of appropriate antibiotic treatment for ventilator-associated pneumonia. Chest 2002;122:262-268.
81. Höffken G, Niederman MS: Nosocomial pneumonia: The importance of a de-escalating strategy

antibiotic treatment of pneumonia in the ICU. Chest 2002;122:2183-2196.
82. Houck PM, Bratzler DW, Nsa W, et al: Timing of antibiotic administration and outcomes for Medicare patients hospitalized with community-acquired pneumonia. Arch Intern Med 2004;164:637-644.
83. Tunkel AR, Hartman BJ, Kaplan SL, et al: Practice guidelines for the management of bacterial meningitis. Clin Infect Dis 2004;39:1267-1284.
84. Aronin SI, Peduzzi P, Quagliarello VJ: Community-acquired bacterial meningitis: Risk stratification for adverse clinical outcome and effect of antibiotic timing. Ann Intern Med 1998; 129:862-869.
85. Dellinger RP, Carlet JM, Masur H, et al: Surviving sepsis campaign guidelines for management of severe sepsis and septic shock. Crit Care Med 2004;32: 858-873.
86. Silverman JA, Mortin LI, VanPraagh AD, et al: Inhibition of daptomycin by pulmonary surfactant: In vitro modeling and clinical impact. J Infect Dis 2004;191:2149-2152.
87. Fuchs PC, Barry AL, Brown SD: In vitro bactericidal activity of daptomycin against staphylococci. J Antimicrob Chemother 2002;49:467-470.
88. King A, Philips I: The in vitro activity of daptomycin against 514 gram-positive aerobic clinical isolates. J Antimicrob Agents Chemother 2001;48:219-223.
89. Wise R, Andrews JM, Ashby JP: Activity of daptomycin against gram-positive pathogens: A comparison with other agents and the determination of a tentative breakpoint. J Antimicrob Chemother 2001;48:563-567.
90. Silverman JA, Perlmutter NG, Shapiro HM: Correlation of daptomycin bactericidal activity and membrane depolarization in *Staphylococcus aureus.* Antimicrob Agents Chemother 2003;47:2538-2544.
91. Arbiet RD, Maki D, Tally FP, et al: The safety and efficacy of daptomycin for the treatment of complicated skin and skin-structure infection. Clin Infect Dis 2004;38:1673-1681.
92. Fowler VG, Boucher HW, Corey GR, et al: Daptomycin versus standard therapy for bacteremia and endocarditis caused by *Staphylococcus aureus.* N Engl J Med 2006;355: 653-665.
93. Lakey JH, Ptak M: Fluorescence indicates a calcium-dependent interaction between the lipopeptide antibiotic LY146032 and phospholipid membranes. Biochemistry 1988;27: 4639-4645.
94. Jung D, Rozek A, Okon M, Hancock REW: Structural transitions as determinants of the action of the calcium-dependent antibiotic daptomycin. Chem Biol 2004;11: 949-957.
95. Raad I, Darouiche R, Vazquez J, et al: Efficacy and safety of weekly dalbavancin therapy for catheter-related bloodstream infection caused by gram-positive pathogens. Clin Infect Dis 2005;40:374-380.
96. Jauregui LE, Babazadeh S, Seltzer E, et al: Randomized, double-blind comparison of once weekly dalbavancin versus twice-daily linezolid therapy for the treatment of complicated skin ans skin structure infections. Clin Infect Dis 2005;41: 1407-1415.
97. Paterson DL: "Collateral damage" from cephalosporin or quinolone antibiotic therapy. Clin Infect Dis 2004;38(Suppl 4):S341-S345.
98. Hota B: Infection control or formulary control: What is the best tool to reduce nosocomial infections due to methicillin-resistant *Staphylococcus aureus?* Clin Infect Dis 2006;42: 785-787.
99. National Nosocomial Infections Surveillance System: National Nosocomial Infections Surveillance (NNIS) System Report, data summary from January 1992 through June 2004, issued October 2004. Am J Infect Control 2004;32:470-485.
100. Bisognano C, Vaudaux P, Rohner P, et al: Induction of fibronectin-binding proteins and increased adhesion of quinolone-resistant *Staphylococcus aureus* by subinhibitory levels of ciprofloxacin. Antimicrob Agents Chemother 2000;44:1428-1437.
101. Blázquez J: Hypermutation as a factor contributing to the acquisition of antimicrobial resistance. Clin Infect Dis 2003;37:1201-1209.
102. Beaber JW, Hochhut B, Waldor M: SOS response promotes horizontal dissemination of antibiotic resistance genes. Nature 2004;427:72-74.
103. Miller C, Thomsen LE, Gaggero C, et al: SOS response induction by β-lactams and bacterial defense against antibiotic lethality. Science 2004;305:1629-1631.
104. McDonald LC, Killgore GE, Thompson A, et al: An epidemic, toxin gene-variant strain of *Clostridium difficile.* N Engl J Med 2005;353:2433-2441.
105. Loo VG, Poirier L, Miller, LA, et al: A predominantly clonal multi-institutional outbreak of *Clostridium difficile*–associated diarrhea with high morbidity and mortality. N Engl J Med 2005;353:2442-2449.
106. Pépin J, Saheb N, Coulombe MA, et al: Emergence of fluoroquinolones as the predominant risk factor for *Clostridium difficile*–associated diarrhea: A cohort study during an epidemic in Quebec. Clin Infect Dis 2005;41: 1254-1260.
107. Trouillet J-L, Chastre J, Vuagnat A, et al: Ventilator-associated pneumonia caused by potentially drug-resistant bacteria. Am J Respir Crit Care Med 1998;157:531-539.
108. CDC NNIS System: National Nosocomial Infections Surveillance (NNIS) system report, data summary. Am J Infect Control 1996;24:380-388.
109. Sanders WE, Sanders CC: *Enterobacter* spp.: Pathogens poised to flourish at the turn of the century. Clin Microbiol Rev 1997;10:220-241.
110. Sanders CC, Sanders WE: Type I β-lactamases of gram-negative bacteria: Interactions with β-lactam antibiotics. J Infect Dis 1986;154:792-800.
111. Lindberg F, Lindquist S, Normark S: Genetic basis of induction and overproduction of chromosomal class I β-lactamase in nonfastidious gram-negative bacilli. Rev Infect Dis 1988;10:782-785.
112. Jacobson KL, Cohen SH, Inciardi JF, et al: The relationship between antecedent antibiotic use and resistance to extended-spectrum cephalosporins in Group I β-lactamase–producing organisms. Clin Infect Dis 1995;21:1107-1113.
113. Chow JW, Fine MJ, Shlaes DM, et al: *Enterobacter* bacteremia: Clinical features and emergence of antibiotic resistance during therapy. Ann Intern Med 1991;115:585-590.
114. Livermore DM: Of *Pseudomonas,* porins, pumps, and carbapenems. J Antimicrob Chemother 2001;47: 247-250.
115. Levy SB: Active efflux mechanisms for antimicrobial resistance. Antimicrob Agents Chemother 1992;695-703.
116. Livermore DM: Multiple mechanisms of antimicrobial resistance in *Pseudomonas aeruginosa:* Our worst nightmare? Clin Infect Dis 2002;34: 634-640.
117. Nikaido H: Antibiotic resistance caused by gram-negative efflux pumps. Clin Infect Dis 1998;27(Suppl 1):S32-S41.
118. Masuda N, Sakagawa E, Ohya S, et al: Substrate specificities of MexAB-OprM, MexCD-OprJ, and MexXY-OprM efflux pumps in *Pseudomonas aeruginosa.* Antimicrob Agents Chemother 2000;44:3322-3327.
119. Quale J, Bratu S, Gupta J, Landman D: Interplay of efflux system, AmpC, and OprD expression in carbapenem resistance of *Pseudomonas aeruginosa* clinical isolates. Antimicrob Agents Chemother 2006;50:1633-1641.
120. Poole K: Multidrug efflux pumps and antimicrobial resistance in *Pseudomonas aeruginosa* and related organisms. J Mol Microbiol Biotechnol 2001;3:255-264.
121. Lister PD, Wolter DJ: Levofloxacin-imipenem combination prevents the emergence of resistance among clinical isolates of *Pseudomonas aeruginosa.* Clin Infect Dis 2005;40: S105-S114.
122. Kohler T, Michea-Hamzehpour M, Epp SF, Pechere JC: Carbapenem activities against Pseudomonas aeruginosa: Respective contributions of OprD and efflux system. Antimicrob Agents Chemother 1999;43:424-427.
123. Chastre J, Fagon J-Y: Ventilator-associated pneumonia. Am J Respir Crit Care Med 2002;165:867-903.
124. Rello J, Paiva JA, Baraibar J, et al: International conference for the development of consensus on the diagnosis and treatment of ventilator-associated pneumonia. Chest 2001;120:955-970.
125. Kollef MH: Ventilator-associated pneumonia: The importance of initial empiric antibiotic selection. Infect Med 2000;17:265-268,278-283.
126. Landman D, Quale JM, Mayorga D, et al: Citywide clonal outbreak of multiresistant *Acinetobacter baumannii* and *Pseudomonas aeruginosa* in Brooklyn, NY. The preantibiotic era has returned. Arch Intern Med 2002;162:1515-1520.
127. Urban C, Segal-Maurer S, Rahal JJ: Considerations in control and treatment of nosocomial infections

due to multidrug resistant *Acinetobacter baumannii.* Clin Infect Dis 2003;36:1268-1274.
128. Hanes SD, Demirkan K, Tolley E, et al: Risk factors for late-onset nosocomial pneumonia caused by *Stenotrophomonas maltophilia* in critically ill trauma patients. Clin Infect Dis 2002;35:228-235.
129. Carmeli Y, Samore MH: Comparison of treatment with imipenem vs. ceftazidime as a predisposing factor for nosocomial acquisition of *Stenotrophomonas maltophilia:* A historical cohort study. Clin Infect Dis 1997;24:1131-1134.
130. Ambler RP, Coulson AF, Frere JM, et al: A standard numbering scheme for the class A beta-lactamases. Biochem J 1991;276:269-270.
131. Bratu S, Landman D, Haag R, et al: Rapid spread of carbapenem-resistant *Klebsiella pneumoniae* in New York City: A new threat to our antibiotic armamentarium. Arch Intern Med 2005;165:1430-1435.
132. Paterson DL, Bonomo RA: Extended-spectrum β-lactamases: A clinical update. Clin Microbiol Rev 2005;18:657-686.
133. Paterson DL, Ko W-C, Von Gottberg A, et al: International prospective study of *Klebsiella pneumoniae* bacteremia: Implications of extended-spectrum β-lactamase production in nosocomial infections. Ann Intern Med 2004;140:26-32.
134. Rodríguez-Baño J, Navarro MD, Romero L, et al: Clinical and molecular epidemiology of extended-spectrum beta-lactamase-producing *Escherichia coli* as a cause of nosocomial infection or colonization: Implications for control. Clin Infect Dis 2006;42:37-45.
135. Paterson DL, Ko WC, Von Gottberg A, et al: Outcome of cephalosporin treatment for serious infections due to apparently susceptible organisms producing extended-spectrum beta-lactamases: Implications for the clinical microbiology laboratory. J Clin Microbiol 2001;39:2206-2212.
136. Paterson DL, Ko W-C, Von Gottberg A, et al: Antibiotic therapy for *Klebsiella pneumoniae* bacteremia: Implications of production of extended-spectrum β-lactamases. Clin Infect Dis 2004;39:31-37.
137. Jacoby GA, Munoz-Price L: The new β-lactamases. N Engl J Med 2005;352:380-391.
138. Craig WA, Bhavnani SM: The inoculum effect: Fact or artifact? Diagn Microbiol Infect Dis 2004;50:229-320.
139. Wang M, Sahm DF, Jacoby GA, Hooper DC: Emerging plasmid-mediated quinolone resistance associated with the *qnr* gene in *Klebsiella pneumoniae* clinical isolates in the United States. Antimicrob Agents Chemother 2004;48:1295-1299.
140. Gruteke P, Goessens W, Van Gils J, et al: Patterns of resistance associated with integrons, the extended-spectrum beta-lactamase SHV-5 gene, and a multidrug efflux pump of *Klebsiella pneumoniae* causing a nosocomial outbreak. J Clin Microbiol 2003;41:1161-1166.
141. Pitout JD, Nordmann P, Laupland KB, Poirel L: Emergence of Enterobacteriaceae producing extended-spectrum β-lactamases (ESBLs) in the community. J Antimicrob Chemother 2005;56:52-59.
142. Dennesen PJW, van der Ven AJ, Kessels AGH, et al: Resolution of infectious parameters after antimicrobial therapy in patients with ventilator-associated pneumonia. Am J Respir Crit Care Med 2001;163:1371-1375.
143. Ibrahim EH, Ward S, Sherman G, et al: Experience with a clinical guideline for the treatment of ventilator-associated pneumonia. Crit Care Med 2001;29:1109-1115.
144. Chastre J, Wolff M, Fagon JY, et al: for the PneumA Trial Group: Comparison of 8 vs 15 days of antibiotic therapy for ventilator-associated pneumonia in adults: A randomized trial. JAMA 2003;290:2588-2598.
145. Burke JP, Pestotnik SL: Computer-assisted prescribing and its impact on resistance. In Andremont A, Brun-Buisson C, McGowan JE (eds): Antibiotic Therapy and Control of Antimicrobial Resistance in Hospitals. Paris, Elsevier, 1999, pp 89-95.
146. Warren DK, Hill HA, Merz LR, et al: A tale of two cities: Does limiting prescribing practices through cycling programs reduce acquisition of antimicrobial resistant infections? (Abstract 223). Fourteenth Annual Meeting of the Society of Healthcare Epidemiology of America, April 19, 2004, Philadelphia.
147. Kollef MH: Is antibiotic cycling the answer to preventing the emergence of bacterial resistance in the intensive care unit? Clin Infect Dis 2006;43: S82-S88.
148. Bergstrom CT, Lo M, Lipsitch M: Ecological theory suggests that antimicrobial cycling will not reduce antimicrobial resistance in hospitals. Proc Natl Acad Sci U S A 2004;101:13285-13290.

Chapter 53

Antifungal and Antiviral Therapy

Luis Ostrosky-Zeichner and John H. Rex

Over the past 15 years, fungal and viral diseases have become progressively more important to the critical care specialist. Increasing populations of immunocompromised hosts with serious fungal and viral infections often require critical care, and patients hospitalized in critical care units are also susceptible to these infections. Effective management of these conditions not only requires use of the appropriate anti-infective agents but in-depth knowledge of their pharmacodynamic/pharmacokinetic properties, as well as awareness of their physiological effects, toxicities, and drug interactions. Recent years have also brought important antifungal and antiviral drug developments, giving the clinician an ever-increasing arsenal of therapeutic choices.

SYSTEMIC ANTIFUNGAL AGENTS

This chapter focuses on systemic antifungal therapy as it is relevant to the critical care setting. Topical therapy of candidiasis and therapy of other systemic fungal infections are omitted or only briefly reviewed. The interested reader is referred to the Infectious Diseases Society of America guidelines on the topic.[1]

Polyenes

Polyenes act by binding to ergosterol in the fungal cytoplasmic membrane, causing ionic leakage and osmotic unstability.[2] Additionally, they cause oxidation of the cytoplasmic membrane.[2] Polyenes are fungicidal in most settings, and the most prominent members of the family are amphotericin B and nystatin. Both drugs have important toxic effects that often limit their use in patients with organ/system failure. Newer formulations of the drugs have been developed to reduce this limitation.

Amphotericin B and Its Lipid Formulations

Amphotericin B is produced by *Streptomyces nodosus* and is one of the oldest and most widely used antifungal agents. Much experience with its use in mycoses and hosts has been reported, and it is usually the comparison standard for new therapies.[3] Because of significant acute and chronic toxicities, there is an extensive anecdotal literature describing ways to ameliorate these toxicities, as well as limitations of all these strategies.[4] The advent of lipid-based formulations of amphotericin B has enhanced our ability to limit toxicities.[5]

Amphotericin B has in vitro and in vivo activity against most isolates of *Candida* spp., *Cryptococcus neoformans, Histoplasma capsulatum, Blastomyces dermatitidis, Mucorales, Coccidioides immitis, Paracoccidioides brasiliensis, Aspergillus* spp., *Fusarium* spp. and *Sporothrix schenckii*.[6] The activity of amphotericin B is so broad that it is almost easier to think of this in terms of the few species that are consistently less susceptible or actually resistant to amphotericin B: *Aspergillus terreus*,[7] *Trichosporon* spp.,[8] and *Pseudallescheria boydii (Scedosporium prolificans)*.[9] One species of *Candida, C. lusitaniae,* readily becomes resistant to the polyenes.[10] Resistance among isolates of *Candida* is otherwise rare.[11,12]

Amphotericin B is hydrophobic and combines with deoxycholate to permit intravenous (IV) administration in an aqueous solvent. Once in the bloodstream, it dissociates and binds to plasma proteins and lipoproteins. It is stored in the liver and other organs and slowly eliminated. Drug metabolism is complex and not affected by renal or liver failure.[3] Hemodialysis or peritoneal dialysis does not remove the drug. Measuring drug levels is possible[13] but not of obvious clinical relevance. Cerebrospinal fluid (CSF) penetration is poor. Although amphotericin B is primarily used in intravenous infusion, it can also be used topically for localized gastrointestinal or urinary infections or instilled directly to treat central nervous system (CNS) infections.

The most common toxicity is the systemic reaction associated with intravenous infusion, thought to be caused by release of inflammatory mediators from monocytes and macrophages and producing fever, hypotension, and on occasion severe dyspnea. Two forms of renal toxicity are seen: (1) a very acute form of renal dysfunction that appears to be related to amphotericin B–induced renal arteriolar constriction[14] and (2) cumulative dose-dependent tubular damage that is almost invariably seen if significant doses are given. The tubular injury is characterized by potassium/magnesium wasting and azotemia. It is generally reversible when the drug is stopped, but it is also particularly aggravated if the patient is volume depleted or given other nephrotoxic drugs. The renal injury also reduces erythropoietin production[15] and thus causes a mild anemia during chronic therapy (the hematocrit will typically fall to approximately 30%). Finally, amphotericin B may precipitate cardiac arrhythmias, especially if the patient is already hypokalemic and hypomagnesemic.[16-19] The deoxycholate formulation of amphotericin B is given intravenously at 0.5 to 1 mg/kg/day, but it can also be administered every other day by doubling the dose. To avoid producing a precipitate, it must be diluted in an electrolyte-free solution at no more than 0.1 mg/mL. It should be administered over no less than 1 hour, and most authorities prefer a 2- to 3-hour infusion.[20] Because of the occasional violent reaction to the drug, an initial test dose of 1 mg of the drug may be given prior to infusing the entire first dose. Premedication with acetaminophen, diphenhydramine, and steroids may be used if the patient develops reactions to the infusion. Volume loading appears to reduce nephrotoxicity, and many authorities give (if possible) 500 to 1000 mL normal saline just prior to each dose of amphotericin B. Administration via a central line is advisable because amphotericin B given peripherally often produces phlebitis.

Treatment goals have been traditionally and arbitrarily cumulative (such as 1 or 2 total g), but a time-based approach is increasingly used for some diseases (e.g., for candidemia, where 2 weeks of therapy at 0.6 to 0.7 mg/kg after the last positive blood culture has been shown to produce a late relapse rate of approximately 1%).[21] Although the importance of therapy in the typical patient is unclear,[22,23] candiduria is sometimes treated with amphotericin B bladder washes. A typical dose is 50 mg of amphotericin B diluted in 1000 mL of water and irrigated over 24 hours. A small number of intracranial fungal infections benefit from intrathecal dosing at 0.1 to 0.5 mg three times per week, but expert advice should be sought if this therapy is considered.

Three lipid-based formulations of the drug are available: amphotericin B colloidal dispersion (ABCD, marketed as Amphotec and Amphocil), amphotericin B lipid complex (ABLC, marketed as Abelcet), and liposomal amphotericin (L-AmB, marketed as AmBisome). The names of these compounds are often confusing. Only one of the drugs (L-AmB) is a true liposome. However, it is not uncommon for physicians to refer to therapy with these compounds in general as therapy with "liposomal amphotericin B." The preferred terminology is "lipid-associated formulation of amphotericin B" (LFAB).[5] When speaking of specific compounds, we find that use of the names ABCD, ABLC, and AmBisome minimizes confusion.

All three LFABs have comparable efficacy among themselves and when compared with regular amphotericin B, but they have significantly less nephrotoxicity.[5,24] They are also thought to be concentrated and distributed in the reticuloendothelial system, theoretically achieving higher tissue delivery and concentration. The lipid carrier does, however, dramatically change the pharmacology and delivery of these compounds, and higher doses than is typical for amphotericin B are both safe and necessary for optimal activity: the licensed doses are 5 mg/kg/day (ABLC), 3 to 6 mg/kg/day (ABCD), and 3 to 5 mg/kg/day (AmBisome). The optimal dose of these compounds is unclear, and the agents appear generally equipotent. Doses of approximately 3 mg/kg/day would appear suitable for treatment of most serious *Candida* infections. Doses of at least 5 mg/kg/day are used for mold infections, with some authors recommending even higher doses.[25-27] However, a recent study showed no advantage to using 10 mg/kg/day over 3 mg/kg/day for invasive aspergillosis and other invasive mold infections.[28]

All three LFABs appear active against the same range of fungal infections that can be treated with amphotericin B. The compounds do differ in their relative toxicities.[24] ABCD appears to have significant administration-related toxicity and is not often used. AmBisome and ABLC are both well tolerated, but AmBisome has been associated with somewhat less nephrotoxicity in some patient settings.[29] Some patients will tolerate one formulation better than another.[30,31]

Because of the cost of the LFABs, there has been great interest in the concept of making a pseudo-LFAB by suspending amphotericin B deoxycholate in commercially available lipid emulsions.[32-34] This practice does not, however, consistently reduce toxicity.[35] This may be because of preparation-dependent precipitation of the amphotericin B noted by some,[36,37] but not all,[38] authors. Most authorities have concluded that further work with this approach should be undertaken as part of a controlled clinical trial that addresses these issues.[39]

The cost of the LFABs is significant, but the counterbalancing reduction in nephrotoxicity is also valuable and should be considered when choosing an LFAB versus a conventional amphotericin B.[40] A recent study of the impact of nephrotoxicity of amphotericin B deoxycholate in patients with invasive aspergillosis suggested that this patient population suffered significant morbidity because of the amphotericin B itself.[41] Use of amphotericin B deoxycholate produces significant nephrotoxicity in about 30%, increasing hospital length of stay and hospitalization costs by nearly $30,000.[42,43] Nevertheless, the context of amphotericin B–induced toxicity should also be considered. A rise of the creatinine to 3 mg/dL in an otherwise well patient who is being treated with amphotericin B for osteoarticular sporotrichosis, for example, may be clinically imperceptible because of the fact that the patient has no other acute medical problems. On the other hand, a rise in creatinine from 1 mg/dL to 2 mg/dL may be disastrous in a surgical patient who is also suffering from nosocomial pneumonia and cardiac insufficiency. No firm guidelines in this area have yet to emerge. We currently believe that an LFAB is appropriate for patients who have failed amphotericin B deoxycholate (FDA indication), who are intolerant of amphotericin B deoxycholate (FDA indication), or who are highly likely to be intolerant (no FDA indication). We define intolerance broadly: a creatinine clearance less than 50% of normal for the patient's age or a fall in creatinine clearance with therapy. Predicting intolerance is difficult, but such factors as concomitant use of highly nephrotoxic agents (e.g., an aminoglycoside) or underlying primary/intrinsic renal disease (e.g., diabetes mellitus) associated with renal dysfunction should be considered.

Flucytosine

Flucytosine (5-FC) is the fluorine analogue of cytosine.[44] It was originally synthesized as an antineoplastic agent, but poor antitumor activity and discovery of its antifungal properties led to its further development as an antifungal agent. 5-FC acts by deamination to 5-fluorouracil and then conversion to a noncompetitive inhibitor of thymidylate synthetase that interferes with fungal deoxyribonucleic acid (DNA) and ribonucleic acid (RNA) synthesis. It has been demonstrated to be effective in cryptococcosis, candidiasis, and chromomycosis, being the drug of choice for the latter infection. Drug resistance in vivo develops quickly, so the standard practice is to combine it with another agent.[45,46] 5-FC is water soluble and has high bioavailability. Protein binding is negligible, and approximately 90% is excreted in urine. Cerebrospinal fluid penetration is good, and both hemodialysis and peritoneal dialysis remove it. 5-FC is teratogenic in rats and therefore contraindicated in pregnancy. Adverse effects include rash, diarrhea, and hepatic dysfunction.

High blood levels (>100 µg/mL) are associated with profound leukopenia and thrombocytopenia.[47] This has prompted the recommendation of monitoring drug levels, renal/liver function, and blood counts in patients receiving 5-FC. Doses of 150 mg/kg/day divided in four doses have usually been suggested, but recent in vivo[48] and human experience[49] suggest that doses of 100 mg/kg/day (again, divided into four doses) may be as effective and better tolerated. Renal failure requires dose adjustment to half the dose if CrCl is 25 to 50 mL/min and a quarter of dose if it falls below 25 mL/min. Patients on hemodialysis should be given the latter dose after dialysis. Combination with amphotericin requires constant monitoring of toxicity parameters and dose adjustment. The target blood level is approximately 50 µg/mL. Most experts would discontinue use of this agent if blood counts start dropping, regardless of the blood levels.

Azole Antifungal Agents

The introduction of this class of drugs was a major advance in antifungal therapy because they offer both IV and oral formulations for the treatment of systemic mycosis. Their widespread use has also prompted the emergence of resistance. Azoles act by blocking the activity of lanosterol demethylase, a cytochrome enzyme in both fungal and mammalian cells. Fungal cell membrane synthesis of ergosterol is inhibited, and other sterol intermediates are substituted in the membrane, resulting in a nonviable cell. This effect is much slower than that of amphotericin, so these drugs are generally regarded as fungistatic. Because these drugs reduce production of the ergosterol to which polyenes must bind to produce their effect, there is a potential for the azoles and polyenes to appear antagonistic. However, these effects are drug, organism, and model dependent and a range of effects may be seen. This area is complex and has recently been reviewed.[50,51] At present, use of such combinations should be avoided outside of a clinical trial. All of the azoles have the ability to interfere with mammalian sterol synthesis. This was most notable with ketoconazole, which can produce gynecomastia and adrenal insufficiency.[52,53] Subsequent azoles have been selected for lack of such effects. All of the azoles can, however, produce hepatic dysfunction. The most common pattern is that of increased transaminases. However, any form of dysfunction may be seen. This can be life threatening if not recognized. The hepatic dysfunction is reversible upon discontinuation of the offending azole.

Another concern with azoles is drug interactions. This becomes particularly important in the critical care setting, where many drugs are being used concomitantly. Table 53-1 summarizes the most important drug interactions that have been reported. The critical interactions generally have to do with drugs cleared by the liver. Some agents (e.g., rifampin and phenobarbital) induce the enzymes that clear the azoles. In other cases the azole interferes with clearance of another agent (e.g., the azoles predictably increase blood levels of cyclosporine). Listing all of the known interactions is impossible. Consultation with a pharmacy specialist is suggested when using azoles in the setting of polypharmacy, particularly in the critical care setting and when caring for patients with multiple comorbidities.

Ketoconazole

Ketoconazole has in vitro activity against dermatophytes, *Candida* spp., *Histoplasma capsulatum, Blastomyces dermatitidis, Coccidioides immitis* and *Sporothrix schenckii.*[54] It also has modest activity against *Aspergillus* spp. and the *Mucorales.* Its oral formulation requires an acid environment for absorption.[55] Once in the circulation, most of it is plasma protein bound and does not penetrate cerebrospinal fluid. As the drug is metabolized by the liver,

Table 53-1. Selected Azole-Drug Interactions*

	Azole Alters Levels of:	Azole Levels Altered by:
Ketoconazole	Astemizole Cisapride Cyclosporine Delavirdine Diazepam Indinavir Midazolam Phenytoin Quinidine Sulfonylureas Tacrolimus Terfenadine Warfarin and coumarins	DDI H_2 blockers Phenobarbital Phenytoin Proton-pump inhibitors Rifampin Sucralfate
Fluconazole	Cisapride Cyclosporine Diazepam Glipizide Glyburide Midazolam Phenytoin Rifabutin Sulfonylureas Tacrolimus Terfenadine Warfarins and coumarins	Rifampin
Itraconazole	Astemizole Cisapride Cyclosporine Diazepam Digoxin Dihydropyridines Lovastatin Methylprednisolone Midazolam Phenytoin Quinidine Ritonavir Sulfonylureas Terfenadine Vinca alkaloids Warfarins and coumarins	Carbamazepine DDI H_2 blockers Phenobarbital Phenytoin Proton-pump inhibitors Rifabutin Rifampin Sucralfate
Voriconazole	Sirolimus Rifabutin Efavirenz Ritonavir Terfenadine Astemizole Cisapride Pimozide Quinidine Cyclosporine Methadone Tacrolimus Phenytoin Warfarin Omeprazole	Rifampin Efavirenz Rifabutin Ritonavir Carbamazepine Phenytoin

*Generally, azoles tend to increase the levels of other drugs, whereas other drugs tend to decrease the level of the azole. This list is not meant to be comprehensive, and the prescriber should consult the full prescribing information. Consultation with a pharmacy specialist is recommended when azoles are going to be used in complex polypharmacy situations.

dose-adjustment is not necessary in renal failure. Side effects include nausea and vomiting, which can be severe, and hepatitis. Inhibition of steroid hormone synthesis occurs at high doses and has the potential for adrenal insufficiency.[56-58] Drug interactions are mainly with H_2 blocker/antacids (which decrease its absorption) and rifampin (which accelerates its metabolism). Ketoconazole also increases levels of cyclosporin A, warfarin, phenytoin, and nonsedating antihistamine agents. The usual dose is 200 to 400 mg/day. Bioavailability problems, together with side effects and drug interactions, have prompted the preferential use of newer triazoles.

Fluconazole

Fluconazole is one of the newer triazoles that has in vitro and in vivo activity mainly against yeast such as *Candida* spp. and *Cryptococcus neoformans*. It also has efficacy against *Coccidioides immitis, Histoplasma capsulatum,* and *Blastomyces dermatitidis*. Unfortunately, resistance (mediated by increased production of target enzymes, efflux pumps, and mutations in target enzyme) has become a problem, particularly in *Candida albicans* (mutation to resistance is seen), *candida glabrata* (has intrinsically lower susceptibility and may become highly resistant), and *candida krusei* (intrinsically highly resistant).[59,60] Nevertheless, fluconazole is still highly active against most strains causing invasive candidiasis and higher doses can be used for organisms that are in the "susceptible–dose dependent" range. Fluconazole is water soluble and is available in oral and IV presentations that produce similar blood levels. Bioavailability is excellent, and it is well absorbed regardless of the gastric contents. It has a long half-life and can be administered in a single daily dose. It exhibits little binding to serum proteins and is widely distributed in all body fluids. CSF penetration is particularly high, making it particularly useful in the treatment of CNS infections such as cryptococcosis and coccidioidomycosis. Fluconazole is excreted by the kidneys, and dosing should be adjusted in proportion to the creatinine clearance. The most common adverse effects are nausea and vomiting. Skin rash is infrequent but can be severe. Hepatitis has also been reported. The usual dose is 400 to 800 mg (or 6 to 8 mg/kg) per day by mouth or intravenously, but doses as high as 2 g/day have been tolerated.[61]

Itraconazole

Itraconazole is a triazole antifungal agent with a wider spectrum than fluconazole. It has in vitro and in vivo activity against *Candida* spp., *Aspergillus* spp., *Histoplasma* spp., *Blastomyces dermatitidis, Sporothrix schenckii, Trichophyton* spp., *Cryptococcus neoformans, Coccidioides immitis,* and *Paracoccidioides brasiliensis*.[62,63] The resistance issues observed for fluconazole are also an issue with itraconazole.[60] Itraconazole was initially available only in a capsule form that has unpredictable bioavailability. Absorption of the capsule formulation is optimized by ingestion with food.[64] Two formulations have been introduced. First, a solution in cyclodextrin for oral administration significantly enhances bioavailability and is now preferred over the capsule for producing maximal blood levels.[65] Second, an IV formulation (again, in a cyclodextrin carrier) is valuable in that it quickly and reliably produces significant blood levels.[66-68] Itraconazole is highly protein bound and has a prolonged half-life. Cerebrospinal fluid penetration is negligible, so it is not generally used for CNS infections. Itraconazole is metabolized by the liver, and dosing does not need to be modified in renal failure. However, the cyclodextrin carrier used in the IV formulation *is* cleared by the kidneys and its behavior in patients with renal dysfunction is not known. Thus this formulation of itraconazole should not be used in patients with a creatinine clearance less than 25 mL/hour.

Adverse effects are mainly gastrointestinal, with nausea, vomiting, and abdominal pain occurring in up to 10% of patients. Hepatitis is uncommon, but liver enzyme monitoring is recommended. Because itraconazole and its major metabolite, hydroxyitraconazole, are inhibitors of CYP3A4, drug interactions are a major issue and the most common ones are summarized in Table 53-1.

The usual oral dose is 100 to 400 mg/day and the oral solution formulation is now preferred. Giving the daily oral dose as two divided doses appears to maximize blood levels. IV dosing is 200 mg twice a day for 2 days and then 200 mg IV every day for a maximum of 14 days. Efficacy is plasma concentration related, and serum levels can be obtained from national reference laboratories. Such testing is warranted if oral itraconazole is being used to treat a serious fungal infection. Although minimal efficacious blood levels have not been defined, the point of testing is to ensure that at least some level is being obtained. Levels of at least 250 ng/mL are desirable.

Voriconazole

Voriconazole is the latest triazole to arrive on the market. It is licensed for the treatment of invasive candidiasis and invasive aspergillosis, as well as for the treatment of *Fusarium* and *Scedosporium* infections. Voriconazole is considered by many experts as the treatment of choice for invasive aspergillosis.[69] Voriconazole was not inferior to amphotericin B followed by fluconazole in a large clinical trial, but it is unknown whether it has any advantages over fluconazole or the echinocandins for treating infections by fluconazole-resistant *C. glabrata*.[70,71] Although it has activity against the endemic mycoses, data are limited at this point, so it is not recommended for routine use in these infections at this time.[72,73]

A relevant gap in its activity is for the *Zygomycetes* (e.g., *Mucor* spp., *Absidia* spp., *Rhizopus* spp.). Although there have been multiple reports of breakthrough *Zygomycetes* infections in patients receiving voriconazole prophylaxis or treatment, a causal relationship has not been established.[74,75] Nevertheless, clinicians should be aware that this drug has no activity against these organisms; thus it should not be used for empirical therapy of mold infections if *Zygomycetes* are in the differential diagnosis.

Voriconazole is available in oral (tablets and suspension) and IV formulations, with 96% bioavailability. Usual dosing is 4 to 6 mg/kg IV every 12 hours or 200 to 300 mg orally every 12 hours. Because voriconazole has nonlinear pharmacokinetics, thus increasing the dose will not necessarily increase blood levels. Routine blood level measurement is not recommended at this time because blood levels clearly associated with specific efficacy and safety margins have not been established. Voriconazole is metabolized by the human hepatic cytochrome P450 enzymes, CYP2C19, CYP2C9 and CYP3A4, and has extensive drug interactions with many drugs commonly used in the critical care setting. Consultation with a pharmacy specialist is recommended for patients on multiple drugs. Like itraconazole, the IV formulation is prepared in a cyclodextrin-based formulation, thus it is not recommended for use in patients with CrCl less than 50 mL/minute. In such patients the PO formulation may be used safely. Adverse events include self-limited visual disturbances; infrequent reports of hepatic insufficiency; and, as with the other azoles, rare reports of arrhythmias and QT prolongation. Monitoring of liver enzymes is recommended during voriconazole therapy.[76-78]

Posaconazole

The triazole posaconazole is in clinical development with promising activity against mold infections, particularly infections by the *Zygomycetes* and *Fusarium*. It has also shown excellent in vitro and in vivo activity against *Candida* spp. with demonstrated efficacy in esophageal disease. It is only available in an oral formulation.[79,80]

Candins

The candin antifungal agents represent an entirely new class of antifungal drugs. Three candins are on the market at this time: caspofungin, micafungin, and anidulafungin. These agents are cyclic lipohexapeptides that act via inhibition of glucan synthesis.[81] Preclinical studies have shown efficacy against all species of *Candida* without any evidence for cross-resistance with polyenes or azoles, *Aspergillus* spp., and selected other fungi.[82,83] Although the target enzyme is present in most fungi, the candins are not active against *C. neoformans* and molds other than *Aspergillus*. The candins appears to be rapidly fungicidal for *Candida* spp., but their activity against *Aspergillus* may be better described as fungistatic.[84] Nonetheless, they are quite active in animal models of both candidiasis and aspergillosis.[85,86] The drugs have a long half-life, permitting once daily dosing and are excreted in the liver. They do not interfere with the cytochrome system and they are not known to be nephrotoxic, having otherwise remarkable safety profiles. At this time, differences between the three drugs appear to be subtle, requiring further study.

Caspofungin

Caspofungin was the first candin on the market. It has excellent in vitro and in vivo activity against *Aspergillus* and *Candida* spp. It has demonstrated efficacy for the treatment of invasive candidiasis, invasive aspergillosis, and empirical therapy of fungal infections in the setting of febrile neutropenia.[87-89]The usual dosing includes loading with 70 mg IV, followed by 50 mg IV every 24 hours. The safety profile is good with mild elevation of liver enzymes. Patients with hepatic insufficiency

(Child-Pugh class B or C) require dosage adjustment to 35 mg/kg IV every 24 hours.[72,90,91] Drug interactions are infrequent, but it is recommended to monitor cyclosporine levels in patients receiving caspofungin.[92]

Micafungin

Although currently only approved by the FDA for the treatment of esophageal candidiasis and prophylaxis of *Candida* infections in stem cell transplant patients, micafungin has excellent in vitro and in vivo activity against *Aspergillus* and *Candida* spp. Clinical data on invasive Aspergillus are limited.[93,94] Although not currently FDA approved for the treatment of invasive candidiasis and candidemia, micafungin has demonstrated efficacy both for the treatment of invasive candidiasis and as a prophylactic agent for fungal infections in allogeneic stem cell transplant recipients.[95-97] The prophylactic dose is 50 mg IV every 24 hours, and the therapeutic dose for invasive candidiasis appears to be between 100 and 150 mg IV every 24 hours. As with the other candins, the most frequent adverse event is mild elevation of liver enzymes. No dosage adjustment is required in the setting of renal insufficiency or moderate hepatic insufficiency. Mild drug interactions have been reported with concomitant use of sirolimus and nifedipine.

Anidulafungin

As with the other candins, anidulafungin has excellent in vitro and in vivo activity against *Aspergillus* and *Candida* spp.[98] It is currently indicated for the treatment of invasive candidiasis, having demonstrated superiority in a clinical trial versus fluconazole. The usual dosing includes a loading dose of 200 mg IV, followed by 100 mg through an intravenous catheter every 24 hours. Anidulafungin does not require dosage adjustment for patients with renal or hepatic failure, and no significant drug interactions are reported.[98-100]

SPECIFIC INDICATIONS AND USES FOR ANTIFUNGALS

Although the precise diagnosis of a fungal infection may be laborious, time consuming, and delayed, therapy should never be withheld in a critically ill patient with suspected or confirmed fungal infection. Empiric therapy will often be started with amphotericin B or one of its lipid preparations and then tailored according to the final identification of the organism. This section presents generally accepted treatment recommendations for the most commonly encountered fungal infections in the critical care setting. Infections by less common fungi may be particularly severe and rapidly progressive and require consultation with an infectious diseases specialist for appropriate treatment. Table 53-2 summarizes the most often encountered fungal diseases in the critical care setting with their generally accepted treatment options. Figure 53-1 presents our approach for the critically ill patient with fungemia.

Candida Infections

Although *C. albicans* remains the most common pathogen in oropharyngeal and cutaneous candidiasis, non-*albicans* species of *Candida* are increasingly frequent

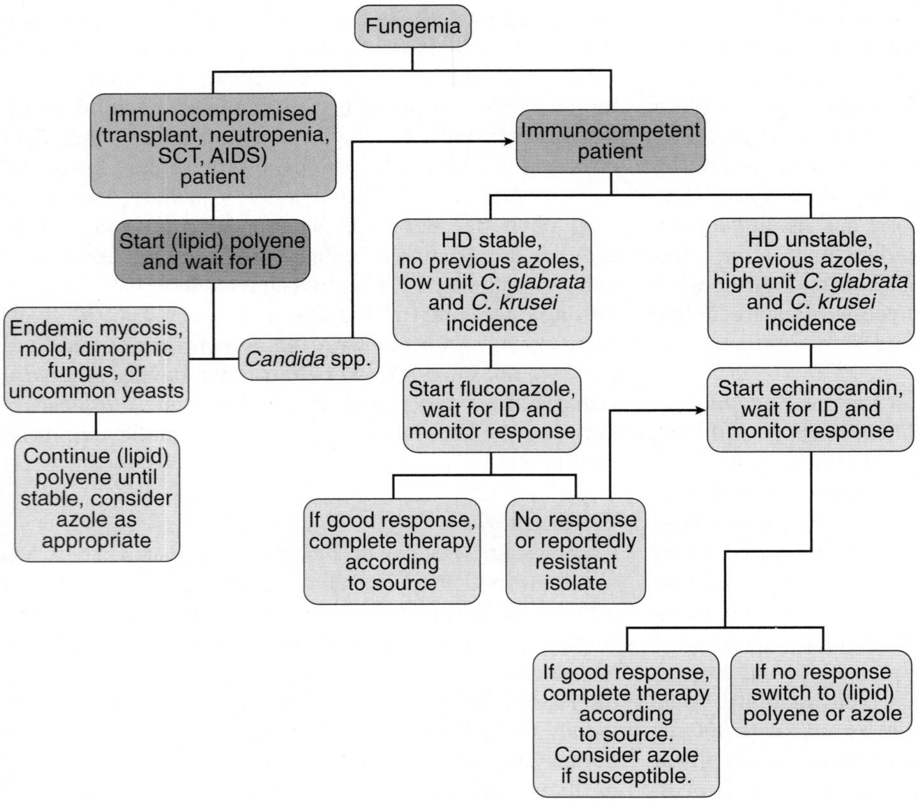

Figure 53-1. Treating the critically ill patient with fungemia. HD, hemodynamically; ID, identification to species level; SCT, stem cell transplant. (Modified from Ostrosky-Zeichner L, Pappas PG: Invasive candidiasis in the intensive care unit. Crit Care Med 2006;34:857-863.)

Table 53-2. Summary of Therapeutic Choices for Fungal Diseases Most Commonly Encountered in the Critical Care Setting

	Therapy of Choice	Alternative Therapy	Duration of Treatment	Comments
Candidiasis				
Oral candidiasis	Nystatin 200,000 U lozenges four times a d or 500,000 U swish and swallow four times a d	Fluconazole 200 mg single dose or 100 mg by mouth daily	3-5 d	
Mucosal nonoral candidiasis	Topical azole	Fluconazole 200 mg first dose and continue 100 mg/d	7-14 d	
Candidemia and most forms of disseminated candidiasis	Amphotericin B 0.5-0.6 mg/kg/d, lipid preparation of amphotericin B 3 mg/kg/d, fluconazole 400 mg every d, voriconazole 4-6 mg/kg every 12 h, caspofungin 50 mg/d, anidulafungin 100 mg/d, or micafungin 100-150 mg/d		14 days following bloodstream clearance for uncomplicated candidemia; until resolution of sites of infection if disseminated	Line removal recommended. Assess for dissemination. A candin or lipid amphotericin B usually preferred as initial therapy if the patient is unstable or infected with a non-*albicans* species. Loading doses recommended for caspofungin and anidulafungin. Micafungin not yet FDA approved for this indication.
Urinary	Fluconazole 200 mg first d and then 100 mg/d or amphotericin B 0.3 mg/kg IV single dose	Amphotericin B bladder washes, 50 mg/1000 mL H_2O in continuous irrigation for 2 d	7-14 d	Asymptomatic funguria does not require treatment. However, it may be a sign of dissemination in compromised hosts. Urinary catheter removal is useful.
Peritonitis	As for disseminated candidiasis			Removal of dialysis catheter is helpful. Surgical débridement if abscess present.
Aspergillosis	Voriconazole 4-6 mg/kg every 12 h	Lipid preparation of amphotericin B 3-5 mg/kg/d	Until resolution of the clinical process and of any associated immunosuppression	May require surgical treatment.
Histoplasmosis	Amphotericin B 0.5-1 mg/kg/d or Liposomal amphotericin B 5 mg/kg/d	Itraconazole 200-400 mg/d	3-12 mo	Lifelong suppression needed in HIV-infected patients.
Cryptococcosis (in HIV-Infected Patients)	Amphotericin B 0.5-0.7 mg/kg/d or lipid preparation of amphotericin B 3-5 mg/kg/d + 5-FC induction 25 mg/kg every 6 h, fluconazole 400 mg/d maintenance	Induction with fluconazole 400 mg/d in stable patients	Managed very differently in HIV-infected (lifelong therapy needed) and uninfected patients (cure is possible). Expert consultation advised.	Consider frequent LP to relieve intracranial pressure. V-P shunts may be necessary.
Zygomycosis	Amphotericin B 0.8-1.5 mg/kg/d or lipid preparation of amphotericin B 3-5 mg/kg/d + surgical débridement + metabolic control			Surgical débridement is critical.

HIV, human immunodeficiency virus; LP, lumbar puncture; V-P, ventriculo-peritoneal.

causes of invasive candidiasis.[101] Guidelines and reviews for therapy of candidiasis in the intensive care setting have recently been published.[102-104] These guidelines are extensive and will not be repeated in detail. Rather, the text focuses on several clinical situations in which candidal infections are particularly challenging for the critical care specialist.

Candidemia and Disseminated Candidiasis

The diagnosis of disseminated candidiasis is always a challenge.[105] No single tool exists to conclusively make this diagnosis. Isolation of *Candida* from the bloodstream is simply the most obvious form of disseminated candidiasis, but clinical experience makes it obvious that disseminated candidiasis can occur in the absence of detectable fungemia.

Candidemia may be treated initially with either fluconazole, voriconazole, amphotericin B (or its lipid preparations), or a candin. In the critically ill and unstable patient, amphotericin B lipid preparations or a candin are preferred because of their broader spectrum of activity and more rapid onset of action.[104,106] Because of their greater safety, candins are increasingly viewed as the initial agents of choice.

The susceptibility of *Candida* to the currently available antifungal agents can generally be predicted if the species of the infecting isolate is known.[10,12,101,107-115] Bloodstream isolates of *C. albicans, C. tropicalis,* and *C. parapsilosis* are generally susceptible to fluconazole and amphotericin B. Isolates of *C. glabrata* and *C. krusei* will often (if not always, as is the case with *C. krusei*) be resistant to fluconazole. Isolates of *C. lusitaniae,* may be resistant to amphotericin B.

Antifungal susceptibility testing is becoming increasingly important as a guide in the treatment of these infections.[116] In particular, detection of fluconazole resistance is valuable because it provides support for continued use of the often more difficult polyenes.

Although all *Candida* species are generally considered to be susceptible to candins, *C. parapsilosis* has higher MICs than the other *Candida* species. This, however, has not translated into reduced activity in clinical trials.[87,117] Once the organism is speciated or if the prevalence of more resistant species is low, therapy may be switched to fluconazole. Fluconazole has demonstrated to be as effective in clearing candidemia as amphotericin B in immunocompetent hosts. Duration of treatment is 14 days following the last positive culture,[21] and if a line is present, removal is highly recommended. If evidence of disseminated candidiasis is found, therapy should be prolonged to at least 4 weeks to ensure proper organ clearance.

Intravenous Catheter in Candidemic Patients

Although long an area of contention, current data strongly suggest that candidemia is often related to (if not primarily propagated by) a central venous catheter. Central venous catheters in particular have been found to be both risk factors for developing candidemia[118-121] and associated with persistent fungemia.[119] Removal of the catheter has been associated with shorter duration of subsequent candidemia[122] and improved patient outcome.[123,124] Unique to the species of *Candida,* candidemia caused by *C. parapsilosis* is almost always caused by a catheter.[125,126] The situation may be different for neutropenic patients, particularly those who have permanent, lower-risk catheters such as Hickman catheters. Such catheters may, of course, become infected, but these patients may also have candidemia because of entry of the organisms from the gut into the bloodstream. This concept is supported both by demonstrations that *Candida* can enter the bloodstream from the gut,[127] by the relative lack of effect of catheter removal in a large cohort of cancer patients,[126] and by the frequent demonstration of gut wall invasion in patients who die with disseminated candidiasis.[128,129] Unfortunately, there is no convincing way to tell if a given catheter is involved. Taking differential quantitative blood cultures through the line and from a peripheral site have been suggested to resolve this problem,[130] but this technique remains controversial.[131] On a practical basis, serious consideration to line removal should be given if fungemia persists for more than a few days.

Mucosal Infections and Colonization

Although there are many risk factors for development of disseminated candidiasis, colonization at one or more nonsterile sites represents an unusually strong risk factor.[132] As discussed earlier, local oral and mucosal candidiasis should thus be considered as a predictor of possible invasive disease in the critically ill or immunocompromised host.[133,134] Esophageal candidiasis does require systemic treatment. Fluconazole is generally preferred here, although amphotericin B and the candins can also be used.

Candiduria

Treatment of asymptomatic candiduria produces only temporary clearing of the urine and is probably not indicated.[22,23] However, candiduria should probably be treated in symptomatic patients, immunocompromised patients, low-birth-weight infants, renal transplant patients, and patients who will undergo urologic manipulation or surgery.[102] If treatment is indicated, systemic therapy with amphotericin or fluconazole is preferred, and amphotericin bladder washes should be reserved for patients with renal insufficiency and low renal clearance. Removal of the urinary catheter is by itself a useful intervention and should always be considered.

Other Forms of Invasive Candidiasis

Many other possible forms of invasive candidiasis exist: meningitis, endocarditis, and osteomyelitis, just to name a few. This area has recently been reviewed,[103] and for most forms of this disease there are few specific data on therapy. The largest body of data will always be anecdotal reports on the use of amphotericin B, and for essentially every form there are at least a few reports of successful therapy with fluconazole. In general, amphotericin B is preferred when the infection is most acute, when data on the nature of the infection are still being generated in the laboratory, or when the patient has previously received azole therapy. Fluconazole provides a good way to step down to an oral agent to complete therapy of infections caused by susceptible isolates. Removal of foreign body and standard surgical drainage are often key as well. An excellent example of the need to remove foreign bodies is found in treatment of dialysis catheter-related peritoneal candidiasis where catheter removal is important. Surgical drainage is, of course, important in candidal peritonitis related to gut injury and fecal spillage.

Cryptococcosis

Treatment of cryptococcosis has recently been reviewed.[135] Cryptococcal meningitis in non–human immunodeficiency virus (HIV)-infected adults continues to be seen sporadically. The majority of the published experience as to treatment is with amphotericin B given for 4 to 6 weeks.[136,137] Because this therapy is curative in approximately two thirds of patients, this approach is warranted. Expert consultation is also appropriate for this relatively uncommon infection.

On the other hand, cryptococcal meningitis in the HIV-infected patient is a well-established and common problem. Meningeal cryptococcosis in this setting should be treated with a 2-week course of IV amphotericin or its lipid preparations,[138,139] followed by lifelong suppression with fluconazole.[140,141] Current trends favor also using 5-FC unless there is a contraindication to its use.[49] Although itraconazole does not penetrate the cerebrospinal fluid, anecdotal evidence has shown that it may be useful in treating CNS disease, although it is apparently less potent as a long-term therapy.[142]

For all forms of cryptococcal meningitis, intracranial hypertension should be aggressively treated with repeated spinal taps or a CSF shunt.[143,144] The addition of steroids and other immune-modulating agents to antifungal therapy has shown promising results in animal models,[145] and clinical trials are being conducted.

Aspergillosis

Treatment of aspergillosis has recently been reviewed.[146,147] Invasive aspergillosis should be considered in any severely immunocompromised patient with an unexplained pulmonary or sinonasal process. Biopsy is normally required for definitive diagnosis, although a new generation of galactomannan-based serodiagnostic tests may prove useful as adjuncts to diagnosis.[148,149] Although amphotericin B has classically been the initial treatment of choice for invasive aspergillosis, the current treatment of choice is voriconazole[69,78] or a lipid preparation of amphotericin B. Aggressive surgical management is necessary and curative in some cases.[105,150] Itraconazole has now been approved for the treatment of aspergillosis in patients who are intolerant of or refractory to amphotericin B.[151] Overall, the outlook for invasive aspergillosis is critically dependent on recovery of immune function. Without this, the prognosis is usually dismal.

Histoplasmosis

The initial treatment of choice for severe acute histoplasmosis is an amphotericin B preparation.[152] Noncritical cases may be treated with itraconazole 200 to 400 mg/day. Fluconazole is only moderately effective and should not be used as primary therapy.[153] Successful treatment results in a decrease of serum and urine *Histoplasma* antigen.[154] Duration of therapy is a function of disease form and underlying immune status. HIV-infected patients with disseminated disease should be treated as acute histoplasmosis and maintained on lifelong suppression with itraconazole. Liposomal amphotericin B has shown excellent efficacy in this setting.[155] Non-HIV-infected patients may require 3 to 12 months of therapy, and expert consultation is generally advised.

Zygomycosis

The treatment of choice for zygomycosis (infections typically caused by *Mucor* spp., *Rhizopus* spp., and *Absidia* spp.) is aggressive surgical débridement and prompt start of high-dose amphotericin B or a lipid preparation.[156] Follow-up therapy with itraconazole or posaconazole may be warranted, and expert consultation is advised. Posaconazole has shown efficacy in this setting.[80] Correction of metabolic abnormalities (acidosis and hyperglycemia) should also be pursued aggressively.

Other Fungal Infections

Other fungal infections such as blastomycosis and fusariosis and infection by *Trichosporon* spp., *Coccidioides immitis, Malassezia furfur,* and *Penicillium* spp. may be occasionally encountered in the critical care setting, particularly when caring for immunocompromised hosts. Although amphotericin B is probably the best empirical drug for any characterized suspected fungal infection, it is not effective against some of these pathogens. Guidelines for treating some of these infections have recently been published.[1] Expert consultation should be promptly obtained.

AREAS OF CONTROVERSY IN ANTIFUNGAL THERAPY

Empiric Antifungal Therapy for the Febrile ICU Patient

Fever in the ICU patient is a complex problem that requires prompt evaluation for many possible sources including infection, atelectasis, pulmonary embolism, drug fever, and thermoregulatory disfunction.[157] Infection by *Candida* should be suspected when the patient has risk factors such as immunocompromise, broad-spectrum antibiotic therapy, parenteral nutrition, steroids, surgery (especially if the gut wall is transected), urinary catheters, and burns.[158,159]

Unfortunately, making a diagnosis of invasive candidiasis is difficult. In the most straightforward scenario, the patient is febrile and has positive blood cultures for *Candida*. On other occasions, biopsy or aspiration is used to make a clear-cut diagnosis of a localized abscess caused by *Candida*. These situations are, however, the exception. Far more common is the scenario of a persistently febrile ICU patient with a combination of the previously mentioned risk factors. In this setting we place great importance on the presence of positive cultures from nonsterile sites such as wounds, sputum, or stool. The key concept is that presence of *Candida* at any of these sites significantly increases the likelihood of developing invasive disease.[132,160] Positive cultures from the urine are also considered in this context (even though that is normally a sterile site). Candiduria in the afebrile patient is generally a clinical nonevent that does not require therapy,[22,23] but candiduria in the febrile ICU patient at the least represents colonization and increased risk of invasive disease and at the worse represents actual upper urinary tract infection. A similar logic applies to *Candida* in the sputum. Pneumonia caused by *Candida* occurs but is generally clinically inapparent.[161] The presence of *Candida* in the sputum more often means that the gut, and thus the patient, are colonized. This, in turn, is a risk factor, as discussed earlier.

In general we seriously entertain usage of empiric antifungal therapy in patients who have been in the ICU for at least 4 days, who have had at least 4 days of broad-spectrum antibiotics, who have an unexplained fever that persists despite these antibiotics, and who have a significant number of the key risk factors listed earlier. In addition, we generally do not start antifungal therapy unless we isolate *Candida* from at least one site. If all of these factors are present, a deliberate trial of empiric therapy is appropriate using a full dose of any of the agents indicated at the beginning of this section. Failure of the fever to break after 3 to 4 days of such therapy should prompt a renewed search for alternate explanations for the fever.

Antifungal Prophylaxis in the ICU

Prevention is always preferred to therapy, and this is certainly true for invasive candidiasis. Although prevention of mucosal disease can be achieved with almost any regimen, prevention of invasive disease has consistently required systemic therapy. Both fluconazole and amphotericin B are effective in the right setting. The key is to select patient populations with a meaningful chance of contracting invasive candidiasis. The value of prophylaxis has been shown convincingly for bone marrow transplantation patients[162,163] and selected liver transplant patients.[164-167] Studies of patients receiving standard chemotherapy for leukemia have shown a trend favoring prophylaxis,[168,169] but the lower rates of disease in the control group lower the statistical power of the studies. To further confuse matters, even a group that sounds homogeneous (e.g., allogeneic bone marrow transplant recipients) really is not—different forms of chemotherapy and degrees of graft-versus-host disease produce different levels of risk. This point was driven home in an editorial emphasizing the range of variation within the category of "neutropenic patient."[170]

For the critical care practitioner, the idea of prophylaxis in the typical non-neutropenic ICU patient is thus a tricky one. Some patient groups are clearly at higher risk. This was nicely shown in a recent study of a group of *highly* selected patients with persistent gastrointestinal leakage.[171] In this group the rate of *Candida* peritonitis was high, and a small placebo-controlled trial was able to show benefit to fluconazole prophylaxis.

In practical terms, three major studies have demonstrated benefits to prophylaxis of invasive candidiasis in the ICU.[171-173] No study or meta-analysis has shown benefits in terms of mortality, however.[174-177] These studies have the limitation of being single-center studies and having limited numbers of patients. Most experts would agree with the fact that routine use of antifungal prophylaxis should be reserved for units with a high incidence of invasive candidiasis or for carefully selected patients at the highest risk.[103] Widespread use of prophylaxis would require major multicenter clinical trials, which have not occurred at this time.[176,177]

Duration of Therapy or Accumulated Dosing

Optimum dose or duration of therapy has not been clearly defined in most fungal infections. Most of the recommended doses and guidelines presented in this chapter have been developed empirically or from extrapolation of other infections or animal models. Response and duration of treatment should be evaluated primarily on a clinical basis when feasible. Surrogate markers such as cell wall antigens or antibody assays, as well as imaging when appropriate, have also been shown to be useful in infections such as cryptococcosis, histoplasmosis, and aspergillosis.

Measurement of Drug Levels

Drug level monitoring is theoretically justified to assure efficacy and avoid toxicity. However, drug level monitoring during antifungal therapy is relatively new and should not be carried out routinely because there is a lack of information on its clinical correlation and meaning. Situations in which drug level monitoring has proved to be useful are (1) itraconazole levels to verify adequate absorption when using the oral forms of this compound and (2) 5-FC levels to watch for possible myelotoxicity.

Susceptibility Testing

In vitro susceptibility testing is an exciting area in antifungal research and development and is finding its way to the clinical setting. Early difficulties included lack of standardized methodology and lack of in vivo correlation to in vitro results. The National Committee for Clinical Laboratory Standards (now Clinical Laboratory Standards Institute) has published a guideline for standardized antifungal susceptibility testing that has been widely adopted[178] as subsequently revised. This methodology is recommended for testing *Candida* and *Cryptococcus* spp., and breakpoints have been developed.[179] Antifungal susceptibility testing is now widely available and should be considered when treating serious *Candida* infections, when treatment failure occurs, or when toxicity or side effects limit the use of a particular drug. It should also be remembered that pharmacology, safety, published experience, and drug interactions must be considered along with susceptibility when selecting a therapy.[102] Mold susceptibility has also been standardized but is not routinely recommended.

ANTIVIRAL AGENTS

Antiviral chemotherapy has made great advances in the past 2 decades. Before then, a diagnosis of a life-threatening viral infection meant mostly supportive therapy and patience. Although still limited, today we have several treatment options for herpetic infections; upper and lower respiratory illness by influenza, cytomegalovirus (CMV), and RSV; and some relatively exotic systemic diseases. Therapy for HIV, hepatitis B, and hepatitis C infection has also made gigantic leaps, but it is usually not undertaken in the critical care setting and is thus beyond the scope of this chapter. Table 53-3 summarizes the currently available non-HIV specific antiviral drugs and their general spectrum.

Acyclovir, Famciclovir, and Valacyclovir

Acyclovir is a nucleoside analogue of guanine that has in vitro and in vivo activity against several viruses in the herpes virus family, particularly against herpes simplex virus type 1 (HSV-1), HSV-2, varicella-zoster virus (VZV), and Epstein-Barr virus (EBV). High concentrations also inhibit CMV. Acyclovir inhibits DNA polymerase causing DNA chain termination.[180-182] Acyclovir is the treatment of choice for severe herpetic infections in immunocompetent and immunocompromised hosts. Resistance caused by viral thymidine kinase mutations or, less often, DNA polymerase mutations may emerge in patients with severe immunocompromise such as transplant recipients and advanced HIV infection during treatment of HSV and VZV infections.[183-185] Acyclovir has also been used for CMV prophylaxis in transplant patients.[186,187] Acyclovir is available in oral, IV, and topical forms. Because bioavailability of the oral form is poor (15% to 21%), high doses are required. Protein binding is less than 20%. Cerebrospinal fluid penetration is low, but acyclovir is active for CNS infections. The topical form is virtually unabsorbed. The half-life is short and the drug is cleared by the kidneys, so dosage adjustment in renal failure and hemodialysis is required. Supplementation is not necessary in peritoneal dialysis. Side effects are uncommon.[188] The main concern with acyclovir therapy is the crystallization of the drug in the renal tubules, leading to renal failure. Aggressive hydration and monitoring of renal function are recommended during IV acyclovir therapy. Oral acyclovir may cause nausea and vomiting. The usual oral dose is 200 to 800 mg orally every 4 hours. The IV dosing range for severe infections is 8 to 12 mg/kg IV every 8 hours. Proven encephalitis is treated with 10 to 12 mg/kg every 8 hours for 14 to 21 days. Doses of up to 20 mg/kg may be more effective in premature infants.[189]

Famciclovir, the prodrug of penciclovir (a guanosine analogue),[190,191] is a well-absorbed oral agent that has shown excellent activity against first-episode or recurrent genital herpes and HSV/VZV infection in both HIV and immunocompetent hosts.[192-194] A dose of 500 mg orally three times a day was shown to be as effective as acyclovir for treatment of herpes zoster.[195]

Valacyclovir, an analogue of acyclovir that has a similar profile of side effects, is now available in oral formulations with the advantage of longer dosing intervals. It appears comparable with acyclovir for treatment of mucocutaneous HSV infections but is more effective in herpes zoster. It is also effective orally for prophylaxis of CMV in renal transplant patients.[196] The dosing range is 500 to 1000 mg orally two to three times a day.[197-199]

Ganciclovir and Valganciclovir

Ganciclovir is another nucleoside analogue of guanine that has a slightly wider antiviral spectrum than acyclovir. It is highly active against CMV, as well as HSV-1, HSV-2, and EBV. Like acyclovir, it acts by interference with DNA polymerase, but it is not an obligate chain terminator. Resistance to ganciclovir by CMV and HSV is increasingly reported. HSV isolates, which are thymidine kinase-deficient and thus resistant to acyclovir, are also resistant to ganciclovir.[185,200] It is mainly indicated in prophylaxis, treatment, and suppression of CMV syndromes in immunocompromised patients.[186,201-205] Ganciclovir is available in oral, intraocular, and IV forms, the first two being useful only in chronic suppression of CMV disease. Once it reaches the bloodstream it has body-wide distribution, low protein binding, and low CNS system penetration.

Table 53-3. Spectrum of Antiviral Agents

	Acyclovir/ Valacyclovir/ Famciclovir	Ganciclovir/ Valganciclovir	Foscarnet	Cidofovir	Amantadine/ Rimantadine	Ribavirin	Oseltamivir/ Zanamivir
HSV-1	++*	++	++	++	0	0	0
HSV-2	++*	++	++	++	0	0	0
VZV	++*	++	++	++	0	0	0
CMV	+/–*	++*	++	++	0	0	0
EBV	+	++	++	++	0	0	0
INFLUENZA A	0	0	0	0	++*	+	++*
INFLUENZA B	0	0	0	0	0	+	++*

*Resistant strains reported.
0, no known activity; +/–, active under specific circumstances; +, active; ++, very active.

Excretion is renal, and dosage adjustment is required in renal failure. Because ganciclovir is removed by hemodialysis, it should be administered after dialysis. Side effects of IV ganciclovir include severe neutropenia (40%), thrombocytopenia (20%), phlebitis, rash, increased liver enzymes, and azotemia. The nephrotoxicity is potentiated by concomitant use of nephrotoxic agents and acyclovir. Ganciclovir should not be used in pregnant women because it is known to be teratogenic. The usual dose in acute infection is 5 mg/kg every 12 hours. Maintenance therapy at 5 mg/kg IV every day should be continued as long as the patient is immunocompromised. Discontinuation of therapy in AIDS patients appears feasible following immune reconstitution.[186,201,206,207] An intraocular delivery system is also available as an adjunct to the treatment of CMV retinitis.

Valganciclovir is an L-valyl ester of ganciclovir that has significantly increased bioavailability over previous oral formulations of ganciclovir, resulting in levels previously unattainable with the traditional formulations. It allows for prophylaxis and treatment of CMV infections with an oral alternative. The usual dose for prophylaxis is 900 mg orally every 24 hours, and for treatment the recommended induction dose is 900 mg orally every 12 hours, followed by a maintenance dose of 900 mg orally every 24 hours. This drug requires adjustment for patients with renal impairment.[208,209]

Cidofovir

Cidofovir is a nucleotide analogue with activity against most herpes viruses. Its activation is not virus enzyme dependent, so it has activity against most acyclovir-resistant HSV and ganciclovir-resistant CMV. Resistant strains have also been reported, and synergy with ganciclovir and foscarnet has been reported. Oral bioavailability is low. Cidofovir is 6% protein bound and excreted by the kidneys.[210,211] Its side effects include neutropenia and nephrotoxicity, which can manifest as proteinuria, azotemia, and a Fanconi-like renal syndrome. Cidofovir has been shown to be teratogenic and mutagenic and is contraindicated in pregnancy. It is currently licensed for CMV retinitis in HIV but has also shown activity against acyclovir-resistant HSV.[212,213] The usual dose is 5 mg/kg every week for 2 weeks, then 5 mg/kg every other week.

Foscarnet

Foscarnet is a pyrophosphate analogue that has antiviral activity against the herpes viruses, HIV, and hepatitis B virus. Its mechanism of action is interference with DNA polymerase or reverse transcriptase to block effective viral replication. Viral isolates that are resistant to ganciclovir or acyclovir are often susceptible to foscarnet, but primary resistance to foscarnet has also been described, particularly in HIV-infected patients.[183,184,214-216] The main therapeutic indication of foscarnet is ganciclovir-resistant CMV disease. Foscarnet is only available in IV formulations and it has body-wide distribution. Protein binding is 15%, and cerebrospinal fluid penetration is good. The drug is excreted almost intact by the kidneys and requires careful dosage adjustment in renal failure. Foscarnet is removed by hemodialysis but should be avoided in patients with severe renal dysfunction. Its main side effect is nephrotoxicity, which occurs in most patients, but is reversible when therapy is stopped.[217] Dosage adjustment should be made by following the creatinine clearance closely. Hypocalcemia and hypercalcemia, as well as phosphate abnormalities, are common, so monitoring of electrolytes is also recommended. The usual dose is 60 mg/kg every 8 hours for CMV infections and 40 mg/kg every 8 hours for treating acyclovir-resistant HSV infections.

Amantadine and Rimantadine

Amantadine is a tricyclic amine inhibitor of influenza A virus. Its mechanism of action involves inhibition of the transmembrane domain of the viral M2 protein, thus preventing viral uncoating during early stages of replication. It has activity against influenza A but no clinical activity against influenza B.[218-221] Resistant strains can be developed in vitro and are also seen in household and nursing home contacts exposed to persons treated for acute influenza. Amantadine is indicated in influenza A prophylaxis and treatment and also for management of Parkinson's disease and drug-induced extrapyramidal reactions. It is well absorbed orally and has body-wide distribution. It is 67% bound to plasma proteins and excreted unchanged in the urine by glomerular filtration and tubular secretion. The usual adult dosage for both prophylaxis and treatment is 100 mg twice a day. The dosage must be reduced in elderly patients and patients with renal insufficiency. In individuals who are 65 or older, the dose should be reduced to 100 mg every day. The dose for a CrCl less than 10 mL/minute is 200 mg per week. The most common adverse events are related to the CNS and correlate directly with high levels. Patients may present with confusion, seizures, hallucinations, and coma. Amantadine also causes gastrointestinal upset.

Rimantadine is another tricyclic amine with similar properties, spectrum, and indications to amantadine.[222,223] The main difference lies in its extensive metabolism by the liver and its minimal renal clearance, but it also requires dosage adjustment in advanced liver and kidney insufficiency (CrCl <10 mL/minute), as well as in the elderly. Its major advantage is less frequent CNS toxicity. The dosage is 100 mg twice a day.

Ribavirin

Ribavirin is a triazole nucleoside analogue that has broad-spectrum antiviral activity. It is effective in vitro against respiratory syncytial virus, influenza A and B, HSV, HIV, hepatitis C virus, and viruses causing hemorrhagic fevers.[193,224-226] Its currently approved clinical indications are treatment of pediatric patients with severe RSV infection and, in combination with injected interferon alfa and ribavirin capsules, treatment of chronic hepatitis C.[227,228] The IV form has been shown to reduce mortality in Korean/Asian hemorrhagic fever with renal syndrome.[231] Its mechanism of action is not fully understood, and intrinsic resistance has not been reported. It is available in oral, aerosolized, and IV formulations. It has high bioavailability through the oral or aerosolized forms and it is metabolized by the liver. Toxicity in the aerosolized formulation consists primarily of severe bronchospasm and cardiac rhythm abnormalities. The IV formulation also causes hemolytic anemia. Use in ventilated patients requires experienced personnel because environmental leaking and diffusion are common.[232] Recommended dosage is 1.1 g/day of ribavirin administered by continuous aerosolization for 12 to 18 hours/day for 3 to 7 days. It should not be combined with other aerosolized medications. Induction of bronchospasm is common, and scheduled use of a bronchodilator may be required during ribavirin therapy.

Oseltamivir

Oseltamivir is a sialic acid neuraminidase inhibitor that has recently become available for the treatment of both influenza A and B.[233-235] Its mechanism of action is inhibition of the viral neuraminidase, causing in turn inhibition of virus release from infected cells and spread in the respiratory tract. Drug resistance has already been reported in vitro in strains with mutations that cause changes in the viral neuraminidase or hemagglutinin. In clinical studies of adults, only 1% to 2% of posttreatment strains showed evidence of mutations with decreased neuraminidase susceptibility. Recent reports have mentioned infrequent resistance in avian-influenza strains.[236,237] Cross-resistance between oseltamivir and zanamivir, the other member of the class, has also been observed in vitro. It is indicated for early treatment of uncomplicated acute influenza A and B. Preventive uses are also under investigation.[238] Major clinical trials have demonstrated that oseltamivir reduces the duration, severity, and rate of complications requiring antibiotic use.[235] Its role in complicated cases such as those seen in the critical care setting is unclear at this time. Oseltamivir is available in an oral form, which has greater than 75% bioavailability. Protein binding is 3% to 42%. The drug is converted to oseltamivir carboxylate, which is eliminated unchanged in the urine. Less than 20% of the dose is eliminated in feces. Dose adjustment is recommended for renal failure and geriatric patients when CrCl is less than 30 mL/minute.[239] The recommended dose in such settings is 75 mg orally every 24 hours for 5 days. Clinically relevant drug interactions have not been identified. Side effects include nausea, vomiting, and abdominal pain, which are usually mild. The recommended dosage is 75 mg orally twice a day for 5 days, and it is recommended that treatment is begun within 2 days of symptom onset.

Zanamivir

Zanamivir is another sialic acid analogue neuraminidase inhibitor that was recently approved for the treatment of both influenza A and B.[233,240] Much like oseltamivir, its mechanism of action is by neuraminidase inhibition with subsequent inhibition of viral release and spread. Resistant strains have also been identified in vitro, and a resistant strain was also recovered from an immunocompromised patient with influenza B after 2 weeks of nebulized treatment.[241,242] It is indicated in acute cases of influenza with early onset of treatment.[234,243-245] Trials on patients with more severe disease are pending. Experience is also building with its use in prophylaxis.[218,246,247] Zanamivir is available in a powder form for oral inhalation. Approximately 4% to 17% of the dose is absorbed, and less than 10% of the drug is protein bound. It is excreted unchanged in the urine, and unabsorbed drug is cleared in the feces. No dosage adjustment in renal or hepatic failure is recommended at this time, but experience is limited. Zanamivir does not have significant drug interactions.[248,249] Bronchospasm may be precipitated particularly in patients with underlying lung disease.[250] The recommended dose is 10 mg (two inhalations) twice a day for 5 days.

SPECIFIC INDICATIONS AND USES FOR ANTIVIRALS

Herpes Simplex Virus and Varicella Zoster

Acyclovir, famciclovir, and valacyclovir are the treatments of choice for virtually all severe herpetic infections.[181,182,193,251-258] The greater oral bioavailability of famciclovir and valacyclovir makes these agents attractive, especially for treatment of VZV. Although primary HSV-1 and HSV-2 infections can be treated orally, immunocompromised patients or severely ill patients will require IV therapy. A high index of suspicion for dissemination should be maintained in immunocompromised patients—mild, localized, or atypical disease may progress to fulminant disease. Duration of therapy in this setting is usually 7 to 14 days.

Herpetic encephalitis has had a substantial decrease in morbidity and mortality since acyclovir was introduced. Being one of the few forms of viral encephalitis for which there is a treatment, empiric use of the drug is justified when viral disease is suspected and until it is ruled out. HSV polymerase chain reaction (PCR) of cerebrospinal fluid is a sensitive and specific test for the diagnosis of this disease. The usual dose is 10 to 12 mg/kg every 8 hours for 14 to 21 days. Visceral infections including esophagitis, hepatitis, pneumonia, and disseminated disease are frequent in immunocompromised patients and should be treated with 5 to 10 mg/kg every 8 hours for 14 to 21 days. HSV may also cause aseptic meningitis without encephalitis in the setting of primary or recurrent genital HSV infection. Unlike the focal necrotizing disease seen with HSV encephalitis, this form of the disease is a mild, self-limited aseptic meningitis with a good prognosis.

Finally, acyclovir-resistant HSV infections, which are an increasing problem in the immunocompromised population,[184,185,259,260] can be treated with foscarnet or cidofovir.

Primary VZV infection (chickenpox) should be treated in all adults, especially in the immunocompromised.[251,254,258,261,262] Reactivation (shingles) should be treated because treatment has been shown to decrease duration and intensity of symptoms.[263,264] Mild cases may be treated with oral famciclovir or valacyclovir. Severe cases (disseminated, immunocompromised patients with involvement of more than one dermatome, or ophthalmic involvement) should be treated with IV acyclovir. Remembering that these patients are contagious and should be suitably isolated using airborne precautions is important. As with HSV, resistant strains may be treated with foscarnet.[265,266]

Cytomegalovirus

CMV infections require treatment in immunocompromised patients. Populations at increased risk of the disease are HIV-infected patients and transplant recipients. In HIV patients, both retinal and visceral involvement are initially treated with IV ganciclovir at 5 mg/kg every 12 hours for 2 weeks.[186,201,202] Valganciclovir is a suitable oral formulation for the treatment of this infection. Various maintenance options are increasingly available (including ganciclovir ocular implants) but are beyond the scope of this chapter. Resistant cases may be treated with foscarnet 60 mg/kg every 8 hours for 2 weeks[207,214] or cidofovir. Clinical and laboratory monitoring while on either of these drugs is essential to avoid therapy-related complications. Refractory cases may be treated with cidofovir.

In the transplant patient the combination of ganciclovir and IV immunoglobulin is now the treatment of choice for CMV pneumonia.[201,267-269] High doses of acyclovir are useful as prophylaxis of CMV in the transplant patient but not in the HIV setting. Ganciclovir-resistant strains should be treated with foscarnet.

Influenza

Clear benefit in the treatment of influenza is seen consistently only when patients are treated early in the course of disease.[233,270-273] Therapeutic options (which can also be used prophylactically) include amantadine/rimantadine, oseltamivir, and zanamivir.[274-279] In patients who present later in the course of the disease, the benefits of therapy are unstudied. Prevention of complications has not been clearly demonstrated. Further trials are required to demonstrate whether one class of drugs is superior to the other and whether these drugs have a role in the critically ill patient. Rapid diagnosis of influenza is now available through different techniques that detect viral components in upper respiratory tract samples. These techniques are useful in detecting and treating infected hospitalized patients early and in regional surveillance of influenza. However, a negative test does not completely rule out influenza and empirical therapy of ambulatory patients with a clinical syndrome strongly suggesting influenza is probably appropriate.

Avian and pandemic influenza have received much attention from the scientific community and the media in the past 2 years. Considerable efforts are being carried out for surveillance, prompt detection, and containment of these diseases.[280-283] Critical care specialists should have increased awareness and involve infection control and public health authorities who have the appropriate epidemiological background when working with particularly severe forms of influenza. Suspected and confirmed cases should be placed on airborne precautions. As mentioned earlier, although there are scarce reports of neuraminidase inhibitor resistance in some avian influenza strains, these viruses appear to be generally susceptible to oseltamivir and zanamivir.[236,237]

An important consideration is vaccination and postexposure prophylaxis in health care personnel working in acute and chronic care facilities. Appropriate vaccination and influenza control measures in both health care personnel and patients have proved to be effective in decreasing disease and even mortality in patients.[284-286]

Other Viruses

Other potentially treatable viral infections that may be encountered in the critical care setting include parvovirus, for which treatment with IV immunoglobulin has shown some beneficial effects[294-296]; enterovirus, for which a drug called pleconaril showed only marginal benefits in the setting of meningitis[297,298]; and hemorrhagic fevers and hantavirus, for which ribavirin may be considered despite definitive proof of efficacy.[226] Dengue and yellow fever can be particularly severe and are most effectively managed with aggressive supportive care.

KEY POINTS

- Amphotericin B and its lipid preparations are the treatments of choice for all critically ill patients with an undiagnosed fungal infection. Once a diagnosis is made, other therapeutic options may be considered.
- Fluconazole has excellent antifungal activity mainly against most yeasts, but resistance is possible and clinically relevant.
- The candins comprise a new class of antifungal agents with activity against *Candida* and *Aspergillus* with proven efficacy and remarkable safety profiles.
- Combinations of antifungals should be approached carefully, being clearly beneficial only in selected entities such as CNS disease and endocarditis.
- Empiric antifungal use and antifungal prophylaxis in the ICU setting remain controversial and should be reserved for carefully selected units and patients.
- Uncommon and serious mycoses require expert consultation.
- Acyclovir and its analogues are the drugs of choice for treatment of HSV and VZV infections. The new oral formulations (famciclovir and valacyclovir) have greater bioavailability and are preferred in ambulatory patients.
- Ganciclovir is the drug of choice for treatment of CMV disease in immunocompromised hosts. Immunoglobulin therapy is added to this in transplant patients with pneumonia.
- Critical care specialists should have a high index of suspicion for avian and pandemic influenza. Suspected or confirmed cases should be placed on airborne precautions and treated with neuraminidase inhibitors.
- Resistance is an increasingly real problem in both antifungal and antiviral therapy.

REFERENCES

1. Sobel JD: Practice guidelines for the treatment of fungal infections. For the Mycoses Study Group. Infectious Diseases Society of America. Clin Infect Dis 2000;30:652.
2. Ghannoum MA, Rice LB: Antifungal agents: Mode of action, mechanisms of resistance, and correlation of these mechanisms with bacterial resistance. Clin Microbiol Rev 1999;12:501-517.
3. Gallis HA, Drew RH, Pickard WW: Amphotericin B: 30 years of clinical experience. Rev Infect Dis 1990;12:308-329.
4. Hoeprich PD: Clinical use of amphotericin B and derivatives: Lore, mystique, and fact. Clin Infect Dis 1992;14(Suppl 1):S114-119.
5. Ostrosky-Zeichner L, Marr KA, Rex JH, Cohen SH: Amphotericin B: Time for a new "gold standard." Clin Infect Dis 2003;37:415-425.
6. Groll AH, Piscitelli SC, Walsh TJ: Clinical pharmacology of systemic antifungal agents: A comprehensive review of agents in clinical use, current investigational compounds, and putative targets for antifungal drug development. Adv Pharmacol 1998;44:343-499.
7. Sutton DA, Sanche SE, Revankar SG, et al: In vitro amphotericin B resistance in clinical isolates of Aspergillus terreus, with a head-to-head comparison to voriconazole. J Clin Microbiol 1999;37:2343-2345.
8. Walsh TJ, Melcher GP, Rinaldi MG, et al: Trichosporon beigelii, an emerging pathogen resistant to amphotericin B. J Clin Microbiol 1990;28:1616-1622.
9. Walsh M, White L, Atkinson K, Enno A: Fungal Pseudallescheria boydii lung infiltrates unresponsive to amphotericin B in leukaemic patients. Aust N Z J Med 1992;22:265-268.
10. Yoon SA, Vazquez JA, Steffan PE, et al: High-frequency, in vitro reversible switching of Candida lusitaniae clinical isolates from amphotericin B susceptibility to resistance. Antimicrob Agents Chemother 1999;43:836-845.
11. Law D, Moore CB, Denning DW: Amphotericin B resistance testing of *Candida* spp: A comparison of methods. J Antimicrob Chemother 1997;40:109-112.
12. Nguyen MH, Clancy CJ, Yu VL, et al: Do in vitro susceptibility data predict the microbiologic response to amphotericin B? Results of a prospective study of patients with Candida fungemia. J Infect Dis 1998;177:425-430.
13. Cleary JD, Chapman SW, Deng J, Lobb CJ: Amphotericin B enzyme-linked immunosorbent assay. Antimicrob Agents Chemother 1996;40:637-641.
14. Sabra R, Branch RA: Mechanisms of amphotericin B-induced decrease in glomerular filtration rate in rats. Antimicrob Agents Chemother 1991;35:2509-2514.
15. Lin AC, Goldwasser E, Bernard EM, Chapman SW: Amphotericin B blunts erythropoietin response to anemia. J Infect Dis 1990;161:348-351.
16. Craven PC, Gremillion DH: Risk factors of ventricular fibrillation during rapid amphotericin B infusion. Antimicrob Agents Chemother 1985;27:868-871.
17. Aguado JM, Hidalgo M, Moya I, et al: Ventricular arrhythmias with conventional and liposomal amphotericin [letter; comment]. Lancet 1993;342:1239.
18. Googe JH, Walterspiel JN: Arrhythmia caused by amphotericin B in a neonate. Pediatr Infect Dis J 1988;7:73.
19. Soler JA, Ibanez L, Zuazu J, Julia A: Bradycardia after rapid intravenous infusion of amphotericin B [letter; comment] [see comments]. Lancet 1993;341:372-373.
20. Oldfield EC III, Garst PD, Hostettler C, et al: Randomized, double-blind trial of 1- versus 4-hour amphotericin B infusion durations. Antimicrob Agents Chemother 1990;34:1402-1406.
21. Rex JH, Bennett JE, Sugar AM, et al: A randomized trial comparing fluconazole with amphotericin B for the treatment of candidemia in patients without neutropenia. N Engl J Med 1994;331:1325-1330.
22. Kauffman CA, Vazquez JA, Sobel JD, et al: Prospective multicenter surveillance study of funguria in hospitalized patients. Clin Infect Dis 2000;30:14-18.
23. Sobel JD, Kauffman CA, McKinsey D, et al: Candiduria: A randomized, double-blind study of treatment with fluconazole and placebo. Clin Infect Dis 2000;30:19-24.
24. Wong-Beringer A, Jacobs RA, Guglielmo BJ: Lipid formulations of amphotericin B: Clinical efficacy and toxicities. Clin Infect Dis 1998;27:603-618.
25. Walsh TJ, Hiemenz JW, Seibel NL, et al: Amphotericin B lipid complex for invasive fungal infections: Analysis of safety and efficacy in 556 cases. Clin Infect Dis 1998;26:1383-1396.
26. Walsh TJ, Hiemenz JW, Seibel N, Anaissie EJ: Amphotericin B lipid complex in the treatment of 225 cases of invasive mycosis. 34th Interscience Conference on Antimicrobial Agents and Chemotherapy, 1994.
27. Walsh TJ, Seibel NL, Arndt C, et al: Amphotericin B lipid complex in pediatric patients with invasive fungal infections. Pediat Inf Dis J 1999;18:702-708.
28. Cornely O, Maertens J, Bresnik M, Herbrecht R: Liposomal amphotericin B (L-AMB) as initial therapy for invasive filamentous fungal infections (IFFI): A randomized-prospective trial of a high loading regimen vs. standard dosing (AmBiLoad trial). Blood 2005;106:900a (Abstract 3222).
29. Wingard JR, White MH, Anaissie EJ, et al: A randomized double blind study of Ambisome and Abelcet in febrile neutropenic patients. San Diego, Calif, Focus on Fungal Infections IX, 1999.
30. Johnson MD, Drew RH, Perfect JR: Chest discomfort associated with liposomal amphotericin B: Report of three cases and review of the literature. Pharmacotherapy 1998;18:1053-1061.
31. Kauffman CA, Wiseman SW: Anaphylaxis upon switching lipid-containing amphotericin B formulations. Clin Infect Dis 1998;26:1237-1238.
32. Ayestaran A, Lopez RM, Montoro JB, et al: Pharmacokinetics of conventional formulation versus fat emulsion formulation of amphotericin B in a group of patients with neutropenia. Antimicrob Agents Chemother 1996;40:609-612.
33. Barquist E, Fein E, Shadick D, et al: A randomized prospective trial of amphotericin B lipid emulsion versus dextrose colloidal solution in critically ill patients. J Trauma 1999;47:336-340.
34. Caillot D, Chavanet P, Casanovas O, et al: Clinical evaluation of a new lipid-based delivery system for intravenous administration of amphotericin B. Eur J Clin Microbiol Infect Dis 1992;11:722-725.
35. Torre D, Banfi G, Tambini R, et al: A retrospective study on the efficacy and safety of amphotericin B in a lipid emulsion for the treatment of cryptococcal meningitis in AIDS patients. J Infection 1998;37:36-38.
36. Trissel LA: Amphotericin B does not mix with fat emulsion. Amer J Health-Syst Pharm 1995;52:1463-1464.
37. Ericsson O, Hallmen A-C, Wikstrom I: Amphotericin B is incompatible with lipid emulsions. Ann Pharmacother 1996;30:298.
38. Owens D, Fleming RA, Restino MS, et al: Stability of amphotericin B 0.05 and 0.5 mg/ml in 20% fat emulsion. Am J Health-Syst Pharm 1997;54:683-686.
39. Cleary JD: Amphotericin B formulated in a lipid emulsion. Ann Pharmacother 1996;30:409-412.
40. Rex JH, Walsh TJ: Editorial response: Estimating the true cost of amphotericin B. Clin Infect Dis 1999;29:1408-1410.
41. Wingard JR, Kubilis P, Lee L, et al: Clinical significance of nephrotoxicity in patients treated with amphotericin B for suspected or proven aspergillosis. Clin Infect Dis 1999;29:1402-1407.
42. Bates DW, Su L, Yu DT, et al: Mortality and costs of acute renal failure associated with amphotericin B therapy. Clin Infect Dis 2001;32:686-693.
43. Bates DW, Su L, Yu DT, et al: Correlates of acute renal failure in patients receiving parenteral amphotericin B. Kidney Int 2001;60:1452-1459.
44. Francis P, Walsh TJ: Evolving role of flucytosine in immunocompromised patients—new insights into safety, pharmacokinetics, and antifungal therapy. Clin Infect Dis 1992;15:1003-1018.
45. Whelan WL: The genetic basis of resistance to 5-fluorocytosine in Candida species and Cryptococcus neoformans. Crit Rev Microbiol 1987;15:45-56.
46. King D, Froggat W, Smith D, et al: Molecular epidemiology of an Amphotericin B, 5-FC resistant strain of *Candida lusitaniae.* 93rd National Meeting of the American Society for Mycrobiology, 1993, p 527.

47. Vermes A, van der Sijs H, Guchelaar HJ: Flucytosine: Correlation between toxicity and pharmacokinetic parameters. Chemotherapy 2000;46:86-94.
48. Lewis RE, Klepser ME, Pfaller MA: In vitro pharmacodynamic characteristics of flucytosine determined by time-kill methods. Diagn Microbiol Infect Dis 2000;36:101-105.
49. Van der Horst CM, Saag MS, Cloud GA, et al: Treatment of cryptococcal meningitis associated with the acquired immunodeficiency syndrome. N Engl J Med 1997;337:15-21.
50. Sugar AS: Use of amphotericin B with azole antifungal drugs: What are we doing? Antimicrob Agents Chemother 1995;39:1907-1912.
51. Sugar AM: Antifungal combination therapy: Where we stand. Drug Resist Updates 1998;1:89-92.
52. Thompson DF, Carter JR: Drug-induced gynecomastia. Pharmacotherapy 1993;13:37-45.
53. Sarver RG, Dalkin BL, Ahmann FR: Ketoconazole-induced adrenal crisis in a patient with metastatic prostatic adenocarcinoma: Case report and review of the literature. Urology 1997;49:781-785.
54. Van Cutsem J: The antifungal activity of ketoconazole. Am J Med 1983;74:9-15.
55. Chin TWF, Loeb M, Fong IW: Effects of an acidic beverage (Coca-Cola) on absorption of ketoconazole. Antimicrob Agents Chemother 1995;39:1671-1675.
56. Khosla S, Wolfson JS, Demerjian Z, Godine JE: Adrenal crisis in the setting of high-dose ketoconazole therapy. Arch Intern Med 1989;149:802-804.
57. Best TR, Jenkins JK, Murphy FY, et al: Persistent adrenal insufficiency secondary to low-dose ketoconazole therapy. Am J Med 1987;82: 676-680.
58. Tucker WS Jr, Snell BB, Island DP, Gregg CR: Reversible adrenal insufficiency induced by ketoconazole. JAMA 1985;253:2413-2414.
59. Rex JH, Rinaldi MG, Pfaller MA: Resistance of Candida species to fluconazole. Antimicrob Agents Chemother 1995;39:1-8.
60. White TC, Marra KA, Bowden RA: Clinical, cellular, and molecular factors that contribute to antifungal drug resistance. Clin Microbiol Rev 1998;11:382-402.
61. Anaissie EJ, Kontonyiannis DP, Huls C, et al: Safety, plasma concentrations, and efficacy of high-dose fluconazole in invasive mold infections. J Infect Dis 1995;172:599-602.
62. Van Cutsem J: The in-vitro antifungal spectrum of itraconazole. Mycoses 1989;32:7-13.
63. Van Cutsem J, Van Gerven F, Janssen PA: Activity of orally, topically, and parenterally administered itraconazole in the treatment of superficial and deep mycoses: Animal models. Rev Infect Dis 1987;9(Suppl 1):S15-32.
64. Hardin TC, Graybill JR, Fetchick R, et al: Pharmacokinetics of itraconazole following oral administration to normal volunteers. Antimicrob Agents Chemother 1988;32:1310-1313.
65. Stevens DA: Itraconazole in cyclodextrin solution. Pharmacotherapy 1999;19:603-611.
66. Boogaerts J, Michaux J-L, Bosly A, et al: Pharmacokinetics and safety of seven days of intravenous (IV) itraconazole followed by two weeks oral itraconazole solution in patients with haematological malignancy. 36th Interscience Conference on Antimicrobial Agents and Chemotherapy, 1996.
67. Vandewoude K, Vogelaers D, Decruyenaere J, et al: Concentrations in plasma and safety of 7 days of intravenous itraconazole followed by 2 weeks of oral itraconazole solution in patients in intensive care units. Antimicrob Agents Chemother 1997;41:2714-2718.
68. Zhou HH, Goldman M, Wu J, et al: A pharmacokinetic study of intravenous itraconazole followed by oral administration of itraconazole capsules in patients with advanced human immunodeficiency virus infection. J Clin Pharmacol 1998;38:593-602.
69. Herbrecht R, Denning DW, Patterson TF, et al: Voriconazole versus amphotericin B for primary therapy of invasive aspergillosis. N Engl J Med 2002;347:408-415.
70. Kullberg BJ, Sobel JD, Ruhnke M, et al: Voriconazole versus a regimen of amphotericin B followed by fluconazole for candidaemia in non-neutropenic patients: A randomised non-inferiority trial. Lancet 2005;366:1435-1442.
71. Ostrosky-Zeichner L, Oude Lashof AM, Kullberg BJ, Rex JH: Voriconazole salvage treatment of invasive candidiasis. Eur J Clin Microbiol Infect Dis 2003;22:651-655.
72. Perfect JR: Use of newer antifungal therapies in clinical practice: What do the data tell us? Oncology (Williston Park) 2004;18:15-23.
73. Perfect JR, Marr KA, Walsh TJ, et al: Voriconazole treatment for less-common, emerging, or refractory fungal infections. Clin Infect Dis 2003;36:1122-1131.
74. Imhof A, Balajee SA, Fredricks DN, et al: Breakthrough fungal infections in stem cell transplant recipients receiving voriconazole. Clin Infect Dis 2004;39:743-746.
75. Marty FM, Cosimi LA, Baden LR: Breakthrough zygomycosis after voriconazole treatment in recipients of hematopoietic stem-cell transplants. N Engl J Med 2004;350:950-952.
76. Boucher HW, Groll AH, Chiou CC, Walsh TJ: Newer systemic antifungal agents: Pharmacokinetics, safety and efficacy. Drugs 2004;64:1997-2020.
77. Donnelly JP, De Pauw BE: Voriconazole-a new therapeutic agent with an extended spectrum of antifungal activity. Clin Microbiol Infect 2004;10(Suppl 1):107-117.
78. Herbrecht R: Voriconazole: Therapeutic review of a new azole antifungal. Expert Rev Anti Infect Ther 2004;2:485-497.
79. Groll AH, Walsh TJ: Posaconazole: Clinical pharmacology and potential for management of fungal infections. Expert Rev Anti Infect Ther 2005;3:467-487.
80. Torres HA, Hachem RY, Chemaly RF, et al: Posaconazole: A broad-spectrum triazole antifungal. Lancet Infect Dis 2005;5:775-785.
81. Kurtz MB, Douglas CM: Lipopeptide inhibitors of fungal glucan synthase. J Med Vet Mycol 1997;35:79-86.
82. Espinel-Ingroff A: Comparison of in vitro activities of the new triazole SCH56592 and the echinocandins MK-0991 (L-743,872) and LY303366 against opportunistic filamentous and dimorphic fungi and yeasts. J Clin Microbiol 1998;36:2950-2956.
83. Del Poeta M, Schell WA, Perfect JR: In vitro antifungal activity of pneumocandin L-743,872 against a variety of clinically important molds. Antimicrob Agents Chemother 1997;41:1835-1836.
84. Petraitis V, Petraitiene R, Groll AH, et al: Antifungal efficacy, safety, and single-dose pharmacokinetics of LY303366, a novel echinocandin B, in experimental pulmonary aspergillosis in persistently neutropenic rabbits. Antimicrob Agents Chemother 1998;42:2898-2905.
85. Abruzzo GK, Flattery AM, Gill CJ, et al: Evaluation of water-soluble pneumocandin analogs L-733560, L-705589, and L-731373 with mouse models of disseminated aspergillosis, candidiasis, and cryptococcosis. Antimicrob Agents Chemother 1995;39:1077-1081.
86. Abruzzo GK, Flattery AM, Gill CJ, et al: Evaluation of the echincocandin antifungal MK-0991 (L-743,872): Efficacies in mouse models of disseminated aspergillosis, candidiasis, and cryptococcosis. Antimicrob Agents Chemother 1997;41:2333-2338.
87. Mora-Duarte J, Betts R, Rotstein C, et al: Comparison of caspofungin and amphotericin B for invasive candidiasis. N Engl J Med 2002;347:2020-2029.
88. Maertens J, Raad I, Petrikkos G, et al: Efficacy and safety of caspofungin for treatment of invasive aspergillosis in patients refractory to or intolerant of conventional antifungal therapy. Clin Infect Dis 2004;39:1563-1571.
89. Walsh TJ, Teppler H, Donowitz GR, et al: Caspofungin versus liposomal amphotericin B for empirical antifungal therapy in patients with persistent fever and neutropenia. N Engl J Med 2004;351:1391-1402.
90. Morrison VA: Echinocandin antifungals: Review and update. Expert Rev Anti Infect Ther 2006;4:325-342.
91. Zaas AK, Alexander BD: Echinocandins: Role in antifungal therapy, 2005. Expert Opin Pharmacother 2005;6:1657-1668.
92. Marr KA, Hachem R, Papanicolaou G, et al: Retrospective study of the hepatic safety profile of patients concomitantly treated with caspofungin and cyclosporin A. Transpl Infect Dis 2004;6:110-116.
93. Jarvis B, Figgitt DP, Scott LJ: Micafungin. Drugs 2004;64:969-982; discussion 83-84.
94. Zaas AK, Steinbach WJ: Micafungin: The US perspective. Expert Rev Anti Infect Ther 2005;3:183-190.
95. Ruhnke M: Comparison of micafungin and liposomal amphotericin B for invasive candidiasis. Abstract M-722c.

Washington, DC, 45th Interscience Conference on Antimicrobial Agents and Chemotherapy, 2005.
96. Ostrosky-Zeichner L, Kontoyiannis D, Raffalli J, et al: International, open-label, noncomparative, clinical trial of micafungin alone and in combination for treatment of newly diagnosed and refractory candidemia. Eur J Clin Microbiol Infect Dis 2005;24:654-661.
97. van Burik JA, Ratanatharathorn V, Stepan DE, et al: Micafungin versus fluconazole for prophylaxis against invasive fungal infections during neutropenia in patients undergoing hematopoietic stem cell transplantation. Clin Infect Dis 2004;39:1407-1416.
98. Vazquez JA: Anidulafungin: A new echinocandin with a novel profile. Clin Ther 2005;27:657-673.
99. Krause DS, Reinhardt J, Vazquez JA, et al: Phase 2, randomized, dose-ranging study evaluating the safety and efficacy of anidulafungin in invasive candidiasis and candidemia. Antimicrob Agents Chemother 2004;48:2021-2024.
100. Pfaller MA: Anidulafungin: An echinocandin antifungal. Expert Opin Investig Drugs 2004;13:1183-1197.
101. Pfaller MA, Jones RN, Messer SA, et al; SCOPE Participant Group: National surveillance of nosocomial blood stream infection due to species of Candida other than Candida albicans: Frequency of occurrence and antifungal susceptibility in the SCOPE program. Diagn Microbiol Infect Dis 1998;30:121-129.
102. Rex JH, Walsh T, Sobel JD, et al: IDSA treatment guidelines for candidiasis. Clin Infect Dis 2000;30:662-678.
103. Pappas PG, Rex JH, Sobel JD, et al: Guidelines for treatment of candidiasis. Clin Infect Dis 2004;38:161-189.
104. Ostrosky-Zeichner L, Pappas PG: Invasive candidiasis in the intensive care unit. Crit Care Med 2006;34:857-863.
105. Rex JH, Walsh TJ, Anaissie EA: Fungal infections in iatrogenically compromised hosts. Adv Intern Med 1998;43:321-371.
106. Edwards JE Jr, Bodey GP, Bowden RA, et al: International conference for the development of a consensus on the management and prevention of severe candidal infections. Clin Infect Dis 1997;25:43-59.
107. Rex JH, Cooper CR Jr, Merz WG, et al: Detection of amphotericin B-resistant Candida isolates in a broth-based system. Antimicrob Agents Chemother 1995;39:906-909.
108. Rex JH, Pfaller MA, Barry AL, et al; NIAID Mycoses Study Group and the Candidemia Study Group: Antifungal susceptibility testing of isolates from a randomized, multicenter trial of fluconazole vs. amphotericin B as treatment of non-neutropenic patients with candidemia. Antimicrob Agents Chemother 1995;39:40-44.
109. Pfaller MA, Bale MJ, Buschelman B, Rhomberg P: Antifungal activity of a new triazole, D0870, compared with four other antifungal agents tested against clinical isolates of Candida and Torulopsis glabrata. Diagn Microbiol Infect Dis 1994;19:75-80.
110. Martinez-Suarez JV, Rodriguez-Tudela JL: Patterns of in vitro activity of itraconazole and imidazole antifungal agents against Candida albicans with decreased susceptibility to fluconazole from Spain. Antimicrob Agents Chemother 1995;39:1512-1516.
111. Wanger A, Mills K, Nelson PW, Rex JH: Comparison of Etest and National Committee for Clinical Laboratory Standards broth macrodilution method for antifungal susceptibility testing: Enhanced ability to detect amphotericin B-resistant Candida isolates. Antimicrob Agents Chemother 1995;39:2520-2522.
112. Rex JH, Lozano-Chiu M, Paetznick V, et al: Susceptibility testing of current Candida bloodstream isolates from Mycoses Study Group (MSG) collaborative study #34: Isolates of *C. krusei* are often resistant to both fluconazole and amphotericin B. Denver, 36th Annual Meeting of the Infectious Diseases Society of America, 1998.
113. Fisher MA, Shen S-H, Haddad J, Tarry WF: Comparison of in vivo activity of fluconazole with that of amphotericin B against *Candida tropicalis, Candida glabrata,* and *Candida krusei.* Antimicrob Agents Chemother 1989;33:1443-1446.
114. Karyotakis NC, Anaissie EJ, Hachem R, et al: Comparison of the efficacy of polyenes and triazoles against hematogenous *Candida krusei* infection in neutropenic mice. J Infect Dis 1993;168:1311-1313.
115. Pfaller MA, Messer SA, Hollis RJ: Strain delineation and antifungal susceptibilities of epidemiologically related and unrelated isolates of Candida lusitaniae. Diagn Microbiol Infect Dis 1994;20:127-133.
116. Ghannoum MA, Rex JH, Galgiani JN: Susceptibility testing of fungi: Current status of the correlation of in vitro data with clinical outcome. J Clin Microbiol 1996;34:489-495.
117. Ostrosky-Zeichner L, Rex JH, Pappas PG, et al: Antifungal susceptibility survey of 2,000 bloodstream Candida isolates in the United States. Antimicrob Agents Chemother 2003;47:3149-3154.
118. Lowder JN, Lazarus HM, Herzig RH: Bacteremias and fungemias in oncologic patients with central venous catheters. Changing spectrum of infection. Arch Intern Med 1982;142:1456-1459.
119. Fraser VJ, Jones M, Dunkel J, et al: Candidemia in a tertiary care hospital: Epidemiology, risk factors, and predictors of mortality. Clin Infect Dis 1992;15:414-421.
120. Wey SB, Mori M, Pfaller MA, et al: Risk factors for hospital-acquired candidemia. A matched case-control study. Arch Intern Med 1989;149:2349-2353.
121. Karabinis A, Hill C, Leclerq B, et al: Risk factors for candidemia in cancer patients: A case-control study. J Clin Microbiol 1988;26:429-432.
122. Rex JH, Bennett JE, Sugar AM, et al: Intravascular catheter exchanges and the duration of candidemia. Clin Infect Dis 1995;21:994-996.
123. Lecciones JA, Lee JW, Navarro EE, et al: Vascular catheter-associated fungemia in patients with cancer: Analysis of 155 episodes. Clin Infect Dis 1992;14:875-883.
124. Nguyen MH, Peacock JE Jr, Tanner DC, et al: Therapeutic approaches in patients with candidemia. Evaluation in a multicenter, prospective, observational study. Arch Intern Med 1995;155:2429-2435.
125. Abi-Said D, Anaissie E, Uzun O, et al: The epidemiology of hematogenous candidiasis caused by different Candida species. Clin Infect Dis 1997;24:1122-1128.
126. Anaissie EJ, Rex JH, Uzun Ö, Vartivarian S: Predictors of adverse outcome in cancer patients with candidemia. Am J Med 1998;104:238-245.
127. Krause W, Matheis H, Wulf K: Fungaemia and funguria after oral administration of Candida albicans. Lancet 1969;i:598-599.
128. Bodey G, Bueltmann B, Duguid W, et al: Fungal infections in cancer patients: An international autopsy survey. Eur J Clin Microbiol Infect Dis 1992;11:99-109.
129. Hughes WT: Systemic candidiasis: A study of 109 fatal cases. Pediatr Infect Dis J 1982;1:11-18.
130. Telenti A, Steckelberg JM, Stockman L, et al: Quantitative blood cultures in candidemia. Mayo Clin Proc 1991;66:1120-1123.
131. Paya CV, Guerra L, Marsh HM, et al: Limited usefulness of quantitative culture of blood drawn through the device for diagnosis of intravascular-device-related bacteremia. J Clin Microbiol 1989;27:1431-1433.
132. Pittet D, Monod M, Suter PM, et al: Candida colonization and subsequent infections in critically ill surgical patients. Ann Surg 1994;220:751-758.
133. Cohen DM, Rex JH: Antifungal therapy. In Schlossberg DM (ed): Current Therapy of Infectious Disease. St. Louis, Mosby-Year Book, 1996, pp 609-612.
134. Martins MD, Rex JH: Antifungal therapy. In Parillo JE (ed): Current Therapy in Critical Care Medicine, 3rd ed. St. Louis, Mosby-Year Book, 1997, pp 295-300.
135. Saag MS, Graybill RJ, Larsen RA, et al: Practice guidelines for the management of cryptococcal disease. Clin Infect Dis 2000;30:710-718.
136. Dismukes WE, Cloud G, Gallis HA, et al: Treatment of cryptococcal meningitis with combination amphotericin B and flucytosine for four as compared with six weeks. N Engl J Med 1987;317:334-341.
137. Bennett JE, Dismukes WE, Duma RJ, et al: A comparison of amphotericin B alone and combined with flucytosine in the treatment of cryptococcal meningitis. N Engl J Med 1979;301:126-131.
138. Leenders AC, Reiss P, Portegies P, et al: Liposomal amphotericin B (AmBisome) compared with amphotericin B both followed by oral fluconazole in the treatment of AIDS-associated cryptococcal meningitis. AIDS 1997;11:1463-1471.
139. Baddour LM, Perfect JR, Ostrosky-Zeichner L: Successful use of

amphotericin B lipid complex in the treatment of cryptococcosis. Clin Infect Dis 2005;40(Suppl 6):S409-413.
140. Van der horst C, Saag M, Cloud G, et al: Part 1. Randomized double blind comparison of amphotericin B plus flucytosine to amphotericin B alone (Step 1) Followed by a comparison of fluconazole to itraconazole (Step 2) in the treatment of acute cryptococcal meningitis in patients with AIDS. 35th Interscience Conference on Antimicrobial Agents and Chemotherapy, 1995.
141. Saag MS, Powderly WG, Cloud GA, et al: Comparison of amphotericin B with fluconazole in the treatment of acute AIDS-associated cryptococcal meningitis. N Engl J Med 1992;326:83-89.
142. Saag MS, Cloud GC, Graybill JR, et al: Comparison of fluconazole versus itraconazole as maintenance therapy of AIDS-associated cryptococcal meningitis. 35th Interscience Conference on Antimicrobial Agents and Chemotherapy, 1995.
143. Denning DW, Armstrong RW, Lewis BH, Stevens DA: Elevated cerebrospinal fluid pressures in patients with cryptococcal meningitis and acquired immunodeficiency syndrome. Am J Med 1991;91:267-272.
144. Rex JH, Larsen RA, Dismukes WE, et al: Catastrophic visual loss due to *Cryptococcus neoformans* meningitis. Medicine (Baltimore) 1993;72: 207-224.
145. Ostrosky-Zeichner L, Soto-Hernandez JL, Angeles-Morales V, et al: Effects of pentoxifylline or dexamethasone in combination with amphotericin B in experimental murine cerebral cryptococcosis: Evidence of neuroexcitatory pathogenic mechanisms. Antimicrob Agents Chemother 1996;40:1194-1197.
146. Stevens DA, Kan VL, Judson MA, et al: Practice guidelines for diseases caused by Aspergillus. Clin Infect Dis 2000;30:696-709.
147. Perfect JR: Management of invasive mycoses in hematology patients: Current approaches. Oncology (Williston Park) 2004;18:5-14.
148. Verweij PE, Denning DW: Diagnostic and therapeutic strategies for invasive aspergillosis. Semin Respir Crit Care Med 1997;18:203-215.
149. Denning DW: Early diagnosis of invasive aspergillosis. Lancet 2000;355:423-424.
150. Denning DW, Stevens DA: Antifungal and surgical treatment of invasive aspergillosis: Review of 2,121 published cases. Rev Infect Dis 1990;12:1147-1201.
151. Denning DW, Lee JY, Hostetler JS, et al: NIAID Mycoses Study Group multicenter trial of oral itraconazole therapy for invasive aspergillosis. Am J Med 1994;97:135-144.
152. Wheat J, Sarosi G, McKinsey D, et al: Practice guidelines for the management of patients with histoplasmosis. Clin Infect Dis 2000;30:688-695.
153. McKinsey DS, Kauffman CA, Pappas PG, et al: Fluconazole therapy for histoplasmosis. Clin Infect Dis 1996;23:996-1001.
154. Buckley HR, Richardson MD, Evans EG, Wheat LJ: Immunodiagnosis of invasive fungal infection. J Med Vet Mycol 1992;30(Suppl 1):249-260.
155. Johnson PC, Wheat LJ, Cloud GA, et al: Safety and efficacy of liposomal amphotericin B compared with conventional amphotericin B for induction therapy of histoplasmosis in patients with AIDS. Ann Intern Med 2002;137:105-109.
156. Roden MM, Zaoutis TE, Buchanan WL, et al: Epidemiology and outcome of zygomycosis: A review of 929 reported cases. Clin Infect Dis 2005;41:634-653.
157. O'Grady NP, Barie PS, Bartlett JG, et al: Practice guidelines for evaluating new fever in critically ill adult patients. Task Force of the Society of Critical Care Medicine and the Infectious Diseases Society of America. Clin Infect Dis 1998;26:1042-1059.
158. Blumberg HM, Jarvis WR, Wenzel RP, the NEMIS Study: Risk factors for Candida bloodstream infection in surgical intensive care units: NEMIS prospective multicenter study. 36th Annual Meeting of the Infectious Diseases Society of America, 1998, Denver.
159. Ostrosky-Zeichner L: New approaches to the risk of Candida in the intensive care unit. Curr Opin Infect Dis 2003;16:533-537.
160. Pelz R, Lipsett PA, Swoboda S, et al: Do surveillance cultures predict fungal infection in critically ill patients? 36th Annual Meeting of the Infectious Diseases Society of America, 1998, Denver.
161. Rodriguez LJ, Anaissie EJ, Rex JH: Pneumonia due to *Candida* species. In Sarosi GA, Davies SF (eds): Fungal Disease of the Lung, 3rd ed. Philadelphia, Lippincott Williams & Wilkins, 2000, pp 115-122.
162. Goodman JL, Winston DJ, Greenfield RA, et al: A controlled trial of fluconazole to prevent fungal infections in patients undergoing bone marrow transplantation. N Engl J Med 1992;326:845-851.
163. Slavin MA, Osborne B, Adams R, et al: Efficacy and safety of fluconazole prophylaxis for fungal infections after bone marrow transplantation—a prospective, randomized, double-blind study. J Infect Dis 1995;171: 1545-1552.
164. Kung N, Fisher N, Gunson B, et al: Fluconazole prophylaxis for high-risk liver transplant recipients. Lancet 1995;349:1234-1235.
165. Tollemar J, Hockerstedt K, Ericzon BG, et al: Liposomal amphotericin B prevents invasive fungal infections in liver transplant recipients. A randomized, placebo-controlled study. Transplantation 1995;59: 45-50.
166. Linden P, Kramer DJ, Mazariegos G, et al: Low-dose amphotericin B for the prophylaxis of serious *Candida* infections in high-risk liver recipients. 36th Interscience Conference on Antimicrobial Agents and Chemotherapy, 1996, New Orleans.
167. Winston DJ, Pakrasi A, Busuttil RW: Prophylactic fluconazole in liver transplant recipients: A randomized, double-blind, placebo-controlled trial. Ann Intern Med 1999;131:729-737.
168. Winston DJ, Chandrasekar PH, Lazarus HM, et al: Fluconazole prophylaxis of fungal infections in patients with acute leukemia. Results of a randomized placebo-controlled, double-blind, multicenter trial. Ann Intern Med 1993;118:495-503.
169. Schaffner A, Schaffner M: Effect of prophylactic fluconazole on the frequency of fungal infections, amphotericin B use, and health care costs in patients undergoing intensive chemotherapy for hematologic neoplasias. J Infect Dis 1995;172:1035-1041.
170. Walsh TJ, Hiemenz J, Pizzo PA: Editorial response: Evolving risk factors for invasive fungal infections—all neutropenic patients are not the same. Clin Infect Dis 1994;18:793-798.
171. Eggimann P, Francioli P, Bille J, et al: Fluconazole prophylaxis prevents intraabdominal candidiasis in high-risk surgical patients. Crit Care Med 1999;27:1066-1072.
172. Garbino J, Lew DP, Romand JA, et al: Prevention of severe Candida infections in nonneutropenic, high-risk, critically ill patients: A randomized, double-blind, placebo-controlled trial in patients treated by selective digestive decontamination. Intens Care Med 2002;28:1708-1717.
173. Pelz RK, Hendrix CW, Swoboda SM, et al: Double-blind placebo-controlled trial of fluconazole to prevent candidal infections in critically ill surgical patients. Ann Surg 2001;233:542-548.
174. Playford EG, Webster AC, Sorrell TC, Craig JC: Antifungal agents for preventing fungal infections in non-neutropenic critically ill and surgical patients: Systematic review and meta-analysis of randomized clinical trials. J Antimicrob Chemother 2006;57:628-638.
175. Shorr AF, Chung K, Jackson WL, et al: Fluconazole prophylaxis in critically ill surgical patients: A meta-analysis. Crit Care Med 2005;33:1928-1935; quiz 36.
176. Ostrosky-Zeichner L: Prophylaxis and treatment of invasive candidiasis in the intensive care setting. Eur J Clin Microbiol Infect Dis 2004;23:739-744.
177. Ostrosky-Zeichner L: Prophylaxis for invasive candidiasis in the intensive care unit: Is it time? Crit Care Med 2005;33:2121-2122.
178. National Committee for Clinical Laboratory Standards: Reference method for broth dilution antifungal susceptibility testing of yeasts; Approved standard NCCLS document M27-A. National Committee for Clinical Laboratory Standards, 1997, Wayne, Pa.
179. Rex JH, Pfaller MA, Walsh TJ, et al: Antifungal susceptibility testing: Practical aspects and current challenges. Clin Microbiol Rev 2001;14:643-658, table of contents.
180. Laskin OL: Acyclovir. Pharmacology and clinical experience. Arch Intern Med 1984;144:1241-1246.
181. Whitley RJ, Gnann JW Jr: Acyclovir: A decade later [published errata appear in N Engl J Med 1993 Mar 4;328:671

and 1997 Dec 4;337:1703]. N Engl J Med 1992;327:782-789.
182. Whitley RJ, Middlebrooks M, Gnann JW Jr: Acyclovir: The past ten years. Adv Exp Med Biol 1990;278:243-253.
183. Safrin S: Treatment of acyclovir-resistant herpes simplex virus infections in patients with AIDS. J Acquir Immune Defic Syndr 1992;5: S29-32.
184. Jacobson MA, Berger TG, Fikrig S, et al: Acyclovir-resistant varicella zoster virus infection after chronic oral acyclovir therapy in patients with the acquired immunodeficiency syndrome (AIDS). Ann Intern Med 1990;112: 187-191.
185. Erlich KS, Mills J, Chatis P, et al: Acyclovir-resistant herpes simplex virus infections in patients with the acquired immunodeficiency syndrome. N Engl J Med 1989;320:293-296.
186. Nichols WG, Boeckh M: Recent advances in the therapy and prevention of CMV infections. J Clin Virol 2000;16:25-40.
187. Meyers JD, Reed EC, Shepp DH, et al: Acyclovir for prevention of cytomegalovirus infection and disease after allogeneic marrow transplantation. N Engl J Med 1988;318:70-75.
188. Laskin OL, Longstreth JA, Saral R, et al: Pharmacokinetics and tolerance of acyclovir, a new anti-herpesvirus agent, in humans. Antimicrob Agents Chemother 1982;21:393-398.
189. Scott LL: Perinatal herpes: Current status and obstetric management strategies. Pediatr Infect Dis J 1995;14:827-832; discussion 32-35.
190. Sacks SL, Wilson B: Famciclovir/penciclovir. Adv Exp Med Biol 1999;458:135-147.
191. Jarvest RL, Sutton D, Vere Hodge RA: Famciclovir. Discovery and development of a novel antiherpesvirus agent. Pharm Biotechnol 1998;11:313-343.
192. Luber AD, Flaherty JF Jr: Famciclovir for treatment of herpesvirus infections. Ann Pharmacother 1996;30:978-985.
193. Keating MR: Antiviral agents for non-human immunodeficiency virus infections. Mayo Clin Proc 1990;74:1266-1283.
194. Faro S: A review of famciclovir in the management of genital herpes. Infect Dis Obstet Gynecol 1998;6:38-43.
195. Tyring SK: Efficacy of famciclovir in the treatment of herpes zoster. Semin Dermatol 1996;15:27-31.
196. Lowance D, Neumayer HH, Legendre CM, et al: Valacyclovir for the prevention of cytomegalovirus disease after renal transplantation. International Valacyclovir Cytomegalovirus Prophylaxis Transplantation Study Group [see comments]. N Engl J Med 1999;340:1462-1470.
197. Perry CM, Faulds D: Valaciclovir: A review of its antiviral activity, pharmacokinetic properties and therapeutic efficacy in herpesvirus infections. Drugs 1996;52:754-772.
198. Stein GE: Pharmacology of new antiherpes agents: Famciclovir and valacyclovir. J Am Pharm Assoc (Wash) 1997;NS37:157-163.
199. Bell AR: Valaciclovir update. Adv Exp Med Biol 1999;458:149-157.
200. Erice A, Chou S, Biron KK, et al: Progressive disease due to ganciclovir-resistant cytomegalovirus in immunocompromised patients. N Engl J Med 1989;320:289-293.
201. Cheung TW, Teich SA: Cytomegalovirus infection in patients with HIV infection. Mt Sinai J Med 1999;66:113-124.
202. Danner SA: Management of cytomegalovirus disease. AIDS 1995;9(Suppl 2):S3-S8.
203. Emanuel D, Cunningham I, Jules-Elysee K, et al: Cytomegalovirus pneumonia after bone marrow transplantation successfully treated with the combination of ganciclovir and high-dose intravenous immune globulin. Ann Intern Med 1988;109:777-782.
204. Goodrich JM, Bowden RA, Fisher L, et al: Ganciclovir prophylaxis to prevent cytomegalovirus disease after allogeneic marrow transplant. Ann Intern Med 1993;118:173-178.
205. Hardy D, Spector S, Polsky B, et al: Combination of ganciclovir and granulocyte-macrophage colony-stimulating factor in the treatment of cytomegalovirus retinitis in AIDS patients. The ACTG 073 Team. Eur J Clin Microbiol Infect Dis 1994;13: S34-40.
206. Holland GN: New strategies for the management of AIDS-related CMV retinitis in the era of potent antiretroviral therapy. Ocul Immunol Inflamm 1999;7:179-188.
207. Whitley RJ, Jacobson MA, Friedberg DN, et al: Guidelines for the treatment of cytomegalovirus diseases in patients with AIDS in the era of potent antiretroviral therapy: Recommendations of an international panel. International AIDS Society-USA. Arch Intern Med 1998;158:957-969.
208. Cvetkovic RS, Wellington K: Valganciclovir: A review of its use in the management of CMV infection and disease in immunocompromised patients. Drugs 2005;65:859-878.
209. Razonable RR, Paya CV: Valganciclovir for the prevention and treatment of cytomegalovirus disease in immunocompromised hosts. Expert Rev Anti Infect Ther 2004;2:27-41.
210. Lalezari JP, Stagg RJ, Jaffe HS, et al: A preclinical and clinical overview of the nucleotide-based antiviral agent cidofovir (HPMPC). Adv Exp Med Biol 1996;394:105-115.
211. Cundy KC, Petty BG, Flaherty J, et al: Clinical pharmacokinetics of cidofovir in human immunodeficiency virus-infected patients. Antimicrob Agents Chemother 1995;39:1247-1252.
212. Safrin S, Cherrington J, Jaffe HS: Clinical uses of cidofovir. Rev Med Virol 1997;7:145-156.
213. Safrin S, Cherrington J, Jaffe HS: Cidofovir. Review of current and potential clinical uses. Adv Exp Med Biol 1999;458:111-120.
214. Jacobson MA, Drew WL, Feinberg J, et al: Foscarnet therapy for ganciclovir-resistant cytomegalovirus retinitis in patients with AIDS. J Infect Dis 1991;163:1348-1351.
215. Pivetti-Pezzi P, Accorinti M, Ciapparoni V, Vullo V: Treatment of clinically resistant cytomegalovirus retinitis in AIDS patients: Combination of intravenous ganciclovir and intravitreal foscarnet. Eur J Ophthalmol 1995;5:199-203.
216. Safrin S, Kemmerly S, Plotkin B, et al: Foscarnet-resistant herpes simplex virus infection in patients with AIDS. J Infect Dis 1994;169:193-196.
217. Jacobson MA: Review of the toxicities of foscarnet. J Acquir Immune Defic Syndr 1992;5:S11-17.
218. Mossad SB: Underused options for preventing and treating influenza. Cleve Clin J Med 1999;66:19-23.
219. Monto AS: Viral respiratory infections in the community: epidemiology, agents, and interventions. Am J Med 1995;99:24S-27S.
220. Monto AS: Using antiviral agents to control outbreaks of influenza A infection. Geriatrics 1994;49:30-34.
221. Long JK, Mossad SB, Goldman MP: Antiviral agents for treating influenza. Cleve Clin J Med 2000;67:92-95.
222. Tominack RL, Hayden FG: Rimantadine hydrochloride and amantadine hydrochloride use in influenza A virus infections. Infect Dis Clin North Am 1987;1:459-478.
223. Wintermeyer SM, Nahata MC: Rimantadine: A clinical perspective. Ann Pharmacother 1995;29:299-310.
224. Crumpacker C, Heagy W, Bubley G, et al: Ribavirin treatment of the acquired immunodeficiency syndrome (AIDS) and the acquired-immunodeficiency-syndrome-related complex (ARC). A phase 1 study shows transient clinical improvement associated with suppression of the human immunodeficiency virus and enhanced lymphocyte proliferation. Ann Intern Med 1987;107:664-674.
225. Gilbert BE, Knight V: Biochemistry and clinical applications of ribavirin. Antimicrob Agents Chemother 1986;30:201-205.
226. McCormick JB, King IJ, Webb PA, et al: Lassa fever. Effective therapy with ribavirin. N Engl J Med 1986;314:20-26.
227. Hall CB, McBride JT, Walsh EE, et al: Aerosolized ribavirin treatment of infants with respiratory syncytial viral infection. A randomized double-blind study. N Engl J Med 1983;308: 1443-1447.
228. Levin MJ: Treatment and prevention options for respiratory syncytial virus infections. J Pediatr 1994;124:S22-S27.
229. Ghosh S, Champlin RE, Englund J, et al: Respiratory syncytial virus upper respiratory tract illnesses in adult blood and marrow transplant recipients: Combination therapy with aerosolized ribavirin and intravenous immunoglobulin. Bone Marrow Transplant 2000;25:751-755.
230. DeVincenzo JP, Hirsch RL, Fuentes RJ, Top FH Jr: Respiratory syncytial virus immune globulin treatment of lower respiratory tract infection in pediatric patients undergoing bone marrow transplantation—a compassionate use experience. Bone Marrow Transplant 2000;25:161-165.
231. Huggins JW, Hsiang CM, Cosgriff TM, et al: Prospective, double-blind, concurrent, placebo-controlled clinical trial of intravenous ribavirin therapy of

hemorrhagic fever with renal syndrome. J Infect Dis 1991;164:1119-1127.
232. Bradley JS, Connor JD, Compogiannis LS, Eiger LL: Exposure of health care workers to ribavirin during therapy for respiratory syncytial virus infections. Antimicrob Agents Chemother 1990;34:668-670.
233. Anonymous: Neuraminidase inhibitors for treatment of influenza A and B infections [published erratum appears in MMWR Morb Mortal Wkly Rep 1999;48:1139]. MMWR Morb Mortal Wkly Rep 1999;48:1-9.
234. Gubareva LV, Kaiser L, Hayden FG: Influenza virus neuraminidase inhibitors. Lancet 2000;355:827-835.
235. Treanor JJ, Hayden FG, Vrooman PS, et al: Efficacy and safety of the oral neuraminidase inhibitor oseltamivir in treating acute influenza: A randomized controlled trial. US Oral Neuraminidase Study Group [see comments]. JAMA 2000;283:1016-1024.
236. Jefferson T, Demicheli V, Di Pietrantonj C, et al: Neuraminidase inhibitors for preventing and treating influenza in healthy adults. Cochrane Database Syst Rev 2006;3:CD001265.
237. Hayden F, Klimov A, Tashiro M, et al: Neuraminidase inhibitor susceptibility network position statement: Antiviral resistance in influenza A/H5N1 viruses. Antivir Ther 2005;10:873-877.
238. Hayden FG, Atmar RL, Schilling M, et al: Use of the selective oral neuraminidase inhibitor oseltamivir to prevent influenza. N Engl J Med 1999;341:1336-1343.
239. He G, Massarella J, Ward P: Clinical pharmacokinetics of the prodrug oseltamivir and its active metabolite Ro 64-0802. Clin Pharmacokinet 1999;37:471-484.
240. Dunn CJ, Goa KL: Zanamivir: A review of its use in influenza. Drugs 1999;58:761-784.
241. Barnett JM, Cadman A, Gor D, et al: Zanamivir susceptibility monitoring and characterization of influenza virus clinical isolates obtained during phase II clinical efficacy studies. Antimicrob Agents Chemother 2000;44:78-87.
242. Gubareva LV, Matrosovich MN, Brenner MK, et al: Evidence for zanamivir resistance in an immunocompromised child infected with influenza B virus. J Infect Dis 1998;178:1257-1262.
243. Hayden FG, Osterhaus AD, Treanor JJ, et al: Efficacy and safety of the neuraminidase inhibitor zanamivir in the treatment of influenzavirus infections. GG167 Influenza Study Group. N Engl J Med 1997;337: 874-880.
244. Matsumoto K, Ogawa N, Nerome K, et al: Safety and efficacy of the neuraminidase inhibitor zanamivir in treating influenza virus infection in adults: Results from Japan. GG167 Group. Antivir Ther 1999;4:61-68.
245. Monto AS, Fleming DM, Henry D, et al: Efficacy and safety of the neuraminidase inhibitor zanamivirin the treatment of influenza A and B virus infections. J Infect Dis 1999;180:254-261.
246. Calfee DP, Peng AW, Cass LM, et al: Safety and efficacy of intravenous zanamivir in preventing experimental human influenza A virus infection. Antimicrob Agents Chemother 1999;43:1616-1620.
247. Monto AS, Robinson DP, Herlocher ML, et al: Zanamivir in the prevention of influenza among healthy adults: A randomized controlled trial [see comments]. JAMA 1999;282:31-35.
248. Cass LM, Efthymiopoulos C, Bye A: Pharmacokinetics of zanamivir after intravenous, oral, inhaled or intranasal administration to healthy volunteers. Clin Pharmacokinet 1999;36:1-11.
249. Freund B, Gravenstein S, Elliott M, Miller I: Zanamivir: A review of clinical safety. Drug Saf 1999;21:267-281.
250. Williamson JC, Pegram PS: Respiratory distress associated with zanamivir [letter]. N Engl J Med 2000;342: 661-662.
251. Balfour HH Jr, Rotbart HA, Feldman S, et al: Acyclovir treatment of varicella in otherwise healthy adolescents. The Collaborative Acyclovir Varicella Study Group [see comments]. J Pediatr 1992;120:627-633.
252. Baker DA: The use of antiviral medications in the treatment of herpes simplex virus infections of women. Int J Fertil Womens Med 1999;44:227-233.
253. Kaplowitz LG, Baker D, Gelb L, et al: Prolonged continuous acyclovir treatment of normal adults with frequently recurring genital herpes simplex virus infection. The Acyclovir Study Group. JAMA 1991;265:747-751.
254. Meyers JD, Wade JC, Shepp DH, Newton B: Acyclovir treatment of varicella-zoster virus infection in the compromised host. Transplantation 1984;37:571-574.
255. Saral R, Burns WH, Laskin OL, et al: Acyclovir prophylaxis of herpes-simplex-virus infections. N Engl J Med 1981;305:63-67.
256. Wade JC, Newton B, McLaren C, et al: Intravenous acyclovir to treat mucocutaneous herpes simplex virus infection after marrow transplantation: A double-blind trial. Ann Intern Med 1982;96:265-269.
257. Wade JC, Newton B, Flournoy N, Meyers JD: Oral acyclovir for prevention of herpes simplex virus reactivation after marrow transplantation. Ann Intern Med 1984;100:823-828.
258. Whitley RJ, Gnann JW: Herpes zoster: Focus on treatment in older adults. Antiviral Res 1999;44:145-154.
259. Burns WH, Saral R, Santos GW, et al: Isolation and characterisation of resistant Herpes simplex virus after acyclovir therapy. Lancet 1982;1:421-423.
260. Crumpacker CS, Schnipper LE, Marlowe SI, et al:: Resistance to antiviral drugs of herpes simplex virus isolated from a patient treated with acyclovir. N Engl J Med 1982;306:343-346.
261. Whitley RJ: Approaches to the treatment of varicella-zoster virus infections. Contrib Microbiol 1999;3:158-172.
262. Whitley RJ, Gnann JW Jr: Therapeutic approaches to the management of herpes zoster. Adv Exp Med Biol 1999;458:159-165.
263. Wood MJ, Johnson RW, McKendrick MW, et al: A randomized trial of acyclovir for 7 days or 21 days with and without prednisolone for treatment of acute herpes zoster [see comments]. N Engl J Med 1994;330:896-900.
264. Whitley RJ, Weiss H, Gnann JW Jr, et al: Acyclovir with and without prednisone for the treatment of herpes zoster. A randomized, placebo-controlled trial. The National Institute of Allergy and Infectious Diseases Collaborative Antiviral Study Group [see comments]. Ann Intern Med 1996;125:376-383.
265. Reusser P: Herpesvirus resistance to antiviral drugs: A review of the mechanisms, clinical importance and therapeutic options. J Hosp Infect 1996;33:235-248.
266. Breton G, Fillet AM, Katlama C, et al: Acyclovir-resistant herpes zoster in human immunodeficiency virus-infected patients: Results of foscarnet therapy. Clin Infect Dis 1998;27:1525-1527.
267. Hadley S, Samore MH, Lewis WD, et al: Major infectious complications after orthotopic liver transplantation and comparison of outcomes in patients receiving cyclosporine or FK506 as primary immunosuppression. Transplantation 1995;59:851-859.
268. Offidani M, Corvatta L, Olivieri A, et al: Infectious complications after autologous peripheral blood progenitor cell transplantation followed by G-CSF. Bone Marrow Transplant 1999;24:1079-1087.
269. Reed EC, Bowden RA, Dandliker PS, et al: Treatment of cytomegalovirus pneumonia with ganciclovir and intravenous cytomegalovirus immunoglobulin in patients with bone marrow transplants. Ann Intern Med 1988;109:783-788.
270. Arden NH: Control of influenza in the long-term-care facility: A review of established approaches and newer options. Infect Control Hosp Epidemiol 2000;21:59-64.
271. Bergen GA, Gompf SG, Sakalosky PA, Sinnott JT: Influenza. More than mom and chicken soup. J Fla Med Assoc 1996;83:19-22.
272. Couch RB: Measures for control of influenza. Pharmacoeconomics 1999;16:41-45.
273. Demicheli V, Jefferson T, Rivetti D, Deeks J: Prevention and early treatment of influenza in healthy adults. Vaccine 2000;18:957-1030.
274. Anonymous: Two neuraminidase inhibitors for treatment of influenza. Med Lett Drugs Ther 1999;41:91-93.
275. Hayden FG: Update on influenza and rhinovirus infections. Adv Exp Med Biol 1999;458:55-67.
276. Hayden FG: Antivirals for pandemic influenza. J Infect Dis 1997;176(Suppl 1):S56-S61.
277. Wenzel RP: Expanding the treatment options for influenza [editorial; comment]. JAMA 2000;283:1057-1059.

278. Shigeta S: Recent progress in anti-influenza chemotherapy. Drugs R D 1999;2:153-164.
279. Peters S: Flu prevention and management. Strategies for the elderly. Adv Nurse Pract 1997;5:57-59.
280. Chang SC, Cheng YY, Shih SR: Avian influenza virus: The threat of a pandemic. Chang Gung Med J 2006;29:130-134.
281. de Jong MD, Hien TT: Avian influenza A (H5N1). J Clin Virol 2006;35:2-13.
282. Fauci AS: Pandemic influenza threat and preparedness. Emerg Infect Dis 2006;12:73-77.
283. Gruber PC, Gomersall CD, Joynt GM: Avian influenza (H5N1): Implications for intensive care. Intensive Care Med 2006;32:823-829.
284. Carman WF, Elder AG, Wallace LA, et al: Effects of influenza vaccination of health-care workers on mortality of elderly people in long-term care: A randomised controlled trial [see comments]. Lancet 2000;355:93-97.
285. Nichol KL: Complications of influenza and benefits of vaccination. Vaccine 1999;17(Suppl 1):S47-S52.
286. Hoffmann CJ, Perl TM: The next battleground for patient safety: Influenza immunization of healthcare workers. Infect Control Hosp Epidemiol 2005;26:850-851.
287. Hall CB, Walsh EE, Hruska JF, et al: Ribavirin treatment of experimental respiratory syncytial viral infection: A controlled double-blind study in young adults. JAMA 1983;249:2666-2670.
288. Knight V, Gilbert BE: Aerosol treatment of respiratory viral disease. Lung 1990;168:406-413.
289. Rodriguez WJ, Parrott RH: Ribavirin aerosol treatment of serious respiratory syncytial virus infection in infants. Infect Dis Clin North Am 1987;1:425-439.
290. Canfield SD, Simoes EA: Prevention of respiratory syncytial virus (RSV) infection: RSV immune globulin intravenous and palivizumab (American Academy of Pediatrics). Pediatr Ann 1999;28:507-514.
291. Moler FW: RSV immune globulin prophylaxis: Is an ounce of prevention worth a pound of cure? [comment]. Pediatrics 1999;104:559-560.
292. Ottolini MG, Porter DD, Hemming VG, et al: Effectiveness of RSVIG prophylaxis and therapy of respiratory syncytial virus in an immunosuppressed animal model. Bone Marrow Transplant 1999;24:41-45.
293. Redding GJ, Braun S, Mayock D: Impact of respiratory syncytial virus immune globulin in 1996-1997: A local controlled comparison. Arch Pediatr Adolesc Med 1999;153:503-507.
294. Marchand S, Tchernia G, Hiesse C, et al: Human parvovirus B19 infection in organ transplant recipients. Clin Transplant 1999;13:17-24.
295. van Elsacker-Niele AM, Kroes AC: Human parvovirus B19: Relevance in internal medicine. Neth J Med 1999;54:221-230.
296. Young NS: Parvovirus infection and its treatment. Clin Exp Immunol 1996;104(Suppl):26-30.
297. Rogers JM, Diana GD, McKinlay MA: Pleconaril. A broad spectrum antipicornaviral agent. Adv Exp Med Biol 1999;458:69-76.
298. Pevear DC, Tull TM, Seipel ME, Groarke JM: Activity of pleconaril against enteroviruses. Antimicrob Agents Chemother 1999;43:2109-2115.

Chapter 54

Critically Ill Immunosuppressed Host

Henry Masur

As the population of patients with cancer, organ transplants, vasculitides, and human immunodeficiency virus (HIV) infection has grown, intensivists are seeing more and more patients with altered immunity. These patients may come to the intensive care unit (ICU) because of life-threatening opportunistic infections, or they may develop life-threatening infection while in the ICU for an unrelated problem. Intensivists must recognize how these patients differ from immunologically normal patients in terms of clinical presentation and management of these infections.

This chapter emphasizes the important ways in which immunosuppressed patients differ from immunologically normal individuals in terms of infectious complications. Clearly, however, immunosuppressed patients also develop complications from their underlying diseases and the drugs used to treat these underlying processes. These noninfectious complications are not the focus of this chapter but are reviewed in Chapter 81.

DEFINITION

Patients who are at increased risk for infectious complications because of a deficiency in any of their host defense mechanisms are referred to as *compromised hosts.* Patients in ICUs are almost universally compromised either by virtue of their underlying disease or by virtue of the invasive devices utilized to support and monitor them. Patients are termed *immunocompromised* or *immunosuppressed* if their defect specifically involves immune response. Often, patients who have deficient inflammatory response (e.g., neutropenia) are grouped into the category of immunocompromised or immunosuppressed, although technically they have a different category of deficient host response. Patients in ICUs are often immunosuppressed as a result of their underlying disease, therapy, or nutritional status. This chapter focuses specifically on patients who are immunocompromised or immunosuppressed.

HOST DEFENSE MECHANISMS

The microbial complications that any patient develops are determined by general, nonspecific barriers; innate immunity; acquired specific immunity; and environmental exposures. Nonspecific barriers include anatomic barriers such as intact skin and mucous membranes; chemical barriers such as gastric acidity or urine pH; and flushing mechanisms such as urinary flow or mucociliary transport. Organisms that breach these barriers encounter nonspecific and innate host factors termed the *acute phase response.* Acute phase responses include trigger molecules and effector molecules. Organisms also encounter acquired specific immune response systems including mononuclear phagocytes and antibodies.[1]

Infections that occur may result from normal flora that colonize mucosal or cutaneous surfaces. Infections may result from abnormal flora that have invaded or replaced normal flora because of environmental exposures, disrupted barriers, or selective pressure of antimicrobial agents. Table 54-1 lists organisms that cause disease when specific anatomic defenses are disrupted in individuals with normal microbial flora.

Infections may also result from common defects in the inflammatory or immunologic systems; examples are detailed in Table 54-2.[1-9] Inflammatory and immunologic barriers can be disrupted by the primary disease process (e.g., tumor can invade the bone marrow, immunologic abnormalities associated with aplastic anemia or collagen vascular disease can destroy cells either in the bone marrow or the periphery). Inflammatory and immunologic mechanisms can also be disrupted by drugs. Cytotoxic drugs, for instance, can reduce neutrophil number and function. Certain monoclonal antibodies can destroy lymphocyte populations or interfere with cytokine attachment to receptor sites. Some agents such as corticosteroids have multiple effects on neutrophils, lymphocytes, and soluble factors. Infections may result from organisms that are usually not pathogenic, but become opportunistic because of poor host defense mechanisms. Opportunistic infections are defined as those that occur with enhanced frequency or severity in a specific patient population compared with a normal patient population. *Pneumocystis jiroveci,* for example, never causes disease

Table 54-1. Normal Flora That Can Cause Disease When Anatomic Barriers Are Disrupted		
Compromised Host Defense: Anatomic Disruption	**Bacteria**	**Fungi**
Oral cavity, esophagus	α-Hemolytic streptococci, oral anaerobes	*Candida* species
Lower gastrointestinal tract	Enterococci Enteric organisms Anaerobes	*Candida species*
Skin	Gram-positive bacilli Staphylococci, streptococci *Corynebacterium, Bacillus* species *Mycobacterium fortuitum, Mycobacterium chelonei*	*Candida* species *Aspergillus*
Urinary tract	Enterococci Enteric organisms	*Candida* species

Table 54-2. Infections Associated with Common Defects in Inflammatory or Immunologic Response		
Host Defect	**Examples of Diseases or Therapies Associated with Defects**	**Common Etiologic Agents of Infections**
Inflammatory Response		
Neutropenia	Hematologic malignancies, cytotoxic chemotherapy, aplastic anemia	Gram-negative bacilli, *Staphylococcus aureus, Candida* species, *Aspergillus* species
Complement System		
C3	Congenital liver disease Systemic lupus erythematosus	*S. aureus, Staphylococcus pneumoniae* *Pseudomonas* species, *Proteus* species
Alternate pathway	Sickle cell disease	*S. pneumoniae, Salmonella*
Immune Response		
T lymphocyte deficiency/ dysfunction	Thymic aplasia, thymic hypoplasia, Hodgkin's disease, sarcoid	*Listeria monocytogenes, Mycobacterium* species, *Candida* species, *Aspergillus* species, *Cryptococcus neoformans, herpes simplex, herpes zoster*
	Human immunodeficiency virus	*Pneumocystis jiroveci,* cytomegalovirus, herpes simplex, *Mycobacterium avium* complex, *C. neoformans, Candida* species
	Mucocutaneous candidiasis	*Candida* species
B-cell deficiency/ dysfunction	Splenectomy, chronic lymphocytic leukemia, hypogammaglobulinemia, chronic lymphocytic leukemia, multiple myeloma, dysgammaglobulinemia	*S. pneumoniae,* other streptococci, *Haemophilus influenzae, Neisseria meningitidis, Babesia sp. Capnocytophaga, Giardia lamblia, P. jiroveci,* enteroviruses
	Selective IgA deficiency	*G. lamblia,* viral hepatitis, *S. pneumoniae, H. influenzae*
Mixed T- and B-cell deficiency/dysfunction	Common variable hypogammaglobulinemia	*P. jiroveci (carinii),* cytomegalovirus, *S. pneumoniae, H. influenzae,* varicella, other bacteria

in immunologically normal individuals but can cause frequent episodes of pneumonia in certain immunosuppressed patients. *Candida* can cause mild mucosal disease in normal patients receiving antibacterial drugs but causes more frequent and more severe mucositis when patients have impaired cell-mediated immunity.

Recognition of which host defense mechanisms are disrupted enables the clinician to focus diagnostic, therapeutic, and prophylactic management and optimize patient outcome. For instance, if a patient presents with severe hypoxemia and diffuse pulmonary infiltrates, a health care provider who recognizes a prior splenectomy as the major predisposition to infection would focus the diagnostic evaluation and the empiric therapy on *Streptococcus pneumoniae* and *Haemophilus influenzae*. By contrast, if the patient's major predisposition to infection were HIV infection with a CD4+ T lymphocyte count below 50 cells/μL, the health care provider would focus on *Pneumocystis jiroveci* and *S. pneumoniae;* if a cytomegalovirus (CMV)-negative patient's major predisposition were a recent allogeneic stem cell transplant from a CMV-positive donor, then CMV would be a prime consideration.[2-9]

Immune competence should ideally be measurable by objective laboratory parameters. In fact, the risk for opportunistic infection in patients with HIV infection can be assessed by clinical laboratories with a high degree of accuracy by measuring the number of circulating CD4+ T lymphocytes.[5] The susceptibility of cancer patients to opportunistic bacterial and *Candida* infections can be assessed by measuring the number of circulating neutrophils.[7,10,11] The predisposition of patients with certain congenital immunodeficiencies can be assessed by measuring serum immunoglobulin levels.[12] Unfortunately, however, for a large number of immunodeficiencies, no objective laboratory measures have been validated as predicting the risk of infection. Moreover, laboratory measures must be interpreted in context. CD4+ T lymphocyte counts have great prognostic value in patients with HIV infection but not in most other patient populations; neutrophil counts are relevant in all patient populations, but low counts are associated with disrupted mucosal surfaces compared with those with intact mucosa. Thus laboratory parameters must be interpreted in the context of the patient's underlying disease—risk is not always easily manageable by measuring one laboratory parameter.

Most importantly, most patients have multiple overlapping predispositions to infection. Knowledge of the infectious complications associated with specific diseases, specific immune defects, and specific laboratory abnormalities is helpful for predicting and managing infectious complications. However, a specific diagnosis should be established in each patient: knowledge of the immune defect helps guide empiric therapy or helps determine therapy if a diagnostic procedure is not safe to perform.

GENERAL APPROACH TO MANAGEMENT

Immunocompromised patients, by definition, are susceptible to a broader array of pathogens than immunocompetent patients. Understanding the specific immune defect can be enormously helpful in understanding the likely location and source of infection. However, the immune defect must be assessed in the context of the specific disease: the clinical manifestations of HIV infection, for instance, are quite different from the clinical manifestations of patients with other diseases that alter cell-mediated immunity such as lymphoma. The immune defect must also be interpreted with the understanding that predisposition to infection is usually multifactorial: in addition to neutropenia or lymphocyte depletion, patients often have impaired mucosal barriers, poor ciliary function, or breaches in their skin (i.e., from catheters) that can increase their risk of infection.

Effective management of opportunistic infections requires understanding of several basic tenets of care.

1. Diseases may present with subtle symptoms and signs, and patients are predisposed to deteriorate precipitously.

   Because immunocompromised patients may lack inflammatory and/or immunologic mediators, the clinical manifestations of infections are often less prominent and less impressive than immunocompetent patients with similar complications. Thus clinicians must recognize that even subtle changes in skin color, catheter site appearance, chest radiograph, or abdominal examination may warrant an aggressive diagnostic evaluation and early institution of broad-spectrum empiric therapy. Although all ICU patients demand prompt attention and vigorous diagnostic and therapeutic management, many types of immunosuppression can be associated with especially precipitous clinical deterioration despite their innocuous presentation.

2. Fever is not invariably present when patients are infected.

   Although fever is not invariably present in any patient population with infection, immunosuppressed patients are notorious for developing infection in the absence of fever. Thus infection must be considered as part of the differential diagnosis among patients with afebrile syndromes that might not appear to be infectious. Conversely, patients with fever may not have infection: Fever may be a manifestation of the underlying disease, an allergic response to a drug, or an underlying neoplastic or collagen vascular disease.

3. Diagnostic evaluation needs to be prompt and definitive.

   As indicated earlier, patients with life-threatening infection may present with subtle symptoms and signs that progress rapidly: these early manifestations merit aggressive attempts to define the anatomy of the lesion and the causative microbial pathogen. Because the spectrum of potential pathogens includes a wide array of microorganisms (e.g., viruses, fungi, protozoa, or bacteria), clinicians must be certain that appropriate specimens are obtained and the appropriate microbiologic and histologic tests are ordered to identify common, as well as uncommon or unusual, pathogens. Invasive diagnostic techniques such as bronchoalveolar lavage or tissue biopsies should be performed with less hesitancy than in immunologically normal patients. Patients often have enhanced risk factors for invasive procedures, such as thrombocytopenia, coagulation factor deficiencies, or compromised organ function. However, the benefit of definitive diagnosis often outweighs these risks when the procedures are performed by experienced operators.

4. The threshold for initiating broad-spectrum empiric therapy should be low.

   Because patients can deteriorate rapidly and because they are susceptible to such a wide array of microbial pathogens, clinicians should have little hesitation in instituting empiric antimicrobial therapy. This therapy must be directed at the full range of bacterial, fungal, viral, protozoal, and helminthic infections to which patients are predisposed. This therapy should be administered promptly, preferably within an hour of suspecting an infectious process. Clinicians should initiate comprehensive regimens: antimicrobial agents can be discontinued or reduced when culture results and clinical events clarify the scenario.

5. Foreign bodies and infectious foci should be addressed.

   Patients may need careful imaging to be certain that they do not have an obstructed viscus or localized collection that should be drained. Such imaging is appropriate even when signs or symptoms are unimpressive. Similarly, patients often have multiple intravascular catheters that may need to be removed, as discussed in Chapter 51.

6. Consideration should be given to augmenting the immune or inflammatory response.

   There may be opportunities to augment immunologic or inflammatory responses by administering pharmacologic or biologic agents such as granulocyte colony-stimulating factor (G-CSF) or intravenous immunoglobulin.[12-15] Eliminating immunosuppressive drugs or reducing the dose can also improve the patient's prognosis.
7. Efficacy and toxicity of therapy should be assessed serially.

   ICU patients characteristically require attentive monitoring to assure the adequacy and safety of therapy. Immunocompromised patients often have multiple prior and concurrent insults to their renal and hepatic function, and they often receive multiple drugs that can produce drug-drug interactions. Thus monitoring the pharmacokinetics and assessing potential toxicities are especially important in these patient populations. Moreover, because response to therapy may be less robust than in immunocompetent patients, antigen titers or PCR titers, as well as serial imaging studies, can be important to assure the adequacy of the management plan. Therapy must often be continued longer than in immunologically normal patients.

MANAGEMENT OF SPECIFIC PATIENT POPULATIONS

Patients with Neutropenia

General Principles

Cytotoxic therapy–induced neutropenia is a major predisposition to infection.[7,11] Counts below 500 cells/mm^3 (the total of polymorphonuclear neutrophils and bands) increase susceptibility to infection in a linear fashion (i.e., the lower the neutrophil count, the greater the degree of susceptibility). The absolute neutrophil count is not the only factor that determines susceptibility, however, because some patients with cyclic neutropenias, drug-induced neutropenias, or HIV-induced neutropenias, for example, are not nearly as susceptible to infection as are cancer patients receiving cytotoxic therapy. Other important contributors to susceptibility, in addition to the absolute neutrophil count, are the duration of neutropenia, the functional capability of neutrophils, the integrity of physical barriers such as the skin and gastrointestinal mucosa, the patient's microbiologic environment (endogenous and exogenous flora), and the status of other immune mechanisms. For example, a patient with vancomycin-induced neutropenia during therapy for a staphylococcal infection may not develop any complications if the neutropenia is brief and defense mechanisms are otherwise intact. A patient with HIV-induced neutropenia may have prolonged or even lifelong neutrophil counts below 500/μL yet suffer few serious bacterial complications.[14] The presence of intact physical defense barriers is a major difference compared with cancer patients, whose skin and mucous membranes are disrupted by cytotoxic therapy in which the skin and gastrointestinal tracts are portals of entry for infections that are not controlled by diminished host immunologic or inflammatory defenses. Thus the patient with HIV infection is usually at a much lower risk for a bacterial infection than is a cancer patient, despite a comparable neutrophil count.

In the 1960s and 1970s, aerobic gram-negative bacilli such as *Escherichia coli, Klebsiella pneumoniae,* and *Pseudomonas aeruginosa* predominated as pathogens in neutropenic patients. Anaerobic bacteria and aerobic gram-positive cocci were recognized less commonly. Aerobic gram-negative bacillus infections were also associated with a poorer outcome than infections from gram-positive cocci. Given the spectrum of pathogenic organisms that were seen in that era, combination therapy was usually advocated.[11,16-24] A number of reasons were proposed to justify combination therapy: (1) broad coverage of potential pathogens; (2) prevention of emergence of resistance; and (3) synergy. In general, these principles are reasonable concepts on which to base a preference for using combination therapeutic regimens. However, no study unequivocally demonstrated that combination therapy provided better outcomes than did monotherapy, assuming that both study arms contained drugs that had activity against the causative organism. In addition, predicting synergy proved difficult.[25]

In the 1990s the spectrum of causative pathogens in neutropenic patients shifted from a predominance of gram-negative bacilli to a majority of gram-positive cocci including streptococci, staphylococci (including oxacillin-resistant *Staphylococcus aureus*), and enterococci (including vancomycin-resistant *enterocci*).[20,24,26] The development of potent broad-spectrum β-lactam and quinolone drugs in the 1980s and 1990s has provided single agents that can probably provide comparable outcomes to combination therapy when used empirically or specifically. In the current era the choice of single or combination regimens is based predominantly on the spectrum of organisms that needs to be covered rather than attempting a strategy of trying to obtain more potency through additive or synergistic combinations.[10,27]

Promptly initiating broad-spectrum antibacterial therapy for all cancer patients who are febrile and who are neutropenic (neutrophil count <500/mm^3) as a result of cytotoxic chemotherapy is standard practice.[7,10,27] For febrile neutropenic patients who have no apparent source of infection, there is no evidence that the initial antibacterial regimen is any more effective if a broad-spectrum antibacterial regimen consisting of two or more drugs is used instead of a single broad-spectrum antibacterial drug. For stable "low-risk" patients outside the ICU, an oral regimen is now considered a reasonable approach.[7,10,17] Such oral regimens would not be used for inpatients in most circumstances and would not be appropriate for high-risk or unstable patients.[7,10] Antifungal and antiviral drugs are generally not used empirically when neutropenic patients are initially treated unless there is a specific reason to have a high suspicion for a fungal or viral process.

Historically, an infectious cause of fever has been found in about two thirds of febrile, neutropenic cancer patients. When a specific causative organism is identified, antimicrobial therapy is modified to include an agent or agents determined to be active by in vitro susceptibility tests and that penetrate to the site of the infection.[10] Combination therapy is advocated by some authorities for the specific (compared with empiric) therapy of either gram-positive or gram-negative bacteria, although, as noted earlier, there are little data for most pathogens that indicate that a combination regimen produces a better outcome than an appropriate single agent. Therapy is generally not narrowed in terms of spectrum, however, because alteration of broad-spectrum coverage to focused therapy has been associated with more complications (e.g., "breakthrough bacteremias") unless the neutropenia resolves. Whenever fever persists, therapy has generally been continued during the entire course of neutropenia because cessation of antimicrobial therapy has been associated with recurrent bacteremia resulting from the initial causative organism or a newly identified pathogen. A 10- to 14-day course of antibacterial therapy is usually the minimum recommended if a causative infection is identified. Therapy is usually stopped promptly when the neutrophil count exceeds 1000 cells/µml if fever resolves and no source was ever identified.

Empiric antibacterial therapy has been a successful strategy for reducing morbidity resulting from bacterial processes but has been associated with the emergence of fungal infections, as well as resistant bacterial pathogens. *Candida* and *Aspergillus* organisms, in particular, have become major causes of morbidity and mortality over the past 2 decades. These fungal processes can be difficult to diagnose because they are not always associated with detectable fungemia. The emergence of fungi as important pathogens, especially in patients with prolonged neutropenia, has led to the recommendation that empiric antifungal therapy be added to neutropenic patients who do not have an identified bacterial process and who do not defervesce within 4 to 7 days of empiric antibacterial therapy.[7,10] Fluconazole or an amphotericin B compound (e.g., liposomal amphotericin B) are often used, although echinocandins or certain other azoles such as voriconazole are being used by some investigators and clinicians.[28-31]

As patients receive chemoprophylaxis with quinolones and/or azoles during periods of intense neutropenia or immunosuppression, breakthrough pathogens are more and more likely to be resistant to the prophylactic agents.[32,33] Thus empiric regimens must be chosen with keen attention to the drugs that patients have received in the recent past, as well as pathogens they have previously been colonized or infected with.[34]

Diagnostic Approach

Patients with fever and neutropenia require aggressive diagnostic efforts to identify the cause of fever so that the appropriate antimicrobial agent is used and appropriate procedures (e.g., surgical drainage, removal of foreign body such as a catheter) can be performed. Regular physical examination is necessary to identify sites that merit more focused investigation: With impaired inflammatory response, findings on examination may be subtle. Knowledge of the specific immunologic defect is important so that when cultures of blood, sputum, urine, or other appropriate body fluids or body sites are performed, special microbiologic approaches can be used to detect viruses, fungi, helminths, protozoa, and bacteria. Imaging studies are also important because intra-abdominal, intrathoracic, intracerebral, or musculoskeletal processes can be clinically subtle and may not be associated with identifiable organisms in the bloodstream. A growing array of antigen, nucleic acid, and gene detection systems including polymerase chain reaction and microarray gene assays are being investigated to facilitate diagnosis. Some antigen or nucleic acid detection systems for blood or other body fluids can be useful for detecting cryptococcus, histoplasma, hepatitis B and C, HIV, mycobacteria, pneumococci, and *Legionella*. Some of these approaches, despite their promising initial reports, are not yet clinically practical because of their level of sensitivity, specificity, or the cost or expertise required to perform them adequately.

Careful attention to antimicrobial susceptibility patterns is also important. Patients are exposed to repeated courses of antimicrobial agents. Patients come into contact with contaminated environments in a variety of health care settings. Resistance is no longer an issue exclusively for aerobic gram-negative organisms but is a concern for anaerobes, gram-positive cocci, viruses, fungi, and protozoa. Clinicians must recognize that pathogens may be resistant when they are acquired by the patient, or they may become resistant during therapy if there is an inducible resistance mechanism or drug concentrations are not adequate to inhibit or kill the organism.

Antimicrobial Therapy

A broad-spectrum agent used as monotherapy for febrile, neutropenic patients should have activity against aerobic gram-positive cocci and aerobic gram-negative bacilli including *P. aeruginosa*.[7,10,19,35] Potential drugs for this indication include certain cephalosporins (e.g., cefepime), carbapenems (e.g., imipenem or meropenem), and β-lactam/β-lactamase combination agents (e.g., piperacillin-tazobactam). Ceftazidime is an option chosen by some, but its poor activity against gram-positive cocci has caused some clinicians to use other agents.[18] Intensivists must recognize, however, that these monotherapy regimens may not be appropriate in an ICU. Patients in ICUs, by definition, are either unstable hemodynamically or have a potentially life-threatening process such as diffuse pneumonia or are "fragile" because of concurrent processes. Thus combination regimens are preferred by many authorities in ICU settings, even though no study clearly documents superior outcomes from such combination regimens. The decade that started in 2000 is an era when microbial resistance is becoming an increasingly important problem for many types of bacteria including aerobic gram-positive cocci and anaerobes, as well as aerobic gram-negative bacilli. Multiple drug empiric regimens are more likely than monotherapy regimens to include an agent with activity against the offending pathogen(s). Thus in a situation in an ICU when failure to use an active drug is more likely to be lethal than in other settings, and when enhanced potency is a logical goal, combination therapy is prudent as an initial management strategy. Thus adding vancomycin or linezolid or daptomycin for better gram-positive coverage, adding a quinolone for better gram-negative bacillus coverage, and adding metronidazole to cefepime would be prudent in this patient population pending results of initial diagnostic studies. Of note, however, is that although this strategy is logical, no study has shown convincingly that such an approach improves outcome.[22]

A substantial number of febrile, neutropenic patients fail to improve in terms of fever or other manifestations. Failure to improve may result from poor immune response, a need for drainage or necessity to remove foreign bodies, the use of drugs without activity against the causative organism, or a noninfectious process including drug allergy (i.e., fever resulting from a drug including an antimicrobial agent). The potential causative processes need to be aggressively reassessed on a regular basis by physical examination, history, cultures, and imaging techniques. Most centers add antifungal therapy empirically at day 4 or day 7 of therapy if patients remain febrile.[10,27,29,36,37] Fluconazole, liposomal amphotericin B, caspofungin, or voriconazole may be used: In some situations fluconazole would be less attractive either because the patient has received fluconazole prophylaxis or because molds are suspected.[28,38,39] The toxicity profile of amphotericin B, even in its liposomal form, has led many clinicians to prefer voriconazole or one of the echinocandins (i.e., caspofungin, micafungin, or anidulafungin).[30,40,41]

After empiric antimicrobial therapy is initiated, the optimal duration of therapy is a complex issue that depends on the type and severity of the infectious process and the duration and severity of immunosuppression, especially the neutropenia. If a causative bacterium is identified, a minimum of 7 to 10 days of therapy is generally advocated, with at least 3 to 4 days being administered after neutropenia has resolved. Longer courses may be required in certain settings. The duration of antifungal therapy is a complex issue and depends on the specific mycosis, the location and extent of disease, and the patient's immune status.[15] This is discussed in Chapter 53. The use of combination therapy for fungal diseases remains controversial.[42,43]

A common problem in febrile, neutropenic patients is managing indwelling intravascular lines.[44-46] In general, these lines can be left in place initially if examination of the site reveals no indication of infection. Blood cultures should be drawn through the catheter. Although some experts advocate drawing a culture through each port of each catheter, obtaining this many blood cultures is often not feasible. If a patient is hemodynamically unstable and fails to respond promptly to fluid administration, it is prudent to remove the line in case an infected catheter is the source of the sepsis. Failure to remove the foreign body in this situation probably increases the likelihood of an unfavorable outcome. Should blood cultures become positive and should the suspicion be high that the catheter is the source, antibacterial therapy may be successful in some settings (e.g., if the pathogen is a bacteria that is relatively sensitive to antibacterial therapy), thus avoiding the need to remove the catheter. Situations suggesting that catheter removal is necessary include hemodynamic instability despite aggressive fluid resuscitation, tunnel infection, or infections resulting from fungi or relatively antibiotic-resistant bacteria such as *P. aeruginosa*.

A major determinant of prognosis is the immunologic status of the patient. Prompt return of neutrophil number to normal improves the outcome. The use of G-CSF or granulocyte-monocyte colony-stimulating factor (GM-CSF), if not contraindicated by the underlying disease, can improve clinical status by hastening the return of neutrophil numbers and function.[12-15,47] Granulocyte transfusions have not been proved useful in most clinical settings because of the inability to administer a large number of cells with adequate frequency.[48] The manipulation of immune response with cytokines, cytokine inhibitors, or immunoglobulins is the subject of considerable investigation: Such interventions may reduce the duration of fever or the incidence of infections when used empirically, but in no setting have they been clearly shown to improve survival when administered after an infection has been documented.

An algorithm for managing fever in neutropenic patients is provided in Figure 54-1. Table 54-3 suggests modifications of standard empiric regimens in certain common clinical scenarios.

Prevention of Infection

Given the experience with frequent and severe infectious complications in cancer patients with neutropenia, it has been logical to attempt to prevent infection.[33] Most microorganisms causing disease in this patient population arise from endogenous gastrointestinal, cutaneous, or respiratory flora. Total protected environments probably reduce frequency of infection, but this approach is expensive and inconvenient. Trying to prove a consistent beneficial impact on survival has been difficult, and thus such isolation is rarely used anymore. Some experts are enthusiastic about placing patients in positive pressure rooms so that pathogens do not enter via particles and droplets from outside the room. This type of isolation has not clearly improved outcome, however, and is not a standard of care.

Prophylactic bacterial therapy has also been controversial.[32] Systemic antibacterial prophylaxis and systemic antifungal prophylaxis have been shown in some studies to reduce the number of infections, but their lack of effect on patient survival, their cost, and their impact on the emergence of resistance have made many clinicians reluctant to use them. Selective gastrointestinal decontamination has not consistently improved survival and thus is not recommended by most authorities in the United States. Antipneumocystis prophylaxis is, in contrast, highly effective in susceptible populations. Prophylaxis for CMV is highly effective in well-defined, high-risk patients (e.g., some recipients of organ transplants who are either sero-

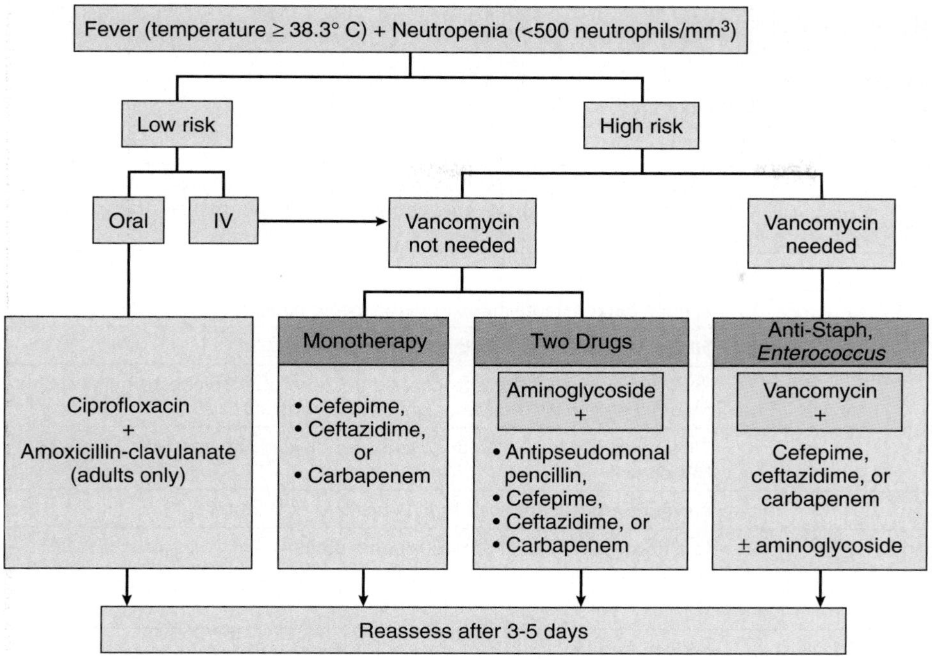

Figure 54-1. Algorithm for management of patients with febrile neutropenia. (From Hughes WT, Armstrong D, Bodey GP, et al: 2002 guidelines for the use of antimicrobial agents in neutropenic patients with cancer. Clin Infect Disease 2002;34:730-751.)

Table 54-3. Modification of Standard Empiric Therapy in Patients with Neutropenia

Clinical Event	Possible Modifications of Standard Empiric Therapy
Breakthrough bacteremia	If gram-positive isolate (e.g., *Staphylococcus aureus*), add vancomycin until susceptibility pattern of isolate is known. If gram-negative isolate, add two new agents likely to have activity until susceptibility pattern of pathogen is known.
Cellulitis or catheter-associated infection	Add vancomycin.
Severe necrotizing mucositis or gingivitis	Add specific antianaerobic agent (e.g., metronidazole, meropenem, imipenem, or piperacillin-tazobactam) plus agent with activity against streptococci; consider acyclovir.
Ulcerative mucositis or gingivitis	Add acyclovir and anaerobic coverage.
Esophagitis	Add fluconazole or caspofungin; consider adding acyclovir.
Pneumonitis, diffuse or interstitial	Add trimethoprim-sulfamethoxazole and azithromycin or levofloxacin or moxifloxacin (plus broad-spectrum antibiotics if the patient is granulocytopenic).
Perianal tenderness	Include anaerobic agents such as metronidazole, imipenem, meropenem, or piperacillin-tazobactam.
Abdominal involvement	Add antianaerobic agent (e.g., metronidazole, meropenem, imipenem, or piperacillin-tazobactam).

positive for CMV or who are seronegative but received a graft from a seropositive donor).[2,4,49] Strategies that reduce the period of immunologic susceptibility (e.g., reduce the duration of neutropenia), such as adding G-CSF to a regimen or reducing the intensity of chemotherapeutic regimens, are promising. Table 54-4 summarizes general strategies of infection prevention in immunosuppressed patients including patients with neutropenia.

Patients with HIV Infection

Because so many patients are receiving highly active antiretroviral therapy (HAART), opportunistic infections are not complicating the course of HIV infection to the same degree that they did in the 1980s and early 1990s.[50-53] Opportunistic infections continue to occur, however, in three groups of HIV-infected patients: (1) those who are unaware of their HIV status until they develop a clinical syndrome; (2) those who are unable or unwilling to receive appropriate therapy; and (3) those who fail HAART and opportunistic infection prophylaxis. Although HAART has dramatically reduced the incidence of opportunistic infections, a surprisingly large fraction of patients either never respond virologically and immunologically or lose their response within the first 12 to 24 months of therapy. These patients, most of whom have dominant viral quasispecies that are highly resistant to currently licensed antiretroviral drugs, will likely experience immunologic decline over the next few years and will again become more susceptible to opportunistic infections.

Table 54-4. Prevention of Infectious Complications in Compromised Patients

Ways to Prevent Acquisition of, Suppress, or Eliminate Microbial Flora	Examples
Isolation	
	Total protective isolation with high-efficiency particulate air filters and absorbable or nonabsorbable antibiotics for bone marrow–transplant recipient
Prophylactic Antibacterial Drugs	
Norfloxacin	Reduce bacterial infections in neutropenic patients
Trimethoprim-sulfamethoxazole	Suppress flora in chronic bronchitis patients
Penicillin	Reduce frequency of streptococcal infections after splenectomy or rheumatic valvular disease or graft-versus-host disease
Rifabutin	Prevention of *Mycobacterium avium* complex in patients with advanced HIV disease
Isoniazid	Prevention of tuberculosis in PPD-positive individuals
Nonabsorbable broad-spectrum agents (i.e., aminoglycoside, plus bacitracin)	Gut decontamination for neutropenic patients
Prophylactic Antiviral Drugs	
Oral acyclovir or valganciclovir, or IV ganciclovir	Reduce frequency of CMV disease following transplantation
Rimantadine, oseltamivir	Prevent influenza
Prophylactic Antifungal Drugs	
Fluconazole	Prevent recurrent candidiasis
Liposomal amphotericin B or voriconazole or caspofungin	Prevent *Candida* or mold infections
Trimethoprim-sulfamethoxazole	Prevent *Pneumocystis* pneumonia
Prophylactic Antiprotozoal/Anthelmintic Drugs	
Albendazole or ivermectin	Prevent disseminated strongyloidiasis in high-risk patients
Augment Host Defenses	
Immunization	Pneumococcal and *Haemophilus* vaccine for patients before splenectomy
Immune serum globulin	Augment levels in deficient patients (e.g., common variable immunodeficiency)
Fresh frozen plasma	Augment complement levels in deficient patients
Neutrophil transfusions	Augment inflammatory response in neutropenic patients or patients with chronic functional neutrophil disorders
Lymphocyte or other mononuclear cell transfusions	Experimental therapies for tumors, various immunodeficiencies
Bone marrow or stem cell transplant	Reconstitute patients with congenital immunodeficiencies or certain acquired cytopenias
Bone marrow human stem cell stimulation	G-CSF or GM-CSF to increase neutrophil or mononuclear cell quantity and function
Gene therapy	Replace genes to allow normal function

AIDS, acquired immunodeficiency syndrome; *CMV,* cytomegalovirus; *G-CSF,* granulocyte colony-stimulating factor; *GM-CSF,* granulocyte-monocyte colony-stimulating factor; *HIV,* human immunodeficiency virus; *PPD,* purified protein derivative.

Spectrum of Clinical Manifestations

Patients with HIV infection develop clinical disease as a result of three basic processes: the direct effect of HIV on specific organs (e.g., cardiomyopathy, enteropathy, dementia); immunologically mediated processes (e.g., glomerulonephritis, thrombocytopenia); or opportunistic infections and tumors that are enabled by HIV-induced immunosuppression.

HIV appears to cause direct organ damage.[50,53-57] This damage may be mediated by cytokines, lymphocytes, monocytes, or inflammatory cells. Cardiomyopathy, for example, can be a profound and lethal process that can lead to ICU admission or complicate other processes.[55] When patients present with or develop pulmonary manifestations such as shortness of breath or diffuse bilateral infiltrates on chest radiograph, cardiogenic causes must be considered. HIV also causes a diffuse pneumonitis,[56] profound encephalopathy,[54] and a diffuse enteropathy.[57] Patients with compatible syndromes need a comprehensive evaluation to look for other specific opportunistic infections or tumors, especially those that can be specifically treated. In all of the HIV-caused syndromes, HIV as the etiology remains a diagnosis of exclusion. The institution of antiretroviral therapy appears to be beneficial for patients with susceptible isolates, although data regarding such effects for these HIV-related entities are largely anecdotal.

HIV-related thrombocytopenia and anemia appear to be immunologically mediated.[58,59] Both can be severe: platelet counts below 10,000/mm^3 and hemoglobins below 10 g/dL can be seen with the expected complications. These disorders are related to the development of antigen-antibody complexes and may improve dramatically with the institution of antiretroviral therapy and a decline in viral load. For thrombocytopenia, intravenous immunoglobulin (or anti RhD antibody), corticosteroids, or splenectomy may also be useful. Hemolytic anemia can also be severe: hemoglobin levels below 5 g/dL can be seen.

The most prominent manifestations of HIV continue to be the opportunistic infections and tumors that occur as a consequence of HIV-induced immunosuppression. The CD4+ T lymphocyte cell number is a useful marker for predicting the occurrence of opportunistic infections in patients with HIV infection.[5,9] This relationship of CD4+ T lymphocyte count to the occurrence of opportunistic infection continues to be as valid in the era of HAART as it was before the licensing of the first antiretroviral agent, zidovudine, in 1987.[60-62] Figure 54-2 demonstrates the typical relationship of CD4+ T lymphocyte counts to the occurrence of opportunistic infections. Knowledge of this relationship permits the focusing of diagnostic, therapeutic, and prophylactic management. For instance, if a patient with HIV infection and a CD4+ T lymphocyte count of 700 cells/µL presents with diffuse pulmonary infiltrates, the diagnostic evaluation and empiric antimicrobial regimen should focus on *S. pneumoniae; H. influenzae; Mycoplasma, Legionella,* and *Chlamydia* organisms, as well as common community-acquired viruses. In contrast, if the same patient had a CD4+ T lymphocyte count of 50 cells/µL, the evaluation and empiric regimen would focus on pneumocystosis and CMV, although the previously mentioned processes that occur at high CD4+ T lymphocyte counts can also occur at lower CD4+ T lymphocyte counts. Keeping in mind that CD4+ T lymphocyte counts are useful predictors of susceptibility to infection is important, but they are not perfect. Occasionally, patients will develop opportunistic infections at "uncharacteristically" high CD4+ T lymphocyte counts. For instance, 5% to 10% of cases of pneumocystosis occur at CD4+ T lymphocyte counts greater than 200 cells/µL.[61] Clinical parameters can provide additional clues; for example, oral candidiasis, a previous opportunistic infection, a prior episode of pneumonia, or high viral load are independent risk factors for the occurrence of *Pneumocystis jiroveci carinii* pneumonia (PCP), and logically for other infections as well.[9]

A frequent question is whether an HIV-infected patient's prior CD4+ T lymphocyte count nadir affects the likelihood of an opportunistic infection occurring if HAART has stimulated a CD4+ T lymphocyte count rise. Specifically, if a patient has a CD4+ T lymphocyte count of 400 cells/µL while receiving HAART and that patient's CD4+ T lymphocyte count was 50 cells/µL before HAART, is that patient at greater risk for developing an opportunistic infection than another patient whose current CD4+ T lymphocyte count is 400 cells/µL but whose nadir before HAART was 250 cells/µL? The data suggest that these two patients have comparable risk (i.e., the current CD4+ T lymphocyte count is the most important predictor of risk and the earlier nadir has only minor influence on opportunistic infection susceptibility).[62]

In evaluating the differential diagnosis of infectious syndromes in patients with HIV (and in every other patient

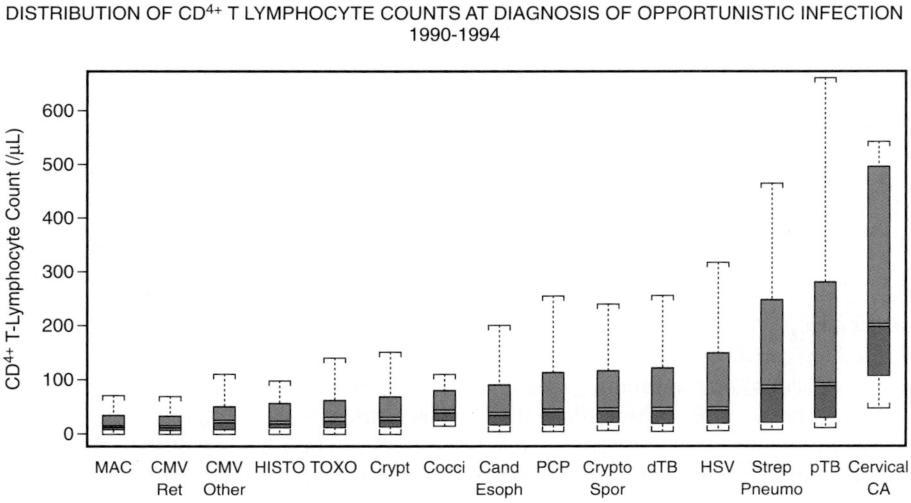

Figure 54-2. CD4+ cell count range for common manifestations of acquired immunodeficiency syndrome. Cand Esoph, *Candida* esophagitis; cervical CA, cervical cancer; CMV Other, other cytomegalovirus diseases; CMV Ret, cytomegalovirus retinitis; Cocci, coccidiorycosis; Crypt, cryptococcosis; Crypto Spor, cryptosporidiosis; dTB, disseminated tuberculosis; HISTO, histoplasmosis; NSV, *herpes simplex virus;* MAC, *Mycobacterium avium* complex; PCP, *Pneumocystic carinii* pneumonia; pTB, pulmonary tuberculosis; Strep Pneumo, *Streptococcus pneumonia;* TOXO, toxoplasmosis.

population as well), geography is an important part of the history. Tuberculosis is always a concern because of the extraordinary susceptibility of HIV-infected patients for developing active disease.[63] In many urban settings in the United States, each pulmonary evaluation should include smears and cultures for *M. tuberculosis*, both to diagnose the appropriate cause of the pulmonary dysfunction and to assist in determining what respiratory precautions are appropriate. In some areas of the country, such as the Ohio River Valley and Indianapolis, histoplasmosis is as common as pneumocystosis in causing diffuse pulmonary infiltrates.[64] In the southwestern United States, coccidioidomycosis must be recognized as a cause of pulmonary infiltrates. The clinical presentations of tuberculosis, histoplasmosis, coccidioidomycosis, and other processes such as CMV can be clinically indistinguishable from PCP. Thus for patients with pulmonary infiltrates in an ICU, prolonged empiric therapy is discouraged in favor of vigorous efforts to establish a specific diagnosis.

HIV-infected patients are admitted to ICUs for several major syndromes: respiratory insufficiency, cerebral dysfunction, septic shock, hepatic or renal failure, and drug toxicities.[50] However, patients with HIV infection also come to ICUs for routine procedures and routine postoperative care. In those situations their management ordinarily requires no extraordinary measures, with two exceptions. First, the staff must be fully aware of how HIV is transmitted, the danger of injuries resulting from sharp objects, and the procedure for managing injuries involving sharp objects contaminated with blood or other biologic fluids from infected or potentially infected patients.[65] Second, drug interactions involving drugs used during procedures and certain antiretroviral drugs can have important clinical consequences.[66,67] Many of the protease inhibitors and the non-nucleoside reverse transcriptase inhibitors that are now the backbone of antiretroviral therapy can inhibit or enhance the metabolism of drugs that depend on the cytochrome P450 system. Thus the half-lives of certain analgesics, sedatives, and hypnotics can be prolonged in HIV-infected patients who are taking ritonavir, for example. This pharmacokinetic effect is also relevant for a host of other therapeutic agents used in the ICU and may affect their efficacy or safety. Clinicians need to be familiar with these interactions when selecting new therapies for procedures or for clinical entities. Table 54-5 summarizes therapeutic and prophylactic approaches to managing patients with HIV-related opportunistic infections.[72]

Respiratory Insufficiency

Patients with HIV infection can develop severe pulmonary dysfunction because of common community-acquired pathogens such as *S. pneumonia, Legionella, Mycoplasma,* and *Chlamydia;* adenovirus; influenza; or respiratory syncytium virus, as well as other opportunistic viruses and fungi. Thus the diagnostic evaluation needs to be comprehensive, emphasizing direct smears of sputum or bronchoalveolar lavage. It is important to recognize that the clinical presentations produced by many causative agents can be similar. For instance, histoplasmosis, tuberculosis, and nonspecific interstitial pneumonitis can present identically to PCP.[50,61,63,64,68] Thus although empiric diagnosis and empiric therapy may be reasonable as initial approaches to some patients with HIV infection and mild pneumonitis, such an approach is usually not appropriate for patients in an ICU.

Evaluation of induced sputum is the first step in the diagnostic approach to PCP. Sensitivity can be 80% to 95% at many hospitals (at some institutions the yield is considerably lower).[69] Specificity should be 100% in an experienced laboratory. Other pathogens, including mycobacteria, fungi, and routine bacteria, can be identified in sputum as well. For intubated patients, respiratory secretions obtained by deep intratracheal suctioning are also likely to be useful, although they have not been as carefully studied as induced sputum. Should the diagnosis not be established by evaluation of sputum or intratracheal secretions, bronchoscopy should be performed. Bronchoalveolar lavage should diagnose almost 100% of cases of PCP, even if patients have received 7 to 10 days of empiric therapy.[70] A diagnosis of PCP is established by visualizing one or more clusters of organisms.

Diagnostic criteria for other opportunistic infections are reviewed in Chapters 12 and 43. In patients with HIV, CMV merits special mention. Culture of sputum or bronchoalveolar lavage does not provide useful information because patients with CD4+ T lymphocyte counts below 100 cells/μL will predictably have CMV present in their secretion independent of whether or not pulmonary disease is present.[71] A diagnosis of CMV pneumonia in this patient population is suggested by cytology and confirmed by the presence of multiple inclusion bodies in lung tissue obtained by transbronchial or open lung biopsy. Similarly, *Mycobacterium avium* complex (MAC) and HSV can often be found in respiratory secretions, but these organisms almost never cause pneumonia in patients with HIV infection. In other patient populations they can clearly cause pneumonia, but the dearth of CMV, MAC, and HSV pneumonia in this patient population emphasizes the point that it is important to know from published literature what the clinical likelihood is for different microbial processes.

Fungal pneumonias other than PCP are generally diagnosed by direct microscopy or culture of respiratory secretions (sputum or lavage). *Candida* organisms almost never cause pneumonia in patients with HIV infection. The frequency of *Cryptococcus, Histoplasma, Blastomyces,* and *Coccidioides* organisms as causes of pneumonia depends on the geographic exposure of the patient. Among these mycoses, antigen detection techniques can be useful for finding *Cryptococcus* and *Histoplasma* organisms.

Mycobacteria frequently infect the respiratory tract of patients with HIV infection. As noted earlier, *M. avium* complex almost never causes pulmonary dysfunction in this patient population. When acid-fast bacilli are seen (as opposed to cultured) in respiratory secretions or tissue, *M. tuberculosis* is almost always the pathogen; *M. kansasii* and other mycobacteria less commonly cause disease. Screening all patients with acid-fast bacillus smears is important for preventing transmission of tuberculosis and

Text continued on p. 1126

Table 54-5. Treatment of HIV-Associated Opportunistic Infections Among Adults

Opportunistic Infections	Preferred Therapy and Duration	Alternative Therapy	Other Options/Issues
Pneumocystis jiroveci Pneumonia (PCP)	Acute therapy ■ Trimethoprim-sulfamethoxazole (TMP/SMX): [15-20 mg TMP and 75-100 mg SMX]/kg body weight/day IV administered q6h or q8h or ■ Same daily dose of TMP/SMX PO in 3 divided doses; or ■ TMP-SMX DS 2 tablets 3 times a day Total duration—21 days Chronic maintenance therapy (Secondary prophylaxis) *First choice:* ■ Trimethoprim-sulfamethoxazole (TMP-SMX) 1 double-strength tablet (DS) PO QD; or ■ TMP-SMX 1 single-strength tablet (SS) PO QD *Alternatives:* ■ Dapsone 50 mg PO twice daily or 100 mg PO daily; or ■ Dapsone 50 mg PO daily plus pyrimethamine 50 mg PO weekly plus leucovorin 25 mg PO weekly; or ■ Dapsone 200 mg PO plus pyrimethamine 75 mg PO plus leucovorin 25 mg PO weekly; aerosolized pentamidine 300 mg every month via Respingard nebulizer (manufactured by Marquest, Englewood, Colorado); or ■ Atovaquone 1500 mg PO QD; or ■ TMP-SMX 1 DS PO TIW	For severe PCP: ■ Pentamidine 4 mg/kg QD infused over at least 60 minutes, some specialists reduce dose to 3 mg/kg IV QD because of toxicities For mild-to-moderate PCP: ■ Dapsone 100 mg PO QD and TMP 15 mg/kg/day PO (3 divided dose); or ■ Primaquine 15-30 mg (base) PO QD and clindamycin 600-900 mg IV q6h to q8h or clindamycin 300-450 mg PO q6h to q8h; or ■ Atovaquone 750 mg PO BID with food	Indications for corticosteroids: Pa_{O_2} <70 mm/Hg at room air; or alveolar-arterial O_2 gradient >35 mm/Hg Prednisone doses (beginning as early as possible and within 72 hours of PCP therapy): 40 mg BID days 1-5, 40 mg QD days 6-10, then 20 mg QD days 11-21 IV methylprednisolone can be administered as 75% of prednisone dose Chronic Maintenance Therapy (Secondary prophylaxis) should be discontinued if $CD4^+$ T lymphocyte count increases in response to ART from <200 to >200 cells/μL for ≥3 months
Toxoplasma gondii encephalitis (TE)	Acute therapy Pyrimethamine 200 mg POx1, then 50 mg (<60 kg body weight) to 75 mg (≥60 kg) PO QD and sulfadiazine 1000 (<60 kg) to 1500 mg (≥60 kg) PO q6h plus leucovorin 10-20 mg PO QD (can increase ≥50 mg) Total duration for acute therapy is at least 6 weeks Chronic maintenance therapy (Secondary prophylaxis) *First choice* ■ Sulfadiazine 500-1000 mg PO QID plus pyrimethamine 25-50 mg PO QD plus leucovorin 10-25 mg by mouth daily *Second choice* ■ Clindamycin 300-450 mg PO every 6-8 hours plus pyrimethamine 25-50 mg PO QD plus leucovorin 10-25 PO QD; or ■ Atovaquone 750 mg PO every 6-12 hours with or without pyrimethamine 25 mg PO QD plus leucovorin 10 mg PO QD	■ Pyrimethamine (leucovorin) and clindamycin 600 mg IV or PO q6h; or ■ TMP-SMX (5 mg/kg TMP and 25 mg/kg SMX) IV or PO bid; or ■ Atovaquone 1,500 mg PO BID with meals (or nutritional supplement) and pyrimethamine (leucovorin); or ■ Atovaquone 1500 mg PO BID with meals (or nutritional supplement) and sulfadiazine 1000-1,500 mg PO q6h; or ■ Atovaquone 1500 mg PO BID with meals; or ■ Pyrimethamine (leucovorin) and azithromycin 900-1200 mg PO QD For severely ill patients who cannot take oral medications TMP-SMX IV and pyrimethamine PO For other regimens with limited experience, see text.	Adjunctive corticosteroids (e.g., dexamethasone) should be administered when clinically indicated for treatment of mass effect attributed to focal lesions or associated edema and discontinued as soon as clinically feasible Anticonvulsants should be administered to patients with a history of seizures Secondary prophylaxis may be discontinued if ■ Free of TE signs and symptoms; and sustained $CD4^+$ T lymphocyte count of >200 cells/μL for >8 months of ART

Table 54-5. Treatment of HIV-Associated Opportunistic Infections Among Adults—cont'd

Opportunistic Infections	Preferred Therapy and Duration	Alternative Therapy	Other Options/Issues
Mycobacterium tuberculosis (MTB)	For drug-sensitive MTB *Initial phase (8 weeks)* Isoniazid (INH) 5 mg/kg body weight (max: 300 mg) PO QD and [rifampin 10 mg/kg (max: 600 mg) PO QD or rifabutin 300 mg PO QD] (or dose adjusted based on concomitant meds) and pyrazinamide (PZA) (dose based on weight) PO QD and ethambutol (EMB) (dose based on weight) PO QD *Continuation phase (19 weeks)* ■ INH 5 mg/kg (max: 300 mg) PO QD and [rifampin 10 mg/kg (max: 600 mg) or rifabutin 300 mg PO QD]; or ■ INH 15 mg/kg (max: 900 mg) PO BIW or TIW plus [rifampin 10 mg/kg (max: 600 mg) or rifabutin 300 mg PO TIW] In patients with delayed clinical or microbiologic response to initial therapy (e.g., sputum culture (+) after 2 months or if cavitary pulmonary lesions are present), total duration up to 9 months	Treatment for drug-resistant MTB: *Resistant to INH* ■ Discontinue INH (and streptomycin, if used) ■ Rifamycin, PZA, and EMB for 6 months; or rifamycin and EMB for 12 months (preferably with PZA during at least first 2 months *Resistant to rifamycin* ■ INH and PZA and EMB and a fluoroquinolone (e.g., levofloxacin 500 mg/day) for 2 months, followed by 10-16 additional months with INH and EMB and fluoroquinolone *Multidrug resistant (MOR) TB—both INH and rifamycin resistant* ■ Therapy should be individualized based on resistance pattern and with close consultation with experienced specialist TB treatment in patients with liver disease *If AST ≥3 times normal before treatment initiation* ■ Standard therapy with frequent monitoring; or ■ Rifamycin and EMB and PZA for 6 months ■ INH and rifamycin and EMB for 2 months, then INH and rifamycin for 7 months *For patients with severe liver disease* ■ Rifamycin and EMB for 12 months (preferably with another agent such as fluoroquinolone for first 2 months)	Treatment by directly observed therapy (DOT) is strongly recommended for all HIV patients Rifabutin has less drug interaction potential and can be used in place of rifampin Rifapenthe administered once weekly can result in development of resistance. It is not recommended among HIV patients Twice weekly intermittent regimen containing rifamycin might lead to rifamycin resistance, particularly among advanced HIV patients with $CD4^+$ T-cell count <100 cells/μL; in this situation, therapy must be administered as daily or three times weekly For paradoxical reaction that is not severe, may be treated with nonsteroidal anti-inflammatory drugs (NSAIDs) without change in TB or HIV medications
Candidiasis (mucosal)	Oropharyngeal candidiasis Initial episodes (7-14 day treatment) ■ Fluconazole 100 mg PO QD; or ■ Itraconazole oral solution 200 mg PO QD; or ■ Clotrimazole troches 10 mg PO 5 times daily; or ■ Nystatin suspension 4-6 mL QID or 1-2 flavored pastilles 4-5 times daily Esophageal candidiasis (14-21 days) ■ Fluconazole 100 mg (up to 400 mg) PO or IV QD; or ■ Itraconazole oral solution 200 mg PO QD ■ Voriconazole 200 mg PO BID ■ Caspofungin 50 mg IV QD Vulvovaginitis ■ Topical azoles (clotrimazole, butoconazole, miconazole, ticonazole, or terconazole) for 7-10 days ■ Topical nystatin 100,000 units/day as vaginal tablet for 14 days ■ Oral itraconzaole 200 mg BID for 1 day or 200 mg QD for 3 days ■ Oral fluconazole 150 mg for 1 dose	Fluconazole-refractory oropharyngeal candidiasis ■ Itraconzaole oral solution ≥200 mg PO QD; or ■ Amphotericin B suspension 100 mg/mL (not available in U.S.)—1 mL PO QID; or ■ Amphotericin B deoxycholate 0.3 mg/kg IV QD Fluconazole-refractory esophageal candidiasis ■ Caspofungin 50 mg IV QD; or ■ Voriconazole 200 mg PO or IV BID ■ Amphotericin B 0.3-0.7 mg/kg IV QD; or ■ Amphotericin liposomal or lipid complex 3-5 mg/kg IV QD	Suppressive therapy—generally not recommended unless patients have frequent or severe recurrences ■ Oropharyngeal candidiasis—fluconazole or itraconazole oral solution may be considered ■ Vuivovaginal candidiasis—daily topical azole for recurrent cases ■ Esophageal candidiasis—fluconazole 100-200 mg QD. Chronic or prolonged use of azoles might promote development of resistance

Cryptococcus neoformans meningitis	Acute infection (induction therapy) ■ Amphotercin B deoxycholate 0.7 mg/kg body weight IV QD and/or flucytosine 25 mg/kg PO QID for 2 weeks; or ■ Liposomal amphotericin B 4 mg/kg IV QD and/or flucytosine 25 mg/kg PO QID for 2 weeks Consolidation therapy ■ Fluconazole 400 mg PO QD for 8 weeks or until CSF cultures are sterile Chronic maintenance therapy (Secondary prophylaxis) ■ Fluconazole 200 mg PO QD;	Induction therapy (alternative) ■ Amphotericin B 0.7 mg/kg/day IV for 2 weeks; or ■ Fluconazole 400-800 mg/day (PO or IV) for less severe disease ■ Fluconazole 400-800 mg/day (PO or IV) and flucytlosine 25 mg/kg PO QID for 4-6 weeks Consolidation therapy (alternative) ■ Itraconazole 200 mg PO BID Chronic maintenance therapy (alternative) ■ Itraconazole 200 mg PO QD—for patients intolerant of or failed fluconazole	Repeated lumbar puncture might be indicated as adjunctive therapy among patients with increased intracranial pressure Discontinuation of antifungal therapy can be considered among patients who remain asymptomatic, with $CD4^+$ T-lymphocyte count >100-200 cells/μL for ≥6 months Some might consider performing a lumbar puncture before discontinuation of maintenance therapy
Histoplasma capsulatum infections	Severe disseminated Acute phase (3-10 days or until clinically improved) ■ Amphotericin B deoxycholate 0.7 mg/kg body weight IV QD; or ■ Liposomal amphotericin B 4 mg/kg IV QD Continuation phase (12 weeks) ■ Itraconazole 200 mg capsule PO BID Less severe disseminated ■ Itraconazole 200 mg capsule PO TID for 3 days, then 200 mg PO BID for 12 weeks Meningitis ■ Amphotericin B deoxycholate or liposomal for 12-16 weeks Chronic maintenance therapy (secondary prophylaxis) ■ Itraconazole capsule 200 mg PO QD	Severe disseminated Acute phase (alternative) ■ Itraconazole 400 mg IV QD Continuation phase (alternative) ■ Itraconazole oral solution 200 mg PO BID ■ Fluconazole 800 mg PO QD Mild disseminated ■ Fluconazole 800 mg PO QD	Acute pulmonary histoplasmosis among HIV-1–infected patients with $CD4^+$ T-lymphocyte count >500 cells/μL might require no therapy Insufficient data to recommend discontinuation of chronic maintenance therapy.
Herpes simplex virus (HSV) disease	Orolabial lesions and initial or recurrent genital HSV Famciclovir 500 mg PO BID or valacyclovir 1 g PO BID or acyclovir 400 mg PO TID for 7-14 days Moderate-to-severe mucocutaneous HSV infections ■ Initial therapy acyclovir 5 mg/kg body weight IV q8h ■ After lesions begin to regress, change to famciclovir 500 mg PO BID or valacyclovir 1 g PO BID or acyclovir 400 mg PO TID; continue therapy until lesions have completely healed HSV keratitis ■ Trifluridine 1% ophthalmic solution, one drop onto the cornea every 2 hours, not to exceed 2 drops per day, for no longer than 21 days HSV encephalitis ■ Acyclovir 10 mg/kg IV q8h for 14-21 days	Acyclovir-resistant HSV ■ Foscarnet 120-200 mg/kg/day IV in 2-3 divided doses until clinical response ■ Cidofovir 5 mg/kg IV weekly until clinical response Alternative for acyclovir-resistant HSV infections ■ Topical trifluridine ■ Topical cidofovir Note: Neither of these topical preparations is commercially available; extemporaneous compounding of these topical products can be prepared using trifluridine ophthalmic solution and cidofovir for intravenous administration	Chronic suppressive therapy with oral acyclovir, famciclovir, or valacyclovir might be indicated among patients with frequent or severe recurrences

Table 54-5. Treatment of HIV-Associated Opportunistic Infections Among Adults—cont'd

Opportunistic Infections	Preferred Therapy and Duration	Alternative Therapy	Other Options/Issues
Varicella zoster virus (VZV) disease	Primary VZV infection (chickenpox) ■ Acyclovir 10 mg/kg body weight IV q8h for 7-10 days ■ Switch to oral therapy (acyclovir 800 mg PO QID or valacyclovir 1 g TID or famciclovir 500 mg TID) after defervescence if no evidence of visceral involvement exists Local dermatomal herpes zoster ■ Famciclovir 500 mg or valacyclovir 1 g PO TID for 7-10 days Extensive cutaneous lesion or visceral involvement ■ Acyclovir 10 mg/kg IV q8h, continue until cutaneous and visceral disease clearly resolved Progressive outer retinal necrosis (PORN) ■ Acyclovir IV 10 mg/kg q8h and foscarnet 80 mg/kg IV q8h		Corticosteroids for dermatomal zoster are not recommended
Coccidioidomycosis	Nonmeningeal infection *Acute phase (diffuse pulmonary or disseminated disease)* ■ Amphotericin B deoxycholate 0.5-1.0 mg/kg body weight IV QD; continue until clinical improvement, usually 500-1,000 mg total dose *Acute phase (milder disease)* ■ Fluconazole 400-800 mg PO QD; or ■ Itraconazole 200 mg PO BID Meningeal Infections ■ Fluconazole 400-800 mg IV or PO QD Chronic maintenance therapy (Secondary prophylaxis) ■ Fluconazole 400 mg PO QD; or ■ Itraconazole 200 mg capsule PO BID	Nonmeningeal infection *Acute phase (diffuse pulmonary or disseminated disease)* ■ Some specialists add azole to amphotericin B therapy Meningeal infection ■ Intrathecal amphoterin B	Insufficient data to recommend discontinuation of chronic maintenance therapy
Invasive aspergillosis	Voriconazole 400 mg IV or PO q12h for 2 days, then 200 mg q12h Duration of therapy based on clinical response	■ Amphotericin B deoxycholate 1 mg/kg body weight/day IV; or ■ Lipid formulations of amphotericin B 5 mg/kg/day IV	Not enough data to recommend chronic suppression or maintenance therapy

Cylomegalovirus (CMV) disease	CMV retinitis For immediate sight-threatening lesions Ganciclovir intraocular implant and valganciclovir 900 mg PO QD *For peripheral lesions* Valganciclovir 900 mg PO BID for 14-21 days, then 900 mg PO QD Chronic maintenance therapy (Secondary prophylaxis) *First choice* ■ Valganciclovir 900 mg PO QD ■ Foscarnet 90-120 mg/kg body weight IV QD CMV esophagitis or colitis ■ Ganciclovir IV or Foscarnet IV for 21-28 days or until signs and symptoms have resolved; oral valganciclovir may be used if symptoms are not severe enough to interfere with oral absorption ■ Maintenance therapy is generally not necessary, but should be considered after relapses CMV pneumonitis ■ Treatment should be considered in patients with histologic evidence of CMV pneumonitis and who do not respond to treatment of other pathogens ■ The role of maintenance therapy is not yet established CMV neurologic disease ■ Ganciclovir IV and Foscarnet IV continue until symptomatic improvement ■ Maintenance therapy should be continued for life	CMV retinitis ■ Ganciclovir 5 mg/kg IV q12h for 14-21 days, then 5 mg/kg IV QD; or ■ Ganciclovir 5 mg/kg IV q12h for 14-21 days, then valganciclovir 900 mg PO QD; or ■ Foscarnet 80 mg/kg IV q8h or 90 mg/kg IV q12h for 14-21 days, then 90-120 mg/kg IV q24h; or ■ Cidofovir 5 mg/kg IV for 2 weeks, then 5 mg/kg every other week; each dose should be administered with IV saline hydration and oral probenecid; or ■ Repeated intravitreal injections with fomivirsen (for relapses only, not as initial therapy) Chronic maintenance therapy ■ Cidofovir 5 mg/kg IV every other week with probenecid 2 g PO 3 hours before the dose followed by 1 g PO 2 hours after the dose, and 1 g PO 8 hours after the dose (total of 4 g); or ■ Fomivirsen 1 vial (330 mg) injected into the vitreous, then repeated every 2-4 weeks	Choice of initial therapy for CMV retinitis should be individualized on the basis of location and severity of the lesion(s), level of immunosuppression, and other factors such as concomitant medications and ability to adhere to treatment Initial therapy among patients with CMV retinitis, esophagitis, colitis, and pneumonitis should include optimization of antiretroviral therapy (ART) Some specialists recommend delaying ART among patients with CMV neurologic disease because of concerns about worsening of condition as a result of immune recovery inflammatory reaction Pre-emptive treatment of patients with CMV viremia without evidence of organ involvement is generally not recommended Maintenance therapy for CMV retinitis can be safely discontinued among patients with inactive disease and sustained $CD4^+$ T lymphocyte (>100-150 cells/μL^3 for ≥8 months); consultation with ophthalmologist is advised Patients with CMV retinitis who discontinued maintenance therapy should undergo regular eye examination for early detection of relapse Ganciclovir intraocular implants might need to be replaced every 6-8 months for patients who remain immunosuppressed with $CD4^+$ T lymphocyte counts <100-150 cells/μL Immune recovery uveitis (IRU) might develop in the setting of immune reconstitution; treatment of IRU; periocular corticosteroids or short courses of systemic steroid. Because of its poor oral bioavailability and with the availability of valganciclovir, oral ganciclovir should not be used

should be considered as part of a routine respiratory evaluation for patients with radiographic infiltrates in most areas of the United States.

Therapy of opportunistic infections is summarized in Table 54-5.[72] While awaiting a specific diagnosis, it is reasonable to initiate empiric therapy in patients ill enough to merit admission to an ICU. For patients with a CD4+ T lymphocyte count greater than 250 to 300 cells/μL, azithromycin and ceftriaxone or azithromycin and ampicillin-sulbactam would be reasonable choices. For patients with CD4+ T lymphocyte counts below 200 to 250 cells/μL, levofloxacin or moxifloxacin plus trimethoprim-sulfamethoxazole or pentamidine plus levofloxacin or moxifloxacin would be potential regimens. If PCP is documented, trimethoprim-sulfamethoxazole is always the drug of choice in patients who can tolerate it. Table 54-5 lists alternatives for sulfa-intolerant individuals. Regardless of which specific antipneumocystis regimen is used, corticosteroid therapy is indicated for any patient who presents with an oxygen pressure (PO_2) below 70 mm Hg or an alveolar-arterial gradient higher than 30 mm Hg.[73-76] Patients with an initial PO_2 lower than 70 mm Hg are the subgroup with substantial mortality for whom corticosteroids have been shown to provide a survival benefit. Corticosteroids may provide more rapid and perhaps more complete resolution of pulmonary manifestations in patients who present with better pulmonary function, but survival in this population is so high that clinical trials have not been able to show survival benefit. Some experts are concerned that corticosteroid use will be associated with reactivation of latent infections such as CMV or tuberculosis. However, reactivation of life-threatening infections has not been associated with this corticosteroid regimen.

How should a patient with AIDS-associated PCP be managed if there is no improvement, or if there is deterioration, after 5 to 10 days of therapy? The median time to improvement in clinical variables is 4 to 8 days; therefore, changes in therapy are probably not warranted before 5 to 10 days. At that point the accuracy of the diagnosis should be reassessed: Consideration should be given to repeat bronchoscopy with transbronchial biopsy to determine if CMV, fungi, mycobacteria, or a nosocomial bacterial process is present. Noninfectious processes such as congestive heart failure or tumor (e.g., Kaposi's sarcoma) must also be considered. If pneumocystosis is the only causative process that can be identified, corticosteroids should be added to the regimen if they have not been already. Whether switching from one antipneumocystis agent to another or whether adding a second agent is helpful has not been determined by clinical trials. Some human pneumocystosis isolates are resistant to sulfonamides, but such testing is available only in a few research centers. Most clinicians add parenteral pentamidine to trimethoprim-sulfamethoxazole. Parenteral trimetrexate or clindamycin-primaquine could be used as salvage regimens as well. Patients who have not improved after 14 to 21 days of therapy with specific chemotherapy plus corticosteroids have an exceedingly poor prognosis.

Should patients with AIDS-related PCP be intubated and provided with mechanical ventilation? Mortality for such patient populations was 70% to 80% in several series in the early 1980s.[77-80] Since that era, supportive care has improved, and treatment modalities for concurrent infectious and noninfectious processes have become more effective. Patient selection for ventilatory support is probably also improving. Patients who have multiple active opportunistic infections, substantial weight loss, and no response to 14 days of therapy have a worse prognosis than ambulating patients who develop respiratory failure the third day of therapy. Thus decisions about ICU support for patients with HIV infection and respiratory failure need to be individualized on the basis of a realistic assessment of prognosis, the availability of resources, and the preference of the individual patient.

A frequent question for any HIV-infected patient in the ICU is whether antiretroviral drugs should be continued or initiated during the critical or life-threatening illness. Although there is no specific study of various strategies, most authorities discourage the use of antiretroviral drugs in the ICU because of drug interactions and drug toxicities. In addition, the initiating HAART can be associated with dramatic "immune reconstitution" syndromes that can complicate the process that brought the patient to the ICU.[81-83] Finally, almost all antiretroviral drugs that are commercially available are oral: In most situations it is better to discontinue all antiretroviral drugs for a few days or weeks or months rather than risk poor absorption and suboptimal serum levels. The latter would enhance the emergence of drug-resistant HIV.

Central Nervous System Dysfunction

An important cause of admitting HIV-infected patients into the ICU is either seizures or altered mental status. Either can result from infectious or neoplastic processes caused by meningeal disease or parenchymal involvement. The differential diagnosis of meningeal disease includes pneumococcal and staphylococcal meningitis, cryptococcal meningitis, tuberculous meningitis, and lymphomatous meningitis, as well as involvement from other endemic mycoses and common community-acquired viral and bacterial processes.[24,84] Diffuse central nervous system parenchymal disease can be caused by HIV itself, by progressive multifocal leukoencephalopathy, and occasionally by herpes viruses such as CMV or herpes simplex virus. Focal mass lesions may be caused by toxoplasmosis or lymphoma. Less often, tuberculosis, fungi, conventional bacterial abscesses, nocardia, and other tumors are the cause of focal lesions. These lesions can be difficult to distinguish clinically and radiologically. The CD4+ T lymphocyte count can help narrow the differential diagnosis, but CSF or brain tissue is usually necessary for definitive diagnosis.

The routine therapies for many of these processes are outlined in Table 54-5. Toxoplasmosis deserves particular mention because of its frequency.[85-87] Toxoplasmosis occurs mainly in patients with HIV infection who have CD4+ T lymphocyte counts below 100 cells/μL, have a positive IgG antibody titer against toxoplasma, and who have not been receiving trimethoprim-sulfamethoxazole or dapsone prophylaxis. Patients present with altered cognition, focal motor or sensory deficits, or seizures. Lesions may be unifocal or multifocal. They usually enhance with contrast, but this is not invariably true. For patients who fit the profile for high risk of toxoplasmosis, and with a compatible presentation, it is reasonable to establish an empiric diagnosis and institute specific therapy with sulfadiazine plus pyrimethamine or, for patients unable to tolerate sulfa, clindamycin plus pyrimethamine. Corticosteroids may be needed for patients with considerable intracerebral edema or elevated intracranial pressure. Antiseizure medication is usually instituted only after a seizure has occurred rather than prophylactically. Most patients improve clinically and radiologically within 7 to 10 days. If patients fail to improve, a stereotactic needle biopsy is appropriate, especially because the prevalence of lymphoma is increasing. Organisms can be difficult to see in brain specimens obtained by this technique.

Hypotension

Patients with HIV infection develop hypotension resulting from the same types of disorders as with non-HIV infected individuals—sepsis from a primary infection or a wound or device (especially an intravascular access device), fluid depletion from vomiting or diarrhea, and hemorrhage from a gastrointestinal lesion are examples of common causes. The evaluation of hypotension in a patient with HIV infection must take into account factors particular to this patient population: It is susceptible to opportunistic infections; it undergoes many procedures that can be associated with infectious complications; and it receives an array of drugs, some of which have cardiovascular effects. Thus evaluating hypotension in this patient population requires a comprehensive and thorough approach. A differential diagnosis of the major causes is shown in Table 54-6. Adrenal function always deserves special attention because several viral processes, fungal and mycobacterial diseases, HIV, and drugs can suppress the adrenal axis and either cause hypotension or exacerbate it.

Table 54-6. Causes of Hypotension in Patients with HIV Infection

Process	Examples of Causes
Distributive Shock	
Septic shock	
Bacterial	*Pneumococcus* or *Haemophilus* organism pneumonia Vascular access infection Surgical wound
Viral	CMV, disseminated VZV
Fungal	*Histoplasma, Coccidioides, Cryptococcus* organisms Vascular access–related candidemia *Pneumocystis jiroveci* pneumonia
Adrenal Insufficiency	Tuberculosis, fungi, CMV, HIV
Oligemic Shock	
Dehydration	Bacterial diarrhea *C. difficile* diarrhea
Gastrointestinal hemorrhage	CMV colitis Gastrointestinal lymphoma
Cardiogenic Shock	
Cardiomyopathy	HIV
Endocarditis	Bacterial pathogens related to IV drug abuse
Extracardiac Obstruction	
Pericardial tamponade	Lymphoma, Kaposi's sarcoma, primary effusion lymphoma Fungus, tuberculosis
Pericardial constriction	Tuberculosis, fungus
Massive pulmonary embolus	Inactivity, inanition

CMV, cytomegalovirus; *HIV,* human immunodeficiency virus; *VZV,* varicella-zoster virus.

Prevention of Opportunistic Infection

Patients with HIV infection typically receive several antimicrobial agents to reduce the likelihood they will acquire opportunistic infections.[9] *Primary prophylaxis* is the term used to indicate strategies that reduce the likelihood of an initial episode of a disease process. *Secondary prophylaxis* is the term used to indicate strategies that prevent recurrences or relapses. *Chronic suppressive therapy* is identical to secondary prophylaxis: This refers to regimens that are continued after the initial therapeutic course to prevent relapses.

All patients with HIV infection and CD4+ T lymphocyte counts below 200 cells/μL typically receive antipneumocystis prophylaxis. Trimethoprim-sulfamethoxazole is the regimen of choice. Patients who actually take this drug have very few breakthroughs of PCP and receive considerable protection against toxoplasmosis and certain routine bacterial infections. Alternative regimens include monthly dapsone, weekly dapsone-pyrimethamine, or daily aerosol pentamidine. Prophylaxis against *M. avium* complex is recommended for patients with CD4+ T lymphocyte counts under 100 cells/μL; clarithromycin and azithromycin are currently the drugs of choice.[9] Many clinicians also use fluconazole or acyclovir prophylaxis to reduce the frequency of fungal and viral processes, respectively, although this is not recommended because of issues of cost, pill burden, and the emergence of resistant pathogens. Isoniazid prophylaxis is important for any patient with a tuberculin skin test that shows more than 5 mm of induration or a history of substantial recent exposure.[9]

Transmission of HIV-Related Pathogens in the ICU

Transmission of tuberculosis from patients to other patients, from patients to staff, or from staff to patients is an urgent concern in ICUs. Patients with HIV infection are extraordinarily susceptible to tuberculosis. Thus an infected patient poses a substantial risk, especially when hospitalized for pneumonia or when undergoing procedures at high risk for producing aerosols such as intubation, bronchoscopy, sputum induction, or aerosol pentamidine treatment. Identifying potentially infected patients early and placing them in appropriate isolation until their tuberculosis status is fully examined is important. In many centers, patients with syndromes compatible with pulmonary or upper airway tuberculosis are maintained in isolation at least until three specimens of respiratory secretions have been examined for tuberculosis. HIV-infected health care practitioners need to carefully assess their risk of acquiring tuberculosis by their exposure in the ICU.

Transmission of HIV

Transmission of HIV is an issue that requires attention in the ICU.[65] No evidence exists that HIV-infected health care professionals can infect patients, regardless of what procedure they perform, outside of two unusual events. HIV patients pose a risk to health care professionals, however. This risk can be substantially reduced by education, by strict monitoring for compliance with universal precautions, and by having proper equipment. Almost all HIV transmission in an occupational setting occurs as a result of injuries involving sharp instruments (e.g., needles, scalpels). The risk of such injuries is about one case of HIV transmission per 250 injuries, but the likelihood of transmission in an individual accident depends on the amount of viremia at the time of the accident (late-stage patients generally have more circulating virus than do early-stage patients) and the nature of the accident. Most authorities recommend immediate prophylaxis if a significant injury occurs involving an HIV-infected patient. Considerable debate exists over the optimal choice of drugs and the optimal duration of therapy, but it is clear that initiating therapy within a period of hours rather than days is best. Many authorities now advocate a HAART regimen for any situation when the patient and health care provider determine that therapy is appropriate, and continue that for 4 to 6 weeks.

Human Stem Cell, Bone Marrow, and Solid Organ Transplant Recipients

Increasingly, ICUs are caring for organ transplant recipients, either in the period immediately after the procedure or during a crisis that occurs days, weeks, months, or years after engraftment. Managing each type of organ transplant recipient has unique features depending on whether bone marrow, kidney, heart, lungs, liver, or other organs are transplanted.[2,6] Laboratory monitoring provides useful predictive information about the status of cellular immunity, humoral immunity, and neutrophil number and function. Ultimately, however, clinical experience is necessary with each type of organ transplant and each immunosuppressive regimen to predict the most likely pathogens, when they most characteristically occur in relation to the transplant procedure, and what influence each immunosuppressive therapy has. An example of the temporal pattern of infectious complications after bone marrow transplantation is shown in Figure 54-3.[9] Although such figures are useful conceptually, however, the immunosuppressive regimens are changing rapidly, and such figures

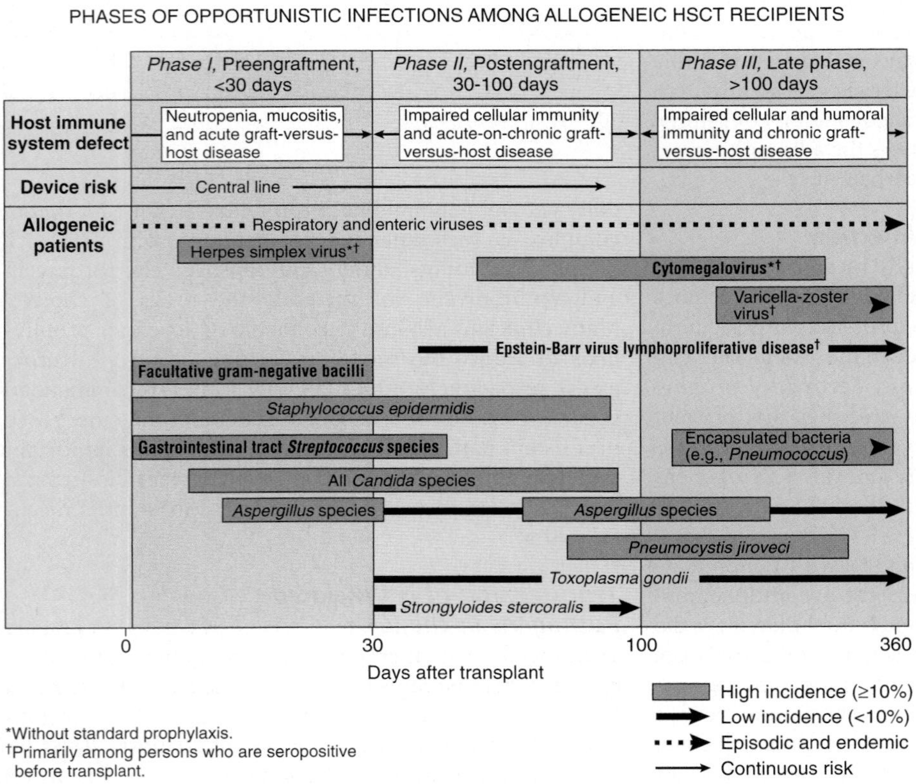

Figure 54-3. Usual sequence of infection after organ transplantation; precise period of susceptibility depends on organ transplanted, immunosuppressive regimen, and concomitant complications. (Adapted from Fishman JA, Rubin RH: Infection in organ-transplant recipients. Infection in organ-transplant recipients. N Engl J Med 1998;338:1741.)

may be misleading when applied to current transplantation protocols.

Organ transplant recipients share a complex interaction between immunosuppression and infection. Immunosuppression is usually necessary in allogeneic transplantation to permit graft survival. The more potent the immunosuppression, the more likely infection is to occur. Strategies that use antimicrobial agents (drugs, vaccines, and other biologic products) aggressively may reduce the risk of and damage from infection in a manner that allows more potent immunosuppression and better graft survival. Such approaches may include prophylactic antibacterial and antiretroviral treatment, as well as prompt empiric therapy for emerging febrile episodes.

Patients receiving hematopoietic stem cell transplantation (HSCT) or solid organ transplants are often receiving antimicrobial prophylaxis. Acyclovir for HSV, valacyclovir for CMV, fluconazole for yeast, voriconazole for yeast and molds, trimethoprim-sulfamethoxazole for PCP, and quinolones for bacteria are used in various combinations at different transplant programs. These agents dictate which organisms will break through to cause disease, and what their antibiotic susceptibility patterns will be.

Several pathogens deserve special mention. CMV is one of the most prominent pathogens for solid organ and bone marrow transplant recipients.[88-90] Most disease is secondary (i.e., disease results from reactivation of a previously acquired, latent infection) in a seropositive organ recipient. In urban areas of the United States, 60% to 70% of the population is seropositive for CMV, and thus 60% to 70% of the transplant recipients will have latent infection that could potentially be reactivated. Some CMV seronegative patients acquire primary infections from a CMV-infected organ or from CMV-infected blood or blood products. A few CMV seropositive individuals develop superimposed CMV disease from CMV acquired through a seropositive donor. Laboratory monitoring of patients for evidence of CMV disease by using a DNA amplification assay, or surveillance of CMV antigen in buffy coat smears, is an important feature in efforts to reduce morbidity and mortality resulting from CMV.[89,91-95] Intensivists need to understand how to interpret these assays in terms of starting empiric, pre-emptive, or definitive therapy. Strategies to reduce the frequency of CMV disease with acyclovir, intravenous or oral ganciclovir (or oral valganciclovir), the investigational agent proganciclovir, or immune globulin are used by many programs. CMV disease can cause substantial morbidity and mortality including fever, hypotension, pneumonitis, hepatitis, glomerulitis, enteritis, and allograft injury. The availability of ganciclovir, foscarnet, and cidofovir has enabled these conditions to be treated successfully in many instances, although all three of these drugs are associated with substantial toxicity. Whether immune globulin (either immune globulin or specific hyperimmune globulin) adds anything to the potency of therapeutic regimens is not clear, although these products are usually administered when they are available.

PCP has been reported in recipients of most types of organ transplants. Most organ transplant programs use PCP prophylaxis.[6,33,96] Trimethoprim-sulfamethoxazole is usually the prophylactic agent of choice because it is more effective than other agents, is well tolerated, and reduces the frequency of urinary tract infections and other potential complications (e.g., disease resulting from *Nocardia, S. pneumoniae,* and *Haemophilus* organisms).

Fungal infections have been common, but the causative pathogens are changing because of changes in prophylactic regimens. With the use of fluconazole, *Candida albicans* infections became less common. Molds, especially *Aspergillus,* became more important pathogens, as did fluconazole-resistant *Candida.* Some programs are now using voriconazole prophylaxis. For such patients, mucormycosis and *non-albicans Candida* are becoming more prominent causes of morbidity. Thus clinicians must know what antifungal prophylaxis has been used in order to anticipate which complications will occur. Mold infections can be difficult to diagnose: serum galactomannan assays can yield specific information, but the test has low sensitivity. Mold infections almost never cause fungemia. Thus diagnosis depends on cultures, which can be highly suggestive if obtained from sources such as bronchoalveolar lavage or biopsy.

Viral respiratory infections require particular mention because some are treatable and most are transmissible. Community-acquired respiratory viruses such as adenoviruses, coronaviruses, or influenza can occur in immunocompetent or immunosuppressed patients. When respiratory infections occur in immunocompromised patients, health care professionals need to be certain that a transmissible virus is not the cause because of the potential to infect other patients, families, or hospital staff. Of the respiratory infections, RSV deserves special attention in HSCT patients. Although RSV can, like other community-acquired viruses, cause disease in any patient population, it is especially lethal in solid organ, bone marrow, and stem cell transplants. Thus RSV must be specifically sought in this patient population, as well as their visitors and health care providers, so that it does not spread to highly susceptible patients.

Similarly, when caring for immunosuppressed patients, attention to *Mycobacterium tuberculosis* is important because this pathogen can also spread to other patients, families, and hospital staff. With more immigrants in the United States and more patients having travel exposure, *M. tuberculosis* needs to be considered in the differential diagnosis and specifically sought by gene probe, smear, or culture where appropriate.

Diagnosis and therapy of opportunistic infections and nosocomial infections should follow the guidelines given in Chapters 43, 51, and 54. In choosing therapies, attention must be focused on the toxicities of antimicrobial agents and how they influence the outcome of the transplanted organ. In addition, drug interactions are important, especially with cyclosporine. Drugs that alter hepatic metabolism, such as rifampin, rifabutin, and fluconazole, can have substantial influence on cyclosporine levels and thus need to be used with careful pharmacologic attention. Finally, clinicians must recognize that new immunosuppressive regimens and changing prophylactic regimens are changing the spectrum of infectious complications. As mentioned earlier, fungal infections are increasingly likely to be caused by species other than *C. albicans: non-albicans Candida, Fusarium,* and *Rhizopus* are recognized with increasing frequency. Similarly, prophylaxis with valganciclovir is reducing CMV disease and pushing disease that does occur later and later in relation to the transplant procedure. Viruses such as HHV-6 and BK virus are causing disease. Thus clinicians need to look for changing spectrum of pathogens, as well as changing manifestations if the morbidity and mortality caused by infection is to be managed optimally.

KEY POINTS

- Knowledge of a patient's specific defects in immunologic and inflammatory response helps predict which opportunistic pathogens are most likely to occur.
- ICUs are increasingly successful in enabling immunosuppressed patients to survive acute crises, especially if the defect in immunologic or inflammatory function is reversible over time or by replacement therapy.
- For neutropenic patients, gram-positive cocci are becoming more frequent than gram-negative bacilli as causes of life-threatening illness.
- Resistance to antimicrobial agents is becoming a major problem including bacteria (e.g., vancomycin-resistant enterococci and penicillin-resistant pneumococci), fungi (e.g., fluconazole-resistant *Candida* organisms), as well as PCP, and viruses (e.g., acyclovir-resistant herpes simplex and ganciclovir-resistant CMV).
- In neutropenic patients, combination therapy should be considered when treating any life-threatening bacterial process.
- A substantial fraction of HIV-infected patients with PCP-related respiratory failure can survive mechanical support and be discharged from the hospital.
- Adjunctive corticosteroid therapy is indicated for respiratory failure related to PCP.
- Tuberculosis is a concern in any immunologically abnormal individual with pulmonary disease but is a special concern in HIV-infected patients. Tuberculosis in these cases often warrants respiratory isolation until appropriate specimens are evaluated for mycobacteria.
- Organ transplant recipients develop opportunistic infections at relatively predictable points depending on the type of transplantation and the specific immunosuppressive regimen used.

REFERENCES

1. Dieffenbach CW, Tramont EC: Innate (general or nonspecific) host defense mechanisms. In Mandell GL, Bennett JE, Dolin R (eds): Principles and Practices of Infectious Diseases, 6th ed. Philadelphia, Elsevier Churchill Livingstone, 2005.
2. Dummer JS, Ho M: Infections in solid organ transplant recipients. In Mandell GL, Bennett CL, Dolin R (eds): Principles and Practice of Infectious Disease, 5th ed. Philadelphia, Elsevier Churchill Livingstone, 2005.
3. Figueroa JE, Densen P: Infectious diseases associated with complement deficiencies. Clin Microbiol Rev 1991;4:359-395.
4. Fishman JA, Rubin RH: Infection in organ-transplant recipients. N Engl J Med 1998;338:1741-1751.
5. Masur H, Ognibene FP, Yarchoan R, et al: CD4 counts as predictors of opportunistic pneumonias in human immunodeficiency virus (HIV) infection. Ann Intern Med 1989;111:223-231.
6. Tolkoff-Rubin NE, Rubin RH: Recent advances in the diagnosis and management of infection in the organ transplant recipient. Semin Nephrol 2000;20:148-163.
7. van Burik JA, Weisdorf D: Infections in recipients of hematopoietic stem cell transplantation. In Mandell GL, Bennett CL, Dolin R (eds): Principles and Practice of Infectious Disease, 5th ed. Philadelphia, Elsevier Churchill Livingstone, 2005.
8. Whimbey E, Kiehn TE, Brannon P, et al: Bacteremia and fungemia in patients with neoplastic disease. Am J Med 1987;82:723-730.
9. Guidelines for the Preventing Opportunistic Infections Among HIV-Infected Persons—2002 Recommendations of the U.S. Public Health Service and the Infectious Diseases Society of America. Available at hppt://www.aidsinfonih.gov
10. Hughes WT, Armstrong D, Bodey GP, et al: 2002 guidelines for the use of antimicrobial agents in neutropenic patients with cancer. Clin Infect Dis 2002;34:730-751.
11. Pizzo PA: Fever in immunocompromised patients. N Engl J Med 1999;341:893-900.
12. Orange JS, Hossny EM, Weiler CR, et al: Use of intravenous immunoglobulin in human disease: A review of evidence by members of the Primary Immunodeficiency Committee of the American Academy of Allergy, Asthma and Immunology. J Allergy Clin Immunol 2006;117(4 Suppl): S525-53.
13. Clark OA, Lyman GH, Castro AA, et al: Colony-stimulating factors for chemotherapy-induced febrile neutropenia: A meta-analysis of randomized controlled trials. J Clin Oncol 2005;23:4198-4214.
14. Kuritzkes DR: Neutropenia, neutrophil dysfunction, and bacterial infection in patients with human immunodeficiency virus disease: The role of granulocyte colony-stimulating factor. Clin Infect Dis 2000;30:256-260.
15. Smith TJ, Khatcheressian J, Lyman GH, et al: 2006 update of recommendations for the use of white blood cell growth factors: An evidence-based clinical practice guideline. J Clin Oncol 2006;24:3187-3205.
16. Cometta A, Calandra T, Gaya H, et al: Monotherapy with meropenem versus combination therapy with ceftazidime plus amikacin as empiric therapy for fever in granulocytopenic patients with cancer. The International Antimicrobial Therapy Cooperative Group of the European Organization for Research and Treatment of Cancer and the Gruppo Italiano Malattie Ematologiche Maligne dell'Adulto Infection Program. Antimicrob Agents Chemother 1996;40:1108-1115.
17. Freifeld A, Marchigiani D, Walsh T, et al: A double-blind comparison of empirical oral and intravenous antibiotic therapy for low-risk febrile patients with neutropenia during cancer chemotherapy. N Engl J Med 1999;341: 305-311.
18. Freifeld AG, Walsh T, Marshall D, et al: Monotherapy for fever and neutropenia in cancer patients: A randomized comparison of ceftazidime versus imipenem. J Clin Oncol 1995;13:165-176.
19. Jandula BM, Martino R, Gurgi M, et al: Treatment of febrile neutropenia with cefepime monotherapy. Chemotherapy 2001;47:226-231.
20. Paul M, Borok S, Fraser A, et al: Additional anti-Gram-positive antibiotic treatment for febrile neutropenic cancer patients. Cochrane Database Syst Rev 2005(3):CD003914.
21. Pizzo PA, Robichaud KJ, Wesley R, et al: Fever in the pediatric and young adult patient with cancer. A prospective study

of 1001 episodes. Medicine (Baltimore) 1982;61:153-165.
22. Rubin M, Hathorn JW, Marshall D, et al: Gram-positive infections and the use of vancomycin in 550 episodes of fever and neutropenia. Ann Intern Med 1988;108:30-35.
23. Sanders JW, Powe NR, Moore RD: Ceftazidime monotherapy for empiric treatment of febrile neutropenic patients: A meta-analysis. J Infect Dis 1991;164:907-916.
24. Wade JC, Schimpff SC, Newman KA, et al: Staphylococcus epidermidis: An increasing cause of infection in patients with granulocytopenia. Ann Intern Med 1982;97:503-508.
25. De Jongh CA, Joshi JH, Newman KA, et al: Antibiotic synergism and response in gram-negative bacteremia in granulocytopenic cancer patients. Am J Med 1986;80(5C):96-100.
26. Murray BE: Vancomycin-resistant enterococcal infections. N Engl J Med 2000;161:397.
27. Glasmacher A, von Lilienfeld-Toal M, Schulte S, et al: An evidence-based evaluation of important aspects of empirical antibiotic therapy in febrile neutropenic patients. Clin Microbiol Infect 2005;11(Suppl 5):17-23.
28. Betts R, Glasmacher A, Maertens J, et al: Efficacy of caspofungin against invasive *Candida* or invasive *Aspergillus* infections in neutropenic patients. Cancer 2006;106:466-473.
29. Klastersky J: Antifungal therapy in patients with fever and neutropenia—more rational and less empirical? N Engl J Med 2004;351:1445-1447.
30. Walsh TJ, Teppler H, Donowitz GR, et al: Caspofungin versus liposomal amphotericin B for empirical antifungal therapy in patients with persistent fever and neutropenia. N Engl J Med 2004;351:1391-1402.
31. Wingard JR, White MH, Anaissie E, et al: A randomized, double-blind comparative trial evaluating the safety of liposomal amphotericin B versus amphotericin B lipid complex in the empirical treatment of febrile neutropenia. L Amph/ABLC Collaborative Study Group. Clin Infect Dis 2000;31:1155-1163.
32. Bucaneve G, Micozzi A, Menichetti F, et al: Levofloxacin to prevent bacterial infection in patients with cancer and neutropenia. N Engl J Med 2005;353:977-987.
33. Centers for Disease Control and Prevention: Guidelines for Preventing Opportunistic Infections Among Hematopoietic Stem Cell Transplant Recipients. Recommendations of CDC, the Infectious Disease Society of America, and the American Society of Blood and Marrow Transplantation. MMWR 2000;49(RR10):1-128.
34. Marty FM, Cosimi LA, Baden LR: Breakthrough zygomycosis after voriconazole treatment in recipients of hematopoietic stem-cell transplants. N Engl J Med 2004;350:950-952.
35. Winston DJ, Ho WG, Bruckner DA, et al: Beta-lactam antibiotic therapy in febrile granulocytopenic patients. A randomized trial comparing cefoperazone plus piperacillin, ceftazidime plus piperacillin, and imipenem alone. Ann Intern Med 1991;115:849-859.
36. Kern WV: Risk assessment and risk-based therapeutic strategies in febrile neutropenia. Curr Opin Infect Dis 2001;14:415-422.
37. White MH, Bowden RA, Sandler ES, et al: Randomized, double-blind clinical trial of amphotericin B colloidal dispersion vs. amphotericin B in the empirical treatment of fever and neutropenia. Clin Infect Dis 1998;27:296-302.
38. Herbrecht R, Denning DW, Patterson TF, et al: Voriconazole versus amphotericin B for primary therapy of invasive aspergillosis. N Engl J Med 2002;347:408-415.
39. Vazquez JA: Review of treatment of zygomycosis with posaconazole in a patient with acute myeloid leukemia. Clin Adv Hematol Oncol 2005;3:777-778.
40. Boogaerts M, Winston DJ, Bow EJ, et al: Intravenous and oral itraconazole versus intravenous amphotericin B deoxycholate as empirical antifungal therapy for persistent fever in neutropenic patients with cancer who are receiving broad-spectrum antibacterial therapy. A randomized, controlled trial. Ann Intern Med 2001;135:412-422.
41. Vazquez JA: Anidulofungin: A new echinocandin with a novel profile. Clin Ther 2005;27:657-673.
42. Marr KA, Boeckh M, Carter RA, et al: Combination antifungal therapy for invasive aspergillosis. Clin Infect Dis 2004;39:797-802.
43. Munoz P, Singh N, Bouza E: Treatment of solid organ transplant patients with invasive fungal infections: should a combination of antifungal drugs be used? Curr Opin Infect Dis 2006;19:365-370.
44. Mermel LA: Prevention of intravascular catheter-related infections. Ann Intern Med 2000;132:391-402.
45. Mermel LA, Farr BM, Sherertz RJ, et al: Guidelines for the management of intravascular catheter-related infections. Clin Infect Dis 2001;32:1249-1272.
46. O'Grady NP, Alexander M, Dellinger EP, et al: Guidelines for the prevention of intravascular catheter-related infections. Centers for Disease Control and Prevention. MMWR Recomm Rep 2002;51(RR-10):1-29.
47. Aapro MS, Cameron DA, Pettengell R, et al: EORTC guidelines for the use of granulocyte-colony stimulating factor to reduce the incidence of chemotherapy-induced febrile neutropenia in adult patients with lymphomas and solid tumours. Eur J Cancer 2006;42:2433-2453.
48. Dale DC, Liles WC: Return of granulocyte transfusions. Curr Opin Pediatr 2000;12:18-22.
49. Kalil AC, Levitsky J, Lyden E, et al: Meta-analysis: The efficacy of strategies to prevent organ disease by cytomegalovirus in solid organ transplant recipients. Ann Intern Med 2005;143:870-880.
50. Huang L, Quartin A, Jones D, et al: Intensive care of patients with HIV infection. N Engl J Med 2006;355:173-181.
51. Morris A, Masur H, Huang L: Current issues in critical care of the human immunodeficiency virus-infected patient. Crit Care Med 2006;34:42-49.
52. Palella FJ Jr, Delaney KM, Moorman AC, et al: Declining morbidity and mortality among patients with advanced human immunodeficiency virus infection. HIV Outpatient Study Investigators. N Engl J Med 1998;338:853-860.
53. Rosen MJ, Narasimhan M: Critical care of immunocompromised patients: Human immunodeficiency virus. Crit Care Med 2006;34(9 Suppl):S245-S50.
54. McArthur JC: Neurologic manifestations of AIDS. Medicine (Baltimore) 1987;66:407-437.
55. Reilly JM, Cunnion RE, Anderson DW, et al: Frequency of myocarditis, left ventricular dysfunction and ventricular tachycardia in the acquired immune deficiency syndrome. Am J Cardiol 1988;62(10 Pt 1):789-793.
56. Suffredini AF, Ognibene FP, Lack EE, et al: Nonspecific interstitial pneumonitis: A common cause of pulmonary disease in the acquired immunodeficiency syndrome. Ann Intern Med 1987;107:7-13.
57. Ullrich R, Zeitz M, Heise W, et al: Small intestinal structure and function in patients infected with human immunodeficiency virus (HIV): Evidence for HIV-induced enteropathy. Ann Intern Med 1989;111:15-21.
58. Louache F, Vainchenker W: Thrombocytopenia in HIV infection. Curr Opin Hematol 1994;1:369-372.
59. Ratner L: Human immunodeficiency virus-associated autoimmune thrombocytopenic purpura: A review. Am J Med 1989;86:194-198.
60. Jones C, Hanson DL, Dworkin MS, et al: Surveillance for AIDS-defining opportunistic illnesses. MMWR 1999;48(SS2):1.
61. Kovacs JA, Masur H: Prophylaxis against opportunistic infections in patients with human immunodeficiency virus infection. N Engl J Med 2000;342:1416-1429.
62. Miller V, Mocroft A, Reiss P, et al: Relations among CD4 lymphocyte count nadir, antiretroviral therapy, and HIV-1 disease progression: Results from the EuroSIDA study. Ann Intern Med 1999;130:570-577.
63. Havlir DV, Barnes PF: Tuberculosis in patients with human immunodeficiency virus infection. N Engl J Med 1999;340:367-373.
64. Wheat LJ, Connolly-Stringfield PA, Baker RL, et al: Disseminated histoplasmosis in the acquired immune deficiency syndrome: Clinical findings, diagnosis and treatment, and review of the literature. Medicine (Baltimore) 1990;69:361-374.
65. Centers for Disease Control and Prevention: Updated U.S. Public Health Service Guidelines for the Management of Occupational Exposures to HIV and Recommendations for Postexposure Prophylaxis. MMWR 2005;54(RR09):1-17.
66. Piscitelli SC, Gallicano KD: Interactions among drugs for HIV and opportunistic infections. N Engl J Med 2001;344:984-996.

67. Piscitelli SC, Rodvold KA: Drug Interactions in Infectious Diseases, 5th ed. Totowa, NJ, Humana Press, 2005.
68. Barnes PF, Steele MA, Young SM, et al: Tuberculosis in patients with human immunodeficiency virus infection. How often does it mimic Pneumocystis carinii pneumonia? Chest 1992;102:428-432.
69. Kovacs JA, Ng VL, Masur H, et al: Diagnosis of *Pneumocystis carinii* pneumonia: Improved detection in sputum with use of monoclonal antibodies. N Engl J Med 1988;318:589-593.
70. Ognibene FP, Shelhamer J, Gill V, et al: The diagnosis of *Pneumocystis carinii* pneumonia in patients with the acquired immunodeficiency syndrome using subsegmental bronchoalveolar lavage. Am Rev Respir Dis 1984;129:929-932.
71. Zurlo JJ, O'Neill D, Polis MA, et al: Lack of clinical utility of cytomegalovirus blood and urine cultures in patients with HIV infection. Ann Intern Med 1993;118:12-17.
72. Treating Opportunistic Infections Among HIV-Infected Adults and Adolescents. Recommendations from CDC, the National Institutes of Health, and the HIV Medicine Association/Infectious Diseases Society of America, 2002. Available at http://www.aidsinfonih.gov
73. National Institute of Health-University of California Expert Panel for Corticosteroids as Adjunctive Therapy for Pneumocystis Pneumonia: Consensus statement on the use of corticosteroids as adjunctive therapy for *Pneumocystis* pneumonia in the acquired immunodeficiency syndrome. N Engl J Med 1990;323:1500.
74. Montaner JS, Lawson LM, Levitt N, et al: Corticosteroids prevent early deterioration in patients with moderately severe *Pneumocystis carinii* pneumonia and the acquired immunodeficiency syndrome (AIDS). Ann Intern Med 1990;113:14-20.
75. Gagnon S, Boota AM, Fischl MA, et al: Corticosteroids as adjunctive therapy for severe Pneumocystis carinii pneumonia in the acquired immunodeficiency syndrome. A double-blind, placebo-controlled trial. N Engl J Med 1990;323:1444-1450.
76. Bozzette SA, Sattler FR, Chiu J, et al: A controlled trial of early adjunctive treatment with corticosteroids for *Pneumocystis carinii* pneumonia in the acquired immunodeficiency syndrome. California Collaborative Treatment Group. N Engl J Med 1990;323:1451-1457.
77. Wachter RM, Russi MB, Bloch DA, et al: *Pneumocystis carinii* pneumonia and respiratory failure in AIDS. Improved outcomes and increased use of intensive care units. Am Rev Respir Dis 1991;143:251-256.
78. Wachter RM, Luce JM, Hopewell PC: Critical care of patients with AIDS. JAMA 1992;267:541-547.
79. el-Sadr W, Simberkoff MS: Survival and prognostic factors in severe *Pneumocystis carinii* pneumonia requiring mechanical ventilation. Am Rev Respir Dis 1988;137:1264-1267.
80. Efferen LS, Nadarajah D, Palat DS: Survival following mechanical ventilation for *Pneumocystis carinii* pneumonia in patients with the acquired immunodeficiency syndrome: A different perspective. Am J Med 1989;87:401-404.
81. Ratnam I, Chiu C, Kandala NB, et al: Incidence and risk factors for immune reconstitution inflammatory syndrome in an ethnically diverse HIV type 1-infected cohort. Clin Infect Dis 2006;42:418-427.
82. Robertson J, Meier M, Wall J, et al: Immune reconstitution syndrome in HIV: Validating a case definition and identifying clinical predictors in persons initiating antiretroviral therapy. Clin Infect Dis 2006;42:1639-1646.
83. Shelburne SA, Visnegarwala F, Darcourt J, et al: Incidence and risk factors for immune reconstitution inflammatory syndrome during highly active antiretroviral therapy. AIDS 2005;19:399-406.
84. Chuck SL, Sande MA: Infections with Cryptococcus neoformans in the acquired immunodeficiency syndrome. N Engl J Med 1989;321:794-799.
85. Cohn JA, McMeeking A, Cohen W, et al: Evaluation of the policy of empiric treatment of suspected Toxoplasma encephalitis in patients with the acquired immunodeficiency syndrome. Am J Med 1989;86:521-527.
86. Luft BJ, Hafner R, Korzun AH, et al: Toxoplasmic encephalitis in patients with the acquired immunodeficiency syndrome. Members of the ACTG 077p/ANRS 009 Study Team. N Engl J Med 1993;329:995-1000.
87. Luft BJ, Remington: Toxoplasmic encephalitis in AIDS. Clin Infect Dis 1992;15:211.
88. Hibberd PL, Tolkoff-Rubin NE, Conti D, et al: Preemptive ganciclovir therapy to prevent cytomegalovirus disease in cytomegalovirus antibody-positive renal transplant recipients. A randomized controlled trial. Ann Intern Med 1995;123:18-26.
89. Paya CV: Prevention of fungal and hepatitis virus infections in liver transplantation. Clin Infect Dis 2001;33(Suppl 1):S47-52.
90. Singh N: Antiviral drugs for cytomegalovirus in transplant recipients: advantages of preemptive therapy. Rev Med Virol 2006;16:281-287.
91. Gane E, Saliba F, Valdecasas GJ, et al: Randomised trial of efficacy and safety of oral ganciclovir in the prevention of cytomegalovirus disease in liver-transplant recipients. The Oral Ganciclovir International Transplantation Study Group [corrected]. Lancet 1997;350:1729-1733.
92. Garrigue I, Boucher S, Couzi L, et al: Whole blood real-time quantitative PCR for cytomegalovirus infection follow-up in transplant recipients. J Clin Virol 2006;36:72-75.
93. Khoury JA, Storch GA, Bohl DL, et al: Prophylactic versus preemptive oral valganciclovir for the management of cytomegalovirus infection in adult renal transplant recipients. Am J Transplant 2006;6:2134-2143.
94. Pescovitz MD: Benefits of cytomegalovirus prophylaxis in solid organ transplantation. Transplantation 2006;82(2 Suppl):S4-8.
95. Snydman DR: Posttransplant microbiological surveillance. Clin Infect Dis 2001;33(Suppl 1):S22-25.
96. Gordon SM, LaRosa SP, Kalmadi S, et al: Should prophylaxis for *Pneumocystis carinii* pneumonia in solid organ transplant recipients ever be discontinued? Clin Infect Dis 1999;28:240-246.

Chapter 55

Specific Infections with Critical Care Implications

Henry S. Fraimow and Annette C. Reboli

Infections and their complications, including severe sepsis and septic shock, are major indications for admission to critical care units worldwide. An enormous variety of infections can result in critical illness, and review of all of these syndromes is beyond the scope of this chapter. The diseases discussed here include the most common infectious syndromes likely to be encountered by critical care specialists, as well as less common infections of particular epidemiologic importance or those conditions in which critical care management is an essential component of management. The topics of community-acquired pneumonia, urinary tract infections, and nosocomial infections are addressed specifically in other chapters.

OVERWHELMING INFECTIONS OF THE CENTRAL NERVOUS SYSTEM

Most patients with serious central nervous system (CNS) infections will require either admission to an intensive care unit (ICU) or the participation of a critical care specialist in their management. This is because of the severity of these infections at the time of presentation, the need for rapid initiation of diagnostic and therapeutic interventions to optimize outcomes, and the potential for rapid progression of these infections with development of fulminant complications. The major acute CNS infectious syndromes include bacterial meningitis, encephalitis, brain abscess, and spinal epidural abscess, although other primary and secondary infectious syndromes can present catastrophically, such as nonbacterial infectious meningitis, suppurative intracranial thrombophlebitis, and mycotic aneurysms. The presentations of all of these infectious syndromes may overlap, and they may also mimic the presentations of noninfectious CNS catastrophes such as stroke or hemorrhage.

Acute Bacterial Meningitis

Epidemiology, Pathogenesis, Risk Factors, and Clinical Presentation

The annual incidence of bacterial meningitis in individuals older than 16 years of age in developed countries is estimated at 4 to 6 cases per 100,000.[1] In studies from the United States and the Netherlands, the predominant organisms in microbiologically confirmed cases of bacterial meningitis were *Streptococcus pneumoniae* (45% to 50%), *Neisseria meningitidis* (30%), and *Listeria monocytogenes* (5%),[2-4] with no pathogen identified in approximately 10% of cases.[1,2] In some studies, rates of culture-negative cases were as high as 25%.[5] Important recent changes in microbiologic etiology of bacterial meningitis reflect the impact of current vaccination strategies. These include the virtual elimination of *Haemophilus influenzae* meningitis in both children and adults and the recent introduction of the conjugated pediatric pneumococcal vaccine that has resulted in decreased rates of invasive childhood pneumococcal disease in children and adults.[6] A new meningococcal vaccine, which has the potential to diminish the rates of meningococcal disease in high risk populations, has also been approved for use in adolescents.[7] Another important trend is the increase in prevalence of nosocomial meningitis.[4] The microbiology of nosocomial meningitis differs from that of community acquired cases, including higher rates of staphylococcal infection and infection due to a variety of aerobic gram negative organisms.

The major route of acquisition of bacterial meningitis follows colonization of the nasopharynx with subsequent hematogenous spread and invasion of cerebrospinal fluid. Less frequently, infection occurs from hematogenous dissemination from distant sites, from other localized intracranial focal infections including sinusitis, mastoiditis, or otitis or is secondary to trauma or neurosurgery. In addition to trauma and contiguous focal infectious processes facilitating invasion of the cerebrospinal fluid (CSF) by bacteria, there are a wide variety of immunologic deficits that result in impaired clearance of encapsulated organisms. These include organism-specific deficits such as terminal complement deficiencies predisposing to meningococcal disease,[7] as well as more general deficits such as immunoglobulin deficiencies, splenectomy, alcoholism, cirrhosis, diabetes mellitus, and human immunodeficiency virus.[2,4] Patients with defects leading to impaired cell-mediated immunity including advanced age and general debility, as well as hematologic malignancies, chemotherapy, and use of tumor necrosis factor (TNF)-α inhibitors, are predisposed to *Listeria* infection.[8]

The presenting symptoms of bacterial meningitis include fever, headache, stiff neck, and altered sensorium. In the recent large series of 696 cases from the Netherlands, 95% had at least two of these four symptoms, although only 44% had all of the classic triad of headache, fever, and stiff neck.[2] Other important presenting symptoms in this cohort included nausea in 74%, focal neurologic deficits in one third of cases, and Glasgow Coma Score of less than 8 in 14% of cases.[2] Rash, especially a petechial or purpural rash that may be an important clue for the diagnosis of meningococcal meningitis, was seen in 26% in this study.[2] The presenting symptoms alone without CSF findings and microbiologic data cannot adequately distinguish between bacterial meningitis and viral or other aseptic meningitis. However, certain features are more suggestive of bacterial rather than viral origin including winter versus summer onset, rapid progression of disease, presentation in shock, and presence of another focal site of bacterial infection such as sinusitis, otitis, or pneumonia. In addition to viruses, other infections including cryptococcosis, tuberculous meningitis, rickettsial diseases, Lyme disease, and syphilis are differential diagnoses of bacterial meningitis.

Diagnostic Strategies and Early Management of Suspected Bacterial Meningitis

The early management of suspected bacterial meningitis requires careful coordination and appropriate sequencing of the procedures necessary for appropriate diagnosis (lumbar puncture and imaging studies) and the interventions necessary for optimal treatment (antibiotics and dexamethasone). Rapid initiation of therapy leads to improved outcomes but may decrease specific microbiologic yield on CSF analysis.[1,5] Similarly, although lumbar puncture can usually be performed safely without any imaging studies, computed tomography (CT) scan may be required to minimize the risk of this procedure, leading to potential delays in institution of antimicrobial therapy.[9] Several recent articles have tried to place these competing urgencies in perspective, using data culled from multiple recent prospective studies and randomized trials.[1,5] One such algorithm for early management of bacterial meningitis is shown in Figure 55-1.

The primary tenet of these algorithms is that the initiation of treatment assumes highest priority and that any delay in performing a lumbar puncture because of the need for imaging before the procedure or because of other patient-specific contraindications should not delay the administration of antibiotic therapy. Brain herniation has been a feared but rare complication of lumbar puncture when performed for diagnosis of suspected meningitis in patients with elevated intracranial pressure.[10] One recent study of a cohort of 301 patients with suspected bacterial meningitis described the relative safety of lumbar puncture without CT scanning in patients without specific clinical contraindications.[9] Criteria for performing imaging prior to lumbar puncture have been proposed and include new-onset seizures, prior CNS disease, immunocompromised state, papilledema, focal neurologic deficits, or moderate to severe impairment of consciousness.[5] Only approximately 45% of patients with bacterial meningitis will have criteria for neuroimaging prior to lumbar puncture, although it is standard practice in many hospitals for all patients with suspected meningitis to undergo imaging first.[1,5] The main purpose of early imaging is to find evidence of brain shift; both noncontrast CT and magnetic resonance imaging (MRI) can be used for this purpose. Considerations for the optimal imaging modality may be different when imaging tests are done to manage subsequent complications of meningitis or to better define space-occupying lesions. Other specific contraindications to lumbar puncture include coagulopathies and presence of local disease such as stasis ulcers, burns, or cellulitis overlying the lumbar puncture site.

The diagnosis of bacterial meningitis relies heavily on analysis of CSF including opening pressure, cell count, protein, glucose and gram stain, and culture. Typically, patients with bacterial meningitis have elevated opening pressures of 200 to 500 mm H_2O, including 40% with opening pressure greater than 400 mm in one recent

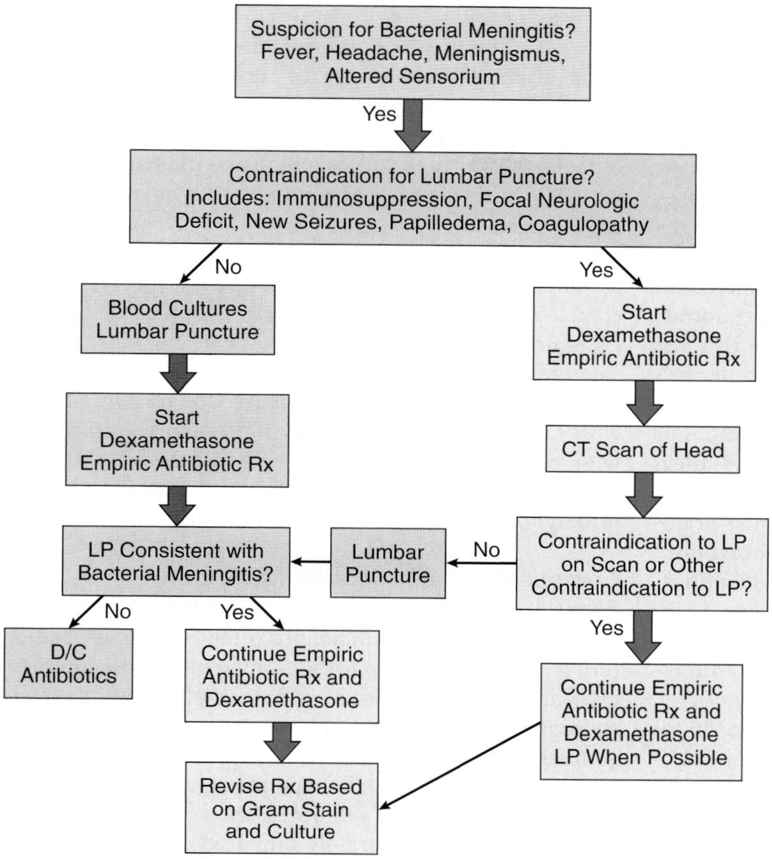

Figure 55-1. Algorithm for early management of suspected bacterial meningitis including when to suspect the diagnosis, determining when imaging should be performed prior to lumbar puncture (LP), and when to initiate or discontinue empiric antibacterial therapy and adjuvant steroids. (Modified with permission from van de Beek D, de Gans J, Tunkel AR, et al: Community-acquired bacterial meningitis in adults. N Engl J Med 2006;354:44-53; and Tunkel AR, Hartman BJ, Kaplan SL, et al: Practice guidelines for the management of bacterial meningitis. Clin Infect Dis 2004;39: 1267-1284.)

cohort.[2,5] White blood cell (WBC) counts may range from 100 to 10,000 cells/mm^3, with most counts in the 1000 to 5000 range; very low CSF WBCs are associated with a worse prognosis.[4,5] Usually a polymorphonuclear (PMN) cell predominance of 80% or greater exists, although up to 10% will have a lymphocytic predominance, particularly early on. CSF-to-serum glucose ratios are less than 0.4, and CSF protein levels are nearly always increased.[5] In studies comparing cohorts of patients with bacterial and viral meningitis, CSF glucose ratios of less than 0.31, total WBC of greater than 2000, and total PMN of greater than 1180 have been predictive of bacterial rather than viral etiology.[11] Gram stains are positive in 60% to 90% of cases of bacterial meningitis, and results on Gram stain are reported to be 97% specific as to etiology.[5] Yield of Gram stain is higher on specimens concentrated by Cytospin. Highest diagnostic yield from Gram staining is for *S. pneumoniae* meningitis; Gram stains in *Listeria* meningitis may reveal organisms in only one third of cases because of the lower inoculum of bacteria in the CSF. However, clinicians should be aware that preliminary "stat" Gram stains done during off-hours are more likely to be misread; thus stains should always be reviewed by trained clinical microbiologists. In untreated patients, cultures will ultimately be positive in up to 90% of cases. Initiation of antibiotic therapy prior to lumbar puncture will not significantly alter cell count, protein, glucose and even Gram stain results but will decrease CSF culture yield by up to 20%.[5] Blood cultures should be performed in all patients with suspected bacterial meningitis, and should be done prior to initiation of antibiotics, even if the lumbar puncture is delayed.

Additional CSF and blood tests have been used to confirm a diagnosis of bacterial meningitis or help distinguish bacterial from viral disease. Latex agglutination tests for bacterial antigens, although initially reported to have good sensitivity and specificity for diagnosis of specific bacterial meningitis pathogens, have more recently been shown to contribute little to the management of most patients with suspected meningitis.[5] Polymerase chain reaction (PCR) of CSF for bacterial deoxyribonucleic acid (DNA) may be useful to confirm an etiologic diagnosis in culture-negative cases but is not routinely available in most hospitals. An elevated CSF lactate of greater than 4.2 mmol/dL is reported to be a sensitive marker for bacterial meningitis, but specificity has been questioned.[12] Elevated serum C-reactive protein (CRP) levels are not specific for bacterial meningitis, but a low CRP has good negative predictive value for bacterial meningitis in patients with abnormal CSF and negative CSF Gram stains.[5] Serum procalcitonin may also prove useful for diagnosis. Additional CSF studies may be useful for diagnosis of other specific infections such as CSF cryptococcal antigen and Venereal Disease Research Laboratory (VDRL) slide test.

Initial antibiotic therapy for suspected bacterial meningitis is most commonly initiated in the absence of culture and even Gram stain data. Initial empiric therapy must include agents active against the most likely pathogens based on the patient's age and underlying illnesses and modified for other specific risk factors such as nosocomial acquisition (Table 55-1). Treatment regimens must take into account local rates of antimicrobial resistance, particularly rates of high-level resistance to penicillin and third-generation cephalosporins in *S. pneumoniae*. Standard regimens include vancomycin administered at doses targeted to achieve adequate CSF levels (serum troughs of 15 to 20 μg/mL) and a third-generation cephalosporin, either ceftriaxone or cefotaxime. In areas with increased rates of resistance to third-generation cephalosporins, rifampin is sometimes added. When there is risk for *Listeria* infection based on age or on other specific risk factors such as alcoholism or altered immunity, high-dose ampicillin is included in the treatment regimen. For patients with nosocomial or postprocedural-related infections, cefotaxime or ceftriaxone may be changed to an agent with improved activity against nosocomial gram-negative organisms including *Pseudomonas aeruginosa*. Antibiotic therapy is modified on the basis of identification and susceptibility data of isolated pathogens. Standard recommended treatment durations are 7 days for meningococcal disease and *H. influenzae*, 10 to 14 days for *S. pneumoniae*, and 21 or more days for *Listeria*.[1,5]

Several recent studies have confirmed the benefits of adjuvant dexamethasone in decreasing mortality and neurologic sequelae in patients with bacterial meningitis.[13,14] In one large, randomized, placebo-controlled trial of 301 adults with suspected bacterial meningitis and cloudy CSF, adjuvant dexamethasone decreased mortality from 15% to 7% and decreased unfavorable outcomes from 25% to 15%.[13] Benefits of corticosteroids were most evident in those with pneumococcal infection and those with a moderately impaired level of consciousness; patients with meningococcal disease had generally better outcomes with or without corticosteroids. The optimal steroid regimen based on published and animal studies appears to be 10 mg of dexamethasone every 6 hours for 4 days and initiated prior to or concurrent with the first dose of antibiotics.[1,5] If steroids are not initiated at the onset of antibiotic therapy, it is unknown at what point initiation of steroids will cease to be beneficial. It is also unknown from the available data whether the net effect of high-dose corticosteroids will prove to be beneficial or harmful in the subset of patients with meningitis and septic shock.

Patients with suspected or confirmed meningococcal meningitis should be placed in isolation to prevent nosocomial transmission via respiratory droplets for the first 24 hours of therapy. Meningococcal prophylaxis is indicated for household and other close contacts of meningococcal cases including first responders. Conversely, patients with Gram stains and clinical presentations consistent with nonmeningococcal disease should also be quickly identified, to eliminate unnecessary use of meningococcal prophylaxis.

Complications of Bacterial Meningitis, Need for ICU Monitoring, and Outcome

Patients with bacterial meningitis often require ICU monitoring either for complications evident at the time of presentation or for observation for complications that may subsequently develop during their course. Criteria for admission to an ICU have been proposed (Table 55-2).[1] These include sepsis and septic shock, respiratory compromise or pulmonary infiltrates, those with high risk of brain herniation, moderately impaired and deteriorating level of consciousness, new or evolving neurologic deficits, and presence of seizures. Some authorities feel that all patients with bacterial meningitis may benefit from intensive monitoring early on for presence of new neurologic signs or subtle seizures and for effective control of agitation.[15] Patients with generally good outcomes can be defined early in their course on the basis of age, Glasgow Coma Score, APACHE II score, absence of focal neurologic abnormalities, and favorable laboratory features, but

Table 55-1. Treatment of Bacterial Meningitis in Adults (Older Than 15 yr)

Host	Most Likely Pathogens	Empiric Antibiotic Therapy	Comments
Age 15 to 50 yr No risk factors*	*Streptococcus pneumoniae, Neisseria meningitidis*	Vancomycin + third-generation cephalosporin†	Adjuvant dexamethasone§
Age 15 to 50 yr plus risk factors*	*S. pneumoniae, N. meningitidis, Listeria monocytogenes, Haemophilus influenzae*	Vancomycin + third-generation cephalosporin† + ampicillin	Adjuvant dexamethasone§
Age older than 50 yr +/− risk factors	*S. pneumoniae, N. meningitidis, L. monocytogenes,* aerobic gram-negative rods	Vancomycin + third-generation cephalosporin† + ampicillin	Adjuvant dexamethasone§
Trauma, postneurosurgical or other nosocomial	*Staphylococcus aureus,* coagulase-negative staphylococci, aerobic gram-negative rods	Vancomycin + *Pseudomonas* active agent‡	Dexamethasone?¶ Consider rifampin for staphylococci

*Risk factors: altered immunity including HIV infection and alcoholism.
†Third-generation cephalosporin: ceftriaxone or cefotaxime; for highly penicillin allergic, alternatives would be aztreonam or a fluoroquinolone.
‡Includes cefepime or ceftazidime, alternatives include aztreonam, meropenem, or ciprofloxacin.
§Consider rifampin if high rates of cephalosporin resistance if dexamethasone is used.
¶Not indicated for post-trauma or shunt-associated meningitis; data for other indications limited.
Modified with permission from van de Beek D, de Gans J, Tunkel AR, et al: Community-acquired bacterial meningitis in adults. N Engl J Med 2006;354:44-53; and Tunkel AR, Hartman BJ, Kaplan SL, et al: Practice guidelines for the management of bacterial meningitis. Clin Infect Dis 2004;39:1267-1284.

Table 55-2. Indications for Intensive Care Monitoring and Management for Bacterial Meningitis

Indication	ICU Management
Sepsis and shock	Hemodynamic support and monitoring, early goal-directed therapy, low-dose corticosteroids
Pulmonary infiltrates or respiratory compromise	Airway management, monitoring of oxygenation, noninvasive or invasive ventilatory support
Glasgow Coma Score <10	Monitoring of examination; monitor for development of increased ICP, hydrocephalus, and seizures
Deteriorating level of consciousness	Monitoring of examination; monitor for development of increased ICP, hydrocephalus, and seizures
New or evolving neurologic deficits	Monitoring of examination; monitor for development of increased ICP, hydrocephalus, and seizures
Evidence of increased ICP	Consider intracranial pressure monitoring; osmotic diuretics
Acute hydrocephalus	Repeated lumbar puncture, lumbar drain, or ventriculostomy
Seizures	Continuous EEG monitoring, antiepileptic agents
Severe agitation	Careful sedation

EEG, electroencephalogram; ICP, intracranial pressure; ICU, intensive care unit.
Modified with permission from van de Beek D, de Gans J, Tunkel AR, et al: Community-acquired bacterial meningitis in adults. N Engl J Med 2006;354:44-53.

these stratification schemes will still fail to identify some patients with more complicated courses.[2,16]

Major complications that occur during the course of bacterial meningitis have been summarized by van de Beek and colleagues[1,2] for cohorts of patients not receiving adjunctive dexamethasone. These include deteriorating level of consciousness, which may be caused by development of meningoencephalitis (15% to 20% of cases), seizures (15% to 23%), brain edema (6% to 10%), or hydrocephalus (3% to 8%). Mannitol, hyperventilation, repeated lumbar taps, prophylactic lumbar drainage, prophylactic ventriculostomy, and other modalities have all been proposed for management of increasing intracranial pressure. Increased pressure is associated with worse prognosis, but no single approach for treatment has been confirmed to be effective in all cases.[1,17] Patients with severely increased pressure with impending herniation may require ventriculostomy with continuous CSF pressure monitoring. All patients should be monitored for seizures including nonfocal seizures that may only manifest as worsening level of consciousness, but routine use of prophylactic antiepileptic medication is not currently recommended.[1,5] Focal neurologic deficits early in the course of meningitis are most often caused by cerebrovascular complications or arteritis secondary to inflammation or less commonly to venous infarcts. The most common late neurologic complication is hearing loss, described in up to 20% of patients overall and in up to 34% of those with pneumococcal meningitis.[1,2] The incidence of hearing loss appears to be significantly decreased in dexamethasone-treated patients.[8,9] Subdural empyema, brain abscess, and hemorrhage are all rare but potentially catastrophic complications of bacterial meningitis.

Repeat lumbar punctures are no longer routinely performed in patients with bacterial meningitis who are improving but are indicated in patients with worsening or suboptimal clinical response at 48 hours.[5] Repeat CSF analysis is also indicated in patients with more resistant organisms such as highly cephalosporin-resistant *S. pneumoniae*, especially when they have been treated with dexamethasone, because steroids may decrease antibiotic penetration into the CSF and delay sterilization.[18] Repeat imaging by MRI or enhanced CT scan should be performed in patients with clinical deterioration or persistent decreased level of consciousness to assess for the complications listed earlier. Overall mortality rates for bacterial meningitis without the use of steroids are reported to be approximately 20%, and an additional 14% will have moderate or major neurologic sequelae.[1] Prognosis for meningococcal meningitis is better than for pneumococcal infection. Late neuropsychiatric cognitive effects are seen in up to 10% of cases of bacterial meningitis.

Encephalitis

The other major CNS infectious syndrome besides bacterial meningitis that may present with fever, headache, altered sensorium, and meningeal signs is acute encephalitis, which is most commonly of viral etiology. Although there is significant overlap between clinical presentations of patients with bacterial meningitis and viral encephalitis, the presentation of viral encephalitis is dominated by evidence of parenchymal brain dysfunction including moderate to severely impaired sensorium, delirium, psychosis, focal neurologic findings, and seizures.[19,20] The presence of meningismus is more variable, but most patients will have some evidence of meningeal enhancement on imaging and inflammatory cells in CSF.

A large number of viruses can cause encephalitis, but management strategies focus on the most common etiologies and those most likely to respond to specific interventions, particularly encephalitis caused by herpes simplex virus (HSV).[20-22] Other important etiologies with worldwide distribution include other herpes group viruses including varicella-zoster virus; Epstein-Barr virus; and cytomegalovirus (CMV), especially in immunocompromised patients.[19,20,21] Influenza virus, mumps, measles, and enteroviruses are also important etiologies of acute viral encephalitis worldwide. Acute HIV infection can also occasionally present as fulminant meningoencephalitis.[21] Acute presentations of progressive multifocal leukoencephaly caused by JC virus are also increasingly reported in HIV-infected and other immunocompromised patients.[23] In addition to viruses seen worldwide, a large variety of vector-borne viruses have regional and seasonal distributions.[19,21] Important pathogens include Eastern, Western, and Venezuela equine encephalitis; Japanese B encephalitis; St. Louis encephalitis; La Crosse encephalitis; and Nipah encephalomyelitis. Recently, West Nile encephalitis emerged as a major pathogen in the United States, first appearing in New York City in 1999 but with cases now distributed throughout the country.[24,25] Rabies, although extremely rare in developed countries, also needs to be considered in the differential diagnosis of fulminant encephalitis, both for its epidemiologic implications and for the potential of survival for patients with this previously universally fatal infection with aggressive ICU management.[26] In addition to viral infections, many atypical bacteria, fungi, and protozoal organisms can present as acute meningoencephalitis. Particularly important to consider early in the differential diagnosis are infections that may respond to specific treatment including rickettsial diseases like Rocky Mountain spotted fever and meningoencephalitis from spirochetal infections including neurosyphilis and Lyme disease.[27,28] Important clues to these diseases include epidemiologic history and associated clinical features such as rash. Data from the California Encephalitis Project, in which cases of suspected infectious encephalitis underwent an aggressive evaluation for a variety of infectious agents, suggest that the etiology of at least 50% to 60% of cases of presumed infectious encephalitis remains undefined.[29]

Herpes simplex encephalitis is the most common sporadic cause of serious viral meningoencephalitis, causing 3% to 10% of cases of infectious encephalitis in adults and with an estimated frequency of about 1000 to 2000 cases per year in the United States.[21,22,29] Ninety percent of cases are caused by HSV type 1, usually occurring in adults as reactivation disease and not primary infection; HSV type 2 commonly causes aseptic meningitis but much less commonly presents as fulminant encephalitis.[22,30] Herpes encephalitis is an acute necrotizing process, typically causing hemorrhagic necrosis with particular predilection for the fronto-temporal lobes and cingulated gyrus. Mortality rates are up to 70% in untreated cases, with 95% of those surviving having serious neurologic sequelae.[21,22] Cases of herpes encephalitis beyond the neonatal period occur throughout life, but the highest case rates occur in younger individuals (younger than 20 years old) and in adults older than age 50 (half of cases). Presentation may include a prodromal viral syndrome in 50% of cases, followed by a generally rapid onset of headache, confusion, and altered level of consciousness. Meningismus, focal neurologic findings, and seizures are also common.[20-22] In one series of patients with encephalitis, of which 37% were caused by HSV, focal CNS disease was much more likely than diffuse CNS disease to be caused by HSV.[31] The approach to cases of suspected herpes encephalitis, as well as other viral or unknown encephalitis, includes early initiation of antiviral therapy and concurrent rapid clinical evaluation that includes imaging, CSF studies, and electroencephalogram (EEG) to establish a diagnosis.[20,22] CT scans can remain normal up to 4 to 5 days into the course, thus MRI is considered the imaging modality of choice. MRI is positive in more than 90% of cases, often showing changes of edema and necrosis in the medial temporal lobes, insular cortex, and cingulate gyrus as soon as 2 to 3 days into the illness.[32] EEGs will be abnormal in nearly all cases, but early findings are nonspecific and the characteristic periodic lateralizing epileptiform discharges are often not seen until later in the course.[22] CSF findings include low- to moderate-grade lymphocytic pleocytosis in 85% and elevated protein in 80%; elevated red blood count and mildly decreased glucose are common but not universal, and cell counts may be completely normal in 8%.[22,30] The International Herpes Management Forum has issued guidelines for confirmation of the diagnosis and for treatment.[22] PCR of CSF for HSV DNA has replaced brain biopsy as the diagnostic method of choice for HSV encephalitis. Based on data from two trials comparing PCR with the gold standard of brain biopsy, sensitivity of PCR was 98% and specificity was 94% for diagnosing HSV encephalitis; the negative predictive value of PCR on CSF obtained more than 72 hours into the course of illness was close to 100% for excluding HSV.[22,33,34] PCR has also expanded understanding of the range of clinical presentations of HSV encephalitis including recognition of less severe cases.[31] Viral culture has low sensitivity for diagnosis in older children and adults and is not recommended, and CSF and serum antibody studies have little role in the diagnosis.[22] Treatment should be initiated on the basis of clinical suspicion pending PCR results using high-dose intravenous (IV) acyclovir at doses of 10 mg/kg every 8 hours and continued for 14 to 21 days, or until PCR results are available or an alternative diagnosis is established. Duration of therapy may be guided in part by repeating CSF PCR at the end of treatment because some experts recommend continuing acyclovir if PCR is still positive.[35]

West Nile Virus Encephalitis

In the 7 years since it first appeared in the Western hemisphere, West Nile virus (WNV) has become a major infectious cause of invasive neurologic disease throughout the United States, with more than 1000 cases from 42 states reported in 2005.[24,36] WNV is a mosquito-borne arbovirus affecting birds, mammals, and humans. Of human cases, 80% are asymptomatic and most of the remainder have West Nile fever, but 1% will develop neuroinvasive disease manifesting as meningitis, encephalitis, and/or a polio-like flaccid paralysis syndrome.[24,25] Risk of encephalitis increases with age or with immunosuppression, particularly organ transplantation, and manifestations can range from mild disorientation to coma and death.[24] Parkinson-like tremors are also commonly reported. The flaccid paralysis syndrome, because of viral infection of anterior horn cells, may have abrupt onset and patients may require prolonged ventilatory support. The fatality rate is 9% for WNV neuroinvasive syndromes, and survivors may have prolonged symptoms. In some patients, flaccid paralysis has not resolved after 1 to 2 years.[24] CSF findings of WNV are similar to those of other viral infections with lymphocytic pleocytosis predominating. Neuroimaging may be normal, but some scans may demonstrate abnormal signal in the basal ganglia, thalamus, and other deep brain structures or abnormal signal in anterior horn cells of the spinal cord.[25,37] Diagnosis is confirmed by the finding of WNV-specific IgM antibodies in CSF and serum or by nucleic acid–based PCR of CSF, serum, or other fluids.[24] Treatment is primarily supportive; multiple interventions including ribavirin, interferon-alpha, immunoglobulin, and others have been tried, but there are currently no good outcome data.

Brain Abscess

Brain abscesses are focal infections of brain parenchyma, occurring from direct spread from local, contiguous infection (ear, sinuses, mastoid, bacterial meningitis); from hematogenous spread of infecting organisms from distant sites; or by direct inoculation from trauma or surgery.[38,39] Modern imaging modalities have improved the initial management and follow-up care of patients with brain abscess, but it is not clear that this has significantly affected overall outcome. Presenting symptoms may be indistinguishable from that of other CNS infections, with fever, headache, and focal neurologic findings predominating.[38-40] Seizures and decreased level of consciousness are also seen. Sepsis was noted in 18% of cases in one recent series.[41] Duration of symptoms prior to presentation is typically much longer than that of bacterial meningitis or viral encephalitis. Microbiology reflects the source of the original infection and most commonly includes streptococci, staphylococci, oral anaerobes, and enteric gram-negative organisms, but multiple other bacterial, fungal, tuberculous, and atypical organisms can also be found.[38-40] In areas of high HIV prevalence, opportunistic brain infections, especially toxoplasmosis, have become more prevalent than typical pyogenic abscesses, and knowledge of HIV status is crucial to initial management of suspected infectious mass lesions.[42]

The diagnosis of brain abscess is suggested by the clinical presentation and imaging findings by either CT or MRI showing enhancing parenchymal lesions usually with surrounding inflammatory changes.[38,39] Radiographic appearance may be indistinguishable from a malignant lesion. Management of suspected abscess includes either stereotactic aspiration or surgical drainage to both establish a microbiologic diagnosis and for primary treatment of the abscess. Smaller lesions (<1 cm) can be treated with antibiotics alone, but larger lesions will require either aspiration or open drainage.[38,39] Several studies suggest that aspiration may result in less residual neurologic deficit than surgical resection.[43] Duration of treatment is until resolution of the abscess on serial imaging studies. Unlike bacterial brain abscesses, toxoplasmosis lesions in patients with AIDS are usually multiple and may respond to empiric toxoplasmosis therapy without need for further invasive diagnostic procedures.[42]

Spinal Epidural Abscess

Spinal epidural infections most commonly arise by contiguous spread of infection into the spinal canal as a complication of vertebral infections or, less commonly, as a complication of epidural procedures such as epidural injections or epidural catheterization.[44-46] Vertebral infections result from hematogenous infection of vertebral bodies or disc space or by direct introduction of organisms from surgery or trauma. In addition to affecting the vertebral bodies and/or intervertebral disc spaces, vertebral osteomyelitis may expand into surrounding paravertebral soft tissues and spinal canal and even on rare occasions into the medullary spinal cord. Paravertebral and epidural infections can rapidly progress, resulting in severe neurologic symptoms from compression of nerve roots or the spinal cord, or by infarction of the spinal cord from inflammation and vasculitis of vertebral arteries.[45,47] Thus an aggressive diagnostic and therapeutic approach is necessary to prevent catastrophic consequences such as irreversible paraplegia and death.

The incidence of spinal epidural infection from large retrospective reviews is reported as approximately 0.2 to 2 cases per 10,000 hospital admissions, but the frequency of this diagnosis may be increasing, perhaps because of improvements in radiographic diagnosis.[45] Incidence in adults increases with age older than 30 years; important predisposing factors include diabetes, injection drug use, alcoholism, immunosuppression, underlying spinal disorders, trauma, invasive procedures, and extraspinal sites of infection that cause significant bacteremia.[45,46] Infections can occur at any level of the spinal cord, although most series report predominance of lumbar involvement. Approximately two thirds of infections are caused by *Staphylococcus aureus,* with a variety of other gram-positive organisms (coagulase-negative staphylococci, *viridans* streptococci, beta-hemolytic streptococci), as well as gram-negative organisms all reported in lesser numbers.[44-46] Granulomatous infections including tuberculosis and brucellosis remain major etiologies of vertebral and epidural infection in many areas of the world.[47] Approximately 10% are culture-negative.[45]

Presenting symptoms are back pain in more than 95% of cases and fever in two thirds of cases; unfortunately these symptoms are extremely nonspecific.[44,45] Thirty percent of cases will present with evidence of early neurologic deficits such as muscle weakness, incontinence, or sensory deficits, and up to one third will have evidence of paralysis on examination.[44-46] Associated laboratory features include leukocytosis in two thirds of cases and elevated ESR in nearly all cases. The most sensitive imaging modality is MRI with gadolinium, with reported sensitivity of greater than 95%, but most infections were also visualized on CT and unenhanced MR.[44,45] Until recently, standard therapy included emergent drainage of the abscess and systemic antibiotic therapy. Over the past 2 decades there has been an emerging literature on more conservative medical management employing percutaneous aspiration and antibiotics without open surgical drainage.[44-46] These reports have suggested that outcomes are similar or better (i.e., less neurologic sequelae) without open surgery.[44] No trials have directly compared treatment modalities, and retrospective analyses do not clearly identify risk factors for worse outcomes with medical therapy alone. Indications for surgery include neurologic progression on treatment or lack of clinical response, thus those managed without surgery require careful monitoring.[44,45] Surgery may also be the preferred treatment for those with more severe neurologic deficits on initial presentation.[44,45]

FULMINANT ENDOVASCULAR INFECTIONS

Infectious endocarditis and other endovascular infections are common causes of bacteremia and sepsis, and these patients are frequently admitted to critical care units for management of sepsis and other complications. Often, the diagnosis of endovascular infection is unsuspected and initiation of appropriate treatment is delayed. Even relatively stable patients with bacterial endocarditis, especially left-sided endocarditis, require careful monitoring and management of potential major complications including heart failure, other cardiac events, and septic emboli. The role of early surgical intervention in improving outcome has become increasingly appreciated in the management of complicated bacterial endocarditis, especially *S. aureus* endocarditis.

Acute Infective Endocarditis

Several recently published large case series have addressed changes in the epidemiology of bacterial endocarditis over the past 2 decades.[48,49] The annual incidence of endocarditis of 5 to 7 cases/100,000 has not changed significantly over time.[48] However, the International Collaboration on Endocarditis Prospective Cohort Study, a multicenter study of 1779 cases from 39 medical centers in 16 countries, has illustrated the recent changes in microbiology and clinical presentation of bacterial endocarditis.[49] In this cohort, as well as other recent cohorts, *S. aureus* rather than *S. viridans* streptococci were the predominant pathogens and increasing numbers of cases were considered either nosocomially acquired or health care associated.[49] *S. aureus* endocarditis is associated with significantly higher mortality, higher rate of stroke, and other systemic embolization and higher rate of sustained bacteremia than endocarditis caused by other organisms.[49-51] The increased antibiotic resistance in organisms causing endocarditis, especially the increasing rates of methicillin-resistant *S. aureus* (MRSA), are reflected in the latest guidelines for diagnosis, treatment, and management of complications of endocarditis from the American Heart Association.[50] Other important recent epidemiologic trends are the decreased importance of congenital valvular and rheumatic disease as predispositions, the increasing age of cases, and the increased role of hemodialysis and indwelling cardiac devices such as pacemakers and implantable defibrillators as risk factors.[49-52]

Infectious endocarditis must be considered in the differential diagnosis of a broad range of clinical syndromes. Fever is the single most common presenting symptom, often accompanied by other constitutional symptoms of anorexia, weight loss, and fatigue. Onset may be acute or subacute. Signs and symptoms may be caused by direct cardiac effects of infection including new or changing heart murmur, worsening congestive heart failure and valvular dysfunction, and onset of heart block from myocardial abscesses.[50,52] The clinical presentation may also be dominated by systemic manifestations of emboli or immune complex disease including such findings as skin lesions, splenomegaly, glomerulonephritis, cerebrovascular events, and other acute vascular embolic events. Patients with acute, fulminant endocarditis, particularly *S. aureus* endocarditis, may present with concurrent cardiogenic and septic shock.

Clinical criteria have been developed and prospectively evaluated for the diagnosis of infective endocarditis.[53,54] The most current version of these, the Modified Duke Criteria for Diagnosis of Infective Endocarditis (Table 55-3), relies primarily on blood culture data and echocardiographic findings as the two major clinical criteria for diagnosis; additional minor clinical criteria (fever, underlying predisposition, embolic phenomena, immunologic phenomena) can also be used as supporting evidence for determining confirmed or suspected cases.[54] Patients with endocarditis have sustained bacteremia; in the absence of prior antibiotic therapy the yield of at least one positive blood culture after three sets are drawn is greater than 90%, and typically multiple cultures are positive. Thus two to three separate sets of blood culture should always be obtained in suspected endocarditis prior to initiation of therapy. Culture-negative cases may be caused by prior antimicrobial therapy or fastidious or difficult-to-cultivate organisms.[50] Follow-up blood cultures are critical to document sterilization of blood and should be repeated frequently until negative. Echocardiography should be performed on all patients with suspected endocarditis.[50,52] When possible, transesophageal echocardiography (TEE) is the preferred modality in adults. Sensitivity of TEE is reported to be as high as 95% for native valve infection compared with 60% to 75% for transthoracic echocardiography (TTE) and is significantly better than TTE for diagnosis of prosthetic valve infection and for detection of complications such as perivalvular abscess that may affect management.[50] In children and uncomplicated adult cases where TTE is diagnostic, TEE may not be necessary. If initial studies are negative, TEE should be repeated in 7 to 10 days if clinical suspicion remains high.[50]

Embolic complications may occur at any time with overall incidence of 20% to 50% in cases of infective endocarditis; risk decreases but still remains significant after initiation of antimicrobial therapy, especially with large vegetations, and remains high for up to 2 to 3 weeks.[50,55,56] Risks for embolization include specific organisms, especially *S. aureus*, *Candida*, HACEK organisms and *Abiotrophia*, increased vegetation size (>10 mm) and mobility as determined by echocardiography; mitral versus aortic valve involvement; and anterior versus pos-

Table 55-3A. Definition of Infective Endocarditis (IE) According to the Modified Duke Criteria
Definite IE
Pathologic Criteria: Microorganisms demonstrated by culture or histological examination of a vegetation, a vegetation that has embolized, or an intracardiac abscess specimen; OR Pathological lesions (as earlier) confirmed by histological examination as showing active endocarditis
Clinical Criteria: 2 *major* criteria OR 1 *major* and 3 *minor* criteria OR 5 *minor* criteria Possible IE: 1 *major* and 1 *minor* criteria OR 3 *minor* criteria
Rejected: Firm alternative diagnosis explaining evidence of IE; OR Resolution of IE syndrome with antibiotic therapy for <4 days; OR No evidence of IE at surgery or autopsy after antibiotic therapy <4 days; OR Does not meet at least minimal criteria for possible IE

Table 55-3B. Definition of Terms Used in the Modified Duke Criteria for the Diagnosis of Infective Endocarditis
Major Criteria
Blood culture positive for IE
Typical organisms consistent with IE (*Viridans* streptococci, *Streptococcus bovis,* HACEK group, *S. aureus,* community-acquired enterococci) from 2 separate blood cultures in absence of a primary focus
Microorganisms consistent with IE from persistently positive blood cultures: at least 2 positive cultures drawn >12 hr apart; or all of 3 or a majority of ≥4 separate cultures drawn over at least 1 hr
Single positive blood culture or positive serology for *Coxiella burnetii*
Evidence of endocardial involvement
Echocardiogram positive for IE defined as follows: oscillating intracardiac mass on valve or supporting structures, in the path of regurgitant jets, or on implanted material in the absence of an alternative anatomic explanation; or abscess; or new partial dehiscence of prosthetic valve; new valvular regurgitation (worsening or changing or pre-existing murmur not sufficient)
Minor Criteria
Predisposition: predisposing heart condition or IDU
Fever: temperature >38° C
Vascular phenomena: major arterial emboli, septic pulmonary infarcts, mycotic aneurysm, intracranial hemorrhage, conjunctival hemorrhages, and Janeway's lesions
Immunologic phenomena: glomerulonephritis, Osler's nodes, Roth's spots, and rheumatoid factor
Microbiological evidence: positive blood culture but does not meet a major criterion as noted earlier or serological evidence of active infection with organism consistent with IE (excludes single positive culture for coagulase-negative staphylococci)
HACEK, *Haemophilus, Actinobacillus, Cardiobacterium, Eikenella, Kingella;* IDU, injection drug use. Modified from Li JS, Sexton DJ, Mick N, et al: Proposed modifications to the Duke Criteria for the Diagnosis of Infective Endocarditis. Clin Infect Dis 2000;30:633-638.

terior location on the mitral valve.[50] More than half of clinically manifesting emboli involve the CNS, most commonly in the middle cerebral artery distribution.[50,55] In addition to emboli, other risks for mortality include congestive heart failure, abnormal mental status, comorbidities, higher APACHE score, and *S. aureus* infection.[49-51] Congestive heart failure appears to have the highest association with mortality.[49-51] Medical therapy (versus surgical therapy) was also associated with higher 6-month mortality in one recent study.[51]

The decision to perform valvular surgery on patients with active endocarditis remains complex. Traditional indications for surgery include refractory congestive heart failure; persistent infection despite optimal antimicrobial therapy; fungal or other difficult-to-treat organisms; one or more emboli during the first weeks of antimicrobial therapy; and valvular complications of dehiscence, perforation, fistula, and large perivalvular abscesses (Table 55-4).[50] Vegetation size and location are also emerging as possible independent indications for surgery.[50] The risk of infecting a new prosthetic valve during surgery for active endocarditis is only 2% to 3%; thus active infection is not a contraindication to surgery for complications associated with high associated mortality.[50] Several studies confirmed

Table 55-4. Possible Indications for Early Surgical Intervention for Acute Infective Endocarditis

Clinical Indications	Refractory congestive heart failure	Most common indication for surgery
	Severe valvular decompensation	Usually acute mitral or aortic insufficiency
	Emboli and recurrent emboli	Especially if 1 or more during first 1 to 2 wk of antimicrobial therapy
	Persistent infection/sepsis	Persistent positive blood cultures after 7 days of optimal antibiotic Rx
	Difficult-to-eradicate organisms	Fungal endocarditis, highly resistant bacteria, ?gram-negative endocarditis
	Extension of infection into myocardium	Evidence of new heart block, echocardiography as later
Echo Indications	Evidence of valve decompensation	Dehiscence, rupture, perforation, fistula, perivalvular abscess
	Vegetation characteristics	>10 mm in size, especially on anterior mitral valve, increase in vegetation size on Rx
Other Possible Indications	Complicated prosthetic valve infection	As defined by TEE findings; high failure rate of medical therapy alone
	?Left-sided *S. aureus* infection	Early surgical Rx may be associated with lower mortality

the decreased mortality of cohorts of patients who were managed with early surgical intervention, especially those with left-sided *S. aureus* endocarditis.[50,52,57] The optimal surgical procedure and the role of more conservative procedures such as vegetation resection remain controversial. The majority of patients who survive an episode of left-sided endocarditis who are not operated on initially will ultimately require valve replacement within the next 15 years.[50]

Anticoagulation in patients with active endocarditis can present difficult management dilemmas. Anticoagulation is relatively contraindicated in active endocarditis because of the risk of hemorrhagic CNS events.[50] In patients already on anticoagulation for mechanical valves or other specific indications, Warfarin should be switched to heparin therapy during the initial phase of therapy, especially in cases in which surgical intervention is being considered. Anticoagulation should be discontinued if possible after acute CNS embolic events. Some evidence suggests that anticoagulation should be stopped in all cases of left-sided *S. aureus* infection for at least the first 2 weeks of therapy because of the high risk of CNS emboli.[58] Neurologic events, most commonly embolic events but also mycotic aneurysms, are the second leading cause of mortality in acute endocarditis after heart failure. Decisions on timing of surgery and management of anticoagulation perioperatively and postoperatively in patients with CNS events are particularly challenging.

Optimal antibiotic therapy for patients with infective endocarditis is outlined in the American Heart Association guidelines.[50] Individual treatment regimens including choice of antibiotic, need for combination therapy, and duration of therapy are based on the organism, susceptibility data, location of infected valve, and whether the infection is complicated or uncomplicated. Left-sided *S. aureus* endocarditis is generally treated for 6 weeks with a parenteral beta-lactam or vancomycin, with or without addition of gentamicin for the initial 3 to 5 days of the treatment course. Oxacillin-resistant staphylococcal infections require vancomycin therapy. Uncomplicated right-sided endocarditis in injection drug users may have a more benign course, and there is evidence for use of shorter courses of therapy and even for use of oral therapy in selected patients. Treatment of *viridans* streptococcal endocarditis is 4 weeks of a beta-lactam or vancomycin, and gentamicin is added for disease caused by relatively penicillin-resistant strains. Selected patients with uncomplicated *viridans* streptococcal infections have been treated with 2 weeks of combination therapy. Beta-lactam therapy for susceptible isolates is always preferred to vancomycin in nonallergic patients. Enterococcal endocarditis is usually treated for 4 to 6 weeks with synergistic combinations of a penicillin or vancomycin and an aminoglycoside, but regimens may need to be modified on the basis of strain resistance patterns. Prosthetic valve infections require longer treatment courses and use of combination therapy, and failure rates of medical therapy of prosthetic valve disease are high.[59]

Device-Related Endovascular Infections

Endovascular infections other than valvular infections have become increasingly common as causes of bacteremia and sepsis. This is related to the increased use of indwelling devices including vascular catheters for chemotherapy and other long-term parenteral therapies, use of accesses for hemodialysis, and the expanding indications for implantable cardiac devices for patients with congestive heart failure and arrhythmias. Infection is the most common serious complication of peripherally inserted central venous catheters (PICCs), tunneled catheters, and totally implanted intravascular devices.[60] Patients presenting with sepsis and focal findings related to the catheter such as tunnel infection, port abscess or cellulitis, those with associated venous thrombosis, or those with concurrent endocarditis or osteomyelitis require removal of the catheter.[60] Management is more difficult in patients with sepsis or bacteremia without local signs of infection where removal of the catheter is not a trivial procedure. Diagnosis of the catheter as the source of a bacteremia can sometimes be made with use of paired central and peripheral blood cultures. Positive central and negative peripheral cultures or central cultures that are positive significantly earlier than peripheral cultures implicate the catheter as the source.[60] The majority of infected permanent catheters require removal; selected uncomplicated catheter infections in nonseptic patients whose bloodstream has sterilized on antibiotics can be treated with catheter retention and antibiotic therapy, especially infections caused by coagulase-negative staphylococci and other less virulent organisms.[60] Algorithms for the management of suspected and confirmed line infections in patients with long-term access devices are shown in Figures 55-2A and 55-2B. Antibiotic lock therapy is a strategy in which antibiotic solutions are used to fill the catheter lumen to maintain high antibiotic concentrations in the catheter and catheter hub. In several trials, antibiotic lock therapy yielded higher rates of catheter salvage than parenteral antibiotics alone.[60] Hemodialysis catheter infections pose particular management challenges because of the high prevalence of infection in these patients and the need to preserve dialysis access. Hemodialysis has emerged as a major risk factor for endocarditis in recent studies. Catheter salvage strategies and guidewire exchange strategies are employed more frequently in hemodialysis catheter–associated infections than in other populations.[61]

Indications for placement of automatic implantable cardioverter-defibrillator devices (AICDs) in patients with cardiac disease have recently been expanded, resulting in increased number of AICDs and increased prevalence of AICD infections.[62,63] Estimates of infection of pacemakers and AICDs range from 1% to 7% including infections in the generator pocket and/or on the leads.[62] Lead infection may be complicated by sepsis and septic shock, suppurative thrombophlebitis, and endocarditis. Lead infections probably occur in less than 1% of implanted devices and almost always require explantation of the device.[62,63] Diagnosis is typically made by blood cultures and TEE, which may show vegetations on the leads or associated endocarditis. The most common organisms are coagulase-negative staphylococci and *S. aureus* in 80% of cases. Experience with transvenous rather than open surgical explantation of infected AICD leads is increasing. Devices should not be replaced until bacteremia has completely resolved.

PRIMARY BACTEREMIAS

In 10% to 30% of patients presenting from the community with bacteremia and sepsis, the primary source of the bacteremia remains unknown, even after careful clinical and radiographic evaluation.[64,65] This includes patients with infections manifesting as a primary bacteremia, as well as those with probable secondary bacteremia from an occult focus. Bacteremia of unknown etiology is associated with higher mortality.[64] Primary bacteremias are more common with certain microorganisms and with specific host predispositions. These syndromes, if unrecognized, have particularly high morbidity and mortality. Patients with impairment in immunoglobulin production or function and impaired or absent splenic function are predisposed to infections with encapsulated organisms such as *S. pneumoniae, N. meningitidis, H. influenzae,* and group B streptococcus.[66] Patients with advanced liver disease and cirrhosis are predisposed to these, as well as a variety of other spontaneous bacteremias.[67] Patients with cell-mediated immune defects may present with other unusual bacteremias such as *Listeria* and *Salmonella* sepsis. Severe neutropenia greatly increases the risk of spontaneous bacteremia and sepsis from endogenous gastrointestinal flora, and the management of fever in neutropenic patients includes empiric initiation of broad-spectrum antibacterial therapy.[68] Several important specific bacteremia syndromes are described as follows.

Meningococcemia and Meningococcal Sepsis

Invasive meningococcal disease can present as either bacterial meningitis or as the syndrome of meningococcemia with meningococcal sepsis without meningitis.[7] The proportion of primary meningococcemia cases depends in part on the serotypes present in the community. The annual incidence of meningococcal disease in the United States is approximately 1 case per 100,000, with mortality of 10% to 14% and significant residual morbidity in up to 20%.[7] Besides young children, adolescents and young adults ages 11 to 19 are at increased risk for meningococcal disease, but risk persists throughout life and is increased in those with certain immune deficiencies such as terminal complement deficiency and cirrhosis.[7,70] Patients with meningococcemia present with fever, headache, malaise, vomiting, and myalgias.[69,70] Most patients will also present with rapid development of a characteristic nonblanching petechial or purpuric rash, but the rash can be maculopapular or absent. Early symptoms that may be important clues to the diagnosis are leg pains and cold hands and feet.[69] If untreated, disease may progress rapidly within 24 hours to fulminant purpura and hemorrhagic shock. The keys to improved outcome are early recognition and aggressive therapy. Early institution of antibiotic therapy with a penicillin or third-generation cephalosporin can significantly improve outcomes. PCR of blood is useful for diagnosis, especially in patients who received antibiotics prior to hospitalization.[7,69] A new tetravalent conjugated polysaccharide vaccine has recently become available in the United States and is now recommended for routine vaccination of adolescents and other high-risk populations.[7]

Primary Pneumococcal Bacteremia

Pneumococcal bacteremia is most commonly a consequence of pneumococcal pneumonia, but 5% to 10% of episodes occur without an identified underlying focus.[71] Severe episodes may present with fulminant sepsis and purpura fulminans clinically indistinguishable from meningococcal sepsis. Important risk factors for pneumococcal sepsis include asplenia and hyposplenism, HIV infection, sickle cell disease, alcoholism, malignancy, and other

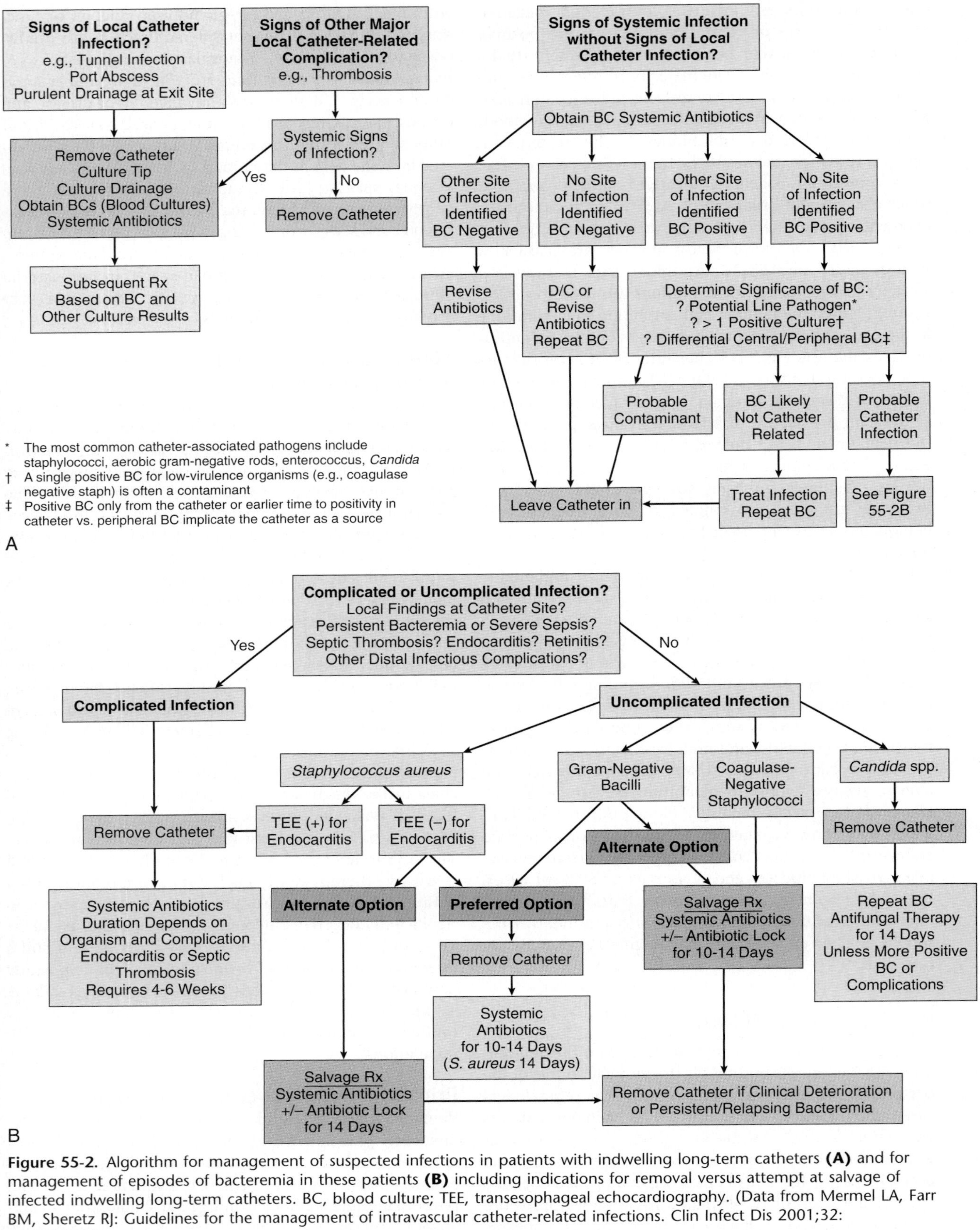

Figure 55-2. Algorithm for management of suspected infections in patients with indwelling long-term catheters **(A)** and for management of episodes of bacteremia in these patients **(B)** including indications for removal versus attempt at salvage of infected indwelling long-term catheters. BC, blood culture; TEE, transesophageal echocardiography. (Data from Mermel LA, Farr BM, Sheretz RJ: Guidelines for the management of intravascular catheter-related infections. Clin Infect Dis 2001;32: 1249-1272.)

immunocompromised states, although this syndrome can occur in otherwise healthy adults and children without predisposing risks.[72] *S. pneumoniae* causes 50% to 90% of cases of the fulminant sepsis syndrome that occurs in postsplenectomy or functionally asplenic patients.[67] Other causes of the postsplenectomy sepsis syndrome include *N. meningitidis; H. influenzae;* and, less commonly, *Capnocytophaga canimorsus, Escherichia coli, Salmonella,* and the vector-borne parasitic infections malaria and babesiosis. Immunization with pneumococcal, meningococcal, and *H. influenzae* vaccines is recommended for those at risk for postsplenectomy sepsis.[67]

Staphylococcus Aureus Bacteremia

S. aureus bacteremia can occur from localized staphylococcal disease such as skin and soft tissue infection or pneumonia, endovascular infection. and endocarditis. It can also be of occult origin. Regardless of the initial source of bacteremia, there is significant risk for development of late complications including endocarditis, bone and joint disease, or other metastatic foci in up to one third of cases.[73] Features associated with complicated *S. aureus* bacteremia include prolonged bacteremia, prolonged fever, and embolic lesions. Longer-course therapy (at least 4 weeks) is recommended for patients with complicated disease, whereas 2 weeks of treatment may be adequate for selected patients with uncomplicated bacteremia.[74] TEE has been recommended to exclude endocarditis in patients with otherwise clinically uncomplicated *S. aureus* bacteremia when short-course therapy is being considered.[73,74]

TOXIN-MEDIATED INFECTIONS

Staphylococcal Toxic Shock Syndrome

S. aureus produces multiple virulence factors that contribute to its success as a human pathogen. These virulence factors potentiate local adherence, tissue invasion, and avoidance of host defenses, all features that are important in the pathogenesis of localized skin and soft tissue infection, pneumonia, bacteremia, and metastatic infections. Staphylococci also produce a variety of exotoxins that are released into the systemic circulation to act at distant sites.[75] Some of these exotoxins are directly pathogenic to specific cells, such as exfoliatoxin B, which causes staphylococcal scalded skin syndrome. Other exotoxins function as potent superantigens, antigens that bypass the intermediate T-cell antigen processing steps by binding directly to Vβ domains on T-cell receptors. This causes direct activation of multiple T-cell classes resulting in unopposed release of large amounts of cytokines including interleukin (IL)-2, IL-4, IL-6, interferon (IFN)-γ, TNF-α, and IL-1β.[75] The resulting "cytokine storm" can lead to septic shock, multiorgan failure, and death.

The most well-studied staphylococcal superantigens are the pyrogenic antigens TSST-1 and TSST-2 and enterotoxins B and C. TSST-1 and TSST-2 are the primary exotoxins causing the staphylococcal toxic shock syndrome.[75] First described in 1979 as a unique syndrome primarily associated with menstruating women using supra-absorbent brands of tampons, staphylococcal toxic shock syndrome is now known to occur potentially from any infection or colonization caused by an exotoxin-producing strain.[76,77] Disease is associated with conditions leading to exotoxin production in a host who lacks preexisting antibodies to TSST-1. The overall incidence of this syndrome, as well as the proportion of cases associated with menstruating women, has decreased since 1980.[76] Toxic shock syndrome is characterized by the acute onset of fever, hypotension, myalgia, scarlatiniform or erythroderma-like rash, nausea, vomiting, diarrhea, and development of multiple-organ failure including renal failure, elevated liver enzymes, and DIC.[76,77] Typically the rash will evolve and cause late desquamation of hands and feet. Specific criteria for the diagnosis of staphylococcal toxic shock syndrome have been described (Table 55-5).[76] Treatment is primarily supportive, but antistaphylococcal agents are administered to treat the underlying staphylococcal colonization or infection; some evidence suggests that immunoglobulin may be beneficial by binding exotoxin and attenuating the cytokine response. Strains producing the staphylococcal enterotoxins A thru I are all also capable of acting as superantigens and can cause toxic shock–like illness. Enterotoxins B and C in particular have been implicated in many nonmenstrual-associated cases.[75]

Streptococcal Toxic Shock Syndrome

Group A β-hemolytic streptococci are also capable of producing a toxic shock–like syndrome analogous to staphylococcal toxic shock syndrome.[78,79] Most often this is seen in the setting of severe bacteremic streptococcal soft tissue infection or with streptococcal necrotizing fasciitis. In one large survey of invasive streptococcal infections in Ontario, 13% were complicated by toxic shock syndrome, and the mortality rate of these infections was 81%.[79] The pathogenesis of this syndrome has been attributed to streptococcal pyrotoxins functioning as superantigens. Binding of streptococcal M protein-fibrinogen complexes to polymorphonuclear cells causing PMN activation and endothelial damage may also be important. Clinical criteria for the diagnosis of streptococcal toxic shock syndrome have been defined (see Table 55-5).[78] In addition to antibiotics that decrease toxin production, such as clindamycin and linezolid, IV immunoglobulin has been used for treatment.[80] Other streptococcal species have also been reported to produce a toxic shock–like illness including *viridans* streptococci, groups B, C, and G β-hemolytic streptococci, and *Streptococcus suis*.

Tetanus

Tetanus is a syndrome of increased muscle rigidity and convulsive spasms caused by a toxin produced by the environmental spore-forming anaerobic bacterium *Clostridium tetani*.[81,82] Since the introduction of routine immunization, tetanus has become increasingly rare, with the number of U.S. cases decreasing from 560 cases in 1947 to only 37 cases in 2002.[82] Clinical disease is caused by contamination of wounds, most commonly traumatic

Table 55-5. Criteria for Diagnosis of Staphylococcal and Streptococcal Toxic Shock Syndromes
Staphylococcal Toxic Shock—CDC Criteria
1. Fever >38.9° C or >102° F
2. Rash (diffuse macular erythroderma)
3. Desquamation 1-2 wk after onset, particularly of the palms and soles
4. Hypotension: systolic blood pressure <90 mm Hg for adults or orthostatic hypotension
5. Multisystem involvement of 3 or more of the following:
Gastrointestinal: vomiting or diarrhea at onset of illness
Muscular: severe myalgia or CPK levels at least 2× upper limit of normal
Mucous membrane: vaginal, oropharyngeal, or conjunctival hyperemia
Renal: BUN or creatinine at least 2× upper limit of normal or >5 leukocytes per high-power field without UTI
Hepatic: total bilirubin, AST or ALT at least 2× upper limit of normal
Hematologic: Platelets ≤100,000/mL
CNS: disoriented or alterations in level of consciousness without focal neurologic signs when fever and hypotension are absent
6. *Negative* results on tests, if obtained
Blood, throat, or cerebrospinal fluid cultures (blood may be positive for *S. aureus*)
Rise in body titer to Rocky Mountain spotted fever, leptospirosis, or measles
Case classification
Probable: 5 of the 6 clinical findings described earlier
Confirmed: all 6 of the findings described earlier including desquamation
Streptococcal Toxic Shock Syndrome A. Isolation of Group A *Streptococcus* 1. From a sterile body site 2. From a nonsterile body site B. Clinical Signs of Severity 1. Hypotension 2. Clinical and laboratory abnormalities (2 or more)
Renal impairment
Coagulopathy
Liver abnormalities
Acute respiratory distress syndrome
Extensive tissue necrosis (i.e., necrotizing fasciitis)
Erythematous rash
Definite Case: A1 plus B (1 + 2)
Probable Case: A2 plus B (1 + 2)
ALT, alanine aminotransferase; AST, aspartate aminotransferase; BUN, blood urea nitrogen; CPK, creatine phosphokinase; UTI, urinary tract infection. Modified from Haijeh RA, Reingold A, Weil A, et al: Toxic shock syndrome in the United States: surveillance update, 1979-1996. Emerg Infect Dis 1999;5:807-810 and Stevens DI: Streptococcal toxic-shock syndrome: Spectrum of disease, pathogenesis, and new concepts in treatment. Emerg Infect Dis 1995;1:69-78.

wounds, with bacterial spores. Spores then germinate and produce toxins including tetanospasmin, a highly potent neurotoxin that inhibits neurotransmitter release, resulting in blockage of inhibitor impulses and unopposed muscle contractions. Cases predominate in the summer or wet season, and disease is now most common in older adults because of either missed primary immunization or waning effects of childhood immunization.[82] The most common syndrome is that of generalized tetanus with descending symptoms of trismus (lockjaw), difficulty swallowing, muscle rigidity, and spasms.[81] Symptoms may persist for several weeks, and complete recovery may take months. Complications include laryngospasm, fractures, hypertension, nosocomial infections, and death. Treatment is primarily supportive, although metronidazole or penicillin may be given to treat potentially infected or colonized wounds. Patients require admission to an ICU for control of rigidity and spasms with benzodiazepines or neuromuscular blocking agents and for ventilator support.[81] Human tetanus immunoglobulin may be administered, but this only binds free toxin, so there may be little benefit by the time of clinical presentation. Routine childhood and adult immunization with tetanus toxoid remains the primary strategy for preventing this rare but often fatal condition. Guidelines for use of immunoglobulin and vaccination in management of potentially infected wounds have been published.[82]

Botulism

Clostridium botulinum is an anaerobic spore-forming bacteria that produces botulinum toxin, a family of closely related but immunologically distinct polypeptide toxins that are among the most potent neurologically acting poisons known.[83] Other, less common clostridial species can also produce botulinum toxin. Botulinum toxin binds irreversibly to synaptic complexes, affecting ganglionic synapses, presympathetic synapses, and neuromuscular junctions. Clinical syndromes include those caused by ingestion of preformed toxin such as food botulism and those resulting from acquisition of the organism and production of toxin in vivo such as infant botulism in very young children and wound botulism from contaminated wounds, most commonly seen in injection drug users. Patients present initially with cranial nerve dysfunction and evolve to descending paralysis without sensory or cognitive effects. Diagnosis is made on clinical grounds; testing of food products or human samples in the United States is performed by the Centers for Disease Control. Treatment is primarily supportive, but both human and equine type-specific antitoxin is available through the CDC: human antitoxin is preferred for infant botulism.[83] Antitoxin is only effective in binding free toxin if given in the first 72 hours. Because of its potency, environmental stability, and potential for aerosolization, botulinum toxin is considered a potential agent of bioterrorism.[83]

Diphtheria

Diphtheria is caused by toxigenic strains of the bacterial species *Corynebacterium diphtheriae*. This disease has become extremely rare in the United States secondary to universal vaccination with diphtheria toxoid vaccine, with an average of one confirmed case per year.[84] Patients with respiratory diphtheria present with sore throat; low-grade fever; occasional neck swelling; and the characteristic grayish adherent membrane covering the tonsils, throat, or nose.[84] Complications include myocarditis, polyneuritis, and airway obstruction, with mortality rates of 5% to 10%. Outbreaks of diphtheria continue to occur in many parts of the world.

SERIOUS SKIN AND SKIN STRUCTURE INFECTIONS

Serious skin and soft tissue infections are characterized by rapidly progressive inflammation and necrosis of skin, subcutaneous fat, and/or fascia. Occasionally, muscle is also involved. Several terms have been used to describe these infections: *necrotizing fasciitis; synergistic cellulitis; synergistic gangrene; nonclostridial cellulitis;* and, when muscle is involved with clostridial infection, *clostridial myonecrosis*.[85] Differentiating among these entities is difficult and somewhat artificial. A variety of features of some of the most important necrotizing skin and soft tissue infections are shown in Table 55-6. Microbiologically, these infections may be caused by a single pathogen

Table 55-6. Differentiating Features of Necrotizing Skin and Soft Tissue Infections

Feature	Progressive Bacterial Synergistic Gangrene	Nonclostridial Anaerobic Cellulitis	Clostridial Myonecrosis (Gas Gangrene)	Necrotizing Fasciitis Type 1	Necrotizing Fasciitis Type 2
Risk factors	Surgery, ileostomy, colostomy, chronic ulceration	Diabetes mellitus	Trauma, surgery	Diabetes mellitus, surgery, perineal infection	Trauma, surgery, none
Microbiology	Microaerophilic streptococci plus *Staphylococcus aureus*	Non–spore-forming anaerobes +/– coliforms, streptococci, *S. aureus*	*Clostridium* spp.	Polymicrobial (Enterobacteriaceae plus anaerobes)	Group A streptococci
Course	Slow	Slow or rapid	Very rapid	Rapid	Very rapid
Pain	++++	+	++++	+++/++++	++++
Gas formation	–	++++	++	++	–
Appearance	Central necrotic ulcer, erythematous periphery	Erythematous skin	Bullae, necrosis	Bullae, skin necrosis	Bullae, necrotic skin and tissue
Drainage	Purulent if present	Purulent	Serosanguineous	"Dishwater," seropurulent	Serous if present
Depth of involvement	Skin, soft tissue	Skin, soft tissue	Muscle	Fascia	Fascia
Systemic toxicity	+/–	+++	++++	+++/++++	++++

–, absent; +/–, occasionally present; +, minimal; ++, mild; +++, moderate; ++++, marked or severe.

such as group A β-hemolytic streptococcus; however, they are more frequently polymicrobial in nature. Risk factors for these infections include diabetes, old age, peripheral vascular disease, malignancy, alcoholism, renal failure, and immunosuppressive therapy. Infection may follow traumatic injuries that become contaminated by soil. The primary traumatic event may be relatively minor. Initial signs and symptoms may be similar to a severe cellulitis. Early findings include fever, tachycardia, moderate to severe pain, and swelling and induration of the skin.[86] Late findings include severe pain or even anesthesia, skin necrosis, hemorrhagic bullae, crepitus, drainage, and signs of systemic inflammatory response syndrome or severe sepsis including multiorgan failure.[86] Laboratory tests usually demonstrate leukocytosis and metabolic acidosis. Plain radiographs may reveal gas in the soft tissues. CT or MRI is useful in delineating extent of disease or the presence of soft tissue gas. Diagnostic evaluation should also include blood cultures, gram staining of tissue exudates, and aerobic and anaerobic cultures obtained at surgery or from a needle aspiration. Incision and exploration or biopsy can even be done at the bedside to obtain material for Gram stain, culture, and histology.

Once a necrotizing soft tissue infection has been identified, prompt therapy is important. Early aggressive surgical débridement is essential.[87] Because most cases of necrotizing skin infection are polymicrobial, empiric antibiotic coverage should be sufficiently broad spectrum to cover gram-positive cocci and gram-negative bacilli and anaerobes. Antibiotic therapy can subsequently be adjusted on the basis of results of cultures and sensitivities.[88] In cases of group A β-hemolytic streptococcal infection, penicillin plus clindamycin is the therapy of choice. Clindamycin is effective in turning off toxin production. Linezolid also has similar activity.[89] Intravenous immunoglobulin (IVIG) is a useful adjuvant therapy for streptococcal toxic shock.[80,90]

Necrotizing Fasciitis

Necrotizing fasciitis is an uncommon, severe infection that causes necrosis of the subcutaneous tissue and fascia with sparing of the underlying muscle. Two types, based on microbiology, are described. In type I, at least one anaerobic species is isolated along with one or more facultative anaerobes and members of the Enterobacteriaceae.[85,91] This form of necrotizing fasciitis most commonly affects the extremities but may involve the abdominal wall, postoperative wounds, perianal area, and groin. It occurs following trauma or a variety of surgical procedures, perirectal abscess, decubitus ulcer, or perforation of the intestines. Patients at increased risk include those with diabetes mellitus, alcoholism, and injection drug use. The involved area is initially erythematous and painful.

Over several days, skin changes include color changes, formation of bullae, and cutaneous gangrene. The involved area becomes anesthetic secondary to thrombosis of small blood vessels and destruction of superficial nerves. Anesthesia may develop before the appearance of skin necrosis and is an important clue to the presence of necrotizing fasciitis rather than simple cellulitis.[86] Subcutaneous gas is often present, and systemic toxicity is common.[91] When the lesion is probed at the bedside or in the operating room, there is no resistance along tissue planes. In type II (also known as hemolytic streptococcal gangrene), group A streptococci are generally isolated alone.[92] These strains usually produce pyrogenic exotoxin A. Periodically, group C or group G streptococci are causative organisms. Infection usually develops at a site of trauma but may occur in the absence of an obvious portal of entry.[91] The involved area is extremely painful, erythematous, and edematous. Infection spreads widely in deep fascial planes with relative sparing of the overlying skin and therefore may not be recognized. This form of necrotizing fasciitis is present in approximately 50% of cases of streptococcal toxic shock syndrome.[92] Over several days, the skin becomes dusky and bullae develop. Bullae then rupture and evolve into an area covered by necrotic eschar, often resembling a third-degree burn. Streptococci can usually be cultured from fluid of the early bullae and frequently from blood. Complications include metastatic abscess formation, and mortality from this infection is high.

Fournier's gangrene is a form of necrotizing fasciitis that involves the male perineum, specifically the scrotum. It is caused by anaerobic streptococci along with other bacteria such as *E. coli; S. aureus;* β-hemolytic streptococci; *Proteus* species; a variety of anaerobes; and, on occasion, *Pseudomonas* species.[93] The first symptoms are commonly scrotal swelling and pain followed by progressive necrosis of scrotal skin and subcutaneous tissues.[93] The patient may appear toxic. Initially the patient may be erroneously diagnosed with an acute abdomen unless the genitalia are examined. Gangrene of the perineum and sometimes the penis may develop. Urgent and aggressive surgery is necessary along with broad-spectrum antibiotics.

Clostridial Myonecrosis

Infection with *Clostridium* species should be suspected when the Gram stain of drainage reveals gram-positive bacilli in a patient who is critically ill. Penicillin G is the drug of choice with or without hyperbaric oxygen. The precise role of hyperbaric oxygen therapy in the treatment of clostridial myonecrosis or in the treatment of necrotizing fasciitis remains controversial. If used, it must be used as an adjunct to aggressive surgery.[94]

Vibrio Infections

Various *Vibrio* species including *Vibrio vulnificus* have caused mild to severe cellulitis in patients who sustained lacerations or puncture wounds when in contact with saltwater in the southeastern United States and the Gulf of Mexico. Septicemia may occur in immunocompromised hosts, especially those with cirrhosis.[95] Increased incidence of *Vibrio* infections has been described as a result of flooding after natural disasters.

Community-Acquired MRSA

During the past few years, community-associated MRSA (CA-MRSA) infections among persons without health care–associated risk factors have emerged in several geographic areas and have become endemic in some areas.[96]

These strains carry the staphylococcal cassette chromosome *mec* type IV element and the gene encoding Panton-Valentine leukocidin, a toxin that promotes tissue destruction.[97,98] Although most CA-MRSA infections are mild skin and soft tissue infections, severe, life-threatening cases of necrotizing fasciitis, myonecrosis, necrotizing pneumonia, and sepsis have occurred.[97,98] For patients with invasive infections caused by CA-MRSA, vancomycin and linezolid are appropriate therapeutic options.[99]

SERIOUS GASTROINTESTINAL AND INTRA-ABDOMINAL INFECTIONS

Bacteremia Associated with Diarrheal Illness

Of the enteric pathogens, *Salmonella* species are most likely to cause bacteremia and serious infection. Enteric fever is usually caused by *Salmonella enterica* serotype typhi and rarely by *Salmonella paratyphi, Salmonella choleraesuis, Yersinia enterocolitica,* or *Campylobacter fetus.*[100] Features of classic typhoidal fever caused by *S. enterica* include sustained fever, bacteremia, headache, and abdominal pain. Physical findings include "rose spots" that are 2- to 4-mm discrete, irregular, blanching pink macules that are often seen on the anterior chest, hepatosplenomegaly, and relative bradycardia. Multiorgan system dysfunction can occur as a consequence of metastatic infection or immune complex deposition.[101] Intestinal bleeding or perforation may occur as a result of hyperplasia of the lymphoid tissue in the terminal ileum. Diarrhea is seen in less than 50% of cases and only early in the illness. Constipation is a frequent later complaint. The following specimens should be sent for culture: stool, blood, or bone marrow. Serologies may provide supportive evidence or may be useful in epidemiologic evaluation.

Therapeutic options include third-generation cephalosporins, fluoroquinolones, or trimethoprim/sulfamethoxazole. Treatment for uncomplicated cases is 12 to 14 days; 30 days of therapy may be necessary for metastatic foci. Metastatic foci are relatively common in the setting of bacteremia. Infection may involve gallbladder, spleen, bone, joints, and the meninges. There is a propensity to infect preexisting intravascular lesions such as atherosclerotic plaques and aneurysms. Sickle cell anemia and the presence of an orthopedic prosthesis are risk factors for osteomyelitis.[101] Meningitis tends to occur in young children.[101]

Peritonitis

Peritonitis is a localized or general inflammation of the peritoneal cavity that is generally caused by bacteria or fungi but may be caused by a variety of noninfectious agents such as gastric contents, talc, or bile salts. Peritonitis is primary when there is infection from an extra-peritoneal source such as the bloodstream.[102] This classification includes spontaneous bacterial peritonitis, which occurs in patients with underlying ascites from cirrhosis or nephrotic syndrome; peritonitis in patients being treated with continuous ambulatory peritoneal dialysis; and tuberculous peritonitis. Secondary peritonitis most often arises from an enteric source or pelvic focus and includes peritonitis following an acute perforation of the gastrointestinal tract, intestinal necrosis, postoperative peritonitis that may be secondary to an anastomotic leak, and posttraumatic peritonitis following blunt or penetrating abdominal trauma. Intestinal ischemia and frank necrotic bowel may be caused by a variety of processes including malignancies, vascular insufficiency, volvulus, or intussusception.[102] Rupture of an abscess in the pancreas, liver, or spleen or, rarely, rupture of a distended gallbladder can also cause peritonitis. Localized lower abdominal peritonitis can also result from gynecologic infections such as salpingitis and endometritis.

Bacterial peritonitis is typically caused by flora of the large intestine including aerobes, with *E. coli* being the most frequent, and anaerobes, of which *Bacteroides fragilis* is the predominant isolate.[103] Common symptoms include localized or generalized abdominal pain, nausea, and vomiting. Treatment with corticosteroids may mask typical signs and symptoms, delaying the diagnosis. Signs may include abdominal rigidity, distention, fever, and an overall toxic appearance. A rigid abdomen may be seen in the early stages of an acute peritonitis, although it may be absent in a peritonitis that progresses more slowly, such as that caused by tuberculosis, or when sterile bile, pancreatic fluid, or urine leak into the peritoneal cavity. As intraperitoneal fluid accumulates, abdominal distention and an ileus occur. The white blood cell count is usually elevated. Bacteremia may occur, and the sepsis syndrome may develop as peritonitis evolves. Aspiration of peritoneal fluid is an essential part of the evaluation for peritonitis. Laparoscopy or laparotomy may be necessary. Studies performed on peritoneal fluid should include a cell count with differential, amylase, Gram stain and aerobic and anaerobic culture, acid-fast smear and culture, and fungal smear and culture.

The primary cause of the peritonitis should be sought and eliminated if possible. Liver function tests and a serum amylase level may define a source in the liver, gallbladder, or pancreas. A plain film of the abdomen or a chest radiograph may reveal free air under the diaphragm in the case of a ruptured viscus. A CT scan of the abdomen may reveal an underlying intra-abdominal abscess or other focal process. Antibiotic therapy to cover gram-negative bacillary organisms and anaerobes should be initiated. Options for empiric therapy include combinations such as a third- or fourth-generation cephalosporin with metronidazole or monotherapy with a β-lactam/β-lactamase inhibitor combination or a carbapenem.[104-107] The optimal duration of therapy is not well defined, although nonbacteremic patients are generally treated for 7 to 10 days.[103] Regimens as short as 2 days of treatment may be adequate in uncomplicated situations with adequate surgical source control and in those with penetrating trauma. Bacteremic patients are generally treated for a total of 14 days using a combination of IV followed by oral therapy.

Spontaneous bacterial peritonitis (SBP) is caused by the translocation of enteric organisms to regional lymph nodes, which produce bacteremia and ultimately seeding of ascitic fluid.[108] Periodically a urinary tract infection may be the source of bacteremia. SBP occurs most commonly in adults with cirrhosis, nephrotic syndrome, or systemic lupus erythematosus.[108,109] Coliforms are the most common pathogens in adults, accounting for 70% of infections, with *E. coli* being the most common isolate followed by *Klebsiella* species. Gram-positive cocci may be seen in up to 20% of cases and anaerobes in less than 5%. Generally SBP is monomicrobial in contrast to the polymicrobial nature of most other forms of peritonitis. Findings of SBP may be subtle, so a high index of suspicion is necessary. Ascites is almost always present.[108] Fever and abdominal pain are seen in the majority of patients. New onset or worsening of hepatic encephalopathy may be seen. Some patients may have abdominal tenderness or rebound tenderness, but these findings are less frequent than in other forms of peritonitis. The most useful diagnostic test is a paracentesis.[108-110] SBP is defined by an ascitic segmented neutrophil count of at least 250 cells/mm^3 with a positive fluid culture and no obvious intra-abdominal source of infection.[109] The pH of ascitic fluid is low in SBP, whereas that of sterile ascitic fluid is the same as in serum.[110] Despite the low sensitivity (≈33%), Gram staining of ascitic fluid should be performed. Patients with other infections of the abdomen, such as tuberculous peritonitis or secondary bacterial peritonitis caused by perforation or peritonitis caused by noninfectious etiologies including pancreatitis or malignancy, also may show elevated neutrophil counts. Presence of a single organism generally confirms the diagnosis of SBP, although gram-negative bacillary organisms may occur as sole pathogens in secondary peritonitis. If mixed gram-positive and gram-negative bacteria are seen, an intestinal perforation is the more likely source.[110] Peritoneal fluid should be cultured aerobically and anaerobically. Blood cultures should also be performed and are positive in about one third of patients with SBP.[109,111] A repeat paracentesis has been advocated to document decrease in cell counts and sterilization of ascitic fluid.[109] Treatment is usually continued for a total of 7 to 10 days, although some experts have suggested that a 5- to 7-day course of IV therapy may be safe and effective.[109,111,112] Most studies show a high mortality rate of 30% to 40% for this syndrome, and after an initial episode of SBP, the probability of recurrence within 1 year is 70%.[108,109]

Intra-Abdominal Abscess

Considering the presence of a potential intra-abdominal abscess in febrile patients without any obvious cause of fever is important, especially if there is a predisposing condition such as diverticulitis, inflammatory bowel disease, or a history of recent abdominal surgery or abdominal trauma. Intra-abdominal abscess formation may complicate either primary or secondary peritonitis. The processes that typically predispose to intra-abdominal abscess formation are the same as those that cause secondary peritonitis and include perforation, complicated acute cholecystitis, suppurative cholangitis, acute appendicitis, diverticulitis, intestinal malignancy, surgical procedures, blunt or penetrating trauma, or an intestinal ischemia from a mesenteric vascular occlusion, an intestinal obstruction, or a volvulus. Most commonly, abscesses are postoperative complications of trauma or of gastrointestinal or biliary surgery.[113] Abscesses can be found anywhere within the abdomen including the retroperitoneal space. Generally their location is in proximity with the original site of contamination, but they may develop at distant sites.[114] One example of distal infection is subphrenic abscess, which may be a consequence of a perforated appendix. Symptoms of intra-abdominal abscess may include fever, chills, anorexia, weight loss, and abdominal pain. Unexplained fever may be the only sign of an occult intra-abdominal abscess. An abdominal CT scan is the imaging modality of choice for diagnosis of abdominal abscess. Drainage is essential to establish the diagnosis, obtain microbiology to target antimicrobial therapy, and achieve therapeutic success. This may be accomplished by the insertion of percutaneous catheters, laparoscopically or operatively.[113,114] Large abscesses cannot be eradicated by antibiotic therapy alone. Criteria for considering percutaneous drainage include the presence of a well-defined fluid collection and a safe percutaneous route of access.[115] Drains should remain in place until drainage volume is minimal, usually less than 10 mL in a 24-hour period.

A repeat CT scan should be performed to demonstrate complete collapse of the abscess cavity.[113] Indications for operative surgical drainage rather than percutaneous drainage include (1) percutaneous drainage cannot be performed safely; (2) percutaneous drainage fails; (3) there are multiple interloop abscesses; (4) there is a coagulopathy; or (5) there is infected pancreatic necrosis. Antibiotic therapy is indicated to treat inflammation in the surrounding tissue and to prevent metastatic infection and sepsis from bacteremia. Antibiotic coverage should be directed at abdominal flora including aerobic and anaerobic organisms even if anaerobes are not isolated.[103,112,113] Mortality with undrained pancreatic, hepatic, or retroperitoneal abscesses is reported to be 45% to 100%.[114] An approach to the management of intra-abdominal abscesses is outlined in Figure 55-3.

Biliary Tract Infections

The biliary tract of healthy individuals is sterile. In acute cholecystitis, infection of the gallbladder is most commonly caused by a number of microorganisms that are generally part of the normal intestinal flora.[116] Most biliary infections are polymicrobial, and anaerobes are more frequently isolated in the elderly and in those with common bile duct manipulation or prior biliary procedures. The source of bacteria is presumed to be the duodenum.[116] Many antibiotics achieve good levels in the bile in the absence of obstruction; however, when obstruction of the hepatic ducts or the common bile duct is present, the levels of such antibiotics are often subtherapeutic. Antibiotic therapy is adjunctive to surgical decompressive therapy. Antibiotics prevent the development of bacteremia, progression of infection, or development of liver abscesses. Cultures of blood and bile should be obtained. Empiric antibiotic therapy should generally be directed at

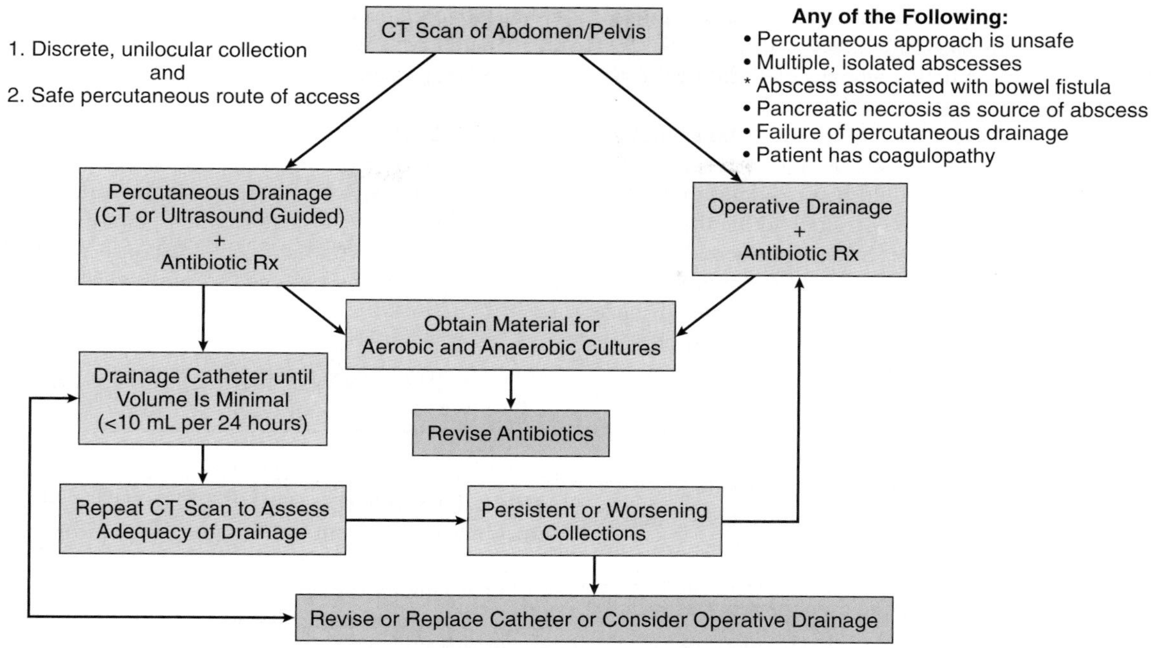

Figure 55-3. Approach to management of intra-abdominal abscesses including indications for consideration of percutaneous versus operative drainage.

gram-negative bacteria. In patients who are critically ill, the elderly, and those with prior common bile duct and complex biliary procedures, antianaerobic and antienterococcal therapy should also be instituted.

Acute acalculous cholecystitis is an acute inflammation of the gallbladder that occurs in the absence of gallstones. Individuals at risk include debilitated, hospitalized patients including those who have had major surgical procedures, prolonged intensive care stays, or hyperalimentation, or predisposing conditions that result in bile stasis, cholecystoparesis, or gallbladder ischemia.[116] The symptoms and findings are similar to those of calculous cholecystitis and include fever, right upper quadrant abdominal pain, nausea, vomiting, leukocytosis, and elevated liver function tests with an obstructive pattern. Diagnostic imaging modalities include ultrasonography, CT scanning, and hepato-iminodiacetic acid (lidofenin) scanning. If an open or laparoscopic cholecystectomy cannot be accomplished because of the patient's underlying condition, then urgent open or percutaneous cholecystostomy should be performed. In addition, broad-spectrum antibiotics should be instituted.

Acute cholangitis is a serious infection with high morbidity and mortality. The most common cause of acute cholangitis is obstruction and subsequent infection associated with stones in the common bile duct, which have usually migrated from the gallbladder. Other causes of biliary tract infection include malignant obstruction of the bile duct secondary to pancreatic cancer, cholangiocarcinoma, cancer of the papilla of Vater, or portahepatic metastases. Periodically biliary strictures, pancreatitis, and infection with the intestinal nematode *Ascaris lumbricoides* can cause obstruction. Bacteria enter the bile duct from the gastrointestinal tract through the blood stream or lymphatics.[117] The most common presenting symptoms are fever, abdominal pain, and jaundice. These symptoms are known as *Charcot's triad.* Septic shock may occur if treatment is delayed. Blood cultures should be obtained, and ultrasound or CT scanning should be performed. Broad-spectrum antibiotics should be initiated, and biliary decompression accomplished either endoscopically with an endoscopic sphincterotomy, via a percutaneous transhepatic biliary drainage procedure, or by surgical decompression. Endoscopic or percutaneous procedures are believed to be the treatment of choice in patients who are seriously ill and at high risk for complications. Elective surgery, which generally includes cholecystectomy and bile duct exploration, can be deferred to a later date when the patient has stabilized.

Pancreatic Infections

Although acute pancreatitis is usually a sterile inflammatory process, infectious complications may occur. In addition, a variety of viral infections (rubella; Coxsackie B virus; mumps; Epstein-Barr virus; cytomegalovirus; and hepatitis A, B, and C), *Mycoplasma pneumoniae;* and parasites such as *A. lumbricoides* have been implicated as causes of pancreatitis.[118] Some patients may develop sterile or infected pancreatic or peripancreatic necrosis or infected pancreatic pseudocysts as complications of acute pancreatitis.[118] Necrosis of either the parenchyma or the duct system occurs in the absence of bacteria and usually occurs very early in the clinical course of severe pancreatitis. Risk for infection increases as necrosis becomes more extensive. Of patients with acute pancreatitis, only approximately 5% develop pancreatic infections; however, the highest mortality from pancreatitis occurs in these patients.[118] The incidence of infection increases over the first few weeks and peaks during the third and fourth weeks. Patients with extensive necrosis, those who are very ill, and those with early infection have the highest mortality.[118] CT scan with high-dose contrast is the most useful modality for predicting who is at risk for the development of infection. Between 40% and 70% of those with more than 30% necrosis seen on CT scan will ultimately become infected.[118] If air bubbles are seen in the region of the pancreas, it should be presumed that infection is present. Clinically, it is extremely difficult to determine whether patients with necrotizing pancreatitis have superimposed infection because sterile pancreatic necrosis may cause leukocytosis and fever even in the absence of infection, and approximately 50% of infected patients may not show early clinical signs of infection. CT-guided aspiration of necrotic pancreatic tissue for Gram stain and aerobic and anaerobic culture is a useful procedure to determine the presence of infection.[118] The microbiology resembles that of the intestinal flora. *E. coli* is seen in 25% of infections, followed by *Pseudomonas* species and *S. aureus*.[102] Fifteen percent of isolated organisms are composed of a variety of anaerobes. Antibiotics that penetrate into pancreatic tissue include the carbapenems, especially imipenem, fluoroquinolones, piperacillin, advanced-generation cephalosporins, and metronidazole.[103]

Clostridium Difficile Colitis

Clostridium difficile causes a spectrum of disease ranging from asymptomatic carriage to a fulminant, relapsing, or life-threatening colitis.[119,120] Antibiotics or chemotherapeutic agents have been associated with alteration of bowel flora and growth of *C. difficile*.[119,120] Diarrhea may develop while a patient is receiving antibiotics or several weeks after completion of a course of antibiotics. Only strains that produce toxins are capable of causing diarrhea or colitis.[119,120] Common symptoms include fever, which may be either low grade or high, crampy abdominal pain, and diarrhea, which is watery, profuse, and foul-smelling. Approximately 50% of patients will have leukocytes in smears of the stool.[119,120] Leukocytosis is common. The diagnosis is established by assaying the stool for *C. difficile* toxin. Complications of severe disease include electrolyte derangements, dehydration, toxic megacolon, and colonic perforation. Some patients may have little or no diarrhea but present with toxic megacolon, colonic perforation, peritonitis, or even septic shock without other localizing symptoms. An emerging strain of *C. difficile* has enhanced toxin production and causes outbreaks of illness with increased severity, lack of response to antibiotic therapy, and frequent relapse.[121] The incidence of colectomy for refractory disease with these infections also appears to be increased. Despite some suggestions to the contrary, metronidazole remains first-line treatment; empiric therapy with oral metronidazole should be started while testing for *C. difficile* toxin is being performed. If patients do not have a favorable response within 3 to 5 days, they should be switched to oral vancomycin.

LIFE-THREATENING INFECTIONS OF THE HEAD AND NECK

Ludwig's Angina, Lateral Pharyngeal Space Infections, and Peritonsillar Abscess

Infections arising from the flora of the mouth and posterior pharynx can involve the fascial planes of the neck and have the potential to progress rapidly and cause serious life-threatening illness.[122,123] In general, these infections are polymicrobial and the microbiology reflects the normal flora of the mouth. They spread rapidly through contiguous fascial spaces and it is essential that they be diagnosed and treated expeditiously to prevent serious sequelae such as airway obstruction, hematogenous infection, and mediastinitis. Potentially life-threatening infections of the head and neck may involve three cervical spaces. Fascial planes both separate and connect these areas. The spaces and infectious manifestations are as follows and representative images are shown in Figure 55-4:

1. The submandibular space may be affected by infection involving the flora of the mouth and tongue. A bilateral cellulitis of the soft tissue, known as *Ludwig's angina*, is the most important type of infection in the submandibular space. Manifestations of this infection include enlargement of the tongue and submandibular swelling. An odontogenic focus is the etiology of 70% to 90% of cases.[123,124]
2. The lateral pharyngeal space consists of an anterior and a posterior compartment divided by the styloid process. The anterior compartment is composed of musculature, and the posterior compartment has nerves

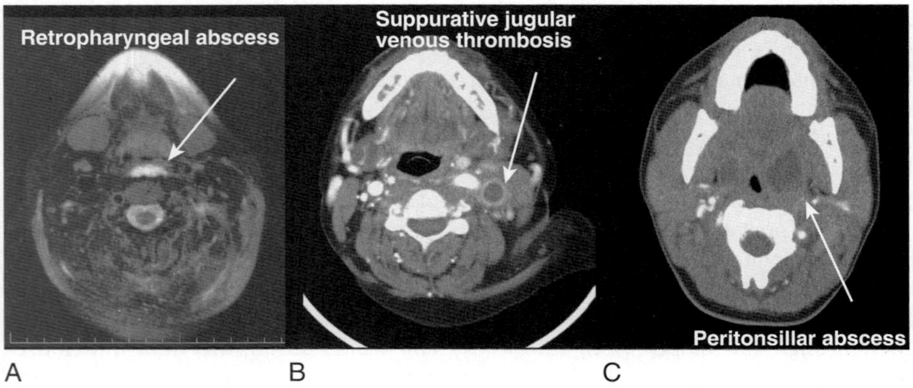

Figure 55-4. Magnetic resonance imaging and computed tomography images showing a variety of life-threatening head and neck infections including retropharyngeal abscess **(A)**, suppurative jugular venous thrombosis **(B)**, and peritonsillar abscess **(C)**. (Images provided by Dr. Joshua Brody, Department of Radiology, the Cooper Health System.)

and blood vessels. Infection in the anterior compartment causes soft tissue swelling that results in unilateral trismus caused by irritation of the internal pterygoid muscle, induration and swelling along the angle of the jaw, bulging of the palatine tonsil into the posterior pharynx, and systemic toxicity. Patients may present with unilateral neck or jaw pain along with ear pain and dysphagia. Pain may worsen when the head is turned because of compression of infected tissue. Dental infection, upper respiratory infection, pharyngitis, and otitis media with mastoiditis may all cause lateral pharyngeal space infection.[125] The carotid sheath is within the posterior compartment and contains the internal carotid artery, the internal jugular vein, the vagus nerve, cranial nerves IX-XII, and lymph nodes. When infection occurs in this space, patients most commonly present with signs of sepsis without localizing signs at the neck. Generally signs and symptoms are related to complications from involvement of the neurovascular structures. The most common complication is suppurative jugular venous thrombosis. Bacteremia and septic emboli may be seen. The carotid artery may also rupture. The carotid sheath is dense and not easily penetrated, so generally arterial erosion is usually a complication of longer duration infections (1 to 2 weeks). Intermittent bleeding from the mouth or nose may precede rupture.[124] Cranial nerve palsies or Horner's syndrome may occur.

3. The retropharyngeal space contains an area that extends from the base of the skull to the diaphragm and hence is a portal for neck infections to extend into the chest. Infections of the retropharyngeal space or prevertebral space may spread as a result of extension through this area. Retropharyngeal space abscesses are relatively uncommon and are most often seen in young children. These abscesses usually result from odontogenic infection, penetrating trauma, or peritonsillar abscess. Peritonsillar abscess, also known as "quinsy," is an unusual complication of acute tonsillitis seen predominantly in adolescents and young adults. Patients usually present with fever, pharyngitis, odynophagia, dysphagia, trismus, drooling, and a muffled voice that has been described as "hot potato" in quality. On examination there is usually swelling of the anterior tonsillar pillars and soft palate. The most common symptoms of retropharyngeal space infection in adults are fever, dysphagia, pharyngeal pain, dyspnea, noisy breathing, and stiff neck. A lateral radiograph of the neck may reveal prevertebral soft tissue swelling. Any deep neck infection has the potential to spread to the mediastinum via the retropharyngeal space. Other potential complications of infection of the oral cavity are aspiration pneumonia and lung abscess.

Because most of these infections originate from an odontogenic focus, the microbiology reflects polymicrobial oral flora and generally includes *Bacteroides* species, aerobic streptococci, microaerophilic streptococci, peptostreptococci, fusobacteria, *Veillonella* species, and *Actinomyces* species. On occasion, enteric gram-negative bacilli, *P. aeruginosa* or *S. aureus* may play a role.[125] Deep neck infections are medical and surgical emergencies. Complications include hematogenous dissemination with sepsis syndrome, airway obstruction, necrotizing pneumonia or empyema, osteomyelitis of the mandible or maxilla, mediastinitis, or intracranial extension and cavernous sinus thrombosis. A contrasted CT scan or MRI of the neck is important to help define the anatomy including the vascular structures and to indicate potential need for drainage. Consultation should be obtained from an otolaryngologist.

Lemierre Syndrome

Lemierre syndrome (postanginal sepsis) is a fulminant infectious syndrome caused by acute oropharyngeal infection that is complicated by secondary septic thrombophlebitis of the internal jugular vein. It is usually seen in healthy adolescents or young adults. *Fusobacterium* species are most commonly implicated. Complications include septicemia, pneumonia, empyema, meningitis, brain abscess, and vocal cord paralysis. This infection may complicate a routine case of infectious mononucleosis.[126] Therapy usually consists of surgical drainage of the focus and broad-spectrum IV antibiotic therapy.

When patients have dyspnea, stridor, or an inability to handle secretions, an artificial airway should be established. Airway obstruction is most likely to occur in infections of the submandibular space. Surgically obtained specimens should be cultured aerobically and anaerobically. For patients with peritonsillar abscess, high-dose IV penicillin is the therapy of choice. Other treatment options include clindamycin or ampicillin-sulbactam. Patients with peritonsillar abscess should undergo incision and drainage to prevent spontaneous rupture, aspiration pneumonia, airway obstruction, or dissection of infection into the lateral retropharyngeal space. Surgical drainage is especially important for infections involving the retropharyngeal and lateral pharyngeal space. Approximately half of cases of Ludwig's angina in the submandibular space can be cured without surgical intervention.[124]

Epiglottitis

Acute infectious epiglottitis is an inflammatory process of the epiglottis, supraglottis, and surrounding soft tissues.[127] Since the near disappearance of invasive *H. influenzae* infections in children following universal immunization, acute epiglottitis has become primarily a disease of adults, with an annual incidence of 1 case/100,000 and peak incidence from ages 40 to 50. Patients present with severe pharyngitis; pain on swallowing; fever; and, less commonly, shortness of breath, hoarseness, and muffled voice. Findings on examination include marked anterior neck tenderness, lymphadenopathy, drooling, and respiratory distress.[127,128] The standard of diagnosis for suspected epiglottitis in adults is visualization of the epiglottis with indirect laryngoscopy.[127] Radiography has low sensitivity and specificity. Treatment includes maintenance of an airway; depending on severity and rapidity of onset of symptoms, this may include emergent tracheostomy, elective intubation, or only close observation in an intensive care unit for the mildest cases.[127] Antibiotics active against the most commonly implicated pathogens, *H. influenzae* and beta hemolytic streptococci, are administered, and corticosteroids are generally recommended.[127,128] Disease may be more aggressive in HIV-infected or other immunocompromised individuals.

Mediastinitis

Acute mediastinitis is an infection of mediastinal structures that can develop from direct extension of pharyngeal and neck infections (descending necrotizing mediastinitis), from esophageal trauma or rupture, or as a complication of cardiothoracic surgical procedures.[129] Descending necrotizing mediastinitis and mediastinitis from esophageal procedures have both become uncommon, and most cases are seen as complications of cardiothoracic surgery procedures or from trauma.[129,130] Symptoms of mediastinitis may initially be mild, but as disease progresses, patients will develop chest pain; dysphagia; and respiratory distress, as well as fever, tachycardia, crepitus, and localized swelling. Sepsis is common. Patients with postcardiothoracic mediastinitis will generally have evidence of local or deep sternal wound infection. Leukocytosis is typical. Plain films may show mediastinal widening; mediastinal air-fluid levels; and subcutaneous, mediastinal, or pericardial air. CT is more sensitive than plain radiographs for diagnosis; contrast esophagography with water-soluble contrast is the optimal study for esophageal perforation.[129]

Treatment of infection related to descending neck infection or esophageal perforation requires broad-spectrum antibiotics directed at oropharyngeal flora including streptococci, oral anaerobes, and gram-negative bacilli and surgical intervention.[129] Mediastinitis following cardiothoracic surgery is most commonly caused by staphylococci, but a large variety of other gram-positive and gram-negative organisms have been implicated. Treatment requires open or closed surgical drainage and antibiotic therapy.[130]

SERIOUS VECTOR-BORNE INFECTIONS

Rocky Mountain Spotted Fever

Tickborne rickettsial diseases cause severe illness and death in otherwise healthy individuals. Although the various rickettsial diseases may have distinct epidemiology and etiology, they are clinically similar.[131] Rocky Mountain spotted fever (RMSF) is caused by *Rickettsia rickettsii,* which is a gram-negative, obligate, intracellular bacteria. Infection is transmitted to humans by a variety of ticks but most frequently by the dog tick, *Dermacentor variabilis.* The incidence is greatest in the southeastern and southcentral United States. The vast majority of cases occur from April to September. Reported risks for infection include living in wooded areas and exposure to dogs. *R. rickettsii* infects endothelial cells, resulting in vasculitis, which leads to the characteristic rash and involvement of the lungs, brain, and other organs.[131-134] Following an incubation period of 3 to 12 days, patients frequently present with fever, rash, and evidence or history of a tick bite, although 30% to 40% of patients do not recall a tick bite.[131] Other symptoms include chills; myalgias; nausea; vomiting; abdominal pain (that may be severe enough to mimic an acute abdomen); diarrhea; headache; photophobia; mental status changes; conjunctival injection; and, periodically, cough or arrhythmias secondary to myocarditis. The rash is classically an erythematous macular rash that appears initially on the ankles/soles and wrists/palms and spreads centripetally to the arms, legs, trunk, neck, and face.[132-134] The lesions evolve to become petechial. The rash typically appears after 2 to 6 days of illness. Although rash is the hallmark of this illness, up to 20% of patients are "spotless" or have an atypical rash at presentation.[135] The most characteristic laboratory abnormality is thrombocytopenia. The white blood cell count is usually normal. More than two thirds of cases have increased band forms. Creatine phosphokinase level may be elevated, as may transaminases and bilirubin.[131] Chest radiograph may reveal infiltrates consistent with pneumonitis or acute respiratory distress syndrome (ARDS). RMSF is frequently a severe illness. Serious complications, in addition to ARDS, include renal failure, disseminated intravascular coagulopathy (DIC), hemophagocytic syndrome, meningoencephalitis, and gangrene.[131]

Rickettsial infections may be difficult to diagnose. The best way to establish the diagnosis of RMSF in patients with a rash is by obtaining a skin biopsy for immunohistochemical or direct immunofluorescent staining. This test has a sensitivity of 70% and specificity of 100%.[132] PCR can also be performed on tissue specimens.[131] Serologies by indirect immunofluorescence or ELISA may also be performed. Empiric treatment with doxycycline should be instituted for suspected RMSF before laboratory confirmation of a diagnosis. Distinguishing RMSF from meningococcemia is especially important. Gastrointestinal symptoms, a pulse-temperature disparity, periorbital edema, edema of the extremities, conjunctival injection, hepatosplenomegaly, and elevated serum transaminases are more likely in RMSF. If there is any doubt as to which infection is present, treatment for both should be instituted empirically.

Ehrlichiosis and Anaplasmosis

Illnesses that cause fever and rash are listed in Table 55-7. Other serious rickettsial diseases are human monocytic ehrlichiosis and human granulocytic anaplasmosis caused by *Ehrlichia chaffeensis* and *Anaplasma phagocytophilium,* respectively.[131] They have a similar presentation, but rash is much less commonly seen than in RMSF. These infections are transmitted by ixodid ticks and are distributed across the United States and Europe. Both are intracellular pathogens that infect leukocytes. Common laboratory abnormalities include leukopenia, relative lymphopenia, presence of atypical lymphocytes, eosinopenia, and thrombocytopenia.[136] Anemia and renal involvement are rare. PCR of serum is now the rapid diagnostic test of choice. Blood smear microscopy might reveal the presence of morulae in infected leukocytes, which is highly suggestive of anaplasmosis or, less commonly,

Table 55-7. Differential Diagnosis of Fever with Maculopapular and/or Petechial Rash	
Rocky Mountain Spotted Fever	***Mycoplasma Pneumoniae* Infection**
Meningococcal disease	Leptospirosis
Enteroviral infection (echovirus and coxsackievirus)	Secondary syphilis
Human herpes virus 6 infection (roseola)	Kawasaki disease
Human parvovirus B19 infection (fifth disease)	Thrombotic thrombocytopenic purpura (TTP)
Epstein-Barr virus infection	Drug reactions
Disseminated gonococcal Infection	Immune complex-mediated illness
Murine typhus	Toxic-shock syndrome
Monocytotrophic ehrlichiosis	Erythema multiforme
Group A *Streptococcus* pharyngitis	Stevens-Johnson syndrome

ehrlichiosis.[131] Serologies can also be diagnostic. Complications include ARDS, bleeding, rhabdomyolysis, and myocarditis.[136]

Malaria

Malaria is a protozoan infection transmitted by female anopheline mosquitoes. The severity of malaria infection depends on a variety of factors including host immunity and age and the species of malaria. Of the four main human pathogens, *Plasmodium falciparum* causes the most serious infection. Chloroquine-resistant *P. falciparum* has spread through many parts of the world. The incubation period of *P. falciparum* is approximately 12 days. It parasitizes all ages of red blood cells and causes the highest degree of parasitemia of any of the species.[137] *P. falciparum* has worldwide distribution and causes a severe illness frequently termed *black water fever*. Common symptoms and signs include fever, chills, headache, myalgia, arthralgia, and hepatosplenomegaly. Other symptoms include jaundice, vomiting, diarrhea, and nonproductive cough.[137] Severe malaria is a multisystem illness with a mortality of up to 25% in the nonimmune, untreated patient.[137] Defining criteria for severe malaria include (1) severe normocytic anemia, (2) renal failure, (3) pulmonary edema, (4) hypoglycemia, (5) shock, (6) DIC, (7) metabolic acidosis and (8) cerebral involvement with coma or generalized seizures. Other signs or symptoms frequently present in severe disease include altered mental status, prostration, jaundice, and high-grade fever.[137,138] Additional laboratory features include thrombocytopenia, elevated transaminases, hyperbilirubinemia, evidence of coagulopathy, elevated BUN and creatinine levels, and macroscopic hemoglobinuria. Parasitemia levels are often high. Patients may develop pulmonary edema, or pulmonary edema may occur after successful treatment of parasitemia. ARDS or secondary infection with bacterial pneumonia may also occur.

The differential diagnosis is broad and includes bacterial sepsis, meningitis, rickettsial infections, pneumonia, viral hemorrhagic fever, leptospirosis, severe influenza, meningococcemia, typhoid fever, and viral hepatitis. The diagnostic test of choice is the thick/thin peripheral blood smear, which confirms the diagnosis. However, patients from an endemic area may occasionally present with another serious illness that may be erroneously attributed to malaria because of incidental parasitemia. Treatment for severe *P. falciparum* malaria consists of IV quinine or IV quinidine.[139,140] When using the latter, the QT interval should be monitored. Adjunctive therapy for severe malaria may include exchange transfusion, although this is controversial.[139] In addition, broad-spectrum antibiotics for bacterial sepsis and/or pneumonia should be given if there is concern for secondary bacterial infection.

Dengue

Hemorrhagic fever is caused by a variety of viruses, and the hallmark is bleeding. Generally dengue has a geographic endemicity, being seen predominantly in Africa, South America, and Asia. Dengue is transmitted by mosquitoes and has no other reservoir except for humans. It is now endemic in at least 112 countries worldwide including many parts of the Caribbean, Mexico, Puerto Rico, and Central America.[141-144] In many areas the mosquito vector is *Aedes aegypti*. This mosquito species has adapted to man-made conditions, and therefore urban transmission is frequent. The virus has four serotypes, each with a number of genotypes.[143] Dengue is generally divided into four clinical syndromes: a mild influenza-like illness; classic dengue (characterized by fever, retro-orbital headache, severe bone pain and myalgia, maculopapular rash, and nausea and vomiting); dengue hemorrhagic fever (DHF); and dengue shock syndrome (DSS).[141] DHF or DSS may manifest after a few days of typical dengue symptoms, and classically symptoms start as the temperature normalizes.[144] Those with DHF have bleeding, petechiae, ascites, pleural effusion, and sometimes encephalopathy. Laboratory features include hemoconcentration, leukopenia, elevated transaminases, and thrombocytopenia.[144] The differential diagnosis includes many of the infectious entities in the differential of malaria. Noninfectious illnesses in the differential include hemolytic-uremic syndrome and thrombotic thrombocytopenic purpura. Diagnosis is established serologically, and treatment is supportive.[143]

SEVERE VIRAL INFECTIONS

Hantavirus Pulmonary Syndrome

Acute infections caused by species of hantavirus are transmitted to humans from rodents and are characterized by nephritis and hemorrhage or a syndrome of acute noncardiogenic pulmonary edema.[145] Four hantaviruses are associated with hantavirus pulmonary syndrome (HPS). This syndrome was first recognized more than a decade ago in the southwestern United States. Rodents, especially deer mice, are the host. Transmission to humans occurs by inhalation of aerosols of rodent urine or feces. Initial symptoms of HPS resemble those of influenza and consist of fever, myalgia, headache, and gastrointestinal symptoms. Two to 15 days later, acute noncardiogenic pulmonary edema and shock develop.[146-148] Laboratory findings at this stage include leukocytosis, hemoconcentration, and thrombocytopenia. Chest radiographic findings include increased vascular markings consistent with pulmonary edema, bilateral infiltrates, and pleural effusions.[149] Treatment is supportive and consists of ventilator support and treatment of shock. This syndrome has a high mortality of 50% to 70%, but those who survive improve rapidly after 5 to 7 days and often have complete recovery within 2 to 3 weeks.

Influenza

Influenza results from infection with influenza A or B virus. Infection occurs in yearly epidemics, typically during the winter in temperate climates, with occasional worldwide epidemics referred to as *pandemics,* which occur when there is antigenic shift (a major antigenic change resulting in a new subtype of influenza A).[150] These viruses are spread from person to person primarily through coughing and sneezing.[151] Onset of symptoms is abrupt and occurs after an incubation period of a day or two.[152] Symptoms include fever, chills, headache, myalgia, sore throat, and malaise.[153] Respiratory symptoms, especially a dry cough, are usually present. As systemic signs and symptoms decrease, respiratory complaints become more prominent. Of these, cough is the most frequent and may persist 1 to 2 weeks after fever resolves. Leukocytosis is common early in the illness, and mild leukopenia may be observed later. Most cases are not associated with any significant complications, but when complications do occur, pulmonary complications are the most frequent. Two types of pulmonary complications are recognized: primary influenza viral pneumonia and secondary bacterial pneumonia.[154] Primary influenza viral pneumonia occurs mainly in individuals with cardiovascular disease or in pregnant women. Rapid progression of fever, cough, dyspnea, and hypoxemia usually occurs. Chest radiographs reveal bilateral findings consistent with pulmonary edema. Patients may develop ARDS. Culture of the sputum fails to reveal significant bacteria, whereas viral cultures yield influenza virus. Mortality of this syndrome is high.

Secondary bacterial pneumonia is more common than primary viral pneumonia. It occurs most often in the elderly or those with preexisting pulmonary disease. Following a classic influenza syndrome and a period of improvement of a few days, there is recrudescence of fever and cough accompanied by sputum production and consolidation on chest radiograph. Gram stain and culture of sputum most often demonstrate *Streptococcus pneumoniae, Haemophilus influenzae,* or *S. aureus.* Other rare complications of influenza include Reye's syndrome, which is an often fatal CNS and hepatic complication, myositis, transverse myelitis, myocarditis, and pericarditis.[155] Influenza virus is readily isolated from nasal or throat specimens, sputum, or tracheal secretions in the first 2 or 3 days of illness. Severe influenza viral pneumonia requires intensive monitoring and support. The neuraminidase inhibitors, inhaled zanamivir and oral oseltamivir, are active against influenza A and B viruses and are effective in treating acute influenza if started early in the illness.[150] Secondary bacterial pneumonia should be treated with antibiotics. Currently, many countries are preparing for a possible avian influenza pandemic.[156] Respiratory syncytial virus is emerging as an important cause of serious illness in the elderly and high-risk adults with clinical manifestations, length of hospital stay, use of ICU, and mortality similar to influenza.[157]

POTENTIAL AGENTS OF BIOTERRORISM

Potential agents of bioterrorism include rare infections that may occur sporadically in specific epidemiologic settings, such as anthrax, as well as diseases considered eradicated, such as smallpox. Features of these illnesses are their potential to cause illness and death, the potential for large-scale dissemination, their ability to cause public disruption, and the requirement for specific public health interventions in the setting of an outbreak. Illness is generally severe, and infected patients are likely to require admission to critical care units. Recognition of these syndromes by clinicians is crucial to triggering the ap-propriate medical, public health, and other governmental response.

Anthrax

Bacillus anthracis, the causative agent of anthrax, is an aerobic, gram-positive, sporulating bacillus. When human infection occurs, spores germinate in blood and tissue. Human infection can be of three types: (1) cutaneous, (2) inhalational, and (3) gastrointestinal.[158] Cutaneous is the most common and characteristically appears as a painless papule that evolves to a vesicular stage and then to a depressed black eschar surrounded by a ring of vesicles. Untreated, it carries a mortality of approximately 20%.[158]

The inhalational form is the form most likely to be encountered in the critical care setting. After an incubation period of generally 1 to 7 days but potentially up to 60 days, patients present with fever, malaise, dry cough, and an influenza-like illness. Progression to severe respiratory distress and septic shock occurs. The hallmark of this infection is a hemorrhagic mediastinitis.[158,159] Mortality has been as high as 85%. In virtually all cases, chest radiographs are abnormal and show either a widened mediastinum and/or pleural effusions. CT scan is particularly sensitive in detecting mediastinal changes.[160] Blood cultures are positive in 70% of cases. Clinical suspicion should be raised by the sudden appearance of multiple cases of severe influenza-like illness with a fulminant course and high mortality. The diagnosis is generally established by culturing the organism from blood, CSF, pleural fluid or vesicular fluid; PCR; or biopsy. Therapy is initially empiric and consists of the combination of ciprofloxacin or doxycycline plus clindamycin and rifampin.[158,159]

Smallpox

Smallpox is caused by the variola virus. This serious infection is highly contagious and fatal in about 30% of cases. Two major clinical forms exist, with the most common being variola major. This is a severe form with extensive rash and high fever. After an incubation period of 12 to 14 days, patients develop high fever, malaise, headache, myalgias, and vomiting. The rash appears initially as small intraoral spots and within 24 hours develops on the face, then spreads to the legs, feet, arms, and hands.[161] The rash appears as papules, which are filled with a thick, opaque fluid and have a depressed center. They evolve into pustules, which are raised, round, and firm to the touch. The differential diagnosis includes varicella. Treatment is supportive. The antiviral cidofovir may have activity.[162]

Plague

The causative agent of plague is *Yersinia pestis,* an aerobic gram-negative bacillus. The three clinical forms are (1) bubonic, (2) pneumonic, and (3) septicemic.[163,164] Pneumonic plague is transmitted person to person through inhalation of contaminated aerosols and is highly contagious. After an incubation period of 2 to 3 days, patients develop fever, chills, headache, hemoptysis, dyspnea, stridor, cyanosis, respiratory failure, circulatory collapse, and bleeding.[163,164] Diagnosis is based on clinical suspicion and cultures, and treatment is with streptomycin and doxycycline.[163,164]

Tularemia

Tularemia is caused by *Franciscella tularensis,* which is a gram-negative coccobacillus. Types of infection include ulceroglandular, typhoidal, and pneumonic. If there were to be an intentional release of this agent, infection would likely occur via the aerosol route.[165,166] Symptoms include cough, substernal pain, abdominal pain, prostration, fever, chills, and headache. Diagnosis is established by culture onto special media or by serology. Treatment is with streptomycin.

Viral Hemorrhagic Fevers

Viral hemorrhagic fevers are caused by several different families of viruses. Symptoms generally include fever, myalgia, hemorrhage, shock, coma, seizures, and possibly renal failure. The diagnosis is established by viral isolation or serologically. Treatment involves supportive care. The antiviral ribavirin may have a role in treatment.[167]

KEY POINTS

- Of patients with bacterial meningitis, 95% will have at least two of the following symptoms: fever, headache, stiff neck, and altered sensorium.
- Morbidity and mortality of bacterial meningitis are decreased with both prompt administration of antibiotics and use of dexamethasone as adjunctive therapy.
- The standard for diagnosis of herpes encephalitis is PCR of CSF, and treatment for suspected herpes encephalitis should be continued until PCR results are back.
- *S. aureus* has become the most common cause of bacterial endocarditis, and *S. aureus* endocarditis is associated with a higher risk of complications and higher mortality.
- Major indications for surgery in acute endocarditis include congestive heart failure, persistent bacteremia and sepsis, ongoing emboli on appropriate antibiotic therapy, and local valvular complications such as dehiscence and perivalvular abscess.
- Staphylococcal and streptococcal toxic shock syndromes are mediated by systemic effects of bacterial exotoxins that trigger massive release of cytokines.
- Necrotizing fasciitis, although uncommon, is a severe infection that causes necrosis of subcutaneous tissue and fascia and requires prompt identification and therapy to minimize morbidity and mortality.
- CA-MRSA is an emerging infection that can cause life-threatening illness including necrotizing skin infections, pneumonia, and sepsis.
- Empiric antibiotic therapy for bacterial peritonitis should be directed at gram-negative bacillary organisms and anaerobes.
- The presence of an intra-abdominal abscess should be entertained in febrile patients without any obvious cause of fever or in the seriously ill patient who is on corticosteroid therapy.
- An emerging strain of *C. difficile* has enhanced toxin production and causes increased severity of illness, poor response to therapy, and frequent relapse.
- Serious infections of the head and neck are polymicrobial and most frequently have an odontogenic source.
- Serious complications of influenza include primary influenza viral pneumonia, bacterial pneumonia, Reye's syndrome, and myocarditis/pericarditis.

REFERENCES

1. van de Beek D, de Gans J, Tunkel AR, et al: Community-acquired bacterial meningitis in adults. N Engl J Med 2006;354:44-53.
2. van de Beek D, de Gans J, Spanjaard L, et al: Clinical features and prognostic factors in adults with bacterial meningitis. N Engl J Med 2004;352:1849-1859.
3. Schuchat A, Robinson K, Wenger JD, et al: Bacterial meningitis in the United States in 1995. N Engl J Med 1997;337:970-976.
4. Durand ML, Calderwood SB, Weber DJ, et al: Acute bacterial meningitis in adults: A review of 493 episodes. N Engl J Med 1993;328:21-28.
5. Tunkel AR, Hartman BJ, Kaplan SL, et al: Practice guidelines for the management of bacterial meningitis. Clin Infect Dis 2004;39:1267-1284.
6. Lexau CA, Lynefield R, Danila R, et al: Changing epidemiology of invasive pneumococcal disease among older adults in the era of pediatric pneumococcal conjugate vaccine. JAMA 2005;294:2043-2051.
7. Bilukha OO, Rosenstein N, National Center for Infectious Diseases, Centers for Disease Control and Prevention (CDC): Prevention and control of meningococcal disease. Recommendations of the Advisory Committee on Immunization Practices (ACIP). MMWR Recomm Rep 2005;54(RR-7):1-21.
8. Mylonakis E, Hohmann EL, Calderwood SB: Central nervous system infection with *Listeria monocytogenes:* 33 years' experience at a general hospital and review of 776 episodes from the literature. Medicine (Baltimore) 1998;77:313-336.
9. Hasbun R, Abrahams J, Jekel J, et al: Computed tomography of the head before lumbar puncture in adults with suspected meningitis. N Engl J Med 2001;345:1727-1733.
10. Korein J, Cravisto H, Leicach M: Reevaluation of lumbar puncture: A study of 129 patients with papilledema or intracranial hypertension. Neurology 1959;9:290-297.
11. Spanos A, Harrell FE Jr, Durack DT: Differential diagnosis of acute meningitis: An analysis of the predictive value of initial observations. JAMA 1989;262:2700-2707.
12. Genton B, Berger JP: Cerebrospinal fluid lactate in 78 cases of adult meningitis. Intensive Care Med 1990;16:196-200.
13. de Gans J, van de Beek D, European Dexamethasone in Adulthood Bacterial Meningitis Study Investigators: Dexamethasone in adults with bacterial meningitis. N Engl J Med 2002;347:1549-1556.
14. van de Beek D, de Gans J, McIntyre P, Prasad K: Steroids in adults with bacterial meningitis: A systematic review. Lancet Infect Dis 2004;4:139-143.
15. Wijdicks EFM: The clinical practice of critical care neurology, 2nd ed. New York, Oxford University Press, 2003, pp 316-328.
16. Flores-Cordero JM, Amaya-Villar R, Rincon-Ferrari MD, et al: Acute community-acquired bacterial meningitis in adults admitted to the intensive care unit: Clinical manifestations, management and prognostic factors. Intensive Care Med 2003;29:1967-1973.
17. Lindvall P, Ahlm C, Ericsson M, et al: Reducing intracranial pressure may increase survival among patients with bacterial meningitis. Clin Infect Dis 2004;38:384-390.
18. Kaplan SL, Mason EO Jr: Management of infections due to antibiotic-resistant *Streptococcus pneumoniae.* Clin Microbiol Rev 1998;11:628-644.
19. Chaudhuri A, Kennedy PGE: Diagnosis and treatment of viral encephalitis. Postgrad Med J 2002;78:575-583.
20. Steiner I, Budka H, Chaudhuri A, et al: Viral encephalitis: A review of diagnostic methods and guidelines for management. Euro J Neurol 205;12:331-343.
21. Whitley RJ, Gnann JW: Viral encephalitis: Familiar infections and emerging pathogens. Lancet 2002;359:507-513.
22. Tyler KL: Herpes simplex virus infections of the central nervous system: Encephalitis and meningitis, including Mollaret's. Herpes 2004;11(Suppl 2):57A-64A.
23. Lima MA, Koralnik IJ: New features of progressive multifocal leukoencephalopathy in the era of highly active antiretroviral therapy and natalizumab. J Neurovirol 2005;11(Suppl 3):52-57.
24. Hayes EB, Sejvar JJ, Zaki SR, et al: Virology, pathology, and clinical manifestations of West Nile Virus disease. Emerg Infect Dis 2005;11:1174-1179.
25. Sejvar JJ, Haddad MB, Tierney BC, et al: Neurologic manifestations and outcome of West Nile virus infection. JAMA 2003;290:511-515.
26. Willoughby RE Jr, Tieves KS, Hoffman GM, et al: Survival after treatment of rabies with induction of coma. N Engl J Med 2005;352:2508-2514.
27. Gunther G, Haglund M: Tick-borne encephalopathies: Epidemiology, diagnosis, treatment and prevention. CNS Drugs 2005;19:1009-1032.
28. Marra CM: Neurosyphilis. Curr Neurol Neurosci Rep 204;4:435-440.
29. Glaser CA, Gilliam S, Schnurr D, et al: In search of encephalitis etiologies: Diagnostic challenges in the California Encephalitis Project, 1998-2000. Clin Infect Dis 2003;36:731-742.
30. Aurelius E, Johansson B, Sköldenberg B, et al: Encephalitis in immunocompetent patients due to Herpes simplex virus type 1 or 2 as determined by two specific polymerase chain reaction and antibody assays of cerebrospinal fluid. J Med Virol 1993;39:179-186.
31. Domingues RB, Tsanaclis AM, Pannuti CS, et al: Evaluation of the range of clinical presentations of herpes simplex encephalitis by using polymerase chain reaction assay of cerebrospinal fluid samples. Clin Infect Dis 1997;25:86-91.
32. McCabe K, Tyler KL, Tanabe J: Diffusion-weighted MRI abnormalities as a clue to the diagnosis of herpes simplex encephalitis. Neurology 2003;61:1015-1016.
33. Aurelius E, Johansson B, Sköldenberg B, et al: Rapid diagnosis of herpes simplex encephalitis by nested polymerase chain reaction assay of cerebrospinal fluid. Lancet 1991;337:189-192.
34. Lakeman FD, Whitley RJ: Diagnosis of herpes simplex encephalitis: Application of polymerase chain reaction to cerebrospinal fluid from brain-biopsied patients and correlation with disease. J Infect Dis 1995;171:857-863.
35. Cinque P, Cleator GM, Weber T, et al: The role of laboratory investigation in the diagnosis and management of patients with suspected herpes simplex encephalitis: A consensus report. The EU Concerted Action on Virus Meningitis and Encephalitis. J Neurol Neurosurg Psychiatry 1996;61:339-345.
36. Centers for Disease Control and Prevention (CDC): West Nile Virus Activity—United States, January 1-December 1, 2005. MMWR Morb Mortal Wkly Rep 2005;54:1253-1256.
37. Li J, Loeb JA, Shy ME, et al: Asymmetric flaccid paralysis: A neuromuscular presentation of West Nile virus infection. Ann Neurol 2003;53:703-710.
38. Calfee DP, Wispelwey B: Brain abscess. Semin Neurol 2000;20:353-360.
39. Mathisen GE, Johnson JP: Brain abscess. Clin Infect Dis 1997;25:763-781.
40. Tonon E, Scotton PG, Gallucci M, et al: Brain abscess: Clinical aspects of 100 patients International J Infect Dis 2006;10:103-109.
41. Lu CH, Chang WN, Lin YC, et al: Bacterial brain abscess: Microbiological features, epidemiological trends and therapeutic outcomes. Q J Med 2002;95:501-509.
42. Mamidi A, DeSimone JA, Pomerantz RJ: Central nervous system infections in individuals with HIV-1 infection. J Neurovirol 2002;8:158-167.
43. Stapleton SR, Bell BA, Uttley D: Stereotactic aspiration of brain abscesses: Is this the treatment of choice? Acta Neurochir (Wien) 1993;121:15-19.
44. Siddiq F, Chowfin A, Tight R, et al: Medical vs. surgical management of spinal epidural abscess. Arch Intern Med 2004;164:2409-2412.
45. Reishaus E, Waldbaur H, Seeling W: Spinal epidural abscess: A meta-analysis of 915 cases. Neurosurg Rev 2000;232:175-202.
46. Maslen D, Jones SR, Crislip MA: Spinal epidural abscess: Optimizing patient care. Arch Intern Med 1993;153:1713-1721.
47. Tsiodras V, Falagas ME: Clinical assessment and medical treatment of spine infections. Clin Orthoped Res 2006;444:38-50.
48. Tleyjeh IM, Steckelberg JM, Murad HS, et al: Temporal trends in infective endocarditis: A population-based study

in Olmsted County, Minnesota. JAMA 2005;293:3022-3028.
49. Fowler VG, Miro JM, Hoen B, et al: *Staphylococcus aureus* endocarditis: A consequence of medical progress. *JAMA* 2005;293:3012-3021.
50. Baddour LM, Wilson WR, Bayer AS, et al: Infective endocarditis: diagnosis, antimicrobial therapy, and management of complications, a statement for healthcare professionals from the Committee on Rheumatic fever, Endocarditis, and Kawasaki disease, Council on Cardiovascular Disease in the Young, and the Councils on Clinical Cardiology, Stroke, and Cardiovascular Surgery and Anesthesia, American Heart association. Circulation 2005;111: e394-e433.
51. Hasbun R, Vikram HR, Barakat LA, et al: Complicated left-sided native valve endocarditis in adults: Risk classification for mortality. JAMA 2003;289:1933-1940.
52. Moreillon P, Que Y-A: Infective endocarditis. Lancet 2004;363: 139-149.
53. Durack DT, Lukes AS, Bright DK: New criteria for diagnosis of infective endocarditis: Utilization of specific echocardiographic findings. Am J Med 1994;96:200-209.
54. Li JS, Sexton DJ, Mick N, et al: Proposed modifications to the Duke criteria for the diagnosis of infective endocarditis. Clin Infect Dis 2000;30:633-638.
55. Heiro M, Nikoskelainen J, Engblom E, et al: Neurologic manifestations of infective endocarditis: A 17-year experience in a teaching hospital in Finland. Arch Intern Med 2000;160:2781-2787.
56. Vilacosta I, Graupner C, San Roman JA, et al: Risk of embolization after institution of antibiotic therapy for infective endocarditis. J Am Coll Cardiol 2002;39:1489-1495.
57. Bishara J, Leibovici L, Gartman-Israel D, et al: Long term outcome of infective endocarditis: The impact of early surgical intervention. Clin Infect Dis 2001;33:1636-1643.
58. Tornos P, Almirante B, Mirabet S, et al: Infective endocarditis due to *Staphylococcus aureus:* Deleterious effect of anticoagulant therapy. Arch Intern Med 1999;159:473-475.
59. Karchmer AW: Infections of prosthetic heart valves. In Waldvogel FA, Bisno A (eds): Infections Associated with Indwelling Medical Devices, 3rd ed. Washington DC, ASM Press, 2000, pp 145-172.
60. Mermel LA, Farr BM, Sheretz RJ: Guidelines for the management of intravascular catheter-related infections. Clin Infect Dis 2001;32:1249-1272.
61. Saxena AK, Panhotra BR: Haemodialysis catheter-related bloodstream infections: Current treatment options and strategies for prevention. Swiss Med Wkly 2005;135:127-138.
62. del Río A, Anguera I, Miró JM, et al: Surgical treatment of pacemaker and defibrillator lead endocarditis: The impact of electrode lead extraction on outcome. Chest 2003;124:1451-1455.
63. Eggimann P, Waldvogel FA: Pacemaker and defibrillator infections. In Waldvogel FA, Bisno A (eds): Infections Associated with Indwelling Medical Devices, 3rd ed. Washington, DC, ASM Press, 2000, pp 247-264.
64. Weinstein MP, Towns ML, Quartey SM, et al: The clinical significance of positive blood cultures in the 1990s: A prospective comprehensive evaluation of the microbiology, epidemiology and outcome of bacteremia and fungemia in adults. Clin Infect Dis 1997;24: 584-602.
65. Leiboici L, Konisberger H, Pitlik SD, et al: Bacteremia and fungemia of unknown origin in adults. Clin Infect Dis 1992;14:436-443.
66. Melles DC, de Marie S: Prevention of infections in hyposplenic and asplenic patients: An update. Neth J Med 2004;62:45-52.
67. Johnson DH, Cunha B: Infections in cirrhosis. Infect Dis Clin North Am 2001;15:363-371.
68. Bow EJ: Management of the febrile neutropenic cancer patient: Lessons from 40 years of study. Clin Microbiol Infect 2005;11(Suppl 5):24-29.
69. Thompson MJ, Ninis N, Perera R, et al: Clinical recognition of meningococcal disease in children and adolescents. Lancet 2006;367:397-403.
70. Rosenstein N, Perkins B, Stephens D, et al: Meningococcal disease. N Engl J Med 2001;344:1378-1388.
71. Trampuz A, Widmer AF, Fluckiger U, et al: Changes in the epidemiology of pneumococcal bacteremia in a Swiss university hospital during a 15-year period, 1986-2000. Mayo Clin Proc 2004;79:604-612.
72. Taylor SN, Sanders CY: Unusual manifestations of invasive pneumococcal infection. Am J Med 1999;107(Suppl 1A):12-27.
73. Fowler VG Jr, Olsen MK, Corey GR, et al: Clinical identifiers of complicated *Staphylococcus aureus* bacteremia. Arch Intern Med 2003;163:2066-2072.
74. Mitchell DH, Howden BP: Diagnosis and management of *Staphylococcus aureus* bacteriemia. Intern Med J 2005;35(Suppl 2):S17-24.
75. McCormick JK, Yarwood JM, Schlievert PM: Toxic shock syndrome and bacterial superantigens: An update. Annu Rev Microbiol 2001;55:77-104.
76. Haijeh RA, Reingold A, Weil A, et al: Toxic shock syndrome in the United States: Surveillance update, 1979-1996. Emerg Infect Dis 1999;5: 807-810.
77. Shands KN, Schmid GP, Dan BB, et al: Toxic-shock syndrome in menstruating women: Association with tampon use and *Staphylococcus aureus* and clinical features in 52 cases. N Engl J Med 1980;303:1436-1442.
78. Stevens DI: Streptococcal toxic-shock syndrome: Spectrum of disease, pathogenesis, and new concepts in treatment. Emerg Infect Dis 1995;1:69-78.
79. Davies HD, McGeer A, Schwartz B, et al: Invasive group A streptococcal infections in Ontario, Canada. Ontario Group A Streptococcal Study Group. N Engl J Med 1996;335:547-554.
80. Kaul R, McGeer A, Norrby-Teglund A, et al: Intravenous immunoglobulin therapy for streptococcal toxic shock syndrome—a comparative observational study. Clin Infect Dis 1999;28:800-807.
81. Richardson JP, Knight AL: The management and prevention of tetanus. J Emerg Med 1993;11:737-742.
82. Nagachinta T, Cortese MM, Roper MH, et al: Tetanus. In Centers for Disease Control and Prevention: Manual for the Surveillance of Vaccine Preventable Diseases. Atlanta, CDC, 2002, pp 1-8.
83. Villar RG, Elliott SP, Davenport KM: Botulism: the many faces of botulinum toxin and its potential for bioterrorism. Infect Dis Clin North Am 2006;20: 313-327.
84. Broder KR, Cortese MM, Iskander JK, et al: Preventing tetanus, diphtheria, and pertussis among adolescents: Use of tetanus toxoid, reduced diphtheria toxoid and acellular pertussis vaccines recommendations of the Advisory Committee on Immunization Practices (ACIP). MMWR Recomm Rep 2006;55(RR-3):1-34.
85. Lewis RT: Necrotizing soft-tissue infections. Infect Dis Clin North Am 1992;6:693-703.
86. Hasham S, Matteucci P, Stanley PRW, et al: Necrotising fasciitis. BMJ 2005;330:830-833.
87. McHenry CR, Piotrowski JJ, Petrinic D, et al: Determinants of mortality for necrotizing soft-tissue infections. Ann Surg 1995;221:558-563.
88. Young MH, Engleberg NC, Mulla ZD, et al: Therapies for necrotizing fasciitis. Expert Opin Biol Ther 2006;6: 155-165.
89. Plosker GL, Figgitt DP: Linezolid: A pharmacoeconomic review of its use in serious Gram-positive infections. Pharmacoeconomics 2005;23: 945-964.
90. Darabi K, Abdel-Wahab O, Dzik WH: Current usage of intravenous immune globulin and the rationale behind it: The Massachusetts General Hospital data and a review of the literature. Transfusion 2006;46:741-753.
91. Vinh DC, Embil JM: Rapidly progressive soft tissue infections. Lancet Infect Dis 2005;5:501-513.
92. Bisno AL, Stevens DL: Streptococcal infections of skin and soft tissues. N Engl J Med 1996;334:240-244.
93. Iorianni P, Oliver GC: Synergistic soft tissue infections of the perineum. Dis Colon Rectum 1992;35:640-644.
94. Jallali N, Withey S, Butler PE: Hyperbaric oxygen as adjuvant therapy in the management of necrotizing fasciitis. Am J Surg 2005;189:462-466.
95. Klontz KC, Lieb S, Schreiber M, et al: Syndrome of Vibrio vulnificus infections: Clinical and epidemiologic features in Florida cases, 1981-1987. Ann Intern Med 1988;109:318-323.
96. Drews TD, Temte JL, Fox BC: Community-associated methicillin-resistant *Staphylococcus aureus:* Review of an emerging public health concern. WMJ 2006;105:52-57.
97. Kluytmans-Vandenbergh MF, Kluytmans JA: Community-acquired methicillin-resistant *Staphylococcus*

aureus: Current perspectives. Clin Microbiol Infect 2006;1:9-15.
98. Kollef MH, Micek ST: Methicillin-resistant Staphylococcus aureus: A new community-acquired pathogen? Curr Opin Infect Dis 2006;19:161-168.
99. Maltezou HC, Giamarellou H: Community-acquired methicillin-resistant *Staphylococcus aureus* infections. Int J Antimicrob Agents 2006;27:87-96.
100. Thielman NM, Guerrant RL: Enteric fever and other causes of abdominal symptoms with fever. In Mandell GL, Bennett JE, Dolin R (eds): Principles and Practice of Infectious Diseases, 6th ed. Philadelphia, Elsevier, 2005, pp 1273-1286.
101. Goldberg MB, Rubin RH: The spectrum of *Salmonella* infection. Infect Dis Clin North Am 1988;2:571-598.
102. Marshall JC, Innes M: Intensive care unit management of intra-abdominal infection. Crit Care Med 2003;31:2228-2237.
103. Gorbach SL: Treatment of intra-abdominal infection. J Antimicrob Chemother 1993;31(Suppl A):67-78.
104. Tellado JM, Wilson SE: Empiric treatment of nosocomial intra-abdominal infections: A focus on the carbapenems. Surg Infect 2005;6:329-343.
105. Blot S, De Waele JJ: Critical issues in the clinical management of complicated intra-abdominal infections. Drugs 2005;65: 1611-1620.
106. Wong PF, Gilliam AD, Kuman S, et al: Antibiotic regimens for secondary peritonitis of gastrointestinal origin in adults. Cochrane Database Syst Rev 2005;18(2):CD004539.
107. Minton J, Stanley P: Intra-abdominal infections. Clin Med 2004;4:519-523.
108. Gilbert JA, Kamath PS: Spontaneous bacterial peritonitis. An update. Mayo Clin Proc 1995;70:365-370.
109. Bhuva M, Ganger D, Jensen D: Spontaneous bacterial peritonitis. An update on evaluation, management, and prevention. Am J Med 1994;97:169-175.
110. Wilcox CM, Dismukes WE: Spontaneous bacterial peritonitis: A review of pathogenesis, diagnosis and treatment. Medicine (Baltimore) 1987;66:447-456.
111. Runyon BA, Hoefs JC: Culture-negative neutrocytic ascites: A variant of spontaneous peritonitis. Hepatology 1984;4:1209-1211.
112. Cheadle WG, Spain DA: The continuing challenge of intra-abdominal infection. Am J Surg 2003;186:15S-22S.
113. Levison ME, Bush LM: Peritonitis and intraperitoneal abscesses. In Mandell GL, Bennett JE, Dolin R (eds): Principles and Practice of Infectious Diseases, 6th ed. Philadelphia, Elsevier, 2005, pp 927-951.
114. Stafford RE, Weigelt JA: Surgical infections in the critically ill. Curr Opin Crit Care 2002;8:449-452.
115. Brolin RE, Nosher JL, Leiman S, et al: Percutaneous catheter versus open surgical drainage in the treatment of abdominal abscesses. Am Surg 1984;50:102-108.
116. Johannsen EC, Madoff LC: Infections of the liver and biliary system. In Mandell GL, Bennett JE, Dolin R (eds): Principles and Practice of Infectious Diseases, 6th ed. Philadelphia, Elsevier, 2005, pp 951-959.
117. Hanau LH, Steigbigel NH: Acute (ascending) cholangitis. Infect Dis Clin North Am 2000;14:521-546.
118. Frey CF: Management of necrotizing pancreatitis. West J Med 1993;159:675-680.
119. Bartlett JG: Antibiotic-associated diarrhea. Clin Infect Dis 1992;15:573-581.
120. Thielman NM, Wilson KH: Antibiotic-associated colitis. In Mandell GL, Bennett JE, Dolin R (eds): Principles and Practice of Infectious Diseases, 6th ed. Philadelphia, Elsevier, 2005, pp 1249-1263.
121. Warny M, Pepin J, Fang A, et al: Toxin production by an emerging strain of *Clostridium difficile* associated with outbreaks of severe disease in North America and Europe. Lancet 2005;366:1079-1084.
122. Chow AW: Life-threatening infections of the head and neck. Clin Infect Dis 1992;14:991-1004.
123. Baker AS, Montgomery WW: Oropharyngeal space infection. Curr Clin Top Infect Dis 1987;8:227-265.
124. Chow AW: Infections of the oral cavity, neck, and head. In Mandell GL, Bennett JE, Dolin R (eds): Principles and Practice of Infectious Diseases, 6th ed. Philadelphia, Elsevier, 2005, pp 787-802.
125. Huang TT, Liu TC, Chen PR, et al: Deep neck infection: Analysis of 185 cases. Head Neck 2004;26:854-860.
126. Sinave CP, Hardy GJ, Fardy PW: The Lemierre syndrome: Suppurative thrombophlebitis of the internal jugular vein secondary to oropharyngeal infection. Medicine 1989;68:85-94.
127. Carey MJ: Epiglottitis in adults. Am J Emerg Med 1996;14:421-424.
128. Frantz TD, Rasgon BM, Quesenberry CP: Acute epiglottitis in adults. Analysis of 129 cases. JAMA 1994;272:1358-1360.
129. Rupp ME: Mediastinitis. In Mandell GL, Bennett JE, Dolin R (eds): Principles and Practice of Infectious Diseases, 6th ed. Philadelphia, Elsevier, 2005, pp 1070-1078.
130. Robiscek F: Post-operative sterno-mediastinitis. Am Surg 2000;66:184-192.
131. Chapman AS: Diagnosis and management of tickborne rickettsial diseases: Rocky Mountain spotted fever, ehrlichiosis, and anaplasmosis—United States. MMWR Recomm Rep 2006;55(RR-4):1-27.
132. Walker DH: Rocky Mountain spotted fever: A seasonal alert. Clin Infect Dis 1995;20:1111-1117.
133. Thorner AR, Walker DH, Petri WA: Rocky Mountain spotted fever. Clin Infect Dis 1998;27:1353-1360.
134. Woodward TE, Cunha BA: Rocky Mountain spotted fever. Infect Dis Pract 1999;23:73-84.
135. Sexton DJ, Corey GR: Rocky Mountain "spotless" and "almost spotless" fever: A wolf in sheep's clothing. Clin Infect Dis 1992;15:439-448.
136. Olano JP, Walker DH: Human ehrlichioses. Med Clin North Am 2002;86:375-392.
137. Murphy GS, Oldfield EC: Falciparum malaria. Infect Dis Clin North Am 1996;10:747-775.
138. Bledsoe GH: Malaria primer for clinicians in the United States. South Med J 2005;98:1197-1204.
139. Miller KD, Greenberg AE, Campbell CC: Treatment of severe malaria in the United States with a continuous infusion of quinidine gluconate and exchange transfusion. N Engl J Med 1989;321:65-70.
140. Baird JK, Hoffman SL: Progress in prevention and treatment of malaria. Curr Opin Infect Dis 1996;9:319-329.
141. Rigau-Perez JG, Clark GG, Gubler DJ, et al: Dengue and dengue hemorrhagic fever. Lancet 1998;352:971-977.
142. Malavige GN, Fernando S, Fernando DJ, et al: Dengue viral infections. Postgrad Med J 2004;80:588-601.
143. Castleberry JS, Mahon Cr: Dengue fever in the Western Hemisphere. Clin Lab Sci 2003;16:34-38.
144. Isturiz RE, Gubler DJ, Brea del Castillo J: Dengue and dengue hemorrhagic fever in Latin America and the Caribbean. Infect Dis Clin North Am 2000;14:121-140.
145. Peters CJ, Mills JN, Spiropoulou C, et al: Hantaviruses. In Guerrant RL, Walker DH, Weller PF (eds): Tropical Infectious Diseases: Principles, Pathogens, and Practice. New York, WB Saunders, 1999, pp 1189-1212.
146. Peters CJ, Simpson G, Levy H: Spectrum of hantavirus infection: Hemorrhagic fever with renal syndrome and hantavirus pulmonary syndrome. Annu Rev Med 1999;50:531-545.
147. Duchin JS, Koster FT, Peters CJ, et al: Hantavirus pulmonary syndrome: A clinical description of 17 patients with a newly recognized disease. The Hantavirus Study Group. N Engl J Med 1994;330:949-955.
148. Peters CJ, Khan AS: Hantavirus pulmonary syndrome: The new American hemorrhagic fever. Clin Infect Dis 2002;34:1224-1231.
149. Ketai LH, Williamson MR, Telepak RJ, et al: Hantavirus pulmonary syndrome: Radiographic findings in 16 patients. Radiology 1994;191: 665-668.
150. Harper SA, Fukuda K, Uyeki TM, et al: Prevention and control of influenza. Recommendations of the Advisory Committee on Immunization Practices (ACIP). MMWR Recomm Rep 2005;54(RR-8):1-40.
151. Murphy BR: Orthomyxoviruses. In Fields KD, Howley PM (eds): Fields Virology. Philadelphia, Lippincott, 1996, pp 1397-1445.
152. Cox NJ, Subbarao K: Influenza. Lancet 1999;354:1277-1282.
153. Nicholson KG: Clinical features of influenza. Semin Respir Infect 1992;7:26-37.
154. Douglas R Jr: Influenza in man. In Kilbourne ED (ed): Influenza Viruses and Influenza. New York, Academic Press, 1975, pp 395-418.
155. Thompson WW, Shay DK, Weintraub E, et al: Influenza-associated

hospitalizations in the United States. JAMA 2004;292:1333-1340.
156. Ferguson NM, Cummings DAT, Cauchemez S, et al: Strategies for containing an emerging influenza pandemic in Southeast Asia. Nature 2005;437:209-214.
157. Falsey AR, Hennessey PA, Formica MA, et al: Respiratory syncytial virus infection in elderly and high-risk adults. N Engl J Med 2005;352:1749-1759.
158. Bartlett JG, Inglesby TV, Borio L: Management of anthrax. Clin Infect Dis 2002;35:851-858.
159. Swartz M: Recognition and management of anthrax—an update. N Engl J Med 2001;345:1621-1626.
160. IDSA Website: Clinical pathway: Inhalational anthrax, 2002. Available at www.idsociety.org.
161. Damon I: Orthopoxviruses: Vaccinia (smallpox vaccine), variola (smallpox), Monkeypox, and Cowpox. In Mandell GL, Bennett JE, Dolin R (eds): Principles and Practice of Infectious Diseases, 6th ed. Philadelphia, Elsevier, 2005, pp 1742-1751.
162. Bray M, Martinez M, Smee DF, et al: Cidofovir protects mice against lethal aerosol or intranasal cowpox virus challenge. J Infect Dis 2000;181:10-19.
163. Perry RD, Fetherston JD: Yersinia pestis—etiologic agent of plague. Clin Microbiol Rev 1997;10:35-66.
164. Inglesby TV, Dennis DT, Henderson DA, et al: Plague as a biological weapon: Medical and public health management. JAMA 2000;283:2281-2290.
165. Franz DR, Jahrling PB, Friedlander AM, et al: Clinical recognition and management of patients exposed to biological warfare agents. JAMA 1997;278:399-411.
166. Dennis DT, Inglesby TV, Henderson DA, et al: Tularemia as a biological weapon: Medical and public health management. JAMA 2001;285:2763-2773.
167. Boria L, Inglesby T, Peters CJ, et al: Hemorrhagic viruses as biological weapons. JAMA 2002;287:2391-2405.

PART

V

RENAL DISEASE AND METABOLIC DISORDERS IN THE CRITICALLY ILL

Chapter

56 Acute Renal Failure

Robert J. Anderson

BACKGROUND AND DEFINITION

Acute renal failure (ARF) is the sudden development of renal insufficiency that leads to retention of nitrogenous waste (urea nitrogen and creatinine) in the body. Despite consensus regarding this broad definition, there are diverse opinions as to the degree of elevation of serum creatinine sufficient to ascribe a diagnosis of ARF.[1-4] These differences in diagnostic criteria, as well as in the populations under study, have led to variances in reported frequency, causes, and outcomes of ARF. In an effort to arrive at a more standard definition of ARF, some recent studies have emphasized the RIFLE criteria.[5-8] These criteria refer to various elements in the developmental pathway of ARF including risk (R), injury (I), failure (F), loss (L), and end stage (E) and are based on both the magnitude of rise in the serum creatinine concentration and the urine output. The RIFLE criteria for the diagnosis of ARF are depicted in Table 56-1. Although further validation of the RIFLE criteria is necessary, these criteria can serve as a reasonable starting point for a more uniform approach to the clinical aspects of ARF. Clearly, better criteria for the uniform definition of ARF are necessary.

Although the precise definition of ARF may remain arguable, experts generally agree on several aspects of contemporary ARF. First, ARF occurs with significant frequency, especially in the hospital and in the intensive care unit (ICU) setting.[1-9] Second, multiple pathophysiologic pathways and clinical events lead to an identical syndrome of ARF.[1-9] Third, timely delineation of the cause of ARF is paramount in designing appropriate therapy.[10-13] Fourth, even when modest in degree, ARF is associated with significant morbidity and mortality.[10,14,15] Fifth, ARF is one of the few causes of complete organ failure that is potentially totally reversible.[1-9] Finally, some studies indicate that a significant percentage of cases of ARF are preventable.[10-13] The high frequency of occurrence, multiple causes, associated morbidity and mortality, and potential reversibility demand an organized approach to ARF. In this chapter we review the incidence, pathogenesis, clinical manifestations, management, and outcome of ARF, especially as it relates to critically ill patients. An overview of contemporary ICU-associated ARF is depicted in Table 56-2.

INCIDENCE

When defined as a modest increase in serum creatinine (e.g., either a 20% increase over basal or an increase of 0.2 to 0.5 mg/dL), the incidence of ICU-associated ARF ranges from 10% to 35%.[1-17] When ARF is defined as severe enough to require renal replacement therapy and either the blood urea nitrogen exceeds 84 mg/dL or the patient is oliguric (<200 mL in 12 hours), a 5.7% prevalence in more than 29,260 patients in ICUs at 54 hospitals shown in 23 countries was found.[9] Figure 56-1 depicts the incidence of ARF in several critically ill populations. The general characteristics of ARF encountered in the ICU are shown in Tables 56-2 and 56-3. Two "types" of ICU-associated ARF can be identified when examined in terms of time of development. In about half of cases, ICU-associated ARF is present at the time of ICU admission, whereas in the remainder of cases it develops during the ICU stay.[18-20]

Table 56-1. RIFLE Criteria for Diagnosis of Acute Renal Failure

	GFR Criteria	Urine Output Criteria	
Risk	Increased SCr × 1.5 or GFR decrease >25%	UO <.5 mL/kg/h × 6 h	**High Sensitivity**
Injury	Increased SCr × 2 or GFR decrease >50%	UO <.5 mL/kg/h × 12 h	
Failure	Increase SCr × 3 GFR decrease 75% or SCr ≥ 4 mg/dL Acute rise ≥ 0.5 mg/dL	UO <.3 mL/kg/h × 24 h or Anuria × 12 h	**High Specificity**
Loss	Persistent ARF = complete loss of kidney function >4 weeks		
ESKD	End-stage kidney disease (>3 months)		

ARF, acute renal failure; ESKD, end-stage kidney disease; GFR, glomerular filtration rate; SCr, serum creatine; UO, urine output.

Table 56-2. Overview of Intensive Care Unit–Associated Acute Renal Failure—Five Representative Studies

	Spain	France	United States	United States	International
Population	13 referring hospitals	20 ICUs	Single center	5 academic ICUs	54 hospitals, 34 countries
Years of study	1991-1992	1991	1991-1992	1999-2001	2000-2001
n	253	360	71	618	1,738
Cause (%)					
Prerenal	18	17	30	36	25
Postrenal	1	4	3	1	3
Renal	81	79	67	63	67
Sepsis related (%)	35	48	30	—	48
Cardiovascular comorbidity (%)	—	—	—	48	—
Liver failure (%)	—	—	—	31	—
Respiratory failure (%)	—	60	—	67	76
Malignant disease (%)	—	—	—	7	—
Mortality (%)	72	58	48	37	60

Table 56-3. Contrast of ICU– and Hospital Ward–Associated Acute Renal Failure (ARF)

	ICU	Non-ICU
No. of Patients	253	495
Age (y)	56	63
Isolated ARF (%)	11	69
Cause (%)		
Prerenal	18	28
Postrenal	1	15
ATN	76	38
Other	3	17
Worsening chronic	8	15
Mortality (%)	72	32
Peak serum creatinine (mg/dL)	5.2	5.8
Required dialysis (%)	71	18
Duration of ARF (d)	13	15

ATN, acute tubular necrosis.
Modified from Liano F, Junco E, Pacual J, et al: The spectrum of acute renal failure in the intensive care unit compared with that seen in other settings. Kidney Int 1998;53(Suppl 66):516.

PATHOGENESIS

General Aspects

The process of urine formation begins with ultrafiltration of the blood delivered to the kidney; proceeds through internal processing of the ultrafiltrate by tubular reabsorption and secretion; and ends by elimination of the formed urine through the ureters, bladder, and urethra. It follows that ARF is the final common pathway for a number of disease processes acting at these different sites. Although somewhat simplistic, from a clinical perspective the initial step when confronted by a patient with ARF is to determine if the renal failure is prerenal (decreased renal perfusion), postrenal (obstruction to urine flow), or renal (disorders of renal vasculature, glomeruli, interstitium, or tubules) in origin (Box 56-1).[1-5] Table 56-2 depicts the causes of ARF in some recently reported series of patients with ICU-associated ARF.[9,19,20] From a practical consideration, the causes of ARF in the ICU differ from those encountered in non-ICU populations (see Table 56-3).[18,19] Also, many cases of ICU-associated ARF have more than a single cause (see Tables 56-2 and 56-3).[9] In a recent international study, ARF occurred in the context of septic shock in 48% of cases and septic shock remains one of

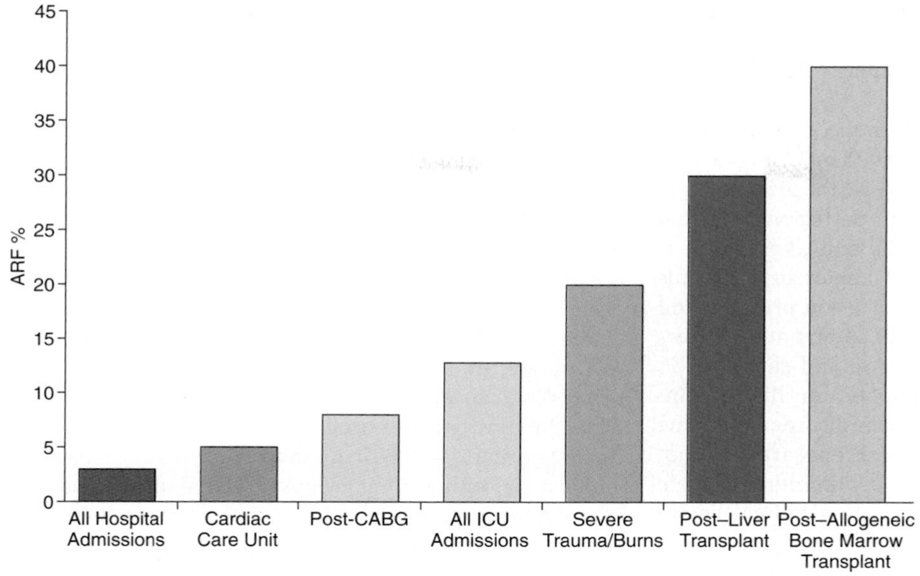

Figure 56-1. Frequency of acute renal failure in selected hospital settings.

Table 56-4. Factors and Settings Associated with ICU-Acquired ARF

Factor/Setting	Frequency (%)
Multiorgan failure	30-75
Sepsis	30-50
Drugs/medications	20-40
Postoperative state	15-30
Impaired cardiac outpatient/hypovolemia	15-30
Pigmenturia	5-15

ARF, acute renal failure; ICU, intensive care unit.

the most common associated/predisposing settings of ICU-acquired ARF.[9,21] Other common associated clinical conditions for ICU-associated ARF (Table 56-4) included major surgery (34%), cardiogenic shock (27%), hypovolemia (26%), medication-related (19%), and in the context of advanced liver disease (6%).[9]

From a pathogenic viewpoint, several mechanisms can operate to impair glomerular filtration.[22,23] The net sum of the Starling physical forces that favor movement of ultrafiltrate from the glomerular capillary (hydrostatic pressure) into the proximal renal tubule usually substantially exceeds the physical forces that oppose filtrate formation (glomerular capillary colloid oncotic pressure and hydrostatic pressure within the renal tubule). A significant reduction in glomerular capillary hydrostatic pressure potentially occurs by a decrease in renal blood flow, marked constriction of the afferent arteriole, or a decrease in efferent arteriolar tone. All of these events can lead to a diminished glomerular filtration rate (GFR) with ARF. A significant rise in proximal tubular hydrostatic pressure, as occurs in obstructive uropathy, also decreases glomerular filtration. Under unusual clinical circumstances, such as after administration of large amounts of mannitol or dextran, glomerular capillary oncotic pressure increases to a sufficient degree to cause a cessation of formation of glomerular filtrate and ARF.

Prerenal Azotemia

Prerenal azotemia caused by extracellular fluid volume loss, extracellular fluid volume sequestration, or a markedly reduced cardiac output is a common cause of ARF, contributing to about 30% to 60% of all cases (see Tables 56-2, 56-3, and 56-4).[9,22,23] This form of ARF, if treated early, is potentially reversible. If it is left untreated, renal ischemia with acute tubular necrosis (ATN) may result. In prerenal azotemia, reduced renal perfusion pressure and afferent arteriolar constriction combine to lower glomerular capillary hydrostatic pressure and the formation of glomerular ultrafiltrate.[22,23] A number of factors are capable of inducing afferent arteriolar constriction, thereby reducing glomerular capillary hydrostatic pressure. These factors include enhanced renal adrenergic neural tone and either locally produced or circulating humoral substances such as norepinephrine, several peptides (angiotensin II, endothelin), and selected lipid-derived substances (endotoxin, thromboxane A_2, leukotrienes, and prostaglandin F_2 alpha-like compounds). The reduced glomerular filtration of prerenal azotemia is usually coupled with avid renal tubular salt and water reabsorption as the kidney attempts to restore its perfusion to normal by expansion of circulating volume. The combined lowering of GFR and increase in tubular reabsorption usually, but not always, leads to an oliguric state in prerenal azotemia.

Three classes of pharmacologic agents—diuretics, nonsteroidal anti-inflammatory drugs (NSAIDs), and drugs that attenuate the renal action of angiotensin II (either angiotensin-converting enzyme inhibitors [ACEIs] or angiotensin II receptor antagonists)—can also induce a form of prerenal azotemia.[10,24,25] The prerenal form of ARF complicating diuretic use is obviously caused by extracellular fluid volume depletion. With NSAIDs, the inhibition of cyclooxygenase leads to a depletion of renal vasodilatory eicosanoids that normally counteract the afferent arteriolar constricting effect of increased renal adrenergic tone and peptide and lipid-derived constrictors. In the presence of abundant renal vasoconstrictor influence, as occurs in edematous disorders, sepsis, heart failure, volume depletion, and hypotensive states, severe afferent arteriolar renal vasoconstriction can occur with NSAIDs, with subsequent reduced glomerular capillary filtration pressure and ARF.

If discontinued quickly, NSAID-induced ARF can be reversible. However, if not discontinued quickly, NSAID-associated ARF can lead to ATN because the afferent arteriolar constriction decreases renal perfusion to renal tubular epithelial cells. With ACEIs and angiotensin II receptor blockers, the reduction of angiotensin II leads to concomitant lowering of renal perfusion pressure and dilation of the efferent arteriole. This combination lowers glomerular capillary filtration pressure and causes ARF. This is particularly likely to happen in high renin-angiotensin II states such as edematous disorders, volume depletion, hypotensive states, bilateral renal artery stenosis, or unilateral renal artery stenosis with either a single kidney or severe disease in the contralateral kidney. Fortunately, the prerenal azotemia that can accompany ACEIs and angiotensin II receptor blockers is usually reversible if the offending agent is quickly stopped because of the fact that a decrease in postglomerular capillary blood flow does not result in ischemia to renal tubular epithelial cells.

Postrenal Azotemia

Postrenal azotemia is a less common cause of ARF, making up 1% to 10% of all cases. Postrenal causes are relatively unusual in the ICU setting, although still present in 1% to 5% of ICU-acquired ARF (see Tables 56-2 and 56-3 and Box 56-1).[9] Postrenal azotemia is almost always treatable. The most frequent cause of extrarenal obstructive uropathy in men is bladder outlet obstruction from prostatic disease. This is particularly common when pharmacologic agents are administered, such as agents with either anticholinergic effects (that decrease detrusor muscle function) or with smooth muscle constrictor properties (that increase sphincter tone). Occasionally, extensive prostatic or bladder cancer can occlude the ureteric orifices. Obstruction to urine flow above the level of the bladder is a less common cause of ARF because both ureters must be occluded. However, an extensive disease process such as retroperitoneal fibrosis or widespread pelvic cancer can occlude both ureters. If one kidney is absent or severely diseased, unilateral ureteric obstruction (by stone, pus, clot, tissue, or ligature) can cause ARF. Obstruction to urine flow can also occur within the kidneys when the distal tubules become occluded with crystals (uric acid, calcium oxalate, acyclovir, methotrexate, indinavir, sulfonamides) or with proteinaceous material (myeloma). In obstructive uropathy either intrarenal or extrarenal blockage of urine flow raises intratubular pressure so that net glomerular filtration pressure is reduced. Glomerular filtration in turn is either markedly reduced or stopped, depending on the degree of obstruction.

Renal Azotemia

Once prerenal and postrenal causes of ARF have been considered, it is appropriate to focus attention on the kidney. When approaching renal causes of ARF, it is helpful to think in terms of the anatomic compartments of the kidney (see Box 56-1). Disorders of the renal vasculature, including both large and small vessels, such as thrombotic occlusion, emboli, malignant hypertension, thrombotic thrombocytopenic purpura (TTP), hemolyticuremic syn-

Box 56-1

Causes and Categories of Acute Renal Failure (ARF)

Prerenal ARF

Extracellular fluid volume loss
Gastrointestinal (vomiting, diarrhea, hemorrhage)
Renal (diuretics, glycosuria)
Skin (burns, heat stroke)

Extracellular fluid sequestration
Gastrointestinal (pancreatitis, post–intra-abdominal surgery, peritonitis)
Early sepsis
Muscle crush injury
Capillary leak syndromes (allergy, interleukin therapy)

Impaired cardiac function
Heart failure
Cardiogenic shock
Pericardial tamponade

Postrenal ARF

Intrarenal obstruction
Crystal deposition (acyclovir, indinavir, sulfonamides, methotrexate, oxalate, uric acid)
Protein deposition (plasma cell dyscrasia)

Extrarenal obstruction
Bladder outlet (prostate and urethral obstruction)
Ureteric (stones, pus, clot, tumor, papilla, ligation, fibrosis)

Renal Causes of ARF

Renal vascular disorders
Large vessel (thrombosis, emboli, aneurysm)
Small vessels (vasculitis, TTP, HUS, DIC, malignant hypertension)
Glomerulonephritis
Interstitial nephritis
Acute tubular necrosis
Ischemia (prolonged prerenal)
Toxins
Pigment

DIC, disseminated intravascular coagulation; HUS, hemolyticuremic syndrome; TTP, thrombotic thrombocytopenia purpura.

drome (HUS), and vasculitis, can all cause ARF. In these disorders a marked reduction in renal blood flow sufficient to reduce glomerular filtration occurs. Acute glomerulonephritis, which destroys the filtering unit of the kidney, can also result in ARF. Acute inflammation of the renal interstitium, as usually results from an allergic drug reaction, also produces ARF. The precise pathogenic mechanisms whereby interstitial inflammation leads to a reduction in GFR remain to be determined. Together, these vascular, glomerular, and interstitial disorders are relatively uncommon causes of hospital-acquired ARF, constituting about 5% to 10% of all such cases. However, these disorders are often amenable to specific therapy.

The most common renal cause of ARF is ATN. Essentially, three major factors predispose an individual to ATN: renal ischemia (prolonged prerenal azotemia), nephrotoxins, and pigmenturia (hemoglobinuria and myoglobinuria). Prolonged renal hypoperfusion (renal ischemia) is the most common setting of ATN. Renal ischemia is commonly associated with shock of any cause, especially septic shock.[21] Great variability in the severity and duration of insults exists to produce ischemic ATN. Early in ischemic ARF the combined influence of a decrease in renal perfusion pressure and afferent arteriolar constriction initiates a reduction of glomerular filtration. Later, a decrease in glomerular capillary permeability, an increase in intratubular hydrostatic pressure caused by obstructing casts and debris shed from ischemic proximal tubular brush border epithelium, and "back-leak" of filtered fluid through leaky tubular epithelium combine to reduce GFR in the maintenance phase of ischemic ATN. The central roles of reduced renal blood flow and tubular obstruction in the pathogenesis of ischemic ATN underlie current clinical therapy, which is directed toward maintaining adequate renal perfusion pressure through use of adequate fluid volume resuscitation and vasoactive drugs.

At the level of the renal tubular epithelial cell, depletion of adenosine triphosphate (ATP) is the initial step in ischemic ATN. The subsequent chronology and mechanisms that lead to renal tubular cell death continue to be debated. Substantial data suggest that ATP depletion leads to disruption of the cytoskeleton, which maintains tight junctions. Tight junctions are the point of cell-to-cell contact and are also responsible for maintenance of normal renal tubular cell polarity. Loss of polarity in early ischemic ATN results in displacement of enzymes such as the sodium pump (Na-K-ATPase), which pumps sodium out of cells, from its basolateral position to an apical (brush border) position. This translocation of Na-K-ATPase may, at least in part, be responsible for the relatively high spot urinary sodium concentration that is the hallmark of ischemic ATN. Also, following ischemia an influx of calcium occurs that results in renal tubular cell calcium overload. This calcium overload may activate several enzyme systems, leading to membrane and organelle disruption and dysfunction. The finding of renal tubular cell calcium overload in many experimental models of ischemia-induced ARF has led to several experimental and clinical trials using calcium channel blockers in an attempt to prevent or attenuate ischemia-induced ATN. However, at present no well-substantiated evidence that calcium channel blockers are of clinical benefit in treating and/or preventing ischemia-related ATN has been established. In the later stages of ischemia when reflow has been established, generation of oxygen-free radicals can occur within the kidney. These free radicals potentially cause lipid peroxidation and destroy cell and organelle membranes. Although some experimental studies suggest that oxygen-free radical scavengers can provide some renal protection, clinical trials of such scavengers have not yet been performed.

The pathophysiological process by which nephrotoxins induce real damage is not clear.[10] Two of the most commonly encountered contemporary nephrotoxins are the aminoglycoside antimicrobials and radiographic contrast agents. Aminoglycosides induce mild (mean rise in serum creatinine of 1 to 3 mg/dL), nonoliguric ATN in 5% to 20% of patients receiving a course of 7 to 10 days of these agents.[26-28] However, even brief exposure in the setting of impaired renal perfusion can induce some renal damage. Aminoglycosides are avidly taken up by proximal tubular brush border epithelium and accumulate within lysozymes, where they bind to acidic phospholipids. The most characteristic feature of experimental aminoglycoside nephrotoxicity is accumulation of the phospholipid from the inhibition of phospholipid degradation. Induction of phospholipidosis and binding to acidic phospholipids by aminoglycosides could exert effects on cellular and organelle membrane properties and enzyme activity. Experimental aminoglycoside nephrotoxicity can also be associated with cellular calcium overload and mitochondria dysfunction.

Radiocontrast agents are remarkably nontoxic in healthy individuals.[29-31] In general, the sicker the patient, the greater the risk of nephrotoxicity. Risk factors for nephrotoxicity from these agents include underlying diabetic nephropathy, prerenal azotemia, concomitant therapy with NSAIDs and exposure to high doses of the contrast agent. Great variability in the severity and duration of the resultant renal failure exists. Radiographic contrast agents can induce marked renal vasoconstriction; some of this vasoconstriction can be attributed to the hypertonicity of these agents, as well as to release of endothelin. Moreover, these agents appear to be directly cytotoxic to renal epithelial cells, and they increase urinary excretion of poorly soluble crystals of uric and oxalic acids. From a clinical perspective, radiographic contrast agent nephrotoxicity can be decreased and/or modestly attenuated by use of either low osmolar or iso-osmolar nonionic agents, as well as by maintenance of good renal perfusion and high urine flow with infusion of a saline solution.

The pathophysiological basis of pigment-induced ARF almost always involves some concomitant element of extracellular volume depletion and renal ischemia.[32-35] Pigmented granular casts obstructing tubular lumina are also a common feature of pigment-induced renal damage. Iron pigments derived from muscle and blood may also play a role in catalyzing formation of free oxygen radicals, which can destroy cell membranes. From a clinical perspective, maintaining adequate extracellular fluid volume and renal perfusion, and perhaps administering mannitol and urinary alkalization (which increases solubility of hemoglobin and myoglobin, thereby reducing cast formation) may provide protection against pigment-associated ARF.[32-35]

CLINICAL MANIFESTATIONS

Retention of Nitrogenous Waste/Elevation in Serum Cystatin C

Of importance is that there are currently no practical, "real-time" methods of diagnosing the presence of ARF. The ability of the clinician to make a "real-time" diagnosis of acute impairment in renal function is key in ameliorating the morbidity and mortality that can accompany ARF. Unfortunately, ARF usually comes to the attention of the clinician through an increasing blood urea nitrogen (BUN) and/or serum creatinine concentration. An increasing BUN and/or serum creatinine often occurs only after substantial loss of GFR has already happened. These nitrogenous waste substances are readily filtered by the kidney and eliminated into the urine. In the absence of glomerular filtration, the BUN usually increases by about 10 to 20 mg/dL/day.

Urea nitrogen is synthesized in the liver, and this synthesis is dependent on protein load. Thus either exogenous (high dietary protein intake) or endogenous (catabolic state, fever, sepsis, corticosteroid therapy, tetracycline administration, or gastrointestinal hemorrhage) protein loading can elevate the BUN without a marked decrease in GFR. Some clinical studies indicate that up to 35% of patients with ARF can be catabolic with a daily rate of rise of BUN of more than 30 mg/dL.[36] Filtered urea nitrogen can be reabsorbed by the renal tubules, especially in states of low urine flow. Thus low urine flow states, as occur with volume depletion, severe heart failure, and obstructive uropathy, can also elevate BUN in the absence of a markedly reduced GFR. The variability in synthesis of urea nitrogen and the non-GFR-related renal factors that influence urinary excretion of urea nitrogen render the BUN a less reliable marker of GFR than the serum creatinine concentration. However, the level of BUN generally correlates quite well with renal failure symptoms.

Creatinine is derived from nonenzymatic hydrolysis of creatine, which is usually released at a constant rate from skeletal muscle. In the absence of glomerular filtration, serum creatinine increases by 1 to 2 mg/dL/day. Serum creatinine is, however, determined by rate of production, volume of distribution, and renal excretion.[37] Thus the serum creatinine concentration may not accurately reflect GFR in the setting of critically ill patients with ARF.[37] If the supply of creatinine into the bloodstream is suddenly increased by skeletal muscle injury (rhabdomyolysis), a striking elevation of serum creatinine may occur. Also, a small amount of creatinine may be secreted into the urine by renal tubules. Some drugs, such as trimethoprim and cimetidine, may interfere with this tubular secretion, thereby slightly increasing serum creatinine concentration. Finally, ketone bodies and cefoxitin can cause chemical interference with the laboratory measurement of creatinine, leading to falsely high values. Generally, the BUN-to–serum creatinine ratio is about 10:1 or 15:1. Several factors can alter this ratio and provide diagnostically helpful clues to the clinician (Table 56-5).

Because relatively large decreases in glomerular filtration rate are associated with potentially only mild or modest increases in serum creatinine concentration (see Chapter 57), other readily available markers of ARF have been sought. Recently, serum cystatin C has been proposed to be a more sensitive marker for decreasing glomerular filtration rate including in ICU patients.[38-40] Cystatin C is a cysteine protease inhibitor released into the bloodstream at a constant rate from all nucleated cells. Cystatin C is readily filtered at the glomerulus and either reabsorbed or catabolized by renal tubular epithelial cells such that little, if any, appears in the urine. In general the serum concentration of cystatin C increases as glomerular filtration rate falls. Whether or not serum cystatin C is a more sensitive marker than serum creatinine in the setting of ARF in ICU patients remains, however, to be determined.[38-40]

Oligoanuria

A second way in which ARF comes to the attention of the clinician is by a decrease in urine flow. Oliguria (often arbitrarily defined as <30 mL/hour or 400 to 700 mL/day) almost always indicates the presence of renal failure.[41] Although oliguria is often considered a cardinal feature of ARF, it is important to emphasize that the majority of cases of ARF currently encountered in medical practice are nonoliguric.[42,43] Moreover, all forms of ARF (prerenal, postrenal, and renal) can be nonoliguric in nature. Although oliguria always suggests the possibility of some cause of ARF, a well-maintained urine output is not a reliable indicator of adequate renal function. Anuria

Table 56-5. BUN-to-Creatinine Ratio

>15-20:1	<15:1
■ Increased urea formation High protein intake Catabolic state (fever, sepsis, tissue necrosis, corticosteroids, sepsis, tetracycline) GI bleed ■ Decreased urea elimination Volume depletion Impaired cardiac output Obstructive uropathy	■ Decreased urea formation Starvation Advanced liver disease Hereditary urea cycle defects ■ Increased urea removal Postdialysis ■ Decreased creatinine elimination Cimetidine Trimethoprim Pyrimethamine ■ False elevation of creatinine Ketones Cefoxitin Levodopa Flucytosine Ascorbic acid ■ Increased creatinine formation Rhabdomyolysis

BUN, blood urea nitrogen; GI, gastrointestinal.

(virtually no urine output) always demands prompt attention. True anuria is most commonly caused by complete obstructive uropathy. Occasionally, cessation of renal blood flow and rapidly progressive glomerulonephritis can cause anuria. Rarely, ATN results in a few hours of anuria.

Detection of Clinical and Biochemical Complications

A third way in which ARF comes to the attention of the clinician, although rarely, is by detection of one of the biochemical or clinical consequences of the loss of renal excretory function. Thus occasionally the development of fluid overload, hyperkalemia, hypocalcemia, hyperphosphatemia, metabolic acidosis, hyperuricemia, anemia, or encephalopathy is the initial manifestation of ARF.

DIAGNOSTIC APPROACH

General Aspects

Appropriate management of ARF depends on accurate assessment of the cause. Thus the first step in approaching the patient with ARF is to determine whether the renal failure is prerenal, postrenal, or renal in origin. Figures 56-2 and 56-3 suggest a diagnostic sequence to follow. An important acknowledgment is that it is not always easy when working with critically ill patients to diagnostically assign an individual to a specific broad category of cause of ARF. Moreover, most cases of ARF encountered in ICU patients have more than a single insult to renal function.[1-4,9,14-20,41-48] The single most common clinical condition predisposing to ARF in ICU patients is sepsis.[9,21] Other common clinical conditions predisposing to ICU-associated ARF include volume depletion, congestive heart failure, use of radiocontrast agents, hemorrhage, or hypotension from any cause. In an older study of ICU-acquired ARF, four risk factors (sepsis, use of aminoglycoside, exposure to contrast agents, and hypotension) were present alone or together in all patients.[49] Clinical conditions predisposing to ARF as acquired in the ICU are listed in Box 56-1 and Table 56-4. One recent study is particularly illustrative of most contemporary series of patients that develop ARF in the ICU.[44] In this study of 487 ICU patients, cardiovascular failure (49%), pulmonary failure (33%), and ARF (16%) were the three most frequent types of organ failure encountered. However, 90% of all ARF patients had failure of organ systems other than the kidneys, and in the vast majority of cases, failure of the other organ systems preceded the onset of ARF.[44] Thus in most cases of ICU-acquired ARF, the kidneys fail after one or more other organ systems have already failed.[4,15-17] In community-acquired ARF, isolated failure of just the kidneys is much more commonly encountered than in hospital-acquired ARF, and a single identifiable cause of renal failure can often be found.[50]

History, Physical Examination, and Record Review

In attempting to identify the cause of ARF, a thorough history, physical examination, and review of the medical record should be the initial steps. The overall clinical setting, recent events in the patient's illness, use of medications, and possible toxic exposures should be noted. A history of vomiting, blood loss, diarrhea, diuretic use, burns, or symptoms compatible with heart failure suggest potential prerenal azotemia. A history of decreased size and force of the urine stream; bladder/prostate/pelvic/intra-abdominal cancer; flank or suprapubic pain; or hematuria or pyuria may suggest postrenal azotemia. History of a systemic disorder, fever, rash, vascular disease, or musculoskeletal complaints is compatible with a renal,

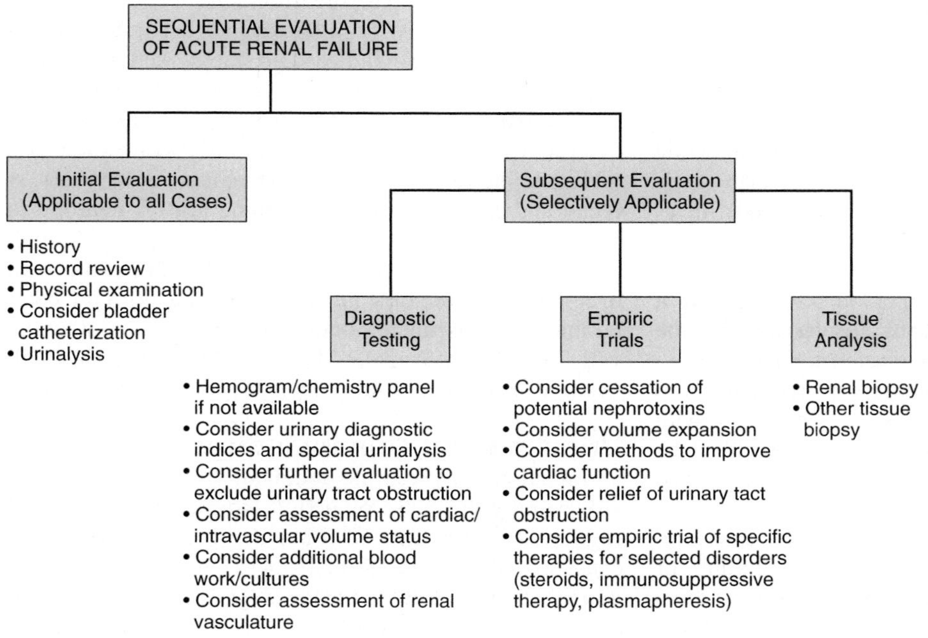

Figure 56-2. Sequential evaluation of acute renal failure.

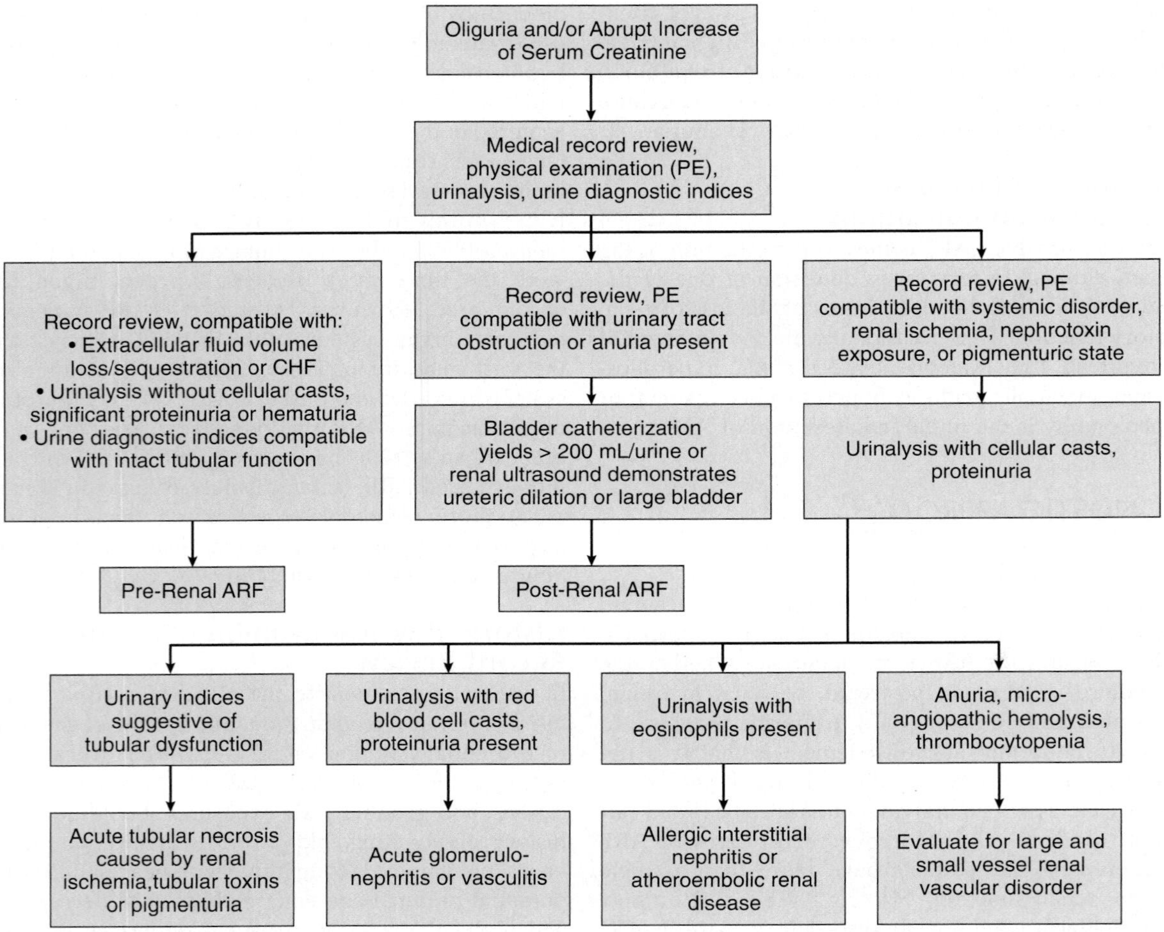

Figure 56-3. Algorithm on approach to the patient with acute deterioration in renal function. ARF, acute renal failure; CHF, congestive heart failure.

vascular, glomerular, or interstitial disorder. Review of the medical record should focus on indices of volume status (serial weights, intake and output, and hemodynamic measurements, when available) to help assess whether prerenal azotemia is present. A review of the medication list to determine exposure to potential nephrotoxins is necessary.[10,42] As noted previously, delineation of the pattern of urine output is often helpful.

The physical examination should focus on detecting evidence of extracellular fluid loss such as orthostatic changes in pulse and blood pressure, dry mucous membranes, decreased skin turgor, longitudinal tongue furrows, and dryness of the axillary and groin areas.[51] A significant (10% to 20%) fall in orthostatic blood pressure with a rise in pulse rate indicates significant intravascular volume depletion. However, orthostatic hypotension is not a sensitive indicator of intravascular volume depletion because it may be absent with acute loss of small volumes or with chronic depletion of large volumes. Examination for neck vein distention, pulmonary rales, ventricular gallops, and pedal edema may indicate the presence of heart failure. Occasionally, a chest radiograph, cardiac index measurement (i.e., echocardiogram or gated blood pool scan), or brain natriuretic peptide level may be necessary to help determine the presence or absence of heart failure. Accurate estimation of extracellular fluid volume status and cardiac output may be difficult on clinical grounds alone, particularly in immobilized, ventilated ICU patients. Thus invasive monitoring (i.e., measurement of left ventricular filling pressure) may be necessary to accurately assess intravascular volume and cardiac status. Abdominal palpation to detect flank, suprapubic, or central abdominal masses may be helpful in assessing the presence of obstructive uropathy and an abdominal aortic aneurysm with possible renal vascular compromise, respectively. A rectal and pelvic examination should always be done to assess for possible causes of obstructive uropathy. Examination of the skin may detect a rash, compatible with drug-induced interstitial nephritis; palpable purpura, compatible with vasculitis; nonpalpable purpura, compatible with TTP and HUS; and livido reticularis, compatible with vascular insufficiency and renal atheroembolic disease.

Urinalysis and Urinary Indices

Examination of the urine sediment is of great value in determining the cause of ARF.[42] Normal urine sediment suggests the presence of either a prerenal or postrenal cause of ARF (Table 56-6). Urinary sediment containing abundant cells, casts, or protein suggests a renal cause of ARF. Specifically, the presence of pigmented granular

Table 56-6. Urine Findings in Acute Renal Failure

Diagnosis	Urine Sediment	U_{Na}/FENa
Prerenal azotemia	Normal or nearly normal (hyaline casts and rare granular casts)	<30 mEq/L; <1%
Postrenal azotemia	Can be normal or can be hematuria, pyuria, and crystals	Not helpful (early prerenal; late resembles ATN)
Renal azotemia		
Vascular disorders	Often has RBC; eosinophiluria can occur with atheroembolic disease	Not helpful (can resemble prerenal)
Glomerulonephritis	RBC, RBC and granular casts; abundant proteinuria	Not helpful (can resemble prerenal)
Interstitial nephritis	Pyuria, WBC casts, eosinophils, and eosinophilic casts	Not helpful (resembles ATN)
Tubular necrosis	Pigmented granular casts, renal tubular epithelial cells, and granular casts	>30 mEq/L, >1%

ATN, acute tubular necrosis; RBC, red blood cell; WBC, white blood cell.

casts or renal epithelial cell casts suggests ATN. Interestingly, experienced nephrologists are more likely to recognize urinalysis features suggestive of ATN or other parenchymal renal diseases than hospital-based laboratories.[53] The presence of white blood cell casts or eosinophil casts (using Hansel's stain of the urinary sediment) suggests acute interstitial nephritis.[42,52] Occasionally atheroembolic disease and glomerulonephritis may also produce eosinophiluria. The presence of red blood cell casts and heavy proteinuria suggests glomerulonephritis or vasculitis. A urine dipstick test that is positive for red blood cells in the absence of red blood cells on microscopic examination suggests the presence of either hemoglobinuria or myoglobinuria.

Analysis of electrolyte composition of the urine may be helpful in differentiating between prerenal azotemia and ATN.[42,52-56] In prerenal azotemia, the tubules avidly reabsorb sodium in an effort to restore extracellular fluid volume and renal perfusion to normal. Thus in prerenal azotemia, spot urine sodium concentrations are usually less than 30 mEq/L, and the fractional excretion of sodium ($U/Pna \div U/P$ creatinine $\times$ 100) is less than 1%. Low urinary sodium excretion in ARF is also seen in states of intense renal vasoconstriction (hepatorenal syndrome, NSAID therapy, soon after a radiocontrast medium is introduced, and the early phase of sepsis and myoglobinuric ARF); with glomerulonephritis; and in diseases that involve the afferent arteriole (hemolytic-uremic syndrome, thrombotic thrombocytopenic purpura). Collectively these disorders are characterized by diminished renal perfusion with intact renal tubular epithelial cell function. By contrast, in ATN the damaged renal tubule cells fail to reabsorb sodium normally, perhaps because of altered cell polarity, with a resultant spot urine sodium greater than 40 mEq/L and a fractional excretion of sodium of more than 1%. Of note is that increased fractional excretion of sodium may occur in prerenal states after diuretic therapy or in the presence of either glycosuria or bicarbonaturia. In patients who have received diuretic therapy, a fractional excretion of urea nitrogen less than 35% may indicate potentially reversible prerenal azotemia.[57] Urinary chemical indices are not of value in determining the presence or absence of obstructive uropathy.

Exclusion of Obstructive Uropathy

For patients in whom the cause of ARF remains unclear or in whom the history or physical examination suggests the possibility of obstructive uropathy, further testing is indicated. The first test should be a bladder catheterization to measure residual volume. A residual volume of more than 100 mL suggests possible bladder outlet obstruction and the need for bladder catheter drainage. If bladder outlet obstruction is not present, occasionally noninvasive testing to examine for ureteric occlusion is indicated. This is most often done by ultrasonography. Rarely, the presence of extensive retroperitoneal disease may give a false-negative ultrasonographic result (so-called *nondilated obstructive uropathy*). Computed tomography (CT) scanning, especially helical or spiral CTs, or magnetic resonance imaging (MRI) may be helpful to delineate the presence or absence and extent of retroperitoneal disease and ureteral occlusion. In some cases, retrograde pyelography may be necessary to definitively exclude ureteric obstruction. Rarely, a trial of percutaneous nephrostomy drainage is used when minimally dilated or nonciliated obstruction is suspected.

Miscellaneous Tests

Sometimes the cause of ARF remains unknown despite careful record review, physical examination, urinalyses, and exclusion of obstructive uropathy. In these cases a review of the hemogram is helpful. The presence of anemia and rouleaux formation may suggest a plasma cell dyscrasia, which often produces ARF. Eosinophilia is compatible with allergic interstitial nephritis, atheroembolic disease, and polyarteritis nodosa. Thrombocytopenia and microangiopathic hemolysis suggest the presence of vasculitis, hemolytic-uremic syndrome, thrombotic thrombocytopenic purpura, disseminated intravascular coagulation (DIC), scleroderma renal crisis, and malignant hypertension—all of which can present as ARF. Standard laboratory data may also prove a diagnostic benefit. An elevated MB (skeletal muscle) fraction of creatine kinase (CK) suggests the possibility of rhabdomyolysis. A disproportionate rate of rise in serum potassium coupled with hyperuricemia, hyperphosphatemia, and high levels of lactic dehydrogenase suggests diffuse tissue destruction, as occurs in ARF complicating tumor lysis syndromes and rhabdomyolysis.

Depending on the clinical presentation, if glomerulonephritis/vasculitis is suspected, serologic testing (complement, antinuclear antibody, anti-DNA, antineutrophilic cytoplasmic antibodies, and antiglomerular basement membrane antibody) may be indicated. Sometimes a cautious trial of extracellular fluid volume expansion may be indicated if volume-depleted prerenal azotemia is possible. If impaired cardiac output is suspected, a trial of maneuvers that decrease preload and afterload and increase cardiac contractility may be considered. Careful follow-up of renal function after cessation of all potential nephrotoxins may be worthwhile. In the case of NSAID and ACEI agent-induced ARF, renal function usually returns rapidly toward normal with drug cessation. Sometimes the possibility of occlusion of renal arterial flow becomes an issue with respect to ARF. In these circumstances renal radionuclide tests, magnetic resonance angiography, and occasionally conventional angiography are indicated.

Renal Biopsy

If the cause of ARF still remains unknown, a percutaneous renal biopsy can be considered.[58] This procedure may reveal the presence of acute glomerulonephritis, vasculitis, or interstitial nephritis, which could respond to corticosteroids or other therapy. The precise indications for a renal biopsy in the setting of ARF have not been firmly established. However, several factors including the lack of clinical or laboratory clues to the cause of the ARF and the presence of features atypical of ATN (proteinuria and red cells or red cell casts on urinalysis, systemic disease, significant hypertension, or the presence of an unexplained pulmonary-renal syndrome) are reasonable indications for ordering a renal biopsy in ARF.[58,59] Experience demonstrates that renal biopsy can be successfully performed in ICU patients undergoing mechanical ventilation.[60]

APPROACH TO MANAGEMENT PREVENTION (Box 56-2)

Maintenance of Renal Perfusion and Urine Flow with Volume Expansion

In general medical-surgical and ICU populations, the major risk factors predisposing to ARF are decreased renal perfusion, nephrotoxins, and septic shock, as noted previously. For example, at the University of Pennsylvania Hospital, the adjusted odds ratios for the development of ARF were 9.4 for volume depletion, 9.0 for congestive heart failure, 5.6 for aminoglycoside use, 4.9 for radiocontrast exposure, and near infinity for septic shock.[61] Thus effects to prevent ARF should be directed at maintaining renal perfusion, avoiding nephrotoxins, and preventing nosocomial infections.

Two approaches are available for maintenance of "renal perfusion" in high-risk populations. The simplest is modest volume expansion. One clinical setting in which ARF may potentially be prevented by volume expansion and maintenance of a high urine flow rate is pigmenturia caused by either myoglobinuria or hemoglobinuria.[62-64] In experimentally induced rhabdomyolysis, extracellular fluid volume status is a critical determinant of renal outcome.[62] For example, experimental rhabdomyolysis dramatically reduces renal blood flow and GFR.[62] Volume expansion within 6 hours of induction of rhabdomyolysis restores renal blood flow and GFR to normal, while volume expansion administered 12 or more hours after rhabdomyolysis restores renal blood flow but not GFR.[56] Empiric observations suggest similar results in humans with muscle crush injury.[63]

The management of fluid volume in patients with septic shock can be a particularly challenging problem.[21,65] Septic shock can be associated with relative vasodilation and venodilation and increased vascular permeability with sequestration of extracellular fluid volume and renal hypoperfusion. Also, cardio-depression commonly occurs in the setting of septic shock. Although many clinicians use modest fluid/volume resuscitation in patients with septic shock, there is significant potential to worsen pulmonary function through induction of pulmonary edema.[21,65] Thus, although fluid challenges can result in stabilization and improvement in renal function in patients with septic shock, persistent fluid challenges should be

Box 56-2

Preventive Strategies to Minimize ARF

Avoid Use of Nephrotoxins
- Recognize agents with nephrotoxic potential
- Recognize high-risk patients
- Avoidance if possible
- Use of smallest dose
- Formulary modifications if available
- Monitor levels if available
- Carefully monitor renal function
- Maintain volume expanded state if possible
- Avoid concurrent administration of more than a single potential nephrotoxin
- Automatic stop orders to help reevaluate need for potential nephrotoxins

Maintain Volume Expanded State and High Urine Flow
- Trauma, burns, major surgery
- Exposure to selected toxins (radiocontrast, cisplatin, acyclovir, high doses of methotrexate, sulfonamides)
- Pigmenturic states

Decrease Risk of Nosocomial Infection
- Minimize use of invasive lines and indwelling catheters
- Avoid aspiration
- Low tolerance to culture

avoided if either no change in renal function or worsening oxygenation occurs.

Modest volume expansion has become standard practice in patients receiving contrast media.[29,66,67] No prospective randomized trial has proved the benefit of fluid administration, and fluid administration may not afford complete protection for high-risk patients.[29,66,67] It has also become standard clinical practice to use modest volume expansion to protect the kidneys from cisplatin-induced nephrotoxicity.[68] Although prospective controlled trials are not available to document efficacy, most oncologists and nephrologists feel strongly that this therapy is of benefit in protecting the kidney from cisplatin-induced decreases in GFR, although newer formulations of cisplatin are less nephrotoxic. Substantial experimental and uncontrolled clinical observations also suggest that maintenance of euvolemia and normal renal perfusion can protect the kidneys from amphotericin-induced nephrotoxicity, although, again, newer formulations of amphotericin may be less nephrotoxic.

Deposition of relatively insoluble crystals within renal tubules with resulting tubular obstruction is another form of ARF that may be preventable by maintenance of a high urine flow rate.[70] Intratubular deposition of uric acid crystals has been clearly demonstrated to be prevented by maintaining a high rate of urine flow in the experimental setting. Although uric acid solubility is enhanced at an alkaline pH, high urine flow appears to be significantly more protective against uric acid nephropathy than alkaline urine pH.[71] Methotrexate, acyclovir, sulfadiazine, and indinavir are therapeutic agents that, when administered in high doses, can occasionally be associated with ARF.[70] Although the mechanisms of the ARF associated with these agents remain to be precisely defined, intratubular precipitation of insoluble parent drug or drug metabolite appears likely. Anecdotal experience suggests that maintaining high urine flow can protect the kidneys from the nephrotoxicity that occasionally follows high doses of these agents, and this is currently standard practice.

Maintenance of Renal Perfusion and Urine Flow with Vasodilators and Diuretics

In addition to volume expansion, use of a variety of renal vasodilators (dopamine, fenoldopam, natriuretic peptides, and other agents) and selected diuretic agents (furosemide and mannitol) has been advocated to prevent ARF in certain high-risk settings. To date, however, small trials have failed to demonstrate benefit of low-dose dopamine to prevent deterioration in renal function in several operative settings including cardiac and high-risk vascular surgery and biliary tract surgery, and larger controlled trials also fail to demonstrate benefit in other settings as well.[42,72-75] Currently, no evidence-based data support a role for prophylactic dopamine in the ICU. More recently, some trials have examined the efficacy of the dopamine DA-1 receptor agonist fenoldopam mesylate on renal function in two populations at high risk for ARF (critically ill cancer patients and septic patients).[76-78] These studies suggest some modest renal functional and length-of-stay benefit, whereas studies in other settings have been less promising.[79] Additional data are necessary to define whether a prophylactic role for fenoldopam in the ICU can be justified. Small trials have suggested some benefit from natriuretic peptides to attenuate and/or ameliorate ARF, but clearly more data are necessary to assess the potential value of these agents in ARF.[80]

Diuretic agents have been utilized in ICU patients in numerous ways in the setting of ARF. Among the rationales for the use of diuretics in patients either at risk or with early ARF are (1) to prevent volume overload; (2) to maintain high urine flow, which could "wash out" debris and cast obstructing tubules, thereby attenuating ARF in patients felt to be at risk for nephrotoxic, pigmenturic, or crystal-associated ARF; (3) to "convert" early oliguric ARF to a nonoliguric state; and (4) perhaps by decreasing renal tubular work and oxygen consumption, to decrease sensitivity to injury. Although some studies suggest that diuretic therapy may increase adverse outcomes in ARF, others fail to find an effect of diuretic agents to increase risk of adverse ARF outcomes.[81,82] Clearly, there is no definitive consensus as to the role and impact of diuretics in the setting of ARF. If diuretics are used and no diuretic response is seen, then continuation should not be done.

Avoidance of Nephrotoxicity

Perhaps up to 15% to 25% of all cases of ARF encountered in the ICU can be attributed, to pharmacologic agent–induced nephrotoxicity.[10,42,61,66,70,83,84] Common nephrotoxins include radiocontrast agents, ACEIs, angiotensin receptor blockers, NSAIDs, and aminoglycosides. Other nephrotoxins that are either less frequently encountered or used in highly selected patient populations include amphotericin B, pentamidine, vancomycin, tetracycline, cisplatin, and high doses of methotrexate and acyclovir, intravenous immunoglobulin (IVIG), and nucleoside inhibitors. General principles involved in avoiding drug-induced nephrotoxicity are (1) recognizing the nephrotoxic potential of selected pharmacologic agents, (2) knowing which patient populations are at high risk for renal toxicity for each potential nephrotoxin, (3) weighing the risk to benefit ratio for use of a potential nephrotoxin in each patient, (4) considering the use of alternative non-nephrotoxic agents, (5) using the smallest effective dose of each potential nephrotoxin for the briefest interval, (6) developing computerized surveillance for symptoms with associated early notification of clinicians for the possible occurrence of drug-related nephrotoxicity,[85] (7) monitoring blood levels when available, and (8) frequently monitoring renal function (serum creatinine).

As noted previously, NSAIDs usually induce ARF by causing intense renal vasoconstriction.[25,86,87] Less frequently, NSAID-induced ARF can be attributed to acute inflammation of the glomerulus and/or interstitium. Patients at high risk for development of NSAID-induced ARF include individuals with volume depletion, shock, hypotension, an edematous disorder, advanced age, and underlying chronic renal failure. Any patient with one or more of these risk factors should be carefully monitored for changes in renal function during NSAID therapy. The same patient population at highest risk for NSAID-induced ARF is also at greatest risk for an abrupt decrease in renal function following ACEI and angiotensin II receptor inhibitor therapy.[24] In addition, patients with bilateral renal artery stenosis or unilateral renal artery stenosis in a solitary kidney are very susceptible for ARF after converting enzyme inhibitor therapy.

Patients at highest risk for developing ARF after exposure to radiocontrast agents include those with diabetic nephropathy, chronic renal insufficiency, underlying poor renal perfusion from volume depletion or heart failure, and exposure to other nephrotoxins and large volumes of contrast material.[29-31] The use of newer, more expensive, low osmotic, nonionic contrast agents exerts a modest protective effect. In patients at risk for contrast nephropathy, the smallest possible dosage of contrast should be used, and repetitive contrast exposure and concomitant nephrotoxins should be avoided. As discussed previously, prophylactic volume expansion may be of benefit. As discussed in Chapter 57, N-acetyl-cysteine and sodium bicarbonate may also be of benefit in selected patients to prevent and/or attenuate radiocontrast-associated ARF.

Risk factors for aminoglycoside nephrotoxicity include high doses; long duration of therapy; decreased renal perfusion; liver disease; concomitant nephrotoxins; and, possibly, advanced age.[26-28] In patients in whom aminoglycoside therapy is being considered, clear guidelines for use and cessation of the agent should be developed, euvolemia and adequate renal perfusion should be maintained, concomitant nephrotoxins should be avoided, dosage should be adjusted to maintain normal plasma levels, and serial measurements of renal function should be made. Once-daily dosing of aminoglycoside exerts bacteriologic cure comparable with standard dosing regimens and perhaps slightly less nephrotoxicity.[83]

It is possible that formulation modification of selected potential nephrotoxic agents can reduce the occurrence of ARF. The two best examples are nonionic contrast and lipid emulsified amphotericin B, which may have modestly reduced nephrotoxicity relative to the standard preparations.

Box 56-3

General Therapeutic Approach in ARF

Correct prerenal factors and maintain euvolemic state.

Attempt to establish a urine output if the patient remains oliguric despite correction of prerenal factors and exclusion of obstructive uropathy.

Provide adequate nutrition.

Carefully monitor all drug therapy.

Monitor for clinical and biochemical complications (see Box 56-4).

Reduce risk for infection (remove invasive lines and bladder catheter as quickly as feasible, and institute prophylactic maneuvers to avoid aspiration of gastric contents).

Use renal replacement therapy when indicated.

TREATMENT (Box 56-3)

Establishing Urine Output—Diuretics and Vasodilators

Once ARF has developed and treatable or reversible prerenal, postrenal, and renal causes have been excluded, the general therapeutic approach outlined in Box 56-3 might be considered. Obviously, optimization of extracellular fluid volume status, cardiac index, and maintenance of perfusion and oxygenation of vital organs is the first consideration.

Once volume status and cardiac output have been optimized and the patient remains oliguric, formerly it was common clinical practice to attempt to make the patient nonoliguric by use of loop diuretics and/or renal vasodilators. However, this issue remains extremely contentious and, in general, has fallen out of favor.[42,88-91] The rationale underlying this therapy is that nonoliguric forms of ATN are associated with significantly less morbidity and mortality and are easier to manage than oliguric forms.[42,43] Moreover, the risk to the patient from a trial of renal vasodilation and/or potent diuretic therapy has generally been assumed to be low. To date, proof is lacking that oliguric forms of ATN can be converted into nonoliguric forms with reduced mortality rates by use of high-dose diuretics.[90,91] If a diuretic response is not seen after one or two doses, diuretic agents should be discontinued.

The use of a renal vasodilator such as dopamine, either alone or combined with high-dose loop diuretics, has been advocated as efficacious in establishing a urine output and attenuating ARF in patients that remain oliguric despite correction of prerenal factors.[42] To date, the efficacy of this approach is supported only by anecdotal data. In studies of oliguric postoperative patients, in which each patient served as his or her own control, low-dose dopamine was clearly capable of inducing a diuretic response but not an effect to increase GFR.[92] Analyses of large databases suggest no benefit to low-dose dopamine to treat either early or more established ARF.[88,89] Use of other vasodilatory peptides has also been studied in the setting of established ARF. Although initial trials with anaritide suggested potential benefit in oliguric ARF, subsequent randomized controlled studies have failed to demonstrate clinical value of either anaritide or of another vasodilatory atrial natriuretic peptides on clinical ARF.[93-95]

Growth Factors/Stem Cells

Selected growth factors have demonstrated significant benefit in the treatment of laboratory models of ARF.[96,97] This benefit results from attenuation of the degree and acceleration in the rate of ARF recovery. One growth factor that improves experimental ARF is insulin-like growth factor 1 (IGF-1). Two studies have examined the clinical utility of IGF-1 in human ARF.[98,99] In 54 patients

Table 56-7. Treatment of Hyperkalemia in Acute Renal Failure

Modality	Onset	Duration	Mechanism
Calcium (10 mL of 10% calcium gluconate for 1-3 doses)	Immediately	Brief (min)	Increases threshold potential
Glucose-insulin-bicarbonate (500 mL of 10%-30% glucose with 10-30 U of insulin and 1-3 ampules of sodium bicarbonate; 100 mL first h, then 20-30 mL/h)	20-60 min	Few h	Intracellular shift of potassium
Albuterol (0.5 mg IV in 5 min or 10-20 mg nebulized and inhaled over 10 min)	30-60 min	1-2 h	Intracellular shift of potassium
Potassium exchange resin (200-500 g sodium polystyrene sulphonate [Kayexalate] plus 70% sorbitol; 20-30 mL and/or 50-100 mL rectal enema)	1-4 h	Few h	Removal of potassium
Hemodialysis	2-3 h	Several h	Removal of potassium

undergoing aortic aneurysm or renal revascularization surgery, half were treated with placebo and half with IGF-1.[98] At 72 hours postoperatively, patients treated with IGF-1 had an approximate 7 mL/minute increase over baseline creatinine clearance, whereas those treated with placebo had a 5 mL/minute decrease in creatinine clearance ($p < 0.05$). A smaller percentage of IGF-1–treated patients demonstrated a postoperative decline in renal function (22%) than placebo-treated patients (33%). By contrast, in a multicenter randomized controlled trial of 72 patients with ARF of diverse origin, no benefit of IGF-1 therapy could be found.[99] Together these data do not support use of this growth factor to treat ARF. Other factors such as thyroxine, hepatocyte growth factor, and bone morphogenic protein have shown promise in animal models of ischemic and toxic ARF, but, to date, efficacy in human trials is lacking.[100] Some experimental data suggests potential benefit of stem cells in the treatment of ARF. However, to date, there are no clinical data with regard to stem cell therapies.[101]

Preventing, Monitoring, and Treating Complications (see Boxes 56-3 and 56-4; Tables 56-7 and 56-8)

Hyperkalemia

Hyperkalemia is an ever-present threat to survival in ARF. Plasma potassium concentrations of more than 5 mEq/L occur in up to 50% and more than 6 mEq/L in up to 30% of patients with ARF.[102] Hyperkalemia occurs because of continued accumulation of potassium in extracellular fluid associated with diminished ability of the kidney to eliminate potassium. Usually the potassium concentration increases by about 0.2 to 0.4 mEq/L/day. Greater increases occur in the presence of continued potassium intake (e.g., intravenous fluids, blood products, and dietary sources) or continued release of potassium from body stores (e.g., hemolysis, tumor lysis, and rhabdomyolysis). Hyperkalemia poses a hazard to patient survival by increasing the resting electrical membrane potential of myocardial conducting tissue. As the resting potential nears the threshold potential, electrocardiographic (ECG) changes (loss of P waves, peaked T waves, bradycardia, left axis deviation, left bundle branch block, wide QRS complex) can occur. These ECG changes are optimally seen in leads V2-4. Eventually a sine wave and asystole result.

Therapeutic alternatives for treating hyperkalemia in ARF are listed in Table 56-7. Mild elevations (<5.5 mEq/L without ECG changes) can best be treated by withdrawing all sources of potassium and continued close ECG and laboratory follow-up. If values increase to more than 6.0 mEq/L, and especially if ECG changes are present, then more active therapy is indicated (see Table 56-7). Intravenous calcium is immediately effective for hyperkalemic emergencies. One or more of the other modalities listed in Table 56-6 can be used when immediate lowering of the potassium level is not necessary.

Box 56-4

Biochemical and Clinical Complications of Acute Renal Failure

Biochemical/Hematologic

- Blood urea nitrogren increases (10-20 mg/dL/day noncatabolic, >30 mg/dL/day catabolic)
- Creatinine increases (1-2 mg/dL/day, except in 20% to 30% of cases of rhabdomyolysis in which increase is greater)
- Potassium increases (0.1-0.5 mEq/L/day)
- Bicarbonate decreases (0-2 mEq/L/day)
- Calcium decreases
- Phosphorus increases
- Uric acid increases
- Hematocrit decreases
- Platelet function decreases

Clinical

- Neuropsychiatric (confusion, disorientation, agitation, asterixis, seizures)
- Cardiovascular (fluid overload, edema, arrhythmias, pericarditis, hypertension)
- Gastrointestinal (anorexia, nausea, vomiting, hiccups, hemorrhage)
- Pulmonary (fluid overload, infection)
- Infectious (intravenous sites, catheters, wounds, lung)

Calcium, Phosphorus, and Magnesium Disorders

Hypocalcemia and hyperphosphatemia are nearly uniform occurrences in ARF.[102-104] The hyperphosphatemia is caused by decreased urinary excretion of phosphorus with continued release of phosphorus from intracellular stores. Usually the increase in serum phosphorus is modest, with peak values in the 4 to 6 mg/dL range. In the presence of diffuse tissue injury (i.e., rhabdomyolysis, tumor lysis syndrome), marked (>9 mg/dL) hyperphosphatemia can occur. Significant hyperphosphatemia can lead to hypocalcemia and tissue deposition of calcium phosphate salts if the calcium times phosphorus product exceeds 60 to 70. Therefore monitoring of serum phosphorus concentration is necessary. Mild elevations can be treated with oral phosphate binders such as aluminum hydroxide and/or calcium carbonate. More marked elevations are usually treated with dialysis.

Hypocalcemia in ARF is usually modest, with values exceeding 6 to 7 mg/dL.[102-104] Hypocalcemia is rarely of clinical significance because the ionized calcium is maintained by metabolic acidemia. However, aggressive correction of acidemia can precipitate tetany and other symptoms of hypocalcemia. The cause of the hypocalcemia is multifactorial. Some can be attributed to hyperphosphatemia with a presumed reciprocal lowering of calcium as a result of calcium phosphate tissue precipitation. The most significant hypocalcemia usually occurs in the presence of profound hyperphosphatemia. Other factors can also contribute to hypocalcemia of ARF. Despite very high parathyroid hormone levels in ARF, parathyroid hormone does not mobilize calcium from bone as it does in normal individuals. This skeletal resistance to parathyroid hormone in ARF may result in part from an impaired ability of the diseased kidney to 1 hydroxylate 25-$(OH)_2$ vitamin D_3, rendering vitamin D active. Thus low levels of the active form of vitamin D_3 (1,25-dihydroxy vitamin D_3) are frequently seen in patients with ARF. Usually lowering serum phosphate concentration when appropriate is the only treatment needed to improve the serum calcium concentration in ARF. If symptoms of hypocalcemia are present, the infusion of calcium gluconate to alleviate these symptoms may be indicated.

Rarely, hypercalcemia complicates the course of ARF. This hypercalcemia usually occurs during the diuretic phase of rhabdomyolysis-associated ARF.[104] The mechanisms of this hypercalcemia are unclear. However, mobilization of calcium salts deposited in damaged tissue combined with normalization of 1,25-dihydroxy vitamin D_3 levels and loss of skeletal resistance to parathyroid hormone may contribute. This hypercalcemia can be treated by dialysis with calcium-free dialysate if necessary.

Hypermagnesemia of modest degree (2 to 4 mg/dL) is frequently seen in ARF.[102,103] This degree of hypermagnesemia is almost always asymptomatic. However, significant symptomatic hypermagnesemia can occur if magnesium-containing antacids are given to patients with ARF.

Hyponatremia

Hyponatremia from excess free water administration in the presence of impaired renal ability to excrete water is common in ARF.[106] This hyponatremia is generally mild and asymptomatic, although a marked reduction in serum sodium concentration that occurs quickly can lead to confusion, disorientation, and seizures. Treatment consists of water restriction. In unusual circumstances, dialytic therapy may be necessary.

Hyperuricemia

Hyperuricemia from continued production concomitant with decreased renal excretion of uric acid usually accompanies ARF. The usual peak uric acid concentration is 9 to 10 mg/dL. Much higher levels of uric acid are seen when ARF accompanies diffuse cell injury, as in rhabdomyolysis, in which case the mean uric acid concentration averages 14 to 15 mg/dL and not infrequently exceeds 20 mg/dL.[34,105] Despite high concentrations of uric acid in the blood, there is little evidence that this temporary hyperuricemia results in harm. The GFR in ARF is usually so low that little uric acid is filtered, and thus intratubular precipitation does not occur. Acute gout is rarely seen in patients with ARF, despite frequent hyperuricemia. Thus the secondary hyperuricemia of ARF is usually not specifically treated. One setting in which hyperuricemia is harmful is acute uric acid nephropathy, which typically occurs after therapy for bulky tumors when there was no pretreatment with xanthine oxidase inhibitors (allopurinol) or aggressive hydration.[105] Almost always the plasma uric acid concentration exceeds 20 mg/dL. Sometimes it is difficult to distinguish whether hyperuricemia is a cause or a consequence of ARF. Hyperuricemia as a cause of renal failure usually requires an acute elevation of plasma

Table 56-8. Treatment Options for Hemorrhagic Diathesis in Acute Renal Failure (ARF)

Treatment	Time of Onset	Duration	Comment
Desmopressin (0.3 g/kg of body weight IV over 30 min)	1-4 h	<8-12 h	Tachyphylaxis with repeated doses
Cryoprecipitate (10 U IV over 15-30 min)	1-4 h	12-14 h	Possible risk of hepatitis
Conjugated estrogens (0.6 mg/kg of body weight IV over 40 min)	12-24 h	Several d with repetitive doses	Not well studied in ARF
Elevation of hematocrit (packed RBCs sufficient to elevate hematocrit level to >30% to 35%)	Few h	Few d	Complications of transfusion

IV, intravenous; RBCs, red blood cells.

uric acid to more than 20 mg/dL and results in oligoanuric ARF with abundant uric acid crystals in the urine.

Metabolic Acidosis

Metabolic acidosis, from continued production of nonvolatile acid combined with inability of the sick kidney to generate new bicarbonate, occurs frequently in ARF. In our experience the decline in plasma bicarbonate concentration that occurs from metabolic acidosis in ARF is usually about 0.5 to 1 mEq/L/day.[43] Approximately 20% of ARF patients develop a bicarbonate concentration of less than 15 mEq/L. This metabolic acidosis is usually associated with an increase in anion gap. In some cases of rhabdomyolysis-associated ARF, a greater anion gap will be seen.[34] The mild nature of the metabolic acidosis that can be attributed to ARF per se usually does not require therapy. However, ARF often occurs in a setting in which excess lactic acid accumulates and following ingestions (e.g., ethylene glycol) that result in marked acidosis.

Anemia

Some degree of anemia usually occurs with ARF.[42] In general, with uncomplicated severe ARF, the hematocrit slowly declines to a nadir of about 30% to 35%, where it remains until renal function improves. The mechanisms underlying the anemia are related, at least in part, to impaired red cell production caused by deficiency of erythropoietin, which is synthesized by the kidney.[107] For example, in a recent study of 20 patients with ARF, radioimmunoassay values for erythropoietin were very low. Several weeks and in some cases months were required for normalization of serum erythropoietin in ARF patients.[107] In one patient with ARF, exogenous recombinant erythropoietin resulted in a brisk reticulocytosis and amelioration of anemia, suggesting a lack of endogenous inhibitors of erythropoiesis in ARF.[107] In other studies, erythropoietin use has not been associated with either a decrease in transfusion requirements or with enhanced renal recovery when given in the context of ARF.[108] Other factors often contribute to the anemia of ARF including frequent blood drawing for laboratory testing, gastrointestinal blood loss, loss of blood during procedures, marrow suppression caused by medications, and loss of red blood cells in dialyzers. Of note, several disease processes that can produce ARF may have prominent hemogram abnormalities such as anemia (plasma cell dyscrasia); eosinophilia (allergic interstitial nephritis, polyarteritis nodosa, atheroembolic disease); and thrombocytopenia (systemic lupus erythematosus, thrombotic thrombocytopenia purpura, hemolytic-uremia syndrome, malignant hypertension, disseminated intravascular coagulation). In general the anemia of ARF develops slowly and is usually well tolerated. Thus not only is specific treatment often not indicated, but it is not likely to be effective.[107-109]

Bleeding

Clinically significant bleeding may complicate the course of 10% to 30% of patients with ARF. For example, Levy and colleagues[14] found that 15% of patients with mild radiocontrast-induced ARF had a bleeding disorder before they developed ARF, and this increased to 27% after the occurrence of ARF. In a large multicenter study, 32% to 42% of patients with ARF had some degree of thrombocytopenia, and 13% to 27% had a coagulapathy.[94]

Usually the coagulopathy results from associated diseases (e.g., liver disease, sepsis, disseminated intravascular coagulation) or treatments (e.g., multiple transfusions, protein C). When ARF results from traumatic and atraumatic rhabdomyolysis, particularly in association with cocaine abuse, thrombocytopenia and disseminated intravascular coagulopathy are especially likely to occur.[110] The ARF state per se may result in a functional defect in platelets, leading to prolongation of the bleeding time and perhaps contributing to clinically relevant coagulopathy.[111-115]

Several therapeutic maneuvers can improve the bleeding time and the coagulopathy that is occasionally seen in ARF states (see Table 56-8). Intravenous administration of desmopressin is the easiest, safest method of shortening the bleeding time.[112] Unfortunately, the effect of desmopressin is short-lived, and patients rapidly become tachyphylactic to repetitive doses. Cryoprecipitate also shortens the bleeding time in renal failure states.[113] Again, the duration is relatively brief. The precise mechanisms whereby desmopressin and cryoprecipitate shorten bleeding time in renal failure are not known. Most data suggest that these agents result in induction (desmopressin) or infusion (cryoprecipitate) of large, multimeric forms of factor VIII-von Willebrand factor aggregates, which enhances binding of platelets to endothelial surfaces.[115] Repeated doses of conjugated estrogen can result in prolonged normalization of the bleeding time in uremia, although the mechanism is not clear.[114] An elevated hematocrit level also shortens the bleeding time in uremia.[113] Finally, dialysis may shorten the bleeding time, but the magnitude of effect and amount of dialysis required to achieve improvement are highly variable.

Infections

Infectious complications are among the most common causes of death in ARF. For example, in an older study infections were judged to be the primary cause of death in 30% to 50% of seriously ill patients with ARF. In most studies of ICU patients with ARF, more than 50% to 75% of patients experience at least one infectious complication.[42] Levy and colleagues[14] found that the frequency of sepsis before and after the development of ARF was 22% and 45%, respectively. Common sources of infections are operative sites, intravascular access lines, the urinary tract, and the lungs. Because of the frequent presence of infection, most ICU patients with ARF are treated with multiple antibiotics for several days. Clinical signs such as fever and leukocytosis are often less pronounced when infection is present in patients with ARF compared with those with normal renal function.[116] To reduce the risk of infection, efforts should be directed at possible prevention of nosocomial infections by removing invasive lines and bladder catheters as soon as possible. Strict aseptic technique and clinical monitoring of line sites are necessary. When infection is suspected, prompt culturing and selective use of antimicrobial agents are indicated. A recent prospective controlled trial also suggests that intravenous gamma globulin may be a helpful therapeutic adjunct in treating ARF.[117] The improved outcome in patients treated with intravenous gamma globulin in this study could not be attributed to a decrease in either number or severity of infections. Confirmation of this study is clearly necessary.

Cardiovascular Complications

Because most patients with ICU-associated ARF are severely ill, hemodynamic instability is commonly encountered. In an oliguric patient with ARF, volume overload with resultant pulmonary edema, peripheral edema, and hypertension is an ever-present threat to well-being and survival.[42] Although pulmonary edema is usually caused by positive fluid balance, decreased colloid oncotic pressure caused by hypoalbuminemia and perhaps increased pulmonary capillary permeability can contribute. Also, many patients at high risk for developing ARF have underlying chronic heart disease. Careful serial clinical evaluation, monitoring of fluid-volume status, body weight, oxygenation, hemodynamic measurements, and chest radiographs are often necessary to help assess volume status in patients with ARF. Several cardiovascular complications such as myocardial infarction; arrhythmias; and, rarely, pericarditis can complicate the course of patients with ARF. In a recent national multicenter study, 22% to 29% of patients with ARF experienced cardiac arrhythmias requiring therapy and 13% to 19% had evidence of myocardial ischemia.[94] The development of any of these cardiovascular complications is a major risk factor for adverse outcome from ARF. Treatment of fluid overload in the setting of ARF depends on the degree of renal impairment. If it is mild nonoliguric ARF, loop diuretics are often effective in reducing positive fluid balance. If the patient has severe oliguric ARF, some type of extracorporeal method of removing volume is necessary.

Pulmonary Complications

In addition to volume overload, several other processes can involve the lungs in patients with ARF. Thus aspiration, infection, and adult respiratory distress syndrome (ARDS) all occur commonly in patients with ARF.[1-17,42] In our experience, patients with ARF have about a 30% chance of developing an infiltrate on chest radiograph.[43] In many series of patients with severe ARF, up to 50% also have respiratory failure sufficient to require mechanical ventilation.[1-17] Allgren and colleagues[94] found that 48% to 55% of ARF patients were intubated and ventilated at the time they developed ARF; Liano and Pascual[18] reported that 28% of ARF patients were intubated and ventilated at the time they developed ARF. Levy and colleagues[14] found that the frequency of respiratory failure was 36% before onset of ARF, and this increased to 78% after ARF occurred. Similar findings have been reported by others.[9,16] Mechanical ventilation is clearly a significant, independent factor associated with increased mortality in patients with ARF.[9]

Several disease processes can cause simultaneous renal and respiratory failure; these include acute glomerulonephritis with volume overload, Goodpasture's syndrome, Wegener's granulomatosis, systemic lupus erythematosus, polyarteritis nodosa, cryoglobulinemia, and renal vein thrombosis with pulmonary emboli.[118] As discussed in the following section, development of a pulmonary complication is one of the most ominous prognostic factors in patients with ARF. Thus strict precautions to guard against the development of aspiration pneumonia are necessary.

Gastrointestinal Complications

Anorexia, nausea, and vomiting are symptoms commonly seen in patients with advanced renal failure. In many series, gastrointestinal hemorrhage, often ascribed to stress gastritis or ulcers, has been reported to occur in 5% to 30% of patients with ARF. Usually gastrointestinal hemorrhage is loosely defined, relatively mild, and easily controlled, but on occasion it may be the cause of death in patients with ARF. Whether the presence of ARF per se is an indication for prophylactic therapy for gastrointestinal bleeding, in the absence of well-recognized indications such as respiratory failure and coagulopathy, is debated.[119] Careful prospective studies are necessary for defining the frequency of occurrence and delineating the cause of gastrointestinal hemorrhage in ARF. Also, extreme caution in using magnesium-containing antacids is necessary in the setting of ARF because of the almost exclusive renal route of elimination of magnesium.

Jaundice frequently occurs during the course of ARF in ICU patients. Liano and colleagues[18] found that 28% of patients with ICU-associated ARF were jaundiced at some time during the course of their illness. The etiologic picture in jaundice is usually multifactorial, with passive hepatic congestion, multiple blood transfusions, sepsis, hypotension, and many medications contributing. A mild increase in amylase also occurs in ARF, and pancreatitis is present in 2% to 10% of patients at the onset of ARF. Because of this amylase elevation, careful clinical assessment and determination of serum lipase levels are often necessary to ascertain whether pancreatitis is present in a patient with ARF.

Neurologic Complications

Neurologic complications such as confusion, disorientation, lethargy, somnolence, coma, myoclonus, asterixis, and seizures can occur as a result of ARF.[42] Levy and colleagues[14] found that the frequency of mental status changes increased from 41% before to 68% after development of ARF. Abnormal consciousness at the time of first visit in patients with ARF was found in 30% of patients reported by Liano and colleagues.[18] Several causes of neurologic dysfunction are often operative in patients with ARF. Most prominent among these are medication-induced encephalopathy, other metabolic disturbances, and primary neurologic disorders such as stroke. Also, several systemic disorders such as vasculitis, endocarditis, TTP, and malignant hypertension can present with simultaneous ARF and neurologic dysfunction.

Medication-Related Complications

Most pharmacologic agents are eliminated, at least in part, by the kidneys. Thus use of standard doses and dosing intervals of many pharmacologic agents in patients with

ARF can lead to accumulation of active drug and/or metabolites, with subsequent drug-induced morbidity and mortality. To avoid medication-induced toxicity in ARF, daily scrutiny of the medication list is essential. All medications not essential for care should be eliminated. A thorough understanding of the pathways of drug metabolism and elimination and the potential side effects of each drug used is mandatory. Excellent, up-to-date resources of this information are readily available.[120] Careful monitoring of clinical and biochemical parameters and drug levels is indicated, especially for agents with narrow therapeutic indices that are eliminated by the kidneys.

NUTRITIONAL CONSIDERATIONS

Nutritional support for patients with ARF must be considered in the overall context of associated comorbid conditions and other aspects of the management of critically ill patients.[2,121-124] Most patients with ARF encountered on general medical-surgical wards are nonoliguric and noncatabolic and have mild renal failure with an increment in serum creatinine less than 2 to 3 mg/dL. In these patients the enteral route of feeding is usually available, and these patients have modestly increased nutritional requirements of about 30 to 35 Kcal/kg/day.[122] About 0.5 to 0.6 g/kg/day of high biologic value protein is necessary. Potassium restriction may be required, depending on the serum potassium concentration. Many ICU patients with ARF are oliguric and have severe renal failure. Moreover, in these patients with ICU-associated ARF, protein catabolic rate is very high.[121-124] The optimal means and outcome of nutritional supplementation in this population of ARF patients are debated.

A key issue regarding nutritional support and supplementation of severe, catabolic ICU-associated ARF is this: Does such support improve clinical outcome? Very early studies were encouraging. In 1973 Abel and colleagues[125] studied 53 patients with severe ARF in a prospective, randomized fashion. Survival of patients treated with L-amino acids and hypertonic glucose was 75% versus 44% in patients treated with hypertonic glucose alone. In a study of 149 patients, Baek and colleagues[126] found a 54% survival rate in patients with ARF treated with glucose and essential amino acids and a 30% survival rate in patients treated with glucose alone. Neither the study by Abel's group nor that of Baek's investigators provided nitrogen balance information. Unfortunately, several smaller prospective trials have not found a survival advantage when ARF patients receiving hyperalimentation therapy with essential and nonessential amino acids were compared with control subjects not receiving amino acid supplementation.[42] Although investigations in these latter studies were unable to confirm the earlier positive outcome results, several consistent findings emerged: (1) exceptionally high catabolic rates are often observed when ARF occurs in a patient who has undergone surgery, had a traumatic injury, or is in multiorgan failure; (2) hyperalimentation can reduce the degree of negative nitrogen balance; (3) it may be difficult to reverse the negative nitrogen balance, even with infusion of large amounts of amino acids and calories; and (4) in experienced hands, hyperalimentation, when combined with dialytic or hemofiltration therapy to maintain euvolemia and electrolyte balance, can be done with a relatively low complication rate. Finally, continuous renal replacement therapy (CRRT) may have significant nutritional implications as well.[123]

From this information, it is clear that nutritional therapy of ARF occurring in the ICU demands that realistic goals be established.[2,123,124,127] Such goals might include calorie and nitrogen support to minimize negative nitrogen balance, calorie and protein delivery in a form and volume that do not introduce complications that outweigh potential benefit, and criteria for assessing efficacy of treatment. For the average 70-kg adult, severe ARF, as encountered in the ICU, requires approximately 30 to 60 Kcal/kg/day, depending on the clinical setting. Whenever possible, the enteral route should be used. The needed calories can be given as dextrose (20% to 70% solution, depending on volume status; 70% provides 2.38 Kcal/mL) and fat (10% or 20%, 250 to 500 mL/wk). Fat provides twice the caloric value per gram of carbohydrate or protein and thus requires smaller volumes; fat should not make up more than 50% to 60% of nonprotein calories. Protein can be given orally as 0.5 to 1 g/kg/day of high-biologic-value protein or intravenously as 10 to 20 g/day of essential amino acids. Supplementation with 10 to 20 g/day of essential or combined essential and nonessential amino acids should be considered once dialysis or hemofiltration is started. The amount of water and electrolytes given must be individualized but should be sufficient to maintain euvolemia and relatively normal plasma concentrations.

The greatest practical concern regarding nutritional management of ARF is fluid volume. The rate of rise of BUN, acidemia, and volume load imposed by parenteral nutrition often leads to earlier and more vigorous dialysis or hemofiltration. Other practical concerns include monitoring for other complications such as line infections, electrolyte disturbances, and metabolic abnormalities. Daily weights and measurements of BUN, glucose, Na^+, K^+, Cl^-, HCO_3^-, CA^{++}, and phosphorus are necessary. Twice-weekly monitoring of Mg^{++}, liver function studies, ammonia, and triglycerides should be done. Finally, means of assessing efficacy should be established. Although nitrogen balance studies are useful investigative tools, the daily rate of rise of BUN is the most practical method of indirectly assessing nitrogen balance. If the daily rate of rise of BUN remains constant or decreases after nutritional therapy, there is probably a reduction in negative nitrogen balance. By contrast, if the rate of rise of BUN increases, either an increase in calorie supply or a decrease in protein load should be considered. Traditional blood parameters including measurements of hepatic secretory proteins such as prealbumin and transferrin are helpful means of assessing protein nutrition status.

RENAL REPLACEMENT THERAPY

The principles of all forms of renal replacement therapy are similar. Fluid removal from a patient occurs when either a hydrostatic (hemodialysis and hemofiltration) or an osmotic (peritoneal dialysis) pressure gradient is induced across a semipermeable membrane that contains the patient's blood. Solute removal from a patient occurs when unwanted solutes are removed either by ultrafiltration (convection) or by diffusion across a semi-permeable membrane (dialysis). In dialysis, solutes diffuse from an area of relatively high concentration (ARF patient's blood) to an area of low concentration (dialysate). Solute diffusion is maintained by continuously moving "fresh" blood and dialysate next to one another on each side of the membrane, thereby preventing equilibration. The rate of solute removal generally increases with increasing blood and dialysate flow rates up to a point at which the relationship flattens. The size of the pores, the thickness of the membrane, and the degree of the hydrostatic-osmotic pressure gradients induced across the membrane are some of the determinants of the ease with which fluid and solutes can be removed. From a practical perspective, renal replacement therapy requires vascular access sufficient to maintain high blood flow and almost always anticoagulation to prevent dialysis or clotting.

Several unresolved, arguable issues regard renal replacement therapy (RRT) for ARF.[2,3] The first is: "When is it necessary?" Generally speaking, about 60% to 80% of patients with oliguric ARF and 15% to 30% of patients with nonoliguric ARF will need some form of renal replacement therapy. No study has adequately addressed timing of initiation of renal replacement therapy. Generally agreed indications include persistent hyperkalemia and/or fluid overload that is unresponsive to medical management; ongoing marked acidosis; symptoms of uremia; and, rarely, bleeding. On the basis of retrospective data, many experts feel that "prophylactic" renal replacement therapy to keep the BUN and creatinine levels below 80 to 100 mg/dL and 8 mg/dL, respectively, can be readily justified. In recent years the trend has been to institute renal replacement therapy much earlier in the course of ARF. For example, in a recent multicenter national study, serum creatinine ranged from 6.5 to 6.9 mg/dL and blood urea nitrogen 86 to 104 mg/dL at institution of dialysis.[94] In some cases early institution of RRT is justified to assist with removal of fluid volume required to maintain nutritional status. It should be kept in mind that an aggressive approach of early commencement of renal replacement therapy does not necessarily equate with an improvement in outcome. One study of 132 critically ill ARF patients found an inverse relationship between serum creatinine concentration at initiation of hemodialysis and mortality.[128] Although these data are subject to at least two interpretations (early dialysis is deleterious; or patients dialyzed earlier are sicker, with more fluid overload and electrolyte disturbances), they do raise concerns. Moreover, intermittent hemodialysis may be associated with hemodynamic instability, which, with potential impairment of renal autoregulatory responses that can occur in ARF, may lead to enhanced ischemic injury.

The modality of RRT for ARF is also debatable, with proponents of both intermittent hemodialysis (IHD) and continuous modes of RRT (CRRT).[2,3,129-142] Continuous modes of renal replacement therapy (which can also be done intermittently) include ultrafiltration only (which can be done arteriovenously without a pump or venovenously with a pump, both now rarely performed); hemofiltration (which is a convective process that can be done arteriovenously or venovenously); and hemodiafiltration (which combines convection and diffusion and can be done arteriovenously and venovenously). Currently, several hybrids of intermittent and continuous modalities are done with acronyms such as SLED (sustained low efficiency dialysis), EDD (extended daily dialysis), and SCD (slow continuous dialysis).[2] At present, most continuous forms of RRT are done venovenously with a pump. Increasing evidence fails to demonstrate that either IHD or CRRT modalities offer significant survival benefits when directly evaluated in comparable patients with ARF, and these modalities should be viewed as complementary rather than competitive.[129-142]

The choice of modality of RRT generally involves availability and comfort level of the practitioners overseeing RRT. Other factors that play major roles in the decision as to either IHD or continuous RRT include the presence of relative hypotension and hemodynamic instability (favors continuous), high patient fluid volume requirements (favors continuous), associated significant cardiac dysfunction (favors continuous), need for urgent treatment of hyperkalemia (favors IHD), need for patient mobility for off-ward testing (favors IHD), and bleeding tendency (favors IHD).[1,2] CRRT modalities, especially hemofiltration techniques that combine dialysis with significant ultrafiltrate volumes to enhance solute clearances, may provide the more intensive treatment necessary to control azotemia in catabolic ICU patients receiving high protein content nutrition. The major disadvantage of CRRT is the need for well-trained ICU nurses to oversee the procedure. A lack of detailed understanding of the CRRT flow sheets and proper procedures for regulating the largely automated controls can lead to problems as a result of significant volume depletion or excess.[131] Occasionally, lactate-based replacement fluid may result in lactate accumulation and worsening acid-base status if the patient has liver disease and is unable to metabolize lactate as a source of base. Because of indwelling catheters and continuous therapy, ambulation and physical therapy may be difficult while the patient is receiving CRRT.

Two technical issues should be noted briefly. First, many clinicians favor biocompatible versus nonbiocompatible membranes in the selection of dialysis membranes for patients with ARF. To date, however, no compelling data suggest that the type of membrane makes a major clinical difference.[2,3] Second, most clinicians prefer a bicarbonate-based over lactate-based dialysate for RRT replacement solutions for patients with ARF because of perceived improved hemodynamic stability.

PREDICTION, PROGNOSIS, AND OUTCOME

To date, a reliable, sensitive, and specific clinical tool that accurately predicts the occurrence of ARF has not been developed.[143-145] From a general perspective, the more ill the patients, the higher the likelihood of development of some form of ARF. Predicting the outcome of ARF is highly dependent on how the disorder is defined and the patient population studied. When all general medical-surgical admissions are studied in epidemiologic surveys, ARF is often defined as an acute increase in the serum creatinine level of at least 0.3 to 1 mg/dL. In this type of study, only about 10% to 20% of patients with ARF require renal replacement therapy, and mortality is relatively low at 10% to 30%. When patients with ARF are selected by reviewing nephrology consultations and hospital discharge diagnosis, the selection bias results in a set of patients in more severe renal failure. In this type of population, 20% to 50% of patients require renal replacement therapy, and mortality rates of 30% to 50% are seen. Most of the prognostic data on ICU patients with ARF are derived from the group of seriously ill individuals requiring renal replacement therapy. In these patients, mortality rates are usually 50% to 90%.

Two key questions regard the outcome from significant ARF. The first is: "Is the outcome improving in recent years with general advances in overall ICU therapies?" Despite major advances in the management of critically ill patients, the majority of data demonstrates that mortality rates of ICU patients with ARF have not improved dramatically over the past 40 years.[146] The lack of improvement in ARF outcome may arise from changes in the characteristics of patients developing ARF, such as older age, increased rate of comorbid conditions, and increased severity and number of associated multiorgan system dysfunctions. Another factor preventing improved outcome is that a real-time method of diagnosis of ARF has not yet been developed to allow early institution of specifically tailored therapy.

A second question regarding ARF outcomes is: "How good are predictive tools in determining outcome in individual cases?" To date, many tools initially developed to assess severity of illness and predict outcome in critically ill patients (e.g., acute physiology and chronic health evaluation or APACHE, simplified acute physiology score or SAPS, the mortality prediction model or MPM, the sequential organ failure assessment or SOFA, the lung injury score or LIS, the number of organs failed or NOF), as well as tools designed specifically to determine outcome in critically ill patients with ARF (the Stuivenberg hospital acute renal failure score or SHARF, the individual severity score-acute tubular necrosis or ISS-ATN, and many others) do not perform sufficiently well to allow use for decision-making in individual ARF patients.[147-157] For many of these predictive instruments, the area under the receiver operating characteristic curve is <0.7 and for some, validation and multi-institutional testing is not available. Clearly, improved predictive instruments for ARF outcome are necessary.

Major outcome determinants of acute renal failure include the cause of the ARF, severity of renal dysfunction, timing of ARF, underlying health of the patient, need for dialysis, and involvement of multiorgan system dysfunction (Box 56-5). Studies have demonstrated that if the renal insult can be identified and easily treated, outcome is improved. Moreover, cases of ARF resulting from prerenal and postrenal causes generally have lower mortality rates than cases with an intrarenal cause of ARF, which has the highest reported mortality (Fig. 56-4). The number of organ systems failed also directly correlates with ARF-related mortality (Fig. 56-5).

Box 56-5

Adverse Prognostic Factors in Acute Renal Failure (ARF) Outcome

Health of the Patient
Advancing age
Advanced underlying primary disease
Chronic health evaluation score >2
Immunosuppressive therapy
Multiple comorbid conditions

Cause and Severity of the ARF
Renal cause of ARF
Abnormal urinalysis
Rise in serum creatinine >2-3 mg/dL
Oliguric state
Requirement for renal replacement therapy

Clinical Conditions Associated with Renal Failure
Increasing severity of illness score
Number of concomitant organ systems failed
Type of concomitant organ systems failed
Presence of hypotension
Sepsis
Catabolic state

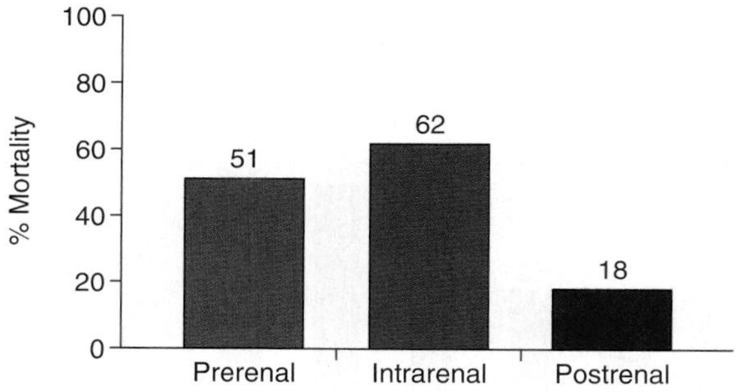

Figure 56-4. Mortality rates based on the cause of acute renal failure in intensive care unit patients. (Modified from Brivet FG, Kleinknecht DJ, Loirat P, et al: Crit Care Med 1996;24:192.)

The severity of the ARF has a major impact on outcome and management. A rise in serum creatinine that is less than 3 mg/dL is associated with lower mortality (10% to 20%) than that reported with larger increments in serum creatinine (50% to 70%).[155] The timing and length of ARF also influence outcome. It has been recognized that the late onset of ARF in the ICU is associated with at least twofold to threefold higher mortality rates. Additionally, nearly all studies have demonstrated a twofold to fourfold increase in mortality when ARF patients are oliguric compared with those that are nonoliguric. The mortality rate associated with nonoliguric ARF is reported on average to be 24%, whereas oliguric ARF averaged 69%.[42] However, it is important to emphasize that the development of nonoliguric ARF can also significantly increase mortality, especially in ICU patients with multiorgan failure and/or chronic disease.

Previously it was felt that the setting in which renal failure occurred (medical versus surgical) was an important determinant of outcome. However, recent studies find that when matched for other prognostic factors, the clinical service in which ARF is encountered has no significant influence on outcome. Advancing age has been reported by several studies to be associated with increased mortality in patients with ARF, yet older age is not uniformly found to be a poor prognostic indicator.[9,19] Furthermore, some experts maintain that advanced age may be a proxy for underlying chronic illness (e.g., cardiovascular disease, chronic renal disease, malignancy), which has been associated with worse outcomes in patients with ARF.

Dialysis is required in about 85% of oliguric patients and 30% of nonoliguric patients with ARF. Finally, the outcome of ARF, particularly as encountered in an ICU, is critically dependent on the number and type of additional organ systems that have failed. Large studies involving several thousand patients from the United States and Europe have clearly demonstrated a significant relationship between the number and duration of organ system failures and ARF outcome. In general, mortality rates for isolated ARF with no other organ system failure are in the range of 7% to 30%.[2,3,19,23,42,147-157] In contrast, dramatic increase in mortality rates of 20% to 40% for each additional organ system that fails has been readily demonstrated by several studies (see Fig. 56-5).[19,158]

Not only is the number of organ systems that concomitantly fail an important determinant of outcome in ARF, but also the type of organ system failure has substantial influence on outcome. Sweet and colleagues[158] were the first to call attention to the devastating consequences on mortality of coexisting respiratory failure and ARF. Numerous studies have subsequently confirmed these observations, demonstrating that one of the most ominous threats to patient survival is the association and/or development of a pulmonary complication. Predictably, the need for ventilatory support is associated with the worst outcomes, and mortality levels as high as 90% have been reported in some series.[9,19,20,23,47,149-161] Other conditions that signify a particularly poor outcome in ICU-acquired ARF are the presence of a cardiovascular complication (hypotension, severe heart failure, or myocardial infarction) and the presence of sepsis. In a recent multinational study, the odds ratio for mortality in patients with ARF complicated by the need for mechanical ventilation was 2.1 and for those requiring either vasopressors or inotropic agents, 2.[9]

Another issue that requires discussion regarding ARF is that of resource use and quality of life.[159,160] Aggregate resource use associated with even uncomplicated forms of ARF exceeds that of many common illnesses and is much higher for complicated cases.[14,160] Moreover, long-term survival and quality of life in individuals who have experienced ARF are not good.[160] Collectively, these issues point strongly to the need for prevention, early diagnosis, and efforts to improve ARF outcomes.

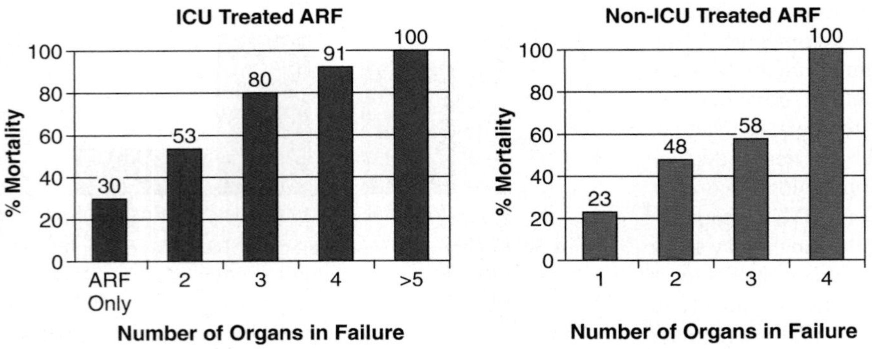

Figure 56-5. Mortality rates based on the cause of acute renal failure (ARF) in ICU and non-ICU patients. (Adapted from Liano F, Junco E, Pascual J, et al: The spectrum of acute renal failure in the intensive care unit compared with that seen in other settings. Kidney Int 1998;53[Suppl 66]:16.)

KEY POINTS

- ARF is commonly encountered in patients admitted to the hospital (1% to 3%) and to the ICU (5% to 20%).
- Preventive strategies and early intervention to attenuate the severity of ARF may help reduce the considerable morbidity and mortality (20% to 80%) associated with this disorder.
- The diagnostic approach to ARF is to first determine whether the renal failure is prerenal, renal, or postrenal in origin.
- A normal result to a urine sediment evaluation suggests either a prerenal or a postrenal cause of ARF. A sediment containing many cells, casts, or protein suggests a renal cause of ARF. ATN often presents with pigmented casts or renal epithelial cells and casts. FeNa greater than 1% or Una greater than 50 mEq/L is suggestive of ATN.
- Indications for renal replacement therapy include persistent hyperkalemia, fluid overload that is not responsive to diuretic therapy, marked acidemia, symptoms of uremia, bleeding (occasionally), and prophylaxis to keep the BUN and creatinine levels less than 100 mg/dL and 10 mg/dL, respectively.
- Several continuous modalities of renal replacement therapy are available, as well as intermittent hemodialysis. These modalities of renal replacement therapy should be considered complementary. The modality used depends on the available technology and expertise and on patient-related factors.
- The prognosis for ARF depends on the underlying health of the patient, the cause and severity of the renal failure, and the patient's overall clinical picture.

REFERENCES

1. Nolan CR, Anderson RJ: Hospital-acquired acute renal failure. J Am Soc Nephrol 1998;7:10.
2. Gill N, Nally JV, Fatica RA: Renal failure secondary to acute tubular necrosis. Chest 2005;128:2847.
3. Kanagasundaram NS, Paganini EP: Acute renal failure on the intensive care unit. Clin Med 2005;5:435.
4. Mehta RL, Pascual MT, Soroko S, et al: Spectrum of acute renal failure in the intensive care unit: The PICARD experience. Kidney Int 2004;66:1613.
5. Jannidis M, Metnitz PG: Epidemiology and natural history of acute renal failure in the ICU. Crit Care Clin 2005;21:239.
6. Bell M, Lijestam E, Grannath F, et al: Optimal follow-up time after continuous renal replacement therapy in actual renal failure patients stratified with the RIFLE criteria. Nephrol Dial Transplant 2004;20:354.
7. Gammill HS, Jeyabalan A: Acute renal failure in pregnancy. Crit Care Med 2005;33:S372.
8. Abosaif NY, Tolber YA, Heap M, et al: The outcome of acute renal failure in the intensive care unit according to RIFLE: Model application, sensitivity, and predictability. Am J Kidney Dis 2005;46:1038.
9. Uchino S, Kellum JA, Bellomo R, et al: Acute renal failure in critically ill patients. JAMA 2005;294:813.
10. Joannidis M: Drug-induced renal failure in the ICU. Int J Artif Organs 2004;27:1034.
11. Bellomo R, Bonventre J, Macias W, et al: Management of early acute renal failure: Focus on post-injury prevention. Curr Opin Crit Care 2005;11:542.
12. Kellum JA, Leblanc M, Gibney RT, et al: Primary prevention of acute renal failure in the critically ill. Curr Opin Crit Care. 2005;11:537.
13. Leblanc M, Kellum JA, Gibney RT, et al: Risk factors for acute renal failure: Inherent and modifiable risks. Curr Opin Crit Care 2005;11:533.
14. Levy EM, Visoli CM, Horwitz RI: The effect of acute renal failure on mortality. JAMA 1996;275:1487.
15. Hegarty J, Middleton RJ, Krebs M, et al: Severe acute renal failure in adults: Place of care, incidence and outcomes. Q J Med 2005;98:661.
16. Bernieh B, Al Hakim M, Boobes Y, et al: Outcome and predictive factors of acute renal failure in the intensive care unit. Transplant Proc 2004;36:1784.
17. d'Avila DO, Cendoroglo NM, dos Santos OF, et al: CE: Acute renal failure needing dialysis in the intensive care unit and prognostic scores. Ren Fail 2004;26:59.
18. Liano F, Pascual J: Epidemiology of acute renal failure: A prospective, multicenter, community-base study. Kidney Int 1996;56:811.
19. Liano F, Junco E, Pascual J, et al: The spectrum of acute renal failure in the intensive care unit compared with that seen in other settings. Kidney Int 1998;53(Suppl 66):16.
20. Brivet FG, Kleinknecht DJ, Loirat P, et al: Acute renal failure in intensive care units—causes, outcome and prognostic factors of hospital mortality: A prospective, multicenter study. Crit Care Med 1996;24:192.
21. Schrier RW, Wang W: Acute renal failure and sepsis. N Engl J Med 2004;351:159.
22. Thadhani R, Pascual M, Bonventre JV: Acute renal failure. N Engl J Med 1996;334:1448.
23. Badr KF, Ichikawa I: Prerenal failure: A deleterious shift from renal compensation to decompensation. N Engl J Med 1988;317:623.
24. Schoolwerth AC, Sica DA, Ballerman BJ, et al: Renal considerations in angiotensin converting enzyme inhibitor therapy. Circulation 2001;104:1985.
25. Cheng HF, Harris RC: Renal effects of non-steroidal anti-inflammatory drugs and selected cyclooygenase-2 inhibitors. Curr Pharm Des 2005;11:1795.
26. Swan SK: Aminoglycoside nephrotoxicity. Semin Nephrol 1997;17:27.
27. Moore RD, Smith CR, Lipskey ED: Risk factors for nephrotoxicity in patients treated with aminoglycosides. Ann Intern Med 1982;73:9.
28. Hatala R, Dinh T, Cook DJ: Once-daily aminoglycoside dosing in immunocompetent adults: A meta-analysis. Ann Intern Med 1996;124:717.
29. Rudnick MR, Kesselheim A, Goldbarb S: Contrast-induced nephropathy: How it develops, how to prevent it. Clev Clinic J Med 2006;73:75.
30. Bagshaw SM, McAlister FA, Manns BJ, et al: Acetylcysteine in the prevention of contrast-induced nephropathy. Arch Intern Med 2006;166:161.
31. Merten GJ, Burgess WP, Gray LV, et al: Prevention of contrast-induced nephropathy with sodium bicarbonate: A randomized controlled trial. JAMA 2004;291:2334.
32. Bywaters EG, Knochel JP: Milestones in nephrology—author commentary. Crush injuries with impairment of renal function commentary. J Am Soc Nephrol 1999;10:321.
33. Eneas JF, Schoenfeld PY, Humphreys MH: The effect of infusion of mannitol-sodium bicarbonate on the clinical course of myoglobinuria. Arch Intern Med 1979;137:801.
34. Gabow PA, Kaehny WD, Kelleher SP: The spectrum of rhabdomyolysis. Medicine 1982;61:41.
35. Brown CV, Rhee P, Chan L, et al: Preventing renal failure in patients with rhabdomyolysis; do bicarbonate and mannitol make a difference? J Trauma 2004;56:1191.
36. Keane WF: The assessment of risk factors in 462 patients with acute renal failure. Am J Kidney Dis 1985;5:97.
37. Moran SM, Meyers BD: Course of acute renal failure studied by a model of creatinine kinetics. Kidney Int 1985;27:920.
38. Villa P, Jiminez M, Soriano MC, et al: Serum cystatin C concentration as a marker of acute renal dysfunction in critically ill patients. Critical Care 2005;9:R139.
39. Mazul-Sunko B, Zarkovic N, Vrkic N, et al: Proatrial natriuretic peptide but not cystatin C is predictive for occurrence of acute renal insufficiency in critically ill septic patients. Nephron 2004;97:c103.
40. Ahlstrom A, Tallgren M, Peltonen S, et al: Evolution and predictive power of serum cystatin C in acute renal failure. Clin Nephrology 2004;62:344.
41. Klahr S, Miller SB: Acute oliguria. N Engl J Med 1998;338:671.
42. Lee VW, Harris DC, Anderson RJ, et al: Acute renal failure. In Schrier RW (ed): Diseases of the Kidney and Urinary Tract, 8th ed. Philadelphia, Lippincott Williams & Wilkins, 2007, p. 986.
43. Anderson RJ, Linas SL, Berns AS, et al: Nonoliguric acute renal failure. N Engl J Med 1979;296:1134.
44. Groeneveld AB, Tran DD, van der Meulen J, et al: Acute renal failure in the medical intensive care unit: predisposing, complicating factors and outcome. Nephron 1991;59:602.
45. Jochimsen F, Schafer JH, Maurer A, et al: Impairment of renal function in medical intensive care: Predictability of acute renal failure. Crit Care Med 1990;18:480.
46. Tran DD, Groeneveld AB, van der Meulen J, et al: Age, chronic disease, sepsis, organ system failure, and mortality in a medical intensive care unit. Crit Care Med 1990;18:474.
47. Behrend T, Miller SB: Acute renal failure in the cardiac care unit: Etiologies, outcomes and prognostic factors. Kidney Int 1999;56:238.
48. McCarthy JT: Prognosis of patients with acute renal failure in the intensive-care unit: A tale of two eras. Mayo Clin Proc 1996;71:117.
49. Menashe PI, Ross SA, Gottlieb JE: Acquired renal insufficiency in critically ill patients. Crit Care Med 1988;16:1106.
50. Kaufman J, Dhakal M, Patel B, et al: Community-acquired acute renal failure. Am J Kidney Dis 1991;17:191.
51. McGee S, Abernathy WB, Dimel DL: Is this patient hypovolemic? JAMA 1999;281:1022.
52. Rabb H: Evaluation of urinary markers in acute renal failure. Curr Opin Nephrol Hypertens 1998;7:681.
53. Tsai JJ, Yeun JY, Kumar VA, et al: Comparison and interpretation or urinalysis performed by a nephrologist versus a hospital-based clinical laboratory. Am J Kidney Dis 2005;46:820.
54. Miller TR, Anderson RJ, Linas SL, et al: Urinary diagnostic indices in acute renal failure. Ann Intern Med 1978;88:47.
55. Steinhausen F: Fractional excretion of trace lithium and uric acid in acute renal failure. J Am Soc Nephrol 1994;4:1429.
56. Han WK, Bonventre JV: Biologic markers for the early detection of acute renal injury. Curr Opin Crit Care 2004;10:476.
57. Carvounis CP, Nisar S, Guro-Razuman S: Significance of the fractional excretion of urea in the differential diagnosis of acute renal failure. Kidney Int 2002;62:2223.

58. Andreucci VE, Fuiano G, Stanziale P, et al: Role of renal biopsy in the diagnosis and prognosis of acute renal failure. Kidney Int 1998;53:591.
59. Richards NT, Darby S, Howie AJ, et al: Knowledge of renal histology alters patient management in over 40% of cases. Nephrology Dialysis Transplant 1994;9:1255.
60. Conlon PJ, Kovalik E, Schwab SJ: Percutaneous renal biopsy of ventilated patients. Clin Nephrol 1995;43:309.
61. Shusterman N, Strom BL, Murray TG, et al: Risk factors and outcome of hospital-acquired acute renal failure. Am J Med 1987;83:65.
62. Reineck HJ, O'Connor GJ, Lifschitz MD: Sequential studies on the pathophysiology of glycerol-induced acute renal failure. J Lab Clin Med 1980;96:356.
63. Sever MS, Vanholder R, Lamiere N: Management of crush-related injuries after disasters. N Engl J Med 2006;354:1052.
64. Better OS, Stein JH: Early management of shock and prophylaxis of acute renal failure in traumatic rhabdomyolysis. N Engl J Med 1990;322:825.
65. Van Besien W, Yegenaga I, Vanholder R, et al: Relationship between fluid status and its management on acute renal failure in intensive care unit patients with sepsis: A prospective analysis. J Nephrology 2005;18:54.
66. Murphy SW, Barrett BJ, Parfrey PS: Contrast nephropathy. J Am Soc Nephrol 2000;11:177.
67. Erley CM: Does hydration prevent radiocontrast-induced acute renal failure? Nephrol Dial Transplant 1999;14:1064.
68. Blachley JD, Hill JB: Renal and electrolyte disturbances associated with cisplatin. Ann Intern Med 1981;95:628.
69. Branch RA, Jackson EK, Jacque E: The prophylactic effect of sodium supplements from co-administration of oral or intravenous saline prophylaxis in the prevention of amphotericin B nephrotoxicity. Klin Wochenschr 1987;65:500.
70. Perazella MA: Crystal-induced acute renal failure. Am J Med 1999;106:459.
71. Conger JD, Falk SA: Intrarenal dynamics in the pathogenesis and prevention of acute urate nephropathy. J Clin Invest 1977;51:786.
72. Prestert G, Druml W, Hiesmayer M: Lack of renoprotective effects of dopamine and furosemide during cardiac surgery. J Am Soc Nephrol 2000;11:99.
73. Jones D, Bellomo R: Renal-dose dopamine: From hypothesis to paradigm to myth and finally, superstition? J Intensive Care 2005;20:199.
74. White JJ, Szerlip HM: Low-dose dopamine; it's like déjà vu all over again. J Intensive Care 2005;29:247.
75. ANZICS Clinical Trials Group: Low-dose dopamine in patients with early renal dysfunction: A placebo-controlled randomized trial. Lancet 2000;356:2139.
76. Samuels J, Finkel K, Gubert M, et al: Effect of fenoldopam mesylate in critically ill patients at risk for acute renal failure is dose dependent. Renal Fail 2005;27:101.
77. Morelli A, Rici Z, Bellomo R, et al: Prophylactic fenoldopam for renal protection in sepsis: A randomized, double-blind, placebo-controlled pilot trial. Crit Care Med 2005;33:2451.
78. Bove T, Landori G, Calabro MG, et al: Renoprotective action of fenoldopam in high-risk patients undergoing cardiac surgery: A prospective, double-blind, randomized clinical trial. Circulation 2005;111:3230.
79. Kellum JA: Prophylactic fenoldopam for renal protection? No, thank you, not for me—not yet at least. Crit Care Med 2005;33:2681.
80. Sward K, Valsson F, Odencrants P, et al: Recombinant human atrial natriuretic peptide in ischemic acute renal failure: A randomized placebo-controlled trial. Crit Care Med 2004;32:1310.
81. Mehta RL, Pacual MT, Soroko S, et al: Diuretics, mortality and nonrecovery of renal function in acute renal failure. JAMA 2002;288:2547.
82. Uchino S, Doig GS, Bellomo R, et al: Diuretics in acute renal failure. Crit Care Med 2004;32:1669.
83. Henrich WL: Nephrotoxicity of several newer agents. Kidney Int 2005;S94:S107.
84. Evenpoel P: Acute toxic renal failure. Best Practices & Research. Clin Anesthesiology 2004;18:37.
85. Rind DM, Safran C, Phillips RS, et al: Effect of computer-based alerts on the treatment and outcomes of hospitalized patients. Arch Intern Med 1994;154:1511.
86. Cheng HF, Harris RC: Renal effects of non-steroidal anti-inflammatory drugs and selected cyclooxygenase-2 inhibitors. Curr Pharm Design 2005;11:1795.
87. Huerta C, Castellsague J, Varas-Lorenzo C, et al: Nonsteroidal anti-inflammatory drugs and risk of ARF in the general population. Am J Kidney Dis 2005;45:531.
88. Chertow GM, Sayegh MH, Allgren RL, et al: Is the administration of dopamine associated with adverse or favorable outcomes in acute renal failure? Am J Med 1997;101:49.
89. Denton MD, Chertow GM, Brady HR: "renal-dose" dopamine for the treatment of acute renal failure: Scientific rationale, experimental studies and clinical trials. Kidney Int 1996;50:4.
90. Duque LA, Fermanian J: Furosemide in acute oliguric renal failure: A controlled trial. Nephron 1976;17:51.
91. Brown CB, Ogg CS, Cameron JS: High dose furosemide in acute renal failure: A controlled trial. Clin Nephrol 1981;15:90.
92. Flancbaum L, Choban PS, Dasta JF: Quantitative effects of low dose dopamine on urine output in oliguric surgical intensive care unit patients. Crit Care Med 1994;22:61.
93. Rahman SN, Kim GE, Matthew AS, et al: Effects of atrial natriuretic peptide in clinical acute renal failure. Kidney Int 1994;445:1731.
94. Allgren RL, Marbury TC, Rahman N, et al: Anaritide in acute tubular necrosis. N Engl J Med 1997;336:828.
95. Meyer M, Pfarr E, Schirmer G, et al: Therapeutic use of the natriuretic peptide ularitide in acute renal failure. Renal Fail 1999;21:85.
96. Hammerman MR: Growth factors and apoptosis in acute renal injury. Curr Opin Nephrol Hypertens 1998;7:419.
97. Schenna FP: Role of growth factors in acute renal failure. Kidney Int 1998;66(Suppl):11.
98. Franklin SE, Moulton M, Sicard G, et al: Insulin-like growth factor I preserves renal function post-operatively. Am J Physiol 1997;272:F257.
99. Hersch R, Kopple J, Lipsett P, et al: Multicenter clinical trial of recombinant human insulin-like growth factor I in patients with acute renal failure. Kidney Int 1999;55:2423.
100. Liu KD: Molecular mechanisms of recovery from acute renal failure. Crit Care Med 2003;31:S572.
101. Bates CM, Lin F: Future strategies in the treatment of acute renal failure: Growth factors, stem cells and other novel therapies. Curr Opin Pediatr 2005;17:215.
102. Dolson GM: Electrolyte abnormalities before and after the onset of acute renal failure. Miner Electrolyte Metab 1991;17:133.
103. Massry SG, Arieff AI, Coburn JW: Divalent ion metabolism in patients with acute renal failure. Kidney Int 1974;5:437.
104. Llach F, Felsenfield AJ, Haussler MR: Pathophysiology of altered calcium metabolism in rhabdomyolsis-induced acute renal failure. N Engl J Med 1981;305:117.
105. Haas M, Ohler L, Watzke H, et al: The spectrum of acute renal failure in tumour lysis syndrome. Nephrol Dialysis Transplant 1999;14:776.
106. Anderson RJ, Chung HM, Kluge R, et al: Hyponatremia: A study of its incidence and the pathogenetic role of vasopressin. Ann Intern Med 1985;102:164.
107. Nielsen OJ, Thaysen JH: Erythropoietin deficiency in acute tubular necrosis. J Intern Med 1990;227:373.
108. du Cheyron D, Parienti JJ, Kekih-Hassen M, et al: Impact of anemia on outcome in critically ill patients with severe acute renal failure. Intensive Care Med 2005;31:1469.
109. Park J, Gage BF, Vijay A: Use of erythropoietin in critically ill patients with acute renal failure requiring renal replacement therapy. Am J Kidney Dis 2005;46:791.
110. Roth D: Acute rhabdomyolysis associated with cocaine intoxication. N Engl J Med 1988;319:673.
111. Janson PS, Jubelier SJ, Weinstein MJ, et al: Treatment of the bleeding tendency in uremia with cryoprecipitate. N Engl J Med 1980;303:1318.
112. Mannucci P, Remuzzi G, Pasineri F, et al: Deamino-8D-arginine vasopressin shortens the bleeding time in uremia. N Engl J Med 1983;308:8.
113. Fernandez F, Goudable C, Sie P, et al: Low hematocrit and prolonged bleeding time in uremic patients:

Effect of red cell transfusions. Br J Haematol 1985;59:139.
114. Vigano G, Gaspari F, Locatelli M, et al: Dose-effect and pharmacokinetics of estrogens given to correct bleeding time in uremia. Kidney Int 1980;34:853.
115. Sagripant A, Barsotti G: Bleeding and thrombosis in chronic uremia. Nephron 1997;75:125.
116. Wolk RJ, Apecella MA: The effects of renal function on the febrile response to bacteremia. Arch Intern Med 1978;138:1084.
117. Keane WF, Hirata-Dulas CA, Bulluck ML, et al: Adjunctive therapy with intravenous human immunoglobulin G improves survival of patients with acute renal failure. J Am Soc Nephrol 1991;2:841.
118. Burkett E, Anderson RJ: Co-existing renal-respiratory failure: How to prevent and how to manage. J Crit Illness 1991;6:118.
119. Saint S, Matthay MA: Risk reduction in the intensive care unit. Am J Med 1998;105:551.
120. Bennett WM: Drug prescribing in renal failure: Dosing guidelines for adults, 3rd ed. Philadelphia, American College of Physicians, 1994.
121. Heyland DK, MacDonald S, Keefe L, et al: Total parenteral nutrition in the critically ill patient. JAMA 1998;280:2013.
122. Star RA: The treatment of acute renal failure. Kidney Int 1998;54:1817.
123. Wooley JA, Btaiche IF, Good KL: Metabolic and nutritional aspects of acute renal failure in critically ill patients requiring continuous renal replacement therapy. Nutr Clin Practice 2005;20:176.
124. Strejc JM: Considerations in the nutritional management of patients with acute renal failure. Hemodialysis Int 2005;9:135.
125. Abel RM, Beck CH, Abbot WM, et al: Improved survival from acute renal failure after treatment with intravenous essential L-amino acids and glucose. N Engl J Med 1973;288:695.
126. Baek S-M, Makabali CCCG, Bryan-Brown CW, et al: The influence of parenteral nutrition on the course of acute renal failure. Surg Gynecol Obstet 1975;141:405.
127. Druml W: Metabolic aspects of continuous renal replacement therapies. Kidney Int 1999;56:556.
128. Chertow GM, Lazarus JM: Intensity of dialysis in established acute renal failure. Semin Dial 1996;9:4476.
129. Palevsky PM, Baldwin I, Davenport A, et al: Renal replacement therapy and the kidney: Minimizing the impact of renal replacement therapy on recovery of acute renal failure. Curr Opin Crit Care 2005;11:548.
130. D'Intini V, Ronco C, Bonello M, et al: Renal replacement therapy in acute renal failure. Best Practice & Research. Clin Anaesthesia 2004;18:145.
131. Ronco C, Ricci Z, Bellomo R, et al: Management of fluid balance in CRRT: A technical approach. Int J Artif Organs 2005;28:765.
132. Augustine JJ, Sandy D, Seifert TH, et al: A randomized, controlled trial, comparing intermittent with continuous venovenous dialysis in patients with ARF. Am J Kidney Dis 2004;44:1000.
133. Tonelli M, Manns B, Feller-Kopman D: Acute renal failure in the intensive care unit: A systematic review of the impact of dialytic modality on mortality and renal recovery. Am J Kidney Dis 2002;40:875.
134. Kellum JA, Angus DC, Johnson JP, et al: Continuous versus intermittent renal replacement therapy: A meta-analysis. Intensive Care Med 2002:28:29.
135. Guerin C, Girard R, Selli JM, et al: Intermittent versus continuous renal replacement for acute renal failure in intensive care unit: Results from a multicentre prospective epidemiological survey. Intensive Care Med 2002;28:1411.
136. Mehta R, McDonald G, Gabbai F, et al: A randomized clinical trial of continuous versus intermittent dialysis for acute renal failure. Kidney Int 2001;60:1154.
137. Swartz RD, Bustami RT, Daley JM, et al: Estimating the impact or renal replacement therapy choice on outcome in severe acute renal failure. Clin Nephrol 2005;63:335.
138. Chang JW, Yang WS, Seo JW, et al: Continuous venovenous hemodiafiltration versus hemodialysis as renal replacement therapy in patients with acute renal failure in the intensive care unit. Scand J Urol Nephrol 2004;38:417.
139. Jacka MJ, Ivancinova X, Gibney RT: Continuous renal replacement therapy improves renal recovery from acute renal failure. Canadian J Anaesthesia 2005;52:327.
140. Gangji AS, Rabbat CG, Margetts PJ: Benefit of continuous renal replacement therapy in subgroups of acutely ill patients; a retrospective analysis. Clin Nephrol 2005;63:267.
141. Uehlinger DE, Jakob SM, Ferrari P, et al: Comparison of continuous and intermittent renal replacement therapy for acute renal failure. Nephrol Dial Transplant 2005;20:1630.
142. Benoit DD, Hoste EA, Depuydt PO, et al: Outcome in critically ill medical patients treated with renal replacement therapy for acute renal failure; comparison between patients with and those without haematological malignancies. Nephrol Dial Transplant 2005;20:552.
143. Chawla LS, Abell L, Mazhari R, et al: Identifying critically ill patients at high risk for developing acute renal failure: A pilot study. Kidney Int 2005;68: 2274.
144. Wu CC, Yeung LK, Tsai WS, et al: Incidence and factors predictive of acute renal failure in patients with advanced liver cirrhosis. Clin Nephrol 2006;65:28.
145. Wijeysundera DN, Karkouti K, Beattie WS, et al: Improving the identification of patients at risk of postoperative renal failure after cardiac surgery. Anesthesiology 2006;104:65.
146. Ympa YP, Sakr Y, Reinhart K, et al: Has mortality from acute renal failure decreased? Am J Med 2005;118:827.
147. Lima EQ, Dirce MT, Castro I, et al: Mortality risk factors and validation of several scoring systems in critically ill patients with acute renal failure. Renal Fail 2005;27:547.
148. Uchino S, Bellomo R, Morimatsu H, et al: External validation of severity scoring systems for acute renal failure using a multinational database. Crit Care Med 2005;33:1961.
149. Batista PB, Cendorogolo NM, dos Santos OF, et al: Evaluation of prognostic indexes in critical acute renal failure patients. Renal Fail 2004;26:545.
150. Dharan KS, John GT, Antonisamy B, et al: Prediction of mortality in acute renal failure in the tropics. Renal Fail 2005;27:289.
151. Schroeder TH, Hansen M, Dinkelaker K, et al: Influence of underlying disease on the outcome of critically ill patients with acute renal failure. Eur J Anaesthesiology 2004;21:848.
152. Lins RL, Elseviers MM, Daelemans R, et al: Re-evaluation and modification of the Stuivenberg Hospital acute renal failure (SHARF) scoring system for the prognosis of acute renal failure: An independent, multicentre study. Nephrol Dial Transplant 2004;19:2282.
153. Wang IK, Wang ST, Chang HW, et al: Prognostic value of acute physiology and chronic health evaluation II and organ system failure in patients with acute renal failure requiring dialysis. Renal Fail 2005;27:663.
154. Abosaif NY, Tolba YA, Heap M, et al: The outcome of acute renal failure in the intensive care unit according to RIFLE: Model application, sensitivity, and predictability. Am J Kidney Dis 2005;46:1038.
155. Hou SH, Bushinsky DA, Wish JB, et al: Hospital-acquired renal insufficiency: A prospective study. Am J Med 1983;74:243.
156. Wyatt CM, Arons RR, Klotman PE, et al: Acute renal failure in hospitalized patients with HIV: Risk factors and impact on in-hospital mortality. AIDS 2006;20:561.
157. Bernieh B, Al Hakim M, Boobes Y, et al: Outcome and predictive factors of acute renal failure in the intensive care unit. Transplant Proc 2004;36:1784.
158. Sweet SJ, Glenney CU, Fitzgibbons JP, et al: Synergistic effect of acute renal failure and respiratory failure in the surgical intensive care unit. Am J Surg 1981;141:492.
159. Ahlstrom A, Tallgren M, Peltonen S, et al: Survival and quality of life of patients requiring acute renal replacement therapy. Intensive Care Med 2005;31:1222.
160. Fisher MJ, Brimhall BB, Lezotte DC, et al: Uncomplicated acute renal failure and hospital resource utilization: A retrospective multicenter study. Am J Kidney Dis 2005;46:1049.

Chapter 57

Chronic Renal Failure

Robert J. Anderson

BACKGROUND

Chronic kidney disease (CKD) is a major health problem.[1,2] Although much of this CKD is "mild" in nature, given the central role of the kidney in maintaining hematopoiesis, fluid, electrolyte, acid-base, and calcium/phosphorus balance, even mild CKD potentially results in enhanced management challenges in critically ill patients. For example, increasing evidence suggests that mild CKD appears to be independently associated with significantly increased cardiovascular and all-cause mortality.[3-9] Moreover, patients with mild to moderate renal insufficiency (serum creatinine of 1.5 to 3 mg/dL) undergoing cardiovascular and general surgery have significantly higher 30-day mortality rates, need for prolonged mechanical ventilation, bleeding complications, and cerebrovascular accidents compared with patients with creatinine levels below 1.5 mg/dL.[10-12] Because patients with mild CKD are predisposed to several medical conditions and represent challenging intensive care unit (ICU) management opportunities, meticulous attention must be paid to identifying patients with CKD.

This chapter presents a brief review of the definition, detection, and prevalence of CKD. The pertinent pathophysiologic features in more advanced CKD are reviewed to help the clinician understand the fluid, electrolyte, and hematologic disturbances frequently observed in patients with CKD. In addition, specific management issues related to the ICU care of patients with all degrees of CKD including those receiving renal replacement therapy (hemodialysis or peritoneal dialysis) are discussed. From a practical perspective, estimating glomerular filtration rate (GFR) in each patient in the ICU and appropriately modifying medical management for the level of renal function is the current standard of care.

DEFINITION AND PREVALENCE

CKD is now defined as kidney damage lasting longer than 3 months and is classified into five stages on the basis of differing levels of kidney damage or decreased GFR, or both (Table 57-1).[13,14] The mildest forms of CKD are those with persistent proteinuria and no decrease in GFR. More severe forms of CKD are associated with a progressive loss in GFR. Population-based studies estimate that the number of Americans affected with CKD exceeds 20 million, of which 8 million or more may have stage 3 or more severe CKD with GFRs less than 60 mL/minute.[1,15] Because many patients with GFR in the 40 to 60 mL/minute range have either no or only minimal increases in their serum creatinine concentrations, much of this CKD may be unrecognized by physicians caring for patients. The increasing incidence of CKD is a worldwide phenomenon.[16]

DIAGNOSIS

An early assessment of the level of renal function is necessary when any patient is admitted to an ICU. The assessment of GFR is of practical importance in helping to risk-stratify patients, as well as in determining appropriate dosing of drugs and in maintaining fluid/electrolyte balance.[17]

Several methods are available for estimating GFR.[17] The steady-state concentration of serum creatinine has traditionally been used to provide an estimate of GFR (Table 57-2). In general, each time the steady-state serum creatinine doubles, the GFR decreases by 50%. For patients older than 60 years of age, the GFR values in Table 57-2 should be reduced by about half. Serum creatinine measurements can vary by as much as 10%, so estimations of GFR are just that: estimations. It must also be kept in

Table 57-1. Criteria for Chronic Kidney Disease (CKD)

Stage of CKD	Renal Function
1	Albuminuria, normal GFR
2	Albuminuria, GFR 60-89 mL/min
3	GFR 30-59 mL/min
4	GFR 15-29 mL/min
5	GFR <15 mL/min

GFR, glomerular filtration rate.

Table 57-2. Estimating Glomerular Filtration Rate (GFR) from the Steady-State Serum Creatinine Concentration

Steady-State Serum Creatinine (mg/dL)	GFR (mL/min)
1	100
2	50
4	25
8	12.5
16	6.25

mind that the determinants of serum creatinine concentration (rate of production, volume of distribution, and renal elimination) often vary in many ICU patients, rendering the serum creatinine concentration as an estimate of GFR less valid because "steady-state" conditions are not operable. Another point evident from Table 57-2 is that relatively large decreases in GFR can be associated with only slight increases in serum creatinine concentration, especially in individuals with a normal baseline serum creatinine concentration. Collectively, these reasons have led many clinicians to seek better methods for estimating GFR in ICU patients.

Creatinine clearance calculations can also be used to estimate GFR in the ICU. Clearance methodology requires a timed urine sample and simultaneous measurements of creatinine in urine and serum. Studies confirm that even brief urine collections (30 minutes in duration), which can be done relatively easily in the ICU setting, can be as reliable as 24-hour urine collections.[18] However, use of timed urine samples with simultaneous measurements of the creatinine concentration in the urine and serum is often not practical in the ICU setting and thus is less frequently done.

A rapid means to estimate GFR is by using a serum creatinine–based formula. One such formula that corrects for age and lean body weight is the Cockcroft-Gault formula[17,19]:

$$\text{Creatinine Clearance} = \frac{(140 - \text{Age}) \times \text{Body weight (kg)}}{72 \times \text{Serum creatinine (mg/dL)}}$$

This formula can be multiplied by 0.85 for women, obese patients, and edematous individuals to better correct for lean body weight. The Cockcroft-Gault formula may be especially useful for estimating GFR in elderly patients. Some type of GFR estimation or measurement, or both, must be done in all elderly patients, for whom large decrements in GFR may be associated with only small increases in the serum creatinine concentration.

The Modification of Diet in Renal Disease (MDRD) study has provided another formula for estimation of GFR that may have greater accuracy compared with other methods including the Cockcroft-Gault formula.[17,20] The formula is as follows:

$$\text{GFR} = 186.3 \times (\text{serum creatinine value in mg/dL})^{-1.154} \times \text{age (years)}^{-0.203} \times 0.742 \text{ (for women)} \times 1.21 \text{ (for blacks)}$$

This method of GFR estimation accounts for factors associated with creatinine production such as age, sex, and ethnicity. Similar to other GFR estimation methods based on serum creatinine measurements, the MDRD study prediction equation also assumes a steady-state situation and is therefore inaccurate for many patients in an ICU setting with a rapidly changing clinical status. This more complex formula may not be applied as easily at the bedside by a busy clinician but, increasingly, is calculated by the central laboratory and made available to clinicians. Formulas like the Cockcroft-Gault and MDRD calculations can provide only ballpark estimates of GFR. Use of these formulas certainly provides a better estimate of GFR than serum creatinine concentration alone, but the estimate may not be precise, especially in the ICU.[20]

Recently, measurement of serum cystatin C has been advocated as a reasonable means of estimating GFR.[21-25] Serum cystatin C is a cysteine proteinase inhibitor that is produced in a constant amount by all nucleated cells. Cystatin C is freely filtered at the glomerulus and nearly completely reabsorbed and catabolized by renal tubular cells so that little, if any, appears in the urine. Cystatin C in serum rises with decreasing GFR. Several studies have demonstrated that serum cystatin C may be more sensitive than serum creatinine for detecting decreases in GFR.[21-25] Whether or not serum cystatin C can outperform serum creatinine-based formulas as estimates of GFR remains to be determined. Although promising, at present, serum cystatin C as a marker for GFR is not in widespread use because of practical considerations such as cost and ease of analysis.

To summarize, an estimate of GFR in each ICU patient is important in guiding clinical management. At present, the serum creatinine concentration is not sufficiently sensitive to serve as an optimal means of estimating GFR. Increasingly, clinical laboratories are using measurements of serum creatinine and data available from hospital databases to provide ICU clinicians a GFR value estimated from one of two formulas. Although these formulas provide a better estimate of GFR than the serum creatinine alone, the lack of steady-state conditions in many ICU patients renders the GFR estimates derived from serum creatinine-based formula as general rather than precise.

CLINICAL IMPLICATONS OF CHRONIC KIDNEY DISEASE

The clinical implications of CKD for the ICU practitioner depend on the level of GRF and the primary and comorbid conditions of the patient. Box 57-1 outlines some of the potential clinical implications of CKD. Applicable to ICU patients, population studies demonstrate that CKD, especially when the GFR is less than 60 mL/min, is recognized to be associated with increased all-cause mortality (including cardiovascular, pulmonary, infectious, cancer and neurologic mortality), increased incidence of cardiovascular disease, worse outcomes from cardiovascular diseases, increased operative morbidity and mortality, and increased frequency of adverse reactions to medications.[3-17,26-33] Collectively, it is no surprise that the presence of CKD is a potentially important determinant of ICU outcomes.[34-37]

Table 57-3 outlines the stages of CKD, the corresponding GFR and serum creatinine concentrations, potential symptoms and signs, biochemical abnormalities, risks for cardiovascular disease, and complications from surgical procedures. Table 57-4 outlines some general ICU considerations for patients with all stages of CKD. For all patients with CKD in the ICU, maintenance of renal function is of primary importance. A checklist of potentially reversible factors that can contribute to further deterioration of renal function in individuals with CKD, especially in the ICU setting, is in Box 57-2.[38]

With regard to stages 1 and 2 of CKD, many individuals can lose from 25% to 50% of their renal function and remain totally asymptomatic. Homeostasis is maintained as individual nephrons increase their secretory and reabsorptive capacities. Measurement of blood urea nitrogen (BUN) and creatinine will usually be normal, especially in the elderly. Important to recognize, however, is that patients with all stages of CKD including stages 1 and 2 have increased risk for cardiovascular disease. Moreover, the presence of stage 2 CKD is clearly associated with an increased frequency of complications (death, congestive heart failure, stroke, cardiac arrest, and reinfarction) after myocardial infarction.[26,31,39]

In patients with stage 3 CKD, management in the ICU potentially becomes more complex. These patients have lost 30% to 70% of renal function and often exhibit impaired ability to eliminate salt and water loads. Some

Box 57-1

Potential Clinical Implications for Patients with Chronic Kidney Disease

- Increased mortality
- Increased frequency of cardiovascular disease
- Adverse cardiovascular disease outcomes
- Adverse operative outcomes
- Increase in adverse reactions/complications from medications

Table 57-3. Clinical Correlations for Patients with Chronic Kidney Disease

Stage	GFR mL/min	Serum Creatinine mg/dL	Symptoms*	Biochemical† Abnormalities	Cardiovascular Risk	Operative Risk
1	Normal	Normal	None	None	Usual	Usual
2	60-89	Normal	None	None	Slight increase	Usual
3	30-59	Normal to 2	Few	Few	Moderate increase	Significant increase
4	15-29	2-6	Some	Frequent	High	High
5	<15	>6	Common	Usual	Very high	High

*Lethargy, fatigue, anorexia, nausea, vomiting, reversal of sleep pattern, muscle fasciculations, neuropathy, bruising/bleeding.
†Anemia, prolonged bleeding time, metabolic acidosis, hypocalcemia, hyperphosphatemia, hyperuricemia, hyperkalemia.

Table 57-4. Overview of ICU Management Issues for Patients with CKD

Stage	Prophylaxis	Medication	Monitoring	Complication
1	Usual	No change	Usual	Usual
2	Usual	No change	Usual	Usual
3	Usual	Common	Renal function, volume, electrolytes, hematocrit	Fluid overload, electrolyte abnormalities, renal function worsening
4	Modified	Usually	Renal function, volume, electrolytes, hematocrit	Fluid overload, electrolyte abnormalities, renal function worsening, infections, bleeding
5	Modified	Always	Renal function, volume, electrolytes, hematocrit, vascular access	Fluid overload, electrolyte abnormalities, renal function worsening, infection, bleeding

CKD, chronic kidney disease; ICU, intensive care unit.

patients in this category may exhibit diminished ability to excrete potassium and have modest anemia. Elimination of many drugs excreted by the kidney will be impaired and require dosage modification.

In patients with CKD stages 4 and 5, the GFR is typically less than 25% of renal function and usually the serum creatinine exceeds 3 to 4 mg/dL. These patients exhibit many of the classic manifestations of decreased kidney function such as hypertension, edema, and fatigue. Ability to eliminate salt, water, and electrolyte loads is impaired. Elimination and metabolism of many pharmacologic agents is decreased, usually requiring dosage modification. Laboratory analyses frequently show a variety of disturbances such as anemia, hyperkalemia, metabolic acidosis, hyperphosphatemia, and hypocalcemia. Platelet function is often impaired, and bleeding with surgical or invasive procedures may be encountered. These patients usually require some form of renal replacement therapy and are at highest risk for an adverse outcome in an ICU setting.

Box 57-2

Factors That Can Contribute to Worsening Renal Function in Patients with Previously Stable Chronic Renal Failure

- Prerenal insults (volume depletion/sequestration, sepsis, hemorrhage, impaired cardiac output, medication-induced hypotension)
- Postrenal problems (obstructive uropathy)
- Renal vascular disorders (emboli, thrombosis)
- Uncontrolled hypertension
- Upper urinary tract infection (which can begin in the lower tract with the common use of Foley catheters in the intensive care unit)
- Nephrotoxin (aminoglycosides, converting enzyme inhibitors, angiotensin II receptor blockers, nonsteroidal anti-inflammatory agents, radiocontrast media, others)
- Hypercalcemia
- Allergic interstitial nephritis

APPROACH TO MANAGEMENT

General Measures (Fig. 57-1)

Once a patient with chronic renal failure (CRF) is admitted to an ICU, a primary concern is preservation of renal function. Worsening of renal function will complicate fluid/electrolyte and drug therapy management of an ICU patient. Moreover, underlying renal disease obviously decreases renal reserve. With such decreased reserve, mild further decreases in renal function may be manifest as acute renal failure, which significantly increases the morbidity and mortality of the hospitalized patient.

One of the major objectives for an ICU clinician is to maximize renal perfusion. Net increases or decreases in renal perfusion are the result of a complex interplay of intravascular volume, arterial blood pressure, cardiac index, and renovascular resistance.

Blood Pressure Control

Appropriate blood pressure management is imperative in patients with CRF to help preserve renal function. Normally the kidney can maintain constant renal blood flow

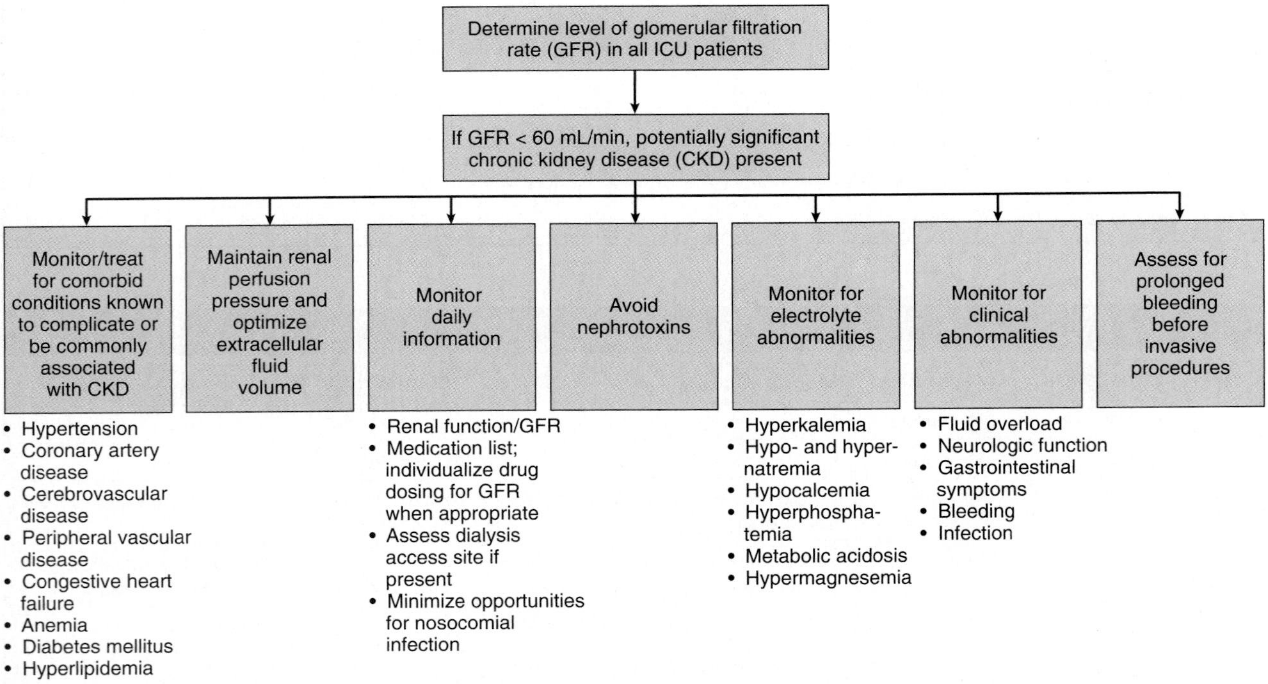

Figure 57-1. Management issues for chronic renal failure patients in the intensive care unit.

and GFR over a wide range of renal perfusion pressures, a phenomenon called *autoregulation*. Patients with long-standing hypertension superimposed on CRF may have impaired autoregulation, increasing the importance of maintaining adequate renal perfusion pressure in patients with renal disease in the ICU. Accordingly, even modest hypotension, such as occurs with intravascular volume contraction, can cause acute worsening of renal function. Appropriately titrated inotropic agents such as dobutamine or vasopressors such as dopamine or norepinephrine may be required to keep the cardiac index and blood pressure within adequate limits.

Conversely, poor control of elevated blood pressure may also worsen renal function in individuals with CKD. A large number of patients with CKD have associated comorbid conditions including hypertension.[40] The reasons that patients with CRF are often hypertensive remain unclear. In some cases essential hypertension results in nephrosclerosis and CKD. In other cases the hypertension appears after the development of renal insufficiency. In the latter case, salt and water retention, enhanced activity of the renin-angiotensin system, increased activity of the sympathetic nervous system, and impairment of endothelial-dependent arterial smooth muscle relaxation may all contribute to the pathogenesis of the hypertensive state.[40-43] Regardless of the cause, patients with CKD often require therapy to maintain control of their blood pressure. No evidence indicates that any single antihypertensive agent is preferable for controlling blood pressure in CKD patients in the ICU.[44] Parenteral therapy may be indicated either when the patient is maintained in a non per os (NPO) status or when acute end-organ involvement is present (e.g., myocardial infarction, congestive heart failure), necessitating a more rapid and accurate control of blood pressure. Consequently, parenteral therapy in such patients requires frequent clinical and arterial pressure monitoring, as well as daily evaluation of renal function. If parenteral therapy with nitroprusside is elected, then careful clinical and laboratory monitoring is necessary to detect potential accumulation of thiocyanate and cyanide.

Vascular Disease and Glycemic Control

Many chronic renal failure patients suffer from chronic hypertension and comorbid conditions such as diabetes mellitus. For example, at least two thirds of all cases of end-stage renal disease (ESRD) are caused by diabetes mellitus or primary hypertensive renal disease. These two diseases cause diffuse atherosclerosis. The chronic renal failure state per se can result in several additional factors that predispose to atherosclerosis such as hyperhomocysteinemia and elevated levels of oxidized low-density lipoproteins.[27,45] The prevalence of left ventricular hypertrophy, coronary artery disease, and congestive heart failure is much higher in patients with CKD than in control populations. Cardiac disease is the single leading cause of death in patients receiving long-term dialysis, accounting for 44% of overall mortality.[45] Thus when dealing with a patient with CKD the prudent clinician must consider such patients particularly susceptible to "vascular" events such as myocardial infarction and stroke and be cognizant of other coexisting medical conditions.[3-15]

Another issue that must be considered in caring for ICU patients with CKD is glycemic control. Recent studies demonstrating that maintenance of glycemic control with intensive insulin therapy may improve outcome in selected ICU patients has led to widespread use of insulin therapy in ICU patients.[46,47] Importantly, one must recognize that patients with CKD, especially those with GFRs less than 30 mL/min, may be especially susceptible to hypoglycemia with insulin therapy. A significant percent of insulin is eliminated by the kidney, and patients with CKD may demonstrate impaired gluconeogenesis and glycogenolysis.[48] Hypoglycemia may occur with renal replacement therapy.[49] In a recent analysis of hypoglycemia occurring in a ICU with patients managed with intensive insulin therapy designed to give a target range of blood glucose of 80 to 110 mg/dL, continuous venovenous hemofiltration with bicarbonate-based buffer substitution fluid was also found to be independently associated with hypoglycemia with an odds ratio of 14.[50] Thus the presence of stage 3 or higher CKD and some conditions of renal replacement therapy demand careful monitoring to prevent potential hypoglycemia in ICU patients receiving insulin infusions.

Fluid and Electrolytes

Sodium

Sodium homeostasis regulates extracellular fluid volume. Extracellular fluid volume is usually normal or mildly increased in the majority of patients with stable CKD at stages 3 to 5.[17,25] CKD patients with superimposed heart failure, hepatic failure, and/or hypoalbuminemia are especially prone to an increase in extracellular fluid volume.

Patients with CKD at stage 3 and above have a limited ability to respond appropriately to excessive amounts and deficits of sodium. To keep total body sodium at relatively normal concentrations, each surviving nephron excretes a greater percentage of filtered sodium. Although urine sodium concentration can be decreased to some extent, the ability of the diseased kidney to conserve sodium is also limited. This salt-losing tendency of some patients with CKD can best be demonstrated when patients are markedly salt restricted. Normal kidneys can produce urine that is essentially sodium-free, whereas diseased kidneys may continue to excrete 20 to 30 mEq/day of sodium.[51] In the ICU meticulous attention to preventing volume depletion is essential because the kidney may no longer be able to reabsorb sodium in response to extracellular fluid volume depletion. Patients with CKD resulting from tubulointerstitial disorders or chronic obstructive uropathy, or both, may be especially prone to a salt-wasting tendency. Some patients in the ICU are therefore at an increased risk for developing volume contraction, leading to decreased cardiac index, decreased renal perfusion, and hence a vicious cycle potentiating renal deterioration.

Increased risk for volume depletion in the ICU is also seen among those with high insensible fluid losses, such as patients with infections, open surgical wounds, burns, and patients receiving mechanical ventilation therapy. Intravascular volume contraction also commonly occurs with postoperative third spacing, as well as with prolonged vomiting and diarrhea. Meticulous monitoring of intake and output, daily weights, and measuring of orthostatic blood pressure and pulse (if possible) are necessary to avoid volume depletion. Patients with superimposed heart failure or hepatic disease may require more invasive monitoring.

Attention must also be directed toward avoiding volume overload. Patients with CKD at stages 3 to 5 are not only limited in their ability to conserve sodium but are often restricted in excreting sodium loads. The upper limits of salt intake correlate directly with remaining renal function. For the euvolemic patient, limiting sodium intake to approximately 80 to 100 mEq/day is appropriate.[52] Patients with CKD caused by glomerular disease such as diabetic glomerulosclerosis appear especially prone to develop sodium retention and volume overload. Because CKD patients often cannot excrete excess sodium, they can easily become fluid overloaded and develop hypertension and peripheral and pulmonary edema if not closely monitored. Therefore daily assessment of volume status in patients with CKD is essential and must include careful attention to 24-hour intake, output, and daily weights. Some patients may require invasive monitoring to ensure protection against volume overload and depletion.

Common sources of sodium in the ICU include sodium-containing intravenous fluids, bicarbonate, antibiotic mixtures, and drips used for infusion such as dopamine and other pressor agents. Orders should specify that all intravenous medications be concentrated and the smallest volume possible administered without saline.

When excess extracellular fluid volume occurs in the ICU patient, it manifests most seriously as pulmonary edema. The effectiveness of treatment of volume overload depends on the degree of renal impairment. Thiazide diuretics have limited natriuretic effect when the GFR is less than 50 mL/minute. Loop diuretics are the agents of choice in individuals with renal insufficiency. In these patients, higher dosages may be required for effective diuresis because of impaired delivery of the drug to its site of action. Typically, maximal natriuretic response occurs with intravenous furosemide boluses of 160 to 200 mg.[53] The total daily dose should not exceed 1 g because of increased risk of ototoxicity. Additionally, studies have demonstrated that continuous intravenous infusion of loop diuretics may be more efficacious than bolus therapy.[54] Infusion rates of furosemide can start at approximately 10 to 15 mg/hour and should not exceed 40 mg/hour. Experts recommend that a loading dose of furosemide be given before a continuous infusion is initiated to decrease the time needed to achieve therapeutic drug concentrations.[53] Other available loop diuretics include torsemide and bumetanide, both of which are available as intravenous formulations.

Metolazone, a potent distal tubule diuretic with some more proximal tubular activity, can be added for patients demonstrating resistance to maximum doses of loop diuretics. Metolazone in oral form can be started at 5 mg/day and increased to a maximum dose of 10 mg/day. This drug is most effective when administered one-half hour before loop diuretics.

In patients with renal failure and a concomitant hypoalbuminemic state, diuretic resistance may pose a significant problem. In a small series of individuals with refractory edema resulting from hypoalbuminemia, increased diuresis was demonstrated with infusion of an albumin-furosemide preparation.[55] However, the significance of this effect is debated and further studies are required before the routine use of albumin in this setting can be advocated. Of important note is that albumin preparations are expensive, have a short half-life, and may result in serious allergic reactions.

Patients with volume overload states that are refractory to high-dose diuretic therapy may require some form of ultrafiltration therapy: continuous venovenous hemodialysis or hemofiltration, hemodialysis, or peritoneal dialysis.

Water

The ability to dilute and concentrate the urine is impaired in patients with CKD at stages 3 and above. Patients with normal kidney function can alter urine osmolality from approximately 50 to 1200 mOsm/kg H_2O. As renal function worsens, urine typically develops a fixed osmolality of approximately 300 mOsm/kg H_2O. When critically ill patients have a fixed urine osmolality, they have a greater tendency to become either hyponatremic when too much water is given or hypernatremic when too little water is given. Both hyponatremia and hypernatremia tend to be hospital- or ICU-acquired electrolyte disturbances.[56,57]

The approach to hyponatremia and hypernatremia in patients with CKD is the same as that in other patients. Because many ICU patients have limited ability to excrete free water because of the presence of CKD and inappropriate secretion of antidiuretic hormone,[56] they will develop hyponatremia when free water intake exceeds the ability of the kidney to excrete free water. Sources of excess water intake include hypotonic intravenous fluids, intravenous medications including antibiotics and drips, and diluted enteral feedings. When patients are noted to have decreasing serum sodium concentration in the face of clinical euvolemia, orders should state that all intravenous fluids be concentrated and hypotonic intravenous fluids avoided.

Hypernatremia develops commonly in patients with CKD who are not receiving adequate water intake.[57] Water deprivation in association with the decreased ability of the kidney to concentrate urine leads to volume contraction and hypernatremia. The amount of free water deficit can be calculated using the following formula:

$$\text{Water deficit} = 0.6 \times \text{Body weight (kg)} \times (P_{Na+} - 140)$$

where P_{Na+} is the patient's plasma sodium concentration.

General recommendations include replacing one third to one half of the water deficit within each 24-hour period for 2 to 3 days. Free water can be most easily replaced through the gastrointestinal tract. Water boluses four times daily are usually well tolerated.

Potassium

Although patients with stable CKD can usually maintain a relatively normal serum potassium concentration until GFR is less than 10% to 20% of normal,[38,58] the clinician needs to be ever-vigilant to prevent potentially fatal hyperkalemia. More than 78% of hospital-acquired hyperkalemia occurs in patients with some degree of advanced CKD.[58] Potassium homeostasis in normal individuals results from a balance among intake, excretion, and transcellular shift of potassium. Total body potassium content in patients with normal kidney function is regulated mainly by excretion by the kidney. Any excess potassium taken in the diet is readily excreted. Patients with more advanced CKD are limited in their renal excretion of potassium. These patients are usually but not always able to stay in potassium balance until close to ESRD through different mechanisms including increased excretion of potassium by the colon and enhanced cellular uptake of potassium.[59]

Cellular uptake of potassium becomes an increasingly important means for maintaining normal serum potassium concentration in patients with CKD. This extrarenal handling of potassium is critical when GFR is less than 25% of normal.[59] Na^+/K^+-ATPase activity is increased in the liver and muscle, so there is increased transport of potassium ions from extracellular fluid into the intracellular space.[59] The intracellular space thus acts like a sponge in soaking up extra potassium.

When hyperkalemia occurs in the ICU, secondary causes must be ruled out.[38] These include increased intake load, decreased excretion, and altered transcellular uptake.[53,61] In the current era, spironolactone is commonly used for the treatment of congestive heart failure and has become a common cause of hyperkalemia, especially in patients with CKD.[62] Box 57-3 contains a checklist to review when patients with CKD present with or develop hyperkalemia in the ICU.

Care must be taken to avoid adding potassium to any IV fluid. In addition, parenteral and enteral nutrition should contain the smallest amount of potassium possible. Substantial potassium can be delivered via blood transfusion. Endogenous "loads" of potassium can occur by release of intracellular contents as seen with tumor lysis syndrome, rhabdomyolysis, and hemolysis. Volume depletion can cause hyperkalemia secondary to both decreased excretion and decreased cellular uptake. Total body excretion of potassium is decreased during volume depletion because there is decreased potassium delivery to both the distal tubule of the kidney and the colonic mucosa.[59] In addition, decreased tissue perfusion associated with volume depletion leads to decreased cellular uptake of potassium by muscle.

Alterations in transcellular movement of potassium can also exacerbate hyperkalemia. Increased tissue release of potassium in metabolic acidosis and with hyperosmolality has been well described.[61] Decreased cellular uptake of potassium can occur in association with insulin deficiency and with the use of nonselective β-blockers, digitalis, and succinylcholine. Various drugs should be used with caution in patients with CKD because hyperkalemia may develop despite previously stable potassium balance. Drugs such as spironolactone, triamterene, or amiloride decrease renal excretion of potassium.[53,61,62] Heparin infusion can also cause hyperkalemia via decreased aldosterone synthesis in the adrenal gland.[52] Nonsteroidal anti-inflammatory drugs, as well as angiotensin-converting enzyme (ACE) inhibitors and angiotensin 2 receptor blockers, can cause hyperkalemia in patients with impaired renal function and therefore should be used only with close monitoring of serum potassium concentration.[61] The diagnosis and management of hyperkalemia are discussed in detail in Chapter 58.

Box 57-3

Secondary Causes of Hyperkalemia in the Intensive Care Unit

Increased Intake
Intravenous fluids, enteral/parenteral nutrition, antibiotics, blood transfusion

Decreased Excretion
Volume depletion; constipation; drugs (triamterene, amiloride, spironolactone, ACE inhibitors, NSAIDs, heparin); renal failure; adrenal deficiency

Transcellular Shift
Increased release of K^+ from cells
Rhabdomyolysis, tumor lysis, hyperosmolality, hyperglycemia, metabolic acidosis

Decreased Uptake of K^+ from ECF
Insulin deficiency, nonselective β-blockers, digitalis, succinylcholine

ACE, angiotensin-converting enzyme; ECF, extracellular fluid; K^+, potassium; NSAIDs, nonsteroidal anti-inflammatory drugs.

Phosphate, Calcium, and Magnesium

Almost all untreated patients with serum creatinine concentrations above 4 mg/dL show evidence of hyperphosphatemia and hypocalcemia. Hypocalcemia is the net result of hyperphosphatemia, decreased intestinal absorption of calcium from decreased intake, impaired kidney synthesis of 1,25-dihydroxyvitamin D, and decreased mobilization of calcium from bone. Hypocalcemia, especially in association with hyperkalemia, can lead to fatal cardiac arrhythmias. Tetany is unusual because concurrent metabolic acidosis often maintains a relatively normal level of ionized calcium. Tetany can be precipitated by acute elevation in blood pH.[60] Administration of an alkaline agent to patients with otherwise stable uremia should therefore be done with caution. Neuromuscular irritability, muscle fasciculations, paresthesias, stridor, seizures, and frank tetany may indicate a decrease in the serum concentration of ionized calcium in patients with CRF.

Marked hyperphosphatemia can lead to tissue deposition of calcium phosphate salts and worsening hypocalcemia when the calcium times phosphorus product exceeds 70. Hyperphosphatemia occurs once the GFR falls to less than 25 mL/min because the kidney can no longer eliminate the daily phosphate load. Tissue destruction with release of intracellular contents, as occurs in rhabdomyolysis and tumor lysis syndrome, may lead to hyperphosphatemia. Moderate hyperphosphatemia can be treated with oral phosphate binders such as calcium carbonate. Markedly elevated phosphorus levels, especially in the presence of hypercalcemia, may require dialysis.

Careful attention to magnesium homeostasis is also necessary in patients with CKD, especially in stages 4 and 5. As in any ICU patient, magnesium depletion may be encountered. However, because the kidney is the primary organ that regulates magnesium excretion, hypomagnesemia is rarely seen. Hypermagnesemia occurs when patients with CKD are given magnesium infusions, magnesium-containing antacids, and/or laxatives.

Metabolic Acidosis

Metabolic acidosis, usually but not invariably with a modest increase in the anion gap, occurs when the serum creatinine exceeds 4 mg/dL. Patients with advanced renal failure caused by diabetes typically display a less severe degree of metabolic acidosis compared with individuals with other forms of renal failure.[63] The majority of patients with stage 4 and 5 stable CKD have a serum bicarbonate level of 12 to 18 mEq/L, with a blood pH of 7.3 or higher.[64] Thus more severe metabolic acidosis in the ICU (bicarbonate concentration <15 mEq/L) mandates a workup for superimposed disease processes associated with metabolic acidosis. The mild metabolic acidosis of CKD rarely requires specific alkalization therapy.

Hematologic Abnormalities

The anemia of CKD is multifactorial and tends to correlate with the degree of renal impairment.[65-70] Decreased red blood cell production secondary to decreased erythropoietin levels results in the classic normochromic/normocytic anemia of renal failure.[65] Generally, a GFR of 30 to 40 mL/minute or less is required for a patient with CKD to have anemia from renal failure per se. Patients with CRF frequently have superimposed iron deficiency as a result of subtle ongoing gastrointestinal blood loss, repeated laboratory testing, and acute or chronic inflammatory conditions. In CKD patients, the recommended target hematocrit level is 11 to 12 g/dL for patients with stages 4 and 5 CKD based on recent studies.[67,68]

The approach to anemia in an ICU patient with CKD requires a thorough evaluation to ensure that no other cause for the anemia is present. A patient who has had an acute drop in hematocrit level should be assessed for the presence of physiologic consequences of anemia (such as tachycardia, orthostatic hypotension, or angina), which would aid in the decision regarding appropriate management.

Patients with advanced CKD are at increased risk of bleeding during even minor procedures because of platelet dysfunction.[70-78] Uremia may not only be the direct cause of coagulopathy but also a marker for comorbid conditions and medications associated with impaired blood clotting. In general, bleeding attributable solely to renal failure occurs only when the BUN exceeds 100 to 200 mg/dL. The mechanism whereby marked CKD causes platelet dysfunction is incompletely understood but is caused by abnormal platelet–platelet and platelet–vessel wall interactions. These abnormal interactions most likely result from a combination of decreased platelet factor III activity, decreased platelet levels of thromboxane A_2, increased prostacyclin within the vascular endothelium, enhanced guanidinosuccinic acid and nitric oxide formation, and impaired von Willebrand complex activity.

Although no studies have been done to date, bleeding times should be considered before any invasive procedures that have the potential for noncompressible bleeding. A prolonged bleeding time can be partially corrected by several different techniques including dialysis, which has been shown to improve bleeding parameters.[72-74] In addition, it has been demonstrated that maintaining a hematocrit level above 30% partially corrects the bleeding diathesis.[75] Intravenous desmopressin; which works quickly (in 1 to 4 hours) but has a brief duration of action (8 to 12 hours); conjugated estrogens, which require at least 12 to 24 hours to work but exert effects for several days; fresh frozen plasma; and cryoprecipitate also help to correct platelet dysfunction.[76-78] Recently, it has been emphasized that individuals with stages 4 and 5 CKD are at higher risk for bleeding with standard doses of a commonly used low molecular weight heparin (enoxaparin).[79]

Complications Associated with Medications

Nearly all drugs and medications are eliminated, at least in part, by the kidney. Moreover, CKD can result in impairment of hepatic drug metabolism and drug protein binding.[32,33,80,81] Accordingly, in patients with CKD in the ICU, extra vigilance is necessary to prevent medication-related complications. Several references are readily available to help adjust drug dosage and intervals appropriately for a patient's level of renal function, and their use is highly recommended.[32,33,80,81] When possible, monitoring of serum drug levels may be helpful.

Another primary objective is to avoid, if possible, the use of any potentially nephrotoxic drugs. The most common causes of nephrotoxin-induced renal deterioration in the ICU include aminoglycosides, radiographic contrast agents, nonsteroidal anti-inflammatory drugs (NSAIDs), and ACE inhibitors.

Aminoglycosides can cause well-described acute renal failure in 5% to 20% of patients.[82-84] Aminoglycoside-induced renal failure tends to manifest as a rise in serum creatinine 7 to 10 days after initiation of therapy. In a patient with CRF, aminoglycoside-induced worsening of renal function can have catastrophic consequences. Risk factors for development of aminoglycoside nephrotoxicity include long duration of therapy, a repeated course of therapy, concomitant use of other nephrotoxic agents, volume depletion, advanced age, liver disease, and renal disease.[82-84] Therefore it is essential that there be clear guidelines for the implementation and cessation of aminoglycosides in patients with CRF. In addition, proper dosing based on estimated or, preferably, measured GFR is important. Because the incidence of renal deterioration increases with higher blood levels of the drugs, aminoglycoside levels should be monitored closely. Unfortunately, most cases of nephrotoxicity occur despite normal drug levels. Decreased renal perfusion may enhance the renal tubular injury seen with normal drug levels.[83] Daily monitoring of serum creatinine is advised when using aminoglycosides.

Some studies suggest that once-daily administration of aminoglycosides may be associated with a decreased frequency of nephrotoxicity compared with multiple-dosing regimens.[84] However, this benefit has not been uniformly demonstrated and has not been well studied in certain populations including patients with renal failure. Accordingly, once-daily administration of aminoglycosides is not routinely recommended in this population.

Intravenous radiocontrast material is another potential nephrotoxic agent that must be used with care in patients with CKD.[85-90] Nephrotoxicity is manifested by a rise in serum creatinine of more than 25% that occurs within 3 to 4 days after exposure to radiocontrast media. Risk factors include underlying diabetic nephropathy, concomitant therapy with nonsteroidal anti-inflammatory agents, the use of large doses of the agents, the presence of prerenal azotemia, and CKD.[85] When using an intravenous radiocontrast medium in a patient with CKD, the smallest possible dose should be used and repeat contrast exposure should be avoided. Newer nonionic low-osmolar contrast agents have replaced ionic, high osmolar agents as standard agents because of lower nephrotoxicity. Some data suggest that newer iso-osmolar agents are even less nephrotoxic, although more data are clearly necessary.

When contrast agents must be given to ICU patients with CKD, care should be taken to ensure modest hydration before dye exposure. Studies support the use of prehydration and posthydration therapy with 0.45% to 0.9% saline solution to prevent contrast-associated nephrotoxicity. A conservative regimen would consist of 0.45% saline solution at 1 mL/kg/hour starting 6 to 12 hours before and continuing for 24 hours after the procedure. Three additional prophylactic modalities can be considered when radiographic contrast must be given to ICU patients with CKD. These include N-acetylcysteine, sodium bicarbonate, and prophylactic hemofiltration.[85-90]

N-acetylcysteine (400 to 600 mg twice a day preprocedure and postprocedure) is safe, easy to use, and inexpensive and may be of some benefit, although not all studies demonstrate clear-cut protection.[86] A single randomized controlled study with a modest number of patients found that sodium bicarbonate (3 ampules added to 1 L of 5% dextrose in water given at 3 mL/kg/hour beginning 1 hour before and continuing to 6 hours following contrast exposure) was significantly protective.[90] Significant amounts of contrast material can be removed by hemodialysis and hemofiltration. Two studies have demonstrated that hemofiltration can significantly reduce the occurrence of contrast nephropathy in patients with advanced stage 4 or 5 CKD.[89,90] Because of the logistical and cost considerations of hemofiltration therapy, additional trials will be helpful to delineate the precise role of hemofiltration therapy in prevention of contrast-induced nephropathy in patients with advanced CKD.

The use of NSAIDs should generally be avoided in a patient with CKD. This is especially true in patients with superimposed volume depletion, hypotension, shock, edematous disorders, sepsis, or advanced age.[91-95] In these conditions GFR is maintained by vasodilation of the afferent arteriole by several different prostaglandins including prostacyclin. Levels of these prostaglandins decrease with the use of NSAIDs, resulting in vasoconstriction of the afferent arteriole. This leads to a significant fall in the GFR, thus predisposing the already damaged kidney to decreased renal perfusion.

NSAIDs can also cause hyperkalemia. Various mechanisms are responsible including decreased GFR, decreased distal sodium delivery with resultant decreased sodium for potassium exchange in the distal nephron, decreased renin and therefore decreased aldosterone secretion, and decreased transport of potassium into cells. It should be emphasized that both the decrease in GFR and the hyperkalemia can occur with all NSAID formulations. Acute renal failure and deterioration of preexisting renal insufficiency have also been reported with the use of the newer NSAIDs, cyclooxygenase-2 inhibitors (COX-2), and therefore these agents should also be avoided in patients with CKD.[95]

ACE inhibitors and angiotensin 2 receptor inhibitors have been demonstrated to protect against the progression of renal insufficiency in patients with various renal diseases. However, ACE inhibitors can worsen renal function in patients with high renin/angiotensin states such as volume depletion, sepsis, edematous disorders, bilateral renal artery stenosis, or unilateral renal artery stenosis in a solitary kidney.[96-100] ACE inhibitors worsen renal function by decreasing mean arterial pressure and therefore renal perfusion pressure, as well as by decreasing vascular resistance at the efferent arteriole. The net effect of these changes is to decrease glomerular capillary hydrostatic pressure and GFR. ACE inhibitors can also cause hyperkalemia by decreasing aldosterone levels and thus decreasing potassium secretion in the distal tubule of the kidney.[73] The renal effects of ACE inhibitors are generally reversible by discontinuing the drug.

Minimizing the Risk of Nosocomial Infections

Patients with CKD may be especially susceptible to nosocomial infections.[81] The precise mechanisms underlying this susceptibility remain unclear. However, it has been well documented that impairment of cellular and humoral immunity and white blood cell dysfunction are present in the uremic state. Additionally, uremia may also alter the clinical manifestations of infection (such as fever), making the diagnosis of infection more difficult.[101] Finally, disruption of normal anatomic barriers to infection via insertion of intravascular and intravesicular catheters often occurs in the ICU setting, further increasing the risk of infection in patients with CKD.

POSTOPERATIVE ISSUES

Recently, it has become increasingly appreciated that CKD, especially at stages 3 and above, is potentially associated with adverse operative outcomes including significantly enhanced mortality and morbidity.[10-12,102,103] The adverse outcomes that occur in patients with CKD are seen with all types of surgical procedures ranging from general surgery through complex cardiovascular operations.[10-12,102,103] The exact level of renal function at which patients are at risk for adverse operative outcomes remains to be better defined. However, patients with basal serum creatinine concentrations of 1.4 mg/dL and higher and creatinine clearances at 40 to 50 mL/minute and lower appear to be clearly at risk for increased operative mortality, as well as all types of morbidity.[10-12,102,103] The mechanism(s) rendering these CKD patients at risk for complications of all types including adverse cardiac, pulmonary, neurologic, bleeding, and infectious outcomes remains to be precisely defined. Many of these postoperative patients will spend some time in an ICU. Thus enhanced awareness and attention of the diverse potential medical complications in this patient group by ICU physicians may be of benefit.

DIALYSIS-RELATED ISSUES

Patients with end-stage CKD who are on maintenance renal replacement therapy pose a special challenge to the ICU clinician.[34-37] For example, four recent studies demonstrate a 9% to 34% mortality rate in patients with end-stage CKD admitted to an ICU.[34-37] Although the conditions precipitating ICU admission for patients with end-stage chronic renal failure are diverse, sepsis, gastrointestinal hemorrhage, fluid overload, cardiovascular events, and electrolyte disturbances account for the majority of ICU admissions. Admissions to ICUs for ESRD patients are often complicated by failure of other organ systems, the development of infections, and need for mechanical ventilation. Indeed, patients on chronic maintenance dialysis therapy have been demonstrated to require prolonged mechanical ventilation in the ICU and may have impaired ventilatory responses to carbon dioxide.[104,105] Of note, commonly used prognostic scoring systems such as Apache II and III, Simplified Acute Physiology Score (SAPS) II, and Sequential Organ Failure Assessment (SOFA) maintain reasonably good predictive performance in patients with end-stage CKD admitted to an ICU.[34-37]

Unlike many patients admitted to the ICU, there is an extensive paper trail for patients receiving long-term renal replacement therapy. One of the best resources of information is records from the patient's dialysis unit. Important information that can be obtained includes medication lists, dry weight, baseline laboratory data, the condition of access sites, baseline electrocardiogram and chest radiographs, and the general health of the patient. In addition, depending on individual state laws and dialysis unit policies, advance directives can usually be found on file. All of the fluid/electrolyte, acid base, hematologic, comorbid, and medication-related issues that complicate diagnosis and treatment of the ICU patient with CRF are magnified in the patient receiving long-term dialysis. Excellent overall reviews are available covering the medical management of long-term dialysis patients.[31,76,81,106]

Infection is a major cause of mortality in patients with end-stage CKD.[76,81,106] It has been demonstrated that septicemia is common among patients on hemodialysis, and vascular access–related infections are responsible for the majority (50% to 90%) of these septicemic episodes.[106-111] The classic signs of inflammation (erythema, swelling, warmth, or tenderness) may be absent in this population and the only presenting manifestation of infection may be fever; therefore in hemodialysis patients fever should prompt the evaluation of possible access-related infection. However, as noted previously, failure of a febrile response is also common among patients with ESRD; thus enhanced clinical vigilance is important when caring for these individuals. Serial blood cultures are the mainstay of diagnosis and should be obtained when patients present with symptoms that might suggest infection. The causative organism in most cases is *Staphylo-coccus aureus.* Initial empiric therapy often includes vancomycin administered as a single dose, which provides therapeutic levels for up to 1 week.

Peritonitis continues to be the most significant complication of peritoneal dialysis and is the cause of death in approximately 2% to 12% of peritoneal dialysis patients.[112-114] Infections related to peritoneal dialysis catheters can occur at the exit site, the tunnel, or within the peritoneum itself. Exit site infections can be observed in 10% to 30% of patients on peritoneal dialysis. A tunnel infection is manifested by swelling, pain, or fever and may be responsible for persistent or recurrent peritonitis. Most common pathogens are *S. aureus* or *Staphylococcus epidermidis.* Recognizing and treating an exit site infection are important to prevent the development of either a tunnel infection or peritonitis. Catheter removal is usually necessary, and an alternative mode of renal replacement therapy must be instituted.

The average incidence of peritonitis is 1.3 to 1.4 episodes per patient per year.[112-114] Diagnosis of peritonitis is based on any two of the following criteria: (1) abdominal tenderness, (2) cloudy dialysate containing more than 100 polymorphonuclear leukocytes per mm^3, with neutrophil predominance of more than 50%, and (3) microorganisms in the peritoneal fluid. The most common pathogens in peritonitis include gram-positive cocci and gram-negative rods. Less common but reported pathogens include fungi, anaerobic bacteria, and mycobacteria. Bacterial peritonitis is most commonly treated with intraperitoneal administration of antibiotics. This mode of treatment achieves high local concentration and permits self-administration of antibiotics in patients who do not require hospitalization. More severely ill patients may require intravenous antibiotic therapy. Aerobic and anaerobic cultures should be obtained before the initiation of therapy. Many acceptable protocols for initial management of peritonitis exist. In general, a cephalosporin plus vancomycin or vancomycin plus another broad-spectrum antimicrobial agent is initially recommended, and a change in antibiotics can be made if necessary, on the basis of culture identification and susceptibility patterns. Catheter removal may be necessary in patients with recurrent or persistent peritonitis.

Maintenance of vascular access is another important issue in the care of a patient on chronic dialysis. Loss of vascular access is a potentially catastrophic problem.[115-119] Arteriovenous fistulas and grafts should be examined daily for palpable thrills or bruits, or both, which confirm graft patency. Occasionally, volume depletion, pericardial tamponade, and intradialytic hypotension can lead to graft thrombosis. Graft occlusion also may be particularly common in the presence of anastomotic stenosis, infection, subclavian stenosis from a previous temporary vascular access, or extrinsic compression from a hematoma. Early diagnosis of diminished graft patency resulting from clotting, infection, or stenosis is critical because a response to local thrombolytic therapy or angioplasty may be possible.

SUMMARY

Patients with CKD pose unique challenges to the critical care physician. Patients with CKD are admitted to the ICU with a wide spectrum of renal impairment. Enhanced clinical vigilance is essential to preserve remaining renal function, as well as to protect these patients from iatrogenic complications. Close attention must be paid to maintaining hemodynamic stability because patients with CKD are less able to tolerate marked changes in volume status and mean arterial blood pressure and often have underlying cardiovascular diseases. Careful monitoring for electrolyte and hematologic abnormalities is essential. Nephrotoxic drugs should be avoided if possible, and drug lists controlled closely to prevent toxicity. Lastly, patients on renal replacement therapy must be observed diligently for access-related complications.

KEY POINTS

- Patients with chronic kidney diseases are at high risk for the development of fluid/electrolyte and other medical problems when in an ICU.
- An early, accurate assessment of the level of renal function is necessary in all ICU patients. This can be optimally done by estimations from formulas such as the Cockcroft-Gault or MDRD formulas.
- Extracellular fluid/volume overload, hypertension and hypotension, hyperkalemia, worsening renal function, infection, hemorrhage, and problems related to medications are the most common complications encountered by chronic kidney disease patients in an ICU.
- Preservation of existing renal function is a major goal when patients with CKD are admitted to an ICU. Nephrotoxins such as radiographic contrast agents, nonsteroidal anti-inflammatory drugs, and aminoglycosides should be used cautiously in patients with CKD.
- Invasive procedures should be minimized in patients with CKD because they are at higher risk of bleeding complications associated with platelet dysfunction.

REFERENCES

1. Coresh J, Astor BC, Greene T, et al: Prevalence of chronic kidney disease and decreased kidney function in the adult US population; Third national health and nutritional examination survey. Am J Kidney Dis 2003;41:1.
2. Coresh J, Byrd-Holt D, Astor BC, et al: Chronic kidney disease awareness, prevalence and trends among U.S. adults, 1999 to 2000. J Am Soc Nephrol 2005;16:180.
3. Henry RM, Kostense PJ, Bos G, et al: Mild renal insufficiency is associated with increased cardiovascular mortality: The Hoorn study. Kidney Int 2002;62:1402.
4. Keith DS, Nichols GA, Gullion CM, et al: Longitudinal follow-up and outcomes among a population with chronic kidney disease in a large managed care organization. Arch Intern Med 2004;164:659.
5. Go AS, Chertow GM, Fan D, et al: Chronic kidney disease and the risks of death, cardiovascular events and hospitalization. N Engl J Med 2004;351:1296.
6. Fried LF, Katz R, Sarnak MJ, et al: Kidney function as a predictor of noncardiovascular mortality. J Am Soc Nephrol 2005;16:3728.
7. Shlipak MG, Sranak MJ, Katz R, et al: Cystatin C and the risk of death and cardiovascular events among elderly persons. N Engl J Med 2005;352: 2049.
8. Shlipak MG, Fried LF, Cushman M, et al: Cardiovascular mortality risk in chronic kidney disease. JAMA 2005;203:1737.
9. O'Hare AM, Bertanthal D, Covinsky KE, at al: Mortality risk stratification in chronic kidney disease: One size for all ages. J Am Soc Nephrol 2006;17:846.
10. Anderson RJ, O'Brien M, MaWhinney S, et al: Mild renal failure is associated with adverse outcome after cardiac valve surgery. Am J Kidney Dis 2000;35:1127.
11. Anderson RJ, O'Brien M, MaWhinney S, et al: Renal failure predisposes patients to adverse outcome after coronary artery bypass surgery. Kidney Int 1999;55:1057.
12. O'Brien MM, Gonzales RG, Shroyer AL, et al: Modest serum creatinine elevation affects adverse outcome after general surgery. Kidney Int 2002;62:585.
13. Levy AS, Coresh J, Balk E, et al: National Kidney Foundation practice guidelines for chronic kidney disease: Evaluation, classification and stratification. Ann Intern Med 2003;39:605.
14. National Kidney Foundation: K/DOQI Clinical Practice Guidelines for Chronic Kidney Disease; Evaluation, Classification and Stratification. Am J Kidney Dis 2002;39:S1.
15. Foley RN, Wang C, Collins AJ: Cardiovascular risk factor profiles and kidney function stage in the US general population: The NHANES III study. Mayo Clin Proc 2005;80: 1270.
16. Barsoum RS: Chronic kidney disease in the developing world. N Engl J Med 2006;354:997.
17. Stevens LA, Coresh J, Greene T, et al: Assessing kidney function-measured

and estimated glomerular filtration rate. N Engl J Med 2006;354:2473.
18. Robert S, Zorowitz BJ, Peterson EL: Predictability of creatinine clearance estimates in critically ill patients. Crit Care Med 1993;21:1487.
19. Cockcroft DW, Gault MH: Prediction of creatinine clearance from serum creatinine. Nephron 1976;16:31.
20. Hoste EA, Damen J, Vanholder RC, et al: Assessment of renal function in recently admitted critically ill patients with normal serum creatinine. Nephrol Dialysis Transp 2005;20:747.
21. Levin A: Cystatin C, serum creatinine and estimates of kidney function: Searching for better measures of kidney function and cardiovascular risk. Ann Intern Med 2005;142:586.
22. Fliser D, Ritz E: Serum cystatin C concentration as a marker or renal dysfunction in the elderly. Am J Kidney Dis 2001:37:79.
23. Newman DJ, Thakkar H, Edwards RG, et al: Serum cystatin C measured by automated immunoassay: A more sensitive marker of changes in GFR than serum creatinine. Kidney Int 1995;47:312.
24. Randers E, Erlandsen EJ: Serum cystatin C as an endogenous marker of renal function—a review. Clin Chem Lab Med 1999;37:389.
25. Coll E, Botey A, Alavarez L, et al: Serum cystatin C as a new marker for noninvasive estimation of glomerular filtration rate and as a marker for early renal impairment. Am J Kidney Dis 2000;36:29.
26. Anavekar NS, McMurray JJ, Velaquez EJ, et al: Relation between renal dysfunction and cardiovascular outcomes after myocardial infarction. N Engl J Med 2004;351:1285.
27. Ritz E: Heart and kidney: Fatal twins? Am J Med 2006:119:5A31S.
28. Weiner DE, Tighioart H, Stark PC, et al: Kidney disease as a risk factor for recurrent cardiovascular disease and mortality. Am J Kidney Dis 2004;44:198.
29. Perazella MA: Increased mortality in chronic kidney disease: A call to action. Am J Med Sci 2006;331:150.
30. Jee SH, Boulware E, Guallar E, et al: Direct, progressive association of cardiovascular risk factors with incident proteinuria. Arch Intern Med 2005;165:2299.
31. Rahman M, Pressel S, Davis BR, et al: Cardiovascular outcomes in high-risk hypertensive subjects stratified by baseline glomerular filtration rate. Ann Intern Med 2006;144:172.
32. Bennett WM: Drug prescribing in renal failure: Dosing guidelines for adults, 3rd ed. Philadelphia, American College of Physicians, 1994.
33. Swan SK: Adjustment of drug dosage in patients with renal insufficiency. In Kelley WM (ed): Textbook of Internal Medicine. New York, Lippincott, 1995.
34. Manhes G, Heng AE, Aublet-Cuvelier B, et al: Clinical features and outcome of chronic dialysis patients admitted to an intensive care unit. Nephrol Transpl Dialysis 2005;20:1127.
35. Dara SI, Afessa B, Bajwa AA, et al: Outcome of patients with end-stage renal disease admitted to the intensive care unit. Mayo Clin Proc 2004;79: 1385.
36. Uchino S, Morimatsu H, Bellomo R, et al: End-stage renal failure patients requiring renal replacement therapy in the intensive care unit: Clinical features and outcome. Blood Purification 2003;21:170.
37. Clermont G, Acker CG, Angus DC, et al: Renal failure in the ICU: Comparison of the impact of acute renal failure and end-stage renal disease on ICU outcomes. Kidney Int 2002;62:986.
38. Rahman M, Smith MC: Chronic renal insufficiency: A diagnostic and therapeutic approach. Arch Intern Med 1998;157:1743.
39. Pinkau T, Hilgers KF, Veelken R, et al: How does minor renal dysfunction influence cardiovascular risk and the management of cardiovascular disease? J Am Soc Nephrol 2004;15:517.
40. Kim KE, Swartz C: Cardiovascular complications of end-stage renal disease. In Schrier RW, Gottschalk CW (eds): Diseases of the Kidney, 5th ed. Boston, Little Brown, 1993.
41. Converse RL, Jaconsen TL, Toto RD, et al: Sympathetic overactivity in patients with chronic renal failure. N Engl J Med 1992;327:1912.
42. Vallance P, Leone A, Calver A, et al: Accumulation of an endogenous inhibitor of nitric oxide synthesis in chronic renal failure. Lancet 1992;339:572.
43. Houston MD: New insights and approaches to reduce end-organ damage in the treatment of hypertension: Subsets of hypertension approach. Am Heart J 1992;123:1337.
44. Ligtenberg G, Blankestijn PF, Oey PL, et al: Reduction of sympathetic hyperactivity by enalapril in patients with chronic renal failure. N Engl J Med 1999;340:1321.
45. Luke RG: Chronic renal failure—a vasculopathic state. N Engl J Med 1998;339:841.
46. Van den Berghe G, Wilmer A, Hermans G, et al: Intensive insulin therapy in the medical ICU. N Engl J Med 2006;354:449.
47. Angus DC, Abraham E: Intensive insulin therapy in critical illness. Am J Resp Crit Care Med 2005;172:1358.
48. Rubenstein AH, Mako ME, Horwitz DL: Insulin and the kidney. Nephron 1975;15:306.
49. Takahashi A, Kubota T, Shibahara N, et al: The mechanism of hypoglycemia caused by hemodialysis. Clin Nephrol 2004;62:362.
50. Vriesendorp TM, van Santen S, DeVries JH, et al: Predisposing factors for hypoglycemia in the intensive care unit. Crit Care Med 2006;34:96.
51. Fine LG, Kurtz I, Woolf AS: Pathophysiology and nephron adaptation in chronic renal failure. In Schrier RW, Gottschalk CW (eds): Diseases of the Kidney, 5th ed. Boston, Little Brown, 1993.
52. Tuso RJ, Nissenson AR, Danovitch GM: Electrolyte disorders in chronic renal failure. In Maxwell M, Kleeman C (eds): Clinical Disorders of Fluid and Electrolyte Metabolism. New York, McGraw-Hill, 1994.
53. Brater DG: Diuretic therapy. N Engl J Med 1998;339:387.
54. Rudy DW, Voelker IR, Greene PK, et al: Loop diuretics for chronic renal insufficiency: A continuous infusion is more efficacious than bolus therapy. Ann Intern Med 1991;115:360.
55. Inoue M, Okajima K, Itoh K, et al: Mechanism of furosemide resistance in analbuminemic rats and hypoalbuminemic patients. Kidney Int 1987;32:198.
56. Anderson RJ, Chung HM, Kluge R, et al: Hyponatremia: A prospective analysis of its epidemiology and the pathogenetic role of vasopressin. Ann Intern Med 1985;102:164.
57. Oh MS, Carroll HJ: Disorders of sodium metabolism: Hyponatremia and hypernatremia. Crit Care Med 1992;20:94.
58. Acker CG, Johnson JP, Palevsky P, et al: Hyperkalemia in hospitalized patients: Causes, adequacy of treatment, and results of an attempt to improve physician compliance with published therapy guidelines. Arch Intern Med 1998;158:917.
59. Martin RS, Panese S, Virginillo M, et al: Increased secretion of potassium in the rectum of humans with chronic renal failure. Am J Kidney Dis 1986;8:105.
60. Knochel JP: Biochemical alterations in advanced uremic failure. In Jacobson HR, Striker GE, Klahr S (eds): The principles and practice of nephrology. Philadelphia, BC Decker, 1991.
61. Weiner ID, Wingo C: Hyperkalemia: A potential silent killer. J Am Soc Nephrol 1998;9:1535.
62. Juurlink DN, Mamdfani MM, Lee DS, et al: Rates of hyperkalemia after publication of the Randomized Aldactone Evaluation Study. N Engl J Med 2004;351:543.
63. Caravaca F, Arrobas M, Pizarro JL, et al: Metabolic acidosis in advanced renal failure: Differences between diabetic and nondiabetic patients. Am J Kidney Dis 1999;33:892.
64. Schwartz WB, Relman AS: Acidosis in renal disease. N Engl J Med 1957;256:1184.
65. Besarab A, Ayyoub F: Anemia in renal disease. In Schrier RW, Gottschalk CW (eds): Diseases of the Kidney, 8th ed. Philadelphia, Lippincott Williams & Wilkins, 2007.
66. McGonigle RJS, Wallen JD, Shadduck RK: Erythropoietin deficiency and inhibition of erythropoiesis in renal insufficiency. Kidney Int 1984;25:437.
67. Drueke TB, Locatelli F, Clyne N, et al: Normalization of hemoglobin level in patients with chronic kidney disease and anemia. N Engl J Med 2006; 355:2071.
68. Singh AK, Szczech L, Tang KL, et al: Correction of anemia with epoietin alfa in chronic kidney disease. N Engl J Med 2006;355:2085.
69. Ifudu O: Care of patients undergoing hemodialysis. N Engl J Med 1998;339:1054.
70. Castaldi PA, Rosenbert MC: The bleeding disorder of uraemia: A qualitative platelet defect. Lancet 1996;1:66.
71. Noris M, Remuzzi G: Uremic bleeding: Closing the circle after 30 years of controversy. Blood 1999;94:2569.

72. Deykin D: Uremic bleeding. Kidney Int 1983;24:698.
73. Lindsay RM, Mourthy AV, Koens F: Platelet function in dialyzed and nondialyzed patients with chronic renal failure. Clin Nephrol 1975;4:52.
74. Remuzzi G, Livio M, Marchiaro G: Bleeders in renal failure: Altered platelet function in chronic uremia only partially connected by hemodialysis. Nephron 1978;22:347.
75. Livio M, Marches D, Remuzzi G, et al: Uremic bleeding: Role of anemia and beneficial effect of red cell transfusion. Lancet 1982;2:1013.
76. Mannucci PM, Remuzzi G, Pusineri F, et al: Deamino-8-D-arginine vasopressin shortens the bleeding time in uremia. N Engl J Med 1983;308:8.
77. Livio M, Mannucci PM, Vigano G, et al: Conjugated estrogens for the management of bleeding associated with renal failure. N Engl J Med 1986;315:731.
78. Mannucci PM, Levi M: Prevention and treatment of major blood loss. N Engl J Med 2007;356:2301.
79. Lim W, Dentali F, Eikelboom JW, et al: Meta-analysis: Low molecular weight heparin and bleeding in patients with severe renal insufficiency. Ann Intern Med 2006;144:673.
80. Manley HJ, Cannella CA, Bailie G, et al: Medication-related problems in ambulatory hemodialysis patients; a pooled analysis. Am J Kidney Dis 2005;46:669.
81. Dember LM: Critical care issues in the patient with chronic renal failure. Crit Care Clin 2002;18:421.
82. Swan SK: Aminoglycoside nephrotoxicity. Semin Nephrol 1997;17:27.
83. Moore RD, Smith CR, Lipskey ED: Risk factors for nephrotoxicity in patients treated with aminoglycosides. Ann Intern Med 1982;73:9.
84. Hatala R, Dinh T, Cook DJ: Once-daily aminoglycoside dosing in immunocompetent adults; a meta-analysis. Ann Intern Med 1996; 124:717.
85. Rudnick MR, Kesselheim A, Goldfarb S: Contrast-induced nephropathy: How it develops, how to prevent it. Clev Clin J Med 2006;73:75.
86. Bagshaw SM, McAlister FA, Manns BJ, et al: Acetylcysteine in the prevention of contrast-induced nephropathy. Arch Intern Med 2006;166:161.
87. Marenzi G, Marana L, Laurie G, et al: The prevention of radiocontrast nephropathy by hemofiltration. N Engl J Med 2003;349:1331.
88. Aspelin P, Aubry P, Franssen SG, et al: Nephrotoxic effects in high risk patients undergoing angiography. A double blind randomized multicenter study of iso-osmolar and low-osmolar non-ionic contrast media. N Engl J Med 2003;119:491.
89. Marenzi G, Mauiri G, Campodoneri J, et al: Comparison of two hemofiltration protocols for prevention of contrast-induced nephropathy in high-risk patients. Am J Med 2006; 119:155.
90. Merten GJ, Burgess WP, Gray LV, et al: Prevention of contrast-induced nephropathy with sodium bicarbonate: A randomized controlled trial. JAMA 2004;291:2334.
91. Murray MD, Brater DC: Effects of NSAIDs on the kidney. Prog Drug Res 1997;49:155.
92. Cheng HF, Harris RC: Renal effects of non-steroidal anti-inflammatory drugs and selected cyclooygenase-2 inhibitors. Curr Pharm Des 2005;11:1795.
93. Huerta C, Castellsague J, Varas-Lorenzo C, et al: Nonsteroidal anti-inflammatory drugs and risk of ARF in the general population. Am J Kidney Dis 2005;45:531.
94. Joannides M: Drug-induced renal failure in the ICU. Int J Artif Organs 2004;27:1034.
95. Perazella MA: Cox 2 inhibitors and the kidney. Hosp Pract (Off Ed) 2001;36:43, 55.
96. Hricik DE, Dunn MJ: Angiotensin-converting enzyme inhibitor-induced renal failure: Causes, consequences and diagnostic uses. J Am Soc Nephrol 1990;1:845.
97. Schoolwerth AC, Sica DA, Ballerman BJ, et al: Renal considerations in angiotensin converting enzyme inhibitor therapy. Circulation 2001;104:1985.
98. Stirling C, Houston J, Robertson S, et al: Diarrhea, vomiting and ACE inhibitors: An important cause of acute renal failure. J Hum Hypertens 2003;17:419.
99. Guo K, Nzerue C: How to prevent, recognize and treat drug-induced nephrotoxicity. Clev Clin J Med 2002;69:289.
100. Johansen TL, Kjar A: Reversible renal impairment induced by treatment with the angiotensin II receptor antagonist candesartan in a patient with bilateral renal artery stenosis. BMC Nephrol 2001;2:1.
101. Wolk PJ, Apecella MA: The effect of renal function on the febrile response to bacteremia, Arch Intern Med 1978;138:1084.
102. Lee TH: Reducing cardiac risk in non-cardiac surgery. N Engl J Med 1999;341:183.
103. Browner WS, Li J, Magano DT: In-hospital and long-term mortality in male veterans following non-cardiac surgery. JAMA 1992;268:228.
104. Nakasuji M, Nishi S, Nakasuji K, et al: Duration of dialysis is a significant predictor of prolonged postoperative mechanical ventilation in dialysis-dependent patients undergoing cardiac surgery. Anesth Analg 2006;102:2.
105. Burgess KR, Burgess EE, Whitelaw WA: Impaired ventilatory response to carbon dioxide in patients with chronic renal failure: Implications for the intensive care unit. Crit Care Med 1994;22:413.
106. Pastan S, Bailey J: Dialysis therapy. N Engl J Med 1998;338:1428.
107. Powe NR, Jaar B, Furth SL, et al: Septicemia in dialysis patients: Incidence, risk factors, and prognosis. Kidney Int 1999;55:1081.
108. Ayus JC, Sheikh-Hamad D: Silent infection in clotted hemodialysis access grafts. J Am Soc Nephrol 1999;9:1314.
109. Tokars JI, Finelli L, Alter M, et al: National surveillance of dialysis-associated diseases in the United States, 2001. Semin Dial 2004;17:310.
110. Stevenson KB, Hannah EL, Lowder CA, et al: Epidemiology of hemodialysis vascular access infections from longitudinal infection surveillance data: Predicting the impact of NKF-DOQI clinical practice guidelines for vascular access. Am J Kidney Dis 2002;39:549.
111. Roberts TL, Obrador GT, St Peter WL, et al: Relationship among catheter insertions, vascular access infections, and anemia management in hemodialysis patients. Kidney Int 2004;66:2429.
112. Piraino B, Bailie GR, Bernardini J, et al: Peritoneal dialysis-related infections recommendations; 2005 update. Perit Dial Int 2005;25:140.
113. Troidle L, Kinkelstein F: Treatment and outcome of CPD-associated peritonitis. Ann Clin Micro Antimicrob 2006;5:6.
114. Vas SI: Microbiologic aspects of chronic ambulatory peritoneal dialysis. Kidney Int 1983;23:83.
115. Butterly DW, Schwab SJ: Catheters access for hemodialysis: An overview. Semin Dial 2001;14:411.
116. Develter W, DeCubber A, Van Biesen W, et al: Survival and complications of indwelling venous catheters for permanent use in hemodialysis patients. Artif Organs 2005;29:399.
117. Allon M, Daugirdas J, Depner TA, et al: Effect of change in vascular access on patient mortality in hemodialysis patients. Am J Kidney Dis 2006;47:469.
118. Huijbregts HJ, Blankestijn PJ: Dialysis access-guidelines for current practice. Eur J Vasc Endovasc Surg 2006;31:284.
119. Parile JL, Ruhter M: Preservation of vascular access. J Am Soc Nephrol 1993;4:997.

Chapter 58

Acid-Base, Electrolyte, and Metabolic Abnormalities

Ahmad Bilal Faridi and Lawrence S. Weisberg

Acid-base, electrolyte, and metabolic disturbances are common in the intensive care unit (ICU). Indeed, critically ill patients often suffer from compound acid-base and electrolyte disorders. Successful evaluation and management of such patients requires recognition of common patterns (e.g., hypokalemia, metabolic alkalosis) and the ability to dissect one disorder from another. This chapter is intended to provide intensivists with the tools they need for diagnosis and treatment of the acid-base, electrolyte, and metabolic disorders encountered in the care of critically ill patients. Space constraints do not permit a comprehensive discussion of such disorders. By reviewing the elements of normal physiology in these areas and presenting a general diagnostic scheme for each condition, we hope to provide readers with a foundation for approaching not only common but also novel and complex disorders.

METABOLIC DISORDERS OF ACID-BASE HOMEOSTASIS

Normal acid-base balance depends on the cooperation of at least two vital organ systems: the lungs and kidneys. The gastrointestinal (GI) tract is also involved in many acid-base disturbances. Multiorgan system involvement, therefore, provides the backdrop for the acid-base disorders commonly seen in critically ill patients.

Normal Acid-Base Physiology

Normal biochemical and physiologic function requires that the extracellular pH be maintained within a narrow range. Although the "normal" range of pH in clinical laboratories is 7.35 to 7.45 pH units, the actual pH in vivo varies considerably less.[1] This tight control is maintained by a complex homeostatic mechanism involving buffers and the elimination of volatile acid by respiration.

The principal extracellular buffer system is the carbonic acid/bicarbonate pair. The equilibrium relationships of the components of this system are illustrated as follows[1]:

$$H_2O + CO_2 \leftrightarrow H_2CO_3 \leftrightarrow H^+ + HCO_3^-$$

From these relationships, the Henderson-Hasselbach equation is derived as follows:

$$pH = pK + \log_{10} \frac{HCO_3^-}{\alpha_{CO2} \times pCO_2}$$

In this equation α_{CO2} is the solubility coefficient of CO_2 (0.03), and pK is the equilibrium constant for this buffer pair (6.1). Rearrangement yields the Henderson equation:

$$H^+ = 24 \times \frac{pCO_2}{HCO_3^-}$$

Apparently, from this equation, disturbances in the proton concentration of the extracellular fluid (and blood) may be caused by perturbation in the numerator, the denominator, or both. Disturbances that affect the pCO_2 primarily are called *respiratory* disturbances, and those that affect the HCO_3^- primarily are called *metabolic.*

Acid-base homeostasis depends on compensation for a primary disturbance. Compensation for a respiratory disturbance is metabolic, and compensation for a metabolic disturbance is respiratory. Furthermore, it is clear from the previous equations that in order to mitigate the change in proton concentration or pH, the direction of the compensation must be the same as the direction of the primary disturbance. Thus consumption of bicarbonate will be accompanied by hyperventilation and a consequent reduction in pCO_2. A simple acid-base disturbance is considered to consist of the primary disturbance *and* its normal compensation. A complex acid-base disturbance consists of more than one primary disturbance. In order to detect complex acid-base disturbances, one must be familiar with both the direction and magnitude of normal compensation (Table 58-1).[2] More than one metabolic disturbance may coexist (e.g., metabolic acidosis, metabolic alkalosis), but only one respiratory disturbance is possible at a time.

This section addresses disorders that affect the metabolic component of acid-base homeostasis: metabolic acidosis and metabolic alkalosis. Respiratory disturbances affecting acid-base balance are discussed elsewhere (see Chapters 14, 38, and 41).

Metabolic Acidosis

Definition and Classification

A metabolic acidosis is a process that, if unopposed, would cause *acidemia* (a high hydrogen ion concentration, or low pH, of the blood) by reducing the extracellular bicarbonate concentration. The extracellular bicarbonate concentration may be reduced by either addition of acid and consequent consumption of bicarbonate or by primary loss of bicarbonate.

An adult eating a normal diet generates 16,000 to 20,000 mmol of acid a day.[3] Almost all of that acid is in the form of carbonic acid, resulting from CO_2 and water generation in the metabolism of carbohydrates and fats. Individuals with normal ventilatory capacity eliminate this prodigious acid load through the lungs, thus the term *volatile acid.* The remainder of the daily acid load, approximately 1 mmol/kg body weight per day, derives from metabolism of phosphate- and sulfate-rich protein (yielding phosphoric and sulfuric acid). These nonvolatile or *fixed acids* are buffered, primarily by extracellular bicarbonate under normal circumstances. The kidneys are responsible for regenerating the consumed bicarbonate by secreting hydrogen ions (protons) in the distal nephron. These secreted protons must be buffered in the tubule lumen in order to allow elimination of the daily fixed acid load within the physiologic constraint of the minimum urinary pH. The urinary buffers are composed of the filtered sodium salts of the phosphoric acid and ammonia, which is synthesized in proximal tubule and "trapped" by acidification in the collecting duct as ammonium (NH_4^+). Under conditions of acid loading, the normal kidney reabsorbs all the filtered bicarbonate in the proximal tubule. Urinary net acid excretion therefore comprises phosphoric acid (so-called *titratable acidity* because it is quantified by titrating the urine with alkali to pH 7.4) and ammonium, less any excreted bicarbonate.[4]

Many factors modify the kidney's capacity to regulate acid-base balance. For example, renal ammoniagenesis is stimulated by acidemia and inhibited by alkalemia and thus participates in a homeostatic feedback loop.[1] Hyperkalemia inhibits, and hypokalemia stimulates renal ammoniagenesis. Hypokalemia further stimulates acid secretion by activating the H^+,K^+-ATPase in the collecting duct. Finally, aldosterone stimulates both proton and K^+ secretion in the collecting duct. For these reasons, hypokalemia tends to perpetuate a metabolic alkalosis, and hyperkalemia a metabolic acidosis.[1]

Metabolic acidosis can be caused by excessive production of fixed acid, decreased renal secretion of fixed acid, or loss of bicarbonate, either through the kidney or through the intestine.[4] The net effect of any of these processes is a reduction in the blood bicarbonate concentration. The plasma *anion gap* helps to distinguish among the various causes of metabolic acidosis. Of course, because of charge neutrality, the sum of the concentration of all cations in the plasma is equal to the sum of all the anions. By convention, however, the anion gap is defined as the difference between the plasma sodium concentration and the sum of

Table 58-1. Expected Compensation for Simple Acid-Base Disorders

Disorder	1° Disturbance	Compensation	Magnitude	Time to Completion
Metabolic acidosis	↓ $[HCO_3^-]$	↓ PCO_2	$1.5 \times [HCO_3^-]+8$	12-24 hr
Metabolic alkalosis	↑ $[HCO_3^-]$	↑ PCO_2	$0.9 \times [HCO_3^-]+9$	12-24 hr
Respiratory acidosis, acute	↑ PCO_2	↑ $[HCO_3^-]$	1 mmol/L/10 mm Hg	<6 hr
Respiratory acidosis, chronic	↑ PCO_2	↑ $[HCO_3^-]$	3.5 mmol/L/10 mm Hg	>5 days
Respiratory alkalosis, acute	↓ PCO_2	↓ $[HCO_3^-]$	2 mmol/L/10 mm Hg	<6 hr
Respiratory alkalosis, chronic	↓ PCO_2	↓ $[HCO_3^-]$	5 mmol/L/10 mm Hg	>7 days

the bicarbonate and chloride concentrations. It represents the concentration of anions that are normally unmeasured by a basic metabolic chemistry panel.[5] The anion gap is normally approximately 10 mmol/L, but it varies widely according to the methods employed by the clinical chemistry laboratory.[6] The anion gap is composed mainly of albumin, along with phosphates, sulfates, and organic anions. Two important pitfalls exist in the interpretation of the anion gap. First, because the anion gap is proportional to the plasma albumin concentration, hypoalbuminemia (common in critically ill patients) will lower the "baseline" anion gap (by approximately 2.5 mmol/L for each g/dL decline in the albumin concentration).[7] Thus profound hypoalbuminemia may falsely lower the anion gap and mask a high anion gap acidosis. Second, alkalemia increases the anion gap by causing lactate generation and by titrating plasma buffers, most notably albumin.[8] (Thus in respiratory alkalosis, the bicarbonate concentration will be low in compensation and the anion gap may be elevated, giving a false impression of a high anion gap metabolic acidosis by inspection of the electrolytes alone.)

If bicarbonate is lost (e.g., through diarrhea) or hydrochloric acid is gained (e.g., renal tubular acidosis or administration of unbuffered amino acid solutions[9]), the bicarbonate concentration falls with a commensurate increase in the plasma chloride concentration; thus the anion gap is unchanged. If, on the other hand, bicarbonate is lost in buffering an organic acid such as lactic acid or a ketoacid, the decrement in the bicarbonate concentration is more or less matched by an increase in the anion gap. Figure 58-1 illustrates these processes.

Table 58-2 lists the causes of hyperchloremic metabolic acidosis. Two diagnoses are of particular interest in the critical care arena. First is the posthypocapnic metabolic acidosis, in which bicarbonate falls in compensation for a chronic respiratory alkalosis. When "normal" minute ventilation is restored, the pH falls until bicarbonate can be retained, giving the appearance of a hyperchloremic metabolic acidosis. This emphasizes the importance of observation over time in the analysis of acid-base status. The second entity of interest is a so-called *dilutional hyperchloremic acidosis*. This is seen in patients who are rapidly resuscitated with large volumes of isotonic saline solution. The acidosis traditionally has been attributed to dilution of blood bicarbonate. Analysis based on physical-chemistry principles may better explain the phenomenon (see later discussion).[10]

The differential diagnosis of high anion gap metabolic acidosis is limited (Table 58-3). The most common cause in critically ill patients is a lactic acidosis. The causes of lactic acidosis are numerous. As shown in Box 58-1, they

Table 58-2. Causes of Hyperchloremic Metabolic Acidosis

Extra-Renal Loss of Base
Diarrhea
Pancreatic fistula
Ureteral diversion
Extra-Renal Gain of Acid
Ammonium chloride
Hydrochloric acid
Sodium chloride
Renal Loss of Base
Type II renal tubular acidosis
Posthypocapnic state
Excretion of organic anions (bicarbonate precursors)
Toluene inhalation (glue sniffing)
Diabetic ketoacidosis
Renal Acid Excretory Defect
Type IV renal tubular acidosis
Chronic kidney disease
Hypoaldosteronism
Urinary tract obstruction
Type I renal tubular acidosis
Sickle cell nephropathy
Lupus nephritis
Renal transplant

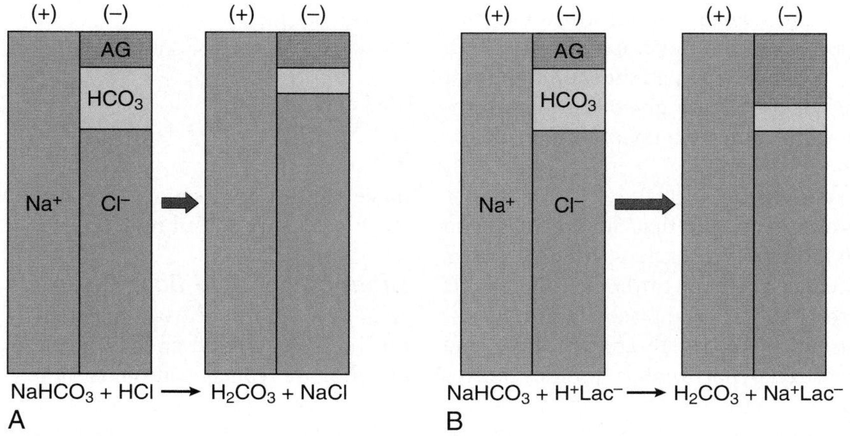

Figure 58-1. The generation of hyperchloremic and anion-gap acidoses. Blocks represent the ionic composition of the plasma, cations (+) to the left and anions (–) to the right. In each panel, the bar to the left represents the basal or normal state. The anion gap (AG) is shown in red. **A,** The change in the ionic composition of the plasma when hydrochloric acid (HCl) is added is demonstrated. The chloride concentration increases as bicarbonate is consumed. **B,** The effect of adding organic acid such as lactic acid (H^+Lac^-), in which case the bicarbonate is consumed and the anion gap increases proportionately, is demonstrated. Cl, chloride; H_2CO_3, carbonic acid; Na, sodium; $NaHCO_3$, sodium bicarbonate.

Table 58-3. Causes of High Anion-Gap Metabolic Acidosis

Ketoacidoses
Diabetic
Alcoholic
Starvation
Intoxications
Methanol
Ethylene glycol
Propylene glycol
Salicylate
Pyroglutamic Acidosis
Congenital
Acquired
Lactic Acidosis (see Box 58-1)
Uremic Acidosis

Box 58-1

Causes of Lactic Acidosis

Type A (Tissue Oxygen Supply:Demand Mismatch)

- Decreased tissue oxygen delivery
  - Shock
  - Hypoxemia
  - Severe anemia
  - Carbon monoxide poisoning
- Increased tissue oxygen demand
  - Grand mal seizure
  - Extreme exercise

Type B (Impaired Tissue Oxygen Utilization)

- Sepsis/Systemic inflammatory response syndrome
- Diabetes mellitus
- Malignancy
- Thiamine deficiency
- Inborn errors of metabolism
- Human immunodeficiency virus infection
- Malaria
- Drugs/toxins
  - Ethanol
  - Metformin
  - Zidovudine
  - Didanosine
  - Stavudine
  - Lamivudine
  - Zalcitabine
  - Salicylate
  - Propofol
  - Niacin
  - Isoniazid
  - Nitroprusside
  - Cyanide
  - Catecholamines
  - Cocaine
  - Acetaminophen
  - Streptozotocin
  - Sorbitol/fructose
- Liver failure
  - Alkalemia

D-Lactic Acidosis

are divided into type A (imbalance between tissue oxygen demand and supply) and type B (impaired oxygen utilization).[5] Diabetic ketoacidosis (see Chapter 59) and intoxications (see Chapter 69) are discussed elsewhere. Two causes of high anion gap acidosis recently added to the differential diagnosis, and of particular relevance to intensivists, are *pyroglutamic acidosis* and intoxication with *propylene glycol.*

Pyroglutamic acid is a metabolic intermediate in the γ-glutamyl cycle, one product of which is glutathione. Pyroglutamic acidosis may be congenital (caused by one of several enzyme deficiencies) or acquired.[8] The acquired syndrome may be caused by acetaminophen (which depletes glutathione, leading to uninhibited pyroglutamic acid synthesis), β-lactam antibiotics, or glycine deficiency. The acidosis may be profound and the anion gap greater than 30 mmol/L.[11] Diagnosis is made by urinary screen for organic acids.

Propylene glycol is a solvent for medications, many of which are commonly infused in critically ill patients, such as lorazepam, nitroglycerin, etomidate, and phenytoin. Propylene glycol is metabolized by alcohol dehydrogenase to lactic acid. High anion gap acidosis has been associated with high- and even low-dose infusions, particularly of lorazepam.[7, 12] Thus development of a high anion gap acidosis in a critically ill patient should prompt a search for a source of propylene glycol because withdrawal of the agent will promptly alleviate the acidosis.

Consequences of Acidemia

Experts have generally accepted that severe acidemia (pH<7.2) is associated with a variety of deleterious effects. Of particular concern are the cardiovascular effects including pressure-resistant arterial vasodilation, venoconstriction, diminished myocardial contractility, and impaired hepatic and renal perfusion.[13] (Some controversy exists as to which of these effects are directly caused by acidemia.[4]) A predisposition to malignant arrhythmias has been reported, in vitro and in animal models. Finally, numerous metabolic derangements have been attributed to the effect of acidemia on key enzymes in metabolic pathways, resulting in sympathetic hyperactivity with diminished catecholamine responsiveness; insulin resistance and suppressed glycolysis; and reduced hepatic lactic acid uptake and metabolism.[14]

Diagnosis of Acid-Base Disorders

Acid-base disorders are revealed most commonly through the basic metabolic chemistry panel, when the plasma bicarbonate concentration is noted to be outside the normal range. If the bicarbonate is low and if the anion gap is clearly elevated on that sample, a diagnosis of high anion gap metabolic acidosis can be made with some confidence, keeping in mind the pitfalls in the interpretation of the anion gap mentioned earlier.[7]

If the bicarbonate is low and the anion gap normal, two possibilities exist: either a hyperchloremic metabolic acidosis or a respiratory alkalosis with metabolic compensation. These two entities can be distinguished by examination of the blood pH and blood gases, a low pH being diagnostic of the former.

If the bicarbonate concentration is high, again there are two alternative diagnoses, requiring blood pH measurement for their differentiation: either a metabolic alkalosis or metabolic compensation for a respiratory acidosis.

Once the primary disturbance has been identified, the astute clinician, recognizing the possibility of a mixed disturbance, is obligated to ask, "Is that all there is?" This question can be answered only by an understanding of the rules of normal compensation for simple acid-base disorders (see Table 58-1).[2] Knowing at least the expected direction of compensation will allow the clinician to diagnose the most obvious mixed disturbances. For example, if the pH is low, the bicarbonate is low, and the pCO_2 is above 40 torr, there is clearly a mixed metabolic and respiratory acidosis. Similarly, if the pH is high, the bicarbonate is high, and the pCO_2 is below 40 torr, the diagnosis is a mixed respiratory and metabolic alkalosis. More subtle mixed disorders can be diagnosed only by understanding not only the expected direction but the expected magnitude of compensation. This will allow one to conclude, for example, whether the hyperventilation in a patient with metabolic acidosis is appropriate (expected compensation), inadequate (a separate respiratory acidosis), or excessive (a separate respiratory alkalosis).

The preceding method permits the diagnosis of simple and dual acid-base disorders. Triple acid-base disorders can be diagnosed only by comparing the change in the anion gap with the change in the plasma bicarbonate concentration. Most simply conceived, the fall in the bicarbonate should equal the rise in the anion gap (see Fig. 58-1). If the rise in the anion gap exceeds the fall in the bicarbonate, a metabolic alkalosis is said to be present in addition to the high anion gap acidosis. Conversely, if the fall in the bicarbonate exceeds the rise in the anion gap, mixed hyperchloremic and high anion gap acidoses are said to coexist. Although this analysis is useful in the case of large discrepancies, in more subtle cases it is confounded by theoretical and practical considerations.[5,15]

The classic approach to acid-base disorders described earlier has been challenged recently by proponents of a physical-chemistry approach described originally by Stewart.[16] According to this method, the pH of the blood depends on the ionization of water by the difference in the concentration of so-called *strong ions* (the strong ion difference, or SID). The main utility of this method in the critical care setting is that it explains the development of a hyperchloremic metabolic acidosis in patients who receive large volumes of isotonic saline.

Treatment of Metabolic Acidosis

Treatment of metabolic acidosis is aimed at reversing the adverse consequences of acidemia. Treatment of hyperchloremic metabolic acidosis is straightforward. In cases of acute metabolic acidosis, treatment depends on successful therapy of the underlying cause (e.g., diarrhea) and correction of the bicarbonate deficit, usually in the form of sodium bicarbonate. One can estimate the bicarbonate deficit as follows:

$$HCO_3\ \text{def.} = (HCO_{3\text{final}} - HCO_{3\text{initial}}) \times (\text{vol. distr. } HCO_3)$$

The difficulty in accurately estimating this value arises from two factors: First, the apparent volume of distribution of bicarbonate varies more than twofold—from 50% of body weight to 100% of body weight—and is inversely proportional to the initial bicarbonate concentration.[17] Second, there are often many simultaneous processes in a critically ill patient that tend to ameliorate or exacerbate the metabolic acidosis, such as vomiting, shock, and liver failure. In order to avoid overshoot alkalemia, it is prudent to estimate the volume of distribution to be 50% of the body weight[14] and to target an increase in the bicarbonate concentration of no more than 8 mmol/L over 12 to 24 hours, depending on the severity of the acidemia.

Sodium bicarbonate is generally considered to be the alkalinizing agent of choice for severe acidemia. Alternative alkalinizing agents such as citrate, acetate, and lactate, which under normal circumstances are oxidized mainly in the liver to bicarbonate, should not be used to treat acidemia in patients with suspected or confirmed hepatic impairment or circulatory compromise. The sodium bicarbonate should be administered as a continuous infusion, the concentration of which should be guided by the patient's serum sodium concentration. Bolus injection of undiluted ampules of sodium bicarbonate (1000 mmol/L) should be used with great restraint and only in patients with the most severe acidemia because of the risk of hyperosmolality. Large volumes of any bicarbonate solution can lead to volume overload, a reduction in the ionized calcium (Ca^{2+}) concentration (see "Hypocalcemia") and increased generation of CO_2. This last effect will tend to cause a respiratory acidosis in patients with ventilatory insufficiency. Plasma electrolytes and blood gases must be monitored frequently to guide adjustments in the composition of the solution and its rate of infusion.

Tris-hydroxymethylaminomethane, or THAM, is an amino alcohol that buffers without generating CO_2. It has the advantage, therefore, of avoiding a superimposed respiratory acidosis. It has been used successfully in animals and humans with various metabolic acidoses.[13,18] It is eliminated by the kidney and thus should be used with caution in the setting of renal insufficiency. Risks include hyperkalemia, hypoglycemia, and hepatic necrosis in neonates.[7]

The treatment of choice for lactic acidosis is reversal of the underlying cause of the acidosis (see Box 58-1). Pending resolution of the underlying disorder, however, the intensivist is often confronted with an unstable patient who is profoundly acidemic. Treatment at this stage is controversial.[5,13] The debate has focused on the potentially deleterious effects of bicarbonate administration in lactic acidosis. In addition to the effects mentioned earlier, bicarbonate in animal models of lactic acidosis has been associated with increased lactate generation, reduction in intracellular pH, increased venous pCO_2, and reduction in cardiac output. (This last effect correlates well with the reduction in ionized

Ca concentration.[13]) Studies in humans likewise show no improvement in cardiac output, morbidity, or mortality with bicarbonate.[13] Continuous hemodialysis (e.g., CVVHD) may be a promising tool for treating lactic acidosis because it provides large amounts of bicarbonate without the risks of volume overload or hypocalcemia. Several cases of successful treatment of metformin-associated lactic acidosis using continuous hemodialysis have been reported.[19,20] Treatment of diabetic ketoacidosis and the acidoses associated with various intoxications are discussed in Chapters 59 and 69, respectively.

Metabolic Alkalosis

Definition and Classification

Metabolic alkalosis is a process leading to accumulation of extracellular bicarbonate that, if unopposed, will result in an increase in the plasma pH (alkalemia). It can be caused by either a gain of bicarbonate or a loss of fixed acid from the extracellular fluid. The etiologies of metabolic alkalosis have been described.[266] In its pure form, it is accompanied by hypoventilation (CO_2 retention).[2]

From a pathophysiologic perspective, metabolic alkalosis is divided into those factors that generate the alkalosis and those factors that maintain or perpetuate it.[21,22] Metabolic alkalosis is generated by addition of bicarbonate to the blood. This can occur either by loss of acid from the body or by addition of exogenous alkali. Loss of acid may be from the stomach (e.g., vomiting or nasogastric suction) or kidney. Renal acid loss is enhanced by a high rate of Na delivery to the distal nephron, high circulating mineralocorticoid levels, K depletion, and high rates of ammoniagenesis.

Because of the kidney's prodigious ability to excrete bicarbonate, however, addition of bicarbonate to the blood is not sufficient to cause a sustained metabolic alkalosis. Some mechanisms to maintain the alkalosis must prevail. The most common mechanism contributing to the maintenance of metabolic alkalosis is volume depletion, either absolute or relative (e.g., congestive heart failure), which (1) reduces glomerular filtration; (2) enhances tubular bicarbonate reabsorption; and (3) causes secondary hyperaldosteronism, further enhancing urinary acidification. Another common perpetuating factor is K depletion, which stimulates proton secretion directly and indirectly by increasing renal ammoniagenesis.[21,22]

Patients with metabolic alkalosis and signs of volume expansion—especially hypertension—usually have excess mineralocorticoid as the explanation for the metabolic alkalosis. Aldosterone and glucocorticoids other than dexamethasone stimulate renal loss of acid and K and thereby generate and maintain the alkalosis.

Causes of metabolic alkalosis are shown in Box 58-2. One entity unique to critically ill patients is the posthypocapnic metabolic alkalosis. This syndrome is caused by abrupt treatment (usually with tracheal intubation and mechanical ventilation) of a chronic respiratory acidosis. The renal bicarbonate retention that compensated for the chronic respiratory acidosis persists (because of volume depletion) after restoration of a normal P_{CO_2}, resulting in the high pH and high plasma bicarbonate characteristic of metabolic alkalosis. The key to the diagnosis is the history and sequential analysis of blood chemistries.[21]

Box 58-2

Causes of Metabolic Alkalosis

Intravascular Volume Depletion, Absolute or "Effective"
- Gastrointestinal acid loss
  - Vomiting or nasogastric suction
  - Villous adenoma
  - Chloride diarrhea
- Renal acid loss
  - Diuretics (loop, thiazide)
  - Bartter syndrome
  - Gitelman's syndrome
  - Magnesium depletion
  - Posthypercapnic state
  - Congestive heart failure
- Hepatic cirrhosis/ascites

Intravascular Volume Expansion
- High renin, high aldosterone
  - Renal artery stenosis
  - Accelerated hypertension
  - Renin-secreting tumor
- Low renin, high aldosterone
  - Primary aldosteronism
- Low renin, low aldosterone
  - Cushing's syndrome or disease
  - Exogenous mineralocorticoid
  - Apparent mineralocorticoid excess syndrome
  - Liddle syndrome
- Renal insufficiency
  - Exogenous alkali load
  - Milk-alkali syndrome

Adapted from Palmer BF, Alpern RJ: Metabolic alkalosis. J Am Soc Nephrol 1997;8:1462-1469.

Clinical Consequences

Alkalemia in critically ill patients is associated with increased mortality.[23] Patients with combined metabolic and respiratory alkalosis have a higher mortality than those with respiratory alkalosis alone, and mortality in alkalemia is roughly proportional to the pH.[23] Although no causal relationship between alkalemia and mortality has been established, the pathophysiology of alkalemia is far from benign.[22]

First, metabolic alkalosis suppresses ventilation, causing CO_2 retention and relative hypoxemia.[24] Second, alkalemia acutely increases hemoglobin's oxygen affinity (Bohr effect). Third, respiratory alkalosis causes vasoconstriction, particularly in the cerebral circulation.[22] All these processes tend to decrease tissue oxygen delivery.[25] (Of note is that chronic alkalemia inhibits 2,3-DPG synthesis, allowing normalization of the oxyhemoglobin desaturation curve, mitigating tissue hypoxia to some extent.) These alterations in tissue oxygen delivery could be responsible at least in part for some of the clinical manifestations of metabolic alkalosis.

Because alkalemia causes a decrease in ionized Ca concentration (see "Calcium" later), many of the neuromuscular manifestations of metabolic alkalosis overlap with those of hypocalcemia including paresthesias, tetany, and a predisposition to seizures.[1] The acutely diminished tissue oxygen delivery to the brain may contribute to initial confusion and obtundation seen with metabolic alkalosis.

Metabolic alkalosis is often accompanied by hypokalemia and hypomagnesemia. Thus there is an association between alkalosis and arrhythmias,[21] but an independent effect of the alkalosis on cardiac arrhythmogenesis has not been established.

Increases in blood lactate concentration may occur in patients with metabolic alkalosis because of upregulation of phosphofructokinase and thus glycolysis and because of tissue hypoxia (see earlier).[8] With severe metabolic alkalosis (arterial pH above 7.55), the tissue hypoxia may be so marked that compensatory hypoventilation will be overridden by hypoxic drive, resulting in a normal to low arterial P_{CO_2} and elevated blood lactate levels (so-called *lactic alkalosis*).[26]

Treatment

Treatment of metabolic alkalosis entails correcting the factors responsible for its maintenance and, if possible, correcting the factor that generated the alkalosis. Once the underlying diagnosis is clear (see Box 58-2), therapy is usually straightforward. If the metabolic alkalosis is maintained by volume contraction, the intravascular volume should be restored to normal, usually with intravenous isotonic saline.[21,22] Potassium (K) should be given, as KCl, to replace any deficits (see "Disorders of Potassium Homeostasis" later) because K depletion perpetuates the metabolic alkalosis. If nasogastric suction cannot be stopped, acid loss can be reduced by the use of H_2-blockers and proton pump inhibitors.

Patients with metabolic alkalosis in the setting of diminished effective circulating volume (e.g., congestive heart failure, hepatic cirrhosis) are often difficult to treat because saline infusion is contraindicated. Such patients may respond to aggressive KCl supplementation. Acetazolamide (a carbonic anhydrase inhibitor) may be of additional benefit by stimulating bicarbonaturia, but care must be taken to avoid exacerbating the hypokalemia typical in such conditions. Another potential complication of acetazolamide administration, particularly in patients with impending ventilatory failure, is worsening of hypercapnia because of inhibition of red blood cell carbonic anhydrase and impaired CO_2 transport.[22] Hydrochloric acid infusion, as a 0.1 to 0.25N solution, has been used with success in patients with severe metabolic acidosis refractory to conventional measures.[22,27] Correction of the metabolic disturbances has been reported with infusion of 0.25N HCl at 100 mL/hour over about 12 hours.[27] Extreme care must be taken to ensure that the infusion catheter is properly positioned within the vena cava because the solution is highly caustic. Plasma chemistries must be monitored frequently in order to avoid overcorrection.

In states of primary mineralocorticoid excess, an aldosterone antagonist such as spironolactone should be used until the underlying abnormality can be corrected. Other K-sparing diuretics such as amiloride and triamterene are useful as well and are essential in managing the rare patient with Liddle syndrome.

DISORDERS OF POTASSIUM HOMEOSTASIS

Normal Potassium Physiology

Disorders of K homeostasis are common in hospitalized patients and may be associated with severe adverse clinical outcomes including death.[28,29] Prevention and proper treatment of hyperkalemia and hypokalemia depend on an understanding of the underlying physiology.

The total body K content of a 70-kg adult is about 3500 mmol, of which only 2% (≈70 mmol) is extracellular.[30] This uneven distribution reflects the large K concentration gradient between the intracellular (Ki ≈ 140 mmol/L) and the extracellular (Ke ≈ 4.5 mmol/L) space, a gradient that is maintained by the intrinsic ion permeabilities of cell membranes and by Na^+,K^+-ATPase, the sodium-K pump.[31] The Ke-to-Ki ratio largely determines the resting membrane potential of cells and thus is crucial for proper function of excitable tissues (muscle and nerve).[31] Small absolute changes in Ke will perturb the ratio significantly. Therefore disturbances of Ke (measured as changes in plasma K concentration, or P_K) may have serious, even lethal, consequences mainly in the form of excitable tissue dysfunction.

Therefore it is not surprising that the extracellular K concentration is tightly regulated. In fact, two separate and cooperative systems participate in K homeostasis. One system regulates *external K balance:* the total-body parity of K elimination with K intake. The other system regulates *internal K balance:* the distribution of K between the intracellular and extracellular fluid compartments. This latter system provides a short-term defense against changes in the P_K that might otherwise result from total-body K losses or gains.

Regulation of Internal Potassium Balance

Internal K balance serves to protect against changes in Ke; K tends to move out of cells during K depletion and into cells following K intake. This process tends to prevent drastic alterations of Ke-to-Ki ratio.[32,33] The factors that influence internal K balance include hormones, acid-base status, plasma tonicity, exercise, and cell integrity (Table 58-4).

Our understanding of the effects of *acid-base balance* on K distribution has undergone considerable revision in recent years.[34,35] The direction and magnitude of an acid-base–related change in P_K clearly depend on the nature and the duration of the disturbance.[36] The most consistent and pronounced relationship between changes in pH and P_K occurs in acute mineral (hyperchloremic) acidosis in

Table 58-4. Factors Affecting Internal K Balance

Factors Causing Cellular K Influx
Insulin
β_2-adrenoceptor agonist (metabolic alkalosis)*
Factors Causing Cellular K Efflux
Cell ischemia/lysis
Exercise
Plasma hypertonicity
α-Adrenoceptor agonist (metabolic acidosis)*

*Factors shown in parentheses have a minor or variable effect. See text.

which there is a strong inverse relationship between these two variables.[34,35] Interestingly, hypokalemia is seen with prolonged mineral acidosis in patients with normal renal function and reflects increased renal K excretion.[35] Unlike mineral acidoses, however, even severe acute organic (high-anion-gap) acidoses are not usually associated with hyperkalemia[37-39] and it is now generally accepted that organic acidoses, like lactic acidosis and ketoacidosis, do not directly affect internal K balance. Nonetheless, factors coincident with the acidosis may alter P_K. For example, mesenteric ischemia may result in both lactic acidosis (from anaerobic metabolism) and hyperkalemia. Even the hyperkalemia so commonly seen in patients with diabetic ketoacidosis does not result from the acidemia; rather, it appears to be a consequence of the characteristic insulin deficiency and hyperglycemia (see "Hypertonicity" later).[37] Respiratory disturbances typically alter P_K less than metabolic disturbances. Alkaloses, respiratory or metabolic, have less effect on P_K than their corresponding acidosis.[34] Bicarbonate administration, which was once thought to reduce the P_K by stimulating cellular K uptake,[40] is now known to have little, if any, immediate effect on internal K balance.[41,42] Nonetheless, longstanding alkalemia causes urinary K losses, which may over time result in profound K depletion.[43]

Hypertonicity, as seen with hypertonic fluid administration[44] or diabetic hyperglycemic states,[45] leads to hyperkalemia, probably as a result of K efflux from cells by way of solvent drag. Lethal hyperkalemia has been attributed to this phenomenon in diabetic patients with ESRD.[46]

Exercise causes a transient shift of K out of cells. Clinically significant hyperkalemia may result from exercise[47,48] (and clinically misleading local venous hyperkalemia results from repeated fist clenching during phlebotomy[49]).

Regulation of External Potassium Balance

In contrast to the prodigious capacity of the kidney to excrete K,[50] renal K conservation is imperfect and explains why significant K depletion and hypokalemia may result from dietary K deficiency alone.[51]

Normally 90% to 95% of dietary K is eliminated through the kidney, and only about 5% to 10% through the intestine. It is the kidney that is almost entirely responsible for matching K output to K intake in order to maintain total body K constant.[52] The majority of K excreted by the kidney derives from K secretion in the distal nephron (connecting tubule and collecting duct).[52] Virtually all regulation of K excretion takes place at this site in the nephron, under the influence of two principal factors: the rate of flow and sodium delivery through that part of the nephron and the effect of aldosterone.[52] K secretion is directly proportional to flow rate and sodium delivery through the distal nephron, explaining in part why diuretic use is often accompanied by hypokalemia.

Bicarbonate delivery to the distal nephron stimulates kaliuresis by increasing the electrochemical "driving force" for K secretion.[52] Other anions that are poorly reabsorbed in the distal nephron (e.g., synthetic penicillins) have a similar effect.[53]

It is well established that aldosterone participates in a homeostatic feedback loop with P_K such that increases in P_K stimulate adrenal aldosterone production, which in turn reduces P_K primarily by stimulating renal K excretion.[52] Hypokalemia is a prominent feature of primary aldosteronism (Conn's syndrome) because the high circulating aldosterone levels are accompanied by volume expansion and thus a high rate of sodium delivery to the distal nephron. When circulating aldosterone levels are high because of volume depletion (secondary aldosteronism), the increase in distal K secretion is offset by a decrease in distal nephron flow, thus mitigating renal K loss. Indeed, it is only when patients with secondary hyperaldosteronism (e.g., congestive heart failure, hepatic cirrhosis) are treated with diuretic drugs that distal nephron flow is increased and hypokalemia may ensue.

Magnesium (Mg) deficiency is associated with renal K wasting and may result in severe K depletion.[54] Because Mg, like Ca, acts to stabilize excitable membranes, the deleterious effects of hypokalemia on the myocardium are magnified by concurrent hypomagnesemia (see "Clinical Manifestations" later).[55]

The effect of dexamethasone (a pure glucocorticoid) to enhance renal K excretion appears to result entirely from hemodynamic changes, which cause an increase in glomerular filtration rate and distal flow rate. All other glucocorticoids tend to further stimulate K secretion in proportion to their mineralocorticoid activity.[52]

Disorders of Potassium Homeostasis

Disorders of K homeostasis may be conveniently divided according to the duration of the disturbance: acute (<48 hours' duration) or chronic. Such a distinction is particularly applicable to the medical intensive care setting in which blood chemistries are sampled frequently and a patient's condition and therapy may change radically over a short time. In addition, the approach to treatment varies according to the acuity of the disturbance. The treatment of acute disturbances is largely independent of their cause, whereas the rational treatment of chronic disturbances depends on understanding their pathogenesis.

Acute Hyperkalemia (Box 58-3)

Excessive Potassium Intake

Given an acute K load, a normal individual will excrete about 50% in the urine and transport about 90% of the

Box 58-3

Causes of Acute Hyperkalemia

Excessive Potassium Intake
- Oral
- Intravenous
- Blood transfusion
- Cardioplegic solutions

Transcellular Potassium Shift
- With acute renal failure
  - Rhabdomyolysis
  - Tumor lysis syndrome
- Tissue infarction
  - Mesenteric limb
- Hypertonicity
  - Hyperglycemia
- Metabolic acidosis
- Drug-induced
  - Digitalis intoxication
  - Succinylcholine
- Hyperkalemic periodic paralysis
- Pseudohyperkalemia
  - Thrombocytosis
  - Leukocytosis
  - In vitro hemolysis
  - Fist-clenching with phlebotomy

remainder into cells over 4 to 6 hours.[56] It is possible to overwhelm this adaptive mechanism such that if too much K is taken in too quickly, significant hyperkalemia will result. Such events are almost always iatrogenic (i.e., overly aggressive K replacement therapy).[57] One's ability to tolerate a K load declines with disordered internal balance (see later) and impaired renal K excretory capacity.[58] In such circumstances, an otherwise tolerable increase in K intake may cause clinically significant hyperkalemia: Doses of oral K supplements as small as 30 to 45 mmol have resulted in severe hyperkalemia in patients with impaired external or internal K homeostasis.[59]

KCl, used as a supplement, is the drug most commonly implicated in acute hyperkalemia.[58,60] Banked blood represents a trivial K load under most circumstances. A unit of blood, either whole or packed cells, contains only about 7 mmol of K.[61] Thus severe hyperkalemia would result only from massive transfusion of compatible blood.[62] Infants[63] or patients with renal insufficiency may develop hyperkalemia from an otherwise tolerable transfusion.

Patients undergoing open heart surgery are exposed to cardioplegic solutions containing KCl typically at about 16 mmol/L,[64] which may lead to clinically significant hyperkalemia in the postoperative period, especially in patients with diabetes mellitus with or without renal failure.[65]

Abnormal Potassium Distribution

Acute hyperkalemia may result from sudden redistribution of intracellular K to the extracellular space. If only 2% of intracellular K were to leak unopposed from cells, P_K would immediately double. Fortunately, such dramatic circumstances are rarely encountered. Nevertheless, smaller degrees of K redistribution commonly result in clinically significant hyperkalemia.

Among the most impressive syndromes associated with acute hyperkalemia are those involving *rapid cell lysis.* The *tumor lysis syndrome* results from treatment of chemosensitive bulky tumors with release of intracellular contents including K into the extracellular fluid.[66] Extreme hyperkalemia, even causing sudden death,[67] has featured prominently in some series of patients. Most of such patients were in renal failure from acute uric acid nephropathy, thus impairing their ability to excrete the K load.[67] *Rhabdomyolysis,* either traumatic or nontraumatic, may result in sudden massive influx of K to the extracellular space.[68] Hyperkalemia is present in about 40% of patients on presentation with rhabdomyolysis[69] and is more common among patients whose course is complicated by oliguric acute renal failure.[70] Rhabdomyolysis is commonly associated with the use of alcohol[69] and cocaine.[71] Extreme hyperkalemia in this latter context has been reported.[72] Statin drugs are frequently associated with rhabdomyolysis,[73] rarely causing extreme hyperkalemia.[74] Other circumstances that may result in redistributive hyperkalemia include severe extensive burns, hemolytic transfusion reactions, and mesenteric ischemia or infarction.

Pharmacologic Agents

Two drugs may rarely cause acute hyperkalemia by redistribution: digitalis glycosides and succinylcholine. Massive digitalis overdose has been associated with extreme hyperkalemia.[75,76] Succinylcholine depolarizes the motor end plate and in normal individuals causes a trivial amount of K leak from muscle, resulting in an increase in P_K by about 0.5 mmol/L.[77] In patients with neuromuscular disorders, muscle damage, or prolonged immobilization, however, muscle depolarization may be more widespread, causing severe hyperkalemia.[78] Prolonged use of nondepolarizing neuromuscular blockers in critically ill patients may predispose to succinylcholine-induced hyperkalemia.[79]

Hyperkalemic Periodic Paralysis

This rare syndrome of episodic hyperkalemia and paralysis is caused by a mutation of the skeletal muscle sodium channel, inherited in an autosomal dominant pattern.[80] Attacks may be precipitated by exercise, fasting, exposure to cold and K administration, and prevented by frequent carbohydrate snacks. Attacks are usually brief, and treatment consists of carbohydrate ingestion. Severe attacks may require intravenous glucose infusions.[81]

Acute Renal Failure Hyperkalemia accompanies acute renal failure in 30% to 50% of cases. It is seen most commonly in oliguric renal failure. Contributing factors include tissue destruction (e.g., tumor lysis syndrome, rhabdomyolysis) and increased catabolism.[82]

Pseudohyperkalemia Pseudohyperkalemia refers to a measured K that is higher than that circulating in the patient's blood. It has a number of possible causes. First, it may be caused by efflux of K out of blood cells in the test tube after phlebotomy. This may be seen in a *serum* specimen in cases of thrombocytosis[83] or leukocytosis,[84] when the clot causes cell lysis in vitro. Today, many clinical laboratories measure electrolytes in plasma (unclotted) specimens. Even under these conditions, extreme leukocytosis may cause pseudohyperkalemia if the specimen is chilled for a long time before the plasma is separated, leading to passive K leak from cells.[85] Hemolysis during specimen collection will falsely raise P_K *or* plasma K concentration by liberating intraerythrocyte K. Second, if the patient's arm is exercised by fist clenching with a tourniquet in place before the specimen is drawn, the sampled blood K concentration will rise significantly as a result of local muscle release of intracellular K.[49]

Acute Hypokalemia

Hypokalemia that develops over hours is virtually always the result of redistribution of K from the extracellular to the intracellular space. The causes of acute hypokalemia are summarized in Box 58-4. Selected causes are discussed as follows.

Treatment of Diabetic Ketoacidosis

It is well recognized that patients presenting in diabetic ketoacidosis (DKA) are always severely total body K depleted, as a result of the glucose-driven osmotic diuresis, poor nutrition, and vomiting during the development of DKA.[37] Paradoxically, most patients in DKA have a normal P_K on admission.[86] Insulin deficiency and hyperglycemia appears to account for the preservation of a normal P_K despite severe total body K depletion.[37] Once therapy for DKA is instituted, however, P_K typically plummets as K is rapidly taken up by cells. K replacement at rates up to 120 mmol per hour have been reported, with total K supplementation of 600 to 800 mmol within the first 24 hours of treatment.[87] Hypokalemia in this setting may lead to respiratory arrest.[88]

Box 58-4

Causes of Acute Hypokalemia

Treatment of Diabetic Ketoacidosis
Refeeding Syndrome
Rapid Cell Production
- Vitamin B_{12} treatment of pernicious anemia
- GM-CSF treatment of leukopenia

Pharmacologic Agents
- β_2-adrenoceptor agonists
- Epinephrine
- Soluble barium salts

Hypokalemic Periodic Paralysis
- Familial
- Sporadic
- Thyrotoxic

Pseudohypokalemia

Refeeding

A situation analogous to DKA arises during aggressive refeeding after prolonged starvation or with aggressive "hyperalimentation" of chronically ill patients. The glucose-stimulated hyperinsulinemia and tissue anabolism shift K into cells, rapidly depleting extracellular K.[89] Death in the setting of refeeding has been reported and may be partly caused by rapid cellular uptake of other ions (e.g., phosphorus, Mg).[90]

Pharmacologic Agents Specific *β_2-adrenoceptor agonists* (e.g., albuterol) may cause electrophysiologically significant hypokalemia, especially when given to patients who are K depleted from the use of diuretic drugs.[91] *Epinephrine,* given IV in a dose about 5% of that recommended for cardiac resuscitation, causes a fall in P_K by about 1 mmol/L.[92] Such a dose achieves plasma levels of epinephrine comparable with those seen after acute myocardial infarction and may explain the transient hypokalemia following resuscitation from cardiac arrest even without the use of exogenous epinephrine (postresuscitation hypokalemia).[93, 94] A rare cause of severe hypokalemia is poisoning with *soluble* barium salts such as chloride, carbonate, hydroxide, and sulfide. Soluble barium salts are used in pesticides and some depilatories, which may be ingested accidentally or intentionally.[95]

Hypokalemic Periodic Paralysis Three forms of this rare syndrome have been described: familial, sporadic, and thyrotoxic.[96,97] All have in common attacks of muscle weakness accompanied by acute hypokalemia caused by cellular K uptake. Death may occur because of ventilatory failure or cardiac dysrhythmias. The *familial* variety—resulting from a skeletal muscle Ca channelopathy[80]—is inherited in an autosomal dominant pattern, with onset of clinical manifestations typically in the second decade of life. Attacks may occur after carbohydrate or salt ingestion or exercise. Administration of K orally or IV will abort an acute attack but is ineffective in preventing attacks.[96] The *sporadic* variety of hypokalemic periodic paralysis is identical to the familial form except for the absence of a hereditary pattern. *Thyrotoxic* periodic paralysis was first described in Asians but is now recognized to be nearly ubiquitous.[97] The usual onset of symptoms is in the third decade. Severe hypophosphatemia may accompany the hypokalemia.[98] Treatment of the disorder is treatment of hyperthyroidism.

Pseudohypokalemia Severe leukocytosis may cause spuriously low plasma K concentrations if blood cells are left in contact with the plasma for a long time at room temperature or higher. This phenomenon results from ongoing cell metabolism in vitro with glucose and K uptake.[54] Unexpected hypokalemia and hypoglycemia in the setting of leukocytosis should alert the clinician to this phenomenon.

Chronic Hyperkalemia

Renal Failure Patients with chronic kidney disease tend to maintain a normal P_K until renal function declines to about 10% of normal.[99] Aldosterone and insulin both appear to play a role in the extrarenal K adaptation in chronic kidney disease.[100] This explains why patients with chronic kidney disease who are mineralocorticoid or insulin deficient, or both, have a particular predisposition to hyperkalemia.[101]

Mineralocorticoid Deficiency Mineralocorticoid deficiency may result from global adrenal insufficiency (Addison's disease) or from selective defects in the renin-angiotensin-aldosterone axis (see Chapter 60). Hyperkalemia in the setting of unexplained hypotension should immediately raise one's suspicion for adrenal insufficiency. A common setting for isolated mineralocorticoid deficiency is the syndrome of *hyporeninemic hypoaldosteronism*.[101] This syndrome is most often seen in elderly patients with diabetes mellitus and moderate renal insufficiency. Hyperkalemia is a universal finding. An associated hyperchloremic metabolic acidosis (type IV renal tubular acidosis) is characteristic.[101] In addition to diabetes mellitus, two other systemic diseases are associated with this syndrome: the acquired immune deficiency syndrome[102,103] and systemic lupus erythematosus.[104]

Aldosterone deficiency may be induced by a variety of pharmacologic agents acting at different sites in the renin-angiotensin-aldosterone axis. β-Adrenoreceptor blockers and, to a greater extent, cyclooxygenase inhibitors (COX-1 and COX-2), predispose patients to hyperkalemia by suppressing renin release.[105] As a general rule, COX inhibitors should be avoided in patients with renal insufficiency or who are otherwise prone to hyperkalemia either because of diabetes or the use of other implicated drugs. Converting enzyme inhibitors and angiotensin receptor blockers decrease aldosterone biosynthesis. These drugs are reported to be implicated in 10% to 38% of hyperkalemia in hospitalized patients.[106] Volume depletion or hypotension, or both, increase the risk of hyperkalemia with all these agents.

High- and low-dose heparin therapy decreases circulating aldosterone levels by selectively inhibiting aldosterone biosynthesis.[107] Hyperkalemia is seen with the use of low-molecular-weight heparins as well, particularly in patients with diabetes mellitus.[108]

Renal K Secretory Defect An isolated defect in renal K secretion (often with a renal tubular acidosis) is associated with sickle cell disease or trait,[109] systemic lupus erythematosus,[104] and after renal transplantation.[110] In this last circumstance, the hyperkalemia is exacerbated by the use of cyclosporine and tacrolimus for immunosuppression.[111,112] A syndrome of hyperkalemic (type IV) distal renal tubular acidosis is seen in patients with urinary tract obstruction.[113]

The so-called *K-sparing diuretics* (spironolactone, eplerenone, amiloride, and triamterene) impair renal K excretion by blocking sodium reabsorption in the distal nephron. Two antibiotics, pentamidine[114] and trimethoprim,[115,116] cause hyperkalemia, occasionally severe, by blocking sodium reabsorption in the distal nephron.

Chronic Hypokalemia

Chronic hypokalemia is virtually always the result of altered external balance: insufficient K intake, excessive K losses, or a combination of the two. Losses are usually either GI or renal.

Inadequate Potassium Intake

Because renal K conservation is not perfect, severe dietary K restriction will cause hypokalemia in 3 to 7 days in normal humans.[51] In one series of hypokalemic hospitalized patients, inadequate K supplementation during IV therapy contributed to the development of severe hypokalemia in 45% of cases and was the sole cause in 6%.[117] Other disorders associated with nutritional hypokalemia include anorexia nervosa, alcoholism, and malignancy.

Excessive Potassium Losses

Hypokalemia may develop as a result of both upper and lower GI fluid losses, but the pathogenesis is quite different in the two situations. With diarrhea, the K is lost from the gut.[118] Gastric fluid losses (e.g., vomiting or gastric suction) are associated with hypokalemia. Paradoxically, however, most of the K losses are renal, not gastric. Gastric fluid K concentration is only 5 to 10 mmol/L. Thus only massive gastric fluid losses would, alone, significantly deplete total body K stores. The gastric fluid losses, however, stimulate renal K secretion in several ways. First, by generating a metabolic alkalosis and increasing bicarbonate delivery to the distal nephron, K secretion is stimulated. The metabolic alkalosis also leads to cellular proton loss and K uptake, which, in renal epithelial cells, enhances K secretion. Finally, the volume contraction that usually accompanies GI fluid losses causes secondary aldosteronism, which further augments urinary K losses. Thus in this situation, urinary K concentration is typically high while urinary chloride concentration is low because of volume contraction. (Urinary sodium losses may be high because of natriuresis obligated by the bicarbonaturia.)

All *diuretics* work by inhibiting sodium and chloride reabsorption by the nephron. Those drugs that act proximal to the K secretory site in the nephron promote a kaliuresis by increasing delivery of fluid distally and causing secondary aldosteronism. Thus hypokalemia frequently accompanies the use of the two most common classes of diuretics: thiazides and loop diuretics.[119] Carbonic anhydrase inhibitors exert an additional kaliuretic effect by shunting bicarbonate-rich, chloride-poor fluid to the distal nephron.[120] Combining two K-wasting diuretics for added diuretic effect (e.g., furosemide plus metolazone) can result in severe hypokalemia. In such cases P_K has been found to fall below 3.5 mmol/L in more than 80% of patients and below 3 mmol/L in more than half.[119]

Various antibiotic agents may cause renal K wasting and thereby hypokalemia. Ninety percent of patients receiving amphotericin B require K supplementation.[121] Penicillin antibiotics, particularly polyanionic derivatives such as carbenicillin and ticarcillin, have been associated with hypokalemia.[122]

Mineralocorticoids predispose to hypokalemia by stimulating renal K excretion. Mineralocorticoid excess may be *primary*[123] (Conn's syndrome) or *secondary* to diminished real or "effective" circulating volume. All glucocorticoid drugs except dexamethasone possess some mineralocorticoid activity. Therefore prolonged administration of these agents can cause severe hypokalemia. In edematous patients with secondary aldosteronism (e.g., congestive heart failure, hepatic cirrhosis) hypokalemia commonly ensues only when diuretic therapy enhances distal nephron flow rate.

Mg deficiency is associated with renal K wasting and may result in severe K depletion (see later). Because Mg, like Ca, acts to stabilize excitable membranes, the deleterious effects of hypokalemia on the myocardium are magnified by concurrent hypomagnesemia.[124] The intensive care setting is fraught with potential causes of hypomagnesemia (see "Disorders of Magnesium Homeostasis" later).

Hypercalcemia causes a salt and water diuresis and is therefore commonly associated with renal hypokalemia (see "Disorders of Calcium Homeostasis" later).[125] In one series, one third of hypercalcemic patients were hypokalemic with no other predisposing factors; the prevalence was 52% in patients with hypercalcemia of malignancy. P_K was inversely proportional to the plasma Ca concentration.[126]

Several inborn tubular transport abnormalities are associated with chronic hypokalemia (and metabolic alkalosis). *Bartter* and *Gitelman's* syndromes are associated with volume contraction and normal blood pressure, and *Liddle* syndrome with hypertension.[127]

Clinical Manifestations of Potassium Imbalance

Alterations in P_K have a variety of adverse clinical consequences, the expression of which may be magnified in the critically ill patient. The most serious of these manifestations are those involving excitable tissues.

Clinical Manifestations of Hyperkalemia

Cardiac Effects

Hyperkalemia depolarizes the cell membrane, slows ventricular conduction, and decreases the duration of the action potential. These changes produce the classic electrocardiographic manifestations of hyperkalemia including (in order of their usual appearance) peaked T waves, prolongation of the PR interval, widening of the QRS complex, loss of the P wave, "sine wave" configuration or ventricular fibrillation, and asystole.[128,129] These electrocardiographic changes may be modified by a multitude of factors such as extracellular fluid pH, Ca concentration, sodium concentration, and the rate of rise of P_K.[128]

Electrocardiographic changes may not accompany changes in P_K. If present, these electrocardiographic changes certainly suggest hyperkalemia. However, in the absence of the classic electrocardiographic changes, the clinician should not be lulled into a false sense of security when evaluating a hyperkalemic patient. Normal electrocardiograms (ECGs) occur despite extreme hyperkalemia,[130] and the first cardiac manifestation of hyperkalemia may be ventricular fibrillation.[131] Consequently, P_K greater than 6.5 mmol/L, even with a normal ECG, should be treated as an emergency (see "Treatment of Potassium Imbalance" later).

Neuromuscular Effects

Hyperkalemia may result in paresthesias and weakness progressing to a flaccid paralysis, which typically spares the diaphragm. Reflexes are depressed or absent. Cranial nerves are rarely involved, and sensory changes are minimal.[132]

Metabolic Effects

Hyperkalemia decreases renal ammoniagenesis, which by itself may produce a mild hyperchloremic metabolic acidosis[133] and will limit the kidney's ability to excrete an acid load and thus prevent correction of a metabolic acidosis.[134]

Clinical Manifestations of Hypokalemia

Although less immediately life threatening than hyperkalemia, hypokalemia has many detrimental effects in critically ill patients. Along with cardiac and neuromuscular manifestations are many more subtle effects.

Cardiac Effects

Hypokalemia hyperpolarizes the cell membrane and prolongs the cardiac action potential.[135] These changes are associated with the following electrocardiographic manifestations: ST segment depression, a decrease in T wave amplitude, and an increase in U wave amplitude.[128,129] However, because all of these are nonspecific, the ECG is an even less reliable index of hypokalemia than it is of hyperkalemia.

Hypokalemia may be associated with an increased incidence of arrhythmias and conduction defects. It is well established that K depletion increases the cardiac toxicity of digitalis glycosides.[136] However, controversy exists as to whether hypokalemia per se induces ventricular arrhythmias in patients not taking digitalis. An increase in benign ventricular ectopy occurs in hypokalemic patients without acute myocardial ischemia.[137] The clinical import of this observation is unclear. In individuals hospitalized with acute myocardial infarction, however, a correlation between hypokalemia and ventricular tachycardia and fibrillation has been observed.[138] The hypokalemia seen in this setting may result from increased cellular K uptake caused by high circulating levels of catecholamines. Because K repletion does not reduce the occurrence of these arrhythmias, it is unlikely that hypokalemia is the sole arrhythmogenic factor.[138]

Neuromuscular Effects

Modest hypokalemia generally presents as weakness, myalgias, muscle fatigue, and "restless" legs. With more severe hypokalemia (<2 mmol/L), paralysis may supervene. This usually involves the extremities but may progress to include the trunk and muscles of ventilation. As with hyperkalemia, cranial nerves typically are spared and sensory function usually remains intact.[54] Importantly, these manifestations may be masked by concomitant hypocalcemia and may only appear when Ca is replenished. Conversely, in patients with hypokalemia and hypocalcemia, tetany may develop only after K replacement.[54] Smooth muscle dysfunction (ileus, gastroparesis) is more commonly seen with hypokalemia than with hyperkalemia.

In addition to the effects of K depletion on the electrical properties of the neuromuscular system, profound hypokalemia may result in muscle injury and frank rhabdomyolysis, even in bed-bound patients.[139]

Miscellaneous Effects

Hypokalemia and K depletion are associated with glucose intolerance,[140] increased protein catabolism, polydipsia and polyuria,[54] and metabolic alkalosis.[141]

Evaluation of Disorders of Potassium Homeostasis

The diagnostic approach to disorders of K homeostasis may be focused by dividing them according to their duration: acute (or of unknown duration) versus chronic.

Evaluation of Acute Hyperkalemia

When P_K rises abruptly or if P_K is high (>6.5 mmol/L) on initial presentation of the patient, the first step is to obtain an ECG to look for electrophysiologic evidence of hyperkalemia. In the presence of such signs, treatment for hyperkalemia should begin urgently (see "Treatment of Potassium Imbalance" later). At the same time, an unclotted blood sample should be obtained, using meticulous phlebotomy technique, for another set of electrolytes, glucose, BUN and creatinine, and CBC. Urine should be tested for heme pigments to exclude acute rhabdomyolysis or hemolysis. The patient's list of medications and diet should be reviewed promptly, looking for exogenous sources of K and drugs that may impair K tolerance (see Box 58-3).

Evaluation of Chronic Hyperkalemia

Figure 58-2 outlines an approach to the patient with hyperkalemia lasting for days. Failure to stimulate cortisol release with a cosyntropin stimulation test (see Chapter 60) supports a diagnosis of Addison's disease. Absent that diagnosis, the patient is likely to have either selective aldosterone deficiency or tubular unresponsiveness to aldosterone, or both. Assessment of the renin-angiotensin-aldosterone axis is most simply done by measuring plasma renin activity (PRA) and aldosterone levels in the basal and diuretic/posture-stimulated state.[101] Tubular unresponsiveness to aldosterone is assessed by measuring the K secretory effect of 9a-fludrocortisone (9a-F, Florinef). One index of the driving force for K secretion that may be useful in this regard is the transtubular K gradient (TTKG), calculated as follows:

$$TTKG = \frac{U_K}{P_K} \times \frac{P_{osm}}{U_{osm}}$$

where P_{osm} and U_{osm} are plasma and urine osmolalities, respectively.[142]

Evaluation of Acute Hypokalemia

Hypokalemia accompanied by serious cardiac or neuromuscular manifestations is an emergency. Likewise, urgent therapy is indicated for profound hypokalemia (P_K <2 mmol/L) even in the absence of clinical complications. In addition, moderate hypokalemia (P_K<3 mmol/L) in patients taking digitalis,[136] and perhaps with acute myocardial ischemia,[138] should be treated urgently because of the risk of ventricular arrhythmias. In all these situations, it is imperative that the blood specimen be obtained and handled properly, especially in patients with leukocytosis, because rapid administration of K to a patient with pseudohypokalemia may cause severe hyperkalemia.

The remainder of the evaluation of acute hypokalemia derives mainly from the patient's history with an emphasis on treatments causing cellular K uptake (e.g., insulin, β-adrenergic agonists) or a rapid increase in tissue anabolism, and a history of periodic paralysis. Patients who are hypokalemic on presentation should be evaluated as if their hypokalemia were acute.

Evaluation of Chronic Hypokalemia

Once acute hypokalemia and transient K redistribution have been excluded, one should next determine whether

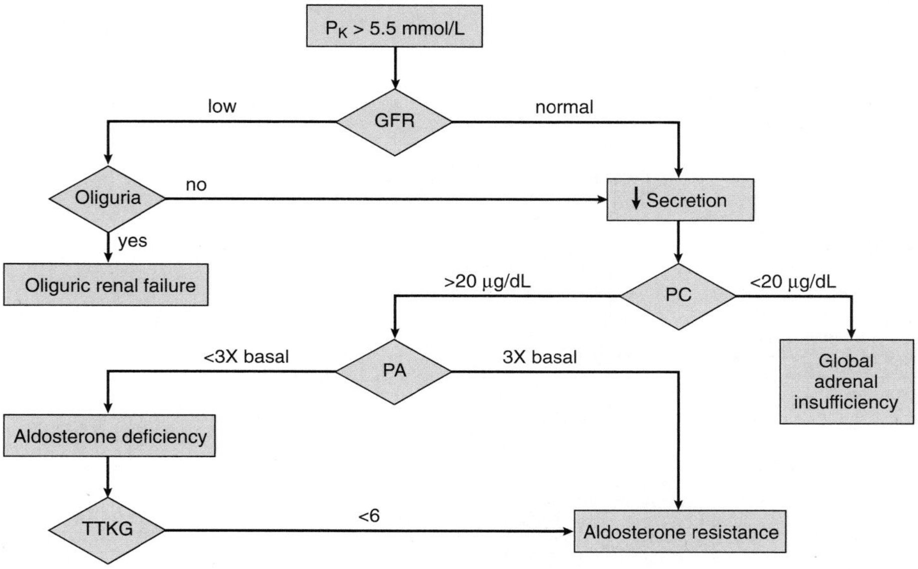

Figure 58-2. Diagnostic evaluation of chronic hyperkalemia. GFR, glomerular filtration rate; PA, stimulated plasma aldosterone (see text); PC, stimulated plasma cortisol (see Chapter 60); TTKG, transtubular potassium gradient (see text).

the kidney is responding appropriately to the K deficit or whether it is contributing to the problem. This is best done by measuring the 24-hour urinary excretion of K during K repletion (Fig. 58-3). K excretion less than 20 mmol per day suggests appropriate renal K conservation and points to extrarenal (lower GI or skin) K losses, recovery from diuretic-induced hypokalemia, or chronically K-deficient diet. Excretion of greater than 20 mmol per day is evidence of inadequate renal K conservation, indicating a renal cause of the hypokalemia. Renal K losses associated with normal systemic blood pressure are most commonly seen with the use of thiazide or loop diuretics and are accompanied by a metabolic alkalosis. Other causes of hypokalemia with metabolic alkalosis in a normotensive patient include gastric fluid loss, Bartter syndrome, and Gitelman's syndrome. These are separable most often by history, but if not, the urinary chloride measurement will be helpful, being low with gastric fluid losses. Renal hypokalemia may accompany a renal tubular acidosis, in which case the plasma bicarbonate will be low.

Mineralocorticoid excess may be the cause if the renal K loss is associated with systemic hypertension, and the renin-aldosterone axis should be studied with basal and saline-suppressed blood hormone measurements. High plasma renin activity and aldosterone levels suggest renal artery stenosis, malignant hypertension, or rarely a renin-secreting tumor. Low plasma renin activity and high aldosterone levels indicate primary aldosteronism. When both plasma renin activity and aldosterone levels are low, one should suspect the syndrome of apparent mineralocorticoid excess, Cushing's syndrome, or rarely Liddle syndrome. Cushing's syndrome caused by ectopic ACTH secretion is often not accompanied by typical cushingoid features.[143]

Treatment of Potassium Imbalance

In general the initial treatment of acute severe K imbalance is independent of the cause of the disturbance, whereas the rational therapy of chronic hyperkalemia or hypokalemia depends on an understanding of its pathogenesis.

Acute Hyperkalemia

In considering when hyperkalemia constitutes an emergency, two points should be kept in mind. First, the electrophysiologic effects of hyperkalemia are directly proportional to both the absolute P_K and its rate of rise.[128] Second, although the electrocardiographic manifestations of hyperkalemia are generally progressive and proportional to the P_K, ventricular fibrillation may be the first electrocardiographic disturbance of hyperkalemia[131]; conversely, a normal ECG may be seen with extreme hyperkalemia.[130] Thus it is apparent that neither the ECG nor the P_K alone is an adequate index of the urgency of hyperkalemia, and that the clinical context must be considered when assessing a hyperkalemic patient. Because most patients manifest hyperkalemic electrocardiographic changes at P_K greater than 6.7 mmol/L,[129] hyperkalemia should be treated emergently for (1) P_K greater than 6.5 mmol/L or (2) electrocardiographic manifestations of hyperkalemia regardless of the P_K.[144]

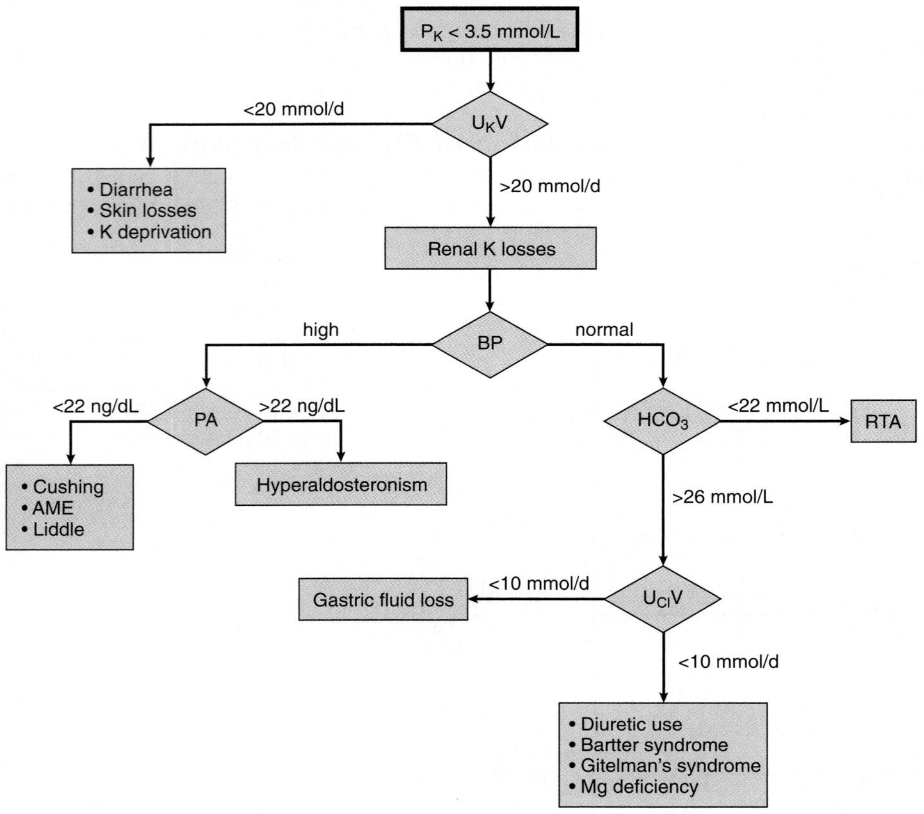

Figure 58-3. Diagnostic evaluation of chronic hypokalemia. AME, syndrome of apparent mineralocorticoid excess; BP, blood pressure; PA, stimulated plasma aldosterone (see text); RTA, renal tubular acidosis; $U_{Cl}V$, urinary chloride excretion; U_KV, urinary potassium excretion.

Therapy of acute or severe hyperkalemia is directed at preventing or ameliorating its untoward electrophysiologic effects on the myocardium. The goals of therapy, in chronologic order, are as follows (Table 58-5):

1. Antagonize the effect of K on excitable cell membranes
2. Redistribute extracellular K into cells
3. Enhance elimination of K from the body

Membrane Antagonism

Calcium

Ca directly antagonizes the myocardial effects of hyperkalemia without lowering P_K.[145] During treatment with Ca, the ECG should be monitored continuously. The dose may be repeated in 5 minutes if there is no improvement in the ECG or if the ECG deteriorates after an initial improvement.[144] Several cases of sudden death in patients given intravenous Ca while also receiving digitalis glycosides have been reported.[146] Although these observations do not provide clear guidance, it may be wise to administer intravenous Ca with caution to patients known or strongly suspected to have toxic levels of digitalis glycosides.

Hypertonic Saline

Intravenous hypertonic sodium chloride has been shown to reverse the electrocardiographic changes of hyperkalemia in patients with concurrent hyponatremia.[147] Whether hypertonic saline is effective in the treatment of eunatremic patients has not been established. Moreover, the extracellular volume load imposed by hypertonic saline argues against its use.

Redistribution of Potassium into Cells

Insulin Insulin reliably lowers P_K in a dose-dependent manner. An intravenous dose of 10 units of regular insulin given as a bolus along with an intravenous bolus of dextrose (25 to 40 g as a 50% solution) to adult patients lowers the P_K by about 1 mmol/L.[148,149] After the initial bolus, a dextrose infusion should be started because a single bolus of 25 g of dextrose has been shown to be inadequate to prevent hypoglycemia at 60 minutes.[148] Continuous insulin infusion apparently has no advantage over a bolus injection.[36] Insulin should be used without dextrose in hyperglycemic patients; indeed, the cause of the hyperkalemia in those patients may be the hyperglycemia itself.[45]

Albuterol P_K has been shown to decline by 0.6 mmol/L after inhalation of 10 mg of albuterol and by about 1 mmol/L after 20 mg in patients with end-stage renal disease.[150] The effect of insulin is additive with that of albuterol, with the combination reported to result in a decline in P_K by about 1.2 mmol/L at 60 minutes.[148] Even among patients not taking β-blockers, up to 40% appear to be resistant to the hypokalemic effect of albuterol.[148,150] For that reason, albuterol should never be used alone for the treatment of urgent hyperkalemia.

Bicarbonate The putative benefits of a bolus injection of sodium bicarbonate in the emergency treatment of hyperkalemia pervaded the literature until the past decade. Ironically, this dogma was based on studies using a prolonged (4 to 6 hours) infusion of bicarbonate.[40] It has now been clearly demonstrated that short-term bicarbonate infusion does not reduce P_K in patients with dialysis-dependent kidney failure, implying that it does not cause K shift into cells.[41,42]

Elimination of Potassium from the Body

Enhanced Renal Elimination Hyperkalemia occurs most often in patients with renal insufficiency. However, renal K excretion may be enhanced even in patients with moderate renal failure by increasing distal nephron flow. This

Table 58-5. Emergency Treatment of Hyperkalemia

Agent	Dose	Onset	Duration	Complications
Membrane Stabilization				
Calcium gluconate (10%)	10 mL IV over 10 min	Immediate	30-60 min	Hypercalcemia
Hypertonic (3%) sodium chloride	50 mL IV push	Immediate	Unknown	Volume overload Hypertonicity
Redistribution				
Insulin (short acting)	10 units IV push, with 25-40 g dextrose (50% solution)	20 min	4-6 hr	Hypoglycemia
Albuterol	20 mg in 4 mL normal saline solution, nebulized over 10 min	30 min	2 hr	Tachycardia Inconsistent response
Elimination				
Loop diuretics				
Furosemide	40-80 mg IV	15 min	2-3 hr	Volume depletion
Bumetanide	2-4 mg IV			
Sodium bicarbonate	150 mmol/L IV at variable rate	Hr	Duration of infusion	Metabolic alkalosis Volume overload
Sodium polystyrene sulfonate (SPS, Kayexalate, Kionex)	15-30 g in 15-30 mL (70% sorbitol orally)	>2 hr	4-6 hr	Variable effect Intestinal necrosis
Hemodialysis		Immediate	3 hr	Arrhythmias

may be accomplished with the *saline* or *sodium bicarbonate infusions* and may be enhanced further by the use of *loop diuretics*. Diuretic-induced volume contraction must be avoided because this will lead to decreased distal nephron flow and reduced K excretion.[144]

Exchange Resin Sodium polystyrene sulfonate (SPS, Kayexalate, Kionex) is a cation exchange resin that exchanges sodium for secreted K in the colon. Each gram of resin binds approximately 0.65 mmol of K in vivo, although the effect is highly variable and unpredictable.[36] The resin causes constipation and hence is almost always given with a cathartic. It is more effective when given orally than by retention enema.[36]

The use of SPS for the treatment of urgent hyperkalemia involves two concerns. The first is its slow effect. When given orally, the onset of action is at least 2 hours and the maximum effect may not be seen for 6 hours or more. One recent study in hemodialysis patients failed to show any effect on P_K after an oral dose of SPS.[151] The second concern with SPS is its possible toxicity. Numerous cases of patients who developed intestinal necrosis after exposure to SPS in sorbitol as an enema[152-154] and orally[155] have been reported. A retrospective study estimated the incidence of colonic necrosis to be 1.8% among postoperative patients.[155]

Dialysis Hemodialysis is the dialytic method of choice for removal of K from the body. P_K falls by over 1 mmol/L in the first 60 minutes of hemodialysis and a total of 2 mmol/L by 180 minutes, after which it reaches a plateau.[36] Rebound always occurs after dialysis, with 35% of the reduction abolished after an hour and nearly 70% after 6 hours.[36] Controversy surrounds whether dialysis for severe hyperkalemia precipitates serious ventricular arrhythmias. Because of this possibility, patients dialyzed for severe hyperkalemia should have continuous electrocardiographic monitoring.[36] The rate of K removal with *peritoneal dialysis* is much slower than with hemodialysis.[36]

Chronic Hyperkalemia

As established previously, chronic hyperkalemia always implies deficient renal K excretion. It follows that the therapy of chronic hyperkalemia is primarily directed toward stimulating renal K excretion while limiting K intake. For all adults with chronic hyperkalemia, daily K intake should be restricted to 60 mmol. All drugs known to impair either internal or external K balance should be eliminated if possible. Finally, all patients with chronic hyperkalemia should be evaluated for occult urinary tract obstruction.

Further therapy of the persistently hyperkalemic patient should be guided by the diagnostic evaluation outlined in Figure 58-2. In cases of mineralocorticoid unresponsiveness or when mineralocorticoid treatment is complicated by fluid overload, a *thiazide* or *loop diuretic* can be added to the regimen. This will restore normal volume status and enhance renal tubular K secretion in many mineralocorticoid-resistant patients. Avoiding diuretic-induced volume depletion is crucial, however, because this will exacerbate the renal K secretory defect.

Patients who fail to respond to the previously mentioned measures with an increase in TTKG and a decrease in P_K may be given sodium bicarbonate to stimulate renal K secretion. This is especially appropriate for patients whose chronic hyperkalemia is accompanied by a renal tubular acidosis (type IV RTA). The usual dose is 1 to 2 mmol bicarbonate per kg body weight per day in 3 or 4 divided doses.[144]

Acute Hypokalemia

A low P_K almost always indicates a large total body K deficit. In fact, P_K decreases by approximately 0.3 mmol/L for each decrement of 100 mmol total body K.[156] But if K is replenished too quickly, the homeostatic mechanisms that defend P_K will be overwhelmed and P_K will rise abruptly. The rate of rise of P_K with K administration can be greatly altered by factors that affect internal K balance. For example, during treatment of DKA with insulin, cellular uptake of K may be massive, obligating enormous replacement doses of K. Conversely, insulin deficiency markedly impairs tolerance to a K load.[56]

See "Evaluation of Acute Hypokalemia" earlier for definitions of urgent hypokalemia. Limited information exists on which to base a rational prescription of KCl in an emergency.[56,157,158]

On the basis of the available literature, we can estimate that nondiabetic patients with normal renal function should respond well to a 1- to 2-hour infusion of KCl at 0.6 mmol per kg per hour given IV in saline. In patients with renal failure of any degree, the infusion rate should be halved (0.3 mmol per kg per hour). Patients with diabetes mellitus not being treated for DKA or hyperglycemia should receive no more than 0.2 mmol per kg per hour, or about 0.1 mmol per kg per hour in the setting of renal failure. For severe hypokalemia, the ECG should be monitored continuously and the infusion stopped immediately if signs of hyperkalemia develop. The maximum increase in P_K is seen at the end of the infusion, and about 50% of the increase is lost over the next 2 to 3 hours when a new steady state is achieved. Thus P_K should be measured at the end of the infusion. If the patient is still dangerously hypokalemic at this point, additional K may be given. If at the end of the infusion P_K is in an acceptable range, the measurement should be repeated 2 to 3 hours later when disposal of K load is complete in order to determine the need for further treatment.[144]

Hypokalemia in the setting of aggressive "refeeding," especially in the treatment of severe DKA, should be treated initially as described earlier. Frequent monitoring of P_K with rapid laboratory turnaround time is critical for proper management.

Hypokalemia that is not life threatening is best treated with oral K replacement. Of importance is recognizing that GI absorption of an oral dose of KCl elixir is essentially complete. Dangerous hyperkalemia can occur in entirely normal individuals following KCl ingestion.[159] The maximum increase in P_K is seen 1.5 to 2 hours after an oral K load. Thus a sensible oral dose of KCl in moderate hypokalemia should probably not exceed the hourly

IV doses proposed earlier. No reason for giving a simultaneous oral and IV K dose exists; serious hyperkalemia may ensue.

Chronic Hypokalemia

Treatment of chronic hypokalemia depends entirely on identifying and, if possible, remediating the cause (see Fig. 58-3). When the cause of the excessive K loss cannot be treated specifically, maintenance K supplementation is necessary.

DISORDERS OF WATER HOMEOSTASIS

Hyponatremia and hypernatremia reflect disorders of water homeostasis. They are common disorders in critically ill patients and are associated with increased morbidity and mortality.[160,161]

Physiology of Water Homeostasis

Normal plasma sodium concentration varies little—even less than the "normal" range of clinical laboratories (135 to 145 mmol/L). This tight regulation depends on the following elements: (1) pituitary secretion of arginine vasopressin (AVP; also known as *antidiuretic hormone,* or ADH) that varies over a wide range in response to physiologic stimuli; (2) kidneys that are capable of responding to circulating vasopressin by varying the urine concentration; (3) intact thirst; and (4) access to water.

Tonicity or *effective osmolality* describes the capacity of particles in solution to effect water movement across a semipermeable membrane like the cell membrane. The normal response to water ingestion (of sufficient magnitude to lower the plasma osmolality even slightly) is the excretion of maximally dilute urine (urine osmolality <100 mOsm/kg). The underlying physiologic sequence is as follows: The plasma *hypotonicity* is sensed by the cells comprising the hypothalamic osmostat. These hypothalamic nuclei then proportionately reduce their synthesis of AVP, leading to diminished AVP release into the circulation by the posterior pituitary. The lower circulating AVP concentration, in turn, results in the insertion of proportionately fewer water channels into the collecting duct of the kidney. This, in turn, creates a more water-impermeable conduit, which allows excretion of the dilute urine elaborated by the more proximal segments of the nephron.[162]

Conversely, plasma hypertonicity leads to higher circulating AVP concentration and proportionately higher water permeability of the collecting duct, as well as the excretion of concentrated urine.[162]

Figure 58-4 shows the relationship among plasma osmolality, plasma AVP concentration, and urine osmolality. The normal "set point" is a plasma osmolality about 285 mOsm/kg. The minimum urine osmolality is about 50 mOsm/kg, and the maximum about 1200 mOsm/kg.[163]

When plasma osmolality rises beyond 290 to 295 mOsm/kg, the *thirst* center of the hypothalamus is stimulated. At that point, neurologically intact individuals with access to water will drink until the plasma osmolality returns to normal.[163]

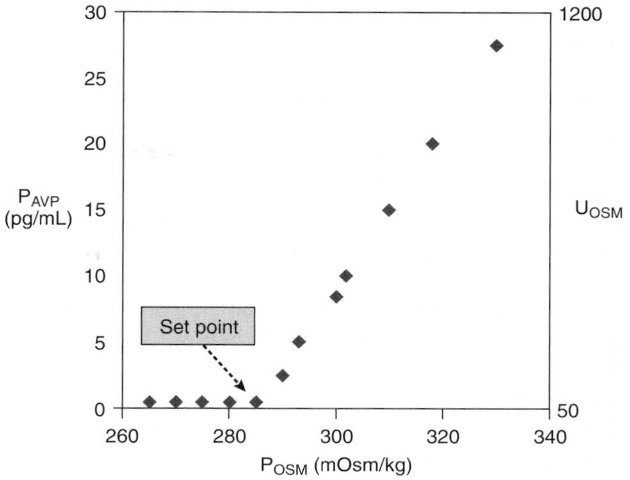

Figure 58-4. Typical example of the relationship between plasma osmolality (P_{osm}), plasma vasopressin concentration (P_{AVP}), and urine osmolality (U_{osm}). P_{AVP} and U_{osm} vary around the *set point* to maintain P_{osm} within the range of normal.

Nonosmotic Vasopressin Release

Importantly, plasma osmolality is not the only determinant of AVP synthesis and release. Low arterial blood pressure and low effective arterial volume powerfully stimulate AVP release.[163] This baroreceptor-mediated AVP release is teleological because water retention is an important component in the defense against hypovolemia. So primal is this circulatory defense that the baroreceptor stimulation predominates over any osmolal effect on AVP release.[163] Thus a volume-contracted or hypotensive individual will have high circulating AVP levels even if his or her plasma osmolality is low. In addition, circulating AVP levels rise with pain, stress, nausea, hypoxia, hypercapnia, and a variety of medications, most notably epinephrine and high doses of narcotic analgesics.[163]

Hyponatremia

Epidemiology and Clinical Manifestations

Hyponatremia (plasma sodium concentration <135 mmol/L) is one of the most common electrolyte disorders, found in approximately 3% of hospitalized patients and up to 30% of patients in ICUs.[160]

The clinical manifestations of hyponatremia are largely attributed to intracellular volume expansion (cellular edema), which occurs only when hyponatremia is associated with hypotonicity. Intracellular volume expansion is of greatest consequence in the brain, where it is translated into increased intracranial pressure because of the rigid calvarium.[164]

The pathophysiology of hypotonic hyponatremia has important implications for its management. Most cells—especially brain cells—have adaptive mechanisms for mitigating tonicity-related volume changes.[164] Cell volume peaks 1 to 2 hours after the onset of acute hypotonicity. Thereafter, solute and water are lost from cells and cell volume returns to normal. After several days of sustained hypotonicity, cell volume is restored nearly to normal.[164]

The morbidity and mortality associated with hypotonic hyponatremia are influenced by several factors including the magnitude and rate of development of the hyponatremia, the patient's age and gender, and the nature and severity of any underlying diseases.[164] The very young and very old, females, and alcoholics appear to be at particular risk.[165] Cell-volume adaptation to hypotonicity may be deficient in premenopausal women, who suffer more frequent and more severe neurologic consequences than men with equivalent degrees of hypotonicity.[166]

Neurologic symptoms usually do not occur until the plasma sodium concentration falls below 125 mmol/L, at which point the patient may complain of anorexia, nausea, and malaise. Between 120 and 110 mmol/L, headache, lethargy, confusion, agitation, and obtundation may be seen. More severe symptoms (seizures, coma) may occur with levels below 110 mmol/L.[167] Focal neurologic findings are unusual but do occur, and transtentorial cerebral herniation has been described in severe cases, especially in young women following surgery.[166] In that setting, hypoxemia is common and often associated with noncardiogenic pulmonary edema.[168] Hypoxia appears to exacerbate the cerebral damage in hyponatremia.[169]

Although symptoms generally resolve with correction of the hypotonicity, permanent neurologic deficits may occur, particularly in acute severe hypotonicity, when the brain's volume-regulatory defenses may be overwhelmed.[166] Profound hypotonicity that develops in less than 24 hours may be associated with residual neurologic deficits and has a 50% mortality rate in some populations.[166] In contrast, when hypotonicity develops more gradually, symptoms are both less common and less severe. Indeed, patients with chronic hyponatremia, even in the range of 115 to 120 mmol/L, may be completely asymptomatic.[164]

Pathophysiology and Differential Diagnosis

Hyponatremia may coexist with a normal, high, or low plasma osmolality. Thus the diagnostic algorithm for hyponatremia (see Fig. 58-2) begins with an assessment of the plasma osmolality (P_{osm}). This may be estimated by the following formula:

$$\text{est. } P_{osm} = (2 \times P_{Na^+}) + \frac{P_{gluc}}{18} + \frac{BUN}{2.8}$$

where P_{gluc} is the plasma glucose concentration and BUN is blood urea nitrogen concentration, both in mg/dL. If there is a suspicion that an unmeasured, osmotically effective solute may be implicated (e.g., mannitol, glycerol), the P_{osm} should be measured directly.

Isotonic hyponatremia (also known as *factitious* or *pseudohyponatremia*) is a laboratory artifact seen with analytic techniques that measure the mass of sodium per unit volume of plasma sampled.[170] It is seen in the presence of marked hypertriglyceridemia or paraproteinemia, when the measurement method involves a predilution step. Direct potentiometry (which uses an ion-selective electrode in undiluted plasma) avoids this problem.[170]

Hypertonic hyponatremia results from the presence in extracellular fluid of abnormal amounts of osmotically effective solutes other than sodium (e.g., glucose, mannitol, glycerol). The osmotic pressure exerted by the nonsodium solute leads to redistribution of water from the intracellular to the extracellular fluid compartment, resulting in cellular dehydration and hyponatremia. The hyponatremia is real (not pseudo-), but it is accompanied by hypertonicity and a decrease in cellular volume.

Hypotonic hyponatremia is almost always caused by an inability of the kidney to excrete sufficient electrolyte-free water to match water intake. This may occur either because the normal diluting capacity of the kidney is overwhelmed by excessive water intake or because the diluting capacity of the kidney is impaired. These alternatives can usually be distinguished by measuring the urine osmolality. A urine osmolality less than 100 mOsm/kg in a patient with hypotonic hyponatremia points to excessive water intake as the cause (Fig. 58-5). It is a prodigious feat for an individual eating a normal diet to overwhelm the normal diluting capacity of the kidney. Estimates are that one can ingest (and excrete) about 20 L of water a day without affecting the plasma osmolality appreciably.[163] Thus patients who develop hyponatremia from so-called *psychogenic* or *primary polydipsia*—usually patients with obsessive-compulsive disorder or psychosis—typically have concurrent urinary diluting defects, either in association with the underlying mental illness or perhaps as a side effect of psychotropic or anticonvulsant medications.[171]

Not all patients with hypotonic hyponatremia and a dilute urine have primary polydipsia. The patient may be ingesting a diet so deficient in protein and salt that he or she excretes very little solute in the urine. In that situation (called *beer potomania* for obvious reasons,[172] although the syndrome has been seen in other patients with very low daily solute intake[173]) the low daily solute excretion limits the total amount of water that can be eliminated even with a maximally dilute urine (i.e., maximum urine volume = solute excretion ÷ minimum U_{osm}). This might reduce the maximum water excretion to only 3 to 4 L/day, a quantity easily exceeded by an enthusiastic beer drinker.

A urine osmolality above 100 mOsm/kg in the face of hypotonic hyponatremia signifies impaired urinary diluting capacity. The concentrated urine usually reflects a high circulating AVP level. Because circulating AVP is affected by systemic hemodynamics and osmolality, assessment of the patient's extracellular fluid volume status and hemodynamics is crucial at this juncture. Hypotonic hyponatremia may be associated with normal, decreased, or increased extracellular volume.

Euvolemic Hyponatremia

Patients with pure water excess appear clinically euvolemic because excess water distributes throughout the total body water space; only one third of total body water is extracellular (and only one twelfth is intravascular). The only evidence of the slight intravascular volume expansion is low blood urea nitrogen and plasma uric acid concentration.[174] The paradigm of euvolemic hyponatremia with a concentrated urine is the syndrome of inappropriate antidiuretic hormone (SIADH), which is characterized

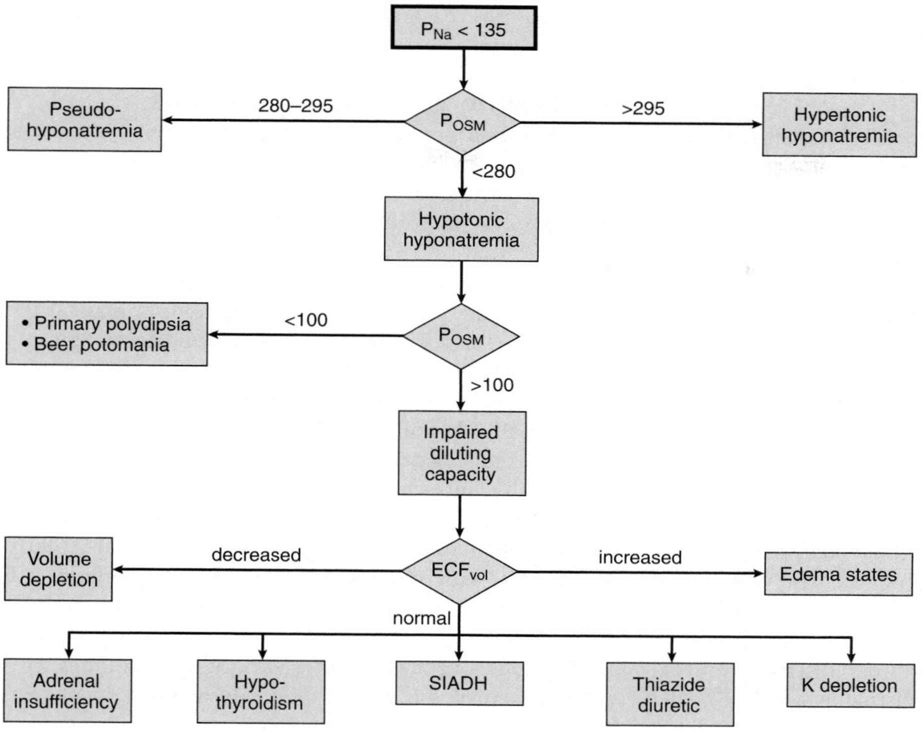

Figure 58-5. Diagnostic evaluation of hyponatremia. ECF_{vol}, extracellular fluid volume status; P_{Na}, plasma sodium concentration; P_{osm}, plasma osmolality (mOsm/kg); SIADH, syndrome of inappropriate antidiuretic hormone secretion.

by elevated circulating AVP (ADH) levels that are inappropriate to vasopressin's two physiologic stimuli (i.e., osmotic or hemodynamic).[175] Hypotonic hyponatremia in patients with SIADH develops to the extent that water ingestion exceeds water eliminated by insensible, GI, and renal routes. Because the normal response to extracellular hypotonicity is the elaboration of maximally dilute urine (urine osmolality <100 mOsm/kg), the urine need only be inappropriately concentrated (i.e., >100 mOsm/kg) to be compatible with a diagnosis of SIADH.

Because hypothyroidism[176] and glucocorticoid insufficiency[177] may impair urinary dilution, patients in whom a diagnosis of SIADH is entertained should undergo appropriate tests of thyroid and adrenocortical function (see Chapter 60).

Once a diagnosis of SIADH is made, its cause must be established because the cause may have important implications in its own right and may be easily remediable. Table 58-6 lists important causes of SIADH. They fall into five major categories: intracranial abnormalities, intrathoracic abnormalities, tumors, drugs, and idiopathic. An important variant of SIADH is the *reset osmostat syndrome,*[178] in which vasopressin levels are regulated normally by tonicity, but around a lower set point than normal. This syndrome is seen most often in patients who are severely debilitated (e.g., malnutrition, metastatic cancer, advanced tuberculosis) and may account for up to one third of cases of SIADH. The diagnosis of reset osmostat syndrome has important therapeutic implications and is discussed later.

Hypovolemic Hyponatremia

The urinary diluting impairment in hypovolemia is mediated both by decreased delivery of fluid to the diluting segments of the nephron and by hemodynamically stimu-

Table 58-6. Causes of SIADH

Intracranial Abnormalities
Infection
Stroke
Hemorrhage
Tumor
Intrathoracic Abnormalities
Malignancy
Pulmonary abscess
Pneumonia
Pleural effusion
Pneumothorax
Chest wall deformity
Drugs
Antidiuretic drugs (vasopressin, 1-deamino-8-D-arginine vasopressin [DDAVP], oxytocin)
Narcotic analgesics
Antidepressant medications
Amiodarone
Major antipsychotic medications
Chlorpropamide and other sulfonylurea drugs
Carbamazepine
Cyclophosphamide
Extracranial Tumors
Small-cell lung carcinoma
Pancreatic cancer
Others
HIV/AIDS
Hereditary
Gain-of-function mutation of vasopressin-2 receptor
Miscellaneous
Guillain-Barré syndrome
Nausea
Stress
Pain
Acute psychosis
Idiopathic

lated vasopressin release. Thus the volume-contracted patient cannot excrete electrolyte-free water normally, and even in the face of modest water ingestion readily may become hyponatremic.

The cause of the volume contraction is usually obvious (e.g., hemorrhage, vomiting, diarrhea, diuretics). When it is not, the urine sodium concentration can be helpful in distinguishing between renal and extrarenal solute losses. Renal losses (e.g., as a result of diuretic medications) are usually reflected by sodium wasting, and extrarenal losses are usually accompanied by sodium conservation (urine sodium concentration <10 mM). Exceptions occur in the recovery phase after diuretic therapy and in metabolic alkalosis because of vomiting. In the latter situation, the urine chloride concentration tends to be low and is the best indicator of extracellular volume depletion.[179,180]

Cerebral salt wasting may be responsible for hypovolemic hyponatremia in patients with intracranial pathology (e.g., tumors, hemorrhage). The pathogenesis of the urinary salt wasting is incompletely understood. The mechanism of hyponatremia in this setting is similar to that of other hypovolemic states. As a hyponatremic syndrome in patients with central nervous system disease, cerebral salt wasting is often difficult to distinguish from SIADH because urinary sodium excretion tends to be high. Particularly confusing in patients with cerebral salt wasting is the finding of hypouricemia, which is thought to reflect impaired solute reabsorption in the proximal tubule.[181] The key features that distinguish cerebral salt wasting from SIADH are volume depletion and urinary sodium excretion inappropriate to the patient's volume status.[181]

The hyponatremia associated with diuretic treatment is multifactorial in origin. Insofar as diuretics produce overt volume depletion, they can cause hyponatremia by the mechanisms discussed earlier. Thiazides have been associated with the development of acute, severe, symptomatic hyponatremia, particularly in small, elderly women, in the absence of overt signs of volume depletion.[182] The cause of this often precipitous syndrome remains uncertain.[183]

Hypervolemic Hyponatremia

Hypervolemic hyponatremia is generally seen in patients who cannot excrete sodium normally because they have either severe renal failure or one of the pathologic edema-forming states (e.g., congestive heart failure, hepatic cirrhosis, the nephrotic syndrome). Patients with advanced chronic kidney disease are predisposed to hyponatremia.[184] Acute oliguric renal failure or end-stage (dialysis-dependent) renal failure will be accompanied by hyponatremia to the extent that water intake exceeds insensible and GI water elimination (see Chapter 56).

Hyponatremia is common in the pathologic edema states, especially congestive heart failure and hepatic cirrhosis. The hormonal milieu of such patients is typical of intravascular volume depletion, even though the absolute intravascular volume is typically increased. Thus these disorders are said to be characterized by reduced effective circulating volume.[185] Because of the perceived intravascular volume depletion, renal diluting ability is compromised for reasons similar to those in hypovolemic hyponatremia.

Management and Complications

Hyponatremia per se requires treatment only when it is associated with hypotonicity. Hypertonic hyponatremia responds to the treatment of the underlying disorder, most commonly a hyperosmolar hyperglycemic state (see Chapter 59).

The therapy of hypotonic hyponatremia must be tailored to (1) the patient's signs and symptoms and (2) the duration of the disorder.[165] Severe hyponatremia (plasma sodium concentration <115 mmol/L) can be life threatening, especially if it develops rapidly.[167,186] The therapy of symptomatic hyponatremia, irrespective of cause, is directed at raising extracellular fluid tonicity to shift water out of the intracellular space, thereby ameliorating cerebral edema. The rate of correction, however, must be carefully regulated. Overly rapid correction, particularly in patients with chronic hyponatremia, in whom cell volume adaptations may be complete, can produce *osmotic demyelination syndrome*.[187,188] Osmotic demyelination syndrome is associated with a variety of sometimes irreversible neurologic deficits (e.g., dysarthria, dysphagia, behavioral disturbances, ataxia, quadriplegia, coma), which typically develop 3 to 10 days after treatment.[189] Additional risk factors for osmotic demyelination include hypokalemia, malnutrition, alcoholism, advanced age, and female sex.[190]

For patients with chronic hyponatremia (>48 hours' duration) or hyponatremia of unknown duration, the plasma sodium concentration should be raised by a maximum of 0.5 mmol/L/hour, 8 to 10 mmol/L in the first 24 hours,[188] and 20 mmol/L over the first 48 hours. Care should be taken to avoid *over*correcting the plasma sodium concentration.[177,189] In grave situations (plasma sodium concentration <105 mmol/L or in the presence of seizure or coma), initial therapy can be more aggressive (targeting a change in the plasma sodium concentration of 1 to 2 mmol/L/hour for the first few hours), but the recommended daily target should not be exceeded.[177,189]

Correction of severe symptomatic hypotonic hyponatremia, regardless of cause, should be accomplished with hypertonic (3%) saline (sodium concentration 513 mmol/L). The volume of 3% saline required can be estimated by the following formula:

$$3\%\text{ saline (L/24 hours)} = \text{target change } P_{Na}\text{ (mmol/L/24 hours)} \times \text{TBW (L)} \div 513$$

For example, in a 70-kg man with a plasma sodium concentration of 105 mmol/L and total body water of 42 L (60% of body weight), the amount of sodium needed to raise the plasma sodium concentration by 10 mmol/L is 10×42, or 420 mmol. Therefore 420÷513 or 0.82 L of 3% saline would be required in the first 24 hours, or 34 mL/hour. Importantly, the calculation provides only a rough guideline. The plasma sodium concentration must be monitored frequently during treatment to adjust the rate of correction. If the rate of correction begins to exceed the target rate, the hypertonic saline infusion should be stopped; rarely, it may be necessary to administer water (enterally or IV) or even desmopressin in order to prevent overly rapid correction.[191] Rapid extracellular volume expansion with hypertonic saline may precipitate pulmonary edema, particularly in patients with underlying heart disease. Thus patients receiving 3% saline should be assessed frequently for evidence of volume overload. One may administer a loop diuretic if necessary, recognizing that this will enhance electrolyte-free water clearance and accelerate the correction. Rarely, administration of isotonic (normal) saline to patients with SIADH paradoxically may *lower* the plasma sodium concentration if the urine osmolality remains high—a process that has been called *desalination.*[192]

The treatment of chronic asymptomatic hypotonicity should be directed at correcting the pathophysiologic mechanisms involved in generating the hypotonic state. Because euvolemic hyponatremia represents pure water excess, treatment depends on restricting water intake to less than the daily water output. Patients with SIADH excrete little or no electrolyte-free water in the urine. Therefore if water intake is limited to less than the amount of insensible water losses (≈10 mL/kg body weight/day), the plasma sodium concentration will slowly rise. Patients with the reset osmostat variant of SIADH characteristically do not develop progressive hypotonicity, and therapy is rarely required.

If the cause of SIADH cannot be corrected and if water restriction is poorly tolerated or ineffective, demeclocycline (a tetracycline antibiotic that increases electrolyte-free water excretion by inhibiting vasopressin-mediated water reabsorption in the collecting duct) can be used. Demeclocycline is contraindicated in patients with renal disease, hepatic cirrhosis, or congestive heart failure because drug-related renal insufficiency has been described in these situations.[193] Conivaptan is the first specific vasopressin (V_2) receptor antagonist (VRA) to be approved by the U.S. Food and Drug Administration for clinical use. Other VRAs are nearing approval. These agents will radically change the management of patients with SIADH in the future.[194]

Therapy of hypovolemic hyponatremia should be directed at restoring intravascular volume with intravenous isotonic saline while identifying and correcting the cause of the excessive solute loss. Volume repletion readily elicits a water diuresis by increasing the delivery of fluid to the renal diluting segments and suppressing vasopressin release. As with all categories of hypotonic hyponatremia, the rate of correction must be carefully controlled.

The treatment of diuretic-induced hyponatremia is straightforward: withdrawing the offending drug, liberalizing salt intake, and replenishing body K stores usually correct the disorder. Severe symptomatic hyponatremia in this setting should be treated with hypertonic saline as detailed earlier. Patients must be watched carefully after correction of the hyponatremia because relapse may occur for up to a week.[183]

Resolution of the hyponatremia associated with any of the pathologic edematous disorders ultimately depends on effective treatment of the underlying disease. Regardless of the specific therapy of the underlying disorder, the mainstay of therapy for the hyponatremic edematous patient remains salt and water restriction. Diuretics are often a double-edged sword in the hyponatremic edematous patient: they may be necessary to treat pulmonary vascular congestion, peripheral edema, and ascites, but if used to excess can produce further decrements in effective arterial blood volume and exacerbate water retention. Strategies directed at increasing effective arterial blood volume (e.g., afterload reduction with angiotensin-converting enzyme inhibitors[195,196]) have had some success in increasing electrolyte-free water excretion and ameliorating hyponatremia in patients with congestive heart failure. VRAs are likely to facilitate treatment of hypervolemic hyponatremia (see earlier).[194]

Hypernatremia

Epidemiology and Clinical Manifestations

Hypernatremia is common in critically ill patients, being present on admission in about 9% of patients, and developing during the course of the ICU stay in another 6%.[197] It is associated with a significantly higher mortality than is seen in patients without hypernatremia.[197]

Sustained hypernatremia develops in patients whose water output exceeds their input. Water ingestion can defend against the development of hypernatremia even when water losses are prodigious. For that reason, hypernatremia on presentation to the hospital occurs most commonly in patients who are incapacitated: those who have impaired thirst sensation, who cannot access water or who cannot express their need for water (e.g., infants and patients with neurologic impairments). Similar predispositions prevail among critically ill patients. Thus the development of hypernatremia in hospitalized patients is considered to be iatrogenic, reflecting an incomplete understanding of the factors that lead to hypernatremia.[197] The increased mortality seen in patients with hypernatremia is probably caused by their underlying vulnerabilities rather than an effect of the hypernatremia itself.[198]

The clinical manifestations of hypernatremia are proportional to the magnitude and rate of rise of the plasma sodium concentration and are attributable to intracellular volume contraction. To counteract cellular volume contraction, cells begin to adapt within minutes by allowing the influx of electrolytes, thus mitigating cell shrinkage. When hypernatremia lasts more than a few hours, brain cells generate new *organic osmolytes.* This leads to further water movement back into brain cells, restoring cell volume nearly to normal after about 3 days.[199] Thus chronic progressive hypernatremia is associated with fewer and milder symptoms than acute severe hypernatremia. Most often, patients with longstanding hypernatremia present with weakness, lethargy, and confusion. Seizure and coma may supervene. Acute severe hypernatremia in infants and small children is associated with intracranial bleeding,[200] presumably caused by brain shrinkage and traction on the penetrating vessels. However,

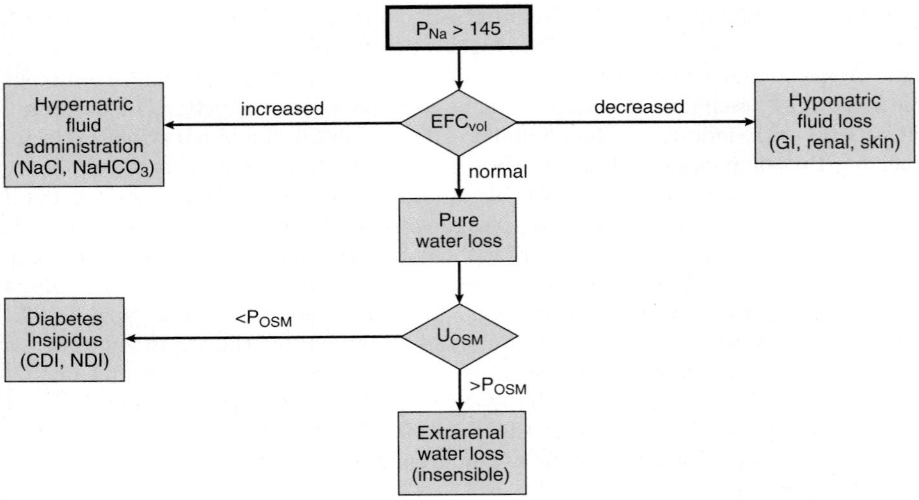

Figure 58-6. Diagnostic evaluation of hypernatremia. See Figure 58-3 legend for abbreviations. CDI, central diabetes insipidus; GI, gastrointestinal; NDI, nephrogenic diabetes insipidus.

some controversy surrounds whether the hypernatremia in that situation is the cause or the effect of the intracranial hemorrhage.[201]

Differential Diagnosis

The plasma sodium concentration reflects the ratio of body sodium content to total body water. Thus hypernatremia (plasma sodium concentration >145 mmol/L) can result from loss of pure water alone, loss of *hyponatric* fluid,* or a gain of sodium or *hypernatric* fluid. Distinguishing among these paths to hypernatremia is important because they have diagnostic and therapeutic implications (Fig. 58-6).

Euvolemic Hypernatremia

Hypernatremic patients who appear euvolemic most likely have pure water loss as an explanation for their hypernatremia. This is because the water is lost from all body compartments proportionately; only $\frac{1}{12}$ of the water loss is intravascular. For example, a 60-kg woman with a 3L pure water loss would experience an intravascular loss of only 250 mL (clinically imperceptible) but would develop a plasma sodium concentration of 155 mmol/L.† Pure water can be lost either through the skin and respiratory tract (so-called *insensible* losses) or in urine.

Insensible losses amount to about 10 mL per kg body weight per day under normal environmental conditions in an afebrile individual with a normal respiratory rate. A hot environment, fever, or rapid respiratory rate may double that rate.[163] Of note is that a patient on a mechanical ventilator using humidified gas will lose no water through the respiratory tract.

The loss of large amounts of dilute, electrolyte-free water in the urine is typical of *diabetes insipidus* (DI). DI may be central (CDI) or nephrogenic (NDI) depending on whether the defect is in vasopressin release from the posterior pituitary or in the renal response to circulating vasopressin, respectively. The causes of DI are shown in Box 58-5. Most cases of CDI, especially those following trauma or intracranial surgery, are self-limited, lasting 3 to 5 days. Of special interest to intensivists is a classic triphasic syndrome that may be seen following severe head trauma:

1. Initially, there is abrupt cessation of vasopressin release from the posterior pituitary, accompanied by polyuria.
2. About a week later, an antidiuretic phase ensues, characterized by urinary concentration and water retention with a tendency toward hyponatremia, lasting 5 to 6 days. This appears to result from the release of stored vasopressin from the degenerating hypothalamic neurons.
3. Persistent CDI recurs when the vasopressin stores are depleted.[202]

Regardless of the cause, patients with DI of either type usually have a plasma sodium concentration within the normal range because their water ingestion matches their urinary water output. They develop hypernatremia only with water deprivation because of mental or physical incapacity or neglect. An awareness of the causes of DI, a careful history, and familiarity with the differential diagnosis of polyuria will prevent hypernatremia in these circumstances.

Hypovolemic Hypernatremia

The loss of salt and water, with the water loss greater than the sodium loss, will lead to hypernatremia and volume depletion, manifested by orthostatic or persistent hypotension and tachycardia, as well as evidence of organ underperfusion (e.g., acute renal failure, lactic acidosis). For example, if the 60-kg woman whose plasma sodium concentration rose to 155 mmol/L (see earlier) had lost the equivalent of half-isotonic saline instead of pure water, her intravascular volume would have contracted by 750 mL, enough to cause at least orthostatic hypotension and tachycardia.

*Hyponatric and hypernatric are used here to refer to a fluid with a sodium concentration less than (or greater than) that of plasma.

†The expected change in serum sodium concentration is calculated as follows: [initial total body water volume] × [serum sodium concentration initial] ÷ [final total body water volume]; 30 L × 140 mmol/L ÷ 27 L = 155 mmol/L.

Box 58-5

Causes of Diabetes Insipidus

Central Diabetes Insipidus
- Posthypophysectomy
- Posttraumatic
- Granulomatous diseases
  - Histiocytosis
  - Sarcoidosis
- Infections
  - Meningitis
  - Encephalitis
- Inflammatory/autoimmune hypophysitis
- Vascular
  - Hypoxia
  - Thrombotic or embolic stroke
  - Hemorrhagic stroke
- Neoplastic
  - Craniopharyngioma
  - Pituitary adenoma
  - Lymphoma
  - Meningioma
- Drugs or toxin
  - Ethanol
  - Snake venom
- Congenital/hereditary

Nephrogenic Diabetes Insipidus
- Drug induced
  - Lithium
  - Demeclocycline
  - Cisplatin
  - Ethanol
- Hypokalemia
- Hypercalcemia
- Vascular
  - Sickle cell anemia
- Infiltrating lesions
  - Sarcoidosis
  - Multiple myeloma
  - Amyloidosis
  - Sjögren's syndrome
- Congenital's
  - Autosomal recessive: aquaporin-2 water channel gene mutations
  - X-linked recessive: AVP v_2 receptor gene mutations

A common cause of hypovolemic hypernatremia is the loss of GI fluids. Most GI fluids have an electrolyte concentration below that of plasma: The concentration of sodium plus K in stool is roughly constant at 110 to 120 mmol/L over a wide range of stool volume.[118] Gastric fluid has an even lower electrolyte concentration—approximately 40 to 50 mmol/L total cation concentration.[203] Diuresis, either osmotic (glucose, mannitol, or urea induced) or medication induced, causes the loss of urine with an electrolyte concentration less than that of plasma, leading to volume contraction and hypernatremia. The loss of sweat, which contains some sodium, can cause hypovolemic hypernatremia in individuals who exercise vigorously in a hot environment. If the cause of the fluid loss is not apparent from the history or physical examination, a urinary chloride concentration less than 10 mmol/L in the face of hypovolemic hypernatremia suggests that the electrolyte loss is extrarenal (cutaneous or GI).

Hypervolemic Hypernatremia

Hypervolemic hypernatremia is relatively uncommon and results from the administration of hypertonic sodium salts to patients without free access to water. Patients show signs of extracellular volume expansion (e.g., hypertension, edema, congestive heart failure, pulmonary edema). In infants, this syndrome has been caused by erroneous preparation of dietary formula using salt instead of sugar; in adult outpatients, it may be caused by ingestion of a concentrated salt solution, usually for its emetic effect.[204] The risk of death is substantial and seems to be proportional to the plasma sodium concentration.[204]

In hospitalized adults, hypervolemic hypernatremia is most often iatrogenic, caused by intravenous administration of undiluted sodium bicarbonate (formulated at 1 mEq/mL or 1000 mmol/L) or sodium chloride (3% [513 mmol/L] or 23.5% [4019 mmol/L]). Not all hypervolemic hypernatremia results from the administration of hypertonic fluids. It may be seen in a volume-expanded patient who then loses hypotonic fluid.[205]

Treatment The initial treatment of the hypernatremic patient depends on his or her volume status. For patients with pure water losses (euvolemic), therapy has two goals: (1) reduction or replacement of ongoing water losses, or both, and (2) replacement of the existing water deficit.

If the water losses are urinary (see Fig. 58-6) and caused by central diabetes insipidus, antidiuretic hormone should be administered. Several formulations are available (Table 58-7). In the acute (postsurgical or posttraumatic) setting, L-arginine vasopressin may be used either subcutaneously or intravenously, although the latter route may be associated with hypertension and coronary spasm and should therefore be used with extreme caution.[206] The advantage of vasopressin in this setting is its short half-life, which allows the physician to repeatedly assess the need for continued hormone replacement, especially when the disorder may be self-limited. Desmopressin (DDAVP) is a synthetic analogue of vasopressin that has no vasoconstrictor properties, thus avoiding the risks of hypertension and myocardial ischemia. The treatment of the urinary water losses associated with nephrogenic diabetes insipidus are best treated with thiazide diuretics with or without cyclooxygenase (COX) inhibitors. Because most of these agents are orally administered, treatment of NDI in the critically ill patient often consists of urinary water replacement until he or she is able to take medications by mouth.

The current body water deficit can be estimated by the following formula:

$$\text{Water deficit (liters)} = \text{TBW}(1 - [140 \div \text{current } P_{Na}])$$

Table 58-7. Pharmacologic Treatment of Central Diabetes Insipidus

Agent	Total Daily Dose	Frequency of Administration	Onset of Action (hr)	Duration of Action (hr)	Comments
Arginine vasopressin, 20 units/mL	5-10 units subcutaneously	Q2-Q4 hr	1-2	2-6	IV route may cause vasoconstriction and coronary spasm
Desmopressin acetate (DDAVP)	10-40 μg intranasal	Daily or bid	1-2	8-12	
10 μg/0.1 mL intranasal 4 μg/mL injection	2-4 μg IV or subcutaneously	Daily or bid	1-2	8-12	

Adapted from Singer I, Oster JR, Fishman LM: The management of diabetes insipidus in adults. Arch Intern Med 1997;157:1293-1301.

where TBW is total body water in liters (estimated as about 0.5×lean body weight [kg] in women and 0.6×lean body weight in men). For example, a 60-kg woman presenting with a plasma sodium concentration of 160 mmol/L is estimated to have a total body water deficit of 30 (1−0.875) or 3.75 L. This formula provides only a rough estimate of the water deficit.

The rate of water replacement should be proportional to the rapidity with which the hypernatremia developed.[199] Thus if the hypernatremia had developed over only a few hours (such as in postsurgical or posttraumatic DI), it can be corrected just as quickly. On the other hand, hypernatremia of more than a day's duration, or of unknown duration, must be corrected slowly in order to avoid cerebral edema. In general, one should aim to correct half the water deficit in the first 24 hours and the remainder over the next 24 to 48 hours.

Water is best administered enterally, as tap water. If that route is unavailable, 5% dextrose in water (D5W) may be used, with the understanding that the capacity to metabolize glucose is limited to about 15 g/hour in a critically ill adult.[207] Thus even in nondiabetic patients the administration of more than 300 mL/hour of D5W is likely to result in hyperglycemia, which may be relatively resistant to insulin administration. Hyperglycemia will exacerbate urinary water losses by causing an osmotic diuresis. Half-normal (0.45%) saline may be a good alternative, as long as one recognizes that only half the administered volume is electrolyte-free water and that the sodium load may cause unwanted volume expansion.

Regardless of the degree of hypernatremia, normal (0.9%) saline should be given intravenously to patients who present with obvious volume depletion, manifested by hypotension, tachycardia, and evidence of impaired tissue perfusion. This is consistent with the first principles of emergency and critical care, prioritizing the adequacy of the circulation. Only after the extracellular volume deficits have been largely corrected may the physician direct his or her attention to the total body water deficit (see earlier).

Patients with hypervolemic hypernatremia need reduction in their extracellular and intravascular volume before their water deficit can be corrected. Failure to do so will exacerbate the volume overload. For patients with adequate renal function, this may be accomplished with the use of diuretic drugs. Loop diuretics tend to cause the excretion of an isotonic urine. Replacement of that urine volume with pure water will allow correction of the hypervolemia and the hypernatremia simultaneously.

Because of the imprecision of the estimation formulas and the failure of the foregoing analysis to take account of other fluids and electrolytes both administered and lost, it is crucial that the plasma electrolytes be monitored frequently during the correction of hypernatremia, especially in view of the dire consequences of overly rapid correction.

CALCIUM

Ca is required for bone mineralization, muscle contraction, nerve conduction, and blood coagulation. It is required for cell division, hormone secretion, phagocytosis, chemotaxis, and activation of numerous intracellular second-messengers.[208] Ca is also responsible for activation of Ca-dependent phospholipases and proteases, generation of free radicals, cytokine release, and inhibition of ATP production in the face of ischemic injury. Thus Ca plays a central role in physiologic, as well as pathologic, conditions.[209]

Normal Calcium Physiology

Ca is the most abundant cation in the body. The total body Ca content of an average adult is approximately 1 kg, 99% of which is found in bones and teeth, with only 1% in plasma and soft tissues.[210] Ca homeostasis is achieved with the cooperation of several organs including the skeleton, gut, and kidney, under the influence of several hormones, mainly vitamin D, parathyroid hormone (PTH), and calcitonin.

Calcium Intake and Absorption

The daily dietary intake of Ca for an average adult in North America is 800 to 1000 mg. The main dietary source of Ca is milk and other dairy products; it is also available in the form of fortified food and Ca-containing supplements. Approximately 20% of dietary Ca is absorbed by the intestines. Intestinal absorptive capacity increases with Ca deprivation and under certain physiologic conditions like growth spurts in children, pregnancy, and lactation.[211] Intestinal absorption occurs via both passive paracellular and active transcellular pathways. Vitamin D increases the active transport of Ca across the intestinal membranes.[210]

Renal Handling of Calcium

The filtered load of Ca (the product of glomerular filtration rate and the plasma concentration of ultrafilterable Ca) is about 10 g per day. Ca balance is maintained when the kidneys excrete about 200 mg/day (the intestinal absorptive load). Thus the fractional excretion of Ca is only about 2%.[210,211] Of the 98% of filtered Ca reabsorbed along the nephron, 60% is reabsorbed in the proximal tubule. Approximately 15% of the filtered Ca is reabsorbed in the thick ascending limb of the loop of Henle (TAL). The reabsorption of Ca in TAL is mostly passive and proportional to the lumen-positive voltage generated by the furosemide-inhibitable NaKCC2 transporter and K recycling via ROMK channels. There is also some active transcellular transport, which is under the influence of PTH and calcitonin.[210,211] In the distal tubule, approximately 10% to 15% of filtered Ca is reabsorbed via active transcellular pathways. The apical membranes of distal convoluted tubules (DCT) and connecting tubules (CNT) contain highly selective epithelial Ca channels (ECaC-1),[210,211] which assists Ca entry into the cells. PTH increases the density and open probability of ECaC-1.[210]

Volume expansion, hypercalcemia, acute and chronic acidosis, and loop diuretics reduce the renal Ca reabsorption and result in hypercalciuria. Conversely, hypocalcemia, alkalosis, PTH, calcitriol, and thiazide diuretics enhance renal Ca reabsorption and cause hypocalciuria.

Regulation of Plasma Calcium

Normal plasma Ca concentration is 8.8 to 10.4 mg/dL. In plasma, Ca exists in two forms: protein-bound and *ultrafilterable* (permeant across the glomerular filtration barrier). Approximately 40% of plasma Ca is bound to plasma proteins (predominantly albumin), cannot cross the biological membranes, and is thus physiologically inert. The ultrafilterable portion of plasma Ca makes up the remaining 60% of plasma Ca and consists of Ca complexed with various anions like citrate, phosphate, and lactate (about 10%) and free, ionized Ca (Ca^{2+})—the biologically active form, accounting for about 50% of plasma Ca.[212]

Plasma ionized Ca concentration is tightly regulated. Several factors play an important role in maintaining plasma Ca^{2+} concentration within a narrow range (about 4.4 to 5.2 mg/dL or 1.1 to 1.3 mmol/L). The principal regulators are PTH, vitamin D_3, and Ca^{2+} itself.

Ca^{2+} acts as a ligand for Ca-sensing receptors (CaSRs) present on the chief cells of the parathyroid glands. A rise in plasma Ca^{2+} concentration results in activation of CaSR, which, in turn, inhibits PTH secretion. Conversely, a fall in Ca^{2+} concentration inhibits CaSR, increasing PTH secretion. PTH mobilizes the Ca from bone stores, stimulates renal Ca reabsorption, and increases the conversion of $25(OH)D_3$ to $1,25(OH)_2D_3$, the most active form of vitamin D_3. Activated vitamin D_3 increases intestinal Ca absorption. All of these systems work in concert to keep the Ca^{2+} levels within physiologic levels.[208]

Plasma Calcium Measurement

Ionized Ca is the physiologically important moiety, yet total Ca is most often measured in clinical laboratories. Under normal circumstances, there is a fairly constant relationship between total and ionized Ca (see earlier), but in critically ill patients this relationship may be disturbed such that total Ca no longer provides a reliable index of the physiologically important Ca concentration. The two major factors affecting the ratio of ionized to total Ca are acid-base status and plasma protein concentration.

Acidemia causes displacement of Ca ions from albumin by protons and results in a relative increase in ionized Ca. Conversely, alkalemia increases Ca binding to albumin, causing a relative fall in ionized Ca levels, whereas total plasma Ca concentration remains unchanged.[208,210]

Changes in the concentration of plasma protein, especially albumin, result in alterations in total Ca concentration: hypoalbuminemia, common in critically ill patients, causes a reduction in total Ca concentration; hyperalbuminemia (e.g., in states of severe volume contraction) tends to cause an increase in total plasma Ca. Numerous formulas have been proposed to adjust the total Ca concentration for changes in plasma albumin concentration.[213] The most commonly used formula is based on the observation that each gram of albumin binds about 0.8 mg Ca at physiologic pH.

Unfortunately, the corrected Ca correlates poorly with Ca^{2+} in various critically ill populations, typically with a low sensitivity for diagnosis of true hypocalcemia.[213-215]

The reasons for this discrepancy include concurrent acid-base disorders; high circulating concentrations of free fatty acids[216]; and infusions of heparin, citrate, and bicarbonate.[215] Therefore in critically ill patients, direct measurement of ionized Ca is recommended for assessing physiologic Ca concentration.

HYPOCALCEMIA

Epidemiology

Hypocalcemia is extremely common in critically ill patients. The prevalence of ionized hypocalcemia is reported to be 60% to 85% among medical, surgical, and trauma ICU patients.[217-220] Risk factors for the development of hypocalcemia in critically ill patients include advanced age, sepsis, acute renal failure, multiple blood transfusion, malnutrition, Mg deficiency, severe shock, and colloid volume resuscitation.[220,221] Mortality is higher in hypocalcemic patients[218,222,223] but does not appear to be independently associated with hypocalcemia.[219,220]

Causes of Hypocalcemia

Causes of hypocalcemia are shown in Box 58-6. Hypocalcemia may be caused by disorders involving the hormonal regulators of Ca homeostasis, PTH and vitamin D; redistribution of Ca; drugs; and miscellaneous influences. Here we discuss causes of particular relevance to the critical care setting.

Box 58-6

Causes of Hypocalcemia

Hypoparathyroidism
- Acquired
  - Parathyroidectomy
  - Infiltrative or malignant disease
- Congenital
- Idiopathic

Vitamin D Deficiency
- Malnutrition
- Malabsorption
- Liver disease
- Kidney disease

Redistribution
- Tissue sequestration
  - Acute pancreatitis
  - Rhabdomyolysis
- Complexation
  - Alkali
    - Citrated blood-product transfusions
    - Citrate anticoagulation in continuous renal replacement therapy
    - Plasmapheresis
    - Bicarbonate infusion for metabolic acidosis
  - Phosphate
    - Tumor lysis syndrome
    - Fleet enemas and phosphate-containing laxatives
    - Rhabdomyolysis
- Ethylenediamine tetra-acetic acid

Drugs
- Cis-platinum
- Bisphosphonates
- Plicamycin

Miscellaneous
- Sepsis/Systemic inflammatory response syndrome
- Hypomagnesemia
- Acute renal failure

Hypoparathyroidism

Parathyroidectomy, for hyperparathyroidism or "incidentally" with thyroidectomy, may cause postoperative hypocalcemia. Risk factors for developing hypocalcemia include subtotal parathyroidectomy and simultaneous thyroidectomy. Profound, long-lasting hypocalcemia may develop, as part of the "hungry bone" syndrome, in which Ca is sequestered into the rapidly remineralizing bone.[224] Hypomagnesemia may contribute to the hypocalcemia (see "Disorders of Magnesium Homeostasis" later).

Vitamin D Deficiency

Vitamin D deficiency is common in elderly, institutionalized patients because of poor dietary intake and inadequate sunlight exposure. Diseases involving liver and small intestine may result in poor absorption of vitamin D. In order to be converted into its most active form, vitamin D requires hydroxylation in liver and kidney. Frequently, critically ill patients suffer from liver and kidney dysfunction, which results in impaired vitamin D synthesis and predisposes the patients to hypocalcemia.[209]

Redistribution

Citrate is useful as a preservative and anticoagulant for blood components precisely because it chelates Ca and thereby inhibits the coagulation cascade. The Ca citrate complex is then metabolized in liver, where citrate is converted into bicarbonate, and ionized Ca is released into the circulation. Massive blood transfusion may result in ionized hypocalcemia because of chelation of Ca by citrate. However, hypocalcemia is transient in patients with normal liver function, and ionized Ca levels return to normal levels within 15 minutes of transfusion.[225] Citrate may also be used for anticoagulation of the dialysis circuit for continuous renal replacement therapy (CVVH and variants).

Under those conditions, Ca is typically infused through a central venous line to prevent hypocalcemia. Inadequate Ca replacement or concomitant liver failure may result in clinically significant hypocalcemia. In the latter case, with citrate accumulation, the total Ca may be misleadingly normal, but the ionized Ca is low.[226,227] Hypocalcemia is frequently reported with plasmapheresis where citrate is used for anticoagulation.[228] Sodium *bicarbonate* to treat metabolic acidosis may cause hypocalcemia from Ca binding to albumin and formation of carbonate complexes. Similarly, abrupt alkalinization from hemodialysis against a bicarbonate bath may precipitate symptomatic hypocalcemia.

Phosphate binds with Ca to form insoluble Ca phosphate complexes. Under normal physiologic conditions, Ca and phosphorus levels are tightly regulated, preventing significant complexation. Any condition that causes acute increase in phosphate levels, however, can cause complexation and resultant ionized hypocalcemia. Examples include endogenous phosphorus overload, as in the tumor lysis syndrome,[66] and exogenous phosphorus overload from laxatives and cathartics.[229-232] Patients with impaired renal function are at particular risk[230] (see "Phosphorus" later).

Hypocalcemia in *rhabdomyolysis* is multifactorial and involves Ca deposition in injured muscles, formation of Ca-phosphate complex because of hyperphosphatemia, and acute renal failure causing decreased synthesis of vitamin D.[233]

Ionized hypocalcemia is reported in up to 85% of patients suffering from acute severe *pancreatitis*.[234] The cause of hypocalcemia in this setting is unclear. Ca has been shown to accumulate in pancreas, liver, and skeletal muscle in an animal model of acute pancreatitis.[235] Low[236] and high[237,238] levels of PTH have been reported. Experimental elevation in free fatty acids, both circulating[239] (as might be seen in the hypertriglyceridemia of acute pancreatitis) and intraperitoneal,[240] have been associated with the hypocalcemia of acute pancreatitis. Finally, high circulating endotoxin levels may have a role.[234]

Drugs

Bisphosphonates are used for the treatment of osteoporosis and hypercalcemia. They act by impairing osteoclast function and reducing osteoclast numbers. Bisphosphonate-induced hypocalcemia has been reported in patients with renal failure, hypoparathyroidism, or vitamin D deficiency.[241] Other drugs such as colchicine, plicamycin (formerly mithramycin), and calcitonin also decrease bone release of Ca.[210]

Sepsis/Systemic Inflammatory Response Syndrome

Hypocalcemia is common in patients suffering from sepsis or systemic inflammatory response syndrome.[218,222] The cause is probably multifactorial.[242] Among the proposed mechanisms are Ca sequestration,[243,244] an effect of inflammatory cytokines,[245] calcitonin precursors,[245,246] hypomagnesemia[247] with inappropriate hypoparathyroidism,[242] and probable PTH resistance.[245,248] Vitamin D deficiency, from malnutrition and inability to hydroxylate vitamin D because of coexisting liver and kidney dysfunction, also has been implicated.[242] The hypocalcemia may serve to protect vulnerable cells from the deleterious effects of Ca during sepsis. Indeed, Ca administration in this setting may be detrimental.[242]

Clinical Manifestations

Hypocalcemia affects predominantly the neuromuscular and cardiovascular systems. Neuromuscular manifestations include paresthesias (perioral and acral), hyperactive reflexes, tetany (carpopedal spasm and other muscle spasm), and seizures.[210] Laryngospasm and bronchospasm may supervene, leading to respiratory arrest.[208] Tetany may be provoked by tapping over the facial nerve and noting ipsilateral facial muscle twitching (Chvostek sign), as well as transiently occluding the brachial artery with a tourniquet and noting carpal spasm (Trousseau sign), although neither of these signs is specific for hypocalcemia. Psychiatric manifestations include anxiety, irritability, confusion, and psychosis.[208]

Cardiovascular findings include a prolonged QT interval and, in severe hypocalcemia, bradycardia, hypotension refractory to fluids and pressors, heart block, heart failure, and cardiac arrest.[209]

Symptoms and signs of hypocalcemia depend on the degree of depression of ionized Ca levels and the rate of decline.[210] Mild hypocalcemia (ionized Ca$>$3.2 mg/dL) is usually well tolerated.

Diagnosis

When hypocalcemia is suspected in a critically ill patient, the diagnosis should be established by direct measurement of ionized Ca levels (see "Plasma Calcium Measurement" earlier). If ionized hypocalcemia is confirmed, plasma Mg and phosphorus should be measured. Further diagnostic evaluation derives from the differential diagnosis (see Box 58-6). Without PTH levels and vitamin D levels, the diagnosis of hypocalcemia remains obscure in the majority of critically ill patients.[218]

Treatment

Therapy of hypocalcemia depends on its severity. Hypocalcemia (ionized Ca$<$3.2 mg/dL) accompanied by serious cardiovascular or neuromuscular signs should be treated urgently. Ca gluconate (10% in 10 mL containing 90 mg elemental Ca) can be given over 5-10 minutes, followed by Ca gluconate infusion (500 to 1000 mg in 500 mL 5% dextrose over 6 hours.[210] Ca chloride (10% in 10 mL containing 272 mg elemental Ca) contains more Ca and can rapidly increase plasma Ca levels, but it is more irritating to the veins and must be given by a central venous catheter. Patients with renal failure, hyperphosphatemia, and serious hypocalcemia may require dialysis.

Patients receiving intravenous Ca should have frequent measurement of the ionized Ca. They should be monitored for side effects of Ca administration including hypertension, skin flushing, nausea, vomiting, and chest pain.

Intravenous Ca should be reserved for patients who have severe hypocalcemia or who are incapable of taking Ca orally. Administration of intravenous Ca can cause complexing with phosphorus and ectopic calcification.

Critically ill patients with mild hypocalcemia (iCa$>$3.2 mg/dL) tend to have few, if any, manifestations. Patients with longstanding or chronic hypocalcemia (e.g., because of vitamin D deficiency or hypoparathyroidism) should receive oral Ca supplementation. Ca is available as the carbonate, citrate, phosphate, and lactate salt. Ca requirement varies between 1 and 4 g elemental Ca daily and must be given in divided doses. Vitamin D can be added with Ca to enhance intestinal absorption.

Several points in the management of hypocalcemia should be borne in mind. First, in cases of concomitant mild hypocalcemia with hyperphosphatemia (e.g., renal failure), the hyperphosphatemia should be corrected using phosphate binders because that alone will often lead to correction of the hypocalcemia. Second, Mg deficits should be corrected because this may restore normal Ca physiology even without Ca supplementation (see "Disorders of Magnesium Homeostasis" later). Finally, concurrent severe metabolic acidosis should await correction of the hypocalcemia because correction of the acidosis will likely worsen the ionized hypocalcemia and precipitate tetany.

HYPERCALCEMIA

Hypercalcemia has been reported in 15% to 30% of critically ill patients[248,249] and thus appears to be less common than hypocalcemia. It is more common in patients with higher severity of illness and in those with concurrent renal failure.[248,249]

Causes of Hypercalcemia

Box 58-7 lists causes of hypercalcemia. About 90% of hypercalcemia in ambulatory and non-ICU patients is caused by only two entities: primary hyperparathyroidism

Box 58-7

Causes of Hypercalcemia

Primary Hyperparathyroidism
Malignancy
- Parathyroid-hormone-related peptide (PTHrP)
- Ectopic parathyroid hormone
- Vitamin D mediated
- Lytic bone lesions

Vitamin D
- Exogenous
- Endogenous

Hyperthyroidism
Adrenal Insufficiency
Rhabdomyolysis, Recovery
Immobilization
Drugs
- Thiazide
- Lithium
- Vitamin D/Calcium supplements
- Vitamin A

and malignancy.[208] The spectrum is a bit broader in critically ill patients.

Primary Hyperparathyroidism

Primary hyperparathyroidism is the most common cause of hypercalcemia, accounting for more than 50% of cases in ambulatory patients. Specific causes include benign adenoma (80% to 90%), hyperplasia (10% to 20%), and carcinoma (1%). Biochemical abnormalities include elevated circulating intact PTH, hypercalcemia, and hypophosphatemia.[208]

Malignancies

Hypercalcemia is rarely the presenting sign of a malignancy; most malignancies are advanced at the time hypercalcemia develops. About 40% of hypercalcemia in hospitalized patients has been associated with cancer.[250] Almost 80% of malignancy-related hypercalcemia is secondary to the secretion of *parathyroid hormone-related peptide* (PTHrP) by the malignant cells.[250] PTHrP is not detected by clinical laboratory assays for PTH. Numerous types of malignancies are associated with PTHrP-mediated hypercalcemia including breast,[251] renal cell, and ovarian carcinomas,[208] and hematologic malignancies.[252]

Increased production of 1,25-$(OH)_2D_3$ by malignant cells is the cause of hypercalcemia in patients with lymphomas.[253,254] Finally, osteolytic bone lesions from advanced cancers like breast, lung, and multiple myeloma frequently result in hypercalcemia.[208]

Rhabdomyolysis

Rhabdomyolysis associated with ARF (acute renal failure) commonly produces hypocalcemia during the initial phase (see "Hypocalcemia" earlier). Approximately 30% of patients, mostly young men, develop hypercalcemia during resolution of the ARF.[255] Release from injured muscles of previously sequestered Ca appears to be the basis for the hypercalcemia.[255,256] PTH is appropriately suppressed according to most,[257,258] but not all,[259] studies. Vitamin D levels may be elevated[257,259] or suppressed[233,258]; its contribution to the syndrome is unclear. Whatever the underlying mechanism, the hypercalcemia is usually mild and self-limited.[255]

Immobilization

Immobilization is associated with hypercalcemia because of increased bone resorption. Risk factors include duration of bed rest, spinal cord injury, multiple skeletal fractures, and underlying disorders leading to increased bone resorption (e.g., Paget disease, malignancy).[260,261] Although hypercalcemia is usually modest and completely reversible with activity, calcitonin and bisphosphonates can be used with success if treatment is required.[260]

Medications

A small percentage (5% to 10%) of patients treated with *lithium* develop hypercalcemia because of lithium-induced hyperparathyroidism.[208] Hyperparathyroidism may or may not be reversible on discontinuation of therapy. *Thiazide diuretics* increase tubular reabsorption of Ca and are well known to cause modest hypercalcemia, which revert to normal on discontinuation of therapy. More severe hypercalcemia should prompt an evaluation for occult hyperparathyroidism. *Vitamin A* may increase osteoclast-mediated bone resorption and cause hypercalcemia.

Clinical Manifestations

Clinical manifestations of hypercalcemia depend on the rate of increase and absolute level of plasma Ca. The most serious manifestations are *neurologic* and *cardiovascular.* Patients may experience muscle weakness, fatigue, depression, and altered mental status. At extremely high levels, stupor and coma may ensue.[208,212] Hypercalcemia causes an increased rate of cardiac repolarization and results in a shortened QT interval. Conduction disturbances and malignant arrhythmias have been reported with hypercalcemia.[262,263]

Hypercalcemia may lead to acute renal failure from volume depletion and renal vasoconstriction and polyuria and polydipsia caused by nephrogenic diabetes insipidus.[208,212] GI symptoms include anorexia, nausea, vomiting, and constipation. Peptic ulcer disease and acute pancreatitis are exceedingly rare, especially in the acute setting.[208]

Diagnosis

The diagnosis of hypercalcemia is often apparent from the history, with an understanding of the differential diagnosis (see Box 58-7). In cases of sustained or unexplained hypercalcemia, assays for intact PTH and vitamin D metabolites are of great value. An assay for PTHrP is rarely necessary in the evaluation of hypercalcemia in a critically ill patient because in most patients with hypercalcemia of malignancy, the cancer is advanced and the diagnosis will be obvious when the PTH and vitamin D levels are shown to be suppressed.

Treatment

The treatment strategy for hypercalcemia depends on the severity of the disturbance and on its underlying cause. Identification of the probable cause of the hypercalcemia is important both for the immediate and long-term management.

Mild hypercalcemia (total Ca ≤ 12 mg/dL or 3 mmol/L) is usually caused by primary hyperparathyroidism, thiazide diuretics, Ca and vitamin D supplements, lithium, and immobilization. Treatment should begin with withdrawal of the offending agent (if possible). Volume deficits should be replaced orally if possible. Early mobilization should be encouraged. Loop diuretics should be avoided in patients with mild asymptomatic hypercalcemia because they may exacerbate the volume depletion, leading to increased renal Ca reabsorption.

The immediate treatment of moderate hypercalcemia (total Ca > 12 mg/dL or 3 mmol/L, and ≤14 mg/dL or 3.5 mmol/L) includes the measures discussed earlier, as well as intravenous volume expansion with isotonic saline. A loop diuretic will enhance renal excretion of Ca, but care must be taken to avoid volume depletion.

Severe hypercalcemia (total Ca > 14 mg/dL or 3.5 mmol/L), even in the absence of signs and symptoms, should be treated as an emergency. Strategies for treatment include (1) enhanced Ca elimination; (2) reduced bone resorption; (3) decreased gut absorption of Ca; and (4) identification and treatment of the underlying cause.

Enhanced Ca Elimination

Forced diuresis is the mainstay of treatment. *Volume expansion* with normal saline should be instituted immediately at a rate of 200 to 300 mL/hour. The net fluid balance in adults should be positive—approximately 2 L in 24 hours. Caution must be taken to avoid symptomatic volume overload in patients with impaired myocardial performance or renal insufficiency, or both.

Once the volume deficit is adequately replaced, *loop diuretics* should be added to enhance renal Ca excretion. A dose of loop diuretic that at least doubles the rate of urine output can be given as often as every 8 hours.

For patients with congestive heart failure unresponsive to diuretics or with advanced kidney failure, *dialysis* should be considered. Hemodialysis against a solution containing 2 mEq/L Ca is effective in decreasing plasma Ca levels. Lower Ca baths are likely to cause hypotension[264] and precipitate tetany.

Reduced Bone Resorption

Several agents are available for the management of hypercalcemia. *Bisphosphonates* inhibit the osteoclast functions and number and inhibit bone turnover. They are well tolerated, although nephrotoxicity may develop if administered too quickly.[212] Pamidronate (60 to 90 mg IV) reduces the plasma Ca in 48 to 72 hours, and the effect may last for a month.[212] Zoledronic acid may be even more efficacious.[265] With the advent of bisphosphonates, two older agents have fallen into disfavor: *Calcitonin* has rapid onset of action, but tachyphylaxis occurs within 48 to 72 hours. *Plicamycin* (formerly mithramycin) has unacceptable liver, renal, and bone marrow toxicity.

Decreased Gut Ca Absorption

If endogenous vitamin D overproduction is implicated in the hypercalcemia (e.g., lymphoma, sarcoidosis), corticosteroids will lower the plasma Ca, at least partly by decreasing gut Ca absorption.

DISORDERS OF MAGNESIUM HOMEOSTASIS

Disorders of Mg balance may be the most commonly seen electrolyte abnormalities in the ICU. Hypomagnesemia, the more common disorder, is seen in 12% of hospitalized patients and up to 65% of critically ill patients.[266-268] Because of Mg's involvement in a host of critical physiologic functions,[269] its derangement can be expected to result in a variety of manifestations.

Normal Magnesium Physiology

The normal adult total body Mg content is approximately 24 g or 2000 mEq, 50% to 60% of which is found in bones and 40% to 50% of which is in the intracellular compartment, mainly muscles and soft tissues. Only about 1% of total body Mg is in the extracellular space, the normal concentration range being 1.8 to 2.3 mg/dL (1.5 to 1.9 mEq/L or about 0.7 to 1 mmol/L).[211] In plasma, 20% to 30% of Mg is bound to protein, mainly albumin, with the rest (70% to 80%) in a form that is filterable across the glomerulus.[211] Mg is taken up slowly into cells, under no known hormonal control.

Mg is a major constituent of chlorophyll, so green vegetables are a good dietary source. Mg is also found in grains, cereals, meat, and seafood.[211,270] The normal adult diet contains about 300 mg of Mg.[271] Under normal circumstances, about one third of that is absorbed in the small bowel; there is some obligatory secretion in that segment as well, along some minor reabsorption downstream in the colon.[266] This results in net absorption of about 100 mg per day. (Mg absorption is highly dependent on dietary Mg content, however, and can increase to up to 70% to 80% of dietary intake under conditions of Mg deprivation.[211]) Unlike Ca absorption, Mg absorption from the intestine does not seem to depend significantly on vitamin D.[211,272] The small intestinal secretion of Mg normally amounts to a loss of only about 20 mg a day. With acute or chronic diarrhea, however, GI losses can be substantial.[211]

The filtered load of Mg (the product of the glomerular filtration rate and the plasma concentration of ultrafilterable Mg) is about 2500 mg per day. In order to maintain external Mg balance, the renal excretion of Mg must equal the intestinal absorption, or about 100 mg per day. Thus the fractional excretion of Mg ($Mg_{excreted} \div Mg_{filtered}$) is about 4% under normal conditions.[211] With Mg depletion, the fractional excretion of Mg can fall to less than 1%, and with Mg loading, can rise to match the excess in the filtered load.[211] This modulation in Mg excretion is largely caused by changes in plasma Mg concentration.

The major site of renal Mg reabsorption (60% to 70% of the filtered load) is the thick ascending limb of the loop of Henle (TAL). This tubular segment is responsible for most of the modulation in Mg excretion. Mg reabsorption here is largely passive and depends on a lumen-positive voltage generated by the (diuretic-inhibitable) NKCC2 channel and K recycling via the ROMK channels.[211] This explains why loop diuretics increase urinary Mg excretion and tend to cause hypomagnesemia. Other factors that inhibit Mg reabsorption in the TAL include volume expansion; hypercalcemia; hypophosphatemia; and, to a lesser extent, metabolic acidosis. Conversely, volume depletion, hypocalcemia, and metabolic alkalosis increase Mg reabsorption. About 10% of filtered Mg is reabsorbed in the distal convoluted tubule. Reabsorption at this site is stimulated by K-sparing diuretics like amiloride.[266]

Mg plays a vital role in cellular physiology. It catalyses more than 300 enzymatic reactions and is an integral part of all ATP-dependent reactions.[269] It is involved in synthesis of proteins; energy-rich compounds, electron and proton transporters; DNA and RNA transcription; translation of mRNA; and regulation of mitochondrial function.[269,273] Evidence indicates that Mg helps regulate intracellular Ca concentration, especially in vascular smooth muscle, and thereby affects vascular tone.[273] In vitro studies suggest a role for Mg in inflammation and immunity, though clinical confirmation is lacking.[273]

Assessment of Body Magnesium Status

Because extracellular Mg accounts for only about 1% of total body Mg, plasma Mg is a poor reflection of body Mg status. Nonetheless, Mg status is most commonly assessed by measuring plasma Mg levels. Like Ca, Mg circulates in the plasma in bound and free (ionized) forms, the latter being the metabolically active form. Determination of ionized Mg is clinically impractical, and there is no reliable correlation with serum albumin concentration. Moreover, the relationship between low ionized Mg concentration and increased morbidity and mortality in critically ill patients has yet to be clearly established.[274-276] Thus the available literature does not support the superiority of the measurement of ionized Mg over the cheaper and widely available total serum Mg levels.

The Mg loading test has been proposed as a more sensitive measure of total body Mg stores than the plasma Mg concentration. In theory, Mg-depleted individuals will translocate more of the administered Mg load into cells and excrete a lower proportion in the urine over 24 hours.[247,266,273] Because the test requires a 24-hour urine collection and must be limited to patients who have normal renal function and who are not on medications that affect Mg excretion (see later), the test is impractical.

Hypomagnesemia

Epidemiology

Patients with malnutrition, chronic alcoholism, congestive heart failure on loop diuretics, patients in the postoperative period (especially after open heart surgery), and patients with cancer are at higher risk than the general ICU population.[266-268,277]

Causes

The causes of hypomagnesemia can be divided into four main categories: (1) insufficient intake, (2) renal loss, (3) extrarenal loss, and (4) redistribution (Box 58-8).

The renal causes can be distinguished from the others by measuring 24-hour urinary Mg excretion or, more practically, the fractional excretion of Mg (FE_{Mg}), calculated as follows[266]:

$$FE_{Mg} = \frac{U_{Mg} \times P_{Cr}}{(0.7 \times P_{Mg}) \times U_{Cr}} \times 100$$

where U_{Mg} and P_{Mg} are the urine and plasma concentrations of Mg, respectively, and U_{Cr} and P_{Cr} are the urine and plasma concentrations of creatinine. (P_{Mg} is multiplied by 0.7 because this represents the ultrafilterable fraction of Mg.) A 24-hour urinary Mg excretion of more than approximately 25 mg, or FE_{Mg} greater than 2%, is consis-

Box 58-8

Causes of Hypomagnesemia

Insufficient Intake
- Mg-deficient parenteral nutrition
- Protein-calorie malnutrition
- Alcoholism

Renal Loss
- Drug induced
  - Loop diuretics
  - Thiazide diuretics
  - Aminoglycosides
  - Amphotericin B
  - Cis-platinum
  - Cetuximab
  - Foscarnet
  - Pentamidine
- Volume expansion
- Osmotic diuresis (e.g., hyperglycemia)
- Alcohol
- Hypercalcemia
- Tubular dysfunction
  - Recovery from acute tubular necrosis
  - Bartter syndrome
  - Gitelman's syndrome

Gastrointestinal
- Small intestine resection
- Inflammatory bowel disease
- Jejunoileal bypass surgery
- Diarrhea
- Steatorrhea
- Malabsorption syndromes

Redistribution
- Acute pancreatitis
- Hungry bone syndrome

tent with renal hypomagnesemia.[208,266] Most hypomagnesemia in critically ill patients is multifactorial.

Deficient Intake

The prevalence of hypomagnesemia in chronic alcoholics is approximately 20% to 30%. Hypomagnesemia in alcoholics is multifactorial and results from decreased dietary intake, increased renal loss, and acute pancreatitis.[266] Parenteral nutrition is an important cause of hypomagnesemia in the ICU. Patients receiving parenteral nutrition have a higher daily Mg requirement for unknown reasons.[208]

Gastrointestinal Losses

Diarrheal fluid contains high concentrations of Mg, up to 16 mg/dL,[208,273] and hypomagnesemia is a common finding in patients suffering from acute or chronic diarrhea from any cause. Because intestinal absorption of Mg occurs primarily in the jejunum and ileum, conditions like celiac disease, inflammatory bowel disease, extensive small bowel resection, and jejunoileal bypass surgery for obesity are frequently associated with intestinal Mg wasting.[266]

Renal Losses

Medications are perhaps the most important cause of renal Mg wasting in critically ill patients. Loop diuretics are commonly used at high doses. Aminoglycosides may cause asymptomatic hypomagnesemia 3 to 4 days after initiation of therapy; typically it resolves after cessation of therapy.[208,278] Almost all patients who receive cisplatin develop renal Mg wasting and hypomagnesemia, which may persist for months after discontinuation of therapy.[279] Most of the patients who receive IV pentamidine therapy develop renal Mg wasting and hypomagnesemia that may last for 1 to 2 months after cessation of the therapy.[208] The renal Mg wasting associated with chronic alcohol use may take up to a month to resolve with abstinence.[266]

Redistribution

Hypomagnesemia is reported in up to 20% of patients with acute pancreatitis.[268,273] The proposed mechanism is saponification of necrotic fat with Mg and Ca. The mechanism of hypomagnesemia with the "hungry bone" syndrome (following parathyroidectomy for hyperparathyroidism) is rapid bone uptake of Mg during remineralization.

Clinical Manifestations

Hypomagnesemia in critically ill patients has been associated with a twofold increase in mortality, even after adjustment for severity of illness.[280] (The observation that Mg supplementation has not been shown to improve outcome[266] suggests that hypomagnesemia may be a marker for pejorative conditions not captured by severity of illness scores.)

The signs and symptoms of hypomagnesemia are cardiovascular, neuromuscular, and metabolic and are shown in Box 58-9.[208,266,269,273] Evidence that hypomagnesemia is associated with arrhythmias in otherwise healthy individuals is scarce. In the setting of acute myocardial ischemia, however, even mild hypomagnesemia has been associated with increased frequency of ventricular arrhythmias.[266] Results of recent large clinical trials, however, have shown no benefit to Mg supplementation in this setting in the absence of overt hypomagnesemia.[273] Torsades de pointes is a malignant ventricular arrhythmia associated with Mg deficiency or drugs that prolong the QT interval. Mg is the treatment of choice. Mg supplementation after cardiopulmonary bypass may reduce the frequency of ventricular ectopy.

Box 58-9

Clinical Manifestations of Hypomagnesemia

Cardiovascular
- Ventricular arrhythmias
  - Torsades de pointes
  - Ventricular fibrillation; premature ventricular contractions
  - Increased digitalis toxicity
- Conduction disturbances
  - Prolonged QT interval
  - Prolonged QRS duration
  - ST depression
  - Peaked T wave

Neuromuscular
- Muscle weakness
- Tetany
- Horizontal and vertical nystagmus
- Choreoathetoid movements
- Seizures

Metabolic
- Hypokalemia, refractory
- Hypocalcemia, refractory

The hypocalcemia associated with hypomagnesemia is caused by both hypoparathyroidism and bone resistance to PTH. The hypokalemia is caused by renal K wasting and will not resolve until the hypomagnesemia is corrected.[281,282]

Treatment

In patients who have malignant cardiac arrhythmias (ventricular fibrillation or torsades de pointes) or seizure attributed to hypomagnesemia, intravenous Mg must be given immediately, 2 g IV of $MGSO_4$ as rapidly as possible (see Chapter 32 for details).

Less urgent cases, but those in which signs and symptoms are present, may be treated with $MGSO_4$ 6 g intravenous in the first 24 hours followed by 3 to 4 g daily for the next 2 to 6 days.[208,266,273] Because translocation of Mg into cells is a slow process, and because urinary excretion is proportional to the plasma Mg level, more rapid infusion rates are associated with urinary Mg wasting that defeats the purpose of the therapy. Effective intravenous infusions should be given over 8 to 12 hours.[266] For patients with impaired renal function, the dose should be reduced by 50% to 75% and serum Mg levels should be monitored frequently. Patients should be monitored closely for symptoms and signs of hypermagnesemia (see later).

Patients with refractory hypokalemia in the setting of hypomagnesemia who are receiving high doses of K must be monitored closely for the development of hyperkalemia once the Mg is being replenished.

For mild asymptomatic hypomagnesemia, patients who can tolerate oral medication should receive oral Mg salts (e.g., $MgCl_2$ 500 mg slow-release tablets, 10 to 12 per day in divided doses). High doses of oral Mg salts may cause diarrhea.

Hypermagnesemia

Causes

Hypermagnesemia is much less common than hypomagnesemia. Patients with normal renal function have prodigious capacity to excrete excess Mg through the kidneys.[208] Thus hypermagnesemia is seen only in patients with compromised renal function receiving enteral or parenteral Mg or in patients with normal renal function receiving massive exogenous Mg (e.g., treatment for preeclampsia and eclampsia).[208] The causes of hypermagnesemia are shown in Box 58-10.

Clinical Manifestations

The clinical manifestations of hypermagnesemia (Box 58-11) are largely caused by the effect of the heart, nerve, and smooth muscle. Initial manifestations, with plasma concentrations of 4 to 6 mg/dL, include nausea and vomiting, hypotension, and flushing. More severe effects including death[283] are seen with levels exceeding 6 mg/dL.

Treatment

Treatment of hypermagnesemia depends on the severity of symptoms and the patient's renal function. Patients with adequate renal function and mild asymptomatic hypermagnesemia require no treatment except to remove all sources of exogenous Mg. The half-time of elimination of Mg is about 28 hours.[208] Mg excretion may be enhanced by saline infusion and the use of loop diuretics.[208] (Care must be taken to prevent hypokalemia and metabolic alkalosis.) Patients with symptomatic hypermagnesemia, especially with cardiovascular manifestations, require urgent treatment. The recommended therapy is Ca gluconate 1 g IV over 5 minutes.

Patients with acute or chronic renal failure and symptomatic hypermagnesemia will require dialysis to remove excess Mg. Hemodialysis removes Mg efficiently, yielding a 30% to 50% reduction in predialysis serum Mg levels after a 3- to 4-hour treatment.[208]

Box 58-10

Causes of Hypermagnesemia

Renal Insufficiency
- Mg-containing antacids (e.g., magnesium aluminum hydroxide)
- Mg-containing laxatives or enemas (e.g., magnesium citrate)

Patients with Normal Renal Function
- Treatment of preeclampsia or eclampsia
- Treatment of hypomagnesemia

Miscellaneous
- Hypothyroidism
- Hyperparathyroidism
- Addison's disease
- Lithium treatment

PHOSPHORUS

Phosphorus has an essential role in normal physiology. It is necessary for skeletal integrity; energy economy (formation of high-energy phosphate bonds); nucleic acid, lipid, and protein structure; cell signaling; and buffering.[211] Not surprisingly, therefore, disorders of phosphorus homeostasis have diverse manifestations.[284-286] Hypophosphatemia is considerably more common in hospitalized and critically ill patients than hyperphosphatemia.

Normal Phosphorus Homeostasis

Total body phosphorus amounts to about 700 g in an adult. About 85% resides in the skeleton, about 15% in soft tissues, and only about 1% in blood.[210] Circulating phosphorus is mostly in the form of inorganic phosphates. The normal plasma concentration of phosphorus is 2.5 to 4.5 mg/dL, also expressed as a phosphate concentration of 0.9 to 1.45 mmol/L. (Phosphate concentration should not be expressed in mEq/L because the average valence of plasma phosphates—a mixture of HPO_4^{2-} and $H_2PO_4^-$—changes with pH.[287]) Of that circulating phosphorus, about 75% is free and ultrafilterable and 25% is protein bound.[211]

Box 58-11

Clinical Manifestations of Hypermagnesemia

Cardiovascular
- Hypotension
- Facial flushing
- Bradycardia
- Sinoatrial or atrioventricular heart block
- Asystole

Gastrointestinal
- Nausea and vomiting
- Ileus

Neuromuscular
- Hyporeflexia
- Flaccid skeletal muscle paralysis
- Respiratory muscle weakness and paralysis
- Lethargy
- Coma

Urinary retention

A normal adult diet includes about 1000 mg of phosphorus per day. Stool contains about 300 mg, so the net absorption (mostly in the small intestine under the influence of vitamin D) is about 70%. The dietary and secreted phosphorus may be bound into insoluble, nonabsorbable salts by cations such as Al^{3+}, Ca^{2+}, and Mg^{2+}. Thus the kidney is responsible for excreting about 700 mg phosphorus per day. Almost all phosphorus reabsorption takes place in the proximal tubule. The most important regulators of renal phosphorus excretion are parathyroid hormone (PTH) and dietary phosphorus content. PTH increases phosphorus excretion.[210] Renal excretion of phosphorus is proportional to the dietary intake. Other factors that increase renal phosphorus excretion include extracellular volume expansion, acute hypercalcemia, diuretics, and glucocorticoids.[210,211] Acid base disorders have a variable effect on phosphorus reabsorption depending on their direction and duration,[210,211] with one exception: Respiratory alkalosis causes a marked decrease in renal phosphorus excretion by causing redistributive hypophosphatemia[285] (see later).

Phosphorus homeostasis depends on PTH and vitamin D. PTH causes phosphaturia by decreasing renal proximal tubule reabsorption. Active vitamin D inhibits PTH release. Vitamin D activation (1-α hydroxylation) is regulated by plasma phosphorus concentration and is inhibited by hyperphosphatemia. Thus hyperphosphatemia inhibits vitamin D activation, which reduces intestinal phosphorus absorption and allows increased PTH secretion, causing phosphaturia and returning plasma phosphorus toward normal. Hypophosphatemia reverses this physiology, allowing increased gut absorption and reduced renal excretion of phosphorus.

Box 58-12

Causes of Hypophosphatemia

Redistribution
- Acute respiratory alkalosis
- Refeeding syndrome
- Treatment of diabetic ketoacidosis
- Hungry bone syndrome (postparathyroidectomy)
- Leukemia

Increased Renal Excretion
- Hyperparathyroidism
- Vitamin D deficiency or resistance
- Volume expansion
- Postobstructive diuresis
- Recovery from acute tubular necrosis
- Fanconi syndrome
- Postrenal transplantation
- Drugs
  - Acetazolamide
  - Corticosteroids
- Inherited disorders

Decreased Intestinal Absorption
- Malnutrition
- Phosphate-binding medications
- Chronic diarrhea
- Chronic alcoholism

Hypophosphatemia

Hypophosphatemia is common in critically ill patients. It has been reported in 29% of adult surgical patients (and 45% of patients with one or more risk factors for hypophosphatemia) and—liberally defined—in 76% of pediatric ICU patients.[288] Patients with malnutrition, uncontrolled diabetes mellitus, sepsis, and chronic alcoholism are at high risk for hypophosphatemia.[289] Hypophosphatemia is associated with a marked increase in mortality in patients with sepsis,[290] and serum phosphorus concentration is inversely correlated with APACHE II after liver resection.[291] In these situations the serum phosphorus concentration is probably a marker of severity of illness. If severe, however, hypophosphatemia itself may cause serious complications.

Causes of Hypophosphatemia

The causes of hypophosphatemia are classically divided into three general categories: (1) redistribution from the extracellular to the intracellular space, (2) increased renal excretion, and (3) decreased intestinal absorption (Box 58-12). Recognizing that many factors have several different effects on phosphorus homeostasis is important.

Redistribution

Respiratory alkalosis causes intracellular phosphate shift (by stimulating glycolysis) and can cause severe symptomatic hypophosphatemia. Respiratory alkalosis is commonly encountered in ICU patients with sepsis and liver failure and in patients requiring mechanical ventilation; in the latter case, the degree of hypophosphatemia is proportional to the pH.[208,292] *Sepsis* is commonly associated with hypophosphatemia, probably because of hyperventilation and respiratory alkalosis. Rapid *refeeding* of patients with malnutrition may result in significant hypophosphatemia because of insulin-mediated intracellular phosphate shift. In one study of ICU patients, refeeding hypophosphatemia developed in 34% of patients after 48 hours of starvation and was predicted by the prealbumin concentration. Profound hypophosphatemia (<1 mmol/dL) occurred in 10% of patients.[293] Patients with anorexia nervosa, uncontrolled diabetes mellitus, chronic malnutrition, and chronic alcoholism are at a particularly high risk of developing refeeding syndrome. *Leukemia* in the leukemic phase[294] and with rapid leukocyte reconstitution after bone marrow transplant[295] has been reported to cause severe redistributive hypophosphatemia.

Diabetic ketoacidosis is associated with phosphorus efflux from cells and increased urinary phosphate excretion, resulting in severe total body phosphorus depletion (often with a deceptively normal presenting serum phosphorus concentration).[285] Initiation of insulin therapy in such patients results in intracellular phosphate shift and can result in profound, symptomatic hypophosphatemia.[285]

Increased Renal Excretion

Any cause of *primary hyperparathyroidism* will cause phosphaturia and tend to cause hypophosphatemia. Hyperparathyroidism caused by hypocalcemia or *vitamin D deficiency or resistance* is similarly associated with hypophosphatemia. The exception is the secondary hyperparathyroidism of chronic kidney disease, in which hyperphosphatemia caused by decreased renal phosphorus elimination is characteristic. *Vitamin D deficiency* or *resistance* also causes hypophosphatemia from decreased intestinal phosphate absorption. Extracellular volume expansion increases the filtered phosphorus load and dilutes the luminal concentration of phosphorus, resulting in phosphaturia. *Ethanol* and *glycosuria* both decrease proximal tubule phosphate reabsorption.[208,285] All *diuretic drugs*, but particularly those with proximal tubular effects like acetazolamide and, to a lesser degree, thiazides, cause phosphaturia.

Decreased Intestinal Absorption

Salts of Al^{3+} and Ca^{2+}, formulated for oral administration as antacids or as phosphate-binding medications, can cause malabsorptive hypophosphatemia. Chronic diarrhea and steatorrhea may reduce intestinal phosphate absorption directly and by way of vitamin D deficiency and cause hypophosphatemia.

The hypophosphatemia commonly associated with *chronic alcohol ingestion* is multifactorial. Dietary phosphorus deficiency, malabsorption, antacid ingestion, hypocalcemia and secondary hyperparathyroidism, hypomagnesemia, and an ethanol-induced renal tubular defect all have been implicated.[285]

Box 58-13

Clinical Manifestations of Hypophosphatemia

Skeletal Muscle
- Weakness
- Rhabdomyolysis

Decreased Cardiac Output

Hematologic
- Erythrocytes
  - Decreased 2,3-DPG
    - Decreased tissue oxygen delivery
  - Spherocytosis
  - Hemolysis
- Impaired leukocyte function
- Impaired platelet function

Neurologic
- Anorexia
- Irritability
- Confusion
- Paresthesias
- Ataxia
- Seizure
- Coma

Skeletal
- Bone pain
- Pseudofractures
- Osteomalacia

Insulin Resistance

Clinical Manifestations

Important clinical manifestations of hypophosphatemia are shown in Box 58-13. Most patients are asymptomatic until plasma phosphorus falls below 1.5 mg/dL or about 0.5 mmol/L. The most severe manifestations such as hemolysis, spontaneous rhabdomyolysis, seizure, and coma are not commonly seen with phosphorus above 1 mg/dL (0.3 mmol/L). Acute clinical manifestations are thought to be largely caused by altered cellular energy economy.[208,210,284,285]

Treatment

The therapy of hypophosphatemia starts with its prevention. In critically ill patients, this depends on recognition and correction of the factors that lead to hypophosphatemia. The astute clinician will be able to anticipate the development of hypophosphatemia (e.g., in refeeding), monitor the patient appropriately, and supplement phosphorus accordingly. Patients on total parenteral nutrition should receive adequate phosphorus for their level of renal function (see Chapter 83).[287]

The exact method of phosphorus supplementation in hypophosphatemia depends on the severity of the disturbance and the patient's underlying condition. In mild to moderate hypophosphatemia (>1.5 mg/dL or about 0.5 mmol/L), oral replacement is usually sufficient. Skim milk is an excellent source of phosphorus and provides 900 mg/L of inorganic phosphate. In patients who cannot tolerate milk, oral sodium phosphate, formulated to provide 250 mg of phosphate in each tablet, can be used. Alternatively, Fleet Phospho-soda can be given to provide 60 mmol of phosphorus per day, divided into three doses of 5 mL each.[210] Supplementation should continue for several days in order to replenish phosphorus deficits adequately. Administration of sufficient doses of oral phosphorus preparations commonly causes diarrhea, limiting its usefulness.

Patients with severe hyperphosphatemia (<1.5 mg/dL) or those for whom the enteral route is not an option require intravenous phosphorus repletion. In such patients, the recommended dose is 2.5 to 5 mg (0.08 to 0.16 mmol) per kg body weight over 6 hours, doses at the higher end of the range being reserved for profound, symptomatic hypophosphatemia.[210,287]

The administered phosphorus can complex with circulating Ca, leading to a decrease in ionized Ca (with attendant hypotension and tetany) and metastatic calcification. The use of K salts of phosphate for repletion of phosphorus deficits has been associated with dangerous hyperkalemia. For that reason, K deficits and phosphorus deficits should be treated separately.[287]

Hyperphosphatemia

Hyperphosphatemia (plasma phosphorus >5 mg/dL or a phosphate concentration >1.6 mmol/L) is usually associated with renal dysfunction. Massive influx of phosphorus into the extracellular space, however, either from endogenous sources or exogenous, can overwhelm normal renal excretory mechanisms and lead to severe hyperphosphatemia.

Causes of Hyperphosphatemia

Hyperphosphatemia may be caused by (1) redistribution of phosphorus from the intracellular to the extracellular space, (2) increased phosphorus intake, and (3) decreased renal excretion of phosphorus (Table 58-8). Importantly, most hyperphosphatemia is multifactorial.

Redistribution

Hyperphosphatemia is a common complication of the *tumor lysis syndrome*.[66] Similarly, rhabdomyolysis is often associated with hyperphosphatemia, especially when it is complicated by acute renal failure.[68,296] Less commonly recognized causes of redistributive hyperphosphatemia include acute and chronic respiratory acidosis, acute pancreatitis,[297] diabetic ketoacidosis,[298] and lactic acidosis.[299]

Increased Intake

Exogenous administration of phosphorus is unlikely to cause hyperphosphatemia unless renal function is compromised. Several cases of potentially life-threatening hyperphosphatemia and hypocalcemia have been reported after the use of phosphate-containing laxatives and enemas, especially in children and the elderly.[229,231,232,300,301] Overly aggressive parenteral phosphorus supplementation can cause hyperphosphatemia. Hypervitaminosis D causes increased intestinal uptake of phosphorus and a decrease in PTH, both of which predispose to hyperphosphatemia.

Decreased Renal Excretion

Acute renal failure is associated with elevated phosphate levels caused by an inability of the kidneys to excrete phosphate load. This is particularly pronounced in patients in whom acute renal failure is caused by the tumor lysis syndrome or rhabdomyolysis. Advanced chronic kidney disease (GFR < 25 mL/min) is commonly associated with hyperphosphatemia. Such patients are particularly susceptible to developing severe and life-threatening hyperphosphatemia if they are exposed to an acute increase in serum phosphate levels. Hypoparathyroidism of any cause is associated with impaired renal phosphorus excretion.

Pseudohyperphosphatemia

Spurious increases in the measured plasma phosphorus concentration are reported to be caused by contamination of the blood sample with phosphate-buffered saline as a diluent for heparin[302] or during sample processing by the laboratory.[303] Even microliter volumes of the contaminant can cause significant elevations in the measured phosphorus.[304] Paraproteinemia can also cause pseudophyperphosphatemia.

Table 58-8. Causes of Hyperphosphatemia

Redistribution
Tumor lysis syndrome
Rhabdomyolysis
Pancreatitis
Respiratory acidosis
Lactic acidosis
Diabetic ketoacidosis
Increased Intake
Phosphate containing enemas and laxatives
Intravenous phosphate
Hypervitaminosis D
Decreased Renal Excretion
Acute renal failure
Chronic kidney disease
Hypoparathyroidism
Pseudohyperphosphatemia

Clinical Manifestations of Hyperphosphatemia

Phosphate complexes with circulating Ca, reducing the concentration of ionized Ca. Thus most of the clinical consequences of hyperphosphatemia are those of hypocalcemia (see earlier). In addition, ectopic deposition of Ca phosphate salts can occur, especially when the Ca-phosphorus product (in mg/dL) exceeds 70.[210] Such ectopic calcification in the heart can cause conduction and rhythm disturbances.[304]

Because phosphate is an "unmeasured ion," hyperphosphatemia causes increases in the anion gap. Extreme hyperphosphatemia can cause shocking elevations in the anion gap. One case of hyperphosphatemia from Phospho-Soda intoxication (serum phosphorus 62.5 mg/dL) was associated with an anion gap of 51 mmol/L.[305] In order to estimate the contribution of phosphorus to the anion gap, one must know not only the plasma concentration of phosphorus but the pH, because the valence of phosphate varies with pH, from 1.8 mEq/mmol at pH 7.4 to 1.6 mEq/L at pH 7.[287] Because extreme hyperphosphatemia can be caused by lactic acidosis or ketoacidosis (see earlier), an elevated anion gap in the setting of hyperphosphatemia should never be attributed to the hyperphosphatemia itself without further investigation.

Treatment of Hyperphosphatemia

Treatment of hyperphosphatemia consists of reducing the phosphate intake and enhancing the removal of excess phosphate. If the patient is on an oral diet, dietary phosphate should be restricted to less than 800 mg per day. Oral phosphate binders can be added with meals to decrease intestinal phosphate absorption.

Patients with normal renal function can be treated with saline diuresis to increase renal phosphate excretion. Acetazolamide can be added to enhance phosphaturia, taking care to avoid metabolic acidosis. Patients with severe hyperphosphatemia with coexisting renal failure may require renal replacement therapy in the form of intermittent or continuous hemodialysis.

KEY POINTS

- Acid-base disorders often provide a window into underlying pathology. Optimal diagnosis of acid-base disorders requires familiarity with the rules of normal compensation, as well as the pitfalls characteristic of critical illness.
- Acute hyperkalemia may result from exogenous K administration or redistribution from cells. Acute hypokalemia is always caused by redistribution.
- Patients, particularly women, are predisposed to catastrophic hyponatremia if hypotonic fluids are administered in the postoperative period.
- The treatment of acute symptomatic hyponatremia is largely independent of its cause, whereas the treatment of chronic hyponatremia depends critically on the underlying pathophysiology.
- Hypernatremia in hospitalized patients should be considered iatrogenic, reflecting insufficient recognition of the causes of water loss and inadequate water replacement in vulnerable patients.
- Plasma Ca concentration, corrected for the plasma albumin concentration, correlates poorly with ionized Ca in critically ill patients. If possible, ionized Ca should be measured directly when considering disorders of Ca homeostasis.
- The clinical manifestations of many metabolic disorders have common features (e.g., hypocalcemia, hypomagnesemia, hyperphosphatemia, metabolic alkalosis) relating to their overlapping pathophysiology.

REFERENCES

1. DuBose TD: Acid-base disorders. In Brenner BM (ed): Brenner & Rector's The Kidney, 7th ed. Philadelphia, Saunders, 2004.
2. Narins RG, Emmett M: Simple and mixed acid-base disorders: A practical approach. Medicine (Baltimore) 1980;59:161-187.
3. Cohen RM, Feldman GM, Fernandez PC: The balance of acid, base and charge in health and disease. Kidney Int 1997;52:287-293.
4. Szerlip HM: Metabolic acidosis. In Greenberg A (ed): Primer on Kidney Diseases, 4th ed. Philadelphia, Saunders, 2005.
5. Ishihara K, Szerlip HM: Anion gap acidosis. Semin Nephrol 1998;18: 83-97.
6. Roberts WL, Johnson RD: The serum anion gap. Has the reference interval really fallen? Arch Pathol Lab Med 1997;121:568-572.
7. Gauthier PM, Szerlip HM: Metabolic acidosis in the intensive care unit. Crit Care Clin 2002;18:289-308, vi.
8. Moe OW, Fuster D: Clinical acid-base pathophysiology: Disorders of plasma anion gap. Best Pract Res Clin Endocrinol Metab 2003;17:559-574.
9. Heird WC, Dell RB, Driscoll JM Jr, et al: Metabolic acidosis resulting from intravenous alimentation mixtures containing synthetic amino acids. N Engl J Med 1972;287:943-948.
10. Gunnerson KJ, Kellum JA: Acid-base and electrolyte analysis in critically ill patients: Are we ready for the new millennium? Curr Opin Crit Care 2003;9:468-473.
11. Dempsey GA, Lyall HJ, Corke CF, et al: Pyroglutamic acidemia: A cause of high anion gap metabolic acidosis. Crit Care Med 2000;28:1803-1807.
12. Arbour R: Propylene glycol toxicity occurs during low-dose infusions of lorazepam. Crit Care Med 2003;31:664-665; author reply 665.
13. Kraut JA, Kurtz I: Use of base in the treatment of severe acidemic states. Am J Kidney Dis 2001;38:703-727.
14. Adrogue HJ, Madias NE: Management of life-threatening acid-base disorders. First of two parts. N Engl J Med 1998;338:26-34.
15. DiNubile MJ: The increment in the anion gap: Overextension of a concept? Lancet 1988;2:951-953.
16. Corey HE: Stewart and beyond: New models of acid-base balance. Kidney Int 203;64:777-787.
17. Fernandez PC, Cohen RM, Feldman GM: The concept of bicarbonate distribution space: The crucial role of body buffers. Kidney Int 1989;36:747-752.
18. Holmdahl MH, Wiklund L, Wetterberg T, et al: The place of THAM in the management of acidemia in clinical practice. Acta Anaesthesiol Scand 2000;44:524-527.
19. Alivanis P, Giannikouris I, Paliuras C, et al: Metformin-associated lactic acidosis treated with continuous renal replacement therapy. Clin Ther 2006;28:396-400.
20. Guo PY, Storsley LJ, Finkle SN: Severe lactic acidosis treated with prolonged hemodialysis: Recovery after massive overdoses of metformin. Semin Dial 2006;19:80-83.
21. Galla JH: Metabolic alkalosis. J Am Soc Nephrol 2000;11:369-375.
22. Palmer BF, Alpern RJ: Metabolic alkalosis. J Am Soc Nephrol 1997;8:1462-1469.
23. Anderson LE, Henrich WL: Alkalemia-associated morbidity and mortality in medical and surgical patients. South Med J 1987;80:729-733.
24. Javaheri S, Shore NS, Rose B, et al: Compensatory hypoventilation in metabolic alkalosis. Chest 1982;81:296-301.
25. Kilmartin JV: Interaction of haemoglobin with protons, CO_2 and 2,3-diphosphoglycerate. Br Med Bull 1976;32:209-212.
26. Bersin RM, Arieff AI: Primary lactic alkalosis. Am J Med 1988;85:867-871.
27. Brimioulle S, Vincent JL, Dufaye P, et al: Hydrochloric acid infusion for treatment of metabolic alkalosis: Effects on acid-base balance and oxygenation. Crit Care Med 1985;13:738-742.
28. Gennari FJ: Disorders of potassium homeostasis. Hypokalemia and hyperkalemia. Crit Care Clin 2002;18:273-288, vi.
29. Stevens MS, Dunlay RW: Hyperkalemia in hospitalized patients. Int Urol Nephrol 2000;32:177-180.
30. Edelman IS, Leibman J: Anatomy of body water and electrolytes. Am J Med 1959;27:256-277.
31. Mount DB, Kambiz Z-N: Disorders of potassium balance. In Brenner B (ed): Brenner & Rector's The Kidney, 7th ed. Philadelphia, Saunders, 2004.
32. Sterns RH, Cox M, Feig PU, et al: Internal potassium balance and the control of the plasma potassium concentration. Medicine (Baltimore) 1981;60:339-354.
33. Sterns RH, Spital A: Disorders of internal potassium balance. Semin Nephrol 1987;7:399-415.
34. Adrogue HJ, Madias NE: Changes in plasma potassium concentration during acute acid-base disturbances. Am J Med 1981;71:456-467.
35. Magner PO, Robinson L, Halperin RM, et al: The plasma potassium concentration in metabolic acidosis: A re-evaluation. Am J Kidney Dis 1988;11:220-224.
36. Ahmed J, Weisberg LS: Hyperkalemia in dialysis patients. Semin Dial 2001;14:348-356.
37. Adrogue HJ, Lederer ED, Suki WN, et al: Determinants of plasma potassium levels in diabetic ketoacidosis. Medicine (Baltimore) 1986;65:163-172.
38. Fulop M: Serum potassium in lactic acidosis and ketoacidosis. N Engl J Med 1979;300:1087-1089.
39. Orringer CE, Eustace JC, Wunsch CD, et al: Natural history of lactic acidosis after grand-mal seizures. A model for the study of an anion-gap acidosis not associated with hyperkalemia. N Engl J Med 1977;297:796-799.
40. Fraley DS, Adler S: Correction of hyperkalemia by bicarbonate despite constant blood pH. Kidney Int 1977;12:354-360.
41. Blumberg A, Weidmann P, Ferrari P: Effect of prolonged bicarbonate

administration on plasma potassium in terminal renal failure. Kidney Int 1992;41:369-374.
42. Blumberg A, Weidmann P, Shaw S, et al: Effect of various therapeutic approaches on plasma potassium and major regulating factors in terminal renal failure. Am J Med 1988;85:507-512.
43. Kassirer JP, Schwartz WB: The response of normal man to selective depletion of hydrochloric acid. Factors in the genesis of persistent gastric alkalosis. Am J Med 1966;40:10-18.
44. Moreno M, Murphy C, Goldsmith C: Increase in serum potassium resulting from the administration of hypertonic mannitol and other solutions. J Lab Clin Med 1969;73:291-298.
45. Goldfarb S, Cox M, Singer I, et al: Acute hyperkalemia induced by hyperglycemia: Hormonal mechanisms. Ann Intern Med 1976;84:426-432.
46. Montoliu J, Revert L: Lethal hyperkalemia associated with severe hyperglycemia in diabetic patients with renal failure. Am J Kidney Dis 1985;5:47-48.
47. Hallen J: K+ balance in humans during exercise. Acta Physiol Scand 1996;156:279-286.
48. McKenna MJ: Effects of training on potassium homeostasis during exercise. J Mol Cell Cardiol 1995;27:941-949.
49. Don BR, Sebastian A, Cheitlin M, et al: Pseudohyperkalemia caused by fist clenching during phlebotomy. N Engl J Med 1990;322:1290-1292.
50. Sebastian A, Schambelan M: Renal hyperkalemia. Semin Nephrol 1987;7:223-238.
51. Squires RD, Huth EJ: Experimental potassium depletion in normal human subjects. I. Relation of ionic intakes to the renal conservation of potassium. J Clin Invest 1959;38:1134-1148.
52. Malnic G, Bailey MA, Giebisch G: Control of renal potassium excretion. In Brenner B (ed): Brenner & Rector's The Kidney, 7th ed. Philadelphia, Saunders, 2004.
53. Brogden RN, Heel RC, Speight TM, et al: Ticarcillin: A review of its pharmacological properties and therapeutic efficacy. Drugs 1980;20:325-352.
54. Weiner ID, Wingo CS: Hypokalemia—consequences, causes, and correction. J Am Soc Nephrol 1997;8:1179-1188.
55. Dyckner T: Relation of cardiovascular disease to potassium and magnesium deficiencies. Am J Cardiol 1990;65:44K-46K.
56. Sterns RH, Guzzo J, Feig PU: The disposition of intravenous potassium in normal man: The role of insulin. Clin Sci (Lond) 1981;61:23-28.
57. Lawson DH: Adverse reactions to potassium chloride. Q J Med 1974;43:433-440.
58. Rimmer JM, Horn JF, Gennari FJ: Hyperkalemia as a complication of drug therapy. Arch Intern Med 1987;147:867-869.
59. Perez GO, Oster JR, Pelleya R, et al: Hyperkalemia from single small oral doses of potassium chloride. Nephron 1984;36:270-271.
60. Ponce SP, Jennings AE, Madias NE, et al: Drug-induced hyperkalemia. Medicine (Baltimore) 1985;64:357-370.
61. Spence RK, Martinez A: Coagulation in trauma: Dilution and massive transfusion. In Spiess BD, Spence RK, Shander A (eds): Perioperative Transfusion Medicine. Philadelphia, Lippincott Williams & Wilkins, 2006.
62. Jameson LC, Popic PM, Harms BA: Hyperkalemic death during use of a high-capacity fluid warmer for massive transfusion. Anesthesiology 1990;73:1050-1052.
63. Baz EM, Kanazi GE, Mahfouz RA, et al: An unusual case of hyperkalaemia-induced cardiac arrest in a paediatric patient during transfusion of a 'fresh' 6-day-old blood unit. Transfus Med 2002;12:383-386.
64. Khoo MS, Braden GL, Deaton D, et al: Outcome and complications of intraoperative hemodialysis during cardiopulmonary bypass with potassium-rich cardioplegia. Am J Kidney Dis 2003;41:1247-1256.
65. Weber DO, Yarnoz MD: Hyperkalemia complicating cardiopulmonary bypass: Analysis of risk factors. Ann Thorac Surg 1982;34:439-445.
66. Locatelli F, Rossi F: Incidence and pathogenesis of tumor lysis syndrome. Contrib Nephrol 2005;147:61-68.
67. Arseneau JC, Bagley CM, Anderson T, et al: Hyperkalaemia, a sequel to chemotherapy of Burkitt's lymphoma. Lancet 1973;1:10-14.
68. Knochel JP: Mechanisms of rhabdomyolysis. Curr Opin Rheumatol 1993;5:725-731.
69. Gabow PA, Kaehny WD, Kelleher SP: The spectrum of rhabdomyolysis. Medicine (Baltimore) 1982;61:141-152.
70. Malinoski DJ, Slater MS, Mullins RJ: Crush injury and rhabdomyolysis. Crit Care Clin 2004;20:171-192.
71. Roth D, Alarcon FJ, Fernandez JA, et al: Acute rhabdomyolysis associated with cocaine intoxication. N Engl J Med 1988;319:673-677.
72. Singhal PC, Faulkner M: Myonecrosis and cocaine abuse. Ann Intern Med 1988;109:843.
73. Antons KA, Williams CD, Baker SK, et al: Clinical perspectives of statin-induced rhabdomyolysis. Am J Med 2006;119:400-409.
74. Hendriks F, Kooman JP, van der Sande FM: Massive rhabdomyolysis and life threatening hyperkalaemia in a patient with the combination of cerivastatin and gemfibrozil. Nephrol Dial Transplant 2001;16:2418-2419.
75. Smith TW, Butler VP Jr, Haber E, et al: Treatment of life-threatening digitalis intoxication with digoxin-specific Fab antibody fragments: Experience in 26 cases. N Engl J Med 1982;307:1357-1362.
76. Woolf AD, Wenger T, Smith TW, et al: The use of digoxin-specific Fab fragments for severe digitalis intoxication in children. N Engl J Med 1992;326:1739-1744.
77. Weisberg LS: The risk of preoperative hyperkalemia. Semin Dial 2003;16:78-79.
78. Martyn JA, Richtsfeld M: Succinylcholine-induced hyperkalemia in acquired pathologic states: Etiologic factors and molecular mechanisms. Anesthesiology 2006;104:158-169.
79. Markewitz BA, Elstad MR: Succinylcholine-induced hyperkalemia following prolonged pharmacologic neuromuscular blockade. Chest 1997;111:248-250.
80. Surtees R: Inherited ion channel disorders. Eur J Pediatr 159 Suppl 2000;3:S199-203.
81. Riggs JE: Periodic paralysis. Clin Neuropharmacol 1989;12:249-257.
82. Anderson RJ, Schrier RW: Acute renal failure. In Schrier RW (ed): Diseases of the Kidney and Urinary Tract, 7th ed. Philadelphia, Lippincott Williams & Wilkins, 2001.
83. Graber M, Subramani K, Corish D, et al: Thrombocytosis elevates serum potassium. Am J Kidney Dis 1988;12:116-120.
84. Bronson WR, DeVita VT, Carbone PP, et al: Pseudohyperkalemia due to release of potassium from white blood cells during clotting. N Engl J Med 1966;274:369-375.
85. Colussi G, Cipriani D: Pseudohyperkalemia in extreme leukocytosis. Am J Nephrol 1995;15:450-452.
86. Beigelman PM: Severe diabetic ketoacidosis (diabetic "coma"). 482 episodes in 257 patients; experience of three years. Diabetes 1971;20:490-500.
87. Murthy K, Harrington JT, Siegel RD: Profound hypokalemia in diabetic ketoacidosis: A therapeutic challenge. Endocr Pract 2005;11:331-334.
88. Krentz AJ, Ryder RE: Hypokalemia-induced respiratory failure complicating treatment of diabetic ketoacidosis. J Diabetes Complications 1994;8:55-56.
89. Solomon SM, Kirby DF: The refeeding syndrome: A review. JPEN J Parenter Enteral Nutr 1990;14:90-97.
90. Weinsier RL, Krumdieck CL: Death resulting from overzealous total parenteral nutrition: The refeeding syndrome revisited. Am J Clin Nutr 1981;34:393-399.
91. Lipworth BJ, McDevitt DG, Struthers AD: Prior treatment with diuretic augments the hypokalemic and electrocardiographic effects of inhaled albuterol. Am J Med 1989;86:653-657.
92. Brown MJ, Brown DC, Murphy MB: Hypokalemia from beta2-receptor stimulation by circulating epinephrine. N Engl J Med 1983;309:1414-1419.
93. Salerno DM: Postresuscitation hypokalemia in a patient with a normal prearrest serum potassium level. Ann Intern Med 1988;108:836-837.
94. Thompson RG, Cobb LA: Hypokalemia after resuscitation from out-of-hospital ventricular fibrillation. JAMA 1982;248:2860-2863.
95. Diengott D, Rozsa O, Levy N, et al: Hypokalaemia in barium poisoning. Lancet 1964;14:343-344.
96. Links TP, Smit AJ, Molenaar WM, et al: Familial hypokalemic periodic paralysis. Clinical, diagnostic and therapeutic aspects. J Neurol Sci 1994;122:33-43.
97. Ober KP: Thyrotoxic periodic paralysis in the United States. Report of 7 cases

and review of the literature. Medicine (Baltimore) 1992;71:109-120.
98. Nora NA, Berns AS: Hypokalaemic, hypophosphatemic thyrotoxic periodic paralysis. Am J Kidney Dis 1989;13: 247-249.
99. van Ypersele de Strihou C: Potassium homeostasis in renal failure. Kidney Int 1977;11:491-504.
100. Tuck ML, Davidson MB, Asp N, et al: Augmented aldosterone and insulin responses to potassium infusion in dogs with renal failure. Kidney Int 1986;30:883-890.
101. DeFronzo RA: Hyperkalemia and hyporeninemic hypoaldosteronism. Kidney Int 1980;17:118-134.
102. Cobbs R, Pepper GM, Torres JG, et al: Adrenocortical insufficiency with normal serum cortisol levels and hyporeninaemia in a patient with acquired immunodeficiency syndrome (AIDS). J Intern Med 1991;230: 179-181.
103. Kalin MF, Poretsky L, Seres DS, et al: Hyporeninemic hypoaldosteronism associated with acquired immune deficiency syndrome. Am J Med 1987;82:1035-1038.
104. Lee FO, Quismorio FP Jr, Troum OM, et al: Mechanisms of hyperkalemia in systemic lupus erythematosus. Arch Intern Med 1988;148:397-401.
105. Whelton A: Renal aspects of treatment with conventional nonsteroidal anti-inflammatory drugs versus cyclooxygenase-2-specific inhibitors. Am J Med 2001;110(Suppl 3A): 33S-42S.
106. Palmer BF: Managing hyperkalemia caused by inhibitors of the renin-angiotensin-aldosterone system. N Engl J Med 2004;351:585-592.
107. Oster JR, Singer I, Fishman LM: Heparin-induced aldosterone suppression and hyperkalemia. Am J Med 1995;98:575-586.
108. Gheno G, Cinetto L, Savarino C, et al: Variations of serum potassium level and risk of hyperkalemia in inpatients receiving low-molecular-weight heparin. Eur J Clin Pharmacol 2003;59:373-377.
109. Batlle D, Itsarayoungyuen K, Arruda JA, et al: Hyperkalemic hyperchloremic metabolic acidosis in sickle cell hemoglobinopathies. Am J Med 1982;72:188-192.
110. DeFronzo RA, Goldberg M, Cooke CR, et al: Investigations into the mechanisms of hyperkalemia following renal transplantation. Kidney Int 1977;11:357-365.
111. Higgins R, Ramaiyan K, Dasgupta T, et al: Hyponatraemia and hyperkalaemia are more frequent in renal transplant recipients treated with tacrolimus than with cyclosporin. Further evidence for differences between cyclosporin and tacrolimus nephrotoxicities. Nephrol Dial Transplant 2004;19:444-450.
112. Woo M, Przepiorka D, Ippoliti C, et al: Toxicities of tacrolimus and cyclosporin A after allogeneic blood stem cell transplantation. Bone Marrow Transplant 1997;20:1095-1098.
113. Batlle DC, Arruda JA, Kurtzman NA: Hyperkalemic distal renal tubular acidosis associated with obstructive uropathy. N Engl J Med 1981;304:373-380.
114. Kleyman TR, Roberts C, Ling BN: A mechanism for pentamidine-induced hyperkalemia: Inhibition of distal nephron sodium transport. Ann Intern Med 1995;122:103-106.
115. Margassery S, Bastani B: Life threatening hyperkalemia and acidosis secondary to trimethoprim-sulfamethoxazole treatment. J Nephrol 2001;14:410-414.
116. Perazella MA: Trimethoprim-induced hyperkalaemia: Clinical data, mechanism, prevention and management. Drug Saf 2000;22:227-236.
117. Halevy J, Gunsherowitz M, Rosenfeld JB: Life-threatening hypokalemia in hospitalized patients. Miner Electrolyte Metab 1988;14:163-166.
118. Fordtran JS, Dietschy JM: Water and electrolyte movement in the intestine. Gastroenterology 1966;50:263-285.
119. Wilcox CS: Metabolic and adverse effects of diuretics. Semin Nephrol 1999;19:557-568.
120. Velazquez H, Giebisch G: Effect of diuretics on specific transport systems: Potassium. Semin Nephrol 1988;8:295-304.
121. Clements JS Jr, Peacock JE Jr: Amphotericin B revisited: Reassessment of toxicity. Am J Med 1990;88: 22N-27N.
122. Neu HC: Carbenicillin and ticarcillin. Med Clin North Am 1982;66:61-77.
123. Blumenfeld JD, Sealey JE, Schlussel Y, et al: Diagnosis and treatment of primary hyperaldosteronism. Ann Intern Med 1994;121:877-885.
124. Whang R, Oei TO, Aikawa JK, et al: Magnesium and potassium interrelationships, experimental and clinical. Acta Med Scand Suppl 1981;647:139-144.
125. Lin SH, Lin YF, Cheema-Dhadli S, et al: Hypercalcaemia and metabolic alkalosis with betel nut chewing: Emphasis on its integrative pathophysiology. Nephrol Dial Transplant 2002;17:708-714.
126. Aldinger KA, Samaan NA: Hypokalemia with hypercalcemia. Prevalence and significance in treatment. Ann Intern Med 1977;87:571-573.
127. Landau D: Potassium handling in health and disease: Lessons from inherited tubulopathies. Pediatr Endocrinol Rev 2004;2:203-208.
128. Fisch C: Relation of electrolyte disturbances to cardiac arrhythmias. Circulation 1973;47:408-419.
129. Surawicz B: Electrolytes and the electrocardiogram. Postgrad Med 1974;55:123-129.
130. Szerlip HM, Weiss J, Singer I: Profound hyperkalemia without electrocardiographic manifestations. Am J Kidney Dis 1986;7:461-465.
131. Dodge HT, Grant RP, Seavey PW: The effect of induced hyperkalemia on the normal and abnormal electrocardiogram. Am Heart J 1953;45:725-740.
132. Weiner ID, Wingo CS: Hyperkalemia: A potential silent killer. J Am Soc Nephrol 1998;9:1535-1543.
133. Tannen RL: Relationship of renal ammonia production and potassium homeostasis. Kidney Int 1977;11:453-465.
134. Szylman P, Better OS, Chaimowitz C, et al: Role of hyperkalemia in the metabolic acidosis of isolated hypoaldosteronism. N Engl J Med 1976;294:361-365.
135. Wong KC, Schafer PG, Schultz JR: Hypokalemia and anesthetic implications. Anesth Analg 1993;77:1238-1260.
136. Steiness E: Diuretics, digitalis and arrhythmias. Acta Med Scand Suppl 1981;647:75-78.
137. Helfant RH: Hypokalemia and arrhythmias. Am J Med 1986;80:13-22.
138. Nordrehaug JE: Malignant arrhythmia in relation to serum potassium in acute myocardial infarction. Am J Cardiol 1985;56:20D-23D.
139. Knochel JP: Rhabdomyolysis and myoglobinuria. Annu Rev Med 1982;33:435-443.
140. Grunfeld C, Chappell DA: Hypokalemia and diabetes mellitus. Am J Med 1983;75:553-554.
141. Jones JW, Sebastian A, Hulter HN, et al: Systemic and renal acid-base effects of chronic dietary potassium depletion in humans. Kidney Int 1982;21:402-410.
142. Zettle RM, West ML, Josse RG, et al: Renal potassium handling during states of low aldosterone bio-activity: A method to differentiate renal and non-renal causes. Am J Nephrol 1987;7:360-366.
143. Beuschlein F, Hammer GD: Ectopic pro-opiomelanocortin syndrome. Endocrinol Metab Clin North Am 2002;31:191-234.
144. Weisberg LS: Potassium homeostasis. In Carlson RW, Geheb MA (eds): Principles and Practice of Medical Intensive Care. Philadelphia, Saunders, 1993.
145. Chamberlain MJ: Emergency treatment of hyperkalaemia. Lancet 1964;18:464-467.
146. Shrager MW: Digitalis intoxication; a review and report of forty cases, with emphasis on etiology. AMA Arch Intern Med 1957;100:881-893.
147. Garcia-Palmieri MR: Reversal of hyperkalemic cardiotoxicity with hypertonic saline. Am Heart J 1962;64:483-488.
148. Allon M, Copkney C: Albuterol and insulin for treatment of hyperkalemia in hemodialysis patients. Kidney Int 1990;38:869-872.
149. Lens XM, Montoliu J, Cases A, et al: Treatment of hyperkalaemia in renal failure: Salbutamol vs. insulin. Nephrol Dial Transplant 1989;4:228-232.
150. Allon M, Dunlay R, Copkney C: Nebulized albuterol for acute hyperkalemia in patients on hemodialysis. Ann Intern Med 1989;110:426-429.
151. Gruy-Kapral C, Emmet M, Santa Nan CA, et al: Effect of single dose resin-cathartic therapy on serum potassium concentration in patients with end-stage renal disease. J Am Soc Nephrol 1998;9:1924-1930.
152. Lillemoe KD, Romolo JL, Hamilton SR, et al: Intestinal necrosis due to sodium polystyrene (Kayexalate) in sorbitol enemas: Clinical and experimental support for the hypothesis. Surgery 1987;101:267-272.

153. Scott TR, Graham SM, Schweitzer EJ, et al: Colonic necrosis following sodium polystyrene sulfonate (Kayexalate)-sorbitol enema in a renal transplant patient. Report of a case and review of the literature. Dis Colon Rectum 1993;36:607-609.
154. Wootton FT, Rhodes DF, Lee WM, et al: Colonic necrosis with Kayexalate-sorbitol enemas after renal transplantation. Ann Intern Med 1989;111:947-949.
155. Gerstman BB, Kirkman R, Platt R: Intestinal necrosis associated with postoperative orally administered sodium polystyrene sulfonate in sorbitol. Am J Kidney Dis 1992;20:159-161.
156. Feig PU, Shook A, Sterns RH: Effect of potassium removal during hemodialysis on the plasma potassium concentration. Nephron 1981;27:25-30.
157. Kruse JA, Carlson RW: Rapid correction of hypokalemia using concentrated intravenous potassium chloride infusions. Arch Intern Med 1990;150:613-617.
158. Sterns RH, Feig PU, Pring M, et al: Disposition of intravenous potassium in anuric man: A kinetic analysis. Kidney Int 1979;15:651-660.
159. Keith NM, Osterberg AE: The tolerance for potassium in severe renal insufficiency: a study of ten cases. J Clin Invest 1947;26:773-783.
160. DeVita MV, Gardenswartz MH, Konecky A, et al: Incidence and etiology of hyponatremia in an intensive care unit. Clin Nephrol 1990;34:163-166.
161. Polderman KH, Schreuder WO, Strack van Schijndel RJ, et al: Hypernatremia in the intensive care unit: An indicator of quality of care? Crit Care Med 1999;27:1105-1108.
162. Knepper M, Gamba G: Urine concentration and dilution. In Brenner B (ed): Brenner and Rector's The Kidney, 7th ed. Philadelphia, Saunders, 2004.
163. Berl T, Verbalis JG: Pathophysiology of water metabolism. In Brenner B (ed): Brenner & Rector's The Kidney, 7th ed. Philadelphia, Saunders, 2004.
164. Verbalis JG: Adaptation to acute and chronic hyponatremia: Implications for symptomatology, diagnosis, and therapy. Semin Nephrol 1998;18:3-19.
165. Lauriat SM, Berl T: The hyponatremic patient: Practical focus on therapy. J Am Soc Nephrol 1997;8:1599-1607.
166. Arieff AI: Hyponatremia, convulsions, respiratory arrest, and permanent brain damage after elective surgery in healthy women. N Engl J Med 1986;314:1529-1535.
167. Sterns RH: Severe symptomatic hyponatremia: Treatment and outcome. A study of 64 cases. Ann Intern Med 1987;107:656-664.
168. Ayus JC, Arieff AI: Pulmonary complications of hyponatremic encephalopathy. Noncardiogenic pulmonary edema and hypercapnic respiratory failure. Chest 1995;107:517-521.
169. Ayus JC, Armstrong D, Arieff AI: Hyponatremia with hypoxia: Effects on brain adaptation, perfusion, and histology in rodents. Kidney Int 2006;69:1319-1325.
170. Weisberg LS: Pseudohyponatremia: A reappraisal. Am J Med 1989;86: 315-318.
171. Illowsky BP, Kirch DG: Polydipsia and hyponatremia in psychiatric patients. Am J Psychiatry 1988;145: 675-683.
172. Fenves AZ, Thomas S, Knochel JP: Beer potomania: Two cases and review of the literature. Clin Nephrol 1996;45: 61-64.
173. Thaler SM, Teitelbaum I, Berl T: "Beer potomania" in non-beer drinkers: Effect of low dietary solute intake. Am J Kidney Dis 1998;31:1028-1031.
174. Beck LH: Hypouricemia in the syndrome of inappropriate secretion of antidiuretic hormone. N Engl J Med 1979;301:528-530.
175. Verbalis JG: Disorders of body water homeostasis. Best Pract Res Clin Endocrinol Metab 2003;17:471-503.
176. Schrier RW, Bichet DG: Osmotic and nonosmotic control of vasopressin release and the pathogenesis of impaired water excretion in adrenal, thyroid, and edematous disorders. J Lab Clin Med 1981;98:1-15.
177. Diederich S, Franzen NF, Bahr V, et al: Severe hyponatremia due to hypopituitarism with adrenal insufficiency: Report on 28 cases. Eur J Endocrinol 2003;148:609-617.
178. DeFronzo RA, Goldberg M, Agus ZS: Normal diluting capacity in hyponatremic patients. Reset osmostat or a variant of the syndrome of inappropriate antidiuretic hormone secretion. Ann Intern Med 1976;84:538-542.
179. Kamel KS, Ethier JH, Richardson RM, et al: Urine electrolytes and osmolality: When and how to use them. Am J Nephrol 1990;10:89-102.
180. Kamel KS, Magner PO, Ethier JH, et al: Urine electrolytes in the assessment of extracellular fluid volume contraction. Am J Nephrol 1989;9:344-347.
181. Palmer BF: Hyponatremia in patients with central nervous system disease: SIADH versus CSW. Trends Endocrinol Metab 2003;14:182-187.
182. Sharabi Y, Illan R, Kamari Y, et al: Diuretic induced hyponatraemia in elderly hypertensive women. J Hum Hypertens 2002;16:631-635.
183. Spital A: Diuretic-induced hyponatremia. Am J Nephrol 1999;19:447-452.
184. Taal M, Luyckx V, Brenner B: Adaptation to nephron loss. In Brenner B (ed): Brenner and Rector's The Kidney, 7th ed. Philadelphia, Saunders, 2004.
185. Schrier RW, Gurevich AK, Cadnapaphornchai MA: Pathogenesis and management of sodium and water retention in cardiac failure and cirrhosis. Semin Nephrol 2001;21:157-172.
186. Sterns RH: The management of symptomatic hyponatremia. Semin Nephrol 1990;10:503-514.
187. Kleinschmidt-DeMasters BK, Norenberg MD: Rapid correction of hyponatremia causes demyelination: Relation to central pontine myelinolysis. Science 1981;211:1068-1070.
188. Martin RJ: Central pontine and extrapontine myelinolysis: The osmotic demyelination syndromes. J Neurol Neurosurg Psychiatry 2004;75(Suppl 3):iii22-28.
189. Gross P: Treatment of severe hyponatremia. Kidney Int 2001;60: 2417-2427.
190. Gross P, Reimann D, Henschkowski J, et al: Treatment of severe hyponatremia: Conventional and novel aspects. J Am Soc Nephrol 2001;12(Suppl 17):S10-14.
191. Adrogue HJ, Madias NE: Hyponatremia. N Engl J Med 2000;342:1581-1589.
192. Steele A, Gowrishankar M, Abrahamson S, et al: Postoperative hyponatremia despite near-isotonic saline infusion: A phenomenon of desalination. Ann Intern Med 1997;126:20-25.
193. Oster JR, Epstein M: Demeclocycline-induced renal failure. Lancet 1977;1:52.
194. Greenberg A, Verbalis JG: Vasopressin receptor antagonists. Kidney Int 2006;69:2124-2130.
195. Elisaf M, Theodorou J, Pappas C, et al: Successful treatment of hyponatremia with angiotensin-converting enzyme inhibitors in patients with congestive heart failure. Cardiology 1995;86: 477-480.
196. Packer M, Medina N, Yushak M: Correction of dilutional hyponatremia in severe chronic heart failure by converting-enzyme inhibition. Ann Intern Med 1984;100:782-789.
197. Palevsky PM, Bhagrath R, Greenberg A: Hypernatremia in hospitalized patients. Ann Intern Med 1996;124:197-203.
198. Snyder NA, Feigal DW, Arieff AI: Hypernatremia in elderly patients. A heterogeneous, morbid, and iatrogenic entity. Ann Intern Med 1987;107:309-319.
199. De Petris L, Luchetti A, Emma F: Cell volume regulation and transport mechanisms across the blood-brain barrier: Implications for the management of hypernatraemic states. Eur J Pediatr 2001;160:71-77.
200. Simmons MA, Adcock EW III, Bard H, et al: Hypernatremia and intracranial hemorrhage in neonates. N Engl J Med 1974;291:6-10.
201. Handy TC, Hanzlick R, Shields LB, et al: Hypernatremia and subdural hematoma in the pediatric age group: Is there a causal relationship? J Forensic Sci 1999;44:1114-1118.
202. Blevins LS Jr, Wand GS: Diabetes insipidus. Crit Care Med 1992;20:69-79.
203. Feldman M: Gastric secretion. In Feldman M (ed): Sleisinger & Fordtran's Gastrointestinal and Liver Diseases. Philadelphia, Elsevier, 2002, p 725.
204. Moder KG, Hurley DL: Fatal hypernatremia from exogenous salt intake: Report of a case and review of the literature. Mayo Clin Proc 1990;65:1587-1594.
205. Kahn T: Hypernatremia with edema. Arch Intern Med 1999;159:93-98.
206. Singer I, Oster JR, Fishman LM: The management of diabetes insipidus in

adults. Arch Intern Med 1997;157:1293-1301.
207. Marsden PA, Halperin ML: Pathophysiological approach to patients presenting with hypernatremia. Am J Nephrol 1985;5:229-235.
208. Pollak MR, Yu ASL: Clinical disturbances of calcium, magnesium, and phosphate metabolism. In Brenner BM (ed): Brenner & Rector's The Kidney, 7th ed. Philadelphia, Saunders, 2004.
209. Zaloga GP: Hypocalcemia in critically ill patients. Crit Care Med 1992;20:251-262.
210. Slatapolsky E, Hruska KA: Disorders of phosphorus, calcium, and magnesium metabolism. In Schrier RW (ed): Diseases of the Kidneys and Urinary Tract, 7th ed. Philadelphia, Lippincott Williams & Wilkins, 2001.
211. Yu ASL: Renal transport of calcium, magnesium, and phosphate. In Brenner BM (ed): Brenner & Rector's The Kidney, 7th ed. Philadelphia, Saunders, 2004.
212. Bushinsky DA, Monk RD: Electrolyte quintet: Calcium. Lancet 1998;352:306-311.
213. Dickerson RN, Alexander KH, Minard G, et al: Accuracy of methods to estimate ionized and "corrected" serum calcium concentrations in critically ill multiple trauma patients receiving specialized nutrition support. JPEN J Parenter Enteral Nutr 2004;28:133-141.
214. Byrnes MC, Huynh K, Helmer SD, et al: A comparison of corrected serum calcium levels to ionized calcium levels among critically ill surgical patients. Am J Surg 2005;189:310-314.
215. Slomp J, van der Voort PH, Gerritsen RT, et al: Albumin-adjusted calcium is not suitable for diagnosis of hyper- and hypocalcemia in the critically ill. Crit Care Med 2003;31:1389-1393.
216. Zaloga GP, Willey S, Tomasic P, et al: Free fatty acids alter calcium binding: A cause for misinterpretation of serum calcium values and hypocalcemia in critical illness. J Clin Endocrinol Metab 1987;64:1010-1014.
217. Chernow B, Zaloga G, McFadden E, et al: Hypocalcemia in critically ill patients. Crit Care Med 1982;10:848-851.
218. Desai TK, Carlson RW, Geheb MA: Prevalence and clinical implications of hypocalcemia in acutely ill patients in a medical intensive care setting. Am J Med 1988;84:209-214.
219. Hastbacka J, Pettila V: Prevalence and predictive value of ionized hypocalcemia among critically ill patients. Acta Anaesthesiol Scand 2003;47:1264-1269.
220. Zivin JR, Gooley T, Zager RA, et al: Hypocalcemia: A pervasive metabolic abnormality in the critically ill. Am J Kidney Dis 2001;37:689-698.
221. Vivien B, Langeron O, Morell E, et al: Early hypocalcemia in severe trauma. Crit Care Med 2005;33:1946-1952.
222. Zaloga GP, Chernow B: The multifactorial basis for hypocalcemia during sepsis. Studies of the parathyroid hormone-vitamin D axis. Ann Intern Med 1987;107:36-41.
223. Carlstedt F, Lind L, Rastad J, et al: Parathyroid hormone and ionized calcium levels are related to the severity of illness and survival in critically ill patients. Eur J Clin Invest 1998;28:898-903.
224. Brasier AR, Nussbaum SR: Hungry bone syndrome: Clinical and biochemical predictors of its occurrence after parathyroid surgery. Am J Med 1988;84:654-660.
225. Denlinger JK, Nahrwold ML, Gibbs PS, et al: Hypocalcaemia during rapid blood transfusion in anaesthetized man. Br J Anaesth 1976;48:995-1000.
226. Meier-Kriesche HU, Finkel KW, Gitomer JJ, et al: Unexpected severe hypocalcemia during continuous venovenous hemodialysis with regional citrate anticoagulation. Am J Kidney Dis 1999;33:e8.
227. Meier-Kriesche HU, Gitomer J, Finkel K, et al: Increased total to ionized calcium ratio during continuous venovenous hemodialysis with regional citrate anticoagulation. Crit Care Med 2001;29:748-752.
228. Weinstein R: Hypocalcemic toxicity and atypical reactions in therapeutic plasma exchange. J Clin Apher 2001;16:210-211.
229. Filho AJ, Lassman MN: Severe hyperphosphatemia induced by a phosphate-containing oral laxative. Ann Pharmacother 1996;30:141-143.
230. Fine A, Patterson J: Severe hyperphosphatemia following phosphate administration for bowel preparation in patients with renal failure: Two cases and a review of the literature. Am J Kidney Dis 1997;29:103-105.
231. Korzets A, Dicker D, Chaimoff C, et al: Life-threatening hyperphosphatemia and hypocalcemic tetany following the use of fleet enemas. J Am Geriatr Soc 1992;40:620-621.
232. Marraffa JM, Hui A, Stork CM: Severe hyperphosphatemia and hypocalcemia following the rectal administration of a phosphate-containing Fleet pediatric enema. Pediatr Emerg Care 2004;20:453-456.
233. Shrestha SM, Berry JL, Davies M, et al: Biphasic hypercalcemia in severe rhabdomyolysis: Serial analysis of PTH and vitamin D metabolites. A case report and literature review. Am J Kidney Dis 2004;43:e31-35.
234. Ammori BJ, Barclay GR, Larvin M, et al: Hypocalcemia in patients with acute pancreatitis: A putative role for systemic endotoxin exposure. Pancreas 2003;26:213-217.
235. Bhattacharya SK, Luther RW, Pate JW, et al: Soft tissue calcium and magnesium content in acute pancreatitis in the dog: Calcium accumulation, a mechanism for hypocalcemia in acute pancreatitis. J Lab Clin Med 1985;105:422-427.
236. Condon JR, Ives D, Knight MJ, et al: The aetiology of hypocalcaemia in acute pancreatitis. Br J Surg 1975;62:115-118.
237. Hauser CJ, Kamrath RO, Sparks J, et al: Calcium homeostasis in patients with acute pancreatitis. Surgery 1983;94:830-835.
238. Izquierdo R, Bermes E Jr, Sandberg L, et al: Serum calcium metabolism in acute experimental pancreatitis. Surgery 1985;98:1031-1037.
239. Warshaw AL, Lee KH, Napier TW, et al: Depression of serum calcium by increased plasma free fatty acids in the rat: A mechanism for hypocalcemia in acute pancreatitis. Gastroenterology 1985;89:814-820.
240. Dettelbach MA, Deftos LJ, Stewart AF: Intraperitoneal free fatty acids induce severe hypocalcemia in rats: A model for the hypocalcemia of pancreatitis. J Bone Miner Res 1990;5:1249-1255.
241. Maalouf NM, Heller HJ, Odvina CV, et al: Bisphosphonate-induced hypocalcemia: Report of 3 cases and review of literature. Endocr Pract 2006;12:48-53.
242. Zaloga GP: Ionized hypocalcemia during sepsis. Crit Care Med 2000;28:266-268.
243. Carlstedt F, Eriksson M, Kiiski R, et al: Hypocalcemia during porcine endotoxemic shock: Effects of calcium administration. Crit Care Med 2000;28:2909-2914.
244. Zaloga GP, Washburn D, Black KW, et al: Human sepsis increases lymphocyte intracellular calcium. Crit Care Med 1993;21:196-202.
245. Lind L, Carlstedt F, Rastad J, et al: Hypocalcemia and parathyroid hormone secretion in critically ill patients. Crit Care Med 2000;28:93-99.
246. Muller B, Becker KL, Kranzlin M, et al: Disordered calcium homeostasis of sepsis: Association with calcitonin precursors. Eur J Clin Invest 2000;30:823-831.
247. Hebert P, Mehta N, Wang J, et al: Functional magnesium deficiency in critically ill patients identified using a magnesium-loading test. Crit Care Med 1997;25:749-755.
248. Lind L, Ljunghall S: Critical care hypercalcemia—a hyperparathyroid state. Exp Clin Endocrinol 1992;100:148-151.
249. Forster J, Querusio L, Burchard KW, et al: Hypercalcemia in critically ill surgical patients. Ann Surg 1985;202:512-518.
250. Walls J, Ratcliffe WA, Howell A, et al: Parathyroid hormone and parathyroid hormone-related protein in the investigation of hypercalcaemia in two hospital populations. Clin Endocrinol (Oxf) 1994;41:407-413.
251. Bundred NJ, Walls J, Ratcliffe WA: Parathyroid hormone-related protein, bone metastases and hypercalcaemia of malignancy. Ann R Coll Surg Engl 1996;78:354-358.
252. Kremer R, Shustik C, Tabak T, et al: Parathyroid-hormone-related peptide in hematologic malignancies. Am J Med 1996;100:406-411.
253. Breslau NA, McGuire JL, Zerwekh JE, et al: Hypercalcemia associated with increased serum calcitriol levels in three patients with lymphoma. Ann Intern Med 1984;100:1-6.
254. Seymour JF, Gagel RF, Hagemeister FB, et al: Calcitriol production in hypercalcemic and normocalcemic patients with non-Hodgkin lymphoma. Ann Intern Med 1994;121:633-640.
255. Meneghini LF, Oster JR, Camacho JR, et al: Hypercalcemia in association with acute renal failure and

rhabdomyolysis. Case report and literature review. Miner Electrolyte Metab 1993;19:1-16.
256. Sperling LS, Tumlin JA: Case report: delayed hypercalcemia after rhabdomyolysis-induced acute renal failure. Am J Med Sci 1996;311:186-188.
257. Akmal M, Bishop JE, Telfer N, et al: Hypocalcemia and hypercalcemia in patients with rhabdomyolysis with and without acute renal failure. J Clin Endocrinol Metab 1986;63:137-142.
258. Hadjis T, Grieff M, Lockhat D, et al: Calcium metabolism in acute renal failure due to rhabdomyolysis. Clin Nephrol 1993;39:22-27.
259. Llach F, Felsenfeld AJ, Haussler MR: The pathophysiology of altered calcium metabolism in rhabdomyolysis-induced acute renal failure. Interactions of parathyroid hormone, 25-hydroxycholecalciferol, and 1,25-dihydroxycholecalciferol. N Engl J Med 1981;305:117-123.
260. Meythaler JM, Tuel SM, Cross LL: Successful treatment of immobilization hypercalcemia using calcitonin and etidronate. Arch Phys Med Rehabil 1993;74:316-319.
261. Stewart AF, Adler M, Byers CM, et al: Calcium homeostasis in immobilization: An example of resorptive hypercalciuria. N Engl J Med 1982;306:1136-1140.
262. Kiewiet RM, Ponssen HH, Janssens EN, et al: Ventricular fibrillation in hypercalcaemic crisis due to primary hyperparathyroidism. Neth J Med 2004;62:94-96.
263. Shah AP, Lopez A, Wachsner RY, et al: Sinus node dysfunction secondary to hyperparathyroidism. J Cardiovasc Pharmacol Ther 2004;9:145-147.
264. Camus C, Charasse C, Jouannic-Montier I, et al: Calcium free hemodialysis: Experience in the treatment of 33 patients with severe hypercalcemia. Intensive Care Med 1996;22:116-121.
265. Major P, Lortholary A, Hon J, et al: Zoledronic acid is superior to pamidronate in the treatment of hypercalcemia of malignancy: A pooled analysis of two randomized, controlled clinical trials. J Clin Oncol 2001;19:558-567.
266. Agus ZS: Hypomagnesemia. J Am Soc Nephrol 1999;10:1616-1622.
267. Reinhart RA, Desbiens NA: Hypomagnesemia in patients entering the ICU. Crit Care Med 1985;13:506-507.
268. Ryzen E, Wagers PW, Singer FR, et al: Magnesium deficiency in a medical ICU population. Crit Care Med 1985;13:19-21.
269. Laurant P, Touyz RM: Physiological and pathophysiological role of magnesium in the cardiovascular system: Implications in hypertension. J Hypertens 2000;18:1177-1191.
270. Fine KD, Santa Ana CA, Porter JL, et al: Intestinal absorption of magnesium from food and supplements. J Clin Invest 1991;88:396-402.
271. Marier JR: Magnesium content of the food supply in the modern-day world. Magnesium 1986;5:1-8.
272. Pointillart A, Denis I, Colin C: Effects of dietary vitamin D on magnesium absorption and bone mineral contents in pigs on normal magnesium intakes. Magnes Res 1995;8:19-26.
273. Tong GM, Rude RK: Magnesium deficiency in critical illness. J Intensive Care Med 2005;20:3-17.
274. Escuela MP, Guerra M, Anon JM, et al: Total and ionized serum magnesium in critically ill patients. Intensive Care Med 2005;31:151-156.
275. Huijgen HJ, Soesan M, Sanders R, et al: Magnesium levels in critically ill patients. What should we measure? Am J Clin Pathol 2000;114:688-695.
276. Soliman HM, Mercan D, Lobo SS, et al: Development of ionized hypomagnesemia is associated with higher mortality rates. Crit Care Med 2003;31:1082-1087.
277. Deheinzelin D, Negri EM, Tucci MR, et al: Hypomagnesemia in critically ill cancer patients: A prospective study of predictive factors. Braz J Med Biol Res 2000;33:1443-1448.
278. Alexandridis G, Liberopoulos E, Elisaf M: Aminoglycoside-induced reversible tubular dysfunction. Pharmacology 2003;67:118-120.
279. Schilsky RL, Anderson T: Hypomagnesemia and renal magnesium wasting in patients receiving cisplatin. Ann Intern Med 1979;90:929-931.
280. Rubeiz GJ, Thill-Baharozian M, Hardie D, et al: Association of hypomagnesemia and mortality in acutely ill medical patients. Crit Care Med 1993;21:203-209.
281. Whang R, Flink EB, Dyckner T, et al: Magnesium depletion as a cause of refractory potassium repletion. Arch Intern Med 1985;145:1686-1689.
282. Whang R, Whang DD, Ryan MP: Refractory potassium repletion. A consequence of magnesium deficiency. Arch Intern Med 1992;152:40-45.
283. Onishi S, Yoshino S: Cathartic-induced fatal hypermagnesemia in the elderly. Intern Med 2006;45:207-210.
284. Fitzgerald F: Clinical hypophosphatemia. Annu Rev Med 1978;29:177-189.
285. Knochel JP: The pathophysiology and clinical characteristics of severe hypophosphatemia. Arch Intern Med 1977;137:203-220.
286. Lotz M, Zisman E, Bartter FC: Evidence for a phosphorus-depletion syndrome in man. N Engl J Med 1968;278:409-415.
287. Lentz RD, Brown DM, Kjellstrand CM: Treatment of severe hypophosphatemia. Ann Intern Med 1978;89:941-944.
288. de Menezes FS, Leite HP, Fernandez J, et al: Hypophosphatemia in children hospitalized within an intensive care unit. J Intensive Care Med 2006;21:235-239.
289. Zazzo JF, Troche G, Ruel P, et al: High incidence of hypophosphatemia in surgical intensive care patients: Efficacy of phosphorus therapy on myocardial function. Intensive Care Med 1995;21:826-831.
290. Shor R, Halabe A, Rishver S, et al: Severe hypophosphatemia in sepsis as a mortality predictor. Ann Clin Lab Sci 2006;36:67-72.
291. Giovannini I, Chiarla C, Nuzzo G: Pathophysiologic and clinical correlates of hypophosphatemia and the relationship with sepsis and outcome in postoperative patients after hepatectomy. Shock 2002;18:111-115.
292. Laaban JP, Grateau G, Psychoyos I, et al: Hypophosphatemia induced by mechanical ventilation in patients with chronic obstructive pulmonary disease. Crit Care Med 1989;17:1115-1120.
293. Marik PE, Bedigian MK: Refeeding hypophosphatemia in critically ill patients in an intensive care unit. A prospective study. Arch Surg 1996;131:1043-1047.
294. Zamkoff KW, Kirshner JJ: Marked hypophosphatemia associated with acute myelomonocytic leukemia. Indirect evidence of phosphorus uptake by leukemic cells. Arch Intern Med 1980;140:1523-1524.
295. Steiner M, Steiner B, Wilhelm S, et al: Severe hypophosphatemia during hematopoietic reconstitution after allogeneic peripheral blood stem cell transplantation. Bone Marrow Transplant 2000;25:1015-1016.
296. Better OS: Traumatic rhabdomyolysis ("crush syndrome")—updated 1989. Isr J Med Sci 1989;25:69-72.
297. Birkenfeld AL, Gollasch M, Gobel U, et al: The phosphorus connection—a puzzling business. Nephrol Dial Transplant 2004;19:1643-1645.
298. Kebler R, McDonald FD, Cadnapaphornchai P: Dynamic changes in serum phosphorus levels in diabetic ketoacidosis. Am J Med 1985;79:571-576.
299. O'Connor LR, Klein KL, Bethune JE: Hyperphosphatemia in lactic acidosis. N Engl J Med 1977;297:707-709.
300. Fass R, Do S, Hixson LJ: Fatal hyperphosphatemia following Fleet Phospo-Soda in a patient with colonic ileus. Am J Gastroenterol 1993;88:929-932.
301. Post SS: Hyperphosphatemic hypocalcemic coma caused by hypertonic sodium phosphate (fleet) enema intoxication. J Clin Gastroenterol 1997;24:192.
302. Ball CL, Tobler K, Ross BC, et al: Spurious hyperphosphatemia due to sample contamination with heparinized saline from an indwelling catheter. Clin Chem Lab Med 2004;42:107-108.
303. Suchin EJ, Cizman B, Connolly BR, et al: Pseudohyperphosphatemia in a hyperphosphatemic hemodialysis patient. Am J Kidney Dis 2002;40:E18.
304. Isotalo PA, Halil A, Green M, et al: Metastatic calcification of the cardiac conduction system with heart block: An under-reported entity in chronic renal failure patients. J Forensic Sci 2000;45:1335-1338.
305. Kirschbaum B: The acidosis of exogenous phosphate intoxication. Arch Intern Med 1998;158:405-408.

Chapter 59

Acute Diabetic Emergencies, Hypoglycemia, and Glycemic Control

Michael Chansky and Ghada Haddad

Diabetes is a group of diseases marked by high levels of blood glucose resulting from defects in insulin production, insulin action, or both. As of 2005 an estimated 7% of the population, or 20.8 million people, had diabetes. The estimated prevalence of diabetes in patients age 60 years or older is 10.3 million, or 20.9%. Even more importantly is the emerging epidemic of type 2 diabetes in children and adolescents. A few years ago, less than 3% of children had type 2 diabetes. It is now estimated that 45% of children with newly diagnosed diabetes mellitus have type 2 diabetes. The increase in prevalence in this age group is directly related to the growing epidemic of obesity, resulting from sedentary lifestyle and high caloric intake.[1] Diabetes was the sixth leading cause of death listed on U.S. death certificates in 2002, but it is likely underreported. Overall, the risk of death among people with diabetes is about twice that of people without diabetes of similar age. Despite rising awareness regarding the importance of diagnosis and therapy, the age-adjusted hospital discharge rate for diabetic ketoacidosis has shown a slight increasing trend. Estimated total diabetes cost in the United States in 2002 was $132 billion.[2] The overall health care environment mandates a coordinated effort of the health care team to improve earlier diagnosis, improve outcomes, and lower costs.

This chapter discusses the diagnosis and management of critically ill adults admitted with or who develop acute diabetic emergencies, management guidelines, and the importance of aggressive glucose control in the intensive care setting. References specific to the care of pediatric patients with diabetic ketoacidosis are available and are therefore not discussed in this chapter.[3-5]

DIABETIC KETOACIDOSIS AND HYPEROSMOLAR HYPERGLYCEMIC STATE

Diabetic ketoacidosis (DKA) and hyperosmolar hyperglycemic state (HHS) are the most serious acute life-threatening complications of diabetes mellitus. Although often described as separate entities, they differ mainly by epidemiology, degree of dehydration, and presence of ketoacidosis. Both conditions are characterized by hyperglycemia, which initiates a significant osmotic diuresis with resultant dehydration and hyperosmolarity, and have a similar approach to diagnosis and treatment. The mortality rate in patients with DKA is less than 5% in experienced centers, whereas the mortality rate of patients with HHS still remains high at approximately 15%.[6] The prognosis of both conditions is substantially worsened at the extremes of age.[7]

Type 1 diabetes mellitus is characterized by autoimmune β-cell destruction, whereas type 2 diabetes has a duel defect of insulin resistance and a relative β-cell secretory deficiency. Both types 1 and 2 diabetics can experience DKA and HHS, but the incidence varies. Patients with an absolute insulin deficiency (type 1) have a higher incidence of DKA than individuals with type 2 diabetes. An absolute insulin deficit leads to production of ketone bodies and metabolic acidosis in DKA, bringing these patients to early medical attention. Patients with HHS appear to have enough circulating portal vein insulin to prevent ketosis but not hyperglycemia. These patients develop insidious profound dehydration in the relative absence of ketonemia. Acidosis, when present, tends to be a combination of lactate and ketones. Most severe hyperglycemic states are diagnosed and initially treated in the emergency department (ED) and then require an intensive care setting.

INCIDENCE AND EPIDEMIOLOGY

Recent data from the United States indicate there were approximately 115,000 hospitalizations for DKA in 2003, with an incidence ranging from 4.6 to 8 per 1000 diabetics.[8] There has been a trend toward increased hospitalization rates. A significant proportion of DKA occurs in patients with type 2 diabetes,[9,10] and approximately 75% of DKA cases occur in adults. The incidence of HHS accounts for less than 1% of all primary diabetic admissions, primarily affects patients with type 2 diabetes, and has a mortality rate ranging from 10% to 50% related to severe underlying illness.[11,12] Mortality is increased in patients older than 65 and in those who present with or develop shock and coma.

Accurate incidence of these syndromes is complicated by considerable overlap that may not be reflected in reported databases. Furthermore, ketosis may go undetected in hyperglycemic patients with a mild metabolic acidosis because β-hydroxybutyrate, the major ketone body formed early in DKA, is not measured by the standard nitroprusside reaction. Numerous studies show that episodes of DKA and HHS are more common in poorly compliant patients, with major risk factors including infrequent or no self-monitoring of glucose at home, high HgbA1c, frequency of omitting insulin[12] or diabetic medicines, and extremes of age.[13] Additional risk factors include poor economic background, lack of insurance or minority status, drug abuse, depression, and the presence of an eating disorder.[7] HHS has a high incidence among elderly institutionalized patients or among those with cognitive deficits who have decreased access to free water and in whom recognition of symptoms may be delayed.

Pathogenesis

DKA and HHS both develop as a consequence of a complete or relative deficiency of insulin, in combination with an excess secretion of the counterregulatory hormones: growth hormone; catecholamines; cortisol; and, most importantly, glucagon in DKA (Fig. 59-1). Insulin, the primary anabolic hormone, is intimately involved in metabolism and storage of glucose, protein, and fat. The relative or complete lack of insulin and excess counterregulatory hormones results in hyperglycemia (because of excess production and underutilization of glucose), osmotic diuresis, prerenal azotemia, severe dehydration in HHS and DKA, a wide-anion gap metabolic acidosis, and ketone formation in DKA (Table 59-1).[7] The reason for lack of ketonemia in HHS is not definitively known, although theories include glucagon resistance and presence of enough portal vein insulin to inhibit hepatic production of ketones but not prevent hyperglycemia.[12]

Insulin

Insulin is normally secreted by the endocrine pancreas β-cells in response to glucose ingestion. Insulin acts at the hepatic level, facilitating uptake of glucose and its conversion to storage glycogen while inhibiting glycogenolysis

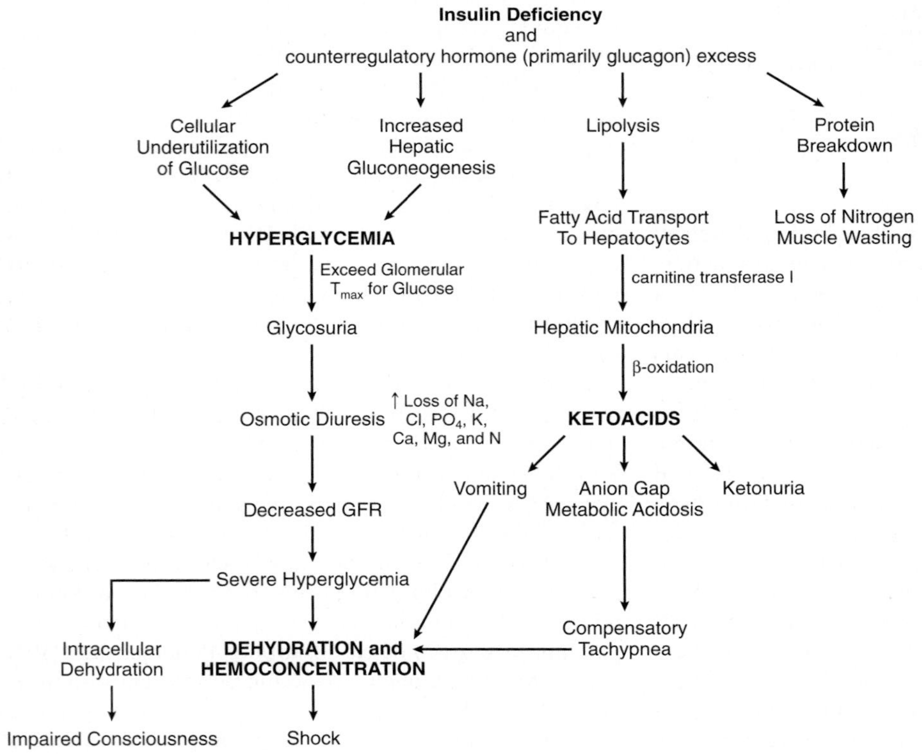

Figure 59-1. Pathogenesis of diabetic ketoacidosis, secondary to relative insulin deficiency and counterregulatory hormone excess. (From Chansky ME, Lubkin CL: Diabetic ketoacidosis. In Tintinalli J, Kelen G, Stapczynski J [eds]: Emergency Medicine, A Comprehensive Study Guide, 6th ed. New York, McGraw-Hill, 2004, p 1290, with permission.)

Table 59-1. Diagnostic Criteria for DKA and HHS

	DKA			
	Mild	Moderate	Severe	HHS
Plasma glucose (mg/dL)	>250	>250	>250	>600
Arterial pH	7.25-7.3	7-7.24	<7	>7.3
Serum bicarbonate (mEq/L)	15-18	10 to <15	<10	>15
Urine ketones*	Positive	Positive	Positive	Small
Serum ketones*	Positive	Positive	Positive	Small
Effective serum osmolality (mOsm/kg)†	Variable	Variable	Variable	>300
Anion gap	>10	>12	>12	Variable
Alteration in sensoria or mental obtundation	Alert	Alert/drowsy	Stupor/coma	

*Nitroprusside reaction method.
†Calculation: 2[measured Na^+] + [glucose]/18.
DKA, diabetic ketoacidosis; HHS, hyperglycemic hyperosmolar syndrome.

and suppressing gluconeogenesis. Insulin affects lipid metabolism by increasing hepatic and adipose storage by producing triglycerides from free fatty acids and glycerol while inhibiting the breakdown of triglycerides. Insulin stimulates uptake of amino acids into skeletal muscle protein while preventing release of amino acids from muscle and hepatic protein sources.

As pancreatic β-cell reserve falters, hyperglycemia can no longer trigger physiologically significant insulin secretion. This loss of the physiologic effect of insulin leads to cellular starvation and secretion of catabolic hormones. Catabolic hormone secretion results in increased gluconeogenesis and breakdown of glycogen, protein, and adipose stores in an attempt to produce a usable cellular fuel. The combination of lack of insulin (underutilization of glucose) and effects of the catabolic hormones (overproduction of glucose) results in hyperglycemia and varying degrees of ketonemia and metabolic acidosis.

Counterregulatory Hormones

Insulin counterregulatory hormones are secreted as a result of stress, illness, or as a consequence of insulin deficiency itself. Elevation of glucagon, catecholamines, cortisol, and growth hormone lead to increased hepatic and renal glucose production and impaired glucose utilization in peripheral tissues, which result in hyperglycemia and parallel changes in osmolarity of the extracellular space. Glucagon is the primary counterregulatory hormone in the pathogenesis of DKA, stimulating both hepatic glycogenolysis and gluconeogenesis.

The combination of insulin deficiency and increased counterregulatory hormones in DKA also leads to the release of free fatty acids into the circulation from adipose tissue and to the unrestrained hepatic fatty acid oxidation to ketone bodies (beta-hydroxybutyrate [BHB] and acetoacetate [AcAc]), with resulting ketonemia and metabolic acidosis. Glucagon is primarily responsible for fatty acid oxidation, exerting its effects by assisting fatty acid transport via the carnitine palmitoyltransferase system located on hepatic mitochondria. The two primary ketone bodies are in equilibrium: $AcAc + NADH \rightleftharpoons BHB + NAD$. Acetoacetate is metabolized to acetone, a third major ketone body present in DKA. These ketoacids are weak acids that overwhelm the body's protein and bicarbonate buffering capacity, leading to an anion gap metabolic acidosis. HHS may differ because circulating portal insulin levels are too low to assist systematic glucose utilization but just adequate enough to prevent lipolysis and ketogenesis.[8]

When persistent hyperglycemia exceeds the renal T_{max} for glucose, an osmotic diuresis is promoted. Loss of sodium, chloride, potassium, magnesium, and phosphate commences, with a subsequent decrease in GFR resulting in more severe hyperglycemia, hyperosmolarity, and dehydration. Significant volume depletion in DKA and HHS activates the renin-angiotensin-aldosterone system, which further exacerbates renal potassium losses. In DKA the kidney retains chloride in exchange for the ketoanions being excreted. This loss of ketoanions represents a loss of bicarbonate, which, when coupled with normal saline (NS) infusion, results in a superimposed hyperchloremic acidosis. Hyperchloremic acidosis can be detected by noting a bicarbonate concentration (HCO_3^-) lower than explainable by the amount the anion gap has increased.

The geriatric population with or without previously recognized diabetes is prone to develop HHS for several reasons. HHS is initiated by a glucosuric diuresis. The euvolemic patient with a normal GFR and an active thirst mechanism can maintain serum glucose levels at the glomular T_{max} for glucose. As intravascular volume contracts and GFR decreases, the safety valve to eliminate glucose is lost, resulting in rising glucose concentration. Excessive water loss in proportion to sodium leads to hyperosmolarity.[11] The kidney itself undergoes many age-related changes that collectively increase the likelihood of developing severe dehydration and hyperosmolarity. An age-related reduction in renal concentrating ability occurs, and mentally impaired patients cannot act on a thirst stimulus.

Renal mass declines, as does GFR, with renal function falling 30% to 50% by age 70 even before coexisting diseases such as hypertensive or diabetic nephropathy are considered.

Precipitating Factors in the Development of DKA and HHS

The most common precipitating factor in the development of DKA or HHS is infection.[8,12] New-onset diabetes may account for up to 30% of patients presenting in DKA, and HHS may be the initial presentation of diabetes in 30% to 40% of this unique patient population. Other factors known to precipitate DKA and HHS include omission of daily insulin injections and a variety of other stressful events such as infection, stroke, myocardial infarction (MI), trauma, pregnancy, hyperthyroidism, pancreatitis, pulmonary embolism, surgery, heat illness, gastrointestinal hemorrhage, substance abuse, and steroid use. Studies have shown that errors in insulin usage are a much more common precipitant of DKA than previously thought, especially in the younger population.[13] Undiagnosed diabetes in the elderly in chronic care facilities is associated with HHS because early symptoms of the disease process often go unrecognized. In approximately 25% of people who develop DKA, no precipitating cause is found.[14]

Clinical Manifestations

The clinical manifestations of HHS and DKA are related directly to the primary metabolic derangements: hyperglycemia and volume depletion with the addition of metabolic acidosis in patients with DKA.[15] Hyperglycemia causes an increased osmotic load with movement of intracellular water into the vascular compartment. The ensuing osmotic diuresis gradually leads to volume loss in addition to renal losses of sodium, chloride, potassium, phosphorus, calcium, and magnesium. Initially able patients may compensate by increasing their fluid intake. In this initial period, polyuria and polydipsia are usually the only symptoms until ketonemia and acidosis develop in DKA or neurologic symptoms develop in HHS.

In DKA, as acidosis progresses the patient develops a compensatory augmented ventilatory response. Increased ventilation is stimulated physiologically by acidemia to diminish the pCO_2 and thus counter the metabolic acidosis. The acidosis combined with the effects of PGI_2 and PGE_2 lead to peripheral vasodilation despite profound levels of volume depletion. Prostaglandin release is also believed to play a role in the often unexplained nausea, vomiting, and abdominal pain that are seen frequently at presentation, especially in children. Vomiting, in addition to the volume depletion, triggers stimulation of aldosterone, exacerbates the potassium losses, and contributes to rapidly progressive volume loss, weakness, and weight loss. As volume depletion progresses, poor absorption of subcutaneous insulin renders its administration ineffective.

Abnormal vital signs may be the only significant physical findings at presentation. Tachycardia and either orthostasis or hypotension may be present. With severe acidemia, Kussmaul respirations (pattern of deep, sighing respirations ± increased respiratory rate) may be observed, or simply an increased respiratory rate noted. On rare occasions the patient may actually present with the chief complaint of shortness of breath. Acetone produces a characteristic fruity odor on the breath detectable by some observers. Infection should be suspected even in the absence of fever. Acute cardiac ischemia or infarction may precipitate DKA or HHS. Diabetics are at risk for silent ischemia, and classic cardiac symptoms may not be present. Elevated creatinine phosphokinase may be associated with rhabdomyolysis, whereas elevated troponins remain specific for acute MI in this setting. Abdominal pain and tenderness may be present and related to gastric dilation, ileus, pancreatitis, or a true surgical emergency such as mesenteric ischemia. Although acute hyperlipidemia may cause pancreatitis in DKA, elevations of traditional markers for pancreatitis (lipase, amylase) may occur in DKA without pancreatitis and are of limited value. In patients with abdominal pain it is prudent to suspect acute pancreatitis in patients with markedly elevated amylase and lipase and to consider computed tomography (CT) of the abdomen to confirm the diagnosis.[16] Mental confusion or coma may be apparent at the time of presentation, although these symptoms are more likely with a serum osmolarity of greater than 340 mOsm/L. If serum osmolarity is less than 340 mOsm/L, one should suspect another etiology of coma than DKA or HHS.

HHS has a reputation for being underrecognized prior to presentation, and the high mortality rate is likely caused by a delay in presentation, failure to treat aggressively, and the high incidence of serious underlying disease.[12,17-19] Unlike in DKA, many patients who develop HHS experience polyuria and polydipsia for days or weeks before coming to medical attention.[20] Insidious dehydration progresses until mental status is altered. The most common reason patients are brought to medical attention is diminished or complete lack of responsiveness.[17] This delay explains the increased severity of dehydration, as compared with patients with DKA. On average, patients diagnosed with DKA present within 3 days of symptom onset, whereas patients with HHS typically present after an average of 12 days.[18,21]

The severity of dehydration in HHS depends on multiple factors including underlying illnesses. Standard signs of dehydration such as poor skin turgor and dry mucous membranes may not be evident. Tachycardia, tachypnea, and hypotension may be present, and patients appear debilitated, weakened, and ill. Silent myocardial ischemia must be considered. Abdominal pain is much less frequent than in DKA, and nausea and vomiting may not be present.[22] Laboratory values may not correctly reflect the degree of dehydration,[21] and in both conditions urine output is maintained by the glucose-mediated osmotic diuresis, which protects against acute renal failure, but may contribute to the underestimation of volume depletion. The degree of altered mental status does correspond with the degree and rate of development of hyperosmolarity. Many neurological symptoms have been described including seizures, hemiparesis, confusion, and coma.[19] A wide variety of severe neurologic findings have been reported: bilateral or unilateral motor hyperreflexia, aphasia, fasciculations, central hyperthermia, hemianopsia, nystagmus, visual loss, visual hallucinations, quadriplegia, dysphagia, and urinary retention.[12]

Differential Diagnosis

DKA and HHS tend to present in different patient populations. Patients with HHS tend to be older, have a more prolonged course, and have prominent mental status changes. Although the exact definition of DKA is variable, patients with a blood glucose greater than 250 mg/dL, bicarbonate level of less than 15 mEq/L, and an arterial or venous pH of less than 7.3 with ketonemia confirms the diagnosis.[7,23] HHS is defined by a serum glucose level of greater than 600 mg/dL, plasma osmolarity greater than 320 mOsm/L, and absent or mild ketoacidosis.[7,19,23]

The differential diagnosis of metabolic coma or change of mental status in a diabetic patient includes HHS, DKA, hypoglycemia, alcoholic ketoacidosis, lactic acidosis, and other causes of wide-anion gap metabolic acidosis. The simplest yet crucial test appropriate for all patients with altered mental status is a fingerstick blood glucose measurement to confirm hypoglycemia or hyperglycemia. Rapid diagnosis can be made in the ED using a glucose reagent strip, urine test strip for ketones, and venous blood gas analysis.[15]

Current evidence indicates that venous and arterial pH have sufficient correlation to be used interchangeably and that arterial blood gas analysis rarely influences the initial treatment and final disposition decisions in patients with DKA.[24-26] It appears that the mean pCO_2 is also significantly correlated between arterial and capillary samples[27] and could be used in acid base analysis. Clinically, an elevated glucose level by reagent strip, presence of ketonuria on dipstick, and a typical metabolic acidosis pattern on the venous blood gas (low pH, low pCO_2) all but confirm the diagnosis of DKA.

Once an anion gap metabolic acidosis is confirmed via serum electrolytes, the differential diagnosis of DKA includes any entity that causes a high-anion-gap metabolic acidosis. These include alcoholic or starvation ketoacidosis, uremia, lactic acidosis, and various ingestions (e.g., methanol, ethylene glycol, aspirin).[28] Alcoholic and starvation ketosis tends to be milder, serum glucose level is low to normal or mildly elevated, and the history is confirmatory. If ingestion cannot be excluded, serum osmolarity or drug-level testing is indicated. Lactic acidosis may occur simultaneously with DKA and HHS, and a serum lactate may be helpful. Type B lactic acidosis rarely occurs in diabetics taking metformin with new-onset renal insufficiency.

The differential diagnosis of altered mental status in the elderly is extensive and focuses primarily on metabolic versus structural etiologies. HHS must be considered when an elderly patient presents to the ED with coma, change in mental status, or severe dehydration. Metabolic etiologies to consider include, but are not limited to, hypoglycemia, electrolyte abnormalities, hypothermia, hyperthermia, myxedema, ingestions, carbon monoxide, acidosis, hepatic failure, and uremia. Structural abnormalities include central nervous system (CNS) hemorrhage, infection, stroke with edema, and trauma. As emphasized earlier, an elevated fingerstick blood glucose level in the setting of altered mental status and dehydration places HHS high on the differential diagnosis and should initiate immediate appropriate therapy.

Diagnostic Criteria and Laboratory Findings

All critically ill patients presenting to the ED or who are already hospitalized with altered mental status, hypotension, nausea and vomiting, acid-base disturbances, acute neurologic deficits, respiratory distress, suspected acute abdominal process, cardiac ischemia, substance abuse, hypothermia, hyperthermia, or infection should be promptly screened via point-of-care testing for hyperglycemia or hypoglycemia. The presence of hyperglycemia should prompt an appropriate history and examination aimed at confirming the diagnosis, identifying precipitating causes, and beginning therapy. Immediate testing for DKA and HHS includes an initial venous (not arterial) blood gas,[24-26] urine dip for glucose and ketones, electrocardiogram (ECG), and definitive blood work and initiation of NS resuscitation. A recent study demonstrated accurate diagnosis of DKA at triage via point-of-care testing for beta-hydroxybutyrate in hyperglycemic patients.[9] A basic metabolic profile is important because it allows calculation of anion gap, serum osmolarity, and initial potassium concentration, which guide further therapy. Table 59-1 lists diagnostic criteria for decompensated diabetes. In addition, a chest radiograph; blood and urine cultures; serum lipase; liver profile; coagulation studies; and, in some cases, cardiac enzymes should be considered.[29] A Foley catheter should be placed in all patients too ill to use a urinal, bed pan, or bathroom. A nasogastric tube is useful in the patient with persistent vomiting or an ileus.

Previously diagnosed or new-onset diabetics who become significantly hyperglycemic and dehydrated may develop either DKA or HHS. The DKA state consists predominantly of dehydration, ketonuria, ketonemia, and anion gap metabolic acidosis. The HHS state consists predominantly of hyperosmolarity and even more marked hyperglycemia and dehydration than DKA, often with a less distinct anion gap metabolic acidosis because of lactate or low-level ketones. However, there is considerable overlap in these two syndromes. Distinguishing these syndromes from each other, as well as other causes of ketosis and anion gap metabolic acidosis, is important.

DKA is confirmed by the presence of hyperglycemia and ketonuria by point-of-care testing, metabolic acidosis demonstrated by an anion gap of greater than 16, a low pH, and low pCO_2 on the venous blood gas in the proper clinical setting (see Table 59-1). Almost all patients with DKA present with a blood glucose level greater than 300 mg/dL. Patients who present just after receiving insulin, have impaired gluconeogenesis (e.g., in alcohol abuse, or liver failure) or have maintained their GFR through fluid intake, may have lower initial serum glucose levels.[23] Elevated serum levels of BHB and AcAc cause ketonuria and metabolic acidosis. The nitroprusside reagent normally used to detect urine and serum ketones detects AcAc but not BHB. Early in the illness mitochondrial NADH accumulates, favoring the formation of BHB. Although the enzymatic test for BHB is reliable, it is not widely used in clinical practice. Paradoxically, as the patient is being treated and clinically improving, measured ketone levels will increase as BHB is converted to AcAc. In addition, false-positive ketone tests can be seen in patients taking sulfhydryl drugs like captopril because of interaction with the nitroprusside reagent.[30] Therefore ketones need only be checked initially in the urine.[15]

Clinically it is better to serially follow the anion gap rather than ketone dilution levels to follow effects of therapy and document improvement in DKA.

Electrolytes must be carefully evaluated for multiple metabolic abnormalities. Presence of an anion gap greater than 16 ($[Na^+] - [Cl^-] + [HCO_3^-]$) confirms a metabolic acidosis, usually because of elevated serum ketones, although other causes of an elevated anion gap (lactic acid, uremia, ingestions) must be considered.[28] One should not use the corrected serum sodium concentration prior to calculating the anion gap. Hyperchloremic acidosis also occurs as described earlier because of ketoanion exchange for chloride in the urine. Metabolic alkalosis may occur secondary to vomiting and osmotic diuresis. Rare patients with DKA may present with normal-appearing $[HCO_3^-]$ or even alkalemia if these alkalotic processes are severe enough to mask the acidosis. In these situations, an elevated anion gap may be the only clue to the presence of an underlying metabolic acidosis.[15]

Although arterial blood gases have been traditionally used to determine precise acid-base status, venous pH and pCO_2 appear to have sufficient agreement as to be clinically interchangeable in patients with DKA who are without respiratory failure.[24-26] Venous phlebotomy avoids painful arterial sticks and eliminates the possibility of arterial compromise or an expanding hematoma. A decreased pCO_2 usually reflects respiratory compensation for the metabolic acidosis and level of serum bicarbonate, as determined in Winter's formula (expected $PaCO_2Pa$ for compensation for metabolic acidosis $= 1.5 \times [HCO_3^-] + 8 \pm 2$).[28] pCO_2 levels lower than explained by the degree of acidosis determined by $[HCO_3^-]$ are caused by a primary respiratory alkalosis, which may be an indicator of pulmonary disease or sepsis. Higher values may imply a concomitant respiratory acidosis.

Total body potassium is severely depleted by renal losses in DKA and HHS. Potassium losses of 3 to 5 mEq/kg occur in DKA, and higher losses of 4 to 6 mEq/kg in HHS (Table 59-2). However, measured serum potassium level is normal or elevated in the majority of patients[7] because of extracellular shift of potassium secondary to acidemia and increased intravascular osmolarity caused by hyperglycemia.[31] Osmotic diuresis leads to marked renal losses of sodium chloride in the urine. Sodium losses of 7 to 10 mEq/kg occur in DKA and 5 to 13 mEq/kg in HHS. It is well described that the presence of hyperglycemia lowers the serum sodium concentration through the body's attempt to maintain normal extracellular osmolarity. Although standard teaching has been to add 1.6 mEq to reported sodium value for every 100 mg of glucose over 100 mg/dL, a reported correction factor of 2.4 appears more accurate, especially for blood glucose levels higher than 400 mg/dL.[32] Urinary losses and total body depletion of phosphorus, calcium, and magnesium also occur, although initial severe hemoconcentration may lead to normal or elevated initial levels. As appropriate therapy with fluids and insulin progress, lower levels of each will be evident.[15] Serum creatinine may be factitiously elevated if the laboratory assay for creatinine and AcAc interfere, although some elevation is expected in prerenal azotemia. Liver function studies, creatine phosphokinase, and amylase[16] are frequently elevated at the time of presentation and normalize during hydration therapy. Although elevated hemoglobin and leukocytosis are often present because of hemoconcentration, an absolute band count of 10,000 μL or more has been shown to reliably predict infection in this population.[33] An initial ECG is important because precipitant myocardial ischemia may be silent, and changes of life-threatening hyperkalemia (absent P-waves, widened QRS complex, tall peaked T-waves) or hypokalemia (diffuse ST depression and prominent U waves) may be present.

Table 59-2. Typical Total Body Deficits of Water and Electrolytes in DKA and HHS

Total water (L)	6	9
Water (mL/kg)*	100	100-200
$[Na^+]$ (mEq/kg)	7-10	5-13
$[Cl^-]$ (mEq/kg)	3-5	5-15
$[K^+]$ (mEq/kg)	3-5	4-6
$[PO_4]$ (mmol/kg)	5-7	3-7
$[Mg^{++}]$ (mEq/kg)	1-2	1-2
$[Ca^{++}]$ (mEq/kg)	1-2	1-2

*Per kilogram of body weight.
DKA, diabetic ketoacidosis; HHS, hyperglycemic hyperosmolar syndrome.

The initial evaluation of the patient with HHS is similar to that of DKA (Figs. 59-2 and 59-3). Identifying any precipitating event and addressing any underlying illness are vital. Typically serum blood glucose concentration in HHS is greater than 600 mg/dL and may exceed 2000 mg/dL.[34] As in DKA, initial serum sodium and potassium concentrations do not necessarily reflect total body losses. Normal or elevated initial serum sodium confirms significant water loss. Correction for initial serum sodium related to hyperglycemia is similar to DKA. Large deficits of potassium are usually encountered, and initial hypokalemia reflects profound total body potassium depletion. All patients with HHS are initially azotemic because of both prerenal and intrinsic renal causes. In one series the average initial blood urea nitrogen (BUN) and creatinine

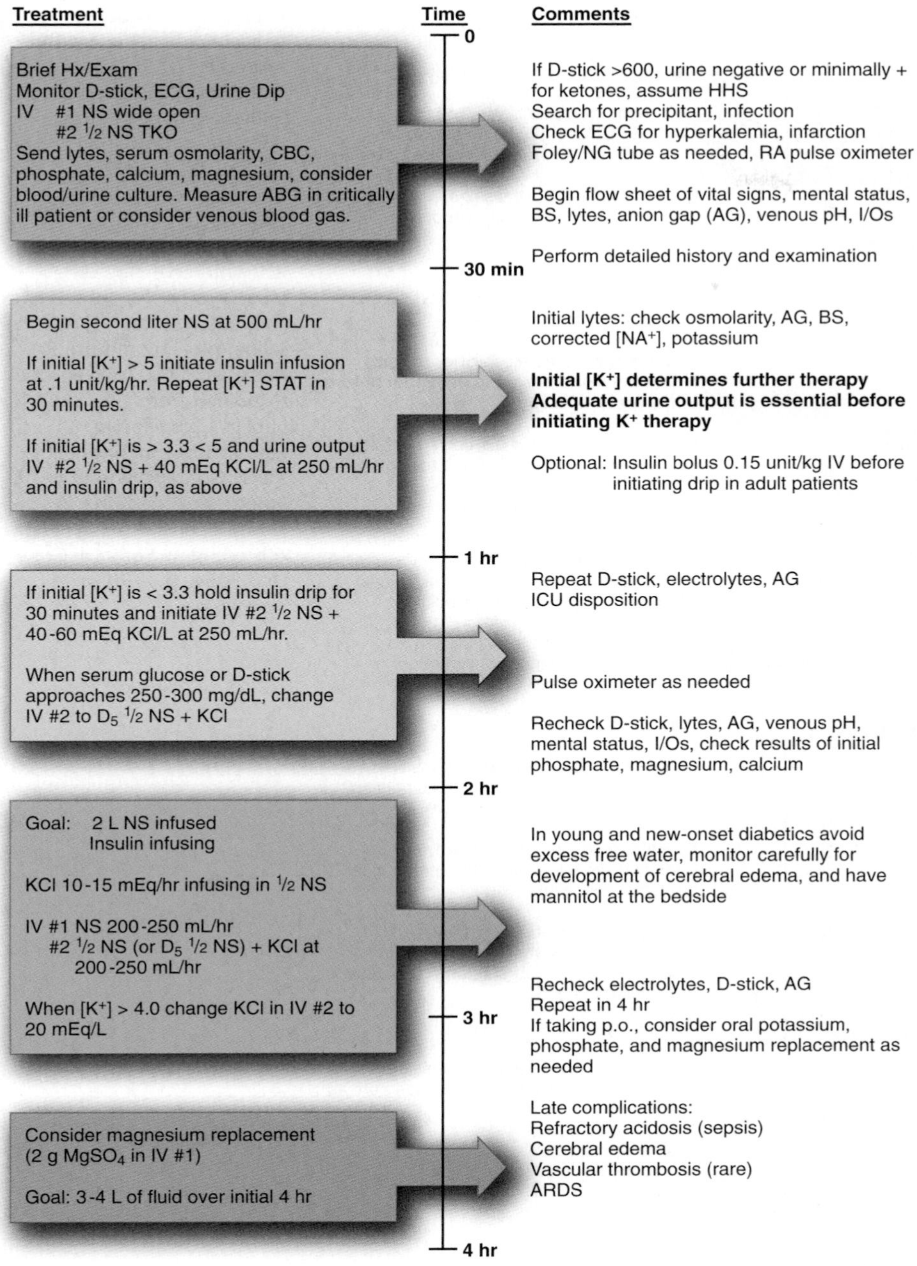
Treatment
Time
Comments
0
Brief Hx/Exam
Monitor D-stick, ECG, Urine Dip
IV #1 NS wide open
#2 1/2 NS TKO
Send lytes, serum osmolarity, CBC, phosphate, calcium, magnesium, consider blood/urine culture. Measure ABG in critically ill patient or consider venous blood gas.
If D-stick >600, urine negative or minimally + for ketones, assume HHS
Search for precipitant, infection
Check ECG for hyperkalemia, infarction
Foley/NG tube as needed, RA pulse oximeter
Begin flow sheet of vital signs, mental status, BS, lytes, anion gap (AG), venous pH, I/Os
Perform detailed history and examination
30 min
Begin second liter NS at 500 mL/hr
If initial [K+] > 5 initiate insulin infusion at .1 unit/kg/hr. Repeat [K+] STAT in 30 minutes.
If initial [K+] is > 3.3 < 5 and urine output IV #2 1/2 NS + 40 mEq KCl/L at 250 mL/hr and insulin drip, as above
Initial lytes: check osmolarity, AG, BS, corrected [NA+], potassium
Initial [K+] determines further therapy
Adequate urine output is essential before initiating K+ therapy
Optional: Insulin bolus 0.15 unit/kg IV before initiating drip in adult patients
1 hr
If initial [K+] is < 3.3 hold insulin drip for 30 minutes and initiate IV #2 1/2 NS + 40-60 mEq KCl/L at 250 mL/hr.
When serum glucose or D-stick approaches 250-300 mg/dL, change IV #2 to D5 1/2 NS + KCl
Repeat D-stick, electrolytes, AG
ICU disposition
Pulse oximeter as needed
Recheck D-stick, lytes, AG, venous pH, mental status, I/Os, check results of initial phosphate, magnesium, calcium
2 hr
Goal: 2 L NS infused
Insulin infusing
KCl 10-15 mEq/hr infusing in 1/2 NS
IV #1 NS 200-250 mL/hr
#2 1/2 NS (or D5 1/2 NS) + KCl at 200-250 mL/hr
When [K+] > 4.0 change KCl in IV #2 to 20 mEq/L
In young and new-onset diabetics avoid excess free water, monitor carefully for development of cerebral edema, and have mannitol at the bedside
Recheck electrolytes, D-stick, AG
Repeat in 4 hr
If taking p.o., consider oral potassium, phosphate, and magnesium replacement as needed
3 hr
Consider magnesium replacement (2 g MgSO4 in IV #1)
Goal: 3-4 L of fluid over initial 4 hr
Late complications:
Refractory acidosis (sepsis)
Cerebral edema
Vascular thrombosis (rare)
ARDS
4 hr

Figure 59-2. Timeline for the typical adult patient with suspected hyperosmolar hyperglycemic state. ABG, arterial blood gas; AG, anion gap; ARDS, acute respiratory distress syndrome; BS, blood sugar; CBC, complete blood cell count; ECG, electrocardiogram; HHS, hyperosmolar hyperglycemic state; ICU, intensive care unit; I/Os, in/outs; IV, intravenous; NG, nasogastric; NS, normal saline; p.o., by mouth; RA, room air; TKO, to keep open. (Modified from Chansky MD, Lubkin CL: Diabetic ketoacidosis. In Tintinalli J, Kelen G, Stapczynski J [eds]: Emergency Medicine, A Comprehensive Study Guide, 6th ed. New York, McGraw-Hill, 2004, p 1290, with permission.)

values were 87 mg/dL and 5.5 mg/dL, respectively. After treatment, the average values had fallen to 24 mg/dL and 2 mg/dL.[17] Effective serum osmolarity should be calculated using the traditional formula; by definition, it is greater than 320 mOsm/kg in patients with HHS.

$$\text{Effective Osmolarity (mOsm/kg water)} = 2[Na^+] + [\text{blood glucose}]/18$$

Urea (BUN) is freely permeable across cell membranes, so it does not create an osmotic gradient between intracellular and extracellular spaces. Excluding the BUN value from the traditional equation is appropriate because azotemia may mask actual hypotonicity of the extracellular fluid.

An anion gap metabolic acidosis is present in about half of patients with HHS.[17] This may be caused by accumulation of lactic acid, smaller concentrations of BHB and AcAc in equilibrium (predominantly BHB), and accumulation of fixed acid metabolites related to azotemia. Hemoconcentration often elevates the initial hemoglobin and hematocrit, and an elevated white blood cell count may suggest a serious underlying infection. As in DKA, an ECG is important to offer immediate potential information regarding $[K^+]$ and identify silent ischemia.

Approach to Management

The approach to management of patients with DKA and HHS has been outlined in detail in several key

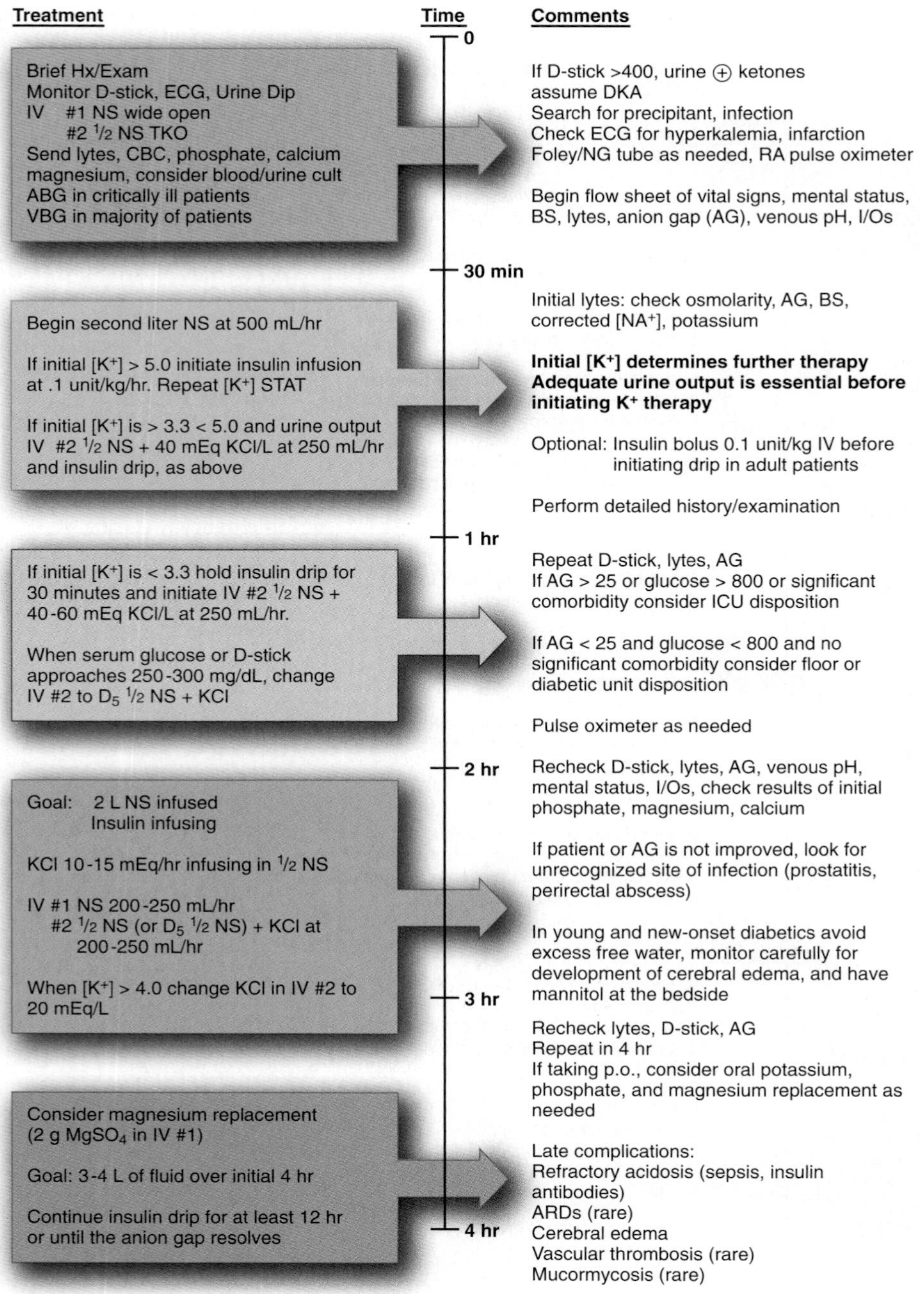
Treatment
Time
Comments
0
Brief Hx/Exam
Monitor D-stick, ECG, Urine Dip
IV #1 NS wide open
#2 1/2 NS TKO
Send lytes, CBC, phosphate, calcium
magnesium, consider blood/urine cult
ABG in critically ill patients
VBG in majority of patients
If D-stick >400, urine ⊕ ketones
assume DKA
Search for precipitant, infection
Check ECG for hyperkalemia, infarction
Foley/NG tube as needed, RA pulse oximeter
Begin flow sheet of vital signs, mental status,
BS, lytes, anion gap (AG), venous pH, I/Os
30 min
Begin second liter NS at 500 mL/hr
If initial [K+] > 5.0 initiate insulin infusion
at .1 unit/kg/hr. Repeat [K+] STAT
If initial [K+] is > 3.3 < 5.0 and urine output
IV #2 1/2 NS + 40 mEq KCl/L at 250 mL/hr
and insulin drip, as above
Initial lytes: check osmolarity, AG, BS,
corrected [NA+], potassium
Initial [K+] determines further therapy
Adequate urine output is essential before
initiating K+ therapy
Optional: Insulin bolus 0.1 unit/kg IV before
initiating drip in adult patients
Perform detailed history/examination
1 hr
If initial [K+] is < 3.3 hold insulin drip for
30 minutes and initiate IV #2 1/2 NS +
40-60 mEq KCl/L at 250 mL/hr.
When serum glucose or D-stick
approaches 250-300 mg/dL, change
IV #2 to D5 1/2 NS + KCl
Repeat D-stick, lytes, AG
If AG > 25 or glucose > 800 or significant
comorbidity consider ICU disposition
If AG < 25 and glucose < 800 and no
significant comorbidity consider floor or
diabetic unit disposition
Pulse oximeter as needed
2 hr
Goal: 2 L NS infused
Insulin infusing
KCl 10-15 mEq/hr infusing in 1/2 NS
IV #1 NS 200-250 mL/hr
#2 1/2 NS (or D5 1/2 NS) + KCl at
200-250 mL/hr
When [K+] > 4.0 change KCl in IV #2 to
20 mEq/L
Recheck D-stick, lytes, AG, venous pH,
mental status, I/Os, check results of initial
phosphate, magnesium, calcium
If patient or AG is not improved, look for
unrecognized site of infection (prostatitis,
perirectal abscess)
In young and new-onset diabetics avoid
excess free water, monitor carefully for
development of cerebral edema, and have
mannitol at the bedside
3 hr
Recheck lytes, D-stick, AG
Repeat in 4 hr
If taking p.o., consider oral potassium,
phosphate, and magnesium replacement as
needed
Consider magnesium replacement
(2 g MgSO4 in IV #1)
Goal: 3-4 L of fluid over initial 4 hr
Continue insulin drip for at least 12 hr
or until the anion gap resolves
4 hr
Late complications:
Refractory acidosis (sepsis, insulin
antibodies)
ARDs (rare)
Cerebral edema
Vascular thrombosis (rare)
Mucormycosis (rare)

Figure 59-3. Timeline for the typical adult patient with suspected DKA. ABG, arterial blood gas; AG, anion gap; ARDS, acute respiratory distress syndrome; BS, blood sugar; CBC, complete blood cell count; DKA, diabetic ketoacidosis; ECG, electrocardiogram; ICU, intensive care unit; I/Os, in/outs; IV, intravenous; NG, nasogastric; NS, normal saline; p.o., by mouth; RA, room air; TKO, to keep open. (Modified from Chansky ME, Lubkin CL: Diabetic ketoacidosis. In Tintinalli J, Kelen G, Stapczynski J [eds]: Emergency Medicine, A Comprehensive Study Guide, 6th ed. New York, McGraw-Hill, 2004, p 1290, with permission.)

references.[3,7,8,11,15,29,35] Many factors including how the patient responds to initial appropriate therapy, age, precipitating and concomitant illnesses, and presence and severity of metabolic acidosis will help determine where subsequent care is appropriate (i.e., intensive care unit, step-down unit, monitored medical floor capable of insulin drips, observation unit, or definitive care prior to discharge in the ED).

Intensive care disposition should be considered for patients with hypotension or oliguria refractory to initial fluid resuscitation, mental obtundation or coma, significant hypokalemia (<3.3 mEq/L initially), anion gap greater than 25 in either syndrome, hypothermia, and any significant medical or surgical comorbidities such as myocardial ischemia, stroke, infection, and age older than 65. Most hospitals require an ICU, step-down unit, or diabetic floor to administer and manage an insulin drip. Transition to subcutaneous insulin should not be considered until the patient can tolerate oral fluids, anion gap is documented to be less than 20, and potassium replacement has been initiated. In general, intravenous (IV) insulin should continue for 1 to 2 hours following administration of subcutaneous insulin to prevent recurrent DKA.

A summary and treatment protocol for the first 4 hours of therapy for patients with suspected HHS and DKA appears in Figures 59-2 and 59-3, respectively. Each patient's therapy will differ, depending on his or her degree of hyperglycemia and dehydration. These two protocols parallel best evidence but cannot be all inclusive. Frequent laboratory testing is necessary to guide further therapy, and a detailed flow chart documenting time; vital signs; laboratory results (chemistries [especially glucose, potassium, osmolarity, and anion gap], venous blood gas, phosphorus, magnesium); fluid intake and output; insulin rates; and mental status is helpful.

When the diagnosis of DKA or HHS is strongly suspected at triage, the patient should be placed in a monitored bed with IV access and an adequate airway ensured. Patients should have at least one large-bore (No. 16 to 18) IV line of NS running wide open, and a second IV line of 0.5% NS to keep the line open. A rapid bedside glucose determination, urine dipstick test for glucose and ketones, ECG, and venous blood gas should be performed as soon as possible. Additional studies described earlier should be sent but, at a minimum, should include a complete blood count, electrolytes, phosphate, magnesium, calcium, and urinalysis. Blood cultures, chest radiograph, liver function tests, and lipase are performed as indicated.

Aggressive fluid therapy should be initiated prior to receiving initial laboratory results.[7] *Volume replenishment is the number one priority in HHS and DKA.* Replacing potassium and/or insulin, phosphate, and magnesium is also crucial. The goals of therapy include safe volume repletion, reversal of the metabolic consequences of insulin insufficiency, correction of electrolyte and acid-base disturbances, recognition and treatment of precipitating causes, and avoidance of complications. Metabolic disturbances should be corrected at about the rate of occurrence, or over 24 to 36 hours. Meeting these goals of therapy requires frequent (every 1 to 2 hours) monitoring of electrolytes (glucose, potassium, anion gap, osmolarity); vital signs; level of consciousness; and volume input/output until recovery is well established. Euglycemia is NOT the endpoint of therapy; it is the resolution of metabolic acidosis via normalization of the anion gap that signifies resolution of DKA. If blood sugar drops to less than 100 mg/dL prior to normalization of the anion gap, a D10 solution should be administered to prevent hypoglycemia while continuing the insulin drip and monitoring serum potassium.

Fluid Administration

Adult HHS patients have profound fluid deficits that average 9 L.[7,19]

Aggressive initial fluid resuscitation with 1 L of 0.9% NS is indicated, whereas the choice of fluids thereafter remains controversial.[7,19,23,36]

NS remains the fluid of choice if the patient displays signs of hypoperfusion. After initial resuscitation, a reasonable plan is to base fluid composition on corrected serum sodium level. If the corrected serum sodium level is high or normal (>135 mEq/L), one should use 0.45% NS infusion, replacing half of the total fluid deficit during the first 12 hours at a rate of approximately 200 to 500 mL per hour, and the remaining deficit over the following 12 to 24 hours.[11,19,23] If the corrected serum sodium is less than 135 mEq/L, one should continue with 0.9% saline. Intravenous fluid resuscitation alone decreases the serum blood glucose level by 25 to 50 mg/dL per hour on average.[23]

In DKA rapid fluid administration is the single most important initial step because fluid helps restore intravascular volume and tonicity, perfuse vital organs, improve glomerular filtration rate, and lower serum glucose and ketone levels. The average adult DKA patient has a water deficit of 100 mL/kg (5 to 10 L) and a sodium deficit of 7 to 10 mEq/kg (see Table 59-2).[7] As in HHS, 0.9% saline is the most frequently recommended fluid for initial resuscitation, even though extracellular fluid is initially hypertonic. NS is felt to prevent an excessively rapid fall in extracellular osmolarity and to have the potential for transfer of excessive water into the CNS manifesting as cerebral edema (a reported clinical issue in children).

On the basis of clinical suspicion and rapid bedside testing alone and prior to initial electrolyte results, the first liter of NS should be administered within the first 30 minutes of triage. After initial resuscitation with 1 to 2 L of 0.9% saline, most authors favor alternating administration of NS with 0.5% NS or using two IV lines—one with NS and one with 0.5% NS. In general the first 2 L are administered rapidly over 0 to 2 hours, the next 2 L over 2 to 6 hours, and an additional 2 L over 6 to 12 hours. This replaces approximately 50% of the total water deficit over the first 12 hours, with the remaining 50% to be replaced over the subsequent 12 hours.[15] Fluid administration lowers glucose and ketone body concentrations prior to insulin therapy.[23] Tissue perfusion improves, as does insulin effectiveness. Blood glucose needs to be carefully monitored, and D5 added to the rehydration solution when the glucose level is 250 to 300 mg/dL. Although a common pitfall is failure to give adequate volume replacement, excess fluid may contribute to the development of adult respiratory distress syndrome and cerebral edema.[37]

Insulin Administration

Initial volume replacement reduces the level of counterregulatory hormones; replaces vital fluid and electrolytes; and, more importantly, makes cells more responsive to insulin. Initial serum potassium concentration determines utilization of insulin and/or potassium as the next therapeutic maneuver. In the rare patient with initial hypokalemia (<3.3 mEq), insulin has been shown to precipitate life-threatening hypokalemic events by shifting potassium intracellularly. Although no studies support the administration of potassium prior to insulin therapy, in the absence of hyperkalemia, the American Diabetes Association recommends that parenteral potassium be administered (10 to 15 mEq/hour) 30 minutes prior to insulin in this patient population.[7]

The approach to insulin therapy is similar in DKA and HHS, with the caveat that many patients diagnosed with HHS have never received insulin, and smaller doses and careful monitoring in combination with adequate fluid resuscitation may prevent dangerous precipitous drops in glucose and osmolarity. Continuous low-dose IV insulin is the accepted therapy of hyperglycemic states.[7] This approach appears to produce a more linear fall in serum glucose and ketone body level, is easy to monitor, and is associated with less severe metabolic complications such as hypoglycemia, hypokalemia, and hypophosphatemia. Patients utilizing an insulin pump should turn off the pump and be treated with IV insulin.

Insulin infusion of 0.1 units/kg/hour should be initiated in patients who have a potassium greater than 3.3 mEq/L, have received at least 1 L of NS, and have adequate urine output.[19,20,23] A one-time IV bolus of regular insulin, 0.15 units/kg, is optional in adults and recommended by many authors but has not been shown to improve recovery or shorten hospital stay. Insulin effects begin almost immediately, as the half-life of IV insulin is 4 to 5 minutes, with an effective biologic half-life at the tissue level of approximately 20 to 30 minutes. Because insulin binds to plastic IV tubing, the first 25 mL of a prepared insulin solution should be discarded and the drip placed into an established IV line via an infusion pump at the port closest to the skin. Frequent monitoring is required to ensure that insulin is being administered in the desired amount and leading to the desired effects. As noted earlier, in the rare patient with initial potassium of less than 3.3 mEq/L, one should hold insulin and administer 10 to 15 mEq/L KCl per hour for 30 minutes or until potassium is documented to be higher than 3.3 mEq/L while continuing on a cardiac monitor. Intravenous administration of higher than 10 mEq/hour often requires a central line for patient comfort.

Intramuscular or subcutaneous administration of regular insulin in DKA and HHS should be avoided.[38] Insulin absorption may be erratic in the volume-depleted patient, delaying achievement of adequate insulin levels. Intramuscular insulin may create deposits of insulin that could be absorbed later, leading to hypoglycemia. Recent studies have evaluated and demonstrated successful outcomes using subcutaneous aspart or lispro insulin in medically stable DKA patients. Stable patients after fluid resuscitation treated with a loading dose of 0.3 U per kg of aspart insulin followed by 0.1 U per kg every hour had no significant difference in outcome compared with IV insulin.[39]

The incidence of nonresponse to low-dose continuous IV insulin is 1% to 2% and usually signifies inadequate fluid administration, infection, or concomitant steroid administration. If the patient fails to respond (i.e., a decrease of serum glucose level by 50 to 70 mg/dL in the first hour), the insulin infusion rate should be doubled.[7]

The goal of insulin therapy in HHS is gradual restoration of osmolarity, whereas in DKA the infusion should be continued until the anion gap has normalized. Hyperglycemia may resolve prior to the anion gap in DKA. When the glucose level has reached 250 to 300 mg/dL, dextrose is added to the IV fluids and serum glucose concentration maintained at this level until hyperosmolarity (in HHS) and the anion gap (in DKA) has resolved. As noted earlier, BHB converts to AcAc during therapy, with an increase in "measurable ketones" in serum and urine despite appropriate therapy. Therefore the anion gap is the most accurate determinant of ongoing recovery and appropriateness of therapy. Most patients with DKA will require at least 12 hours of insulin therapy, allowing for an overlap period in which subcutaneous insulin can be initiated preceding discontinuation of IV insulin.

Potassium

Initial potassium concentration may not reliably predict total body potassium stores because of profound total body potassium deficits in the range of 3 to 5 mEq/kg in DKA and potentially larger deficits in HHS. Only 2% of total-body potassium is intravascular and thus measurable.

In DKA this severe deficiency is caused by insulin deficiency, metabolic acidosis, osmotic diuresis, aldosterone-mediated renal losses, and vomiting. Initial serum concentration is usually normal or high because of intracellular exchange of potassium for hydrogen ions during acidosis and severe volume depletion. Initial hypokalemia, although rare, signifies severe total body potassium deficits and may necessitate large amounts of IV or oral potassium during the first 24 to 36 hours of therapy.

The goal of potassium replacement in DKA and HHS is to maintain a normal extracellular potassium concentration during the acute phase of therapy and replace the intracellular deficit over a period of days. During initial therapy with fluids and insulin, serum potassium concentration will reliably fall, primarily because of the action of insulin promoting reentry of potassium into cells, dilution of extracellular fluid, correction of acidosis, and increased urinary loss of potassium. Rapid development of hypokalemia may result in fatal cardiac arrhythmias, respiratory paralysis,[40] paralytic ileus, and rhabdomyolysis. The development of severe hypokalemia is potentially the most life-threatening electrolyte derangement during the treatment of DKA.[7]

Early potassium replacement is now a standard approach in patients with HHS and DKA. Potassium therapy is not initiated until the patient has received NS resuscitation, the initial electrolytes reflect a serum potassium of less than 5.0 mEq/L, and adequate urine output is demonstrated. As a general guideline, an *initial* serum potassium level greater than 3.3 mEq/L and less than 5 mEq/L (prior to fluid resuscitation and IV insulin) calls for 10 to 15 mEq of KCl per hour in IV fluid for at least 4 hours. Because rapid shifts of potassium occur during this initial phase of treatment, serum potassium concentration should be monitored at least every 1 to 2 hours. Oliguria (fortunately quite rare because of the protective osmotic diuresis) necessitates careful adjustment of potassium administration and closer monitoring.

Initial serum potassium greater than 5 mEq/L usually reflects a more severe acidemia in DKA and volume depletion in HHS. ECG changes consistent with hyperkalemia may be present prior to initiation of therapy. Intravenous potassium replacement is withheld until the serum potassium level is documented to be below 5 mEq/L and adequate urine flow is established. NS and insulin therapy alone will lower the serum potassium concentration rapidly to safe levels. Ketoacid clearance in DKA and correction of the acidosis lowers serum potassium concentration as well. In general, for each 0.1 change in pH, serum potassium changes approximately 0.5 mEq/L inversely.

As discussed earlier, initial hypokalemia in HHS and especially DKA reflects large total body potassium deficits and mandates potassium therapy prior to insulin. In this rare setting, potassium should be given intravenously at 10 to 15 mEq/hour either until serum potassium is demonstrated to be above 3.3 mEq or for 30 minutes prior to insulin administration. No advantage to using potassium phosphate over potassium chloride has been documented in the literature; excessive use of potassium phosphate may result in hypocalcemia[8] or metastatic precipitation of calcium phosphate in tissue.

The goal is to maintain serum potassium levels within the normal range of 4 to 5 mEq/L and avoid life-threatening hyperkalemia or hypokalemia. Oral potassium replacement is safe and equally effective to IV therapy and should be used as soon as the patient can tolerate oral fluids. During the first 24 hours 100 mEq of potassium chloride may be required, and rarely up to 500 mEq is necessary to maintain normal range potassium concentration.[15]

Phosphate

Phosphate plays an integral role in the conversion of energy from adenosine triphosphate (ATP) and in the delivery of oxygen at the tissue level. Phosphate, like potassium, is primarily intracellular and shifts to the extracellular compartment during DKA. Serum levels often are normal or increased on presentation and do not reflect the total body phosphate deficits secondary to enhanced urinary losses.[14] Similar to glucose and potassium, phosphate reenters the intracellular space during fluid resuscitation and insulin therapy, resulting in low phosphate concentrations. Hypophosphatemia is usually most severe 24 to 48 hours into continuous insulin therapy and should be closely monitored during the initial phases of DKA and HHS therapy. Severe hypophosphatemia (defined as <1 mg/dL), has been associated with a variety of clinical disorders including hypoxia, rhabdomyolysis, hemolysis, respiratory failure, and cardiac dysfunction.[41] Fortunately, all are extremely rare during therapy of DKA.[38]

The role of phosphate replacement during the treatment of DKA and HHS remains controversial. No clinical trial has demonstrated significant benefits from routine IV phosphate therapy in DKA.[8,14] However, to avoid cardiac and skeletal muscle weakness and respiratory depression caused by hypophosphatemia, careful phosphate replacement may sometimes be indicated in patients with cardiac dysfunction, anemia, or respiratory depression and in those seriously ill patients with serum phosphate concentration less than 1 mg/dL.[8] When absolutely necessary, in an intensive care setting 20 to 30 mEq/L potassium phosphate can be added to replacement fluids. No current studies are available on the use of phosphate in the treatment of HHS, although careful monitoring and following the same principles as in DKA are appropriate. Administration of IV phosphate has been associated with severe electrolyte disturbances including hypocalcemia and hypomagnesemia,[42] as well as metastatic calcification in tissue. As with potassium therapy, hypophosphatemia can be corrected safely and effectively with oral replenishment, which may lead to diarrhea.[15] Serum phosphate, calcium, and magnesium levels should be monitored during therapy of DKA and HHS, but the routine early use of parenteral phosphate replacement has not been established.

Magnesium

Magnesium is stored primarily in bone and excreted in the urine. Ongoing osmotic diuresis may cause significant depletion of magnesium stores and hypomagnesemia in HHS and DKA. Specific symptoms of hypomagnesemia are difficult to recognize and overlap with symptoms caused by deficiencies of calcium, potassium, and sodium. Paresthesias, tremor, carpopedal spasm, agitation, seizures, and cardiac dysrhythmias all are reported symptoms.[8] Monitoring magnesium and calcium levels at presentation and 24 hours into therapy is appropriate in patients with HHS and DKA, and specific therapy should be considered if the serum magnesium concentration is less than 1.2 mg/dL or symptoms develop that are suggestive of hypomagnesemia. Magnesium can safely be given parenterally as magnesium sulfate or orally in the form of magnesium oxide.

Bicarbonate

Although bicarbonate has no role in the therapy of HHS, the use of bicarbonate in DKA has been debated for decades. The metabolic acidosis, decreased bicarbonate level, and anion gap found in DKA will resolve with appropriate fluid, insulin, and potassium therapy described earlier. Bicarbonate is still recommended in many texts for arbitrary pH levels. To date, not a single study clearly demonstrates improved clinical outcomes using bicarbonate in the treatment of DKA. Mortality in DKA does not appear to be related to the level of bicarbonate on presentation. Routine use of supplemental bicarbonate in the treatment of DKA is not recommended.[14,15,43,44] Children with initial pH values as low as 6.73 have been shown to recover promptly from DKA with appropriate therapy without bicarbonate.[45]

Severe metabolic acidosis may be associated with numerous deleterious cardiovascular effects including impaired contractility of the heart, vasodilation, and hypotension. Theoretical advantages of bicarbonate include improved myocardial contractility, elevated ventricular fibrillation threshold, improved catecholamine tissue response, and decreased work of breathing.[45] These theoretical advantages seem outweighed by the apparent disadvantages of bicarbonate including worsening hypokalemia by enhancing renal excretion, paradoxical CNS acidosis, worsening intracellular acidosis, impaired oxygen delivery to the tissues, shifting the oxyhemoglobin curve to the left, hypertonicity and sodium overload, delayed recovery from ketosis,[43] elevation of lactate levels, and possible precipitation of cerebral edema.[45]

Severe metabolic acidosis on presentation (pH < 7) in the absence of a respiratory acidosis and worsening pH despite aggressive appropriate therapy for DKA should prompt the clinician to rule out other causes of metabolic acidosis (e.g., consider lactate from sepsis, bowel infarction, methanol ingestion). Many authors continue to recommend bicarbonate administration in adult patients with pH less than 6.9[8,35] to protect against the cardiac and neurologic effects. The potential benefits of bicarbonate in the elderly with cardiovascular instability and DKA must be balanced against the potential disadvantages, and pH monitored closely during therapy.[7,14]

Complications

Critically ill patients with DKA or HHS must have precipitating illnesses addressed aggressively. Of the factors responsible for precipitating DKA, infection and MI are not, surprisingly, major contributors to mortality. Patients with high initial osmolarity, BUN, and glucose have higher mortality. Additional factors that reduce survival are older age, prolonged hypotension or coma, and underlying renal and cardiovascular disease.

Causes of death in DKA and HHS include infections, vascular thromboses, refractory shock, and cerebral edema.[46] Patients with significant hyperosmolarity may develop mesenteric thromboses, adult respiratory distress syndrome (ARDS), disseminated intravascular coagulation, and multiple system organ failure. Patients at risk for vascular disease who present with severe dehydration are at risk for deep venous thrombosis, and administration of prophylactic anticoagulation should be considered.

Major complications related to therapy of DKA and HHS include hypoglycemia, hypokalemia, hypophosphatemia, ARDS, and cerebral edema. As emphasized, the overall goal of therapy in both disorders is gradual return to normal metabolic balance, which will mitigate these possible outcomes to some extent.[15] Careful monitoring and appropriate replenishment during the acute phase of illness is important to prevent the complications of hypoglycemia and disorders of potassium, phosphate, and magnesium.

Hypoxemia and, rarely, ARDS may complicate the treatment of DKA. Hypoxemia is attributed to aggressive fluid resuscitation and a reduction in colloid osmotic pressure combined with an increase in left atrial end-diastolic pressure, leading to increased lung water content and decreased pulmonary compliance. Patients with DKA who have a wide alveolar-arterial oxygen gradient noted on initial arterial blood gas or patients with rales on examination may be at higher risk for development of ARDS[7] and should have their fluid rate decreased and be closely monitored for hypoxia.

Cerebral edema is rare in adults treated for these two syndromes. In DKA, cerebral edema tends to occur between 4 and 12 hours after the start of therapy but may develop as late as 48 hours into therapy.[37] It is often described when the patient appears to be improving clinically and biochemically.[14,37] Studies have demonstrated mild, asymptomatic cerebral edema in children with DKA at the time of presentation and during therapy.[47,48] The true incidence of cerebral edema is unknown but has been estimated to occur between 0.5 and 1 per 100 episodes of DKA in children.[3,14] Mortality of cerebral edema in patients recovering from DKA ranges in reports from 25% to 70%, and the neurological sequelae of survivors is often severe.[3] Pathogenesis of cerebral edema is unknown and has been the subject of intense interest in the pediatric literature. The rate of fluid administration, change in serum glucose concentration, and change in serum osmolarity have not reliably been shown to be risk factors for development of cerebral edema in children.[3] One hypothesis is that during the hyperosmolar and hyperglycemic state, brain cells produce enzymatically active osmolar particles or idiogenic osmoles that protect cells from further loss of water and shrinkage. During therapy with fluids and insulin, water moves into brain cells faster than idiogenic osmoles can dissipate, promoting cellular swelling.[14,37] Multiple studies and reviews have found no specific presentation or treatment variables that predict or contribute to the development of cerebral edema.[37,47] Young age and new-onset diabetics in DKA are the only true identified potential risk factors. In a large retrospective study of cerebral edema in children, risk factors identified included a low arterial partial pressure of CO_2, a high BUN on presentation, slow rate of increase of Na^+ during therapy, and use of bicarbonate during therapy,[47] although these results have never been duplicated in a prospective trial. Other studies have identified excessive initial fluid administration of greater than 4 L/m^2 of body surface area per day, initial "corrected" hypernatremia, and initial fall in Na^+ during therapy as possible risk factors.[37,48,49] Recent literature has suggested a vasogenic mechanism for cerebral edema in contrast to the traditional osmotic cellular swelling model.[50]

Approximately half of the patients who develop cerebral edema have premonitory symptoms of severe headache, incontinence, change in arousal or behavior, pupillary changes, blood pressure changes, seizures, bradycardia, or disturbed temperature regulation.[15] Development of a severe headache during therapy of DKA or other neurologic symptoms should be taken extremely seriously, especially in younger, new-onset diabetics. Because of the rarity of cerebral edema, data are limited regarding the effectiveness of pharmacologic interventions for treatment.[3] Immediate availability of mannitol (1 to 2 g/kg) should be at the bedside of high-risk patients and used with the first onset of any neurologic symptom that could be attributed to cerebral edema prior to confirmatory CT scan of the head. Other aggressive measures such as intubation, hyperventilation, and fluid restriction may be necessary, although it is recommended to maintain the pCO_2 at levels expected for a compensated metabolic acidosis.[3] Hypertonic saline has been used and reported in pediatric patients[51] and may be useful in patients with a dropping serum sodium concentration during therapy.

Persistent anion gap metabolic acidosis refractory to routine therapy may be secondary to unrecognized infection (lactic acidosis), insulin antibodies, or improper preparation or administration of the insulin drip.[15] Shock unresponsive to fluid resuscitation should raise suspicion of sepsis and prompt early goal-directed therapy or clinically unapparent MI.

Hyperchloremic nonanion gap metabolic acidosis develops in virtually all patients treated for DKA because bicarbonate equivalents are lost in the urine as ketone bodies and replaced with the volume expander sodium chloride. This emphasizes the importance of monitoring the anion gap during therapy of DKA, not the serum bicarbonate concentration. The nonanion gap metabolic acidosis will typically resolve in patients with normal renal function over 24 to 48 hours because bicarbonate is regenerated through enhanced renal acid excretion.[20]

Arterial thrombotic disease is often cited either as a precipitating factor or complication of DKA and HHS. Many clinical features of DKA and HHS predispose to thrombosis: dehydration and volume contraction, low cardiac output, increased blood viscosity, and the frequent presence of underlying atherosclerosis. Thrombosis typically begins hours or days after admission.[46] Late arterial thrombosis may occur in any muscular artery, although the cerebral vessels appear to be most susceptible.[38] No controlled trial has been performed looking at prophylactic dosages of heparin, most likely because of the rarity of thrombosis. Heparin may be useful in elderly patients or those with severe hyperosmolality in conjunction with prophylactic gastric acid suppression.

Mucormycosis is an opportunistic fungal infection seen in patients with leukemia, lymphoma, immunosuppression, and diabetes. Pulmonary or rhinocerebral mucormycosis is most likely to develop in patients with poorly controlled diabetes mellitus and those recovering from DKA. Development of a fever during the recovery phase of DKA or HHS should prompt a thorough evaluation, and symptoms referable to the chest or nasal turbinates or sinuses (typically a bloody discharge) should be taken seriously. This organism tends to invade the elastic lamina of blood vessels and can lead to extensive tissue destruction. Even with early aggressive débridement and antifungal therapy, the prognosis is poor.

Diabetic Ketoacidosis and Pregnancy

In the United States more than 8 million women have pregestational diabetes.[52] As a result of the epidemic of obesity, the majority of diabetes now seen in pregnancy is caused by type 2 diabetes.[53] Diabetic ketoacidosis occurs in 1% to 2% of all pregnancies complicated by pregestational diabetes.[54] The incidence is highest in the second and third trimesters because of an increase in insulin resistance related to a high level of human placental lactogen, progesterone, and cortisol.[55] This diabetogenic state of pregnancy accounts for the increased requirement of insulin throughout pregnancy, particularly in the 28th through 32nd weeks of gestation.[56] Lack of appropriate insulin adjustment could also contribute to the higher incidence of DKA observed during this time.[57] Although maternal mortality of DKA is similar to the nonpregnant state,[57] fetal mortality is significantly higher, ranging from 10% to 35%.[54,58] Early recognition and prompt treatment can prevent fetal death. DKA could be the first manifestation of diabetes in pregnancy[59-61]; in one reported case of DKA in a pregnant woman without prior history of diabetes, a 5-hour delay in initiating treatment resulted in fetal death.[60] DKA should be suspected in pregnant women presenting with abdominal pain, nausea, vomiting, and altered mental status. Laboratory findings include high anion gap acidosis, ketosis, and hyperglycemia[62]; however, up to 36% of women may have a serum glucose less than 200 mg/dL. Vomiting and decreased caloric intake such as seen in pregnancy can lead to euglycemic ketoacidosis. After a prolonged fast, the liver is depleted of glycogen and produces ketones rather than glucose; in addition, the glomerular filtration rate is increased in pregnancy, resulting in an increased amount of filtered glucose; therefore the presence of normoglycemia should not exclude the diagnosis of DKA.[54] In addition, the diagnosis of DKA should not be based solely on the presence of ketones because ketone bodies can be detected in the serum and urine of normal pregnant women.[63] Continuous monitoring of fetal heart rate often demonstrates absent accelerations and late decelerations,[64] which are reversed after treatment.[65] The most common precipitating factors of DKA in pregnancy are poor compliance with insulin therapy, infection,[66] insulin pump failure, treatment with β-sympathomimetic tocolytic agents, and corticosteroid use.[62,67] In addition, new-onset diabetes is seen in almost 30% of women presenting with DKA.[61,68] Management of diabetic ketosis in pregnancy is similar to that in patients who are not pregnant, with particular attention to replacement of glucose and potassium.

Summary

DKA and HHS are serious disease states that often present to EDs or develop in the hospital. Initial diagnosis and therapy is often started in the ED, with critical care physicians consulted shortly thereafter. Following airway protection, initial attention is directed toward fluid resuscitation and identifying any precipitating illness, particularly infections and myocardial infarction. Initial serum potassium concentration determines the next priority of therapy: insulin in patients with K^+ greater than 3.3 mEq/L and potassium chloride in the rare subset of patients with K^+ less than 3.3 mEq/L. Careful attention and monitoring therapy and electrolytes, osmolarity, potassium, anion gap, and venous pH will prevent common complications of therapy, specifically hypokalemia and hypoglycemia. Despite best practice, patients with HHS have a high mortality primarily related to significant underlying illness.

HYPOGLYCEMIA

Incidence

Hypoglycemia is the most common endocrine medical emergency.[69] It is most frequently encountered in diabetic patients treated with insulin and/or oral agents. Most episodes of hypoglycemia are usually mild and self-treated;

however, the clinical spectrum can vary from mild to severe, requiring third-party intervention, and can even be fatal. Between 1989 and 1991 there were 75,000 hospitalizations per year for hypoglycemia in the United States, and nearly 17,000 of them were for hypoglycemic coma.[70]

As emerging evidence supports that tighter glycemic control improves clinical outcomes in diabetic patients, the goal of near normalization of HbA1c is becoming the standard of care; however, this goal is often achieved at the expense of more hypoglycemic events. Hypoglycemia, especially in insulin-treated patients, becomes the limiting factor in the management of type 1 and type 2 diabetes and has associated morbidity and mortality.[71,72]

Is It True Hypoglycemia?

The diagnosis of hypoglycemia should not be made solely on the basis of plasma glucose measurement.[73] A true definition of hypoglycemia is not well established and has ranged from 45 to 70 mg/dL. In normal women, fasting glucose can be as low as 40 mg/dL and in men as low as 55 mg/dL. Pathology should be strongly suspected if blood glucose is less than 45 mg/dL, especially if the individual experiences clinical symptoms at that time. The finding of a low serum glucose concentration in an otherwise totally asymptomatic patient should also raise the possibility of pseudohypoglycemia that could occur if the blood sample was collected in a tube that does not contain an antiglycolytic agent or if there is an increase in consumption of glucose seen in samples of patients with leukemia or hemolytic anemia.[73]

Clinical Manifestations

The clinical manifestations of hypoglycemia are typically divided into two categories: the sympathoadrenal and neuroglycopenic symptoms (Table 59-3). The initial symptoms of sweating, palpitations, anxiety, and tremor occur as the plasma glucose concentration falls below 60 mg/dL. These symptoms provide a protective response in individuals to correct the hypoglycemia. Symptoms of cognitive dysfunction become apparent with a serum glucose less than 50 mg/dL, but it is clear that recent episodes of hypoglycemia can alter this threshold so that greater reduction in serum glucose concentration is required before hormonal response and symptoms are manifest.[74] In the Diabetes Control and Complication Trial (DCCT), one third of all severe hypoglycemic episodes during waking hours were associated with mild symptoms preventing the patients from taking adequate corrective action.[75] The reverse could also occur (i.e., a diabetic patient may be symptomatically hypoglycemic at a normal serum glucose concentration if his or her diabetes control is poor). In this instance, one would have to gradually improve control to prevent hypoglycemic symptoms.

In addition to the symptoms listed in Table 59-3, hypoglycemia could cause cardiovascular manifestations such as elevated systolic blood pressure, tachycardia, and increased frequency of premature atrial and ventricular contractions.[76] Angina with transient ECG changes, ST elevation, and T wave inversion have been reported with hypoglycemia; this has occurred with normal coronaries on catheterization.[77] The adrenergic symptoms of hypoglycemia are often blunted in diabetics with neuropathy or patients receiving β-adrenergic blockers.

Table 59-3. Clinical Symptoms of Hypoglycemia

Sympathoadrenal	Neuroglycopenic
Tremor	Tiredness or drowsiness
Palpitations	Difficulty thinking
Diaphoresis	Confusion
Nervousness	Blurred vision
Anxiety or apprehension	Slurred speech
Hunger	Dizziness, weakness
Pallor	Abnormal or belligerent behavior
	Seizure
	Coma or death

Physiologic Response to Hypoglycemia

Maintenance of the plasma glucose concentration is critical to survival because the brain relies almost exclusively on glucose as a source of energy but cannot synthesize or store it. This issue becomes even more important as tight glycemic control becomes the standard of care in diabetic patients, exposing them to more hypoglycemia with potential risk of brain function impairment.

In a normal subject, as the plasma glucose falls below approximately 80 mg/dL, endogenous insulin secretion will decrease. This response, however, cannot occur in diabetic patients in whom insulin is given exogenously; therefore the counterregulatory hormones play a major role in the defense against hypoglycemia.[78] When the plasma glucose concentration falls below 70 mg/dL, release of the most important counterregulatory hormones, glucagon and epinephrine, occurs; if the hypoglycemia is severe and persistent, release of cortisol and growth hormone also occurs. Glucagon stimulates hepatic glycogenolysis and favors gluconeogenesis. Epinephrine stimulates hepatic and renal glucose production, decreases clearance of glucose by muscle, and also mobilizes gluconeogenetic precursors. This hormonal response typically precedes the onset of hypoglycemic symptoms. The initial symptoms of sweating, anxiety, and heart palpitations occur at a serum glucose level below 60 mg/dL, providing warning signs of hypoglycemia, which allows the patient to seek corrective measures. Once the serum glucose is less than 50 mg/dL, cognitive dysfunction occurs. If the serum glucose continues to fall without treatment, more severe neurological symptoms such as convulsions, coma, and death can occur. In type 1 diabetic and advanced type 2 diabetic patients, the physiologic response to hypoglycemia as described earlier is altered; as glucose level falls, therapeutic insulin levels do not fall, and thus the response of glucagon and epinephrine secretion is blunted. This results in lack of recognizable warning symptoms or what is known as *hypoglycemic unawareness*.[74,78-80] This lack of hormonal response is more often seen in patients who have recurrent prior episodes of hypoglycemia. However, the strict avoidance of hypoglycemia for 2 weeks can restore neurohumoral response. Iatrogenic hypoglycemia is the result of the interplay of insulin excess and compromised glucose counterregulation.[79]

The incidence of severe hypoglycemic episodes in one study of insulin-dependent diabetics was as high as 91% in patients with complete unawareness, 69% in those with partial unawareness, and only 18% in patients with normal awareness.[82] Aggressive glycemic therapy also contributes to defective counterregulation. A prospective study of long-term intensive insulin therapy in type 1 diabetes found that the frequency of hypoglycemia and the lack of awareness symptoms were much higher in those who had an HbA1c less than 6% as compared with those with an HbA1c between 6% and 8%.[83] These observations often preclude intensive insulin therapy in some patients. Reviewing the risk factors for hypoglycemia and discussing ways of risk factor reduction with individual patients are important.

Prevalence of Hospital Hypoglycemia

Hypoglycemia is a major barrier to glucose control as shown in the Diabetes Control and Complication Trial (DCCT): in type 1 diabetics receiving intensive insulin therapy, there was a threefold increase in the risk of hypoglycemia, especially nocturnal hypoglycemia.[72,84] The mortality rate in hypoglycemic hospitalized patients varied from 22.2% to 27% in observational series including diabetic patients.[85,86] Although the mortality rate in hospitalized diabetic patients with hypoglycemia is higher, some investigators showed that hypoglycemia was not an independent factor for mortality. In a case control study among 5404 inpatients 70 years or older, 281 (5.2%) had documented hypoglycemia. Compared with a randomly selected nonhypoglycemic group ($n = 281$), there were more women than men; sepsis was 10 times more common ($P < .001$); malignancy was 2.8 times more common ($P = .04$); the mean serum albumin level was lower; and the mean serum creatinine and alkaline phosphatase levels were higher ($P < .001$ for both). Diabetes was known in 42% of the hypoglycemic group and in 31% of the nonhypoglycemic group ($P = .03$); 70 patients in the hypoglycemic group were taking sulfonylureas or insulin. In-hospital mortality and 3-month mortality were about twice as high in the hypoglycemic group ($P < .001$). However, multivariate analysis of mortality found that sepsis, low albumin level, and malignancy were independent predictors, whereas hypoglycemia was not an independent predictor for mortality.[87]

Prevention of Hospital Hypoglycemia

The most common causes of hypoglycemia in the hospital are decreased caloric intake and the lack of insulin dose adjustment despite lowering of glucose level. Common events that trigger hypoglycemia in the hospital follow:

- Sudden non per os (NPO) status or decrease in oral intake
- Interruption of total parenteral nutrition or enteral feeding
- Intravenous dextrose discontinued
- Transportation off unit floor or ward causing meal delay
- Reduction in corticosteroid dose

Box 59-1

Predisposing Conditions for Hospital Hypoglycemia

Renal failure
Liver disease
Sepsis
Malnutrition
Shock
Congestive heart failure
Total parenteral nutrition
Patient inability to self-report symptoms
Hypoglycemic unawareness
Alcoholism
Old age
Tapering of glucocorticoid dose
Adrenal insufficiency
Hypopituitarism

A list of conditions that predispose to inpatient hypoglycemia is provided in Box 59-1.[88]

Identifying risk factors and reacting to these triggering events is an important part in preventing hypoglycemia. Administering IV glucose is important if feeding is interrupted, as is decreasing the dose of insulin in patients with renal failure, in type 1 diabetics with hypoglycemic unawareness, in patients on a tapered dose of glucocorticoid, and in those transitioning from IV or enteral feeding to regular meal frequency. Close monitoring of blood glucose in these instances is required.

Diagnostic Approach

The first step in evaluating a patient with suspected hypoglycemia is to document low blood glucose when the patient is symptomatic. The most useful classification of the causes of hypoglycemia is based on whether the patient appears healthy or ill (Table 59-4).[89] It is not uncommon to see hypoglycemia in critically ill patients with multiorgan failure (often associated with sepsis and renal insufficiency); the presence of spontaneous hypoglycemia in an otherwise healthy outpatient should prompt further evaluation of rare causes such as insulinoma. The possibility of drug-induced hypoglycemia in healthy individuals should also always be carefully sought because this could occur from surreptitious use, a suicide attempt, or a pharmacist inadvertently dispensing the drug. In diabetic patients the most common and obvious cause of hypoglycemia is overtreatment with insulin. In a study analyzing 137 episodes of hypoglycemia (serum glucose <49 mg/dL) occurring in 94 adult patients hospitalized during a 6-month period at a tertiary care hospital, 45% of the patients had diabetes mellitus, and administered insulin was implicated in 90% of episodes in diabetics.[90] However, the recent shift in the use of new insulin analogues including the short-acting analogues glulisine, lispro, and aspart[91] and the long-acting basal insulins such as glargine and detemir[92] causes less hypoglycemic events

Table 59-4. Clinical Classification of Hypoglycemia in Adults

Healthy-Appearing Patient	Ill-Appearing Patient
Type 1 or 2 diabetic: inappropriate insulin or oral agent; concurrent use of alcohol/β-blockers or ACE inhibitors	Renal failure Sepsis Hepatic disease Congestive heart failure
Cardiac patient: drug use of disopyramide, cibenzoline	Large non–β–cell tumors (fibroma, sarcoma) Hypopituitarism, hypoadrenalism
Drug use: ethanol, salicylates, quinine, haloperidol	Starvation, anorexia nervosa
Insulinoma Factitious use of insulin or sulfonylurea Autoimmune hypoglycemia Dispensing error (substitution of sulfonylurea drug) Ackee fruit poisoning	Drug use: Co-trimoxazole in renal failure Pentamidine for *Pneumocystis* Quinine in malaria Topical salicylates in renal failure

ACE, angiotensin-converting enzyme.
Modified from Service FJ: Hypoglycemic disorders. N Engl J Med 1995; 332:1144-1152.

compared with human regular or NPH. Most cases of sulfonylurea overdose occur in the elderly, in whom decreased renal clearance and hepatic dysfunction are contributing factors.

Glyburide causes the highest incidence of hypoglycemia among sulfonylurea users. In a 4-year retrospective study of 14,000 patients 65 years or older with type 2 diabetes treated with different sulfonylurea drugs, the incidence of serious hypoglycemia was rare but was the highest in those treated with glyburide.[93] The hypoglycemic effect of glyburide can last more than 24 hours.[94] The short-acting insulin secretagogues repaglinide and nateglinide have a potential for causing hypoglycemia but to a lesser magnitude compared with glyburide. Monotherapy with metformin or thiazolidinediones (pioglitazone or rosiglitazone) should not cause hypoglycemia. The second most important factor identified causing hypoglycemia in hospitalized patients was renal failure, even in nondiabetics. Others included malnutrition, liver disease, heart failure, sepsis, treatment of hyperkalemia, shock, and total parenteral nutrition with insulin.[90]

Excess alcohol consumption by diabetics treated with insulin or oral agents can result in profound hypoglycemia.[95] In type 1 diabetes, even moderate consumption of alcohol in the evening has been associated with hypoglycemia after breakfast the next morning.[96] Ethanol primarily inhibits gluconeogenesis and also inhibits cortisol and growth hormone response and delays epinephrine response to hypoglycemia. Alcohol-induced hypoglycemia in nondiabetic individuals typically follows a binge of moderate to heavy alcohol consumption during which the person eats little food. The patient often presents to the ED in a comatose state and may be hypothermic. The mortality rate in these hospitalized patients could be as high as 10%.[97] One study revealed that 18% to 52% of patients admitted to the ED with sustained hypoglycemia had alcohol intoxication.[97] Some chronic alcoholics present with alcohol ketoacidosis resembling diabetic ketoacidosis. This is a more indolent process that often occurs several days after alcohol consumption and poor diet. These patients often present with vomiting, severe abdominal pain, and an anion gap metabolic acidosis secondary to ketones and concurrent metabolic alkalosis, which may nearly normalize pH. Alcohol level may be minimal or absent because none may have been consumed for several days before admission. Plasma glucose levels are usually normal or modestly elevated but can be severely low. An elevated osmolal gap is also seen because of acetone accumulation and the presence of ethanol.[98] Lactic acidosis could also be seen because of hypoperfusion. This medical emergency should be treated with thiamine injection followed by IV 5% glucose in NS to prevent development of Wernicke encephalopathy. Patients with severe hypoglycemia can present to the ED with the same neuroglycopenic symptoms of an intoxicated individual; therefore it is important to always check point-of-care blood glucose in patients suspected of intoxication to exclude severe hypoglycemia and prevent potential fatal complications if left untreated.

Hypoglycemia could also be caused by large mesenchymal and epithelial tumors such as sarcoma, mesothelioma, fibroma, hemangiopericytoma, and hepatoma. The cause of hypoglycemia in these tumors is related to the production of a humoral insulin growth factor II (IGF II), as well as consumption of glucose by these large tumors. The diagnosis of these non–islet cell tumors is based on the findings of an elevated IGF II with suppressed level of insulin and C peptide.[99] Box 59-2 addresses diagnostic testing of hypoglycemia in ill-appearing adults.

The diagnosis of a hypoglycemic disorder in a healthy-appearing subject should be strongly suspected if all three criteria of Whipple's triad are present:

Box 59-2

Diagnostic Testing for Hypoglycemia in Ill-Appearing Adult Patients

Glucose level, when patient is symptomatic
Tests directed to underlying disease
Optional tests based on clinical suspicion
Blood and other cultures
Adrenocorticotropic hormone/cortisol, while hypoglycemic
Liver function tests
Thyroid profile/thyroid-stimulating hormone
Insulin-like growth factor II (rarely needed)

Modified from Service FJ: Endocrine clinics. Endo Metab Clin North Am 1999;28:519-532.

- The recognition that the patient's symptoms could be caused by hypoglycemia
- Documentation that the patient's serum glucose concentration is low when the symptoms are present.
- Relief of symptoms by administration of glucose.

The most important diagnostic test is obtaining a serum glucose while the patient is symptomatic. If the serum glucose at that time is normal, no further evaluation is necessary. If the serum glucose is below 60 mg/dL during symptoms consistent with hypoglycemia, further evaluation is necessary to exclude the possibility of insulinoma or factitious intake of insulin or other drugs. The 72-hour fast should then be done[100] in a non-ICU setting. If the patient develops hypoglycemia, it is important to measure insulin at the time of hypoglycemia. Plasma insulin concentration of 3 mIU/mL when the plasma glucose concentration is below 55 mg/dL while the patient is symptomatic indicates an excess of insulin consistent with insulinoma. Measurement of plasma C-peptide is important to distinguish an exogenous from an endogenous source of hyperinsulinemia. When serum glucose is less than 45 mg/dL, a C-peptide value of 0.6 ng/mL or above is indicative of insulinoma. Screening for the presence of sulfonylureas in the blood should also be obtained. Emphasizing that random measurement of C-peptide and insulin is of little diagnostic value is important. The measurement of these hormones should be done simultaneously and is only of diagnostic usefulness when obtained at a time of documented hypoglycemia. If a patient develops a spontaneous episode of hypoglycemia and is symptomatic, measurement of plasma insulin C peptide and proinsulin should be done at that time, obviating the need for a 72-hour fast (Box 59-3).

Approach to Management

Patients should be taught how to recognize warning signs and symptoms of hypoglycemia and educated on factors that predispose to hypoglycemia such as missing a meal, timing of insulin (which should be given before rather than after a meal), and the effect of exercise on lowering blood sugar (which can last several hours after the exercise is over). The importance of blood glucose monitoring should be emphasized, as well as the need to carry glucose tablets, especially in potentially dangerous situations such as driving a car.

The initial treatment should be with 15 to 20 g of glucose, in the form of glucose tablets or an equivalent such as 4 oz of orange juice or soda, 6 jelly beans, or 8 lifesaver candies. This should be followed by ingestion of complex carbohydrates if a meal is not taken shortly after.

In patients who are confused with poor coordination and difficulty swallowing, glucose gel can be inserted in the buccal mucosa. In the home setting when a patient is unconscious or in a hospitalized patient without IV access, 1 mg glucagon administered subcutaneously or intramuscularly is the best treatment. Nausea and vomiting are the major side effects of glucagon. Treatment with parenteral glucagon at home requires that a family member be able to locate the glucagon emergency kit and administer it. When the patient is alert enough to swallow, administration of glucose following glucagon treatment is recommended.

In the hospital or ED an IV bolus of 25% to 50% dextrose has been the standard treatment of choice with repeat blood sugar monitoring. One should use caution in administering highly concentrated IV dextrose because extravasation-induced hand amputation has been reported with the use of D50.[101] In non–life-threatening cases of hypoglycemia, it might be prudent to give a more diluted solution such as 50 to 100 mL of 20% dextrose to prevent tissue toxicity, as well as compensatory hyperglycemia. Continuous delivery of glucose is often required in cases of hypoglycemia because of long-acting sulfonylurea or long-acting insulin, especially in the presence of renal failure. Doses as high as 80 g of glucose per hour may be required for up to 60 or more hours.[102] Patients should be monitored for at least 24 hours to prevent recurrence of hypoglycemia. In insulinoma cases that are not surgically resectable, administration of diazoxide is recommended.

Box 59-3

Diagnostic Testing for Hypoglycemia in Healthy-Appearing Adult Patients

Glucose level, when patient is symptomatic
Sulfonylurea levels (first and second generation)
Alcohol level
Drug screen
Electrolytes, blood urea nitrogen, creatinine
Insulin/C-peptide level while patient is hypoglycemic
Formal 72-hour fast

Modified from Service FJ: Endocrine clinics. Endo Metab Clin North Am 1999;28:519-532.

GLUCOSE CONTROL IN THE INTENSIVE CARE UNIT

As the epidemic of diabetes rises, so does the number of diabetic patients admitted to the hospital. In the year 2000, 12.4% of hospital discharges in the United States listed diabetes as a diagnosis.[103] The number of diabetics discharged from the hospital has increased by more than 50% during the 1990s[104] with an estimated direct care cost of 40 billion dollars in 2001.[105] Adults with diabetes are six times more likely to be hospitalized than those without diabetes[106] because of concurrent cardiovascular and infectious complications or surgical problems. Yet inpatient glycemic control in most hospitals remains far from optimal, partly because the care of diabetes becomes secondary to the care of the acute illness.

Hyperglycemia and Poor Outcome

Several studies have established the association between hyperglycemia and adverse outcomes. Umpierrez[107] reviewed 1886 patients on general medical and surgical units with fasting blood glucose levels of more than 126 mg/dL or random blood glucose levels of more than 200 mg/dL; after adjusting for confounding factors, patients with new hyperglycemia had an 18-fold increase in hospital mortality and those with known diabetes had a 2.7-fold increase in mortality compared with the normoglycemic group. Hyperglycemic patients also had a longer length of stay, greater risk of infection, and more subsequent nursing home care.[107] In a large prospective study of patients undergoing coronary bypass grafting, diabetic patients were found to have a higher mortality rate compared with nondiabetic patients and a higher incidence of stroke.[108] In 1826 critically ill patients, mortality was directly correlated with increased blood sugar above 80 mg/dL. Patients with a mean glucose level between 80 and 99 mg/dL had a 9.6% hospital mortality; those between 100 and 119 mg/dL had a 12.2% mortality; and those greater than 300 mg/dL had up to 42.5% mortality.[109] A meta-analysis of 26 studies in patients with cerebral vascular accident showed an increased mortality in patients with blood glucose levels greater than 110 to 126 mg/dL and worse functional recovery with blood glucose greater than 121 to 144 mg/dL.[110]

Does Intensive Insulin Improve Outcome?

The importance of tight glycemic control in hospitalized patients is gaining more acceptance since the publication of a landmark trial by Van Der Berghe and colleagues[111] in 2001. In this trial 1548 surgical ICU patients on mechanical ventilation were randomized to intensive insulin infusion to keep the blood glucose between 80 and 110 mg/dL or conventional therapy to maintain blood glucose between 180 and 200 mg/dL. In comparison with conventional therapy, the intensive insulin treatment group had a 42% reduction in ICU mortality, 34% reduction in overall hospital mortality, 46% reduction in risk of infection, 41% reduction in acute renal failure requiring dialysis, 50% reduction in number of red blood cell transfusions, and 44% decrease in critical illness polyneuropathy.[111] The beneficial effect of insulin therapy seems to be caused by meticulous glucose control rather than insulin treatment or insulin dose.[112]

In the Diabetes and Insulin-Glucose infusion in Acute Myocardial Infarction (DIGAMI) study, the investigators randomly assigned 620 diabetic patients with acute myocardial infarction to a control group versus an infusion group that received IV insulin for 24 hours followed by multidose subcutaneous insulin for at least 3 months. At hospital discharge the mean glucose value was 162 mg/dL in the control group and 148 mg/dL in the infusion group. After 1 year, mortality was reduced by 28% in the intensely treated group[113,114] and 11% after 3.4 years follow-up.[115] In another study of diabetic patients undergoing coronary artery bypass grafts, the mortality was reduced from 5.3% to 2.5% in patients on intensive glycemic control.[116]

Two prospective studies did not show the benefit of the DIGAMI 2 trial,[117] perhaps because of the lack of strict adherence to the use of insulin during the 3 years of follow-up. Also in a second recent prospective study by Van Der Berghe and colleagues,[112] of 1200 medical ICU patients randomly assigned to insulin infusion with a goal of blood glucose between 80 and 110 mg/dL versus conventional therapy (blood glucose around 200 mg/dL), there was no statistical difference in mortality, in contrast to the previous study in the surgical ICU by the same author. However, the study did show reduction in morbidity such as prevention of acquired kidney injury, earlier weaning from mechanical ventilation, and early discharge from the medical ICU and hospital.[118] The findings of these studies, however, do not offset the strong evidence from epidemiologic data and large prospective randomized trials that successfully supports the benefit of intensive glycemic control.

The American Diabetes Association (ADA) published a comprehensive review on glycemic control and hospital outcomes and recommendations on how best to achieve these goals.[119]

What Is the Target Glucose Level for Hospitalized Patients?

On the basis of new evidence that intensive glucose control is beneficial in the hospital setting, a consensus development conference in 2004 sponsored by the American Association of Clinical Endocrinologists, in conjunction with the American Diabetes Association and Critical Care Society, established the following goals[120]:

- Preprandial less than 110 mg/dL
- Peak postprandial less than 180 mg/dL
- Critically ill surgical patients 80 to 110 mg/dL

In 2005 the ADA proposed a target goal in critically ill patients of less than 180 mg/dL and as close to 110 mg/dL as possible.[121]

Achieving the Goal

Insulin is the drug of choice for treatment of hyperglycemia in the intensive care setting and perioperative period. In contrast to oral agents, it is safer and easily titrated under rapidly changing circumstances. Metformin in particular should not be given to critically ill patients who are at higher risk of developing lactic acidosis because of concern over altered renal function, hypoxia, congestive heart failure, septicemia, liver failure, and the potential need for contrast radiograph studies. Thiazolidinediones should be avoided in patients with increased intravascular volume because they could worsen congestive heart failure and should not be given to patients with hepatic dysfunction. Sulfonylureas have a long duration of action and can cause hypoglycemia in patients with poor PO intake or with renal failure.[122] The widely used insulin sliding scales, when prescribed alone, are usually ineffective. They do not provide any basal insulin but only treat hyperglycemia after the fact instead of preventing the occurrence of hyperglycemia, resulting in erratic glucose control.[123,124] A sliding scale should never be used as a sole therapy in type 1 diabetic patients who are NPO. Patients with type 1 diabetes require basal insulin at all times (even when not eating) along with dextrose to prevent diabetic ketoacidosis. Insulin coverage scale should always be used in conjunction with at least one injection of basal insulin or multiple doses of short- or intermediate-acting insulin. If frequent correction doses are required, the next day's scheduled dose of insulin should be increased to prevent hyperglycemia. Also, the dose of insulin in the sliding scale should vary according to weight and insulin sensitivity.

The subcutaneous insulin requirement in most patients should be given in a scheduled dose that will provide 50% basal insulin and 50% bolus or prandial insulin. Basal insulin is provided by long-acting insulin preparation such as neutral protamine Hagedorn (NPH), lente, detemir, and glargine, given once or twice a day to suppress hepatic neoglucogenics and control fasting glucose, as well as premeal blood glucose. Basal insulin can also be provided via an insulin pump delivering continuous fast-acting insulin. This pattern of delivery is mostly used in type 1 diabetes. In glucocorticoid therapy, the prandial component seems to be increased up to 70% of the total dose of insulin administered. Patients receiving high-dose IV glucocorticoid will often require IV insulin infusion.[125]

Insulin analogues lispro, aspart, and glulisine are preferred for prandial coverage, as well as correction dose therapy. They are typically provided as a premeal bolus to cover the extra requirement after food. They have a rapid onset of action within 15 minutes and provide better postprandial coverage and less post absorptive hypoglycemia in comparison with regular insulin.[126] They are also commonly used in insulin pumps (Table 59-5).

In total parenteral nutrition (TPN), the use of a separate IV insulin infusion is the best option because it often achieves the target goal within 24 hours compared with adding an incremental dose of insulin in the TPN, which takes many days to achieve the target goal.[125] Once control is obtained, 66% to 100% of the total units of insulin infused intravenously over 24 hours should be added to the TPN bag.

Table 59-5. Insulin Preparations and Effects

Insulin Preparation	Onset of Action	Peak Action	Duration of Action
Standard			
Regular (soluble)	30-60 min	2-3 hr	8-10 hr
NPH (isophane)	2-4 hr	4-10 hr	12-18 hr
Zinc insulin (Lente)	2-4 hr	4-12 hr	12-20 hr
Analogues			
Lispro	5-15 min	30-90 min	4-6 hr
Aspart	5-15 min	30-90 min	4-6 hr
Glulisine	5-15 min	30-90 min	4-6 hr
Glargine	2-4 hr	Peakless	20-24 hr

In enteral feeding only one small study of 34 patients has reported glycemic outcomes in patients with type 2 diabetes receiving different enteral formula[127]; those on a lower carbohydrate formula had a slightly lower HbA1c after 3 months but did not reach statistical significance. In continuous enteral feeding once- or twice-daily injection of insulin glargine or detemir is appropriate with correction dose of short-acting insulin every 4 to 6 hours while the glargine dose is being increased. Another option would be to use IV insulin as described with TPN. For patients receiving only an overnight tube feed, NPH with regular insulin as a single injection at the time of enteral feeding provides good coverage. A major caution of using insulin in this situation, particularly long-acting ones, is the risk of hypoglycemia should feeding get interrupted—thus the need for IV glucose in the interim.

Perioperative Insulin Requirements

For type 1 diabetes, one should give half to two thirds of the standard outpatient long-acting insulin in the morning and start a 5% dextrose solution at 75 to 100 mL/hour before and after surgery. Dialysis patients should receive 10% dextrose at a lower rate. Basal insulin should always be given the night before to achieve optimal glucose control before surgery. If prior fasting blood glucose has been trending low, the dose of basal insulin at night should be reduced by 20%. An alternative would be IV insulin. In critically ill patients continuous subcutaneous insulin infusion through a pump should be discontinued and replaced by IV insulin because of the erratic absorption and variable perfusion of the subcutaneous tissue. In addition, patients may not be alert to self-manage the administration of insulin through the pump.

For type 2 diabetes, basal insulin should be given the night before and could be withheld the morning of surgery. If the patient is back by lunch time, two thirds of the scheduled morning dose should be given then. A small dose of short-acting insulin could be given on the morning of the procedure if fasting blood glucose is greater than 180 to 200 mg/dL.

Intravenous insulin therapy remains the best method to achieve rapid glycemic control in critically ill patients. It is often necessary in patients who have uncontrolled diabetes and widely fluctuating blood glucose on subcutaneous insulin injection; in patients with diabetic ketoacidosis, a hyperglycemic hyperosmolar state, myocardial infarction; in patients who have had postoperative coronary bypass surgery; during general perioperative care and high-dose glucocorticoid therapy; and in critically ill patients. We recommend the protocol in Table 59-6. Requirements of IV insulin are often higher in patients undergoing cardiopulmonary bypass surgery, organ transplantation, TPN, glucocorticoid therapy, and sepsis.[128] Lower infusion rates are usually necessary in renal and hepatic failure, in a subset of type 1 diabetics with increased sensitivity to regular insulin, and in patients with hypoglycemic unawareness.[129] Alternate IV insulin protocols are available.[116,130]

Table 59-6. Intravenous Insulin Therapy Protocol

General Guidelines: **Goal Blood Glucose (BG) = ——** (Usually 80-180 mg/dL)

- **Standard drip:** 100 Units/100 mL 0.9% NaCl via an infusion device.
- Surgical patients who have received an oral diabetes medication within 24 hr should start when BG > 120 mg/dL. All other patients can start when BG ≥ 70.
- Insulin infusions should be discontinued when a patient is eating AND has received first dose of subcutaneous insulin.

Intravenous Fluids:

- Most patients will need 5-10 g of glucose/hr
  - D_5W or $D_5W1\backslash 2NS$ at 100-200 mL/hr or equivalent (e.g., TPN, enteral feeds)

Initiating the Infusion:

- **Algorithm 1:** Start here for most patients.
- **Algorithm 2:** For patients not controlled with Algorithm 1, or start here if s/p CABG, s/p solid organ transplant or islet cell transplant, receiving glucocorticoids, or patient with diabetes receiving >80 units/day of insulin as an outpatient.
- **Algorithm 3:** For patients not controlled on Algorithm 2. NO PATIENTS START HERE without authorization from the endocrine service.
- **Algorithm 4:** For patients not controlled on Algorithm 3. NO PATIENTS START HERE.
- Patients not controlled with the above algorithms need an endocrine consult.

Algorithm 1		**Algorithm 2**		**Algorithm 3**		**Algorithm 4**	
BG	Units/hr	BG	Units/hr	BG	Units/hr	BG	Units/hr
<60 = Hypoglycemia (See below for treatment)							
<70	Off	<70	Off	<70	Off	<70	Off
70-109	0.2	70-109	0.5	70-109	1	70-109	1.5
110-119	0.5	110-119	1	110-119	2	110-119	3
120-149	1	120-149	1.5	120-149	3	120-149	5
150-179	1.5	150-179	2	150-179	4	150-179	7
180-209	2	180-209	3	180-209	5	180-209	9
210-239	2	210-239	4	210-239	6	210-239	12
240-269	3	240-269	5	240-269	8	240-269	16
270-299	3	270-299	6	270-299	10	270-299	20
300-329	4	300-329	7	300-329	12	300-329	24
330-359	4	330-359	8	330-359	14	>330	28
>360	6	>360	12	>360	16		

Moving from Algorithm to Algorithm:

- *Moving Up:* An algorithm failure is defined as BG outside the goal range (see above goal), and the BG does not change by at least 60 mg/dL within 1 hr.
- *Moving Down:* When BG is <70 mg/dL × 2

Patient Monitoring

- Check capillary BG every hour until it is within goal range for 4 hr, then decrease to every 2 hr for 4 hr, and if remains stable may decrease to every 4 hr.
- Hourly monitoring may be indicated for critically ill patients even if they have stable BG

Treatment of Hypoglycemia **(BG < 60 mg/dL)**

- Discontinue insulin drip AND
- Give $D_{50}W$ IV
  - Patient awake: 25 mL (1/2 amp)
  - Patient not awake: 50 mL (1 amp)
- Recheck BG every 20 min and repeat 25 mL of $D_{50}W$ IV if <60 mg/dL. Restart drip once BG is >70 mg/dL × 2 checks. Restart drip with lower algorithm (see Moving Down).

Notify the physician:

- For any BG change >100 mg/dL in 1 hr.
- For BG >360 mg/dL
- For hypoglycemia that has not resolved within 20 min of administering 50 ml of $D_{50}W$ IV and discontinuing the insulin drip.

BG, blood glucose; CABG, coronary artery bypass grafting; NS, normal saline; TPN, total parenteral nutrition.
Adapted with permission from Trence D, Kelly J, Hirsh I: The rationale and management of hyperglycemia for in-patients with cardiovascular disease: Time for a change. J Clin Endocrinol Metab 2003;88:2430-2437. Copyright 2003, The Endocrine Society.

KEY POINTS

- DKA, HHS, and hypoglycemia are life-threatening disorders of glucose metabolism.
- Considerable overlap occurs in clinical and laboratory presentations of DKA and HHS.
- Identifying and treating precipitating causes such as infection, major illnesses, and inadequate insulin therapy are essential.
- Diagnosis in the ED should be suspected at triage using point-of-care testing for blood glucose, urine ketones, ECG, and venous blood gas.
- Initial therapy of DKA and HHS requires replacement of fluids (initiated prior to laboratory results), insulin and/or potassium, electrolytes, and any precipitating etiology identified.
- Initial potassium concentration determines timing of insulin therapy.
- Insulin is given by continuous infusion, with an optional bolus. Lower rates of insulin are usually given in HHS.
- Bicarbonate therapy is not recommended in the routine treatment of DKA.
- Insulin infusion should not be stopped when euglycemia is obtained but only when the anion gap normalizes.
- The diagnosis of hypoglycemia should be made when the serum glucose is low and the patient is symptomatic.
- Excess insulin and defective counterregulatory response are the most common causes of hypoglycemia. In critically ill patients, sepsis and renal failure play a major role.
- Intensive intravenous insulin therapy with the goal of blood glucose 80 to 110 mg/dL reduces morbidity and mortality in surgical ICU patients.
- Use of insulin sliding scale alone without scheduled basal insulin is ineffective; type 1 diabetics always require basal insulin even when they are NPO.
- Frequent insulin dose adjustment is often necessary in hospitalized patients, and intravenous insulin is the best therapy in critically ill patients.

REFERENCES

1. American Diabetes Association: Type 2 diabetes in children and adolescents. Diabetes Care 2000;23:381-389.
2. Centers for Disease Control and Prevention: National diabetes fact sheet: General information and national estimates on diabetes in the United States, 2005. Atlanta, U.S. Department of Health and Human Services, Centers for Disease Control and Prevention, 2005.
3. American Diabetes Association: Diabetic ketoacidosis in infants, children, and adolescents. Diabetes Care 2006;29:5.
4. Ellis EN: Concepts of fluid therapy in diabetic ketoacidosis and hyperosmolar hyperglycemic nonketotic coma. Pediatr Clin North Am 1990;37:313-321.
5. Gottschalk ME, Ros SP, Zeller WP: The emergency management of hyperglycemic-hyperosmolar nonketotic coma in the pediatric patient. Pediatr Emerg Care 1996;12:48-51.
6. Kitabchi AE, Umpierrez GE, Murphy MB, et al: Management of hyperglycemic crises in patients with diabetes. Diabetes Care 2001;24: 131-154.
7. American Diabetes Association: Hyperglycemic crisis in patients with diabetes mellitus. Diabetes Care 2002;25:S100-S108.
8. American Diabetes Association: Hyperglycemic crises in diabetes. Diabetes Care 2004;27(Suppl 1): S94-102.
9. Naunheim R, Jang TJ, Banet G, et al: Point-of-care test identifies diabetic ketoacidosis at triage. Acad Emerg Med 2006;13:683-685.
10. Westphal SA: The occurrence of diabetic ketoacidosis in non-insulin dependent diabetes and newly diagnosed diabetic adults. Am J Med 1996;101:19-24.
11. Stoner GD: Hyperosmolar hyperglycemic state. Am Fam Physician 2005;71:1723-1730.
12. English P, Williams G: Hyperglycaemic crises and lactic acidosis in diabetes mellitus. Postgrad Med J 2004;80: 253-261.
13. Thompson CJ, Cummings F, Chalmers J, et al: Abnormal insulin treatment behavior: A major cause of ketoacidosis in the young adult. Diabet Med 1995;12:429.
14. Lebovitz HE: Diabetic ketoacidosis. Lancet 1995;345:767.
15. Chansky ME, Lubkin CL: Diabetic ketoacidosis. In Tintinalli JE, Kelen GD, Stapczynski JS (eds): Tintinalli's Emergency Medicine: A Comprehensive Study Guide, 6th ed. New York, McGraw-Hill, 2004, pp 1287-1294.
16. Nair S, Yadav D, Pitchumoni CS: Association of diabetic ketoacidosis and acute pancreatitis: Observations in 100 consecutive episodes of DKA. Am J Gastroenterol 2000;95:10, 2795-2800.
17. Arieff AI, Carroll HJ: Nonketotic hyperosmolar coma with hyperglycemia: Clinical features, pathophysiology, renal function, acid-base balance, plasma-cerebrospinal fluid equilibrium and the effects of therapy in 37 cases. Medicine 1972;51:73-94.
18. Gerich JE, Martin MM, Recant L: Clinical and metabolic characteristics of hyperosmolar nonketotic coma. Diabetes 1971;20:228-238.
19. Trence DL, Hirsch IB: Hyperglycemic crisis in diabetes mellitus Type 2. Endocrinol Metab Clin North Am 2001;30:817-831.
20. Chiasson JL, Aris-Jilwan N, Belanger R, et al: Diagnosis and treatment of diabetic ketoacidosis and the hyperglycemic hyperosmolar state. Can Med Assoc J 2003;168:859-866.
21. Arieff AI, Carroll HJ: Cerebral edema and depression of sensorium in nonketotic hyperosmolar coma. Diabetes 1974;23:525-531.
22. Umpierrez G, Freire AX: Abdominal pain in patients with hyperglycemic crises. J Crit Care 2002;17:63-67.
23. Umpierrez GE, Khajavi M, Kitabchi AE: Review: Diabetic ketoacidosis and hyperglycemic hyperosmolar nonketotic syndrome. Am J Med Sci 1996;311:225-233.
24. Ma OJ, Rush MD, Godfrey MM, et al: Arterial blood gas results rarely influence emergency physician management of patients with suspected diabetic ketoacidosis. Acad Emerg Med 2003;10:836-841.
25. Kelly AM: The case for venous rather than arterial blood gases in diabetic ketoacidosis. Emerg Med Australas 2006;18:64-67.
26. Kreshak A, Chen EH: Arterial blood gas analysis: Are its values needed for the management of diabetic ketoacidosis? Ann Emerg Med 2005;45:5.
27. Hale PJ, Nattrass M: A comparison of arterial and non-arterialized capillary blood gases in diabetic ketoacidosis. Diabet Med 1988;5:76-78.
28. Emmett M, Nairns RG: Clinical use of the anion gap. Medicine 1977;56: 38-54.
29. Chansky ME, Riggs RL: Hyperosmolar hyperglycemic state. In Wolfson AB (ed): Harwood-Nuss' Clinical Practice of Emergency Medicine, 4th ed. Philadelphia, Lippincott Williams & Wilkins, 2005, pp 846-849.
30. Csako G, Elin RJ: Unrecognized false positive ketones from drugs containing

free sulfhydryl group. JAMA 1993;269:1634.
31. Adrogue HJ, Lederer ED, Suki WN, et al: Determinants of plasma potassium levels in diabetic ketoacidosis. Medicine 1986;65:163.
32. Hillier TA, Abbott RD, Barrett EJ: Hyponatremia: Evaluating the correction factor for hyperglycemia. Am J Med 1999;106:399.
33. Slovis CM, Mork BGC, Slovis RJ, et al: Diabetic ketoacidosis and infection: Leukocyte count and differential as early predictors of serious infection. Am J Emerg Med 1987;5:1.
34. Filbin MR, Brown DF, Nadel ES: Hyperglycemic hyperosmolar nonketotic coma. J Emerg Med 2001;20:285-290.
35. Trachtenbarg DE: Diabetic ketoacidosis. Am Fam Physician 2005;71:1705-1714.
36. Feig PU, McCurdy DK: The hypertonic state. N Engl J Med 1977;297:1444-1454.
37. Edge J: Cerebral oedema during treatment of diabetic ketoacidosis: Are we any nearer finding a cause? Diabetes Metab Res Rev 2000;16:316.
38. Foster DW, McGarry JD: The metabolic derangements and treatment of diabetic ketoacidosis. N Engl J Med 1989;309:159.
39. Umpierrez GE, Cuervo R, Karabell A, et al: Treatment of diabetic ketoacidosis with subcutaneous insulin aspart. Diabetes Care 2004;27:1873-1878.
40. Dorin RI, Crapo LM: Hypokalemic respiratory arrest in diabetic ketoacidosis. JAMA 1987;257:1517-1518.
41. Knochel JP: The pathophysiology and clinical characteristics of severe hypophosphatemia. Arch Intern Med 1977;137:203.
42. Winter RJ, Harris CJ, Phillips LS, Green OC: DKA: Induction of hypocalcemia and hypomagnesemia by phosphate therapy. Am J Med 1979;67:897-900.
43. Okuda Y, Adrogue HJ, Field JB, et al: Counterproductive effects of sodium bicarbonate in diabetic ketoacidosis. J Clin Endocrinol Metab 1996;81:314.
44. Viallon A, Zeni F, Lafond P, et al: Does bicarbonate therapy improve the management of severe diabetic ketoacidosis? Crit Care Med 1999;27:2690.
45. Green SM, Rothrock SG, Ho JD, et al: Failure of adjunctive bicarbonate to improve outcome in severe pediatric diabetic ketoacidosis. Emerg Med 1998;31:41.
46. Clements RS Jr, Vourganti B: Fatal diabetic ketoacidosis: Major causes and approaches to their prevention. Diabetes Care 1978;1:314-325.
47. Glaser N, Barnett P, McCaslin I, et al: Risk factors for cerebral edema in children with diabetic ketoacidosis. N Engl J Med 2001;344:264.
48. Hale PM, Rezvani I, Braunstein AW, et al: Factors predicting cerebral edema in young children with diabetic ketoacidosis and new onset type I diabetes. Acta Paediatr 1997;86:626.
49. Krane EJ, Rockoff MA, Wallman JK, Wolfsdorf JI: Subclinical brain swelling in children during treatment of diabetic ketoacidosis. N Engl J Med 1985;312:1147-1151.
50. Glaser NS, Wooton-Gorges SL, Marcin JP, et al: Mechanism of cerebral edema in children with diabetic ketoacidosis. J Pediatr 2004;145:164-171.
51. Kamat P, Vats A, Gross M, Checchia PA: Use of hypertonic saline for the treatment of altered mental status associated with diabetic ketoacidosis. Pediatr Crit Care Med 2003;4:239-242.
52. Lethbridge-Cejku M, Schiller JS, Bernadel L: Summary health statistics for US adults: National Health interview Survey, 2002. National Center for Health Statistics. Vital Health Stat 2004;10:1-160.
53. Narayan KM, Boyle JP, Thompson TJ, et al: Lifetime risk for diabetes mellitus in the United States. JAMA 2003;290:1884-1890.
54. Cullen MT, Reece EA, Homko CJ, et al: The changing presentations of diabetic ketoacidosis during pregnancy. Am J Perinatology 1996;13:449-451.
55. Ryan EA: Hormones and insulin resistance during pregnancy. Lancet 2003;362:1777-1778.
56. Steel JM, Johnstone FD, Hume R, et al: Insulin requirements during pregnancy in women with type I diabetes. Obstet Gynecol 1994;83:253-258.
57. Ramin K: Diabetic ketoacidosis in pregnancy. Obstet Gynec Clin North Am 1999;26:481-488.
58. Chauhan SP, Perry KG Jr, McLaughlin BN, et al: Diabetic ketoacidosis complicating pregnancy. J Perinatol 1996;16:173-175.
59. Sills IN, Rappaport R: New onset IDDM presenting with diabetic ketoacidosis in a pregnant adolescent. Diabet Care 1994;17:904-905.
60. Carroll MA, Yeomans E: Diabetic ketoacidosis in pregnancy. Crit Care Med 2005;33(Suppl 10):347-353.
61. Kamalakannan D, Baskar V, Barton DM, et al: Diabetic ketoacidosis in pregnancy. Postgrad Med 2003;79:699-714.
62. Montoro MN: Diabetic ketoacidosis in pregnancy. In Reece A, Coustan D, Gabbe S (eds): Diabetes in Women: Adolescence, Pregnancy, and Menopause, 3rd ed. Philadelphia, Lippincott Williams & Wilkins, 2004, pp 345-350.
63. Laffel L: Ketone bodies: A review of physiology, pathophysiology and application of monitoring to diabetes. Diab Metab Res Rev 1999;15:412-426.
64. ACOG Practice Bulletin No. 60. Pregestational Diabetes Mellitus. Obstet Gynecol 2005;105:675-685.
65. Hagay ZJ, Weissman A, Lurie S, et al: Reversal of fetal distress following intensive treatment of maternal diabetic ketoacidosis. Am J Perinatol 1994;11:430-432.
66. Montoro MN, Myers VP, Mestman JH, et al: Outcome of pregnancy in diabetic ketoacidosis. Am J Perinatol 1993;10:17-20.
67. Bedalov A, Balasubramanyam B: Glucocorticoid induced ketoacidosis in gestational diabetes: Sequela of the acute treatment of preterm labor. Diabetes Care 1997;20:922-924.
68. Cunningham FG, McDonald PC, Gant NP: Diabetes. In Cunningham FG, Williams JW (eds): Williams' Obstetrics, 20th ed. Stamford, Conn, Appleton & Lange, 1997.
69. Service FJ: Hypoglycemia. Med Clin North Am 1995;79:1.
70. Fishbein H, Palumbo PJ: Acute metabolic complications in diabetes. In National Diabetes Data Group: Diabetes in America, ed 2. Bethesda, Md, National Institutes of Health, 1995.
71. Cryer PE: Hypoglycemia: The limiting factor in the glycemic management of type 1 and type 2 diabetes. Diabetologia 2002;4:937-948.
72. Cryer PE, Davis SN, Shamoon H: Hypoglycemia in diabetes. Diabetes Care 2003;26:1902-1912.
73. Macaron CI, Kadri A, Macaron Z: Nucleated red blood cells and artifactual hypoglycemia. Diabetes Care 1981;4:113-115.
74. Cryer PE: Diverse causes of hypoglycemia-associated autonomic failure in diabetes. N Engl J Med 2004;350:2272-2279.
75. The DCCT Research Group. Epidemiology of severe hypoglycemia in the diabetes control and complication trial. Am J Med 1991;90:450-459.
76. Shimada R, Nakashima T, Nunoi K, et al: Arrhythmia during insulin-induced hypoglycemia in a diabetic patient. Arch Intern Med 1984;144:1068.
77. Bowman CE, MacMahon DG, Mourant AJ: Hypoglycemia and angina. Lancet 1985;1:639.
78. Cryer PE: Mechanism of hypoglycemia associated autonomic failure and its component syndromes in diabetes. Diabetes 2005;54:3592-3602.
79. Segal SA, Panamore DS, Cryer PE: Hypoglycemia associated autonomic failure in advanced type 2 diabetes. Diabetes 2002;51:724-733.
80. Cryer PE: Mechanism of sympathoadrenal failure and hypoglycemia in diabetes. J Clin Invest 2006;116:1470-1473.
81. Lingenfelser T, Budtner U, Tobis M, et al: Improvement of impaired counterregulatory hormone response and symptoms perception by short term avoidance of hypoglycemia in insulin dependent diabetes. Diabetes Care 1995;18:321-325.
82. Hepburn DA, Patrick AW, Eadington DW, et al: Unawareness of hypoglycemia in insulin treated diabetic patients: Prevalence and relationship to autonomic neuropathy. Diabetes Med 1990;7:711-717.
83. Pampanelli S, Fanelli C, Lalli C, et al: Long term intensive insulin therapy in IDDM: Effects on HA1c risk for severe and mild hypoglycaemia, status of counterregulation and awareness of hypoglycaemia. Diabetologia 1996;39:677-686.
84. The Diabetes Control and Complications Trial Research Group: The effect of intensive treatment of diabetes on the development and progression of long-term complications in insulin-dependent diabetes mellitus. N Engl J Med 1993;329:977-986.
85. Stagnaro-Green A, Barton MK, Linekin PL, et al: Mortality in hospitalized patients with hypoglycemia and severe hyperglycemia. Mt Sinai J Med 1995;62:422-426.

86. Fischer KF, Lees JA, Newman JH: Hypoglycemia in hospitalized patients: Causes and outcomes. N Engl J Med 1986;315:1245-1250.
87. Kagansky N, Levy S, Rimon E, et al: Hypoglycemia as a predictor of mortality in hospitalized elderly patients. Arch Intern Med 2003;163:1825-1829.
88. Braithwate SS, Buie MM, Thompson CL, et al: Hospital hypoglycemia: Not only treatment but also prevention. Endocrine Pract 2004;10(Suppl 2):89-99.
89. Service FJ: Classification of hypoglycemic disorders. Endo Metab Clin North Am 1999;28:555.
90. Fisher KF, Lees JA, Newman JN, et al: Hypoglycemia in hospitalized patients: Causes and outcomes. N Engl J Med 1986;315:1245.
91. Sunder M, Lindberg F, Beederson MP: Insulin aspart (B28-asp-insulin): A fast acting analog of human insulin absorption kinetics and action profile compared with regular human insulin in healthy non diabetic subjects. Diabetes Care 1999;Sept:1501.
92. Hermansen K, Fontaine P, Kukoljak K, et al: Insulin analogues (insulin detemir and insulin aspart) versus traditional human insulins. Diabetologia 2004;47:622-629.
93. Shorr RI, Ray WA, Daugherty JR: Individual sulfonylureas and serious hypoglycemia in older people. J Am Geriatr Soc 1996;44:751-755.
94. Jonsson A, Rydberg T, Ekberg G, et al: Slow elimination of glyburide in NIDDM subjects. Diabetes Care 1994;17:142-145.
95. Melander A, Lebovitz HE, Faber OK: Sulfonylureas: Why, which, and how? Diabetes Care 1990;13(Suppl 3): 18-25.
96. Turner BC, Jenkins E, Kerr D: The effect of evening alcohol consumption on next morning glucose control in type 1 diabetes. Diabetes Care 2001;24:1888-1893.
97. Marks V, Teale JD: Drug induced hypoglycemia. Endocrinol Metab Clin North Am 1999;28:555-577.
98. Schelling JR, Howard RL, Winter SD, Linas SL: Increased osmolal gap in alcoholic ketoacidosis and lactic acidosis. Ann Intern Med 1990;113:580-582.
99. Moller N, Blum WF, Mengel A, et al: Basal and insulin stimulated substrate metabolism in tumor induced hypoglycemia; evidence of increased muscle glucose uptake. Diabetologia 1999;34:17-20.
100. Service FJ, Natt N: The prolonged fast. J Clin Endocrinol Metab 2000;85: 3973.
101. Collier A, Steedman DJ, Patrick AW, et al: Comparison of intravenous glucagon and dextrose in the treatment of severe hypoglycemia in the accident and emergency department. Diabetes Care 1987;10:712-715.
102. Feher MD, Grout P, Kennedy A, et al: Hypoglycemia in an inner city accident and emergency department: A 12-month survey. Arch Emerg Med 1989;6:183.
103. Tierney E: Data from the National Hospital Discharge Survey Database 2000, Center of Disease Control and Prevention, Division of Diabetes Translation, Atlanta, 2003. Personal Communication.
104. Centers for Disease Control and Prevention: National diabetes fact sheet: General information and national estimates on diabetes in the United States, 2003. Atlanta, U.S. Department of Health and Human Services, Centers for Disease Control and Prevention, 2004.
105. Hogan P, Dall T, Nikolov P: Economic cost of diabetes in the US in 2002. Diabetes Care 2003;26:917-932.
106. Roman SH, Harris MI: Management of diabetes mellitus from a public health perspective. Endocrinol Metab North Am 1997;26:443-474.
107. Umpierrez GE, Isaacs SD, Bazargan N, et al: Hyperglycemia: An independent marker of in hospital mortality in patients with undiagnosed diabetes. J Clin Endocrinol Metab 2002;87:978-982.
108. Thourani V, Weintraub W, Stein B, et al: Influence of diabetes mellitus on early and late outcome after coronary artery bypass grafting. Ann Thorac Surg 1999;67:1045-1052.
109. Krinsley JS: Association between hyperglycemia and increased hospital mortality in a heterogeneous population of critically ill patients. Mayo Clin Proc 2003;278:1471-1478.
110. Capes SE, Hunt D, Malmberg K, et al: Stress hyperglycemia and prognosis of stroke in non diabetic and diabetic patients: A systemic overview. Stroke 2001;32:2426-2432.
111. Van Der Berghe G, Wouters P, Weekers F, et al: Intensive insulin therapy in critically ill patients. N Engl J Med 2001;345:1359-1367.
112. Van Der Berghe G, Wouter PJ, Weekers F, et al: Outcome benefit of intensive insulin therapy in the critically ill: Insulin dose versus glycemic control. Crit Care Med 2003;31:359-366.
113. Malmberg K, Norhammar A, Wedel H,Ryden L: Glycometabolic state at admission; Important risk marker of mortality in conventionally treated patients with diabetes mellitus and acute myocardial infarction. Circulation 1999;99:2626-2632.
114. Malmberg K, Ryden L, Efendic S, et al: Randomized trial of insulin-glucose infusion followed by subcutaneous insulin treatment in diabetic patients with acute myocardial infarction (DIGAMI study): Effects on mortality at one year. J Am Coll Cardiol 1995;26:57-65.
115. Malmberg K, for the DIGAMI Study Group: Prospective randomized study of intensive insulin treatment on long term survival after acute myocardial infarction in patients with diabetes mellitus. BMJ 1997;314:1512-1515.
116. Furnary AP, Wu Y, Bookin So, et al: Effect of hyperglycemia and continuous intravenous insulin infusions on outcome of cardiac surgical procedures: The Portland Diabetic Project. Endocr Pract 2004;10(Suppl 2):21-33.
117. Malmberg K, Ryden L, Wedel H: Intense metabolic control by means of insulin in patients with diabetes mellitus and acute myocardial infarction(DIGAMI 2): Effects on mortality and morbidity. Eur Heart J 2005;26:650-661.
118. Van Den Berghe G, Wilmer A, Hermans G: Intensive insulin therapy in the medical ICU. N Engl J Med 2006;354:449-461.
119. Clement S, Braithwaite SS, Magee MF, et al: Management of diabetes and hyperglycemia in hospitals. Diabetes Care 2004;27:553-591.
120. American College of Endocrinology Position Statement on Inpatient Diabetes and Metabolic Control. Endocr Pract 2004;10(Suppl 2):4-9.
121. American Diabetes Association Standards of medical care in diabetes. Diabetes Care 2005;28: S4-S36.
122. Miller C, Phillips L, Ziemer D, et al: Hypoglycemia in patients with type 2 diabetes. Arch Intern Med 2001;161:1653-1659.
123. Shagan BP: Does anyone here know how to make insulin work backwards? Pract Diabetes 1990;9:1-4.
124. Queale WS, Seidler AJ, Brancati FL: Glycemic control and sliding scale insulin use in medical inpatients with diabetes mellitus. Arch Intern Med 1997;157:545-552.
125. Hirsh IB, Paauw DS: Diabetes management in special situations. Endocr Metab Clin North Am 1997;26:631-645.
126. Hirsh IB: Insulin analogues. N Engl J Med 2005;352:174-183.
127. Craig ID, Nicholson S, Silverstone FA, et al: Use of a reduced-carbohydrate, modified-fat enteral formula for improving metabolic control and clinical outcomes in long-term care residents with type 2 diabetes: Results of a pilot trial. Nutrition 1998;14: 529-534.
128. Marks JB, Hirsh IB: Surgery and diabetes mellitus. In De Fronzo RA (ed): Current Therapy of Diabetes Mellitus. St Louis, Mosby, 1998, pp 88-1011.
129. Rossini AA, Thompson MJ, Gottlieb PA, et al: Irwin and Rippe's Intensive Care Medicine, 4th ed. Philadelphia, Lippincott-Raven, 1999.
130. Goldberg PA, Siegal MD, Sherwin RS, et al: Implementation of a safe and effective insulin infusion protocol in a medical intensive care unit. Diabetes Care 2004;27:461-467.

Chapter 60

Adrenal Insufficiency in the Critically Ill Patient

Robert W. Taylor

Adrenal diseases are infrequent primary admitting diagnoses to the intensive care unit (ICU). However, patients with unrecognized or previously diagnosed disease of the hypothalamic-pituitary-adrenal (HPA) axis may demonstrate severe decompensation in the setting of other critical illness.

Adrenal insufficiency (AI) is by far the most common adrenal disorder seen in the ICU and is the focus of this chapter. It occurs more frequently in critically ill patients than in general hospitalized patients and represents a true emergency that requires rapid diagnosis and treatment. If missed, the condition can be lethal. In addition, because critical illness is often the precipitant of overt AI, the intensivist may have the first and only chance to make the diagnosis.[1]

Primary AI results from a subtotal or complete destruction of the adrenal cortex (>90%) and results in cortisol, aldosterone and androgen deficiency. Multiple causes of primary AI include autoimmune destruction (Addison's disease), polyendocrine deficiency syndrome, infections (e.g., tuberculosis, fungus), vascular compromise, primary or metastatic cancer, amyloidosis, and surgical removal of the adrenal glands.

Secondary adrenal insufficiency is much more common than primary adrenal insufficiency and can be traced to a lack of adrenorticotropic hormone (ACTH). Without ACTH to stimulate the adrenal glands, production of cortisol falls but aldosterone secretion remains intact. The most common cause of secondary adrenal insufficiency is the inadvertent abrupt withdrawal of therapeutic exogenous corticosteroids. Another cause of secondary adrenal insufficiency is the surgical removal of benign, or noncancerous, ACTH-producing tumors of the pituitary gland (Cushing's disease). In this case the source of ACTH is suddenly removed, and replacement hormones must be taken until normal ACTH and cortisol production resumes.

Less commonly, secondary adrenal insufficiency occurs when the pituitary gland reduces or ceases production of ACTH. This can occur for a variety of reasons including tumors or infections of the area, loss of blood flow to the pituitary, radiation for the treatment of pituitary tumors, total or subtotal removal of the hypothalamus, and surgical removal of the pituitary gland.

The concept of relative adrenal insufficiency has recently emerged.[2,3] In this condition the measured serum cortisol may actually be normal or high but still inadequate for the current physiologic stress. In addition, the patient may not be able to compensate for additional stresses.

Because the presenting signs, symptoms, and laboratory abnormalities of AI may be nonspecific, a high index of suspicion is necessary to make the diagnosis.[4] In addition, steroid medications (derived from adrenal glucocorticoid hormones) are commonly used in the care of the critically ill. For these reasons the intensivist must understand clinical problems associated with the HPA axis and the use of glucocorticoid hormones.

INCIDENCE AND PREVALENCE

The actual incidence of acute AI is not known. The reported occurrence rate in critically ill patients varies from zero to 28%[5] and depends on the criteria used to make the diagnosis. The adrenal gland, therefore, possesses a great functional reserve; AI is a relatively uncommon disorder.[6]

At least 90% of both adrenal glands must be destroyed before clinical and biochemical manifestations of AI occur. Tissue hypoxia, a relatively common disorder in critically ill patients, has little effect on the synthesis of cortisol. Secondary AI may be more common than primary AI. The clinical presentation of secondary AI is relatively nonspecific and often resembles other conditions common in the ICU. Hence it is not uncommon to attribute the clinical features resulting from acute AI to commonly seen medical conditions in the ICU.[7]

Pathogenesis

To understand the pathogenesis of adrenal diseases one must understand the physiology of the adrenal glands and the causes that result in the disruption of the physiologic process.

Pathophysiology

The adrenal glands are pyramid shaped, each weighing about 5 to 10 g, and located just superior to their respective kidneys. The left adrenal gland is usually slightly more cephalad than the right. Each adrenal gland is composed of an inner medulla and outer cortex. These layers are embryologically, anatomically, and physiologically distinct. The adrenal cortex is responsible for the secretion of multiple steroid hormones. The adrenal medulla is responsible for the secretion of catecholamines.

The adrenal cortex is composed of three zones: the outer zona glomerulosa, inner zona fasciculata, and zona reticularis. The zona glomerulosa secretes the mineralocorticoid aldosterone in response to angiotensin, ACTH, and a high circulating potassium concentration. The zona fasciculata and zona reticularis secrete glucocorticoids and adrenal androgens.

The principal mineralocorticoid is aldosterone, which is regulated not only by ACTH but also by serum sodium and potassium levels and by the renin-angiotensin system.[8,9] Mineralocorticoids exert their primary effect on distal renal tubule cells, resulting in renal sodium retention at the expense of potassium loss in the urine. A third major class of adrenal steroids is the sex hormones: dehydroepiandrosterone (DHEA), DHEA-sulfate, and androstenedione. Like the glucocorticoids, ACTH primarily regulates these steroid hormones. They function mainly as precursors for the primary circulating androgen, testosterone, and also may undergo separate conversion to estrogen hormones. In critically ill patients, glucocorticoids are the steroid hormones of greatest concern and therefore remain the focus of the remainder of this discussion.

Glucocorticoid synthesis is regulated by (1) a negative feedback mechanism involving cortisol and adrenal steroids, (2) a diurnal rhythm, and (3) stress. The hypothalamus and the pituitary gland closely regulate adrenal hormone production. Corticotropin-releasing hormone (CRH) is produced in the hypothalamus and acts on specialized cells in the pituitary, stimulating production of ACTH, which serves, in turn, to stimulate adrenal cortical cells to produce numerous steroid hormones including cortisol. Adrenal hormones have a negative influence at the level of the hypothalamus and the pituitary, inhibiting CRH and ACTH release. The adrenal gland in turn ceases its secretory activity until the cortisol concentration returns to normal. When serum cortisol levels are below normal, secretion of CRH and ACTH increases, stimulating the adrenal glands to produce cortisol until its level normalizes. Therefore abnormalities in circulating serum levels of adrenal steroid hormone can be caused by either adrenal or hypothalamic pituitary disease. Because ACTH possesses alpha-melanocyte stimulating hormone activity, excessive production of ACTH is associated with hyperpigmentation.

Cortisol is normally secreted in a diurnal pattern. The circulating cortisol level is increased in the morning hours, at approximately 8 AM. Serum cortisol concentrations decrease throughout the remainder of the day.[10] Similarly, the serum cortisol response to ACTH stimulation also varies in a circadian rhythm. Afternoon responsiveness is much greater because of the decreased circadian level of cortisol at that time. In addition, cortisol is secreted in a series of pulses rather than in a continuous fashion. These factors contribute to make interpretation of a random cortisol level and the ACTH-stimulated value difficult.

"Stress" (exemplified by sepsis, major surgery, or trauma) also affects glucocorticoid synthesis.[11-13] The *stress response* is characterized by continuous ACTH secretion despite a high serum cortisol concentration. Stress overrides all other regulatory mechanisms of cortisol secretion by the adrenal cortex and increases cortisol secretion irrespective of the time of day or the current serum cortisol concentration. The mechanism by which the HPA axis is regulated during stress is not clearly understood. Periventricular neurons in the hypothalamus respond to stress by increasing the levels of CRH messenger ribonucleic acid (mRNA).[14,15] It has been shown that production of cytokines interleukin-1 (IL-1), interleukin-6 (IL-6), and tumor necrosis factor-alpha (TNF-α) also play an important role in the regulation of the HPA axis.[16-20] The cortisol secretion that occurs because of the activation of the HPA axis causes an inhibitory effect not only on the secretion of CRH and ACTH but also on the liberation of interleukins.[21] Thus there is a functional loop between immune activation and regulation of the HPA axis during stress.

The stress response is biphasic including an early phase in which both ACTH and cortisol are elevated and a late phase in which the serum cortisol level is elevated but the serum ACTH level is paradoxically low.[9] This is explained by the fact that endothelin and atrial natriuretic peptide are both elevated in severe illnesses. Endothelin increases cortisol production by the adrenals, whereas the atrial natriuretic peptide inhibits ACTH production by acting at the hypothalamic-pituitary level.

Acute respiratory failure causes a 50% to 100% rise in serum cortisol concentration. A twofold to sixfold rise occurs with septic shock and following surgical procedures and trauma. The rise in serum cortisol correlates positively with severity of illness[7] and negatively with survival.[8]

The normal daily output of cortisol by the adrenal glands is 20 to 30 mg. The normal adrenal gland secretes about 10 to 12 times the normal daily output of cortisol when under maximal physiologic stress. Hence approximately 200 to 300 mg of hydrocortisone or its equivalent is considered a daily "stress dose" of glucocorticoid.

GLUCOCORTICOID ACTIONS

Cardiovascular Effects

Glucocorticoids help to maintain vascular tone and cardiac contractility. The presence of glucocorticoids is important to the physiologic effects of catecholamines on vascular smooth muscle. Glucocorticoids affect blood pressure by different mechanisms including direct action of glucocorticoids on the vasculature, permissive effects of the glucocorticoids on the vasopressor action of catecholamines, and glucocorticoid-induced decrease in the levels of prostaglandin E2 and kallikrein (vasodilators).[22] Glucocorticoids increase the synthesis of β-adrenergic receptors, reverse β-2 receptor dysfunction, and increase the coupling of the receptor with the second messenger system.[23]

Two hemodynamic states have been described during acute AI:

1. Low cardiac output, high systemic vascular resistance shock caused by both decreased myocardial contractility and decreased preload
2. High cardiac output, low systemic vascular resistance shock, which mimics septic shock.[24] It appears that patients with AI present initially with a combination of cardiogenic shock and hypovolemic shock. Intravascular volume expansion with intravenous fluids results in an increase in cardiac output and a lowering of systemic vascular resistance. The hemodynamic profile that one sees depends on the timing of pulmonary artery catheter placement during the course of treatment in an individual patient. Thus the hypotension of AI can mimic cardiogenic, hypovolemic, or septic shock (depending on when the hemodynamic assessment was made) and may be poorly responsive or unresponsive to treatment with fluids and vasopressors in the absence of glucocorticoid therapy.

Metabolic Effects

Glucocorticoid hormones have profound influence on carbohydrate metabolism. A major action is on gluconeogenesis. Glucocorticoids increase hepatic glycogen and glucose by inducing the synthesis of hepatic enzymes and increasing the availability of gluconeogenic substrates. This is because of glucocorticoid-induced proteolytic activity on peripheral tissues, which causes mobilization of glycogenic amino acid precursors from peripheral supporting structures such as bone, skin, muscle, and connective tissue because of protein breakdown and inhibition of protein synthesis. Glucocorticoids decrease the peripheral uptake and utilization of glucose. They have a permissive effect on other hormones such as glucagon and catecholamines, thus serving to increase the circulating glucose concentration, which in turn increases insulin secretion.

Glucocorticoids also affect fat and protein metabolism. They increase lipolysis both directly and indirectly by action on other hormones. Glucocorticoids regulate fatty acid mobilization by enhancing activation of cellular lipase by lipid-mobilizing hormones (e.g., catecholamines, pituitary peptides). They elevate free fatty acid levels in the plasma and enhance any tendency to ketosis. Glucocorticoids stimulate peripheral protein metabolism, using the amino acid products as gluconeogenic precursors. Glucocorticoids inhibit RNA synthesis in most body tissues, but in the liver they stimulate RNA synthesis.

Renal Effects

Glucocorticoids bind to the mineralocorticoid receptors in renal tubules and increase sodium reabsorption and excretion of potassium and hydrogen ion. Glucocorticoids also increase free water excretion by inhibiting the release of antidiuretic hormone (ADH).

Immunologic Effects

Glucocorticoids contribute to the regulation of the inflammatory response by altering both the quality and quantity of macrophages and leukocytes. Glucocorticoids increase the number of circulating neutrophils by 2000 to 5000 cells/mm^3, usually showing a peak effect by 4 to 6 hours following administration of a single dose. Although they increase the number of neutrophils in the peripheral circulation, glucocorticoids cause a decrease in the actual number of lymphocytes, monocytes, eosinophils, and basophils. The decrease in circulating lymphocytes is primarily caused by a redistribution of T-lymphocytes from the circulating pool into the lymphoid tissue. *The most important immunosuppressive effect of glucocorticoids is their ability to improve recruitment of neutrophils, monocytes, and macrophages into an area of inflammation.* Thus despite the apparent increase in the number of neutrophils in the intravascular compartment, the net effect of glucocorticoids is a decrease in the cellular defense mechanism. Glucocorticoids also decrease the proliferation of T-lymphocytes and natural killer cells and improve macrophage activity. They also affect humoral immunity by increasing release of effector substances, antigen processing, and antibody formation by B-lymphocytes.

Glucocorticoids mediate anti-inflammatory effects by stabilizing lysosomal membranes. They also decrease the release of inflammatory mediators like histamine, cytokines, and prostaglandins.

The immunologic actions of glucocorticoids are only significant in circumstances in which they are present in supraphysiological amounts such as markedly increased endogenous production or exogenous administration.

Gastrointestinal Effects

It has been postulated that CRH inhibits the release of motilin, a duodenal hormone that is responsible for the initiation of peristaltic contractions, which begin in the stomach and propagate distally. Glucocorticoids decrease CRH production and thus inhibit gastric and intestinal motility. This could explain the vomiting, constipation, and abdominal pain seen in cortisol deficiency.

Calcium Metabolism

Glucocorticoids lower serum calcium levels by several mechanisms. They inhibit calcium absorption from the gut, decrease renal calcium reabsorption (which results in hypercalciuria), and promote shift of calcium from the extracellular compartment to the intracellular compartment. Osteoporosis occurs in approximately 50% of patients who require long-term glucocorticoids.[25]

Other Effects

Glucocorticoids have many other effects. These include the ability to produce significant mood changes and even psychosis in some patients. Glucocorticoids have an association with cataract formation and increased intraocular pressure. They also affect the production and action of a number of other hormones including insulin, thyroid hormones, and gonadal hormones.

Aldosterone secretion is regulated mainly by the renin-angiotensin system. The most potent modulator of this system is renal perfusion. Potassium also affects aldosterone secretion independent of its effect on the renin-angiotensin system. Hyperkalemia inhibits production of renin but increases the synthesis of aldosterone. Aldosterone increases sodium reabsorption in the collecting tubules and at the same time causes potassium and hydrogen ion excretion. This is mediated by the Na-K pump in the presence of the enzyme Na, K-ATPase and results in sodium and water retention and an increase in intravascular volume.

Hyperkalemia, hyponatremia, non–anion gap metabolic acidosis, hemoconcentration, and hypovolemia provide important clinical clues to the diagnosis of primary AI. Because ACTH is not a potent regulator of aldosterone secretion, secondary AI is usually not associated with hyperkalemia. Hyponatremia and hypovolemia may be present in secondary AI but not to the degree found in primary AI. The renin-angiotensin system is activated during AI and serves as a defense mechanism to improve the low intravascular volume and the altered vasomotor tone that results from aldosterone and cortisol deficiency.[26,27]

Box 60-1

Causes of Primary Adrenal Insufficiency

- Autoimmune (idiopathic) 80% (most common cause)
- Infectious
  - Tuberculosis (second most common cause)
  - Pneumococcus
  - Histoplasmosis
  - Coccidioidomycosis
  - Blastomycosis
  - Meningococcus
  - Cryptococcosis
  - Candidiasis
  - Torulopsis
  - Cytomegalovirus
- Acquired immune deficiency syndrome
- Neoplasia
- Metastatic carcinoma
- Lymphoma
- Infiltrative diseases
  - Amyloidosis
  - Sarcoidosis
  - Hemochromatosis
- Adrenal hemorrhage
- Sepsis
- Anticoagulants
- Coagulopathy
- Trauma
- Prior surgery
- Difficult pregnancy
- Metastatic carcinoma
- Vasculitis
- Postadrenal venography
- Medications
  - Ketoconazole
  - Phenytoin
  - Phenobarbital
  - Rifampin
  - Etomidate
  - Fluorouracil
  - Metyrapone
- Miscellaneous
  - Irradiation
  - Bilateral adrenalectomy
- Congenital conditions

ETIOLOGY AND PATHOGENESIS

Causes of primary AI have been previously discussed and are shown in Box 60-1.

Autoimmune Disease

Autoimmune disease (Addison's disease) is currently the most common cause of primary AI and accounts for approximately 80% of cases. For many years tuberculosis was the most common cause. AI may occur as isolated disease or as part of a polyglandular autoimmune syndrome associated with thyroiditis, diabetes mellitus (Schmidt's syndrome), hypogonadism, vitiligo, and pernicious anemia.[28-30] Autoimmune AI is more common in women than men and usually occurs in the third to fifth decades of life. The mean duration of symptoms before diagnosis is approximately 3 years. In this disorder high levels of circulating autoantibodies attack the cytoplasm of adrenal cortical cells and inhibit synthesis of glucocorticoids.[28,29]

Infectious Disease

Tuberculosis

The second most common cause of primary AI is adrenal gland destruction by *Mycobacterium tuberculosis.* This currently accounts for less than 20% of cases.[31] This usually occurs in the presence of tuberculosis elsewhere in the body, especially with involvement of the lungs, genitourinary system, and gastrointestinal system. AI is usually manifest years after the initial presentation of tuberculosis.[32] The mean duration of symptoms of AI prior to diagnosis is 6 to 9 months. AI secondary to tuberculosis occurs with equal frequency in males and females. In contrast to autoimmune adrenalitis, tuberculosis-induced adrenal disease is not associated with other endocrine diseases. In addition, with tuberculosis the adrenal glands are enlarged and may be calcified. In contrast, the adrenal glands in autoimmune adrenalitis are usually atrophied and noncalcified.

Fungal Disease

Fungal disease can also cause primary AI. *Histoplasma capsulatum* is the most common organism. As seen in tuberculosis, fungal infection is usually disseminated and involves organs other than the adrenal glands. Adrenal involvement may be seen during the active phase or may develop years later after the disease has become "inactive." Sarosi and colleagues[33] reported that more than 50% of patients with disseminated histoplasmosis had AI and it was the most common cause of death.

Acquired Immune Deficiency Syndrome

Patients with acquired immune deficiency syndrome (AIDS) are at risk of developing AI by several different mechanisms. Fungal infections are more common in this patient population, and disseminated disease may involve the adrenal glands. Similarly, mycobacterial infection, cytomegalovirus infection, and Kaposi sarcoma may cause involvement of the adrenals in up to 50% of patients.[3] In addition, sepsis and spontaneous adrenal hemorrhage are also seen in this group of patients. As HIV patients survive longer, an increased incidence of AI is likely.

Neoplasia

Neoplastic metastasis to the adrenal glands has been found on autopsy in 27% to 40% of patients who die of malignancy.[34-37] Yet metastatic carcinoma accounts for less than 1% of cases of primary AI.[34] This is explained by the tremendous functional reserve possessed by the adrenal glands. More than 90% of the adrenal gland must be destroyed before hypofunction occurs. Many patients with metastasis to the adrenals do not develop hormonal deficiency.[38] The most common neoplasms to involve the adrenals are lung cancer, breast cancer, melanoma, and lymphoma.[39] AI usually occurs in the setting of widespread metastatic disease and is rarely the initial manifestation of malignancy.

Medications

Certain medications can cause AI. Of particular interest to the intensivist are ketoconazole, phenytoin, phenobarbital, rifampin, and etomidate. Ketoconazole decreases glucocorticoid production and is also a glucocorticoid receptor antagonist. Etomidate decreases glucocorticoid production. Phenytoin, rifampin, and barbiturates increase the catabolism of glucocorticoids. These medications can precipitate acute AI by decreasing glucocorticoid production or function in a patient who has compromised adrenal reserve.

Adrenal Hemorrhage

Adrenal hemorrhage is an important but uncommon cause of AI in the ICU. The association of adrenal hemorrhage with fulminant sepsis was first described with *Neisseria meningitidis* (Waterhouse-Friderichsen syndrome). Infections with *Streptococcus pneumoniae, Pseudomonas* species, and *Haemophilus influenzae* type B can also cause this syndrome.

Besides the infectious etiologies, other conditions may predispose to adrenal hemorrhage including severe illness (particularly cardiac disease), coagulopathy, anticoagulant therapy, thromboembolism, burns, and trauma.[40] Under these circumstances the typical signs and symptoms of AI are often mistaken for those of other common conditions. Typical settings include the patient who is in the first or second postoperative week or a patient who has been started recently on anticoagulation therapy. Common findings include abdominal, back, flank, or chest pain; nausea; vomiting; fever; altered mental status; orthostatic hypotension; and a sudden drop in hematocrit. The hemodynamic crisis associated with adrenal hemorrhage occurs 1 to 3 days after the initial hemorrhage.

Etiology of Secondary Adrenal Insufficiency

Causes of secondary AI have been discussed previously and are shown in Box 60-2. Secondary AI occurs because of a decrease in ACTH caused by either hypothalamic-pituitary disease or suppression of the HPA axis as a result of glucocorticoid therapy. The most common cause today is discontinuation of corticosteroid therapy. Chronic glucocorticoid therapy leads to HPA axis suppression with resulting secondary AI if glucocorticoids are abruptly discontinued. With the exception of AI because of discontinuation of chronic glucocorticoid therapy, secondary adrenocortical insufficiency is much less common than primary AI. Isolated ACTH deficiency is rare, and ACTH is the last pituitary hormone to be impaired by enlarging sellar and suprasellar tumors.

Most patients admitted to the ICU with secondary AI have recently received steroid therapy or have taken steroids within the year prior to admission. No clear evidence indicates that detailing the duration or dose of steroid therapy predisposes patients to adrenal suppression. Doses of 25 mg of prednisone twice a day for 2 days, 12.5 mg per day for 6 months, or 5 mg per day for 5 years have all been shown to cause adrenal suppression. On the other hand, studies have shown that prednisone less than 40 mg per day every morning for 5 to 7 days did not cause adrenal suppression.[41]

As a practical guideline, all patients who have taken 40 mg of prednisone per day or its equivalent for a period greater than 2 or 3 weeks should be considered to be adrenal insufficient until proved otherwise. If glucocorticoids have been given to a patient for more than 1 to 2 weeks, they should be tapered off to allow time for the adrenal glands to recover function. AI can occur in response to stress as long as 1 year after steroids are discontinued.[42] All of these patients should be evaluated for

Box 60-2

Causes of Secondary Adrenal Insufficiency

Glucocorticoid therapy (most common cause of secondary AI)
Neoplastic
- Pituitary adenoma
- Meningioma
- Craniopharyngioma
- Metastatic carcinoma
- Breast
- Lung
- Gastrointestinal
- Lymphoma
- Leukemia

Vascular
Pituitary apoplexy
Sheehan's syndrome
Sickle cell
Intracranial aneurysm
Cavernous sinus thrombosis
Vasculitis
Eclampsia
Infection
- Tuberculosis
- Fungal infection
- Malaria
- Actinomycosis
- Viruses

Autoimmune disorders
Infiltrative disorders
Sarcoidosis
Hemochromatosis
Irradiation
Head trauma and pituitary surgery
Isolated adrenocorticotropic hormone deficiency

adrenal function and should be treated with stress doses of steroids during the interim period.

CLINICAL FEATURES OF ADRENAL INSUFFICIENCY

Common symptoms and signs of AI are shown in Box 60-3. The symptoms, signs, and general laboratory data seen in AI are nonspecific. However, when taken together they form a pattern of findings that should suggest the possibility of AI. Patients with acute AI share many characteristics with patients who have chronic AI, but the symptoms are usually more severe in the acute setting. Virtually all patients complain of weakness, fatigue, and loss of appetite. They also complain of nausea and diarrhea with occasional vomiting and abdominal pain. Infrequently, patients note myalgias, arthralgias, and dizziness caused by orthostatic hypotension. Weight loss can occur. The classic presentation of acute AI is a patient with unexplained hemodynamic instability who is unresponsive to intravascular volume resuscitation and use of vasopressors. Patients with primary AI may have hyperpigmentation of the tongue, buccal mucosa, palmar creases, and scar tissue. This is caused by increased production of ACTH from the pituitary. Hyperpigmentation is notably absent in secondary AI. If the underlying problem is autoimmune adrenalitis, the patient may have vitiligo, pernicious anemia, or one of the other associated endocrinopathies.

Box 60-3

Common Symptoms and Signs of Adrenal Insufficiency

Symptoms
- Weakness
- Fatigue
- Anorexia
- Gastrointestinal symptoms (nausea, vomiting, abdominal pain, diarrhea, constipation, and weight loss)
- Orthostatic symptoms
- Myalgias
- Arthralgias

Signs
- Weight loss
- Orthostatic hypotension
- Hyperpigmentation
- Vitiligo
- Confusion/psychosis

DIAGNOSIS

The diagnosis of AI demands a high index of suspicion. The classic symptoms, signs, and laboratory findings of AI are not commonly seen. The consequences of missing the diagnosis can be lethal, but if the diagnosis is made the condition can usually be treated easily. If the diagnosis of AI is being considered, the patient's history should be carefully reviewed for use of steroids (especially in the past year), exposure to tuberculosis, use of anticoagulant therapy, presence of sepsis, or history of cancer that may have metastasized to the adrenals. Patients on high doses of steroids can develop AI when subjected to stress.

Laboratory Findings

Laboratory evaluation of patients with suspected AI is essential. In a patient with acute worsening of a chronic hypoadrenal state, the common laboratory findings shown in Box 60-4 are more likely to be present and are likely to be more pronounced. Electrolyte abnormalities depend on the type of deficiency: a combined glucocorticoid and mineralocorticoid deficiency (typically seen in primary AI) or an isolated glucocorticoid deficiency (characteristic of secondary AI).

Patients who have a combined deficiency may show hyponatremia, hyperkalemia, decreased serum bicarbon-

Box 60-4

Common Laboratory Findings in Adrenal Insufficiency

- Hyponatremia
- Hyperkalemia
- Acidosis
- Prerenal azotemia
- Hypoglycemia
- Lymphocytosis
- Eosinophilia

ate, and increased blood urea nitrogen (BUN). This is primarily caused by the mineralocorticoid deficiency, which leads to renal sodium loss, potassium retention, and dehydration with acidosis and prerenal azotemia. Patients with secondary adrenocortical deficiency usually have milder electrolyte abnormalities. Their normal adrenal glands are able to produce sufficient amounts of mineralocorticoid even in the absence of ACTH stimulation. They usually have mild hyponatremia with normal potassium levels, and they show little evidence of dehydration. Patients with AI may also have hypoglycemia. This occurs as a result of increased utilization of glucose and decreased gluconeogenesis in the face of glucocorticoid deficiency.

Diagnostic Tests

When there is a high suspicion of AI, hormonal testing is necessary to confirm the diagnosis. The laboratory evaluations most commonly used to detect AI in the critically ill patients are the random serum cortisol level and the rapid ACTH stimulation test.

Serum Cortisol Level

The biochemical diagnosis of AI is controversial. It is based on the demonstration of decreased cortisol production. Most clinical laboratories routinely measure total rather than free cortisol levels. Experts have recently suggested that measurement of free cortisol levels makes more physiologic sense.[43] In addition, variability of cortisol assays can confound the diagnosis of AI.[44]

Given the controversy in diagnosis, the following recommendations are made. A randomly measured serum cortisol level that exceeds 44 μg/dL makes the diagno-sis of adrenocortical deficiency unlikely.[45] Serum cortisol levels increase significantly in patients with normal adrenal function who are in shock and critically ill. The finding of a random serum cortisol level of less than 10 μg/dL in this setting is highly suggestive of compromised adrenal function and should prompt treatment or a confirmatory ACTH stimulation test.[45]

One must be careful in the interpretation of random serum cortisol levels in patients treated with several commonly used drugs in the ICU. Propofol produces a temporary reduction in serum cortisol levels. However, it does not seem to inhibit adrenal responsiveness to ACTH. Etomidate, on the other hand, is associated with a reduced serum cortisol concentration despite ACTH stimulation.[46]

Rapid ACTH Stimulation Test

The ACTH stimulation test measures the response of the adrenal gland to stimulation by exogenous ACTH. This test can be performed at any time of the day because the normal diurnal variation of cortisol is lost in the setting of critical illness. A blood sample is drawn, and a baseline serum cortisol level is measured. Cosyntropin (synthetic ACTH) 250 μg is then administered intravenously. Although controversial, some studies have shown that a low dose of ACTH (1 to 5 μg) produces a similar response as the 250 μg dose.[47,48] Repeat samples are drawn at 60 minutes.

An increase in serum cortisol of less than 9 μg/dL following 250 μg of cosyntropin is highly suggestive of AI irrespective of the baseline cortisol level. An increase in serum cortisol of greater than 17 μg/dL suggests adrenal competence.[45]

The rapid ACTH stimulation test is a relatively simple test for evaluating AI.[49] It does not, however, differentiate between primary and secondary AI. To differentiate between primary and secondary AI, a basal plasma ACTH determination is made. A serum cortisol measurement is then made following a continuous 48-hour infusion of ACTH. An increased basal ACTH (>250 pcg/mL) or a serum cortisol level (<20 μg/dL) after 48 hours of ACTH stimulation is compatible with primary AI. On the other hand, a decreased basal ACTH and a high cortisol after ACTH administration suggest secondary AI.

Relative Adrenal Insufficiency

Despite no conclusive evidence of benefit, in the 1950s, 1960s, and into the 1970s cortisol at low doses over days was often used in patients with severe manifestations of sepsis to counter the assumption that AI was present. This was based on autopsy studies that revealed adrenal necrosis in patients dying with severe infection. The subsequent recognition of the systemic effects of inflammation in sepsis and the discovery that the majority of patients in septic shock had normal or increased cortisol levels led to a paradigm shift in treating septic shock with massive doses of steroids given for a short period of time. This was based on animal studies showing that large doses of steroids given prior to boluses of endotoxin or gram-negative bacteria prevented mortality.[44] Clinical trials testing the utility of several large doses of steroids in patients with septic shock failed to show benefit.[50,51]

One study in patients with septic shock demonstrated that regardless of baseline cortisol level, the inability to raise the cortisol level following ACTH stimulation by at least 10 μg/dL signified poor prognosis.[52] This failure of ACTH to increase cortisol level by 10 μg/dL was labeled by the authors as "relative AI." Of this poor prognostic group, the higher the baseline cortisol level with failure to produce a 10 μg/dL increase, the worse the prognosis. The concept of relative AI exists when the measured serum cortisol is normal or high but still inadequate for the current physiologic stress.

Once the diagnosis of AI is made, a search for the etiology should be initiated as the patient is being stabilized. To rule out tuberculosis, a PPD skin test must be placed and a chest radiograph performed. An abnormal prothrombin time, partial thromboplastin time, or platelet count may point to an unsuspected coagulopathy suggesting the possibility of adrenal hemorrhage. Antiadrenal antibodies are found in about 70% of patients with autoimmune adrenal disease and in less than 0.1% of normals.[53] Computed tomography scanning of the abdomen is useful in determining the size and presence of calcification of the adrenal glands. Adrenal calcification can be seen in 53% of cases of tuberculosis.[54]

MANAGEMENT OF ADRENAL INSUFFICIENCY

Management of AI can be best accomplished by identifying the degree of acuteness and severity of the patient's illness at the time of presentation.[55]

Preexisting Adrenal Insufficiency

Patients who are known to have AI or who have received glucocorticoid therapy in the past year should receive stress doses of corticosteroids during critical illnesses and during surgical procedures. Hydrocortisone 100 mg IV bolus is administered followed by 100 mg as an intravenous infusion every 6 to 8 hours. Isotonic saline is administered intravenously in volumes sufficient to support blood pressure. Five percent dextrose in isotonic saline may be used in the hypoglycemic patient. Once the acute insult has resolved, the hydrocortisone should be tapered to a maintenance dose. The replacement dose is usually 5 mg of prednisone or 30 mg of hydrocortisone each day.

Patients with known AI scheduled for operation should continue the existing steroid dose prior to surgery. The morning of the operation hydrocortisone 100 mg is given intravenously. During the operation a 100-mg hydrocortisone infusion is given. Following surgery 100 mg of hydrocortisone is administered intravenously every 8 hours during the first postoperative day. The dose is then tapered back to the baseline steroid dose over the next 3 to 4 days.

Adequate instruction is important in this group of patients. Patients with AI should be advised to wear a medical alert bracelet. These patients should be provided with a parenteral form of glucocorticoid and taught to self-administer the drug in case of emergency. They should be taught about the clinical situations in which increased amounts of glucocorticoids are required.

Hemodynamically Stable Patient

A patient who is suspected of having AI and who is hemodynamically stable should be managed in the following manner. A serum cortisol level and a rapid ACTH stimulation test should be performed prior to initiation of stress doses of corticosteroids. Hypovolemia should be treated with 5% dextrose in isotonic saline. If the diagnosis of AI is confirmed, hydrocortisone 100 mg should be administered as an intravenous infusion every 6 to 8 hours.

Hemodynamically Unstable Patient

Acute AI is a life-threatening emergency and requires immediate and aggressive therapy to ensure prompt recovery. A patient who is suspected of having AI and who is hemodynamically unstable should be managed in the following manner. Immediate glucocorticoid therapy and intravenous administration of isotonic fluids are warranted. Blood should be obtained for baseline serum cortisol concentration, electrolytes, glucose, BUN, and creatinine.

Dexamethasone 4 mg should be given intravenously. Dexamethasone is preferred as the initial glucocorticoid because unlike hydrocortisone, it does not interfere with the cortisol assay and thus the ACTH stimulation test can still be performed without interference. Although dexamethasone contains no mineralocorticoid activity, vigorous hydration with isotonic saline allows the patient to tolerate this lack of mineralocorticoid activity for the 1 hour that is required to perform the rapid ACTH stimulation test. After the ACTH stimulation test has been performed, hydrocortisone should be substituted for dexamethasone. Hydrocortisone has sufficient mineralocorticoid activity to make concurrent use of mineralocorticoid replacement unnecessary. The dose of hydrocortisone is 100 mg IV bolus followed by 100 mg IV every 6 hours. After the patient has stabilized, the hydrocortisone is tapered at 10 to 15 mg per day until a maintenance dose of 30 mg per day is achieved.

Vigorous intravascular volume expansion with saline- and glucose-containing solutions is recommended. Volume resuscitation is usually initiated with 0.9% normal saline and 5% dextrose solution. This helps to restore intravascular volume and prevent hypoglycemia. The patient's fluid, electrolyte, and glucose status should be carefully monitored during resuscitation. In general, patients with acute AI have a deficit that is approximately 20% of their extracellular space. Adequate resuscitation usually requires approximately 3 L of a glucose-containing saline solution. The rapidity of infusion depends on the patient's hemodynamic status and the presence or absence of underlying cardiovascular disease. A pulmonary artery catheter may be helpful in monitoring hemodynamic status and guiding fluid therapy. Vasopressors may be necessary in the initial stages to maintain an adequate blood pressure to ensure tissue perfusion. In general, if the hypotension is caused by AI, improvement in blood pressure should be seen within 6 hours of corticosteroid therapy.

Mineralocorticoid administration is usually not required initially during acute AI, because the large doses of hydrocortisone provide adequate mineralocorticoid activity. Once the acute event has resolved and the hydrocortisone is tapered to less than 100 mg per day, mineralocorticoids should be started. Fludrocortisone is recommended at a dose of 0.05 to 0.20 mg per day. Excess mineralocorticoids can cause congestive heart failure, hypokalemia, and metabolic alkalosis.

In patients with concurrent hypothyroidism, glucocorticoid replacement should begin prior to thyroid hormone replacement. Administration of thyroid hormone increases the metabolism of glucocorticoids. Thus treatment with thyroid hormone before glucocorticoid therapy might worsen the hypoadrenal state and precipitate AI.

Reversal of the underlying cause of adrenal dysfunction is an important aspect of treatment. The precipitation of acute adrenal failure is provoked by another acute process and thus the causes of both primary and secondary AI should be sought. Prophylactic use of antibiotics is not beneficial, but specific infections should be treated aggressively with appropriate antibiotic therapy.

Severe Sepsis and Septic Shock

Several clinical trials suggest that replacement of hydrocortisone decreases the need for vasopressor support in patients with septic shock.[56,57] In patients with septic shock with blood pressure that is poorly responsive to vasopressors following adequate fluid resuscitation, intravenous corticosteroids (hydrocortisone 200 to 300 mg/day) in 3 or 4 divided doses or by continuous infusion is recommended. Fludrocortisone 50 μg/day administered enterally is recommended by some.[56] Initial treatment with dexamethasone should be considered until the diagnosis of AI is confirmed in this setting. Dexamethasone does not interfere with the ACTH stimulation test. Treatment should continue for approximately 7 days. To date, no studies document an improved outcome with corticosteroid use in the absence of septic shock (Fig. 60-1).

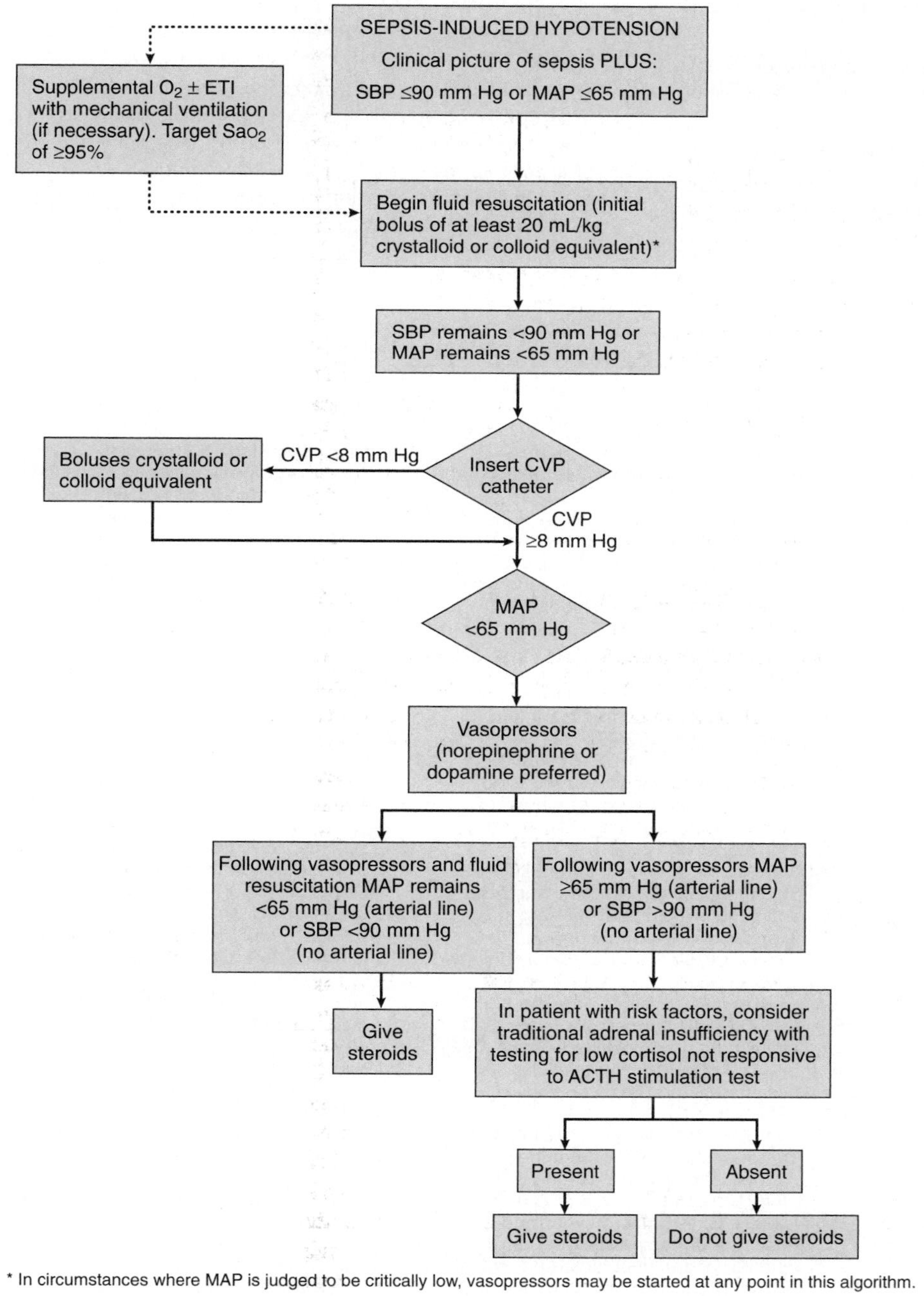

Figure 60-1. Algorithm for management of severe sepsis/septic shock. CVP, central venous pressure; ETI, endotracheal intubation; MAP, mean arterial pressure; SBP, systolic blood pressure.

SUMMARY

Management of acute AI involves prompt diagnosis and immediate treatment to prevent cardiovascular collapse and death. A high index of suspicion is necessary because the condition can be lethal if missed. Therapy with stress doses of corticosteroids should be initiated even before the confirmation of the diagnosis when there is a high index of suspicion. The side effects of a short course of high-dose corticosteroids in a critically ill patient are minor compared with the possible consequence of cardiovascular collapse and death.

KEY POINTS

- AI is a true emergency and requires rapid diagnosis.
- Common symptoms of AI include weakness, fatigue, and loss of appetite.
- The classic presentation of acute AI is a patient with unexplained hemodynamic instability who is unresponsive to intravascular volume resuscitation and use of vasopressors. AI can mimic cardiogenic, hypovolemic, or septic shock.
- Secondary AI is more common than primary AI. The most common cause of secondary AI is discontinuation of corticosteroid therapy.
- Patients who have taken 40 mg of prednisone per day or its equivalent for a period greater than 2 or 3 weeks during the past year should be considered to be adrenal insufficient until proved otherwise.
- Autoimmune disease is currently the most common cause of primary AI and accounts for approximately 80% of cases. The second most common cause of primary AI is adrenal gland destruction by *Mycobacterium tuberculosis.*
- Ketoconazole, pherytoin, phenobarbital, rifampin, and etomidate can cause AI.
- When there is a high suspicion of AI, hormonal testing is necessary to confirm the diagnosis.
- Therapy with stress doses of corticosteroids should be initiated even before the confirmation of the diagnosis when there is a high index of suspicion. The side effects of a short course of high-dose corticosteroids in a critically ill patient are minor compared with the possible consequence of cardiovascular collapse and death.

REFERENCES

1. Cooper MS, Stewart PM: Corticosteroid insufficiency in acutely ill patients. N Engl J Med 2003;348:727-734.
2. Soni A, Pepepr GM, Wyrwinski PM, et al: Adrenal insufficiency occurring during septic shock: Incidence, outcome, and relationship to peripheral cytokine levels. Am J Med 1995;98:266-271.
3. Rothwell PM, Udwasia ZF, Lawler PG: Cortisol response to corticotrophin and survival in septic shock. Lancet 1991;337:582-583.
4. Babich DJ: Clinical problem solving: Identifying Addison's disease. N Engl J Med 1996;334:1403.
5. Jurney TH, Cockrell JL, Lindbergh JS, et al: Spectrum of serum cortisol response to ACTH in patients. Chest 1987;92:292.
6. Mason SA, Meade TW, Lee JAH, et al: Epidemiological and clinical picture of Addison's disease. Lancet 1968;2:744.
7. Span LFR, Hermus ARMM, Bartelink AKM, et al: Adrenocortical function: An indicator of severity of disease and survival in chronically ill patients. Intensive Care Med 1992;18:93.
8. Jurney TH, Cockrell JL, Lindberg JS, et al: Spectrum of cortisol response to ACTH in patients: Correlation with degree of illness and mortality. Chest 1987;92:292.
9. Vermes I, Beishuizen A, Hampsink RM, et al: Dissociation of plasma ACTH and cortisol levels in critically ill patients. Possible role of endothelin and atrial natriuretic hormone. J Clin Endocrinol Metab 1995;80:1238.
10. Horrocks PM, Jones AF, Ratcliffe WA, et al: Pattern of ACTH and cortisol pulsatility over 24 hours in normal males and females. Clin Endocrinol 1990;32:127.
11. Chernow B, Alexander HR, Smallridge RC, et al: Hormonal responses to graded surgical stress, Arch Intern Med 1987;147:1273.
12. Nto T, Fukata J, Tam S, et al: Biphasic changes in hypothalamo-pituitary-adrenal function during the early recovery period after major abdominal surgery. J Clin Endo Metabolism 1991;73:111.
13. Ellis MJ, Schmidli RS, Livesey JH, et al: Plasma corticotropin releasing factor and vasopressin responses to hypoglycemia in normal man. Clin Endocrinol 1990;32:93.
14. Wittert GA, Stewart DE, Graves MP, et al: Plasma corticotropin releasing factor and vasopressin responses to exercise in normal man. Clin Endocrinol 1991;35:311.
15. Bartanusz V, Jezova D, Bertini LC, et al: Stress induced increase in vasopressin and corticotropin releasing factor expression in hypophysiotropic paraventricular neurons. Endocrinology 1993;132:895.
16. Gllard WO, Turnhill D, Sappino P, Muller AF: Tumor necrosis factor alpha inhibits the hormonal response of the pituitary gland to hypothalamic releasing factors. Endocrinology 1990;127:101.
17. Darling G, Goldstein DS, Stull R, et al: Tumor necrosis factor: Immune endocrine interaction. Surgery 1989;106:1155.
18. Jaattela M, Ilvesmaki V, Voutilnen R, et al: Tumor necrosis factor as a potent inhibitor of adrenocorticotropin induced cortisol production and steroidogenic P450 enzyme gene expression in cultured human fetal adrenal cells. Endocrinology 1991;128:623.
19. Sharp BM, Matta SG, Peterson PK, et al: Tumor necrosis factor alpha is a potent ACTH secretagogue: Comparison to interleukin 1 beta. Endocrinology 1989;124:3131.
20. Bateman A, Singh A, Kral T, Solomon S: The immune hypothalamo-pituitary axis. Endocrinol Rev 1989;10:92.
21. Besedovsky H, Delrey A, Sorkin E, Dinarello CA: Immunoregulatory feedback between interleukin 1 and glucocorticoid hormone. Science 1986;233:652.
22. Stewart PM: The adrenal cortex. In Kronenberg HM, Melmed S, Polonsky KS (eds): Textbook of Endocrinology, 10th ed. Philadelphia, Saunders, 2003, pp 491-551.
23. Svedmyr N: Action of corticosteroids on beta-adrenergic receptors. Am Rev Respir Dis 1990;141:S31.
24. Bouachour G, Tirot P, Varache N, et al: Hemodynamic changes in acute AI. Intensive Care Med 1994;20:138.
25. Luckert BP, Rsz LG: Glucocorticoid induced osteoporosis: Pathogenesis and management. Ann Intern Med 1990;112:352.
26. Munck A, Náray-Fejes-Tóth A: Glucocorticoid physiology. In DeGroot L, Jameson JL (eds): Endocrinology, 5th ed. Philadelphia, Saunders, 2005, pp 2287-2309.
27. Schwartz J, Keil LC, Masseli J, Reid I: Role of vasopressin in regulating blood pressure in AI. Endocrinology 1983;112:234.
28. Bright GM, Singh I: Adrenal autoantibodies bind to adrenal

subcellular fractions enriched in cytochrome c reductase and 5′ nucleotidase. J Clin Endocrinol Metab 1990;70:95.
29. De Bellis, Bizzarro A, Rossi R, et al: Remission of subclinical adrenocortical failure in subjects with adrenal autoantibodies. J Clin Endocrinol Metab 1993;76:1002.
30. Loriaux DL: The polyendocrine deficiency syndromes. N Engl J Med 1985;312:1568.
31. Irwine WJ, Barnes EW: AI. Clin Endocrinol Metab 1972;1:549.
32. Guttma PH: Addison's disease. Arch Pathol 1930;10:742.
33. Sarosi GA, Voth DW, Dahl BA, et al: Disseminated histoplasmosis: Results of long term follow up. A CDC cooperative mycoses study. Ann Intern Med 1971;75:511.
34. Knowlton AI: Adrenal insufficiency in the intensive care setting. J Intensive Care Med 1989;4:35.
35. Dluhy RG: The growing spectrum of HIV related endocrine abnormalities. J Clin Endocrinol 1990;70:563.
36. Redman BG, Pazdur R, Zingas AP, Loredo R: Prospective evaluation of AI in patients with adrenal metastasis. Cancer 1987;60:103.
37. Irwine W: Autoimmunity in endocrine disease. Proc R Soc Med 1974;67:548.
38. Kung AWC, Pun KK, Lam K, et al: Addisonian crisis as presenting feature in malignancies. Cancer 1990;65: 177.
39. Redman BG, Pazdur R, Zingas AP, Loredo R: Prospective evaluation of AI in patients with adrenal metastasis. Cancer 1987;60:103.
40. Rao RH, Vagnucci AH, Amico JA: Bilateral massive adrenal hemorrhage: Early recognition and treatment. Ann Intern Med 1989;110:227.
41. Christy NP, Wallace EZ, Jler JW: Comparative effects of prednisone and cortisone in suppressing the response of the adrenal cortex to exogenous adrenocorticotropin. J Clin Endocrinol Metab 1956;16:1059.
42. Graber AL, Ney RL, Nicholson WE, et al: Natural history of pituitary-adrenal recovery following long term suppression with corticosteroids. J Clin Endocrinol 1956;25:11.
43. Hamrahain AH, Oseni TS, Awafah BM, et al: Measurement of serum free cortisol in critically ill patients. N Engl J Med 2004;350:1629-1639.
44. Cohen J, Ward G, Prins J, et al: Variability of cortisol assays can confound the diagnosis of adrenal insufficiency in the critically ill population. Intensive Care Med 2006;32:1901-1911.
45. Annane D, Maxime V, Ibrahin F, et al: Diagnosis of adrenal insufficiency in severe sepsis. Am Rev Respir Dis 2006;174:1319-1326.
46. Jackson WL: Should we use etomidate as an induction agent for endotracheal intubation in patients with septic shock? A critical appraisal. Chest 2005;127: 1031-1038.
47. Dickstein G, Shechner C, Nicholson WE, et al: Adrenocorticotropin stimulation test: Effects of basal cortisol level, time of day, and suggested new sensitive low dose test. J Clin Endocrinol Metab 1991;72:773.
48. Crowley S, Hindmarsh C, Honour JW, Brook CGD: Reproducibility of the cortisol response to stimulation with dose of ACTH: The effect of basal cortisol levels and comparison of low dose with high dose secretory dynamics. Endocrinology 1993;136:167.
49. Motsay GJ, Alho A, Jaeger T, et al: Effects of corticosteroids on the circulation in shock: Experimental and clinical results. Fed Proc 1970;29: 1861-1873.
50. Sprung CL, Caralis PV, Marcial EH, et al: The effects of high-dose corticosteroids in patients with septic shock. N Engl J Med 1984;311:1137-1143.
51. Bone RC, Fisher CJ, Clemmer TP, et al, and the Methylprednisolone Severe Sepsis Study Group: A controlled clinical trial of high-dose methylprednisolone in the treatment of severe sepsis and septic shock. N Engl J Med 1987;317:653-658.
52. Annane D, Sébille V, Troché G, et al: A 3-level prognostic classification in septic shock based on cortisol levels and cortisol response to corticotropin. JAMA 2000;283:1038-1045.
53. Nerup J: Addison's disease—a review of some clinical, pathological and immunological features. Dan Med Bull 1974;21:201.
54. Doppman JL, Gill JR, Nienhuis AW, et al: CT findings in Addison's disease. J Comput Assist Tomogr 1982;6:757.
55. Lamberts SWJ, Bruining HA, Dejong FH: Drug therapy: Corticosteroid therapy in severe illness. N Engl J Med 1997;337:1285-1292.
56. Annane D, Sebille V, Charpentier C, et al: Effect of treatment with low doses of hydrocortisone and fludrocortisone on mortality in patients with septic shock. JAMA 2002;288:862-871.
57. Briegel J, Forst H, Haller M, et al: Stress doses of hydrocortisone reverse single-center study. Crit Care Med 1999;27:723-732.

Chapter 61

Thyroid Disorders

Susan S. Braithwaite

This chapter addresses nonthyroidal illness syndrome and critical illnesses or complications during critical illness that are manifestations of thyroid disease.

THYROID PHYSIOLOGY

The actions of thyroid hormones are profound and multisystemic, influencing differentiation and development, growth, calorigenesis, rate of metabolic processes, cardiovascular action, and neurologic irritability. Changes of thyroid hormone production or circulating thyroid hormone concentration, even when they occur abruptly, are slow to exert their full effect on the intact organism.

Cellular Effects of Thyroid Hormone

Thyroid hormone action is initiated by the binding of nuclear hormone receptors activated by 3,5,3′-triiodothyronine (T_3) to nuclear thyroid hormone response elements, where the hormone-receptor complex acts as a transcription factor.[1] In addition, T_3 exerts rapid nontranscriptional extranuclear effects that are especially important in cardiovascular physiology. Thyroxine (T_4) acts as a prohormone for T_3 and itself is only weakly interactive with thyroid hormone receptors. The compound 3,3′,5′-triiodothyronine (reverse T_3) is almost devoid of metabolic activity. Unfortunately, clinical laboratory markers for assessing cellular effects of thyroid hormone, such as angiotensin-converting enzyme (ACE) or sex hormone-binding globulin levels, are of limited utility.

Peripheral and Intrathyroidal Conversions of T_4 and T_3

Normally about 80% of circulating T_3 and probably greater than 90% of circulating reverse T_3 are derived from circulating T_4. Quantitatively, the most important sites for peripheral conversion of T_4 to T_3 are the liver, kidney, and skeletal muscle. Peripheral production of T_3 is modulated by the availability of T_4.

Thyroid hormone deiodinations are catalyzed by iodothyronine selenodeiodinases, having three isoforms, identified as deiodinases types 1, 2, and 3 (D1, D2, and D3). Rapid advancement of knowledge of the subcellular location (cell membranes, endoplasmic reticulum) and tissue distribution (thyroid, pituitary, central nervous system, and peripheral tissues) of each enzyme in normal and pathologic states has occurred.[2-8] Peripheral conversions of T_4 to T_3 and reverse T_3 to T_2 are catalyzed by D1 and D2, and conversion of T_3 to T_2 is catalyzed by D3. Sulfation of T3 enhances susceptibility of T_3 to inactivating deiodination.

The D1 enzyme is subject to substrate inhibition (T_4), and it is inhibited noncompetitively by propylthiouracil.[2] The D1 activity in liver is downregulated during nonthyroidal illness, whereas D3 in contrast, not normally active in liver or skeletal muscle, is induced in these tissues in nonthyroidal illness.[6] The net effect in nonthyroidal illness is a reduction of circulating T_3 (Fig. 61-1).

Hormone Transport

Circulating T_4 is carried about 64% to 68% by thyroxine-binding globulin (TBG), 11% to 13% by transthyretin, and 9% to 20% by albumin. T_3 is carried 80% by TBG, 9% by transthyretin, and 11% by albumin.[1,9,10] A small

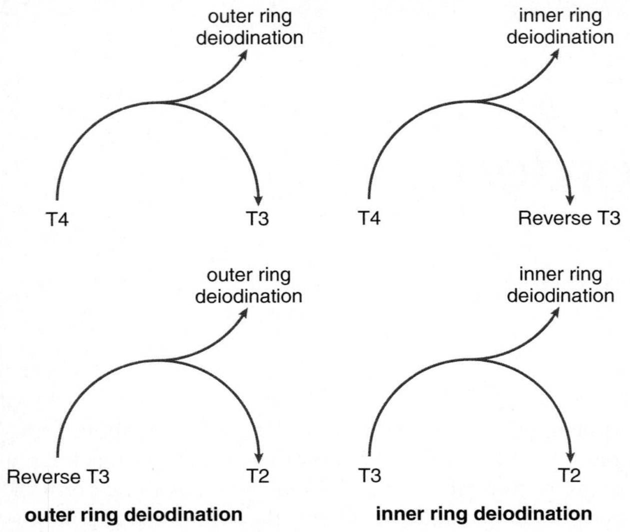

Figure 61-1. D1 catalyzes both outer and inner ring deiodinations, whereas D2 catalyzes outer ring deiodination and D3 inner ring deiodination. Outer ring deiodination of the prohormone T_4 to T_3 is an activating step. Inner ring deiodination, resulting in conversion of T_4 to reverse T_3, and conversion of T_3 to T_2, is an inactivating step. In critical illness, outer ring deiodination by D1 is reduced, contributing to the findings of low T_3 and high reverse T_3, and the D3 enzyme activity responsible for inner ring deiodination is abnormally increased, contributing to increased removal of T_3.

fraction is transported by lipoproteins.[11] About 0.03% of circulating T_4 and 0.3% of T_3 is free or unbound. TBG is produced by the liver, and transthyretin by the liver and choroid plexus. The approximate half-lives of circulating transport proteins are transthyretin, 2 days; TBG, 5 days; and albumen, 15 days.[10] The circulating concentrations of thyroxine binding globulin are increased normally during pregnancy. The free hormone hypothesis is accepted as correct with respect to T_3 and T_4—that only the unbound fraction of circulating hormone gains access to peripheral tissues and pituitary, determines metabolic status, or participates in feedback inhibition of the pituitary.

Expressed in molar units, the normal serum concentrations of thyroid hormone are T_4 64 to 154 nmol/L, T_3 1.2 to 2.9 nmol/L, free T_4 13 to 39 pmol/L, and free T_3 3.8 to 10 pmol/L.[12] Unbound circulating hormone remains in a dynamic equilibrium with hormone provided by thyroid output, carried on transport proteins, or taken up or released by peripheral tissues. The half-life of circulating hormone is about 1 week for T_4 and 1 day for T_3.[1] Deiodination occurs in many tissues, and iodothyronine moieties are excreted in bile. Some enterohepatic recirculation of iodothyronine occurs.

Thyroid Function

Thyroid function is regulated by cyclic-AMP dependent events initiated by binding of thyroid-stimulating hormone (thyrotropin; TSH) to the thyroid follicular cell membrane TSH receptor. TSH stimulation leads to consumption of colloid and the release of thyroglobulin (TG), T_4, T_3, and reverse T_3. Thyroid autoregulation is influenced by the availability of iodine.

Pituitary and Hypothalamic Function

Pituitary TSH and hypothalamic thyrotropin-releasing hormone (TRH) are ultimately necessary for regulation of adequate thyroid hormonogenesis and thyroid hormone secretion. On the principle of feedback inhibition and in the absence of central disease, an inverse relationship is expected between circulating levels of TSH and T_4.

DIAGNOSTIC APPROACH TO THYROID DISEASE

History, Physical Examination, and Record Review

In critical illness, ambiguity of thyroid function tests is commonplace. The obstacles to laboratory assessment enhance the importance of record review, history, and physical examination, which will usually yield multisystemic positive findings when overt thyroid dysfunction is present.[13]

Case-Finding by Screening

Ambulatory patients who should be screened and periodically monitored for thyroid dysfunction include those with a history of previous thyroid surgery or radioactive iodine therapy; deterioration of cardiac function or weight loss; and those receiving lithium, amiodarone, or α-interferon. Routine screening of older women is defensible. In the ambulatory setting, TSH measurement is effective monoscreening for potentially subtle abnormalities of thyroid function. If the TSH level is abnormal, to confirm thyroid status and establish severity of dysfunction it is necessary to make a redetermination of TSH level accompanied by an estimate of free T_4.

Because of the variability of observed TSH results among hospitalized patients, TSH assessment should not be ordered as monoscreening.[14-25] Measurements of total and free T_4 and sometimes T_3 should accompany TSH determinations, but the results are assay dependent and may be misleading in critically ill patients.[6-8,26-88] In a meta-analysis of earlier studies, the frequency of thyroid disease ascertainable by screening hospitalized patients was similar to that among outpatients, about 1% to 2%.[76] In the hospital the relatively low case-finding rate and the confounding effect of nonthyroidal illness have been viewed as impediments to general screening of unselected patients, except possibly among elderly women.[55,56] However, one study in which TSH and free thyroxine index were performed on sera drawn at the time of admission from 364 consecutive patients suggested that the rate of nonthyroidal illness syndrome (7.4%) was exceeded by the combined rates of unsuspected thyroidal failure (5.8%), subclinical hypothyroidism (6%), and hyperthyroidism (2%).[60] Clinical suspicion including emergency presentation with atrial fibrillation should, of course, result in screening.[83]

Among critical care patients, the case-finding rate for thyroid disease during screening is not known with confidence.

Assays and Imaging

Simultaneity of Sampling of Trophic and Target Hormone

In unstable patients, sampling of TSH, thyroid hormone concentrations, and any assessments of hormone binding should occur simultaneously.

Thyroid-Stimulating Hormone

The indication for measuring TSH is to support a diagnosis of primary hypothyroidism or hyperthyroidism. Reasons for misleading TSH results,[20] some of which apply to critically ill patients, include nonequilibrium conditions in which thyroid status has recently fluctuated, acute psychiatric illness, nonthyroidal illness syndrome, central causes of hyperthyroidism or hypothyroidism, and the effects of medication.

The claim has been made that second- and third-generation TSH assays differentiate between nonthyroidal illness syndrome and thyrotoxicosis. However, the distribution of TSH results in nonthyroidal illness syndrome may overlap with the range seen in thyrotoxicosis.[23,24] Conversely, in mild cases of subclinical thyrotoxicosis, for example in nodular thyroid disease at the earliest stages of autonomy, TSH suppression may be minimal, below normal, and at concentrations sometimes associated with nonthyroidal illness but greater than 0.1 μIU/mL, the threshold below which hyperthyroidism is normally suspected.

Estimates of Free Thyroxine

The indication for ordering a free T_4 rather than total T_4 assay is to assess thyroid function in the presence of suspected abnormalities of thyroid hormone transport or to clarify the significance of an abnormal total T_4 result in a patient whose clinical condition appears euthyroid. A normal result of a free T_4 determination is reassuring. However, in critically ill patients assays that estimate free T_4 sometimes yield low results that cannot be verified by an equilibrium dialysis method.[34,37,43,48,52,74] On the other hand, drugs and circulating inhibitors of T_4 binding to transport proteins sometimes cause free T_4 assays to yield high results. Therefore in the care of critically ill patients the utility of most commercial methods for determining free T_4 levels is limited.

Total Thyroxine

The indication for ordering a total T_4 assay is to demonstrate and quantitate the severity of hypothyroidism or hyperthyroidism. In the care of a critically ill patient, a normal total T_4 level is a reassuring finding for two reasons. First, the patient is probably euthyroid. Second, nonthyroidal illness syndrome, if present, is not of sufficient severity to present with its adverse prognostic indicator, low T_4. The institutional turnaround time for a total T_4 assay may be faster than for a free T_4.

T_3 Uptake and Calculated Free T_4 Index

The T_3 uptake, together with a determination of total T_4, is used in index methods to estimate free T_4 (Table 61-1).

Table 61-1. Use of Total T_4 and T_3 Uptake to Calculate Free Thyroxine Index

	Total T_4	T_3 Uptake	FTI
Normal	nl	nl	nl
Increased binding sites	↑	↓	nl
Reduced binding sites	↓	↑	nl
Hyperthyroid	↑	↑	↑
Hypothyroid	↓	↓	↓

When the serum of the patient is exposed to a solid-phase substance with affinity for thyroid hormone, the uptake of labeled T_3 by the solid-phase substance is inversely proportional to unoccupied binding sites of the thyroid hormone transport proteins of the patient's serum. The free T_4 index is a unitless number derived from the product of the T_3 uptake and the T_4. Conditions with increased availability of transport protein binding sites include estrogen therapy or pregnancy; conditions with reduced binding by transport proteins include nonthyroidal illness syndrome. In hyperthyroidism and hypothyroidism there are no major changes in the concentration of transport proteins, but the supply of hormone from the thyroid is altered. The altered supply affects the dynamic equilibrium among free hormone, hormone bound to transport proteins, and hormone available to tissues. Transport protein binding sites are hypersaturated or hyposaturated with thyroid hormone in hyperthyroidism and hypothyroidism, respectively, and total T_4 or total T_3 measurements usually correctly reflect thyroid status.

In critically ill patients with hypothyroxinemia, the free T_4 index is frequently misleading.[31] Nevertheless, when hypothyroxinemia exists but its interpretation is uncertain, it is advantageous to review a second independent assay such as the T_3 uptake or direct measurement of transport proteins to see whether qualitatively the result is consistent with the diagnosis of nonthyroidal illness syndrome. Elevation of T_3 uptake suggests reduced hormone binding to transport proteins, consistent with nonthyroidal illness syndrome. Nonelevated T_3 uptake accompanied by hypothyroxinemia in the face of nonthyroidal illness suggests the possibility of intrinsic hypothyroidism. The use of total T_4, T_3 uptake, and calculated free T_4 index is being replaced by widespread use of assays that directly estimate free T_4.

Free T_4 by Equilibrium Dialysis or Ultrafiltration

In critical care medicine the indication for ordering a free T_4 evaluation by equilibrium dialysis or ultrafiltration is the concern that other free T_4 methods might yield false low results.

Total T_3

The main indication for measuring total T_3 is suspicion of T_3 toxicosis or hyperthyroidism in patients lacking hyperthyroxinemia. If the TSH is suppressed to less than 0.1 μIU/mL but hyperthyroxinemia is absent, measurement of T_3

is necessary. T_3 is also measured to evaluate for amiodarone-induced hyperthyroidism. Measurement of T_3 should not be employed to evaluate the possibility of hypothyroidism. Under intense TSH stimulation the failing thyroid preferentially secretes T_3 rather than T_4 so that patients with T_4 reduction may maintain normal T_3 levels. Assuming hyperthyroidism is not suspected, in nonthyroidal illness syndrome it is not important to measure T_3 unless the caregiver is engaged in research or is committed to using T_3 therapy for some affected patients.

Free T_3

The indication for ordering the free T_3 test is to confirm or exclude T_3 toxicosis or amiodarone-induced hyperthyroidism in patients suspected of having thyroid transport abnormalities.

Reverse T_3

The indication for ordering reverse T_3 is to differentiate intrinsic hypothyroidism from nonthyroidal illness syndrome, in which there are low and potentially high concentrations of reverse T_3, respectively.[29,31,41] Slow laboratory turnaround and frequency of normal results in nonthyroidal illness syndrome limit the usefulness of reverse T_3 measurement.[40]

Patients with chronic renal failure who have low T_3 do not invariably have high reverse T_3 levels,[33,35] and patients with HIV have low reverse T_3.[53]

Serum Albumin

When low T_4 levels are present, a finding of concomitant hypoalbuminemia usually permits the caregiver tentatively to attribute the low T_4 results to reduction of circulating transport proteins. Hypoalbuminemia is highly associated with nonthyroidal illness syndrome.[75,86] A low serum albumin level often, but not always, predicts low TBG.

Thyroxine-Binding Globulin

The transport protein TBG can be directly measured, and the result can be used together with a determination of T_4 as one method of calculating a free thyroxine index. TBG levels are increased in hepatitis, hepatoma, and HIV.[53]

Antithyroid Peroxidase (Antimicrosomal) and Antithyroglobulin Antibodies

In the critical care setting the principal indication for antithyroid antibody determination is to evaluate the significance of a TSH elevation. In sufficient titer, positive antibodies strongly suggest autoimmune thyroid disease.

Radioiodine Uptake and Thyroid Scan

The utility of the radioactive iodine uptake and thyroid scan is to identify the cause of hyperthyroidism to help decide between therapeutic alternatives and, before radioactive iodine therapy, to guide dosing decisions. The radioactive iodine uptake is a number, expressed as a percent uptake counted 24 hours after administration of a small dose of radioactive iodine, and the scan provides an image. The radioactive iodine uptake test helps differentiate low-uptake forms of hyperthyroidism (amiodarone- or iodine-induced hyperthyroidism, thyroiditis, factitious hyperthyroidism, and others) from high-uptake forms of hyperthyroidism (Graves' disease, toxic adenoma, and toxic multinodular goiter). These tests often are postponed until 4 to 6 weeks after the last use of an iodinated contrast medium.

Ultrasonography and Computed Tomography

The indication for thyroid ultrasonography is to obtain information about the size, texture, and nodularity of the thyroid and to evaluate other structures in the neck. Examination of the thoracic inlet in cases of large compressive goiters is best accomplished with computed tomography.

"Best Panel" for Critically Ill Patients

An approach to diagnosis of thyroid disease is summarized in Box 61-1. If the free T_4 assay yields high results as a consequence of nonthyroidal illness syndrome, unavailability of a total T_4 determination would create a risk of misinterpretation. A panel rather than a single test is drawn at the outset. The initial "best panel" is whichever one of the following has the faster turnaround time or weekend availability, or both, at the laboratory used by the institution:

- TSH, total T_4, and T_3 uptake (with calculated free thyroxine index)
- TSH, total T_4, free T_4 estimate by any other method

These panels will yield unambiguous results in most cases of critical illness that are caused or complicated by preexisting clinically significant primary hypothyroidism or hyperthyroidism. Furthermore, the finding of normal

Box 61-1

"Best Panel" and Follow-up Studies for Critically Ill Patients

Initial "Best Panel" for Suspected Thyroid Disease
TSH
Total T_4
T_3 uptake
or
TSH
Total T_4
Free T_4

Confirming Panel for Suspected Hyperthyroidism
Reserved for patients with normal free T_4 and suppressed TSH or for amiodarone-treated patients
TSH
Total and free T_3

Confirming Panel That Sometimes Differentiates Suspected Nonthyroidal Illness Syndrome from Central Hypothyroidism
TSH
Free T_4 by equilibrium dialysis or ultrafiltration

TSH and normal or elevated free T_4 suggests the absence of both hypothyroidism and hyperthyroidism.

If clinical examination suggests hyperthyroidism and marked suppression of a second or third generation TSH is present, but if hyperthyroxinemia cannot be demonstrated, then the next step is to draw simultaneously the following:

- TSH, total and free T_3

If the free T_4 and TSH considered as a hormone pair appear discordant (both values high or both values low), and if the explanation or management is not straightforward, a consultation should be obtained. However, in the setting of nonthyroidal illness, if low T_4, low free T_4 estimate, and normal or low TSH are demonstrated during screening, to discount the diagnosis of secondary hypothyroidism it is sometimes helpful to order the following:

- TSH, T_4, free T_4 by equilibrium dialysis

Demonstration of nonthyroidal illness syndrome is seldom the rationale for ordering thyroid function testing. However, if the physician wants to demonstrate changes characteristic of nonthyroidal illness, quantitate its severity, predict prognosis, or demonstrate sequential changes of that syndrome, the "best panel" would be one of the following, which can be ordered shortly after the onset of nonthyroidal illness and repeated at nadir and during recovery:

- TSH, T_4, free T_4 by equilibrium dialysis, total and free T_3, or
- TSH, T_4, free T_4 by equilibrium dialysis, total and free T_3, reverse T_3

Table 61-2. Thyroid Function Test Abnormalities Induced by Medication in Euthyroid Individuals

Abnormality	Medication
Low TSH	Dopamine and congeners Glucocorticoids
High T_4, high free T_4, low T_3	Amiodarone
High free T_4	Heparin Salicylates and congeners Furosemide
High T_4	Estrogen Oral contraceptives Tamoxifen
Low T_4	Salicylates and congeners Glucocorticoids
Low T_4 and low free T_4	Phenytoin Carbamazepine
Thyroid Dysfunction Induced by Medication	
Hypothyroidism or hyperthyroidism	Iodides Amiodarone α-Interferon
Hypothyroidism	Lithium

Box 61-2

Possible Outcomes of Amiodarone Therapy

Euthyroidism
Normal TSH
High T_4 and free T_4
Low T_3

Hypothyroidism
High TSH
Normal or low T_4 and free T_4

Hyperthyroidism
Low TSH
High T_3 and free T_3

MEDICATION EFFECTS

When unexpected thyroid function test results suggest the possibility of drug interferences, a medication review should be conducted.[89] Common medication effects are summarized in Table 61-2 and Box 61-2. Drugs that affect thyroid test results often are capable of inducing one or more of the following: suppression of TSH (dopaminergic drugs,[90,91] glucocorticoids[92]); inhibition of peripheral conversion of T_4 to T_3 (glucocorticoids,[93] β-blockers, iodinated contrast agents, amiodarone, propylthiouracil); reduction of transport proteins (glucocorticoids); elevation of transport proteins (estrogen, oral contraceptives, tamoxifen); displacement of thyroid hormone from transport proteins (heparin, salicylates and congeners, furosemide, phenytoin, carbamazepine)[94-102]; both induction of hyperthyroidism and inhibition of thyroid function (iodine,[103] amiodarone,[104-130] α-interferon); or inhibition of thyroid function (lithium, thionamides). In the case of interferon and amiodarone, a possible sequence is hyperthyroidism followed by hypothyroidism.[115,123]

NONTHYROIDAL ILLNESS SYNDROME

Nonthyroidal illness syndrome is a constellation of thyroid function abnormalities of uncertain clinical significance, not all of which are expressed in each case, that occur with acute psychiatric illness, starvation, congestive heart failure, chronic renal failure, postoperative status, trauma, and other critical illnesses.[131-133]

History and Incidence

Historically, nonthyroidal illness syndrome was recognized when laboratory techniques were developed to measure circulating thyroid hormone concentrations, evaluate transport of thyroid hormones, and measure TSH levels. In the absence of intrinsic thyroid disease, apparent thyroid-related abnormalities (as seen by laboratory results) resolve after recovery from nonthyroidal illness; thus the term *euthyroid sick syndrome* was initially used to refer to the constellation of observed thyroid function test abnormalities. Because of growing suspicion that affected patients might experience actual thyroid hormone deficiency, most physicians now refer to the same findings as *nonthyroidal illness syndrome*. When intrinsic pituitary or thyroid disease is judged to be absent, the standard of care has been to observe the patient without treatment. Although there is increasing interest in evaluating T_3 therapy for nonthyroidal illness syndrome, it is expected that differences in outcome resulting from such treatment will be small and difficult to demonstrate.[132]

Among hospitalized patients, intrinsic thyroid disease is less common than nonthyroidal illness syndrome.[14,40,56,76,134] The prevalence of nonthyroidal illness syndrome among patients with psychiatric disease is about 10.2%, often manifesting as elevated TSH or elevated T_4.[22,25] Low T_3 is reported in 18% of patients with moderate to severe heart failure,[71] 66% of elderly hospitalized patients,[55] and 81% of an infected subgroup of elderly postoperative patients.[75] Low T_4 is reported in 24% of critically ill patients.[38]

Pathogenesis

In the evolution of nonthyroidal illness syndrome, reduction of circulating T_3 is the first and most consistently observed finding,[26,27,55] and the apparent mechanism is a marked reduction in peripheral production of T_3 from T_4, as well as enhanced sulfation and deiodination of T_3.[5,6,30,41] Failure to metabolize reverse T_3 results in concomitant elevations of reverse T_3.[29,31,41] Decreased activity of the D1 enzyme and abnormally increased activity of the D3 enzyme are implicated as the causes of reduced peripheral T_3.[6,44,135-138]

Although early data in nonthyroidal illness syndrome suggested that reductions of total T_3 were accompanied by reductions of free T_3,[40] recent studies suggest that the results are method dependent and free T_3 levels may be normal in some patients.[68,70,73,74]

A subgroup of patients with low T_3 also has subnormal T_4 levels. These are usually patients with disease of greater severity and longer duration, usually with reduction of transport protein concentration. There is a reduced rate of T_4 exit from serum but increased fractional disposal of T_4, possibly reflecting decreased binding of T_4 to vascular and extravascular sites.[28,33] In nonthyroidal illness syndrome inhibitors of hormone binding to transport proteins such as nonesterified fatty acids are recognized.[37] The action of serine proteases present at inflammatory sites may cleave TBG, causing release of T_4.[139] Free T_4 elevations are sometimes demonstrated, often accompanied by low or low normal total T_4,[31] but there is controversy on the importance of the free T_4 elevation in vivo and suspicion that at least some instances represent artifact, such as could be introduced by nonselective β-blockers, furosemide, or free fatty acids produced through the action of heparin-induced lipoprotein lipase activity.[39,44,47,96-99,101,108,110,111] Low free T_4 is demonstrated among other patients with nonthyroidal illness syndrome.[15,43] However, most patients including those with low T_4 have normal free T_4.[40,49,52,74]

The question of the true levels of circulating free T_4 remains unresolved, dogged by issues of assay artifact and heterogeneity within the patient population. With respect to the question of greatest importance—whether tissue concentrations and effects of thyroid hormone are appropriate for the altered milieu created by nonthyroidal illness—the answer is unknown.[7,140]

Several lines of evidence suggest that inhibition of thyroidal, pituitary, and hypothalamic function occurs in nonthyroidal illness syndrome. Cytokines, although they do not appear to inhibit peripheral conversion of T_4 to T_3, may inhibit thyroidal production of hormone; however, an early decline in T_3 occurs during abdominal surgery independent of IL-6 or TNF-α.[80,141-147] The more severely ill patients with nonthyroidal illness syndrome, usually those having low T_4 levels, as well as low T_3, may have low circulating levels of TSH.[15,17,21,24,148] It has been proposed that lipopolysaccharide or cytokine induction by lipopolysaccharide may cause increased D2 activity and therefore local excess of T_3 in the hypothalamus, resulting in suppression of TSH.[148] During recovery following nonthyroidal illness or TNF-α administration, there is often overshoot of TSH into the mildly elevated range, and then eventually normalization of TSH levels.[17,146]

Presently it is unknown whether nonthyroidal illness syndrome is adaptive or maladaptive. In starvation, low T_3 syndrome may promote protein sparing.[149] Human trials have not been conducted with a sufficient number of randomized, critically ill human subjects to resolve the question of whether thyroid hormone therapy is beneficial. In a nonrandomized study of patients with sepsis, T_3 was used to reduce dopamine dependence.[150] Treatment with T_3 for human burn injury showed no benefit.[151] In a small study of critically ill patients with low T_3 and low T_4, therapy with T_4 did not correct the low T_3 or improve the prognosis,[152] and thyroxine may increase mortality among acute renal failure patients.[153]

A special niche may exist for the use of T_3 after correction of any reversible ischemia in treatment of cardiac patients who require hemodynamic support.[54,71,154-163] Low T_3 levels are observed in the setting of advanced heart failure,[82,84,87] after revascularization, and after myocardial infarction.[54,71] Use of intravenous T_3 shows promise as an inotrope and vasodilator.[161,164] In the setting of advanced heart failure, coronary bypass or valve surgery, correction of congenital heart lesions, or in the treatment of transplantation donors and recipients, the benefits that have been attributed to intravenous T_3 therapy include improvement of cardiac index with reduction of systemic vascular resistance,[161,164] a reduction in postoperative episodes of atrial fibrillation,[158] reduction in estimated mortality among high-risk patients,[160] a reduced requirement for inotropic support and mechanical devices,[160,162,163] a lower incidence of postoperative myocardial ischemia,[163] and improved cardiac allograft function.[154] Whether the apparently beneficial cardiac effects of T_3 administration are pharmacologic effects or at least partially the effects of physiologic replacement of a true hormone deficiency are unclear. On the other hand, high levels of triiodothyronine have been identified as a risk factor for coronary events.[165] Overall, the use of triiodothyronine for cardiac indications has not gained widespread acceptance.

Clinical Manifestations

Nonthyroidal illness syndrome is usually recognized as a constellation of laboratory findings discovered on thyroid function testing. Patients usually appear clinically euthyroid.

Diagnostic Approach

The finding of an isolated reduction of T_3, with normal or elevated free T_4 and without abnormality of total T_4 or TSH, suggests early or mild nonthyroidal illness syndrome. For low T_3 syndrome, no further evaluation is necessary.

The additional finding of a low T_4 together with low T_3 suggests nonthyroidal illness syndrome of greater severity.[52] Some cases of low total T_4 are caused by transport protein deficiency alone, whereas others may result from TSH suppression. If the free T_4, as evaluated by equilibrium dialysis, is low, the differential diagnosis includes the less common condition of central hypothyroidism. Before recovery, biochemical differentiation is often not possible between nonthyroidal illness syndrome and central hypothyroidism. In fact, nonthyroidal illness syndrome may be one cause of central hypothyroidism.

TSH suppression resulting from severe nonthyroidal illness itself often is accompanied by low T_4 and low T_3 and is observed during the advanced or subacute stages of critical illness, not usually at the onset or during recovery. During recovery from nonthyroidal illness the TSH often is mildly elevated above the normal ambulatory reference range, and the free T_4 is normal. The differential diagnosis includes subclinical primary hypothyroidism.

After recovery from nonthyroidal illness syndrome, thyroid function tests are normal.

Approach to Management

Although future research may bring about changes in the standard of care, at the present time for nonthyroidal illness syndrome most experts recommend observation without thyroid hormone treatment, with reevaluation of thyroid function tests after recovery.[166] The philosophy of nontreatment would imply that there is no obligation to order thyroid tests unless thyroid disease is suspected. If the patient is euthyroid and free of reversible myocardial ischemia, treatment with thyroid hormone will probably do no harm. Treatment is offered when caregivers believe the clinical evaluation and results of thyroid tests do not permit exclusion of intrinsic disease of the thyroid, pituitary, or hypothalamus.

Therapeutic Alternatives

For nonthyroidal illness syndrome a proposed regimen is to administer T_3 orally or intravenously in divided doses of 50 to 75 μg/day and T_4 initially at a low dosage. Hormone levels might be measured every 48 hours, aiming for a trough T_3 level of 70 to 100 ng/dL.[79] Among dopamine-treated patients, it may be possible to overcome pituitary TSH inhibition through the use of repeated doses of the hypothalamic peptide thyrotropin-releasing hormone (TRH).[91] These proposed approaches have not been adequately studied for safety or efficacy in patients having nonthyroidal illness syndrome.

Among patients with severely impaired left ventricular performance, the use of intravenous T_3 as an alternative to standard therapy (such as dopamine) and the compatibility or usefulness of T_3 in combination with other inotropic and vasodilating regimens require further research.

Prognosis

Normal T_3 is a favorable prognostic indicator,[66] whereas the biochemical findings of low T_3 or other findings of nonthyroidal illness syndrome predict worse outcomes of critical illness in general.*

HYPOTHYROIDISM AND MYXEDEMA COMA

Hypothyroidism

History and Incidence

Among outpatients in iodine-replete regions, the prevalence of newly diagnosed hypothyroidism is up to 3 or 4 per 1000.[167-170] An age-related increase of incidence of hypothyroidism exists, and the prevalence is higher in women. The appearance of overt hypothyroidism is predicted by prior isolated TSH elevation and positive antithyroid antibodies.[171] The prevalence of amiodarone-induced hypothyroidism has been variably reported, but it may be seen in up to 22% of treated patients from iodine-sufficient regions,[106] and its occurrence may be predicted by the presence of positive antibodies.[105]

Pathogenesis

The most common mechanisms of hypothyroidism are autoimmune destruction (Hashimoto's thyroiditis) or previous surgery or radioiodine ablation therapy for hyperthyroidism. Lithium, α-interferon, iodine,[103] and amiodarone[106,107,114] can induce hypothyroidism. Patients with antithyroid antibodies may be at special risk of iodine- or amiodarone-induced hypothyroidism. The manifestations of hypothyroidism are dependent not only on the severity of hormone deficiency by laboratory testing but also the duration of hypothyroidism.

Patients with severe hypothyroidism have reduced calorigenesis and oxygen consumption. Many metabolic processes proceed at a markedly reduced rate. Glycosaminoglycan metabolism is impeded, resulting in widespread tissue deposition of hyaluronan. A contributory factor in the production of generalized edema is transcapillary albumin escape.[172] Slowing of the metabolism of lipoproteins results in secondary hyperlipidemia. There is reduced conversion of carotene to vitamin A. The slow metabolism of drugs contributes to the marked propensity of hypothyroid patients to experience the effects of overdosage, especially with respect to digoxin, narcotics, sedatives, and analgesics. Perhaps because of reduced clearance of vitamin K–dependent factors, however, there is resistance to warfarin.

Reduced ventilatory responses to hypoxia and hypercapnia appear to have a dominantly central mechanism, and there may be upper airway obstruction.[173-178] The effusions of myxedema contain high concentrations of

*Data from references 27, 28, 37, 42, 45, 46, 51, 54, 59, 63, 66, 67, 72, 85.

protein and cholesterol. Pericardial effusion is more characteristic than pericardial tamponade.[179-183] Vasoconstriction with or without hypertension exists. The mechanisms of resistance to catecholamine effects are complex and controversial. There is reduced responsiveness to adrenergic stimuli but actual elevation of circulating norepinephrine concentration. In the heart the activities of the calcium-activated ATP-ase of the sarcoplasmic reticulum, phospholamban, malic enzyme, and other proteins are regulated by thyroid hormone. Myocardial contractility, oxygen consumption, ejection time, diastolic ventricular compliance, stroke volume, heart rate, and cardiac index are reduced. However, unlike in congestive heart failure, the left ventricular end-diastolic pressure is not elevated in myxedema and the cardiac index increases in response to exercise.[184-190] An increased occurrence of coronary artery disease may exist.[166,191-197] Hypomotility of the bowels is common. There may be coexistent iron losses as a result of menorrhagia or gastrointestinal bleeding. Malabsorption of vitamin B_{12} and folic acid may occur. A reduction in atrial natriuretic factor production may occur,[198] as well as a reduction of the glomerular filtration rate. The kidney cannot excrete a water load effectively, but antidiuretic hormone deficiency cannot be consistently implicated when hyponatremia and defective intrarenal mechanisms are suspected.[199-201] Calcium loading can result in hypercalcemia. Hyperuricemia commonly results from underexcretion of uric acid. Pituitary overproduction of prolactin but retarded responsiveness of the pituitary-adrenal axis to appropriate challenges in myxedema may occur.

Clinical Manifestations

An adult patient with long-standing hypothyroidism will have multisystemic findings. Constitutional symptoms include cold intolerance, fatigue, constipation, and weight gain, the latter not invariably observed and usually modest. Dry, brittle hair may be noted. Sleep apnea may occur. Women may have galactorrhea or menorrhagia. Myopathic and arthritic complaints can lead to misdiagnosis of a primary rheumatic disorder. Patients may have carpal tunnel syndrome. A history of somnolence, dementia, syncope, or seizures may exist.

Hypertension may be attributable to myxedema. The thyroid is often atrophic but may be goitrous. The following characteristics often permit clinical diagnosis: a deep, husky quality of the voice; slow mode of speech; involuntary blepharoptosis; torpid expression; facial bloating; eyelid and infraorbital edema; sallowness, facial pallor; hearing loss; bradycardia, distant muffled heart tones; cool, dry, coarse skin; nonpitting edema of the supraclavicular fossae, hands, legs, and feet; bruising; and the delayed relaxation of deep tendon reflexes. The patient may present with adynamic ileus.

Despite the reduction of glomerular filtration rate, the serum creatinine and BUN are normal. Macrocytic anemia may be present with or without B_{12} deficiency, and iron deficiency is common. The sedimentation rate is modestly elevated. Unless a CK is measured, abnormal AST and ALT levels of muscle origin may be misinterpreted as representative of liver dysfunction. An electrocardiogram (ECG) may show sinus bradycardia, first-degree AV block, low voltage QRS complexes, and nonspecific T-wave changes.

Diagnostic Approach

The TSH level of patients with untreated primary hypothyroidism can be lowered into the normal range by critical illness, but only rarely.[202] Sometimes the severity of TSH elevation is blunted by the myxedema itself, with extreme hypothyroxinemia accompanied by TSH levels that may be less than 20 μIU/mL. In most cases of advanced hypothyroidism the TSH will be above the normal reference range and the T_4 and free T_4 will be low. Therefore in general, during nonthyroidal illness the laboratory diagnosis of coexistent primary hypothyroidism is straightforward (Fig. 61-2).

Milder cases of hypothyroidism potentially can be confused with the recovery phase of nonthyroidal illness syndrome, when transitory TSH elevation commonly occurs. The patient should be examined for goiter. The finding of subnormal free T_4, positive antithyroid peroxidase antibodies, or TSH above 20 μIU/mL sometimes signifies intrinsic thyroid disease.[17,18] Outpatient reassessment should occur.

In critically ill patients the diagnosis of secondary hypothyroidism is not straightforward. When a low free T_4 level by equilibrium dialysis and low TSH level are present, the question arises of whether the findings signify central hypothyroidism for any reason other than nonthyroidal illness syndrome. The most pressing immediate need would be to recognize and treat cortisol deficiency or pituitary mass effect. History of prior reproductive dysfunction, examination of cranial nerve function and mental status, and measurements of cortisol and other pituitary and target gland hormones may suggest preexisting pituitary dysfunction with or without tumor or the new occurrence of pituitary apoplexy. The diagnosis of pituitary tumor or apoplexy is confirmed by pituitary MRI or CT scanning.

Approach to Management

Precautions in the Care of the Hypothyroid Patient

The patient who has not yet been rendered euthyroid by therapy is at risk of water intoxication by overly vigorous intravenous fluid administration. There is risk of oversedation and CNS suppression from sedative and analgesic drugs, which are metabolized and excreted abnormally slowly in the presence of hypothyroidism. These drugs and digitalis should be given with caution, in reduced dosage. Warfarin sensitivity may increase during treatment.

Standard Therapy for Hypothyroidism

Replacement therapy for hypothyroidism can be provided as T_4 or T_3, each of which is available for oral or intravenous administration, but T_4 is the preferred hormone for ambulatory patients and most hospitalized patients.[203-216] Normally production of T_3 from T_4 occurs rapidly. Because of the prolonged half life of T_4, after each daily dose or

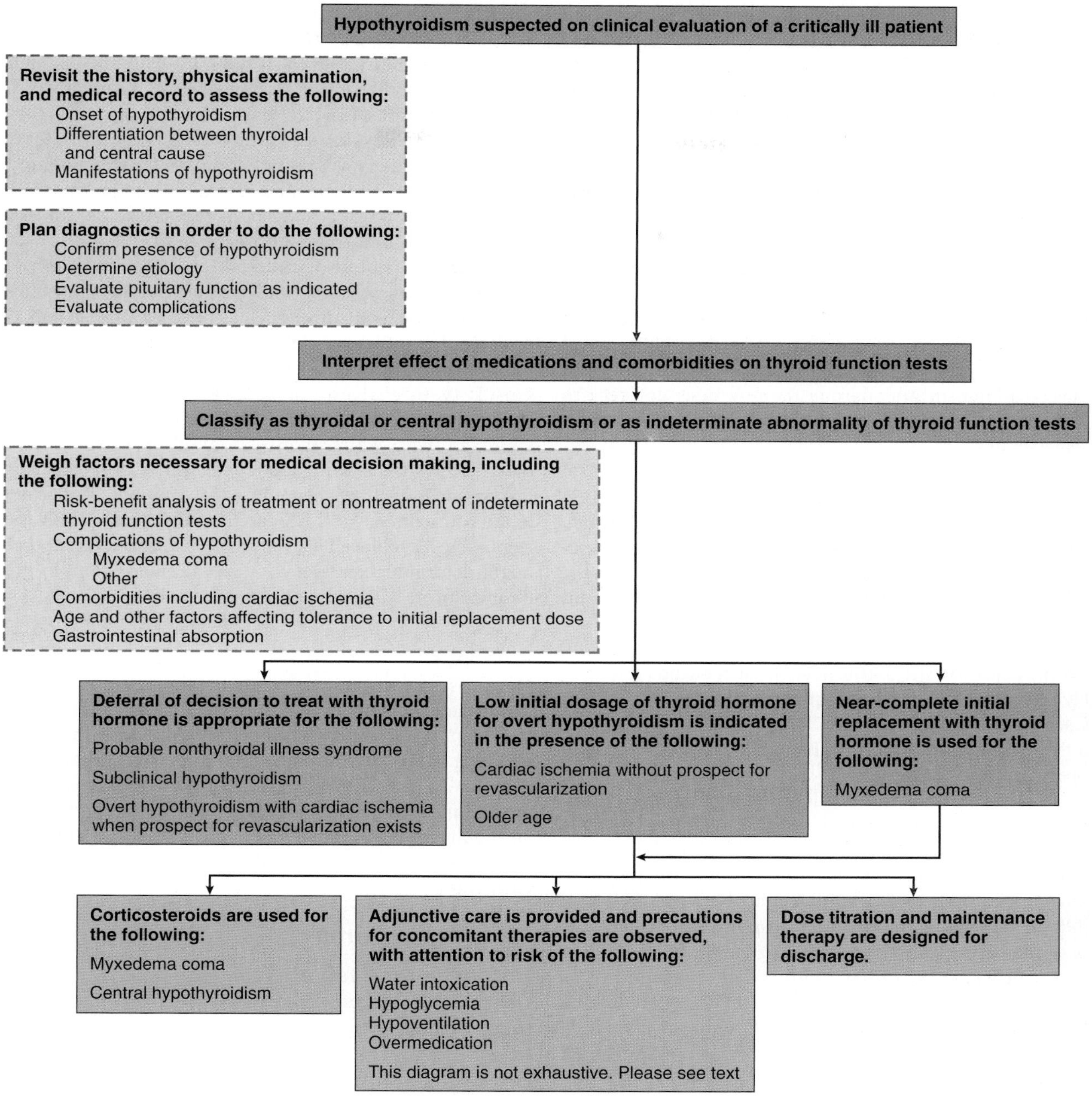

Figure 61-2. Approach to management for hypothyroidism.

after short-term interruption of chronic T_4 therapy there are stable blood levels of T_4 and T_3.[207,208] An ambulatory hypothyroid patient, when treated with T_4 in dosage sufficient to maintain euthyroidism (normal TSH), often has normal T_3 but blood levels of T_4 slightly above the mean for a euthyroid patient.[212] A patient whose T_4 dose requirement was established before hospitalization generally should be maintained on the same dose, if it can be given orally. The oral absorption of thyroxine is impeded by intestinal disease or concomitant administration of iron, sucralfate, cholestyramine, colestipol, calcium, and other drugs.[214] Enteric administration of thyroxine should be separated from these drugs by at least 2 to 4 hours. For patients whose oral intake will be curtailed for a prolonged interval, approximately 50% to 70% of the established daily dose of thyroxine may be administered as a single daily intravenous bolus.[205]

To initiate therapy, patients with abrupt development of hypothyroidism or young patients may be started on full replacement doses of levothyroxine. Those with long-standing severe untreated hypothyroidism are started at 0.05 mg/day or, for older patients or those with coronary artery disease, 0.025 mg/day. Increments of 0.025 mg for older patients are made at about 3-week intervals until it is estimated that the patient is close to full replacement, then the free T_4 and TSH levels are rechecked. After a dosage adjustment of T_4 therapy, 6 weeks is necessary before biochemical reevaluation will reflect a steady-state condition. After upward titration of the dose, the average adult requirement for hypothyroidism is about 0.112 mg/day levothyroxine orally. For elderly patients the dose is lower than for younger patients,[209,212] and for subclinical or early hypothyroidism, the dose of T_4 necessary to normalize the TSH may be as low as 0.05 to 0.075 mg/day.

After levothyroxine treatment there will be increased whole-body oxygen consumption and myocardial workload. If coronary artery disease is present, the demand for increased myocardial oxygen consumption may not be met.

It may be stated anecdotally that atrial arrhythmias are no contraindication to providing replacement therapy for hypothyroidism.[139,141] Development of hypothyroidism during lithium or amiodarone therapy does not require drug discontinuation but may require thyroid hormone replacement.

Subclinical hypothyroidism refers to persistent TSH elevation with normal free T_4 and absence of characteristic symptoms of hypothyroidism. In the ambulatory setting, when antithyroid antibodies are present, the high risk of progression to overt hypothyroidism justifies therapy. Mild or subclinical hypothyroidism is not likely to present short-term risks to a critically ill patient.

Preparation of the Patient with Untreated Hypothyroidism for Emergency Surgery or Cardiac Surgery

Subclinical hypothyroidism has not been shown to increase operative risk.[143] For patients with overt hypothyroidism, elective surgery should be deferred until euthyroidism is attained. For emergency surgery, younger patients without coronary disease should be prepared as if they already had myxedema coma, using a preoperative intravenous bolus of levothyroxine between 200 and 500 μg, depending on age and transport protein status, as described later (see "Myxedema Coma"), and providing hydrocortisone coverage, with other precautions as described earlier (see "Precautions in the Care of the Hypothyroid Patient"). Emergency surgery should be deferred for 24 to 48 hours after treatment if possible.[143]

Patients who are candidates for correction of reversible myocardial ischemia generally should undergo revascularization before one attempts to treat their hypothyroidism. The risks of immediate thyroid hormone replacement before noncardiac surgery should be weighed against the probably acceptable risks of successful operation without thyroxine pretreatment.[166,217-236]

A protocol for patients with correctable coronary artery disease might be to use light preoperative analgesia and sedation, avoid water intoxication, administer glucose as small volumes of concentrated dextrose solutions, be prepared to support ventilation for prolonged intervals postoperatively, provide hydrocortisone 100 mg every 8 hours on the first postoperative day, taper and discontinue hydrocortisone over 5 to 7 days, and initiate intravenous levothyroxine 0.05 mg daily in the immediate postoperative period.

Therapeutic Alternatives

For patients receiving oral therapy, T_3 in dosage sufficient to maintain euthyroidism results in daily peaks and troughs of blood levels of T_3, low levels of T_4, and incomplete suppression of TSH.[207] Earlier studies suggested that some patients developed adverse fluctuating symptoms during such therapy with T_3 or during combination therapy with T_3 and T_4. For critically ill patients, impairment of conversion of T_4 to T_3 may be a theoretical reason for inclusion of T_3 in a treatment regimen.[210]

Critically ill patients with coexistent untreated intrinsic hypothyroidism pose a special problem because they may develop adverse outcomes such as reduced cardiac index, prolonged ventilatory dependency, respiratory deconditioning, hypertension or hypotension, hyponatremia, sensitivity to analgesic or sedative drugs, altered consciousness, or progression to myxedema coma. One approach, with which there is limited experience, is to treat such patients with immediate full T_4 replacement intravenously rather than the usual cautious T_4 dosage initiation regimen.[206,211] Research on indications for T_3 or aggressive T_4 replacement and patient characteristics that might determine candidacy for rapid replacement, in the absence of myxedema coma, is necessary.

Prognosis

New onset of angina, myocardial infarction, or sudden death may occur within days or weeks after initiation of treatment for hypothyroidism.[203,204] Mental retardation resulting from untreated neonatal hypothyroidism is not completely reversible. Secondary hyperlipidemia and most clinical manifestations of juvenile hypothyroidism and adult myxedema are reversible after therapy, although some features, such as anemia, may require months for correction.

Myxedema Coma

History and Incidence

Our present-day knowledge of myxedema coma derives from isolated case reports and small retrospective series.[235,237-256] Historically the low doses of thyroid hormone normally used to initiate treatment of uncomplicated hypothyroidism, when administered enterally for myxedema coma, failed to prevent fatalities. The mortality rate was probably higher than 80%. In 1964 it was demonstrated that intravenous replacement with 500 μg levothyroxine, a dose calculated to nearly replete body stores of thyroxine, improved the rate of survival.[242] Triiodothyronine for intravenous injection later became commercially available.

Pathogenesis

Myxedema coma arising in the community can generally be divided into episodes that arise spontaneously and those that arise in connection with a precipitating illness or event. Those arising spontaneously tend to occur during the colder months of the year. Precipitating factors may include congestive heart failure, pneumonia or other infection, bleeding, administration of hypotonic fluids, sedative and analgesic drugs, or anesthesia and surgery. The particular risk of hypoventilation probably is increased by the presence of heart failure, obesity, pleural or other restrictive disease, chronic obstructive lung disease, neuromuscular disease, or exposure to drugs that reduce respiratory drive.[174,175]

Clinical Manifestations and Diagnosis

Myxedema coma presents with a constellation of findings including physical evidence of advanced hypothyroidism, stupor, bradycardia, hypotension, hypothermia, alveolar hypoventilation, obstipation, or ileus, and sometimes water intoxication or hypoglycemia.[248] Patients are often elderly. The condition if untreated progresses to fatal hypotension.

In the cases of myxedema coma arising spontaneously in the community, stupor progresses over several days, and families report that the number of hours spent sleeping has gradually increased to include most of a 24-hour period. Seizures have been reported.[245] In history taking it is important to ask whether the patient with suspected myxedema coma formerly was diagnosed with hypothyroidism or formerly was treated with radioactive iodine or surgery for overactive thyroid. On physical examination overt manifestations of myxedema are apparent. The patient often can be aroused and will make monosyllabic responses to questioning before lapsing back into stupor. Breathing is stertorous. Some patients with an infectious process may not have a fever. The most ominous sign of impending myxedema coma for a hypothyroid patient under inpatient observation is progressive hypothermia.

In contrast to patients with nonthyroidal illness syndrome, the laboratory evaluation will demonstrate low free T_4 and high TSH in the majority of true cases. Myxedema coma resulting from pituitary failure is uncommon.[251]

Approach to Management

Before initiating therapy for myxedema coma, the caregiver should question whether the hypothyroid patient is experiencing a self-limited consequence of a definable precipitating event. Stupor may be induced by sedatives and analgesics, especially opiates, and may resolve without rapid thyroid hormone replacement. Hyponatremia may be induced by intravenous therapy. Short-term ventilatory dependency may result from surgery. Yet each of these complications by itself does not require rapid replacement of thyroid hormone therapy unless conservative management fails.

A blood sample should be withdrawn for determination of TSH, free T_4, and serum cortisol levels before treatment is initiated. In the presence of progressive hypothermia and with a clinical picture of advanced myxedema, therapy should be initiated before the return of the results of thyroid function tests. If the TSH level is not elevated, the diagnosis of myxedema coma must be questioned. The needed initial dose of levothyroxine is unlikely to cause adverse effects, should the laboratory studies unexpectedly suggest euthyroidism or nonthyroidal illness syndrome.

The patient should be treated in an intensive care unit. Complications during treatment of myxedema coma include gastrointestinal bleeding and intracranial hemorrhage, which may result from coagulopathy resulting from myxedema itself. Pressors are generally ineffective in combating hypotension and may precipitate arrhythmia. Efforts at rewarming the patient may precipitate shock as a result of vasodilation in an individual whose cardiac output cannot match the demand. Treatment should include fluid restriction, avoidance of hypotonic fluids, administration of glucose as concentrated solutions if required, avoidance of pressors, and use of ordinary blankets for rewarming. Respiration should be supported as needed to treat alveolar hypoventilation.

The author uses a 500-μg T_4 intravenous bolus only for those patients without nonthyroidal illness syndrome whose myxedema coma arose in the community without obvious precipitating cause and who are known to have normal serum albumin and absence of cardiac risk factors. If the patient is hypoalbuminemic or the serum albumin is unknown, or if the patient has cardiac risk factors, an initial 200- to 300-μg T_4 intravenous bolus should be used for myxedema coma, and, if coexistent precipitating illness is present, combination therapy with T_3 should be considered (see the following). If an albumin level is subsequently reported normal and if the patient demonstrates no arrhythmia or manifestations of cardiac ischemia, 100 μg of levothyroxine can be added every several hours to bring the cumulative dose up to 500 μg in the first 24 hours. Such replacement provides protection against relapsing hormonal deficiency in a way that short-acting T_3 monotherapy cannot.[243] The oral route is unsatisfactory for initial therapy because of the likelihood of ileus or delayed absorption. After intravenous treatment, T_4 can be withheld for several days until the patient is able to take medication orally or 50 μg of T_4 daily can be administered intravenously beginning on the second day. Hydrocortisone 100 mg every 8 hours is given during the first 24 hours. Glucocorticoids are tapered and discontinued before discharge. There should be a low threshold for evaluation for the presence of coronary artery disease.

Therapeutic Alternatives

Arguments in favor of intravenous T_4 as monotherapy include its long history of successful use, its ability to prevent relapsing of hypothyroidism, avoidance of supranormal levels of T_3, and the observation that in the absence of intercurrent illness T_3 levels become normal within 24 hours.

Theoretical controversy continues to exist on whether to include intravenous T_3 in the initial treatment plan. Some authorities recommend using both hormones at the outset, especially if coexistent illnesses are present that might impede conversion of T_4 to T_3.[251,252] Additional arguments in favor of including triiodothyronine relate to the delayed conversion of T_4 that is seen in hypometabolic patients and the more rapid effect on tissues when T_3 therapy is used.[210] On the other hand, it has been speculated that some cases of mortality were caused by relatively high T_3 levels attained early in therapy.[249] In combination therapy, the recommended intravenous doses are approximately 10 to 20 μg of T_3 initially and 10 μg of T_3 every 8 to 12 hours on the first day, combined with an initial loading dose of about 200 to 250 μg T_4. This treatment is followed by approximately 100 μg of T_4 daily intravenously on the second day and 50 μg T_4 daily thereafter.

Prognosis

Patient findings associated with fatality have included old age, cerebrovascular bleeding or myocardial infarction during treatment[237,249,250,253] or suspected coronary events after recovery.[242] In a series of 11 cases the level of consciousness, Glasgow score, and APACHE II score were predictive of mortality.[255] Treatment factors associated with mortality may include overly gradual oral regimen of replacement of thyroid hormone, high replacement doses of thyroid hormone (T_3 doses=75 μg/day, T4 doses=500 μg/day), or high measured levels of triiodothyronine during treatment.[237,249,253] Within 6 to 36 hours most patients treated with thyroxine in sufficient dosage experience a rise of temperature and blood pressure; improvement of mentation; and, through peripheral conversion of T_4, correction of low T_3 levels.

HYPERTHYROIDISM, THYROID STORM, THYROCARDIAC CRISIS, AND CORONARY ARTERY SPASM

Hyperthyroidism

Prevalence and Incidence

The prevalence of overt hyperthyroidism is between 0.5% and 2% in women, with an annual incidence rate of 0.4 per 1000 women and 0.1 per 1000 men.[170,257] Of interest in the Wickham study in England was the apparent lack of effect of age on incidence.[258] However, age-related incidence depends on the cause of hyperthyroidism. In Sweden the overall incidences of Graves' disease, toxic multinodular goiter, and toxic adenoma were 17.7, 5.4, and 2.7/100,000/year, respectively, but the peak age-specific incidence of toxic multinodular goiter and toxic adenoma occurred in the 80-plus age group: 31.5/100,000/year.[259] In the ambulatory setting among adult patients, the overall prevalence of subclinical hyperthyroidism (isolated TSH suppression) is 0.5% to 6.3 %, with variability dependent on population under study, inclusion or exclusion of patients with thyroid disease, and definition of threshold TSH for inclusion.[168-170] Hyperthyroidism may occur in up to 9.6% or more of patients treated with amiodarone; the incidence is greater in relatively iodine-deficient regions.[105]

Pathogenesis

The commonest causes of hyperthyroidism in the United States are Graves' disease, toxic multinodular goiter, and toxic adenoma. In the hyperthyroidism of Graves' disease, the TSH receptor/G protein/adenylyl cyclase complex is activated by abnormal thyroid-stimulating immunoglobulins with affinity for the TSH receptor. The associated phenomena of orbitopathy and dermopathy also are thought to result from autoimmune processes. In some cases of hyperthyroidism resulting from toxic adenoma, a G protein mutation is demonstrable that results in activation of the membrane adenylyl cyclase associated with the TSH receptor complex. Plummer's disease (toxic multinodular goiter) is most commonly seen in older patients and represents a late outcome in the natural history of euthyroid multinodular goiter. Because of TSH suppression, internodular thyroidal tissue is metabolically inactive in accumulating iodine.

Hyperthyroidism can be produced by glandular destruction, as in thyroiditis. In susceptible individuals, especially those from iodine-deficient regions of the world or with preexisting nodular thyroid disease, hyperthyroidism can be produced by iodine (Jod-Basedow phenomenon).[103] Two different mechanisms of hyperthyroidism are possible during amiodarone therapy: iodine-induced hyperthyroidism and thyroiditis.[116] Therapy with α-interferon can produce persisting hyperthyroidism or a low-uptake thyroiditis-like picture with transitory hyperthyroidism.

In general intense activation of the TSH receptor complex results in an increased ratio of T_3 to T_4 resulting from direct thyroidal T_3 secretion. The augmentation of thyroidal T_3 release of hyperthyroid patients may result in part from enhancement of the thyroidal type II 5′-deiodinase activity.[260] The altered ratio of T_3 to T_4 is not observed in destructive hyperthyroidism.[261]

Of special interest to the intensivist are the enhanced target organ response to sympathoadrenal stimuli in hyperthyroidism and the cardiac manifestations of hyperthyroidism.[262-264]

Clinical Manifestations

Intubation and central lines may prevent adequate palpation of the thyroid. If thyroidal bruit is detected on auscultation of the upper poles of the lateral lobes of the thyroid, the diagnosis of Graves' disease essentially is assured. The eyes, nails, and pretibial skin should be examined for evidence of orbitopathy, onycholysis, fine skin quality (smooth elbows), or dermopathy ("pretibial myxedema"). The remainder of the physical examination is likely to yield findings that are suggestive of hyperthyroidism but nonspecific, such as hyperhidrosis, atrial arrhythmia, hyperdynamic heart, precordial lift, systolic ejection murmur, S3 gallop, restlessness, hyperkinesia, agitation, or briskness of Achilles reflexes. A different spectrum of symptoms and signs has been reported in the elderly, who may appear apathetic or depressed, and among whom the average number of thyrotoxic symptoms may be as low as two, with dominance of weight loss, proximal myopathy, tremor, and cardiac manifestations such as heart failure, sinus tachycardia, or atrial fibrillation.[265-267]

Diagnostic Approach

Laboratory Diagnosis of Hyperthyroidism

The laboratory findings will include TSH below 0.1 μIU/mL and usually elevation of total and free T_4. If the T_4

level is normal and TSH is below 0.1 μIU/mL, elevated T_3 will identify T_3 toxicosis. Diagnosis of amiodarone-induced hyperthyroidism requires demonstration of low TSH and high T_3.

T4 Hyperthyroidism

High T_3 is a sensitive finding for diagnosis of hyperthyroidism, often detectable earlier in the course of the disease than high T_4. The finding of high T_4 without high T_3, although atypical of hyperthyroidism, sometimes occurs after surgery, during exposure to substances that block conversion of T_4 to T_3, among the elderly or the critically ill, or sporadically.[32,268-271] In a hyperthyroxinemic patient the finding of a normal sensitive TSH level is reassuring evidence against hyperthyroidism. For patients with TSH suppression, evaluation of high T_4 might include free T_3 determination[32] and follow-up hormonal studies after recovery; these sometimes corroborate the prior suspicion of hyperthyroidism but may demonstrate resolution of hyperthyroxinemia or persistence of euthyroid hyperthyroxinemia, a laboratory constellation that has a small differential diagnosis.

Subclinical Hyperthyroidism

When there are normal T_4 and T_3 levels but unexplained suppression of TSH, the diagnosis of subclinical hyperthyroidism is sometimes considered. When the TSH level is below normal but greater than 0.1 μIU/mL, the diagnosis of hyperthyroidism is made with less confidence. Nevertheless, patients with toxic nodular goiters in the early years of their disease may have TSH suppressions that are only marginal, and yet the diagnosis of subclinical hyperthyroidism can be suspected by thyroid palpation and confirmed by finding autonomous nodularity on thyroid scanning. Stable TSH suppression over several months, in the absence of drug effects, pituitary or hypothalamic disease, or concomitant hypothyroxinemia, suggests hyperthyroidism.

Determining the Cause of Hyperthyroidism

The history and physical examination often suggest the cause of hyperthyroidism. Confirming procedures, the radioactive iodine uptake and thyroid scan, usually are omitted or postponed until recovery. In high-uptake forms of hyperthyroidism, a 24-hour radioiodine uptake evaluation sometimes yields intermediate range or normal results, suggesting mild disease or an unrecognized source of exogenous iodide. In toxic adenoma and toxic multinodular goiter, a normal uptake is common.

Approach to Management

Therapeutic Modalities in Hyperthyroidism

For patients with biochemical evidence of subclinical or overt hyperthyroidism who are receiving exogenous thyroid hormone replacement therapy, a dose reduction should be made. An exception would be a patient treated with thyroid hormone for differentiated thyroid cancer. If endogenous hyperthyroidism was recognized before hospitalization, and if biochemical euthyroidism had been maintained until the time of admission by use of a stable dosage of antithyroid medication, the established dose probably should be maintained during the critical illness.

One issue confronting the critical care physician is selection of untreated patients with suspected endogenous hyperthyroidism for antithyroid treatment, observation, or further study. Most patients with untreated overt hyperthyroidism should be treated. If a diagnosis of untreated subclinical hyperthyroidism is made or suspected by clinical evaluation, assuming the cause is not likely to be transitory, indications for treatment include atrial fibrillation, other atrial arrhythmias, other cardiac disorders, or evidence of accelerated bone loss. Other factors influencing the decision to treat include older age, presence of symptoms, or risk factors for cardiac or skeletal disease. Asymptomatic patients without these risks usually can be observed for several months before treatment to ensure stability of the TSH suppression. A reasonable threshold for treatment is persistent suppression of TSH below 0.1 μIU/mL.

The drugs used in treatment of hyperthyroidism include the thionamides propylthiouracil and the longer-acting drug methimazole.[272-277] Thionamides inhibit the coupling of iodothyronine moieties on thyroglobulin and organification of iodide, thus preventing storage and synthesis of thyroid hormone. Additionally, by inhibiting the type I iodothyronine 5′-deiodinase, propylthiouracil reduces peripheral production of T_3 from T_4.[2,272] To initiate therapy it is common practice to start with a relatively higher dose than will be required for maintenance and also to choose a dosage on the basis of the apparent clinical severity of hyperthyroidism and size of the thyroid gland. Thus the initial daily dosage might be propylthiouracil 50 to 200 mg every 8 hours or methimazole up to 20 mg every 8 hours. After control is achieved methimazole is usually converted to once-daily therapy and sometimes given in doses as little as 5 mg daily. Propylthiouracil must be continued in divided dosage to prevent escape. Equivalent doses are propylthiouracil 100 mg and methimazole 10 mg. Potential but uncommon adverse effects include agranulocytosis, hepatic injury, and a rheumatic syndrome.

During hyperthyroidism β-blocker therapy is the preferred method of controlling tachycardia and peripheral manifestations of sensitivity to catecholamines. Among the β-blockers, there is the greatest experience with propranolol, which exerts not only cardioprotective but also peripheral effects that benefit the thyrotoxic patient. The metabolism of propranolol is enhanced, and blood levels are highly variable in hyperthyroidism. Other β-blockers have been used, and some advocate cardioselective agents.[278-288] Most patients requiring enteral propranolol should begin with 20 to 40 mg four times per day.

Treatment of low-uptake causes of hyperthyroidism consists of β-blockers. In severe and protracted cases of amiodarone-induced hyperthyroidism propylthiouracil is used, but there is unlikely to be a full response. For amiodarone-induced thyroiditis, glucocorticoids may be beneficial,[112] and the course of the hyperthyroidism sometimes may be transitory.[115,123]

Definitive treatment of hyperthyroidism consists of radioactive iodine or surgery. Use of radioiodine therapy is inappropriate for low-uptake hyperthyroidism. Sometimes surgery is the best option available for treatment of resistant cases of amiodarone-induced hyperthyroidism.[109] Postoperatively amiodarone may be reinstituted.

Precautions in the Care of the Hyperthyroid Patient

Thyrotoxic patients display enhanced susceptibility to sympathetic stimuli and adrenergic drugs. They may be volume depleted and may not tolerate excessive diuresis. Before administering contrast, the physician should consider whether needed radioactive iodine uptake or thyroid scanning tests can be deferred. Administration of a thionamide should precede use of iodinated substances.

Preparation of the Patient with Uncontrolled Hyperthyroidism for Emergency Surgery

Before emergency surgery, the risk of thyroid storm obligates the caregiver to prepare the patient with antithyroid treatment.[289] For newly diagnosed patients with endogenous hyperthyroidism, preoperatively 600 to 1200 mg of propylthiouracil daily should be given in divided dosage. At least 2 hours after the first dose of propylthiouracil, the patient should receive iodide, ipodate, or iopanoic acid (as described later in the treatment of thyroid storm). In the absence of contraindications, propranolol orally in a dosage up to 20 to 40 mg four times per day should be started. The regimen should be continued in the immediate postoperative period by use of a nasogastric tube if necessary. Before discharge the propylthiouracil dose should be tapered. Unless the patient has an unusual severity of hyperthyroidism or large size of the thyroid gland, an appropriate discharge dose of propylthiouracil usually would be 50 to 200 mg every 8 hours. Glucocorticoids also may have a role in preoperative preparation.

Therapeutic Alternatives

For patients who cannot take oral medications, antithyroid drugs can be prepared for rectal administration.[273,274] Patients with a history of minor skin reactions to one thionamide may be treated with the other. Patients with a history of hepatocellular jaundice during propylthiouracil therapy may be treated with methimazole.[275,276] Lithium has been used for control of hyperthyroidism for patients unable to use propylthiouracil or methimazole, starting at a dose of 300 mg twice per day.[290,291] The ability of the radiographic contrast agents iopanoic acid and ipodate to inhibit thyroid hormone release, peripheral conversion of T_4, and possibly nuclear binding of T_3 has been exploited in certain hyperthyroid states including cases of destructive hyperthyroidism and in thionamide intolerance.[292-296] The use of radiographic contrast agents usually should be adjunctive to thionamides and β-blocker therapy. Instances of escape after prolonged use of iodinated substances have been reported.[294] Therefore if a radiographic contrast agent is used as an antithyroid medication without antecedent and concomitant thionamide medication, some patients will require thyroidectomy as soon as reasonable control has been obtained. Recommended daily doses are ipodate 500 to 1000 mg orally or iopanoic acid 500 mg twice daily.[289,295-298]

For patients with contraindications to the use of β-blockers, older regimens included guanethidine or reserpine, which are seldom used at present. For control of heart rate in patients with reversible airway disease, diltiazem is an alternative to β-blockers.[299]

Prognosis

After a treatment course with thionamides administered for as long as 18 to 24 months, a variably reported percentage of patients with Graves' disease (probably <50%) will be in remission. Some will develop hypothyroidism as a result of Hashimoto's disease. With toxic adenoma, remission of hyperthyroidism is uncommon. With toxic multinodular goiter, hyperthyroidism is persistent. Low-uptake forms of hyperthyroidism are self-limited conditions, and hyperthyroidism usually resolves within 6 months. If there is an offending drug, it should be discontinued. However, storage of amiodarone in adipose tissue may prolong the episode of thyroid dysfunction (Fig. 61-3).

Thyroid Storm

History and Incidence

Thyroid storm is a clinically defined and potentially lethal complication of hyperthyroidism.[271,279,287,300-343] Initially this entity was recognized as a lethal complication of thyroidectomy for hyperthyroidism that had been performed in unprepared patients.[300] In an early series, two thirds of the patients died[301]; postmortem examinations were not illuminating. As it was recognized that patients had to be rendered euthyroid before thyroidectomy, the incidence of storm after thyroidectomy declined, and the literature began to focus on nonsurgical precipitating factors.[303,304] As early as 1960, after the use of reserpine and glucocorticoids was added to therapy with antithyroid medication and iodide, it was reported that the mortality rate from thyroid storm had been reduced from 60% or 70% to 25%.[304] In 1966 the importance of initiating thionamide therapy before iodide administration was emphasized.[305] By employing guanethidine as reported in 1969[306] or reserpine therapy reported in 1970,[307] the mortality of thyroid storm in small series was as low as 7% and 0%, respectively. By the mid-1970s the use of propranolol had largely replaced earlier methods of attaining sympathetic blockade.

Thyroid storm is a relatively infrequent reason for admission to critical care units. Even before the existence of modern antithyroid therapy, the estimated incidence of thyroid storm among patients hospitalized for hyperthyroidism was only 7%.[304]

Pathogenesis

Graves' hyperthyroidism is the commonest thyroid disorder identified with thyroid storm, but storm has also been associated with toxic multinodular goiter, amiodarone-

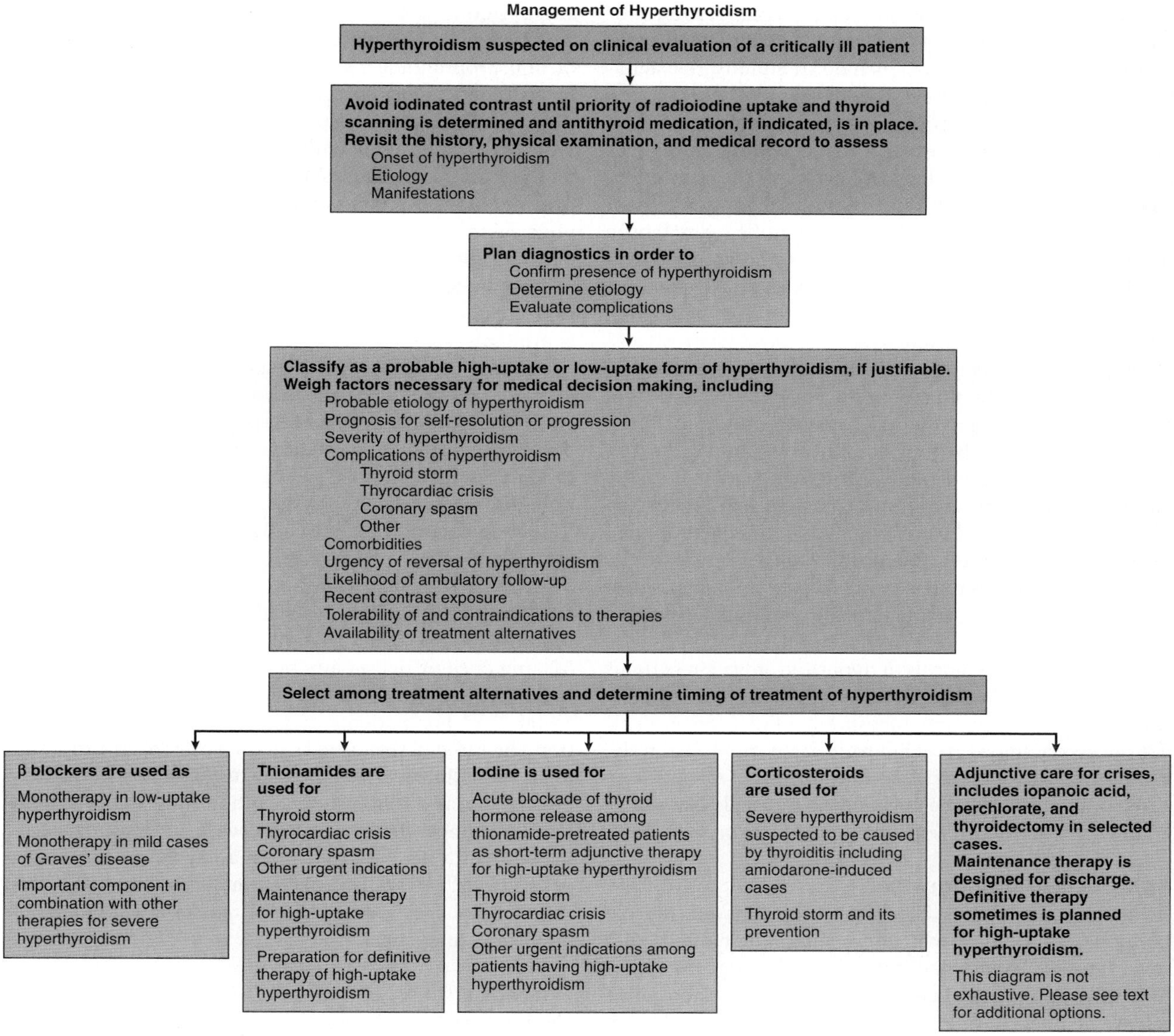
Management of Hyperthyroidism
Hyperthyroidism suspected on clinical evaluation of a critically ill patient
Avoid iodinated contrast until priority of radioiodine uptake and thyroid scanning is determined and antithyroid medication, if indicated, is in place.
Revisit the history, physical examination, and medical record to assess
Onset of hyperthyroidism
Etiology
Manifestations
Plan diagnostics in order to
Confirm presence of hyperthyroidism
Determine etiology
Evaluate complications
Classify as a probable high-uptake or low-uptake form of hyperthyroidism, if justifiable.
Weigh factors necessary for medical decision making, including
Probable etiology of hyperthyroidism
Prognosis for self-resolution or progression
Severity of hyperthyroidism
Complications of hyperthyroidism
Thyroid storm
Thyrocardiac crisis
Coronary spasm
Other
Comorbidities
Urgency of reversal of hyperthyroidism
Likelihood of ambulatory follow-up
Recent contrast exposure
Tolerability of and contraindications to therapies
Availability of treatment alternatives
Select among treatment alternatives and determine timing of treatment of hyperthyroidism
β blockers are used as
Monotherapy in low-uptake hyperthyroidism
Monotherapy in mild cases of Graves' disease
Important component in combination with other therapies for severe hyperthyroidism
Thionamides are used for
Thyroid storm
Thyrocardiac crisis
Coronary spasm
Other urgent indications
Maintenance therapy for high-uptake hyperthyroidism
Preparation for definitive therapy of high-uptake hyperthyroidism
Iodine is used for
Acute blockade of thyroid hormone release among thionamide-pretreated patients as short-term adjunctive therapy for high-uptake hyperthyroidism
Thyroid storm
Thyrocardiac crisis
Coronary spasm
Other urgent indications among patients having high-uptake hyperthyroidism
Corticosteroids are used for
Severe hyperthyroidism suspected to be caused by thyroiditis including amiodarone-induced cases
Thyroid storm and its prevention
Adjunctive care for crises, includes iopanoic acid, perchlorate, and thyroidectomy in selected cases.
Maintenance therapy is designed for discharge.
Definitive therapy sometimes is planned for high-uptake hyperthyroidism.
This diagram is not exhaustive. Please see text for additional options.

Figure 61-3. Approach to management for hyperthyroidism.

induced hyperthyroidism,[320] and rarely massive exogenous thyroid hormone overdosage.[302,315,338] Precipitating factors precede development of thyroid storm in the majority of cases. Identifiable events include infection, trauma,[321] parturition, diabetic ketoacidosis,[332] pulmonary embolism,[304] surgery,[300,301] withdrawal of inorganic iodide,[301] administration of radioactive iodine,[303,311,311] pseudoephedrine administration,[317] discontinuation of antithyroid medication,[303] or a lapse in care. In the absence of thionamide therapy, administration of iodine-containing compounds floods the gland with iodine, but inhibition of hormone release may be incomplete or temporary, and thyroid storm may occur during continued administration of iodine.[301] Recently instituted or incompletely effective thionamide therapy does not necessarily protect against storm induced by radiation thyroiditis.[314] Reliance on lithium[313] or propranolol[279] monotherapy of hyperthyroidism as preoperative preparation may be responsible for thyroid storm.

In thyroid storm the T_3 and total T_4 levels are not different from levels in uncomplicated cases of hyperthyroidism, but the dialyzable fraction of T_4 (the percentage that is free) is higher.[309,310] This finding has been taken to support the idea that the medical illness may cause acute unbinding of thyroid hormone from transport proteins.

Clinical Manifestations and Diagnosis

The definition of thyroid storm has come to include a constellation of fever greater than 100°F, tachycardia out of proportion to fever, and exaggerated manifestations of thyrotoxicosis affecting at least two other of the following systems: cardiac, gastrointestinal, or neurologic.[304] A clinical scoring system has been proposed in which identification of a precipitating factor is one diagnostic criterion.[316] Cardiac findings may include marked tachycardia out of proportion to fever, atrial arrhythmia, and heart failure. Gastrointestinal symptoms include hyperdefecation, diarrhea, vomiting, abdominal pain, an acute condition of the abdomen,[322] duodenal obstruction,[323] and jaundice or liver failure,[326,328] usually as a result of right-sided heart failure. Neurologic features include tremulousness, agitation, hyperkinesia, muscle weakness, delirium, apathy, prostration, or obtundation. Brisk contraction and relaxation time often are observed when deep tendon reflexes are elicited. Fever is the hallmark of the condition, sometimes as high as 106°F. As a practical matter, even if another underlying cause of fever is identified, any febrile patient (temperature >100°F) who has known hyperthyroidism with marked tachycardia or exaggerated manifestations of hyperthyroidism is best treated as having impending thyroid storm.

The question often arises whether a previous history of hyperthyroidism should create suspicion of thyroid storm as a diagnosis of a patient's present condition. If the patient has become hypothyroid after definitive therapy (surgery or radioactive iodine), or if for several weeks the patient has been receiving and continues to receive an effective and stable dose of thionamide medication, and recent test results are in the normal range, assuredly the diagnosis is not thyroid storm. However, a history of medical treatment is not reassuring without verification of its effect.

The laboratory diagnosis of hyperthyroidism in patients having storm is based on demonstration of TSH suppression and free T_4 elevation. Measurement of T_3 generally is not necessary unless free T_4 levels are normal.[308] Rarely, in the presence of coexisting illness, the T_4 may be elevated but total T_3 may be normal.[271] No specific laboratory finding defines the presence of thyroid storm, however.

Approach to Management

Although thionamides block the synthesis of thyroid hormone, this effect will not benefit the patient until several weeks later, when thyroid glandular stores of preformed hormone have been discharged. To block hormone release acutely, iodide is administered. Thionamide pretreatment is essential to induce a biosynthetic blockade that will prevent flooding of the gland with iodide, with the attendant future risk of exacerbation of hyperthyroidism. Glucocorticoid therapy is employed to correct potential relative adrenal insufficiency. β-blockers combat cardiac sensitivity to catecholamines and reduce central and peripheral neurologic manifestations of hyperthyroidism. Propylthiouracil, glucocorticoids, and propranolol block conversion of T_4 to T_3.

A common starting regimen is an initial propylthiouracil dose of 400 mg, and thereafter a continued dose of 200 mg is given every 4 hours, or 1200 mg daily in divided dosage, orally or by nasogastric tube. Beginning 2 hours after the first dose of propylthiouracil, saturated solution of potassium iodide is administered, 5 drops every 6 hours. Propylthiouracil normally is administered enterally, but the rectal route for administration has been described.[319,344] Hydrocortisone is administered in a dose of 100 mg every 8 hours. Propranolol 0.5 to 1 mg intravenously is cautiously provided with monitoring of blood pressure and rhythm while awaiting the effects of orally administered propranolol; the dose may be increased to 2 to 3 mg over 15 minutes if tolerated.[316] The needed dose of oral propranolol may be 40 to 80 mg every 6 hours. For patients having evidence of heart failure or hypotension or developing these findings during treatment, β-blockers must be given with great caution, and alternative methods of controlling heart rate and rhythm should be considered.[329] Digoxin is used for atrial fibrillation. The underlying cause of thyroid storm must be identified and treated, cultures made, and in general empiric antibiotics provided until infection is excluded. Fluid and electrolyte replacement are necessary, and administration of vitamins is prudent.

Often, propylthiouracil is tapered by the time of discharge to 450 to 600 mg daily in divided dosage, the glucocorticoids are tapered and discontinued, and the iodide dose is reduced to 2 drops three times per day. The iodide therapy is discontinued within 2 weeks. Anticipating potential financial, philosophic, or emotional barriers to follow-up care and definitive therapy is important.

Therapeutic Alternatives

For thyroid storm the doses of alternative medications are lithium 300 mg every 6 hours[318] and ipodate therapy 500 mg once or twice daily or iopanoic acid.[298] The route of administration of iodide may be sublingual or rectal.[319,323] For patients at risk of cardiac decompensation, the rapid-acting drug esmolol may replace propranolol as initial intravenous therapy, used while awaiting the effects of orally administered cautious doses of propranolol.[287] Adjuncts to therapy, reserved for resistant cases, include peritoneal dialysis, plasma exchange, or plasmapheresis.[312,314,340,342] Thyroidectomy also has been used successfully for iodine-induced storm and failure of medical management.[327,334,337]

Prognosis

Clinical markers suggesting a poor prognosis include delay in therapy, coma, jaundice, and shock. Normalization of temperature, drop of heart rate, and improved mental status are favorable signs. With treatment as described earlier, a sharp reduction of circulating thyroid hormone concentration is observable by the second hospital day, but it may be several days before adequate stabilization of clinical manifestations is seen.[318]

Thyrocardiac Crisis and Coronary Artery Spasm

Thyrocardiac crises can be divided into the following major problems: atrial arrhythmias; congestive heart failure without atrial arrhythmia; and the rare risks of myocardial infarction, ventricular arrhythmia, and sudden death. Coronary artery spasm is increasingly recognized as a potentially reversible complication of uncontrolled hyperthyroidism, sometimes seen in young women.

Incidence

Among ambulatory patients with atrial fibrillation, screening for thyroid dysfunction is not performed consistently.[345] Among white patients hospitalized for atrial fibrillation in Birmingham, England, the frequency of hyperthyroidism was 7.5% (no cases were found among black or Asian patients).[346] Emergency presentation with atrial fibrillation justifies screening for hyperthyroidism.[83,347]

Thyrocardiac crises without storm include rhythm disturbances and congestive heart failure, and these are relatively more common than thyroid storm.[264,348-360] Preexisting heart disease and age older than 60 are risk factors for manifestations of thyrocardiac disease.[349,351,357] Among 462 patients with hyperthyroidism who had no associated organic heart disease and who were referred for radioactive iodine, a 1958 study reported the prevalence to be atrial fibrillation 10%, congestive heart failure with atrial fibrillation 5%, and congestive heart failure with sinus rhythm 0.6%.[349] In a study of unselected hyperthyroid patients, the prevalence was atrial fibrillation 9% and congestive heart failure 6%.[351] In the Framingham Heart Study, for persons with TSH=0.1 μIU/mL compared with persons with normal TSH, the relative risk of atrial fibrillation was 3.1 (95% confidence interval, 1.7 to 5.5). Among patients with TSH suppression of less severity (i.e., >0.1 μIU/mL), the risk for atrial fibrillation was comparable with the risk among people with normal TSH.[361] In one study, high levels of triiodothyronine predicted subsequent cardiac events.[165]

The cardiovascular and cerebrovascular mortality of patients with history of radioiodine therapy for hyperthyroidism and with subclinical hyperthyroidism may be increased.[362-365] However, the occurrence of coronary ischemic events during hyperthyroidism is surprisingly low. In an early series of unselected hyperthyroid patients, 2 of 200 died as a result of myocardial infarction.[351]

Pathogenesis

Whereas the full evolution of most manifestations of thyroid hormone excess requires time, sudden onset of thyrocardiac effects may complicate any form of hyperthyroidism, even fleeting or recent-onset thyrotoxicosis, such as that resulting from subacute thyroiditis or overdosage of thyroid hormone.

Structural and regulatory proteins in the heart are encoded by genes regulated by T_3.[264] Despite the low levels of circulating catecholamines, the physiology of a hyperthyroid patient resembles a hyperadrenergic state.[366] Increased blood volume and heart rate in hyperthyroidism and shortening of systolic contraction and diastolic relaxation times occur, and contractile reserve is reduced. The patient with thyroid heart disease has a high left ventricular ejection fraction at rest, high cardiac output, subnormal response to exercise, and sometimes rate-related heart failure.[264,348,354] The appearance of atrial fibrillation may be predicted by increased signal-averaged P-wave duration.[359] Hyperthyroidism promotes cholesterol reduction.

Small numbers of patients in whom coronary spasm has been recognized have been reported.[367-374] Among patients with uncontrolled hyperthyroidism including young patients, there are reports of sudden death or ventricular arrhythmia[262,264,368,371,375] and myocardial infarction.[373,376-381]

Clinical Manifestations

Atrial fibrillation, heart failure, and coronary vasospasm are potentially seen without the complete picture of thyroid storm—in particular, without fever. Chest discomfort is not an uncommon complaint among patients with hyperthyroidism, even among the young, and usually has benign significance. Characteristic anginal symptoms are uncommon. Sinus tachycardia is the commonest arrhythmia in uncomplicated hyperthyroidism.

Approach to Management

β-Blockade is part of the therapy unless contraindications are present. In treating atrial fibrillation digoxin is used, and for congestive heart failure digoxin and furosemide are used. β-Blockade may result in hypotension and should be instituted with careful monitoring if some degree of systolic cardiac dysfunction may be present. For patients with tachycardia-related congestive heart failure, the use of β-blockers in doses equivalent to 20 mg propranolol every 6 hours may be well tolerated, and the dose may be titrated up to 40 or 80 mg every 6 hours. However, in low-output heart failure or heart disease of other causes complicated by hyperthyroidism, administration of β-blockers must be approached with caution if these agents are used at all.[234] Diltiazem also must be used with caution because it may have negative inotropic effects. Thionamides should be given in relatively high dosage, such as 400 mg propylthiouracil initially followed by 200 mg every 8 hours. Two hours after the first dose of propylthiouracil, SSKI 5 drops every 6 hours may be started. Iodide is tapered to 2 drops three times per day before discharge and is discontinued after 7 to 14 days. Patients in atrial fibrillation resulting from hyperthyroidism generally should receive anticoagulation therapy according to the same criteria as other patients. For thyrocardiac crises, treatment with glucocorticoids is seldom indicated. Future outpatient administration of radioactive iodine will usually be desirable.

The frequency of spontaneous conversion to sinus rhythm is greater if relatively large ablative doses of radioactive iodine are used, sufficient to bring about prompt development of hypothyroidism.[233] Radiation thyroiditis or interruption of antithyroid medication to permit radioiodine administration can cause patient destabilization. If antithyroid medication is reinstituted after radioiodine treatment, any recurrence of hyperthyroidism is usually corrected within 4 to 6 weeks.

Patients who do not spontaneously convert to sinus rhythm generally should be rendered euthyroid before elective cardioversion is attempted; otherwise, there is a greater risk of relapse of atrial fibrillation after cardioversion. It has been suggested that because no spontaneous conversions occurred more than 16 weeks after attainment of euthyroidism, the ideal timing for elective cardioversion is at that time.[232] Hyperthyroid patients are more sensitive to warfarin than others. The immediate risks of anticoagulation sometimes must be weighed against the desirability of postponing elective cardioversion.

In cases of anginal pain and coronary vasospasm, aggressive medical treatment of vasospasm and hyperthyroidism are indicated.

Prognosis

Even in young adult patients, atrial fibrillation may be complicated by thromboembolism resulting in fatal or disabling cerebrovascular accidents.[352,353,360]

About 37% to 61% of patients may experience spontaneous conversion of atrial fibrillation after attainment of euthyroidism, mostly within 6 weeks.[349,355] Absence of congestive heart failure is a favorable prognostic predictor of spontaneous conversion. Other patients may be successfully cardioverted. The absence of other heart disease, short duration of atrial fibrillation, and younger age predict successful conversion and maintenance of sinus rhythm.

As a result of treatment of hyperthyroidism, a patient with heart failure caused by thyrotoxic heart disease experiences improved ability to augment cardiac output during exercise.[231] With treatment of thyrotoxicosis alone, about 41% of patients with congestive heart failure and thyrotoxicosis who receive radioactive iodine experience relief of heart failure.[349] No body of literature exists on predictors of myocardial infarction, ventricular arrhythmia, or sudden death. For the rare patient having hyperthyroidism and anginal chest pain caused by coronary artery spasm, isolated published case reports emphasize reversibility of anginal symptoms after successful treatment of hyperthyroidism.

Lipid status should be reevaluated after correction of hyperthyroidism.

KEY POINTS

- Low TSH is attributable to dopamine or glucocorticoid therapy in some critically ill patients.
- High free T_4 is attributable to furosemide, heparin, or sepsis in some critically ill patients.
- Thyroid function test abnormalities that resolve after recovery are common in critical illness (nonthyroidal illness syndrome).
- Low T_3 is the earliest finding of nonthyroidal illness syndrome, resulting from impaired activation of T_4 (peripheral conversion of T_4 to T_3) and enhanced deactivation of T_3 (conversion of T_3 to T_2).
- Low transport protein concentrations, low total T_4, and low TSH are seen in more longstanding or severe cases of nonthyroidal illness syndrome.
- Biochemical differentiation between nonthyroidal illness syndrome and intrinsic hypofunction of the pituitary or hypothalamus may be impossible until after recovery.
- Because it is unknown whether the changes of nonthyroidal illness syndrome are detrimental to the patient, the present-day standard of care does not require thyroid hormone treatment.
- T_3 has inotropic and vasodilatory effects.
- The rise of total T_4 and T_3 into the normal range that occurs during recovery from severe nonthyroidal illness syndrome is accompanied by TSH elevation above the normal ambulatory range.
- Findings of low T_4, low free T_4, and high TSH generally signify hypothyroidism.
- Findings of high T_4, high free T_4, and low TSH generally signify hyperthyroidism.
- Myxedema coma, thyroid storm, and thyrocardiac crisis are diagnosed by clinical evidence of the emergency condition and biochemical verification of thyroid status and are often appropriately treated in a critical care unit. Coronary vasospasm, reversible with medical management, may occur during hyperthyroidism.

REFERENCES

1. De Groot LJ: Thyroid hormone transport, cellular uptake, metabolism, and molecular action. In De Groot LJ, Larsen PR, Hennemann G (eds): The Thyroid and Its Diseases, 6th ed. New York, Churchill Livingstone, 1996, pp 61-111.
2. Mandel SJ, Berry MJ, Kieffer JD, et al: Cloning and in vitro expression of the human selenoprotein, type I iodothyronine deiodinase. J Clin Endocrinol Metab 1992;75: 1133-1139.
3. Salvatore D, Bartha T, Harney JW, Larsen PR: Molecular biological and biochemical characterization of the human type 2 selenodeiodinase. Endocrinology 1996;137:3308-3315.
4. Hosoi Y, Murakami M, Mizuma H, et al: Expression and regulation of type II iodothyronine deiodinase in cultured human skeletal muscle cells. J Clin Endocrinol Metab 1999;84: 3293-3300.
5. Bianco AC, Salvatore D, Gereben B, et al: Biochemistry, cellular and molecular biology, and physiological roles of the iodothyronine selenodeiodinases. Endocr Rev 2002;23:38-89.
6. Peeters RP, Wouters PJ, Kaptein E, et al: Reduced activation and increased inactivation of thyroid hormone in tissues of critically ill patients. J Clin Endocrinol Metab 2003;88:3202-3211.
7. Peeters RP, van der Geyten S, Wouters PJ, et al: Tissue thyroid hormone levels in critical illness. J Clin Endocrinol Metab 2005;90:6498-6507.
8. Peeters RP, Kester MHA, Wouters PJ, et al: Increased thyroxine sulfate levels in critically ill patients as a result of a decreased hepatic type I deiodinase activity. J Clin Endocrinol Metab 2005;90:6460-6465.
9. Robbins J: Thyroid hormone transport proteins and the physiology of hormone binding. In Braverman LE, Utiger RD (eds): Werner & Ingbar's The Thyroid: A Fundamental and Clinical Text, 8th ed. Philadelphia, Lippincott Williams & Wilkins, 2000, pp 105-120.
10. Benvenga S: Thyroid hormone transport proteins and the physiology of hormone binding. In Braverman LE, Utiger RD (eds): Werner & Ingbar's The Thyroid: A Fundamental and Clinical Text, 9th ed. Philadelphia, Lippincott Williams & Wilkins, 2005, pp 97-108.
11. Benvenga S, Cahnmann HJ, Gregg RE, Robbins J: Characterization of the binding of thyroxine to high density lipoproteins and apolipoproteins A-I.

PART

VI NEUROLOGIC DISEASE IN THE CRITICALLY ILL

Chapter 62

Coma

Igor Ougorets and John J. Caronna

Altered states of consciousness are a common reason for visits to the emergency department and admission to intensive care units (ICUs). Few patients are more difficult to manage than the unconscious ones because the potential causes of an altered mental status are considerable and the time for diagnosis and effective intervention is short.

Consciousness may be defined as the state of awareness of the self and the environment. The phenomenon of consciousness depends on two intact and interdependent physiologic and anatomic components: (1) arousal (or wakefulness) and its underlying neural substrate; the ascending reticular activating system (ARAS) and diencephalon; and (2) awareness, which requires the functioning cerebral cortex of both hemispheres. Most disorders that acutely disturb consciousness are in fact impairments of arousal that create circumstances under which the brain's capacity for consciousness cannot be accurately assessed. In other words, failure of arousal renders it impossible to test awareness.

Alterations of arousal may be transient, lasting only several seconds or minutes (following seizures, syncope, and cardiac dysrhythmia) or sustained, lasting several hours or longer. Four terms are used to describe disturbed arousal of a patient. *Alert* refers to a normal state of arousal. *Stupor* describes a state of spontaneous unarousability in which strong external stimuli can transiently restore wakefulness. Stupor implies evidence that at least a limited degree of appropriate cognitive activity accompanies the arousal, even if transient. *Coma* is characterized by an uninterruptible loss of the capacity for arousal. The eyes are closed, sleep-wake cycles disappear, and even vigorous stimulation produces no evidence of appropriate psychological reaction. At best, only reflex responses can be elicited. *Lethargy* describes a range of behavior between arousal and stupor. Only the terms *alert* and *coma* have enough precision to be used without further qualification; possibly coma has gradations in depth, but this cannot be accurately assessed once the patient is no longer responsive to external stimuli. Stupor and coma reflect an acute or subacute brain insult. Altered consciousness reflects either diffuse and bilateral cerebral dysfunction, failure of the brainstem-thalamic ARAS, or both. All alterations in arousal should be regarded as acute and potentially life-threatening emergencies.

The evaluation of a comatose patient demands a systematic approach with appropriate, directed diagnostic and therapeutic endeavors. Patient evaluation and treatment must occur simultaneously. Urgent steps are required to prevent or minimize permanent brain damage from reversible causes. Effective treatment demands an understanding of the pathophysiology of consciousness and the ways in which it may be deranged.

ANATOMY, PATHOLOGY, AND PATHOPHYSIOLOGY

Consciousness depends on an intact ARAS in the brainstem and adjacent thalamus, which acts as the alerting or awakening element of consciousness, and functioning cerebral cortex, which determines the content of that consciousness.[1] The ARAS lies within a more or less isodendritic core that extends from the medulla through the tegmentum of the pons to the midbrain and paramedian thalamus. The system is continuous caudally with the reticular intermediate gray matter of the spinal cord and rostrally with the subthalamus, hypothalamus, anterior thalamus, and basal forebrain.[2] The ARAS itself arises within the rostral pontine tegmentum and extends across the mesencephalic tegmentum and its adjacent intrathalamic nuclei. ARAS functions and interconnections are considerable and probably contribute more than only a cortical arousal system. The specific role of the various links from the reticular formation to the thalamus has yet to be fully identified.[3] Furthermore, the cerebral cortex feeds back on the thalamic nuclei to contribute an important self-cycling loop that amplifies arousal mechanisms.[4,5]

The ascending arousal system contains cholinergic, monoaminergic, and γ-aminobutyric acid (GABA) neurotransmitters, none of which has been identified as the singular "arousal neurotransmitter."[6,7] It follows that acute structural damage to or metabolic-chemical derangements of either the ascending brainstem-thalamic activating system or the thalamo-cortico-thalamic loop are capable of altering the aroused, attentive state. Consciousness depends on the continuous interaction between the mechanisms that provide arousal and awareness. The brainstem and thalamus provide the activating mechanism, and the cerebrum provides full cognition and self-excitation. Content of consciousness can best be regarded as an amalgam or integration of all cognitive function that resides in the thalamo-cortical circuits of both hemispheres. Altered awareness arises from disruption of this cortical activity by diffuse pathology. Focal lesions of the cerebrum can produce profound deficits such as aphasia, alexia, amnesia, and hemianopsia, but only diffuse bilateral damage, sparing the ARAS and diencephalon, can lead to wakeful unawareness. Thus there are two kinds of altered consciousness: (1) altered arousal caused by dysfunction of the ARAS-diencephalon and (2) altered awareness caused by bilateral diffuse cerebral hemisphere dysfunction.

Four major pathologic groupings can cause such severe, global, acute reductions of consciousness[1,8]:

1. In the presence of diffuse or extensive multifocal bilateral dysfunction of the cerebral cortex, the cortical gray matter is diffusely and acutely depressed or destroyed. Concurrently, cortical-subcortical physiologic feedback excitatory loops are impaired with the result that brainstem autonomic mechanisms temporarily become profoundly inhibited, producing the equivalent of acute "reticular shock" below the level of the lesion.
2. Direct damage to a paramedian upper brainstem and posterior-inferior diencephalic ascending arousal system blocks normal cortical activation. Anatomically, the affected structures lie predominantly in the paramedian gray matter, extending rostrally from the level of the nucleus parabrachialis of the pontine tegmentum as far as the ventral posterior hypothalamus and adjacent pretectal area.
3. Widespread disconnection of the cortex from subcortical activating mechanisms acts pathophysiologically to produce effects similar to both previously mentioned conditions.
4. Diffuse disorders, usually metabolic in origin, concurrently affect both the cortical and subcortical arousal mechanisms, although to a different degree according to the cause.

STRUCTURAL LESIONS CAUSING COMA

Intracranial mass lesions that produce coma may be located in the supratentorial or infratentorial compartments. From either location, impaired arousal or coma can be produced by compression of the brainstem-hypothalamic activating mechanisms secondary to swelling and displacement of deep lying intracranial contents. Coma may occur either because of obstructed axoplasmic flow or sustained neuronal depolarization caused by ischemia or hemorrhage. Factors that contribute to the degree of loss of arousal include the rate of development, location, and ultimate size of the lesion (Fig. 62-1). Cerebral mass lesions that distort the intracranial anatomy alter the cerebrospinal fluid circulation and brain blood supply, resulting in an increased bulk of the injured tissue and a reduction in intracranial compliance. Intercompartmental pressure gradients that result in herniation syndromes are not necessarily associated with large increases in intracranial pressure (ICP). Recently sustained or evolving mass lesions that disturb cerebral vascular autoregulation can produce abrupt but short-lasting vasodilation. Vasodilatation, in turn, causes recurrent increases in intracranial pressure (pressure waves), thereby further compromising cerebral blood supply to injured regions.

Two herniation syndromes demonstrate the mechanism by which *supratentorial lesions* produce coma. The rate

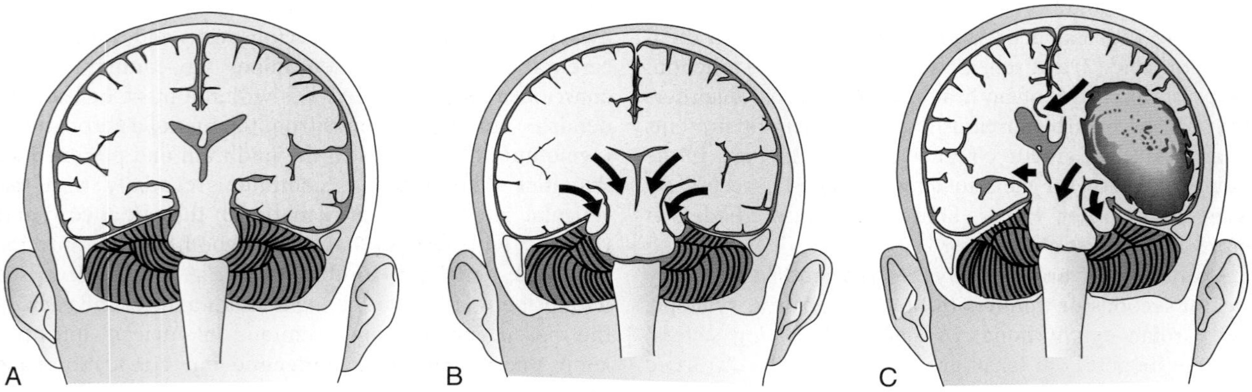

Figure 62-1. **A,** Coronal view of the relationship of supratentorial and infratentorial compartments. **B,** Central transtentorial herniation: The brain is swollen; the diencephalon is compressed and elongated; and the medial temporal lobes are forced along the brainstem through the tentorial notch. **C,** Uncal and transtentorial herniation: The cingulate gyrus is herniated under the falx cerebri; the uncus herniates through the tentorial notch, and the brainstem is compressed and shifted laterally and downward.

of evolution of a mass dictates whether the anatomic distortion precedes (in slowly evolving lesions) or parallels the patient's deterioration of wakefulness. Downward transtentorial herniation can be central or predominantly unilateral. Central herniation is caused by caudally displaced deep midline supratentorial masses, large space-occupying hemisphere lesions, or large unilateral or bilateral compressive extra-axial lesions, and results in compression of the ARAS. The progressive rostral-caudal pathologic and clinical stages of the herniation syndromes were outlined by Plum and Posner.[1] Pathologically, bilateral symmetric displacement of the supratentorial contents occurs through the tentorial notch into the posterior fossa. Alertness is impaired early, pupils become small (to 3 mm) and reactive, and bilateral upper motor neuron signs develop. The clinical manifestations are periodic, crescendo-decrescendo (Cheyne-Stokes) breathing, grasp reflexes, roving eye movements, or depressed oculocephalic reflexes. In the absence of effective therapy at this diencephalic stage, herniation progresses caudally to compress the midbrain, leading to a coma and fixed, midposition (3- to 5-mm) pupils, signifying both sympathetic and parasympathetic interruption. Spontaneous eye movements cease, and oculovestibular and oculocephalic reflexes become difficult to elicit. Spontaneous extensor posturing may occur. Once this stage is reached, full recovery becomes unlikely. As the caudal compression-ischemia process advances, pontine and medullary function fail, leading to absent reflex eye movements and bizarre breathing patterns. Finally, autonomic cardiovascular and respiratory functions cease when medullary centers are destroyed.

Uncus herniation results from laterally placed hemisphere lesions, particularly of the temporal lobes, that cause side-to-side cerebral displacement and transtentorial herniation. Focal hemisphere dysfunction (contralateral hemiparesis, aphasia, seizures) precedes unilateral (usually ipsilateral) paralysis of the third cranial nerve. An early sign of uncus herniation is an ipsilateral or (less often) contralateral enlarged pupil that responds sluggishly to light followed by a fixed, dilated pupil and an oculomotor palsy characterized by an eye turned downward and outward.[1] The ipsilateral posterior cerebral artery may become compressed as it crosses the tentorium with resulting ipsilateral occipital lobe ischemia. Unchecked, the temporal lobe compresses the midbrain, with loss of consciousness and bilateral or contralateral extensor posturing. Ipsilateral to the intracranial lesion, a hemiparesis may develop if the opposite cerebral peduncle becomes compressed against the contralateral tentorial edge (Kernohan's notch phenomenon). As herniation progresses, abnormal brainstem signs become symmetric and herniation proceeds in the same pattern seen with central herniation, as rostro-caudal brainstem displacement progresses.

Infratentorial lesions cause coma by displacement, compression, or direct destruction of the pontomesencephalic tegmental activating system. Displacement of the medulla downward sufficient to push the brainstem and cerebellar tonsils into the foramen magnum causes cardiorespiratory collapse. Acute intrinsic lesions of the brainstem, usually hemorrhagic or ischemic, cause abrupt onset of coma and are associated with abnormal neuro-ophthalmologic findings. Pupils may be pinpoint as a result of disruption of pontine sympathetic pathways, or they may be dilated as a result of destruction of the third cranial nerve nuclei or intra-axial exiting fibers. Dysconjugate eye movements and nystagmus occur, and vertical eye movements are relatively spared. Ocular bobbing signifies pontine damage. Upper motor neuron signs develop, and patients may become quadriplegic; flaccidity in the upper extremities and flexor withdrawal responses in the lower extremities often accompany midbrain-pontine damage.

Pathologically, *basilar artery occlusion* leads to asymmetric ischemia of the brainstem, affecting the ARAS, the neighboring densely packed neuropil, and the descending and ascending motor and sensory tracts. Thrombosis of the rostral basilar artery leads to infarction of the midline thalamic nuclei and coma without other obvious brainstem signs. Hemorrhage into the ventral pons sometimes spares consciousness but produces neuro-ophthalmologic signs and motor dysfunction. Extension of the hemorrhage into the rostral pontine tegmentum results in stupor, coma, or death. *Basilar artery migraine* may produce altered consciousness by interfering with arterial blood flow in basilar artery tributaries. Rapidly developing, extensive central *pontine myelinolysis* may cause coma by extension into the pontine tegmentum. Other intrinsic brainstem lesions (e.g., tumor, abscess, granuloma, demyelination) tend to progress slowly and usually spare arousal mechanisms but may reduce attention and other cognitive functions, leading to severe psychomotor retardation.

Extra-axial posterior fossa lesions cause coma by direct compression of the ARAS in the brainstem and in the diencephalon by upward transtentorial herniation. Compression of the pons may be difficult to distinguish from intrinsic lesions but is often accompanied by headache, vomiting, and hypertension caused by a Cushing reflex. Upward herniation at the midbrain level is initially characterized by coma, reactive miotic pupils, asymmetric or absent caloric eye responses, and extensor posturing; caudal-rostral brainstem dysfunction then occurs, with midbrain failure and midposition, fixed pupils.[9] Causes of brainstem compression include cerebellar hemorrhage, infarction, and abscess; rapidly expanding cerebellar or fourth ventricular tumors; or, less commonly, infratentorial epidural or subdural hematomas. Drainage of the lateral ventricles aimed at relieving obstructive hydrocephalus associated with posterior fossa masses may potentially precipitate acute upward transtentorial herniation.[10,11]

Downward herniation of the cerebellar tonsils through the foramen magnum causes acute medullary dysfunction and abrupt respiratory and circulatory collapse. Less severe impaction of the tonsils in the foramen magnum may lead to obstructive hydrocephalus and consequent bihemispheric dysfunction with an altered arousal. Accompanying manifestations include headache, nausea, vomiting, lower cranial nerve signs, vertical nystagmus, ataxia, and irregular breathing. Lumbar puncture in this setting carries a risk of catastrophic consequences.[10]

NONSTRUCTURAL DISORDERS CAUSING COMA

Nonstructural disorders such as metabolic or toxic disturbances produce coma by diffusely depressing the function of the brainstem and cerebral arousal mechanisms. The precise anatomic locus of metabolic brain disease has not been defined. The onset of coma can be abrupt, as with toxic drug ingestion, surgical-level anesthesia, or cardiac arrest, or it may evolve slowly after a period of confusion and inattention. The chief manifestations of metabolic encephalopathy are disturbances in arousal and cognitive function. Other findings, depending on the cause of encephalopathy, may include abnormalities of the sleep-wake cycle, autonomic disturbances, and abnormal respiratory pattern. The most helpful distinguishing clinical feature of a diffuse encephalopathy is the preservation of the pupillary light response, the only exceptions being an overdose of anticholinergic agents, near-fatal anoxia, or malingering. Lack of pupillary reactivity requires a search for an underlying structural lesion. The neurologic examination in metabolic encephalopathy shows a decreased level of arousal and a widespread cognitive decline. Comatose patients without brainstem or hemisphere function and no known cause for unconsciousness must be assumed to have suffered accidental or intentional self-poisoning. Metabolic disturbances of arousal and thinking particularly affect elderly patients who suffer from serious systemic illnesses or who have undergone complicated surgery.

Metabolic encephalopathy is characterized clinically by multilevel central nervous system dysfunction. At onset, abnormalities in cognition are at least as severe as the disturbance of arousal. Misperception, disorientation, multimodality hallucinations, defects in concentration and memory, or occasionally hypervigilance may progress to stupor and coma. The patient's level of arousal and consciousness often fluctuates between examinations. Motor abnormalities, if present, are usually bilateral and symmetric. Patients often manifest tremor, asterixis, and multifocal myoclonus. Spontaneous motor activity ranges from hypoactivity (in cases of sedating drug or endogenous metabolic disturbances) to hyperactivity (after drug withdrawal or overdose of stimulating agents, such as cocaine and phencyclidine). Seizures occasionally occur, particularly after alcohol or drug withdrawal, and particularly in patients with a cortical pathologic condition. Focal seizures may occur even without structural disease in patients with hyperglycemia or hypoglycemia, hepatic encephalopathy, uremia, abnormal calcium levels, or toxin ingestion. Autonomic dysregulation including hypothermia occurs with hypoglycemia, myxedema, and sedative drug overdose. Hyperthermia occurs in withdrawal states, particularly delirium tremens, anticholinergic drug overdose, infection, neuroleptic malignant syndrome, or malignant hyperthermia.

The metabolic needs of the brain depend on the oxidation of glucose to carbon dioxide and water. Certain fatty acids and ketone bodies can supply part of the metabolic needs in emergency circumstances, but these alternate fuels never provide an entirely sufficient substrate to meet all energy requirements. Normal cerebral blood flow (CBF) is around 55 mL/100 g of tissue/minute. At a CBF below 20 mL/100 g/minute oxygen delivery becomes insufficient for normal levels of oxidative metabolism, and cerebral glycolytic rate increases. At CBF levels between 16 and 20 mL/100 g/minute, the patient loses consciousness and an electroencephalogram (EEG) will demonstrate suppression resulting from synaptic failure. The cortical evoked response is abolished at a CBF below about 15 mL/100 g/minute. At a CBF of about 8 mL/100 g/minute, the energy-requiring membrane pump fails and the membrane potential collapses. Unless CBF is restored promptly, irreversible neuronal injury will ensue. The threshold for ischemic neuronal injury is time dependent: Complete cessation of CBF leads to loss of consciousness in 8 seconds, and EEG suppression occurs at 10 to 12 seconds. ATP exhaustion and ionic pump failure occurs in 120 seconds. Selective neuronal damage starts after periods as brief as 5 minutes, and severe neuronal damage occurs after 20 to 30 minutes. Brain necrosis or infarction starts within 1 to 2 hours.

Under physiologic conditions, glucose is the brain's only substrate and crosses the blood-brain barrier by facilitated transport. The normal brain uses about 5.5 mg of glucose/100 g/minute. If there is hypoglycemia, defined in adults as a blood glucose concentration below 40 mg/dL, symptoms and signs of encephalopathy result.

The cerebral cortex is more vulnerable than the brainstem to the effects of hypoglycemia. The neurologic presentation of hypoglycemia can vary from focal motor or sensory deficits to coma. Acute symptoms of hypoglycemia are better correlated with the rate at which blood glucose levels decrease than with the degree of hypoglycemia. The blood glucose level at which cerebral metabolism fails and symptoms develop varies among individuals, but in general, confusion occurs at levels below 30 mg/dL and coma below 10 mg/dL. The brain stores about 2 g of glucose and glycogen. For this reason, a patient in hypoglycemic coma may survive 90 minutes without suffering irreversible brain damage.

The cause of metabolic coma from hypoglycemia is not well understood. The disorder cannot solely be attributed to glucose starvation of neurons. Rather than such an internal catabolic death, evidence suggests that neurons are killed by external factors. At the time when the EEG reveals isoelectric activity, endogenous neurotoxins are produced and released by the brain into tissue and cerebrospinal fluid. The distribution of necrotic neurons in hypoglycemia, unlike that in ischemia, is related to white matter and cerebrospinal fluid pathways. The toxins act first by disrupting dendritic trees, sparing the intermediate axons, an indication of excitotoxic neuronal injury. The mechanism of excitotoxic neuronal necrosis involves hyperexcitation and culminates in cell membrane rupture. During hypoglycemia, the synthesis of amino acids such as γ-aminobutyric acid, glutamate, glutamine, and alanine, as well as acetylcholine, is suppressed. Whether reduction of these molecules or alteration in nerve synaptic transmission significantly contributes to the onset of coma associated with severe hypoglycemia is not established.

The pathophysiologic processes in other metabolic encephalopathies have not been established precisely and are discussed elsewhere.[1] Hepatic encephalopathy is caused not solely by ammonia intoxication but also by the accumulation of neurotoxins such as short- and medium-chain fatty acids, mercaptans, and phenols. Altered neurotransmission occurs because of the accumulation of benzodiazepine-like substances, the imbalance of serotonergic and glutaminergic neurotransmission, and the accumulation of false neurotransmitters. The identity of the neurotoxin in uremic encephalopathy is uncertain and includes urea itself, guanidine and related compounds, phenols, aromatic hydroxyacids, amines, various peptide "middle molecules," myoinositol, parathormone, and amino acid imbalance. The cause of the dysequilibrium syndrome may entail more than osmotic water shifts from plasma into brain cells, and reduction in cortical potassium, with intracellular acidosis resulting from increased production of organic acids in the brain, has been reported. The pathogenesis of pancreatic encephalopathy involves patchy demyelination of brain white matter as a result of liberated enzymes from a damaged pancreas, disseminated intravascular coagulation, or fat embolism.

The mechanism of action of exogenous toxins or drugs depends partly on the structure and partly on the dose. Sedatives produce depression before they irrepressibly damage the nervous system, making prompt diagnosis and effective treatment particularly important.

DIFFERENTIAL DIAGNOSIS

Several different behavioral states are clinically similar to, and can be confused with, coma. Differentiating such states from true coma has important diagnostic, therapeutic, and prognostic implications. Moreover, coma is not a permanent state; patients who survive initial coma may evolve through and into these altered behavioral states. All patients who survive beyond the stage of acute systemic complications reawaken and either proceed to recovery (with no disability or varying degrees of disability) or survive in a vegetative state.

The *vegetative state* can be defined as wakefulness without awareness and is the consequence of various diffuse brain insults.[1,12] It may be a transient phase through which patients in coma pass if the cerebral cortex recovers more slowly than the brainstem. Clinically, vegetative patients appear to be awake and to have cyclical sleep patterns; however, such individuals do not show evidence of cognitive function or learned behavioral responses to external stimuli. Vegetative patients show spontaneous eye opening and eye movements and stereotypic facial and limb movements; however, they do not demonstrate speech or comprehension, and they lack purposeful activity. Vegetative patients generate normal body temperature and usually have normally functioning cardiovascular, respiratory, and digestive systems, but they are incontinent of urine and feces. The vegetative state should be termed *persistent* at 1 month after injury and *permanent* at 3 months after a nontraumatic injury or 12 months after a traumatic injury.[13,14] Extended observation of the patient is required to assess behavioral responses to external stimulation and to demonstrate cognitive unawareness. An EEG is never isoelectric but shows various patterns of rhythm and amplitude that are inconsistent from one patient to the next. Normal EEG sleep-wake patterns are absent.

In the *locked-in syndrome,* patients retain or regain arousability and self-awareness, but because of extensive bilateral paralysis (i.e., differentiation) can no longer communicate except in severely limited ways. Such patients suffer bilateral ventral pontine lesions with quadriplegia, horizontal gaze palsies, and lower cranial nerve palsies; voluntarily, they are capable only of vertical eye movements or blinking, or both.[1] Sleep may be abnormal, with marked reduction in non-REM and REM sleep phases. The most common cause is pontine infarction resulting from basilar artery thrombosis, but also pontine hemorrhage, central pontine myelinolysis, and brainstem mass lesions. Neuromuscular causes include severe, acute inflammatory demyelinating polyradiculoneuropathies; myasthenia gravis; botulism; and neuromuscular blocking agents. In these peripheral disorders, upward gaze is not selectively spared.

Akinetic mutism describes a rare subacute or chronic state of altered behavior in which an alert-appearing patient is both silent and immobile but not paralyzed.[15] External evidence of mental activity is unobtainable. The patient usually lies with eyes opened and retains cycles of self-sustained arousal, giving the appearance of vigilance. Skeletal muscle tone can be normal or hypertonic but is usually not spastic. Movements are rudimentary even in response to unpleasant stimuli. Affected patients are usually doubly incontinent. Lesions that result in akinetic mutism may vary widely. One pattern consists of bilateral damage to frontal lobe or limbic-cortical integration with relative sparing of motor pathways. Vulnerable areas involve both basal medial frontal areas. Somewhat similar behavior also can follow incomplete lesions of the deep gray matter (paramedian reticular formation of the posterior diencephalon and adjacent midbrain), but such patients usually suffer double hemiplegia and act slowly yet are not completely akinetic or noncommunicative.

Catatonia is a symptom complex associated most often with psychiatric disease. This behavioral disturbance is characterized by stupor or excitement and variable mutism, posturing, rigidity, grimacing, and catalepsy. Catatonia can be caused by a variety of illnesses, both psychiatric (affective more than psychotic) disorders and structural or metabolic diseases (toxic and drug-induced psychosis, encephalitis, and alcoholic degeneration). Psychiatric catatonia may be difficult to distinguish from organic disease because patients often appear lethargic or stuporous rather than totally unresponsive. Such patients also may have a variety of endocrine or autonomic abnormalities. Patients in catatonic stupor do not move spontaneously and appear unresponsive to the environment despite what appears to be a normal level of arousal and consciousness. This impression is supported by normal results on neurologic examination and a subsequent recall of most events that occurred during the unresponsive period. Patients usually lie with eyes opened and may not blink to visual threat, but one can usually elicit optokinetic responses. The pupils are semidilated and reactive to light, oculocephalic reflexes are absent, and vestibulo-ocular testing evokes normal nystagmus. Patients may hypersalivate and be doubly incontinent. Passive movement of the limbs meets with waxy flexibility, and catalepsy is seen in 30% of patients. Choreiform jerks of the extremities and facial grimaces are common. The EEG, both of catatonic excitement and stupor, most often shows a reactive, low-voltage, fast-normal record rather than the slow record of a comatose patient.

APPROACH TO COMA

The initial approach to stupor and coma is based on the principle that all alterations in arousal are acute life-threatening emergencies (Fig. 62-2). Urgent steps are required to prevent or minimize permanent brain damage from reversible causes. Patient evaluation and treatment must occur simultaneously. Serial examinations are necessary with accurate documentation to determine a change in state of the patient. Accordingly, management decisions (therapeutic and diagnostic) must be made. The clinical approach to an unconscious patient logically entails the following steps: (1) emergency treatment; (2) history (from relatives, friends, and emergency medical personnel); (3) general physical examination; (4) neurologic profile, the key to categorizing the nature of coma; and (5) specific management.

Emergency Management

Initial assessment must focus on the vital signs to determine the appropriate resuscitation measures; the diagnostic process begins later. Urgent and sometimes empiric therapy must be given to avoid additional brain insult.

Oxygenation

Oxygenation must be ensured by establishing an airway for ventilation of the lungs. The threshold for intubation should be low in a comatose patient, even if respiratory function is sufficient for proper ventilation and oxygenation; the level of consciousness may deteriorate, and breathing may decompensate suddenly and unexpectedly. An open airway must be ensured and protected from aspiration of vomitus and blood. If severe neck injury is a possibility or has not been excluded, intubation should be performed by the most skilled practitioner without extension of the patient's neck. A brief neurologic examination is mandatory before the sedation required for intubation is given.

The key points of a rapid neurologic examination are the following[16]:

- Hand drop from over the head (to assess for malingering or hysterical loss of consciousness)
- Pupillary size and response to light

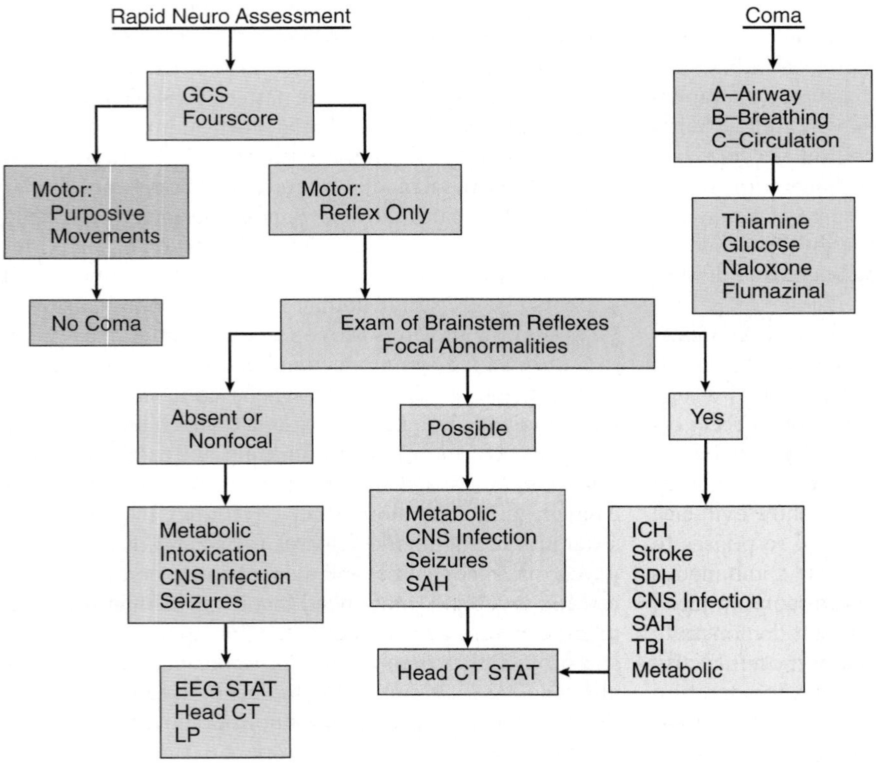

Figure 62-2. Emergency assessment and management of coma. CNS, central nervous system; CT, computed tomography; EEG, electroencephalogram; GCS, Glasgow Coma Score; ICH, intracerebral hemorrhage; SAH, subarachnoid hemorrhage; SDH, subdural hematoma; STAT, immediately; TBI, traumatic brain injury.

- Abnormal eye movements (active dysconjugate, unilaterally paralytic, passively induced, or not at all)
- Grimacing, withdrawal from noxious stimulation
- Abnormal plantar response (unilateral or bilateral Babinski's sign)

Mask-bag-assisted ventilation should continue during the examination if necessary. Signs of arousal or inadequate sedation include dilated, reactive pupils, copious tears, diaphoresis, tachycardia, and systemic hypertension.

Intubation

The preferred route of emergency intubation is orotracheal, which can be performed rapidly, safely, and reliably with in-line stabilization of the neck in patients with suspected cervical spine injury.

Intubation causes intense reflexive cardiovascular stimulation that may lead to a deleterious elevation of ICP. Therefore the patient should be adequately sedated during intubation. Etomidate should be a first choice in the patient with suspected raised ICP; it reliably facilitates induction in less than 1 minute with a duration of action of 4 to 6 minutes. Propofol is another anesthetic agent without the potential to increase ICP. Both medications result in a dose-dependent decrease of cerebral metabolic rate that reduces CBF and ICP.

Respiration/PEEP

The effect of positive end-expiratory pressure (PEEP) on ICP is not predictable for a number of reasons. Lung and pleural pressures are transmitted to the CSF column through intravertebral spaces and the vertebral venous plexus, and to the jugular venous system through the superior vena cava. The effect of PEEP on ICP depends on both intracranial and pulmonary compliance. ICP response is not limited to PEEP but is related more closely to mean airway pressure, which can be raised by many factors other than PEEP including peak airway pressure and inspiratory time. Of note, the position of the patient's head and upper body can significantly affect ICP. A nasogastric tube should be placed to facilitate gastric lavage and prevent regurgitation.

Circulation

Circulation must be maintained to ensure adequate cerebral perfusion. The appropriate resuscitation fluid is lactated Ringer's solution; normal saline solution is also used when high ICP is suspected. A mean systemic arterial pressure of about 100 mm Hg is adequate and safe for most patients. While obtaining venous access, blood samples should be collected for anticipated tests and more (Box 62-1). Hypotension is treated by replacing any blood volume loss, and vasoactive agents are used (preferably dopamine). Elevated blood pressure should be judiciously managed with hypotensive agents that do not substantially raise ICP by their vasodilating effect (labetalol, hydralazine, or nicardipine are the favored agents for managing uncontrollable hypertension). For most situations, a systolic blood pressure of 150 to 160 mm Hg and a diastolic pressure of 90 to 100 mm Hg is maintained. Urine output should be at least 0.5 mL/kg/hour; accurate measurement requires bladder catheterization.

Box 62-1

Emergency Laboratory Tests of Metabolic Coma

Immediate Tests

- Venous blood
  - Glucose
  - Electrolytes (Na, K, Cl, CO_2, PO_4)
  - Urea and creatinine
  - Osmolality
- Arterial blood (check color)
  - pH
  - PO_2
  - PCO_2
  - HCO_3
  - HbCO (if available)
- Cerebrospinal fluid
  - Gram stain
  - Cell count
  - Glucose
- Electrocardiogram

Deferred Tests (Initial Sample, Process Later)

- Venous blood
  - Sedative and toxic drugs
  - Liver function
  - Coagulation studies
  - Thyroid and adrenal function
  - Blood cultures
  - Viral titers
- Urine
  - Sedative and toxic drugs
  - Culture
- Cerebrospinal fluid
  - Protein
  - Culture
  - Viral and fungal titers

Glucose and Thiamine

Hypoglycemia is a frequent cause of altered consciousness; glucose (25 g as a 50% solution) should be administered intravenously immediately after blood is drawn for baseline values. Empiric glucose treatment will prevent hypoglycemic brain damage, and it outweighs the theoretical risks of additional harm to the brain in hyperglycemic, hyperosmolar, or anoxic coma. Thiamine (100 mg) must be given with the glucose infusion to prevent precipitation of Wernicke's encephalopathy in malnourished, thiamine-depleted patients. Rarely, an established thiamine deficiency can cause coma.

Seizures

Repeated generalized seizures damage the brain and must be stopped. Initial treatment should include intravenous benzodiazepine lorazepam (2 to 4 mg/kg). Seizure control can be maintained with intravenous phenytoin (18 mg/kg at a rate of 25 mg/min). Seizure breakthrough requires additional administration of benzodiazepine.

Sedation

Careful and mild sedation should be given to an agitated, hyperactive patient to prevent self-injury. A quiet patient facilitates ventilator support and diagnostic procedures. Small doses of intravenous benzodiazepines, intravenous haloperidol (1 mg as often as hourly until the desired effect is achieved), or intravenous morphine (2 to 4 mg) are appropriate. In a supported patient the effects set in quickly, can be reversed, and are short lasting.

Reversal of Drug Overdose

Consider specific antidotes: drug overdose is the largest single cause (30%) of coma in the emergency department. Most drug overdoses can be treated by supportive measures alone. Certain antagonists, however, specifically reverse the effects of coma-producing drugs. Intravenous naloxone (0.4 to 2 mg) is the antidote for opiate coma. The reversal of narcotic effect may precipitate acute withdrawal phenomena in an opiate addict. In suspected opiate coma the minimum amount of naloxone should be administered to establish the diagnosis by pupillary dilation and to reverse depressed breathing and coma. One should not attempt to completely reverse all drug effects with the first dose. Intravenous flumazenil reverses all benzodiazepine-induced coma. It follows, therefore, that coma unresponsive to administration of 5 mg flumazenil in divided doses given over 5 minutes is not caused by benzodiazepine overdose. Recurrent sedation can be prevented with 1 mg flumazenil every 20 minutes.[17] The sedative effects of drugs with anticholinergic properties, particularly tricyclic antidepressants, can be reversed with 1 to 2 mg physostigmine intravenously. Pretreatment with 0.5 mg atropine will prevent bradycardia. Only full awakening is characteristic of an anticholinergic drug overdose because physostigmine has nonspecific arousal properties. Physostigmine has a short duration of action (45 to 60 minutes), and its use may have to be repeated.

Body Temperature

Body temperature may require adjustment: hyperthermia is dangerous because it increases brain metabolic demand and, at extreme levels, denatures brain proteins.[18] Elevated temperature greater than 104°F (40°C) requires nonspecific cooling measures, even before the underlying cause is determined and treated. In 2002 European and Australian groups published two independent studies showing that lowering the body temperature to 33°Celsius for 12 or 24 hours in comatose survivors of cardiac arrest resulted in doubling the number of patients being discharged home or to a rehabilitation facility. Protective effect of moderate hypothermia could be explained by avoiding the death of neurons in vulnerable regions of the brain by diminishing numerous deleterious biochemical mechanisms after the restoration of spontaneous circulation. Hyperthermia can indicate infection but may be caused by intracranial hemorrhage, anticholinergic drug intoxication, or heat exposure. A body temperature of less than 93°F (34°C) should be slowly elevated to above 95°F (35°C) to prevent cardiac dysrhythmia. Hypothermia accompanies profound sepsis, sedative/hypnotic drug overdose, near-drowning, hypoglycemia, or Wernicke's encephalopathy.

History

Once vital functions have been protected and the patient's condition is stable, clues to the cause of coma must be sought by interviewing relatives, friends, bystanders, or medical personnel who may have observed the patient before or during the decline in consciousness. The history should include the following:

- Witnessed events: head injury; seizure; details of a motor vehicle accident; circumstances under which the patient was found
- Evolution of coma: abrupt or gradual; headache; progressive or recurrent weakness; vertigo; nausea and vomiting
- Recent medical history: surgical procedures; infections; current medication
- Medical history: epilepsy; head injury; drug or alcohol abuse; stroke; hypertension; diabetes; heart disease; cancer; uremia
- Psychiatric history: depression; suicide attempts; social stresses
- Access to drugs: sedatives; psychotropic drugs; narcotics; illicit drugs; drug paraphernalia; empty medicine bottles

General Physical Examination

A systematic, detailed examination is helpful and necessary in the approach to the comatose patient who is in no condition to describe prior or current medical problems. This examination is an extension of the initial evaluation and includes the following:

- Repeated assessment of vital signs to determine efficacy of resuscitation measures
- External evidence of trauma
- Evidence of acute or chronic medical illnesses
- Evidence of ingestion or self-administration of drugs (needle marks, alcohol on breath)
- Evaluation for nuchal rigidity; care is required if neck injury is possible or has not been excluded

Neurologic Profile

Establishing the nature of the coma is critical for appropriate management. This requires the following:

- Correct interpretation of neurologic signs that reflect the integrity (or impairment) of various functional levels of the brain
- Determining whether the pattern and evolution of these signs are best explained by a supratentorial or infratentorial structural lesion, a metabolic-toxic encephalopathy, or a psychiatric cause (Box 62-2 and Table 62-1)

Box 62-2

Neurologic Profile—A Modified Glasgow Coma Scale

Verbal Response
Oriented speech
Confused conversation
Inappropriate speech
Incomprehensible speech
No speech

Eye Opening
Spontaneous
Response to verbal stimuli
Response to noxious stimuli
None

Motor Response
Obeys
Localizes
Withdraws (flexion)
Abnormal flexion
Abnormal extension
None

Pupillary Reaction
Present
Absent

Spontaneous Eye Movement
Orienting
Roving conjugate
Roving dysconjugate
Miscellaneous abnormal movements
None

Oculocephalic Response
Normal (unpredictable)
Full
Minimal
None

Oculovestibular Response
Normal (nystagmus)
Tonic conjugate
Minimal or dysconjugate
None

Deep Tendon Reflexes
Normal
Increased
Absent

Table 62-1. Correlation between Levels of Brain Function and Clinical Signs

Structure	Function	Clinical Sign
Cerebral cortex	Conscious behavior	Speech (including any sounds) Purposeful movement Spontaneous To command To pain
Brainstem activating and sensory pathways (reticular activating system)	Sleep/wake cycle	Eye opening Spontaneous To command To pain
Brainstem motor pathways	Reflex limb movements	Flexor posturing (decorticate) Extensor posturing (decerebrate)
Midbrain CN III	Innervation of ciliary muscle and certain extraocular muscles	Pupillary reactivity
Pontomesencephalic MLF	Connects pontine gaze center with CN III nucleus	Internuclear ophthalmoplegia
Upper pons CN V CN VII	 Facial and corneal Facial muscle innervation	 Corneal reflex-sensory Corneal reflex-motor response Blink Grimace
Lower pons CN VIII (vestibular portion) connects by brainstem pathways with CN III, IV, VI	 Reflex eye movements	 Doll's eyes Caloric responses
Pontomedullary junction pressure	Spontaneous breathing Maintained blood pressure	Breathing and blood pressure do not require mechanical or chemical support
Spinal cord	Primitive protective responses	Deep tendon reflexes Babinski response

CN, cranial nerve; MLF, medial longitudinal fasciculus.

The clinical neurologic functions that provide the most useful information in making a categoric diagnosis are outlined in Box 62-3. These indices are easily and quickly obtained. Furthermore, they have a high degree of inter-examiner consistency and, when applied serially, accurately reflect the patient's clinical course. Once the cause of coma can be assigned to one of these categories, specific radiographic, electrophysiologic, or chemical laboratory studies can be used to make a disease-specific diagnosis and to detect existing or potential complications (Fig. 62-3).

Specific Management

Supratentorial Mass Lesions

If the presumed cause of coma is a supratentorial mass, the severity and rate of evolution of signs must be determined. A relatively stable patient next requires an emergency head CT scan or magnetic resonance imaging (MRI). The priority in deep coma or in established or threatening transtentorial herniation is to apply medical treatment of intracranial hypertension. Brief hyperventilation to a $PaCO_2$ between 25 and 30 mm Hg is the most rapid method to lower elevated ICP. This is achieved by adjusting the ventilation rate to 10 to 16/minute and tidal volume to 12 to 14 mL/kg. The vasoconstrictive effect is transient (lasting less than an hour), so an osmotic agent must be administered concurrently. Sustained hyperventilation below 30 to 35 mm Hg removes all future value of this procedure.

Two types of osmotic agents remain in current use: mannitol and hypertonic saline solutions. For years, mannitol has been used in the setting of increased ICP caused by a variety of conditions such as stroke and head trauma. Although its mechanism of action has never been fully elucidated, experts widely believe that mannitol creates an osmotic gradient which mediates its effects on ICP. Other postulated mechanisms of action are free radical scavenging effects and increases in cerebral blood flow. The use of hypertonic solutions (2%, 3%, and 23.4% sodium chloride) were initially used for in-the-field resuscitation of patients with multisystem trauma and later for treatment of increased ICP caused by conditions such as brain tumors or isolated traumatic brain injury. Recently, hypertonic solutions have been used as osmotic therapy for brain edema in the neurocritical arena.

Box 62-3

Characteristics of Categories of Coma

Supratentorial Mass Lesion Affecting the Diencephalon/Brainstem
Initial focal cerebral dysfunction
Dysfunction progresses rostral to caudal
Signs reflect dysfunction at one level
Signs often asymmetric

Infratentorial Structural Lesion
Symptoms of brainstem dysfunction or sudden onset coma
Brainstem signs precede/accompany coma
Cranial nerve and oculovestibular dysfunction
Early onset of abnormal respiratory patterns

Metabolic-Toxic Coma
Confusion/stupor precede motor signs
Motor signs usually symmetric
Pupil responses generally preserved
Myoclonus, asterixis, tremulousness, and generalized seizures common
Acid-based imbalance common with compensatory ventilatory changes

Psychogenic Coma
Eyelids squeezed shut
Pupils reactive or dilated, unreactive (cycloplegics)
Oculocephalic reflex unpredictable; nystagmus on caloric tests
Motor tone normal or inconsistent
No pathologic reflexes
Awake-pattern EEG

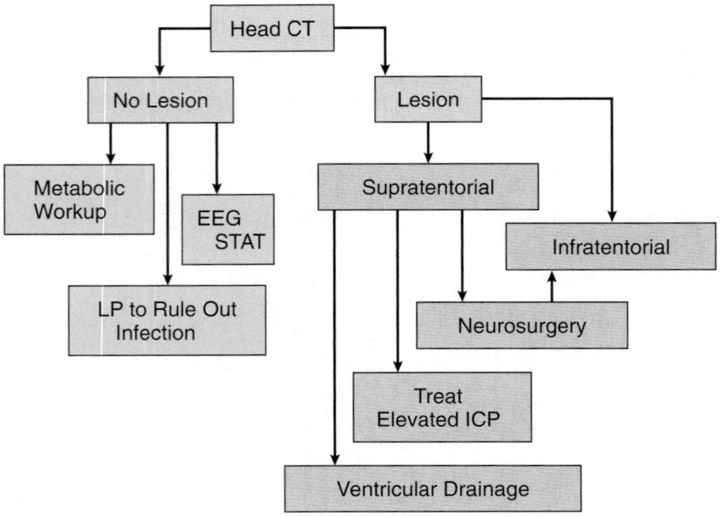

Figure 62-3. Specific management of coma using head computed tomography (CT) scans. EEG, electroencephalogram; ICP, intracranial pressure; LP, lumbar puncture; STAT, immediately.

A dose of 1 to 2 mL/kg of 23.4% sodium chloride should be administered via a central line over 20 to 30 minutes. Serial serum sodium concentration monitoring is required to avoid a rapid rise with a limit of serum sodium concentration increase by 12 mEq/L over 24 hours or 0.5 to 1 mEq/L/hour. All these patients must have an ICP monitor to assess and guide response to therapies before the administration of 23.4% saline or immediately after. On a case-by-case basis, the clinical response to 23.4% may be enough to assess the positive response to the treatment. Standing orders should not be used; the primary endpoint of its administration is the acute treatment of the neurologic emergency while other measures are rapidly instituted. The rapid achievement of a hyperosmolar state using 23.4% saline should not be considered a secondary endpoint because there is evidence that a favorable acute clinical response may occur even in the absence of induced hypernatremia. Additional doses of 23.4% saline may be administered as needed following the initial ICP response to therapy. As part of the hyperosmolar therapy in these patients, the institution of therapy with 2% or 3% NaCl at 1 to 2 mL/kg/hour should be considered for prolonged ICP control if indicated.

The endpoint of therapy is a serum sodium concentration range of 145 to 155 mEq/L, which closely corresponds to a serum osmolarity of 310 to 315 mOsm/L. Serum electrolytes should be frequently monitored (every 6 to 8 hours) throughout the length of therapy and 24 hours after discontinuation in order to assess goals of treatment (induced hypernatremia) and possible complications such as hypokalemia and hyperchloremic metabolic acidosis. Daily CXR should be obtained to assess for congestive heart failure.

Improvement of intracranial pressure elevation (clinically or by ICP monitoring) will dictate the duration of the induced hypernatremic state.

Corticosteroids are not indicated in the emergent, empiric management of elevated ICP because their full effects are observed only after a few hours. Furthermore, because steroid drugs are effective only for certain lesions (e.g., edema around a brain tumor or abscess), their use can be delayed until a diagnosis has been made with the aid of neuroimaging studies. Following initial ICP management, a head CT or MRI is required. The scan will demonstrate the nature of the supratentorial lesion and associated mass effect. Arrangements must be made to evacuate promptly an epidural or subdural hematoma. Intraparenchymal masses that acutely affect the brainstem ARAS and present with coma are best managed nonsurgically. If steroid agents are indicated, a dexamethasone bolus should be given (up to 100 mg intravenously), followed by 6 to 24 mg every 6 hours.

The patient's vital signs and neurologic condition require repeated evaluation. The head should be kept elevated at 30 degrees. Administration of mannitol (0.5 to 1.5 mg/kg) may be repeated, if necessary, every 4 to 6 hours. Serum electrolytes and fluid balance must be monitored.

When patients with presumed increased ICP do not respond clinically as expected to medical management or when obstructive hydrocephalus complicates a supratentorial mass lesion, we favor placement of a ventriculostomy into the lateral ventricle. The ventriculostomy allows accurate measurement of intraventricular ICP and provides a method for CSF drainage, if necessary. The placement of a ventriculostomy allows calculation of cerebral perfusion pressure (mean systemic arterial pressure minus ICP), a critical determinant of cerebral blood flow and therefore of oxygen and substrate delivery. Monitoring of ICP also allows adjustment of therapeutic interventions before clinical deterioration occurs in patients with diminished intracranial compliance. Drainage of CSF aims to relieve high ICP to maintain cerebral perfusion pressure (>60 mm Hg) and to improve intracranial compliance. After increased ICP has responded to emergency management and the patient's condition has stabilized, definitive treatment of the mass lesion is required as deemed appropriate.

Infratentorial Lesions

The evolution of neurologic symptoms and signs and the neurologic examination generally give sufficient information to localize the lesion to the posterior fossa; the lesions themselves may be intrinsic or extrinsic to the brainstem.

Treatment of a presumed extrinsic compressive lesion of the brainstem entails measures that decrease ICP, as outlined earlier. Patients who are stuporous or show signs of progressive brainstem compression from a cerebellar hemorrhage or infarction require urgent evacuation. Intrinsic brainstem lesions are best treated conservatively; an uncompleted stroke may benefit from a thrombolytic or an anticoagulant, or both. Posterior fossa tumors are managed initially with osmotic agents and steroids; definitive treatment includes surgery or irradiation, or both. The placement of a ventricular catheter for acute hydrocephalus must be considered cautiously and in consultation with a neurosurgeon; there is danger of a potentially fatal upward transtentorial herniation.[11]

Metabolic Toxic Coma

The task of the physician in first contact with the patient in metabolic coma is to preserve and protect the brain from permanent damage. Metabolic and toxicologic studies must be performed on the first blood drawn (see Box 62-1). Treatable conditions that quickly and irreversibly damage the brain are discussed next.

Hypoglycemia

As noted earlier, glucose (50 mL of a 50% intravenous solution) should be administered during emergency treatment before blood results return from the laboratory. Prolonged hypoglycemic coma that has considerably damaged the brain will not be reversed by a glucose load; a glucose bolus may transiently worsen hyperglycemic, hyperosmolar coma. By contrast, the osmolar load of intravenous glucose may transiently decrease elevated ICP and lighten nonhypoglycemic coma. A glucose infusion is necessary to prevent recurrent hypoglycemia.

Acid-Base Imbalance

The hyperventilating comatose patient with acute, severe metabolic acidosis and threatening cardiovascular collapse requires emergency treatment. For accurate assessment an arterial blood gas is required. An intravenous infusion of $NaHCO_3$ (1 mEq/kg of body weight) can be lifesaving. Simultaneously, a search for and specific treatment of the cause must be conducted.

Hypoxia

Suspected or proven carbon monoxide poisoning requires hyperoxygenation with 100% oxygen to facilitate excretion of this toxin. Blood pressure and cardiac rhythm abnormalities should be closely monitored and corrected. Idiopathic and drug-induced methemoglobinemia is treated with methylene blue (1 to 2 mg/kg intravenously over a few minutes; a repeat dose is given after 1 hour if needed). Anemia alone does not cause coma but exacerbates other forms of hypoxia. Transfusion of packed red cells or whole blood is appropriate for severe anemia (hematocrit level <25%). Cyanide poisoning causes histotoxic hypoxia of the brain. Treatment entails amylnitrite (vapor or crushed ampule inhaled every minute) and sodium nitrite (300 mg intravenously), followed by sodium thiosulphate (12.5 g intravenously).

Acute Bacterial Meningitis

A lumbar puncture must be considered in any unconscious patient with fever or signs of meningeal irritation, or both. If possible, an emergency head CT should be performed before lumbar puncture on a comatose patient to rule out unexpected mass lesions. Increased ICP is present in all cases of bacterial meningitis, but a lumbar puncture is not contraindicated when this diagnosis is suspected. Cerebral herniation seldom, if ever, occurs except in small children with *Haemophilus influenzae* meningitis.[19] Clinical correlates of impending herniation demand a more cautious approach to lumbar puncture: coma or rapidly deteriorating level of arousal, focal neurologic signs, and tonic or prolonged fits. (Papilledema is rare in acute bacterial meningitis.) Should unexpected herniation occur after lumbar puncture, treatment with hyperventilation and intravenous mannitol is indicated. Appropriate antibiotic treatment should be initiated while awaiting the results of a spinal fluid Gram stain. If the Gram stain test is negative yet a bacterial cause is suspected, empiric, broad-spectrum antibiotic treatment with a third-generation cephalosporin and vancomycin is appropriate to continue.

Drug Overdose

Certain general principles apply to all patients suspected of having ingested sedative drugs.[20,21] Most drug overdose is treated by emergency treatment (already discussed) and supportive measures (Table 62-2). Once vital signs are stable, attempts should be made to remove, neutralize, or reverse the effects of the drug. Patients in coma from recent drug ingestion require gastric lavage after endotracheal intubation. A large, preferably double-lumen, gastric tube must be placed orally. The lavage is performed with the patient in the head-down position on the left side. Lavage is performed with a 200- to 300-mL bolus of tap water or half normal saline solution and is continued until the return is clear. After lavage, 1 or 2 tablespoons of activated charcoal are passed down the lavage tube. With meticulous supportive measures, patients with uncomplicated drug-induced coma should recover without neurologic deficit. Recovery from coma resulting from massive doses of barbiturates or glutethimide can be hastened by hemodialysis.

Constant vigilance and attention to the patient's condition, with timely and appropriate diagnostic and therapeutic evaluation, ensures the best possible outcome of metabolic coma. Effective care demands meticulous attention to maintaining tissue perfusion and oxygenation; documenting and anticipating acute neurologic events (particularly diminished cerebral perfusion, herniation, or seizures); aggressive, rapid treatment of initial or subsequent infections; and preventing agitation. Deep venous thrombosis can be decreased with subcutaneous heparin (5000 U every 8 to 12 hours) and full-length pneumatic compression leg boots. Enteral or parenteral feeding within 36 to 48 hours is required to satisfy nutritional needs. Corneal injury can be prevented by protecting the eyes with lubricants and taping the lids shut.

ROLE OF SPECIAL INVESTIGATIONS

Neurodiagnostic Imaging

Once the patient with an altered mental status is appropriately resuscitated and stabilized, further investigation may be necessary to document the location of the lesion and provide guidance for therapeutic intervention. CT and MRI provide an anatomic assessment of the CNS and provide helpful information for defining the localization of lesions that produce coma.

CT scanning is currently the most expedient imaging technique and gives the most rapid information about possible structural lesions with the least risk to the patient. The value of the CT scan to demonstrate mass lesions, hemorrhage, and hydrocephalus is well established. Axial cuts (10 mm for the cerebral hemispheres and 5 mm for the posterior fossa) are sufficient initially; intravenous iodinated contrast highlights areas of blood-brain barrier breakdown such as tumor, abscess, and subacute strokes and may be necessary to better define such lesions. The CT scan is indispensable in the management of acute head injury and acute stroke and can delineate calvarial fractures and intracranial hematomas (epidural, subdural, intraparenchymal, intraventricular, and subarachnoid), which may require immediate neurosurgical intervention. The CT scan shows tissue shifts caused by intracranial intercompartmental pressure gradients, but compared with MRI it may underestimate the anatomy of herniation and its associated syndromes.[10] Certain lesions such as early infarction (<12 hours' duration), encephalitis, and isodense subdural hemorrhage may be difficult to

Table 62-2. Neurologic Manifestations of Common Drug Poisoning

Drug	Signs and Symptoms	Diagnostic Test	Treatment
Carbon monoxide	Confusion; agitation; headache; convulsions; coma, respiratory failure; cardiovascular collapse	History Carboxyhemoglobin level	Remove patient from area; 100% oxygen until carboxyhemoglobin levels fall to <5% Hyperbaric oxygen if central nervous system affected Treat cerebral edema with hyperventilation, diuretics, and cerebrospinal fluid drainage, if necessary
Salicylate	Tinnitus; hyperpnea; confusion; convulsions; coma; hyperthermia	Blood	Supportive care; gastric lavage; charcoal; systemic alkalinization; hemodialysis for coma or seizures
Cyanide	Agitation; confusion; headache; vertigo; hypertension; hypotension; seizures; paralysis; apnea; coma	Blood	Amyl nitrate; sodium nitrate; sodium thiosulfate; 100% oxygen; hyperbaric oxygen for refractory signs Vitamin B_{12} injection
Anticonvulsants Phenytoin, carbamazepine, phenobarbital (see barbiturates), valproic acid, primidone, ethosuximide, felbamate, clonazepam (see benzodiazepines)	Drowsiness; ataxia; nystagmus; tremulousness; coma; dysrhythmias with carbamazepine or phenytoin overdose	Blood Ammonia level in patients taking valproic acid	Supportive care; gastric lavage; charcoal; watch for withdrawal seizures
Sedative Hypnotics Benzodiazepines, barbiturates, chloral hydrate, meprobamate, ethchlorvynol (Placidyl)	Confusion; lethargy; ataxia; nystagmus; hypothermia; dysarthria; respiratory depression; coma Pupillary reactions preserved except in instances of deep barbiturate coma Possible withdrawal seizures	Blood	Supportive care; gastric lavage; flumazenil for benzodiazepine overdose; hemoperfusion for extreme barbiturate intoxication
Methaqualone	Agitation; hypertonic; hyperreflexia; ataxia; hallucinations; convulsions	Blood	As above
Ethanol	Confusion; agitation; delirium; ataxia; nystagmus; dysarthria; coma	Blood; breath	Supportive care; lavage if within 1 hr of ingestion; thiamine; glucose
Opioids	Lethargy; small reactive pupils; hypothermia; hypotension; urinary retention; shallow, irregular respirations; convulsions	Urine Response to naloxone	Naloxone, 0.4 mg IV or IM; continuous naloxone infusion, if necessary Supportive care with intubation as needed Lavage if overdose is by ingestion
Stimulants Amphetamine, methylphenidate, cocaine	Hypervigilance; paranoia; violent behavior; tremulousness; dilated pupils; hyperthermia; tachycardia or arrhythmia, focal neurologic signs secondary to CNS stroke or hemorrhage; seizures	Blood, urine	Supportive care; sedation with benzodiazepines Treat hypertensive crisis with sodium nitroprusside or labetalol Watch for rhabdomyolysis

Continued

Table 62-2. Neurologic Manifestations of Common Drug Poisoning—cont'd

Drug	Signs and Symptoms	Diagnostic Test	Treatment
Psychedelics			
LSD, mescaline, PCP	Delirium; delusions; marked agitation; hallucinations; hyperactivity; dilated pupils; hyperreflexia; nystagmus	Blood Measure PCP levels in gastric juice	Gastric lavage; charcoal; benzodiazepines and haloperidol for sedation
Antidepressants			
Tricyclic antidepressants	Anticholinergic effects: dry mouth; agitation; restlessness; ataxia; tachycardia or arrhythmias; hyperthermia; hysteria; convulsions; mydriasis	Blood, urine	Cardiac monitoring; gastric lavage; charcoal; mild systemic alkalinization Physostigmine for refractory arrhythmias Anticonvulsants for seizures
Monoamine oxidase inhibitors	Drowsiness; ataxia; seizures; hypertensive crisis; hypotension with severe overdose		Symptomatic care; gastric lavage; avoid narcotics
Neuroleptics	Dystonia; drowsiness; coma; convulsions; hypotension; miosis; tremor; hypothermia; neuroleptic malignant syndrome	Urine	Gastric lavage; treat extrapyramidal signs with diphenhydramine or benztropine mesylate; treat neuroleptic malignant syndrome with dantrolene or bromocriptine
Lithium	Lethargy; weakness; polyuria; polydipsia; ataxia; tremulousness; seizures; coma	Blood	Hemodialysis for delirium, seizures, or coma
Methanol, ethylene glycol	Drunkenness; hyperventilation; stupor; convulsions; coma Blindness with methanol use	Blood	Symptomatic care; gastric lavage; ethanol infusion; hemodialysis For methanol intoxication, supportive care
Antihistamines	Anticholinergic effects: dry mucosa; flushed skin; hyperthermia; dilated pupils; delirium; hallucinations; seizures; coma		Supportive care; gastric lavage; control of seizures with benzodiazepines; physostigmine for life-threatening anticholinergic effects
Organophosphates	Cholinergic crisis: cramps; excessive secretions; diarrhea; bronchoconstriction; later, tremulousness; fasciculations; weakness; convulsions; hypertension; tachycardia; confusion; anxiety; coma	Red blood cell cholinesterase level	Symptomatic care; decontamination; atropine; pralidoxime

visualize. A pathologic condition of the posterior fossa may be somewhat obscured by bone artifact inherent in the CT technique. Raised ICP is suggested by effacement of cortical sulci, a narrow third ventricle, and obliteration of the suprasellar or quadrigeminal cisterns, but it cannot be otherwise quantified.

MRI may be performed, depending on the clinical setting and the stability of the patient's condition. The use of MRI is limited in the urgent setting of coma evaluation because of the length of time required to perform the imaging, image degradation by even a slight movement of the patient, and the relative inaccessibility of the patient for emergencies that may occur during the imaging process. Nevertheless, MRI provides superb visualization of the posterior fossa and its contents, which is useful when intrinsic brainstem lesions are suspected as the cause of coma.[10] The MRI images anatomic lesions such as those resulting from acute stroke, encephalitis, central pontine myelinolysis, and traumatic shear injury with greater resolution and at an earlier time than CT scanning. The injection of the paramagnetic substance, gadolinium, helps delineate areas of blood-brain barrier breakdown and may augment the sensitivity of this scanning technique. The "diffusion" technique detects changes in the hydrogen atom (free water) distribution between the intracellular and extracellular spaces and can demonstrate ischemic brain virtually immediately. Sagittal MRI views are particularly useful in documenting the degree of supratentorial or infratentorial herniations and may enable intervention before clinical deterioration occurs (Fig. 62-4).[10]

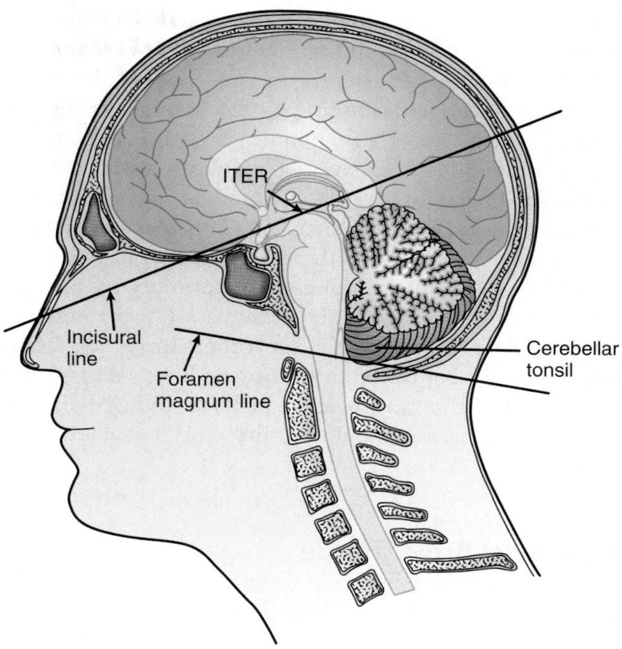

Figure 62-4. Midsagittal view of a normal adult brain. The opening of the tentorium of the cerebellum or anterior cerebellar notch lies along a line (incisural line) defined anteriorly by the anterior tubercle of the sella turcica and posteriorly by the junction of Galen's vein, the inferior sagittal sinus, and the confluence of the straight sinus. The proximal opening of the aqueduct of Sylvius, the ITER *(arrow),* lies within 2 mm of the incisural line. The foramen magnum line is defined between the inferior tip of the clivus anteriorly and the bony base of the posterior lip of the foramen magnum.

Newer MRI techniques allow functional imaging of the CNS by measurement of cerebral blood flow to a particular region. Future application of this technique may allow rapid determination of diminished cerebral blood flow such as occurs in stroke or vasospasm and will probably be useful in assessing the effect of therapeutic interventions.

Electroencephalography

The EEG is a qualitative indicator of cerebral function that sometimes gives useful additional information in the evaluation of an unresponsive patient. With metabolic and toxic disorders, the EEG changes generally reflect the degree and severity of altered arousal or delirium characterized by a decreased frequency of the background rhythm and the appearance of diffuse slow activity in the theta (4 to 7 Hz) or delta (1 to 3 Hz) range, or both. Bilaterally synchronous and symmetric, medium- to high-voltage broad triphasic waves are seen in various metabolic encephalopathies, most often in hepatic coma. Rapid beta activity (>13 Hz) in a comatose patient suggests the ingestion of sedative hypnotics such as barbiturates and benzodiazepines. Acute, focally destructive lesions show focal slow activity; when periodic lateralized epileptiform discharges appear acutely in one or both temporal lobes, herpes simplex encephalitis must be strongly considered. A nonreactive, diffuse alpha pattern in a comatose patient usually implies a poor prognosis and is most often seen after anoxic insults to the brain or acute, destructive pontine tegmental damage.[22,23] A normally reactive EEG in an unresponsive patient suggests psychiatric disease; however, a relatively normal EEG can accompany the locked-in syndrome, some examples of akinetic mutism, and catatonia, all of which can be caused by structural brain lesions. Attempts to correlate the pattern and frequency spectra of postresuscitative EEG with neurologic outcome have been unsatisfactory because the predictive value of the EEG is at best 88% accurate.[24] At present the most useful information regarding patient prognosis is still obtained by the correct interpretation of physical signs.

Nonconvulsive generalized status epilepticus and repeated complex partial seizures may produce altered levels of awareness or arousal; the EEG is an indispensable tool in the diagnosis and management of both these disorders. Continuous EEG monitoring optimizes management of status epilepticus as clinical assessment is insufficiently sensitive to detect continued electrographic seizures. Furthermore, continuous EEG monitoring in the intensive care unit setting has shown an unsuspected high incidence of electrographic seizure activity in critically ill neurologic patients.[25,26]

Jugular Venous Oximetry

Changes in jugular venous oxygen saturation measure the relationship between cerebral metabolic rate and cerebral blood flow.[27] Placement of a fiberoptic catheter into the internal jugular vein provides continuous measurements of venous oxygen saturation. Jugular venous oximetry catheters should be inserted on the side of dominant venous drainage with the tip position high in the jugular bulb. The most common complications are malposition and carotid puncture. Normal jugular venous oxygen saturation is 50% to 75%. Less than 50% indicates critical ischemia; greater than 75% indicates hyperemia. This form of monitoring offers the potential to minimize secondary insults after traumatic brain injury by providing warning of cerebral ischemia. Other applications include monitoring after other forms of brain injury and during neurosurgical procedures. When used with other continuous measurements including ICP, the approach to the treatment of brain injury becomes more logical.

Assessing Brain Tissue

Brain tissue PO_2 monitoring using polarographic parenchymal microprobes was introduced in the mid-1990s. Studies have shown that in severe TBI patients, brain tissue PO_2 correlates with CPP and low brain tissue PO_2 is associated with poor outcome. The role of this parameter for patient management, nevertheless, has not been clearly defined. Normal brain tissue PO_2 values in cerebral white matter range between 20 and 40 mm Hg, and values below 10 to 15 mm Hg are considered critical. The probe is placed into the white matter of the frontal lobes.

Monitoring of brain tissue PO_2 could be useful in order to monitor and guide potentially harmful treatment interventions such as hyperventilation. Brain tissue PO_2 monitoring may also allow us to better define certain patient groups that may benefit from a management that does not blindly follow the ICP treatment protocol. For example, patients may have compromised brain tissue PO_2 despite normal ICP and CPP values and, therefore, should be treated more aggressively with interventions aimed at increasing cerebral perfusion and oxygenation. Conversely, there may be patients who tolerate ICP and CPP values that are within the critical zone and, therefore, should be spared the potentially harmful use of ICP treatment interventions.

Quantitative monitoring of parenchymal cerebral blood flow (CBF) has become available using thermal diffusion technology. Critical values for cerebral white matter CBF are below 10 to 18 mL/100 g/minute. Inadequate CBF is an important cause of secondary brain damage, but the interpretation of absolute numbers of CBF can be problematic because the thresholds for ischemia and hyperemia are variable after different mechanisms of brain injury. We have found CBF monitoring more helpful in determining the status of cerebral autoregulation and identifying patients at risk for cerebral ischemia from arterial hypotension.

Microdialysis monitoring adds another set of variables to ever-increasing information collected bedside in the ICU. Microdialysis is a technique for sampling the chemistry of the interstitial fluid. Monitoring of intracerebral biochemistry with microdialysis has reached a stage where it is feasible to perform in the ICU settings. The goal is to predict irreversible damage before it occurs and leave a therapeutic time window for interventions by sampling markers of ischemia and cell damage. Microdialysis catheters implanted in relevant positions in relation to the affected brain tissue contribute important information on the development of ischemia (lactate/pyruvate ratio), and microdialysis helps in determination of how seriously it affects brain tissue and the necessity to intervene. After interventions, microdialysis shows the resulting effects on brain chemistry.

Transcranial Doppler Ultrasonography

Transcranial Doppler (TCD) ultrasonography allows noninvasive measurement of blood flow velocity in basal cerebral arteries.[28] The high dynamic resolution provided and the confirmed correlation with other hemodynamic modalities have encouraged increasing numbers of neurointensivists to adopt the technique. Its importance in early detection of vasospasm in subarachnoid hemorrhage is now clearly established; increased flow velocity can be documented before neurologic deterioration, thus allowing early institution of therapy. Velocity also increases when there is augmentation of flow as a result of collateral contributions to other vascular territories or supply to a large arteriovenous malformation. At the time of brain death, a characteristic and diagnostic pattern of flow has been noticed using TCD in large basal intracranial vessels.[29] An oscillating reverbatory movement has been observed in the flow velocity waveforms. The diagnosis is based on the finding of the reflux phenomenon during late systole following anterograde injection of blood into the vascular tree.

Evoked Potentials

Evoked potentials (EPs) are used to follow the level of functioning of the CNS in comatose patients.[30] Clinical use of brainstem auditory evoked potentials (BAEPs) and short latency somatosensory evoked potential (SEP) responses arises from the close correlation between EP waveform and specific anatomic structures. The SEP shows special promise in the intensive care unit because components generated supratentorially in the thalamus and primary sensory cortex can be identified and followed over time. Shifts of intracranial structures that lead to herniation syndromes are reflected in abnormalities in SEPs, whereas BAEPs are generated entirely at or below the lower midbrain and are less often affected. EPs have the advantage of being less affected than EEG readings by sedative medications and septic or metabolic encephalopathies, factors that frequently confound interpretations in comatose patients.

Anatomic specificity and physiologic and metabolic immutability are the basis of clinical utility of EPs. Abnormalities demonstrated by these tests, however, are etiologically nonspecific and must be carefully integrated into the clinical situation by a physician familiar with their clinical use. Studies have shown that all patients with anoxic coma and bilaterally absent SEPs died or remained in a persistent vegetative state.[31] In traumatic coma, absent SEPs may be a less definitive prognostic indicator because recovery of consciousness has been reported in some patients.[40] Also, caution is necessary in the interpretation of SEPs to ensure that the absence is not caused by technical problems. Repeat SEPs are also useful in following patients' progress. A progressive decline in amplitude appears to be associated with a poor prognosis. Furthermore, a comatose patient with motor response of flexor posture or, better, with an initial poor prognostic EEG pattern but normal SEPs, may have the potential for recovery and should be supported until the patient's condition has changed to a more prognostically definitive category.[32]

PROGNOSIS

A complete evaluation of a comatose patient must include an estimate of prognosis. The outcome in a given comatose patient cannot be predicted with absolute certainty. Available serial data are not sufficiently specific or selective to help in establishing the prognosis in an individual patient. Guidelines on the outcome of coma have been compiled on the basis of serial examinations (Table 62-3). Although the status of the comatose patient on admission is valuable in providing early, informed discussion with relatives of patients and medical colleagues, that moment in most instances does not provide sufficient information to withhold immediate therapy. However, the early establishment of a highly probable outcome ideally should be made within 24 hours after hospital admission to ration intensive care services and protect families from false hope in futile cases. A logical and sensible approach to prognostication includes an etiological subcategorization into medical, drug-induced, and traumatic coma.

Factors that are useful in determining the outcome of medical coma include the cause, depth, and duration of coma. Certain clinical signs, particularly those involving brainstem, motor, and verbal function, are the most helpful and best validated predictors (confidence interval 0.95).[33-36]

Overall, only 15% of patients in established *medical coma* for 6 hours will make a good or moderate recovery; others will die (61%), remain vegetative (12%), or become permanently dependent on others for daily living (11%). Prognosis depends on the cause of medical coma. Patients in coma resulting from a stroke, subarachnoid hemorrhage, or cardiorespiratory arrest have only about a 10% chance of achieving independent function. Thirty-five percent of patients will achieve moderate to good recovery if coma is caused by other metabolic reasons including infection, organ failure, and biochemical disturbances. As noted earlier, almost all patients who reach the hospital after sedative overdose or other exogenous agents will recover moderately or completely.

The depth of coma affects the individual prognosis. Patients who open their eyes in response to noxious stimuli after 6 hours of coma have a 20% chance of making a good recovery, compared with 10% if the eyes remain closed.

The longer coma persists, the less likely are the chances for recovery; 15% of patients in coma for 6 hours make a good or moderate recovery, compared with only 3% who remain unconscious at 1 week.[33,34] Coma following head trauma has a somewhat better prognosis (see later).

The severity of signs of brainstem dysfunction on admission inversely correlates with the chance of good recovery in medical coma. Absent pupillary responses at any time after onset and, except in barbiturate or phenytoin poisoning, absent caloric-vestibular reflexes 1 day after onset indicate a poor prognosis (<2% recovery). Except for sedative drug poisoning, no patient with absent pupillary light reflexes, corneal reflexes, oculocephalic or caloric responses, or lack of a motor response to noxious stimulation at 3 days after onset is likely to ever regain independent function. In a prospective study of 500 patients in medical coma, a uniform group of 210 patients suffered anoxic injury: 52 of these had no pupillary reflex at 24 hours; all of these patients died. By the third day, 70 were left with a motor response worse than withdrawal, and all died. By the seventh day, the absence of roving eye movements was seen in 16 patients, all of whom died.[33,34]

Patients likely to recover to functional independence will within 1 to 3 days speak words, open their eyes to noise, show nystagmus on caloric testing, or have spontaneous eye movements. More than 25% of patients with anoxic injury who show roving conjugate eye movements

Table 62-3. Trauma Scale

Glasgow Coma Scale Total	
14-15	5
11-13	4
8-10	3
5-7	2
3-4	1
Respiratory Rate	
10-24/min	4
25-35/min	3
>35/min	2
1-9/min	1
None	0
Respiratory Expansion	
Normal	1
None	0
Systolic Blood Pressure	
>89 mm Hg	4
70-89 mm Hg	3
50-69 mm Hg	2
0-49 mm Hg	1
No pulse	0
Peripheral Perfusion (Capillary Refill)	
Normal	2
Delayed	1
None	0
Total Trauma Score—Sum of the Individual Scores*	

*Scores <10 represent <60% chance of survival.

within 6 hours of the onset of coma or who show withdrawal responses to pain or eye opening to pain will recover independence and make a moderate or good recovery. The use of combinations of clinical signs helps to improve the accuracy of prognosis: at 24 hours the absence of a corneal response, pupillary light reaction, or caloric or doll's eye response is not compatible with recovery to independence.

Postanoxic convulsive status epilepticus or myoclonic status epilepticus (MSE), or both, reflect a poor prognosis. Some patients recover consciousness but remain handicapped. Most die or become vegetative.[37,38] Associated clinical findings such as loss of brainstem reflexes or eye-opening at the onset of myoclonic jerks, as well as sinister EEG patterns such as suppression or burst-suppression, confirm a grim neurologic outcome in this group. Autopsy studies show that cerebral and cerebellar damage can be ascribed to the initial ischemic hypoxic event; there is no evidence that status epilepticus further contributes to this damage. We initially treat patients with an intravenous loading dose of a major anticonvulsant (phenytoin 13 to 18 mg/kg at 25 mg/minute and/or phenobarbital 20 mg/kg at 50 mg/minute). MSE is generally resistant to therapy; we give intermittent doses of benzodiazepines (lorazepam 2 to 4 mg or clonazepam 0.5 mg) intravenously as needed to suppress particularly severe myoclonus that interferes with ventilatory support. Anesthetic agents are rarely indicated and are unlikely to alter outcome.

The most accurate prediction of outcome in a patient in medical coma is obtained from the use of a combination of clinical signs, and little is added by more sophisticated testing other than in identifying the cause of coma.[33,34] Within the first week it is difficult to justify the withdrawal of therapy from patients in medical coma unless they are already brain dead or lack all signs of brainstem function. After that, the probability of being able to predict the quality of life increases steadily.

Recently, a multisociety task force of neurologists and neurosurgeons obtained a large body of data concerning the persistent vegetative state (PVS); these data provide guidelines to outcomes in patients remaining vegetative 1 month after severe head trauma or coma-producing medical illness (mostly anoxic).[14]

Among adults with head trauma who were in a vegetative state at 1 month (n=106, 33%), 15% remained vegetative and 28% suffered severe disability at 1 year. Among children who were in a vegetative state for 1 month following traumatic injury (n=106, 9%), 29% remained in a PVS and 35% were severely disabled at 1 year; only 27% attained moderate to good recovery.

Nontraumatic (medical) coma results were even worse. Among 169 adults with nontraumatic brain injury who were vegetative at 1 month, 53% died within a year, 32% remained vegetative, and only 14% made a moderate to good recovery. The outcome of 45 children in similar circumstances showed 22% dead, 65% still vegetative, and only 6% who had made a moderate to good recovery at 1 year.

In a fraction of patients it is possible to predict within the first week those who will recover, those who will die in coma or enter a vegetative state, and those who will survive with severe disability. It is well established that patients in anoxic coma who are in a vegetative state at 1 month will never recover their full preanoxic physical or cognitive function.

Patients in coma resulting from *exogenous agents* (except carbon monoxide poisoning) carry an overall good prognosis if circulation and respiration are protected by avoiding or correcting cardiac dysrhythmia, aspiration pneumonia, and respiratory arrest. Despite absent brainstem reflexes or electrocerebral silence on EEG, patients with deep sedative drug intoxication have the potential for complete recovery. Therefore in an emergent situation, patients in a coma of uncertain cause should be supported vigorously until the precise cause of coma has been fully established.

The outcome of *traumatic coma* is generally better than for medical coma, and prognostic criteria are somewhat different[14,39,40]: (1) Many patients with head injury are young. (2) Prolonged posttraumatic unconsciousness of up to several months does not always preclude a satisfactory outcome. (3) Compared with the initial degree of neurologic abnormality, patients in traumatic coma recover more completely than patients in medical coma. Patients in coma for longer than 6 hours after head injury have a 40% chance to recover to moderate disability or better at 6 months. The most reliable predictors of outcome at 6 months include the following:

- Patient age (worse outcome can be predicted with increasing age, especially in those older than 60 years)
- Depth and duration of coma (an inverse correlation with Glasgow coma score)
- Pupil reaction and eye movements (absence at 24 hours predicts death or a vegetative state in 90% of patients)
- Motor response in the first week of injury (see Box 62-1)
- An independent poor prognostic indicator is sustained, uncontrollably increased ICP (>20 mm Hg)

Additional factors play a role in the eventual outcome from traumatic coma. Specific lesions such as subdural hematoma that result in coma can have a less than 10% recovery rate.[41] In studies of blunt trauma injuries, comatose patients with increased plasma glucose, hypokalemia, or elevated blood leukocyte counts were associated with lower Glasgow coma scale scores and an increased probability of death.[42]

Factors that appear to have little influence on outcome include the following:

- Cause of head injury
- Skull fractures
- Lateralization of damage to one hemisphere
- Extent of extracranial injury

Anecdotal reports of patients who have suffered coma as a result of head trauma and in whom an improvement from the vegetative state has been recognized after months are difficult to validate. It seems possible that such patients were not truly vegetative but rather in a state of profound disability, but with cognition, at the beginning of the observation.[43]

The prognostic guidelines for medical and traumatic coma should be applied with care. One must be sure that evaluation and interpretation of clinical signs are correct. In addition, the effect of anticholinergic agents used during resuscitation on pupillary reactivity and the effect of paralytic agents on motor response must be excluded.

The ability to predict prognosis following coma can benefit the patient, family, and physician. Families can be spared both the emotional and financial burdens of caring for individuals with an insignificant chance of independent function and quality of life. Physicians can then properly allocate limited resources to patients with the potential to benefit from advanced medical care.

KEY POINTS

- Coma is a state of pathologic unresponsiveness from which the patient cannot be aroused. The eyes are closed, and only reflex responses can be elicited from the patient with vigorous stimulation.
- The cause of coma is diverse and follows neuronal damage to both cerebral hemispheres or to the reticular activating system in the diencephalon and brainstem.
- Supratentorial mass lesions cause intercompartmental brain shifts known as cingulate, central (transtentorial), or uncal herniation.
- Lesions below the tentorium involve the brainstem arousal system directly or impair its function by compression.
- Alteration in cognitive function is the earliest manifestation of metabolic encephalopathy. Each disease process yields a specific clinical picture.
- The brain uses oxygen to metabolize glucose. It cannot store oxygen and survives only a few minutes after its oxygen supply is reduced below critical levels.
- During hypoglycemia (blood glucose concentration <40 mg/dL), encephalopathy results secondary to cerebral cortex or brainstem dysfunction, or both.
- Initial attention must focus on the restoration of respiratory, hemodynamic, and metabolic homeostasis; a search directed at the cause of coma begins thereafter. A comatose patient's recovery depends on appropriate treatment of the underlying disorder.
- Deeply comatose patients without brainstem and hemisphere function and with no known cause for coma must be assumed to have taken poison or a drug, either accidentally or intentionally.
- Status epilepticus is characterized by repetitive seizures without regaining consciousness. It can result in permanent brain damage and requires immediate attention.
- The neurologic examination consists of an assessment of the level of arousal determined by eye opening, verbal responses, and reflex or purposeful movements in response to noxious stimulation of the face, arms, and legs. Neuro-ophthalmologic function is evaluated by spontaneous eye movements, pupillary size and response to light, oculocephalic (doll's eyes), and oculovestibular (ice water caloric) responses. Vegetative function is assessed by the respiratory pattern.
- EEG, head CT, and MRI are tools to help establish the cause of coma.
- Placement of a ventriculostomy allows accurate measurement of intraventricular ICP and provides a method for drainage of CSF if needed.

REFERENCES

•1. Plum F, Posner JB: The Diagnosis of Stupor and Coma, ed 3. Philadelphia, FA Davis, 1980.
2. Brodal A: Neurological Anatomy in Relation to Clinical Medicine, ed 3. Oxford, Oxford University Press, 1981.
3. Steriade M, McCarly RW: Brain Stem Control of Wakefulness and Sleep. New York, Plenum, 1990.
4. McCormick DA, Von Krosigk M: Corticothalamic activation modulates thalamic firing through glutamate "metabotropic" receptors. Proc Natl Acad Sci 1992;89:2774.
5. Sejnowski TJ, McCormick DA, Steriade M: Thalamocortical oscillations in sleep and wakefulness. In Arbib MA (ed): The Handbook of Brain Theory and Neural Networks. Cambridge, Mass, MIT Press, 1995.
6. Kales A: Pharmacology of Sleep. Handbook of Experimental Pharmacology Series, vol 116. Berlin, Springer-Verlag, 1995.
7. Tinuper P: Idiopathic recurring stupor: A case with possible involvement of the gamma aminobutyric acid (GABA)ergic system. Ann Neurol 1992;31:503.
8. Plum F: Coma. In Adelman G, Smith BH (eds): Encyclopedia of Neuroscience, ed 2. Amsterdam, Elsevier Science, 1999.
9. Cuneo RA, Caronna JJ, Pitts L, et al: Upward transtentorial herniation: seven cases and a literature review, Arch Neurol 1979; 36:618.
•10. Reich JB, Sierra J, Camp W, et al: Magnetic resonance imaging measurements and clinical changes accompanying transtentorial and foramen magnum brain herniation. Ann Neurol 1993;33:159.
11. Kase CS, Wolf PA: Cerebellar infarction: Upward transtentorial herniation after ventriculostomy. Stroke 1993;24:1096.
12. Jennett WB, Plum F: The persistent vegetative state: A syndrome in search for a name. Lancet 1972;1:734.
13. Council on Scientific Affairs and Council on Ethical and Judicial Affairs: Persistent vegetative state and the decision to withdraw or withhold life support. JAMA 1990;263:426.
14. Multi-Society Task Force on PVS: Medical aspects of the persistent vegetative state: Statement of a multi-society task force. N Engl J Med 1994;330:1499.
15. Cairns H: Disturbances of consciousness with lesions of the brain stem and diencephalon. Brain 1952;75:109.
16. Goldberg S: The Four Minute Neurologic Exam. Miami, Fla, Medmaster, 1992.
17. Winkler E, Shlomo A, Kriger D, et al: Use of flumazenil in the diagnosis and treatment of patients with coma of unknown etiology. Crit Care Med 1993;21:538.
18. Hund EF, Lehman-Horn F: Life-threatening hyperthermic syndromes. In Hacke W (ed): Neurocritical Care. Berlin, Springer-Verlag, 1994.
19. Rennick G, Shann F, de Campo J: Cerebral herniation during bacterial

meningitis in children. Br Med J 1993;306:953.
20. Howell JM, Altieri M, Jagoda AS, et al: Emergency Medicine. Philadelphia, WB Saunders, 1998.
21. Ellenhorn MJ, Schonwald S, Ordog G, et al: Ellenhorn's Medical Toxicology: Diagnosis and Treatment of Human Poisoning, ed 2. Baltimore, Williams & Wilkins, 1997.
22. Austin EG, Walkus RJ, Longstreth WT: Etiology and prognosis of alpha coma. Neurology 1988;38:773.
•23. Synek VM: Prognostically important EEG coma patterns in diffuse anoxic and traumatic encephalopathies in adults. J Clin Neurophysiol 1988;5:161.
24. Edgren E, Hedstrend U, Nordin M, et al: Prediction of outcome after cardiac arrest. Crit Care Med 1987;15:820.
25. Young GB, Jordan KG, Doig GS: An assessment of non-convulsive seizures in the intensive care unit using continuous EEG monitoring: An investigation of variables associated with mortality. Neurology 1996;47:83.
26. Lowenstein DH, Aminoff MJ: Clinical and EEG features of status epilepticus in comatose patients. Neurology 1992;42:100.
27. Souter MJ, Andrews PJD: A review of jugular venous oximetry. Intensive Care World 1996;13:32.
28. DeWitt LD, Wechsler LR: Transcranial Doppler. Stroke 1988;19:915.
•29. Ropper AH, Kehne SM, Wechsler LR: Transcranial Doppler in brain death. Neurology 1987;37:1733.
30. Chiappa KH, Hoch DB: Electrophysiologic monitoring. In Ropper AH (ed): Neurological and Neurosurgical Intensive Care, ed 3. New York, Raven Press, 1993.
31. Chen R, Bolton CF, Young GB: Prediction of outcome in patients with anoxic coma: A clinical and electrophysiologic study. Crit Care Med 1996;24:672.
32. Lindsay K, Pasaoglu A, Hirst D, et al: Somatosensory and auditory brainstem conduction after head injury: A comparison with clinical features in prediction of outcome. Neurosurgery 1990;26:278.
•33. Levy DE, Bates D, Caronna JJ, et al: Prognosis in non-traumatic coma. Ann Intern Med 1981;94:293.
•34. Levy DE, Caronna JJ, Singer BH, et al: Predicting outcome from hypoxic-ischemic coma. JAMA 1985;253:1420.
35. Edgren E, Hedstrand U, Sutton-Tyrrel K, et al: Assessment of neurological prognosis in comatose survivors of cardiac arrest. Lancet 1994;343:1055.
36. Longstreth WT, Diehr P, Init S: Prediction of awakening after out of hospital cardiac arrest. N Engl J Med 1983;308:1378.
37. Young GB, Gilbert JJ, Zochodine DW: The significance of myoclonic status epilepticus in postanoxic coma. Neurology 1990;40:1843.
38. Wijdecks EFM, Parisi JE, Scarborough FW: Prognostic value of myoclonus status in comatose survivors of cardiac arrest. Ann Neurol 1994;35:239.
•39. Jennett B, Teasdale G, Braakman R, et al: Prognosis of patients with severe head injury. Neurosurgery 1979;4:283.
40. Marshall LF, Gautille T, Klauber MR, et al: The outcome of severe head injury. J Neurosurg 1991;75(Suppl): 28.
•41. Gennarelli TA, Spielman GM, Langfitt TW, et al: Influence of the type of intracranial lesion on outcome from severe head injury. J Neurosurg 1982;56:26.
42. Kassum DA, Thomas EJ, Wang CJ: Early determinations of outcome in blunt injury. Can J Surg 1984;27:64.
43. Rosenberg GA, Johnson SF, Brenner RP: Recovery of cognition after prolonged vegetative state. Ann Neurol 1977;2:167.
44. Wijdicks EF, Bamlet WR, Maramattom BV, et al: Validation of a new coma scale: The FOUR score. Ann Neurol 2005;58:585-593.

Chapter 63

Neurologic Criteria for Death in Adults

Joseph A. Karam and John M. Luce

The task of determining brain death is a highly complicated matter that varies according to state law and local hospital policies. This has led to considerable confusion among health care professionals regarding what constitutes brain death. This chapter summarizes the available data to reduce this confusion. It begins with a historical overview of how death has been conceptualized and defined. It then discusses the present-day concept of brain death and describes how brain death is legally defined. It next offers a practical approach to diagnosing brain death in adult patients. Brain death then is contrasted with the persistent vegetative state (PVS). The chapter ends with a discussion of how to deal with organ donation, brain death, and other issues with the families of brain-dead patients.

HISTORICAL OVERVIEW

Throughout the history of humankind, descriptions of death have been recorded both in medical and in nonmedical contexts. Along with these descriptions, the recognition of death progressed from observational to diagnostic. It was not until the mid-18th century that physician involvement in the diagnosis of death became commonplace. Indeed, in the writings of Hippocrates (the Hippocratic Corpus), physician involvement at the end of life is frowned on. For centuries, the diagnosis of death was left to the family and undertakers and centered on circulation and respiration. By the middle of the 18th century, validity testing modalities such as soap bubbles or feathers placed under the nose to detect respiration, total body submersion in water, or trumpeting directly into the decedent's ear were used to confirm death.[1,2] The invention of the stethoscope in 1816 and its subsequent evolution added to the expertise for the confirmation of cardiopulmonary death. Ethical and philosophical questions about what constituted life and death were not of practical importance, because after respiration and circulation ceased, the brain inevitably failed soon afterward.

The introduction of the modern positive-pressure mechanical ventilator in the early 1950s was the most significant technological advance that mandated a new definition of death.[3] Although mechanical ventilation had been available before this in the form of the iron lung, such ventilators were impractical in an acute situation such as a cardiac arrest. The introduction of positive-pressure ventilation meant that endotracheal intubation and mechanical ventilation could be performed in a few minutes. This advance allowed many patients to be saved who otherwise would have died. The ventilator revolutionized the care of the critically ill patient, but it created new problems.

As positive-pressure ventilation rapidly became more commonplace, a subgroup of patients in irreversible coma came to be recognized, surviving on the ventilator for days, weeks, or even longer. In these patients, who had suffered either primary or secondary neurologic insult, spontaneous respirations were supplanted by mechanical support. As skill with the management of the ventilator progressed, it became evident that some comatose patients would not be breathing at all except with the assistance of a ventilator. By the late 1950s, C. M. Fisher in the United States and Jouvet in France had begun to study this group of patients and found that a skilled neurologic examination[3] and electrocerebral silence, as shown by electroencephalogram (EEG),[4] could accurately predict poor neurologic outcomes in this subgroup of patients.

Although these studies provided the medical basis for defining brain death by clinical and electroencephalographic criteria, the legal definition of death in the early 1960s was still based on the absence of pulse and respirations. However, the growing number of hospitalized patients without neurologic function on ventilators, coupled with advances in organ transplantation techniques, mandated a change to include neurologic criteria to determine death for legal purposes.[3] In 1963, several neurologists at the Massachusetts General Hospital proposed that a patient be certified as dead despite cardiac function using the following clinical criteria: deep coma, dilated unreactive pupils, absence of corneal and oculovestibular reflexes to ice water calorics, paralysis of the limbs, apnea for 30 minutes, and an isoelectric EEG tracing in all leads for 30 minutes.[5] Despite this initial proposal, the first widely accepted criteria for defining brain death were not published until 1968.[6]

CONCEPT OF BRAIN DEATH

In 1968, the "Report of the Ad Hoc Committee of the Harvard Medical School to Examine the Definition of Brain Death" was published in the *Journal of the American Medical Association.*[6] The primary purpose of this report was to define irreversible coma as a new criterion for death. The committee was composed of well-respected academic neurologists who drew from the large experience of the clinical stroke service of the Harvard Medical School affiliate hospitals. The committee defined brain death using the "whole brain concept" by stating that a brain that no longer functions and has no possibility of functioning again is for all purposes dead.[6]

The committee then set out to establish clinical characteristics of the permanently nonfunctioning brain. The clinical criteria were (1) total unawareness and complete unresponsiveness, (2) absence of any movement or spontaneous respiration, and (3) absence of brainstem (and usually spinal) reflexes. The committee also noted that an isoelectric EEG was of great confirmatory value and when available should be used. Both clinical and EEG assessment should be repeated after 24 hours, and presence of hypothermia (a temperature lower than 90° F [32.2° C]) or central nervous depressant drugs should be ruled out. Only a physician should make this assessment; if the findings were consistent with brain death, death should be declared and the ventilator should be turned off.[6]

In 1976, the Medical Royal Colleges and their faculties in the United Kingdom developed their criteria for brain death.[7] This definition of brain death was based on the lower brain concept of brain death, or brainstem death. Because the reticular activating system resides in the brainstem and is necessary for consciousness, death of the brainstem implies permanent unconsciousness and, in the opinion of the Royal College investigators, was the medical definition of brain death. The Royal College group specified the following conditions under which the diagnosis of brain death should be considered: (1) the patient should be deeply comatose with no evidence for the presence of depressant drugs or metabolic or endocrine causes of coma and should have a temperature greater than 35° C; (2) he or she must be on a ventilator because spontaneous respirations were inadequate or absent in the absence of drugs that could depress ventilation; and (3) the structural cause and irreversibility of the brain damage should not be in doubt.

If these conditions were met, the following findings on specific diagnostic tests confirmed brain death: (1) pupils fixed and unreactive to light; (2) absence of corneal, vestibular-ocular, and gag reflexes; (3) absence of motor movements in response to stimulation of somatic areas within the cranial nerve distribution; and (4) absence of respiratory movements after the arterial partial pressure of carbon dioxide ($PaCO_2$) has risen above the threshold for stimulation of respiration. The Royal College guidelines did not require the use of an EEG or other confirmatory tests, although the investigators recognized the possiblity of indications for their use. Additionally, it recognized that spinal reflexes may be preserved in brain-dead patients.

Although these two working groups provided the first guidelines for brain death determination, the validity of their conclusions had never been formally tested. With advances in organ transplantation and the increased need for harvesting perfused organs, it was crucial that such validity be established. This was done in 1977, when the National Institute of Neurological and Communicative Disorders and Stroke (part of the National Institutes of Health [NIH]) organized a multicenter study to test the accuracy of clinical criteria in the assessment of brain death.[8] As with the Harvard criteria, the NIH study used the whole brain concept of death, stating that cerebral death implies total destruction of the brain so that evidence of both volitional and reflex responsiveness is absent.

This study enrolled 503 patients with coma and apnea and tested the validity of clinical and EEG criteria in establishing brain death. Of 187 patients with cerebral unresponsiveness, apnea, and electrocerebral silence on initial examination, 185 (99%) died. The two patients who met these criteria and survived were patients with drug intoxication. Because of the ramifications of diagnosing a live patient as brain dead, however, additional criteria were added. The study group maintained that it was better to have redundant tests for brain death than to falsely diagnose a patient as brain dead. Accordingly, to diagnose brain death, this group required that reversible causes such as sedative drugs, hypothermia, shock, and other remedial causes be first excluded by laboratory and radiologic examinations. Then, on the basis of the clinical experience of their members, both study groups concluded that brain death could be safely established if cerebral unresponsiveness, apnea, dilated pupils, absent cephalic reflexes, and electrocerebral silence were present for 30 minutes at least 6 hours after the ictus. Additionally, if any doubt existed regarding the validity of one of the prerequisites or the standards, or if a shorter period of observation was necessary, a confirmatory test documenting the absence of cerebral blood flow was recommended. Recently, the reliability of the clinical diagnosis of brain death when made by experienced examiners using established criteria was reconfirmed.[9]

Multiple criteria exist worldwide for diagnosing brain death. Because of confusion over which criteria should be used, a Presidential Commission was formed to examine this issue and provide a more uniform standard in the United States for the determination of brain death. In 1981, the "Report of the Medical Consultants on the

Diagnosis of Death to the President's Commission for the Study of Ethical Problems in Medicine and Biomedical and Behavioral Research" was published.[10] As with previous U.S. criteria, it used the whole brain concept of death and stated that brain death was present with irreversible loss of all brain function, both brainstem function and cortical function. The proposed criteria for brain death included unresponsiveness and unreactivity, absence of brainstem function, absence of brainstem respiratory reflexes, and evidence of irreversibility.[10] The President's Commission described apnea testing and suggested that a $PaCO_2$ greater than 60 mm Hg was necessary to demonstrate the absence of respiratory drive in the normothermic patient. The Commission explicitly stated that occurrence of seizures or decerebrate or decorticate posturing, but not spinal reflexes, was incompatible with the diagnosis of brain death.

The President's Commission specified that for brain death to be deemed irreversible, the cause of brain death should be known; reversible causes such as drugs, hypothermia, metabolic disorders, and shock should be excluded; and no improvement in the neurologic condition should occur during a period of observation. The duration of this period of observation was left to the clinical judgment of the physician. An observation period of from 6 to 12 hours was recommended, depending on whether a confirmatory test such as an EEG or cerebral blood flow study was performed, but could be shorter in certain circumstances. Observation for 24 hours was recommended in cases of anoxic brain damage.[10]

In 1995, the American Academy of Neurology published practice parameters for determining brain death in adults.[11] Brain death was selected as a topic for practice parameters because of the need for standardization of the neurologic examination criteria for the diagnosis of brain death, differences in clinical practice in performing the apnea test, and controversies over appropriate confirmatory laboratory tests.[11,12] This document outlines the clinical criteria for brain death and the procedures of testing in patients older than 18 years.[11] The recommendations for diagnosis in neonates and children have been published as a position paper by the American Academy of Pediatrics[13]; in addition, a review is available.[14]

BRAIN DEATH AND THE LAW

In 1970 Kansas became the first state to recognize that a legal determination of death can be made by establishing brain death.[15] Other states followed with similar statutes recognizing brain death. The exact wording of these statutes varied, however. These early statutes allowed medical professionals to use "ordinary standards of medical practice" to determine when death occurred, based on the cessation of either cardiopulmonary or brain function.[16]

In an attempt to standardize the various state legal definitions of death, the President's Commission for the Study of Ethical Problems in Medicine and Biomedical and Behavioral Research drafted the Uniform Determination of Death Act.[17] Published in 1981, this document was developed by the Commission working directly with delegates from national and state law associations and the American Medical Association. The act states: "An individual who has sustained either 1) irreversible cessation of circulatory and respiratory functions, or 2) irreversible cessation of all functions of the entire brain, including the brainstem, is dead. A determination of death must be made in accordance with accepted medical standards."

Although this model provided the legal foundation for defining brain death as death, the specific medical criteria for establishing the diagnosis were left unspecified.[10] "Accepted medical standards" were the criteria used to establish brain death in the Uniform Determination of Death Act. What constitutes these medical standards is a matter of law, determined by the trial courts on the basis of expert testimony regarding medical care given by physicians with similar training practicing under similar circumstances.[16]

Today all states and the District of Columbia have statutes for determining brain death based on the Uniform Determination of Death Act.[16] Most of these statutes use "accepted medical standards" as the criterion to establish brain death. Certain state statutes, however, differ in minor but important ways. Some require that brain death be determined by more than one physician, and some require that the hospital attempt to notify the next of kin before declaration of brain death.[16] In addition, state regulations differ with regard to details of brain death determination, or lack thereof. Ultimately, it becomes the responsibility of the individual hospital to develop policy and procedure for brain death determination that falls within the state regulations. It is important for physicians to know the state and hospital requirements for brain death.

DIAGNOSING BRAIN DEATH

As is evident from the preceding sections, minor differences exist among the various published medical criteria for brain death. Furthermore, although most states base their statutes on the Uniform Determination of Death Act, some variability in such statutes exists. These differences often lead to confusion when a member of the medical profession is faced with having to declare brain death in a comatose patient. To make matters worse, a survey published in 2004 by Powner and associates found that variation still exists among institutional policies with regard to the determination of brain death.[18] The position paper by the American Academy of Neurology on brain death may be consulted as a useful reference.[11,12] The following approach is offered as a general guideline in assessing a patient for brain death. More specific guidelines depend on individual state laws and local hospital policies.

Initiation of Brain Death Determination

Brain death can be considered in circumstances when catastrophic neurologic injury has occurred. Although trauma may be the most commonly considered cause, other sources of neurologic injury include hypertensive or aneurysmal hemorrhage, compressive brain tumors, and anoxic brain injury. Many of the patients evaluated on the basis of diagnosis alone will not meet the screening criteria on the initial examination, and continued resuscitation and evaluation will be necessary.

Although organ donation has played an important role in the evolution and the history of concept of brain death, it may be a consideration but should never be the driving force in the initiation of brain death determination. The separation of organ donation and brain death consideration is an important concept and certainly important for the patient's family to understand. Brain death may be a difficult concept for the layperson to understand, which is compounded by the inevitable stress of the current situation of a dying family member. Trust between the medical staff and the family can quickly erode if the family's perception is that the care team does not have their loved one's best interests in mind at all times.

Early conversations with the patient's family are a must. A good deal of education and reinforcement will be required about the nature of brain death and the fact that once brain death has occurred, the patient is declared dead and the time of death is recorded at the pronouncement.

Who Can Make the Determination of Brain Death?

The determination of brain death should be made by a physician who has experience in the neurologic assessment of comatose patients and the legal requirements for brain death. It is generally recommended (or required in some states) that this determination be carried out by an attending physician. At some clinical centers, testing must be carried out by a physician who has had training in neurology or neurosurgery.[19] In instances in which the patient is a potential organ donor, it is strongly recommended that the physician making the determination not be directly involved with the organ transplantation team; otherwise, a clear conflict of interest would be apparent.[20] Additionally, the physician should have no legal or economic conflicts of interest. Although most state statutes do not require that a neurosurgeon or a neurologist make the diagnosis, in cases in which a doubt about the diagnosis exists, consultation with an expert is recommended. As previously mentioned, some states require that the determination be made by two physicians.

What Are the Actual Criteria for Brain Death?

As stated in the Uniform Determination of Death Act, the criteria for brain death are based on "accepted medical standards." This would allow for the application of new technologies as they are developed and tested. Because actual criteria are not specified, and published criteria differ, how is a physician to be sure that he or she is practicing within medical standards? Such assurance is best obtained by examining the essential features of all current published criteria and applying them carefully in the context of local standards and legal statutes. All published brain death criteria share four common elements that need to be considered: (1) irreversibility, (2) absence of neurologic function, (3) apnea, and, although they are controversial, (4) additional confirmatory tests.[11] Again, the position paper by the American Academy of Neurology provides useful guidance for making this determination in adults.[11,12] Figure 63-1 outlines proposed guidelines for determining brain death.

Irreversibility

The central theme in irreversibility is recognition of a specific mechanism for the neurologic devastation and anatomic findings that are consistent with the mechanism. This concept has several features.

First, the cause of brain death should be established and be deemed sufficient to account for the neurologic picture. Severe head injury, intracerebral hemorrhage, and subarachnoid hemorrhage are the most common causes. Encephalitis, anoxic-ischemic encephalopathy, and meningitis are less common causes.[21] Evidence of reversible brain damage should be sought with computed tomography (CT) or magnetic resonance imaging when appropriate.[20] A normal CT scan should cast doubt on the diagnosis of brain death, and the diagnosis should be made only when a high degree of certainty exists about the mechanism that led to brain death.[21] If the CT scan is normal and definite evidence of an acute central nervous system catastrophe is lacking, a cerebrospinal fluid examination is warranted to evaluate for blood, inflammatory mediators, or protein and glucose abnormalities.[21] Reversible factors such as hypothermia (temperature lower than

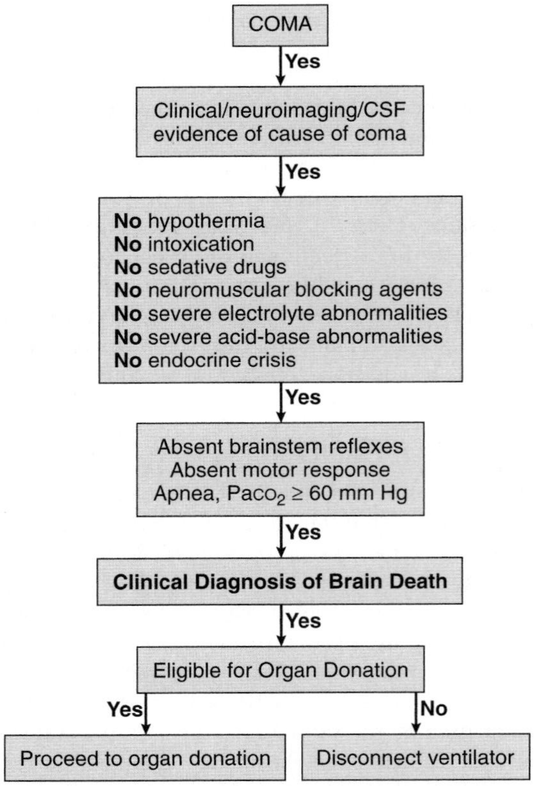

Figure 63-1. Algorithm incorporating proposed guidelines for the clinical diagnosis of brain death. CSF, cerebrospinal fluid. (Redrawn from Wijdicks EFM: Determining brain death in adults. Neurology 1995;45:1003.)

32.2° C or 90° F), shock, metabolic or endocrine disorders, acid-base disorders, drug intoxication and poisoning, or neuromuscular blocking drugs should be excluded. Finally, irreversibility is assumed if the neurologic examination shows no improvement over time.

The actual period of observation is a matter of clinical judgment.[10] Many standards use 6 hours as a minimum period, and most extend this observation period to 24 hours in cases of anoxic injury. No minimal observation period has been defined, however, and in certain instances (e.g., gross head trauma with brain avulsion), shorter periods of observation are sufficient. Similarly, no published guidelines are available on what serum levels of barbiturates or level of electrolyte or renal or hepatic abnormalities negate the diagnosis of brain death. Although the diagnosis of brain death should not be made in the presence of toxic levels of central nervous system depressants, clinicians disagree on whether brain death can be declared on clinical grounds when a therapeutic level of these drugs is present. Again, at present, this remains a matter of clinical judgment. Generally, the higher the drug level or the greater the metabolic abnormality, the longer the observation period should be. Alternatively, a confirmatory test demonstrating absent cerebral blood flow can be employed to establish irreversibility in cases where the role of potentially reversible disorders is unclear.[10,22,23]

The overarching concept is that of "certainty." For the declaration of brain death, interval examinations and use of different examiners attempt to ensure the consistency of the examination. Measurements of drug levels, electrolytes, body temperature, and so on attempt to ensure that none of these parameters is significant enough to impair the brainstem examination.

Absence of Neurologic Function

The cardinal clinical feature of brain death is the total absence of function of the entire brain (including brainstem) on neurologic examination. Box 63-1 lists the criteria for brain death from the American Academy of Neurology's position paper.[11] The patient should be unreceptive and in unresponsive coma. He or she should not react to stimuli, and motor responses of the limbs to painful stimuli should be absent (such responses should be differentiated from spinal reflexes). The presence of seizures or decerebrate or decorticate posturing negates the diagnosis of whole brain death.[9] Approximately one third of brain-dead patients will retain spinal stretch reflexes, so deep tendon or Babinski reflexes may be elicited.[8,24] Additionally, spontaneous movements of the limbs from spinal mechanisms have been reported and consist of rapid flexion of the arms, raising of all limbs or one limb off the bed, jerking of one leg, and walking-like movements.[21] Likewise, respiratory-type movements (shoulder elevation and adduction, back arching, intercostal expansion without significant tidal volumes) may occur and do not themselves indicate brainstem function.[11] Neurologic consultation is indicated when uncertainty exists about whether movement is of spinal or central origin.

All brainstem function should be absent. The pupils should be fixed and unreactive to a bright light. Although pupils were classically described as fixed and dilated in death, most pupils are in middle position (4 to 6 mm), but measurements of position may range from 4 to 9 mm.[21] Therefore, it is the unreactivity, not the size of the pupil, that is the crucial finding. It is important to remember, however, that most medication overdoses cause small pupils; the physician must be absolutely sure that presence of any of these medications has been excluded when the pupils are small. Corneal reflexes and oropharyngeal reflexes (to both gag and tracheal suction) should be absent. The patient should not grimace in response to painful stimuli. In patients with preexisting severe pupillary abnormalities or facial trauma, it may be difficult to test these reflexes, and additional confirmatory tests may be required. No movement of the eyes should occur in response to movement of the head or to the irrigation of each external auditory canal with 50 mL of ice water.

Finally, sweating, blushing, tachycardia, normal blood pressure without pharmacologic support, sudden increases in blood pressure, and lack of evidence of diabetes insipidus are occasionally seen in the brain-dead patient, and their presence (or absence) should not be interpreted as evidence of brainstem function.

Apnea

Complete apnea must exist for a diagnosis of brain death. Furthermore, because mechanical ventilation may remove the stimulus for spontaneous respiration, it is necessary to allow the $PaCO_2$ to rise to a level high enough to stimulate respiration by performing an apnea test. The $PaCO_2$ threshold for respiratory stimulation is not well defined in brain-injured patients and may be as high as 60 mm Hg. Apnea testing, as described next, cannot always be accomplished in every patient. Occasionally, coexisting lung disease causes the patient to experience O_2 desaturation before the $PaCO_2$ can rise to adequate levels. Additionally, apneic testing may be difficult in patients with chronic obstructive lung disease (COPD). Because the $PaCO_2$ in these patients often is already elevated, a $PaCO_2$ of 60 mm Hg may not provide a sufficient stimulus to breathe. These patients again require a rise in $PaCO_2$ of 20 mm Hg from their baseline to ensure an adequate stimulus for respiratory drive; unfortunately, this often is difficult to achieve. Some clinicians believe that certain patients with COPD require a hypoxic stimulus for ventilation, and this can be tested only by achieving an oxygen (O_2) tension (PaO_2) of 50 mm Hg.[25] As a general concept, hypoxemia should never be allowed in patients with neurologic dysfunction because of the possibility of worsening a potentially reversible injury. The presumption of reversibility of any brain injury should prevail during the testing period. In cases in which apnea testing cannot be completed, other confirmatory tests for brain death should be employed.

Apnea testing can be performed in a variety of ways.[26] However, because apnea testing can result in hypoxemia, thereby worsening a potentially reversible neurologic insult, the following prerequisites are suggested: core temperature of 36.5° C or greater, systolic blood pressure of 90 mm Hg or greater, euvolemia (or positive fluid balance in the previ-

Box 63-1

Diagnostic Criteria for Clinical Diagnosis of Brain Death

A. Prerequisites. Brain death is the absence of clinical brain function when the proximate cause is known and demonstrably irreversible.

1. Clinical or neuroimaging evidence of an acute central nervous system catastrophe that is compatible with the clinical diagnosis of brain death.
2. Exclusion of complicating medical conditions that may confound clinical assessment (no severe electrolyte, acid-base, or endocrine disturbance).
3. No drug intoxication or poisoning
4. Core temperature=32° C (90° F)

B. The three cardinal findings in brain death are coma or unresponsiveness, absence of brainstem reflexes, and apnea.

1. Coma or unresponsiveness—no cerebral motor response to pain in all extremities (nail bed pressure and supraorbital pressure).
2. Absence of brainstem reflexes.
   a. Pupils
      i. No response to bright light
      ii. Size: midposition (4 mm) to dilated (9 mm)
   b. Ocular movement
      i. No oculocephalic reflex (testing only when no fracture or instability of the cervical spine is apparent)
      ii. No deviation of the eyes to irrigation in each ear with 50 mL of cold water (allow 1 minute after injection and at least 5 minutes between testing on each side)
   c. Facial sensation and facial motor response
      i. No corneal reflex to touch with a throat swab
      ii. No jaw reflex
      iii. No grimacing to deep pressure on nail bed, supraorbital ridge, or temporomandibular joint
   d. Pharyngeal and tracheal reflexes
      i. No response after stimulation of the posterior pharynx with tongue blade
      ii. No cough response to bronchial suctioning
3. Apnea testing performed as follows:
   a. Prerequisites
      i. Core temperature ≥36.5° C or 97° F
      ii. Systolic blood pressure ≥90 mm Hg
      iii. Euvolemia. *Option:* Positive fluid balance in the previous 6 hours
      iv. Normal $Pa{CO_2}$. *Option:* Arterial $Pa{CO_2}$ ≥40 mm Hg
      v. Normal $Pa{O_2}$. *Option:* Preoxygenation to obtain arterial $Pa{O_2}$ ≥200 mm Hg
   b. Connect a pulse oximeter and disconnect the ventilator.
   c. Deliver 100% O_2, 6 L/min, into the trachea. *Option:* Place a cannula at the level of the carina.
   d. Look closely for respiratory movements (abdominal or chest excursions that produce adequate tidal volumes).
   e. Measure $Pa{O_2}$, $Pa{CO_2}$, and pH after approximately 8 minutes and reconnect the ventilator.
   f. If respiratory movements are absent and arterial pressure is ≥60 mm Hg (*option:* 20 mm Hg increase in $Pa{CO_2}$ over a baseline normal $Pa{CO_2}$), the apnea test result is positive (i.e., it supports the diagnosis of brain death).
   g. If respiratory movements are observed, the apnea test result is negative (i.e., it does not support the clinical diagnosis of brain death), and the test should be repeated.
   h. Connect the ventilator if, during testing, the systolic blood pressure becomes ≤90 mm Hg or the pulse oximeter indicates significant oxygen desaturation,or cardiac arrhythmias are present; immediately draw an arterial blood sample and analyze arterial blood gas. If $Pa{CO_2}$ is ≥60 mm Hg or $Pa{CO_2}$ increase is ≥20 mm Hg over baseline normal $Pa{CO_2}$, the apnea test result is positive (it supports the clinical diagnosis of brain death); if $Pa{CO_2}$ is <60 mm Hg or $Pa{CO_2}$ increase is <20 mm Hg over baseline normal $Pa{CO_2}$, the result is indeterminate, and an additional confirmatory test can be considered.

From Report of the Quality Standards Subcommittee of the American Academy of Neurology: Practice parameters for determining brain death in adults (summary statement). Neurology 1995;45:1012.

ous 6 hours), normal $Pa{CO_2}$ ($Pa{CO_2}$ of 40 mm Hg or greater), and a normal $Pa{O_2}$ with an option of preoxygenation to obtain a $Pa{O_2}$ of 200 mm Hg or greater.[11] An arterial blood gas should be obtained before disconnection of the ventilator to ensure the foregoing criteria have been met.

The preferred method to test for apnea involves preoxygenation and passive (apneic) oxygenation.[24] The test should always begin at a normal pH and $Pa{CO_2}$ level. The patient should be preoxygenated for at least 10 minutes with 100% O_2 before testing. Heart rate and rhythm, O_2 saturation, and blood pressure should be continually monitored. Ideally, end-tidal pressure of carbon dioxide also should be monitored. After preoxygenation, the respirator is disconnected and the patient is placed on a T piece with 100% O_2. Additionally, many physicians place a catheter carrying 100% O_2 at 6 L per minute in the endotracheal tube proximal to the carina, to help prevent hypoxia. The patient is observed closely for respiratory movements (abdominal or chest excursions that produce adequate tidal volumes). After approximately 8 minutes, PaO_2, $PaCO_2$, and pH are measured and the ventilator is reconnected. If respiratory movements are absent at this time and $PaCO_2$ is 60 mm Hg or greater (or the $PaCO_2$ has increased 20 mm Hg over a baseline normal $PaCO_2$), the apnea test result is positive (i.e., it supports the diagnosis of brain death). If respiratory movements are observed, the apnea test result is negative (i.e., it does not support the clinical diagnosis of brain death). The test should be repeated at some future time if the findings on clinical examination continue to be consistent with brain death. If during testing, the systolic blood pressure becomes 90 mm Hg or less the pulse oximeter indicates significant oxygen desaturation, or cardiac arrhythmias are present, the ventilator is immediately reconnected and an arterial blood sample is drawn for blood gas analysis. If $PaCO_2$ is 60 mm Hg or greater or $PaCO_2$ increase is 20 mm Hg or more over baseline normal $PaCO_2$, the apnea test result is positive (it supports the clinical diagnosis of brain death). If $PaCO_2$ is less than 60 mm Hg or the $PaCO_2$ increase is less than 20 mm Hg above baseline normal $PaCO_2$, the result is considered indeterminate. The apnea test may be repeated with a longer duration of observation (as long as the patient remains stable and maintains good oxygen saturation) or an additional confirmatory test may be considered.

Additional Confirmatory Tests

Brain death is a clinical diagnosis. The use of confirmatory tests for the diagnosis of brain death is controversial. The President's Commission did not require their routine use in situations in which the foregoing criteria of irreversibility, absence of brain function, and apnea are met.[10] However, the Commission did recommend their use when brainstem reflexes are not testable, when the cause of brain death is not fully established, or when it is desirable to shorten the period of observation.[10] Most institutions follow these recommendations and use confirmatory tests only in special circumstances.

A variety of confirmatory tests presently are used to support the diagnosis of brain death. It should be emphasized that any of the suggested confirmatory tests may produce similar results in patients with catastrophic brain damage who do not (yet) fulfill the clinical criteria of brain death.[11] These tests can provide strong evidence of brain death, but all have their limitations and must be applied only when other clinical criteria for brain death are satisfied. They can be broadly classified into two categories: those that evaluate cerebral function and those that evaluate intracranial blood flow. Blood flow to the brainstem itself is not qualified separately by any testing method and is not required by the American Academy of Neurology practice parameters.

An EEG may be extremely helpful in evaluating a patient with suspected brain death. Cerebral activity seen on an EEG implies functioning brain tissue and refutes the diagnosis of brain death. Once found, it cannot be ignored. Electrocerebral silence, defined as the absence of any EEG activity of cerebral origin greater than 2 μV in amplitude during a 30-minute recording, done as recommended by the Ad Hoc Committee on EEG Criteria for Cerebral Death, is the EEG finding in brain death. In the NIH study of brain death, if all patients with drug-induced comas were eliminated, no patients recovered after having a 30-minute isoelectric EEG.[8] Therefore, in the absence of drugs, an isoelectric EEG provides good supportive evidence for the diagnosis of brain death. The EEG is not infallible, however, and the diagnosis of brain death should not be based solely on a single isoelectric EEG. Patients with drug-induced coma, cerebral trauma, hypothermia, and encephalitis have recovered after a single isoelectric EEG.[8,27,28] Additionally, the EEG often is difficult to perform in the artifact-rich environment of today's intensive care unit (ICU) and is subject to observer error in about 3% of records.[8]

The usefulness of somatosensory evoked potentials (SEPs) in the evaluation of brain death is controversial.[29] SEPs test the integrity of the sensory pathways. For this evaluation, a repetitive stimulus (usually electrical) is applied to a sensory nerve in the upper or lower extremity, and various waves generated by anatomic structures in the spinal cord, lemniscal pathways, and cortex are recorded. These evoked potentials are not ablated by barbiturates but are limited in that they test only one anatomic pathway. The most common SEP finding in brain death is the presence of a response over the cervical spinal cord with the absence of all later responses.[30,31] Unfortunately, some patients who are not brain dead but in a PVS exhibit similar findings, and in rare instances, patients with this pattern have survived with normal neurologic function.[32] For these reasons, the use of SEPs is not advocated in the evaluation of brain death.

Cerebral angiography documenting no intracerebral filling at the level of the carotid bifurcation or circle of Willis is the most sensitive confirmatory test for brain death. However, this technique is cumbersome, expensive, and seldom used clinically.

Transcranial Doppler ultrasonography (TCD) has been used over the past 2 decades to evaluate cerebral blood flow, and its application as a confirmatory test in the diagnosis of brain death has been the subject of several studies and the focus of an international task force.[33-36] Comparison of TCD with angiography revealed a strong correlation between both methods in determining the absence of intracranial blood flow.[35,37] TCD uses low-frequency ultrasound to visualize or insonate the major vessels of the intracranial and extracranial arterial tree. The anterior, middle and posterior cerebral arteries all are accessed via a transtemporal window while the vertebral arteries are insonated via a transoccipital window. The internal carotid artery is insonated through a transocular window. Bilateral evaluation is mandatory. The flow velocities can be affected by significant changes in cardiac output, $PaCO_2$, and hematocrit. Even in competent hands, the initial absence of Doppler signals cannot be interpreted as consistent with brain death because of absence of temporal insonation windows or other technical or transmission problems. Reported TCD findings in patients with brain death are absent or reversal of flow in diastole and a sharp systolic upstroke, or small spike waveforms either above or both above and below the baseline at the

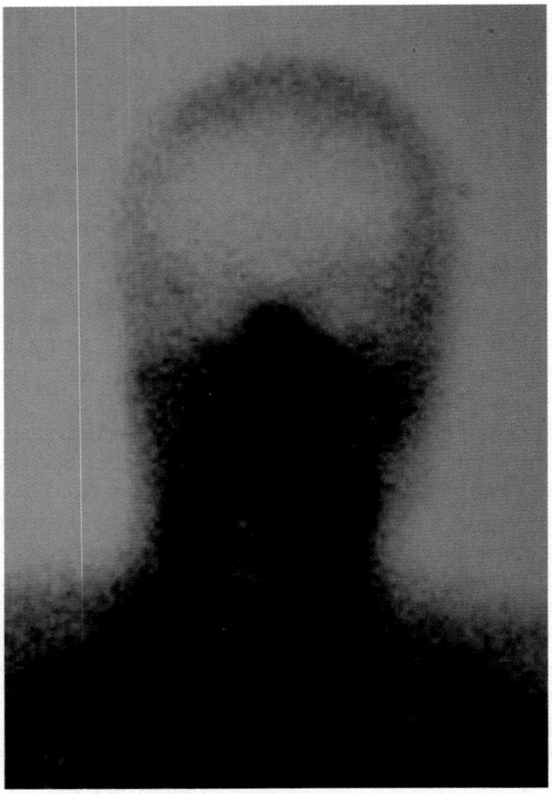

Figure 63-2. Technetium-99m brain scan showing the classic "hollow skull phenomenon."

beginning of systole.[38,39] This latter pattern of small systolic peaks in early systole without diastolic flow or reverberating flow indicates very high vascular resistance associated with greatly increased intracranial pressure and is the TCD finding in brain death used in the American Academy of Neurology's position paper.[11]

The technetium-99m hexamethylpropyleneamineoxime (technetium-99m HM-PAO) brain scan also is used as a confirmatory test for brain death.[11] In brain death, no uptake of isotope is seen in the brain parenchyma ("hollow skull phenomenon") (Fig. 63-2). Although large, well-controlled trials have not been performed, sensitivity has been reported to be 94%, with a specificity of 100%.[40] Additionally, the correlation between cerebral angiography and technetium-99m HM-PAO scanning was found to be excellent in one study.[41]

It should be noted that in rare cases, cerebral blood flow may be maintained in the presence of brain death. Such cases present very great difficulty in diagnosis and may require additional confirmatory testing.[42] With craniectomy becoming a more commonly practiced therapy to relieve intracranial hypertension, this conundrum may become more commonplace.

PERSISTENT VEGETATIVE STATE

Although knowledge of the medical and legal criteria for declaring brain death is important for physicians caring for severely brain-injured patients, a diagnosis of brain death is actually made in relatively few instances.[12] A much more common scenario in today's ICU is that in which a patient has suffered a severe anoxic or traumatic brain injury and is left in a deep coma but with partially preserved brainstem function. When clinical improvement does not occur, this condition is termed the *persistent vegetative state* (PVS). The exact prevalence of the PVS in the United States is unknown, but the number of affected patients is estimated to be in excess of 15,000.[43] The care of patients in the PVS can be extremely difficult and emotionally trying because of uncertainty about the prognosis and about the major ethical and legal issues that may arise. Additionally, much confusion still remains among physicians as to how to diagnose the PVS. Because the PVS is similar in some respects to brain death and is a common ICU problem, it is important to define it precisely and to characterize appropriate care of these patients.

Brain death and PVS share many common features. Both are caused by death of neurons in the brain, and both necessarily are secondary to disorders capable of causing neuronal loss. In both conditions, the potential for cognition is totally and permanently lost.[44] They differ, however, in several important ways: (1) brain death is death of the entire brain including the brainstem, whereas PVS is caused by the total loss of forebrain functions; and (2) patients with a diagnosis of brain death are dead both legally and medically; patients with PVS are not.

In 1994 and 1995, the Multispecialty Task Force on PVS and the Quality Standards Subcommittee of the American Academy of Neurology reviewed all of the literature on the PVS and issued a series of reports and guidelines.[45-47] These documents have been instrumental in summarizing current knowledge about the PVS and in helping physicians rationally address management issues in patients with severe brain injury. The Multispecialty Task Force defines the *vegetative state* as "a clinical condition of complete unawareness of the self and the environment, accompanied by sleep-wake cycles, with either complete or partial preservation of hypothalamic and brainstem autonomic functions. In addition, patients in a vegetative state show no evidence of sustained, reproducible, purposeful, or voluntary behavioral responses to visual, auditory, tactile, or noxious stimuli; show no evidence of language comprehension or expression; have bowel and bladder incontinence; and have variably preserved cranial nerve and spinal reflexes."[48]

The *persistent* vegetative state is defined as a vegetative state present at 1 month after acute traumatic or nontraumatic brain injury, or present for at least 1 month in patients with degenerative or metabolic disorders or developmental malformations.[45-47]

The *permanent* vegetative state means an irreversible state—a definition, as with all clinical diagnoses in medicine, based on probabilities, not absolutes.[45-47] A patient in a PVS becomes permanently vegetative when irreversibility can be established with a high degree of clinical certainty (i.e., when the chance of regaining consciousness is exceedingly rare).

The Multispecialty Task Force found that the PVS can be diagnosed on clinical grounds with a high degree of medical certainty in most adult and pediatric patients after careful, repeated neurologic examinations. The Task Force investigtors recommend that the diagnosis of PVS be established by a physician who, by reason of training and experience, is competent in neurologic function assessment and diagnosis. Additionally, they found that reliable criteria do not exist for making a diagnosis of PVS in infants younger than 3 months of age, except in patients with anencephaly. Adjunctive diagnostic studies may support the diagnosis of PVS, but none adds to diagnostic specificity with certainty.[45-47]

Three major categories of diseases in adults and children may result in PVS. In studies of these categories (described later on), the Multispecialty Task Force found that the clinical course and outcome of PVS patients were highly correlated with its specific etiology.[45-47] An additional classification of neurologic status related to the PVS is the minimally conscious state, described next.

Minimally Conscious State

Recent years have seen an effort to further characterize patients in a poorly responsive state. This effort has led to recognition of the diagnosis of a *minimally conscious state* (MCS).[49] These patients differ from those in a PVS in having some preservation of environmental awareness. Patients can be said to be in this state if they demonstrate one or more of the following: (1) ability to follow simple commands; (2) capability of gesture or verbal yes-or-no answers, regardless of accuracy; (3) intelligible verbalization; or (4) purposeful behavior in response to external stimuli such as smiling or crying, vocalizations or gestures, reaching for objects, touching or holding objects, or pursuit eye movements. Although initially met with some skepticism,[50] MCS has become an accepted diagnosis. The definition of this condition and the prognosis for affected persons are likely to evolve as new data are gathered.[51]

Acute Traumatic and Nontraumatic Brain Injury

In patients who have suffered acute brain injury, the PVS usually evolves within 1 month of injury from a state of eyes-closed coma to a state of wakefulness without awareness with sleep-wake cycles and preserved brainstem functions. As described later on, however, the prognosis differs significantly for traumatic and for nontraumatic brain injury.

Degenerative and Metabolic Disorders of the Brain

Many degenerative and metabolic nervous system disorders inevitably progress toward an irreversible vegetative state. For patients in whom neurologic function is severely impaired but who retain some degree of awareness, a temporary encephalopathy (i.e., resulting from medication or infection) must be corrected before establishing that the patient is in PVS. If the vegetative state persists for several months, recovery of consciousness is unlikely.

Severe Developmental Malformations of the Nervous System

The developmental vegetative state is a form of PVS present in some infants and children with severe congenital malformations of the nervous system. These children do not acquire awareness of the self or the environment. This diagnosis can be made at birth only in infants with anencephaly. For children with other severe malformations who appear vegetative at birth, observation for 3 to 6 months is recommended to determine whether awareness is acquired. A majority of such infants who are vegetative at birth remain vegetative; those who acquire awareness usually recover only to a severe disability.

Having extensively reviewed all available literature on PVS, the Multispecialty Task Force looked at prognosis for recovery in these various categories.[45-47] Recovery from PVS was defined in terms of recovery of consciousness and recovery of function. Recovery of consciousness was verified when a patient showed reliable evidence of awareness of self and the environment, consistent appearance of voluntary behavioral responses to visual and auditory stimuli, and interaction with others. Recovery of function was verified when a patient became mobile and was able to communicate and learn, perform adaptive skills and self-care, and participate in recreational or vocational activities. On the basis of the available data, the Multispecialty Task Force found that recovery of consciousness from posttraumatic PVS after 12 months in adults and children is unlikely. Recovery from nontraumatic PVS after 3 months is exceedingly rare. Several individual case reports, however, describe verified late recoveries of consciousness from traumatic (beyond 12 months) or nontraumatic (beyond 3 months) injury.[52,53]

On the basis of these findings, the Quality Standards Subcommittee of the American Academy of Neurology recommended the following diagnostic standards for adults in the PVS:

- The vegetative state is diagnosable. It is defined as being persistent at 1 month.
- The PVS can be judged to be permanent 12 months after traumatic injury.
- The PVS can be judged to be permanent for nontraumatic injury after 3 months.
- The chance for recovery after these periods is exceedingly low, and recovery is almost always to a severe disability.[45]

Much has been written in the past decade regarding certain aspects of care of the patient in the PVS.[14-17,21,44,54-57] Advances in the law through landmark decisions in the Quinlan case, the Brophy case, the Jobes case, and others have supported the patient's right to forego medical support, including fluid and nutrition, when further care is not considered beneficial.[58-61] In 2005 the Terri Schiavo case ignited national and international debate and brought the diagnosis of persistent vegetative state into public discussions.[62,63] Because of the complex ethical, legal, and moral issues involved in withdrawal of support from these patients, the American Academy of Neurology has published recommendations on the management and care of the PVS patient.[45,55,64] These recommendations reaffirm that patients in PVS should receive appropriate medical, nursing, or home care to maintain their personal dignity and hygiene.[45] Furthermore, these guidelines state that physicians caring for PVS patients have the responsibility of discussing with the family or surrogates the probabilities of the patient's attaining the various stages of recovery or remaining in a PVS.

Additionally, physicians and the family must determine appropriate levels of treatment relative to the administration or withdrawal of the following:

- Medications and other commonly ordered treatments
- Supplemental oxygen and use of antibiotics
- Complex organ-sustaining treatments such as dialysis
- Administration of blood products
- Artificial hydration and nutrition

The guidelines also state that "once PVS is considered to be permanent, a 'Do Not Resuscitate' (DNR) order is appropriate. A DNR order includes no ventilatory or cardiopulmonary resuscitation. The decision to implement a DNR order, however, may be made earlier in the course of the patient's illness if there is an advance directive or agreement by the appropriate surrogate of the patient and the physician (or physicians) responsible for the care of the patient."[45]

Additionally, the American College of Chest Physicians and the Society for Critical Care Medicine have issued ethical and moral guidelines for the initiation, continuation, and withdrawal of care.[65] Although local laws may vary, these documents are extremely helpful in guiding individual decisions regarding the care of PVS patients.

BRAIN DEATH AND ORGAN DONATION

One of the major factors that led to much of today's legislation on brain death was the need for well-perfused organs for donation. Despite legislation such as the Uniform Anatomical Gift Act and the Uniform Determination of Death Act, the need for organs is still increasing.[66,67] Patients in ICUs provide 98% of donated organs.[30] Many potential organ donations, however, are lost because of the failure to recognize potential donors and approach the family for permission to use the deceased patient's organs and because of inadequate donor management in the ICU before organ procurement.

Some physicians are reluctant to approach family members regarding donation for fear of subjecting them to additional stresses.[68] Follow-up studies with donor families, however, have found that in many instances the donation actually lessened their grief.[66,67] The physician's attitude and approach to the request for donation are critical factors in the organ donation process. Positive characteristics of the request that appear to be related to family consent include (1) the certainty of the brain death declaration, (2) an informative and sensitive request, (3) the presence of other family members for support, (4) knowledgeable and supportive medical personnel, (5) the presence of a donor card signed by the deceased, and (6) an appropriately timed request.[69] With regard to this last point, it has been shown that family approval is much more likely with a clear temporal separation between the explanation of death or the certainty of family acceptance of death and the request for donation.[70] Additionally, family permission is more likely if the physician first makes the declaration of brain death and then the organ transplantation team makes the request for organ donation. This approach separates the roles of each group and minimizes the perception that the physician is being influenced by other factors (such as the need by another patient for an organ) to make the brain death pronouncement prematurely.

As a result of the continued shortage of viable organs for transplantation, there is renewed interest in donations from non–heart-beating donors. Non–heart-beating donation is the process by which organs are recovered from patients after the pronouncement of death by *cardiopulmonary criteria.* Although these patients typically are severely brain-injured, it is important to realize that they are not brain dead. The ethical and social issues surrounding this controversial topic are beyond the scope of this chapter and are considered elsewhere.[71-74]

INTERACTIONS WITH THE FAMILY

There are few situations in clinical medicine in which effective communication is more vital than in dealing with family and friends during discussions of brain death, the PVS, and organ donation. It is the physician's responsibility to ensure that effective communication occurs. Ideally, this role is best accomplished by the physician. However, if he or she is not comfortable with this role or is not a good communicator, the assistance of a facilitator should be enlisted. Chaplains, psychologists, nurses, social workers, or members of the hospital ethics committee may serve in this role.

The following guidelines have been proposed for effective communication with families.[25] First, an environment that fosters communication should be created. These discussions should be in an office or lounge and should be free of interruptions. They should not take place in a hospital corridor. The discussion should not be rushed, and the family should be encouraged to ask questions and express their feelings. Communication should be kept simple until it is clear that more detail will be helpful rather than overwhelming. Asking the family to summarize its understanding of the situation at the end of the discussion is a good way to be sure the communication has been effective. Because questions often arise after the discussion is complete, the family should be assured that the physician is amenable to further talks and should be encouraged to approach him or her with their concerns and questions.

In cases of suspected brain death, it is helpful for the physician to raise this possibility with the family while performing the brain death evaluation. This prepares them for the possibility and allows them to notify other family members. After brain death is diagnosed, the family should be notified in simple terms that the patient is dead. Privacy, religious and emotional support, and an opportunity for the family to visit the body should be ensured. The patient should then be taken to the operating room if organ donation is being performed. Otherwise, the patient should be removed from the ventilator. Generally, this should be done after the family has left because possible spinal-mediated movements may be misinterpreted by the family and further upset them.

SUMMARY

Brain-dead patients in the United States are considered dead both medically and legally. The essentials of the brain death determination lie in (1) establishing irreversibility through a compatible history, the exclusion of reversible disorders, and a period of observation; (2) a neurologic examination demonstrating unresponsiveness and the absence of brainstem reflexes; (3) demonstrating apnea to an adequate CO_2 stimulus; and (4) the use of additional tests in infants and children or when there is doubt about the diagnosis.

It is critical that the physician be knowledgeable about local and state brain death statutes because these may show minor but important differences. Finally, special care and time must be given to the families in addressing the various medical and ethical issues related to management of patients with severe neurologic injuries.

KEY POINTS

- Until the advent of the mechanical ventilator, death was defined by the cessation of cardiac and respiratory function. With the invention of the modern ventilator, a new definition of death based on the cessation of neurologic function was necessary. Brain-dead patients are medically and legally dead.
- The concept of brain death in the United States is based on the whole brain concept, which states that a brain that no longer functions and has no possibility of functioning again is for all purposes dead.
- Essential clinical characteristics of brain death include the following: (1) Demonstration that the cause of the brain death is irreversible by excluding all reversible causes and by an appropriate period of observation. (2) Total absence of function of the entire brain including brainstem on neurologic examination. The patient should be unreceptive and totally unresponsive and should not react to stimuli or exhibit spontaneous movement of any kind. The presence of seizures negates the diagnosis of brain death. (3) Demonstration of apnea.
- The use of confirmatory tests for the diagnosis of brain death in adults is controversial and at the discretion of the treating physician. Such tests are recommended when brainstem reflexes or the presence of apnea cannot be fully evaluated or when it is desirable to shorten the period of observation.
- The legal criteria for diagnosing brain death vary from state to state. Although most such criteria are based on the Uniform Determination of Death Act, it is important for physicians to be aware of their state's statutes. The Uniform Determination of Death Act uses "accepted medical standards" as the medical criteria to establish brain death.
- A common problem in ICUs is the management of patients in the PVS. The PVS is a form of eyes-open, permanent unconsciousness in which the patient has periods of wakefulness and physiologic sleep-wake cycles but at no time is aware of self or the environment.
- Guidelines are available for dealing with the many complex ethical, legal, and moral issues involved with the care of these patients. Although local laws regarding the care of the PVS patient may vary, these documents are extremely helpful in guiding individual decisions regarding the care of these patients.
- Special care and time must be given to the families of these patients in addressing the various medical and ethical issues surrounding brain death and the PVS.

REFERENCES

1. Powner DJ, Ackerman BM, Grenvik A: Medical diagnosis of death in adults: Historical contributions to current controversies. Lancet 1996;348:1219-1223.
2. Farrell MM, Levin MF: Brain death in the pediatric patient: Historical, sociological, medical, religious, cultural, legal, and ethical considerations. Crit Care Med 1993;21(12):1951-1965.
3. Fisher CM: The neurologic examination of the comatose patient. Acta Neurol Scand 1969;45(suppl 36):1.
4. Jouvet M: Diagnostic electro-sous-cortico-graphique de la mort du systeme nerveux central au cours de certain comas. Electroencephalogr Clin Neurophysiol 1959;11:805-808.
5. Schwab R, Potts F, Bonazzi A: EEG as an aid in determining death in the presence of cardiac activity (ethical, legal, and medical aspects). Electroencephalogr Clin Neurophysiol 1963;15:147.
6. Ad Hoc Committee of the Harvard Medical School to Examine the Definition of Brain Death: A definition of irreversible coma. JAMA 1968;205:337-340.
7. A Statement issued by the Honorary Secretary of the Conference of Medical Royal Colleges and Their Facilities in the United Kingdom. BMJ 1976;2:1187-1188.
8. National Institute of Neurologic and Communicative Disorders and Stroke: An appraisal of the criteria of cerebral death: A summary statement. JAMA 1977;237:982-986.
9. Flowers W Jr, Patel BR: Accuracy of clinical evaluation in the determination of brain death. South Med J 2000;93:203-206.
10. Medical Consultants on the Diagnosis of Death to the President's Commission for the Study of Ethical Problems in Medicine and Biomedical and Behavioral Research: Guidelines for the determination of death. JAMA 1981;246:2184-2186.
11. Report of the Quality Standards Subcommittee of the American Academy of Neurology: Practice parameters for determining brain death in adults (summary statement). Neurology 1995;45:1012-1014.
12. Wijdicks E: Determining brain death in adults. Neurology 1995;45:1003-1011.
13. American Academy of Pediatrics: Report of Special Task Force: Guidelines for the determination of brain death in children. Pediatrics 1987;80:298-300.
14. Lynch J, Eldadah M: Brain-death criteria currently used by pediatric intensivists. Clin Pediatr 1992;31:457-460.
15. Frist W, Fanning W: Donor management and matching. Cardiol Clin 1990;8:55-71.
16. Diringer M: When to stop treatment: Concepts in brain death and withdrawal of futile lifesustaining interventions. Paper presented at the Annual Meeting of the American Academy of Neurology: Critical Care and Emergency Neurology, San Diego, Calif, 1992.
17. President's Commission for the Study of Ethical Problems in Medicine and Biomedical and Behavorial Research:

A Report of the Medical, Legal, and Ethical Problems in Medicine and Biomedical and Behavioral Research. U.S. Government Printing Office, Washington. DC, 1981.
18. Powner D, Hernandez M, Rives T: Variability among hospital policies for determining brain death in adults. Crit Care Med 2004;32(6):1284-1288.
19. Linde-Zwirble M, Bishop B, Menker J: Management of the organ donor: A first step in transplantation. Crit Care Nurs Q 1991;13:19-24.
20. Gentleman D, Easton J, Jennett B: Brain death and organ donation in a neurosurgical unit: Audit of recent practice. BMJ (Clin Res Ed) 1990;301:1203-1206.
21. Wijdicks E: The Clinical Practice of Critical Care Neurology. Lippincott-Raven, Philadelphia, 1997.
22. Prager M: Care of organ donors. Int Anesthesiol Clin 1991;29:1-16.
23. Darby JM, Stein K, Grenvik A, et al: Approach to management of the heartbeating "brain dead" organ donor. JAMA 1989;261:2222-2228.
24. Robertson K, Cook D: Perioperative management of the mutiorgan donor. Anesth Analges J 1990;70: 546-556.
25. Ruark J, Raffin T: Initiating and withdrawing life support: Principles and practice in adult medicine. N Engl J Med 1988;318:25-30.
26. Earnest M, Beresford H, McIntyre H: Test for apnea in suspected brain death: Methods used by 129 clinicians. Neurology 1986;36:542-544.
27. Bricolo A, Benati A, Mazza C: Prolonged isoelectric EEG in a case of post-traumatic coma. Electroencephalogr Clin Neurophysiol 1971;31:174.
28. Tentler R, Sadove M, Beck D: Electroencephalographic evidence of cortical "death" followed by full recovery: Protective action of hypothermia. JAMA 1957;164:1667.
29. Aminoff MJ: The use of somatosensory evoked potentials in the evaluation of the central nervous system. Neurol Clin 1988;6:809.
30. Goldie W, Chiappa KH, Young RR, et al: Brainstem auditory and short-latency somatosensory evoked responses in brain death. Neurology 1981;31: 248-256.
31. Belsh J, Chokroverty S: Short-latency evoked potentials in brain dead patients. Electroencephalogr Clin Neurophysiol 1987;68:75.
32. Newlon P, Greenberg RP, Enas GG, et al: Effect of therapeutic phenobarbital coma on multimodality evoked potentials recorded from severely head injured patients. Neurosurgery 1983;12:613-619.
33. Petty G, Wiebers D, Meissner I: Transcranial Doppler ultrasonography: Clinical applications in cerebrovascular disease. Mayo Clin Proc 1990;65:1350-1364.
34. Hadani M, Bruk B, Ram Z, et al: Application of transcranial Doppler ultrasonography for the diagnosis of brain death. Intensive Care Med 1999;25:822-828.
35. Ducrocq X, Braun M, Debouverie M, et al: Brain death and transcranial Doppler: Experience in 130 cases of brain patients. J Neurol Sci 1998;160: 46-46.
36. Ducrocq X, Nassler W, Moritake K, et al: Consensus opinion on diagnosis of cerebral circulatory arrest using Doppler-sonography: Task Force Group on cerebral death of the Neurosonology Research Group of the World Federation of Neurology. J Neurol Sci 1998;159: 145-150.
37. DeFreitas G, Andre C: Sensitivity of transcranial Doppler for confirming brain death: A prospective study of 270 cases. Acta Neurol Scand 2006;113(6):426-432.
38. Petty G, Mohr JP, Pedley TA, et al: The role of transcranial Doppler in confirming brain death: Sensitivity, specificity, and suggestions for performance and interpretation. Neurology 1990;40:300-303.
39. Ropper A, Kehne S, Wechsler L: Transcranial Doppler in brain death. Neurology 1987;37:1733-1755.
40. George M: Establishing brain death: The potential role of nuclear medicine in the search for a reliable confirmatory test. Eur J Nucl Med 1991;18:75-77.
41. Laurin N, Driedler AA, Hurwite GA, et al: Cerebral Perfusion Imaging with technetium-99m HM-PAO in brain death and severe central nervous system injury. J Nucl Med 1989;30:1627-1635.
42. Flowers W Jr, Bharti R: Persistence of cerebral blood flow after brain death. South Med J 2000;93:364-367.
43. Hirsch J: Raising conciousness. J Clin Invest 2005;115:1102 (Editorial).
44. Young B, Blume W, Lynch A: Brain death and the persistent vegetative state: Similarities and contrasts. Can J Neurol Sci 1989;16:388-393 (Editorial).
45. Practice parameters: Assessment and management of patients in the persistent vegetative state (summary statement). Neurology 1995;45:1015-1018.
46. Multi-Society Task Force on PVS: Medical aspects of the persistent vegatative state (1). N Engl J Med 1994;330:1499-1508.
47. Multi-Society Task Force on PVS: Medical aspects of the persistent vegetative state (2). N Engl J Med 1994;330:1572-1579.
48. Ashwal S, Cranford R, Rosenberg J: Commentary on the practice parameters for the persistent vegetative state. Neurology 1995;45:859-860.
49. Giacino P, Ashwal S, Childs N, et al: The minimally conscious state. Definition and diagnostic criteria. Neurology 2002;58:349-353.
50. Shewmon D: The minimally concious state: Definition and diagnostic criteria. Neurology, 2002;58:506 (letter).
51. Wijdicks E, Cranford R: Clinical diagnosis of prolonged states of impaired consciousness in adults. Mayo Clin Proc 2005;80(8):1037-1046.
52. Rosenberg G, Johnson S, Brenner R: Recovery of cognition after prolonged vegetative state. Ann Neurol 1977;2:167.
53. Shuttleworth E: Recovery to social and economic independence from prolonged postanoxic vegetative state. Neurology 1983;33:372-374.
54. Sprung C: Changing attitudes and practices in forgoing life-sustaining treatments. JAMA 1990;263:2211-2215.
55. Munsat T, Stuart W, Cranford R: Guidelines on the vegetative state. Commentary on the American Academy of Neurology Statement (editorial). Neurology 1989;39:123-124.
56. Golden G: Medical-legal aspects of neurologic problems. Current Prob Pediatr 1991;21:259-281.
57. Singer P, Siegler M: Elective use of life-sustaining treatments in internal medicine. Adv Intern Med 1991;36:57-79.
58. In the matter of Karen Quinlan. NJ Superior 277, 348 A2d 801, 1975.
59. Brophy *v.* New England Sinai Hospital Inc. 497 NE2d 626, 1986.
60. Matter of Jobes. 529 A2d 434, 1987.
61. In re Conroy. 486 A2d 1209, 1985.
62. Hook C, Mueller P: The Terri Schiavo saga: The making of a tragedy and lessons learned. Mayo Clin Proc 2005;80(11):1449-1460.
63. Wijdicks E: Minimally concious vs. persistent vegetative state: The case of Terry (Wallis) vs Terri (Schiavo). Mayo Clin Proc 2006;81(9):1155-1158.
64. Executive Board of the American Academy of Neurology: Position of the American Academy of Neurology on certain aspects and management of the persistent vegetative state patient. Neurology 1989;39:125-126.
65. American College of Chest Physicians/ Society for Critical Care Medicine Consensus Panel: Ethical and moral guidelines for the inititaion, continuation, and withdrawal of intensive care. Chest 1990;97:949-958.
66. Bartucci M: Organ donation: A study of the donor family perspective. J Neurosci Nurs 1987;19:305-359.
67. Morton J, Leonard D: Cadaver nephrectomy: An operation on the donor's family. BMJ (Clin Res Ed) 1979;1:239.
68. River E, Busc SM, Birens BA, et al: Organ and tissue procurement in the acute care setting: Principles and practice. Ann Emerg Med 1990;19: 78-85.
69. Perkins K: The shortage of cadaver donor organs for transplantation: Can psychology help? Am Psychol 1987;42:921-930.
70. Garrison R, Bently FR, Raque GH, et al: There is an answer to the shortage of organ donors. Surg Gynecol Obstet 1991;173:391-396.
71. Sanchez-Fructuoso A, Prats D, Torrente J, et al: Renal transplantation from non-heart beating donors: A promising alternative to enlarge the donor pool. J Am Soc Nephrol 2000;11:350-358.
72. Edwards JM, Hasz RD, Jr, Robertson YM: Non-heart beating organ donation: Process and review. AACN Clin Issues 1999;10:293-300.
73. DuBois J: Ethical assessments of brain death and organ procurement policies: A survey of transplant personnel in the United States. J Transplant Coord 1999;9:210-218.
74. Campbell G, Sutherland F: Non-heart beating organ donors as a source of kidneys for transplantation: A chart review. Can Med Assoc J 1999;160:1573-1576.

Chapter 64

Stroke

Thomas R. Mirsen

BACKGROUND

Stroke has a major impact in the United States, with an estimated yearly incidence of 731,100 new and recurrent strokes[1] from 1993-1994. In 1997, 821,760 stroke admissions occurred in this country.[2] Stroke constitutes the third leading cause of death and is a major cause of disability.[3] Although stroke is a lesser cause of disability than heart disease,[4] the population of stroke survivors continues to increase, in part because of a fall in mortality.[5] Stroke has not been emphasized in the critical care setting historically because of the limited scope of interventions in the past. In the early 1990s, neurologic diseases, including but not limited to stroke, comprised a mere 6% to 7% of admissions to critical care units.[6] Now there is acute treatment for stroke, namely the use of t-PA for ischemic stroke within 3 hours of symptom onset,[7] as well as intra-arterial (IA) thrombolysis for as long as 6 hours following stroke onset.[8] A clot removal device (MERCI)[9] has been approved, and thrombolytic agents that may be usable within a longer time window of 9 hours are being studied.[10] The great danger with the use of these agents is the risk of intracerebral hemorrhage. Frequent monitoring, as often as every 15 minutes following administration of a thrombolytic, is standard for patients so treated, and observation in a critical care unit is required.

Consequently, critical care physicians need to learn about this condition, which has become a regular part of their professional lives, particularly in centers that devote themselves to the care of stroke patients. In one critical care unit with which the author is familiar, ischemic stroke accounts for 3% of the primary admissions and hemorrhagic stroke for 5.4%.[11]

INTRODUCTION

This chapter reviews the general diagnosis and treatment of ischemic stroke. It describes the following:

- The specific interventions available
- Their rationale and utility
- New developments in the area
- The reasons for critical care consultation

Stroke is traditionally defined as a focal neurologic deficit of presumed vascular onset, lasting 24 hours or longer, as opposed to transient ischemic attack (TIA), which is an episode shorter than 24 hours in duration.[12] Many TIAs actually last for less than 60 minutes.[13]

Stroke symptoms including retinal TIA *(amaurosis fugax)*, arise either from the territory fed by the internal carotid artery or from the vertebrobasilar system. The carotid, through its major branches, the anterior (ACAs) and middle cerebral arteries (MCAs), provides blood to the major portion of the cerebral hemispheres. The vertebrobasilar system, in contrast, perfuses the brainstem and cerebellum, as well as the inferior and medial aspects of the occipital and temporal lobes. Blood supply to the thalamus stems from both systems, such that thalamic infarction may result from thrombosis in either system.

Carotid symptoms, as listed in Box 64-1, primarily consist of hemisensory loss, hemiparesis, or retinal ischemia (monocular blindness). Left hemispheric ischemia, generally in the perisylvian area, may result in varying degrees of aphasia.[14] Involvement of the sensory association areas within the right parietal lobe can produce the phenomenon of neglect.[15] In neglect, a stimulus is felt when it is alone but not in the presence of a competing stimulus. For example, a touch on the left hand or an object in the left visual field may be perceived when alone, but not when another stimulus is simultaneously presented, generally on the right side (double simultaneous stimulation). In that instance the right-sided stimulus alone is perceived. In extreme circumstances, affected individuals may not recognize the left side of the body as being theirs *(anosognosia)*, as described memorably by Oliver Sacks in *The Man Who Mistook His Wife for a Hat*.[16]

Box 64-1 lists symptoms resulting from ischemia in the vertebrobasilar territory, which includes the cerebellum, brainstem, and the medial aspect of the occipital lobe, as well as the inferomedial portions of the temporal lobe. As

Box 64-1

Stroke Symptoms

Carotid Distribution

1. Hemiparesis
2. Hemisensory loss
3. Aphasia
4. Retinal ischemia
5. Neglect
6. Homonymous hemianopsia

Vertebrobasilar Distribution

1. Motor dysfunction—crossed or bilateral
2. Sensory loss—crossed or bilateral
3. Gait ataxia
4. Homonymous hemianopsia
5. Diplopia, dysphagia, dysarthria, vertigo, hiccups—none of these alone qualify as stroke/TIA symptoms
6. Combinations of the above

Symptoms Not Considered Vascular in Origin

1. Syncope or presyncope
2. Dizziness, wooziness, giddiness
3. Impaired vision associated with alteration of consciousness
4. Any of these in isolation: amnesia, confusion, vertigo, diplopia, dysphagia, dysarthria
5. Tonic and/or clonic motor activity
6. March of sensory or motor deficits
7. Focal symptoms in association with migraine
8. Bowel or bladder incontinence

Modified from Hachinski V, Norris JW: The Acute Stroke. Philadelphia, FA Davis, 1985.

Box 64-2

Common Seizure Symptoms

Incontinence
Tongue-biting
Tonic movements
Clonic movements
Jacksonian march (sensory, motor, or both)
Automatisms (grimacing, chewing)

a result, vertebrobasilar ischemia can produce cranial nerve dysfunction, nystagmus, cerebellar dysmetria, ataxia, and long tract signs such as sensory loss or motor impairment. These may involve one or both sides of the body. Memory disorders and visual field deficits also occur. In extreme circumstances, when the basilar artery becomes occluded, coma and/or quadriparesis may develop, although the presentation may vary, as described by Kubik and Adams[17] in 1946. As a result of coma or quadriparesis, mechanical ventilation may be required, and the prognosis in such patients is grim. In one study,[18] 22 of 25 patients died, and the other 3 lingered in the “locked-in syndrome.”[19] This frightening manifestation of basilar occlusion, secondary to pontine infarction, leaves patients chronically limited to eye blinking as their sole means of communication.

Differentiating between carotid and vertebrobasilar symptoms is important. There exists intervention to repair carotid stenosis, which is most effective following stroke or TIA in the distribution of the affected vessel. Failure to recognize symptoms as originating from the vertebrobasilar territory may lead to unwarranted intervention for carotid narrowing.

Likewise, one must not label complaints that are not cerebrovascular in nature as stroke (see Box 64-1). Syncope, wooziness, and the like usually reflect systemic hypotension as opposed to focal ischemia. The still widespread practice of studying carotid vessels—most often through ultrasound—following the development of syncope should be abandoned because syncope does not result from ischemic stroke.

Item 4 under “Symptoms Not Considered Vascular in Origin” (see Box 64-1) draws attention to the fact that certain symptoms may represent stroke when associated with other symptoms, but not in isolation. Vertigo, for instance, can result from disease of the semicircular canals. If other complaints or findings referable to the posterior fossa of the brain (brainstem and cerebellum) coexist, such as those listed in Box 64-1 under “Vertebrobasilar Distribution,” the symptoms may indeed localize there. Similarly, amnesia alone may follow a seizure or result from transient global amnesia as opposed to stroke, and so on.

The items listed in Box 64-2 reflect the presence of seizures. Seizure onset may be unwitnessed, and in the hospital only postictal deficits, such as aphasia or hemiparesis, may be observed. The appearance of any number of positive phenomena will draw attention to the correct diagnosis of seizure. These phenomena contrast with the abolition of normal function that happens with stroke and instead represent abnormal activity resulting from the uncontrolled electrical discharges that underlie seizures. Occasionally, however, limb shaking may represent carotid ischemia, usually as the result of hemodynamic compromise in the territory of the ipsilateral carotid artery.[20] A comprehensive classification of epilepsy types and symptoms appears in Dreifuss.[21]

Migraine can also be associated with focal neurologic complaints. Commonest among these are visual complaints including scotomas, whether scintillating or not. The most dramatic manifestation is hemiplegic migraine, which raises the fear of intracerebral hemorrhage at first presentation. Aphasia and paresthesia are also described. Silberstein and colleagues[22] have reviewed the manifestations of migraine.

Box 64-3 lists those entities that most frequently mimic stroke. Hypoglycemia may produce focal neurologic deficits. Occasionally a mass lesion such as tumor or subdural hematoma may present with fluctuating deficits or be revealed by seizure activity that may itself be confused with stroke. In the case of subdural hematoma in the

Box 64-3

Stroke Mimics

Intracerebral hemorrhage
Seizure
Migraine
Hypoglycemia
Tumor

elderly, the inciting trauma may have been minor or forgotten. Headache may be prominent, mild, or even absent. Mass lesions and hemorrhage are frequently marked by confusion, decreased level of consciousness, or headache, but if the lesion is small, these symptoms may not appear. Consequently, blood sugar measurements and computed tomography (CT) scans (without contrast) are obligatory in all instances of suspected stroke. Within the first 6 hours of the event, CT may well be negative, even in instances of major infarction such as that involving the entire middle cerebral artery watershed. Thus CT finds its greatest utility not in confirming the clinical diagnosis but in excluding the presence of small hemorrhages. Neurologists have relied on clinical findings to diagnose stroke, especially in the hyperacute phase (0 to 6 hours), when CT is least helpful.

Advances in Radiology

With the advent of diffusion-weighted imaging (DWI), magnetic resonance imaging (MRI) scans (Fig. 64-1) can now be used to detect acute cerebral ischemia within the initial 6-hour period following symptom onset.[23] This allows the clinician to confirm or exclude the presence of stroke in doubtful cases. Most commonly, such circumstances involve the possibility of a new lesion in a previously injured area of the brain. For example, in the case of a new seizure originating from the hemisphere affected by a prior stroke, DWI can show whether the new event is seizure alone or caused by a new stroke. By the same token, if a newly delirious or febrile patient should manifest worsening of a preexisting neurologic deficit, DWI will clarify whether the worsening stems from the intercurrent injury or from a coincident new stroke. DWI can also reveal silent areas of cerebral ischemia, which sometimes appear simultaneously with the clinically eloquent area of injury that presents symptomatically as stroke. The coincident development of ischemia in different vascular territories may indicate the presence of an unusual mechanism of infarction, such as vasculitis, hypercoagulable state, or cardiac source of emboli. MRI has been proven just as effective as CT in detecting intracerebral hemorrhage,[24] thus potentially removing an extra step (the initial head CT) from the stroke evaluation. Unfortunately, MRI is less immediately available than CT, requires more time and cooperation from the patient, and may not be feasible in the face of claustrophobia or of ferromagnetic implants/fragments within the body.

Both CT and MRI technology can delineate the cerebral vasculature in detail, starting from the aortic arch and extending to the vicinity of the circle of Willis. Computed tomographic angiography (CTA) has been shown to be reliable in studying the intracranial vasculature[25] and the extracranial segment of the carotid artery (Fig. 64-2).[26] Magnetic resonance angiography (MRA) is superior to ultrasound in detecting carotid artery stenosis in the neck[27] and is effective as well intracranially[28] (Figs. 64-3

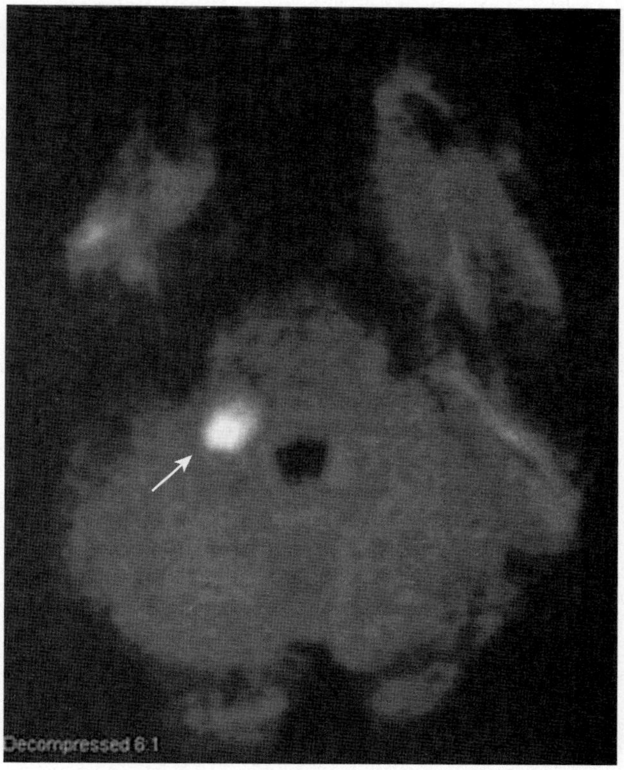

Figure 64-1. Cerebral infarction as shown by diffusion-weighted imaging (DWI, *arrow*) on magnetic resonance imaging. Hyperdensity in the right middle cerebellar peduncle is demonstrated.

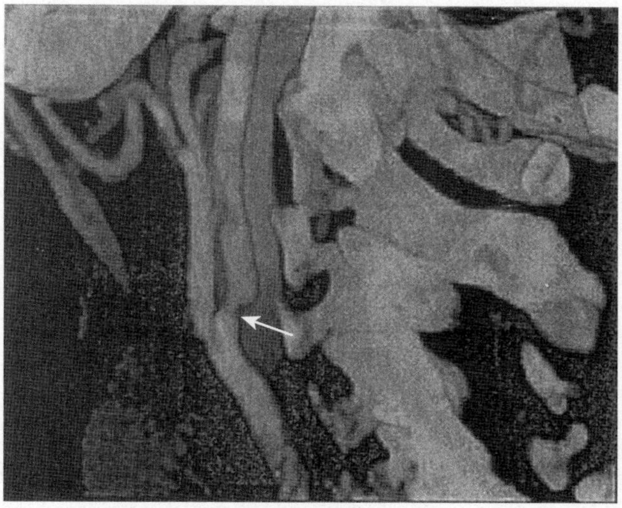

Figure 64-2. CT angiogram of the extracranial carotid artery. An area of stenosis *(arrow)* is shown in the internal carotid artery.

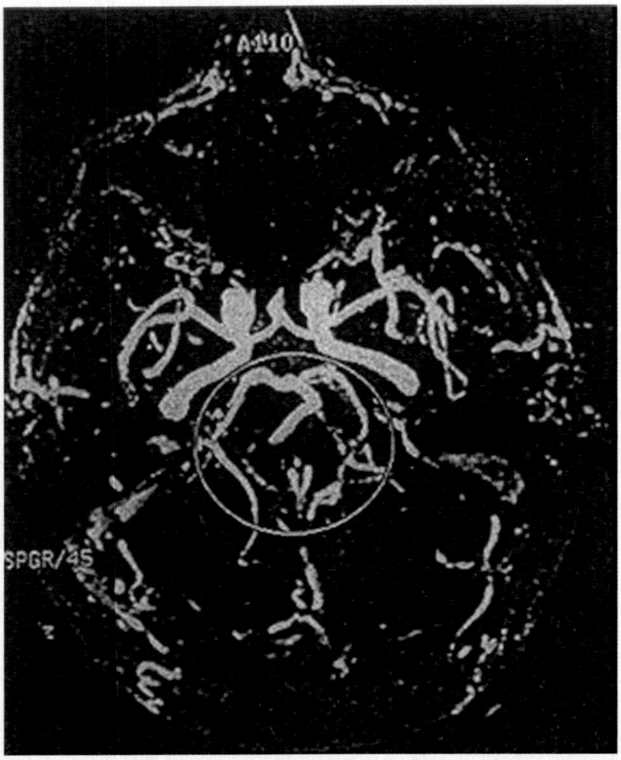

Figure 64-3. Magnetic resonance angiogram demonstrating circle of Willis *(highlighted)* and its vertebrobasilar component *(circle).*

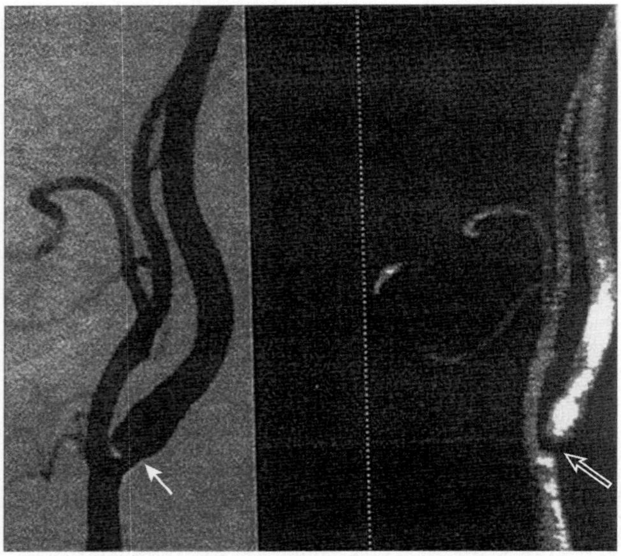

Figure 64-4. Shown are magnetic resonance angiography *(left)* and computed tomographic angiography *(right)* of the extracranial carotid artery in a patient with internal carotid artery stenosis *(arrows)* located above the common carotid bifurcation.

and 64-4), although its specificity and sensitivity in both instances are likely to improve. CTA has its own limitations, namely the difficulty in performing the study in patients with contrast-dye allergies. Because of these new techniques, the performance of conventional cerebral angiography is limited to specific indications, as outlined in Box 64-4.

Box 64-4

Indications for Conventional Cerebral Angiography

To ascertain the precise degree of arterial stenosis, most often of the extracranial carotid artery, in doubtful cases
To detect and map intracranial aneurysms and arteriovenous malformations
To determine patterns of collateral flow in the brain
To diagnose vasculitis
To detect intraluminal thrombus
To enable intra-arterial thrombolysis or mechanical clot extraction
For the performance of carotid angiography and stenting

Thrombolysis in Stroke

The era of thrombolysis in acute stroke began with the publication of the NINDS t-PA trial in 1995.[7] This groundbreaking study was the first to demonstrate a beneficial effect of t-PA when given to patients presenting within 3 hours of the onset of the event. Depending on the criteria used to determine favorable outcome at 3 months, roughly an additional 11% to 13% of subjects receiving t-PA recovered with little or no disability. If one uses the National Institutes of Health stroke scale (NIHSS) (Table 64-1) score, a reliable measure[29] to measure disability, the improvement was from 20% with minimal or no disability with placebo to 31% with t-PA. This was counterbalanced by an increase in the rate of intracerebral hemorrhage (ICH), from 0.6% in the placebo group to 6.4% in the t-PA cohort. Half the subjects in the placebo group who suffered ICH died, whereas the mortality rate from ICH in the t-PA cohort was 2.9% (less than half). Hemorrhage following t-PA use does not necessarily occupy the same area of the brain affected by the initial thrombosis.[30]

Strict inclusion (Box 64-5) and exclusion (Box 64-6) criteria are applied to attempt to minimize the risk of ICH. The safety and efficacy of thrombolysis have not been analyzed in children. The time of onset of symptoms is taken to be the last time that the patient was seen to be normal. For example, an individual who went to sleep at 10 PM and awoke at 6 AM, immediately hemiplegic, will not qualify for t-PA therapy. One who awoke at 4 AM, went back to sleep, and awoke again at 6 AM with stroke symptoms may be treated with t-PA, but only up to 7 AM. A person who awoke at 6 AM, was briefly normal, and developed stroke symptoms at 6:05 AM may be treated until 9:05 AM.

The blood glucose must be determined before initiating t-PA therapy to avoid misdiagnosing hypoglycemia as stroke (see Box 64-3). A CT scan of the head is essential to look for a mass, most often an intracerebral hemor-

Table 64-1. National Institutes of Health Stroke Scale

1a. Level of consciousness (LOC)	Alert	0
	Drowsy	1
	Stuporous	2
	Coma	3
1b. LOC questions	Answers both correctly	0
	Answers one correctly	1
	Incorrect	2
1c. LOC commands	Obeys both correctly	0
	Obeys one correctly	1
	Incorrect	2
2. Best gaze	Normal	0
	Partial gaze palsy	1
	Forced deviation	2
3. Visual field	No visual loss	0
	Partial hemianopsia	1
	Complete hemianopsia	2
	Bilateral hemianopsia	3
4. Facial palsy	Normal	0
	Minor	1
	Partial	2
	Complete	3
5. Motor arm	No drift	0
	Drift	1
	Some effort against gravity	2
	No effort against gravity	3
	Plegia	4
6. Motor leg	No drift	0
	Drift	1
	Some effort against gravity	2
	No effort against gravity	3
	Plegia	4
7. Limb ataxia	Absent	0
	Present in upper or lower	1
	Present in both	2
8. Sensory	Normal	0
	Partial loss	1
	Dense loss	2
9. Best language	No aphasia	0
	Mild to moderate aphasia	1
	Severe aphasia	2
	Mute	3
10. Dysarthria	Normal articulation	0
	Mild to moderate dysarthria	1
	Near unintelligible or worse	2
11. Extinction and inattention	No neglect	0
	Partial neglect	1
	Complete neglect	2

Box 64-5

Thrombolysis Inclusion Criteria

Ischemic stroke with clearly defined time of onset
Neurologic deficit measurable using the NIH stroke scale
CT scan of the brain without evidence of intracerebral hemorrhage
Age 18 years or older

Box 64-6

Thrombolysis Exclusion Criteria

Stroke or serious head injury within the past 3 months
Major surgery within the previous 14 days
Prior history of intracerebral hemorrhage
Systolic blood pressure >185 or diastolic blood pressure >110
Rapid neurologic improvement or minor deficit
Symptoms suggestive of subarachnoid hemorrhage
Gastrointestinal or genitourinary hemorrhage within the previous 21 days
Lumbar puncture or arterial puncture at noncompressible site within the previous 7 days
Biopsy of an internal organ within the previous 7 days
Seizure at onset of stroke
Anticoagulation or heparin use within 48 hours before treatment and elevated PTT
Prothrombin time greater than 15 or INR greater than 1.7
Platelet count less than 100,000
Blood glucose less than 50 or greater than 400
Recent use of low-molecular-weight heparin
Large myocardial infarction in the past 3 months
CT with hypodensity involving >⅓ of the cerebral hemisphere

CT, computed tomography; INR, internal normalized ratio; PTT, partial thromboplastin time.
Modified from Adams H, Adams R, Del Zoppo G, et al: Guidelines for the early management of patients with ischemic stroke. 2005 Guidelines Update. Stroke 2005;36:916-923.

rhage or subdural hematoma. The CT must also be scrutinized for the presence of early ischemic changes, such as sulcal effacement, hypolucency within the brain, or loss of definition between structures within the brain, or for the presence of a hyperdense middle cerebral artery, suggestive of thrombosis.[31] Whether ischemic changes on CT predict a heightened risk of hemorrhagic transformation is controversial.[30,32] However, CT findings appear more commonly among subjects with scans performed relatively late in the course of their stroke.[32] Hence their appearance should prompt re-evaluation of the time of onset of the stroke because it suggests that the stroke occurred earlier than initially thought. Prior intracerebral hemorrhage (ICH), recent stroke, and hypertension at presentation are believed to increase the risk of sustaining ICH. Avoiding systemic bleeding, which may result in hypotension, worsening of the neurologic deficit, and even death, is also important. Extremes of blood glucose or the presence of a coincident seizure make the neurologic deficit seem worse than it is, rendering calculation of a risk-benefit ratio more difficult.

Two blood tests must be checked before embarking on thrombolysis: a blood sugar, as mentioned earlier, and a platelet count. If the patient is on anticoagulant therapy, the prothrombin time/international normalized ratio or partial thromboplastin time must be available before deciding whether to proceed with treatment. If a patient is not known to be receiving anticoagulants at baseline, but the coagulation profile proves abnormal, the infusion must be stopped if thrombolysis is still ongoing at the time that the abnormal value returns. If a patient is receiving low-molecular-weight heparin, there is no rapid way of determining the degree of anticoagulation, and intervention must be withheld.

If the blood pressure is elevated (>180 systolic or 110 diastolic), a modest dosage of labetalol, 5-10 mg IV, may be given and repeated if necessary, up to a maximum dosage of 40 mg. Nitropaste is a less exact alternative but has the advantage that it can be removed. If the blood pressure subsequently rebounds to the undesirable range, t-PA should not be given. Although a small bolus is acceptable, as noted earlier, *continuous IV infusions of labetalol, nicardipine, or IV nitrates may not be given in order to allow for administration of t-PA*. If the pressure should rise above 180 systolic or 105 diastolic subsequent to starting the t-PA infusion, it is paramount to bring it down by whatever means possible including IV infusions of antihypertensive agents (Table 64-2). In this context, it is worth emphasizing that blood pressure should only be treated acutely when there exists a specific indication for doing so, as defined on the table.

t-PA should not be given in the presence of a deficit mild enough that reasonable recovery may be expected within 3 months. However, there is not a clear cutoff based on the NIH stroke scale to identify those patients whose deficits are too mild to warrant intervention. The choice falls to the treating physician. For instance, a partial hemisensory loss, facial palsy, or mild dysarthria would not normally warrant treatment with t-PA when appearing in isolation. A hemianopsia in a bedridden elderly subject residing in a nursing facility may not be considered deserving of thrombolysis by some physicians. However, an active middle-aged person with a job, car, and family presenting with an isolated hemianopsia would probably be treated more aggressively by most doctors. The most difficult choices exist in the setting of mild motor or speech deficits. Such deficits may recover well, but a percentage of subjects will worsen while in the hospital and then no longer be candidates for rescue using

Table 64-2. Approach to Elevated Blood Pressure in Acute Ischemic Stroke

Blood Pressure Level, mm Hg	Treatment
A. Not eligible for thrombolytic therapy	
Systolic ≤220 OR diastolic ≤120	Observe unless other end-organ involvement (e.g., aortic dissection, acute myocardial infarction, pulmonary edema, hypertensive encephalopathy) Treat other symptoms of stroke (e.g., headache, pain, agitation, nausea, vomiting) Treat other acute complications of stroke including hypoxia, increased intracranial pressure, seizures, or hypoglycemia
Systolic >220 OR diastolic 121-140	Labetalol 10-20 mg IV over 1-2 min May repeat or double every 10 min (max dose 300 mg) OR Nicardipine 5 mg/hr IV infusion as initial dose; titrate to desired effect by increasing 2.5 mg/hr every 5 min to max of 15 mg/hr Aim for a 10%-15% reduction in blood pressure
Diastolic >140	Nitroprusside 0.5 μg/kg/min IV infusion as initial dose with continuous blood pressure monitoring Aim for a 10%-15% reduction in blood pressure
B. Eligible for thrombolytic therapy	
Pretreatment Systolic >185 OR diastolic >110	Labetalol 10-20 mg IV over 1-2 min May repeat 1 time or nitropaste 1-2 inches
During/after treatment	
1. Monitor blood pressure	Check blood pressure every 15 min for 2 hr, then every 30 min for 6 hr, and finally every hour for 16 hr
2. Diastolic >140	Sodium nitroprusside 0.5/μg/kg/min IV infusion as initial dose and titrate to desired blood pressure
3. Systolic >230 OR diastolic 121-140	Labetalol 10 μg IV over 1-2 min May repeat or double labetalol every 10 min to maximum dose of 300 mg or give initial labetalol dose, then start labetalol drip at 2-8 mg/min OR Nicarpidine 5 mg/h IV infusion as initial dose and titrate to desired effect by increasing 2.5 mg/h every 5 min to maximum of 15 mg/h; if blood pressure is not controlled by labetalol, consider sodium nitroprusside
4. Systolic 180-230 OR diastolic 105-120	Labetalol 10 mg IV over 1-2 min May repeat or double labetalol every 10-20 min to maximum dose of 300 mg or give initial labetalol dose, then start labetalol drip at 2-8 mg/min

From Adams H, Adams R, Del Zoppo G, et al: Guidelines for the early management of patients with ischemic stroke. 2005 Guidelines Update. Stroke 2005;36:916-923.

thrombolysis. Unfortunately, we presently lack a tool to predict which subjects will worsen during their acute hospital stay and which will remain stable or improve rapidly.

Subjects who have been on antiplatelet agents such as aspirin before their event may receive t-PA, but no anticoagulants or antiplatelet agents may be given for the 24 hours following the start of t-PA therapy. Arterial punctures, nasogastric tubes, and catheterization should be avoided unless they are essential to care, in order to minimize the risk of bleeding.

Hypotension may develop, raising the concern of systemic hemorrhage. Of course, hypotension may have a variety of other causes. The most feared event following t-PA use is the development of ICH. The presenting signs and symptoms appear in Box 64-7. Most are self-explanatory. Hypertension is a compensatory response to increased intracranial pressure, to maintain cerebral perfusion, and bradycardia occurs secondary to hypertension.

The steps to be taken with suspected ICH appear in Box 64-8. It is relatively uncommon for neurosurgeons to intervene on hemorrhages in the setting of t-PA because of the risk of further bleeding into the surgical bed. Systemic hemorrhage is handled in a similar fashion, but transfusion may also be necessary. Platelets should be administered if the count is significantly decreased (<50,000).

The benefit of t-PA is greatest in the instances of the smallest vascular occlusions (lacunar, as opposed to cortical, infarcts). Older subjects with particularly severe strokes are most likely to have a poor outcome, but even in this group t-PA remains beneficial overall.[34] The sooner t-PA is administered, the higher the likelihood of successful recovery, as shown by a meta-analysis[35] of thrombolysis trials. A residual benefit of t-PA exists, as far out as 6 hours from the ictus. However, two studies[36,37] that specifically examined treatment beyond 3 hours failed to show a benefit of administration of t-PA within a 5- or 6-hour time frame. No doubt there exists a subgroup of subjects presenting beyond 3 hours that remains amenable to treatment, but this group cannot be identified. Studies are under way[38] to use MR technology, specifically perfusion-diffusion mismatch, to discriminate among subjects who may or may not benefit from thrombolysis beyond the 3-hour window.

Box 64-7

Signs and Symptoms of Intracerebral Hemorrhage

New neurologic deficits
Worsening of existing neurologic deficits
Headache
Nausea, vomiting
Decreased level of consciousness, coma
Marked hypertension
Bradycardia

Box 64-8

Management of Suspected Intracerebral Hemorrhage Following Use of tPA

Discontinue the t-PA infusion if it remains in progress
STAT CT of the head (noncontrast)
STAT PT, PTT, platelet count, fibrinogen
Type and cross
Consult neurosurgery
Administer fresh frozen plasma or cryoprecipitate (4 to 8 units)

CT, computed tomography; PT, prothrombin time; PTT, partial thromboplastin time.

Various authors have identified different predictors of ICH following treatment with t-PA. Levy and colleagues[39] cited the dosage of t-PA given, the age of the subjects, and diastolic hypertension as pertinent factors. Larrue and colleagues[30] also found age to heighten the risk of development of ICH, but not the degree of hypertension nor the time to treatment. It has become clear that t-PA can be given safely in the community[40] and that complication rates of t-PA use can be lowered to a satisfactory level by careful adherence to the exclusion criteria.[41]

Intra-arterial thrombolysis can be used to treat acute ischemic stroke beyond the 3-hour time window for IV t-PA. Basilar thrombosis has been treated as late as 24 hours after the onset of symptoms using this approach.[42] Other subjects with occlusion of the proximal (M1 or M2) segments of the middle cerebral artery have been successfully treated between 3 and 6 hours following stroke onset. The utility of this approach rests on the PROACT II trial,[8] a study using a novel agent, pro-urokinase (pro-UK). In contrast to the IV t-PA trial, aspirin was allowed in the first 24 hours following stroke onset and heparin was used acutely following pro-UK to prevent vascular reocclusion. To enter the study, the upper age limit was 85 years of age and the minimum NIHSS score was 11.

The trial showed a 40% rate of favorable neurologic outcome at 3 months following IA thrombolysis, as opposed to 25% in the control group. The rate of ICH with clinical deterioration at 24 hours following study entry was 10% in the pro-UK group, as opposed to 2% in the placebo group. Although pro-UK itself has not been approved for use in this country, IA t-PA is used for subjects who cannot be treated within 3 hours with IV t-PA. Inclusion and exclusion criteria for the use of IA t-PA, as employed at one center, appear in Boxes 64-9 and 64-10.[43] Apparent predictors of hemorrhagic transformation of cerebral infarct in patients subjected to IA thrombolysis appear in Box 64-11.[44] In another study,[45] 36 subjects underwent IA thrombolysis for stroke within 2 weeks of major surgery (mean time from surgery to treatment of 21.5 hours). Nine of the subjects (25%) died, but only three died of hemorrhagic complications, suggesting that IA thrombolysis may be considered following major surgery when IV thrombolysis is contraindicated. The smaller dosage of thrombolytic (0.2 mg/kg vs. 0.9 mg/kg) used may render the IA approach

Box 64-9

Intra-arterial tPA: Inclusion Criteria

Patient must be between 18 and 85 years of age
National Institutes of Health stroke scale score between 11 and 30
Angiographic complete occlusion (TIMI 0) or penetration with minimal perfusion (TIMI 1) of the apparent symptom-related M1 or M2 segment of the MCA or of the basilar artery
Diagnosis of ischemic stroke causing measurable neurological deficit (defined as impairment of language, motor function, cognition and/or gaze, vision or neglect) characterized by the sudden onset of acute focal neurologic deficit presumed to be due to cerebral ischemia after exclusion of hemorrhage by CT scan.
Onset of symptoms within 6 hours of IA t-PA administration. (Consider if patient presents within 4½ hours of stroke.) In event of basilar thrombosis, the time window is 12 hours.

Note: "time of onset" of stroke is the point at which change in baseline neurological function occurred. If time not known, e.g., the patient awakens from sleep with new symptoms, the last time the patient was observed to be neurologically intact is considered the time of onset.
MCA, middle cerebral artery; TIMI, thrombolysis in myocardial infarction.

safe in this setting. Intra-arterial thrombolysis is also used when cardiac catheterization is complicated by stroke, in large part because of immediate access to the vascular tree. This approach, although reasonable, has not been studied systematically.[46]

The use of a 0.6 mg/kg systemic bolus of IV t-PA acutely, followed by IA thrombolysis if shown necessary by immediate angiography, is being assessed.[47] Although efficacy data are not yet available, so far the rate of symptomatic ICH is low at 6%.[48]

Neurointerventionists attempt to heighten the effectiveness of local thrombolytics by using catheters to mechanically disrupt clots. Such an approach is difficult to assess in a standardized fashion. Its most dedicated proponents use the MERCI device, designed to extract clot via the endovascular approach without thrombolysis.[10] The MERCI device has not undergone randomized trials. Available data consist of a series of patients treated with the device compared with historical controls. The data focus on the rate of recanalization of the occluded vessel and only secondarily on clinical outcome. The limitations of such an analysis are all too obvious and are discussed in detail elsewhere.[49] Mechanical clot extraction may find a niche distinct from thrombolysis in the acute treatment of ischemic stroke, but that role remains to be defined by further study.

Symptomatic Carotid Disease

Carotid endarterectomy dramatically reduces stroke risk in patients with cerebral or retinal ischemia who prove to

Box 64-10

Intra-arterial t-PA: Exclusion Criteria

Related to the Acute Stroke:

NIHSS score greater than 30 (for MCA symptoms)
Patient with only minor stroke symptoms or major symptoms that are rapidly improving
Lacunar infarction
Seizure at onset of stroke symptoms
Presentation suggestive of SAH, even if CT is normal
Hypertension; SBP greater than 180 or DBP greater than 100 on repeated measures prior to study entry or requiring aggressive antihypertensive therapy to reduce BP to within limits
Presumed septic embolus

Preceding Events:

History of stroke within 3 months
History of intracerebral hemorrhage, SAH, AV malformation, or aneurysm
History of intracranial tumor, except for small coincidental meningioma
Lumbar puncture or arterial puncture at a noncompressible site within 7 days
Biopsy of parenchymal organ within 30 days
Trauma within 30 days, with internal injury or ulcerative wounds
Major surgery within 30 days (**relative** contraindication)
Gastrointestinal or genitourinary hemorrhage within 30 days
Head trauma within 90 days

Coexisting Conditions:

Pregnant or lactating woman
Known serious sensitivity to contrast agents
Bleeding tendency (e.g., ↑PT or PTT >1½ × control, coagulation factor deficiency, oral anticoagulant therapy with PT >15 or INR >1.7)
Baseline: GLU less than 50 or greater than 400
Baseline PLT less than 100,000
Baseline Hct less than 25

CT Scan Exclusions:

High-density lesion consistent with any degree of hemorrhage
Significant mass effect with midline shift
Subarachnoid hemorrhage
Parenchymal hypodensity and/or effacement of cerebral sulci in greater than 33% of the MCA territory
Carotid dissection, vasculitis, occlusion of internal carotid or anterior cerebral arteries

AV, arteriovenous; BP, blood pressure; CT, computed tomography; DBP, diastolic blood pressure; GLU, glucose; Hct, hematocrit; MCA, middle cerebral artery; NIHSS, National Institutes of Health stroke scale; PLT, platelet; PT, prothrombin time; PTT, partial thromboplastin time; SAH, subarachnoid hemorrhage; SBP, systolic blood pressure.

Box 64-11

Predictors of Hemorrhagic Transformation of Cerebral Infarction after IA t-PA

Higher NIHSS score
Longer time to arterial recanalization
Hyperglycemia
Lower platelet count

Box 64-12

High-Risk Criteria for Entry into the SAPPHIRE Trial

Clinically significant heart disease: congestive heart failure, abnormal stress test, or need for open-heart surgery
Severe pulmonary disease
Contralateral carotid artery occlusion
Contralateral laryngeal nerve palsy
Previous radical neck surgery
Previous radiation therapy to the neck
Carotid restenosis following prior endarterectomy
Age older than 80 years

harbor a significant carotid stenosis ipsilateral to the affected cerebral hemisphere. Two separate randomized controlled trials[50,51] have shown similar results. In NASCET,[51] the risk of stroke fell from 26% over 2 years in the nonsurgical group to 9% over 2 years in the surgical group, with a surgical morbidity and mortality of 5.6%. A more modest benefit was seen in men with stenoses between 50% and 69%, namely a reduction in stroke risk from 22.2% over 5 years without surgery to 14.9% over 5 years with surgery. This is an absolute reduction of the stroke rate of 7.3% over 5 years, as opposed to an absolute reduction of 17% over 2 years in the group with stenosis greater than 70%. Superior surgical skill is necessary in order to lower the surgical morbidity and mortality to a point that the procedure remains beneficial in this cohort.

In order for endarterectomy to be beneficial, there must be a reasonable expectation of survival without other major disability over a 5-year period. Thus subjects with moderately advanced dementia, hepatic failure, or renal failure are generally not considered suitable candidates.

Other considerations help determine which patients carry an increased risk of poor outcome acutely from endarterectomy. As far back as 1975, Sundt and colleagues[52] recognized that poor or unstable neurologic status, as well as cerebral ischemia within 24 hours of surgery, identified a group at high surgical risk. These authors also related high risk to the following: congestive heart failure, recent cardiac ischemia, marked hypertension, emphysema, age older than 70, and severe obesity. The presence of a contralateral carotid occlusion places subjects at extremely high risk of stroke if left untreated but also carries a high morbidity and mortality acutely.[53]

The likelihood of stroke in patients with carotid stenosis rises steadily with increasing severity of stenosis greater than 70%[54] and then decreases again as the stenosis reaches 94% to 99%. However, surgery appears to remain beneficial in this range.[55] In addition, hemispheric symptoms predict roughly twice the danger of stroke as do isolated retinal symptoms.[56] The presence of ulceration in conjunction with stenosis, as detected angiographically, increases the risk of stroke. This effect is most marked when associated with the highest degrees of stenosis and becomes progressively more modest as the degree of stenosis decreases toward 70%.[57]

Recently, a meta-analysis[58] showed that men benefit more from carotid surgery than women, presumably because of a poorer prognosis if left untreated. In contrast to Sundt and colleagues'[52] prior findings, there is a greater benefit of the procedure in persons older than 75 years, undoubtedly because of a worse natural history. The most important finding to emerge from this report, however, is the dramatic benefit when endarterectomy is performed within 2 weeks of the sentinel event, which diminishes rapidly if surgery is delayed. Presumably, the patients go on to stroke while waiting for surgery if left untreated for any time. The previously established surgical practice, to wait for 4 to 6 weeks following stroke or TIA before proceeding with surgery, has become untenable. Where severe disability exists, endarterectomy may be reasonably delayed in order to see if sufficient recovery occurs to warrant intervention. However, carotid revascularization, whether by means of endarterectomy or, as discussed later, carotid angioplasty and stenting, should be undertaken acutely in the absence of major neurologic disability.

Protected carotid angioplasty and stenting (CAS) has been compared with carotid endarterectomy in a controlled, randomized trial.[59] Study participants were 18 years old or older and had either a greater than 50% symptomatic stenosis or a greater than 80% asymptomatic stenosis. They were at high risk, as defined by at least one of the factors listed in Box 64-12.

SAPPHIRE showed a trend favoring CAS for the incidence of death and major ipsilateral stroke, both in the year following intervention. These gains fell short of statistical significance, perhaps because the study was terminated prematurely. The CAS group benefited significantly as far as reduction of hospital length of stay (by 1 day) and reduction in the incidence of laryngeal nerve palsy. Lastly, there was a significant decline in the rate of myocardial infarction (MI) at 1 month following intervention in the CAS group when compared with endarterectomy, caused primarily by a fall in the incidence of non Q-wave MI. Some of this benefit may reflect the use of clopidogrel in addition to aspirin for 2 to 4 weeks following treatment in the CAS group, whereas the endarterectomy subjects received only aspirin. In summary, the study showed that CAS was not inferior to endarterectomy and was suggested to be superior in some ways in this group. The durability of these results is not known because of limited follow-up. A more important question involves the necessity of intervention. The authors do not systematically distinguish between symptomatic and asymptomatic subjects in their report. Is the benefit of stenting, or any intervention, more evident in one group in particular? Do the patients with significant systemic illness (cardiac or pulmonary disease) survive long enough to warrant the initial risk of any intervention? There is no control group treated with medical therapy alone for comparison.

In conclusion, SAPPHIRE establishes CAS as a practical alternative to endarterectomy in a somewhat heterogeneous high-risk population. It is intuitively attractive because it is less invasive. The clinician must still decide who will benefit from the procedure on an individual basis. CAS will find an important role in the management of subjects with symptomatic carotid stenosis who are awaiting coronary artery bypass surgery. The requisite use of clopidogrel following stenting will mandate a delay of 6 weeks before proceeding with surgery. CAS also may supplant endarterectomy in the treatment of asymptomatic carotid disease, even in low-risk patients. The benefit of surgery in this setting is modest enough[62] that even a mild increase in surgical morbidity and mortality can erase it. As the less invasive procedure, CAS, if durable, may be preferable.

Subsequently published studies, SPACE[60] and EVA-3S,[61] have been used to cast doubt on the efficacy of CAS. Thirty-day results from SPACE suggest that CAS is less effective than CEA, but the difference is small and the follow-up limited. EVA-3S suggests that the complication rate of CAS is much higher (9.6%) than the complication rate of CEA (3.6%), but these results may be peculiar to that trial. The surgeons had a low complication rate, whereas the complication rate of CAS was unusually high. SPACE has its own flaws. The severity of stenosis was assessed by carotid ultrasound alone, without further validation. Distal protection devices were employed in only a quarter of the CAS patients. Although the authors state that the incidence of periprocedural stroke was not affected by the use of such devices, it is not clear how the decision was taken to use them. Also, SAPPHIRE and the newer trials are not directly comparable. SAPPHIRE focused on a high-risk population and included asymptomatic subjects, whereas SPACE and EVA-3S compared CEA and CAS in all symptomatic candidates for revascularization. CAS may indeed be beneficial in one setting but not the other.

Anticoagulation in Stroke

Anticoagulants occupy an important but limited place in stroke therapy. The acute use of heparin in unselected stroke patients was studied some years ago but not justified.[63] More recently, the treatment with warfarin of subjects presenting with symptomatic intracranial stenosis has proven no better than therapy with high-dose (1300 mg daily) aspirin. This use of warfarin produced increased morbidity, in part because of an increased risk of major hemorrhage, primarily gastrointestinal.[64] When warfarin is given to unselected stroke patients in a population including a slight majority of subjects with lacunar stroke, it confers no advantage relative to aspirin.[65] Whether warfarin reduces the incidence of stroke among subjects with a decreased ejection fraction (<35%) is the focus of an ongoing trial.[66]

Warfarin clearly prevents stroke among subjects suffering from nonrheumatic atrial fibrillation, even if they have never had a stroke or TIA.[67] The risk of stroke falls by 68%, a robust and consistent effect that aspirin cannot equal. Individuals younger than 65 years of age with atrial fibrillation who have no significant vascular risk factors are at low risk and do not need anticoagulation. Such individuals are rare in clinical practice. The risk of systemic hemorrhage and of ICH with warfarin use in this setting is low. A combination of clopidogrel and low-dose aspirin has recently[68] proven inferior to warfarin in stroke prevention among patients with atrial fibrillation. The bleeding risk was actually lower with warfarin than with the antiplatelet combination.

Individuals with atrial fibrillation who sustain a minor stroke or TIA have a high stroke risk (12% per year), which falls to 4% per year upon treatment with warfarin. A 2.8% yearly risk of all bleeding complications with warfarin exists, as opposed to 0.7% with placebo. Aspirin is nearly as safe as placebo, but it reduces the stroke risk only modestly.[69] It remains uncertain when in the course of stroke to initiate anticoagulant therapy. A randomized trial[70] has compared a form of low-molecular-weight heparin (dalteparin) to 160 mg of aspirin in patients with stroke and atrial fibrillation. Treatment began within 30 hours of stroke onset, and the risk of recurrent stroke at 14 days was determined. This proved to be 8%. Dalteparin was equivalent to aspirin. This study was not powered to demonstrate a more modest beneficial effect of dalteparin, which may or may not be present. Nevertheless, this study urges caution on those who would treat completed stroke acutely with anticoagulants. The exclusion criteria for the study serve as a guideline as to when *not* to treat with anticoagulants. Patients with severe strokes and those with marked elevation of blood pressure were not entered. Acute anticoagulation in the face of stroke should be withheld if there is a sizable infarct as measured by the NIHSS (perhaps a score of ≥12) or on CT (>⅓ of MCA territory), which could progress to herniation and death as a result of hemorrhage into the infarct bed. The 185/110 cutoff used in the NINDS t-PA trial may give some idea of the range of hypertension that would cause one to withhold acute treatment with anticoagulants.

In contrast, one should move quickly to anticoagulation following a TIA occurring in conjunction with atrial fibrillation or any other recognized indication for anticoagulation. Minor strokes that begin with potentially devastating deficits but go on to resolve substantially should receive anticoagulation if its use is indicated. These recommendations seem appropriate in view of the high risk of stroke recurrence in atrial fibrillation, as cited above.[69]

Other indications for anticoagulation appear in Box 64-13. Some, such as the presence of rheumatic heart

Box 64-13

Indications for Anticoagulation in Stroke

Atrial fibrillation, with or without rheumatic heart disease
Prosthetic heart valve
Deep venous thrombosis, with or without the potential for paradoxical embolus
Hypercoagulable state
Venous sinus thrombosis
Arterial dissection

Box 64-14

Causes of Hypercoagulable States

Protein C deficiency
Protein S deficiency
Antithrombin III deficiency
Factor V Leiden
Prothrombin gene mutation
Antiphospholipid antibodies
Lupus anticoagulant

disease with atrial fibrillation, prosthetic heart valve, or deep venous thrombosis (DVT), are long established. Anticoagulation carries more urgency when a DVT coexists with a communication across the atrial septum, such as patent foramen ovale (PFO), because there is risk of both recurrent stroke and pulmonary embolism.

Venous sinus thrombosis is an uncommon condition that manifests with headache and papilledema, as well as focal symptoms, and often leads to intracerebral hemorrhage.[71] Diagnosis is by magnetic resonance venography.[72] Treatment is with heparin acutely, even in the presence of intracerebral hemorrhage.[73] More recent reports have established the safety of low-molecular-weight heparin followed by 3 months of warfarin therapy for this condition, although only a trend toward favorable outcome emerged.[74] Retrograde thrombolysis through the venous system with t-PA in conjunction with intravenous heparin is effective in more serious cases.[75]

Spontaneous dissection of the carotid and vertebral arteries is the subject of a review by Schievink.[76] This is a significant cause of stroke in younger individuals. Carotid dissection often presents with neck pain, radiating to the head, and with components of Horner's syndrome (ptosis, miosis, and anhidrosis). Vertebral dissection presents with pain in the neck or back of the head initially. Either may proceed to cerebral infarction or to retinal infarction in the case of carotid dissection. MRA diagnoses carotid dissection quite accurately, and vertebral dissection less so.[77] Anticoagulation is commonly employed but has not been subjected to a rigorous trial. The presence of dissection does not appear to contraindicate the performance of thrombolysis by whatever route.[78]

Box 64-14 lists the hypercoagulable states.[79] Most of these correlate chiefly to the development of venous thrombosis including the most recently discovered mutation of the prothrombin gene.[80] Antiphospholipid antibodies and the lupus anticoagulant may produce both venous and arterial thrombosis. The duration of anticoagulation rests on the judgment of the treating physician. Three to six months of therapy are commonly undertaken if the episode of thrombosis is isolated.

Antiplatelet Agents in Stroke

Secondary stroke prevention continues to depend on aspirin, as it has for many years. A meta-analysis carried out in 1994[81] showed that antiplatelet therapy, primarily with aspirin, reduces the risk of stroke, MI, and vascular death in aggregate by 25%. This analysis did not discriminate among those subjects treated primarily for heart disease and those treated for cerebral ischemia. A similar analysis[82] focusing only on the latter found a lesser benefit of aspirin, on the order of 13%. The optimal dosage of aspirin remains unknown. One study[83] failed to show a difference in outcome when comparing dosages of 30 mg and 283 mg. Another study[84] revealed no difference in efficacy between 300 mg and 1200 mg of aspirin a day. In both reports, the lesser dosage led to fewer significant bleeding episodes.

The limited effect of aspirin on stroke recurrence, coupled with the seeming failure of increases in dosage to further reduce stroke risk, led to a search for other antiplatelet agents. Ticlopidine enjoyed brief popularity but was found to produce agranulocytosis ($<1500/mm^3$) in 2.4% of subjects, which was severe ($<450/mm^3$) in 0.8%.[85] Thrombotic thrombocytopenic purpura, fatal in 4 of 13 cases, also occurred.[86] Both the need for regular blood monitoring and the risk of a severe and potentially fatal complication led to the virtual abandonment of this agent.

Another thienopyridine, clopidogrel, was studied in the CAPRIE trial.[87] It exhibited minimal benefit compared with aspirin in preventing vascular events both in patients presenting with stroke and in those manifesting with MI. Nevertheless, it was approved for use primarily on the strength of its ability to reduce the development of vascular events in subjects presenting with peripheral arterial disease. It has won wide support and has subsequently proven quite useful, administered together with aspirin, in the treatment of unstable angina[88] and acute MI[89,90] and following stent placement in the coronary vessels.[91]

Physicians have used clopidogrel in conjunction with aspirin for stroke prevention in the expectation that the combination would prove superior to clopidogrel in isolation. However, a comparison between the use of 75 mg of aspirin together with 75 mg of clopidogrel and the use of clopidogrel alone revealed no benefit of combination therapy, just a heightened risk of GI hemorrhage.[92] Another study[93] failed to show a benefit of combination therapy when compared with the use of aspirin alone in preventing stroke, MI, or vascular death. In addition, the risk of "moderate" hemorrhage was increased in the group receiving combination therapy. Patients, in order to enter this study, had to have either established vascular disease or, in a minority, multiple vascular risk factors. The study as published does not assess the risks or benefits of combination therapy relative to aspirin in subjects randomized for stroke alone. Nevertheless, the results do not support the chronic use of combination therapy in the prevention of acute vascular syndromes and death of vascular origin. Perhaps combination therapy may be useful in the setting of acute cerebral ischemia, as it is for acute coronary syndromes with ST-segment elevation.[89,90] Certainly the use of aspirin is recognized as beneficial in acute stroke when instituted within 48 hours,[94] and one may imagine, on the basis of the cardiac data, that clopidogrel may also benefit stroke acutely. However, no studies have evaluated this issue.

An alternative to the use of aspirin or clopidogrel is the combination of low-dose aspirin in conjunction with extended-release dipyridamole (ASA + ER/DP). The initial aspirin and dipyridamole study, ESPS,[95] showed a striking benefit of the combination of 990 mg of aspirin and 75 mg of dipyridamole daily in reducing stroke, by 38%. This result raised the question of whether the high aspirin dosage or the addition of dipyridamole was responsible for the dramatic improvement in outcome. A second trial, ESPS-2,[96] revealed a similar benefit using a regimen of 50 mg of aspirin and 400 mg of ER/DP per day. The effect of the two agents was additive. However, there was no improvement in mortality or in the rate of MI in any of the treatment groups (ASA, ER/DP, or ASA + ER/DP) when compared with placebo in ESPS-2. This contrasts with the results of ESPS, in which combination therapy did reduce both the rate of vascular death and, in the intention-to-treat analysis, that of MI. Thus both the active regimen used in ESPS and the combination therapy used in ESPS-2 significantly reduced the rate of recurrent stroke. However, only in ESPS, which used a much higher aspirin dosage, was there a reduction in the rate of MI and vascular death.

This disparity raises the question of whether the bar was set too low in ESPS-2 as far as aspirin dosing was concerned. Perhaps an increased aspirin dosage in the aspirin-only and aspirin + dipyridamole groups, whether 81 or 325 mg daily, would have reduced the relative benefit derived from the addition of extended-release dipyridamole to aspirin. The recently published ESPRIT trial[97] attempts to answer this question. In this study patients were randomized, unblinded, to either aspirin or the combination of aspirin and high-dose dipyridamole. A significant dropout rate occurred with the latter combination, caused by a high rate of headache secondary to dipyridamole, but it proved superior to aspirin alone in the prevention of the triad of stroke, MI, and vascular death. The main criticism of this study is the relatively low dose of aspirin used, anywhere from 30 to 325 mg, with a median dosage of 75 mg. One wonders whether a similar benefit could be achieved with a higher aspirin dosage of 325 mg daily alone. The rate of gastrointestinal hemorrhage might rise consequently, but there would be significant savings in the cost of medication. As already noted, previous studies[83,84] have not revealed significant differences in outcome on the basis of the aspirin dosage used but the numbers enrolled in these trials are relatively modest and differences cannot be definitively excluded.

Lastly, a randomized trial is under way comparing ASA + ER/DP to clopidogrel in the prevention of stroke, MI, and death among patients presenting with stroke.[98] If clopidogrel proves superior in prevention of MI and ASA + ER/DP is better for stroke prevention, clinicians may find themselves in a quandary when selecting antiplatelet agents.

In conclusion, the area of antiplatelet therapy for stroke remains in evolution. Clopidogrel remains the drug of choice under certain circumstances (Box 64-15). The combination of low-dose aspirin and high-dose ER/DP has taken an important step toward acceptance with the publication of the ESPRIT trial, although tolerability of this regimen remains a problem. The absence of a "high-dose," aspirin-only arm in this study provides ammunition for skeptics. Clinicians often change therapy from one antiplatelet agent to another following the development of a cerebral ischemic event, but one must expect a significant failure rate with any of these agents. Whether such a strategy is beneficial is unclear. Aspirin will remain the agent of choice for many patients, especially those with poor insurance or limited funds. Combination therapy with aspirin and dipyridamole will be widely used in individuals with cerebral vascular disease who are at risk for the development of gastrointestinal hemorrhage.

Patent Foramen Ovale

Patent foramen ovale (PFO) is a recently recognized cause of cardiac embolization to the brain. PFO is detected by 2-D echocardiography with injection of agitated saline or a transesophageal study. In one report it appeared in 18% of young controls and in 40% of subjects with cryptogenic stroke. PFO was more common as well in younger as opposed to older patients with cryptogenic stroke (stroke of unknown origin following standard evaluation).[99] The combination of PFO with atrial septal aneurysm in stroke patients younger than the age of 55 is associated with a high (15.2% over 4 years) risk of recurrent stroke.[100] Others[101] have found a large diameter (>4 mm) of the PFO

Box 64-15

Indications for the Use of Clopidogrel Following Cerebral Ischemia

Recent acute coronary syndromes
Recent stent placement
Absolute aspirin intolerance including aspirin allergy
Coexistent symptomatic peripheral arterial disease

to predict increased risk of stroke recurrence. PFO can be treated with warfarin, aspirin, surgical closure, and now endovascular closure. No data suggest conclusively that one treatment surpasses the others,[102] although trials are under way comparing endovascular closure to medical management.

Massive Hemispheric Cerebral Infarct

Infarction of the entire middle cerebral artery territory leads to the development of the "malignant MCA" syndrome.[103] This major injury leads to death in 78% of cases in the first week after the ictus, as the result of cerebral edema leading to transtentorial herniation, and the survivors are quite disabled. Brain swelling peaks at 3 to 5 days following stroke onset.

The presence of early CT changes, namely hypodensity of more than 50% of the MCA territory, indicates a poor prognosis.[104] In the absence of appropriate intervention, midline displacement of the pineal gland greater than 4 mm predicts death reliably. Large volume of infarction (Fig. 64-5) and displacement of the septum pellucidum also indicate a poor outcome.[105] At initial presentation, aphasia or neglect may be present, depending on the hemisphere affected. Characteristically, the patients display hemiplegia and a dense hemisensory loss, although the leg may be relatively spared. Quite often, there is a forced eye deviation and hemianopsia may coexist. Mortality is higher in older individuals with this syndrome,[106] but transtentorial herniation is a more significant cause of death among younger subjects with ischemic stroke.[107] Presumably younger individuals have less cerebral atrophy and less room within the cranial vault to accommodate brain swelling, so they proceed more quickly to herniation and death.

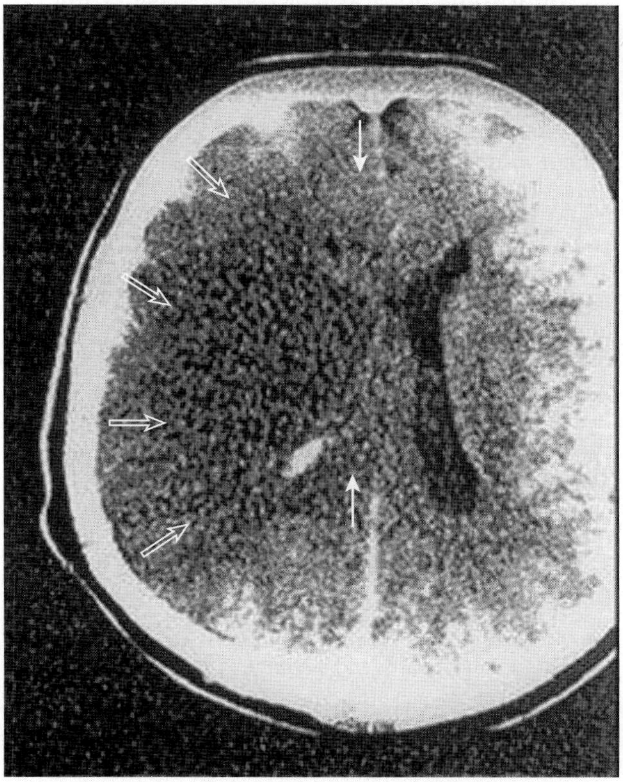

Figure 64-5. Massive middle cerebral artery (MCA) infarct. Hypolucency of the entire right MCA territory *(open arrows)* and compression of the right lateral ventricle *(white arrows)* are demonstrated.

Treatment of this syndrome has so far proved disappointing, as reviewed by different authors.[108-110] The review by Wijdicks[110] is particularly comprehensive. Standard therapies include hyperventilation and the administration of intravenous mannitol. Mannitol is a dehydrating agent, an osmotic diuretic, which aims at reducing cerebral volume and thus intracranial pressure (ICP). It is given initially at a dosage of 1 g/kg, followed by recurrent dosing four times daily with 0.25 to 0.5 g/kg. The goal of therapy is a serum osmolality of 315 to 320 mOsm/L. Mechanical ventilation with hyperventilation produces hypocarbia, which leads to cerebral vasoconstriction, reduced cerebral blood volume, and decreased ICP. The target range for $Pa{CO_2}$ is not well defined. Steiner and colleagues[109] state that lowering $P{CO_2}$ from "35 to 29 mm Hg lowers ICP by 25% to 30% in most subjects." The benefit of these interventions in clinical practice appears to be short-lived. Because hyperventilation is associated with decreased blood flow, it should be viewed as a temporizing measure only.

More promising therapies include hypothermia and decompressive hemicraniectomy. Hypothermia in one pilot trial[111] lowered ICP temporarily when instituted within 14 hours of onset of major MCA stroke. Hypothermia has also been employed[112] shortly after thrombolysis. The use of a device placed in the inferior vena cava lowers body temperature much more quickly than surface cooling,[113] although there is a concern regarding the development of deep venous thrombosis. However, in the absence of large randomized controlled studies there are no definitive conclusions regarding the safety and efficacy of hypothermia.

Much the same is true of decompressive hemicraniectomy with durotomy. This surgery, championed by the group at Heidelberg, Germany,[114,115] appears beneficial when compared with medical treatment,[114] particularly when intervention occurs before the appearance of signs of incipient herniation.[115] However, the surgically treated patients in these two reports differed significantly from the control patients. The surgical patients were younger, and subjects with large left hemispheric infarcts producing global aphasia were not considered for surgery. Some, if not all, of the benefit in the surgically treated group may be explained by this imbalance between the control and treated groups. Results from two randomized trials (DESTINY and HeaDDFIRST) have not been published in their entirety, although preliminary information from these trials, favoring surgical intervention, has reached the medical public through the Internet.[116] A larger randomized trial is necessary.

Surgical intervention also exists for cerebellar infarction, which, when large, may expand and place pressure on the brainstem.[117] Both ventriculostomy to relieve hydrocephalus acutely and decompressive craniotomy are

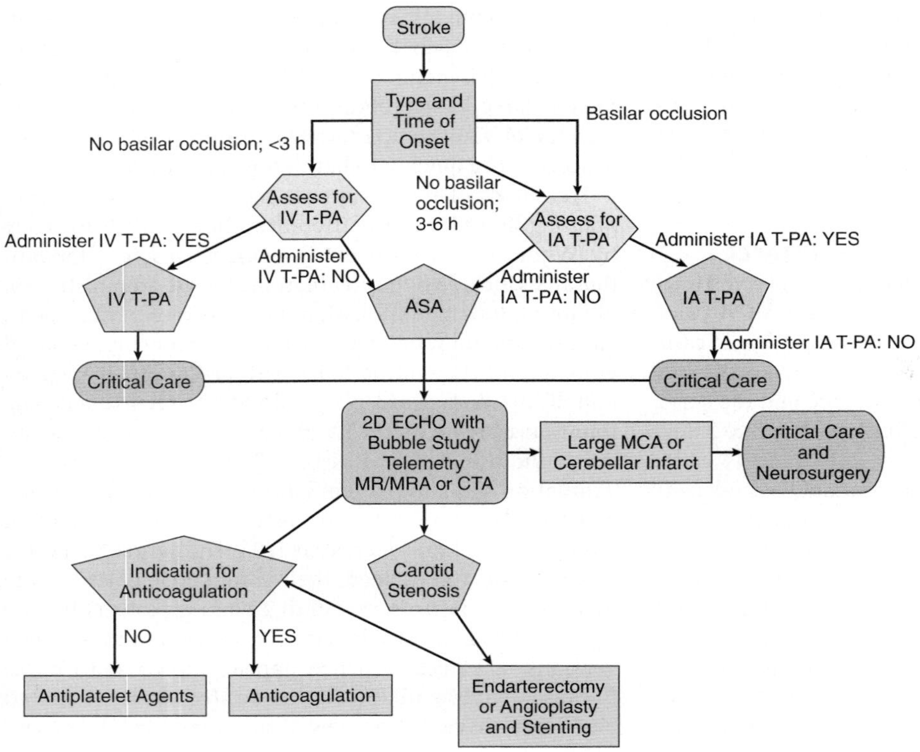

Figure 64-6. Critical care approach for management of stroke patients.

employed. The main determinant of survival and recovery is the absence of coma on presentation. Surgery is the accepted treatment, but the exact timing of intervention remains uncertain.[118]

Critical Care Consultation

Critical care consultation for stroke patients is indicated for the following reasons (Box 64-16, Fig. 64-6).

SUMMARY

In conclusion, stroke therapy is advancing significantly. Thrombolysis, both intravenous and IA, has developed over the past 20 years. Technological advances in radiology have far improved the capacity to image both small infarcts and blood vessels. Endarterectomy has become established in the treatment of carotid disease, and angioplasty and stenting may well follow. The role of anticoagulation is clearer, although it often remains uncertain when to initiate its use and when to discontinue it. No longer is aspirin the only antiplatelet agent available to the clinician. New entities, such as PFO, are being recognized, and their meaning weighed. Decompressive surgery can save lives that would otherwise be lost. Hypothermia may soon join these other therapies in the physician's armamentarium. Much of this activity has taken place in the critical care unit. One may hope that the next 20 years will bring further revelations, enabling the treatment of many more stroke patients in the acute phase and introducing what has so long been lacking—treatment for stroke in evolution. As our means for intervention increase, so will the role of critical care in reducing death and disability from stroke.

Box 64-16

Indications for Critical Care Consultation

- Intubation and mechanical ventilation
- Administration of continuous infusions of antihypertensive agents
- Administration of pressor agents
- Monitoring not feasible in other settings
- Intraventricular drainage
- Induction and maintenance of hypothermia

KEY POINTS

- Determine time of onset of all new strokes.
- Consider intravenous thrombolysis with t-PA if within 3 hours of onset.
- Consider IA thrombolysis for basilar thrombosis or if within 6 hours of stroke onset.
- Observe published guidelines for blood pressure control.
- Use MRI and MRA or CT and CTA to visualize the brain and its vasculature.
- Proceed promptly to carotid endarterectomy or carotid angioplasty and stenting.
- Apply anticoagulants when indicated.
- Use antiplatelet agents according to specific indications.
- Treat malignant MCA infarction with craniectomy.
- Consider surgical intervention for large cerebellar infarcts.

REFERENCES

1. Broderick J, Brott T, Kothari R, et al: The Greater Cincinnati/Northern Kentucky Stroke Study: Preliminary first-ever and total incidence rates of stroke among blacks. Stroke 1998;29:415-421.
2. Fang J, Alderman MH: Trend of stroke hospitalization, United States, 1988-1997. Stroke 2001;32:2221-2226.
3. Thom T, Haase N, Rosamond W, et al: Heart disease and stroke statistics—Update. Circulation 2006;113: e85-e151.
4. Centers for Disease Control and Prevention (CDC): Prevalence of disabilities and associated health conditions among adults: United States, 1999. MMWR 2001;50: 120-125.
5. Muntner P, Garrett E, Klag MJ, et al: Trends in stroke prevalence between 1973 and 1991 in the US population 25 to 74 years of age. Stroke 2002;33: 1209-1213.
6. Groeger JS, Guntupalli KK, Strosberg M, et al: Descriptive analysis of critical care units in the United States: Patient characteristics and intensive care unit utilization. Crit Care Med 1993;21: 279-291.
7. The National Institute of Neurological Disorders and Stroke t-PA Stroke Study Group: Tissue plasminogen activator for acute ischemic stroke. N Engl J Med 1995;333;1581-1587.
8. Furlan A, Higashida R, Wechsler L, et al: Intra-arterial prourokinase for acute ischemic Stroke. The PROACT II Study: A randomized controlled trial. JAMA 1999;282:2003-2011.
9. Smith WS, Sung G, Starkman S, et al: Safety and Efficacy of Mechanical Embolization in Acute Ischemic Stroke: Results of the MERCI Trial. Stroke 2005;36:1432-1438.
10. Furlan AJ, Eyding D, Albers GW, et al: Dose Escalation of Desmoteplase for Acute Ischemic Stroke (DEDAS). Evidence of safety and efficacy 3 to 9 hours after stroke onset. Stroke Mar 30 2006: Epub ahead of print.
11. Dellinger RP: Personal communication.
12. Albers GW, Caplan LR, Easton JD, et al: Transient ischemic attack-proposal for a new definition. N Engl J Med 2002;347:1713-1716.
13. Pessin MS, Duncan GW, Mohr JP, et al: Clinical and angiographic features of carotid transient ischemic attacks. N Engl J Med 1977;296:358-362.
14. Caplan D: Aphasia. In Heilman KM, Valenstein E (eds): Clinical Neuropsychology, 4th ed. Oxford, Oxford University Press, 2003, pp 14-34.
15. Heilman KM, Watson RT, Valenstein E: Neglect and related disorders. In Heilman KM, Valenstein E (eds): Clinical Neuropsychology, 4th ed. Oxford, Oxford University Press, 2003, pp 296-346.
16. Sacks O: The Man Who Fell Out of Bed. In: The Man Who Mistook His Wife for a Hat. New York, Simon & Schuster, 1998.
17. Kubik CS, Adams RD: Occlusion of the basilar artery—a clinical and pathological study. Brain 1946;69: 73-124.
18. Wijdicks EFM, Scott JP: Outcome in patients with acute basilar artery occlusion requiring mechanical ventilation. Stroke 1996;27:1301-1303.
19. Plum F, Posner JB: The Diagnosis of Stupor and Coma, 3rd ed. Philadelphia, FA Davis, 1980, p 9.
20. Baquis GD, Pessin MS, Scott RM: Limb shaking—a carotid TIA. Stroke 1985;16:444-448.
21. Dreifuss FE: Classification of epileptic seizures. In Engel J, Pedley TA (eds): Epilepsy: A Comprehensive Textbook. Philadelphia, Lippincott-Raven, 1997, pp 517-524.
22. Silberstein SD, Lipton RB, Goadsby PJ: Headache in Clinical Practice, 2nd ed. London, Martin Dunitz Ltd., 2002, pp 69-111.
23. Tong DC, Yenari MA, Albers GW, et al: Correlation of perfusion- and diffusion-weighted MRI with NIHSS score in acute (<6.5 hour) ischemic stroke. Neurology 1999;50:864-869.
24. Fiebach JB, Schellinger PD, Gass A, et al, for the Kompetenznetzwerk Schlaganfall B5: Stroke magnetic resonance imaging is accurate in hyperacute intracerebral hemorrhage: A multicenter study on the validity of stroke imaging. Stroke 2004;35: 502-506.
25. Knauth M, von Kummer R, Jansen O, et al: Potential of CT angiography in acute ischemic stroke. Am J Neuroradiol 1997;18:1001-1010.
26. Koelemay MJW, Nederkoorn PJ, Reitsma JB, Majoie CB: Systematic review of CT angiography for assessment of carotid artery disease. Stroke 2004;35:2306-2312.
27. Johnston DCC, Goldstein LB: Clinical carotid endarterectomy decision making: Noninvasive vascular imaging versus angiography. Neurology 2001:56:1009-1015.
28. Tomanek AI, Coutts SB, Demchuk AM, et al: MR angiography compared to conventional selective angiography in acute stroke. Canad J Neurol Sci 2006;33:58-62.
29. Brott T, Adams HP Jr, Olinger CP, et al: Measurements of acute cerebral infarction: A clinical examination scale. Stroke 1989;20:864-870.
30. Larrue V, von Kummer R, del Zoppo, et al: Hemorrhagic transformation in acute ischemic stroke. Potential contributing factors in the European Cooperative Acute Stroke Study. Stroke 1997;28:957-960.
31. Von Kummer R, Bozzao C, Manelfe C: Early CT Diagnosis of Hemispheric Brain Infarction. Berlin, Springer Verlag, 1995.
32. Patel SC, Levine SR, Tilley BC, et al: Lack of clinical significance of early ischemic changes on computed topography in acute stroke. JAMA 2001;286:2830-2838.
33. Adams HP, Adams R, Del Zoppo G, et al: Guidelines for the early management of patients with ischemic stroke. 2005 Guidelines Update. Stroke 2005;36:916-921.
34. The NINDS t-PA Stroke Study Group: Generalized efficacy of t-PA for acute stroke. Subgroup analysis of the NINDS t-PA stroke trial. Stroke 1997;28:2119-2125.
35. The ATLANTIS, ECASS, and NINDS rt-PA Study Group Investigators: Association of outcome with early stroke treatment: Pooled analysis of ATLANTIS, ECASS, and NINDS rt-PA stroke trials. Lancet 2004;363: 768-774.
36. Hacke W, Kaste M, Fieschi C, et al: Randomised double-blind placebo-controlled trial of thrombolytic therapy with intravenous alteplase in acute ischaemic stroke (ECASS II). Lancet 1998;352:1245-1251.
37. Clark WM, Wissman S, Albers GW, et al: Recombinant tissue-type plasminogen activator (alteplase) for ischemic stroke 3 to 5 hours after symptom onset: The ATLANTIS study—a randomized controlled trial. JAMA 1999;282:2019-2026.
38. Davis SM, Donnan GA, Butcher K, et al: Selection of thrombolytic therapy beyond 3 hours using magnetic resonance imaging. Curr Opin Neurol 2005;18:47-52.
39. Levy DL, Brott TG, Haley EC, et al: Factors related to intracranial hematoma formation in patients receiving tissue-type plasminogen activator for acute ischemic stroke. Stroke 1994;25:291-297.
40. Graham GD: Tissue plasminogen activator for acute ischemic stroke in clinical practice. A meta-analysis of safety data. Stroke 2003;34: 2847-2850.
41. Katzan IL, Hammer MD, Furlan AJ, et al: Quality improvement and tissue-type plasminogen activator for acute ischemic stroke: A Cleveland update. Stroke 2003;34:799-800.
42. Levy EI, Firlik AD, Wisniewski S, et al: Factors affecting survival rates for acute vertebrobasilar artery occlusions treated with intra-arterial thrombolytic therapy: A meta-analytical approach. Neurosurgery 1999;45:539-548.
43. Kasner SE, personal communication.
44. Kidwell CS, Saver JL, Carneado J, et al: Predictors of hemorrhagic transformation in patients receiving intra-arterial thrombolysis. Stroke 2002;33:717-724.
45. Chalela JA, Katzan I, Liebeskind DS, et al: Safety of intra-arterial thrombolysis in the postoperative period. Stroke 2001;32:1365-1369.
46. Khatri P, Kasner SE: Ischemic strokes after cardiac catheterization: Opportune thrombolysis candidates? Arch Neurol 2006;63:817-821.
47. The Interventional Management of Stroke Investigators: Combination intravenous and intra-arterial recanalization for acute ischemic stroke: The Interventional Management of Stroke Study. Stroke 2004;34:904-911.
48. The IMS Study Investigators: Hemorrhage in the Interventional Management of Stroke Trial. Stroke 2006;37:847-851.
49. Becker KJ, Brott TG: Approval of the MERCI clot retriever: A critical view. Stroke 2005;36:400-402.
50. European Carotid Surgery Trialists' Collaborative Group: Randomised trial

of endarterectomy for recently symptomatic carotid stenosis: Final results of the MRC European Carotid Surgery Trial (ECST). Lancet 1998;351:1379-1387.
51. North American Symptomatic Carotid Endarterectomy Trial Collaborators: Beneficial effect of carotid endarterectomy in symptomatic patients with high-grade carotid stenosis. N Engl J Med 1991;325:445-453.
52. Sundt TM Jr, Sandok BA, Whisnant JP: Carotid endarterectomy. Complications and preoperative assessment of risk. Mayo Clin Proc 1975;50:301-306.
53. Gasecki AP, Eliasziw M, Ferguson GG, et al: Long-term prognosis and effect of endarterectomy in patients with symptomatic severe carotid stenosis and contralateral carotid stenosis or occlusion: Results from NASCET. North American Symptomatic Carotid Endarterectomy Trial (NASCET) Group. J Neurosurg 1995;83:778-782.
54. Streifler JY, Eliasziw M, Benavente OR, et al: The risk of stroke in patients with first-ever retinal vs. hemispheric transient ischemic attacks and high-grade carotid stenosis. North American Symptomatic Carotid Endarterectomy Trial. Arch Neurol 1995;52:246-249.
55. Morgenstern LB, Fox AJ, Sharpe BL, et al: The risks and benefits of carotid endarterectomy in patients with near-occlusion of the carotid artery. Neurology 1997;48:911-915.
56. Benavente OR, Eliasziw M, Streifler JY, et al: Prognosis after transient monocular blindness associated with carotid artery stenosis. N Engl J Med 2001;345:1084-1090.
57. Eliasziw M, Streifler JY, Fox AJ, et al: Significance of plaque ulceration in symptomatic patients with high-grade carotid stenosis. North American Symptomatic Carotid Endarterectomy Trial. Stroke 1994;25:304-308.
58. Rothwell PM, Eliasziw M, Gutnikov, SA, et al: Endarterectomy for Symptomatic Carotid Stenosis in Relation to Clinical Subgroups and Timing of Surgery. Lancet 2004;363:915-924.
59. Yadav JS, Wholey MH, Kuntz RE, et al: Protected carotid-artery stenting versus endarterectomy in high-risk patients. N Engl J Med 2004;351: 1493-1501.
60. The SPACE Collaborative Group: 30 day results from the SPACE trial of Stent-Protected Angioplasty versus Carotid Endarterectomy in Symptomatic Patients: A randomised non-inferiority trial. Lancet 2006;368:1239-1247.
61. Mas J-L, Chatellier G, Beyssen B, et al, for the EVA-3S Investigators: Endarterectomy versus stenting in patients with symptomatic severe carotid stenosis. N Engl J Med 2006;355:1660-1671.
62. Executive Committee for the Asymptomatic Carotid Atherosclerosis Study: Endarterectomy for asymptomatic carotid artery stenosis. JAMA 1995;273:1421-1428.
63. Duke RJ, Bloch RF, Turpie AG, et al: Intravenous heparin for the prevention of stroke progression in acute partial stable stroke. Ann Intern Med 1986;105:825-828.
64. Mohr JP, Thompson JLP, Lazar RM, et al: A comparison of warfarin and aspirin for the prevention of recurrent ischemic stroke. N Engl J Med 2001;345:1444-1451.
65. Chimowitz MI, Lynn MJ, Howlett-Smith H, et al: Comparison of warfarin and aspirin for symptomatic intracranial arterial stenosis. N Engl J Med 2005;352:1305-1316.
66. Pullicino P, Thompson JL, Barton B, et al, on behalf of the WARCEF Investigators: Warfarin versus Aspirin in patients with Reduced Cardiac Ejection Fraction (WARCEF): Rationale, objectives, and design. J Card Fail 2006;12:39-46.
67. Risk factors for stroke and efficacy of antithrombotic therapy in atrial fibrillation. Analysis of pooled data from five randomized controlled trials. Arch Int Med 1994;154:1449-1457.
68. ACTIVE Writing Group on Behalf of the ACTIVE Investigators: Clopidogrel plus Aspirin versus Oral Anticoagulation for Atrial Fibrillation in the Atrial Fibrillation Clopidogrel Trial with Irbesartan for Prevention of Vascular Events (ACTIVE W): A randomized controlled trial. Lancet 2006;367:1903-1912.
69. EAFT (European Atrial Fibrillation Trial) study group: Secondary prevention in non-rheumatic atrial fibrillation after transient ischaemic attack or minor stroke. Lancet 1993;342:1255-1262.
70. Berge E, Abdelnoor M, Nakstad PH, Sandset PM, on behalf of the HAEST Study Group: Low molecular-weight heparin versus aspirin in patients with acute ischemic stroke and atrial fibrillation: A double-blind randomised study. Lancet 2000;355:1205-1210.
71. De Bruijn SFTM, de Haan RJ, Stam J, for the Cerebral Venous Sinus Thrombosis Study Group: Clinical features and prognostic factors of cerebral venous sinus thrombosis in a prospective series of 59 patients. J Neurol Neurosurg Psychiatr 2001;70:105-108.
72. Vogl TJ, Bergman C, Villringer A, et al: Dural sinus thrombosis: Value of venous MR angiography for diagnosis and follow-up. Am J Roentgenol 1994;162:1191-1198.
73. Einhaupl KM, Villringer A, Meister W, et al: Heparin treatment in sinus venous thrombosis. Lancet 1991;338:596-600.
74. De Bruijn SFTM, Stam J, for the Cerebral Venous Sinus Thrombosis Study Group: Randomized, placebo-controlled trial of anticoagulant treatment with low-molecular-weight heparin for cerebral sinus thrombosis. Stroke 1999;30:484-488.
75. Frey JL, Muro GJ, McDougall CG, et al: Cerebral venous thrombosis. Combined intrathrombus rtPA and intravenous heparin. Stroke 1999;30:489-494.
76. Schievink WI: Current concepts: Spontaneous dissection of the carotid and vertebral arteries. N Engl J Med 2001;344:898-906.
77. Levy C, Laissy JP, Raveau V, et al: Carotid and vertebral artery dissections: Three-dimensional time-of-flight MR angiography and MR imaging versus conventional angiography. Radiology 1994;190: 97-103.
78. Arnold M, Nedeltchev K, Sturzenegger M, et al: Thrombolysis in patients with acute stroke caused by cervical artery dissection: Analysis of nine patients and review of the literature. Arch Neurol 2002;59:549-553.
79. Thomas DP, Roberts HR: Hypercoagulability in venous and arterial thrombosis. Ann Intern Med 1997;26:638-644.
80. Poort SR, Rosendaal FR, Reitsma PH, Bertina RM: A common genetic variation in the 3'-untranslated region of the prothrombin gene is associated with elevated plasma prothrombin levels and an increase in venous thrombosis. Blood 1996;88:3698-3703.
81. Antiplatelet Trialists' Collaboration: Collaborative overview of randomized trials of antiplatelet treatment: Part 1: Prevention of death, MI and stroke by prolonged antiplatelet therapy in various categories of patients. BMJ 1994;308:81-106.
82. Algra A, Van Gijn J: Aspirin at any dose above 30 mg offers only modest protection after cerebral ischemia. J Neurol Neurosurg Psychiatr 1996;60:197-199.
83. The Dutch TIA Study Group: A comparison of two doses of aspirin (30 mg vs. 283 mg a day) in patients after a transient ischemic attack or minor ischemic stroke. N Engl J Med 1991;325:1261-1266.
84. Farrell B, Goodwin J, Richard S, et al: The United Kingdom transient ischemic attack (UK-TIA) aspirin trial: Final results. J Neurol Neurosurg Psychiatr 1991;54:1044-1054.
85. Ticlid (Ticlopidine hydrochloride tablets). Complete Prescribing Information. Roche Pharmaceuticals, Nutley, NJ, March 2001.
86. Chen DK, Kim JS, Sutton DMC: Thrombotic thrombocytopenic purpura associated with ticlopidine use: A report of three cases and review of the literature. Arch Intern Med 1999;159:311-314.
87. CAPRIE Steering Committee: A randomized, blinded trial of Clopidogrel versus Aspirin in Patients at Risk of Ischemic Events (CAPRIE). Lancet 1996;348:1329-1339.
88. The Clopidogrel in Unstable Angina to Prevent Recurrent Events Trial Investigators: Effects of Clopidogrel in Addition to Aspirin in Patients with Acute Coronary Syndrome without ST-Segment Elevation. N Engl J Med 2001;345:494-502.
89. Chen ZM, Jiang LX, Chen YP, et al: Addition of clopidogrel to aspirin in patients with acute myocardial infarction: Randomized placebo-controlled trial. Lancet 2005;366: 1607-1621.
90. Sabatine MS, Cannon CP, Gibson CM, et al: Addition of clopidogrel to aspirin and fibrinolytic therapy for myocardial infarction with ST-segment elevations. N Engl J Med 2005;352: 1179-1189.
91. Mehta SM, Yusuf S, Peters RJG, et al: Effects of pre-treatment with clopidogrel and aspirin followed by long-term therapy in patients

undergoing percutaneous coronary intervention: The PCI-CURE Study. Lancet 2001;358:527-533.
92. Diener HC, Bogousslavsky J, Brass LM, et al: Aspirin and clopidogrel compared with clopidogrel alone after recent ischaemic stroke or transient ischaemic attack in high-risk patients (MATCH): Randomized, double-blinded, placebo-controlled trial. Lancet 2004;364:331-337.
93. Bhatt DL, Fox KA, Hacke W, et al: Clopidogrel and aspirin versus aspirin alone for the prevention of atherothrombotic events. N Engl J Med 2006;354:1706-1717.
94. Chen ZM, Sandercock P, Pan HC, et al: Indications for early aspirin use in acute ischemic stroke: A combined analysis of 40,000 randomized patients from the Chinese Acute Stroke Trial and the International Stroke Trial. Stroke 2000;31:1240-1249.
95. ESPS Group: European Stroke Prevention Study. Stroke 1990;21:1122-1130.
96. Diener HC, Cunha L, Forbes C, et al: European Stroke Prevention Study 2. Dipyridamole and acetylsalicylic acid in the secondary prevention of stroke. J Neurol Sci 1996;143:1-13.
97. The ESPRIT Study Group: Aspirin Plus Dipyridamole versus Aspirin Alone After Cerebral Ischemia of Arterial Origin (ESPRIT). Lancet 2006;367: 1665-1673.
98. http://www.profess.study.com
99. Di Tullio M, Sacco RL, Gopal A, et al: Patent foramen ovale as a risk factor for cryptogenic stroke. Ann Intern Med 1992;117:461-465.
100. Mas J-L, Arquizan C, Lamy C, et al: Recurrent cerebrovascular events associated with patent foramen ovale, atrial septal aneurysm, or both. N Engl J Med 2001;345:1740-1746.
101. Schuchlenz HW, Weihs W, Horner S, Quehenbeger F: The association between the diameter of a patent foramen ovale and the risk of embolic cerebrovascular events. Am J Med 2000;109:456-462.
102. Messe SR, Silverman IE, Kizer JR, et al: Practice parameter: Recurrent stroke with patent foramen ovale and atrial septal aneurysm. Report of the Quality Standards Subcommittee of the American Academy of Neurology. Neurology 2004;62: 1042-1050.
103. Hacke W, Schwab S, Horn M, et al: "Malignant" middle cerebral artery territory infarction: Clinical course and prognostic signs. Arch Neurol 1996;53:309-315.
104. Wijdicks EF, Diringer MN: Middle cerebral artery territory infarction and early brain swelling: Progression and effect of age on outcome. Mayo Clin Proc 1998;73:829-836.
105. Biller J, Adams HP Jr, Bruno A, et al: Mortality in acute cerebral infarction in young adults: A ten-year experience. Angiology 1991;42:224-230.
106. Krieger DW, Demchuk AM, Kasner SE, et al: Early clinical and radiological predictors of fatal brain swelling in ischemic stroke. Stroke 1999;30: 287-292.
107. Pullicino PM, Alexandrov AV, Shelton JA, et al: Mass effect and death from severe acute stroke. Neurology 1997;49:1090-1095.
108. Hofmeijer J, van der Worp B, Kapelle LJ: Treatment of space-occupying cerebral infarction. Crit Care Med 2003;31:617-625.
109. Steiner T, Ringleb P, Hacke W: Treatment options for large hemispheric stroke. Neurology 2001;57(Suppl 2):S61-S68.
110. Wijdicks EFM: Management of massive hemispheric cerebral infarct: Is there a ray of hope? Mayo Clin Proc 2000;75:945-952.
111. Schwab S, Schwarz S, Spranger M, et al: Moderate hypothermia in the treatment of patients with severe middle cerebral artery infarction. Stroke 1998;29:2461-2466.
112. Krieger DW, De Georgia MA, Abou-Chebl A, et al: Cooling for acute ischemic brain damage (COOL AID): An open pilot study of induced hypothermia in acute ischemic stroke. Stroke 2001;32:1847-1854.
113. De Georgia MA, Krieger DW, Abou-Chebl A, et al: Cooling for acute ischemic brain damage (COOL AID): A feasibility trial of endovascular cooling. Neurology 2004;63: 312-317.
114. Rieke K, Schwab S, Krieger D, et al: Decompressive surgery in space-occupying hemispheric infarction: Results of an open, prospective trial. Crit Care Med 1995;23:1576-1587.
115. Schwab S, Steiner T, Aschoff A, et al: Early hemicraniectomy in patients with complete middle cerebral artery infarction. Stroke 1998;29:1888-1893.
116. Berrie C: Decompressive surgery for treatment of malignant infarction of the middle cerebral artery: Presented at the European Stroke Conference. Doctor's Guide Dispatch: May 24, 2006.
117. Hornig CR, Rust DS, Busse O, et al: Space-occupying cerebellar infarction. Clinical course and prognosis. Stroke 1994;25:372-374.
118. Jauss M, Krieger D, Hornig C, et al, for the GASCIS Study Centers: Surgical and Medical Management of Patients with Massive Cerebellar Infarctions: Results of the German-Austrian Cerebellar Infarction Study. J Neurol 1999;246: 257-264.

Chapter 65

Acute Neuromuscular Respiratory Failure in Myasthenia Gravis and Guillain-Barré Syndrome

Osman Samil Kozak and Eelco F. M. Wijdicks

Acquired causes of neuromuscular weakness have been recognized more frequently in today's intensive care unit (ICU).[1] Recognition of critical illness polyneuropathy also has increased, but the role of this entity in respiratory failure remains poorly defined. In most instances, neuromuscular weakness–induced acute respiratory failure treated in the ICU involves Guillain-Barré syndrome (GBS) or an exacerbation of previously diagnosed myasthenia gravis (MG). The management of patients with these disorders is challenging and demanding, with uncertainty about modes of ventilation, timing of tracheostomy, and long-term care. New information has become available that can guide physicians in the timing of intubation. This chapter provides a comprehensive overview of optimal management for respiratory failure resulting from GBS and MG and reviews the underlying pathophysiology.

PATHOPHYSIOLOGY OF NEUROMUSCULAR RESPIRATORY FAILURE

In neuromuscular respiratory failure, ventilatory function is compromised through two mechanisms: (1) respiratory muscle weakness or fatigue (involving mainly the diaphragm but later the intercostals) and (2) oropharyngeal weakness, which leads to obstruction of upper airway and inability to clear secretions. Although neuromuscular respiratory failure usually is associated with generalized weakness, up to 20% of patients do not have limb weakness on presentation of respiratory compromise.[2]

Neuromuscular weakness of the respiratory muscles is characterized by the inability to generate or maintain normal respiratory pressures. Pulmonary studies typically reveal a pure ventilatory defect with otherwise normal pulmonary parenchyma, which becomes compromised with development of atelectasis. The degree of involvement of the inspiratory and the expiratory muscles is variable, and the clinical manifestations reflect the compromise of both muscle groups.

During respiration, lungs can be expanded and contracted in two ways: by downward and upward movement of the diaphragm, to lengthen and shorten the chest cavity, and by elevation and depression of the ribs, to increase and decrease the anteroposterior diameter of the chest. Normal quiet breathing is accomplished almost entirely by the first of the two methods—by the movement of the diaphragm. In neuromuscular respiratory failure, ventilation remains intact until diaphragm involvement becomes significant. The first indication of diaphragmatic weakness is alveolar hypoventilation and impaired CO_2 exchange. These changes are followed by an increase in respiratory rate as a compensatory mechanism to attempt to maintain minute ventilation. Later, accessory muscles of ventilation are recruited in response to increased ventilatory demand. Paradoxical breathing, also known as thoracoabdominal asynchrony, occurs with severe respiratory weakness. Typically, the abdomen and chest expand and contract in a synchronized fashion. During inspiration, a downward movement of diaphragm pushes the abdominal contents down and out as the rib margins are lifted and moved out, causing both chest and abdomen to rise. With diaphragmatic weakness or paralysis, the diaphragm moves up rather than down during inspiration, and the abdomen moves in, contracting during chest rise. This is known as "paradoxical breathing" and can be visualized with fluoroscopy (Fig. 65-1).

Although the upper airway muscles do not contribute directly to chest expansion or collapse, they are essential

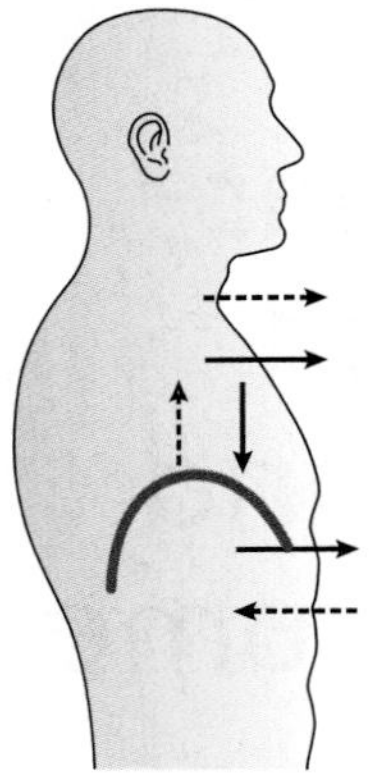

Figure 65-1. Paradoxical breathing in neuromuscular respiratory failure.

Box 65-1

Pathophysiologic Changes with Neuromuscular Failure

- Normal respiratory function is present with VC of 65 mL/kg.
- Poor cough is evident with accumulation of secretions and with VC of 30 mL/kg.
- With VC of 20 mL/kg, the sigh mechanism is impaired, and atelectasis and hypoxia develop.
- Sigh is lost with VC of 15 mL/kg, and atelectasis and shunting appear.
- Hypoventilation starts with VC of 10 mL/kg.
- Hypercapnia develops with VC between 5 and 10 mL/kg.

FVC, forced vital capacity; VC, vital capacity.

for keeping the airways open during respiration. They play an important role in preventing collapse of the pharynx during inspiration and preventing aspiration during swallowing. With the exception of laryngeal muscles, these muscles have a higher proportion of fast fibers and therefore a lower fatigue resistance than the diaphragm.

Ventilatory drive response to an increase in CO_2 in patients with GBS and MG has been studied and was found to be unlikely to contribute to hypoventilation during ventilatory failure.[3] Ventilatory drive increases during acute hypoventilation, and the ventilatory drive response to CO_2 remains intact, even when the minute ventilation response to CO_2 is poor.

CLINICAL EVALUATION OF NEUROMUSCULAR RESPIRATORY FAILURE

Vital capacity (VC), the volume of exhaled air after maximal inspiration, normally is 60 to 70 mL/kg and in normal persons is determined primarily by the size of the thorax and lungs. Reduction of VC to 30 mL/kg is associated with weak cough, accumulation of oropharyngeal secretions, atelectasis, and hypoxemia. Another measure of respiratory muscle strength is the ability to generate negative pressure with inspiratory effort. In normal persons, respiratory muscles cause pleural and alveolar pressures to change by approximately 3 cm H_2O during the breathing cycle. Maximal pressure generation can be determined by blocking the upper airway and recording mouth pressure changes during inspiratory effort. Maximal negative inspiratory pressures (NIPs) generated by adults average −114 cm H_2O in young men and −67 cm H_2O in young women (normal, exceeding −70 cm H_2O). Forced expiratory pressures average 160 cm H_2O in young men and 95 cm H_2O in young women (normal, greater than 100 cm H_2O). This means that the respiratory muscles are capable of generating more than 30 times the amount of force necessary for tidal breathing.[4] NIP measures the strength of the diaphragm and other muscles of inspiration and reflects the ability to maintain normal lung expansion and avoid atelectasis. Positive expiratory force (PEF) measures strength of the muscles of expiration, and correlates with strength of cough and ability to clear secretions from the airway[3] (Box 65-1).

A simple bedside test, asking patients to count to 20 without the need of an additional respiration, may identify early weakness.

CLINICAL PRESENTATION OF GUILLAIN-BARRÉ SYNDROME

Guillain-Barré syndrome is an acute, monophasic, inflammatory, demyelinating polyneuropathy, also known as acute inflammatory demyelinating polyneuropathy (AIDP). Its incidence is 1 to 2 cases per 100,000 people and remains fairly constant across the globe. GBS commonly is precipitated by an infection, but the immunopathogenesis has remained elusive since its original description in 1916. *Campylobacter jejuni*, cytomegalovirus, Epstein-Barr virus, and *Mycoplasma pneumoniae* predominate as preceding infection pathogens.[5]

The diagnosis of GBS often is straightforward. Severe back pain and limb paresthesias, starting in the ankles and wrists, with a "tight band" feeling are typical presenting signs. The paresthesias gradually scatter over the limbs and move proximally. Ascending motor paralysis is the classic feature but may not be observed in many variants of GBS. Weakness begins in the more proximal muscles, causing difficulty with climbing stairs and getting out of a chair, and is notable 1 or 2 days after the onset of paresthesias. It is characteristically symmetric and accompanied by depressed or absent deep tendon reflexes. Facial and oropharyngeal muscles also are affected in 50% of the cases, and weakness of these muscle groups may be the initial manifestation. Dysautonomia occurs in up to 70% of the cases, mainly manifested as arrhythmias, hypotension or hypertension, urinary retention, and ileus.[6] Although paresthesias often are the presenting symptom, sensory modalities remain normal to mildly impaired. Symptoms and signs may progress for up to 4 weeks. Recovery often starts after the second week. Progression over 8 weeks alters the diagnosis to chronic inflammatory demyelinating polyneuropathy (CIDP). CSF analysis typically shows high protein with a normal white blood cell count (the historical albuminocytologic dissociation). More than 10 cells per is unusual and occurs in association with Lyme disease and AIDS.[7] Electrophysiologic studies are essential not only for diagnosis but also for prognosis, accomplished by determining the extent of axonal involvement and demyelination.

Respiratory failure, if it occurs in GBS, commonly appears within 1 week after the onset of paresthesias.[8] The clinical signs and symptoms include staccato speech; ability to speak only short sentences, small tidal volume with increased respiratory rate, tachycardia, and diaphoresis.

CLINICAL PRESENTATION OF MYASTHENIA GRAVIS

MG is an autoimmune disease of defective neurotransmission leading to fatigable muscle weakness. The incidence is 0.5 to 5 cases per 100,000 people. Its pathogenesis can be briefly summarized as an antibody reaction at the antigen epitopes of the acetylcholine receptor, eventually leading to destruction and simplification of the junctional fold and widening synaptic cleft.[9] Onset may be at any age but tends to be earlier in females (mean 28 years) than in males (mean 42 years). MG results in either transient or persistent weakness or abnormal fatigability of any or all of the skeletal muscles, but in more than half of the cases the initial symptoms involve the eyes.[10] In a majority of patients, no precipitating factor can be identified; in a few, MG appears to be precipitated by a viral or bacterial infection, physical trauma, surgical procedures (particularly thyroidectomy), pregnancy and delivery, or exposure to drugs with neuromuscular blocking action such as quinidine, penicillamine, or procainamide.

Myasthenic crisis is defined as weakness resulting from myasthenia that is severe enough to necessitate mechanical ventilation or airway protection. The need for ventilatory asssistance usually follows onset of weakness of diaphragmatic or accessory respiratory muscles, but mechanical ventilation also may become necessary because of airway collapse from oropharyngeal muscle weakness, stridor from vocal cord weakness, or the inability to clear secretions.[11] Myasthenic crisis requires urgent evaluation and treatment. It affects 8% to 27% of patients with MG and tends to occur soon after diagnosis, usually within the first 2 years (in 74% of the cases).[2,12] The mortality rate for myasthenic crisis has declined from 70% in the 1920s to 5% after the 1980s with discovery and application of acetylcholinesterase compounds, mechanical ventilation, immunosuppressive agents, and, more recently, plasma exchange and intravenous immunoglobulin (IVIG). Despite the decrease in mortality, however, the duration of myasthenic crisis has not changed and continues to average 2 weeks.[2]

RESPIRATORY FAILURE IN GUILLAIN-BARRÉ SYNDROME AND MYASTHENIA GRAVIS

Arterial blood gas (ABG) analysis performed early after development of a rapid, shallow breathing pattern may show a decreased arterial partial pressure of carbon dioxide (Pa_{CO_2}). This change is followed by progressive inspiratory muscle weakness, leading to hypoventilation and hypercapnia. The P_{CO_2} in alveolar gas or arterial blood is inversely related to the alveolar ventilation. If the alveolar ventilation is halved, the P_{CO_2} doubles while the CO_2 production rate remains constant. Microatelectasis and alveolar collapse also can develop in patients unable to take deep breaths, leading to ventilation-perfusion mismatching and decreased arterial partial pressure of oxygen (Pa_{O_2}). It is important to recognize that in patients with neuromuscular respiratory failure and imminent respiratory arrest, ABG analysis results often remain unimpressive until severe respiratory muscle weakness or total failure develops.

Because in myasthenic crisis most of the identified causes are related to infection or medications, physical examination, chest x-ray imaging, complete blood count, and blood and other cultures (depending on the presentation) should be part of the workup.

Respiratory insufficiency and failure to clear secretions are the major consequences of inspiratory and expiratory muscle weakness, respectively. Although often overlooked, therapies to augment secretion clearance and cough are important in patients with neuromuscular weakness. The first step in evaluation of respiratory status is assessment of clinical features along with repeated pulmonary function tests. Frequent (at least four times daily) assessment of pulmonary function should be instituted. This typically includes VC and maximum NIP.

MANAGEMENT OF MYASTHENIA GRAVIS

In patients with known MG, other causes of respiratory dysfunction, such as pulmonary embolism and cardiac failure, should be considered in the appropriate setting. Otherwise, the evaluation is relatively straightforward and is geared toward identifying the typical causes of crisis. Known causes of myasthenic crisis include respiratory tract infection, aspiration pneumonitis, surgery (especially thymectomy), changes in medication, and emotional stress. Changes in medication may relate to the recent addition of a corticosteroid, a dose reduction, or overtreatment with acetylcholinesterase inhibitors. In approximately one third of crises, a precipitant cannot be identified.[2] A careful review of medications, including over-the-counter preparations, is mandatory.

The issue of cholinergic crisis is controversial. Cholinergic crisis is believed to occur as a result of overtreatment with acetylcholinesterase inhibitors. It may manifest with copious respiratory secretions and fasciculations from nicotinic toxicity. Historically, when the treatment of MG was limited to use of acetylcholinesterase inhibitors, overdose could lead to MG crisis, but this entity is now infrequently encountered, and its importance may have been overstated.[10] In a retrospective review of 73 episodes of myasthenic crisis, no instances of cholinergic crisis were identified.[2] To avoid any confusion during the acute management of myasthenic crisis, it is recommended to discontinue acetylcholinesterase inhibitors during invasive mechanical ventilation. During noninvasive mechanical ventilation (NMV), this decision should be made on a case-by-case base, depending on the patient's response to acetylcholinesterase inhibitors.

The mainstay of immunotherapy for the short-term treatment of MG is plasma exchange. Plasma exchange directly removes acetylcholine receptor (AChR) antibodies from the circulation, and clinical improvement roughly correlates with the degree of elimination as reflected in AChR antibody levels. Although widely used and considered effective, plasmapheresis for crisis has not been compared with placebo in a controlled trial. It was first introduced in 1976 as a short-term therapy for acute exacerbations of MG.[13] A total of four to six exchanges typically are done over 2 weeks, and 2 to 4 L of plasma is removed with each exchange. Improvement usually is noted within days, although some patients may not show evidence of response until weeks after therapy. Effects last approximately 1 to 12 weeks. IVIG also is widely used in the management of MG. Its mechanism of action in MG is less certain, but it is believed to work by introduction of anti-idiotype antibodies and reduced AChR antibody production achieved through negative feedback. It often is employed in a dose of 0.4 g per kg of body weight given over 5 days (total dose of 2 g per kg), although a recent randomized clinical trial found no significant superiority of 2 g per kg over 1 g per kg of IVIG in MG exacerbation.[14] Trials comparing plasma exchange and IVIG found more rapid onset of improvement in clinical measures of MG, as well as earlier time to extubation, with early (in the first 2 weeks) institution of plasmapheresis, but did not find any significant difference on long-term follow-up evaluation.[6,15] One study found plasma exchange also to be effective in patients in whom IVIG has failed.[16] Among neuromuscular disease experts, plasma exchange is preferred as first-line therapy in MG crisis. Plasma exchange and IVIG also can be quite useful to prevent deterioration preoperatively in patients undergoing thymectomy or other surgery.

Major complications of plasma exchange are problems with vascular access (including infection, local thrombosis, and vascular perforation), hypotension, transient electrolyte disturbances, and heparin-induced thrombocytopenia. IVIG often is better tolerated. Side effects related to IVIG treatment are often mild and include headache, chills, fever, and nausea. These manifestations are related to the rate of infusion. Major side effects independent of infusion rate are acute renal failure, thrombotic events, and anaphylaxis.

High-dose steroids can transiently worsen the neuromuscular weakness associated with MG during early stages of treatment in up to 50% of patients. For this reason, during myasthenic crisis, it is recommended to start steroids only after initiation of plasma exchange or IVIG treatments and then to continue until a remission occurs.[17]

Major medical complications secondary to myasthenic crisis are related to days on mechanical ventilation. Fever is the most common complication (occurring in 70% of patients), followed by pneumonia (in 50%) and atelectasis (in 40%).

Thymectomy is indicated in cases of thymoma-associated MG, but in cases without thymoma demonstrated on computed tomography or magnetic resonance imaging of the chest, treatment with thymectomy is controversial. Empiric thymectomy in the elderly is likely to be less effective because of atrophy of the thymus, so many experts do not recommend surgery for patients older than 60 years of age. Postoperative myasthenic crisis is not uncommon. In a recent retrospective study, predictors of postoperative myasthenic crisis were preoperative bulbar symptoms, preoperative serum antiacetylcholine receptor antibody level greater than 100 nmol/L, and intraoperative blood loss greater than 1 L.[18] Delaying thymectomy until immunosuppressive treatment has been initiated and bulbar symptoms are resolved may be beneficial in avoiding postoperative myasthenic crisis. Sekine and colleagues reported reduced risk of post-thymectomy myasthenic crisis in patients who received alternate-day high-dose prednisolone preoperatively.[19] Improvement after thymectomy may not be seen for months or even years.

MANAGEMENT OF GUILLAIN-BARRÉ SYNDROME

The management of patients with GBS can be challenging because of its unpredictable course with potential for rapid deterioration, leading to respiratory failure. Any patient without clear-cut evidence of stable neuromuscular status on initial evaluation or presentation will require admission and observation in an ICU. However, only one in three patients will deteriorate significantly enough to mandate further or prolonged ICU monitoring and possibly intubation.

Main modalities of acute treatment are plasma exchange and IVIG, both of which are recommended for nonambulatory patients with GBS who present within 4 weeks of onset. Large multicenter trials have established the effectiveness of plasma exchange in GBS.[20,21] Earlier clinical improvement, reduced need for mechanical ventilation, and faster recovery have been shown. A systematic review of six randomized trials in 2002 found that plasma exchange was superior to supportive care.[22] Plasma exchange was most effective when started within 7 days of symptom onset; however, an improvement in outcome was still observed if treatment was instituted up to 30 days after onset of symptoms in the North American study. Two plasma exchanges are superior to none in mild GBS, and four exchanges are superior to two in moderately severe GBS. However, six exchanges were not superior to four in severe GBS requiring mechanical ventilation.

No randomized trials have been conducted to compare IVIG with placebo for the treatment of GBS but IVIG was shown to be as effective as plasma exchange for the treatment of GBS by a 2006 meta-analysis of five trials.[23] Analysis found no significant difference between plasma exchange and IVIG in disability scores at 4 weeks. Combining IVIG with plasma exchange also has been tried and was found not to have additional benefit.[24] Corticosteroids alone have no significant benefit in GBS. Intravenous methylprednisolone in combination with IVIG may hasten recovery but does not significantly affect the long-term outcome.[25-27]

NONINVASIVE VENTILATION: BILEVEL POSITIVE AIRWAY PRESSURE

Traditionally, patients with acute neuromuscular respiratory failure are ventilated by invasive mechanical ventilation. Prolonged endotracheal intubation, however, is associated with discomfort and with ventilator-associated complications.[2] In both MG and GBS, mortality and morbidity are strongly tied to the duration of invasive mechanical ventilation. Noninvasive ventilation is being used increasingly to manage acute deterioration in patients with neuromuscular failure.[28,29] Downsides of noninvasive ventilation are, in the patients with associated bulbar weakness, upper airway collapse with increased airway resistance and lack of airway protection from secretions.[30]

Noninvasive mechanical ventilation (NMV) using bilevel positive airway pressure (BiPAP) ventilation (inspiration and expiration pressure application) in acute respiratory failure caused by MG was shown to be effective in a group of patients with MG from the Mayo Clinic.[28] NMV averted endotracheal intubation in 11 cases of severe MG exacerbation, even in the presence of bulbar weakness. In this study, presence of hypercapnia ($Paco_2$ greater than 50 mm Hg) at onset predicted NMV failure and subsequent intubation. Of interest, bedside pulmonary function tests did not predict the outcome of NMV ventilation trials. The investigators claimed that NMV could prevent intubation in 70% of trials.

In contrast with the findings with MG, data on use of NMV in GBS are scarce. One study warned against its use because improvement following initiation of NIV masked the slow deterioration of GBS.[31]

MECHANICAL VENTILATION: ENDOTRACHEAL INTUBATION

Guillain-Barré Syndrome

Mechanical ventilation is required in 20% to 30% of patients with GBS.[32-34] The decision of when to intubate patients with respiratory failure caused by GBS has been discretionary. It requires a clinical choice between premature intubation, with secondary risk of tracheal and pulmonary injury, and watchful observation, which could lead to the need for emergency intubation. Emergency intubation was found to be associated with prolonged time on mechanical ventilation and, when associated with respiratory arrest, with anoxic brain injury.[35] Several clinical factors have been proposed to predict when to intervene. Predictive factors for intubation include rapid progression, dysautonomia, bilateral facial palsy, and oropharyngeal weakness.[36] Serial measurements on pulmonary function testing are essential in anticipating the need for mechanical ventilation. A vital capacity of less than 20 mL/kg, a maximum inspiratory pressure (PImax) of less than 30 cm H_2O, and a maximum expiratory pressure (PEmax) of less than 40 cm H_2O (20/30/40 rule) suggest the need for mechanical ventilation[36] (Fig. 65-2). Elective intubation should be anticipated. Profound abnormalities

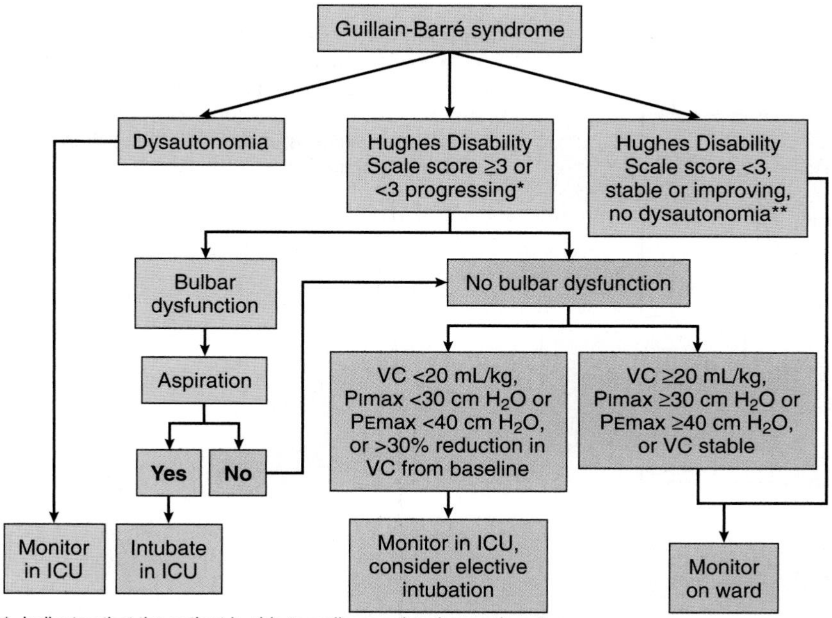

* Indicates that the patient is able to walk unassisted more than 5 m.
** Indicates that the patient is unable to walk unassisted more than 5 m or is bedridden or mechanically ventilated.

Figure 65-2. Flowchart based on clinical and respiratory factors in the management of Guillain-Barré syndrome. ICU, intensive care unit; PEmax, maximum expiratory pressure; PImax, maximum inspiratory pressure; VC, vital capacity.

of phrenic nerve conduction time and findings on diaphragmatic electromyography may predict the need for mechanical ventilation.[37]

Duration of mechanical ventilation in patients with GBS ranged from 18 to 49 days in large clinical series.[38-40] Inspiratory pressures and ABGs immediately preceding intubation did not predict the need for prolonged ventilation.[34] IVIG and plasma exchange have been shown to reduce the duration of ventilation in randomized trials.[21,40] A majority of complications in GBS occur during this stage. Prolonged intubation (14 days) was found to be associated with increased morbidity and mortality, mainly due to increased risk of ventilator-associated pneumonia and longer duration of mechanical ventilation.[41] Aggressive respiratory therapy, including frequent suctioning and use of ventilatory strategies aiming at minimizing atelectasis, should be emphasized. If no improvement is noted, aggressive respiratory management should include tracheostomy to allow more efficient bronchial clearing and reduction in the work of breathing imposed by the endotracheal tube.

Tracheostomy and its timing is a debated topic. The need for tracheostomy is more likely in the elderly and in the presence of pre-existing pulmonary disease.[34] A majority of patients with GBS-associated neuromuscular failure and mechanical ventilation undergo tracheostomy (up to 89%).[41] Tracheostomy should be postponed until the third week in patients who show some clinical improvement. This provides a period of assessment during which neuromuscular respiratory function may improve in response to treatment, and up to 50% of these patients (those showing improvement) could be spared from tracheostomy by waiting until the third week. Percutaneous tracheostomy may allow transfer of unstable patients to the operating room, thereby decreasing incidence of wound infection and providing better cosmetic results.[42]

Myasthenia Gravis

Invasive mechanical ventilation in patients with MG can be avoided in a majority of cases with early implementation of rapid immunomodulatory treatments and noninvasive ventilation.[28] Frequent pulmonary function tests are important to monitor the progression of respiratory function (Fig. 65-3). Although several parameters traditionally have been suggested for intubation (VC less than 15 mL/kg, NIP less than –30), the fluctuating nature of the disease and frequently associated facial muscle weakness give these parameters limited positive predictive power.[12,43] Ventilatory support is unlikely to be needed when VC is more than 20 mL/kg. Assessment of respiratory function should use a range of criteria including symptoms of breathlessness, paradoxical abdominal wall motion, bulbar nerve palsy, and ABG analysis to look for presence of hypercapnia or hypoxia. Patients with P_{CO_2} greater than 50 mm Hg usually are unresponsive to noninvasive ventilation and should be managed with endotracheal intubation. Hypercapnia alone usually but not always is a mandatory indication for mechanical ventilation, and this decision should take into consideration the patient's ease of respiration and level of consciousness and stability of Pa_{CO_2}.[12]

Patients in whom Anti-MuSK antibodies can be demonstrated have a greater risk for the development of respiratory compromise.[44]

EXTUBATION TRIALS

Weaning from mechanical ventilation should be guided by improvement in strength and normalization of values

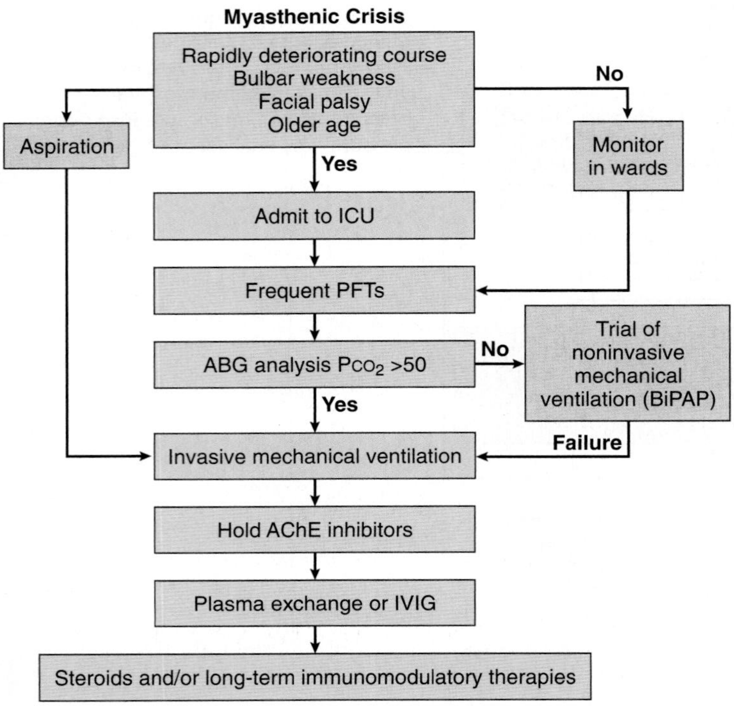

Figure 65-3. Clinical flowchart for the management of myasthenic crisis. ABG, arterial blood gas; AChE, acetylcholinesterase; BiPAP, bilevel positive airway pressure; ICU, intensive care unit; IVIG, intravenous immunoglobulin; PFTs, pulmonary function tests.

on serial pulmonary function tests. Diaphragmatic weakness may reverse before extremity weakness; thus, the timing of weaning should not be gauged solely by recovery of extremity muscle strength.

The weaning process in patients with MG often is challenging because of the fluctuating nature of the disease. Reintubation is not uncommon. Older age, pneumonia, and atelectasis are major risk factors for poor outcome.[45] In a review of 26 episodes of myasthenic crisis, the reintubation rate was 27%. In selected patients, noninvasive ventilation can be used for bridging during the weaning process to prevent reintubation.[28] Weaning trials may begin when VC exceeds 10 to 15 mL/kg, NIP exceeds −20 cm H_2O, and oxygenation is adequate on inspired oxygen concentrations (FiO_2) of 4% or less.

It is important to reintroduce cholinesterase inhibitors before extubation trials are initiated. Weaning methods may vary. Patients can be switched to continuous positive airway pressure (CPAP) with pressure support ventilation (PSV) and the level decreased 1 to 3 cm H_2O each day. A decrease in tidal volume and an increase in respiratory and heart rates are indicators of fatigue. Once the patient demonstrates good endurance at low pressure support (5 cm H_2O), usually for more than 2 hours, extubation can be accomplished. After extubation, incentive spirometry is helpful to reduce the risk of atelectasis and re-intubation.[46]

In GBS, weaning from mechanical ventilation should be undertaken as early as possible because of the number of significant complications related to prolonged intubation.[44,47] After intubation, however, respiratory function parameters often continue to fall. Reducing intermittent mandatory ventilation rate or reducing pressure support level can be used as weaning approaches, at the discretion of the treating physician.[8,48] The weaning process can be initiated once VC reaches 25 mL/kg and spontaneous tidal volumes of 10 to 12 mL/kg are attained. NIP exceeding −50 cm H_2O and VC improvement by 4 mL/kg from preintubation to pre-extubation are associated with successful extubation.[49] Extubation often is delayed if dysautonomia is still present. Electrophysiologic testing can be helpful in decisions for extubation. Established risk factors for poor outcome in GBS are electrophysiologic evidence of axonal degeneration, preceding diarrheal illness, and rapid disease progression.[40]

KEY POINTS

- Clinical examination and pulmonary function tests form the basis of assessment in patients with neuromuscular respiratory failure.
- VC less than 20 mL/kg, NIP less than −30 cm H_2O, and PEF less than 40 cm H_2O usually will indicate the need for mechanical ventilation in patients with GBS (20/30/40 rule).
- In myasthenic crisis, pulmonary function tests have a limited positive predictive value. Respiratory support is unlikely to be needed when VC is more than 20 mL/kg.
- NIV is the first-line treatment in respiratory failure secondary to MG when P_{CO_2} levels are less than 50 mm Hg and definitive therapy is rapidly initiated. This can prevent intubation up to 70% of the time.
- NIV is not beneficial in respiratory failure secondary to GBS and can even be detrimental by masking further respiratory decline.
- Timing for tracheostomy in GBS is unclear, but waiting for 2 to 3 weeks in patients showing improvement may prevent the need for tracheostomy in up to 50% of cases.
- Both IVIG and plasma exchange probably are equal in efficacy for the treatment of GBS, although relapse rates may differ.
- In treatment of ventilatory failure secondary to MG, plasma exchange is superior to use of IVIG. Plasma exchange or IVIG must be followed by long-term immunosuppression.

REFERENCES

1. Lacomis D, Petrella JT, Giuliani MJ: Causes of neuromuscular weakness in the intensive care unit: A study of ninety-two patients. Muscle Nerve 1998;21:610-617.
2. Thomas CE, Mayer SA, Gungor Y, et al: Myasthenic crisis: Clinical features, mortality, complications, and risk factors for prolonged intubation. Neurology 1997;48:1253-1260.
3. Borel CO, Teitelbaum JS, Hanley DF: Ventilatory drive and carbon dioxide response in ventilatory failure due to myasthenia gravis and Guillain-Barré syndrome. Crit Care Med 1993;21:1717-1726.
4. Hicks GH: Cardiopulmonary Anatomy and Physiology. Philadelphia, WB Saunders, 2000.
5. Hadden RD, Karch H, Hartung HP, et al: Preceding infections, immune factors, and outcome in Guillain-Barré syndrome. Neurology 2001;56:758-765.
6. Ronager J, Ravnborg M, Hermansen I, Vorstrup S: Immunoglobulin treatment versus plasma exchange in patients with chronic moderate to severe myasthenia gravis. Artif Organs 2001;25:967-973.
7. Fulgham JR, Wijdicks EF: Guillain-Barré syndrome. Crit Care Clin 1997;13:1-15.
8. Henderson RD, Lawn ND, Fletcher DD, et al: The morbidity of Guillain-Barré syndrome admitted to the intensive care unit. Neurology 2003;60:17-21.
9. Engel AG: Myasthenia gravis and myasthenic syndromes. Ann Neurol 1984;16:519-534.
10. Engel AG: Myasthenia Gravis and Myasthenic Disorders. Oxford: Oxford University Press, 1999.
11. Keesey JC: "Crisis" in myasthenia gravis: An historical perspective. Muscle Nerve 2002;26:1-3.
12. Thieben MJ, Blacker DJ, Liu PY, et al: Pulmonary function tests and blood gases in worsening myasthenia gravis. Muscle Nerve 2005;32:664-667.
13. Dau PC, Lindstrom JM, Cassel CK, et al: Plasmapheresis and immunosuppressive drug therapy in myasthenia gravis. N Engl J Med 1977;297:1134-1140.
14. Gajdos P, Tranchant C, Clair B, et al: Treatment of myasthenia gravis exacerbation with intravenous immunoglobulin: A randomized double-blind clinical trial. Arch Neurol 2005;62:1689-1693.
15. Qureshi AI, Choudhry MA, Akbar MS, et al: Plasma exchange versus intravenous immunoglobulin treatment in myasthenic crisis. Neurology 1999;52:629-632.
16. Stricker RB, Kwiatkowska BJ, Habis JA, Kiprov DD: Myasthenic crisis. Response to plasmapheresis following failure of

intravenous gamma-globulin. Arch Neurol 1993;50:837-840.
17. Mahalati K, Dawson RB, Collins JO, Mayer RF: Predictable recovery from myasthenia gravis crisis with plasma exchange: Thirty-six cases and review of current management. J Clin Apher 1999;14:1-8.
18. Watanabe A, Watanabe T, Obama T, et al: Prognostic factors for myasthenic crisis after transsternal thymectomy in patients with myasthenia gravis. J Thorac Cardiovasc Surg 2004;127:868-876.
19. Sekine Y, Kawaguchi N, Hamada C, et al: Does perioperative high-dose prednisolone have clinical benefits for generalized myasthenia gravis? Eur J Cardiothorac Surg 2006;29:908-913.
20. Osterman PO, Fagius J, Lundemo G, et al: Beneficial effects of plasma exchange in acute inflammatory polyradiculoneuropathy. Lancet 1984;2:1296-1299.
21. Plasmapheresis and acute Guillain-Barré syndrome. The Guillain-Barré Syndrome Study Group. Neurology 1985;35:1096-1104.
22. Raphael JC, Chevret S, Hughes RA, Annane D: Plasma exchange for Guillain-Barré syndrome. Cochrane Database Syst Rev 2002(2):CD001798.
23. Hughes RA, Raphael JC, Swan AV, van Doorn PA: Intravenous immunoglobulin for Guillain-Barré syndrome. Cochrane Database Syst Rev 2006(1):CD002063.
24. Randomised trial of plasma exchange, intravenous immunoglobulin, and combined treatments in Guillain-Barré syndrome. Plasma Exchange/ Sandoglobulin Guillain-Barré Syndrome Trial Group. Lancet 1997;349:225-230.
25. Hughes RA, Swan AV, van Koningsveld R, van Doorn PA: Corticosteroids for Guillain-Barré syndrome. Cochrane Database Syst Rev 2006(2):CD001446.
26. Hughes RA: Ineffectiveness of high-dose intravenous methylprednisolone in Guillain-Barré syndrome. Lancet 1991;338:1142.
27. Hughes RA, van der Meche FG: Corticosteroids for treating Guillain-Barré syndrome. Cochrane Database Syst Rev 2000(2):CD001446.
28. Rabinstein A, Wijdicks EF: BiPAP in acute respiratory failure due to myasthenic crisis may prevent intubation. Neurology 2002;59:1647-1649.
29. Wijdicks EF: Noninvasive mechanical ventilation in acute neurologic disorders. Rev Neurol Dis 2005;2:8-12.
30. Rabinstein AA, Wijdicks EF: Warning signs of imminent respiratory failure in neurological patients. Semin Neurol 2003;23:97-104.
31. Wijdicks EF, Roy TK: BiPAP in early Guillain-Barré syndrome may fail. Can J Neurol Sci 2006;33:105-106.
32. Rees JH, Thompson RD, Smeeton NC, Hughes RA: Epidemiological study of Guillain-Barré syndrome in southeast England. J Neurol Neurosurg Psychiatry 1998;64:74-77.
33. Ropper AH: Severe acute Guillain-Barré syndrome. Neurology 1986;36: 429-432.
34. Lawn ND, Wijdicks EF: Tracheostomy in Guillain-Barré syndrome. Muscle Nerve 1999;22:1058-1062.
35. Wijdicks EF, Henderson RD, McClelland RL: Emergency intubation for respiratory failure in Guillain-Barré syndrome. Arch Neurol 2003;60:947-948.
36. Lawn ND, Fletcher DD, Henderson RD, et al: Anticipating mechanical ventilation in Guillain-Barré syndrome. Arch Neurol 2001;58:893-898.
37. Zifko U, Chen R, Remtulla H, et al: Respiratory electrophysiological studies in Guillain-Barré syndrome. J Neurol Neurosurg Psychiatry 1996;60:191-194.
38. Ropper AH, Kehne SM: Guillain-Barré syndrome: Management of respiratory failure. Neurology 1985;35:1662-1665.
39. Gracey DR, McMichan JC, Divertie MB, Howard FM Jr: Respiratory failure in Guillain-Barré syndrome: A 6-year experience. Mayo Clin Proc 1982;57:742-746.
40. Efficiency of plasma exchange in Guillain-Barré syndrome: Role of replacement fluids. French Cooperative Group on Plasma Exchange in Guillain-Barré syndrome. Ann Neurol 1987;22:753-7561.
41. Ali MI, Fernandez-Perez ER, Pendem S, et al: Mechanical ventilation in patients with guillain-barre syndrome. Respir Care 2006;51:1403-1407.
42. Griggs WM, Myburgh JA, Worthley LI: A prospective comparison of a percutaneous tracheostomy technique with standard surgical tracheostomy. Intensive Care Med 1991;17:261-263.
43. Rieder P, Louis M, Jolliet P, Chevrolet JC: The repeated measurement of vital capacity is a poor predictor of the need for mechanical ventilation in myasthenia gravis. Intensive Care Med 1995;21:663-638.
44. Rabinstein AA: Update on respiratory management of critically ill neurologic patients. Curr Neurol Neurosci Rep 2005;5:476-482.
45. Rabinstein AA, Mueller-Kronast N: Risk of extubation failure in patients with myasthenic crisis. Neurocrit Care 2005;3:213-215.
46. Varelas PN, Chua HC, Natterman J, et al: Ventilatory care in myasthenia gravis crisis: Assessing the baseline adverse event rate. Crit Care Med 2002;30:2663-2668.
47. Wijdicks EF, Borel CO: Respiratory management in acute neurologic illness. Neurology 1998;50:11-20.
48. Borel CO, Guy J: Ventilatory management in critical neurologic illness. Neurol Clin 1995;13:627-644.
49. Nguyen TN, Badjatia N, Malhotra A, et al: Factors predicting extubation success in patients with Guillain-Barré syndrome. Neurocrit Care 2006;5:230-234.

Chapter 66

Seizures in the Critically Ill

Thomas P. Bleck

Seizures complicate the clinical course in approximately 3% of adult patients admitted to intensive care units (ICUs) for non-neurologic conditions,[1] and more frequently in specialized neuroscience ICUs.[2] The medical and economic impact of seizures in these patients confers a significance to these events out of proportion to their incidence. Seizures often are the first indication of a central nervous system (CNS) complication in these patients, making their rapid etiologic diagnosis mandatory. Furthermore, because epilepsy is a common disorder (affecting about 2% of the general population), patients with pre-existing seizure disorders occasionally will require ICU admission for intercurrent conditions. The intensivist usually manages the initial treatment of these patients, so he or she must be familiar with the indications and risks of the potential therapies as they affect the already critically ill patient. In addition, the patient who develops status epilepticus (SE), whether already in the ICU or not, will often require the care of a critical care specialist in addition to a neurologist.

HISTORY

Although seizures have been recognized at least since Hippocratic times, their relatively high rate of occurrence in critically ill patients has only recently been recognized. Precipitation of seizures as a side effect of critical care treatments (e.g., as a complication of lidocaine infusion for ventricular arrhythmias) also is a recent phenomenon.

The first recorded description of SE is by Gavasetti in 1586.[3,4] Sir Thomas Willis described the complications of untreated SE in 1667:

> . . . as to what further belongs to the prognostication of the Disease, if it end not about the time of ripe age, neither can be driven away by the use of medicines, there happens yet a diverse event in several sick Patients, for it either ends immediately in Death, or is changed into some other Disease, to wit, the Palsie, stupidite, or melancholly, for the most part incurable. As to the former, whenas the fits are often repeated, and every time grow more cruell, the animal functions are quickly debilitated; and from thence, by the taint, by degrees brought on by the Spirits, and the Nerves serving the Praecordia, the vital function is by little and little enervated, till at length, the whole body languishing, and the pulse is loosned, and at length ceasing, at last the vital flame is extinguished.[5]

Attempts at treating SE in the 19th century included use of bromide,[6] morphine,[7] and ice applications. Barbiturates were introduced in 1912, followed by the identification and use of phenytoin in 1937; these were the first rational treatments for SE.[8] Paraldehyde gained brief prominence in the next decades.[9] The most recent major improvement was the use of benzodiazepines, pioneered by the French in the 1960s.[10]

EPIDEMIOLOGY

Few data are available concerning the epidemiology of seizures in ICU patients. A 10-year retrospective study of all ICU patients at the Mayo Clinic reported approximately 7 patients with seizures per 1000 ICU admissions.[11] In a 2-year prospective study in a medical ICU, the observed rate was approximately 35 patients with seizures per 1000 admissions.[1] These studies are not strictly comparable, beause the patient populations and methods of detection differed. The incidence of seizures probably is higher in pediatric ICUs than in medical ICUs.[12-14]

Certain ICU patients appear to be at increased risk for seizures, but the degree of that increased risk has not been quantitated. Patients with renal failure or with an altered blood-brain barrier who receive imipenem-cilastatin are an obvious example, but other patients receiving this combination antibiotic or a γ-aminobutyric acid (GABA) antagonist such as penicillin occasionally experience seizures. Transplant recipients, especially those receiving cyclosporine, appear to have an increased risk for convulsions. Patients who rapidly become hypo-osmolar from any etiologic disorder also are at risk. Patients with nonketotic hyperglycemia have a high likelihood of partial seizures; this is a rare instance of a metabolic disorder producing focal neurologic syndromes.[15] Less commonly, diabetic ketoacidosis also may produce partial seizures.[16]

The epidemiology of SE is somewhat better understood. Estimates of the incidence of generalized convulsive SE (GCSE) in the United States range from 50,000 cases per year[17] to 250,000 cases per year[18]; most workers assume about 60,000 cases per year is correct. Some portion of this discrepancy may be due to differences in definitions. The larger estimate comes from the only population-based data available, however, and may be more accurate. Similarly large variations occur in mortality estimates, ranging from 1% to 2% in the former study to 22% in the latter. This disagreement stems, at least in part, from a conceptual discordance: The smaller number attempts to determine mortality directly attributable to SE, whereas the larger figure reflects the overall mortality rate for patients in SE, in whom death frequently was a consequence of the cause of the underlying disease, rather than of SE itself. In the study reporting the higher SE incidence,[18] for example, anoxia was the cause of SE in adults with the highest mortality. In many of the reports surveyed in the earlier review, these patients would not have been included.

A number of important risk factors have emerged from the Richmond study. When SE lasted longer than 1 hour, the mortality rate was 32%; when it lasted less than 1 hour, the mortality rate was only 2.7%. SE caused by anoxia was associated with a mortality rate of about 70% in adults, but the corresponding rate in children was less than 10% (the researchers have not yet described the functional capabilities of the survivors). After the age of 12 months, the mortality for SE rose with increasing age. In this study, the commonest cause of SE in adults was stroke, followed thereafter by withdrawal from anticonvulsant drug therapy; cryptogenic (or idiopathic) SE; and SE related to ethanol withdrawal, anoxia, and metabolic disorders. Systemic infection was the most commonly diagnosed cause of SE in children; this was followed by congenital abnormalities, anoxia, metabolic disorders, anticonvulsant drug withdrawal, CNS infections, and trauma. Although brain tumors were seldom the cause of SE in children, such patients experienced a nearly 50% mortality rate.

Towne and colleagues demonstrated that 8% of an unselected series of comatose medical ICU patients had unsuspected nonconvulsive status epilepticus.[19]

Hospital-based series of patients with SE usually are subject to considerable selection bias regarding etiology. The data in Table 66-1, based on 20 years of experience at the San Francisco General Hospital,[20-22] are of great interest, because almost all patients with SE in the city of San Francisco with onset of seizures outside of the hospital will be transported to this institution.

Between 6% and 12% of epilepsy patients present with SE,[23] and approximately 20% of patients with a seizure disorder will experience an episode of SE within 5 years of their first seizure.[17]

Table 66-1. Causes of Status Epilepticus at the San Francisco General Hospital

	1970-1980 (%) *N*=98		1980-1989 (%) *N*=152	
Causative Disorder/Condition	**Prior Seizures**	**No Prior Seizures**	**Prior Seizures**	**No Prior Seizures**
Ethanol-related	11	4	25	12
Anticonvulsant noncompliance	27	0	41	0
Drug toxicity	0	10	5	10
Refractory epilepsy	(category not used)		8	0
CNS infection*	0	4	2	10
Trauma	1	2	2	6
Tumor	0	4	2	7
Metabolic*	3	5	2	4
Stroke*	4	11	2	5
Anoxia*	0	4	0	6
Other	11	5	3	5

*Conditions most likely to result in admission to the intensive care unit.
CNS, central nervous system.
Adapted from Aminoff MJ, Simon RP: Status epilepticus: Causes, clinical features and consequences in 98 patients. Am J Med 1980;69:657-666; Lowenstein DH, Alldredge BK: Status epilepticus in an urban public hospital in the 1980s. Neurology 1993;42:483-488; and Bleck TP: Status epilepticus. Univ Rep Epilepsy 1992;1:1-7.

NOSOLOGY AND SEMIOLOGY

Numerous systems have evolved for the classification of seizures; the most frequently used system today is that of the International League Against Epilepsy[24] (Box 66-1). This schema allows classification based primarily on clinical criteria, without inferences about etiology. It is important because of its predictive value for etiology, prognosis, and treatment decisions in ICU patients. *Simple partial* seizures occur focally in the cerebral cortex, without taking over either the limbic system or subcortical nuclei. The patient remains aware of the environment during the ictus and, except for the seizure itself, appears unchanged. Bilateral limbic system dysfunction results in a *complex partial* seizure; the patient's awareness and ability to interact with the environment are diminished (but not always completely abolished). *Automatisms* are movements that the patient evidently makes without being aware of them; typical automatisms include swallowing, masticatory movements, and fumbling with nearby items.

Box 66-1

International Classification of Epileptic Seizures

I. Partial seizures (seizures beginning locally)
  A. Simple partial seizures (SPSs) (consciousness not impaired)
    1. With motor symptoms
    2. With somatosensory or special sensory symptoms
    3. With autonomic symptoms
    4. With psychic symptoms
  B. Complex partial seizures (CPSs) (with impairment of consciousness)
    1. Beginning as SPS and progressing to impairment of consciousness
      a. Without automatisms
      b. With automatisms
    2. With impairment of consciousness at onset
      a. With no other features
      b. With features of SPS
      c. With automatisms
  C. Partial seizures (simple or complex), secondarily generalized
II. Primary generalized seizures (bilaterally symmetric, without localized onset)
  A. Absence seizures
    1. True absence ("petit mal")
    2. Atypical absence
  B. Myoclonic seizures
  C. Clonic seizures
  D. Tonic seizures
  E. Tonic-clonic seizures ("grand mal") (GTC)
  F. Atonic seizures
III. Unclassified seizures

From Commission on Classification and Terminology of the International League Against Epilepsy: Proposal for revised clinical and electroencephalographic classification of epileptic seizures. Epilepsia 1981;22:489-501.

Secondary generalization implies invasion of either the other hemisphere (with loss of consciousness) or, more commonly, subcortical structures, with the development of a generalized convulsion.

Primary generalized seizures seem to arise from the entire cerebral cortex and the diencephalon at the same time; no focal phenomena are visible. Consciousness is lost from the start of the seizure. True *absence* seizures usually are confined to childhood; they consist of the abrupt onset of a blank stare usually lasting 5 to 15 seconds, without lateralizing phenomena, from which the patient abruptly returns to normal. Atypical absence usually is seen in children who have the Lennox-Gastaut syndrome. *Myoclonic* seizures begin with brief, bilaterally synchronous jerks without an initial change in consciousness, followed by a generalized convulsion. They occur in several of the genetic epilepsies but in the ICU are more commonly the consequence of anoxia or metabolic disturbances.[25] *Clonic* seizures involve repetitive movements; they may be generalized (with synchronous movements of all extremities and both sides of the face) or partial (e.g., involving one side of the face and the arm of the same side). *Tonic* seizures are episodes of tonic extension of the arms, legs, and trunk; they must be distinguished from decerebrate rigidity and from tetanic spasms.[26] *Tonic-clonic* seizures begin with tonic extension, followed by a brief phase of rapid vibration of the extremities, evolving into bilaterally synchronous clonus, and concluding with a postictal phase in which incontinence is common and brief apnea occasionally is noted. They may be primarily generalized or, more commonly, occur as the manifestation of spread of a partial seizure. Only those seizures that are known to involve progression through the tonic and clonic stages should be called tonic-clonic.

When seizures occur in ICU patients, clinical judgment is required to apply this classification system. Patients whose consciousness is already altered by drugs, hypotension, sepsis, or intracranial pathology may be difficult to diagnose regarding the simple versus complex nature of their partial seizures.

SE is classified by a somewhat similar system, with alterations to match the observable clinical phenomena[27] (Box 66-2). Again, the ability to use clinical observation without inferences about etiology is important. *Generalized convulsive* SE (GCSE) is the type most commonly encountered in ICUs and poses the greatest risk to the patient. GCSE may either be primarily generalized, as in the intoxicated patient, or represent secondary generalization, as in the patient with a brain abscess in whom GCSE develops. *Tonic* SE usually is seen in children or adolescents with a history of severe CNS dysfunction. *Nonconvulsive* SE (NCSE) in the ICU most commonly is the consequence of partially treated GCSE. Some authors use the nonconvulsive designation as a general term for any SE involving altered consciousness without convulsive movements. Although conceptually useful, this blurs the distinctions among absence SE, partially treated GCSE, and *complex partial* SE (CPSE), which have different causes and treatments. *Epilepsia partialis continua* (EPC) is a special form of partial SE in which a small area of the

Box 66-2

Clinical Classification of Status Epilepticus

I. Generalized seizures
  A. Generalized convulsive SE (GCSE)
    1. Primary generalized SE
      a. Tonic-clonic SE
      b. Myoclonic SE
      c. Clonic-tonic-clonic SE
    2. Secondarily generalized SE
      a. Partial seizure with secondary generalization
      b. Tonic SE
  B. Nonconvulsive SE (NCSE)
    1. Absence SE (petit mal status)
    2. Atypical absence SE (e.g., in Lennox-Gastaut syndrome)
    3. Atonic SE
    4. NCSE as a sequel of partially treated GCSE
II. Partial SE
  A. Simple partial SE
    1. Typical
    2. Epilepsia partialis continua (EPC)
  B. Complex partial SE (CPSE)
III. Neonatal SE

Adapted from Ettinger AB, Shinnar S: New-onset seizures in an elderly hospitalized population. Neurology 1993;43:489.

body makes repetitive movements, sometimes for months or years after a CNS insult.

PATHOGENESIS

With clinical SE, the list of potential causative disorders is long and varied. The relative frequencies of etiologic disorders depend on the definition of SE used (for example, if repetitive, stereotypical myoclonic activity after a cardiorespiratory arrest is considered to represent SE, then the frequency of such events as a cause of SE will rise).

The reported "causes" of SE can be separated, if imperfectly, into predispositions and precipitants. *Predispositions* are relatively fixed conditions that increase the likelihood of SE, such as a brain tumor, in the presence of a precipitant. *Precipitants,* by contrast, are transient conditions that can produce SE in most, if not all, people, but will tend to cause seizures more readily in patients with predispositions to SE.

For experimental purposes, the nosologic division of SE into partial (focal) or generalized based on the type of seizures produced works well, as does the recognition of convulsive and nonconvulsive seizure types. An important point is that these are models of *acute SE;* they are not chronic conditions that occasionally produce SE, as are many of the afflictions of patients. Nevertheless, they have substantial explanatory power for understanding the neuronal and systemic processes of SE, for studying its consequences, and for predicting responses to therapy.

PATHOPHYSIOLOGY

The causes and effects of SE at the cellular, brain, and systemic levels are interrelated, but individual analysis is useful for understanding them and their therapeutic implications. One must first understand the consequences of a single seizure and then contrast this information with the effects of prolonged or frequent seizures merging into SE. Longer durations of SE produce more profound alterations with an increasing likelihood of permanence, and of becoming refractory to treatment. Figure 66-1 illustrates the variety of processes involved in a single seizure and in the transition to SE.[28]

At the cellular level, occurrence of a seizure follows the opening of ion channels coupled to excitatory amino acid (EAA) receptors. Although the endogenous ligands of these channels are glutamate and aspartate, the channels are named for synthetic compounds that potently activate them. From the standpoint of the intensivist concerned with SE, three channels are particularly important because their activation may raise intracellular free calcium to toxic concentrations. The first primarily conduct sodium ions (the AMPA channels). The second are the *N*-methyl-D-aspartate (NMDA) channels, which admit sodium and calcium when the cell has been depolarized (which relieves the resting blockade of the ionophore by magnesium). The third, the metabotropic or ACPD channels, mobilize calcium from intracellular stores via coupling to G protein–linked second messengers.

These EAA systems normally are crucial for learning and memory. Many drugs that block these systems, such as ketamine and phencyclidine, are too toxic to use as chronic anticonvulsants. However, the deleterious consequences of SE, and the brief period during which they would be needed, suggest that similar agents may prove to have a role in the management of SE. Counterregulatory ionic events also are triggered by the epileptiform discharge; the most important is activation of inhibitory interneurons, which feed back to the bursting cells via $GABA_A$ synapses.

The cellular consequences of the excessive EAA channel activation include (1) accumulation of toxic concentrations of free intracellular calcium; (2) activation of autolytic enzyme systems; (3) production of oxygen free radicals; (4) generation of nitric oxide, which both enhances subsequent excitation and serves as a toxin; (5) phosphorylation of several enzyme and receptor systems, making seizures likely; and (6) increasing intracellular osmolality, thereby producing neuronal swelling. If ATP production should fail (because substrate becomes inadequate, or is diverted into EAA-related events), membrane ion exchange systems stop functioning, and the neuron swells further. These events are responsible for the neuronal damage associated with SE

Many other important biophysical and biochemical alterations occur during and after SE. The intense neuronal activity activates immediate-early genes and produces heat shock proteins, providing strong indications of the deleterious effects of SE, and providing insight into the mechanisms by which neurons protect themselves.[29]

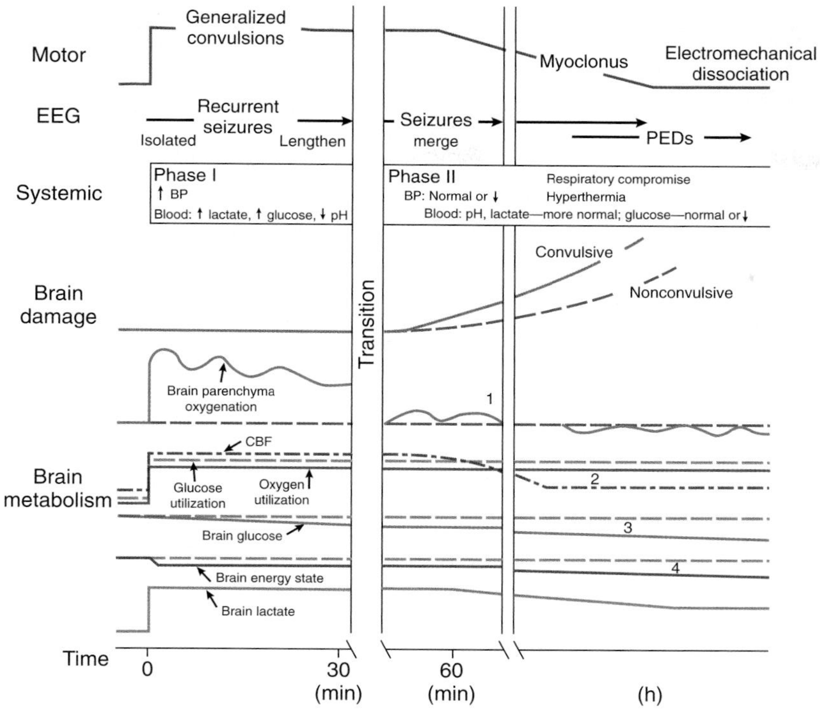

Figure 66-1. Pathophysiology of status epilepticus (SE): Summary of pathophysiologic events during experimental SE. Note that the abscissa is discontinuous. *Numerals within figure:* 1, loss of cortical responsiveness to changes in oxygen tension; 2, a fall in cerebral blood flow; 3, depletion of brain glucose; 4, a decline in the total brain energy state. BP, blood pressure; CBF, cerebral blood flow; EEG, electroencephalogram; PEDs, periodic epileptiform discharges. (Adapted from Lothman EW, Bertram EH: Epileptogenic effects of status epilepticus. Epilepsia 1993;34[Suppl 1]:S59-S70.)

Wasterlain's group summarized the many mechanisms through which SE damages the nervous system.[30]

Absence SE is an exception among these conditions. It appears to consist of rhythmically increased inhibition and does not produce clinical sequelae or neuropathologic abnormalities.

The mechanisms that terminate seizure activity are uncertain. In view of the relative rarity of SE in a population in which at least 1 in 50 patients has had a seizure, it can be inferred that these mechanisms generally are effective. The leading candidates for seizure-terminating systems are inhibitory mechanisms, primarily GABAergic neuronal aggregates. This hypothesis receives strong support from the clinical observation that human SE frequently follows withdrawal from GABA agonists (e.g., benzodiazepines).

The electrical phenomena of SE at the whole brain level, as seen on the scalp electroencephalogram (EEG), reflect the seizure type that initiates SE (Fig. 66-2). Thus, absence SE begins with a generalized 3-Hz wave-and-spike EEG pattern. During the course of SE, some slowing of this rhythm usually is observed, but the wave-and-spike characteristic persists. By contrast, GCSE goes through the sequence of electrographic changes outlined in Table 66-2. The initial high-frequency discharge becomes progressively less well formed over minutes; this decay implies that neuronal activity becomes less synchronous. Whether this indicates that inhibitory systems are attempting to terminate SE, or the occurrence of a progressive decay in the ability of synaptic mechanisms to maintain synchrony or global deterioration in neuronal function, remains to be determined.

The repetitive firing that characterizes SE alters the extracellular microenvironment. The most important change probably is the elevation of the extracellular potassium concentration. Although extruding potassium is an effective strategy to maintain normal electronegativity, the excessive amounts of potassium ejected during SE overcome the ability of astrocytes to buffer it. Patients with cerebral edema, glial scarring, or alien tissue lesions have extracellular space abnormalities that impair the potassium buffering ability of glial cells. Raising extracellular potassium is a potent epileptogenic stimulus.

The tremendously increased cellular activity of SE elevates tissue demand for oxygen and glucose. To meet this demand, cerebral blood flow initially increases threefold or greater. However, after about 20 minutes, energy supplies become exhausted. This accentuates the demand for local catabolism in order to support ion pumps (in a vain attempt to restore the internal milieu during the flood of sodium and calcium). Many researchers believe that this is the major cause of epileptic brain damage in GCSE. Other forms of SE may not be subject to such severe hypercatabolism, but still pose a risk.

When partial seizures generalize, subcortical structures begin to play an active role in the clinical phenomena observed. Spread of the electrical activity into the substantia nigra and other subcortical regions appears to be necessary before a tonic-clonic convulsion occurs.

The brain contains intrinsic systems that terminate seizure activity; both local GABAergic interneurons and inhibitory thalamic neurons are involved. Whether these systems have evolved, at least in part, for protection against seizures or whether this effect is an epiphenomenon of some other physiologic function is unresolved.

SE also can produce cerebral edema, which follows ictal damage to the blood-brain barrier.

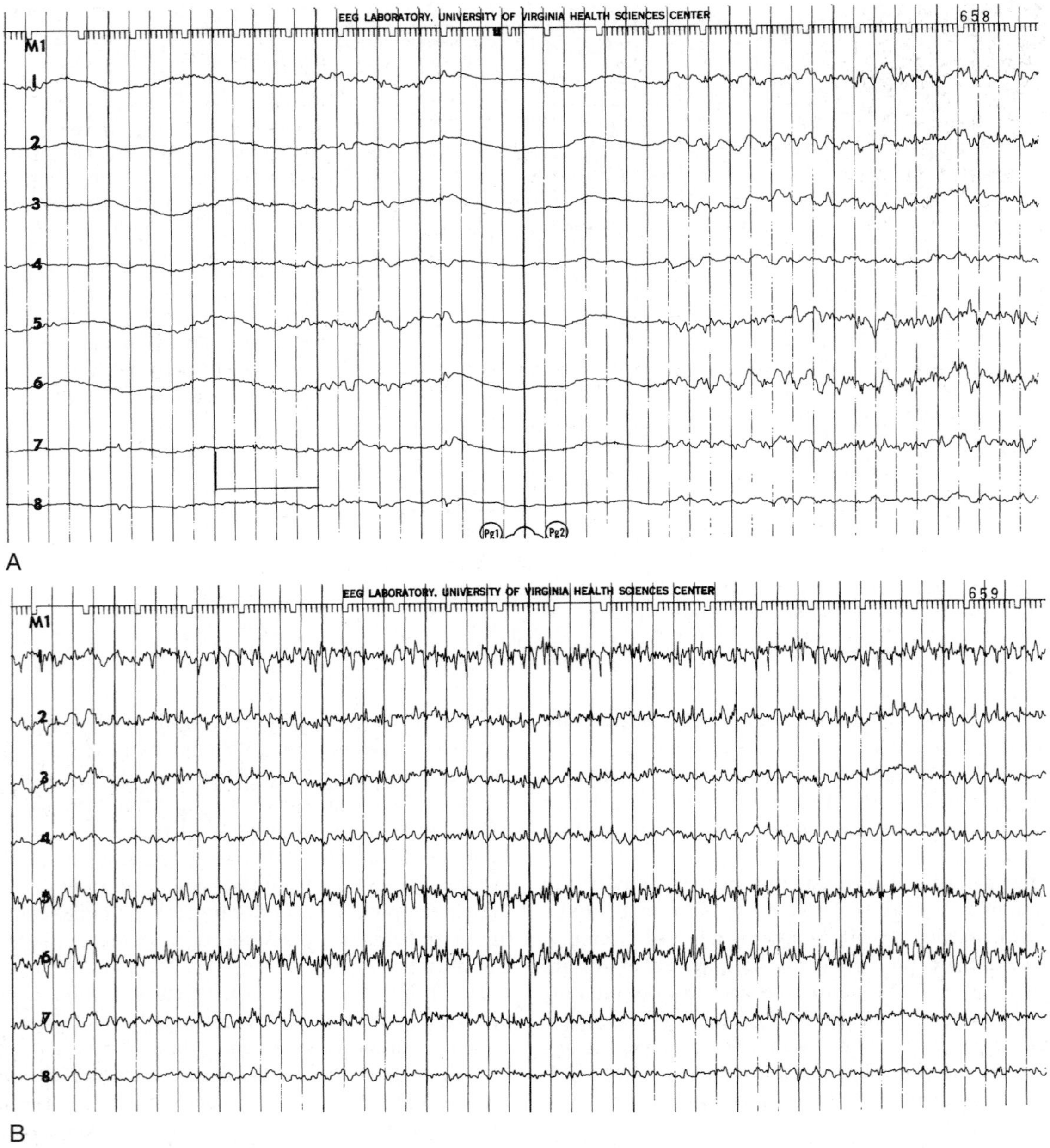

Figure 66-2. Electroencephalographic recording during status epilepticus. **A,** Onset of the seizure; **B-D,** Evolution of the seizure. *Montage:* longitudinal, bipolar; channels 1 to 4, left temporal; and channels 5 to 8, left parasagittal. *Calibration:* vertical, 50 μV; horizontal, 1 s.

Prolonged SE produces chronic neuropathologic changes. Before the 1970s, these changes often were attributed to the systemic effects of SE (e.g., hypoxia and hyperthermia). It is now clear, however, that SE itself produces these changes even in patients who are paralyzed, ventilated, and maintained at normal temperature and blood pressure. The hippocampus, which is one of the most important areas for memory function, contains the most susceptible neurons, but the cerebral cortex also is vulnerable. These regions express high densities of EAA receptors and may be relatively deficient in systems for handling unusual elevations of free intracellular calcium. Cells that contain nitric oxide synthase seem relatively protected.

In addition to damaging the CNS, GCSE produces serious, often life-threatening systemic effects.[31] Pressures in the systemic arterial system (under sympathetic control) and in the pulmonary arterial system (raised via efferents from pontine and medullary centers) are dramatically elevated from the moment of seizure onset. Epinephrine and cortisol release prompts further elevations of systemic arterial pressure and also produces hyperglycemia. Increased muscular work raises the circulating lactate concentration. Respiration becomes ineffective; both airway obstruction and diaphragmatic contraction impede air movement. The consequent hypoxia further elevates lactate levels. Ventilatory failure impairs CO_2 excretion,

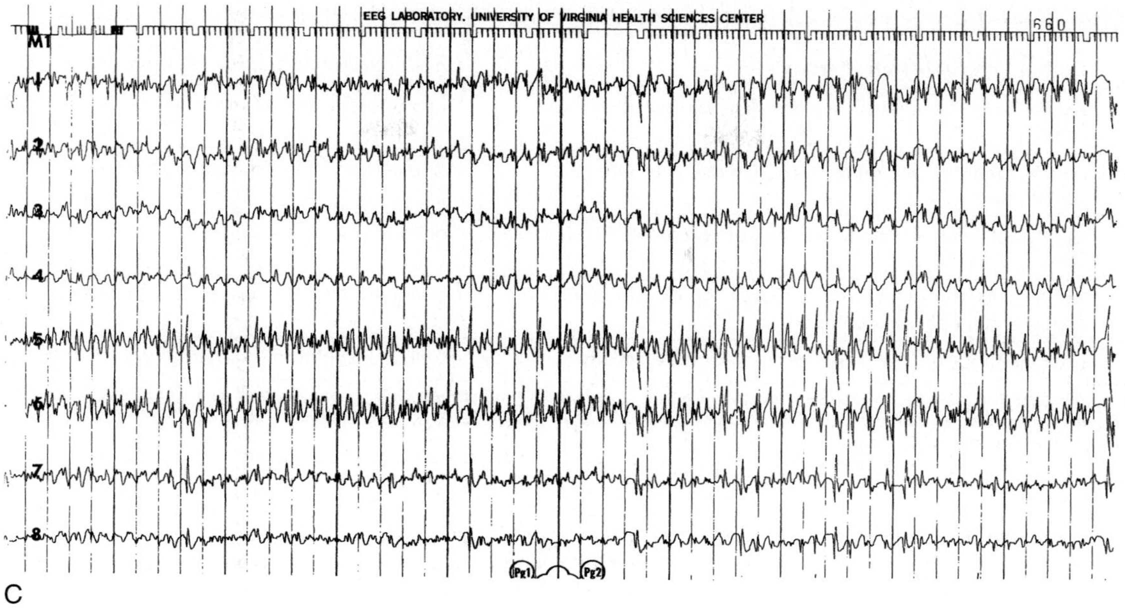

C

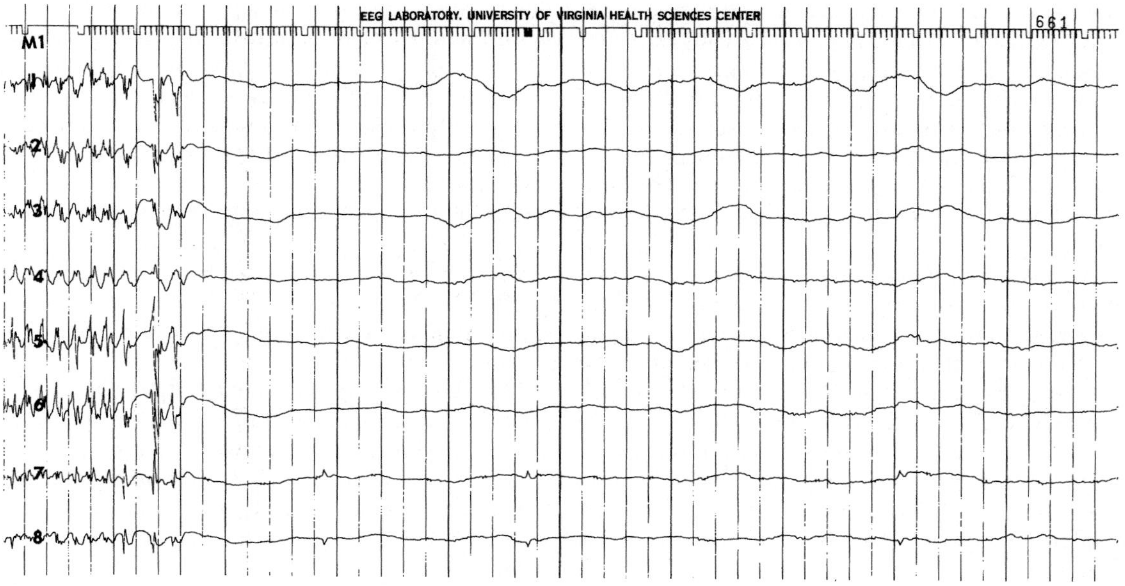

D

Figure 66-2, cont'd

while CO_2 production increases markedly, adding a respiratory component to the acidosis. In GCSE, the arterial blood pH frequently falls below 7.0. The muscular work accelerates heat production; when coupled with decreased dermal blood flow (produced by sympathetic stimulation), GCSE can quickly raise the core temperature to 40° C or higher.

If GCSE is not completely controlled within the first 20 minutes, motor activity begins to diminish in intensity, and ventilation usually improves. Therefore, even without treatment, the metabolic acidosis begins to reverse. Core temperature may continue to climb, however, probably reflecting hypothalamic dysfunction. The initial hyperglycemia diminishes; after an hour or more, hepatic gluconeogenesis may fail, and hypoglycemia develops.

Patients with GCSE frequently suffer secondary complications as well. Aspiration of oral or gastric contents commonly leads to chemical pneumonitis, with bacterial pneumonia often following. Rhabdomyolysis is common and occasionally is followed by acute renal failure. Compression fractures, joint dislocations, and tendon avulsions are other common sequelae of GCSE.

CLINICAL MANIFESTATIONS

Recognition of Seizures

Because of the close observation patients receive in the critical care setting, most seizures are witnessed. The partial onset of a secondarily generalized convulsion, a

Table 66-2. Electrographic-Clinical Correlations in Generalized Convulsive Status Epilepticus

Stage	Typical Clinical Manifestations*	Electroencephalographic Features
1	Tonic-clonic convulsions; hypertension and hyperglycemia common	Discrete seizures with interictal slowing
2	Low or medium amplitude clonic activity, with rare convulsions	Waxing and waning of ictal discharges
3	Slight, but frequent, clonic activity, often confined to the eyes, face, or hands	Continuous ictal discharges
4	Rare episodes of slight clonic activity; hypotension and hypoglycemia become manifest	Continuous ictal discharges punctuated by flat periods
5	Coma without other manifestations of seizure activity	Periodic epileptiform discharges on a flat background

*Clinical manifestations may vary considerably, depending on the underlying neuropathophysiologic process (and its anatomy), systemic diseases, and medications. In particular, stages of the electrographic progression may be so brief as to be overlooked. Partial treatment of status epilepticus may dissociate the clinical and electrographic features.

finding of important diagnostic significance, is more likely to be seen and properly described in the ICU than on regular hospital floors or in the community. Three problems occur with ICU seizure recognition: (1) complex partial seizures in patients with already impaired awareness, (2) seizures in patients receiving neuromuscular junction blockade, and (3) the misinterpretation of movement disorders and psychiatric disturbances as seizures. (In any ICU patient who exhibits abnormal movements or unexplained changes in awareness, thiamine deficiency should be excluded immediately by giving thiamine.)

ICU patients often have altered awareness in the absence of seizures, reflecting their underlying condition, complications of those conditions (such as septic encephalopathy[32]), and drugs that depress alertness (intentionally or not). Although clonic motor activity in these patients remains visible, it may be difficult to tell whether a subsequent further decline in alertness reflects a seizure or some other process. In this situation, an EEG is required to make the diagnosis of a complex partial seizure. The detailed interpretation of EEGs is beyond the scope of this chapter; nonetheless, the intensivist can easily learn to recognize basic seizure types and other important EEG abnormalities in critically ill patients.[33]

Patients receiving neuromuscular junction blocking agents will not manifest any of the usual signs of seizures. Becaise most such patients receive concomitant sedation with GABA agonists (e.g., benzodiazepines), the likelihood of seizures is small. The autonomic signs of seizures (hypertension, tachycardia, pupillary dilation) are not readily distinguished from the effects of pain or the patient's response to inadequate sedation. Thus, any patient who manifests these findings and who has a potential reason for seizures (e.g., intracranial pathology) should have an EEG to exclude this possibility. Until prospective trials of EEG monitoring are performed, the actual incidence of this problem will remain unknown.

Many sorts of abnormal movements occur in patients with severe metabolic disturbances or anoxic brain damage. Some of them can be distinguished from seizures by observation; such movements frequently are evoked or exacerbated by sensory stimuli and sometimes can be suppressed by changing the patient's posture. These interventions have little effect on seizures. If any doubt about the nature of such movements persists, an EEG should be performed. Psychiatric disturbances in the ICU occasionally resemble complex partial seizures; a routine portable EEG will be diagnostically adequate if the problem is continually present. Prolonged EEG monitoring may be required if the problem is intermittent, in order to capture the episode.

During therapeutic cooling for patients in coma after cardiac arrest, seizures may be difficult to detect clinically, especially when neuromuscular junction blockade is used.[34] EEG monitoring should be considered in such cases while more experience is accumulated.

Manifestations of Status Epilepticus

The neurologic manifestations of SE depend on the type of SE and, for the partial forms, the area of cortex from which the abnormality arises. Box 66-2 summarizes the types of SE encountered in clinical practice. The varieties of SE seen most frequently among ICU patients are considered next.

Primary GCSE usually begins as tonic extension of the trunk and extremities, without any preceding focal ictal activity. If the patient was awake before onset, no aura is reported, and consciousness is immediately lost. After several seconds of tonic extension, the extremities begin to vibrate; this phase gives way to clonic (rhythmic) extension of the extremities, with flexion occurring during each brief relaxation. Usually, this clonic phase will wane in intensity over 1 to 3 minutes. With further development of SE, the patient may then repeat the cycle of tonic activity followed by clonic movements, or may continue to have intermittent bursts of clonic activity without recovery between. Less commonly encountered forms of GCSE are *myoclonic SE,* in which bursts of brief myoclonic jerks increase in intensity until a convulsion occurs, and *clonic-tonic-clonic SE,* in which a period of clonic activity precedes the first tonic contraction. Myoclonic SE is especially common in patients with anoxic encephalopathy or metabolic disturbances, particularly renal failure.

Secondarily generalized SE in the ICU begins with a partial (focal) seizure, which progresses to a tonic-clonic convulsion. Even under the watchful eye of the ICU staff, the initial focal clinical activity may be overlooked. Because this type of seizure constitutes very strong evidence of a structural brain lesion, care should be taken to elicit evidence of any lateralized movement. *Tonic SE* is almost always confined to patients (usually children) with serious pre-existing cerebral disorders. Its importance in critical care practice follows from the observation that benzodiazepines may *precipitate* tonic SE; paradoxically, these agents also are used to treat it.

Several forms of *generalized nonconvulsive SE* are recognized. Of greatest importance to intensivists is NCSE as a sequel of inadequately treated GCSE. In this circumstance, a patient with GCSE is treated with one or more anticonvulsants, often in inadequate doses, after which visible convulsive activity stops. However, the patient does not awaken (or otherwise return to baseline), and SE is actually continuing. As a general rule, patients are expected to begin to awaken within 15 to 20 minutes after the successful termination of SE; many will regain consciousness much faster. Those who have not begun to awaken after 20 minutes should be assumed to have entered NCSE. This form of SE is sometimes termed "subtle SE," and careful observation often will reveal low-amplitude clonic activity in some part of the body (most commonly the face or the hands). Most investigators view NCSE as an extremely dangerous problem because the neuronally destructive effects of SE continue unabated, often for several hours. *This condition requires emergent treatment under EEG monitoring* to prevent further cortical damage. There are no clinical criteria that indicate when therapy has finally become effective.

The usual form of *partial SE* in the ICU follows a stroke or may be seen in patients with rapidly expanding cerebral masses (e.g., abscesses). Although clonic motor activity is the most easily recognized form, the seizure will take on the functional characteristics of the adjacent functional tissue. Thus, somatosensory or special sensory manifestations may occur; the ICU patient who is already neurologically impaired may not be able to report these symptoms. Aphasic SE may occur if the seizure begins in a language area; this must be distinguished from a stroke. Physical examination usually reveals at least some mild lateralizing findings.

As noted earlier, *EPC* is a special type of partial SE in which repetitive movements are confined to a small portion of the body (typically the thumb); these movements may occur over months or years. It is the type of SE most commonly associated with nonketotic hyperosmolar hyperglycemia and does not respond to conventional anticonvulsant treatment.

Complex partial SE manifests as a state of diminished awareness, although frank loss of consciousness is rarely noted. The patient may exhibit automatisms, but commonly the diagnosis comes as a surprise when an EEG is obtained.

DIAGNOSTIC APPROACH

The Patient with New-Onset Seizures in the Intensive Care Unit

When a patient already in an ICU has a seizure, the staff has a natural tendency to try in some way to stop the ictus. This may, unfortunately, lead to both diagnostic obscuration and iatrogenic complications. Beyond trying to protect the patient from harm, very little can be done with sufficient rapidity to influence the course of the seizure. In particular, padded tongue blades (or similar items) should not be placed in the mouth, because they are more likely to obstruct the airway than to preserve it. Similarly, the seizure activity in most patients will have stopped before any medication, even administered into a pre-existing intravenous line, can reach the brain in an effective concentration. A common scenario is the administration of intravenous diazepam, which begins to take effect after the seizure is over; the patient is now both postictal and pharmacologically sedated and becomes apneic.

The most important "intervention" during a single seizure is careful observation. This is the best time to collect evidence of a partial onset, which implies structural brain disease. The postictal examination is similarly valuable; language, motor, sensory, or reflex abnormalities after an apparently generalized convulsion also should be viewed as evidence of focal pathology.

In addition to the standard historical information to be requested from the patient and family members after a seizure, several special predispositions specific to the ICU must be investigated. Medications are an important cause of ICU seizures, especially in patients with diminished renal or hepatic function, or with damage to the blood-brain barrier. Imipenem-cilastatin is a common cause of seizures in this setting, but other antibiotics also may be offenders. The neurotoxic desmethyl metabolite of meperidine accumulates in renal failure; it also may produce seizures in patients with normal renal function. A complete list of potentially epileptogenic drugs is beyond the scope of this chapter; the medications of any patient who experiences a seizure should be reviewed with this possibility in mind.

Drug withdrawal is another common problem. Although ethanol withdrawal is the most common offender, discontinuing any hypnosedative agent (e.g., barbiturates, benzodiazepines, other sedatives) may prompt convulsions 24 to 96 hours later. This may be a particular problem in the ICU, where such agents may be withheld from patients because the staff is afraid that the drug's effects will obscure the neurologic examination.

The physical examination should be conducted with special emphasis on the points described for the postictal examination. In addition, evidence of cardiovascular disease (as a source for cerebral emboli) or systemic infection should be sought. Careful examination of the skin and fundi sometimes is revealing. The presence of papilledema is obviously important, but its absence does not exclude increased intracranial pressure.

In addition to routine biochemical studies, screening for drugs of abuse should be performed on patients with unexplained seizures. Cocaine has emerged as a prominent cause of seizures in many urban hospitals.[35] One area of controversy involves the importance of divalent cation disturbances in adult seizures. In my experience, hypocalcemia is rarely a cause of seizures beyond the neonatal period, and its discovery should not be the end of the diagnostic work-up. Hyperparathyroidism has been linked anecdotally to seizures, with the inference that parathormone is neurotoxic. Similarly, hypomagnesemia has an unwarranted reputation as a cause of seizures, especially in the malnourished alcoholic patient.

The need for imaging studies in critically ill patients who experience seizures has been an area of contention. In a prospective study of neurologic complications in medical ICU patients, 38 of 61 patients (62%) with seizures had a vascular, infectious, or neoplastic explanation for their fits. This is in contrast with the retrospective general ICU experience of Wijdicks and Sharbrough, in which very few patients were found to have structural problems. Until this discrepancy can be resolved, I recommend that computed tomography (CT) or magnetic resonance imaging (MRI) be performed in all ICU patients with new seizures, with a few exceptions. Hypoglycemia and nonketotic hyperosmolar hyperglycemia commonly will produce seizures (even partial seizures), and such patients can be treated for their metabolic disturbance and observed if there is no other indication of neurologic disease. With currently available technology, almost all patients can be transported to undergo CT scanning. Although MRI is preferable diagnostically in most situations and does not use potentially nephrotoxic contrast, the magnetic field precludes use of infusion pumps and other metallic devices (nonferromagnetic ventilators are available). Whether to administer contrast for a CT depends on the clinical setting and on the appearance of the plain scan.

The EEG is a vital diagnostic tool for the seizure patient. Partial seizures usually are associated with EEG abnormalities, which begin in, and may remain confined to, the area of cortex producing the seizures. Primary generalized seizures, by contrast, appear to start over the entire cortex at once. Areas of postictal slowing or depressed amplitude provide clues to the focal etiology of the seizures, and interictal epileptiform activity helps to classify the type of seizure and guide subsequent treatment. In patients who do not begin to awaken soon after seizures have apparently been controlled, an emergent EEG is necessary to exclude NCSE.

The need for a lumbar puncture (LP) depends on the clinical situation. In view of the common causes of seizures in the critical care setting, patients who need cerebrospinal fluid (CSF) analysis will usually require a CT scan before the LP. If a CNS infection is suspected in such patients, empiric antibiotic treatment should be strongly considered while these studies are being performed, rather than waiting for the scan to be performed and CSF to be obtained.

The Patient Presenting with or Developing Status Epilepticus

In contrast with the ICU patient with a single or a few seizures, the patient in SE will require concomitant diagnostic and therapeutic efforts. The first issue is to make a diagnosis of SE. Although 20 minutes of continuous or recurrent seizure activity usually is used as the definition of SE, the clinician should not stand at the bedside with a stopwatch timing this period before starting treatment. Because most seizures stop within 2 or 3 minutes, it is reasonable to begin treatment after 5 minutes of continuous seizure activity, or after the second or third seizure occurring without recovery between the spells. The types of treatment available are discussed in the following section.

SE has a limited differential diagnosis. GCSE may rarely be confused with decerebrate posturing, but the evolutionary nature of the former and the stimulus sensitivity of the latter make their clinical distinction straightforward. Generalized tetanus patients are awake during their spasms and almost always flex their arms rather than extending them.[26] The distinction of seizures from movement disorders and psychiatric conditions is discussed earlier.

EEG monitoring frequently is useful in SE,[36] but treatment should not be delayed to obtain an EEG when the diagnosis is apparent. A variety of EEG findings may be present, depending on the type of SE and its duration (see Table 66-2). The most typical pattern early in SE is that of rhythmic, high-frequency (greater than 12 Hz) activity that increases in amplitude and decreases in frequency, finally terminating abruptly and leaving postictal low-amplitude slowing in its wake. Patients with CPSE often lack such organized discharges but may instead demonstrate waxing and waning rhythmic activity in one or several head regions. Such a pattern requires a high index of suspicion in order to correctly diagnose CPSE; a diagnostic trial of an intravenous benzodiazepine often is necessary. Patients in whom refractory SE develops, or who experience seizures during neuromuscular blockade, will require continuous EEG monitoring. The technology to perform such monitoring outside of specialized epilepsy centers is only now becoming available.

MANAGEMENT APPROACH

The Patient with New-Onset Seizures in the Intensive Care Unit

Deciding whether to administer anticonvulsants to an ICU patient who experiences a single seizure or a few seizures requires a provisional etiologic diagnosis, an estimate of the likelihood of seizure recurrence, and an understanding of the utility and limitations of available anticonvulsants. For example, the patient who experiences a seizure during ethanol withdrawal probably will not benefit from chronic anticonvulsant treatment, and the administration of phenytoin will not prevent more withdrawal convulsions during the same episode. Such a patient may need prophylaxis against delirium tremens with benzodiazepines, but the seizures themselves seldom require treatment. The patient who has a seizure during barbiturate or benzodiazepine withdrawal, by contrast, usually should receive short-term treatment (usually with lorazepam) to prevent the development of SE. Seizures occurring as a result of drug intoxications or metabolic disturbances should similarly be treated for a brief period but do not necessitate chronic anticonvulsant therapy.

The ICU patient with CNS pathology who has even a single seizure probably should be started on a chronic anticonvulsant regimen, with the decision to continue medication reviewed before hospital discharge. It is now apparent that initiating anticonvulsant therapy after the first *unprovoked* (e.g., not drug- or withdrawal-related) seizure helps delay the onset of subsequent seizures but does not change their eventual incidence.[37] Starting treatment after the first seizure in a critically ill patient who has a condition predictive of seizure recurrence may be even more important if the patient's problems include a coagulopathy, myocardial ischemia, or another condition that would be seriously complicated by a convulsion.

In the ICU setting, phenytoin given as a loading dose of 20 mg per kg, no faster than 50 mg per minute, followed by an initial maintenance dose of 5 mg per kg per day, is often chosen to prevent subsequent seizures because of its relative ease of administration. Slowing the infusion rate to less than 25 mg per minute usually can prevent hypotension and cardiac arrhythmias, which may complicate its rapid intravenous administration. Because of the possible precipitation of third-degree atrioventricular (AV) block, an external cardiac pacemaker should be available when patients with conduction abnormalities receive intravenous phenytoin. Patients who are not actively seizing can be loaded enterally over 6 to 12 hours. Although fosphenytoin is safer than phenytoin if it extravasates, this agent does not have less cardiovascular toxicity. Fosphenytoin can also be used for intramuscular loading; phenytoin (pH 12) should not be administered intramuscularly because it produces myonecrosis.

The total phenytoin serum concentration should be kept in the "therapeutic" range of 10 to 20 μg per mL while the patient is in the ICU, unless further seizures occur; the level may then be increased until signs of toxicity occur. If the patient is unable to express these signs (e.g., ataxia) because of his or her underlying condition or its treatment, failure to prevent seizures at a concentration of 25 μg per mL usually is an indication to add phenobarbital (see later on). Although the usual goal of chronic anticonvulsant treatment is to administer the smallest dose of a tolerated single agent, which completely controls seizures, such an approach often is impossible in the critical care environment. When the patient is more stable, an attempt to decrease minor side effects or to convert to monotherapy may then be made.

Phenytoin normally is approximately 90% protein bound. Patients with renal dysfunction will have lower total phenytoin levels for a given dose, because the drug is displaced from its binding sites, but the free (unbound) level is not affected. Thus, in renal failure patients, and perhaps in others who are receiving highly protein-bound drugs (which will compete for phenytoin-binding sites), it may be advantageous to measure free phenytoin levels. Because only the free fraction is significantly metabolized, the dose need not be altered with changing renal function. Calculations of the unbound concentration based on the serum albumin concentration are unreliable. The half-time for phenytoin clearance in patients with normal liver function varies from about 20 hours for the intravenous form to over 24 hours for the extended-release oral capsules. Hence, a new steady-state serum concentration will take 4 to 6 days to establish. The drug need not be given more often than every 12 hours; the dosage interval for the enteral forms depends on the preparation, but may be even longer. Hepatic dysfunction will mandate a decrease in the maintenance dose; if the serum albumin is very low, the loading dose can be reduced as well.

Hypersensitivity to phenytoin is the major adverse effect of concern to the intensivist. This allergy may be manifested solely as fever but more commonly includes a rash and eosinophilia. Febrile reactions appear to be more common with intravenous than with enteral loading. Stevens-Johnson syndrome occurs rarely. The diagnosis and management of adverse reactions to phenytoin and other anticonvulsants have been reviewed.[38] Phenytoin is associated with a number of long-term adverse effects in patients with subarachnoid hemorrhage[39]; whether this is true in other patient groups remains to be determined.

Phenobarbital, in a loading dose of 10 to 20 mg per kg, followed by an initial maintenance dose of 1.5 mg per kg per day, remains useful as an anticonvulsant for patients who cannot tolerate phenytoin, or who have breakthrough seizures after *adequate* phenytoin loading. The target level for phenobarbital in ICU patients should be 20 to 40 μg per mL. Either hepatic or renal dysfunction may affect phenobarbital metabolism. The half-time for phenobarbital clearance is approximately 96 hours. Thus, maintenance doses of this agent need be given only once a day, and a steady-state level will take approximately 3 weeks to be established. Sedation is the major adverse effect; allergy is rare.

Carbamazepine, one of the most useful chronic anticonvulsants, is seldom given to critically ill patients because its insolubility has precluded a parenteral formulation. Oral loading with carbamazepine in conscious patients may produce coma lasting several days. It should be recalled as a cause of hyponatremia in patients receiving it chronically. Patients on carbamazepine in whom diplopia develops may benefit from switching to oxcarbazepine.

The place of the newer anticonvulsants in critical care is not well established. Levetiracetam has gained substantial popularity because of its limited drug interactions; it is now available for oral or intravenous administration. It is excreted predominantly by the kidney, so the dose must be adjusted in renal insufficiency. The usual dose for seizure prevention is between 500 and 1500 mg per day. The role of serum concentrations for assessment of efficacy or toxicity is not yet established. Lamotrigine and topiramate are seldom helpful to commence in the ICU setting because they should not be given in loading doses (except for topiramate as a potential agent in SE, discussed next).

Status Epilepticus

Figure 66-3 is a management algorithm for status epilepticus. GCSE constitutes an obvious medical emergency; unfortunately, NCSE and CPSE also require emergent treatment but are less straightforward to recognize. *In a patient with any of these three conditions, the clinician must move quickly to stop seizures in order to prevent further brain destruction.*[40] A suggested management protocol for these conditions is presented in Box 66-3. Patients with simple partial SE or EPC appear to be at substantially less risk for the development of widespread cerebral damage and also appear less likely to respond to the aggressive approach outlined in Box 66-3. In this group, correction of underlying problems (such as nonketotic hyperosmolar hyperglycemia) is most important. Of the available anticonvulsants, phenobarbital seems most likely to be efficacious. These patients often are loaded with phenytoin in the hope that this agent will prevent secondary generalization, but the actual value of this practice is unknown.

Some frequent errors in the use of medications to terminate SE include (1) use of inadequate doses of potentially effective agents and, conversely, (2) continued administration of drugs which are ineffective in the patient being treated. The first point most frequently applies to phenytoin; the proverbial "gram of Dilantin" is not adequate for patients weighing more than 50 kg.

Specific Agents

Benzodiazepines

Lorazepam is the agent of first choice for terminating SE. A study in the Veterans Affairs (VA) medical system compared lorazepam, diazepam followed by phenytoin, phenytoin alone, and phenobarbital as first-line agents, and demonstrated that lorazepam is the definitive agent of first choice.[41] The advantages of lorazepam over phenytoin include (1) its longer duration of action against SE (4 to 14 hours, as opposed to 20 minutes) and (2) a higher initial response rate (65%, compared with 45%). One study concluded that children receiving phenytoin for SE were far more likely to require intubation for ventilatory failure than comparable children receiving lorazepam.[42] In Europe, midazolam or clonazepam often is used initially. Midazolam is exceptionally useful for management of refractory SE, but it is hampered by tachyphylaxis.[43] Respiratory depression is the major adverse effect of all agents in this class when administered intravenously, especially in combination with barbiturates.

Preliminary data from the VA cooperative trial indicates that the use of other conventional agents after failure of the first one is very unlikely to terminate SE.

Hydantoins

Phenytoin is an effective anti-SE agent but cannot be delivered rapidly enough to be used as a first-line agent. Its major advantage is a very long duration of action once an adequate dose has been administered (the 20 mg per kg loading dose reliably produces a total serum

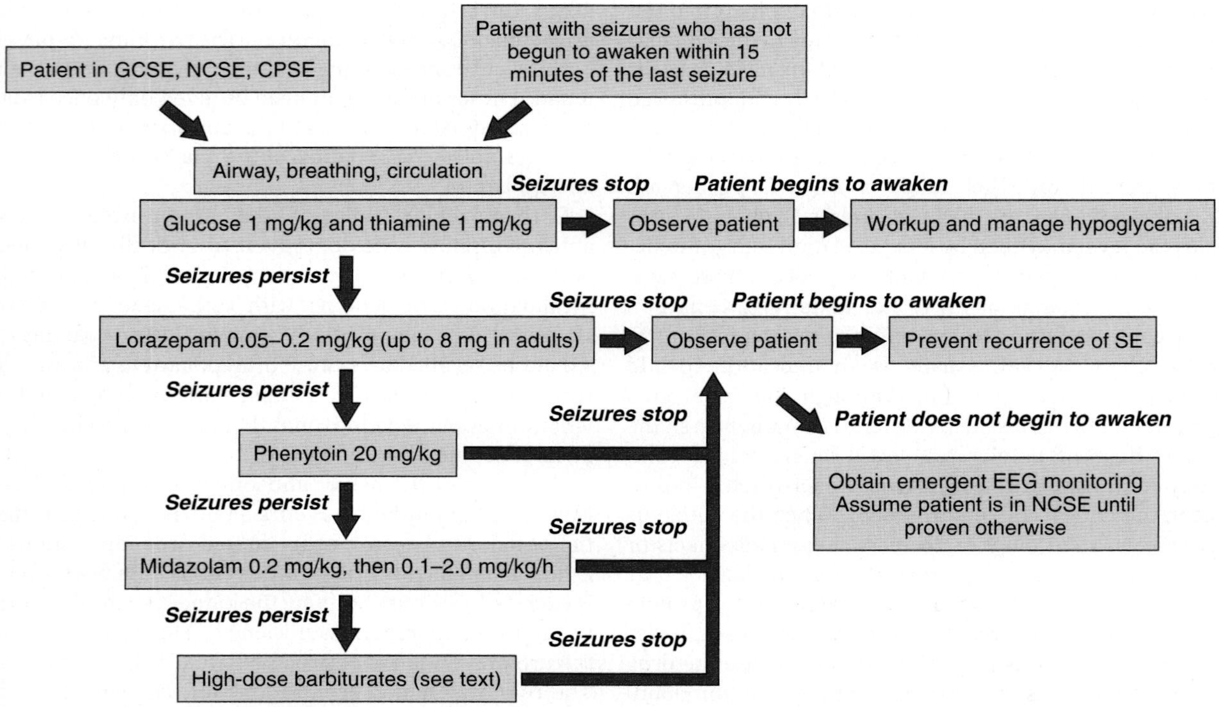

Figure 66-3. Management algorithm for status epilepticus (SE). CPSE, complex partial SE; EEG, electroencephalogram; GCSE, generalized convulsive SE; NCSE, nonconvulsive SE.

Box 66-3

Suggested Therapeutic Sequence for Terminating Status Epilepticus

I. Establish airway. Often the most rapid way to accomplish this is to rapidly terminate SE. If endotracheal intubation under neuromuscular junction blockade is necessary, use a nondepolarizing agent such as rapacuronium (1.5 mg/kg) or vecuronium (0.1 mg/kg). If increased intracranial pressure is a concern, premedicate with lidocaine (1 mg/kg) or thiopental (4 to 5 mg/kg). If these agents are used, the patient should be considered still to be in SE until neuromuscular transmission is re-established, or an EEG demonstrates that SE is no longer present.

II. Determine blood pressure. If the patient is hypotensive, begin volume replacement or vasoactive agents as clinically indicated. GCSE patients who present with hypotension will usually require admission to a critical care unit. (Hypertension should not be treated until SE is controlled, because terminating SE usually will substantially correct blood pressure, and many of the agents used to terminate SE can produce hypotension.)

III. Unless the patient is known to be normoglycemic or hyperglycemic, administer dextrose (1 mg/kg) and thiamine (1 mg/kg).

IV. Terminate SE. The following sequence of pharmacologic agents is recommended (see text for discussion of these and alternative agents). Be cognizant of the potential for these drugs to eliminate the visible convulsive movements of GCSE while leaving the patient in nonconvulsive SE. Patients who do not begin to respond to external stimuli 15 minutes after the apparent termination of GCSE should be considered at risk for nonconvulsive SE and undergo emergent EEG monitoring.

   A. Lorazepam 0.1 mg/kg at 0.04 mg/kg/minute. This drug should be diluted in an equal volume of the solution being used for intravenous infusion, because it is quite viscous. Most adult patients who will respond will have done so by a total dose of 8 mg. The latency of effect is debated, but lack of response after 5 minutes should be considered a failure.

   B. If SE persists, administer midazolam 0.2 mg/kg as a bolus, followed by an infusion of 0.1 to 2.0 mg/kg/hour to achieve seizure control (as determined by EEG monitoring). Intubation of the patient should be done at this stage if this has not already been accomplished. Patients reaching this stage should be treated in a critical care unit.

   C. Should the patient not be controlled with midazolam, administer propofol at a dose of 50 to 250 μg/kg/minute. Prolonged infusions of propofol have hemodynamic consequences similar to pentobarbital. Alternative agents include valproate, ketamine, and levetiracetam.

   D. If propofol fails, use pentobarbital 12 mg/kg at 0.2 to 0.4 mg/kg/minute as tolerated, followed by an infusion of 0.25-2.0 mg/kg/hour as determined by EEG monitoring (with a goal of burst suppression). Most patients will require systemic and pulmonary arterial catheterization, with fluid and vasoactive therapy as indicated to maintain blood pressure. Other complications of this treatment are discussed in the text.

V. Prevent recurrence of SE. The choice of drugs depends greatly on the etiology of SE and the patient's medical status and social support. In general, patients not previously receiving anticonvulsants whose SE is easily controlled often respond well to chronic treatment with phenytoin or carbamazepine. By contrast, others (e.g., patients with acute encephalitis) will require two or three anticonvulsants at "toxic" levels (e.g., phenobarbital at greater than 100 μg per mL) to be weaned from midazolam or pentobarbital, and may still have occasional seizures.

VI. Treat complications.

   A. Rhabdomyolysis should be treated with a vigorous saline diuresis to prevent acute renal failure; urinary alkalinization may be a useful adjunct. If definitive treatment of GCSE takes longer than expected because of hypotension or arrhythmias, neuromuscular junction blockade under EEG monitoring might be considered.

   B. Hyperthermia usually remits rapidly after termination of SE. External cooling usually suffices if the core temperature remains elevated. In rare instances, cool peritoneal lavage or extracorporeal blood cooling may be required. High dose pentobarbital generally produces poikilothermia.

   C. The treatment of cerebral edema secondary to SE has not been well studied. When substantial edema is present, the SE and cerebral edema both may be manifestations of the same underlying condition. Hyperventilation and mannitol may be valuable if edema is life-threatening. Edema due to SE is vasogenic, so steroids may be useful as well.

concentration above 20 μg per mL for 24 hours). Adding an additional dose of 5 mg per kg if 20 mg per kg fails to terminate SE sometimes is useful.[44] Concerns about its intravenous administration have already been discussed. If the patient is no longer in SE during phenytoin administration, the slower rate should be employed.

Phenytoin is highly insoluble and must be dissolved in sodium hydroxide and propylene glycol at a pH greater than 11 to remain in solution. Therefore, extravasation can produce severe necrosis. The drug also can cause thrombophlebitis, which may result in the "purple glove syndrome."[45]

Fosphenytoin is a phenytoin prodrug, which is converted to phenytoin with a half-time of approximately 7 minutes. It is prescribed in "phenytoin equivalents," so the loading dose remains 20 mg per kg of body weight. The maximal recommended rate of infusion is 150 mg per minute, but it should be started more slowly and increased to this rate if tolerated. No difference has been found in the potential for cardiovascular toxicity between phenytoin and fosphenytoin. Because it is water-soluble, extravasation of fosphenytoin does not pose the problem of skin and soft tissue necrosis inherent in the very alkaline vehicle of phenytoin.

Hydantoins should not be used in absence SE because they may worsen the condition.

Barbiturates

Phenobarbital has long been one of the major anti-SE agents. Some clinicians have advocated it as a first-line drug,[46] but it is rarely used in this role today. It has classically been a third-line agent for control of SE, after a benzodiazepine and phenytoin. Its utility in SE is diminished by the length of time required to obtain a therapeutic effect in patients in whom benzodiazepine and phenytoin therapies have already failed. It remains an important agent in patients with simple partial SE, and in preparing patients to be withdrawn from high-dose pentobarbital.

Pentobarbital and thiopental commonly are reserved for the control of refractory SE. Although these agents will be effective if used in large enough doses, side effects often limit their use[47] or may even be fatal.[48] They are important when other rapidly available modalities have failed (see Box 66-3).

Valproate

Intravenous valproate, given in a dose of 20 to 30 mg per kg, has gained popularity for the treatment of SE because it does not appear to produce respiratory depression or marked sedation. It has been reportedly successful in case series[49,50] and may be more effective than phenytoin.[51] Hypotension may occur with large doses.[52] This drug should be avoided if the patient may have an inborn error of metabolism affecting the liver, because it may precipitate fulminant hepatic failure.[53] Valproate has a number of drug interactions, which limits its utility in the ICU.[54]

Lidocaine

Lidocaine, in a dose of 1 mg per kg given intravenously, may occasionally be of value in patients in SE who do not respond to conventional treatment. The appropriate role of this drug has not been defined, but because it is readily available in ICUs, a reasonable approach may be to try this agent after a benzodiazepine and phenytoin have failed, before use of more definitive but difficult therapies. Its use should not delay the start of more definitive agents should it fail. Unfortunately, lidocaine is more often proconvulsant than anticonvulsant.

Isoflurane and Desflurane

The inhalational anesthetics isoflurane and desflurane sometimes are effective in controlling refractory SE,[55] even when other agents have failed,[56] perhaps because they can block interneuronal gap junctions as well as affecting synaptic transmission. The difficulties involved in delivering the gas (such as the requirement for an anesthesia machine) and the need for a gas-scavenging system essentially confine their use to the operating suite or the recovery area.[57] They do not have any proven advantages over the intravenously administered anticonvulsants and can raise intracranial pressure.

Propofol

Propofol has been reported to be effective in refractory SE in doses up to 250 μg per kg per minute[58] but has not been prospectively compared with other drugs. It theoretically offers a lower risk of respiratory depression and more rapid recovery of consciousness after the agent is stopped. I use it in SE patients in whom midazolam therapy has failed or who have become resistant to midazolam.[59]

Ketamine

Although only anecdotal evidence and small case series are available, ketamine appears to be a useful agent for the termination of refractory SE.[60] Its NMDA-blocking effect distinguishes it from the other agents discussed here and carries theoretical advantages in terms of brain protection.[61] Its intrinsic sympathomimetic effect makes it a useful choice in hypotensive patients, and it does not markedly impair ventilation. When the tidal volume is maintained constant, it does not increase intracranial pressure. The appropriate dose in SE has not been established; I use a loading dose of 1 to 4.5 mg per kg, with an infusion of 10 to 50 μg per kg per minute.

Levetiracetam

Levetiracetam is now available for intravenous use, but its role in SE remains to be determined. The effective dose in adults is reported to be between 1 and 3 g per day.[62] Oral administration may be useful for maintenance.[63]

Etomidate

Successful treatment of a few cases of SE with etomidate has been reported, but the drug also has an uncertain role in SE.[27] Although this agent generally is well tolerated for short periods, adrenal suppression poses a substantial problem when prolonged infusions are administered.

Controversial Management Issues

Controversy remains regarding the long-term neurologic consequences of two clinical conditions: periodic lateralized epileptiform discharges (PLEDs) and EPC. PLEDs are an EEG phenomenon usually seen in the setting of large acute strokes or rapidly expanding mass lesions (e.g., tumors or abscesses). Less commonly, acute metabolic or toxic disorders will "reactivate" PLEDs in the vicinity of an old lesion. The EEG activity signifies the repetitive, synchronous firing of large numbers of neurons near the lesion; contralateral myoclonic jerking of the hand or face occasionally may be seen. Expert opinion is divided regarding the possibly epileptic nature of these phenomena. Patients who have clinical seizures (i.e., other than the myoclonic jerks) should receive anticonvulsants. The myoclonic movements associated with PLEDs are difficult to suppress without resorting to high-dose barbiturates or benzodiazepines. The available data do not suggest that suppressing the electrical phenomenon improves outcome.

EPC usually is diagnosed in a patient who demonstrates an isolated repetitive movement (usually of the hand or face), often following an infectious or vascular insult, or in the setting of nonketotic hyperglycemia.[64] The movement may persist for months or years. Most patients receive anticonvulsants to prevent spread of the discharge, but these agents seldom affect EPC itself. Attempts at treatment with high-dose barbiturates result in short-term suppression of the movement, but the abnormality usually returns as the drug levels decline. One report suggests that isoflurane (used in that case to control secondarily generalized SE) may be helpful.[65]

Another area of contention concerns the periodic epileptiform discharges occasionally seen after respiratory or cardiac arrest. Because experimental studies show that neurons in anoxic animals exhibit epileptiform behavior, some investigators have raised the possibility that these discharges are a form of SE and should therefore be treated. Although this possibility has not been systematically studied in humans, the lack even of anecdotes of neurologic improvement with anticonvulsant treatment suggests that currently available anticonvulsant drugs do not improve patient outcome in this condition. If it is associated with myoclonus that the family finds disconcerting, suppression of the movements with neuromuscular junction blockers may be useful. High-dose barbiturates or benzodiazepines also will stop the movements, but they obscure the neurologic examination and complicate the possible diagnosis of death by neurologic criteria. These drugs do not improve prognosis in post-anoxia patients.

Patients with refractory SE due to encephalitis and other disorders associated with prolonged CNS inflammation may need treatment for weeks or even months and still make good neurologic recovery.[66] Thus, no duration over which aggressive therapy is required by itself indicates that treatment should not be continued.

If drug therapy for refractory SE fails, a limited experience with neurosurgical treatment provides some options. Focal resections,[67] multiple subpial transections,[68] and vagus nerve stimulators[69] have been used.

PROGNOSIS

Wijdicks and Sharbrough reported that 34% of patients experiencing a seizure in any ICU at the Mayo Clinic died during that hospitalization.[11] In a prospective study of neurologic complications in medical ICU patients,[1] having even one seizure while in the unit for a non-neurologic reason approximately doubled the patient's in-hospital mortality risk. This effect on prognosis appeared to be due to the effect of the *etiology* of the ictus, rather than the seizure itself.

Three major factors determine the outcome of SE: the type of SE, its etiology, and its duration. In general, GCSE carries the worst prognosis for neurologic recovery as a consequence of SE itself; myoclonic SE following an anoxic episode carries a very poor prognosis for survival. CPSE is associated with some risk of limbic system damage, usually manifested by memory dysfunction. Simple partial SE may produce neuronal damage, but this is difficult to discern from the effect of the lesion that commonly produces this form of SE. At the far end of the spectrum, absence SE does not seem to carry a risk of neurologic deterioration.

Most studies of SE outcome have concentrated on mortality in GCSE. Hauser[17] summarized the data available in 1990, showing mortality rates for SE to range from 1% to 53%. The few studies that attempted to distinguish the mortality due to SE from that due to the underlying disease attributed rates of 1% to 7% to SE and 2% to 25% to the etiologic disorder.

The Medical College of Virginia population-based studies have analyzed the mortality risks for various aspects of GCSE.[18] SE duration of longer than 1 hour was associated with an almost 10-fold increase in mortality when compared with SE lasting less than 1 hour. Other etiologic disorders and conditions associated with marked increases in mortality were anoxia, intracranial hemorrhages, tumors, infections, and trauma. Mortality in childhood SE is much lower, probably reflecting the differences in precipitants.[70]

Very few data are available regarding the functional status of survivors of GCSE, and there are none that reliably allow a distinction between the effects of SE and those of the specific etiologic disorder. A review of intellectual impairment as an outcome of SE concluded that intellectual abilities probably did decline as a consequence of SE.[71] In my own clinical experience, survivors of SE frequently have memory and behavioral disorders out of proportion to any structural damage produced by the cause of their seizures. This observation is supported by a wealth of experimental data and argues strongly for the rapid and effective control of SE.

The prognosis for CPSE is less certain, but case reports of severe memory deficits after prolonged CPSE have appeared.[72]

The effect of the treatment of SE on the risk of subsequent epilepsy is uncertain. Experimental studies suggest that SE does lower the threshold for subsequent seizures.[73]

KEY POINTS

- Seizures are one of the most common neurologic complications in the course of a critical illness, occurring in approximately 35 patients per 1000 ICU admissions.
- Approximately 8% of comatose ICU patients without any history of apparent seizure activity are found to be in nonconvulsive SE.
- Treatment of GCSE with a conventional anticonvulsant succeeds in at most 65% of cases. Lorazepam is the most efficacious of the established agents; phenytoin is inferior to it for this purpose but remains a useful agent to prevent seizure recurrence. The roles of newer intravenously available drugs such as valproate and levetiracetam remain to be established.
- Approximately 20% of patients who receive treatment for GCSE stop convulsing but remain in SE. EEG monitoring is necessary to detect the SE and manage the patient.
- High-dose midazolam, propofol, and pentobarbital are useful agents for the control of refractory SE.

REFERENCES

1. Bleck TP, Smith MC, Pierre-Louis JC, et al: Neurologic complications of critical medical illnesses. Crit Care Med 1993:21:98-103.
2. Varelas PN, Mirski M: Treatment of seizures in the neurologic intensive care unit. Curr Treat Options Neurol 2007;9:136-145.
3. Gavassetti M: Libri duo. Alter de rebus praeter naturum: Alter de indicationibus curativus. Venice, 1586. Quoted by Hunter RA: Status epilepticus. History, incidence and problems. Epilepsia 1959/1960;1:162-188.
4. Hunter RA: Status epilepticus. History, incidence and problems. Epilepsia 1959/1960;1:162-188.
5. Willis T: Pathologiae cerebri et nervosi generis specimen. In quo agitur de morbis convulsivis et de scorbuto. 1667. Translated by S. Pordage. London, Dring, 1681, p. 18. Quoted by Hunter RA: Status epilepticus. History, incidence and problems. Epilepsia 1959/1960;1:162-188.
6. Wilks S: Bromide and iodide of potassium in epilepsy. Med Times Gaz (Lond) 1861;2:635-636.
7. Gowers WR: Epilepsy and Other Chronic Convulsive Diseases: Their Causes, Symptoms,and Treatment. London, J. & A. Churchill, 1881.
8. Bleck TP, Klawans HL: Mechanisms of epilepsy and anticonvulsant action. In Klawans HL, Goetz CG, Tanner CM (eds): Textbook of Clinical Neuropharmacology. New York, Raven Press, 1992, pp 23-30.
9. Weschler IS: Intravenous injection of paraldehyde for control of convulsions. JAMA 1940;114:2198.
10. Gastaut H, Naquet R, Poiré R, Tassinari CA: Treatment of status epilepticus with diazepam (Valium). Epilepsia 1965;6:167-182.
11. Wijdicks EFM, Sharbrough FW: New-onset seizures in critically ill patients. Neurology 1993;43: 1042-1044.
12. Hussain N, Appleton R, Thorburn K: Aetiology, course and outcome of children admitted to paediatric intensive care with convulsive status epilepticus: A retrospective 5-year review. Seizure 2007;Feb 8 (Epub ahead of print).
13. Valencia I, Lozano G, Kothare SV, et al: Epileptic seizures in the pediatric intensive care unit setting. Epileptic Disord 2006;8:277-284.
14. Saengpattrachai M, Sharma R, Hunjan A, et al: Nonconvulsive seizures in the pediatric intensive care unit: Etiology, EEG, and brain imaging findings. Epilepsia 2006;47:1510-1518.
15. Chung SJ, Lee JH, Lee SA, et al: Co-occurrence of seizure and chorea in a patient with nonketotic hyperglycemia. Eur Neurol 2005;54:230-232.
16. Placidi F, Floris R, Bozzao A, et al: etotic hyperglycemia and epilepsia partialis continua. Neurology 2001;57:534-537.
17. Hauser WA: Status epilepticus: Epidemiologic considerations. Neurology 1990;40(Suppl 2):9-13.
18. DeLorenzo RJ, Towne AR, Pellock JM, et al: Status epilepticus in children, adults, and the elderly. Epilepsia 1992;33(Suppl 4):S15-S25.
19. Towne AR, Waterhouse EJ, Boggs JG, et al: Prevalence of nonconvulsive status epilepticus in comatose patients. Neurology 2000;54:340-345.
20. Aminoff MJ, Simon RP: Status epilepticus: Causes, clinical features and consequences in 98 patients. Am J Med 1980;69:657-666.
21. Lowenstein DH, Alldredge BK: Status epilepticus in an urban public hospital in the 1980s. Neurology 1993;42:483-488.
22. Bleck TP: Status epilepticus. Univ Rep Epilepsy 1992;1:1-7.
23. Ettinger AB, Shinnar S: New-onset seizures in an elderly hospitalized population. Neurology 1993;43:489-492.
24. Commission on Classification and Terminology of the International League Against Epilepsy: Proposal for revised clinical and electroencephalographic classification of epileptic seizures. Epilepsia 1981;22:489-501.
25. Bleck TP: Metabolic encephalopathy. In Weiner WJ, Shulman LM (eds): Emergent and Urgent Neurology, 2nd ed. Philadelphia, Lippincott, 1999, pp 223-253.
26. Bleck TP, Brauner JS: Tetanus. In Scheld WM, Whitley RJ, Durack DT (eds): Infections of the Central Nervous System, 2nd ed. New York, Lippincott-Raven, 1997, pp 629-653.
27. Bleck TP: Status epilepticus. In Klawans HL, Goetz CG, Tanner CM (eds): Textbook of Clinical Neuropharmacology, 2nd ed. New York, Raven Press, 1992, pp 65-73.
28. Lothman EW: The biochemical basis and pathophysiology of status epilepticus. Neurology 1990;40(Suppl 2):13-23.
29. Lowenstein DH, Simon RP, Sharp FR: The pattern of 72-kDa heat shock protein-like immunoreactivity in the rat brain following fluothyl-induced status epilepticus. Brain Res 1990;531:173-182.
30. Wasterlain CG, Fujikawa DG, Penix L, Sankar R: Pathophysiological mechanisms of brain damage from status epilepticus. Epilepsia 1993;34(Suppl 1):S37-S53.
31. Walton NY: Systemic effects of generalized convulsive status epilepticus. Epilepsia 1993;34(Suppl 1): S54-S58.
32. Bleck TP: Neurologic alterations in sepsis. In Fein AM, Abraham E, Balk R, et al (eds): Textbook of Sepsis and Multiorgan Failure. Media, PA, Williams & Wilkins, 1997, pp 236-242.
33. Bleck TP, Hirsch LJ, Vespa PM: Electroencephalography in the intensive care unit. In Engel JE, Pedley T (eds): Epilepsy: A Comprehensive Textbook, 2nd ed. Philadelphia, Lippincott Williams & Wilkins (in press).
34. Geocadin RG, Koenig MA, Stevens RD, Peberdy MA: Intensive care for brain injury after cardiac arrest: Therapeutic hypothermia and related neuroprotective strategies. Crit Care Clin 2006;22:619-636.
35. Rowbotham MC; Lowenstein DH: Neurologic complications of cocaine use. Annu Rev Med 1990;41:417-422.
36. Ross C, Blake A, Whitehouse WP: Status epilepticus on the paediatric intensive care unit—the role of EEG monitoring. Seizure 1999;8:335-338.
37. First Seizure Trial Group: Randomized clinical trial of the efficacy of antiepileptic drugs in reducing the risk of relapse after a first unprovoked tonic-clonic seizure. Neurology 1993;43:478-483.
38. Smith MC, Bleck TP: Toxicity of anticonvulsants. In Klawans HL, Goetz CG, Tanner CM (eds): Textbook of Clinical Neuropharmacology, 2nd ed. New York, Raven Press, 1992, pp 45-64.
39. Naidech AM, Kreiter KT, Janjua N, et al: Phenytoin exposure is associated with functional and cognitive disability after subarachnoid hemorrhage. Stroke 2005;36:583-587.
40. Alldredge B, Treiman DM, Bleck TP, Shorvon SD: Treatment of status

epilepticus. In Engel JE, Pedley T (eds): Epilepsy: A Comprehensive Textbook, 2nd ed. Philadelphia, Lippincott Williams & Wilkins (in press).
41. Treiman DM, Meyers PD, Walton NY, et al: A comparison of four treatments for generalized convulsive status epilepticus. Veterans Affairs Status Epilepticus Cooperative Study Group. N Engl J Med 1998;339:792-798.
42. Chuilli DA, Ternfrup TE, Kanter RK: The influence of diazepam or lorazepam on the frequency of endotracheal intubation in childhood status epilepticus. J Emerg Med 1991;9:13-17.
43. Kumar A, Bleck TP: Intravenous midazolam for the treatment of refractory status epilepticus. Crit Care Med 1992;20:483-488.
44. Osorio I, Reed RC: Treatment of refractory generalized tonic-clonic status epilepticus with pentobarbital anesthesia after high-dose phenytoin. Epilepsia 1989;30:464-471.
45. O'Brien TJ, Cascino GD, So EL, Hanna DR: Incidence and clinical consequence of the purple glove syndrome in patients receiving intravenous phenytoin. Neurology 1998;51:1034-1039.
46. Shaner DM, McCurdy SA, Herring MO, Gabor AJ: Treatment of status epilepticus: A prospective comparison of diazepam and phenytoin versus phenobarbital and optional phenytoin. Neurology 1988;38:202-206.
47. Yaffe K, Lowenstein DH: Prognostic factors of pentobarbital therapy for refractory generalized status epilepticus. Neurology 1993;43:895-900.
48. Bleck TP: High-dose pentobarbital treatment of refractory status epilepticus: A meta-analysis of published studies. Epilepsia 1992;33:5.
49. Venkataraman V, Wheless JW: Safety of rapid intravenous infusion of valproate loading doses in epilepsy patients. Epilepsy Res 1999;35:147-153.
50. Sinha S, Naritoku DK: Intravenous valproate is well tolerated in unstable patients with status epilepticus. Neurology 2000;55:722-724.
51. Misra UK, Kalita J, Patel R: Sodium valproate vs phenytoin in status epilepticus: A pilot study. Neurology 2006;67:340-342.
52. White JR, Santos CS.:Intravenous valproate associated with significant hypotension in the treatment of status epilepticus. J Child Neurol 1999;14:822-823.
53. Krahenbuhl S, Brandner S, Kleinle S, et al: Mitochondrial diseases represent a risk factor for valproate-induced fulminant liver failure. Liver 2000;20:346-348.
54. Spriet I, Meersseman W, De Troy E, et al: Meropenem-valproic acid interaction in patients with cefepime-associated status epilepticus. Am J Health Syst Pharm 2007;64:54-58.
55. Mirsattari SM, Sharpe MD, Young GB: Treatment of refractory status epilepticus with inhalational anesthetic agents isoflurane and desflurane. Arch Neurol 2004;61:1254-1259.
56. Kofke WA, Bloom MJ, Van Cott A, Brenner RP: Electrographic tachyphylaxis to etomidate and ketamine used for refractory status epilepticus controlled with isoflurane. J Neurosurg Anesthesiol 1997;9:269-272.
57. Bleck TP: Therapy for status epilepticus. Clin Neuropharmacol 1983;6:255-268.
58. Stecker MM, Kramer TH, Raps EC, et al: Treatment of refractory status epilepticus with propofol: Clinical and pharmacokinetic findings. Epilepsia 1998;39:18-26.
59. Prasad A, Worrall BB, Bertram EB, Bleck TP: Propofol and midazolam in the treatment of refractory status epilepticus. Epilepsia 2001;42:380-386.
60. Sheth RD, Gidal BE: Refractory status epilepticus: Response to ketamine. Neurology 1998;51:1765-1766.
61. Mazarati AM, Wasterlain CG: *N*-methyl-D-asparate receptor antagonists abolish the maintenance phase of self-sustaining status epilepticus in rat. Neurosci Lett 1999;265:187-190.
62. Falip M, Carreno M, Amaro S, et al: Use of levetiracetam in hospitalized patients. Epilepsia 2006;47:2186-2188.
63. Rossetti AO, Bromfield EB: Determinants of success in the use of oral levetiracetam in status epilepticus. Epilepsy Behav 2006;8:651-654.
64. Schomer DL: Focal status epilepticus and epilepsia partialis continua in adults and children. Epilepsia 1993;34(Suppl 1):S29-S36.
65. Hughes DR, Sharpe MD, McLachlan RS: Control of epilepsia partialis continua and secondary generalized status epilepticus with isoflurane. J Neurol Neurosurg Psychiatry 1992;55:739-740.
66. Mirski MA, Williams MA, Hanley DF: Prolonged pentobarbital and phenobarbital coma for refractory generalized status epilepticus. Crit Care Med 1995;23:400-404.
67. Ng YT, Kerrigan JF, Rekate HL: Neurosurgical treatment of status epilepticus. J Neurosurg 2006;105(5 Suppl):378-381.
68. Costello DJ, Simon MV, Eskandar EN, et al: Efficacy of surgical treatment of de novo, adult-onset, cryptogenic, refractory focal status epilepticus. Arch Neurol 2006;63:895-901.
69. Patwardhan RV, Dellabadia J Jr, Rashidi M, et al: Control of refractory status epilepticus precipitated by anticonvulsant withdrawal using left vagal nerve stimulation: A case report. Surg Neurol 2005;64:170-173.
70. Neville BG, Chin RF, Scott RC: Childhood convulsive status epilepticus: Epidemiology, management and outcome. Acta Neurol Scand 2007;115:21-24.
71. Dodrill CB, Wilensky AJ: Intellectual impairment as an outcome of status epilepticus. Neurology 1990;40(Suppl 2):23-27.
72. Treiman DM, Delgado-Escueta AV: Complex partial status epilepticus. Adv Neurol 1983;34:69-81.
73. Lothman EW, Bertram EH: Epileptogenic effects of status epilepticus. Epilepsia 1993;34(Suppl 1):S59-S70.

Chapter 67

Head Injury

Alan R. Turtz and H. Warren Goldman

In the context of critical care medicine, the management of severe head injuries remains the Achilles heel of neurosurgery, as borne out by our own observations over 3 decades of practice at academic centers. Although revolutionary advances now allow imaging of the brain and spinal cord with greatly improved speed and anatomic detail, translation of this resource into better outcomes has been disappointing. The search for a neuroprotective agent that can consistently prevent the deadly cascade of events that leads to irreparable brain damage remains for future investigators as of this writing.

Key to optimizing clinical outcomes has been the recognition that the time from injury to surgery must be as short as possible to minimize the secondary manifestations of serious brain trauma. Other valuable lessons from clinical experience reported in the literature are that glucocorticoids have no significant therapeutic benefit in managing severe head injuries, and that hyperventilation, very effective in reducing high intracranial pressure (ICP), must be used judiciously; otherwise, it may become more harmful than helpful.

It also has been demonstrated that the management of serious brain trauma requires specialty teams consisting of experienced neurosurgeons, traumatologists, and intensivists (specifically, neurointensivists) working together in a dedicated unit equipped and staffed to optimally care for these patients. In the absence of such facilities, outcomes suffer.[1-3]

Finally, the introduction of a simple-to-use and highly predictable neurologic status scoring system, the Glascow Coma Scale (GCS), has enabled meaningful multidisciplinary communication from the accident scene through intensive care and beyond, resulting in efficient and timely triage and treatment of these patients in very tenuous condition.

INCIDENCE

The incidence of head injury in the United States is approximately 200 per 100,000 population per year.[4] Based on a U.S. population of 250 million, approximately 500,000 people are estimated to sustain a head injury every year that is severe enough to prompt them to seek medical attention. Of these, 40,000 to 50,000 die before hospital admission.[4] The peak incidence of head injury occurs at 15 to 24 years of age.[5] A secondary peak has been noted for infants and the elderly. Head injury remains the most common cause of death in young adults and is two to three times more common in males.[4,7-8] The incidence of head injury is inversely proportional to socioeconomic status.[6] Motor vehicle accidents account for more than 50% of head injuries in the United States. Approximately 13% to 15% of head injuries are the result of gunshot wounds. In the United States more than one half of all motorcycle accidents result in death (15% of all deaths are the result of vehicular accidents) or major head injury. Helmets have been proved to reduce this problem significantly.[9]

In other countries, different injury patterns have been found. Pedestrian head injuries are frequent in Nigeria and certain parts of England.[4-6,8-10] In some regions of South Africa, penetrating knife injury to the brain is very common.[11]

DIAGNOSTIC APPROACH

The presenting neurologic condition of patients with head injuries is the primary factor in determining the initial management and prognosis. When a detailed history is unavailable, it is important to keep in mind that loss of consciousness may have preceded and in fact caused the traumatic event, such as aneurysmal subarachnoid hemorrhage (SAH), hypoglycemia, intoxication, or syncope. Level of consciousness is one of the most important neurologic considerations in managing a head-injured patient. Neurosurgical patients generally have an alteration in level of consciousness from either brainstem or bilateral cerebral hemispheric involvement. This may be secondary to poor perfusion due to high ICP or brainstem compression, both of which require neurosurgical intervention. Therefore, an accurate tool to measure level of consciousness is essential. Many clinical assessment tools are available for use in the critical care setting.[12-24]

Glasgow Coma Scale

Ideally, using the GCS, a nurse, medical student, paramedic, physician assistant, intensivist, trauma surgeon, emergency medicine physician, neurologist, and neurosurgeon all should obtain the same score when assessing a patient. The GCS system is not perfect, but it has proved itself to be, overall, a practical, straightforward grading system that can be used by health professionals in various fields and at different levels to produce reliable results.[25-30] The GCS has become the most widely used assessment tool and is considered the gold standard for evaluation of patients with head injuries.[12]

The GCS is a measure of level of consciousness and does not take into account focal deficits. It is based on eye opening,[1-4] verbal response,[1-5] and motor response[1-6] (Table 67-1). A patient with a normal level of consciousness should have the highest possible score of 15. The lowest score possible is 3, not 0 as might be expected. An intubated patient technically gets a 1 for verbal response and is assigned 1T (for *t*ube) for the verbal score. It is important to identify the score for each observed variable tested. For example, a typical score for an intubated patient with decorticate posturing probably would be E1+V1T+M3=5T (where E denotes eye opening, V is verbal response, and M is motor response). It also is important to realize the shortcoming of this system in evaluating patients with dementia or aphasia. A point to keep in mind is that the GCS attempts to put a numerical value on level of consciousness, with 15 being representative of normal. If a demented patient from a nursing home presents with a normal level of consciousness after a fall but doesn't know what day it is, the GCS would be calculated as E4+V4+M6=14. A GCS score of 14 describes a patient with an abnormal level of consciousness but fails to accurately communicate this particular patient's condition. Likewise, clinicians must use caution when applying the GCS to patients with aphasia. Conversely, patients with profound focal deficits and a normal level of consciousness should have a GCS score of 15. Another problematic case is that of a quadriplegic patient with a normal level of consciousness who is able to blink the eyes or stick out the tongue to command, thereby giving a top score of 6 on the motor assessment.

Table 67-1. Glasgow Coma Scale

Component	Score
Eye opening	
Spontaneously	4
To voice	3
To pain	2
No response	1
Verbal	
Oriented	5
Disoriented	4
Inappropriate	3
Incomprehensible sounds	2
No response	1
Motor	
Following commands	6
Localizing to pain	5
Withdrawing to pain	4
Abnormal flexion	3
Abnormal extension	2
No response	1

The GCS has been used to predict outcome.[31] The motor score itself has predictive value as well.[32] The GCS score should be calculated after hemodynamic and pulmonary resuscitation and without sedatives or muscle relaxants.[33]

Aggressive implementation of early sedation and intubation in severely head-injured patients compromises the ability to determine an accurate GCS score.[34]

Computed Tomography Classification: Marshall Classification

A useful classification of brain injuries by findings on computed tomography (CT) has been devised by Marshall and colleagues. This CT classification, presented in Table 67-2, can serve as a guide in describing scans and has strong predictive power.[34,35]

Maas and associates have proposed a scoring system with better predictive power (Table 67-3), with a sum total adjusted to be consistent with the GCS.[34] Table 67-4 presents a mortality prediction chart based on this classification.

This scoring system is best used as one piece of data in the overall clinical assessment in considering a patient's prognosis.[36]

Prediction of Outcomes

Severe brain injury outcomes can be accurately predicted using four variables: age, Glasgow Coma Scale score on admission (especially motor score), CT characteristics, and presence of ischemic and hemodynamic secondary insults. Using these four predictors, numerous investigators have used statistical modeling techniques to predict up to 80% or more of outcomes.[37]

Head injuries generally are classified as mild (GCS score of 13 to 15), moderate (GCS score of 9 to 12), or severe,[3-8] although the evidence may be sufficient to include a GCS score of 13 in the moderate category.[38]

CT scanning is the diagnostic imaging study of choice in trauma. Plain x-ray films of the skull are rarely indicated as a screening study for head-injured patients. Outcomes with the strategy of obtaining CT scans in all head-injured patients are superior to those with other

Table 67-2. Marshall Computed Tomography Classification

Category	Definition
Diffuse injury I (no visible pathology)	No visible intracranial pathology seen on computed tomography scan
Diffuse injury II	Cisterns are present with midline shift of 0-5 mm and/or: • lesion densities present • no high- or mixed-density lesion >25 cm^3 • may include bone fragments and foreign bodies
Diffuse injury III (swelling)	Cisterns compressed or absent with midline shift of 0-5 mm; no high- or mixed-density lesion >25 cm^3
Diffuse injury IV (shift)	Midline shift >5 mm; no high- or mixed-density lesion >25 cm^3
Evacuated mass lesion	Any lesion surgically evacuated
Nonevacuated mass lesion	High- or mixed-density lesion >25 cm^3; not surgically evacuated

From Marshall LF, Marshall SB, Klauber MR, et al: A new classification of head injury based on computerized tomography. J Neurosurg 1991;75:S14-S20.

Table 67-3. Prognostic Score Chart for Probability of Mortality in Patients with Severe or Moderate Traumatic Brain Injury by Computed Tomography Characteristics

Predictor	Score
Basal cisterns	
Normal	0
Compressed	1
Absent	2
Midline shift	
No shift or shift ≤5 mm	0
Shift >5 mm	1
Epidural mass lesion	
Present	0
Absent	1
Intraventricular blood or tSAH	
Absent	0
Present	1
Sum score*	+1

*The sum score can be used to obtain the predicted probability of mortality (see Table 67-4). The authors chose to add plus 1 to make the grading numerically consistent with the grading of the motor score of the GCS and with the Marshall CT classification.
tSAH, traumatic subarachnoid hemorrhage.

management strategies. The incidence of missed surgical lesions in mildly head-injured patients by CT scanning is 0.028%.[39-42]

PRIMARY HEAD INJURY

Primary head injury can be defined as the damage that occurs at the moment of impact and can take the form of skull fractures, surface contusions and lacerations, diffuse axonal injury, or diffuse vascular injury.[42] Some authors include the contusions and hematomas that form as a direct and immediate effect of the impact as part of the primary injury as well.[43] These hemorrhages may manifest with significant mass effect requiring surgical intervention.

Table 67-4. Computed Tomography Classification by Prediction Score

Score	Mortality Rate (%)
1	0
2	6.8
3	16
4	26
5	53
6	61

Emergent neurosurgical intervention is designed to prevent permanent damage to the central nervous system (CNS) in general and to the reticular activating system in particular. Located in the brainstem, the reticular activating system is what allows a meaningful, awake condition; if it is destroyed, the patient will be vegetative. The surgical management of head-injured patients typically is driven by the presence of pathologic masses (hematomas) in anatomic spaces. These spaces are best described by reviewing the anatomic layers.

In virtually all cases of head injury seen in clinical practice, the pathogenic mechanism is an impact. The first layer involved is the scalp, the layers of which are best remembered by the pneumonic SCALP: S for skin, C for connective tissue, A for galea aponeurosis, L for the loose connective tissue layer, and P for periosteum. The scalp is the thickest skin in the body and absorbs some of the energy delivered to the head during impact. The scalp has a rich blood supply with relatively large blood vessels situated in the space where the connective tissue meets the galea. A large laceration has the potential for heavy blood loss and needs to be managed with local, direct pressure until surgical repair can be accomplished. Care must be taken in applying pressure if there is an underlying depressed skull fracture or, especially, a skull defect as is seen in missile injuries. It should be noted that an unattended, serious scalp laceration does have the potential for blood loss to the point of hemodynamic instability, but this is the only exception to the rule that an adult cannot lose enough blood from any intracranial hemorrhage to cause hypovolemic shock and hemodynamic instability. Blood clots within the scalp usually are limited to the loose connective tissue layer and are referred to as subgaleal hematomas, which may be a feature of massive injuries or a sign of coagulopathy but rarely require treatment other than direct pressure if active bleeding is suspected. A cephalohematoma is a blood clot that expands in the potential space between the periosteum and the skull; this lesion is limited to neonates.

Skull Fractures

The next layer involved in trauma is the skull, composed of outer and inner tables with the intervening vascular diploic space. Skull fractures are best considered as involving the cranial vault or the skull base. Cranial vault fractures are further divided into linear or depressed and open or closed. In general, closed, linear fractures of the cranial vault do not require any specific treatment.

Basilar skull fractures typically are linear and involve the anterior cranial base and the petrous part of the temporal bone. These fractures have the potential for an associated dural laceration adjacent to potentially contaminated paranasal sinuses, or the external ear canal if the tympanic membrane is disrupted. This allows the potential for a cerebrospinal fluid (CSF) fistula to develop, as well as meningitis. Clinical signs of a fracture of the petrous portion of the temporal bone include hemotympanum with or without tympanic membrane disruption, hearing loss, CSF otorrhea, and Battle sign. The cranial nerves that course through the temporal bone include the facial, acoustic, and vestibular nerves; therefore, associated vestibular dysfunction or facial weakness may be noted (Fig. 67-1). Anterior cranial base fractures may be associated with "raccoon eyes," anosmia, and CSF rhinorrhea. It is important to remember that when a fracture of the floor of the anterior cranial base is suspected, a nasogastric tube should not be inserted, because of the risk of intracranial penetration (Fig. 67-2).

The use of prophylactic antibiotics in basilar skull fractures has been debated but generally is not recommended. When CSF leak does occur, the break in the tissue usually will heal with conservative treatment over the course of a week, unless the defect is very large or a bony spicule is identified. Keeping the patient's head elevated and possibly using external CSF diversion after a few days are reasonable nonoperative methods; however, if the leak persists, surgical repair is indicated.[44]

Most depressed skull fractures occur in men younger than 30 years of age.[45]

Despite very little literature to support any particular management strategy, closed depressed skull fractures generally are operated on if the extent of depression is greater than the full thickness of the adjacent skull, with the theoretical benefits of improved cosmetic result, a decrease in late-onset post-traumatic epilepsy, and a reduction in the incidence of persistent neurologic deficit.[46] Most depressed skull fractures, however, are open[45] (Fig. 67-3)—meaning that a scalp laceration with galeal disruption overlying the fracture is present.

Open depressed skull fractures may be associated with significant morbidity and mortality.[45,47] Infection rates are reported to be between 1.9% and 10.6%,[46-50] with neurologic morbidity and mortality rates of approximately 11% each[46] and an incidence of late epilepsy up to 15%.[51]

By convention, open depressed cranial vault fractures are treated surgically, with débridement and elevation, primarily to attempt to decrease the incidence of infection. Open depressed cranial fractures may be treated nonoperatively if clinical and radiographic examination reveals no evidence of dural penetration, significant intracranial hematoma, depression greater than 1 cm, frontal sinus involvement, gross cosmetic deformity, wound infection, pneumocephalus, or gross wound contamination.[46]

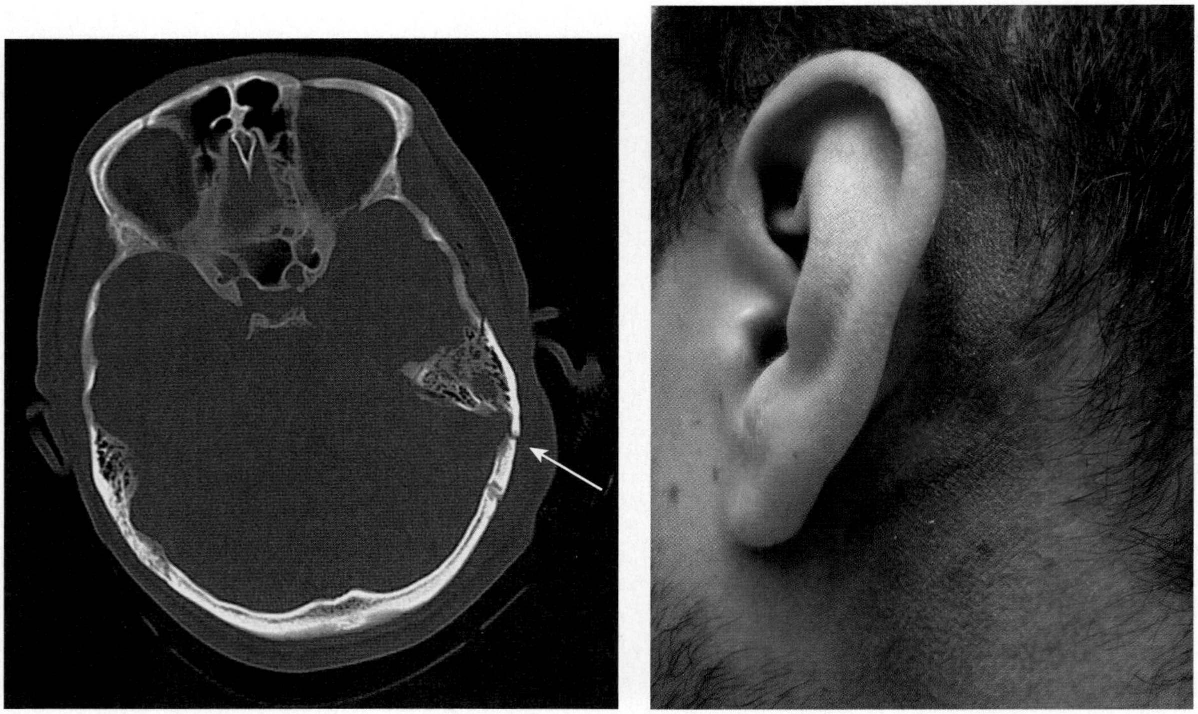

A B

Figure 67-1. A, Axial computed tomography image demonstrating skull base fracture *(arrow)* through the petrous portion of the temporal bone. **B,** Battle sign.

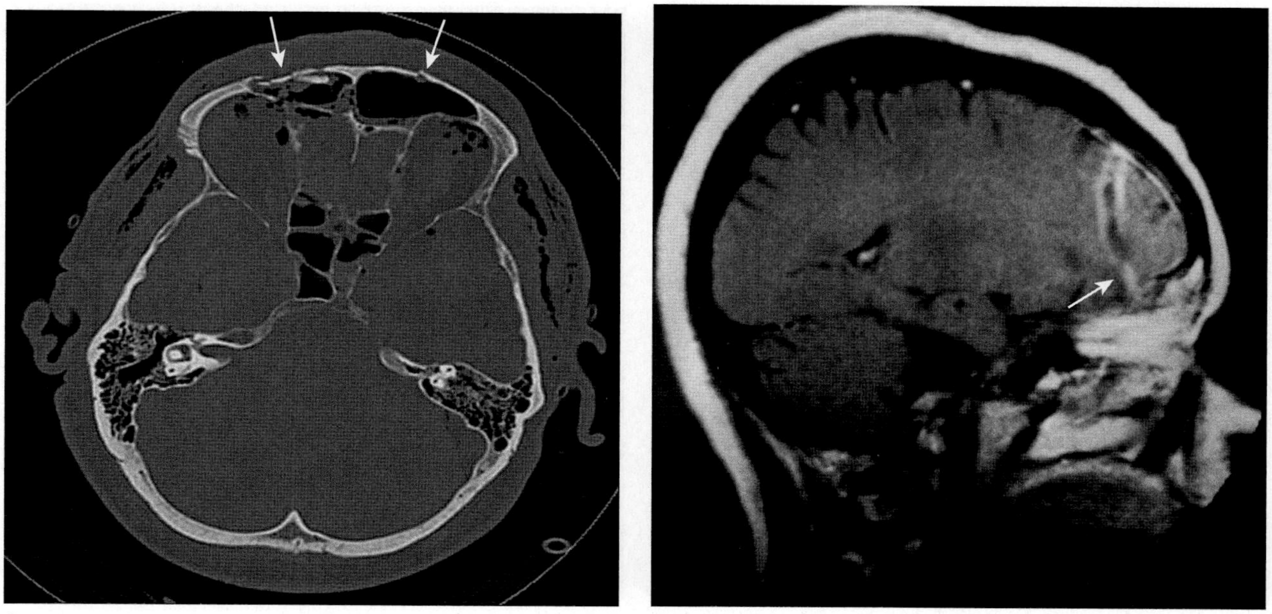

A B

Figure 67-2. A, Preoperative axial computed tomography image demonstrates multiple anterior cranial base fractures involving the cribriform plate and posterior wall of the frontal sinus *(arrows)* in a 50-year-old man who fell off a ladder onto his face. The patient sustained minimal brain injury from the impact because the facial and anterior frontal sinuses absorbed much of the energy, cushioning the brain during impact, much like an air bag. **B,** Image from a preoperative sagittal T1 MRI study without contrast demonstrates the tract of a nasogastric tube through the frontal lobe in a 42-year-old woman with an anterior cranial base defect *(arrow).*

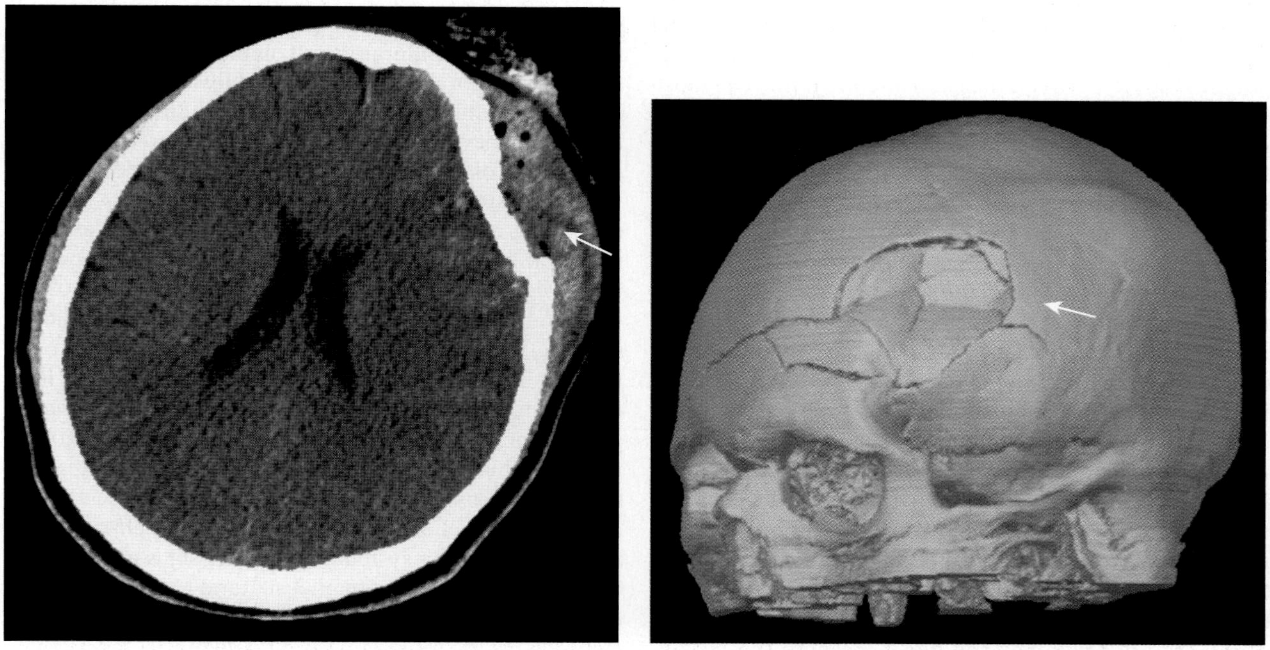

A B

Figure 67-3. Depressed skull fracture. **A,** Brain window *(arrow).* **B,** Computed tomography three-dimensional reconstruction also demonstrates the depressed skull fracture *(arrow).*

A special type of depressed fracture is fracture of the frontal sinus. Depression of the fracture may require surgery to prevent CNS infection and CSF leak (Fig. 67-4). Another special type of depressed fracture involves a major dural venous sinus (see Fig. 67-4). Under these circumstances, the risks associated with surgery are increased, and elevation of the fracture fragment generally is reserved for significant compromise of venous drainage.[44]

Epidural Hematoma

The next anatomic layer after the skull is the dura, which is the periosteum of the inner table of the skull and, as

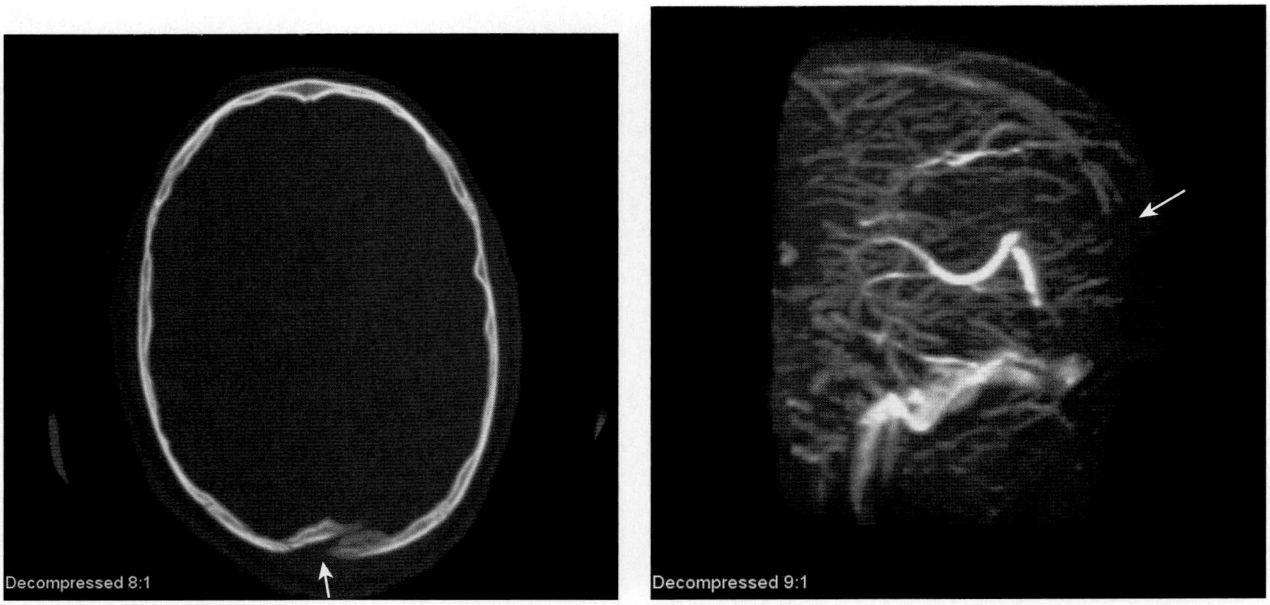

A B

Figure 67-4. Depressed skull fracture requiring urgent decompressive surgery. The patient was a 32-year-old man hit on the back of the head by a metal beam at a construction site who presented with a deteriorating level of consciousness. **A,** Axial computed tomography scan demonstrates an open depressed skull fracture *(arrow)* at the level of the superior sagittal sinus (SSS) that extended down to the confluence of the transverse and SSS. **B,** Sagittal magnetic resonance venogram demonstrates occlusion of venous outflow *(arrow)* at the level of the fracture, which necessitated emergency surgical decompression and repair of the SSS.

such, is tightly adherent to the bone. The potential space between the inner table of the skull and the dura is the *epidural space.* Epidural hematomas (EDHs) form in this potential space between the skull and the dura. The most common mechanism for the development of an EDH is a motor vehicle crash (in 53% of the cases), followed by falls (in 30%) and assault (in 8%).[52-60] Typically, bleeding results from damage to the middle meningeal artery, but an EDH also can occur from injury to the middle meningeal vein, diploic veins, or the venous sinuses.[60]

EDHs generally occur in the temporal and temporoparietal regions (Figure 67-5).[52,57,61-64] A useful way to describe the development of an EDH is to follow the events that take place when a patient presents with an initial lucid interval following brief loss of consciousness after head trauma. A lucid interval occurs when a patient initially is rendered unconscious from a concussive head injury that causes a linear skull fracture involving the middle meningeal artery or one of its branches. The middle meningeal artery is a dural vessel that runs half in the dura and half through the groove in the inner table of the skull. When a fracture extends across the bony groove of the artery, it will tear and bleed. Because the dura is tightly adherent to the inner table of the skull, significant force is needed to push the dura off the inner table. An arterial hemorrhage generally has enough pressure to strip the dura off the bone, converting the potential epidural space into a mass. The bony attachment of the dura becomes progressively stronger with age; therefore, the dura of a younger patient requires less force to push it off the bone than would be required in an older patient. Not surprisingly, the mean age of patients with EDH is between 20 and 30 years of age,[53-55,63-70] and EDHs are unusual in patients older than 50.[60]

The growing epidural mass commonly compresses the anterior temporal lobe which usually will not cause a major detectable neurologic deficit early in the course in the emergency department. During this so-called lucid component of the lucid interval, the patient regains consciousness from the concussive injury while the EDH is expanding and compressing the relatively silent anterior temporal lobe. The medial part of the temporal lobe, the uncas, lies just lateral to the brainstem at the level of the third cranial nerve (oculomotor nerve), which runs alongside the tentorial edge. When the EDH enlarges to the point at which it pushes the uncas of the temporal lobe over the tentorial edge, rapid development of a third nerve palsy, along with brainstem compression, is possible—which, at this level, will cause a contralateral hemiparesis from direct compression of the cerebral peduncle and a decrease in level of consciousness from the effect on the reticular activating system. The classic signs at this point are coma with a dilated pupil ipsilateral to the EDH and a contralateral hemiparesis. Occasionally, instead of directly compressing the ipsilateral cerebral peduncle, the herniating uncas can shift the brainstem into the contralateral tentorial edge, a relatively sharp rigid structure. This can damage the brainstem on the side opposite the EDH and cause a hemiparesis ipsilateral to the side of the hematoma. This is known as Kernihan's notch phenomenon.

Taking a general view, the patient goes from unconscious at the time of impact from a concussive injury, to awake, to unconscious again secondary to brainstem compression—hence the term *lucid interval.* The lucid interval

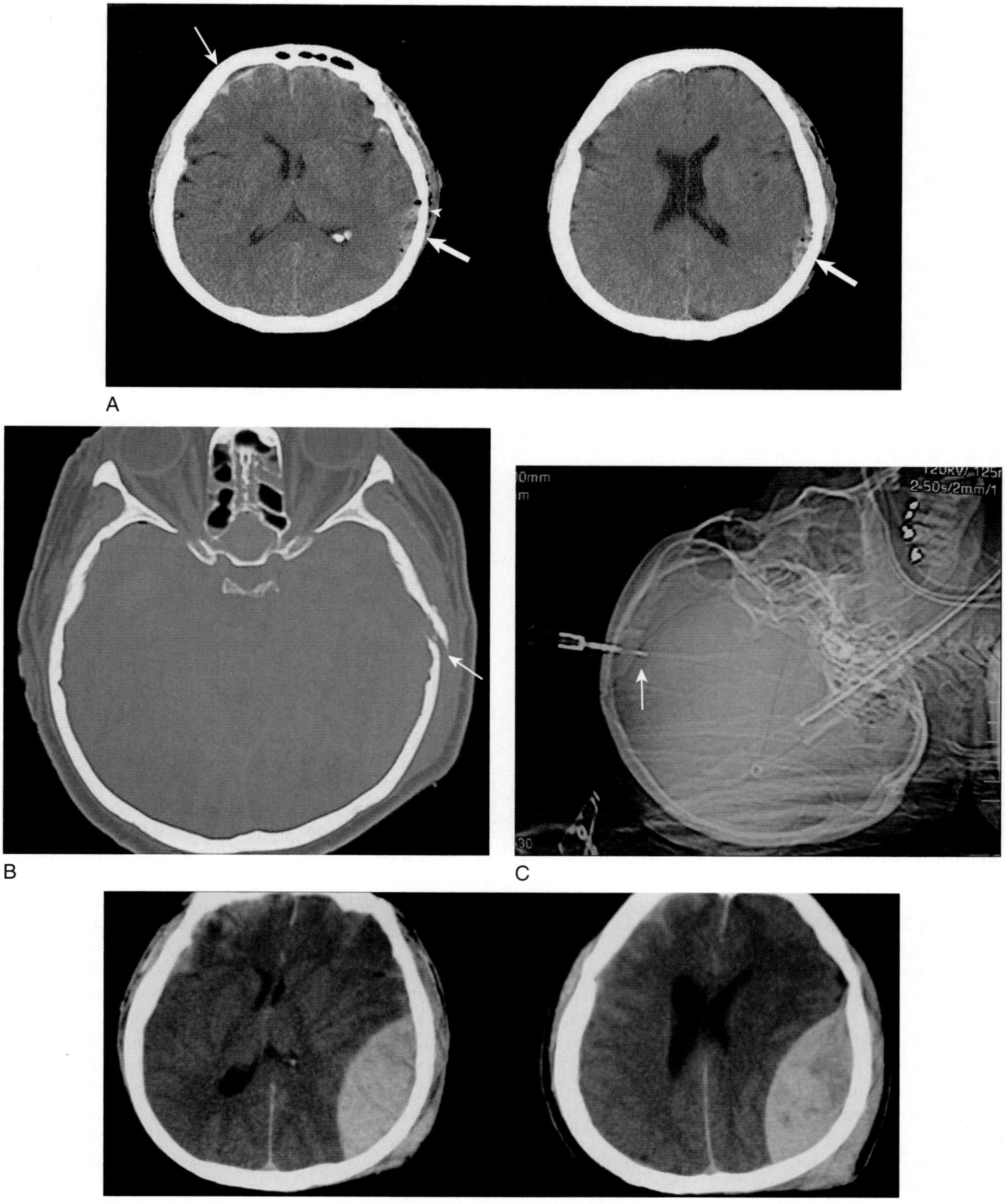

Figure 67-5. The patient was a 58-year-old female pedestrian who was hit by a car and unconscious at the accident scene. She was combative on presentation, pharmacologically paralyzed and intubated in the trauma bay. **A,** Computed tomography (CT) image shows a small left temporal epidural hematoma without significant mass effect *(large arrow).* Note the right frontal traumatic subarachnoid hemorrhage *(small, thin arrow)* and the small amount of air *(arrowhead)* from the associated open, linear fracture *(arrow),* seen in **B.** There is no significant mass effect, and an intracranial pressure monitor *(arrow)* was placed, seen in **C.** ICP steadily increased shortly after placement, and immediate follow-up CT scans, shown in **D,** reveal marked expansion of the epidural hematoma with mass effect and shift requiring emergency craniotomy.

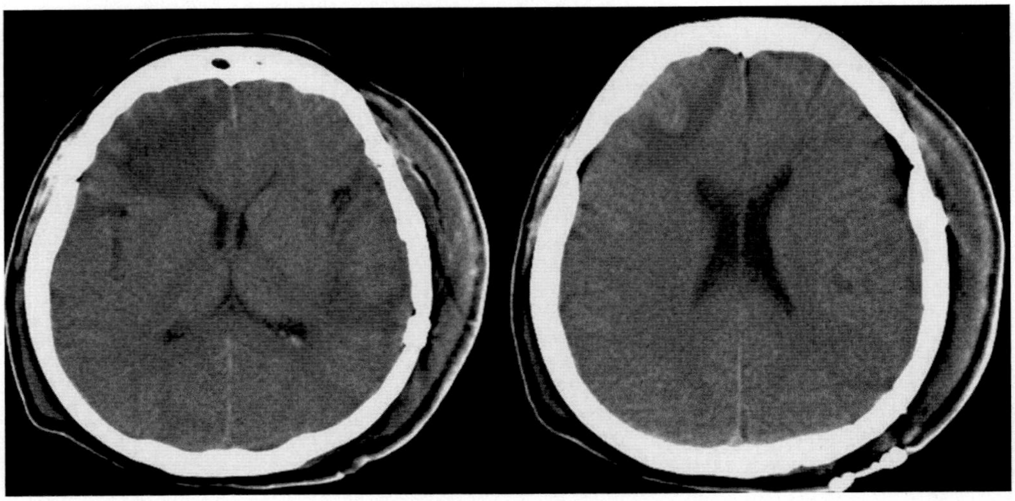

E

Figure 67-5, cont'd E, Postoperative CT scans reveal adequate decompression of surgical clot, with subsequent development of edema on the right side of the brain.

is observed in close to half of the patients undergoing surgery for EDH.[52,55,60,65,69,71-73]

Pupillary abnormalities occur in approximately 20% to 30% of patients with surgical EDH.[52,54,59,60,67] Cranial fractures are present in between 70% and 95% of the cases.[54,60,68,70,74,75] Associated intracranial lesions are found in 30% to 50% of adults with surgical EDHs,[52,54,55,57-60,63-67,73,76,77] and subdural or parenchymal lesions in association with EDH lower the chance of a good outcome.[60]

The overall mortality rate (for all ages and GCS scores) is approximately 10%.[54,55,64,65,68,72,73,78,79] The time lapse between the onset of pupillary abnormalities and surgery determines outcome,[61,66,80] but the single most important predictor of outcome in patients operated on for EDH is the GCS score on admission and before surgery.[52,53,55,61,81-83]

Not all EDHs, however, require surgery. No prospective randomized trials have been conducted to compare surgical treatment with nonoperative management, nor should there be. Available data describe nonsurgical management in selected cases. In one study, approximately 10% of the total number of EDHs were treated nonoperatively. All were conscious with a GCS score greater than 11 and a midline shift on CT scan of less than 10 mm. None of these nonoperative hematomas was in the temporal region.[84]

Another study reported findings in a group of 57 selected patients treated nonoperatively with an initial GCS score of 10 or higher, with maximum hematoma thickness less than 13 mm, with 5 clots located in the temporal region, but only one patient had a midline shift on CT.[53]

An interesting approach for dealing with thin, acute EDHs in an early stage has been reported in a small, isolated series of patients using endovascular techniques to occlude the middle meningeal artery.[85] Surgical decision making for an acute EDH is based on GCS score, pupillary findings, comorbid conditions, CT findings, age, and, in delayed decisions, ICP. Guidelines for the surgical management of acute EDH published in 2006 recommend surgical evacuation of an EDH less than 30 mL in volume. Smaller hematomas in patients with a GCS score greater than 8 and without focal deficits, clot thickness less than 15 mm, and less than 5 mm of midline shift may be considered for nonoperative management. Close neurologic monitoring and serial CT scanning are essential. Of importance, a temporal location for an EDH is associated with failure of nonoperative management and should lower the threshold for surgery.[60]

Because time between neurologic deterioration and surgery is critical, the question of whether a patient with an acute EDH should receive treatment at the nearest hospital or should be transferred to a trauma center is important. The issue is whether or not a non-neurosurgeon should operate on a patient deteriorating from an acute EDH as a true emergency. One suboptimally controlled study reported worse outcomes in a small group of patients who underwent emergency operations by non-neurosurgeons and attributed this mainly to the technical inadequacy of the operation.[59,60] Other studies have documented worse outcomes in patients transferred from outlying hospitals for surgery.[52,73] The take-home message is that EDHs are extra-axial hemorrhages located adjacent to the brainstem that can represent a true neurosurgical emergency, and that rapid, competent decompression makes a difference.

Subdural Hematoma

Proceeding deep to the skull, the next space is the subdural space. Unlike the potential epidural space, the subdural space is a real space. It is a compartment that follows the contour of the brain, which is how it appears on a CT scan (Fig. 67-6). Anatomically, bridging veins course through the subdural space from the cerebral hemispheres to the superior sagittal sinus. As the brain accelerates within the skull after impact, these veins can stretch and tear.[86]

The source of bleeding also can be from a cortical artery[87,88] or vein. These hematomas typically form over the surface or between the cerebral hemispheres, along the tentorium, or between the temporal lobe and base of the skull.

An acute subdural hematoma (SDH), as defined by Bullock and colleagues, appears within 14 days of injury,[60] although some authors consider an SDH to be subacute when signs and symptoms develop between 3 and 20 days after trauma.[89]

Acute SDHs consist of clotted blood, which is fibrous and often adherent to adjacent tissue. The blood remains clotted for several days. After this time, the clot gradually and progressively lyses, resulting in a mixture of clot and fluid. After several weeks, the clot is liquified and becomes a chronic SDH. Chronic SDHs may manifest weeks or months after what may have been mild or insignificant trauma. Chronic SDHs occur more often in elderly patients and those individuals who have more intracranial space because of cortical atrophy. These hematomas often become surrounded by a membrane, and the collection of fluid may slowly grow in size because of repeated small bleeds or accumulation of fluid transudate from the membrane.[86]

The incidence of acute SDHs is approximately 20% in severe traumatic brain injury,[60,90-93] and the mean age is between 31 and 47 years, with most of the patients being men.[60,94-97] The mechanism of injury differs between age groups, with patients older than 65 more commonly presenting after a fall, and younger patients being involved more often in a motor vehicle crash,[60,98-100] which, among comatose patients with acute SDH, is the most common mechanism of injury.[60,91,93,101]

Between 37% and 80% of patients with acute SDH present with a GCS score of 8 or lower,[60,65,71,94,97,102] and the overall mortality rate is between 40% and 60%.[60,66,92,95,96,104-106] Mortality rates among comatose patients requiring surgery are somewhat higher, with reported rates between 57% and 68%.[60,76,81,91,92,101,106] Acute subdural hematomas frequently are associated with other brain injuries,[97,102] which is one of the reasons why the mortality rate is relatively high.

A simple acute SDH is a subdural, extra-axial hematoma without any other associated brain injury (Fig. 67-7). A complex SDH is associated with parenchymal injury (Fig. 67-8).[108] Fewer than half of acute SDHs requiring surgery are isolated, simple lesions.[60,97,102]

One useful method to identify the presence of associated injury is to measure the thickness of the subdural clot relative to the amount of brain shift on the CT scan. If the amount of shift is directly proportional to the thickness of the extra-axial clot, the injury is likely to be simple

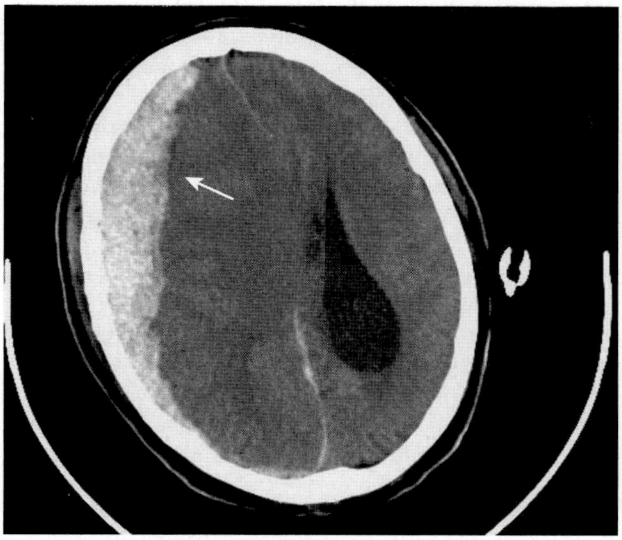

Figure 67-6. Axial computed tomography scan demonstrating a typical acute subdural hematoma *(arrow)*. Note that the hematoma expands the subdural space and follows the contour of the brain as it generates severe extra-axial mass effect and shift.

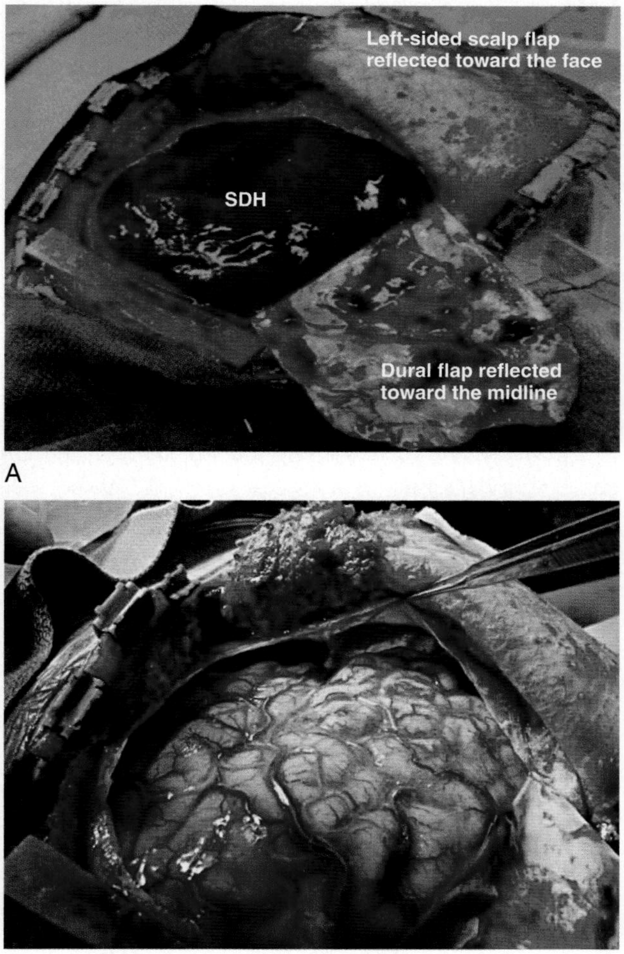

Figure 67-7. A, Intraoperative view of a solid subdural hematoma (SDH) on the surface of the brain. **B,** Decompressed brain with demonstration of evacuated subdural space.

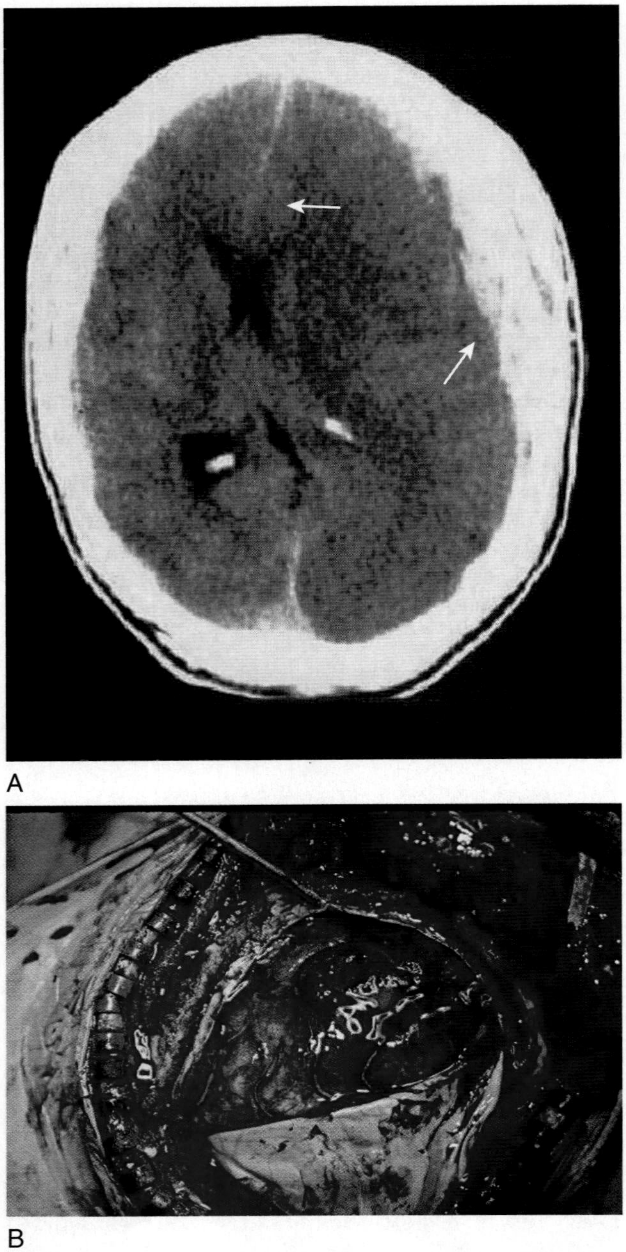

Figure 67-8. **A,** Computed tomography scan of acute, complex left-sided subdural hematoma (SDH) *(lower arrow)* with mass effect *(upper arrow)* out of proportion to the size of the clot, indicating more than just the effect of an extra-axial compressive mass—that is, intrinsic, parenchymal brain injury with edema. **B,** Intraoperative photograph of decompressed brain reveals hemorrhagic, inflamed, and edematous brain swelling out through the cranial defect. Compare with the intraoperative photograph of the simple SDH in Figure 67-7.

and only the brain compressed. However, if the amount of shift is more than expected as indicated by the size of the hematoma, then additional parenchymal brain injury probably is present under the clot, causing additive mass effect. Not surprisingly, the mortality for complex injuries is higher than that for simple SDHs.[107,108]

In addition to the obvious compressive effects that an SDH generates, the available evidence points to a direct toxic effect of the blood itself on the underlying cortex, thereby compounding the problem.[109,110]

Age is an important factor in acute SDHs. There is a significant increase in poor outcome among patients older than 60 years of age with severe head injury in general.[93,98-101,111,112] Older patients with an acute SDH and a low GCS score do especially poorly.[98-101,111,112]

Decision for immediate surgery is dependent on GCS score, age, pupillary examination, comorbidities, CT findings, and salvageability with respect to the patient's level of injury. In addition to all of these factors, decision making for delayed surgery is dependent on clinical course and ICP.[60]

On the basis of a contemporary search of the literature, Bullock and colleagues found that CT parameters of a midline shift greater than 5 mm and a clot thickness greater than 10 mm were independent factors requiring surgery in salvageable patients. They also identified a select group of comatose patients with smaller SDHs that could be managed nonoperatively if the patients remained neurologically stable with normal pupils and ICP of 20 mm or less.[60]

Traumatic Subarachnoid Hemorrhage

The subarachnoid space is a CSF-filled compartment within which are the major cerebral blood vessels. The CSF within the subarachnoid space fills the basal cisterns and interdigitates into the cortical sulci. Traumatic SAH can be caused by bleeding of cortical arteries, veins, or brain surface cerebral contusions.[113]

In contrast with hemorrhages in other locations, SAH is not a discrete surgical clot that requires evacuation. Trauma is the most common cause of SAH; a ruptured aneurysm is the most common cause of a spontaneous SAH. Aneurysmal SAH generally involves the suprasellar cistern, where the circle of Willis lies. Traumatic SAH can be found as small-volume hemorrhages in the sylvian fissures and especially in the interpeduncular cistern. Traumatic SAH also commonly involves the cerebral convexity and can fill cortical sulci, which can sometimes mimic sulcal effacement[114] (Fig. 67-9A).

Occasionally, the distribution of the hemorrhage may be hard to differentiate from an aneurysmal hemorrhage. Under this circumstance, a vascular study should be obtained (see Fig. 67-9B). Cerebral vasospasm following aneurysmal SAH is a common, well-described problem with an unclear pathogenesis. Increasing evidence suggests that SAH from trauma also may cause clinically significant cerebral vasospasm, which may be responsible for ischemia and infarction.[115,116]

Clearly the incidence of clinically relevant cerebral vasospasm is less than what is seen in aneurysmal SAH; however, post-traumatic SAH may cause ischemia during the acute as well as the delayed phase.[115,117]

In severe nonpenetrating head injury, the degree of SAH can be predictive of outcome,[118-119] and although traumatic SAH can be an isolated finding, it is commonly associated with other intracranial injuries.[120]

Traumatic SAH can be a marker of severe primary injury and the amount of blood can also be an

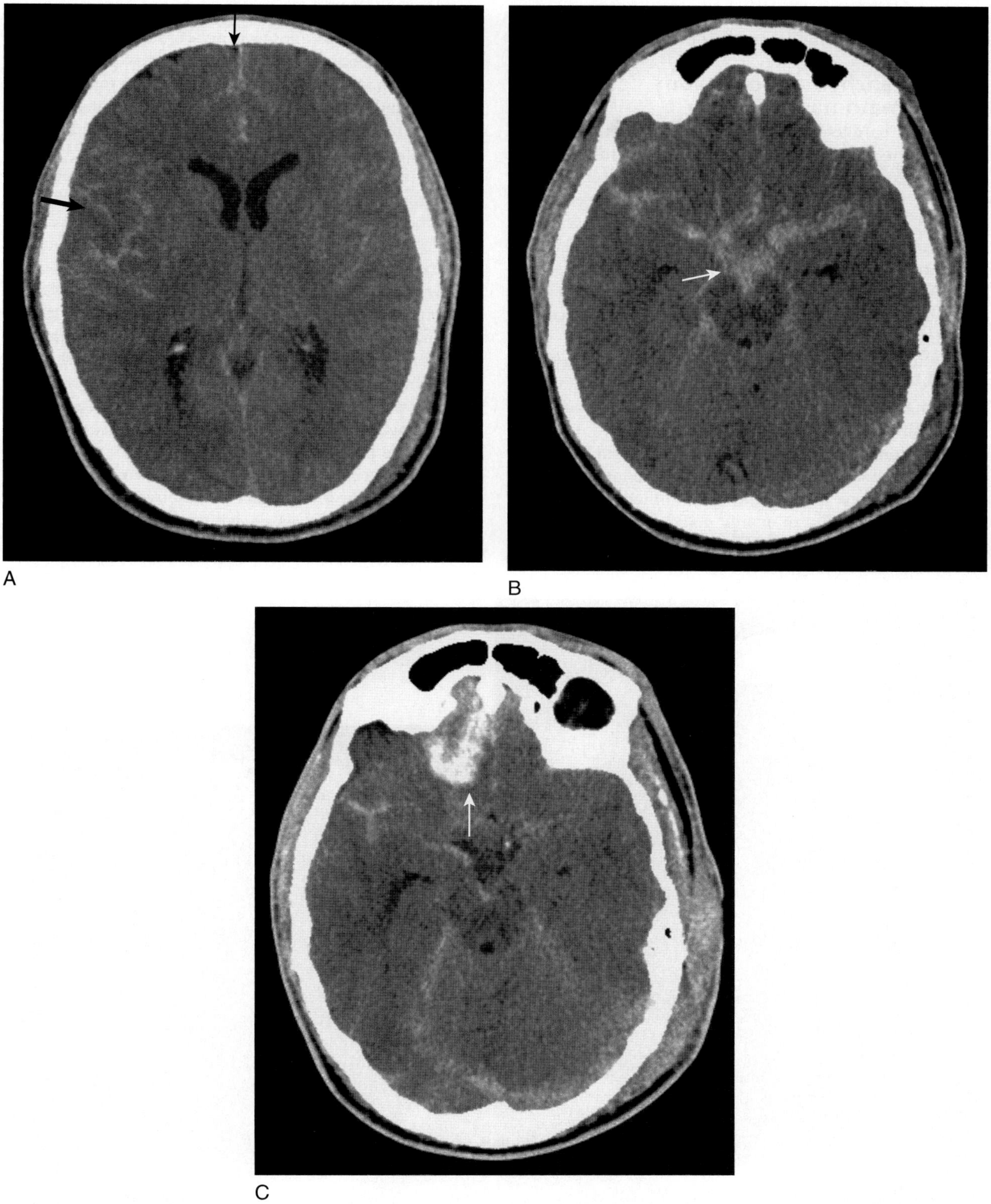

Figure 67-9. The patient was a 25-year-old man who sustained a brain injury in a motorcycle accident. **A,** Computed tomography (CT) scan immediately after the accident demonstrates traumatic SAH in cortical sulci *(thick arrow)* and anterior interhemispheric fissure *(thin arrow)*. **B,** CT scan at the level of the circle of Willis reveals a distribution of subarachnoid blood *(arrow)* throughout the suprasellar cistern, a pattern similar to that seen with a ruptured aneurysm. Findings on an immediate cerebral angiogram to rule out an aneurysm were normal. **C,** Follow-up CT scan obtained 8.5 hours later demonstrates an intraparenchymal contusion *(arrow)* that was not seen on the initial study, with rapid clearing of the traumatic SAH in the suprasellar cistern.

independent predictor of the development and progression of intraparenchymal contusions[113] (see Fig. 67-9C).

Intraparenchymal Contusions and Hematomas

Traumatic parenchymal mass lesions are common and are reported in 13% to 35% of severe traumatic brain injury.[121-127] Contusions consist of heterogeneous areas of necrosis, pulping, infarction, hemorrhage, and edema.[89,128,129] Hemorrhagic contusions are mixtures of blood and edematous cerebral parenchyma that also have a heterogeneous appearance on CT.[89] Contusions commonly occur in the frontal and temporal lobes both at the poles and on the inferior surfaces as a result of contact with the rough, bony skull base[130] (Fig. 67-10A).

Contusions typically involve the crests of the gyri but in more severe injury may extend into the substance of the white matter. If the pia-arachnoid is torn, contusions are classified as cortical lacerations.[130-132]

Contusions represent one end of a spectrum of injury on which hematomas, which are well-defined, homogeneous collections of blood, are the other end (see Fig. 67-10B). The amount of energy delivered may have only been enough to cause failure of small vessels, resulting in contusions. If more energy is delivered, failure of larger vessels may occur, resulting in hematomas. Alternatively, the hemorrhagic component of a contusion may continue to bleed and coalesce into a more discrete hematoma. In general, the most common traumatic parenchymal lesions are contusions,[89] and they tend to evolve.[122,126,127,133,134]

Risk factors for the progression of intraparenchymal hemorrhage include the presence of SAH (see Fig. 67-9C), and subdural hematoma, as well as the size of the clot on the initial CT scan. Enlargement of contusions occurs approximately 40% of the time, which justifies early follow-up CT scanning.[135] In addition to the problem of progressive enlargement of existing contusions is a phenomenon of delayed appearance of traumatic intracerebral contusions (DITCH). DITCH is defined as a new contusion identified on a CT scan in an area of brain that was normal on the admission CT scan. These delayed hemorrhages are reported to occur in up to 7% of patients with severe head injuries.[90]

Contusions can be subdivided into two groups. *Coup* contusions occur in the brain tissue under the impact site and usually are associated with an acceleration injury.

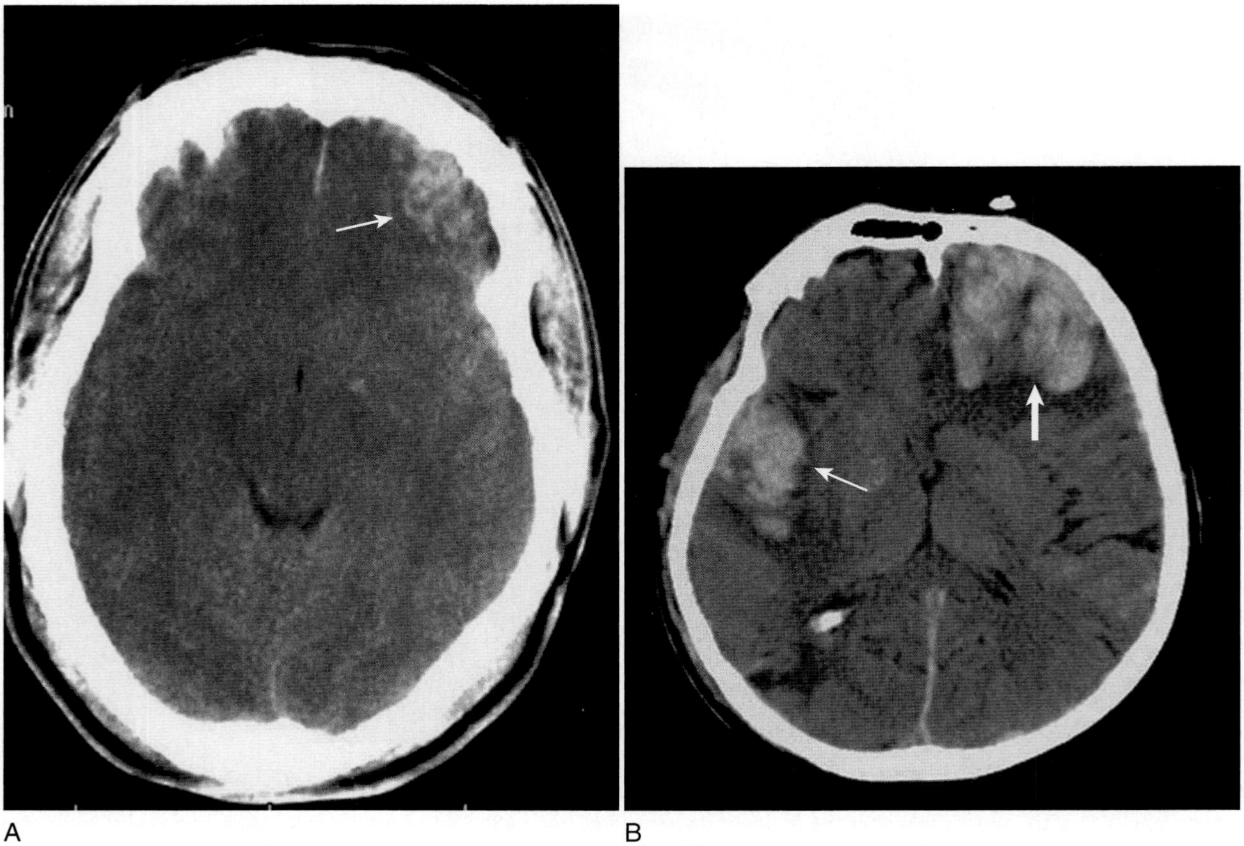

Figure 67-10. A, Computed tomography (CT) scan demonstrates a typical left frontal basal contusion *(arrow)* where the brain interfaces with the rough base of the anterior cranial fossa. **B,** CT scan demonstrates left frontal *(thick arrow)* and right temporal hemorrhagic *(thin arrow)* contusions. The floor of the middle (temporal) fossa also is quite rough. This scan also illustrates the continuum from contusion to hematoma. Note the large, homogeneous areas within the contusions that could be classified as hematomas.

Contrecoup contusions are located away from the point of impact and usually are associated with a deceleration injury.[130,131,136-138]

Understanding the biomechanics of how a contrecoup contusion develops is useful. In general, biologic tissues tolerate strain better if they are deformed slowly rather than quickly. For example, a 150-mL hematoma with accumulation of blood over minutes is likely to be lethal, whereas a 150-mL slow-growing meningioma may have no appreciable effect on the patient's level of consciousness. In trauma, the cause of tissue damage may be any of three types of induced strains: compression, tension, and shear. The skull, brain, and blood vessels will tolerate compression better than tension, and tension better than shear. These strains are induced by contact or inertia (relative to acceleration-deceleration), or both. Contact injuries are a result of impact, which may cause inward deformation of the skull with local effects, and of shock waves, which can produce remote effects. As a consequence of contact the head is set in motion, which leads to inertial injury. Inertial injuries may cause damage by differential acceleration of the skull and brain. In addition, acceleration-deceleration can independently produce strains in the brain itself. The two clinically relevant types of acceleration are translational (when the brain moves in a straight line) and angular. Most injuries are a combination of both.[139]

These effects are best illustrated by a case example of a 37-year-old man who falls from a height onto the back of his head and presents with a deteriorating level of consciousness. His CT scan (Fig. 67-11) reveals soft tissue swelling at the point of impact in the right occipital region with a small underlying hemorrhage, as well as a large, hemorrhagic contusion in the left frontal lobe. The mechanism involved is primarily translational (linear) deceleration. The skull stops suddenly as it hits the ground, but the brain continues to move toward the impact site, where compression is induced (Fig. 67-12).

As the brain is moving toward the inner table of the skull at the impact site, it also is moving away from the skull on the opposite side, creating regions of low pressure and tensile strains. Contributing to the extensive tissue damage in the left frontal lobe also may be movement of the brain across the rough surface of the anterior cranial base.[89,139]

The same amount of energy is delivered to the brain in nearly a straight line, with the compressive injury at the point of impact resulting in much less damage than the contrecoup injury caused by tension. In view of the dramatic differential susceptibilities of the brain and blood vessels to compressive and tensile strains induced in trauma, it is understandable that diffuse injuries can be caused by seemingly less violent trauma when the head undergoes an injury with a large component of angular acceleration-deceleration. This is the motion that can induce shearing strains, which the tissues tolerate poorly (see "Diffuse Axonal Injury" later on).

Surgical decision making is more straightforward for epidural and subdural types of hematoma, in which the extra-axial mass causing compression is simply on the surface of the brain. Contusions and hematomas, however, are intra-axial masses intimately associated with surrounding regions of brain that may be salvageable. It is one thing to surgically evacuate an extra-axial hematoma *compressing* the dominant frontal lobe, and quite another to operate on a large contusion *within* the dominant frontal lobe.

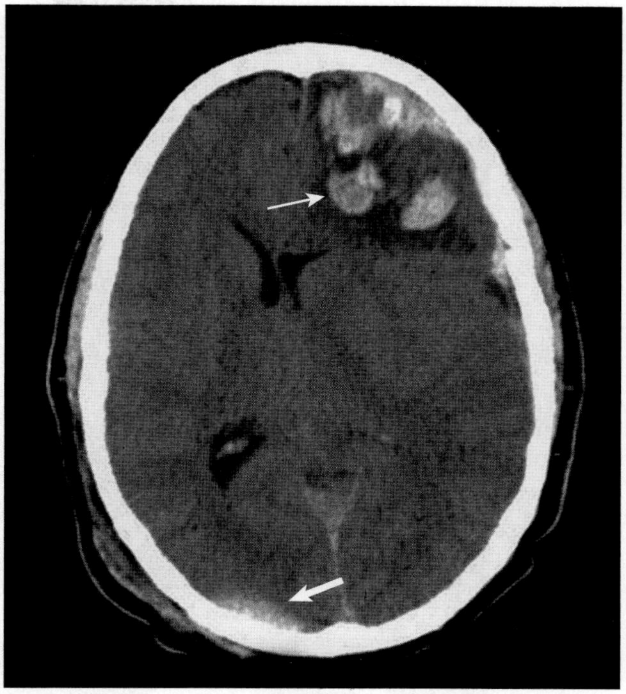

Figure 67-11. Computed tomography scan demonstrates a relatively small right occipital hemorrhage *(thick arrow)* underlying the point of impact as confirmed by the overlying soft tissue swelling of the scalp and a large, left frontal hemorrhagic contrecoup contusion *(thin arrow).*

In 2006, guidelines were published after a thorough review of the relevant, but scientifically weak literature. The reviewers reported that patients with parenchymal mass lesions and signs of progressive neurologic deterioration referable to the lesion, medically refractory intracranial hypertension, or signs of mass effect on CT scan should be treated operatively. Patients with GCS scores of 6 to 8 with frontal or temporal contusions greater than 20 cc in volume with midline shift of at least 5 mm or cisternal compression on CT scan, and patients with any lesion greater than 50 cc in volume should receive operative treatment. Patients with parenchymal mass lesions who do not show evidence of neurologic compromise, whose ICP is controlled, and who demonstrate no significant signs of mass effect on CT scan may be managed nonoperatively with intensive monitoring and serial imaging. For patients with refractory intracranial hypertension and diffuse parenchymal injury with clinical and radiographic evidence for impending transtentorial herniation, the guidelines also recommended, as treatment options, subtemporal decompression, temporal lobec-

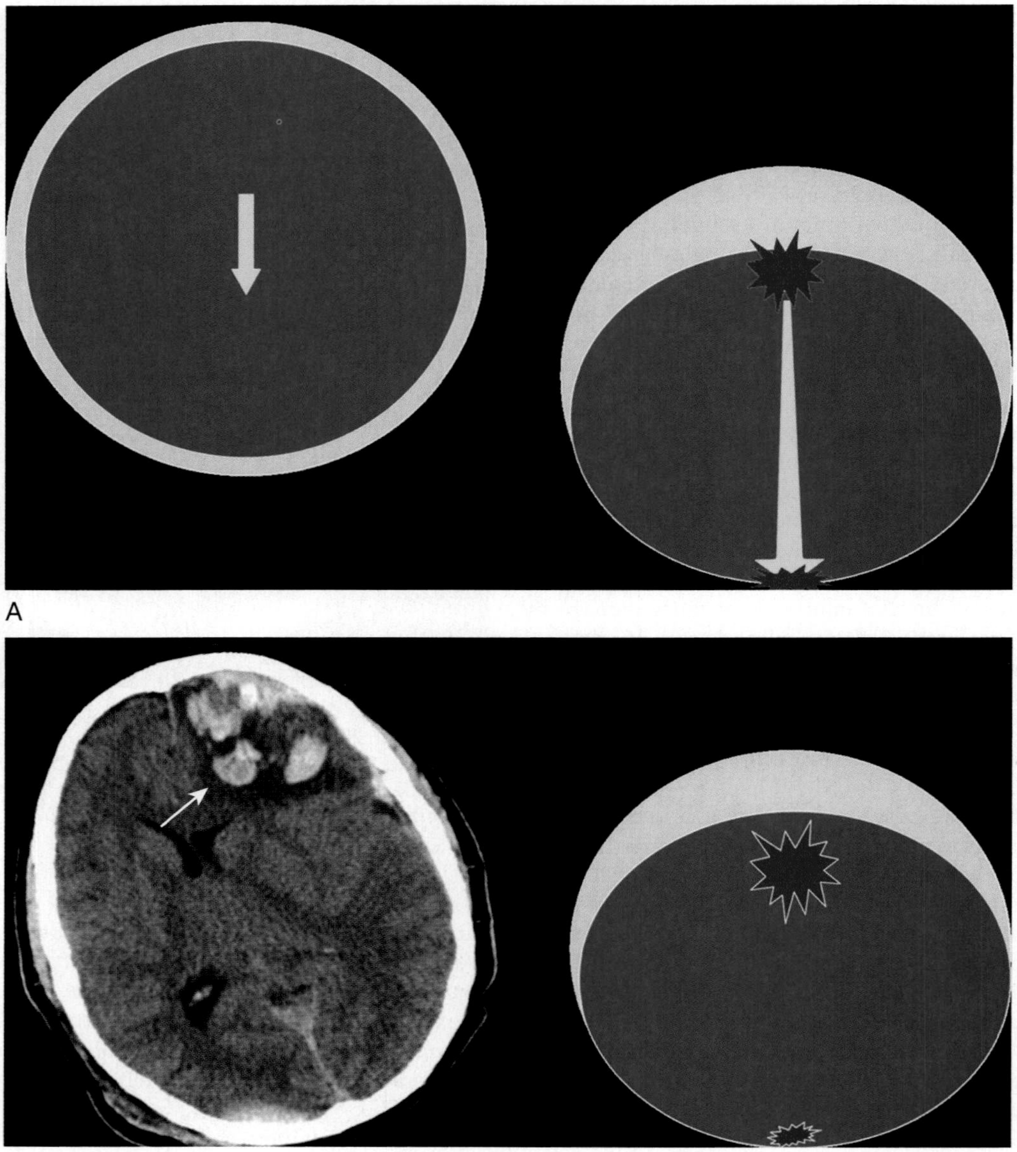

A

B

Figure 67-12. A, Schematic representing the head falling in a straight line. Rapid deceleration of the skull occurs as the brain continues to move toward the impact site. The energy is applied in a linear trajectory, resulting in a compressive strain generated at the impact site and a tensile strain at the opposite point *(right diagram).* The same energy delivered to the brain results in more damage by tension than compression. **B,** A comparison of this schematic with that for a similar mechanism of injury would demonstrate why a contrecoup contusion (*arrow* on computed tomography scan, *left*) generally is more severe than the injury sustained as a result of compression at the point of impact.

tomy, or hemispheric decompressive craniectomy (Fig. 67-13). With regard to timing of surgery, the literature supports a bifrontal decompressive craniectomy within 48 hours of injury as a treatment option for patients with diffuse, medically refractory post-traumatic cerebral edema and resultant intracranial hypertension.[127]

Hypothalamic-Pituitary Injury

Injury to the pituitary and hypothalamus can complicate head injury. A prolonged loss of consciousness often is reported in patients with such injuries. Up to 80% of cases are associated with a fracture through the skull base. Injuries include (in decreasing order of frequency) pericapsular hemorrhage, hypothalamic infarction, posterior pituitary hemorrhage, anterior pituitary infarction, and rupture of the infundibulum.[140-142] Clinically measurable decreases in pituitary hormone production are not seen until at least 75% of the gland is destroyed. Complete loss of production requires destruction of at least 90% of the gland.

Derangements in pituitary function can result in decreased production of any of the pituitary hormones. Of particular clinical significance is impairment of adrenocorticotropic hormone release that can result in second-

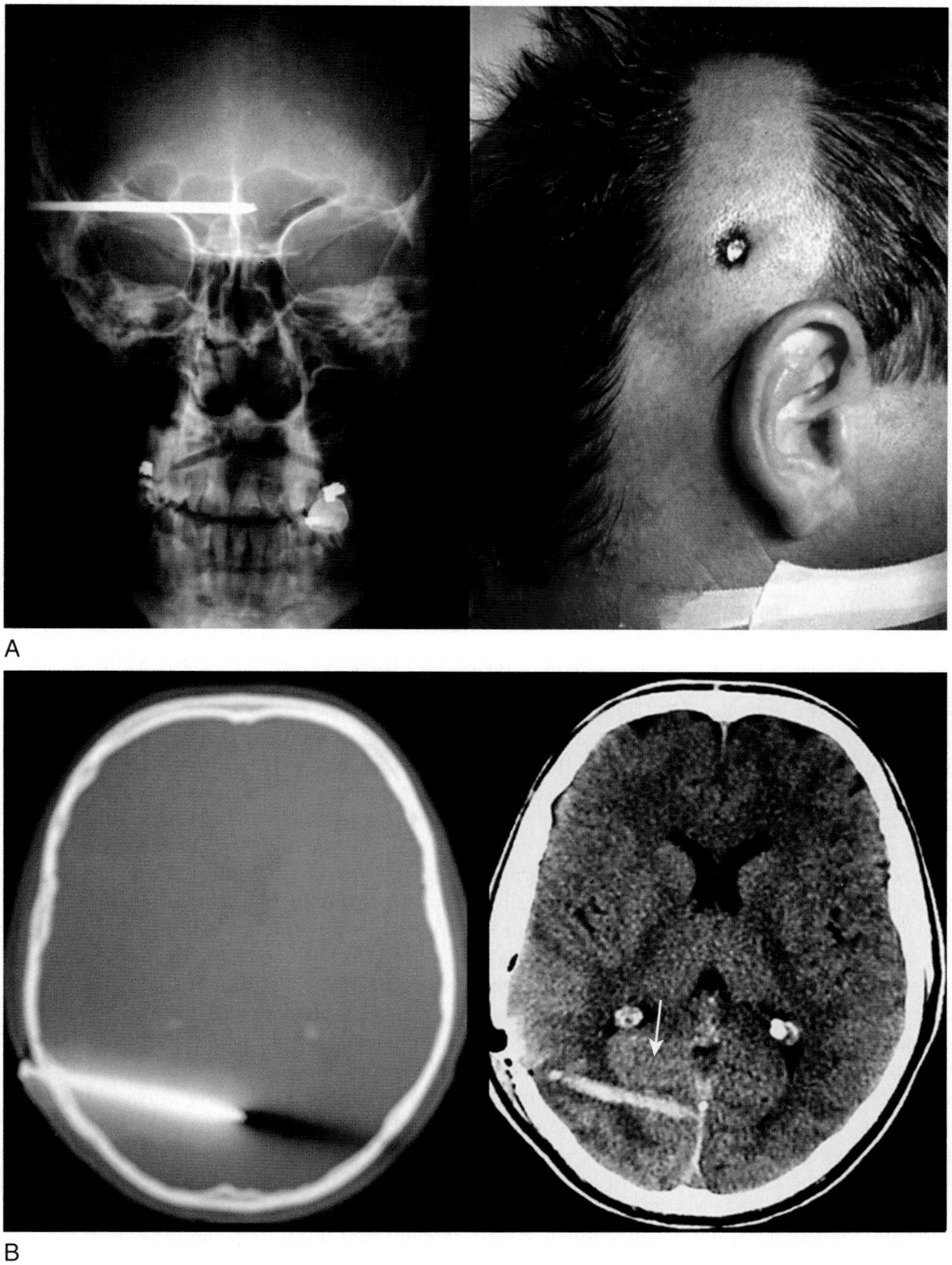

Figure 67-13. A 32-year-old man presented awake and alert after accidental discharge of a nail gun to the head while working at a construction site. **A,** *Left,* An anteroposterior radiograph of the skull demonstrates the nail. *Right,* On this intraoperative photograph, the head of the nail can be seen indenting the surface of the scalp. **B,** Preoperative bone-windowed computed tomography (CT) scan *(left)* and immediate postoperative brain-windowed CT scan *(right)* demonstrate the blood-stained tract after removal.

ary adrenal insufficiency (Addison's disease). Physiologic stressors such as trauma, surgery, or infection can result in addisonian crisis, with potentially life-threatening results. Diabetes insipidus has been reported in a significant number of severe head injuries, with a high percentage of cases remaining permanent.[143] Injuries to the pituitary often are not suspected in the acute period, and the diagnosis of hypopituitarism is therefore often delayed (Fig. 67-14).

Diffuse Axonal Injury

The term *diffuse axonal injury* (DAI) describes brain damage in a group of patients who become immediately unconscious or go into coma at the time of the head

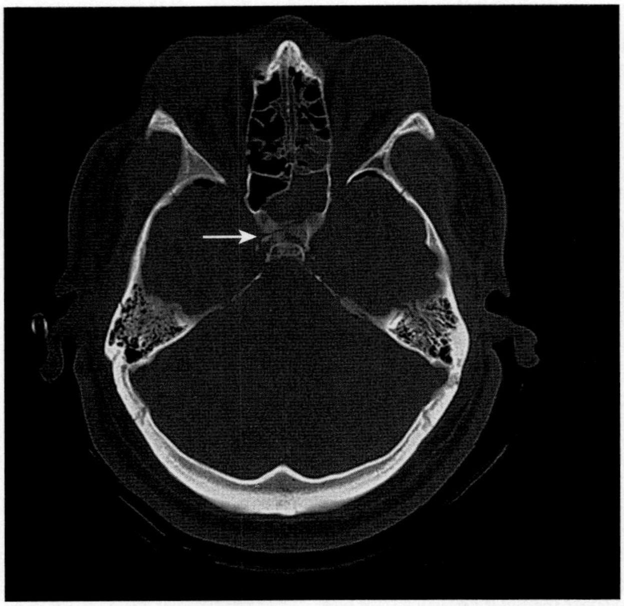

Figure 67-14. Computed tomography scan through the skull base in bone window demonstrating fractures through the sella turcica *(arrow)*.

trauma.[81] Depending on the severity of the injury, patients may have mild, moderate, or severe DAI. A large number of patients with severe head injury will have DAI. Because of the gradient acceleration difference of certain brain areas during primary impact, shearing forces at the gray-white junction, corpus callosum, or brainstem may occur.[131,144] The result of these forces will be diffuse tearing of axons and small blood vessels. These lesions initially may be hemorrhagic, but as they become chronic, shrinking, softening, and scarring ensue, often with cyst formation.[42,145] The lesions usually are microscopic but can be large and macroscopic. Although small, focal, petechial hemorrhages may be visualized, the initial CT scan often is normal.[146] Most of the clinical and experimental studies support that the diffuse injury occurs at the time of initial impact and is not the result of other adverse factors, such as decreased brain oxygenation, increased ICP, or brain swelling,[145,147] although these factors tend to accentuate the amount of damage.

The term *gliding contusions* originally was introduced by Lindenberg and Freytag[148] to describe hemorrhagic lesions in parasagittal white matter; this brain injury concept has been reanalyzed.[149] Gliding contusions frequently are found in association with DAI and acute subdural hematomas. Two mechanisms have been considered in relation to the formation of these contusions. First, during angular acceleration, more movement and displacement of the cortical gray matter occur than of the deep white matter; accordingly, most of the tissue injury occurs at the gray-white junction because shearing strains predominate. The second mechanism involves excessive displacement of the bridging veins during brain acceleration. Patients with severe DAI who survive may be profoundly disabled, but some patients with mild or moderate DAI may recover with mild or no disability.[81] The importance of recognizing DAI in the initial evaluation cannot be overstressed; this will affect the management and outcome. Clinically, these patients will have impaired consciousness secondary to bicortical damage, possibly in association with unremarkable imaging findings and normal ICP.

Penetrating Brain Injury

It is estimated that between 6000 to 7000 people die each year in the United States from gunshot wounds to the brain.[130-139,150-152]

Classification

Low-velocity penetrating brain injuries include wounds from nail guns, arrows, and knives and some types of gunshot wounds (Fig. 67-15). Gunshot wounds are divided into low-velocity injuries, such as from civilian handguns and shrapnel, and high-velocity injuries, from rifles and military weapons[152] (see Table 67-1).

A recent Israeli report described an intermediate type of injury from spherical bolts whereby the ball bearings used by suicide bombers, having unique ballistics, may cause a type of "stab wound" injury to the brain.[152]

Ballistics

The biomechanics of penetrating brain injury (PBI) are important and require an understanding of the dynamics of projectiles—that is, ballistics. Ballistics can be divided into three phases. The first phase, internal ballistics, deals with the source of the projectile and its intrinsic dynamics (e.g., rifle, bomb). External ballistics, the second phase, focuses on the flight of the projectile itself and the deviation of its longitudinal axis relative to the line of flight, referred to as yaw motion. Collision of the projectile with any object during this external phase will change the speed, angle, and yaw. The third phase is referred to as terminal ballistics, which is the physical interaction between the projectile and the body.[152]

As the projectile directly crushes tissue, it forms a permanent cavity, and as surrounding tissue is compressed, a temporary cavity also is formed. As the missile breaks through the skull, secondary projectiles of bone fragments may be generated, causing independent, secondary permanent and temporary cavities.[152-156]

Terminal ballistics are influenced by many factors, such as size, shape, and stability of the penetrating object; however, most authors (but not all) believe that entrance velocity is the most important factor in determining the degree of tissue damage.[152,153,155,157-159] Experimental evidence has demonstrated an immediate increase in ICP with a pressure wave transmitted throughout the cranial cavity, which probably accounts for the transient respiratory arrest observed in PBI.[152,160] High-velocity injuries (velocity greater than 320 meters per second) cause shock waves that emanate from the front of the missile. These shock waves can reflect off the inside of the skull and summate, producing significant pressure gradients with remote effects.

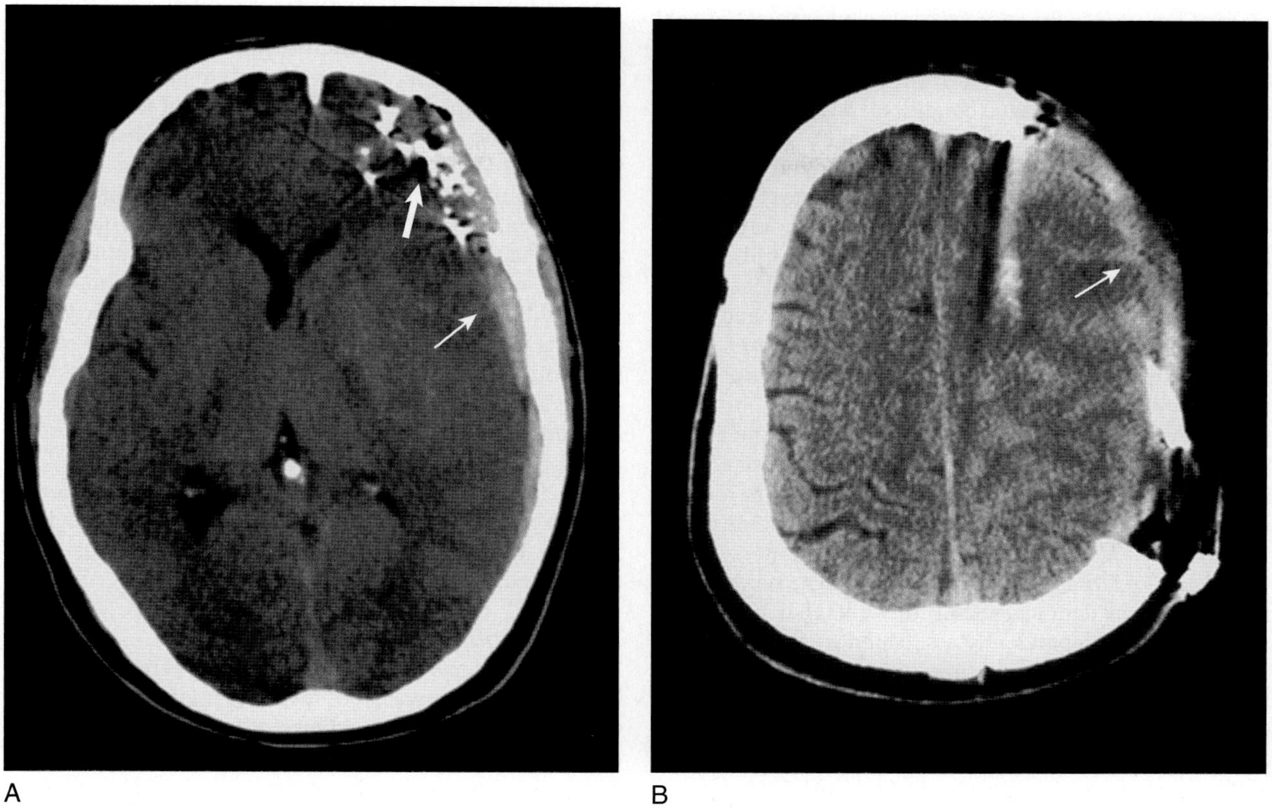

Figure 67-15. The patient was a 27-year-old man with a self-inflicted gunshot wound to the head who presented with a deteriorating level of consciousness. The patient put the muzzle of a handgun to the right medial orbital roof. The bullet traversed the frontal sinus and traveled through the left frontal lobe. **A,** Computed tomography (CT) scan demonstrates bullet fragments *(thick arrow)* and an associated left frontotemporal acute subdural hematoma *(thin arrow),* requiring surgical evacuation and hemicraniectomy for anticipated swelling. **B,** Postoperative CT scan demonstrates edematous hemisphere herniating out through the cranial defect *(arrow).* There was damage to the anterior cranial base with contamination secondary to involvement of the frontal sinus. Surgical repair of the skull base was delayed because of the anticipated cerebral edema, and the patient was placed on antibiotics. When the cerebral swelling resolved, there was no evidence of CSF rhinorrhea or infection. The patient never required the delayed repair of the anterior cranial base anticipated. He made an excellent neurologic recovery and returned to work as a professional recruiter several months after replacement of his cranial bone flap.

Initial Resuscitation

Initial resuscitation in the trauma bay should be in accordance with current recommendations for head-injured patients in general. During this initial resuscitation, it is important to recognize that hypotension in PBI either is a terminal event or related to other injuries. Once resuscitation has been accomplished, a CT scan is essential. Although skull films seldom add to the information obtained from a CT scan,[152] our group has found plain films to be very helpful in PBI, particularly in industrial accidents, in which the shape of the penetrating object may be unknown.

Surgical Management

Most of what is known about the surgical management of PBI comes from the battlefield, beginning with World War I, when Harvey Cushing, the father of American neurosurgery, described his technique of en bloc craniectomy under aseptic conditions; thorough débridement of scalp, bone, brain, metal, and bone fragments; and watertight closure of the scalp. Using this management strategy nearly 100 years ago, in the absence of antibiotics, Cushing reported a significant drop in postoperative mortality from 55% to 28%.[161,162]

Mortality decreased even further in World War II, primarily because neurosurgical personnel were present in forward military hospitals and antibiotics were introduced. The operative approach, however, was largely the same: that of radical débridement. Treatment consisted of four tiers: emergent life-saving maneuvers through hemostasis and cerebral decompression; prevention of infection through extensive débridement; preservation of nervous tissue through prevention of meningocerebral scars; and restoration of anatomic structures through accurate closure of the dura and scalp. Although untested against other management strategies, this approach became the standard of treatment for PBI by default. Indeed, in the U.S. military, thorough débridement of intracranial bone and metal fragments was official military policy through the Vietnam War.[165]

The overall mortality rate from PBI sustained during relatively modern wartime conditions ranges from 8% to 43% and generally is considered to be in the 20% range.[162-171] The mortality rate from military gunshot wounds has been reported to be 2.5 to 4 times more than from shrapnel.[162-165,170] Of interest, mortality rates from wartime PBIs in the U.S. military from World War II through the Vietnam War did not change significantly,[172] which is consistent with the relatively unchanged management strategy of complete removal of intracranial bone or metal fragments, using repeated surgery as necessary.[173]

Aggressive débridement was intended to reduce complications such as infection, epilepsy, and cerebral edema. However, studies reveal that additional surgery to remove retained fragments results in significant morbidity and mortality.[170,174,175]

The use of broad-spectrum antibiotics in recent wars has resulted in data suggesting that retained bone fragments are not independently associated with an increased risk of infection. Therefore, aggressive débridement is no longer supported.[162,176] The use of broad-spectrum antibiotics in PBI has now become universal.[152]

Multiple studies have looked at post-PBI epilepsy and reported an incidence of 22% to 53%.[167,177,178] Several studies suggest that it is not necessary to remove all bone fragments in order to decrease the chance of developing epilepsy, but the value of removing metal fragments in this regard remains unclear.[162,167,169,177,178] In military PBI, it appears that vigorous débridement is associated with increased morbidity and mortality and is not necessary to prevent infection, has no obvious efficacy in preventing epilepsy, and does not appear to improve survival.[162]

A CSF leak resulting from a PBI is the variable most highly correlated with intracranial infection.[162,166,167,170,179-182] One study found that most CSF leaks appeared within 2 weeks of the injury and less than half of them closed spontaneously. The incidence of infecti\on was approximately 10 times higher in the group with CSF fistulas than in the group without leaks, and the mortality was greater as well.[181] Because CSF leaks are the primary predictor of the development of intracranial infection.[167,169,171] it is important to fix or prevent a CSF leak; therefore, a watertight closure of the scalp entry wound is necessary.[181]

To accomplish this objective, a wide range of surgical interventions are available. Small entrance wounds without underlying surgical pathology may be cleaned up and closed in the emergency department.[182] Complex entry wounds or those with underlying surgical pathology will require more extensive surgical manipulation, which may include extending the incision to allow vigorous superficial débridement; complete excision of devitalized tissues including muscle, fascia, and periosteum; extension and débridement of the bony entry or exit site by craniectomy; and similarly generous débridement of the dural opening with watertight closure, using grafting as necessary.[161,168,170,172,183,184]

Predictive Factors

Increased mortality in penetrating head injury is associated with increasing age, suicide attempts, hypotension, coagulopathy (particularly with lower GCS scores), respiratory distress, low GCS score, bilateral fixed and dilated pupils, high ICP, and cisternal effacement on CT scan. Mortality also is increased with traumatic injuries in which a missile tract perforates the skull (through-and-through injury) or with injuries that involve both hemispheres, multiple lobes, or the ventricular system.[162]

In civilian gunshot wounds to the head, a specific vector analysis from Los Angeles County demonstrated a region of involvement that resulted in 100% fatality and is designated as the zona fatalis. This region comprises the midbody of the ventricle, the body of the corpus callosum, and the cingulum.[184]

No effect has been demonstrated for weapon caliber on outcome, independent of total kinetic energy, and no relation between midline shift and outcome has been established.[162]

Special Problems

Special problems that may be encountered with PBI include those associated with craniofacial entrance wounds: an increased incidence of hematoma formation, direct vascular injury, extensive contamination due to paranasal sinus involvement (see Fig. 67-15), and CSF fistulas.[152]

Other special problems include dural venous sinus involvement, tangential wounds, and traumatic aneurysms, with 0.4% to 0.7% of all intracranial aneurysms being caused by penetrating trauma.[185]

In PBI, mechanical loading of the cerebral vasculature, by either the contact forces of the projectile or the shearing forces of a pulsating temporary cavity, may cause partial or complete transection of an arterial wall. Such damage can result in SAH or formation of intracerebral and intraventricular hematomas.[162,186,187]

Damage to the arterial wall also may cause the development of a traumatic intracranial aneurysm (TICA). TICAs are primarily false aneurysms, which could heal or change in size over time, but they are especially vulnerable to rupture and can lead to delayed traumatic intracerebral hematoma or SAH, or both.[185,188-190]

Patients with an increased risk of vascular injury include cases in which the trajectory passes through or near the sylvian fissure, supraclinoid carotid, cavernous sinus, or a major venous sinus. The development of substantial and otherwise unexplained SAH or delayed hematoma also should prompt consideration of a vascular injury.[162]

Cerebral angiography (CTA or conventional) remains the usual technique to detect intracranial aneurysms.[187,189,191] Because a majority of traumatic intracranial aneurysms are not true aneurysms, excluding the aneurysm by clipping may not be possible and may require trapping between clips on the parent vessel.[162]

Course in the Intensive Care Unit

Not surprisingly, intracranial hypertension is common after PBI.[181,192-194] Early ICP monitoring should be considered when the ICU clinician is unable to assess the patient's neurologic status accurately; if the need to evacuate a mass lesion is unclear; or if CT scanning suggests elevated ICP.[162] Another practical use for ICP monitoring is ongoing assessment of a patient with a depressed level of consciousness to look for an early sign of progressive intracranial pathology, which may require repeated imaging and surgical decompression.[181,192,194]

Cerebral autoregulation may be defective after PBI[181,192,194]; cerebral edema can appear extremely rapidly, contributing to medically refractory intracranial hypertension. Systemic hypertension may exacerbate intracranial hypertension after PBI.[162]

Treatment is not necessarily futile, and some patients with intracranial hypertension can be managed successfully and survive with acceptable morbidity.[181,192,194,195] However, the literature does not clearly relate successful treatment of intracranial hypertension after PBI to an improved outcome. Not enough good data are available to guide management strategies for intracranial hypertension after PBI. It cannot be assumed that the intracranial pathology is the same as in nonpenetrating traumatic brain injury. Because of the paucity of data, however, treatment generally follows the methods for nonpenetrating traumatic brain injury as outlined in Guidelines for the Management of Severe Traumatic Brain Injury.[162,196]

Harrington and Apostolides have proposed a treatment algorithm for patients with gunshot wounds to the head. Patients who have lesions causing mass effect and a post-resuscitation GCS score of 7 or greater undergo surgery, and patients with a GCS score of 3 or 4 with bilaterally fixed pupils after resuscitation receive no treatment beyond wound closure. In patients with GCS scores of 5 or 6, treatment should be individualized, depending on pupillary findings and other conditions.[197]

SECONDARY HEAD INJURY

Basic Concepts

Management of primary head injury generally entails the surgical management of head-injured patients and typically is driven by the presence of pathologic masses (hematomas) in anatomic spaces. Management of secondary head injury usually involves the nonsurgical management of these patients and deals with the pathologic derangement of physiologic processes.

The three functional volumetric compartments in the head are blood, brain, and CSF. The volumes of these three functional compartments are approximately 1200 mL for brain, 150 mL for CSF, and roughly 150 mL for the variable blood compartment. The total volume of the intracranial compartment is relatively fixed and relatively incompressible. Therefore, if volume is added to one of these three compartments, a compensatory loss of volume from another compartment will occur; otherwise, ICP will rise. To illustrate this point, a pressure-volume curve for the intracranial compartment is shown in Figure 67-16. Initially, as volume is added to the system, no significant change in pressure occurs. With cerebral edema, for example, as the brain compartment increases in volume, venous capacitance vessels collapse, which moves blood volume out of the system; therefore, overall net volume does not change and ICP remains stable. As the brain continues to swell and increase in volume, the ventricles become smaller as CSF moves out of the system, again keeping overall net volume and ICP relatively stable. At some point the system loses this buffering capacity, and as more injury-related volume accumulates, ICP starts to rise. The rise in ICP is gradual, progressive, and nonlinear. As the system continues to get stressed with additional volume, it progressively loses compliance and, in effect, gets stiffer. The result is that increasingly smaller volumes introduced into the system result in higher changes in ICP. Using MRI methods to study cerebral edema, Marmarou and colleagues noted a rise in ICP when edema was only 1% higher than the normal water content of brain tissue. These investigators also showed that when water content increased in a contused hemisphere, ICP increased exponentially. These findings demonstrate the importance of small changes in intracranial volume, particularly when the buffering capacity of the system has been exhausted.[198]

Increased ICP may be associated with mass effect secondary to unbalanced forces, causing direct, mechanical compressive damage to involved structures. This condition generally necessitates surgical decompression in the operating room. Increased ICP also may result in inadequate perfusion. This condition generally requires medical management in the ICU (Fig. 67-17).

The heart delivers blood at a given mean arterial blood pressure (MABP), the systemic perfusion pressure, to the base of the skull. The blood pressure then has to overcome whatever pressure is inside the head for blood flow to get in, and whatever is left over will be the pressure that perfuses the brain—that is, cerebral perfusion pressure (CPP). Simple in concept and calculation, CPP is defined as the mean arterial blood pressure minus ICP ($CPP = MABP - ICP$). It is the physiologic variable that defines the pressure gradient driving cerebral blood flow (CBF) and metabolic delivery and is therefore closely related to ischemia.[199]

Technically, the MABP should be measured as the mean carotid pressure with the arterial line transducer zeroed at the level of the foramen of Monro (as opposed to the right atrium),[200] but this approach is not common in clinical practice. Normal values generally are considered to be 60 to 80 mm Hg for CPP and approximately 10 mm Hg or less for ICP.

The ultimate cause of secondary injury is typically ischemic, and the fundamental goal in dealing with severe traumatic brain injury is to ensure adequate CBF relative to the metabolic demand of the brain. It is, however, impractical to continuously measure CBF at the bedside. Fortunately, CBF is dependent on CPP—which can easily and continuously be measured at the bedside. Therefore, a fundamental management strategy for treating a head-injured patient is to maintain adequate CPP by lowering ICP, accomplished by reducing intracranial volume.

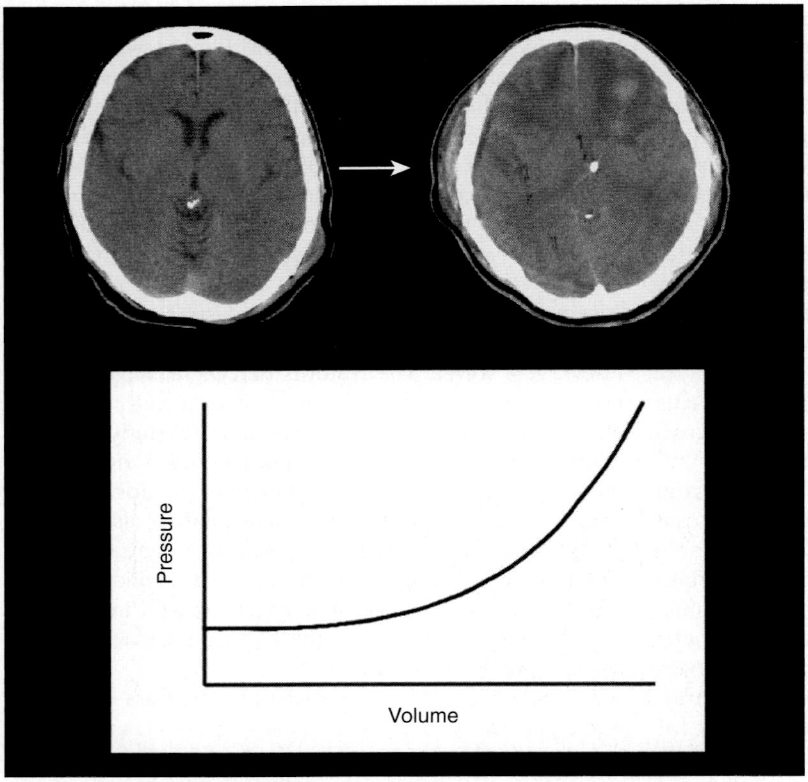

Figure 67-16. Pressure-volume curve of the intracranial compartment using cerebral edema as an example (see text). The computed tomography (CT) scan above the graph on the *left* is an image of a normal brain. The CT scan on the *right* demonstrates severe cerebral edema in a trauma patient with obliteration of most of the subarachnoid space, reducing cerebrospinal fluid (CSF) volume to make room for the swelling brain. Initially, as CSF moves out of the system, overall net volume does not change significantly. This part of the process is represented by the flat part of the curve toward the *left* and reflects the buffering capacity of the brain to respond to gradual increases in volume.

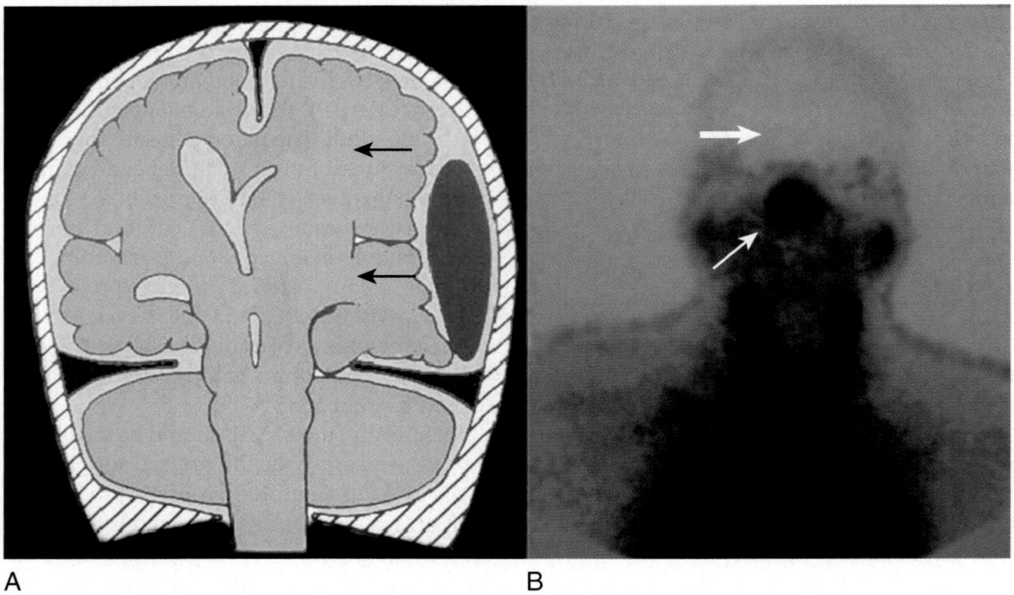

Figure 67-17. A, Increased intracranial pressure can be associated with unbalanced forces causing mass effect, shift, and possibly herniation. The resultant pathostructural changes from such unbalanced forces *(arrows)* usually are managed surgically. With increased intracranial pressure, cerebral perfusion may be impaired, with the end result of ischemia—the ultimate secondary injury. Intractable intracranial hypertension and inadequate perfusion can lead to brain death, as demonstrated by the nuclear flow study shown in **B.** Note the absence of flow to the brain *(thick arrow),* compared with the overly generous blood supply to the face, sometimes referred to as the "hot nose sign" *(thin arrow).*

Surgical methods for reducing intracranial volume include evacuating an intracranial hematoma, removing part of the frontal or temporal lobe, and placing a ventriculostomy to drain CSF. Other methods for reducing intracranial volume are applicable in the ICU setting, where management strategies are directed at treating volume in the blood and brain compartments.

Cerebral Blood Volume

In discussing cerebral blood volume, it is useful to divide this topic into the arterial and venous compartments.

Arterial Blood Compartment

Blood Pressure

Systemic blood pressure has a direct effect on arterial cerebral blood volume. Normally, CBF will remain relatively constant over a wide range of perfusion pressures as cerebrovascular resistance (CVR) automatically adjusts. The autoregulation curve (Fig. 67-18) demonstrates the relationship among CBF, perfusion pressure, and cerebrovascular resistance. As MABP goes up, CVR increases in order to maintain a stable CBF.

The CVR increases by vasoconstriction, which reduces the volume of blood in the brain. Conversely, as MAPB drops, CVR goes down by means of vasodilation, which increases the volume of blood in the brain. This is a very powerful system; a cerebral arteriole has the ability to change its diameter by up to 200%. It also is quite fast, responding to sudden changes in pressure within 3 to 5 seconds.

Most people have had the experience of suddenly jumping out of bed after having been recumbent for several hours and then feeling the "lights going out" as the cerebral vasculature rapidly dilates in response to the sudden drop in perfusion pressure and CBF; after several seconds, the lights come back on as cerebrovascular status is restored, as reflected by flattening of the autoregulation curve.

A normal MABP for a young, healthy adult is approximately between 70 and 90 mm Hg, and a normal ICP generally is considered to be approximately 10 mm Hg or less, which is consistent with a normal range of CPP values between 60 and 80 mm Hg. Although the normal ranges are at the low end of the autoregulation curve, there is the ability to autoregulate between perfusion

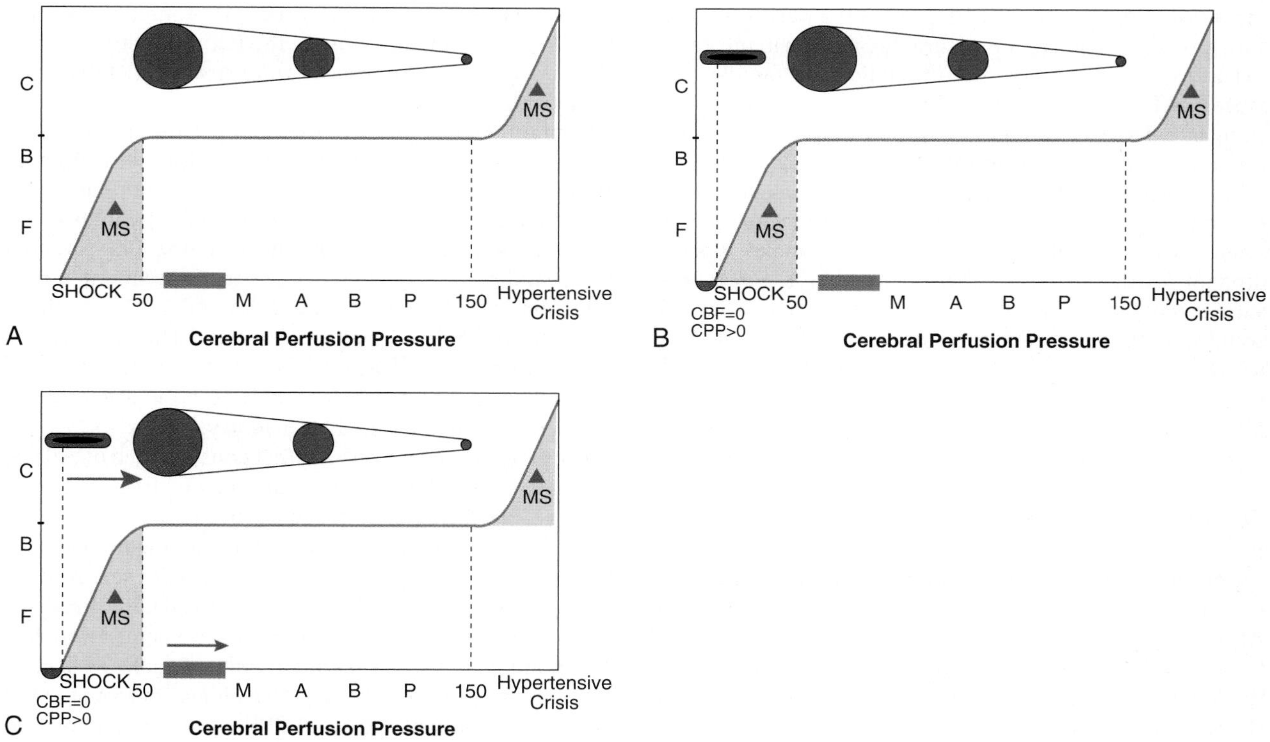

Figure 67-18. A, The autoregulation curve demonstrates how the brain maintains a relatively constant CBF over a wide range of perfusion pressures by changing the caliber (resistance) of the cerebral vasculature, which necessarily leads to changes in intracranial volume. Under normal circumstances, when ICP is negligible, the MABP is equivalent to CPP; however, when ICP is elevated, it is the CPP that is "read" by the brain. CPP will drive CBF, causing changes in cerebrovascular resistance, unless overridden by other superimposed processes such as hyperventilation, which may be pathologic or intentionally altered for a therapeutic effect. Although we have the ability to autoregulate over a wide range of perfusion pressures, the normal range is at the lower end of the curve *(horizontal green bar).* **B,** The normal resting state of the cerebrovasculature is collapsed. These vessels have critical opening and closing pressures that are slightly different from each other. With the vessel open, it typically will collapse at a slightly lower pressure than is required to open it from a collapsed state. **C,** After a significant injury, the potential exists to increase the critical closing pressure, which could shift the autoregulation curve to the right. CBF, cerebral blood flow; CPP, cerebral perfusion pressure; MABP, mean arterial blood pressure; MS, mental status.

pressures ranging from 50 to 150 mm Hg. It is clear from the autoregulation curve that CBF becomes a direct, linear function of MABP when outside the ability of the cerebrovascular bed to maximally dilate (MABP less than 50 mm Hg) or constrict (MABP greater than 150 mm Hg).

The normal range of 50 to 150 mm Hg is not rigidly fixed, and individual variations are common. A hypotensive patient with a MABP of 20 mm Hg clearly is in shock, but what about a 21-year-old athlete who has just had surgery for a ruptured appendix with an MABP of 45 mm Hg? Clearly a clinical assessment is necessary in borderline situations, and one of the most important indicators of shock is a change in mental status. In this example, if the athlete demonstrates a change in mental status, he is likely to be off his autoregulation curve and in shock.

At the other end of the spectrum is systemic hypertension. Is a 74-year-old patient with long-standing hypertension who presents with a MABP exceeding 150 mm Hg by a few points having a hypertensive crisis? Again, a change in mental status may be the indicator that autoregulatory capacity has been exceeded, and the patient may be diagnosed with hypertensive encephalopathy.

CVR often is increased by trauma. At the beginning of the autoregulation curve, CBF is zero at a perfusion pressure greater than zero. A measurable pressure in the vessel exists, yet no blood flow occurs, indicating vascular collapse (see Fig. 67-18). The cerebrovasculature in its resting state is collapsed; it takes a certain amount of energy (pressure) to open the vessels. These vessels each have critical opening and closing pressures. After a head injury, free radicals can be released, which tend to make biologic tissues less compliant. This in turn may make it more difficult for the vessels to stay open—that is, more pressure is required to keep the vessels from closing, which could shift the autoregulation curve to the right (see Fig. 67-18).[201-204] This is the theoretical basis for the studies that led to the earlier recommendations to keep the minimum CPP in head-injured patients above normal values—that is, at 70 mm Hg or greater.[205]

Cerebral Perfusion Pressure

A low perfusion pressure jeopardizes ischemic regions of the brain. Increasing intravascular hydrostatic pressure by increasing CPP can help improve cerebral perfusion. Although CPP can be manipulated and enhancement of CPP may help to avoid both global and regional ischemia, the level at which CPP is best maintained is not entirely clear,[205] and considerable interest has been directed toward attempts to determine the optimum CPP for a head-injured patient.

Some studies suggest that increasing CPP to greater than 70 mm Hg leads to improved outcomes.[206]

A combination of studies of traumatic brain injury in which CPP was actively maintained at approximately 70 mm Hg in patients with a GCS score less than 8 reported a mean mortality rate of 21%, which was substantially less than the 40% mortality rate reported for similar patients in the Traumatic Coma Data Bank (TCDB). Good recovery and moderate disability rates were 54% in the patients whose CPP values were maintained in the 70 mm Hg range, compared with the 37% reported in the TCDB. However, it could not be concluded that the improved outcomes in these studies were a result of CPP management because none of the reported studies was randomized, prospective trials of this treatment[199,204,207-211]; and in some, another treatment was actually the focus of the study.[207,208]

In a prospective study of 21 patients with severe traumatic brain injury in whom brain tissue PO_2 ($BtiO_2$) was monitored, ischemic episodes during the first week after injury were associated with unfavorable neurologic outcomes. Elevation of the CPP improved $BtiO_2$, but raising CPP above 68 mm Hg did not cause a further increase in $BtiO_2$. In the investigators' analysis, a CPP greater than 60 mm Hg emerged as the most important factor determining a sufficient $BtiO_2$.[199,212]

Another prospective, controlled trial of 189 adult patients with a motor GCS score of 5 or lower within 12 hours of head injury randomized patients to an "ICP-targeted protocol" in which CPP was kept above 50 mm Hg; or to a "CBF-targeted protocol" in which CPP was kept above 70 mm Hg. The investigators in this study found no significant difference in outcome. In this trial, the mean CPP for patients managed in the CBF-targeted protocol was 76 mm Hg and for those in the ICP-targeted protocol, 72 mm Hg. These differences were small but statistically significant.[213]

Contant and associates used data from this trial to examine risk factors for acute respiratory distress syndrome (ARDS) and consequences of its development. The risk of ARDS was five times greater among patients in the CBF-targeted group than in those in the ICP-targeted group and was associated with a more frequent use of epinephrine and a higher dose of dopamine.[199,214] Patients in whom ARDS developed were two and a half times more likely to develop refractory intracranial hypertension[214] and almost three times more likely to be in a vegetative state or dead at 6 months after injury.[214,215]

These outcomes may be a direct consequence of ARDS, and the related therapeutic limitations of treating raised ICP and low CPP in the presence of ARDS.[199]

Analysis of data from a study investigating the value of a neuroprotective agent in 427 patients with severe traumatic brain injury revealed that the critical CPP threshold was 60 mm Hg. Although CPPs that were persistently less than 60 mm Hg were associated with a significant decline in outcomes, no effect on neurologic outcomes was observed for patients who had CPPs that were higher, and specifically no difference between those who averaged 60 mm Hg compared with those at 70 mm Hg or higher.[199,216]

In 1995 and 2000 the Brain Trauma Foundation in cooperation with the American Association of Neurological Surgeons and the Joint Section for Trauma and Critical Care published guidelines for the management of severe head injury. From the data available, based on the theoretical need to increase the minimum CPP because of a change in critical closing pressures (see Fig. 67-18), the guidelines recommended maintaining a minimum CPP of 70 mm Hg or greater—10 mm Hg above the accepted norm. In 2003, this group updated the recommendation for CPP management, and current evidence supports a guideline that CPP should be maintained at a minimum of 60 mm Hg. In the absence of cerebral ischemia, aggressive attempts to maintain CPP above 70 mm Hg with fluids and pressors should be avoided because of the risk of ARDS.[199]

Carbon Dioxide

Carbon dioxide is a powerful regulator of cerebrovascular resistance. At any given physiologic perfusion pressure, PCO_2 can act rapidly and severely to affect CBF in a linear fashion by vasodilating or vasoconstricting the cerebrovascular bed. For every mm Hg change in $PaCO_2$, a 3% change in CBF can occur.[118]

Allowing the $PaCO_2$ to rise to levels between 60 and 80 mm Hg can result in a doubling of CBF, through vasodilation with a concomitant increase in cerebral blood volume (CBV). Conversely, aggressive hyperventilation of a patient down to a PCO_2 of 20 mm Hg or less can result in CBF's being cut in half, along with a reduction in CBV. Hyperventilation was a mainstay in the therapeutic management strategy of treating head-injured patients because it had such immediate and measurable effects on ICP. Lowering $PaCO_2$ causes rapid vasoconstriction, resulting in reduced CBV, which translates to reduced intracranial volume, which lowers ICP and increases CPP. However, hyperventilation reduces ICP by taking blood *away* from the brain, when the goal is to prevent ischemia. As seen on the autoregulation curve, the cerebrovasculature is fine-tuned to the existing perfusion pressure, providing a normal level of CBF. Aggressive hyperventilation can override the normal effect of MABP and cause a marked increase in CVR to the point at which a very high perfusion pressure would be needed to match the degree of severe vasoconstriction induced in order to maintain a normal level of CBF. This is the mechanism involved when a normal person hyperventilates, vasoconstricts, and becomes lightheaded as CBF falls. It is important to recognize that this individual has a normal MABP, ICP, and CBF before the $PaCO_2$ decreases.

Despite the fact that hyperventilation lowers ICP, the degree of vasoconstriction can be disproportionate relative to the enhancement in CPP. For example, at an MABP of 80 mm Hg with an ICP of 30 mm Hg and a CPP of 50 mm Hg, aggressive hyperventilation could reduce ICP to 15 by reducing intracranial volume, thereby improving CPP to 65. But aggressive hyperventilation can cause severe vasoconstriction. At maximal vasoconstriction, the cerebrovascular bed would need an MABP of 150 mm Hg with a normal ICP in order to maintain a normal CBF.

The data on CBF in severely head-injured patients indicate that phases of CBF change over time after traumatic brain injury, with hypoperfusion occurring in the first 24 hours.[223] Multiple studies have identified brain ischemia in up to 35% of serious head injuries within the first 12 hours.[199,118-222] It appears that this reduction happens almost immediately. Mean CBF values measured less than 4 hours after head injury in adults were 32 mL per 100 g per minute in survivors and 20 mL per 100 g per minute in nonsurvivors (normal CBF is 55 mL per 100 g per minute).[223] Low cerebral blood flow, to ischemic levels (less than 18 mL per 100 g per minute), was observed in 31% of patients with severe head injury measured an average of 3 hours after trauma.[199,224]

Because of the consistent data regarding reduced CBF early after trauma, attempts at further reductions using hyperventilation have come under close scrutiny. Some evidence suggests that hyperventilation carries a particular risk of causing cerebral hypoxia when PCO_2 is 30 mm Hg or less, or within the first 24 hours[225,226] because of a further reduction of an already low CBF.[224] It has become clear that hyperventilation decreases $BtiO_2$ because of decreased CBF in most patients, which negates the perceived benefit of improving intracranial and cerebral perfusion pressures.[212,225,226-231]

On the basis of principles reflecting a *high* degree of clinical certainty, the Brain Trauma Foundation (BTF) in 1995 and 2000 recommended that in the absence of increased ICP, chronic prolonged hyperventilation therapy (PCO_2 of 25 mm Hg or less) should be avoided after severe traumatic brain injury.[232]

On the basis of principles reflecting a *moderate* degree of clinical certainty, this group recommended that the use of prophylactic hyperventilation (PCO_2 less than 35 mm Hg) therapy during the first 24 hours after severe traumatic brain injury should be avoided because it can compromise cerebral perfusion during a time when CBF is reduced. On the basis of principles for which there is *unclear* clinical certainty, the group recommended that hyperventilation therapy may be necessary for brief periods during acute neurologic deterioration, or for longer periods in the presence of intracranial hypertension refractory to sedation, paralysis, CSF drainage, and osmotic diuretics.[233]

Oxygen

Within a normal physiologic range, oxygen causes little or no change in CBF (Fig. 67-19). Beyond a PaO_2 of approximately 300 mm Hg, CBF can begin to wane. Oxygenation does become very important at PaO_2 levels considered to be hypoxic. Below a PaO_2 of 60 mm Hg in most

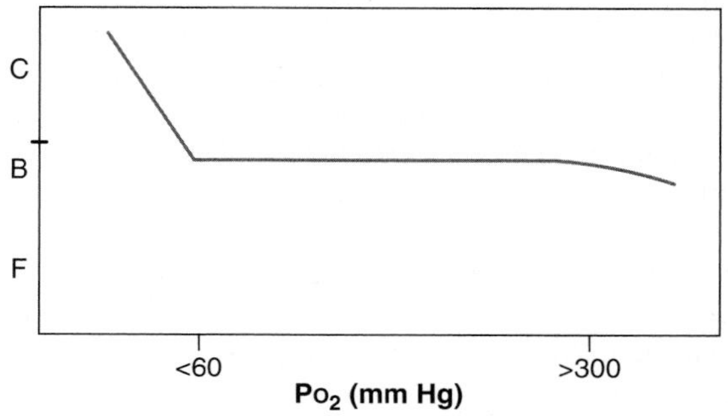

Figure 67-19. Graph demonstrating the relationship of cerebral blood flow (CBF) to oxygen (PO_2). Within a physiologic range, oxygen is of no use as a therapeutic tool. The cerebral vasculature will vasodilate under hypoxic conditions, so hypoxia must be avoided.

head-injured patients, the cerebrovasculature can vasodilate rapidly, causing an increase in CBV with poorly oxygenated blood, with an attendant increase in intracranial volume and pressure.

With careful clinical monitoring, our group has observed ICP spikes as a result of acute oxygen desaturation before a change in the pulse oximeter reading. With a moderate degree of clinical certainty, the BTF has recommended that hypoxia, defined as apnea or cyanosis in the field or a PaO_2 less than 60 mm Hg, must be scrupulously avoided or corrected immediately. Therefore, in contrast with $PaCO_2$, manipulation of PaO_2 is not a useful tool for medical management of a head-injured patient, and hypoxia must be avoided.[199]

In view of the powerful effects of hypoxia and hypercarbia, it is no surprise that early intubation in significant head injury is important.

Metabolism

Under normal circumstances, the cerebral metabolic rate of oxygen ($CMRO_2$) is directly related to CBF; this is referred to as a coupled relationship. As metabolic demand increases, the cerebrovasculature will vasodilate to supply an appropriate increase in CBF; and, conversely as $CMRO_2$ decreases, the cerebrovasculature will vasoconstrict to maintain a coupled relationship between supply and demand. As demand exceeds supply and the ability of the brain to extract more oxygen wanes, ischemia develops. Therefore, whatever increases the $CMRO_2$ will cause an appropriate vasodilatory response in the brain with its attendant increase in CBV and, potentially, ICP, with a resultant decrease in CPP. Clearly, if the primary event is an increase in demand and the end result is a reduction in supply, the gap between supply and demand increases, and with it the potential for ischemia. Under physiologic conditions whereby the $CMRO_2$ is coupled to CBF, various clinical states will demonstrate an appropriate balance of the two. For example, a comatose patient will have low $CMRO_2$, and a patient having a generalized seizure will have a high $CMRO_2$.

The metabolic state of the brain is sensitive to changes in temperature; lower temperatures lower $CMRO_2$, and vice versa. Recognition of this relationship has led to interest in using hypothermia as a therapeutic tool in severe head injury, both as a way to lower ICP and as a neuroprotectant strategy by reducing demand in the face of limited supply. Unfortunately, results have been discouraging. A recent Cochrane review of therapeutic hypothermia for head injury looked at 14 trials with more than 1000 participants and found no evidence that hypothermia is beneficial in the treatment of head injury, and that it increased the risk of pneumonia nearly twofold.[234]

Clifton and associates found that ICP was lower in patients managed with hypothermia, but no improvement in outcome was observed, and the complication rate was higher than in a normothermic group. These investigators concluded that lowering body temperature to 33° C within 8 hours after injury was not effective in improving outcomes in patients with brain injuries.[235] Despite the absence of convincing evidence that hypothermia improves outcome in adults, it can be a useful adjunct to standard treatments for controlling elevated ICP.[236]

Alternatively, even though it does not appear that therapeutic hypothermia is helpful, *hyperthermia* is believed to be *harmful* to a severely head-injured patient.[237] As the temperature rises, so does the $CMRO_2$, with a concomitant increase in CBV. If the patient has lost enough compliance that small changes in intracranial volume can result in big changes in ICP (see Fig. 67-16), CPP will fall.

A frequent scenario is development of a fever in a trauma patient with a high ICP and poor compliance who is barely meeting metabolic needs. Metabolic requirements increase as CBV and ICP increase and CPP decreases, widening the gap between supply and demand, resulting in ischemia.

Another consideration in the management of $CMRO_2$ is drug effect. Pentobarbital is the gold standard drug for reducing cerebral metabolism and can be used in cases of refractory intracranial hypertension to induce a barbiturate coma. A condition of *burst suppression* is achieved, meaning that the continuous EEG recording demonstrates periods of an isoelectric tracing (straight line) interrupted by bursts of cortical electrical activity. This therapy results in vasoconstriction appropriate for the degree of reduction in metabolism, with an attendant decrease in ICP. This has the theoretical advantage of improving supply to a brain with reduced metabolic demands. However, despite the evidence for cerebral protection in experimental models, little clinical evidence is available to suggest that barbiturates improve outcome after severe head injuries in humans. Other drugs that reduce the $CMRO_2$ and CBF are other barbiturates such as thiopental, as well as the substituted phenol propofol, the hypnotic agent etomidate, and the water-soluble short-acting benzodiazepine midazolam.[237]

Viscosity

When autoregulation is intact, lowering viscosity of the blood improves flow dynamics and results in an appropriate increase in CVR to maintain a constant, normal CBF.[238-241]

This vasoconstriction reduces intracranial volume. From a rheologic standpoint, there is an advantage to lowering viscosity by hemodilution, but this is at the expense of oxygen-carrying capacity. Reducing the hematocrit from 45% to 30% can theoretically double CBF, yet oxygen-carrying capacity would be reduced by only a third. By generalizing experimental and clinical data involving ischemia and hematocrit, it is reasonable to consider an optimum hematocrit of approximately 30% to 35%.[248]

A common mechanism for lowering viscosity in traumatic head injury is the use of mannitol, which causes an immediate influx of extravascular water, leading to hemodilution. The vasoconstriction resulting from this reduction in viscosity allows the same CBF and oxygen delivery to be maintained by means of smaller vessels and with a lower intracranial volume (see later section, "Hyperosmolar Therapy." In addition, mannitol will dehydrate the red blood cells themselves by about 15%, which further improves blood flow dynamics.[243]

Venous Blood Compartment

In general, vascular organization of most organ systems is anatomically similar—for example, the renal artery travels with the renal vein. The brain, however, has two entirely different anatomic systems for arterial supply and venous drainage. The paired carotid and vertebral arteries provide the arterial supply to the brain but have no corresponding venous counterparts. Blood leaves the brain through cortical and deep draining veins that empty into the superior sagittal, transverse, and sigmoid sinuses. These dural sinuses are open, semirigid structures that empty into bilateral jugular veins, which communicate directly with the right heart through the superior vena cava. There are no valves in this entire venous system. This means that right heart pressures are in direct continuity with the superior sagittal sinus within the intracranial compartment. When measured with the subject lying supine, ICP cannot be lower than central venous pressure. Of more importance, right heart pressures will be directly transmitted to the intracranial compartment, a relevant dynamic involved with a Valsalva maneuver.

During a Valsalva maneuver, intrathoracic pressure elevates and venous return to the right heart goes down. Decreased venous return means decreased venous outflow from the brain. This results in a rapid, instantaneous increase in CBV as the arterial side continues to supply the brain with blood that is not getting physiological draining. A Valsalva maneuver also will decrease cardiac output along with a decrease in venous return, but it is a disproportionate change. A common neurosurgical practice is to have the anesthesiologist induce a controlled Valsalva maneuver toward the end of a brain operation during the final stages of hemostasis, just before beginning the closure. Intrathoracic pressure is elevated to approximately 30 mm Hg for 10 seconds as the surgeon looks for any areas of bleeding while the brain immediately physically and visibly swells as it engorges with blood. An intrathoracic pressure of 30 mm Hg will overcome a normal CVP and essentially interrupt venous outflow from the brain. The concomitant decrease in cardiac output with a pressure of 30 mm Hg will have much less of an effect than on the venous side; therefore, a relatively large volume of arterial blood will continue to fill the brain. Even a normal brain with normal compliance will immediately "feel" the effect of decreased venous outflow because it happens faster than the buffering capacity of the brain can handle (see Fig. 67-16). In fact, one of the mechanisms the brain will use to buffer increases in volume is to collapse venous capacitance vessels, which, in the case of decreased venous outflow from the brain, becomes part of the problem, not the solution.

Other common ways in which venous outflow from the brain can be compromised is with anything that interferes with jugular venous drainage such as a tight-fitting rigid cervical collar or thrombosis from an internal jugular line. It is not uncommon to have dominant venous outflow on one side and, following head rotation to that side, increased resistance to venous outflow. Obviously, gravity also will have a role, with head elevation enhancing venous outflow from the brain. We generally keep our patients with the head elevated at 30 degrees, with neck straight and free of lines, with a good-fitting cervical collar that is not too tight.

Brain Compartment

Another functional volumetric compartment is the brain itself. One of the consequences of traumatic brain injury is an acute increase in total brain water.[244]

The volume of the brain parenchyma can be affected by therapeutic dehydration induced with the use of osmotic agents. These agents can be used to treat cerebral edema in an effort to remove a pathologic accumulation of fluid. Dehydration also can be used to manipulate the volume status of an otherwise normal but threatened brain compartment in order to emergently manage an increase in ICP as a temporizing measure before surgery, such as with extra-axial hematoma or hydrocephalus. The agents most commonly used to effect these changes are mannitol and hypertonic saline.

Cerebral Edema

By definition, brain edema is an abnormal accumulation of fluid within the brain parenchyma that produces a volumetric enlargement of the brain tissue.[198] The three types of cerebral edema are vasogenic, neurotoxic, and cytotoxic. *Vasogenic* edema occurs when the blood-brain barrier opens, resulting in movement of vascular fluid into the extracellular spaces of the brain.[245] Neurotoxic edema involves astrocytic and dendritic swelling secondary to the neurotoxic effects of excitatory amino acids, particularly glutamate, seen with reperfusion.[198] Cytotoxic edema results from retention of water within swollen cells, most commonly found in stroke, in which interruption of energy supply leads to pump failure and an intracellular increase in sodium and water.[198]

It is *ischemia,* associated with energy failure at the level of mitochondria, that contributes to cytotoxic brain edema and intracranial hypertension.[244-252] Earlier studies lead to the general acceptance that traumatic brain swelling was primarily a result of vascular engorgement, which caused increased ICP.[253-257] Although opinions differ, more recent work has demonstrated that cerebral edema may be primarily responsible for brain swelling, not vascular engorgement.[249,258] Marmarou and colleagues have used sophisticated MRI techniques to demonstrate that traumatic brain edema is predominantly a cellular phenomenon in both focal and diffuse brain injury.[198]

Although cellular edema predominates, it is likely that edema formation in head injury is complicated, with time-dependent contributions of both vasogenic and cytotoxic mechanisms. Experimental evidence points to transient compromise of the blood-brain barrier occurring immediately after injury, with resultant vasogenic edema. Studies indicate early closure of the blod-brain barrier, after which cytotoxic, cellular edema predominates.[198,259-261]

Hyperosmolar Therapy

Mannitol

Mannitol, an inert six-carbon alcohol of the corresponding sugar mannose, causes cellular dehydration by increasing serum osmolarity. The use of mannitol in head-injured patients to lower ICP is based on two mechanisms of action of this drug: It establishes an osmotic gradient across the blood-brain barrier to reduce water content,[262,263] and it causes cerebral vasoconstriction through rheologic effects that decrease blood viscosity and enhance CBF and MABP (see earlier section, "Viscosity").[243,264,265] This vascular mechanism of action has a strong, independent effect, such that CBF can be enhanced even when ICP is not substantially reduced.[266,267]

With head-injured patients, mannitol is used in two clinical scenarios. The first is that of a comatose trauma patient with a surgical clot, when mannitol is given on the way to the operating room to buy time until emergent decompression is accomplished. Generally, higher doses of up to 1.2 to 1.4 g per kg can be given in this scenario.[268,269]

The second clinical scenario is one of cerebral edema, when mannitol is given to control ICP. Unlike with its use for emergency surgical clots, there is no consensus on the optimal dosing regimen of mannitol in the ICU to manage ICP. Doses ranging from 0.25 g per kg to 1.0 g per kg may be effective. Mannitol can be given in response to high ICP, or it can be used prophylactically regardless of ICP, using serum osmolarity as an end point of treatment,[270] although some evidence indicates that it is most effective when used in the presence of high ICP or low perfusion pressure.[265,271]

Regardless of how mannitol is used, because of its osmotic diuresis, replacement of urinary water and electrolyte losses is critical, to avoid hypovolemia and hypotension. Mannitol typically is given as a bolus at a rate not to exceed 0.1 g per kg per minute, in order to avoid hypotension.[270] Caution should be exercised in patients with a propensity toward congestive heart failure, because the early effects of bolus administration cause intravascular volume expansion.[270]

Mannitol can extravasate into the interstitium of the brain, with breakdown of the blood-brain barrier, which may be a cause of cerebral edema. This is thought to be less of an issue with bolus dosing as opposed to continuous infusion.[272] Because of this particular concern with mannitol toxicity, many clinicians prefer to use the smallest doses of mannitol necessary, and to administer it only for proven intracranial hypertension.[273]

Another concern is renal failure, which is a rare complication of mannitol therapy. It is generally believed that the kidneys are at risk above a serum osmolarity of 320 mOsm per L[274,275]; however, kidney damage may in fact be due to high serum concentrations of mannitol itself, as opposed to high serum osmolarity. It is suggested that keeping the osmolar gap (measured serum osmolarity minus calculated serum osmolarity) below 55 mOsm per kg of H_2O may be better than using serum osmolarity alone to direct mannitol therapy.[270,275]

To summarize, mannitol therapy in the ICU is effective given as boluses for elevated ICP while keeping the patient normovolemic and hyperosmolar with an osmolar gap less than 55 mOsm per kg.

Furosemide, a loop diuretic, has some effectiveness for removing extracellular fluid from the brain. Although it does not work as fast as mannitol, furosemide commonly is used in conjunction with that agent because of a synergistic effect on ICP.[276]

Hypertonic Saline

In many ICUs, *hypertonic saline* is being used with increasing frequency for the treatment of raised ICP in patients with traumatic brain injury.[277] It is known that patients with hypotension after severe traumatic brain injury have twice the mortality rate of normotensive patients[278]; therefore, aggressive resuscitation with intravenous fluids is recommended in the current guidelines for the management of patients with severe traumatic brain injury.[279] However, the real concern for the development of cerebral edema is reason enough to limit the amount of free water available to the injured brain during this early period. The use of hypertonic saline, both to increase mean arterial pressure and to decrease ICP, is a logical and promising approach to limit secondary injury and improve neurologic outcome.

The rapid infusion of a small volume of hypertonic solution originally was designed for the prehospital treatment of hemorrhagic shock,[280-283] and a recent trial found a trend toward a reduction of ICP in a double-blind, randomized, controlled trial of prehospital fluid resuscitation using hypertonic saline in comatose and hypotensive head-injured patients (although no improvement in outcome was demonstrated).[284]

The rapid infusion of small volumes of hypertonic solution leads to an osmotic gradient that mobilizes parenchymal fluid into the vascular compartment,[285,286] resulting in hemodilution, endothelial shrinkage, and improved blood flow in the microcirculation,[287,288] as well as improved cardiac output.[280,281,289] Hypertonic saline has been shown to reduce brain bulk and ICP[290-293] and to be effective in lowering ICP both in bolus form and as a maintenance fluid.[2940-296]

It is widely believed that the mechanism of action of both hypertonic saline and mannitol in reducing ICP is their hyperosmolar properties, although additional mechanisms are likely to be in play. Some authors have found hypertonic saline to be more effective than mannitol in selected patients.[297,298]

Concerns about central pontine myelinolysis and acute renal failure appear to be unfounded on the basis of clinical experience; however, a rebound effect may occur in some patients.[299] A recent trial also reported no episodes of acute anemia or hypokalemia associated with 23.4% saline administration, nor were there any episodes of convulsions, congestive heart failure, or coagulopathy after the administration of hypertonic saline.[297]

In the United States, 3% sodium chloride is readily available. An initial dose of 1.5 to 3.0 mL per kg with a target for a serum sodium concentration of approximately 155 mEq per L is reasonable,[293] although 23.4% saline has been shown to be safe and effective in the treatment of intracranial hypertension.[297] As with hyperosmolar therapy for mannitol, it is important to maintain a normovolemic state at all times during treatment.

Cerebrospinal Fluid Compartment

CSF is produced mostly by the choroid plexus located in the ventricles. CSF flows from the lateral ventricles (first two ventricles) through the foramina of Monro into the third ventricle, and from there the fluid moves through the aqueduct of Sylvius to the fourth ventricle. From the fourth ventricle, CSF moves out of the ventricular system through the foramen of Magendie in the midline and the foramina of Lushka laterally. CSF then enters the subarachnoid space of the brain and spinal cord and circulates around the surface of the cerebellum and brainstem as it comes up through the tentorial hiatus, thus forming the basal cisterns. The clear and colorless fluid migrates over the cerebral hemispheres toward the midline, where, through a semiactive process, it is transported from the subarachnoid space into the superior sagittal sinus.

CSF is made at a continuous rate of approximately 0.3 mL per minute. With a total volume of approximately 150 mL (roughly 10% of intracranial volume), the entire CSF volume is replaced three times a day. A little less than one third of the total volume is in the ventricular system.

In severe head injury, CSF can be displaced out of the intracranial compartment as pressure differences between the superior sagittal sinus and the intracranial compartment increase (see Fig. 67-16). The spinal CSF compartment also is an important physiologic sink, and this contribution of CSF flow to ICP is another justification for nursing traumatic brain–injured patients with the head elevated.[298]

A standard way of managing the CSF compartment in the trauma patient is by draining CSF through an indwelling ventricular catheter (ventriculostomy). This has proved to be a relatively safe and effective tool in lowering intracranial volume and pressure, although ventricles in younger trauma patients commonly are smaller and harder to access and have less CSF to drain. Ventricular drainage is discussed further in Chapter 17.

SPECIFIC TREATMENT CONSIDERATIONS

Craniectomy

Craniectomy is an alternative to the medical and direct surgical methods for reducing intracranial volume. This is a surgical strategy for managing a dangerous increase in intracranial volume by expanding the size of the intracranial compartment. The necessary expansion is accomplished by removing a large portion of the skull and opening the dura (see Fig. 67-13).

Intractable intracranial hypertension despite maximal medical therapy is associated with a high risk of morbidity and death.[299-301] In one multicenter trial, an 86% mortality rate was found among patients whose condition failed to respond to an induced pentobarbital coma[302]—the last line of defense in medical management. Similarly, a significant relationship has been recognized between an ICP higher than 25 mm Hg and a poor outcome.[303]

Because of these ominous facts, craniectomy to increase the space available for the swollen brain has been used to lower ICP, although early outcome studies of hemicraniectomy yielded poor results.[304-306] More contemporary experiences, however, have achieved better results. In 2006 Aarabi and colleagues reviewed 10 reports published since 1988, with a total of 323 patients treated with decompressive craniectomy for post-traumatic brain swelling and intractable intracranial hypertension, and calculated a collective mortality rate of 22.3%, with good outcomes in 48.3%, with the rest of the patients (29.4%) remaining severely disabled or vegetative. These results compared favorably with six previous reports in which mortality rates ranged from 42% to 100% when ICP greater than 20 mm Hg remained refractory to medical management. Reported complications included subgaleal collections, which resolved over the course of weeks to months; delayed wound healing; bone flap resorption and infections; increased swelling and hemorrhagic contusions; and parenchymal lucencies, possibly due to ischemia.[10,216,285,299,303,307-316]

In addition to the demonstrated improvement in outcome, contrast-enhanced ultrasonography recently has been used to assess cerebral perfusion after decompressive craniectomy and found an average fivefold improvement in microvascular blood flow.[317] A technical point worth emphasizing is that a decompressive craniectomy must be sufficiently large in order to be helpful.[318]

Management of Intracranial Hypertension

Acute, severe traumatic brain injury is a dynamic process with the potential for dangerous changes that can evolve over hours to days; therefore, all patients need to be observed closely. Ideally, ongoing assessment by neurologic examination should be at least hourly. In most patients with a GCS score of 8 or less, however, airway protection mechanisms will be impaired, necessitating intubation and, therefore, sedation, which makes an accurate neurologic assessment problematic. An ICP measuring device usually is needed at this point to adequately monitor the patient, in lieu of a reliable examination (see Chapter 17 on ICP monitoring).

The medical management of intracranial hypertension in the ICU generally occurs after surgical decompression of hematomas causing unbalanced forces, or in patients without a surgical lesion. This management strategy generally is divided into tiers of therapy. The first tier is sedation, analgesia, and intubation without hyperventilation, keeping the head elevated and the neck straight and uncompressed. The routine use of paralytics may increase the risk of pulmonary complications; therefore, muscle relaxants should be used for ICP control when sedation is inadequate.[319] If ICP exceeds 20 mm Hg[320] despite these maneuvers, moving to the next level of care is indicated, which includes CSF drainage if a ventriculostomy is being used, mannitol, or hypertonic saline. Beyond the first 24 hours, mild hyperventilation to keep P_{CO_2} in the mid 30s can be used. Throughout the clinical course it also is necessary to maintain an adequate CPP of at least 60 mm Hg by ensuring normovolemia and a safe MABP. If ICP is refractory to these treatments, the next step is use of decompressive hemicraniectomies or barbiturate coma (or both). Historically, surgical decompression has been reserved as a radical, end-of-the-line treatment after the patient has failed to respond to burst suppression barbiturate coma; however, craniectomy is moving up in the treatment algorithm of most centers (Fig. 67-20).

When ICP goes up, it is important to understand why and then try to correct the underlying problem if possible. In any given head-injured patient in whom the brain has lost its buffering capacity, with resultant poor compliance, small increases in intracranial volume can cause a significant rise in pressure. When ICP rises, CPP goes down. This usually will result in a decrease in CVR and vasodilation, with its attendant increase in cerebral blood volume and increase in intracranial volume. This of course leads to a further increase in ICP, and the cycle perpetuates itself. This is the mechanism of a plateau wave.[243]

In managing these patients, *it is critical to try and determine the source of the problem.* Perhaps the patient became hypovolemic and the blood pressure dropped, or a ventilator change caused hypercarbia or hypoxia. Maybe the patient is inadequately sedated or having an unrecognized seizure while pharmacologically paralyzed. The problem may be as simple as a high fever or a rigid cervical collar compressing the jugular veins. Whatever is driving this process must be corrected to break this dangerous plateau wave.

If the cause cannot be determined, a new CT scan may need to be taken, and therapeutic maneuvers should be employed to help turn things around, such as increasing sedation, further head elevation, ventricular drainage, administration of mannitol or hypertonic saline, pressors when needed, and brief periods of gentle hyperventilation.

Anticoagulation

It is intuitive that severe coagulopathy is associated with increased mortality after head injury.[321-323] Penetrating or blunt brain injury can be associated with the massive release of thromboplastin from neuronal tissue, thereby initiating the coagulation process, which evolves to an exaggerated fibrinolytic response and disseminated intravascular coagulopathy (DIC).[322] This brain injury–induced coagulopathy may lead to significant secondary injury and delay the invasive monitoring necessary for the aggressive management of intracranial hypertension.[330] The criteria for the diagnosis of DIC include abnormal clotting studies, thrombocytopenia, low fibrinogen, and, in some cases, elevation in levels of products of fibrinolysis (D-dimer or fibrin degradation products).[325] The DIC caused by head trauma is relatively common and frequently is detected by a prolonged prothrombin time and elevated international normalized ratio (INR). Its presence may be an indication for more intense clinical observation and follow-up CT scanning. An important component of DIC is coagulation; however, in the setting of active bleeding, anticoagulation is not indicated. The therapeutic focus is on hemostasis and replacement of diluted or consumed blood elements and components.[326-327]

Typical treatment of coagulopathy consists of fresh frozen plasma (FFP) administration; however, use of FFP can be problematic. This product takes time to administer, so that a relatively large volume of fluid may be given to a head-injured patient when it is important to avoid hypervolemia. Other concerns are the possibility of blood-borne disease transmission and, as reported in a rare case, transfusion-related acute lung injury. Another important issue is the variable effect FFP can have on brain injury–induced coagulopathy, such that it ultimately may fail to correct the coagulopathy.

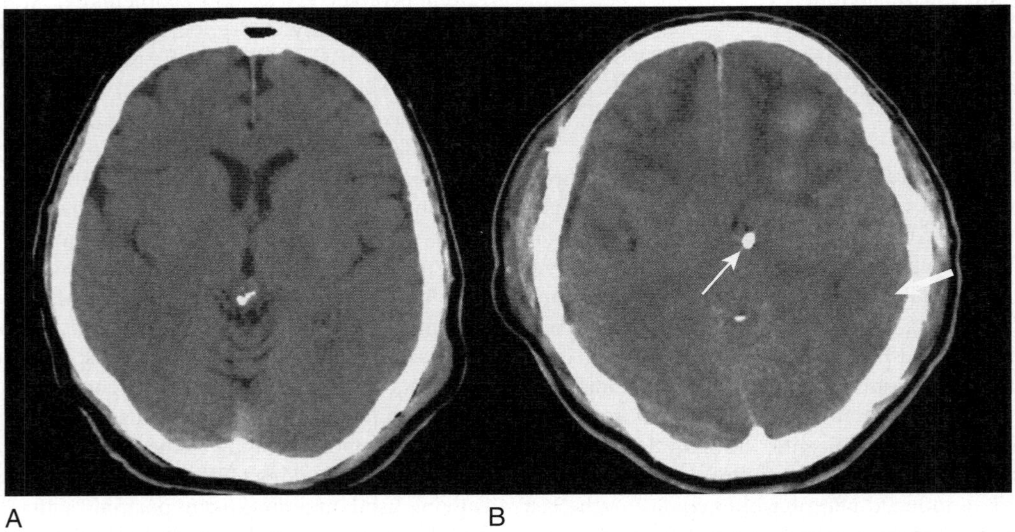

Figure 67-20. A, Computed tomography (CT) image of a normal brain. **B,** CT scan of the brain of a patient with severe traumatic brain injury and medically intractable intracranial hypertension. Between the poorly controlled cerebral edema and the indwelling ventriculostomy, almost no cerebrospinal fluid can be identified on the scan, which shows complete obliteration of cortical sulci *(thick arrow)* and basal cisterns *(thin arrow).* Given the absence of shift, bilateral hemicraniectomies were required.

Preliminary data indicate that recombinant activated factor VII (rFVIIa) provides a rapid and successful correction of coagulopathy in head-injured patients.[324] Originally developed for treatment of hemophiliacs, rFVIIa also may be helpful in reversing the effects of anticoagulants and antiplatelet drugs.[324,328-338] It is a vitamin K–dependent glycoprotein, similar to the human plasma–derived factor VIIa, which appears to promote hemostasis by activating the extrinsic pathway of the coagulation cascade.[339] Its mechanism of action is not fully understood but includes interaction with platelets or tissue factor to augment thrombin generation and platelet activation.[328,330,332,333] Factor VIIa seems to be the bottleneck, the critical factor most depleted when patients are profoundly anticoagulated.[340] The use of rFVIIa to correct a coagulopathy before neurosurgical intervention was reported in 1998 in a hemophiliac patient with an EDH requiring craniotomy for evacuation.[341] Although not specifically evaluated for use in DIC, rFVIIa has been administered to neurosurgical patients in whom DIC was likely to be present.[327,336] Recombinant FVIIa has been used in the absence of hemophilia for neurosurgical emergencies such as EDH and SDH, SAH and intracerebral hemorrhage, tumor resection, and during placement of ICP monitors.[331,334,336,338] A recent retrospective study found improved outcomes, without complications, when rFVIIa was used for coagulopathic patients requiring urgent neurosurgical intervention.[342] The incidence of thrombosis after rFVIIa is low, but thrombosis is an extremely important potential complication[332,336,337,343,344] and of particular concern in DIC.[326] Precise dosing for conditions other than hemophilia has not been confirmed[330]; at this time, rFVIIa is approved by the FDA only for use in hemophilia; other uses are considered off-label.

In addition to the coagulopathy induced by a brain injury, neurosurgeons and intensivists often are faced with managing patients with traumatic intracranial hemorrhage who are pharmacologically anticoagulated. The use of these drugs is expected to increase as the population ages.[327] These patients must have normal coagulation rapidly restored to prevent further bleeding and to make surgical intervention possible. One of the more common drugs encountered in clinical practice is warfarin; a typical scenario is one in which an elderly patient on warfarin sodium (Coumadin) falls and hits her head. It takes about 4 days to normalize coagulation if warfarin is stopped. With vitamin K, full reversal begins 4 to 6 hours after administration and takes about 24 hours to lower the INR. FFP contains vitamin K–dependent factors, is rapidly effective, and is given intravenously. Recombinant factor VIIa also can be used to normalize coagulation in these patients.[327,334,345,346]

In hospitalized patients on heparin, reversal occurs approximately 60 minutes after an intravenous infusion is stopped. If it needs to be reversed faster, protamine is recommended. Desmopressin also has been recommended to reverse the effects of heparin. Subcutaneous heparin is usually not reversed.[327]

With low-molecular-weight heparin (LMWH), a partial thomboplastin time (PTT) is variably altered and not a reliable measure of its effect. Reversal of LMWH effect with protamine is variable in humans.[327]

A common situation is the presentation of a head-injured patient on an antiplatelet agent such as aspirin or other nonsteroidal anti-inflammatory drug (NSAID). Acetylsalicylic acid (ASA) inhibits platelet aggregation for the life of the affected platelet, which is approximately 10 days. This occurs even at the lowest dose of 81 mg per day. A period of 5 to 6 days typically is needed after stopping aspirin to replace approximately half of the circulating platelets (10% per 24 hours). The effect of ASA on platelets is complete and irreversible. If treatment is necessary, platelet transfusion is given to provide unaffected platelets so long as no ASA remains in the circulation. Desmopressin (DDAVP) may secondarily improve platelet adhesion to endothelial defects and is therefore also recommended to overcome aspirin-induced platelet dysfunction. Other NSAIDs have various anticoagulant effects. If significant NSAID use has occurred before a neurosurgical emergency, the same interventional strategy may apply. Data confirming efficacy in counteracting an anticoagulant effect, however, are not available.[327]

Other antiplatelet agents include adenosine diphosphate (ADP) and glycoprotein receptor–blocking agents. Clopidogrel and ticlopidine irreversibly alter platelet aggregation[347-350] through a mechanism that is additive to the antiplatelet effects of aspirin. The platelets are permanently affected; once the drug is stopped, recovery of normal platelet function requires about a week until new platelets are produced. Rapid correction requires platelet transfusion, and DDAVP also may have a beneficial, short-term effect.[327]

Abciximab, eptifibatide, and tirofiban are highly effective in generating 80% to 95% reversible inhibition in platelet aggregation.[347,348,350-353] Stopping the medication allows return of normal platelet function in approximately 48 hours for abciximab and in 4 to 8 hours for the others. Platelet transfusion increases the proportion of unaffected platelets and is the primary intervention.[327]

Fibrinolytic and thrombolytic agents disrupt formed clots.[353-355] These drugs have a prolonged half-life and frequently are used in combination with heparin or other agents to ensure continued therapeutic anticoagulation. Because circulating fibrinogen is decreased during thrombolysis, cryoprecipitate, a source of concentrated fibrinogen, is the basis for reversing treatment.[327] Although these agents have well-recognized applications for cardiac[356] and neurologic[357,358] problems, their use generally is not seen in patients presenting with head injury.

Hypothermia also is known to cause and worsen coagulation abnormalities,[330,359] the treatment for which is rewarming. Certain medical conditions also may affect coagulation, which may be important as underlying factors in patients with a head injury. DDAVP increases the release of factor VIII and von Willebrand factor and is used to treat mild hemophilia A, von Willebrand disease, and chronic renal and liver disease, as well as acquired and congenital platelet disorders.[359,360-363]

DDAVP has a significant antidiuretic effect and will increase free water reabsorption in the kidney, potentially leading to overhydration and hyponatremia. This may cause serious problems in a severely head-injured patient with cerebral edema, poor compliance, and high ICP.

Unintended, iatrogenic worsening of coagulopathy may result with use of hetastarch solutions, which often are administered to increase intravascular volume. These solutions may lower von Willebrand factor levels and alter platelet function. Low-molecular-weight hetastarch preparations are available that may cause less severe changes; however, if the patient requires correction of a coagulation abnormality, these solutions should be avoided if possible.[363-366]

Nutritional Support

Replacement of 140% of resting metabolic expenditure in nonparalyzed patients and 100% resting metabolic expenditure in paralyzed patients using enteral or parenteral formulas containing at least 15% of calories as protein by the seventh day after injury is recommended.[3,367]

Role of Steroid Therapy

On the basis of class 1 evidence originating from a prospective randomized trial comparing dexamethasone and placebo in 300 head-injured patients, dexamethasone was found to be ineffective in improving outcome or reducing ICP in patients with severe brain injury.[3,310] Therefore, the use of steroids is not recommended in the management of head-injured patients.

CONCLUSIONS

The management of traumatic brain injury will remain for the foreseeable future a major medical and surgical challenge. Despite concentrated basic research directed at elucidating the metabolic factors that mediate the transition from primary to secondary tissue damage, nothing has been found that might have clinical efficacy. As the percentage of the population older than 70 years of age continues to rise, ICU physicians will face an ethical dilemma of dealing with brain hemorrhages in this age group. Subdural hematoma in an 86-year-old with mild dementia on warfarin sodium (Coumadin) for atrial fibrillation is becoming one of the most common presentations in an active trauma center. At present, intensivists are left with the application of best protocol–driven critical care management, supported by a high index of suspicion for surgically correctable lesions, the judicious use of decompressive hemicraniectomy, and a societal commitment to protective and preventive programs.

KEY POINTS

- The management of severe head injuries remains a major challenge to neurosurgeons.
- The time from injury to surgery must be as short as possible to minimize the secondary manifestations of serious brain trauma.
- Hyperventilation, although very effective in reducing high ICP, must be used judiciously; otherwise, it may become more harmful than helpful. Glucocorticoids have no significant therapeutic benefit in managing severe head injuries.
- A simple-to-use and highly predictable neurologic status scoring system, the GCS, has enabled meaningful multidisciplinary communication from the accident scene through intensive care and beyond, resulting in efficient and timely triage and treatment of these patients.
- Mannitol is used in head-injured patients to lower ICP. This drug exerts its beneficial effect through two mechanisms of action: It establishes an osmotic gradient across the blood-brain barrier to reduce water content, and it causes cerebral vasoconstriction through blood flow dynamic effects that decrease blood viscosity and enhance CBF and MABP.
- The use of hypertonic saline to increase mean arterial pressure and decrease ICP is a logical and promising approach to limit secondary injury and improve neurologic outcome.
- Craniectomy can be used to increase the space available for the swollen brain, thereby lowering ICP.

REFERENCES

1. Varelas PN, Eastwood D, Yun HJ, et al: Impact of a neurointensivist on outcomes in patients with head trauma treated in a neurosciences intensive care unit. J Neurosurg 2006;104:713-719.
2. Smith RF, Frateschi L, Sloan EP, et al: The impact of volume on outcome in seriously injured trauma patients: Two years' experience of the Chicago Trauma System. J Trauma 1990;30: 1066-1076.
3. Bullock R, Chestnut R, Clifton G, et al: Guidelines for the management of severe traumatic brain injury. A joint initiative of The Brain Trauma Foundation, The American Association of Neurological Surgeons, Congress of Neurological Surgeons, Joint Section on Neurotrauma and Critical Care. 2001.
4. Kraus JF: Epidemiology of head injury. In Cooper PR (ed): Head Injury. Baltimore, Williams & Wilkins, 1993.
5. Frankowski RF, Anneges JF, Whitman S: Epidemiologic and descriptive studies, Part I: The descriptive epidemiology of head trauma in the United States. In Becker DP, Povlishock JT (eds): Central Nervous System Trauma Status Report. Bethesda, MD, National Institute of Health (NINCDS), 1985.
6. Cooper JD, Tabaddor K, Hauser WA: The epidemiology of head injury in the Bronx. Neuroepidemiology 1983;2:70.
7. U.S. Department of Health and Human Sciences, Public Health Service: Interagency Head Injury Task Force Report. Bethesda, MD, National Institute of Health, National Institute of Neurological Disorders and Stroke, 1989.
8. Sosin DM, Sacks JJ, Smith SM: Head injury-associated deaths in the United States from 1979-1986. JAMA 1989;262:2251.
9. Kerr JA, Kay DW, Lassman LP: Characteristics of patients, type of accident, and mortality in a consecutive series of head injuries admitted to a neurosurgical unit. Br J Prev Soc Med 1971;25:179.
10. Kraus J, Fife DK, Conroy C: Incidence, severity, and outcome of brain injuries involving bicycles, Am J Public Health 1987;77:76.
11. Du Trevor MD, Van Dellen JR: Penetrating stab wounds to the brain:

The timing of angiography in patients with the weapon already removed. Neurosurgery 1992;31:905.
12. Oyesiku NM: What is the best way to assess and classify head-injured patients? In Valadka AB, Andrews BT (eds): Neurotrauma. New York, Thieme Medical Publications, 2005, pp 8-14.
13. Teasdale G, Jennet B: Assessment of coma and impaired consciousness: A practical scale. Lancet 1974;2: 81-84.
14. Starmark JE, Stalhammer D, Holmgren E, et al: A comparison of the Glasgow Coma Scale and the Reaction Level Scale (RLS85). J Neurosurg 1988;69: 699-706.
15. Stalhammer D, Starmark JE, Holmgren E, et al: Assessment of reponsiveness in acute cerebral disorders: A multicentre study on the reaction level scale (RLS85). Acta Neurchir (Wien) 1988;90:73-80.
16. Benzer A, Mitterschiffthaler G, Marosi M, et al: Prediction of nonsurvival after trauma: Innsbruck Coma Scale. Lancet 1991;338:977-978.
17. Sugiura K, Muraoka K, Chishiki T, et al: The Edinburgh-2 coma scale: A new scale for assessing impaired consciousness. Neurosurgery 1983;12:411-415.
18. Sugiura K, Muraoka K, Kanazawa C, et al: A clinical study on a system of assessment of impaired consciousness (the second report). No To Shinkei 1978;30:1025-1029.
19. Sugiura K, Kanazawa C, Sato S, et al: A clinical study on a system of assessment of impaired consciousness (the first report). No To Shinkei 1977;29:879-883.
20. Stanczak DE, White JG III, Gouview WD, et al: Assessment of level of consciousness following severe neurologic insult: A comparison of the psychometric qualities of the Glasgow Coma Scale and the Comprehensive Level of Consciousness Scale. J Neurosurg 1984;60:955-960.
21. Salcman M, Schepp RS, Ducker TB: Calculated recovery rates in severe head trauma. Neurosurgery 1981;8:301-308.
22. Born JD, Albert A, Hans P, et al: Relative prognostic value of best motor response and brain stem reflexes in patients with severe head injury. Neurosurgery 1985;16:595-601.
23. Born JD: The Glasgow-Liege Scale: Prognostic value, and evolution of motor response and brain stem reflexes after severe head injury. Acta Neurochir (Wien) 1988;91:1-11.
24. Yen JK, Bourke RS, Nelson LR, et al: Numerical grading of clinical neurological status after serious head injury. J Neurol Neurosurg Psychiatry 1978;41:1125-1130.
25. Teasdale G, Knill-Jones R, van der Sande J: Observer variability in assessing impaired consciousness and coma. J Neurol Neurosurg Psychiatry 1978;41:603-610.
26. Braakman R, Avezaat CJ, Maas AI, et al: Inter observer agreement in the assessment of the motor response of the Glasgow Coma Scale. Clin Neurol Neurosurg 1977;80:100-106.
27. Ingersoll GL, Leyden DB: The Glasgow Coma Scale for patients with head injuries. Crit Care Nurse 1987;7:26-32.
28. Rowley G, Fielding K: Reliability and accuracy of the Glasgow Coma Scale with experienced and inexperienced users. Lancet 1991;337:535-538.
29. Fielding K, Rowley G: Reliability of assessments by skilled observers using the Glasgow Coma Scale. Aust J Adv Nurs 1990;7:13-17.
30. Jennett B, Teasdale G, Galbraith S, et al: Severe head injuries in three countries. J Neurol Neurosurg Peychiatry 1977;40:291-298.
31. Teasdale G, Jennett B: Assessment and prognosis of coma after head injury. Acta Neurochir (Wien) 1976;34:45-55.
32. Jagger J, Jane JA, Rimel R: The Glasgow Coma Scale: To sum or not to sum? Lancet 1983;2:97.
33. The Brain Trauma Foundation, The American Association of Neurological Surgeons, The Joint Section on Neurotrauma and Critical Care: Management and prognosis of severe traumatic brain injury. Glascow Coma Scale score. J Neurotrauma 2000;17:563-571.
34. Maas AI, Hukkelhoven CW, Marshall LF, Steyerberg EW: Prediction of outcome in traumatic brain injury with computed tomographic characteristics: A comparison between the computed tomographic classification and combinations of computed tomographic predictors. Neurosurgery 2005;57:1173-1182.
35. Marshall LF, Marshall SB, Klauber MR, et al: A new classification of head injury based on computerized tomography. J Neurosurg 1991;75: S14-S20.
36. Valadka AB: Comment. Neurosurgery 2005;57:1181.
37. Bullock MR: Comment. Neurosurgery 2005;57:1181.
38. Stein SC: Minor head injury: 13 is an unlucky number. J Trauma 2001;50: 759-760.
39. Dacey RG Jr, Alves WM, Rimel RW, et al: Neurosurgical complications after apparently minor head injury: Assessment of risk in a series of 610 patients. J Neurosurg 1986;65: 203-210.
40. Culotta VP, Sementilli ME, Gerold K, et al: Clinicopathological heterogenicity in the classification of mild head injury. Neurosurgery 1996;38:245-250.
41. Stein SC, Burnett MG: When are computed tomography scans and skull x-rays indicated for patients with minor head injury? In Valadka AB, Andrews BT (eds): Neurotrauma. New York, Thieme Medical Publications, 2005, pp 19-24.
42. Graham DI, Gennarelli TA: Pathology of brain damage after head injury. In Cooper PR, Golfinos JG (eds): Head Injury, 4th ed. New York, McGraw-Hill, 2000, pp 133-153.
43. Firlik AD, Marion DW: Intracranial pressure physiology and pathophysiology. In Cooper PR, Golfinos JG (eds): Head Injury, 4th ed. New York, McGraw-Hill, 2000, pp 221-228.
44. Golfinos JG, Cooper PR: Skull fracture and post-traumatic cerebrospinal fluid fistulae. In Cooper PR, Golfinos JG (eds): Head Injury, 4th ed. New York, McGraw-Hill, 2000, pp 155-174.
45. Braakman R: Depressed skull fracture: Data, treatment, and follow-up in 225 consecutive cases. J Neurol Neurosurg Psychiatry 1972;34:395-402.
46. Bullock MR, Chestnut R, Ghajar J: Surgical management of depressed cranial fractures. Neurosurgery (Suppl) 2006;58:S2-56–S2-60.
47. Wylen EL, Willis BK, Nanda A: Infection rate with replacement of bone fragment in compound depressed skull fractures. Surg Neurol 1999;51:452-457.
48. Jennett B, Miller J: Infection after depressed fracture of skull. Implications for management of nonmissile injuries. J Neurosurg 1972;36:333-339.
49. Mendelow AD, Campbell D, Tsementzis SA, et al: Prophylactic antimicrobial management of compound depressed skull fracture. J R Coll Surg Edinb 1983;28:80-83.
50. van den Heever CM, van der Merwe DJ: Management of depressed skull fractures. Selective conservative management of nonmissile injuries. J Neurosurg 1989;71:186-190.
51. Jennett B, Miller J, Braakman R: Epilepsy after nonmissile depressed skull fracture. J Neurosurg 1974;41:208-216.
52. Bricolo A, Pasut L: Extradural hematoma: Toward zero mortality. A prospective study. Neurosurgery 1984;14:8-12.
53. Cucciniello B, Martellotta N, Nigro D, Citro E: Conservative management of extradural haematomas. Acta Neurochir (Wien) 1993;120:47-52.
54. Kuday C, Uzan M, Hanci M: Statistical analysis of the factors affecting the outcome of extradural haematomas: 115 cases. Acta Neurochir (Wien) 1994;131:203-206.
55. Lee E, Hung Y, Wang L, et al: Factors influencing the functional outcome of patients with acute epidural hematomas: Analysis of 200 patients undergoing surgery. J Trauma 1998;45:946-952.
56. Meier U, Heinitz A, Kintzel D: Surgical outcome after severe craniocerebral trauma in childhood and adulthood. A comparative study [in German]. Unfallchirurg 1994;97:406-409.
57. Mohanty A, Kolluri V, Subbakrishna D, et al: Prognosis of extradural haematomas in children. Pediatr Neurosurg 1995;23:57-63.
58. Servadei F, Faccani G, Roccella P, et al: Asymptomatic extradural hematomas. Results of a multicenter study of 158 cases in minor head injury. Acta Neurochir (Wien) 1989;96:39-45.
59. Wester K: Decompressive surgery for "pure" epidural hematomas: Does neurosurgical expertise improve the outcome? Neurosurgery 1999;44:495-500.
60. Bullock RM, Chestnut R, Ghajar J, et al: Surgical management of acute epidural hematomas. Neurosurgery 2006;58(suppl):S2-7–S2-15.
61. Cohen J, Montero A, Israel Z: Prognosis and clinical relevance of anisocoria craniotomy latency for

epidural hematoma in comatose patients. J Trauma 1996;41:120-122.
62. Maggi G, Aliberti F, Petrone G, Ruggiero C: Extradural hematomas in children. J Neurosurg Sci 1998;42:95-99.
63. Paterniti S, Fiore P, Macri E, et al: Extradural haematoma. Report of 37 consecutive cases with survival. Acta Neurochir (Wien) 1994;131:207-210.
64. Rivas J, Lobato R, Sarabia R, et al: Extradural hematoma: Analysis of factors influencing the courses of 161 patients. Neurosurgery 1988;23:44-51.
65. Cordobes F, Lobato R, Rivas J, et al: Observations on 82 patients with extradural hematoma. Comparison of results before and after the advent of computerized tomography. J Neurosurg 1981;54:179-186.
66. Haselsberger K, Pucher R, Auer L: Prognosis after acute subdural or epidural haemorrhage. Acta Neurochir (Wien) 1988;90:111-116.
67. Jamjoom A: The influence of concomitant intradural pathology on the presentation and outcome of patients with acute traumatic extradural haematoma. Acta Neurochir (Wien) 1992;115:86-89.
68. Jamjoom A: The difference in the outcome of surgery for traumatic extradural hematoma between patients who are admitted directly to the neurosurgical unit and those referred from another hospital. Neurosurg Rev 1997;20:227-230.
69. Jones N, Molloy C, Kloeden C, et al: Extradural haematoma: Trends in outcome over 35 years. Br J Neurosurg 1993;7:465-471.
70. Sullivan T, Jarvik J, Cohen W: Follow-up of conservatively managed epidural hematomas: Implications for timing of repeat CT. AJNR Am J Neuroradiol 1999;20:107-113.
71. van den Brink WA, Zwienenberg M, Zandee SM, et al: The prognostic importance of the volume of traumatic epidural and subdural haematomas revisited. Acta Neurochir (Wien) 1999;141:509-514.
72. Otsuka S, Nakatsu S, Matsumoto S, et al: Study on cases with posterior fossa epidural hematoma: Clinical features and indications for operation. Neurol Med Chir (Tokyo) 1990;30:24-28.
73. Poon W, Li A: Comparison of management outcome of primary and secondary referred patients with traumatic extradural hematoma in a neurosurgical unit. Injury 1991;22:323-325.
74. Hunt J, Hill D, Besser M, et al: Outcome of patients with neurotrauma: The effect of a regionalized trauma system. Aust N Z J Surg 1995;65:83-86.
75. Pillay R, Peter J: Extradural haematomas in children. S Afr Med J 1995;85:672-674.
76. Lobato R, Cordobes F, Rivas J, et al: Outcome from severe head injury related to the type of intracranial lesion. A computerized tomography study. J Neurosurg 1983;59:762-774.
77. Seelig J, Marshall L, Toutant S, et al: Traumatic acute epidural hematoma: Unrecognized high lethality in comatose patients. Neurosurgery 1984;15:617-620.
78. Cook R, Dorsch N, Fearnside M, Chaseling R: Outcome prediction in extradural haematomas. Acta Neurochir (Wien) 1988;95:90-94.
79. Heinzelmann M, Platz A, Imhof H: Outcome after acute extradural haematoma, influence of additional injuries and neurological complications in the ICU. Injury 1996;27:345-349.
80. Sakas D, Bullock M, Teasdale G: One-year outcome following craniotomy or traumatic hematoma in patients with fixed dilated pupils. J Neurosurg 1995;82:961-965.
81. Gennarelli T, Spielman G, Langfitt T, et al: Influence of the type of intracranial lesion on outcome from severe head injury. J Neurosurg 1982;56:26-32.
82. Lobato R, Rivas J, Cordobes F, et al: Acute epidural hematoma: An analysis of factors influencing the outcome of patients undergoing surgery in coma. J Neurosurg 1988;68:48-57.
83. Uzan M, Yentur E, Hanci M, et al: Is it possible to recover from uncal herniation? Analysis of 71 head injured cases. J Neurosurg Sci 1998;42:89-94.
84. Bullock R, Smith R, van Dellen JR: Nonoperative management of extradural hematoma. Neurosurgery 1985;16:602-606.
85. Suzuki S, Endo M, Kurata A, et al: Efficacy of endovascular surgery for the treatment of acute epidural hematomas. Am J Neuroradiol 2004;25:1177-1180.
86. Gennarelli TA, Thibault LE: Biomechanics of acute subdural hematoma. J Trauma 1982;22:680-686.
87. Drake CG: Subdural hematoma from arterial rupture. J Neurosurg 1961;8:597.
88. Shenkin HA: Acute subdural hematoma: Review of 39 consecutive cases with high incidence of cortical artery rupture. J Neurosurg 1982;57:254-257.
89. Cooper PR: Post-traumatic intracranial mass lesions. In Cooper PR, Golfinos JG (eds): Head Injury, 4th ed. New York, McGraw-Hill, 2000, pp 293-348.
90. Ersahin Y, Mutluer S: Posterior fossa extradural hematomas in children. Pediatr Neurosurg 1993;19:31-33.
91. Seelig J, Becker D, Miller J, et al: Traumatic acute subdural hematoma: Major mortality reduction in comatose patients treated within four hours. N Engl J Med 1981;304:1511-1518.
92. Servadei F, Nasi M, Cremonini A, et al: Importance of a reliable admission Glasgow Coma Scale score for determining the need for evacuation of posttraumatic subdural hematomas: A prospective study of 65 patients. J Trauma 1998;44:868-873.
93. Wilberger JJ, Harris M, Diamond D: Acute subdural hematoma: Morbidity, mortality, and operative timing. J Neurosurg 1991;74:212-218.
94. Dent D, Croce M, Menke P, et al: Prognostic factors after acute subdural hematoma. J Trauma 1995;39:36-42.
95. Gabl M, Mohsenipour I, Benedetto K: Acute posttraumatic subdural hematoma in advanced age [in German]. Unfallchirurgie 1989;15:273-278.
96. Koc R, Akdemir H, Oktem I, et al: Acute subdural hematoma: Outcome and outcome prediction. Neurosurg Rev 1997;20:239-244.
97. Massaro F, Lanotte M, Faccani G, Triolo C: One hundred and twenty-seven cases of acute subdural haematoma operated on. Correlation between CT scan findings and outcome. Acta Neurochir (Wien) 1996;138:185-191.
98. Howard MA 3rd, Gross AS, Dacey RJ Jr, Winn HR: Acute subdural hematomas: An age-dependent clinical entity. J Neurosurg 1989;71:858-863.
99. Cagetti B, Cossu M, Pau A, et al: The outcome from acute subdural and epidural intracranial haematomas in very elderly patients. Br J Neurosurg 1992;6:227-231.
100. Jamjoom A: Justification for evacuating acute subdural haematomas in patients above the age of 75 years. Injury 1992;23:518-520.
101. Kotwica Z, Brzezinski J: Acute subdural haematoma in adults: An analysis of outcome in comatose patients. Acta Neurochir (Wien) 1993;121:95-99.
102. Servadei F, Nasi M, Giuliani G, et al: CT prognostic factors in acute subdural haematomas: The value of the "worst" CT scan. Br J Neurosurg 2000;14:110-116.
103. Fell D, Fitzgerald S, Moiel R, Caram P: Acute subdural hematomas. Review of 144 cases. J Neurosurg 1975;42:37-42.
104. Hatashita S, Koga N, Hosaka Y, Takagi S: Acute subdural hematoma: Severity of injury, surgical intervention, and mortality. Neurol Med Chir (Tokyo) 1993;33:13-18.
105. Zumkeller M, Behrmann R, Heissler H, Dietz H: Computed tomographic criteria and survival rate for patients with acute subdural hematoma. Neurosurgery 1996;39:708-712.
106. Domenicucci M, Strzelecki J, Delfini R: Acute posttraumatic subdural hematomas: "Intradural" computed tomographic appearance as a favorable prognostic factor. Neurosurgery 1998;42:51-55.
107. Jamieson KG, Yelland JDN: Surgically treated traumatic subdural hematomas. J Neurosurg 1972;37:137-149.
108. Stone JL, Rifai MHS, Sugar O, et al: Subdural hematomas. I. Acute subdural hematomas: Progress in definition, clinical pathology, and therapy. Surg Neurol 1983;19:216-231.
109. Miller JD, Bullock R, Graham DJ, et al: Ischemic brain damage in a model of acute subdural hematoma. Neurosurgery 1990;27:433-439.
110. Yilmazlar S, Kuday C, Oz B, et al: Blood degradation products play a role in cerebral ischemia caused by acute subdural hematoma. J Neurosurg Sci 1997;41:379-385.
111. Brain Trauma Foundation: Early indicators of prognosis in severe traumatic brain injury. J Neurotrauma 2000;17:535-627.
112. Kotwica Z, Jakubowski J: Acute head injuries in the elderly. An analysis of 136 consecutive patients. Acta Neurochir (Wien) 1992;118:98-102.
113. Chieregato A, Fainardi E, Morselli-Labate AM, et al: Factors associated with neurological outcome and lesion

progression in traumatic subarachnoid hemorrhage. Neurosurgery 2005;56:671-680.
114. Britt PM, Heiserman JE: Imaging evaluation. In Cooper PR, Golfinos JG (eds): Head Injury, 4th ed. New York, McGraw-Hill, 2000, pp 361-396.
115. Chandler JP, Batjer HH, Kuznits S, et al: Intracranial and cervical vascular injuries. In Cooper PR, Golfinos JG (eds): Head Injury, 4th ed. New York, McGraw-Hill, 2000, pp 361-396.
116. Sander D, Kligelhofer J: Cerebral vasospasm following post-traumatic subarachnoid hemorrhage evaluated by transcranial Doppler ultrasonography. J Neurol Sci 1993;11:1.
117. Marshall LF, Bruce DA, Bruno L, et al: Vertebrobasilar spasm: A significant cause of neurologic deficit in head injury. J Neurosurg 1978;48:560-564.
118. Greene KA, Jacobawitz R, Marciano FF, et al: Impact of traumatic subarachnoid hemorrhage on outcome in nonpenetrating head injury. Part II: Relationship to clinical course and outcome variables during acute hospitalization. J Trauma 1996;41:964-971.
119. Greene KA, Marciano FF, Johnson BA, et al: Impact of traumatic subarachnoid hemorrhage on outcome in nonpenetrating head injury. Part I: A proposed computerized tomography grading scale. J Neurosurg 1995;83:445-452.
120. Kakarieka A: Review of traumatic subarachnoid hemorrhage. Neurol Res 1997;19:230-232.
121. Bullock R, Golek J, Blake G: Traumatic intracerebral hematoma: Which patients should undergo surgical evacuation? CT scan features and ICP monitoring as a basis for decision making. Surg Neurol 1989;32: 181-187.
122. Lobato RD, Gomez PA, Alday R, et al: Sequential computerized tomography changes and related final outcome in severe head injury patients. Acta Neurochir (Wien) 1997;139:385-391.
123. Miller JD, Butterworth JF, Gudeman SK, et al: Further experience in the management of severe head injury. J Neurosurg 1981;54:289-299.
124. Nordstrom C, Messeter K, Sundbarg G, Wahlander S: Severe traumatic brain lesions in Sweden. Part I: Aspects of management in non-neurosurgical clinics. Brain Inj 1989;3:247-265.
125. Singounas E: Severe head injury in a paediatric population. J Neurosurg Sci 1992;36:201-206.
126. Soloniuk D, Pitts LH, Lovely M, Bartkowski H: Traumatic intracerebral hematomas: Timing of appearance and indications for operative removal. J Trauma 1986;26:787-794.
127. Bullock RM, Chestnut R, Ghajar J, et al: Surgical management of traumatic parenchymal lesions. Neurosurgery 2006;58(suppl):S2-25–S2-46.
128. Schonauer M, Schisano G, Cimino R, et al: Space occupying contusions of cerebral lobes after closed brain injury: Considerations about 51 cases. J Neurosurg Sci 1979;23:279-288.
129. Evans JP, Scheinker IM: Histological studies of the brain following head trauama. II. Post-traumatic petechial and massive intracerebral hemorrhage. J Neurosurg 1946;3:101-113.
130. Graham DI, Gennarelli: Pathology of brain damage after head injury. In Cooper PR, Golfinos JG (eds): Head Injury, 4th ed. New York, McGraw-Hill, 2000, pp 134-153.
131. Adams JH, Graham DI, Genuarelli TA: Contemporary neuropathological considerations regarding brain damage after head injury. In Becker DP, Povlishock JT (eds): Central Nervous System Trauma: Status Report. National Institute of Neurological and Communicative Disorders and Stroke, National Institutes of Health, Bethesda, MD, 1985.
132. Ribas G, Jane JA: Traumatic contusions and intracerebral hematomas. J Neurotrauma 1992;9(suppl 1):S265.
133. Servadei F, Murray GD, Penny K, et al: The value of the "worst" computed tomographic scan in clinical studies of moderate and severe head injury. European Brain Injury Consortium. Neurosurgery 2000;46:70-75.
134. Servadei F, Nanni A, Nasi M, et al: Evolving brain lesions in the first 12 hours after head injury: Analysis of 37 comatose patients. Neurosurgery 1995;37:899-906.
135. Chang EF, Meeker M, Holland MC: Acute traumatic intraparenchymal hemorrhage: Risk factors for progression in the early post-injury period. Neurosurgery 2006;58:647-656.
136. Adams JH, Graham DI, Gennarelli TA: Neuropathology of acceleration induced head injury in the subhuman primate. In Grossman RG, Gildenberg PL (eds): Head Injury: Basic Clinical Aspects. New York, Raven Press, 1992.
137. Courville CB: Coup-contrecoup mechanism of craniocerebral injuries-some observations, Arch Surg 1942;4:19.
138. Ommaya AK, Grubb RL, Nauman RA: Coup and contrecoup injury: Observations on the mechanics of visible brain injuries in the rhesus monkey, J Neurosurg 1971;35:305.
139. Gennarelli TA, Thibault LE: Biomechanics of head injury. In Wilkins RH, Rengachary SS (eds): Neurosurgery. New York, McGraw-Hill, 1985, pp 1531-1536.
140. Daniel PM, Treip CS: The pathology of the pituitary gland in head injury. In Gardner-Hill H (ed): Modern Trends in Endocrinology. London, Butterworth, 1961.
141. Crompton MR: Hypothalamic and pituitary lesions. In Vinken PJ, Bruyn GN (eds): Handbook of Clinical Neurology. Injuries of the Brain and Skull, part I. Amsterdam, North-Holland, 1975.
142. Landau H, Adin I, Spitz IM: Pituitary insufficiency following head injury. Israel J Med Sci 1978;14:785.
143. Edwards OM, Clark JDA: Post-traumatic hypopituitarism. Six cases and a review of the literature. Medicine 1986;65:281.
144. Blumbergs PC, Jones NR, Nath JB: Diffuse axonal injury in head trauma. J Neurol Neurosurg Psychiatry 1989;52:838.
145. Gennarelli TA, Thibault LE, Adams JH, et al: Diffuse axonal injury and traumatic coma in the primate. Ann Neurol 1982;12:564.
146. Levi L, Guilburd, Lemberger A, et al: Diffuse axonal injury: Analysis of 100 patients with radiological signs. Neurosurgery 1990;27:429.
147. Gennarelli TA: Head injury in man and experimental animals—clinical aspects. Acta Neuroclin 1983;32(suppl):1.
148. Lindenberg R, Freytag E: A mechanism of cerebral contusions: A pathologic anatomic study. Arch Pathol 1960;69:440.
149. Michaud LJ, Rivara FP, Grady MS, et al: Predictors of survival and severity of disability after severe brain injury in children. Neurosurgery 1992;31:254.
150. Sosin DM, Sacks JJ, Smith SM: Head injury associated deaths in the United States from 1979 to 1986. JAMA 1989;262:2251-2255.
151. Wintemute GJ: The relationship between firearm design and firearm violence: Handguns in the 1990's. JAMA 1996;275:1749-1753.
152. Harrington T, Apostolides P: Penetrating brain injury. In Cooper PR, Golfinos JG (eds): Head Injury, 4th ed. New York, McGraw-Hill, 2000, pp 349-359.
153. Roth J, Mayo A, Elran H, Razon N, et al: Brain injuries caused by spherical bolts. J Neurosurg 2005;102:864-869.
154. Allen IV, Scott R, Tanner JA: Experimental high-velocity missile head injury. Injury 1982;14:183-193.
155. Jahrsdoerfer RA, Johns ME, Cantrell RW: Penetrating wounds of the head and neck. Arch Otolaryngol 1979;105:721-725.
156. Marion DW (ed): Traumatic Brain Injury. New York, Thieme Medical Publishers, 1999.
157. Fackler ML: Wound ballistics. A review of common misconceptions. JAMA 1988;259:2730-2736.
158. Mendelson JA: The relationship between mechanisms of wounding and principles of treatment of missile wounds. J Trauma 1991;31:1181-1202.
159. Lindsey D: The idolatry of velocity, or lies, damn lies, and ballistics. J Trauma 1980;20:1068-1069.
160. Carey ME, Sarna GS, Farrell JB: Experimental missile wound to the brain. J Neurosurg 1989;71:754-764.
161. Cushing H: A study of a series of wounds involving the brain and its enveloping structures. Br J Surg 1918;5:558-684.
162. Walters BC, Aarabi B, Chestnut RM, et al: Methodology for development of guidelines for the management of penetrating brain injury. J Trauma 2001;51:S16-S25.
163. Levi L, Borovich B, Guilburd JL, et al: Wartime neurosurgical experience in Lebanon, 1982-85, I: Penetrating craniocerebral injuries. Isr J Med Sci 1990;26:548-554.
164. Levi L, Borovich B, Guilburd JL, et al: Wartime neurosurgical experience in Lebanon, 1982-85. II: Penetrating craniocerebral injuries. Isr J Med Sci 1990;26:555-558.
165. Aarabi B: Surgical outcome in 435 patients who sustained missile head

wounds during the Iran-Iraq war. Neurosurgery 1990;27:692-695.
166. Ameen A: The management of acute craniocerebral injuries caused by missiles: Analysis of 110 consecutive penetrating wounds of the brain from Basrah. Injury 1984;16:88-90.
167. Brandvold B, Levi L, Feinsod M, George ED: Penetrating craniocerebral injuries in the Israeli involvement in the Lebanese conflict, 1982-85. J Neurosurg 1990;72:15-21.
168. Carey ME, Young HF, Mathis JL: The neurosurgical treatment of craniocerebral missile wounds in Vietnam. Surg Gynecol Obstet 1972;135:386-390.
169. Gonul E, Baysefer A, Kahraman S, et al: Causes of infections and management results in penetrating craniocerebral injuries. Neurosurg Rev 1997;20:177-181.
170. Hammon WM, Kempe LG: Analysis of 2187 consecutive penetrating wounds of the brain from Vietnam. J Neurosurg 1971;34:127-131.
171. Taha JM, Haddad FS, Brown JA: Intracranial infection after missile injuries to the brain: Report of 30 cases from the Lebanese conflict. Neurosurgery 1991;29:864-868.
172. Carey ME, Young HF, Rish BL, Mathis JL: Follow-up study of 103 American soldiers who sustained a brain wound in Vietnam. J Neurosurg 1974;41:542-549.
173. Rosegay H: Craniocerebral injuries. In Ravitch MM (ed): Current Problems in Surgery: Military Surgical Practices of the United States Army in Vietnam. Chicago: Year Book Medical Publishers, 1966.
174. Chaudhri KA, Choudhury AR, al Moutaery KR, Cybulski GR: Penetrating craniocerebral shrapnel injuries during "Operation Desert Storm": Early results of a conservative surgical treatment. Acta Neurochir (Wien) 1994;126:120-123.
175. Martin J, Campbell EH: Early complications following penetrating wounds of the skull. J Neurosurg 1946;2:58-73.
176. Aarabi B, Taghipour M, Alibaii E, Kamgarpour A: Central nervous system infections after military missile head wounds. Neurosurgery 1998;42:500-509.
177. Caveness WF, Walker AE, Ashcroft PB, et al: Incidence of posttraumatic epilepsy in Korean veterans as compared with those from World War I and World War II. J Neurosurg 1962;19:122-129.
178. Salazar AM, Jabbari B, Vance SC, et al: Epilepsy after penetrating head injury, I: Clinical correlates—a report of the Vietnam Head Injury Study. Neurology 1985;35:1406-1414.
179. Rish BL, Caveness WF, Dillon JD, et al: Analysis of brain abscess after penetrating craniocerebral injuries in Vietnam. Neurosurgery 1981;9: 535-541.
180. Aarabi B: Comparative study of bacteriological contamination between primary and secondary exploration of missile head wounds. Neurosurgery 1987;20:610-616.
181. Nagib MG, Rockswold GL, Sherman RS, Lagaard MW: Civilian gunshot wounds to the brain: Prognosis and management. Neurosurgery 1986;18:533-537.
182. Suddaby L, Weir B, Forsyth C: The management of .22 caliber gunshot wounds of the brain: A review of 49 cases. Can J Neurol Sci 1987;14:268-272.
183. Byrnes DP, Crockard HA, Gordon DS, Gleadhill CA: Penetrating craniocerebral missile injuries in the civil disturbances in Northern Ireland. Br J Surg 1974;61:169-176.
184. Kim KA, Wang MY, McNatt SA, et al: Vector analysis correlating bullet trajectory to outcome after civilian through-and-through gunshot wound to the head: Using imaging cues to predict fatal outcome. Neurosurgery 2005;57:737-747.
185. Aarabi B: Management of traumatic aneurysms caused by high velocity missile head wounds. Neurosurg Clin North Am 1995;6:775-797.
186. Aldrich EF, Eisenberg HM, Saydjari C, et al: Predictors of mortality in severely head-injured patients with civilian gunshot wound: A report from the NIH Traumatic Coma Data Bank. Surg Neurol 1992;38:418-423.
187. Levy ML, Rezai A, Masri LS, et al: The significance of subarachnoid hemorrhage after penetrating craniocerebral injury: Correlations with angiography and outcome in civilian population. Neurosurgery 1993;32:532-540.
188. Aarabi B: Traumatic aneurysms of brain due to high velocity missile head wounds. Neurosurgery 1988;22:1056-1063.
189. Haddad FS, Haddad GF, Taha J: Traumatic intracranial aneurysms caused by missiles: Their presentation and management. Neurosurgery 1997;28:1-7.
190. Amirjamshidi A, Rahmat H, Abbassioun K: Traumatic aneurysms and arteriovenous fistulas of intracranial vessels associated with penetrating head injuries occurring during war: Principles and pitfalls in diagnosis and management—a survey of 31 cases and review of the literature. J Neurosurg 1996;84:769-780.
191. Jinkins JR, Dadsetan MR, Sener RN, et al: Value of acute-phase angiography in the detection of vascular injuries caused by gunshot wounds to the head: Analysis of 12 cases. AJR Am J Roentgenol 1992;159:365-368.
192. Crockard HA: Early intracranial pressure studies in gunshot wounds of the brain. J Trauma. 1975;15:339-347.
193. Lillard PL: Five years experience with penetrating craniocerebral gunshot wounds. Surg Neurol 1978;9:79-83.
194. Sarnaik AP, Kopec J, Moylan P, et al: Role of aggressive intracranial pressure control in management of pediatric craniocerebral gunshot wounds with unfavorable features. J Trauma 1989;29:1434-1437.
195. Miner ME, Ewing-Cobbs L, Kopaniky DR, et al: The results of treatment of gunshot wounds to the brain in children. Neurosurgery 1990;26:20-25.
196. Guidelines for the management of severe traumatic brain injury. Brain Trauma Foundation, American Association of Neurological Surgeons, Joint Section on Neurotrauma and Critical Care. J Neurotrauma 2000;17:451-627.
197. Harrington T, Apostolides P: Penetrating brain injury. In Cooper PR, Golfinos JG (eds): Head Injury, 4th ed. New York, McGraw-Hill, 2000, pp 349-359.
198. Marmarou A, Signoretti S, Fatouros PP, et al: Predominance of cellular edema in traumatic brain swelling in patients with severe head injuries. J Neurosurg 2000;104:720-730.
199. The Brain Trauma Foundation, The American Association of Neurological Surgeons, The Congress of Neurological Surgeons The Joint Section on Neurotrauma and Critical Care: Update notice, guidelines for the management of severe traumatic brain injury: cerebral perfusion pressure. New York, The Brain Trauma Foundation, copyright 2000. Updated CPP Guidelines approved by the AANS on March 14, 2003.
200. Rosner MJ, Coley IB: Cerebral perfusion pressure, intracranial pressure, and head elevation. J Neurosurg 1986;65:636-641.
201. Bouma GJ, Muizelaar JP: Relationship between cardiac output and cerebral blood flow in patients with intact and with impaired autoregulation. J Neurosurg 1990;73:368-374.
202. Bruce DA, Langfitt TW, Miller JD, et al: Regional cerebral blood flow, intracranial pressure, and brain metabolism in comatose patients. J Neurosurg 1973;38:131-144.
203. Hoff JT: Cerebral perfusion pressure, autoregulation and the PVI reflection point. In Betz AL (ed): Intracranial Pressure VII. Berlin, Springer-Verlag, 1988, pp 829-833.
204. Fortune JB, Feustel PJ, Weigle CGM, et al: Continuous measurement of jugular venous oxygen saturation in response to transient elevations of blood pressure in head-injured patients. J Neurosurg 1994;80:461-468.
205. The Brain Trauma Foundation, The American Association of Neurological Surgeons, The Congress of Neurological Surgeons The Joint Section on Neurotrauma and Critical Care: Guidelines for cerebral perfusion pressure. New York, The Brain Trauma Foundation, copyright 1995, pp 8-1–8-10.
206. Rosner MJ, Rosner SD, Johnson AH: Cerebral perfusion pressure: Management protocol and clinical results. J Neurosurg 1995;83:949-962.
207. Clifton GL, Allen S, Barrodale P, et al: A phase II study of moderate hypothermia in severe brain injury. J Neurotrauma 1993;10:263-271.
208. Marion DW, Penrod LE, Kelsey SF, et al: Treatment of traumatic brain injury with moderate hypothermia. N Engl J Med 1997;336:540-546.
209. Rosner MJ, Daughton S: Cerebral perfusion pressure management in head injury. J Trauma 1990;30: 933-941.
210. Yoshida A, Shima T, Okada Y, et al: Outcome of patients with severe head injury—evaluation by cerebral perfusion pressure. In Nakamura N,

Hashimoto T, Yasue M (eds): Recent Advances in Neurotraumatology. Hong Kong, Springer-Verlag, 1993, pp 309-312.
211. Marshall LF, Gautille T, Klauber MR, et al: The outcome of severe closed head injury. J Neurosurg 1991;75:S28-S36.
212. Kiening KL, Hartl R, Unterberg AW, et al: Brain tissue pO_2-monitoring in comatose patients: implications for therapy. Neurol Res 1997;19:233-240.
213. Robertson CS, Valadka AB, Hannay HJ, et al: Prevention of secondary ischemic insults after severe head injury. Crit Care Med 1999;27:2086-2095.
214. Contant CF, Valadka AB, Gopinath SP, et al: Adult respiratory distress syndrome: A complication of induced hypertension after severe head injury. J Neurosurg 2001;95:560-568.
215. Bratton SL, Davis RL: Acute lung injury in isolated traumatic brain injury. Neurosurgery 1997;40:707-712.
216. Juul N, Morris GF, Marshall SB, et al: Intracranial hypertension and cerebral perfusion pressure: Influence on neurological deterioration and outcome in severe head injury. The Executive Committee of the International Selfotel Trial. J Neurosurg 2000;92:106.
217. Martin NA, Patwardhan RV, Alexander MJ, et al: Characterization of cerebral hemodynamic phases following severe head trauma: Hypoperfusion, hyperemia, and vasospasm. J Neurosurg 1997;87:9-19.
218. Chestnut RM, Marshall LF, Klauber MR, et al: The role of secondary brain injury in determining outcome from severe head injury. J Trauma 1993;34:216-222.
219. Stocchetti N, Furlan A, Volta F: Hypoxemia and arterial hypotension at the accident scene in head injury. J Trauma 1996;40:764-767.
220. Bouma GJ, Muizelaar JP, Choi PG, et al: Cerebral circulation and metabolism after severe traumatic brain injury: The elusive role of ischemia. J Neurosurg 1991;75:685-693.
221. Vigue B, Ract C, Benayed M, et al: Early $SjvO_2$ monitoring in patients with severe brain trauma. Intensive Care Med 1999;25:445-451.
222. Eker C, Asgeirsson B, Grande PO, et al: Improved outcome after severe head injury with a new therapy based on principles for brain volume regulation and preserved microcirculation. Crit Care Med 1998;26:1881-1886.
223. Schroder ML, Muizelaar JP, Kuta AJ, et al: Thresholds for cerebral ischemia after severe head injury: Relationship with late CT findings and outcome. J Neurotrauma 1996;13:17-23.
224. Bouma GJ, Muizelaar JP, Stringer WA, et al: Ultraearly evaluation of regional cerebral blood flow in severely head-injured patients using xenon-enhanced computerized tomography. J. Neurosurg 1992;77:360-368.
225. Carmona Suazo JA, Maas AI, van den Brink WA, et al: CO_2 reactivity and brain oxygen pressure monitoring in severe head injury. Crit Care Med 2000;28:3268-3274.
226. Dings J, Meixensberger J, Amschler J, et al: Brain tissue PO_2 in relation to cerebral perfusion pressure, TCD findings and TCD-CO_2 reactivity after severe head injury. Acta Neurochir (Wien) 1996;138:425-434.
227. KL, Sarrafzadeh AS, Stover JF, Unterberg AW: Should I monitor brain tissue PO_2? In Valadka AB, Andrews BT (eds): Neurotrauma. New York, Thieme Medical Publishers, 2005, pp 62-67.
228. Imberti R, Bellinzona G, Langer M: Cerebral tissue PO_2 and $SjvO_2$ changes during moderate hyperventilation in patients with severe traumatic brain injury. J Neurosurg 2002;96:97-102.
229. Zhi DS, Zhang S, Zhou LG: Continuous monitoring of brain tissue oxygen pressure in patients with severe head injury during moderate hypothermia. Surg Neurol 1999;52:393-396.
230. Dings J, Meixensberger J, Amschler J, et al: Continuous monitoring of brain tissue PO_2: A new tool to minimize the risk of ischemia caused by hyperventilation therapy. Zentralbl Neurochir 1996;57:177-183.
231. Schneider GH, Sarrafzadeh AS, Kiening KL, et al: Influence of hyperventilation on brain tissue PO_2, PCO_2, and pH in patients with intracranial hypertension. Acta Neurochir Suppl (Wien) 1998;71:62-65.
232. Unterberg AW, Kiening KL, Hartl R, et al: Multimodal monitoring in patients with head injury: Evaluation of the effects of treatment on cerebral oxygenation. J Trauma 1997;42: S32-S37.
233. Muizelaar JP, Marmarou A, Ward JD, et al: Adverse effects of prolonged hyperventilation in patients with severe head injury: A randomized clinical trial. J. Neurosurg 1991;75:731-739.
234. Brain Trauma Foundation, American Association of Neurological Surgeons, Joint Section on Neurotrauma and Critical Care: Management and prognosis of severe traumatic brain injury: Part I: Guidelines for the management of severe traumatic brain injury. New York, Brain Trauma Foundation, 2000, pp 105-118.
235. Alderson P, Gadkary C, Signorini DF: Therapeutic hypothermia for head injury. Update of Cochrane Database Syst Rev 2002(1);CD001048. Cochrane Database Syst Rev 2004(4);CD001048.
236. Clifton GL, Miller ER, Choi SC, et al: Lack of effect of induction of hypothermia after acute brain injury. N Engl J Med 2001;344:556-563.
237. Clifton GL: Is keeping cool still hot? An update on hypothermia in brain injury. Curr Opin Crit Care 2004;10:116-119.
238. Guy L, Ludbrook GL: Sedation and anesthesia. In Reilly P, Bullock R (eds): Head Injury. London, Chapman & Hall, 1997, pp 364-383.
239. Kee DB, Wood JH: Rheology of the cerebral circulation. Neurosurgery 1984;15:125-131.
240. Korosue K, Heros RC: Mechanism of cerebral blood flow augmentation by hemodilution in rabbits. Stroke 1992;23:1487-1492.
241. Muizelaar JP, Wei EP, Kontos HA, et al: Cerebral blood flow is regulated by changes in blood pressure and blood viscosity. Stroke 1986;17:44-48.
242. Muizelaar JP, Wei EP, Kontos HA, Becker DP: Mannitol causes compensatory cerebral vasoconstriction and vasodilation in response to blood viscosity changes. J Neurosurg 1983;59:822-828.
243. Deutsch H, Ullman JS: What is the optimal hematocrit and hemoglobin for head injured patients? In Valadka AB, Andrews BT (eds): Neurotrauma. New York, Thieme Medical Publishers, 2005, pp 88-90.
244. Klatzo I: Evolution of brain edema concepts. Acta Neurochir Suppl 1994;60:3-6.
245. Rosener MJ: Pathophysiology and management of increased intracranial pressure. In Andrews BT (ed): Neurosurgical Intensive Care. San Francisco, McGraw-Hill, 1993, pp 57-112.
246. Aarabi B, Hesdorffer D, Ahn E, et al: Outcome following decompressive cranietomy for malignant swelling due to severe head injury. J Neurosurg 2006;104:469-479.
247. Bergsneider M, Wu C, Huang H, et al: Early abnormalities of regional brain metabolism following human traumatic brain injury: FDG and O-15 PET studies of hyperglycolysis, metabolic depression and ischemia. Paper presented at the American Association of Neurolgical Surgeons Annual Meeting, April 16-21, 2005, New Orleans.
248. Cruz J, Jaggi JL, Hoffstad OJ: Cerebral blood flow, vascular resistance, and oxygen metabolism in acute brain trauma: Redefining the role of cerebral perfusion pressure? Crit Care Med 1995;23:142-1417.
249. Marmarou A: Pathohysiology of traumatic brain edema: Current concepts. Acta Neurochir Suppl 2003;86:7-10.
250. Marmarou A, Fatouros PP, Barzo P, et al: Contribution of edema and cerebral blood volume to traumatic brain swelling in head injured patients. J Neurosurg 2000;93:183-193.
251. Robertson CS, Gopinath Sp, Uzura M, et al: Metabolic changes in the brain during transient ischemia measured with microdialysis. Neurol Res 1998;20(Suppl 1):S91-S94.
252. Verweij BH, Muizelaar JP, Vinas FC, et al: Impaired cerebral mitochondrial function after traumatic brain injury in humans. J Neurosurg 2000;93: 815-820.
253. Zauner A, Daugherty WP, Bullock MR, Warner DS: Brain oxygenation and energy metabolism: Part 1—biological function and pathophysiology. Neurosurgery 2002;51:289-302.
254. Langfitt TW: Etiology and management of acute brain swelling. W V Med J 1966;62:49.
255. Langfitt TW, Marshall WJ, Kassell NF, Schutta HS: The pathophysiology of brain swelling produced by mechanical trauma and hypertension. Scand J Clin Lab Invest Suppl 1968;102:xiv.
256. Langfitt TW, Tannanbaum HM, Kassell NF: The etiology of acute brain swelling following experimental brain injury. J Neurosurg 1966;24:47-56.

257. Langfitt TW, Weinstein JD, Kassell, NF: Cerebral vasomotor paralysis as a cause of brain swelling. Trans Am Neurol Assoc 1964:89:214-215.
258. Langfitt TW, Weinstein JD, Sklar FH, et al: Contribution of intracranial blood volume to three forms of experimental brain swelling. Johns Hopkins Med J 1968;122:261-270.
259. Kita H, Marmarou A: The cause of acute brain swelling after the closed head injury in rats. Acta Neurochir Suppl (Wien) 1994;60:452-455.
260. Barzo P, Marmarou A, Fatouros P, et al: Magnetic resonance imaging–monitored acute blood-brain barrier changes in experimental traumatic brain injury. J Neurosurg 1996;85:1113-1121.
261. Barzo P, Marmarou A, Fatouros P, et al: Contribution of vasogenic and cellular edema to traumatic brain swelling measured by diffusion weighted-imaging. J Neurosurg 1997;87:900-907.
262. Stroop R, Thomale UW, Pauser S, et al: Magnetic resonance imaging studies with cluster algorithm for characterization of brain edema after controlled cortical impact (CCII). Acta Neurochir Suppl 1998;71:303-305.
263. Marshall LF, Smith RW, Rauscher LA, et al: Mannitol dose requirements in brain-injured patients. J Neurosurg 1978;48:169-172.
264. Nath F, Galbraith S: The effect of mannitol on cerbral white matter water content. J Neurosurg 1986;65:41-43.
265. Burke AM, Quest DO, Chien S, et al: The effects of mannitol on blood viscosity. J Neurosurg 1981;55:550-553.
266. Rosner MJ, Coley I: Cerebral perfusion pressure: A hemodynamic mechanism of mannitol and the postmannitol hemogram. Neurosurgery 1987;21:147-156.
267. Bruce DA, Langfitt TW, Miller JD, et al: Regional cerebral blood flow, intracranial pressure, and brain metabolism in comatose patients. J Neurosurg 1973;38:131-144.
268. Muizelaar JP, Lutz HA III, Becker DP: Effect of mannitol on ICP and CBF and correlation with pressure autoregulation in severely head-injured patients. J Neurosurg 1984;61:700-706.
269. Cruz J, Minoja G, Okuchi K: Improving clinical outcomes from acute subdural hematomas with the emergency preoperative administration of high doses of mannitol: A randomized trial. Neurosurgery 2001;49:864-871.
270. Cruz J, Minoja G, Okuchi K: Major clinical and physiological benefits of early high doses of mannitol for intraparenchymal temporal lobe hemorrhages with abnormal pupillary widening: A randomized trial. Neurosurgery 2002;51:628-638.
271. Schrot RJ, Muizelaar JP: Is there a "best" way to give mannitol? In Valadka AB, Andrews BT (eds): Neurotrauma. New York, Thieme, 2005, pp 142-147.
272. Mendelow AD, ZTeasdale GM, Russell T, et al: Effect of mannitol on cerebral blood flow and cerebral perfusion pressure in human head injury. J Neurosurg 1985;63:43-48.
273. Kaufmann AM, Cardoso ER: Aggravation of vasogenic cerebral edema by multiple-dose mannitol. J Neurosurg 1992;77:584-589.
274. Chestnut RM: Medical management of intracranial pressure. In Cooper PR, Golfinos JG (eds): Head Injury, 4th ed. New York, McGraw-Hill, 2000, pp 229-263.
275. Becker D, Vries J: The alleviation of increased intracranial pressure by the chronic administration of osmotic agents. In Brock M, Dietz H (eds): Intracranial Pressure. Berlin, Springer-Verlag, 1972, pp 309-315.
276. Dorman HR, Sondheimer JH, Cadnapaphornchai P: Mannitol induced acute renal failure. Medicine (Baltimore) 1990;69:153-159.
277. Wilberger JE: Emergency care and initial evaluation. In Cooper PR, Golfinos JG (eds): Head Injury, 4th ed. New York, McGraw-Hill, 2000, pp 27-40.
278. Maas A: Effects of 23.4% sodium chloride solution in reducing intracranial pressure in patients with traumatic brain injury: A preliminary study. Neurosurgery 2005;57:736 (Comment).
279. U.S. National Institutes of Health: Rehabilitation of persons with traumatic brain injury: NIH Consensus Statement 1998. Available at: http://consensus.nih.gov/cons/109/109_intro.htm (accessed on July 31, 2006).
280. Bullock RM, Chesnut RM, Clifton GL, et al: Management and prognosis of severe traumatic brain injury. J Neurotrauma 2000;17:449-553.
281. Bitterman H, Triolo J, Lefer AM: Use of hypertonic saline in the treatment of hemorrhagic shock. Circ Shock 1987;21:271-283.
282. de Felippe J Jr, Timoner J, Velasco IT, et al: Treatment of refractory hypovolaemic shock by 7.5% sodium chloride injections. Lancet 1980;2:1002-1004.
283. Kreimeier U, Bruckner UB, Niemczyk S, Messmer K: Hyperosmotic saline dextran for resuscitation from traumatic-hemorrhagic hypotension: Effect on regional blood flow. Circ Shock 1990;32:83-99.
284. Nakayama S, Sibley L, Gunther RA, et al: Small-volume resuscitation with hypertonic saline (2,400 mOsm/liter) during hemorrhagic shock. Circ Shock 1984;13:149-159.
285. Cooper DJ, Myles PS, McDermott FT, et al: Prehospital hypertonic saline resuscitation of patients with hypotension and severe traumatic brain injury: A randomized controlled trial. JAMA 2004;291:1350-1357.
286. Miller JD, Becker DP, Ward JD, et al: Significance of intracranial hypertension in severe head injury. J Neurosurg 1977;47:503-516.
287. Velasco IT, Pontieri V, Rocha e Silva M Jr, Lopes OU: Hyperosmotic NaCl and severe hemorrhagic shock. Am J Physiol 1980;239:664-673.
288. Mazzoni MC, Borgstrom P, Arfors KE, Intaglietta M: Dynamic fluid redistribution in hyperosmotic resuscitation of hypovolemic hemorrhage. Am J Physiol 1988;255: H629-H637.
289. Messmer K, Kreimeier U: Microcirculatory therapy in shock. Resuscitation 1989;18(suppl): 51-61.
290. Maningas PA: Resuscitation with 7.5% NaCl in 6% dextran-70 during hemorrhagic shock in swine: Effects on organ blood flow. Crit Care Med 1987;15:1121-1126.
291. Gemma M, Cozzi S, Tommasino C, et al: 7.5% hypertonic saline versus 20% mannitol during elective neurosurgical supratentorial procedures. J Neurosurg Anesthesiol 1979;9:329-334.
292. Munar F, Ferrer AM, de Nadal M, et al: Cerebral hemodynamic effects of 7.2% hypertonic saline in patients with head injury and raised intracranial pressure. J Neurotrauma 2000;17:41-51.
293. De Vivo P, Del Gaudio A, Ciritella P, et al: Hypertonic saline solution: A safe alternative to mannitol 18% in neurosurgery. Minerva Anestesiol 201;67:603-611.
294. Prough DS: Should I use hypertonic saline to treat high intracranial pressure? In Valadka AB, Andrews BT (eds): Neurotrauma. New York, Thieme, 2005, pp 148-151.
295. Fisher B, Thomas D, Peterson B: Hypertonic saline lowers raised intracranial pressure in children after head trauma. J Neurosurg Anesthesiol 1992;4:4-10.
296. Suarez JI, Qureshi AI, Bhardwaj A, et al: Treatment of refractory intracranial hypertension with 23.4% saline. Crit Care Med 1998;26:1118-1122.
297. Khanna S, Davis D, Peterson B, et al: Use of hypertonic saline in the treatment of severe refractory posttraumatic intracranial hypertension in pediatric traumatic brain injury. Crit Care Med 2000;28:1144-1151.
298. Ware ML, Nemani VM, Meeker M, et al: Effects of 23.4% sodium chloride solution in reducing intracranial pressure in patients with traumatic brain injury: A preliminary study. Neurosurgery 2005;57:727-736.
299. Vialet R, Albanese J, Thomachot L, et al: Isovolume hypertonic solutes (sodium chloride or mannitol) in the treatment of refractory posttraumatic intracranial hypertension: 2 mL/kg 7.5% saline is more effective than 2 mL/kg 20% mannitol. Crit Care Med 2003;31:1683-1687.
300. Vassar MJ, Perry CA, Holcroft JW: Analysis of potential risks associated with 7.5% sodium chloride resuscitation of traumatic shock. Arch Surg 1990;125:1309-1315.
301. Marion DA (comment), Poca MA, Sahuquillo J, et al: Posture-induced changes in intracranial pressure: A comparative study in patients with and without a cerebrospinal fluid block at the craniovertebral junction. Neurosurgery 2006;58:899-906.
302. Marshall LF, Smith RW, Shapiro HM: The outcome of aggressive treatment in severe head injuries. Part I: The significance of intracranial pressure monitoring. J Neurosurg 1979;50:20-25.

303. Eisenberg HM, Frankowski RF, Contant CF, et al: High-dose barbiturate control of elevated intracranial pressure in patients with severe head injury. J Neurosurg 1988;69:15-23.
304. Clifton GL, Miller ER, Choi SC, Levin HS: Fluid thresholds and outcome from severe brain injury. Crit Care Med 2002;30:739-745.
305. Clark K, Nash TM, Hutchison GC: The failure of cicumferential craniectomy in acute traumatic cerebral swelling. J Neurosurg 1968;29:367-371.
306. Cooper PR, Rovit RL, Ransohoff J: Hemicraniectomy in the treatment of acute subdural hematoma: A reappraisal. Surg Neurol 1976;5:25-28.
307. Kjellberg RN, Prieto A Jr: Bifrontal decompressive craniotomy for massive cerebral edema. J Neurosurg 1971;34:488-493.
308. Polin RS, Shaffrey ME, Bogaev CA, et al: Decompressive bifrontal craniectomy in the treatment of severe refractory posttraumatic cerebral edema. Neurosurgery 1997;41:84-94.
309. Albanese J, Leone M, Alliez JR, et al: Decompressive craniectomy for severe traumatic brain injury: Evaluation of the effects at one year. Crit Care Med 2003;1:2535-2538.
310. De Lucca GP, Volpin L, Fornezza U, et al: The role of decompressive craniectomy in the treatment of uncontrollable post-traumatic intracranial hypertension. Acta Neurochir Suppl 2000;76:401-404.
311. Gaab MR, Rittierodt M, Lorenz M, Heissler HE: Traumatic brain swelling and operative decompression: A prospective investigation. Acta Neurochir Suppl 1990;51:326-328.
312. Gower DJ, Lee KS, McWhorter JM: Role of subtemporal decompression in severe closed head injury. Neurosurgery 1988;23:417-422.
313. Guerra WK, Gaab MR, Dietz H, et al: Surgical decompression for traumatic brain swelling: Indications and results. J Neurosurg 1999;90:187-196.
314. Schneider GH, Bardt T, Lanksch WR, Unterberg A: Decompressive craniectomy following traumatic brain injury: ICP, CPP, and neurological outcome. Acta Neurochir Suppl 2002;81:77-79.
315. Taylor A, Butt W, RosenfeldJ, et al: A randomized trial of early decompressive craniectomy in children with traumatic brain injury and sustained intracranial hypertension. Childs Nerv Syst 2001;17:154-162.
316. Whitfield PC, Patel H, Hutchinson PJ, et al: Bifrontal decompressive craniectomy in the management of posttraumatic intracranial hypertension. Br J Neurosurg 2001;15:500-507.
317. Marmarou A, Anderson RL, Ward JD, et al: Impact of ICP instability and hypotension on outcome in patients with severe head trauma. J Neurosurg 1991;75(Suppl):S59-S66.
318. Heppner P, Ellegala DB, Durieux M, et al: Contrast ultrasonographic assesssment of cerebral perfusion in patients undergoing decompressive craniectomy for traumatic brain injury. J Neurosurg 2006;104:738-745.
319. Grady MS: Decompressive craniectomy. J. Neurosurg 2006;104:467-468 (Editorial).
320. Hsiang JK, Chestnut RM, Crisp CB, et al: Early, routine paralysis for intracranial pressure control in severe head injury: Is it necessary? Crit Care Med 1994;22:1471-1476.
321. Sahuquillo J: At what level should I start treating elevated intracranial pressure? In Valadka AB, Andrews BT (eds): Neurotrauma. New York, Thieme, 2005, pp 135-141.
322. Part II: Prognosis in penetrating brain injury. J Trauma 2001;51(2 Suppl): S62.
323. Tien R, Chesnut RM: Medical management of the traumatic brain-injured patient. In Cooper PR, Golfinos JG (eds): Head Injury, 4th ed. New York, McGraw-Hill, 2000, pp 457-482.
324. Vajkoczy P, Schurer L, Munch E, Schmiedek P: Penetrating craniocerebral injuries in a civilian population in mid-Europe. Clin Neurol Neurosurg 1999;101:175-181.
325. Morenski JD, Tobias JD, Jimenez DF: Recombinant activated factor VII for cerebral injury-induced coagulopathy in pediatric patients. Report of three cases and review of the literature. J Neurosurg 2003;98:611-616.
326. Bakhtiari K, Meijers JC, deJonge E, Levi M: Prospective validation of the International Society of Thrombosis and Haemostasis scoring system for disseminated intravascular coagulation. Crit Care Med 2004;32:2416-2421.
327. Hardy JF, de Moerloose, P, Samama M: Massive transfusion and coagulopathy: Pathophysiology and implication for clinical management. Can J Anesth 2004;51:293-310.
328. Powner DJ, Hartwell EA, Hoots WK: Counteracting the effects of anticoagulants and antiplatelet agents during neurosurgical emergencies. Neurosurg 2005;57:823-831.
329. Allen GA, Hoffman M, Roberts HR, Monroe DM: Recombinant activated factor VII: Its mechanism of action and role in the control of hemorrhage. Can J Anesth 2002;49:S7-S14.
330. Fewel ME, Park P: The emerging role of recombinant-activated factor VII in neurocritical care. Neurocrit Care 2004;1:19-29.
331. Grounds M: Recombinant factor VIIa (rFVIIa) and its use in severe bleeding in surgery and trauma: A review. Blood Rev 2003;17:S11-S21.
332. Karadimov D, Binev K, Nachkov Y, Platikanov V: Use of activated recombinant factor VII (NovoSeven) during neurosurgery. J Neurosurg Anesthesiol 2003;15:330-332.
333. Key NS: Recombinant FVIIa for intractable hemorrhage: More questions than answers. Transfusion 2003;43:1649-1651.
334. Lau HK: The interaction between platelets and factor VII/VIIa. Transfus Apheresis Sci 2003;28:279-283.
335. Lin J, Hanigan WC, Tarantino M, Wang J: The use of recombinant activated factor VII to reverse warfarin-induced anticoagulation in patients with hemorrhages in the central nervous system: Preliminary findings. J Neurosurg 2003;98:737-740.
336. Mayer SA: Ultra-early hemostatic therapy for intracerebral hemorrhage. Stroke 2003;34:224-229.
337. Park P, Fewel ME, Garton HJ, et al: Recombinant activated factor VII for the rapid correction of coagulopathy in nonhemophilic neurosurgical patients. Neurosurgery 2003;53: 34-39.
338. Roberts HR: Recombinant factor VIIa (NovoSeven) and the safety of treatment. Semin Hematol 2001;38:48-50.
339. Veshchev I, Elran H, Salame K: Recombinant coagulation factor VIIa for rapid preoperative correction of warfarin-related coagulopathy in patients with acute subdural hematoma. Med Sci Monit 2002;8: CS98-CS100.
340. Roberts HR: Thoughts on the mechanism of action of FVIIa. Presented at 2nd Symposium on New Aspects of Hemophilia Treatment, Copenhagen, 1991, pp 153-156.
341. Penning-Van Beest FJ, Gomez Garcia EB, Van Der Meer FJ, et al: Levels of vitamin K–dependent procoagulant and anticoagulant proteins in over-anticoagulated patients. Blood Coagul Fibrinolysis 2002;13:733-739.
342. Lusher J, Ingerslev J, Roberts H, Hedner U: Clinical experience with recombinant factor VIIa: A review. Blood Coagul Fibrinolysis 1998;9:119-128.
343. Roitberg B, Emechebe-Kennedy O, Amin-Hanjani S, et al: Human recombinant factor VII for emergency reversal of coagulopathy in neurosurgical patients: A retrospective comparative study. Neurosurgery 2005;57:832-836.
344. Hedner U, Erhardtsen E: Potential role for rFVIIa in transfusion medicine. Transfusion 2002;42:114-124.
345. O'Connell NM, Perry DJ, Hodgson AJ, et al: Recombinant FVIIa in the management of uncontrolled hemorrhage. Transfusion 2003;43:1711-1716.
346. Deveras RA, Kessler CM: Reversal of warfarin-induced excessive anticoagulation with recomninant human factor VIIa concentrate. Ann Intern Med 2002;137:884-888.
347. Sorensen B, Johansen P, Nielsen GL, et al: Reversal of the international normalized ratio with recombinant activated factor VII in central nervous system bleeding during warfarin thromboprophylaxis: Clinical and biochemical aspects. Blood Coagul Fibrinol 2003;14:469-477.
348. Kam PC, Nethery CM: The thienopyridine derivatives (platelet adenosine diphosphate receptor antagonists), pharmacology and clinical developments. Anaesthesia 2003;58:28-35.
349. Kovesi T, Royston D: Is there a bleeding problem with platelet-active drugs? Br J Anaesth 2002;88: 159-163.
350. Mannucci PM: Desmopressin (DDAVP) in the treatment of bleeding disorders: The first twenty years. Haemophilia 2000;6(Suppl 1):60-67.
351. Patrono C, Coller B, FitzGerald GA, et al: Platelet-active drugs: The relationships among dose,

effectiveness, and side effects. Chest 2004;126(3 Suppl):234S-264S.
352. Li YF, Spencer FA, Becker RC: Comparative efficacy of fibrinogen and platelet supplementation on the in vitro reversibility of competitive glycoprotein IIb/IIIa receptor–directed platelet inhibition. Am Heart J 2001;142:204-210.
353. Schroeder WS, Gandhi PJ: Emergency management of hemorrhagic complications in the era of glycoprotein IIb/IIIa receptor antagonists, clopidogrel, low molecular weight heparin, and third-generation fibrinolygic agents. Curr Cardiol Report 2003;5:310-317.
354. Sane DC, Califf RM, Topol EJ, et al: Bleeding during thrombolytic therapy for acute myocardial infarction: Mechanisms and management. Ann Intern Med 2989;111:1010-1022.
355. Warkentin TE, Crowther MA: Reversing anticoagulants both old and new. Can J Anesth 2002;49:S11-S25.
356. Menon V, Harrington RA, Hochman J, et al: Thrombolysis and adjunctive therapy in acute myocardial infarction. Chest 2004;126(3 Suppl):549S-575S.
357. Albers GW, Amarenco P, Easton JD, et al: Antithrombotic and thrombolytic therapy of ischemic stroke. Chest 2004;126(Suppl 3): 483S-512S.
358. Ng PP, Higashida RT, Cullen SP, et al: Intrarterial thrombolysis trials in acute ischemic stroke. J Vasc Interv Radiol 2004;15(1 Pt 2):S77-S85.
359. DeLoughery TG: Coagulation defects in trauma patients: Etiology, recognition, and therapy. Crit Care Clin 2004;20:13-24.
360. Kaufmann JE, Vischer UM: Cellular mechanisms of the hemostatic effects of desmopressin (DDAVP). J Thromb Haemost 2003;1:682-689.
361. Lethagen S: Desmopessin in mild hemophilia A: Indications, limitations, efficacy, and safety. Semin Thromb Hemost 2003;29:101-106.
362. Samama CM, Bastien O, Forestier F, et al for the Expert Group: Antiplatelet agents in the perioperative period: Expert recommendations of the French Society of Anesthesiology and Intensive Care (SFAR) 2001: Summary statement. Can J Anesth 2002;49: S26-S35.
363. de Jonge E, Levi M: Effects of different plasma substitutes on blood coagulation: A comparative review. Crit Care Med 2001;29: 1261-1267.
364. de Jonge E, Levi M, Buller HR, et al: Decreased circulating levels of von Willebrand factor after intravenous administration of a rapidly degradable hydroxyethyl starch (HES 2000/0.5/6) in healthy human subjects. Intensive Care Med 2001;27:1825-1829.
365. Gan TJ, Bennett-Guerrero E, Phillips-Bute B, et al: Hextend, a physiologically balanced plasma expander for large volume use in major surgery: A randomized phase III clinical trial. Anesth Analg 1999;88:992-998.
366. Neff TA, Doelberg M, Jungheinrich C, et al: Repetitive large-dose infusion of the novel hydroxyethyl starch 130/0.4 in patients with severe head injury. Anesth Analg 2003;96:1453-1459.
367. Rapp RP, Young B, Twyman D, et al: The favorable effect of early parenteral feeding on survival in head-injured patients. J Neurosurg 1983;58: 907-912.

PART

VII PHYSICAL AND TOXIC INJURY IN THE CRITICALLY ILL

Chapter 68

Critical Care Management of the Severely Burned Patient

Jeffrey R. Saffle

Patients suffering major burn injuries present unique challenges in both the types and magnitude of management problems. Fluid resuscitation, pulmonary dysfunction, metabolic stress, and infections complicating major burns may equal or surpass similar problems in other intensive care unit (ICU) populations, and treatment is further complicated by abnormal drug pharmacology, severe pain, and psychosocial stress, all superimposed on the need for multiple major surgical procedures and physical therapy.

This chapter provides an overview of the critical care management of burned adults. The reader will find it apparent that in many areas, existing literature is neither comprehensive nor rigorously evidence based.[1] In providing a rationale for treatment, therefore, it is often necessary to extrapolate from studies in other disorders, particularly trauma. This may or may not be valid, particularly in such burn-specific areas as fluid resuscitation, inhalation injury, and nutritional support. These issues are discussed as they arise, but readers need to interpret this information for themselves.

INCIDENCE AND SURVIVAL FROM BURN INJURY

The incidence of burn injury has declined in the United States throughout recent decades. From the 1960s to the early 1990s, reported burns decreased from 10.2 to approximately 4.2 injuries per 1000 Americans annually, or about 1.25 million injuries[2]; hospitalizations decreased from more than 90,000 to approximately 52,000/year; and deaths decreased at least 40%, from 9000 to 5500/year. These trends are likely continuing.

Simultaneously, survival from burns has improved dramatically. During World War II, burns of 40% total body surface area (TBSA) produced a 50% mortality; today similar mortality is seen with burns of more than 80% TBSA.[3] Survival is lower—though still improved—for the elderly and even higher for children and young adults.[4] These accomplishments are caused by cumulative advances in fluid resuscitation, critical care, nutrition, surgery, and skin substitutes. However, it has been the organization of specialized burn centers around a consolidated *team* of experts that has made this success possible.

Survival from burns has been repeatedly shown to depend on three factors: (1) patient age, (2) burn size, and (3) the presence of inhalation injury. Pulmonary damage from smoke inhalation is itself a serious injury and can as much as double mortality from cutaneous burns alone.[3,5] Ryan and colleagues[6] found that burn size 40% or greater of TBSA, age 60 years or more, and inhalation injury contributed to mortality in a stepwise manner; patients with all three had mortality of 90% (Table 68-1).[6]

This information supports two important observations about current burn treatment. First, mortality for most patients is now so low that almost no injury precludes survival. The practice of intentionally withholding treatment should now be rare and based on predicted *quality* of life rather than survival itself. Second, this success has focused ongoing research and interest in the rehabilitation of patients who increasingly survive catastrophic injuries. Functional outcomes of burn treatment including quality of life and return to work are now the most relevant measures of successful care for all patients.[7,8]

PATHOPHYSIOLOGY OF BURNS

Although the term "burn" strictly denotes injury caused by heat from flames, scalding liquids, and so on, other agents including chemicals, electrical current, ionizing radiation, and friction produce nearly identical coagulative necrosis of tissues. The amount of necrosis is determined by the intensity of the source of injury (e.g., temperature, voltage, pH) and the duration of contact. Similarly, the clinical severity of a burn is a function of

Table 68-1. Risk Factors for Mortality from Burn Injuries

No. Risk Factors	Age >60 yr	Burns Size ≥40% TBSA	Inhalation Injury	No. Patients	No. Deaths	Mortality (%)
0	No	No	No	1314	3	0.2
1	No	No	Yes	112	5	4
1	No	Yes	No	31	1	3
1	Yes	No	No	75	4	5
2	No	Yes	Yes	79	21	27
2	Yes	No	Yes	31	12	39
2	Yes	Yes	No	1	0	0
3	Yes	Yes	Yes	22	21	95
Totals				1665	67	4.0

This table indicates the three risk factors universally accepted to affect burn patient mortality, their prevalence, and relative contribution to mortality. These data are similar to those from many modern burn centers. Overall mortality is only 4%, and most patients are relatively young and have limited burn wounds, placing them at little risk of dying.

Modified with permission from Ryan CM, Schoenfeld DA, Thorpe WP, et al: Objective estimates of the probability of death from burn injuries. N Engl J Med 1998;338:362-366.

the depth and extent of injury. These determine what skin structures are destroyed, the magnitude of response, and the ability of the wound to heal. Accurate assessment of burn wounds is essential in determining appropriate treatment and in predicting outcome.

The epidermis serves as a unique barrier to moisture, bacteria, and chemicals. The epidermis is metabolically active and richly vascularized, with rapid cell proliferation and turnover. Burns limited to the epidermis are characterized by redness, mild to moderate pain, and limited inflammatory response. Burns extending into the dermis (second degree, or partial-thickness burns) vary greatly in appearance and severity. Superficial dermal burns exhibit erythema and pain, with fluid-filled blisters and a wet wound surface. As damage penetrates more deeply into the dermis, coagulative necrosis effectively seals off the skin surface from fluid leakage; instead, edema collects beneath the wound. The most severe burns destroy the entire dermis, producing full-thickness or third-degree burns. Such injuries may be a variety of colors but are invariably dry and relatively insensate. The coagulated dermis is constricted and rigid; as fluid accumulates beneath it, tissue pressure can increase to a dangerous degree, causing vascular compromise and compartmental compression (see later).

Coagulation necrosis of skin generates intense inflammation that persists even after wound coverage is attained and produces protean systemic manifestations. Immediate release of inflammatory mediators causes widespread loss of capillary integrity and depletion of intravascular volume, as well as depressed myocardial contractility, increased peripheral vascular resistance, and systemic hypoperfusion. This shock state can be rapidly lethal, but if patients are supported adequately, their cardiovascular response reverses within 24 to 48 hours and is thereafter characterized by increased cardiac output and decreased vascular resistance. This process is fueled by a complex cascade of local and systemic inflammatory mediators and also stimulates sustained release of epinephrine, cortisol, and glucagon, which generate hypermetabolism, autocannibalism of body protein stores, and glucose intolerance that persists well into rehabilitation (see "Metabolic Support" later).

The second important consequence of burn injury is the burn wound itself. Burned skin quickly accumulates a coating of tenacious "eschar," composed of dried serum and necrotic dermis. Minor burn injuries can often be allowed to heal spontaneously as eschar sloughs and new epidermis emerges from hair follicles and sweat glands to cover the wounds. But the eschar that covers deep or extensive injuries is extremely susceptible to infection, which has historically been a major cause of death from burns. Prompt removal of eschar and coverage with intact skin is essential to control sepsis, ameliorate inflammation, reduce scarring, and optimize functional long-term outcomes.

ACUTE CARE OF THE BURNED PATIENT

Acute burn treatment is usually divided into three phases. The first 48 hours following injury constitute *acute resuscitation,* focused on initial assessment, airway support, and fluid replacement. The *wound coverage phase* then ensues, in which the major focus of treatment is surgical excision and closure of burn wounds. Ventilator management, metabolic support, control of infection and pain, physical therapy, and other supportive measures are essential adjuncts to surgery during this period. The goals of the final, *rehabilitation phase* include scar control, optimizing function, and return to independent living. This period can last for months and continue long past discharge. Obviously, these phases overlap: Many units begin surgical excision even before resuscitation is completed, and several aspects of rehabilitation—physical therapy, psychosocial support, nutrition—should start essentially at the time of injury.

RESUSCITATION PHASE

Initial Assessment

Initial assessment of burn victims should follow the universally accepted protocol of The American College of Surgeons' Advanced Trauma Life Support (ATLS) course.[9] In doing so, attention must be paid to a number of burn-specific issues, but it must also be remembered that unsuspected injuries of other types can always be present, emphasizing the importance of systematic patient evaluation.

Primary Survey: Inhalation Injury

In burn patients, assessment of airway, breathing, and circulation must include evaluation for signs and symptoms of inhalation injury. Carbon monoxide (CO) poisoning and asphyxia cause the vast majority of scene and emergency department fatalities and up to 80% of fire-related deaths.[10,11] Immediate intubation and ventilation with high-flow oxygen are imperative to treat these conditions and to salvage neurologic and functional outcomes.

Inhalation injury should be suspected in all victims of flame burns. A fire occurring within an enclosed space is the most important clue to the presence of inhalation injury, particularly if the patient was unconscious or trapped. Other signs and symptoms include facial burns, singed nasal hairs or eyebrows, wheezing or stridor, carbonaceous sputum, hoarseness, or anxiety. These findings are highly suggestive of inhalation injury and should alert the examiner to the likelihood of this complication, as well as the possible need for airway support.[12]

Inhalation injury is classically considered to consist of three distinct entities: CO poisoning, upper airway injury, and lower airway injury (the "true" inhalation injury). Although these mechanisms can overlap and patients frequently present with a combination of all three, this classification is worthwhile because of the different pathologic processes and time courses with which these injuries present.

Carbon Monoxide Poisoning

CO is a byproduct of incomplete combustion, and its highest concentrations occur in indoor fires, where its effects may be amplified by flame-induced depletion of available oxygen ("asphyxia").[13] CO is not a pulmonary toxin; rather, its extremely high affinity for hemoglobin displaces oxygen binding, producing systemic hypoxia despite normal oxygen tension. The most common symptoms are mental status changes varying from headache to coma; CO toxicity should be suspected in anyone with confusion or loss of consciousness following a fire. Patients may present without burn injuries, airway compromise, or respiratory distress and may be overlooked easily. Classic "cherry red cyanosis" is absent in many victims or can be obscured by soot or burns. Importantly, *pulse-oximetry is inaccurate* in the presence of this compound, which leads to falsely elevated readings. For this reason, all burn victims exposed to smoke should be immediately treated with high-flow oxygen. Blood gases should be drawn for determination of carboxyhemoglobin concentration, but treatment should never await results. Patients are at greatest risk on presentation, and immediate application of oxygen usually provides definitive treatment. As reviewed in Chapter 49, the use of hyperbaric oxygen for acute CO poisoning is controversial; it should probably be reserved for severe cases with neurologic compromise, when its use will not interfere with other essential components of acute burn evaluation and treatment.

Smoke contains many other toxic chemicals including cyanide. If inhaled in significant quantities, cyanide toxicity can produce coma, metabolic acidosis, and cardiovascular collapse. Cyanide poisoning has been documented in burn victims and does not always correlate with CO exposure.[14] Because blood levels cannot be obtained immediately, empiric treatment using cyanide antidote kits has been performed in patients with unusually severe acidosis or shock.[15] However, this appears to be a rare clinical problem, and routine treatment is not advocated.[16]

Upper Airway Injury

Patients with extensive or deep burns to the face, or who have breathed substantial quantities of hot gases or soot, are at risk of airway occlusion from pharyngeal or supraglottic edema and from chemical and thermal burns of the pharynx, epiglottis, and larynx. Much of this problem is caused by facial swelling and can thus occur even in the absence of smoke exposure such as in children with scald burns or injuries associated with "priming the carburetor." Edema formation can be extremely rapid and is progressive for at least 24 hours. For these reasons, patients must be followed serially and intubated early and electively if evidence of progressive airway compromise occurs. Figure 68-1 illustrates such a case.

Indications for Intubation

Awareness of the risk of acute airway compromise following burn injury has led to a liberal attitude toward intubation, which is probably appropriate. "When in doubt, intubate" expresses many physicians' attitude toward this problem. However, strict adherence to this dictum has sometimes led to indiscriminant intubation of patients with even minor facial burns, which is unnecessary and risks complications of its own. Suspicion of inhalation injury does not itself mandate intubation, and airway compromise can be life threatening even in the absence of inhalation injury. Indications for elective intubation, as in all trauma patients, are based on *symptoms* found on initial assessment. They include altered mental status, refractory hypoxemia, and signs of impending airway obstruction including wheezing, stridor, dyspnea, tachypnea, and progressive facial swelling. Tracheostomy or cricothyroidotomy as emergency procedures should rarely be necessary if intubation is performed in a timely manner and can be extremely difficult to perform in the setting of massive head and neck swelling.

Pulmonary ("True") Inhalation Injury

Exposure of the bronchi and small airways to toxic smoke produces chemical injury to the epithelium, which over

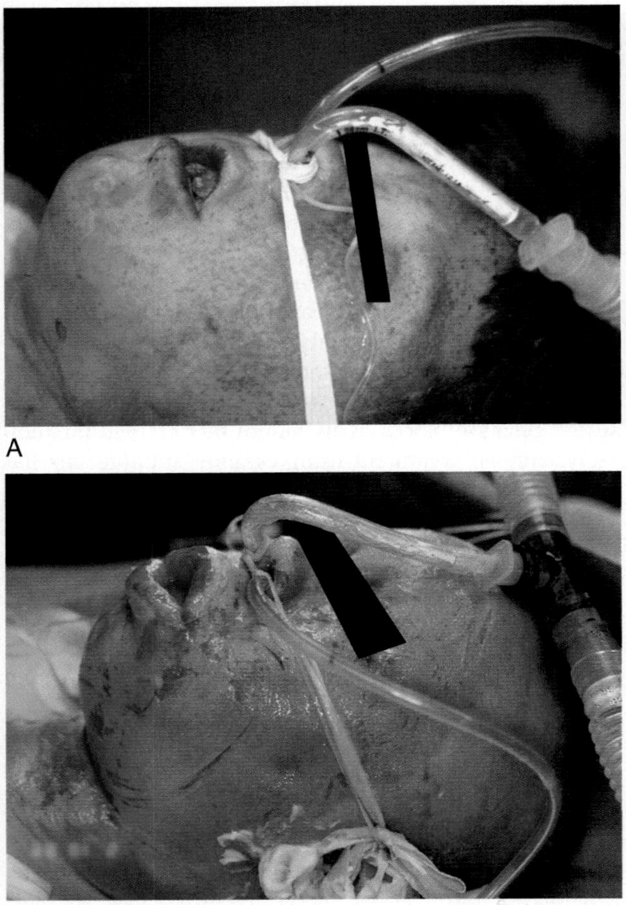

A

B

Figure 68-1. **A,** This 12-year-old was burned playing with matches and gasoline, sustaining burns to 60% total body surface area including his entire face. On presentation, he was alert and breathing comfortably. Arterial blood gases (including carboxyhemoglobin) and chest radiograph were normal. On the basis of the extent and location of his injuries, elective nasotracheal intubation was performed. **B,** Six hours later, the patient displayed massive facial edema. Eyes were swollen shut, and oral excursion was severely restricted. If he had lost his endotracheal tube at this point, his airway could not have been maintained. Of note is that the tube was tied around his head securely, not taped in position. Such a patient needs to remain intubated for at least 3 to 5 days until most of the edema resolves.

time produces mucosal sloughing, mucous plugging, bronchiectasis, ventilation-perfusion mismatch, and often severe pulmonary infection. However, this chemical reaction is not immediate, and its effects are rarely apparent on presentation. Initial chest radiographs are usually normal.[17] Patients with immediate respiratory distress, stridor, or hypoxemia are much more likely to have upper airway injury. In the absence of symptoms, patients suspected of having inhalation injury can be followed expectantly; however, this diagnosis greatly increases the risk of subsequent respiratory distress and mandates hospital admission and close observation. In addition to the symptoms listed previously, visual inspection of the trachea and

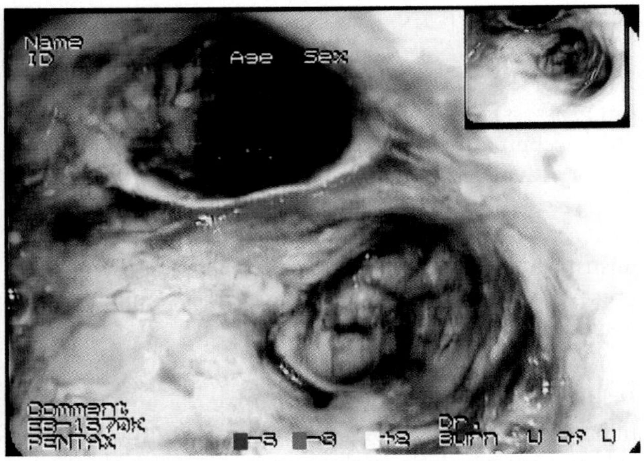

Figure 68-2. Bronchoscopic appearance of the carina of a man who was dragged unconscious from a burning house. Carbonaceous deposits are apparent in his trachea and more extensively in the mainstem bronchi. This finding is diagnostic of inhalation injury.

bronchi using fiberoptic bronchoscopy is accurate; findings of carbonaceous debris, erythema, mucosal sloughing, or bronchorrhea are diagnostic of inhalation injury (Fig. 68-2).[18] Many centers perform this procedure with an endotracheal tube loaded on the bronchoscope and proceed with immediate intubation if inhalation injury is confirmed. Inhalation injury is discussed later and in Chapter 47.

Secondary Survey

Following the primary survey, a thorough, head-to-toe examination is performed. Burn victims frequently suffer other trauma, which can be obscured by overlying burns (see later). During this evaluation, an estimate must be made of the extent and depth of burn injuries. Much of the subsequent care of a patient with a major burn injury is based on this assessment including fluid resuscitation, nutritional requirements, surgery, and even in selected cases the decision to provide aggressive treatment. For these reasons, the burn wound should be documented as accurately as possible, preferably by an experienced clinician. This is best done after burns are thoroughly washed and débrided. Rough estimates of burn size are often made using the rule of nines; more accurate, detailed documentation can be done using the Lund and Browder chart (Fig. 68-3). Computerized programs are also becoming popular, such as the Sage Diagram (www.sagediagram.com). In evaluating smaller injuries, another useful rule is that the area of the patient's palm (with fingers) equals about 1% of his or her TBSA.

Burns and Multiple Trauma

The remarkable variety of etiologies of burn injury make it obvious that trauma of all types can occur with burns. Mechanisms that favor such combined injuries include explosions (blasts, falls, projectile wounds); electrocutions (tetany-induced fractures); falls from heights; fires in motor vehicle or airplane crashes; and escaping fires (soft tissue trauma from window glass or falls).

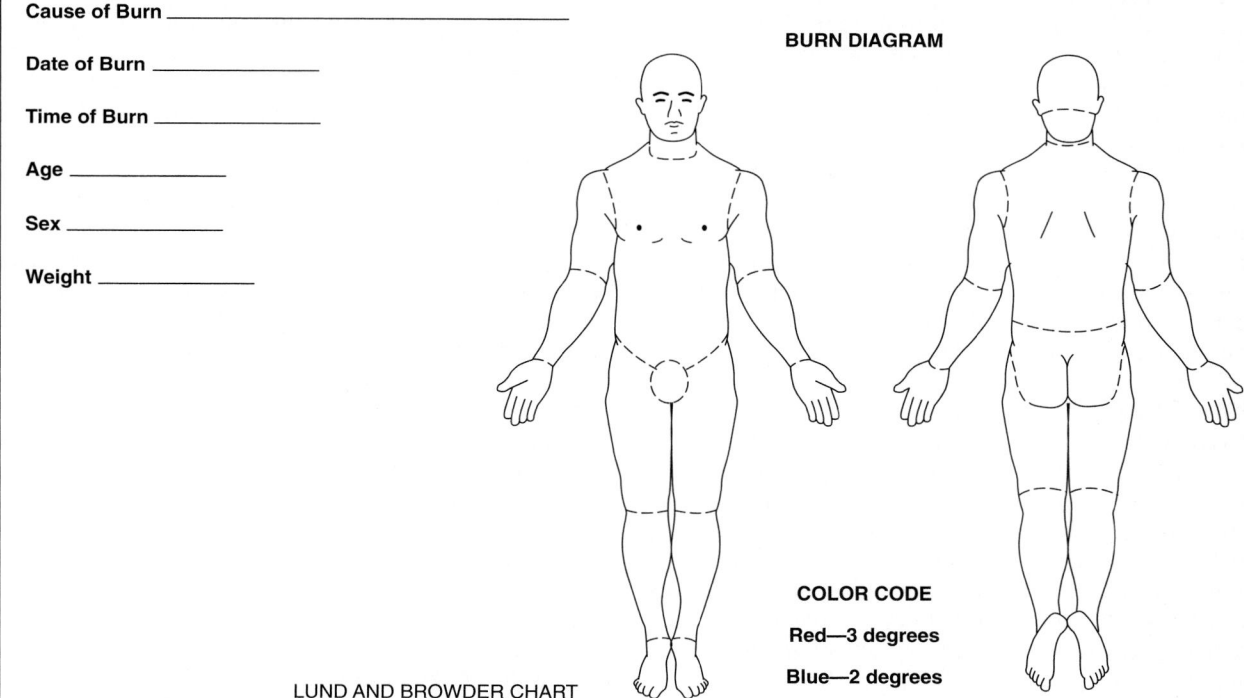

BURN ESTIMATE AND DIAGRAM
AGE VERSUS AREA

Area	Birth 1 yr	1–4 yr	5–9 yr	10–14 yr	15 yr	Adult	2 degrees	3 degrees	Total	Donor Areas
Head	19	17	13	11	9	7				
Neck	2	2	2	2	2	2				
Ant. Trunk	13	13	13	13	13	13				
Post. Trunk	13	13	13	13	13	13				
R. Buttock	2 1/2	2 1/2	2 1/2	2 1/2	2 1/2	2 1/2				
L. Buttock	2 1/2	2 1/2	2 1/2	2 1/2	2 1/2	2 1/2				
Genitalia	1	1	1	1	1	1				
R. U. Arm	4	4	4	4	4	4				
L. U. Arm	4	4	4	4	4	4				
R. L. Arm	3	3	3	3	3	3				
L. L. Arm	3	3	3	3	3	3				
R. Hand	2 1/2	2 1/2	2 1/2	2 1/2	2 1/2	2 1/2				
L. Hand	2 1/2	2 1/2	2 1/2	2 1/2	2 1/2	2 1/2				
R. Thigh	5 1/2	6 1/2	8	8 1/2	9	9 1/2				
L. Thigh	5 1/2	6 1/2	8	8 1/2	9	9 1/2				
R. Leg	5	5	5 1/2	6	6 1/2	7				
L. Leg	5	5	5 1/2	6	6 1/2	7				
R. Foot	3 1/2	3 1/2	3 1/2	3 1/2	3 1/2	3 1/2				
L. Foot	3 1/2	3 1/2	3 1/2	3 1/2	3 1/2	3 1/2				
						TOTAL				

Cause of Burn ______________________

Date of Burn __________

Time of Burn __________

Age __________

Sex __________

Weight __________

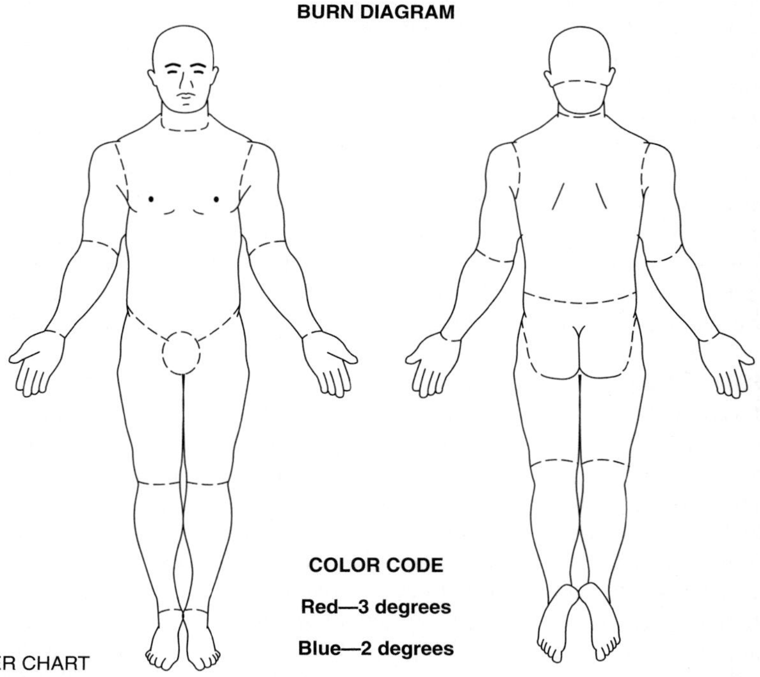

LUND AND BROWDER CHART

Figure 68-3. The Lund and Browder chart is in widespread use in burn centers for diagramming and calculating burn extent and depth. The chart divides the body into small areas and gives the relative percent total body surface area for each area for different age groups. With a little practice, physicians can estimate burns quite accurately. To do so, they should evaluate wounds after they have been washed and débrided. Each area should be inspected carefully, and the physician should attempt to distinguish between partial- and full-thickness burn wounds. Total burn size is calculated by adding individual body areas.

Medical problems that impair consciousness or sensation including drug/alcohol intoxication, seizures, strokes, paralysis, and diabetes predispose patients to burns from stoves, heaters, scalding showers, etc. Combined burn/trauma injuries are particularly likely following assault or child abuse and should increase suspicion for such occurrences.[19]

The combined mortality of burns and trauma appears to be at least additive compared with either injury alone.[20,21] Whether such patients are treated in burn centers, trauma units, or medical ICUs, the same principles of care apply. First, thorough evaluation of all potential injuries according to ATLS guidelines is imperative. Diagnosis of other trauma can be challenging in burn patients. The discoloration, pain, and swelling of burn wounds, for example, can make underlying fractures difficult to detect,[22] whereas burns of the torso and accompanying inhalation injury can conceal a pneumothorax or other injuries. For this reason, it is important not to focus too heavily on burn injuries in completing the secondary survey and to maintain a high index of suspicion for multiple trauma.

Second, care should be provided by a multispecialty team with expertise in managing all injuries. Third, treatment of many traumatic injuries will take priority over definitive burn care. Because fresh burn wounds are initially—and *briefly*—free of bacteria, repair of lacerations and operative fixation of fractures should be performed immediately, and no later than 12 to 24 hours postburn.[23,24] This approach will permit definitive repair of fractures while minimizing infections, permit early mobilization, and facilitate access to burn wounds for dressings and surgery. Other emergent procedures including craniotomy and laparotomy are also best performed before massive edema and inevitable wound contamination develop. These interventions can be performed safely, provided essential components of burn care are also provided. These include definitive airway management, patient temperature control, and aggressive fluid resuscitation, which should be continued through surgery. Close coordination between the burn center and trauma center will optimize outcome for these patients.

Burn Shock

Once initial evaluation is completed, the primary focus of burn treatment is fluid resuscitation. The goals of resuscitation are to support organ function while avoiding complications of overadministration or underadministration of fluid.[25] This can be a real challenge, given the huge fluid shifts and cardiovascular abnormalities that accompany acute burns. Development of effective protocols for resuscitation represents one of the major advancements in burn care in this century.

Burn shock resembles ischemia-reperfusion and other injuries, although the magnitude of the fluid losses that result are unique to burns. Burn shock is manifested within cells, within tissues, and systemically. At the cellular level, burn injury impairs membrane ATP-ase activity and reduces transmembrane potential,[26,27] resulting in increased intracellular sodium and extracellular potassium concentrations, cellular swelling, and acidosis. This process begins immediately in burned tissue and also occurs in unburned areas in proportion to burn size. Fluid resuscitation only partially corrects these abnormalities, which may require several days to resolve completely as local inflammation subsides.

Far more obvious clinically is increased capillary permeability, producing massive tissue edema at the expense of intravascular volume. This process is initiated by a profound local inflammatory response. Histamine release occurs almost instantly, increasing local perfusion and initiating capillary leakage.[28] Serotonin potentiates the vasoconstrictive effects of massive catecholamine secretion.[27,29] TNF-α elaborated by local macrophages produces myocardial depression and activates a number of other mediators and local vasodilators.[30] Prostaglandins, leukotrienes, oxygen radicals, products of platelet activation and coagulation, and a cascade of cytokines also contribute to these abnormalities.[31,32] A variety of alterations in local blood flow combine to increase arteriolar tone and pressure, while producing dilation of post-capillary venules, resulting in local capillary perfusion becoming less selective and greatly increased. These effects also favor edema formation.

The forces that control transcapillary fluid flux are summarized in Starling's equation[33]; their alterations in burn injury have been reviewed by Demling[34] and are summarized in Table 68-2. The greatest edema formation occurs almost immediately within the wound, caused by near-total permeability to even very large (350 Å) molecules,[35] permitting protein-rich plasma to pour into the interstitium.[36] Maximum protein extravasation occurs within the first hour of injury and is quite transient, but both its duration and magnitude are proportional to burn size.[37,38]

As capillary integrity is restored within 8 to 12 hours, continued edema formation in all tissues depends increasingly on changes in oncotic pressure and interstitial compliance. This is the major cause of edema in unburned tissues, although altered capillary permeability plays a role as well.[39] The rapid loss of intravascular proteins, further diluted by crystalloid resuscitation,[40] eliminates the oncotic pressure gradient ($\pi p - \pi i$ in Table 68-2), which is important for maintaining intravascular volume. Depletion of plasma proteins alone can mimic burn edema, and infusions of albumin or dextran can almost completely prevent edema in unburned tissues.[41,42] This process acts in concert with alterations in the interstitium, normally composed of collagen and hyaluronic acid molecules that are densely coiled to limit fluid influx and act as a safety valve to edema formation.[43] Burn injury disrupts this configuration, increasing compliance and producing osmotically active molecular fragments, generating negative ("sucking") interstitial pressure,[44] which also causes extremely rapid fluid sequestion.[39] Although this gradient is neutralized within a few hours, compliance continues to increase as interstitial gel is hydrated, allowing liters of fluid to accumulate with little change in hydrostatic pressure[45] and permitting edema to persist for weeks following injury.

Table 68-2. Starling Forces and Capillary Permeability (See Demling[33])
Starling's Formula: $Q = Kf\,(Pcap - Pi) + \sigma\,(\pi p - \pi i)$

Symbol	Definition	Alteration in Burn Injury
Q	Net rate of fluid passage across the capillary membrane	Increased dramatically as a result of changes in all component forces
Kf	Filtration coefficient; consists of two components: Surface area of the capillary system; Compliance of the interstitium	Increased as a result of increased local blood flow, perfusing more capillaries. Increased because of alterations in molecular configuration (see text)
Pcap	Capillary hydrostatic pressure	Increased as a result of arterial vasoconstriction
Pi	Interstitial hydrostatic pressure	Decreased, secondary to changes in molecular configuration of the interstitium (see text)
σ	Reflection coefficient—describes the permeability of the capillary to macromolecules. Ordinarily this is quite limited; a coefficient of 1 indicates that no protein can pass across the membrane; a coefficient of zero implies total permeability. For normal skin, this value is approximately 0.9.	Greatly increased permeability to even large molecules. In burned skin, this value approximates 0.3. This effect appears largely limited to burned tissues; generation of edema formation in nonburned tissues depends more on changes in colloid oncotic pressure and interstitial compliance.
πp	Plasma colloid oncotic pressure. Each gram of albumin generates approximately 4 mm/Hg of oncotic pressure; normal πp is 20 mm/Hg.	Progressively reduced. Most direct leakage of albumin is into burned tissues, but as this occurs, πp is reduced systemically. This is further diluted by crystalloid resuscitation.
πi	Interstitial colloid oncotic pressure	Reduced slightly, but this is limited because of changes in interstitial compliance
Pcap − Pi	The difference in hydrostatic pressure across the capillary membrane. The greater the gradient, the more rapid the flow of fluid. Normal gradient is 10-12 mm/Hg.	Increased because of increased hydrostatic pressure; little or no increase in interstitial pressure
$\pi p - \pi i$	The difference in oncotic pressure across the capillary membrane	Reduced because of dilution of plasma proteins, little change in interstitial pressure

Adapted with permission from Ryan CM, Schoenfeld DA, Thorpe WP, et al: Objective estimates of the probability of death from burn injuries. N Engl J Med 1998;338:362-366.

Systemically, cardiac output (QT) falls within minutes of injury, reaching 50% to 60% of normal within an hour, whereas systemic vascular resistance (SVR) increases dramatically. Both changes occur far faster than the depletion of intravascular volume,[36,46] regardless of fluid resuscitation. Release of catecholamines and other vasoactive mediators clearly increases SVR, but the decrease in QT is harder to explain. Researchers have long postulated existence of a "myocardial depressant factor,"[47] although no such substance has been isolated. It seems more likely that QT is impaired by the combination of increased SVR, volume depletion, and actions of TNF-α, endotoxin, and other chemicals. One clinically important side effect of capillary permeability is hemoconcentration—a marked rise in hematocrit as plasma is sieved out of the bloodstream into the interstitium. This process increases blood viscosity and further impairs QT.

Cardiac output begins to recover within a few hours of injury and requires 12 to 24 hours to return to normal even with vigorous resuscitation. Systemic vascular resistance follows an opposite course, peaking quickly, then declining to near normal within 24 to 48 hours (Fig. 68-4). Following these initial changes a chronic hyperdynamic circulation is maintained, with cardiac output persisting well above normal, and marked vasodilation and decreased SVR.

Fluid Resuscitation of Burn Patients

Before World War II, patients with even moderate burns usually died within a few days of progressive shock and renal failure. In 1942 Cope and Moore designed the first formal resuscitation regimen to treat victims of the Cocoanut Grove nightclub fire, with substantial improvements in survival.[27] With continued refinements in resuscitation, today almost all patients can be resuscitated successfully, and renal failure complicating fluid resuscitation is rare. A host of formulas have been used, almost all based on body weight and burn size, with various combinations of crystalloid and colloid solutions. An archetype for such regimens, and unquestionably the most widely used, is the Parkland formula, designed by Baxter.[26] He demonstrated that a volume of lactated Ringer's (LR) solution equal to 4 mL per kilogram body weight for each percent TBSA burned (4 mL/kg/%TBSA), given in the first 24 hours after injury, would maintain urine output of 50 to 70 mL/hour, replete blood volume, and restore cellular transmembrane potential and cardiac output in most patients. Half this calculated volume is given in the first 8 hours postburn, and the remainder over the next 16 hours. The IV rate is adjusted hourly to maintain urine output and decreased gradually until a maintenance rate is reached at approximately 24 hours.

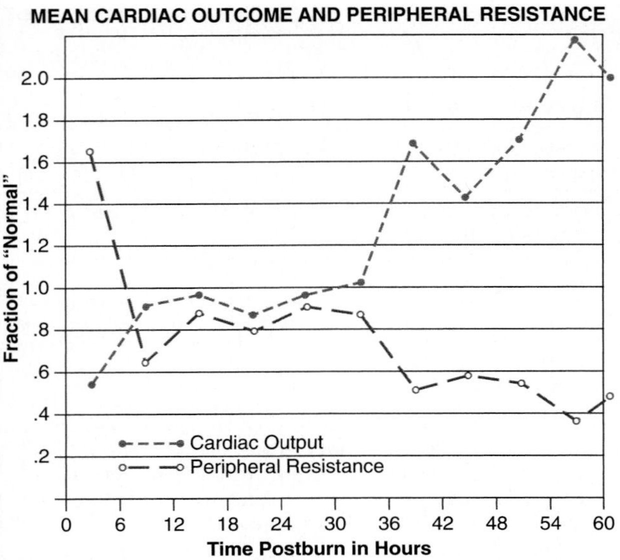

Figure 68-4. Graph showing characteristic postburn changes in cardiac output and peripheral vascular resistance in a group of seven patients (mean burn size 64.5% total body surface area [TBSA]) resuscitated with the Brooke formula (LR, 1.5 mL/kg/percent TBSA, albumin, 0.5 mL/kg/percent TBSA, plus 2000 mL dextrose/water in the first 24 hours). Cardiac output falls acutely, before blood volume has changed appreciably, then rebounds gradually, with return to normal by 24 to 36 hours, and thereafter remaining above normal. Peripheral vascular resistance shows an opposite effect. (From Pruitt BA Jr, Mason AD Jr, Moncrief JA: Hemodynamic changes in the early postburn patient: The influence of fluid administration and of a vasodilator (hydralazine). J Trauma 1971;11:36-46.)

Maintenance requirements for burn patients are also increased because of ongoing evaporative and metabolic losses. A variety of formulas to estimate these requirements have been developed as well. A popular formula is that developed by Warden[48]:

24 hour maintenance fluid requirements
= Evaporative water losses + normal insensible losses

Evaporative water losses: $(35 + \%\text{TBSA burn}) \times M^2 \times 24$

Normal insensible losses: $(1500 \times M^2)$ per 24 hours

M^2 = body surface area in square meters

This equation forms the basis of modern burn resuscitation. But despite widespread acceptance of the principles of fluid replacement, disagreement persists over almost every aspect of practical management, fueled by lack of definitive clinical data. These issues include the following.

Monitoring and End Points of Resuscitation

Far more important than the formula used to calculate fluids—which dictates primarily where to *start* infusions—successful resuscitation demands meticulous monitoring and adjustment based on patient response. Traditional burn resuscitation relies almost exclusively on hourly urine output for this purpose, so the amount of fluid required for resuscitation depends partly on the urine output targeted. Baxter used an output of 50 to 70 mL/hour; several other formulas that accept outputs of 0.5 mL/kg/hour (1 mL/kg/hour in children) call for LR infusion rates between 2 and 3 mL/kg/%TBSA and are also in widespread use.[25,27]

Several patient groups are known to routinely require more resuscitation fluid than predicted by the Parkland formula. These include patients with inhalation injury,[49] in whom inflammatory response is heightened; children, whose ratio of body surface area to mass is larger; patients with secondary injuries including multiple trauma and electrical burns; patients in whom onset of resuscitation is substantially delayed[4]; and patients with alcohol or drug abuse.[50] In addition, inexperienced clinicians often make substantial errors in estimating burn size, which can result in significant underestimation or overestimation of fluid requirements.[51] Careful monitoring of resuscitation and individualized fluid therapy can obviate these problems and result in all patients receiving the resuscitation they need.

Clinicians have long accepted the consensus that patients should receive as little fluid as possible to maintain organ perfusion.[52] Baxter stated that even with the exceptions listed earlier, more than 80% of patients could be successfully resuscitated by strict adherence to the Parkland formula. But despite this tenet, in recent years a widespread tendency to give increasing quantities of fluid for resuscitation has been observed, a phenomenon termed *fluid creep*.[53] For example, Cancio and colleagues[54] found that 63% of their recent patients received more than 4 mL/kg/%TBSA for resuscitation (mean of 6.1 ± 0.22 mL/kg/%TBSA), despite being held to modest urine output. Other authors have documented fluid requirements exceeding Parkland predictions in up to 100% of patients.[55-57] The potential complications of fluid creep are far from benign and include increased extremity and abdominal compartment syndromes, worsening pulmonary dysfunction, and more frequent and prolonged endotracheal intubation.

This departure from tradition is probably caused by several influences. First, fluid requirements correlate at least somewhat with burn size.[54] In Baxter's initial series of 277 patients, 89% of those with burns 60% or greater of TBSA died.[36] However, modern survival is much better and may owe some of its success to persisting with aggressive fluid resuscitation beyond the confines of the Parkland formula. This experience has likely influenced regimens for smaller injuries as well.

Second, it is probable that fluid creep perpetuates itself. Overly zealous initial fluid administration—often performed in the field—increases the early depletion of serum proteins, generating a vicious cycle of reduced oncotic pressure and enhanced edema, which in turn increases crystalloid requirements. This mechanism also helps explain an apparent increase in resuscitation failure, in which fluid volumes required to maintain urine output actually escalate despite adequate or excessive crystalloid administration.[58] The use of colloid-containing fluids can arrest this cycle and restore oncotic pressure but adds to overall fluid requirements.

Perhaps most obviously, fluid creep is encouraged by resuscitation trends in other ICU populations. Traditional resuscitation formulas including Parkland's do not prevent significant deficits in vascular volume and cardiac output, which persist until the end of 24 hours.[36] The routine observation of hematocrits as high as 70% is consistent with this concept. In this sense, such formulas succeed in their goal of requiring the least fluid possible.

In contrast, resuscitation in other shock states is now aggressively directed at achieving physiologic goals—normalizing lactic acid (LA) and base deficit (BD) and optimizing oxygen delivery (VO_2), pulmonary wedge pressure, and cardiac output (QT).[59,60] When these parameters are measured in burn patients, traditional resuscitation is obviously deficient. Jeng and colleagues[61] found that both LA and BD remained elevated despite resuscitation to traditional endpoints of urine output and blood pressure in a group of 53 burn patients.[61] Dries and Waxman demonstrated that such a regimen failed to reflect changes in QT and VO_2,[62] whereas Schiller and colleagues[63] found that resuscitation to optimize VO_2 and QT was associated with improved survival in a group of patients with severe burns. As goal-directed resuscitation becomes increasingly accepted in critical care, burn care clinicians may be inclined to monitor these parameters and respond to abnormalities in QT, VO_2, LA, or BD by increasing fluid support.

However, it remains unclear how valid this approach is in burn patients. Although it is accepted that patients' ability to achieve optimal values of QT and VO_2 correlates strongly with outcome, it is far less clear whether exaggerated fluid infusion, invasive monitoring, or inotropic support can change nonresponders into responders and thus improve survival.[64] Both Kaups and colleagues[56] and Choi and colleagues[57] found that elevated BD (>6 mmol/L) was associated with increased fluid requirements in burn patients, but they were unable to determine if resuscitation aimed at normalizing BD was effective or beneficial. In other studies of goal-directed therapy, attaining target values of QT, VO_2, or wedge pressure routinely required more fluid—as much as four times Parkland calculations—without obvious improvement in survival.[65,66] Because complications such as abdominal compartment syndrome appear directly related to the fluid volume administered,[67,68] the benefits to be gained by this form of resuscitation may be overshadowed by the complications.

Clearly, the optimal method of monitoring and delivering burn resuscitation has yet to be determined. Although fluid creep is widespread, most burn centers still base fluid administration primarily on urine output. Invasive hemodynamic monitoring does not appear to be indicated for routine use. However, it may be helpful in guiding therapy and avoiding over- or under-resuscitation in individuals who are clearly failing to respond to traditional resuscitation, including some elderly patients and those with massive injuries or cardiac disease, associated multiple trauma, or severe pulmonary dysfunction.

Composition of Crystalloids: Hypertonic Resuscitation

Given the indiscriminant nature of initial postburn capillary leakage, crystalloids are clearly the fluids of choice. The effective component of crystalloid is sodium,[69] which has led to use of hypertonic saline solutions to satisfy capillary and cellular leakage while minimizing fluid volume and the complications of edema.[70,71] When solutions containing up to 300 mEq sodium per liter have been compared with LR in burn resuscitation, each regimen results in delivery of almost identical quantities of sodium, whereas the amount of free water is inversely proportional to sodium content.[72] Hypertonic saline solutions have been advocated for children[73] and the elderly,[74] who tolerate under- and over-resuscitation poorly, as well as for patients with head injuries,[75] and for field and combat resuscitation in which weight of available solutions must be minimized.[76,77]

Hypertonic saline resuscitation carries the risk of significant hypernatremia, hyperchloremia, acidosis, and hyperosmolarity and probably requires more careful monitoring than LR-based regimens. In addition, savings in initial fluid requirements may be balanced by increased free water retention later.[78] Hypertonic saline has been associated with increased mortality in at least one study, possibly related to increased renal failure.[78] However, it is still used selectively in some burn centers[71,79] and remains an option in acute burn management.

Crystalloid versus Colloid

As discussed earlier, colloids are no more efficacious than crystalloids in early burn shock; certainly they are more expensive.[46] For this and other reasons, colloid use in resuscitation of all types has been condemned.[80] However, it is apparent that capillary integrity is largely restored by the end of 24 hours postinjury, and colloids given at this time can effectively expand plasma volume, restore oncotic pressure, and reduce secondary edema in unburned tissue[26,42] including possible prevention of abdominal compartment syndrome.[81]

Colloids used in burn resuscitation have included albumin, plasma protein fraction (Plasmanate), fresh frozen plasma, and synthetic colloids dextran and hetastarch. Routine albumin administration is a component of some traditional resuscitation regimens including the Evans and Brooke formulas.[27,46] In a widely quoted randomized trial, Goodwin and colleagues found that albumin-based resuscitation required less total fluid than LR alone (2.98 vs. 3.81 mL/kg/%TBSA; $p<0.05$) but was associated with a sustained increase in extravascular lung water.[82] Critics have also pointed out that routine albumin supplementation has no apparent benefits.[83] Nonetheless, albumin remains a popular colloid; its current use varies among burn centers from routine administration within 8 to 12 hours of injury,[41,48] to selective use in problem resuscitations, to near-total interdiction. Fresh frozen plasma has also been used successfully[84]; its colloid effects probably explain much of the efficacy of plasma exchange therapy in complex burn resuscitations.[85] However, its routine use is now less widespread because of concerns over infectious risks, availability, and cost.

Both low-molecular-weight dextran and hetastarch have been used in burn resuscitation regimens, sometimes combined with hypertonic saline, and appear to be as effective as albumin in maintaining oncotic pressure and reducing edema in unburned tissues.[42,86,87] They offer advantages of long shelf life, availability, freedom from disease transmission, and lower cost. However, hetastarch has been associated with dose-dependent development of coagulopathy and bleeding, as well as rare anaphylactic reactions that may limit its use in large volumes.[88]

Colloid use appears unnecessary for resuscitation of most patients with uncomplicated injuries. With increasing burn size, the benefits of colloid administration, restricted to use after the first 8 to 12 hours postburn, may be significant in reducing total fluid requirements and the complications of excessive edema formation. Some centers have developed protocols utilizing LR for the first hours postinjury, followed by hypertonic saline or colloid, or both, to reduce edema as resuscitation is completed.[48] This area of resuscitation is extremely controversial and will benefit from randomized, multicenter trials.

Pharmacologic Manipulation of Resuscitation

As understanding of the pathophysiology of burn shock has increased, a number of investigators have attempted to reduce its severity by blocking some of its specific chemical mediators. These efforts have included use of vasodilators such as hydralazine, histamine blockade using cimetidine, the serotonin antagonist ketanserin, and anti-inflammatory drugs such as hydrocortisone and ibuprofen.[34,46,89-91] The antioxidant vitamin C, given in high doses in the early postburn period, has been shown to decrease fluid requirements in clinical burn resuscitation.[92] Many of these efforts have succeeded to a limited extent, although none has found its way into widespread clinical use. The possibility of developing an effective cocktail to ameliorate the effects of burn shock holds promise for the future.

Practicing Effective Resuscitation

As the preceding sections illustrate, a bewildering array of regimens (and opinions) are in current use for burn resuscitation. In attempting to practice resuscitation effectively, the clinician must decide on a protocol that is uniform and easy to apply by nurses yet flexible enough to permit individualized therapy and provide appropriate "escapes" for patients who are unstable.

An example of the protocol used at the University of Utah is included as Figure 68-5. The protocol is based on the Parkland formula but contains an option for the use of LR/albumin to arrest escalating fluid requirements. It requires nurses to adjust infusions on the basis of hourly urine output but mandates that physicians be contacted if worrisome parameters develop. We have found this protocol effective in resuscitating the vast majority of patients without frequent input from physicians. Figure 68-6 shows the theoretical course of a patient resuscitated with such a protocol. Similar protocols are in use in a number of burn centers.

Complications of Edema

Although the quantity of edema in both burned and unburned tissue is affected by fluid resuscitation, it is also true that substantial swelling is inevitable and occurs regardless of the resuscitation regimen used. Swelling within the face, eyes, extremities, and torso can have catastrophic consequences if untreated, and it is essential to remember that *edema is progressive for 24 hours following burn injury;* an area that is soft and pliable on admission may become tensely swollen within hours or overnight. Clinicians must be aware of the potential for these complications, follow serial examinations, and treat them as they develop.

Facial Swelling

Full-thickness facial burns can swell massively and produce complete airway obstruction within an hour or two of injury, as illustrated in Figure 68-1. As discussed under initial assessment, endotracheal intubation is essential in this setting and should be performed early and electively.

Continued facial swelling may preclude safe extubation for several days following injury. Accidental extubation in this period can be disastrous, so tubes must be secured as carefully as possible, and patients may require heavy sedation or paralysis, or both, to ensure that their tubes remain undisturbed. As edema begins to resolve within 48 to 72 hours, extubation should not be attempted until patients can open their eyes and breathe spontaneously, until an obvious air leak can be demonstrated when the ET tube cuff is deflated, and until the clinician feels they could be reintubated successfully. Early tracheostomy may provide a more comfortable and secure airway for patients with large injuries.

Ocular Swelling

Elevated intraocular pressure (IOP) has been documented in burn patients and appears to correlate with resuscitation volume. No data exist on the consequences of this phenomenon, but the risk of optic nerve ischemia and permanent visual loss may exist. Lateral canthotomy has been recommended for patients with persistently high IOPs.[93] Although not routinely practiced, measurement of IOP during acute burn resuscitation may be warranted in patients with severe facial injuries and eyelid edema.

Extremity Compartment Syndromes

Burns probably constitute the most common cause of extremity compartment syndromes. The pathophysiology is identical to that which accompanies fractures, crush injuries, and so on, with the notable exception that in burn patients the constricting layer is the eschar, not the underlying fascia. Therefore incision through the burn wound—escharotomy—is usually all that is necessary to relieve compression.

Failure to diagnose circulatory embarrassment of a burned extremity can lead to catastrophic ischemia, myonecrosis, and amputation. Because this diagnosis can be especially difficult in burn patients, a high index of suspicion and performance of *serial* examinations are essential.

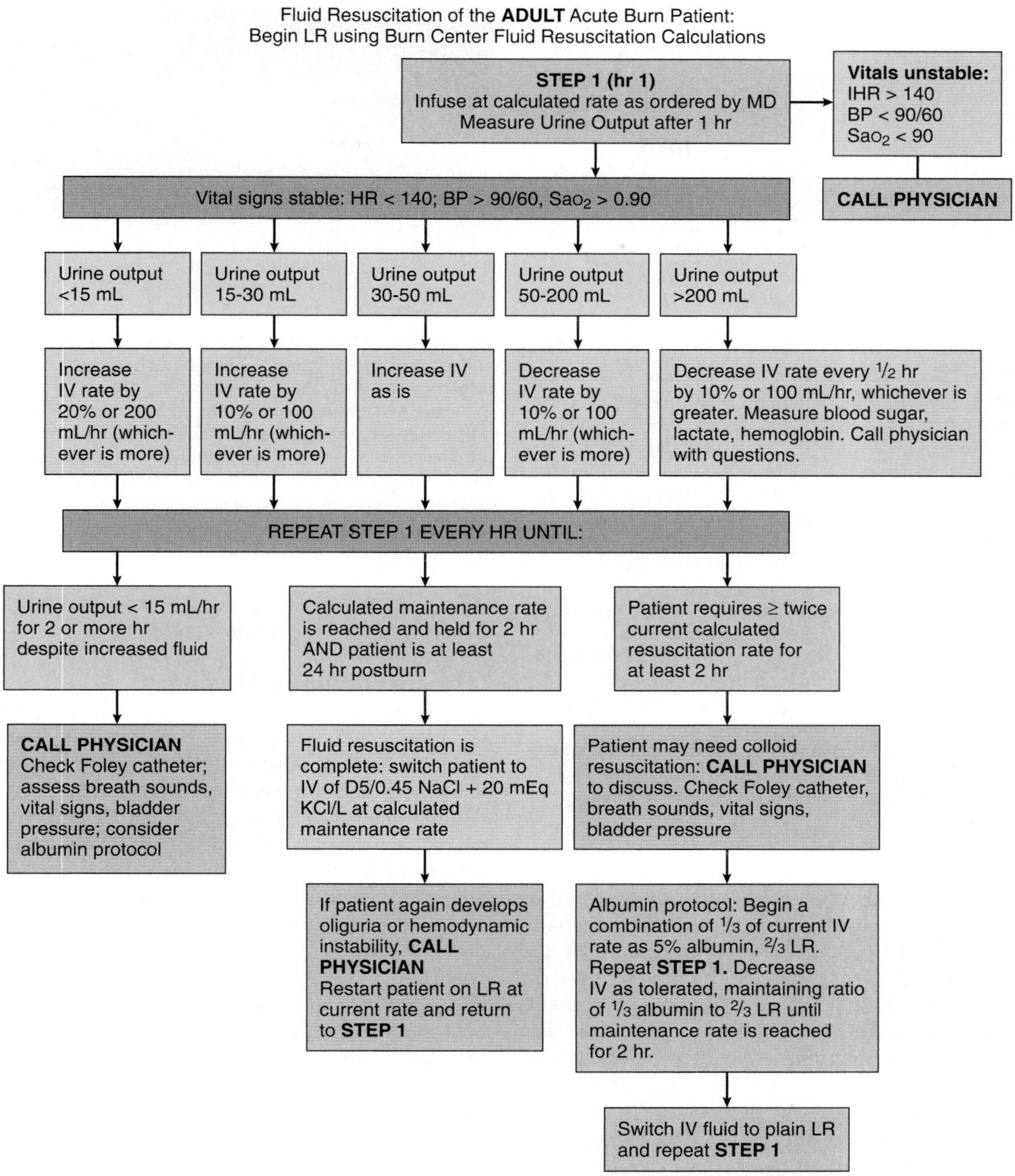

Figure 68-5. Burn fluid resuscitation protocol used at the University of Utah. Physicians order an initial infusion rate of lactated Ringer's solution based on Parkland calculations and indicate the target maintenance rate. Nursing staff measures hourly urine output and increase or decrease fluids on the basis of this response. If patients develop unexpected changes in vital signs or fail to respond appropriately, physicians are contacted. An option for the use of colloid-containing resuscitation is included for patients whose requirements fail to decline. This regimen permits close titration of fluids without requiring hourly physician input. BP, blood pressure; HR, heart rate; IHR, heart rate; IV, intravenous; LR, lactated Ringer's solution.

Classic findings of pain, paralysis, and so on (the "five Ps") may not be apparent beneath burn injuries or be impossible to assess in intubated patients and can develop insidiously in extremities that are soft on initial presentation. Significant compression is most likely following full-thickness, circumferential extremity burns, but compartment syndromes can develop in the absence of either of these findings or even in unburned extremities in patients who require excessive resuscitation volumes, particularly children. Limb-threatening compression can exist despite persistent palpable or Doppler pulses.[94] In addition, findings of paralysis or numbness may indicate irreversible nerve damage, and extremities should be decompressed before such symptoms develop.

Some authorities perform escharotomies on the basis of a general impression of extremity swelling, or even prophylactically. However, many clinicians use measurements of intramuscular pressure to help overcome the

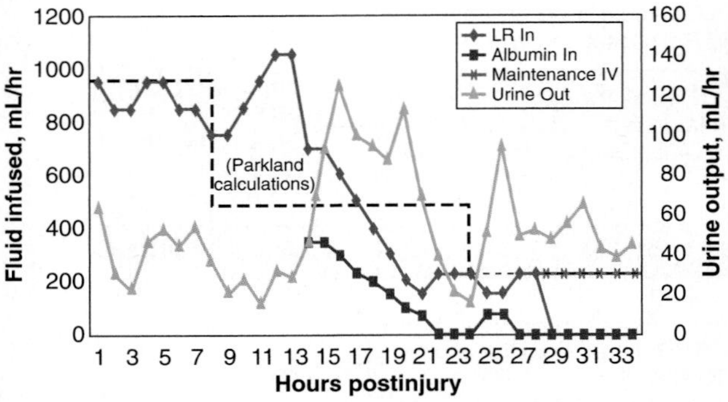

Hour	1	6	12	18	24	30
Hct, %	48	52	56	50	46	36
LA, mg/dL	4.5	5.0	5.4	4.8	3.6	2.2

Figure 68-6. Graphic representation of the theoretical course of fluid resuscitation for an 82-kg man with burns to 46% total body surface area who receives resuscitation according to the protocol in Figure 68-5. Parkland calculations *(dashed black line)* predict a total of (4×82×46) 15,088 mL in the first 24 hours. Half is given over the first 8 hours, or 943 mL/hr; the rate is cut in half after 8 hours. Initial fluid administration *(blue line)* is approximately equal to these predictions; however, requirements begin to increase at 9 to 10 hours postinjury. When they exceed twice the calculated rate for this time period (471 mL/hr), fluids are switched to a combination of two-thirds LR and one-third 5% albumin. This results in rapid increase in urine output, permitting fluids to be decreased incrementally. Albumin is discontinued at hour 22, but progressively falling urine output results in its reinstitution at hour 24. Urine output again responds and is sustained while the patient is switched to a maintenance regimen. Values of hematocrit and lactic acid are indicated in the box.

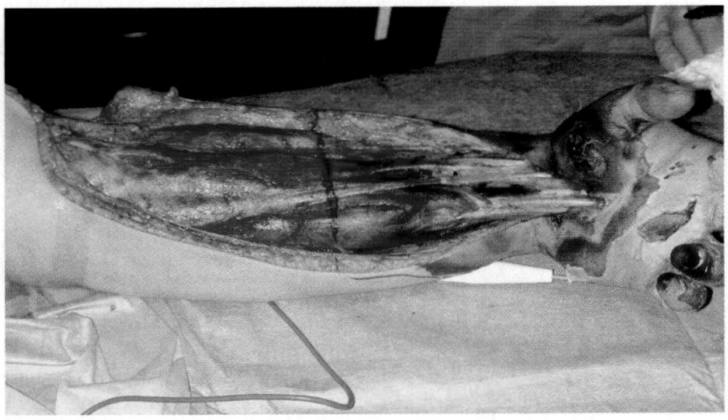

Figure 68-7. Massively swollen forearm following high-voltage electrocution injury. Simple escharotomy of the distal forearm and hand failed to decompress the extremity, so extensive fasciotomy was performed to above the elbow. The skin edges are widely separated by edema. Proximal forearm muscles are viable, but tissues distal to the drawn line—the line of anticipated amputation—are clearly necrotic. The wrist and fingers are "frozen" in flexion caused by contraction of damaged muscles.

limitations of physical examination listed earlier. This procedure is easily done by inserting a large-bore (18-gauge) needle attached to a pressure transducer through the eschar into the underlying muscle. The muscles must be entirely relaxed during this procedure, and pressure allowed to equilibrate to a steady state. Pressures that exceed 30 cm/H_2O compromise capillary perfusion and mandate decompression.[95] Measurements should be repeated to document successful decompression following incisions; pressures that remain elevated following escharotomy indicate the need to deepen or extend incisions or to proceed with fasciotomy. This may be particularly likely in patients with very deep burns, associated trauma, or electrical injury (Fig. 68-7).

Swollen extremities should be initially treated with elevation and avoidance of constricting dressings. If escharotomies are necessary, they can often be done at the bedside using electrocautery and appropriate analgesia. Longitudinal incisions should run the length of the burn wound and be placed medially and laterally on the supinated limb to avoid major nerves and vessels and facilitate resurfacing with skin grafts. Incisions must penetrate through the burn until the wound edges pop open, and pressure is clearly relieved. Incisions in burned hands should extend at least to the metacarpal-phalangeal joints; performance of individual digit escharotomies has some support,[96] but is often omitted. As an alternative, the use of enzymatic débriding agents to provide "chemical escharotomy" is popular in some centers.[97]

Torso Compartment Syndromes

Recent awareness of massive abdominal swelling as a cause of cardiorespiratory compromise has led to protocols for monitoring intra-abdominal pressure and performing decompressive laparotomy in many ICU populations. In burn patients, increased occurrence of abdominal compartment syndrome (ACS) likely reflects the widespread trend toward fluid creep, as discussed earlier,[67] although it can clearly develop in the absence of excessive resuscitation. Like other edema-related complications, intra-abdominal hypertension develops progressively throughout fluid resuscitation and often presents suddenly with oliguria, hypotension, and respiratory embarrassment that can be life threatening.

Patients with major (≥25% TBSA) burns or extensive torso injuries, or both, or those who require large resuscitation volumes (≥500 mL/hour[68]) should have routine monitoring of bladder pressures.[68,98] The finding of intra-abdominal hypertension in the absence of clinical symptoms does not mandate laparotomy but should prompt other measures to reduce abdominal pressures.[99] In patients with deep burns of the chest or abdomen, performance of torso escharotomy—sometimes repeatedly—will often relieve pressures, improve ventilation, and obviate laparotomy. There is evidence that both hypertonic saline and colloid-based resuscitation prevent development of ACS[71,81]; in addition, a bolus of albumin or Hespan can sometimes arrest increasing bladder pressures or even decrease them. Removal of peritoneal fluid with dialysis catheters has also been effective.[100] Unfortunately, many patients with ACS present with diffuse intraperitoneal and retroperitoneal swelling, rather than free peritoneal fluid; diagnostic ultrasound can make this decision and guide catheter placement if free fluid is seen.

Although the mortality of ACS in burn patients is high,[101] this is likely caused as much by the severity of the underlying burn as by this complication itself. Delayed performance of decompressive laparotomy may potentiate ongoing shock and "oxygen debt" and even lead to intestinal necrosis, whereas prompt decompression will both improve survival and reduce ongoing resuscitation requirements.[102] Patients in whom other measures fail or symptoms progress rapidly should undergo immediate decompressive laparotomy, at the bedside if necessary. Open abdomens are difficult to manage in burn patients; the widely used vacuum-assisted closure dressings[103] may be impossible to secure over burn eschar. Placement of temporary mesh silos may be the best way to manage exposed viscera. As edema resolves, every effort should be made to reduce eviscerated contents and obtain fascial closure through repeated wound revisions. Figure 68-8 illustrates a patient in whom numerous complications of edema—massive facial swelling, extremity compartment syndromes, and ACS—have occurred simultaneously. This is not uncommon in the modern treatment of massive burn injuries.

Acute Renal Failure

As mentioned previously, development of effective protocols for fluid resuscitation has greatly reduced acute renal failure (ARF) during initial burn treatment. ARF may still develop if resuscitation is delayed or inadequate,[104] particularly in patients with high-voltage electrical injuries or extremely deep burns, in whom pigment-induced nephropathy from myoglobin/hemoglobin is possible. Patients with visibly red or black urine should have resuscitation increased to produce urine outputs of 50 to 100 mL/hour. A one-time initial dose of an osmotic diuretic such as mannitol to stimulate urine production, as well as alkalinization of the urine by adding bicarbonate to IV fluids, is also widely practiced.[105,106]

ARF in burn patients is now most often a late complication of infection or dehydration.[107] Established ARF has a high mortality, primarily from underlying sepsis and multiple organ failure. Clearly its prevention is the best management strategy, through meticulous attention to fluid resuscitation and infection control. When ARF develops, patients should be treated with dialysis according to standard indications. Continuous veno-venous or arteriovenous hemofiltration can be particularly effective in managing large fluid volumes in patients who tolerate intermittent dialysis poorly.[108] Nutritional support should not be reduced in this setting; rather, patients should continue to receive the calories and protein they require and undergo dialysis as needed.

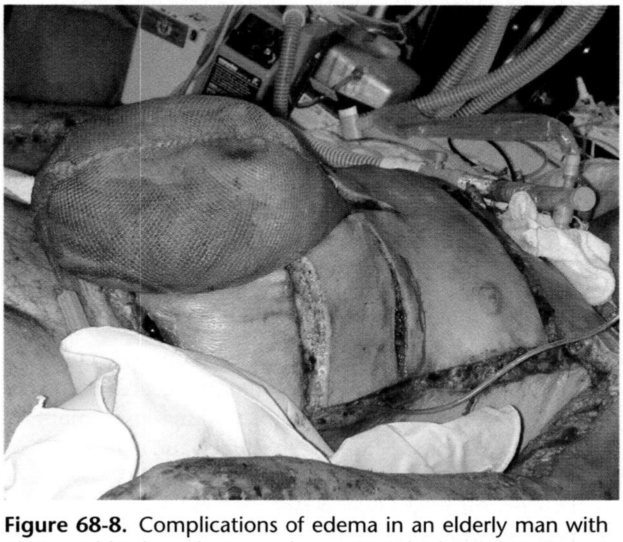

Figure 68-8. Complications of edema in an elderly man with 70% total body surface area burns. Facial edema is massive; tracheostomy has been performed to provide secure, long-term airway support. Escharotomies on upper extremities and multiple torso escharotomies have resulted in increased swelling and separation of wound edges. Despite these measures, abdominal compartment syndrome necessitated bedside laparotomy and placement of a synthetic mesh "silo" to contain eviscerated abdominal contents. As edema resolved over several days, viscera were gradually returned to the abdomen, and the silo trimmed until closure of the fascia was possible. The other escharotomy wounds were covered with skin grafts.

Electrolyte Abnormalities

Although almost any disturbance of serum chemistries can occur during and following burn resuscitation, several characteristic patterns are seen. Most frequent are disturbances in serum sodium concentration. Massive resuscitation with LR (sodium content 130 mEq/L) may itself produce mild hyponatremia but also markedly increases total body sodium content. The formula given previously for maintenance fluids following resuscitation provides only an estimate of these requirements; individuals vary substantially, and fluid needs can also be shifted up or down by fever, wound closure, ventilator support, hyperglycemia-induced diuresis, and other abnormalities. Following resuscitation, urine output will be less sensitive to fluid balance because of an obligatory diuresis generated by the huge amounts of sodium given during resuscitation, and serum sodium concentration will reflect free water balance. Progressive hyponatremia should prompt a reduction in total free water intake, whereas hypernatremia should be treated with increased free water. Dehydration can develop insidiously, with progressive increases in serum sodium and blood urea nitrogen despite adequate daily urine output.

Hyperkalemia may occur immediately postburn, caused by cellular injury, acidosis, and volume contraction. This is usually short lived and rarely requires treatment unless renal function is also impaired. With effective fluid resuscitation, potassium levels often drop below normal and patients may require substantial supplementation. Aldosterone levels are elevated following burn injury and contribute to chronic hypokalemia and alkalosis.[109] Potassium supplementation is also required as part of the "refeeding" effect of aggressive nutritional support.

Hypophosphatemia is extremely common following burns and has multiple etiologies including catecholamine secretion, metabolic alkalosis, impaired renal phosphate absorption, and increased excretion during post-resuscitation diuresis.[110] Phosphate levels typically reach a nadir 2 to 5 days after injury and rebound slowly afterward. Significant hypophosphatemia can lead to cardiac dysfunction, reduced red blood cell survival, and neurologic abnormalities, particularly during refeeding. Substantial phosphate supplementation may be necessary throughout the wound coverage phase of burn treatment.

Decreased levels of magnesium, like potassium and phosphate, may all result from fluid resuscitation, increased aldosterone secretion, and consumption during glucose metabolism and protein synthesis and may potentiate each other as well. Routine monitoring and replacement of electrolytes should be performed at least until patients no longer require intravenous fluids.

WOUND COVERAGE PHASE

Surgical Treatment of Burn Patients

Although effective fluid resuscitation has reduced *acute* mortality of burned patients, aggressive surgery has produced the greatest advancement in *overall* survival from burns. Early excision of wounds and coverage with skin or skin substitutes removes burn eschar as a major source of infection, shortens hypermetabolism, relieves pain, improves functional results, and permits earlier mobilization and preservation of muscle mass.

As discussed previously, burn eschar left in place eventually separates from underlying tissue through the action of leukocyte enzymes. Bacterial infection assists this process, and burn eschar is an ideal medium for bacterial growth. In the era before routine excision, many patients died from sepsis while awaiting eschar separation and experienced unremitting pain and prolonged muscle wasting, which was often fatal in itself. Surgical excision of burns was first practiced in the early 20th century but was associated with high mortality from blood loss and anesthesia. Beginning in the 1970s, increasingly aggressive protocols for excision of major burns have produced improved survival and decreased length of stay[111,112] and are now considered standard of care. A detailed discussion of these techniques is beyond the scope of this chapter. However, intensivists must be aware of the principles of surgical treatment and be able to support patients preoperatively and postoperatively.[113]

Indications and Timing of Surgery

The larger the burn injury, the more critical the need for early excision. Patients with small (<10% to 15% TBSA) burns can be followed for up to 14 days while wounds "declare" themselves, but when burn size exceeds 25% to 30% TBSA, a widely accepted goal is removal of essentially all of the burn wound within 7 days of injury. Herndon and colleagues[114] excise the entire wound in a single procedure even while fluid resuscitation is ongoing,[114] but most units practice a staged approach, removing 15% to 20% TBSA at each operation.

Type of Procedure

Excision of full-thickness skin and subcutaneous tissue, called "fascial excision," is rapid, is relatively bloodless, and creates a reliable bed for skin grafting. It is often practiced in the elderly and for particularly deep burns. However, fascial excisions are disfiguring and cause substantial problems with joint stiffness and pain. Far more common today is tangential excision, in which thin slices of tissue are removed until a viable bed of dermis or subcutaneous fat is reached. This requires more skill and time and produces more blood loss, but long-term results are unquestionably superior.

Wound Coverage

Excised burn wounds left uncovered will eventually desiccate and develop a new layer of necrotic tissue—in essence, a second eschar—with attendant problems of metabolic stress, pain, and susceptibility to infection. The ultimate goal of all burn surgery is autografting, or coverage with the patient's own skin. Burns excised within 7 to 10 days of injury are usually quite clean and are often excised and autografted in one procedure, providing prompt wound closure and facilitating early mobility. If donor sites are limited, autografts can be meshed to expand and cover more area. In recent years, use of a variety of skin substitutes has become standard when donors are not available or if burns appear infected or poorly vascularized. Most simply, excised wounds can be covered with antibiotic wet soaks to maintain tissue viability and combat infection. However, the most widely used technique is coverage with cadaver allograft skin obtained from tissue banks. Like autograft, allograft permits vascular ingrowth and take—sometimes for weeks—although this tissue is always eventually rejected. Allograft placement reduces bacterial colonization and pain; retards wound contraction; creates a clean, vascular bed; and serves as a test for subsequent autografting. Cultured epithelial autografts ("cultured skin") can be used to cover extensive areas but are expensive, fragile, and prone to loss from infection. They are best used over a scaffolding of intact or allograft dermis, and meticulous wound preparation is essential for success. Various synthetic and processed skin substitutes are also regularly used in acute burn care. These include synthetic dermis (Integra, Integra, Inc., Plainsboro, NJ), acellular dermal matrix (Alloderm, LifeCell Corp., Branchburg, NJ), amniotic membrane, and collagen-bound polymer membranes (Biobrane and Transcyte, Smith and Nephew, Inc., Hull, UK). Products still in development combine synthetic dermis with cultured epidermis, providing the potential for future one-step complete skin replacement.[115] All of these products require experience and skill to utilize successfully.

Hemodynamic Support

During and after fluid resuscitation blood pressure is sustained by elevated catecholamine levels, blood volume may remain below normal, and hematocrit artificially high. With induction of anesthesia, adrenergic blockade and vasodilation can produce sudden hypotension as this ongoing, hidden hypovolemia and anemia are revealed. In addition, surgical excision of old or infected burn wounds may stimulate bacteremia and potentiate hemodynamic instability.[116] The surgical team should prepare for these contingencies by continuing liberal fluid infusions during surgery and anticipating blood loss. Major burn excisions produce significant bleeding, which is often underestimated by surgeons. The blood loss resulting from excision of 1% of the body surface area of an adult has been estimated at approximately 100 mL.[117] Use of tourniquets for excision, performance of staged excisions, and use of subdermal clysis of epinephrine-containing solutions—the Pitkin procedure—can all help reduce intraoperative bleeding.[118]

Temperature Control

Although burn patients often display low-grade fever secondary to hypermetabolism, they also have accelerated evaporative heat loss. In the operating room, exposure of wounds for surgery and suppression of metabolism increases the risk of hypothermia, which can be difficult to correct. Temperature should be monitored carefully, patient warming devices should always be used in the OR, and the room itself kept warm. Limiting operations to 2 to 3 hours is also helpful in avoiding hypothermia.

Burn Pharmacology and Anesthesia

As mentioned in Chapter 47, depolarizing muscle relaxants (succinylcholine) should not be used in patients with acute burn injuries,[119] but burn patients are also relatively resistant to nondepolarizing agents and frequently require increased dosage. Induction agents that produce vasodilation, such as propofol, may potentiate hypotension and should be used with caution. Ketamine maintains hemodynamic stability and can be used effectively in surgery or for bedside procedures and dressing changes. Pharmacokinetics and dynamics of many other drugs are also significantly altered in burn patients.[120] Blood volume is chronically increased following resuscitation, and some degree of minor capillary leakage persists. Decreased serum albumin reduces binding of many drugs including benzodiazepines, further increasing volume of distribution. Increased renal blood flow increases clearance of some drugs including many antibiotics, necessitating monitoring and individualized dosing.[121]

Pain Control

Pain management is notoriously difficult in burn patients, who often require remarkable quantities of narcotics and sedatives throughout their hospital course. Although altered pharmacology undoubtedly plays a role in this process, the most important factors contributing to the increased narcotic and sedative needs of burn patients are the extreme levels of sustained pain produced by burn injuries, as well as tachyphylaxis, which develops during long-term administration of opioids. Patient-controlled analgesia (PCA) can be effective, but use may be limited by impaired consciousness and hand function.[122] Nonopioid analgesics such as ibuprofen and Toradol can be useful adjuncts in patients with cutaneous injuries. Finally, behavior modifications such as relaxation therapy, hypnosis, and virtual reality can be extremely helpful in overcoming the anxiety of dressing changes and physical therapy. Careful assessment of pain and anxiety, as well as individualized dosing regimens, are essential for successful management of burn patients.[123]

Pulmonary Management

Pulmonary complications are extremely common in burn patients and constitute a substantial component of patient support. A variety of different pulmonary processes can occur; they can demand simultaneous treatment and be difficult to sort out. Initial airway compromise, discussed previously, can be isolated and self-limited but leads frequently to long-term complications from pulmonary infection and inflammation. Adult respiratory distress syndrome (ARDS) can occur in the absence of inhalation injury, or components of both disorders can coexist and complement each other. Pulmonary edema or large pleural effusions can complicate fluid resuscitation. Aspiration, narcotic-induced respiratory depression, atelectasis and immobilization from bed rest, associated chest trauma, pulmonary thromboembolism, barotrauma, and pneumothorax/hemothorax following central line placement are all encountered in the management of major burns.

Chapter 47 provides a detailed discussion of the pathophysiology and treatment of inhalation injury. No effective treatment for inhalation injury exists; management is expectant and directed at its complications. In fact, the most important reason to diagnose inhalation injury is probably to anticipate increased likelihood of acute lung injury and the need for ventilatory support. Recent evidence suggests that inadequate fluid resuscitation may actually accentuate pulmonary damage.[124] Burn patients with inhalation injuries require increased volumes of fluid[49] and should be resuscitated as aggressively as other burn patients, and to the same end points. Pulmonary artery catheterization may be helpful in patients with severe lung injuries who require high ventilator pressures. Although colloid-based resuscitation may be associated with persistently increased extravascular lung water,[82] this does not appear to be the case with crystalloid, even in patients with inhalation injury given substantially more than Parkland requirements.[66]

A number of reports have focused on techniques to improve oxygenation in burn patients with severe acute lung injury: extracorporeal membrane oxygenation[125]; inhaled nitric oxide[126]; and novel ventilator strategies such as high-frequency volume diffusive[127]; oscillation[128]; or percussive ventilation.[129] However, these modalities are limited in their availability and usefulness, and clear-cut indications for each have not been developed. The use of permissive hypercapnia may be beneficial,[130] although other protective lung strategies have not been evaluated in burns. The vast majority of burn patients can be managed effectively with conventional ventilation techniques, and death purely from hypoxia is rare.

At present, multiple organ failure is the most common cause of death in burn patients.[131,132] Respiratory failure is the most common organ failure encountered and is almost invariably present in patients who die.[133] Pneumonia, in turn, is probably the most frequent source of respiratory failure and certainly the most common practical problem in pulmonary management of burn patients. This pneumonia is usually ventilator associated; intubation facilitates contamination of the lower airways already primed for infection by the mucosal sloughing, mucous plugging, and atelectasis caused by inhalation of chemical irritants.

Pneumonia can be particularly severe and persistent in burn patients, and frequent cultures and aggressive antibiotic treatment—sometimes for prolonged periods—are necessary for successful treatment. A number of other strategies aimed at improving pulmonary function have also been utilized in this setting. Meticulous attention to pulmonary toilet including humidified oxygen, frequent suctioning, and chest physiotherapy should be used in all cases. Strategies that have been effective in other populations have included elevation of the head of the bed, closed suction techniques, postpyloric feeding, and frequent oral care.[134] The use of heparin and acetylcysteine aerosols—sometimes combined with bronchodilators—to liquefy and mobilize casts and debris has been associated with reduced ventilator dependence and mortality in pediatric patients.[135] Improved mobilization of secretions may also be the mechanism by which percussive or oscillatory ventilation is beneficial.[129] Fiberoptic bronchoscopy and bronchoalveolar lavage can be used both for diagnosis of pneumonia and as a therapeutic maneuver to clear tenacious plugs and improve ventilation.[12] Based on limited evidence, neither corticosteroids nor prophylactic antibiotics appear to be helpful in treating respiratory failure or preventing pneumonia.[136] Performance of tracheostomy in patients who fail initial attempts at extubation may or may not reduce infections,[137] but it unquestionably provides a more comfortable and secure airway for long-term ventilator support.

Cardiovascular Complications and Care

As mentioned earlier, the typical immediate response to burn injury consists of reduced cardiac output and increased peripheral resistance, followed by gradual return of both values to near-normal at the end of resuscitation, after which markedly elevated cardiac output and reduced peripheral resistance persists through wound coverage and into rehabilitation (see Fig. 68-3). This response is so predictable that invasive hemodynamic monitoring is rarely necessary during fluid resuscitation and may result in markedly increased fluid requirements. Swan-Ganz pulmonary artery catheters, inotropic support, and measurements of oxygen delivery and consumption should be reserved for problem or complicated patients, or those who fail to respond as predicted to fluid resuscitation.

Catecholamine stimulation of cardiac function often results in hypertension, which can be difficult to manage, as well as sustained tachycardia and tachyarrhythmias. β-Blockade is useful in treating these problems and may be indicated for routine administration as well. β-Blockers are tolerated well in this situation and may even contribute to improved outcomes.[138]

Hypotension can also occur in burn patients during acute care. Obligatory postresuscitation diuresis coupled with increased evaporative and metabolic fluid losses favors development of occult volume depletion. Increased serum sodium, progressive azotemia, and sustained tachycardia can all provide clues to this diagnosis. Multiple fluid boluses may be required to treat this problem and are usually well tolerated. Persistent hypotension should lead to a search for sepsis. Invasive monitoring may be helpful in this setting as well; however, the classic hemodynamic picture of sepsis—increased cardiac output and reduced peripheral resistance—is also the characteristic postburn response, so that such monitoring will likely be more useful in guiding therapy than in diagnosis.

Adrenal Insufficiency

Recent studies have demonstrated a surprisingly high frequency of absolute or relative adrenal insufficiency in critical-care patients, which may greatly increase the mortality from shock and sepsis.[139] However, the quoted incidence of this problem has varied greatly, depending on the diagnostic criteria used[140] and on the populations studied.[140-143] No systematic evaluation of adrenal insufficiency has been conducted in burn patients. This complication appears to be rare,[144] but may be more common than previously suspected, and is diagnosed fairly frequently when sought. Adrenal insufficiency should be considered in burn patients with refractory hypotension.

Infection Control

Burn Wound Infections

Historically, overwhelming burn wound sepsis was the major cause of death in patients who survived resuscitation. Over the past 50 years, use of systemic and topical antibiotics, coupled with surgical excision and skin grafting, has resulted in a dramatic decrease in this problem. However, infection in burn wounds including skin grafts remains an important source of morbidity and mortality. As with other infections, development of increasingly effective antibiotics has been matched by rapid adaptation and evolution of microbial pathogens. Initial experience with antibiotics in World War II controlled *Streptococcus* and *Staphylococcus* infections, but these were supplanted by gram-negatives, particularly *Pseudomonas*. In the 1960s and 1970s, development of silver nitrate solution, mafenide acetate (Sulfamylon), and silver sulfadiazine (Silvadene, Thermazene, SSD) were effective in combating these infections, but microflora continued to evolve. Today, burn wound infections are increasingly caused by multiply-resistant gram-negatives, *Acinetobacter*, methicillin-resistant *Staphylococcus*, *Candida*, and fungi.[145] Individual patients display a similar progression of bacterial flora, from relatively straightforward gram-positive infections initially, to increasingly resistant and uncommon gram-negatives, yeast, and fungi as therapy and antibiotic administration continues.

Established principles of infection control remain a critical component of burn patient care. Essentially every open wound should be treated with topical agents until healed. The time-tested topical agents sulfadiazine and mafenide remain effective against a wide range of bacteria and still constitute first-line agents for acute burn treatment despite some limitations. Silver sulfadiazine has been associated with neutropenia, although this is often a normal phenomenon in the early postburn period (see later) and appears reversible. Mafenide acetate inhibits carbonic anhydrase and can produce significant metabolic acidosis if used on large areas for prolonged periods. Mafenide use has also been linked to emergence of fungal infections.[146] A number of additional topical agents are now available for specific indications, including silver-containing dressings (Acticoat, Acquacel-Ag); cerium-silver nitrate; combinations of polymyxin, neosporin, and bacitracin; mupirocin (Bactroban); chlorhexidine; Betadine; and others. Broad-spectrum agents (sulfadiazine, silver nitrate, mafenide, Acticoat) should be used in the early postburn period and on large wounds; this therapy can be tapered in smaller injuries and as wounds heal. Agents may also need to be adjusted on the basis of culture results and wound appearance. Silver nitrate, silver-eluting agents, and topical antifungals such as nystatin and amphotericin are effective against yeast and mold infections, whereas antibiotic solutions including mafenide are widely used to soak fresh skin grafts and some skin substitutes. The "melting graft syndrome" has been attributed to chronic infection with *Staphylococcus* species[147]; topical mupirocin may be particularly effective in this setting.

In addition to topical antibiotics, physical cleansing of all wounds is a major component of effective care. Unhealed wounds should be washed and gently débrided at least daily, and wounds inspected carefully. Findings suggestive of invasive infection include green or black discoloration, purulent exudate, extending erythema or tissue necrosis, conversion of superficial-appearing burns to deep wounds, development of satellite lesions (ecthyma gangrenosum), or loss of vascularized skin grafts. Any of these findings should prompt careful culturing of wounds, escalating or changing topical and systemic antibiotics, and possibly surgery.

Surface cultures of burn wounds can be used to identify dominant organisms but cannot distinguish between invasive infection and colonization. Burn wound biopsies can be obtained for quantitative culture; bacterial counts of 10^6 per gram of tissue or more have been used as a criterion for invasive burn wound sepsis. However, false-positive results are frequent; wounds may be heavily colonized without bacterial invasion, and biopsies must be obtained in exactly the right place. Histologic findings of penetration of organisms into viable tissue and capillaries remain a valid diagnostic finding.[145] However, many centers lack an experienced pathologist to read these samples accurately. As a result, routine biopsies are now used less frequently than in the past. Daily examination of wounds and clinical suspicion remain the most important tools for prompt diagnosis of burn wound infection. Once diagnosis is made, burn wound sepsis is best treated by aggressive, total wound excision, broad-spectrum systemic coverage, and topical antibiotic soaks in preparation for allograft or autograft placement. Burn wound sepsis is an extremely serious complication and should involve every member of the burn team.

Other Infections

Modern methods of infection prevention and control have contributed to decreased rates of many types of infections in burn patients. With the decline in burn wound infections, pneumonia, discussed previously, has emerged as the most common infection in burn patients. Central venous catheter infections also remain a constant threat. Burn victims have the highest incidence of catheter-related candidemia of any hospitalized group.[148] Bacterial endocarditis is a rare but dreaded complication that usually presents following prolonged hospitalization. Central venous catheters contribute to occurrence of right-sided valvular lesions, particularly if lines are allowed to reach the atrium or ventricle.[149] However, neither routine catheter changes nor rewires have been shown to decrease infectious risks.[150] Adherence to widely accepted principles of catheter placement and care[151] and prompt removal of catheters in the face of fever or leukocytosis, or when catheters are no longer necessary, should be practiced. Improved wound management, nutrition, and hygiene have all but eliminated such historically important infections as suppurative thrombophlebitis, chondritis of the ear, and suppurative parotitis as clinical problems.

Diagnosis of infection can be difficult in burn patients. Fever, leukocytosis, and tachycardia are all normal consequences of acute burn injury, but these should decline within 48 to 72 hours. Thereafter, low-grade fever may be sustained, but any increase in temperature above 38.5°C or increases in white blood cell count or heart rate should prompt an evaluation for infection. The once-ubiquitous policy of obtaining routine "surveillance" cultures of blood, urine, sputum, or wounds is now controversial. Such cultures have relatively low yield and a high incidence of false-positivity.[152] Few units still obtain routine burn wound biopsies; some use swab cultures to detect colonization and to track dominant flora for epidemiologic reasons. Cultures of blood, sputum, urine, stool, nasal mucosa, and so on should be obtained when clinically indicated and suspicion of infection exists.

Systemic prophylactic antibiotics have not been shown to reduce burn-wound or other infections and should not be used.[153,154] As in all ICU patients, antibiotic use should be guided by the clinical situation and culture results. As noted previously, because of altered blood volume, renal function, hepatic function, and clearance, burn patients often exhibit abnormal drug kinetics. Increased antibiotic dosing and careful monitoring of antibiotic efficacy is essential and illustrates the value of the clinical pharmacist as a member of the burn team. Isolation of burn patients through universal precautions and separation of infected patients by cohort nursing should be practiced as routine components of infection control. The practice of selective digestive decontamination in burn patients is controversial; although some centers report benefits,[155] and some no effect,[156] from this time-consuming technique, it is not routinely practiced in U.S. burn centers.

Metabolic Support and Gastrointestinal Management

Hypermetabolism of Burn Injury

Burns induce the greatest hypermetabolic response of any injury. This response typically follows the ebb and flow pattern described more than 70 years ago,[157] in which initial reduced energy expenditure is followed by increasing metabolism that peaks 10 to 14 days after injury, then tapers slowly as wound healing progresses. The degree of hypermetabolism correlates with burn size but appears to level off with burns of 40% to 50% TBSA, above which no further increase is seen.[158] This response is generated by sustained secretion of catecholamines, cortisol, and glucagon that rise almost immediately postburn and persist until after wounds are closed. Together these hormones accelerate catabolism through breakdown of skeletal muscle, reduced uptake of fats, and opposition to the effects of insulin.[159,160] The result is obligatory muscle wasting to support gluconeogenesis; lipids have little protein-sparing effect, and even exogenous glucose is limited in its ability to prevent protein wasting.[161]

In the 1970s patients frequently demonstrated calorie and protein consumption that exceeded twice normal for prolonged periods and caused fatal inanition within a few weeks of injury.[162-165] Modern burn treatment including aggressive excision and skin grafting has not altered the *nature* of this hypermetabolism but has clearly reduced its *magnitude* and duration.[166] Use of skin substitutes, control of sepsis and pain, mechanical ventilation, and maintaining high ambient temperature all reduce energy requirements.[158,167] However, significant hypermetabolism persists well after burn wounds are closed, and careful nutritional support is an important adjunct to rehabilitation of burn patients (Fig. 68-9).[168]

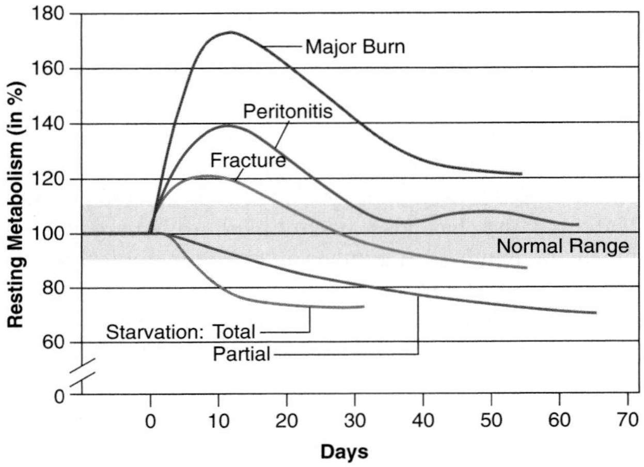

Figure 68-9. Alterations in resting metabolic rate produced by various disease states. Although starvation results in a decrease in resting energy expenditure, all injuries increase metabolism and protein catabolism. Major burns produce the greatest increases, and for the longest duration. This classic figure was produced in 1979; modern advances in burn care have not reduced the nature of this hypermetabolic response but have reduced the magnitude. Today, peak energy expenditure following a major burn is estimated at between 120% and 150% of normal metabolic rate. The duration of hypermetabolism is unchanged. (Long CL, Geiger JW, Schiller WR, Blakemore WS: Metabolic response to injury and illness: Estimation of energy and protein needs from indirect calorimetry and nitrogen balance. JPEN J Parenter Enteral Nutr 1979;3:454, with permission from the American Society for Parenteral and Enteral Nutrition [A.S.P.E.N.]. A.S.P.E.N. does not endorse the use of this material in any form other than its entirety.)

Route and Timing of Nutritional Support

The superiority of enteral nutrition is widely accepted[169] and may be especially true for burn patients. Enteral nutrition nourishes bowel mucosa, preserves blood supply, reduces permeability, and improves associated immune function.[170-172] In trauma and ICU patients, early and aggressive enteral nutrition appears to decrease infectious complications, whereas total parenteral nutrition (TPN) has been asso-ciated with increased infectious mortality in burn patients[173,174] and also promotes development of fatty liver.[175] TPN should be avoided in burn patients; it may be preferable to withhold nutrition entirely for limited periods, rather than use TPN.

Enteral feeding should begin as quickly as practical following injury, especially if patients will not be able to eat within 5 to 7 days. In contrast to early studies,[176] immediate enteral feedings do not reduce hypermetabolism[177] but do decrease calorie deficit and improve nitrogen balance.[178,179] Feedings can be started within a few hours of injury and continued even through surgical procedures.[180] Use of promotility agents has not been studied in burn patients.[181,182] It is also unclear whether small intestinal feedings are superior to gastric feedings; both can have complications, and both require careful monitoring.

Energy Requirements

Dozens of regimens have been used to estimate caloric needs of burn patients including the famous Curreri formula.[183] However, static formulas cannot accommodate the major fluctuations that occur over time and among individuals of different ages and burn sizes.[184] And as modern burn treatment has reduced hypermetabolism, older formulas overestimate requirements significantly.[185] Current recommended caloric intake for adults with major burns is 120% to 150% of Harris-Benedict estimates of basal needs.[186] Many centers also use indirect calorimetry to measure energy expenditure and to detect significant underfeeding or overfeeding.[187] Regardless, support should still be increased during periods of peak energy expenditure to avoid underfeeding and reduced later to avoid overfeeding.

Whatever the regimen chosen, the practical difficulties of delivering nutritional support are substantial.[188,189] Interruptions in feedings, fluctuations in energy consumption caused by fever and activity, and delivery of empty calories in glucose solutions all frustrate attempts to tailor individual nutrition exactly. This may explain why the superiority of indirect calorimetry-based nutrition has not been proved.[184] Involvement of the *team* including a dietician in implementing, assessing, and adjusting feedings are probably all more important than adherence to predetermined estimations.[190]

Table 68-3 lists some popular, commercially available enteral formulas that can be used in burn patients. Specific components of effective enteral formulas include the following:

Carbohydrates and Glucose Control

The catabolic hormonal environment of burn injury makes carbohydrates the preferred energy source but also causes significant problems with hyperglycemia. Recent studies have demonstrated the value of meticulous glucose control in ICU populations,[191] in reducing organ failure, length of stay, and inflammation.[192] These benefits are likely seen in burn patients as well,[193] but hormonally mediated resistance to insulin—the so-called diabetes of injury—makes attaining control a major challenge, even in patients who are not diabetic before injury. Many burn units are developing protocols for blood sugar control, which requires frequent (or continuous) dosing of insulin and careful monitoring. Oral hypoglycemics appear helpful in this effort[194]; in addition, giving limited calories as fat helps reduce the glucose burden required by these metabolically active patients. However, some "specialty" formulas designed for use in pulmonary failure or diabetes contain more fat calories than is optimal for burn patients (see Table 68-3).

Fat

A certain (small) quantity of dietary fat is essential. However, lipolysis is suppressed in burn patients, as is ability to utilize exogenous fat as an energy source. Fat intake should be restricted to less than 30% of total nonprotein calories, or about 1 gm/kg/day[195] or even less.[196,197] Withholding fat entirely from TPN for substantial periods may be beneficial.[169,198] In addition, products high in ω-3 fatty acids (FFAs) and correspondingly low in ω-6 FFAs may improve glucose control and reduce infections.[199,200] Most clinical experience has been obtained with use of immune-enhancing diets (see later) in which the effects of individual components have been difficult to assess.

Protein

Accelerated proteolysis is a key component of burn-induced hypermetabolism and often its most problematic consequence. A major goal of nutrition is to reduce or replace these losses, which can exceed ½ pound of lean body mass per day. Provision of adequate calories will not eliminate increased muscle breakdown,[201] so increased dietary protein must be provided as well. As with calories, protein utilization increases with burn size[202,203]; increasing dietary protein has resulted in reduced infections and mortality in patients with major injuries.[204] Current recommendations in burn patients are 1.5 to 2 g of protein per kg body weight per day (up to 3 g/kg/day in children),[187,190,205] which corresponds to a nonprotein calorie-to-nitrogen ratio of 100 : 1 or less. Nitrogen balance should be monitored regularly; other nutritional markers are discussed later.

Specific Amino Acids

The amino acids arginine (ARG) and glutamine (GLU) play enhanced roles in critical illness; both are depleted rapidly following burns and are considered conditionally essential in burn patients.[201,206] Glutamine is important in energy transport, as a precursor of glutathione,[207] and as a nutrient for enterocytes, helping to preserve bowel integrity and limit permeability.[208-210] In burn patients provision of up to 25 g GLU/day, given parenterally[211] or enterally,[212] has been associated with improved visceral protein levels and reduced infectious mortality and length of stay. GLU supplementation is not routinely practiced, although it has been recommended.[169] GLU is almost totally absent from TPN, which may explain many of the benefits of enteral nutrition in burn patients.

Arginine enhances natural killer cell function and nitric oxide (NO) synthesis, promoting inflammation and resistance to infection.[213,214] Specific studies of ARG supplementation have not been performed in burn patients; instead, ARG has been incorporated into complex immune-enhancing diets (IEDs) containing ω-3 FFAs, ARG, GLU, RNA, and so on.[215] These diets have shown benefits in surgical populations[216] but deleterious or no effects in patients with sepsis or pneumonia,[217] for which ARG has been blamed.[218] Little data are available on IEDs in burn patients,[219] but the mixed results in other groups suggest that components should be studied separately before incorporating them into cocktails with even more unpredictable effects. Widespread use of IEDs has been questioned[169]; at present, other high-protein stress formulas are recommended for burn patients, many of which contain increased ARG and GLU.

Other Nutrients

A number of micronutrients including vitamins A, C, and D; iron, and zinc are important in wound healing and may be depleted following burn injury,[220] so some supplementation has been recommended.[221] Many centers simply administer multivitamins, which is probably adequate.[159,222] Commercial enteral stress formulas also contain far more than recommended daily allowances of many vitamins and trace elements.

Monitoring Nutritional Support

Because burn injury alters many parameters of nutritional status, monitoring nutrition can be as difficult as providing it. For example, substantial weight gain is inevitable following fluid resuscitation,[223] whereas aggressive feeding can increase body fat even as protein stores are depleted.[224,225] As a result, patients have often lost more lean body mass than is reflected by weight alone.[226] Nitrogen balance studies can be useful, but sedation and bed rest make attaining positive nitrogen balance difficult,[227] emphasizing the need to continue physical therapy even during acute care. Serum protein markers are often distorted; levels of albumin,[228] prealbumin, and transferrin[187,229] fall quickly following injury and recover only slowly even with appropriate nutrition. Burn-induced anergy confounds use of delayed-type hypersensitivity testing. Perhaps the best marker of nutritional adequacy in burn patients is their overall status including vital signs, wound healing, and functional improvement. Body weight,

Table 68-3. Commercially Available Formulas for Enteral Nutrition of Burned Adults

			Contents (per 1000 Kcal)								
			Carbs		Protein			Fat			
Brand Name (Manufacturer)	mL	%RDI per 1000 mL	Gm	%Kcal	Gm	%Kcal	Cal:N2	Gm	%Kcal	ω6: ω3	Comments
Immune-Enhancing and Healing Adult Formulas											
Crucial (Nestle)	667	100	90	36	63	25	67:1	45	39	2:1	Elemental, hypertonic, concentrated Enhanced with arginine
Impact (Novartis)	1000	67	130	53	56	22	71:1	28	25	1.4:1	Widely used immune-enhancing formula; supplemented with arginine; high in ω-3 FFAs
Replete (Nestle)	1000	100	113	45	63	25	75:1	34	30	3:1	Inexpensive, high-protein formula
TraumaCal (Mead-Johnson)	667	33	95	38	55	22	91:1	45	40	6.3:1	High-protein, concentrated. Relatively high proportion of ω-6 FFAs
Standard Adult Formulas											
Isocal-HN (Mead-Johnson)	943	80	117	46	42	17	125:1	43	37	N/a	Isotonic all purpose feeding,without fiber
Jevity (Ross)	943	67	146	54	42	17	125:1	33	29	4.2:1	Isotonic, with fiber
Specialty Adult Formulas											
Nepro (Ross)	500	52	111	43	35	14	154:1	48	43	N/a	Widely-used renal failure formula; low in potassium, phosphorus, protein. Can be supplemented with protein for burn patients.
Glucerna (Ross)	1000	70	96	34	42	17	125:1	54	49	10.8:1	Low-carbohydrate formula for diabetics; relies on high-fat content, which is of limited efficacy in burn patients
Pulmocare (Ross)	667	70	71	28	42	17	125:1	62	55	4:1	Customized formula for pulmonary failure relies on high fat content to avoid excessive VCO_2; limited efficacy in burn patients
Peptamen (Nestle)	1000	67	127	51	40	16	131:1	39	33	7:1	Semi-elemental, isotonic

FFAs, free fatty acids; N/a, not available.

nitrogen balance, and protein markers may be most useful in tracking trends in individuals.[230]

Modulation of Hypermetabolism

Burn-related hormonal changes create tremendous problems in nutritional support but also provide mechanisms by which hypermetabolism can be manipulated and at least partially controlled. Recent studies have shown promising results and suggest that manipulation of the metabolic response to injury may become routine in the future. Various approaches have been used including β-blockade with propranolol, low-dose insulin infusions, use of counter-regulatory hormones such as insulin-like growth factor-1 (IGF-1), or anabolic agents such as testosterone and oxandrolone.[231] Use of propranolol appears to be a safe, low-cost way to ameliorate the cardiovascular response to acute burn injury and to reduce hypermetabolic muscle wasting during acute burn care.[232] Administration of the synthetic oral androgen oxandrolone has been shown to reduce muscle breakdown, speed rehabilitation, and lead to decreased length of stay in hospitalized patients.[233,234] Although none of these therapies is now routine, they are becoming much more widespread. Recommendations for their routine use will need to await larger controlled trials to demonstrate efficacy.

Gastrointestinal Complications in Burn Patients

Burn patients can develop a host of abdominal and gastrointestinal problems. Although the incidence of most GI complications has decreased dramatically with improved resuscitation and control of infection, several problems are frequent or serious enough to deserve discussion.

Acute Cholecystitis

Cholecystitis—usually acalculous—can have a number of causes including gallbladder ischemia from shock and dehydration,[235] biliary stasis from narcotics and TPN, bile pigment loads from hemolysis and transfusion, and bacterial seeding from sepsis. With more effective control of these factors, acute cholecystitis is now rare; a recent review documented just 20 cases among 10,762 acutely burned patients (0.18%), with progressive declines in recent years.[236] Fever, leukocytosis, feeding intolerance, and abdominal pain are characteristic findings, although they may be difficult to sort out in acutely ill, ventilated patients. Ultrasound and CT scanning are preferred for confirmation of diagnosis; biliary scintigraphy can have a high false-positive rate. Treatment has traditionally consisted of prompt cholecystectomy, although bedside placement of cholecystostomy tubes under ultrasound guidance can provide definitive treatment in many patients.[237] With prompt diagnosis, mortality from this complication should be low.

Hepatic Enzyme Elevation

A number of liver enzyme abnormalities can occur following burn injury. Initially, hemolysis and ileus can contribute to a cholestatic picture, which should resolve within a few days of injury. Some degree of chronic fatty infiltration of the liver may be inevitable in patients with major burns, and mild enzyme elevations are often seen. This problem is aggravated by use of TPN and overfeeding, although it can develop in the absence of these.[175] Severe hepatic steatosis may be both a cause and consequence of sepsis, and it correlates with increased mortality.

Pancreatitis

Pancreatitis can also result from systemic hypoperfusion. In contrast to cholecystitis, however, the incidence of pancreatitis may be increasing because more severely injured patients now survive burn shock. Ryan and colleagues[238] documented hyperamylasemia in 40% of patients with large burns, often in association with septic events. These patients had increased mortality and length of stay,[238] although pancreatic pseudocysts and abscesses were quite rare. Pancreatic enzymes should be measured in patients with feeding intolerance, abdominal pain, or nausea; in many cases, transient bowel rest and fluid support will be effective treatment. Use of TPN should be avoided unless pancreatitis is unusually severe and prolonged.

Gastrointestinal Bleeding

Although the time-honored eponym "Curling's ulcer" has sometimes been considered a unique entity, burn patients develop the same stress ulcerations that occur in other acutely ill patients. Mucosal erosions and atrophy have been demonstrated within 72 hours of burn injury, which can progress to large (often multiple) ulcerations of the prepyloric area, or duodenum. Their primary cause is thought to be impaired gastric mucosal perfusion from shock or sepsis; the role of *Helicobacter pylori* infection is unclear.[239,240] Modern treatment strategies including aggressive fluid resuscitation, suppression or neutralization of gastric acid, and early enteral feeding have resulted in a dramatic decline in incidence of this complication, from as high as 86% in early postmortem studies[241] to less than 2% today. Bleeding is more frequent with large injuries and in patients with coagulopathy, prolonged mechanical ventilation, and sepsis. Aggressive evaluation of any observed gastrointestinal bleeding should be undertaken. Most patients can be controlled with endoscopic maneuvers and continuous proton-pump inhibitors. Surgery for acute upper GI bleeding is now rarely required.[242]

Ileus and Intestinal Necrosis

Ileus occurs routinely following acute burns, and oral intake should be withheld at least until resuscitation is completed. Impaired intestinal motility can be aggravated by narcotics, infections, and ventilatory support. Severe colonic ileus (Ogilvie's syndrome) can occur in this setting,[243] and concomitant enteral feeding can cause bowel distention, ischemia, and bacterial overgrowth, ultimately leading to necrosis and perforation. Although rare, this catastrophic complication can be difficult to detect and causes death in more than 50% of patients.[244,245] For this reason, feedings should be monitored carefully and held if obstipation, distention, or pain become significant.

CT scanning can confirm bowel dilation or free air, in which case immediate laparotomy is mandatory.

Diarrhea

Diarrhea is extremely common with enteral feedings and can be a major problem in management. The cause is often multifactorial[246] including high osmotic loads, overfeeding, enteral medications, and infections including cytomegalovirus and *Clostridium difficile*.[247] Treatment options include enteral opiates such as Imodium or paregoric or use of fiber-containing products. However, fiber can clog small diameter tubes and has been blamed for intestinal distention and necrosis,[248] whereas slowing intestinal transit can potentiate infectious diarrhea. Often simply holding feedings for a few hours will suffice; diarrhea unresponsive to simple measures should prompt a search for infectious causes, inside or outside of the bowel.[249]

Hematologic Considerations

Red Blood Cells

The hemoconcentration that accompanies burn shock can result in hematocrits as high as 70%. This increases blood viscosity, producing sludging and contributing to increased vascular resistance. As resuscitation proceeds, hematocrits fall progressively and are usually below normal by the end of 48 hours. Thereafter, anemia often persists or worsens until wound coverage is obtained. Several mechanisms contribute to this finding.[250] First, burn injury destroys red cells directly; significant acute hemolysis can occur within minutes of injury, even while hematocrits are increased by loss of plasma volume. This may be manifested by hemoglobinuria or jaundice, or both. Burn injury also induces persistent changes in red cell morphology resulting in spherocytosis, increased membrane fragility, and shortened red cell survival. Erythropoietic response is blunted, apparently at the stem cell level.[251] This is not caused by erythropoietin deficiency, as stores are often supranormal, and erythropoietin supplementation is not helpful.[252] Acute hemorrhage from surgery and more gradual blood loss from wound débridements add to these effects.

The issue of appropriate transfusion "trigger" is controversial in burn patients. No systematic trial of transfusion thresholds has been performed, and no standard is universally accepted,[253] although limited evidence supports the practice of conservative transfusion in burn patients as in other ICU populations. In a multicenter review, Palmieri and colleagues[254] found that transfusion number correlated with both mortality and infectious episodes in major burns, which supports the concept that transfusions be based on physiologic assessment and not given routinely. Aggressive early excision probably increases transfusion requirements,[255] although these may be reduced by "total excision" performed within 24 hours of injury.[256] Other strategies used to reduce surgical blood loss have been reviewed previously.

White Blood Cells (WBCs)

Immediately postburn, leukocytosis and WBC demargination are nonspecific components of the stress response. As with red cells, WBC numbers decline following resuscitation, reaching a nadir that is often well below normal on postburn days 2 to 5. In the past, this has been attributed to use of silver sulfadiazine but appears to occur regardless of whether this topical agent is used and resolves spontaneously even if the drug is continued. After this period, WBC levels reflect systemic infection and stress. Leukocytosis is common with acute infections, but neutropenia is a far more ominous finding in severe sepsis and may suggest bone marrow failure. Granulopoiesis is accelerated following injury and is mediated at least partially by catecholamines. Treatment with colony-stimulating factors has not been routinely practiced.

Platelets

Platelets and coagulation factors are also consumed in the early postburn period; platelet counts below 100,000/mm^3 and coagulopathy are common for the first few days, and supplementation may be necessary, particularly if major excisions are performed. Subsequently, both rebound to supranormal levels. During wound coverage, patients may demonstrate platelet counts in excess of 1,000,000/mm^3, and fibrinogen levels may exceed twice normal. These are reactive abnormalities and do not require treatment.[257] Platelet counts are a sensitive indicator of infection; a falling platelet count occurring after the first few days should suggest sepsis and is associated with a poor prognosis.

Thromboembolism

Systemic inflammation, a hypercoagulable state, and frequent immobilization might all suggest that thromboembolic complications are common in burn patients. In fact, reported incidences of clinically apparent deep venous thrombosis (DVT) and pulmonary embolism (PE) are low.[258] However, prospective evaluation of burn patients suggests an incidence of DVT/PE similar to that of other moderate to high-risk populations.[259] At present, no consensus exists on the issue of DVT prophylaxis in burn patients. Some centers use it routinely, whereas many centers provide it for "high-risk" patients including the obese, patients with large burns, lower extremity burns, or femoral venous lines.

REHABILITATION

Although the focus of this chapter is the acute care of burn patients, it must be remembered that "rehabilitation begins at the time of injury." The physical therapist is an essential member of the *acute* burn team, and therapy should begin before resuscitation is completed. Physical therapy, mobilization, and prevention of skin breakdown and muscle wasting can have profound effects on the overall success of acute burn care. Immobility and inactivity result in rapid depletion of muscle mass and function; other complications include demineralization of bone and pathologic fractures,[260] myositis ossificans, and extensive contracture formation. Therapeutic exercise regimens, beginning during acute care and continuing beyond hospital discharge, can result in improved function and well-being and increased return to independent living.[261]

KEY POINTS

- Carbon monoxide poisoning and asphyxia are the most immediate causes of death in burn patients exposed to smoke. High-flow oxygen should be administered to all patients immediately.
- Acute airway obstruction can occur at any time during the first 24 hours of injury, even in the absence of smoke inhalation. Early and elective endotracheal intubation should be performed in patients who develop wheezing, stridor, dyspnea, or significant facial swelling.
- Following initial assessment, fluid resuscitation is the primary goal of initial burn treatment. Fluid resuscitation should be instituted using a formula based on body weight and burn size such as the Parkland formula and adjusted to maintain urine output of 0.5 to 1 mL/hour.
- During the first 8 to 12 hours postburn, crystalloid solutions such as LR should be the sole fluids used for burn resuscitation. After that time, the addition of colloid-containing solutions may be helpful in limiting edema in unburned tissues.
- Invasive hemodynamic monitoring with Swan-Ganz catheters and inotropic fluid support should be reserved for problem patients who are not responding to standard fluid resuscitation.
- Edema in both burned and unburned tissue is progressive throughout fluid resuscitation and may progress rapidly. Intubation should be performed if facial swelling is severe or increasing.
- Extremities with full-thickness or circumferential burns should be monitored with measurements of intramuscular pressure, and escharotomies performed if pressures exceed 30 cm/H_2O. Fasciotomies should be performed if pressures fail to improve with escharotomy.
- Torso compartment syndromes can present with sudden and life-threatening hypotension, oliguria, and respiratory distress. Bladder pressures should be measured in patients with extensive torso injuries. Torso escharotomies should be performed initially, but decompressive laparotomy may be required in patients with progressive compromise.
- Multiple trauma in burn patients can be managed using standard approaches, as long as fluid resuscitation is continued.
- Surgical excision and skin grafting of burn wounds requires specialized attention to fluid support, blood loss, temperature control, and drug pharmacology.
- Pain control is often difficult in burn patients, who often require increased quantities of narcotics. Routine pain assessment and individualized dosing is necessary for successful pain control.
- Acute lung injury is the most common organ failure in burn patients, and pneumonia is the most common infection. Meticulous pulmonary toilet, ventilator support, and antibiotic treatment guided by culture results are all important components of care.
- Burn wound infections remain common in burn patients. Careful wound cleansing, débridement, and examination should be performed daily. Burn wound biopsies can be used to confirm diagnosis and direct therapy, but clinical evaluation remains the most important method for diagnosing these infections.
- Suspected or confirmed burn wound sepsis requires immediate excision of the wound, along with topical and systemic antibiotics.
- Aggressive nutritional support of burn patients is an essential component of care. Enteral nutrition should be started immediately after injury and consist of a high-calorie, high-protein diet that is relatively low in fat. Commercially available tube feedings also contain sufficient vitamins and trace elements for effective support. Use of "immune-enhancing diets" is controversial.
- Gastrointestinal complications of burn injury can include acalculous cholecystitis, pancreatitis, ileus, and ischemic necrosis of the bowel.
- Prophylaxis against deep venous thrombosis is not routinely practiced in burn patients but is probably indicated for patients with a prior history of thromboembolism, patients with extensive lower extremity injuries, or those who are obese.
- Rehabilitation is an essential component of burn treatment and should begin with initial care.

REFERENCES

1. Saffle JR (ed): Practice guidelines for burn care. Published as a supplement to the Journal of Burn Care and Rehabilitation. J Burn Care Rehabil 2001;22:S1-69.
2. Brigham PA, McLoughlin E: Burn incidence and medical care use in the United States: estimates, trends, and data sources. J Burn Care Rehabil 1996;17:95-107.
3. Saffle JR, Davis B, Williams P: Recent outcomes in the treatment of burn injury in the United States: A report from the American Burn Association Patient Registry. J Burn Care Rehabil 1995;16(3 Pt 1):219-232; discussion 88-89.
4. Wolf SE, Rose JK, Desai MH, et al: Mortality determinants in massive pediatric burns. An analysis of 103 children with > or =80% TBSA burns (> or =70% full-thickness). Ann Surg 1997;225:554-565; discussion 65-69.
5. Shirani KZ, Pruitt BA Jr, Mason AD Jr: The influence of inhalation injury and pneumonia on burn mortality. Ann Surg 1987;205:82-87.
6. Ryan CM, Schoenfeld DA, Thorpe WP, et al: Objective estimates of the probability of death from burn injuries. N Engl J Med 1998;338:362-366.
7. Salisbury R: Burn rehabilitation: Our unanswered challenge. The 1992 presidential address to the American Burn Association. J Burn Care Rehabil 1992;13:495-505.
8. Pereira C, Murphy K, Herndon D: Outcome measures in burn care. Is mortality dead? Burns 2004;30:761-771.
9. Chapter 1: Initial assessment and management. In Manual of Advanced Trauma Life Support. Chicago, American College of Surgeons, 2004, pp 1-10.
10. Birky MM, Clarke FB: Inhalation of toxic products from fires. Bull N Y Acad Med 1981;57:997-1013.
11. Zikria BA, Weston GC, Chodoff M, Ferrer JM: Smoke and carbon monoxide poisoning in fire victims. J Trauma 1972;12:641-645.
12. Fitzpatrick J, Cioffi W: Diagnosis and treatment of inhalation injury. In Herndon D (ed): Total Burn Care. Philadelphia, WB Saunders, 2002, pp 232-241.

13. Fein A, Leff A, Hopewell PC: Pathophysiology and management of the complications resulting from fire and the inhaled products of combustion: Review of the literature. Crit Care Med 1980;8:94-98.
14. Silverman SH, Purdue GF, Hunt JL, Bost RO: Cyanide toxicity in burned patients. J Trauma 1988;28:171-176.
15. Kirk MA, Gerace R, Kulig KW: Cyanide and methemoglobin kinetics in smoke inhalation victims treated with the cyanide antidote kit. Ann Emerg Med 1993;22:1413-1418.
16. Barillo DJ, Goode R, Esch V: Cyanide poisoning in victims of fire: Analysis of 364 cases and review of the literature. J Burn Care Rehabil 1994;15:46-57.
17. Wittram C, Kenny JB: The admission chest radiograph after acute inhalation injury and burns. Br J Radiol 1994;67:751-754.
18. Masanes MJ, Legendre C, Lioret N, et al: Fiberoptic bronchoscopy for the early diagnosis of subglottal inhalation injury: Comparative value in the assessment of prognosis. J Trauma 1994;36:59-67.
19. Varghese TK, Kim AW, Kowal-Vern A, Latenser BA: Frequency of burn-trauma patients in an urban setting. Arch Surg 2003;138:1292-1296.
20. Hawkins A, Maclennan PA, McGwin G Jr, et al: The impact of combined trauma and burns on patient mortality. J Trauma 2005;58:284-288.
21. Santaniello JM, Luchette FA, Esposito TJ, et al: Ten year experience of burn, trauma, and combined burn/trauma injuries comparing outcomes. J Trauma 2004;57:696-700; discussion 1.
22. Chang CH, Holmes JF, Mower WR, Panacek EA: Distracting injuries in patients with vertebral injuries. J Emerg Med 2005;28:147-152.
23. Saffle JR, Schnelby A, Hofmann A, Warden GD: The management of fractures in thermally injured patients. J Trauma 1983;23:902-910.
24. Purdue GF, Hunt JL: Multiple trauma and the burn patient. Am J Surg 1989;158:536-539.
25. Chapter 3: Shock and fluid resuscitation. In Manual of Advanced Burn Life Support. Chicago, American Burn Association, 2001, pp 33-40.
26. Baxter C: Fluid volume and electrolyte changes in the early post-burn period. Clin Plast Surg 1974;1:693-703.
27. Warden G: Fluid resuscitation and early management. In Herndon D (ed): Total Burn Care. Philadelphia, WB Saunders, 2002, pp 88-97.
28. Friedl HP, Till GO, Trentz O, Ward PA: Roles of histamine, complement and xanthine oxidase in thermal injury of skin. Am J Pathol 1989;135:203-217.
29. Carvajal HF, Brouhard BH, Linares HA: Effect of antihistamine-antiserotonin and ganglionic blocking agents upon increased capillary permeability following burn trauma. J Trauma 1975;15:969-975.
30. Sherwood E, Traber D: The systemic inflammatory response syndrome. In Herndon D (ed): Total Burn Care. Philadelphia, WB Saunders, 2002, pp 257-270.
31. Kramer G, Lund T, Herndon D: Pathophysiology of burn shock and burn edema. In Herndon D (ed): Total Burn Care. Philadelphia, WB Saunders, 2002, pp 78-85.
32. Youn YK, LaLonde C, Demling R: The role of mediators in the response to thermal injury. World J Surg 1992;16:30-36.
33. Starling E: On the absorption of fluids from the connective tissue spaces. J Physiol (Lond) 1986;19:312-326.
34. Demling RH: The burn edema process: Current concepts. J Burn Care Rehabil 2005;26:207-227.
35. Arturson G: Microvascular permeability to macromolecules in thermal injury. Acta Physiol Scand Suppl 1979;463:111-122.
36. Baxter CR, Shires T: Physiological response to crystalloid resuscitation of severe burns. Ann N Y Acad Sci 1968;150:874-894.
37. Birke G, Liljedahl SO, Plantin LO: Distribution and losses of plasma proteins during the early stage of severe burns. Ann N Y Acad Sci 1968;150:895-904.
38. Carvajal HF, Linares HA, Brouhard BH: Relationship of burn size to vascular permeability changes in rats. Surg Gynecol Obstet 1979;149:193-202.
39. Leape LL: Initial changes in burns: Tissue changes in burned and unburned skin of rhesus monkeys. J Trauma 1970;10:488-492.
40. Zetterstrom H, Arturson G: Plasma oncotic pressure and plasma protein concentration in patients following thermal injury. Acta Anaesthesiol Scand 1980;24:288-294.
41. Demling RH, Kramer G, Harms B: Role of thermal injury-induced hypoproteinemia on fluid flux and protein permeability in burned and nonburned tissue. Surgery 1984;95:136-144.
42. Demling RH, Kramer GC, Gunther R, Nerlich M: Effect of nonprotein colloid on postburn edema formation in soft tissues and lung. Surgery 1984;95: 593-602.
43. Guyton AC: Interstitial fluid pressure. I. Pressure-volume curves of interstitial space. Circ Res 1965;16:452-460.
44. Tanaka H, Lund T, Wiig H, et al: High dose vitamin C counteracts the negative interstitial fluid hydrostatic pressure and early edema generation in thermally injured rats. Burns 1999;25:569-574.
45. Miserocchi G, Negrini D, Passi A, De Luca G: Development of lung edema: Interstitial fluid dynamics and molecular structure. News Physiol Sci 2001;16:66-71.
46. Pruitt BA Jr, Mason AD Jr, Moncrief JA: Hemodynamic changes in the early postburn patient: The influence of fluid administration and of a vasodilator (hydralazine). J Trauma 1971;11:36-46.
47. Hilton JG, Marullo DS: Effects of thermal trauma on cardiac force of contraction. Burns Incl Therm Inj 1986;12:167-171.
48. Warden GD: Burn shock resuscitation. World J Surg 1992;16:16-23.
49. Navar PD, Saffle JR, Warden GD: Effect of inhalation injury on fluid resuscitation requirements after thermal injury. Am J Surg 1985;150:716-720.
50. Yowler CJ, Fratianne RB: Current status of burn resuscitation. Clin Plast Surg 2000;27:1-10.
51. Saffle JR, Edelman L, Morris SE: Regional air transport of burn patients: A case for telemedicine? J Trauma 57:57-64; discussion 2004.
52. Schwartz SI: Supportive therapy in burn care. Consensus summary on fluid resuscitation. J Trauma 1979;19(11 Suppl):876-877.
53. Friedrich JB, Sullivan SR, Engrav LH, et al: Is supra-Baxter resuscitation in burn patients a new phenomenon? Burns 2004;30:464-466.
54. Cancio LC, Chavez S, Alvarado-Ortega M, et al: Predicting increased fluid requirements during the resuscitation of thermally injured patients. J Trauma 2004;56:404-413; discussion 13-14.
55. Engrav LH, Colescott PL, Kemalyan N, et al: A biopsy of the use of the Baxter formula to resuscitate burns or do we do it like Charlie did it? J Burn Care Rehabil 2000;21:91-95.
56. Kaups KL, Davis JW, Dominic WJ: Base deficit as an indicator or resuscitation needs in patients with burn injuries. J Burn Care Rehabil 1998;19:346-348.
57. Choi J, Cooper A, Gomez M, et al: The 2000 Moyer Award. The relevance of base deficits after burn injuries. J Burn Care Rehabil 2000;21:499-505.
58. Cancio LC, Reifenberg L, Barillo DJ, et al: Standard variables fail to identify patients who will not respond to fluid resuscitation following thermal injury: Brief report. Burns 2005;31:358-365.
59. Tuchschmidt JA, Mecher CE: Predictors of outcome from critical illness. Shock and cardiopulmonary resuscitation. Crit Care Clin 1994;10:179-195.
60. Fiddian-Green RG, Haglund U, Gutierrez G, Shoemaker WC: Goals for the resuscitation of shock. Crit Care Med 1993;21(2 Suppl):S25-31.
61. Jeng JC, Lee K, Jablonski K, Jordan MH: Serum lactate and base deficit suggest inadequate resuscitation of patients with burn injuries: Application of a point-of-care laboratory instrument. J Burn Care Rehabil 1997;18:402-405.
62. Dries DJ, Waxman K: Adequate resuscitation of burn patients may not be measured by urine output and vital signs. Crit Care Med 1991;19: 327-329.
63. Schiller WR, Bay RC, Garren RL, et al: Hyperdynamic resuscitation improves survival in patients with life-threatening burns. J Burn Care Rehabil 1997;18(1 Pt 1):10-16.
64. Velmahos GC, Demetriades D, Shoemaker WC, et al: Endpoints of resuscitation of critically injured patients: Normal or supranormal? A prospective randomized trial. Ann Surg 2000;232:409-418.
65. Barton RG, Saffle JR, Morris SE, et al: Resuscitation of thermally injured patients with oxygen transport criteria as goals of therapy. J Burn Care Rehabil 1997;18(1 Pt 1):1-9.
66. Holm C, Tegeler J, Mayr M, et al: Effect of crystalloid resuscitation and inhalation injury on extravascular lung water: Clinical implications. Chest 2002;121:1956-1962.
67. Oda J, Yamashita K, Inoue T, et al: Resuscitation fluid volume and

abdominal compartment syndrome in patients with major burns. Burns 2006;32:151-154.
68. Britt RC, Gannon T, Collins JN, et al: Secondary abdominal compartment syndrome: Risk factors and outcomes. Am Surg 2005;71:982-985.
69. Moylan JA, Mason AD Jr, Rogers PW, Walker HL: Postburn shock: A critical evaluation of resuscitation. J Trauma 1973;13:354-358.
70. Monafo WW, Halverson JD, Schechtman K: The role of concentrated sodium solutions in the resuscitation of patients with severe burns. Surgery 1984;95:129-135.
71. Oda J, Ueyama M, Yamashita K, et al: Hypertonic lactated saline resuscitation reduces the risk of abdominal compartment syndrome in severely burned patients. J Trauma 2006;60:64-71.
72. Caldwell FT, Bowser BH: Critical evaluation of hypertonic and hypotonic solutions to resuscitate severely burned children: A prospective study. Ann Surg 1979;189:546-552.
73. Bowser-Wallace BH, Caldwell FT Jr: A prospective analysis of hypertonic lactated saline v. Ringer's lactate-colloid for the resuscitation of severely burned children. Burns Incl Therm Inj 1986;12:402-409.
74. Bowser-Wallace BH, Cone JB, Caldwell FT Jr: Hypertonic lactated saline resuscitation of severely burned patients over 60 years of age. J Trauma 1985;25:22-26.
75. Cooper DJ: Hypertonic saline resuscitation for head injured patients. Crit Care Resusc 1999;1:161.
76. Thomas SJ, Kramer GC, Herndon DN: Burns: Military options and tactical solutions. J Trauma 2003;54(5 Suppl): S207-218.
77. Vassar MJ, Perry CA, Gannaway WL, Holcroft JW: 7.5% sodium chloride/dextran for resuscitation of trauma patients undergoing helicopter transport. Arch Surg 1991;126:1065-1072.
78. Huang PP, Stucky FS, Dimick AR, et al: Hypertonic sodium resuscitation is associated with renal failure and death. Ann Surg 1995;221:543-554; discussion 54-57.
79. Griswold JA, Anglin BL, Love RT Jr, Scott-Conner C: Hypertonic saline resuscitation: efficacy in a community-based burn unit. South Med J 1991;84:692-696.
80. Roberts I, Alderson P, Bunn F, et al: Colloids versus crystalloids for fluid resuscitation in critically ill patients. Cochrane Database Syst Rev 2004;(4): CD000567.
81. O'Mara MS, Slater H, Goldfarb IW, Caushaj PF: A prospective, randomized evaluation of intra-abdominal pressures with crystalloid and colloid resuscitation in burn patients. J Trauma 2005;58:1011-1018.
82. Goodwin CW, Dorethy J, Lam V, Pruitt BA Jr: Randomized trial of efficacy of crystalloid and colloid resuscitation on hemodynamic response and lung water following thermal injury. Ann Surg 1983;197:520-531.
83. Greenhalgh DG, Housinger TA, Kagan RJ, et al: Maintenance of serum albumin levels in pediatric burn patients: A prospective, randomized trial. J Trauma 1995;39:67-73; discussion 4.
84. Du GB, Slater H, Goldfarb IW: Influences of different resuscitation regimens on acute early weight gain in extensively burned patients. Burns 1991;17:147-150.
85. Kravitz M, Warden GD, Sullivan JJ, Saffle JR: A randomized trial of plasma exchange in the treatment of burn shock. J Burn Care Rehabil 1989;10:17-26.
86. Guha SC, Kinsky MP, Button B, et al: Burn resuscitation: Crystalloid versus colloid versus hypertonic saline hyperoncotic colloid in sheep. Crit Care Med 1996;24:1849-1857.
87. Waters LM, Christensen MA, Sato RM: Hetastarch: An alternative colloid in burn shock management. J Burn Care Rehabil 1989;10:11-16.
88. Wiedermann CJ: Hydroxyethyl starch—can the safety problems be ignored? Wien Klin Wochenschr 2004;116: 583-594.
89. Tanaka H, Wada T, Simazaki S, et al: Effects of cimetidine on fluid requirement during resuscitation of third-degree burns. J Burn Care Rehabil 1991;12:425-429.
90. Holliman CJ, Meuleman TR, Larsen KR, et al: The effect of ketanserin, a specific serotonin antagonist, on burn shock hemodynamic parameters in a porcine burn model. J Trauma 1983;23:867-871.
91. Bjork J, Arturson G: Effect of cimetidine, hydrocortisone superoxide dismutase and catalase on the development of oedema after thermal injury. Burns Incl Therm Inj 1983;9:249-256.
92. Tanaka H, Matsuda T, Miyagantani Y, et al: Reduction of resuscitation fluid volumes in severely burned patients using ascorbic acid administration: A randomized, prospective study. Arch Surg 2000;135:326-331.
93. Sullivan SR, Ahmadi AJ, Singh CN, et al: Elevated orbital pressure: Another untoward effect of massive resuscitation after burn injury. J Trauma 2006;60:72-76.
94. Smith DJ Jr, Bendick PJ, Madison SA: Evaluation of vascular compromise in the injured extremity: A photoplethysmographic technique. J Hand Surg (Am) 1984;9:314-319.
95. Saffle JR, Zeluff GR, Warden GD: Intramuscular pressure in the burned arm: Measurement and response to escharotomy. Am J Surg 1980;140:825-831.
96. Salisbury RE, Taylor JW, Levine NS: Evaluation of digital escharotomy in burned hands. Plast Reconstr Surg 1976;58:440-443.
97. Krieger Y, Rosenberg L, Lapid O, et al: Escharotomy using an enzymatic débridement agent for treating experimental burn-induced compartment syndrome in an animal model. J Trauma 2005;58:1259-1264.
98. Fusco MA, Martin RS, Chang MC: Estimation of intra-abdominal pressure by bladder pressure measurement: Validity and methodology. J Trauma 2001;50:297-302.
99. Hong JJ, Cohn SM, Perez JM, et al: Prospective study of the incidence and outcome of intra-abdominal hypertension and the abdominal compartment syndrome. Br J Surg 2002;89:591-596.
100. Latenser BA, Kowal-Vern A, Kimball D, et al: A pilot study comparing percutaneous decompression with decompressive laparotomy for acute abdominal compartment syndrome in thermal injury. J Burn Care Rehabil 2002;23:190-195.
101. Jensen AR, Hughes WB, Grewal H: Secondary abdominal compartment syndrome in children with burns and trauma: A potentially lethal complication. J Burn Care Res 2006;27:242-246.
102. Hobson KG, Young KM, Ciraulo A, et al: Release of abdominal compartment syndrome improves survival in patients with burn injury. J Trauma 2002;53:1129-1133; discussion 33-34.
103. Miller PR, Meredith JW, Johnson JC, Chang MC: Prospective evaluation of vacuum-assisted fascial closure after open abdomen: Planned ventral hernia rate is substantially reduced. Ann Surg 2004;239:608-614; discussion 14-16.
104. Barrow RE, Jeschke MG, Herndon DN: Early fluid resuscitation improves outcomes in severely burned children. Resuscitation 2000;45:91-96.
105. Colic M, Ristic L, Jovanovic M: Emergency treatment and early fluid resuscitation following electrical injuries. Acta Chir Plast 1996;38:137-141.
106. Abassi ZA, Hoffman A, Better OS: Acute renal failure complicating muscle crush injury. Semin Nephrol 1998;18:558-565.
107. Holm C, Horbrand F, von Donnersmarck GH, Muhlbauer W: Acute renal failure in severely burned patients. Burns 1999;25:171-178.
108. Tremblay R, Ethier J, Querin S, et al: Veno-venous continuous renal replacement therapy for burned patients with acute renal failure. Burns 2000;26:638-643.
109. Dolecek R: Endocrine changes after burn trauma—a review. Keio J Med 1989;38:262-276.
110. Mozingo D, Mason A: Hypophosphatemia. In Herndon D (ed): Total Burn Care. Philadelphia, WB Saunders, 2002, pp 309-315.
111. Burke JF, Bondoc CC, Quinby WC: Primary burn excision and immediate grafting: A method shortening illness. J Trauma 1974;14:389-395.
112. Herndon DN, Barrow RE, Rutan RL, et al: A comparison of conservative versus early excision. Therapies in severely burned patients. Ann Surg 1989;209:547-552; discussion 52-53.
113. Saffle J: Role of surgical management. In Webb A, Shapiro M, Singer M, Suter P (eds): Oxford Textbook of Critical Care. Oxford, England, Oxford Medical Publishers, 1999, pp 774-776.
114. Muller M, Herndon D: Operative wound management. In Herndon D (ed): Total Burn Care. Philadelphia, WB Saunders, 2002, pp 170-182.
115. Supp DM, Boyce ST: Engineered skin substitutes: Practices and potentials. Clin Dermatol 2005;23:403-412.

116. Mozingo DW, McManus AT, Kim SH, Pruitt BA Jr: Incidence of bacteremia after burn wound manipulation in the early postburn period. J Trauma 1997;42:1006-1010; discussion 10-11.
117. Budny PG, Regan PJ, Roberts AH: The estimation of blood loss during burns surgery. Burns 1993;19:134-137.
118. Warden GD, Saffle JR, Kravitz M: A two-stage technique for excision and grafting of burn wounds. J Trauma 1982;22:98-103.
119. MacLennan N, Heimbach DM, Cullen BF: Anesthesia for major thermal injury. Anesthesiology 1998;89:749-770.
120. Jaehde U, Sorgel F: Clinical pharmacokinetics in patients with burns. Clin Pharmacokinet 1995;29:15-28.
121. Weinbren MJ: Pharmacokinetics of antibiotics in burns patients. J Antimicrob Chemother 2001;47:720.
122. Rovers J, Knighton J, Neligan P, Peters W: Patient-controlled analgesia in burn patients: A critical review of the literature and case report. Hosp Pharm 1994;29:106, 108-111.
123. Faucher L: Modern pain management in burn care. Problems in General Surgery: Burns 2003;20:80-87.
124. Herndon DN, Traber DL, Traber LD: The effect of resuscitation on inhalation injury. Surgery 1986;100:248-251.
125. Thompson JT, Molnar JA, Hines MH, et al: Successful management of adult smoke inhalation with extracorporeal membrane oxygenation. J Burn Care Rehabil 2005;26:62-66.
126. Musgrave MA, Fingland R, Gomez M, et al: The use of inhaled nitric oxide as adjuvant therapy in patients with burn injuries and respiratory failure. J Burn Care Rehabil 2000;21:551-557.
127. Carman B, Cahill T, Warden G, McCall J: A prospective, randomized comparison of the Volume Diffusive Respirator vs conventional ventilation for ventilation of burned children. 2001 ABA paper. J Burn Care Rehabil 2002;23:444-448.
128. Cartotto R, Ellis S, Smith T: Use of high-frequency oscillatory ventilation in burn patients. Crit Care Med 2005;33(3 Suppl):S175-181.
129. Cortiella J, Mlcak R, Herndon D: High frequency percussive ventilation in pediatric patients with inhalation injury. J Burn Care Rehabil 1999;20:232-235.
130. Sheridan RL, Kacmarek RM, McEttrick MM, et al: Permissive hypercapnia as a ventilatory strategy in burned children: Effect on barotrauma, pneumonia, and mortality. J Trauma 1995;39:854-859.
131. Saffle JR, Sullivan JJ, Tuohig GM, Larson CM: Multiple organ failure in patients with thermal injury. Crit Care Med 1993;21:1673-1683.
132. Fitzwater J, Purdue GF, Hunt JL, O'Keefe GE: The risk factors and time course of sepsis and organ dysfunction after burn trauma. J Trauma 2003;54:959-966.
133. Hollingsed TC, Saffle JR, Barton RG, et al: Etiology and consequences of respiratory failure in thermally injured patients. Am J Surg 1993;166:592-596; discussion 6-7.
134. Baxter AD, Allan J, Bedard J, et al: Adherence to simple and effective measures reduces the incidence of ventilator-associated pneumonia. Can J Anaesth 2005;52:535-541.
135. Desai MH, Mlcak R, Richardson J, et al: Reduction in mortality in pediatric patients with inhalation injury with aerosolized heparin/N-acetylcystine [correction of acetylcystine] therapy. J Burn Care Rehabil 1998;19:210-212.
136. Levine BA, Petroff PA, Slade CL, Pruitt BA Jr: Prospective trials of dexamethasone and aerosolized gentamicin in the treatment of inhalation injury in the burned patient. J Trauma 1978;18:188-193.
137. Saffle JR, Morris SE, Edelman L: Early tracheostomy does not improve outcome in burn patients. J Burn Care Rehabil 2002;23:431-438.
138. Arbabi S, Ahrns KS, Wahl WL, et al: Beta-blocker use is associated with improved outcomes in adult burn patients. J Trauma 2004;56:265-269; discussion 9-71.
139. Marik PE, Zaloga GP: Adrenal insufficiency in the critically ill: A new look at an old problem. Chest 2002;122:1784-1796.
140. Marik PE, Zaloga GP: Adrenal insufficiency during septic shock. Crit Care Med 2003;31:141-145.
141. Cooper MS, Stewart PM: Corticosteroid insufficiency in acutely ill patients. N Engl J Med 2003;348:727-734.
142. Burchard K: A review of the adrenal cortex and severe inflammation: Quest of the "eucorticoid" state. J Trauma 2001;51:800-814.
143. Barquist E, Kirton O: Adrenal insufficiency in the surgical intensive care unit patient. J Trauma 1997;42:27-31.
144. Sheridan RL, Ryan CM, Tompkins RG: Acute adrenal insufficiency in the burn intensive care unit. Burns 1993;19:63-66.
145. Pruitt BA Jr, McManus AT, Kim SH, Goodwin CW: Burn wound infections: Current status. World J Surg 1998;22:135-145.
146. Becker WK, Cioffi WG Jr, McManus AT, et al: Fungal burn wound infection. A 10-year experience. Arch Surg 1991;126:44-48.
147. Matsumura H, Meyer NA, Mann R, Heimbach DM: Melting graft-wound syndrome. J Burn Care Rehabil 1998;19:292-295.
148. Jarvis WR: Epidemiology of nosocomial fungal infections, with emphasis on Candida species. Clin Infect Dis 1995;20:1526-1530.
149. Sasaki TM, Panke TW, Dorethy JF, et al: The relationship of central venous and pulmonary artery catheter position to acute right-sided endocarditis in severe thermal injury. J Trauma 1979;19:740-743.
150. Kealey GP, Chang P, Heinle J, et al: Prospective comparison of two management strategies of central venous catheters in burn patients. J Trauma 1995;38:344-349.
151. O'Grady NP, Alexander M, Dellinger EP, et al: Guidelines for the prevention of intravascular catheter-related infections. The Hospital Infection Control Practices Advisory Committee, Center for Disse Control and Prevention, U.S. Pediatrics 2002;110:e51.
152. Keen A, Knoblock L, Edelman L, Saffle J: Effective limitation of blood culture use in the burn unit. J Burn Care Rehabil 2002;23:183-189.
153. Sheridan RL, Weber JM, Pasternack MS, Tompkins RG: Antibiotic prophylaxis for group A streptococcal burn wound infection is not necessary. J Trauma 2001;51:352-355.
154. Boss WK, Brand DA, Acampora D, et al: Effectiveness of prophylactic antibiotics in the outpatient treatment of burns. J Trauma 1985;25:224-227.
155. Mackie DP, van Hertum WA, Schumburg T, et al: Prevention of infection in burns: Preliminary experience with selective decontamination of the digestive tract in patients with extensive injuries. J Trauma 1992;32:570-575.
156. Barret JP, Jeschke MG, Herndon DN: Selective decontamination of the digestive tract in severely burned pediatric patients. Burns 2001;27:439-445.
157. Cuthbertson D: The disturbance of metabolism produced by bony and nonbony injury with notes of certain abnormal conditions of bone. Biochem J 1930;24:1244-1263.
158. Hart DW, Wolf SE, Chinkes DL, et al: Determinants of skeletal muscle catabolism after severe burn. Ann Surg 2000;232:455-465.
159. Kudsk K, Brown R: Nutritional support. In Mattox K, Feliciano D, Moore E (eds): Trauma. New York, McGraw-Hill, 2000, pp 1369-1405.
160. Bessey P, Jiang Z, Johnson D, et al: Posttraumatic skeletal muscle proteolysis: The role of the hormonal environment. World J Surg 1989;13:465-470.
161. Long C, Kinney J, Geiger C: Nonsuppressibility of gluconeogenesis by glucose in septic patients. Metabolism 1976;25:193.
162. Long C, Schaffel N, Geiger C, et al: Metabolic response to injury and illness: Estimation of energy and protein needs from indirect calorimetry and nitrogen balance. JPEN J Parenter Enteral Nutr 1979;3:452-456.
163. Wilmore D, Long J, Mason A, et al: Catecholamines: Mediators of the hypermetabolic response to thermal injury. Ann Surg 1974;180:653-658.
164. Newsome T, Mason A, Pruitt B: Weight loss following thermal injury. Ann Surg 1973;178:215-217.
165. Wilmore D: Nutrition and metabolism following thermal injury. Clin Plast Surg 1974;1:603-619.
166. Rutan T, Herndon D, VanOsten T, Abston S: Metabolic rate alterations in early excision and grafting versus conservative treatment. J Trauma 1986;26:140-146.
167. Royall D, Fairholm L, Peters WJ, et al: Continuous measurement of energy expenditure in ventilated burn patients: An analysis. Crit Care Med 1994;22:399-406.
168. Mittendorfer B, Hildreth MA, Desai MH, Herndon DN: The 1995 Clinical Research Award. Younger pediatric

patients with burns are at risk for continuing postdischarge weight loss. J Burn Care Rehabil 1995;16:589-595.
169. Heyland DK, Dhaliwal R, Drover JW, et al: Canadian clinical practice guidelines for nutrition support in mechanically ventilated, critically ill adult patients. JPEN J Parenter Enteral Nutr 2003;27:355-373.
170. Magnotti L, Deitch E: Burns, bacterial translocation, gut barrier function, and failure. J Burn Care Rehabil 2005;26:383-391.
171. Andel H, Rab M, Andel D, et al: Impact of duodenal feeding on the oxygen balance of the splanchnic region during different phases of severe burn injury. Burns 2002;28:60-64.
172. Saito H, Trocki O, Alexander J, et al: The effect of route of nutrient administration on the nutritional state, catabolic hormone secretion and gut mucosal integrity after burn injury. JPEN J Parenter Enteral Nutr 1987;11:1-7.
173. Herndon D, Stein M, Rutan T, et al: Failure of TPN supplementation to improve liver function, immunity, and mortality in thermally injured patients. J Trauma 1987;27:195-204.
174. Herndon D, Barrow R, Stein M, et al: Increased mortality with intravenous supplemented feeding in severely burned patients. J Burn Care Rehabil 1989;10:309-313.
175. Barret JP, Jeschke MG, Herndon DN: Fatty infiltration of the liver in severely burned pediatric patients: Autopsy findings and clinical implications. J Trauma 2001;51:736-739.
176. Mochizuki H, Trocki O, Dominioni L, et al: Mechanism of prevention of postburn hypermetabolism and catabolism by early enteral feeding. Ann Surg 1984;200:297-310.
177. Peck MD, Kessler M, Cairns BA, et al: Early enteral nutrition does not decrease hypermetabolism associated with burn injury. J Trauma 2004;57:1143-1149.
178. Moore E, Jones T: Benefits of immediate jejunostomy feeding after major abdominal trauma—a prospective, randomized study. J Trauma 1988;26:874-881.
179. Gottschlich M, Jenkins M, Mayes T, et al: The 2002 Clinical Research Award: An evaluation of the safety of early vs delayed enteral support and effects on clinical nutritional, and endocrine outcomes after severe burns. J Burn Care Rehabil 2002;23:401-415.
180. Jenkins M, Gottschlich M, Mayes T, et al: Enteral feeding during operative procedures. J Burn Care Rehabil 1994;15:199-205.
181. Komenaka IK, Giffard K, Miller J, Schein M: Erythromycin and position facilitated placement of postpyloric feeding tubes in burned patients. Dig Surg 2000;17:578-580.
182. Booth CM, Heyland DK, Paterson WG: Gastrointestinal promotility drugs in the critical care setting: A systematic review of the evidence. Crit Care Med 2002;30:1429-1435.
183. Curreri P, Richmond D, Marvin J, Baxter C: Dietary requirements of patients with major burns. J Am Diet Assoc 1974;65:415-417.
184. Saffle J, Medina E, Raymond J, et al: Use of indirect calorimetry in the nutritional management of burn patients. J Trauma 1985;25:32-39.
185. Dickerson RN, Gervasio JM, Riley ML, et al: Accuracy of predictive methods to estimate resting energy expenditure of thermally-injured patients. JPEN J Parenter Enteral Nutr 2002;26:17-29.
186. Harris J, Benedict F: A Biometric Study of Basal Metabolism in Man. Washington, DC, Carnegie Institute of Washington, 1919.
187. Peck M: Practice guidelines for burn care: Nutritional support. J Burn Care Rehabil 2001;22:59S-66S.
188. Adam S, Batson S: A study of problems associated with the delivery of enteral feed in critically ill patients in five ICUs in the UK. Intensive Care Med 1997;23:261-266.
189. De Jonghe B, Appere-De-Vechi C, Fournier M, et al: A prospective survey of nutritional support practices in intensive care unit patients: What is prescribed? What is delivered? Crit Care Med 2001;29:8-12.
190. Saffle J, Hildreth M: Metabolic support of the burned patient. In Herndon D (ed): Total Burn Care, 2nd ed. New York, WB Saunders, 2002, pp 271-287.
191. van den Berghe G, Wouters P, Weekers F, et al: Intensive insulin therapy in the critically ill patients. N Engl J Med 2001;345:1359-1367.
192. Solano T, Totaro R: Insulin therapy in critically ill patients. Curr Opin Clin Nutr Metab Care 2004;7:199-205.
193. Wu X, Thomas SJ, Herndon DN, et al: Insulin decreases hepatic acute phase protein levels in severely burned children. Surgery 2004;135:196-202.
194. Gore DC, Wolf SE, Sanford A, et al: Influence of metformin on glucose intolerance and muscle catabolism following severe burn injury. Ann Surg 2005;241:334-342.
195. Demling R, Signe P: Metabolic management of patients with severe burns. World J Surg 2000;24:673-680.
196. Garrel D, Razi M, Lariviere R: Improved clinical status and length of care with low-fat nutrition support in burn patients. JPEN J Parenter Enteral Nutr 1995;19:482-491.
197. Mochizuki H, Trocki O, Dominioni L, et al: Optimal lipid content for enteral diets following thermal injury. JPEN J Parenter Enteral Nutr 1984;8:638-646.
198. Battistella FD, Widergren JT, Anderson JT, et al: A prospective, randomized trial of intravenous fat emulsion administration in trauma victims requiring total parenteral nutrition. J Trauma 1997;43:52-58; discussion 8-60.
199. Huschak G, Zur Nieden K, Hoell T, et al: Olive oil based nutrition in multiple trauma patients: A pilot study. Intensive Care Med 2005;31:1202-1208.
200. Alexander J, Saito H, Trocki O, Ogle C: The importance of lipid type in the diet after burn injury. Ann Surg 1986;204:1-8.
201. Soeters PB, van de Poll MC, van Gemert WG, Dejong CH: Amino acid adequacy in pathophysiological states. J Nutr 2004;134(6 Suppl):1575S-1582S.
202. Prelack K, Cunningham J, Sheridan R, Tompkins R: Energy and protein provisions for thermally injured children revisited: An outcome-based approach for determining requirements. J Burn Care Rehabil 1997;18:117-181.
203. Matsuda T, Kagan R, Hanumadass M, Jonasson O: The importance of burn wound size in determining the optimal calorie:nitrogen ratio. Surgery 1983;94:562-568.
204. Alexander JW, MacMillan BG, Stinnett JD, et al: Beneficial effects of aggressive protein feeding in severely burned children. Ann Surg 1980;192:505-517.
205. Waymack J, Herndon D: Nutritional support of the burned patient. World J Surg 1992;16:80-86.
206. Yu YM, Ryan CM, Castillo L, et al: Arginine and ornithine kinetics in severely burned patients: Increased rate of arginine disposal. Am J Physiol Endocrinol Metab 2001;280:E509-517.
207. Novak F, Heyland DK, Avenell A, et al: Glutamine supplementation in serious illness: A systematic review of the evidence. Crit Care Med 2002;30:2022-2029.
208. Souba W: Glutamine: A key substrate for the splanchnic bed. Ann Rev Nutrition 1991;11:285-289.
209. De-Souza DA, Greene LJ: Intestinal permeability and systemic infections in critically ill patients: Effect of glutamine. Crit Care Med 2005;33:1125-1135.
210. Wischmeyer PE: Can glutamine turn off the motor that drives systemic inflammation? Crit Care Med 2005;33:1175-1178.
211. Wischmeyer PE, Lynch J, Liedel J, et al: Glutamine administration reduces gram-negative bacteremia in severely burned patients: A prospective, randomized, double-blind trial versus isonitrogenous control. Crit Care Med 2001;29:2075-2080.
212. Zhou YP, Jiang ZM, Sun YH, et al: The effect of supplemental enteral glutamine on plasma levels, gut function, and outcome in severe burns: A randomized, double-blind, controlled clinical trial. JPEN J Parenter Enteral Nutr 2003;27:241-245.
213. Barbul A, Larzarrow S, Efron O: Arginine enhances wound healing and lymphocyte immune response in humans. Surgery 1990;108:331-335.
214. Kirk S, Barbul A: Role of arginine in trauma, sepsis, and immunity. J Parenter Enteral Nutr 1990;14:226S-2269S.
215. Gottschlich M, Jenkins M, Warden G, et al: Differential effects of three enteral dietary regimens on selected outcome variables in burn patients. J Parenter Enteral Nutr 1990;14:225-236.
216. Heys S, Walker L, Smith I, Eremin O: Enteral nutritional supplementation with key nutrients in patients with critical illness and cancer: A meta-analysis of randomized controlled trials. Ann Surg 1999;229:467-477.
217. Heyland DK, Samis A: Does immunonutrition in patients with sepsis do more harm than good? Intensive Care Med 2003;29:669-671.

218. Luiking YC, Poeze M, Ramsay G, Deutz NE: The role of arginine in infection and sepsis. JPEN J Parenter Enteral Nutr 2005;29(1 Suppl):S70-74.
219. Saffle J, Wiebke G, Jennings K, et al: Randomized trial of immune-enhancing enteral nutrition in burn patients. J Trauma 1997;42:793-802.
220. Gamliel Z, DeBiasse M, Demling R: Essential microminerals and their response to burn injury. J Burn Care Rehabil 1996;17:264-272.
221. Gottschlich M, Warden G: Vitamin supplementation in the patient with burns. J Burn Care Rehabil 1990;11:275-279.
222. Shippee R, Wilson S, King N: Trace mineral supplementation of burn patients: A national survey. J Amer Diet Assoc 1987;87:300-303.
223. Gump F, Kinney J: Energy balance and weight loss in burned patients. Arch Surg 1971;103:442-448.
224. Streat S, Beddoe A, Hill G: Aggressive nutritional support does not prevent protein loss despite fat gain in septic intensive care patients. J Trauma 1987;27:262-266.
225. Hart DW, Wolf SE, Herndon DN, et al: Energy expenditure and caloric balance after burn: increased feeding leads to fat rather than lean mass accretion. Ann Surg 2002;235:152-161.
226. Zdolsek HJ, Lindahl OA, Angquist KA, Sjoberg F: Non-invasive assessment of intercompartmental fluid shifts in burn victims. Burns 1998;24:233-240.
227. LeBlanc A, Gogia P, Schneider V, et al: Calf muscle area and strength changes after five weeks of horizontal bed rest. Am J Sports Med 1988;16:624-629.
228. Rettmer R, Williamson J, Labbe R, Heimbach D: Laboratory monitoring of nutrition status in burn patients. Clin Chem 1992;38:334-337.
229. Manelli J, Abdetii C, Botti G, Golstein M: A reference standard for plasma proteins is required for nutritional assessment of adult burn patients. Burns 1998;24:337-345.
230. Williamson J: Actual burn nutrition care practices: A national survey (Part II). J Burn Care Rehabil 1989;10:185-194.
231. Pereira CT, Herndon DN: The pharmacologic modulation of the hypermetabolic response to burns. Adv Surg 2005;39:245-261.
232. Herndon DN, Hart DW, Wolf SE, et al: Reversal of catabolism by beta-blockade after severe burns. N Engl J Med 2001;345:1223-1229.
233. Wolf SE, Edelman LS, Kemalyan N, et al: Effects of oxandrolone on outcome measures in the severely burned: A multicenter prospective randomized double-blind trial. J Burn Care Res 2006;27:131-139; discussion 40-41.
234. Demling RH, DeSanti L: Oxandrolone induced lean mass gain during recovery from severe burns is maintained after discontinuation of the anabolic steroid. Burns 2003;29:793-797.
235. Glenn F, Becker CG: Acute acalculous cholecystitis. An increasing entity. Ann Surg 1982;195:131-136.
236. Arnoldo BD, Hunt JL, Purdue GF: Acute cholecystitis in burn patients. J Burn Care Res 2006;27:170-173.
237. Sheridan RL, Ryan CM, Lee MJ, et al: Percutaneous cholecystostomy in the critically ill burn patient. J Trauma 1995;38:248-251.
238. Ryan CM, Sheridan RL, Schoenfeld DA, et al: Postburn pancreatitis. Ann Surg 1995;222:163-170.
239. Maury E, Tankovic J, Ebel A, Offenstadt G: An observational study of upper gastrointestinal bleeding in intensive care units: Is *Helicobacter pylori* the culprit? Crit Care Med 2005;33:1513-1518.
240. Robert R, Gissot V, Pierrot M, et al: *Helicobacter pylori* infection is not associated with an increased hemorrhagic risk in patients in the intensive care unit. Crit Care 2006;10:R77.
241. Czaja A, McAlhany J, Pruitt B: Acute gastroduodenal disease after thermal injury. N Engl J Med 1984;18:925-929.
242. Chung D, Robie D, Hernandez A, et al: Surgical management of complications of burn injury. In Herndon D (ed): Total Burn Care. Philadelphia, WB Saunders, 2002, pp 442-451.
243. Kadesky K, Purdue GF, Hunt JL: Acute pseudo-obstruction in critically ill patients with burns. J Burn Care Rehabil 1995;16(2 Pt 1):132-135.
244. Marvin R, McKinley B, McQuiggan M, et al: Nonocclusive bowel necrosis occurring in critically-ill trauma patients receiving enteral nutrition manifests no reliable clinical signs for early detection. Am J Surg 2000;179:7-12.
245. Kowal-Vern A, McGill V, Gamelli R: Ischemic necrotic bowel disease in thermal injury. Arch Surg 1997;1132:440-443.
246. Eisenberg P: Causes of diarrhea in tube-fed patients: A comprehensive approach to diagnosis and management. Nutr Clin Pract 1993;8:119-123.
247. Grube B, Heimbach C, Marvin J: Clostridium difficile diarrhea in critically ill burn patients. Arch Surg 1987;122:655-661.
248. Scaife CL, Saffle JR, Morris SE: Intestinal obstruction secondary to enteral feedings in burn trauma patients. J Trauma 1999;47:859-863.
249. Wolf S, Jeschke M, Rose J, et al: Enteral feeding intolerance: An indicator of sepsis-associated mortality in burned children. Arch Surg 1997;132:1310-1313.
250. Shankar R, Amin C, Gamelli R: Hematologic, hematopoietic, and acute phase response. In Herndon D (ed): Total Burn Care. Philadelphia, WB Saunders, 2002, pp 331-346.
251. Wallner SF, Vautrin R: The anemia of thermal injury: Mechanism of inhibition of erythropoiesis. Proc Soc Exp Biol Med 1986;181:144-150.
252. Still JM Jr, Belcher K, Law EJ, et al: A double-blinded prospective evaluation of recombinant human erythropoietin in acutely burned patients. J Trauma 1995;38:233-236.
253. Palmieri TL, Greenhalgh DG: Blood transfusion in burns: What do we do? J Burn Care Rehabil 2004;25:71-75.
254. Palmieri TL, Caruso DM, Foster KN, et al: Effect of blood transfusion on outcome after major burn injury: A multicenter study. Crit Care Med 2006;34:1602-1607.
255. Ong YS, Samuel M, Song C: Meta-analysis of early excision of burns. Burns 2006;32:145-150.
256. Desai MH, Herndon DN, Broemeling L, et al: Early burn wound excision significantly reduces blood loss. Ann Surg 1990;211:753-759; discussion 9-62.
257. Valade N, Decailliot F, Rebufat Y, et al: Thrombocytosis after trauma: Incidence, aetiology, and clinical significance. Br J Anaesth 2005;94:18-23.
258. Rue LW III, Cioffi WG Jr, Rush R, et al: Thromboembolic complications in thermally injured patients. World J Surg 1992;16:1151-1154; discussion 5.
259. Wibbenmeyer LA, Hoballah JJ, Amelon MJ, et al: The prevalence of venous thromboembolism of the lower extremity among thermally injured patients determined by duplex sonography. J Trauma 2003;55:1162-1167.
260. Klein GL, Herndon DN, Goodman WG, et al: Histomorphometric and biochemical characterization of bone following acute severe burns in children. Bone 1995;17:455-460.
261. Celis MM, Suman OE, Huang TT, et al: Effect of a supervised exercise and physiotherapy program on surgical interventions in children with thermal injury. J Burn Care Rehabil 2003;24:57-61; discussion 56.

Chapter 69

Poisonings

Janice L. Zimmerman and Maria Rudis

Poisonings may result from intentional or unintentional ingestion, inhalation, or contact. Toxic complications can also result with therapeutic use of medications. Although mortality from toxin exposures is low, patients requiring hospitalization are often cared for in the intensive care unit (ICU). Limited evidence-based information on management of poisonings is available because the variety of drugs and doses that patients are exposed to limit the ability to conduct clinical trials of specific interventions. Animal and human volunteer studies with nontoxic amounts of drugs fail to fully replicate the clinical situations that are commonly encountered. Most therapy is based on extrapolation of data from animal models, human volunteer studies, case reports, pharmacokinetic information, known pathophysiology, and consensus opinion. Toxicologists and local poison control centers are valuable sources of additional information for the clinician.

The approach to the poisoned patient requires an organized evaluation and management plan that often requires the input of emergency physicians, primary care physicians, and intensivists. The basic steps include initial resuscitation and stabilization, diagnosis, gastrointestinal (GI) decontamination and toxin elimination, institution of specific antidotes or interventions, and supportive care. After a discussion of pharmacokinetic issues pertinent to poisonings, this chapter addresses these components of management in regard to poisonings most likely to be encountered in ICU patients.

PHARMACOKINETICS AND TOXICOKINETICS

In the poisoned patient, pharmacokinetic and dynamic principles aid in the assessment of the likelihood of toxicity, the onset and duration of effects, and the effectiveness of therapeutic modalities designed to enhance elimination of the drug or toxins. *Pharmacokinetics* is the term used to describe the absorption, distribution, metabolism, and elimination of drugs in the body when administered in therapeutic doses. Pharmacodynamics is the relationship between the concentration of a drug in a measurable compartment and the pharmacologic effect exerted at the site of action. Toxicokinetics and toxicodynamics are terms applied to evaluate the pharmacokinetics and dynamics, respectively, of substances in situations in which a toxic dose is given or a toxic effect is seen. Pharmacokinetic parameters are described under controlled situations for most therapeutic agents, but these parameters cannot be applied to toxicology because often there is an unknown time of ingestion, an unknown amount or course of ingestion, and ingestion of multiple agents.[1,2]

Absorption

The rate and extent of drug absorption determine toxicity. The rate of absorption will determine the onset of effects, and the extent absorbed will determine, in part, the severity of toxicity. Factors affecting drug absorption include physical characteristics such as solubility; molecular weight; dissolution rate; and the presence of adsorbent substances like activated charcoal, as well as physiologic variables including gastric emptying time, intestinal motility, tissue perfusion, and first-pass metabolism. Most substances are absorbed by passive diffusion primarily in the small intestine because of the large surface area, high permeability, and extensive blood flow. Disease states or factors that prolong gastric emptying time (e.g., congestive heart failure, concurrent ingestion of opioids, anticholinergic agents) decrease the rate of absorption and delay the onset of action. The pharmacologic effect of an ingested drug may result in decreased blood pressure or reduced cardiac output, in turn resulting in hypoperfusion to organs of elimination and the gastrointestinal (GI) tract. These factors will result in unpredictable absorption patterns. Delayed and prolonged absorption may also occur because of concretion formation in the stomach (e.g., overdoses of salicylates, iron, sustained-release drugs).

First-pass metabolism is the proportion of the dose metabolized or eliminated during one pass through the liver before it reaches the general circulation. The bioavailability of drugs with a high hepatic extraction ratio such as cyclic antidepressants, phenothiazines, opioids, and many β-blockers is increased because of saturation of these metabolic or elimination pathways. Increased bioavailability of high extraction ratio drugs may also be observed in patients with hepatic dysfunction. In a patient exposed to cytochrome P_{450} enzyme inhibitors, the metabolic clearance will be reduced for acetaminophen, opioids, diazepam, and theophylline. Conversely, exposure to inducers of the hepatic enzyme mixed function oxidase system such as phenytoin, phenobarbital, and cigarette smoking will increase first-pass metabolism and bioavailability.

Distribution

After a substance is in the blood compartment, distribution throughout the body depends on tissue perfusion, pH, protein and tissue binding, and lipid solubility. Changes in plasma concentration during the distribution phase primarily reflect movement within the various body fluids and tissues rather than elimination from the body. The postdistribution plasma concentrations reflect the amount of substance in the body and the extent of distribution.

The rate of distribution will be affected by factors that decrease blood pressure and cardiac output. Changes in systemic and urinary pH can modify drug movement from the plasma compartment into specific tissue sites. For example, acidemia increases the proportion of nonionized salicylate, which is the form capable of entering the brain. Acidification of urine when basic substances are involved is not recommended because of the risk of metabolic acidosis and the potential of precipitating myoglobinuria. During periods of hypoperfusion, the response of the autonomic nervous system results in more drug being distributed to the central nervous system (CNS) and myocardium, resulting in exaggeration of toxicities.

The volume of distribution (Vd) is not a real volume but the size of a single compartment that would be created when one assumes that all of the drug or toxin in the body exists at the same concentration as it does in plasma. A Vd greater than 1 L/kg indicates that the substance distributes outside the plasma compartment into other body fluids or tissues. As this volume increases (e.g., cyclic antidepressants 10 to 50 L/kg), the concentration in tissues is higher than in the plasma. The Vd only indicates the extent of distribution of a substance, not the precise location. The Vd may be used to estimate the plasma concentrations when a known amount of substance has been ingested by the following formula:

$$\text{Maximum plasma concentration} = \frac{\text{Amount of drug ingested}}{\text{Vd}\,(\text{L/kg}) \times \text{weight}\,(\text{kg})}$$

Plasma concentrations taken before completion of distribution (equilibrium) will not reflect tissue concentrations at the sites of pharmacologic activity or potential toxicity. Clinicians must be cognizant of the meaning of sampling during the distribution phase. An antidote may also change the Vd. Fab fragments for digoxin toxicity bind plasma digoxin and reduce the Vd.

Protein and Tissue Binding

The distribution of substances is also affected by binding to plasma proteins and tissues. With the exception of salicylates and nonsteroidal anti-inflammatory drugs, most drugs do not saturate their binding sites until toxic levels are reached. Generally, substances that are extensively bound to proteins (>90%) have a small Vd and are confined predominantly to the plasma compartment. Only unbound substances are free to diffuse across cellular membranes and equilibrate with receptor sites in tissues to exert pharmacologic and toxicologic effects. Most laboratories measure total drug concentrations (i.e., bound and unbound drug).

Physiologic and pathologic conditions can alter drug protein binding through the alteration of affinity of substances for plasma proteins and the alteration of the concentration of plasma proteins available for binding. For example, in patients with normal protein binding, the therapeutic range of phenytoin is 10 to 20 μg/mL, of which 10% is free unbound drug. If a patient with hypoalbuminemia overdoses on phenytoin, toxic effects may occur with plasma phenytoin levels significantly lower than 20 μg/mL. A much greater proportion of the total phenytoin is free to exert toxic effects.

The major determinant of toxicity is the amount of drug or toxin that is physically present to bind to receptor sites, which are usually located in highly vascular tissue compartments. Little is known about tissue binding changes in poisonings because of limited ability to measure drug or toxin concentrations at receptor sites. Tissue binding may be affected by disease states but may also be modified by therapeutic interventions in the intoxicated patient. In cyclic antidepressant overdose, serum alkalinization alters the tissue distribution and concentration of drug at its binding to sodium channels.

Lipid Solubility

The physicochemical properties of a substance determine the extent to which it distributes into the peripheral compartment. Highly lipophilic substances such as organophosphate insecticides penetrate membranes easier. Generally, they have a longer duration of action because they accumulate in fat tissue and slowly leach out as the plasma concentration decreases. The effects may be further prolonged if the victim has a proportionately larger fat-to-water ratio.

Elimination

Drug or toxin elimination is an extremely complex and dynamic process. It is affected by changes in vital signs or tissue perfusion and is modified by changes in absorption, binding, and distribution. Elimination also changes with age, presence of hepatic enzyme inducers or inhibitors, and altered organ function during critical illness. Chronic ingestion of ethanol has been shown to induce the cytochrome P_{450} mixed-function oxidase system that may increase the production of toxic metabolites of acetaminophen. Septic shock decreases function of the cytochrome P_{450} isozymes.

Clearance is useful to evaluate elimination in a poisoned patient and is defined as the volume of blood that is cleared of drug per unit of time. The elimination of a substance may be a result of metabolic processes, renal excretion, chelation, or binding to activated charcoal. The total body clearance (Cl_t) is equal to the sum of all of the clearance processes, such that:

$$Cl_t = Cl\ renal + Cl\ hepatic + Cl\ activated\ charcoal + Cl\ chelation$$ [1]

The two major organs of elimination are the kidneys and liver, but the GI tract may also function in this capacity in the poisoned patient. Renal elimination is critical for eliminating renally cleared active drugs or toxins, metabolites, chelated toxins, or drugs bound to Fab fragments. Many substances eliminated by the kidney are nephrotoxins as well. Patients with preexisting renal insufficiency or acute renal failure induced directly or indirectly by the offending agent may require extracorporeal removal. Antidotes such as deferoxamine, digoxin-specific Fab fragments, and cyanide antidotes may also require renal elimination.

The GI tract may serve as an organ of elimination when the toxin or its metabolites undergo significant enteroenteric or enterohepatic circulation. The intrinsic hepatic clearance of drugs or toxins involves two phases. Phase I includes oxidation-reduction, hydrolysis, and conjugation with sulfhydryl or amide groups. The induction of the hepatic microsomal enzyme system by multiple potential agents increases the clearance of theophylline. Phase II pathways include reactions such as acetylation, sulfation, and glucuronidation. These reactions increase the polarity and thus the water solubility of substances and increase renal or biliary excretion. Drugs or toxins that are primarily metabolized in the liver by phase I oxidation, such as diazepam, are affected by cirrhosis and other liver diseases. Drugs eliminated by phase II conjugation reactions, such as lorazepam, do not appear to be affected by liver disease.

RESUSCITATION AND STABILIZATION

The initial management of seriously ill poisoned patients requires assessment of airway patency, breathing difficulties, circulatory problems, and the level of consciousness. These issues, along with immediate resuscitation interventions, are usually addressed in the emergency department but may be continued in the ICU (Box 69-1).

DIAGNOSIS

History

In the case of an unknown ingestion, a complete history should be obtained regarding the substance or substances ingested, quantity ingested, time of the ingestion, form of medication (regular or sustained-release), and chronicity of the ingestion to determine the significance of the presenting symptoms. Every attempt should be made to quantify the amount ingested (e.g., number of pills used versus those missing from container, size of spills on floor). Specifically, the clinician should inquire about the patient's baseline mental and health status and the medical, occupational, and social history. A detailed medication history should include information about over-the-counter, prescription, and alternative or herbal medications. Intentional ingestions often involve multiple coingestants or alcohol, or both. Additional or corroborating information should be obtained from family, friends, paramedics, or witnesses, if available. Family and paramedics should be advised to bring in all available containers found at the site.

Physical Examination

The initial physical examination should evaluate vital signs and neurologic findings that may provide valuable physiologic clues to the toxicologic etiology. Many toxic substances affect the autonomic nervous system, which is responsible for changes in vital signs mediated by the

Box 69-1

Approach to Resuscitation and Stabilization of the Poisoned Patient

Assess Airway and Breathing
Supplemental oxygen
Intubation and mechanical ventilation for airway protection, hypoventilation, or hypoxemia

Assess Hemodynamic Status
Isotonic fluids for hypotension
Treat significant arrhythmias

Assess Mental Status[4]
50% glucose (25 to 50 g IV)
Thiamine (100 mg IV)
Naloxone (0.4 to 2 mg IV or IM initially)
Flumazenil (not routinely recommended)*

*See section on benzodiazepines for further information.

sympathetic and parasympathetic pathways. Meticulous attention to these initial and subsequent clinical signs is of paramount importance in identifying patterns or changes suggesting a particular drug or group of drugs (Table 69-1). Changes in the clinical examination after a therapeutic intervention or the administration of an antidote should be noted. Continued monitoring and reevaluation are necessary because drug effects may not be present on initial examination.

Altered mental status is common in a toxicologic emergency. A detailed assessment of neurologic status should be made to determine if there is any alteration in level (stupor/coma) or content of consciousness (confusion/delirium). The evaluation should include an assessment of pupillary reactivity, ocular movements, and motor responses. Ruling out structural versus toxic or metabolic reasons for the altered state is important. In the patient with confusion or delirium, the clinician should assess orientation, presence of hallucinations, and behavior. Drug-induced seizures are often difficult to treat and may respond only to specific antidotal therapy. In general, benzodiazepines are more effective in terminating drug-induced seizures than other agents.

Table 69-1. Drug Effects on Vital Signs

Increased	Decreased
Blood Pressure	
Amphetamines	Antihypertensive agents
Anticholinergics	Cyanide
Cocaine	Cyclic antidepressants
Ephedrine	Ethanol
	Opioids
	Organophosphates/carbamates
	Sedative-hypnotics
Heart Rate	
Amphetamines	β-blockers
Anticholinergics	Calcium channel blockers
Carbon monoxide	Digitalis glycosides
Cocaine	Gamma hydroxybutyrate
Cyanide	Organophosphates/carbamates
Cyclic antidepressants	Sedative-hypnotics
Ethanol	
Theophylline	
Respiratory Rate	
Alcohols	Barbiturates
Amphetamines	Ethanol
Anticholinergics	Gamma hydroxybutyrate
Carbon monoxide	Isopropanol
Hydrocarbons	Opioids
Organophosphates/carbamates	Sedative-hypnotics
Salicylates	
Theophylline	
Temperature	
Amphetamines	Barbiturates
Anticholinergics	β-blockers
Cocaine	Carbon monoxide
Cyclic antidepressants	Ethanol
Lithium	Hypoglycemic agents
Salicylates	Opioids
Theophylline	Sedative-hypnotics

Pupils should be assessed for size and reactivity, and ocular movements should be evaluated for the presence of sustained nystagmus. Agents associated with miosis include organophosphates/carbamates (mydriasis also seen), other cholinergic agents, opioids, acetone, clonidine, phencyclidine, and nicotine. Both anticholinergics and sympathomimetics may cause mydriasis; the pupils are reactive to light with cocaine but unreactive in diphenhydramine overdose. The assessment may be complex in the setting of multiple coingestants, whereby the response may be blocked or partially manifested. Horizontal nystagmus is commonly seen with alcohols, lithium, carbamazepine, solvents, and primidone. Phenytoin, sedative-hypnotics, and phencyclidine may cause a combination of vertical, horizontal, or rotatory nystagmus.

The clinical examination should also include evaluation of bowel sounds (decreased/hyperactive), skin (wet/dry), and mucosa (secretions).

Toxidromes

A complex of signs and symptoms may be identified by physical examination and grouped into a toxic syndrome, or "toxidrome." In most cases, recognition of this toxic pattern is more important than identifying a specific offending agent. Identifying a toxidrome enables the clinician to initiate the assessment, derive a differential diagnosis, and formulate a treatment plan. The most typical toxidromes are listed in Table 69-2.[5] Importantly, the clinician should note that patients may not present with a classic toxidrome, but rather some components of a toxidrome.

Laboratory

A laboratory test for a patient exposed to toxic agents should be helpful in monitoring, diagnostically confirming, or screening. Select laboratory examinations may be used in the immediate management of the critically ill patient to determine the three gaps of toxicology—the anion gap, the osmolar gap, and oxygen saturation gap. An arterial blood gas (ABG) will identify hypoxemia or hypoventilation, as well as acid-base abnormalities. Agents associated with a gap in oxygen saturation (>5% difference between measured and calculated saturation) include carbon monoxide, cyanide, hydrogen sulfide, and methemoglobin. In these exposures, a pulse oximeter inaccurately reflects the oxygen saturation of tissues. Determination of electrolytes with blood urea nitrogen (BUN) and creatinine will detect abnormalities and allow calculation of the anion gap. An osmolar gap (>10 mOsm) may be caused by any small particle (toxin) that increases the measured osmolarity as measured by freezing point depression. Such agents include ethanol, ethylene glycol, glycerol, iodine, isopropanol, mannitol, methanol, and sorbitol. An electrocardiogram (ECG) should be obtained when indicated to assess potential cardiac toxicity.

A qualitative drug screen is a combination of tests that serves to identify common drugs encountered in overdoses. However, a "tox screen" is usually unnecessary because the results rarely change management and many toxins are not detectable. Quantitative determination of

Table 69-2. Toxidromes

Group	Vital Signs BP	HR	RR	T	Mental Status	Pupil Size	Peristalsis	Diaphoresis	Other
Adrenergic (sympathomimetic) agents	↑	↑	↑	↑	Altered	↑	↑	↑	Flushing, potential for seizures
Anticholinergic agents	±	↑	±	↑	Altered	↑	↓	↓	Dry mucous membranes, thirst, flushing, urinary retention
Cholinergic (muscarinic, nicotinic) agents	±	±	—	—	Altered	±	↑	↑	Salivation, lacrimation, urination, emesis, bronchorrhea, fasciculations
Opioids	↓	↓	↓	↓	Altered	↓	↓	↓	Hyporeflexia
Sedative-hypnotics or ethanol	↓	↓	↓	↓	Altered	±	↓	↓	Hyporeflexia

↑, Increases; ↓, decreases; ±, variable; —, change unlikely.
Adapted from Goldfrank LR, Flomenbaum NE, Lewin NA, et al: Vital signs and toxic syndromes. In Goldfrank LR, Flomenbaum NE, Lewin NA, et al (eds): Goldfrank's Toxicologic Emergencies, ed 7. New York, McGraw-Hill, 2002.

drug/toxin concentrations is indicated by history and clinical examination to monitor the treatment or course of a patient, diagnose clinically inapparent or delayed toxicity, or define indications for specific interventions. Serum concentration measurements may be required as criteria for therapy or to assess the effectiveness of therapy. Because of the ubiquity of acetaminophen in over-the-counter preparations and the potential for significant morbidity and mortality, a level should be obtained in any suspected polydrug ingestion.

GASTROINTESTINAL DECONTAMINATION

Gastrointestinal decontamination in the poisoned patient can be considered with gastric emptying procedures (ipecac-induced emesis, gastric lavage), adsorption of drugs (activated charcoal), and increasing transit through the GI tract (cathartics, whole bowel irrigation). Although most of these procedures are initiated or completed before ICU admission, the clinician should have an understanding of the current evidence, recommendations, and controversies. In general, there is less use of most GI decontamination interventions today. The choice of GI decontamination technique depends on the substance ingested, potential for deterioration in respiratory and mental status, severity of symptoms, dose, and time since ingestion. A single strategy for all ingestions cannot be recommended.

Ipecac, which contains emetic alkaloids, stimulates gastric mucosal sensory receptors and the chemoreceptor trigger zone in the brain to produce vomiting. The amount of ingested drug removed by ipecac-induced emesis is highly variable, and no benefit of ipecac has been confirmed even when administered less than 60 minutes after ingestion. Experts recommend that ipecac should not be administered routinely in the management of poisoned patients.[7] Ipecac is contraindicated in patients with evident or potential decrease in level of consciousness or when corrosive substances or hydrocarbons are ingested. Complications associated with ipecac administration include aspiration pneumonitis, esophageal rupture, Mallory-Weiss tear, pneumomediastinum, and protracted vomiting that can delay administration of activated charcoal. Currently, ipecac is not used when managing adult poisoning victims.

Gastric lavage with a large bore (36- to 40-French) orogastric tube has been used to empty the stomach in overdose patients, but utilization is decreasing. After insertion of the tube, lavage is accomplished with 100- to 200-mL aliquots of normal saline or water until no pill fragments are retrieved. Intubation is required before the procedure to protect the airway in patients with a depressed level of consciousness or potential for sedation. Complications include aspiration pneumonitis, esophageal perforation, and cardiovascular instability. Gastric lavage is contraindicated with ingestions of substances such as acid, alkali, or hydrocarbons where the risk of aspiration is increased. Patients with a risk of GI perforation or severe bleeding diathesis or who are combative should also not be subjected to gastric lavage. No clear benefit of gastric lavage exists, even when instituted in obtunded patients presenting within 1 hour of ingestion.[6] Gastric lavage should not be employed routinely in the management of poisoned patients.[8] It may be considered for use when a patient ingests a life-threatening amount of poison, and lavage can be instituted within 60 minutes of ingestion (or it is likely that toxin is present in the stomach). Clinical judgment in weighing risks and benefits should guide the decision to undertake gastric lavage in an individual patient.

Single-dose activated charcoal is the most frequently used intervention for GI decontamination. Activated charcoal potentially adsorbs the toxin in the GI tract and minimizes systemic absorption. The optimum dose of activated charcoal has not been established by well-designed studies, but the usual dose for adults is 1 g/kg. Activated charcoal is not effective in adsorbing iron, lithium, cyanide, strong acids and bases, alcohols, and some hydrocarbons. Activated charcoal is contraindicated if the patient has a depressed level of consciousness without airway protection, when administration increases the risk of aspiration, or the patient is known or suspected to have a GI perforation. Few complications are associated with the appropriate use of single-dose activated charcoal. Emesis has been reported but may be related to the concomitant cathartic used with charcoal or the ingested toxin. One clinical study examined the benefit of activated charcoal versus no intervention and found no improvement in outcomes.[10] Volunteer studies suggest that the greatest benefit of activated charcoal may be within 1 hour of ingestion.[9] The clinician must take into account the time since ingestion when deciding to administer single-dose activated charcoal.

Cathartics have been used in poisonings on the basis of the principle that absorption and overall bioavailability of the agent are decreased by reducing contact time in the GI tract. Sorbitol (70% solution with activated charcoal) is the most commonly used cathartic, but magnesium citrate and magnesium sulfate have also been used. No clinical studies have demonstrated beneficial effects of cathartics in poisoned patients. A cathartic alone has no role in the management of poisonings, and even the routine use of a cathartic in combination with activated charcoal cannot be recommended.[11] If a cathartic is used, only a single dose should be administered. A cathartic should not be administered in patients with ileus, GI obstruction or perforation, or hemodynamic instability. Complications of cathartics include nausea, vomiting, and abdominal cramping. Multiple doses of magnesium-containing cathartics may result in significant dehydration and electrolyte abnormalities.

Whole bowel irrigation (WBI) has been proposed as a technique to prevent absorption of poisons by rapidly expelling the bowel contents. WBI involves the enteral administration of large volumes (1 to 2 L/hour in adults) of polyethylene glycol electrolyte solution; this is continued until the rectal effluent is clear or elimination of the toxin has been confirmed. During the procedure, the head of the bed should be elevated to 45 degrees to decrease the likelihood of vomiting and aspiration. No clinical trials have assessed the impact of WBI on patient outcomes. Currently, there are no established indications for WBI, but it may be considered for potentially toxic ingestions of sustained-release or enteric-coated drugs, iron, and illicit drug packets.[13] Other applications of WBI are of theoretical benefit. WBI is contraindicated in the presence of ileus, GI obstruction or perforation, hemodynamic instability, or intractable vomiting. In the patient with decreased level of consciousness or respiratory depression, the airway must be protected before instituting WBI.

ENHANCED ELIMINATION

Multiple-dose activated charcoal (MDAC) therapy involves the repeated administration of oral-activated charcoal to enhance elimination of drugs already absorbed into the body by functioning as an adsorbent "sink" at several sites in the gut.[3] First, it can interrupt enterohepatic circulation of drugs or metabolites that are actively secreted into bile. Secondly, it can adsorb drugs or metabolites that enter the gut by active secretion or passive diffusion and prevent reabsorption. Finally, it may prevent desorption of drugs, particularly acidic substances that bind two to three times less avidly to activated charcoal in the alkalotic milieu of the intestinal lumen than in the acidic environment of the stomach. Drugs with a prolonged elimination half-life after overdose and small Vd are particularly likely to have elimination enhanced significantly by MDAC.

One suggested regimen for administering MDAC is to follow the initial dose of activated charcoal with 0.5 to 1 g/kg every 4 hours. Alternatively, it is possible to administer charcoal as an aqueous solution by continuous infusion via a nasogastric tube at a rate of 0.25 to 0.5 g/kg/hour (not $<$12.5 g/hour). Additionally, the smaller doses (and volumes) administered more frequently may reduce the likelihood of vomiting. It may still be necessary to give an antiemetic intravenously to ensure satisfactory administration. The dosing schedule will be dictated by clinical parameters such as patient cooperation, degree of obtundation, the presence of ileus, and the presence and severity of vomiting. MDAC should be continued until the patient's clinical condition and laboratory parameters including drug plasma concentrations are improving. MDAC administration should be monitored carefully for the development of constipation, obstruction, and for the prevention of aspiration.

No evidence has yet demonstrated convincingly that MDAC reduces morbidity and mortality in poisoned patients.[13] However, MDAC should be considered if the patient has ingested a life-threatening amount of carbamazepine, dapsone, phenobarbital, quinine, or theophylline and may obviate the need for invasive extracorporeal techniques. Some evidence suggests that MDAC may also increase the elimination of salicylates. MDAC is not effective with digoxin, meprobamate, methotrexate, phenytoin, cyclic antidepressants, or valproic acid.[14]

Forced diuresis involves the intravenous (IV) administration of large volumes of isotonic fluids and diuretics to enhance net renal excretion of drug or metabolite. This method is of limited clinical benefit and should not be used because of the potential for fluid overload and acid-base disturbances.

Urinary alkalinization is beneficial in increasing renal clearance of weak acids such as salicylates and phenobarbital/primidone. These weak acids are ionized at alkaline urine pH, trapped in the renal tubules, and not reabsorbed. Alkalinization can be initiated by adding 88 to 132 mEq sodium bicarbonate to 1 L of D_5W. Urine pH should be tested every hour, and the rate of the bicarbonate infusion should be titrated to achieve a urine pH of 7.5 to 8.5. This degree of alkalinization is difficult if metabolic acidosis is present. Hypokalemia is likely and requires correction to achieve urinary alkalinization. Fluid and electrolyte losses should be replaced. Increasing the urine pH with carbonic anhydrase inhibitors such as acetazolamide is not recommended because metabolic acidosis will worsen.

Hemodialysis is useful to increase the clearance of certain drugs and metabolites, as well as correct metabolic acidosis induced by some substances. The concentration gradient of the unbound toxin provides the driving force for clearance. The following criteria should be applied to a drug to determine the potential for enhanced elimination by hemodialysis: low Vd (<1 L/kg), single-compartment kinetics, low endogenous clearance (<4 mL/min/kg), molecular weight less than 500 daltons, water soluble, and low plasma protein binding. Drugs for which hemodialysis should be considered early in the presentation of the intoxication include methanol, ethylene glycol, salicylates, lithium, boric acid, and thallium. Hemodialysis should also be considered after heavy metal chelation in patients with renal failure. For hemodialysis to be performed, blood pressure and cardiac reserve must be adequate to tolerate blood flow through the dialyzer and fluid removal. The usual complications of hemodialysis may occur, particularly if the patient is unstable.

Hemoperfusion is a form of extracorporeal removal whereby whole blood is passed through an adsorbent-containing (charcoal) cartridge. In general, if a compound is well adsorbed by activated charcoal, then charcoal hemoperfusion clearance will exceed that of hemodialysis. Contrary to hemodialysis, substances with a high degree of plasma protein binding can be removed. Charcoal hemoperfusion is the preferred modality for elimination of carbamazepine, phenobarbital, phenytoin, and theophylline. Lithium and other heavy metals are not well removed by hemoperfusion. Charcoal hemoperfusion is generally performed for 4 to 6 hours at flow rates of 250 to 400 mL/minute. The risks of hemoperfusion are similar to those of hemodialysis. Additionally, hypoglycemia, hypocalcemia, and hypothermia may occur.

Intermittent renal replacement therapies frequently need to be continued for more than 6 hours to eliminate toxin. The pharmacokinetics of many drugs in overdose change from first order, whereby a constant fraction of a substance is removed per unit time, to zero order, in which a constant amount of toxin is removed per unit time, irrespective of concentration. After hemodialysis (or hemoperfusion) is instituted, the kinetics will revert to first order because of the rapid removal of drug from plasma. Continuous renal replacement therapies (e.g., continuous arteriovenous hemofiltration [CAVH], continuous venovenous hemofiltration [CVVH]) are a newer modality of extracorporeal drug removal in the treatment of poisoning. Clearance rates achieved with these techniques are considerably lower than those achieved with hemodialysis. Clearance rates may be significantly increased by having a dialysis solution running countercurrent to the blood flow (hemodiafiltration, CAVHD, CVVHD). Such therapy may be instituted after hemodialysis or hemoperfusion to further remove drug after it slowly redistributes from tissue to blood. This is an attractive option for agents such as lithium or procainamide. Continuous renal replacement techniques may be advantageous in hemodynamically unstable patients who cannot tolerate conventional hemodialysis or hemoperfusion. Despite many case reports demonstrating significant drug clearance, there are no data demonstrating that these techniques affect outcome. Attention must be paid to the undesirable removal of other therapeutic agents such as antibiotics.

SPECIFIC POISONINGS

Acetaminophen

Acetaminophen (*N*-acetyl-*p*-aminophenol [APAP]) is present in more than 200 prescription and over-the-counter medications and is frequently a coingestant with other drugs. Because APAP overdose may result in significant hepatotoxicity and mortality that is preventable, it is important to recognize and initiate appropriate therapy. APAP is metabolized in the liver by the mixed function oxidase system to the toxic metabolite, *N*-acetyl-*p*-benzoquinoneimine (NAPQI), which results in cell injury and death. The clinical course of APAP toxicity has been divided into stages on the basis of the development of hepatotoxicity (Table 69-3).

If possible, an estimate of the quantity and dosage form of APAP ingested and the time of ingestion should be obtained. In adults, hepatic toxicity may occur after ingestion of more than 7.5 to 10 g during 8 hours or less. Fatalities are infrequent with overdoses of less than 15 g. For patients with a single, acute ingestion, an acetaminophen level should be obtained at least 4 hours after ingestion. Liver enzymes should be evaluated if the APAP level indicates potential toxicity or the clinical examination suggests hepatic injury. If the time of ingestion is unknown, an APAP level should be obtained on admission. An APAP

Table 69-3. Stages of Acetaminophen Toxicity

Stage	Time Course (after ingestion)	Characteristics
I	0-24 hr	Asymptomatic; nausea, vomiting; normal LFTs
II	24-72 hr	Right upper quadrant pain; abnormal LFTs
III	72-96 hr	Encephalopathy, jaundice, bleeding, renal dysfunction; maximal hepatic injury, synthetic dysfunction
IV	4 days-2 wk	Recovery of liver function

LFT, liver function tests.

level and liver function tests should be determined in patients presenting late, patients with multiple ingestions over time, or chronic ingesters of APAP.

No evidence indicates that gastric lavage is beneficial in APAP overdose. Although there are no data to support the efficacy of activated charcoal, it does adsorb acetaminophen, and it is reasonable to administer charcoal up to 4 hours after ingestion. Acetaminophen is absorbed within 2 to 4 hours, so later use of charcoal is not warranted. Administration of activated charcoal will not interfere with subsequent administration of oral N-acetylcysteine therapy.

N-acetylcysteine (NAC) is the antidote for APAP poisoning, but the optimal route and duration of treatment are debated.[14,15] NAC limits toxicity by combining with NAPQI and by serving as a precursor of glutathione, which inactivates NAPQI. For patients with a single, acute ingestion of APAP, the serum acetaminophen level assessed at least 4 hours after ingestion is compared with the Rumack-Matthew nomogram. Treatment with NAC is initiated in the United States if the value falls above the lower possible hepatotoxicity line. Only the initial APAP level is used in making the decision to initiate or continue NAC treatment. Subsequent levels are unnecessary unless extended-release preparations are ingested (see following). The Rumack-Matthew nomogram is not applicable for patients with multiple ingestions of APAP over time, chronic ingesters, or those ingesting extended-release forms. If acetaminophen levels are not available, NAC treatment should be initiated if more than 150 mg/kg or 10 g acetaminophen is ingested. For extended-release APAP, a second level 4 hours after an initial nontoxic level should be evaluated to assess for delayed absorption. If the second value is above the lower line on the Rumack-Matthew nomogram, NAC is initiated.

NAC is most effective in preventing toxicity if administered within 8 hours of ingestion. NAC therapy can be initiated pending results of the acetaminophen level if the patient is presenting late or APAP level results will be delayed. The oral regimen for NAC includes a loading dose of 140 mg/kg followed by 17 oral maintenance doses of 70 mg/kg administered 4 hours apart. A nasogastric tube may be placed for administration, and antiemetic therapy may be necessary to control vomiting. If the patient vomits the loading dose or any maintenance dose within 1 hour of administration, the dose should be repeated. IV NAC is administered as a loading dose of 150 mg/kg over 15 minutes followed by 50 mg/kg infused over 4 hours and then 100 mg/kg infused over 16 hours. Anaphylactoid reactions may occur in 14% to 18% of patients with IV NAC. Oral and IV regimens of administering NAC are similar in efficacy.[16] If the patient has a serum APAP level in the potentially toxic range, the aspartate aminotransferase (AST) or alanine aminotransferase (ALT) should be evaluated daily. If abnormal, additional tests such as bilirubin, prothrombin time, creatinine, BUN, blood glucose, and electrolytes should also be obtained. In patients with elevated liver enzymes, NAC may be continued beyond the full course of therapy until enzymes are decreasing.

Chronic ingesters of APAP or patients with multiple ingestions over time are problematic when determining the need to administer NAC. Presentation beyond 19 hours after ingestion makes the APAP level essentially useless, and there are no established guidelines for administration of NAC in these circumstances. A marker of toxicity that may be useful is the evaluation of AST and ALT. If enzymes are elevated at the time of presentation (>50 IU/L) or the APAP level is greater than 10 μg/mL (>10 micromol/L), a course of NAC may be strongly considered.[17] A course of NAC may also benefit patients with hepatic failure caused by APAP.

Patients with potential toxicity from APAP should be monitored for signs and symptoms of hepatic failure. This includes evaluating mental status and frequently assessing blood glucose. In cases where fulminant hepatic failure develops, appropriate consultation with a hepatologist should be obtained. Transplant may be an option in severe cases.

Alcohols

Methanol and ethylene glycol are toxic alcohols that have similar properties. Toxicity can occur through ingestion, inhalation, or dermal absorption. Cardiopulmonary and CNS symptoms are common, and both agents can produce an anion gap metabolic acidosis and an osmolar gap. However, absence of an osmolar gap or anion gap does not exclude a toxic ingestion. The osmolar gap may be normal if all alcohol is metabolized to acid metabolites, and an anion gap may be normal when metabolism of alcohol has not yet produced acid metabolites (e.g., concomitant ethanol ingestion). If toxic alcohol ingestion is suspected, regardless of whether the patient is symptomatic, blood should be immediately sent for serum methanol, ethylene glycol, and ethanol levels, and definitive treatment initiated immediately. Significant toxicity is associated with methanol and ethylene glycol levels greater than 50 mg/dL. Not uncommonly, the pH will be less than 7 with a serum bicarbonate level below 10 mEq/L and an anion gap higher than 35 mEq/L. The severity of these abnormalities appears to be directly correlated with the likelihood of survival.

Methanol is found in windshield washer fluid, solvents, and bootleg whiskey. It is broken down through alcohol dehydrogenase to formaldehyde, which is metabolized by aldehyde dehydrogenase to formic acid. Uncoupling of the mitochondrial oxidative metabolism produces lactic acid. The metabolic derangements are caused by lactic and formic acid; the latter is responsible for ocular disturbances. When methanol is ingested, peak levels occur within 30 to 60 minutes but there is often a latent period of about 24 hours (range 1 to 72 hours) before the development of toxic symptoms or metabolic acidosis. GI (abdominal pain, nausea, vomiting); CNS (dizziness, headache, seizures, coma); and ocular toxicities (blurred vision, photophobia, retinal edema, disc hyperemia, blindness) are seen.

Ethylene glycol is found in antifreeze and deicing solutions. Ethylene glycol causes an acidemia as a result of conversion to glycolic and oxalic acid. Oxalate crystals in the urine may be detected with a Wood's lamp or on microscopic examination, or they may not be present. Three classic phases of ethylene glycol toxicity have been described: neurologic, cardiopulmonary, and renal. During the first 0.5 to 12 hours after ingestion, ethylene glycol produces transient inebriation without the usual odor of ethanol, along with GI symptoms (nausea, vomiting). After toxic metabolites form (4 to 12 hours after ingestion), a metabolic acidosis develops along with CNS depression. The CNS symptoms may progress to coma associated with hypotonia, hyporeflexia, and occasionally seizures, meningismus, and cerebral edema. In the second stage (12 to 24 hours after ingestion), tachycardia and hypertension often occur along with progression of metabolic acidosis. Hypoxia may result from aspiration, heart failure, or acute respiratory distress syndrome. Death is most common in this stage. In the third stage (24 to 72 hours after ingestion), oliguria, flank pain, acute tubular necrosis, and renal failure develop.

Practice guidelines are available for the treatment of ethylene glycol and methanol intoxication.[18,19] If the patient has symptoms and is significantly acidemic, sodium bicarbonate may be administered to enhance formate and oxalate elimination by ion trapping. Management is dictated by frequent pH determinations, but fluid overload and hyperosmolarity may become significant problems as a result of bicarbonate administration. Hydration is helpful because ethylene glycol is well excreted by the kidney as long as renal function is maintained. The definitive treatment of intoxication with methanol or ethylene glycol is hemodialysis to remove the alcohol and toxic metabolites and to correct metabolic abnormalities. Hemodialysis should be considered for the following conditions: deteriorating vital signs despite intensive supportive care, significant metabolic acidosis (pH$<$7.25 to 7.3), blood level of methanol or ethylene glycol higher than 25 mg/dL, or any evidence of renal failure or electrolyte imbalances unresponsive to conventional therapy.[18,19]

Antidotal treatment of significant poisoning involves inhibition of alcohol dehydrogenase to prevent metabolism of the alcohols to toxic metabolites with ethanol or fomepizole. Ethanol (IV or oral) allows preferential metabolism of ethanol over methanol and ethylene glycol. Ethanol should be administered to maintain a blood level of 100 to 150 mg/dL. A loading dose should be followed by a maintenance infusion according to the established dosing requirements for nondrinkers, drinkers, and during hemodialysis (Table 69-4). Problems encountered during ethanol administration include CNS depression, hypoglycemia, dehydration, and fluctuating serum concentrations. A second IV line using 0.9% sodium chloride may be necessary to avoid development of hyponatremia because of the large free water content and significant hypertonicity (1713 mOsm/L) of the 10% ethanol solution. Advance notice should be given to the pharmacy to allow sufficient time to locate enough ethanol for administering and preparing the solution. If IV ethanol is not available, oral ethanol can be used.

Table 69-4. Intravenous Administration of 10% Ethanol

	Weight					
	10 kg	15 kg	30 kg	50 kg	70 kg	100 kg
Loading Dose*						
Loading dose of 0.8 g/kg of 10% ethanol (mL infused over 1 hr as tolerated)†	80	120	240	400	560	800
***Maintenance Dose*‡**						
***Infusion Rate (mL/hr for Various Weights)*§**						
Normal Maintenance Range						
80 mg/kg/hr	8	12	24	40	56	80
110 mg/kg/hr	11	16	33	55	77	110
130 mg/kg/hr	13	19	39	65	91	130
Approximate Maintenance Dose for Chronic Alcoholic						
150 mg/kg/hr	15	22	45	75	105	150
Range Required During Hemodialysis						
250 mg/kg/hr	25	38	75	125	175	250
300 mg/kg/hr	30	45	90	150	210	300
350 mg/kg/hr	35	53	105	175	245	350

*A 10% vol/vol concentration yields approximately 100 mg/mL.
†For a 5% concentration, multiply the amount by 2.
‡Infusion to be started immediately after the loading dose. Concentrations above 10% are not recommended for intravenous administration. The dose schedule is based on the premise that the patient initially has a zero ethanol level. The aim of therapy is to maintain a serum ethanol level of 100 to 150 mg/dL, but constant monitoring of the ethanol level is required because of wide variations in endogenous metabolic capacity. Ethanol will be removed by hemodialysis. Prolonged ethanol administration may lead to hypoglycemia.
§Rounded to the nearest milliliter.
From Reith DM, Dawson AH, Epid, D, et al: Relative toxicity of beta blockers in overdose. J Toxicol Clin Toxicol 1996;34:273.

Fomepizole (4-methylpyrazole), a competitive inhibitor of alcohol dehydrogenase, is approved for use in ethylene glycol and methanol overdose (Table 69-5). It is easier to administer than ethanol and does not cause sedation. Fomepizole administration should be considered instead of ethanol if the patient develops altered consciousness, seizures, or a significant metabolic acidosis. Although fomepizole appears to be equally effective, there are no data to demonstrate its comparative efficacy or cost-effectiveness. Administration of ethanol or fomepizole should continue after dialysis until the serum ethylene glycol or methanol concentration is undetectable or less than 20 mg/dL or acidosis is resolved and the patient is asymptomatic. In the absence of renal dysfunction and a significant metabolic acidosis, the use of fomepizole potentially could obviate the need for hemodialysis, even though the serum ethylene glycol or methanol concentration exceeds 50 mg/dL. If patients with high serum concentrations of ethylene glycol are not treated with hemodialysis, then their acid-base balance should be monitored closely and hemodialysis instituted if a metabolic acidosis develops.[18]

Additional therapeutic measures for ethylene glycol ingestions may include thiamine 100 mg IV and pyridoxine 50 mg every 6 hours until the ethylene glycol level is zero and no acidosis persists. If the patient becomes hypocalcemic as a result of precipitation of calcium oxalate crystals, calcium should be replaced. In methanol overdose, it may be reasonable to also administer IV folate (folinic or folic acids) at 50 to 75 mg IV every 4 hours for at least 24 hours to provide the cofactor for enhancing formic acid elimination.

Isopropyl alcohol is also a commonly ingested alcohol, particularly in chronic alcoholics with no access to ethanol. It is found in rubbing alcohol in a concentration of 70%. Oral absorption occurs rapidly (within 0.5 hour), and it undergoes metabolism to acetone, carbon dioxide, and water. Symptoms may include severe abdominal pain, GI bleeding, nausea, and vomiting. Isopropyl alcohol is two to three times more potent than ethanol as a CNS depressant, and acetone is comparable with ethanol. Patients frequently present with headache, lethargy, ataxia, or coma. Respiratory depression occurs secondary to the CNS depression. Laboratory findings include an osmolar gap without a metabolic acidosis. Patients may, however, have a fruity odor on their breath, and ketonemia and ketonuria may also be present. Treatment is supportive with fluid administration for significant dehydration. Hemodialysis should be considered when isopropyl alcohol levels exceed 400 to 500 mg/dL, evidence of hypoperfusion exists, coma is present, or a failure to respond to supportive therapy is noted.

Table 69-5. Dosing Schedule of Fomepizole during Hemodialysis

Dose at Beginning of Dialysis	
<6 hr since last dose	Do not administer dose
>6 hr since last dose	Give next scheduled dose
Dose During Dialysis	
Give dose every 4 hr	
Dose at Completion of Dialysis	
<1 hr since last dose	No additional dose
1-3 hr since last dose	Administer half of next scheduled dose
>3 hr since last dose	Administer next scheduled dose
Maintenance Dose Off Dialysis	
12 hr after last dose	

From Roberts JR, Hedges J (eds): Clinical Procedures in Emergency Medicine. Philadelphia, WB Saunders, 1985.

Amphetamines/Methamphetamines

Amphetamines, methamphetamines, and related agents have enjoyed varying popularity as drugs of abuse. In general, these drugs cause release of catecholamines, which result in a sympathomimetic/adrenergic toxidrome characterized by tachycardia, hyperthermia, agitation, hypertension, and mydriasis. Hallucinations (visual and tactile) and acute psychoses are frequently observed. The acute adverse consequences are similar to those seen with cocaine abuse (see following) and include myocardial ischemia and arrhythmias, seizures, intracranial hemorrhage, stroke, rhabdomyolysis, necrotizing vasculitis, and death.[20] Long-term use of these drugs may result in dilated cardiomyopathy.

Methamphetamine hydrochloride in a crystalline form called "ice," "crank," or "crystal" is one of the most popular drugs in this class. It has high purity and can be orally ingested, smoked, insufflated nasally, or injected intravenously. An amphetamine-like drug—3-4-methylenedioxymethamphetamine—is a designer drug commonly known as Ecstasy, XTC, or MDMA that acts simultaneously as a stimulant and hallucinogen.[21] It results in serotonin release in the brain with inhibition of serotonin reuptake and has been reported to produce serotonin syndrome. Complications are usually a result of the drug effects and nonstop physical activity. Complications include hyperthermia, hyponatremia, rhabdomyolysis, renal failure, cardiac collapse, cerebral infarction/hemorrhage, and multiple organ failure. MDMA and other amphetamines will usually be detected on qualitative toxicology assays of urine.

Management of amphetamine intoxication is primarily supportive. Gastric lavage is not recommended because absorption after oral ingestion is usually complete when patients present. Activated charcoal may be considered if a recent oral ingestion is known to have occurred. Further interventions are dependent on patient complaints and clinical findings. A careful assessment for complications should be made including measurement of core temperature, obtaining an ECG, and evaluating laboratory data for evidence of renal dysfunction and rhabdomyolysis. IV hydration for possible rhabdomyolysis is warranted in individuals with known exertional activities pending creatine phosphokinase (CPK) results. Benzodiazepines, often in high doses, should be used for controlling agitation. Haloperidol should be reserved for patients who do not have an adequate response to benzodiazepines.

Benzodiazepines

Although ingestions are relatively common, fatalities from benzodiazepines alone are rare. Benzodiazepine overdose results in a typical sedative-hypnotic toxidrome characterized by depressed level of consciousness, respiratory depression, hyporeflexia, and possibly hypotension and bradycardia. The clinical manifestations may be exacerbated by concomitant ingestion of other agents with sedating properties, such as ethanol or antidepressants. Alprazolam is commonly seen in overdoses and may result in greater toxicity than other benzodiazepines.[22] Flunitrazepam is a benzodiazepine not approved for use in the United States that has been associated with sexual assault. Diagnosis of benzodiazepine ingestion is primarily based on the history and clinical manifestations. Many benzodiazepines can be detected in qualitative urine toxicology assays, but a negative test does not rule out ingestion. If warranted, gas chromatography/mass spectrometry can be requested for definitive detection.

Managing benzodiazepine ingestions should be guided by the clinical presentation of the patient. The airway is assessed and stabilized if necessary. Activated charcoal is the primary method of GI decontamination for recent ingestions. Supportive care with intubation and mechanical ventilation may be necessary for patients with significant toxicity. Hypotension should be initially treated with volume infusion.

Flumazenil is a competitive benzodiazepine receptor antagonist that will reverse the sedative effects of benzodiazepines. It may be a helpful diagnostic tool in evaluating an overdose patient but should not be routinely used as a substitute for adequate airway protection.[23] An initial dose of 0.2 mg is administered IV over 30 seconds, followed in 30 seconds by a dose of 0.3 mg if needed. Additional doses of 0.5 mg are given at 1-minute intervals to a total of 3 mg. A dose greater than 1 mg is seldom necessary in overdose victims. The short half-life of flumazenil (0.7 to 1.3 hours) makes resedation likely because of the longer half-life of benzodiazepines. Continuous monitoring must be instituted if flumazenil is used to arouse the patient. Flumazenil use has been associated with seizures in patients with chronic benzodiazepine use and when cyclic antidepressants are present.[22] It is best to avoid flumazenil in those situations and in patients with a seizure disorder or when a drug capable of causing seizures has been ingested. Slow titration of flumazenil (0.1 mg/min) and limiting the total dose to 1 mg may minimize the risk of seizures. If seizures occur with flumazenil, benzodiazepines (often in higher doses) may be effective.

β-Blockers

β-Adrenergic blockers differ in their lipid solubility, oral availability, first-pass effect, protein binding, metabolism, β-1 selectivity, and intrinsic sympathomimetic activity. Clinical findings with β-blocker toxicity include bradycardia, atrioventricular conduction abnormalities (QRS prolongation), and hypotension. With the exception of sotalol, ventricular fibrillation and other dysrhythmias are not usually seen. The more lipophilic β-adrenergic antagonists such as propranolol, metoprolol, acebutolol, and timolol cause delirium, coma, and seizures even in the absence of hypotension. Hypoglycemia is rare in adults. Toxicity occurs early, generally within 6 hours of ingestion. Ingestion of sotalol or extended-release preparations may result in delayed toxicity, and these patients should be observed for 24 hours or longer if absorption is delayed.[23] Propranolol is associated with the highest mortality, which likely reflects its greater frequency of use and greater toxicity attributable to membrane stabilizing effects.[23] Bradydysrhythmia and asystole usually precede death.

GI decontamination with gastric lavage may be considered if there is a large ingestion of propranolol and the patient presents within the first hour, even if symptoms are absent. Because of the risk of vagal stimulation, pretreatment with atropine may be indicated. WBI may be considered in ingestions of sustained-release preparations. Extracorporeal removal is ineffective for lipid-soluble β-blockers because of the large Vd. Hemodialysis may be rarely used for atenolol, a water-soluble β-blocker.

Initial treatment of bradycardia and hypotension consists of atropine and isotonic fluids. If the patient is unresponsive to these measures, then glucagon 2 to 5 mg IV should be administered followed by a dose of 10 mg if necessary. If there is a response, a continuous infusion should be started at the response dose per hour (usually 5 to 10 mg/hour). Glucagon stimulates cyclic adenosine monophosphate (cAMP) by bypassing adrenergic receptors.[26] Although no clinical trials have been performed in humans, clinical experience suggests that it may be equally or more effective than vasopressors. Adverse effects of glucagon include nausea, vomiting, hyperglycemia, and hypocalcemia. After cardiac glycoside ingestion (e.g., digoxin) has been excluded, calcium salts may be effective in reversing hypotension. Calcium chloride 10% (1 g by slow IV push) may be administered, and up to 3 g is recommended.

Ventricular pacing is the next step, although it may increase the heart rate without increasing cardiac output or blood pressure. If calcium administration and pacing fail, catecholamine infusions should be initiated. The combination of dobutamine and norepinephrine may allow for titration of desired effects against cardiac output and blood pressure. Very large doses may be required because the β-adrenergic receptors are blocked; as a result, tachyarrhythmias are likely. Alternatively, phenylephrine may be used in conjunction with dobutamine. Epinephrine has been shown to be more effective than isoproterenol.[26] Infusion of any vasoactive agent should be started at usual doses but rapidly escalated to achieve a clinical response, but it should be stopped if there is a further fall in blood pressure. Phosphodiesterase inhibitors such as amrinone, milrinone, and enoximone have been reported to be as effective as glucagon in animal models and cases of human ingestions.[27] These agents may be useful in patients who fail glucagon, although the long half-lives prevent easy titration and may cause further hypotension through peripheral vasodilation. Because of these potential problems, the use of catecholamines and phosphodiesterase inhibitors should be guided by invasive monitoring whenever possible. Recently, high-dose insulin infusions together with glucose drips to maintain euglycemia have been shown to be effective.[28] The beneficial effect may be caused in part by the metabolic effects of decreasing cardiac uptake of free fatty acids and increasing carbohydrate use. Careful monitoring of glucose and potassium is required. Intraaortic balloon pump or cardiopulmonary bypass are potential options in the unstable patient unresponsive to other interventions and may be necessary to maintain circulation until drug is metabolized.

Calcium Channel Blockers

Calcium channel blockers selectively inhibit calcium movement in cardiac or vascular smooth muscle membranes during the slow inward phase of excitation-contraction. These agents have varying degrees of negative inotropic effect (verapamil), vasodilatory effect (nifedipine, diltiazem), depression of rate of discharge of the sinus node, and slowed conduction through the atrioventricular node (verapamil, diltiazem). All are well absorbed with clinically significant protein binding (80%) and a Vd greater than 1 L/kg. All undergo extensive hepatic metabolism, many through the cytochrome P_{450} system, and have varying degrees of active metabolites.

Signs and symptoms of toxicity occur within 6 hours for regular formulations but are delayed 6 to 18 hours for sustained-release preparations.[29] Gastric concretions often form, acting as a further reservoir for sustained absorption. Nausea, vomiting, and hypotension are usually accompanied by bradycardia (with verapamil and diltiazem) or reflex tachycardia with nifedipine. Heart block may include first-degree block; Wenckebach block; third-degree atrioventricular (AV) block; and AV dissociation, particularly with verapamil and diltiazem but less commonly with nifedipine. Hypoperfusion secondary to decreased cardiac output may lead to cardiac, mesenteric, renal, and cerebral ischemia, and mild metabolic acidosis. The patient may present with CNS symptoms such as lethargy, confusion, and coma. Hyperglycemia occurs occasionally.

Activated charcoal is the preferred method of GI decontamination in recent ingestions. Because of the hepatic metabolism of calcium channel blockers, the parent and active metabolites exhibit enterohepatic circulation. However, once absorbed, calcium channel blockers decrease cardiac output and may lead to mesenteric ischemia and diminished bowel motility, which is a relative contraindication to MDAC. WBI may be considered for removing sustained release preparations.

As with β-blockers, initial treatment of calcium channel blocker overdose should be aimed at treating hypotension and significant conduction defects. Heart block may require atropine, calcium, or glucagon. Calcium chloride is of limited benefit for either hypotension or bradycardia, but a brief, aggressive attempt should be made after digoxin has been excluded as a potential coingestant. If a metabolic acidosis is present, calcium gluconate should be used. Although there are no trials demonstrating the superiority of glucagon over calcium or vasopressors, glucagon has been reported to be beneficial and should be used early in a symptomatic patient.[31] Glucagon is dosed as in β-blocker overdoses. A continuous infusion of glucagon can be titrated to maintain blood pressure, cardiac output, and sinus rhythm. Insulin-glucose infusions have also been evaluated as an adjunctive treatment in severe cases.[31] As with β-blocker overdose, large doses of vasopressors and inotropes may be required. A transvenous pacer may be effective. Refractory hypotension may require intra-aortic balloon pump or cardiopulmonary bypass. Another agent that increases calcium influx through blocking potassium channels is 4-aminopyridine, which is currently experimental.

Carbon Monoxide

Carbon monoxide (CO) poisoning may be accidental or intentional and continues to be a common cause of morbidity in the United States. Sources of CO include motor vehicle exhaust fumes, poorly functioning heating systems, and inhaled smoke. CO binds to hemoglobin with an affinity 200 to 250 times greater than oxygen. Toxicities result from impaired release of oxygen at the tissue level, causing cell hypoxia and possibly direct CO-mediated damage at the cellular level. The clinical manifestations of CO poisoning are nonspecific and may suggest other illnesses unless exposure is known or suspected. Headache, nausea, and vomiting are common. Cellular hypoxia may also result in confusion, angina, arrhythmias, syncope, and seizures. Tachycardia and tachypnea are frequently present as compensatory mechanisms for hypoxia. Classic findings of cherry red lips, cyanosis, and retinal hemorrhages occur rarely. Symptoms can range from mild to severe, and carboxyhemoglobin levels do not necessarily correlate with symptom severity. After recovery from acute CO exposure, delayed neuropsychiatric sequelae may occur.

Diagnosis requires a high level of suspicion. Carboxyhemoglobin levels can be measured in venous or arterial blood and must be interpreted carefully. Carboxyhemoglobin levels may be as high as 10% in smokers and are higher in urban compared with rural areas. An elevated level of carboxyhemoglobin may often be diagnostic, but a normal level does not rule out the diagnosis. The carboxyhemoglobin level may have decreased because of removal of the patient from the exposure and intervention with oxygen before hospital arrival.

Management of CO poisoning includes a detailed evaluation of neurologic and cardiorespiratory status. Acid-base status should be determined and an ECG examined for evidence of ischemia or arrhythmia. Oxygen is the antidote and shortens the half-life of carboxyhemoglobin by competing for binding with hemoglobin. High-concentration oxygen should be instituted as soon as possible and continued until the carboxyhemoglobin level has decreased to normal. Pulse oximetry overestimates arterial oxygenation because carboxyhemoglobin is misinterpreted as oxyhemoglobin. Analysis of arterial blood by co-oximetry is required for an accurate assessment of oxygen content. Intubation may be necessary in patients exposed to CO from fire. Hyperbaric oxygen therapy shortens the half-life of carboxyhemoglobin to 15 to 30 minutes compared with 40 to 80 minutes when patients breathe 100% oxygen. However, controversy exists over the specific indications for instituting hyperbaric oxygen therapy in CO poisoning.[32,33] Coma has been used as an indication for hyperbaric oxygen therapy; other suggested indications include a period of unconsciousness, neurologic findings other than headache, carboxyhemoglobin level greater than 40%, pregnancy with carboxyhemoglobin level greater than 15%, cardiac ischemia or arrhythmia, history of ischemic heart disease with carboxyhemoglobin level greater than 20%, and symptoms that do not resolve with normobaric oxygen after 4 to 6 hours. Hyperbaric oxygen treatment may decrease postexposure cognitive deficits.[34]

Cocaine

Cocaine is a common drug of abuse in the United States and results in significant morbidity and mortality.[35] Cocaine hydrochloride is water soluble and used intravenously or by intranasal insufflation. Crack or rock cocaine is the alkaloid form primarily abused by inhalation. Both forms of cocaine are rapidly absorbed from all mucosal surfaces and undergo hydrolysis by plasma cholinesterase. The metabolites benzoylecgonine and ecgonine methyl ester are excreted in the urine and can be detected by qualitative urine assays. The metabolites of cocaine may be detectable in urine for 24 to 36 hours after use, but prolonged detection has occurred in frequent users of high doses. Cocaine is a sympathetic stimulant resulting in characteristic clinical findings of tachycardia, dilated pupils, hypertension, hyperthermia, and agitation. The sympathetic stimulation also results in multiple complications (Table 69-6). Complications such as myocardial ischemia or cerebral infarction may occur several days after the last use of cocaine. Complications of transporting cocaine in body cavities may include rupture of packets with drug absorption and bowel obstruction.

No specific antidote exists for cocaine. Treatment is primarily aimed at detecting complications, intervening as indicated, and preventing further injury. Benzodiazepines should be used liberally for control of agitation. Haloperidol is reserved for overt psychosis because of its potential for lowering the seizure threshold.

No large clinical trials have evaluated therapeutic strategies for myocardial ischemia resulting from cocaine. Aspirin should be administered if the risk of intracranial hemorrhage is low because a significant number of patients have thrombotic occlusion as the etiology of ischemia. Benzodiazepines and nitroglycerin are first-line agents for relief of chest pain, but small clinical studies have yielded conflicting results on the benefit of combining the agents.[36,37] α-Blockers such as phentolamine and calcium channel blockers have been recommended as second-line treatment for unrelieved pain but are rarely necessary.[38] The use of β-blockers in the management of myocardial ischemia is debated. There is a potential concern of worsening vasospasm or hypertension because of unopposed stimulation of alpha receptors. However, β-blockers have been used, particularly in the setting of myocardial infarction without complications. It may be appropriate to avoid administration of β-blockers in patients manifesting acute sympathomimetic findings, but the benefits of these agents should be considered in other patients with ongoing myocardial ischemia. Reperfusion interventions should be considered for patients with myocardial infarction. Primary percutaneous angioplasty is usually preferred, especially when the diagnosis may be in doubt. Thrombolytic therapy has been used safely in cocaine-associated MI and may be considered if invasive reperfusion is not available.[39]

Table 69-6. Complications Associated with Cocaine Use

Cardiovascular	***Renal***
Myocardial ischemia, infarction	Renal infarction
Dysrhythmias	Renal failure
Aortic dissection, rupture	Scleroderma renal crisis
Hypertension	
Atherosclerosis	***Gastrointestinal***
Cardiomyopathy	Mesenteric ischemia, infarction
Vasculitis	GI perforations
Central Nervous System	***Metabolic***
Seizures	Hyperthermia
Cerebral infarction	Rhabdomyolysis
Transient ischemic attack	Weight loss
Intracranial hemorrhage (intraparenchymal, intraventricular, subarachnoid)	Multiple organ failure
	Other
Cerebral vasculitis	Deep venous thrombosis
Cognitive dysfunction	Skin ischemia
	Dystonic reactions
Pulmonary	
Bronchospasm	
Barotrauma	
Noncardiogenic edema	
Pulmonary hypertension	
Pulmonary hemorrhage, hemoptysis	

Cerebral complications should be managed by standard interventions specific for the injury. Seizures are best managed with benzodiazepines. A significant number of patients with intracranial hemorrhage have underlying vascular malformations that may require specific intervention.[40,41] Severe hyperthermia is managed as heat stroke with either conductive or evaporative cooling. When there is suspicion of rhabdomyolysis, IV hydration should be instituted immediately pending assessment of renal function and CPK levels. Asymptomatic transporters of cocaine packets should be managed conservatively with activated charcoal, possible WBI, and supportive care. Surgery is reserved for patients exhibiting manifestations of cocaine poisoning or GI perforation or obstruction.[42] The potential for suicidal intent should be recognized in cocaine abusers, and psychiatric consultation may be appropriate after stabilization.

Cyanide

Inhalation or ingestion of cyanide is rare but can produce severe poisoning rapidly leading to death. A history of potential cyanide exposure is extremely important in suggesting the diagnosis because rapid cyanide assays are not available and clinical manifestations are nonspecific.[43] Cyanide exposure may occur from incomplete combustion of products containing carbon and nitrogen in fires, industrial processes such as electroplating, metal refining, photography, fumigation, and gold or silver extraction. Cyanogenic substances are also found in a variety of plants, although severe toxicity is rare. Iatrogenic cyanide intoxication may occur during nitroprusside administration.

Cyanide is a nonspecific inhibitor of enzymes; inhibition of mitochondrial cytochrome oxidase results in anaerobic metabolism with decreased adenosine triphosphate (ATP) production, lactic acidosis, and decreased oxygen utilization. Clinical characteristics of acute cyanide poisoning are rapid deterioration, loss of consciousness, anion gap metabolic acidosis, and cardiopulmonary failure. CNS signs and symptoms include headache, anxiety, agitation, confusion, seizures, and coma. Cardiovascular responses manifest as initial bradycardia and hypertension, followed by hypotension with reflex tachycardia that can progress to terminal bradycardia and hypotension. Ventricular dysrhythmias and myocardial ischemia also occur. Pulmonary findings include cardiogenic and noncardiogenic pulmonary edema. GI symptoms of abdominal pain, nausea, and vomiting are less common. A bitter almond odor from vomitus or gastric contents is described in cyanide poisonings but may not be present and is often not detectable by health care personnel.

Early diagnosis, rapid administration of antidote, and aggressive supportive care are necessary to stabilize patients with severe cyanide poisoning. A cyanide level may be requested for confirmation, but results will not be available to guide immediate care. Intubation and mechanical ventilation are usually required. Fluids or inotropes and vasopressors may be indicated for hypotension. If the poison was ingested, gastric lavage may be indicated but should not delay the administration of antidote. As soon as cyanide poisoning is suspected, a cyanide antidote kit or equivalent should be used. The kit contains amyl nitrite ampules, 3% sodium nitrite, and 25% sodium thiosulfate. Amyl nitrite is an immediate source of nitrite that oxidizes hemoglobin to methemoglobin, which has a higher affinity for cyanide than cytochrome oxidase. Cyanmethemoglobin is formed, which eventually dissociates, but at such a rate that cyanide can be metabolized by hepatic rhodanase. The ampules are crushed in a gauze sponge and initially intermittently inhaled. This is followed by IV administration of 300 mg of sodium nitrite (10 mL 3% solution) as soon as possible. The optimum methemoglobin level that should be achieved is unknown, but clinical responses have occurred with levels of 3.6% to 9.2%. The second component of the antidote package is 25% sodium thiosulfate (12.5 g for adults), which provides sulfur for conversion of cyanide to thiocyanate by hepatic rhodanese. Thiocyanate is then excreted by the kidneys.

Hydroxocobalamin, a vitamin B_{12} precursor administered at an initial dose of 4 g, is commonly used in Europe for acute cyanide poisoning and is now available in the United States. It displaces cyanide from the cytochrome oxidase and forms cyanocobalamin, which is then excreted in the urine or metabolized by hepatic rhodanese. Another potential treatment used in Europe is 4-dimethylaminophenol (4-DMAP), which is administered at a dose of 3 mg/kg to induce methemoglobin. Thiosulfate is administered with hydroxocobalamin and 4-DMAP. Hyperbaric oxygen has also been proposed for treating cyanide toxicity, but data supporting efficacy are not available.

Cyclic Antidepressants

Deaths caused by overdose with cyclic antidepressants are declining because of the increasing use of newer, safer antidepressants. The principal toxicities of cyclic antidepressants result from central and peripheral anticholinergic activity, α-adrenergic antagonism, and inhibition of norepinephrine reuptake. They also exert a membrane-depressant local anesthetic effect on the myocardium by blocking rapid sodium influx during phase 0 of the action potential. Primary toxicities include depressed level of consciousness, wide-complex dysrhythmias, seizures, and hypotension. Anticholinergic effects include mydriasis, fever, dry skin, delirium, tachycardia, ileus, and urinary retention. Life-threatening events usually occur within 6 hours of ingestion, most often in the first 2 hours.[44] Several electrocardiographic criteria have been proposed to predict complications: QRS duration greater than 0.1 second correlates with risk of seizures, QRS duration greater than 0.16 second correlates with increased risk of dysrhythmias, and the presence of an R wave in aVR greater than 3 mm predicts seizures and dysrhythmias.[45,46] However, the performance of these criteria in predicting complications including death is relatively poor.[47]

If wide-complex dysrhythmias (or ECG changes described previously), hypotension, or seizures are present, stabilization requires immediate alkalinization of the blood and sodium loading with sodium bicarbonate.[48] Sodium bicarbonate should be administered in 50 to 100 mEq (1 to 2 mEq/kg) boluses to alkalinize the blood pH to 7.5 to 7.55. Clinical end points are normalization (narrowing) of the QRS complex, reestablishment of an adequate blood pressure, or termination of seizure activity. Alkalinization appears to decrease the free drug by increasing protein binding and shifting the concentration gradient away from tissues back into the main compartment. Sodium loading may have a greater benefit by overcoming the blockade of the myocardial sodium channels. The bolus doses of sodium bicarbonate should be immediately followed with a continuous infusion, which can be prepared by adding 150 mEq $NaHCO_3$ (sodium bicarbonate) to 1 L of D_5W. This should be titrated to the desired blood pH, QRS interval, and blood pressure. The infusion may be discontinued after 4 to 6 hours if the width of the QRS complex remains less than 100 ms without the administration of sodium bicarbonate. Hyperventilation to achieve blood alkalinization may be less effective but useful in patients who cannot tolerate the sodium and volume load or in those who develop pulmonary edema from treatment with sodium bicarbonate.[49] Hyperventilation without the administration of sodium bicarbonate may also be considered for patients with cerebral edema, head trauma, or poorly controlled congestive heart failure. Hypertonic saline has been effective in treating cardiac toxicity refractory to initial blood alkalinization.[50,51]

If torsades de pointes is associated with QT prolongation, magnesium sulfate 1 to 2 g IV over 2 to 5 minutes should be administered. Hypotension refractory to volume expansion is best treated with a direct-acting catecholamine such as norepinephrine or phenylephrine in the setting of depleted norepinephrine stores.[52] An inotropic agent such as dobutamine can be added if hypotension is the result of depressed myocardial contractility and decreased cardiac output. If hypotension remains refractory to fluids and vasopressors, the use of an intra-aortic balloon pump should be considered as a temporizing measure.

After the patient with a known or suspected cyclic antidepressant overdose has been stabilized and the airway protected, activated charcoal is indicated. Gastric lavage should only be performed if the patient is seriously ill and the ingestion occurred within 1 hour of presentation. A second dose of activated charcoal may be given in several hours if it seems plausible that the drug still remains in the GI tract in the case of a massive ingestion or hypotension. MDAC to enhance elimination is not warranted given the extremely large Vd (10 to 50 L/kg) and the low-protein binding of cyclic antidepressants.[13] Forced diuresis, hemodialysis, and hemoperfusion are ineffective. Physostigmine should also be avoided because of the potential anticholinergic toxicity of seizures and asystole.

If the patient has had altered mental status, seizures, or cardiac dysrhythmia, the patient should remain in the ICU for 12 hours after all supportive therapeutic interventions have been discontinued. If the patient remains asymptomatic with a normal ECG and a normal pH during this phase of observation, the patient may then transfer for additional care.

Digoxin

The cardiac glycosides inhibit active transport of Na^+ and K^+ across cell membranes by reversibly binding onto a specific site on the Na^+,K^+-ATPase. The alterations in cardiac rate and rhythm occurring in digitalis toxicity can produce almost every type of dysrhythmia. Toxicity results from the complex influence of digitalis on the electrophysiologic properties of the heart, as well as the cumulative result of the direct, vagotonic, and antiadrenergic actions of digitalis. Toxicity should be suspected if there is evidence of increased automaticity (ectopic rhythms) and depressed conduction (prolonged PR interval, AV node blockade, decreased QT interval). Early in acute intoxication, depression of SA or AV node function may be reversed by atropine, but atropine subsequently does not reverse the direct and vagomimetic actions of the drug. Noncardiac manifestations of acute digitalis intoxication include anorexia, confusion, nausea or vomiting, and rising K^+ concentrations.

GI decontamination of digoxin overdose consists of activated charcoal, if the timing is appropriate. MDAC may be beneficial given the 35% enterohepatic and enteroenteric recirculation of digoxin.[3] Steroid-binding resins such as cholestyramine and colestipol have also been used to prevent further absorption from the GI tract and reduce serum half-life in the same manner as charcoal. Forced diuresis, hemoperfusion, and hemodialysis are not effective in hastening the elimination of digoxin because of the large Vd (4 to 10 L/kg). Only 1% of total body stores of digoxin is in the serum; of that, 25% is protein bound.

The treatment for life-threatening digitalis toxicity is administration of digoxin-specific antibody fragments. Administration of digoxin-specific antibody fragments results in a sharp decrease in free digoxin levels, an increase in total serum digoxin, an increase in renal excretion of digoxin bound to Fab, and a decrease of serum potassium toward normal. The time to response is approximately 30 minutes (range 20 to 90 minutes). Indications for administration of digoxin-specific antibody fragments include severe ventricular dysrhythmias, progressive bradydysrhythmias unresponsive to atropine, potassium concentration greater than 5 mEq/L in the setting of suspected digoxin toxicity, rapidly progressive cardiac or GI symptoms, a rising potassium concentration, serum digoxin concentration greater than 15 ng/mL at any time or more than 10 ng/mL at steady state, ingestion of more than 10 mg of digoxin in a previously healthy adult, and to establish the diagnosis. In the event that digoxin-specific fragments are not immediately available, phenytoin (50 mg/minute up to 1000 mg) or lidocaine may be administered until control of the dysrhythmia is achieved. Atropine may work for severe supraventricular bradydysrhythmias or varying degrees of AV block if administered early. β-Blockers may be used for supraventricular and ventricular tachycardias. Magnesium sulfate may be an effective temporizing measure for the treatment of ventricular dysrhythmias in the absence of digoxin-specific antibodies, even in the presence of hypermagnesemia. All class Ia drugs are contraindicated. Isoproterenol should be avoided because there is an increased risk of ventricular ectopy in the presence of toxic digoxin levels. External or transvenous pacemakers have limited value in this setting.[53]

Hypokalemia, hyperkalemia, and hypomagnesemia can exacerbate digitalis cardiotoxicity and should be normalized. When hyperkalemia exists with toxic digoxin levels and ECG evidence of potassium toxicity, the serum potassium should be treated with conventional interventions if digoxin-specific Fab fragments are not immediately available. Calcium chloride, in the presence of digitalis toxicity, can theoretically be disastrous because intracellular hypercalcemia already exists. Intractable ventricular fibrillation or tachycardia may result.

After digoxin-specific antibodies have been administered, serum digoxin levels are no longer reliable because they represent free and bound digoxin. The digoxin-specific antibodies are effective even in anephric patients. In renal insufficiency, the Fab half-life is prolonged tenfold with no change in Vd. Fab concentrations remain detectable for 2 to 3 weeks. Although there is no dissociation of the complex, in renal insufficiency, free digoxin levels rebound (redistribution from tissue sites) and Fab fragments leave the vascular space over 7 to 14 days.[54] During this time symptoms may recur and a second dose may be necessary.

Gamma Hydroxybutyrate

Gamma hydroxybutyrate (GHB), a naturally occurring substance found in the brain and peripheral tissues, has been banned in the United States except for the treatment for narcolepsy. It is one of several agents characterized as a "date rape" drug and has been promoted to build muscle, improve performance, produce euphoria, induce fat loss, and enhance sleep. Several deaths have been attributed to GHB and related agents.[55] The drug is usually available as a colorless, odorless liquid with a mild, salty taste that is easy to mask in drinks. GHB is rapidly absorbed from the stomach (usually within 10 to 15 minutes) and readily crosses the blood-brain barrier. It is metabolized to carbon dioxide and water without active metabolites. Stimulatory effects occur from resulting increased dopamine levels in the brain and sedative effects by potentiation of endogenous opioids. The manifestations of GHB toxicity are dose related and include agitation, coma, seizures, respiratory depression, and vomiting.[56] Other effects include amnesia, tremors, myoclonus, hypotonia, hypothermia, decreased cardiac output, and bradycardia. Coma and respiratory depression may be potentiated by the concomitant use of ethanol. GHB is not routinely detected by urine toxicology assays but can be detected in plasma or urine by gas chromatographic–mass spectrophotometric techniques. Diagnosis is usually determined by the clinical course and history of exposure elicited after the patient recovers. Gamma butyrolactone (GBL), also known as 2 (3H)-furanone dihydro, and 1,4 butanediol (BD), also called tetramethylene glycol, have been abused with the same adverse effects as GHB including death. Both agents are metabolized in the body to GHB.

No antidote for GHB, GBL, or BD exists. The primary management for ingestion of these drugs is supportive care with particular attention to airway protection. In some cases, intubation and mechanical ventilation are required. Gastric lavage and activated charcoal are not indicated because of the small amounts involved and the rapid absorption. Naloxone and flumazenil are of no benefit. Patients with mild intoxication may be observed in the emergency department and released after symptoms resolve. A rapid recovery of consciousness from an obtunded condition is frequently observed. In patients requiring intubation and mechanical ventilation, symptoms can be expected to resolve within 2 to 96 hours unless complications such as aspiration or anoxic injury have occurred. The concomitant use of alcohol may prolong the CNS depression. Although physostigmine has been used to awaken patients with GHB intoxication, its use is not recommended.

A withdrawal syndrome has been described in patients who frequently ingest high doses of GHB (every 1 to 3 hours).[57] Mild symptoms such as anxiety, insomnia, nausea, vomiting, and tremors begin within 6 hours of the last dose and may progress to severe delirium with autonomic instability (usually mild) requiring hospitalization and sedation. The duration of symptoms requiring treatment may be as long as 2 weeks. Benzodiazepines are the initial choice for management, and high doses may be required. Propofol and barbiturates have also been used successfully.

Isoniazid

Isoniazid (INH) toxicity produces altered mental status, seizures refractory to standard therapy, coma, an anion gap metabolic acidosis, and hepatic toxicity. The neurotoxicity of INH is the result of vitamin B_6 (pyridoxine) depletion, which is a necessary cofactor in the synthesis and metabolism of amino acids such as GABA, the major inhibitory neurotransmitter in the CNS. In the liver, toxicity is mediated directly by the products of INH metabolism. Patients are usually symptomatic within 30 to 45 minutes of ingestion, although symptoms may be delayed for up to 2 hours when peak absorption occurs. Ingestion of less than 1.5 g in adults is usually associated with mild toxicity, although greater than 10 g may be fatal. Seizures occur with more than 20 mg/kg but may occur with lesser ingestions in susceptible patients. Patients who are asymptomatic after an ingestion of INH should be observed for 6 hours because toxicity usually develops in this time. The treatment of choice is intensive supportive care with airway protection and the administration of pyridoxine 5 g IV (1 g every 2 to 3 minutes) or a dose equivalent to the amount of INH ingested. When the airway is secured and seizures controlled, gastric lavage may be considered and activated charcoal administered. Hemoperfusion or hemodialysis may be considered, particularly in patients with renal insufficiency or those with persistent symptoms despite adequate therapy.

After the initial dose of pyridoxine is administered, a continuous infusion of pyridoxine is beneficial because it is rapidly cleared from the body. If seizures recur, then a repeat dose of 5 g may be administered. If no parenteral form of pyridoxine is available, pyridoxine tablets may be crushed and administered enterally as a slurry in the same dose. Phenytoin is not indicated because it acts on sodium channels and is therefore not effective.

Lithium

Although lithium is commonly used to treat bipolar affective disorders, its narrow therapeutic index predisposes to toxicity. After oral ingestion, lithium is absorbed within 1 to 2 hours, reaching peak blood levels in 2 to 4 hours with regular preparations or in 4 to 12 hours with sustained release preparations. Lithium does not bind to plasma proteins and is excreted almost entirely by the kidneys. Toxicity may occur with acute, acute on chronic, or chronic ingestions. Drugs that increase lithium reabsorption (ACE inhibitors, thiazides, nonsteroidal anti-inflammatory drug), sodium restriction, volume depletion, and intrinsic renal dysfunction increase the risk of toxicity. Lithium levels do not necessarily correlate with toxic symptoms. With an acute ingestion, the patient may be asymptomatic with a lithium level of 6 to 8 mmol/L. In chronic lithium ingestion, a high total-body lithium burden results in more immediate toxicity at lower serum levels.

The clinical presentation of patients with lithium toxicity varies with the type of ingestion. In an acute ingestion, nausea, vomiting, and diarrhea occur early with CNS symptoms developing later because of a delay in tissue distribution. In chronic ingestions, neurologic abnormalities are usually the major presenting manifestations. Patients with acute on chronic ingestions may manifest GI and neurologic symptoms. Neurologic abnormalities include tremor, hyperreflexia, agitation, fasciculations, clonus, and altered mental status. Confusion may be followed by lethargy, coma, and seizures. The tremor, hyperreflexia, and clonus usually precede altered mental status. Lithium can impair urine-concentrating ability in acute ingestions and cause nephrogenic diabetes insipidus and renal dysfunction in chronic ingestions that result in volume depletion. Although myocardial dysfunction and rhythm abnormalities have been reported in lithium toxicity, they occur rarely. Lithium toxicity may produce flattened or inverted T-waves and U-waves on electrocardiogram.

Lithium toxicity is confirmed by assessment of the serum lithium level. A lithium level should be assessed immediately and 2 hours later to evaluate for increasing levels. Levels higher than 2.5 mmol/L in a chronic ingestion or higher than 4 mmol/L in an acute ingestion are potentially life-threatening. Renal function and volume status should also be assessed.

Management decisions in treating lithium toxicity may depend on the type of ingestion (acute versus chronic) and the product ingested (regular versus sustained release). Lithium is not adsorbed by activated charcoal, but charcoal may be administered if other drugs are ingested or suspected. A forced diuresis is not effective in enhancing lithium excretion, but isotonic saline should be administered to replete and maintain intravascular volume and promote adequate urine output.[58] Diuretics can worsen lithium toxicity and should be avoided. WBI has been proposed for GI decontamination with acute or acute on chronic ingestions, ingestion of sustained release products, or when serial lithium levels are rising. Despite lack of proven clinical benefit, this approach may be considered with appropriate precautions. Hemodialysis is effective in removing lithium, but controversy exists on the indications for treatment and duration of therapy. Proposed indications that have not been validated include renal dysfunction, severe neurologic dysfunction, inability to tolerate fluid replacement, lithium level higher than 4 mmol/L in an acute overdose, and lithium level higher than 2.5 mmol/L in chronic toxicity. The lithium level, duration of exposure, and severity of clinical symptoms should be balanced against risks of the procedure before initiating hemodialysis. Hemodialysis clears lithium only from the plasma, and a rebound increase can develop from drug redistribution. A lithium level should be assessed immediately after hemodialysis and 6 to 8 hours later. Repeat dialysis can be considered if the lithium level increases or neurologic toxicity persists at that time. Although a lithium level of 1 mmol/L is often recommended as the end point for hemodialysis, no systematic investigations have established the ideal end point for optimal outcome. Because of redistribution of lithium, improvement of neurologic toxicity lags behind the decrease in plasma level. Prolonged monitoring of lithium levels may be necessary, especially when sustained release preparations are ingested. Continuous arteriovenous and venovenous hemodiafiltration have also been used to remove lithium and may be associated with less rebound.[59] These techniques result in a slower lithium clearance compared with hemodialysis and are not recommended if hemodialysis is available and can be tolerated. Sodium polystyrene sulfonate resin has been proposed to bind and remove lithium, but it is not currently recommended and may result in hypokalemia, hypernatremia, and fluid overload. Aminophylline and low-dose dopamine infusions have also been proposed to enhance lithium excretion, but no evidence of clinical efficacy exists and they should not be used.[58]

Opioids

Illicit and prescription opioids can result in a toxidrome characterized by depressed level of consciousness, respiratory depression, and miosis. However, manifestations may be variable depending on the drug used and presence of other drugs or alcohol. Miosis is not seen with meperidine, propoxyphene, and tramadol toxicity. Additional clinical findings may include hypotension, pulmonary edema, bronchospasm (heroin), ileus, nausea, vomiting, and pruritus. Seizures may be a manifestation of toxicity with meperidine and propoxyphene. Although all opioids are associated with toxicity, heroin purity and use have increased resulting in overdoses and fatalities. Heroin is rapidly absorbed by all routes of administration including IV, intranasal, intramuscular, subcutaneous, and inhalation. Most fatal overdoses occur with IV administration. IV fentanyl (some times extracted from analgesic patches) is also associated with fatalities. Oral opioids are available illicitly or by prescription, and toxicity depends on the potency of the agent, dose ingested, and tolerance of the individual. Diagnosis of an opioid overdose is made by characteristic clinical findings, exposure history, qualitative toxicology assay, and response to naloxone. Qualitative assays may not detect all opioid derivatives (e.g., fentanyl).

The immediate priorities in a patient with opioid toxicity are support of ventilation, correction of hypotension if present, and reversal of the toxic effects with an opioid antagonist. If reversal of respiratory depression cannot be accomplished quickly, intubation may be necessary. Likewise, isotonic fluids should be administered for hypotension. Gastric lavage may be considered for significant oral ingestions that occur a short time before presentation.

Naloxone, a potent competitive opioid antagonist, is the antidote for opioid toxicity. It can be administered intravenously, intramuscularly, by sublingual injection, or through an endotracheal tube. The initial dose of naloxone in a suspected opioid overdose is 0.4 to 2 mg; the lower dose should be considered in patients suspected of chronic addiction to avoid precipitating acute withdrawal symptoms. The goal of therapy is to restore adequate spontaneous respirations rather than complete arousal. Doses of naloxone up to 10 to 20 mg may be required to reverse the effects of synthetic opioids such as propoxyphene, pentazocine, methadone, and fentanyl. The effects of naloxone last approximately 60 to 90 minutes, necessitating continued observation of the patient for resedation. Patients may require continuous infusion of naloxone to maintain adequate respirations, particularly with long-acting opioids. The dose for infusion is typically one half to two thirds of the initial amount of naloxone that reversed the respiratory depression administered on an hourly basis. Adjustments of the dose should be made to achieve clinical end points and avoid withdrawal symptoms. Nalmefene, a long-acting opioid antagonist, has also been used to treat opioid overdoses, but prolonged withdrawal symptoms may be a concern.[60] The potential for acetaminophen toxicity should be considered in patients ingesting opioids formulated with acetaminophen. Patients should also be observed for potential complications of opioid overdose including aspiration pneumonitis and noncardiogenic pulmonary edema. Noncardiogenic pulmonary edema is usually self-limited (24 to 36 hours) and managed with supportive care that may include intubation and mechanical ventilation.[61] Other complications that may be related to injection drug use include wound botulism, endocarditis, rhabdomyolysis, and compartment syndrome.

Organophosphate and Carbamate Agents

Organophosphates and carbamates are cholinesterase inhibitors and are usually a component of insecticides. However, nerve agents used in chemical warfare such as sarin and VX are also organophosphate compounds. Cholinesterase inhibitors exert toxicity by blocking the activity of acetylcholinesterase resulting in acetylcholine accumulation at cholinergic receptors. When organophosphates or carbamates bind to acetylcholinesterase, they form a conjugate that is infinitely more stable than the acetylcholine-acetylcholinesterase conjugate. Carbamate enzyme spontaneously degrades in minutes to hours so that the enzyme is eventually regenerated (reversible binding). Also, because they are quaternary ammonium compounds, carbamates do not penetrate the CNS, resulting in limited toxicity. Most carbamate poisonings spontaneously resolve within 24 to 48 hours and do not have significant morbidity or mortality. Phosphorylated or phosphonylated enzymes, however, degrade over days to weeks, making acetylcholinesterase essentially inactive (irreversible binding). For the physiologic enzyme activity to return, new enzyme must be generated or antidote given. After the acetylcholinesterase is phosphorylated over 24 to 48 hours, "aging" occurs, and the enzyme can no longer spontaneously hydrolyze and is permanently inactivated.[62]

Organophosphates may be absorbed by virtually any route including transdermal, transconjunctival, inhalation, across the GI or genitourinary mucosa, and through direct injection. Onset of systemic symptoms may occur in 5 minutes with inhalation, and most patients will develop symptoms within 12 hours of ingestion, unless exposure to fat-soluble organophosphates (e.g., fenthion, clorfenthion) has occurred or if significant metabolic activation must occur (e.g., parathion). Signs and symptoms of cholinesterase poisoning are listed in Table 69-7. Pulmonary toxicity from bronchorrhea, bronchospasm, and respiratory depression is the primary concern.[63]

Early intubation is usually indicated with significant toxicity, and succinylcholine should be avoided because of prolonged paralysis. Initially, atropine 2 to 4 mg is given and repeated every 5 minutes. If there are no CNS symptoms, glycopyrrolate may be substituted. The end point of atropinization is clearing of secretions. Tachycardia is not a contraindication to atropine use because it may represent hypoxia and autonomic stimulation. The tachycardia may resolve with improved oxygenation. In massive exposures, hundreds of milligrams of atropine may be required over days or weeks. A continuous infusion of atropine should be initiated at 0.05 mg/kg/hour and titrated to effect. After the patient is adequately stabilized, atropine must be carefully and slowly withdrawn because secretions will likely return if the drug is still bound to acetylcholinesterase or leaches from fat stores.

Atropine does not reverse nicotinic effects, and patients with significant respiratory muscle weakness require the

Table 69-7. Signs and Symptoms of Cholinesterase Poisoning

Muscarinic Effects	Nicotinic Effects	CNS Effects
Salivation	Muscle fasciculations, cramping, weakness	Restlessness
Lacrimation	Diaphragmatic fatigue	Headache
Urination	Respiratory failure	Tremor
Diarrhea	Areflexia	Drowsiness
Nausea, vomiting	Paralysis	Confusion, delirium
Bronchorrhea	Tachycardia	Slurred speech
Bronchoconstriction	Mydriasis	Ataxia
Miosis		Seizures
Bradycardia		Psychosis
		Respiratory depression

use of pralidoxime (2-PAM). 2-PAM is a nucleophilic oxime that regenerates acetylcholinesterase at muscarinic, nicotinic, and CNS sites. It may also prevent continued toxicity by scavenging the remaining organophosphate molecules. Treatment with 2-PAM may be most effective when started early. It may have benefit beyond the 48-hour aging limit, although the mechanisms have not been clearly elucidated. It should be continued as long as atropine is continued. The evidence for benefit of any oxime in pesticide poisoning is limited.[64] Pralidoxime is usually administered as a loading dose (1 to 2 g in NS 500 mL administered over 30 minutes) and then as a continuous infusion at 200 to 500 mg/hour to maintain serum levels higher than 4 μg/L.[65] Other dosing regimens have also been proposed.[63] 2-PAM may also be protective against the development of the intermediate syndrome and other long-term neurologic sequelae.

In addition to acute toxicity, organophosphates may cause persistent effects, which may manifest while the patient is in the ICU and last several weeks to months. These include organophosphate-induced delayed neurotoxicity and delayed polyneuropathy that occur 1 to 3 weeks after exposure.[66] Recovery may occur gradually or not at all. The third complication is intermediate syndrome.[67] Clinically, 24 to 96 hours after resolution of an acute, severe cholinergic crisis, patients develop acute respiratory paralysis, weakness in the bulbar musculature, nuchal weakness, proximal limb weakness, and depressed reflexes. Electromyography studies show decremental conduction with repetitive nerve stimulation and suggest both presynaptic and postsynaptic nerve impairment. Recovery takes 2 to 4 times longer than the development.

Salicylates

Salicylates should be considered as a potential etiology if a metabolic acidosis with an anion gap of unknown cause is present. Uncoupling of mitochondrial oxidative phosphorylation results in metabolic acidosis, stimulation of medullary respiratory centers resulting in tachypnea and respiratory alkalosis, and hyperthermia. Initial symptoms include tinnitus and nausea or vomiting. Systemic acidosis promotes penetration of salicylate into the CNS, resulting in a depressed level of consciousness, coma, and seizures. Coagulopathy, transient hepatotoxicity, and hypoglycemia may also develop. Noncardiogenic pulmonary edema occurs more frequently in chronic salicylate toxicity than in acute overdose.

Activated charcoal can be used for GI decontamination. Salicylates in large ingestions can result in gastric concretions providing a depot for continued absorption. A salicylate ingestion is toxic if symptoms are present, if more than 150 mg/kg has been ingested, or if levels are higher than 35 mg/dL at 6 hours after ingestion. The Done nomogram was developed in pediatric ingestions and does not provide good clinical correlation with toxicity in adults. Acute intoxication with salicylate levels in excess of 35 mg/dL at 6 hours after ingestion should be treated with sodium bicarbonate to alkalinize the urine to a pH 7 to 8, which increases the renal clearance of salicylate metabolites through ion trapping. Hypokalemia will develop with correction of metabolic acidosis and must be corrected for urine alkalinization to be achieved. Alkalemia shifts the gradient of movement of salicylate from brain and tissues to blood. Large therapeutic and toxic doses resulting in levels greater than 35 mg/dL result in saturation of several elimination pathways, resulting in zero-order pharmacokinetics, prolonged elimination, decreased protein binding, and larger Vd. If levels continue to rise, a second dose of activated charcoal is controversial.[13]

Fluid status must be closely observed, along with coagulation, complete blood counts, arterial blood gases, electrolytes, and urine pH. Hemodialysis may be required for levels greater than 100 mg/dL in an acute ingestion, seizures, persistent alteration in mental status, refractory acidosis, persistent electrolyte abnormalities despite adequate therapy, or fluid overload resulting from sodium bicarbonate therapy. Additional indications for hemodialysis may include congestive heart failure (relative), noncardiogenic pulmonary edema, hepatotoxicity with coagulopathy or renal insufficiency.

Selective Serotonin Reuptake Inhibitors

Selective serotonin reuptake inhibitors (SSRIs) and related antidepressants are frequently prescribed for depression and other disorders. They have decreased lethality and few adverse cardiovascular effects compared with cyclic antidepressants. Most fatalities involving SSRIs involve coingestion of other substances. Manifestations of an acute SSRI overdose may include nausea, vomiting, dizziness, blurred vision, and rarely CNS depression. Seizures and a wide QRS occur rarely but may be more likely with citalopram and bupropion, a unicyclic antidepressant. A syndrome characteristic of SSRIs is the serotonin syndrome, which may occur after a single dose, high dose, overdose, or when combined with other serotonergic agents. The pathophysiology is related to excessive stimulation of central and peripheral serotonergic receptors. Clinical manifestations include altered mental status ranging from agitation to coma, autonomic dysfunction including diaphoresis, tachycardia, hyperthermia, unstable blood pressure, and diarrhea, and neuromuscular abnormalities that may range from tremors to myoclonus and rigidity.[68] Severe cases may be complicated by rhabdomyolysis, renal failure, disseminated intravascular coagulation, or acute respiratory distress syndrome.

Management of an acute overdose of SSRIs is largely supportive. Gastric lavage is not warranted because of the low toxicity of these compounds, but use of activated charcoal may be considered. An ECG should be obtained to assess for the rare occurrence of a wide QRS or other abnormality. Although clinical experience is limited, there are reports of sodium bicarbonate administration resulting in a narrowing of the QRS. The treatment of serotonin syndrome is primarily supportive therapy after discontinuing the precipitating agents. Intubation and mechanical ventilation may be necessary for patients with significant alteration of mental status. Benzodiazepines are useful for control of agitation and external cooling for sustained hyperthermia. Rarely, neuromuscular blockers may be necessary for control of muscle rigidity or tremor. The syndrome usually resolves in 24 to 72 hours. Treatment of patients with serotonin antagonists has been proposed, but experience is limited to case reports. Cyproheptadine in varying dose regimens (12 to 32 mg/24 hour) has been most commonly recommended as a treatment option. Currently there is no role for the use of bromocriptine or dantrolene.[68]

Valproic Acid

Use of valproic acid (VPA) is increasing for seizure disorders, psychiatric disorders, migraine prophylaxis, and neuropathic pain and has resulted in increased reports of toxicity with therapeutic doses and overdoses.[69] The most common manifestation of toxicity is CNS depression with higher drug levels associated with an increased incidence of coma and respiratory depression requiring intubation. Cerebral edema may occur 48 to 72 hours after overdoses and may be related to hyperammonemia that occurs in the absence of hepatotoxicity. Massive VPA ingestions can result in refractory hypotension. Pancreatitis has been associated with both chronic ingestion and acute overdose. Metabolic abnormalities of VPA toxicity include hypernatremia, anion gap metabolic acidosis, hypocalcemia, and acute renal failure. Serial VPA levels should be obtained because of delayed peak serum levels in overdose. Patients may be comatose with normal serum VPA concentrations caused by unmeasured metabolites. An ammonia level should be obtained in patients with altered level of consciousness. Activated charcoal should be administered if the patient presents early after ingestion. Multiple-dose activated charcoal may be beneficial because of a potential enterohepatic recirculation of drug, but routine use is not currently recommended. Because the percentage of VPA that is protein bound is decreased at high serum concentrations, hemoperfusion, combined hemodialysis-hemoperfusion, or high flux hemodialysis may be considered in patients with persistent hemodynamic instability or metabolic acidosis. No antidote exists for VPA toxicity, but L-carnitine supplementation has been proposed for patients with VPA toxicity and hyperammonemia on the basis of observations that chronic VPA therapy has been associated with carnitine deficiency. However, there is no evidence that L-carnitine alters clinical outcome.

Herbal Medicines/ Nutritional Supplements

Herbal and nutritional products are categorized as dietary supplements and can be marketed without testing for safety or efficacy. Although some herbs and supplements may have inherent toxicity, poisoning may result from product misuse, contamination of the product, or through interaction with other medications.[70,71] Patients and their families should always be questioned regarding use of nutritional supplements, herbal preparations, or natural remedies when considering possible toxin exposure as an etiology of clinical abnormalities. Adverse effects resulting from these products should be reported to the U.S. Food and Drug Administration. Table 69-8 contains a partial list of toxicities that may result in or complicate critical illness.

Management is usually supportive. A digoxin level should be obtained in any patient demonstrating digoxin toxic symptoms. The level may not correlate with clinical findings because numerous cardiac glycosides will not cross-react in the digoxin immunoassay. With significant toxicity, digoxin-specific antibodies should be administered.

Toxicity from ingestion of herbal preparations and nutritional supplements may result from product contaminants. Products may contain heavy metals, unlisted drugs, or other ingredients. The California Department of Health Services, Food and Drug Branch, screened 260 Asian patent medicine products and found 32% contained undeclared pharmaceuticals or heavy metals.[72] Unusual symptoms or toxidromes in patients ingesting such products may require the assistance of the local health department or toxicologist to identify a possible toxin. Additional information about specific agents can be found at www.herbmed.org or www.mskcc.org/aboutherbs.

Table 69-8. Toxicities of Selected Herbal and Alternative Agents

Aconite	Bradycardia, ventricular tachycardia and fibrillation, hypersalivation, GI disturbances, muscle weakness
Cardiac glycosides (digoxin-like factors)	Arrhythmias, GI disturbances, visual disturbances
Ephedrine (ma huang)	Sympathomimetic syndrome, intracranial hemorrhage, seizures, arrhythmias, myocardial infarction, stroke, hepatic failure, death
Ephedrine-free supplements (Synephrine, octopamine)	Myocardial ischemia, syncope, stroke
Ginkgo	Bleeding (cerebral or extracerebral)
Ginseng	Hypoglycemia, potential bleeding
Garlic	Bleeding
Kava kava	Hepatic failure, potentiation of anesthetics

KEY POINTS

- Evaluating and managing the poisoned patient involves resuscitation and stabilization, diagnosis, GI decontamination and toxin elimination, institution of specific antidotes or interventions, and supportive care.
- Pharmacokinetic and dynamic principles aid in assessing the likelihood of toxicity, the onset and duration of effect, and the effectiveness of therapeutic modalities designed to enhance elimination of the drug or toxin.
- In the poisoned patient with altered mental status, hypertonic dextrose, thiamine, and naloxone should be considered for administration.
- Patterns of signs and symptoms identified by physical examination may often suggest a toxidrome that is associated with classes of toxins.
- Single-dose activated charcoal is currently the most common technique used for gastrointestinal decontamination.
- Recognition of potential acetaminophen toxicity is essential for appropriate treatment and prevention of morbidity.
- Findings of bradycardia and hypotension should suggest possible ingestion of a β-blocker or calcium channel blocker.
- Cyclic antidepressant toxicity with increased QRS duration or wide complex tachyarrhythmia requires immediate alkalinization of the blood with sodium bicarbonate or hyperventilation.
- The decision to initiate hemodialysis for lithium toxicity should take into account the lithium level, duration of exposure, and severity of clinical symptoms.
- Herbal medicines and nutritional supplements can result in significant toxicities including cardiac and cerebrovascular.

REFERENCES

1. Weisman RS, Smith C, Goldfrank LR: Toxicokinetics: Applying pharmacokinetic principles to the poisoned patient. In Hoffman RS, Goldfrank LR (eds): Critical Care Toxicology. New York, Churchill Livingstone, 1991.
2. Dawson AH, Whyte IM: Therapeutic drug monitoring in drug overdose. Br J Clin Pharmacol 1999;48:278.
3. Levy G: Gastrointestinal clearance of drugs with activated charcoal. N Engl J Med 1982;307:676.
4. Hoffman RS, Goldfrank LR: The poisoned patient with altered consciousness. JAMA 1995;274:562.
5. Goldfrank LR, Flomenbaum NE, Lewin NA, et al: Vital signs and toxic syndromes. In Goldfrank LR, Flomenbaum NE, Lewin NA, et al (eds): Goldfrank's Toxicologic Emergencies, ed 7. New York, McGraw-Hill, 2002.
6. Pond SM, Lewis-Driver DJ, Williams GM, et al: Gastric emptying in acute overdose: A prospective randomized controlled trial. Med J Aust 1995;163:345.
7. American Academy of Clinical Toxicology; European Association of Poisons Centres and Clinical Toxicologists: Position paper: Ipecac syrup. J Toxicol Clin Toxicol 2004;42:133.
•8. American Academy of Clinical Toxicology; European Association of Poisons Centres and Clinical Toxicologists: Position paper: Gastric lavage. J Toxicol Clin Toxicol 2004;42:933.
9. American Academy of Clinical Toxicology and European Association of Poisons Centres and Clinical Toxicologists: Position paper: Single-dose activated charcoal. Clin Toxicol 2005;43:61.
10. Cooper GM, Le Couteur DG, Richardson D, Buckely NA: A randomized clinical trial of activated charcoal for the routine management of oral drug overdose. QJM 2005;98:655.
11. American Academy of Clinical Toxicology; European Association of Poisons Centres and Clinical Toxicologists: Position paper: Cathartics. J Toxicol Clin Toxicol 2004;42:243.
12. American Academy of Clinical Toxicology; European Association of Poisons Centres and Clinical Toxicologists: Position paper: Whole bowel irrigation. J Toxicol Clin Toxicol 2004;42:843.
13. American Academy of Clinical Toxicology; European Association of Poison Centres and Clinical Toxicologists: Position Statement and practice guidelines on the use of multi-dose activated charcoal in the treatment of acute poisoning. J Toxicol Clin Toxicol 1999;37:731.
14. Smilkstein MJ, Bronstein AC, Linden C, et al: Acetaminophen overdose: A 48-hour intravenous N-acetylcysteine treatment protocol. Ann Emerg Med 1991;20:1058.
15. Prescott L: Oral or intravenous N-acetylcysteine for acetaminophen poisoning? Ann Emerg Med 2005;45:409.
16. Brok J, Buckley N, Gluud C: Interventions for paracetamol (acetaminophen) overdose. Cochrane Database Syst Rev 2006;Issue 2;CD003328.
17. Daly FFS, O'Malley GF, Heard K, et al: Prospective evaluation of repeated suprtherapeutic acetaminophen (paracetamol) ingestion. Ann Emerg Med 2004;44:393.
18. Barceloux DG, Krenzelok EP, Olson K, Watson W: American Academy of Clinical Toxicology practice guidelines on the treatment of ethylene glycol poisoning. J Toxicol Clin Toxicol 1999;37:537.
19. Barceloux DG, Bong GR, Krenzelok EP, et al: American Academy of Clinical Toxicology practice guidelines on the treatment of methanol poisoning. J Toxicol Clin Toxicol 2002;40:415.
20. Lineberry TW, Bostwick JM: Methamphetamine abuse: a perfect storm of complications, Mayo Clin Proc 2006;81:77.
21. de la Torre R, Farré M, Roset PN, et al: Human pharmacology of MDMA, pharmacokinetics, metabolism, and disposition. Ther Drug Monit 2004;26:137.
22. Isbister GK, O'Regan G, Sibbritt D, Whyte IM: Alprazolam is relatively more toxic than other benzodiazepines in overdose. Br J Clin Pharmacol 2004;58:88.
23. Seger DL: Flumazenil-treatment or toxin. J Toxicol Clin Toxicol 2004;42:209-216.
24. Reith DM, Dawson AH, Epid D, et al: Relative toxicity of beta blockers in overdose. J Toxicol Clin Toxicol 1996;34:273.
25. Love JN, Litovitz TL, Howell JM, Clancy C: Characterization of fatal beta blocker ingestion: A review of the American Association of Poison Control Centers Data from 1985 to 1995. J Toxicol Clin Toxicol 1997;35:353.
26. White CM: A review of potential cardiovascular uses of intravenous glucagon administration. J Clin Pharmacol 1999;39:442.27.
27. Love JN, Leasure JA, Mundt DJ, et al: A comparison of amrinone and glucagon therapy for cardiovascular depression associated with propranolol toxicity in a canine model. J Toxicol Clin Toxicol 1992;30:399.
28. Kerns W, Schoroeder D, Williams C, et al: Insulin improves survival in a canine model of acute beta-blocker toxicity. Ann Emerg Med 1997;29:748.
29. Ramoska EA, Spiller HA, Myers A: Calcium channel blocker toxicity. Ann Emerg Med 1990;19:649.
30. Mahr NC, Valdes A, Lamas G: Use of glucagon for acute intravenous diltiazem toxicity. Am J Cardiol 1997;79:1570.
31. Shepherd G, Klein-Schwartz W: High-dose insulin therapy for calcium-channel

blocker overdose. Ann Pharmacother 2005;39:923.
32. Domachevsky L, Adir Y, Grupper M, Keynan Y: Hyperbaric oxygen in the treatment of carbon monoxide poisoning. Clin Toxicol 2005;43:181.
33. Juurlink DN, Buckley NA, Stanbrook MB, et al: Hyperbaric oxygen for carbon monoxide poisoning. Cochrane Database Syst Rev 2005;(1): CD002041.
34. Weaver LK, Hopkins RO, Chan KJ, et al: Hyperbaric oxygen for acute carbon monoxide poisoning. N Engl J Med 2002;347:1057.
35. Shanti CM, Lucas CE: Cocaine and the critical care challenge. Crit Care Med 2003;31:1851.
36. Baumann BM, Perrone J, Hornig SE, et al: Randomized, double-blind, placebo-controlled trial of diazepam, nitroglycerin, or both for treatment of patients with potential cocaine-associated acute coronary syndromes. Acad Emerg Med 2000;7:878-885.
37. Honderick T, Williams D, Seaberg D, Wears R: A prospective, randomized, controlled trial of benzodiazepines and nitroglycerine or nitroglycerine alone in the treatment of cocaine-associated acute coronary syndromes. Am J Emerg Med 2003;21:39-42.
38. Hollander JE: The management of cocaine-associated myocardial ischemia. N Engl J Med 1995;333: 1267.
39. Hollander JE, Burstein JL, Hoffman RS, et al: Cocaine-associated myocardial infarction. Clinical safety of thrombolytic therapy. Chest 1995;107:1237-1241.
40. Nolte KB, Brass LM, Fletterick CF: Intracranial hemorrhage associated with cocaine-abuse: A prospective autopsy study. Neurology 1996;46:1291.
41. Fessler RD, Esshaki CM, Stankewitz RC, et al: The neurovascular complications of cocaine. Surg Neurol 1997;47:339-345.
42. Traub SJ, Hoffman RS, Nelson LS: Body packing—the internal concealment of illicit drugs. N Engl J Med 2003;349:2519.
43. Hall AH, Rumack BH: Clinical toxicology cyanide. Ann Emerg Med 1986;15:1067.
44. Callaham M, Kassel D: Epidemiology of fatal tricyclic antidepressant ingestion: Implications for management. Ann Emerg Med 1985;14:1.
45. Boehnert M, Lovejoy FH Jr: Value of the QRS duration versus the serum drug level in predicting seizures and ventricular arrhythmias after an acute overdose of tricyclic antidepressants. N Engl J Med 1985;313:474.
46. Liebelt EL, Francis PD, Woolf AD: ECG lead AVR versus QRS interval in predicting seizures and arrhythmias in acute tricyclic antidepressant toxicity. Ann Emerg Med 1995;26:195.
47. Bailey B, Buckley NA, Amre DK: A meta-analysis of prognostic indicators to predict seizures, arrhythmias, or death after tricyclic antidepressant overdose. J Toxicol Clin Toxicol 2004;42:877.
48. Liebelt EL: Targeted management strategies for cardiovascular toxicity from tricyclic antidepressant overdose. The pivotal role for alkalinization and sodium loading. Pediatr Emerg Care 1998;14:293.
49. Pentel PR, Benowitz NL: Tricyclic antidepressant poisoning—management of arrhythmias. Med Toxicol 1986;1:101.
50. McCabe JL, Cobaugh DJ, Menegazzi JJ, et al: Experimental tricyclic antidepressant toxicity: A randomized, controlled comparison of hypertonic saline solution, sodium bicarbonate, and hyperventilation. Ann Emerg Med 1998;32:329.
51. McKinney PE, Rasmussen R: Reversal of severe tricyclic antidepressant-induced cardiotoxicity with intravenous hypertonic saline solution. Ann Emerg Med 2003;42:20.
52. Tran TP, Panacek EA, Rhee KJ, et al: Response to dopamine vs norepinephrine in tricyclic antidepressant-induced hypotension. Acad Emerg Med 1997;4:864.
53. Taboulet P, Baud FJ. Bismuth C, et al: Acute digitalis intoxication: Is pacing still appropriate? J Toxicol Clin Toxicol 1993;31:261.
54. Ujhelyi MR, Robert S: Pharmacokinetic aspects of digoxin-specific Fab therapy in the management of digitalis toxicity. Clin Pharmacokinet 1995;28:483.
55. Zvosec DL, Smith SW, McCutcheon JR, et al: Adverse events, including death, associated with the use of 1,4-butanediol. N Engl J Med 2001;344:87.
56. Snead OC, Gibson KM: Gamma-hydroxybutyric acid. N Engl J Med 2005;352:2721.
57. Dyer JE, Roth B, Hyma BA: Gamma-hydroxybutyrate withdrawal syndrome. Ann Emerg Med 2001;37:147.
58. Scharman EJ: Methods used to decrease lithium absorption or enhance elimination. J Toxicol Clin Toxicol 1997;35:601.
59. LeBlanc M, Raymond M, Bonnardeaux A, et al: Lithium poisoning treated by high performance continuous arteriovenous and venovenous hemodiafiltration. Am J Kidney Dis 1996;27:365.
60. Kaplan JL, Marx JA, Calabro JJ, et al: Double-blind, randomized study of nalmefene and naloxone in emergency department patients with suspected narcotic overdose. Ann Emerg Med 1999;34:42.
61. Sporer KA, Dorn E: Heroin-related noncardiogenic pulmonary edema. Chest 2001;120:1628.
62. Peter JV, Cherian AM: Organic insecticides. Anaes Intens Care 2000;28:11.
63. Leikin JB, Thomas RG, Walter FG, et al: A review of nerve agent exposure for the critical care physician. Crit Care Med 2002;30:2346.
64. Buckley NA, Eddleston M, Szinicz L: Oximes for organophosphate pesticide poisoning. Cochrane Database of Systematic Reviews 2005;Issue 1;CD005085.
65. Eddleston M, Szinicz L, Eyer P, Buckley N: Oximes in acute organophosphorous pesticide poisoning: A systematic review of clinical trials. Q J Med 2002;95:275.
66. Abou-Donia MB, Lapadula DM: Mechanisms of organophosphorus ester-induced delayed neurotoxicity: Type I and type II. Annu Rev Pharmacol Toxicol 1990;30:405.
67. Senanayake N, Karalliede L: Neurotoxic effects of organophosphorus insecticides: An intermediate syndrome. N Engl J Med 1987;316:761.
68. Boyer EW, Shannon M: The serotonin syndrome. N Engl J Med 2005;352:1112.
69. Sztajnkrycer MD: Valproic acid toxicity: Overview and management. J Toxicol Clin Toxicol 2002;40:789.
70. De Smet PAGM: Herbal remedies. N Engl J Med 2002;347:2046.
71. Ang-Lee MK, Moss J, Yuan C-S: Herbal medicines and perioperative care. JAMA 2001;286:208.
72. Ko RJ: Adulterants in Asian patent medicines (letter). N Engl J Med 1998;339:847.

Chapter 70

Hypothermia, Hyperthermia, and Rhabdomyolysis

Sanjay Subramanian, J. Christopher Farmer, and Christopher McFadden

Severe hypothermia and hyperthermia are major causes of morbidity and mortality in critically ill patients, both as primary disorders and as comorbid manifestations of other clinical conditions. For example, in some centers, major trauma victims who also present with significant hypothermia suffer increased mortality compared with patients matched for diagnosis and severity of illness indices.[1] Similarly, cocaine intoxication is rapidly becoming the leading cause of heatstroke in urban centers and is a major factor in the development of other significant organ system complications.[2]

Prompt recognition of these disorders is particularly important because outcome is adversely affected by any delays in institution of therapy. Central neuronal damage increases exponentially as time required for cooling a heatstroke victim passes. By contrast, efforts to resuscitate a severely hypothermic patient may be prematurely halted if the core body temperature is not accurately measured (many glass and digital thermometers do not measure below 35° C). In fact, elderly patients may be misdiagnosed (e.g., presumed intra-abdominal sepsis) unless a clinical suspicion for hypothermia is maintained.

HYPOTHERMIA

HISTORY AND INCIDENCE

Hypothermia has a long, well-established relationship with the military. Numerous testimonies predating the birth of Christ relate the effects of hypothermia on various military campaigns. In the early 1800s, Napoleon's chief surgeon noted that hypothermia victims placed farthest from the fire were the most likely patients to die. More recently, the Germans during World War II recognized the absolute lethality of immersion hypothermia to U-boat crews patrolling the North Atlantic Ocean. Tragically, preventive research was carried out using people interred in German concentration camps.

During the period 1999 to 2002, a total of 4607 death certificates in the United States had hypothermia-related diagnoses listed as the underlying cause of death (annual incidence: 4 per 1 million population).[3] A majority of cases occur in urban areas and are especially concentrated among elderly patients, alcoholics, and others with chronic debilitating diseases.[3,4] For patients older than 65 years of age, the Centers for Disease Control and Prevention (CDC) has reported higher mortality rates among racial minorities in the United States, an observation that underscores the impact of socioeconomic status on exposure risk and access to health care in these urban populations.[5] These CDC figures, however, almost certainly underestimate the true incidence of accidental hypothermia, owing to the failure to recognize the diagnosis and the subsequent attribution of death to other causes, particularly in patients without obvious environmental exposure histories.

PATHOGENESIS

Accidental hypothermia is defined as an unintentional fall in core body temperature to less than 35° C. Hypothermia generally develops because of (1) altered central thermoregulation, (2) an inability to produce sufficient metabolic heat to maintain core temperature, or (3) unalterably increased heat losses.

Hypothermia results when the amount of body heat dissipated exceeds the heat produced by normal and compensatory metabolic activities. At rest, most heat is generated by energy-consuming processes within the viscera. However, periods of exercise shift heat-generating activity to the skeletal muscle. Shivering is the most effective involuntary heat-generating activity in normal people. Elderly, alcoholic, and chronically ill patients have impaired heat-generating capacity owing to reduced lean body mass, impaired mobility, inadequate diet, and reduced shivering in response to cold.[6] When this diminished heat-generating capacity is coupled with impaired central thermoregulation, hypothermia develops quickly. The impact of these physiologic observations is highlighted by a study from Britain in the early 1970s that found a 12% incidence of clinically inapparent hypothermia during routine epidemiologic screening of the elderly.[7]

Numerous conditions and disorders are associated with altered central thermoregulation. These include drug–induced alteration in central dopaminergic tone (e.g., from phenothiazines, barbiturates, lithium, or α-blockers), central nervous system (CNS) disease states (e.g., Parkinson's disease, stroke, multiple sclerosis), and diseases that impair central thermoregulation (e.g., alcoholism, advanced age, diabetes mellitus, uremia, hypothyroidism, hypopituitarism, hypoadrenalism). Under these circumstances, hypothermia develops because the affected person's perception of ambient temperature is altered; the patient does not dress warmly, seek relief from a cold environment, or adjust home heating accordingly.[7] In the absence of exposure to climatic extremes, hypothermia develops subacutely. Yet another very important precipitating factor is sepsis. Hypothermia in septic patients carries a worse prognosis. The pathomechanism of sepsis-induced hypothermia is unclear and may be related to cytokine-induced hypothalamic dysregulation of temperature.

Operative patients also are at risk for the development of hypothermia. When the air-to-skin temperature gradient exceeds 4° C, substantial radiant thermal loss rapidly follows.[8] In addition, the concurrent use of anesthesia blunts most normal physiologic responses to cold stress. Postoperative hypothermia is a common occurrence and can become clinically significant if unrecognized. These effects become magnified in patients requiring aggressive volume resuscitation, such as trauma victims. In a patient admitted to a medical ICU with massive gastrointestinal hemorrhage, for example, the required aggressive volume resuscitation and blood product administration commonly overwhelm blunted heat generation mechanisms if these fluids are not appropriately warmed. For this purpose, the Level 1 Fluid Warmer (Level 1 Technologies, Inc., Rockland, Mass.) is considered the gold standard device of its kind. The fluid warmer is an effective heat exchanger, allows rapid fluid administration, and has a reliable filtering system (mandatory requirements of any warming system). Fluid warmers must be used in all patients requiring massive volume and blood product resuscitation, to prevent serious complications due to hypothermia.

The development of exposure-related hypothermia is more straightforward. Glycogen depletion and physical exhaustion are common co-variables. Although these patients are generally healthy and have thermoregulatory mechanisms, ongoing cold exposure, metabolic depletion, and fatigue lead to hypothermia.[9,10]

Box 70-1 lists disorders and conditions associated with hypothermia.

CLINICAL MANIFESTATIONS

Core temperature is best ascertained using a full-range rectal probe thermometer, because glass thermometers frequently do not register or become inaccurate below 35° C. Core temperatures measured using invasive hemodynamic monitors such as pulmonary artery catheters are accurate; however, use of these catheters generally should be avoided because they may precipitate arrhythmias in patients who have irritable myocardium.

Classification of Hypothermia

Clinical manifestations vary but predictably worsen with stepwise decrements in core body temperature For this reason, accidental hypothermia frequently is classified as mild (core body temperature 32° to 35° C), moderate (core body temperature 28° to 32° C), or severe (core body temperature less than 28° C). The progression of symptoms often is insidious, with nonspecific complaints such as nausea, dizziness, dyspnea, or chills. When it is not recognized, hypothermia may progress rapidly to produce more serious sequelae. The foregoing classification schema identifies the progressive syndromes of hypothermia, provides an aid to identify patients at risk for end-organ damage, and guides the tempo of corrective measures.

Mild hypothermia is defined clinically by a core temperature between 32° and 35° C. Affected patients usually are not seriously ill and present with hemodynamically stable vital signs. In fact, heart rate, blood pressure, and respiratory rate typically are increased with the metabolic

Box 70-1

Conditions and Diseases Associated with Hypothermia

- Chronic medical disorders
  - Heart failure
  - Renal failure
  - Chronic hepatic insufficiency
  - Alcoholism/Wernicke's encephalopathy
- Central nervous system abnormalities
  - Tumor/mass lesion
  - Stroke
  - Paraplegia
  - Parkinson's disease
  - Multiple sclerosis
  - Sarcoidosis
- Dermatologic disorders
  - Burns
  - Generalized cutaneous psoriasis/ichthyosis
  - Exfoliative dermatitis
- Endocrine/metabolic
  - Panhypopituitarism
  - Hypoadrenalism
  - Diabetes mellitus with neuropathy
  - Hypothyroidism
  - Physical/metabolic exhaustion (substrate depletion)
  - Anorexia nervosa/protein malnutrition
- Drugs
  - Ethanol
  - Phenothiazines
  - Tricyclic antidepressants
  - Barbiturates
  - Paralytic muscle relaxants
  - Lithium (in toxic doses)
  - Clonidine
  - Anticholinergic drugs (e.g., bethanechol, atropine)

demands of increased thermogenesis. Shivering, which can be mistaken for rigors, should be seen in this temperature range unless thermoregulation is impaired by an underlying defect. Mental status generally is intact but may be mildly to moderately impaired, ranging from lethargy to confusion within this temperature range. Finally, most laboratory screening variables remain within normal limits at this point. Clearly, these findings are nonspecific, and the true diagnosis may be easily missed unless an exposure history is obtained.

Moderate hypothermia (28° to 32° C) is more serious. Hypotension is common, as are arrhythmias such as atrial fibrillation, reentrant supraventricular tachycardias, and increased ventricular ectopy. Shivering is notably absent, and overall muscle tone is rigid. Affected patients often are obtunded or incoherent. Pupillary dilation generally is present below a core temperature of 30° C. Again, the diagnosis of hypothermia could be easily missed. For example, although these findings are consistent with hypothermia, drug intoxication also is a significant etiologic consideration (e.g., with tricyclic antidepressants). A careful clinical history and an increased index of suspicion are key to making the correct diagnosis.

In *severe hypothermia,* patients have a core temperature less than 26° to 28° C and may appear dead. Vital signs usually are not present, and demonstrable neurologic function is absent, including deep tendon, oculocephalic, and corneal reflexes. Ventricular fibrillation is present in more than 50% of patients. Laboratory abnormalities (discussed later) become more profound and may include hemoconcentration and findings indicative of rhabdomyolysis.

End-Organ Effects

Central Nervous System Effects

CNS electrical activity decreases as hypothermia progresses and the core temperature falls below 33° C. At mild levels of hypothermia, dysarthria, bradykinesia, confusion, and impaired judgment and memory can be seen. CNS vascular autoregulation is lost at temperatures below 25° C, with a concomitant decrease in cerebral blood flow. Owing to decreased cerebral metabolism, however, the ischemic threshold is higher than in normothermic persons. As the core body temperature falls below 32° C, patients often stop complaining of cold, and shivering stops. Muscular rigidity develops, and patients become frankly obtunded.[11] As mentioned, severe hypothermia may be associated with complete cessation of observable CNS function, including brainstem reflexes. An electrically silent electroencephalogram (EEG) is typical in most patients with core temperatures below 25° C. CNS metabolic activity is profoundly depressed below 25° C, and the probability of enduring cerebral hypoperfusion without sustaining ischemic brain injury increases dramatically.[12,13] "Brain death" in hypothermic patients, even after cardiac arrest, should not be diagnosed until a normal core temperature is restored and CNS function remains absent. Complete recovery has been reported in patients who present with core body temperatures below 25° C and in full cardiac arrest, many without CNS sequelae. Hypothermia also has an effect on the autonomic nervous system secondary to delay in neural conduction velocities, which may explain the profound orthostasis observed in these patients and the emphasis on avoiding head-up position during transport.

Cardiovascular Effects

With mild hypothermia there is an initial tachycardia and peripheral vasoconstriction, which progresses to atropine-refractory bradycardia and a consequent fall in cardiac output when the core temperature drops below 32° C. Systemic vascular resistance (SVR) may remain elevated on account of reflex vasoconstriction, hemoconcentration, and increased viscosity. Bradycardia and decreased cardiac output mirror an overall decline in metabolic rate and O_2 consumption. Conduction abnormalities, such as heart block, often are observed. In addition, cardiac contraction and stroke volume decrease as body temperature drops. At 28° C the cardiac output drops to less than 50% of baseline function and the heart rate falls to 30 to 40 beats per minute. Rates inconsistent with the temperature should prompt a search for coexistent hypoglycemia, hypovolemia, or drug ingestion.

Myocardial irritability also increases as the core temperature drops.[14] Ventricular fibrillation is more common below 27° C and may be precipitated by physical movement, instrumentation, acid base changes, or changes in P_{O_2} or P_{CO_2}. At temperatures less than 24° C there is a high risk of asystole. One study has suggested that asystole may be a primary manifestation of hypothermia, with fibrillation occurring during rewarming.[15]

Pulmonary Effects

Respiratory rate typically increases in patients with mild hypothermia, reflecting an overall state of increased metabolic activity. With worsening hypothermia, there is also depression of the ventilatory drive, and at temperatures below 34° C, sensitivity to P_{CO_2} stimulation is attenuated. Cold-induced bronchorrhea and bronchospasm have been described and, when combined with a blunted cough reflex, may produce significant atelectasis. Blunting of the cough reflex also increases the risk of aspiration of gastric contents in patients who present with severe hypothermia. Noncardiogenic pulmonary edema due solely to hypothermia has been controversially described.[16,17] In this setting, worsening hypoxemia, localized or diffuse infiltrates on the chest radiograph, and decreased pulmonary compliance without another apparent explanation generally signal the development of either pneumonia or the acute respiratory distress syndrome (ARDS). Finally, a leftward shift of the oxygen-hemoglobin dissociation curve occurs, resulting in impaired oxygen delivery.

Gastrointestinal and Hepatic Effects

Gastrointestinal hypomotility rapidly develops in patients with progressive hypothermia and typically is manifested as an ileus. Shallow gastrointestinal ulceration (Wischnevsky's ulcers), punctate hemorrhages, and erosions commonly are found in autopsy studies. Hepatic and pancreatic function also decreases as hypothermia worsens. Animal models have shown decreased insulin secretion and biochemical function below core temperatures of 30° C.[18] At this temperature range, hepatic clearance of drugs also is impaired. The liver also loses the capability to convert lactate to bicarbonate and glucose via gluconeogenesis (the Cori cycle). Therefore, lactated Ringer's solution should not be administered to severely hypothermic patients because it may worsen a pre-existing metabolic acidosis by further depressing cardiac function.[19] Pancreatitis has been reported in 20% to 30% of cases during autopsy, and hyperamylasemia is found in more than 50% of cases.[20]

Renal Effects

When core temperature declines, renal metabolic activity decreases, as do renal perfusion and glomerular filtration rate. Tubular reabsorption of water and solutes declines because of decreased cellular activity or resistance to antidiuretic hormone (ADH) effects. In patients with mild to moderate hypothermia, tubular dysfunction tends to predominate, and the kidneys excrete large amounts of hyposthenuric urine (the so-called cold diuresis). Diminished tubular secretion of hydrogen ions also results in acidosis. Thus, intravascular volume frequently is depleted by the time severe hypothermia occurs. Oliguria commonly is seen in severe hypothermia and may be due to prerenal factors (poor cardiac output, volume depletion) or acute tubular necrosis, with or without superimposed rhabdomyolysis. Clinically, acute renal failure is seen in approximately 40% of patients with accidental hypothermia.

Hematologic Effects

Hemoconcentration induced by plasma extravasation frequently is seen in patients with moderate to severe hypothermia, with the hematocrit increasing by approximately 2% for each one-degree decline in temperature. Bone marrow suppression resulting in thrombocytopenia, granulocytopenia, erythroid hypoplasia, and sideroblastic anemia have been described.[21,22] Thrombocytopenia may be further compounded by splenic sequestration. Qualitative platelet dysfunction also has been observed and is the result of a temperature-dependent decrease in platelet production of thromboxane B_2.[23] The bleeding tendency in hypothermic patients is further compounded by a coagulopathy due to cold inactivation of coagulation enzymes. Because the prothrombin time and other laboratory measures are performed at 37° C, laboratory evaluation may not reflect clinical bleeding tendency in this setting.[24,25] Elevated cryofibrinogen levels have been described in patients with hypothermia in the setting of *Escherichia coli* sepsis, diabetes, and malignancy. The use of heparin, which can polymerize cryofibrinogen, thereby causing severe hyperviscosity, may be considered a relative contraindication in this setting.

Disseminated intravascular coagulation (DIC) develops in some patients with severe hypothermia. Diagnostic criteria suggesting the need for therapeutic intervention are the same as in other patients: (1) coagulopathy, (2) hypofibrinogenemia, (3) thrombocytopenia, and (4) clinical bleeding. DIC may be difficult to distinguish from cold-induced coagulopathy and bleeding. Nevertheless, therapy is the same—warm the patient and provide blood product support as needed.

Laboratory Findings

Serum chemistries should be checked initially and repeated during resuscitation. There is no prototypical laboratory pattern for patients with hypothermia. Both hyper- and hypokalemia can be seen (hyperkalemia occurs in association with rhabdomyolysis). Hyperglycemia is common in some forms of acute, severe hypothermia, such as immersion, and probably is due to the initial catecholamine response. By contrast, patients in whom hypothermia develops subacutely often present with hypoglycemia (as a result of glycogen depletion and the stress of prolonged shivering and thermogenesis). Increased serum transaminases and azotemia often are observed in moderate and severe cases of hypothermia. Finally, hyperamylasemia may reflect underlying pancreatitis and has been reported to correlate with both severity of hypothermia and, ultimately, mortality.

Finally, much discussion has centered on the interpretation of arterial blood gas results.[26,27] To review, the oxyhemoglobin dissociation curve shifts leftward as body temperature falls. In addition, measured pH is falsely low and Pa_{O_2} and Pa_{CO_2} are falsely high unless arterial gas solubility coefficients are corrected for temperature. However, arterial blood gas machines are calibrated at 37° C (they also warm the blood specimen to 37° C before measurement), which yields higher O_2 and CO_2 levels and lower pH values than the real values for the patient's hypothermic state. In any case, the clinical impact of these inaccuracies probably is minimal in most patients.[28] The notable exception is in patients with a severe acidosis requiring acid-base or CO_2 manipulation. For these patients, the pH should be corrected for temperature to avoid overenthusiastic use of bicarbonate or hyperventilation, which may in fact increase the predisposition to ventricular fibrillation, especially during rewarming. Box 70-2 outlines the mathematics involved in temperature correction for determination of arterial blood gases.

Electrocardiographic Changes

Hypothermia produces a spectrum of abnormalities on the electrocardiogram (ECG) reflecting a variety of conduction abnormalities. The most distinctive is a repolarization abnormality called the Osborn J wave (Fig. 70-1), a notch and deflection at the QRS-ST junction previously considered pathognomonic for hypothermia. This may, however, also be seen in other conditions such as subarachnoid hemorrhage and myocardial ischemia. Although the Osborn wave may be present in up to 80% of cases, an increasing number of reports, including a recent summary of eight normothermic patients with the finding, cast doubt on the assertion that it is pathognomonic for hypothermia.[29] Other ECG changes seen in severely hypothermic patients include T wave inversion; progressive prolongation of the PR, QRS, and QT intervals; bradycardia (a late finding); and the ventricular and supraventricular ectopic rhythms mentioned earlier.[30] Spontaneous ventricular fibrillation is the most common nonperfusing cardiac rhythm; asystole is much less common.

Box 70-2

Temperature Correction Factors for Arterial Blood Gas (ABG) Specimens*

ABG Component Correction Factor

$pH + 0.015\,(37 - T_c)$

$Pa_{O_2} - 0.072\,(37 - T_c) \times Pa_{O_2}$

$Pa_{CO_2} - 0.044\,(37 - T_c) \times Pa_{CO_2}$

Example

A patient presents with a core temperature of 32° C with the following ABG values: pH=7.12, Pa_{CO_2}= 52 mm Hg, and Pa_{O_2}=52 mm Hg. Corrections for temperature are as follows:

$pH = 7.12 + [0.015\,(37 - 32)] = 7.195$

$Pa_{O_2} = 52 - [0.072\,(37 - 32) \times 52] = 33.28$ mm Hg

$Pa_{CO_2} = 52 - [0.044\,(37 - 32) \times 52] = 40.56$ mm Hg

These corrections also may be used for hyperthermia.

*ABG values not corrected for temperature in significantly hypothermic patients yield falsely low pH and falsely elevated Pa_{CO_2} and Pa_{O_2} values.
T_c, core temperature.

APPROACH TO MANAGEMENT

Restoration of normal body temperature is the crux of therapy for hypothermia. Therapeutic options for warming are numerous, with increasingly invasive methods employed in more severe cases. All therapies should be aggressively continued until the patient is completely rewarmed. Attempts to identify nonsurvivors before return of core temperature to at least 33° to 34° C are unreliable. In addition, the diverse complications discussed earlier must be concurrently sought out and addressed.

Supportive Measures Including Pharmacologic Adjuncts

All therapeutic efforts in critically ill patients begin with the establishment and maintenance of airway, breathing, and circulation—the ABCs. Airway-protective reflexes commonly are absent or impaired in patients with moderate to severe hypothermia. In this situation, endotracheal intubation will provide a secure airway and, in cold environs, a means to limit continued heat loss through the respiratory system. Oxygenation is rarely a problem unless acute lung injury or significant pneumonia develops. Minute ventilation demands in a hypothermic patient can be quite dynamic while temperature rises, metabolic processes accelerate, and perfusion is re-established. In one study, CO_2 production in nonparalyzed postoperative cardiac patients increased by as much as 65% as their core temperatures returned to normal.[31] Support of circulation begins with an accurate assessment of intravascular volume status, and this should be considered the highest priority after rewarming efforts are begun. All subsequent resuscitation variables will be directly affected by this assessment.

Intravascular volume status determination in patients with significant hypothermia can be problematic. "Cold diuresis" typically leads to significant volume depletion.

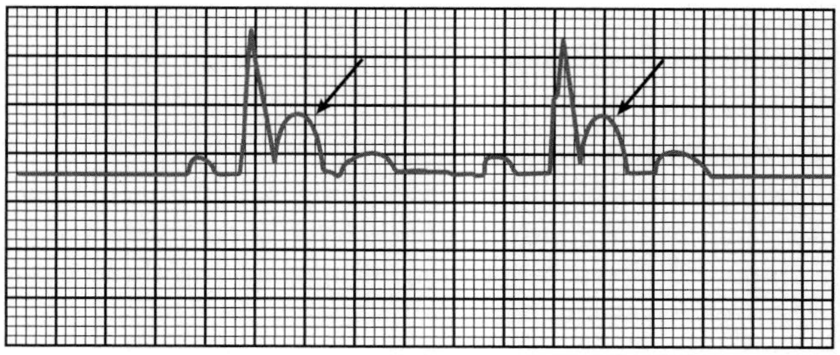

Figure 70-1. Portion of an electrocardiographic tracing from a patient with hypothermia showing the Osborn J wave *(arrows)*.

In addition, cardiac contractile function often is depressed in patients because of the direct effects of severe hypothermia. This can be further exacerbated in patients with significant pre-existing cardiac disease. Finally, clinical evidence of vasoconstriction and extremity hypoperfusion is not discriminatory. Of note, placing a pulmonary artery catheter to sort out these confounding variables may incite ventricular ectopy, or worse. Therefore, judicious administration of intravenous fluids to expand intravascular volume should be initiated in hemodynamically unstable patients. The clinical response (or lack thereof) provides the bedside intensivist with important diagnostic clues about a patient's actual volume status. Insertion of a pulmonary artery catheter should be reserved for those few patients in whom a reasonable estimate of intravascular volume status after volume loading cannot be made, or when severe, pre-existing cardiac dysfunction is strongly suspected in the face of hemodynamic instability.

Intravascular volume expansion always begins with warmed fluids (36° to 40° C). Because hypothermic patients typically have some degree of increased vascular tone, vasopressors should be employed only when further volume expansion appears deleterious. Use of inotropes may be considered in situations in which significant impairment of ventricular performance is likely. In the setting of severe hypothermia, markedly reduced intracellular metabolism renders advanced cardiac life support (ACLS) pharmacologic interventions ineffective until the core temperature exceeds 28° to 30° C.[32] Furthermore, the heart generally cannot sustain rhythmic electrical function until this same temperature threshold is surpassed. Basic cardiopulmonary resuscitation should therefore be continued until these temperature thresholds are met, and then ACLS protocols should be initiated. Prima facie evidence of efficacy for any antiarrhythmic drug in these patients is lacking. Currently, the drug of choice for the augmentation of electrical defibrillation is bretylium tosylate, in contrast with the usual first-line approach with lidocaine hydrochloride.[33] Epinephrine and vasopressin have improved coronary perfusion in hypothermic animal studies and may have a role. Magnesium sulfate also has been used successfully. Procainamide may increase the incidence of ventriccular fibrillation. The successful use of amiodarone to control ventricular fibrillation in a normothermic patient with prominent Osborn waves raises the question of its future application in refractory fibrillation in hypothermia.[34] External transthoracic and transvenous temporary pacemaker devices have, at best, limited demonstrable efficacy.

Rewarming

The optimal technique for rewarming is controversial, and no randomized controlled trials have been conducted to compare different rewarming strategies. The three basic types of rewarming are

- Passive external rewarming
- Active external rewarming
- Active core rewarming

Passive external warming techniques are appropriate for mild hypothermia. These include minimizing heat loss by warming the room, removing wet clothing, and wrapping an insulating layer around the patient (e.g., a blanket). In a mildly hypothermic patient, rewarming is accomplished by augmenting heat generation above that of the basal metabolic rate. These mechanisms (predominantly shivering) may increase and allow the body's own normal heat-generating mechanisms to restore the core temperature. The rewarming rates vary, ranging from 0.5° to 2.0° C per hour.

Active external rewarming techniques should be considered in hypothermic patients who present with the following:

1. A core temperature less than 32° C
2. Hemodynamic instability
3. Known pre-existing medical conditions that alter thermoregulation/thermogenesis (e.g., myxedema, physical exhaustion with metabolic depletion)
4. Failure to respond to passive rewarming techniques

Active external rewarming techniques range from hot water bottles or chemical packs (heat production capability less than 45° C) to heating blankets to submersion tanks in the emergency department. These all are potentially useful and can greatly speed patient rewarming. Currently, forced air warming devices seem to be the most efficacious method of active external rewarming; the rate of temperature rise is approximately 2.5° C.[35,36] Active external rewarming, however, carries some risks that should be considered before implementation. Many therapies, such as immersion, make timely medical intervention difficult or impossible if complications develop. Additionally, indiscriminant application of external heat sources can sometimes cause severe local burns to vasoconstricted dermis. An additional potential risk of external rewarming in severely hypothermic patients is hemodynamic instability, which may be associated with a phenomenon called core temperature afterdrop.

Afterdrop refers to an initial paradoxical drop in the core temperature associated with external rewarming. As a patient begins to warm and vasodilate, cold acidotic blood is returned from the extremities or periphery to the core. One commonly quoted study noted that patients with mild hypothermia who underwent external rewarming experienced a drop in mean arterial pressure and SVR.[37] The clinical relevance of this phenomenon has more recently been questioned, however, as reports of active external rewarming from severe hypothermia without observed afterdrop become more common. Generally, core temperature afterdrop should be avoided if possible. Most authors agree that in patients with stable, moderate hypothermia, active external rewarming is best applied conservatively and in combination with an active core rewarming technique, such as infusion of heated intravenous fluids.

Active core rewarming usually is used for rewarming severely hypothermic patients. The techniques have included the use of warmed intravenous fluids; heated, humidified gases administered through the ventilator circuit; gastric, rectal, peritoneal, pleural, or mediastinal lavage; hemodialysis; and arteriovenous, venovenous, and cardiac bypass.

As mentioned, intubation and ventilation with warmed (40° to 44° C), humidified air can be an important adjunct to initial management in exposure cases, but the contribution of this approach to active warming in a controlled environment has recently been called into question. The relative contribution of heat convection from heated air versus warm room air to raising core body temperature has been found to be less significant than initial reports had promised. As a general rule, rewarming techniques that rely on conduction more efficiently transfer bio-heat and raise the core body temperature more quickly than do convection-based methods.

The traditional techniques of rectal and gastric lavage are limited in efficacy owing to the small surface areas involved, the risk of perforated viscus, the risk of gastric aspiration, and possible colonic absorption of excess free water. By contrast, warmed peritoneal or pleural lavage also may be employed. Although bleeding complications, perforations, and organ injury have been reported, these methods can rapidly raise core temperatures at rates of 2° to 4° C per hour. Peritoneal lavage is instituted through a peritoneal dialysis catheter using heated dialysate at 40° C and offers the additional advantage of controlling serum potassium levels. Thoracic lavage involves placement of anterior and posterior chest tubes and infusion of heated saline through the anterior tube with gravity-dependent drainage through the posterior tube. All of these methods are contraindicated in the setting of abdominal or thoracic trauma or recent surgical procedures.

The preferred method of rewarming patients with life-threatening hypothermia is extracorporeal warming of blood cycled through a heated arteriovenous or a venovenous hemofiltration circuit. Numerous studies have demonstrated feasibility, and even reduced morbidity and mortality, in specific settings with these systems.[38,39] In this regard, continuous venovenous hemofiltration (CVVH) offers the advantages of more consistent flow rates, generally less complicated vascular access, and the ability to rapidly correct intravascular volume deficits. These methods have been feasible even in juvenile animal models, suggesting utility in the pediatric population.[40] The possible requirement of systemic heparinization, however, may limit the use of CVVH to non-trauma patients.

In patients without a perfusing cardiac rhythm, cardiopulmonary bypass remains the standard of care for rewarming and restoring blood flow. Core temperatures can be rapidly increased by up to 9° C per hour using this method.[41-43] Cardiopulmonary bypass has been used with success in patients with deep hypothermia, resulting in survival with minimal cerebral impairment.[44] Theoretical advantages of this technique include (1) a higher degree of CNS and organ system perfusion, (2) prevention of shock from peripheral vasodilation by earlier core rewarming, and (3) rapid correction of hypothermia-associated metabolic abnormalities. Furthermore, the reported successful use of a heparin-coated bypass apparatus makes this modality potentially useful in trauma situations, in which anticoagulation would further exacerbate coagulopathy.[45] Unfortunately, the technique is clearly not available at all facilities. If bypass is not available, venovenous rewarming offers an alternative that may be employed with minimal disruption of life support measures.

Additional therapeutic interventions should be considered in patients with known endocrine disorders. Intravenous levothyroxine may be necessary in patients with hypothyroidism and suspected myxedema. Similarly, intravenous hydrocortisone may be required for patients with known or suspected adrenal insufficiency.

Pneumonia is a common complication of severe hypothermia; however, empiric antibiotics do not lessen the incidence or severity of the disease. Deep vein thrombosis also is a common complication of severe hypothermia; appropriate prophylaxis should always be considered and instituted, as in other critically ill, at-risk patients. Finally, the presence of occult traumatic injuries should be aggressively sought in all patients with hypothermia.

HYPERTHERMIA

HISTORY AND INCIDENCE

Innumerable military campaigns throughout history were lost as a result of heat illness, long before the enemy ever raised a weapon. In modern times, the Israeli Six-Day War during the late 1960s provides the best example of the ravages of heat illness. The Israeli army had forced water consumption policies, by the clock, including strict disciplinary measures for evidence of heat injury due to negligence. By contrast, the Egyptian army did not have well-enforced policies. In the end, while the Israeli army's heat injury statistics were negligible, more than 50% of the Egyptian soldiers in the same locale suffered from heat illnesses that rendered them unable to effectively perform their expected tasks.

Heatstroke and hypothermia have been identified as the environmental diseases least frequently monitored by epidemiology systems in the United States. Serious heat illness has received considerable recent attention owing to catastrophic heat waves in the United States and Europe, the deaths of high-profile athletes, and military deployments. A recent study documented heat illness hospitalizations and deaths for the U.S. Army from 1980 through 2002. In this study, 5246 were hospitalized, and 37 died from heat illness.[46]

The exact incidence of heatstroke in the United States is unknown. The CDC reported that between the years 1987 and 1988, 1092 death certificates listed excessive heat as either a primary or a secondary cause.[47] It is suspected that a number of other heat-related severe illnesses and deaths occur each year that are attributed to other causes. Guidelines from the National Association of Medical Examiners suggest that in cases in which the measured antemortem body temperature at the time of collapse was 105° F (40.6° degrees C) or higher, the cause of death should be certified as heatstroke or hyperthermia. Deaths also may be certified as heatstroke or hyperthermia with lower body temperatures when cooling has been attempted before arrival at the hospital or when the clinical history includes mental status changes and elevated liver and muscle enzymes.[48]

PATHOGENESIS

Heatstroke is a complex syndrome of end-organ dysfunction initiated by hyperthermia that occurs when heat accumulation in the body overwhelms heat-dissipating mechanisms. The diagnosis should be considered in patients with core body temperatures greater than 41° C, or in patients with a core temperature of 40.6° C and concomitant mental status changes. Because anhidrosis is a late finding and sweating may be observed in severely hyperthermic patients, diaphoresis should not be considered a discriminatory finding. Heatstroke traditionally is subdivided into exertional and nonexertional causes. Box 70-3 outlines examples of disease and conditions within each of these categories. To understand the pathogenesis of heatstroke, the systemic and cellular responses to heat stress must be appreciated. These responses include thermoregulation (with acclimatization), an acute-phase response, and a response that involves the production of heat shock proteins.

Thermoregulation

At basal metabolic levels, less than 100 kcal of metabolic heat is generated per hour. However, when physical activity increases, heat production may rise as high as 900 kcal per hour. This level of heat production is capable of raising the core body temperature by 1° C every 5 to 8 minutes. Heat is dissipated via evaporation, conduction or radiation, and convectional losses. Cutaneous vasodilation results in heat loss through all of these physical mechanisms except evaporation. Unfortunately, when the ambient temperature exceeds body temperature, only evaporative losses associated with perspiration actually dissipate heat. Perspiration can produce a maximum rate of heat loss of approximately 400 to 650 kcal per hour in acclimatized persons. When heat production exceeds this threshold, body temperature quickly begins to rise.

Acclimatization

Acclimatization is a physiologic term that collectively describes various adaptive responses to repeated heat stress. Many of these responses are directed at conserving plasma volume. They include decreased total sweat sodium concentration and nonreflexively increased aldosterone secretion. In addition, acclimatized people tend to drink greater volumes of water and have measurable increases in extracellular fluid volume beyond that of nonacclimatized persons. Ultimately, maximum cardiac output and stroke volume increase, while maximum heart rate and O_2 consumption decrease (improved efficiency per unit of metabolic work expended).[49] Similarly, the net amount of heat generated per unit of work expended also decreases.

Acute-Phase Response

The acute-phase response, involving endothelial cells, leukocytes, and epithelial cells, protects body tissues from heat-induced tissue injury. A variety of immunomodulatory and inflammatory cytokines are released in response to increased endogenous or environmental heat, including interleukin-6 (IL-6), tumor necrosis factor-α (TNF-α), IL-10, IL-12, and interferon.

Heat Shock Response

Cells respond to heat by production of inducible heat shock proteins that help induce a state of tolerance to heat stress. These proteins function as molecular chaperones that bind to partially folded or misfolded proteins and thereby prevent their irreversible denaturation. Heat shock proteins also may help regulate the baroreceptor reflex response during heat stress, abating hypotension and bradycardia.

Box 70-3

Conditions and Diseases Associated with Heatstroke

Clinical Cause/Associated Condition

Exertional

Environmental: high ambient temperatures/humidity

Physiologic: lack of conditioning, inadequate acclimatization, or overexertion

Nonexertional

Environmental: high ambient temperatures/humidity, lack of air conditioning, lack of shrubbery/trees around dwelling, height of home above ground level

Physiologic: age older than 65 years, alcoholism, congestive heart failure, renal failure, diabetes mellitus, chronic obstructive pulmonary disease, dementia, schizophrenia, cystic fibrosis, thyrotoxicosis, hypokalemia, dehydration

Drugs: alcohol, antidopaminergics, anticholinergics, amphetamines, β-blockers, butyrophenones, cocaine, diuretics, hallucinogens, tricyclic anti-depressants

PREDISPOSING FACTORS

The epidemiology of heatstroke parallels that of hypothermia—nonexertional heatstroke is seen in elderly, alcoholic, or otherwise debilitated patients in urban areas. By contrast, exertional heatstroke develops in otherwise healthy people who overexert themselves in exceedingly hot or humid conditions. Like hypothermia, heatstroke most often develops in patients with impaired thermoregulation. Antidopaminergic drugs, alcohol, and primary CNS disorders are common denominators in many patients.[49] A number of environmental and socioeconomic conditions have been associated in recent years with heatstroke.[50,51] A lack of air conditioning and a lack of trees or shrubbery around homes are commonly observed in patients presenting with heatstroke. People who are apartment bound, particularly those on higher floors, also appear to be at higher risk during summer heat waves. Finally, elderly patients not only have diminished temperature perception but also do not produce the same volume of sweat, placing them at higher risk for the development of heatstroke.

Many drugs, "recreational" and prescription, are associated with an increased risk of hyperthermia and deserve further emphasis. Cocaine causes generalized sympathetic activation and loss of response to environmental cues. It is rapidly becoming a leading cause of heatstroke in many urban emergency departments. β-Blockers, on the other hand, have been implicated in heatstroke through a drug-mediated direct decrease in sweat gland production. Diuretics decrease baseline circulating plasma volume, leading to decreased sweat production. Hypokalemia decreases sweat gland output as well, and barbiturates can even cause sweat gland necrosis. When a heat wave arrives in an urban area, any one or several of the foregoing factors combined can lead to outbreaks of heat injury.

PRESENTATION AND CLINICAL MANIFESTATIONS

Nonexertional heatstroke may manifest insidiously.[52] An urban setting and the recognized presence of a heat wave may be the best available diagnostic clues. Some form of CNS dysfunction is nearly universal in patients with nonexertional heatstroke. The spectrum of dysfunction ranges from increased irritability and confusion to stupor and coma. Hyperpyrexia often is the most specific physical finding. In many cases, the presentation of an elderly patient with an altered mental status, irritability, and a high fever suggests sepsis. However, epidemiologic associations, concurrent debilitating disease, and the impact of medications that limit thermoregulation should be considered before limiting therapy to empiric antibiotics and antipyretic medications.

Exertional heatstroke typically occurs more suddenly, and with a more self-evident clinical history.[53] Severe dehydration, anhidrosis, and extreme hyperpyrexia are common. Affected persons appear hyperdynamic, with tachycardia, increased cardiac output, and peripheral arterial vasodilation. CNS dysfunction is somewhat less common in this patient subset. Initially, thermoregulation is intact in patients with exertional hyperthermia. At high core body temperatures, however, metabolic activity overwhelms normal heat dissipation mechanisms, and clear-cut disruption of normal thermoregulation may then appear. Hyperthermia is further accelerated by the loss of effective sweating for evaporative heat dissipation. Myocardial dysfunction with depression of left ventricular ejection fraction also has been described after heatstroke, which resolves with treatment.[54]

In addition to alterations of consciousness, hallucinations, focal neurologic deficits, various cranial nerve abnormalities, and opisthotonos are well described. Seizures occur in greater than half of these patients and may be related strictly to core body temperature, or to concomitant disorders of free water–electrolyte balance. Decerebrate posturing also is rarely observed in some patients without other known mechanisms of acute brain injury. Many patients may suffer residual defects such as dementia, personality changes, focal deficits, cerebellar changes or pyramidal findings. Nevertheless, many patients also proceed to complete recovery, suggesting that early findings should not deter acute management.[51]

DIAGNOSTIC APPROACH

In addition to CNS dysfunction, rhabdomyolysis is a frequent feature of exertional hyperthermia. Manifestations sometimes include tender, edematous muscles and "Coke-colored" urine, but the condition more commonly is defined by elevation in total creatine kinase (CK), serum aldolase, uric acid, or serum potassium (alone or in combination). Hyperkalemia in this situation may be life-threatening.

Acute renal failure occurs in up to one third of patients with heatstroke.[54,55] It is considerably more common in patients in whom rhabdomyolysis is a feature (i.e., with myoglobinuria or urate nephropathy). However, direct heat injury and renal hypoperfusion also may contribute. Acute tubular necrosis in heatstroke typically manifests with oliguria, non-nephrotic range proteinuria, and abundant granular cast formation.

Evidence of hepatocellular injury is present to some degree in essentially all patients with heatstroke and is attributed principally to a direct toxic effect of hyperthermia on hepatocytes.[56] Elevation of serum transaminases is a cardinal feature of this toxicity and often is observed within 30 minutes of syndrome onset. So prevalent is this finding that the absence of transaminitis should cast serious doubt on the diagnosis of heatstroke. Histologic changes including centrilobular necrosis have been observed within 24 hours of heat injury and evolve over the ensuing days. Transaminase and lactate dehydrogenase levels typically peak on the third or fourth hospital day, and depending upon the extent of injury, these changes may be accompanied by increased alkaline phosphatase levels, hyperbilirubinemia, and a prolonged prothrombin time. Overall, fulminant hepatic necrosis is rare; however, hepatic insufficiency contributes to late morbidity and mortality in patients who survive the initial resuscitation.[57] Prolongation of coagulation times also may be due to DIC. Although DIC also is rare, it is a marker of poor prognosis when present. Clinical manifestations of DIC range from isolated laboratory abnormalities to generalized bleeding. In patients with heatstroke, DIC may exacerbate hepatic injury and is associated with the development of ARDS. In fact, the co-development of DIC and ARDS in patients with heatstroke is predictive of a high mortality (>75%). Qualitative coagulation function (including platelet function) also may be impaired by heat injury. The clinical effects of these impairments are variable.

A range of electrolyte abnormalities related to renal failure and dehydration in heatstroke victims are well described. These include hyponatremia, hypocalcemia, hypokalemia (hyperkalemia in patients with acute tubular necrosis and/or rhabdomyolysis), hypophosphatemia, and hypomagnesemia. Of these, hyponatremia and free water excess may produce severe neurologic effects including central pontine myelinolysis (CPM). CPM has been reported in patients with heatstroke who receive aggressive prehospital resuscitation with hypotonic solutions. Serum osmolality should be carefully monitored during volume resuscitation, and intravenous solutions should be modified accordingly. Severe lactic acidosis is especially common in patients with exertional heat injury.[58] Finally, arterial blood gas results are influenced by temperature in a fashion opposite that described with hypothermia (see Box 70-2).

APPROACH TO MANAGEMENT

Duration of extreme hyperpyrexia is the single most important determinant of morbidity and mortality in all patients with heatstroke (both exertional and nonexertional). Therefore, expeditious cooling should be initiated simultaneously with other basic and advanced life support modalities. Indeed, a review of outcomes data for heatstroke victims during the Chicago heat wave of 1995 suggested that computed tomography imaging of the brain contributed little to patient management and simply delayed efforts to rapidly cool the patient.[59] General supportive measures and specific measures for cooling the patient are discussed next.

Supportive Measures

Intravascular volume restoration must be individualized. In general, patients with exertional hypothermia are severely hypovolemic. Hemodynamic monitoring has demonstrated that patients may manifest two distinct responses to heatstroke: (1) a hyperdynamic response with an elevated cardiac index (CI) and depressed SVR and (2) a hypodynamic response with depressed CI and elevated SVR.[55] Although the hypodynamic response may be more common in older patients with pre-existing medical problems and classic heatstroke, severe hyperthermia can lead to myocardial dysfunction even in young, healthy adults without pre-existing cardiac disease. Overzealous volume resuscitation in this setting can produce significant pulmonary congestion. The rapid restoration of an adequate perfusion pressure without pressor support is a reasonable goal, and if this is achieved, further volume resuscitation should proceed at a more measured pace. Pulmonary artery catheterization is recommended early in the clinical course for patients with unclear cardiovascular physiology. Finally, isoproterenol traditionally has been considered the inotrope of choice for patients with severely depressed myocardial performance. Its lack of α-activity ensures that heat dissipation is not impeded. Dobutamine may be a more rational choice, however, because it has considerably fewer myocardial irritant and arrhythmogenic properties.

Seizures are treated according to standard guidelines. Benzodiazepines are used for acute, ongoing convulsive activity. Dilantin is useful for added control or prophylaxis; however, hypotension with rapid intravenous infusion should be anticipated. Barbiturates also are effective antiseizure drugs, but should be reserved as second-line therapeutic agents because of their theoretical impediment to sweat formation and heat dissipation.

Acute renal failure should be approached aggressively in patients with rhabdomyolysis. Intravascular volume repletion should be promptly accomplished, with continued infusion of volume to produce forced diuresis. Mannitol or loop diuretics may be of value to maintain appropriate urine output. Hyperkalemia management may be challenging. The clinician should not hesitate to administer glucose, insulin, and calcium in patients with ECG changes. Subsequent sodium polystyrene sulfonate (Kayexalate) dosing may also be required.

Cooling Measures

Effective heat dissipation depends on the rapid transfer of heat from the core to the skin and from the skin to the external environment. In persons with hyperthermia, transfer of heat from the core to the skin is facilitated by active cutaneous vasodilation. Therapeutic cooling techniques are therefore aimed at accelerating the transfer of heat from the skin to the environment without compromising the flow of blood to the skin, which can be accomplished by increasing the temperature gradient between the skin and the environment (for cooling by conduction) or by increasing the gradient of water-vapor pressure between the skin and the environment (for cooling by evaporation), as well as by increasing the velocity of air adjacent to the skin (for cooling by convection).

Core body temperature should be rapidly cooled to a goal of 38° to 39° C. The most effective approaches to lowering the core temperature are immersion and evaporative methods. Of these, efficacy data related to ice-water immersion modalities historically have been better defined, with observed cooling rates of up to 0.13° C per minute. Similar efficacy has been noted with cool-water immersion as well, which should be less uncomfortable for both patient and staff members. Unfortunately, water immersion is not practical for many critically ill patients. Monitoring and treatment for arrhythmias, seizures, and other sequelae are problematic while the patient is immersed in a tub.

Evaporative techniques are quite effective and allow the ICU patient to be placed on a bed or other supportive surface and treated accordingly. The patient is repeatedly wetted with tepid water (not alcohol) or sprayed with water mist while warm air from a fan is blown across the body surface. Evaporative cooling by this method has shown a faster cooling rate in a canine model than that for immersion, reaching rates as high as 0.32° C per minute.[60] An aggressive approach to cooling the heatstroke victim, whatever the approach, is most important. Other adjuncts to cooling include rectal, intraperitoneal, and gastric lavage with iced saline. These techniques are effective at rapidly lowering core temperature but are cumbersome and generally unnecessary and may lead to unwanted iatrogenesis.

Efforts to cool a patient should be discontinued when the core temperature falls to 38° to 39°C. At that point, a continued fall by 1° or 2°C is expected. Dantrolene sodium has been used in some patients but was found to be ineffective in a double-blinded randomized study.[61,62] Chlorpromazine may be useful in patients in whom shivering develops during active cooling efforts; however, if neuroleptic malignant syndrome (NMS) is in the differential diagnosis (and it often is), meperidine may be a better option than an antidopaminergic agent in patients with normal renal function.

Specific Hyperthermic Syndromes

Malignant hyperthermia (MH) and NMS deserve special emphasis because of their potentially catastrophic impact on critically ill patients, particularly when they are not promptly recognized. MH is associated with use of certain anesthetic agents and can lead to profound skeletal muscle contraction and the subsequent development of life-threatening hyperthermia and other complications. NMS is caused by a variety of antipsychotic drugs and also leads to sustained muscular contraction and hyperthermia.

Box 70-4

Anesthetics Associated with the Development of Malignant Hyperthermia and Neuroleptic Malignant Syndrome

Malignant Hyperthermia

Volatile Anesthetics
Cyclopropane, diethyl ether, enflurane, ethylene, halothane, isoflurane, methoxyflurane, sevoflurane

Muscle Relaxants
Succinylcholine, decamethonium

Neuroleptic Malignant Syndrome

Phenothiazines
Fluphenazine, chlorpromazine, levomepromazine, thioridazine, trimeprazine, trifluoroperazine, prochlorperazine

Butyrophenones
Haloperidol, bromoperidol, droperidol

Dibenzoxepine
Loxapine

Dopamine-Depleting Drugs
Alpha-methyltyrosine, tetrabenzamine

Dopaminergic Agent Withdrawal
Levodopa-carbidopa, amantadine

MALIGNANT HYPERTHERMIA

MH develops in approximately 1 of 15,000 patients who undergo surgical procedures requiring general anesthesia. The vast majority of cases are associated with either halothane or succinylcholine use; however, a variety of other drugs also have been implicated. Box 70-4 outlines these agents by type. Unlike in heatstroke, endogenous heat production is solely responsible for the observed hyperpyrexia. MH constitutes a true medical emergency because of the rapid tempo at which severe sequelae evolve. Better recognition of this syndrome and modern treatment techniques, however, have reduced mortality rates from 70% to approximately 10% in recent years.

PATHOGENESIS

MH results from a rapid, sustained increase in myoplasmic Ca^{++} levels in response to halogenated anesthetics and depolarizing neuromuscular blocking agents. Susceptibility to MH results from mutations in calcium channel proteins that mediate excitation-contraction coupling, with the ryanodine receptor calcium release channel (RyR1) representing the major locus. The mode of inheritance appears to be autosomal dominant, with variable penetrance. The phenomenon occurs in persons who have a mutation in the ryanodine type 1 receptor, resulting in a defective protein in the skeletal muscle sarcoplasmic reticulum membrane.[63] The uncontrolled rise in the myoplasmic Ca^{++} concentration disables the troponin inhibition of actin and myosin, resulting in uncontrolled muscle tetany. This surge in muscle metabolic activity causes thermogenesis to increase exponentially and is rapidly followed by total body rigidity and extreme hyperpyrexia.

Numerous familial myopathies (such as Evans myopathy, King-Denborough syndrome, and central core disease) have been associated with the reaction.[64,65] Curiously, this genetic predisposition does not translate into the predictable development of MH. That is, an initial challenge with an anesthetic drug that leads to MH does not consistently predict whether or not MH will occur with future exposures to the same drug. Measured contraction in caffeine or halothane preparations of muscle biopsy specimens is the most reliable predictor of risk for MH.

PRESENTATION

MH is characterized by the triad of (1) severe hyperthermia, (2) muscle rigidity, and (3) metabolic acidosis. MH usually is an acute and rapidly progressive process; however, many reports suggest that the syndrome may vary considerably in severity and rate of progression. In the anesthesia setting, capnography may provide the earliest clue of impending MH, as end-tidal CO_2 rises in response to the increased metabolic rate. Clinical harbingers of impending MH include masseter muscle rigidity or trismus and tachycardia, which is reported to occur in greater than 95% of patients.[64] Cyanosis, increased blood pressure, and increased respiratory rate all may be observed with the onset of the reaction as the hypermetabolic response is triggered.

Muscle rigidity may explosively progress from localized masseter contraction to diffuse rigidity of skeletal muscle groups. When uninterrupted, this process will lead to progressive, severe hyperthermia. Extreme hyperpyrexia is considered a late finding in MH. Mortality has been related to peak core body temperature, reflecting both MH severity and delayed recognition. With progressing rigidity, a mixed metabolic and respiratory acidosis may occur, along with a variety of other electrolyte abnormalities, including hyperkalemia, hypercalcemia, and hypermagnesemia. Severe chest wall rigidity may even prevent adequate mechanical ventilation, leading to life-threatening hypoxemia and hypoventilation. Rhabdomyolysis is reflected in elevated CK levels, usually greater than 1500 and often greater than 10,000 U per L. Myoglobinuria may produce acute tubular necrosis with oliguric renal failure and severe DIC. High fever may result in myocardial dysfunction, pulmonary edema, and cerebral edema.

DIAGNOSIS

Susceptibility to MH can be identified unequivocally only by an in vitro muscle test. Fascicles of muscle obtained from the thigh by biopsy are exposed to halothane and separately to increasing concentrations of caffeine in vitro. The muscle contractures are increased in persons who are susceptible to MH. This test is now widely used to identify susceptibility to MH in patients who have had a reaction to inhaled halogenated anaesthetics or suxamethonium that is suggestive of MH. If the test results in the propositus are positive, testing can be offered to first-degree relatives for genetic counseling. Patients whose biopsied muscle demonstrates a contracture to 3% halothane of 0.5 g or more and a contracture to 2 mmol/L caffeine of 0.2 g or more are considered to be susceptible to MH.[66] An in vitro contracture test is the gold standard for diagnosing susceptibility to MH. Two different protocols are used. European laboratories use the protocol devised by Ellis in Leeds with incremental doses of halothane up to 2% and incremental doses of caffeine. In the United States, a single dose of 3% halothane and incremental doses of caffeine are used. The two protocols give essentially the same results.[67]

TREATMENT

By far, the most important measure for MH is the immediate cessation of any suspected triggering agents. If anesthesia must be maintained, nontriggering agents should be used. Agents considered safe in MH include barbiturates, narcotics, benzodiazepines, and propofol, to name only a few. Nondepolarizing neuromuscular blockers such as vecuronium or atracurium, although also considered safe in these patients, will do nothing to abort the MH reaction beause the primary pathology resides within the skeletal muscle cell itself—beyond the neuromuscular junction.

In addition to discontinuing offending agents, sodium dantrolene should be administered intravenously at a dose of 2 to 3 mg per kg every 5 to 10 minutes. Sodium dantrolene initially was tested as an antimicrobial; however, dantrolene was found to produce muscle weakness by blocking the Ca^{++} efflux from the sarcoplasmic reticulum. The agent is capable of reversing the MH reaction by lowering myoplasmic Ca^{++} concentrations. Doses of 10 mg per kg often are recommended, but as much as 20 mg per kg has been required in some case reports. The onset of action usually is within 2 to 3 minutes, with initial responses including muscle relaxation, decreasing heart rate, and decreasing core body temperature. Muscle weakness may follow drug administration, but this should never limit proper therapy. After the initial response, dantrolene may be dosed orally at 1 mg/kg every 6 hours for 24 to 48 hours. Late recurrences of MH have been reported if inadequate dantrolene dosing occurs. Intravenous preparations of dantrolene contain significant amounts of mannitol, which may produce a subsequent osmotic diuresis. Although this reaction may be desirable in patients with rhabdomyolysis, volume and electrolyte management should take this effect into account.

Systemic cooling may be best achieved in these complex patients with evaporative techniques, cooling blankets, cold saline infusion, or ice packs. Because of its similar actions on myoplasmic Ca^{++} concentration, procainamide was the drug of choice for this syndrome before the advent of dantrolene therapy. Cardiac dysrhythmias not responding to electrolyte correction may be safely treated with procainamide or lidocaine. Numerous reports suggest that intravenous calcium may be safely infused for toxic hyperkalemia. Diltiazem and verapamil may interact with dantrolene to produce hyperkalemia; therefore these agents should be avoided. Although the effects of MH on cardiac muscle remain unclear, some authors advocate that cardiac glycosides also should be avoided because they increase intracellular Ca^{++} concentration.

NEUROLEPTIC MALIGNANT SYNDROME (NMS)

NMS is an idiosyncratic reaction to neuroleptic drugs and other antidopaminergic agents. A number of drugs that are known to be associated with NMS are listed in Box 70-4. The syndrome is characterized by muscle rigidity and altered mental status, followed by autonomic instability and hyperthermia. However, temperature elevations generally are less extreme than in MH and are not as life-threatening.

NMS is reported to occur in up to 2% to 3% of all patients receiving neuroleptic medications. The reaction typically develops within a few days of initiating therapy and almost always appears within the first 30 days. Curiously, NMS also occurs rarely in some patients after many years on a stable dosing regimen. Of importance, NMS also can occur in response to the withdrawal of central dopaminergic agonists such as bromocriptine or levodopa-carbidopa.

PATHOPHYSIOLOGY

Some investigators suspect that the genetic predisposition to MH also defines patients at risk for NMS, but most work has failed to demonstrate a relationship between

NMS and altered sarcolemmal membrane calcium permeability. Unlike in MH, patients with NMS appear to have both increased heat production and impaired central thermoregulation, compromising heat dissipation. In these patients, a decrease in central dopaminergic tone also results in extrapyramidal signs of skeletal muscle rigidity and tremor and may account for alterations in mental status due to effects in the mesolimbic system and mesocortical pathways.[68] Finally, even though altered central thermoregulation may contribute to hyperthermia in NMS, rapid resolution of fever after administration of neuromuscular relaxing agents or dantrolene suggests that hyperthermia is due primarily to increased heat generation by skeletal muscle rigidity.

PRESENTATION

NMS should be considered when fever, muscular rigidity, catatonia, or dystonia occur in the setting of neuroleptic drug administration. Recent reviews have suggested the following criteria for the diagnosis of NMS: treatment with neuroleptics within 7 days; hyperthermia with core temperatures greater than 38° C; muscle rigidity; exclusion of other systemic or drug-related illness; and any five of the following: altered mental status, tachycardia, hypertension or hypotension, tachypnea or hypoxia, diaphoresis or sialorrhea, tremor, incontinence, CK elevation or myoglobinuria, leukocytosis, or metabolic acidosis.[68,69]

Altered mental status commonly precedes the onset of other symptoms and may manifest as confusion or agitation. More severe cases may progress to obtundation or coma, or may manifest as a mute catatonia that is difficult to differentiate from lethal catatonia. Muscle rigidity typically involves the neck, shoulders, and limbs but may compromise ventilation if chest wall involvement is severe. Other neuromuscular findings are diverse and may include dysarthria, dyskinesias, ataxia, or tremors.

Autonomic findings typically include diaphoresis, hypertension, and tachycardia. However, hypotension may develop in some patients. Fever is a late finding and usually occurs in the range of 38° to 42° C. When fever exceeds 42° C, it may cause end-organ damage like that seen in other hyperthermia syndromes.

Rhabdomyolysis occurs often, though it usually is of a milder caliber than that observed in MH or exertional heatstroke. Elevations in serum transaminases, BUN, and serum creatinine often are seen, as well as a leukocytosis.

TREATMENT

When NMS is suspected, the offending drug should be discontinued immediately and supportive measures initiated. Volume resuscitation, physical measures for cooling, and monitoring of cardiopulmonary and renal parameters should be instituted immediately. Pharmacologic options for the treatment of NMS are more numerous than for other hyperthermia syndromes, because they may be directed toward restoring central dopaminergic tone or reducing peripheral rigidity until the neuroleptic effects subside.

Dopamine agonists such as bromocriptine, amantadine, and levodopa-carbidopa have been successfully employed in NMS.[68,70] These agents act to directly increase central dopaminergic tone, thereby antagonizing the various effects of neuroleptic dopamine blockade. Regimens include bromocriptine, 2.5 mg given orally every 8 hours (up to 10 to 20 mg per dose has been used) for up to 10 days before tapering, or amantadine, 100 mg given orally every 8 hours. If a levodopa-carbidopa combination is used, it should be dosed four times a day owing to its shorter half-life. Some authors advocate avoiding central dopamine agonists if the diagnosis is unclear or if psychosis remains in the differential diagnosis, to avoid acutely exacerbating the psychotic state or contributing to a lethal catatonia.

Sodium dantrolene has been successfully used in numerous small series. The muscle relaxation that occurs helps to reduce temperature and decrease the sequelae of prolonged rigidity. Neuromuscular blockers also are effective at decreasing skeletal muscle tone, and in patients with high fever and autonomic instability, these agents offer a rapid means of establishing therapeutic effects. Combinations of central dopamine agonists and peripheral-acting agents have not as yet demonstrated a significant advantage over either treatment alone. Electroconvulsive therapy (ECT) has been used in a number of reports, but its advantages over supportive care alone have not been adequately assessed.[70] Furthermore, the need for anesthesia presents an additional hazard that may complicate management in these patients.

Airway-protective reflexes should be vigilantly assessed because dystonia and impaired bulbar functions increase the risk of gastric aspiration in patients with NMS. Morbidity and mortality in these cases often arises from pulmonary complications such as aspiration, pneumonia, ARDS, or pulmonary embolism. Cardiac complications such as arrhythmias or myocardial infarction in more fulminant cases also contribute to mortality in these patients. As in all of the hyperthermia syndromes, worsening rhabdomyolysis and acute renal failure have been identified as signs of poor prognosis.

RHABDOMYOLYSIS

Rhabdomyolysis is a pathologic state in which the necrosis of muscle cells, resulting from trauma, toxins, medications, or other causes, leads to an excess of intracellular solutes in the extracellular compartments. Target organ damage can range from minimal to severe, depending on the degree of necrosis; the main consequences are metabolic abnormalities and acute renal failure. Current understanding of the pathophysiology of rhabdomyolysis has evolved with emphasis on early diagnosis and treatment, often in the setting of major catastrophes. The first report in the English literature, describing four cases of crush injury in Britain during World War II, was recently republished.[71]

EPIDEMIOLOGY

The incidence of rhabdomyolysis is dependent on the population undergoing analysis and the diagnostic criteria being used. It is recognized as a major cause of mortality following severe musculoskeletal injury from trauma.[72] After the 1999 Marmara earthquake in Northwestern Turkey, 8.9% of hospitalized patients required renal replacement therapy for crush-related injuries.[73] Recently, a particular focus has been the ability of the hydroxymethylglutaryl–coenzyme A (HMG-CoA) reductase inhibitor class of medications to cause rhabdomyolysis. Although probably a class-related phenomenon, the incidence of rhabdomyolysis is not equivalent for all medications and is increased with the addition of other specific agents—in particular, gemfibrozil or cyclosporine.[74] Additional causes of rhabdomyolysis are listed in Box 70-5.[75]

The epidemiology of rhabdomyolysis is limited by a lack of uniformity regarding the critical value in CK elevation needed to make a diagnosis. Values used may range from 1000 to 10,000 U/L, although values in the range of 5000 to 10,000 are most common.[76] From an intensivist's perspective, CK elevations of less than 5000 should not be associated with myoglobin-induced renal failure.

Box 70-5

Causes of Rhabdomyolysis*

- Trauma/crush injuries
- Prolonged immobilization
- Electrical injury
- Excessive muscular activity
- Excessive exertion
- Malignant hyperthermia
- Neuroleptic malignant syndrome
- Infections
  - Sepsis
  - Viral myositis
- Medications†
  - Hydroxymethylglutaryl–coenzyme A reductase inhibitors
  - Gemfibrozil
  - Paraphenylenediamine (hair dye)
  - Phenothiazines
  - Theophylline
- Toxins
  - Cocaine
  - Carbon monoxide
  - Amphetamines
  - Alcohol
  - *Tricholoma equestre* (wild mushrooms)
  - Hemlock
- Metabolic myopathies
  - Carnitine palmitoyl transferase deficiency
  - Mitochondrial respiratory chain deficiencies
  - McArdle disease
  - Phosphofructokinase deficiency

*In addition to the listed causes, risk factors include excessive heat, hyponatremia, hypophosphatemia, and hypokalemia.
†Additional medications have been associated with rhabdomyolysis.

PATHOPHYSIOLOGY

The primary event in rhabdomyolysis is muscle cell necrosis, resulting in the accumulation of sodium and calcium intracellularly; disruption of the cell membrane and excessive requirements for ATP accelerate this insult.[77,78] After the necrosis-inducing insult, intracellular substances including potassium, uric acid, phosphorus, lactic acid, and myoglobin are released from the cells. Under normal circumstances, haptoglobin binds any free myoglobin, thereby prohibiting filtration across the glomerulus. As the haptoglobin binding is overwhelmed, free myoglobin is filtered and presented to the renal tubular cells, leading to one potential cause for acute renal failure. This process involves free radical toxicity. Additional causes include volume depletion, renal vasoconstriction, renal tubular cell damage, and subsequent tubular obstruction.[75] The observation that myoglobin and tubular protein casts are more prone to precipitation at a lower pH is the rationale for the emphasis on achieving an alkaline diuresis.[79]

Research has suggested that it is the reperfusion of ischemic muscle, as much as the ischemia itself, that produces a high burden of oxygen free radicals with subsequent cellular lipid membrane injury.[80] As renal function worsens, particularly when accompanied by intravascular volume depletion and renal failure, patients cannot excrete the high load of metabolites associated with muscle death, especially potassium. Amazingly, little information is available on the non-renal toxicity of free myoglobin.

Myoglobin release occurs across a spectrum of physical injuries from moderate exercise to lethal crush injuries. Myoglobinemia was noted in 39% of a cohort of Marine recruits, illustrating the frequency of mild muscle cell necrosis with strenuous exercise.[81] Obviously, not all such injuries lead to acute renal failure. Beyond the actual amount of muscle necrosis, the development of acute renal failure is most dependent on the degree of volume depletion present during the initial insult and the rapidity with which it is restored. Many of the syndromes that lead to the development of rhabdomyolysis, such as very strenuous exercise, crush injuries, or intoxications, are accompanied by volume depletion.

CLINICAL PRESENTATION

Patients with rhabdomyolysis present with a variety of symptoms. Often the history includes injury, weakness, or muscle pain. Dark red or brown urine may or may not be present, depending on the amount of muscle necrosis and delay from injury. Frequently, the history is limited owing to altered sensorium; clues include unexplained acidosis, hyperkalemia, hyperuricemia, hypocalcemia, elevations in CK not consistent with myocardial infarction, or unexplained renal failure. Recurrent presentations warrant an evaluation for a metabolic myopathy.[82]

In most instances, serum CK will increase during the initial 48 hours of hospitalization. In a retrospective review of patients admitted to an ICU with rhabdomyolysis, defined as a CK greater than 10,000 U/L, significantly higher CK levels were associated with renal failure.[83] In the group with renal failure, the mean CK levels were 47,194 U/L and 55,366 at admission and peak, respectively; in the group without renal failure, the same levels were 17,531 U/L and 28,643 U/L.

Although myoglobin is the most important protein in terms of nephrotoxicity, serum CK is routinely used in clinical practice as a marker of disease severity. This inconsistency is due to the widespread availability of the CK assay. Myoglobin clearance is faster than CK clearance whether or not renal failure is present.[84] Consequently, CK levels when used to monitor for disease activity may not correlate with the timing of the renal injury. Acute renal failure associated with peak CK levels less than 5000 U/L should not be attributed to rhabdomyolysis unless the diagnosis was made substantially after the peak period of muscle cell necrosis; in this scenario, the CK levels will have decreased from a previously undocumented level. The renal insult would have occurred with the previous CK and myoglobin elevations.

The change in serum creatinine in non-rhabdomyolysis oliguric acute renal failure is usually not more than 1 mg/dL per 24 hours. In rhabdomyolysis, creatinine enters the intravascular compartment at a higher rate owing to cell lysis, yielding an unusually rapid rise in serum creatinine. In an early report, Grossman and colleagues noted a rise in creatinine frequently greater than 2.5 mg/dL.[85] These authors also noted the impressive rate of recovery from rhabdomyolysis-induced acute renal failure seen in a majority of patients.

SPECIFIC TREATMENT REQUIREMENTS

The most important intervention to limit renal complications of crush-related injuries is early and aggressive volume resuscitation. Delays in initiation of intravenous fluid are associated with a requirement for renal replacement therapy in a higher proportion of patients.[86] The damaged muscle cells provide a large reservoir for fluid sequestration; as a result, large volumes of intravenous fluids have to be given and, ideally, should be instituted as early as possible, even on site, before victims of crush injuries are freed, for example.[87]

A debate exists in the medical literature regarding the ideal type of volume resuscitation. As previously mentioned, alkaline diuresis has been shown in animal models to decrease the formation of myoglobin casts and subsequent acute renal failure.[79] Similarly, a mannitol diuresis has been proposed to promote free radical scavenging, with the ability to limit acute renal failure.[88,89] These treatments have not been validated in a well-designed, prospective trial. Retrospective studies suggest no benefit with the addition of mannitol or alkaline diuresis over saline alone.[90] In addition, there are potential risks to volume expansion with bicarbonate-based solutions or mannitol-based diureses. These include the increased risk of calcium-phosphate complex formation, hypocalcemia, and the development of a hyperosmolar state when renal failure limits mannitol excretion. Finally, mannitol may increase the risk of renal failure in certain populations.[91] In summary, volume expansion, irrespective of the type of agent, is the most important treatment modality.

The focus on adequate diuresis is appropriate but presumes that myoglobin-induced renal damage is ongoing. Intensivists often encounter patients whose myoglobin load is falling and whose renal insult has already occurred. Although the creatinine may continue to rise, the onset of oliguria suggests limited benefit from further aggressive volume resuscitation, if adequate intravascular volume has been restored. In fact, given the good prognosis for acute renal failure, overzealous volume resuscitation only risks pulmonary compromise. Nonetheless, it is worthwhile to note that necrotic muscles can absorb significant volume; as a result, the amount of intravenous fluids needed to attain euvolemia may be surprisingly large.[92]

Historically, extremely aggressive volume resuscitation was pursued with an initial diuresis goal of up to 12 liters per day in patients with intact renal function. Less aggressive volume resuscitation may be equally protective, although data supporting this approach are lacking. The focus on diuresis downplays the importance of establishing and maintaining adequate intravascular volume. A central venous pressure line or other means to monitor intravascular pressure may be more useful to determine adequate resuscitation. It also is likely that the rapidity with which volume status is restored, irrespective of the type or quantity of diuresis, is the key determininant. Unfortunately, these guidelines have been poorly studied in a prospective format.

In the setting of acute renal failure requiring renal replacement therapy, the ideal modality is the one most easily accessible, in patients with stable hemodynamics. Options include hemodialysis, peritoneal dialysis, and continuous modalities. Although continuous renal replacement modalities provide the best theoretical protection from ongoing metabolic and volume complications, the superiority of such modalities has not been verified in rigorous trials. Moreover, use of continuous techniques without anticoagulation in trauma patients may be less effective. In cases associated with large-scale injuries such as earthquakes, the remaining infrastructure often dictates which dialytic modality can and should be provided.[72,93]

Historically, peritoneal dialysis has not been considered adequate in its ability to remove the large solute load present with rhabdomyolysis.[94] Nonetheless, if it is the only available modality, its potential may be improved with more modern techniques such as frequent exchanges with a cycler. It should be noted that no renal replacement method has the capability of removing myoglobin, owing to the size of the molecule. In view of the rapid extrarenal clearance of myoglobin, it is unclear whether therapy focused on myoglobin clearance will be superior to current care. A novel approach recently evaluated the use of super high-flux (SHF) membranes to clear myoglobin while the patient undergoes continuous veno-venous hemofiltration.[95] The investigators demonstrated a fivefold increase in myoglobin removal but did acknowledge the potential for the removal of albumin, clotting factors, and protein-bound medications.

Beyond cardiovascular support, hypocalcemia may provide challenging management choices. Calcium entry into necrotic muscle cells often causes profound hypocalcemia. Calcium supplementation should be reserved for those patients with symptomatic hypocalcemia, because hypercalcemia is a frequent finding during disease recovery.[96]

Additional issues include close monitoring for limb ischemia due to compartment syndromes induced by muscle damage and worsened by fluid sequestration. Intracompartmental pressure monitoring may predict the need for intervention, although research has suggested that additional factors, most importantly hypotension and the difference between mean arterial pressure and intracompartmental pressures, influence whether compartment syndrome develops or not.[97] The history of, rationale for, and disappointing results with early and aggressive fasciotomy have recently been described.[98] Mannitol is postulated to "decompress" intracompartmental edema in acute muscle compartment syndromes. Animal data support an acute reduction in intracompartmental pressures[99]; long-term tissue protection and human outcomes have not been validated.

In summary, rhabdomyolysis is a frequent, treatable disorder. Extensive metabolic research has yielded a number of clues about the cause of the major comorbid condition associated with rhabdomyolysis, acute renal failure. Therapy should emphasize aggressive and early volume resuscitation. Renal replacement therapy may be necessary to assist in managing the metabolic complications in patients with acute renal failure; patients have a good prognosis for recovery of rhabdomyolysis-induced acute renal failure.

KEY POINTS

- A high index of clinical suspicion for hypothermia is required because many thermometers in clinical use are not calibrated below 35°C, and hypothermia may be confused with other conditions.
- In the United States, severe hypothermia is most commonly seen in (1) the elderly, (2) debilitated patients with chronic medical diseases that are associated with impaired central thermoregulation, and (3) alcoholics.
- Patients often present to the critical care unit with severe hypothermia after prolonged or complicated surgical procedures.
- Initial resuscitation is directed primarily toward the return of core temperature to normal, as well as toward the maintenance of the ABCs. *Corollary:* All resuscitative efforts should ethically continue until the temperature exceeds at least 32° to 33°C.
- Passive external rewarming techniques should be used only in patients with mild hypothermia and relatively intact thermogenesis mechanisms.
- Invasive core rewarming (i.e., cardiopulmonary bypass) is the most efficacious therapeutic approach for hypothermia victims presenting without spontaneous respiration or perfusing cardiac rhythm.
- Aspiration pneumonia, DIC, and gastrointestinal stress ulceration are serious and common complications associated with hypothermia.
- Exertional heatstroke is seen in otherwise healthy persons who overexert themselves during times of increased ambient temperature and humidity (skeletal muscle heat production outstrips heat-dissipating capacity).
- Classic (nonexertional) heatstroke develops in chronically ill and debilitated patients with altered central thermoregulation.
- Physical findings other than fever are nonspecific so that the diagnosis of heatstroke is not always readily apparent.
- Severity of organ system damage is most directly related to the duration of hyperpyrexia, rather than to the absolute temperature elevation. *Corollary:* The patient must be cooled as rapidly as possible; seconds count.
- Immersion and evaporative techniques are equally effective methods of rapidly lowering the core temperature.
- Common complications include CNS dysfunction, hepatic dysfunction, DIC, acute tubular necrosis, and rhabdomyolysis.
- The predisposition to malignant hyperthermia (MH) is inherited as an autosomal dominant trait with variable penetrance and occurs as often as 1 of 15,000 patients who receive general anesthesia.
- After the administration of anesthetic drugs, MH develops rapidly as trismus, followed by whole body rigidity, CO_2 production, intense hyperpyrexia, and profound chest wall noncompliance or inability to ventilate.
- Keys to successful therapy of MH include rapid recognition and abortion of the anesthetic drug sequence and emergent administration of dantrolene sodium.
- Neuroleptic malignant syndrome (NMS) is seen in patients receiving a wide variety of neuroleptic drugs, often as antipsychotic therapy in the ICU, and most typically is characterized by fever, altered mental status, muscular rigidity or dystonia, and rhabdomyolysis.
- Therapy consists of discontinuation of the offending drug, supportive measures, and central dopamine agonists or skeletal muscle relaxants.

REFERENCES

1. Jurkovich GJ, Greiser WB, Luterman A, et al: Hypothermia in trauma victims: An ominous predictor of survival. J Trauma 1987;27:1019-1024.
2. Mueller PD, Olson KR: Cocaine. Emerg Med Clin North Am 1990;8:481.
3. Centers for Disease Control and Prevention: Hypothermia-related deaths. MMWR Morb Mortal Wkly Rep 2006;55:282-284.
4. Miller JW, Danzl DF, Thomas DM: Urban accidental hypothermia; 135 cases. Ann Emerg Med 1980;16:1042.
5. Centers for Disease Control and Prevention: Hypothermia-related deaths, Virginia-November 1996–April 1997. MMWR Morb Mortal Wkly Rep 1997;46:1157.
6. Collins KJ, Exton-Smith AN, Fox RH, et al: Accidental hypothermia and impaired temperature homeostasis in the elderly. BMJ 1977;1:353-356.
7. Gautam P, Ghosh S, Mandal A, Vargas E: Hypothermia in the elderly: Sociomedical characteristics and the outcome in 86 patients. Public Health 1989;103:15.
8. English MJ, Farmer C, Scott WA: Heat loss in exposed volunteers. J Trauma 1990;30:422.
9. Danzl DF, Pozos RS Hamlet MP: Accidental hypothermia. In Auerbach P, Geehr R (eds): Management of Wilderness and Environmental Emergencies, 2nd ed. St. Louis, Mosby, 1989.
10. Martyn JW: Diagnosing and treating hypothermia. Can Med J 1981;125: 1089.
11. Danzl DF, Pozos RS: Accidental hypothermia. N Engl J Med 1994;331:1756-1760.
12. Golden F: Mechanisms of body cooling in submersed victims. Resuscitation 197;35:107.
13. Schneider SM, Danzl DF: Hypothermia: From recognition to rewarming. Emerg Med Rep 1992;13:1.
14. Bartley B, Crnkovich DJ, Usman AR, et al: How to recognize hypothermia in critically ill patients. J Crit Illness 1996;11:118.
15. Southwick FS, Dalglish PH: Recovery after prolonged cardiac arrest in profound hypothermia. JAMA 1980;243:1250-1253.
16. O'Keefe KM: Noncardiogenic pulmonary edema from accidental hypothermia. Col Med 1980;77:106-107.
17. Morales CF, Strollo PJ: Noncardiogenic pulmonary edema associated with accidental hypothermia. Chest 1993;103:971-973.
18. Smith OLK: Insulin response in rats acutely exposed to cold. Can J Physiol Pharmacol 1984;62:92.
19. Davenport A, Will EJ, Davison AM: Hyperlactataemia and metabolic acidosis during hemofiltration using lactate-buffered fluids. Nephron 1991;59:461-465.
20. Maclean D, Murison J, Griffiths PD: Acute pancreatitis and DKA in accidental hypothermia. BMJ 1973;4:757-761.
21. O'Brien RC, Amess JAL, Mollin DL: Recurrent thrombocytopenia, erythroid hyperplasia, and sideroblastic anemia-associated with hypothermia. Br J Hematol 1982;51:451-456.
22. Rosenkranz L: Bone marrow failure and pancytopenia in two patients with hypothermia. South Med J 1985:78;358-359.
23. Valeri CR, Feingold J, Cassidy G, et al: Hypothermia-induced reversible platelet dysfunction. Ann Surg 1987;205:175-181.
24. Rohrer MJ, Natale AM: Effect of hypothermia on the coagulation cascade. Crit Care Med 1992;20:1402-1405.
25. Reed RL, Johnson TD, Hudson JD, et al: The disparity between hypothermic coagulopathy and clotting studies. J Trauma 1992;33:465-470.
26. Ream AK Reitz BA, Silverberg G: Temperature correction of Pa_{CO_2} and pH in estimating acid-base status: An example of the emperor's new clothes? Anesthesiology 1982;56;41.
27. Hansen JE, Sue DY: Should blood gas measurements be corrected for the patient's temperature? N Engl J Med 1980;303:341.
28. Delaney KA, Howland MA, Vassallo S, Goldfrank LR: Assessment of acid-base disturbances in hypothermia and their physiologic consequences. Ann Emerg Med 1989;18:72.
29. Patel A, Getsos JP, Moussa G, et al: The Osborn wave of hypothermia in normothermic patients. Clin Cardiol 1994;17:273-276.
30. Solomon A, Barish RA, Brown B, Tso E: The electrocardiographic features of hypothermia. J Emerg Med 1989;7:169.
31. Zwischenberger JB, Kirsh MM, Dechert RE, et al: Suppression of shivering decreases oxygen consumption and improves hemodynamic stability during postoperative rewarming. Ann Thorac Surg 1987;43:428-431.
32. Steinman AM: The hypothermic code: CPR controversy revisited. J Emerg Med Serv 1983;10:32.
33. Dronen S, Nowak RM, Tomlanivich MC: Bretylium tosylate and ventricular fibrillation in hypothermia. Ann Intern Med 1986;105:624.
34. Kalla J, Yan GX, Marinchak R: Ventricular fibrillation in a patient with prominent J (Osborn) waves and ST segment elevation in the inferior electrocardiographic leads: A Brugada syndrome variant? J Cardiovasc Electrophysiol 2000;11:95-98.
35. Kornberger E, Schwarz B, Linder KH, et al: Forced air surface rewarming in patients with severe accidental hypothermia. Resuscitation 1999;41:105-111.
36. Steele MT, Nelson MJ, Sessler DI, et al: Forced air speeds rewarming in accidental hypothermia. Ann Emerg Med 1996;27:479-484.
37. Hayward JS, Eckerson JD, Kemna D: Thermal and cardiovascular changes during three methods of resuscitation from mild hypothermia. Resuscitation 1984;11:21-33.
38. Gregory JS, Bergstein JM, Aprehamian C, et al: Comparison of three methods of rewarming from hypothermia: Advantages of extracorporial blood rewarming. J Trauma 1991;319:1247-1251.
39. Gentilello LM, Cobean RA, Offner PJ, et al: Continuous arteriovenous rewarming: Rapid reversal of hypothermia in critically ill patients. J Trauma 1999;32:316-325.
40. Seigler RS, Golding E, Blackhurst MS: Continuous venovenous rewarming: Results from a juvenile animal model. Crit Care Med 1998;26:2016-2020.
41. Vretnar DF, Urschel JD, Parrott JC, et al: Cardiopulmonary bypass resuscitation for accidental hypothermia. Ann Thorac Surg 1994;58:895-898.
42. Gentilello LM, Moujaes S: Treatment of hypothermia in trauma victims: Thermodynamic considerations. J Intensive Care Med 1995;10:5-14.
43. Gentilello LM: Advances in the management of hypothermia. Surg Clin North Am 1995;75:243-256.
44. Walpoth BH, Walpoth-Aslan BN, Mattle HP, et al: Outcome of survivors of accidental deep hypothermia and circulatory arrest treated with extracorporeal blood warming. N Engl J Med 1997;337:1500-1505.
45. von Segesser LK, Garcia E, Turina M: Perfusion without systemic heparinization for rewarming in accidental hypothermia. Ann Thorac Surg 1991;52:560-561.
46. Carter R 3rd, Cheuvront SN, Williams JO, et al: Epidemiology of hospitalizations and deaths from heat illness in soldiers. Med Sci Sports Exerc 2005;37:1338-1344.
47. Centers for Disease Control and Prevention: Monitoring environmental disease—United States, 1997. JAMA 1998;280:688-689.
48. Heat-related deaths—Philadelphia and the United States. MMWR Morb Mortal Wkly Rep1994;43:453-455.
49. Kilbourne EM, Choi, K, Jones TS, et al: Risk factors for heat stroke. A case control study. JAMA 1982;247:3332.
50. Donoghue ER, Graham MA, Jentzen JM, et al: Criteria for the diagnosis of heat-related deaths: National Association of Medical Examiners. Position paper. National Association of Medical Examiners Ad Hoc Committee on the Definition of Heat-Related Fatalities. Am J Forensic Med Pathol 1997;18:11-14.
51. Richards D, Richards R, Schofield J: Management of heat exhaustion in Sydney's, the sun city-to-surf fun runners. Med J Aust 1979;2:457.
52. Nadel ER: Temperature regulation and hyperthermia during exercise. Clin Chest Med 1984;5:13-20.
53. Schvartz E, Shapiro Y, Magazanik A, et al: Heat acclimatization, physical fitness and response to exercise in temperate and hot environment. J Appl Physiol 1977;43:678.
54. Rousseau JM, Villevieille T, Schiano P, et al: Reversible myocardial dysfunction after exertional heat stroke. Intensive Care Med 2001;27:328-329.
55. Tucker LE, Stanford J, Graves B, et al: Classical heatstroke: Clinical and laboratory assessment. Southern Med J 1985;78:20.
56. Amundson DE: The spectrum of heat related injury with compartment syndrome. Milit Med 1989;154:450.

57. Jacobsen TD, Krenzelok EP, Shicker L, et al: Environmental injuries. Dis Mon 1997;43:809-907.
58. Bouchama A, Devol EB: Acid-base alterations in heatstroke. Intensive Care Med 2001;27:680-685.
59. Dematte JE, O'Mara K, Buescher J, et al: Near-fatal heat stroke during the 1995 heat wave in Chicago. Ann Intern Med 1998;129:179-181.
60. White DJ, Kamath R, Nucci R, et al: Evaporation versus iced peritoneal lavage treatment of heatstroke: Comparative efficacy in a canine model. Am J Emerg Med 1993;11:1-3.
61. Bouchama A, Cafege A, Devol EB, et al: Ineffectiveness of dantrolene sodium in the treatment of heatstroke. Crit Care Med 1991;19:176-180.
62. Zucherman GB, Singer LP, Rubin DH, et al: Effects of dantrolene on cooling times and cardiovascular parameters in an immature porcine model of heatstroke. Crit Care Med 1997;25:135-139.
63. Quane KA, Healy JM, Keating KE, et al: Mutations in the ryanodine receptor gene in central core disease and malignant hyperthermia. Nat Genet 1993;5:51-55.
64. Brandon BW: The genetics of malignant hyperthermia. Anesthesiol Clin North Am 2005;23:615-619.
65. Denborough M: Malignant hyperthermia. Lancet 1998;352: 1131-1136.
66. Moulds RFW, MA Denborough MA: Identification of susceptibility to malignant hyperthermia. BMJ 1974;2:245-247.
67. European Malignant Hyperpyrexia Group: A protocol for the investigation of malignant hyperpyrexia (MH) susceptibility. Br J Anaesth 1984;56:1267-1269.
68. Chan TC, Evans SD, Clark RF: Drug-induced hyperthermia. Crit Care Clin 1997;13:785-808.
69. Caroff SN, Mann SC: Neuroleptic malignant syndrome. Med Clin North Am 1993;77:185.
70. Balzan MV: The neuroleptic malignant syndrome: A logical approach to the patient with temperature and rigidity. Postgrad Med J 1998;74:72-76.
71. Bywaters EG, Beall D: Crush injuries with impairment of renal function. J Am Soc Nephrol 1998;9:322-332.
72. Sever MS, Vanholder R, Lameire N: Management of crush-related injuries after disasters. N Engl J Med 2006;354:1052-1063.
73. Sever MS, Erek E, Vanholder R, et al: Renal replacement therapies in the aftermath of the catastrophic Marmara earthquake. Kidney Int 2002;62:2264-2271.
74. Ballantyne CM, Corsini A, Davidson MH, et al: Risk for myopathy with statin therapy in high-risk patients. Arch Intern Med 2003;163:553-564.
75. Huerta-Alardin AL, Varon J, Marik PE: Bench-to-bedside review: Rhabdomyolysis—an overview for clinicians. Crit Care 2005;9:158-169.
76. Allison RC, Bedsole DL: The other medical causes of rhabdomyolysis. Am J Med Sci 2003;326:79-88.
77. Knochel JP: Mechanisms of rhabdomyolysis. Curr Opin Rheumatol 1993;5:725-731.
78. Malinoski DJ, Slater MS, Mullins RJ: Crush injury and rhabdomyolysis. Crit Care Clin 2004;20:171-192.
79. Zager RA: Studies of mechanisms and protective maneuvers in myoglobinuric acute renal injury. Lab Invest 1989;60:619-629.
80. Harris K, Walker PM, Mickle DA, et al: Metabolic response of skeletal muscle to ischemia. Am J Physiol 1986;250(2 Pt 2):H213-H220.
81. Olerud JE, Homer LD, Carroll HW: Incidence of acute exertional rhabdomyolysis. Serum myoglobin and enzyme levels as indicators of muscle injury. Arch Intern Med 1976;136: 692-697.
82. Lofberg M, Jankala H, Paetau A, et al: Metabolic causes of recurrent rhabdomyolysis. Acta Neurol Scand 1998;98:268-275.
83. de Meijer AR, Fikkers BG, de Keijzer MH, et al: Serum creatine kinase as predictor of clinical course in rhabdomyolysis: A 5-year intensive care survey. Intensive Care Med 2003;29:1121-1125.
84. Lappalainen H, Tiula E, Uotila L, Manttari M: Elimination kinetics of myoglobin and creatine kinase in rhabdomyolysis: Implications for follow-up. Critic Care Med 2002;30: 2212-2215.
85. Grossman RA, Hamilton RW, Morse BM, et al: Nontraumatic rhabdomyolysis and acute renal failure. N Engl J Med 1974;291:807-811.
86. Gunal AI, Celiker H, Dogukan A, et al: Early and vigorous fluid resuscitation prevents acute renal failure in the crush victims of catastrophic earthquakes. J Am Soc Nephrol 2004;15:1862-1867.
87. Vanholder R, Sever MS, Erek E, Lameire N: Rhabdomyolysis. J Am Soc Nephrol 2000;11:1553-1561.
88. Odeh M: The role of reperfusion-induced injury in the pathogenesis of the crush syndrome. N Engl J Med 1991;324:1417-1422.
89. Zager RA: Rhabdomyolysis and myohemoglobinuric acute renal failure. Kidney Int 1996;49:314-326.
90. Brown CVR, Rhee P, Chan L, et al: Preventing renal failure in patients with rhabdomyolysis: Do bicarbonate and mannitol make a difference? J Trauma 2004;56:1191-1196.
91. Visweswaran P, Massin EK, Dubose TD Jr: Mannitol-induced acute renal failure. J Am Soc Nephrol 1997;8:1028-1033.
92. Better OS, Stein JH: Early management of shock and prophylaxis of acute renal failure in traumatic rhabdomyolysis. N Engl J Med 1990;322:825-829.
93. Sever MS, Erek E, Vanholder R, et al for the Marmara Earthquake Study Group: Treatment modalities and outcome of the renal victims of the Marmara earthquake. Nephron 2002;92:64-71.
94. Nolph KD, Whitcomb ME, Schrier RW: Mechanisms for inefficient peritoneal dialysis in acute renal failure associated with heat stress and exercise. Ann Intern Med 1969;71:317-336.
95. Naka T, Jones D, Baldwin I, et al: Myoglobin clearance by super high-flux hemofiltration in a case of severe rhabdomyolysis: A case report. Crit Care 2005;9:R90-R95.
96. Akmal M, Goldstein DA, Telfer N, et al: Resolution of muscle calcification in rhabdomyolysis and acute renal failure. Ann Intern Med 1978;89:928-930.
97. Heppenstall RB, Sapega AA, Izant T, et al: Compartment syndrome: A quantitative study of high-energy phosphorus compounds using ^{31}P-magnetic resonance spectroscopy. J Trauma 1989;29:1113-1119.
98. Better OS, Rubinstein I, Reis DN: Muscle crush compartment syndrome: Fulminant local edema with threatening systemic effects. Kidney Int 2003;63:1155-1157.
99. Better OS, Zinman C, Reis DN, et al: Hypertonic mannitol ameliorates intracompartmental tamponade in model compartment syndrome in the dog. Nephron 1991;58:344-346.

PART

VIII ADMINISTRATIVE, ETHICAL, AND PSYCHOLOGICAL ISSUES IN CARE OF THE CRITICALLY ILL

Chapter 71

Intensive Care Unit Administration and Performance Improvement

Sean Townsend and Carolyn Bekes

Delivery of critical care services continues to represent a disproportionate share of health care expenditures relative to the proportion of patients who use these services. The federal Medicare program has become the largest provider of health care insurance in the United States and in 2002 accounted for nearly 30% of annual payments to hospitals.[1] An analysis of Medicare admissions in 2000 determined that cases involving a stay in an intensive care unit (ICU) cost nearly three times as much as those limited to the general care wards. Nevertheless, only 83% of the cost of the care of ICU patients was reimbursed, compared with 105% for patients cared for on the general care floors.[2]

Against this lean background, ICU administrators must plan for expected needs, improve on the efficiency and quality of care, and adequately staff their organizations. Additional challenges include coping with a pending reduction in the size of the critical care workforce concomitant with an increase in the proportion of patients utilizing these resources. Administrators must respond to pressures from external organizations to meet higher standards of care delivery. These tasks are not insurmountable. The ICU leadership in cooperation with administration is uniquely positioned to respond to these problems. In the ICU, the relatively small number of ICU beds, a compartmentalized physical plant, and the large degree of control that leaders can exert over the environment make it a fertile ground for change.

Accordingly, the principal consideration for ICU administrators becomes a question of what type of structure and leadership their ICU will need to accomplish its mission. Typically, ICUs have been structured along the lines of tertiary, large community, and small community hospitals. These hospitals have different aims and goals and differing capacities to respond to acuity in the care of patients. Likewise, most ICUs have a designated ICU director with roles and responsibilities commensurate with those goals. Standards of care for typical arrangements have been described in the literature.[3] An essential function of ICU administration is to determine and specifically articulate the ICU's relationship to these standards.

Once an ICU's structure and leadership is well established, administrators may turn their attention to addressing the challenges presented by economic, market, and technological forces. Increasingly, well-run ICUs have striven to promote an ICU culture that aims for efficiency while continuously improving the quality of care provided to patients. Performance improvement seeks to integrate best scientific practice into the care of critically ill patients. Regardless of the type of structure and leadership selected for a particular ICU, a focus on quality improvement can optimize function and build efficiencies to care for critically ill patients.

THE PRESENT-DAY CRITICAL CARE LANDSCAPE

In order to describe an agenda for administrators and leaders of ICUs, a critical appraisal of the current state of affairs in critical care delivery is essential. This section begins with a survey of what is known about the scope, size, and structure of the critical care landscape today. Then, the available best practice guidelines for ICU administration in any hospital environment are reviewed as a basis for quality improvement in the field of critical care.

Three studies form the basis of current understanding of critical care in the United States today. The first study was completed by Groeger and colleagues in 1992 and aimed to gather data about available technology, staffing, administrative policies, and bed capacities of ICUs in the United States.[4] These data were reanalyzed in 1993 with the intent of gathering information about occupancy, admission characteristics, patients' ages, and types of therapy used in ICUs in the United States.[5]

In this study, survey data were obtained from 1706 hospitals registered with the American Hospital Association. Information was obtained for 32,850 ICU beds with 25,871 patients from 2876 separate ICUs. The response rate to the survey mailing was 40%, which resulted in an estimate of 6000 ICUs and 72,000 ICU beds nationally. Findings included that the number of ICU beds per hospital increases with overall hospital size. The average ICU size, nationally, was 11.7±7.8 beds per unit. Thirty-six percent of the units were located within the hospital's department of medicine; 23% had no departmental affiliation. The perception of whether the medical director of the ICU supervised daily activities varied directly with unit size. Overall, an internist directed 63% of all ICUs, and in 44% of all units, the medical director was board certified in critical care medicine. Sixty-one percent of medical directors served part-time, and 51% were unpaid for their activities.

The study also concluded that most ICUs surveyed were combined medical-surgical-coronary care units. As indicated by the patient sample, 10% of ICU patients were in hospitals with less than 100 beds, 40% in hospitals with 100 to 300 beds, 30% in hospitals with 300 to 500 beds, and 20% in hospitals with more than 500 beds.

A second study completed in 2000 was published as a joint effort on behalf of the American Thoracic Society (ATS), the American College of Chest Physicians (ACCP), and the Society of Critical Care Medicine (SCCM).[6] The Committee on Manpower for the Pulmonary and Critical Care Societies (COMPACCS) study estimated current and future requirements for adult critical care and pulmonary medicine physicians in the United States. Angus and coworkers, on behalf of the COMPACCS group, extended their inquiry in 2006 to profile the organization and distribution of ICU patients and services in the United States.[7]

The initial COMPACCS study concluded that in 1997, intensivists provided care to 36.8% of all ICU patients and that intensivist level care was more common in regions with high managed care penetration. The 2006 update estimated that there were 5980 ICUs in the United States, caring for approximately 55,000 patients per day. Sixty-five percent of ICUs were combined medical-surgical ICUs; 71% were located in nonteaching community hospitals; and 62% of all ICUs were located in hospitals with fewer than 300 beds.

Other important findings in the initial COMPACCS study included projections related to physician demand in the critical care workforce. Supply was expected to equal demand until 2007, when demand is expected to grow rapidly as the population ages rapidly. The supply of critical care physicians will remain near constant during the rising demand, however, producing a shortfall of 22% of demand by 2020 and 35% by 2030.

The third study, a 2006 report to Congress from the U.S. Department of Health and Human Services' Health Services and Resource Administration (HSRA), updated the findings in COMPACCS with respect to the critical care workforce.[8] The analysis had been requested by the U.S. Senate in response to the physician shortfalls noted in the COMPACCS study. The HRSA report essentially reaffirmed the emerging crisis described in the COMPACCS study. The HSRA workforce analysis indicated that the growth and aging of the population alone will increase demand for adult intensivist services by at least 38% between 2000 and 2020. If the proportion of ICU patients whose care is directed by an intensivist increases from the present 30% to 60%, demand may reach 129% of the expected supply. Similarly, critical care nursing availability remains a seller's market, and recruitment and retention strategies are paramount to maintain high-quality nursing care (Box 71-1).

Box 71-1

Reasons for Nursing Turnover and Retention Strategies

Why Nurses Leave

- Increased market demand
- Heavy workload/inadequate staffing
- Better pay elsewhere
- More flexible scheduling elsewhere
- Better career/developmental opportunities elsewhere
- More desirable work culture elsewhere
- Better benefits elsewhere
- Inadequate managerial skills
- Physician relationships
- Better employer reputation elsewhere

Retention Strategies

- Enhancing supplemental pay plans
- Increasing base pay
- Retention bonuses
- Variable pay/incentives
- Flexible scheduling/shifts
- Addressing staffing needs using rotations/float pools
- Staffing support using unlicensed personnel
- New clinical advancement programs
- Enhanced continuing education
- Regular staff input/surveys
- New processes to assist in delivery of care
- Changing patient care delivery model
- Increasing staff understanding of organizational mission, goals and initiatives
- Management training/skill building
- Enhancing collaboration with support departments
- Physician relations programs
- New work environment/culture initiatives

From Medical Economics 2000;77:33.

Despite expected reductions in available manpower, calls for increased access to intensivists continue. These solicitations are based on multiple studies demonstrating mortality and cost-savings benefits to critically ill patients receiving care by intensivists. Young and Birkmeyer estimated that in the context of 360,000 deaths occurring each year in ICUs, 54,000 lives may be saved annually with intensivist staffing.[9] Similarly, Pronovost and colleagues have estimated that more than $5 billion could be saved annually.[10] A report generated for the Agency for Healthcare Research and Quality (AHRQ) notes that these benefits alone underestimate the potential improvement in the quality of care in terms of fewer complications, avoiding inappropriate utilization, decreased patient suffering, and better end-of-life care.[11]

Recently, a consortium of Fortune 500 companies that spend in excess of $45 billion annually on health care for their employees formed to leverage their purchasing power to improve the quality of care, forming what is known as The Leapfrog Group. This powerful group has specifically called for (1) the use of computerized physician order entry, (2) the oversight of critical care physicians in the care of ICU patients, and (3) the use of evidence-based hospital referral systems. The influence of this group on both payers and health systems alike has contributed to the increasing demand for intensivists to care for critically ill patients. Unfortunately, the 2006 update to the COMPACCS study suggests that this need has gone essentially unmet. Loosely defining Leapfrog-compliant intensivist coverage for 80% of critically ill patients and the presence of 24-hour in-house physician coverage, Angus and colleagues found that only one in four ICUs had 80% intensivist coverage, and that half had no intensivist coverage. Very few hospitals provided in-house physician coverage during off hours: 20% during weekend days, 12% during weekday nights, and 10% during weekend nights. Overall, only 4% of adult ICUs in the United States appeared to meet even a liberal interpretation of Leapfrog standards.

On the basis of the information cited in these studies, several conclusions can be drawn with reasonable certainty. Of the 6000 ICUs in the United States, more than half are combined medical-surgical units located in hospitals with fewer than 300 beds. These ICUs are in predominantly nonteaching facilities and care for 50% of the critically ill patients in the United States at any given time. Collectively, fewer than half of the medical directors in the United States are board certified in critical care medicine, and only one third of critically ill patients benefit from treatment by intensivists. Most ICU directors are part-time employees, and about half are unpaid for their work. Although savings of tens of thousands of lives and perhaps billions of dollars may be possible annually with intensivist staffing, even a liberal model to assess compliance with Leapfrog standards shows virtually no market penetration. All estimates completed to date suggest that these statistics will only darken as a shortage of critical care–trained physicians becomes more apparent with the aging of the U.S. population.

IDEALIZED DESIGN FOR CRITICAL CARE PRACTICE

In the face of an emerging demand-driven crisis in critical care, the task of effective ICU administration will only become a more difficult challenge. Nevertheless, efforts must be made to adapt care delivery patterns to the emerging demand crisis. Failure to develop new patterns of critical care delivery will ensure inadequate care for thousands of patients for years to come. In the absence of renewed planning, failure probably will evolve slowly, first affecting vulnerable populations, such as the uninsured and those located in rural areas. As time passes, a larger and larger proportion of Americans will receive less than the ideal standard of care.

As solutions to this crisis emerge, a key first step is to halt further deterioration in present practice. Effective coordinating and communication strategies in the ICU and with other areas can help to mitigate further erosion in practice standards and will be a prerequisite to reform (Boxes 71-2 and 71-3). Strategies to refine critical care

Box 71-2

Examples of Best Practices for Coordinating Care in the Intensive Care Unit

Within the Intensive Care Unit

- Specific guidelines and protocols for medical and nursing care
- Physician credentialing for selected procedures (e.g., intubation, invasive monitoring)
- Updated protocols for limiting life-supporting therapy
- Physician rounds made early, facilitating communications and planning by nurses
- Orientation, written guidelines, and close supervision for residents
- Rounds and conferences with pharmacist, dietitian, radiologist
- Emphasis on decentralized services (satellite pharmacy, laboratory, and radiograph viewing) or close to ICU
- Guidelines for nursing change of shift report

Between the Intensive Care Unit and Other Areas

- New nurses oriented to emergency, recovery, step-down units
- Standardized nursing reports for patients transferred from ICU; interunit conferences for long-term, complex cases
- Floor care for hopelessly ill or chronically ventilated patients with a do-not-resuscitate order and other treatment limits
- Direct phone line from visiting area to unit clerk
- Administrative and support services with emphasis on importance of satisfying "internal" customers

From Zimmerman JE, Shortell SM, Rousseau DM, et al: Improving intensive care: Observations based on organizational case studies in nine intensive care units: A prospective, multicenter study. Crit Care Med 1993;21:1443.

Box 71-3

Examples of Best Communication Practices

- Bulletin boards used to highlight important messages
- Communication books for facilitating information transfer
- Regular, consistent staff meetings with a set agenda and staff input
- Brief, group change-of-shift report followed by individual bedside reports
- Nurse manager available to staff through regular visits on all shifts
- Working paging systems; immediate response 24 hours a day, 7 days a week
- Charting systems that are user friendly, clear, and readily available
- Daily rounds promoting high levels of interaction between nurses and physicians
- Multidisciplinary forums for information sharing
- Social workers used to facilitate communication with patients' families
- Open visiting hours for family members
- Rotating shifts for orienting new nurses
- Standard evaluation form for registry/agency nurses

From Zimmerman JE, Shortell SM, Rousseau DM, et al: Improving intensive care: Observations based on organizational case studies in nine intensive care units: A prospective, multicenter study. Crit Care Med 1993;21:1443.

Box 71-4

Levels of Critical Care

Level I critical care: Level I critical care centers have ICUs that provide comprehensive care for a wide range of disorders requiring intensive care.[3] They require the continuous availability of sophisticated equipment, specialized nurses, and physicians with critical care training. Support services including pharmacy services, respiratory therapy, nutritional services, pastoral care, and social services are comprehensive. Although most of these centers fulfill an academic mission in a teaching hospital setting, some may be community-hospital based.

Level II critical care: Level II critical care centers have the capability to provide comprehensive critical care but may not have resources to care for specific patient populations (e.g., cardiothoracic surgery, neurosurgery, trauma). Although these centers may be able to deliver high-quality care to most critically ill patients, transfer agreements must be established in advance for patients with specific problems. The ICUs in level II centers may or may not have an academic mission.

Level III critical care: Hospitals that have level III capabilities have the ability to provide initial stabilization of critically ill patients, but they are limited in the ability to provide comprehensive critical care. These hospitals require written policies addressing the transfer of critically ill patients to critical care centers that are capable of providing the comprehensive critical care required (level I or level II). These facilities may continue to admit and care for a limited number of ICU patients for whom care is routine and consistent with hospital and community resources.

Adapted from Haupt MT, Bekes CE, Brilli RJ, et al: Guidelines on critical care services and personnel: Recommendations based on a system of categorization of three levels of care. Crit Care Med 2003;3:267-268.

delivery and meet predicted needs are already evident in the literature. It will be necessary to take advantage of efficiencies that have proved effective in analogous settings such as trauma care. Likewise, it is appropriate to build on current designs to streamline access to critical care by adopting best practice guidelines. Hospital systems will need to collaborate on the care of critically ill patients in order to distribute critical care equitably as a resource, a social commodity. Finally, a realignment of values among health care leaders to build and reinforce a culture of efficiency, safety, and continuous improvement may stave off mediocrity.

Rational Model for Critical Care Delivery

A rational model for delivery of critical care should attempt to balance the needs of the community with access to the highest-quality critical care services within that area. The American College of Surgeons (ACS) set the precedent for national practice standards for specific sets of critically ill patients when trauma centers were organized. When patients sustain injury with possible trauma, their care is initiated at appropriate trauma centers, depending on readiness and capacity to deliver care. Each designated level of classification (levels I to IV) has associated standards designated by the ACS. The structure has redefined the care of trauma patients and has been associated with improved outcomes and decreased mortality rates.[12,13]

A similar approach is possible with regard to the more general category of critical care delivery. The American College of Critical Care Medicine (ACCM) of the Society of Critical Care Medicine has developed a system to segregate hospitals into specific categories based on readiness and capacity to deliver critical care services (Box 71-4). These guidelines were first published in 1999 and revised in 2003.[3] Application of these guidelines is an essential first step in developing efficiencies in the provision of critical care to patients. Appropriate application will allow facilities to take advantage of collaborative relationships and to ensure a streamlined approach to critical care delivery.

Although the ACCM guidelines set the stage for ideal function of hospitals within each classification, there remains a substantial performance gap between compliance with the guidelines and actual practice. To coordinate a hospital's provision of critical care services effectively, administrators should define their mission, thereby determining the range of services that their hospital seeks to offer patients. In doing so, it is instrumental to consider the population the hospital serves, the services provided by neighboring hospitals, and the subspecialties of the staff physicians. Other factors that may be informative in redesign include a list of common diagnoses in patients presenting for treatment and an assessment of the acuity of illness that is routinely treated.[3]

Even hospitals that appear to have well-integrated strategies can benefit from review of operating procedures. As part of the overall strategy for transition of hospitals into this operating model and as facilities' aims and goals and new care patterns are put into practice, it is reasonable to expect a large number of hospitals to be in transition at any given time. In addition, some degree of resistance to regionalization at the local level can be anticipated. Local hospital administrators will not want to forego revenue, community physicians will not want to "lose" patients to the referral hospital, and communities may resist loss of local services.

The specific standards that define level I and level II care are summarized in Box 71-5. Many hospitals will not be able to maintain these standards, and overlap with level II or level III critical care facilities may be considerable. Level II hospitals capable of providing comprehensive care for most diagnoses should attempt to emulate the level I guidelines for most conditions. For instance, a level II institution may not have the resources for optimal treatment of severe burns, but that facility may provide excellent surgical, cardiac, and post-transplantation

Box 71-5

Intensive Care Unit Leadership

A. A physician Unit Director is required. In general, the director should meet the guidelines for the definition of an intensivist as published by the Society of Critical Care Medicine. Specific requirements for the Unit Director include:
   1. Training, interest, and time availability to give clinical, administrative, and educational direction to the ICU
   2. Board certification in critical care medicine
   3. Time and commitment to maintain active and regular involvement in the care of patients in the unit
   4. Expertise necessary to oversee the administrative aspects of unit management, including formation of policies and procedures, enforcement of unit policies, and the education of unit staff
   5. The ability to ensure the quality, safety, and appropriateness of care in the ICU
   6. Availability (of either the Director or a similarly qualified surrogate) to the unit 24 hours a day, 7 days a week for both clinical and administrative matters
   7. Active involvement in local or national critical care societies
   8. Hospital privileges to perform relevant invasive procedures
   9. Active involvement as an advisor and participant in the organization of the care of the critically ill patient in the community as a whole
   10. Participation in the education of unit staff, other physicians, house staff, and medical staff as indicated
   11. Participation in scholarly activity (case reports, clinical and/or basic research)
   12. Active participation in the review of the appropriate utilization of ICU resources in the hospital

B. A Nurse Manager is appointed to provide precise lines of authority, responsibility, and accountability for the delivery of high-quality patient care. Specific requirements for the Nurse Manager include:
   1. An RN with a BSN or preferably an MSN degree
   2. Certification in critical care or equivalent graduate education
   3. At least 2 years of experience working in a critical care unit
   4. Previous management experience, including experience with health information systems, quality improvement risk management activities, and health care economies
   5. Preparation to participate in the on-site education of critical care unit nursing staff and physicians-in-training
   6. Ability to foster a cooperative atmosphere with regard to the training of nurses, physicians, respiratory therapists, and other personnel involved in the care of critical care unit patients
   7. Regular participation in ongoing continuing nursing education
   8. Ability to participate in, and foster cooperation for, scholarly activity in the ICU (e.g., presentations, clinical research)
   9. Knowledge about current advances in the field of critical care nursing
   10. Participation in strategic planning and redesign efforts

From Haupt M, Bekes CE, Bayly RW, et al: Critical care services and personnel: Recommendations based on a system of categorization into two levels of care. American College of Critical Care Medicine of the Society of Critical Care Medicine. Crit Care Med 1999;27:422.

medical care. Such a facility should aim to meet level I standards for conditions other than severe burns.

For level II or III institutions, a critical requirement of the guidelines is to establish agreements for transfer of patients for higher levels of care. It should be a usual practice in such facilities to stabilize patients with the intention to invoke established agreements to transfer to collaborating facilities.[14] Although completing transfers may be routine for ICU staff, the requirement for agreements established in advance with collaborating institutions to accept transfers may be novel. In order to develop the efficiencies that will be necessary in the emerging critical care environment, these types of prenegotiated arrangements will be necessary to ensure access to needed care.

The requirement to transfer also implies a burden of review on level II and level III centers to understand the treatment options available at more advanced centers with respect to a wide array of diagnoses. Although many administrators may assume that their clinicians maintain a full understanding of treatment options outside their facility, this assumption may be faulty. It is therefore appropriate with respect to specific diagnoses to develop codified procedures that demarcate established points in care suitable for transfer. These procedures may be incorporated as part of the envisioned interhospital agreement to coordinate transfers. Bed availability in the tertiary hospital may require alternative solutions in times of high occupancy.

Committing the national critical care infrastructure to reorganization in line with the ACCM guidelines will not shield critical care providers and their patients from evolving demographic and market forces. However, by advancing institutions' understanding of their own critical care infrastructure, needs, and capacity, and by establishing agreements for transfer between hospitals, the initiative will facilitate the movement toward regionalization of care. A study commissioned by the SCCM in 1994 suggested that regionalization of critical care services probably is beneficial to patients, in part by promoting access to larger academic institutions and resources, increasing subspecialty availability, and providing expertise in the care of the critically ill.[15]

In trauma systems, studies suggest that considerable efficiencies have been obtained with regionalization. Both mortality rates and hospital lengths of stay have decreased.[12,16] Transition to level I ACS status has incurred increased costs at some centers, whereas other centers indicate that certification reduced costs.[17,18] Beyond the financial impact of regionalization, the transition to a regional trauma system has promoted interhospital cooperation and promoted more effective resource utilization.[19,20]

Financial Modeling of Critical Care

The need for a transition to more rational structures in the provision of critical care services implies that hospitals will require an accurate accounting of costs and revenues as changes are made. In addition, as discussed next, quality improvement programs in the ICU rely on an accurate understanding of costs to measure benefit (or harm) from programs intended to improve the quality of care. A variety of financial models exist to assess costs in the ICU.[21,22] A given hospital's cost accounting system may determine whether the ICU is viewed as generating a profit or a loss. Traditional methods have focused on the ICU as a cost center but not as a venue that may be revenue generating.[23] Even in cases in which an ICU may always represent a net loss of revenue for an institution, understanding the revenue streams can permit optimization and diminish losses.

STATE OF CRITICAL CARE REIMBURSEMENT

The federal Healthcare Financing Administration, which formerly administered Medicare and Medicaid, was renamed in 2001 the Centers for Medicaid and Medicare Services (CMS). Data from CMS's Medicare Provider Analysis and Review (MEDPAR) database remain the single best public source to support understanding of the financial horizon for hospital administrators. Contributing 30% of annual payments to hospitals in 2002, Medicare is the single largest payor in the U.S. health care system.[1]

In 2004 Cooper and Linde-Zwirble analyzed all hospital admissions during 2000 as available in the MEDPAR database to determine the incidence, cost, and payment for ICU services among Medicare beneficiaries.[24] Their findings suggested that more than one fifth of all Medicare cases involved the use of ICU stays. Caring for ICU patients cost hospitals nearly three times as much as floor patients—$14,135 versus $5571. However, ICU cases were paid at a rate only twice that of floor cases—$11,704 versus $5835. This means that only 83% of costs were paid for ICU patients, compared with 105% for floor patients, generating an annual $5.8 billion loss to hospitals when ICU care is required.

Focus on Expenditures and Revenues

In view of the dramatic overall losses that hospitals sustain relative to expenditures on critical care patient services, a natural instinct among ICU administrators is to cut costs by reducing services. Hospital costs are best analyzed as either fixed or variable costs and as either direct or indirect expenditures. Fixed costs represent expenditures related to buildings, equipment, and certain labor costs; variable costs include items dependent on the volume of hospital operations, such as pharmaceutical expenditures and patient care supplies.

Reducing services is a flawed method to contain costs, however, because the fixed costs (and some variable costs) associated with the provision of critical care remain high and the differential savings achieved by limiting access to these services is small. Typically, direct patient care costs can be accounted to individual patients whose care generated those costs, and indirect patient care costs are averaged across all patients admitted to critical care. The indirect costs are not reduced when access to available services is limited. Reliable savings stem from elimination of services, rather than limiting access to or frequency of utilization of services.[25]

Moreover, the availability of sufficient services to care for the population at large remains essential. In line with the need to develop a more rational distribution of critical care delivery as outlined earlier, eliminating unnecessary services due to duplication in the community is appropriate. Once unnecessary or underutilized services have been eliminated, the next most appropriate steps to maximize ICU efficiency involve turning attention away from cost-cutting measures and toward revenue-enhancing strategies.

Critical Care as a Product Line

Bekes and colleagues have described a business plan for the critical care division of their hospital.[23] The plan isolated the major sources of critical care patients and their relative profit or loss for the division. In this analysis, using the usual cost accounting methods employed by the hospital, hospital-to-hospital transfers appeared to generate the most revenue. Focusing on this source of revenue as a unique "product line" enabled these clinician-investigators to promote these services more widely in the surrounding community.

Viable "products" may vary from institution to institution. Factors that may influence whether a particular service offered by the ICU is profitable or not include the availability of critical care resources in the community, the presence or absence of a stable network of hospitals for referrals, and the organizing structure of the institution (academic versus community, tertiary care versus otherwise, and so on). Presuming that the gap in reimbursement for critical care services noted in the Medicare data reflects patterns from other payors, many institutions may not be able to demonstrate a profit from their ICU regardless of identifiable sources of revenue. Nevertheless, in order to stave off losses of even greater magnitude, efforts to identify sources of revenue within critical care units will be essential as the health care market evolves.

CRITICAL CARE QUALITY IMPROVEMENT

Several market forces, as described earlier, in combination with clinicians' drive to provide the best possible care for ICU patients in a safe environment, have created a new paradigm in critical care delivery: quality improvement. Although quality improvement in health care may not seem novel to practitioners involved in the day-to-day delivery of critical care, the field, much like critical care as a specialty, is relatively new. Many organizations and participants have begun to outline the scope of the field, but at present the boundaries of critical care quality improvement are defined only by a consensus of the involved parties. Critical care quality improvement initiatives are less than reified, however, and they are increasingly becoming the lens through which many intensivists view their daily work in the ICU.

Background

In 1999, the Institute of Medicine (IOM) of the National Academies published a landmark report, *To Err Is Human: Building a Safer Health System.* The National Academies bring together committees of experts in all areas of scientific and technological endeavor to address critical national issues and give advice to the federal government and the public. The IOM report was widely hailed as groundbreaking in view of its documentation of the ways in which the health care system harms patients. Some of the findings about the American health care system included the following (1) tremendous gaps exist between medical knowledge and practice; (2) adverse events harm patients far too often; (3) too many people do not get the care they need; and (4) the system propagates waste by permitting fragmentation of care and utilization inefficiencies.[26] In *To Err is Human,* the IOM also estimated that despite incurring costs that are 40% greater than those for the next most expensive nation in terms of health care, 44,000 to 98,000 Americans die each year as a result of errors in their health care.

In 2003, in an exhaustive review of nearly 7000 patient charts across all regions of the United States, McGlynn and colleagues reported that the average defect rate, defined as the percent of cases in which care consistent with 439 indicators of quality was not delivered, approached 45% nationally.[27] Stated otherwise, patients receive the care indicated slightly more than one half of the time. These investigators concluded that the deficits identified in adherence to recommended processes for basic care posed a continuing immediate danger to the health of the American public.

Donabedian Framework

Building on work begun by Donabedian, the IOM published *Crossing the Quality Chasm: A New Health System for the 21st Century* in 2001. The report outlined fundamental changes that must be made in order to improve health care in the United States. Donabedian had described three components of quality care: structure, process, and outcome, each of which must be addressed to effectively control and manage quality in health care settings.[28] He proposed that each overarching concept of control should be monitored using specific tools (Table 71-1). The IOM report also refined Donabedian's seven attributes of high-quality health care, proposing instead six primary aims: safety, effectiveness, patient-centeredness, timeliness, efficiency, and equity.[29]

Table 71-1. Relations between Quality Areas and Management Tools with Their Relative Importance

	Management Tools		
Quality Area	Standards	Guidelines	Indicators
Structures	+++	+	+
Processes	++	+++	++
Results/outcomes	+	++	+++

Reproduced from Frutiger A, Moreno R, Carlet J, et al for the Working Group on Quality Improvement of the European Society of Intensive Care Medicine: A clinician's guide to the use of quality terminology. Intensive Care Med 1998;24:860-863.

Quality Improvement Landscape

Based on formidable critiques of the quality of the U.S. health care system, a variety of organizations either willingly have taken up the challenge to improve health care or, through legislation, have been empowered to improve the delivery of health care in the United States. All of these efforts have led to creation of agencies or activities with relevance to the ICU.

Agency for Healthcare Research and Quality

Funding for health services research is achieved primarily through grant applications to the AHRQ. Lucian Leape and Donald Berwick report that the Center for Quality Improvement and Safety, a division of AHRQ, has emerged as a leader in education, training, convening agenda setting workshops, disseminating information, developing measures, and facilitating the setting of standards.[30] AHRQ supports and funds efforts to evaluate best practices, medical errors, and development of patient safety indicators. The agency also has articulated an agenda that promotes the advancement of evidence-based best practices.

In 2001, Congress appropriated $50 million in annual funding for general patient safety research through AHRQ. Within 3 years these funds were assigned to an information technology focus. Leape and Berwick, key health care quality opinion leaders, lamented that this initial funding and subsequent reversal both legitimized health services research and at the same time starved these new researchers of the ability to undertake additional efforts.[30]

National Quality Forum

The National Quality Forum (NQF) has maintained close alignment with the platform advanced by the AHRQ. The NQF is a private, not-for-profit membership organization created to develop and implement a national strategy for health care quality measurement and reporting. The group seeks to improve American health care through endorsement of consensus-based national standards for measurement and public reporting of health care performance data. Working with a broad base of health care interests including governmental agencies, insurers, and various medical associations, the NQF has prevailed upon hospitals to report compliance rates with their measures. In 2002 the NQF published a list of 30 evidence-based best practices ready for implementation. This list of practices was expanded in 2005.

The Joint Commission

The Joint Commission (JC), formerly the Joint Commission on Accreditation of Healthcare Organizations (JCAHO), evaluates and accredits nearly 15,000 health care organizations and programs in the United States. The Commission, commonly misunderstood to be a governmental agency, is an independent not-for-profit organization. This body seeks to continuously improve the safety and quality of care provided to the public through the provision of health care accreditation and support for services that foster performance improvement in health care organizations.[31]

In 2003, after NQF's publication of evidence-based safe practices, the JC required hospitals to implement 11 of these practices.[32] The JC also has taken a special interest in developing a set of ICU core measures that are at present part of its library of supplemental measures.[33] Reserve measures, unlike the core measures previously proposed by the JC to satisfy its ORYX* performance measurement requirements for accreditation, are available for hospitals that are seeking a set of voluntary measures to monitor ICU care.

The ICU JC reserve measures included six measures:

ICU 1: Ventilator pneumonia (VAP) prevention—patient positioning
ICU 2: Stress ulcer disease (SUD) prophylaxis
ICU 3: Deep vein thrombosis (DVT) prophylaxis
ICU 4: Central line–associated bloodstream infection rate
ICU 5: CU length of stay, risk-adjusted
ICU 6: Hospital mortality for ICU patients, risk-adjusted[34]

Reporting of the JCAHO ICU core measures was stopped July 1, 2005, after a decision was taken to align the measure set with those under development at CMS and a new entity, the Surgical Care Improvement Project (SCIP). SCIP is a collaboration among CMS, the Centers for Disease Control and Prevention (CDC), and more than 20 surgical organizations. Under this arrangement, JCAHO has agreed to refocus the ICU reserve measures to apply primarily to surgical care. Ultimately, once these standards are evaluated and approved through the NQF consensus process, they will satisfy ORYX performance measurement standards.[35]

Alignment of Efforts

The alignment of forces interested in promoting evidence-based standards of care has led to efforts to establish a single set of applicable measures for hospitals. Although NQF appears to remain the ultimate clearing house for the endorsement of national standardized measures, the Hospital Quality Alliance (HQA) has been instrumental in decreasing fragmentation in the development of national measures for quality of care. The HQA is a public-private collaboration including the CMS, the American Hospital Association, the Federation of American Hospitals, and the Association of American Medical Colleges. The HQA is supported by the AHRQ, NQF, JCAHO, American Medical Association, American Nurses Association, National Association of Children's Hospitals and Related Institutions, Consumer-Purchaser Disclosure Project, AFL-CIO, AARP, and U.S. Chamber of Commerce.[36]

The Leapfrog Group: Purchasers and Payers

The Leapfrog Group is a coalition of more than 160 large private employers and public purchasers that joined in 2000 to obtain leverage in health care purchasing decisions for employees. This powerful alliance purchases benefits for more than 34 million Americans and has strongly

*ORYX is the name of the Joint Commission's initiative to integrate performance measures into the accreditation process.

encouraged the adoption of a number of safer practices in hospitals, including computerized physician order entry systems, proper staffing of intensive care units, and the concentration of highly technical surgery services in high-volume centers. The group aims to "leapfrog" over key barriers as goals of their purchasing directives in order to overcome the poor value in the health care marketplace.[37] The most recent "leap" has focused on implementation of the NQF's Safe Practices.

Leapfrog relies on a survey of hospital quality and safety to inform its leadership about adherence to Leapfrog standards nationally. Completion of the survey is voluntary; however, it is required for certification of Leapfrog compliance.

The Institute for Healthcare Improvement

The Institute for Healthcare Improvement (IHI) is a not-for-profit organization with the self-declared aim of leading the improvement of health care throughout the world. Founded in 1991, The IHI has as its mission the acceleration of change in health care by cultivating promising concepts for improving patient care and turning those ideas into action. The IHI has championed the use of collaborative methods to produce improvement in health care and boasts a membership organization of more than 200 hospitals. These facilities benefit from initiatives to improve patient safety, to enhance the reliable delivery of quality care, and to refocus emphasis onto patient-centered care. The IHI has sought to develop idealized designs for specific aspects of health care, such as outpatient practice and critical care. Most recently, the IHI coordinated the 100,000 Lives Campaign to reduce mortality in hospitals throughout the United States. More than 3000 organizations shared in implementing a multifaceted platform of interventions. The IHI projected success of the project based on statistical estimates over an 18-month period.

Sponsored Statewide and Integrated Health System Collaboratives

As a national quality agenda has become better articulated, several critical care quality improvement projects have emerged at the state level. In Michigan, for instance, The Michigan Health and Hospital Association's (MHA) Keystone Center for Patient Safety & Quality was created in March 2003. In collaboration with patient safety experts at Johns Hopkins University, MHA launched Keystone: ICU. Keystone: ICU enjoys the participation of at least 120 ICUs and 70 hospitals. Johns Hopkins University and MHA estimate that the Keystone: ICU project saved 1574 lives, more than 84,000 ICU days, and greater than $175 million.[38,39] This initiative has been expanded to other states such as New Jersey and Rhode Island. Group purchasing organizations such as VHA and Premier, Inc. have launched similar national initiatives in critical care quality improvement available to their membership.

Pay for Performance

Beyond specific programs and agencies dedicated to critical care quality improvement, a growing interest has developed in harnessing economic forces to drive the health care quality agenda forward. The public health and policy literature is now replete with references to pay-for-performance initiatives. Private and public insurers, health care purchasing organizations, and quality improvement thought leaders have pressed for the establishment of pay-for-performance plans to drive the market toward meeting evidence-based standards.[40,41] Hospital accreditation bodies, physicians' groups, and hospital associations have responded with guidelines to ensure the fairness of pay-for-performance plans, however, most recognize the inevitable increase in such initiatives.[42,43]

Pay for performance has been variously described. One iteration refers to direct payments to physicians from hospitals, or less commonly from insurers, as a reward for high-quality performance. For example, the most recent general practitioner contract in the United Kingdom includes 146 performance measures across seven areas of practice. This contract rewards performance in accordance with the measures with financial incentives.[44] First-year results were recently reported: physicians exceeded projections of their performance and achieved a mean of 91% compliance with clinical guidelines. This resulted in payments estimated at $700 million more than expected.[45] Despite the seeming success of this program, there is no means to detect whether physicians' compliance efforts also may have detracted from quality in unmeasured patterns of care.[46]

Specific Quality Improvement Interventions in Critical Care

Several intervention-specific quality improvement initiatives in critical care have emerged in the past decade. Many organizations have committed resources to implement such initiatives based in part on high-profile campaigns to improve care and new regulatory or accreditation standards. Some of the strategies for ICU quality improvement benefit from standardized measures available through the NQF and others; however, as practitioners take notice of the growing imperative to change the way critical care is delivered, many cutting-edge initiatives are moving forward without a consensus on which quality indicators should be applied. Often, specific interventions are coupled to strategies that advance more general goals such as developing a culture of safety in the ICU to prevent harm.

Shewart Model for Process Improvement

Critical care quality improvement initiatives typically have been executed in the setting of collaborative efforts as initially championed by the IHI and adapted by other groups. The precise mechanisms of implementation for these initiatives vary, but most sponsored quality improvement initiatives encourage the use of small-scale experiments to test new ideas. The principle calls for organizations to make the process of scientific prediction a part of routine work and was first advanced in 1931 by Walter Shewart, a pioneer in industrial quality control. Shewart advocated the use of iterative "plan-do-check-act" (PDCA) cycles to systematically test new ideas, evaluate their results, and, if successful, implement them.[47] More

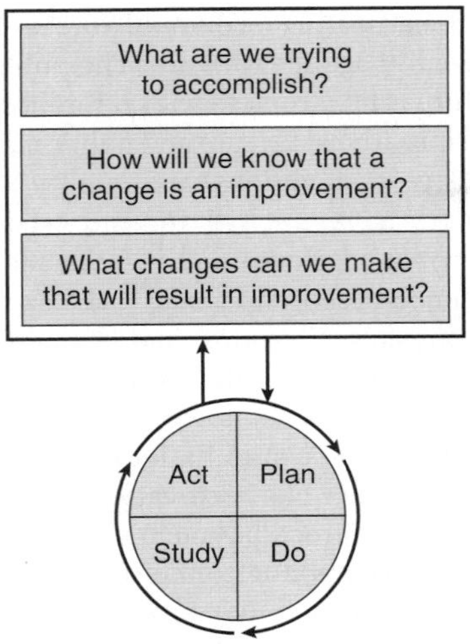

Figure 71-1. Institute for Healthcare Improvement (IHI) model for quality improvement. (From Langley GL, Nolan KM, Nolan TW, et al: The improvement guide: A practical approach to enhancing organization performance. Associates in Process Improvement.)

recently, the IHI has advocated a similar structure known as the Model for Improvement[48] (Fig. 71-1).

Decreasing Ventilator-Associated Pneumonia Rates

Reducing mortality due to VAP requires an organized process that guarantees the early recognition of pneumonia along with the uniform and consistent application of the best evidence-based practices. Despite variability in clinical definitions to establish valid criteria to diagnose VAP, institutions have devoted considerable effort to combating VAP rates. The most recent evidence suggests the selection of diagnostic criteria may be irrelevant to outcomes. The Centers for Disease Control and Prevention (CDC), however, has offered a clinical definition of VAP that has been widely adopted by the quality organizations cited earlier.[49]

The prototypical collaborative effort to decrease VAP rates has been use of the "ventilator bundle" promulgated by the IHI. The IHI ventilator initiative was initially launched to describe a pattern of best practices for ventilated patients, not to decrease VAP rates. A careful review of the literature on the care of ventilated patients produced four well-evidenced recommendations: elevation of head of the bed to 30 degrees, provision of a daily awakening or "sedation vacation," application of deep vein thrombosis prophylaxis, and provision of peptic ulcer disease prophylaxis. Although not components of IHI's ventilator bundle, several other practices with varying supporting evidence have become commonly applied as well, including the use of oral care techniques and subglottic suctioning.

Between July 2002 and January 2004, multidisciplinary improvement teams from 61 health care organizations participated in an IHI collaborative that included use of the ventilator bundle. Thirty-five of these teams consistently collected data on ventilator bundle element adherence and VAP rates. An average 44.5% reduction in the incidence of VAP was observed in these groups.[50] Sixteen units were medical-surgical ICUs, where the average VAP rate decreased from 5.5 to 2.7 cases per 1000 ventilator days.[50] By comparison, the nationwide VAP rate for medical-surgical ICUs reported by the CDC for the January 2002 to June 2003 period was approximately 6.0 per 1000 ventilator days.[51]

Decreasing Central Line–Associated Bloodstream Infection Rates

In an effort similar to that for decreasing VAP rates, decreasing central line–associated bloodstream infections (CLABSIs) has been a national priority in critical care quality improvement. The CDC has produced a standard measure that defines prevention of these infections as part of the National Healthcare Safety Network's (NHSN) patient safety component protocol.[52]

A typical approach to preventing CLABSIs has been advocated by the IHI and includes four elements of care: proper hand hygiene, use of chlorhexadine for skin antisepsis, routine application of maximal barrier precautions, and optimal site selection. In 2004, Berenholtz and colleagues reported that in using a similar strategy, the rate of CLABSIs fell from 11.3 to 0 per 1000 catheter days.[53] These results were estimated to have prevented 43 catheter-related bloodstream infections, 559 additional days in the ICU, and 8 deaths.[53] Cost savings were estimated to be $1,824,447.[53]

Deploying Rapid Response Teams

The rapid response team (RRT)—sometimes referred to in the literature as a medical emergency team—is a team of nurses and other health care professionals (respiratory therapists, pharmacists, emergency department personnel, and others) who bring critical care expertise to the bedside. The teams may or may not include physicians. The essential concept is intervening to prevent harm when nursing staff is urgently concerned about a patient's well-being. The key goal is to act before "failure to rescue" occurs and a patient has suffered a cardiac or respiratory arrest.[54]

The evidence supporting RRT adoption is mixed. Nevertheless, many hospitals have detected the need to have such a team to respond to urgent patient issues when physicians or housestaff may not be readily available. Several facilities that have implemented RRTs have reported a reduction in cardiac arrests and deaths, as well as a reduction in ICU and hospital bed-days among survivors of cardiac arrest.[55-57] Despite these findings, a single comprehensive negative trial has been published on the effects of MET/RRTs. Eleven hospitals functioned as usual, and 12 introduced an MET system. The investigators concluded that although the introduction of the MET system led to an increase in calls to the team, it did not substantially affect the incidence of cardiac arrest, unplanned ICU admissions, or unexpected death.[58]

Resuscitation and Treatment for Severe Sepsis or Septic Shock

Unique among projects to improve the quality of care for critically ill patients, the Surviving Sepsis Campaign (SSC) was formed in 2003 with the joint cooperation of the SCCM, the European Society of Intensive Care Medicine (ESICM) and the International Sepsis Forum (ISF). The campaign spearheaded the development and publication of the first evidence-based guidelines for the treatment of severe sepsis and septic shock in 2004[59] and later that year, in partnership with the IHI, transformed into a global performance improvement initiative replete with a bundle strategy, process, and outcomes measures.[60] The SSC has a 5-year goal to reduce mortality due to severe sepsis by 25% and has participants from around the globe.

Establishing Multidisciplinary Rounds

Multidisciplinary rounds enable all members of the team caring for critically ill patients to come together formally and offer their expertise as cases in the ICU are reviewed. Multidisciplinary rounds have been established in critical care units with various structures, either nurse-led or physician-led, meeting daily or regularly during the week.

Experience with applying multidisciplinary rounds suggests that although initial meetings may be wide-ranging and unstructured, they can become a vital adjunct to patient care. Specifically, they provide an opportunity for disciplines to share their knowledge of patient care needs and focus the entire care team on common goals. Surveys of institutional perceptions of the state of safety in ICUs have led to establishment of multidisciplinary rounds.[61] These rounds are a mainstay of the effort to change the culture of ICUs from compartmentalized care based upon a single discipline's knowledge to a more holistic approach integrating the talents of the many services caring for critically ill patients.[62]

Assessing Daily Patient Goals

Daily goals assessment allows all parties involved in the care of patients to formally keep track of plans established on either patient care rounds or multidisciplinary rounds and to verify their completion. This typically has been achieved in critical care units by using a daily goals worksheet completed by the rounding team.

One such tool was evaluated by Johns Hopkins University, the VHA, and the IHI in a prospective study. The tool was designed to facilitate explicit communication in the ICU, allow for independent redundancy to monitor key practices, empower nursing to carry out clear plans, increase nurse morale, and avoid duplicate work. The worksheets aimed to reduce ICU length of stay and mortality while increasing the care team's understanding of the daily goals for patients in the ICU. In addition, the worksheets were used to document specific items that must be accomplished for patients to leave the ICU; to identify the greatest safety risk to a particular ICU patient; to institute a reminder system that identifies key processes for patients on ventilators; to document the scheduled laboratory tests for a patient; to compile information about the age, number, and sites of catheters; and to organize daily work flow to include communication with the family.

All patients admitted to a 16-bed surgical oncology ICU were eligible for inclusion. The outcome variables assessed were ICU length of stay and percent of ICU residents and nurses who understood the goals of care for patients in the ICU. Baseline measurements were compared with measurements of understanding after implementation of a daily goals form. At baseline, less than 10% of residents and nurses understood the goals of care for the day. After implementing the daily goals form, greater than 95% of nurses and residents understood the goals of care for the day. After implementation of the ICU Daily Goals Worksheet, ICU length of stay decreased from a mean of 2.2 days to 1.1 days.[63]

Open versus Closed Intensive Care Units: Intensivist-Led Model

A prime example of a structural change (as in the Donabedian model described earlier) that may lead to improvement in the quality of care includes the establishment of an intensivist-led ICU service in medical ICUs. Although in other ICUs, such as neurosurgical units or pediatric units, it is commonly expected that the attending physician is an intensivist trained in that specialty, this has not been the rule in medical ICUs. Typically, mixed medical-surgical ICUs in the United States are "open" in that any physician on staff may admit patients to the ICU and write orders for care of that patient. A recent well-developed literature suggests that "closed" ICUs in which only medical intensivists care for medical patients may be associated with decreased morbidity, mortality, and length of stay.[64] Reorganizing ICU physician services in one organization by implementing an intensivist infrastructure has resulted in a 14% absolute risk reduction in mortality.[65]

Despite these findings, a number of barriers exist to adopting a "closed" model of care. These include excess inpatient bed capacity; reimbursement strategies that provide an incentive for nonintensivists to stay involved in ICU care; internal political barriers among the medical staff that hamper closure; and the growth of the hospitalist movement and an associated unwillingness to relinquish control of patients when admitted to ICU. Some intensivists have adopted a "consultative" model, rather than providing 24-hour patient coverage.[66]

CULTURE TRANSFORMATION AND ORGANIZATIONAL LEARNING

The ultimate goal of clinical quality improvement work of any sort remains that of creating a culture of enduring change that can absorb new initiatives and sustain gains earned in prior improvement efforts. Underscoring the long-term strategy of ICU culture change in describing improvement initiatives cannot be overestimated. If insufficient attention is paid to the context in which improvement efforts are set into motion, an environment unfamiliar with testing changes and hostile to deviations from routine will frustrate the project itself. To this end, as clinical initiatives are advanced, concern must be maintained for executing projects so as to encourage collaboration and cooperation among the persons who work in the ICU. Typically, these strategies involve crafting of change teams, devising and testing protocols to incorporate the concerns of the front-line users of the protocols, and adapting to local cultural needs and traditions while bringing in new ideas. In the course of this work, colleagues cease contemplating their work as discrete projects that can be finalized. Instead, they learn to constantly revise protocols and strategies in response to feedback from the front-line users. If these ideals are maintained in the rollout of key initiatives and structural changes, often a change in mindset from an organization of independent actors to one in which collaborative efforts promote organizational learning can take hold. Unfortunately, to make these cultural transformations gracefully, no scientific procedure is available that can guide the way. The talents of committed and patient people are essential.

KEY POINTS

- Critical care represents a disproportionate share of health care expenditures relative to the proportion of patients who access these services.
- Present trends suggest that demand for critical care physician and nursing care will exceed supply in the next 20 years.
- Administrative solutions to an emerging critical care crisis are possible and rely on efficiencies that may be obtained in care delivery.
- Market forces and clinicians' drive to provide the best possible care for ICU patients have created a new paradigm in critical care delivery: quality improvement.
- A variety of interventions have been identified to reduce mortality in critical care but need to be reliably implemented.

REFERENCES

1. Medicare Payment Advisory Committee (MedPAC): A Data Book: Health Care Spending and the Medicare Program. Washington, DC, June 2005, p 80.
2. Cooper LM, Linde-Zwirble WT: Medicare intensive care unit use: Analysis of incidence, cost, and payment. Crit Care Med 2004;32:2247-2253.
3. Haupt MT, Bekes CE, Brilli RJ, et al: Task Force of the American College of Critical Care Medicine, Society of Critical Care Medicine. Guidelines on critical care services and personnel: Recommendations based on a system of categorization of three levels of care. Crit Care Med 2003;31:2677-2683.
4. Groeger JS, Kalpalatha KG, Strosberg M, et al: Descriptive analysis of intensive care units in the United States. Crit Care Med 1992;20:846.
5. Groeger JS, Kalpalatha KG, Strosberg M, et al: Descriptive analysis of intensive care units in the United States: Patient characteristics and intensive care unit utilizations. Crit Care Med 1993;21:279.
6. Angus DC, Kelley MA, Schmitz RJ, et al: Current and projected workforce requirements for care of the critically ill and patients with pulmonary disease: Can we meet the requirements of an aging population? JAMA 2000;284:2762-2770.
7. Angus DC, Shorr AF, White A, et al on behalf of the Committee on Manpower for Pulmonary and Critical Care Societies (COMPACCS): Critical care delivery in the United States: Distribution of services and compliance with Leapfrog recommendations. Crit Care Med 2006;34:1016-1024.
8. U.S. Department of Health and Human Services Health Services and Research Administration: The critical care workforce: A study of the supply and demand for critical care physicians. Washington, DC, Health Services and Research Administration, 2006. Available at: ftp://ftp.hrsa.gov/bhpr/nationalcenter/criticalcare.pdf
9. Young M, Birkmeyer J: Potential reduction in mortality rates using an intensivist model to manage intensive care units. Eff Clin Pract 2000;3:284-289.
10. Pronovost PJ, Waters H, Dorman T: Impact of critical care physician workforce for intensive care unit physician staffing. Curr Opin in Crit Care 2001;7:456-459.
11. Rothschild JM: "Closed" intensive care units and other models of care for critically ill patients. In Making Health Care Safer: A Critical Analysis of Patient Safety Practices. AHRQ Evidence Report/Technology Assessment No. 43. Rockville, MD, Agency for Healthcare Research and Quality, 1999, p 413.
12. Cayten CJ, Quervalu I, Agarwal N: Fatality analysis reporting system demonstrates association between trauma system initiatives and decreasing death rates. J Trauma 1999;46:751-756.
13. Mullins RJ, Veum-Stone J, Hedges JR, et al: Influence of a statewide trauma system on location and hospitalization and outcome of trauma patients. J Trauma 1996;40:536-546.
14. Guidelines Committee of the American College of Critical Care Medicine, Society of Critical Care Medicine and American Association of Critical-Care Nurses Transfer Guidelines Task Force: Guidelines for the transfer of critically ill patients. Crit Care Med 1993;21: 931-937.
15. Thompson DR, Clemmer TP, Applefeld JJ, et al: Regionalization of critical care medicine: Task Force Report of the American College of Critical Care Medicine. Crit Care Med 1994;22:1306-1313.
16. Rutledge R, Fakhry SM, Meyer A, et al: An analysis of the association of trauma centers with per capita hospitalizations and death rates from injuries. Ann Surg 1993;218:512-524.
17. Dailey JT, Teter H, Cowley RA: Trauma center closures: A national assessment. J Trauma 1992;33:539-549.
18. DiRusso S, Holly C, Kamath R, et al: Preparation and achievement of American College of Surgeons level I trauma verification raises hospital performance and improves patient outcome. J Trauma 2001;51:294-299.
19. Guss DA, Meyer FT, Neuman TS, et al: Impact of a regionalized trauma system in San Diego County. Ann Emerg Med 1989;18:1141-1145.
20. Schwab W, Frankel HL, Rotondo MF, et al: The impact of true partnership between a university level I trauma center and a community level II trauma center of patient transfer practices. J Trauma 1998;44:815-819.
21. Noseworthy TW, Konopad E, Shustack A, et al: Cost accounting of adult intensive care: Methods and human and capital inputs. Crit Care Med 1996;24:1168-1172.
22. Edbrooke DL, Stevens VG, Hibbert CL, et al: A new method of accurately identifying costs of individual patients in intensive care: The initial results. Intensive Care Med 1997;23:645-650.
23. Bekes CE, Dellinger RP, Brooks D, et al: Critical care medicine as a distinct product line with substantial financial profitability: The role of business planning. Crit Care Med 2004;32:1207-12014.
24. Cooper LM, Linde-Zwirble WT: Medicare intensive care unit use: Analysis of incidence, cost, and payment. Crit Care Med 2004;32:2247-2253.
25. Roberts RR, Frotos PW, Ciavarella GG, et al: Distribution of variable vs. fixed costs of hospital care. JAMA 1999;281:644.
26. Kohn LT, Corrigan JM, Donaldson MS (eds); Committee on Quality of Health Care in America, Institute of Medicine: To Err Is Human: Building a Safer Health System. Washington, DC, National Academies Press, 1999.
27. McGlynn EA, Asch SM, Adams J, et al: The quality of health care delivered to adults in the United States. N Engl J Med 2003;348:2635-2645.
28. Donabedian A: Aspects of Medical Care Administration: Specifying Requirement for Health Care. Cambridge, MA, Harvard University Press, 1973.
29. Committee on Quality of Health Care in America, Institute of Medicine: Crossing

the Quality Chasm: A New Health System for the 21st Century. Washington, DC, National Academies Press, 2001.
30. Leape LL, Berwick DM: Five years after To Err Is Human: What have we learned? JAMA 2005;293:2384-2390.
31. Joint Commission on Accreditation of Healthcare Organizations: Joint Commission facts. Available at: http://www.jointcommission.org/AboutUs/joint_commission_facts.htm (accessed September 18, 2006).
32. Joint Commission on Accreditation of Healthcare Organizations: Joint Commission announces national patient safety goals. Available at: http://www.jcaho.org/news_room/latest_from_jcaho/npsg.htm (accessed December 3, 2002).
33. Joint Commission on Accreditation of Healthcare Organizations: Joint Commission measure reserve libary. Available at: http://www.jointcommission.org/PerformanceMeasurement/MeasureReserveLibrary/Spec+Manual+-+ICU.htm (accessed September 18, 2006).
34. Joint Commission on Accreditation of Healthcare Organizations: Specifications manual for national hospital quality measures—ICU. Available at: http://www.jointcommission.org/NR/rdonlyres/F9F58E03-D7EB-40CF-9189-4243273F6ff5/0/ICUManualPDF.zip (accessed September 18, 2006).
35. Joint Commission on Accreditation of Healthcare Organizations: ICU notification. Available at: http://www.jointcommission.org/NR/rdonlyres/9A4EB4A8-B229-4A5F-AF28-F14D9961C113/0/ICUNotificationtomeasurementsystems.pdf (accessed July 1, 2005).
36. U.S. Department of Health and Human Services, Centers for Medicare and Medicaid Services: Hospital quality alliance. Available at: http://www.cms.hhs.gov/HospitalQualityInits/15_HospitalQualityAlliance.asp (accessed September 18, 2006).
37. Galvin RS, Delbanco S, Milstein A, et al: Has the Leapfrog group had an impact on the health care market? Health Aff (Millwood) 2005;24:228-233.
38. Available at: http://www.leapfroggroup.org/about_us/how_leapfrog_works (acessed July 28, 2005).
39. Robeznieks A: ICU effort saved lives, money: Organizers. More than 70 hospitals took part in the Keystone: ICU program. Mod Health Care 2005;35:16.
40. Berwick DM, DeParle NA, Eddy DM, et al: Paying for performance: Medicare should lead. Health Aff (Millwood) 2003;22:8-10.
41. Fong T: Unfulfilled potential. More performance pay would improve care: NCQA. Mod Health Care 2004;34:12.
42. Pilonero T: JCAHO performance pay guidelines hard to meet. Health Care Strateg Manage 2005;23:1, 13-15.
43. Romano M: AMA sets some ground rules. Detailed conditions outlined for pay-for-performance. Mod Health Care 2005;35:17.
44. Eggleston K: Multitasking and mixed systems for provider payment. J Health Econ 2005;24:211-223.
45. Galvin R: Pay-for-performance: Too much of a good thing? Health Aff 2006;25:w412-w419.
46. Newhouse, JP: Pricing the Priceless: A Health Care Conundrum. Cambridge, MA, MIT Press, 2002, p 203.
47. Shewart W: Economic Control of Quality of Manufactured Product. Milwaukee, IL, ASOC Quality Press, 1980.
48. Langley GL, Nolan KM, Nolan TW, et al: The Improvement Guide: A Practical Approach to Enhancing Organizational Performance. San Francisco, Jossey-Bass, 1996,
49. National Healthcare Safety Network (NHSN) Patient Safety Component Protocol. Centers for Disease Control and Prevention. Available at: http://www.azhha.org/public/uploads/CDC%20PS%20Protocol.pdf (accessed December 25, 2006).
50. Resar R, Pronovost PJ, Haraden C, et al: Using a bundle approach to improve ventilator care processes and reduce ventilator-associated pneumonia. Jt Comm J Qual Saf 2005;31:243-248.
51. National Nosocomial Infections Surveillance (NNIS) System Report. Data summary from January 1992 through June 2003, issued August 2003. Am J Infect Control 2003;31:448-498.
52. National Healthcare Safety Network (NHSN) Patient Safety Component Protocol, Centers for Disease Control and Prevention. Available at: http://www.azhha.org/public/uploads/CDC%20PS%20Protocol.pdf (accessed December 25, 2006).
53. Berenholtz SM, Pronovost PJ, Lipsett PA, et al: Eliminating catheter-related bloodstream infections in the intensive care unit. Crit Care Med 2004;32:2014-2020.
54. Hillman K, Parr M, Flabouris A, et al: Redefining in-hospital resuscitation: The concept of the medical emergency team. Resuscitation 2001;48:105-110.
55. Buist MD, Moore GE, Bernard SA, et al: Effects of a medical emergency team on reduction of incidence of and mortality from unexpected cardiac arrests in hospital: Preliminary study. BMJ 2002;324:387-390.
56. Bellomo R, Goldsmith D, Uchino S, et al: A prospective before-and-after trial of a medical emergency team. Med J Austr 2003;179:283-287.
57. Priestley G, Watson W, Rashidian A, et al: Introducing critical care outreach: A ward-randomised trial of phased introduction in a general hospital. Intensive Care Med 2004;30:1398-1404.
58. Hillman K, Chen J, Cretikos M, et al: Introduction of the medical emergency team (MET) system: A cluster-randomised controlled trial. Lancet 2005;365:2091-2097.
59. Dellinger RP, Carlet JM, Masur H et al: Surviving Sepsis Campaign guidelines for management of severe sepsis and septic shock. Crit Care Med 2004;32:858-873.
60. Levy MM, Pronovost PJ, Dellinger RP et al: Sepsis change bundles: Converting guidelines into meaningful change in behavior and clinical outcome. Crit Care Med 2004;32(11 Suppl):S595-S597.
61. Pronovost PJ, Weast B, Holzmueller CG, et al: Evaluation of the culture of safety: Survey of clinicians and managers in an academic medical center. Qual Saf Health Care 2003;12:405-410.
62. Vazirani S, Hays RD, Shapiro MF, et al: Effect of a multidisciplinary communication and collaboration on physicians and nurses. Am J Crit Care 2005;14:1, 71-77.
63. Pronovost P, Berenholtz S, Dorman T, et al: Improving communication in the ICU using daily goals. J Crit Care 2003;1871-1875.
64. Pronovost PJ, Angus DC, Dorman T, et al: Physician staffing patterns and clinical outcomes in critically ill patients: A systematic review. JAMA 2002 Nov 6;288:2151-2162.
65. Pronovost P, Berenholtz S: A practical guide to measuring performance in the intensive care unit. Research Series, Vol. 2. Irving, Tex, VHA, 2002.
66. Gipe B: ICU administration. In Parrillo JE, Dellinger RP (eds): Critical Care Medicine: Principles of Diagnosis and Management in the Adult, 2nd ed. St. Louis, Mosby, p 1560.

Chapter 72

Ethical Considerations in Managing Critically Ill Patients

Marion Danis, Ezekiel Emanuel, and Henry Silverman

Critical illnesses and the interventions necessary to address them pose many ethical dilemmas for clinicians. Therefore, it is not surprising that critical care physicians encounter ethical dilemmas more often than do general internists.[1] The most frequent predicaments relate to end-of-life care, including decisions about termination of medical treatment, respect for patient autonomy, and conflicts among various parties involved in patient care. Less frequent quandaries stem from concerns about equitable use of resources, truth-telling, religious and cultural differences, and professional conduct.

The first section of this chapter focuses on ethical considerations in the everyday operation of the intensive care unit (ICU). The second section discusses the difficult ethical issues involved in decisions at the end of life. The third section discusses ethical questions involved in research in the ICU. Clinical practice and clinical research are fundamentally distinct enterprises, with different aims and different ethical requirements. In research, the interests of the patient are not the sole priority; but at the same time, the human subjects of ICU research must be protected.

THE DOCTOR-PATIENT RELATIONSHIP

Critical illness stresses the relationship between patients and hospital staff members caring for them. Patients with life-threatening illness often are frightened and feel isolated. Physicians and nurses often must make crucial decisions quickly and despite uncertainty about the consequences of various options. In addition, key decisions frequently must be made while patients are cognitively impaired or unable to communicate. Thus, a combination of the disease process and medical interventions often deprives patients of the power to control their lives.

As a rule, clinicians should follow the same ethical guidance in critical care situations as in less stressful contexts[2]: They should treat patients with respect. They should deal honestly with patients and should not reveal confidences entrusted to them, unless the well-being of others is threatened. They should act in good faith, keep promises and commitments, and try faithfully to meet fiduciary responsibilities to patients.

At the same time, ICU staff must balance competing moral obligations that may limit or override obligations to fidelity to one particular patient, such as the needs of other patients who are currently under their care or may need their care in the future. Various models of decision making have been proposed—ranging from an *informative* model, in which patients make the decisions quite independently after the clinician has offered sufficient information, to a more *paternalistic* model, in which clinicians make decisions based on their judgment of what is in the best interest of the patient.[3] The most commonly accepted model today is a *deliberative* model, in which the clinician gives the patient information about his or her condition and the medical options, along with their advantages and disadvantages, and the patient explains his or her values and preferences, and together they reach a treatment decision. Yet this model must be adapted to the extreme circumstance of critical illness.[4,5]

Clinicians in the ICU should assess each patient's cognitive ability, provide information, and involve the patient or the patient's family in decisions about his or her treatment to the extent feasible.

Most physicians do not follow the same model with every patient or in every encounter. Regardless of the model adopted, clinicians should heed the elements of good ethical practice when making their decisions (Box 72-1). ICU clinicians also should be attentive to the many facets of patients' lives that influence their views and preferences. For example, patients' families play a large role in shaping their experiences and beliefs and in supporting them, particularly when they are sick. Ethicists in North America initially took an approach to patient autonomy that ignored the family, but more recent thought has recognized the importance of the family's supportive role.[6,7]

Clinicians also should be sensitive to the needs of the family when a patient is sick.[8] Among these, according to a recent study, are the need to talk about negative feelings such as guilt and anger; to talk about the possibility of the patient's death; to be told what to expect before they go into the ICU for the first time; to visit at any time; to talk to the same nurse every day; to receive explanations that are understandable; to feel that there is hope; to have good food available in the hospital; to be assured that it is all right to leave the hospital for a while; and to feel accepted by the staff.[9]

Members of the ICU staff also should take note of the religious affiliation and cultural identity of their patients. However, they should not stereotype patients and presume to know what patients want based on their affiliation, but rather should be ready to inquire about each patient's views and should be respectful of diverse beliefs[10,11] (Box 72-2).

Communication with Patients

From an ethical standpoint, communication is an important component of respect for patients; it is an indispensable ingredient for learning about patients' needs, values, and preferences. Many factors undermine communication with patients and with families in the ICU: insufficient time for staff members and patients to get to know one another and develop a trusting relationship, discomfort or fear of talking about illness and death, focus on the patient's physiologic function, and lack of a conducive setting for communication. However, taking time to talk to patients and families on a daily basis is a crucial element of respectful care.

Often, the ICU clinician must convey bad news. Recommendations for breaking bad news include the following[12]:

- Use a location that is comfortable, quiet, and private.
- Set aside adequate time for discussion.
- Check what the patient or family already knows.
- Give some warning that there will be unfortunate news.

Box 72-1

Elements of Good Ethical Practice in Medical Decisions in the Intensive Care Unit

- Careful assessment of the patient's condition
- Evaluation of the risks and benefits of therapeutic options
- Clear communication with the patient or proxy to inform about options and identify plan of care
- Identification and respect for a competent patient's or proxy's preferences
- Plan of care based on clinical assessment and mutually identified goals
- Toleration of uncertainty when making decisions
- Toleration of disagreement between parties
- Ongoing dialogue to resolve difficult situations

Box 72-2

Guiding Questions for Attending to Diverse Perspectives of Critically Ill Patients

Language
- What language do the patient and family prefer to use to discuss illness and disease? How openly do they wish to discuss diagnosis, prognosis, and death itself?

Religion
- What is their religious background and how avid is their religious affiliation?
- What do the patient and family think about the sanctity of life, and how do they conceive of death?
- Do they believe in miracles? Do they believe in an afterlife? Do they believe the body should be handled in a certain way after death?

Social, Political, and Historical Context
- Do any of the following factors affect the attitudes of the patient and family: the patient's status in the family, country of origin, or experiences such as poverty, refugee status, past discrimination, or lack of access to care?

Beliefs about Illness
- What do the patient and family believe are the causal agents in illness, and how do these relate to the dying process?

Decision-Making Style
- Who makes decisions about matters of importance in the family?
- Are the patient and family fatalistic about the course of events, or do they wish to take active control of events?

Social Support and Resources
- What resources, including community and religious leaders, family members, and language translators, are available to aid in the complex effort of interpreting cultural dimensions of a patient's illness?

Adapted from Koenig B, Gates-Williams J: Understanding cultural differences in caring for dying patients. West J Med 1995;163:244-249.

- Let the patient's desire for information guide the discussion.
- Elicit and address the patient's reactions and concerns.
- Foster an appropriate level of hope.
- Be honest, caring, and empathic.

Communication with ventilated patients is particularly difficult. Clinicians should make every effort to use techniques designed to overcome communication barriers with ventilated patients.[13]

Decision Making for Cognitively Impaired Patients

Because many patients are, or may become, cognitively impaired, clinicians should frequently and repeatedly assess patients' capacity to understand their situation and make decisions. When patients are capable of decision making, they should be involved to the extent that they desire. Patients who have not prepared advance directives should be asked if they would like to prepare such a directive and should be asked to designate someone to hold durable power of attorney for them.

When such a conversation is not possible and no advance directive exists, clinicians should be aware that most states have laws that determine who has legal decision-making status for persons who have not assigned durable power of attorney. When no family member or other surrogate is available to make decisions on behalf of a decisionally incapacitated patient who needs emergency treatment, the physician in charge should carefully document the pressing necessity for treatment even without consent.

Collaborative Care

Care in the ICU is provided by a multidisciplinary team; good collaboration among its members is essential. Paying attention to the perspectives of all team members and respecting their skills and clinical judgment are ethically important and are associated with improved clinical outcomes.[14] Collaboration is valuable not only for individual patients' care but also to achieve optimal function of the unit as a whole.[15]

Avoiding Conflicts in the Intensive Care Unit

Because of the high stakes and emotional tension surrounding the care of critically ill patients, conflicts often arise among patient, family members, and staff. Strategies for avoiding conflict are worth pursuing because it often is difficult to resolve conflicts once they have arisen.

Conflict avoidance tactics should include the following: giving frequent information to families about patients' status, including realistic assessment of outcomes; acknowledging uncertainty regarding predictions, so that forecasts that do not come to pass are not an undue source of disappointment; coordinating the provision of information among ICU staff members, so that the patient and family receive consistent information about the patient's status and plans for care; and eliciting patient and family concerns.

Justice-Related Issues

Because critical care is expensive and limited in supply, clinicians should deliver critical care services in a manner that distributes the benefits fairly. Much of the ethics literature has focused attention on making decisions that will allocate critical care resources justly. The issue is one of distributive justice; it arises most frequently when clinicians decide whether to admit or discharge patients from the ICU, and when they face triage decisions during periods in which resources are limited. Less obvious instances obtain whenever a clinician considers whether to use a marginally beneficial intervention.

Several dominant, contending theories of distributive justice provide plausible underpinnings for making such decisions. *Utilitarian* theory is based on the tenet that one should act in a manner that promotes the greatest happiness for the greatest number of people. An act is morally right if it brings about a greater amount of good than any other possible act under the circumstances. Such an assessment is *consequentialist* in that it is based on expected outcome. *Egalitarianism* is another prominent contender. This view holds that all humans are equal and should be treated equally in similar circumstances. *Social contract* theory holds that a just arrangement can be identified by asking rational persons to consider what scheme they would agree to if they had no idea whether or when it might be applied to themselves.

The ethical theory most commonly applied to decisions about admission, discharge, and triage is a utilitarian one. In other words, those patients who are expected to gain the most benefit from intensive care are considered the ones who should receive it. Accordingly, patients who are so severely ill that they are likely to die despite intervention, and patients who are so minimally sick that ICU care will not add to the likelihood of their survival, should not receive ICU care. Patients whose conditions are chronic and devastating, such as those in a permanent vegetative state, often are included among patients who should not receive ICU care for any acute life-threatening events, because their underlying illnesses are not amenable to improvement.

Of interest, Baker and Strosberg have argued that the assumption that triage is based on a utilitarian theory of justice is not correct.[16] They point out that triage was developed by Larrey, surgeon general of Napoleon's army, as a strategy for systematically handling the wounded so that those who had to be attended to first got care without regard to rank, in keeping with the French Revolutionary commitment to liberty, equality, and fraternity. Baker and Strosberg suggest that an egalitarian form of triage is advantageous because the public is likely to voluntarily comply with it. Persons with normal "rational self-interest" would agree with it because it improves everyone's chances of survival. The chances of survival of the fatally wounded and the slightly wounded would not be significantly altered by deferred treatment. This optimal arrangement thus also is compatible with a social contract theory of justice.[17]

Although triage strategies have relied on the probability of survival, some authors have argued that this is too crude an outcome measure to guide triage. Englehardt and Rie have suggested that critical decisions to admit, continue care, or discharge patients should be based on a more complete formula that includes probability of successful outcome, quality of life, predicted length of life remaining, and cost of therapy.[18]

Admission Criteria

The Task Force on Guidelines of the Society of Critical Care Medicine (SCCM) and the American College of Critical Care Medicine (ACCM) has published recommendations for ICU admission and discharge.[19,20] Each ICU should create a specific policy that explicitly articulates admission and discharge criteria and defines the services that it provides to the population served. Compliance with the policy should be monitored, and the policy should be revised as needed. Any decision to deny a patient admission should be made by clinicians who are familiar with expert opinion and relevant literature and should use established guidelines. Standardized criteria and guidelines facilitate fair rationing because they enhance the likelihood that patients will be treated similarly.

Discharge Criteria

Discharge decisions should be guided by an assessment that less care is necessary and should take patient safety into account. Decisions to transfer a patient from the ICU to other hospital facilities should always be accompanied by good communication with the receiving team to avoid oversights and errors in care.[21] Straightforward indications would include, at one extreme, improvement in medical condition that obviates the need for further intensive therapy or, at the other extreme, a decision to end intensive care because of impending death. The ethically challenging aspect of discharge criteria involves the question of discharge when a patient's probability of survival is expected to be only minimally improved by remaining in the ICU, but the probability is not zero.

Triage

Triage decisions should be made explicitly and without bias. Ethnicity, race, gender, social status, sexual preference, and financial status should not be considered.[20] Factors that are appropriate to consider include probability of survival; likely functional outcome; age; chronic underlying conditions; marginal benefit to be gained; and preferences expressed by the patient or surrogate.[22] When the ICU is full, patients already in the ICU should not necessarily be given priority if someone else stands to benefit more from the care.[23] Like many ethically difficult decisions, triage decisions can be made more manageable by thinking proactively, every day, about the disposition of patients. For example, ICU physicians should regularly review the status of all patients in the unit to assess their degree of readiness for discharge in case the need for new admissions arises.[21] Application of this kind of strategy should involve cooperation with other patient care units in the hospital to arrange smooth transfer.

Even when policies are in place for fair triage through an admission approval process by a designated individual, attempts to circumvent admission rules by seeking permission from ICU clinicians or administrators who are on duty in the ICU, are fairly common.[24] Therefore, policies should be designed to anticipate—and resist—such backdoor efforts.

In addition to decisions about admission, discharge, and triage, ICU physicians frequently must deal with the question of whether to offer or withhold treatments from patients with ultimately fatal injuries or illnesses. The ethical reasoning behind decisions to ration possibly beneficial interventions should be clear in the clinician's mind[25]; this issue is discussed more fully later in the section on termination of medical care.

Because expected benefit is a crucial factor in decision making, it is important for critical care physicians to understand the limits of prognostic guidelines for patients with life-threatening illnesses.[26] Physicians should recognize the degree of uncertainty that surrounds mortality estimates. Although it is useful to consider a patient's expected outcome, and to use this prognosis to guide decisions, a false sense of certainty can lead to mistakes. Furthermore, communicating prognostic information with a false sense of certainty can lead to misunderstanding and subsequent distrust on the part of families. Prognostic scoring systems can serve as a useful baseline on which to build treatment recommendations, but firm thresholds should not be set. For a patient with a very uncertain prognosis, trying different treatments for short periods can avoid extended inappropriate treatments without denying care that has a minute chance of working. Medical decision making requires more than functional assessment and prediction. Scoring systems can provide an unbiased measure to help inform physicians' decisions, but such measures should not be adopted as absolute guides.[26]

Disparity in Use and Outcome of Intensive Care

Critical care clinicians should be aware that a number of studies show a pattern of disparity in use of intensive care that are the result of forces outside the ICU itself. Patients of lower socioeconomic status have higher mortality.[27] Patients who lack health insurance are less likely to be admitted to hospitals; once hospitalized, however, they are more likely to be admitted to the ICU and more likely to die in the hospital.[28] Patients with private attending physicians are likely to stay longer in the ICU. Intensive care providers should try to prevent inequitable use of resources in the delivery of critical care services.

Ethics Consultation in the Intensive Care Unit

In view of the many ethical dilemmas that arise in the ICU, proactive ethics consultation can be useful for reducing conflicts over treatment and for planning wise use of resources, as supported by good evidence.[29]

THE ETHICS OF END-OF-LIFE CARE

Historical Perspective

The first suggestion that physicians should withhold medical interventions from terminally ill patients probably dates to Hippocrates' injunction to "refuse to treat those [patients] who are overmastered by their disease, realizing that in such cases medicine is powerless."[30] In 1835, Jacob Bigelow urged members of the Massachusetts Medical Society to withhold "therapies"—such as cathartics and emetics—from hopelessly ill patients.[31] In 1848, John Warren, the surgeon who performed the first operation with ether anesthesia, urged that ether should be used "in mitigating the agonies of death."[32] In 1958, Pope Pius XII, in response to questions about resuscitating patients and maintaining comatose patients on respirators, stated that physicians had no obligation to use such "extraordinary" means to forestall death.[33] In 1976, the *Quinlan* case recognized a patient's right to refuse life-sustaining treatments.[34]

More recently, some groups have advocated broadening the right to refuse medical care to include euthanasia and physician-assisted suicide. Simultaneously, as highlighted in the *Schiavo* case, others have tried to restrict the right of surrogate decision makers to refuse medical treatments for patients who are mentally incapacitated. Finally, ethicists have recognized that a right to terminate care is not the sole concern. This recognition has led to a focus on providing optimal end-of-life care, instead of on patients' rights to engage in treatment decisions.

For physicians to understand acceptable practices for the termination of care, it is most useful to consider four topics: (1) legal standards; (2) advance care documents; (3) end-of-life care practices; and (4) euthanasia and physician-assisted suicide.

Legal Standards Regarding Termination of Medical Care

The Right to Refuse Medical Interventions

In its 1990 *Cruzan* decision, the U.S. Supreme Court recognized that competent patients have a constitutional right to refuse medical care[35] (Table 72-1). This was reaffirmed in later suicide cases. As Chief Justice William Rehnquist put it:

> [A]lthough *Cruzan* is often described as a "right to die" case . . . we were, in fact, more precise: we assumed that the Constitution granted competent persons a "constitutionally protected right to refuse lifesaving hydration and nutrition." . . . [A] liberty interest in refusing unwanted medical treatment may be inferred from our prior decisions.[36]

Competent patients need not be terminally ill to exercise this right to refuse interventions; they have the right regardless of health status. Moreover, the right applies both to withholding proposed treatments and to discontinuing initiated treatments. This does not, however, imply that patients have a correlative right to demand treatment.[37,38]

In theory, the right of patients to refuse medical therapy can be limited by state interests in the preservation of life, prevention of suicide, protection of third parties such as children, and preserving the integrity of the medical profession.[38] In practice, these interests almost never override the right of competent patients, or of incapacitated patients who have left explicit advance directives.

Although mentally incapacitated patients have the same right, the Supreme Court allowed states to impose restrictions on how explicit and specific the patient's prior wishes have to be.[35] The Court's consistent refusal to intervene in the *Schiavo* case on behalf of her parents' desire to continue nutrition and hydration is reaffirmation of this right even for mentally incapacitated patients.

Medical Interventions That May Be Stopped

Every medical intervention, including artificial nutrition and hydration, may be terminated under some conditions (see Table 72-1). Court decisions have sanctioned the withholding or withdrawal of respirators, chemotherapy, blood transfusions, hemodialysis, and major surgical operations. In *Cruzan,* the U.S. Supreme Court definitively stated that artificial nutrition and hydration can be withheld or withdrawn under the guidelines that apply to other medical treatments.[35]

In cases in which a patient's wishes may conflict with those of the family, the patient's right to refuse care is determinative. If mentally incapacitated patients have drawn up living wills or other advance care documents, the wishes in these directives are determinative.

If an incapacitated patient has not prepared an advance care directive, the patient's family usually is considered the most appropriate surrogate decision maker. In the 1980s, many court decisions affirmed the view that when patients have had explicit but unrecorded conversations with family, friends, or others about their wishes, these conversations should be used as decision-making guides. However, empirical studies suggest that spouses and other family members generally do not know the preferences of patients regarding the termination of life-sustaining treatments and may not make the same decision that the patient would have made.[39,40]

In *Cruzan,* the U.S. Supreme Court held that there is no constitutional requirement that families be permitted to exercise the right of mentally incapacitated patients to terminate care when the patients have not left explicit statements of their preferences.[35] Of importance, however, the Court did not delineate uniform national rules regarding who should decide for mentally incapacitated patients. Instead, the Court permitted each state to make the rules it deemed best. The Court also endorsed, as legally acceptable but not required, Missouri's requirement that the "evidence of the incompetent's wishes as to the withdrawal of treatment be provided by *clear and convincing* evidence" (emphasis added).

Recently, several state supreme courts have limited the right of families to decide for incompetent patients when there is no advance care directive or formal appointment of a surrogate decision maker.[41,42] These courts have accepted the proposition that when a patient is in a

Table 72-1. Major Legal Cases Regarding the Withholding or Withdrawing of Medical Interventions

Case and Citation	Year	State	Facts	Decision
In re Quinlan 70 N.J. 10	1976	NJ	21-year-old woman in a persistent vegetative state dependent on a respirator, artificial nutrition, and hydration.	The right to privacy includes a right to refuse medical care and extends to incompetent patients. Patient's guardian can withdraw her respirator. No need for judicial review in most cases.
Superintendent of Belchertown v. Saikewicz 373 Mass 728	1977	MA	67-year-old retarded man with a mental age of 2 years 8 months who had always lived in a state institution developed acute myelomonocytic leukemia. Did he have to receive chemotherapy?	All persons, including incompetent persons, have the right to refuse medical treatment. Using substituted judgment, the court determined that the patient would not want chemotherapy.
In re Eichner (Brother Fox) 52 N.Y. 2d 262	1981	NY	83-year-old priest was in a persistent vegetative state after a cardiac arrest. Before the event, he had publicly stated that he would not want to be respirator-dependent if he were vegetative.	Patients have the right to determine the course of their own medical care. Patient's wishes were known, even if not expressed in writing. Respirator should be withdrawn.
In re Conroy 98 N.J. 321	1985	NJ	84-year-old bedridden, totally impaired woman with organic brain syndrome fed by a nasogastric tube. Her nephew requested removal of the tube.	Nasogastric tube feedings are medical interventions that can be withdrawn.
Brophy v. New England Sinai Hospital 398 Mass 417	1986	MA	49-year-old man in persistent vegetative state after a ruptured aneurysm; maintained by gastric tube feedings. He had no written living will but had explicitly stated that he would never want to live on life support systems.	Common law and the constitutional right of privacy give a person the right to refuse medical treatment. The patient's wishes are clearly known from explicit conversations. The gastric tube can be withdrawn.
Bouvia v. Superior Court 225 Cal Rptr 297	1986	CA	29-year-old mentally competent woman with cerebral palsy that left her almost completely immobile and totally unable to care for herself. She requests that a nasogastric tube to supplement her inadequate oral intake be withdrawn.	The patient has the "right to refuse any medical treatment even that which may save or prolong her life."
In re Jobes 108 N.J. 394	1987	NJ	32-year-old woman in permanent vegetative state, receiving J-tube feedings. Her husband and parents request withdrawal of the feedings. She left no clear written or verbal indication of her wishes.	Incompetent patients have the right to refuse medical care even if they have left no clear indication of their wishes. Using substituted judgment the family can exercise her right to withdraw the J-tube feedings.

Cruzan v. Director of Missouri Department of Health 110 S. Ct. 2841	1990	U.S.	33-year-old woman in persistent vegetative state maintained by gastric tube nutrition and hydration. Her parents requested that these tube feedings be terminated.	By 8 to 1, the Supreme Court ruled that patients have a constitutional right to refuse medical care and that this applies to artificial nutrition and hydration. If there was no clear and convincing written or verbal statement of the patient's wishes, states could regulate how families exercise the right.
In re Helga Wanglie Fourth Judicial District PX-91-283. Minnesota (Hennepin County)	1991	MN	85-year-old woman in a persistent vegetative state. After months, physicians suggested withdrawal of life-sustaining treatment because the patient was receiving no benefit. The family refused withdrawal.	The husband should represent the patient's interests, and his refusal to discontinue the respirator is binding.
Wendland v. Wendland 110 Cal Rptr 2d. 412	2001	CA	42-year-old conscious man with severe cognitive impairments, hemiparesis, and limited communication who was not terminally ill required feeding tube. The feeding tube fell out and needed to be replaced. After authorizing replacement of the feeding tube 3 times, wife refused replacement.	Patients have a right to refuse all medical treatments including life-sustaining treatments. This right can be exercised for mentally incompetent patients through advance care directives. For patients who are terminally ill, in persistent vegetative state, or comatose who have not completed an advance care directive, proxies who have not been formally appointed can terminate interventions. However, for mentally incompetent but conscious patients, "clear and convincing" evidence of the patient's wishes is needed before life-sustaining treatment can be stopped.
In re guardianship of Schiavo No. 90-20-8GD–003, 2000 WL 34546715 (Fla. Cir Ct Feb 11, 2000)	2005	FL	In Feb. 1990, Terri Schiavo collapsed in her apartment. She was resuscitated but left in persistent vegetative state not requiring a respirator but receiving artificial nutrition and hydration. Many attempts were made to rehabilitate her, including thalamic stimulation. In May 1998, her husband filed a motion to remove the nasogastric tube. This engendered conflict between her husband and parents. Her parents claimed she would not want feedings ended and that her husband should not be the guardian. In 2000, a judge heard case about her medical condition and wishes, and who should be her guardian. The judge ruled she was in a persistent vegetative state, her husband could make decisions for her, and she made oral declarations indicating she would not want to be kept alive in persistent vegetative state. In 2003, Florida legislature passed "Terri's Law" to give the governor power to intervene. Over 7 years, 14 appeals, and 5 suits in Federal District Court led to removal and reinsertion of the feeding tube 3 times. In March 2005, feeding tube was removed and Terri Schiavo died.	Terri Schiavo's husband is the rightful guardian, there is oral evidence of patient's wishes, and based on her wishes, her husband has the authority to make the decision to remove the feeding tube. Terri's law violates the Florida constitution.

persistent vegetative state, comatose, or terminally ill, family members, even if not formally appointed as surrogate decision makers, can withdraw life-sustaining treatments based on prior conversations with the patient or their understanding of the patient's values. However, they have refused to permit family members who have not been formally appointed as proxies to terminate life-sustaining treatments for mentally incapacitated but conscious patients who can interact minimally.[41] Even explicit statements by the patient that relate to not wanting to be on life support or in a vegetative state, courts have argued, do not meet the standard of "clear and convincing" evidence.[41] The *Schiavo* case suggests the possibility that these limitations will be extended to other patients, including terminally ill cancer patients. These limits and the controversy over the *Schiavo* case emphasize the value of having patients complete formal advance care directives, specifying their wishes regarding life-sustaining treatments and who they want to be their surrogate decision maker.

Occasionally families want patients in a coma, in a persistent vegetative state, or with anencephaly to be maintained with life-sustaining treatments, although the treating physicians object to providing such care.[43] In the *Wanglie* case, the family of an elderly woman in a persistent vegetative state wanted her respirator continued. The court ruled that the family had a right to decide what treatments the patient should receive.

Criteria for Stopping Medical Interventions

Competent patients have the right to refuse medical care and can use whatever criteria they deem acceptable; it is their values that guide the choice.[44] Similarly, when mentally incapacitated patients have left advance directives that specify the interventions they want or do not want, their values determine their choices.

For mentally incapacitated patients who appointed a surrogate decision maker but did not give specific indications of their wishes, or who never completed an advance care directive, four guiding decision criteria have been proposed: (1) the ordinary- versus extraordinary care distinction, (2) futile care, (3) substituted judgment, and (4) best interests.

Some patients may be incompetent to make decisions and also lack a surrogate decision maker. Although clear guidelines regarding decisions to limit treatment under such circumstances are lacking, clinicians should seek the opinion of a second physician or an ethics consultant before withdrawing life support.[25]

Ordinary/Extraordinary Care

Following Pope Pius XII's and Roman Catholic teachings, some ethicists advocate a distinction between ordinary and extraordinary care: Ordinary care is considered to be mandatory, whereas extraordinary care may be withheld or withdrawn.[33] One commentator explained this distinction as follows:

> *Ordinary* means of preserving life are all medicines, treatments, and operations, which offer a reasonable hope of benefit for the patient and which can be obtained and used without excessive expense, pain, or inconvenience. . . . *Extraordinary* means of preserving life mean all medicines, treatments, and operations, which cannot be obtained without excessive expense, pain, or other inconvenience, or which, if used, would not offer reasonable hope of benefit.[45]

Many ethicists and courts have concluded that this distinction is too vague and has "too many conflicting meanings" to be helpful in guiding surrogate decision makers and physicians.[37,38,46,47] As one lawyer noted, ordinary and extraordinary are "extremely fact-sensitive, relative terms. . . . What is ordinary for one patient under particular circumstances may be extraordinary for the same patient under different circumstances, or for a different patient under the same circumstances."[47] Thus, the ordinary versus extraordinary distinction should not be used to justify decisions about stopping treatment.[38]

Futile Treatments

In the late 1980s and early 1990s, some argued that physicians could ethically terminate futile treatments.[48] Unfortunately, the term *futile* has been used inconsistently.[49-52] Physiologic futility means that an intervention will have no physiologic effect. Some have defined a qualitatively futile treatment as one that "fails to end a patient's total dependence on intensive medical care."[48] Quantitative futility occurs "when physicians conclude (either through personal experience, experiences shared with colleagues, or consideration of reported empirical data) that in the last 100 cases, a medical treatment has been useless."[48] In general, it is now agreed that there is no objective standard of futility; the term merely conceals subjective value judgments about when a treatment is "not beneficial."[49-52]

Some hospitals have enacted "unilateral do-not-resuscitate" policies to allow clinicians to provide a do-not-resuscitate order in cases where consensus cannot be reached with families and there is medical opinion that resuscitation would be futile. Texas, Virginia, Maryland, and California have enacted so-called medical futility laws.[53] These laws protect physicians from liability if they terminate life-sustaining treatments against family wishes.

In Texas, if the medical team and the hospital ethics committee believe that interventions should be terminated, but the patient's family disagrees, the hospital is supposed to seek another institution willing to provide treatment.[53] If, after 10 days, this fails, then the hospital and the physician may unilaterally withdraw treatments determined to be futile; however, the family may appeal to a state court. Early data suggest that the law increases futility consultations with the ethics committee, and that most families concur with withdrawal decision.[53]

Substituted Judgment

Many courts advocate use of the substituted judgment criterion. Substituted judgment holds that the surrogate decision maker should try to imagine what the patient would do if the patient were competent.[46] That is, the surrogate should try to "ascertain the incompetent person's actual interests and preferences" and to make the decision that "would be made by the incompetent person, if that person were competent."[54]

Most surrogates, even close family members, cannot accurately predict what the patient would want.[3,40] Therefore, in the absence of specific guidance from the patient, substituted judgment involves surmising what a patient would want, rather than a guaranteed fulfillment of the patient's wishes.[38,55] Of note, patients who were surveyed varied regarding the extent to which they want families to strictly adhere to their personal wishes in making end-of-life decisions on their behalf.[56]

Best Interests

The best-interests criterion holds that the surrogate should evaluate treatments by balancing their benefits and risks and should select those treatments in which the benefits maximally outweigh the burdens of treatment.[37,38] Legally, this standard is considered "objective" because it does not rely on imagining what the patient would choose but rather is consistent with an externally defined standard.[37] The President's Commission for the Study of Ethical Problems in Medicine and Biomedical and Behavioral Research—a landmark advisory group that laid the groundwork for U.S. regulation of medical research in the 1970s—endorsed this standard, as have several courts.[37,57]

For the best-interests standard to work, there must be some "objective, societally shared criteria" about what constitutes benefits and burdens.[57] However, as is made clear by many court cases involving conflict between family members, or between family members and the medical team, no objective way of determining benefits and burdens, and how they should be balanced, has been recognized. One court suggested that burdens should be determined solely by levels of pain.[37] However, many people consider a permanent vegetative state to be a serious burden that they want to avoid, even if they do not feel pain. In the absence of an objective best-interests standard, families largely decide what constitutes a benefit or burden from their estimation of a patient's personal values.

As a matter of practice, physicians rely on family members to make decisions that they feel are best and only object if these decisions seem to demand treatments that the physician considers nonbeneficial. Without a perfect solution to the problems raised by proxy decision making, this approach may be the most reasonable one in difficult circumstances.

Advance Care Documents and Durable Powers of Attorney

The living will was first proposed in 1967. In 1976, after the *Quinlan* decision, California enacted the first living will law. By 2007, all states but Massachusetts and Michigan had enacted laws authorizing the use of living wills—and in these two states, courts have recognized living will documents as legally enforceable expressions of patients' wishes.[58] These living wills may have some legal limitations. For instance, in 25 states, the living will is not valid if a woman is pregnant (Table 72-2).

Table 72-2. 25 States in Which Living Wills Are Not Valid If the Woman Is Pregnant

Alabama	Indiana	Pennsylvania
Arkansas	Iowa	Rhode Island*
California	Kentucky	South Dakota
Colorado	Minnesota	Texas
Connecticut	Missouri	Utah
Georgia	North Dakota	Washington
Hawaii	Ohio*	Wisconsin
Idaho	Oklahoma	Wyoming
Illinois		

*Not valid only if fetus could develop sufficiently for a live birth.

There are two types of advance care planning documents: living wills and proxy statements. *Living wills* or instructional directives are advisory documents specifying the patient's preferences to specific care decisions. State-specific forms that people can fill in to draw up advance directives are available on the Internet.[59] Some advance directives, such as The Medical Directive, enumerate different scenarios and interventions for the patient to choose from.[60] Among these, some are for general use and others are designed for use by patients with a specific disease, such as cancer.[61] Less specific directives can be general statements of not wanting life-sustaining interventions or forms that describe the values that should guide specific terminal care decisions. Of importance, a person does not have to use a state-specific form because "a living will or health care power of attorney that does not strictly follow the statutory [state] form is also valid in most states" and the U.S. Supreme Court has ruled that a person has a constitutional right to refuse medical treatments.[58]

The health care *proxy statement,* sometimes called a durable power of attorney for health care, specifies a person selected by the patient to make decisions. Often, a combined directive includes both instructions and the designation of a proxy; the directive should clearly indicate whether the specified patient preferences or the proxy's choice should take precedence if they conflict.[60]

Many states permit clear and explicit verbal statements to be legally binding even if not written down.[58] However, such statements must be very explicit. In the *Wendland* case, a 42-year-old man suffered permanent brain damage and hemiparesis in a car accident.[41] The California Supreme Court ruled that when the patient is conscious and there is no advance care directive, there must be "clear and convincing" evidence of the patient's view, in order to permit withdrawal of a feeding tube.[41] "Clear and convincing" evidence requires prior comments to refer to the specific intervention in the specific circumstances of the patient, not a similar health state.

In 1984, California passed the first law recognizing the appointment of a designated proxy for health care decisions; by 2007, all 50 states and the District of Columbia had enacted statutes recognizing the durable power of attorney for health care decisions. There are some limitations. For instance, although most states permit proxies to terminate life-sustaining treatments, Alaska prohibits such decisions by proxies. In other states, orally appointed proxies are limited to a particular hospitalization or episode of illness. Nevertheless, it appears that any properly-filled-out, formal advance care document or durable power of attorney designation, whether or not it conforms to a state's specific document, is protected by the U.S. Constitution and must be honored.[35]

End-of-Life Care Practices

Data on end-of-life care practices indicate that withholding or withdrawing life-sustaining treatment is routine and occurs in more than 90% of all deaths. In addition, most physicians have become significantly more comfortable with stopping medical treatments. For instance, approximately one third of patients in the United States—and about 60% of cancer patients—die receiving hospice care and forgo life-sustaining medical interventions.[59,62] Furthermore, more than 85% of Americans die without cardiopulmonary resuscitation.[63] Similarly, data indicate that 90% of patients who die in ICUs do not receive resuscitation efforts, and 90% die after medical interventions are withheld or withdrawn.[64-66]

Despite polling data showing that approximately 80% of Americans endorse the use of advance directives, and passage in 1990 of the federal Patient Self-Determination Act (PSDA), which requires hospitals and other health care facilities to inform patients about their right to complete an advance care directive, the proportion of Americans who have completed such documents is low. Before the *Schiavo* case, approximately 20% of Americans had a written advance care directive of some type—the same level as in 1990, the year of the *Cruzan* decision. After the *Schiavo* decision, about 30% of Americans have a written advance care directive.

Of greater importance, even when advance care directives have been prepared, they frequently are not in the patient's medical record, and the patient's physician may not be aware of the existence or content of the document.[67,68] In addition, recent studies suggest that most advance directives are either proxy forms or standard living wills, and that few have any specific directions from the patient.[69] Finally, all studies confirm that proxies and family members tend to be poorly informed about patients' wishes regarding end-of-life care and therefore are unlikely to make decisions as the patient would.[3,40]

Caring for Dying Patients in the Intensive Care Unit

Critical care clinicians have a particularly challenging responsibility when taking care of patients whose chances of survival are uncertain. Under such circumstances, clinicians need to understand how to use prediction tools such as the Acute Physiology and Chronic Health Evaluation (APACHE) tool or the Simplified Acute Physiology Score (SAPS) system, or SAPS II, to estimate the likelihood of survival. Awareness of the limited predictive ability of these tools is important for the ICU physician, who at the same time will use them to trigger decisions and interventions as part of a systematic approach to improving care.[70]

While prognosis is uncertain, clinicians are advised to attend to the dual goals of prolonging life and palliating symptoms. As a patient's prognosis becomes increasingly worse, consideration needs to be given to withholding or withdrawing life-sustaining treatments. Useful guidelines for withdrawing life support are shown in Box 72-3.

Because decisions to limit life support should be shared with patients or their families, clinicians should be familiar with the important components of discussing these decisions. These components are summarized in Box 72-4.

Critically ill patients require relief of symptoms regardless of their prognosis. It is increasingly recognized that the goals of care are both to prolong life and to alleviate suffering. Once a patient is thought to be dying, the focus of care increasingly shifts to palliative care. Critical care clinicians should aim to deliver high-quality palliative care (Box 72-5).

Assisted Suicide and Euthanasia

Historical Perspective

The ethics of euthanasia have been a contentious issue since the beginning of medicine. The Hippocratic Oath requires doctors to pledge never to "give a deadly drug to anybody if asked for it, nor . . . make a suggestion to this effect."[30] In ancient Greece and Rome, this position was the minority view; physicians commonly participated in euthanasia and physician-assisted suicide.

The modern debate about euthanasia can be dated from 1870, when a nonphysician, Samuel Williams, argued for euthanasia in front of the Birmingham Speculative Club.[71] The growing acceptance of terminating life-sustaining care, the legalization of euthanasia in the Netherlands and Belgium, the Kevorkian suicide machine, and the 1988 publication in *JAMA* of the article "It's over, Debbie"[72]—in which a hospital resident recounted his administering

Box 72-3

Guiding Principles of Withdrawing Life Support

1. The goal of withdrawing life sustaining treatment is to remove treatments that are no longer desired or do not provide comfort to the patient.
2. The withholding of life-sustaining treatments is morally and legally equivalent to their withdrawal.
3. Actions with the sole goal of hastening death are morally and legally problematic.
4. Any treatment can be withheld or withdrawn.
5. Withdrawal of life-sustaining treatment is a medical procedure.
6. *Corollary to principles 1 and 2:* When circumstances justify withholding a life-sustaining treatment, consideration should be given to withdrawing current life-sustaining treatment.

From Rubenfeld GD, Gordon SW: Principles and practice of withdrawing life-sustaining treatments in the ICU. In Curtis JR, Rubenfeld GD (eds): Managing Death in the Intensive Care Unit. New York, Oxford University Press, 2001.

Box 72-4

Components of a Discussion about End-of-Life Care in the Intensive Care Unit

Making Preparations before a Discussion about End-of-Life Care

Review previous knowledge about the patient and family.
Review previous knowledge about the patient's attitudes and reactions.
Review your knowledge of the disease—prognosis, treatment options.
Review your own personal feelings, attitudes, biases, and grief.
Plan the location and setting: a quiet private place.
Have advance discussion with the family about who will be present.

Holding a Discussion about End-of-Life Care in the Intensive Care Unit

Introduce everyone present.
If appropriate, set the tone in a nonthreatening way: "This is a discussion I have with all my patients."
Find out what the patient and family understand.
Find out how much the patient and family want to know.
Be aware that some patients do not want to discuss end-of-life care.
Discuss prognosis frankly in a way that is meaningful to the patient.
Do not discourage all hope.
Avoid temptation to give too much medical detail.
Make it clear that withholding life-sustaining treatment is not withholding caring.
Use repetition to show that you understand what the patient or family member is saying.
Acknowledge strong emotions and use reflection to encourage patients or families to talk about their emotion.
Tolerate silence.

Finishing a Discussion of End-of-Life Care in the Intensive Care Unit

Achieve common understanding of the disease and treatment issues.
Make a recommendation about treatment.
Ask if there are any questions.
Ensure that a basic follow-up plan is in place, and make sure the patient or appropriate family member knows how to reach you for questions.

Modified from Curtis JR, Patrick DL: How to discuss dying and death in the ICU. In Curtis JR, Rubenfeld GD (eds): Managing Death in the Intensive Care Unit. New York, Oxford University Press, 2001.

Box 72-5

Quality Measures for Palliative and End-of-Life Care

Patient and Family-Centered Decision Making

Assessment of the patient's decisional capacity
Documentation of a surrogate decision maker within 24 hours
Documentation of the presence and, if present, contents of advance directive
Documentation of the goals of care
Communication within team and with the patient and the family
Documentation of timely physician communication with the family
Documentation of timely interdisciplinary clinician-family conference

Continuity of Care

Transition of key information with transfer of the patient out of the ICU
Policy of continuity of nursing service
Emotional and practical support for patient and family
Open visitation policy for family members
Documentation that psychosocial support has been offered

Symptom Management and Comfort Care

Documentation of pain assessment and management
Documentation of respiratory distress assessment and management
Protocol for analgesia and sedation in terminal withdrawal or mechanical ventilation
Appropriate medications available during withdrawal of mechanical ventilation

Spiritual Support for Patients and Family

Documentation that spiritual support was offered
Emotional and organizational support for clinicians
Opportunity to review experience of caring for dying patients by ICU clinicians

From Mularski RA, Curtis JR, Billings JA, et al: Proposed quality measures for palliative care in the critically ill: A consensus from the Robert Wood Johnson Foundation Critical Care Workgroup. Crit Care Med 2006;34:S404-S411.

a fatal morphine overdose to a dying cancer patient—all have stimulated the contemporary debate about the value of euthanasia and physician-assisted suicide.

Definitions

The term *euthanasia* is imprecise. So-called passive euthanasia is actually the withdrawal or withholding of life-sustaining medical interventions and is widely accepted as both ethical and legal. "Indirect euthanasia"—such as increasing narcotic dosage to ease a patient's pain, even if this has the consequence of hastening the patient's death—also is a misnomer; it generally has been deemed both ethical and legal for more than 100 years.[71] Almost all commentators agree that involuntary and nonvoluntary active euthanasia are unethical because they end the life of a patient without consent. Consequently, the focus of debate is on physician-assisted suicide and voluntary, active euthanasia. To avoid confusion, use of the term *euthanasia* should be restricted to voluntary, active euthanasia.

Ethical Standards Regarding Euthanasia and Assisted Suicide

Proponents typically cite four reasons to justify physician-assisted suicide or euthanasia.[71,73] First, they claim that euthanasia ensures patients' autonomy. Different people have different values. How a person dies is essential to that person's values. Therefore, to respect patients' autonomy, it is mandatory to respect their wishes regarding the manner and timing of their death, through euthanasia and physician-assisted suicide.[74,75] Second, for some patients, dying causes pain and suffering. A main purpose of euthanasia or physician-assisted suicide is a comfortable, quick death. Hence, euthanasia or physician-assisted suicide furthers beneficence, which is one of the major principles of medical ethics.[74,75] Third, euthanasia and physician-assisted suicide are morally equivalent to terminating life-sustaining treatments. The goal is the same: a peaceful, painless death. Furthermore, there is no difference between an act of omission and an act of commission.[75] Finally, the potential adverse consequences of legalization are speculative.

Opponents of euthanasia and physician-assisted suicide offer four parallel but opposite arguments. First, autonomy does not justify euthanasia or physician-assisted suicide.[76-78] Autonomy does not mean a person should be permitted to do anything he or she wishes. Both Kant and Mill thought that a person's autonomy could be limited to prevent voluntary dueling or slavery. Similarly, because euthanasia and physician-assisted suicide are aimed at ending autonomy, they can be limited without infringing autonomy. Second, many terminally ill patients receive inadequate treatment for pain, fatigue, and depression. With proper treatment, few people would experience pain and suffering of a level sufficient to justify euthanasia or physician-assisted suicide. Third, acts of omission and acts of commission are not equivalent. The ethical validity of an act does not depend solely on its final result but also stems from the intention of the person performing it. When physicians stop a medical intervention, they are stopping unwanted bodily intrusion, not trying to end a person's life; euthanasia and physician-assisted suicide do aim to end a person's life.[36,76-78] Finally, permitting euthanasia and physician-assisted suicide would have a variety of well-documented adverse consequences. These include disruption of the doctor-patient relationship, intrusion of the courts, and possibly extension of euthanasia to children, mentally incapacitated patients, and others.[78]

Legal Aspects of Euthanasia and Physician-Assisted Suicide

Although the U.S. Supreme Court has upheld the right of patients to reject medical treatment, the Court ruled unanimously in 1997 that there is no constitutional right to euthanasia or physician-assisted suicide.[36] The majority view—written by Chief Justice Rehnquist—drew a distinction between the right to withdraw or withhold life-sustaining treatments as a liberty interest in being free of unwanted bodily invasion and the right to physician-assisted suicide, which does not contain a liberty interest.[36] The unanimity of the ruling suggests that it is unlikely to be overturned in the future.

Of importance, the Supreme Court did permit individual states to legalize these interventions. Oregon has enacted the Death with Dignity Act, which permits physician-assisted suicide. This law has several requirements including the following: the patient must be a resident of Oregon; the patient must make two oral requests, separated by a 15-day waiting period; the patient must make a written request witnessed by two people; the physician and another consultant must confirm the patient's diagnosis and terminal prognosis; and the physician and another consultant must confirm that the patient is mentally competent and not suffering from depression or other psychiatric impairment.[79]

The Netherlands and Belgium have legalized both euthanasia and physician-assisted suicide. Their legislation included the following safeguards: The patient must have unbearable pain and suffering that cannot be medically relieved; the patient must be competent and must repeatedly request to have his or her life ended; and the physician must consult a second physician.[80]

For a brief period the Northern Territory of Australia had legalized euthanasia, but this was rescinded by the national legislature.[81] In Switzerland assisted suicide is legal, and the assitance need not be provided by a physician.[82]

Empiric Data Regarding Euthanasia and Physician-Assisted Suicide

Polling data indicate that a majority of the American public is willing to support euthanasia and physician-assisted suicide in hypothetical cases and for terminally ill patients with extreme pain. Support declines if euthanasia or physician-assisted suicide is being carried out for reasons other than pain.[73]

Less than 10% to 20% of terminally ill patients actually consider euthanasia or physician-assisted suicide for themselves. In Oregon approximately 0.1% of deaths are by physician-assisted suicide,[79] in The Netherlands about 3.5% of deaths are by euthanasia or physician-assisted suicide,[83] and in Belgium about 1.8% of deaths.[84] In both The Netherlands and Oregon, more than 70% of patients using these interventions are dying of cancer; less than 5% of deaths by euthanasia or physician-assisted suicide involve patients with AIDS or amyotrophic lateral sclerosis.[79,83,84]

Pain is not a primary motivator for patients' requests for or interest in euthanasia or physician-assisted suicide. Data obtained for patients with cancer, human immunodeficiency virus infection or acquired immunodeficiency syndrome (HIV/AIDS), and amyotrophic lateral sclerosis in the United States, and for patients with cancer in The Netherlands and patients who were euthanized in the Northern Territory when it was legal, indicate that depression, hopelessness, and psychological distress are the primary factors.[73,81,85-87] In a recent study from The Netherlands, depressed terminally ill cancer patients were four times more likely to request euthanasia.[88] Euthanasia and physician-assisted suicide are not always painless and quick approaches to dying.[89]

Studies report that between 12% and 54% of physicians will receive a request for euthanasia or physician-assisted suicide during their careers, whether or not they are practicing in an area in which euthanasia is legal.

Responding to a Request for Euthanasia or Physician-Assisted Suicide

After receiving a request for euthanasia or physician-assisted suicide, health care providers should carefully clarify the request with empathetic, open-ended questions to help elucidate the underlying cause—for example: "What makes you want to consider this option?" Expressing either moral opposition to or moral support for the act tends to be counterproductive, either appearing judgmental or seeming to endorse the idea that the patient's life is worthless. Health care providers must reassure the patient of their continued care and commitment. The patient should be educated about alternative, less controversial options, such as symptom management and withdrawal of any unwanted treatments. Physicians also should discuss the realities of euthanasia and physician-assisted suicide, because the patient may have misconceptions about their effectiveness and the legal implications of the choice.

In addition, the physician should re-evaluate the patient's condition—not just for physical and psychological symptoms but also for lack of social support and spiritual fulfillment and need for care, which are strongly associated with interest in euthanasia and physician-assisted suicide. The physician should reassess whether additional interventions are required, including psychiatric evaluation, palliative care consultations, availability of skilled or unskilled home health care, and pastoral services. Obviously, the patient and family should be reassured that the physician will not abandon them and will provide care and attend to the patient's symptoms and needs.

RESEARCH IN CRITICALLY ILL PATIENTS

Research involving critically ill patients in the ICU presents special ethical challenges. Clinical medicine aims at providing optimal medical care for individual patients. Clinical research lies outside of the context of the doctor-patient relationship; it is designed to answer a scientific question, with the aim of promoting the medical good of future patients. Research abuses occur when the interest of advancing science is allowed to outweigh that of protecting the human subject of research. Adherence to ethical principles for research serves to minimize the possibility of such abuses.

History and the Fundamentals of Human Research Ethics

Before the 19th century, medical research was conducted on a small scale and was largely therapeutic in intent. Among the first documented experiments with human subjects were vaccination trials in the 1700s. In these early trials, many physicians used themselves or their family members as test subjects.

Even these early practices were not without some formulations of research ethics. In 1865, the French physiologist Claude Bernard wrote that the first principle of medical morality "consists in never performing on man an experiment which might be harmful to him to any extent, even though the result might be highly advantageous to science."[90] Louis Pasteur is reported to have "agonized" over treating humans, even though he was confident of the results obtained through animal trials. He finally did so only when he was convinced that the death of the first test subject "appeared inevitable."[91]

The rise of the experimental method in medicine in the late 19th century led to an acceleration of the progress of medicine. Clinical trials became large-scale endeavors, and many trials targeted vulnerable groups of persons who could not protect their own interests, such as orphans, the mentally ill, and prisoners. During this era, no formal codes of research ethics existed to guide physicians in their experiments.

In the 20th century, the medical experiments conducted by German physicians on concentration camp prisoners during World War II ushered in a new era of research ethics. After the war, 23 Nazi doctors and scientists were put on trial at Nuremberg for the torture and murder of concentration camp inmates who were used as research subjects. Most were convicted and either condemned to death by hanging or sentenced to prison terms ranging from 10 years to life.[92]

When the Nuremberg judges issued their verdict in August 1947, they included in their legal judgment 10 points describing the elements of ethical research with humans. These points became known as the Nuremberg Code,[93,94] and they formed the basis of the research ethics codes that are used internationally today.

The Nuremberg Code's first principle was stated as a basic human right: "The voluntary consent of the human subject is absolutely essential." Another basic right of research subjects was the right to withdraw from the experiment at any time. The other eight principles aimed to protect the welfare of human subjects by insisting, for example, that only qualified scientists conduct the research, that physical and mental suffering are avoided, and that risks are balanced against the importance of the scientific problem to be solved.

In the United States, the fundamental ethical guidelines for medical research were set out in 1974 by the National Commission for the Protection of Human Subjects in Biomedical and Behavioral Research, which was created by Congress after a series of ethical scandals in the 1960s and 1970s. In its *Belmont Report,* the Commission outlined three basic ethical principles for the conduct of medical research: *respect for persons; beneficence;* and *justice*[95] (Table 72-3).

Respect for Persons. Respect for persons requires that people should be treated as autonomous agents and that those with diminished capacity, such as children or the mentally ill, are entitled to special protection. To respect autonomy is to give weight to a person's considered opinions and choices. To show lack of respect for autonomy is to repudiate a person's considered judgments, to deny the person the freedom to act on those considered judgments, or to withhold information necessary to make a considered judgment, when there are no compelling reasons to do so. Respect for persons is manifested in the *informed consent* process, in which potential subjects are provided with information about the experiment and then are allowed to decide whether to participate.

Beneficence/Nonmaleficence. Treating people in an ethical manner means not only respecting their decisions but also making efforts to secure their well-being. Such treatment falls under the principle of beneficence, which obliges physician-researchers to (1) do no harm and (2) maximize possible benefits and minimize possible harms. Beneficence requires that investigators and members of institutional review boards (IRBs) analyze the risks and benefits to the subjects, making sure that anticipated risks are proportional to the potential benefits. Risk should be minimized as much as possible.

Justice. Justice requires that the benefits and burdens of research be distributed equitably. Subjects should not be chosen simply because they are available and easy to manipulate. In addition, subjects who are likely to benefit from a study should not be excluded. Finally, whenever research supported by public funds leads to the development of therapeutic devices and procedures, these should be available not only to the wealthy but to all society; and such research should not unduly involve groups who are unlikely to benefit from the research.

The U.S. federal regulations and most international regulations governing research with human beings are largely based on these principles.

Putting Principles into Practice: Applications

Although ethics codes and regulations exist to ensure the ethical conduct of research, what is needed is a systematic and coherent framework for evaluating the ethics of human subject research that incorporates all relevant ethical considerations. Stemming from the principles of research ethics, several *requirements* have been proposed to ensure the ethical conduct of research (see Table 72-3). Several of these requirements that are particularly pertinent to the conduct of clinical trials involving critically ill patients are addressed next.

Scientific Validity

Clinical trials must be designed to answer valuable scientific questions with the necessary methodologic rigor to validly claim any scientific conclusions. The large number of therapeutic interventions required in the care of the critically ill creates special challenges in the conduct of clinical trials in the ICU.

The ideal clinical trial establishes whether therapeutic interventions work and determines the overall benefits and risks of each alternative. This is achieved by limiting

Table 72-3. Principles and Derived Requirements for Ethical Research

Respect for Persons	Beneficence; Nonmaleficence	Justice
Persons should be treated as autonomous agents Persons with diminished autonomy need protection **Informed Consent** Disclosure of information Understanding of information Voluntariness of decisions Surrogate consent for vulnerable persons	Minimize possible harms Maximize societal and potential individual benefits **Social Value** Research will lead to knowledge that will improve societal health **Scientific Validity** Research will produce reliable and valid data **Favorable Risk/Benefit** Risks are identified Risks are minimized Benefits are maximized Risks are reasonable to potential benefits to subject and society **Independent Review** Persons free from controlling influences review research to enhance implementation of ethical requirements and enhance subject protection	Fairness in distribution of risks and potential benefits of research to all groups Fairness in selection of subjects **Fair Subject Selection** Vulnerable subjects are not targeted for enrollment because of their compromised position Aims of research dictate subject selection Selected subjects are likely to be recipients of future benefits When possible, less burdened groups of persons should bear the risks of research

the effects of chance, bias, and confounding. The need for scientific rigor also must be balanced against other requirements of clinical trials, such as protection of subjects' rights and welfare as well as minimizing the cost and the number of subjects necessary for enrollment to achieve significant results.[96]

An important ethical construct in clinical trials is that of clinical *equipoise*.[97] This notion refers to a state of uncertainty in the community of expert physicians concerning the relative benefits and harms of the interventions being tested. The presence of clinical equipoise serves two important goals.[98] The first is to ensure that the welfare and integrity of research subjects are not knowingly sacrificed for the interests of future patients. When neither of the interventions in the study groups dominates the other in terms of perceived safety and efficacy, it is ethically permissible to allow a subject's care to be determined by random selection. The other goal is to ensure that the research will yield reliable, generalizable information that can be applied to disturb clinical equipoise. The randomized controlled trial (RCT) is a formal method of resolving uncertainty about scientific knowledge, although well-conducted observational cohort and case-control studies also can provide valuable information to disturb equipoise and might lead to better human subject protections.[99,100]

Informed Consent

Informed consent is the ethical prerequisite for all clinical trials involving human beings. The informed consent process respects subjects' autonomy and ensures that they are not to be used merely as a means to another's end.[101] It also provides research subjects a mechanism to protect themselves.[102,103] Valid informed consent consists of three major elements: disclosure of information, subject competence to make a decision, and voluntariness of the decision.[104]

Disclosure of Information

The basic elements of information that should be communicated to potential subjects and their surrogates include a full description of any reasonably foreseeable risks or discomforts a subject may experience, and full disclosure of other procedures or courses of treatment that are available[105,106] (Box 72-6). Some of these elements are absent in many informed consent forms, including those used in critical care clinical trials.[107,108] Recommendations for writing informed consent forms for critical care studies have been published.[109]

Box 72-6

Required Basic Elements of Informed Consent

Element 1: Description of Research

a. Purpose of the research
b. A statement that the study involves research
c. Expected duration of the subject's participation
d. Description of the procedures to be followed and identification of any procedures that are experimental

Element 2: Risk

Description of any reasonably foreseeable risks or discomforts to the subject

Element 3: Benefits

Description of benefits that might reasonably be expected from the research:
a. To the subject
b. To others

Element 4: Alternatives

Disclosure of alternative procedures or courses of treatment, if any, that might be advantageous to the subject

Element 5: Confidentiality

Assurance of confidentiality

Element 6: Risk Management

For research involving more than minimal risk, if research injury occurs:
a. An explanation as to whether any compensation is available
b. An explanation as to whether any medical treatments are available

Element 7: Contact Information

a. An explanation of whom to contact for answers to questions about the research
b. An explanation of whom to contact for questions about the research subjects' rights
c. An explanation of whom to contact in the event of a research-related injury

Element 8: Voluntariness

a. Voluntariness of participation
b. Assurance that subject may discontinue participation without penalty or loss of benefits to which the subject is otherwise entitled

Competence

In order to give valid informed consent, potential trial subjects must be able to understand information, to understand or appreciate their situation and its consequences, to rationally consider information in light of their underlying values, and to commit to a decision.

Subjects enrolled in clinical trials often have limited understanding of the research to which they provided consent.[110,111] Many subjects have difficulty understanding the concept of randomization, the notion of a placebo design, and the risks in a study. Understanding is less complete in severely ill patients than in healthier patients.[112] Investigators should make special efforts to ensure that potential subjects understand these elements of informed consent.

Investigators also should keep in mind that written descriptions of the research may not be effective—particularly if the written material is so long and technical that potential subjects do not read it fully. Information given verbally can enhance understanding by giving subjects the opportunity to engage in a dialogue with the investigator. The opportunity for such a dialogue, however, may not be present for patients receiving ventilatory support.

The so-called *therapeutic misconception* is of particular concern. Patients and families have a strong tendency to inaccurately attribute therapeutic intent to the research.[113] However, the goal of clinical trials is not to provide direct benefits to subjects[95,114]; the primary goal of research is to generate generalizable knowledge for future patients. Physician-investigators should explicitly refute such a "therapeutic misconception" and should dispel any notion that a clinical trial is designed to or will provide patients with direct benefits, or that the research substitutes for clinical care.

Finally, the research community often assumes that subjects derive benefits solely from participating in a research study—even if they are receiving inert placebo—because of the extra monitoring and superior care associated with academic "centers of excellence." Such an "inclusion benefit," however, has not been proved.[115,116]

Voluntariness

Valid informed consent requires that patients' decisions to enroll in clinical trials are free from coercion—including a fear, justified or not, that they may be harmed in some way if they do not enroll in the clinical trial.[95] The institutional setting of the research may be a source of subtle or covert coercion. Critically ill patients often lack decisional capacity. Patients may feel they have little choice but to participate in research when "their doctor" asks them to do so—particularly if their treating physician occupies the dual role of clinician-investigator. Accordingly, someone other than the treating physician should obtain informed consent from patients.[117,118]

Another factor that may affect voluntariness is the presence of undue influence, which occurs when offers to induce enrollment, such as financial payments or free medical care, are of such magnitude that they influence subjects' decisions.[119]

Surrogate Consent

Ethically acceptable research may proceed with critically ill patients who are—or are at risk of becoming—decisionally impaired, if the investigators receive appropriate proxy consent.[186,187] U.S. and European standards require surrogate decision makers to be legally authorized to provide such consent. In the United States, the legal representative for the patient is determined by the applicable laws of the state—although precisely what this means is still uncertain in many states.

If possible, surrogate decision makers should follow the "substituted judgment" standard: They should make a good-faith judgment of what the subjects would have decided if capable of making a decision themselves. As discussed earlier, however, surrogates often do not know patients' previous preferences.[120,121] Therefore, they also should consider what would be in the best interests of the patient.

Finally, studies have shown high levels of anxiety and psychological distress in family members of critically ill patients. This might impair their ability to give adequate informed consent for research participation for incapacitated patients.[122,123]

If subjects who were entered into a trial through proxy consent regain decisional capacity during the trial, investigators should obtain their informed consent for continuing their participation.[124] Such retrospective consent should be sought even when the research procedures have been completed, because subjects have a right to know that they have participated in a trial and that further data may be collected. Whether subjects should be given the right to withdraw the data obtained from them when they were unconscious is an emerging issue. This is a sound proposal, ethically speaking, but from a methodologic standpoint, it is arguable because it could ruin the comparability of study groups.

Subject Vulnerability

Patients can be "vulnerable" because of intrinsic factors, such as lack of capacity to make decisions, or because of situations that threaten voluntary choice, such as coercive settings or undue inducements.

Additional protections for vulnerable people and groups should be based on the level of risk of the procedures that will be involved.[125-127] For example, ethics guidelines and regulatory agencies[128,129] recommend that investigators should outline a specific plan to assess the capacity of any potential subject when groups that may include decisionally impaired persons are targeted for research. Patients who are receiving mechanical ventilation would fall in this category. Such assessments can consist of asking potential subjects several questions to test their understanding of the research involved. Formal methods of assessing capacity also are available.[130]

For research involving possibly beneficial procedures that pose more than minimal risk, additional protections for vulnerable subjects could include designating independent monitors to witness the informed consent process or to determine when it might be appropriate to withdraw the subject from the study.[131,132] The subject's legally authorized representative should ordinarily fill this role of a participation monitor.[131]

When the procedures do not offer a prospect of direct benefit to the patient, commentators have argued that the risk should be capped at the level of minimal risk.[133,134] This position reflects the concern that vulnerable subjects should not be put at undue risk for the sake of society and that such research is exploitative. However, advocating such a risk ceiling would seriously impair important research. Instead of restricting such research, a desirable alternative might be to institute a safeguard for this risk level, such as the "necessity requirement." Such a safeguard would provide that decisionally impaired subjects can be enrolled in research only when their participation is scientifically necessary—for example, when the desired information cannot be obtained by enrolling adults who can consent. To provide supplemental protection, some guidelines reinforce the necessity requirement with a "subject condition" requirement, under which the research must involve a condition from which the subject suffers.

The most controversial category is research that presents more than a minor increment above minimal risk. The risks associated with bronchoscopy in critically ill patients receiving mechanical ventilation to obtain bronchoalveolar lavage samples, performed solely for research purposes, might be an example of this level of risk.

Waiver of Informed Consent

In some circumstances, the informed consent requirement can be waived—but only when an IRB finds that all of the following conditions are met[135]:

- The research involves no more than minimal risk to the subjects.
- The waiver or alteration of informed consent requirements will not adversely affect the rights and welfare of the subjects.
- The research could not practicably be carried out without the waiver or alteration.
- Whenever appropriate, the subjects will be provided with additional pertinent information after participation.

Under U.S. regulations, research may be characterized as minimal risk if "the probability and magnitude of harms or discomforts anticipated in the research are not greater in and of themselves than those ordinarily encountered in daily life or during the performance of routine physical or psychological examinations or tests."[136] In other words, the types of minimal risks that are considered socially acceptable, such as in driving to work or crossing a street, or those encountered in routine physical or psychological evaluations, are acceptable in research.

Under these federal regulations, a waiver of informed consent requirements would be acceptable in a chart review of several thousand patient records to determine the recurrence rates of cancer after radiation treatment. Such a project would pose minimal risk to subjects, would not include any identifiable information, and would include data regarding some patients who are dead and probably some whose current addresses are unknown.

A waiver would be inappropriate, however, for a project that obtains extra samples of bronchoalveolar lavage fluid for research purposes from patients undergoing bronchoscopy and lavage for clinical purposes. Even though this procedure poses minimal risk, obtaining informed consent from subjects before the bronchoscopy would not be impracticable and would be respectful of their human rights.

Methodologic Issues

Some research methods and techniques also can raise ethical issues that are not encountered in the clinical treatment of ICU patients. Some examples follow.

Placebo Controls

The distinction between clinical research and clinical practice is particularly pronounced in placebo-controlled trials, in which one group of trial subjects receives a placebo treatment—in effect, no treatment at all—even though a proven effective treatment exists for the medical condition under investigation. Placebo controls have been used in trials of critical care treatments for a wide range of conditions, including asthma and pulmonary hypertension.[137,138]

Critics of placebo-controlled trials contend that when effective treatments exist, placing patients in a placebo group is not only unethical but also unwise. They argue that no scientific or clinical value derives from determining whether an investigational drug is better than an inert placebo; instead, they say, an experimental treatment should be compared with a standard treatment, to demonstrate which is better.[139,140]

Advocates of placebo-controlled studies argue that such studies are not only ethical but indeed necessary under many circumstances.[141-143] For example, an experimental therapy may have fewer side effects or may be more effective for particular subgroups of patients, but these effects might not be recognized in active-control trials. Moreover, demonstrating that a new treatment is equivalent to an existing treatment may not prove that the new treatment is effective; both treatments could be ineffective. And comparing an experimental treatment with an existing treatment would require many more patients in each arm of the study than are necessary for a placebo-controlled trial.

To be sure, a placebo-controlled trial would be unethical when life-saving—or at least life-prolonging—treatment is available, and if patients assigned to receive placebo would be substantially more likely to suffer serious harm than those assigned to receive the investigational agent. Such trials involving diseases that are less serious, however, may be ethically appropriate if compelling methodologic reasons exist to conduct a placebo-controlled trial, and if the known harm associated with forgoing standard of care treatment in the placebo group would be mild to moderate in degree and reversible.

Pragmatic versus Explanatory Studies

An important decision in designing a clinical trial is whether the focus of the trial is to be pragmatic or explanatory. Pragmatic studies measure the efficacy of an intervention in routine clinical practice. Explanatory trials measure the efficacy under ideal conditions, often using carefully defined subjects.[144,145]

Pragmatic studies seek to maximize external validity to ensure that the results can be generalized. Therefore, investigators enroll patients with few exclusion criteria and relax restrictions on physicians' choice of co-interventions. Commonly, the subjects in the control group receive therapy that is identical or similar to standard care. "Usual care" control groups have been used in several important critical care studies,[146-150] including those involving mechanical ventilation,[151-153] and have proved to be extremely informative in such studies.[154]

Explanatory studies seek to maximize internal validity. They impose constraints on study and nonstudy interventions in both the experimental and the control groups to reduce sources of variation, thereby maximizing the ability to detect differences in outcome. However, to change clinical practice, such control groups should be representative of usual care practices. Surveys and observational studies of clinicians' practice patterns would help ensure that such control groups reflect usual care. An international trial evaluating two target ranges for glycemic control in ICU patients has taken such an approach.[155]

Analyzing Risks and Benefits

Assessment of the potential risks involves three steps.[156] First, the risks and discomforts of the trial must be identified; these include not only the physical risks but also psychological, economic, and social risks, including those that might emanate from breaches of confidentiality. Second, the risks must be minimized by changing the study design if possible—for example, excluding subjects who are at substantially higher risk, replacing invasive procedures with less risky procedures, or providing enhanced safety monitoring. Finally, the risks must be reasonable when weighed against potential benefits to the subjects and to society. In weighing risks and benefits, some ethicists have found it useful to use a component analysis, which distinguishes between procedures with potential for benefiting subjects and procedures that merely answer a scientific question, without offering a potential direct benefit to subjects.[157,158]

Within a component analysis, a study should be acceptable only if the risk of each component of the research—that is, each procedure the researchers will carry out—is justified separately. Components that do not benefit the subject but are designed solely to answer a research question are justified if the risks are reasonable in relation to the potential to generate scientific knowledge—a so-called risk-knowledge calculus. Procedures that may directly benefit the subject must meet an additional standard of equipoise: There must be genuine uncertainty about whether the balance of risks and potential benefits of the experimental intervention are superior to those of accepted practice.

The evidence used to evaluate the separate risks and benefits of each component is fraught with uncertainty; therefore, investigators should be more conservative in estimating the degree of risks than in projecting potential benefits.

Justifying risks by the separate components of the study does not imply that there is no upper limit to acceptable risk.[125] Without an absolute risk threshold, the degree of permissible risk may be tied to the severity of the subjects' condition, for example, and trials involving high-risk procedures may wrongly be considered ethically sound.

Research Performed in the Emergency Setting

An IRB can grant a waiver of informed consent for research on novel therapies in emergency situations, such as cardiac arrest, stroke, severe arrhythmias, and life-threatening traumatic injury. Patients with these conditions cannot give consent, and the narrow time window in which treatment must be given often does not afford sufficient time to obtain consent from a legal representative.

In a trial assessing the safety and efficacy of an infusion of low-dose steroid in severe septic shock,[159] patients initially were supposed to be randomized to a treatment group within 3 hours from the beginning of shock. Written informed consent had to be obtained from patients or their families. It soon became clear that, given the informed consent requirement, the trial could not be completed within a reasonable period of time. Subsequently, the hospital's IRB approved a waiver of informed consent and increased the maximum time between the beginning of septic shock and randomization to the study treatment group from 3 to 8 hours, thereby yielding sufficient recruitment.

Various countries and regions have differing regulations governing such research. In 1996, the U.S. government specified several mechanisms under which research involving incapacitated subjects in emergency situations can be allowed without informed consent of a legally authorized representative.[230] But these procedures have been criticized as unnecessarily complicated and burdensome, and possible revisions were under consideration in 2007.[161-163]

A European Directive regarding clinical research on drugs contains no provisions for waiver of informed consent for research in emergencies. Some European countries, however, provide for possible waivers in their own regulations.[164]

Research in the emergency setting has been performed in other countries under less ambiguous and burdensome regulations. For example, in Australia, the Saline versus Albumin Fluid Evaluation (SAFE) study randomized subjects with evidence of volume depletion to receive either albumin or normal saline.[150] Australia's National Statement on Ethical Conduct in Research Involving Humans allows an ethics committee to approve research without prior consent provided that (1) inclusion in the research is not contrary to the interest of the patient; (2) the research is intended to be therapeutic, and the research intervention poses no more risk than that inherent in the patient's condition and alternative methods of treatment; (3) the research is based on valid scientific hypotheses that support a reasonable possibility of benefit over standard care; and (4) as soon as reasonably possible, the patient or the patient's relatives or legal representatives, or both, will be informed of the patient's inclusion in the research and of the option to withdraw from the research without any reduction in quality of care.[165]

Regulations in Canada stipulate that research in the emergency setting may proceed under the following conditions: if a serious threat to the prospective subject requires immediate intervention,[166] if no standard efficacious care exists or the research offers a real possibility of direct benefit to the subject in comparison with standard care, or if the risk of harm is not greater than that involved in standard efficacious care or is clearly justified by direct benefit to the subject.

Monitoring for Subject Safety

The welfare of human subjects of clinical trials is overseen not just by IRBs and research ethics committees, which approve protocols before a trial can begin, but also by data and safety monitoring boards (DSMBs) which monitor data from ongoing trials, particularly large, multicenter trials.[167] The role of DSMBs is to collect data that otherwise might not be aggregated until much later in a trial and to watch for unexpected adverse results that might necessitate halting the trial—or unexpected beneficial results that might justify making the experimental therapy more widely available.

Investigators should be vigilant in observing and reporting adverse events to their research ethics committees and other regulatory agencies. Although interpretation of individual adverse events may be problematic for IRBs, these ethics committees do need to conduct effective continuing reviews. DSMBs should review individual reported adverse events, as well as aggregate data on mortality or other outcome trends. By using preplanned statistical analyses, DSMBs can determine when trials should be stopped early to avoid continued exposure of subjects to inferior treatments.

CONCLUSIONS

The ethical conduct of research in the critical care setting is complex, evolving, and fraught with hazards to persons who participate in such research. Heightened awareness of the principles and requirements that govern such research would enhance the ability of the research community to conduct such research ethically and to maintain the public trust in the research endeavor.

KEY POINTS

- The goals of the ICU team are to resolve life-threatening illness, to prolong life, and to relieve suffering.
- ICU providers should understand concepts of biomedical ethics including beneficence, nonmaleficence, autonomy, justice, truth telling, and confidentiality.
- When a diagnostic or therapeutic option is not medically indicated, a physician should not make it available.
- Given the likelihood that critically ill patients may be unable to participate in life-sustaining treatment decisions, clinicians should make efforts to promote advance care planning—use of advance directives—and should anticipate the need for limited treatment orders in advance of life threatening events.
- Competent patients have the legal right to refuse medical treatments, even if physicians believe that such treatments are indicated. Patients do not, however, have a correlative right to demand treatment.
- Withholding or withdrawing life-sustaining treatment—with the informed consent of the patient or surrogate decision maker, or in compliance with advance directives—is both valid and quite common. However state laws regulating the authority of surrogate decision makers vary.
- Active euthanasia—for example, administering a fatal overdose of a narcotic with the express purpose of ending life—and physician-assisted suicide are illegal in most states but are the subject of intense ethical debate. According to published studies, between 12% and 54% of U.S. physicians receive a request for euthanasia or physician-assisted suicide at some time in their careers.
- Research lies outside of the context of the doctor-patient relationship. In medical practice, physicians' primary obligation is to protect the best interests of their patients. Researchers have dual interests: an interest in testing a research hypothesis to advance medical science and an interest in protecting the rights and welfare of human subjects. Physicians engaged in clinical research should make certain that their patients understand the difference.

REFERENCES

1. DuVal G, Clarridge B, Gensler G, Danis M: A national survey of U.S. internists' experiences with ethical dilemmas and ethics consultation. J Gen Intern Med 2004;19:251-258.
2. Beauchamp TL, Childress JF: Principles of Biomedical Ethics, 5th ed. New York, Oxford University Press, 2001.
3. Emanuel EJ, Emanuel LL: Four models of the physician-patient relationship. JAMA 1992;267:2221-2226.
4. Cohen CB: Can autonomy and equity coexist in the ICU? Hastings Cent Rept 1986;October:39-41.
5. Cook D: Patient autonomy versus paternalism. Crit Care Med 2001;29: N24-N25.
6. Nelson JL, Nelson HL: Guided by intimates. Hastings Cent Rep 1993;23:14-15.
7. Kuczewski MG: Reconceiving the family. The process of consent in medical decision making. Hastings Cent Rep 1996;26:30-37.
8. Davidson JE, Powers K, Hedayat KM, et al: Clinical practice guidelines for support of the family in the patient-centered intensive care unit: American College of Critical Care Task Force 2004-2005. Crit Care Med 2007; 5:2-18.
9. Browning G, Warren NA: Unmet needs of family members in the medical intensive care waiting room. Crit Care Nurs Q 2006;29:86-95.
10. Koenig B, Gates-Williams J: Understanding cultural differences in caring for dying patients. West J Med 1995;163:244-249.
11. Danis M: Role of ethnicity, race, religion, and socio-economic status in end of life care in the ICU. In Curtis JR, Rubenfeld GD (eds): The Transition from Cure to Comfort: Managing Death in the Intensive Care Unit. Oxford, Oxford University Press, 2000.
12. Mir NU: Breaking bad news: Practical advice for busy doctors. Hosp Med 2004;65:613-615.
13. Lingren VA, Ames NJ: Caring for patients on mechanical ventilation: What research indicates is best practice. Am J Nurs 2005;105: 50-60.
14. Jain M, Miller L, Belt D, et al: Decline in ICU adverse events, nosocomial infections and cost through a quality improvement initiative focusing on teamwork and culture change. Qual Safety Health Care 2006;15:235-239.
15. Mills AE, Spencer EM: Values based decision making: A tool for achieving the goals of healthcare. HEC Forum 2005;17:18-32.
16. Baker R, Strosberg M: Triage and equality: An historical reassessment of utilitarian analyses of triage. Kennedy Inst Ethics J 1992;2:103-123.
17. Swenson MD: Scarcity in the intensive care unit: Principles of justice for rationing ICU beds. Am J Med 1992;92:551-555.
18. Engelhardt HT, Rie MA: Intensive care units, scarce resources, and conflicting

principles of justice. JAMA 1986; 255:1159-1164.
19. Task Force on Guidelines, Society of Critical Care Medicine: Recommendations for intensive care unit admission and discharge criteria. Crit Care Med 1988;16:807-808.
20. Task Force of the American College of Critical Care Medicine, Society of Critical Care Medicine: Guidelines for intensive care unit admission, discharge, and triage. Crit Care Med 1999;27:633-638.
21. Dawson JA: Admission, discharge, and triage in critical care. Critical Care Clinics;9:555-574, 1993.
22. Teres D: Civilian triage in the intensive care unit: The ritual of the last bed. Crit Care Med 1993;21:598-606.
23. Terry P, Rushton CH: Allocation of scarce resources: Ethical challenges, clinical realities. Am J Crit Care 1996;5:326-330.
24. Cooper AB, Joglekar AS, Gibson J, et al: Communication of bed allocation decisions in a critical care unit and accountability for reasonableness. BMC Health Serv Res 2005;5(67),.
25. Truog RD, Brock DW, Cook DJ, et al: Rationing in the intensive care unit. Crit Care Med. 2006;34:958-963; quiz 971.
26. Knaus W: Ethical implications of risk stratification in the acute care setting. Cambridge Q Healthcare Ethics 1993;2:193-196.
27. Latour J, Lopez V, Rodriguez M, et al: Inequalities in health in intensive care patients. J Clin Epidemiol 1991;44:889-894.
28. Danis M, Linde-Zwirble WT, Astor A, et al: How does lack of insurance affect use of intensive care? A population-based study. Crit Care Med 2006;34:2043-2048.
29. Schneiderman LJ, Gilmer T, Teetzel HD, et al: Effects of ethics consultation on nonbeneficial life-sustaining treatments in the intensive care setting: A randomized controlled trial. JAMA 2003;290:1166-1172.
30. Hippocrates: The art. In Jones WHS (ed): Hippocrates. The Loeb Classical Library. Cambridge, MA, Harvard University Press, 1923.
31. Bigelow J: Self-limited disease: Address to the Massachusetts Medical Society, May 27, 1835. In Nature in Disease. Boston, Ticknor and Fields, 1854.
32. Warren J: Etherization, with Surgical Remarks. Boston, Ticknor & Co, 1848.
33. Pope Pius XII: The prolongation of life. In Reiser SJ, Dyck AJ, Curran WJ (eds): thics in Medicine. Cambridge, MA, MIT Press, 1977.
34. In re Quinlan, 70 N.J. 10 (1976).
35. Cruzan v. Director of Missouri Department of Health, 110 S. Ct. 2841 (1990).
36. Washington v. Glucksberg, 117 S. Ct. 2302 (1997).
37. In re Conroy, 98 N.J. 321 (1985).
38. Emanuel EJ: A review of the ethical and legal aspects of terminating medical care. Am J Med 1988; 84:291-301.
39. Emanuel EJ, Emanuel LL: Proxy decision making for incompetent patients. An ethical and empirical analysis. JAMA 1992;267:2067-2071.
40. Shalowitz DI, Garrett-Mayer E, Wendler D: The accuracy of surrogate decision makers: A systematic review. Arch Intern Med 2006;166:493-497.
41. Wendland v. Wendland, 110 Cal. Rptr. 2d 412 (2001).
42. In re Martin, 538 N.W.2d 399 (Mich. 1995).
43. Miles SH: Informed demand for "non-beneficial" medical treatment. N Engl J Med 1991;325:512-515.
44. Bouvia v. Superior Court, 225 Cal. Rptr. 297 (1986).
45. Kelly G: Medico-moral Problems. St. Louis, The Catholic Hospital Association, 1958.
46. Brophy v. New England Sinai Hospital, 398 Mass. 417 (1986).
47. Meisel A: Legal myths about terminating life support. Arch Intern Med 1991;151:1497-1502.
48. Schneiderman LJ, Jecker NS, Jonsen AR: Medical futility: Its meaning and ethical implications. Ann Intern Med 1990;112:949-954.
49. Truog RD, Brett AS, Frader J: The problem with futility. N Engl J Med 1992;326:1560-1564.
50. Veatch RM: Why physicians cannot determine if care is futile. J Am Geriatr Soc 1994;42:871-874.
51. Helft PR, Siegler M, Lantos J: The rise and fall of the futility movement. N Engl J Med 2000;343:293-296.
52. Curtis JR, Park DR, Krone MR, Pearlman RA: Use of the medical futility rationale in do-not-attempt-resuscitation orders. JAMA 1995;273:124-128.
53. Fine RL, Mayo TW: Resolution of futility by due process: Early experience with the Texas Advance Directives Act. Ann Intern Med 2003;138:743-746.
54. In re Mary Moe, 385 Mass. 555 (1982).
55. In re Storar 52 N.Y. 2d 363 (1981).
56. Sehgal A, Galbraith A, Chesney M, et al: How strictly do dialysis patients want their advance directives followed? JAMA 1992;267:59-63.
57. The President's Commission for the Study of Ethical Problems in Medicine and Biomedical and Behavioral Research: Deciding to forego life-sustaining treatment. Washington, DC, U.S. Government Printing Office, 1983.
58. Meisel A, Snyder L, Quill T for the American College of Physicians–American Society of Internal Medicine End-of-Life Care Consensus Panel: Seven legal barriers to end-of-life care: Myths, realities, and grains of truth. JAMA 2000;284:2495-2501.
59. www.nhpco.org.
60. www.medicaldirective.org.
61. Berry SR, Singer PA: The cancer specific advance directive. Cancer 1998;82:1570-77.
62. Emanuel EJ, Ash A, Yu W, et al: Managed care, hospice use, site of death, and medical expenditures in the last year of life. Arch Intern Med 2002;162:1722-1728.
63. Vitelli CE, Cooper K, Rogatko A, et al: Cardiopulmonary resuscitation and the patient with cancer. J Clin Oncol 1991;9:111-115.
64. Prendergast TJ, Claessens MT, Luce JM: A national survey of end-of-life care for critically ill patients. Am J Respir Crit Care Med 1998;158:1163-1167.
65. Faber-Langendoen K: A multi-institutional study of care given to patients dying in hospitals. Ethical and practice implications. Arch Intern Med 1996;156:2130-2136.
66. Prendergast TJ, Luce JM: Increasing incidence of withholding and withdrawal of life support from the critically ill. Am J Respir Crit Care Med 1997;Jan;155(1):15-20.
67. Teno J, Lynn J, Wenger N, et al: Advance directives for seriously ill hospitalized patients: effectiveness with the patient self-determination act and the SUPPORT intervention. SUPPORT Investigators. Study to Understand Prognoses and Preferences for Outcomes and Risks of Treatment. J Am Geriatr Soc 1997;45:500-507.
68. Danis M, Southerland LI, Garrett JM, et al: A prospective study of advance directives for life-sustaining care. New Engl J Med 1991;324:882-888.
69. Teno JM, Stevens M, Spernak S, et al: Role of written advance directives in decision making: Insights from qualitative and quantitative data. J Gen Intern Med 1998;13:439-446.
70. Kollef MH: Outcome prediction in the ICU. In Curtis JR, Rubenfeld GD (eds): Managing Death in the Intensive Care Unit. New York, Oxford University Press, 2001.
71. Emanuel EJ: Euthanasia: Historical, ethical, and empiric perspectives. Arch Intern Med 1994;154:1890.
72. A piece of my mind: It's over, Debbie. JAMA 1988;259:272.
73. Cassel CK, Meier DE: Morals and moralism in the debate over euthanasia and assisted suicide. N Engl J Med 1992;327:1280-1384.
74. Rachels J: The End of Life: Euthanasia and Morality. New York, Oxford University Press, 1986.
75. Brock DW: Voluntary active euthanasia. Hastings Cent Rep 1992;22:10-22.
76. Callahan D: When self-determination runs amok. Hastings Cent Rep 1992;22:52-55.
77. Kass LR: Is there a right to die? Hastings Cent Rep 1993;23:34-43.
78. Singer PA, Siegler M: Euthanasia—a critique. N Engl J Med 1990;322: 1881-1883.
79. The Oregon Death with Dignity Act. Available at: http://www.oregon.gov/DHS/ph/pas/index.shtml.
80. Deliens L, van der Wal G: The euthanasia law in Belgium and the Netherlands. Lancet 2003;362:1239.
81. Kissane DW, Street A, Nitschke P: Seven deaths in Darwin: Case studies under the Rights of the Terminally Ill Act, Northern Territory, Australia. Lancet 1998;352:1097.
82. Hurst SA, Mauron A: Assisted suicide and euthanasia in Switzerland: Allowing a role for non-physicians. BMJ 2003;326:271-273.
83. Onwuteaka-Philipsen BD, van der Heide A, Koper D, et al: Euthanasia and other end-of-life decisions in the Netherlands in 1990, 1995, and 2001. Lancet 2003;362:395.
84. van der Heide A, Deliens L, Faisst K, et al: End-of-life decision-making in six European countries: Descriptive study. Lancet 2003;362:345, 2003.

85. Breitbart W, Rosenfeld BD, Passik SD: Interest in physician-assisted suicide among ambulatory HIV-infected patients. Am J Psychiatry 1996;153: 238.
86. Ganzini L, Johnston WS, McFarland BH, et al: Attitudes of patients with amyotrophic lateral sclerosis and their care givers toward assisted suicide. N Engl J Med 1998;339:967.
87. Emanuel EJ, Fairclough DL, Daniels ER, et al: Euthanasia and physician-assisted suicide: Attitudes and experiences of oncology patients, oncologists, and the public, Lancet 1996;347:1805.
88. van der Lee ML, van der Bom JG, Swarte NB, et al: Euthanasia and depression: A prospective cohort study among terminally ill cancer patients. J Clin Oncol 2005;23: 6607-6612.
89. Groenewoud JH, van der Heide A, Onwuteaka-Philipsen BD, et al: Clinical problems with the performance of euthanasia and physician-assisted suicide in The Netherlands. N Engl J Med 2000;342:551.
90. Bernard C: An Introduction to the Study of Experimental Medicine. London, Macmillan & Co, Ltd, 1865 (first English translation, 1927).
91. Rothman DJ: Strangers at the Bedside: A History of How Law and Bioethics Transformed Medical Decision Making. New York: Basic Books; 1991.
92. Mitscherlich A, Mielke F: Epilogue: Seven were hanged. In Annas GJ, Rodin MA (eds): The Nazi Doctors and the Nuremberg Code—Human Rights in Human Experimentation. New York, Oxford University Press, 1992, pp 105-107.
93. International Military Tribunal: Trials of war criminals before the Nuremberg Military Tribunals under Control Council law no. 10. Washington, DC, U.S. Government Printing Office, 1950.
94. World Medical Association: Declaration of Helsinki: Ethical principles for medical research involving human subjects. Ferney-Voltaire, France, World Health Organization, 1964.
95. National Commission for the Protection of Human Subjects of Biomedical and Behavioral Research: The Belmont Report: Ethical principles and guidelines for the protection of human subjects of research. Washington, DC, U.S. Government Printing Office, 1979.
96. Silverman HJ, Miller FG: Control group selection in critical care randomized controlled trials evaluating interventional strategies: An ethical assessment. Crit Care Med 2004;32:852-857.
97. Freedman B: Equipoise and the ethics of clinical research. N Engl J Med 1987;317:141-145.
98. London AJ, Kadane JB: Placebos that harm: Sham surgery controls in clinical trials. Statist Meth Med Res 2002; 11:413-427.
99. Dreyfuss D: Is it better to consent to an RCT or to care? Intensive Care Med 2005;31:345-355.
100. Concato J, Shah N, Horwitz RI: Randomized, controlled trials, observational studies, and the hierarchy of research designs. N Engl J Med 2000;342:1887-1892.
101. Kant I: Groundwork for the Metaphysics of Morals. New Haven, Yale University Press, 2002.
102. Lidz WW, Appelbaum PS: The therapeutic misconception. Problems and solutions. Med Care 2002;40: V55-V63.
103. Dresser R: The ubiquity and utility of the therapeutic misconception. Soc Phil Policy Found 2002;19:271-294.
104. Silverman HJ: Ethical considerations of ensuring an informed and autonomous consent in research involving critically ill patients. Am J Respir Crit Care Med 1996;154: 582-586.
105. 45 CFR 46 116 (d)(1-4): Protection of Human Subjects;. Rev. June 18 1991.
106. International Conference on Harmonisation of Technical Requirements for Registration of Pharmaceuticals for Human Use (ICH) adopts Consolidated Guideline on Good Clinical Practice in the Conduct of Clinical Trials on Medicinal Products for Human Use. Int Dig Health Legis 1997;48(2):231-234.
107. Silverman HJ, Hull SC, Sugarman J: Variability among institutional review boards' decisions within the context of a multicenter trial. Crit Care Med 2001;29:235-241.
108. ACHRE (Advisory Committee on Human Radiation Experiments): Advisory Committee on Human Radiation Experiments, Final Report. Washington, DC, U.S. Government Printing Office, 1995.
109. Silverman HJ, Luce JM, Lanken PN, et al: for the NHLBI Acute Respiratory Distress Syndrome Clinical Trials Network (ARDSnet): Recommendations for informed consent forms for critical care clinical trials. Crit Care Med 2005;33:867-882.
110. Estey A, Wilkin G, Dossetor J: Are research subjects able to retain the information they are given during the consent process? Health Law Rev 1994;3:37-41.
111. Williams FF, French JK, White HD for the HERO-2 Consent Substudy Investigators: Informed consent during the clinical emergency of acute myocardial infarction (HERO-2 consent substudy): A prospective observational study. Lancet 2003; 361:918-922.
112. Schaeffer MH, Krantz DS, Wichman A, et al: The impact of disease severity on the informed consent process in clinical research. Am J Med 1996;100: 261-268.
113. Appelbaum PS, Roth LH, Lidz CW, et al: False hopes and best data: Consent to research and the therapeutic misconception. Hastings Cent Rep 1987;17:20-24.
114. Miller FG, Rosenstein DL: The therapeutic orientation to clinical trials. N Engl J Med 2003;348:1383-1386.
115. Clemens JD, Frederik FP, van Loon L, et al: Nonparticipation as a determinant of adverse health outcomes in a field trial of oral cholera vaccines. Am J Epidemiol 1992;135:865-874.
116. Peppercorn JM, Weeks JC, Cook EF, et al: Comparison of outcomes in cancer patients treated within and outside clinical trials: Conceptual framework and structured review. Lancet 2004;363:263-270.
117. World Medical Association: World Medical Association Declaration of Helsinki: Ethical principles for medical research involving human subjects. HIV Clin Trials 2001;(2):92-95.
118. Morin K, Rakatansky H, Riddick FA, et al: Managing conflicts of interest in the conduct of clinical trials. JAMA 2002;287:78-84.
119. Hawkins JS, Emanuel EJ: Clarifying confusions about coercion. Hastings Cent Rep 2005;35:16-19.
120. Sulmasy DP, Terry PB, Weisman CS, et al: The accuracy of substituted judgments in patients with terminal diagnoses. Ann Intern Med 1998;128:621-629.
121. Coppolino M, Ackerson L: Do surrogate decision makers provide accurate consent for intensive care research? Chest 2001;119: 603-612.
122. Jones C, Skirrow P, Griffiths R, et al: Post-traumatic stress disorder-related symptoms in relatives of patients following intensive care. Intensive Care Med 2004;30:456-460.
123. Pochard F, Azoulay E, Chevret S, et al: Symptoms of anxiety and depression in family members of intensive care unit patients: Ethical hypothesis regarding decision-making capacity. Crit Care Med 2001;29:1893-1897.
124. Silverman HJ, Luce JM, Schwartz J: Protecting subjects with decisional impairment in research. The need for a multifaceted approach. Am J Respir Crit Care Med 2004;169:10-14.
125. National Bioethics Advisory Commission (NBAC): Ethical and policy issues in research involving human participants. Rockville, MD: U.S. Government Printing Office, 2001.
126. Tri-Council Policy Statement: Ethical conduct for research involving humans. Available at: http://wwwcsualbertaca/~wfb/ethics/ethics-epdf#search=%22tri-council%20policy%20statement%22 1998.
127. Directive 2001/20/EC of the European Parliament and of the Council of 4 April 2001 on the approximation of the laws, regulations and administrative provisions of the member states relating to the implementation of good clinical practice in the conduct of clinical trials on medicinal products for human use. Off J Eur Communities 2001;L121: 33-44.
128. Compliance determination letters. Available at: http://ohrp.osophs.dhhs.gov/detrm_letrs/jul2000.htm.
129. University of California Office of the President Office of Research: Guidance on surrogate consent for research. Available at: http://www.llnl.gov/HumanSubjects/pdfs/surrogate.pdf; 2002 (accessed September 22, 2003).
130. Saks ER: Competency to decide on treatment and research. The MacArthur Capacity Instruments. In National Bioethics Advisory Commission (ed): Research Involving Persons with Mental Disorders That May Affect Decisionmaking Capacity.

Vol II: Commissioned Papers. Rockville, MD, National Bioethics Advisory Commission, 1999.
131. National Bioethics Advisory Commission: Research Involving Persons with Mental Disorders That May Affect Decisionmaking Capacity. 2 vols. Rockville, MD, U.S. Government Printing Office, 1998.
132. Keyserlingk EW, Kogan GK, Gauthier S: Proposed guidelines for the participation of persons with dementia as research subjects. Perspect Biol Med 1995;38:319-361.
133. Karlawish JHT: Research involving cognitively impaired adults. N Engl J Med 2003;348:1289-1392.
134. Keyserlingk EW, Kogan GK, Gauthier S: Proposed guidelines for the participation of persons with dementia as research subjects. Perspect Biol Med 1995;38:319-361.
135. 45 CFR 46 116 (d)(1-4): Protection of Human Subjects. Rev. June 18, 1991.
136. 45 CFR 46. 102(i): Protection of Human Subjects. Rev. June 18, 1991.
137. Onder RF: The ethics of placebo-controlled trials: The case of asthma. J Allergy Clin Immunol 2005;115:1228-1234.
138. Barst RJ, Langleben D, Frost A, et al: Sitazsentan therapy for pulmonary arterial hypertension. Am J Respir Crit Care Med 2004;169:441-447.
139. Freedman B: Placebo-controlled trials and the logic of clinical purpose. IRB 1990;12:1-6.
140. Freedman B, Weijer C, Glass KC: Placebo orthodoxy in clinical research I: Empirical and methodological myths. J Law Med Ethics 1996;24:243-251.
141. Temple RT, Ellenberg SS: Placebo-controlled trials and active-control trials in the evaluation of new treatments. Part 1: Ethical and scientific issues. Ann Intern Med 2000;133:455-463.
142. Temple R, Ellenberg SE: Placebo-controlled trials and active-control trials in the evaluation of new treatments. Part 2: Ethical and scientific issues. Ann Intern Med 2000;133:464-470.
143. Miller FG: The ethics of placebo-controlled trials—a middle ground. N Engl J Med 2001;345:915-919.
144. Hebert PC, Cook DJ, Wells G, Marshall J: The design of randomized clinical trials in critically ill patients. Chest 2002;121:1290-1300.
145. Sackett DL: Why randomized controlled trials fail but needn't: 2. Failure to employ physiological statistics, or the only formula a clinician-trialist is ever likely to need (or understand!). CMAJ 2001;165:1226-1237.
146. Gutierrez G, Palizas F, Doglio G, et al: Gastric intramucosal pH as a therapeutic index of tissue oxygenation in critically ill patients. Lancet 1992;339:195-199.
147. Sandham JD, Hull RD, Brant RF, et al: A randomized, controlled trial of the use of pulmonary-artery catheters in high-risk surgical patients. N Engl J Med 2003;348:5-14.
148. Richard C, Warszawski J, Anguel N, et al for the French Pulmonary Artery Catheter Study Group: Early use of the pulmonary artery catheter and outcomes in patients with shock and acute respiratory distress syndrome. A randomized controlled trial. JAMA 2003;290:2713-2720.
149. Harvey S, Harrison DA, Singer M, et al: Assessment of the clinical effectiveness of pulmonary artery catheters in management of patients in intensive care (PAC-Man): A randomized controlled trial. Lancet 2005;366: 472-477.
150. The SAFE Study Investigators: A comparision of albumin and saline for fluid resuscitation in the intensive care unit. N Engl M Med 2004;350: 2247-2256.
151. Krishnan JA, Moore D, Roveson C, et al: A prospective, controlled trial of a protocol-based strategy to discontinue mechanical ventilation. Am J Respir Crit Care Med 2004;169:673-678.
152. Randolph AG, Wjypij D, Venkataraman ST, et al: Efect of mechanical ventilator weaning protocols on respiratory outcomes in infancts and children: A randomized controlled trial. JAMA 2002;288:2561-2568.
153. Ely EW, Baker AM, Duagan DP, et al: Effect on the duration of mechanical ventilation of identifying patients capable of breathing spontaneously. N Engl J Med 1996;335:1864-1869.
154. The Ethical Conduct of Clinical Research Involving Critically Ill Patients in the United States and Canada. Am J Respir Crit Care Med 2004;170: 1375-1384.
155. The NICE-SUGAR Study Investigators: A multi-centre, open label, randomised controlled trial of two target ranges for glycaemic control in intensive care unit (ICU) patients. Available at: http://controlled-trialscom/isrctn/trial/ ISRCTN0498275/0/04968275html 2005 (accessed Feb. 5, 2006).
156. Emanuel EJ, Wendler D, Grady C: What makes clinical research ethical? JAMA 2000;283:2701-2711.
157. Weijer C: The ethical analysis of risk. J Law Med Ethics 2000;28:344-361.
158. McRae AD, Weijer C: Lessons from everyday lives: A moral justification for acute care research. Crit Care Med 2002;30:1146-1151.
159. Annane D, Outin H, Fisch C, Bellissant E: The effect of waiving consent on enrollment in a sepsis trial. Intensive Care Med 2004;30:321-324.
160. U.S. Department of Health and Human Services: Protection of human subjects: Informed consent and waiver of informed consent requirements in certain emergency research. Final rules. Fed Reg 1996;61:51500-51533.
161. Nichol G, Huszti E, Rokosh J, et al: Impact of informed consent requirements on cardiac arrest research in the United States: Exception from consent or from research? Resuscitation 2004;62:3-23.
162. Hiller KM, Haukoos JS, Heard K, et al: Impact of the Final Rule on the rate of clinical cardiac arrest research in the United States. Acad Emerg Med 2005;12:1091-1098.
163. Guidance for Institutional Review Boards, Clinical Investigators, and Sponsors: Exception from informed consent requirements for emergency research—draft. Available at: http:// www.fda.gov/OHRMS/DOCKETS/98fr/ 06d-0331-gdl0001.pdf
164. Lemaire F: Waiving consent for emergency research. Eur J Clin Invest 2005;35:287-289.
165. National Health and Medical Research Council: National statement on ethical conduct in research involving humans. Canberra, Australia, National Health and Medical Research Council, 1999.
166. Tri-Council Policy Statement: Ethical conduct for research involving humans. Available at: http:// wwwcsualbertaca/~wfb/ethics/ethics-epdf#search=%22tri-council%20policy %20statement%22 1998.
167. Morse MA, Califf RM, Sugarman J: Monitoring and ensuring safety during clinical research. JAMA 2001:285:1201-1205.

Chapter 73

Delirium, Sleep, and Mental Health Disturbances in Critical Illness

Pratik Pandharipande, James Jackson, and E. Wesley Ely

OVERVIEW

Advances in clinical medicine have resulted in improvements in patient outcomes in a host of medical conditions, such as acute respiratory distress syndrome (ARDS) and sepsis. Both the lay public and health care professionals are now becoming increasingly concerned not only with survival but also with the preservation of cognitive abilities, prevention of functional decline, and the quality of life among patients who survive critical illness.[1-5] In a recent survey, the potential of being left cognitively impaired was the major determinant of patients' treatment preferences at the end of life, with 9 of every 10 patients preferring death to severe cognitive impairment.[6] Similarly, in a report from the international "Surviving Intensive Care" 2002 Roundtable Conference held in Brussels,[7] the need for future investigations in neurocognitive abnormalities among survivors of intensive care received the strongest recommendation from the international panel of experts. Physicians and health care providers in intensive care units (ICUs) are accustomed to recognizing multiple organ dysfunction syndrome (MODS),[8-11] with therapy focused on the causes and treatment of respiratory, cardiovascular, renal, and hepatic dysfunction. There is a dearth of understanding and research, however, on the syndrome of brain dysfunction in the ICU. This chapter focuses on the cognitive and mental health disturbances of critical illness, with emphasis on delirium and sleep disturbances during critical illness as well as a brief discussion on post-traumatic stress disorder (PTSD), long-term cognitive impairment (LTCI), and depression after critical illness.

ACUTE BRAIN DYSFUNCTION OR DELIRIUM

Delirium

Delirium is defined by American Psychiatric Association's *The Diagnostic and Statistical Manual of Mental Disorders,* 4th revised edition (DSM IV),[12] as a disturbance of consciousness with inattention, accompanied by a change in cognition or perceptual disturbance that develops over a short time (hours to days) and fluctuates over time. Many different terms have been used to describe this spectrum of cognitive impairment in critically ill patients, including ICU psychosis, ICU syndrome, acute confusional state, septic encephalopathy, and acute brain failure.[13-15] The current consensus of many authorities is to consistently use the unifying term *delirium* and subcategorize according to the level of alertness (hyperactive, hypoactive, or mixed).[16] This is the approach that we will be taking in this chapter.

Prevalence and Subtypes

The prevalence of delirium in medical ICU cohort studies has been reported to be between 20% and 80%,[17-19] depending on the severity of illness and the delirium detection instrument used. Similarly, delirium is seen in about 70% of mechanically ventilated trauma and surgical ICU patients.[20] Unfortunately, delirium goes unrecognized by the clinician in a majority of the patients experiencing this complication,[21,22] and it may be incorrectly attributed to dementia, depression, or just an "expected" occurrence in the critically ill, elderly patient.[21] Peterson and associates[23] reported on delirium subtypes from a cohort of ventilated and nonventilated ICU patients in whom delirium was monitored. They found the rates of these subtypes in the ICU to be 1.6% for hyperactive, 43.5% for hypoactive, and 54.1% for mixed.[24]

Hyperactive delirium, which is rare in the pure form and associated with a better overall prognosis,[25] is characterized by agitation, restlessness, attempting to remove catheters or tubes, hitting, biting, and emotional lability.[16,26] This subtype is often referred to as "ICU psychosis." *Hypoactive delirium,* on the other hand, is very common and in many circumstances actually more deleterious for the patient in the long run.[25] Unfortunately, it remains unrecognized in 66% to 84% of patients, whether being treated in the ICU, hospital ward, or emergency department.[22,27-29] This delirium subtype is characterized by withdrawal, flat affect, apathy, lethargy, and decreased responsiveness.[25,30,31] Some authorities continue to refer to the hypoactive delirium as "encephalopathy" and the hyperactive subtype as "delirium or ICU psychosis." Because of the fluctuating nature of delirium, patients may present with a *mixed* clinical picture or may sequentially experience both of these subtypes. Most critical care providers would report that hyperactive delirium is far more common, perhaps because affected patients attract attention because of their immediate threat to self and others. Unless routine monitoring for delirium is implemented, the majority of delirium episodes, especially the "quiet" (hypoactive) form, will be missed.

Prognostic Significance

In non-ICU populations, the development of delirium in the hospital is associated with an in-hospital mortality of 25% to 33%, prolonged hospital stay, and three times greater likelihood of discharge to a nursing home.[32-34] In a three-site study of non-ICU medical patients, delirium was found to be an independent predictor of the combined outcome of death or nursing home placement.[35] McCusker and colleagues[36] found a 2.11 adjusted hazard ratio for dying in association with the development of delirium. This mortality increase has now been shown independent of dementia status.[37] Furthermore, three prospective studies have found that delirium was associated with a higher risk for dementia during the 2 to 3 years after hospitalization in non-ICU patient populations.[38-40]

Among medical ICU patients, delirium has been shown to be a strong predictor of longer duration of mechanical ventilation, longer length of ICU stay, higher costs, prolonged neuropsychological dysfunction, and even death.[41-44] The development of delirium is associated with a threefold increase in risk of death after data were controlled for pre-existing comorbidities, severity of illness, coma, and the use of sedative and analgesic medications.[41] These data also showed that delirium is not simply a transition state from coma to normal, because delirium occurred just as often among patients who never had coma as it did among patients with coma and persisted in 11% of patients at the time of hospital discharge.

Pathophysiology

The mechanisms of delirium remain a very promising area of neuroscientific study and likely relate to those factors leading to long-term cognitive impairment, which are as follows:

Neurotransmitters: From a neuroscience perspective, delirium is thought to be related to imbalances in the synthesis, release, and inactivation of neurotransmitters modulating the control of cognitive function, behavior, and mood.[25,31] Three of the neurotransmitter systems involved in the pathophysiology of delirium are dopamine, gamma-aminobutyric acid (GABA), and acetylcholine.[14,45,46] Whereas dopamine increases excitability of neurons, GABA and acetylcholine decrease neuronal excitability.[14] An imbalance in one or more of these neurotransmitters results in neuronal instability and unpredictable neurotransmission. In general, an excess of dopamine and depletion of acetylcholine are two major physiologic problems believed to be central to delirium. Other neurotransmitter systems thought to be involved in the development of delirium are serotonin imbalance, endorphin hyperfunction, and increased central noradrenergic activity.[25,45]

Inflammatory mediators: Other factors thought to be mechanistically deliriogenic in ICU patients are inflammatory abnormalities induced by endotoxin and cytokines.[47-50] The inflammatory mediators produced in sepsis, such as tumor necrosis factor-alpha (TNF-α), interleukin-1, and other cytokines and chemokines, initiate a cascade that leads to endothelial damage, thrombin formation, and microvascular compromise.[51] Animal models show that these inflammatory mediators cross the blood-brain barrier,[52] increase vascular permeability in the brain,[53] and result in electroencephalography (EEG) changes consistent with those seen in septic patients with delirium.[54,55] Release of inflammatory mediators may occur from (1) decreased cerebral blood flow, a result of the formation of microaggregates of fibrin, platelets, neutrophils, and erythrocytes in the cerebral microvasculature, (2) cerebral vasoconstriction occurring in response to α_1-adrenergic receptor activity[56]; or (3) interference with neurotransmitter synthesis and neurotransmission.[57]

Impaired oxidative metabolism: One hypothesis attempts to explain acute delirium as a behavioral manifestation of a "widespread reduction of cerebral oxidative metabolism resulting in an imbalance of neurotransmission."[58] On the basis of a series of investigations in which they evaluated delirious patients using EEG, Engel and Romano[59] postulated that delirium is a state of "cerebral insufficiency," that is, a global failure of cerebral oxidative metabolism. Their work showed that delirium is associated with diffuse slowing on EEG, a finding believed to represent a reduction in brain metabolism.

Cholinergic deficiency: Blass and colleagues[60] offered a possible link between the state of cerebral insufficiency proposed by Engel and Romano[59] and the hypothesis of cholinergic blockade by suggesting that impaired oxidative metabolism in the brain results in a cholinergic deficiency. The finding that hypoxia impairs acetylcholine synthesis supports this hypothesis.[61] This reduction in cholinergic function leads to an increase in the level of glutamate, dopamine, and norepinephrine in the brain. Additionally, serotonin and gamma GABA levels are reduced; all of these changes contribute to delirium.

Large neutral amino acid in delirium: Changes in the plasma levels of various amino acid precursors of cerebral neurotransmitters may affect their function, thus contributing to the development of delirium.[62] The amino acid entry into the brain is regulated by a sodium-independent large neutral amino acid transporter type 1 (LAT1).[63] The essential amino acid tryptophan, which is the precursor for serotonin, competes with several large neutral amino acids (LNAAs), such as tyrosine, phenylalanine, valine, leucine, and isoleucine, for transport across the blood-brain barrier via the LAT1 transporter.[63] This competition determines its uptake into the brain.[63] Another amino acid that may play an important role in the pathogenesis of delirium is phenylalanine.[58] Like tryptophan, phenylalanine competes with the other LNAAs (tyrosine, tryptophan, valine, leucine, and isoleucine) for transport across the blood-brain barrier. An increase in the cerebral uptake of tyrosine and phenylalanine compared with the other LNAAs leads to greater availability of precursors for both dopamine and norepinephrine, two neurotransmitters that have been implicated in the pathogenesis of delirium.[58]

It is important to realize that although delirium may occur as a result of perturbations in other organ systems, the brain responds to systemic infections and injury with an inflammatory response of its own that also involves cytokine production, cell infiltration, and tissue damage.[64,65] Reports indicate that local inflammation in the brain and subsequent activation of these central nervous system immune responses are accompanied by manifestations of systemic inflammation,[46,66,67] including production of large amounts of peripherally produced tumor necrosis factor-alpha, interleukin-10, and interferon-γ.[64,68-70] Thus, it is postulated that the brain can become an engine of inflammation, driving the development, resolution, or both, of multiple organ dysfunction syndrome.

Risk Factors for Delirium

Although non-ICU cohort studies have identified numerous risk factors for the development of delirium,[34] only a few studies have examined these factors in the ICU population. Baseline risk factors that predispose patients to a greater degree of vulnerability for delirium include Alzheimer's disease, chronic illness, advanced age, and depression.[14,71,72] Dubois and coworkers[73] found that preexisting hypertension and smoking (presumably because of relative hypoperfusion and nicotine withdrawal, respectively) were significantly associated with the development of ICU delirium. Another investigation reported that preexisting dementia was a significant risk factor for development of delirium in the post-ICU period.[18]

Precipitating and iatrogenic risk factors represent areas of potential modification and, thus, intervention for delirium prevention and treatment. Precipitating factors are hypoxia, metabolic disturbances, electrolyte imbalances, withdrawal syndromes, acute infection (systemic and intracranial), seizures, dehydration, hyperthermia, sleep deprivation, head trauma, vascular disorders, and intracranial space-occupying lesions.[14,71,72]

In practical terms, the risk factors for delirium can be divided into the following categories: (1) host factors, (2) the acute illness itself, and (3) iatrogenic or environmental factors (Table 73-1). Although delirium may be a function of patients' specific underlying illness, it may also be due to medical management issues and thus may have preventable causes. Of these risk factors, sedative and analgesic medications and sleep deprivation appear to be the leading iatrogenic and hence possibly preventable risk factors for delirium. There are conflicting data on the association of anticholinergics, corticosteroids, histamine H_2 antagonists, and anticonvulsants with the development of delirium in ICU patients.[21,74-76] These agents are not discussed here.

Sedatives and Analgesic Agents Contributing to Delirium

Sedative and analgesic medications are routinely administered to patients undergoing mechanical ventilation, in accordance with widely recognized clinical practice guidelines by the Society of Critical Care Medicine (SCCM),[77] in order to reduce pain and anxiety. Investigations have shown that continuous intravenous sedation is associated with prolonged mechanical ventilation and greater morbidity.[78] Similarly, associations between psychoactive medications and worsening cognitive outcomes have been reported in postoperative patients. Marcantonio and colleagues,[79] studying postoperative patients in whom delirium developed, found an association between use of benzodiazepines and meperidine and the occurrence of delirium. Dubois and coworkers[73] have shown that opiates (morphine and meperidine) administered either intravenously or via an epidural catheter may be associated with the development of delirium in medical/surgical ICU patients. Studies such as these have generated concern about whether such drugs were actually responsible for the development of delirium or were given as a result of delirium.

Table 73-1. Selected Risk Factors for Delirium in ICU Patients

Host factors	Age Baseline comorbidities Baseline cognitive impairment Genetic predisposition (?)
Acute illness	Sepsis Hypoxemia* Global severity of illness score Metabolic disturbances
Iatrogenic or environmental factors	Metabolic disturbances* Anticholinergic medications* Sedative and analgesic medications* Sleep disturbances*

*Potentially modifiable factor.

Our group has studied this temporal relationship between the administration of sedatives and analgesics and delirium.[80] To do so, one must make repeated cognitive assessments and must be able to assess the risk factors a patient is exposed to in between these assessments in order to study which of these factors is associated with a transition or a change in cognitive status to or from normal, delirium, or coma. In our study, lorazepam was found to be an independent risk factor for daily transition to delirium, and fentanyl, morphine, and propofol were associated with higher but not statistically significant odds ratios for such transition (Fig. 73-1).[80] Increasing age and Acute Physiology and Chronic Health Evaluation II (APACHE II) scores were also independent predictors of transitioning to delirium (Figs. 73-2 and 73-3).[80] Similar associations between another benzodiazepine, midazolam, and transition to delirium have been found in another study conducted in our trauma and surgical ICU patients.[20]

At this time it is not clear whether this association between benzodiazepines, and possibly opioids, and delirium is related to the pharmacokinetic properties of the agents or the pharmacodynamics of the drug. Benzodiazepines and propofol have high affinity for the GABA receptor in the central nervous system.[81] This GABA-mimetic effect can alter levels of numerous neurotransmitters believed to be deliriogenic.[57,82] Novel sedative agents that are GABA receptor sparing may help reduce some of the cognitive dysfunction seen in ICU patients. It is important to note that the data for opioids and delirium are not as consistent as those for the benzodiazepines. Although meperidine has been associated with delirium in most of the published studies, evidence for both fentanyl and morphine has been less convincing.[73,79,83] Morrison and colleagues[83] conducted a prospective observational trial in patients who had undergone hip surgery and found that patients whose pain was well controlled with morphine were less likely to demonstrate delirium than those who received other opioids. These investigations point to the importance of the judicious use of psychoactive medications, with focus on adequate analgesia.[84] One hopes that ongoing randomized controlled trials will pave the way to development of sedation and analgesic guidelines for the prevention or reduction of the occurrence of delirium due to administration of these psycho-active drugs.

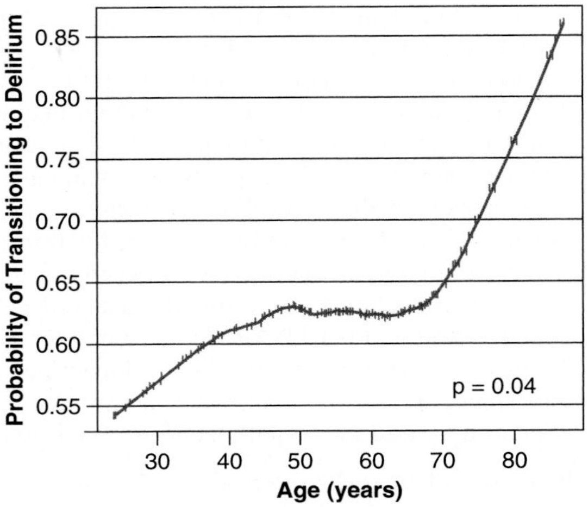

Figure 73-2. Age versus the probability of transitioning to delirium. The most notable finding related to age was that probability of transitioning to delirium increased dramatically for each year of life after 65 years. (With permission from Lippincott Williams & Wilkins. Pandharipande P, Shintani A, Truman P, et al: Lorazepam is an independent risk factor for transitioning to delirium in intensive care unit patients. Anesthesiology 2006;104:21-26.)

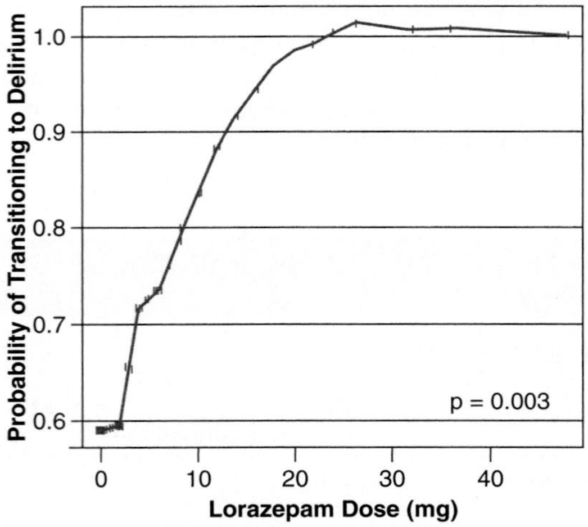

Figure 73-1. Lorazepam dose versus probability of transitioning to delirium. The probability of transitioning to delirium increased with the dose of lorazepam administered in the previous 24 hours. This *incremental* risk was large at low doses and plateaued at around 20 mg/day. (With permission from Lippincott Williams & Wilkins. Pandharipande P, Shintani A, Truman P, et al: Lorazepam is an independent risk factor for transitioning to delirium in intensive care unit patients. Anesthesiology 2006;104:21-26.)

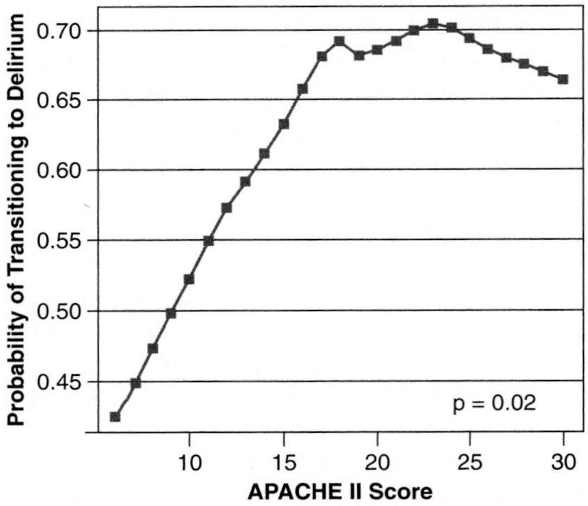

Figure 73-3. Severity of illness versus the probability of transitioning to delirium. The probability of transitioning to delirium increased dramatically for each additional point in APACHE II severity of illness score until it reached a plateau score of 18. (With permission from Lippincott Williams & Wilkins. Pandharipande P, Shintani A, Truman P, et al: Lorazepam is an independent risk factor for transitioning to delirium in intensive care unit patients. Anesthesiology 2006;104:21-26.)

Diagnosis

The development of tools such as the Intensive Care Delirium Screening Checklist (ICDSC)[17] and the Confusion Assessment Method for the ICU (CAM-ICU)[19] have allowed for the rapid diagnosis of delirium in patients by nonpsychiatric physicians and other health care personnel even while such patients are mechanically ventilated. The Society of Critical Care Medicine has proposed guidelines for more routine and more diligent monitoring of delirium using reliable and validated scales.[77]

Diagnosis of delirium is a two-step process. Level of arousal is first measured with the use of a standardized sedation scale, like the Richmond Agitation-Sedation Scale (RASS) (Fig. 73-4).[85,86] This is a 10-point scale with scores ranging from +4 to –5, score of 0 denoting a calm and alert patient. Positive RASS scores denote positive or aggressive symptomatology ranging from +1 (mild restlessness) to +4 (dangerous agitation). The negative RASS scores differentiate between response to verbal commands (scores –1 to –3) and physical stimulus (scores –4 and –5). If the patient's RASS score is –4 or –5 or not arousable by verbal commands, no further evaluation for delirium is performed, because the patient is comatose and is unable to be assessed for delirium. For patients who are arousable (RASS scores of –3 and higher), delirium can be assessed with the ICDSC[17] or by the CAM-ICU.[19] The ICDSC assesses eight features of delirium: altered level of consciousness, inattention, disorientation, hallucinations, psychomotor agitation/retardation, inappropriate mood/speech, sleep/wake cycle disturbance, and symptom fluctuation. The sensitivity and specificity of this tool are 99% and 64%, respectively.[17] The CAM-ICU, which can be performed in about 60 to 90 seconds,[87] is comprised of four features that assess the following: acute change or fluctuation of mental status (feature 1), inattention (feature 2), disorganized thinking (feature 3), or an altered level of consciousness (feature 4).

To be diagnosed as delirious, a patient must have a RASS score of –3 or higher, with an acute change or fluctuation in mental status (feature 1), accompanied by inattention (feature 2) and either disorganized thinking (feature 3) or an altered level of consciousness (feature 4). A complete description of the CAM-ICU as well as training materials, including translations and clinical vignettes, can be found at our website (www.icudelirium.org).

Prevention and Management

Primary Prevention and Nonpharmacologic Approaches

In a trial of 852 general medical patients older than 70 years,[88] implementation of strategies for primary prevention of delirium resulted in a 40% reduction in the odds for development of delirium (15% in controls vs. 9.9% in the intervention patients). The protocol focused on optimization of risk factors via the following methods: repeated reorientation of the patient by trained volunteers and nurses, provision of cognitively stimulating

Linking Sedation and Delirium Monitoring:
A Two Step Approach to Assess Consciousness

Step One: Sedation Assessment
The Richmond Agitation and Sedation Scale: The RASS

Score	Term	Description	
+4	Combative	Overly combative, violent, immediate danger to staff	
+3	Very agitated	Pulls or removes tube(s) or catheter(s); aggressive	
+2	Agitated	Frequent non-purposeful movement, fights ventilator	
+1	Restless	Anxious but movements not aggressive vigorous	
0	Alert and calm		
–1	Drowsy	Not fully alert, but has sustained awakening (eye-opening/eye contact) to *voice* **(≥10 seconds)**	Verbal Stimulation
–2	Light sedation	Briefly awakens with eye contact to *voice* **(<10 seconds)**	
–3	Moderate sedation	Movement or eye opening to *voice* **(but no eye contact)**	
–4	Deep sedation	No response to voice, but movement or eye opening to *physical* stimulation	Physical Stimulation
–5	Unarousable	No response to *voice or physical* stimulation	

If RASS is –4 or –5, then **Stop** and **Reassess** patient at later time
If RASS is above –4 (–3 through +4) then **Proceed to Step Two**

Step Two: Delirium Assessment

Feature 1: Acute onset of mental status changes or a fluctuating course

And

Feature 2: Inattention

And

Feature 3: Disorganized thinking OR **Feature 4:** Altered level of consciousness

= DELIRIUM

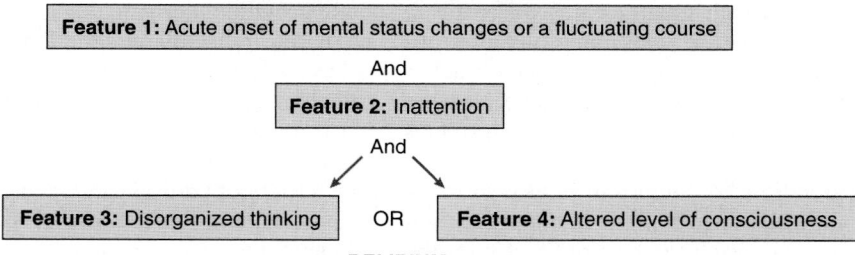

Figure 73-4. Richmond Agitation-Sedation Scale (RASS) and the Confusion Assessment Method for the ICU (CAM-ICU). This sedation scale and delirium instrument can be used together as a two-step approach to assess consciousness and diagnose delirium. Patients are considered to have delirium if they have RASS scores of –3 and higher and are assessed by CAM-ICU as "positive" by having both features 1 and 2 and either feature 3 or feature 4. (Data from references 19, 85, 86, and 148.)

activities for the patient three times per day, a nonpharmacologic sleep protocol to enhance normalization of sleep/wake cycles, early mobilization activities and range of motion exercises, timely removal of catheters and physical restraints, institution of the use of eyeglasses and magnifying lenses, use of hearing aids and earwax disimpaction, and early correction of dehydration.[88] Unfortunately, this intervention did not show sustained benefit during the 6 months of follow-up.[89] Later studies of delirium were unable to reproduce this success in reducing the incidence of delirium.[90,91]

Milisen and associates[92] and Lundstrom and coworkers,[93] who studied the implementation of multifactorial and multidisciplinary educational strategies, reported decreases in the duration and severity of delirium in patients cared for by staff who had received delirium-specific education.[92,93] Milisen and associates[92] measured the impact on delirium of implementing a nurse-led intervention program that involved delirium education for the nursing staff, systematic cognitive screening, availability of consultative services from a delirium resource nurse, and scheduled pain protocol on delirium. These researchers reported that although the program had no effect on the incidence of delirium, the duration and severity of delirium were significantly lower.[92] Lundstrom and coworkers[93] reported that in patients on a ward where the staff participated in specific educational activities focused on delirium and where the bedside nursing care was reorganized to provide more continuity of patient-centered care, duration of delirium and hospital stay were shorter and mortality was lower than in control patients. Cole and colleagues[91] found no difference in delirium rates between patients cared for by an intervention nurse and patients who received standard care. All of these nonpharmacologic, "protocolization of care" studies focused on non-ICU patient populations. Clearly such investigations must be designed and conducted in the ICU (rather than simply extrapolated from non-ICU studies).

Although primary prevention of delirium is preferred, some delirium is inevitable in the ICU. In patients exhibiting delirium, the basic tenets of patient management, such as restoration of sleep/wake cycles, timely removal of catheters, early mobilization, minimization of unnecessary noise/stimuli, and frequent reorientation, should be applied liberally. Additionally, it should be emphasized that although sedative and analgesic agents have a very important role in patient comfort, health care professionals must also strive to achieve the right balance of administering these drugs through greater focus on reducing unnecessary or overzealous use. Instituting daily interruption of sedatives and analgesics, protocolizing their delivery, and instituting target-based sedation have all been shown to improve patient outcomes, although the studies reporting these results have not specifically looked at delirium rate or duration.[94-96] Studies have also shown a benefit for pain control using morphine in the prevention of delirium, because pain itself can be a risk factor for the development of delirium. Family involvement can also be very helpful in reorienting and soothing some delirious patients. It is important to teach family members about the fluctuating course of delirium as well as how they can detect it. Preventive and management strategies for delirium in the ICU represent an important area for future investigation.

Pharmacologic Therapy

Medications should be used for delirium only after adequate attention has been given to correction of modifiable contributing factors (e.g., sleep disturbance, restraints), as discussed previously. It is important to remember that delirium could be a manifestation of an acute, life-threatening problem that requires immediate attention (such as hypoxia, hypercarbia, hypoglycemia, metabolic derangement, or shock). After such concerns have been addressed, pharmacologic management should be considered. It should be recognized that although agents used to treat delirium are intended to improve cognition, they all have psychoactive effects that may further cloud the sensorium and promote a longer overall duration of cognitive impairment. Therefore, until we have outcomes data that confirm beneficial effects of treatment, these drugs should be used judiciously in the smallest possible dose and for the shortest time necessary, a practice *infrequently* adhered to in most ICUs. Indeed, some cases prove refractory to all "cocktail" approaches to sedation and delirium therapy, and in these cases, a trial of complete cessation of all psychoactive drugs should be considered. Some reports have described the utility of dexmedetomidine (an α_2 agonist) as an adjunct to assist with weaning patients from all psychoactive medications.[97] Preliminary results from a prospective, randomized, yet unblinded trial in postoperative patients who had undergone cardiac surgery showed that sedation with dexmedetomidine at sternal closure was associated with an 8% incidence of postoperative delirium compared with 50% for either propofol or benzodiazepines.[98]

Benzodiazepines, which are used most commonly in the ICU for sedation, are not recommended for the management of delirium because of the likelihood of oversedation, exacerbation of confusion, and respiratory suppression. However, they remain the drugs of choice for the treatment of delirium tremens (and other withdrawal syndromes) and seizures. The amnestic qualities of benzodiazepines make these agents especially useful when noxious or unpleasant procedures are required. It is likely, however, that residual accumulation of these drugs may lead to prolonged delirium long after they have been discontinued. In certain populations, particularly elderly patients with underlying dementia, benzodiazepines may increase confusion and agitation. In such cases, one may try to take advantage of the sedative effects of haloperidol in lieu of continuing the benzodiazepine therapy.

Currently, no drugs are approved by the U.S. Food and Drug Administration (FDA) for the treatment of delirium. The Society of Critical Care Medicine guidelines[77] recommend haloperidol as the drug of choice, with the acknowledgment that this recommendation is based on sparse outcomes data from nonrandomized case series and anecdotal reports (i.e., level C data). Nevertheless, haloperidol is a butyrophenone "typical" antipsychotic, which is the most widely used neuroleptic agent for delirium.[99] It does not suppress the respiratory drive and works as a dopamine receptor antagonist by blocking the δ_2 opioid receptor, resulting in treatment of positive symptomatology (hallucinations, unstructured thought patterns, etc.) and producing a variable sedative effect.

In the non-ICU setting, the recommended starting dose of haloperidol is 0.5 to 1.0 mg orally or parenterally, with repeated doses every 20 to 30 minutes until the desired effect is achieved. In the ICU, a recommended starting dose would be 2 to 5 mg every 6 to 12 hours (intravenously or orally), with maximal effective doses usually in the neighborhood of 20 mg/day. This dose range will usually be adequate to achieve the "theoretically optimal" 60% δ_2 receptor blockage[100] while avoiding complete δ_2 receptor saturation associated with the adverse effects cited later. Because of the urgency of the situation in many ICU patients—due to the potential for inadvertent removal of central lines, endotracheal tubes, or even aortic balloon pumps—much higher doses of haloperidol or a sedative are often used. Unfortunately, there are few data from formal pharmacologic investigations to guide dosage recommendations in the ICU. Once calm, the patient can usually be managed with much lower maintenance doses of haloperidol.

Neither haloperidol nor similar agents (i.e., droperidol and chlorpromazine) have been extensively studied for ICU use.[77] Newer "atypical" antipsychotic agents (e.g., risperidone, ziprasidone, quetiapine, and olanzapine) may also prove helpful for delirium.[101] The rationale behind use of the atypical antipsychotics rather than haloperidol (especially in hypoactive/mixed subtypes of delirium) is theoretical and centers on the fact that they affect not only dopamine but also other potentially key neurotransmitters such as serotonin, acetylcholine, and norepinephrine.[101-104] The use of haloperidol has been reported to have a mortality benefit in a retrospective analysis of critically ill, mechanically ventilated patients.[105] Kalisvaart and associates[106] showed that low-dose haloperidol prophylaxis reduced the duration and severity of delirium in elderly patients recovering from hip surgery, even though the actual prevalence of delirium was not reduced. Skrobik and colleagues[101] reported that olanzapine and haloperidol were equally efficacious in treating ICU delirium in both medical and surgical patients but that olanzapine had fewer side effects. The results of this initial study in ICU patients should be tested in larger, more robust trials with a placebo group. Kato and coworkers[107] reported a case study that suggests that genotyping may affect the choice of antipsychotic drugs. They showed that a patient with the CYP2D6 genotype had persistent delirium and demonstrated severe extrapyramidal symptoms when treated with risperidone. When quetiapine (metabolized by CYP3A4) was used instead, the patient's delirium cleared within 2 days without side effects. This case report is not proof of a positive effect of antipsychotics, yet it is interesting and suggests that pharmacogenetics may play an important role in medication choices in the near future. Adequately powered prospective, randomized controlled trials of these agents are not available to date and must be performed to provide clinicians with evidence-based guidelines for preventing and treating delirium.

Adverse effects of typical and atypical antipsychotics include hypotension, acute dystonias, extrapyramidal effects, laryngeal spasm, malignant hyperthermia, glucose and lipid dysregulation, and anticholinergic effects such as dry mouth, constipation, and urinary retention. Perhaps the most immediately life-threatening adverse effect of antipsychotics is torsades de pointes, and these agents should not be given to patients with prolonged QT intervals unless absolutely necessary. Patents who receive substantial quantities of typical or atypical antipsychotics or coadministered arrhythmogenic drugs should be monitored closely with electrocardiography. In early 2005, the FDA issued an alert that atypical antipsychotic medications are associated with a mortality risk among elderly patients. This warning was supported by a meta-analysis of a large volume of data from outpatient treatment of patients with dementia who were experiencing psychotic symptoms that resulted in their receiving antipsychotic medications.[108] Similar associations with higher stroke risk and mortality have been reported by other investigators.[109,110] Subsequently, other studies have suggested that this higher risk of death in non-ICU elderly patients treated with antipsychotics may not be limited to the atypical antipsychotic agents; Schneider and colleagues[109] found that the conventional antipsychotic haloperidol had an even higher mortality risk.

Protocols and evidence-based strategies for prevention and treatment of delirium will no doubt emerge as more evidence becomes available from ongoing randomized clinical trials of both nonpharmacologic and pharmacologic strategies. To assist readers in developing a delirium management algorithm in their respective clinical arenas, we have provided an empiric protocol largely based on the current Society of Critical Care Medicine clinical practice guidelines (Fig. 73-5). At this time, we have few data as to which antipsychotic medications are most suitable for delirium. The nonpharmacologic interventions recommended in this protocol have shown beneficial results in non-ICU patients, but the extrapolation to ICU populations is speculative. Nevertheless, such data emphasize the need for more research in this area and underscore the importance of exercising caution in the treatment of delirium. We wish to emphasize that protocols such as these must be updated regularly with new data and also individualized at each medical center to form an integrated approach to delirium monitoring, sedation targeting, and delirium management in critically ill ICU patients.

SLEEP DISRUPTION IN THE CRITICALLY ILL

The sleep cycle is divided into rapid eye movement (REM) sleep and non–rapid eye movement (NREM) sleep.[111] NREM sleep is further divided into four stages according to an increasing depth of sleep.[111] A normal sleep cycle lasts approximately 90 minutes, cycling continuously between REM and NREM sleep. Stages 3 and 4 of the NREM sleep represent slow-wave or more restful sleep.[111]

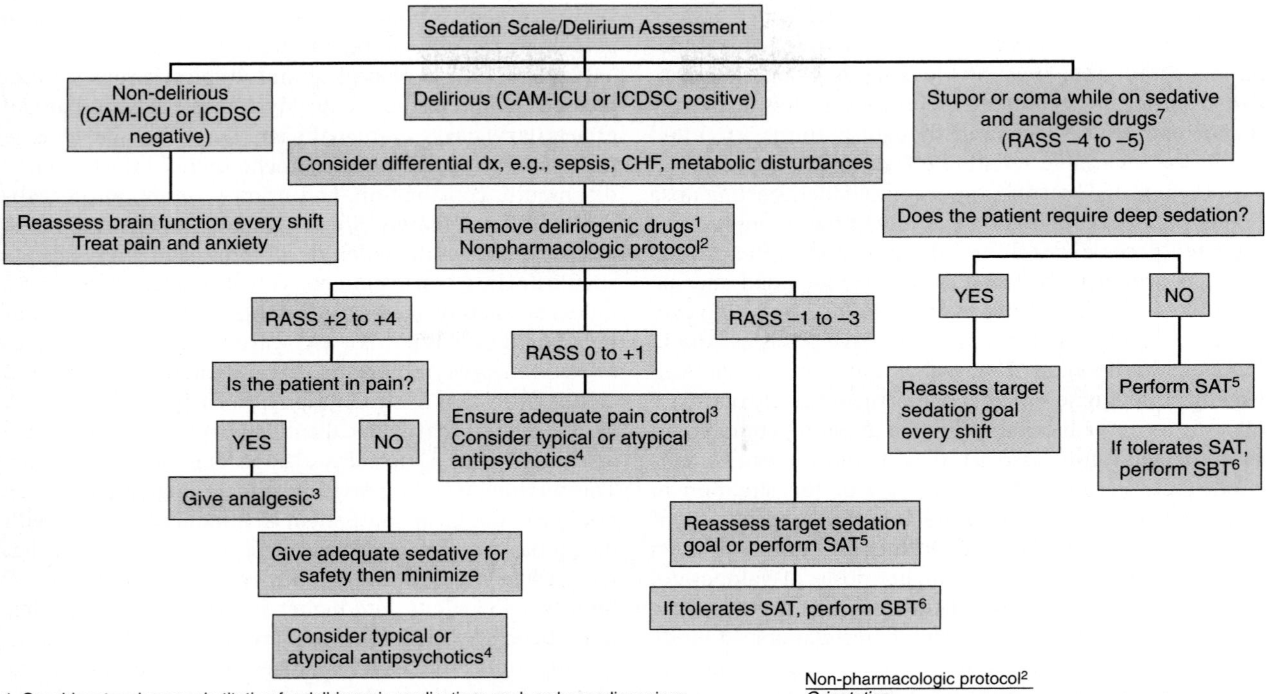

1. Consider stopping or substituting for deliriogenic medications such as benzodiazepines, anticholinergic medications (metochlorpromide, H2 blockers, promethazine, diphenhydramine), steroids, etc.
2. See non-pharmacologic protocol—at right
3. Analgesia—Adequate pain control may decrease delirium. Consider intermittent narcotics if feasible. Assess with objective tool.
4. Typical or atypical antipsychotics—While tapering or discontinuing sedatives, consider haloperidol 2 to 5 mg IV initially (0.5–2 mg in elderly) and then q 6 hours. Guideline for max haloperidol dose is 20 mg/day due to ~60% D_2-receptor saturation. May also consider using any of the atypicals (e.g. olanzapine, quetiapine, risperidone, ziprasidone, or abilifide). Discontinue if high fever, QTc prolongation, or drug-induced rigidity.
5. Spontaneous Awakening Trial (SAT)—Stop sedation or decrease infusion (especially benzodiazepines) to awaken patient as tolerated.
6. Spontaneous Breathing Trial (SBT)—CPAP trial if on ≤50% and ≤8 PEEP and Sats 90%
7. Sedatives and analgesics may include benzodiazepines, propofol, dexmedetomidine, fentanyl, or morphine.

Non-pharmacologic protocol[2]

Orientation
- Provide visual and hearing aids
- Encourage communication and reorient patient repetitively
- Have familiar objects from patient's home in the room
- Attempt consistency in nursing staff
- Allow television during day with daily news
- Non-verbal music

Environment
- Sleep hygiene: Lights off at night, on during day. Sleep aids (zolpidem, mirtazipine)?
- Control excess noise (staff, equipment, visitors) at night
- Ambulate or mobilize patient early and often

Clinical parameters
- Maintain systolic blood pressure >90 mm Hg
- Maintain oxygen saturations >90%
- Treat underlying metabolic derangements and infections

Figure 73-5. Delirium protocol. This empiric protocol, which is based largely on the current Society of Critical Care Medicine's clinical practice guidelines, is the algorithm we use to treat delirium in our ICUs. We wish to emphasize that such protocols need to be updated regularly with new data and also individualized at each medical center. Specific recommendations about the choice of antipsychotics to treat delirium have not been described, because limited data are available regarding the appropriate drug to use in ICU patients. The nonpharmacologic interventions recommended in this protocol have been shown to have beneficial results in non-ICU patients, but the extrapolation to ICU populations is speculative. CAM-ICU, Confusion Assessment Method for the ICU; ICDSC, Intensive Care Delirium Screening Checklist; RASS, Richmond Agitation-Sedation Scale. Sats, saturations.

Critically ill patients have severe sleep deprivation with disruption of sleep architecture. The average amount of sleep in the ICU has been measured to be about 2 hours out of 24 hours, with less than 6% of it spent in REM sleep. In a study by Cooper and associates,[112] the majority of the patients had abnormal sleep patterns. The causes of sleep deprivation in the ICU have been extensively reported. They consist of excessive noise and lighting, patient care activities such as procedures and baths, metabolic consequences of critical illness, mechanical ventilation, and the sedative and analgesic medications that are administered to these patients.[113] This disturbance in duration and quality of sleep has detrimental effects on protein synthesis, cellular and humoral immunity, and energy expenditure, resulting in respiratory and hemodynamic effects as well as cognitive function.[113,114] Studies that have looked at sleep disturbances due to noise, patient activities, and light have found that only about 30% of the sleep arousals were a result of these environmental factors, suggesting that other patient factors or management issues play an important role.[115] Of these, it is interesting that the psychoactive medications are common risk factors for both delirium and sleep disturbances, whereas sleep deprivation can itself lead to delirium.

Neurotransmission in Sleep

The ventrolateral preoptic (VLPO) nucleus in the anterior hypothalamus is the major area of the brain that controls sleep induction and maintenance.[116] Its major neurotransmitter is GABA, and during the awake state, the GABA release from the VLPO nucleus is inhibited by norepinephrine (NE) from the locus ceruleus.[116] With the inhibition of GABA, neurotransmitters such as orexin, serotonin, histamine, and acetylcholine are released, resulting in a state of wakefulness (Fig. 73-6). During NREM sleep, norepinephrine release diminishes, thus removing the inhibi-

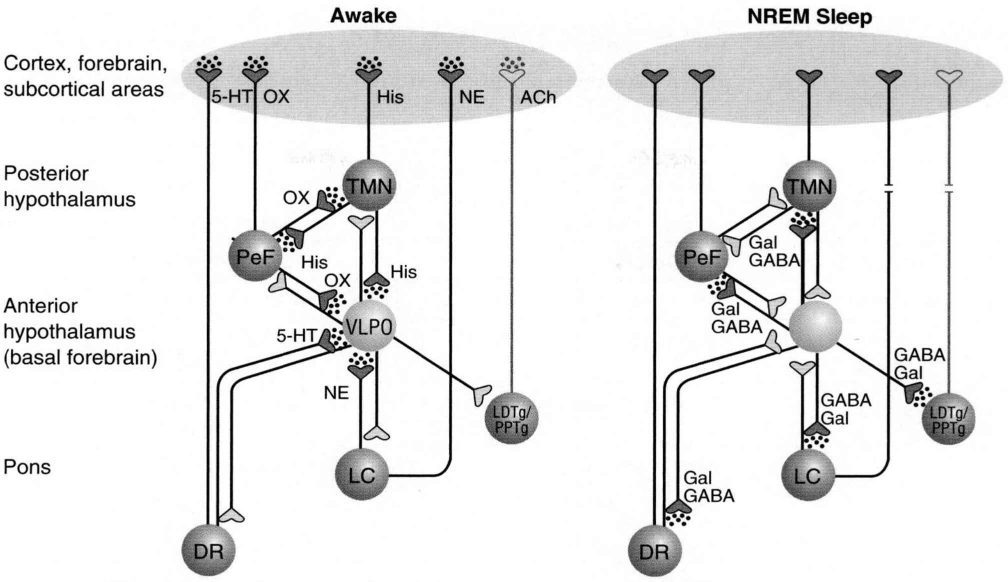

Figure 73-6. Neurotransmitter mechanism for wakefulness and non–rapid eye movement (NREM) sleep. The ventrolateral preoptic (VLPO) nucleus in the anterior hypothalamus is the major area of the brain that controls sleep induction and maintenance. Its major neurotransmitter is gamma-aminobutyric acid (GABA), and during the awake state, GABA release from the VLPO nucleus is inhibited by norepinephrine (NE) from the locus ceruleus (LC). With the inhibition of GABA, neurotransmitters such as orexin (OX), serotonin (5-HT), histamine (His), and acetylcholine (ACh) are released, resulting in a state of wakefulness. During NREM sleep, there is a hierarchical sequence of changes in which inhibition of the LC disinhibits the VLPO nucleus to release GABA and galanin (Gal) at the projections that terminate at the tuberomamillary nucleus (TMN). These inhibitory neurotransmitters inhibit firing of the TMN projections to the cortical and subcortical regions. LDTg, laterodorsal tegmental nucleus; PPTg, pedunculopontine tegmental nucleus. (With permission from Dr. Mervyn Maze and Elsevier, Inc. From Analgesics: Receptor ligands: Alpha 2 adrenergic receptor agonists. In Evers AS, Maze M: Anesthetic Pharmacology: Physiologic Principles and Clinical Practice. St. Louis, Churchill Livingstone, 2004.)

tory effect on release of GABA from the VLPO nucleus. Firing of GABA neurons inhibits the neurotransmitters of wakefulness (orexin, serotonin, histamine and acetylcholine), resulting in NREM sleep (see Fig. 73-6). REM sleep, on the other hand, is facilitated by neurons in the pons that release acetylcholine. Studies show that serotonin and norepinephrine inhibit these neurons, suppressing REM sleep.

Sedative and analgesic medications are routinely administered to critically ill patients to promote sleep. However, although patients appear sedated, their sleep architecture is often adversely affected.[111] Benzodiazepines and propofol prolong stage 2 NREM sleep while decreasing slow-wave sleep and REM sleep. Opioids, on the other hand, increase stage 1 NREM sleep while decreasing slow-wave and REM sleep. Numerous other medications routinely administered to critically ill patients affect sleep architecture. These include antiarrhythmic agents, inotropes and vasopressors, antibiotics, antidepressants, steroids, anticonvulsants, and bronchodilators.[111] The effects of these drugs on sleep patterns are summarized in Table 73-2.

Although they lack anxiolytic properties, ω_1 receptor agonists such as zolpidem may preserve REM as well as slow-wave sleep.[117] Similarly, mirtazapine, a noradrenergic and specific serotonergic antidepressant, has been studied in healthy volunteers and shown to improve sleep efficiency reducing the number and duration of awakenings.[118] The slow-wave sleep time was also increased, whereas stage 1 sleep time was reduced significantly. This agent had no significant effect on REM sleep variables.[119] An investigation of the use of dexmedetomidine (an α_2 agonist) in rats shows that it mimics and increases NREM sleep[116] but decreases REM sleep. By acting on the locus ceruleus, dexmedetomidine inhibits NE release of norepinephrine, thus causing GABA output from the VLPO nucleus and inhibition of the neurotransmitters of wakefulness to produce a NREM sleep pattern. In contrast, benzodiazepines and propofol exert their sedative action on the VLPO nucleus to increase GABA and decrease the neurotransmitters such as orexin, histamine, and serotonin but without affecting norepinephrine release from the locus ceruleus. Further clinical trials are required to ascertain the role of these medications in improving the quality and quantity of sleep in critically ill patients and to see whether such improvement may better the cognitive outcomes in ICU patients.

POST-TRAUMATIC STRESS DISORDER

Definition and Diagnostic Criteria

The DSM-IV[12] defines PTSD as a potentially debilitating psychiatric condition that develops as the result of exposure to a traumatic occurrence, in which the person experienced, witnessed, or was confronted with an event or events that involved actual or threatened death or serious

Table 73-2. Drugs Commonly Used in the ICU and Their Effects on Sleep Patterns

Drug Class or Individual Drug	Sleep Disorder Induced or Reported	Possible Mechanism
Benzodiazepines	↓REM, ↓SWS	Gamma aminobutyric acid type A (GABA[A]) receptor stimulation
Opioids	↓REM, ↓SWS	μ opioid receptor stimulation
Clonidine	↓REM	α_2-adrenergic receptor stimulation
Nonsteroidal anti-inflammatory drugs	↓TST, ↓SE	Prostaglandin synthesis inhibition
Norepinephrine/epinephrine	Insomnia, ↓REM, ↓SWS	α_1-adrenergic receptor stimulation
Dopamine	Insomnia, ↓REM, ↓SWS	δ_2 opioid receptor stimulation/α_1-adrenergic receptor stimulation
β-blockers	Insomnia, ↓REM, nightmares	Central nervous system β-blockade by lipophilic agents
Amiodarone	Nightmares	Unknown mechanism
Corticosteroids	Insomnia, ↓REM, ↓SWS	Reduced melatonin secretion
Aminophylline	Insomnia, ↓REM, ↓SWS, ↓TST, ↓SE	Adenosine receptor antagonism
Quinolones	Insomnia	GABA(A) receptor inhibition
Tricyclic antidepressants	↓REM	Antimuscarinic activity and α_1-adrenergic receptor stimulation
Selective serotonin reuptake inhibitors	↓REM, ↓TST, ↓SE	Increased serotonergic activity
Phenytoin	↑Sleep fragmentation	Inhibition of neuronal calcium influx
Phenobarbital	↓REM	Increased GABA(A) activity
Carbamazepine	↓REM	Adenosine receptor stimulation and/or serotonergic activity

REM, rapid eye movement (sleep); SE, sleep efficiency; SWS, slow-wave sleep; TST, total sleep time.
Reproduced with permission from Bourne RS, Mills GH: Sleep disruption in critically ill patients—pharmacological considerations. Anaesthesia 2004;59:374-384.

injury, or a threat to the physical integrity of self or others and that generates intense feelings of fear, helplessness, or horror in the person exposed to the trauma. This condition is characterized by a constellation of symptoms in the following three domains:

- Symptoms of re-experiencing (e.g., intrusive thoughts and upsetting recollections of the trauma, recurrent dreams or nightmares, and flashbacks)
- Symptoms of avoidance and emotional numbing (e.g., efforts to avoid conversations, places, and thoughts associated with the trauma; detachment from others; and a restricted range of affect)
- Symptoms of increased arousal (e.g., sleep disruption, hypervigilance, and exaggerated startle response)

These symptoms must meet two criteria to be diagnosed as PTSD, as follows:

1. Symptoms must cause significant impairment in social, occupational, or other important functional domains.
2. Symptoms must be present for at least 1 month after exposure to the traumatic event or events.

Prevalence of Intensive Care Unit–Related Post-Traumatic Stress Disorder

The prevalence rates reported in studies on PTSD after critical illness vary widely (5% to >50%) and differ according to whether the specific outcome in question is a diagnosis of PTSD or merely the presence of PTSD symptoms. In the eight investigations that focused on the identification of subjects with PTSD (as opposed to those with PTSD symptoms), prevalence rates ranged from 9.7% to approximately 40%.[119] Prevalence of PTSD differed depending on the time of assessment, with higher rates identified in closer proximity to the time of hospital discharge. In investigations that included serial evaluations, patients generally demonstrated a decrease in symptoms over time. For example, Kapfhammer and colleagues[120] reported that 43.5% of study subjects had PTSD at discharge (although according to the DSM-IV, PTSD cannot be diagnosed until 4 weeks after exposure to the "traumatic stressor"), whereas 23.9% suffered from PTSD an average of 8 years later. Prevalence rates tend to be higher among some specific ICU populations, such as patients with sepsis or ARDS (25% to 40% at follow-up), in comparison with general medical ICU cohorts.[120]

Risk Factors for Post-Traumatic Stress Disorder

A number of subject characteristics appear to raise the risk of PTSD symptoms or an actual diagnosis of PTSD, although consensus among the studies reviewed is limited. Reported risk factors include delusional memories of the

ICU, a greater number of traumatic memories of the ICU, longer ICU length of stay or duration of mechanical ventilation or both, younger age, prior mental health history, female gender, and higher levels of sedation and neuromuscular blockade.[121] No studies have investigated the association between delirium and PTSD.

Conceptual Explanations for Post-Traumatic Stress Disorder after Critical Illness

Although the stresses associated with ICU hospitalization may differ from events typically described as "traumatic experiences," there are a variety of conceptual explanations for the development of PTSD following critical illness. They include (1) profound feelings of helplessness associated with the experience of critical illness, (2) high rates of pre-existing psychiatric morbidity that may characterize ICU patients,[122] (3) cognitive impairment, including decreased working memory, which may limit individual abilities to suppress intrusive thoughts,[122] and (4) multiple traumatic episodes associated with anxiety, panic, or pain that occur during ICU hospitalization, such as intubations, extubations, nightmares, and respiratory distress.[123,124]

The frequency of anxiety-provoking episodes during ICU hospitalization might partly explain the association between higher levels of sedation and increased PTSD symptoms, in that anxious patients may receive more sedatives. Brewin and Holmes[125] suggest that immobilization with incomplete sedation promotes a dissociative experience that may be a PTSD risk factor.

A significant percentage of patients treated in the ICU have chronic medical illnesses,[126,127] which may increase anxiety or susceptibility to anxiety reactions. The presence of such stressors may have a cumulative effect on an individual's coping resources, leading to a greater vulnerability to PTSD. This concept is bolstered by evidence from numerous studies as well as the theoretical work of Turner and Lloyd,[128] which supports the notion that healthy coping responses are impeded by the "accumulated burden of adversity" associated with illness or disease.[129-131] Although the contribution of cumulative illness to the development of PTSD has not been assessed in ICU populations, investigations support an association between accumulated medical burden and higher risk of PTSD. For example, accident victims (without chronic medical illnesses) who are admitted to the trauma ICU have a lower prevalence of PTSD than their medical ICU counterparts (with multiple chronic diseases).[132] Alternatively, patients with chronic cardiovascular disease who have undergone cardiac surgery have relatively high rates of PTSD, which correlate positively with preoperative disease severity.[123]

The relationship between cognitive function and PTSD is a subject of ongoing debate, particularly as it relates to the role of memory in mediating the development of PTSD.[133] The importance of specific, *explicit memories* (memories pertaining to facts and events, which are accessible to consciousness)[134,135] in the generation and maintenance of PTSD is difficult to estimate because they are the basis for nightmares, flashbacks, and intrusive thoughts and contribute to symptoms of avoidance and reexperiencing. Although a detailed treatment of these issues is beyond the scope of this chapter, we briefly discuss several key findings from the literature as they relate to ICU populations.

The preponderance of evidence suggests that the absence of episodic memory for a traumatic event is protective against the development of PTSD, because a majority of studies have shown that the risk of PTSD is markedly lower in individuals unable to recall a traumatic event than in those with explicit memory of it.[136-140] The literature is not unanimous and is narrow in scope, with virtually all relevant studies having been conducted on victims of motor vehicle accidents or other traumas with concomitant traumatic brain injury.[141] Theories of information processing suggest that traumatic memories can be encoded *implicitly* during periods of impaired consciousness and may provide the basis for the generation of PTSD symptoms even if patients are not consciously aware of the memories.[142-145] Additionally, during periods of impaired consciousness, the encoding of emotional experiences such as panic and severe pain appear to be sufficient for the generation of PTSD symptoms.[146]

Many ICU patients report little if any conscious awareness of their critical illness, although as Jones and associates[147] have reported, delusional memories, often with violent and paranoid themes, are pervasive among such patients. Distorted and fragmentary memories may be vestiges of the nightmares, hallucinations, or delusions induced by critical illness, a variety of medications, or other causes and may be particularly likely to occur during delirium, which is ubiquitous in critically ill, mechanically ventilated patients.[15,148] Sedative medications may constitute one factor that mediates the development of delusional memories.[149] Delusional memories may exist in the absence of factual memories, which provide markers of reality and may serve to orient the patient. For example, daily sedative interruption has been found to be associated with fewer symptoms of PTSD,[150] suggesting that even limited factual memories from brief awakening may reduce PTSD. In addition, delusional memories tend to be stable over time and are significantly more persistent than factual memories.[151] Delusional memories may be more refractory to the normal cognitive processes of habituation and reappraisal because they are not well integrated into the long-term memory. Although research is limited, the presence of delusional memories of the ICU is associated with higher levels of anxiety and PTSD.[152,153]

LONG-TERM COGNITIVE IMPAIRMENT AFTER CRITICAL ILLNESS

Medical and surgical management of critical illnesses can, and frequently does, result in de novo neurocognitive impairments. Approximately one third or more of ICU survivors have long-term cognitive impairment (LTCI).[154] It is difficult to make comparisons among studies owing to differences in definitions of neurocognitive sequelae, administered neuropsychological tests, time to follow-up, patient population, study design (prospective vs. retrospective), and inclusion of a control group. Nevertheless, current data suggest that neurocognitive impairments are extremely common in survivors of critical illness.

Currently, 10 cohort studies totaling approximately 455 patients have assessed LTCI after critical illness.[154-164] The populations of the patient cohorts include patients with ARDS, acute lung injury, and respiratory failure in the ICU[154,155,159,161-164] as well as two studies in general ICU patients.[156,160] The time to neurocognitive assessments was variable, with the majority occurring during the first year after hospital discharge. Three studies assessed patients more than 1 year later. A prospective longitudinal study monitored patients at hospital discharge and then at 1 and 2 years after hospital discharge,[165] and two retrospective studies assessed the patients at approximately 6 years after hospital discharge.[159,163]

The evidence from the 10 cohorts suggests that 25% to 78% of ICU survivors experience neurocognitive impairments.[154-164] Among specific populations, such as patients with ARDS, the prevalence of LTCI is even greater; it may be as high as 78% at hospital discharge, 46% at 1 year,[155] and 25% at 6 years.[163] Hopkins and colleagues[155] assessed ARDS patients' premorbid estimated intelligence quotient (IQ) and found it was significantly higher than the patients' measured IQ at hospital discharge. However, the patients' measured IQ improved to their premorbid level by 1-year follow-up, with no additional improvement at 2 years. The finding that patients recovered over time with regard to intelligence does not necessarily suggest a comparable recovery in all cognitive domains, because data from traumatic and anoxic brain injury literature suggests that some neurocognitive abilities are more likely to improve than others.[166]

A 2004 study found that neurocognitive impairments occur in 70% of ARDS patients at hospital discharge, 45% at 1 year, and 47% at 2 years.[165] The neurocognitive test scores of the ARDS survivors with neurocognitive sequelae (≈50% of survivors) fell below the sixth percentile of the normal distribution of cognitive function. These ARDS survivors had marked difficulty with tasks that require executive function, memory, attention, or quick mental processing. The neurocognitive impairments in critically patients are similar to those reported in medical ICU survivors[154] after carbon monoxide poisoning[167] and several years after elective coronary artery bypass graft surgery.[168]

In addition to ARDS survivors, neurocognitive impairments have been reported in the general population of critically ill patients. Jackson and colleagues,[154] evaluating 34 medical ICU survivors at 6 months, found that 33% had LTCI (using a very conservative definition of impairment as 2 test scores 2 standard deviations below the mean or 3 test scores 1.5 standard deviations below the mean). The neurocognitive impairments were similar to those reported in ARDS survivors; they included mental processing speed, memory, language, and visuospatial abilities. Additional support for cognitive impairment in the general critically ill population comes from a prospective cohort of 32 critically ill patients who underwent long-term mechanical ventilation (>5 days). The patients were evaluated at hospital discharge and 6 months later.[157] Of the patients who received long-term mechanical ventilation, 91% at hospital discharge and 41% at 6 months had impairments in attention, memory, mental processing speed, and executive function.[157]

It is hoped that ongoing investigations will provide information about the risk factors for the development of LTCI and help guide interventions for prevention of the rather debilitating sequelae of critical illness that affect a person's quality of life.

DEPRESSION

Many ICU survivors experience significant affective symptoms, such as depression and anxiety.[169] The prevalence and severity of affective disorders, including symptoms of depression and anxiety in ICU survivors, range from less than 10% to 58%.[119,154,155,162,170] Depression has been reported to occur in up to 30% of ICU survivors,[154] and it is estimated that 47% have clinically significant anxiety.[169] Indeed, the high rates of depression among ICU survivors may be related to the cognitive impairment they experience, although this issue has not been eva-luated in ICU cohorts. Affective disorders such as depression, PTSD, and anxiety may adversely affect test performance, especially if severe.[171,172] Moderate to severe depression may result in decreased effort and low motivation, which may in turn lower neuropsychological test scores in cognitive domains such as psychomotor speed and attention.[173,174] Moderate to severe anxiety, however, may lead to increased distractibility and blocked thoughts or words.[175,176] In some cases, severe depression may mimic symptoms of cognitive impairment, although there are important differences between these conditions. In general, individuals with depression retain the ability to learn and do not forget as rapidly, do not display significant decrements in language, are inconsistent with regard to orientation to time and date, and are typically more self-aware than their cognitively impaired counterparts.[177-179]

A variety of instruments are available for use in the assessment of affective function. Tools such as the Geriatric Depression Scale-Short Form (GDS-SF),[180] the Beck Depression Inventory (BDI),[181] the Center for Epidemiologic Studies Depression Scale (CES-D),[182] and the Hospital Anxiety-Depression Scale (HADS)[183] assess depression. Anxiety can be assessed with the Hospital Anxiety-Depression Scale (HADS)[183] or the Beck Anxiety Inventory (BAI).[184] Discussion of these tools is beyond the scope of this chapter.

KEY POINTS

- Delirium is a disturbance of consciousness with inattention, accompanied by a change in cognition or perceptual disturbance, that develops over a short time and has a fluctuating course.
- The prevalence of delirium in medical and surgical ICU cohort studies has been reported to be 20% to 80%, depending on the severity of illness and the delirium detection instrument used.
- Delirium is independently associated with longer duration of mechanical ventilation, longer ICU stays, higher costs, and, more importantly, a threefold higher risk of dying within 6 months.
- The development of tools such as the Intensive Care Delirium Screening Checklist and the Confusion Assessment Method for the ICU have allowed for the rapid diagnosis of delirium in patients by nonpsychiatric physicians and health care personnel even during mechanical ventilation.
- Sedative and analgesic medications and sleep disturbances in the ICU may be modifiable risk factors of delirium.
- Critically ill patients often have severe sleep deprivation with disruption of sleep architecture.
- The average amount of sleep in ICU patients has been measured to be about 2 hours in a 24-hour period, less than 6% of which is REM sleep.
- PTSD is a potentially debilitating psychiatric condition, which develops in 5% to 50% of ICU survivors as the result of exposure to a traumatic occurrence that generates intense feelings of fear, helplessness, or horror.
- Medical and surgical management of critical illnesses can lead to long-term neurocognitive impairments in approximately one third of ICU survivors, significantly affecting quality of life.
- Many ICU survivors experience significant affective symptoms, such as depression and anxiety.

REFERENCES

1. Comarow A: You're never too old: Surgery on patients of 80, 90, and up? It's gaining acceptance. US News World Rep 2004;137:83-88.
2. National Research Council: The Aging Mind: Opportunities in Cognitive Research. Washington, DC, National Academy Press, 2000.
3. Mehta KM, Yaffe K, Covinsky KE: Cognitive impairment, depressive symptoms, and functional decline in older people. J Am Geriatr Soc 2002;50:1045-1050.
4. Inouye SK, Peduzzi PN, Robison JT, et al: Importance of functional measures in predicting mortality among older hospitalized patients. JAMA 1998;279:1187-1193.
5. Inouye SK, Bogardus ST, Baker DI, et al: The Hospital Elder Life Program: A model of care to prevent cognitive and functional decline in older hospitalized patients. J Am Geriatr Soc 2000;1697-1706.
6. Fried TR, Bradley EH, Towle VR, Allore H: Understanding the treatment preferences of seriously ill patients. N Engl J Med 2002;346:1061-1066.
7. Angus DC, Carlet J: Surviving intensive care: A report from the 2002 Brussels Roundtable. Intensive Care Med 2003;29:368-377.
8. Bone RC, Grodzin CJ, Balk RA: Sepsis: A new hypothesis for pathogenesis of the disease process. Chest 1997;112:235-243.
9. Bone RC: Sepsis, the sepsis syndrome, multiorgan failure: A plea for comparable definitions. Ann Intern Med 1991;114:332-333.
10. Bone RC: Multiple system organ failure and the sepsis syndrome. Hosp Pract 1991;26:101-109.
11. Russell JA, Singer J, Bernard G, et al: Changing pattern of organ dysfunction in early human sepsis is related to mortality. Crit Care Med 2000;28:3405-3411.
12. American Psychiatric Association: Diagnostic and Statistical Manual Of Mental Disorders, 4th ed, text rev. Washington, DC, American Psychiatric Association, 2000.
13. Granberg A, Engberg B, Lundberg D: Intensive care syndrome: A literature review. Intensive Crit Care Nurse 1996;12:173-182.
14. Webb JM, Carlton EF, Geeham DM: Delirium in the intensive care unit: Are we helping the patient? Crit Care Nurs Q 2000;22:47-60.
15. Ely EW, Siegel MD, Inouye SK: Delirium in the intensive care unit: An under-recognized syndrome of organ dysfunction. Semin Respir Crit Care Med 2001;22:115-126.
16. Milisen K, Foreman MD, Godderis J, et al: Delirium in the hospitalized elderly: Nursing assessment and management. Nurs Clin North Am 1998;33:417-436.
17. Bergeron N, Dubois MJ, Dumont M, et al: Intensive Care Delirium Screening Checklist: Evaluation of a new screening tool. Intensive Care Med 2001;27:859-864.
18. McNicoll L, Pisani MA, Zhang Y, et al: Delirium in the intensive care unit: Occurrence and clinical course in older patients. J Am Geriatr Soc 2003;51:591-598.
19. Ely EW, Inouye SK, Bernard GR et al: Delirium in mechanically ventilated patients: Validity and reliability of the confusion assessment method for the intensive care unit (CAM-ICU). JAMA 2001;286:2703-2710.
20. Pandharipande P, Cotton B, Costabile S, Ely EW: Prevalence of delirium in surgical ICU patients. Crit Care 2005;33:167-S.
21. Francis J, Martin D, Kapoor WN: A prospective study of delirium in hospitalized elderly. JAMA 1990;263:1097-1101.
22. Inouye SK: The dilemma of delirium: Clinical and research controversies regarding diagnosis and evaluation of delirium in hospitalized elderly medical patients. Am J Med 1994;97:278-288.
23. Peterson JF, Truman BL, Shintani A, et al: The prevalence of hypoactive, hyperactive, and mixed type delirium in medical ICU patients (abstract). J Am Geriatr Soc 2003;51:S174.
24. Peterson JF, Pun BT, Dittus RS et al: Delirium and its motoric subtypes: A study of 614 critically ill patients. J Am Geriatr Soc 2006;54:479-484.
25. Meagher DJ, Trzepacz PT: Motoric subtypes of delirium. Semin Clin Neuropsychiatry 2000;5:75-85.
26. O'Keeffe ST, Lavan JN: Clinical significance of delirium subtypes in older people. Age Ageing 1999;28:115-119.
27. Marcantonio ER, Goldman L, Mangione CM, et al: A clinical prediction rule for delirium after elective noncardiac surgery. JAMA 1994;271:134-139.
28. Sanders AB: Missed delirium in older emergency department patients: A quality-of-care problem. Ann Emerg Med 2002;39:338-341.
29. Hustey FM, Meldon SW: The prevalence and documentation of impaired mental status in elderly emergency department patients. Ann Emerg Med 2002;39:248-253.
30. Meagher DJ, Hanlon DO, Mahony EO, et al: Relationship between symptoms and motoric subtype of delirium. J Neuropsychiatry Clin Neurosci 2000;12:51-56.
31. Justic M: Does "ICU psychosis" really exist? Crit Care Nurse 2000;20:28-37.
32. Inouye SK, Schlesinger MJ, Lydon TJ: Delirium: A symptom of how hospital care is failing older persons and a window to improve quality of hospital care. Am J Med 1999;106:565-573.
33. Levkoff SE, Evans DA, Liptzin B, et al: Delirium: The occurrence and persistence of symptoms among elderly hospitalized patients. Arch Intern Med 1992;152:334-340.

34. American Psychiatric Association: Practice guideline for the treatment of patients with delirium. Am J Psychiatry 1999;156:1-20.
35. Inouye SK, Rushing JT, Foreman MD, et al: Does delirium contribute to poor hospital outcomes? A three-site epidemiologic study. J Gen Intern Med 1998;13:234-242.
36. McCusker J, Cole M, Abrahamowicz M, et al: Delirium predicts 12 month mortality. Arch Intern Med 2002; 162:457-463.
37. Fick DM, Agostini JV, Inouye SK: Delirium superimposed on dementia: A systematic review. J Am Geriatr Soc 2002;50:1723-1732.
38. Rockwood K, Cosway S, Carver D: The risk of dementia and death after delirium. Age Ageing 1999;28: 551-556.
39. Rahkonen T, Luukkainen-Markkula R, Paanilla S, Sulkava R: Delirium episode as a sign of undetected dementia among community dwelling subjects: A 2 year follow up study. J Neurol Neurosurg Psychiatry 2000;69: 519-521.
40. McCusker J, Cole M, Dendukuri N, et al: Delirium in older medical inpatients and subsequent cognitive and functional status: a prospective study. CMAJ 2001;165:575-583.
41. Ely EW, Shintani A, Truman B, et al: Delirium as a predictor of mortality in mechanically ventilated patients in the intensive care unit. JAMA 2004;291: 1753-1762.
42. Lin SM, Liu CY, Wang CH, et al: The impact of delirium on the survival of mechanically ventilated patients. Crit Care Med 2004;32:2254-2259.
43. Milbrandt EB, Deppen S, Harrison PL, et al: Costs associated with delirium in mechanically ventilated patients. Crit Care Med 2004;32:955-962.
44. Ely EW, Gautam S, Margolin R, et al: The impact of delirium in the intensive care unit on hospital length of stay. Intensive Care Med 2001;27: 1892-1900.
45. Crippen D: Treatment of agitation and its comorbidities in the intensive care unit. In Hill NS, Levy MM (eds): Ventilator Management Strategies for Critical Care. New York, Marcel Dekker, 2001, pp 243-284.
46. Pavlov VA, Wang H, Czura CJ, et al: The cholinergic anti-inflammatory pathway: A missing link in neuroimmunomodulation. Mol Med 2003;9:125-134.
47. Fulkerson W, MacIntyre N, Stamler J, Crapo J: Pathogenesis and treatment of the adult respiratory distress syndrome. Arch Intern Med 1996;156:29-38.
48. Bellingan G: The pulmonary physician in critical care—6: The pathogenesis of ALI/ARDS. Thorax 2002;57: 540-546.
49. Arvin B, Neville LF, Barone FC, Feurstein GZ: Brain injury and inflammation: A putative role for TNF-alpha. Ann N Y Acad Sci 1995;116:62-71.
50. Fink MP, Evans TW: Mechanisms of organ dysfunction in critical illness: Report from a round table conference held in Brussels. Intensive Care Med 2002;28:369-375.
51. Wheeler AP, Bernard GR: Treating patients with severe sepsis. N Engl J Med 1999;340:207-214.
52. Papadopoulos MC, Lamb FJ, Moss RF, et al: Faecal peritonitis causes oedema and neuronal injury in pig cerebral cortex. Clin Sci (Lond) 1999; 96:461-466.
53. Huynh HK, Dorovini-Zis K: Effects of interferon-gamma on primary cultures of human brain microvessel endothelial cells. Am J Pathol 1993;142:1265-1278.
54. Krueger JM, Walter J, Dinarello CA, et al: Sleep-promoting effects of endogenous pyrogen (interleukin-1). Am J Physiol 1984;246:R994-R999.
55. Papadopoulos MC, Davies DC, Moss RF, et al: Pathophysiology of septic encephalopathy: A review. Crit Care Med 2000;28:3019-3024.
56. Breslow MJ, Miller CF, Parker SD, et al: Effect of vasopressors on organ blood flow during endotoxin shock in pigs. Am J Physiol 1987;252:H291-H300.
57. Van Der Mast RC: Pathophysiology of delirium. J Geriatr Psychiatry Neurol 1998;11:138-145.
58. Lipowski ZJ: Delirium: Acute Confusional States, rev ed. New York, Oxford University Press, 1990.
59. Engel GL, Romano J: Delirium, a syndrome of cerebral insufficiency. J Chronic Dis 1959;9:260-277.
60. Blass JP, Gibson GE, Duffy TE, Plum F: Cholinergic dysfunction: A common denominator in metabolic encephalopathies. In Pepeu G, Ledinsky H (eds): Cholinergic Mechanisms: Phylogenetic Aspects, Central and Peripheral Synapses, and Clinical Significance. New York, Plenum Press, 1981, pp 921-928.
61. Gibson GE, Peterson C, Sansone J: Decreases in amino acids and acetylcholine metabolism during hypoxia. J Neurochem 1981;37: 192-201.
62. Van Der Mast RC, Fekkes D, Moleman P, Pepplinkhuizen L: Is postoperative delirium related to reduced plasma tryptophan? Lancet 2003;338: 851-852.
63. Wurtman RJ, Hefti F, Melamed E: Precursor control of neurotransmitter synthesis. Pharmacol Rev 1980;32: 315-335.
64. Perry VH, Andersson B, Gordon S: Macrophages and inflammation in the central nervous system. Trends Neurosci 1993;16:268-273.
65. Rothwell NJ, Luheshi G, Toulmond S: Cytokines and their receptors in the central nervous system: Physiology, pharmacology and pathology. Pharmacol Ther 1996;69:85-95.
66. Czura CJ, Friedman SG, Tracey KJ: Neural inhibition of inflammation: The cholinergic anti-inflammatory pathway. J Endotoxin Res 2003;9:409-413.
67. Munford RS, Tracey KJ: Is severe sepsis a neuroendocrine disease? Mol Med 2002;8:437-442.
68. Woiciechowsky C, Asudullah K, Nestler D, et al: Sympathetic activation triggers systemic interleukin-10 release in immunodepression induced brain injury. Nat Med 1998;4:808-813.
69. Woiciechowsky C, Schoening B, Daberkow N, et al: Brain IL-1 beta induces local inflammation but systemic anti-inflammatory response through stimulation of both hypothalamic-pituitary-adrenal axis and sympathetic nervous system. Brain Res 1999;816:563-571.
70. Nicholson TE, Renton KW: The role of cytokines in the depression of CYP1A activity using cultured astrocytes as an in vitro model of inflammation in the CNS. Drug Metab Dispos 2002;30:42-46.
71. Francis J: Drug-induced delirium: Diagnosis and treatment. CNS Drugs 1996;5:103-114.
72. Inouye SK, Charpentier PA: Precipitating factors for delirium in hospitalized elderly persons: Predictive model and interrelationship with baseline vulnerability. JAMA 1996;275:852-857.
73. Dubois MJ, Bergeron N, Dumont M, et al: Delirium in an intensive care unit: A study of risk factors. Intensive Care Med 2001;27:1297-1304.
74. Lipowski ZJ: Delirium in the elderly patient. N Engl J Med 1989;320: 578-582.
75. Inouye SK, Viscoli CM, Horwitz RI, et al: A predictive model for delirium in hospitalized elderly medical patients based on admission characteristics. Ann Intern Med 1993;119:474-481.
76. Francis J, Kapoor WN: Delirium in hospitalized elderly. J Gen Intern Med 1990;5:65-79.
77. Jacobi J, Fraser GL, Coursin DB, et al: Clinical practice guidelines for the sustained use of sedatives and analgesics in the critically ill adult. Crit Care Med 2002;30:119-141.
78. Kollef MH, Levy NT, Ahrens TS, et al: The use of continuous i.v. sedation is associated with prolongation of mechanical ventilation. Chest 1998;114:541-548.
79. Marcantonio ER, Juarez G, Goldman L, et al: The relationship of postoperative delirium with psychoactive medications. JAMA 1994;272: 1518-1522.
80. Pandharipande P, Shintani A, Truman P, et al: Lorazepam is an independent risk factor for transitioning to delirium in intensive care unit patients. Anesthesiology 2006;104:21-26.
81. Mihic S, Harris R: GABA and the GABAA receptor. Alcohol Health Res World 1997;21:127-131.
82. Van Der Mast RC: Delirium: The underlying pathophysiological mechanisms and the need for clinical research. J Psychosom Res 1996;41:109-113.
83. Morrison RS, Magaziner J, Gilbert M, et al: Relationship between pain and opioid analgesics on the development of delirium following hip fracture. J Gerontol A Biol Sci Med Sci 2003;58:76-81.
84. Pandharipande P, Ely EW: Narcotic-based sedation regimens for critically ill mechanically ventilated patients. Crit Care 2005;9:247-248.
85. Sessler CN, Gosnell M, Grap MJ, et al: The Richmond Agitation-Sedation Scale: Validity and reliability in adult intensive care patients. Am J Respir Crit Care Med 2002;166:1338-1344.
86. Ely EW, Truman B, Shintani A, et al: Monitoring sedation status over time in ICU patients: Reliability and validity

of the Richmond Agitation-Sedation Scale (RASS). JAMA 2003;289: 2983-2991.
87. Pun BT, Gordon SM, Peterson JF, et al: Large-scale implementation of sedation and delirium monitoring in the intensive care unit: A report from two medical centers. Crit Care Med 2005;33:1199-1205.
88. Inouye SK, Bogardus ST Jr., Charpentier PA, et al: A multicomponent intervention to prevent delirium in hospitalized older patients. N Engl J Med 1999;340: 669-676.
89. Bogardus ST, Desai MM, Williams CS, et al: The effects of a targeted multicomponent delirium intervention of postdischarge outcomes for hospitalized older adults. Am J Med 2003;114:383-390.
90. Marcantonio ER, Flacker JM, Wright RJ, Resnick NM: Reducing delirium after hip fracture: A randomized trial. J Am Geriatr Soc 2001;49:516-522.
91. Cole MG, McCusker J, Bellavance F, et al: Systematic detection and multidisciplinary care of delirium in older medical inpatients: A randomized trial. CMAJ 2002;167:753-759.
92. Milisen K, Foreman MD, Abraham IL, et al: A nurse-led interdisciplinary intervention program for delirium in elderly hip-fracture patients. J Am Geriatr Soc 2001;49:523-532.
93. Lundstrom M, Edlund A, Karlsson S, et al: A multifactorial intervention program reduces the duration of delirium, length of hospitalization, and mortality in delirious patients. J Am Geriatr Soc 2005;53:622-628.
94. Kollef MH, Levy NT, Ahrens T, et al: The use of continuous IV sedation is associated with prolongation of mechanical ventilation. Chest 1999;114:541-548.
95. Brook AD, Ahrens TS, Schaiff R, et al: Effect of a nursing implemented sedation protocol on the duration of mechanical ventilation. Crit Care Med 1999;27:2609-2615.
96. Kress JP, Pohlman AS, O'Connor MF, Hall JB: Daily interruption of sedative infusions in critically ill patients undergoing mechanical ventilation. N Engl J Med 2000;342:1471-1477.
97. Siobal MS, Kallet RH, Kivett VA, Tang JF: Use of dexmedetomidine to facilitate extubation in surgical intensive-care-unit patients who failed previous weaning attempts following prolonged mechanical ventilation: A pilot study. Respir Care 2006;51:492-496.
98. Maldonado JR, van der Starre PJ, Wysong A: Post-operative sedation and the incidence of ICU delirium in cardiac surgery patients. Anesthesiology 2003;99:A465.
99. Ely EW, Stephens RK, Jackson JC, et al: Current opinions regarding the importance, diagnosis, and management of delirium in the intensive care unit: A survey of 912 healthcare professionals. Crit Care Med 2004;32:106-112.
100. Kapur S, Remington G, Jones C, et al: High levels of dopamine d2 receptor occupancy with low-dose haloperidol treatment: a pet study. Am J Psychiatry 1996;153:948-950.
101. Skrobik Y, Bergeron N, Dumont M, Gottfried SB: Olanzapine vs haloperidol: Treating delirium in a critical care setting. Intensive Care Med 2004;30:444-449.
102. Tune L: The role of antipsychotics in treating delirium. Curr Psychiatric Rep 2002;4:209-212.
103. Foreman M, Milisen K, Marcantonia EM: Prevention and treatment strategies for delirium. Prim Psychiatry 2004;11:52-58.
104. Alao AO, Soderberg M, Pohl EL, Koss M: Aripiprazole in the treatment of delirium. Int J Psychiatry Med 2005;35:429-433.
105. Milbrandt EB, Kersten A, Kong L, et al: Haloperidol use is associated with lower hospital mortality in mechanically ventilated patients. Crit Care Med 2005;33:226-229.
106. Kalisvaart KJ, de Jonghe JF, Bogaards MJ, et al: Haloperidol prophylaxis for elderly hip-surgery patients at risk for delirium: A randomized placebo-controlled study. J Am Geriatr Soc 2005;53:1658-1666.
107. Kato D, Kawanishi C, Kishida I, et al: Delirium resolving upon switching from risperidone to quetiapine: Implication of the CYP2D6 genotype. Psychosomatics 2005;46:374-375.
108. Wang PS, Schneeweiss S, Avorn J, et al: Risk of death in elderly users of conventional vs. atypical antipsychotic medications. N Engl J Med 2005;353:2335-2341.
109. Schneider LS, Dagerman KS, Insel P: Risk of death with atypical antipsychotic drug treatment for dementia: Meta-analysis of randomized placebo-controlled trials. JAMA 2005;294:1934-1943.
110. Sink KM, Holden KF, Yaffe K: Pharmacological treatment of neuropsychiatric symptoms of dementia: A review of the evidence. JAMA 2005;293:596-608.
111. Bourne RS, Mills GH: Sleep disruption in critically ill patients—pharmacological considerations. Anaesthesia 2004;59:374-384.
112. Cooper AB, Thornley KS, Young GB, et al: Sleep in critical ill patients requiring mechanical ventilation. Chest 2000;117:809-818.
113. Gabor JY, Cooper AB, Crombach SA, et al: Contribution of the intensive care unit environment to sleep disruption in mechanically ventilated patients and health subjects. Am J Respir Crit Care Med 2003;167:708-715.
114. Helton MC, Gordon SH, Nunnery SL: The correlation between sleep deprivation and the intensive care unit syndrome. Heart Lung 1980;9: 464-468.
115. Freedman NS, Gazendam J, Levan L, et al: Abnormal sleep/wake cycles and the effect of environmental noise on sleep disruption in the intensive care unit. Am J Respir Crit Care Med 2001;163:451-457.
116. Nelson LE, Lu J, Guo T, et al: The $alpha_2$-adrenoceptor agonist dexmedetomidine converges on an endogenous sleep-promoting pathway to exert its sedative effects. Anesthesiology 2003;98:428-436.
117. Langtry HD, Benfield P: Zolpidem: A review of its pharmacodynamic and pharmacokinetic properties and therapeutic potential. Drugs 1990;40:291-313.
118. Aslan S, Isik E, Cosar B: The effects of mirtazapine on sleep: A placebo controlled, double-blind study in young healthy volunteers. Sleep 2002;25:677-679.
119. Schelling G, Stoll C, Haller M, et al: Health-related quality of life and posttraumatic stress disorder in survivors of the acute respiratory distress syndrome. Crit Care Med 1998;26:651-659.
120. Kapfhammer HP, Rothenhausler HB, Krauseneck T, et al: Posttraumatic stress disorder and health-related quality of life in long-term survivors of acute respiratory distress syndrome. Am J Psychiatry 2004;161:45-52.
121. Ozer EJ, Best SR, Lipsey TL, Weiss DS: Predictors of posttraumatic stress disorder and symptoms in adults: A meta-analysis. Psychol Bull 2003;129:52-73.
122. Brewin CR, Smart L: Working memory and suppression of intrusive thoughts. J Behav Ther Exp Psychiatry 2005;36:61-68.
123. Stoll C, Kapfhammer HP, Rothenhausler HB, et al: Sensitivity and specificity of a screening test to document traumatic experiences and to diagnose post-traumatic stress disorder in ARDS patients after intensive care treatment. Intensive Care Med 1999;25:697-704.
124. Murray MJ, Cowen J, Deblock H, et al: Clinical practice guidelines for sustained neuromuscular blockade in the adult critically ill patient. Crit Care Med 2002;30:142-156.
125. Brewin CR, Holmes EA: Psychological theories of posttraumatic stress disorder. Clin Psychol Rev 2005;23: 339-376.
126. Zilberberg MD, Epstein SK: Acute lung injury in the medical ICU: Comorbid conditions, age, etiology, and hospital outcome. Am J Respir Crit Care Med 1998;157:1159-1164.
127. Rosenberg AL, Hofer TP, Hayward RA, et al: Who bounces back? Physiologic and other predictors of intensive care readmission. Crit Care Med 2001;29:511-518.
128. Turner RJ, Lloyd DA: Lifetime traumas and mental health: The significance of cumulative adversity. J Health Soc Behav 2005;36:360-376.
129. Alonzo AA: The experience of chronic illness and post-traumatic stress disorder: The consequences of cumulative adversity. Soc Sci Med 2000;50:1475-1484.
130. Lloyd DA, Turner RJ: Cumulative adversity and posttraumatic stress disorder: Evidence from a diverse community of young adults. Am J Orthopsychiatry 2003;73:381-391.
131. Miranda J, Green BL: The need for mental health services research focusing on poor young women. J Ment Health Policy Econ 1999;2:73-80.
132. Schnyder U, Moergeli H, Trentz O, et al: Prediction of psychiatric

morbidity in severely injured accident victims at one-year follow-up. Am J Respir Crit Care Med 2001;164:653-656.
133. Foreman M, Milisen K: Improving recognition of delirium in the elderly. Prim Psychiatry 2004;11:46-50.
134. Squire L: Declarative and non-declarative memory: Multiple brain systems supporting learning and memory. J Cogn Neurosci 1992;4:232-243.
135. Parkin A: Human memory. Curr Biol 1999;9:582-585.
136. Sbordone R, Liter J: Mild traumatic brain injury does not produce post traumatic stress disorder. Brain Injury 1995;9:405-412.
137. Sbordone R, Seyraniniana GD, Ruff RM: Are the subjective complaints of traumatically brain injured patients reliable? Brain Injury 1998;12:505-512.
138. Malt U: The long term psychiatric consequences of accidental injury. Br J Psychiatry 1988;153:810-818.
139. Ursano R, Fullerton C, Epstein R: Acute and chronic posttraumatic stress disorder in motor vehicle victims. Am J Psychiatry 1999;156:589-595.
140. Bontke C, Rattok J, Boake C: Do patients with mild brain injury have post-traumatic stress disorder too? J Head Trauma Rehabil 1996;11:95-102.
141. Klein E, Caspi Y, Gil S: The relation between memory of the traumatic brain injury and PTSD: Evidence from studies of traumatic brain injury. Can J Psychiatry 2003;48:28-33.
142. Bryant RA: Posttraumatic stress disorder and traumatic brain injury: Can they co-exist? Clin Psychol Rev 2001;21:931-948.
143. Brewin CR: A cognitive neuroscience account of posttraumatic stress disorder and its treatment. Behav Res Ther 2001;39:373-393.
144. Brewin CR, Dalgleish T, Joseph S: A dual representation theory of posttraumatic stress disorder. Psychol Rev 1996;103:670-686.
145. Schacter DL, Chiu CYP, Ochsner KN: Implicit memory: A selective review. Neuroscience 1993;16:159-182.
146. Sessler C: Top ten list in sepsis. Chest 2001;120:1390-1393.
147. Jones C, Griffiths RD, Humphris G: Disturbed memory and amnesia related to intensive care. Memory 2000;8:79-94.
148. Ely EW, Margolin R, Francis J, et al: Evaluation of delirium in critically ill patients: Validation of the confusion assessment method for the intensive care unit (CAM-ICU). Crit Care Med 2001;29:1370-1379.
149. Capuzzo M, Valpondi V, Cingolani E, et al: Post-traumatic stress disorder-related symptoms after intensive care. Minerva Anestesiol 2005;71:167-179.
150. Kress JP, Gehlbach B, Lacy M, et al: The long-term psychological effects of daily sedative interruption on critically ill patients. Am J Respir Crit Care Med 2003;168:1457-1461.
151. Capuzzo M, Valpondi V, Cingolani E, et al: Application of the Italian version of the Intensive Care Unit Memory tool in the clinical setting. Crit Care 2004;8:R48-R55.
152. Jones C, Griffiths RD, Humphris G, Skirrow PM: Memory, delusions, and the development of acute posttraumatic stress disorder-related symptoms after intensive care. Crit Care Med 2001;29:573-577.
153. Jones C, Skirrow PM, Griffiths RD, et al: Rehabilitation after critical illness: A randomized, controlled trial. Crit Care Med 2003;31:2456-2461.
154. Jackson JC, Hart RP, Gordon SM, et al: Six-month neuropsychological outcome of medical intensive care unit patients. Crit Care Med 2003;31: 1226-1234.
155. Hopkins RO, Weaver LK, Pope D, et al: Neuropsychological sequelae and impaired health status in survivors of severe acute respiratory distress syndrome. Am J Respir Crit Care Med 1999;160:50-56.
156. Jones C, Griffiths RD, Slater T, et al: Significant cognitive dysfunction in non-delirious patients identified during and persisting following critical illness. Intensive Care Med 2006;32:923-926.
157. Hopkins RO, Jackson JC, Wallace C: Neurocognitive impairments in ICU patients with prolonged mechanical ventilation (abstract). J Int Neuropsychol Soc 2005;11(Suppl 1):60.
158. Hopkins RO: Relationship of cognitive dysfunction to quality of life. J Int Neuropsychol Soc 2003;10:1005-1017.
159. Suchyta MR, Hopkins RO, White J, et al: The incidence of cognitive dysfunction after ARDS (abstract). Am J Respir Crit Care Med 2004;169:A18.
160. Sukantarat KT, Burgess PW, Williamson RC, Brett SJ: Prolonged cognitive dysfunction in survivors of critical illness. Anaesthesia 2005;60:847-853.
161. Marquis KA, Curtis JR, Caldwell E, et al: Neuropsychological sequelae in survivors of ARDS compared with critically ill control patients (abstract). Am J Respir Crit Care Med 2000;161: A383.
162. Al-Saidi F, McAndrews MP, Cheung AM, et al: Neuropsychological sequelae in ARDS survivors (abstract). Am J Respir Crit Care Med 2003;167: A737.
163. Rothenhausler HB, Ehrentraut S, Stoll C, et al: The relationship between cognitive performance and employment and health status in long-term survivors of the acute respiratory distress syndrome: Results of an exploratory study. Gen Hosp Psychiatry 2001;23:90-96.
164. Christie JD, Biester RC, Taichman DB, et al: Formation and validation of a telephone battery to assess cognitive function in acute respiratory distress syndrome survivors. J Crit Care 2006;21:125-132.
165. Hopkins RO, Weaver LK, Chan KJ, Orme JF Jr: Quality of life, emotional, and cognitive function following acute respiratory distress syndrome. J Int Neuropsychol Soc 2004;10:1005-1017.
166. Whitley E, Ball J: Statistics review 1: Presenting and summarising data. Crit Care Forum 2002;6:66-71.
167. Weaver LK, Hopkins RO, Chan KJ, et al: Hyperbaric oxygen for acute carbon monoxide poisoning. N Engl J Med 2002;347:1057-1067.
168. Newman MF, Kirchner JL, Phillips-Bute B, et al: Longitudinal assessment of neurocognitive function after coronary-artery bypass surgery. N Engl J Med 2001;344:395-402.
169. Scragg P, Jones A, Fauvel N: Psychological problems following ICU treatment. Anaesthesia 2001;56:9-14.
170. Skodol AE: Anxiety in the medically ill: Nosology and principles of differential diagnosis. Semin Clin Neuropsychiatry 1999;4:64.
171. Brandes D, Ben-Schachar G, Gilboa A, et al: PTSD symptoms and cognitive performance in recent trauma survivors. Psychiatry Res 2002; 110:231-238.
172. Ravnkilde B, Videbech P, Clemmensen K, et al: Cognitive deficits in major depression. Scand J Psychol 2002;43:239-251.
173. Massman PJ, Delis DC, Butters N, et al: The subcortical dysfunction model of memory deficits in depression: Neuropsychological validation in a subgroup of patients. J Clin Exp Neuropsychol 1992;14:687-706.
174. Richards PM, Ruff RM: Motivational effects on neuropsychological functioning: Comparison of depressed versus nondepressed individuals. J Consult Clin Psychol 1989;57: 396-402.
175. Buckelew SP, Hannay HJ: Relationships among anxiety, defensiveness, sex, task difficulty, and performance on various neuropsychological tasks. Percept Motor Skills 1986;63:711-718.
176. Eysenck MW: Anxiety and cognitive functioning: A multifaceted approach. In Lister RG, Weingartner HJ (eds): Perspectives of Cognitive Neuroscience. New York, Oxford University Press, 2003.
177. Hart RP, Kwentus JA, Taylor JR, Harkins SW: Rate of forgetting in dementia and depression. J Consult Clin Psychol 1997;55:101-105.
178. McGlynn SM, Schacter DL: Unawareness of deficits in neuropsychological syndromes. J Clin Exp Neuropsychol 1989;11:143-205.
179. Jones RD, Tranel D, Benton A, Paulsen J: Differentiating dementia from pseudo-dementia early in the clinical course: Utility of neuropsychological tests. Neuropsychology 1992;6:13-21.
180. Sheikh JL, Yesavage JA: Geriatric Depression Scale (GDS): Recent evidence and development of a shorter version. Clin Gerontol 1986;5:165-173.
181. Beck AT: BDI-II Depression Inventory Manual, 2nd ed. New York, Harcourt Brace, 1996.
182. Radloff LS: The CES-D Scale: A self report depression scale for research in the general population. Applied Psychological Measurement 1977;1:385-401.
183. Zigmond AS, Snaith RP: The hospital anxiety and depression scale. Acta Psychiatr Scand 1983;67:361-370.
184. Beck AT, Brown G, Steer RA: An inventory for assessing clinical anxiety: Psychometric properties. J Consult Clin Psychol 1988;56:893-897.

Chapter 74

Severity Scoring Systems: Tools for the Evaluation of Patients and Intensive Care Units

Rui P. Moreno and Philipp G. H. Metnitz

When you can measure a phenomenon about which you are talking and express it in numbers, you know something about it. But, when you can not express it in numbers, your knowledge is vague and unsatisfactory. It may be the beginning of knowledge, but you progressed very little toward the state of science.

Lord Kelvin (1824-1907)

The goal of intensive care is to provide the highest quality of treatment in order to achieve the best outcomes for critically ill patients. Although intensive care medicine has developed rapidly over the years, scientific evidence pointing to optimal treatments and practices is minimal. Moreover, intensive care faces new economic challenges, increasing the need to provide evidence on both the *effectiveness* (the probability of benefit to patients from a medical technology applied for a given medical problem under average conditions of use) and *efficiency* (effectiveness of an intervention with respect to the resources used) of care. Intensive care is a complex process that is carried out on a very heterogeneous population and is influenced by variables that include cultural background and differences in structure and organization of health care systems. It is therefore extremely difficult to reduce the quality of intensive care to something measurable, to quantify it, and then to compare it between different institutions.

Although quality encompasses a variety of dimensions, the main interest to date focuses on effectiveness and efficiency. Other issues are less relevant if the care being provided is either ineffective or harmful. The priority must be to evaluate effectiveness. The instrument available to measure effectiveness in intensive care is outcomes research. The starting point for this research was the high degree of variability in medical processes identified in the first part of the 20th century, when epidemiological research was developing. The variation in clinical practice—including the lack of standardization—led to the search for "optimal" therapy.

The undertaking of randomized controlled trials in intensive care is fraught with ethical and other difficulties. For this reason, observational studies to evaluate the effects of intensive care treatment frequently are employed. Outcomes research provides the methods necessary to compare different groups of patients and institutions. Risk adjustment (also called case mix adjustment) is the method of choice to standardize different groups of patients. The purpose of risk adjustment is to take into account all of the characteristics of patients known to affect their outcome, irrespective of the treatment received.

This chapter describes the different methods and systems currently available for assessing and comparing severity of illness and outcome in critically ill patients. Starting with a short historical outline of the development of scoring systems over time is presented first, followed by a discussion of how such systems have been designed and constructed. Available systems with their applications and limitations are described next. Finally, potential applications of these systems, both at patient level and at ICU level, are reviewed.

HISTORICAL PERSPECTIVE

Scoring systems have been in broad use in medicine for several decades. In 1953 Virginia Apgar[1] published a simple scoring tool, the first general severity score designed to be applicable to a general population of newborn children. It was composed of five variables, easily evaluated at the bedside, that reflect cardiopulmonary and central nervous system function. Its simplicity and accuracy have never been improved on, and any child born in a hospital today receives an Apgar score at 1 and 5 minutes after birth. More than 50 years ago Dr. Apgar commented on the state of research in neonatal resuscitation: "Seldom have there been such imaginative ideas, such enthusiasms and dislikes, and such unscientific observations and study about one clinical picture." She suggested that part of the solution to this problem would be a "simple, clear classification or grading of newborn infants which can be used as the basis for discussion and comparison of the results of obstetric practices, types of maternal pain relief and the effects of resuscitation." Some 30 years later, physicians working in intensive care units (ICUs) found themselves saying the same thing about the state of adult critical care.

Efforts to improve risk assessment during the 1960s and 1970s were directed at improving clinicians' ability to quickly select patients most likely to benefit from promising new treatments. For example, Child and Turcotte[2] created a score to measure the severity of liver disease and estimate mortality risk for patients undergoing portosystemic shunting. In 1967 Killip and Kimball classified the severity of acute myocardial infarction by the presence and severity of signs of congestive heart failure.[3]

In 1974 Teasdale and Jennette introduced the Glasgow Coma Scale (GCS) for reproducibly evaluating the severity of coma.[4] The usefulness of the GCS has been confirmed by the consistent relationship between poor outcome and a reduced score among patients with a variety of diseases. The GCS is reliable and easy to perform, but problems with the timing of evaluation, the use of sedation, interobserver variability, and its use in prognostication have caused controversy.[5] Nevertheless, the GCS remains the most widely used neurologic measure for risk assessment.

The 1980s saw an explosive increase in the use of new technology and therapies in critical care. The rapidity of change and the large and growing investment in these high-cost services prompted demands for better evidence for the indications and benefit of critical care. In response, several researchers developed systems to evaluate and to compare severity of illness and outcome in critically ill patients. The first of these systems was the Acute Physiology and Chronic Health Evaluation (APACHE) system, published by Knaus and associates in 1981,[6] followed soon after by the Simplified Acute Physiology Score (SAPS) from Le Gall and coworkers.[7] The APACHE system subsequently was updated to APACHE II,[8] and another system—the Mortality Probability Models (MPM)—joined the group.[9]

By the beginning of the 1990s, multiple systems were available to describe and classify ICU populations, to compare ICU patients with respect to severity of illness, and to predict mortality within the ICU. These systems performed well, but concerns included errors in prediction caused by differences in patient selection and also lead-time bias (the effect of time and previous therapeutic interventions on the calculation of the score). Other concerns were related to adequacy of size of the database and data accrual methods. These concerns, in part, led to the development of revised systems such as APACHE III,[10] the SAPS II,[11] and the MPM II,[12] all published between 1991 and 1993.

During the mid-1990s, the need to quantify not only mortality but also morbidity in specific groups of patients became evident and led to the development of organ dysfunction scores, such as the Multiple Organ Dysfunction Score (MODS),[13] the Logistic Organ Dysfunction System (LODS) score,[14] and the Sequential Organ Failure Assessment (SOFA) score.[15]

SEVERITY OF ILLNESS ASSESSMENT AND OUTCOME PREDICTION

The evaluation of severity of illness in the critically ill patient is made through the use of severity scores and prognostic models. Severity scores are instruments that aim at stratifying patients by severity of illness, assigning to each patient an increasing score as illness severity increases; apart from this stratification ability, prognostic models aim at predicting a certain outcome (usually the vital status at hospital discharge) on the basis of a given set of prognostic variables and a certain modeling equation.

The development of these types of systems, applicable to heterogeneous groups of critically ill patients, started in the 1980s (Table 74-1). The first general severity of illness score applicable to most critically ill patients was the APACHE.[6] Developed at George Washington University Medical Center in 1981 by Knaus and coworkers, the APACHE system demonstrated the ability to evaluate, in an accurate and reproducible form, the severity of disease in this population.[16-18] Two years later, Le Gall and coworkers published a simplified version of this model, the SAPS.[19] This model soon became very popular in Europe, especially in France. Another simplification of the original APACHE system, the APACHE II, was published in 1985 by the same authors of the original model.[8] This system introduced the possibility to predict mortality, using for this purpose the selection of a major reason for ICU admission from a list comprising 50 operative and nonoperative diagnoses. Additional contributions for increasing prognostic ability comprise the MPM,[20] developed by Lemeshow using logistic regression techniques. Further developments in this field include the third version of the APACHE system (APACHE III)[10] and the second versions of the SAPS (SAPS II)[11] and of the MPM (MPM II).[12] All use multiple logistic regression to select and weight the variables and can compute the probability of in-hospital mortality for groups of critically ill patients. It has been demonstrated that they perform better than their previous counterparts[21,22] and, as of the end of the last century, represent the state of the art in this field.

Because of the lack of ongoing calibration of these models, performance of these instruments slowly

Table 74-1. General Severity Scores and Outcome Prediction Models

Characteristic	APACHE	SAPS	APACHE II	MPM*	APACHE III	SAPS II	MPM II†	SAPS 3	APACHE IV
Year	1981	1984	1985	1988	1991	1993	1993	2005	2006
No. of countries	1	1	1	1	1	12	12	35	1
No. of ICUs	2	8	13	1	40	137	140	303	104
No. of patients	705	679	5,815	2,783	17,440	12,997	19,124	16,784	110,558
Method of variable selection/weighting	Panel of experts	Panel of experts	Panel of experts	Multiple logistic regression	Multiple logistic regression	Multiple logistic regression	Multiple logistic regression	Multiple logistic regression	Multiple logistic regression
Variables									
Age	No	Yes	Yes	Yes	Yes	Yes	Yes	Yes	Yes
Origin	No	No	No	No	Yes	No	No	Yes	Yes
Surgical status	No	No	Yes	Yes	Yes	Yes	Yes	Yes	Yes
Chronic health status	Yes	No	Yes	Yes	Yes	Yes	Yes	Yes	Yes
Physiology	Yes	Yes	Yes	Yes	Yes	Yes	Yes	Yes	Yes
Acute diagnosis	No	No	Yes	No	Yes	No	Yes	Yes	Yes
Number of variables	34	14	17	11	26	17	15‡	20	142
Score	Yes	Yes	Yes	No	Yes	Yes	No	Yes	Yes
Mortality prediction	No	No	Yes	Yes	Yes	Yes	Yes	Yes	Yes

*These models are based on previous versions developed by Lemeshow and colleagues.[9,222]

†The numbers presented are those for the admission component of the model (MPM II_0). MPM II_{24} was developed from data for 15,925 patients from the same ICUs.

‡MPM II_{24} uses only 13 variables.

ICU, intensive care unit.

Data from APACHE, Acute Physiology and Chronic Health Evaluation; SAPS, Simplified Acute Physiology Score; MPM, Mortality Probability Models.

deteriorates as time passes. Changes occurring over time in the baseline characteristics of admitted patients, the circumstances of ICU admission, and the availability of general and specific therapeutic measures have the potential to produce an increasing gap between actual mortality and predicted mortality.[23] An increase in mean age of the admitted patients, a larger number of chronically sick patients and immunosuppresed patients, and an increase in the number of admissions due to sepsis was noted in the last years of the previous decade.[24,25] Although most of the models kept an acceptable discrimination, their calibration (or prognostic accuracy) deteriorated to a point at which major changes were needed.

Use of these instruments outside their sampling space was responsible for some misapplication of the instruments, especially for risk adjustment in clinical trials,[26,27] as demonstrated recently.[28]

A new generation of general outcome prediction models has now been developed: the MPM III, developed in the IMPACT database in the United States[29]; new models based on computerized analysis by hierarchical regression, developed by some authors of the APACHE systems[30]; the APACHE IV model[31]; and the SAPS 3 admission model, developed by hierarchical regression using a worldwide database.[32,33] Models based on other statistical techniques such as artificial neural networks and genetic algorithms have been proposed.[34,35] These approaches have been reviewed recently[36] and are summarized later in the chapter.

Recalibrating and Expanding Existing Models

All of the existing general outcome prediction models use logistic regression equations to estimate the probabilities of a given outcome in a patient with a certain set of predictive variables. Consequently, the first approach to improve the calibration of a model when the original model is not able to adequately describe the population is to customize the model.[37] Several methods and suggestions have been proposed for this exercise,[38] based usually on one of two strategies:

- *First level customization,* or the customization of the logit, introducing slight modifications in the logistic equation (without changing the weights of the constituent variables) such as proposed by Le Gall or Apolone.[39,40]
- *Second level customization,* or the customization of the coefficients of all the variables in the model as described for the MPM II_0 model.[37]

Both of these methods have been used in the past, with some success in increasing the prognostic ability of the models.[37,41] Both fail, however, when the problem with the score lies in discrimination (of observations with a positive outcome from those with a negative outcome) or in poor performance in subgroups of patients (poor uniformity of fit).[42] The addition of new variables to an existing model may be useful in this context.[43,44] This approach may lead to very complex models, requiring the collection of special data with a considerable increase in cost and time expenditure. The tradeoff between the burden of data collection and accuracy should be addressed on a case-by-case basis. It should be noted that the aim of first level customization—which is nothing more than a mathematical translation of the original logit in order to get a different probability of mortality—is to improve the calibration of a model and not to improve discrimination. This approach should therefore not be considered when the improvement of this parameter is considered important.

Also of potential value would be a third level of customization, through introduction in the model of new prognostic variables and recalculation of the weights and coefficients for all variables, but this technique straddles both of the other approaches, customizing a model and building a new predictive model. All of these approaches have been tried recently.

In France, Le Gall and colleagues customized the SAPS II model, using a retrospective database containing input for 77,490 patients hospitalized in 106 French ICUs in France between January 1, 1998, and December 31, 1999.[45] On the basis of these data, the investigators evaluated the goodness of fit (calibration and discrimination) of the original SAPS II model, of a customized SAPS II, and of an expanded SAPS II developed in the training set by adding six admission variables: age, sex, length of pre-ICU hospital stay, patient location before ICU admission, clinical category, and presence or absence of drug overdose. They concluded that the calibration of the original SAPS II calibration was poor, with marked underestimation of observed mortality, whereas discrimination was good. Customization improved calibration but had poor uniformity of fit, and discrimination was unchanged from that reported originally.[37] The expanded SAPS II exhibited good calibration, good uniformity of fit, and better discrimination than in the original model. It should be noted that some ICUs had better and others worse risk-adjusted mortality with the expanded SAPS II than with the customized SAPS II. The investigators concluded that customization improved the statistical qualities of the model but gave poor uniformity of fit. Adding simple variables to create an expanded SAPS II model led to better calibration, discrimination, and uniformity of fit.

Also in France, Aegerter and colleagues performed a retrospective analysis of prospectively collected data for a multicenter database including 33,471 patients from 32 ICUs belonging to the Cub-Rea* database.[46] On the basis of this dataset, these investigators estimated two logistic regression models based on SAPS II: one model using first level customization (having only the SAPS II score as independent variable) and a second model reevaluating the original items of SAPS II with integration of the preadmission location and chronic comorbid conditions. Again, the more complex model had better calibration than the original SAPS II for in-hospital mortality, but its discrimination was not significantly higher. Second level customization and integration of new items improved uniformity of fit for various categories of patients except for diagnosis-related groups. The rank order of ICUs was modified according to the model used.

*Cub-Rea, Collége des Utilisateurs de Base de Donnees en Réanimation.

Finally, in the United Kingdom, Harrison and colleagues used a massive database with input for 141,106 patients from a total of 163 adult general critical care units in England, Wales, and Northern Ireland, during the period December 1995 to August 2003, participating in the ICNARC* database.[47] These researchers compared the published versions of the APACHE II,[8] APACHE II UK,[48] APACHE III,[10] SAPS II,[11] and MPM II,[12] demonstrating that all models showed good discrimination but imperfect calibration. Recalibration of the models was performed by the Cox method with re-estimation of the coefficients, leading to improved discrimination and calibration, although all models still showed significant departure from perfect calibration.

New Models Available

Two other general outcome prediction models have been developed and published: the SAPS 3 admission model in 2005 and the APACHE IV in 2006. A third model, the MPM III, is available, but results are soon to be published.

The SAPS 3 Admission Model

Developed by a group of investigators working on behalf of the SAPS 3 Outcomes Research Group, the SAPS 3 model was published in 2005.[32,33] The study used a total of 19,577 patients consecutively admitted to 307 ICUs all over the world from October 14 to December 15, 2002. This multinational database was designed to reflect the heterogeneity of current ICU case mix and typology throughout the world, including areas outside of Western Europe and the United States.

The SAPS 3 database reflects important differences in patients' and health care systems' baseline characteristics that are known to affect outcome. These include, for example, differences in genetic makeup and in lifestyle and related factors; heterogeneous distribution of major diseases within different regions; issues such as access to the health care system in general and to intensive care in particular; and differences in availability and use of major diagnostic and therapeutic measures within the ICU. Although the integration of ICUs outside Europe and the United States surely has increased representativeness, the extent to which the SAPS 3 database reflects case mix in ICUs worldwide cannot be determined.

On the basis of data collected at ICU admission (±1 hour), the researhers developed regression coefficients by using multilevel logistic regression to estimate the probability of hospital death. The final model, which comprises 20 variables, exhibited good discrimination, without major differences across patient typology, and calibration was satisfactory. Customized equations for major areas of the world were devised and demonstrate overall goodness of fit. Of interest, determinants of hospital mortality changed remarkably from the early 1990s,[10] with chronic health status and circumstances of ICU admission being responsible for almost three fourths of the prognostic power of the model.

*ICNARC, Intensive Care National Audit and Research Centre.

To provide all interested intensivists with the ability to calculate and use SAPS 3 scores, an electronic tool kit for this purpose is available free of charge at the original publisher's website (www.springer.com). Included are complete and detailed descriptions of all variables, as well as additional information on SAPS 3 performance. Moreover, the SAPS 3 Outcomes Research Group provides several additional resources at the project website (www.saps3.org).

The APACHE IV Model

In early 2006, Zimmerman, one of the authors of the original APACHE models, in collaboration with colleagues from Cerner Corporation (in Vienna, Virginia), published the APACHE IV model.[31] The study was based on a database of 110,558 consecutive admissions during 2002 and 2003 to 104 ICUs in 45 U.S. hospitals participating in the APACHE III database. The APACHE IV model uses the worst values during the first 24 hours in the ICU and a multivariate logistic regression procedure to estimate the probability of in-hospital death.

Predictor variables were similar to those in APACHE III, but new variables were added and different statistical modeling has been used. The accuracy of APACHE IV predictions was analyzed in the overall database and in major patient subgroups. APACHE IV had good discrimination and calibration. For 90% of 116 ICU admission diagnoses, the ratio of observed to predicted mortality was not significantly different from 1.0. Predictions were compared with those for the APACHE III versions developed 7 and 14 years previously: Little change was observed in discrimination, but aggregate mortality was systematically overestimated as model age increased. When examined across disease, predictive accuracy was maintained for some diagnoses but for others seemed to reflect changes in practice or therapy. A predictive model for risk-adjusted ICU length of stay also was published by the same goup.[49]

More information about the model and about the possibility of determining the probability of death for individual patients is available at the website of Cerner Corporation (www.criticaloutcomes.cerner.com).

The MPM III Model

The MPM III originally was described by Higgins and coworkers in 2005.[29] This model was developed using data from U.S. ICUs participating in the Project IMPACT database, but no data evaluating its behavior have been published.

DEVELOPING PREDICTIVE MODELS

Selecting the Target Population

Most of the existing general predictive models are not applicable to all ICU patients. Data for patients with burns, patients hospitalized with coronary ischemia (or to rule out myocardial infarction), young patients (younger than 16 or 18 years of age), post–cardiac surgery patients, and patients with a very short length of ICU stay were explicitly excluded from the development of a majority of systems. This limitation is especially important in evaluating specialized ICUs, with a predefined homogeneous case mix, but also can be important in evaluating general ICUs. In many cases, the application of exclusion criteria leads to an analysis of only a small proportion of the admitted patients, resulting in significant modeling errors for general use.

Outcome Selection

Outcome selection identifies the end point of interest. At a minimum, the selected outcome should have the following characteristics:

- A relatively common event
- Ease of definition, recognition, and measurability
- Clinical relevance
- Independence from therapeutic decisions

Mortality meets all of these criteria; however, confounding factors must be considered with use of mortality as an outcome. The location of the patient at the time of death can considerably reduce hospital mortality rates. For example, in a study of 116,340 ICU patients, a significant decline in the ratio of observed to predicted mortality was attributed to a decrease in hospital mortality as a result of earlier transfer of patients with a high severity of illness to skilled nursing facilities.[50] In the APACHE III study, a significant regional difference in mortality was due entirely to variations in hospital length of stay.[51] Variations in any of these factors will lead to differences between observed and predicted mortality that have little to do with case mix or effectiveness of therapy. Increases in the use of advance directives, do-not-resuscitate orders, and limitation or withdrawal of therapy all potentially increase hospital mortality.

Improvements in therapy, such as the use of thrombolysis in myocardial infarction or steroids in *Pneumocystis jiroveci* pneumonia and the acquired immunodeficiency syndrome,[52] can dramatically reduce hospital mortality. Predictive instruments for measuring long-term mortality provide accurate prognostic estimates within the first month of hospital discharge, but their accuracy falls off considerably thereafter, because other factors, such as human immunodeficiency virus infection or malignancy, dominate the long-term survival pattern. Accordingly, mortality is the most useful outcome for designing general severity of illness scores and predictive instruments.

Other outcome measures represent important issues in improving ICU care. These include the following:

- Morbidity and complication rates
- Organ dysfunction
- Resource use
- Duration of mechanical ventilation, use of pulmonary artery catheters
- Quality of life after ICU or hospital discharge
- Length of stay in the ICU

Case mix adjustment is indispensable for studying morbidity, resource utilization, and length of stay. Although these outcomes are difficult to define and are sensitive to local conditions, they are related to the cost of care and have therefore been useful in measuring and comparing ICU efficiency.

Current outcome prediction models aim to predict survival status at hospital discharge. It is, however, incorrect to use them to predict other outcomes, such as the survival status at ICU discharge or vital status 28 days after ICU admission. Such inappropriate application will result in gross underestimation of mortality rates.[53]

Data Collection

The next step in the development of a general outcome prediction model is the evaluation, selection, and registration of the predictive variables. At this stage, major attention should be given to variable definitions, as well as to the time frames for data collection.[54-56] Very frequently, models have been applied incorrectly; the most common errors have been identified as

- The definitions of the variables
- The time frames for the evaluation and registration of the data
- The frequency of measurement and registration of the variables
- The applied exclusion criteria
- Data handling before analysis

It should be noted that all existing models have been calibrated for nonautomated (manual) data collection. The use of electronic patient data management systems (with high sampling rates) has been demonstrated to have a significant impact on the results[57,58]: The higher the sampling rate, the more outliers will be found, and the higher the scores will be.

The evaluation of intra- and interobserver reliability should always be described and reported, together with the frequency of missing values.

Selection of Variables

The number of variables used in severity and prognostic systems is influenced by the data collection burden, statistical considerations, measurement reliability, and frequency. Variable selection reflects a balance between adding variables with a diminishing impact on outcome and limiting variables to the strongest predictors to ease data collection and minimize processing errors. Variables should have the following characteristics:

- Readily available and clinically relevant
- Demonstrate plausible relationship to outcome and easily defined and measured
- Independent of treatment processes
- Verifiable by checks of data accuracy

Initial selection of variables can be either deductive (subjective), using terms that are known or suspected to influence outcome, or inductive (objective) using any deviation from homeostasis or normal health status. The deductive approach employs a group of experts who supply a consensus regarding the measurements and events most strongly associated with the outcome. This approach is faster and requires less computational work; APACHE I and SAPS I both started this way. A purely inductive strategy, used by MPM, begins with the database and tests candidate variables with a plausible relationship to outcome. In the SAPS 3 model, several complementary methods have been used, such as logistic regression on mutually exclusive categories built using smoothed curves based on LOWESS[59] and regression trees (MART).[60]

As a practical matter, neither technique is used exclusively; all systems now use a combination of these techniques. Variables that have been used in severity and prognostic systems include the following:

- Age
- Chronic disease status or comorbid conditions
- Circumstances of ICU admission
- Physiologic measures
- Reasons for ICU admission and admitting diagnoses
- CPR or mechanical ventilation before ICU admission
- Location and length of stay before admission
- Emergency surgery and operative status

Predictor variables should be easily defined and reliably measured to ensure uniform data collection and minimize scoring variations. For statistical purposes, variables are considered dichotomous (e.g., surgery or not), categoric (e.g., disease classification or patient location before admission), or continuous (blood pressure or heart rate). With very large sample sizes, some continuous variables may be rendered dichotomous or categoric if it is discovered that strong and biologically sound threshold values exist beyond which their numeric value has no additional significance.

Assigning weights for ICU admission diagnosis or reason for ICU admission (e.g., asthma versus acute respiratory distress syndrome) will significantly augment prognostic accuracy because a similar extent of physiologic derangement reflects substantial variations in mortality risk for different diseases. Of interest, circumstances of ICU admission, such as the planned or unplanned character of the admission, have been demonstrated to be very important. Systems that include weights for admitting diagnosis must include sufficient numbers of patients in each disease category to perform statistical analyses. Predictive instruments that ignore admitting diagnosis reduce the data collection burden but perform poorly in ICUs with a case mix that differs significantly from that for the development database.

Location and length of stay before ICU admission accounts, at least partly, for lead-time bias, which has an important impact on outcome. For example, a patient who received treatment for 2 days and then was admitted to the ICU is at greater risk for death than a patient with the same diagnosis and severity of illness admitted from the emergency department.

The accuracy of any scoring system depends on the quality of the database from which it was developed. Even with well-defined variables, significant interobserver variability is reported.[61,62]

In calculating the scores, several practical issues should be considered.[63,64] First, when multiple measurements of the same variables are available, which value should be used? It is true that for many of the more simple variables, several measurements will be taken during any 24-hour period. Should the lowest, highest, or an average be taken as the representative value of that day? By general consensus, for the purposes of the score, the worst value in any 24-hour period should be considered. Second, what about missing values? Should the last known value repeatedly be considered as representative until a new value is obtained, or should the mean value between two successive values be taken? Both options make assumptions that may influence the reliability of the score. The first option assumes that knowledge of the evolution of values with time is absent, and the second assumes that changes usually are fairly predictable and regular. The second option seems preferable, because values may be missing for several days and repeating the last known value may involve considerable error in calculation. In addition, changes in most of the variables measured (platelet count, bilirubin, urea) usually are, in fact, fairly regular, moving up or down in a systematic manner.

Validation of the Model

All predictive models developed for outcome prediction need to be validated to demonstrate their ability to predict the outcome under evaluation. Three aspects should be evaluated in this context: the first aspect is *calibration,* or degree of correspondence between the predictions of the model and observed results. The second is *discrimination,* or capability of the model to distinguish observations with a positive outcome from those with a negative outcome. The third is *uniformity of fit* of the model—the performance in various subgroups of patients. The calibration and discrimination components taken together have been named *goodness of fit.*

Goodness of Fit: Calibration and Discrimination

As noted, goodness of fit comprises calibration and discrimination as evaluated in the analyzed population.

Calibration evaluates the degree of correspondence between the estimated probabilities of mortality and the actual mortality in the analyzed sample. Four methods usually are proposed: observed-to-estimated (O/E) mortality ratio, Flora's Z score,[65] Hosmer-Lemeshow goodness of fit tests,[66-68] and calibration curves.

O/E mortality ratios are calculated by dividing the observed mortality (in other words, the number of deaths) by the predicted mortality (the sum of the probabilities of mortality of all patients in the sample). In a perfectly calibrated model this value should be 1.

Hosmer-Lemeshow goodness of fit tests are two chi-square statistics proposed for the formal evaluation of the calibration of predictive models.[66-68] In the Hosmer-Lemeshow H test, patients are classified into 10 groups according to their probabilities of death. Then, a chi-square statistic is used to compare the observed number of deaths and the predicted number of survivors with the observed number of deaths and the observed number of survivors in each of the groups. The formula is:

$$\hat{C}_g = \hat{H}_g = \sum_{i=1}^{g} \frac{(o_1 - e_1)^2}{e_1(1-\bar{\pi}_1)}$$

with g being the number of groups (usually 10), o_1 the number of events observed in group 1, e_1 the number of events expected in the same group and $\bar{\pi}_1$ the mean estimated probability, always in group 1. The resulting statistic is then compared with a chi-square table with 8 degrees of freedom (model development) or 10 degrees of freedom (model validation), in order to know if the observed differences can be explained exclusively by random fluctuation. The Hosmer-Lemeshow $\hat{C}$ test is similar, with the 10 groups containing equal numbers of patients. Hosmer and Lemeshow demonstrated that the grouping method used on the $\hat{C}$ statistics behaves better when most of the probabilities are low.[66]

These tests are now considered by most experts to be mandatory for the evaluation of calibration,[69] although subject to criticism by some.[70,71] It should be stressed that the analyzed sample must be large enough to have the power to detect the lack of agreement between predicted and observed mortality rates.[38]

Calibration curves also are used to describe the calibration of a predictive model. These types of graphics compare observed and predicted mortality. They can, however, be misleading, because the number of patients usually decreases from left to right (on moving from low probabilities to high probabilities), and as a consequence, even small differences in high-severity groups appear visually more important than small differences in low-probability groups. It should be stressed that calibration curves are not a formal statistical test.

Discrimination evaluates the capability of the model to distinguish between patients who die and patients who survive. This evaluation can be made using a nonparametric test such as Harrell's C index, using the order of magnitude of the error.[72] This index measures the probability that, for any two patients chosen randomly, the one with the greater probability will have the outcome of interest (death). This index is directly related with the area under the receiver operating characteristic (ROC) curve and can be obtained as the parameter of the Mann-Whitney-Wilcox statistic.[73] Additional calculations can be used to compute the confidence interval of this measure.[74]

The concept of the area under the ROC curve is derived from psycho-physic tests. In an ROC curve, a series of 2×2 contingency tables are built, ranging from the smallest to the largest score value. For each table, the rate of true-positives (or sensitivity) and the false-positive rate (or 1 minus the specificity) are calculated. The final plot of all possible pairs of rates of true-positives versus false-positives, then, gives the ROC curve.

The interpretation of the area under the ROC curve is easy: A virtual model with a perfect discrimination would have an area of 1.0, and a model with a discrimination no better than chance an area of 0.5. Discriminative abilities of an ROC curve are said to be satisfactory with a value for this area greater than 0.70. General outcome prediction models usually have areas greater than 0.80.

Several methods have been described to compare the areas under two (or more) ROC curves,[75-77] but they can be misleading if the shapes of the curves are different.[78]

Other measures based on classification tables have been used, describing sensitivity, specificity, positive and negative predictive values, and the correct classification rates. Because these calculations must use a fixed cutoff (usually 10%, 50%, or 90%), however, their value is limited.

The relative importance of calibration and discrimination depends on the intended use of the model. Some authors advise that for group comparison, calibration is especially important,[79] and that for decisions involving individual patients, both parameters are important.[80]

Uniformity of Fit

The evaluation of calibration and discrimination in the analyzed sample is now current practice. More complex is the identification of subgroups of patients in which the behavior of the model is not optimal. The presence of such subgroups, can be viewed as an influential observation in model building, and their contribution to the global error of the model can be very large.[81]

The most important subgroups are related to the case mix characteristics that can be eventually related to the outcome of interest. Such characteristics may include the following:

- The intrahospital location before ICU admission
- The surgical status
- The degree of physiologic reserve (age, comorbid conditions)
- The acute diagnosis (including the presence, site, and extent of infection on ICU admission)

Although some authors, such as Rowan and Goldhill in the United Kingdom[48,82] and Apolone and Sicignano in Italy,[40,83] have suggested that the behavior of a model can depend to a significant extent on the case mix of the sample, no consensus exists about the subpopulations for which such analysis should be mandatory.[42]

Updating Severity Scores

Changes in the characteristics of the populations, changes in the therapy of major diseases, and the introduction of new diagnostic methods all imply modifications that result in necessary updates. Moreover, the use of a model outside its development population can eventually imply its modification and adaptation.

Using a Severity of Illness Score

Calculating a Severity of Illness Score

Using the original score sheets (or a well-developed and validated computer software program), a score is assigned to each variable, depending on its deviation from normal values. The arithmetic sum of these variable scores (the sum score) represents the severity score for that patient, which is then used in the equation to predict hospital mortality. As described earlier, this approach was not chosen by the MPM systems, in which the variables are used directly to calculate a probability of death in the hospital by a logistic regression equation.

Transforming the Score into a Probability of Death

The transformation of the severity score into a probability of death in the hospital uses a logistic regression equation. The dependent variable (hospital mortality), y, is related to the set of independent (predictive) variables by the equation

$$\text{logit} = b_0 + b_1x_1 + b_2x_2 \ldots b_kx_k$$

with b_0 being the intercept of the model, x_1 to x_k the predictive variables, and b_1 to b_k the estimated regression coefficients. The probability of death is then given by:

$$\text{Probability of death} = \frac{e^{\text{logit}}}{1+e^{\text{logit}}}$$

with the logit being y as described before. The logistic transformation included in this equation allows the S-shaped relationship between the two variables to become linear (on the logit scale). In the extremes of the score (very low or very high values), changes in the probability of death are small; for intermediate values, even small changes in the score are associated with very large changes in the probability of death. This ensures that outliers do not overly influence the prediction.

Application of a Severity of Illness Score

All existing models aim at predicting an outcome (vital status at hospital discharge) based on a given set of variables: They estimate the outcome for a patient with a certain clinical condition (defined by the registered variables), treated in a hypothetical reference ICU. Several issues, however, need to be taken into account in order to apply one of the previously described models in another population:

- Patient selection
- Evaluation and registration of the predictive variables
- Evaluation and registration of the outcome.
- Computation of the severity score
- Transformation of the score in a probability of death

After validation, the utility and applicability of a model must be evaluated. Literature is full of models developed in large populations that failed when applied within other contexts.[40,41,48,84-88] Thus, this question can be answered only by validating the model in its final population. The potential applications of a model—and consequently its utility—are different for individual patients and for groups.[89]

Evaluating Individual Patients

Some evidence suggests that statistical methods behave better than clinicians in predicting outcome,[90-97] or that they can help clinicians in the decision-making process.[98-100] This opinion is, however, controversial,[101-103] especially for decisions to withdraw or to withhold therapy.[104] Moreover, the application of different models to the same patient frequently results in very different predictions.[105] Thus, application of these models to individual patients for decision making is not recommended.[106]

It should not be forgotten that such statistical models are probabilistic in nature. A well-calibrated model applied to an individual patient may, for example, predict a hospital mortality rate of 46% for that person. The actual meaning of this statistic, however, is that for a group of 100 patients with a similar severity of illness, 46 patients are predicted to die; it makes no statement about whether the individual patient is included in the 46% who will eventually die or in the 54% who will eventually survive.

It should be noted that severity scores have been proposed for uses as diverse as determination of the use of total parenteral nutrition[107] or the identification of futility in intensive care medicine.[108] Some authors have demonstrated that knowledge of predictive information will not have an adverse effect on the quality of care, helping at the same time to decrease the consumption of resources and to increase the availability of beds.[109]

One area for which the scientific community agrees that these models are useful is in the stratification of patients for inclusion into clinical trials and for the comparison of the balance of randomization to different groups.[110]

Evaluating Groups of Patients

At the group level, general outcome prediction models have been proposed for two objectives: distribution of resources and performance evaluation. Several studies were published describing methods to identify and to characterize patients with a low risk of mortality.[111-115] These patients, who require only basic monitoring and general care, eventually could be transferred to other areas of the hospital.[100,116] It could, however, also be argued that these patients have a low mortality because they have been monitored and cared for in an ICU.[117] Also, the use of current instruments is not recommended for the purpose of triage in the emergency department.[118] Moreover, the use of early physiologic indicators outside the ICU has been questioned.[119]

Patient costs in the ICU depend on the amount of required (and utilized) nursing workload. Patient characteristics (diagnosis, degree of physiologic dysfunction) are not the only determinants. Costs depend also on the practices and policies in a given ICU. Focusing attention on the effective use of nursing workload[120] or the dynamic evolution of the clinical course[121,122] seems a more promising strategy than those approaches based exclusively on the condition of the patient during the first hours in the ICU or in the O/E length of stay in the ICU.[51,123,124]

On the other hand, general outcome prediction models have been proposed to identify patients who require more resources.[125] Unfortunately, these patients only rarely can be identified at ICU admission, because their degree of physiologic dysfunction during the first 24 hours in the ICU tends to be moderate, although variable.[126-128] Even if someday these patients can be well identified, the question of what to do with this information remains.

Another important area in which these types of models have been used is in evaluation of ICU performance.

Several investigators proposed the use of standardized mortality ratios (SMR) for performance evaluation, assuming that current models can take into account the main determinants of mortality.[129] The SMR is calculated by dividing the observed mortality by the averaged predicted mortality (the sum of the individual probabilities of mortality for all of the patients in the sample). Additional computations can be made to estimate the confidence interval for this ratio.[130]

The interpretation of the SMR is easy: A ratio lower than 1 implies a performance better than that in the reference population, and a ratio greater than 1 a performance worse than in the reference population. This methodology has been used for international comparison of ICUs,[17,48,62,85,131,132] comparison of hospitals,[16,51,86,87,123,129,133,134] ICU evaluation,[135-138] management evaluation,[134,139,140] and the influence of organization and management factors on performance of the ICU.[141]

Before application of this methodology, six questions should always be answered:

1. Is it possible to evaluate and register all of the data needed for application of the models?
2. Can the models be used in the large majority of ICU patients?
3. Are existent models able to control for the main patient characteristics related to mortality?
4. Has the reference population been well chosen and are the models well calibrated to this population?
5. Is the sample size sufficient for meaningful differences to be identified?
6. Is vital status at ICU discharge the main performance indicator?

Each of these assumptions has been questioned, and no definitive answer exists at present. Most investigators, however, believe that performance is multidimensional and consequently should be evaluated in several dimensions.[23,142] The problem of sample size seems especially important with respect to the risk of a type II error (in other words, to say that there are no differences when in fact they exist).

The comparison between observed and predicted might make more sense if done separately in low-, intermediate-, and high-risk patients, because the performance of an ICU can change according to the severity of the condition of the admitted patients. This approach was advocated in the past on the basis of theoretical concerns[143-145] but was used in only a small number of studies.[141,146] Multilevel modeling, with varying slopes, can be an answer for the developers of such models.[23,147]

ORGAN DYSFUNCTION/FAILURE SCORING SYSTEMS

Organ failure scores are designed to describe organ dysfunction, not to predict survival. In the development of organ function scores, three important principles need to be remembered.[15] First, organ failure is not a simple all-or-nothing phenomenon; rather, a spectrum or continuum of organ dysfunction exists, ranging from very mild alteration in function to total organ failure. Second, organ failure is not a static process, and the degree of dysfunction may vary during the course of disease so that scores need to be calculated repeatedly. Third, the variables chosen to evaluate each organ need to be objective, simple, and available but reliable, routinely measured in every institution, specific to the organ in question, and independent of patient variables, so that the score can be easily calculated on any patient in any ICU. Interobserver variability in scoring can be a problem with more complex systems,[56,148] and the use of simple, unequivocal variables can avoid this potential problem. Ideally, scores should be independent of therapeutic variables, as stressed by Marshall and associates,[13] but, in fact, this is virtually impossible to achieve, because all factors are more or less treatment dependent. For example, the PaO_2/FIO_2 ratio is dependent on ventilatory conditions and use of positive end-expiratory pressure, platelet count may be influenced by platelet transfusions, urea levels are affected by hemofiltration, and so on.

The process of organ function description is relatively new, and general agreement is lacking on which organs to assess and which parameters to use. Numerous scoring systems have been developed for assessing organ dysfunction,[13-15,149-157] differing in the organ systems included in the score, the definitions used for organ dysfunction, and the grading scale used.[64,158] A majority of scores include six key organ systems—cardiovascular, respiratory, hematologic, central nervous, renal, and hepatic—with other systems, such as the gastrointestinal system, less commonly included. Early scoring systems assessed organ failure as either present or absent, but this approach is very dependent on where the limits for organ function are set, and newer scores consider organ failure as a spectrum of dysfunction. Most scores have been developed in the general ICU population, but some are aimed specifically at the septic patient.[15,150,151,155,156] In this section, three of the more recently developed systems are discussed in some detail. The main difference among them is in the definition of cardiovascular system dysfunction (Table 74-2).

Multiple Organ Dysfunction Score

The MODS (Multiple Organ Dysfunction Score) system was developed using a literature review of clinical studies of multiple organ failure from 1969 to 1993.[13] Optimal descriptors of organ dysfunction were identified and validated against a clinical database. Six organ systems were chosen, and a score of 0 to 4 was allotted for each organ according to function (with 0 indicating normal function and 4, most severe dysfunction), with a maximum score of 24. With MODS, the worst score for each organ system in each 24-hour period is taken for calculation of the aggregate score. A high initial MODS correlated with ICU mortality, and the delta MODS (calculated as the MODS over the whole ICU stay less the admission MODS) was even more predictive of outcome.[13] In a study of 368 critically ill patients, the MODS was found to better describe outcome groups than the APACHE II or the organ failure score, although the predicted risk of mortality was similar for all scoring systems.[159] The MODS has

Table 74-2. Organ Dysfunction/Failure Scoring Systems

Organ System	MODS*	SOFA†	LODS‡
Respiratory	PaO_2/FIO_2 ratio	PaO_2/FIO_2 ratio Mechanical ventilation	PaO_2/FIO_2 ratio Mechanical ventilation
Cardiovascular	Pressure-adjusted heart rate	Mean arterial pressure Use of vasoactive agents	Systolic arterial pressure Heart rate
Renal	Creatinine	Creatinine Urinary output	Creatinine Urinary output Urea
Hematologic	Platelets	Platelets	Platelets Leukocytes
Neurologic	Glasgow Coma Scale score	Glasgow Coma Scale score	Glasgow Coma Scale score
Hepatic	Bilirubin	Bilirubin	Bilirubin Prothrombin time

LODS, Logistic Organ Dysfunction System; MODS, Multiple Organ Dysfunction Score; SOFA, Sequential Organ Failure Assessment.
*From Marshall JC, Cook DA, Christou NV, et al: Multiple organ dysfunction score: A reliable descriptor of a complex clinical outcome. Crit Care Med 1995;23:1638-1652.
†From Vincent J-L, Moreno R, Takala J, et al: The SOFA (Sepsis-Related Organ Failure Assessment) score to describe organ dysfunction/failure. Intensive Care Med 1996;22:707-710.
‡From Le Gall JR, Klar J, Lemeshow S, et al: The logistic organ dysfunction system. A new way to assess organ dysfunction in the intensive care unit. JAMA 1996;276:802-810.

been used to assess organ dysfunction in clinical studies of various groups of critically ill patients, including those with severe sepsis.[160-163]

Sequential Organ Failure Assessment Score

The SOFA (Sequential Organ Failure Assessment) scoring system was developed in 1994 during a consensus conference organized by the European Society of Intensive Care and Emergency Medicine, in an attempt to provide a means of quantitatively and objectively describing the degree of organ failure over time in individual patients and in groups of patients with sepsis.[15] Initially termed the "Sepsis-Related Organ Failure Assessment Score," the score was then renamed the Sequential Organ Failure Assessment following the recognition that it could be applied equally to nonseptic patients.

In devising the score, the participants of the conference decided to limit to six the number of systems studied: respiratory, coagulation, hepatic, cardiovascular, central nervous system, and renal. A score of 0 is given for normal function through to 4 for most abnormal, and the worst values on each day are recorded. Individual organ function can thus be assessed and monitored over time, and an overall global score also can be calculated. A high total SOFA score (SOFA max) and a high delta SOFA (the total maximum SOFA minus the admission total SOFA) have been shown to be related to a worse outcome,[121,164] and the total score has been shown to increase over time in nonsurvivors compared with survivors.[164] The SOFA score has been used for organ failure assessment in several clinical trials, including one in patients in septic shock.[165-168]

Logistic Organ Dysfunction System Score

The LODS (Logistic Organ Dysfunction System) was developed in 1996 using multiple logistic regression applied to selected variables from a large database of ICU patients.[14] To calculate the score, each organ system receives points according to the worst value for any variable for that system on that day. If no organ dysfunction is present, the score is 0, rising to a maximum of 5. Because the relative severity of organ dysfunction differs between organ systems, the LODS score allows for the maximum 5 points to be awarded only to the neurologic, renal, and cardiovascular systems. For maximum dysfunction of the pulmonary and coagulation systems, a maximum of 3 points can be given for the most severe levels of dysfunction, and for the liver, the most severe dysfunction only receives 1 point. Thus, the total maximum score is 22. The LODS score is designed to be used as a once-only measure of organ dysfunction in the first 24 hours of ICU admission, rather than as a repeated assessment measure. The LODS is quite complex and seldom used; nevertheless, it has been used to assess organ dysfunction in clinical studies.[169]

Comparison of Scoring Systems

The main difference among the three described models is the method chosen for the evaluation of the cardiovascular dysfunction: SOFA uses blood pressure and the level of adrenergic support; MODS uses a composed variable (the pressure-adjusted heart rate: heart rate×central venous pressure/mean arterial pressure) and mean arterial pressure; and LODS score uses the heart rate and the systolic blood pressure. A comparison analysis, published only as an abstract, was presented at the 10th Annual Congress of the European Society of Intensive Care Medicine (Paris, 1997), and the results seem to indicate a greater discriminative capability of MODS and SOFA scores over LODS score.[170] Owing to the small size of the sample, however, this result requires further validation.

Mixed models, integrating organ failure assessment scores and and general severity scores, have been published[154,171] but never gained widespread acceptance.

SCORING SYSTEMS FOR SPECIFIC CLINICAL CONDITIONS

Several scoring systems have been developed to be applied on subsamples of patients with specific clinical conditions, such as cardiac surgery, sepsis, trauma, and acute renal failure. This section briefly reviews the most important of these systems.

Septic Patients

In several areas, use of the scoring systems discussed earlier can be beneficial in patients with septic shock, as in other groups of critically ill patients.[172] First, they can be invaluable in the classification and stratification of patients for enrollment in clinical trials of new antisepsis treatments. Mortality prediction scores can be used to stratify groups of patients and assess outcome in terms of mortality, and organ dysfunction scores can help evaluate the effects of new treatments on morbidity, thereby changing the emphasis of outcome measure from mortality to morbidity. Of importance, improved morbidity must be associated with a reduced, or trend to reduced, mortality. Second, such scoring systems can be used to describe patient populations in epidemiologic studies for comparison of patients over time or from different institutions. Third, estimated probabilities of mortality and actual outcomes can be compared to create an SMR. SMRs from a cross section of different ICUs or from the same ICU over time could then be used to facilitate resource allocation.

Before these scores can be used to compare ICU performances in different geographic areas or populations, however, they may need to be customized to the local population, and their use as a management instrument is limited.[173] Also, doubts exist about the appropriateness of the SMR as performance indicator.[42,174,175]

Although these scores are useful in the prediction of mortality for a group of patients, they have not been validated to provide a precise prediction of outcome in individual patients. Clinical decisions concerning individual patient care should not be based exclusively on any scoring system, although such scores may provide valuable information to be used in addition to clinical assessment,[107,176,177] even in septic patients.[178]

As current understanding of the pathophysiologic mechanisms underlying sepsis has advanced, some authors have proposed that the inclusion of biologic markers of disease in scoring systems may be useful in certain categories of patients, such as those with sepsis.[179,180] One biologic scoring system developed by Casey and coworkers[181] measured levels of lipopolysaccharide and the cytokines tumor necrosis factor-α (TNF-α and interleukins IL-1 and IL-6 and devised a total lipopolysaccharide-cytokine score that correlated well with mortality in their population of 97 patients with sepsis syndrome. The accuracy of cytokine levels in the diagnosis of sepsis is controversial, however, and further study is needed to better define sepsis markers before such scores can be included in currently available disease severity scoring systems.

The most recent scoring system for the evaluation of septic patients was developed from a European multicenter study.[182] The Risk of Infection to Severe Sepsis and Shock Score (RISSC) was developed to examine the incidence of risk factors worsening sepsis in infected patients. The study found the incidence of worsening sepsis to be 20% at day 10 and 24% at day 30. Several factors were identified to be independently associated with the risk of worsening sepsis. The investigators concluded that the RISSC score may be a valuable tool to stratify septic patients.

Trauma Patients

Several different scoring systems have been developed for the evaluation of trauma patients. Principally, two different principles have been followed: One principle is apparent in the morphologic classification of the underlying traumatic injury as it has been proposed already by the Committee on Injury Scaling—the so-called Abbreviated Injury Scale (AIS). This score classifies each injury according to the body region, the anatomic structures involved, and the level of injury. It has been revised several times and currently is available as the AIS 2005 revision (at www.carcrash.org). Subsequently, Baker and colleagues proposed the Injury Severity Score (ISS), based on the AIS.[183] It uses the AIS to score the three most severely injured body regions.

A second principle applies in physiology-based scores developed to quantify the underlying physiologic deviation for a trauma patient. Main representatives of this category are the Trauma Score developed by Champion and associates[184] and its successor, the Revised Trauma Score (RTS).[185] The latter system includes the Glasgow Coma Scale, systolic blood pressure, and respiratory rate at the time of the admission to the emergency department.

The most successful score—the Trauma and Injury Severity Score (TRISS)[186]—was, however, again developed by Champion and associates and in fact is derived from a combination of two different principles. TRISS was the result of merging two existing systems, morphologic and physiologic, for trauma assessment: the Injury Severity Score and the RTS.[185] It uses the ISS to describe the anatomic injury, the RTS to describe the physiologic malfunction, and, in addition, age as a variable to calculate a predicted probability of survival.

A major problem with the TRISS results from the fact that the underlying database—namely, the Major Trauma Outcome Study (MTOS)—was a pure Anglo-American database, which poorly translates into different settings. Trauma patterns are, for example, completely different in European trauma centers. Additionally, another reported problem is a lack of prognostic accuracy in elderly patients presenting with various physiologic derangements and chronic diseases, independent from the traumatic injury.[187]

General severity of illness scores, such as the SAPS II, on the other hand, work well in adjustment of physiologic derangement but provide no means to describe the severity of trauma and therefore also do not perform well in trauma patients.[188] Specialists in trauma care have expressed reservations about the accuracy of these methodologies,[189,190] and comparisons between trauma ICUs have been rendered difficult by the malperformance of TRISS, as well as SAPS II, in trauma patients: Because the TRISS score yields unrealistically high survival probabilities, these departments perform less well than expected. A recent study by Reiter and colleagues thus tried to evaluate the combination of a general severity of illness score with the TRISS method.[191] These investigators showed that the combination of both systems was superior in predicting outcome (i.e., survival at hospital discharge). If such a methodology could be of use for the assessment of trauma, ICUs would need further clarification with prospective studies.

In 1990, Champion and associates published another system for the assessment of trauma patients, the ASCOT (A Severity Characterization of Trauma) score.[192] The score was later validated and used in different settings. Although ASCOT was found to be superior to the TRISS in predicting outcome,[70,193,194] its prognostic performance was found to be low in other settings.[195,196] Further modifications of TRISS-like methodology have been published by various groups.[197-199]

Glance and colleagues recently published a retrospective cohort study, using more than 91,000 admissions from 69 hospitals from the National Trauma Databank.[200] They used TRISS and ASCOT methodologies to calculate O/E ratios for each center and found a substantial disagreement between the two methods in identifying quality outliers. Moreover, these investigators found both methods to be poorly calibrated in this population.[200] Accordingly, they concluded that it is currently impossible to use one of these systems to determine "best practice" for trauma care and recommended to update the existing sysytems.

Cardiac Surgical Patients

Several models have been developed to risk-stratify patients who require cardiac surgery.[201-204] The most widely used system was the Parsonnet score, which was developed using a database of 3500 admissions and prospectively validated in a single-center study. It used 14 variables shown to be significant in a univariate regression analysis. The Parsonnet score remained the gold standard for preoperative risk assessment more than a decade.

Several models to assess the perioperative risk for cardiac surgery patients have been developed from hospital or regional databases, such as the Society of Thoracic Surgeons National Cardiac Surgery Database, the New York State Database, or the Veteran Affairs Database.[205-208] A majority of these models, however, have been neither developed nor validated for use in the ICU.

In 1999 the results of a multicenter European study were published: the European System for Cardiac Operative Risk Evaluation (EuroSCORE).[209] A total of 19,030 patients from 128 centers who underwent cardiac surgery were included in this study. The score was constructed using multiple logistic regression analysis of 68 preoperative and 29 operative risk factors. The final score consisted of 20 variables that allowed, for the first time, a quick assessment of the patient's operative risk. The EuroSCORE has meanwhile been validated in a variety of settings.[210-213] Moreover, it has been found useful to assess costs and resource use among patients undergoing cardiac surgery,[214] and to evaluate the incidence of readmission in this population.[215] In addition, EuroSCORE was found to be a good predictor for complications in the perioperative setting[216] and to be associated with long-term outcome after cardiac surgery.[217]

The EuroSCORE system exists now in two versions: additive and logistic. After the initial score was published, the authors added a version that was developed with logistic regression methods and recently published the coefficients.[218]

A review by Gogbashian and colleagues suggested that the additive EuroSCORE may not be well calibrated: Overestimation of mortality in low-risk patients and underestimation in high-risk patients were consistently found.[219] Accordingly, these investigators concluded that using the additive EuroSCORE has the effect of penalizing those centers that take on high risk-cases. Moreover, they suggested that a systematic review of the prognostic performance of the logistic EuroSCORE should be undertaken as soon as studies using this score become available.

DIRECTIONS FOR FURTHER RESEARCH

Recent years have seen the development of a new generation of general outcome prediction models. More complex than their old counterparts, relying heavily on computerized data registry and analysis (although scores with the SAPS 3 model can be still calculated easily by hand), and incorporating a more extensive array of the reasons and circumstances responsible for ICU admission, these instruments now need to be evaluated outside their development populations.

The selection of a severity scoring system remains largely subjective and dependent on the reference database chosen by the user: the U.S. centers participating in the APACHE III database or a more heterogeneous sample of ICUs across all major regions of the globe. The absence of any fee for use of the SAPS 3 model and the availability of equations specific for each region of the world should be weighed against participation in a pay-for-use continuous database program that provides greater professional support and analysis of the data.

No matter which model is chosen, users should keep in mind that the accuracy of these models is dynamic and should be periodically retested, and that when accuracy deteriorates the models must be revised or updated. Also, their use should be complementary and not alternative to the use of clinical evaluation, because both predictive methods are prone to error,[220] especially in the individual patient.[221]

KEY POINTS

- Scoring systems have been broadly used in medicine for several decades, both for clinical research and for the evaluation of ICU effectiveness.
- The evaluation of severity of illness in the critically ill patient is made through the use of severity scores and prognostic models. Severity scores are instruments that aim at stratifying patients according to their severity, assigning to each patient an increasing score as illness severity increases; in addition to the stratification process, prognostic models aim at predicting a certain outcome based in a given set of prognostic variables and a specific modeling equation.
- Different systems are available to describe and classify ICU populations, to compare severity of illness and to predict mortality in the patients. These systems perform globally well, but there are still concerns about errors in prediction caused by differences in patient selection, lead-time bias, sample size, representativeness of the databases used to develop the systems and poor calibration within patient subgroups and across geographic locations.
- The most widely used general outcome prognostic systems for adults are APACHE II and III, the SAPS II, and the MPM II. Newer published models are the APACHE IV and the SAPS 3.
- At patient-level, severity scores and prognostic models have been used for purposes as diverse as to determine the use of total parenteral nutrition, the identification of futility in intensive care medicine, the use of new therapies in sepsis, the stratification of patients for inclusion into clinical trials or the analysis of the balance of randomization in different groups during clinical trials. At group level, general outcome prediction models have been proposed for allocation of resources and performance evaluation, though the use of the observed to expected mortality ratio or standardized mortality ratio.
- Organ failure scoring systems are designed to measure the presence and degree of organ dysfunction or failure in critically ill patients. Most models evaluate six key organ systems, cardiovascular, respiratory, hematologic, central nervous, renal, and hepatic, with other systems, such as the gastrointestinal system, less commonly included. All of them use a combination of physiologic and therapeutic variables to assess organ dysfunction or failure.
- Several scoring systems have been developed to be applied in more specific populations with specific clinical conditions, such as cardiac surgery or trauma. Models specifically developed to be used in neonates or children also are available.
- The choice between existing systems remains largely subjective and will depend on the reference database selected by the user: the U.S. centers participating in the APACHE III database or a more heterogeneous sample of ICUs across all major regions of the globe. Complexity, cost, and the existence of equations specific for each region of the world should be weighted, as well as participation in a continuous database program for professional support and analysis of the data. No matter which the model is chosen, accuracy should be periodically retested, and as it deteriorates, the model must be revised or updated. The use of such models should be complementary and not alternative to the use of clinical evaluation.

REFERENCES

1. Apgar V: A proposal for a new method of evaluation of the newborn infant. Anesth Analg 1953;32: 260-267.
2. Child CG, Turcotte JG: Surgery and portal hypertension. Major Probl Clin Surg 1964;1:1-85.
3. Killip TK 3rd, Kimball JT: Treatment of myocardial infarction in a coronary care unit. Am J Cardiol 1967;20:457-464.
4. Teasdale G, Jennett B: Assessment of coma and impaired consciousness. Lancet 1974;2:81-84.
5. Bastos PG, Sun X, Wagner DP, et al: Glasgow Coma Scale score in the evaluation of outcome in the intensive care unit: Findings from the Acute Physiology and Chronic Health Evaluation III study. Crit Care Med 1993;21:1459-1465.
6. Knaus WA, Zimmerman JE, Wagner DP, et al: APACHE—Acute Physiology And Chronic Health Evaluation: A physiologically based classification system. Crit Care Med 1981;9:591-597.
7. Le Gall J-R, Loirat P, Alperovitch A: Simplified acute physiological score for intensive care patients. Lancet 1983;2:741.
8. Knaus WA, Draper EA, Wagner DP, Zimmerman JE: APACHE II: A severity of disease classification system. Crit Care Med 1985;13:818-829.
9. Lemeshow S, Teres D, Pastides H, et al: A method for predicting survival and mortality of ICU patients using objectively derived weights. Crit Care Med 1985;13:519-525.
10. Knaus WA, Wagner DP, Draper EA, et al: The APACHE III prognostic system. Risk prediction of hospital mortality for critically ill hospitalized adults. Chest 1991;100:1619-1636.
11. Le Gall JR, Lemeshow S, Saulnier F: A new Simplified Acute Physiology Score (SAPS II) based on a European/North American multicenter study. JAMA 1993;270:2957-2963.
12. Lemeshow S, Teres D, Klar J, et al: Mortality Probability Models (MPM II) based on an international cohort of intensive care unit patients. JAMA 1993;270:2478-2486.
13. Marshall JC, Cook DA, Christou NV, et al: Multiple organ dysfunction score: A reliable descriptor of a complex clinical outcome. Crit Care Med 1995;23:1638-1652.
14. Le Gall JR, Klar J, Lemeshow S, et al: The logistic organ dysfunction system. A new way to assess organ dysfunction in the intensive care unit. JAMA 1996;276:802-810.
15. Vincent J-L, Moreno R, Takala J, et al: The SOFA (Sepsis-related Organ Failure Assessment) score to describe organ dysfunction/failure. Intensive Care Med 1996;22:707-710.
16. Knaus WA, Draper EA, Wagner DP, et al: Evaluating outcome from intensive care: A preliminary multihospital comparison. Crit Care Med 1982;10:491-496.
17. Knaus WA, Le Gall JR, Wagner DP, et al: A comparison of intensive care in the U.S.A. and France. Lancet 1982;642-646.
18. Wagner DP, Draper EA, Abizanda Campos R, et al: Initial international use of APACHE: An acute severity of disease measure. Med Dec Making 1984;4:297.
19. Le Gall JR, Loirat P, Alperovitch A, et al: A simplified acute physiologic score for ICU patients. Crit Care Med 1984;12:975-977.
20. Lemeshow S, Teres D, Avrunin J, Gage RW: Refining intensive care unit outcome by using changing probabilities of mortality. Crit Care Med 1988;16:470-477.

21. Castella X, Artigas A, Bion J, for the The European/North American Severity Study Group: A comparison of severity of illness scoring systems for intensive care unit patients: Results of a multicenter, multinational study. Crit Care Med 1995;23:1327-1335.
22. Bertolini G, D'Amico R, Apolone G, et al: Predicting outcome in the intensive care unit using scoring systems: Is new better? A comparison of SAPS and SAPS II in a cohort of 1,393 patients. Med Care 1998;36:1371-1382.
23. Moreno R, Matos R: The "new" scores: What problems have been fixed, and what remain? Curr Opin Crit Care 2000;6:158-165.
24. Angus DC, Linde-Zwirble WT, Lidicker J, et al: Epidemiology of severe sepsis in the United States: Analysis of incidence, outcome and associated costs of care. Crit Care Med 2001;29:1303-1310.
25. Martin GS, Mannino DM, Eaton S, Moss M: The epidemiology of sepsis in the United States from 1979 through 2000. N Engl J Med 2003;348:1546-1554.
26. Bernard GR, Vincent J-L, Laterre P-F, et al: Efficacy and safety of recombinant human activated protein C for severe sepsis. N Engl J Med 2001;344:699-709.
27. Ely EW, Laterre P-F, Angus DC, et al: Drotrecogin alfa (activated) administration across clinically important subgroups of patients with severe sepsis. Crit Care Med 2003;31:12-19.
28. Moreno R, Metnitz P, Jordan B, et al: SAPS 3 28 days score: A prognostic model to estimate patient survival during the first 28 days in the ICU. Intensive Care Med 2006;32:S203 (Abstract).
29. Higgins T, Teres D, Copes W, et al: Preliminary update of the Mortality Prediction Model (MPM_0). Crit Care 2005;9:S97 (Abstract).
30. Render ML, Kim M, Deddens J, et al: Variation in outcomes in Veterans Affairs intensive care units with a computerized severity measure. Crit Care Med 2005;33:930-939.
31. Zimmerman JE, Kramer AA, McNair DS, Malila FM: Acute Physiology and Chronic Health Evaluation (APACHE) IV: Hospital mortality assessment for today's critically ill patients. Crit Care Med 2006;34:1297-1310.
32. Metnitz PG, Moreno RP, Almeida E, et al: SAPS 3. From evaluation of the patient to evaluation of the intensive care unit. Part 1: Objectives, methods and cohort description. Intensive Care Med 2005;31:1336-1344.
33. Moreno RP, Metnitz PG, Almeida E, et al: SAPS 3. From evaluation of the patient to evaluation of the intensive care unit. Part 2: Development of a prognostic model for hospital mortality at ICU admission. Intensive Care Med 2005;31:1345-1355.
34. Dybowski R, Weller P, Chang R, Gant V: Prediction of outcome in critically ill patients using artificial neural network, synthesised by genetic algorithm. Lancet 1996;347:1146-1150.
35. Engoren M, Moreno R, Reis Miranda D: A genetic algorithm to predict hospital mortality in an ICU population. Crit Care Med 1999;27:A52.
36. Moreno R, Afonso S: Ethical, legal and organizational issues in the ICU: Prediction of outcome. Curr Opin Crit Care 2006;12:619-623.
37. Moreno R, Apolone G: The impact of different customization strategies in the performance of a general severity score. Crit Care Med 1997;25:2001-2008.
38. Zhu B-P, Lemeshow S, Hosmer DW, et al: Factors affecting the performance of the models in the mortality probability model and strategies of customization: A simulation study. Crit Care Med 1996;24:57-63.
39. Le Gall J-R, Lemeshow S, Leleu G, et al: Customized probability models for early severe sepsis in adult intensive care patients. JAMA 1995;273:644-650.
40. Apolone G, D'Amico R, Bertolini G, et al: The performance of SAPS II in a cohort of patients admitted in 99 Italian ICUs: Results from the GiViTI. Intensive Care Med 1996;22:1368-1378.
41. Metnitz PG, Valentin A, Vesely H, et al: Prognostic performance and customization of the SAPS II: Results of a multicenter Austrian study. Intensive Care Med 1999;25:192-197.
42. Moreno R, Apolone G, Reis Miranda D: Evaluation of the uniformity of fit of general outcome prediction models. Intensive Care Med 1998;24:40-47.
43. Knaus WA, Harrell FE, Fisher CJ, et al: The clinical evaluation of new drugs for sepsis. A prospective study design based on survival analysis. JAMA 1993;270:1233-1341.
44. Knaus WA, Harrell FE, LaBrecque JF, et al: Use of predicted risk of mortality to evaluate the efficacy of anticytokine therapy in sepsis. Crit Care Med 1996;24:46-56.
45. Le Gall1 J-R, Neumann A, Hemery F, et al: Mortality prediction using SAPS II: An update for French intensive care units. Crit Care 2005;9:R645-R652.
46. Aegerter P, Boumendil A, Retbi A, et al: SAPS II revisited. Intensive Care Med 2005;31:416-423.
47. Harrison DA, Brady AR, Parry GJ, et al: Recalibration of risk prediction models in a large multicenter cohort of admissions to adult, general critical care units in the United Kingdom. Crit Care Med 2006;34:1378-1388.
48. Rowan KM, Kerr JH, Major E, et al: Intensive Care Society's APACHE II study in Britain and Ireland—II: Outcome comparisons of intensive care units after adjustment for case mix by the American APACHE II method. BMJ 1993;307:977-981.
49. Zimmerman JE, Kramer AA, McNair DS, et al: Intensive care unit length of stay: Benchmarking based on Acute Physiology and Chronic Health Evaluation (APACHE) IV. Crit Care Med 2006;34:2517-2529.
50. Sirio CA, Shepardson LB, Rotondi AJ, et al: Community-wide assessment of intensive care outcomes using a physiologically based prognostic measure: Implications for critical care delivery from Cleveland Health Quality Choice. Chest 1999;115:793.
51. Knaus WA, Wagner DP, Zimmerman JE, Draper EA: Variations in mortality and length of stay in intensive care units. Ann Intern Med 1993;118:753-761.
52. Montaner JSG, Lawson LM, Levitt N, et al: Corticosteroids prevent early deterioration in patients with moderate severe *Pneumocystis carinii* pneumonia and the acquired immunodeficiency syndrome. Ann Intern Med 1990;113:14-20.
53. Moreno R, Miranda DR, Matos R, Fevereiro T: Mortality after discharge from intensive care: The impact of organ system failure and nursing workload use at discharge. Intensive Care Med 2001;27:999-1004.
54. Abizanda Campos R, Balerdi B, Lopez J, et al: Fallos de prediccion de resultados mediante APACHE II. Analisis de los errores de prediction de mortalidad en pacientes criticos. Med Clin Barc 1994;102:527-531.
55. Fery-Lemmonier E, Landais P, Kleinknecht D, Brivet F: Evaluation of severity scoring systems in ICUs: Translation, conversion and definition ambiguities as a source of inter-observer variability in APACHE II, SAPS, and OSF. Intensive Care Med 1995;21:356-360.
56. Rowan K: The reliability of case mix measurements in intensive care. Curr Opin Crit Care 1996;2:209-213.
57. Bosman RJ, Oudemane van Straaten HM, Zandstra DF: The use of intensive care information systems alters outcome prediction. Intensive Care Med 1998;24:953-958.
58. Suistomaa M, Kari A, Ruokonen E, Takala J: Sampling rate causes bias in APACHE II and SAPS II scores. Intensive Care Med 2000;26:1773-1778.
59. Cleveland WS: LOWESS: A program for smoothing scatterplots by robust locally weighted regression. Am Stat 1981;35:54.
60. Ridgeway G: The state of boosting. Comput Sci Statist 1999;31:172-181.
61. Damiano AM, Bergner M, Draper EA, et al: Reliability of a measure of severity of illness: Acute physiology and chronic health evaluation II. J Clin Epidemiol 1992;45:93-101.
62. Moreno R, Reis Miranda D, Fidler V, Van Schilfgaarde R: Evaluation of two outcome predictors on an independent database. Crit Care Med 1998;26:50-61.
63. Guyatt GH, Meade MO: Outcome measures: Methodologic principles. Sepsis 1997;1:21-25.
64. Marshall JD, Bernard G, Le Gall J-R, Vincent J-L: The measurement of organ dysfunction/failure as an ICU outcome. Sepsis 1997;1:41.
65. Flora JD: A method for comparing survival of burn patients to a standard survival curve. J Trauma 1978;18:701-705.
66. Hosmer DW, Lemeshow S: Applied Logistic Regression. New York, John Wiley & Sons, 1989.
67. Lemeshow S, Hosmer DW: A review of goodness of fit statistics for use in the development of logistic regression models. Am J Epidemiol 1982;115:92-106.
68. Hosmer DW, Lemeshow S: A goodness-of-fit test for the multiple

logistic regression model. Comm Stat 1980;A10:1043-1069.
69. Hadorn DC, Keeler EB, Rogers WH, Brook RH: Assessing the Performance of Mortality Prediction Models. Santa Monica, CA, RAND/UCLA/Harvard Center for Health Care Financing Policy Research, 1993.
70. Champion HR, Copes WS, Sacco WJ, et al: Improved predictions from a severity characterization of trauma (ASCOT) over trauma and injury severity score (TRISS): Results of an independent evaluation. J Trauma 1996;40:42-49.
71. Bertolini G, D'Amico R, Nardi D, et al: One model, several results: The paradox of the Hosmer-Lemeshow goodness-of-fit test for the logistic regression model. J Epidemiol Biostatistics 2000;5:251-253.
72. Harrell FE Jr, Califf RM, Pryor DB, et al: Evaluating the yield of medical tests. JAMA 1982;247:2543-2546.
73. Hanley J, McNeil B: The meaning and use of the area under a receiver operating characteristic (ROC) curve. Radiology 1982;143:29-36.
74. Ma G, Hall WJ: Confidence bands for receiver operating characteristic curves. Med Decis Making 1993;13:191-197.
75. Hanley J, McNeil B: A method of comparing the areas under receiver operating characteristic curves derived from the same cases. Radiology 1983;148:839-843.
76. McClish DK: Comparing the areas under more than two independent ROC curves. Med Decis Making 1987;7:149-155.
77. DeLong ER, DeLong DM, Clarke-Pearson DL: Comparing the areas under two or more correlated receiver operating characteristic curves: A nonparametric approach. Biometrics 1988;44:837-845.
78. Hilden J: The area under the ROC curve and its competitors. Med Decis Making 1991;11:95-101.
79. Schuster DP: Predicting outcome after ICU admission. The art and science of assessing risk. Chest 1992;102: 1861-1870.
80. Kollef MH, Schuster DP: Predicting intensive care unit outcome with scoring systems. Underlying concepts and principles. Crit Care Clin 1994;10:1-18.
81. Miller ME, Hui SL: Validation techniques for logistic regression models. Stat Med 1991;10: 1213-1226.
82. Goldhill DR, Withington PS: The effects of casemix adjustment on mortality as predicted by APACHE II. Intensive Care Med 1996;22: 415-419.
83. Sicignano A, Carozzi C, Giudici D, et al: The influence of length of stay in the ICU on power of discrimination of a multipurpose severity score (SAPS). Intensive Care Med 1996;22: 1048-1051.
84. Castella X, Gilabert J, Torner F, Torres C: Mortality prediction models in intensive care: Acute Physiology and Chronic Health Evaluation II and Mortality Prediction Model compared. Crit Care Med 1991;19:191-197.
85. Sirio CA, Tajimi K, Tase C, et al: An initial comparison of intensive care in Japan and United States. Crit Care Med 1992;20:1207-1215.
86. Bastos PG, Sun X, Wagner DP, et al for the Brazil APACHE III Study Group: Application of the APACHE III prognostic system in Brazilian intensive care units: A prospective multicenter study. Intensive Care Med 1996;22:564-570.
87. Moreno R, Morais P: Outcome prediction in intensive care: Results of a prospective, multicentre, Portuguese study. Intensive Care Med 1997;23:177-186.
88. Rivera-Fernandez R, Vazquez-Mata G, Bravo M, et al: The Apache III prognostic system: Customized mortality predictions for Spanish ICU patients. Intensive Care Med 1998;24:574-581.
89. Moreno R: From the evaluation of the individual ptient to the evaluation of the ICU. Réanimation 2003;12:47S-48S.
90. Perkins HS, Jonsen AR, Epstein WV: Providers as predictors: Using outcome predictions in intensive care. Crit Care Med 1986;14:105-110.
91. Silverstein MD: Prediction instruments and clinical judgement in critical care. JAMA 1988;260:1758-1759.
92. Dawes RM, Faust D, Mechl PE: Clinical versus actuarial judgement. Sci Med Man 1989;243:1674-1688.
93. Kleinmuntz B: Why we still use our heads instead of formulas: Toward an integrative approach. Psychol Bull 1990;107:296-310.
94. McClish DK, Powell SH: How well can physicians estimate mortality in a medical intensive care unit? Med Decis Making 1989;9:125-132.
95. Poses RM, Bekes C, Winkler RL, et al: Are two (inexperienced) heads better than one (experienced) head? Averaging house officers prognostic judgement for critically ill patients. Arch Intern Med 1990;150: 1874-1878.
96. Poses RM, Bekes C, Copare FJ, et al: The answer to "what are my chances, doctor?" depends on whom is asked: Prognostic disagreement and inaccuracy for critically ill patients. Crit Care Med 1989;17:827-833.
97. Winkler RL, Poses RM: Evaluating and combining physicians' probabilities of survival in an intensive care unit. Manag Sci 1993;39:1526-1543.
98. Chang RWS, Lee B, Jacobs S, Lee B: Accuracy of decisions to withdraw therapy in critically ill patients: Clinical judgement versus a computer model. Crit Care Med 1989;17:1091-1097.
99. Knaus WA, Rauss A, Alperovitch A, et al: Do objective estimates of chances for survival influence decisions to withhold or withdraw treatment? Med Decis Making 1990;10:163-171.
100. Zimmerman JE, Wagner DP, Draper EA, Knaus WA: Improving intensive care unit discharge decisions: Supplementary physician judgment with predictions of next day risk for life support. Crit Care Med 1994;22:1373-1384.
101. Branner AL, Godfrey LJ, Goetter WE: Prediction of outcome from critical illness: A comparison of clinical judgement with a prediction rule. Arch Intern Med 1989;149:1083-1086.
102. Kruse JA, Thill-Baharozin MC, Carlson RW: Comparison of clinical assessment with APACHE II for predicting mortality risk in patients admitted to a medical intensive care unit. JAMA 1988;260:1739-1742.
103. Marks RJ, Simons RS, Blizzard RA, et al: Predicting outcome in intensive therapy units—a comparison of APACHE II with subjective assessments. Intensive Care Med 1991;17:159-163.
104. Knaus WA, Wagner DP, Lynn J: Short-term mortality predictions for critically ill hospitalized adults: science and ethics. Sci Med Man 1991;254: 389-394.
105. Lemeshow S, Klar J, Teres D: Outcome prediction for individual intensive care patients: Useful, misused, or abused? Intensive Care Med 1995;21: 770-776.
106. Suter P, Armagandis A, Beaufils F, et al: Predicting outcome in ICU patients: Consensus conference organized by the ESICM and the SRLF. Intensive Care Med 1994;20:390-397.
107. Chang RW, Jacobs S, Lee B: Use of APACHE II severity of disease classification to identify intensive-care-unit patients who would not benefit from total parenteral nutrition. Lancet 1986;1:1483-1486.
108. Atkinson S, Bihari D, Smithies M, et al: Identification of futility in intensive care. Lancet 1994;344:1203-1206.
109. Murray LS, Teasdale GM, Murray GD, et al: Does prediction of outcome alter patient management? Lancet 1993;341:1487-1491.
110. Gattinoni L, Brazzi L, Pelosi P, et al: A trial of goal orientated hemodynamic therapy in critically ill patients. N Engl J Med 1995;333:1025-1032.
111. Henning RJ, McClish D, Daly B, et al: Clinical characteristics and resource utilization of ICU patients: Implementation for organization of intensive care. Crit Care Med 1987;15:264-269.
112. Wagner DP, Knaus WA, Draper EA: Identification of low-risk monitor admissions to medical-surgical ICUs. Chest 1987;92:423-428.
113. Wagner DP, Knaus WA, Draper EA, et al: Identification of low-risk monitor patients within a medical-surgical ICU. Med Care 1983;21:425-433.
114. Zimmerman JE, Wagner DP, Knaus WA, et al: The use of risk predictors to identify candidates for intermediate care units. Implications for intensive care unit utilization. Chest 1995;108:490-499.
115. Zimmerman JE, Wagner DP, Sun X, et al: Planning patient services for intermediate care units: Insights based on care for intensive care unit low-risk monitor admissions. Crit Care Med 1996;24:1626-1632.
116. Strauss MJ, LoGerfo JP, Yeltatzie JA, et al: Rationing of intensive care unit services. An everyday occurrence. JAMA 1986;255:1143-1146.
117. Civetta JM, Hudson-Civetta JA, Nelson LD: Evaluation of APACHE II for cost containment and quality assurance. Ann Surg 1990;212:266-276.

118. Jones AE, Fitch MT, Kline JA: Operational performance of validated physiologic scoring systems for predicting in-hospital mortality among critically ill emergency department patients. Crit Care Med 2005;33: 974-978.
119. MERIT Study Investigators: Introduction of the medical emergency team (MET) system: A cluster-randomised controlled trial. Lancet 2005;365:2091-2097.
120. Moreno R, Reis Miranda D: Nursing staff in intensive care in Europe. The mismatch between planning and practice. Chest 1998;113:752-758.
121. Moreno R, Vincent J-L, Matos R, et al: The use of maximum SOFA score to quantify organ dysfunction/failure in intensive care. Results of a prospective, multicentre study. Intensive Care Med 1999;25:686-696.
122. Clermont G, Kaplan V, Moreno R, et al: Dynamic microsimulation to model multiple outcomes in cohorts of critically ill patients. Intensive Care Med 2004;30:2237-2244.
123. Zimmerman JE, Shortell SM, Knaus WA, et al: Value and cost of teaching hospitals: A prospective, multicenter, inception cohort study. Crit Care Med 1993;21:1432-1442.
124. Rapoport J, Teres D, Lemeshow S, Gehlbach S: A method for assessing the clinical performance and cost-effectiveness of intensive care units: A multicenter inception cohort study. Crit Care Med 1994;22:1385-1391.
125. Teres D, Rapoport J: Identifying patients with high risk of high cost. Chest 1991;99:530-531.
126. Cerra FB, Negro F, Abrams J: APACHE II score does not predict multiple organ failure or mortality in post-operative surgical patients. Arch Surg 1990;125:519-522.
127. Rapoport J, Teres D, Lemeshow S, et al: Explaining variability of cost using a severity of illness measure for ICU patients. Med Care 1990;28:338-348.
128. Oye RK, Bellamy PF: Patterns of resource consumption in medical intensive care. Chest 1991;99:695-689.
129. Knaus WA, Draper EA, Wagner DP, Zimmerman JE: An evaluation of outcome from intensive care in major medical centers. Ann Intern Med 1986;104:410-418.
130. Hosmer DW, Lemeshow S: Confidence interval estimates of an index of quality performance based on logistic regression estimates. Stat Med 1995;14:2161-2172.
131. Rapoport J, Teres D, Barnett R, et al: A comparison of intensive care unit utilization in Alberta and Western Massachusetts. Crit Care Med 1995;23:1336-1346.
132. Wong DT, Crofts SL, Gomez M, et al: Evaluation of predictive ability of APACHE II system and hospital outcome in Canadian intensive care unit patients. Crit Care Med 1995;23:1177-1183.
133. Le Gall JR, Loirat P, Nicolas F, et al: Utilisation d'un indice de gravité dans huit services de réanimation multidisciplinaire. Presse Med 1983;12:1757-1761.
134. Zimmerman JE, Rousseau DM, Duffy J, et al: Intensive care at two teaching hospitals: An organizational case study. Am J Crit Care 1994;3:129-138.
135. Chisakuta AM, Alexander JP: Audit in intensive care. The APACHE II classification of severity of disease. Ulster Med J 1990;59:161-167.
136. Marsh HM, Krishan I, Naessens JM, et al: Assessment of prediction of mortality by using the APACHE II scoring system in intensive care units. Mayo Clin Proc 1990;65:1549-1557.
137. Turner JS, Mudaliar YM, Chang RW, Morgan CJ: Acute Physiology and Chronic Health Evaluation (APACHE II) scoring in a cardiothoracic intensive care unit. Crit Care Med 1991;19:1266-1269.
138. Oh TE, Hutchinson R, Short S, et al: Verification of the acute physiology and chronic health evaluation scoring system in a Hong Kong intensive care unit. Crit Care Med 1993;21:698-705.
139. Zimmerman JE, Shortell SM, Rousseau DM, et al: Improving intensive care: Observations based on organizational case studies in nine intensive care units: A prospective, multicenter study. Crit Care Med 1993;21:1443-1451.
140. Shortell SM, Zimmerman JE, Rousseau DM, et al: The performance of intensive care units: does good management make a difference? Med Care 1994;32:508-525.
141. Reis Miranda D, Ryan DW, Schaufeli WB, Fidler V (eds): Organization and Management of Intensive Care: A Prospective Study in 12 European Countries. Vol 29. Berlin/Heidelberg, Springer-Verlag, 1997.
142. Moreno R, Matos R: New issues in severity scoring: Interfacing the ICU and evaluating it. Curr Opin Crit Care 2001;7:469-474.
143. Teres D, Lemeshow S: Using severity measures to describe high performance intensive care units. Crit Care Clin 1993;9:543-554.
144. Teres D, Lemeshow S: Why severity models should be used with caution. Crit Care Clin 1994;10:93-110.
145. Teres D, Lieberman S: Are we ready to regionalize pediatric intensive care? Crit Care Med 1991;19:139-140.
146. Pollack MM, Alexander SR, Clarke N, et al: Improved outcomes from tertiary center pediatric intensive care: A statewide comparison of tertiary and nontertiary care facilities. Crit Care Med 1990;19:150-159.
147. Goldstein H, Spiegelhalter DJ: League tables and their limitations: Statistical issues in comparisons of institutional performance. J R Stat Soc A 1996;159:385-443.
148. Polderman KH, Thijs LG, Girbes AR: Interobserver variability in the use of APACHE II scores. Lancet 1999;353:380 (Letter).
149. Fry DE, Pearlstein L, Fulton RL, Polk HC: Multiple system organ failure. The role of uncontrolled infection. Arch Surg 1980;115:136-140.
150. Elebute EA, Stoner HB: The grading of sepsis. Br J Surg 1983;70:29-31.
151. Stevens LE: Gauging the severity of surgical sepsis. Arch Surg 1983;118:1190-1192.
152. Goris RJA, te Boekhorst TP, Nuytinck JKS, Gimbrère JSF: Multiple-organ failure. Generalized autodestructive inflammation? Arch Surg 1985;120:1109-1115.
153. Knaus WA, Draper EA, Wagner DP, Zimmerman JE: Prognosis in acute organ-system failure. Ann Surg 1985;202:685-693.
154. Chang RW, Jacobs S, Lee B: Predicting outcome among intensive care unit patients using computerised trend analysis of daily Apache II scores corrected for organ system failure. Intensive Care Med 1988;14:558-566.
155. Meek M, Munster AM, Winchurch RA, et al: The Baltimore Sepsis Scale: Measurement of sepsis in patients with burns using a new scoring system. J Burn Care Rehabil 1991;12:564.
156. Baumgartner JD, Bula C, Vaney C, et al: A novel score for predicting the mortality of septic shock patients. Crit Care Med 1992;20:953.
157. Bernard GR, Doig BG, Hudson G, et al: Quantification of organ failure for clinical trials and clinical practice. Am J Respir Crit Care Med 1995;151: A323 (Abstract).
158. Bertleff MJ, Bruining HA: How should multiple organ dysfunction syndrome be assessed? A review of the variations in current scoring systems. Eur J Surg 1997;163:405-409.
159. Jacobs S, Zuleika M, Mphansa T: The multiple organ dysfunction score as a descriptor of patient outcome in septic shock compared with two other scoring systems. Crit Care Med 1999;27:741-744.
160. Gonçalves JA, Hydo LJ, Barie PS: Factors influencing outcome of prolonged norepinephrine therapy for shock in critical surgical illness. Shock 1998;10:231-236.
161. Maziak DE, Lindsay TF, Marshall JC, et al: The impact of multiple organ dysfunction on mortality following ruptured abdominal aortic aneurysm repair. Ann Vasc Surg 1998; 12:93-100.
162. Pinilla JC, Hayes P, Laverty W, et al: The C-reactive protein to prealbumin ratio correlates with the severity of multiple organ dysfunction. Surgery 1998;124:799-805.
163. Staubach KH, Schroder J, Stuber F, et al: Effect of pentoxifylline in severe sepsis: Results of a randomized, double-blind, placebo-controlled study. Arch Surg 1998;133:94-100.
164. Vincent J-L, de Mendonça A, Cantraine F, et al: Use of the SOFA score to assess the incidence of organ dysfunction/failure in intensive care units: Results of a multicentric, prospective study. Crit Care Med 1998;26:1793-1800.
165. Di Filippo A, De Gaudio AR, Novelli A, et al: Continuous infusion of vancomycin in methicillin-resistant staphylococcus infection. Chemotherapy 1998;44:63-68.
166. Fiore G, Donadio PP, Gianferrari P, et al: CVVH in postoperative care of liver transplantation. Minerva Anestesiol 1998;64:83-87.
167. Briegel J, Forst H, Haller M, et al: Stress doses of hydrocortisone reverse hyperdynamic septic shock: A

prospective, randomized, double-blind, single-center study. Crit Care Med 1999;27:723-732.
168. Hynninen M, Valtonen M, Markkanen H, et al: Interleukin 1 receptor antagonist and E-selectin concentrations: A comparison in patients with severe acute pancreatitis and severe sepsis. J Crit Care 1999;14:63-68.
169. Soufir L, Timsits JF, Mahe C, et al: Attributable morbidity and mortality of catheter-related septicemia in critically ill patients: A matched, risk-adjusted, cohort study. Infect Control Hosp Epidemiol 1999;20:396-401.
170. Moreno R, Pereira E, Matos R, Fevereiro T: The evaluation of cardiovascular dysfunction/failure in multiple organ failure [abstract]. Intensive Care Med 1997; 23:S153.
171. Timsit JF, Fosse JP, Troche G, et al: Accuracy of a composite score using daily SAPS II and LOD scores for predicting hospital mortality in ICU patients hospitalized for more than 72 h. Intensive Care Med 2001;27:1012-1021.
172. Meade MO, Cook DJ: A critical appraisal and systematic review of illness severity scoring systems in the intensive care unit. Curr Opin Crit Care 1995;1:191.
173. Reis Miranda D, Moreno R: ICU models and their role in management and utilization programs. Curr Opin Crit Care 1997;3:183-187.
174. Boyd O, Grounds M: Can standardized mortality ratio be used to compare quality of intensive care unit performance? Crit Care Med 1994;22:1706-1708 (Letter).
175. Moreno R: Performance of the ICU. Are we able to measure it? In Vincent JL (ed): 1998 Yearbook of Intensive Care and Emergency Medicine. New York, Springer-Verlag, 1998, pp 729-743.
176. Hopfel AW, Taaffe CL, Herrmann VM: Failure of APACHE II alone as a predictor of mortality in patients receiving total parenteral nutrition. Crit Care Med 1989;17:414-417.
177. Esserman L, Belkora J, Lenert L: Potentially ineffective care. A new outcome to assess the limits of critical care. JAMA 1995;274:1544-1551.
178. Moreno R, Matos R, Fevereiro T, Pereira ME: À procura de um índice de gravidade na sépsis. Rev Port Med Intensiva 1999;8:43-52.
179. Carlet J, Nicolas F: Specific severity of illness scoring systems. Curr Opin Crit Care 1995;1:233.
180. Abecasis PB: Quantificação das alterações sistémicas como índice prognóstico em Medicina Intensiva. Lisbon, Universidade Nova de Lisboa, 1997.
181. Casey LC, Balk RA, Bone RC: Plasma cytokine and endotoxin levels correlate with survival in patients with the sepsis syndrome. Ann Intern Med 1993;119:771.
182. Alberti C, Brun-Buisson C, Chevret S, et al: Systemic inflammatory response and progression to severe sepsis in critically ill infected patients. Am J Respir Crit Care Med 2005;171:461-468.
183. Backer S, O'Neill B, Haddon Jr W, Long WN: The injury severity score: A method for describing patients with multiple injuries and evaluating emergency care. J Trauma 1974;14:187-196.
184. Champion HR, Sacco WJ, Carnazzo AJ, et al: Trauma score. Crit Care 1981;9:672-676.
185. Champion HR, Sacco WJ, Copes WS, et al: A revision of the Trauma Score. J Trauma 1989;29.
186. Champion HR, Sacco WJ, Hunt TK: Trauma severity scoring to predict mortality. World J Surg 1983;7:4-11.
187. Pickering SAW, Esberger D, Moran CG: The outcome following major trauma in the elderly. Predictors of survival. Injury 1999;30:703-706.
188. Sicignano A, Giudici D: Probability model of hospital death for severe trauma patients based on the Simplified Acute Physiology Score I: Development and validation. J Trauma 1997;43:585-589.
189. Unertl K, Kottler BM: [Prognostic scores in intensive care]. Anaesthesist 1997;46:471-480.
190. Barbieri S, Michieletto E, Feltracco P, et al: [Prognostic systems in intensive care: TRISS, SAPS II, APACHE III]. Minerva Anestesiol 2001;67:519.
191. Reiter A, Mauritz W, Jordan B, et al: Improving risk adjustment in critically ill trauma patients: The TRISS-SAPS score. J Trauma 2004;57:375-380.
192. Champion HR, Copes WS, Sacco WJ, et al: A new characterization of injury severity. J Trauma 1990;30:539-545.
193. Markle J, Cayten CG, Byrne DW, et al: Comparison between TRISS and ASCOT methods in controlling for injury severity. J Trauma 1992;33:326-332.
194. Hannan EL, Mendeloff J, Farrell LS, et al: Validation of TRISS and ASCOT using a non-MTOS trauma registry. J Trauma 1995;38:83-88.
195. Gabbe BJ, Cameron PA, Wolfe R, et al: Predictors of mortality, length of stay and discharge destination in blunt trauma. Austr N Z J Surg 2005;75:650-656.
196. Hannan EL, Farrell LS, Cayten CG: Predicting survival of victims of motor vehicle crashes in New York state. Injury 1997;28:607-615.
197. Schall LC, Potoka DA, Ford HR: A new method for estimating probability of survival in pediatric patients using revised TRISS methodology based on age-adjusted weights. J Trauma 2002;52:235-241.
198. Davis EG, MacKenzie EJ, Sacco WJ, et al: A new "TRISS-like" probability of survival model for intubated trauma patients. J Trauma 2003;55:53-61.
199. Osler TM, Rogers FB, Badger GJ, et al: A simple mathematical modification of TRISS markedly improves calibration. J Trauma 2002;53:630-634.
200. Glance LG, Osler TM, Dick AW; Evaluating trauma center quality: Does the choice of the severity-adjustment model make a difference? J Trauma 2005;58:1265-1271.
201. Parsonnet V, Dean D, Bernstein A: A method for uniform stratification of risk for evaluating the results of surgery in acquired adult heart disease. Circulation 1989;79:I3-I12.
202. Higgins TL, Estafanous FG, Loop FD, et al: Stratification of morbidity and mortality outcome by preoperative risk factors in coronary artery bypass patients. A clinical severity score. JAMA 1992;267:2344-2348.
203. Roques F, Gabrielle F, Michel P, et al: Quality of care in adult heart surgery: Proposal for a self-assessment approach based on a French multicenter study. Eur J Cardiothorac Surg 1995;9: 439-440.
204. Tuman KJ, McCarthy RJ, March RJ, et al: Morbidity and duration of ICU stay after cardiac surgery. A model for preoperative risk assessment. Chest 1992;102:36-44.
205. Shroyer AL, Plomondon ME, Grover FL, Edwards FH: The 1996 coronary artery bypass risk model: The Society of Thoracic Surgeons Adult Cardiac National Database. Ann Thorac Surg 1999;67:1205-1208.
206. Hannan EL, Kilburn H Jr, O'Donnell JF, et al: Adult open heart surgery in New York State. An analysis of risk factors and hospital mortality rates. JAMA 1990;264:2768-2774.
207. Grover FL, Shroyer AL, Hammermeister KE: Calculating risk and outcome: The Veterans Affairs database. Ann Thorac Surg 1996;62:S6-S11.
208. O'Connor GT, Plume SK, Olmstead EM, et al: Multivariate prediction of in-hospital mortality associated with coronary artery bypass graft surgery. Northern New England Cardiovascular Disease Study Group. Circulation 1992;85:2110-2118.
209. Nashef SA, Roques F, Michel P, et al: European System for Cardiac Operative Risk Evaluation (EuroSCORE). Eur J Cardiothorac Surg 1999;16:9-13.
210. Kawachi Y, Nakashima A, Toshima Y, et al: Risk stratification analysis of operative mortality in heart and thoracic aorta surgery: Comparison between Parsonnet and EuroSCORE additive model. Eur J Cardiothorac Surg 2001;20:961-966.
211. Sergeant P, de Worm E, Meyns B: Single centre, single domain validation of the EuroSCORE on a consecutive sample of primary and repeat CABG. Eur J Cardiothorac Surg 2001;20:1176-1182.
212. Kurki TS, Jarvinen O, Kataja MJ, et al: Performance of three preoperative risk indices; CABDEAL, EuroSCORE and Cleveland models in a prospective coronary bypass database. Eur J Cardiothorac Surg 2002;21:406-410.
213. Nashef SA, Roques F, Hammill BG, et al: Validation of European System for Cardiac Operative Risk Evaluation (EuroSCORE) in North American cardiac surgery. Eur J Cardiothorac Surg 2002;22:101-105.
214. Sokolovic E, Schmidlin D, Schmid ER, et al: Determinants of costs and resource utilization associated with open heart surgery. Eur J Cardiothorac Surg 2002;23:574-578.
215. Chung DA, Sharples LD, Nashef SA: A case-control analysis of readmissions to the cardiac surgical intensive care unit. Eur J Cardiothorac Surg 2002;22:282-286.

216. Gurler S, Gebhard A, Godehardt E, et al: EuroSCORE as a predictor for complications and outcome. Eur J Cardiothorac Surg 2003;51:73-77.
217. De Maria R, Mazzoni M, Parolini M, et al: Predictive value of EuroSCORE on long term outcome in cardiac surgery patients: A single institution study. Heart 2005;91:779-784.
218. Roques F, Michel P, Goldstone AR, Nashef SA: The logistic EuroSCORE. Eur Heart J 2003;24:881-882 (Letter).
219. Gogbashian A, Sedrakyan A, Treasure T: EuroSCORE: A systematic review of international performance. Eur J Cardiothorac Surg 2004;25:695-700.
220. Sinuff T, Adhikari NKJ, Cook DJ, et al: Mortality predictions in the intensive care unit: Comparing physicians with scoring systems. Crit Care Med 2006;34:878-885.
221. Booth FV, Short M, Shorr AF, et al: Application of a population-based severity scoring system to individual patients results in frequent misclassification. Crit Care 2006;9:R522-R529.

Chapter 75

Education and Training in Critical Care

Nandan Gautam, Hannah Reay, and Julian Bion

All critically ill and injured persons receive care from integrated teams of dedicated experts directed by trained and present intensivist physicians. Multiprofessional teams use knowledge, technology and compassion to provide timely, safe, effective and efficient patient-centred care.[1]

This laudable mission statement for education and training from the Society of Critical Care Medicine (SCCM) demonstrates the gap between aspiration and reality. In the United States, only one in three critically ill patients receives intensivist-directed care.[2] Staffing and funding constraints combined with limitations on hours of work both in the United States[3] and in Europe[4] are creating challenges for health services.[5] These challenges are also an opportunity to examine new ways of working and learning and to revisit the whole ethos of medical education: a life-long process for improving the care that we offer to our patients.

THE GOAL: TRAINING ASPIRATIONS FOR CRITICAL CARE MEDICINE

The purpose of any medical education program should be to integrate knowledge, skills, attitudes, and behavior within a sound ethical and professional framework that encourages reflective life-long learning, with the aim of producing competent and caring practitioners who possess both team-working and leadership capacities. To achieve this objective requires a firm focus on the needs of patients and confident and effective structures and processes for training and education. This in turn requires adequate resources for training and visible recognition by universities and governments of the importance of medical education.

How best to deliver this education is a matter of active debate. The structures in place for training and assessment are varied and closely allied to strong domestic traditions and imperatives. This has led to wide diversity in specialty ownership of critical care, in the format and duration of training programs, and in methods of assessment and accreditation.[6] This diversity may represent a richness of choice for trainees, but absence of an international (or in some cases, national) standard for the content and outcomes of training in intensive care medicine (ICM) lacks logic.

THE CHALLENGE: THE TRAINING ENVIRONMENT

Training and clinical delivery of care are necessary companions; changes in the health service will therefore inevitably have an impact on medical education. In the last 15 years, health systems worldwide have seen that patients' expectations of safe and reliable health care are not always satisfied.[7,8] It is reasonable for patients to expect that their care should be delivered by fully trained specialists and not by less experienced individuals or those in training grades. However, this expectation is made difficult to satisfy by cost pressure, rationing, increased throughput, staffing limitations, and reduced hours of work for trainees. These challenges are a particular problem for acute and emergency care, including critical care,[9] but it is in precisely these areas that some of the most innovative solutions may be found in terms of developing physician assistants and transdisciplinary team working and new ways of delivering medical education to supplement apprenticeship-style training and evaluation.

Physician assistants or extended-role nurse practitioners, including respiratory therapists, screening endoscopists,[10] nurse anesthetists, and advanced critical care practitioners, work within fairly well-defined pathways of responsibility.[11] Critical care outreach, medical emergency teams,[12] and the United Kingdom's hospital at night[13] teams all involve senior nurses with diagnostic and management training. In the United States, growth of the hospitalist movement[14] into a new specialty demonstrates how the clinical demands of acutely ill patients can have an impact on training and education. The National Organization of Nurse Practitioner Faculties has developed a national program of competencies that includes diagnostic algorithms and treatment based on protocols,[15] and many of the competencies are centered around management of acutely ill or physiologically unstable patients.

Acutely ill patients are necessarily cared for by multiple teams involving physicians, nurses, and allied health care professionals. Cancer teams are well accustomed to this style of working, but the environment of acute and emergency care makes this a very different concept, more akin to the armed forces in combat than the more leisured approach of elective clinical care. Itinerant team handoffs require not only good communication skills but also the capacity of each member to detect rapidly changing clinical conditions in patients whom they will not have met before. Continuity of care requires continuity of perspective if the care is not to become fragmented. This needs to be supplemented by objective measures of physiologic deterioration, which requires a much stronger focus in medical training on clinical assessment of acutely ill patients, starting at undergraduate level.[16,17] Critical care has a major contribution to make in this hospital-wide focus on training in the management of acutely ill patients.

CURRENT TRAINING IN INTENSIVE CARE MEDICINE

Critical care medicine developed as a consequence of the polio epidemics of the 1950s. The introduction of tracheal intubation and mechanical positive-pressure ventilation meant that anesthesia became dominant in many of the early training programs. The safety record of anesthesia combined with better technology and drugs has enabled increasingly complex surgery and has extended the role of the anesthetist into postoperative intensive care. Respiratory physicians also have a traditional association with critical care, particularly in the United States, where they remain the most numerous specialists within critical care medicine.[18] Principles of ICM are a mandatory component of many specialty training programs worldwide, but the extent to which this training is recognized as specialist ICM training varies. Specialists from primary disciplines such as surgery and internal and emergency medicine (and pediatrics) participate in critical care, but not all are permitted to undertake specialist ICM training.

In a survey of 41 countries carried out by the CoBaTrICE Collaboration under the aegis of the European Society for Intensive Care Medicine (ESICM), 54 different ICM training programs were identified (37 within the European region) that ranged in duration from 3 months to 6 years (most frequently 2 years).[6] Entry criteria were significantly different between some countries with regard to the structure and format of the training program. Nursing surveys demonstrate similar diversity in their training programs.[19,20]

Most countries observe one or more of the following models of ICM training: primary specialty (critical care training directly after medical school), subspecialty (critical care training as an exclusive component of a primary discipline), or supraspecialty training (common critical care training shared by multiple primary specialties).[6]

In *primary specialty* training, ICM is regarded as a fully independent specialty with a separate training program accessed directly from the undergraduate level. This may be undertaken in addition to a complementary primary specialty, commonly anesthesia or internal medicine.

Subspecialty refers to ICM training within a parent specialty and exclusive to it. In the majority of such systems, ICM training can be accessed only through anesthesia. Other disciplines, such as internal medicine and surgery, may offer their own subspecialty training in ICM. These separate routes may be related to each other but are administered differently and often have different components. Certification will reflect the base specialty but often documents subspecialty status also.

Supraspecialty training is the most common model. Here, a primary specialty is chosen and intensive care training is grafted onto it, either in a modular or in single-block format. Certification in ICM requires certification in the primary specialty also. It allows a number of specialties to access common ICM training. In practice, however, the specialties remain predominantly anesthesiology, internal medicine, and respiratory medicine.

Although there are similarities between curricula, at present only 6% of programs define the outcomes of training in terms of the competencies expected of a specialist in ICM.[6] There is tacit acknowledgment that the terms "attending," "consultant," and "specialist" may have administrative and logistic equivalence within individual countries and that a "good" specialist in one country is likely to be as well equipped with knowledge and skills as a good specialist in another, but there is little evidence to prove this.

Effort has been made to harmonize standards of ICM training through the provision of guidelines and recommendations. Minimum requirements have been identified for training, duration of training programs, core curricula of theoretical knowledge and procedural experience, and criteria for training committees and for the accreditation of training centers.[21-26] A common approach to the assessment of ICM training via a multidisciplinary European diploma has been developed,[27] and there are a growing number of joint educational initiatives, consensus statements, and practice guidelines (for example, see De Lange and colleagues[23] and Dellinger and coworkers[28]) that indicate common themes and the pursuit of common outcomes within ICM training. However, until completion of the CoBaTrICE project in 2006 (see later), there had been no formal international consensus about the core competencies that define a specialist in ICM.[6]

Specialist status in all these schemes is obtained through some combination of time spent in the program, competency-based assessments, case reports, submission of diploma theses, oral (viva voce) examination, and clinical examination. There does not as yet exist an enforced recertification process in any country, nor an agreed standard for benchmarking intensive care units or training programs.

MOVING TOWARD COMPETENCY-BASED TRAINING IN INTENSIVE CARE MEDICINE

Competencies are a method for describing the knowledge, skills, attitudes, and behavior expected of specialists in terms of what they are able to do. Several national regulatory bodies for physicians have started to modify their training programs from syllabus-based examination-driven systems to programs based on competencies assessed in the workplace. The growing popularity of a competency-based approach to general medical training is reflected across all stages of undergraduate and postgraduate training in these countries.[29-35] The challenge for trainers and trainees is to develop robust methods for workplace-based assessment and to create the necessary flexibility within training programs to allow time-based training to be replaced by programs in which trainees acquire competencies at different rates.

The United Kingdom developed a comprehensive competency-based program for ICM in 2001,[36] and this approach has now been replicated through an international partnership of professional organizations and critical care clinicians working together to harmonize training in ICM worldwide. The CoBaTrICE Collaboration was formed in 2003 to define outcomes of specialist ICM training and to develop an internationally acceptable competency-based training program in ICM for Europe (CoBaTrICE) and, through collaboration, with other world regions.[37] The underlying principle of this initiative was the concept that an ICM specialist trained in one country should have the same core skills and abilities as one trained in another, thereby ensuring a common standard of clinical competence. This follows the European Union ethos of free movement of professionals and mutual recognition of medical qualifications between member states.[38] Competency-based training makes convergence possible by defining the outcomes of specialist training—a common "end product"—rather than enforcing rigid structures and processes of training. A minimum standard of knowledge, skills, attitudes, and behavior is defined a priori and applied to existing structures and processes of training; acquisition and assessment of competence occur during training in the workplace.

DEFINING CORE COMPETENCIES

The CoBaTrICE project has used consensus techniques—an extensive international consultation process using a modified online Delphi involving more than 500 clinicians in more than 50 countries, an 8-country postal survey of patients and relatives, and an expert nominal group—to define the core competencies required of a specialist in ICM.[39] These competencies have been linked to a comprehensive syllabus, relevant educational resources, and guidance for the standardized assessment of competence in the workplace via a dedicated website.[37] After its launch in September 2006, many national training programs are adopting CoBaTrICE; implementation and long-term evaluation of the CoBaTrICE program will be necessary to assess its impact on individuals' competence and harmonization of ICM training.

EVOLVING PROFESSIONAL ROLES: IMPLICATIONS FOR TRAINING

The CoBaTrICE Delphi demonstrated the importance that intensive care clinicians attach not only to the acquisition of procedural technical skills but equally to aspects of professionalism—communication skills, attitudes and behavior, governance, team working, and judgment.[39] The intensivist is clearly perceived as an "acute general practitioner," a family doctor with added technical ability. This raises questions about the traditional model for physician training and practice. Thinking more about the skills of the team than individual components is appropriate. Competency-based training makes this possible by explicitly identifying which skills are shared in common and which are peculiar to specific disciplines. Thus, weaning from ventilation,[40] instigation of renal replacement, nutritional support, prophylaxis for venous thromboembolism, or chest pain management pathways,[41] among others, can be nurse led and protocol driven, with the intensivist providing a strategic, integrating, and continuity role as much as a technical one. Opportunities for collaboration between critical care physicians and hospitalists can also be clarified in this manner. In this model, hierarchies become flatter, practitioners become more patient focused, and the intensivist's leadership skills must include the capacity for collaborative decision making while continuing to assume final responsibility for patient care. As nonphysician roles increase and extend, it is essential that the schemes for training be coordinated and better integrated with those for physicians.[42] As stated earlier, this process should start at the undergraduate level for maximum effect.[17]

PRACTICAL IMPLICATIONS OF COMPETENCY-BASED TRAINING

Concerns about competency-based training include the risk of setting a minimum "craftsman's" standard instead of encouraging "professional" excellence and that "being a good doctor" is too complex to be defined by lists of skills or activities.[43-45] The answer to these concerns is that it is our responsibility as senior clinicians and educators to provide role models that amplify the safe standard set by competency training. A minimum safe standard is where professional training starts, not where it ends.

The *duration of training* is determined by the acquisition of competencies, not by a fixed and arbitrary period in training, although training programs will of course need to continue to set a minimum time. The practical implication is that some trainees may not meet the expected targets and will require remedial training or more focused attention. The key to this is adequate supervision by "trained trainers" supported by all senior staff. Monitoring progress is essential to avoid discovering problems too late for effective remediation, such as at the end of training, or after specialist accreditation through adverse events or clinical complaints.

Documentation is a crucial component of training because it provides the evidence on which the trainee makes the case for being accepted as competent or, indeed, excellent. Portfolios are the responsibility of the trainee but require review by the trainer designated as mentor or supervisor for that trainee. This personal relationship is very important because shorter training times and reduced hours of work can make it difficult for trainers and trainees to interact with sufficient frequency for reliable assessment by all senior staff.

Maintenance of competence has important implications for specialists in terms of continuing accreditation and appraisal. Standards for recertification vary widely[46]; the process is routine in Australia, New Zealand, Canada, and the United States. Methods vary between specialty boards in the United States, with multiple choice examination often being used,[47] but with formal approval by the Accreditation Council for Continuing Medical Education. The majority of European countries have voluntary systems of education credits, and only the Netherlands has a mandatory system of recertification. The United Kingdom is currently revising proposals for the regulation and professional development of physicians; the probable outcome will be a mandated system that links appraisal, professional development, and recertification.[48]

Access to educational materials is another important consideration. Service pressures and budgetary constraints mean that education will need to be delivered locally, supplemented by distance-learning programs combined with self-assessment. To work well, education needs to be integrated with the clinical and training environment, be available in a timely manner, and be placed in context—for example, during a ward round or immediately after seeing a patient with a particular condition. Computers and clinical decision support systems can provide this, but careful collaborative development by information technology experts, clinicians, and educators is required. Linking educational resources to competencies is a necessary step in building and maintaining competency-based systems of training.[37] The Internet allows both peer-reviewed and entirely unedited repositories of knowledge to be created, many of which are excellent, but some of which require critical evaluation.

Box 75-1

Workplace-Based Assessment Methods

Direct Observation

- Direct observation of skills (e.g., DOPS, OSATS)[50,51,60]
  Direct observation of a physician performing diagnostic and interventional procedures during normal ("routine") clinical practice—used to assess the doctor-patient interaction and the process as a whole, not just the procedure itself
- Clinical evaluation exercise (CEX)[52,53]
  A "snapshot" observation of a normal ("routine") clinical encounter
- Audiovisual records
  Assessment of real-time videoed consultations by using a structured rating scale
- Multisource feedback (MSF)[49,54-56]
  Patients' or colleagues' views of the physician's professional attitudes and behavior in day-to-day practice are collected on a structured rating form; completed forms are returned to a central point and summarized. Feedback is then provided during a meeting between the doctor and the reviewer. MSF is also termed 360-degree assessment, peer assessment, or team assessment of behavior

Case Reviews and Analysis

- Case-based discussion or chart-stimulated recall[57,58]
  Use of an actual written record to focus structured discussion about a case
- Structured case histories[59]
  A written report summarizing a case that has been encountered and, with reference to the relevant literature, reflects on the management of this case

DOPS, Directly Observed Procedural Skills; OSATS, Objective Structured Assessment of Technical Skills.
Data from references 49-61.

ASSESSMENT

Workplace-based assessment of competence (Box 75-1) is not generally problematic for the majority of trainees, but the potential complexity of assessment becomes apparent when there is a trainee in difficulty or when an adverse assessment results in litigation or revelations of serial malpractice later in life. Why was the problem not detected earlier? Whose responsibility is it to undertake assessment? How should it be performed? How often should assessments be made? How reliable and repeatable are the methods used, and how does one deal with disagreement between different trainers?

For any program of training, a system of evaluation must exist to test the validity of the teaching method, the content, and its application.[62] If the curriculum is to have an assessment component, it too requires regular evaluation to ensure that it remains valid, that is, repeatable and consistent between observers. The ultimate test is whether the curriculum and method of testing lead to improvements in health care. Miller's hierarchy of learning (Fig. 75-1) suggests that whereas undergraduate training is more focused on the acquisition of knowledge,[63] postgraduate training places increasing importance on performance, and assessment strategies must therefore focus at the "action" or "does" level. Assessments need to take into account the trainees' abilities and previous experience, the complexity of the tasks that they perform, and the context.[64] In a variation of the Miller pyramid, the route to becoming a true specialist might be a training ladder as illustrated in Figure 75-2. Step 1 (the novice) is the acquisition of knowledge. Step 2 (the trainee) is the period of training, which will vary in duration and intensity, depending on needs. Step 3 (the competent new specialist) suggests competence, but step 4 (the expert) is more akin to the specialists whom we would all like treating us and requires experience and further training beyond basic competencies. The steps are not truly rigid because in reality, skills and knowledge are learned together and experiences and practice occur at all stages in training. This schema is equally applicable to all disciplines.

Definitions of competencies serve to guide the assessment process. Descriptions of what physicians should be able to do create a benchmark against which judgments can be made of clinical performance ("does"). A range of methods and tools may be used to assess training, but assessment of physicians' performance at work is still in its infancy.[65] Assessment must go beyond technical skills to include aspects of professionalism, attitudes, and behavior: communication skills, familiarity with current knowledge, shared decision making, respect for autonomy, and compassion. One way of making these assessments of professionalism is with "360-degree assessment," also called multisource feedback.[49] This involves actively seeking the opinion of others on the team, both one's peers and junior colleagues and, where appropriate, patients and relatives, about one's performance.

During training these assessments should be formative—that is, they should contribute to learning and be not a final pass/fail judgment. This traditional "apprentice-master" model requires frequent observation during routine clinical work by an experienced trainer and works well for the majority of trainees. However, they may need to be supplemented by formal methods involving more objective assessment of performance (Table 75-1). The assessments should be documented in the trainee's portfolio and combined with annual appraisal.

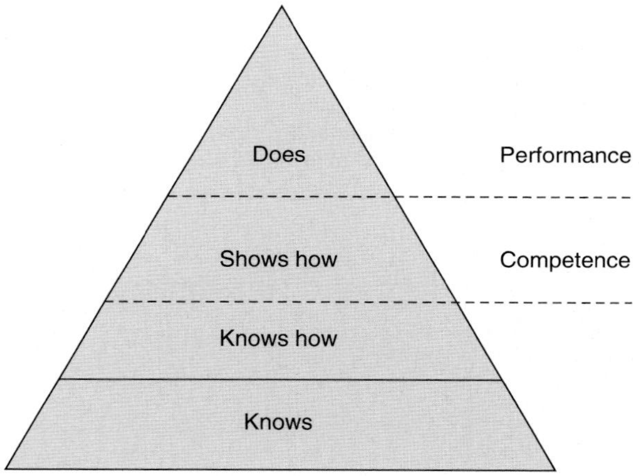

Figure 75-1. Miller's hierarchy. (Redrawn from Miller GE: The assessment of clinical skills and competence/performance. Acad Med 1990;65:563-567.)

Institutions need to allow protected time for trainers to be trained in formal assessment techniques and time to carry them out within employment contracts. It is important that all members of the team contribute to teaching and to training assessments; it cannot be the sole responsibility of one individual.

DELIVERING TRAINING AND ASSESSMENT IN THE WORKPLACE: ROLE OF SIMULATORS

An article in the New York Times[66] in December 1999 informed the American public that attempts at cardiopulmonary resuscitation were prolonged to allow interns to practice specific procedures before or after death. It has also been disclosed that patients under anesthesia or heavy sedation have undergone internal examinations by students,[67] thus raising questions of consent and morality.[68] The need to gain a basic level of proficiency before undertaking procedures on patients has encouraged the development of life-like manikins and increasingly sophisticated simulators. The advanced life support (ALS) and advanced cardiac life support (ACLS) courses[69-71] have provided a useful basis for this development by combining both training and assessment; the highly successful Fundamentals of Critical Care Support course developed by the SCCM is another example.

Modern medical simulators come in various guises, from simple anatomic models, to part task trainers, to complex virtual reality systems (see Table 75-1). Intermediate- and high-fidelity human patient manikins are becoming increasingly popular, although many remain underused. However, the most important part of a simulator is probably not the manikin and its functionality, but the thought and experience that go into creating realistic scenarios.

Simulated cases lend themselves well to acute care settings. Here, a number of discrete interventions carried

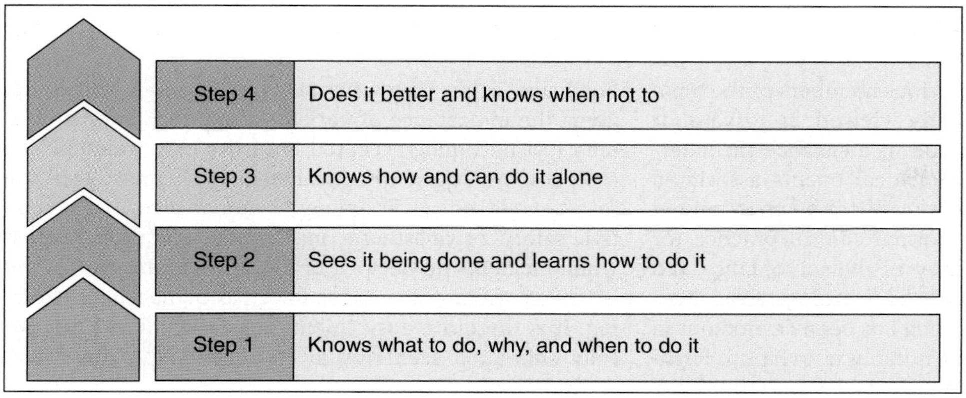

Figure 75-2. Steps in postgraduate training.

Table 75-1. Broad Categories of Simulators Used in Medicine

Item	Description	Example	Uses	Relative Cost
Diagrams and static models	Basic anatomic representations	Circulatory system	Largely illustrative	Low
Part task trainers	Anatomically correct models that have simple moving parts demonstrating one or more processes	Airway manikin with inflatable bladders representing lungs	Clinical skills and procedural training to look at individual tasks	Low
Computer simulations	Computer- or Web-based programs that can re-create physiologic processes and the responses to interventions	ACLS Sim*	Rehearsal of treatment algorithms and practice in applying knowledge	Low
Complex task trainers	Anatomically correct models with a number of elements that can be manipulated and respond to manipulation to produce physiologically credible effects	Resusci-Annie† ALS training manikins with inflatable lungs, rhythm generators for electrocardiographic analysis	More complex scenario-based training when multiple interventions are required	Medium
Intermediate-fidelity manikins	Anatomically correct human manikins that have automated and instructor-driven responses to a range of interventions	Instructor driven manikins Laerdal Sim Man‡	Complex multiuser scenario-based training and assessment	Medium to high
High-fidelity manikins	These have response algorithms that can mimic the physiologic responses of numerous patient types to a range of interventions and environmental changes	Instructor- and algorithm-driven manikins Meti Human patient simulator§	Complex multiuser scenario-based training and assessment	High
Virtual reality	Simple VR trainers exist that largely resemble complex task trainers. Experimental systems will ultimately be able to re-create any clinical situation in any environment	Training and assessing complex tasks Full-blown re-creations of events True telemedicine		Very High

*ACLS Sim is a computer screen–based Advanced Cardiac Life Support training program that tests applied knowledge of resuscitation treatment algorithms. Available at www.acls.net/sim.htm
†Resusci-Annie is an ALS trainer manikin made by Laerdal Medical AS, Stavanger, Norway. Available at www.laerdal.com.
‡Sim Man is the universal patient simulator made by Laerdal Medical AS, Stavanger, Norway. Available at www.laerdal.com.
§Meti-HPS is the human patient simulator made by Medical Education Technologies, Inc., Sarasota, FL. Available at www.meti.com.
From Gautam N: Uses of Human Patient Simulators for Critical Care Training [thesis for diploma in intensive care medicine]. ICBTICM, 2004.

out on a single "patient" by various members of the team can be evaluated, subsequently viewed in private or during group discussion, and be of assistance in understanding team working. Rare critical events associated with high mortality or morbidity will not be encountered with sufficient frequency in normal clinical practice for all clinicians to gain proficiency in their avoidance and management, but they can easily be incorporated in simulations.[72] Critical incident training has been carried out in industry for many years, most notably in aviation. High-fidelity aircraft simulators have been in routine use by flight and cabin crews for many years. It is surprising, given the importance of patient safety, that simulation is only just becoming accepted in health care training. The most common cause of critical incidents in anesthesia, the safest of all medical disciplines, is human error.[73] The relative safety of anesthesia may lead to unpreparedness when incidents do occur[74]; in these situations, simulation offers particular advantages for crisis management training. It is therefore easy to envisage a significant role for fully simulated scenarios in certification processes and revalidation.[75]

SUMMARY

Critical care medicine provides important training opportunities for all clinicians and is an ideal environment in which to gain proficiency in technical skills, team working, ethics, and professionalism. Training in ICM should start at the undergraduate level to maximize these opportunities. A universal set of core competencies can be expanded according to local requirements and be used to foster shared team-based skills in acute care across different disciplines. Health care systems need to invest in education in the workplace, with access to information integrated with clinical work, support for trainers, and the development of workplace-based methods for assessment. Portfolios should become reflective life-long learning documents for specialists, as much as for trainees.

KEY POINTS

- Critical care training is heterogeneous in access, process, and certification.
- There appears to be growing consensus on the core knowledge and skills needed to practice intensive care.
- Internationally recognized competency-based training should ensure a minimum knowledge and skill base for specialists and allow meaningful comparisons.
- Continuous workplace assessments and appraisals will be needed for revalidation.
- Service delivery pressures will require greater use of specialist nonphysician grades to operate within protocol-driven frameworks. Competency-based training will allow integration of their training with that of physicians.
- Simulators and simulated environments will increasingly be used for team training and to adequately prepare staff to deal with uncommon situations.
- The reduced length of training will lead to better trained but less experienced individuals entering the specialist workforce. This emphasizes the need for continuing medical education integrated with clinical practice and formal "protected" training sessions conducted by experienced clinical educators.
- There are significant resource implications associated with life-long training and assessment schemes with mutual recognition across international borders.

REFERENCES

1. Vision statement of the Society of Critical Care Medicine: Available at www.sccm.org (accessed April 2006).
2. Angus DC, Kelley MA, Schmitz RJ, et al, for the Committee on Manpower for Pulmonary and Critical Care Societies (COMPACCS): Current and projected workforce requirements for care of the critically ill and patients with pulmonary disease. Can we meet the requirements of an aging population? JAMA 2000;284:2762-2770.
3. ACGME duty hours requirements: Available at http://www.acgme.org/acWebsite/dutyHours/dh_Lang703.pdf (accessed Dec. 2006).
4. European working time directive: Available at http://www.incomesdata.co.uk/information/worktimedirective.htm (accessed Dec. 2006).
5. Nowak D: Doctors on strike—the crisis in German health care delivery. N Engl J Med 2006;355:1520-1522.
6. Barrett H, Bion JF, on behalf of the CoBaTrICE Collaboration: An international survey of training in adult intensive care medicine. Intensive Care Med 2005;31:552-561.
7. Kohn LT, Corrigan JM, Donaldson MS (eds): To Err Is Human: Building a Safer Health System. Washington, DC, National Academy Press, 2000.
8. Blendon RJ, DesRoches CM, Brodie M, et al: Views of practicing physicians and the public on medical errors. N Engl J Med 2002;347:1933-1940.
9. Bion JF, Heffner J: Improving hospital safety for acutely ill patients. A Lancet quintet. I: Current challenges in the care of the acutely ill patient. Lancet 2004;363:970-977.
10. Lahad A, Levy-Lahad E, Bryant J, et al: Nurse practitioners as endoscopists. N Engl J Med 1994;330:1534-1535.
11. Department of Health: The national Education and Competence Framework for Advanced Critical Care Practitioners. London, Department of Health, 2006. Available at http://www.dh.gov.uk/assetRoot/04/13/73/64/04137364.pdf (accessed Dec. 2006).
12. Bellomo R, Goldsmith D, Uchino S: A prospective before-and-after trial of a medical emergency team. Med J Aust 2003;179:283-287.
13. MacDonald R: The hospital at night. BMJ Career Focus 2004;328:19s.
14. Wachter RM: Hospitalists in the United States: Mission accomplished or work-in-progress. N Engl J Med 2004;350:1935-1936.
15. National Panel for Acute Care Nurse Practitioner Competencies: Acute Care Nurse Practitioner Competencies. Washington, DC, National Organization of Nurse Practitioner Faculties, 2004.
16. Hall P, Weaver L: Interdisciplinary education and teamwork: A long and winding road. Med Educ 2001;35:867-875.
17. Perkins GD, Barrett H, Bullock I, et al: The Acute Care Undergraduate Teaching (ACUTE) Initiative: Consensus development of core competencies in acute care for undergraduates in the United Kingdom. Intensive Care Med 2005;31:1627-1633.
18. Graduate Medical Education. JAMA 2005;294:1129-1143.
19. Scholes J, Endacott R, Chellel A: A formula for diversity: A review of critical care curricula. J Clin Nurs 2000;9:382-390.
20. Baktoft B, Drigo E, Hohl ML, et al: A survey of critical care nursing in Europe. Connect: The World of Critical Care Nursing 2003;2(3):85-87.
21. Vincent JL, Baltopoulos G, Bihari D, et al (ESICM Task Force): Guidelines for training in intensive care medicine. Intensive Care Med 1994;20:80-81.
22. Thijs LG, Baltopoulos G, Bihari D, et al (ESICM & ESPNIC Task Force): Guidelines for a training program in intensive care medicine. Intensive Care Med 1996;22:166-172.
23. De Lange S, Van Aken H, Burchardi H: European Society of Intensive Care Medicine statement: Intensive care medicine in Europe—structure, organisation and training guidelines of the Multidisciplinary Joint Committee of Intensive Care Medicine (MJCICM) of the European Union of Medical Specialists (UEMS). Intensive Care Med 2002;28:1505-1511.
24. American College of Critical Care Medicine of the Society of Critical Care Medicine: Guidelines for advanced training for physicians in critical care. Crit Care Med 1997;25:1601-1607.
25. Dorman T, Angood PB, Angus DC, et al: Guidelines for critical care medicine training and continuing medical education. Crit Care Med 2004;32:263-272.
26. Society of Critical Care Medicine: Guidelines for the definition of an intensivist and the practice of critical care medicine. Crit Care Med 1992;20:540-542.

27. European Society of Intensive Care Medicine (ESICM): European Diploma of Intensive Care Medicine. Available at http://www.esicm.org/PAGE_europeandiploma (accessed Nov 2006).
28. Dellinger RP, Carlet JM, Masu H, et al (for the Surviving Sepsis Campaign Management Guidelines Committee): Surviving Sepsis Campaign Guidelines for management of severe sepsis and septic shock. Crit Care Med 2004;32:858-873.
29. Royal College of General Practitioners (RCGP): Available at http://www.rcgp.org.uk/education/education_home/curriculum/gp_curriculum_documents.aspx (accessed Nov. 2006).
30. Intercollegiate Surgical Curriculum Project (ISCP): Available at http://www.iscp.ac.uk/Home.aspx (accessed Nov 2006).
31. General Medical Council: Draft Recommendations on Undergraduate Medical Education. London, General Medical Council, 2001.
32. RCPSC: Royal College of Physicians and Surgeons of Canada. Extract from the CanMEDS 2000 Project Societal Needs Working Group report. Med Teacher 2000;22:549-554.
33. RCPSC: Royal College of Physicians and Surgeons of Canada. CanMEDS 2005 Framework: Available at http://www.healthcare.ubc.ca/residency/CanMEDS_2005_Framework.pdf (accessed Dec. 2006).
34. ACGME: Accreditation Council for Graduate Medical Education. ACGME Outcome project: Available at http://www.acgme.org/outcome/project/proHome.asp (accessed Nov. 2006).
35. AAMC: Association of American Medical Colleges. Report 1: Learning Objectives for Medical Student Education. Guidelines for Medical Schools. Medical School Objectives Project. Washington, DC, Association of American Medical Colleges, 1998.
36. The Intercollegiate Board for Training in Intensive Care Medicine (IBTICM): The CCST in intensive care medicine competency based training and assessment. Part I: A reference manual for trainees and trainers. London, IBTICM, 2001: Available at http://www.rcoa.ac.uk/ibticm/docs/CBTPart1.pdf (accessed Dec. 2004).
37. CoBaTrICE website: Available at http://www.cobatrice.org (accessed Dec. 2006).
38. Lonbay J: Reflections on education and culture in European community law. In Craufurd-Smith R (ed): Culture and European Union Law. Oxford, Oxford University Press, 2004.
39. The CoBaTrICE Collaboration: Development of core competencies for an international training programme in intensive care medicine. Intensive Care Med 2006;32:1371-1382.
40. Gregory P, Marelich GP, Murin S, et al: Protocol weaning of mechanical ventilation in medical and surgical patients by respiratory care practitioners and nurses: Effect on weaning time and incidence of ventilator-associated pneumonia. Chest 2000;118:459-467.
41. Gomez MA, Anderson JL, Karagounis LA, et al: An emergency department–based protocol for rapidly ruling out myocardial ischemia reduces hospital time and expense: Results of a randomized study (ROMIO). J Am Coll Cardiol 1996;28:25-33.
42. Ross F, Southgate L: Learning together in medical and nursing training: Aspirations and activity. Med Educ 2000;34:739-743.
43. Harden RM, Crosby JR, Davis MH: AMEE Guide 14: Outcome based education: Part 1—an introduction to outcome-based education. Med Teacher 1999;21:7-14.
44. Leung W: Competency based medical training: Review. BMJ 2002;325:693-695.
45. Gonczi A: Review of international trends and developments in competency based education and training. In Argulles A, Gonczi A (eds): Competency Based Education and Training: A World Perspective. Balderas, Mexico, Noriega Editores, 2000.
46. Peck C, McCall M, McLaren B, et al: Continuing medical education and continuing professional development: International comparisons. BMJ 2000;320:432-435.
47. Brennan TA: Recertification for internists—one "grandfather's" experience. N Engl J Med 2005;353:1989-1992.
48. Chief Medical Officer: Good Doctors, Safer Patients. Proposals to Strengthen the System to Assure and Improve the Performance of Doctors and to Protect the Safety of Patients. A Report by the Chief Medical Officer. London, Department of Health, 2006.
49. Evans R, Elwyn G, Edwards A: Review of instruments for peer assessment of physicians. BMJ 2004;328:1240.
50. Modernising Medical Careers, DOPS (Direct Observation of Procedural Skills): Available at http://www.mmc.nhs.uk/pages/assessment/dops (accessed July 2007).
51. Healthcare Assessment and Training, DOPS: Available at http://www.hcat.nhs.uk/assessment/DOPS.htm (accessed July 2007).
52. Modernising Medical Careers, Mini-CEX (Clinical Evaluation Exercise): Available at http://www.mmc.nhs.uk/pages/assessment/minicex (accessed July 2007).
53. Norcini JJ, Blank LL, Duffy FD, et al: The miniCEX: A method for assessing clinical skills. Ann Intern Med 2003;138:476-481.
54. TAB: Available at http://www.mmc.nhs.uk/pages/assessment/msf (accessed July 2007).
55. Mini-PAT: Available at http://www.hcat.nhs.uk/assessments/min-epat (accessed July 2007).
56. Ramsey PG, Wenrich MD, Carline JD, et al: Use of peer ratings to evaluate physician performance. JAMA 1993;269:1655-1660.
57. Modernising Medical Careers, CbD (Case-based Discussion): Available at http://www.mmc.nhs.uk/pages/assessment/cbd (accessed July 2007).
58. Healthcare Assessment and Training, CbD: Available at http://www.hcat.nhs.uk/assessments/cbd (accessed July 2007).
59. The Intercollegiate Board for Training in Intensive Care Medicine (IBTICM): The CCST in Intensive Care Medicine—Competency Based Training and Assessment: Part II (version 6): Available at http://www.rcoa.ac.uk/ibticm/docs/CBTPart2.pdf (accessed March 2007).
60. Accreditation Council for Graduate Medical Education (ACGME) Outcome project (2000): Toolbox of assessment methods: Available at http://www.acgme.org/Outcome/assess/Toolbox.pdf (accessed March 2007).
61. Davies H: Work based assessments. BMJ Career Focus 2005;331:88-89.
62. Gaba DM, Small S: How can full environment-realistic patient simulators be used for performance assessment? Newslett Am Soc Anesthiol 1997;10.
63. Miller GE: The assessment of clinical skills and competence/performance. Acad Med 1990;65(9 Suppl):S63-S67.
64. Ringsted C, Skaarup AM, Henriksen AH, et al: Person-task-context: A model for designing curriculum and in-training assessment in postgraduate education. Med Teacher 2006;28:70-76.
65. Norcini JJ: Current perspectives in assessment: The assessment of performance at work. Med Educ 2005;39:880-889.
66. Grady G: Doctors' practice on the dying should be stopped. New York Times, December 30, 1999.
67. Singer P: Intimate examinations and other ethical challenges in medical education. BMJ 2003;326:62-63.
68. Ziv A, Wolpe PR: Simulation-based medical education: An ethical imperative. Acad Med 2003;78:783-788.
69. Resucitation Council (UK): Available at http://www.resus.org.uk (accessed June 2006).
70. American Heart Association: Available at http://www.americanheart.org (accessed June 2006).
71. Bullock I (ed): Advanced Life Support Instructor Manual. London, Resuscitation Council, 2001.
72. Chopra V, Gesink BJ, de Jong J, et al: Does training in a simulator lead to improvement in performance? Br J Anaesth 1994;73:293-297.
73. Gaba DM, Maxwell M, DeAnda A: Anaesthetic mishaps: Breaking the chain of accident evolution. Anesthesiology 1987;66:670-676.
74. Gaba DM, Fish KJ, Howard SK: Crisis Management in Anaesthesiology. London, Churchill Livingstone, 1994.
75. Howard SK, Gaba DM, Fish KJ, et al: Anaesthesia crisis resource management training: Teaching anaesthesiologists to handle critical incidents. Aviat Space Environ Med 1992;63:763-770.

PART

IX

OTHER CRITICAL CARE DISORDERS AND ISSUES IN CARE OF THE CRITICALLY ILL

Chapter 76

Diagnosis and Management of Liver Failure in the Adult

Nick Murphy

Liver failure is most often encountered as a result of decompensation of chronic liver disease but can also occur de novo in patients with previously normal livers. These patients are often described as having fulminant or acute liver failure (ALF), depending on the definition used.

Liver failure is characterized by a constellation of physical signs and symptoms including jaundice, coagulopathy, and encephalopathy. Not all of these must be present for a diagnosis to be made, but as the syndrome progresses they are usually present to varying degrees. Liver failure progresses to multiple organ failure and ultimately death in a large proportion of patients, and supportive care plus removal of the primary cause is the mainstay of treatment. Liver transplantation is indicated in a small group. Liver support systems are being actively investigated and may someday be able to bridge a patient to recovery or transplantation.

DECOMPENSATION OF CHRONIC LIVER DISEASE

The pathological basis of acute decompensation in chronic liver disease or acute-on-chronic liver failure (AoCLF) is incompletely understood but is thought to be precipitated by systemic inflammation.[1] Patients with well-compensated cirrhosis may appear to decompensate following a defined event. The precipitants can be split into two types: (1) those caused by direct liver insult such as ischemia, a toxic insult such as alcohol, or a superimposed viral infection; and (2) those in which the liver is affected as a bystander in a systemic inflammatory process, such as following an episode of sepsis or a gastrointestinal bleed. This is contrasted to the progressive liver failure of end-stage cirrhosis. Both present with similar clinical pictures, but in AoCLF there remains the possibility of improvement and reversibility.[1] Differentiating between the two is difficult, but the presence of a precipitating factor and history can be useful. In patients with end-stage liver cirrhosis there is often a history of gradual deterioration in biochemical parameters, clinical status, and other organ function. Organ support in this setting is of dubious utility because it is almost always futile.

One group has proposed a working definition for AoCLF as "acute deterioration in liver function over a period of 2 to 4 weeks, usually associated with a precipitating event, leading to severe deterioration in clinical status, with jaundice and hepatic encephalopathy and/or hepatorenal syndrome (HRS), with a high SOFA/APACHE II score."[1]

FACTORS PRECIPITATING AoCLF

Alcoholic Hepatitis

Alcoholic hepatitis (AH) is a common manifestation of alcohol abuse. Among heavy drinkers, 20% to 30% will present with AH at some time. The clinical picture is variable, from a relatively mild syndrome associated with loss of appetite, nausea, and vomiting with right upper quadrant pain to severe life-threatening liver decompensation. Overall, following first presentation, 35% to 50% of patients will die within the first month of diagnosis.[2] It usually presents following a bout of heavy drinking and often occurs on a background of cirrhosis. Patients frequently deteriorate after stopping alcohol. In patients without cirrhosis, abstinence and nutritional support can lead to a marked improvement in liver function over time.

Features suggestive of malnutrition such as muscle wasting and vitamin deficiency are seen commonly. In severe decompensation, other intercurrent illnesses such as pneumonia or urinary tract infection or a gastrointestinal bleed are often present. Systemic inflammation may be the precipitant of decompensation in these patients.[3]

In AH liver enzymes are moderately raised with an aspartate aminotransferase (AST) rarely greater than 300 U/L. The ratio of AST to alanine aminotransferase (ALT) is usually raised to greater than 2.[4] A high white cell count and bilirubin are also typical. The liver is usually enlarged and fatty on ultrasound. Portal hypertension often complicates the clinical picture, presenting as worsening of ascites. Assessment of filling pressures can be difficult if ascites is tense. Further hemodynamic monitoring is recommended if there is any doubt regarding filling status or if cardiac output is thought to be compromised.

Strictly speaking, liver biopsy is required to make the diagnosis of AH and is often performed to assess the extent of fibrosis, although it is not required for acute management demonstrated under light microscopy, the Mallory's hyaline and a neutrophil infiltration (the amount of which is a marker of severity and prognosis), necrosis of hepatocytes, collagen deposition, and fatty change.

The prognosis of patients with AH depends on the severity of the disease. Risk stratification is important, both in defining the indications for the use of specific pharmacologic agents aimed at the interruption of progression and in clinical research. Serum markers and liver histology provide the best means for risk stratification. In many cases, however, biopsy is precluded because of the risks of bleeding. Serum bilirubin, coagulation parameters, and creatinine have been shown to predict outcome and have been combined into several scoring systems including the discriminative function (DF); Child-Turcotte-Pugh (CTP); and, most recently, the Mayo end-stage liver disease (MELD) score. Of these, the MELD score appears to offer the best prediction of mortality because of the inclusion of renal function (creatinine), as well as liver function, because renal deterioration in this setting has a particularly poor prognosis.[5] Standard critical care prognostic scores have also been used to assess the prognosis of patients with decompensated chronic liver disease of any cause. The sequential organ failure score (SOFA) has been shown to provide useful prognostic information.[1]

In early disease, abstinence and good nutrition including supplementation with B vitamins is the mainstay of management. In severe disease, progression to hepatic encephalopathy and organ failure can be rapid. In addition to general supportive care, specific therapies have been used in an attempt to halt and reverse the hepatic inflammation and prevent the fall into multiple organ failure and ultimately death. Of these, corticosteroids and pentoxifylline have been the most extensively studied.[6]

Portal Hypertensive Bleeding

Portal hypertension is a significant complication of chronic liver disease leading to the formation of portosystemic collateral vessels. Of these, the most clinically significant are those that occur in the wall of the stomach and esophagus. In patients with portal hypertension as a result of cirrhosis, the development of gastrointestinal varices occurs in approximately 60% at the time of diagnosis.[7] The incidence of first acute bleed in an unselected patient is relatively low at about 5% per year but can be catastrophic when it occurs.[8] The mortality associated with the event has fallen over the past 20 years from approximately 30% to 50% to about 20%, and control of the initial bleeding episode is achieved in about 90% of patients.[9] Half of this mortality occurs in the first 5 days following an acute bleed. Approximately half of this is because of uncontrolled bleeding, whereas the rest is caused by multiple organ failure. This pattern remains the same when mortality in the first 6 weeks following the first bleed is examined.[9]

Control of bleeding episodes is via direct endoscopic therapy, usually in the form of band ligation in the case of esophageal varices.[8] Terlipressin, a synthetic analogue of vasopressin, can be used as an adjunct to band ligation. Terlipressin induces splanchnic vasoconstriction, reduces portal pressure, and has been shown to reduce mortality.[10] Some data indicate that somatostatin may reduce the amount of blood transfused, but the evidence is weak.[11] Uncontrolled bleeding caused by either failed endoscopic or pharmacologic therapy or when resources do not allow immediate endoscopic therapy may be managed with balloon tamponade of stomach or esophageal varices. Primary control of esophageal varices is usually successful, but balloons should not be inflated for more than 12 hours because of the risks of mucosal necrosis. Care should be exercised when inserting and inflating a Sengstaken-Blackmore or Minnesota tube because perforation of the esophagus is usually fatal in this setting. Following control with the insertion of a balloon tamponade device, further endoscopic therapy, surgical shunting, or transjugular intrahepatic portosystemic stent-shunts (TIPS) may be attempted. Of the shunt procedures used, TIPS is the most commonly attempted, where technical skills are available. The procedure involves decompressing the portal circulation into the hepatic vein via a stent inserted percutaneously through the liver via the internal jugular vein. The procedure is a successful salvage therapy for controlling bleeding but can induce certain complications: (1) volume overload as a result of portal shunting into the right atrium, which can induce heart failure; (2) bypass of the portal circulation, resulting in ischemic liver injury; (3) rarely, liver failure; and (4) worsening of encephalopathy grade, the most common complication, resulting in failure to wake from the procedure, extended ventilation, and the risk of hospital-acquired infection. No controlled trials of TIPS as salvage therapy in this setting have occurred, and it is unclear what role TIPS has in the management of acute bleeding varices because it may just result in prolongation of the dying process. Despite better prevention of rebleeding when compared with endoscopic therapy in patients with bleeding varices, a mortality benefit cannot be shown with TIPS.[12]

Coagulation abnormalities are commonly present in patients with acutely bleeding varices, and abnormalities in clotting factors have been shown to be independent prognostic factors in patients with esophageal varices. Attempts to treat coagulation abnormalities with clotting components should be undertaken during an acute bleed to include fresh frozen plasma (FFP) and platelets targeted to correct abnormal partial thromboplastin time (PTT) and platelet count. Activated factor VII has also been investigated in this setting. The authors showed that in patients with worse cirrhosis, as defined by Child-Pugh grade B and C, rFVIIa increased the chances of controlling the bleeding.[13]

Bleeding from varices is associated with infection. Among cirrhotic patients with bleeding varices, 35% to 60% have documented infection over the following 2 weeks.[14] The use of antibiotic prophylaxis has been shown to reduce the incidence of infection in this group of patients and to improve short-term mortality.[14] Infection is proposed to be the precipitant to an acute increase in portal pressure that may trigger bleeding.[15]

Bacterial Peritonitis

Patients with chronic liver disease are at increased risk of infection. The immunosuppression associated with chronic liver disease is incompletely understood but relates to a range of factors including an impaired innate and adaptive immune response.[16,17]

In patients with ascites as a result of cirrhosis, decompensation is often caused by infection. Bacterial peritonitis is a common and severe complication. It is often spontaneous, without any obvious source. It has generally been caused by gram-negative bacteria, although gram-positive bacteria including methicillin-resistant *Staphylococcus aureus* (MRSA) are increasingly being recognized as a pathogen, especially in the hospital setting.[18] In any patient with ascites and decompensation of liver disease, spontaneous bacterial peritonitis (SBP) should be suspected. Diagnosis is demonstrated by an absolute leukocyte count in ascitic fluid of greater than 250/mm^3. Antibiotics should be started as soon as SBP is suspected, following blood culture and a diagnostic ascitic tap. Empiric broad-spectrum coverage for gram-negative bacteria and MRSA should be started until cultures are available. Resolution of infection is signaled by the resolution of clinical signs and by a drop in the ascitic neutrophil count.

Renal failure is a significant complication of SBP in patients with cirrhosis and is discussed later.

SUPPORTIVE MANAGEMENT IN CRITICAL CARE

The presentation of acute-on-chronic liver failure (AoCLF) will depend on the precipitating event or events, but the clinical picture and pattern of organ failure will on the whole look similar.

Hyperbilirubinemia and the resulting jaundice are almost universal, as are other biochemical manifestations of poor liver function. Plasma protein production is deranged, leading to a prolongation of prothrombin time and hypoalbuminemia. Thrombocytopenia caused by hypersplenism and sepsis is also characteristic.

The pattern of circulatory changes associated with cirrhosis is distinctive. Hypotension and an increase in cardiac output are typical, resulting in a hyperdynamic circulation. Peripheral vasodilation is, however, not distributed evenly and occurs mainly in the splanchnic circulation as a result of sinusoidal portal hypertension. Splanchnic vasodilation results in effective arterial underfilling with the resulting activation of compensatory mechanisms.[19] During decompensation circulatory changes become more pronounced with an increase in portal pressure, systemic vasodilation worsens, and blood pressure drops further and becomes less responsive to vasopressor support. Recent work shows that cardiac output actually falls in those who develop hepatorenal failure, as does cardiac filling pressures and pulmonary artery pressure. These changes point toward some form of cardiac depressant factor associated with decompensation.[19] A reduction in intrarenal blood flow occurs because of the activation of compensatory mechanisms designed to maintain arterial volume, such as the renin-angiotensin system and sympathetic nervous system. This results in a further reduction in glomerular filtration rate (GFR) and urine output.

Hepatorenal syndrome (HRS) is a severe and progressive reduction in renal function in patients with severe liver disease. It presents in two clinical patterns. Initially HRS is potentially reversible as the kidneys are functionally normal; however, the longer the circulatory changes last without re-establishing the GFR, the less likely the kidneys will recover and the distinction between HRS and acute tubular neurosis (ATN) becomes less clear. Type 1 HRS is characterized by the rapid decline in renal function defined as a 100% increase in serum creatinine to a level greater than 221 mmol/L or a 50% reduction in 24-hour creatinine clearance to a level less than 20 mL/minute in less than 2 weeks.[20] In most patients there is a precipitating event, whereas in others it occurs in close proximity to an event such as the resolution of SBP. Type 2 HRS is characterized by a less severe and more gradual reduction in renal function associated with diuretic resistant ascites and hyponatremia. The diagnosis is made by the exclusion of other causes and is based on criteria developed by the International Ascites Club.[20]

Until recently there was no effective treatment for patients with HRS other than liver transplantation. HRS represents the consequence of circulatory changes associated with severe liver disease. Observational studies show that countering the compensatory changes that promote intrarenal vasoconstriction with use of systemic and selective vasoconstrictors plus plasma volume expansion with albumin can lead to significant improvement in renal function. The aim of therapy is to focus vasoconstriction on the dilated splanchnic vessels, resulting in a redistribution of the blood volume back into the systemic arterial circulation. Over time this results in suppression of the compensatory mechanisms, a reduction in plasma renin activity, sympathetic activity, and circulating catecholamines with an associated increase in GFR, sodium excretion, and urine output.[21] Many different vasoconstrictors have been tried in this setting. The drug most commonly studied is terlipressin, which is often given with 20% human albumin solution (HAS). This approach has been subjected to a randomized controlled clinical trial in which the addition of albumin was associated with an improvement in outcome.[22] Evidence suggests that vasoconstrictor therapy, with or without plasma volume expansion, results in an improvement in renal function in about 50% to 70% of patients with type 1 HRS.[21]

Hepatic encephalopathy (HE) is almost universal during decompensation of chronic liver disease and is characterized by loss of normal day/night differentiation, confusion, somnolence, asterixis, hyperreflexia, and progression to coma. It is reversible in the event of recovery of liver function or removal of the precipitating event. The etiology of hepatic encephalopathy is incompletely understood but probably relates to an inability of the failing liver to clear circulating toxins and to minor degrees of cerebral edema.[23]

Ammonia production in the gut is important in the pathogenesis of HE. This is usually cleared from the portal circulation in the liver. The mainstays of treatment are colonic cleansing with enemas and enteral disaccharides such as lactulose. Both procedures have been shown to improve encephalopathy grades. The restriction of protein, once fashionable in patients with liver disease, is contraindicated. The majority of these patients are malnourished, and adequate enteral nutrition is essential.[24]

Patients with AoCLF and high grades of HE will require intubation and ventilation, not because of hypoxia but to allow airway protection. Airway protection is most frequently necessary in patients with bleeding esophageal or gastric varices requiring endoscopic therapy for large-volume hematemesis in the presence of HE and difficult or prolonged endoscopic procedure. Patients with AoCLF are usually exquisitely sensitive to sedative and anesthetic agents. Even small doses of benzodiazepines can cause prolonged coma. Care should be exercised in their use, and shorter-acting agents such as propofol are preferred.

Large-volume paracentesis should be considered in any patient with tense ascites. Evidence indicates that large-volume paracentesis improves lung mechanics and oxygenation in nonventilated patients, but data in ventilated patients are lacking.[25-27] Hepatic hydrothorax is a persistent pleural effusion that is almost always associated with ascites, usually on the right side of the chest. It can be massive in size containing many liters of fluid and is thought to be caused by communication from the peritoneum. Management can be difficult. Direct drainage with thoracocentesis is usually inadvisable because the fluid accumulation is persistent, leading to a continued need for chest tube placement with the risk of infection. Management should be directed at the ascites. This includes diuretics, salt restriction, and paracentesis. TIPS can be used to control both ascites and hydrothorax but is associated with worsening encephalopathy grade in some patients.[28]

Adrenal dysfunction in patients with septic shock is well recognized, and evidence indicates that steroid replacement therapy can increase shock reversal and improve outcome.[29,30] A debate is ongoing over the role of steroid therapy in patients with a normal response to ACTH stimulation. It has been recently shown that hypotensive patients with decompensated cirrhosis have a high incidence of adrenal suppression. Patients with adrenal suppression have worse hepatic and renal function, more organ failure, and a higher intensive care unit (ICU) and hospital mortality.[29,31] Adrenal function may also deteriorate during critical care admission, so repeat testing has been recommended.[29] In patients with cirrhosis and septic shock admitted to the ICU with adrenal insufficiency as defined by a suboptimal response to ACTH stimulation, replacement of hydrocortisone (50 mg every 6 hours) results in a higher incidence of shock resolution and hospital survival when compared with historical controls.[32]

CRITICAL CARE OUTCOME IN AoCLF

Despite ICU care, the outcome in patients with decompensated cirrhosis is poor. In one study overall cumulative mortality rates were 36% in the critical care unit, 46% in the hospital, and 56% at 6-month follow-up.[33]

In patients who require organ support within the critical care environment, a number of observations can be made. Derangement of acute physiology at admission is a predictor of outcome as it is for unselected patients admitted to the ICU.[34] In addition, the number of organs requiring support is also predictive of outcome.[33,35] Patients with cirrhosis and three organ systems requiring support have a mortality in excess of 90%.[35] Severity of liver disease at admission has a significant bearing on outcome irrespective of indication for admission to the ICU.[35,36]

ACUTE (FULMINANT) LIVER FAILURE

ALF is a syndrome manifest by the rapid cessation of normal function in individuals with previously normal livers. The rate of decline in function dictates the manner in which the syndrome manifests and influences the outcome. The etiology is the main influence on the rate of progression and the likelihood of spontaneous recovery.[37]

The pathologic basis of massive hepatic necrosis was described in detail by Lucké and Mallory following World War II in 1946.[38] The presence of the American army in East Asia and Africa resulted in exposure to both epidemic and serum hepatitis, and data regarding the clinical course of the syndrome and pathology were collated via the army medical services.

In 1970 Trey and Davidson introduced the term *fulminant hepatic failure* (FHF) to encompass the current clinicopathologic understanding of the syndrome.[39] This definition was an attempt to encapsulate the clinical course and to differentiate it from decompensation of chronic liver disease. They described a syndrome of rapidly progressing liver failure (within 8 weeks) in which the defining point was the onset of hepatic encephalopathy following the onset of symptoms in someone without previous liver disease. They make the point that the syndrome is potentially reversible in some patients. This definition is still used today; however, it has become clear that this definition is too narrow and that subgroups exist.

Speed of progression to encephalopathy from the onset of jaundice or other initial symptoms is used to define subgroups. This is because the rate of progression of the syndrome is directly related to the etiology of the underlying cause of liver failure. For example, patients with significant acetaminophen-induced hepatotoxicity will generally present with liver failure within 7 days of ingestion, unless ingestion is staggered over a period of time in which the timing of liver insult is difficult to define. Patients often present with cardiovascular collapse and renal failure before they become encephalopathic. In contrast, patients presenting with sero-negative hepatitis (unknown etiology, non–A/non–B [NANB] hepatitis) can have a prolonged illness, over a period of months, resulting in a patient who is deeply jaundiced with evidence of portal hypertension such as ascites at the onset of encephalopathy. It is the two extreme ends of the syndrome that split the group into hyperacute, acute, and subacute liver failure. Interestingly, it is the hyperacute group that has the best chance for spontaneous recovery, although this group has the highest risk of cerebral edema. The subacute group has the worse prognosis with medical management alone (Box 76-1).[37]

Etiology of Acute Liver Failure

Worldwide, particularly in the developing world, approximately 95% to 100% of patients presenting with ALF will have viral hepatitis.[40] Within the United Kingdom and United States, paracetamol hepatotoxicity is the leading cause of ALF. This is followed by liver failure of unknown etiology or seronegative hepatitis.[41,42]

The pattern of ALF within the United Kingdom and United States has been changing over the past 30 years.[41,42] Until the late 1990s the rate of hospital admission caused by paracetamol ingestion had risen year by year. In the United Kingdom paracetamol overdose (POD) is usually caused by deliberate self-harm. In contrast, U.S. data suggest that more than half of all patients with ALF caused by POD were caused by therapeutic misadventure. Some doubts have been expressed regarding this interpretation because some of the patients in the misadventure group may actually be occult suicide attempts.[42,43] In 1998 legislation was introduced in the United Kingdom to restrict the over-the-counter sale of paracetamol to 16 tablets from most retail outlets and 32 tablets from pharmacies in the form of blister packs. Since then the rates of admissions to the hospital, severe liver toxicity, and transplantation for POD have fallen.[44]

Box 76-1

Hyperacute, Acute, and Subacute Liver Failure

- Hyperacute liver failure
  - Jaundice to encephalopathy within 7 days—usually because of paracetamol hepatotoxicity
- Acute liver failure
  - Jaundice to encephalopathy from 8 to 28 days
- Subacute liver failure
  - Jaundice to encephalopathy from 29 days to 6 months

In the United Kingdom and United States the incidence of acute hepatitis A virus (HAV) and hepatitis B virus (HBV) infection has fallen dramatically since the 1980s.[41,45] Less than 1% of acute hepatitis A or B progresses to ALF.[41] In the United States and United Kingdom a proportion of the total number of admissions with ALF caused by viral hepatitis has fallen steadily and is currently responsible for less than 5% of all admissions in the United Kingdom and 11% in the United States.[41,45]

Indeterminate hepatitis (non–A to E hepatitis, sero-negative ALF, non–A/non–B hepatitis) is often presumed to be viral in origin and is the most common presentation excluding POD in the United Kingdom and United States and viral hepatitis in the developing world. It is a diagnosis of exclusion and, as diagnostic capabilities improve, it is falling in incidence in some centers.[41]

Acetaminophen (Paracetamol)

Acetaminophen-induced liver failure is the cause of the vast majority of hyperacute liver failure. Acetaminophen poisoning is a common cause of presentation to acute and emergency departments in the United Kingdom and United States; however, the case progression to ALF following paracetamol ingestion is rare at just 0.6% of all presentations in the United Kingdom.[46]

In the mid 1960s the main mechanisms of paracetamol-induced liver injury were elucidated. The scheme outlined by various groups revealed that the production of electrophilic quinone imine (N-acetyl-p-benzoquinone imine, NAPQI), which covalently binds to hepatic proteins, was central to the resultant centrolobular necrosis seen following poisoning. The two major pathways for paracetamol metabolism are the glucuronidation and sulfation of the phenolic group with the metabolites produced excreted in the urine. In therapeutic doses approximately 80% of the drug is metabolized via these two pathways, and 5% to 10% is excreted unchanged in the urine. The remainder is metabolized via the hepatic mixed function oxidase, cytochrome P450, to produce NAPQI.

Following poisoning the half-life of acetaminophen is greatly prolonged because of the saturation of glucuronidation and sulfate conjugation. As a result there is an increase in the quantity of NAPQI produced. NAPQI is extremely reactive in biologic systems and has a short half-life. Following poisoning, reaction of NAPQI occurs within the centrilobular portions of the liver and leads to necrosis in experimental models. It reacts with cellular constituents in a covalent and noncovalent manner. The exact mechanisms by which NAPQI induces cell death are incompletely understood but include the deactivation of critical cellular proteins; induction of reactive oxygen species, and activation of Kupffer cells.[47] The loss of regulatory protein function results in abnormal calcium homeostasis and resultant energy failure within the cell and mitochondria.[47] Other events such as noncovalent interaction with intracellular signaling and lipid peroxidation also contribute to the toxicity of this molecule. Following this primary toxic phase there is a secondary or extrinsic phase. This extrinsic phase is equated with the recruitment of immune cells to the liver. The liver is one of the major immune organs of the body. Up to 35% of the liver is made up of nonparenchymal cells, including endothelium, Kupffer cells, and resident lymphocytes. These, together with macrophages within the liver, perform a major role in immune regulation and in the filtering of antigens from the gut contents via the portal circulation. They are also implicated in the pathologic processes that occur following liver insult. Massive activation of immune cells in response to the intrinsic cellular damage induces the release of cytokines and chemokines both locally and into the systemic circulation.[48,49]

Immune effects following the direct toxic effects of NAPQI result in the secondary effects of poisoning such as the release of cytokines from the liver and induction of organ failure.

Following a significant intake of paracetamol the symptoms over the following 24 hours, irrespective of amount ingested, are usually nausea and vomiting. The minimum dose that can induce hepatic damage appears to be about 125 mg/kg. This represents 15 500-mg tablets in a 60-kg individual, although hepatic necrosis has been recorded at much lower doses, especially if associated with hepatic enzyme induction. Doses above 250 mg/kg (30 500-mg tablets in a 60-kg individual) will often produce damage, and doses in excess of 350 mg/kg invariably produce significant damage.[50] During the following 4 to 5 days, if liver failure ensues, there is a gradual worsening of the patient's general condition. Those with significant overdose should be admitted to the hospital and monitored closely.

The antidote for acetaminophen poisoning is N-acetylcysteine (NAC). It provides complete protection against hepatotoxicity if given within 12 hours of nonstaggered ingestion.[51] Within 12 hours, if the time from ingestion is known with certainty and a plasma acetaminophen level is obtained, reference can be made to nomogram to see if the potential for hepatotoxicity is present. The nomograms are unreliable if the time from ingestion is uncertain or if there was staggered ingestion over a period of time, as often occurs with therapeutic misadventure or repeated overdose. The use of alcohol often accompanies POD, making timing unreliable. Situations that alter normal cytochrome P450 function such as drug induction (chronic ethanol use, phenytoin, and isoniazid) again render the information unreliable.[52] The use of the nomogram as the only basis for the decision to withhold NAC therapy is to be discouraged because of the uncertainty associated with this timing and the catastrophic potential if NAC is erroneously withheld.

The main effect of NAC is to increase hepatic glutathione production. This promotes the conjugation of NAPQI and its subsequent excretion. In addition, NAC may act as an antioxidant within and outside the liver. It is most effective if given within the first 8 hours following overdose but is effective to a lesser degree later. Some evidence indicates that NAC is effective when administered to the patient up to 72 hours following poisoning, although the mechanism of action is unclear and probably relates to antioxidant effects rather than to any effect on acetaminophen metabolism.[53] The role of NAC in established ALF from any etiology is more controversial and, despite widespread use, its role is not established.[54,55]

Viral Hepatitis

Both epidemic and serum hepatitis were recognized well before the viral etiology was discovered. The seminal work of Lucké and Mallory in 1946 described 196 patients who died of ALF following both epidemic hepatitis and serum hepatitis, related to the administration of blood products during World War II.[38]

ALF following acute viral hepatitis is uncommon with a reported incidence of 0.2% to 4% depending on the underlying etiology.[56] Liver failure following viral hepatitis tends to run an acute or hyperacute course with the onset of encephalopathy occurring within days or weeks of the first symptoms.[57]

Hepatitis A is now rare in the United States and Western Europe but is a common form of acute enterally transmitted hepatitis in the developing world, where it is mainly a mild and self-limiting illness of children.[57,58] The progression to ALF is the lowest of all the hepatotrophic viruses. In the West the incidence of ALF following hepatitis A appears to be higher than in the endemic areas. It occurs more commonly in adults and is more severe. Persistent infection with hepatitis A has also been reported[59] and can even recur following liver transplantation.[60] Diagnosis is made on the basis of IgM antibodies at the time of hospitalization, although false negatives can occur.[61]

Hepatitis B may lead to ALF in several settings. It occurs most commonly following acute infection but can occur following an acute increase in viral replication following immunosuppressive therapy such as cancer chemotherapy or steroids, as well as with coinfection with other viral agents such as delta virus. The host immune response is thought to be responsible for the severity of reaction to the virus, subsequent clearance, and the induction of ALF. This can be seen following the withdrawal of immunosuppressive therapy when there is an active immune response to the increased viral load. In acute infection surface antigen (HBsAg) is often negative, but IgM antibodies to the viral core (HBcAb) are usually positive. Mutations to the precore stop codon or the core promoter region of the viral genome may be associated with a higher incidence of ALF.[62] These particular genes code for HBeAg, and lack of this antigen is associated with a more profound immune response. A high incidence of ALF has been associated with outbreaks of acute hepatitis B in the setting of intravenous drug use and chronic hepatitis C infection.[63]

Hepatitis C as a cause of ALF is rare in Northern Europe and the United States but has been described.[64] A wide spectrum of clinical presentation is associated with acute infection with the more florid presentation associated with a more rapid clearance rate, suggesting that the magnitude of the initial immune response is important.[65] Liver failure associated with acute infection appears to be more common in India and the Far East.[66] Acute infection may contribute to decompensation in patients with preexisting liver disease, and hepatitis C seropositivity may predispose to liver failure when coinfection with another hepatotrophic virus is present.[66]

Hepatitis E is likely the most common cause of ALF worldwide and is certainly true for the Indian subcontinent.[66] In the Far East acute hepatitis B infection is the most common cause of ALF because of the high levels of endemicity.[67]

The existence of hepatitis E was inferred before serological evidence was available by a process of exclusion. It was long assumed that most, if not all, epidemic enteric hepatitis was caused by the A virus. When serological markers for hepatitis A became available in the early 1980s, it was apparent that the majority of waterborne epidemic hepatitis was caused by other agents, producing a syndrome clinically similar to hepatitis A.[68] Hepatitis E does not produce a chronic infection, and in the vast majority it is a self-limiting infection that occurs most commonly in young adults, in contrast to hepatitis A, which is primarily an infection of children. The incidence of hepatitis E associated with ALF is small with a case-related mortality reported at about 0.5% to 4% in the general population but with a much higher mortality in pregnancy, as high as 20% in the third trimester. Pregnancy itself appears to be a risk factor for ALF, with a quarter of all infected female patients reported as pregnant in one series. However, this may not be particular to hepatitis E but rather because of the high incidence of epidemic hepatitis E in a relatively immunosuppressed state.[66] In the West, travel to endemic areas is a risk factor but sporadic cases are now being seen more commonly in the developed world. Some of these cases have been associated with contact with animals.[69]

Sero-negative hepatitis is the second most common cause of ALF worldwide in most published series. In Northern Europe and the United States it comes in behind paracetamol toxicity, and in the developing world it is second to acute viral hepatitis (Figs. 76-1 and 76-2).

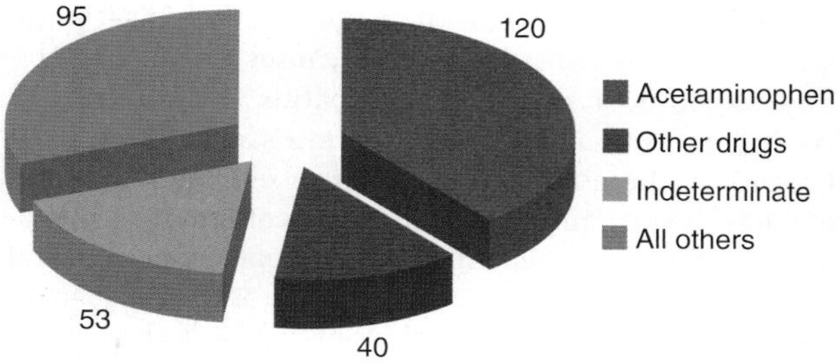

Figure 76-1. Etiology of acute liver failure in the United States 1998-2001 based on 17 centers. (From Ostapowicz G, Fontana RJ, Schiodt FV, et al: Results of a prospective study of acute liver failure at 17 tertiary care centers in the United States. Ann Intern Med 2002;137:947-954.)

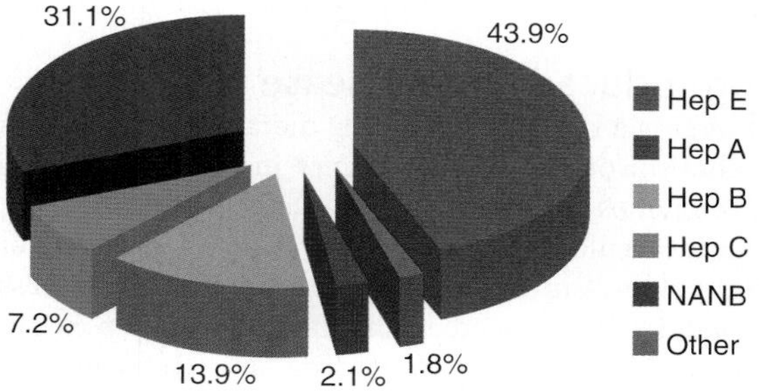

Figure 76-2. Etiology of acute liver failure in an Indian center 1989-1996. NANB, non–A to E hepatitis or seronegative hepatitis. (From Khuroo MS, Kamili S: Aetiology and prognostic factors in acute liver failure in India. J Viral Hepat 2003;10:224-231.)

Sero-negative hepatitis can be conveniently thought of as a single entity. In reality it is probably an amalgam of various causes including acute presentations of autoimmune hepatitis, idiosyncratic drug reactions, and viruses.[70,71] Sero-negative hepatitis has a variable clinical presentation including a slow insidious onset of general malaise, jaundice, and ascites followed by progressive signs and symptoms of liver failure. At presentation the patient may be deeply jaundiced and already have ascites and splenomegaly. Sero-negative hepatitis can also present with a hyperacute picture. The pattern of signs, symptoms, and organ failure is dictated by the rate of progression. In subacute sero-negative hepatitis the presenting clinical picture can be similar to that of decompensated chronic liver disease, causing occasional diagnostic difficulty. A liver biopsy is sometimes necessary to differentiate between the two.

Acute Presentation of Autoimmune Hepatitis

Autoimmune hepatitis can occur at any time of life from childhood until old age. It is more common in women, with a male-to-female ratio of 1:3. Presentation can be asymptomatic, discovered following routine laboratory testing, or, more commonly, presentation is jaundice and general malaise. In rare cases autoimmune hepatitis can present as ALF.[72] Unfortunately there are no serologic tests with sufficient sensitivity or specificity to make the diagnosis certain. Patterns of markers in the right clinical setting and in the absence of other causes may be useful.[73] The diagnosis of autoimmune hepatitis in the setting of ALF is difficult, and a degree of uncertainty often lasts. Classically there is a combination of elevated immunoglobulin levels, autoantibodies, and confirmatory histological evidence of hepatitis in the absence of active viral markers. Elevation of autoantibodies is often seen in patients with ALF because of other causes such as drug-induced liver disease.[72] Liver failure should be assessed in the same way as for other etiologies, and once signs of encephalopathy become apparent standard prognostic criteria apply. The role of steroids is unproven but should be considered in patients prior to the onset of encephalopathy. Once listed for transplantation, steroid use is controversial because of the increased risk of infection.

Drug-Induced Liver Disease

The liver is a major site for drug metabolism in the body. Metabolism of xenobiotics occurs in a series of specialized enzymes that increase the water solubility of lipophilic molecules by the incorporation of polar groups. Drug metabolism often involves a number of processes. Intermediates produced during the process are sometimes more toxic than the parent drug and can cause liver damage by a number of mechanisms.

Drug-induced liver disease may be caused by a known dose-dependent toxicity as with paracetamol. Alternatively, unpredictable, rare, idiosyncratic reactions can occur with any drug with a frequency of about 1 in 1000 to 1 in 100,000 patient prescriptions.[52] Drug-induced liver failure can mimic all forms of acute and chronic liver disease. However, the predominant clinical presentation consists of either acute hepatitis or cholestatic liver disease. The former has a reported mortality of 10% irrespective of the drug implicated.

The patterns of injury associated with these idiosyncratic reactions relate to the mechanism of damage and the cells involved.[74] Many patterns have been described, but it is massive hepatic necrosis that most often presents as ALF. Liver failure associated with severe cholestasis and veno-occlusive disease is also seen.[74]

Liver injury is usually seen within 6 months following the initiation of therapy. Even if the diagnosis of drug-induced liver failure is considered, a search for other possible etiologies should be performed. Although any drug is capable of inducing liver injury, more common causes include herbal remedies and recreationally used drugs such as "Ecstasy" and cocaine. If suspected, a comprehensive history with a timetable of drug initiation should be constructed. Management includes stopping the offending drug and supportive care. Transplantation should be considered once liver failure occurs because the outcome from drug-induced liver failure, other than that induced by paracetamol, can be poor.[75] Presentation profiles for various drugs causing ALF are shown in Table 76-1.[52]

Pregnancy-Induced Liver Disease

In general, pregnancy-associated liver failure has the best prognosis when compared with all other causes of ALF, and prompt recovery can be expected with delivery of the fetus in most cases, if recognized early enough.

Table 76-1. Idiosyncratic Drug Reactions and the Cells That Are Affected[52]

Type of Reaction	Effect on Cells	Examples of Drugs
Hepatocellular	Direct effect or production by enzyme–drug adduct leads to cell dysfunction, membrane dysfunction, cytotoxic T-cell response	Isoniazid, trazodone, diclofenac, nefazodone, venlafaxine, lovastatin
Cholestasis	Injury to canalicular membrane and transporters	Chlorpromazine, estrogen, erythromycin and its derivatives
Immunoallergic	Enzyme–drug adducts on cell surface induce IgE response	Halothane, phenytoin, sulfamethoxazole
Granulomatous	Macrophages, lymphocytes infiltrate hepatic lobule	Diltiazem, sulfa drugs, quinidine
Microvesicular fat	Altered mitochondrial respiration, β-oxidation leads to lactic acidosis and triglyceride accumulation	Didanosine, tetracycline, acetylsalicylic acid, valproic acid
Steatohepatitis	Multifactorial	Amiodarone, tamoxifen
Autoimmune	Cytotoxic lymphocyte response directed at hepatocyte membrane components	Nitrofurantoin, methyldopa, lovastatin, minocycline
Fibrosis	Activation of stellate cells	Methotrexate, excess vitamin A
Vascular collapse	Causes ischemic or hypoxic injury	Nicotinic acid, cocaine, methylenedioxymethamphetamine
Oncogenesis	Encourages tumor formation	Oral contraceptives, androgens
Mixed	Cytoplasmic and canalicular injury, direct damage to bile ducts	Amoxicillin–clavulanate, carbamazepine, herbs, cyclosporine, methimazole, troglitazone

From Lee WM: Drug-induced hepatotoxicity. N Engl J Med 2003;349:474-485.

Pregnancy-associated liver failure can present in several ways including the syndromes of preeclampsia and the HELLP syndrome (hemolysis, elevated liver function tests, and low platelets); liver rupture; and acute fatty liver of pregnancy. Any cause of ALF can occur during pregnancy and, in particular, viral hepatitis can be particularly fulminant in its course. This is especially true for hepatitis E and herpes simplex virus infection.

Although originally thought to be a variant of preeclampsia, there is evidence that HELLP syndrome may be a separate entity and, in fact, more related to acute fatty liver of pregnancy.[76] Both HELLP and preeclampsia appear to be related to an endothelial injury, possibly immunologically initiated with activation of the coagulation and complement cascades and an imbalance of prostaglandin and thromboxane resulting in increased vascular tone, microangiopathic hemolytic anemia, and vascular thrombosis.[77] HELLP is thought to occur in approximately 1 in every 1000 live deliveries, and patients usually present in the third trimester with nonspecific signs often seen in preeclampsia such as weight gain caused by edema and hypertension. In addition, right upper quadrant pain accompanied by nausea and vomiting is commonly seen. Laboratory abnormalities include hyperbilirubinemia caused by liver dysfunction and evidence of hemolysis. Transaminases are modestly raised, and the platelet count is usually less than 100,000. Liver biopsy, although commonly normal in preeclampsia, shows specific changes of periportal necrosis and fibrin microthrombi. Microvascular steatosis may also be present.[77] The liver failure associated with HELLP is manifest as a prolonged prothrombin time and ascites. Renal failure is common. Maternal mortality is low, but fetal mortality is high, between 20% and 60%.[77,78] Treatment of choice is delivery of the baby. Conservative therapy is associated with an increase in both maternal and fetal complications.

Spontaneous rupture of the liver can occur in the setting of both preeclampsia and the HELLP syndrome, although it can occur de novo. It often presents with sudden onset of right upper quadrant pain accompanied by signs of hypovolemia or shock and is more common in multiparous women.[77] Spontaneous rupture of the liver has a high maternal and fetal mortality. Its pathogenesis is unclear, but it appears that periportal hemorrhage associated with the HELLP syndrome may occur close to the capsule, resulting in lifting and bleeding into the potential space. These areas of the capsule then coalesce and rupture. Management of this devastating complication includes prompt delivery of the fetus, local surgical control with packs, and aggressive management of the accompanying coagulopathy. Embolization of any feeding vessels in the liver may be of utility if such skills are available. Hepatectomy followed by liver transplantation can be life saving and has been performed.

Acute fatty liver of pregnancy (AFLP) occurs during the third trimester of pregnancy and should be considered in any patient exhibiting signs of liver dysfunction. It is uncommon, with an incidence of approximately 1 in 6659 live births.[79] If left untreated, maternal and fetal mortality are high. The treatment of choice is delivery, and prompt recovery can then be expected. There is usually a prodromal illness over a couple of weeks with nonspecific symptoms progressing to jaundice and encephalopathy. Symptoms and signs of preeclampsia or the HELLP syndrome are seen in one third of cases, and there is some evidence of a common etiology caused by a fetal fatty acid metabolism disorder.[76] Diagnosis is critical and should be differentiated from viral hepatitis or hepatic failure because of other causes. Liver biopsy can aid in the diagnosis and can be performed via the jugular route if coagulopathy precludes the conventional approach. Characteristic zone 3 microvesicular steatosis is seen. Delivery is the best treatment if diagnosed early. Characteristic features include normoblasts on blood smears and high serum urate. Bleeding can be a major problem during operative delivery. On occasion transplantation may be the only viable option.

Wilson's Disease

Wilson's disease is a rare autosomal recessive disorder resulting from copper toxicity with primarily brain and liver manifestation. It usually presents in the second or third decade of life, although it can present from early childhood until late middle age.[80] The disease can present with predominantly liver or neurologic symptoms. Neurologic symptoms relate to the distribution of copper to the basal ganglia and result in movement disorders. Patients presenting with liver disease may present with an active hepatitis, established cirrhosis, or ALF. Other signs such as Kayser-Fleisher rings are associated but not pathognomonic for Wilson's disease. These are greenish-brown rings in the cornea resulting from deposition of copper.

ALF caused by Wilson's disease can present at any age but commonly presents in the early 20s. High urinary copper excretion is possibly the most predictable laboratory finding, although the patient may be anuric on presentation. A low serum ceruloplasmin is an additional indicator, but again it is unreliable in ALF. A high serum bilirubin in combination with modest elevations of transaminases and alkaline phosphatase is often seen, as is intravascular hemolysis, contributing to the raised bilirubin level. Patients with severe liver failure caused by Wilson's disease have an almost 100% mortality without liver transplantation, which should be considered as soon as the diagnosis is made.[80] Experts debate whether liver failure secondary to Wilson's disease is truly ALF—it does not fit the definition because cirrhosis is invariably present on liver biopsy at the time of presentation. Nevertheless, many patients have not been diagnosed at this point, and the presentation is often acute and catastrophic. In this sense the timing of the onset and the lack of previous symptoms place fulminant Wilson's disease in the ALF group.

Neoplastic Infiltration

Infiltration into the liver can occur with some cancers, resulting in liver failure. In the majority the diagnosis is apparent as part of end-stage carcinomatosis, but rarely infiltration into the liver can occur de novo and be the initial presentation. This occurs typically with lymphomas but has been reported with other forms of cancer. Hepatosplenomegaly and a raised alkaline phosphatase are often present. Other stigmata including palpable lymphadenopathy and marrow or peripheral blood film changes may be present. Imaging may be diagnostic, especially with massive hepatomegaly.

Budd-Chiari Syndrome

ALF secondary to Budd-Chiari syndrome is usually fatal without transplantation. The syndrome is defined as outflow obstruction to the hepatic veins, and the underlying pathogenesis is thrombosis in the majority, but tumor invasion or vascular membrane obstruction may be the cause. This is a rare disorder that occurs predominantly in young adults and affects more women than men. Overall, 5-year survival varies from 50% to 80% in different series.[81] Many patients with the syndrome have a predisposing disease state, either congenital or acquired, leading to a clotting abnormality such as a malignancy, myeloproliferative disorders, protein C or S deficiency, polycythemia rubra vera, lupus anticoagulant, antithrombin III deficiency, or antiphospholipid syndrome.[82] The fulminant form of the syndrome in which the patient develops encephalopathy within 8 weeks of the onset of symptoms is rare, and it is much more common for Budd-Chiari syndrome to present in a subacute form over a 3- or 4-month period, characterized by ascites, abdominal pain and hepatomegaly, jaundice, coagulopathy, raised AST, and alkaline phosphatase. Others present with signs of portal hypertension including refractory ascites and variceal bleeding and relatively intact hepatocellular function. The diagnosis is made with a combination of clinical presentation and imaging including Doppler ultrasound studies of the hepatic vessels, plus or minus liver histology, usually via the jugular route because of coagulopathy. The management of the syndrome depends on the manner in which it presents and the underlying cause. Medical management of the syndrome involves the use of anticoagulants and diuretics in an attempt to control ascites.

Thrombolysis can be attempted in selected patients with recent-onset disease.[83] In patients in whom there is progression to signs and symptoms of liver cell failure, some sort of portosystemic shunting procedure may reduce symptoms and prevent progression of the disease, allowing time for collateral vessels to develop. Transjugular intrahepatic portosystemic stent-shunt (TIPS) is most often attempted unless there is evidence of a hypertrophied caudate lobe and IVC compression, making mesoatrial shunting a better option. In patients with signs of liver failure, care must be used when considering a TIPS procedure because this can precipitate decompensation and rapid progression to ALF.[84] Liver transplantation is ultimately the only option in many patients in whom there is a failure of medical and shunt therapy, as well as in the fulminant presentation of the syndrome.[85] Anticoagulation is usually necessary in the immediate postoperative period.

Veno-Occlusive Disease of the Liver

Veno-occlusive disease (VOD) of the liver is a relatively common complication of myeloablative chemotherapy induction regimens in preparation for bone marrow transplantation (BMT), being seen in up to 54% in some series.[86] It was first described in children following the ingestion of herbal teas in South Africa. Pathologically it results from the nonthrombotic fibrous occlusion of centrolobular hepatic venules, and it represents a nonspecific response to certain noxious stimuli. Certain induction regimens such as high-dose cyclophosphamide and total body irradiation are implicated in the pathogenesis. The more aggressive induction regimens appear to result in a higher incidence of VOD. Recent reduction in incidence may be caused by a reduction in the use of myeloablative regimens and better monitoring of plasma drug concentrations.[87] The symptoms of VOD usually occur within 2 weeks of BMT. The development of jaundice, hepatomegaly, abdominal pain, and encephalopathy in the setting of recent BMT strongly suggests the diagnosis. Severe cases are characterized by evidence of hepatocellular necrosis and a high AST concentration. In 25% of cases, which are characterized as severe, the syndrome is progressive, leading to ALF.[88] Treatment options in these patients are limited because the outcome is poor with medical management or liver transplantation, although there is hope that newer therapies such as defibrotide, if initiated early before the onset of multiple organ failure, may improve the outlook.[87]

Ischemic Hepatitis

In patients with chronic congestive heart failure (CCHF), liver congestion is common. This is usually manifest as mild abnormalities of liver function tests, a prolonged prothrombin time, and mild ascites in some. Hepatic congestion is usually clinically inapparent unless jaundice is present, which can occur following multiple bouts of CCHF. Chronic congestion can lead to fibrosis and ultimately cirrhosis in some patients. Acute rises in serum transaminase and prolongation in prothrombin time, representing acute hepatic necrosis, most commonly develop in patients with CCHF when there is a sudden drop in cardiac output because of an event such as an arrhythmia or myocardial infarction (MI). It is relatively uncommon for the liver to become involved during shock states because of the huge redundancy in blood supply and the ability of the portal system to compensate for any reduction in hepatic arterial flow. If, however, portal flow is already compromised because of passive congestion, an acute drop in hepatic blood flow can result in ischemia. Ischemic hepatitis occurs uncommonly without a recognizable precipitant, but it can occur because of a silent MI or arrhythmia, for example. It can occur before the diagnosis of CCHF has been made or be the primary diagnostic event in a younger patient with cardiomyopathy. Clinically, severe ischemic hepatitis becomes apparent between 24 and 48 hours following an event and is manifest as huge rises in serum transaminase (up to 10 to 20 times normal). There is prolongation of the prothrombin time, encephalopathy, hypoglycemia, jaundice, and renal failure. The syndrome is usually self-limiting once the hemodynamic disturbance has receded, and there is a rapid fall in serum transaminases (usually 50% in the first 72 hours).[89] Occasionally there is progressive liver cellular failure leading rapidly to death. Management should be aimed at investigating and supporting the cardiovascular system.

Heat Stroke

Exertional heat stroke may occur in new recruits to the army or police force engaging in physical initiation programs. It can also occur in unacclimatized athletes in hot conditions or with drug overdoses such as cocaine. It is a potentially devastating syndrome that can lead to multiple organ failure and death. Liver involvement is usually seen as part of multisystem disorder. It ranges from mild involvement to ALF and is seen to develop during the first few days following the event. Management is supportive, and the majority improve over a period of days to weeks. Liver transplantation has been used in severe cases, but the outcome is poor because of coincident organ failure.[90]

Mushroom Poisoning

Many types of poisonous fungi in the world are responsible for various disorders that can be classified according to the type of poisoning and the timing of onset.[91]

A number of Fungi are associated with the induction of liver failure following ingestion. Of these the most common and most deadly are of the genus *Amanita*. *Amanita*-associated hepatotoxicity follows a triphasic response after ingestion. The first is a self-limiting, nonspecific, gastrointestinal upset that occurs within the first 6 to 24 hours. Nausea and vomiting, abdominal cramps, and diarrhea are often seen, and mushroom poisoning can mimic food poisoning. This is followed by a period of recovery and a few days later by progressive liver failure.

Management is essentially supportive. Although many specific therapies have been tried in the treatment of *Amanita* toxicity such as high-dose penicillin, silibinin, cimetidine, and NAC, none has been shown to improve outcome. Liver transplantation should be considered for patients with severe liver failure, and standard criteria apply.[91]

CLINICAL COURSE AND EARLY MANAGEMENT OF ACUTE LIVER FAILURE

History and Examination

The presentation and clinical course of ALF depends on its etiology and the rate of progression of the syndrome. This varies widely from admission via an emergency department following a paracetamol overdose or acute viral hepatitis versus admission from a hepatology outpatient department in a patient with progressive jaundice and ascites. Because of its relative rarity, the diagnosis can often be missed during initial contact; this may detrimentally influence the outcome.

The history will initially focus on the rate of progression of the illness and any clues to the etiology. The first symptoms are often the onset of jaundice (typically noticed by a relative). Any history of foreign travel or high-risk behavioral activity (IV drug use or unprotected intercourse) associated with the contraction of viral hepatitis should be investigated. A thorough drug history should be taken for prescribed and recreational drug use for the preceding 6 to 10 weeks. Drug therapy or recreational use that can induce or inhibit hepatic enzymes should be noted. If the patient or patient's relatives cannot provide this information, the patient's primary care physician should be contacted for help.

The history may be self-evident in the case of paracetamol hepatotoxicity, especially if the patient is self-presenting following deliberate self-harm. However, therapeutic misadventure, which is a relatively common cause of hepatotoxicity, may not be obvious unless considered by the physician. Any patient presenting with coma should have a drug screen including paracetamol.

Subacute liver failure is, by definition, a more insidious onset. Jaundice is often preceded by nonspecific symptoms of fatigue and general malaise. Abnormal liver enzymes will often be revealed during initial workup. Subsequent investigations will include viral, iron, copper, and genetic studies and, in addition, attempt to rule out decompensation of chronic liver disease as a cause of the current symptoms and signs. Liver biopsy may be considered in subacute liver failure.

Initial Resuscitation and Emergency Care

Patients presenting with acute or hyperacute liver failure tend to follow a similar course irrespective of etiology. Initial therapy and emergency care will be dictated by the condition of the patient at presentation. Liver failure is a multisystem disease and can progress rapidly to multiple organ failure.

Patients presenting with rapidly progressive hepatic encephalopathy via the emergency care system will often be intubated and ventilated at the time of, or shortly after, admission. The emergency physicians often perform a head CT scan because of diagnostic uncertainty.[50] The symptoms and signs of hepatic encephalopathy in ALF are subjectively different from those seen in decompensated chronic liver disease or in patients with stable chronic encephalopathy. Agitation and aggressive behavior are more common in ALF. This may be based on an increased turnover of the excitatory neurotransmitter glutamate in ALF associated with an acute increase in cerebral ammonia uptake.[92]

The West Haven criteria, designed to assess coma grade in patients with cirrhosis, are often applied to patients with ALF and are useful because of their familiarity.[93] However, once the patient becomes unconscious at grade IV encephalopathy, the scale does not provide any further information and is too crude to provide a clinically useful description of the level of consciousness. The Glasgow Coma Score, although not assessed specifically in this setting, is useful in relating clinical information to others.[23] Encephalopathy grade can progress quickly, especially with hyperacute presentation. Intubation and sedation are recommended once grade III encephalopathy is achieved because of the attendant risks to airway and possibilities of raised intracranial pressure (ICP) (Fig. 76-3).

Early contact with a regional liver center should be made for any patient with signs of acute severe liver dysfunction because serial blood results and clinical signs can be relayed to the center over the phone. Patients with paracetanol hepatotoxicity can often be managed over the phone, but plans for transfer can be made well in advance if necessary. As liver failure progresses over the next several days, a number of organ systems may become affected.

Following the safe and appropriate management of airway and breathing, focus can be directed to the correction of any circulatory dysfunction. Patients with ALF can progress rapidly to circulatory shock. The circulatory changes associated with ALF are predictable, usually associated with systemic vasodilation and relative hypovolemia. This can be profound and can require significant volume resuscitation. Underestimating the amount of fluid required in the early stages of ALF is easy, and the use of prognostic markers is unreliable before adequate circulatory function is restored. Monitoring at this stage should include a central venous catheter and direct arterial access for both blood pressure monitoring and for repeated blood tests. Care must be given to serum electrolytes because they often become deranged during this initial period. In particular, hyponatremia and hypophosphatemia are common.[94-96] This may be because of excess quantities of hypotonic fluid administration. A typical flow sheet of investigations of a patient presenting with paracetamol poisoning from a referring hospital is shown in Table 76-2.

Regardless of etiology, patients with significant liver damage or signs of secondary organ dysfunction should be managed within the ICU. The speed at which patients deteriorate can be rapid, and it is not uncommon for hepatic encephalopathy to progress from grade 0 to grade IV over several hours.

For prognostic reasons it is important not to correct any biochemical coagulopathy at this stage if possible. Despite quite significant prolongation of prothrombin

Table 76-2. Investigation of Acetaminophen Overdose*

Dates	7/10/2003	8/10/2003 AM	8/10/2003 PM	9/10/2003 AM
INR	2.08	3.17	3.79	6.2
Bilirubin	12	37		35
AST/ALT	273/223	8535/4254		15734/10060
Alk Phos				100
ALB	52	45		30
Glucose	4.1		7.5	5.2
Urea		5.5		3.0
Creatinine		86	83	128
pH		7.38	7.41	7.39
Lactate			5.4	

*A 20-year-old female intravenous drug user who took a 250-tablet overdose (500 mg acetaminophen tablets) the day before presentation at hospital. She received n-acetylcysteine 25 hours following overdose. The patient was transferred and listed for transplantation.
ALB, albumin; ALT, alanine aminotransferase; AST, aspartate aminotransferase; INR, international normalized ratio.

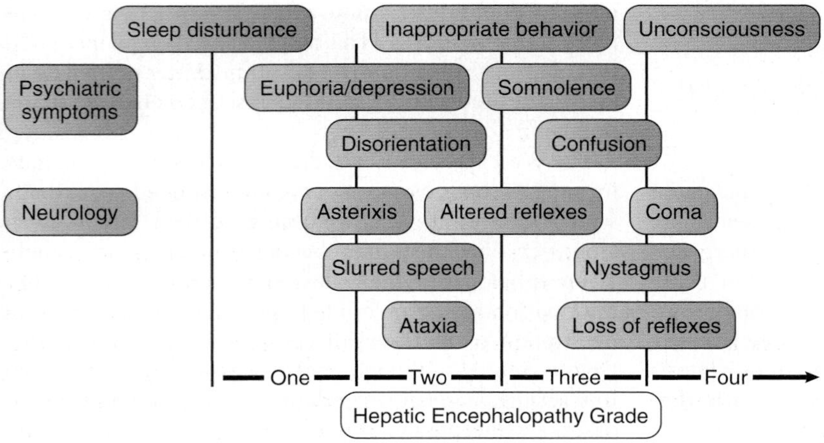

Figure 76-3. Hepatic encephalopathy grade in acute liver failure.

time, bleeding from line sites is uncommon in the initial stages of ALF. In fact, evidence indicates that the patients are prothrombotic in vivo.[97]

Investigation in a Patient with Suspected Acute Liver Failure

Initial investigations provide a baseline from which important diagnostic and prognostic information is taken. Serial blood test measurements should be performed as severity and prognosis are assessed over time from initial presentation (Table 76-3). Dependent on the manner and speed of presentation, a complete blood count, clotting, liver function tests, arterial blood gases, and ammonia should be performed twice daily, if not more often, in the early stages to assess progression of the illness. A liver ultrasound scan to assess liver size should be performed.

Transfer Criteria Guide

ALF is a sporadic syndrome with a case incidence of about 2000 per year in the United States.[98] Management is complex, and liver transplantation is the only effective therapy in severe cases. Transfer to a unit with experience in the management of these patients, preferably one with a liver transplant program, will provide optimal care. Deciding when or whether to transfer a patient with acute liver dysfunction is often difficult, and this will vary according to etiology and presentation. The best-described clinical course is that following severe paracetamol poisoning after a deliberate overdose.[37] Staggered overdose and therapeutic misadventure are less well defined, but the clinical and laboratory signs of severe disease are still present.

The following list of criteria for transfer is based on expert opinion; it has not been subjected to rigorous study and errs on the side of caution.[99]

- International normalized ratio (INR) greater than 3 in nonparacetamol etiologies
- A prothrombin time in seconds greater than hours since paracetamol overdose (e.g., INR 2.6 at 24 hours, 4.9 at 48 hours, 7.8 at 72 hours postoverdose)
- If the INR is still rising from day 3 and 4 following a timed paracetamol overdose
- If there is an elevated creatinine (>200 μmol/L) with a significantly raised INR (>3) or acidosis in any patient with ALF
- Significant hypoglycemia in any patient with ALF
- Any evidence of encephalopathy in any patient with ALF
- Anyone who is hypotensive (mean arterial pressure <60 mm Hg) following fluid resuscitation (mean blood pressure = systolic + 2 × diastolic/3)
- Anyone who has evidence of a persistent metabolic acidosis (pH <7.3), a significant base deficit (<–3), or a raised lactate following volume resuscitation

In patients with a subacute presentation, it is better to transfer them before they have progressed to grade II encephalopathy because of the additional complications associated with transferring ventilated patients.

Table 76-3. Initial Investigation and Common Findings in ALF

Investigations	Common Findings
Complete blood count	Platelets often low
Urea and electrolytes	Serum sodium often low, especially in paracetamol hepatotoxicity Urea often low because of reduced production Serum creatinine is a useful prognostic marker
Liver enzymes	AST/ALT variable, high in paracetamol toxicity Bilirubin a prognostic marker in nonparacetamol liver failure; can also be high in Wilson's disease because of hemolysis
Phosphate	Often low, especially in paracetamol toxicity Poor prognostic sign if high—suggests lack of regeneration
Magnesium	Often low
Prothrombin time, INR	Sensitive indicator of liver function Has prognostic significance in all forms of acute liver failure May improve with vitamin K if deficient
Viral serology for all known hepatotrophic viruses	
Urinary copper, plasma ceruloplasmin if Wilson's disease is suspected	Ceruloplasmin level often low but can be normal Urine copper usually high
Arterial ammonia	Has some prognostic value and may be an indicator of cerebral edema in patients at risk
Arterial whole blood lactate	Sensitive marker for liver function, particularly in paracetamol toxicity High levels indicative of poor prognosis
Serum glucose	Hypoglycemia common
Beta HCG in women	Unwanted pregnancy can be a precipitant of deliberate self-harm

HCG, human chorionic gonadotropin; INR, international normalized ratio.

Patients with acute or hyperacute liver failure showing signs of early encephalopathy should be intubated and ventilated prior to transfer. This can occasionally result in disagreement between referring hospitals and receiving liver units on how the transfer should be managed. Many anecdotal stories from liver units around the world have described patients who became unmanageable during transfer, in planes, helicopters, and road ambulances, resulting in injury to patients and staff.

Heroic transfers are almost always inappropriate. Patients should not be considered for transfer if they are on rapidly accelerating inotropic support, have severe hypoxemia, or already have fixed dilated pupils. In these cases, subjecting a patient to dying in an ambulance is pointless.

MANAGEMENT

Supportive Care

Airway and Ventilation

Patients with ALF who reach grade II or III encephalopathy require intubation and ventilation. This is usually necessary to provide safe management in the setting of increasing agitation, protection of the airway from stomach contents, or transfer from peripheral hospitals. In patients with severe liver failure it can be expected that encephalopathy grade will progress, so waiting until some predefined stage before intubation often delays adequate resuscitation and monitoring.

Controlled ventilation to a normal $PaCO_2$ is recommended at this stage. The use of hyperventilation is not indicated without further monitoring.[100,101]

Circulation

The circulatory changes associated with ALF can be profound.[102] The pathologic basis for this is incompletely understood but similar in many ways to changes observed in patients with a systemic inflammatory response caused by sepsis or trauma. The pattern observed depends on the etiology and rate of onset of the syndrome. In hyperacute liver failure caused by paracetamol overdose, patients can develop fulminant peripheral cardiovascular collapse that can be an early mode of death.[103] Others with a more subacute onset can develop peripheral vascular changes similar to those with decompensated chronic liver disease and hepatorenal failure. Loss of vascular tone results in peripheral vasodilation. When compounded by vomiting, especially in POD, this results in both relative and actual hypovolemia and hypotension.

Fluid resuscitation should be commenced as soon as possible after presentation and should be directed by invasive monitoring. The type of fluid used for resuscitation has not been subjected to a controlled trial in this setting, but it has been shown that hypertonic saline infusion reduces the incidence of intracranial hypertension in patients with ALF.[94] Hypoglycemia should be avoided.

If mean arterial pressure remains less than 65 mm Hg following adequate fluid resuscitation, a vasopressor should be started. Norepinephrine is the vasopressor of choice because it induces vasoconstriction without the induction of lactate production, as often seen with the use of epinephrine, although epinephrine has been used successfully in this setting.

Vasopressin and its longer-acting analogue terlipressin have been used as vasopressors in septic and cardiogenic shock.[104,105] Terlipressin results in profound systemic vasoconstriction and has the potential to result in worsening oxygen delivery and consumption. It has been shown to increase intracranial hypertension in ALF due to an increase in cerebral blood volume because of the breakdown in cerebrovascular autoregulation.[106] Because of its relatively long half-life and difficulty with dosing, as well as the association with increased intracranial hypertension, the use of terlipressin cannot be recommended.

The majority of patients presenting with ALF are young adults, and as a result comorbid cardiac dysfunction is usually absent. Cardiac depression has been reported in association with POD.[103] On occasion cardiac disease can present as ALF in the case of ischemic hepatitis, as discussed previously.

Relative adrenal insufficiency has been shown to occur in patients with septic shock, decompensated chronic liver disease, and ALF.[29,31,107,108] The use of stress doses of corticosteroids has been shown to reduce norepinephrine requirements in patients with ALF.[109]

Renal Failure

Renal failure is common in ALF, with a reported incidence of up to 70%.[110] Paracetamol toxicity causes direct renal tubular dysfunction, possibly by affecting membrane protein function. Occasionally renal failure is the predominant organ affected.[111,112] As a result, renal failure can be expected in this setting. Although it is most commonly associated with POD, the incidence in other etiologies such as Wilson's disease, because of the direct toxic effects of copper, is also high.

Consensus is lacking regarding the classification and definition of renal dysfunction in the critically ill, although attempts are being made to remedy this situation.[113] The term *acute tubular necrosis* is inadequate in the setting of critical illness because it fails to describe the full spectrum of renal dysfunction. This is even truer in the setting of ALF. In addition, the use of the term *hepatorenal syndrome* in ALF is also inappropriate because this definition does not adequately describe the often rapid clinical deterioration. This is not to say that altered systemic and renal hemodynamics do not contribute to the pathophysiology of renal failure as they do in critical illness in general. In the subacute presentation of this syndrome early renal dysfunction can be similar to that seen in end-stage chronic liver disease, with sodium and water retention in the absence of intrinsic renal damage.[114]

Management of renal failure is essentially the same as in ALF and other forms of multiple organ failure and consists of maintenance of intravascular volume, cardiac output, and mean arterial pressure.[98]

Extracorporeal renal support is necessary in most patients with ALF at some time. Continuous veno-venous hemofiltration (CVVH) is the most efficient and safest method for renal support and should be started early.[115] Indications for the early use of renal support are not just limited to oliguria. CVVH has been shown to improve hemodynamic stability in patients with critical illness and has been used as salvage therapy in patients on high dose vasopressor. Survival advantage relative to dose has also been shown.[116] In addition it can be used to induce hypothermia in the setting of raised ICP. It also enables the infusions of large quantities of blood products and drugs, often required during intensive care, helping to maintain fluid balance. High-volume hemofiltration (4000 mL/hour ultrafiltrate exchange) has been studied in ALF and shown to reduce serum lactate, base deficit, and norepinephrine requirements, when compared with historical controls, although survival benefit has not been shown.[117]

Patients with liver failure do not tolerate the lactate load associated with lactate-buffered replacement fluid during CVVH. In fact, the rapid infusion of lactate can induce a systemic acidosis in this setting.[118] Also, the infusion of large quantities of lactate containing fluid reduces the utility of serum lactate as one of the most important prognostic indicators.[119] As a consequence the use of bicarbonate hemofiltration is recommended.[120]

CVVH can often be performed successfully without anticoagulation in ALF. Paradoxically, patients with ALF appear to be hypercoagulable, in vivo, despite prolonged coagulation parameters. This may be because of a reduction in protein C production.[97] If required, a loading dose of 2000 units of heparin and thereafter 500 to 1000 units an hour depending on the activated clotting time can be used if needed to allow CVVH. If bleeding is a problem or there is severe thrombocytopenia, epoprostenol should be instituted (2.5 to 5 ng/kg/min) either alone or in association with low-dose heparin (100 units/hour). Blood flow rates of 200 mL/min and above will help with filter life.

Cerebral Edema

Etiology

Cerebral edema was noted and commented on in the seminal clinicopathologic review of servicemen presenting with fulminant epidemic hepatitis during the East Asian campaign of World War II.[38] However, the recognition that cerebral edema was a distinct clinical entity and cause of death associated with ALF did not become clear until much later.[121,122]

The recognition that brain swelling is an important component of ALF is now well established. Management strategies place the risk of intracranial hypertension (IHT) at the forefront of care and prophylactic therapy. Monitoring and treatment and are widely debated in the literature.[123,124]

The pathology of cerebral edema and intracranial hypertension in ALF is not completely understood, but in recent years progress has been made into the processes involved.[125] Ammonia has long been implicated as important in hepatic encephalopathy and, as the evidence mounts, increasingly recognized as an important factor in the etiology of cerebral edema in ALF.[126] Recent work has shown that whole blood ammonia predicts outcome and the chances of cerebral herniation.[127,128] Electron-microscopic analysis of postmortem brain biopsy, together with gravimetric analysis of brain water content in animal models has shown that swelling occurs in the gray matter and that astrocytes are the main target.[129,130] Ammonia is detoxified in astrocytes by combining with glutamate to produce glutamine. Astrocytes are the only cell type in the brain that contain glutamine synthetase, and this normal pathway maintains the ratio of glutamate to glutamine within astrocytes and neurons. The raised serum ammonia induces a buildup of glutamine within astrocytes, increasing the osmotic potential, absorption of water, and volume. Evidence of this effect can be inferred by the fact that inhibition of glutamine synthetase, which catalyzes the reaction, prevents brain swelling in experimental models.[131] An osmotic effect may not be the only mechanism by which glutamine induces cellular swelling, but circumstantial evidence indicates that it occurs to some extent. In subacute and chronic liver disease there is time for adaptation to the increase in astrocyte osmotic potential by the excretion of intracellular osmolytes such as myo-inositol.[132] In ALF there is no time for adaptation because of the rapid increase in intracellular glutamine. Recently, however, the direct correlation between astrocyte glutamine levels and cell volume has been questioned. Experimental data have not been able to show a correlation between the two, with peak glutamine levels occurring before cellular volume reaches its maximum.[133,134] Clinical study using cerebral microdialysis has shown abnormal glutamate/glutamine trafficking within the brain extracellular space, with initial high levels of glutamate but then a reduction to low levels without any correlation with ICP.[92] Extracellular lactate concentration was shown to rise prior to surges in ICP, however.[92]

A breakdown in cellular energy metabolism induced by an increase in intracellular glutamine and ammonia is another possible mechanism for the cellular swelling. Impairment of alpha-ketoglutarate dehydrogenase and pyruvate dehydrogenase induced by oxidative stress and ammonia results in a breakdown in astrocyte energy production and an increase in glycolysis. This is supported by an increase in extracellular lactate and brain lactate flux in clinical studies.[92,100] Mitochondrial dysfunction induced by ammonia may also play a role.[126]

In addition to the cytotoxic edema seen early in ALF, changes in cerebral blood volume may play an important role in the development of intracranial hypertension. Cerebral blood flow shows wide variation in patients with ALF, and the normal close relationship between cerebral metabolism and flow appears to be lost.[135] In animal models of liver failure a gradual increase in cerebral blood flow occurs, but this situation is less clear in human studies.[125,136] Cerebral metabolism is generally reduced in high-grade encephalopathy and there is a breakdown in vascular autoregulation. Evidence indicates that relative or absolute cerebral hyperemia can contribute to intracranial hypertension.[106,137] An increase in cerebral blood flow may induce intracranial hypertension by a number of mechanisms and induce further cerebral swelling. This could occur because of an increased flux of potentially toxic metabolites such as ammonia or by an increase in cerebral water content because of an increase in cerebrovascular hydrostatic pressure. Neither hypothesis has been proved, and the evidence indicates that the blood-brain barrier is relatively intact in ALF, suggesting that hydrostatic or vasogenic edema is uncommon.[130] Autoregulation is lost in ALF.[136,138] The cause is unknown, but a gradual cerebral vasoparesis concurs with clinical observation. Autoregulation can be restored by hyperventilation and mild hypothermia but not by the use of indomethacin.[139] It has been suggested that the increase in astrocyte glutamine plays a role in this gradual vasoparalysis and loss of autoregulation by the induction of local nitric oxide or carbon monoxide.[125] It is relatively common to find a patient with a high ICP and jugular venous oxygen saturation above 80%. This suggests a state of luxury perfusion (unregulated blood supply in excess of demand) in which an increase in cerebral blood volume in an already swollen brain accounts for the associated increase in ICP.[140]

Management

In the management of IHT in ALF it is important to target those at risk. IHT remains a leading cause of death despite advances in the understanding of etiology and management of patients.[141,142] Monitoring the brain is difficult and invasive. Despite investigation a reliable noninvasive method for the evaluation of cerebral blood flow, cerebral oxygenation, and ICP remains elusive.[143] Important points must be considered when managing a patient with ALF and possible raised ICP:

- Prediction of patients at risk of IHT
- How to monitor the brain
- Prophylactic management
- Treatment of established IHT

Predicting Intracranial Hypertension

In ALF the development of cerebral edema is seen in patients with the shortest time between the development of jaundice and the onset of encephalopathy.[37] A fulminating presentation, lack of time for cerebral adaptation, and systemic burden of a necrotic liver appear to be the likely reasons. Patients with paracetamol toxicity make up the largest number in this group. Other etiologies can fall into the hyperacute group including patients with ALF caused by hepatotrophic viruses, particularly hepatitis B. In contrast, patients with subacute liver failure caused by non-A or non-B hepatitis have a smaller risk.

The incidence of IHT following paracetamol toxicity has fallen since the mid-1980s.[144] However, it still represents a significant complication in this setting. Recent work from King's College Hospital (KCH) in London suggests an incidence of 20% to 30% in all patients with ALF.[141] Data from our own unit suggest that intracranial hypertension is implicated in the death of 25% of all patients with ALF and 35% of those following paracetamol-induced toxicity.[142]

Young age has consistently been found to be a risk factor.[121,141] Arterial ammonia concentration has been shown to correlate with death and cerebral herniation.[127,128,145] Recent commentary suggests that arterial ammonia should be measured serially in all patients with ALF, and ICP monitoring be instituted if the concentration is greater or equal to 150 μmol/L.[140]

Monitoring the Brain

A number of monitoring devices and methods can be undertaken to screen for raised ICP or cerebral ischemia or both. Some of these are more invasive than others, and the possible risks and benefits need to be understood.

Computed tomography is a standard investigation tool in any patient with suspected intracranial pathology. Cerebral edema can be recognized in CT scans of patients with ALF. The severity correlates crudely to encephalopathy grade, but the correlation between imaging and severity of ICP measurement is poor.[146,147] As little additional information is gained, careful consideration should be undertaken before transporting this sick group of patients to the CT scanner. Occasionally, if there are diagnostic difficulties or a suspected complication of ICP bolt insertion, CT scanning might be considered.

Functional brain imaging using single positron emission tomography (SPECT) has been used to investigate the distribution of cerebral blood flow in ALF, and MRI scanning has been used to investigate the distribution of intracerebral water, but neither has found a place in clinical practice.[101,148]

In patients with suspected IHT the direct monitoring of cerebral oxygenation and blood flow are appealing, but current methods have technical and clinical limitations. Tissue PO_2 and interstitial metabolites, using intra-parenchymal probes, have been investigated in traumatic brain injury and to a limited extent in ALF.[92,149] They have the advantage in traumatic injury of providing localized information around the area of injury. The use of cerebral microdialysis (sampling of the cerebral interstitial fluid using a micro-coaxial catheter with a semi-permeable membrane) remains a research tool in ALF at present.

Methods used for the estimation of global cerebral oxygenation include the sampling of jugular venous (JV) blood for oxygen saturation and products of metabolism such as lactate. A JV saturation of less than 55% suggests an ischemic brain. This can be caused by a reduction in blood flow in excess of demand because of brain swelling or cerebral vasoconstriction caused by hypocarbia, if the patient is being hyperventilated. An increase in demand because of seizure activity can also manifest as a reduction in JV saturation.[150] High JV saturation (>80%) may represent a hyperemic brain, and steps can be taken to reduce cerebral blood volume if ICP is raised. High JV saturation is often seen as a terminal event and may represent a complete loss of oxygen extraction by the brain (Fig. 76-4).

Near infrared spectroscopy is a noninvasive technique used to assess the oxygen content of various organs. It can be used to determine cerebral oxygenation and changes in cerebral perfusion in ALF and warrants further investigation.[151]

Noninvasive measurement of cerebral blood flow using transcranial Doppler has been investigated in ALF and found to be predictive of changes in cerebral blood flow induced by hyperventilation; however, the technique does not provide data on cerebral oxygenation and so cannot be recommended without the addition of a JV catheter.[152]

The recognition that ICP is raised in a significant proportion of patients with ALF and that this is implicated in significant morbidity and mortality has led to the use of

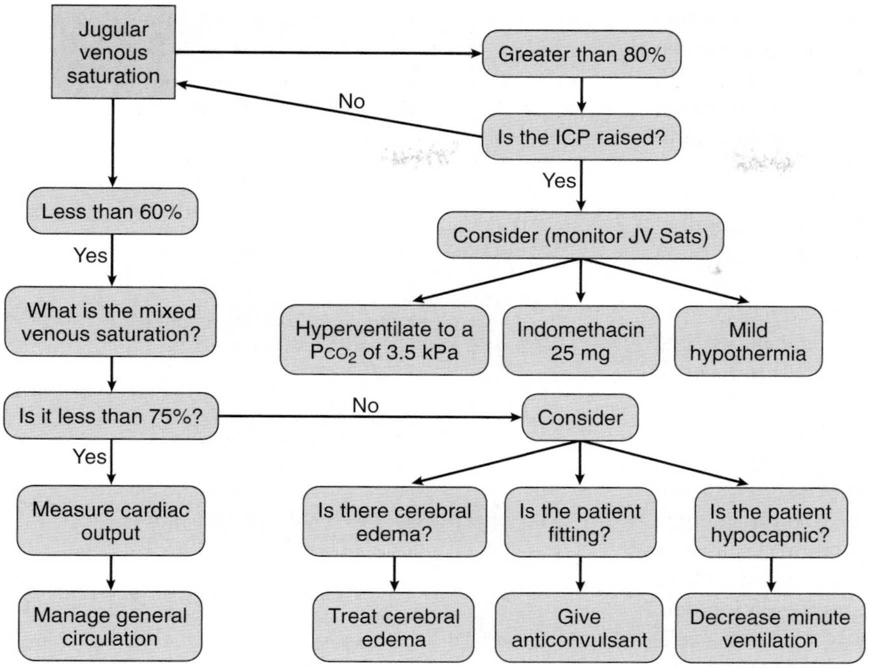

Figure 76-4. Monitoring cerebral oxygenation with jugular bulb sampling. Sats, oxygen saturation.

direct measurement of ICP with various forms of monitoring.[121,153] These techniques, although fully supported internationally in traumatic brain injury, are controversial in the field of ALF, and a dichotomy of opinion remains in most countries with some units using them and others not.[123,124,154,155]

Controversy revolves around the lack of evidence of improved outcome with the monitoring of ICP and the risk of intracranial bleeding complicating insertion. The reported risk of bleeding, from survey data, is between 10% and 20% overall, the majority of which is not clinically significant. Mortality is reportedly between 1% and 3% (Alistair Lee, Edinburgh, personal communication).[153,155] The risk of bleeding following placement is higher than that seen following traumatic brain injury. Uncontrolled evidence indicates that activated factor VII can reduce this risk.[156]

Proving that ICP monitoring improves survival in ALF has not been possible, because a randomized controlled clinical trial has not been performed to evaluate it. However, it is generally accepted that medical intervention can reduce ICP and prevent cerebral ischemia and brain herniation in patients with ALF.[140] Published data suggest that the intervention rate is increased in patients with ICP monitors compared with those without them, and monitoring increases the length of survival in the critical care unit, if not overall survival.[157] The majority of patients with ALF die of multiple organ failure because of sepsis, however. Intervention to reduce ICP may just prevent early cerebral death.

Although the risks of monitoring are documented, the risks of not monitoring are less clear. Without monitoring ICP there are tendencies toward therapeutic paralysis because of uncertainty and toward managing all patients as if they had raised ICP. The reassurance of a normal ICP enables a reduction in sedation and paralysis. It allows tracheal suctioning and other nursing care without the uncertainty of worsening an unknown ICP. With ICP monitoring, modest increases in ICP can be treated early before clinical signs suggest impending brain herniation. Monitoring ICP permits the calculation of cerebral perfusion pressure and together with the monitoring of JV oxygen saturation allows a more complete picture of cerebral perfusion and oxygenation. The use of ICP monitoring has been advocated in the setting of liver transplantation for ALF and, of course, facilitates continued clinical research into the management of cerebral edema.

Prophylactic Measures

In patients at high risk of cerebral edema a number of prophylactic interventions have been shown to reduce the incidence of intracranial hypertension.

Serum sodium is often low in patients with ALF. In a consecutive group of patients with ALF from POD admitted to KCH liver ICU, 65% were hyponatremic on arrival (Will Bernal, personal communication). Hyponatremia is associated with a poor outcome in ALF.[158] On the basis of retrospective data showing an inverse relationship between ICP and serum sodium in patients with ALF, moderate hypernatremia was investigated as a possible prophylactic intervention.[94,159] Maintaining serum sodium between 145 and 155 mmol/L using hypertonic saline was found to reduce ICP from baseline and reduce the incidence of surges in ICP.[94] Hypothermia improves outcome following out-of-hospital cardiac arrest and has been investigated in patients with traumatic brain injury. Early reports suggest that hypothermia can reduce ICP and ammonia production in patients with ALF. Prophylactic hypothermia is currently being investigated in this setting. Simple measures such as raising the head of the bed to a 30-degree angle and avoidance of excessive stimulation are also prudent.

Cerebral Perfusion Pressure

In traumatic brain injury there is a consensus of opinion supporting the use of cerebral perfusion pressure (CPP) as a treatment goal.[160] In ALF the concept of CPP-directed therapy is less useful. To assume a correlation with cerebral blood flow, there must be a consistent cerebrovascular resistance and this is not the case in ALF.[161] This is because of the loss of cerebrovascular autoregulation, and attempts to increase cerebral perfusion are often unsuccessful because the use of a vasopressor results in an increase in ICP as brain blood volume increases.[106,162] However, this is not to say that CPP should be ignored entirely but that the safe lower limit of CPP has yet to be defined because there are many reports of patients surviving with normal cerebral function despite a low CCP.[163] The normal lower limit of cerebral autoregulation is reached at a mean arterial blood pressure of about 50 mm Hg, below which flow becomes pressure dependent. In patients with absent autoregulation, such as in ALF, CCP should probably be maintained above 40 mm Hg (the normal lower limit of autoregulation with an ICP ≤10 mm Hg), but no data exist to back this statement up. Maintenance of CPP in ALF is best achieved by decreasing ICP and aiming for a mean arterial pressure with fluid and vasopressor that does not increase ICP above 25 mm Hg. Attempting to improve cerebral oxygen balance is also attractive in this setting. This may be attempted with intravenous indomethacin (has been shown to improve CPP without compromising cerebral oxygenation), hypothermia, increased sedation, and hyperventilation.[139,164-166] Monitoring cerebral oxygenation is useful during such maneuvers.[161]

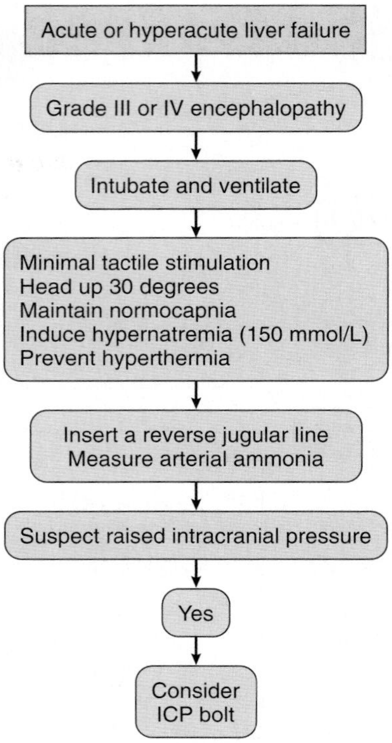

Figure 76-5. Initial management of patient with high-grade encephalopathy.

Treatment of Established Intracranial Pressure

In patients at risk of or with suspected cerebral edema, prophylactic measures should be instituted. The clinical team must decide whether to insert an ICP bolt. If inserted, there is the potential to manage ICP.

ICP is normally less than 15 mm Hg in an adult. The definition of IHT is not precise and will vary between patients. Available data are derived from patients with traumatic brain injury (TBI) in whom observational studies suggest that intervention to reduce pressure should be instituted between 20 and 25 mm Hg, although pupillary abnormalities and brain herniation can occur at lower pressures.[167] No studies have investigated treatment threshold in ALF, so similar thresholds to TBI are used.

The management of IHT is usually escalated along standard algorithms (Figs. 76-5 and 76-6). One should elevate the patient to an angle of 30 degrees and avoid tight straps around the neck to encourage venous drainage. ICP tends to increase during nursing intervention. If this takes more than a couple of minutes to recover, it can suggest poor intracranial compliance. Treatment is usually instituted for a sustained rise in ICP (>5 to 10 mm Hg minutes) or clinical signs suggesting cerebral ischemia or impending herniation. Sedation should be increased. Propofol is probably the agent of choice.[143] Osmotherapy is the mainstay of treatment following these simple measures. Mannitol as a rapid infusion (0.5 to 1 g/kg) has been shown to reduce ICP reliably in ALF.[168] The dose can be repeated, but care must be used in renal failure because of accumulation and multiple administrations can result in a hyperosmolar syndrome. Plasma osmolality should be monitored if multiple doses are used. Current practice is to remove 500 mL of ultrafiltrate via CVVH following each bolus dose of mannitol. Bolus doses of 20 mL hypertonic saline (30%) have a similar effect to mannitol in this setting (personal observation). Hypertonic saline has a higher reflectance coefficient at the blood brain barrier (BBB) compared with mannitol, and there appears to be less tachyphylaxis to multiple administration.[94]

In patients with a raised ICP and cerebral hyperemia, suggested by a jugular venous oxygen saturation of 80% or greater (luxury perfusion), short-term hyperventilation will induce cerebral vasoconstriction and reduce blood volume. This maneuver has not been shown to impair cerebral oxygenation, but close monitoring of cerebral oxygenation should be employed if it is attempted.[166] Short-term hyperventilation has not been shown to improve outcome in ALF but does prolong survival in the ICU.[169] Hyperventilation may be life saving and buy time for definitive treatment (transplantation). Indomethacin induces cerebral vasoconstriction and reduces ICP in patients with both TBI and ALF without impairing cerebral oxygenation, although confirmatory studies are necessary.[139]

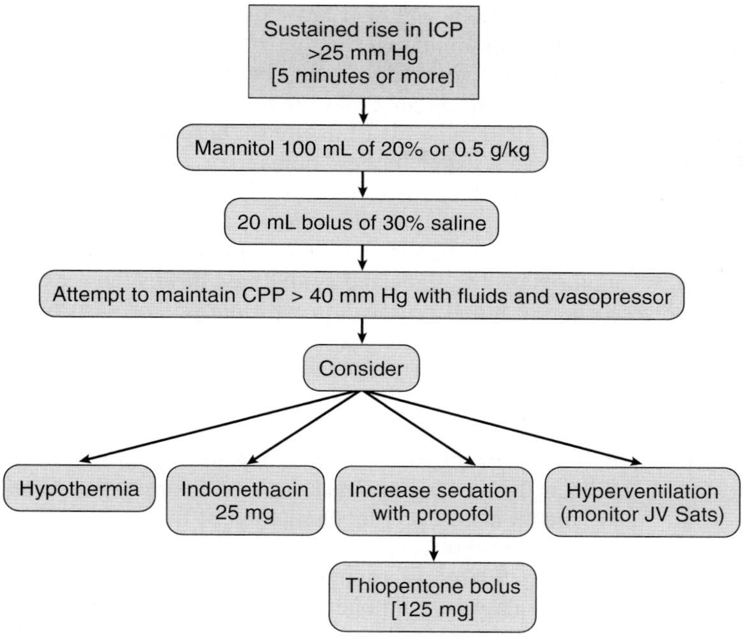

Figure 76-6. Management of a sustained rise in intracranial pressure (ICP). Sats, oxygen saturation.

Seizures

Ammonia toxicity and cerebral edema are associated with seizure activity, and it has been recognized that subclinical seizures occur more commonly than previously thought.[150] The use of mechanical ventilation assisted by sedatives and muscular paralysis can mask clinical signs. Seizures, which adversely affect cerebral oxygen consumption and may contribute to cerebral edema, are a cause of low jugular oxygen saturation. It has been suggested that prophylactic phenytoin be used in all patients with ALF and high-grade encephalopathy. Others have questioned this approach because of the significant side effects and apparent lack of effect on outcome.[170] If confirmed, seizure activity should be managed along standard management guidelines.

Infection and Immunosuppression

Patients with ALF have multiple immune defects and are susceptible to infections.[171] Infection is a common cause of progression and complications in ALF.[172] Antibiotic prophylaxis has been shown to reduce the incidence of infection and enable transplantation to proceed but has not been shown to improve survival. Selective decontamination of the digestive tract has not been shown to be superior to IV antibiotics alone.[171,173]

Current practice is to prescribe broad-spectrum antibacterial and antifungal medication to patients with ALF depending on local sensitivities. The general trend is that gram-positive infections occur earlier than gram-negative infections. Early gram-negative infections tend to be less resistant endogenous bacteria, followed later by resistant hospital-acquired organisms.[174]

Nutrition

Within the general intensive care literature there is a consensus toward enteral nutrition (EN) as the route of choice.[175] Additional data on which to base decisions in patients with ALF are scarce. However, wide regional variation exists in the prescribing of parenteral nutrition (PN) compared with EN. The reason for this is unclear because EN is associated with a reduction in infectious complications.[175] However, some centers clearly prefer PN.[176]

Nutritional requirements in ALF are not well understood. Energy expenditure is raised during ALF. This is surprising considering the normal contribution of the liver, a large metabolically active organ, on the overall energy expenditure, illustrated by the effects of hepatectomy on energy expenditure during elective liver transplantation.[177] Organ-specific lactate production exists in both the liver and lungs, as well as evidence of a systemic inflammatory response in many patients.[172,178,179] The cause of systemic inflammation in ALF is activation of inflammatory cells (leukocytes and endothelium) and the release of systemic cytokines. This may be initiated by infection.[172] Patients in the early stages of ALF are markedly catabolic with insulin resistance despite the frequent presence of a hypoglycemic state.[180] The Harris-Benedict equation is inaccurate in ALF, and indirect calorimetry should be used if energy requirements are sought.

Hypoglycemia is common because of the failure of both glycogenolysis and gluconeogenesis. Massive hepatic necrosis can result in a precipitous fall in serum glucose concentration. For this reason an infusion of 50% glucose should be used at least until feeding is established. Low-volume, high concentrations of glucose are preferred to reduce the infusion of large quantities of water and the resultant hyponatremia if lower concentrations are used.

Serum amino acids are consistently deranged during liver failure. A low or normal concentration of glutamine, branched chain amino acids, and tryptophan is found, and there tends to be an increase in other amino acids.[181] High brain concentration of ammonia is thought to contribute to cerebral edema and encephalopathy in ALF. Manipulation of ingested amino acids has been investigated in an attempt to reduce ammonia concentration. L-ornithine and L-arginine (LOLA) infusions encourage alternate pathway metabolism and reduce hepatic encephalopathy in chronic liver disease.[182] LOLA has been investigated in animal models of ALF and has resulted in normalization of plasma ammonia concentration, significant delay in the onset of encephalopathy, and a reduction in brain water concentration.[183] This simple treatment method has not been investigated in ALF but would seem to warrant further investigation. NAC is primarily used as a glutathione precursor and antidote in paracetamol poisoning but is used widely in patients with ALF induced by other causes and later in its subsequent course. Evidence is lacking for its use outside the first 24 hours post paracetamol poisoning.

Little evidence suggests that protein restriction has any role in ALF, and protein requirements based on total calorie ingestion should be used. Some authorities have suggested that lactulose therapy may reduce ammonia concentration and increase survival time in patients with ALF, but this needs confirmation and cannot be recommended at this time.[184]

Serum electrolytes are often deranged in the early stages of ALF. Hypophosphatemia is common in patients with ALF and is a good prognostic sign. High or normal phosphate may indicate a lack of hepatic regeneration and renal impairment.[95] Hypomagnesemia is also common and should be corrected.

ARTIFICIAL LIVER SUPPORT

At present, liver transplantation is the only form of definitive therapy for severe hepatic failure. However, the scarcity of organs and potential for delay in transplantation, together with a proportion of patients who will make a full recovery if supported while the liver regenerates, suggest that there would be a role for some kind of liver support system.

The liver is a complex organ and, to be an ideal liver replacement, any system must support a wide range of biosynthetic and metabolic functions (Box 76-2). Any working system will also have to counter the systemic effects of the dying liver.[185]

Artificial liver support can be split into two main approaches. In the first there is an attempt to simulate or replace all or most liver functions. These systems include hepatocytes from either human or animal sources. Another view of liver failure suggests that toxins either excreted by the dying liver or not metabolized because of an acute reduction in function are responsible for the majority of the signs and symptoms. In this view extracorporeal blood purification with dialysis or adsorption techniques are employed, and serum proteins not produced are replaced with plasma.

Box 76-2

Liver Functions

- Excretion of bilirubin, cholesterol, hormones, and drugs
- Metabolism of fats, proteins, and carbohydrates
- Enzyme activation
- Storage of glycogen, vitamins, and minerals and regulation of glucose levels
- Synthesis of plasma proteins such as albumin, clotting factors, and bile production
- Blood detoxification and purification
- Immune regulation

Biologic Systems

Biologic systems consist of a bioreactor within which the cellular biomass is contained and a mechanism of separating the biomass from the circulation of the patient. They require an extracorporeal system to deliver blood or plasma to the bioreactor and may also contain an adsorption or dialysis component. Data from liver resection suggests that approximately 250 mL of liver by volume is required to prevent death from liver failure. This typically represents 20% to 30% of liver mass.[186] More may be necessary to counter the effects of a dying necrotic liver.

Possible cell types to use as the biomass include animal or human primary hepatocytes or other forms of cell line with hepatocyte phenotype. Primary hepatocytes outperform other cell lines but are of limited availability and tend to have a time-dependent loss of hepatic phenotype. In addition, scaling up production with primary hepatocytes is difficult because they do not readily undergo cell division under laboratory conditions. Instead they must be directly seeded into the bioreactor either immediately following harvest or following a period of storage and cryopreservation. Human cells are limited in availability but can be obtained from unused livers and cutdown grafts. Theoretically, animal cells are readily available but uncertainty about possible cross infection from animal pathogen to the patient with organisms such as porcine endogenous retrovirus and incompatibility of secreted antigens render them far from ideal. Therefore regulatory authorities are often reluctant to sanction their use.

Immortalized cell lines that proliferate in culture, although retaining some liver-specific functionality, can be used in an attempt to overcome the limitations of primary hepatocytes. Many lines have been created by retroviral transfection with regulatory genes that stimulate cell division. The insertion of "terminator" genes that give the cells a limited life or enable switching off of the immortalizing gene have also been developed to improve safety.[187] Other sources of immortal and readily cultured cells are tumor derived, such as the ubiquitous Hep G2/C3A hepatoblastoma line. Finally, stem cell sources appear to offer the most hope in terms of a readily available and functional supply of differentiated hepatocytes.[188]

Clinical trials in the use of bioartificial liver support have been relatively disappointing. The bio-artificial liver uses porcine hepatocytes and a charcoal column in series. The largest trial published so far in the field was powered for survival advantage in ALF and primary nonfunction following liver transplantation.[189] The study was terminated early by the data and safety monitoring board because the trial was likely to be futile on the basis of the results at interim analysis.[189] Post hoc analysis suggested some effect in the ALF group alone. The Extracorporeal Liver Assist Device (ELAD) system uses the Hep G2/C3A hepatoblastoma line and has been investigated in a number of phase 1 studies designed to report safety and activity.[190,191] The most recent study was a randomized controlled study, not powered for mortality, which showed a trend for improved survival in the treatment group.[191] Other small case series and controlled trials with various systems have been reported over the past 10 years.[192-194]

Nonbiologic Systems

Many of the molecules that accumulate within the blood during ALF are small or middle sized.[185] These can be targeted by a variety of extracorporeal purification techniques including dialysis through various types of membrane and adsorption onto carriers such as charcoal, resins, or albumin.

Nonbiologic systems are attractive because they are relatively inexpensive (compared with biologic systems) and logistically much easier to implement.

Early work with hemodialysis was unsuccessful and was largely abandoned with the conclusion that the toxemia of ALF was not solely caused by small water-soluble molecules. The advent of synthetic membranes in the 1970s rekindled the interest in convective therapy for ALF. These allowed larger molecules to pass through compared with the cuprophane alternatives. Opolon[195] reported clinical improvement with the use of high-permeability membrane hemodialysis and hemofiltration in patients with ALF. Hemofiltration, as a form of renal support, is used in most liver critical care units as part of general supportive care, and there is some evidence that increased convective exchange, with high volume (>35 mL/kg/hour) hemofiltration, is associated with improved hemodynamic stability and improved encephalopathy scores.[117,195]

Charcoal hemoperfusion has been investigated extensively. Initial trials were encouraging, but later larger randomized controlled trials were unable to show an improvement in outcome.[110] Large-volume plasma exchange showed some improvement in hemodynamics and other parameters in initial studies.[196] The therapy is logistically difficult to perform and, like total exchange transfusion, is an inefficient method of clearing the toxemia of ALF.

In an attempt to improve the efficacy of dialysis techniques, adsorbents have been added to the dialysis fluid to widen the range of molecules removed. The two most extensively studied are charcoal suspension in the BioLogic-DT system and 20% albumin in the molecular adsorbent recirculating system (MARS).

Both the BioLogic-DT and MARS have been shown to improve blood pressure, increase vascular resistance, and improve short-term encephalopathy scores in patients with AoCLF. The results of studies into their utility in ALF is less clear-cut, with inconsistent results from small uncontrolled series and case reports. With MARS therapy there appears to be an increase in peripheral vascular resistance and concomitant reduction in cardiac index in the short term. There does not appear to be any consistent effect on IHT.[197,198] Similar results have been reproduced with high-volume hemofiltration, pointing to the need for comparative randomized controlled trials.[117]

A meta-analysis of all randomized controlled trials in nonbiologic liver support concluded that there was an improvement in short-term mortality in AoCLF but that this could not be shown in ALF.[199,200]

LIVER TRANSPLANTATION

When and Whom to Transplant

Liver transplantation for ALF was used sporadically during the 1980s but has gained pace since then and now has a huge impact. It remains the only definitive form of therapy for some patients.

Timing is important, and in those with severe liver injury there is a window of opportunity beyond which transplantation often becomes futile because of deteriorating organ function.[201] It was recognized early in the history of transplantation for ALF that the challenge was to develop robust prognostic indicators. These must be sensitive, early enough to provide maximum advantage to the patient, and specific enough not to result in unnecessary transplants.

A "super-urgent" designation exists in the national transplant sharing scheme in the United Kingdom, and a similar "category 1A" designation exists in the United States—see http://www.unos.org/ for details. These categories recognize the role of early transplantation in ALF and the detrimental effect of delay in this setting.

In the United Kingdom the super-urgent designation (Table 76-4) is closely linked to the prognostic score developed in KCH in the late 1980s using retrospective multivariate analysis with prospective validation.[202] The prognostic criteria have been subsequently validated in other centers and shown to be robust.[203] Other criteria have been developed.[204]

The criteria are not perfect. First, despite their good specificity (i.e., if the patient achieves criteria that they are likely to die), the sensitivity and negative predictive value are not as good and a substantial proportion of patients will die without ever reaching transplant criteria. In addition, awaiting positive criteria can lead to delay in listing and worsening of organ failure, which often then precludes listing. This contributes to the fact that published rates of transplantation in those who reach criteria are only 50% following POD.[205] Clinical practice has changed since this designation was first defined. For example, it is rare to see a patient following POD with a

Table 76-4. Prognostic Indicators for Liver Transplantation

Category 1:	Paracetamol: pH <7.25 more than 24 hours after overdose and after fluid resuscitation
Category 2:	Paracetamol: Coexisting prothrombin time >100 sec or INR >6.5, serum creatinine >300 μmol/L or anuria, grade 3-4 encephalopathy
Category 3:	Paracetamol: Serum lactate >3.5 mmol/L on admission or >3 mmol/L more than 24 hours after overdose and after fluid resuscitation
Category 4:	Paracetamol: Two of three criteria from category 2 with clinical evidence of deterioration (e.g., increased ICP, FIO_2 >50%, increasing inotrope requirements) in the absence of clinical sepsis
Category 5:	Etiology: Hepatitis A, hepatitis B, idiosyncratic drug reaction, seronegative hepatitis; prothrombin time >100 seconds or INR >6.5 and any grade of encephalopathy
Category 6:	Etiology: Hepatitis A, hepatitis B, idiosyncratic drug reaction, seronegative hepatitis. Any grade of encephalopathy and any three from the following: unfavorable etiology (idiosyncratic drug reaction, seronegative hepatitis), age older than 40 years, jaundice to encephalopathy time >7 days, serum bilirubin >300 μmol/L, prothrombin time >50 seconds or INR >3.5
Category 7:	Etiology: Acute presentation of Wilson's disease, acute presentation of Budd-Chiari syndrome. Combination of coagulopathy and any degree of encephalopathy
Category 8:	Hepatic artery thrombosis within 14 days of liver transplantation
Category 9:	Early graft dysfunction with at least two of the following: AST >10,000, INR >3, serum lactate >3 mmol/L, absence of bile production
Category 10:	Acute liver failure in children: Multisystem disorder in which severe acute impairment of liver function with or without encephalopathy occurs in association with hepatocellular necrosis in a child with no recognized underlying chronic liver disease. Children with leukemia/lymphoma, hemophagocytosis and disseminated intravascular coagulopathy are excluded. Criteria: INR >4 or grade 3-4 encephalopathy. If paracetamol overdose, adult criteria apply. See categories 1-4

AST, aspartate aminotransferase; ICP, intracranial pressure; INR, international normalized ratio.

pH less than 7.3 or a creatinine greater than 300 mmol/L because of improved resuscitation and early renal support at the referring hospital. Because of these factors, ongoing efforts to establish markers that increase sensitivity and occur even earlier in the course of the syndrome, while maintaining good specificity and not reducing the positive predictive value to unacceptable levels leading to unnecessary transplants, continue.

Serum phosphate levels are higher in nonsurvivors following both POD and other causes of ALF.[95,206] However, there appears to be an unacceptable overlap and others have suggested that the use of serum phosphate does not provide any additional benefit to existing markers.[96,207,208] Other factors investigated include α-fetoprotein levels and nuclear magnetic resonance analysis of peripheral blood.[95,209] Acute physiology scoring as a basis for prediction has also been used.[210]

The liver plays a central role in lactate metabolism. In fact, in patients with severe liver necrosis the liver changes from being a consumer of lactate to being a net producer.[178] Arterial blood lactate levels have been shown to improve the sensitivity and maintain the specificity if added to the original KCH criteria and are achieved earlier in the course of the syndrome.[119]

On the practical issue of actually managing patients with FHF, some room for clinical interpretation has been included in the super-urgent listing rules. For example, a group of patients does not achieve KCH criteria but subsequently dies, usually of cerebral edema or multiple organ failure secondary to sepsis.[142,211] These patients often have worse acute physiology scores compared with survivors.[205,210] As a result, the U.K. super-urgent criteria allow an assessment of deteriorating acute physiology on the basis of cardiovascular, respiratory, or cerebral pathology. Similarly, the UNOS 1A criteria allow for patients "not expected to survive a further 7 days."

Outcome from Transplantation

In Europe the 1-year survival rate following transplantation for ALF is worse than that seen in chronic liver disease. The excess mortality is in the first month or so post transplant. This represents the severity of organ dysfunction seen prior to transplantation in ALF. Following this initial period, the curve flattens and the survival rate is actually better than that of patients with chronic liver disease (Fig. 76-7). This probably represents a younger age group and less disease recurrence. A huge degree of heterogeneity occurs in ALF, and those transplanted with sero-negative hepatitis display a better survival profile than patients transplanted for other causes, although they exhibit a similar early mortality while in the ICU.[71]

A tremendous amount of research effort has been put into the search for prognostic criteria on which to base the decision to transplant patients with ALF; however, much less information is available about the prediction of mortality following transplantation. This is important because decisions to withdraw from the waiting list on the basis of severity are difficult.

Both recipient and donor factors apparently help predict the outcome from transplantation in ALF.[71,205,212,213] In theory the severity of illness and organ dysfunction prior to transplantation should predict outcome. However, because unstable patients tend to be either not listed or withdrawn from the waiting list, there is inherent bias in retrospective analysis. Age of the recipient is a significant factor—certainly for seronegative ALF but also in POD, in which age is often used to exclude listing.[205] In nonparacetamol ALF, serum creatinine at the time of

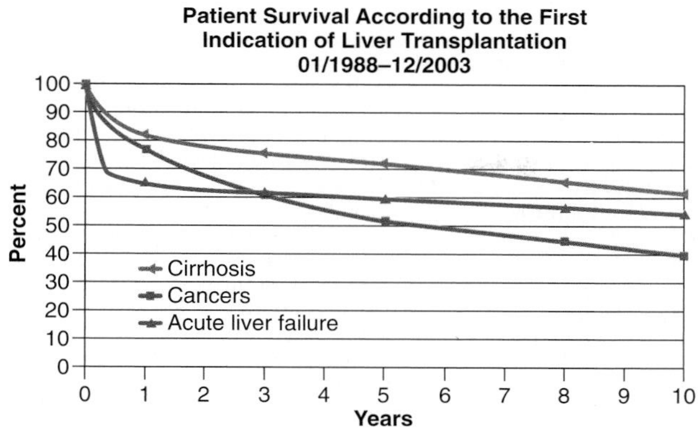

Figure 76-7. Patient survival according to the first indication for liver transplant. (From European Liver Transplant Registry: Available at http://www.eltr.org).

transplantation is a predictor of 2-month survival. Following POD, time from ingestion to transplantation has been shown to be a good predictor of 2-month survival; all patients transplanted later than 6 days from ingestion died. APACHE III score at transplantation and the severity of metabolic acidosis are also predictive.[212]

Donor factors found to be important are the use of reduced size grafts in paracetamol-induced ALF and evidence of early graft dysfunction as defined by a high AST or INR in the early postoperative period. In addition, a high donor body mass index (BMI) is a risk factor for death in sero-negative hepatitis.[71,205]

The conclusions from these data are difficult to interpret with confidence but suggest that older recipients with severe preoperative organ dysfunction are less able to tolerate poor early graft function, often seen with marginal grafts. Therefore in order to achieve the best graft and patient survival, there should be matching of the organ to the recipient, as has been suggested in both chronic liver disease and ALF.[213,214] This is not often an option because of time constraints.

Auxiliary Transplantation

Auxiliary partial liver transplantation has many theoretical advantages compared with standard orthotopic transplantation in ALF. It can be performed orthotopically (in the same place as the original liver) or heterotopically (in the left iliac fossa). Today it is always performed as a partial orthotopic transplant with a native left lobe in situ in adults and a right lobe in children using an adult left lobe graft, depending on size.

It provides the potential to support the patient during the acute phase of liver failure, enabling the regeneration of the native liver. This is attractive because in a number of patients immunosuppressive drugs can be withdrawn, allowing the graft to atrophy or be removed and eliminating the risks associated with lifelong immunosuppression. Data on this procedure have been accumulating over the past 10 years. Initial reports suggested that the procedure was associated with a high incidence of technical problems, primary dysfunction, and retransplantation. Later reports, however, suggest that many of these issues are resolving with greater experience, and better patient selection and graft selection. The best outcome has been seen in patients younger than 40 years of age with either acute viral hepatitis or paracetamol hepatotoxicity in whom 1-year graft and patient survival is similar to standard transplantation for ALF. Withdrawal of immunosuppression can be achieved in 30% to 70% of patients transplanted.[215-217]

Living-Related Lobe Donation

In many countries the only chance of transplantation for ALF is in a living-related donation of a liver lobe. This is most often performed in children, in whom an adult left lobe can often be used. In adults a right lobe is usually required, increasing the risk to the donor. With the worldwide shortage of donor organs, living-related transplantation for ALF is widely accepted in many but not all countries. Significant issues related to living-related transplantation in ALF include donor mortality of 1% and major morbidity of 40% to 60%. Adequately preparing the donor, medically and psychologically, in a time of acute crisis also has ethical implications.[218]

KEY POINTS

- Liver failure progresses to multiple organ failure and ultimately death in a large proportion of patients, and supportive care is the mainstay of therapy.
- AoCLF is seen much more commonly than acute (fulminant) liver failure and is often complicated by portal hypertension, leading to the formation of portosystemic collateral vessels, ascites, and hepatorenal failure. Therapy is aimed at the prevention of sepsis and aggressive management of the circulation.
- Worldwide, particularly in the developing world, approximately 95% to 100% of patients presenting with ALF will have viral hepatitis.[40]
- Acetaminophen poisoning is the most common cause of ALF in northern Europe and the United States. It can be treated successfully, in the majority of patients with NAC, if given within the first 12 hours of nonstaggered ingestion.[51]
- Liver failure following viral hepatitis tends to run an acute or hyperacute course with the onset of encephalopathy occurring within days or weeks of the first symptoms.[57]
- The presentation and clinical course of ALF depends on its etiology and the rate of progression of the syndrome.
- The West Haven criteria, designed to assess coma grade in patients with cirrhosis, are often applied to patients with ALF and are useful because of their familiarity.
- Cerebral edema often complicates severe acute and hyperactive liver failure and remains a leading cause of death.
- Management of ALF is complex, and liver transplantation is the only effective therapy in severe cases.

REFERENCES

1. Sen S, Williams R, Jalan R: The pathophysiological basis of acute-on-chronic liver failure. Liver 2002;22(Suppl 2):5-13.
2. Mathurin P: Is alcoholic hepatitis an indication for transplantation? Current management and outcomes. Liver Transpl 2005;11(Suppl 2):S21-24.
3. Hines IN, Wheeler MD: Recent advances in alcoholic liver disease III. Role of the innate immune response in alcoholic hepatitis. Am J Physiol Gastrointest Liver Physiol 2004;287: G310-14.
4. Sorbi D, Boynton J, Lindor KD: The ratio of aspartate aminotransferase to alanine aminotransferase: Potential value in differentiating nonalcoholic steatohepatitis from alcoholic liver disease. Am J Gastroenterol 1999;94:1018-1022.
5. Dunn W, Jamil LH, Brown LS, et al: MELD accurately predicts mortality in patients with alcoholic hepatitis. Hepatology 2005;41:353-358.
6. Mathurin P: Corticosteroids for alcoholic hepatitis—what's next? J Hepatol 2005;43:526-533.
7. D'Amico G, Pagliaro L, Bosch J: The treatment of portal hypertension: A meta-analytic review. Hepatology 1995;22:332-354.
8. Goulis J, Burroughs A: Portal hypertensive bleeding. In McDonald JW, Burroughs A, Feagan BG (eds): Evidence-Based Gastroenterology and Hepatology, 2nd ed. Oxford, Blackwell Publishing, 2004, pp 453-485.
9. D'Amico G, De Franchis R: Upper digestive bleeding in cirrhosis. Post-therapeutic outcome and prognostic indicators. Hepatology 2003;38: 599-612.
10. Ioannou G, Doust J, Rockey DC: Terlipressin for acute esophageal variceal hemorrhage. Cochrane Database Syst Rev 2003(1):CD002147.
11. Gotzsche PC, Hrobjartsson A: Somatostatin analogues for acute bleeding oesophageal varices. Cochrane Database Syst Rev 2005(1): CD000193.
12. Khan S, Tudur Smith C, Williamson P, Sutton R: Portosystemic shunts versus endoscopic therapy for variceal rebleeding in patients with cirrhosis. Cochrane Database Syst Rev 2006(4): CD000553.
13. Bosch J, Thabut D, Bendtsen F, et al: Recombinant factor VIIa for upper gastrointestinal bleeding in patients with cirrhosis: A randomized, double-blind trial. Gastroenterology 2004;127:1123-1130.
14. Bernard B, Grange JD, Khac EN, et al: Antibiotic prophylaxis for the prevention of bacterial infections in cirrhotic patients with gastrointestinal bleeding: A meta-analysis. Hepatology 1999;29:1655-1661.
15. Goulis J, Patch D, Burroughs AK: Bacterial infection in the pathogenesis of variceal bleeding. Lancet 1999;353:139-142.
16. Wong F, Bernardi M, Balk R, et al: Sepsis in cirrhosis: Report on the 7th meeting of the International Ascites Club. Gut 2005;54:718-725.
17. Wasmuth HE, Kunz D, Yagmur E, et al: Patients with acute on chronic liver failure display "sepsis-like" immune paralysis. J Hepatol 2005;42:195-201.
18. Fernandez J, Navasa M, Gomez J, et al: Bacterial infections in cirrhosis: Epidemiological changes with invasive procedures and norfloxacin prophylaxis. Hepatology 2002;35:140-148.
19. Ruiz-del-Arbol L, Monescillo A, Arocena C, et al: Circulatory function and hepatorenal syndrome in cirrhosis. Hepatology 2005;42:439-447.
20. Arroyo V, Gines P, Gerbes AL, et al: Definition and diagnostic criteria of refractory ascites and hepatorenal syndrome in cirrhosis. International Ascites Club. Hepatology 1996;23:164-176.
21. Moreau R, Lebrec D: The use of vasoconstrictors in patients with cirrhosis: Type 1 HRS and beyond. Hepatology 2006;43:385-394.
22. Ortega R, Gines P, Uriz J, et al: Terlipressin therapy with and without albumin for patients with hepatorenal syndrome: Results of a prospective, nonrandomized study. Hepatology 2002;36(4 Pt 1):941-948.
23. Vaquero J, Chung C, Cahill ME, Blei AT: Pathogenesis of hepatic encephalopathy in acute liver failure. Semin Liver Dis 2003;23:259-269.
24. Mizock BA: Nutritional support in hepatic encephalopathy. Nutrition 1999;15:220-228.
25. Gupta D, Lalrothuama, Agrawal PN, et al: Pulmonary function changes after large volume paracentesis. Trop Gastroenterol 2000;21:68-70.
26. Byrd RP Jr, Roy TM, Simons M: Improvement in oxygenation after large volume paracentesis. South Med J 1996;89:689-692.
27. Duranti R, Laffi G, Misuri G, et al: Respiratory mechanics in patients with tense cirrhotic ascites. Eur Respir J 1997;10:1622-1630.
28. Gur C, Ilan Y, Shibolet O: Hepatic hydrothorax—pathophysiology, diagnosis and treatment—review of the literature. Liver Int 2004;24: 281-284.
29. Marik PE: Adrenal-exhaustion syndrome in patients with liver disease. Intensive Care Med 2006;32:275-280.
30. Annane D, Sebille V, Charpentier C, et al: Effect of treatment with low doses of hydrocortisone and fludrocortisone on mortality in patients with septic shock. JAMA 2002;288:862-871.
31. Tsai MH, Peng YS, Chen YC, et al: Adrenal insufficiency in patients with cirrhosis, severe sepsis and septic shock. Hepatology 2006;43:673-681.
32. Fernandez J, Escorsell A, Zabalza M, et al: Adrenal insufficiency in patients with cirrhosis and septic shock: Effect of treatment with hydrocortisone on survival. Hepatology 2006;44: 1288-1295.
33. Wehler M, Kokoska J, Reulbach U, et al: Short-term prognosis in critically ill patients with cirrhosis assessed by prognostic scoring systems. Hepatology 2001;34:255-261.
34. Aggarwal A, Ong JP, Younossi ZM, et al: Predictors of mortality and resource utilization in cirrhotic patients admitted to the medical ICU. Chest 2001;119:1489-1497.
35. Cholongitas E, Senzolo M, Patch D, et al: Risk factors, sequential organ failure assessment and model for end-stage liver disease scores for predicting short term mortality in cirrhotic patients admitted to intensive care unit. Aliment Pharmacol Ther 2006;23:883-893.
36. Rabe C, Schmitz V, Paashaus M, et al: Does intubation really equal death in cirrhotic patients? Factors influencing outcome in patients with liver cirrhosis requiring mechanical ventilation. Intensive Care Med 2004;30: 1564-1571.
37. O'Grady JG, Schalm SW, Williams R: Acute liver failure: Redefining the syndromes. Lancet 1993;342:273-275.
38. Lucke B, Mallory T: Fulminant form of epidemic hepatitis. Am J Pathol 1946;22:867-945.
39. Trey C, Davidson CS: The management of fulminant hepatic failure. Prog Liver Dis 1970;3:282-298.
40. Dhiman RK, Seth AK, Jain S, et al: Prognostic evaluation of early indicators in fulminant hepatic failure by multivariate analysis. Dig Dis Sci 1998;43:1311-1316.
41. Bernal W: Changing patterns of causation and the use of transplantation in the United Kingdom. Semin Liver Dis 2003;23:227-237.
42. Lee WM: Acute liver failure in the United States. Semin Liver Dis 2003;23:217-226.
43. Ostapowicz G, Fontana RJ, Schiodt FV, et al: Results of a prospective study of acute liver failure at 17 tertiary care centers in the United States. Ann Intern Med 2002;137:947-954.
44. Hawton K, Simkin S, Deeks J, et al: UK legislation on analgesic packs: Before and after study of long term effect on poisonings. BMJ 2004;329:1076.
45. Schiodt FV, Balko J, Schilsky M, et al: Thrombopoietin in acute liver failure. Hepatology 2003;37:558-561.
46. Jones A: Over-the-counter analgesics: A toxicology perspective. Am J Ther 2002;9:245-257.
47. James LP, Mayeux PR, Hinson JA: Acetaminophen-induced hepatotoxicity. Drug Metab Dispos 2003;31:1499-1506.
48. Bernal W, Donaldson P, Underhill J, et al: Tumor necrosis factor genomic polymorphism and outcome of acetaminophen (paracetamol)-induced acute liver failure. J Hepatol 1998;29:53-59.
49. Bernal W, Langley P, Wendon J: Circulating markers of endothelial activation in acetaminophen induced acute liver failure. Critical Care 1998;2(Suppl 1):P009.
50. Makin A, Williams R: Acetaminophen-induced acute liver failure. In Lee W, Williams R (eds): Acute Liver Failure. Cambridge, England, Cambridge University Press, 1997, pp 32-42.
51. Prescott LF, Illingworth RN, Critchley JA, et al: Intravenous N-acetylcysteine: The treatment of choice for

paracetamol poisoning. BMJ 1979;2: 1097-1100.
52. Lee WM: Drug-induced hepatotoxicity. N Engl J Med 2003;349:474-485.
53. Keays R, Harrison PM, Wendon JA, et al: Intravenous acetylcysteine in paracetamol induced fulminant hepatic failure: A prospective controlled trial. BMJ 1991;303:1026-1029.
54. Jones AL: Recent advances in the management of late paracetamol poisoning. Emergency Medicine Australasia 2000;12:14-21.
55. Sklar GE, Subramaniam M: Acetylcysteine treatment for non-acetaminophen-induced acute liver failure. Ann Pharmacother 2004;38:498-500.
56. O'Grady JG: Acute liver failure. Postgrad Med J 2005;81:148-154.
57. Schiodt FV, Davern TJ, Shakil AO, et al: Viral hepatitis-related acute liver failure. Am J Gastroenterol 2003;98: 448-453.
58. Chadha MS, Walimbe AM, Chobe LP, Arankalle VA: Comparison of etiology of sporadic acute and fulminant viral hepatitis in hospitalized patients in Pune, India during 1978-81 and 1994-97. Indian J Gastroenterol 2003;22: 11-15.
59. Schiff ER: Atypical clinical manifestations of hepatitis A. Vaccine 1992;10(Suppl 1):S18-20.
60. Fagan E, Yousef G, Brahm J, et al: Persistence of hepatitis A virus in fulminant hepatitis and after liver transplantation. J Med Virol 1990;30:131-136.
61. Liaw YF, Yang CY, Chu CM, Huang MJ: Appearance and persistence of hepatitis A IgM antibody in acute clinical hepatitis A observed in an outbreak. Infection 1986;14: 156-158.
62. Sato S, Suzuki K, Akahane Y, et al: Hepatitis B virus strains with mutations in the core promoter in patients with fulminant hepatitis. Ann Intern Med 1995;122:241-248.
63. Garfein RS, Bower WA, Loney CM, et al: Factors associated with fulminant liver failure during an outbreak among injection drug users with acute hepatitis B. Hepatology 2004;40: 865-873.
64. Farci P, Alter HJ, Shimoda A, et al: Hepatitis C virus-associated fulminant hepatic failure. N Engl J Med 1996;335:631-634.
65. Vogt M, Lang T, Frosner G, et al: Prevalence and clinical outcome of hepatitis C infection in children who underwent cardiac surgery before the implementation of blood-donor screening. N Engl J Med 1999;341:866-870.
66. Acharya SK, Panda SK, Saxena A, Gupta SD: Acute hepatic failure in India: A perspective from the East. J Gastroenterol Hepatol 2000;15:473-479.
67. Cheng VC, Lo CM, Lau GK: Current issues and treatment of fulminant hepatic failure including transplantation in Hong Kong and the Far East. Semin Liver Dis 2003;23:239-250.
68. Emerson SU, Purcell RH: Running like water—the omnipresence of hepatitis E. N Engl J Med 2004;351:2367-2368.
69. Wu JC, Chen CM, Chiang TY, et al: Clinical and epidemiological implications of swine hepatitis E virus infection. J Med Virol 2000;60: 166-171.
70. Gow P, Hathaway M, Gunson B, et al: Association of fulminant non-A non-B hepatitis with homozygosity for HLA A1-B8-DR3. J Gastroenterol Hepatol 2005;20:555-561.
71. Wigg AJ, Gunson BK, Mutimer DJ: Outcomes following liver transplantation for seronegative acute liver failure: Experience during a 12-year period with more than 100 patients. Liver Transpl 2005;11:27-34.
72. Manns MP, Vogel A: Autoimmune hepatitis, from mechanisms to therapy. Hepatology 2006;43(Suppl 1): S132-144.
73. Vergani D, Alvarez F, Bianchi FB, et al: Liver autoimmune serology: A consensus statement from the committee for autoimmune serology of the International Autoimmune Hepatitis Group. J Hepatol 2004;41:677-683.
74. Bissell DM, Gores GJ, Laskin DL, Hoofnagle JH: Drug-induced liver injury: Mechanisms and test systems. Hepatology 2001;33:1009-1013.
75. Devlin J, O'Grady J: Indications for referral and assessment in adult liver transplantation: A clinical guideline. British Society of Gastroenterology. Gut 1999;45(Suppl 6):VI1-VI22.
76. Ibdah JA, Bennett MJ, Rinaldo P, et al: A fetal fatty-acid oxidation disorder as a cause of liver disease in pregnant women. N Engl J Med 1999;340:1723-1731.
77. Guntupalli SR, Steingrub J: Hepatic disease and pregnancy: An overview of diagnosis and management. Crit Care Med 2005;33(10 Suppl): S332-339.
78. Hamid SS, Jafri SM, Khan H, et al: Fulminant hepatic failure in pregnant women: Acute fatty liver or acute viral hepatitis? J Hepatol 1996;25:20-27.
79. Castro MA, Fassett MJ, Reynolds TB, et al: Reversible peripartum liver failure: A new perspective on the diagnosis, treatment, and cause of acute fatty liver of pregnancy, based on 28 consecutive cases. Am J Obstet Gynecol 1999;181:389-395.
80. Brewer GJ, Askari FK: Wilson's disease: Clinical management and therapy. J Hepatol 2005;42(Suppl):S13-21.
81. Murad SD, Valla DC, de Groen PC, et al: Determinants of survival and the effect of portosystemic shunting in patients with Budd-Chiari syndrome. Hepatology 2004;39:500-508.
82. Menon KV, Shah V, Kamath PS: The Budd-Chiari syndrome. N Engl J Med 2004;350:578-585.
83. Slakey DP, Klein AS, Venbrux AC, Cameron JL: Budd-Chiari syndrome: Current management options. Ann Surg 2001;233:522-527.
84. Mancuso A, Fung K, Mela M, et al: TIPS for acute and chronic Budd-Chiari syndrome: A single-centre experience. J Hepatol 2003;38:751-754.
85. Mentha G, Giostra E, Majno PE, et al: Liver transplantation for Budd-Chiari syndrome: A European study on 248 patients from 51 centres. J Hepatol 2006;44:520-528.
86. McDonald GB, Hinds MS, Fisher LD, et al: Veno-occlusive disease of the liver and multiorgan failure after bone marrow transplantation: A cohort study of 355 patients. Ann Intern Med 1993;118:255-267.
87. MacQuillan GC, Mutimer D: Fulminant liver failure due to severe veno-occlusive disease after haematopoietic cell transplantation: A depressing experience. QJM 2004;97:581-589.
88. Baron F, Deprez M, Beguin Y: The veno-occlusive disease of the liver. Haematologica 1997;82:718-725.
89. Naschitz JE, Slobodin G, Lewis RJ, et al: Heart diseases affecting the liver and liver diseases affecting the heart. Am Heart J 2000;140:111-120.
90. Hadad E, Ben-Ari Z, Heled Y, et al: Liver transplantation in exertional heat stroke: A medical dilemma. Intensive Care Med 2004;30:1474-1478.
91. Diaz JH: Syndromic diagnosis and management of confirmed mushroom poisonings. Crit Care Med 2005;33:427-436.
92. Tofteng F, Jorgensen L, Hansen BA, et al: Cerebral microdialysis in patients with fulminant hepatic failure. Hepatology 2002;36:1333-1340.
93. Atterbury CE, Maddrey WC, Conn HO: Neomycin-sorbitol and lactulose in the treatment of acute portal-systemic encephalopathy. A controlled, double-blind clinical trial. Am J Dig Dis 1978;23:398-406.
94. Murphy N, Auzinger G, Bernel W, Wendon J: The effect of hypertonic sodium chloride on intracranial pressure in patients with acute liver failure. Hepatology 2004;39:464-70.
95. Schmidt LE, Dalhoff K: Serum phosphate is an early predictor of outcome in severe acetaminophen-induced hepatotoxicity. Hepatology 2002;36:659-665.
96. Macquillan GC, Seyam MS, Nightingale P, et al: Blood lactate but not serum phosphate levels can predict patient outcome in fulminant hepatic failure. Liver Transpl 2005;11:1073-1079.
97. Yamaguchi M, Gabazza EC, Taguchi O, et al: Decreased protein C activation in patients with fulminant hepatic failure. Scand J Gastroenterol 2006;41:331-337.
98. Polson J, Lee WM: AASLD position paper: The management of acute liver failure. Hepatology 2005;41: 1179-1197.
99. O'Grady J: Acute liver failure. J R Coll Physicians Lond 1997;31:603-607.
100. Wendon JA, Harrison PM, Keays R, Williams R: Cerebral blood flow and metabolism in fulminant liver failure. Hepatology 1994;19:1407-1413.
101. Strauss GI, Hogh P, Moller K, et al: Regional cerebral blood flow during mechanical hyperventilation in patients with fulminant hepatic failure. Hepatology 1999;30:1368-1373.
102. Ellis A, Wendon J: Circulatory, respiratory, cerebral, and renal derangements in acute liver failure: Pathophysiology and management. Semin Liver Dis 1996;16:379-388.
103. McCormick PA, Treanor D, McCormack G, Farrell M: Early death

from paracetamol (acetaminophen) induced fulminant hepatic failure without cerebral oedema. J Hepatol 2003;39:547-551.
104. Landry DW, Levin HR, Gallant EM, et al: Vasopressin deficiency contributes to the vasodilation of septic shock. Circulation 1997;95:1122-1125.
105. Dunser MW, Mayr AJ, Ulmer H, et al: Arginine vasopressin in advanced vasodilatory shock: A prospective, randomized, controlled study. Circulation 2003;107:2313-2319.
106. Shawcross DL, Davies NA, Mookerjee RP, et al: Worsening of cerebral hyperemia by the administration of terlipressin in acute liver failure with severe encephalopathy. Hepatology 2004;39:471-475.
107. Harry R, Auzinger G, Wendon J: The clinical importance of adrenal insufficiency in acute hepatic dysfunction. Hepatology 2002;36:395-402.
108. Annane D: Glucocorticoids in the treatment of severe sepsis and septic shock. Curr Opin Crit Care 2005;11:449-453.
109. Harry R, Auzinger G, Wendon J: The effects of supraphysiological doses of corticosteroids in hypotensive liver failure. Liver Int 2003;23:71-77.
110. O'Grady JG, Gimson AE, O'Brien CJ, et al: Controlled trials of charcoal hemoperfusion and prognostic factors in fulminant hepatic failure. Gastroenterology 1988;94:1186-1192.
111. Trumper L, Coux G, Monasterolo LA, et al: Effect of acetaminophen on the membrane anchoring of Na+, K+ATPase of rat renal cortical cells. Biochim Biophys Acta 2005;1740:332-339.
112. Cobden I, Record CO, Ward MK, Kerr DN: Paracetamol-induced acute renal failure in the absence of fulminant liver damage. Br Med J (Clin Res Ed) 1982;284:21-22.
113. Bellomo R, Ronco C, Kellum JA, et al: Acute renal failure—definition, outcome measures, animal models, fluid therapy and information technology needs: The Second International Consensus Conference of the Acute Dialysis Quality Initiative (ADQI) Group. Crit Care 2004;8: R204-212.
114. Bal C, Longkumer T, Patel C, et al: Renal function and structure in subacute hepatic failure. J Gastroenterol Hepatol 2000;15:1318-1324.
115. Davenport A: The management of renal failure in patients at risk of cerebral edema/hypoxia. New Horiz 1995;3:717-724.
116. Honore PM, Joannes-Boyau O, Merson L, et al: The big bang of hemofiltration: The beginning of a new era in the third millennium for extra-corporeal blood purification! Int J Artif Organs 2006;29:649-659.
117. Bernal W, Wong T, Wendon J: High-volume continuous veno-venous haemofiltration in hyper-acute liver failure: A pilot study. Critical Care 2000;3(Suppl 1):P212.
118. Davenport A, Will EJ, Davison AM: Hyperlactataemia and metabolic acidosis during haemofiltration using lactate-buffered fluids. Nephron 1991;59:461-465.
119. Bernal W, Donaldson N, Wyncoll D, Wendon J: Blood lactate as an early predictor of outcome in paracetamol-induced acute liver failure: A cohort study. Lancet 2002;359:558-563.
120. Davenport A: Dialysate and substitution fluids for patients treated by continuous forms of renal replacement therapy. Contrib Nephrol 2001:313-322.
121. Ware AJ, D'Agostino AN, Combes B: Cerebral edema: A major complication of massive hepatic necrosis. Gastroenterology 1971;61:877-884.
122. Hanid MA, Mackenzie RL, Jenner RE, et al: Intracranial pressure in pigs with surgically induced acute liver failure. Gastroenterology 1979;76:123-131.
123. Julia A, Wendon FSL: Intracranial pressure monitoring in acute liver failure. A procedure with clear indications. Hepatology 2006;44:504-506.
124. Jacques Bernuau FD: Intracranial pressure monitoring in patients with acute liver failure: A questionable invasive surveillance. Hepatology 2006;44:502-504.
125. Blei AT: The pathophysiology of brain edema in acute liver failure. Neurochem Int 2005;47:71-77.
126. Norenberg MD, Rao KV, Jayakumar AR: Mechanisms of ammonia-induced astrocyte swelling. Metab Brain Dis 2005;20:303-318.
127. Clemmesen JO, Larsen FS, Kondrup J, et al: Cerebral herniation in patients with acute liver failure is correlated with arterial ammonia concentration. Hepatology 1999;29:648-653.
128. Bhatia V, Singh R, Acharya SK: Predictive value of arterial ammonia for complications and outcome in acute liver failure. Gut 2005;55: 98-104.
129. Traber PG, Dal Canto M, Ganger DR, Blei AT: Electron microscopic evaluation of brain edema in rabbits with galactosamine-induced fulminant hepatic failure: Ultrastructure and integrity of the blood-brain barrier. Hepatology 1987;7:1272-1277.
130. Kato M, Hughes RD, Keays RT, Williams R: Electron microscopic study of brain capillaries in cerebral edema from fulminant hepatic failure. Hepatology 1992;15:1060-1066.
131. Takahashi H, Koehler RC, Brusilow SW, Traystman RJ. Inhibition of brain glutamine accumulation prevents cerebral edema in hyperammonemic rats. Am J Physiol 1991;261(3 Pt 2): H825-829.
132. Cordoba J, Gottstein J, Blei AT: Glutamine, myo-inositol, and organic brain osmolytes after portocaval anastomosis in the rat: Implications for ammonia-induced brain edema. Hepatology 1996;24:919-923.
133. Zwingmann C, Chatauret N, Leibfritz D, Butterworth RF: Selective increase of brain lactate synthesis in experimental acute liver failure: Results of a [H-C] nuclear magnetic resonance study. Hepatology 2003;37:420-428.
134. Jayakumar AR, Rao KV, Murthy Ch R, Norenberg MD: Glutamine in the mechanism of ammonia-induced astrocyte swelling. Neurochem Int 2006;48:623-628.
135. Blei AT, Larsen FS: Pathophysiology of cerebral edema in fulminant hepatic failure. J Hepatol 1999;31:771-776.
136. Larsen FS, Adel Hansen B, Pott F, et al: Dissociated cerebral vasoparalysis in acute liver failure. A hypothesis of gradual cerebral hyperaemia. J Hepatol 1996;25:145-151.
137. Aggarwal S, Obrist W, Yonas H, et al: Cerebral hemodynamic and metabolic profiles in fulminant hepatic failure: Relationship to outcome. Liver Transpl 2005;11:1353-1360.
138. Strauss G, Hansen BA, Kirkegaard P, et al: Liver function, cerebral blood flow autoregulation, and hepatic encephalopathy in fulminant hepatic failure. Hepatology 1997;25:837-839.
139. Tofteng F, Larsen FS: The effect of indomethacin on intracranial pressure, cerebral perfusion and extracellular lactate and glutamate concentrations in patients with fulminant hepatic failure. J Cereb Blood Flow Metab 2004;24:798-804.
140. Tofteng F, Larsen FS: Management of patients with fulminant hepatic failure and brain edema. Metab Brain Dis 2004;19:207.
141. Bernal W, Wendon J: Intracranial hypertension in acute liver failure; prevalence and risk factors for development. Hepatology 2004;40(Suppl 4):162A-266A.
142. Boeckx NK, Haydon G, Rusli F, Murphy N: Multiorgan failure is the commonest cause of death in fulminant hepatic failure: A single centre experience. Liver Int 2004;24:702-703.
143. Jalan R: Intracranial hypertension in acute liver failure: Pathophysiological basis of rational management. Semin Liver Dis 2003;23:271-282.
144. Makin AJ, Wendon J, Williams R: A 7-year experience of severe acetaminophen-induced hepatotoxicity (1987-1993). Gastroenterology 1995;109:1907-1916.
145. Tofteng F, Hauerberg J, Hansen BA, et al: Persistent arterial hyperammonemia increases the concentration of glutamine and alanine in the brain and correlates with intracranial pressure in patients with fulminant hepatic failure. J Cereb Blood Flow Metab 2006;26:21-27.
146. Wijdicks EF, Plevak DJ, Rakela J, Wiesner RH: Clinical and radiologic features of cerebral edema in fulminant hepatic failure. Mayo Clin Proc 1995;70:119-124.
147. Munoz SJ, Robinson M, Northrup B, et al: Elevated intracranial pressure and computed tomography of the brain in fulminant hepatocellular failure. Hepatology 1991;13:209-212.
148. Ranjan P, Mishra AM, Kale R, et al: Cytotoxic edema is responsible for raised intracranial pressure in fulminant hepatic failure: In vivo demonstration using diffusion-weighted MRI in human subjects. Metab Brain Dis 2005;20:181-192.
149. Nortje J, Gupta AK: The role of tissue oxygen monitoring in patients with acute brain injury. Br J Anaesth 2006;97:95-106.

150. Ellis AJ, Wendon JA, Williams R: Subclinical seizure activity and prophylactic phenytoin infusion in acute liver failure: A controlled clinical trial. Hepatology 2000;32:536-541.
151. Nielsen HB, Tofteng F, Wang LP, Larsen FS: Cerebral oxygenation determined by near-infrared spectrophotometry in patients with fulminant hepatic failure. J Hepatol 2003;38:188-192.
152. Strauss GI, Moller K, Holm S, et al: Transcranial Doppler sonography and internal jugular bulb saturation during hyperventilation in patients with fulminant hepatic failure. Liver Transpl 2001;7:352-358.
153. Blei AT, Olafsson S, Webster S, Levy R: Complications of intracranial pressure monitoring in fulminant hepatic failure. Lancet 1993;341:157-158.
154. The Brain Trauma Foundation. The American Association of Neurological Surgeons. The Joint Section on Neurotrauma and Critical Care. Indications for intracranial pressure monitoring. J Neurotrauma 2000;17:479-491.
155. Vaquero J, Fontana RJ, Larson AM, et al: Complications and use of intracranial pressure monitoring in patients with acute liver failure and severe encephalopathy. Liver Transpl 2005;11:1581-1589.
156. Shami VM, Caldwell SH, Hespenheide EE, et al: Recombinant activated factor VII for coagulopathy in fulminant hepatic failure compared with conventional therapy. Liver Transpl 2003;9:138-143.
157. Keays RT, Alexander GL, Williams R: The safety and value of extradural intracranial pressure monitors in fulminant hepatic failure. J Hepatol 1993;18:205-209.
158. Tandon BN, Joshi YK, Tandon M: Acute liver failure. Experience with 145 patients. J Clin Gastroenterol 1986;8:664-668.
159. Murphy ND, Wendon J: Serum sodium is inversely proportional to intracranial pressure in acute liver failure. Crit Care 1999;3(Suppl 1):P220.
160. Brain Trauma Foundation, American Association of Neurological Surgeons, Joint Section on Neurotrauma and Critical Care: Guidelines for cerebral perfusion pressure. J Neurotrauma 2000;17:507-511.
161. Toftengi F, Larsen FS: Management of patients with fulminant hepatic failure and brain edema. Metab Brain Dis 2004;19:207-214.
162. Jalan R, Olde Damink SW, Deutz NE, et al: Restoration of cerebral blood flow autoregulation and reactivity to carbon dioxide in acute liver failure by moderate hypothermia. Hepatology 2001;34:50-54.
163. Davis MA, Mutimer D, Lowes J, et al: Recovery despite impaired cerebral perfusion in fulminant hepatic failure. Lancet 1994;343:1329-1330.
164. Jalan R, Olde Damink SW, Deutz NE, et al: Moderate hypothermia in patients with acute liver failure and uncontrolled intracranial hypertension. Gastroenterology 2004;127: 1338-1346.
165. Wijdicks EF, Nyberg SL: Propofol to control intracranial pressure in fulminant hepatic failure. Transplant Proc 2002;34:1220-1222.
166. Strauss GI, Moller K, Larsen FS, et al: Cerebral glucose and oxygen metabolism in patients with fulminant hepatic failure. Liver Transpl 2003;9:1244-1252.
167. Brain Trauma Foundation, American Association of Neurological Surgeons, Joint Section on Neurotrauma and Critical Care: Intracranial pressure treatment threshold. J Neurotrauma 2000;17:493-495.
168. Canalese J, Gimson AE, Davis C, et al: Controlled trial of dexamethasone and mannitol for the cerebral oedema of fulminant hepatic failure. Gut 1982;23:625-629.
169. Ede RJ, Gimson AE, Bihari D, Williams R: Controlled hyperventilation in the prevention of cerebral oedema in fulminant hepatic failure. J Hepatol 1986;2:43-51.
170. Bhatia V, Batra Y, Acharya SK: Prophylactic phenytoin does not improve cerebral edema or survival in acute liver failure—a controlled clinical trial. J Hepatol 2004;41:89-96.
171. Rolando N, Philpott-Howard J, Williams R: Bacterial and fungal infection in acute liver failure. Semin Liver Dis 1996;16:389-402.
172. Rolando N, Wade J, Davalos M, et al: The systemic inflammatory response syndrome in acute liver failure. Hepatology 2000;32(4 Pt 1):734-739.
173. Rolando N, Gimson AES, Wade JJ, et al: Prospective controlled trial of selective parenteral and enteral antimicrobial regimen in fulminant hepatic failure. Hepatology 1993;17:196-201.
174. Wade J, Rolando N, Philpott-Howard J, Wendon J: Timing and aetiology of bacterial infections in a liver intensive care unit. J Hosp Infect 2003;53:144-146.
175. Gramlich L, Kichian K, Pinilla J, et al: Does enteral nutrition compared to parenteral nutrition result in better outcomes in critically ill adult patients? A systematic review of the literature. Nutrition 2004;20:843-848.
176. Schutz T, Bechstein WO, Neuhaus P, et al: Clinical practice of nutrition in acute liver failure—a European survey. Clin Nutr 2004;23:975-982.
177. Walsh TS, Wigmore SJ, Hopton P, et al: Energy expenditure in acetaminophen-induced fulminant hepatic failure. Crit Care Med 2000;28:649-654.
178. Murphy ND, Kodakat SK, Wendon JA, et al: Liver and intestinal lactate metabolism in patients with acute hepatic failure undergoing liver transplantation. Crit Care Med 2001;29:2111-2118.
179. Walsh TS, McLellan S, Mackenzie SJ, Lee A: Hyperlactatemia and pulmonary lactate production in patients with fulminant hepatic failure. Chest 1999;116:471-476.
180. Clark SJ, Shojaee-Moradie F, Croos P, et al: Temporal changes in insulin sensitivity following the development of acute liver failure secondary to acetaminophen. Hepatology 2001;34:109-115.
181. Strauss GI, Knudsen GM, Kondrup J, et al: Cerebral metabolism of ammonia and amino acids in patients with fulminant hepatic failure. Gastroenterology 2001;121: 1109-1119.
182. Kircheis G, Wettstein M, Dahl S, Haussinger D: Clinical efficacy of L-ornithine-L-aspartate in the management of hepatic encephalopathy. Metab Brain Dis 2002;17:453-462.
183. Rose C, Michalak A, Rao KV, et al: L-ornithine-L-aspartate lowers plasma and cerebrospinal fluid ammonia and prevents brain edema in rats with acute liver failure. Hepatology 1999;30:636-640.
184. Alba L, Hay JE, Angulo P, Lee WM: Lactulose therapy in acute liver failure. J Hepatology 2002;36:33A.
185. Atillasoy E, Berk PD: Extracorporeal liver support: Historical background and critical analysis. In Lee WM, Williams R (eds): Acute Liver Failure. Cambridge, England, Cambridge University Press, 1997, pp 223-244.
186. Shirabe K, Shimada M, Gion T, et al: Postoperative liver failure after major hepatic resection for hepatocellular carcinoma in the modern era with special reference to remnant liver volume. J Am Coll Surg 1999;188:304-309.
187. Kobayashi N, Noguchi H, Totsugawa T, et al: Insertion of a suicide gene into an immortalized human hepatocyte cell line. Cell Transplant 2001;10:373-376.
188. Selden C, Hodgson H: Cellular therapies for liver replacement. Transpl Immunol 2004;12:273-288.
189. Demetriou AA, Brown RS Jr, Busuttil RW, et al: Prospective, randomized, multicenter, controlled trial of a bioartificial liver in treating acute liver failure. Ann Surg 2004;239:660-667; discussion 7-70.
190. Ellis AJ, Hughes RD, Wendon JA, et al: Pilot-controlled trial of the extracorporeal liver assist device in acute liver failure. Hepatology 1996;24:1446-1451.
191. Millis MJ, Kramer DJ, O'Grady JG, et al: Results of phase I trial of the extracorporeal liver assist device for patients with fulminant hepatic failure. Am J Transplantation 2001;1(Suppl 1):391.
192. van de Kerkhove MP, Di Florio E, Scuderi V, et al: Phase I clinical trial with the AMC-bioartificial liver. Int J Artif Organs 2002;25:950-959.
193. Sauer IM, Kardassis D, Zeillinger K, et al: Clinical extracorporeal hybrid liver support—phase I study with primary porcine liver cells. Xenotransplantation 2003;10:460-469.
194. Samuel D, Ichai P, Feray C, et al: Neurological improvement during bioartificial liver sessions in patients with acute liver failure awaiting transplantation. Transplantation 2002;73:257-264.
195. Opolon P: High-permeability membrane hemodialysis and hemofiltration in acute hepatic coma: Experimental and clinical results. Artif Organs 1979;3:354-360.
196. Larsen FS, Hansen BA, Jorgensen LG, et al: High-volume plasmapheresis and acute liver transplantation in fulminant hepatic failure. Transplant Proc 1994;26:1788.

197. Lai WK, Haydon G, Mutimer D, Murphy N: The effect of molecular adsorbent recirculating system on pathophysiological parameters in patients with acute liver failure. Intensive Care Med 2005;31: 1544-1549.
198. Schmidt LE, Wang LP, Hansen BA, Larsen FS: Systemic hemodynamic effects of treatment with the molecular adsorbents recirculating system in patients with hyperacute liver failure: A prospective controlled trial. Liver Transpl 2003;9:290-297.
199. Liu JP, Gluud LL, Als-Nielsen B, Gluud C: Artificial and bioartificial support systems for liver failure. Cochrane Database Syst Rev 2004(1):CD003628.
200. Khuroo MS, Khuroo MS, Farahat KL: Molecular adsorbent recirculating system for acute and acute-on-chronic liver failure: A meta-analysis. Liver Transpl 2004;10:1099-1106.
201. O'Grady JG, Wendon J, Tan KC, et al: Liver transplantation after paracetamol overdose. BMJ 1991;303:221-223.
202. O'Grady JG, Alexander GJ, Hayllar KM, Williams R: Early indicators of prognosis in fulminant hepatic failure. Gastroenterology 1989;97:439-445.
203. Anand AC, Nightingale P, Neuberger JM: Early indicators of prognosis in fulminant hepatic failure: An assessment of the King's criteria. J Hepatol 1997;26:62-68.
204. Bernuau J, Goudeau A, Poynard T, et al: Multivariate analysis of prognostic factors in fulminant hepatitis B. Hepatology 1986;6:648-651.
205. Bernal W, Wendon J, Rela M, et al: Use and outcome of liver transplantation in acetaminophen-induced acute liver failure. Hepatology 1998;27:1050-1055.
206. Baquerizo A, Anselmo D, Shackleton C, et al: Phosphorus as an early predictive factor in patients with acute liver failure. Transplantation 2003;75:2007-2014.
207. Bernal W, Wendon J: More on serum phosphate and prognosis of acute liver failure. Hepatology 2003;38:533-534.
208. Ng KL, Davidson JS, Bathgate AJ: Serum phosphate is not a reliable early predictor of outcome in paracetamol induced hepatotoxicity. Liver Transpl 2004;10:158-159.
209. Dabos KJ, Newsome PN, Parkinson JA, et al: Biochemical prognostic markers of outcome in non-paracetamol-induced fulminant hepatic failure. Transplantation 2004;77:200-205.
210. Mitchell I, Bihari D, Chang R, et al: Earlier identification of patients at risk from acetaminophen-induced acute liver failure. Crit Care Med 1998;26:279-284.
211. Makin AJ, Wendon J, Williams R: A 7-year experience of severe acetaminophen-induced hepatotoxicity (1987-1993). Gastroenterology 1995;109:1907-1916.
212. Devlin J, Wendon J, Heaton N, et al: Pretransplantation clinical status and outcome of emergency transplantation for acute liver failure. Hepatology 1995;21:1018-1024.
213. Haydon GH, Hiltunen Y, Murphy N, et al: A new model to maximize the utility of liver allografts in patients with fulminant non-A non-B hepatitis. Hepatology 2004;40(Suppl 1):552A.
214. Haydon GH, Hiltunen Y, Lucey MR, et al: Self-organizing maps can determine outcome and match recipients and donors at orthotopic liver transplantation. Transplantation 2005;79:213-218.
215. Chenard-Neu MP, Boudjema K, Bernuau J, et al: Auxiliary liver transplantation: Regeneration of the native liver and outcome in 30 patients with fulminant hepatic failure—a multicenter European study. Hepatology 1996;23:1119-1127.
216. Girlanda R, Vilca-Melendez H, Srinivasan P, et al: Immunosuppression withdrawal after auxiliary liver transplantation for acute liver failure. Transplant Proc 2005;37:1720-1721.
217. van Hoek B, de Boer J, Boudjema K, et al: Auxiliary versus orthotopic liver transplantation for acute liver failure. EURALT Study Group. European Auxiliary Liver Transplant Registry. J Hepatol 1999;30:699-705.
218. Neuberger J, Price D: Role of living liver donation in the United Kingdom. BMJ 2003;327:676-679.

Chapter 77

Gastrointestinal Bleeding

Louis Chaptini and Steven Peikin

Gastrointestinal (GI) bleeding encompasses a wide range of diagnoses with multiple types of lesions and bleeding that can occur virtually anywhere in the GI tract. Acute GI bleeding is often an emergency that can be alarming to both the patient and physician. Management and the outcome of GI bleeding depend on both the severity of the bleeding and any comorbid conditions present at the time of the bleeding. Acute GI bleeding often requires close monitoring and management in an intensive care unit (ICU). Management of such bleeding relies on a team approach that involves the expertise of an intensivist, gastroenterologist (endoscopist), radiologist, and surgeon.

More than 300,000 annual hospitalizations in the United States are attributed to GI bleeding.[1] Upper GI bleeding accounts for most of these hospitalizations, with an incidence rate of 100 cases per 100,000,[1] whereas the incidence of lower GI bleeding is estimated at 20 to 27 cases per 100,000.[2,3] Mortality rates vary depending on the source of the bleeding. Most nonvariceal upper GI bleeding studies document mortality rates approximating 10%.[4,5] These rates have not changed over the past 2 decades despite the evolution of acid suppression therapy, which is probably explained by an aging population with increased comorbid diseases. Mortality rates for lower GI bleeding are usually in the range of 5%.[6,7]

CLINICAL PRESENTATION

Initial Evaluation and Resuscitation

The clinical findings in a patient with GI bleeding are crucial in determining the site, cause, and rate of bleeding. The first step in clinical evaluation is to assess the severity of the bleeding. This is done primarily by measuring hemodynamic parameters in an attempt to quantify the amount of blood volume lost (Table 77-1).[8] Because bleeding can represent a dynamic ongoing situation, continuous monitoring of hemodynamics is necessary to guide resuscitation efforts and provide key prognostic information. In patients with GI bleeding, two large-bore intravenous catheters should be placed immediately on arrival to restore euvolemia.

The hematocrit at initial evaluation may not reflect the severity of the bleeding because very recent loss of both plasma and red cells leads to a percentage of red cells in the remaining blood (which defines the hematocrit) that is close to the same value. The hematocrit drops when hemodilution occurs as extravascular fluid enters the vascular space to restore volume, a process that may take up to 72 hours (Fig. 77-1).[9]

The rapidity of blood and colloid infusion depends in part on the patient's cardiovascular condition. Placement of a central venous pressure catheter can help one base decisions on more objective findings. The amount of blood transfused depends on the clinical situation: raising the hematocrit to 30% is appropriate in elderly patients, whereas a hematocrit of 20% to 25% is acceptable in young, otherwise healthy patients; in patients with portal hypertension, it should not exceed 27% to 28%.[8] In patients with conditions associated with defects in platelet or coagulation factors, these substances should be replaced. Patients requiring massive transfusion of packed red blood cells require fresh frozen plasma and platelets. Hypocalcemia can develop in these patients because of the large amount of citrate received with massive transfusion, and thus calcium replacement should be considered, especially in individuals with end-stage liver disease and heart failure, in whom citrate metabolism may be impaired.[10]

History and Clinical Findings

After hemodynamic stabilization is achieved, a careful history and clinical examination are imperative to make

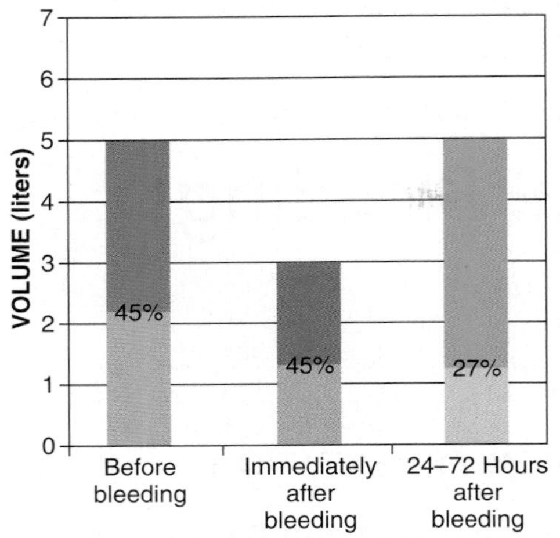

Figure 77-1. Plasma volumes *(solid bars),* red blood cell volumes *(pale bars),* and hematocrit values (%) before bleeding and after blood loss of 2 L. A baseline hematocrit level of 45% is assumed. (From Rockey DC: Gastrointestinal bleeding. In Feldman M, Friedman LS, Sleisenger MH [eds]: Sleisenger and Fordtran's Gastrointestinal and Liver Disease, 7th ed. Philadelphia, Saunders, 2002, pp 221-248.)

Table 77-1. Hemodynamics, Vital Signs, and Blood Loss

Hemodynamics and Vital Signs	% Blood Loss (Fraction of Intravascular Volume)	Bleeding Type
Shock (resting hypotension)	20-25	Massive
Postural (orthostatic tachycardia or hypotension)	10-20	Moderate
Normal	<10	Minor

From Rockey DC: Gastrointestinal bleeding. Gastroenterol Clin North Am 2005;34:581-588.

a preliminary assessment of the location and cause of the bleeding. Important historical features in the evaluation of GI bleeding are shown in Box 77-1.[8]

Hematemesis typically points to an upper source of bleeding, proximal to the ligament of Treitz. In rare cases, hematemesis can be a sign of swallowed blood from oral, pharyngeal, or nasal bleeding. Melena is defined as black tarry stool with a glistering sheen and results from degradation of blood in the GI tract. At least 50 mL of blood in the upper GI tract is required to cause melena, although volumes up to 100 mL may be clinically silent.[11] Melena usually indicates upper GI bleeding, but its source may be the small bowel and sometimes even the proximal part of the colon when the volume of blood is too small to cause hematochezia. Coffee-ground emesis is typically a sign of recent, but currently inactive upper GI bleeding, and its appearance is caused by the acid's effect on blood in the lumen. Hematochezia is generally associated with colonic bleeding but can also be caused by more proximal bleeding. Proximal bleeding in association with hematochezia is usually more hemodynamically significant.

Box 77-1

Historical Features in the Assessment of Gastrointestinal Bleeding

Age
Previous bleeding
Previous gastrointestinal disease
Previous surgery
Underlying medical disorder (especially liver disease)
Nonsteroidal anti-inflammatory drugs
Abdominal pain
Change in bowel habits
Weight loss or anorexia
History of oropharyngeal disease

From Rockey DC: Gastrointestinal bleeding. Gastroenterol Clin North Am 2005;34:581-588.

Other symptoms at initial evaluation can help in narrowing the differential diagnosis. Abdominal pain before or at the time of the bleeding episode can be a sign of underlying peptic ulcer disease (PUD), mesenteric or colonic ischemia, perforation, or even intestinal infarction. Multiple episodes of vomiting and retching preceding the bleeding episode should alert one to the presence of a Mallory-Weiss tear.

A previous history of bleeding from PUD, esophageal or gastric varices, diverticulosis, or vascular ectasia puts these diagnoses high on the differential diagnosis list. A history of abdominal vascular surgery adds aortoenteric fistula to this list. In patients with known liver disease, the possibility of bleeding from conditions associated with portal hypertension, such as esophageal or gastric varices and portal gastropathy, should be raised. One should also look for risk factors for chronic liver disease, such as a history of chronic alcohol abuse and chronic hepatitis.

GI bleeding in elderly patients is usually caused by conditions less commonly encountered in younger patients (i.e., diverticulosis, vascular ectasia, ischemic colitis), whereas in younger patients, bleeding from sources such as varices, ulcer disease, and esophagitis is more common.

Ingestion of aspirin and other nonsteroidal anti-inflammatory drugs (NSAIDs) increases the risk of bleeding from PUD. In patients taking anticoagulant medications, bleeding most often results from underlying GI pathology such as ulcer disease or vascular ectasia, even in the setting of a supratherapeutic international normalized ratio, and should not be attributed to the anticoagulation itself.

Other medical conditions present at the time of the bleeding can have a large impact on the resuscitation efforts and subsequent management. Bleeding patients with a history of coronary artery disease are at increased risk for myocardial infarction, and restoration of volume and oxygenation should be an immediate goal. Patients with pulmonary disease may need airway intubation before sedation when endoscopy is being contemplated.

Physical examination should look for evidence of chronic liver disease such as spider angiomas, gynecomastia, splenomegaly, and ascites. The presence of these signs suggests the possibility of portal hypertension. Telangiectases of the skin or mucous membranes and lips raise the possibility of hereditary hemorrhagic telangiectasia (Osler-Weber-Rendu disease). Acanthosis nigricans can be a sign of GI malignancy (especially gastric cancer). The presence of purpura suggests vascular diseases such as Henoch-Schönlein purpura or polyarteritis nodosa. Tenderness with or without peritoneal signs on abdominal examination may indicate PUD, ischemia, or perforation. The abdominal examination should include percussion and palpation to look for organomegaly and masses. Bedside examination of the character of the stool is a necessary measure that provides critical information about the source and severity of the bleeding episode. Bright red blood per rectum, maroon-colored stools, and melena suggest active bleeding, whereas brown stools indicate less aggressive bleeding.

A nasogastric tube is commonly inserted on arrival in patients with upper (and sometimes lower) GI bleeding. A bloody aspirate suggests, with some degree of certainty, an upper source of bleeding because false-positive results are rare and generally related to nasogastric trauma.[12] In contrast, a nonbloody aspirate does not exclude an upper source, even in the presence of bile-colored aspirate, but suggests nonactive upper or lower GI bleeding. Besides localization of bleeding, nasogastric aspiration has been used to predict the presence of high-risk lesions such as an oozing or spurting lesion or a nonbleeding visible vessel. In one study, investigators demonstrated that a bloody aspirate was significantly associated with and had the highest specificity for high-risk lesions when compared with a coffee-ground and clear/biliary aspirate.[13] In the setting of hematochezia with hemodynamic instability, extremely brisk upper bleeding should be suspected, and a positive nasogastric aspirate can confirm upper GI bleeding. Testing for occult blood in a nasogastric aspirate is indicated rarely and may be helpful only when the coffee-ground appearance of the aspirate is caused by food or dark bile. A common practice is to perform a tap water gastric lavage when bloody or coffee-ground material is found and to consider the bleeding active if the effluent does not clear after 250 to 500 mL of lavage. However, this approach has not been validated, and some data discourage the use of nasogastric lavage to assess the activity of bleeding.[14]

Diagnostic Tests

The initial laboratory evaluation in patients with GI bleeding should include a complete blood count, liver enzymes, prothrombin time, blood urea nitrogen (BUN), and creatinine. As mentioned earlier, the first hematocrit level may be falsely reassuring, so management decisions should rely on other parameters such as hemodynamics and the nature of the bleeding. A high white blood cell count should alert one to the presence of ischemia or infarction. Thrombocytopenia can be a sign of portal hypertension, and a critically low platelet count, as well as a high prothrombin time, should be addressed immediately by transfusion of platelets and fresh frozen plasma. An elevation in the BUN level out of proportion to creatinine is compatible with upper GI bleeding but may also be seen with intravascular volume depletion from any source of bleeding. In one study, this ratio was significantly higher in patients with upper GI bleeding than in those with lower GI bleeding (22.5 ± 11.5 versus 15.9 ± 8.2; $P = .001$); however, the degree of overlap shows the poor discriminatory value of this ratio.[15]

After initial resuscitation and stabilization, a diagnostic plan should be initiated. Several diagnostic tools are available, including endoscopy, radionuclide imaging, and angiography. These tests are aimed at detecting the location, source, and activity of bleeding. Other tests may be necessary in specific clinical situations, such as computed tomography scanning when abdominal pain is a prominent complaint to rule out ischemia, infarction, and perforation. Endoscopy and to some extent angiography have the advantage of allowing both diagnosis and therapy.

Therapeutic Options

In addition to controlling the current episode of bleeding, treatment is also aimed at preventing recurrent bleeding. The available forms of therapy are pharmacologic, endoscopic, angiographic, and surgical. They are often complementary and require a multidisciplinary team approach. Use of these different modalities varies with the specific cause and source of bleeding.

Advances in potent acid suppression with the advent of proton-pump inhibitors (PPIs) and the progress made in endoscopic technology have revolutionized the management of GI bleeding. Effective acid suppression has an established role in decreasing bleeding recurrence. Different endoscopic treatment modalities can be used alone or in combination during endoscopy and have been shown to decrease bleeding recurrence. Such modalities include injection, cautery, and mechanical therapy.

Detailed approaches to the diagnostic and therapeutic options will be highlighted in specific sections of this chapter.

UPPER GASTROINTESTINAL BLEEDING

Differential Diagnosis

Nonvariceal Bleeding

Nonvariceal upper GI bleeding remains a significant cause of mortality and morbidity despite recent advances in pharmacologic and endoscopic therapy. The cause of nonvariceal bleeding encompasses a large array of diagnoses involving multiple organs above the ligament of Treitz and at times outside the GI tract. The causes and frequency of nonvariceal bleeding are listed in Table 77-2.[16]

Peptic Ulcer Disease

PUD traditionally refers to gastric and duodenal ulcers, gastritis, and duodenitis. A number of population-based and prospective studies rank PUD as the most common source of acute upper GI bleeding, with PUD representing up to 50% of all such cases.[17] However, recent analysis from the Clinical Outcomes Research Initiative (CORI) database reported that the most common endoscopic finding in persons with acute upper GI bleeding was "mucosal abnormality" (40%), and gastric or duodenal ulcers were found in 20.6%.[18] Eradication of *Helicobacter pylori* and extensive use of PPIs are probably responsible for this observed decline in the frequency of PUD.

The most important factors predisposing to ulcer disease include acid, *H. pylori* infection, and NSAIDs; however, the role of some of these risk factors in inducing ulcer bleeding remains unclear. Indirect evidence regarding the role of acid in ulcer bleeding comes from data showing that acid suppression by PPIs in patients with active or recent bleeding reduces the risk for rebleeding.[19] Despite the firm association between *H. pylori* and PUD, its role in bleeding is controversial. Some authors suggested an increase in the likelihood of bleeding in patients infected with *H. pylori* (relative risk of approximately 1.5),[20,21] whereas others showed a decrease in the incidence of *H. pylori* in patients with actively bleeding ulcers.[22] Evidence of the association between NSAIDs and ulcer bleeding is strong and comes from both placebo-controlled and case-control studies.[23,24]

The pathogenesis of bleeding from an ulcer involves aneurysmal dilation with an intense arteritis associated with a marked inflammatory response.[25] When eroding into large vessels, ulcers can cause catastrophic bleeding. This most commonly occurs in the posterior portion of the duodenal bulb, where ulcers can erode directly into the pancreaticoduodenal artery.

Table 77-2. Causes of Nonvariceal Upper Gastrointestinal Bleeding

Diagnosis	Incidence (%)
Peptic ulcer	30-50
Mallory-Weiss tear	15-20
Erosive gastritis or duodenitis	10-15
Esophagitis	5-10
Malignancy	1-2
Angiodysplasia or vascular malformations	5
Other	5

From Ferguson CB, Mitchell RM: Nonvariceal upper gastrointestinal bleeding: Standard and new treatment. Gastroenterol Clin North Am 2005;34:607-621.

Other Sources of Nonvariceal Upper Gastrointestinal Bleeding

Mallory-Weiss tears (MWTs) are mucosal and occasionally submucosal lacerations caused by sudden increases in pressure within the cardia and lower esophagus produced by retching. MWTs are responsible for 5% to 15% of upper GI bleeding.[17] The majority of upper GI bleeding caused by MWTs stops spontaneously and does not require any blood transfusion or endoscopic treatment. However, some cases are severe enough to require endoscopic hemostasis and occasionally angiography with embolization or even surgery. A history of retching on arrival at the emergency department is not always present.[26] Endoscopically, tears are usually 1.5 to 2 cm in length and occur at the gastroesophageal junction or, most commonly, in the proximal part of the stomach (Fig. 77-2).

Angiodysplasia, also referred to as arteriovenous malformation or vascular ectasia, is another source of upper GI bleeding and accounts for approximately 5% to 10% of cases.[17] It occurs in inherited syndromes such as heredi-

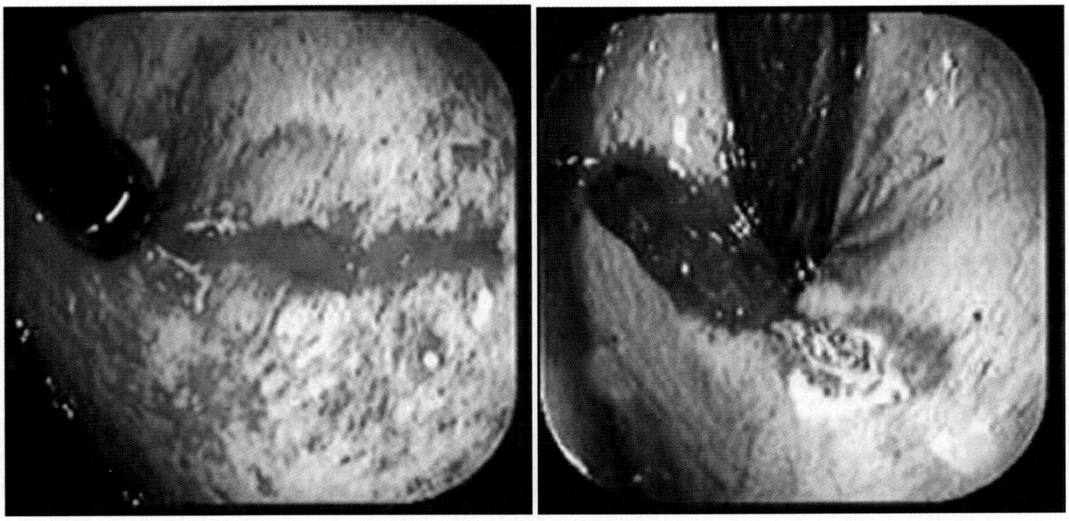

A B

Figure 77-2. A, Mallory-Weiss tear in the cardia of the stomach. Active bleeding is seen. **B,** The same tear seen in **A** after injection with epinephrine and coagulation. The bleeding is controlled. (From Schmulewitz N, O'Connor JB: Esophageal disease caused by medication, radiation and internal trauma. In DiMarino AJ, Benjamin S [eds]: Gastrointestinal Disease: An Endoscopic Approach, 2nd ed. Thorofare, NJ, Slack, 2002, pp 245-262.)

tary hemorrhagic telangiectasia (Osler-Weber-Rendu syndrome) and blue rubber bleb nevus syndrome, but most cases are acquired.[27] The association of angiodysplasia with medical conditions such as renal failure, aortic stenosis, connective tissue disease (scleroderma), and von Willebrand's disease has been recognized, but the evidence for these associations is limited.[17,28]

Dieulafoy's lesion is an under-recognized cause of upper GI bleeding and is described as a visible vessel protruding from a small mucosal defect without any underlying ulcer.[17] It has also been called "caliber-persistent artery" in submucosal tissue. Bleeding from Dieulafoy's lesion represents less than 5% of cases of upper GI bleeding.[29,30] The lesion is generally located on the lesser curvature within 6 cm of the gastroesophageal junction and can be difficult to detect because of its small size and normal surrounding mucosa (Fig. 77-3).[28]

Benign and malignant neoplasms are responsible for less than 5% of upper GI bleeding.[31] Bleeding can be the initial symptom of tumors originating from the esophagus, stomach, or small intestine. These neoplasms can be primary malignancies, such as adenocarcinoma of the esophagus, stomach, or duodenum; squamous cell carcinoma of the esophagus; and gastric or duodenal lymphomas. Gastrointestinal stromal cell tumors (GISTs), carcinoid tumors, and lipomas are examples of benign tumors that can cause upper GI bleeding.[17]

Upper GI bleeding from an aortoenteric fistula is very rare but should be considered in the appropriate clinical setting (such as a patient with a history of aortic aneurysm repair). Fistulas are generally located in the third portion of the duodenum. Patients will frequently have a small hemorrhage first, known as a "herald bleed," that occurs before a major hemorrhage.[32]

Another rare cause of upper GI bleeding is hemobilia. It can occur after liver biopsy or hepatobiliary tree instrumentation (such as with endoscopic retrograde cholangiopancreatography [ERCP]) or from biliary tumors.

Hemosuccus pancreaticus is an uncommon cause of upper GI bleeding that occurs secondary to pseudoaneurysm formation and rupture into the pancreatic duct as a complication of a pancreatic pseudocyst in patients with chronic pancreatitis.[33]

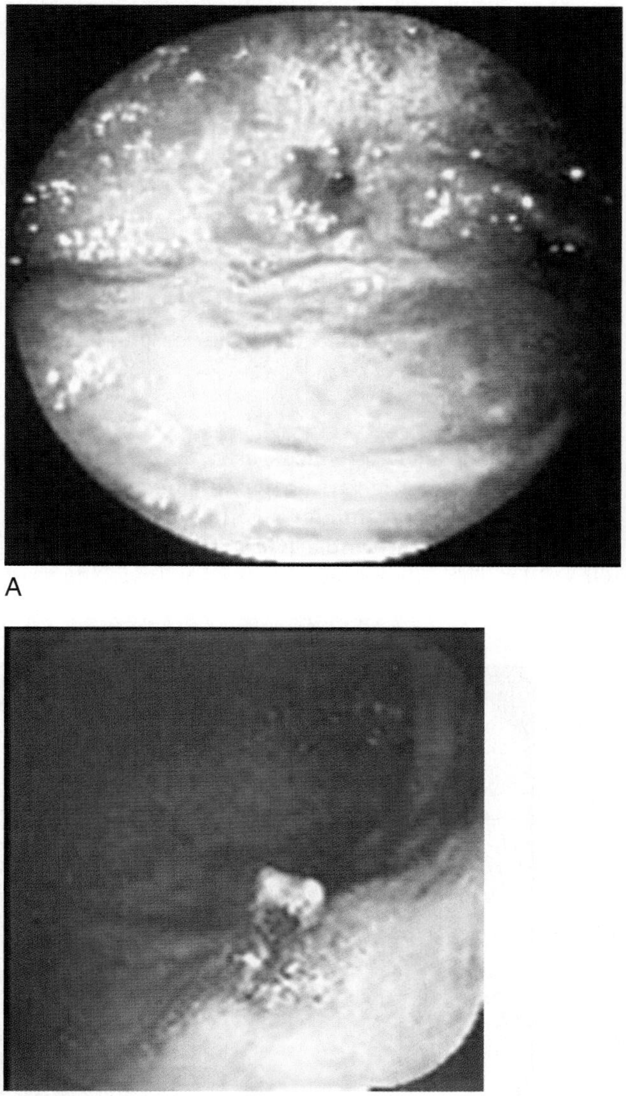

A

B

Figure 77-3. A and **B,** Endoscopic appearance of a Dieulafoy lesion in the proximal part of the stomach. (From Bashir RM, Al-Kawas FH: Vascular lesions of the stomach. In DiMarino AJ, Benjamin S [eds]: Gastrointestinal Disease: An Endoscopic Approach, 2nd ed. Thorofare, NJ, Slack, 2002, pp 535-550.)

Bleeding Secondary to Portal Hypertension

Portal hypertension is defined by a hepatic venous pressure gradient (HVPG) greater than 5 mm Hg. HVPG represents the difference between portal vein pressure and free hepatic vein pressure. Portal hypertension is most commonly related to cirrhosis but can be secondary to a variety of other conditions. It has been classified as prehepatic, hepatic, and posthepatic, depending on the location of the obstruction to flow. Examples of noncirrhotic portal hypertension include portal vein thrombosis, Budd-Chiari syndrome, and constrictive pericarditis. In the presence of portal hypertension, the development of portosystemic collateral venous drainage results in the formation of varices. Varices develop most commonly in the distal portion of the esophagus and the stomach. Ectopic varices can be seen in the duodenum, jejunum, or colon; at the level of stomas (ileostomy and colostomy); and in the anorectal region.

Most portal hypertensive bleeding results from ruptured esophageal varices, but clinically significant bleeding can also be secondary to gastric varices, portal gastropathy, and ectopic varices.

Esophageal Varices

The incidence of varices among all cirrhotic patients is around 50%. However, if monitored long enough, varices eventually develop in most cirrhotics.[34] Variceal hemorrhage occurs in a third of cirrhotic patients with varices. Although portal hypertension is defined by an HVPG greater than 5 mm Hg, Garcia-Tsao and colleagues showed that varices do not develop and hence do not bleed as long as the HVPG is less than 12 mm Hg.[35] However, once this threshold is reached, there is poor correlation between the pressure gradient and the risk for bleeding. Other risk factors associated with variceal bleeding include the degree of liver disease (provided by Child's classification), variceal location and size (higher risk near the gastroesophageal junction and with large varices), and the presence of particular endoscopic signs (red wale markings suggestive of dilated longitudinal venules, cherry-red spots, and hematocystic spots consisting of small red dots or a reddish blister-like formation on the variceal surface and the white or purple nipple sign on a varix) (Fig. 77-4).[34,36]

Gastric Varices

Sarin and colleagues classified gastric varices into two groups: isolated gastric varices (IGVs) and gastroesophageal varices (GEVs) (continuous with esophageal varices and extending to the cardia [GEV 1] or to the fundus [GEV 2]).[37] The authors found that GEV 1 was the most common type of gastric varices but IGV was the type that bleeds the most. Overall, gastric varices bleed less commonly but more severely than esophageal varices do.[34]

Diagnostic Evaluation

Endoscopic Examination

After the initial evaluation, resuscitation, and stabilization of a patient with upper GI bleeding, effort is directed at localization and treatment of the hemorrhage. Endoscopy has become the preferred diagnostic and therapeutic modality for upper GI bleeding because of its accuracy and low complication rate. With its use, a specific diagnosis can be achieved in 95% of patients. The use of promotility agents such as erythromycin (250 mg by intravenous bolus or 3 mg/kg over a 30-minute period) before the endoscopic examination can significantly improve mucosal visibility by promoting gastric motility and emptying of gastric contents.[38,39]

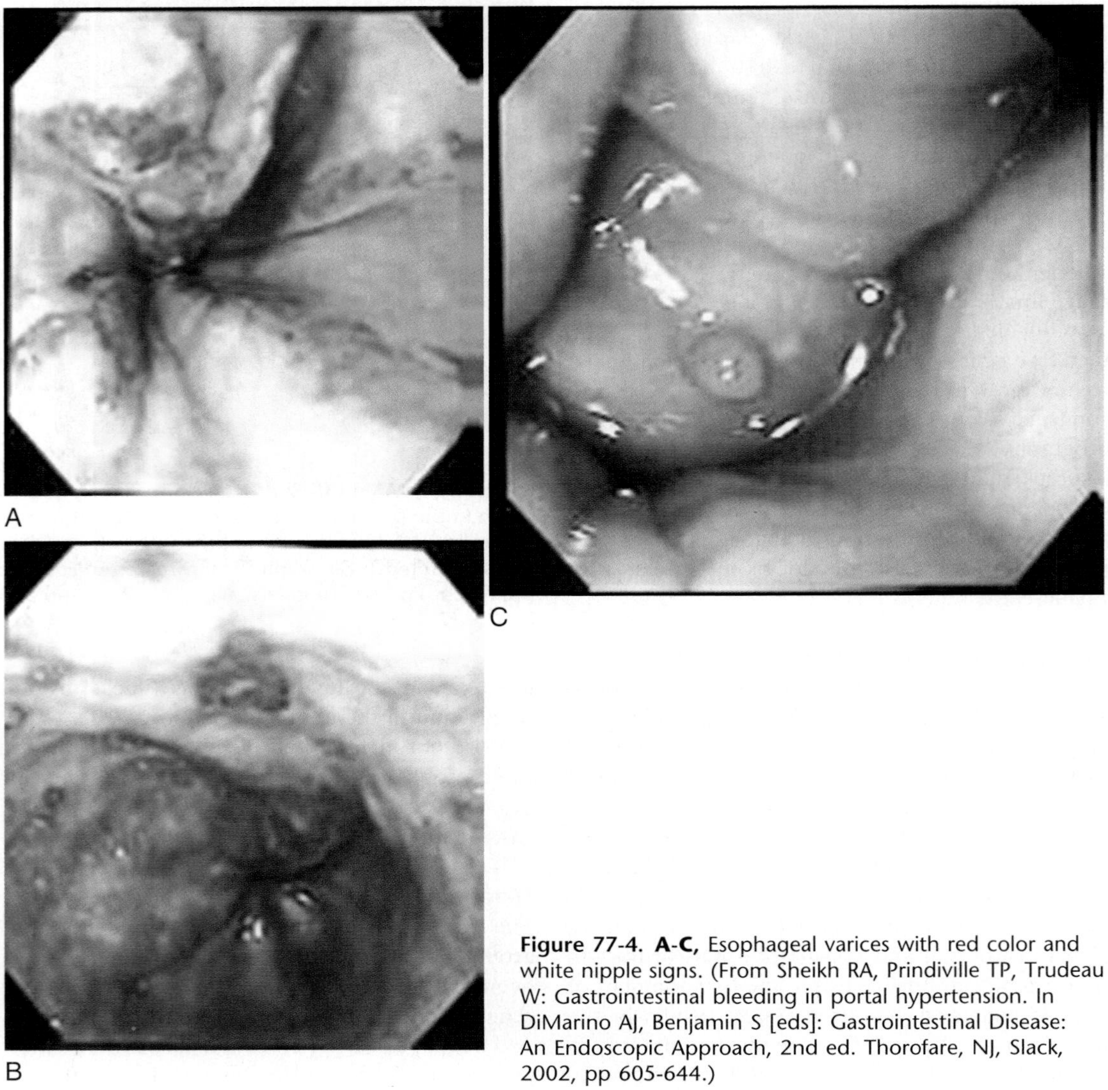

Figure 77-4. A-C, Esophageal varices with red color and white nipple signs. (From Sheikh RA, Prindiville TP, Trudeau W: Gastrointestinal bleeding in portal hypertension. In DiMarino AJ, Benjamin S [eds]: Gastrointestinal Disease: An Endoscopic Approach, 2nd ed. Thorofare, NJ, Slack, 2002, pp 605-644.)

The optimal timing of endoscopy remains a balance between clinical need and resources and is still subject to controversy.[16] Emergency endoscopy is generally performed in patients with orthostasis, tachycardia, shock, and signs of continued bleeding who cannot be hemodynamically stabilized.[40] When performed early (within 24 hours of arrival), endoscopy has been shown to have an impact on the length of hospital stay and blood transfusion requirements and may reduce the likelihood of rebleeding or surgical intervention in high-risk patients.[16,41,42]

One major role of endoscopy is to identify stigmata of recent hemorrhage known to correlate well with an increased risk for rebleeding and thus a need for endoscopic therapy. Rates of rebleeding with these specific endoscopic findings are summarized in Table 77-3.[41]

Nonendoscopic Assessment

When endoscopy is not able to be performed or has not yielded a definitive diagnosis, angiography and radionuclide imaging may be useful alternatives. Such endoscopic failures are most often related to anatomic situations (i.e., strictures or surgical alterations) preventing full endoscopy. Esophagography and upper GI series are no longer used as part of the diagnostic evaluation of patients with upper GI bleeding.

Therapeutic Alternatives

Nonvariceal Bleeding

Pharmacotherapy

Acid suppression has been shown to play a role in the inactivation of pepsin, optimization of platelet function, and inhibition of fibrinolysis. Subsequently, clot stabilization and ulcer healing may be more effective and rapid within a less acidic environment. This constitutes the rationale for acid suppressive therapy in patients with bleeding peptic ulcers. Several trials studied the effect of acid suppression with either H_2 receptor antagonists (H_2RAs) or PPIs, with or without endoscopic treatment, on rates of rebleeding, surgery, and death.

Table 77-3. Stigmata of Ulcer Hemorrhage and Risk for Recurrent Bleeding without Endoscopic Therapy

Stigmata	Risk for Recurrent Bleeding without Therapy
Active arterial (spurting) bleeding	Approaches 100%
Nonbleeding visible vessel ("pigmented protuberance")	Up to 50%
Nonbleeding adherent clot	30%-35%
Ulcer oozing (without other stigmata)	10%-27%
Flat spots	<8%
Clean-based ulcers	<3%

From ASGE Standards of Practice Committee: ASGE guideline: The role of endoscopy in acute non-variceal upper GI-hemorrhage. Gastrointest Endosc 1999;49:145-152.

One meta-analysis of the use of H_2RAs in acute upper GI bleeding demonstrated a modest benefit in reducing rates of rebleeding, surgery, and death.[43] However, other more recent trials and a meta-analysis have failed to show similar effects,[44] thus leading to a consensus group opinion that the available data do not support the use of H_2RAs in patients with ulcer bleeding.[45]

Recent emphasis has shifted to PPIs. These agents have a number of advantages over H_2RAs, including more prolonged and profound acid suppression and lack of tachyphylaxis. A number of studies investigating PPIs in different doses and different routes of administration (oral, intravenous bolus, continuous intravenous infusion) were conducted in recent years. In these studies PPIs were used with or without endoscopic hemostasis, in the presence of specific bleeding or nonbleeding lesions, and were compared with placebo and H_2RAs. Two recent meta-analyses provided strong support for the use of PPIs in peptic ulcer bleeding by showing a significant decrease in ulcer rebleeding and surgery, regardless of the dosing regimen and mode of administration.[46,47] Only one of these meta-analyses showed a significant decrease in mortality.[47] Despite the extensive data supporting the use of PPIs in bleeding ulcer patients, it is still unclear which route of administration, which dose, which agent, and what duration of therapy are most appropriate and effective. Based on a number of selected trials, a consensus panel on nonvariceal upper GI bleeding recommended the use of an intravenous bolus followed by continuous infusion of a PPI after successful endoscopic therapy.[45] The use of a continuous infusion is supported by data showing that maintenance of intragastric pH at greater than 6 after endoscopic hemostasis is associated with the lowest rebleeding rates and that this goal can be achieved only by bolus administration of a PPI followed by a constant infusion.[48]

Other agents with different mechanisms of action have been studied in patients with upper GI bleeding. One meta-analysis showed that tranexamic acid, an antifibrinolytic agent, has positive effects on reduction of rebleeding, surgery, and mortality, but the studies included were conducted without endoscopic therapy.[49,50] Furthermore, the use of tranexamic acid has been associated with increased rates of thrombotic events.[50] A reduction in splanchnic blood flow with somatostatin and its analogues (such as octreotide) is an attractive measure in patients with upper GI bleeding and has been the subject of several trials, with conflicting results.[45,51,52] To date, the available data are not convincingly in favor of using these agents in patients with nonvariceal upper GI bleeding, even though some authors find them useful in patients who are bleeding uncontrollably while awaiting endoscopy or surgery or in whom surgery is contraindicated.[45]

Endoscopic Therapy

Endoscopic therapy for nonvariceal upper GI bleeding in patients with high-risk lesions has been shown to reduce the rate of rebleeding, need for surgery, and mortality.[53] It is indicated in patients with active bleeding, spurting arterial vessels, and nonbleeding visible vessels in an underlying ulcer.[41] Recent data have also shown benefit in removal and endoscopic treatment of adherent clots (as opposed to observation alone).[54,55] Different forms of endoscopic therapy include injection technique, thermal technique, and mechanical technique. In many cases a combination of these modalities is used to treat a single bleeding lesion or one at high risk of bleeding.

Injection therapy results in hemostasis, probably from a combination of vascular tamponade and pharmacologic effect of the injected agent. Agents used for injection include normal saline solution, epinephrine, and sclerosants such as ethanol, ethanolamine, and polidocanol. In addition to the local tamponade effect of normal saline solution and epinephrine, the latter has a vasoconstricting effect. Sclerosant agents work by causing direct tissue injury and thrombosis.[41] Another class of agents used during injection therapy includes thrombin, fibrin, and cyanoacrylate glue. These agents create a primary tissue seal at the bleeding site. Epinephrine at a concentration of 1:10,000 or 1:20,000 is the most commonly used agent, sometimes in conjunction with other agents or techniques.

Thermal therapy consists of the delivery of heat to the mucosa, which results in edema, coagulation of tissue proteins, and contraction of arteries. When heat is delivered through a contact probe, an additional effect is achieved by mechanical compression of the target artery before delivery of the heat.

Thermal energy can be delivered through noncontact techniques such as the Nd:YAG and argon lasers and argon plasma coagulation (APC). The laser technique has been abandoned because of its high cost and the high risk of complications associated with its use. In APC, the argon gas forms a plasma and acts as an electrical conductor of the current, thereby resulting in coagulation of superficial tissues. Despite comparable results with the heater probe technique when used for ulcer bleeding,[56] APC is used primarily for the treatment of superficial lesions such as vascular abnormalities.[41]

Contact thermal techniques refer to the delivery of heat through direct contact of the mucosa with heater probes or electrocautery probes (monopolar and bipolar probes). The heater probe is an aluminum cylinder that delivers a programmed amount of energy (heat) through its end or sides to the tissue. The catheter tip can also be used to apply firm pressure on the bleeding point or the visible vessel. Electrocautery probes use an electrical current that passes from the electrode tip through the patient's body to a grounding plate (monopolar) or flows between two or more electrodes at the probe tip (bipolar or multipolar). The advantage of the bipolar (multipolar) probe is that the concentration of current at the level of the tip results in less depth of tissue injury and lower potential for perforation.

Mechanical therapy refers to the use of a device that causes physical tamponade of a bleeding site. Such devices include metallic clips, sewing devices, rubber band ligation, and endoloops. Metallic clips are the most studied of these devices and have shown variable success, probably because of the difficulty encountered with their placement. Some authors have suggested the use of clips in combination with other endoscopic treatments.[45]

The choice of endoscopic therapy depends on the stigmata of ulcer hemorrhage and the experience of the endoscopist. Monotherapy (with either injection or thermal techniques) and combination therapy have been the subject of several randomized controlled trials. Meta-analyses looking at injection or thermal endoscopic therapies showed statistically significant relative decreases in rebleeding rates and mortality.[57,58] Combination therapy with both injection and thermal therapy has been shown to be superior to medical therapy[59,60] and, furthermore, to either treatment alone.[61]

Angiographic Therapy

Angiography can be useful as a potential diagnostic and therapeutic modality in specific cases of upper GI bleeding when endoscopy cannot be performed or fails to reveal the bleeding site and when endoscopic hemostasis is unsuccessful. It is also considered in patients who are poor surgical candidates.

Angiographic or "transcatheter" intervention in cases of upper GI bleeding involves two techniques: infusion of vasoconstricting medication and mechanical occlusion (embolization) of the arterial supply responsible for the hemorrhage. Vasopressin infusion induces vasoconstriction and results in cessation of bleeding in 70% to 80% of cases initially, but rebleeding occurs in up to 20%. Complications can range from problems related to arterial access to pulmonary edema and myocardial depression.[62] Vasopressin infusion has lost favor with the advent of embolization. Transcatheter embolization has become the mainstay for the radiographic treatment of nonvariceal upper GI bleeding and comes second after endoscopic therapy in most centers.[63] The embolic material used can be temporary (such as a gelatin sponge and autologous clot) or permanent (such as coils). Clinical success with embolization ranges from 52% to 91%. Potential complications of embolization include ischemia and perforation.[63]

Surgical Therapy

When endoscopic hemostasis fails to control the bleeding or when hemorrhage recurs after successful control of bleeding, surgical intervention provides an alternative therapeutic option. The main goal of surgery is control of active bleeding and prevention of exsanguination, with a secondary aim to prevent recurrent ulceration. The choice of operation depends on the location of the bleeding lesion and the surgeon's expertise. Truncal vagotomy with antrectomy and vagotomy with pyloroplasty are examples of operations performed in cases of nonvariceal upper GI bleeding. Total gastrectomy is rarely indicated. Because recurrent ulcers can be prevented by avoiding NSAIDs, eliminating *H. pylori* if present, or administering prophylactic PPI therapy, most ulcer operations for acute bleeding focus on oversewing the ulcer rather than performing the more definitive surgeries just listed.

Variceal Bleeding

Pharmacotherapy

Pharmacologic agents used in the treatment of acute variceal bleeding are aimed at reducing portal pressure by either decreasing portal blood flow or reducing intrahepatic resistance. Infusion of vasoactive agents constitutes an adjunct to endoscopic therapy and often precedes endoscopy when suspicion of variceal bleeding is high.

Vasopressin, terlipressin, somatostatin, and somatostatin analogues (octreotide and lanreotide) all induce constriction of the splanchnic vasculature and result in a decrease in portal blood flow. Vasopressin causes systemic vasoconstriction, as well as splanchnic vasoconstriction, and can lead to adverse effects such as myocardial ischemia and infarction and cerebrovascular accidents.[64] These dangerous side effects led to the combination of vasopressin with other agents and the search for analogues with a better safety profile.

In one study, the combination of vasopressin with nitroglycerin resulted in a reduction in side effects and improved efficacy over vasopressin alone.[64] Nitroglycerin, a potent venous dilator, decreases the hemodynamic side effects of vasopressin and at the same time reduces intrahepatic resistance, thereby resulting in a further reduction in portal pressure.

Terlipressin is a synthetic analogue of vasopressin with a longer duration of action and fewer side effects than vasopressin. Unlike other vasoactive agents, terlipressin has been shown to reduce mortality when compared with placebo.[65] At present, terlipressin is not available in the United States.

Somatostatin is a naturally occurring peptide that induces splanchnic vasoconstriction without affecting the systemic circulation and thus results in a decrease in portal pressure. When compared with vasopressin, somatostatin was equivalent in bleeding control but had significantly fewer side effects.[66] Further data suggested that somatostatin has the greatest effect when used in conjunction with endoscopic therapy.[67,68] Octreotide, a somatostatin analogue, is approved for use in variceal bleeding in the United States. Initial results regarding its efficacy have been inconsistent,[68] but a meta-analysis by Corley and associates was able to demonstrate its efficacy in controlling acute variceal bleeding when compared with placebo and other vasoactive agents.[69] At present, because of its excellent safety profile and easy availability, octreotide (50-μg bolus followed by a 50-μg/h continuous infusion for 3 to 5 days) is almost always used in conjunction with endoscopic therapy.

The use of prophylactic antibiotics in patients with variceal bleeding has been shown to decrease mortality in several randomized controlled trials.[67] The rationale behind antibiotic prophylaxis derives from the fact that bacterial infection is present in up to 20% of patients with cirrhosis who are admitted with variceal bleeding and that infection develops in as many as 50% of patients while hospitalized.[70] Mortality is significantly higher in infected cirrhotic patients than in noninfected cirrhotics.[71,72] Furthermore, infected cirrhotic patients have a higher rate of variceal rebleeding.[73] This is probably due to the presence of cytokines and endotoxins that induce hematologic abnormalities such as platelet dysfunction and activation of the coagulation and fibrinolytic systems.[67] Despite the fact that antibiotic prophylaxis is strongly recommended in bleeding cirrhotic patients and has become the standard of care, the optimal choice of antibiotic and duration of therapy are still unclear. Benefit was demonstrated with quinolones, cephalosporins, nonabsorbable antibiotics, and other agents. We tend to administer quinolone intravenously (followed by the oral route as soon as the patient's condition allows) for a total of 7 to 10 days. If a patient was taking quinolone orally for prophylaxis of spontaneous bacterial peritonitis, intravenous cephalosporin is used (because of concern over quinolone resistance). In conclusion, it should be emphasized that according to the current body of literature, antibiotic prophylaxis has been consistently associated with improved survival rates, an outcome not achieved with most vasoactive agents.

The use of recombinant factor VIIa in cirrhotic patients with upper GI bleeding has been attractive because cirrhotic patients will often have deficiencies in coagulation factors and factor VII in particular. In a randomized controlled trial investigating the use of this factor, Bosch and coworkers[74] demonstrated benefit in the rate of rebleeding only in the subgroup of patients with advanced cirrhosis (Child-Pugh grades B and C). Further studies are needed before routine use of this therapy can be recommended.

Endoscopic Therapy

Endoscopic sclerotherapy and endoscopic band ligation are the mainstay of therapy for acute variceal bleeding. These procedures are successful in achieving hemostasis in 80% to 90% of patients.[67]

Sclerotherapy consists of intravariceal or paravariceal injection of a sclerosant agent such as sodium tetradecyl sulfate or ethanolamine. These agents provoke a severe inflammatory reaction within or around the varix that leads to variceal thrombosis and obliteration. Despite its high effectiveness in controlling bleeding, the complication rate with sclerotherapy can be as high as 40%.[75] Complications range from local effects, such as deep ulcers causing rebleeding, odynophagia, and in some cases perforation, to bacteremia and systemic complications such as pleural and pericardial effusion. Esophageal stricture is the most common long-term side effect of sclerotherapy. Once the acute bleeding is controlled, repeated sessions of sclerotherapy are required to eradicate the varices and prevent rebleeding.

Endoscopic band ligation is comparable to sclerotherapy in achieving initial hemostasis.[76] A ligating device is attached to the tip of the endoscope, and elastic rings are placed over the targeted varix (Fig. 77-5). With the availability of multiband ligating devices, 5 to 10 bands can be deployed in one session. Band ligation has a lower rate of complication (including the rebleeding rate in some but not all studies[77]) than sclerotherapy does, but it can be difficult to perform during acute bleeding.[67] Superficial mucosal ulceration occurs when the elastic ring and

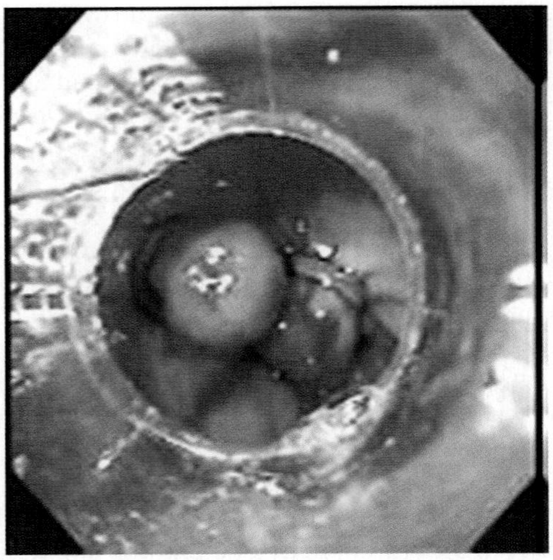

Figure 77-5. Esophageal varices immediately after band ligation. (From Bashir RM, Al-Kawas FH: Vascular lesions of the stomach. In DiMarino AJ, Benjamin S (eds): Gastrointestinal Disease: An Endoscopic Approach, 2nd ed. Thorofare, NJ, Slack, 2002, pp 245-262.)

underlying tissue slough off. Transient chest discomfort and dysphagia are common after band ligation. Band ligation also has the advantage of achieving eradication of varices with fewer endoscopic sessions than typically needed for sclerotherapy.[77]

Balloon Tamponade

The use of balloon tamponade in the control of active variceal bleeding comes as a last resort when other forms of therapy are not available or fail to achieve hemostasis. Three balloons have been used for this purpose: the Minnesota tube, the Sengstaken-Blakemore tube, and the Linton-Nachlas tube. Control of bleeding with these tubes depends on patient selection, the concomitant use of other therapies, and the experience of the staff using them. With the advent of other therapies and the increasing experience of endoscopists in sclerotherapy and endoscopic banding, experience in the use of tamponade balloons decreased substantially. A major concern with the use of these tubes is the high risk of rebleeding after deflation of the balloon, in addition to the risk of esophageal rupture. Balloon tamponade should be used only as a temporary means of stabilization and as a bridge to a more definitive form of therapy.

Transjugular Intrahepatic Portosystemic Shunt

The transjugular intrahepatic portosystemic shunt (TIPS) procedure involves the creation of a low-resistance channel between the portal vein and the hepatic vein through which blood is shunted from the portal to the systemic circulation. Via an angiographic technique, an expandable metal stent is deployed across this channel and results in a significant decrease in portal pressure. This technique allows the creation of a portosystemic shunt without requiring general anesthesia and major surgery. TIPS is indicated in situations in which acute variceal bleeding is refractory to endoscopic and pharmacologic therapy. It has been shown to control bleeding in more than 90% of patients, with a rebleeding rate of less than 20%.[78,79] However, the mortality rate after the TIPS procedure in the setting of acute uncontrollable variceal bleeding is between 30% and 40%.[67] A major complication associated with this procedure is the development of encephalopathy in 10% to 20% of patients. Stenosis and complete occlusion of the shunt occur in 5% to 15% of the cases, requiring revision.

Surgical Therapy

Surgical creation of portosystemic shunts has been used for decompression of the portal system to treat and prevent variceal bleeding. The various forms of surgical shunts include portocaval shunts, distal splenorenal shunts, and partial shunts. Revascularization of the esophagus is another surgical option for the treatment of variceal bleeding. Interest in surgery has declined over the years because of the advent of the less invasive endoscopic and TIPS procedures. At present, surgery is considered only when medical and endoscopic therapy fails to control bleeding and TIPS is not available.[67]

STRESS-RELATED MUCOSAL DISEASE

The term stress-related mucosal disease (SRMD) covers a spectrum of conditions ranging from superficial mucosal damage to focal deep mucosal damage (stress ulcers). The terms *stress ulcer, stress gastritis, stress erosions,* and *stress lesions* are used interchangeably in the literature.

SRMD is defined as mucosal abnormalities of the upper GI tract that occur with extreme physiologic stress, typically in the ICU.

The incidence of endoscopically documented gastric lesions in patients in the ICU ranges from 74% to 100%.[80] The lesions are typically, but not exclusively, located in the fundus and body of the stomach. However, most of these lesions are of little significance because healing occurs rapidly. Clinically evident bleeding, defined as blood in a nasogastric aspirate, hematemesis, and melena, occurs in 5% to 25% of patients in the ICU. Clinically important bleeding, however, is defined as overt bleeding associated with one of the following within 24 hours of the onset of the bleeding: a drop in systolic blood pressure of greater than 20 mm Hg, an increase in the pulse rate of more than 20 beats per minute and a 10–mm Hg drop in systolic blood pressure, or a decrease in hemoglobin of greater than 2 g/dL requiring blood transfusion and failure of hemoglobin to increase by the number of units transfused minus 2 g/dL.[81] Clinically important bleeding affects only 3% to 6% of critically ill patients.[82]

The pathogenesis of SRMD involves a disruption in the balance between aggressive and protective factors that leads to gastric mucosal damage. Adequate microcirculation in the upper GI tract is the most important defense mechanism against luminal aggressors such as acid and enzyme secretion, as well as infection. The role of the microcirculation is to provide nutrients and eliminate toxic oxygen-derived free radicals. In the presence of severe physiologic stress, disruption of intramucosal blood flow leads to a number of events, including the formation of toxic oxygen-derived radicals, a decrease in the synthesis of cytoprotective prostaglandins and mucus production, and a reduction in bicarbonate secretion resulting in an increase in intramural acidity (Fig. 77-6).[80,82] These events create a favorable setting for mucosal injury and ulceration.[83,84] Subsequent reperfusion also plays a major role in the development of lesions.[84]

Identification of critically ill patients at risk for significant bleeding from SRMD has been the subject of several studies. A landmark study by Cook and associates[81] demonstrated a significant increase in the risk for bleeding from SRMD in patients requiring mechanical ventilation for more than 48 hours and in those with coagulopathy (defined as thrombocytopenia [platelet count <50,000/mL^3], an international normalized ratio above 1.5, or a partial thromboplastin time more than 2.0 times the control value) (Table 77-4). Other risk factors such as shock, sepsis, renal failure, liver failure, and glucocorticoids were identified, but the association with bleeding was not statistically significant. Risk factors associated with the presence of SRMD (not necessarily bleeding) include recent major surgery, major trauma, severe burns (Curling's ulcers), head trauma or coma (Cushing's ulcers), and multiple organ failure.[85-87] Further understanding of the risk factors associated with bleeding from SRMD will help in directing prophylactic therapy to patients who will benefit most from this therapy.[88]

The reported mortality rates in critically ill patients with bleeding from SRMD ranges from 46% to 77%.[81,89,90] These high rates are most likely due to the underlying disease and not directly related to GI bleeding. However, they reveal the importance of significant bleeding as a sign of the degree of severity of the primary illness.

Prophylaxis

As mentioned earlier, the risk for bleeding from SRMD is significantly increased in patients undergoing prolonged

Table 77-4. Risk Factors for Upper Gastrointestinal Bleeding in Critically Ill Patients

	Simple Regression		Multiple Regression	
	Odds Ratio	*P* Value	Odds Ratio	*P* Value
Respiratory failure	25.5	<0.001	15.6	<.001
Coagulopathy	9.5	<0.001	4.3	<.001
Hypotension	5.0	.03	3.7	.08
Sepsis	7.3	<0.001	2.0	.17
Hepatic failure	6.5	<0.001	1.6	.27
Renal failure	4.6	<0.001	1.6	.26
Enteral feeding	3.8	<0.001	1.0	.99
Glucocorticoid administration	3.7	<0.001	1.5	.26
Organ transplantation	3.6	.006	1.5	.42
Anticoagulant therapy	3.3	.004	1.1	.88

From Cook DJ, Fuller HD, Guyatt GH, et al: Risk factors for gastrointestinal bleeding in critically ill patients. N Engl J Med 1994;330:377-381.

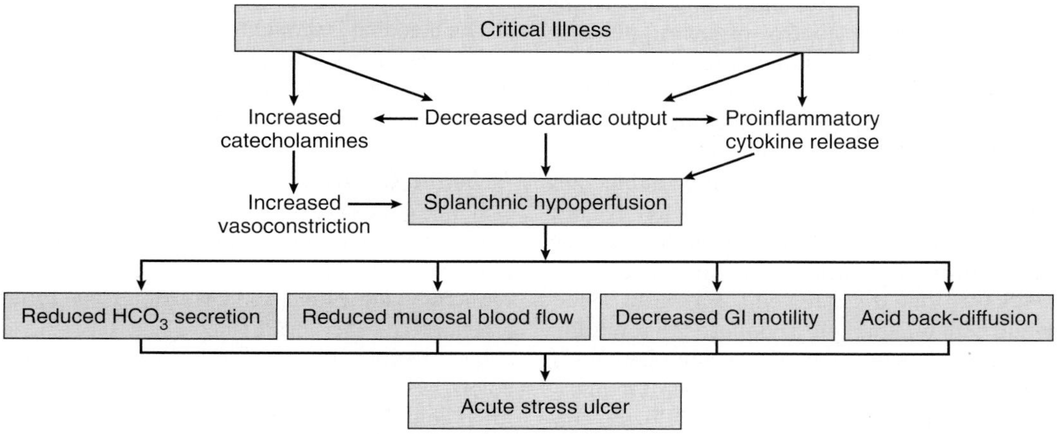

Figure 77-6. Pathophysiology of stress ulcers. (From Mutlu GM, Mutlu EA, Factor P: GI complications in patients receiving mechanical ventilation. Chest 2001;119:1222-1241.)

mechanical ventilation and in those with coagulopathy. Such patients should benefit from the different forms of prophylaxis available.

The role of enteral nutrition in prophylaxis for SRMD is controversial.[91,92] The rationale behind the use of enteral nutrition derives from its ability to improve blood flow to the stomach and sustain mucosal immunity and integrity.[93] However, experimental data in hemodynamically compromised animals showed an increase in tissue hypoxia when enteral nutrition was administered.[94] Furthermore, in one study the degree of acid suppression was reduced in patients receiving H_2RAs or PPIs with concomitant enteral feeding.[95]

When compared with placebo, antacids have been shown to decrease bleeding in patients with SRMD.[96] However, antacids require frequent dosing and monitoring of pH and are not practical to use, especially with the advent of other effective agents for prophylaxis.

Sucralfate works by coating the gastric mucosa and forming a thin protective layer between the mucosa and the gastric acid in the lumen without affecting acid secretion and intragastric pH. The use of sucralfate for prevention of bleeding in patients with SRMD gained interest because of theoretical concern about gram-negative bacterial overgrowth when the pH of the stomach is increased by the use of H_2RAs or PPIs, which can potentially lead to nosocomial pneumonia. Conflicting results were reported regarding this issue, but a large trial by Cook and colleagues in which ranitidine and sucralfate were compared showed no significant difference in the development of nosocomial pneumonia.[97] In this same trial, the incidence of clinically important bleeding was significantly lower with ranitidine. Other studies demonstrated comparable efficacy between sucralfate and antacids and H_2RAs in terms of prevention of SRMD.[98,99] One drawback to the use of sucralfate is that it may decrease the absorption of other concomitantly administered oral drugs.

Intravenous H_2RAs are the most widely used pharmacologic agents for the prophylaxis of bleeding in patients with SRMD. Meta-analysis of studies looking at the role of H_2RAs in SRMD demonstrated a decrease in the incidence of clinically important bleeding.[96] Furthermore, H_2RAs were more effective than antacids in preventing bleeding.[96,100] Despite better control of gastric pH with continuous infusion of H_2RAs, bolus infusion has been shown to be as effective in preventing bleeding.[96,101] One major concern is the development of tolerance to H_2RAs when administered for a prolonged period.

PPIs are gaining wider use in the prevention of bleeding from SRMD because of their ease of dosing, effective and predictable acid suppression, lack of need for regular gastric pH monitoring, and lack of tolerance as encountered with H_2RAs.[93] One trial showed a significant reduction in bleeding with omeprazole as opposed to ranitidine (6.3% versus 31.4%, respectively; $P < .05$), but patients in the ranitidine group had a higher number of risk factors.[102] A recent trial comparing immediate-release PPI with continuous infusion of H_2RA showed a slightly lower (but not significantly different) incidence of clinically important bleeding with PPI therapy.[103] Larger randomized studies comparing PPIs with H_2RAs are needed to establish clearer guidelines regarding the prophylaxis of bleeding in patients with SRMD.

Treatment

Endoscopy is the principal diagnostic and therapeutic procedure used in patients with bleeding from SRMD. The same endoscopic techniques used for hemostasis in peptic ulcer bleeding are used in SRMD when an actively bleeding lesion is found. Surgery is reserved for patients with uncontrolled hemorrhage and usually involves vagotomy. oversewing of bleeding sites, and in rare cases, subtotal or total gastrectomy.[93] In poor surgical candidates with severe uncontrolled hemorrhage, angiography may be a useful diagnostic and therapeutic option.

LOWER GASTROINTESTINAL BLEEDING

Differential Diagnosis

Lower GI bleeding is defined as bleeding that originates from a source distal to the ligament of Treitz. It is caused by a diverse range of bleeding sources and can range from trivial to life-threatening bleeding. It can also be acute, arbitrarily defined as less than 3 days' duration and possibly resulting in hemodynamic compromise, or chronic, extending over a period of several days or longer and usually less severe in terms of the amount of blood loss.[104] Sources of lower GI bleeding and their incidence from several large studies are listed in Table 77-5.[105-112]

Diverticular Bleeding

Diverticular bleeding, the most common source of lower GI bleeding, accounts for up to 40% of cases.[104] Diverticular disease is more common in the elderly. It affects up to two thirds of people older than 80 years. Only 3% to 15% of patients with diverticulosis experience diverticular bleeding.[104]

Patients with diverticular bleeding typically have painless hematochezia. Most patients will stop bleeding spontaneously, but the bleeding can recur in 10% to 40% of cases.[113]

The bleeding is thought to occur after repetitive trauma to the vasa recta (nutrient arteries) that stretch over the diverticular dome.[114] NSAIDs have been associated with increased risk for diverticular bleeding.[115]

Ischemic Colitis and Other Forms of Colitis

Ischemic colitis accounts for up to 19% of lower GI bleeding.[104] It results from a sudden reduction in mesenteric blood flow. As opposed to acute mesenteric ischemia, this reduction is transient and reversible. The typical regions affected are the "watershed" areas of the colon: the splenic flexure, the rectosigmoid junction, and the right colon. Ischemia is precipitated by any event that compromises colonic blood flow. Clinically, patients have a sudden onset of abdominal pain, followed by hematochezia within

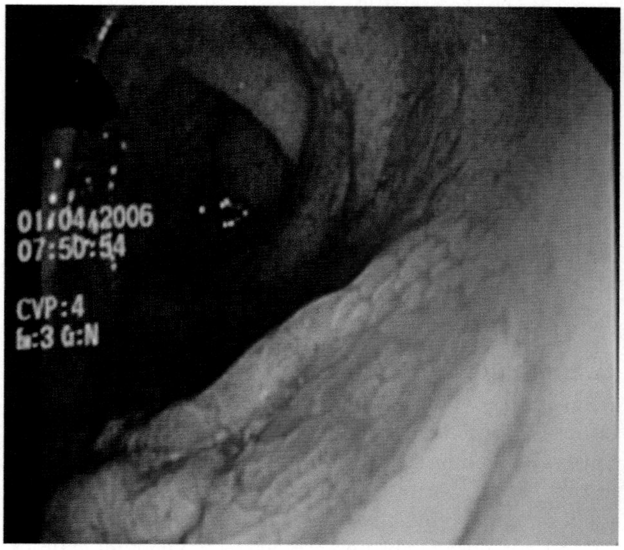

A

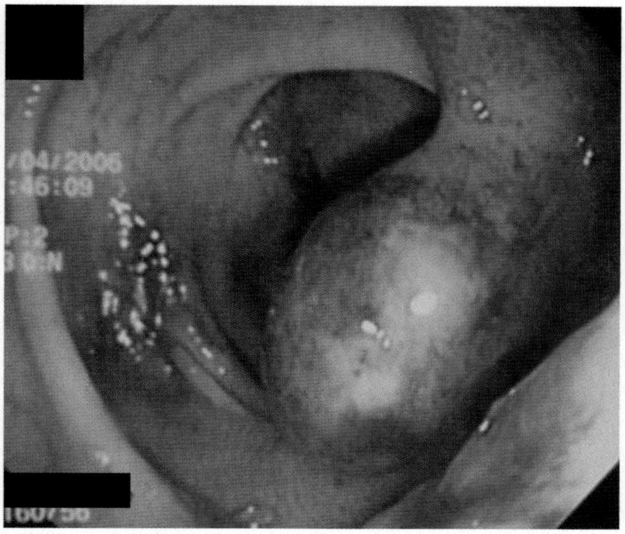

B

Figure 77-7. **A** and **B,** Ischemic colitis.

Table 77-5. Sources of Lower Gastrointestinal Bleeding

Study	Diverticulosis, No. (%)	Angiodysplasia, No. (%)	Cancer/ Polyp, No. (%)	Colitis/ Ulcers,* No. (%)	Anorectal,† No. (%)	Others,‡ No. (%)	Unknown, No. (%)	Totals
Jensen and Machicado[106]	13 (20)	24 (37)	9 (14)	7 (11)	3 (5)	3 (5)	5 (8)	64
Longstreth[107]	91 (41)	6 (3)	20 (9)	35 (16)	10 (5)	31 (14)	26 (12)	219
Farrands and Taylor[108]	30 (29)	6 (6)	38 (36)	20 (19)	5 (5)	5 (5)	1 (1)	105
Bramley et al.[109]	60 (24)	17 (7)	25 (10)	52 (21)	22 (9)	11 (4)	64 (25)	251
Colacchio et al.[110]	98 (55)	13 (7)	14 (8)	11 (6)	5 (3)	5 (3)	32 (18)	178
Richter et al.[111]	51 (48)	13 (12)	12 (11)	6 (6)	3 (3)	7 (6)	15 (14)	107
Rossini et al.[112]	60 (15)	16 (4)	122 (30)	92 (22)	0 (0)	47 (11)	72 (18)	409
Totals	403 (33)	95 (8)	240 (19)	223 (18)	48 (4)	109 (8)	215 (16)	1333

*Includes inflammatory bowel disease, infectious colitis, ischemic colitis, radiation colitis, vasculitis, and inflammation of unknown origin.
†Includes hemorrhoids, anal fissure, and idiopathic rectal ulcers.
‡Includes postpolypectomy bleeding, aortocolonic fistula, trauma from fecal impaction, and anastomotic bleeding.
From Zuckerman GR, Prakash C: Acute lower intestinal bleeding. Part II: Etiology, therapy, and outcomes. Gastrointest Endosc 1999;49:228-238.

24 hours. Endoscopically, ischemia is suspected in the presence of bluish hemorrhagic nodules from submucosal bleeding, cyanotic or necrotic mucosa with hemorrhagic ulcerations, or segmental distribution with an abrupt transition between injured and normal mucosa (Fig. 77-7).[104] Most cases of ischemic colitis resolve spontaneously with supportive treatment. Rare cases require surgery (if peritoneal signs are present) or develop chronic ischemic colitis with stricture formation. Ischemic colitis is a common cause of lower GI bleeding in patients in the ICU because of the frequent hemodynamic instability in this setting.[116]

Infectious colitis, radiation colitis, and inflammatory bowel diseases can also result in bloody diarrhea, but the bleeding is rarely severe.

Angiodysplasia

Estimates of angiodysplasia as a source of lower GI bleeding vary widely and reach 37% in some reports.[107] Current data suggest that acute bleeding caused by angiodysplasia is less frequent than previously thought, with most cases demonstrating iron deficiency anemia and occult blood loss.[114] These lesions are seen predominantly in the elderly. They appear endoscopically as red, flat lesions

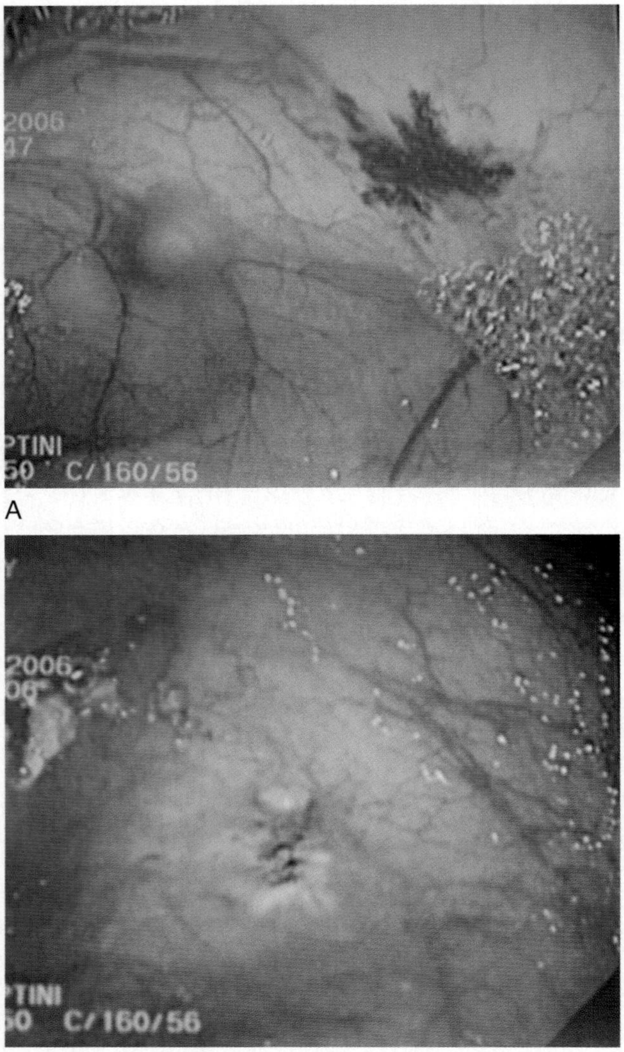

A

B

Figure 77-8. A, Angiodysplasia in the cecum. **B,** Same lesion after thermal therapy (electrocauterization).

with ectatic blood vessels radiating from a central feeding vessel, usually in the right colon (Fig. 77-8). Overt bleeding from angiodysplasia is usually brisk and painless and cannot be distinguished from diverticular bleeding. Endoscopic treatment is highly effective and safe and prevents bleeding episodes from recurring.

Other Sources of Lower Gastrointestinal Bleeding

Acute significant bleeding from colonic neoplasia and polyps is uncommon despite reports in which it accounts for up to 36% of cases.[111] Cancer and polyps are thought to bleed from erosions on the surface.

Postpolypectomy bleeding occurs in 1% to 6% of patients undergoing colonoscopic polypectomy.[114] Bleeding can be immediate or delayed up to 3 weeks after the procedure. Risk factors for postpolypectomy bleeding include large size, sessile morphology, and right colonic location.[117]

Anorectal sources of lower GI bleeding include hemorrhoids, anorectal fissures, stercoral ulcers, and proctitis. Hemorrhoids can cause significant bleeding and may sometimes require endoscopic or surgical intervention. Bleeding from rectal ulcers is common in elderly bedridden patients and in critically ill patients.[105]

Small bowel sources of lower GI bleeding include angiodysplasia (most frequent), lymphoma, small bowel ulcers, and Crohn's disease.[114] Small bowel lesions are typically more difficult to identify and require more diagnostic procedures.[118]

Diagnostic Evaluation

Colonoscopy

After initial evaluation, stabilization, and exclusion of an upper GI source, management shifts to localization of the lower GI bleeding site. Colonoscopy is an attractive choice in this setting because it offers the best opportunity for early diagnosis and subsequent management. In the past, colonoscopy used to be performed in an expectant manner, after cessation of bleeding and colonic preparation. Concern about poor visibility, the potential for complications, and the adverse effects of bowel preparation in the setting of bleeding is behind the reluctance in performing "urgent" colonoscopy. More recently, early colonoscopy has gained interest in the management of lower GI bleeding. Several reports have shown that early (or urgent) colonoscopy is safe and has high diagnostic yield in patients with hematochezia.[119-123] The definition of "urgent" varied in these reports, from within 8 hours to within 24 hours of initial evaluation. This approach was also associated with shorter hospital stay.[124] Bowel preparation is generally recommended before urgent colonoscopy to improve visibility and prevent complications related to poor visibility. Polyethylene glycol lavage solution by mouth or through a nasogastric tube is commonly used in these cases. It can be administered at a rate of approximately 1 L every 30 to 45 minutes.[104] Some authors have proposed the use of colonoscopy without bowel preparation and have shown high diagnostic yield with this approach.[125] Despite the fact that urgent colonoscopy improves the diagnostic yield and leads to more frequent endoscopic therapy, there is still controversy regarding its impact on important outcomes such as mortality, rebleeding, and the need for surgery.[121,123] Jensen and colleagues[121] showed that urgent colonoscopy with endoscopic treatment in a group of patients with active diverticular bleeding (versus a historical group that did not receive endoscopic treatment) may prevent recurrent bleeding and the need for surgery. A more recent randomized trial compared urgent colonoscopy with a standard care algorithm in which radionuclide scanning, followed, if positive, by angiography, was used in patients with suspected active bleeding versus expectant colonoscopy in those without active bleeding. This trial showed that a definite source of bleeding was found more often in urgent colonoscopy patients. However, no difference in mortality, surgery, and rebleeding was found in the two groups.[123] In our opinion, the decision about the timing of colonoscopy should be based on individual experience and local expertise.

Radionuclide Scanning

The use of radionuclide scanning (also known as a technetium-labeled red blood cell scan) in patients with lower GI bleeding is highly controversial. It has been used for several decades as a method for localization of the bleeding source.[114] A main advantage of radionuclide scanning is its sensitivity for bleeding at a rate as low as 0.05 to 0.1 mL/min, in addition to its noninvasive nature.[114] On the other hand, this diagnostic modality lacks therapeutic capability, has variable accuracy, and may delay other diagnostic and therapeutic procedures. A common practice in the setting of ongoing lower GI bleeding is to perform radionuclide scanning as a screening test before angiography and in some cases as a guide to surgery. The problem with this approach is the inconsistent and widely variable accuracy and the high rate of false-positive results in different reports.[114,126,127] Prospective randomized studies of radionuclide scanning are needed to help answer questions regarding its usefulness.

Angiography

Angiography is less sensitive than radionuclide scanning in the detection of active bleeding. It can detect bleeding at a rate of 0.5 to 1.0 mL/min. In addition to its role in accurate localization of bleeding lesions, angiography offers therapeutic possibilities. As with radionuclide scanning, the ability of angiography to detect the bleeding source varies widely among studies, from 20% to 70%.[114] This variation is due to several factors, including patient selection (higher diagnostic yield in patients with positive radionuclide scanning), the severity and intermittent nature of the bleeding, procedural delay, and venous or small vessel bleeding.[114] Angiography is usually performed in patients with ongoing lower GI bleeding with or without a positive radionuclide scan. This sequence in management was the standard approach to ongoing bleeding up until recently, when colonoscopy started gaining interest in the setting of acute bleeding (as opposed to expectant elective colonoscopy). When angiographic therapy fails or is not available after localization of the bleeding, the findings are used to guide surgical resection. Angiography can cause serious complications such as contrast reactions, arterial thrombosis and dissection, and catheter site infection and bleeding. Thus, it should be used in carefully selected patients.

Therapeutic Alternatives

Endoscopic Therapy

Data on the effectiveness of endoscopic therapy for lesions causing lower GI bleeding are limited. However, the experience from published series suggests that this form of therapy is likely to be beneficial. Methods of endoscopic hemostasis are similar to those used for upper GI bleeding and include injection therapy, thermal therapy (APC and heater and electrocautery probes), and mechanical therapy (hemoclips). Unlike endoscopic treatment of upper GI bleeding, data comparing each of these modalities for lower GI bleeding are not available. On average, 10% to 15% of patients undergoing urgent colonoscopy receive endoscopic treatment.[128]

Angiographic Therapy

When angiography identifies the bleeding site in cases of lower GI bleeding, hemostasis can be achieved by the intra-arterial infusion of vasopressin or superselective embolization. Infusion of vasopressin can control bleeding in up to 91% of cases,[128] but complications develop in 10% to 20% and include arrhythmia, pulmonary edema, and ischemia.[128] Furthermore, rebleeding occurs in as many as 50% of cases.[128] In early studies, transcatheter embolization carried a high risk for bowel infarction, but current superselective techniques using smaller catheters with various agents (gelatin sponge, microcoils, and polyvinyl alcohol particles) appear to be more effective and safer than the old techniques. Selective embolization initially controls the bleeding in up to 100% of patients with lower GI bleeding, but rebleeding rates are 15% to 40%.[128] Since the advent of these new techniques, embolization has become the preferred modality when angiographic therapy is contemplated.

Surgical Therapy

Surgery is indicated in cases of recurrent bleeding (especially diverticular) and massive ongoing bleeding with high transfusion requirements (generally more than 6 units of packed red blood cells in a 24-hour period).[104] Accurate localization of the site of bleeding preoperatively is crucial so that segmental rather than subtotal colectomy can be performed. Unfortunately, the accuracy of radionuclide scanning in localization of the bleeding is variable, and hence it should not be used as a guide for surgery. Colonoscopy and angiography may be used as a guide for surgery in cases in which bleeding is initially identified and possibly treated through these modalities and then recurs and requires surgery.

OBSCURE GASTROINTESTINAL BLEEDING

Obscure GI bleeding is bleeding that persists or recurs without an obvious source identified on upper and lower endoscopy. Obscure bleeding can be occult (positive fecal occult blood testing without frank recognizable blood loss) or overt (clinically evident). Obscure bleeding can be very challenging to the physician and, in cases of overt massive bleeding, life-threatening to the patient. The initial approach to the problem is the same as with upper and lower GI bleeding and includes resuscitation and stabilization, followed by a search for the source.

Differential Diagnosis

Missed lesions on upper and lower endoscopy should be considered first in the work-up of obscure bleeding. Causes difficult to identify on routine endoscopy include hemosuccus pancreaticus, hemobilia, aortoenteric fistula, Dieulafoy's ulcer, and extraesophageal varices. Small bowel lesions are another source of obscure bleeding and include tumors (lymphomas, carcinoids, adenocarcinomas), vascular ectasia, NSAID-induced ulcers, Meckel's diverticulum and other less common causes.[129]

Diagnostic Evaluation

Repeat upper and lower endoscopy is usually warranted at least once after the index endoscopy, with the uncommon and subtle lesions just listed kept in mind. When the patient has active ongoing bleeding, radionuclide scanning and angiography should be considered. In young patients, Meckel's scan may be helpful. If all these tests are negative, the focus should shift to evaluation of the small bowel. Radiographic, endoscopic, and surgical modalities are used for this purpose.

Small bowel follow-through (SBFT) and enteroclysis (which is a modified form of SBFT) should be performed only when Crohn's disease or malignancy is suspected. These modalities have lost favor with the advent of capsule endoscopy (except in cases in which there may be narrowing of the small bowel). Small bowel enteroscopy can be very helpful in identifying and, in some cases, treating lesions in the small bowel that are responsible for obscure bleeding. Unfortunately, it can examine only 50 to 150 cm of small bowel.[130] Recently, studies from Japan have demonstrated high diagnostic yield with double-balloon enteroscopy, a modality that uses longer scopes, overtubes, and balloons to examine the entire small bowel.[131] These results need to be validated in larger prospective studies.

Capsule endoscopy gained large interest in evaluation of the small bowel because of its ability to examine the entire small bowel and its noninvasive nature. It consists of swallowing a pill-sized camera with sufficient battery life to image the entire small bowel. Studies have supported the role of capsule endoscopy in the evaluation of

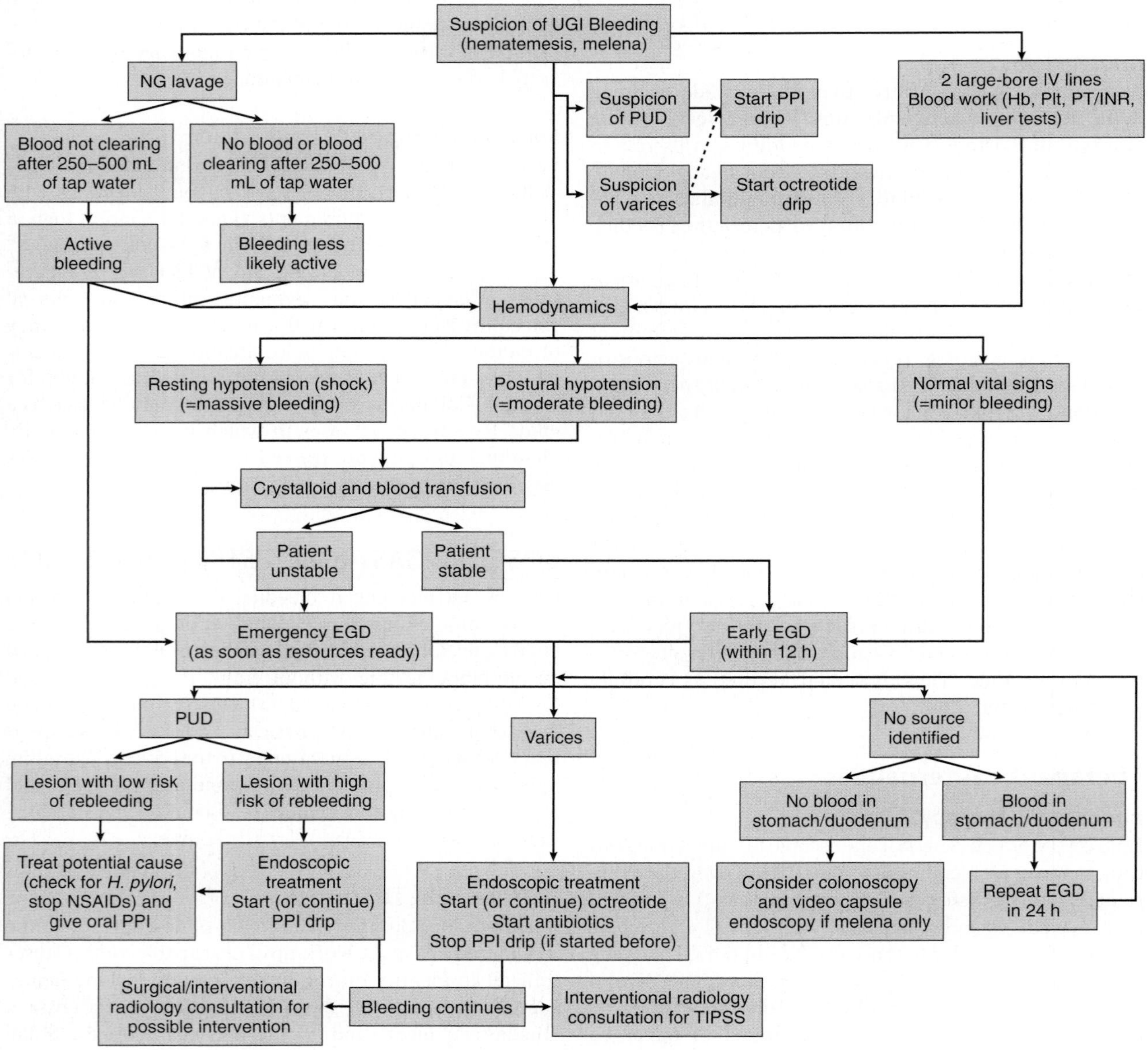

A

Figure 77-9. A, Approach to managing upper gastrointestinal bleeding in critical care patients.

obscure GI bleeding with an overall diagnostic yield of 55% to 70%.[129] The diagnostic yield is even higher when it is administered to patients with ongoing bleeding (87% to 92%).[132,133] In our opinion, effort should be made to perform capsule endoscopy in patients with obscure overt bleeding while still in the hospital instead of waiting until discharge (which is the current standard practice in most centers). Capsule endoscopy is contraindicated in patients in whom narrowing of the small bowel is suspected. While the capsule is still in the body, magnetic resonance imaging cannot be performed.

Exploratory laparotomy is generally the last option in the evaluation of obscure GI bleeding. When combined with intraoperative enteroscopy, the diagnostic yield reaches 50% to 100%.[129]

CONCLUSION

In summary, acute GI bleeding is a life-threatening emergency that requires a quick response and a coordinated team approach. Acute management is the same regardless of the source of bleeding (Fig. 77-9) and should be orches-

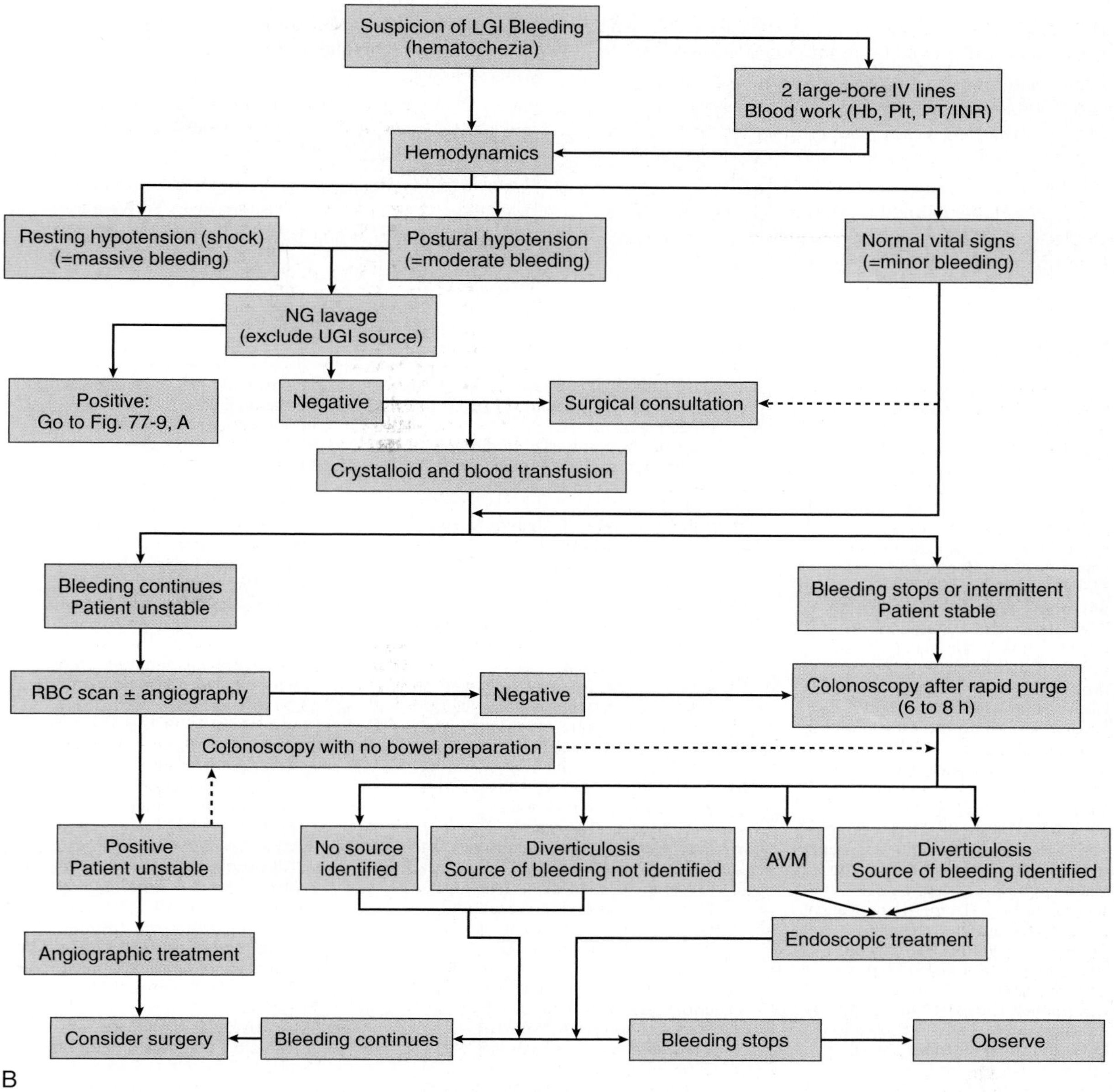

Figure 77-9, cont'd. B, Approach to managing lower gastrointestinal bleeding in critical care patients. AVM, arteriovenous malformation; EGD, esophagogastroduodenoscopy; Hb, hemoglobin; INR, international normalized ratio; LGI, lower gastrointestinal; NG, nasogastric; NSAIDs, nonsteroidal anti-inflammatory drugs; Plt, platelets; PPI, proton-pump inhibitor; PT, prothrombin time; PUD, peptic ulcer disease; RBC, red blood cell; TIPSS, transjugular intrahepatic portosystemic stent shunt; UGI, upper gastrointestinal.

trated by a critical care team. The prime direction in resuscitation should be restoration of euvolemia. Once a source is suspected, specific management and therapeutic options are considered, and specialists such as gastroenterologists, interventional radiologists, and surgeons may get involved. Prevention of bleeding from SRMD is indicated in a specific population of critically ill patients. Endoscopy plays a major role in the diagnosis and management of acute GI bleeding. Endoscopic therapy with standard and innovative techniques has been shown to have a major impact on the prognosis of bleeding patients.

KEY POINTS

- The history gives important clues regarding the etiology of the acute GI bleeding and helps direct initial management.
- Management of GI bleeding relies on a team approach involving an intensivist, endoscopist, radiologist, and surgeon.
- The prime direction of evaluation and resuscitation in a bleeding patient should be restoration of euvolemia.
- Stress-related mucosal disease is a common source of upper GI bleeding in physiologically stressed patients, and prophylaxis with acid suppressants should be given to patients with coagulopathy and those undergoing prolonged mechanical ventilation.
- PPIs in drip form should be given to patients with upper GI bleeding after endoscopic treatment of lesions with a high risk of rebleeding.
- Antibiotic therapy decreases mortality in patients with variceal bleeding. It should be given empirically along with vasoactive agents (octreotide).
- Several forms of endoscopic therapy are effective for nonvariceal bleeding, including injection, thermal and mechanical therapy.
- Endoscopic band ligation is the most commonly used and preferred technique for the treatment of bleeding varices.
- Early colonoscopy has become an attractive choice in lower GI bleeding because of its diagnostic and therapeutic abilities.
- Videocapsule endoscopy has an important role in the evaluation of patients with obscure overt GI bleeding, and efforts should aim at performing it in hospitalized patients.

REFERENCES

1. Longstreth GF: Epidemiology of hospitalization for acute upper gastrointestinal hemorrhage: A population based study. Am J Gastroenterol 1995;90:206-210.
2. Longstreth GF: Epidemiology and outcome of patients hospitalized with acute lower gastrointestinal hemorrhage: A population based study. Am J Gastroenterol 1997;92:419-424.
3. Bramley PN, Masson JW, McKnight G, et al: The role of an open-access bleeding unit in the management of colonic hemorrhage. A 2-year prospective study. Scand J Gastroenterol 1996;31:764-769.
4. Yavorski RT, Wong RK, Maydonovitch C, et al: Analysis of 3,294 cases of upper gastrointestinal bleeding in military medical facilities. Am J Gastroenterol 1995;90:568-573.
5. Rockall TA, Logan RF, Devlin HB, et al: Variation in outcome after acute upper gastrointestinal haemorrhage. The National Audit of Acute Upper Gastrointestinal Haemorrhage. Lancet 1995;346:346-350.
6. Zuckerman GR, Prakash C: Acute lower intestinal bleeding, Part I: Clinical presentation and diagnosis. Gastrointest Endosc 1998;48:606-617.
7. Zuckerman GR, Prakash C: Acute lower intestinal bleeding, Part II: Etiology, therapy, and outcomes. Gastrointest Endosc 1999;49:228-238.
8. Rockey DC: Gastrointestinal bleeding. Gastroenterol Clin North Am 2005;34:581-588.
9. Rockey DC: Gastrointestinal bleeding. In Feldman M, Friedman LS, Sleisenger MH (eds): Sleisenger and Fordtran's Gastrointestinal and Liver Disease, 7th ed. Philadelphia, Saunders, 2002, pp 221-248.
10. Kruskall MS, Mintz PD, Bergin JJ, et al: Transfusion therapy in emergency medicine. Ann Emerg Med 1988;17:327-335.
11. Schiff L, Stevens RJ, Shapiro N, et al: Observations on the oral administration of citrate blood in man. Am J Med Sci 1942;203:409.
12. Luk GD, Bynum TE, Hendrix TR: Gastric aspiration in localization of gastrointestinal hemorrhage. JAMA 1979;241:576-578.
13. Aljebreen AM, Fallone CA, Barkun AN: Nasogastric aspirate predicts high-risk endoscopic lesions in patients with acute upper-GI bleeding. Gastrointest Endosc 2004;59:172-178.
14. Cuellar RE, Gavaler JS, Alexander JA, et al: Gastrointestinal tract hemorrhage. The value of a nasogastric aspirate. Arch Intern Med 1990;150:1381-1384.
15. Chalasani N, Clark WS, Wilcox CM: Blood urea nitrogen to creatinine concentration in gastrointestinal bleeding: A reappraisal. Am J Gastroenterol 1997;92:1796-1799.
16. Ferguson CB, Mitchell RM: Nonvariceal upper gastrointestinal bleeding: Standard and new treatment. Gastroenterol Clin North Am 2005;34:607-621.
17. Esrailian E, Gralnek IM: Nonvariceal upper gastrointestinal bleeding: Epidemiology and diagnosis. Gastroenterol Clin North Am 2005;34:589-605.
18. Lieberman D, Fennerty MB, Morris CD, et al: Endoscopic evaluation of patients with dyspepsia: Results from the national endoscopic data repository. Gastroenterology 2004;127:1067-1075.
19. Hasselgren G, Lind T, Lundell L, et al: Continuous intravenous infusion of omeprazole in elderly patients with peptic ulcer bleeding. Results of a placebo-controlled multicenter study. Scand J Gastroenterol 1997;32:328-333.
20. Kuyvenhoven JP, Veenendaal RA, Vandenbroucke JP: Peptic ulcer bleeding: Interaction between non-steroidal anti-inflammatory drugs, *Helicobacter pylori* infection, and the ABO blood group system. Scand J Gastroenterol 1999;34:1082-1086.
21. Labenz J, Peitz U, Kohl H, et al: *Helicobacter pylori* increases the risk of peptic ulcer bleeding: A case control study. Ital J Gastroenterol Hepatol 1999;31:110-115.
22. Hosking SW, Yung MY, Chung SC, et al: Differing prevalence of *Helicobacter* in bleeding and nonbleeding ulcers. Gastroenterology 1992;102:A85.
23. Roderick PJ, Wilkes HC, Meade TW: The gastrointestinal toxicity of aspirin: An overview of randomised controlled trials. Br J Clin Pharmacol 1993;35:219-226.
24. Bjorkman DJ: Current status of nonsteroidal anti-inflammatory drug (NSAID) use in the United States: Risk factors and frequency of complications. Am J Med 1999;107:3-8; discussion 8-10.
25. Swain CP, Storey DW, Bown SG, et al: Nature of the bleeding vessel in recurrently bleeding gastric ulcers. Gastroenterology 1986;90:595-608.

26. Schmulewitz N, O'Connor JB: Esophageal disease caused by medication, radiation and internal trauma. In DiMarino AJ, Benjamin S (eds): Gastrointestinal Disease: An Endoscopic Approach, 2nd ed. Thorofare, NJ, Slack, 2002, pp 245-262.
27. Machicado GA, Jensen DM: Upper gastrointestinal angiomata: Diagnosis and treatment. Gastointest Endosc Clin North Am 1991;1:241-262.
28. Bashir RM, Al-Kawas FH: Vascular lesions of the stomach. In DiMarino AJ, Benjamin S (eds): Gastrointestinal Disease: An Endoscopic Approach, 2nd ed. Thorofare, NJ, Slack, 2002, pp 535-550.
29. Romaozinho JM, Pontes JM, Lerias C, et al: Dieulafoy's lesion: Management and long-term outcome. Endoscopy 2004;36:416-420.
30. Park CH, Joo YE, Kim HS, et al: A prospective, randomized trial of endoscopic band ligation versus endoscopic hemoclip placement for bleeding gastric Dieulafoy's lesions. Endoscopy 2004;36:677-681.
31. Savides TJ, Jensen DM, Cohen J, et al: Severe upper gastrointestinal tumor bleeding: Endoscopic findings, treatment, and outcome. Endoscopy 1996;28:244-248.
32. Busuttil RW, Rees W, Baker JD, et al: Pathogenesis of aortoduodenal fistula: Experimental and clinical correlates. Surgery 1979;85:1-13.
33. Elton E, Howell DA, Amberson SM, et al: Combined angiographic and endoscopic management of bleeding pancreatic pseudoaneurysms. Gastrointest Endosc 1997;46:544-549.
34. Luketic VA, Sanyal AJ: Esophageal varices. I. Clinical presentation, medical therapy, and endoscopic therapy. Gastroenterol Clin North Am 2000;29:337-385.
35. Garcia-Tsao G, Groszmann RJ, Fisher RL, et al: Portal pressure, presence of gastroesophageal varices and variceal bleeding. Hepatology 1985;5:419-424.
36. Sheikh RA, Prindiville TP, Trudeau W: Gastrointestinal bleeding in portal hypertension. In DiMarino AJ, Benjamin S (eds): Gastrointestinal Disease: An Endoscopic Approach, 2nd ed. Thorofare, NJ, Slack, 2002, pp 605-644.
37. Sarin SK, Lahoti D, Saxena SP, et al: Prevalence, classification and natural history of gastric varices: Long-term follow up study in 568 patients with portal hypertension. Hepatology 1992;16:1343-1349.
38. Frossard JL, Spahr L, Queneau PE, et al: Erythromycin IV bolus infusion in acute upper gastrointestinal bleeding: A randomized, controlled, double-blind trial. Gastroenterology 2002;123:17-23.
39. Coffin B, Pocard M, Panis Y, et al: Erythromycin improves the quality of EGD in patients with acute upper GI bleeding: A randomized controlled study. Gastrointest Endosc 2002;56:174-179.
40. Eisen GM, Dominitz JA, Faigel DO, et al: American Society for Gastrointestinal Endoscopy. Standards of Practice Committee. An annotated algorithmic approach to upper gastrointestinal bleeding. Gastrointest Endosc 2001;53:853-858.
41. ASGE Standards of Practice Committee: ASGE guideline: The role of endoscopy in acute non-variceal upper-GI hemorrhage. Gastrointest Endosc 2004;60:497-504.
42. Cooper GS, Chak A, Way LE, et al: Early endoscopy in upper gastrointestinal hemorrhage: Associations with recurrent bleeding, surgery, and length of hospital stay. Gastrointest Endosc 1999;49:145-152.
43. Collins R, Langman M: Treatment with histamine H_2 antagonists in acute upper gastrointestinal hemorrhage. Implications of randomized trials. N Engl J Med 1985;313:660-666.
44. Levine JE, Leontiadis GI, Sharma VK, et al: Meta-analysis: The efficacy of intravenous H_2-receptor antagonists in bleeding peptic ulcer. Aliment Pharmacol Ther 2002;16:1137-1142.
45. Barkun A, Bardou M, Marshall JK: Nonvariceal Upper GI Bleeding Consensus Conference Group. Consensus recommendations for managing patients with nonvariceal upper gastrointestinal bleeding. Ann Intern Med 2003;139:843-857.
46. Leontiadis GI, Sharma VK, Howden CW: Systemic review and meta-analysis of proton pump inhibitor therapy in peptic ulcer bleeding. BMJ 2005;300:568-575.
47. Bardou M, Toubouti Y, Benhaberou-Brun D, et al: Meta-analysis: Proton-pump inhibition in high-risk patients with acute peptic ulcer bleeding. Aliment Pharmacol Ther 2005;21:677-686.
48. Julapalli VR, Graham DY: Appropriate use of intravenous proton pump inhibitors in the management of bleeding peptic ulcer. Dig Dis Sci 2005;50:1185-1193.
49. Henry DA, O'Connell DL: Effects of fibrinolytic inhibitors on mortality from upper gastrointestinal haemorrhage. BMJ 1989;298:1142-1146.
50. Rivkin K, Lyakhovetskiy A: Treatment of nonvariceal upper gastrointestinal bleeding. Am J Health Syst Pharm 2005;62:1159-1170.
51. Imperiale TF, Birgisson S: Somatostatin or octreotide compared with H_2 antagonists and placebo in the management of acute nonvariceal upper gastrointestinal hemorrhage: A meta-analysis. Ann Intern Med 1997;127:1062-1071.
52. Lin HJ, Wang K, Perng CL, et al: Octreotide and heater probe thermocoagulation for arrest of peptic ulcer hemorrhage. A prospective, randomized, controlled trial. J Clin Gastroenterol 1995;21:95-98.
53. Cook DJ, Guyatt GH, Salena BJ, et al: Endoscopic therapy for acute nonvariceal upper gastrointestinal hemorrhage: A meta-analysis. Gastroenterology 1992;102:139-148.
54. Bini EJ, Cohen J: Endoscopic treatment compared with medical therapy for the prevention of recurrent ulcer hemorrhage in patients with adherent clots. Gastrointest Endosc 2003;58:707-714.
55. Kahi CJ, Jensen DM, Sung JJ, et al: Endoscopic therapy versus medical therapy for bleeding peptic ulcer with adherent clot: A meta-analysis. Gastroenterology 2005;129:855-862.
56. Cipolletta L, Bianco MA, Rotondano G, et al: Prospective comparison of argon plasma coagulator and heater probe in the endoscopic treatment of major peptic ulcer bleeding. Gastrointest Endosc 1998;48:191-195.
57. Sacks HS, Chalmers TC, Blum AL, et al: Endoscopic hemostasis. An effective therapy for bleeding peptic ulcers. JAMA 1990;264:494-499.
58. Cook DJ, Guyatt GH, Salena BJ, et al: Endoscopic therapy for acute nonvariceal upper gastrointestinal hemorrhage: A meta-analysis. Gastroenterology 1992;102:139-148.
59. Bleau BL, Gostout CJ, Sherman KE, et al: Recurrent bleeding from peptic ulcer associated with adherent clot: A randomized study comparing endoscopic treatment with medical therapy. Gastrointest Endosc 2002;56:1-6.
60. Tekant Y, Goh P, Alexander DJ, et al: Combination therapy using adrenaline and heater probe to reduce rebleeding in patients with peptic ulcer haemorrhage: A prospective randomized trial. Br J Surg 1995;82:223-226.
61. Chung SS, Lau JY, Sung JJ, et al: Randomised comparison between adrenaline injection alone and adrenaline injection plus heat probe treatment for actively bleeding ulcers. BMJ 1997;314:1307-1311.
62. Sherman LM, Shenoy SS, Cerra FB: Selective intraarterial vasopressin: Clinical efficacy and complications. Ann Surg 1979;189:298-302.
63. Miller M Jr, Smith TP: Angiographic diagnosis and endovascular management of nonvariceal gastrointestinal hemorrhage. Gastroenterol Clin North Am 2005;34:735-752.
64. D'Amico G, Pagliaro L, Bosch J: The treatment of portal hypertension: A meta-analytic review. Hepatology 1995;22:332-354.
65. Ioannu GN, Doust J, Rockey D: Systematic review: Terlipressin in acute oesophageal variceal hemorrhage. Aliment Pharmacol Ther 2003;17:53-64.
66. D'Amico G, Pagliaro L, Bosch J: Pharmacologic treatment of portal hypertension: An evidenced approach. Semin Liver Dis 1999;19:475-505.
67. Zaman A, Chalasani N: Bleeding caused by portal hypertension. Gastroenterol Clin North Am 2005;34:623-642.
68. Villanueva C, Ortiz J, Sabat M, et al: Somatostatin alone or combined with emergency sclerotherapy in the treatment of acute esophageal variceal bleeding: A prospective randomized trial. Hepatology 1999;30:384-389.
69. Corley DA, Cello JP, Adkisson W, et al: Octreotide for acute esophageal variceal bleeding: Meta-analysis. Gastroenterology 2001;120:946-954.
70. Soares-Weiser K, Brezis M, Tur-Kaspa R, et al: Antibiotic prophylaxis for cirrhotic patients with gastrointestinal bleeding. Cochrane Database Syst Rev 2002;CD002907.
71. Bleichner G, Boulanger R, Squara P, et al: Frequency of infections in

cirrhotic patients presenting with acute gastrointestinal hemorrhage. Br J Surg 1986;73:724-726.
72. Caly WR, Strauss E: A prospective study of bacterial infections in patients with cirrhosis. J Hepatol 1993;18: 353-358.
73. Bernard B, Cadranell JF, Valla D, et al: Prognostic significance of bacterial infection in bleeding cirrhotic patients: A prospective study. Gastroenterology 1995;108:1828-1834.
74. Bosch J, Thiabut D, Bendtsen F, et al: Recombinant factor VIIa for upper gastrointestinal bleeding in patients with cirrhosis: A randomized, double-blind trial. Gastroenterology 2004;127:1123-1130.
75. Heaton ND, Howard ER: Complications and limitations of injection sclerotherapy in portal hypertension. Gut 1993;34:7-10.
76. Steigmann GV, Goff JS, Michaletz-Onody P, et al: Endoscopic sclerotherapy as compared with endoscopic ligation for bleeding esophageal varices. N Engl J Med 1992;326:1527-1532.
77. Avgerinos A, Armonis A, Manolakpoulos S, et al: Endoscopic sclerotherapy versus variceal ligation in the long-term management of patients with cirrhosis after variceal bleeding: A prospective randomized study. J Hepatol 1997;26:1034-1041.
78. Burroughs AK, Patch D: Transjugular intrahepatic portosystemic shunt. Semin Liver Dis 1999;19:457-473.
79. Vangeli M, Patch D, Burroughs AK: Salvage TIPS for uncontrolled variceal bleeding. J Hepatol 2003;37: 703-704.
80. Mutlu GM, Mutlu EA, Factor P: GI complications in patients receiving mechanical ventilation. Chest 2001;119:1222-1241.
81. Cook DJ, Fuller HD, Guyatt GH, et al: Risk factors for gastrointestinal bleeding in critically ill patients. N Engl J Med 1994;330:377-381.
82. Martindale RG: Contemporary strategies for the prevention of stress-related mucosal bleeding. Am J Health Syst Pharm 2005;62(Suppl 2):S11-S17.
83. Itoh M, Guth PH: Role of oxygen-derived free radicals in hemorrhagic shock–induced gastric lesions in the rat. Gastroenterology 1985;88: 1162-1167.
84. Yasue N, Guth PH: Role of exogenous acid and retransfusion in hemorrhagic shock–induced gastric lesions in the rat. Gastroenterology 1988;94: 1135-1143.
85. Czaja AJ, McAlhany JC, Pruitt BA Jr: Acute gastroduodenal disease after thermal injury. An endoscopic evaluation of incidence and natural history. N Engl J Med 1974;291: 925-929.
86. Goodman AA, Frey CF: Massive upper gastrointestinal hemorrhage following surgical operations. Ann Surg 1968;167:180-184.
87. Brown TH, Davidson PF, Larson GM: Acute gastritis occurring within 24 hours of severe head injury. Gastrointest Endosc 1989;35:37-40.
88. Schuster DP: Stress ulcer prophylaxis: In whom? With what? Crit Care Med 1993;21:4-6.
89. Cook DJ, Griffith LE, Walter SD, et al: The attributable mortality and length of intensive care unit stay of clinically important gastrointestinal bleeding in critically ill patients. Crit Care 2001;5:368-375.
90. Zuckerman GR, Shuman R: Therapeutic goals and treatment options for prevention of stress ulcer syndrome. Am J Med 1987;83:29-35.
91. Stollman N, Metz DC: Pathophysiology and prophylaxis of stress ulcer in intensive care unit patients. J Crit Care 2005;20:35-45.
92. MacLaren R, Jarvis CL, Fish DN: Use of enteral nutrition for stress ulcer prophylaxis. Ann Pharmacother 2001;35:1614-1623.
93. Harty RF, Ancha HB: Stress ulcer bleeding. Curr Treat Options Gastroenterol 2006;9:157-166.
94. Kles KA, Wellig MA, Tappenden KA: Luminal nutrients exacerbate intestinal hypoxia in the hypoperfused jejunum. JPEN J Parenter Enteral Nutr 2001;25:246-253.
95. Smith JS, Karlstadt R, Blatcher, et al: Gastric pH from NPO to enteral-fed period with intermittent intravenous (IV) pantoprazole (P) vs continuously infused cimetidine (C). Am J Gastroenterol 2002;97:S47-S48.
96. Cook DJ, Reeve BK, Guyatt GH, et al: Stress ulcer prophylaxis in critically ill patients. Resolving discordant meta-analysis. JAMA 1996;275:308-314.
97. Cook D, Guyatt G, Marshall J, et al: A comparison of sucralfate and ranitidine for the prevention of upper gastrointestinal bleeding in patients requiring mechanical ventilation. Canadian Critical Care Trials Group. N Engl J Med 1998;388:791-797.
98. Szabo S, Hollander D: Pathways of gastrointestinal protection and repair: Mechanisms of action of sucralfate. Am J Med 1989;86:23-31.
99. Tryba M: Sucralfate versus antacids or H_2-antagonists for stress ulcer prophylaxis: A meta-analysis on efficacy and pneumonia rate. Crit Care Med 1991;19:942-949.
100. Macdougall BRD, Bailey RJ, Williams R: H_2-receptor antagonists and antacids in the prevention of acute gastrointestinal hemorrhage in fulminant hepatic failure: Two controlled trials. Lancet 1977;19:617-619.
101. Baghaie AA, Mojtahedzadeh M, Levine RL, et al: Comparison of the effect of intermittent administration and continuous infusion of famotidine on gastric pH in critically ill patients: Results of a prospective randomized, crossover study. Crit Care Med 1995;23:687-691.
102. Levy MJ, Seelig CB, Robinson NJ, et al: Comparison of omeprazole and ranitidine for stress ulcer prophylaxis. Dig Dis Sci 1997;42:1255-1259.
103. Conrad SA, Gabrielli A, Margolis B, et al: Randomized, double-blind comparison of immediate-release omeprazole oral suspension versus intravenous cimetidine for the prevention of upper gastrointestinal bleeding in critically ill patients. Crit Care Med 2005;33:1-6.
104. Davila RE, Rajan E, Adler DG, et al: ASGE guideline: The role of endoscopy in the patient with lower-GI bleeding. Gastrointest Endosc 2005;62:656-660.
105. Zuckerman GR, Prakash C: Acute lower intestinal bleeding. Part II: Etiology, therapy, and outcomes. Gastrointest Endosc 1999;49:228-238.
106. Jensen DM, Machicado GA: Diagnosis and treatment of severe hematochezia: The role of urgent colonoscopy after purge. Gastroenterology 1988;95: 1569-1574.
107. Longstreth GF: Epidemiology and outcome of patients hospitalized with acute lower gastrointestinal hemorrhage: A population-based study. Am J Gastroenterol 1997;92: 419-424.
108. Farrands PA, Taylor I: Management of acute lower gastrointestinal haemorrhage in a surgical unit over a 4-year period. J R Soc Med 1987;80: 79-82.
109. Bramley PN, Masson JW, McKnight G, et al: The role of an open-access bleeding unit in the management of colonic hemorrhage: A 2-year prospective study. Scand J Gastroenterol 1996;31:764-769.
110. Colacchio TA, Forde KA, Patsos TJ, et al: Impact of modern diagnostic methods on the management of active rectal bleeding—ten year experience. Am J Surg 1982;143: 607-610.
111. Richter JM, Christensen MR, Kaplan LM, et al: Effectiveness of current technology in the diagnosis and management of lower gastrointestinal hemorrhage. Gastrointest Endosc 1995;41:93-98.
112. Rossini FP, Ferrari A, Spandre M, et al: Emergency colonoscopy. World J Surg 1989;13:190-192.
113. McGuire HH Jr: Bleeding colonic diverticula. A reappraisal of natural history and management. Ann Surg 1994;220:653-656.
114. Strate LL: Lower GI bleeding: Epidemiology and diagnosis. Gastroenterol Clin North Am 2005;34:643-664.
115. Laine L, Connors LG, Reicin A, et al: Serious lower gastrointestinal clinical events with nonselective NSAID or coxib use. Gastroenterology 2003;124:288-292.
116. Lin CC, Lee YC, Lee H, et al: Bedside colonoscopy for critically ill patients with acute lower gastrointestinal bleeding. Intensive Care Med 2005;31:743-746.
117. Sorbi D, Norton I, Conio M, et al: Postpolypectomy lower GI bleeding: Descriptive analysis. Gastrointest Endosc 2000;51:690-696.
118. Prakash C, Zuckerman GR: Acute small bowel bleeding: A distinct entity with significantly different economic implications compared with GI bleeding from other locations. Gastrointest Endosc 2003;58:330-335.
119. Chaudhry V, Hyser MJ, Gracias VH, et al: Colonoscopy: The initial test for acute lower gastrointestinal bleeding. Am Surg 1998;64:723-728.
120. Kok KY, Kum CK, Goh PM: Colonoscopic evaluation of severe hematochezia in an Oriental population. Endoscopy 1998;30:675-680.

121. Jensen DM, Machicado GA, Jutabha R, et al: Urgent colonoscopy for the diagnosis and treatment of severe diverticular hemorrhage. N Engl J Med 2000;342:78-82.
122. Angtuaco TL, Reddy SK, Drapkin S, et al: The utility of urgent colonoscopy in the evaluation of acute lower gastrointestinal tract bleeding: A 2-year experience from a single center. Am J Gastroenterol 2001;96:1782-1785.
123. Green BT, Rockey DC, Portwood G, et al: Urgent colonoscopy for evaluation and management of acute lower gastrointestinal hemorrhage: A randomized controlled trial. Am J Gastroenterol 2005;100:2395-2402.
124. State LL, Syngal S: Timing of colonoscopy: Impact on length of hospital stay in patients with acute lower intestinal bleeding. Am J Gastroenterol 2003;98:317-322.
125. Chaudhry V, Hyser MJ, Gracias VH, et al: Colonoscopy: The initial test for acute lower gastrointestinal bleeding. Am Surg 1998;64:723-728.
126. Hunter JM, Pezim ME: Limited value of technetium 99m–labeled red cell scintigraphy in localization of lower gastrointestinal bleeding. Am J Surg 1990;159:504-506.
127. Voeller GR, Bunch G, Britt LG: Use of technetium-labeled red blood cell scintigraphy in the detection and management of gastrointestinal hemorrhage. Surgery 1991;110: 799-804.
128. Green BT, Rockey DC: Lower gastrointestinal bleeding management. Gastroenterol Clin North Am 2005;34:665-678.
129. Lin S, Rockey DC: Obscure gastrointestinal bleeding. Gastroenterol Clin North Am 2005;34: 679-698.
130. Carey EJ, Fleischer DE: Investigation of the small bowel in gastrointestinal bleeding—enteroscopy and capsule endoscopy. Gastroenterol Clin North Am 2005;34:719-734.
131. Yamamoto H, Kita H, Sunada K, et al: Clinical outcomes of double-balloon endoscopy for the diagnosis and treatment of small-intestinal diseases. Clin Gastroenterol Hepatol 2004;2:1010-1016.
132. Pennazio M, Santucci R, Rondonotti E, et al: Outcome of patients with obscure gastrointestinal bleeding after capsule endoscopy: Report of 100 consecutive patients. Gastroenterology 2004;126:643-653.
133. Carey EJ, Leighton JA, Heigh RI, et al: Single center outcomes of 260 consecutive patients undergoing capsule endoscopy for obscure GI bleeding. Gastroenterology 2004;126: A96.

Chapter 78

Acute Pancreatitis

John C. Marshall

Acute pancreatitis is a complex disease with a highly variable clinical course. It is responsible for more than 200,000 hospital admissions each year in the United States[1] and has an annual incidence of 10 to 80 cases per 100,000 in the developed world.[2-5] Incidence rates have been increasing over the past few decades.[6] For reasons that are unknown, there is seasonal variation in rates of the disease, the incidence being maximal in the spring and fall.[7] For the majority of patients with pancreatitis, the disease is benign and self-limited; it results in a hospital stay of only several days with no significant lasting sequelae. In 20% to 30% of affected patients, however, it is severe enough to lead to admission to an intensive care unit (ICU) or high-dependency unit and a complicated clinical course with a mortality risk that may exceed 30%.[1,8] These latter patients can present the intensivist with formidable challenges during the course of their illness, but if they recover, as most do, such patients can return to their premorbid state of health with no significant diminution in quality of life.

The prognosis for patients with severe acute pancreatitis has improved considerably over the 30 years since Ranson proposed his widely used severity criteria. In the mid 1970s, the mortality for patients with severe pancreatitis approached 100%[9]; today, the risk is less than half that figure. This improved outcome can be ascribed in part to general improvement in the care of critically ill patients and, more importantly, fundamental changes in the approach to the medical and surgical care of patients with acute pancreatitis, which in turn reflects an evolving understanding of the pathophysiology of the disease.

DEFINITIONS AND TERMINOLOGY

Pancreatitis is an acute inflammatory disorder that arises as a consequence of the activation of pancreatic digestive enzymes within the parenchyma of the gland and surrounding tissues of the peritoneal cavity and retroperitoneum. Its evolution and complications are quite variable and give rise to terminology that is both confusing and imprecise. The most widely used classification system is that known as the Atlanta classification, devised in 1992 (Table 78-1).[10] Its reproducibility, however, is poor,[11] and it is easier to conceptualize the disease as a spectrum of overlapping abnormalities resulting from the leakage of activated pancreatic enzymes, the host response to local tissue injury, and the superimposed complication of infection of what is initially a sterile process (Fig. 78-1).

In the mildest form of the disease, leakage of activated enzymes is minimal, and the most prominent manifestation is pancreatic edema secondary to a local inflammatory process. In more severe cases, pancreatic ductal disruption results in leakage of pancreatic enzymes. If the leakage occurs anteriorly into the peritoneal cavity, fluid collections will be evident. The local peritoneal inflammatory response triggers coagulation and fibrin deposition, which walls the collection off and creates a pseudocyst—so called because it is a fluid collection that lacks an epithelial lining. Drainage of pancreatic ascites through the diaphragm can create a pleural effusion; typically, this is seen on the left. Marked elevation of the amylase level in pleural fluid establishes the collection as pancreatic juice rather than a reaction to an inflammatory process on the abdominal side of the diaphragm. Alternatively, if leakage is into fatty tissues of the retroperitoneum, necrosis predominates, although small loculated fluid collections are frequently present. Often in patients with severe acute pancreatitis, computed tomography (CT) shows evidence of both intraperitoneal and retroperitoneal involvement. The older term "hemorrhagic pancreatitis" describes the sequelae of extension of retroperitoneal necrosis into blood vessels of the retroperitoneum. Extraperitoneal tracking of the resulting hematoma gives rise to Grey

Table 78-1. The Atlanta Classification System for Acute Pancreatitis

Term	Definition
Acute pancreatitis	Acute inflammation of the pancreas with variable involvement of peripancreatic and remote tissues
Mild acute pancreatitis	Edema of the pancreas; benign clinical course with minimal organ dysfunction and full recovery
Severe acute pancreatitis	Evidence of pancreatic necrosis; complications of infection, pseudocyst; clinical course characterized by organ failure
Acute fluid collection	Pancreatic or peripancreatic fluid, evident early in course of disease and lacking a wall
Pancreatic pseudocyst	Contained collection of pancreatic juice within a capsule of fibrous tissue and arising after an episode of acute pancreatitis
Pancreatic necrosis	Diffuse or focal loss of viability of pancreatic parenchyma or peripancreatic fat, evident as nonenhancing tissue on a contrast-enhanced CT scan
Pancreatic abscess	Localized collection of pus within the pancreas or peripancreatic region and containing little or no necrotic material

CT, computed tomography.
Adapted from Bradley EL: A clinically based classification system for acute pancreatitis. Arch Surg 1993;128:586-590.

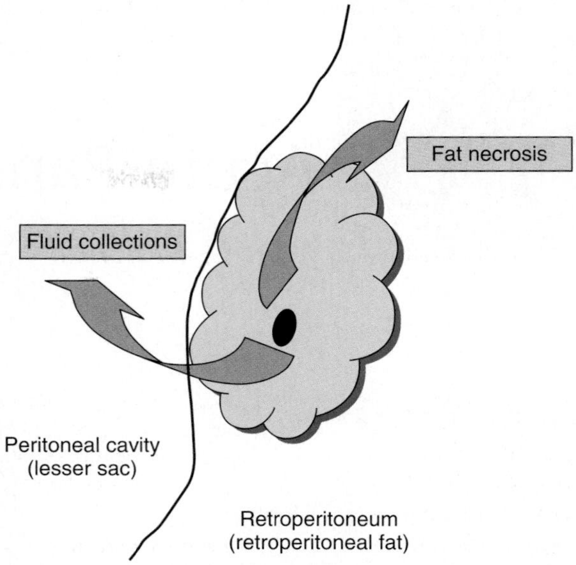

Figure 78-1. Disruption of the pancreatic ductal system results in leakage of activated digestive enzymes into peripancreatic tissues. When the predominant direction is anterior into the lesser sac, the result is one or more fluid collections that either resolve or coalesce to form a pseudocyst. Leakage posteriorly into fatty tissues of the retroperitoneum results in fat necrosis.

Turner's sign when the ecchymosis is evident in the flanks and Cullen's sign when it tracks anteriorly through the falciform ligament to the umbilicus.[12]

Both necrotic tissue and fluid collections can become secondarily infected with bacteria and fungi from the gastrointestinal tract, the former giving rise to infected pancreatic or peripancreatic necrosis and the latter to an infected pseudocyst or pancreatic abscess—the latter terms being largely interchangeable.

PATHOGENESIS

Acute pancreatitis arises in the pancreas through the leakage of activated pancreatic enzymes into pancreatic and peripancreatic tissue. The characteristic clinical syndrome, however, reflects the activation of a massive systemic inflammatory response to the local tissue injury.

Beyond its role as an endocrine organ, the pancreas plays a fundamental role in the digestion of foodstuff through the production of enzymes that degrade the major constituents of ingested food—protein (proteases), fat (lipases), starch (amylase), and nucleic acids (nucleases). Pancreatic enzymes are synthesized by the acinar cells lining the pancreatic ductal system and released from the cell as inactive zymogens.[13] They pass via the pancreatic duct into the lumen of the duodenum, where they are activated by mucosal enzymes such as enterokinase and thus become capable of degrading their target substrates. Under normal circumstances, activation is actively inhibited within the pancreas itself through sequestration of newly synthesized enzymes within zymogen granules and further inhibited through the local action of a specific inhibitor of trypsin activation called serine protease inhibitor of the Kazal type (SPINK).[14] The importance of normal mechanisms that inhibit trypsin activation is underlined by the observation that genetic mutations in the *SPINK* gene associated with reduced activity have been implicated in the pathogenesis of hereditary pancreatitis.[15]

Acute pancreatitis arises through the activation of pancreatic enzymes within the pancreas itself, possibly through the activity of lysosomal hydrolases in the acinar cell; the activated enzymes initiate autodigestion of the pancreas and surrounding tissue.[16,17] Activation of trypsinogen to trypsin appears to be a critical event during early pathogenesis of the acute process,[18,19] and an increase in intracellular calcium concentration may contribute to the activation of trypsinogen.[20] Trypsinogen can also be activated by lysosomal cathepsin B within the acinar cell.[21] Pancreatic acinar cells can die by either necrosis or apoptosis. Necrotic death is characterized by cell lysis, with leakage of intracellular constituents into the surrounding microenvironment, and the activation of an acute inflammatory response. Neutrophil recruitment in response to the local tissue injury has been implicated in the amplification of cellular damage in acute pancreatitis.[22-24] Apoptotic death, in contrast, is noninflammatory. Cells are degraded into membrane-bound vesicles that are taken up by fixed tissue macrophages. Phagocytosis of an apoptotic cell not only prevents the local activation of inflammation but also triggers transcriptional programs in the phagocytosing cell that are anti-inflammatory and reparative in nature, with upregulation of counterinflammatory cytokines such as interleukin-10 (IL-10).[25] The local cellular injury in acute pancreatitis can also be conceptualized as an imbalance between necrotic and apoptotic cell death. Activation of caspases—the intracellular enzymes that mediate apoptosis—attenuate the severity of pancreatitis,[26] whereas severe pancreatitis is associated with reduced levels of IL-10.[27]

Activated pancreatic enzymes injure not only cells of the pancreas but also those of surrounding tissue. Fat cells appear to be particularly vulnerable, and the disease tends to be more severe in the obese because of the greater amount of peripancreatic fat necrosis.[28] However, the degradative effects of pancreatic enzymes and the secondary tissue injury resulting from the host response can injure other structures in the vicinity of the pancreas, in particular the transverse colon, as well as major vessels such as the splenic artery and vein.[29] Pancreatitis rapidly evolves from an inflammatory disease of the pancreas to a chemical burn of the retroperitoneum.

The pathogenesis of the clinical syndrome is further complicated by the presence of the gastrointestinal tract immediately adjacent to the pancreas (Fig. 78-2). The head of the pancreas lies within the curve of the duodenum and immediately behind the stomach above and the transverse colon below. Damage to terminal feeding vessels in the colonic fat caused by activated pancreatic enzymes can result in focal perforation of the colon, with leakage of colonic bacteria into the peritoneal cavity.[30] Although the stomach and duodenum are only lightly colonized in health, the local ileus induced by the acute pancreatic inflammation promotes proximal gut overgrowth with enteric bacteria.[31] Finally, changes in gut mucosal barrier function arising from local inflammation and the absence of enteral nutrients promote the translocation of luminal bacteria and bacterial products such as endotoxin into the injured or necrotic peripancreatic tissue.[32]

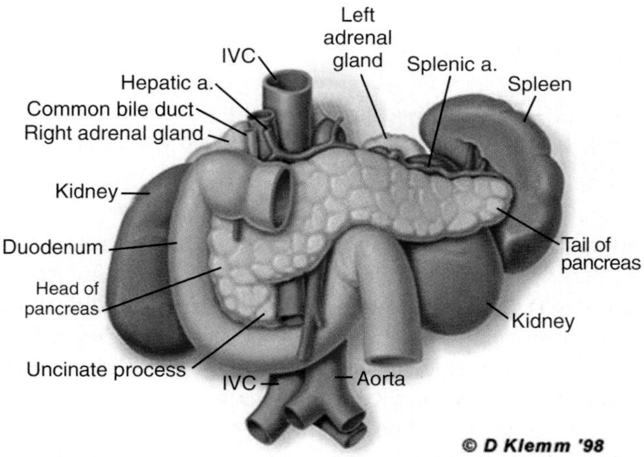

Figure 78-2. The pancreas is a retroperitoneal organ that lies posterior to the stomach, within the curve of the duodenum. It is in the immediate proximity of a number of large blood vessels, including the splenic artery and vein, the superior mesenteric artery and vein, and the portal vein. IVC, inferior vena cava.

Ultimately in more severe cases, the clinical syndrome evolves as a result of a systemically activated inflammatory response, with the same changes in microvascular blood flow, endothelial permeability, and release of inflammatory mediators that characterize bacterial sepsis.[33]

ETIOLOGY AND RISK FACTORS

Acute pancreatitis has many causes, although 75% of cases in the developed world result from either alcohol or gallstones (Table 78-2). The mechanism of alcohol-induced pancreatitis is unclear. The acinar cell of the pancreas is capable of metabolizing alcohol and also appears to be the primary target of alcohol-mediated pancreatic injury.[34] In vitro studies show that alcohol reduces the sensitivity of isolated acini to zymogen activation by cholecystokinin.[35] Gallstone pancreatitis appears to be the consequence of a transient acute increase in pancreatic ductal pressure associated with the passage of a small gallstone through the sphincter of Oddi in patients with a common channel for the bile and pancreatic ducts.[36] True obstruction of the duct is uncommon, and approximately 90% of patients will be found to have gallstones in their stool, thus implicating passage of the stone rather than an obstructing mechanism as the cause of the resulting pancreatic inflammation. The list of drugs implicated in the etiology of acute pancreatitis is long[37]; some of the more prominent associations are shown in Table 78-2.

Genetic factors have been associated with the development of acute pancreatitis. A polymorphism in the secre-

Table 78-2. Causes of Acute Pancreatitis

Congenital	
Anatomic abnormalities	Pancreas divisum, choledochocele, periampullary diverticulum
Familial pancreatitis	
Cystic fibrosis	
Hereditary angioedema	
Acquired	
Toxic	Alcohol, scorpion venom
Obstructive	Gallstones, duodenojejunal intussusception
Metabolic	Hypercalcemia, hypertriglyceridemia
Trauma	Blunt/penetrating
Drugs	Induced by ERCP
	Operative
	Thiazides, corticosteroids
Ischemia	Low-flow state
Infectious	Mumps, HIV, CMV, other viral infections, *Salmonella,* ascariasis, tuberculosis, brucellosis, leptospirosis
Autoimmune disease	Systemic lupus erythematosus
Idiopathic	

CMV, cytomegalovirus; ERCP, endoscopic retrograde cholangiopancreatography; HIV, human immunodeficiency virus.

tory trypsin inhibitor *(SPINK1)* gene is associated with an increased risk for acute pancreatitis,[38] as are mutations in the cystic fibrosis transmembrane conductance regulator *(CFTR)* gene.[39] Polymorphisms in the genes for tumor necrosis factor-α (TNF-α) and heat shock protein 70 have also been linked to an increased risk for acute pancreatitis,[40] although the association is less clear.

CLINICAL PRESENTATION AND DIAGNOSIS

Acute pancreatitis is typically manifested as severe acute epigastric pain that radiates to the back because of the retroperitoneal position of the pancreas. Nausea and vomiting are common associated symptoms. From the perspective of the intensivist, the predominant manifestations of severe acute pancreatitis are those that reflect hemodynamic instability secondary to an activated systemic inflammatory response. These manifestations can evolve with alarming rapidity, and the severity of the process is frequently not appreciated until it is quite advanced.

The cause of shock in a patient with acute pancreatitis is multifactorial. Initially, the acute inflammatory process in the retroperitoneum elicits local inflammation with outpouring of fluid into the relatively confined space of the retroperitoneum or into the peritoneal cavity itself. Intra-abdominal inflammation evokes secondary ileus within the gastrointestinal tract, and fluid is sequestered here, thereby increasing the relative intravascular volume deficit. Nausea, vomiting, and a reluctance to take fluids by mouth further exacerbate this fluid deficit. As the process evolves, a systemic inflammatory response to the local abdominal process results in diffuse vasodilation and capillary leak syndrome. In aggregate, the effective loss of intravascular volume can be enormous, and thus the initial resuscitation may require large volumes of intravenous fluid. Acute hypocalcemia may also contribute to the clinical picture of cardiovascular compromise. Indeed, the classic prognostic criteria articulated by Ranson (Box 78-1) emphasize the importance of acute inflammation (white blood cell count) and the secondary hemodynamic (fluid sequestration, base excess, blood urea nitrogen, and hematocrit) and metabolic (glucose, calcium) sequelae in determining the ultimate prognosis.

The diagnosis of pancreatitis is usually straightforward and based on the combination of clinical manifestations and characteristic biochemical findings of elevations in circulating levels of amylase and lipase, the latter being somewhat more accurate diagnostically.[41] The diagnosis can be confirmed and the severity of the disease evaluated by CT (Fig. 78-3) according to the grading system developed by Balthazar (Table 78-3).[42]

An initial assessment of the severity of the disease is useful primarily in deciding the optimal venue for early management of the patient because at least some of the delayed morbidity of acute pancreatitis can be reduced through aggressive initial resuscitation and support. A variety of approaches have been used to quantify disease severity. Ranson identified 11 variables—5 at initial evaluation and 6 over the ensuing 48 hours—that correlated in a graded fashion with the ultimate risk for mortality (see Box 78-1). The Glasgow-Imrie criteria are a modification of Ranson's scale and represent an alternative model of severity scoring. In head-to-head studies, APACHE (Acute Physiology, Age, and Chronic Health Evaluation) II—a generic severity-of-illness scale—performs at least as well as the Ranson or Glasgow-Imrie criteria in predicting hospital survival.[43] Moreover, even simpler scales appear to provide comparable prognostic information.[19,44] A variety of biochemical measures, including C-reactive protein, procalcitonin, IL-6, and trypsinogen activation peptide, are purported to differentiate mild and severe

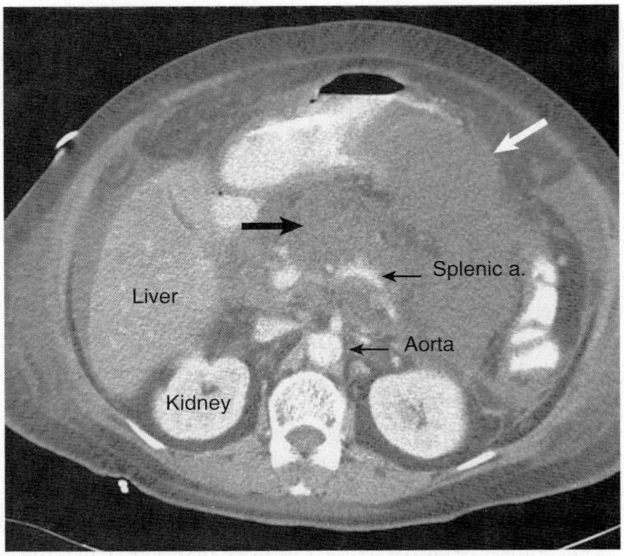

Figure 78-3. Computed tomography findings in severe acute pancreatitis (Balthazar grade E). Note the combination of pancreatic necrosis *(black arrow)* and fluid and debris *(white arrow)* and the intimate relationship of the inflamed pancreas to the splenic artery.

Box 78-1

Ranson's Criteria for Acute Pancreatitis

On Admission
Age >55 years
White cell count >16,000/μL
Blood sugar >11.1 mmol/L (200 mg/dL)
LDH>350 IU/L
AST>250 IU/L

Over the First 48 Hours
Po_2<60 mm Hg
Estimated fluid sequestration >6 L
Calcium <2.00 mm/L (8 mg/dL)
Hematocrit fall <10%
BUN rise >1.8 mmol/L (5 mg/dL)
Base excess >–4 mEq/L

AST, aspartate aminotransferase; BUN, blood urea nitrogen; LDH, lactate dehydrogenase.

Table 78-3. Balthazar's Grading of Computed Tomography Findings in Acute Pancreatitis

Grade	Findings
A	Normal pancreas
B	Pancreatic enlargement
C	Pancreatic or peripancreatic inflammation
D	Single peripancreatic fluid collection
E	2 or more pancreatic collections and/or retroperitoneal air

From Balthazar EJ: CT diagnosis and staging of acute pancreatitis. Radiol Clin North Am 1989;27:19-37.

pancreatitis early during the clinical evolution of the disease[45-47]; their clinical utility is unclear, however. Persistence of the clinical manifestations of systemic inflammation beyond 48 hours is also associated with subsequent organ dysfunction and higher mortality.[48] Precision in prognostication is far less important than early recognition of patients in whom close monitoring and aggressive resuscitation can alter the clinical course, and a low threshold for management in a more controlled and monitored setting is an important factor in reducing the complications of pancreatitis.[49]

Box 78-2

Common Microbial Isolates in Pancreatic and Peripancreatic Infections

Gram-Negative Aerobes
Escherichia coli
Klebsiella
Pseudomonas
Proteus
Enterobacter

Gram-Positive Aerobes
Enterococcus
Staphylococcus aureus
Staphylococcus epidermidis

Anerobes
Bacteroides

Fungi
Candida

EARLY MANAGEMENT OF CRITICALLY ILL PATIENTS WITH ACUTE PANCREATITIS

Initial Resuscitation

Intravascular fluid deficits early in the course of pancreatitis can be substantial. Early aggressive fluid resuscitation is the cornerstone of initial successful management.[50] Volume status should be monitored with a urinary catheter and central venous catheter, and although studies in the specific setting of pancreatitis have not been performed, there is every reason to believe that the principles of goal-directed resuscitation should be followed.[51] There are no data to support a preference for colloids or crystalloids during resuscitation; the key, however, is to administer sufficient volumes rapidly enough to restore adequate circulating volume.[52] Typically, this consists of many liters of fluid, and not infrequently, the sickest patients will receive more than 10 to 15 L of fluid resuscitation over the first 24 hours. Such aggressive resuscitation is best carried out within the well-monitored environment of the ICU.

Although aggressive fluid resuscitation can minimize later complications such as pancreatic necrosis and acute renal failure, in patients with increased vascular permeability it carries a high risk of complications related to interstitial edema. Frequently, patients will require endotracheal intubation and mechanical ventilation. The development of abdominal compartment syndrome is a relatively common and underdiagnosed complication of resuscitated acute pancreatitis.[53] Intra-abdominal pressure can be measured by passing a urinary catheter into the bladder. Normal pressures approximate central venous pressure, whereas pressures greater than 20 cm H_2O indicate intra-abdominal hypertension, and pressures greater than 30 cm H_2O indicate a compartment syndrome and carry an increased risk for ischemic injury because of impairment of visceral venous drainage. In severe cases, management requires abdominal decompression by laparotomy. The need for laparotomy in patients with acute pancreatitis may be avoided by the use of continuous venovenous hemofiltration[54] or decompressive anterior abdominal fasciotomy.[55]

Infection Prophylaxis

Infection is a common complication of acute necrotizing pancreatitis, and its development is associated with an increased risk for morbidity and mortality.[56] In critically ill patients with severe acute pancreatitis, these infections may arise within the injured or necrotic peripancreatic tissue or at distant sites as nosocomial infection.

The characteristic microbial flora of peripancreatic infection includes organisms normally resident within the gastrointestinal tract[57] and organisms that characteristically colonize the proximal gastrointestinal tract of critically ill patients (Box 78-2).[31] Anaerobes may be present but are uncommon, whereas organisms such as *Candida*,[58,59] enterococci, and coagulase-negative staphylococci are encountered with increasing frequency. This infecting flora reflects the role of the gastrointestinal tract as the reservoir of organisms inducing superinfection during acute pancreatitis.[60]

Infection of necrotic tissue in the retroperitoneum can arise by any of several routes. Bacteremic spread from a distant site, retrograde passage up the pancreatic duct, and direct extension through a defect in the adjacent gastrointestinal tract are all plausible mechanisms. However, the most significant mechanism of infection appears to occur as a consequence of the translocation of viable microorganisms across an anatomically intact gastrointestinal tract, either the colon or the small intestine. Bacterial translocation is readily demonstrable in animal models of acute pancreatitis,[61,62] and indirect evidence suggests that the phenomenon contributes to infectious complications in human pancreatitis.[60] Patients with severe pancreatitis, for example, have higher rates of proximal gut colonization with the same enteric organisms that produce infection,[63] and intestinal colonization invariably precedes the development of invasive infection.[64] Moreover, suppression of pathologic gut colonization reduces the risk of infection.[65]

Host-microbial interactions within the gastrointestinal tract are complex,[66,67] and the changes that occur in pancreatitis are much more than a state of generalized leakiness. Colectomy, for example, increases rates of small bowel microbial colonization and bacterial translocation.[68] Furthermore, the anaerobic flora of the gut provides a barrier to intestinal mucosal colonization with pathogenic aerobes and serves to inhibit bacterial translocation.[69] Thus, anaerobes are uncommonly found in pancreatic infections, and isolation of an anaerobic organism from an area of infected pancreatic necrosis is highly suggestive of a physical breach in the gastrointestinal tract.

Infection of pancreatic necrosis is a relatively late event that occurs maximally during the second or third week after onset of the acute disease.[70] However, circulating bacterial DNA[71] or endotoxin from gram-negative bacteria[72] can be detected early during the course of the disease.

The role of antibiotic prophylaxis, however, is controversial. A meta-analysis of randomized controlled trials of prophylactic antibiotics for patients with acute pancreatitis concluded that prophylaxis can improve survival, without significantly altering rates of pancreatic infection.[73] Nonetheless, a consensus conference of critical care organizations has recommended that routine antibiotic prophylaxis not be used in the absence of more compelling evidence from randomized controlled trials.[49] This push for conservatism is driven by three principal factors—the low methodologic quality of trials supporting antibiotic prophylaxis, concern regarding the adverse ecologic consequences of prolonged broad-spectrum antibiotic administration, and the increasing use of an alternative prophylactic strategy, enteral feeding.[74] One of the most influential studies of prophylactic antibiotics in pancreatitis, for example, reported a significant improvement in survival associated with antibiotic prophylaxis in a cohort of 60 patients[75]; in that study, however, antibiotic use had no impact on rates of pancreatic infection, and fully three quarters of patients in the control arm received antibiotics early in the course of their disease. Prevention of pathologic gut colonization through the use of selective digestive tract decontamination has been shown to decrease rates of pancreatic infectious complications[65] and reduce the mortality associated with gram-negative infections.[76] Whether antifungal prophylaxis is efficacious is also controversial.[77,78]

Nutritional Support

In contrast to the persistent controversy regarding the utility of antibiotic prophylaxis in severe acute pancreatitis, it is now generally accepted that patients do better and, in particular, experience less infectious and inflammatory morbidity if they are fed enterally rather than parenterally. Enteral feeding is associated with maintenance of epithelial barrier function and reduced rates of translocation of endotoxin and viable bacteria in experimental animals.[79,80] A meta-analysis of six trials that recruited more than 200 patients found a lower rate of infectious complications (relative risk, 0.45; 95% confidence interval [CI], 0.26 to 0.78), reduced need for operative intervention (relative risk, 0.48; 95% CI, 0.22 to 1.0), and shorter hospital stay (mean, 2.9 days; 95% CI, 1.6 to 4.3 days; $P<.001$), along with an insignificant trend toward improved survival.[81]

Current guidelines recommend early institution of enteral feeding in patients with severe acute pancreatitis, supplemented, as needed, with parenteral support to meet full nutritional requirements.[49,82,83] Although the presence of gastric ileus in acute pancreatitis has resulted in a preference for the nasojejunal rather than the nasogastric route of feeding, there is no evidence of the inferiority of nasogastric feeding in recent clinical trials.[84,85] Similarly, there is no compelling evidence at present to favor any particular nutritional formulation.

Adjuvant Therapy

Despite a substantial body of literature suggesting a benefit for a variety of different adjuvant treatments in preclinical models, there is no evidence of benefit for any specific therapy in human disease. A systematic review of the use of cimetidine found no evidence that suppression of gastric acid secretion improved outcome, but rather a trend to a higher risk for complications.[86] Pooled data from small studies have suggested that somatostatin or octreotide can improve survival in patients with severe acute pancreatitis,[87] but data from larger, more robust trials are lacking. Protease inhibitors have also been suggested to reduce mortality in moderate to severe pancreatitis.[88]

Platelet-activating factor (PAF) is a potent proinflammatory lipid mediator that has been implicated in the local and remote manifestations of acute pancreatitis.[89] Inhibition of PAF with the administration of either a receptor antagonist[90] or recombinant PAF acetylhydrolase—the enzyme responsible for degrading PAF[91]—results in attenuation of injury in animal models. Unfortunately, despite early promise in phase II clinical trials,[92,93] a phase III trial failed to show any benefit for adjuvant treatment with the PAF receptor antagonist lexipafant in 290 patients with severe acute pancreatitis.[94]

Activated protein C (drotrecogin alfa activated) is a recombinant version of an endogenous anticoagulant that has been shown to improve survival in patients with severe sepsis.[95] Activated protein C improves multiple parameters in experimental pancreatitis,[96] and based on the clinical similarity of sepsis and acute pancreatitis, it may ultimately prove efficacious for patients with necrotizing pancreatitis as well.[97] This role has not been studied, and at present its indication in pancreatitis is limited to patients with infectious complications such as infected pancreatic necrosis.[49]

Other strategies such as inhibition of TNF or blockade of IL-1 have shown promise in preclinical models but have not been evaluated in human disease.[98]

Endoscopic Retrograde Cholangiopancreatography in Acute Gallstone Pancreatitis

Gallstone pancreatitis is caused by a gallstone that has migrated from the gallbladder into the common bile duct and has produced, at least transiently, obstruction of the pancreatic duct. This pathogenetic mechanism raises the possibility that measures to relieve the obstruction at the level of the sphincter of Oddi might reduce the severity of the disease. This possibility has been evaluated in at least four clinical trials, the pooled data from which suggest benefit for patients with severe pancreatitis in reducing subsequent complications.[99] It is unclear whether the benefit extends to all patients or simply to the subset of patients with persistent common bile duct obstruction and concomitant cholangitis.[100,101]

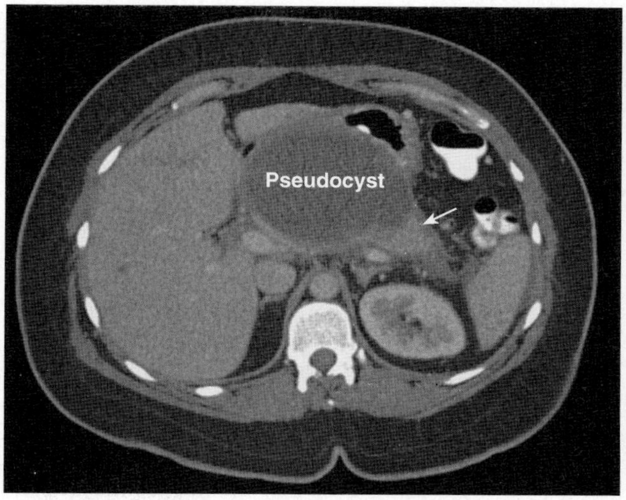

Figure 78-4. A maturing pancreatic pseudocyst, evident as a well-circumscribed fluid collection in the lesser sac that is compressing the residual pancreas *(arrow).*

MANAGEMENT OF LATE COMPLICATIONS OF SEVERE ACUTE PANCREATITIS

It is apparent from the foregoing that the early management of a patient with severe acute pancreatitis is focused primarily on adequate resuscitation and organ support. Early lethal postresuscitation complications are uncommon[102] and include intestinal ischemia (typically secondary to a low-flow state or mesenteric venous thrombosis after delayed resuscitation)[103] or bleeding secondary to erosion into a major vessel. In the absence of these catastrophic and fortunately rare complications, the subsequent management of a critically ill patient with acute pancreatitis involves optimal intensive care,[104] close monitoring, and patience.

Pancreatic Pseudocysts

Serial evaluation by CT shows that the diffuse fluid collections evident in early pancreatitis coalesce to form discrete cyst-like collections contained within an organized capsule of fibrin that are termed pseudocysts. Typically, they arise in the lesser sac, between the pancreas and the posterior wall of the stomach (Fig. 78-4). Management is expectant in the absence of complications,[105] and rarely is intervention required in the ICU. The most common symptom precipitating drainage is persistent pain or symptoms of gastric obstruction. Other important complications include infection and hemorrhage into the cyst.

The classic approach to the management of a pancreatic pseudocyst involved waiting until the fibrous capsule of the cyst had matured and then draining the cyst into the back wall of the stomach. Open surgical pseudocyst gastrostomy has largely given way to less invasive approaches involving cyst gastrostomy by radiologic image-guided,[106] endoscopic,[107] or laparoscopic approaches.[108] A pseudocyst forms as a result of injury to the main pancreatic duct or one of its branches and persists because of obstruction to the flow of pancreatic juice through the duct. If the obstruction continues, external drainage will result in a persistent pancreaticocutaneous fistula. Thus, regardless of how it is accomplished, drainage into the stomach avoids this complication by replacing the external fistula with an internal fistula that is without clinical importance. Open surgery may be required for massive hemorrhage; angiographic embolization of the bleeding vessel is another alternative.[109]

Infected Necrosis and Pancreatic Abscess

One of the most significant advances in the treatment of severe pancreatitis has been the adoption of a policy of surgical conservatism in managing patients with suspected pancreatic or peripancreatic infection. Case series demonstrate improved survival rates when surgery is delayed,[110-114] and a single randomized trial showed that delaying surgical intervention for at least 2 weeks in patients with necrotizing pancreatitis improves clinical outcomes.[115] The improved outcomes can be attributed to a reduced frequency of major bleeding complications associated with the débridement of necrotic, infected retroperitoneal tissue.

Just as serial evaluation reveals localization of pancreatic fluid collections, serial study of areas of pancreatic necrosis shows that they too coalesce with time and become more circumscribed. Importantly, a wall of granulation tissue develops between the areas of necrosis and viable surrounding tissue. It is this clear demarcation between viable and nonviable tissue that renders operative intervention safe and obviates the need for repeat surgery or open abdominal approaches. Typically, the process of demarcation takes 3 to 4 weeks or longer to occur; thus, surgical intervention, if contemplated, should be deferred. A strategy of surgical conservatism in a patient with clinical manifestations of sepsis and ongoing organ dysfunction may appear counterintuitive, but it is both well tolerated and safer than the alternative.[116]

There is general consensus that the indication for operative intervention in a patient with severe pancreatitis is infected necrosis; sterile necrosis should be managed conservatively.[111,117,118] The diagnosis of infection of pancreatic necrosis can be challenging to establish because clinical manifestations of systemic inflammation are common in an acutely ill patient with pancreatitis, even in the absence of infection, as are nosocomial infections in sites other than the necrotic retroperitoneal tissue. A diagnosis of infection may be suggested by a new elevation in levels of procalcitonin[119,120] or by CT findings of air in the necrotic tissue (Fig. 78-5). However, definitive diagnosis of infection is best established by CT-guided fine-needle aspiration of the peripancreatic necrotic tissue.[121]

Documentation of infection on a fine-needle aspirate is not an absolute indication for operative intervention. Antibiotics should be administered as guided by the results of culture and sensitivity, and then source control options should be evaluated. Early in the course of the disease, before the demarcation of necrotic and viable tissue, percutaneous drainage of the fluid component of the collection can be a temporizing measure until operative intervention is safer (see Fig. 78-5). Percutaneous drainage alone may be curative,[122,123] and there is even an evolving literature indicating that some patients with infected pancreatic necrosis can be successfully managed nonoperatively.[124,125]

Surgical management of infected pancreatic necrosis entails débridement of the necrotic retroperitoneal tissue and drainage of the resulting cavity. Approaches span the surgical spectrum from minimal-access techniques[126-128] to open abdominal approaches.[129,130] In general, the optimal approach is the one that entails the least anatomic and physiologic upset to the patient. Open laparotomy can be performed with either a midline or a bilateral subcostal incision. With the aid of a recent CT scan to guide the dissection, the infected retroperitoneal necrosis is approached either through the gastrocolic omentum and the lesser sac or through the inferior aspect of the transverse mesocolon. Dissection is performed largely blindly and bluntly, with evacuation of necrotic retroperitoneal fat and pus. Soft drains are left in the resulting cavity to provide egress for pancreatic juice, and the abdomen can usually be closed primarily. If there is evidence of significant involvement of the mesocolon or preoperative cultures yield anaerobic organisms, a proximal diverting ileostomy may be added to minimize contamination from the adjacent colon. If the patient is likely to require a prolonged ICU stay, an operative feeding jejunostomy can facilitate nutritional support.

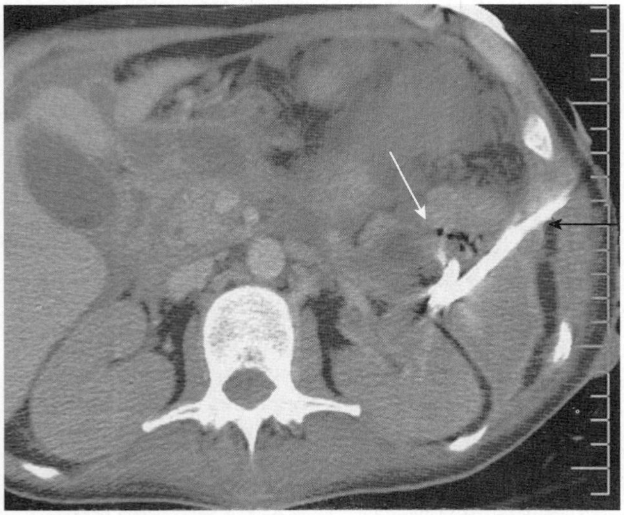

Figure 78-5. Infected pancreatic necrosis *(white arrow).* The fluid component of the collection was decompressed with a percutaneously placed drain *(black arrow)* to allow delayed laparoscopic débridement.

Laparoscopic techniques have the added advantage of permitting direct visualization of the abscess cavity,[128,131,132] but may be challenging if there is extensive or multiloculated areas of necrosis. Infected necrosis can also be approached via the flank by using a nephroscope or laparoscope to aid in visualization of the abscess contents.[133] Further insight into the role of minimally invasive approaches should emerge from several ongoing clinical trials.[108,134] The role of open abdominal approaches in the management of infected pancreatic necrosis is diminishing as surgical practice shifts to delayed intervention with more minimally invasive techniques.[135]

Peritoneal lavage with the objective of evacuating activated pancreatic enzymes enjoyed a period of popularity,[136] but it is now used less frequently. Some authors recommend continuous postoperative lavage after pancreatic necrosectomy,[135] although the benefits of this approach are unproven.

Vascular Complications of Necrotizing Pancreatitis

Vascular complications of acute pancreatitis include both thrombosis and hemorrhage.[137,138] Thrombosis of the splenic, superior mesenteric, and portal vessels develops as a consequence of the prothrombotic effects of the adjacent inflamed pancreas and reduced flow before full resuscitation. Less commonly, more distant vessels such as the inferior vena cava or renal veins may thrombose. Venous thrombosis may give rise to portal venous gas on CT; in the absence of clinical findings dictating a need for emergency intervention, both the venous thrombosis and the associated CT findings can be managed conservatively.[139] Treatment consists of anticoagulation; intestinal infarction secondary to venous thrombosis in patients with acute pancreatitis carries prohibitive mortality, even with surgery.

Erosion of the retroperitoneal inflammatory process into a major artery can produce bleeding into either the peritoneal cavity or the gut lumen, in which case it is manifested as gastrointestinal hemorrhage. Commonly involved vessels include the splenic artery, the gastroduodenal artery, and the pancreaticoduodenal arcade.[140] Operative exposure is challenging in patients with acute retroperitoneal inflammation, and whenever feasible, bleeding is best managed by angiographic embolization.[109]

LONG-TERM OUTCOME AND QUALITY OF LIFE

Acute necrotizing pancreatitis can be an enormously challenging process to treat (Fig. 78-6). ICU and hospital stays are often prolonged, and in addition to operative procedures undertaken during the acute episode, there is frequently a need for later intervention to close a stoma, repair an incisional hernia, or excise the gallbladder. Yet there is ample evidence that patients who survive their acute illness return to a health-related quality of life that is no different from that of age-matched controls.[141-144] Abnormalities in both endocrine and exocrine function are commonly evident at follow-up,[145] and diabetes develops in approximately a third of survivors of severe necrotizing pancreatitis.[146]

CONCLUSIONS

Necrotizing pancreatitis is a challenging, but enormously satisfying disease to manage. Current management approaches are supportive, with treatment directed at correcting complications of the disease process. Adjunctive treatment strategies that target the pathologic host inflammatory response are not yet available but should emerge over the coming decade. Although the outcome is heavily dependent on disease severity, with early and aggressive resuscitation, optimal supportive care in an ICU, and judicious and delayed intervention to manage infected necrosis, the overwhelming majority of patients survive and are rehabilitated to an excellent quality of life.

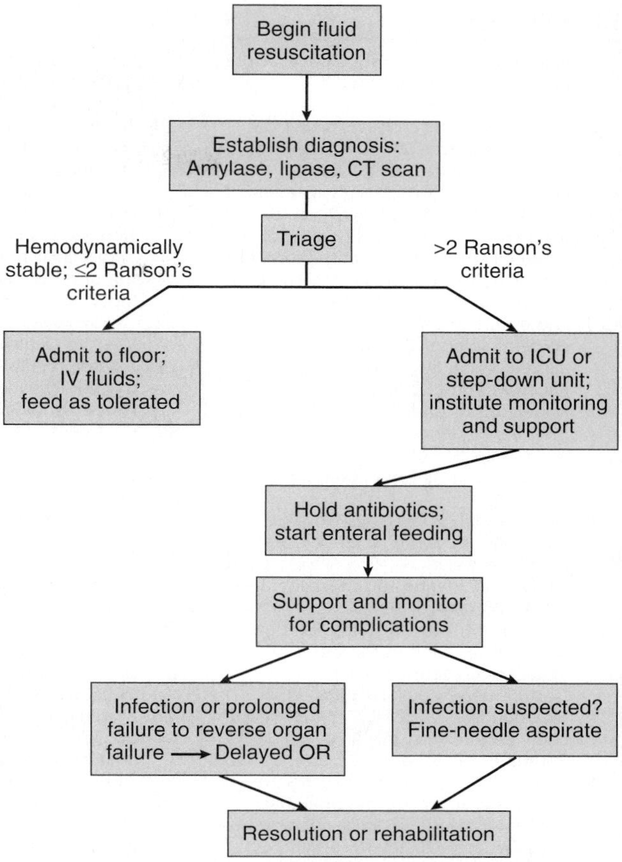

Figure 78-6. Approach to the patient with acute pancreatitis. CT, computed tomography; ICU, intensive care unit; IV, intravenous; OR, operation.

KEY POINTS

- The initial manifestation of severe acute pancreatitis can be subtle; early objective quantification of disease severity is important in guiding the intensity of resuscitation and informing decisions regarding patient disposition.
- Aggressive fluid resuscitation is the cornerstone of successful management. Large volumes of intravenous fluid must often be given, and the development of acute respiratory failure with a need for endotracheal intubation and admission to an ICU is neither uncommon nor undesirable.
- The role of prophylactic antibiotics is controversial; in the absence of more compelling evidence of efficacy, their use is discouraged.
- Nutritional support should be instituted early and by the enteral route, with parenteral nutrition reserved for patients who cannot meet their caloric needs by the enteral route.
- There is, at present, no established role for other adjuvant treatments, and management after resuscitation is entirely supportive.
- Serial CT scans can document the severity of the disease and monitor its progression; CT-guided fine-needle aspiration is the diagnostic technique of choice to identify infected necrosis.
- Management of infected necrosis consists of the administration of systemic antibiotics guided by culture and delayed surgical intervention. There is an increasing role for minimally invasive techniques of pancreatic débridement and even for nonoperative management of infected necrosis.
- Despite the complexity and morbidity of the acute episode, long-term health-related quality of life for survivors of acute necrotizing pancreatitis is excellent.

REFERENCES

1. Whitcomb DC: Clinical practice. Acute pancreatitis. N Engl J Med 2006;354:2142-2150.
2. Shahen NJ, Hansen RA, Morgan DR, et al: The burden of gastrointestinal and liver diseases, 2006. Am J Gastroenterol 2006;101:2128-2138.
3. Frey CF, Zhou H, Harvey DJ, et al: The incidence and case-fatality rates of acute biliary, alcoholic, and idiopathic pancreatitis in California, 1994-2001. Pancreas 2006;33:336-344.
4. Yadav D, Lowenfels AB: Trends in the epidemiology of the first attack of acute pancreatitis: A systematic review. Pancreas 2006;33:323-330.
5. Andersson R, Anderrson B, Haraldsen P, et al: Incidence, management and recurrence rate of acute pancreatitis. Scand J Gastroenterol 2004;39:891-894.
6. Goldacre MJ, Roberts SE: Hospital admission for acute pancreatitis in an English population, 1963-98: Database study of incidence and mortality. BMJ 2004;328:1466-1469.
7. Gallerani M, Boari B, Salmi R, et al: Seasonal variation in the onset of acute pancreatitis. World J Gastroenterol 2004;10:3328-3331.
8. Swaroop VS, Chari ST, Clain JE: Severe acute pancreatitis. JAMA 2004;291:2865-2868.
9. Ranson JHC, Rifkind KM, Turner JW: Prognostic signs and nonoperative peritoneal lavage in acute pancreatitis. Surg Gynecol Obstet 1976;143:209-219.
10. Bradley EL: A clinically based classification system for acute pancreatitis. Arch Surg 1993;128:586-590.
11. Besselink MG, van Santvoort HC, Bollen TL, et al: Describing computed tomography findings in acute necrotizing pancreatitis with the Atlanta classification: An interobserver agreement study. Pancreas 2007;33:331-335.
12. Sugimoto M, Takada T, Yasuda H, et al: MPR-hCT imaging of the pancreatic fluid pathway to Grey-Turner's and Cullen's sign in acute pancreatitis. Hepatogastroenterology 2005;52:1613-1616.
13. Pandol SJ: Acute pancreatitis. Curr Opin Gastroenterol 2006;22:481-486.
14. Liddle RA: Pathophysiology of SPINK mutations in pancreatic development and disease. Endocrinol Metab Clin North Am 2006;35:345-356.
15. Halangk W, Lerch MM: Early events in acute pancreatitis. Clin Lab Med 2005;25:1-15.
16. Gorelick FS, Otani T: Mechanisms of intracellular zymogen activation. Baillieres Best Pract Res Clin Gastroenterol 1999;13:227-240.
17. van Acker GJ, Perides G, Steer ML: Co-localization hypothesis: A mechanism for the intrapancreatic activation of digestive enzymes during the early phases of acute pancreatitis. World J Gastroenterol 2006;12:1985-1990.
18. Bhatia M, Wong FL, Cao Y, et al: Pathophysiology of acute pancreatitis. Pancreatology 2005;5:132-144.
19. Spitzer AL, Barcia AM, Schell MT, et al: Applying Ockham's razor to pancreatitis prognostication: A four-variable predictive model. Ann Surg 2006;243:380-388.
20. Petersen OH, Sutton R: Ca^{2+} signalling and pancreatitis: Effects of alcohol, bile and coffee. Trends Pharmacol Sci 2006;27:113-120.
21. Halangk W, Lerch MM, Brandt-Nedelev B, et al: Role of cathepsin B in intracellular trypsinogen activation and the onset of acute pancreatitis. J Clin Invest 2000;106:773-781.
22. Gukovskaya AS, Vaquero E, Zaninovic V, et al: Neutrophils and NADPH oxidase mediate intrapancreatic trypsin activation in murine experimental acute pancreatitis. Gastroenterology 2002;122:974-984.
23. Raraty MG, Murphy JA, Mcloughlin E, et al: Mechanisms of acinar cell injury in acute pancreatitis. Scand J Surg 2005;94:89-96.
24. Shields CJ, Winter DC, Redmond HP: Lung injury in acute pancreatitis: Mechanisms, prevention, and therapy. Curr Opin Crit Care 2002;8:158-163.
25. Serhan CN, Savill J: Resolution of inflammation: The beginning programs the end. Nat Immunol 2005;6:1191-1197.
26. Mareninova OA, Sung KF, Hong P, et al: Cell death in pancreatitis: Caspases protect from necrotizing pancreatitis. J Biol Chem 2006;281:3370-3381.
27. Laveda R, Martinez J, Munoz C, et al: Different profile of cytokine synthesis according to the severity of acute pancreatitis. World J Gastroenterol 2005;11:5309-5313.
28. Martinez J, Johnson CD, Sanchez-Paya J, et al: Obesity is a definitive risk factor of severity and mortality in acute pancreatitis: An updated meta-analysis. Pancreatology 2006;6:206-209.
29. Flati G, Salvatori F, Porowska B, et al: Severe hemorrhagic complications in pancreatitis. Ann Ital Chir 2007;66:233-237.
30. van Minnen LP, Besselink MG, Bosscha K, et al: Colonic involvement in acute pancreatitis. A retrospective study of 16 patients. Dig Surg 2004;21:33-40.
31. Marshall JC, Christou NV, Meakins JL: The gastrointestinal tract. The "undrained abscess" of multiple organ failure. Ann Surg 1993;218:111-119.
32. Penalva JC, Martinez J, Laveda R, et al: A study of intestinal permeability in relation to the inflammatory response and plasma endocab IgM levels in patients with acute pancreatitis. J Clin Gastroenterol 2004;38:512-517.
33. Cuthbertson CM, Christophi C: Disturbances of the microcirculation in acute pancreatitis. Br J Surg 2006;93:518-530.
34. Apte MV, Pirola RC, Wilson JS: Molecular mechanisms of alcoholic pancreatitis. Dig Dis 2005;23:232-240.
35. Gorelick FS: Alcohol and zymogen activation in the pancreatic acinar cell. Pancreas 2003;27:305-310.
36. Acosta JM, Ledesma CL: Gallstone migration as a cause of acute pancreatitis. N Engl J Med 1974;290:484-487.
37. Trivedi CD, Pitchumoni CS: Drug-induced pancreatitis: An update. J Clin Gastroenterol 2005;39:709-716.
38. Tukiainen E, Kylanpaa ML, Kemppainen E, et al: Pancreatic secretory trypsin inhibitor (SPINK1) gene mutations in patients with acute pancreatitis. Pancreas 2005;30:239-242.
39. Bishop MD, Freedman SD, Zielenski J, et al: The cystic fibrosis transmembrane conductance regulator gene and ion channel function in patients with idiopathic pancreatitis. Hum Genet 2005;118:372-381.
40. Balog A, Gyulai Z, Boros LG, et al: Polymorphism of the TNF-alpha, HSP70-2, and CD14 genes increases susceptibility to severe acute pancreatitis. Pancreas 2005;30:46-50.
41. Smith RC, Southwell-Keely J, Chesher D: Should serum pancreatic lipase replace serum amylase as a biomarker of acute pancreatitis? Aust N Z J Surg 2005;75:399-404.
42. Balthazar EJ: Acute pancreatitis: Assessment of severity with clinical and CT evaluation. Radiology 2002;223:603-613.
43. Yeung YP, Lam BY, Yip AW: APACHE system is better than Ranson system in the prediction of severity of acute pancreatitis. Hepatobiliary Pancreat Dis Int 2006;5:294-299.
44. Ueda T, Takeyama Y, Yasuda T, et al: Simple scoring system for the prediction of the prognosis of severe acute pancreatitis. Surgery 2007;141:51-58.
45. Rau B, Schilling MK, Beger HG: Laboratory markers of severe acute pancreatitis. Dig Dis 2004;22:247-257.
46. Papachristou GI, Whitcomb DC: Inflammatory markers of disease severity in acute pancreatitis. Clin Lab Med 2005;25:17-37.
47. Neoptolemos JP, Kemppainen EA, Mayer JM, et al: Early prediction of severity in acute pancreatitis by urinary trypsinogen activation peptide: A multicentre study. Lancet 2000;355:1955-1960.
48. Mofidi R, Duff MD, Wigmore SJ, et al: Association between early systemic inflammatory response, severity of multiorgan dysfunction and death in acute pancreatitis. Br J Surg 2006;93:738-744.
49. Nathens AB, Curtis JR, Beale RJ, et al: Management of the critically ill patient with severe acute pancreatitis. Crit Care Med 2004;32:2524-2536.
50. Tenner S: Initial management of acute pancreatitis: Critical issues during the first 72 hours. Am J Gastroenterol 2004;99:2489-2494.
51. Rivers E, Nguyen B, Havstad S, et al: Early goal-directed therapy in the treatment of severe sepsis and septic shock. N Engl J Med 2001;345:1368-1377.
52. Brown A, Baillargeon JD, Hughes MD, et al: Can fluid resuscitation prevent pancreatic necrosis in severe acute pancreatitis? Pancreatology 2002;2:104-107.
53. De Waele JJ, Hoste E, Blot SI, et al: Intra-abdominal hypertension in

patients with severe acute pancreatitis. Crit Care 2005;9:R452-R457.
54. Sun ZX, Huang HR, Zhou H: Indwelling catheter and conservative measures in the treatment of abdominal compartment syndrome in fulminant acute pancreatitis. World J Gastroenterol 2006;12:5068-5070.
55. Leppaniemi AK, Hienonen PA, Siren JE, et al: Treatment of abdominal compartment syndrome with subcutaneous anterior abdominal fasciotomy in severe acute pancreatitis. World J Surg 2006;30:1922-1924.
56. Isenmann R, Rau B, Beger HG: Bacterial infection and extent of necrosis are determinants of organ failure in patients with acute necrotizing pancreatitis. Br J Surg 2007;86:1020-1024.
57. Schmid SW, Uhl W, Friess H, et al: The role of infection in acute pancreatitis. Gut 1999;45:311-316.
58. Shanmugam N, Isenmann R, Barkin JS, et al: Pancreatic fungal infection. Pancreas 2007;27:133-138.
59. Isenmann R, Schwarz M, Rau B, et al: Characteristics of infection with *Candida* species in patients with necrotizing pancreatitis. World J Surg 2002;26:372-376.
60. Ammori BJ: Role of the gut in the course of severe acute pancreatitis. Pancreas 2003;26:122-129.
61. Scwarz M, Thomsen J, Meyer H, et al: Frequency and time course of pancreatic and extrapancreatic bacterial infection in experimental acute pancreatitis in rats. Surgery 2000;127:427-432.
62. Kouris GJ, Liu Q, Rossi H, et al: The effect of glucagon-like peptide 2 on intestinal permeability and bacterial translocation in acute necrotizing pancreatitis. Am J Surg 2001;181:571-575.
63. McNaught CE, Woodcock NP, Mitchell CJ, et al: Gastric colonisation, intestinal permeability and septic morbidity in acute pancreatitis. Pancreatology 2002;2:463-468.
64. Luiten EJ, Hop WC, Endtz HP, et al: Prognostic importance of gram-negative intestinal colonization preceding pancreatic infection in severe acute pancreatitis. Results of a controlled clinical trial of selective decontamination. Intensive Care Med 1998;24:438-445.
65. Luiten EJ, Hop WCJ, Lange JF, et al: Controlled clinical trial of selective decontamination for the treatment of severe acute pancreatitis. Ann Surg 1995;222:57-65.
66. Hooper LV, Gordon JI: Commensal host-bacterial relationships in the gut. Science 2001;292:1115-1118.
67. Alverdy JC, Laughlin RS, Wu L: Influence of the critically ill state on host-pathogen interactions within the intestine: Gut-derived sepsis redefined. Crit Care Med 2003;31:598-607.
68. van Minnen LP, Nieuwnhuijs VB, de Bruijn MT, et al: Effects of subtotal colectomy on bacterial translocation during experimental acute pancreatitis. Pancreas 2006;32:110-114.
69. Marshall JC: Lipopolysaccharide: An endotoxin or an exogenous hormone? Clin Infect Dis 2005;41(Suppl 7): S470-S480.
70. Beger HG, Bittner R, Block S, et al: Bacterial contamination of pancreatic necrosis. A prospective clinical study. Gastroenterology 1986;91:433-438.
71. de Madaria E, Martinez J, Lozano B, et al: Detection and identification of bacterial DNA in serum from patients with acute pancreatitis. Gut 2005;54:1293-1297.
72. Buttenschoen K, Berger D, Hiki N, et al: Endotoxin and antiendotoxin antibodies in patients with acute pancreatitis. Eur J Surg 2000;166:459-466.
73. Villatoro E, Bbassi C, Larvin M: Antibiotic therapy for prophylaxis against infection of pancreatic necrosis in acute pancreatitis. Cochrane Database Syst Rev 2006;4:CD002941.
74. Targarona Modena J, Barreda Cevasco L, Arroyo Basto C, et al: Total enteral nutrition as prophylactic therapy for pancreatic necrosis infection in severe acute pancreatitis. Pancreatology 2006;6:58-64.
75. Sainio V, Kemppainen E, Puolakkainen P, et al: Early antibiotic treatment in acute necrotising pancreatitis. Lancet 1995;346:663-667.
76. Luiten EJ, Hop WC, Lange JF, et al: Differential prognosis of gram-negative versus gram-positive infected and sterile pancreatic necrosis: Results of a randomized trial in patients with severe acute pancreatitis treated with adjuvant selective decontamination. Clin Infect Dis 1997;25:811-816.
77. De Waele JJ, Vogelaers D, Blot S, et al: Fungal infections in patients with severe acute pancreatitis and the use of prophylactic therapy. Clin Infect Dis 2003;37:208-213.
78. Hoerauf A, Hammer S, Muller-Myhsok B, et al: Intra-abdominal *Candida* infection during acute necrotizing pancreatitis has a high prevalence and is associated with increased mortality. Crit Care Med 1998;26:2010-2015.
79. Kotani J, Usami M, Nomura H, et al: Enteral nutrition prevents bacterial translocation but does not improve survival during acute pancreatitis. Arch Surg 1999;134:287-292.
80. Qin HL, Su ZD, Hu LG, et al: Effect of early intrajejunal nutrition on pancreatic pathological features and gut barrier function in dogs with acute pancreatitis. Clin Nutr 2002;21:469-473.
81. Marik PE, Zaloga GP: Meta-analysis of parenteral nutrition versus enteral nutrition in patients with acute pancreatitis. BMJ 2004;328:1407.
82. Meier R, Ockenga J, Pertkiewicz M, et al: ESPEN guidelines on enteral nutrition: Pancreas. Clin Nutr 2006;25:275-284.
83. McClave SA, Chang WK, Dhaliwal R, et al: Nutrition support in acute pancreatitis: A systematic review of the literature. JPEN J Parenter Enteral Nutr 2006;30:143-156.
84. Eatock FC, Chong P, Menezes N, et al: A randomized study of early nasogastric versus nasojejunal feeding in severe acute pancreatitis. Am J Gastroenterol 2005;100:432-439.
85. Eckerwall GE, Axelsson JB, Andersson RG: Early nasogastric feeding in predicted severe acute pancreatitis: A clinical, randomized study. Ann Surg 2006;244:959-967.
86. Morimoto T, Noguchi Y, Sakai T, et al: Acute pancreatitis and the role of histamine-2 receptor antagonists: A meta-analysis of randomized controlled trials of cimetidine. Eur J Gastroenterol Hepatol 2002;14:679-686.
87. Anriulli A, Leandro G, Clemente R, et al: Meta-analysis of somatostatin, octreotide and gabexate mesilate in the therapy of acute pancreatitis. Aliment Pharmacol Ther 1998;12:237-245.
88. Seta T, Noguchi Y, Shimada T, et al: Treatment of acute pancreatitis with protease inhibitors: A meta-analysis. Eur J Gastroenterol Hepatol 2004;16:1287-1293.
89. Liu LR, Xia SH: Role of platelet-activating factor in the pathogenesis of acute pancreatitis. World J Gastroenterol 2006;12:539-545.
90. Formela LJ, Wood LM, Whittaker M, et al: Amelioration of experimental acute pancreatitis with a potent platelet-activating factor antagonist. Br J Surg 1994;81:1783-1785.
91. Hofbauer B, Saluja AK, Bhatia M, et al: Effect of recombinant platelet-activating factor acetylhydrolase on two models of experimental acute pancreatitis. Gastroenterology 1998;115:1238-1247.
92. Kingsnorth AN, Galloway SW, Formela LJ: Randomized, double-blind phase II trial of lexipafant, a platelet-activating factor antagonist, in human acute pancreatitis. Br J Surg 1995;82:1414-1420.
93. McKay CJ, Curran F, Sharples C, et al: Prospective placebo-controlled randomized trial of lexipafant in predicted severe acute pancreatitis. Br J Surg 1997;84:1239-1243.
94. Johnson CD, Kingsnorth AN, Imrie CW, et al: Double blind, randomised, placebo controlled study of a platelet activating factor antagonist, lexipafant, in the treatment and prevention of organ failure in predicted severe acute pancreatitis. Gut 2001;48:62-69.
95. Bernard GR, Vincent J-L, Laterre PF, et al: Efficacy and safety of recombinant human activated protein C for severe sepsis. N Engl J Med 2001;344: 699-709.
96. Yamanel L, Mas MR, Comert B, et al: The effect of activated protein C on experimental acute necrotizing pancreatitis. Crit Care 2005;9: R184-R190.
97. Jamdar S, Siriwardena AK: Drotrecogin alfa (recombinant human activated protein C) in severe acute pancreatitis. Crit Care 2005;9:321-322.
98. Granger J, Remick D: Acute pancreatitis: Models, markers, and mediators. Shock 2005;24(Suppl 1): 45-51.
99. Ayub K, Imada R, Slavin J: Endoscopic retrograde cholangiopancreatography in gallstone-associated acute pancreatitis. Cochrane Database Syst Rev 2004;4:CD003630.
100. Folsch UR, Nitsche R, Ludtke R, et al: Early ERCP and papillotomy compared with conservative treatment for acute biliary pancreatitis. N Engl J Med 1997;336:237-242.

101. Oria A, Cimmino D, Ocampo C, et al: Early endoscopic intervention versus early conservative management in patients with acute gallstone pancreatitis and biliopancreatic obstruction: A randomized clinical trial. Ann Surg 2007;245:10-17.
102. Gloor B, Muller CA, Worni M, et al: Late mortality in patients with severe acute pancreatitis. Br J Surg 2001;88:975-979.
103. Hirota M, Inoue K, Kimura Y, et al: Non-occlusive mesenteric ischemia and its associated intestinal gangrene in acute pancreatitis. Pancreatology 2003;3:316-322.
104. Dellinger RP, Carlet JM, Masur H, et al: Surviving sepsis campaign guidelines for management of severe sepsis and septic shock. Crit Care Med 2004;32:858-873.
105. Pitchumoni CS, Agarwal N: Pancreatic pseudocysts. When and how should drainage be performed? Gastroenterol Clin North Am 1999;28:615-639.
106. Ferrucci JT 3rd, Mueller PR: Interventional approach to pancreatic fluid collections. Radiol Clin North Am 2003;41:1217-1226.
107. Baron TH: Endoscopic drainage of pancreatic fluid collections and pancreatic necrosis. Gastrointest Endosc Clin N Am 2003;13:743-764.
108. Kellogg TA, Horvath KD: Minimal-access approaches to complications of acute pancreatitis and benign neoplasms of the pancreas. Surg Endosc 2003;17:1692-1704.
109. Beattie GC, Hardman JG, Redhead D, et al: Evidence for a central role for selective mesenteric angiography in the management of the major vascular complications of pancreatitis. Am J Surg 2003;185:96-102.
110. Aultman DF, Bilton DB, Zibari GB, et al: Nonoperative therapy for acute necrotizing pancreatitis. Am Surg 1997;63:1114-1117.
111. Ashley SW, Perez A, Pierce EA, et al: Necrotizing pancreatitis: Contemporary analysis of 99 consecutive cases. Ann Surg 2001;234:572-580.
112. Hartwig W, Maksan SM, Foitzik T, et al: Reduction in mortality with delayed surgical therapy of severe pancreatitis. J Gastrointest Surg 2002;6:481-487.
113. Gotzinger P, Wamser P, Exner R, et al: Surgical treatment of severe acute pancreatitis: Timing of operation is crucial for survival. Surg Infect 2003;4:205-211.
114. Hungness ES, Robb BW, Seeskin C, et al: Early debridement for necrotizing pancreatitis: Is it worthwhile? J Am Coll Surg 2002;194:740-744.
115. Mier J, Leon EL, Castillo A, et al: Early versus late necrosectomy in severe necrotizing pancreatitis. Am J Surg 1997;173:71-75.
116. Bradley EL 3rd, Allen K: A prospective longitudinal study of observation versus surgical intervention in the management of necrotizing pancreatitis. Am J Surg 1991;161:19-25.
117. Rau B, Pralle U, Uhl W, et al: Management of sterile necrosis in instances of severe acute pancreatitis. J Am Coll Surg 1995;181:279-288.
118. Buchler MW, Gloor B, Muller CA, et al: Acute necrotizing pancreatitis: Treatment strategy according to the status of infection. Ann Surg 2000;232:619-626.
119. Olah A, Belagyi T, Issekutz A, et al: Value of procalcitonin quick test in the differentiation between sterile and infected forms of acute pancreatitis. Hepatogastroenterology 2005;52:243-245.
120. Riche FC, Cholley BP, Laisne MJ, et al: Inflammatory cytokines, C reactive protein, and procalcitonin as early predictors of necrosis infection in acute necrotizing pancreatitis. Surgery 2003;133:257-262.
121. Rau B, Pralle U, Mayer JM, et al: Role of ultrasonographically guided fine-needle aspiration cytology in the diagnosis of infected pancreatic necrosis. Br J Surg 1998;85:179-184.
122. Freeny PC, Hauptmann E, Althaus SJ, et al: Percutaneous CT-guided catheter drainage of infected acute necrotizing pancreatitis: Techniques and results. AJR Am J Roentgenol 1998;170: 969-975.
123. Zorger N, Hamer OW, Feuerbach S, et al: Percutaneous treatment of a patient with infected necrotizing pancreatitis. Nat Clin Pract Gastroenterol Hepatol 2005;2:54-57.
124. Olah A, Belagyi T, Bartek P, et al: Alternative treatment modalities of infected pancreatic necrosis. Hepatogastroenterology 2007;53:603-607.
125. Runzi M, Niebel W, Goebell H, et al: Severe acute pancreatitis: Nonsurgical treatment of infected necroses. Pancreas 2005;30:195-199.
126. Adamson GD, Cuschieri A: Multimedia article. Laparoscopic infracolic necrosectomy for infected pancreatic necrosis. Surg Endosc 2003;17:1675.
127. Ammori BJ: Laparoscopic transgastric pancreatic necrosectomy for infected pancreatic necrosis. Surg Endosc 2002;16:1632.
128. Horvath KD, Kao LS, Wherry KL, et al: A technique for laparoscopic-assisted percutaneous drainage of infected pancreatic necrosis and pancreatic abscess. Surg Endosc 2001;15: 1221-1225.
129. Bradley EL: A fifteen-year experience with open drainage for infected pancreatic necrosis. Surg Gynecol Obstet 1993;177:215-222.
130. Fernandez-del Castillo C, Rattner DW, Makary MA, et al: Debridement and closed packing for the treatment of necrotizing pancreatitis. Ann Surg 1998;228:676-684.
131. Parekh D: Laparoscopic-assisted pancreatic necrosectomy: A new surgical option for treatment of severe necrotizing pancreatitis. Arch Surg 2006;141:895-902.
132. Zhou ZG, Zheng YC, Shu Y, et al: Laparoscopic management of severe acute pancreatitis. Pancreas 2003;27: e46-e50.
133. Connor S, Raraty MG, Howes N, et al: Surgery in the treatment of acute pancreatitis—minimal access pancreatic necrosectomy. Scand J Surg 2005;94:135-142.
134. Besselink MG, van Santvoort HC, Nieuwenhuijs VB, et al: Minimally invasive "step-up approach" versus maximal necrosectomy in patients with acute necrotising pancreatitis (PANTER trial): Design and rationale of a randomised controlled multicenter trial [ISRCTN38327949]. BMC Surg 2006;6:6.
135. Besselink MG, de Bruijn MT, Rutten JP, et al: Surgical intervention in patients with necrotizing pancreatitis. Br J Surg 2006;93:593-599.
136. Ranson JHC, Berman RS: Long peritoneal lavage decreases pancreatic sepsis in acute pancreatitis. Ann Surg 1990;211:708-718.
137. Balachandra S, Siriwardena AK: Systematic appraisal of the management of the major vascular complications of pancreatitis. Am J Surg 2005;190:489-495.
138. Mortele KJ, Mergo PJ, Taylor HM, et al: Peripancreatic vascular abnormalities complicating acute pancreatitis: Contrast-enhanced helical CT findings. Eur J Radiol 2004;52:67-72.
139. Iannitti DA, Gregg SC, Mayo-Smith WW, et al: Portal venous gas detected by computed tomography: Is surgery imperative? Dig Surg 2003;20: 306-315.
140. Testart J, Boyet L, Pperrier G, et al: Arterial erosions in acute pancreatitis. Acta Chir Belg 2001;101:232-239.
141. Bosscha K, Reijnders K, Jacobs MH, et al: Quality of life after severe bacterial peritonitis and infected necrotizing pancreatitis treated with open management of the abdomen and planned re-operations. Crit Care Med 2001;29:1539-1543.
142. Halonen KI, Pettila V, Leppaniemi AK, et al: Long-term health-related quality of life in survivors of severe acute pancreatitis. Intensive Care Med 2003;29:782-786.
143. Soran A, Chelluri L, Lee KK, et al: Outcome and quality of life of patients with acute pancreatitis requiring intensive care. J Surg Res 2000;91:89-94.
144. Cinquepalmi L, Boni L, Dionigi G, et al: Long-term results and quality of life of patients undergoing sequential surgical treatment for severe acute pancreatitis complicated by infected pancreatic necrosis. Surg Infect 2006;7(Suppl 2):S113-S116.
145. Symersky T, van Hoorn B, Masclee AA: The outcome of a long-term follow-up of pancreatic function after recovery from acute pancreatitis. JOP 2006;7:447-453.
146. Connor S, Alexakis N, Raraty MG, et al: Early and late complications after pancreatic necrosectomy. Surgery 2005;137:499-505.

Chapter 79

Hemorrhagic and Thrombotic Disorders

Neil A. Lachant

Disorders of blood coagulation commonly occur in critically ill patients and become problematic in a variety of ways. Hemorrhage or thrombosis may be the dominant concern or may seriously complicate the management of other pathologic processes. Many of these disorders are complex and may quickly become life-threatening. Management of hemorrhage or thrombosis in critically ill patients requires weighing the answers to two questions: How threatening is the problem? and How dangerous is the treatment? The information in this chapter is intended to offer some guidance in this task.

APPROACH TO A CRITICALLY ILL PATIENT WITH HEMORRHAGE OR THROMBOSIS

The history taker must be a detective interviewing the patient, family members, and outside health care providers. Depending on the situation, useful information may include a personal or family history of a known bleeding disorder; bleeding after previous trauma, surgery, or dental procedures; a personal history of recent bleeding, bruising, or menorrhagia; and a history of liver or kidney disease, malabsorption, or recent chemotherapy. Perhaps the most challenging is obtaining a medication history, particularly as it may relate to covert heparin exposure. The use of anticoagulants, antiplatelet agents, aspirin, and nonsteroidal anti-inflammatory drugs (NSAIDs) should be determined. Recently started or intermittently used medications (e.g., quinine) that may cause thrombocytopenia should be elicited. In a hypercoaguable patient, a personal or family history of a known thrombophilic defect, thrombosis, recurrent miscarriage, or stillbirth may be useful.

The physical examination can be used to assess active problems, although physical signs of hemorrhage or thrombosis can be subtle. Petechiae or purpura may develop only in dependent areas in a bedridden patient. Likewise, the edema associated with thrombosis may be missed in a leg that has remained horizontal, and tenderness may go undetected if the patient's mental status is altered. The digits and skin should be carefully examined for signs of ischemia or necrosis.

LABORATORY TESTS OF COAGULATION

The integrity of the coagulant mechanisms is routinely tested by a limited set of in vitro assays based on the clotting time of plasma (Fig. 79-1). Screening coagulation tests may shed light on the cause of active bleeding or warn of potential hemorrhagic problems, but no screening laboratory test will predict thrombosis. The prothrombin time (PT) reflects the cascade of reactions traditionally called the "extrinsic" pathway, whereas the activated partial thromboplastin time (APTT) reflects the "intrinsic" pathway.

Once a coagulopathy has been identified, the next step is to determine whether it is due to a factor deficiency or a circulating inhibitor. In the inhibitor or mixing study, the patient's plasma is mixed with an equal volume of normal pooled plasma. Normalization of the PT or APTT in such a "mixing study" reflects a deficiency of one or more coagulation factors. It also implies that administration of plasma to the patient should correct the coagulopathy. A more specific diagnosis requires special factor assays. If there is partial or no correction in the mixing study, an inhibitor is suspected—most often contaminating heparin or a lupus anticoagulant.

The thrombin time (TT) measures the rate of conversion of fibrinogen to insoluble fibrin polymer after thrombin is added to plasma. A prolonged TT may be due to an inhibitor of thrombin (e.g., heparin, direct thrombin inhib-

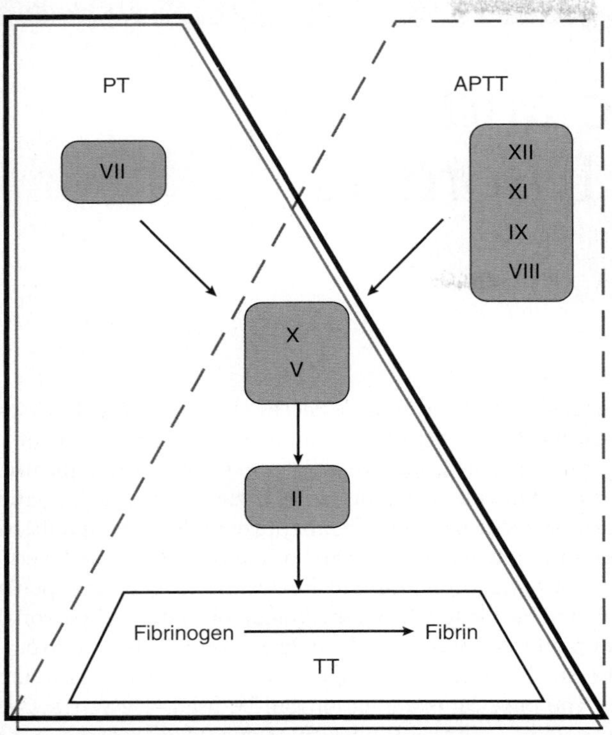

Figure 79-1. Coagulation factors evaluated in routine coagulation assays. APTT, activated partial thromboplastin time; PT, prothrombin time; TT, thrombin time.

Box 79-1

Common Causes of Thrombocytopenia in Critically Ill Patients

Decreased Production
Drugs (e.g., thiazides, linezolid)
Ethanol
Liver disease
Right heart failure

Increased Destruction/Consumption
Bacteremia
Sepsis
Drugs
Disseminated intravascular coagulation
Massive bleeding/transfusions
Pulmonary artery catheter
Intra-aortic balloon pump
Ventricular assist device
Idiopathic thrombocytopenic purpura
Burns
Post-transfusion purpura
Thrombotic thrombocytopenic purpura
Antiphospholipid syndrome

Splenic Sequestration
Portal hypertension

itor [DTI]), hypofibrinogenemia or dysfibrinogenemia, fibrin degradation products (FDPs), and rarely paraproteins.

The only specific coagulation factor that is routinely measured is fibrinogen.

The template bleeding time (BT) has been used to assess in vivo platelet function in patients with normal platelet counts. It may be a useful test to screen for disorders of platelet function. However, the concept of using the BT to predict surgical bleeding is archaic.

DISORDERS OF PLATELETS

Thrombocytopenia

Mechanisms and General Management

Thrombocytopenia is common in the intensive care unit (ICU). It has been estimated that 23% to 41% of patients in the ICU have a platelet count less than 100,000/μL and 10% to 17% have one less than 5,000/μL.[1] Thrombocytopenia may be due to decreased production, shortened survival in the circulation, splenic sequestration, consumption from bleeding, or hemodilution. Common causes of thrombocytopenia in the ICU are shown in Box 79-1. Bacteremia and sepsis, either clinically evident or occult, are the most common causes of thrombocytopenia in the ICU.[2] In complex, acutely ill patients, many of these mechanisms may operate simultaneously.

Frequently, thrombocytopenia must be managed without a specifically defined etiology. As a general approach, the patient's medications should be reviewed for potentially causative agents that can be discontinued.[3] Inhibitors of platelet function should be avoided. If there is evidence of bleeding or if invasive procedures are anticipated, platelet transfusions should be given, unless contraindicated, to elevate the platelet count above 50,000/μL. In life-threatening situations, the goal should be a platelet count higher than 100,000/μL. In nonbleeding patients, maintenance of a platelet count above 10,000/μL (20,000/μL with fever or infection) with prophylactic transfusions is usually adequate.[4]

Pseudothrombocytopenia

Pseudothrombocytopenia is a laboratory artifact.[5] The platelet count is factitiously lowered because of the presence of naturally occurring antibodies that cause platelet agglutination in the presence of ethylenediaminetetraacetic acid (EDTA) at room temperature. The diagnosis is suspected by finding platelet clumps on the peripheral blood smear. Repeating the platelet count with a different anticoagulant such as citrate will generally produce a normal platelet count.

Drug-Induced Thrombocytopenia

Although a large number of drugs have been associated with thrombocytopenia, a limited number have evidence-based data to support a causal role in the development of thrombocytopenia.[3,6,7] Medications commonly used in the ICU that can cause thrombocytopenia are shown in Box

Box 79-2

Drugs Commonly Causing Thrombocytopenia in the Intensive Care Unit

Abciximab	Linezolid
Amiodarone	Procainamide
Amphotericin B	Quinidine
Cimetidine	Quinine
Clopidogrel	Ranitidine
Digoxin	Tirofiban
Eptifibatide	Trimethoprim-sulfamethoxazole
Heparin	
Hydrochlorothiazide	Vancomycin

79-2. Drug-induced thrombocytopenia most commonly occurs 7 to 21 days after exposure to the offending agent. Clinical manifestations can range from an asymptomatic decrease in platelets to life-threatening bleeding. The diagnosis is established by finding (1) a temporal relationship between starting the drug and the fall in the platelet count, (2) having no alternative diagnosis, and (3) having the platelet count recover after removal of the putative offending agent. Unfortunately, this is usually difficult to establish in the typical ICU patient. Treatment is based on removing the offending agent and initiating a drug of another class if possible. Though often used, steroids in general have not been shown to hasten the rate of platelet recovery. In severe thrombocytopenia with bleeding such as seen with quinine-induced thrombocytopenia, intravenous immunoglobulin (IVIG) (1 g/kg/d for 2 days) and platelet transfusion are beneficial.

Glycoprotein IIb/IIIa Inhibitors

All platelet glycoprotein (GP) IIb/IIIa inhibitors have been associated with severe thrombocytopenia that can occur within hours of exposure, although the thrombocytopenia from abciximab may develop up to 2 weeks after exposure.[6] These patients are usually concomitantly exposed to heparin, thus making heparin-induced thrombocytopenia (HIT) the main differential diagnosis. Bleeding is very uncommon with HIT because of the strong prothrombotic state. Conversely, with GP IIb/IIIa inhibitor–associated thrombocytopenia, bleeding or hematoma formation may occur, especially at the site of the sheath. A platelet count less than 20,000/µL and clinical bleeding are indications for platelet transfusion. The use of IVIG and corticosteroids is not evidence based.

Idiopathic Thrombocytopenic Purpura

Idiopathic thrombocytopenic purpura (ITP) is an immune-mediated thrombocytopenia that results from autoimmune destruction of IgG-coated platelets in the reticuloendothelial system, primarily the spleen.[8] Thrombopoiesis is not generally increased significantly. ITP is an isolated thrombocytopenia. Anemia, if present, may be autoimmune (Evans syndrome) or due to bleeding and iron deficiency. The differential diagnosis of isolated thrombocytopenia includes pseudothrombocytopenia, immune thrombocytopenia secondary to systemic lupus, human immunodeficiency virus (HIV) infection, hepatitis C, and drug-induced thrombocytopenia.[8,9]

Guidelines for the diagnosis and management of ITP have been developed.[10,11] Patients with ITP characteristically do not need therapy until the platelet count is lower than 20,000 to 30,000/µL unless bleeding is present. Corticosteroid therapy (prednisone, 1 mg/kg/d, or pulse dexamethasone, 40 mg/d for 4 days monthly) is the usual initial therapy for a general medical patient with ITP.[12] Individuals with ITP in the ICU usually have severe or life-threatening bleeding. Several modalities should be used in concert to raise the platelet count in urgent situations (methylprednisolone [Solu-Medrol], 1 g/d for 3 days, and IVIG, 1 g/kg/d for 2 days). Although platelets may be destroyed quickly, platelet transfusions should still be used as initial therapy. The response to platelet transfusion may improve after IVIG is given. Anti-Rh_0(D) IgG (WinRho), 50 to 75 µg/kg, has also been used.[13] Because the dose of WinRho must be reduced in face of anemia, its use may be problematic in a patient with severe bleeding. Anti-Rh_0(D) IgG is ineffective in Rh-negative patients and after splenectomy. ε-Aminocaproic acid may be useful for mucosal bleeding and severe menorrhagia.

Post-transfusion Purpura

Post-transfusion purpura is a rare condition characterized by acute, severe immune-mediated thrombocytopenia. It occurs in human platelet antigen-1–negative individuals who receive human platelet antigen-1 (HPA-1) positive platelets (most commonly as a contaminant in packed red blood cells [RBCs]). These individuals have previously been sensitized to the HPA-1 antigen through prior transfusion or pregnancy. Usually 7 to 10 days after re-exposure to HPA-1, an anamnestic response occurs and results in a severe, precipitous decline in the platelet count. Petechiae and bleeding are common. IVIG and plasma exchange are effective.[14]

Washout Thrombocytopenia

Thrombocytopenia may occur after 1 blood volume has been replaced in less than 24 hours (usually <2 hours) or with fluid resuscitation of a bleeding patient in the absence of transfusion. Platelets should not be given empirically based on the number of units of fresh frozen plasma (FFP) and RBCs given to a patient with massive bleeding. Rather, the clinician should be vigilant for the development of thrombocytopenia and transfuse platelets when thrombocytopenia develops.

Acquired Platelet Dysfunction

Medication-Induced Abnormalities

A variety of medications used in intensive care have effects on platelet function. Aspirin irreversibly acetylates cyclooxygenase (COX), which inhibits platelet function for the life of the platelet (7 to 10 days). The effect of aspirin can be overcome with platelet transfusion or the infusion of DDAVP (desmopressin). Platelet inhibition by

NSAIDs has most clearly been associated with increased bleeding. The effect of NSAIDs, such as ibuprofen, is reversible and disappears as the drug is cleared, generally within 24 to 48 hours. The risk of bleeding from NSAIDs is lowest with ibuprofen and greatest with ketorolac. The thienopyridine clopidogrel tightly binds the platelet adenosine diphosphate receptor. Clopidogrel should be withheld for 5 days before elective surgery or invasive procedures.[15] In the emergency setting, platelet transfusion can be used, but platelet function may not be fully restored because of circulating clopidogrel metabolites, which have a half-life of 8 hours and bind to the transfused platelets. COX-2 inhibitors do not affect platelet function.

Renal Failure

The hemorrhagic diathesis of renal failure arises from an acquired platelet defect, partly as a result of a variety of metabolic derangements related to uremic toxins.[16,17] Bleeding may worsen when the hematocrit falls below 30%.[18] This is related to a rheologic phenomenon in which rapidly flowing RBCs normally gravitate to the center of the streaming blood and force the platelets toward the vessel wall.

Uremic bleeding is uncommon in the modern era of dialysis.[18] An unexpected "coagulopathy" (isolated prolonged APTT) may develop as a result of delayed clearance of heparin after dialysis. The TT is prolonged in face of normal fibrinogen. If available, an anti-Xa assay will show the presence of heparin. The APTT returns to normal as the heparin is cleared. For clinical bleeding, intravenous DDAVP (0.3 μg/kg given over a 30-minute period) is often therapeutic.[17,19] In this circumstance, when the hematocrit is less than 30%, the patient should be transfused with packed RBCs.[17,18] Erythropoietin can accomplish the same goal but takes longer.[20] An alternative to desmopressin is cryoprecipitate (10 bags every 12 to 24 hours).[17,21] Intravenous conjugated estrogen, 0.6 mg/kg/day for 5 days, is also effective, and oral estrogen therapy may be beneficial as well.[17]

COMPLEX THROMBOHEMORRHAGIC DISORDERS

Heparin-Induced Thrombocytopenia

HIT is a paradoxical condition in which modest thrombocytopenia may be associated with devastating thromboses. Thus, the physician needs to be vigilant for the development of HIT in any patient receiving heparin. HIT has been associated with all types of heparin (unfractionated [UFH] and low-molecular-weight [LMWH] heparin), at any dose, and by any route, including flushes and heparin-coated pulmonary artery catheters.[1,22] The incidence of HIT has been estimated to be 0.8% in general medical patients receiving LMWH and less than 1% of patients in the ICU.[23,24] HIT occurs in three time intervals. Classic HIT takes place 5 to 15 days after the initiation of heparin. Rapid-onset HIT develops hours to 1 to 2 days after heparin is started and occurs in individuals who have preformed circulating antibodies from a previous exposure to heparin, usually in the last 2 months. Classic and rapid-onset HIT may be manifested as thrombocytopenia with or without thrombosis. Delayed-onset HIT occurs an average of 12 days after the discontinuation of heparin and is manifested as isolated thrombosis. The thrombocytopenia of HIT is usually modest with an average platelet count of 50,000 to 60,000/μL.[25] Severe thrombocytopenia (<10,000/μL) should suggest an alternative diagnosis. HIT may be associated with a normal platelet count if there is a baseline thrombocytosis (e.g., postoperatively). HIT may be manifested as isolated thrombocytopenia or thrombocytopenia with potentially devastating thromboses (HITT). Venous complications include deep venous thrombosis (DVT), pulmonary embolism, cerebral sinus thrombosis, adrenal hemorrhage, and skin necrosis at the heparin injection site. Arterial complications include iliofemoral artery thrombosis, digital ischemia, myocardial infarction, stroke, and mesenteric artery thrombosis.

HIT is an immune-mediated process in which the heparin–platelet factor 4 complex becomes immunogenic. Antibodies are formed that activate platelets via the FcγIIa receptor and cause the release of thrombogenic microparticles. These antibodies can also activate monocytes and endothelial cells.[26]

The diagnosis of HIT is clinicopathologic. HIT should be thought of in appropriate clinical situations (Box 79-3). The "4 T" score has been used to predict the likelihood (pretest probability) of HIT (Table 79-1).[27] The decision to initiate therapy for HIT should be based on the clinical likelihood of the diagnosis. Laboratory testing should be undertaken for retrospective corroboration of the pretest likelihood of HIT. The complexities of HIT antibody testing are reviewed elsewhere.[28] As a general rule of thumb, a strongly positive enzyme-linked immunosorbent assay (ELISA) and strongly positive serotonin release assay (SRA) in the presence of a high pretest probability confirm the diagnosis of HIT, whereas a negative ELISA and a negative SRA make the diagnosis of HIT unlikely

Box 79-3

Clinical Situations to Suspect Heparin-Induced Thrombocytopenia

Current use of heparin or heparin exposure within 40 days and at least one of the following:
- Platelets <100,000/μL
- Platelets <50% of baseline or <50% of the maximum level if reactive thrombocytosis is present
- Platelets less than baseline 5 days after open heart surgery
- New arterial or venous thrombotic event
- Inflammation or necrosis at heparin injection sites
- Acute allergic or anaphylactic reaction to a heparin bolus

Recent admission to a hospital, nursing, or rehabilitation facility plus
- A new venous thromboembolic event
- A new arterial ischemic event

Table 79-1. Determining the Pretest Probability of Heparin-Induced Thrombocytopenia: The 4 T's

Points	Thrombocytopenia	Timing of Onset of Thrombocytopenia (or Other Serious Sequelae of HIT)*	Thrombosis or Other Sequelae	OTher Causes of Thrombocytopenia
2	>50% decrease and nadir >20,000/μL	Day 5-10 or ≤1 day with recent heparin (past 30 days)	Proven new thrombosis, skin necrosis, or acute systemic reaction to heparin bolus	None evident
1	30%-50% decrease or nadir of 10,000-19,000/μL	>Day 10 or timing unclear or <1 day with recent heparin (past 31-100 days)	Progressive or recurrent thrombosis, erythematous skin lesions, suspected thrombosis (not proven)	Possible
0	<30% decrease or nadir of <10,000/μL	<Day 4 (no recent heparin)	None	Definite

Pretest probability score: 0 to 3 points=low (<5%), 3 to 5 points=intermediate (physician judgment), 6 to 8 points=high (>80%).
*First day of heparin exposure=day 0.
Adapted from Lo GK, Juhl D, Warkentin TE, et al: Evaluation of pretest clinical score (4 T's) for the diagnosis of heparin-induced thrombocytopenia in two clinical settings. J Thromb Haemost 2006:4:759.

Table 79-2. Anticoagulants Doses

	Dosage			
		Therapeutic		
Anticoagulant	Prophylactic	Initial	Maintenance	Therapeutic Level
Unfractionated heparin	5000 U SC q8h	80 U/kg by IV bolus	18 U/kg/h by continuous IV infusion	APTT range corresponding to 0.3-0.7 U/mL
Enoxaparin	40 mg SC qd	1 mg/kg SC q12h	Continue at initial dose	0.5-1.0 U/mL obtained 3.5-4.0 h after the dose
Fondaparinux	2.5 mg SC qd	<50 kg: 5 mg SC qd 50-100 kg: 7.5 mg SC qd >100 kg: 10 mg SC qd	Continue at initial dose	None
Argatroban	None	No bolus	2 μg/kg/min CI 0.5 μg/kg/min CI (liver disease)	APTT 1.5-3.0 × patient's baseline
ICU*	None	No bolus	1 μg/kg/min CI 0.5 μg/kg/min CI (liver disease)	None
Lepirudin (Ccr ≥ 60 mL/min)	25 mg SC q12h	0.4 mg/kg	0.15 mg/kg/hr CI	APTT 1.5-2.5× midnormal APTT
ICU*				
No life-threatening thrombosis	25 mg SC q12h	No bolus	0.5-1.0 mg/kg/hr CI	None
Life-threatening thrombosis	None	0.2 mg/kg	0.5-1.0 mg/kg/hr CI	None

APTT, activated partial thromboplastin time; CI, continuous infusion; qd, each day; SC, subcutaneously.
*Suggested dose modification in ICU patients. Selleng K, Warkentin TE, Greinacher A. Heparin-induced thrombocytopenia in intensive care patients. Crit Care Med 2007;35:1165-1176

with a low pretest probability. In other situations, clinical judgment prevails in establishing or excluding a diagnosis of HIT, especially because ELISA and SRA testing from commercial labs has not been validated in clinical studies.[1,28,29]

Once the diagnosis of HIT is thought to be likely, all heparin should be discontinued. Heparin-coated pulmonary artery catheters should be replaced with noncoated catheters. Catheters for dialysis or apheresis should be locked with 4% citrate or tissue plasminogen activator. The patient's chart and bedside should be labeled *heparin allergy*. Platelet transfusions should be avoided except in the event of life-threatening bleeding, given the anecdotal observations of acute thrombosis occurring after platelet transfusion. A patient with life- or limb-threatening arterial thrombosis should be evaluated for surgical intervention. Otherwise, anticoagulation with a DTI (i.e., argatroban, lepirudin) should be initiated (Table 79-2) in all patients unless contraindicated. Once the diagnosis of HIT is entertained in a patient treated with UFH, LMWH is also contraindicated. Conversion to warfarin can be considered after a minimum of 5 days of DTI therapy if the platelet count has returned to normal (suggesting that the process has cooled off and the patient is no longer hyperprothrombotic) and no future invasive procedures are planned. Simply discontinuing heparin therapy and not starting a DTI is inappropriate because occult thrombosis may have already developed.[30] Starting or continuing warfarin monotherapy is also contraindicated because of the risk of venous limb gangrene as a result of lowering the natural anticoagulants proteins C and S.[31] If invasive procedures are needed (e.g., tracheostomy, pacemaker), it is best to delay them, if medically safe, until the platelet count is normal to minimize the risk for the development of thrombosis during the time that DTI therapy has to be withheld. Vena cava filters should be avoided because of the risk for vena cava thrombosis. Patients with active HIT may need invasive procedures such as percutaneous coronary intervention (PCI). Argatroban has been approved by the Food and Drug Administration (FDA) for use during PCI in patients with HIT.[32] Though not FDA approved, bivalirudin has been used safely in this situation.[33] In a patient who has active HIT or persistent HIT antibodies and who needs open heart surgery, medical management is recommended until antibody testing becomes negative. If urgent surgery is needed, bivalirudin is most commonly used.[34] Use of lepirudin is limited by the lack of access to the Ecarin clotting time assay needed to monitor the degree of anticoagulation. Another scenario is a patient with a past history of HIT who needs open heart surgery. As long as the patient is currently heparin antibody negative, heparin can be used during bypass and a DTI started as soon as it is surgically safe postoperatively.[35]

Thrombotic Thrombocytopenic Purpura

Thrombotic thrombocytopenic purpura (TTP) is a relatively rare disorder whose hallmark is thrombocytopenia and microangiopathic hemolytic anemia (MAHA). The classic pentad of TTP (thrombocytopenia, MAHA, neurologic signs, renal dysfunction, and fever) occurred in only 52% of patients. The diagnosis of TTP should be considered in any patient with unexplained thrombocytopenia and MAHA, even if other features of the classic pentad are absent.[36] TTP is the clinical manifestation of a heterogeneous group of underlying disorders driven by different pathophysiologic processes. Although most cases of TTP are idiopathic, TTP may be associated with exposure to certain drugs (e.g., ticlopidine, clopidogrel, quinine, mitomycin C, gemcitabine, cyclosporine), pregnancy, HIV infection and bone marrow transplantation.[37,38] The morphologic hallmark of TTP is hyaline thrombi in precapillary arterioles composed primarily of platelets.[39] Classic TTP is due to an immune-mediated deficiency of a metalloproteinase, ADAMTS13, that cleaves ultralarge multimers of von Willebrand factor (vWF) into smaller multimers that are less platelet reactive.[39] Deficiency of this enzyme allows ultralarge forms of vWF that are normally sequestered in the endothelium to bind platelets and form microthrombi in the circulation. Conversely, the TTP associated with bone marrow transplantation, as well as another clinically related thrombotic microangiopathy, hemolytic-uremic syndrome, has normal ADAMTS13 activity.[39] Organ dysfunction is due to microvascular thrombosis. Commonly involved organs are the brain, kidneys, heart, and pancreas. It is critical to establish the diagnosis quickly because TTP can be rapidly fatal if not properly treated. Patients may have what appears to be pancreatitis yet suddenly die of heart block. Because of the proclivity of TTP to rapidly progress, all patients should initially be treated in the ICU.

The core laboratory features of TTP are those of MAHA (more than two schistocytes per oil immersion field on a peripheral smear, increased reticulocytes, increased lactate dehydrogenase). The diagnosis of TTP can easily be established in a patient with MAHA, thrombocytopenia, and neurologic dysfunction (the classic triad). It should also tentatively be made in the presence of MAHA and thrombocytopenia with other no obvious cause. Although ADAMTS13 testing is commercially available, establishing the diagnosis of TTP should not be delayed while waiting for these results. The differential diagnosis includes disseminated intravascular coagulation (DIC), severe vasculitis, eclampsia, HELLP syndrome (hemolysis, elevated liver enzymes, and low platelet count), malignant hypertension, and sepsis.[40]

Once the diagnosis of TTP is thought to be likely, therapy should be initiated quickly because of the proclivity of the disease to progress rapidly. Platelet transfusions should be avoided except in face of life-threatening bleeding because of anecdotal reports of patients acutely decompensating after platelet transfusions. Unless a patient has excellent peripheral veins, a large-bore catheter will need to be placed, even in those with severe thrombocytopenia. The mainstay and only evidence-based component of therapy for TTP is daily plasma exchange.[41] Most commonly, 1.5 plasma volumes are exchanged daily with FFP. A clue that TTP is the correct diagnosis is the color of the plasma removed from the first plasmapheresis. A red or brown color suggests free hemoglobin from intravascular hemolysis. If plasma exchange cannot be initiated in a timely manner, infusion of 30 mL/kg of FFP daily can be a temporizing maneuver.[41] Corticosteroids (e.g., prednisone, 1 mg/kg/d) are commonly used as well. The use of antiplatelet agents, which may increase the risk of bleeding, and vincristine is controversial.[42] Because of the tendency of patients to rapidly deteriorate, my non–evidence-based, personal approach has been to use dipyridamole, 250 mg/m^2/d orally divided into four daily doses, and vincristine, 2 mg, in patients with significant neurologic dysfunction. In patients who do not respond to initial therapy, rituximab is an attractive second-line therapy.[43]

Disseminated Intravascular Coagulation

DIC is always a manifestation of an underlying severe pathologic process. Although the potential initiating disease processes are myriad (Box 79-4), they all lead to the production of thrombin, which stimulates platelet activation and converts fibrinogen to fibrin, thereby leading

Box 79-4

Common Causes of Disseminated Intravascular Coagulation

Acute

- Infection
  - Bacteria
  - Fungus
  - Virus
- Complications of pregnancy
  - Abruptio placentae
  - Amniotic fluid embolus

Chronic

- Neoplasia
  - Adenocarcinoma
  - Acute promyelocytic leukemia
- Liver disease
- Retained dead fetus

Localized

- Aortic aneurysm
- Cavernous hemangioma

to the formation of microthrombi; if severe enough, the microthrombi can lead to organ dysfunction.[44-47] In the process, natural anticoagulant proteins are consumed and fibrinolytic mechanisms are activated. Circulating FDPs, along with the consumption of platelets and coagulation factors, lead to a bleeding diathesis. The balance between these competing processes results in the clinical manifestations in any particular individual. The hallmarks of acute DIC are microvascular thrombosis and acute hemorrhage, whereas those of chronic DIC secondary to cancer are larger vessel thrombosis.

The clinical manifestations of DIC are protean. Microvascular thrombosis produces an ischemia that affects many tissues, including the brain (delirium, coma), skin (digital gangrene, purpura fulminans), kidney, lungs (adult respiratory distress syndrome), gastrointestinal tract (mucosal ulceration), and blood (MAHA). The bleeding associated with DIC is global and due to the combination of depletion of coagulation factors, thrombocytopenia, inhibitory effects of FDPs on coagulation and platelet function, and tissue necrosis with ulceration. Common manifestations are intracerebral bleeding, oozing at lines and venipuncture sites, hematuria, epistaxis, gingival bleeding, and gastrointestinal bleeding.

There are no strict, evidence-based laboratory criteria for the diagnosis of DIC.[48] The diagnosis is based on the combination of identifying an underlying predisposition, clinical features, and laboratory testing. The most common laboratory features of DIC are thrombocytopenia, elevated FDP or D-dimer levels, and decreased fibrinogen. (The PT and APTT may or may not be prolonged, depending on the degree of baseline elevation of coagulation factors as acute-phase reactants, the rate of consumption of coagulation factors, and the amount of FDPs released.

Table 79-3. Original IST Scoring System for Overt DIC and the Modified ISTH Scoring System for Overt DIC in Severe Sepsis

Test	Score
Platelet count (per μL)	
≥100,000	0
50,000-99,999	1
<50,000	2
D-dimer (μg/mL)	
≤0.39 (upper limit of normal)	0
0.40-4.0	2
>4.0	3
Prothrombin time prolongation (s)	
≤3	0
>3 but <6	1
≥6	2
Fibrinogen (mg/dL)	
>100	0
<100	1

Original International Society of Thrombosis and Haemostasis (ISTH) score: (platelets+D-dimer+PT+fibrinogen) ≥5=overt DIC.
Modified ISTH score: (platelets+D-dimer+PT) ≥5=overt DIC in severe sepsis.
Adapted from Taylor FB, Toh C-H, Hoots WK, et al: Towards definition, clinical and laboratory criteria, and a scoring system for disseminated intravascular coagulation. Thromb Haemost 2001;86:1327; and Dhainaut J-F, Yan SB, Joyce DE, et al: Treatment effects of drotrecogin alfa (activated) in patients with severe sepsis with or without overt disseminated intravascular coagulation. J Thromb Haemost 2003;2:1924.

An absolute decrease in fibrinogen is very suggestive of DIC. However, fibrinogen activity in the normal range may still be consistent with DIC because fibrinogen is an acute-phase reactant and its level may be inappropriately low for the underlying physiologic state.[49] Serial measurement of fibrinogen to look for a decrease is often useful. Schistocytes are seen in half the cases. The natural anticoagulants antithrombin III (AT-III), protein C, and protein S are decreased, and thrombin-antithrombin complexes are increased, but their levels cannot usually be measured in real time.

Though not prospectively validated, the International Society of Thrombosis and Haemostasis (ISTH) has developed a scoring system for the identification of overt DIC by using four commonly available tests (platelets, fibrinogen, FDPs or soluble fibrin monomer, and fibrinogen) to address these issues.[46] This scoring system was modified (fibrinogen was excluded because data were not available and quantification of D-dimer replaced qualitative elevations in FDPs or soluble fibrin monomer) and retrospectively applied to prospective data collected from patients with severe sepsis in the PROWESS trial (Table 79-3).[47] Twenty-nine percent of evaluable patients met the criteria for overt DIC. Overt DIC was an independent predictor of all-cause mortality at day 28.[47] Though intriguing, this scoring system should be used with caution in the general ICU population. These data were retrospectively derived from a population of patients with severe sepsis and stringently defined entry criteria. Coagulation tests were performed in a central laboratory using single methods for PT and D-dimer. Prospective studies are needed to validate this scoring system in diverse causes of DIC using a variety of commercially available methods, especially given the variability in PT based on the reagents used.

It is important to remember that all these laboratory abnormalities can be caused by other disease processes. Vitamin K deficiency, a heparin-contaminated blood sample, or a lupus anticoagulant can cause a coagulopathy, whereas concomitant elevations in FDP can develop after surgery or trauma and levels may increase as a result of extravascular fibrin(ogen)olysis related to metastatic tumors.[50,51] Microangiopathies cause thrombocytopenia and RBC fragmentation. Liver failure can produce a constellation of laboratory abnormalities indistinguishable from those observed in DIC: reduced procoagulant and anticoagulant synthesis mistaken for factor consumption, hypersplenism causing thrombocytopenia, and reduced clearance of FDPs mimicking increased FDP production.[52]

The most important principle in the management of DIC is to treat the underlying cause as vigorously as possible.[53-55] If treatment of the primary disease is unsuccessful, the mortality rate associated with DIC is very high.[47,56,57] Hypothermia and acidosis should be corrected because they interfere with the function of the coagulation factors that are present. Specific interventions depend on the cause of the DIC, the clinical manifestations (bleeding, thrombosis), the tempo of the process (acute versus chronic), and the overall goals of therapy.

If the diagnosis is suspected only because of laboratory abnormalities, management should be conservative. Alternative, potentially correctable processes should be kept in mind, such as vitamin K deficiency and drug-induced thrombocytopenia.

If clinically significant bleeding becomes apparent, a patient with overt DIC should receive blood component therapy (FFP, platelet concentrates, and cryoprecipitate if fibrinogen is less than 100 mg/dL). A realistic goal is to keep the fibrinogen level greater that 150 mg/dL, the APTT close to normal, and the platelet count greater than 50,000/μL.

The role of heparin is controversial in patients with acute, decompensated DIC. Heparin may be helpful for ischemic manifestations (e.g., digital ischemia, skin necrosis). A continuous infusion at a rate of 7 U/kg/h is a reasonable starting dose. Similarly, low-dose heparin infusions may be considered when the platelet count and fibrinogen level do not rise despite aggressive replacement.

Other treatment modalities have been tried in DIC. Although FFP contains AT-III, the use of AT-III concentrates produced no significant decrease in mortality.[58] The role of activated protein C will be discussed in detail in the chapter on sepsis.[47] Because of the intense fibrin(ogen)olytic activity in DIC, antifibrinolytic agents (ε-aminocaproic acid and tranexamic acid) have been administered in an attempt to reduce bleeding. In general, however, failure rates have been quite high, and in some cases serious thrombosis has occurred because the lysis of diffuse microthrombi was suppressed.[54,59]

DISORDERS OF HEMOSTASIS

It has been estimated that 16% of ICU patients have bleeding caused by a coagulation defect and another 66% have abnormal coagulation test results.

Artifacts

Though not a true coagulopathy, a common cause of an unexplained prolongation of the APTT is unsuspected heparin in the line from which the blood was drawn. Heparin may stick to lines even though 10 mL of blood has been drawn before the coagulation studies. Because venous access is often an issue in the ICU, blood for coagulation studies should be drawn by venipuncture if at all possible. A prolonged TT with a normal fibrinogen level is a clue to the diagnosis. If available, a heparin level (anti-Xa assay) will confirm the diagnosis.

Coagulation Factor Abnormalities

Acquired Deficiencies of Procoagulants

Vitamin K Deficiency

Vitamin K is essential for the post-translational modification (γ-carboxylation) of factors II, VII, IX, and X, protein C, and protein S. All vitamin K–dependent proteins contain glutamic acid moieties that must undergo γ-carboxylation for the molecule to be functional. The daily requirement of vitamin K is 50 μg. Normally, daily intake of vitamin K is 200 μg from the diet and 200 μg from intestinal flora. Thus, vitamin K deficiency occurs with loss of both dietary intake and alteration of intestinal flora. Vitamin K stores last approximately 1 week.

Because factor VII has the shortest half-life (approximately 4 hours), early vitamin K deficiency is manifested by a prolonged PT with a normal APTT. As factors II, IX, and X become depleted, the APTT will be prolonged as well. Vitamin K deficiency is common in critically ill patients and may result in serious bleeding.[60] Treatment of vitamin K deficiency depends on the clinical situation. In a nonbleeding patient, vitamin K should be given enterally if the gut is working. Subcutaneous vitamin K should be avoided if the gut is working because of its erratic absorption, especially in face of impaired tissue perfusion and because anaphylactic reactions have been reported with subcutaneous vitamin K.[61] In a bleeding patient, FFP will correct the coagulopathy most quickly. In critically ill patients with an urgent need for vitamin K replacement, phytonadione may be administered intravenously if the benefits are thought to outweigh the risk of anaphylaxis. Vitamin K should be given no faster than 1 mg/min with cardiorespiratory monitoring because anaphylactic reactions can occur even at this slow infusion rate.[61] In patients with normal hepatic function, the coagulopathy should begin improving within 6 to 12 hours.

Liver Disease

The alteration in hemostasis in liver disease is complex. All the hemostatic factors except for vWF and plasminogen activator inhibitor-1 are synthesized in the liver. Loss of the ability to synthesize factor VII is disproportionately greater in patients with liver disease than in those undergoing anticoagulation with warfarin. Accordingly, the significance (bleeding risk) of a prolonged international normalized ratio (INR) in face of liver disease is not as great as the same level of INR with warfarin therapy, thus making the autoanticoagulation of liver disease promulgated among house staff a myth.[62]

Hepatic dysfunction most commonly causes a hemorrhagic diathesis. As a rough guide, the ability to synthesize coagulation factors becomes impaired when albumin falls to approximately 2.5 g/dL. Similar to vitamin K deficiency, the earliest abnormality is a reduction in factor VII, which produces an isolated prolongation of the PT. In more severe liver disease, the other coagulation factors become deficient with progressive prolongation of the PT and APTT. Factor V and fibrinogen do not usually decrease significantly until the liver failure is preterminal or fulminant.[52] Dysfibrinogenemia may also occur. In contrast, the activities of factor VIII and vWF are normal or elevated. AT-III, proteins C and S, and plasminogen are also decreased, thereby impairing the antithrombotic and fibrinolytic mechanisms. There is also reduced hepatic clearance of activated procoagulants and FDPs. Thrombocytopenia may develop as a result of decreased platelet production secondary to decreased thrombopoietin production. With portal hypertension, there may be splenic sequestration of platelets. Advanced liver disease may also be complicated by vitamin K deficiency from malnutrition and decreased vitamin K absorption as a result of cholestasis.

A variety of approaches have been used to treat a coagulopathic patient with liver disease. If the patient is not bleeding, a trial of vitamin K can be given for 3 days to see whether the coagulopathy corrects. Because all patients with liver disease have some degree of biliary obstruction and fat malabsorption, the subcutaneous route is preferred over oral administration of vitamin K. Although the risk of anaphylaxis with intravenous vitamin K is low, it is not generally recommended empirically in a patient with liver disease because of the low likelihood that vitamin K will completely correct the coagulopathy.[61] If bleeding is a problem, FFP should be administered. On average, a unit of FFP increases all coagulation factors by 6% to 7%. A typical patient with the coagulopathy of liver disease may have approximately 10% to 15% of normal levels of coagulation factors. If a factor level of 50% of normal is needed for hemostasis, 6 units of FFP should correct the coagulopathy. Remember to check the PT and APTT immediately after the FFP is administered. Given the short half-life of factor VII, waiting until the next morning's routine blood draw will probably produce a prolongation of at least the PT and give the impression that the coagulopathy is uncorrectable. A subsequent infusion of FFP every 6 to 12 hours as volume status permits may maintain adequate factor levels, but even the most vigorous plasma infusion may not normalize the PT because of the short half-life of factor VII. Fortunately, factor VII levels as low as 10% to 15% are sufficient for hemostasis.

Massive Transfusion

Massive volume replacement (>1 blood volume in <24 hours) may not give the liver sufficient time to replace coagulation factors. FFP should not be given empirically based on the number of units of RBCs given to a patient with massive bleeding. Rather, the clinician should be vigilant for the development of this coagulation defect and infuse FFP when the defect develops.

Acquired Circulating Inhibitors

Factor VIII Inhibitors

Factor VIII inhibitors may cause severe bleeding or an unexplained prolongation of the APTT in a patient with no previous history of bleeding or coagulopathy. The APTT is markedly prolonged with a normal PT, TT, fibrinogen level, and BT. The mixing study does not correct. The diagnosis is made by assaying the activities of factors VIII, IX, XI, and XII. Hematomas should not be drained except in severe circumstances (e.g., compartment syndrome) because of the risk for bleeding, even with therapy. Treatment options depend on the severity of the inhibitor. A low-titer inhibitor (<5 Bethesda units) may be treated with factor VIII infusion (200 U/kg every 8 to 12 hours). For a high-titer antibody (>5 Bethesda units), the treatment options are recombinant human factor VIIa (rH-VIIa; NovoSeven) and virally inactivated concentrates containing activated coagulation factors (e.g., Autoplex, Feiba). The dose of rH-VIIa is 90 μg/kg, which can be repeated every 2 hours until the bleeding stops. rH-VIIa does carry a risk of thrombotic and ischemic events in individuals with severe coagulopathy.[63] Coagulation studies are not used to adjust the dosage, but the PT is always shorter than control values. The dose of activated concentrate varies with the product but is in the range of 50 to 100 U/kg, repeated every 8 to 12 hours. A total of 500 units of heparin can be added to each bag to prevent phlebitis in the vein used for infusion. The clinical response is monitored rather than the APTT.

Factor V Inhibitor

Topical thrombin (a.k.a. fibrin glue) is ubiquitously used in the operating room. Bovine thrombin is contaminated with bovine factor V. Approximately 7 to 10 days after the use of fibrin glue, the PT and APTT may be prolonged as a result of the development of antibodies against bovine factor V and rarely factor II. Bleeding is uncommon because platelet factor V is protected from the antibody.

Inherited Deficiencies of Procoagulants

Management of critically ill patients with inherited coagulopathies requires specialized expertise. A hematologist or coagulationist should be consulted.

von Willebrand's Disease

von Willebrand's disease (vWD) is the most common inherited coagulation disorder. Synthesized in the vascular endothelium and megakaryocytes, vWF is the ligand that binds to the platelet GP Ib/IX/V complex and promotes platelet adhesion in vivo. Factor VIII procoagulant, which is synthesized by the liver, circulates bound to vWF as a complex. Unbound factor VIII is unstable and unable to participate in coagulation. vWF is a complex multimeric protein, with the largest molecular weight forms having the greatest platelet-binding capacity.

vWD is inherited in an autosomal dominant manner with partial penetrance. Clinical bleeding often starts in childhood and may improve after puberty. Because vWF is critical for platelet adhesion, the bleeding associated with vWD is typical of that seen in disorders of platelet function. Easy bruising, menorrhagia, and bleeding after dental extraction are common. Spontaneous bleeding into joints and soft tissues is uncommon. Bleeding can occur with invasive procedures.

The laboratory features of vWD are those of both a platelet disorder and a coagulopathy. The classic screening pattern is that of a prolonged APTT with a normal PT and a prolonged BT. Laboratory confirmation of the diagnosis of vWD may be difficult. The classic pattern is a decrease in factor VIII activity, vWF activity, and von Willebrand antigen. Platelet aggregation studies show an impaired response to ristocetin. Control of the level of vWF in vivo is complex. Lower levels of vWF activity are seen in women than in men, in younger than in older individuals, and in those with blood group O as opposed to blood groups A, B, and AB. Unfortunately, commercial laboratories do not give normal ranges based on age, sex, and blood group. In the past it has been difficult to know where to draw the line between normal individuals and those with blood group O and between individuals with blood group O and those with inherited vWD. As a general rule, vWF activity lower than 20% is diagnostic of inherited vWD. Those with vWF activity of 20% to 50% may have blood group O vWD. Individuals with similar levels of vWF because of inherited vWD or associated with blood group O have a similar predisposition to bleeding.[64] von Willebrand multimer analysis is used to subtype vWD. Type I vWD is most common. Multimer analysis shows all molecular weight sizes of von Willebrand antigen present, albeit at decreased concentrations. Type I vWD is due to impaired secretion of von Willebrand protein from endothelial cells. Type II vWD is due to abnormal subunit structure. The hallmark of type IIA and type IIB vWD is the absence of large- and intermediate-weight forms on electrophoresis. In type IIB, loss of the higher molecular weight forms is due to an increased affinity of vWF for the platelet GP Ib/IX/V receptor, which results in increased plasma clearance of vWF. These individuals may have thrombocytopenia. Type IIB vWD is associated with platelet hyper-responsiveness to a low concentration of ristocetin. The use of DDAVP is contraindicated. Individuals with type III vWD usually have severe bleeding, and von Willebrand protein is very low to absent on multimer analysis.

Patients with vWD in the ICU most commonly have had major surgery, closed head trauma, major trauma, or life-threatening hemorrhage. The goal of therapy is to increase vWF activity and factor VIII activity to 100% of normal and to maintain them above 50%. Historically, cryoprecipitate (which contains approximately 100 units of vWF per bag) was the treatment of choice for vWD. However, the risk of viral infection with untreated plasma products has made this option less desirable. Two virally inactivated "factor VIII" concentrates are rich enough in vWF to be of clinical use for treating vWD. Humate-P and Alphanate are available in the United States. The other brands of factor VIII concentrate do not contain enough vWF to be of clinical value. The rH-VIII used in hemophilia A is of no benefit in vWD. Each vial of "factor VIII" concentrate is labeled with the number of units of factor VIII and vWF because it varies from lot to lot. The number of units of factor VIII and vWF are not the same. "Factor VIII" concentrates should be given as a bolus of 40 to 50 U/kg of vWF followed by 20 to 25 U/kg every 12 hours. Peak and trough levels of vWF and factor VIII should be obtained to help guide therapy. Doses should be rounded to the size of the nearest vial, if possible, so that these expensive factors are not wasted. In mild cases of type I vWD, desmopressin may be adequate for promoting hemostasis. Repeat doses may be given every 12 hours, although patients may become tachyphylactic because of the exhaustion of vWF stores in the Weibel-Palade bodies of the endothelium. Patients should be monitored for hyponatremia, especially if large volumes of fluid are given. In general, DDAVP is less useful in the ICU because it may not be known a priori if a patient is a DDAVP responder. In addition, given that the response to serial doses of DDAVP is less predictable, the use of DDAVP may be problematic if factor VIII and vWF levels are not available on site.

Factor VIII Deficiency

Factor VIII deficiency (hemophilia A) is an X-linked recessive disorder that occurs in approximately 1 in 10,000 white males. Women are obligate carriers. However, women can be hemophilic if they are homozygotes or double heterozygotes or have disproportionate inactivation of the wild-type X chromosome (poor lyonization). A negative family history of bleeding does not exclude a diagnosis of hemophilia A because approximately 30% of affected males have a spontaneous mutation. Hemophilia A produces lifelong bleeding that does not improve with puberty. Bleeding characteristically occurs in the joints, soft tissues, and gastrointestinal tract.

The laboratory features of hemophilia A are a prolonged APTT with a normal PT and BT. The prolonged APTT corrects in the mixing study. Specific factor assays show a decrease in factor VIII activity with normal activity of factors IX, XI, and XII. Although the platelet count should be normal, individuals with hemophilia A complicated by hepatitis C or HIV infection may have a concomitant immune thrombocytopenia.

For major surgery, closed-head trauma, major trauma, or life-threatening hemorrhage, the factor VIII level should be raised to 100% and then maintained continuously above 50% for the first 5 to 7 days and above 40% for an additional 5 to 7 days. Peak and trough factor VIII levels should be obtained after the first dose and at least daily. rH-VIII is the treatment of choice for hemophilia A. Because it is not plasma derived, rH-VIII does not carry a risk of viral infection. Giving 1 unit of factor VIII per kilogram should raise plasma factor VIII activity by 2%. Thus, the initial dose should be 50 U/kg followed by

25 U/kg every 8 hours. In an emergency situation if rH-VIII is not available, virally inactivated factor VIII would be the treatment of choice. The dosing schema is similar to that of rH-VIII. In an emergency situation in a smaller facility that does not stock hemostatic factors on site, cryoprecipitate could be used at a dose of two bags per 5 kg followed by one bag per 5 kg every 8 hours until rH-VIII becomes available. Similar to vWD, DDAVP can be given for the treatment of mild or moderate factor VIII deficiency in known DDAVP responders.

Factor IX Deficiency

Except for the rate of spontaneous mutations, the clinical picture of factor IX deficiency (hemophilia B) is indistinguishable from that of hemophilia A. The laboratory features are similar except that specific factor assays show decreased factor IX activity and normal factor VIII activity. The treatment of choice for factor IX deficiency is rH-IX. Because of differences in the volume of distribution in comparison to rH-VIII, the initial loading dose of rH-IX is 1 U/kg followed by half the dose every 12 hours. At least 30% of individuals require a higher dose. Thus, it is not unreasonable to start with a dose of 1.25 to 1.5 U/kg, especially in a patient whom you do not want to underdose. Peak and trough levels should be monitored similarly to hemophilia A. If rH-IX is not available in an emergency situation, virally inactivated factor IX concentrate is the next choice. The initial dose is 100 units of factor IX per kilogram, followed by 50 U/kg every 12 hours. DDAVP and cryoprecipitate are not effective.

Factor XI Deficiency

Factor XI deficiency is an autosomal recessive disorder most commonly seen in Ashkenazi Jews. The bleeding history is variable and ranges from menorrhagia to bleeding with delivery or surgery. Individuals with factor XI deficiency may be seen in the ICU because factor XI deficiency is not protective against myocardial infarction, which may lead to a need for emergency cardiac catheterization and coronary intervention.[65] FFP (10 to 20 mL/kg followed by 3 to 6 mL/kg every 6 hours) is the treatment of choice. Clopidogrel has been given safely after coronary stenting.

DEEP VENOUS THROMBOSIS

DVT is common in critically ill patients. Lower extremity DVT has been documented in 32% of major trauma cases and 28% of patients in medical intensive care.[66,67] Most patients admitted to the ICU have multiple predisposing risk factors, including recent surgery, trauma, sepsis, malignancy, immobilization, stroke, advanced age, heart or respiratory failure, previous venous thromboembolism, pregnancy, and indwelling catheters.[68-73]

DVT Prophylaxis

All patients admitted to the ICU should be evaluated for their risk for DVT. Because of the nature of illnesses requiring intensive care, essentially all patients will be candidates for DVT prophylaxis. The perceived risk of thrombosis and bleeding needs to be assessed in each patient. Recent guidelines have been suggested.[74] In patients with a high bleeding risk, graded compression stockings and intermittent pneumatic compression devices are recommended. In high-risk patients (orthopedic surgery, major trauma), LMWH is recommended. For all others, either UFH or LMWH is an option. Intermittent pneumatic compression devices can also be added to anticoagulation when the risk for thrombosis is particularly great.[75]

Therapy for DVT

In a non–critical care patient, venous thromboembolism is routinely treated with at least 5 days of UFH, LMWH or fondaparinux (see Table 79-2), followed by varying durations of anticoagulation with warfarin. In an ICU patient, intravenous UFH is the safest mode of anticoagulation. LMWH has the disadvantage of being only partially reversed with protamine, and fondaparinux has no antidote.[76] In unstable patients, warfarin can be very difficult to regulate because of drug interactions and erratic oral intake. Furthermore, warfarin can be quickly reversed only with plasma transfusions.

Inferior Vena Cava Filter

It has been estimated that 80% of pulmonary emboli develop as a result of DVT in the lower extremities via the inferior vena cava (IVC). IVC filter placement is accepted as indicated in the following two situations: patients who have a contraindication to anticoagulation (e.g., recent intracranial hemorrhage or stroke, recent neurologic or ophthalmologic surgery, active gastrointestinal hemorrhage, cerebral metastasis considered to be high risk for bleeding [e.g., melanoma, renal cell, seminoma])[77] and patients with recurrent pulmonary embolism despite therapeutic anticoagulation. Although there are no evidence-based studies to support their use, placement of prophylactic IVC filters has been suggested by some in the following situations: free-floating iliofemoral DVT, trauma patients, and patients with poor cardiac reserve. IVC filters do not eliminate all risk of emboli, and they promote thrombosis in the lower extremities, particularly that related to percutaneous femoral insertion sites.[70,73]

CATASTROPHIC ANTIPHOSPHOLIPID SYNDROME

Catastrophic antiphospholipid syndrome is an uncommon disorder manifested as multiple organ dysfunction secondary to microvascular thrombi. The diagnosis should be considered in patients with an acute onset of more than three of the following: respiratory failure, stroke or other neurologic impairment, abnormal liver function, renal impairment, skin infarction, and thrombocytopenia. Laboratory testing should show evidence of antiphospholipid antibodies. Though not evidence based, empiric therapy has centered around the combined use of high-dose corticosteroids, anticoagulation, and plasma exchange.

ANTICOAGULANTS

Heparin and Heparin Derivatives

Heparin

Heparin is a glycosaminoglycan that anticoagulants blood by greatly augmenting the activity of AT-III.[78] Complexes of heparin and AT-III inhibit not only thrombin but also factor Xa and other procoagulant proteases as well. For clinical purposes, two kinds of heparin are available: "standard" or UFH and its derivatives LMWH. The first five sugars of heparin bind to AT-III, and the number of additional sugars determines the differences in their protein binding and pharmacokinetics.[78]

Unfractionated Heparin

Binding of heparin to AT-III varies markedly between individuals. Thus, the anti-IIa property of heparin is measured by the APTT. Because the anti-IIa and anti-Xa properties of UFH are equivalent, UFH can be monitored by the APTT.

The goal of therapeutic heparinization is to maintain the APTT in a range that corresponds to a heparin level of 0.3 to 0.7 U/mL.[78] Given the marked variability in APTT response to heparin because of differences in reagents and laboratory equipment, this range needs to be determined in each laboratory. The old-fashioned goal of an APTT ratio of 1.5 to 2.5 times the control value correlates very poorly with the anti-Xa heparin assay and should not be used. The dose of heparin is based on weight. No adjustments are needed for obesity, hepatic dysfunction, or renal impairment. Because not all hospitals have a heparin protocol, an adaptation of the Raschke nomogram is shown in Table 79-4.[79] The hemoglobin and platelet count should be monitored daily as surveillance for occult bleeding and incipient HIT. Excessive anticoagulation with heparin can often be managed by simply discontinuing the drug temporarily. In cases of serious bleeding, heparin can be reversed immediately with intravenous protamine sulfate.[78] One milligram of protamine will neutralize 100 units of heparin. If bleeding occurs during the constant infusion, the amount of heparin given during the previous 2 hours should be used. Thus, a patient bleeding after a 5000-unit heparin bolus will need 50 mg of protamine, whereas a patient undergoing a 1250-U/h infusion will need only 25 mg of protamine. Protamine should be given slowly over a 1- to 3-minute period to minimize the risk for hypotension and bradycardia. The risk for anaphylaxis is increased in those who have received protamine zinc insulin or who have had a vasectomy.

Table 79-4. Heparin Nomogram

Anti-Xa (U/mL)	APTT
Initial dose	80 U/kg bolus, then 18 U/kg/h
<0.15	80 U/kg bolus, increase by 4 U/kg/h
0.15-0.29	40 U/kg bolus, increase by 2 U/kg/h
0.30-0.70	No change
0.71-0.85	Decrease infusion by 2 U/kg/h
>0.85	Hold 1 h, decrease infusion by 3 U/kg/h

Adapted from Raschke RA, Reilly BM, Guidry JR, et al: The weight based heparin dosing nomogram compared with a "standard care" nomogram: A randomized controlled trial. Ann Intern Med 1993;119:874.

Low-Molecular-Weight Heparin

The properties of LMWH vary significantly from those of UFH.[78] The anti-Xa–to–anti-IIa ratio of LMWH is approximately 4. Thus, LMWH does not significantly affect the APTT. There is little protein binding, which allows predictable renal excretion. In a normal-sized adult (50 to 150 kg) with normal renal function, monitoring is not necessary. If monitoring is necessary, anti-Xa activity should be measured 3.5 to 4.0 hours after a dose. The therapeutic range for enoxaparin, 1 mg/kg every 12 hours, is 0.5 to 1.0 U/mL. The properties of the different LMWH formulations are not the same. Their kinetics and dosing are not interchangeable.[78] Enoxaparin needs to be reduced in dose in patients with renal impairment (creatine clearance <30 mL/min) and should not be used in those with end-stage renal disease (creatine clearance <10 mL/min). Anti-Xa levels should be checked in adults weighing less than 50 kg and more than 150 kg. LMWH is only 60% reversible by protamine.[78] If bleeding occurs within 8 hours of the LMWH injection, a protamine dose of 1 mg per 100 anti-Xa units should be given. Because of the kinetics of LMWH, a second protamine dose of 0.5 mg per 100 anti-Xa units should be given if the bleeding persists.[78]

Pentasaccharide

Fondaparinux is a derivative of the first five sugars of heparin. Because of its small size, it inactivates Xa only via its interaction with AT-III. Fondaparinux is approved for the treatment of DVT and pulmonary embolism and for DVT prophylaxis in orthopedic and abdominal surgery. As a result of its 18- to 21-hour half-life, its use in the ICU is limited because it is not rapidly cleared in a patient population that needs frequent interventions and procedures and that has a high risk of bleeding. It does not prolong the PT, APTT, or TT. It can be detected in the anti-Xa assay calibrated for fondaparinux. Its anticoagulant effect is not reversed by protamine. A bleeding patient who has received fondaparinux should be supported by transfusion. rH-VIIa can be tried.

Alternatives to Heparin

Several other parenteral anticoagulants are available. However, because of their expense they are generally reserved for the treatment of patients with HITT or with HIT to prevent thrombosis. Although none of them have an antidote, rH-VIIa has anecdotally been used off-label to stop bleeding.

Direct Thrombin Inhibitors

Argatroban is an arginine analogue. It has a short half-life (about 40 minutes) that allows rapid dose adjustments. It is metabolized in the liver, and the half-life increases to around 140 minutes with hepatic dysfunction. Because of its short half-life, an initial bolus is not needed. Argatroban is monitored by the APTT but also has a significant effect on the PT.[80] As an estimate, argatroban monotherapy will approximately double the INR and can markedly prolong the INR with concomitant warfarin. As long as the APTT is therapeutic, this exaggerated increase in INR does not increase the bleeding risk.

Hirudin is a recombinant protein originally extracted from the salivary glands of leeches.[81] It can be given subcutaneously or intravenously as a bolus followed by a continuous infusion. It is monitored with the APTT. The half-life of intravenous lepirudin is 80 to 180 minutes, but it extends to days in patients with severe renal failure. It should not be used in those with sulfite sensitivity. Although hirudin can be removed by hemofiltration, the filters are not approved for use in the United States.[82]

Heparinoids

Danaparoid is a mixture of sulfated glycosaminoglycans, distinct from heparin, that produces an anticoagulant effect primarily by enhancing the activity of antithrombin. It is usually given subcutaneously in a dose based on body weight and requires no laboratory monitoring.[83] However, if monitoring is necessary, such as during renal failure, anti-Xa activity must be determined because danaparoid has little effect on the APTT or PT. Though no longer available in the United States, danaparoid is available in Canada and Europe.

Warfarin

Warfarin is the oral anticoagulant used in North America.[78] Unlike the parenteral anticoagulants, it does not inhibit procoagulant enzyme activity. Rather, it acts by antagonizing vitamin K. Warfarin prolongs the PT more readily than the APTT because of its effect on factor VII, which has a particularly short half-life. Prolongation of the PT is often seen within the first 24 to 48 hours after initiation of warfarin. The initial rise in PT, however, does not reflect the therapeutic effect of the drug because the important natural anticoagulants, proteins C and S, are also rapidly reduced. Four to 5 days is required for the other vitamin K–dependent procoagulants to drop to antithrombotic levels.

Sensitivity to warfarin is variable and affected by many factors common in critically ill patients, such as poor nutrition (vitamin K deficiency), liver dysfunction, and coadministration of medications that can affect warfarin pharmacokinetics. It is monitored by a variation of the PT, the INR, which adjusts for in vitro factors that cause the PT to vary among different laboratories. It is not uncommon for patients to become over-anticoagulated with warfarin. An approach to warfarin reversal is shown in Box 79-5.[78]

Box 79-5

Reversal of Warfarin

Inr<5.0, No Bleeding
- Lower dose or
- Omit dose and restart at a lower dose

INR>5.0 but <9.0, No Significant Bleeding
- Omit 1 or 2 doses and restart at a lower dose, or
- Omit dose and give vitamin K, 1 to 2.5 mg orally, or
- For rapid reversal (e.g., surgery), vitamin K, 3 to 5 mg orally
  INR should decrease in 24 hours
  Give another 1 to 2 mg if the goal is not reached

INR>9.0, No Significant Bleeding
- Hold warfarin and
- Give vitamin K, 5 to 10 mg orally
  The INR should be significantly reduced in 24 to 48 hours
  Give additional vitamin K orally if needed
  Resume warfarin when the INR is therapeutic

Any INR>3.0, Serious Bleeding
- Hold warfarin
- Vitamin K, 10 mg by slow intravenous infusion
- Repeat vitamin K every 12 hours as needed
- If urgent correction needed
  Fresh frozen plasma or
  Recombinant human factor VIIa

Any Inr, Life-Threatening Bleeding
- Hold warfarin
- Recombinant human factor VIIa
- Vitamin K, 10 mg intravenously

Adapted from Hirsch J, Raschke R: Heparin and low molecular weight heparin: The seventh ACCP conference on antithrombotic and thrombolytic therapy. Chest 2004;126:188S.

KEY POINTS

- Hemorrhagic and thrombotic complications in a critically ill patient can usually be anticipated and avoided by careful history taking and physical examination. Routine laboratory tests (platelet count, PT, APTT, TT, fibrinogen) are helpful in evaluating hemorrhagic disorders but not thrombotic disorders.
- Vitamin K deficiency is a relatively common coagulopathy in critically ill patients, and it is easily treated if recognized.
- von Willebrand's disease, the most common inherited coagulopathy, varies highly in clinical severity. Humate-P and Alphanate are the only "factor VIII" concentrates that are therapeutic.
- The bleeding diathesis of uremia can improve with several different treatments, including dialysis, DDAVP, intravenous administration of estrogens, and cryoprecipitate.

- Idiopathic thrombocytopenic purpura in adults is usually chronic. If life-threatening, several modalities are available for urgent elevation of the platelet count.
- Disseminated intravascular coagulation is always a secondary disease process. Treatment must be focused on the underlying cause. If bleeding occurs, blood components should be given. Heparin is generally reserved for clinically evident thrombosis.
- Thrombotic thrombocytopenic purpura is a clinical diagnosis associated with multiple inciting events. It is often fatal unless recognized early and treated with plasma exchange.
- Heparin-induced thrombocytopenia with thrombosis may be life-threatening. It should be looked for in any patient with thrombocytopenia who has been exposed to heparin. It can be managed with direct thrombin inhibitors.
- Deep venous thrombosis is common in critically ill patients. Prophylactic treatment should be considered for every patient in the ICU. Intravenous unfractionated heparin is often the safest treatment of established deep venous thrombosis in the critical care setting.

REFERENCES

1. Napolitano LM, Warkentin TE, Almahameed A, et al: Heparin-induced thrombocytopenia in the critical care setting: Diagnosis and management. Crit Care Med 2006;34:2898-2911.
2. Stephan F, Hollande J, Richard O, et al: Thrombocytopenia in a surgical ICU. Chest 1999;115:1363-1370.
3. George JN, Raskob GE, Shah SR, et al: Drug-induced thrombocytopenia: A systematic review of published case reports. Ann Intern Med 1998;129:886-890. Available at http://moon.ouhsc.edu/jgeorge
4. Norfolk DR, Ancliffe PJ, Contreras M, et al: Consensus conference on platelet transfusion, Royal College of Physicians of Edinburgh, 27-28 November 1997. Br J Haematol 1998;101:609-617.
5. Bizzaro N: EDTA-dependent pseudothrombocytopenia: A clinical and epidemiological study of 112 cases, with 10-year follow-up. Am J Hematol 1995;50:103-109.
6. Huxtable LM, Tafreshi MJ, Rakkar ANS: Frequency and management of thrombocytopenia with the glycoprotein IIb/IIIa receptor antagonists. Am J Cardiol 2006;97:426-429.
7. Von Drygalski A, Curtis BR, Bougie DW, et al: Vancomycin-induced immune thrombocytopenia. N Engl J Med 2007;356:904-910.
8. Beardsley DS: ITP in the 21st century. In Berliner N, Linker C, Schiffer CA (eds): Hematology. American Society of Hematology Education Program, 2006, pp 402-407. Available free online at http://asheducationbook.hematologylibrary.org/
9. Cole JL, Marzec UM, Gunthel CJ, et al: Ineffective platelet production in thrombocytopenic human immunodeficiency virus–infected patients. Blood 1998;91:3239-3246.
10. McMillan R: Therapy for adults with refractory chronic immune thrombocytopenic purpura. Ann Intern Med 1997;126:307-314.
11. The American Society of Hematology ITP Practice Guideline Panel: Diagnosis and treatment of idiopathic thrombocytopenic purpura: Recommendations of the American Society of Hematology. Ann Intern Med 1997;126:319-326.
12. Andersen JC: Response of resistant idiopathic thrombocytopenic purpura to pulsed high-dose dexamethasone therapy. N Engl J Med 1994;330:1560-1564.
13. Newman GC, Novoa MV, Fodero EM, et al: A dose of 75 μg/kg/d of IV anti-D increases the platelet count more rapidly and for a longer period of time than does 50 μg/kg/d in adults with immune thrombocytopenic purpura (ITP). Br J Haematol 2001;112;1076-1078.
14. McCrae KR, Herman JH: Posttransfusion purpura: Two unusual cases a literature review. Am J Hematol 1996;52:205-211.
15. Ascione R, Ghosh A, Rogers CA, et al: In-hospital patients exposed to clopidogrel prior to CABG: A word of caution. Ann Thorac Surg 2005;79:1210-1216.
16. Eberst ME, Berkowitz LR: Hemostasis in renal disease: Pathophysiology and management. Am J Med 1994;96:168-179.
17. Hedges SJ, Dehoney SB, Hooper JS, et al: Evidence-based treatment recommendations for uremic bleeding. Nat Clin Pract Nephrol 2007;3:138-153.
18. Fernandez F, Goudable C, Sie P, et al: Low hematocrit and prolonged bleeding time in uraemic patients: Effect of red cell transfusions. Br J Haematol 1985;59:139-148.
19. Mannucci PM, Remuzzi G, Pusineri F, et al: Deamino-8-D-arginine vasopressin shortens the bleeding time in uremia. N Engl J Med 1983;308:8-12.
20. Moia M, Mannucci PM, Vizzotto L, et al: Improvement in the haemostatic defect of uraemia after treatment with recombinant human erythropoietin. Lancet 1987;2:1227-1229.
21. Janson PA, Jubelier SJ, Weinstein MJ, et al: Treatment of the bleeding tendency in uremia with cryoprecipitate. N Engl J Med 1980;303:1318-1322.
22. Laster J, Silver D: Heparin coated catheters and heparin-induced thrombocytopenia. J Vasc Surg 1988;7:667-672.
23. Prandoni P, Siragusa S, Girolami B, et al: The risk of heparin-induced thrombocytopenia in medical patients treated with low-molecular-weight heparin: A prospective cohort study. Blood 2005;106:3049-3054.
24. Selleng K, Warkentin TE, Greinacher A: Heparin-induced thrombocytopenia in intensive care patients. Crit Care Med 2007;35:1165-1176.
25. Warkentin TE: Heparin-induced thrombocytopenia: Pathogenesis and management. Br J Haematol 2003;116:535-555.
26. Warkentin TE: Heparin-induced thrombocytopenia: Diagnosis and management. Circulation 2004;110:e454-e458.
27. Lo GK, Juhl D, Warkentin TE, et al: Evaluation of pretest clinical score (4 T's) for the diagnosis of heparin-induced thrombocytopenia in two clinical settings. J Thromb Haemost 2006;4:759-765.
28. Warkentin TE, Sheppard J-AI: Testing for heparin-induced thrombocytopenia antibodies. Trans Med Rev 2006;20:259-272.
29. Menajovsky LB: Heparin-induced thrombocytopenia: Clinical manifestations and management strategies. Am J Med 2005;118:21S-30S.
30. Wallis DE, Workman DK, Lewis BE, et al: Failure of early heparin cessation as treatment for heparin-induced thrombocytopenia. Am J Med 1999;106:629-635.
31. Warkentin TE, Elavathil LJ, Hayward CPM, et al: The pathogenesis of venous limb gangrene associated with heparin-induced thrombocytopenia. Ann Intern Med 1997;127:804-812.
32. Lewis BE, Maathai WH Jr, Cohen M, et al: Argatroban anticoagulation during percutaneous coronary artery intervention in patients with heparin-induced thrombocytopenia. Cathet Cardiovasc Interv 2002;57:177-184.
33. Mahaffey KW, Lewis BE, Wildermann NM, et al: Anticoagulant therapy with bivalirudin to assist in the performance of percutaneous coronary intervention in patients with heparin-induced thrombocytopenia (ATBAT study): Main results. J Invas Cardiol 2003;15:611-616.
34. Greinacher A: The use of direct thrombin inhibitors in cardiovascular surgery in patients with heparin-induced thrombocytopenia. Semin Thromb Haemost 2004;30:315-327.
35. Warkentin TE, Kelton JG: Temporal aspects of heparin induced thrombocytopenia. N Engl J Med 2001;344:1286-1292.
36. George JN: Thrombotic thrombocytopenic purpura. N Engl J Med 2006;354:1927-1935.

37. Thompson CE, Damon LED, Ries CA: Thrombotic microangiopathies in the 1980s: Clinical features, response to treatment, and the impact of the human immunodeficiency virus epidemic. Blood 1992;80:1890-1895.
38. Moake JL, Byrnes JJ: Thrombotic microangiopathies associated with drugs and bone marrow transplantation. Hematol Oncol Clin North Am 1996;10:485-497.
39. Moake JL: Thrombotic microangiopathies. N Engl J Med 2002; 347:589-600.
40. Martin JN, Stedman CM: Imitators of preeclampsia and HELLP syndrome. Obstet Gynecol Clin North Am 1991;18:181-198.
41. Rock GA, Shumak KH, Buskard NA, et al: Comparison of plasma exchange with plasma infusion in the treatment of thrombotic thrombocytopenic purpura. N Engl J Med 1991;325:393-397.
42. Ziman A, Mitri M, Klapper E, et al: Combination vincristine and plasma exchange as initial therapy in patients with thrombotic thrombocytopenic purpura: One institution's experience and review of the literature. Transfusion 2005;45:41-49.
43. Fakhouri F, Vernant J-P, Veyradier A, et al: Efficiency of prophylactic and curative treatment with rituximab in ADAMTS 13–deficient thrombotic thrombocytopenic purpura: A study of 11 cases. Blood 2005;106:1932-1937.
44. Levi M, ten Cate H: Disseminated intravascular coagulation. N Engl J Med 1999;341:586-592.
45. Gando S, Kameue T, Nanzaki S, et al: Disseminated intravascular coagulation is a frequent complication of systemic inflammatory response syndrome. Thromb Haemost 1996;75:224-228.
46. Taylor FB, Toh C-H, Hoots WK, et al: Towards definition, clinical and laboratory criteria, and a scoring system for disseminated intravascular coagulation. Thromb Haemost 2001;86:1327-1330.
47. Dhainaut J-F, Yan SB, Joyce DE, et al: Treatment effects of drotrecogin alfa (activated) in patients with severe sepsis with or without overt disseminated intravascular coagulation. J Thromb Haemost 2003;2:1924-1933.
48. Marder VJ, Feinstein DI, Colman RW, et al: Consumptive thrombohemorrhagic disorders. In Colman RW, Marder VJ, Clowes AW, et al (eds): Hemostasis and Thrombosis: Basic Principles and Clinical Practice, 5th ed. Philadelphia, Lippincott Williams & Wilkins, 2006, 1571-1600.
49. Spero AJ, Lewis JH, Hasiba U: DIC: Findings in 346 patients. Thromb Haemost 1980;43:28-33.
50. Bongard O, Wicky J, Peter R, et al: D-dimer plasma measurements in patients undergoing major hip surgery: Use in the prediction and diagnosis of postoperative proximal vein thrombosis. Thromb Res 1994;74:487-493.
51. Dvorak HF, Senger DR, Dvorak AM, et al: Regulation of extravascular coagulation by microvascular permeability. Science 1985;227: 1059-1061.
52. Martinez J, Barsigian C: Coagulopathy of liver failure and vitamin K deficiency. In Loscalzo J, Schafer AI (eds): Thrombosis and Hemorrhage, 2nd ed. Baltimore, Williams & Wilkins, 1998, 987-1004.
53. Rubin RN, Colman RW: Disseminated intravascular coagulation: Approach to treatment. Drugs 1992;44:963-971.
54. Kitchens CS: Disseminated intravascular coagulation. In Alving BM (ed): Blood Components and Pharmacologic Agents in the Treatment of Congenital and Acquired Bleeding Disorders. Bethesda, MD, AABB Press, 1999, 151-165.
55. Feinstein DI: Treatment of disseminated intravascular coagulation. Semin Thromb Hemost 1988;14:351-362.
56. Gando S, Nakanishi Y, Tedo I: Cytokines and plasminogen activator inhibitor-1 in posttrauma disseminated intravascular coagulation: Relationship to multiple organ dysfunction syndrome. Crit Care Med 1995;23:1835-1842.
57. Fourrier F, Chopin C, Goudemand J, et al: Septic shock, multiple organ failure, and disseminated intravascular coagulation. Chest 1992;101:816-823.
58. Warren BL, Eid A, Singer P, et al: Caring for the critically ill patient. High-dose anti-thrombin III in severe sepsis: A randomized controlled trial. JAMA 2001;286:1869-1878.
59. Gralnick HR, Greipp P: Thrombosis with epsilon aminocaproic acid therapy. Am J Clin Pathol 1971;56:151-154.
60. Alperin JB: Coagulopathy caused by vitamin K deficiency in critically ill, hospitalized patients. JAMA 1987;258:1916-1919.
61. Fiore LD, Scola MA, Cantillon CE, et al: Anaphylactoid reactions to vitamin K. J Thrombosis Thrombolysis 2001;11: 175-183.
62. Deitcher SR: Interpretation of the international normalized ratio (INR) in patients with liver disease. Lancet 2002;359:47-48.
63. Abshire T, Kenet G: Recombinant factor VIIa: Review of efficacy, dosing regimens and safety in patients with congenital and acquired factor VIII or IX inhibitors. J Thromb Haemost 2004;2:899-909.
64. Federici AB: Diagnosis of inherited von Willebrand disease: A clinical perspective. Semin Thromb Haemost 2006;32:555-565.
65. Salomon O, Stenberg DM, Dardick R, et al: Inherited factor XI deficiency confers no protection against myocardial infarction. J Thromb Haemost 2003;1:658-661.
66. Kudsk KA, Fabian TC, Baum S, et al: Silent deep vein thrombosis in immobilized multiple trauma patients. Am J Surg 1989;158:515-519.
67. Hirsch ER, Ingenito EP, Goldhaber SZ: Prevalence of deep venous thrombosis among patients in medical intensive care. JAMA 1995;274:335-337.
68. Geerts W, Cook D, Selby R, et al: Venous thromboembolism and its prevention in critical care. J Crit Care 2002;17:95-104.
69. Joynt GM, Kew J, Gomersall CD, et al: Deep venous thrombosis caused by femoral venous catheters in critically ill adult patients. Chest 2000;117:178-183.
70. Blebea J, Wilson R, Waybill P, et al: Deep venous thrombosis after percutaneous insertion of vena caval filters. J Vasc Surg 1999;30:821-828.
71. Gilon D, Schechter D, Rein AJJT, et al: Right atrial thrombi are related to indwelling central venous catheter position: Insights into time course and possible mechanism of formation. Am Heart J 1998;135:457-462.
72. Ducatman BS, McMichan JC, Edwards WD: Catheter-induced lesions of the right side of the heart. JAMA 1985;253:791-795.
73. Gould JR, Carloss HW, Skinner WL: Groshong catheter–associated subclavian venous thrombosis. Am J Med 1993;95:419-423.
74. Geerts WH, Pineo GF, Heit JA, et al: Prevention of venous thromboembolism: The seventh ACCP Conference on Antithrombotic and Thrombolytic Therapy. Chest 2004;126:338S-400S.
75. Paiement G, Wessinger SJ, Waltman AC, et al: Low-dose warfarin versus external pneumatic compression for prophylaxis against venous thromboembolism following total hip replacement. J Arthroplasty 1987;2:23-26.
76. Gram J, Mercker S, Bruhn HD: Does protamine chloride neutralize low molecular weight heparin sufficiently? Thromb Res 1988;52:353-359.
77. Gerber DE, Grossman SA, Streiff MB: Management of venous thromboembolism in patients with primary and metastatic brain tumors. J Clin Oncol 2006;24:1310-1318.
78. Hirsch J, Raschke R: Heparin and low molecular weight heparin: The seventh ACCP conference on antithrombotic and thrombolytic therapy. Chest 2004;126:188S-203S.
79. Raschke RA, Reilly BM, Guidry JR, et al: The weight based heparin dosing nomogram compared with a "standard care" nomogram: A randomized controlled trial. Ann Intern Med 1993;119:874-881.
80. Hursting MJ, Alford KL, Becker J-CP, et al: Novastan (brand of argatroban): A small-molecule, direct thrombin inhibitor. Semin Thromb Hemost 1997;23:503-516.
81. Greinacher A, Janssens U, Berg G, et al: Lepirudin (recombinant hirudin) for parenteral anticoagulation in patients with heparin-induced thrombocytopenia. Circulation 1999;100:587-593.
82. Fischer K-G, van de Loo A, Bohler J: Recombinant hirudin (lepirudin) as anticoagulant in intensive care patients treated with continuous hemodialysis. Kidney Int 1999;56(Suppl 72):S46-S50.
83. Danhof M, de Boer A, Magnani HN, et al: Pharmacokinetic considerations on Orgaran (Org 10172) therapy. Haemostasis 1992;22:73-84.

Chapter 80

Use of Blood Components in the Intensive Care Unit

Judith A. Luce

SOURCE AND PROVISION OF BLOOD COMPONENTS

Most patients admitted to an intensive care unit (ICU) require the administration of one or more blood components during their stay. Such patients exhibit great diversity in conditions necessitating care in the ICU, age, underlying medical problems, and integrity of physiologic compensatory mechanisms. All these patients, however, share the need for optimized oxygen-carrying capacity and tissue perfusion. Ongoing blood loss resulting from injuries, surgical wounds, invasive monitoring equipment, and blood sampling requirements, coupled with inadequate marrow function and, in some, red cell destruction, makes red cell transfusion a necessity for many ICU patients. Additionally, many patients are susceptible to the development of hemostatic disorders requiring the administration of such blood components as plasma, cryoprecipitate, or platelet concentrates.

Blood components should be considered drugs because they exert potent therapeutic responses yet are also capable of causing significant adverse effects. The Food and Drug Administration (FDA) regulates blood component preparation, testing, and administration.[1]

Unlike pharmaceutical agents, however, blood components have fewer objective indications for use and no therapeutic index relating dose to safety. It is not as simple to monitor the efficacy and continuing need for a blood component as it is to determine the blood level of a drug. In addition, the risks associated with transfusion cannot be known in advance and may be lethal; such risks include medical errors, as well as infectious and immunologic hazards. Unlike pharmaceutical agents, these prescribed products require documentation of patient consent and indication for use.

Although the American blood supply is now safer than ever before, zero-risk transfusion is not achievable, even if blood components could be sterilized. The process of donor selection and screening has become increasingly stringent, an evolution that began in response to the well-defined risks of transfusion-transmitted hepatitis and human immunodeficiency virus (HIV) infection. Although the value of maximizing recipient safety is unarguable, increasing donor selectivity has its price. As more tests are added and more conditions placed on the donor, the number of usable donations has declined. This trend has led to occasional regional and seasonal blood shortages and, rarely, outright inability to provide certain blood components. Clinicians who prescribe blood components must be aware of these uncertainties in availability and contribute by using blood products appropriately while the national blood banking system seeks strategies to ensure an adequate, safe blood supply.

Donor screening strategies to ensure recipient safety take several forms.[1,2] American blood donors are voluntary donors; cash payment was eliminated in the 1970s after studies linked professional donors with transmission of hepatitis. Confidential questionnaires were initiated to limit transmission of HIV and hepatitis and to allow voluntary self-exclusion and involuntary exclusion of donors who pose an increased risk of transmitting infectious agents. Multiple specific serologic and biochemical tests are performed to detect the potential for transmission of HIV and other retroviruses, hepatitis, and syphilis. Any donor who indicates high-risk behavior or who tests repeatedly positive is placed on a permanent deferral list.

Some patients may insist on blood obtained from relatives or friends. This practice is termed *directed* or *designated donation.* These selected donors must undergo the same rigorous questioning and testing as volunteer donors. Some studies have found an increased frequency of hepatitis markers in the blood of directed donors when compared with blood drawn from unselected volunteers, but others suggest that designated donors may be no different from new volunteers.[3,4] There continues to be no consensus about whether directed donors are, as a group, as safe as volunteer donors.[5,6] Institutional policies about the acceptability and processing of directed donations vary widely. In any case, supporting ICU patients who require large-volume transfusion with directed donations is unlikely to be advantageous or practical.

BLOOD COMPONENT THERAPY

The basic principle of blood component therapy is prescription of the specific blood product needed to meet the patient's requirement. A single whole blood (WB) donation can be separated into its composite parts, or components, which can be distributed to several recipients with differing physiologic needs. Component therapy thus meets the clinical requirements of increased safety, efficacy, and conservation of limited resources. As the variety of blood product components increases, however, the complexity of transfusion medicine also increases.

A WB donation is typically separated into red blood cells (RBCs), a platelet concentrate, and fresh frozen plasma (FFP) within hours of its collection. The plasma may be further processed into cryoprecipitate and supernatant (cryopoor) plasma.

Whole Blood and Red Blood Cells

One unit of WB measures approximately 500 mL, including 63 mL of citrate anticoagulant/preservative solution. Each unit of WB supplies about 200 mL of RBCs and 300 mL of plasma for volume replacement. WB is refrigerated for 21 to 35 days, depending on the preservative used. After less than 24 hours of refrigerated storage in this preservative and bag system, platelet and granulocyte function is lost. With further storage, levels of the "labile" coagulation factors V and VIII decrease.[7] Some blood centers offer modified WB, which is produced by removal of the platelet or cryoprecipitate fraction and return of the supernatant plasma to the red cells. This permits provision of the more labile components to patients with specific needs, with the remainder forming a product having a composition essentially the same as cold-stored WB. However, the growing need for specialized blood components has resulted in processing the majority of blood donations into components, thus limiting the availability of WB and modified WB.

RBCs, or in common usage, "packed" red cells (PRBCs), are the blood component most commonly transfused to increase red cell mass. PRBCs are derived from the centrifugation or sedimentation of WB and removal of most of the plasma/anticoagulant solution. If collected into citrate-phosphate-dextrose-adenine solution, the volume is approximately 250 mL, the hematocrit (Hct) is 70% to 80%, and the storage life is 35 days. Extended additive solutions permit storage up to 42 days but increase the volume to 300 mL and decrease the Hct to 60%. These extended storage units are commonly used and easier to transfuse because of lower viscosity, but they may pose a problem because of their larger volume.

The transfusion of leukocyte-reduced RBCs may benefit certain patients. Transfusion of blood components containing leukocytes may lead to febrile reactions, a greater propensity for alloimmunization, platelet alloimmunization, and transmission of pathogens carried by leukocytes, such as cytomegalovirus (CMV). Leukocyte reduction, as defined by the FDA, requires filtration of the blood component by a special filter.[1] Filtration may be performed either at the time of blood donation and processing or later at the time of transfusion ("bedside filtration"). Filtration before storage conveys the benefit of removing white blood cells (WBCs) before they can deteriorate and elaborate cytokines and other unwanted substances during storage.[8] Because of proven and theoretical benefits of leukocyte reduction of blood components (discussed later in the section covering the adverse effects of transfusion), many European countries and Canada require that all transfusions be leukocyte reduced, a process called *universal leukoreduction* (ULR). Some institutions in the United States have also made that decision, but either method of leukocyte reduction adds significantly to the cost of each transfusion ($25 to $30), and the benefits of this measure when applied globally have yet to be quantified.[9]

Washing PRBCs involves recentrifuging to remove the plasma/preservative solution from the unit. However, washing may take an hour or more, limits subsequent storage time, and causes some loss of RBCs. Washing is also not an effective method of leukoreduction. There are very few indications for the use of washed RBCs, although some recipients with plasma reactions may benefit. PRBCs can be frozen in cryoprotective solution and stored for extended periods. Frozen RBCs are generally limited to units of special value, such as those with a rare RBC antigen profile or autologous blood donations that need to be stored for future use. A rare-donor registry of frozen PRBCs exists to assist in providing blood to patients with complex or multiple alloantibodies to red cell antigens. Significant advanced planning is necessary to acquire and thaw frozen PRBCs for transfusion, thus limiting their use in acute situations.

WB and PRBCs suffer some cell loss during storage. The current technology of bag and preservative solutions attempts to optimize cell quality and quantity by using strict criteria to determine the length of allowable storage time. Nonetheless, as red cell metabolism decreases progressively, a "storage lesion" results,[10] with accumulation of a variety of undesirable substances and loss of cellular function. Over time in storage, a slow rise in the concentration of potassium, lactate, aspartate aminotransferase, lactate dehydrogenase, ammonia, phosphate, and free hemoglobin and a slow decrease in pH and bicarbonate concentration occur. Cytokines and inflammatory mediators such as interleukin-1, interleukin-6 and tumor necrosis factor also accumulate. The pH of freshly stored blood in citrate solution is 7.16, which declines to approximately 6.73 at the end of the unit's shelf life. As potassium leaks from red cells during storage, levels as high as 25 mEq/L may result. However, each unit transfused supplies at most 7 mEq of potassium, which is well tolerated under most circumstances.

During the storage period there is also a progressive decrease in RBC-associated 2,3-diphosphoglycerate (2,3-DPG) and adenosine triphosphate (ATP).[10] A decrease in 2,3-DPG increases the affinity of hemoglobin for oxygen, which shifts the oxygen dissociation curve to the left and decreases oxygen delivery to tissues. There is little evidence, however, that this transient increase in oxygen affinity has clinical importance. After infusion, 2,3-DPG gradually increases as the transfused red cells circulate, with 25% recovery in 8 hours and full replacement by 24 hours.[11] Decreased ATP during storage diminishes the viability of red cells after transfusion and is one of the chief factors limiting storage time. There is no currently available storage or rejuvenation solution that optimizes these cellular constituents.

The majority of blood transfusions are in the form of PRBCs, the component indicated for normovolemic patients or those for whom intravascular volume constraints are necessary. The use of WB may be desirable for patients who require both increased oxygen-carrying capacity and volume resuscitation because of a large and ongoing hemorrhage; however, the availability of WB is generally limited. Resuscitation is effectively achieved with the use of PRBCs and crystalloid solutions. Each unit of PRBCs or WB is expected to raise the hemoglobin level by 1 g/dL and the Hct by 3% in stable, nonbleeding, average-sized adults. Although some studies have demonstrated a slight superiority of fresh WB over components when used during cardiac surgery in selected patients,[12] the benefits of fresh blood remain controversial, and current testing and processing requirements limit general availability.

Indications for Red Cell Transfusion

Despite a long tradition of transfusion of RBCs in critically ill patients, the precise indications for transfusion remain a source of controversy, and specific transfusion practices may vary widely among clinicians. Before the major randomized studies of RBC transfusion policies, a survey of transfusion practice showed that about half of ICU patients were receiving red cell transfusions,[13] and another showed that if the ICU stay was longer than a week, the rate of transfusion was 85%.[14] The total number of transfusions was high, and ICU practice was characterized by high rates of transfusion.[15]

The reasons for the controversies are clear: RBCs should be transfused only to enhance tissue oxygen delivery, but the underlying physiology of anemia, the complex adaptations to anemia, and the potential advantages and disadvantages to particular groups of patients are not as well understood. Compensatory mechanisms for acute and chronic anemia are diverse and complex.[16,17] All work in concert to maintain oxygenation within the microcirculation. Cardiovascular adjustments leading to increased cardiac output include decreased afterload and increased preload resulting from changes in vascular tone, increased myocardial contractility, and elevated heart rate. Lowered blood viscosity permits improved flow of erythrocytes within capillaries. Blood flow is redistributed to favor critical organs with higher oxygen extraction. Pulmonary mechanisms, though contributing relatively little to short-term oxygenation demands, exert potent effects on related metabolic variables. Finally, the hemoglobin molecule can undergo biochemical and conformational changes to enhance unloading of oxygen at the capillary level. All these mechanisms contribute to an "oxygen reserve" capacity that exceeds baseline requirements by approximately fourfold.[16]

No experimental model exists that encompasses the diversity of physiologic compensations for hypoxia. Experiments carried out in animals and case reports in patients refusing transfusion indicate that an extremely low Hct is tolerated if tissue perfusion is adequate.[18-20] Certain objective, though indirect, measurements of tissue oxygenation exist and are available to clinicians caring for patients monitored invasively in the ICU. Mixed venous oxygen content ($P\bar{v}O_2$) and cardiac output can be measured in patients undergoing pulmonary artery catheterization; arterial oxygen content can also be measured directly. The oxygen extraction ratio (ER) can be calculated directly, and in the presence of normal or high cardiac output it is a measure of tissue oxygen extraction and, indirectly, the adequacy of tissue oxygen delivery. The total body ER at baseline is about 25%. A falling $P\bar{v}O_2$ and an ER increasing to greater than 50% have been proposed as indicators of the need for red cell transfusion.[21]

There have been only 10 randomized trials of transfusion policy in the ICU, and only 1 of them was large enough to draw specific, statistically significant conclusions.[22] The Canadian Critical Care Trials Group compared a liberal (target hemoglobin, 10 to 12 g/dL) with a restrictive (target hemoglobin, 7 to 9 g/dL) red cell transfusion policy in patients stratified for disease severity. At 30 days from randomization, the restrictive strategy was at least as good as, if not better than ($P = .11$) the liberal strategy, and overall hospital mortality was significantly lower in the restrictive strategy group ($P = .05$). For patients younger than 55 years and for patients with lower (<20) APACHE (Acute Physiology, Age, and Chronic Health Evaluation) II scores, the restrictive strategy was clearly superior. In addition, liberal transfusion was not associated with shorter ICU stays, less organ failure, or shorter hospital stays; longer mechanical ventilation times and cardiac events were more frequent in the liberal strategy group. A later subgroup analysis of patients with cardiovascular disease, though small enough to have statistical doubt, suggested that a more liberal transfusion strategy was probably appropriate for patients with severe ischemic coronary disease.[23] This observation has some support in experimental studies of the effects of anemia in laboratory animals with coronary occlusion.[24] The Canadian study has highlighted the many and complex issues involved in transfusion decision making in the ICU.

Since publication of the Canadian study, several large reports have examined the use of red cell transfusions in critical care units. Vincent and colleagues[25] surveyed European ICUs and found that the transfusion rate in 3534 patients was 37% during the ICU stay and 12.7% after the stay. The mean pretransfusion hemoglobin level was 8.4 g/dL. Corwin and colleagues[26] studied 284 ICUs in the United States a year later and found great similarity: nearly 50% of patients received transfusions, and the mean threshold hemoglobin level was 8.6 g/dL. A single large Scottish teaching hospital reported a more parsimonious practice: the rate of transfusion was still 52% in its ICU patients, but the total volume of blood used was slightly smaller and the mean pretransfusion hemoglobin level was only 7.8 g/dL.[27] All these authors have concluded that ICU practice has not fully embraced the guidelines of the Canadian clinical trial. In contrast, 18 hospitals in Australia and New Zealand have reported on transfusion in 1808 consecutive ICU admissions, and although the authors found a median pretransfusion hemoglobin concentration of 8.2 g/dL, the rate of transfusion was lower, at only 19.7% of patients, 60% of whom were bleeding.[28] The "inappropriate" transfusion rate was 3%. The authors speculate that the practitioners may have been influenced by publication of the Canadian study and their own regional survey of transfusion practices. Nonetheless, they agree that full implementation of the Canadian guidelines in their clinical setting might be controversial.

The literature on RBC transfusion in the setting of surgery, particularly surgery with the use of blood products, is growing. A mounting body of data illustrate the human tolerance of a low Hct during and after surgery. A recent randomized trial of RBC transfusion strategy in orthopedic surgery demonstrated no significant differences in outcome between a restrictive (8 g/dL) and a liberal (10 g/dL) transfusion threshold and included monitoring for silent myocardial ischemia preoperatively and postoperatively.[29] Provided that adequate perfusion of the microcirculation is maintained, purposeful maintenance of a low Hct during surgery, a technique called *normovolemic hemodilution,*[30] can be a powerful tool in minimizing blood loss and the attendant need for red cell transfusion.

Table 80-1 summarizes guidelines proposed by the National Institutes of Health,[31] the American Society of Anesthesiologists,[32] and the American College of Physicians[33] relative to the transfusion of RBCs. These guidelines have been provided with the intent of establishing parameters, not with the intent of substituting for the individual clinician's judgment. The art of medical decision making in transfusion, as in other areas of medicine, lies in determination of the appropriate treatment for the individual patient.

Table 80-1. Indications for Red Cell Transfusion

To increase the oxygen-carrying capacity based on the hemoglobin level:	
Hb ≤ 60-70 g/L	Acute anemia: transfusion frequently required Chronic anemia: transfusion may be necessary if the patient is symptomatic, there is limited cardiopulmonary reserve, or bleeding is present
Hb > 60-70 g/L but ≤100 g/L	Hb adequate for the majority of patients; transfuse only if the patient is symptomatic, is actively bleeding, or has limited cardiopulmonary reserve Physiologic parameters in critical care: extraction ratio exceeding 50%, fall in $\dot{V}O_2$ to less than 50% of baseline or $P\bar{v}O_2$ to less than 25 mm Hg
Hb > 100 g/L	Few patients require transfusion

Hb, hemoglobin; $P\bar{v}O_2$, mixed venous oxygen content; $\dot{V}O_2$, oxygen consumption.

Platelets

A platelet concentrate *(random-donor platelets)* is obtained by centrifugation from a unit of donated WB. Each unit contains a minimum of 55×10^{10} platelets suspended in about 50 mL of plasma. Platelets are stored at room temperature to avoid loss of function from refrigeration and are constantly agitated to maximize gas exchange. The length of storage varies with the container used, but most systems permit 5-day storage. Because of this limited storage time and the increasing demand for this component, platelets are often subject to supply shortages. Some loss of viability and platelet numbers occurs during storage, but 5-day-old platelets still effect hemostasis. Once the bags are entered for pooling before transfusion, the platelets must be administered within 4 hours.

Each unit of platelets is expected to increase the platelet count by 10×10^9/L in a typical 70-kg adult. The usual dose is 6 units, or 1 U/10 kg of body weight. A 1-hour post-transfusion platelet count should be obtained to determine the adequacy of response. The following equation, which relates platelet number and body size to the post-transfusion increment, can be used to assess the effectiveness of the transfusion:

$$\text{Corrected count increment (CCI)} = \frac{\text{Observed rise in platelet count} \times \text{Body surface area } (\text{m}^2)}{\text{Number of platelet units transfused}}$$

A CCI of 10×10^9/L or higher can be considered a good response, whereas a CCI of 5×10^9/L or lower indicates a poor response to transfusion.[34]

ABO-compatible platelets are desirable but not essential. When ABO-mismatched platelets are given, removal of some of the incompatible plasma can be carried out at the time of pooling for transfusion. Likewise, volume reduction may be necessary for patients at risk for fluid overload from the 300 to 500 mL of plasma present in 6 to 10 units of platelets. Nonetheless, the remaining plasma is a good source of stable coagulation factors and contains diminished but still potentially beneficial amounts of factors V and VIII. There is no contraindication to the use of Rh-positive platelets in Rh-negative patients; if given to women with future childbearing potential, Rh immune globulin (RhIG) may be used prophylactically against the small risk of Rh alloimmunization from red cells that may be contained in the platelet concentrate.

Plateletpheresis (common terms: *single-donor platelets, apheresis platelets*) involves separating and removing platelets from one donor by cytapheresis during a $1\frac{1}{2}$- to 2-hour procedure on an automated device and then retransfusing the remainder of the blood back into the donor. Each collection contains an equivalent of 6 to 10 units of platelet concentrates. Single-donor platelets are suspended in about 300 mL of plasma, so the same ABO and volume considerations discussed earlier pertain. Single-donor platelets offer the clear benefit of reducing the risk of multiple-donor exposure to the recipient. Single-donor platelets may also be the only available alternative for recipients who have been alloimmunized by previous platelet transfusions because they may be human leukocyte antigen (HLA) or platelet antigen matched to the recipient. The use of apheresis platelets now exceeds the use of pooled random-donor platelets; however, use of this product in emergency situations is limited by the availability of volunteer donors.[35]

Indications for Platelet Transfusion

Platelet transfusions are indicated for patients bleeding because of thrombocytopenia or functional platelet defects.[36] Guidelines for transfusion continue to evolve, and the current guidelines merely provide a desirable range for platelet counts, assuming normal platelet function (Table 80-2). There is ample evidence that bleeding medical or surgical patients with platelet counts of 50×10^9/L or above will not benefit from transfusion if thrombocytopenia is the only abnormality. For critical invasive procedures in which even a small amount of bleeding could lead to loss of vital organ function or death, maintaining the platelet count at 50×10^9/L or greater is typically preferred. The presence of other factors that diminish platelet function, such as certain drugs, foreign intravascular devices (e.g., intra-aortic balloon pump or membrane oxygenator), infection, or uremia, may alter this requirement upward. Patients at risk for small but strategically important hemorrhage, such as neurosurgical patients, may need to be maintained at counts of 80 to 100×10^9/L.

Table 80-2. Conservative Indications for Prophylactic Platelet Transfusion

Platelet Count $\times10^9$/L	Clinical Situation
0-5	Spontaneous bleeding likely, transfusion warranted
6-10	With fresh minor hemorrhage or fever, rapidly falling count
11-20	With concomitant coagulation disorder, heparin therapy, or planned minor invasive procedure
21-50	With major bleeding, surgical procedure
>50	Bleeding unlikely to be caused by thrombocytopenia unless a qualitative platelet defect is present

Patients without hemorrhage who have platelet counts of 5×10^9/L or lower appear to be at increased risk for significant hemorrhage. Indications for transfusion to patients with counts above 10×10^9/L are less well established; thus, the majority of guidelines propose prophylactic platelet transfusion to prevent hemorrhage at a threshold of 10×10^9/L. The bleeding time is not a useful procedure in this situation because it is usually prolonged at counts below 80×10^9/L, may be insufficiently reproducible, and correlates poorly with the risk for bleeding.[37]

Patients undergoing cardiac bypass surgery experience a drop in platelet count and often acquire a transient platelet functional defect from damage associated with the bypass apparatus.[38] Most patients do not experience platelet-associated bleeding, however, so prophylactic transfusion in the absence of bleeding is not warranted. In a patient who continues to bleed postoperatively, more likely causes are a localized, surgically correctable lesion or failure to reverse heparinization. If these conditions are excluded, empiric transfusion of platelets may be justified.

Patients thrombocytopenic by virtue of immunologic destructive processes such as idiopathic thrombocytopenic purpura (ITP) receive little benefit from platelet transfusions because the transfused platelets are rapidly removed from the circulation. In the event of life-threatening hemorrhage or an extensive surgical procedure, transfusion may prove beneficial for its short-term effect. Transfusion may be accomplished effectively by pretreatment with high-dose immunoglobulin or high-dose anti-D antiserum (RhIG).[39,40] Platelet transfusion has been reported to be deleterious in thrombotic thrombocytopenic purpura (TTP),[41] in the related hemolytic-uremic syndrome, and in heparin-induced thrombocytopenia. Cautious administration, in cases of life-threatening thrombocytopenic bleeding only, is prudent.

Prophylactic platelet transfusion for thrombocytopenia secondary to underproduction remains controversial. The common practice of transfusion to maintain the platelet count above 20×10^9/L derives from data published in 1962, which demonstrated an increase in spontaneous bleeding in leukemic patients at that level.[42] However, critical evaluation of the data reveals that serious hemorrhage was not greatly increased until counts fell to 5×10^9/L or lower and that these patients received aspirin for fever, which might have compromised platelet function and enhanced the bleeding.

A somewhat more recent study quantitating stool blood loss in aplastic anemia patients defined a bleeding threshold at platelet counts of 5 to 10×10^9/L.[43] A prospective study of a more conservative transfusion protocol found that major bleeding episodes occurred on 1.9% of days with counts of less than 10×10^9/L and on only 0.07% of days with counts of 10 to 20×10^9/L.[44] The trigger for prophylactic platelet transfusion in the 5 to 10×10^9/L range, however, applies primarily to stable thrombocytopenic patients. Factors such as fever, use of anticoagulant or antiplatelet drugs, and invasive procedures must be considered when generating a treatment plan for individual patients. Patients experiencing rapid drops in platelet count may be at greater risk than those at steady state and thus may benefit from transfusion at higher counts. Benefits to the patient with more judicious use of platelet transfusion include decreased donor exposure, which lessens the risk of transfusion-transmitted disease; fewer febrile and allergic reactions that may complicate the hospital course; and the potential delay or prevention of alloimmunization to HLA and platelet antigens.[45]

The development of refractoriness to platelet transfusions is a serious event heralded by a falling CCI. Poor response to platelet transfusions can be seen in patients with other reasons for platelet consumption, including splenomegaly, fever, trauma and crush injury, burns, disseminated intravascular coagulation (DIC), concomitant drugs, or transfusion of platelets of substandard quality.[46] These factors should be sought and corrected if possible. Alloimmunization is characterized by the development of anti-HLA or platelet-specific antibodies, with resultant immune platelet destruction. As many as 70% of patients receiving multiple red cell or platelet transfusions become immunized.[45] Leukocyte depletion of transfused components can prevent or delay this phenomenon, but it is important to use leukoreduced components early in the course of transfusion therapy.[45,47] When patients fail to achieve expected increments after platelet transfusion, provision of ABO-specific platelet concentrates that are less than 48 hours old may improve the response. If no improvement is seen and the aforementioned medical conditions are excluded, the patient should be screened for HLA antibodies or be HLA typed and provided with HLA-compatible single-donor platelets. Alternatively, platelet crossmatching with the patient's serum can be carried out. There is no advantage to unmatched single-donor platelets in this situation.

Plasma-Derived Components

Plasma

Standard FFP is prepared by centrifugation of WB and is frozen within 8 hours of blood donation.[1,2] FFP may be stored frozen for 1 year. The usual volume is about 250 mL, depending on the donor's Hct. The most common method of thawing before transfusion is soaking in a 37° C water bath, which requires about 30 to 45 minutes. Once thawed, FFP can be stored refrigerated for a maximum of 24 hours. When prepared and stored in this manner, FFP supplies all the constituents in the amounts normally present in circulating plasma, including stable and labile coagulation factors, complement, albumin, and globulins. By convention, the coagulation factors are present in concentrations of 1 U/mL. Crossmatching to the recipient is not performed, but FFP must be ABO compatible.

Standard FFP is as likely to transmit hepatitis, HIV, and most other transfusion-related infections as cellular components are. New FFP products have recently been introduced in response to concern about the transmission of infectious diseases. One such product is solvent-detergent–treated FFP.[48] Solvent-detergent treatment is a means of viral inactivation that removes the infectivity of lipid-enveloped viruses, such as hepatitis B and C and HIV. Because the product is derived from pooled plasma, with as many as 2500 donors in each lot, it has the potential to actually increase recipient exposure to pathogens not inactivated by the solvent-detergent method, such as hepatitis A and parvovirus B19, and be more vulnerable to any newly emerging non–lipid-enveloped agent. A variety of other techniques for reducing pathogen exposure in FFP have been developed, including exposure to low pH or vapor heating and treatment with ultraviolet irradiation, gamma irradiation, or psoralens and light to inactivate pathogens by inducing DNA damage.[49]

Because none of the FFP products is entirely free from the risk of disease transmission or other adverse effects and because infection-reducing modifications add significantly to the cost of the components, FFP should be used judiciously.[50] It should be administered only to provide coagulation factors or plasma proteins that cannot be obtained from safer sources. FFP is commonly used to treat *bleeding* patients with acquired deficiency of multiple coagulation factors, as in liver disease, DIC, or dilutional coagulopathy, or to treat patients with congenital deficiency of a coagulation factor or other protein for which concentrates or safer sources do not exist. FFP may be indicated for emergency reversal of the coagulopathy induced by warfarin anticoagulants when more concentrated products are not available or for the provision of protein C or S in patients who are deficient and suffering acute thrombosis. FFP should be administered as boluses as rapidly as feasible so that the resulting factor levels allow hemostasis. The use of FFP infusions without adequate bolus administration is not helpful. FFP should not be used for volume expansion or wound healing or as a nutritional source of protein. FFP does not reverse anticoagulation induced by heparin and in theory might exacerbate bleeding by supplying more antithrombin, heparin's cofactor.

Prophylactic administration of FFP does not improve patient outcome in the setting of massive transfusion or cardiac surgery unless there is bleeding with an associated documented coagulation abnormality.[51,52] Patients do not usually bleed as a result of coagulation factor insufficiency when the international normalized ratio (INR) is less than about 2.0, and even then the results are not always predictable.[53] The partial thromboplastin time (PTT) is not useful in predicting procedural bleeding risk.[54] FFP is often requested prophylactically before an invasive procedure when the patient exhibits mild prolongation in coagulation studies. Most of these procedures may be carried out safely without transfusing FFP.[53,55]

FFP is probably the most misused blood component, as illustrated by retrospective surveys.[56] Coagulation factors are normally present in the blood far in excess of the minimum levels required for hemostasis. As little as 10% of the normal plasma concentration of several factors will effect hemostasis. Conversely, FFP treatment of acquired multiple deficiencies, as in hepatic failure, is often ineffective because many patients cannot tolerate the infusion volumes required to achieve hemostatic levels of coagulation factors, even transiently.[57] The plasma half-life of transfused factor VII is only 2 to 6 hours. It may be impossible to administer sufficient FFP every few hours without encountering intravascular volume overload. Finally, in some instances, transfusion of seemingly adequate volumes may still fail to correct the coagulopathy.[58] Careful documentation of both the need for FFP and the adequacy and outcomes of therapy is essential.[59]

Cryoprecipitate

Cryoprecipitate is manufactured by thawing and centrifuging FFP below 6°C and resuspending the precipitated proteins in about 15 mL of supernatant plasma.[1,2] Each bag is a concentrated source of factor VIII (80 to 120 units), von Willebrand factor (vWF) (50% of original plasma content), fibrinogen (250 mg), factor XIII (30% of original plasma content), and fibronectin. Cryoprecipitate offers the advantage of transfusing more specific protein and less total volume than the equivalent dose of FFP does. It has been used to treat patients with inherited coagulopathies, such as hemophilia A, von Willebrand disease, or factor XIII deficiency. In the critical care setting, it is more commonly used to replenish fibrinogen, especially in bleeding patients with hypofibrinogenemia caused by dilutional or consumptive coagulopathy. Cryoprecipitate also reportedly improves hemostasis in uremic patients, presumably by reversing the functional platelet defect,[60] but desmopressin acetate (DDAVP)[61] or conjugated estrogens exert similar effects and should be used preferentially to avoid potential transfusion-transmitted disease.

The usual dose of cryoprecipitate to treat hypofibrinogenemia is 10 bags/units to start, then 6 to 10 bags/units every 8 hours or as necessary to keep the fibrinogen level above 100 mg/dL. Each bag/unit of cryoprecipitate carries a risk of disease transmission equivalent to that of 1 unit of blood. For this reason, commercial factor VIII concentrates, recombinant or treated to inactivate viruses, are preferred over cryoprecipitate for treating hemophilia A patients.

Immune Globulin Preparations

Immune serum globulin (IG), RhIG, and hyperimmune globulins for diseases such as hepatitis B and varicella zoster are obtained by fractionation of pooled plasma, followed by chromatography, delipidation, and other steps to remove aggregates and infectious agents. Intravenous IG (IVIG) is available in solution or lyophilized form, with protein content varying by mode of preparation. The available products vary slightly in the amounts of IgA and IgM contained in them, which are mostly present in only trace quantities.

IG preparations can be used to provide passive antibody prophylaxis or to supply IG in certain immunodeficiency states. Hyperimmune globulins may be used to treat active infections in immunosuppressed hosts. Recent applications have exploited IG's immunomodulatory effects in treating a wide variety of disorders with an immune basis. The specific mechanism of action of IVIG in such conditions has not yet been identified, but possibilities include interference with macrophage Fc receptor function, neutralization of anti-idiotypic antibodies, and interference with the incorporation of activated complement fragments into immune complexes. A recent review more completely discusses the effects of IVIG on the immune system and its potential uses.[62]

RhIG is prepared from pools of plasma obtained from donors sensitized to the red cell antigen D from the Rh group. The standard-dose vial contains primarily IgG anti-D, with a protein content of 300 µg in 1 mL. This dose will protect against 15 mL of D^+ red cells or 30 mL of WB.[63] RhIG carries no risk of virus transmission. Although RhIG is used primarily in obstetrics, it may also be indicated to prevent alloimmunization in Rh-negative patients receiving small amounts of Rh-positive red cells, as in platelet concentrates. Routine prophylaxis against large numbers of red cells, as in a unit of Rh-positive WB or PRBCs given by accident to an Rh-negative recipient, is not reliable and usually involves the administration of large amounts, but instances of its effective use in these circumstances have been reported. Higher doses of intravenous RhIG have been used in the treatment of ITP.

Plasma-Derived Colloid Solution

Plasma-derived colloids include human serum albumin (HSA), available in 5% and 25% solutions, and plasma protein fraction (PPF), available in a 5% solution. Both are derived from pooled donor plasma but are essentially pathogen-free. HSA is composed of at least 96% albumin, whereas PPF is subjected to fewer purification steps and contains at least 83% albumin, with correspondingly more globulins. The 5% solutions are iso-oncotic, whereas the 25% solution of HSA is hyperoncotic and requires infusion with crystalloid solutions.

Potential clinical indications for colloid solutions include hypovolemic shock, hypotension associated with hypoproteinemia in patients with liver failure or protein-losing conditions, as a replacement solution in plasma exchange or exchange transfusion, and to facilitate diuresis in fluid-overloaded hypoproteinemic patients. Albumin solutions are not indicated as a nutritional source to raise serum albumin. Their use in some indications, particularly for resuscitation, has become controversial, and pulmonary edema has been reported in association with their infusion.[64]

Although albumin solutions are reasonably safe products to administer, expense and limited availability restrict their use. Anaphylactic reactions have been reported in less than 0.1% of recipients. The use of PPF has been associated with severe hypotensive episodes, with Hageman factor fragments or prekallikrein activator being demonstrated,[65] thus making PPF a less desirable resuscitation fluid and contraindicated in cardiac surgery.

Granulocytes

Granulocyte concentrates for transfusion are obtained from a single donor by cytapheresis methods, which generally involve the administration of hydroxyethyl starch and corticosteroids to the donor to improve granulocyte yield. Granulocyte colony-stimulating factor (G-CSF) has been added to some collection regimens and increases both cell counts and granulocyte survival substantially. Each collection should contain at least 10^{10} granulocytes[1,2] and is suspended in approximately 200 mL of plasma. A significant number of red cells are present, so crossmatching for the recipient is required. Because of the potential risk for graft-versus-host disease (GVHD), granulocytes are usually collected from HLA-matched donors. Granulocytes are stored at room temperature and must be transfused within 24 hours of collection, although sooner is better because of rapid deterioration of the cells.

Patients who may benefit from granulocyte transfusions include those who are neutropenic (absolute neutrophil count of less than 0.5×10^9/L) and those who are unresponsive to appropriate antibiotic treatment but in whom bone marrow recovery is expected to occur. A course of therapy generally involves daily infusion for 4 to 7 days. Granulocytes have been used for progressive fungal infections in immunosuppressed granulocytopenic patients, in patients with defective leukocytes (e.g., chronic granulomatous disease), and in the neonatal ICU for neonatal sepsis. Randomized trials had suggested that granulocyte transfusions under these circumstances can reduce mortality, but such trials have not been conducted for more than 2 decades.[66] Effective antibiotic regimens and the significant adverse effects associated with the use of granulocyte concentrates, including pulmonary insufficiency related to alloimmunization and CMV infection, have limited their use in recent years.

TRANSFUSION REACTIONS

The decision to transfuse blood components, like any therapeutic maneuver, must be made with full awareness of the potential risk to the recipient, as well as the expected benefits. Public expectations of a zero-risk blood supply help raise the acuity of physicians' decisions. For some patients, the benefit from transfusion is so obvious that the associated risks pale in comparison to the consequences of withholding transfusion. However, the clinician's knowledge of the incidence and management of adverse reactions to transfusion is vital, not only to ensure the best patient care but also to provide appropriate patient education and true informed consent.

Almost every patient who receives an allogeneic blood transfusion will experience some adverse reaction if such universal effects as immunomodulation and bone marrow suppression are considered. Measurable reactions to transfusion occur in about 20% of patients; more serious adverse responses may be expected in only 1% to 2% of transfusions.[67] The nature of these adverse reactions ranges from those that are common but clinically unimportant to those that may cause significant morbidity or death (Table 80-3).

Acute Transfusion Reactions

Transfusion in the ICU is a common and often lightly regarded event. However, because the signs and symptoms of severe, life-threatening reactions are frequently indistinguishable from those of troublesome, but less significant reactions, every transfused patient who experiences a significant change in condition, such as an elevation in temperature, change in pulse or blood pressure, dyspnea, or pain, must be promptly and fully evaluated to identify the cause of the reaction and to institute treatment when necessary. The basic approach to all acute reactions should be to maintain a high index of suspicion for acute hemolytic reactions by stopping the transfusion immediately, maintaining venous access with intravenous fluids, and informing the blood bank laboratory immediately so that the appropriate transfusion reaction protocol can be instituted and post-transfusion specimens obtained. Early recognition of severe transfusion reactions may be lifesaving.

Acute Hemolysis

The most feared reaction to blood transfusion is intravascular hemolysis, caused by the recipient's complement-fixing antibodies attaching to donor RBCs with resultant RBC lysis. ABO incompatibility is most often implicated

Table 80-3. Frequency of Transfusion Reactions

Complication	Estimated Frequency/Unit
Acute hemolytic transfusion reactions	1/250,000-1/1 million
Delayed hemolytic transfusion reactions	1/1000
Anaphylaxis	1/150,000
Febrile, nonhemolytic reaction	1/100-200
Allergic/urticarial reaction	1/200
Transfusion-related acute lung injury	1/8000
Human immunodeficiency virus	1/1.2-2.4 million
Hepatitis B	1/60,000-1/200,000
Hepatitis C	1/800,000-1/1.6 million
Bacterial infection from red blood cells	1/500,000
Bacterial infection from platelets	1/2000
Alloimmunization to red blood cells	1/100
Graft-versus-host disease	Rare (?)

in these incidents. Intravascular hemolysis is still the single most common acute cause of fatalities associated with the transfusion episode.[68] In addition to hemolysis, complement activation stimulates the release of inflammatory mediators and cytokines and thereby leads to hypotension and vascular collapse. Activation of the coagulation system may result in DIC. Acute renal failure may also occur, presumably on the basis of immune complex interactions. Morbidity and mortality are directly related to the quantity of incompatible blood transfused, which is why prompt recognition and cessation of transfusion cannot be overemphasized.

Misidentification of the patient, or "clerical error," at any time beginning with the process of specimen acquisition through release of the unit and initiation of infusion is the major cause of acute intravascular hemolysis.[69,70] This reaction is more likely to occur in critical care settings, such as the ICU, operating room, and emergency department, than anywhere else in the hospital. It is far preferable to transfuse uncrossmatched group O red cells than to chance ABO incompatibility caused by improper patient and specimen identification procedures.

The most common clinical sign of hemolysis is fever, with or without chills.[71] Other common signs and symptoms include back or flank pain, anxiety, nausea, lightheadedness, dyspnea, and hemodynamic instability. In a comatose or anesthetized patient, many of these symptoms will not be evident; therefore, signs such as hypotension, hemoglobinuria, and diffuse oozing from puncture sites or incisions may be the only notable features.

Immediate management of hemolytic transfusion reactions must include cessation of the transfusion; the remainder of care is supportive. Rapid verification of patient and unit identification must be made, not only to confirm the suspected reaction but also to prevent a second patient from receiving a reciprocally incompatible unit if a clerical error has been made. Desired end points of supportive care include maintenance of blood pressure, high urine output, and support of coagulopathy or further blood loss. Steroids, heparin, or other specific pharmacologic interventions have no role in treatment.

Anaphylaxis

Anaphylactic reactions to blood transfusions are fortunately rare but may be life-threatening. The usual cause is recipient antibody to a component of plasma that the patient lacks, most commonly antibody to IgA in IgA-deficient individuals.[72] Signs and symptoms include severe malaise and anxiety, flushing, dizziness, dyspnea, bronchospasm, abdominal pain, vomiting, diarrhea, hypotension, and eventually shock. Fever and hemolysis do not occur. Management includes immediate cessation of transfusion and standard therapy for anaphylaxis. If anti-IgA antibodies are determined to be the cause of this reaction, the patient must receive blood components donated by IgA-deficient individuals or, if unavailable, specially prepared washed RBCs and platelet concentrates. Plasma-derived preparations, such as albumin, and IG contain varying amounts of IgA and pose a substantial risk in these patients.

Febrile Nonhemolytic Reactions

Febrile nonhemolytic reactions (FNHRs) are the most commonly occurring immediate transfusion reaction. These reactions are annoying to the clinician, patient, and transfusion service alike in that they can cause significant discomfort and, because they share certain manifestations with acute hemolytic reactions, must be investigated in every instance. FNHRs occur in approximately 0.5% to 1.0% of transfusion episodes.[73] The etiologic factors are probably complex and multiple, but many reactions are caused by the release of cytokines and pyrogens, either within the transfused unit of blood or as a result of recipient antibodies to donor leukocytes. Clinical signs include fever, with or without chills, usually beginning 1 to 2 hours after the start of the transfusion but occasionally delayed up to 4 to 6 hours. Multiparous women and patients who are multiply transfused are particularly prone to FNHRs. The transfusion must be stopped and the appropriate transfusion reaction evaluation instituted. Antipyretics such as acetaminophen may be administered. Though commonly used, antihistamines such as diphenhydramine are neither preventive nor therapeutic. Once acute hemolysis is excluded, transfusion of a new unit may be instituted. Most patients will not experience a second such reaction.[73] If repeated reactions become problematic, leukocyte-depleted blood components may be supplied. The implementation of ULR results in a reduction in the frequency of all fevers seen after transfusion by only about 12%.[74]

Allergic and Urticarial Reactions

Hives and pruritus are relatively common adverse effects of transfusion.[68] They are a hypersensitivity reaction localized to the skin, and their cause is unknown but may include both donor and recipient characteristics. These reactions consist of localized or generalized urticaria beginning shortly after the start of transfusion without other signs or symptoms of anaphylaxis or hemolysis. The transfusion should be temporarily stopped, and antihistamines may be administered. If the hives resolve in a short time, the same unit of blood may be cautiously restarted. If repeated urticarial reactions occur, premedication with antihistamines may be effective, or blood components washed to remove plasma may be required.

Volume Overload

Intravascular volume overexpansion is particularly likely to occur in critical care patients with limited cardiac reserve. Aside from the inherent volume of the blood components, the intravenous normal saline concurrently administered adds to the volume load. Unfortunately, normal saline solution is the only intravenous fluid that may be administered with blood components. With careful attention to transfusion requirements and the use of volume reduction maneuvers available to the transfusion service, volume overload can be minimized in most instances. The frequency of this complication of transfusion is not reported.

IMMUNOLOGIC EFFECTS OF TRANSFUSION

Delayed Hemolytic or Serologic Reactions

Delayed hemolysis is an uncommon but probably under-recognized reaction to transfusion that results from the stimulation of a primary or secondary (anamnestic) recipient antibody response to foreign RBC antigens. These antibodies are undetected at the time of transfusion but increase after transfusion in a manner analogous to the vaccination "booster" effect. These reactions typically occur 3 to 14 days after transfusion but are unrecognized because of the lack of a clear temporal association with transfusion. Fever, chills, and an unexplained decline in Hct are the usual signs.[75] Transient elevation in bilirubin and lactate dehydrogenase may also occur. The diagnosis is established by a positive direct antiglobulin (Coombs) test resulting from recipient antibody coating donor RBCs. The antibody may be identified by eluting it from the RBCs or by demonstrating it within the recipient's serum. The specificity of the antibody is often against such RBC antigens as the Rh family, Kidd, Duffy, or Kell systems. Hemolysis may not occur, but if it does, it is likely to be extravascular and only rarely causes renal failure or DIC.

Prevention of these reactions is difficult. Alloimmunization to foreign RBC antigens occurs in approximately 1% of transfusions.[67] Detection of delayed antibodies is the purpose for requiring a new blood bank specimen every 72 hours if the patient has recently been transfused. Permanent transfusion records should record the occurrence of delayed antibodies, even though they may not be apparent at a later crossmatch. Access to transfusion databases is critical for the care of patients with a past history of transfusion.

Transfusion-Related Acute Lung Injury

Transfusion-related acute lung injury (TRALI) is an uncommon (0.02%)[76] but serious adverse effect of transfusion that has only recently been gaining recognition. Similar reactions have been called *pulmonary leukoagglutinin reaction* or *noncardiogenic pulmonary edema.* These reactions consist of acute respiratory distress syndrome (ARDS), which develops 1 to 6 hours after transfusion. Signs and symptoms include bilateral pulmonary infiltrates, hypoxemia, fever, and occasionally hypotension. Monitored patients are found to have normal or low pulmonary wedge pressure and central venous pressure, as contrasted with patients experiencing volume overload. If adequate respiratory support and oxygenation are established promptly, spontaneous resolution generally occurs within 1 to 4 days. Deaths have nonetheless occurred, particularly with a delay in diagnosis.[77,78]

Episodes of TRALI appear to have several possible causative mechanisms. Some cases may be caused by donor antibodies reacting with recipient neutrophil or HLA antigens.[79] Plasma factors related to blood storage have also been implicated, such as lipid substances from deterioration of donor cell membranes that prime recipient neutrophils, which then damage the pulmonary vasculature and lead to increased capillary permeability and an ARDS-like syndrome.[80] Other clinical factors may contribute to increased risk, such as cardiac bypass surgery or other procedures. In the antibody model at least, the implicated antibody is unique to the donor and the afflicted recipient will probably not experience another such reaction, provided that the recipient is not exposed to the same donor. TRALI is undoubtedly under-recognized in the critical care setting and may frequently be confused with fluid overload or cardiogenic pulmonary edema.

Transfusion-Associated Graft-versus-Host Disease

Transfusion-associated GVHD (TA-GVHD) is a well-documented, but probably under-recognized, highly lethal immunologic complication of blood transfusion.[81] Immunocompromised patients infused with blood components containing viable donor lymphocytes are at risk for engraftment of the allogeneic lymphocytes and ensuing rejection of recipient (host) tissues. Transfusion recipients who are at highest risk include neonates, especially the very premature, bone marrow and organ transplant recipients, and leukemia and lymphoma patients. TA-GVHD has also been reported in patients after cardiac surgery who received designated donor blood from relatives; presumably, the HLA antigenic differences between donor and recipient were insufficient to stimulate a recipient immune response but sufficient to elicit a donor immune response.[82] The onset of TA-GVHD is usually within 8 to 30 days after transfusion, and it is manifested as fever and rash, followed by diarrhea and evidence of liver and bone marrow injury. TA-GVHD differs from that seen in bone marrow transplantation (BMT) by its involvement of the marrow and by far greater mortality. Treatment is largely ineffective, and mortality exceeds 90%.

Irradiation of blood components at 25 Gy prevents TA-GVHD by eliminating the donor lymphocyte mitogenic response. All cellular blood components should be irradiated before transfusion to high-risk patients. The functions of the cellular components of blood are unaffected, although damage to RBC membranes limits postirradiation storage of PRBCs.[83] Blood donated by a relative for any patient should be irradiated, as should HLA-matched or crossmatched platelet products.

Transfusion-Associated Immunosuppression

Allogeneic blood transfusion has been shown to modulate and suppress the recipient's immune response, an effect first noted with kidney transplantation.[84] Immunosuppression in a critical care setting is generally undesirable, but whether transfusion has a significant impact is debated. Ongoing clinical issues center around two areas of controversy: the putative association between blood transfusion and increased numbers of postoperative infections and increased and more rapid rates of tumor recurrence in surgical oncology patients with certain malignancies. There has been no resolution of either issue despite a few prospective trials having been performed. The largest prospective trial of colorectal cancer resection, for example, is negative,[85] but a meta-analysis of the extant data suggests that an adverse effect on recurrence does exist.[86] Similarly, most of the randomized trials of postoperative or critical care unit infections are too small to indicate an effect of transfusion, but all point in the direction of an adverse effect.[87,88] Controversy will continue until larger randomized trials are conducted.

The precise mechanism of the immunosuppression induced by allogeneic transfusion has not yet been delineated, and several mechanisms may be involved.[89] Alterations identified in laboratory and clinical transfusion recipients have included depression of the T-helper/T-suppressor lymphocyte ratio, decreased natural killer cell activity, diminished interleukin-2 generation, formation of anti-idiotype antibodies, impairment of phagocytic cell function, and chronic persistence of donor lymphocytes (microchimerism), suggestive of low-level GVHD. Difficulties in analysis of human data arise because patients requiring blood transfusions have conditions that themselves induce immune changes. There is some evidence, bolstered by the results of two large clinical trials, to suggest that leukocyte reduction of blood components reduces or eliminates this immunosuppressive effect.[90] Proponents of this viewpoint argue that for this reason, ULR would benefit most patients receiving blood transfusions and lead to fewer infections, tumor recurrences, and other related putative risks of transfusion, all potentially resulting in saving lives and cost. Prospective trials will be extremely important.[91]

Transfusion-Transmitted Infectious Diseases

Public awareness of transfusion-associated acquired immunodeficiency syndrome (AIDS) has done more to revolutionize transfusion practice than any other transfusion risk by resulting in more conservative blood use, more stringent donor selection criteria, and improved screening tests. The result is that viral transmission rates are now difficult to measure, and the risk of transfusion-related infectious diseases is lower than ever.[92] The current best estimate is that 3 to 4 units per 10,000 will transmit some kind of infection[93] if agents such as CMV or Epstein-Barr virus are included. Bacterial infection has become the most common infectious risk thanks to increasingly sensitive donor screening tests, including nucleic acid testing (NAT) to detect viral DNA or RNA, which has shortened the infectious period and reduced the risk for post-transfusion hepatitis (PTH) and other viral infections.

Microbial and Endotoxin Contamination

Several fatalities are reported yearly from the transfusion of blood components contaminated with viable, proliferating bacteria, with or without the accumulation of endotoxin.[94] Platelet concentrates, because they must be stored at room temperature, are particularly prone to bacterial growth, with a reported incidence of 6 in 10,000 transfusions.[95] Organisms isolated from platelets and implicated in fatal transfusion reactions include *Staphylococcus* and *Streptococcus* species and gram-negative bacilli. Fatalities resulting from bacterial contamination of refrigerated RBCs have occurred as well and more often involve cryophilic bacteria. RBC transfusions contaminated by *Yersinia enterocolitica* have been consistently reported for a decade.[96] Transfusion reactions caused by bacterial or endotoxin contamination are fortunately quite rare, but mortality exceeds 60%.

Signs and symptoms of reactions caused by microbial contamination overlap those of hemolytic transfusion reactions and consist primarily of fever and hypotension, along with other signs of endotoxic shock. If recognized promptly, a Gram stain of the implicated unit can be prepared immediately and, if positive, appropriate antibiotic and supportive therapy instituted. Autologous blood components may also be contaminated at the time of collection; therefore, reactions occurring in patients who are receiving their own blood should not be dismissed but instead should be evaluated as fully as though the patients had received allogeneic blood.

Hepatitis

The success of viral screening measures is most clearly illustrated by the fall in the risk for PTH over the past 2 decades. Although PTH continues to be a significant cause of morbidity and mortality, the nature of PTH has changed through the years with the stepwise institution of various donor screening measures. The elimination of paid donors in 1972 and the successive introduction of immunologic tests for hepatitis B have resulted in a steady reduction in the rates of PTH caused by hepatitis B virus (HBV) to approximately 17 per million units of transfused blood products. Although about 30% to 40% of HBV transmissions will result in acute hepatitis, chronic HBV infection develops in less than 10% of such patients. In contrast, the risk for chronic hepatitis C virus (HCV) infection after transfusion is higher, nearly 50%, and the long-term risk for cirrhosis- or hepatocellular carcinoma–related mortality is about 15% over more than 20 years after PTH secondary to HCV.[97,98] The clinical course of hepatitis A is generally milder, and the lack of a chronic carrier state means that with donor screening for symptoms of the acute illness, the risk of transmission is much lower, estimated at less than one in a million units.[99]

The prevalence of hepatitis B surface antigenemia among first-time blood donors is 0.7%, and the prevalence of hepatitis C antibodies in donors is approximately 0.1% to 0.5%. At this time, given the sensitivity of current screening assays, including the latest generation of enzyme immunoassays (EIAs) and NAT, the current risk of PTH resulting from HCV is believed to be about 1 in 150,000 or less.[100] Although HBV is still implicated in PTH (attributable to the seronegative "window" period in newly infected donors), the risk of transfusion-associated hepatitis B is about 1 in 200,000 units.[100]

Retroviruses

Retroviruses, RNA-based viruses characterized by their reverse transcriptase and integration into the host genome, and lentiviruses, a subset of retroviruses, are ubiquitous in animals and were initially identified in humans in the early 1980s. Those known to be capable of transmission by transfusion are HIV-1, HIV-2, and human T-cell leukemia/lymphoma virus (HTLV) I and II.

Transfusion-associated AIDS was initially reported in late 1982.[101] The first report of an associated viral agent did not appear until late in 1983, and in March 1985 the screening enzyme-linked immunosorbent assay (ELISA) to detect antibody to HIV-1 was licensed and immediately incorporated into the blood-screening process. Improved confidential donor screening appeared to decrease the risk of infectious units appearing in the donor pool.[102,103] The discovery that heat treatment reduced transmission resulted in a reduction in transmission by plasma products, especially to persons with hemophilia. Clinical AIDS developed in more than 90% of recipients of infected blood products, and the vast majority succumbed to the disease. Removal of donor units with seropositivity by ELISA was insufficient to prevent transmission of HIV-1; several hundred cases were reported annually after introduction of the ELISA test. Subsequent development of an assay for the p24 antigen and then NAT has lowered the risk of transfusion-associated HIV-1 infection to less than one in a million (see Table 80-3).

Despite donor screening and sensitive assays, including EIA, NAT, and p24 antigen, an extremely small, but finite risk of HIV-1 transmission by screened blood transfusions remains. This risk is largely due to the seronegative "window" period experienced by newly infected donors, which is estimated to be an average of 16 days.[100]

A second retrovirus, HIV-2, first described in residents of countries in West Africa and subsequently detected in migrants to western Europe, causes an immunodeficiency syndrome similar to that caused by HIV-1. Although very few cases of HIV-2 have been reported in the United States[104,105] and there have been no reported transfusion-transmitted cases, experience with other retroviruses suggests that screening may prevent the majority of potential transmission. Therefore, donated blood is now screened by an assay for the presence of antibody to HIV-2.

The retrovirus HTLV-I is the causative agent of adult T-cell leukemia (ATL) and is strongly implicated in the chronic, progressive neurologic disorder termed *tropical spastic paraparesis* or *HTLV-I–associated myelopathy* (TSP/HAM). HTLV-II has been linked to hairy cell leukemia, but no transfusion-transmitted cases have been reported. The virus exhibits strong serologic cross-reactivity with HTLV-I such that screening assays fail to distinguish between antibodies to either virus.

Transfusion-transmitted HTLV-I has been demonstrated.[106] TSP/HAM has developed in a small percentage of infected transfusion recipients, but no transfusion-associated cases of ATL have been seen. Approximately 0.025% of donors in the United States are seropositive for HTLV-I and HTLV-II[107]; further testing reveals the majority of them to be HTLV-II. Donated blood is currently screened for antibodies to HTLV-I and HTLV-II. The estimated risk of HTLV transmission by screened negative blood is believed to be 1 in 250,000 to 2 million.

Cytomegalovirus

CMV is a human herpesvirus that establishes latent infection in the host's tissues, particularly leukocytes, and is transmitted by all cellular blood components.[108] Seropositivity, or the presence of antibody, denotes previous exposure to the virus but does not confer protective immunity. Secondary reinfection or reactivation of latent infection can occur. Antibodies to CMV persist for life and serve as a marker indicating the potential for transmission of live virus.

Immunocompetent recipients of transfused CMV-positive blood experience minimal morbidity and mortality. The majority are asymptomatic, whereas a heterophile-negative mononucleosis syndrome may develop in a few. Immunocompromised patients, however, may suffer life-threatening manifestations such as severe interstitial pneumonitis, gastroenteritis, hepatitis, or disseminated disease. Several groups of patients are at particular risk (Box 80-1),[109] and these patients should receive blood incapable of transmitting the virus. Other patients may benefit from CMV-negative blood as well, such as seronegative solid organ transplant recipients or autologous BMT patients. Screening of donated blood for CMV is not routinely done but can be performed quickly if necessary. Because the prevalence of donor seropositivity is quite high in some regions (50% to 70%), CMV-seronegative blood may not be readily available. Blood that is leukocyte depleted ("CMV safe") may be as effective as seronegative blood in the prevention of CMV transmission, although a recent meta-analysis of clinical trials comparing the two methods suggests that CMV-negative blood products might have a slight advantage over leukocyte-depleted products.[110]

Parasites

Many blood-borne parasites may be transmitted by transfusion, although this is a rare occurrence in the United States because of donor screening questions and the low endemicity of implicated agents.[111] Changing immigration patterns and worldwide travel, however, make transfusion-transmitted parasites an increasing concern.

On a worldwide basis, malaria is the most important transfusion-transmitted infective organism, although only about three cases occur in the United States each year. Such infections are manifested by delayed fever, chills,

Box 80-1

Patients for Whom Cytomegalovirus-Safe Blood Components Are Strongly Recommended

- Seronegative pregnant women
- Seronegative premature infants weighing less than 1200 g
- Seronegative allogeneic or autologous bone marrow transplant recipients
- Seronegative transplant recipients of seronegative organs

diaphoresis, and hemolysis, often masked by underlying medical conditions. Fatalities have occurred. Babesiosis, a tick-borne disease, is endemic in regions of the United States, especially the northeast, with a seroprevalence of about 4%. Transfusion-transmitted cases have been reported, with asplenic or immunocompromised patients being particularly susceptible. With increases in the number of Latin American immigrants to the United States, American trypanosomiasis (Chagas' disease), which is endemic in Latin American countries, has emerged as a potential pathogen. Other parasitic diseases that have been transmitted by transfusion include toxoplasmosis, leishmaniasis, and Lyme disease.

Emerging Infections in Transfusion Medicine

Parvovirus B19 has now been recognized as a pathogen capable of transmission by transfusion, with typical clinical findings and the potential for severe hematologic complications. Cases of Epstein-Barr virus infection with a typical mononucleosis-like illness have been reported after transfusion. West Nile virus has also been transmitted by transfusion. H2N1 influenza, severe acute respiratory syndrome (SARS), and other new viral infections should be capable of transmission by transfusion, although cases have not been reported and the prevalence of asymptomatic disease is unknown. A rising area of concern is the transmission of prion disease, either Jacob-Creutzfeldt disease or bovine spongiform encephalopathy (BSE). Donor referral criteria were implemented in 1987 for these diseases, and transmission of BSE has been reported in the United Kingdom.

SPECIAL TRANSFUSION SITUATIONS IN THE CRITICAL CARE SETTING

Massive Transfusion

Massive transfusion is defined as the administration of blood components in excess of one blood volume within a 24-hour period. In an average adult (70 kg), this represents approximately 10 units of WB or equivalent PRBCs, crystalloid solution, and other components. Massive transfusion, especially in the range of 20 or more units of blood products, causes complications not generally seen in usual transfusion practice: accumulation of undesirable substances present within banked blood and dilutional depletion of normal blood constituents that are lacking in stored units. Trauma victims, surgical patients undergoing extensive procedures, and patients with vascular or coagulation disorders may be massively transfused in the critical care setting. Survival of the massive transfusion episode is determined more by the nature and degree of the patient's injuries or medical conditions than by the transfusions themselves, but the presence of adverse effects of massive transfusion can complicate patients' courses in the ICU.

Transfusion of large quantities of stored blood deficient in functional platelets often results in hemostatic defects or outright thrombocytopenia. Circulating platelets consistently decrease in inverse proportion to the amount of blood administered, with the hemostatically significant level of 50×10^9/L reached after 20 U.[112,113] Functional defects have also been noted, and the bleeding time is prolonged.[114] Despite these laboratory changes, severe diffuse bleeding develops in less than 20% of massively transfused patients, and no laboratory studies predict those who will. Prophylactic platelet transfusion has not been shown to be of benefit.[115] Platelet counts may return to hemostatically effective levels quickly in patients with normal marrow function.

Currently, resuscitation of massively bleeding patients is most often accomplished with PRBCs in combination with crystalloid solution. This should result in hemodilution to about 60% of normal plasma factor levels after the transfusion of about 10 units; this factor level can effect normal hemostasis. In reality, however, crystalloids may be given in excess of PRBCs, so after 10 units is transfused, less plasma protein may remain. Bleeding is unlikely until prothrombin time (PT)/INR and PTT prolongations exceed 1.5 to 1.8 times the midpoint normal range, the equivalent of an INR approaching 2.0.[113] As with platelets, prophylactic administration of FFP has not proved effective in preventing diffuse bleeding.[116] Thus, the decision to transfuse should be made on an individual basis, as determined by the presence of bleeding or unacceptable risk in patients with documented abnormalities in coagulation.

One new area of controversy in the treatment of patients with massive hemorrhage is the use of recombinant activated factor VII. This new agent was created for the treatment of hemophiliac patients with high titers of antibodies to factor VIII, which makes them unable to benefit from transfusion of recombinant factor VIII. Activated factor VII bypasses that problem by binding to tissue factor and directly activating thrombin and hence generating fibrin.[117] It is extremely expensive, has a short half-life, and carries a risk of inducing pathologic thrombosis, with potentially grave consequences. Nevertheless, in numerous case reports, this new agent appears to potentially be beneficial if used early in the resuscitation of massively injured patients. Unfortunately, its unsupervised use has also resulted in thrombotic complications and relative lack of success, both of which suggest that carefully controlled clinical trials are appropriate.[118]

Blood preservative solutions contain excess citrate, which anticoagulates stored blood by binding ionized calcium. WB contains approximately 1.8 g of citrate/citric acid per unit in the plasma fraction. Patients with normal liver function can metabolize the citrate load in 1 unit of WB in 5 minutes, but hepatic impairment may extend removal to 15 minutes or longer. Toxicity may result when citrate is administered in excess of the metabolic rate, thereby causing a decrease in ionized calcium levels.[119] Although paresthesias, cramps, and myoclonus accompany citrate excess, the chief danger of hypocalcemia is depression of myocardial contractility and potential prolongation of the QT interval. Because the effects of citrate are transient and the use of PRBCs containing little residual citrated plasma is far more common than massive transfusion with WB, routine administration of calcium is not indicated; clinically significant rebound hypercalcemia may result. Calcium infusion should be limited to hypoperfused patients with hepatic or cardiac failure who manifest citrate toxicity, and careful monitoring is essential.

As potassium leaks from RBCs during storage, up to 7 mEq of extracellular potassium may accumulate in each unit. However, dangerous levels of potassium rarely develop in adults from stored blood; the potassium level is more likely to be determined by the patient's acid-base status.[117] Studies of massively transfused patients have demonstrated a wide range of potassium levels, with hypokalemia seen as frequently as hyperkalemia. Because of the many physiologic mechanisms altered during resuscitation, including those of the respiratory, renal, cardiac, and hepatic systems, it is impossible to predict the net effect of massive transfusion on serum potassium levels.

The pH of banked blood drops during storage, from 7.16 at the time of collection to as low as 6.73 after several weeks of storage. Administration of large quantities of acidic blood, together with the metabolic acidosis common in these patients before resuscitation, would lead one to expect worsening acidosis as the outcome of massive transfusion. However, patients are more likely to exhibit metabolic alkalosis at the end of the transfusion episode,[120,121] partly because of improved tissue perfusion and the metabolism of citrate and lactate to bicarbonate. Patients in renal failure may be unable to handle the bicarbonate load and require dialysis. Acidosis persisting after transfusion suggests inadequate tissue perfusion.[119] Empiric administration of bicarbonate to counter the acid load is not warranted and may contribute to the deleterious effects of hypercapnia in patients with impaired ventilation.

As discussed previously, the level of RBC-associated 2,3-DPG in banked blood declines during storage, which increases the affinity of hemoglobin for oxygen and thereby results in decreased oxygen off-loaded to tissues. Even in massively transfused patients, it has been difficult to document a clinical impact of this shift, and no reliable method for restoring red cell 2,3-DPG has been developed.

WB and PRBCs are stored at approximately 4°C and require 30 to 45 minutes to warm to room temperature. Elective transfusions at standard flow rates are tolerated without the need to warm the blood; however, core body temperature, measured by esophageal probe, can fall to 30°C or lower with the administration of large volumes of cold blood over a period of 1 to 2 hours.[122] Adverse effects of hypothermia include a decreased heart rate and myocardial contractility, cardiac arrhythmias, increased affinity of hemoglobin for oxygen resulting in decreased tissue oxygen delivery, DIC, and impaired ability to metabolize the citrate load of stored blood. Both blood warmers and patient warming may be instituted during massive transfusion, and patient core temperature should be monitored during such resuscitative efforts.

Whether massive transfusion in and of itself is a cause of ARDS is another source of controversy. There are certainly theoretical reasons why massive transfusion might precipitate ARDS: all cellular transfusions contain damaged or activated WBCs, cell membranes, aggregated platelets, and microthrombi, all of which are capable of lodging in and damaging pulmonary capillaries. Despite this possibility, neither microfiltration of transfusions nor routine leukocyte depletion has shown a significant impact on the incidence of ARDS in massively transfused patients.[123] Certainly, other causes of ARDS exist in patients who undergo massive transfusion, and the possibility of volume overload and TRALI should be considered in the evaluation of patients with hypoxia and diffuse pulmonary infiltrates after massive transfusion. Management of such patients is supportive, consistent with the overall management of massive transfusion.[124,125]

Autoimmune Hemolytic Anemia

Patients with autoimmune hemolytic anemia (AIHA) have an autoantibody, usually of broad specificity, that fixes itself to their RBCs and triggers extravascular immune-mediated destruction. Patients with AIHA have a positive direct antiglobulin test[126] (DAT, commonly known as the Coombs test) and varying degrees of hemolysis, and their autoantibodies cause agglutination of RBCs from all donors during crossmatching. If the hemolysis is brisk, patients may require red cell transfusion to support oxygen needs before medical management of the AIHA is effective. Hence, transfusion is difficult because agglutination during crossmatching interferes with proper definition of compatible units of RBCs and because the transfused RBCs are themselves subject to the same immune hemolysis as the host RBCs. Many blood banks have methods for depletion of autoantibodies from the recipient's plasma and elution of antibodies from RBCs to arrive at a proper crossmatch.[127] Although such crossmatches are time consuming and not generally available on an emergency basis, they can be lifesaving. Criteria for transfusion should remain the same as for other recipients.

Necessary Transfusion of Incompatible Blood

RBCs are crossmatched for red cell antigens in the ABO and $Rh_0(D)$ group and for other red cell antigens when antibodies are present. However, there are several hundred other red cell antigens in the human family, and with repeated transfusion recipients may become alloimmunized to other antigens. Generally, alloimmunization occurs in approximately 1% of transfusions,[68] but the prevalence of alloantibodies is higher in chronically transfused, relatively immunocompetent patients, especially African Americans, whose distribution of red cell antigens has significant variation from the white population. Alloimmunization rates of 30% or higher may be found in chronically transfused patients with hemoglobinopathies who have not received RBCs matched to potent minor antigens such as Kell, Duffy, and Lewis. Alloimmunization may present difficulties in crossmatching of blood, to the point that compatible blood must be obtained from rare-donor registries, if at all. Other patients present unresolved serologic problems in that the alloantibody is never precisely identified yet the majority of blood available for transfusion is incompatible. The delay engendered by working with multiple or unidentified antibodies may be unacceptable in some critical care situations in which the need for oxygen-carrying capacity leaves no choice but to transfuse incompatible blood. The behavior of these antibodies in the laboratory may assist in predicting the clinical outcome of the incompatible transfusion.[128] Special procedures such as clearance studies,[129] flow cytometry[130] and in vivo crossmatching (cautious administration of a small aliquot of blood, with subsequent observation of serum and urine for evidence of hemolysis) are useful if time permits.

Emergency transfusion of type O, Rh-negative uncrossmatched blood is generally reserved for the resuscitation of trauma patients, for whom the delay in crossmatching may be life-threatening. The risks of alloimmunization are generally accepted as low. Even Rh-positive type O RBCs may be used because rates of alloimmunization to $Rh_0(D)$ are low under the circumstances of emergency transfusion.[128,131]

Transfusion in Patients with Disseminated Intravascular Coagulation

DIC can present the clinician with difficult therapeutic choices. This common disorder in critically ill patients may be manifested as severe hemorrhage or thrombosis. Therapy is primarily directed at alleviating the cause and supporting the patient. Supportive therapy includes the transfusion of components needed to correct the bleeding diathesis caused by the consumption of platelets and fibrinogen, in addition to PRBCs to restore oxygen-carrying capacity. Platelets and fibrinogen (as cryoprecipitate) are the most useful components needed to repair the coagulopathy, but their use risks merely "fueling the fire" and increasing the microthrombosis of DIC. Heparin anticoagulation is controversial[132,133] and may increase the risk of bleeding, especially if depleted factors are not replenished. No definitive clinical trials have endorsed the routine use of heparin, and randomized trials of other components and coagulation inhibitors have uniformly been negative. In general, the use of heparin and antifibrinolytic agents has been confined to the most severe and protracted cases of DIC.[134]

Hepatic Failure

Cirrhotic patients or those with fulminant hepatic failure have a variety of hemostatic disorders that complicate transfusion management of a bleeding patient.[135] Hepatic synthesis of coagulation factors may be markedly diminished, thereby necessitating replacement by FFP or cryoprecipitate. Patterns of factor diminution may vary between acute hepatic necrosis and chronic cirrhosis.[136] Associated hemodynamic alterations may make it impossible to administer the volumes required for effective hemostasis, however, and any effect is transient. The use of factor concentrates or antifibrinolytic agents may precipitate thrombosis. Activation of fibrinolysis and decreased clearance of activated factors may produce or mimic chronic DIC, thus further exacerbating the factor deficiencies and impairing coagulation. Abnormal platelet function and thrombocytopenia may contribute to the coagulopathy of liver disease, with concomitant splenomegaly reducing the effectiveness of platelet transfusions.

Uremia

Bleeding in uremic patients is exacerbated by an acquired platelet defect, in part secondary to dialyzable circulating molecules soluble in platelet membranes. Platelet-associated vWF and plasma high-molecular-weight vWF multimers have also been shown to be decreased,[137] which may explain the benefit shown by DDAVP[138] and cryoprecipitate in shortening the bleeding time and improving hemostasis in some uremic patients. Raising the Hct by red cell transfusion in anemic patients has also been shown to shorten the bleeding time, presumably as a result of blood vessel wall–laminar blood flow interaction. Transfusion of platelets in the absence of thrombocytopenia is unlikely to be of benefit because the transfused platelets rapidly become dysfunctional. More aggressive hemodialysis is the most widely accepted method of reducing platelet dysfunction.

Bone Marrow Transplantation

BMT patients are vulnerable to the severe infectious and toxic side effects of ablative treatment and hence may be cared for in critical care units. These patients may have intensive red cell and platelet transfusion requirements and need specialized products such as CMV-negative and irradiated blood components. A blood bank problem uniquely encountered in BMT is the need to switch the patient's ABO group because of an ABO-mismatched transplant, thus necessitating an exchange transfusion of red cells and plasma-containing products (i.e., platelet concentrates) of differing ABO type to avoid hemolysis of donor and recipient cells. BMT patients may also manifest an increased rate of delayed hemolytic reactions[139] as donor "passenger" lymphocytes recognize recipient or transfused red cell antigens. Patients should be monitored particularly closely between days 10 and 20 after a minor-mismatched allogeneic transplant, and aggressive transfusion should be undertaken if the hemoglobin level falls and the DAT result becomes positive.

ALTERNATIVES TO TRANSFUSION OF BLOOD COMPONENTS

The safest transfusion is one that is not given. Therefore, alternatives to blood component therapy continue to be sought and are valuable adjuncts in some instances. It is possible to limit homologous blood exposure by the appropriate use of pharmacologic agents that promote hemostasis and the administration of recombinant hematopoietic growth factors or biologic growth modifiers to stimulate marrow hematopoiesis.

Blood Substitutes

Only one substitute for RBC transfusions has been approved in the United States, a polyfluorocarbon oxygen carrier with significant limitations as a blood substitute.[140] Other preparations that have been explored in clinical trials are cell-free hemoglobin solutions cross-linked or polymerized by chemical manipulation to prevent rapid clearance from the circulation. They are intended to provide short-term oxygen-carrying capacity for acutely ill patients and have the advantage of not requiring cross-matching or infection control. Although these proposed products may have a longer shelf-life and are easier to transport, their drawbacks are many. Most have a circulatory half-life of only about 24 hours. The oxygen dissociation curve for these substitutes is also frequently not favorable: either a high FIO_2 is required to "load" these molecules or they are less likely to deliver oxygen efficiently at lower PO_2 levels.[141]

Because the hemoglobin source is reclaimed bovine or human red cells, it is unlikely that patients who do not accept blood components because of their religious beliefs (Jehovah's Witnesses) will accept these types of hemoglobin solutions. One product in development uses recombinant technology to generate hemoglobin, and it is hoped that this solution may be acceptable to these patients.

The licensed perfluorocarbon solutions have failed to demonstrate any utility as intravascular oxygen carriers because of their unfavorable P-50 (oxygen half-saturation pressure) and oxygen off-loading characteristics. They are finding limited application in regional oxygenation during angioplasty or stent placement procedures and a more novel use in "liquid ventilation." This involves the ventilation of intubated patients experiencing severe pulmonary compromise with superoxygenated perfluorocarbon solutions in place of oxygen-enriched air.[142]

Desmopressin

The synthetic vasopressin analogue DDAVP increases plasma factor VIII:c and promotes the release of vWF from endothelial stores.[143] DDAVP has provided effective hemostasis in bleeding patients with mild hemophilia A and type I von Willebrand's disease and has been used as prophylaxis for patients undergoing surgery. DDAVP reportedly improves platelet function in some patients with qualitative platelet disorders associated with uremia,[136] cirrhosis, and aspirin ingestion. Studies of its efficacy in cardiopulmonary bypass procedures are conflicting, but a subset of these patients may benefit. The chief drawback to its use is tachyphylaxis, which develops in essentially all cases after short-term repeated administration.

Antifibrinolytic Agents

The lysine analogues ε-aminocaproic acid and tranexamic acid inhibit fibrinolysis by blocking the binding of plasminogen and plasmin to fibrin. These antifibrinolytic agents may decrease bleeding and thus the need for homologous blood components in patients with hemophilia, thrombocytopenia, and systemic fibrinolysis. A novel and effective use of tranexamic acid involves administration as a mouthwash in preparation for oral surgery in patients with hemophilia or those receiving oral anticoagulant therapy.[144] The most serious side effect of these agents when systemically administered is thrombosis; thus, it is important to use them appropriately and monitor the patient carefully during their use.

Aprotinin is a naturally occurring bovine serine protease inhibitor that acts on plasma serine proteases such as plasmin, kallikrein, trypsin, and some coagulation proteins. Aprotinin has been shown to reduce blood loss in patients undergoing cardiopulmonary bypass surgery[145] by inhibiting fibrinolysis and preventing platelet damage. However, more recent reports of renal injury and long-term mortality may mean an end to its use.[146] Aprotinin has been used extensively in liver transplantation, which involves high blood loss. Repeated administration poses the risk of anaphylaxis and renal dysfunction.

Vitamin K

When time permits, vitamin K is the preferred agent to reverse the coagulopathy induced by oral anticoagulants. Normalization of the PT can be seen in as few as 6 to 12 hours. Additionally, selected cirrhotic patients may exhibit improvement in the PT when treated with therapeutic doses of vitamin K. Many patients in critical care units exhibit a prolonged PT, especially if dietary supplements are limited and broad-spectrum antibiotic therapy is given. Vitamin K is a safe and effective agent for reversing this effect.

Hematopoietic Growth Factors

Recombinant erythropoietin (EPO) has dramatically reduced the red cell transfusion requirements of patients in chronic renal failure. EPO also has applications in the adjunctive treatment of the anemia of premature infants and the anemia of chronic disease, especially rheumatoid arthritis, cancer, and AIDS. Studies of its efficacy in reducing perioperative red cell transfusion requirements by increasing the yield of predeposited autologous blood or stimulating bone marrow synthesis after surgery have shown benefit in reducing blood transfusion, although preoperative planning and autologous deposits are required.[147] In contrast and probably because the impact of EPO is not immediate, the efficacy of EPO in the ICU is unproven and awaits the results of large clinical trials.

Recombinant growth factors such as granulocyte-macrophage colony-stimulating factor (GM-CSF) and G-CSF stimulate marrow production of leukocytes by enhancing several different granulocyte and macrophage functions. These agents are finding application in reducing the neutropenic period in BMT and cancer chemotherapy by increasing the leukocyte count in hypoproliferative marrow conditions. These myeloid growth factors are replacing granulocyte transfusions for their few remaining indications.

Cell Salvage Technology

Cell salvage equipment has been in clinical use for several decades, and although cell salvage is clearly capable of rescuing otherwise "lost" red cells, its full impact on transfusions has been poorly documented. Cell salvage generally consists of collection of shed blood from a clean, uncontaminated operating field, followed by removal of the cellular elements and retransfusion into the patient. Cell salvage has been used both intraoperatively and postoperatively, especially in cardiac surgery. Although the clinical studies of cell salvage have many flaws, the overall success of this therapy in reducing transfusion has resulted in its wide application.[148] Risks include bacterial contamination, febrile reactions, triggering of DIC, and coagulopathy as a result of dilution. When combined with acute intraoperative hemodilution, this technology is also potentially cost saving.[149]

Therapeutic Apheresis

The word *apheresis* is derived from the Greek *aphairein,* "to take away"; thus, therapeutic hemapheresis is performed to remove unwanted plasma constituents (plasmapheresis) or blood cells (cytapheresis). Automated cell separators use centrifugation or membrane filtration to remove and concentrate the selected blood element. Many of the same devices used to prepare apheresis blood components for transfusion are used to perform patient procedures, so therapeutic apheresis is often administered under the auspices of the transfusion medicine service. Rapid removal of plasma or cells may find several applications in intensive care practice (Box 80-2).

The goal of plasmapheresis, or plasma exchange (PE), is to remove or reduce the levels of an undesirable plasma constituent or, alternatively, by means of plasma replacement, to supply a missing substance. The agent to be removed by PE is thought to be an autoantibody in some of the neurologic, renal, or hematologic conditions treated in this manner.[150] Immunomodulation by PE is another explanation for its effect, a theory indirectly supported by the equivalent efficacy of IVIG therapy for several of these disorders.[151] PE for the amelioration of hyperviscosity from either excess IgM in Waldenström's macroglobulinemia or excess Ig in multiple myeloma is an effective temporizing measure in the treatment of these conditions.[152] Plasmapheresis with PE is the standard therapy for TTP.[153]

Box 80-2

Critical Care Indications for Emergency Hemapheresis

Plasmapheresis
- Symptomatic hyperviscosity
- Thrombotic thrombocytopenic purpura
- Neurologic diseases: myasthenia gravis, Guillain-Barré syndrome
- Uncontrolled systemic vasculitis with critical end-organ injury

Cytapheresis
- Symptomatic leukocytosis
- Symptomatic thrombocythemia
- Sickle cell anemia crisis (pulmonary or central nervous system manifestations)

Unfortunately, few controlled trials of PE exist, although anecdotal reports abound. PE is seldom the definitive treatment of most of these conditions and is used most appropriately as a short-term adjunct to other medical modalities. The kinetics of PE predicts that a one-volume exchange removes 65% of a given plasma constituent if the blood volume does not change or additional synthesis or mobilization of the substance does not occur. Two or three volume exchanges remove 87% and 95%, respectively. Highly protein-bound, intravascularly concentrated substances are most efficiently removed, whereas substances with a large volume of distribution such as IgG, active synthesis, or large extravascular stores are removed at less than predicted rates. The usual short-term intense course of PE schedules five one-volume exchanges (approximately 3 L in normal-sized adults) over a 7-day period. The appropriate replacement fluid in most conditions is an albumin-saline mixture, which provides oncotic support without the risk of disease transmission borne by FFP. PE in patients with TTP uses replacement with FFP to supply the plasma protease that is consumed during the disease.

Side effects of PE are relatively common (10% to 30% of procedures) but generally minor and are related to vascular access, temporary discomfort, or vasomotor symptoms.[154] Patient death is rarely due to the procedure itself but is largely of cardiopulmonary causes. Plasma proteins such as coagulation factors, immunoglobulins, and complement will be removed by PE, and laboratory test results of coagulation and electrolytes may be deranged in the hours after PE. Clinical bleeding is rarely observed. Most coagulation factors do not fall below hemostatic levels and recover within hours, with the exception of fibrinogen, which may require several days for complete replenishment.

Leukapheresis may be required to urgently reduce the WBC count in patients with acute myeloid or lymphoblastic leukemia or chronic myelogenous leukemia with peripheral counts of 100×10^9/L or greater. Each procedure is expected to drop the count by a third, but the effect is short lived. Leukapheresis should be reserved for use only as an adjunct to chemotherapy in patients with pulmonary or cerebral leukostasis or for cytoreduction before chemotherapy in patients at risk for severe tumor lysis syndrome.

Plateletpheresis may be beneficial as short-term therapy in patients with symptomatic thrombocythemia manifested as cerebral or myocardial ischemia, pulmonary emboli, or gastrointestinal bleeding. Each procedure should effect a 50% reduction in the platelet count. Cytotoxic therapy should be started concomitantly as the definitive treatment.

LEGAL ISSUES IN TRANSFUSION MEDICINE

Litigation related to blood transfusion has become prominent, particularly after the epidemic of transfusion-associated AIDS.[155] Most states regulate blood banking and medical practice, but blood products are regarded as a service, not as a commodity, so standard product liability does not pertain to blood components.[156] However, negligence in the course of preparing, testing, transferring, crossmatching, or administering blood products is still a potential cause for legal action. Every clinician who orders transfusions must be aware that blood components, like drugs, are approved for specific uses and that the indications should be clearly documented in the medical record.

The informed consent of the patient is an important area of potential liability. The Joint Commission on Accreditation of Healthcare Organizations (JCAHO) has required written patient consent for blood transfusions since 1996. What constitutes adequate informed consent and who is responsible for advising the patient are still in contention. Elements of informed consent include an understanding of the need for transfusion, its risks and benefits, and the alternatives, including the risk of not undergoing transfusion, as well as the opportunity to ask questions. Whether the clinician documents informed consent with an individual progress note in the patient record or with a standardized form is generally established as institutional policy. Similarly, institutions vary with respect to policies for consenting adults who are temporarily incompetent, such as sedated patients in the ICU.

A competent adult patient may refuse blood transfusion, and Jehovah's Witnesses commonly do so for religious reasons. Case law is clear in upholding this right of the patient,[157] which extends to care given at such time as the patient may become incompetent (i.e., comatose) after such refusal was expressed before becoming incompetent. Courts will usually order a lifesaving transfusion for minors. Exceptions have been made in the case of some "emancipated minors" who are at the age of reason. Most states have evoked a "special interest" in the welfare of a fetus in ordering transfusions to pregnant women.

The advent of sentinel event reviews and other quality management procedures for patient safety has had an impact on transfusion practice as well. Procedures for patient identification before surgical procedures, including devices such as bar code readers, have also been applied to transfusion practice. However, annual sentinel event reviews reporting transfusion errors have remained constant according to JCAHO records.[158]

KEY POINTS

- Blood components should be prescribed like drugs. Appropriate blood component therapy requires that the specific blood product needed for a clear indication be prescribed, with avoidance of a formulaic approach.
- Red blood cells should be transfused only to increase oxygen-carrying capacity. Transfusion decisions should be based on individual patient physiology. The majority of patients with hemoglobin levels greater than 60 or 70 g/L will not require transfusion unless they have limited cardiopulmonary reserve or active bleeding.
- Platelet transfusions are indicated for patients who are bleeding because of thrombocytopenia or functional platelet defects. Guidelines for platelet transfusion are also conservative. Prophylactic platelet transfusion remains controversial and is not warranted in many situations.
- Fresh frozen plasma is indicated for the repletion of coagulation factors in bleeding patients deficient in those factors or to provide specific plasma proteins that cannot be obtained from safer sources.
- Cryoprecipitate is a concentrated source of fibrinogen and selected coagulation factors. Cryoprecipitate may be more helpful in correcting the hypofibrinogenemia of dilutional or consumptive coagulopathy than fresh frozen plasma.
- Adverse reactions to blood components occur in 1% to 2% of transfusion episodes. Adherence to routine protocols for the evaluation of transfusion reactions may save lives.
- Acute hemolytic reactions are the leading cause of immediate transfusion fatalities. Prevention of these reactions requires strict adherence to transfusion and patient identification procedures.
- Transmission of infectious agents by transfusion has been markedly reduced, and bacterial infection is now the most common infectious complication of transfusion.
- Adverse effects unique to massive transfusion are likely to occur in the ICU and complicate the management of critically ill or severely injured patients. Component therapy for such patients should remain conservative. The emerging role of activated factor VII in the treatment of these patients requires further evaluation.
- Informed consent for blood transfusion is a standard of practice. A competent adult has the legal right to refuse blood transfusion. Consent in critically ill patients remains subject to individual institution policies.

REFERENCES

1. U.S. Department of Health and Human Services, Food and Drug Administration: The Code of Federal Regulations, 21 CFR Parts 600, 606, 640. Washington, DC, U.S. Government Printing Office, 1999.
2. Standards for Blood Banks and Transfusion Services, 21st ed. Bethesda, MD, American Association of Blood Banks, 2002.
3. Starkey JM, Mactherson JL, Bolgiano DC, et al: Markers for transfusion-transmitted disease in different groups of blood donors. JAMA 1989;262:3452-3454.
4. Whyte G, Coghlan P: Comparative safety of units donated by autologous, designated and allogeneic (homologous) donors. Transfus Med 1996;6:209-211.
5. Page PL: Directed blood donations: Con. Transfusion 1989;29:65-69.
6. Goldfinger D: Directed blood donations: Pro. Transfusion 1989;29:70-74.
7. Nilsson L, Hedner U, Nilsson IM, et al: Shelf-life of bank blood and stored plasma with special reference to coagulation factors. Transfusion 1983;23:377-381.

8. Shanwell A, Kristiansson M, Remberger M, et al: Generation of cytokines in red cell concentrates during storage is prevented by prestorage white cell reduction. Transfusion 1997;37:678-684.
9. Vamvakas EC, Blajchman MA: Universal WBC reduction: The case for and against. Transfusion 2001;41:691-712.
10. Latham JT, Bove JR, Weirich FL: Chemical and hematological changes in stored CPDA-1 blood. Transfusion 1982;22:158-159.
11. Valeri CR, Hirsch NM: Restoration in vitro of erythrocyte adenosine triphosphate, 2,3-diphosphoglycerate, potassium ion, and sodium ion concentrations following the transfusion of acid-citrate-dextrose stored human red blood cells. J Lab Clin Med 1969;73:722-733.
12. Manno CS, Hedberg KW, Kim HC, et al: Comparison of the hemostatic effects of fresh whole blood, stored whole blood, and components after open heart surgery in children. Blood 1991;77:930-936.
13. Littenberg B, Corwin HL, Gettinger A, et al: A practice guideline and decision aide for blood transfusion. Immunohematology 1995;11:88-94.
14. Corwin HC, Parsonnet KC, Gettinger A: RBC transfusion in the ICU: Is there a reason? Chest 1995;108:767-771.
15. Groeger JS, Guntapalli KK, Strosberg M, et al: Descriptive analysis of critical care units in the United States: Patient characteristics and intensive care unit utilization. Crit Care Med 1993;21:279-291.
16. Finch CA, Lenfant C: Oxygen transport in man. N Engl J Med 1972;286: 407-415.
17. Hebert PC, Van der Linden P, Biro G, et al: Physiologic aspects of anemia. Crit Care Clin 2004;20:187-212.
18. Wilkerson DK, Rosen AL, Gould SA, et al: Oxygen extraction ratio: A valid indicator of myocardial metabolism in anemia. J Surg Res 1987;42:629-634.
19. Weiskopf RB, Viele MK, Feiner J, et al: Human cardiovascular and metabolic response to acute, severe isovolemic anemia. JAMA 1998;279:217-221.
20. Spence RK, Alexander JB, Del Rossi AJ, et al: Transfusion guidelines for cardiovascular surgery: Lessons learned from operations in Jehovah's Witnesses. J Vasc Surg 1992;16: 825-829.
21. Levine E, Rosen A, Sehgal L, et al: Physiologic effects of acute anemia: Implications for a reduced transfusion trigger. Transfusion 1990;30:11-14.
22. Hebert PC, Wells G, Blajchman MA, et al: A multicenter, randomized, controlled clinical trial of transfusion requirements in critical care. N Engl J Med 1999;340:409-417.
23. Hebert PC, Yetisir E, Martin C, et al: Is a low transfusion threshold safe in critically ill patients with cardiovascular diseases? Crit Care Med 2001;29:227-234.
24. Levy PS, Chavez RP, Crystal GJ, et al: Oxygen extraction ratio: A valid indicator of transfusion need in limited coronary vascular reserve? J Trauma 1992;32:769-773.
25. Vincent JL, Baron J-F, Reinhart K, et al, for the ABC Investigators: Anemia and blood transfusion in critically ill patients. JAMA 2002;288:1499-1507.
26. Corwin HL, Gettinger A, Pearl RG, et al: The CRIT study: Anemia and blood transfusion in the critically ill—current clinical practice in the United States. Crit Care Med 2004;32:39-52.
27. Chohan SS, McArdle F, McClelland DBL, et al: Red cell transfusion practice following the Transfusion Requirements in Critical Care (TRICC) study: Prospective observational cohort study in a large UK intensive care unit. Vox Sang 2003;84:211-218.
28. French CJ, Bellomo R, Finfer SR, et al: Appropriateness of red blood cell transfusion in Australasian intensive care practice. Med J Aust 2002;177:548-551.
29. Grover M, Talkwalkar S, Casbard A, et al: Silent myocardial ischaemia and haemoglobin concentration: A randomized controlled trial of transfusion strategy in lower limb arthroplasty. Vox Sang 2006;90:105-112.
30. Weiskopf RB: Mathematical analysis of isovolemic hemodilution indicates that it can decrease the need for allogeneic blood transfusion. Transfusion 1995;35:37-41.
31. NIH Consensus Conference: Guidelines for perioperative red blood cell transfusions. JAMA 1988;260: 2700-2703.
32. American Society of Anesthesiologists Task Force: Practice guidelines for blood component therapy. Anesthesiology 1996;84:732-747.
33. Welch HG, Meehan KR, Goodnough LT: Prudent strategies for elective red blood cell transfusion. Ann Intern Med 1992;116:403-406.
34. Daly PA, Schiffer CA, Aisner J, et al: Platelet transfusion therapy. One-hour posttransfusion increments are valuable in predicting the need for HLA-matched preparations. JAMA 1980;243:435-438.
35. Waxman DA: Volunteer donor apheresis. Ther Apher 2002;6:77-81.
36. National Institutes of Health Consensus Conference: Platelet transfusion therapy. Transfus Med Rev 1987;1:195-200.
37. Harker LA, Slichter SI: The bleeding time as a screening test for evaluation of platelet function. N Engl J Med 1972;287:155-159.
38. Gelb AB, Roth RI, Levin J, et al: Changes in blood coagulation during and following cardiopulmonary bypass: Lack of correlation with clinical bleeding. Am J Clin Pathol 1996;106:87-99.
39. Bierling P, Farcet JP, Dvedari N, et al: Gamma globulin for idiopathic thrombocytopenic purpura. N Engl J Med 1982;307:1150-1151.
40. Scaradavou A, Woo B, Woloski BM, et al: Intravenous anti-D treatment of immune thrombocytopenic purpura: Experience in 272 patients. Blood 1997;89:2689-2700.
41. Harkness DR, Byrnes JJ, Lian EC-Y, et al: Hazard of platelet transfusion in thrombotic thrombocytopenic purpura. JAMA 1981;246:1931-1933.
42. Gaydos LA, Freireich EI, Mantel N: The quantitative relation between platelet count and hemorrhage in patients with acute leukemia, N Engl J Med 1962;266:905-909.
43. Slichter SI: Controversies in platelet transfusion therapy. Annu Rev Med 1980;31:509-540.
44. Gmur J, Burger J, Schanz U, et al: Safety of stringent prophylactic platelet transfusion policy for patients with acute leukemia. Lancet 1991;338:1223-1226.
45. Howard JE, Perkins HA: The natural history of alloimmunization to platelets. Transfusion 1978;18: 496-503.
46. Bishop JF, McGrath K, Wolf MM, et al: Clinical factors influencing the efficacy of pooled platelet transfusions. Blood 1988;71:383-387.
47. Heal JM, Blumberg N: Optimizing platelet transfusion therapy. Blood Rev 2004;18:149-165.
48. Klein HG, Dodd RY, Dzik WH, et al: Current status of solvent/detergent-treated frozen plasma. Transfusion 1998;38:102-107.
49. Solheim BG, Seghatchian J: Update on pathogen reduction technology for therapeutic plasma: An overview. Transfus Apher Sci 2006;35:83-90.
50. National Institutes of Health Consensus Conference: Fresh frozen plasma: Indications and risks. JAMA 1985;253:551-553.
51. Casbard AC, Williamson LM, Murphy MF, et al: The role of prophylactic fresh frozen plasma in decreasing blood loss and correcting coagulopathy in cardiac surgery: A systematic review. Anaesthesia 2004;59:550-558.
52. Manucci PM, Federici AB, Sirchia G: Hemostasis testing during massive blood replacement: A study of 172 cases. Vox Sang 1982;42:113-123.
53. Holland L, Sarode R: Should plasma be transfused prophylactically before invasive procedures? Curr Opin Hematol 2006;13:447-451.
54. Eckman MH, Erban JK, Singh SK, et al: Screening for the risk for bleeding or thrombosis. Ann Intern Med 2003;138:15-24.
55. McVay PA, Toy PTCY: Lack of increased bleeding after liver biopsy in patients with mild hemostatic abnormalities. Am J Clin Pathol 1990;94:747-753.
56. Snyder AJ, Gottschall JL, Menitove JE: Why is fresh-frozen plasma transfused? Transfusion 1986;26:107-112.
57. Spector I, Corn M, Ticktin HE: Effect of plasma transfusions on the prothrombin time and clotting factors in liver disease. N Engl J Med 1966;275:1032-1037.
58. Ciavarella D, Reed RL, Counts RB, et al: Clotting factor levels and the risk of diffuse microvascular bleeding in the massively transfused patient. Br J Haematol 1987;67:365-368.
59. Gajic O, Dzik WH, Toy P: Fresh frozen plasma and platelet transfusion for nonbleeding patients in the intensive care unit: Benefit or harm? Crit Care Med 2006;34(5 Suppl): S170-S173.
60. Janson PA, Jubelirer SJ, Weinstein JM, et al: Treatment of the bleeding tendency in uremia with

cryoprecipitate. N Engl J Med 1980;303:1318-1322.
61. Mannucci PM: Desmopressin: A nontransfusional form of treatment for congenital and acquired bleeding disorders. Blood 1988;72:1449-1455.
62. Jolles S, Sewell WAC, Misbah SA: Clinical uses of intravenous immunoglobulin. Clin Exp Immunol 2005;142:1-11.
63. American College of Obstetricians and Gynecologists: Prevention of D Isoimmunization, Technical Bulletin No 147. Washington, DC, 1990.
64. Alderson P, Bunn F, Lefebvre C, et al: Human albumin solution for resuscitation and volume expansion in critically ill patients. Cochrane Database Syst Rev 2004;4:CD001208.
65. Alving BM, Hojima Y, Pisano JJ, et al: Hypotension associated with prekallikrein activator (Hageman-factor fragments) in plasma protein fraction. N Engl J Med 1978;299:66-70.
66. Stanworth SJ, Massey E, Hyde C: Granulocyte transfusions for treating infections in patients with neutropenia or neutrophil dysfunction. Cochrane Database Syst Rev 2005;3:CD005339.
67. Walker RH: Special report: Transfusion risks. Am J Clin Pathol 1987;88: 374-378.
68. Sazama K: Transfusion errors: Scope of the problem, consequences, and solutions. Curr Hematol Rep 2003;2:518-521.
69. Linden JV, Wagner K, Voytovich AE, et al: Transfusion errors in New York State: An analysis of 10 years' experience. Transfusion 2001;40:1207-1213.
70. JCAHO: Blood transfusion errors: Preventing future occurrences: Available at http://www.jointcommission.org/SentinelEvents/SentinelEventAlert/sea_10.htm, 1999.
71. Pineda AA, Brzica SM, Taswell HF: Hemolytic transfusion reaction. Mayo Clin Proc 1978;53:378-390.
72. Pineda AA, Taswell HF: Transfusion reactions associated with anti-IgA antibodies: Report of four cases and review of the literature. Transfusion 1975;15:10-15.
73. Menitove JE, McElligott MC, Aster RH: Febrile transfusion reaction: What blood component should be given next? Vox Sang 1982;42:318-321.
74. Hebert PC, Fergusson D, Blajchman MA, et al: Clinical outcomes following institution of the Canadian universal leukoreduction program for red blood cell transfusions. JAMA 2003;289:1941-1949.
75. Pineda AA, Taswell HF, Brzica SM: Delayed hemolytic transfusion reaction: An immunologic hazard of blood transfusion. Transfusion 1978;18:1-7.
76. Rana R, Fernandez-Perez ER, Khan SA, et al: Transfusion-related acute lung injury and pulmonary edema in critically ill patients: A retrospective study. Transfusion 2006;46:1465-1468.
77. Toy P, Popovsky MA, Abraham E, et al, for the NHLBI Working Group on TRALI: Transfusion-related acute lung injury: Definition and review. Crit Care Med 2005;33:721-726.
78. Moore SB: Transfusion-associated acute lung injury (TRALI): Clinical presentation, treatment and prognosis. Crit Care Med 2006;35(5 Suppl): S114-S117.
79. Nicolle AL, Chapman CE, Carter V, et al: Transfusion-related acute lung injury caused by two donors with anti-human leucocyte antigen class II antibodies: A look-back investigation. Transfus Med 2004;14:225-230.
80. Goldman M, Webert KE, Arnold DM, et al, for the TRALI Consensus Panel: Proceedings of a consensus conference: Towards an understanding of TRALI. Transfus Med Rev 2005;19:2-31.
81. Vogelsang GB, Hess AD: Graft-versus-host disease: New directions for a persistent problem. Blood 1994;84:2061-2067.
82. Ohto H, Anderson KC: Survey of transfusion-associated graft-versus-host disease in immunocompetent recipients. Transf Med Rev 1996;10:31-43.
83. Davey RJ, McCoy NC, Yu M, et al: The effect of prestorage irradiation on post-transfusion red cell survival. Transfusion 1992;32:525-528.
84. Opelz G, Terasaki PI: Improvement of kidney-graft survival with increased numbers of blood transfusion. N Engl J Med 1978;299:799-803.
85. Heiss MM, Mempel W, Delanoff D, et al: Blood transfusion–modulated tumor recurrence: First results of a randomized study of autologous versus allogeneic blood transfusion in colorectal cancer surgery. J Clin Oncol 1994;12:1859-1867.
86. Vamvakas EC: Transfusion-associated cancer recurrence and postoperative infection: Meta-analysis of randomized, controlled clinical trials. Transfusion 1996;36:175-186.
87. Shorr AF, Jackson WL: Transfusion practice and nosocomial infection: Assessing the evidence. Curr Opin Crit Care 2005;11:468-472.
88. Banbury MK, Brizzio ME, Rajeswaran J, et al: Transfusion increases the risk of postoperative infection after cardiovascular surgery. J Am Coll Surg 2006;202:131-138.
89. Smith DM: Immunosuppressive effects of blood transfusion. Clin Lab Med 1992;12:723-741.
90. Fergusson D, Khanna MP, Tinmouth A, et al: Transfusion of leukoreduced red blood cells may decrease postoperative infections: Two meta-analyses of randomized controlled trials. Can J Anaesth 2004;51:417-424.
91. Blajchman MA: Transfusion immunomodulation or TRIM: What does it mean clinically? Hematology 2005;10(Suppl 1):208-214.
92. Goodnough LT: Risks of blood transfusion. Anesthesiol Clin North Am 2005;23:241-252.
93. Gunter K, Luban N: Transfusion-transmitted cytomegalovirus and Epstein-Barr virus diseases. In Rossi EC, Simon TL, Moss GL, et al (eds): Principles of Transfusion Medicine, 2nd ed. Baltimore, Williams & Wilkins, 1996.
94. Klein HG, Dodd RY, Ness PM, et al: Current status of microbial contamination of blood components: Summary of a conference. Transfusion 1997;37:95-101.
95. Morrow JF, Braine HG, Kickler TS, et al: Septic reactions to platelet transfusions: A persistent problem. JAMA 1991;266:555-558.
96. Centers for Disease Control and Prevention (CDC): Red blood cell transfusions contaminated with *Yersinia enterocolitica*—United States, 1991-1997, and initiation of a national study to detect bacteria-associated transfusion reactions. MMWR Morb Mortal Weekly Rep 1997;46(24): 553-555.
97. Conry-Cantilena C, van Raden M, Gibble J, et al: Routes of infection, viremia, and liver disease in blood donors found to have hepatitis C infection. N Engl J Med 1996;334:1691-1696.
98. Tong MJ, El-Farra NS, Reikes AR, et al: Clinical outcomes after transfusion-associated hepatitis C. N Engl J Med 1995;332:1463-1466.
99. Dodd RY: Adverse consequences of blood transfusion: Quantitative risk estimates. In Nance ST (ed): Blood Supply: Risks, Perceptions, and Prospects for the Future. Bethesda, MD, American Association of Blood Banks, 1994, pp 1-24.
100. Dodd RY, Notari EP, Stramer SL: Current prevalence and incidence of infectious disease markers and estimated window-period risk in the American Red Cross blood donor population. Transfusion 2002;42:975-979.
101. Centers for Disease Control and Prevention (CDC): Possible transfusion-associated acquired immune deficiency syndrome (AIDS): California. MMWR Morb Mortal Wkly Rep 1982;31(48): 652-654.
102. Silvergleid AJ, Leparc GF, Schmidt PJ: Impact of explicit questions about high-risk activities on donor attitudes and donor referral patterns. Results in two community blood centers. Transfusion 1989;29:362-364.
103. Petersen LR, Lackritz E, Lewis W, et al: The effectiveness of the confidential unit exclusion option. Transfusion 1994;34:865-869.
104. O'Brien TR, George JR, Holmberg SD: Human immunodeficiency virus type 2 infection in the United States: Epidemiology, diagnosis, and public health implications. JAMA 1992;267:2775-2779.
105. Centers for Disease Control and Infection (CDC): Update: HIV-2 infection among blood and plasma donors—United States, June 1992-June 1995. MMWR Morb Mortal Wkly Rep 1995;44(32):603-606.
106. Sullivan MT, Williams AE, Fang CT, et al: Transmission of human T-lymphotropic virus types I and II by blood transfusion. Arch Intern Med 1991;151:2043-2048.
107. Manns A, Wilks RJ, Murphy EL, et al: A prospective study of transmission by transfusion of HTLV-I and risk factors associated with seroconversion. Int J Cancer 1992;51:886-891.
108. Tegtmeier GE: Post-transfusion cytomegalovirus infections. Arch Pathol Lab Med 1989;113:236-245.
109. Sayers MH, Anderson KC, Goodnough LT, et al: Reducing the risk for transfusion-transmitted

cytomegalovirus infection. Ann Intern Med 1992;116:55-62.
110. Vamvakas EC: Is white blood cell reduction equivalent to antibody screening in preventing transmission of cytomegalovirus by transfusion? A review of the literature and meta-analysis. Transfus Med Rev 2005;19:181-199.
111. Shulman I: Transmission of parasitic infections by blood transfusion. In Rossi EC, Simon TL, Moss GL, et al (eds): Principles of Transfusion Medicine, 2nd ed. Baltimore, Williams & Wilkins, 1996.
112. Counts RB, Haisch C, Simon TL, et al: Hemostasis in massively transfused trauma patients. Ann Surg 1979;190:91-99.
113. Leslie SD, Toy PTCY: Laboratory hemostatic abnormalities in massively transfused patients given red blood cells and crystalloid. Am J Clin Pathol 1991;96:770-773.
114. Harrigan C, Lucas CE, Ledgerwood AM, et al: Serial changes in primary hemostasis after massive transfusion. Surgery 1985;98:836-844.
115. Reed RL, Heimbach DM, Counts RB, et al: Prophylactic platelet administration during massive transfusion. Ann Surg 1986;203:40-48.
116. Ciavarelia D, Reed RL, Counts RB, et al: Clotting factor levels and the risk of diffuse rnicrovascular bleeding in the massively transfused patient. Br J Haematol 1987;67:365-368.
117. Hedner U, Erhardtsen E: Potential role of recombinant factor VIIa as a hemostatic agent. Clin Adv Hematol Oncol 2003;1:112-119.
118. Ganguly S, Spengel K, Tilzer LL, et al: Recombinant factor VIIa: Unregulated continuous use in patients with bleeding and coagulopathy dues not alter mortality and outcome. Clin Lab Haematol 2006;28:309-312.
119. Kahn RC, Jascott D, Carlon GC, et al: Massive blood replacement: Correlation of ionized calcium, citrate, and hydrogen ion concentration. Anesth Analg 1979;58:274-278.
120. Schweizer O, Howland WS: Potassium levels, acid-base balance and massive blood replacement. Anesthesiology 1962;23:735-740.
121. Collins JA, Simmons RL, James PM, et al: Acid-base status of seriously wounded combat casualties: Resuscitation with stored blood. Ann Surg 1971;173:6-18.
122. Boyan CP, Howland WS: Blood temperature: A critical factor in massive transfusion. Anesthesiology 1961;22:559-564.
123. Snyder EL, Underwood PS, Spivack M, et al: An in vivo evaluation of microaggregate blood filtration during total hip replacement. Ann Surg 1979;190:75-79.
124. Nathens AB: Massive transfusion as a risk factor for acute lung injury: Association or causation? Crit Care Med 2006;34:(Suppl):S144-S150.
125. Stainsby D, MacLennan S, Thomas D, et al: Guidelines on the management of massive blood loss. Br J Haematol 2006;135:634-641.
126. Petz LD: Autoimmune hemolytic anemia. Hum Pathol 1983;14: 251-255.
127. Garratty G, Petz LD: Approaches to selecting blood for transfusion to patients with autoimmune hemolytic anemia. Transfusion 2002;42:1390-1392.
128. Lozano M, Cid J: The clinical implications of platelet transfusions associated with ABO or Rh(D) incompatibility. Transfus Med Rev 2003;17:57-68.
129. Mollison PL: Survival curves of incompatible red cells: An analytical review. Transfusion 1986;26:43-50.
130. Stussi G, Huggel K, Lutz HU, et al: Isotype-specific detection of ABO blood group antibodies using a novel flow cytometric method. Br J Haematol 2005;130:954-963.
131. Schmidt PJ, Leparc GF, Samia CT: Use of Rh positive blood in emergency situations. Surg Gynecol Obstet 1988;167:229-233.
132. Bolan CD, Alving BM: Pharmacologic agents in the management of bleeding disorders. Transfusion 1990;30:541-551.
133. Rubin RN, Coleman RW: Disseminated intravascular coagulation. Approach to treatment. Drugs 1992;44:963-971.
134. Saba HI, Morelli GA: The pathogenesis and management of disseminated intravascular coagulation. Clin Adv Hematol Oncol 2006;4:919-926.
135. Amitrano L, Guardascione MA, Francaccio V, et al: Coagulation disorders in liver disease. Semin Liver Dis 2002;22:83-96.
136. Kerr R: New insights into haemostasis in liver failure. Blood Coagul Fibrinolysis 2003;14(Suppl 1):S43-S45.
137. Gralnick HR, McKeown LP, Williams SB, et al: Plasma and platelet von Willebrand factor defects in uremia. Am J Med 1988;85:806-810.
138. Manucci PM, Remuzzi G, Pusineri F, et al: Deamino-8-D-arginine vasopressin shortens the bleeding time in uremia. N Engl J Med 1983;308:8-12.
139. Hows J, Beddow K, Gordon-Smith E, et al: Donor-derived red blood cell antibodies and immune hemolysis after allogeneic bone marrow transplantation. Blood 1986;67:177-181.
140. Gould SA, Rosen AL, Sehgal LR, et al: Fluosol-DA as a red-cell substitute in acute anemia. N Engl J Med 1986;314:1653-1656.
141. Klein HG: The prospect for red cell substitutes. N Engl J Med 2000;342:1666-1668.
142. Lemaire F: Low-dose perfluorocarbon: A revival for partial liquid ventilation? Crit Care Med 2007;35:662-663.
143. Mannucci PM, Canciani MT, Rota L, et al: Response of factor VIII/von Willebrand factor to DDAVP in healthy subjects and patients with haemophilia A and von Willebrand's disease. Br J Haematol 1981;47:283-293.
144. Sindet-Petersen S, Ingerslev J, Ramstrom G, et al: Management of oral bleeding in haemophiliac patients [letter]. Lancet 1988;2:566.
145. Bidstrup BP, Hunt BJ, Sheikh S, et al: Amelioration of the bleeding tendency of preoperative aspirin after aortocoronary bypass grafting. Ann Thorac Surg 2000;69:541-547.
146. Mangano DT, Miao Y, Vuylsteke A, et al, for Investigators of the Multicenter Study of Perioperative Ischemia Research Group: Mortality associated with aprotinin during 5 years following coronary artery bypass graft surgery. JAMA 2007;297: 471-479.
147. Alghamdi AA, Albanna MJ, Guru V, et al: Does the use of erythropoietin reduce the risk of exposure to allogeneic blood transfusion in cardiac surgery? A systematic review and meta-analysis. J Card Surg 2006;21:320-326.
148. Carless PA, Henry DA, Moxey AJ, et al: Cell salvage for minimizing perioperative allogeneic blood transfusion. Cochrane Database Syst Rev 2006;4:CD001888.
149. Davies L, Brown TJ, Haynes S, et al: Cost-effectiveness of cell salvage and alternative methods of minimizing perioperative allogeneic blood transfusion: A systematic review and economic model. Health Technol Assess 2006;10:iii-iv, ix-x, 1-210.
150. Rahman T, Harper L: Plasmapheresis in nephrology: An update. Curr Opin Nephrol Hypertens 2006;15:603-609.
151. National Institutes of Health Consensus Conference: The utility of therapeutic plasmapheresis for neurological disorders. JAMA 1986;256:1333-1337.
152. Zarkovic M, Kwaan HC: Correction of hyperviscosity by apheresis. Semin Thromb Hemost 2003;29:535-542.
153. Bell WR, Braine HG, Ness PM, et al: Improved survival in thrombotic thrombocytopenic purpura–hemolytic uremic syndrome. N Engl J Med 1991;325:398-402.
154. Yeo FE, Bohen EM, Yuan CM, et al: Therapeutic plasma exchange as a nephrological procedure: A single-center experience. J Clin Apheresis 2005;20:208-216.
155. Kern JM, Croy BB: A review of transfusion-associated AIDS litigation: 1984 through 1993. Transfusion 1994;34:484-491.
156. Weinberg PD, Hounshell J, Sherman LA, et al: Legal, financial, and public health consequences of HIV contamination of blood and blood products in the 1980s and 1990s. Ann Intern Med 2002;136:312-319.
157. Goldman EB, Oberman HA: Legal aspects of transfusion of Jehovah's Witnesses. Transfus Med Rev 1991;5:263-270.
158. Joint Commission on Accreditation of Hospitals and Healthcare Organizations: Sentinel event statistics: Available at http://www.jointcommission.org/SentinelEvents/Statistics/

Chapter 81

Intensive Care of the Cancer Patient

Brendan D. Curti and Dan L. Longo

The diagnosis of malignancy in the United States has become common over the past 50 years, although the age-adjusted incidence and death rates for all cancer sites combined have been declining since 1992. The annual incidence of new invasive cancers in the United States in 2006 was nearly 1.4 million, with 565,000 deaths.[1] Although metastatic solid tumors, such as breast and colon carcinoma, are not curable with current technologies, the number of tumor types that can be cured with intensive treatment has markedly increased over the last 2 decades. Examples of curable metastatic malignancies include acute lymphoblastic leukemia, acute and chronic myeloid leukemia, Hodgkin's and non-Hodgkin's lymphoma, germ cell tumors, ovarian cancer, Wilms' tumor, and Ewing's sarcoma.[2-8] Long-term remissions have been achieved with immunotherapy in some malignancies that previously had a particularly poor prognosis, such as metastatic melanoma and renal cell carcinoma.[9,10] It is now estimated that approximately 65% of all individuals in whom cancer is diagnosed are alive after 5 years, as compared with less than 20% 50 years ago.[1] Much of the improved prognosis can be attributed to advances in medical imaging and early diagnosis, more sophisticated cancer surgical techniques, and the adjuvant treatment of cancer before recurrence or metastasis has occurred. For the treatment of metastatic malignancies, a measure of success has come from the ability to deliver chemotherapy, radiation therapy, immunotherapy, or combination regimens with increased dose intensity.[5,11,12] Progress in supportive care and intensive care medicine has allowed oncologists to treat their patients aggressively and support them despite the toxicities inherent in dose-intense treatment modalities. A greater understanding of the mechanisms of these toxicities has also improved care and patient outcomes.

This chapter describes specific oncologic clinical entities and cancer treatment toxicities that require intensive care management. The discussion of these problems is organized according to organ system because cancers are best understood as systemic diseases that can directly or indirectly influence all organ systems. The pathophysiology that gives rise to these clinical circumstances is increasingly understood and is being used as the basis for treatment recommendations. Aspects unique to biologic therapies and bone marrow transplantation are treated in separate sections. The ethical aspects of treating cancer patients in the intensive care unit (ICU) are also discussed.

METABOLIC AND ENDOCRINE COMPLICATIONS

Endocrine syndromes associated with malignancies have been described for many years.[13] These problems may be manifested as solitary laboratory derangements, such as hypercalcemia or hyperphosphatemia, or they can represent clinical syndromes, such as Cushing's syndrome in small cell lung cancer. Metabolic disorders can also arise as a consequence of cancer treatment. This is most often seen with chemotherapy for rapidly growing tumors such as leukemias or lymphomas. Abrupt changes in metabolic variables have also been observed after interleukin-2 (IL-2)-based immunotherapy and the rapid in vivo expansion of lymphocytes.[14] The most common of these clinical entities are tumor lysis syndrome (TLS), hypercalcemia, oncogenic osteomalacia, syndrome of inappropriate secretion of antidiuretic hormone (SIADH), adrenal failure, pheochromocytoma, tumor-induced hypoglycemia, and chemotherapy-induced metabolic disturbances.

Tumor Lysis Syndrome

Case reports of metabolic and electrolyte abnormalities after chemotherapy for rapidly growing tumors such as Burkitt's lymphoma and leukemias were first published in the 1950s.[15] Bertino and colleagues in the 1970s proposed a mechanism that linked these metabolic observations.[16] More recently, TLS has been observed in patients with solid tumors, such as metastatic breast cancer, small cell lung cancer, and medulloblastoma. It has also been observed in patients receiving immunotherapy, such as IL-2 and rituximab.[17,18] TLS after treatment of solid tumors is relatively rare.

The syndrome is characterized by hyperuricemia, hyperkalemia, hyperphosphatemia, and hypocalcemia.[16] Electrolyte abnormalities can appear as soon as 6 hours after the administration of chemotherapy and persist for 5 to 7 days after treatment. The hyperuricemia comes from the massive release of intracellular nucleic acids and their metabolism by xanthine oxidase into uric acid. Urate crystals can form in the renal collecting ducts and result in oliguric and anuric renal failure. Similarly, potassium and phosphate are released from lysing tumor cells, and renal excretion of these intracellular ions is impaired by hyperuricemia. Serum calcium levels drop from ectopic calcium deposition; this becomes more likely as the calcium-phosphorus product increases. Calcium deposition is favored by a calcium-phosphorus product greater than 60 and becomes severe when the product is higher than 75. The clinical manifestations of TLS depend on which electrolyte derangement predominates. Tetany, confusion, hypotension, dysrhythmias, and sudden death have been reported with TLS. The most effective management approach for this syndrome is to anticipate its occurrence and intervene prospectively. Patients at greatest risk for TLS are those with a diagnosis of a rapidly growing lymphoma or leukemia with high blast counts and pretreatment levels of lactate dehydrogenase greater than 1500 U/dL and uric acid greater than 10 mg/dL. Pretreatment azotemia is also a poor prognostic sign. Azotemia may be exacerbated by uric acid nephropathy, which is more common with uric acid levels exceeding 20 mg/dL. It is unlikely that TLS will occur in patients at risk in whom metabolic changes do not develop within 48 hours after receiving chemotherapy. Guidelines for prophylaxis and treatment of TLS are given in Box 81-1.

Hypercalcemia

Hypercalcemia is the most common metabolic abnormality that occurs in cancer patients. Approximately 10% to 20% of all cancer patients have hypercalcemia at some point in their malignancy. The clinical symptoms of hypercalcemia are nonspecific and include lethargy, confusion, nausea, and anorexia. Frequently, the clinical symptoms

Box 81-1

Treatment Recommendations in Tumor Lysis Syndrome

When No Metabolic Aberration Exists

- Allopurinol: 300 mg qd, reduce to 100 mg qd after 3 days of chemotherapy
- Hydration: 3000 mL/d, 0.45% saline
- Initiate chemotherapy within 24 to 48 hours of admission
- Monitor serum chemistry values every 12 to 24 hours

When Metabolic Aberration Exists

- Allopurinol as above; reduce the dose if hyperuricemia is controlled or for renal insufficiency
- Hydration with 5% dextrose in water with 2 ampules of $NaCO_3$ per liter; add nonthiazide diuretics as needed
- Urinary alkalization to keep urine pH higher than 7.0; may discontinue when the serum uric acid level is normal
- Postpone chemotherapy until uric acid is decreased and electrolytes are stable
- Monitor serum chemistry values every 6 to 8 hours
- If serum uric acid is greater than 8 mg/dL and/or serum creatinine is greater than 1.6 mg/dL, add rasburicase, 0.2 mg/kg intravenously daily (contraindicated in the setting of glucose-6-phosphate dehydrogenase deficiency)
- Replace calcium with a slow intravenous infusion of calcium gluconate (if symptomatic or for electrocardiographic changes)
- Treat hyperkalemia and hyperphosphatemia with exchange resins and phosphate binders, respectively

Criteria for Hemodialysis in Patients Unresponsive to the Above

- Serum potassium greater than 6.0 mEq/L
- Serum uric acid greater than 20 mg/dL
- Serum phosphorus greater than 10 mg/dL
- Fluid overload unresponsive to diuretics
- Symptomatic hypercalcemia

in cancer patients may be subtle because the onset of hypercalcemia is gradual. The mechanism that underlies all cases of cancer-related hypercalcemia is increased calcium resorption from bone. This increase in resorption can be due to the local action of tumor in bone or to the production of bone-resorbing hormones and cytokines by tumor cells remote from bone (humoral hypercalcemia). Normally, increased circulating calcium results in decreased production of parathyroid hormone (PTH). When PTH levels decrease, bone resorption and renal tubular reabsorption of calcium decline. In addition, low PTH levels cause a decrease in vitamin D production; thus, gut absorption of calcium is lowered. Although PTH levels are suppressed in cancer patients with hypercalcemia, the destructive action of tumor deposits in bone or the action of tumor-produced hormones on bone maintains the high calcium resorption rates. This is accomplished through osteoclast activation and proliferation from factors produced by the tumor, such as IL-1, tumor necrosis factor (TNF), prostaglandin E_2, granulocyte-macrophage colony-stimulating factor (GM-CSF), transforming growth factor-α, platelet-derived growth factor, and PTH-related peptides.[19-22] The most common promoter of hypercalcemia in patients with solid tumors is PTH-related peptide.[23] Malignancies that frequently cause hypercalcemia include multiple myeloma, breast carcinoma, epidermoid lung carcinoma, and renal cell carcinoma. Hypercalcemia in lymphoma and leukemia is probably not associated with PTH-related peptide but instead with the overproduction of activated vitamin D.[23,24]

Cardiac dysfunction and renal dysfunction are the most serious end-organ effects of hypercalcemia. Electrocardiographic changes include prolongation of the PR and QRS intervals and shortening of the QT interval. Bradydysrhythmias and bundle branch blocks become more frequent with serum calcium levels greater than 16 mg/dL. These abnormalities may progress to complete heart block and asystole. Renal dysfunction may also occur because increased serum calcium induces a diuretic effect, which can cause moderate to severe dehydration and prerenal azotemia. This can result in acute tubular necrosis if untreated.

Management of any symptomatic hypercalcemic patient should begin with intravenous hydration, which may increase renal blood flow and enhance calciuresis.[25] Renal excretion of calcium can be enhanced with furosemide diuresis, although no randomized trials exist to support its use in hypercalcemia. These measures should be viewed as temporizing steps until definitive treatment has been implemented. The bisphosphonates zoledronic acid, pamidronate, etidronate, and clodronate have been shown to be highly effective in the long-term treatment of hypercalcemia of malignancy. These agents work by binding to the hydroxyapatite in bone and preventing calcium resorption, although they may also have much more complicated effects on the cell cycle and bone turnover.[26] A commonly used bisphosphonate regimen is a single dose of pamidronate (60 to 90 mg intravenously over a 2- to 4-hour period) or zoledronic acid (4 mg intravenously over a 15-minute period). Doses may be repeated in 3 to 4 days if the calcium level does not decline. In addition, therapy directed at controlling the tumor should be implemented. Gallium nitrate should be tried in patients with hypercalcemia unresponsive to bisphosphonates.[27] Calcitonin, glucocorticoids, or mithramycin can also be tried in patients unresponsive to first-line therapies. Dialysis may be necessary if renal compromise is severe. Treatment recommendations are summarized in Table 81-1.

Table 81-1. Agents Used for the Management of Hypercalcemia

Drug	Dosage
Pamidronate	90 mg IV over 2-h period
Zoledronic acid	4 mg IV over 15-min period
Gallium nitrate	200 mg/m^2 by continuous infusion for 5 d
Calcitonin	400 IU SQ q8h
Mithramycin	25 μg/kg IV once or twice per week

Oncogenic Osteomalacia

Oncogenic osteomalacia is a rare syndrome characterized by severe hypophosphatemia, high serum alkaline phosphatase, aminoaciduria, glycosuria, low levels of 1,25-dihydroxyvitamin D, and normal serum calcium. The syndrome is the result of humoral inhibition of activation of 25-hydroxyvitamin D. Patients complain of bone pain and muscle weakness. Hemolysis from hypophosphatemia is a possible sequela of this syndrome. Tumors that give rise to oncogenic osteomalacia are usually vascular mesenchymal tumors, such as hemangiopericytoma. Treatment involves surgical removal of the tumor and phosphate supplementation.

Syndrome of Inappropriate Secretion of Antidiuretic Hormone

SIADH is associated with carcinoid tumors, lymphoma, and carcinomas originating in the lung, prostate, esophagus, head and neck, adrenal gland, and pancreas. Cerebral metastasis from any tumor can also give rise to SIADH. Clinical findings are mainly neurologic and range from mild confusion to coma and seizures. Because the clinical findings are secondary to water intoxication and hyponatremia, treatment involves water restriction (500 mL/day) and control of the primary tumor. More aggressive treatment should be started with 0.9% or 3% saline solution and furosemide diuresis for patients with neurologic deficits from hyponatremia. The rate of intravenous fluid supplementation should be adjusted according to the urinary excretion of sodium and potassium. Correction of severe hyponatremia (sodium <125 mEq/L) should take place over a span of 7 to 10 days. Too rapid correction can lead to serious neurologic sequelae such as central pontine myelinosis. Patients who fail to respond to water restriction can be treated with demeclocycline (600 to 1200 mg daily), which blocks the peripheral action of ADH.

Adrenal Failure

Cancers of the lung, breast, kidney, stomach, and pancreas and melanoma are the tumors that metastasize most often to the adrenal glands. It is estimated that more than 90% of adrenal tissue must be destroyed before clinical manifestations of adrenal insufficiency appear. The clinical signs and symptoms of hypoadrenalism include weakness, gastrointestinal complaints, postural hypotension, dehydration, and electrolyte disturbances. The typical electrolyte profile is hyponatremia, hyperkalemia, and a mild anion gap acidosis.

The diagnosis can be made with a cosyntropin stimulation test. Plasma cortisol levels are determined before the injection of cosyntropin (0.25 mg intravenously) and 30 and 60 minutes afterward. A normal response is an increase in plasma cortisol of at least 7.0 mg/dL in 60 minutes. If the cortisol response to cosyntropin stimulation is suboptimal, physiologic doses of glucocorticoids should be administered (cortisone acetate, 25 mg every morning and 12.5 mg every evening). Mineralocorticoid supplementation is required in some patients (fludrocortisone, 0.05 to 0.1 mg daily). If the diagnosis of adrenal insufficiency is highly suspected, treatment should begin immediately after completion of the cosyntropin test. For patients in adrenal crisis with circulatory collapse, hydrocortisone should be given at stress doses (100 mg intravenously every 8 hours). This dose of hydrocortisone should also be adequate to supplement mineralocorticoid-deficient patients. It should be remembered that patients receiving glucocorticoids as part of their chemotherapy regimen (usually lymphoma or myeloma patients) may have baseline adrenal suppression and might require bolus glucocorticoid doses during episodes of febrile neutropenia or sepsis.

Pheochromocytoma

Pheochromocytoma is most commonly associated with the multiple endocrine neoplasia syndrome. The clinical features of this tumor are related to episodic catecholamine release and include hypertension, severe headache, cardiac dysrhythmias, pallor, perspiration, and rarely, hypotension. Patients can also have a multisystem crisis characterized by encephalopathy, hyperpyrexia, and hemodynamic instability.[28] The diagnosis is made by measuring urinary catecholamine metabolites. An elevated vanillylmandelic acid level is accurate approximately 90% of the time in making the diagnosis.[29] In patients with borderline catecholamine levels, pheochromocytoma can often be diagnosed with the clonidine suppression test.[30] Localization of pheochromocytoma can be difficult because the tumor can arise anywhere between the base of the brain and the scrotum and can be multicentric. Magnetic resonance imaging (MRI) and computed tomography (CT) are helpful in visualizing adrenal abnormalities. Nuclear medicine studies with *meta*-[^{111}I]iodobenzylguanidine (MIBG) can be used if CT is negative. MIBG scans are sensitive and specific in detecting ectopic adrenal medullary tissue.[31] Positron emission tomography (PET) can detect sites of disease not apparent on CT or MIBG and can aid in surgical planning.[32] Surgical extirpation of the tumor is the only effective treatment. Preoperative control of catechol secretion is necessary and can be achieved with α-adrenergic blockade (phenoxybenzamine, 10 mg orally two or three times daily). Tachycardia can be controlled with β-blockers, but these medications should be started only after phenoxybenzamine. Patients in hypertensive crisis can be managed with α-methyltyrosine or calcium channel blockers such as nifedipine or nicardipine.[33-35]

Tumor-Induced Hypoglycemia

Functional endocrine tumors can give rise to a variety of clinical syndromes. Most of these problems can be managed outside the ICU; however, tumor-induced hypoglycemia can cause serious consequences, including coma, seizures, and focal neurologic deficits. A number of different mechanisms can give rise to hypoglycemia. Autonomous insulin production is most commonly associated with islet cell tumors, whereas production of insulin-like growth factors (IGF-I or IGF-II) is seen with non–islet cell tumors.[36] Slow-growing mesenchymal tumors such as leiomyosarcoma, mesothelioma, and fibrosarcoma are the most common non–islet cell tumors that cause hypoglycemia.

Treatment should be focused on control of the tumor. Insulinomas are frequently benign and can be cured by surgical removal. For unresectable malignancies, hypoglycemic episodes can often be reduced with supportive measures such as dietary modification with frequent meals. Insulinomas may respond to diazoxide, an inhibitor of insulin secretion. Glucagon infusions may be beneficial in some patients.[37]

Chemotherapy-Induced Metabolic Disturbances

A number of chemotherapy drugs can cause potentially severe electrolyte disturbances. Cyclophosphamide is associated with hyponatremia from SIADH. Vinca alkaloids may also cause SIADH. Cisplatin and carboplatin can cause renal tubular defects resulting in hypokalemia and hypomagnesemia, which can be severe enough to require intravenous replacement. Mithramycin lowers serum calcium by a mechanism that is thought to involve inhibition of the effect of PTH on osteoclasts. Although mithramycin can be used for the treatment of hypercalcemia, it can also cause hypocalcemia in patients with normal serum calcium. Cetuximab, a humanized murine antibody directed against the epidermal growth factor receptor (EGFR) and used to treat colon carcinoma and head and neck cancer, is associated with severe and symptomatic hypomagnesemia from inappropriate urinary excretion.[38] Cetuximab may interact with EGFR in the loop of Henle and thereby block resorption of magnesium and cause secondary hypokalemia and hypocalcemia.

CARDIAC COMPLICATIONS IN CANCER PATIENTS

Cardiac dysfunction in cancer patients can be secondary to direct mechanical effects of the tumor on the heart, pericardium, or great vessels. Certain chemotherapy drugs, immunotherapy agents, and radiation can also cause treatment-related cardiac problems. Both emergency and chronic clinical entities are discussed.

Superior Vena Cava Syndrome

Obstruction of blood flow through the superior vena cava (SVC) can be caused by fibrosis, thrombosis, external compression, or invasion of the vessel by tumor. SVC syndrome can also be caused by thrombus secondary to a central venous access device, which is now a common fixture of oncologic care. Malignancies that involve the mediastinum, such as lung carcinoma and lymphoma, are the most common causes of this syndrome. Facial and upper extremity edema, facial plethora, headache, and tachypnea are the most common clinical findings. Collateral venous channels may be found on the chest or abdomen. Death from SVC syndrome is rare, but life-threatening respiratory compromise and elevated intracranial pressure can occur. Therapy for SVC syndrome depends on the underlying malignancy; thus, a biopsy is mandatory for optimal management of these patients. If lymphoma or small cell lung carcinoma is the cause of SVC syndrome, initiation of the appropriate chemotherapy regimen can rapidly shrink the mediastinal mass and is the treatment of choice. For tumors not responsive to chemotherapy, radiation therapy given with high initial fractions (3 to 4 Gy/d) can provide symptomatic relief in more than 80% of patients.[39] Thrombolysis has been studied only in catheter-associated SVC syndrome and is effective in this setting.[40]

Cardiac Tamponade

Although primary tumors of the heart have been described, pericardial tamponade is far more frequent. Causes of cardiac tamponade in cancer patients include metastatic tumors of the breast and lung, melanoma, lymphoma, and leukemia. Tamponade may occur through either encasement of the heart by tumor or production of a malignant pericardial effusion. The clinical manifestations of tamponade include decreased exercise tolerance, shortness of breath, and cough. Voltage may be decreased on the electrocardiogram with a pulsus alternans pattern present. Muffled heart tones, a pericardial rub, or an increased paradoxical pulse (i.e., decrease in systolic blood pressure on inspiration exceeding 10 mm Hg) may be present on physical examination. Echocardiography is extremely useful in confirming the diagnosis of tamponade if it is suspected on physical examination. Diastolic collapse of the right atrium or right ventricle on echocardiography is an indicator of hemodynamic compromise.[41,42] Swan-Ganz catheterization may be helpful in confirming the presence of significant tamponade.

Pericardiocentesis for relief of tamponade is indicated on an emergency basis when echocardiographic or clinical evidence of hemodynamic compromise is present. Intravenous infusions of normal saline at high flow rates (100 to 500 mL/h) may be required to support the patient until a drainage procedure is performed. Although rapid reversal of cardiac filling problems can be accomplished with this procedure, a long-term solution is required. Creation of a pericardial window can prevent the reaccumulation of fluid in more than 90% of patients.[43] The mechanism by which pericardial windows work is probably not by creating an opening for fluid outflow but rather by inducing an inflammatory response that seals the potential space between the pericardium and epicardium. This mechanism has been confirmed in a limited number of autopsies after pericardial window procedures.[44] Sclerosing agents such as tetracycline and bleomycin have also been used to prevent reaccumulation of pericardial fluid.[45] Sclerosants may be instilled into the pericardial space after adequate drainage has been accomplished and appear to have a success rate comparable to that of pericardial window procedures.

Treatment-Induced Cardiac Dysfunction

A number of medications used to treat cancer have cardiac toxicities that can be life-threatening. Cumulative doses of doxorubicin greater than 450 mg/m^2 are associated with an increased risk (≈5%) for congestive heart failure (CHF). The heart damage caused by this drug is thought to be due to iron-dependent generation of free radicals, which secondarily cause oxidative damage to lipid membranes and intracellular organelles.[45] This toxicity can occur acutely or months after drug administration. It is more prevalent in older patients and those with a history of coronary artery disease, hypertension, or chest radiation therapy. Initial management with diuretics, digoxin, and angiotensin-converting enzyme inhibitors is usually of benefit, but the heart failure can be progressive. Preventive strategies, such as liposomal encapsulation of the drug and the use of dexrazoxane to prevent oxygen radical formation, may diminish the cardiac toxicity of doxorubicin.[46-48] Other anthracyclines, such as mitoxantrone and epirubicin, may be associated with a lower incidence of heart failure. Furthermore, weekly low-dose boluses or continuous-infusion methods of administration of doxorubicin appear to reduce the incidence of clinically significant heart damage. Although anthracycline-induced cardiac damage has generally been considered irreversible, some studies suggest that some improvement in cardiac function may occur with aggressive medical management.[49] Paclitaxel, which is commonly used in ovarian, breast, and lung carcinoma, is associated with bradydysrhythmias. This problem was seen in several of the phase I studies with the drug but is usually asymptomatic.[50,51] Ventricular tachycardia, myocardial infarction, and cardiac ischemia have also been reported. Cyclophosphamide, which is commonly used in breast cancer, lymphoma, and stem cell transplant–conditioning regimens, is associated with sporadic instances of CHF that may be severe and occur within a few days of cyclophosphamide administration, especially at high doses. Hemorrhagic myocarditis with myonecrosis was seen on autopsy specimens from these patients. These events appear to be unrelated to the cumulative dose or method of administration. CHF from ifosfamide has also been reported.[52] CHF is usually seen approximately 2 weeks after high doses of the drug and appears more frequently in patients with concurrent renal insufficiency. Medical management successfully reverses the heart failure in most patients. CHF is also associated with trastuzumab, an antibody to HER-2/neu, used commonly in the management of breast carcinoma. The incidence of CHF after trastuzumab therapy in a large randomized trial was between 3% and 4%, and it was more common in patients with antecedent cardiac disease, older patients, and those with a diminished ejection fraction after anthracycline-containing chemotherapy.[53] Most patients with trastuzumab-induced cardiac dysfunction have improved symptoms with appropriate medical management of CHF and discontinuation of trastuzumab.

Radiation therapy delivered to the chest for the treatment of Hodgkin's disease, lung malignancies, breast cancer, or other neoplasms can result in a number of cardiac toxicities, including radiation pericarditis with tamponade, myocardial fibrosis, and premature coronary artery disease. The toxic effects of radiation therapy are secondary to microvessel fibrosis and may take up to 20 years to appear.[54] After mantle field radiation therapy, the risk for fatal myocardial infarction is more than three times greater than in age-matched controls.

PULMONARY COMPLICATIONS IN CANCER PATIENTS

Many of the same mechanical issues that influence cardiac dysfunction are likewise pertinent to pulmonary problems with an underlying neoplasm. Chemotherapy and radiation therapy can also cause lasting and sometimes fatal pulmonary complications. Many of these conditions are difficult to diagnose and can be confused with other clinical entities, such as opportunistic infections. Indeed, pneumonia is the most common pulmonary disorder requiring intensive care in cancer patients. A number of acute and chronic pulmonary manifestations are discussed.

Lymphangitic Tumor Involvement

Interstitial lung processes in cancer patients may be due to a variety of infectious insults but can also be caused by direct lymphangitic spread of the tumor. The symptoms of lymphangitic involvement are nonspecific and include dyspnea, nonproductive cough, and hypoxemia. Pulmonary hypertension and cor pulmonale can also be present. The diagnosis can be established by open lung or transbronchial biopsy. Pulmonary microvascular cytology of cells obtained with a wedged pulmonary artery catheter may be a less invasive way to make the diagnosis of lymphangitic carcinomatosis.[55] The prognosis of this condition is generally poor, with a life expectancy of 1 to 6 months. Appropriate chemotherapy or hormonal treatment should be implemented when the site of the primary malignancy is diagnosed.

Treatment-Induced Pulmonary Dysfunction

A number of chemotherapy agents and radiation therapy can cause chronic pneumonitis leading to pulmonary fibrosis. The chemotherapeutic agents most likely to cause this problem are bleomycin and mitomycin, but other alkylators, nitrosoureas, antimetabolites, gemcitabine, and vinca alkaloids can cause pulmonary dysfunction. Although acute hypersensitivity reactions can occur with procarbazine and methotrexate,[56] the most common mechanism for both chemotherapy- and radiation-induced lung damage is oxygen free radical formation. Both alveolar and microvascular damage can occur through this mechanism. The pathophysiology is similar to oxygen toxicity and can be exacerbated by oxygen. For this reason, cancer patients in need of supplemental oxygen should receive the lowest possible fractional concentration of oxygen that produces a hemoglobin oxygen saturation of greater than 90%. Irreversible lung damage can occur if excessive oxygen is administered to patients receiving bleomycin or radiation therapy. Clinical assessment is crucial to patient management because there are no sensitive or accurate tests to predict the onset or course of bleomycin-induced pulmonary toxicity. The resting diffusion capacity has been used, but it is suboptimal for monitoring patients.[57] Treatment recommendations are based on the recognition of three distinct clinical entities:

1. Asymptomatic radiographic changes. Such patients do not require treatment.
2. Radiation- or chemotherapy-induced pneumonitis; pulmonary infiltrates in association with fever, cough, and shortness of breath. Glucocorticoids are the treatment of choice. The mechanism of glucocorticoid action may involve reducing inflammation and microvessel damage through inhibition of leukotriene synthesis, inducing granulocyte demargination from endothelial cells, and direct toxicity to lymphocytes.
3. Chronic pulmonary fibrosis, cor pulmonale, or pulmonary hypertension from chemotherapy or radiation therapy. No therapy has proved effective.

Diffuse Interstitial Pneumonitis

The differential diagnosis of diffuse pulmonary infiltrates in cancer patients is extensive. Infectious causes include bacterial, viral, fungal, and protozoal pathogens. Noninfectious causes of diffuse pulmonary infiltrates are neoplasms, autoimmune disease, cardiac failure, leukostasis, pulmonary hemorrhage, and radiation- or chemotherapy-induced pneumonitis. Making a diagnosis on clinical grounds is difficult because the radiographic and physical examination findings are virtually indistinguishable among these diverse entities. Performing an open lung biopsy is often the only way to confirm a diagnosis; however, empiric treatment may result in equally good patient outcomes. A randomized study compared immediate open lung biopsy followed by therapy directed at the diagnosis and empiric antibiotics alone without biopsy to treat diffuse pulmonary infiltrates in cancer patients.[58] The antibiotic regimen included trimethoprim-sulfamethoxazole (20 mg/kg/d intravenously) and erythromycin (30 mg/kg/d intravenously, divided into four daily doses). A broad-spectrum antibiotic was added if the patient was neutropenic at the time of diagnosis. There was no significant difference in the outcome of patients managed by these two methods; however, those who underwent open lung biopsy had a greater complication rate. Empiric antibiotics are appropriate initial management for diffuse interstitial infiltrates, but patients who do not improve after 4 days of empiric therapy should undergo open lung biopsy.

The decision to place a patient with a cancer diagnosis on ventilator support is often controversial for medical staff and families. It is generally recognized that such patients have a poor prognosis, with a mortality rate approaching 80%. A large multicenter trial prospectively examined prognostic variables for cancer patients requiring ventilatory support.[59] Factors having a statistically significant negative influence on survival were a diagnosis of leukemia, allogeneic stem cell transplantation, progressive cancer, cardiac dysrhythmia, the presence of disseminated intravascular coagulation (DIC), and a need for vasopressor support. Previous surgery with curative intent was protective and probably relates to a selection bias for patients with physiologic reserve sufficient to tolerate surgery. Although this model is similar to other prognostic models used in the ICU, it differs in its emphasis on cancer-specific factors. In general, assessment of the potential reversibility of the organ dysfunction is the critical variable. Most iatrogenic toxicities are reversible, and patients placed in danger by the treatment can generally be supported to recovery. Similarly, the organ dysfunction from treatable malignancies should be assumed to be reversible. However, when more than three organ systems are failing, the chance of recovery is very small. The decision to place a cancer patient on ventilator support is highly individualized, but such models can assist in counseling families about level-of-care issues.

Hemoptysis

Hemoptysis can be an initial sign of cancer, especially endobronchial lesions of non–small cell lung cancer. Patients with significant hemoptysis and airway compromise can be palliated with a variety of bronchoscopic techniques, including argon or neodymium : yttrium-aluminum-garnet (Nd : YAG) laser, photodynamic therapy, stent placement, endoluminal brachytherapy, or combinations of these techniques.[60] External beam radiation, pulmonary artery embolization, and blood pressure control can also be effective in controlling hemoptysis.

Bevacizumab, a monoclonal antibody against vascular endothelial growth factor, has been used with chemotherapy agents to increase the overall response time to progression in lung cancer. Bevacizumab can also cause significant and life-threatening hemoptysis, especially in patients with squamous cell lung cancer.[61] The mechanism of hemoptysis after bevacizumab is collapse of the tumor vasculature resulting in tumor cavitation in proximity to major blood vessels. Because cancer outcomes can be improved with bevacizumab, we endorse an aggressive approach in supporting patients who experience hemoptysis as a result of this vascular-targeting agent.

INFECTIOUS COMPLICATIONS IN CANCER PATIENTS

Pancytopenia is perhaps the most common sequela of dose-intense chemotherapy regimens. Fever in the setting of neutropenia is a life-threatening complication of many chemotherapies, whether given with adjuvant, palliative, or curative intent. The microbial pathogens that infect neutropenic patients have changed over the last 20 years. Previously, *Pseudomonas aeruginosa* was one of the most common organisms in this setting, but staphylococci, streptococci, and vancomycin-resistant organisms have become increasingly prevalent.[62] Improved broad-spectrum antibiotics and hematopoietic growth factors have greatly improved the outcome of febrile neutropenic patients,[63,64] many of whom can be managed easily without intensive care interventions. Despite these advances, a substantial percentage of patients who die during chemotherapy still succumb to neutropenic infections. This section focuses on septic shock and the infections that commonly occur as complications of cancer treatment. Infections that arise as a consequence of the severe immune system compromise after bone marrow transplantation are covered separately.

Febrile Neutropenia and Septic Shock

Despite appropriate broad-spectrum antibiotics, approximately 10% of febrile neutropenic patients progress to septic shock. The pathogenesis of the circulatory changes in septic shock may be similar to those that take place after IL-1 or IL-2 administration (see later). Patients in septic shock have elevated nitrate levels.[65] In a randomized, double-blind, placebo-controlled trial of 12 patients testing N^G-monomethyl-L-arginine (L-NMMA) as a nitric oxide inhibitor, significant increases in mean arterial pressure, systemic vascular resistance, pulmonary vascular resistance, and central venous pressure were seen with L-NMMA.[66] L-NMMA cannot be advocated for the routine treatment of septic shock because decreases in cardiac output were also observed; thus, tissue perfusion may be compromised with this agent.

Other strategies have been tried in an attempt to prevent the circulatory collapse and end-organ changes that occur during sepsis. Most of these strategies involve blocking cytokine receptors; however, clinical results have been mixed, and additional investigation is required before they become accepted treatment.[67,68] Activated recombinant protein C (drotrecogin alfa) has been shown to diminish mortality in severe sepsis and was approved by the Food and Drug Administration for this indication.[69] The mechanism of action of drotrecogin involves modulation of the inflammatory process that causes endovascular injury and end-organ damage. There is a risk of severe bleeding after drotrecogin, and it should not be used unless there is multiple organ failure from sepsis.

Despite a growing number of drugs that may influence the pathophysiology of shock, pressor agents such as phenylephrine, dopamine, dobutamine, and norepinephrine remain standard treatment of the hemodynamic consequences of shock.

NEUROLOGIC COMPLICATIONS IN CANCER PATIENTS

Brain or spinal cord metastases can often be managed outside the ICU but may require acute intervention if there is evidence of increased intracranial pressure or spinal cord compression. Seizure management in cancer patients is also discussed.

Spinal Cord Compression

The tumors that most often cause spinal cord compression from epidural metastases or bone destruction are carcinomas of the lung, breast, and prostate and multiple myeloma. The level of spinal cord involvement determines the clinical neurologic deficit. Cervical cord compression can cause quadriplegia or respiratory arrest; thoracic involvement can result in paraplegia, and lumbar involvement can give rise to loss of bladder and bowel function. If the problem is detected when local or radicular pain is the only symptom, treatment with glucocorticoids, radiation therapy, or laminectomy can be highly effective. If the patient has a neurologic deficit, such as an inability to walk, the chance of significant improvement is less than 10%.[70] MRI is the diagnostic test of choice for diagnosing epidural metastases. Glucocorticoids should be started on an emergency basis in patients with myelopathy (dexamethasone, 10 mg followed by 4 mg every 6 hours) and imaging obtained as soon as possible. The maximal effect of dexamethasone in alleviating symptoms may not be achieved at total doses of 24 mg/day. If clinical improvement from glucocorticoids is suboptimal, doubling the dose each day up to a maximum total dose of 200 mg/d may improve control of symptoms until definitive therapy is implemented.[71] The standard of care for cord compression had been glucocorticoids and radiation therapy; however, a randomized trial has shown benefit with decompressive surgery followed by radiation therapy.[72] Eighty-four percent of patients randomized to receive surgery and radiation therapy maintained the ability to walk, as compared with 57% in the radiation-alone group. Better palliation of pain and duration of ambulation were maintained in the surgery group. This study has been criticized for possible biases in patient assignment and because the outcome of the radiation-alone group was poorer than would normally be expected. Furthermore, the potential morbidity associated with an anterior approach to surgical cord decompression was de-emphasized in the authors' interpretation of their results. Nevertheless, surgery can be an effective control measure and is no longer reserved solely for patients with obvious displaced fractures of the vertebrae.

Brain Metastases and Hemorrhage

Tumor metastatic to the brain may be a localized problem amenable to surgical resection with good results.[73] Patients with significant peritumoral edema and increased intracranial pressure may suffer brain herniation if acute measures are not taken. Therapy includes high-dose glucocorticoids (dexamethasone, 10 mg followed by 4 mg intravenously every 6 hours), intubation and mechanical hyperventilation to maintain an arterial partial pressure of carbon dioxide ($PaCO_2$) between 25 and 30 mm Hg, and mannitol diuresis (1.0 to 1.5 g/kg intravenously as a 20% solution). Patients who do not respond may benefit from higher glucocorticoid doses (dexamethasone, 25 to 50 mg every 6 hours). After stabilizing the patient with these acute interventions, definitive treatment with radiation therapy or surgery can be started. Prophylactic anticonvulsants are often administered; however, this intervention has scant supportive data and should be withheld in most patients until a seizure has occurred.[74] Frontal lobe tumor deposits and brain metastases from melanoma are two situations in which prophylactic phenytoin should be considered. Newer radiation techniques such as gamma knife radiosurgery can also be effective in controlling or eradicating brain metastatic disease, although this modality is more appropriate for patients with good functional status.

Dose-intensive therapy for acute leukemias is associated with prolonged thrombocytopenia and the possibility of intracranial hemorrhage. It was previously thought that such events were highly associated with platelet counts lower than 20,000/μL[75]; however, the threshold for platelet transfusion used in most medical centers is now 10,000/μL based on a randomized trial that showed no difference in patient outcome with the more stringent threshold.[76] Other events, such as sepsis and fever, contribute to the likelihood of bleeding with thrombocytopenia. Patients with solid tumors are also less likely than those with leukemia to bleed as a consequence of thrombocytopenia. In cancer patients with suspected intracranial bleeding and thrombocytopenia, the platelet count should be maintained above 50,000/μL. The best strategy to maintain adequate hemostatic function with platelet transfusion support is controversial because platelet kinetics are complex.[77,78] Transfusion strategies range from frequent transfusion of a small number of platelet units, continuous infusion of platelets, to less frequent administration of large numbers of platelet units. We advocate frequent dosing or continuous infusion of platelets in actively bleeding thrombocytopenic patients who have poor increments after transfusion as a result of platelet sensitization. The blood bank should identify human leukocyte antigen (HLA)-matched platelet donors for such patients and maintain an adequate supply of the HLA-matched platelets. Single-donor platelets are more effective than pooled platelets in this setting.

Uncontrolled Seizures

In 15% to 30% of patients in whom brain metastases develop, the initial sign is a generalized seizure.[79] Metabolic disturbances, such as hyponatremia from SIADH, may also cause seizures in cancer patients. Acute control can be achieved with intravenous diazepam (5 mg every 5 to 10 minutes, up to 30 mg). Standard measures to protect the airway, prevent aspiration, and avoid limb injury should also be implemented. After acute control has been attained, phenytoin should be started (15 mg/kg intravenously at a maximum rate of 50 mg/min, then maintenance doses of 300 mg/d). Phenytoin levels should be checked because glucocorticoids given for brain metastases can increase the rate of phenytoin metabolism. Phenytoin upregulates the P-450 system in the liver, which may accelerate the metabolism of certain chemotherapy agents such as paclitaxel and docetaxel.[80,81] Antiseizure agents that do not influence P-450 cytochromes, such as gabapentin, should be used in patients requiring taxane-based chemotherapy.

Seizures, coma, and other neurologic complications can occur with a variety of chemotherapy and biologic agents. Most of these toxicities improve with cessation of the causative agent and supportive care. Ifosfamide-induced neurotoxicity has a unique mechanism related to changes in mitochondrial fatty acid oxidation and the accumulation of glutaric acid metabolites.[82] Treatment with methylene blue (200 to 300 mg orally or intravenously daily), an electron-accepting drug, can reverse and prevent neurologic toxicity during ifosfamide infusion.[83]

GASTROINTESTINAL COMPLICATIONS IN CANCER PATIENTS

Bowel obstruction is still a common cause of morbidity and mortality in cancer patients. Lymphomatous bowel involvement is relatively common in lymphoma patients with acquired immunodeficiency syndrome (AIDS).[84] Management of these problems can often be accomplished with meticulous standard care; however, intensive support may be needed for emergency surgical or medical conditions arising from gastrointestinal complications.

Tumor-Induced Emergencies

For most tumor types, obstruction may be related to a localized constricting or obstructing lesion that is readily amenable to surgical correction. In women with ovarian cancer, the obstruction is often related to loss of peristalsis in long segments of bowel because of diffuse wall invasion by malignancy. Little can be done with surgical intervention in such circumstances. Improvement hinges on the availability of effective chemotherapy. Bowel obstruction or perforation can occur from primary or metastatic tumors. If the patient has peritoneal signs of an acute abdomen, emergency exploratory surgery is indicated.[85] For less clear-cut manifestations, abdominal radiographs, CT scans, and endoscopy may be helpful. These patients can be managed initially with bowel rest, nasogastric suction, and anaerobic antibiotic coverage until a diagnosis is made. Somatostatin can provide palliation in some patients, probably by increasing intestinal water resorption.[86]

Biliary obstruction can occur from primary tumors of the pancreas, bile ducts, or gallbladder but is more commonly associated with tumors metastatic to the porta hepatis, such as breast carcinoma, melanoma, or lymphoma. Ascending cholangitis and sepsis are possible sequelae if bile drainage is not accomplished. A percutaneous or endoscopic approach can be used to decompress the bile ducts on an emergency basis. Effective treatment of the primary tumor should be implemented when possible. If the tumor is unlikely to respond to chemotherapy or radiation therapy, palliation with an internal stent or an operative biliary diversion procedure is indicated.

Hemorrhage of an abdominal viscus can occur in association with chemotherapy or as a result of an uncontrolled tumor. Identifying the source of the bleeding can be accomplished with endoscopy, CT, angiography, or labeled red blood cell studies. Bleeding from ulcers or mucosal irritation from chemotherapy can usually be managed medically or with endoscopic control via a heater probe or Nd:YAG laser. If a tumor deposit is the cause, surgical control of the site should be considered. If the patient is not a surgical candidate, an angiographic embolization procedure may provide effective palliation.

Chemotherapy-Induced Gastrointestinal Dysfunction

Typhlitis (ileocecal syndrome) is seen most often in patients with leukemia who are receiving induction chemotherapy. It usually develops after more than 7 days of neutropenia and consists of watery diarrhea, abdominal distention, and right-sided abdominal tenderness. Bowel rest and antibiotics may be successful in treating this condition, but surgery is required for repeated sepsis, bowel necrosis, or perforation. This syndrome can occur on subsequent cycles of chemotherapy; thus, a colonic diversion procedure may be needed to complete chemotherapy.

A number of chemotherapeutic agents can cause decreases in bowel motility and ileus. Examples of such medications are vincristine and cytosine arabinoside. Supportive care of the ileus is usually successful, but toxic megacolon can occur and is an indication for surgical management.

A particularly difficult management problem is the severe constipation that can accompany the use of opioid analgesics in patients with advanced cancer. Prophylactic measures are very important, including the use of stool softeners and osmotic laxatives and maintaining patient activity as much as possible. Even with optimal prophylaxis, results are often unsatisfactory.

Gastrointestinal Lymphomas

Lymphoma manifested as a gastric or intestinal mass is common in AIDS patients and in those with B-cell lymphomas arising in mucosa-associated lymphatic tissue (MALT) of the stomach secondary to *Helicobacter pylori* infection. This situation warrants extreme caution because perforation of an abdominal viscus is a possible life-threatening complication of potentially curative chemotherapy. Because perforation is a major concern in these patients, initial surgical resection is advocated by some authors.[87,88] Others have noted low rates of abdominal catastrophe in patients treated with chemotherapy and radiation therapy alone.[89] Perforation is rare in patients with MALT lymphoma who achieve a tumor response with antibiotics or radiation therapy.[90] Patients with extensive gastric involvement by lymphoma who undergo chemotherapy should start treatment in the hospital with surgical consultation to monitor for possible perforation or obstruction. Perforation is more common in patients with small intestinal involvement by lymphomas with aggressive histology than in patients with gastric or colon involvement.

GENITOURINARY COMPLICATIONS IN CANCER PATIENTS

Intensive care interventions for genitourinary tract problems may be required for the sequelae of obstruction or primary renal dysfunction. Tumors arising locally, metastatic tumors, and certain chemotherapy drugs can give rise to genitourinary problems. Both tumor-induced and chemotherapy toxicities are discussed.

Tumor-Induced Genitourinary Dysfunction

Obstructive uropathy resulting in hydronephrosis can occur at the bladder outlet or anywhere along the path of the ureter. Bladder outlet problems are most commonly caused by local tumor invasion from cervical, prostate, bladder, rectosigmoid, or ovarian neoplasms. Metastatic deposits from gastric, breast, or pancreatic malignancies can also obstruct the bladder outlet. Tumors that arise from retroperitoneal structures or metastasize to the retroperitoneum can cause ureteral obstruction. Examples of tumors that commonly have a retroperitoneal focus are Hodgkin's and non-Hodgkin's lymphoma, testicular tumors, and axial sarcomas. Primary tumors of the ureter can also cause obstruction. If the obstruction and resulting hydronephrosis are of short duration, percutaneous drainage and decompression are recommended. If a concurrent infection is present, decompression is mandatory and constitutes an oncologic emergency. After a period of 48 to 72 hours, a ureteral stent can be placed via an anterograde or retrograde approach. Furosemide renal scanning can be used to confirm the presence of kidney function if there is a question about the reversibility of the functional impairment of the obstructed kidney.[91] After stenting, appropriate radiation therapy, chemotherapy, or hormonal treatment should be implemented for control of the malignancy.

Renal function can also be compromised indirectly by malignancies. Nephrotic syndrome is seen in association with several solid tumors, such as colon, gastric, ovarian, and breast carcinoma. Lymphomas, especially those of T-cell origin, and chronic lymphocytic leukemia can also cause nephrotic syndrome and other glomerulopathies. Multiple myeloma and Waldenström's macroglobulinemia can produce amyloid and cryoglobulin deposits in the kidneys and result in acute tubular necrosis or interstitial nephritis. Recurrent and chronic pyelonephritis is common in patients with myeloma. Dialysis may be necessary to support the patient until effective antitumor therapy is given.

Chemotherapy-Induced Genitourinary Complications

Hemorrhagic cystitis can be caused by acrolein, a metabolite of cyclophosphamide and ifosfamide. This problem can usually be prevented with adequate hydration, bladder irrigation, or the use of thiol-based chemoprotectants such as mesna. Administration of mesna is mandatory for ifosfamide treatment. If the hemorrhagic cystitis is severe and unresponsive to supportive measures and saline bladder irrigation, formalin bladder instillation can be performed under general anesthesia.[92] A 1% formalin solution should be used, but bladder fibrosis and strictures may occur despite this low concentration. Care must be taken to avoid reflux of the formalin up the ureters. Urinary diversion and cystectomy may be required for uncontrolled bleeding.

Table 81-2. Leucovorin Rescue for Methotrexate Toxicity

Methotrexate drug levels above 5×10^{-7} M 48 h after infusion require additional leucovorin rescue as follows:

Drug Level	Dose of Leucovorin
5×10^{-7}	15 mg/m² q6h×8 doses
1×10^{-6}	100 mg/m² q6h×8 doses
2×10^{-6}	200 mg/m² q6h×8 doses

Drug levels should be determined every 48 hours and the leucovorin dose adjusted until the drug concentration is less than 5×10^{-8} M.

Methotrexate, an antifolate chemotherapeutic agent, can precipitate in renal tubules and cause acute tubular necrosis if adequate hydration and urinary alkalinization are not achieved before therapy. If renal toxicity occurs, leucovorin rescue should be started, based on serum levels of methotrexate (see Table 81-2 for details of prevention or reversal of methotrexate toxicity). Intravenous fluids containing bicarbonate, furosemide, and mannitol may be helpful in preventing oliguric renal failure.

HEMATOLOGIC COMPLICATIONS IN CANCER PATIENTS

Although clinical prodromes for leukemias may evolve over a period of weeks or months, treatment of these disorders, once diagnosed, is often urgent and requires intensive care support. This support is needed not only to treat a number of well-known disease-related complications but also to manage chemotherapy toxicities because some of the most dose-intense drug regimens are used against these malignancies.

Hyperleukocytosis

Large numbers of leukemic blasts may be present in acute leukemias or in the late stages of chronic leukemias. When the number of circulating myeloblasts is greater than 100,000 cells/μL, the viscosity of blood increases because white blood cells are much less deformable than red blood cells. Patients with chronic lymphocytic leukemia can tolerate higher circulating numbers of malignant cells (e.g., 100,000 to 300,000 cells/μL) without consequence. In acute leukemia, the blasts may invade and weaken the vessel wall, thereby leading to hemorrhage. Hyperleukocytosis chiefly affects the microvasculature in the lungs and the central nervous system. Symptoms can range from mild shortness of breath and blurred vision to pulmonary congestion, hypoxia, intracranial hemorrhage, and TLS. Rapid institution of leukapheresis can often decrease leukocyte counts by 20% to 50%.[93] Although the improvement may be transient, chemotherapy for the underlying leukemia can be accomplished with greater safety and perhaps a lesser degree of TLS.

All-*trans*-retinoic acid (ATRA), used in the treatment of acute promyelocytic leukemia (APL), induces differentiation of leukemic cells.[94] ATRA is associated with a leukocytosis syndrome characterized by fever, dyspnea, and interstitial lung infiltrates on the chest radiograph, which can progress to acute respiratory distress syndrome (ARDS).[95] ARDS may be secondary to the accumulation of differentiated leukemic blasts and their release of cytokines such as IL-2 into the lung. Leukapheresis is ineffective in this setting; however, the early implementation of glucocorticoids is beneficial (dexamethasone, 10 to 20 mg/d in divided doses).

Disseminated Intravascular Coagulation

DIC can be associated with a variety of solid tumors, including carcinoma of the prostate, lung, breast, and gastrointestinal tract and melanomas. However, DIC is the hallmark of the clinical manifestation of APL. The leukemic blasts in APL manufacture procoagulants that are released into the circulation, particularly after cytotoxic chemotherapy.[96] The use of ATRA for treating APL has lessened the severity of DIC in this illness, but a new complication has been added (discussed previously). To manage DIC in APL, serial determinations of fibrin split products and fibrinogen levels should be made. Replacement of fibrinogen can be accomplished with cryoprecipitate (1 bag per 2 kg of body weight initially, followed by 1 bag per 10 to 15 kg of body weight daily). If DIC worsens after cryoprecipitate, intravenous heparin can be started but should be used cautiously. Antifibrinolytic agents, such as ε-aminocaproic acid, should be avoided because they can block the normal dissolution of thrombi and increase organ damage.

The most effective approach to DIC is prevention. Given the reciprocal serious complications associated with using ATRA alone or cytotoxic chemotherapy in the treatment of APL, the DIC and ATRA syndromes are best prevented by using ATRA and combination chemotherapy together so that the mass of cells differentiating in response to ATRA can be reduced by the cytotoxic chemotherapy to levels that do not result in sticking and sludging in the lungs.

BIOLOGIC THERAPY

Advances in molecular biology have made large quantities of cytokines, monoclonal antibodies, and chimeric molecules available for clinical use and testing. Examples of biologically active compounds that have been approved for patient use or are in clinical trials include the interferons (α, β, and γ), interleukins (IL-2, IL-11, IL-12, IL-18), colony-stimulating factors (GM-CSF), monoclonal antibodies (anti–HER-2/neu [trastuzumab, Herceptin], anti-CD20 [rituximab, Rituxan]), and antibody-radioisotope conjugates (tositumomab [Bexxar]). Intensive basic science and clinical research efforts are ongoing to realize the full potential of these molecules. Although their role in the treatment of cancer, infectious disease, and immune disorders is a work in progress, much has been learned about their clinical toxicities. Most are not associated with toxicities that require intensive or emergency care aside from very rare hypersensitivity reactions. Hypotension limits the dose of some of these agents, particularly IL-2 and IL-12. Mechanisms of cytokine-induced hypotension are discussed next, followed by a more extensive review of other IL-2 toxicities because it has been approved for clinical use in metastatic melanoma and renal cell carcinoma.[9,10]

Interleukin-2 Therapy–Induced Hypotension

The causes of IL-2–induced hypotension and vascular leak are increasingly being understood. It is known that cytokines such as IL-1 and IL-2 cause relaxation of the endothelium via induction of nitric oxide.[65,97] Clinical data also support the notion that nitrate levels are greatly elevated in patients treated with IL-2.[98] Nitric oxide can be produced by vascular endothelial cells, macrophages, hepatocytes, and central nervous system neurons. It is synthesized from arginine by nitric oxide synthase (NOS), a nicotinamide adenine dinucleotide phosphate–dependent enzyme.[99] Nitric oxide is thought to diffuse through vascular endothelial cells and act on pericytes and myocytes to cause blood vessel relaxation. This process is mediated through cyclical guanosine monophosphate (cGMP). Increased levels of cGMP induce a sequence of modifications of the myosin light chain in smooth muscle that result in muscle relaxation and blood vessel dilation.[100] There are a number of ways to manipulate nitric oxide synthesis pathways or block the effects of nitric oxide after it is made. Arginine analogues such as L-NMMA, N^G-nitro-L-arginine methyl ester, and N^G-amino-L-arginine competitively bind to NOS and inhibit nitric oxide production. Clinical trials are investigating the effectiveness of these agents on IL-2–induced hypotension, although preliminary results have been disappointing with this strategy. Another approach to inhibit nitrates involves the inhibition of tetrahydrobiopterin synthesis in macrophages. Elevated neopterin levels, a marker of macrophage activation, have been measured in patients receiving IL-2 or IL-12.[14,101,102] Neopterin is a by-product of tetrahydrobiopterin synthesis, which in turn is a necessary cofactor for nitrate production.[95] Sepiapterin reductase inhibitors such as *N*-acetylserotonin and *N*-acetyl-*m*-tyramine, decrease tetrahydrobiopterin production as shown in in vitro experiments.[103] Manipulation of this pathway has not yet been tested in humans.

Although IL-2 induces the synthesis of nitric oxide, other mechanisms may also be operative in IL-2–induced hypotension and vascular leak. Adhesion of activated lymphocytes to vascular endothelium after the administration of IL-2 has been shown to cause vascular leak in a rabbit model.[104] Furthermore, it was shown in this model that both lymphocyte adhesion and vascular leak were decreased by intravenous dextran sulfate infusions. Other in vitro evidence supports the hypothesis that dextrans inhibit lymphocyte-endothelial interactions.[105,106] Dextrans with a molecular weight of 450,000 to 500,000 D were the most effective in blocking these lymphocyte-endothelium interactions. The vascular toxicity from IL-12 treatment is also largely dependent on natural killer (NK) cell trafficking.[107] In a murine model, abrogation of IL-12–induced vascular collapse was achieved by eliminating NK cells. In humans, other cytokines mediate the vascular and immunologic effects of IL-12, most notably interferon-γ.[101]

The hemodynamic physiology of IL-2–induced hypotension is essentially the same as warm shock[108]; thus, effective support for these patients requires the use of parenteral α-adrenergic agonists such as phenylephrine or dopamine.[109] Recommendations for treating cytokine-induced hypotension are given in Table 81-3. Fluid administration, though of transient benefit, often exacerbates the pulmonary capillary leak seen with IL-2. IL-2 infusions can be continued, despite hypotension, with appropriate pressor management. In our clinical experience, phenylephrine doses of up to 200 μg/min are well tolerated while continuing IL-2. If the patient requires more than this level of pressor support, IL-2 doses are withheld until the capillary leak has improved sufficiently to warrant a decrease in phenylephrine to less than 100 μg/min.

As illustrated previously, many of the mediators of cytokine-induced hypotension are also central to the pathophysiology of septic shock. Thus, advances in the treatment of immunotherapy-related toxicities may translate into improvements in general intensive care medicine. There are a number of other systemic toxicities that complicate cytokine therapy. IL-2 will be used to illustrate these problems because clinical experience with it is more extensive than with other cytokines and it is also the only interleukin approved for cancer treatment.

Table 81-3. Schema for the Treatment of Cytokine-Induced Hypotension

Blood Pressure (BP) (mm Hg)	Treatment
80<BP<90 (asymptomatic)	500-mL 0.9% saline bolus followed by IV saline at 150 mL/h Phenylephrine, 50 μg/min IV titrated up to 200 μg/min to maintain systolic BP>90
70<BP<80	Maintain or consider an increase in phenylephrine and add dopamine; titrate to a maximum of 20 μg/kg/min to maintain systolic BP>90
BP<70 or 70<BP<80 on the maximal phenylephrine dose	Consider infusion of norepinephrine, methylprednisolone
BP unresponsive to above or cardiac sequelae of hypotension	Hetastarch, 500-mL IV bolus, then 250 mg IV q6h; methylene blue, 1-3 mg/kg IV over 5-min period, followed by infusion at the same rate per hour if the bolus increases BP

Interleukin-2 Toxicities and Their Management

Pulmonary Capillary Leak

The clinical manifestations of IL-2–related pulmonary toxicity often do not correlate with the severity of the radiologic findings. Between 70% and 80% of patients receiving IL-2 have some radiographic abnormality, which may consist of pleural effusions, diffuse infiltrates, or focal infiltrates.[110,111] These findings do not correlate with the degree of systemic capillary leak but occur more frequently in the presence of concurrent bacteremia and pretreatment pulmonary compromise as manifested by decreased forced expiratory volume in 1 second (FEV_1).

Pulmonary capillary leak with IL-2 may be mediated by infiltration of the lungs with neutrophils and systemic increases in thromboxane B_2.[112] Because clinically significant pulmonary capillary leak cannot be anticipated by radiographic findings, relatively minor symptoms such as tachypnea need to be carefully evaluated in patients receiving IL-2. Pulse oximetry is sometimes helpful but can be falsely low in patients concurrently receiving phenylephrine for IL-2–induced hypotension; therefore, arterial blood gas analysis may be required for these patients. Hypoxemia should be treated with oxygen supplementation, which can be delivered initially by nasal cannula or Venturi mask. Worsening hypoxemia may sometimes respond to diuresis; however, intubation may be required in some patients. A key to the ventilatory management of IL-2–induced lung toxicity is to reverse the pulmonary edema through positive end-expiratory pressure and enhancement of renal function. Although high partial pressures of oxygen may be required in the initial treatment of these patients, prolonged oxygen exposure may exacerbate IL-2 toxicity.[109] For this reason, rapid titration of oxygen to maintain an arterial partial pressure of oxygen of 60 mm Hg or greater is recommended. If diffuse pulmonary infiltrates worsen and an ARDS-like syndrome develops, parenteral glucocorticoids should be considered. A large body of literature suggests that glucocorticoids are contraindicated in the management of ARDS.[113] There has been no controlled study of glucocorticoid use in patients receiving cytokines. Some evidence suggests that glucocorticoids improve IL-2–related toxicities, but no randomized trials have been performed.[114] It has been our experience that individual patients with severe IL-2 pulmonary toxicity usually improve with the use of glucocorticoids. The beneficial effect of glucocorticoids may be mediated by the lysis of activated lymphocytes that have been stimulated by IL-2.[115]

Renal and Liver Dysfunction

Hypotension and the systemic capillary leak associated with IL-2 also create renal and liver toxicities. The renal dysfunction typically consists of oliguria and prerenal azotemia with elevated blood urea nitrogen and creatinine.[116,117] Creatinine levels greater than 6.0 mg/dL or 530 μmol/L are often tolerated without modifying IL-2 doses because recovery is rapid after IL-2 treatment is completed. The associated oliguria mandates meticulous fluid management because the pulmonary toxicity may be exacerbated by fluid overload. Low-dose dopamine (2 to 5 μg/kg/min) is often helpful to maintain urine output but does not change the degree of IL-2–induced azotemia.[118] Furosemide or other nonthiazide diuretics can be tried but are infrequently effective and may exacerbate IL-2–related hypotension.

Liver toxicity from IL-2 is usually manifested as hyperbilirubinemia and elevations in hepatocellular enzymes.[109] Liver synthetic functions may be impaired with some IL-2 regimens.[14] This phenomenon may be related to diminished hepatic protein synthesis with inducible nitrate production.[119] Disturbances in liver function rarely cause discontinuation of IL-2 therapy or need specific medical intervention. Even bilirubin levels higher than 10 mg/dL are generally followed by complete recovery after IL-2 administration is stopped.

Cardiac Rhythm Disturbances and Myocardial Infarction

IL-2 is associated with a variety of cardiac problems, including nonspecific ST or T wave changes, dysrhythmias (most commonly supraventricular tachycardia, but ventricular tachycardia can also occur), myocarditis, pericarditis, and myocardial ischemia or infarction. The rhythm disturbances and inflammatory conditions may be secondary to infiltration of the myocardium or pericardium by lymphocytes.[120] Any cardiac toxicity (with the exception of sinus tachycardia) should be treated initially by discontinuation of IL-2. Supraventricular tachycardia may respond to adenosine (12 mg by rapid intravenous bolus) and is our agent of choice when IL-2–induced hypotension is present. If hypotension is present and adenosine is ineffective, intravenous diltiazem at doses between 0.15 and 0.45 mg/kg should be considered (as long as the QRS complex is not prolonged >0.12 second) because the incidence of hypotension appears to be less than with other calcium channel blockers.[121] Other cardiovascular events should be managed with the same medical and intensive care interventions used for any other acute cardiac patient.

Hypothyroidism

Hypothyroidism occurs in approximately 10% of patients who receive IL-2 and may be related to antitumor responses.[122] Although hypothyroidism rarely requires acute or intensive care, it may complicate the management of other IL-2 toxicities, such as pulmonary dysfunction. It should be considered in patients requiring ventilatory support after IL-2 who have difficulty recovering their respiratory mechanics. The mechanism of injury appears to be autoimmune destruction of the thyroid. A small fraction of patients may have signs and symptoms of hyperthyroidism because autoimmune destruction may transiently lead to increases in release of thyroid hormone.

Adoptive Cell Transfer and Its Toxicity

A number of immune cell types have been used to treat cancer patients, including lymphokine-activated killer cells, ex vivo activated T cells, tumor-infiltrating lymphocytes, peptide-pulsed or gene-modified dendritic cells, and donor leukocyte infusions.[123-126]

Adoptive cellular therapy with activated lymphocytes may cause pulmonary toxicity. These effects are often acute and develop during cell infusion.[127] When dyspnea occurs during cell infusion, the problem can be managed by slowing or stopping the cell infusion. If more severe toxicity ensues, management should be similar to that described for the pulmonary toxicities of IL-2. Glucocorticoids should be routinely administered for adoptive cell–related pulmonary toxicity that requires intubation.[114]

Allergic and Anaphylactic Reactions to Monoclonal Antibodies

Allergic reactions to monoclonal antibodies occur in 10% to 15% of patients, probably because some agents are chimeric mouse proteins. Molecular engineering to "humanize" these antibodies appears to have diminished the allergic reactions and development of human antimouse antibodies, which can potentially limit the beneficial effect of the monoclonals. However, even humanized antibodies can produce shortness of breath, tachycardia, and hypotension, especially with the first infusion. The symptoms may result from activation of complement by the antibody and are safely managed by slowing or temporarily stopping the antibody infusion. When the symptoms abate, the antibody infusion can be resumed at half the initial rate. Mild allergic manifestations, such as urticaria and pruritus, can be managed with oral antihistamines. We advocate a stepwise approach, starting with H_1 blockers (diphenhydramine, 50 mg every 4 hours, alternating with hydroxyzine, 50 mg). H_2 blockers (ranitidine, 150 mg every 12 hours) may be added if the urticaria worsens. Pharyngeal and laryngeal edema can occur, with or without bronchospasm. Clinical manifestations of upper airway edema include drooling, phonation changes, and a sensation of throat pain or tightness. For these more severe symptoms, cessation of treatment with the antibody is recommended. Parenteral antihistamines should be started, along with inhaled β_1-agonists, if bronchospasm is present. Fiberoptic endoscopic examination of the hypopharynx should be performed to determine the extent of the edema. If repeat fiberoptic examination after 4 to 6 hours shows resolution of the edema, resumption of the antibody at the lower dose or a reduced flow rate can be considered. If the laryngeal edema worsens, intubation may be necessary to protect the airway.

There are rare patients who experience an anaphylactic reaction with circulatory collapse after monoclonal antibody treatment or other immunotherapy. This response is not always predicted by test doses of the antibody. The prognosis for these individuals in our clinical experience is poor, with a mortality rate approaching 100% despite the prompt implementation of intensive care support. Agents that reverse nitrate production or receptor antagonists for IL-1 or TNF may eventually prove useful in the management of this syndrome.

SPECIAL CONSIDERATIONS IN BONE MARROW TRANSPLANTATION

High-dose chemotherapy with stem cell support is central to managing many oncologic disorders, including leukemia, myeloma, and lymphoma. It has been used in other illnesses, such as collagen vascular diseases, aplastic anemia, and hemoglobinopathies. A number of life-threatening toxicities are unique to this form of dose-intense therapy and require intensive care management. The pathophysiology and treatment recommendations for these entities are discussed later.

Acute and Chronic Graft-versus-Host Disease

Graft-versus-host disease (GVHD) is most commonly seen in the setting of allogeneic transplantation but can be observed after syngeneic and autologous transplants. It is well documented that GVHD can reduce recurrence rates in leukemia[128]; it also lowers overall survival after transplantation. The prerequisites for GVHD are that the graft include a population of immunologically competent T cells, the graft recipient must be unable to destroy these cells, and tissue antigens must be present in the recipient that are not present in the donor.[129]

The clinical manifestations of GVHD include rash (maculopapular or diffusely erythematous), liver function abnormalities, and gastrointestinal symptoms such as diarrhea, nausea, vomiting, and ileus.[128] These toxicities are graded (I to IV) on a semiquantitative basis. Grade I or II GVHD has relatively little morbidity, but grade IV GVHD carries a 100% mortality rate. Treatment of established GVHD requires suppression of the immune system. The means for accomplishing this goal are relatively nonspecific at present. The drugs most commonly used to suppress GVHD are glucocorticoids, cyclosporine, tacrolimus, and methotrexate, which are generally used in combination. Other agents to modulate GVHD, such as engineered T cells, anti–T-cell antibodies, mycophenolate mofetil, and thalidomide, are in clinical trials. Treatment with gamma globulins may also be beneficial in the prophylaxis of GVHD.[130] The mechanism of action of gamma globulin is unknown but may involve binding to Fc receptors, which may prevent T cells from recognizing target tissues.

Veno-occlusive Disease

Hepatic veno-occlusive disease (VOD) is a clinical syndrome characterized by weight gain (fluid), tender hepatomegaly, and elevations of hepatocellular enzymes and bilirubin. The syndrome is due to endothelial toxicity from high-dose chemotherapy and results in a local hypercoagulable state with tissue factor synthesis, downregulation of thrombomodulin, and release of von Willebrand factor with the resultant formation of blood clots in the veins.[131] The incidence of VOD can be diminished with the prophylactic use of heparin.[132] Agents used in the treatment of established VOD include tissue plasminogen activator,[133] antithrombin III,[134] antioxidant therapy,[135] and a transjugular intrahepatic portosystemic stent shunt.[136] Intensive support is often needed for patients with VOD. Despite aggressive treatment, mortality with severe established VOD approaches 100%.[137] Patients with milder disease may recover with supportive measures. Early recognition and intervention are key factors influencing outcome.

Infectious Complications of Stem Cell Transplantation

Different facets of immune function return at varying intervals after bone marrow transplantation.[138] The type of infection that occurs at a given time depends on what parts of the immune system are still compromised after transplantation. Integumentary and mucosal barriers are disrupted in the period immediately after myeloablative chemotherapy. For this reason, aerobic bacteria and *Candida* organisms are the most likely pathogens early in the course. Neutrophil numbers are decreased for the first 2 to 4 weeks after receiving a transplant, although the use of colony-stimulating factors shortens the neutrophil recovery period. Until neutrophil numbers increase, herpes simplex virus, *Candida, Aspergillus,* and bacterial infections are common. It should be noted that the full chemotactic function of neutrophils does not return for 100 days after transplantation. The defects in cellular and humoral immunity persist for 1 to 3 months after transplantation. These T- and B-cell problems may lengthen if GVHD occurs. Fungal and cytomegalovirus (CMV) infections predominate in this period.[139,140] From 3 months to 1 year after transplantation, T cells remain dysfunctional, and disordered immunoregulation may occur. Varicella zoster, hepatitis C, *Pneumocystis carinii* pneumonia, and pneumococcal pneumonia are the most common infections until T-cell function has recovered. The immune deficits may be moderated by antigen-specific immunity conferred by the transplanted marrow and the use of gamma globulin infusions, which are now routinely given after allogeneic transplantation. Antibiotic recommendations in patients with bone marrow transplants are similar to those for other febrile neutropenic cancer patients. Individual recommendations should take into account the frequency of specific microorganisms isolated at a given institution. Trimethoprim-sulfamethoxazole and fluoroquinolone antibiotics (e.g., ciprofloxacin) are routinely used for the prophylaxis of *Pneumocystis* organisms and gram positive infections, respectively. Amphotericin remains the antifungal agent of choice for documented or suspected *Candida* infections. Fluconazole can also be used for the treatment of oral or esophageal candidiasis. *Aspergillus* is very difficult to treat and requires high doses of amphotericin (1.5- to 2.0-g total dose), itraconazole, or the combination of voriconazole and caspofungin. CMV responds poorly to single-agent therapy, but the combination of ganciclovir and gamma globulin infusion improves outcomes in these patients. Death rates from CMV pneumonitis approached 80% before use of the combination regimen. The use of CMV-negative donors and elimination of CMV-contaminated leukocytes from platelet and red blood cell transfusions with leukocyte filters have reduced mortality from CMV.

In the future, cytotoxic T-lymphocyte (CTL) clones may be available for the treatment of specific opportunistic infections. Adoptive transfer of a specific CTL clone against CMV has been tested in patients. Augmentation of antiviral activity was conferred with these infusions.[141] This strategy may prove useful in reducing the number of life-threatening infections in bone marrow transplantation, human immunodeficiency virus, and other immunodeficiency states.[142]

CODE STATUS AND INTENSIVE CARE IN CANCER PATIENTS

The high cost of intensive care and the demands placed on these precious resources by all medical and surgical subspecialties mandate that critical care interventions be meted out wisely. Certainly, there are patients who are saved by these technologies, as well as others on whom much money and effort are spent without a good medical outcome. Because cost containment has become imperative in the practice of medicine, certain illnesses with a poor prognosis, including cancer, are perceived by the public and often by medical staff as relative contraindications to cardiopulmonary resuscitation or intensive care interventions.[143] There is also a perception that a disproportionate amount of health care resources are spent on the intensive care of patients with incurable cancer. These perceptions must be placed in the appropriate context. Although several studies have shown that cardiopulmonary resuscitation in patients with cancer has a low success rate (less than 10%), as defined by the number of patients discharged alive from the hospital,[144,145] this is not a convincing argument for rationing critical care for cancer patients. The success rate for noncancer diagnoses in similar studies has also been unimpressive (<5%).[146] Hospital utilization studies do not support the notion that a disproportionate amount of special care resources are used in terminally ill cancer patients.[147] The central determination in each case should hinge on the answer to a single question: "Is it likely that these abnormalities are reversible?" For nearly all iatrogenic toxicities, the answer is generally yes. For patients with curable tumor types, every effort should be made to support the patient until the long-term prognosis of the underlying tumor can be ascertained. Given that about 65% of individuals with a cancer diagnosis are cured of their disease, intensive care interventions are justified, particularly in support of dose-intense treatment modalities.

When viewed in the context of other underlying medical conditions, a cancer diagnosis is neither medically nor ethically a contraindication to intensive care management. The wishes of the individual and the family are central in establishing an appropriate level of care for any patient. It is now mandated by law that hospitals inquire about advance directives before any hospital admission. Public awareness of these issues is increasing, and many cancer patients now have such directives, which include living wills, "do not resuscitate" orders, and guidelines that specify the level of care to be provided in certain circumstances (e.g., antibiotics only, no intravenous feeding). These directives can be helpful to the physician and the patient's family, although they sometimes complicate medical management in clinical situations in which reversible conditions exist whose care might require violating a directive.[148] Patient education and strong support from social work and pastoral and legal services can assist the physician in arriving at the appropriate level of care for each individual.

SUMMARY AND CONCLUSIONS

Intensive care management is central to the success of any dose-intense cancer treatment modality. Support of treatment toxicities is justified given the growing improvement in outcome for cancer diagnoses. Understanding of the pathophysiology of a number of clinical entities, such as septic shock and cytokine-induced hypotension, will provide the basis for more rational and effective management of many of these toxicities. However, it is even more important to develop cancer treatments that attack the malignancy and spare the host. This level of therapeutic sophistication is attainable through our increasing knowledge of the molecular basis of malignancy and the physiology of tumors. Even when the goal of therapeutic specificity in oncology is achieved, intensive care will still be salient in the support of patients with the end-organ sequelae of malignancy.

KEY POINTS

- TLS occurs most frequently in rapidly growing lymphomas or leukemias with high myeloblast or lymphoblast counts. The most effective management strategy is to anticipate the occurrence of TLS and initiate allopurinol, hydration, and intensive monitoring before metabolic aberrations occur.
- Hypercalcemia is the most common metabolic disturbance in cancer patients. Intravenous hydration and bisphosphonates are the initial treatments of hypercalcemia.
- SIADH in cancer patients is often accompanied by neurologic findings. The initial treatment is fluid restriction.
- Treatment of SVC syndrome depends on the underlying histologic diagnosis; therefore, biopsy is mandatory in previously undiagnosed patients. If SVC syndrome is

secondary to lymphoma or small cell lung cancer, chemotherapy is the treatment of choice. Radiation therapy with high initial dose fractions can be palliative in more than 80% of patients with malignancies unresponsive to chemotherapy.

- Central nervous system or spinal metastases can often be managed on an outpatient basis with dexamethasone and radiation treatment. Individual patients may benefit from higher doses of dexamethasone (up to 200 mg/d), and surgery with radiation can achieve significant palliation for some patients.
- DIC is observed in a number of solid tumors and is the hallmark of APL. Serial levels of fibrin split products and fibrinogen will determine the amount of cryoprecipitate needed to replace the consumed coagulation proteins. Heparin can be used in patients who do not respond to cryoprecipitate.
- Febrile neutropenia can often be managed outside the ICU with appropriate broad-spectrum antibiotic support. The choice of antibiotics should take into account the microbial pathogens most prevalent in the treating institution.
- Hypotension caused by IL-2 and other cytokines has a pathophysiology similar to that of septic shock, with the induction of nitric oxide and other vasoactive mediators. Phenylephrine is an effective pressor agent for IL-2–induced hypotension. Glucocorticoids may be useful in patients with circulatory collapse or ARDS from IL-2 or other immunotherapy.
- The types of infections that occur after bone marrow transplantation are related to the recovery of different parts of immune function after transplantation. Aerobic bacteria and *Candida* infections are most prevalent early, when mucosal barriers are disrupted by myeloablative chemotherapy. Herpes simplex, *Candida,* bacterial, and *Aspergillus* infections are common until neutrophil recovery has occurred. Varicella zoster, hepatitis C, and *P. carinii* infections are observed up to 3 months after transplantation until cellular immune function recovers.
- A cancer diagnosis is not a contraindication to intensive care management. Dose-intense treatment modalities mandate intensive support and have resulted in improved outcomes for patients with malignancies.

REFERENCES

1. Jemal A, Siegel R, Ward E, et al: Cancer statistics, 2006. Ca Cancer J Clin 2006;56:106.
2. Pui CH, Evans WE: Acute lymphoblastic leukemia. N Engl J Med 1998;339:605.
3. Sawyers CL: Chronic myeloid leukemia. N Engl J Med 1999;340:1330.
4. Löwenberg B, Downing JR, Burnett A: Acute myeloid leukemia. N Engl J Med 1999;341:1051.
5. Philip T, Guglielmi C, Hagenbeek A, et al: Autologous bone marrow transplantation as compared with salvage chemotherapy in relapses of chemotherapy-sensitive non-Hodgkin's lymphoma. N Engl J Med 1995;333:1540.
6. Bosl GJ, Motzer RJ: Testicular germ-cell cancer. N Engl J Med 1997;337:242.
7. Coppes MJ, de Kraker J, van Dijken PJ, et al: Bilateral Wilms' tumor: Long-term survival and some epidemiological features. J Clin Oncol 1989;7:310.
8. Hayes FA, Thompson EI, Meyer WH, et al: Therapy for localized Ewing's sarcoma of bone. J Clin Oncol 1989;7:208.
•9. Atkins MB, Lotze MT, Dutcher JP, et al: High-dose recombinant interleukin-2 therapy for patients with metastatic melanoma: Analysis of 270 patients treated between 1985 and 1993. J Clin Oncol 1999;17:2105.
10. Fisher RI, Rosenberg SA, Sznol M, et al: High-dose aldesleukin in renal cell carcinoma: Long-term survival update. Cancer J Sci Am 1997;3:S70.
11. Longo DL: Chemotherapy for advanced aggressive lymphoma: More is better . . . isn't it? J Clin Oncol 1990;8:952.
12. Cassileth PA, Harrington DP, Appelbaum FR, et al: Chemotherapy compared with autologous or allogeneic bone marrow transplantation in the management of acute myeloid leukemia in first remission. N Engl J Med 1998;339:1649.
•13. de Bustros BA, Baylin SB: Hormone production by tumours: Biologic and clinical aspects. Clin Endocrinol Metab 1985;14:221.
14. Curti BD, Longo DL, Ochoa AC, et al: Treatment of cancer patients with ex vivo anti-CD3–activated killer cells and interleukin-2. J Clin Oncol 1993;11:652.
15. Holland JF, Sharpe W, Mamrod LM: Urate excretion in patients with acute leukemia. J Natl Cancer Inst 1959;23:1097.
16. Cadman EC, Lundberg WB, Bertino JR: Hyperphosphatemia and hypocalcemia accompanying rapid cell lysis in a patient with Burkitt's lymphoma and Burkitt cell leukemia. Am J Med 1977;62:283.
17. Castro MP, Van Auken J, Spencer-Cisek P, et al: Acute tumor lysis syndrome associated with concurrent biochemotherapy of metastatic melanoma: A case report and review of the literature. Cancer 1999;85:1055.
18. Yang H, Rosove MH, Figlin RA: Tumor lysis syndrome occurring after the administration of rituximab in lymphoproliferative disorders: High-grade non-Hodgkin's lymphoma and chronic lymphocytic leukemia. Am J Hematol 1999;62:247.
19. Dewhirst FE, Stashenko PP, Mole JE, et al: Purification and partial sequence of human osteoclast-activating factor: Identity with interleukin 1 beta. J Immunol 1985;135:2562.
20. Stashenko P, Dewhirst FE, Peros WJ, et al: Synergistic interactions between interleukin 1, tumor necrosis factor, and lymphotoxin in bone resorption. J Immunol 1987;138:1464.
21. Stern PH, Krieger NS, Nissenson RA, et al: Human transforming growth factor-alpha stimulates bone resorption in vitro. J Clin Invest 1985;76:2016.
22. Seyberth HW, Segre GV, Morgan JL, et al: Prostaglandins as mediators of hypercalcemia associated with certain types of cancer. N Engl J Med 1975;293:1278.
•23. Wysolmerski JJ, Broadus AE: Hypercalcemia of malignancy: The central role of parathyroid hormone–related protein. Annu Rev Med 1994;45:189.
24. Fetchick DA, Bertolini DR, Sarin PS, et al: Production of 1,25-dihydroxyvitamin D_3 by human T cell lymphotrophic virus-I–transformed lymphocytes. J Clin Invest 1986;78:592.
25. Blythe WB, Gitelman HJ, Welt LG: Effect of expansion of the extracellular space on the rate of urinary excretion of calcium. Am J Physiol 1968;214:52.
•26. Mundy GR, Yoneda T: Bisphosphonates as anticancer drugs. N Engl J Med 1998;339:398.
27. Bertheault-Cvitkovic F, Tubiana-Hulin M, Chevalier B, et al: Gallium nitrate (GN) vs pamidronate (APD) for acute control of cancer-related hypercalcemia (CRH): Interim results of a randomized, double-blind, multi-national study (Meeting abstract). Proc Annu Meet Am Soc Clin Oncol 1995;14:A369.
28. Newell KA, Prinz RA, Pickleman J, et al: Pheochromocytoma multisystem crisis. A surgical emergency. Arch Surg 1988;123:956.
29. Sheps SG, Jiang NS, Klee GG, et al: Recent developments in the

diagnosis and treatment of pheochromocytoma. Mayo Clin Proc 1990;65:88.
30. Bravo EL, Tarazi RC, Fouad FM, et al: Clonidine-suppression test: A useful aid in the diagnosis of pheochromocytoma. N Engl J Med 1981;305:623.
31. Shapiro B, Copp JE, Sisson JC, et al: Iodine-131 metaiodobenzylguanidine for the locating of suspected pheochromocytoma: Experience in 400 cases. J Nucl Med 1985;26:576.
32. Mann GN, Link JM, Pickett CA, et al: [^{11}C]metahydroxyephedrine and [^{18}F]fluorodeoxyglucose positron emission tomography improve clinical decision making in suspected pheochromocytoma. Ann Surg Oncol 2006;13:187.
33. Perry RR, Keiser HR, Norton JA, et al: Surgical management of pheochromocytoma with the use of metyrosine. Ann Surg 1990;212:621.
34. Chimori K, Miyazaki S, Nakajima T, et al: Preoperative management of pheochromocytoma with the calcium-antagonist nifedipine. Clin Ther 1985;7:372.
35. Proye C, Thevenin D, Cecat P, et al: Exclusive use of calcium channel blockers in preoperative and intraoperative control of pheochromocytomas: Hemodynamics and free catecholamine assays in ten consecutive patients. Surgery 1989;106:1149.
36. Daughaday WH, Emanuele MA, Brooks MH, et al: Synthesis and secretion of insulin-like growth factor II by a leiomyosarcoma with associated hypoglycemia. N Engl J Med 1988;319:1434.
37. Samaan NA, Pham FK, Sellin RV, et al: Successful treatment of hypoglycemia using glucagon in a patient with an extrapancreatic tumor. Ann Intern Med 1990;113:404.
38. Schrag D, Chung KY, Flombaum C, et al: Cetuximab therapy and symptomatic hypomagnesia. J Natl Cancer Inst 2005;97:1791.
39. Armstrong BA, Perez CA, Simpson JR, et al: Role of irradiation in the management of superior vena cava syndrome. Int J Radiat Oncol Biol Phys 1987;13:531.
40. Gray BH, Olin JW, Graor RA, et al: Safety and efficacy of thrombolytic therapy for superior vena cava syndrome. Chest 1991;99:54.
41. Chandraratna PA: Echocardiography and Doppler ultrasound in the evaluation of pericardial disease. Circulation 1991;84:I303.
42. Hutchison SJ, Smalling RG, Albornoz M, et al: Comparison of transthoracic and transesophageal echocardiography in clinically overt or suspected pericardial heart disease. Am J Cardiol 1994;74:962.
43. Sugimoto JT, Little AG, Ferguson MK, et al: Pericardial window: Mechanisms of efficacy. Ann Thorac Surg 1990;50:442.
44. Cormican MC, Nyman CR: Intrapericardial bleomycin for the management of cardiac tamponade secondary to malignant pericardial effusion. Br Heart J 1990;63:61.
45. Myers CE, McGuire WP, Liss RH, et al: Adriamycin: The role of lipid peroxidation in cardiac toxicity and tumor response. Science 1977;197:165.
46. Speyer JL, Green MD, Sanger J, et al: A prospective randomized trial of ICRF-187 for prevention of cumulative doxorubicin-induced cardiac toxicity in women with breast cancer. Cancer Treat Rev 1990;17:161.
47. Hortobagyi GN, Frye D, Buzdar AU, et al: Decreased cardiac toxicity of doxorubicin administered by continuous intravenous infusion in combination chemotherapy for metastatic breast carcinoma. Cancer 1989;63:37.
48. Swain SM, Whaley FS, Gerber MC, et al: Cardioprotection with dexrazoxane for doxorubicin-containing therapy in advanced breast cancer. J Clin Oncol 1997;15:1318.
49. Moreb JS, Oblon DJ: Outcome of clinical congestive heart failure induced by anthracycline chemotherapy. Cancer 1992;70:2637.
50. Rowinsky EK, Donehower RC: Paclitaxel (Taxol) [published erratum appears in N Engl J Med 1995;333:75]. N Engl J Med 1995;332:1004.
51. Rowinsky EK, McGuire WP, Guarnieri T, et al: Cardiac disturbances during the administration of taxol. J Clin Oncol 1991;9:1704.
52. Quezado ZM, Wilson WH, Cunnion RE, et al: High-dose ifosfamide is associated with severe, reversible cardiac dysfunction. Ann Intern Med 1993;118:31.
53. Tan-Chiu E, Yothers G, Romond, E, et al: Assessment of cardiac dysfunction in a randomized trial comparing cyclophosphamide followed by paclitaxel, with or without trastuzumab as adjuvant therapy in node-positive, human epidermal growth factor receptor 2–overexpressing breast cancer: NSABP B-31. J Clin Oncol 2005;23:7811.
54. Adamson IY, Bowden DH: Endothelial injury and repair in radiation-induced pulmonary fibrosis. Am J Pathol 1983;112:224.
55. Masson RG, Krikorian J, Lukl P, et al: Pulmonary microvascular cytology in the diagnosis of lymphangitic carcinomatosis. N Engl J Med 1989;321:71.
•56. Cooper JAJ, White DA, Matthay RA: Drug-induced pulmonary disease. Part 1: Cytotoxic drugs. Am Rev Respir Dis 1986;133:321.
57. McKeage MJ, Evans BD, Atkinson C, et al: Carbon monoxide diffusing capacity is a poor predictor of clinically significant bleomycin lung. New Zealand Clinical Oncology Group. J Clin Oncol 1990;8:779.
•58. Browne MJ, Potter D, Gress J, et al: A randomized trial of open lung biopsy versus empiric antimicrobial therapy in cancer patients with diffuse pulmonary infiltrates. J Clin Oncol 1990;8:222.
•59. Groeger JS, White PJ, Nierman DM, et al: Outcome for cancer patients requiring mechanical ventilation. J Clin Oncol 1999;17:991.
60. Santos RS, Raftopoulos Y, Keenan RJ, et al: Bronchoscopic palliation of primary lung cancer: Single or multimodality therapy? Surg Endosc 2004;18:931.
61. Johnson DH, Fehrenbacher L, Novotny WF, et al: Randomized phase II trial comparing bevacizumab plus carboplatin and paclitaxel with carboplatin and paclitaxel alone in previously untreated locally advanced or metastatic non–small-cell lung cancer. J Clin Oncol 2004;22:2184.
•62. Hughes WT, Armstrong D, Bodey GP, et al: 1997 guidelines for the use of antimicrobial agents in neutropenic patients with unexplained fever. Clin Infect Dis 1997;25:551.
63. Hartmann LC, Tschetter LK, Haberman TM, et al: Granulocyte colony-stimulating factor in severe chemotherapy-induced afebrile neutropenia. N Engl J Med 1997;336:1776.
•64. Freifeld A, Marchigiani D, Walsh T, et al: A double-blind comparison of empirical oral and intravenous antibiotic therapy for low-risk febrile patients with neutropenia during cancer chemotherapy. N Engl J Med 1999;341:305.
65. Kilbourn RG, Griffith OW: Overproduction of nitric oxide in cytokine-mediated and septic shock. J Natl Cancer Inst 1992;84:827.
66. Petros A, Lamb G, Leone A, et al: Effects of a nitric oxide synthase inhibitor in humans with septic shock. Cardiovasc Res 1994;28:34-39.
67. Bone RC, Balk RA, Fein AM, et al: A second large controlled clinical study of E5, a monoclonal antibody to endotoxin: Results of a prospective, multicenter, randomized, controlled trial. The E5 Sepsis Study Group [published erratum appears in Crit Care Med 1995;23:1616]. Crit Care Med 1995;23:994.
68. Ziegler EJ, Fisher CJJ, Sprung CL, et al: Treatment of gram-negative bacteremia and septic shock with HA-1A human monoclonal antibody against endotoxin. A randomized, double-blind, placebo-controlled trial. The HA-1A Sepsis Study Group. N Engl J Med 1991;324:429.
69. Bernard GR, Vincent JL, Laterre PF, et al: Efficacy and safety of recombinant human activated protein C for severe sepsis. N Engl J Med 2001;344:699.
70. Gilbert RW, Kim JH, Posner JB: Epidural spinal cord compression from metastatic tumor: Diagnosis and treatment. Ann Neurol 1978;3:40.
71. Renaudin J, Fewer D, Wilson CB, et al: Dose dependency of Decadron in patients with partially excised brain tumors. J Neurosurg 1973;39:302.
72. Patchall RA, Tibbs PA, Regine WF, et al: Direct decompressive surgical resection in the treatment of spinal cord compression caused by metastatic cancer: A randomized trial. Lancet 2005;366:643.
73. Patchell RA, Tibbs PA, Walsh JW, et al: A randomized trial of surgery in the

treatment of single metastases to the brain. N Engl J Med 1990;322:494.
74. Cohen N, Strauss G, Lew R, et al: Should prophylactic anticonvulsants be administered to patients with newly-diagnosed cerebral metastases? A retrospective analysis. J Clin Oncol 1988;6:1621.
75. Beutler E: Platelet transfusions: The 20,000/microliter trigger. Blood 1993;81:1411.
•76. Rebulla P, Finazzi G, Marangoni F, et al: A multicenter randomized study of the threshold for prophylactic platelet transfusions in adults with acute myeloid leukemia. Gruppo Italiano Malattie Ematologiche Maligne dell'Adulto. N Engl J Med 1997;337:1870.
77. Harker LA, Roskos L, Cheung E: Effective and efficient platelet transfusion strategies that maintain hemostatic protection. Transfusion 1998;38:619.
78. Hersh JK, Hom EG, Brecher ME: Mathematical modeling of platelet survival with implications for optimal transfusion practice in the chronically platelet transfusion–dependent patient. Transfusion 1998;38:637.
•79. Posner JB: Management of central nervous system metastases. Semin Oncol 1977;4:81.
80. Cresteil T, Monsarrat B, Alvinerie P, et al: Taxol metabolism by human liver microsomes: Identification of cytochrome P450 isozymes involved in its biotransformation. Cancer Res 1994;54:386.
81. Royer I, Monsarrat B, Sonnier M, et al: Metabolism of docetaxel by human cytochromes P450: Interactions with paclitaxel and other antineoplastic drugs. Cancer Res 1996;56:58.
82. Kupfer A, Aeschlimann C, Wermuth B, et al: Prophylaxis and reversal of ifosfamide encephalopathy with methylene-blue. Lancet 1994;343:763.
•83. Pelgrims J, De Vos F, Van den Brande J, et al: Methylene blue in the treatment and prevention of ifosfamide-induced encephalopathy: Report of 12 cases and a review of the literature. Br J Cancer 2000;82:291.
84. Kaplan LD, Abrams DI, Feigal E, et al: AIDS-associated non-Hodgkin's lymphoma in San Francisco. JAMA 1989;261:719.
•85. Stellato TA, Shenk RR: Gastrointestinal emergencies in the oncology patient. Semin Oncol 1989;16:521.
86. Mulvihill SJ, Pappas TN, Fonkalsrud EW, et al: The effect of somatostatin on experimental intestinal obstruction. Ann Surg 1988;207:169.
87. Paulson S, Sheehan RG, Stone MJ, et al: Large cell lymphomas of the stomach: Improved prognosis with complete resection of all intrinsic gastrointestinal disease. J Clin Oncol 1983;1:263.
88. Fleming ID, Mitchell S, Dilawari RA: The role of surgery in the management of gastric lymphoma. Cancer 1982;49:1135.
89. Rosen CB, van Heerden JA, Martin JKJ, et al: Is an aggressive surgical approach to the patient with gastric lymphoma warranted? Ann Surg 1987;205:634.
90. Bayerdörffer E, Neubauer A, Rudolf B, et al: Regression of primary gastric lymphoma of mucosa-associated lymphoid tissue type after cure of *Helicobacter pylori* infection. Lancet 1995;345:1591.
91. Mesrobian HG, Perry JR: Radionuclide diuresis pyelography. J Urol 1991;146:601.
92. Brown RB: A method of management of inoperative carcinoma of the bladder. J Urol 1968;40:489.
93. Cuttner J, Holland JF, Norton L, et al: Therapeutic leukapheresis for hyperleukocytosis in acute myelocytic leukemia. Med Pediatric Oncol 1983;11:76.
94. Degos L, Dombret H, Chomienne C, et al: All-*trans*-retinoic acid as a differentiating agent in the treatment of acute promyelocytic leukemia. Blood 1995;85:2643.
•95. Frankel SR, Eardley A, Lauwers G, et al: The "retinoic acid syndrome" in acute promyelocytic leukemia. Ann Intern Med 1992;117:292.
96. Warrell RP Jr, de The H, Wang ZY, et al: Acute promyelocytic leukemia. N Engl J Med 1993;329:177.
97. Kilbourn RG, Belloni P: Endothelial cell production of nitrogen oxides in response to interferon gamma in combination with tumor necrosis factor, interleukin-1, or endotoxin. J Natl Cancer Inst 1990;82:772.
98. Ochoa JB, Curti B, Peitzman AB, et al: Increased circulating nitrogen oxides after human tumor immunotherapy: Correlation with toxic hemodynamic changes. J Natl Cancer Inst 1992;84:864.
99. Marletta MA: Nitric oxide synthase: Function and mechanism. Adv Exp Med Biol 1993;338:281.
100. Rapoport RM, Draznin MB, Murad F: Endothelium-dependent vasodilator- and nitrovasodilator-induced relaxation may be mediated through cyclic GMP formation and cyclic GMP–dependent protein phosphorylation. Trans Assoc Am Physicians 1983;96:19.
101. Atkins MB, Robertson MJ, Gordon M, et al: Phase I evaluation of intravenous recombinant human interleukin 12 in patients with advanced malignancies. Clin Cancer Res 1997;3:409.
102. Tayeh MA, Marletta MA: Macrophage oxidation of L-arginine to nitric oxide, nitrite, and nitrate. Tetrahydrobiopterin is required as a cofactor. J Biol Chem 1989;264:19654.
103. Smith GK, Duch DS, Edelstein MP, et al: New inhibitors of sepiapterin reductase. Lack of an effect of intracellular tetrahydrobiopterin depletion upon in vitro proliferation of two human cell lines. J Biol Chem 1992;267:5599.
104. Ohkubo C, Bigos D, Jain RK: Interleukin 2 induced leukocyte adhesion to the normal and tumor microvascular endothelium in vivo and its inhibition by dextran sulfate: Implications for vascular leak syndrome. Cancer Res 1991;51:1561.
105. Ley K, Lundgren E, Berger E, et al: Shear-dependent inhibition of granulocyte adhesion to cultured endothelium by dextran sulfate. Blood 1989;73:1324.
106. Kornfeld H, Berman JS, Beer DJ, et al: Induction of human T lymphocyte motility by interleukin 2. J Immunol 1985;134:3887.
107. Carson WE, Yu H, Dierksheide J, et al: A fatal cytokine-induced systemic inflammatory response reveals a critical role for NK cells. J Immunol 1999;162:4943.
108. Lee RE, Lotze MT, Skibber JM, et al: Cardiorespiratory effects of immunotherapy with interleukin-2. J Clin Oncol 1989;7:7.
109. Margolin KA, Rayner AA, Hawkins MJ, et al: Interleukin-2 and lymphokine-activated killer cell therapy of solid tumors: Analysis of toxicity and management guidelines. J Clin Oncol 1989;7:486.
110. Saxon RR, Klein JS, Bar MH, et al: Pathogenesis of pulmonary edema during interleukin-2 therapy: Correlation of chest radiographic and clinical findings in 54 patients. AJR Am J Roentgenol 1991;156:281.
•111. Vogelzang PJ, Bloom SM, Mier JW, et al: Chest roentgenographic abnormalities in IL-2 recipients. Incidence and correlation with clinical parameters. Chest 1992;101:746.
112. Welbourn R, Goldman G, Kobzik L, et al: Involvement of thromboxane and neutrophils in multiple-system organ edema with interleukin-2. Ann Surg 1990;212:728.
113. Meduri GU, Belenchia JM, Estes RJ, et al: Fibroproliferative phase of ARDS. Clinical findings and effects of corticosteroids. Chest 1991;100:943.
114. Vetto JT, Papa MZ, Lotze MT, et al: Reduction of toxicity of interleukin-2 and lymphokine-activated killer cells in humans by the administration of corticosteroids. J Clin Oncol 1987;5:496.
115. Crabtree GR, Gillis S, Smith KA, et al: Mechanisms of glucocorticoid-induced immunosuppression: Inhibitory effects on expression of Fc receptors and production of T-cell growth factor. J Steroid Biochem 1980;12:445.
116. Kozeny GA, Nicolas JD, Creekmore S, et al: Effects of interleukin-2 immunotherapy on renal function. J Clin Oncol 1988;6:1170.
117. Guleria AS, Yang JC, Topalian SL, et al: Renal dysfunction associated with the administration of high-dose interleukin-2 in 199 consecutive patients with metastatic melanoma or renal carcinoma. J Clin Oncol 1994;12:2714.
118. Cormier JN, Hurst R, Vasselli J, et al: A prospective randomized evaluation of the prophylactic use of low-dose dopamine in cancer patients receiving interleukin-2. J Immunother 1997;20:292.
119. Curran RD, Ferrari FK, Kispert PH, et al: Nitric oxide and nitric oxide–generating compounds inhibit hepatocyte protein synthesis. FASEB J 1991;5:2085.

120. Kragel AH, Travis WD, Feinberg L, et al: Pathologic findings associated with interleukin-2–based immunotherapy for cancer: A postmortem study of 19 patients. Hum Pathol 1990;21:493.
121. Dougherty AH, Jackman WM, Naccarelli GV, et al: Acute conversion of paroxysmal supraventricular tachycardia with intravenous diltiazem. IV Diltiazem Study Group. Am J Cardiol 1992;70:587.
122. Jacobs EL, Clare-Salzler MJ, Chopra IJ, et al: Thyroid function abnormalities associated with the chronic outpatient administration of recombinant interleukin-2 and recombinant interferon-alpha. J Immunother 1991;10:448.
123. Clark JW, Smith JWI, Steis RG, et al: Interleukin 2 and lymphokine-activated killer cell therapy: Analysis of a bolus interleukin 2 and a continuous infusion interleukin 2 regimen. Cancer Res 1990;50:7343.
124. Curti BD, Ochoa AC, Powers GC, et al: A phase I trial of anti-CD3–stimulated $CD4^+$ T cells, infusional interleukin-2 and cyclophosphamide in patients with advanced cancer. J Clin Oncol 1998;16:2760.
125. Collins RH, Shpilberg O, Drobyski WR, et al: Donor leukocyte infusions in 140 patients with relapsed malignancy after allogeneic bone marrow transplantation. J Clin Oncol 1997;15:433.
126. Yannelli JR, Hyatt C, McConnell S, et al: Growth of tumor-infiltrating lymphocytes from human solid cancers: Summary of a 5 year experience. Int J Cancer 1996;65:413.
127. Sznol M, Dutcher JP, Atkins MB, et al: Review of interleukin-2 alone and interleukin-2/Lak clinical trials in metastatic malignant melanoma. Cancer Treat Rev 1994;16(Suppl A):29.
•128. Deeg HJ: Prophylaxis and treatment of acute graft-versus-host disease: Current state, implications of new immunopharmacologic compounds and future strategies to prevent and treat acute GVHD in high-risk patients. Bone Marrow Transplant 1994;114(Suppl 4):S56.
129. Billingham RE: The biology of graft-versus-host reactions. Harvey Lect 1966;62:21.
130. Sullivan KM, Kopecky KJ, Jocom J, et al: Immunomodulatory and antimicrobial efficacy of intravenous immunoglobulin in bone marrow transplantation. N Engl J Med 1990;323:705.
•131. Bearman SI: The syndrome of hepatic veno-occlusive disease after marrow transplantation. Blood 1995;85:3005.
•132. Attal M, Huguet F, Rubie H, et al: Prevention of hepatic veno-occlusive disease after bone marrow transplantation by continuous infusion of low-dose heparin: A prospective, randomized trial. Blood 1992;79:2834.
133. Bearman SI, Lee JL, Baron AE, et al: Treatment of hepatic venocclusive disease with recombinant human tissue plasminogen activator and heparin in 42 marrow transplant patients. Blood 1997;89:1501.
134. Morris JD, Harris RE, Hashmi R, et al: Antithrombin-III for the treatment of chemotherapy-induced organ dysfunction following bone marrow transplantation. Bone Marrow Transplant 1997;20:871.
135. Nattakom TV, Charlton A, Wilmore DW: Use of vitamin E and glutamine in the successful treatment of severe veno-occlusive disease following bone marrow transplantation. Nutr Clin Prac 1995;10:16.
136. Levy V, Azoulay D, Rio B, et al: Successful treatment of severe hepatic veno-occlusive disease after allogeneic bone marrow transplantation by transjugular intrahepatic portosystemic stent-shunt (TIPS). Bone Marrow Transplant 1996;18:443.
•137. McDonald GB, Hinds MS, Fisher LD, et al: Veno-occlusive disease of the liver and multiorgan failure after bone marrow transplantation: A cohort study of 355 patients. Ann Intern Med 1993;118:255.
138. Lum LG: Recapitulation of immune ontogeny: A vital component for the success of bone marrow transplantation. Cancer Treat Res 1990;50:27.
139. Wingard JR: Fungal infections after bone marrow transplant. Biol Blood Marrow Transplant 1999;5:55.
140. Wingard JR: Viral infections in leukemia and bone marrow transplant patients. Leuk Lymphoma 1993;11(Suppl 2):115.
•141. Walter EA, Greenberg PD, Gilbert MJ, et al: Reconstitution of cellular immunity against cytomegalovirus in recipients of allogeneic bone marrow by transfer of T-cell clones from the donor. N Engl J Med 1995;333:1038.
142. Greenberg PD, Finch RJ, Gavin MA, et al: Genetic modification of T-cell clones for therapy of human viral and malignant diseases. Cancer J Sci Am 1998;4(Suppl 1):S100.
143. Lawrence VA, Clark GM: Cancer and resuscitation. Does the diagnosis affect the decision? Arch Intern Med 1987;147:1637.
144. Vitelli CE, Cooper K, Rogatko A, et al: Cardiopulmonary resuscitation and the patient with cancer. J Clin Oncol 1991;9:111.
145. Schapira DV, Studnicki J, Bradham DD, et al: Intensive care, survival, and expense of treating critically ill cancer patients. JAMA 1993;269:783.
146. Gray WA, Capone RJ, Most AS: Unsuccessful emergency medical resuscitation—are continued efforts in the emergency department justified? N Engl J Med 1991;325:1393.
147. Studnicki J, Schapira DV, Straumfjord JV, et al: A national profile of the use of intensive care by Medicare patients with cancer. Cancer 1994;74:2366.
148. Ewer MS, Taubert JK: Advance directives in the intensive care unit of a tertiary cancer center. Cancer 1995;76:1268.

Chapter 82

Critical Care Medicine in Pregnancy

Stephen E. Lapinsky

Management of the critically ill pregnant patient is a situation with which few intensive care physicians gain significant expertise. The usual clinical approach may be altered by the physiologic changes induced by pregnancy, by the relatively uncommon pregnancy-specific conditions, and by limitations on therapy produced by the presence of a fetus (Fig. 82-1).

PHYSIOLOGIC CHANGES IN PREGNANCY

The pregnant woman undergoes a number of physiologic changes affecting various systems relevant to critical care management. From a respiratory perspective, the upper airways develop edema and hyperemia, which may be relevant during endotracheal intubation. Changes in lung volumes occur, with a 10% to 25% decrease in functional residual capacity (FRC), whereas total lung capacity decreases only minimally as the thoracic cage widens to compensate.[1] Forced expiratory volume in 1 second (FEV_1) is not altered by the pregnant state. Lung compliance remains unchanged, but chest wall and total respiratory compliance are reduced.[2]

The rising progesterone level stimulates an increase in ventilation. Tidal volume and minute ventilation increase from the first trimester, reaching 20% to 40% above baseline by term (Table 82-1).[3] A mild respiratory alkalosis is produced with compensatory renal excretion of bicarbonate ($Pa{CO_2}$ 28 to 32 mm Hg; HCO_3^- 18 to 21 mEq/L). Oxygen consumption increases because of the demands of the fetus and maternal metabolic processes, reaching levels up to 33% above baseline by term. Arterial PO_2 remains normal throughout pregnancy, but mild hypoxemia caused by an increased alveolar-arterial oxygen tension difference may develop in the supine position, as FRC diminishes near term.

Maternal blood volume and cardiac output increase through pregnancy, reaching a peak at 30% to 50% above baseline levels by about 28 weeks (Fig. 82-2).[4] Hemodynamic measurements by pulmonary artery catheter in the near-term patient demonstrate this increased cardiac output, with a reduced systemic vascular resistance and pulmonary vascular resistance (see Table 82-1).[5] During labor and continuing into the immediate postpartum period, cardiac output is further augmented by the return of 300 to 500 mL of blood to the central circulation.[6]

Oxygen delivery to the fetus is dependent on the maternal arterial oxygen content and the uterine blood flow. Maternal hypotension; alkalosis (e.g., hyperventilation); and endogenous or exogenous catecholamines can vasoconstrict the uterine artery and adversely affect fetal oxygenation.[7] Uterine blood flow is also reduced transiently by uterine contractions. Although umbilical venous blood returning to the fetus has a relatively low oxygen tension, a high oxygen content is maintained by the left shift of the oxygen dissociation curve of fetal hemoglobin.

Glomerular filtration rate increases early in pregnancy, reaching a value 50% above prepregnancy levels in the second trimester, and remains elevated throughout pregnancy (see Fig. 82-2).[8] The normal serum creatinine level is therefore in the range of 0.5 to 0.7 mg/dL (45 to 60 µmol/L). As pregnancy progresses, mild uteric dilation and mild hydronephrosis may occur as a result of uterine compression and smooth muscle relaxation.

Pregnancy is associated with a reduced lower esophageal sphincter pressure, reaching a nadir at 36 weeks. The position of the stomach is displaced, further decreasing the effectiveness of the gastroesophageal sphincter and

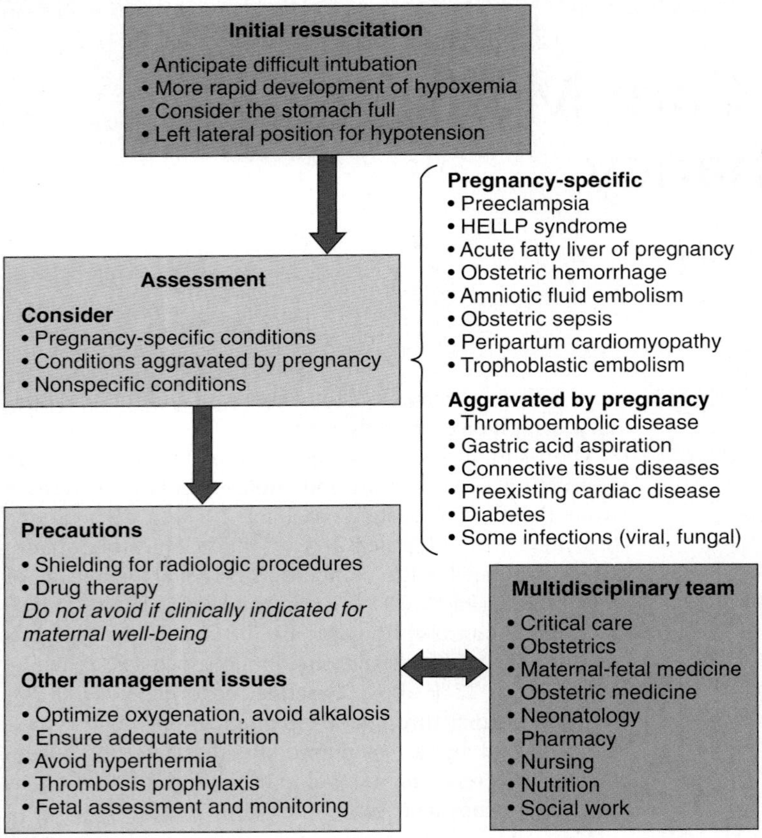

Figure 82-1. Approach to the assessment and management of the critically ill obstetric patient.

Table 82-1. Physiologic Changes in Late Pregnancy

Parameter	Change
Respiratory	
Functional residual capacity	Decreased 10%-25%
Minute ventilation	Increased 20%-40%
Arterial partial pressure of oxygen	No change
Arterial partial pressure of carbon dioxide	Reduced to 28-32 mm Hg
Serum bicarbonate	Reduced to 18-21 mEq/L
Cardiac	
Heart rate	Increased 10%-30%
Pulmonary capillary wedge pressure	No change
Cardiac output	Increased 30%-50%
Systemic vascular resistance	Decreased 20%-30%
Pulmonary vascular resistance	Decreased 20%-30%
Renal	
GFR	Increased 50%
Creatinine	Decreased (24-68 μmol/L; 0.29-0.77 mg/dL)

reducing gastric emptying. The pregnant woman should therefore always be considered at risk for aspiration of stomach contents, regardless of the time elapsed since her last meal.

The increase in plasma volume is associated with a lesser increase in red cell mass causing a physiologic anemia, with a hematocrit of 32% to 34% by the third trimester. A mild leukocytosis occurs with white cell count rising further during labor. Platelet counts are usually unchanged, although a condition of benign mild thrombocytopenia may occur.[9] Procoagulant factors rise, contributing to the hypercoagulable state of pregnancy. The erythrocyte sedimentation rate (ESR) rises related to increased levels of plasma globulins.

CRITICAL CARE MANAGEMENT

General Care

Positioning

In the supine position the gravid uterus produces mechanical effects on the vena cava and aorta, reducing central venous return. This results in a decrease in cardiac output and hypotension. This "supine hypotensive syndrome" should be considered in hemodynamically unstable patients.[10] Pregnant patients should be positioned on their left side, or at least with the right hip slightly elevated.

Nutrition

During starvation, maternal body stores are protected at the expense of the fetus and inadequate nutrition may result in intrauterine growth retardation and fetal loss. Growth restriction before 26 weeks' gestation may lead to fetal neurological impairment. Caloric requirements in pregnancy increase by about 300 Kcal per day, and protein

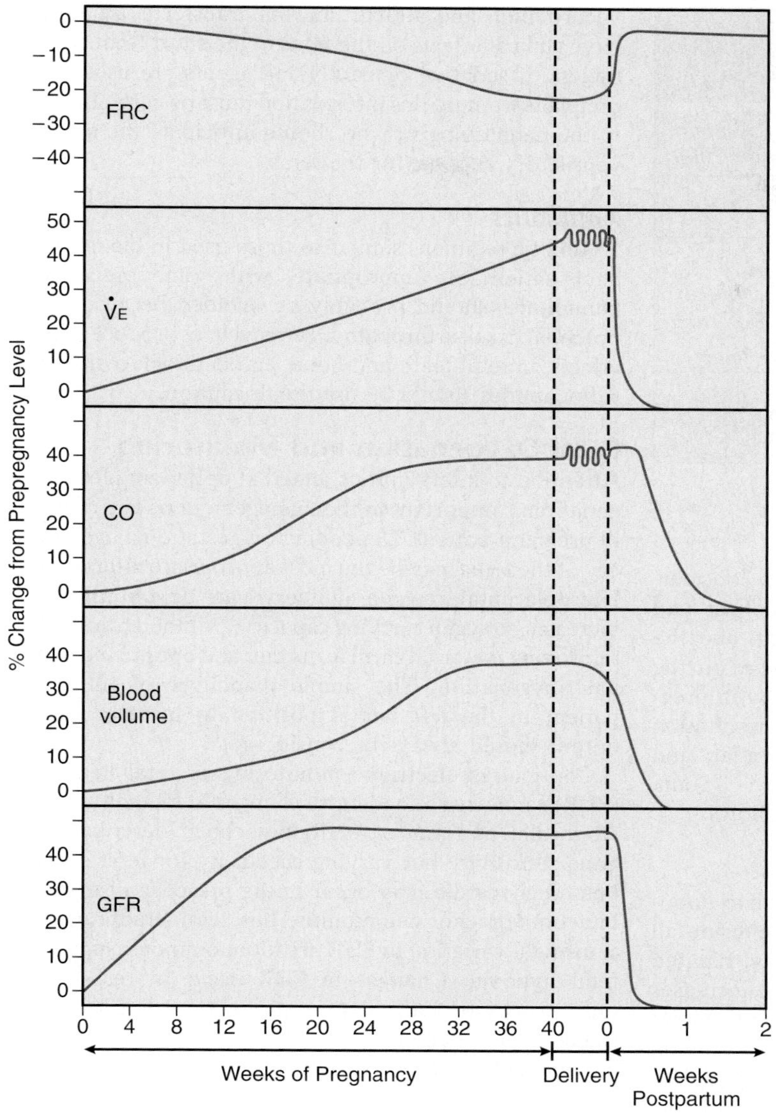

Figure 82-2. Physiologic changes in pregnancy: graphic representation of some of the physiologic changes occurring in pregnancy. CO, cardiac output; FRC, functional residual capacity; GFR, glomerular filtration rate; V̇E, minute ventilation. (From Lapinsky SE, Kruczynski K, Slutsky AS: Critical care in the pregnant patient. Am J Respir Crit Care Med 1995;152:427-455.)

intake should be augmented by 20% to 50%. Several nutrients have an increased requirement in pregnancy including iron, folate, and calcium. Total parenteral nutrition (TPN) has been used successfully to provide nutritional support during pregnancy, in the patient in whom enteral nutrition is not possible. Blood glucose should be measured frequently in view of the predisposition to hyperglycemia.

Thrombosis Prophylaxis

Pregnancy increases the risks of venous thrombosis caused by hypercoagulability and venous stasis. Antithrombotic measures including physical interventions and heparin prophylaxis should be considered.

Radiologic Procedures and Fetal Risk

Radiologic investigations are often essential for the assessment and management of the critically ill pregnant patient. Although there are potential risks of exposing the fetus to ionizing radiation, fetal well-being depends on maternal recovery and appropriate radiologic procedures should not be avoided. Techniques such as shielding the abdomen with lead and using a well-collimated x-ray beam can effectively reduce exposure. With these precautions, estimated fetal radiation exposure can be limited to safe levels for most procedures, although investigations such as abdominal-pelvic computed tomography (CT) will obviously cause significant fetal radiation exposure (Table 82-2).[11]

The adverse effects of fetal exposure to radiation include oncogenicity and teratogenicity. A twofold increased risk of childhood leukemia may result from fetal exposure in the range of 20 to 50 mGy (2 to 5 rads). Most intensive care unit (ICU) procedures can be carried out well below these levels of exposure to the fetus (see Table 82-2). Teratogenicity does not appear to occur at these radiation doses, requiring radiation exposure greater than 50 to 100 mGy (5 to 10 rads). Every effort should nonetheless be made to minimize uterine exposure, particularly in the first trimester.

Table 82-2. Risk of Fetal Radiation Exposure Resulting from Radiologic Studies in the Critically Ill Pregnant Patient

Investigation	Fetal Radiation Exposure (mGy)
Chest radiograph (with abdomen shielded)	0.01
Ventilation-perfusion scan:	
Perfusion	0.1-1
Ventilation	0.1-0.4
CT pulmonary angiogram	0.1-1
CT pelvis and abdomen	30-50
Radiation effect on the fetus:	
Teratogenicity	50-100
Oncogenicity	20-50

Drug Therapy in Pregnancy

Pharmacotherapy during pregnancy requires consideration of the altered drug clearance, metabolism and volume of distribution of drugs in pregnancy, and the potential pharmacologic and teratogenic effects on the embryo. A detailed description of drug therapy in pregnancy is beyond the scope of this chapter. Consultation with an obstetrician and pharmacist is essential, and several excellent resources are available.[12,13] Some common ICU drugs are discussed briefly as follows.

Catecholamines

Catecholamines commonly used in the ICU such as dobutamine, dopamine, norepinephrine, and epinephrine all have the potential to reduce uterine blood flow. Limited animal and human data suggest that ephedrine increases maternal blood pressure without reducing uterine blood flow. Nonpharmacologic maneuvers such as volume replacement and left lateral positioning are essential to the management of hypotension, and the rapidity of correction of blood pressure may be more important than the specific inotropic agent used. If vasopressor therapy is required to support maternal hemodynamics, this therapy should not be withheld because of concerns for potential adverse effects on the fetus.

Sedation, Analgesia, and Neuromuscular Blockade

Little data exist on the preferred drugs for prolonged sedation, analgesia, or neuromuscular blockade in pregnancy. Benzodiazepine use in early pregnancy has been associated with a small risk of congenital malformations, mainly cleft lip and palate. Midazolam crosses the placenta to a lesser degree than diazepam, which can accumulate in the fetus at levels greater than in the mother. Although no data exist on the prolonged use of propofol in pregnancy, it has been used as an induction agent for caesarean section. Congenital malformations have not been demonstrated with use of narcotic analgesics such as morphine, meperidine, and fentanyl. The majority of nondepolarizing neuromuscular blocking agents have been shown to cross the placenta including pancuronium, vecuronium, and atracurium, but transfer is unlikely to have clinical effects on the fetus in the short term. Nevertheless, if sedative or paralyzing agents are used in the pregnant woman, this information must be communicated to the neonatologist, who should anticipate the need for ventilatory support for the fetus.

Antibiotics

Antibiotic regimens similar to those used in the nonpregnant patient are appropriate, with some precautions. Quinolones should probably be avoided because of the potential risk of arthropathy. Tetracyclines produce adverse effects on fetal teeth and bone, and aminoglycosides and sulfonamides should be used with caution.

Fetal Oxygenation and Monitoring

Attention to interventions aimed at optimizing fetal oxygenation is important in the management of any critically ill pregnant patient. Depending on gestational age, delivery of the fetus may be the most appropriate intervention. Uteroplacental oxygen delivery can be optimized by increasing oxygen carrying capacity, by blood transfusion, improving maternal cardiac output, and optimizing maternal oxygenation. The simple maneuver of tilting the patient to the left lateral position to increase cardiac output should always be considered.[10]

Continuous electronic monitoring of fetal heart rate (FHR) can be used to identify changes in fetal physiology. Abnormal patterns of FHR have been described with good sensitivity but varying specificity for fetal distress. Fetal tachycardia may occur in the presence of maternal infection or chorioamnionitis, but fetal bradycardia or sinusoidal variation in FHR are more ominous, suggesting fetal hypoxia. Changes in FHR occur in response to uterine activity. Early decelerations coinciding with contractions are benign, but late decelerations beginning beyond the peak in contraction and persisting after the contraction may indicate fetal compromise, particularly if associated with a reduced beat-to-beat variation. Fetal compromise may occur as a result of uteroplacental or fetal pathology but may also indicate maternal illness with reduced uterine oxygen delivery. The fetus may be further assessed by an ultrasound biophysical profile that evaluates factors such as spontaneous movement, breathing action, and amniotic fluid volume. A normal biophysical profile carries a good prognosis.

Hemodynamic Monitoring

In general the indications for use of the pulmonary artery catheter are similar to those in nonobstetric patients, and pregnancy is not a contraindication to invasive hemodynamic monitoring. An awareness of the normal cardiovascular physiologic changes in pregnancy (discussed earlier) is necessary in order to correctly interpret the hemodynamic data obtained.

Ventilatory Support

Noninvasive Ventilation

Noninvasive ventilation avoids the adverse effects of endotracheal intubation, such as airway trauma, the increased risk of nosocomial pneumonia, and the complications associated with sedation. This modality is ideally suited to short-term ventilatory support, which is the case in many obstetric complications that reverse rapidly. The major concern with mask ventilation in pregnancy is the risk of aspiration because of the increased intraabdominal pressure, delayed gastric emptying, and reduced lower esophageal sphincter tone accompanying pregnancy. Noninvasive ventilation should therefore be reserved for the patient who is alert, protecting her airway, and who has an expectation of a relatively brief requirement for mechanical ventilatory support.

Airway Management

Failed intubation is more common in the obstetric population than in other anesthetic intubations.[14] The reduced oxygen reserve caused by diminished functional residual capacity and increased oxygen consumption produces rapid desaturation in response to apnea or hypoventilation.[15] Preoxygenation with 100% oxygen is beneficial, but respiratory alkalosis must be avoided. In view of the delayed gastric emptying and elevated intraabdominal pressure, the pregnant patient should always be considered to have a full stomach and appropriate precautions should be taken. Upper airway hyperemia and edema may reduce visualization and increase the risk of bleeding. Nasal intubation should be avoided, and a smaller endotracheal tube may be required.

Mechanical Ventilation

The normal $Pa{CO_2}$ of about 30 mm Hg in late pregnancy should be considered in the interpretation of arterial blood gases when decisions are made to institute ventilatory support. Data on the prolonged mechanical ventilation of pregnant patients are limited. Hyperventilation should be avoided because this adversely affects uterine blood flow[16] because of the resulting alkalemia as well as the effect of positive pressure ventilation in reducing cardiac output. The current ventilatory approach of avoiding excessive lung stretch by pressure limitation and permissive hypercapnia has not been assessed in pregnancy. The usual pressure limits (e.g., plateau pressure of 35 cm H_2O) may not be applicable in the near-term patient, where chest wall compliance is reduced. Transpulmonary pressures may not be elevated at a plateau pressure of 35 cm H_2O, and higher ventilatory pressures may be acceptable in pregnant patients near term. Although late pregnancy is associated with a mild respiratory alkalosis, maternal hypercapnia up to 60 mm Hg in the presence of adequate oxygenation does not appear to be detrimental to the fetus.[17] Fetal acidemia with associated fetal heart rate changes may be noted. If marked respiratory acidosis results from permissive hypercapnia, treatment with bicarbonate may improve maternal and fetal acidemia.

Cardiopulmonary Resuscitation

Cardiopulmonary resuscitation requires only minor modifications from standard protocols.[18] Electrical cardioversion and defibrillation may be performed in pregnancy, but fetal monitoring leads should be removed to prevent electrical arcing. Management in the supine position may cause aortocaval compression, resulting in impaired venous return and inadequate cardiac output. A left lateral tilt, a wedge under the right hip, or manual displacement of the uterus to the left should be used. Appropriate pharmacologic therapy should not be withheld if clinically indicated. Perimortem cesarean section may save the fetus when initial attempts at resuscitation have failed in a woman with a fetus at a viable gestation. Data suggest that infant survival without neurologic sequelae is highest if the postmortem cesarean section is initiated within four minutes of cardiac arrest.[19]

PREGNANCY-SPECIFIC CONDITIONS REQUIRING INTENSIVE CARE UNIT CARE

Preeclampsia

Preeclampsia is a pregnancy-induced condition occurring after 20 weeks' gestation, characterized by hypertension and proteinuria.[20] The cause remains unknown but is likely related to a placental abnormality producing a diffuse maternal endothelial effect, which leads to vasospasm and reduced organ perfusion (Fig. 82-3). Preeclampsia and its complications account for 20% to 50% of obstetric admissions to the ICU.[21-23] Less common multisystem diseases should be considered in the differential diagnosis including systemic lupus erythematosus (SLE), thrombotic thrombocytopenic purpura (TTP), and hemolytic-uremic syndrome (HUS) (Table 82-3). Complications of preeclampsia may result in critical illness including pulmonary edema, cerebral edema, renal failure, hypertensive crisis, seizures (eclampsia), and the HELLP syndrome (microangiopathic hemolytic anemia, thrombocytopenia, and hepatic involvement).[24]

The only specific treatment is delivery of the fetus and placenta. Delivery is always in the best interest of the mother, but timing may depend on fetal maturity. The role of antihypertensive therapy is to prevent maternal hyper-

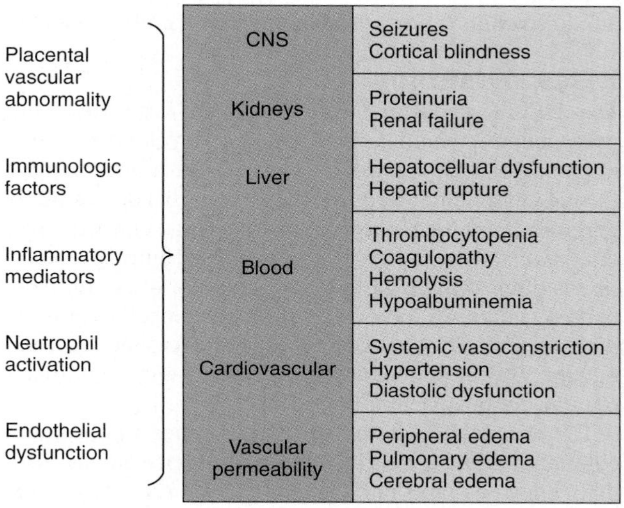

Figure 82-3. Pathophysiology and multiorgan effects of preeclampsia.

Table 82-3. Differential Diagnosis of Pregnancy-Related Complications

	Pregnancy Specific	Nonspecific
1. Hypertension	Preeclampsia Secondary hypertension (renal, pheochromocytoma)	Essential hypertension
2. Thrombocytopenia	Preeclampsia HELLP syndrome Acute fatty liver of pregnancy SLE	TTP ITP Sepsis
3. Abnormal liver enzymes	Preeclampsia HELLP syndrome Acute fatty liver of pregnancy Cholestasis of pregnancy	Viral hepatitis Drug-induced hepatitis Budd-Chiari syndrome
4. Renal dysfunction	Preeclampsia Acute fatty liver of pregnancy Idiopathic postpartum renal failure SLE	Sepsis Hypovolemia/hemorrhage TTP/HUS
5. Pulmonary edema	Preeclampsia Peripartum cardiomyopathy Tocolytic pulmonary edema Amniotic fluid emboli	Valvular heart disease Ischemic heart disease ARDS Aspiration

HUS, hemolytic-uremic syndrome; ITP, idiopathic thrombocytopenic purpura; SLE, systemic lupus erythematosus; TTP, thrombotic thrombocytopenic purpura.

tensive complications, and it does not alter the natural history of the condition or benefit the fetus.[25] Commonly used agents include intravenous hydralazine or labetalol, as well as oral calcium antagonists. Rapid reduction in blood pressure should usually be avoided because of the risk of reducing uteroplacental perfusion. Magnesium sulfate is used for seizure prophylaxis and treatment, giving an initial intravenous bolus (2 to 4 g) followed by an infusion of 2 to 3 g/hour. Toxic magnesium levels may occur, particularly in the presence of renal dysfunction, producing respiratory muscle weakness and cardiac conduction defects. Hypocalcemia may be noted during magnesium infusion and should not routinely be corrected because this would negate the therapeutic effects of magnesium. Fluid management in preeclampsia usually requires careful volume expansion, but excessive fluid administration can cause pulmonary or cerebral edema.

HELLP Syndrome

The HELLP syndrome is a condition associated with preeclampsia, characterized by the development of a microangiopathic hemolytic anemia and a consumptive thrombocytopenia. Reduced hepatic perfusion results in periportal and focal parenchymal necrosis, elevated liver enzymes, and rarely hepatic rupture. The clinical presentation is often with epigastric or right upper quadrant pain, nausea, vomiting, or evidence of bleeding. Features of preeclampsia do not occur in all patients, and approximately 30% of patients with HELLP develop the disease only in the postpartum period.

The diagnosis is based on the presence of thrombocytopenia ($<100 \times 10^9$/L), with a moderate elevation of liver enzymes, and microangiopathic hemolytic anemia (increased lactate dehydrogenase, bilirubin, abnormal blood smear). Many patients are found to have a more widespread coagulation defect than just thrombocytopenia. White blood cell count may be elevated, and hypoglycemia is uncommon, in contrast to acute fatty liver of pregnancy.

Management includes early delivery if the fetus is viable, blood product support, and management of associated preeclampsia. Dexamethasone initiated prior to delivery has been reported to produce more rapid recovery of thrombocytopenia in some studies but does not affect outcome.[26,27] Delivery may require platelet support, and if cesarean section is necessary, hemorrhage should be anticipated and adequate drains should be inserted. Epidural anesthesia is usually contraindicated in the presence of thrombocytopenia.

The maternal complications of HELLP include hemorrhage, ARDS, and acute renal failure. An uncommon but catastrophic consequence of the HELLP syndrome is hepatic subcapsular hemorrhage, which occurs in about 2% of patients and can progress to hepatic rupture. Hepatic rupture should be considered in any preeclamptic with sudden shock or acute abdominal pain. Management requires aggressive hemodynamic and blood product support, urgent delivery, and invasive control of the hemorrhage with embolization or laparotomy with packing of the liver. Hemorrhage without rupture may be managed conservatively if the patient remains hemodynamically stable.

Significant overlap exists between HELLP and other multisystem conditions and thrombotic microangiopathies (see Table 82-3). A response to plasmapheresis may be noted in some patients, possibly representing those with TTP or HUS rather than HELLP. Plasmapheresis is recommended for patients with delayed postpartum resolution when severe thrombocytopenia, hemolysis, or organ dysfunction persist more than 72 hours following delivery. The maternal mortality for women with HELLP syndrome is reported between 1% and 3% (with isolated reports as high as 25%) and with a significant perinatal mortality at 8% to 60%.

Acute Fatty Liver of Pregnancy

Acute fatty liver of pregnancy (AFLP) is an uncommon condition affecting about 1 in 15,000 pregnancies. Although early reports described acute fulminant hepatic failure with a high maternal and fetal mortality rate, the condition is now usually recognized at an earlier stage, allowing early delivery and a significantly improved outcome.[28] Maternal mortality has been reported at 0% to 18% with fetal loss of 23% to 60%. The etiology of this condition is unknown, but an association with a fetal inborn error of metabolism (L-CHAD deficiency) has been described.[29] Pathologically, diffuse fatty infiltration of the liver occurs with necrosis and inflammation being mild or absent.

Patients usually present toward the end of the third trimester with a range of onset from as early as 30 weeks' gestation up until the puerperium. Prodromal symptoms of malaise, anorexia, and vomiting may precede the onset of jaundice by 1 to 2 weeks. Abdominal pain may occur, which may be diffuse or localized to the right upper quadrant. Laboratory investigations demonstrate a moderate elevation in transaminase levels (e.g., 300 to 600 units), in contrast with the higher levels occurring in acute hepatitis. The white blood cell count is often elevated and thrombocytopenia and fragmented red blood cells may be demonstrated. Features of hepatic dysfunction such as hypoalbuminemia, hypoglycemia, and coagulopathy occur in more severe cases.

The differential diagnosis of liver disease in pregnancy is wide, and the multisystemic effects of AFLP may resemble systemic lupus, thrombotic thrombocytopenic purpura, or hemolytic-uremic syndrome (see Table 82-3).

The definitive treatment is delivery of the fetus, and early recognition of this condition is responsible for an improved outcome. Because the presentation is usually close to term, the decision is usually easy and carries little additional risk for the fetus. However, AFLP is associated with placental insufficiency because of fibrin deposition, producing increased fetal loss. It has been reported that this process may be exacerbated by therapeutic coagulation factor replacement. Supportive therapy is similar to that for other causes of fulminant hepatic failure including correction of coagulation abnormalities and hypoglycemia. Hepatic encephalopathy requires attention to airway protection, dietary protein restriction, bowel sterilization, and oral or rectal lactulose administration. Transient worsening of hepatic function may occur following delivery with improvement usually beginning within 2 to 3 days. A small subset of patients continue to deteriorate following delivery, and liver transplantation may be indicated. Complications such as hemorrhage, pancreatitis, renal failure, diabetes insipidus, and infection should be sought and treated.

Amniotic Fluid Embolism

Amniotic fluid embolism is a catastrophic cardiopulmonary complication of pregnancy, carrying a mortality rate of 10% to 86%.[30] It usually occurs in association with labor and delivery but may be precipitated by uterine trauma or manipulations. Amniotic fluid enters the venous circulation and particulate contents or humoral factors produce acute pulmonary hypertension, as well as acute left ventricular dysfunction.[31] The pregnant woman develops sudden onset of dyspnea, hypoxemia, and cardiovascular collapse. The presenting feature may sometimes be seizures related to cerebral hypoxia or acute fetal hypoxia and distress. Many patients with amniotic fluid embolism die within the first hour. No specific diagnostic test is available, and the diagnosis of amniotic fluid embolism is based on a typical clinical picture and exclusion of other conditions such as septic shock, pulmonary thromboembolism, abruptio placentae, tension pneumothorax, or a myocardial ischemic event.

Treatment involves routine resuscitative and supportive measures including mechanical ventilation and inotropic therapy. A role for corticosteroids has been suggested on the basis of the hypothesis that the process may involve an anaphylactoid reaction to amniotic fluid contents.[30] Survivors of the initial process may develop DIC and acute respiratory distress syndrome (ARDS). Neurologic damage caused by the initial hypotension and hypoxemia is common.

Obstetric Hemorrhage

Uterine blood flow reaches 600 mL/minute near term, subjecting the pregnant patient to the risk of devastating blood loss. Antepartum hemorrhage occurs from disruption of the placenta, such as with placental abruption or a low lying placenta (placenta previa) as the cervix dilates. Most hemorrhage occurs postpartum because of uterine atony, cervical or vaginal lacerations, related to antepartum hemorrhage, or associated with coagulopathy. The pregnant woman is physiologically prepared for blood loss and tolerates the loss from a normal vaginal delivery (600 mL) or cesarean section (1000 mL). However, excessive blood loss will result in hypovolemic shock with compromise to fetus and vital organs. The pregnant woman is particularly susceptible to hypoperfusion injury to the kidney. A high incidence of myocardial ischemia has been noted in pregnant women with hemorrhagic shock.

Supportive management of obstetric hemorrhage is similar to any cause of hemorrhage and involves rapid volume replacement, supplemental oxygen administration, and red cell and blood product support for an associated dilutional coagulopathy. Various pharmacologic agents are utilized to control uterine bleeding. Intramuscular administration of methylergonovine (0.2 mg) may be useful in the presence of uterine atony but is contraindicated in the presence of hypertension.[32] Oxytocin is infused intravenously in a dose greater than that used for augmentation of labor, up to 100 mU/minute (e.g., 40 U in 1000 mL normal saline at 150 mL/hour). This dose may produce an antidiuretic effect and cause hyponatremia. A prostaglandin F_{2a} analogue (carboprost tromethamine—Hemabate) given intramuscularly (0.25 mg, repeated every 15 to 90 minutes to maximum 2 mg) or intramyometrially, is effective in controlling hemorrhage.[32,33] Side effects include vomiting, hypertension, bronchoconstriction, and increased intrapulmonary shunt. Isolated reports suggest that recombinant Factor VIIa may be useful in the management of severe obstetric hemorrhage.[34] If pharmacologic methods fail to control bleeding, radiologic transcatheter embolization of the internal iliac or uterine artery is usually effective.[35] Surgical exploration with arterial ligation or hysterectomy may become necessary.

Peripartum Cardiomyopathy

Cardiac failure may occur in the absence of preexisting heart disease because of peripartum cardiomyopathy. This idiopathic condition presents in the last month of pregnancy or within 5 months of delivery, with an incidence of approximately 1 in 3500 live births.[36] The clinical presentation is usually after 36 weeks' gestation (in contrast to women with preexisting cardiac disease) and involves the gradual onset of symptoms of heart failure. The diagnosis is by the demonstration of left ventricular systolic dysfunction and by the exclusion of other causes of cardiomyopathy. During labor and the early postpartum period, tachycardia and increased cardiac output may precipitate acute pulmonary edema.

Treatment is similar to other patients with cardiac failure, although angiotensin-converting enzyme (ACE) inhibitors should be avoided before delivery. Anticoagulation is essential because of the hypercoagulable state of pregnancy and the high incidence of thrombotic complications. A subset of patients may have an inflammatory myocarditis, and immunosuppressive therapy may be considered in those who do not improve after 2 weeks of standard treatment.[36] Although a high mortality rate has been described (10% to 50%), about half of patients recover normal ventricular function.[37]

Tocolytic Pulmonary Edema

β-Adrenergic blockers can be used to inhibit uterine contractions in preterm labor, although this is less frequently used because studies demonstrated a lack of fetal benefit from this practice. A complication of this β-agonist therapy in pregnancy is the development of acute pulmonary edema.[38] Treatment involves discontinuing the β-agonist and supportive treatment including diuresis and oxygen therapy. Failure of the pulmonary edema to resolve within 24 hours should prompt a search for an alternative diagnosis (Table 82-4).

Gestational Trophoblastic Disease

Pulmonary hypertension and pulmonary edema may occur in the setting of benign hydatidiform mole, as a result of trophoblastic pulmonary embolism. This most commonly occurs during evacuation of the uterus, with a higher incidence of pulmonary complications in the woman later in pregnancy.[39] With supportive treatment resolution occurs within 48 to 72 hours. Molar pregnancy may also be associated with choriocarcinoma, which can produce multiple, discrete, pulmonary metastases.

CONDITIONS NOT SPECIFIC TO PREGNANCY

Septic Shock

The pregnant woman is at risk of pregnancy-related infections, as well infections not specific to pregnancy. Some increased susceptibility to certain infections may occur, possibly related to changes in cell-mediated immunity. *Listeria monocytogenes* infection, disseminated herpesvirus infections, varicella, and coccidioidomycosis infections may be more common or more severe. Human immunodeficiency virus infections should always be considered. Obstetric sepsis in the antepartum period produces chorioamnionitis, but most obstetric sepsis occurs in the postpartum period. The most common location of infection is the placental site, causing endometritis, which can spread to a peritonitis. Episiotomy sites or cesarean

Table 82-4. Differential Diagnosis of Acute Respiratory Distress in Pregnancy

Disorder	Distinguishing Features
Pregnancy Specific	
Amniotic fluid embolism	Cardiorespiratory collapse, seizures, DIC
Pulmonary edema secondary to preeclampsia	Hypertension, proteinuria
ARDS secondary to obstetric sepsis	Evidence of obstetric sepsis, shock
Tocolytic pulmonary edema	Tocolytic administration, rapid improvement
Peripartum cardiomyopathy	Gradual onset, cardiac gallop, cardiomegaly
Trophoblastic embolism	Nodular infiltrate, molar pregnancy
Risk Increased by Pregnancy	
Aspiration pneumonitis	Vomiting, aspiration
Venous thromboembolism	Evidence of DVT, positive $\dot{V}/\dot{Q}$ scan, leg Dopplers, CT angiogram
Pneumomediastinum	Occurs during delivery, subcutaneous emphysema
Valvular heart disease	Pulmonary edema, cardiac murmur, cardiomegaly
ARDS secondary to sepsis	Evidence of sepsis (e.g., pyelonephritis)
Unrelated to Pregnancy	
Asthma	Features similar to nonpregnant patient
Pneumonia	

ARDS, acute respiratory distress syndrome; DIC, disseminated intravascular coagulopathy; DVT, deep venous thrombosis; $\dot{V}/\dot{Q}$, ventilation-perfusion.

section wounds may also become infected. Infections often involve a mixed flora, with microorganisms originating from the vagina (e.g., anaerobes, group B streptococci), intestine (gram-negative organisms, enterococci, anaerobes), sexual transmission (e.g., *Neisseria gonorrhoeae*), or hematogenous spread (e.g., *Listeria*, group A streptococci).[40]

Management of septic shock is similar to that in the nonpregnant patient, with prompt resuscitation with volume expansion. If inotropic therapy is necessary in the antepartum patient, the effects of such drugs on uteroplacental perfusion should be considered. Adequate specimens for culture should be obtained including amniocentesis in the antepartum patient. Ultrasonography may be valuable to identify a source of localized infection and exclude retained products of conception.

Initial empiric antibiotic therapy should provide broad gram-negative, gram-positive, and anaerobic cover. Common regimens use drugs such as ampicillin, gentamicin, and clindamycin; ampicillin/sulbactam; ticarcillin-clavulanate; piperacillin and gentamicin; or carbapenems.[41] Urgent delivery may be required for management of chorioamnionitis with sepsis syndrome. Activated protein C can be considered in the postpartum patient.

A poor response to antibiotic therapy may indicate a resistant organism (e.g., *Enterococcus*), a localized abscess, myometrial microabscesses, or septic pelvic thrombophlebitis. Gas in the subcutaneous tissues or uterine wall suggests clostridial gas gangrene. Patients with retained products or devitalized tissue are at significant risk. Toxic shock caused by *Staphylococcus aureus* or *Clostridium sordelli* may occur, often associated with septic abortion. Surgical evacuation of the uterus or laparotomy with débridement or even hysterectomy may be required. Puerperal ovarian vein thrombophlebitis may complicate endometritis, presenting with acute deterioration with fever. The diagnosis can be confirmed with CT or magnetic resonance imaging scanning, and treatment requires anticoagulation and antibiotic therapy. Surgical intervention with venous ligation or excision may be required.

Group A streptococcal necrotizing fasciitis and toxic shock syndrome have been reported to occur unexpectedly following an uncomplicated pregnancy and delivery.[42] Management includes antibiotic therapy with penicillin and clindamycin and early surgical intervention. Intravenous immunoglobulin (2 g/kg) may be beneficial.

Acute Respiratory Distress Syndrome in Pregnancy

The pregnant patient is at risk of developing acute lung injury from pregnancy-associated complications and other conditions (see Table 82-4).[43] The pregnant patient appears to be at increased risk of developing pulmonary edema because of the cardiovascular changes and the reduced albumin level occurring in pregnancy.

Management is similar to that in the nonpregnant patient. Adequate maternal oxygenation is essential for fetal well-being, and delivery may benefit both the mother and the fetus.[44] Survival from ARDS is as good as or better than that in the general population, likely because of these patients' young age, lack of comorbidity, and the reversibility of many of the predisposing conditions.

Pulmonary Thromboembolic Disease

Pulmonary thromboembolism is a leading cause of maternal mortality. Although the risk is significantly increased in pregnant women because of increased coagulation factors, hormonally medicated venous stasis, and local pressure effects, the incidence is relatively low at about 1 per 1000 deliveries. Pulmonary embolism occurs most frequently in the early postpartum period.

Investigation of suspected pulmonary embolism is not different from that in the nonpregnant patient, with duplex ultrasound as the initial investigation. False positives may occur with Doppler alone because of venous obstruction by the gravid uterus. Ventilation-perfusion scanning and CT pulmonary angiography can be performed with low risk of fetal exposure (see Table 82-2).[11]

Warfarin is generally avoided in pregnancy because of the risk of a first trimester embryopathy and central nervous system abnormalities with second- and third-trimester exposure. Heparin does not cross the placenta and can be readily reversed, and low molecular weight heparins are safe and effective in pregnancy although less easy to reverse acutely.[45] Thrombolysis has been used successfully in pregnancy but should be limited to life-threatening situations. Transvenous inferior vena caval filters have been used in the pregnant patient, although there is a risk of dislodgment because of venous dilation and pressure effects.

Asthma

The hormonal changes of pregnancy can affect asthma variably, with worsening, improvement, or no substantial change occurring. Asthma is a common condition, and acute asthmatic attacks are therefore an important cause of respiratory compromise in pregnancy. In assessment of the patient with a severe acute attack, the reduced $Pa{CO_2}$ occurring in late pregnancy should be considered; a normal $Pa{CO_2}$ level associated with acidosis may imply respiratory failure. Treatment is similar to the nonpregnant patient, including β-agonists and corticosteroids. Although there is a natural reluctance to prescribe drug therapy in these patients, pregnancy is not an absolute contraindication to systemic corticosteroid therapy.[46] Uncontrolled asthma is more dangerous to the fetus than appropriate drug therapy, and management should highlight the importance of adequate oxygenation.

Cardiac Disease

Overt or occult preexisting heart disease may produce acute cardiac decompensation as the blood volume and cardiac output increase during pregnancy. Women with prior cardiac events, cyanosis, or pulmonary hypertension are at particular risk. Patients with mitral and aortic stenosis are at risk of developing hemodynamic deterioration as the physiologic changes peak at about 28 weeks, although mild to moderate regurgitant valvular disease is generally well tolerated.[47] The onset of atrial fibrillation or severe hypertension can precipitate sudden hemodynamic deterioration even in those women with less severe cardiac disease.

Patients with moderate to severe mitral stenosis are likely to experience hemodynamic deterioration during the third trimester or during labor. Treatment is similar to the nonpregnant patient using digoxin and β-blockers to control heart rate and diuretics to reduce left atrial pressure.[48] Angiotensin-converting enzyme inhibitors should be avoided. Most patients with mitral stenosis can undergo vaginal delivery with consideration to invasive hemodynamic monitoring during labor and the early postpartum period. Epidural anesthesia is usually better tolerated hemodynamically than general anesthesia during labor and delivery. Electrical cardioversion can be performed safely if indicated.

Severe aortic stenosis is associated with significant risk during pregnancy,[48] with symptoms such as dyspnea, angina, or syncope appearing from late in the second trimester. Percutaneous aortic balloon valvuloplasty can be performed during pregnancy. Spinal and epidural anesthesia during labor may adversely affect hemodynamics because of the vasodilatory effects. Although antibiotic prophylaxis is not usually indicated for routine deliveries, prophylaxis is often administered because uncomplicated delivery cannot always be anticipated.[48]

Ischemic heart disease is uncommon in pregnancy but may be missed because of masking of the symptoms, signs, and cardiac enzyme levels by pregnancy. Coronary artery dissection may occur, particularly in the immediate postpartum period. Aortic dissection may occur related to hypertension, aortic coarctation, or Marfan's syndrome and is associated with significant maternal and fetal mortality.[49]

Woman with cyanotic congenital heart disease, particularly those with associated pulmonary hypertension, are at significant risk during pregnancy. Because of the inability of the right ventricle to tolerate the increases in cardiac output, primary or secondary pulmonary hypertension is associated with a high mortality rate in pregnancy.[50] Treatment with vasodilators including prostacyclin and nitric oxide has been described, with or without invasive hemodynamic monitoring. These patients should be managed in a center with expertise and experience in this area.

Trauma

The anatomic and physiologic changes of pregnancy may alter the manifestations and severity of traumatic injury. Uterine injury can produce severe hemorrhage because of the high uterine blood flow and may precipitate placental abruption or rarely uterine rupture. Uterine rupture manifests with maternal shock, abdominal pain, and palpable fetal parts. Penetrating injury to the abdomen predominantly affects the uterus in later pregnancy, but because intraabdominal viscera are compressed in the upper abdomen, minor injury may result in significant damage.[51] Fractures of the pelvis can produce severe retroperitoneal hemorrhage because of dilation of pelvic veins.

Maternal trauma is associated with a significant increase in fetal loss, due to maternal shock or hypoxia, placental injury, or direct fetal injury.[52] Direct fetal injury resulting from blunt trauma usually involves head injury related to maternal pelvic fracture. Other fetal injuries may occur following blunt or penetrating trauma, sometimes with minimal maternal injury. A high fetal mortality occurs in the presence of maternal burns to greater than 30% of the body surface area. Placental abruption is an important cause of fetal demise,[51] and may present with vaginal bleeding, abdominal cramps, uterine tenderness, amniotic fluid leakage, and unexplained fetal distress or maternal hypovolemia. Placental abruption is often complicated by DIC due to release of thromboplastin into the maternal circulation.

Evaluation of the pregnant trauma patient should include a detailed abdominal examination, but physical signs may be affected by changing organ position and the reduced peritoneal sensitivity that occurs in pregnancy.[53] Initial investigations should include blood type including Rh status. Ultrasound is useful for evaluation of the fetus for injury and biophysical profile and to assess intra-abdominal organ damage. Ultrasound-guided paracentesis or diagnostic peritoneal lavage (by open technique, above the uterus) may aid in detecting bowel perforation or intraperitoneal hemorrhage. Transplacental hemorrhage of fetal blood into the maternal circulation may occur and can result in fetal exsanguination and maternal Rh sensitization. Fetomaternal hemorrhage is detected by the Kleihauer-Betke test, which identifies fetal cells in the maternal blood smear, and can estimate the volume of fetal hemorrhage by the percentage of red cells of fetal origin. Fetal evaluation includes heart rate assessment by auscultation (possible from 20 weeks) or Doppler probe. Obstetric consultation and continuous fetal cardiotocography are important when the fetus is at a viable gestation.

Care of the severely injured pregnant patient requires a multidisciplinary approach involving the emergency physician, trauma surgeon, obstetrician, intensivist, and neonatologist. Initial resuscitation follows usual principles with efforts directed primarily at stabilizing the mother. Fluid replacement may need to be given more rapidly than in nonpregnant women because of the physiologic increase in plasma volume, and maternal blood pressure and heart rate may not be reliable predictors of the degree of hemorrhage.[53] Left lateral positioning to prevent supine hypotensive syndrome is an important consideration in the hypotensive patient. Rh-negative mothers with abdominal trauma should receive Rh immune globulin even in the presence of a negative Kleihauer-Betke test. Higher doses of Rh immune globulin will be necessary in the presence of significant feto-maternal hemorrhage.

In the unstable mother, management of maternal injuries takes precedence over fetal distress because correction of maternal hemodynamics is beneficial to the fetus. The fetus is extremely vulnerable to hypotension and hypoxemia, and uterine blood flow will be markedly reduced when maternal circulation is compromised. If the mother is stable, cesarean section may be appropriate if the fetus is considered viable, the limits of viability being largely dependent on the level of neonatal care available.

KEY POINTS

- The reduced FRC and increased oxygen consumption in pregnancy result in rapid oxygen desaturation during apnea or intubation.
- Although there is a risk to the fetus from radiologic procedures and drug therapy, necessary investigations and treatment should not be withheld, with appropriate precautions.
- The various pregnancy-specific conditions should be considered in the differential diagnosis of a critically ill pregnant woman including preeclampsia, HELLP syndrome, acute fatty liver of pregnancy, and amniotic fluid embolism.
- Hypotension may occur in the supine position in late pregnancy because of aortocaval compression—the clinician should position the hypotensive pregnant patient in the left lateral position.
- Management of preeclampsia, the commonest cause of ICU admission, involves delivery of the fetus, seizure prophylaxis with magnesium sulfate, correction of fluid balance, and treatment of hypertension if clinically significant.

REFERENCES

1. Elkus R, Popovich J: Respiratory physiology in pregnancy. Clin Chest Med 1992;13:555-565.
2. Marx GF, Murthy PK, Orkin LR: Static compliance before and after vaginal delivery. Br J Anaesth 1970;42:1100-1104.
3. Rees GB, Pipkin FB, Symonds EM, Patrick JM: A longitudinal study of respiratory changes in normal human pregnancy with cross-sectional data on subjects with pregnancy-induced hypertension. Am J Obstet Gynecol 1990;162:826-830.
4. Mabie WC, DiSessa TG, Crocker LG, et al: A longitudinal study of cardiac output in normal human pregnancy. Am J Obstet Gynecol 1994;170: 849-856.
5. Clark SL, Cotton DB, Lee W, et al: Central hemodynamic assessment of normal term pregnancy. Am J Obstet Gynecol 1989;161:1439-1442.
6. Robson SC, Dunlop W, Boys RJ, Hunter S: Cardiac output during labour. BMJ 1987;295:1169-1171.
7. Assali NS: Dynamics of the uteroplacental circulation in health and disease. Am J Perinatol 1989;6:105-109.
8. Baylis C: Glomerular filtration rate in normal and abnormal pregnancies. Semin Nephrol 1999;19:133-139.
9. Schwartz KA: Gestational thrombocytopenia and immune thrombocytopenias in pregnancy. Hematol Oncol Clin North Am 2000;14:1101-1116.
10. Kinsella SM, Lohmann G: Supine hypotensive syndrome. Obstet Gynecol 1994;83:774-788.
11. Lowe SA: Diagnostic radiography in pregnancy: Risks and reality. Aust N Z J Obstet Gynaecol 2004;44:191-196.
12. Briggs GG, Freeman RK, Yaffe SJ (eds): Drugs in Pregnancy and Lactation, 7th ed. Baltimore, Lippincott Williams & Wilkins, 2005.
13. Hospital for Sick Children, Toronto. Available at http://www.motherisk.org Accessed July 18, 2007.
14. King TA, Adams AP: Failed tracheal intubation. Br J Anaesth 1990;65:400-414.
15. Archer GW, Marx GF: Arterial oxygen tension during apnoea in parturient women. Br J Anaesth 1974;46:358-360.
16. Levinson G, Shnider SM, deLorimier AA, Steffenson JL: Effects of maternal hyperventilation on uterine blood flow and fetal oxygenation and acid-base status. Anesthesiology 1974;40: 340-347.
17. Ivankovic AD, Elam JO, Huffman J: Effect of maternal hypercarbia on the newborn infant. Am J Obstet Gynecol 1970;107:939-946.
18. 2005 American Heart Association Guidelines for Cardiopulmonary Resuscitation and Emergency Cardiovascular Care. Part 10.8: Cardiac arrest associated with pregnancy. Circulation 2005;112(Suppl I): IV-150-IV-153.
19. Strong TH, Lowe RA: Perimortem cesarean section. Am J Emerg Med 1989;7:489-494.
20. Anonymous. Report of the National High Blood Pressure Education Program Working Group on high blood pressure in pregnancy. Am J Obstet Gynecol 2000;183:S1-S22.
21. Lapinsky SE, Kruczynski K, Seaward G, et al: Critical care management of the obstetric patient. Can J Anaesth 1997;44:325-329.
22. Hazelgrove JF, Price C, Pappachan VJ, et al: Multicenter study of obstetric admissions to 14 intensive care units in southern England. Crit Care Med 2001;29:770-775.
23. Karnad DR, Lapsia V, Krishnan A, Salvi VS: Prognostic factors in obstetric patients admitted to an Indian intensive care unit. Crit Care Med 2004;32:1294-1299.
24. Weinstein L: Syndrome of hemolysis, elevated liver enzymes, and low platelet count: A severe consequence of hypertension in pregnancy. Am J Obstet Gynecol 1982;142:159-167.
25. von Dadelszen P, Ornstein MP, Bull SB, et al: Fall in mean arterial pressure and fetal growth restriction in pregnancy hypertension: A meta-analysis. Lancet 2000;355:87-92.
26. Matchaba P, Moodley J: Corticosteroids for HELLP syndrome in pregnancy. The Cochrane Database of Systematic Reviews Issue 1. 2004;CD002076.
27. Fonseca JE, Mendez F, Catano C, Arias F: Dexamethasone treatment does not improve the outcome of women with HELLP syndrome: A double-blind, placebo-controlled, randomized clinical trial. Am J Obstet Gynecol 2005;193:1591-1598.
28. Knox TA, Olans LB: Liver disease in pregnancy. N Engl J Med 1996;335:569-576.
29. Ibdah JA, Bennett MJ, Rinaldo P, et al: A fetal fatty-acid oxidation disorder as a cause of liver disease in pregnant women. N Engl J Med 1999;340:1723-1731.
30. Clark SL, Hankins GD, Dudley DA, et al: Amniotic fluid embolism: Analysis of the national registry. Am J Obstet Gynecol 1995;172:1158-1167.
31. Clark SL, Cotton DB, Gonik B, et al: Central hemodynamic alterations in amniotic fluid embolism. Am J Obstet Gynecol 1988;158:1124-1126.
32. Shevell T, Malone FD: Management of obstetric hemorrhage. Semin Perinatol 2003;27:86-104.
33. Hayashi RH, Castillo MS, Noah ML: Management of severe postpartum hemorrhage with a prostaglandin F_{2a} analogue. Obstet Gynecol 1984;63:806-814.
34. Segal S, Shemesh IY, Blumenthal R: Treatment of obstetric hemorrhage with recombinant activated factor VII (rFVIIa). Arch Gynecol Obstet 2003;268:266-267.
35. Hansch E, Chitkara U, McAlpine J, et al: Pelvic arterial embolization for control of obstetric hemorrhage: A five-year experience. Am J Obstet Gynecol 1999;180:1454-1460.
36. Pearson GD, Veille JC, Rahimtoola S, et al: Peripartum cardiomyopathy: National Heart, Lung, and Blood Institute and Office of Rare Diseases (National Institutes of Health) workshop recommendations and review. JAMA 2000;283:1183-1188.
37. O'Connell JB, Costanzo-Nordin MR, Subramanian R, et al: Peripartum cardiomyopathy: clinical, hemodynamic, histologic and prognostic characteristics. J Am Coll Cardiol 1986;8:52-56.
38. Pisani RJ, Rosenow EC III: Pulmonary edema associated with tocolytic therapy. Ann Intern Med 1989;110:714-718.
39. Twiggs LB, Morrow CP, Schlaerth JB: Acute pulmonary complications of

molar pregnancy. Am J Obstet Gynecol 1979;135:189-194.
40. Lapinsky SE, Seaward PGR: Sepsis in the gynecological and obstetric patient. In Fein A, Abraham EM, Balk R, et al (eds): Sepsis and Multiorgan Failure: Mechanisms for Treatment Strategies. Baltimore, Williams & Wilkins, 1997, pp 419-430.
41. Ledger WJ: Post-partum endomyometritis diagnosis and treatment: A review. J Obstet Gynaecol Res 2003;29:364-373.
42. Silver RM, Heddleston LN, McGregor JA, Gibbs RS: Life-threatening puerperal infection due to group A streptococci. Obstet Gynecol 1992;79:894-896.
43. Bandi VD, Munnur U, Matthay MA: Acute lung injury and acute respiratory distress syndrome in pregnancy. Crit Care Clin 2004;20:577-607.
44. Daily WH, Katz AR, Tonnesen A, Allen SJ: Beneficial effect of delivery in a patient with adult respiratory distress syndrome. Anesthesiology 1990;72:383-386.
45. Bates SM, Greer IA, Hirsh J, Ginsberg JS: Use of antithrombotic agents during pregnancy: The Seventh ACCP Conference on Antithrombotic and Thrombolytic Therapy. Chest 2004;126:627S-644S.
46. Guy ES, Kirumaki A, Hanania NA: Acute asthma in pregnancy. Crit Care Clin 2004;20:731-745.
47. Ray P, Murphy GJ, Shutt LE: Recognition and management of maternal cardiac disease in pregnancy. Br J Anaesth 2004;93:428-439.
48. Siu SC, Colman JM: Heart disease and pregnancy. Heart 2001;85:710-715.
49. Zeebregts CJ, Schepens MA, Hameeteman TM, et al: Acute aortic dissection complicating pregnancy. Ann Thorac Surg 1997;64:1345-1348.
50. Weiss BM, Zemp L, Seifert B, Hess OM: Outcome of pulmonary vascular disease in pregnancy: A systematic overview from 1978 through 1996. J Am Coll Cardiol 1998;31:1650-1657.
51. Pearlman MD, Tintinalli JE, Lorenz RP: A prospective controlled study of outcome after trauma during pregnancy. Am J Obstet Gynecol 1990;162:665-671.
52. Drost TF, Rosemurgy AS, Sherman HF, et al: Major trauma in pregnant women: Maternal/fetal outcome. J Trauma 1990;30:574-578.
53. Pearlman MD, Tintinalli JE, Lorenz RP: Blunt trauma during pregnancy. N Engl J Med 1990;323:1609-1613.

Chapter 83

Nutrition Support

Richard G. Barton

MALNUTRITION

Malnutrition is a disorder in body composition in which inadequate macronutrient (protein, carbohydrate, and fat) or micronutrient (vitamins, minerals, and trace elements) intake results in decreased body mass, reduced organ mass, and most importantly, decreased organ function. Although malnutrition is most frequently associated with a risk for immune dysfunction–related infection, wound healing/fascial dehiscence, and breakdown of surgical anastomoses, it can affect virtually all organ systems when severe. Skeletal muscle wasting, decreased myocardial mass, diastolic cardiac dysfunction and decreased sensitivity to inotropic agents, respiratory insufficiency/need for prolonged mechanical ventilation, renal cortical atrophy, and loss of gastrointestinal absorptive/barrier functions have all been associated with malnutrition.

Malnutrition can occur as a result of combined protein-calorie deficiency (marasmus), predominantly protein deficiency (kwashiorkor), and deficiencies in specific micronutrients, as well as altered metabolism arising from a disease state such as sepsis, burns, or trauma. Critically ill patients may suffer from a combination of these causes. Malnutrition is thought to be present in as many as 25% to 50% of patients on hospital admission and may affect an additional 25% to 30% of patients during their hospital stay. In older, retrospective studies, malnourished patients are thought to have a twofold to fourfold increase in morbidity (primarily infectious and wound complications) and as much as a threefold to sixfold increase in mortality.[1-4] In multivariate analysis of postoperative patients, malnutrition has been associated with gastrointestinal anastomotic leakage.[5] More recently, the National Surgical Quality Improvement Program (NSQIP) has shown preoperative serum albumin, a measure of chronic nutritional status, to be an independent predictor of mortality in a study of more than 400,000 surgical patients and specifically in patients undergoing colectomy, proctectomy, transurethral resection of bladder tumors, and major lung resection.[6-9] Malnutrition becomes particularly important in critically ill patients, in whom the combination of bed rest and catabolic illnesses such as sepsis, multiple trauma, burns, pancreatitis, and acute respiratory distress syndrome hasten the malnutrition, loss of lean body mass, and organ system dysfunction.

The purpose of this chapter is to contrast starvation and stress metabolism with emphasis on protein, carbohydrate, and fat metabolism; review the basic concepts of nutrition support with regard to energy and substrate requirements; discuss routes of nutrition support; provide an overview of organ-specific nutrition and immunonutrition; briefly summarize nutritional assessment and monitoring; and discuss the complications of nutrition support and their prevention.

STARVATION VERSUS STRESS METABOLISM

Starvation is a clinical situation that develops whenever nutrient supply is inadequate to meet nutrient demand. It is characterized by a specific metabolic adaptive response aimed at preserving lean body mass, as well as by decreased energy expenditure, utilization of alternative fuel sources, and reduced protein wasting. During the initial 12 to 24 hours of starvation, glycogen is the primary oxidative fuel source. Thereafter, gluconeogenesis increases temporarily and glucose synthesized from amino acids becomes the primary fuel source for the production of "obligate" glucose for use by tissues such as the brain and, to some degree, the liver and skeletal muscle. Over time, gluconeogenesis decreases as these organs adapt to ketone bodies as the primary oxidative fuel source, and in the fully adapted starved state, fatty acids, ketones, and glycerol become the primary fuel source in all tissues except the brain and red blood cells. The respiratory quotient (i.e., the ratio of carbon dioxide produced to oxygen consumed) is 0.6 to 0.7 as a result of the use of fat as the primary fuel source. Ultimately, rates of net protein catabolism and ureagenesis are decreased, relative to the fed state, during starvation. From a clinical perspective, it is important to understand that the metabolic response to starvation is reversible with feeding.

Stress metabolism is a generalized response whereby energy and substrate are mobilized to support inflammation, immune function, and tissue repair. It occurs in response to a variety of stimuli such as sepsis, multiple trauma, burns, pancreatitis, bone marrow transplantation, and major surgery. This mobilization of energy and substrate occurs at the expense of lean body mass. It is driven by endocrine hormones such as cortisol, glucagon, and catecholamines, as well as by a multitude of inflammatory mediators. The stress response is often related to some degree of perfusion deficit (shock) and resultant microcirculatory injury. Clinically, the response is characterized by increased energy expenditure and increased oxygen consumption. The stress response is further characterized by hyperglycemia, elevated lactate, and increased urinary nitrogen excretion. The respiratory quotient is often elevated in the range of 0.80 to 0.95 as a result of the use of a mixed oxidative fuel source. Loss of lean body mass occurs more rapidly than with simple starvation because skeletal muscle protein stores become the "fuel" for the stress response. Most importantly, the malnutrition associated with stress metabolism is less responsive to nutrition support than is starvation metabolism. Reversal of stress-associated malnutrition is dependent not only on the provision of adequate nutrients but also on elimination of the underlying stress response (i.e., control of infection, stabilization of fractures, grafting of burns, or resolution of the inflammatory state). Starvation and stress metabolism are summarized in Table 83-1.

Carbohydrate Metabolism in Critical Illness

Carbohydrate metabolism in critical illness is characterized clinically by hyperglycemia, often described as being due to "insulin resistance" based on increased blood glucose levels in the presence of high circulating levels of insulin. In fact, cellular glucose uptake and oxidation in the critically ill are increased,[10-12] and hyperglycemia is associated with increased glucose production, decreased insulin-mediated glucose uptake, and increased non–insulin-mediated glucose uptake.[10,13]

Table 83-1. Starvation versus Stress Hypermetabolism

Characteristic	Starvation	Hypermetabolism
Energy expenditure	Decreased	Increased
Respiratory quotient	Low (0.7)	High (0.85)
Response to feeding	+++	+
Mediator activation	+	+++
Primary fuels	Fat	Mixed
Gluconeogenesis	+	+++
Proteolysis	+	+++
Protein synthesis	+	++
Ureagenesis/urinary urea nitrogen	+	+++
Ketone formation	++++	+

Glucose production is increased primarily by increased hepatic gluconeogenesis, to a lesser extent by renal gluconeogenesis,[14] and by increased glycogenolysis. Increased glucose production occurs under the influence of glucagon, catecholamines, and cortisol, with glucagon being the most important stimulant of hepatic gluconeogenesis and epinephrine being the primary stimulant of glycogenolysis.[15,16] The hormonal changes observed in critical illness appear to be mediated by cytokines in both the central nervous system and peripheral tissues. Interleukin-1 (IL-1) stimulates the release of adrenocorticotropic hormone, which in turn favors the release of cortisol and glucagon, and tumor necrosis factor (TNF) stimulates increased secretion of glucagon.[17-19] Gluconeogenic substrates include lactate and alanine, as well as glutamine, glycine, serine, and glycerol. The amino acids used for gluconeogenesis are derived largely from proteolysis in skeletal muscle.

Glucose uptake into cells is regulated by a process of facilitated transport in which a carrier protein promotes the movement of glucose across the cell membrane down its concentration gradient. Three isoforms of this glucose carrier protein (glucose transporter 1 [GLUT-1], GLUT-2, and GLUT-4) are thought to be important in glucose transport.[20] Non–insulin-mediated glucose uptake is dependent on the GLUT-1 isoform, whereas insulin-mediated glucose transport is dependent on the GLUT-4 isoform. During stress, total body glucose uptake is increased, but largely via non–insulin-mediated pathways.[13] Non–insulin-mediated glucose uptake is particularly important in the central nervous system and in tissues rich in macrophages and neutrophils (e.g., lung, liver, intestine, spleen, wound), which use glucose for energy and in the process generate the respiratory burst.[10,21-23] Inflammatory cytokines may promote the uptake of glucose by increasing the synthesis, plasma membrane concentration, or activity of the glucose transporter.[24,25] Insulin-mediated glucose transport is suppressed in the liver, heart, and skeletal muscle.[26-29] Hepatic insulin resistance is characterized by elevated circulating levels of insulin-like growth factor–binding protein-1.[26,27] The mechanisms of insulin resistance are incompletely understood, although proinflammatory cytokines may alter insulin receptor signaling.[23,30,31]

The net result of these alterations in carbohydrate metabolism in critical illness is hyperglycemia inasmuch as the liver seems to be unresponsive to high levels of circulating insulin and glucose and continues to synthesize glucose via gluconeogenesis. In other tissues, non–insulin-mediated glucose uptake is enhanced and results in increased glycolytic oxidation to pyruvate and a stoichiometric rise in lactate.[10,11] Although hyperlactatemia is usually thought of as being reflective of anaerobic metabolism, it can be indicative of glycolytic flux and the level of metabolic stress when observed in conjunction with elevated pyruvate.[10]

Fat Metabolism in Critical Illness

In both starvation and stress metabolism, fat metabolism is characterized by increased lipolysis and decreased lipogenesis as fat stores are mobilized for energy. In the stressed state there is a marked increase in lipolytic activity in adipose tissue as a result of catecholamine-mediated stimulation of β_2-receptors; cytokines may also participate in this process.[32,33] Fatty acids are released from adipose tissue in quantities that exceed the amount oxidized, and approximately half of these fatty acids are re-esterified in the liver.[29,34] In this triglyceride–fatty acid cycle, triglycerides and fatty acids are shunted back and forth between the liver and adipose tissue in an apparently futile pathway.[35]

Stress fat metabolism is further characterized by increased oxidation of fatty acids of all chain lengths and decreased plasma levels of medium- and long-chain essential fatty acids relative to the quantities of oleic acid. The latter may reflect preferential oxidation of essential fatty acids, suppressed mobilization because of hyperinsulinemia, or conversion of ω-6 fatty acids to inflammatory mediators.

Hypertriglyceridemia is common in critically ill patients, particularly in the presence of multiple organ dysfunction, and results from the combination of increased hepatic triglyceride production and decreased clearance.[36,37] Hepatic steatosis has classically been attributed to overfeeding because triglycerides are constructed from fatty acids synthesized from excess carbohydrate. This theory has been called into question inasmuch as a substantial proportion of hepatic triglyceride may be synthesized from recycled fatty acids rather than from fatty acids synthesized de novo from carbohydrate.[38] It is possible that fatty infiltration of the liver reflects a cytokine-mediated defect in triglyceride secretion that represents an organ-specific response to critical illness rather than an adverse effect of carbohydrate overfeeding.[39,40] Regardless of the immediate source of the fatty acids used in triglyceride synthesis, experience suggests that clinically apparent fatty infiltration of the liver can be prevented by avoiding overfeeding.

Ketonemia is common in starvation, whereas ketogenesis is decreased in stress metabolism.[41] Acetoacetate continues to be used as an oxidative fuel source, although the reduction of β-hydroxybutyrate to acetoacetate is impaired.[42] With the development of multiple organ dysfunction, there is a progressive decrease in the acetoacetate-to–β-hydroxybutyrate ratio.[43] This alteration in hepatic redox potential reflects a disturbance in the cellular energy charge that may be associated with hepatic mitochondrial damage by toxic oxygen radicals and other inflammatory mediators.[44]

Protein Metabolism in Critical Illness

Protein synthesis is increased in the stressed state relative to that seen in starvation. Protein breakdown is markedly increased in comparison to the synthetic rate, thereby resulting in net protein catabolism and a rapid decrease in lean body mass.[41,45] There is a net efflux of amino acids from skeletal muscle as protein breakdown via the ubiquitin-proteosome pathway of protein degradation is accelerated by catecholamines, cortisol, and cytokines.[46-50] Amino acid uptake by skeletal muscle is impaired despite excess amino acids circulating in the bloodstream early in the course of stress metabolism; the situation deteriorates further as plasma concentrations of specific amino acids such as leucine begin to fall.[51] Decreased plasma glutamine is known to have deleterious effects on immune function and gastrointestinal barrier function.[52,53] Although it has long been thought that the accelerated protein catabolism associated with critical illness is unresponsive to the provision of amino acids or other fuel sources, the fact that muscle amino acid uptake is in part compromised by decreased plasma levels of specific amino acids suggests the possibility that protein catabolism during stress may be attenuated with the provision of appropriate nutrition support.[54]

Amino acids mobilized from skeletal muscle are redistributed to other areas of the body to support immune function, wound healing, and tissue repair, as well as for the hepatic synthesis of acute-phase proteins, presumably in an attempt to enhance survival. It has recently been demonstrated that endotoxemia induces significant increases in protein synthesis in the liver, spleen, kidney, jejunum, diaphragm, lung, and skin at the expense of skeletal muscle catabolism.[55] Amino acids such as alanine, glutamine, glycine, and serine are used as gluconeogenic substrate, and branched-chain amino acids (leucine, isoleucine, and valine) can be used as an oxidative fuel source, particularly in skeletal muscle. The net result of stress protein metabolism is a rapid decrease in lean body mass that exceeds that associated with bed rest or simple starvation, along with increased ureagenesis, azotemia, and increased urinary nitrogen excretion.

INDICATIONS FOR NUTRITION SUPPORT

Nutrition support should be considered once hemorrhage has been controlled, devitalized tissue débrided, fractures stabilized, and the patient resuscitated from shock. Limited data are available regarding the appropriate timing for the institution of nutrition support, although there are suggestions in the literature that early enteral feeding, within 24 to 72 hours of admission, may help decrease postburn and postinjury hypermetabolism and reduce infectious complications. In general, nutrition support should be considered for any patient who is malnourished on admission to the intensive care unit (ICU), for any patient who is likely to become malnourished during a long and complicated ICU stay, and for any patient who has not eaten for 5 to 7 days.

GOALS OF NUTRITION SUPPORT

The goals of nutrition support in a critically ill patient are to minimize the effects of starvation, provide appropriate doses of macronutrients and micronutrients, modulate the metabolic processes of the disease to some extent, minimize complications of nutrition support, and, it is hoped, improve outcomes. More specifically, the goals of nutrition support in the critically ill or injured are to provide sufficient calories to meet the energy requirements of the hypermetabolic state while avoiding the complications associated with overfeeding, provide sufficient protein to attain nitrogen balance or minimize the nitrogen deficit, provide electrolytes to maintain normal levels while taking into account excessive losses or impaired excretion, and provide appropriate vitamins and trace elements with consideration of disease-specific requirements.

NUTRITION SUPPORT IN CRITICAL ILLNESS

Calories

In any metabolic state, energy requirements must be met to minimize the use of stored energy reserves and to decrease the loss of lean body mass. In the setting of adapted starvation, the protein-sparing effect of an adequate caloric intake is well recognized; however, in the stressed state, protein catabolism is only partially responsive to caloric intake and continues to a significant degree regardless of caloric intake.[41,45,54] Overfeeding is of particular concern in a critically ill patient because it can result in excess carbon dioxide production and ventilator dependence,[56] lipogenesis and fatty infiltration of the liver,[57-59] and hyperglycemia with its attendant hyperosmolar and infectious complications.[23,60-62]

The daily caloric requirement depends on total energy expenditure (TEE), which is the sum of basal energy expenditure (BEE), diet-induced thermogenesis (DIT), and activity energy expenditure (AEE). BEE is the caloric expenditure of a person in the recumbent position who has fasted for at least 10 hours. DIT is the energy expended to perform all aspects of food consumption, including eating and hydrolysis and absorption of nutrients, and may account for 15% to 40% of TEE. Resting energy expenditure (REE) is the energy expenditure of a recumbent person who is not fasting and is the sum of BEE and DIT. These relationships can be expressed by the following equations:

$$\text{REE} = \text{BEE} + \text{DIT}$$

$$\text{TEE} = \text{REE} + \text{AEE}$$

Caloric requirement can be estimated by using a number of formulas or measured with indirect calorimetry. Most commonly, BEE is estimated with the Harris-Benedict equations, which are based on sex, age, height, and weight and then multiplied by stress and activity factors to estimate caloric requirement. The Harris-Benedict equations are as follows:

$$\text{For males: BEE} = 66.42 + (13.75 \times \text{Wt [kg]}) + (5.0 \times \text{Ht [cm]}) - (6.77 \times \text{Age [yr]})$$

$$\text{For females: BEE} = 655.10 + (9.65 \times \text{Wt [kg]}) + 1.85 \times \text{Ht [cm]}) - (4.68 \times \text{Age [yr]})$$

Classically, REE is then estimated by multiplying the calculated BEE by a stress factor ranging from 1.0 in a stable, mechanically ventilated patient to 2.0 in a patient with a 50% total body surface area burn. Stress factors for patients with multiple trauma or sepsis fall somewhere between the two extremes. TEE is estimated by multiplying REE by an activity factor of 1.2 to 1.3 for ambulatory patients. The caloric requirement is decreased to varying degrees (6% to 30%) in mechanically ventilated patients receiving narcotics or sedatives and is reduced by as much as 33% in chemically paralyzed patients.[63] In nonventilated postoperative patients or in patients with decreased lung compliance as a result of chronic lung disease, energy expenditure related to the work of breathing may increase. Although estimation of energy expenditure is relatively accurate in healthy people, it is much less reliable in critically ill patients because of the heterogeneity of the metabolic response and variations in sedation, work of breathing, and physical activity. Most critically ill patients should receive calories to supply 100% to 120% of calculated BEE. Estimation of energy expenditure in obese patients is particularly difficult. If indirect calorimetry is unavailable, 25 to 30 kcal/kg can be provided to an obese patient based on obesity-adjusted weight; obesity-adjusted weight = ideal body weight + (actual body weight − ideal body weight) × 0.25.[64] Hypocaloric feeding may decrease ventilator days and length of ICU stay in obese patients.[65]

Indirect calorimetry can be used to measure REE and does not require the addition of estimated stress factors. REE is based on measured oxygen consumption and carbon dioxide production and is calculated according to the Weir equation: $\text{REE} = (3.94 \times \dot{V}O_2) + (1.1 \times (\dot{V}CO_2)$, where $\dot{V}O_2$ = oxygen consumption and $\dot{V}CO_2$ = carbon dioxide production. Even when not used routinely, indirect calorimetry can still be helpful in assessing the energy needs of obese patients, to rule out overfeeding in patients with seemingly excessive ventilatory demands, in severely malnourished patients, and in patients with apparently high levels of metabolic stress.

In general, critically ill patients should receive 25 to 30 kcal/kg/d, with sedated mechanically ventilated patients receiving closer to 25 kcal/kg/d. Chemically paralyzed patients generally require 20 kcal/kg/d.[63]

Carbohydrate

Carbohydrate is usually the primary source of calories in human beings. The maximum rate of glucose oxidation is approximately 5 mg/kg/min, or 7.2 g/kg/d.[66] In stressed patients, part of this maximally tolerated glucose load will be provided by glucose synthesized endogenously from amino acids via gluconeogenesis. In a severely hypermetabolic patient, gluconeogenesis may provide as much as 4 mg/kg/min of glucose[67] and result in significant hyperglycemia when large exogenous glucose loads are administered. Insulin tends to be ineffective in controlling this hyperglycemia, in part because glucose oxidation may already be maximal, endogenous insulin levels are already high, and insulin-mediated glucose uptake in the liver and other tissues is suppressed in a septic and hypermetabolic patient.[26-29] Complications of excess glucose administration include (1) hyperglycemia and its attendant hyperosmolar/infectious complications, (2) excess carbon dioxide production, and (3) ventilator dependence and hepatic steatosis. In general, glucose should initially be provided at a rate of 5 g/kg/d or approximately 20 kcal/kg/d. Carbohydrate should generally constitute 60% to 70% of nonprotein calories in a hypermetabolic patient (Table 83-2).

Fat

In a hypermetabolic patient, fat should constitute 15% to 40% of daily caloric intake, both to prevent essential fatty acid deficiency and to meet caloric needs in the face of a fixed capacity to oxidize glucose. In the starved state, as little as 2% to 5% of calories can be provided as fat, primarily to prevent essential fatty acid deficiency. Substituting lipid calories for carbohydrate calories can reduce carbon dioxide production, although avoiding excess calories in general is probably most important in minimizing carbon dioxide production and ventilator dependence. Complications of excess lipid administration, particularly when given parenterally, include hyperlipemia, immunosuppression, and hypoxemia as a result of both impaired oxygen diffusion and ventilation-perfusion mismatching. In general, a hypermetabolic patient should receive 15% to 40% of calories as fat, not to exceed 1.0 to 1.5 g/kg/d (see Table 83-2).[68]

Protein

Protein needs in a hypermetabolic patient are increased in comparison to those in a patient with simple starvation. Protein catabolism in a stressed patient has long been thought to be unresponsive to protein or amino acid administration or glucose infusion,[69] and attainment of nitrogen balance is thought to depend largely on the support of stress protein synthesis.[45,54,70,71] However, recent evidence suggests that protein catabolism may be attenuated by the provision of appropriate nutrition support.[55] Regardless of the specific mechanisms involved, lean body mass decreases during catabolic illness because of bed rest and inactivity. Amino acids are redistributed from skeletal muscle to support hepatic protein synthesis, the cellular inflammatory response, and gluconeogenesis and are used as oxidative fuel sources. Although the recommended dietary allowance (RDA) for protein in healthy adults is 0.8 g/kg/d,[72] a septic or injured patient may require 1.2 to 2.0 g/kg/d to promote nitrogen balance or at least minimize the nitrogen deficit. Provision of more than 2.0 g/kg/d of protein rarely promotes nitrogen balance and usually results simply in increased urinary nitrogen excretion (see Table 83-2).

To meet the protein requirements of the stressed state and at the same time avoid excess calories and its attendant complications, an injured or septic patient may require nutrition support with a nonprotein calorie-to-nitrogen ratio of 80 or 100 : 1, as compared with a patient with starvation metabolism, who may tolerate a nonprotein calorie-to-nitrogen ratio of 150 : 1 or higher. The higher protein needs of a patient with catabolic illness can be met with custom-compounded total parenteral nutrition (TPN) or with numerous commercially available enteral formulas specifically designed for such patients (Table 83-3).

Table 83-2. Nutrition Support in a Hypermetabolic Patient

Nutrient	General Recommendation
Total calories	25-30 kcal/kg/d or BEE×1.2-2.0 or REE by IDC
Glucose	5 g/kg/d or 20 kcal/kg/d or 60%-70% of calories
Fat	15%-40% of calories or Less than 1 g/kg/d
Amino acids or protein	1.2-2.0 g/kg/d
Trace elements and vitamins	RDA
Electrolytes	Maintain normal levels

BEE, basal energy expenditure; IDC, indirect calorimetry; RDA, recommended daily allowance; REE, resting energy expenditure.

Electrolytes, Vitamins, and Trace Elements

Fluid and electrolytes should be provided to maintain adequate urine output and normal serum electrolyte levels. Typical daily electrolyte requirements include sodium, 60 to 100 mEq/d, potassium, 60 to 100 mEq/d, magnesium, 10 to 20 mEq/d, calcium, 10 to 15 mEq/d, chloride, 80 to 120 mEq/d, and phosphorus, 20 to 30 mmol/d. Intravenous amino acid formulations contain acetate, but additional acetate can be added in the setting of metabolic acidosis. Particular attention should be paid to the intracellular electrolytes (potassium, phosphorus, and magnesium), which are required for attainment of nitrogen balance[73] and serum levels of which can fall precipitously when nutrition support is initiated.

The requirements for vitamins and trace elements in critical illness are largely unknown, and in general the RDA for both should be provided. Patients with prolonged diarrhea or large burns or those undergoing dialysis have increased trace element loss and vitamin requirements, and deficiencies can develop if intake is inadequate. The daily requirement for zinc in adult patients receiving TPN ranges from 2.5 to 4.0 mg/d. Additional zinc is recommended in patients with burns, ileostomy, or excessive small intestinal loss. Patients receiving TPN should be given chromium, 10 to 15 μg/d, copper, 0.5 to 1.5 mg/d, and manganese, 0.15 to 0.8 mg/d. Requirements for iodine, selenium, and molybdenum have not been established. Initial limitation of trace elements should be considered in patients with renal failure. Routine supplementation of vitamins is necessary in patients receiving TPN. Typically, one ampule of a standard multivitamin

Table 83-3. Enteral Nutrition Formulas

Type	General Information	Sample Formulas	Concentration (kcal/mL)	Osmolality	Nonprotein Calorie-Nitrogen Ratio	Protein (g/1000 kcal)	Carbohydrate (% kcal)	Fat (% kcal)
Intact Protein								
Standard	Some may be taken by mouth; generally lactose free, low residue, and isotonic	Ensure	1.5	525	125:1	41.8	54.3	29
		Osmolite	1.06	300	153:1	35	57	29
		Isosource	1.2	490	149:1	44.2	57	29
		Nutren	1.5	510	131:1	40	45	39
High protein	Similar to above formulas except contain >45 g protein/L	Replete	1.0	300-350	75:1	62.4	45	30
		TraumaCal	1.5	560	91:1	54.7	38	40
		Isosource VHN	1.0	300	77:1	62	50	25
		Promote	1.0	340	75:1	62.5	52	23
Fluid concentrated	Calorically dense (1.5-2.0 cal/mL), lactose free, moderate-to-high osmolality	Nutren 2.0	2.0	745	131:1	40	39	45
		Deliver 2.0	2.0	640	144:1	37.5	40	45
		TwoCal HN	2.0	690	125.1	41.8	43.2	40.1
Immunity enhancing	May contain fiber, MCT, fish oil, added vitamins/minerals; 22%-25% protein	Immun-Aid	1.0	460	53:1	80	48	20
		Impact	1.0	375	71:1	56	53	25
		Impact with Glutamine	1.3	630	64:1	60	46	30
		Perative	1.3	385	97:1	52.1	54.5	25
Diabetic	33%-40% carbohydrate, contains fiber, standard to high protein	DiabetiSource	1.0	360	100:1	50	36	44
		ReSource Diabetic	1.06	300-320	79:1	59.4	36	40
		Glucerna	1.0	355	125:1	41.8	34.3	49
		Glytrol	1.0	380	114:1	45	40	42
Hepatic	High BCAA, 1.2-1.5 cal/mL	NutriHep Diet	1.5	690	209:1	26.7	77	12
		Hepatic-Aid II	1.2	560	148:1	36.8	57.3	27.7
Pulmonary	40%-55% fat, lactose free	NutriVent	1.5	330-450	116:1	45	55	55
		NovaSource	1.5	650	102:1	50.1	40	40
		Respalor	1.5	400	102:1	50	40	40
		Oxepa	1.5	493	125:1	41.6	28.1	55.2
		Pulmocare	1.5	475	125:1	41.7	28.2	55.1
Renal	2 cal/mL, low to standard protein, low to no electrolytes	Renalcal	2.0	600	338:1	17.2	58.1	35
		Suplena	2.0	600	393:1	15	51	43
		Magnacal Renal	2.0	570	180:1	37.5	40	45
		NovaSource	2.0	700-960	140:1	37	40	45
Hydrolyzed Protein								
Immunity enhancing	Standard to high protein, may have added vitamins/minerals or amino acids	Crucial	1.5	490	67:1	62.7	36	39
		Criticare HN	1.06	650	149:1	35.8	81.5	4.5
		AlitraQ	1.0	575	94:1	52.5	65.7	13.2
GI compromised	Mix of peptides and amino acids, >40% fat as MCT	Peptamen	1.0	270-380	131:1	40	51	33
		Peptamen VHP	1.0	300-430	75:1	62.5	42	33
		Reabilan	1.0	350	175:1	31.5	52.5	35
		Reabilan HN	1.33	490	117:1	43.8	47.5	35
		SandoSource Peptide	1.0	490	100:1	50	65	15
		Vital HB	1.0	500	125:1	41.7	73.8	9.5
Crystalline amino acids	Powdered form, 8%-18% protein, <6% fat	Vivonex T.E.N.	1.0	630	149:1	38	82	3
		Vivonex Plus	1.0	650	115:1	45	76	6

BCAA, branched-chain amino acid; MCT, medium-chain triglyceride.

preparation is added to TPN daily. Vitamin K, which is light sensitive, must be added separately in a light-impermeable bag or given by another route once or twice weekly. Burned patients routinely receive supplements of vitamins A and C and folic acid. Excessive doses of vitamin C should be avoided in renal failure because of the accumulation of oxalate. Vitamin A accumulates and should not be supplemented beyond the RDA.[74]

ROUTE OF ADMINISTRATION

Nutrition support can be delivered enterally (via the gastrointestinal tract) or parenterally (via the intravenous route). The preferred route has been the subject of considerable controversy and a substantial body of literature during the past 40 years.

Both routes have advantages and disadvantages, and nitrogen balance can be achieved by either route. TPN does not require an intact or functioning gastrointestinal tract, it is convenient to use, and its use virtually guarantees that the nutrients prescribed will be administered and that these nutrients will appear in the bloodstream. Disadvantages of parenteral nutrition include cost, procedure (central venous catheter) related complications, and an increased likelihood of metabolic complications, including hyperglycemia. Enteral nutrition is much less expensive, is more physiologic, is associated with fewer metabolic complications such as electrolyte abnormalities and hyperglycemia, and has long been thought to preserve gut mucosal integrity and barrier function better than parenteral nutrition does. Disadvantages of enteral nutrition include the requirement for an intact and functioning gastrointestinal tract, procedural (feeding tube placement) related complications, pulmonary aspiration, malabsorption, feeding intolerance (pain, vomiting, bloating, diarrhea), and as a result, an inability to deliver the entire nutrient prescription.

The gastrointestinal tract is a major interface between the host and the environment and not only regulates the ingestion and absorption of nutrients but is also responsible for defending the host against noxious microorganisms and toxins. Malnutrition impairs gastrointestinal barrier function,[75,76] as does the lack of luminal nutrients independent of general nutritional status.[77-80] Enteral nutrition has been shown to promote mucosal growth, improve absorptive capacity, alter digestive enzyme production, improve gut mucosal weight, generate DNA and protein synthesis, and improve the efficiency of nutrient utilization.[81] Several animal studies have demonstrated decreased mortality after an infectious challenge when nutrition was provided enterally as opposed to parenterally.[82-84] In the 1980s, several small trials in high-risk surgical patients failed to demonstrate the superiority of enteral to parenteral nutrition in terms of organ failure, mortality, or infectious complications.[85-89] Subsequently, two randomized prospective trials in trauma patients did demonstrate significantly fewer infectious complications in patients fed enterally.[90,91] A meta-analysis of eight randomized trials of enteral versus parenteral nutrition involving 230 patients demonstrated significantly fewer total complications and infectious complications in patients fed enterally.[92] In a more recent meta-analysis of 13 randomized trials, enteral nutrition was associated with significantly fewer infections than parenteral nutrition was.[93]

As a result of the studies just mentioned, enteral nutrition has become the standard of care. This concept could be questioned. In the studies mentioned, as many as 15% of patients did not tolerate enteral nutrition. In other studies, patients fed enterally received 33% to 68% of their caloric requirements,[94-97] thus demonstrating that not all patients can be successfully fed enterally. Whether luminal nutrients are as important in adult humans as in animals has been called into question. Bacterial translocation occurs rarely in humans[98,99] and does not appear to be affected by the route of nutrition.[98] More recent studies comparing enteral with parenteral nutrition in humans have failed to show a reduction in sepsis or infectious complications in patients fed enterally.[100-102] In several of the studies mentioned in previous paragraphs, many of the patients managed with parenteral nutrition received significantly more calories and had a higher incidence of hyperglygemia[93] than did their enterally fed counterparts. In a study in which parenterally fed patients had a higher incidence of sepsis, twice as many patients receiving parenteral nutrition had hyperglycemia as enterally fed patients.[103] More recently, in a large prospective trial comparing tight glucose control with standard glucose control, patients with tight glucose control had significantly less morbidity, infectious complications, and mortality.[62] Further analysis of these data revealed that when glucose was tightly controlled, there was no difference in infection when patients were nourished parenterally rather than enterally.[104] These data suggest that control of hyperglycemia may be as important as the route of nutrition in minimizing infectious complications.

In summary, because it is less costly and associated with fewer metabolic complications and a lower incidence of infection, the enteral route continues to be the recommended route for nutrition support. Many critically ill patients, however, do not tolerate enteral nutrition, and parenteral nutrition can probably be used more liberally, particularly if hyperglycemia is prevented.

TYPES OF NUTRITIONAL FORMULAS

Parenteral nutrition is most commonly administered as a three-in-one solution of dextrose, lipid, and amino acids. TPN order forms typically allow the physician to order "standard" or custom solutions, fluid-restricted solutions, and in some cases, disease-specific solutions such as renal failure or hepatic failure solutions. Electrolytes can usually be added in standard stock concentrations or individually. Electrolytes should be added with care and according to pharmacy recommendations, both to prevent precipitation of calcium and phosphate in the solution and to avoid discarding a bag of TPN because the patient's electrolyte levels are suddenly dangerously high. Vitamins and trace elements are generally added in standard quantities but can be supplemented. H_2 blockers for stress ulcer prophylaxis and regular insulin can also be added.

Enteral formulas are usually premixed with a fixed nonprotein calorie-to-nitrogen ratio, and the needs of a specific patient are generally met by changing the formula. Protein and carbohydrate supplements can be added at the bedside to alter premixed formulas. Enteral formulas can be classified numerous ways, including the form in which protein is provided (e.g., intact protein, hydrolyzed protein [chemically defined or peptide], or crystalline amino acids [elemental]), the quantity of protein contained, the caloric density of the formula, and the disease state for which they were designed. Examples of different formulas are shown in Table 83-3. More detailed information is available elsewhere.[105]

Intact protein solutions contain protein as caseinate or soy isolate–based products that are lactose and gluten free and low in residue. Such solutions contain 45% to 60% of calories as carbohydrate (oligosaccharides), 20% to 35% of calories as long-chain fats (e.g., linoleic acid), and 15% to 20% of calories as protein. Intact formulas are usually isosmotic and may contain 1 to 2 kcal/mL of solution. Some formulas contain fiber as a means to improve diarrhea or glycemic control. Hydrolyzed formulas provide protein as peptides or amino acids, are generally low in fat, and are designed for patients with gut dysfunction or malabsorption.[106] Elemental solutions contain protein exclusively as amino acids and are intended for similar indications. Controlled studies comparing hydrolyzed or elemental formulas with intact formulas have not demonstrated improved tolerance or outcomes.

High-protein formulas contain more than 45 g protein per 1000 kcal and are designed for patients with increased protein needs, such as patients with catabolic illness.

Calorie-dense formulas are designed for patients in whom fluid restriction is required. They are generally relatively low in protein and not ideal for a stressed patient.

Specialty formulas are products designed to meet the nutritional requirements of patients with specific disease states. None has been consistently shown to improve outcomes when compared with conventional formulas.

Pulmonary failure formulas are designed for patients with acute respiratory failure associated with chronic lung disease. They contain at least 50% of calories as fat and thus reduce CO_2 production and decrease the work of breathing relative to high-carbohydrate formulas. Few data suggest a benefit with specific pulmonary formulas, and avoiding overfeeding is probably more important in reducing ventilatory demand.[107]

Hepatic failure formulas were developed for patients with encephalopathy. They contain high concentrations of branched-chain amino acids and reduced concentrations of aromatic amino acids. Although these solutions have been shown to correct the abnormal amino acid profile characteristic of patients with liver failure,[108,109] it is less clear that they actually treat hepatic encephalopathy.[109]

Renal failure formulas have reduced concentrations of electrolytes and decreased protein content to minimize nitrogenous waste in patients with renal failure. Patients with acute renal failure frequently have associated catabolic illness and as a result need more protein rather than less. Although these formulas may be useful in patients not yet being dialyzed, they are often inappropriate for patients with catabolic illness who are undergoing dialysis.

Immunity-enhancing enteral formulas have received considerable attention in the past 15 years. These formulas have been supplemented with various combinations of specific nutrients, including branched-chain amino acids, arginine, ω-3 polyunsaturated fatty acids, nucleotides, glutamine, and antioxidants, and are aimed at improving immune function and reducing inflammation in critically ill patients. Formulas supplemented with *branched-chain amino acids* stimulate hepatic protein synthesis more effectively than conventional formulas do and appear to benefit various indices of immunocompetence.[110] *Arginine* is a nonessential amino acid that appears to stimulate lymphocyte proliferation[111] and reduce mortality from peritonitis in animal models,[112] improve wound healing in humans,[113] and be a precursor for the synthesis of nitric oxide, which in turn is a modulator of hepatic protein synthesis and vascular tone. *ω-3 fatty acids* are incorporated into the phospholipid fraction of cell membranes and converted to trienoic prostaglandins and pentaenoic leukotrienes, which are less "inflammatory" than their ω-6 counterparts. ω-3 fatty acids have been shown to decrease prostaglandin E_2, TNF, and IL-1 production in rat Kupffer cells[114] and alter TNF and IL-1 production in human monocytes.[115] Furthermore, ω-3 fats have been shown to be beneficial in animal models of chronic inflammation and in humans with psoriasis[116] and rheumatoid arthritis.[117] *Nucleotides* may stimulate natural killer cells and T lymphocytes. *Glutamine* is an important fuel for enterocytes and cells of the immune system. Considered a nonessential amino acid, glutamine may become conditionally essential when skeletal muscle stores and plasma levels become depleted during catabolic illness, thereby resulting in adverse effects on gut barrier and immune function.[118-120] Glutamine has been shown to improve nitrogen balance and decrease bacterial translocation in animals.[121-123] It also promotes the synthesis of glutathione, an important antioxidant. A recent meta-analysis of 14 randomized trials in which glutamine-supplemented nutrition was compared with standard nutrition demonstrated reduced infectious morbidity and mortality with glutamine supplementation, particularly in parenterally nourished surgical patients.[124] *Antioxidants* such as vitamins A, E, and C, selenium, and *N*-acetylcysteine offer the potential to reduce oxidant injury but have not been studied individually in critically ill patients in terms of clinical outcomes.[125]

Numerous studies comparing immunity-enhancing enteral nutrition with conventional nutrition have produced contradictory results. In a recent meta-analysis of 22 studies (2419 patients) in which enteral nutrition supplemented with various combinations of arginine, ω-3 fatty acids, glutamine, and nucleotides was compared with conventional enteral nutrition, the supplemented patients had decreased infectious morbidity but no difference in mortality when compared with patients receiving the control diet.[126] The majority of studies demonstrating benefit involved elective surgery patients and not critically ill patients. In a more recent study comparing immunity-enhancing enteral nutrition with parenteral nutrition, enrollment of septic patients was stopped after interim analysis revealed fourfold higher mortality in septic patients receiving immunonutrition.[127] In the subsequently published and largest (597 patients) randomized trial to date, immunonutrition had no benefit in terms of infectious morbidity, length of stay, number of ventilator days, or mortality.[128] The use of immunity-enhancing enteral formulas, at least as they currently exist, is probably not justified in critically ill patients. Glutamine, administered as the dipeptide, may be beneficial, particularly in parenterally fed patients.

NUTRITIONAL ASSESSMENT AND MONITORING

The history and physical examination remain the mainstay of nutritional assessment, although they are perhaps more useful in the ambulatory setting or in patients with chronic malnutrition.[129] Pertinent historical information includes height and weight, a history of recent weight change, genetic background, recent nutritional intake, and a history of pathology that might affect nutrient intake, absorption, or tolerance. The physical examination might, on occasion, demonstrate abnormal end-organ function that reflects malnutrition, but more commonly it is useful for the assessment of body mass and detection of specific nutrient deficiencies. Signs and symptoms of selected vitamin and mineral deficiencies are presented in Tables 83-4 and 83-5.

Anthropometric measurements such as triceps skin fold thickness (SFT), midarm circumference (MAC), and arm muscle area, which is derived from SFT and MAC, can be used to estimate fat mass and lean body mass.[130] Although serial measurements may be useful in certain patients over long periods, SFT measurements are less reliable in the elderly because of changes in fat distribution and skin compressibility associated with aging[130,131] and are inaccurate in patients with peripheral edema.[132] In general, these measurements are not practical for nutritional monitoring in a recumbent, critically ill patient.[133]

Visceral protein levels have long been used in nutritional assessment and monitoring and can be useful in the

Table 83-4. Selected Vitamin Deficiencies

Vitamin	Function	Signs of Deficiency
Niacin (B_5)	Component of the coenzymes NAD and NADP, which play a role in oxidation-reduction reactions. These enzymes play a role in the oxidative catabolism of carbohydrates, proteins, lipids and the biosynthesis of fatty acids	Pellagra, dermatitis, headaches, loss of memory, dementia, glossitis, diarrhea
Folate (B_9)	Transfer of single-carbon units; DNA synthesis	Megaloblastic anemia, diarrhea, glossitis
Cyanocobalamin (B_{12})	Maintains normal folate metabolism; coenzyme in reactions involving isomerizations and reductions; participates in the metabolism of fat, carbohydrate, and protein and in myelin synthesis	Pernicious anemia, glossitis, peripheral neuropathy, spinal cord degeneration
Thiamine	Carbohydrate metabolism coenzyme in oxidative decarboxylation	Paresthesias, impaired memory, nystagmus, congestive heart failure, Wernicke-Korsakoff syndrome
Riboflavin (B_2)	Electronic transport as flavin nucleotides	Mucositides, dermatitis, cheilosis, vascularization of the cornea, photophobia, decreased vision, lacrimation, impaired wound healing
Pyridoxine (B_6)	Coenzyme in transformations of amino acids	Neuritis, dermatitis, convulsions
Pantothenic acid	Precursor of coenzyme A (Krebs cycle)	Headache, fatigue, malaise, insomnia, vomiting, abdominal cramps
Biotin	Coenzyme for carboxylation reactions	As with other B vitamins (normally synthesized and absorbed from gut)
Ascorbic acid	Reducing agent, wound healing, integrity of blood vessels, folate metabolism	Enlargement and keratosis of hair follicles, impaired wound healing, anemia, ecchymosis, lethargy, depression, bleeding
A	Normal vision, mucopolysaccharide synthesis, protease release, entry of macrophages and leukocytes into an acute wound, immune stimulation, mucosal integrity	Dermatitis, keratomalacia, xerophthalmia, night blindness
D	Calcium and phosphorus homeostasis	Rickets, osteomalacia
E	Antioxidant	Hemolysis
K	Clotting factors II, VII, IX, X	Bleeding

Table 83-5. Selected Mineral Deficiencies

Trace Element	Function	Signs of Deficiency
Chromium	Glucose tolerance; possible role in maintenance of normal serum lipid levels	Elevated serum lipids, insulin-resistant glucose intolerance
Copper	Metalloenzyme biochemical processes, component of ceruloplasmin, connective tissue metabolism, melanin formation	Anemia, neutropenia, leukopenia, depigmentation of skin
Iron	Constituent of hemoglobin, myoglobin, and the cytochrome enzymes	Microcytic hypochromic anemia, fatigue, faulty digestion, decreased serum iron
Zinc	Essential for the function of many enzymes and a component of lipid, protein, carbohydrate, and nucleic acid metabolism; cell replication and connective tissue synthesis	Dermatitis; impaired wound healing; alopecia; depressed cell-mediated immunity, taste acuity, and dark adaptation; sexual retardation; depressed visceral protein status
Cobalt	Biologic methylation	Pernicious anemia, methylmalonic aciduria
Manganese	Oxidative phosphorylation, fatty acid metabolism, protein and mucopolysaccharide synthesis	Growth retardation, bony abnormalities, central nervous system dysfunction

appropriate clinical setting. They are affected by a number of variables other than nutritional status, such as hydration state and gastrointestinal and urinary losses, and must therefore be used cautiously in a critically ill patient.

Albumin is contained in a large body pool (4 to 5 g/kg) and has a half-life of 20 days, so it is insensitive to acute changes and responds slowly to nutritional therapy. Serum albumin levels are decreased in nephrotic syndrome, enteropathies, hepatic failure, and dialysis (particularly peritoneal dialysis), as well as in the setting of acute volume expansion. Levels may be increased in the presence of dehydration, hypercortisolemia, and anabolic hormones such as insulin, growth hormone, and estrogen. Although serum albumin levels are useful in predicting surgical mortality and monitoring nutritional status over the long term, they are much less useful in monitoring a critically ill patient.[134]

Transferrin is contained in a smaller body pool and has a shorter half-life than albumin does (8 to 10 days), so it is a more sensitive indicator of nutritional status. It is subject to the same influences as mentioned for albumin and, in addition, is affected inversely by serum iron levels.[135]

Retinol-binding protein is a specific carrier involved in vitamin A transport and is linked with thyroxine-binding prealbumin in a constant molar ratio.[136] It has a 12-hour half-life and is sensitive to synthesis and utilization rates. Levels rise in patients with renal disease[137] and with excess vitamin A administration and are reduced in patients with liver disease, cystic fibrosis, hyperthyroidism, and vitamin A deficiency.

Transthyretin (thyroxine-binding prealbumin) is involved in the transport of thyroid hormone and is a carrier for retinol-binding protein. It has a small body pool and a short half-life (2 to 3 days) and as such may be a sensitive indicator of nutritional status.[138,139] Levels are affected by the same variables that affect albumin and transferrin. Levels are low in patients with hyperthyroidism, cystic fibrosis, chronic illness, and acute stress. Because of its short half-life and ease of measurement, transthyretin is the visceral protein of choice for nutritional assessment and monitoring, although its use in a critically ill patient is controversial. During catabolic illness, hepatic protein synthesis is reprioritized, under the influence of cytokines, with increased synthesis of acute-phase reactant proteins and decreased synthesis of visceral proteins.[140-142] Transthyretin levels fall early in the course of catabolic illness and rise with the subsequent decrease in acute-phase reactant proteins as a result of reversal of the reprioritized hepatic protein synthesis.[134] The association of this response with specific nutrients,[143-148] nitrogen balance,[65,149-153] and outcomes[152,154,155] has been variable. Whether transthyretin levels are reflective of appropriate nutrition support or simply a reflection of the course and severity of the inflammatory response is unclear. Regardless of the mechanisms involved, it is generally accepted that an initial transthyretin level lower than 50 mg/L or failure to increase by 40 mg/L per week is associated with a poor prognosis.[139]

Nitrogen balance is the nutritional parameter most consistently associated with improved outcomes, and nitrogen balance studies are used routinely in many ICUs to monitor nutrition support. Ideally, positive nitrogen balance is the goal, but minimizing the nitrogen deficit in a critically ill patient is probably more realistic when one considers the fact that proteolysis in the skeletal muscle compartment, which constitutes 70% of body protein stores, is likely to exceed protein synthesis related to the inflammatory response and wound healing, simply because of the size of the compartments involved. Nitrogen balance is calculated as

$$\text{Nitrogen balance (g)} = \text{Nitrogen intake (g)} - \text{Nitrogen output (g)}$$

$$\text{Nitrogen intake (g)} = \text{Protein or amino acid intake (g)}/6.25$$

$$\text{Nitrogen output (g)} = \text{Urinary nitrogen losses (g)} + 2\text{ g (stool and skin losses)}$$

Urinary nitrogen consists of several components, including urea, creatinine, uric acid, ammonia, and amino acids. In health, urea constitutes 90% of urinary nitrogen, whereas in catabolic states, urea may represent as little as 70% of urinary nitrogen. Measurement of total urinary nitrogen (TUN) is complex and not done in most hospitals, whereas urinary urea nitrogen (UUN) is measured routinely. When UUN is used in the calculation of urinary nitrogen excretion, an additional 20% of the UUN is added to account for nonurea nitrogen losses. In the absence of abnormal stool or skin losses, nitrogen output is calculated as

$$\text{Nitrogen output (g)} = \text{TUN (g/24 h)} + 2\text{ g (stool and skin losses)}$$

or

$$\text{Nitrogen output (g)} = \text{UUN (g/24 h)} + 20\%\ \text{UUN} + 2\text{ g (stool and skin losses)}$$

Classically, measurement of urinary nitrogen excretion involves a 24-hour urine collection, but recent evidence suggests that a carefully collected 12- or even 6-hour urine collection can be obtained and normalized to a 24-hour period.[156] Nitrogen balance is usually calculated weekly.

Numerous techniques for assessment and monitoring of energy balance have been studied, but no method is ideal. Continuous whole-body calorimetry is accurate[157-159] but not practical in patients confined to the ICU. The doubly labeled water technique has been used to assess energy expenditure in healthy individuals over extended periods, but it depends on steady-state CO_2 and water turnover and a stable body water pool,[157,160] thus rendering critically ill patients poor candidates for this technique.[157,161,162] Nuclear magnetic resonance spectroscopy using ^{31}P can be performed to assess relative adenosine triphosphate, creatine phosphate, and inorganic phosphate in muscle and has proved useful in assessing and monitoring energetics in animals and humans.[163-165] It is expensive and currently not practical for clinical use.

Indirect calorimetry is used to determine the heat produced by oxidative processes by measuring oxygen consumption and carbon dioxide production, which are then used to calculate REE via the abbreviated Weir equation.[166,167] Indirect calorimetry is widely used at the bedside, convenient, relatively inexpensive, and accurately estimates REE when compared with standard predictive formulas.[168-174] Perhaps the greatest weakness of indirect calorimetry is that it is performed on patients at rest and therefore does not account for energy expenditure during periods of activity. Many clinicians will increase caloric input by 20% to 25% above measured REE to account for physical activity, particularly in patients who are agitated, ambulatory, or involved in intense physical therapy.[175-177]

Inadequate[95,178-185] or excessive caloric intake[56,62,63,186-189] has been associated with poor outcomes in critically ill patients. Current recommendations are to provide 25 to 30 kcal/kg/d or to base the provision of calories on REE measured by indirect calorimetry.[190] The author uses the former as a starting point to initiate nutrition support and performs indirect calorimetry weekly and as needed based on the patient's clinical course.

In addition to the nutrition-specific monitoring techniques mentioned, the usual laboratory values should be monitored for fluid and electrolyte composition, hepatic function, infection, and any coagulopathy that might reflect vitamin K deficiency. In a critically ill patient, serum electrolytes (Na^+, K^+, Cl^-, and HCO_3^-) should be determined daily and as needed. Special attention should be paid to the intracellular electrolytes (K^+, Mg^{++}, and $PO_4^=$), which are required for the attainment of nitrogen balance[73] and can fall precipitously when nutrition support, particularly glucose, is initiated. Rapid uptake into cells can result in dangerously low serum levels acutely. Intracellular electrolyte levels should be measured before starting nutrition support, 1 or 2 days after starting support, and at least weekly thereafter. Liver function and coagulation parameters should be evaluated weekly and as needed. Glucose should be measured every 6 hours initially and then as needed; it can be measured as often as 2 hours when continuous insulin infusions are being used (Fig. 83-1).

Complications of Nutrition Support

Complications of nutrition support include those related to the route of nutrition support and those related to nutrition support in general and are discussed in the following paragraphs. Perhaps the most important problem with nutrition support is failure to achieve therapeutic goals. Recommendations for appropriate doses of protein and calories, electrolytes, vitamins, and trace elements are discussed in previous paragraphs.

Complications of Enteral Nutrition Support

Complications specific to enteral nutrition support include mechanical or technical complications, gastrointestinal complications, and aspiration pneumonia.

Mechanical and technical complications of enteral nutrition include feeding tube misplacement, gastrointestinal perforation, sinusitis, otitis media, ulceration of the nasal septum, and obstruction of the feeding tube. Proper placement of feeding tubes in the gastrointestinal tract should be confirmed radiographically or with pH testing before feeding is initiated. Auscultatory techniques for confirmation of proper tube placement are unreliable.[191] Nasally placed feeding tubes are a potential cause of sinusitis or otitis media (or both), particularly when stiff, large-bore nasogastric tubes are used as feeding tubes. Soft, small-caliber tubes such as Miller-Frederick or Dobbhoff tubes seem to cause sinusitis less frequently. In mechanically ventilated patients, feeding tubes may be placed orally to minimize the incidence of sinusitis.[192] Perforation of the esophagus or other parts of the gastrointestinal tract is a disastrous complication and seems to occur most frequently in the setting of stricture, obstructing tumor, or abnormal anatomy as a result of surgery. In these situations, tube placement under fluoroscopic guidance or endoscopic tube placement should be considered. Dislodgment of the feeding tube is a frequent and frustrat-

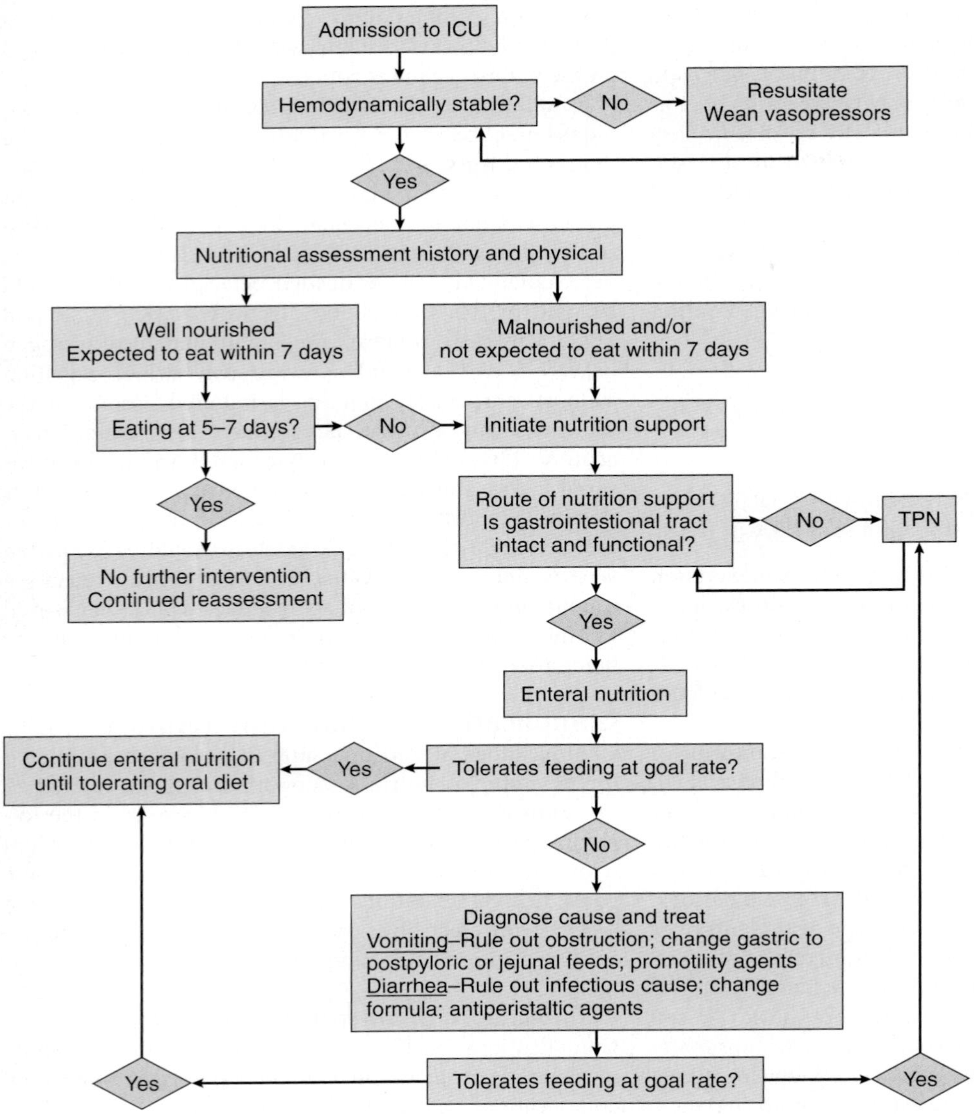

Figure 83-1. Approach to administering nutritional support to a critical care patient. ICU, intensive care unit; TPN, total parenteral nutrition.

ing problem and can be disastrous when the tube dislodged is a recent, surgically placed tube such as a gastrostomy or jejunostomy tube. When a surgically placed tube has been present for longer than 1 to 2 weeks, the stomach or intestine should be adherent to the abdominal wall and the tube can usually be replaced through the existing tract, as long as the tube is replaced within a few hours before the tract begins to close. A radiograph with contrast enhancement should be used to verify replacement of the tube in the appropriate location. Dislodgment of a surgically placed tube within a week of placement can result in peritonitis from spillage of enteral formula or gastrointestinal contents into the abdominal cavity. Care should be taken to properly secure all feeding tubes either with sutures and tape or with commercially available fixation systems, and tubes should be protected with appropriate patient restraints and caregiver attention when the patient is being moved. Feeding tube obstruction occurs most frequently when tubes are not routinely flushed or when crushed medications are delivered through the tube. Tubes should be flushed every 6 hours and after every medication dose. Numerous techniques have been used to clear obstructed tubes, including flushing with cola, pancreatic enzymes, cranberry juice, and streptokinase, although none is universally successful. Clearing a nasoenteric tube with a stylet or wire carries the risk of perforating the gastrointestinal tract and should be avoided unless done under fluoroscopic guidance to ensure that the stylet remains within the tube lumen.

Gastrointestinal complications such as abdominal distention, nausea, vomiting, diarrhea, and constipation occur in approximately 60% of critically ill patients receiving nutrition support.[193] Gastrointestinal motility is often decreased in these patients,[193,194] although gastric stasis and high gastric residual volumes occur more frequently than decreased small intestinal motility does.[194] Potential causes of gastroparesis include increased sympathetic tone, elevated intracranial pressure, opiates, benzodiazepines, dopamine, hyperglycemia, recent abdominal surgery, and pancreatitis. Prokinetic agents such as metoclopramide may restore gastric motility and allow gastric feeding.[195] Postpyloric feeding tube placement will often allow the continuation of enteral nutrition. Advancement of the feeding tube into the proximal jejunum facilitates enteral nutrition in patients with pancreatitis.[100]

Diarrhea occurs in as many as 70% of critically ill patients.[193] Potential causes include antibiotics and other drugs, hyperosmolar formulas, infected solutions, hypoalbuminemia, chronic malnutrition and disuse mucosal atrophy, intolerance to lactose or other nutrients, pancreatic insufficiency, biliary fistula, and short-gut syndrome.

Clostridium difficile overgrowth is perhaps the most serious cause of antibiotic-associated diarrhea, and stool should be assayed for *C. difficile* toxin in every case of persistent diarrhea in the critically ill. *C. difficile* enterocolitis should be treated with appropriate antibiotics. Antibiotics may also cause diarrhea by eliminating the bacteria that ferment dietary fiber into short-chain fatty acids. Short-chain fatty acids are important for maintaining colonic mucosal integrity and enhance water and electrolyte absorption.[196] Enteral formulas should be replaced daily to avoid bacterial contamination of the solution.

A change in formula or more gradual institution of nutrition support can be used to overcome problems caused by nutrient intolerance, disuse atrophy, and short-gut syndrome. Semielemental or peptide formulas may reduce diarrhea in patients with mucosal atrophy. H_2 blockers can be used to decrease the contribution of gastric secretions to diarrhea in patients with short-gut syndrome. Drugs with the potential to cause diarrhea should be identified and eliminated if possible. Pancreatic insufficiency should be treated with commercially available pancreatic enzymes. Diarrhea secondary to a biliary fistula may be improved with reinfusion of bile into the intestine distal to the fistula. Once correctable causes of diarrhea have been identified and eliminated, Kaopectate can be given for symptomatic relief. Antiperistaltic agents such as Imodium or opiates should be avoided until infectious causes of diarrhea have been ruled out. Fiber may be used to thicken stool and lessen perineal irritation, but it may be associated with constipation and fecal impaction in critically ill patients. Intractable diarrhea may warrant the discontinuation of enteral nutrition and the initiation of parenteral nutrition.

Aspiration pneumonia is the major infectious complication of enteral nutrition. Bolus feeding carries a higher risk of aspiration than continuous feeding does. Gastric residual volume, which has traditionally been used to assess gastric feeding tolerance, does not appear to correlate with risk for aspiration.[197] Gastric feeding is routinely used in many ICUs, but because a nasogastric tube is one of the leading causes of aspiration, gastric feeding should probably be done with a soft, small-caliber tube designed for feeding. The risk of aspiration associated with gastric feeding may be lower when done via a percutaneous gastrostomy tube,[197] which avoids compromising the function of the gastroesophageal junction and swallowing mechanics. Multiple studies have compared the risk of aspirating gastric versus postpyloric feedings, but the results have been contradictory.[155,198,199] In a recent meta-analysis of seven randomized trials, small bowel feeding was associated with a lower risk of aspiration pneumonia than was gastric feeding.[200] Nursing protocols for the bedside placement of postpyloric feeding tubes have been developed,[201,202] although placement under fluoroscopic guidance is more likely to be successful and is cost-effective.[203] The semirecumbent body position has been shown to significantly reduce aspiration pneumonia as compared with the supine body position.[204]

Complications of Parenteral Nutrition Support

The primary complications of parenteral nutrition include mechanical or technical complications and infectious complications. Mechanical and technical complications are related to central venous catheter placement and include pneumothorax, arterial injury, hemothorax, hydrothorax, cardiac arrhythmia, and cardiac perforation with tamponade. The incidence of severe complications with subclavian vein catheterization is 1% to 3%, with an overall complication rate of 5%.[205] The incidence of complications with jugular venous catheterization ranges from 0.1% to 4.2%.[206] Jugular venous catheterization under ultrasound guidance is increasingly being recommended.[207-210] Jugular or subclavian vein thrombosis is a postprocedural complication that is manifested as neck or arm swelling and should be managed by catheter removal and anticoagulation; thrombolytics have also been recommended.[211]

Catheter infection and catheter-associated bloodstream infection are the major infectious complications of parenteral nutrition and occur in 2% to 8% of patients with central venous catheters. The most common infecting organisms are coagulase-negative staphylococci, *Staphylococcus aureus,* and *Candida* species. Infection is more likely when parenteral nutrition is administered through a multilumen catheter than through a single-lumen catheter,[212] although the incidence of infection may be reduced when parenteral nutrition is infused through a dedicated port.[213] Jugular and femoral catheters have higher rates of infection than do subclavian catheters.[214] Dedicated central line care teams and regular dressing change protocols may reduce the incidence of catheter infection.[213] Antibiotic-coated or antibiotic-impregnated catheters are expensive but appear to be effective in reducing catheter-related bloodstream infections.[215] Guidewire exchange is associated with a decreased incidence of technical complications but an increased incidence of catheter infections.[216] Although the possibility of catheter infection increases with time, routine catheter exchange is probably not indicated.[215] Catheters should be replaced, ideally at a fresh site, for obvious site infection, for the evaluation and treatment of fever of unknown origin, and after any positive blood culture. If guidewire exchange is used and the removed catheter proves to be infected, the new catheter often becomes infected during the exchange and should in turn be removed and replaced at a fresh site.

Metabolic Complications of Nutrition Support

Common metabolic complications of nutrition support include hyperglycemia, hepatobiliary complications, disturbances in water and electrolyte balance, and acid-base abnormalities. Though more common in patients receiving parenteral nutrition, metabolic complications can occur with either form of nutrition support.

Hyperglycemia occurs frequently in critically ill patients receiving nutrition support and is most common in diabetic patients and those with catabolic illness.

Complications related to hyperglycemia include infection, hyperosmolarity, and osmotic diuresis. The first step in the control of blood sugar is avoidance of overfeeding, as discussed previously. In surgical patients, blood glucose should probably be maintained in the range of 80 to 120 mg/dL by administering intermittent or continuously infused insulin.[62] Although the benefits of tight glucose control in medical patients are less clear, a large recent trial suggests that normoglycemia is associated with decreased renal failure, decreased ventilator days, and reduced ICU and hospital length of stay.[217] Symptomatic hypoglycemia has been reported in children after sudden withdrawal of TPN but is rare in adults, and weaning of TPN in adults is not usually necessary.[218]

Hepatobiliary complications of nutrition support include hepatic steatosis (fatty infiltration of the liver) and intrahepatic and extrahepatic cholestasis. Progression to chronic liver disease occurs in premature infants[219] but is rare in adults. Hepatic steatosis may develop after 7 to 21 days of parenteral nutrition and is characterized initially by elevated transaminases. Usually asymptomatic, fatty infiltration can, in severe cases, be accompanied by hepatomegaly and right upper quadrant abdominal pain. Histologically, mild cases are characterized by periportal fat infiltration and severe cases by centrilobular infiltration. Overfeeding, hyperinsulinemia, essential fatty acid deficiency, and carnitine deficiency may predispose to fatty infiltration. Cholestasis occurs later in the course of parenteral nutrition and is characterized by elevations in bilirubin and alkaline phosphatase. Histologically, periportal or pericentral canalicular bile plugging, bile staining of surrounding hepatocytes, and lymphocytic triaditis characterize cholestasis. Cholelithiasis has been linked to long-term TPN use. Gallstone formation is almost certainly related to the lack of enteral feeding and the resultant lack of neural and hormonal stimulation of gallbladder contraction. Other potential but unproven causes of cholestasis include overfeeding, the production of toxic bile acids by intestinal bacteria, hormones, endotoxin, and taurine deficiency.[42,220-223] Management of hepatobiliary complications is aimed at prevention. Overfeeding should be avoided. Cyclical TPN and enteral feeding, even if only partial, may help prevent cholestasis. A trial of oral neomycin and metronidazole may be helpful.[223]

Serum electrolyte levels should be monitored and electrolytes added to or eliminated from TPN as indicated, with consideration of excess losses or abnormal accumulation. Hypernatremia or hyponatremia can be managed by increasing or decreasing free water. Particular attention should be paid to the intracellular electrolytes potassium, magnesium, and phosphorus. In malnourished individuals, these electrolytes rapidly move intracellularly when nutrition support is initiated. Termed the refeeding syndrome, serum levels of these intracellular electrolytes fall precipitously, with hypophosphatemia resulting in hemolysis, rhabdomyolysis, and heart failure with hypokalemia and hypomagnesemia leading to cardiac arrhythmias.[224,225] Serum levels of intracellular electrolytes should be corrected before and, in particular, 24 hours after the institution of nutrition support. Abnormally high levels of the intracellular electrolytes are of concern in renal failure and often need to be reduced or eliminated from TPN solutions. Hyperkalemia and hypomagnesemia may lead to weakness and cardiac arrhythmia, and hyperphosphatemia may result in hypotension, hypocalcemia, and metastatic calcification. Hyperphosphatemia is often treated with oral phosphate binders such as calcium carbonate.

Metabolic acidosis related to nutrition support is most commonly due to excess chloride administration and resultant renal bicarbonate losses, but it can also occur as a result of thiamine deficiency with resultant lactic acidosis.[226,227]

KEY POINTS

- Malnutrition is a significant contributor to morbidity and mortality in critically ill patients.
- Distinguishing stress metabolism from starvation metabolism is critical to the provision of appropriate nutrition support.
- Critically ill patients may require more energy but are less able to tolerate glucose than starved patients are and require a significant portion of calories as fat.
- Critically ill patients require increased protein to achieve nitrogen balance.
- Enteral nutrition is less costly, more physiologic, associated with fewer metabolic disturbances, and may be associated with fewer infections than parenteral nutrition is and remains the preferred route for nutrition support.
- Parenteral nutrition is acceptable when enteral nutrition cannot be used, particularly if blood glucose is tightly controlled.
- Nutrition support should be closely monitored to avoid complications.

REFERENCES

1. Seltzer MH, Bastidas JA, Cooper DM, et al: Instant nutritional assessment. JPEN J Parenter Enteral Nutr 1979;3:157-159.
2. Reinhardt GF, Myscofski JW, Wilkens DB, et al: Incidence and mortality of hypoalbuminemic patients in hospitalized veterans. JPEN J Parenter Enteral Nutr 1980;4:357-359.
3. Detsky AS, Baker JP, O'Rourke K, et al: Perioperative parenteral nutrition: A meta-analysis. Ann Intern Med 1987;107:195-203.
4. Reilly JJ Jr, Hull SF, Albert N, et al: Economic impact of malnutrition: A model system for hospitalized patients. JPEN J Parenter Enteral Nutr 1988;12:371-376.
5. Golub R, Golub RW, Cantu R Jr, et al: A multivariate analysis of factors

contributing to leakage of intestinal anastomoses. J Am Coll Surg 1997;184:364-372.
6. Khuri SF, Daley J, Henderson W, et al: The Department of Veterans Affairs' NSQIP: The first national, validated, outcome-based, risk-adjusted, and peer-controlled program for the measurement and enhancement of the quality of surgical care. National VA Surgical Quality Improvement Program. Ann Surg 1998;228: 491-507.
7. Longo WE, Virgo KS, Johnson FE, et al: Risk factors for morbidity and mortality after colectomy for colon cancer. Dis Colon Rectum 2000;43:83-91.
8. Hollenbeck BK, Miller DC, Taub D, et al: Risk factors for adverse outcomes after transurethral resection of bladder tumors. Cancer 2006;106:1527-1535.
9. Harpole DH Jr, DeCamp MM Jr, Daley J, et al: Prognostic models of thirty-day mortality and morbidity after major pulmonary resection. J Thorac Cardiovasc Surg 1999;117:969-979.
10. Mizock BA: Alterations in carbohydrate metabolism during stress: A review of the literature. Am J Med 1995;98:75-84.
11. Wolfe RR, Jahoor F, Herndon DN, et al: Isotopic evaluation of the metabolism of pyruvate and related substrates in normal adult volunteers and severely burned children: Effect of dichloroacetate and glucose infusion. Surgery 1991;110:54-67.
12. Long CL, Spencer JL, Kinney JM, et al: Carbohydrate metabolism in man: Effect of elective operations and major injury. J Appl Physiol 1971;31: 110-116.
13. Lang CH, Dobrescu C: Gram-negative infection increases noninsulin-mediated glucose disposal. Endocrinology 1991;128:645-753.
14. Stumvoll M, Meyer C, Mitrakou A, et al: Renal glucose production and utilization: New aspects in humans. Diabetologia 1997;40:749-757.
15. McGuinness OP, Shau V, Benson EM, et al: Role of epinephrine and norepinephrine in the metabolic response to stress hormone infusion in the conscious dog. Am J Physiol 1997;273:E674-E681.
16. Chu CA, Sindelar DK, Neal DW, et al: Comparison of the direct and indirect effects of epinephrine on hepatic glucose production. J Clin Invest 1997;99:1044-1056.
17. Jahoor F, Herndon DN, Wolfe RR: Role of insulin and glucagon in the response of glucose and alanine kinetics in burn-injured patients. J Clin Invest 1986;78:807-814.
18. Roh M, Moldawer L, Ekman L, et al: Stimulatory effect of interleukin-1 upon hepatic metabolism. Metabolism 1986;35:419-424.
19. Petit F, Bagby GJ, Lang CH: Tumor necrosis factor mediates zymosan-induced increase in glucose flux and insulin resistance. Am J Physiol 1995;268:E219-E28.
20. Pessin JE, Bell GI: Mammalian facilitative glucose transporter family: Structure and molecular regulation. Annu Rev Physiol 1992;54:911-930.
21. Wilmore D: The wound as an organ. In Little RA, Frayn KN (eds): The Scientific Basis for the Care of the Critically Ill. Manchester, UK, Manchester University Press, 1986.
22. Haji-Michael PG, Ladriere L, Sener A, et al: Leukocyte glycolysis and lactate output in animal sepsis and ex vivo human blood. Metabolism 1999;48:779-785.
23. McCowen KC, Malhotra A, Bistrian BR: Stress-induced hyperglycemia. Crit Care Clin 2001;17:107-124.
24. Meszaros K, Lang CH, Bagby GJ, et al: Tumor necrosis factor increases in vivo glucose utilization of macrophage-rich tissues. Biochem Biophys Res Commun 1987;149:1-6.
25. Bird TA, Davies A, Baldwin SA, et al: Interleukin 1 stimulates hexose transport in fibroblasts by increasing the expression of glucose transporters. J Biol Chem 1990;265:13578-13583.
26. Van den Berghe G, Wouters P, Weekers F, et al: Reactivation of pituitary hormone release and metabolic improvement by infusion of growth hormone–releasing peptide and thyrotropin-releasing hormone in patients with protracted critical illness. J Clin Endocrinol Metab 1999;84:1311-1323.
27. Van den Berghe G, Baxter RC, Weekers F, et al: A paradoxical gender dissociation within the growth hormone/insulin-like growth factor I axis during protracted critical illness. J Clin Endocrinol Metab 2000;85:183-192.
28. Wolfe RR, Durkot MJ, Allsop JR, et al: Glucose metabolism in severely burned patients. Metabolism 1979;28:1031-1039.
29. Wolfe RR, Herndon DN, Jahoor F, et al: Effect of severe burn injury on substrate cycling by glucose and fatty acids. N Engl J Med 1987;317: 403-408.
30. Grimble RF: Inflammatory status and insulin resistance. Curr Opin Clin Nutr Metab Care 2002;5:551-559.
31. Marette A: Mediators of cytokine-induced insulin resistance in obesity and other inflammatory settings. Curr Opin Clin Nutr Metab Care 2002;5:377-383.
32. Herndon DN, Nguyen TT, Wolfe RR, et al: Lipolysis in burned patients is stimulated by the beta 2-receptor for catecholamines. Arch Surg 1994;129:1301-1304; discussion 1304-1305.
33. Hardardottir I, Grunfeld C, Feingold KR: Effects of endotoxin and cytokines on lipid metabolism. Curr Opin Lipidol 1994;5:207-215.
34. Wolfe RR: Herman Award Lecture, 1996: Relation of metabolic studies to clinical nutrition—the example of burn injury. Am J Clin Nutr 1996;64: 800-808.
35. Wolfe R: The role of triglyceride–fatty acid cycling and glucose cycling in thermogenesis and amplification of net substrate flux in human subjects. In Muller JM, Danforth E, Burger AG, et al (eds): Hormones and Nutrition in Obesity and Cachexia. New York, Springer Verlag, 1989.
36. Wolfe RR, Shaw JH, Durkot MJ: Effect of sepsis on VLDL kinetics: Responses in basal state and during glucose infusion. Am J Physiol 1985;248: E732-E740.
37. Lanza-Jacoby S, Sedkova N, Phetteplace H, et al: Sepsis-induced regulation of lipoprotein lipase expression in rat adipose tissue and soleus muscle. J Lipid Res 1997;38:701-710.
38. Aarsland A, Chinkes D, Wolfe RR: Contributions of de novo synthesis of fatty acids to total VLDL-triglyceride secretion during prolonged hyperglycemia/hyperinsulinemia in normal man. J Clin Invest 1996;98:2008-2017.
39. Feingold KR, Serio MK, Adi S, et al: Tumor necrosis factor stimulates hepatic lipid synthesis and secretion. Endocrinology 1989;124:2336-2342.
40. Wolfe BM, Walker BK, Shaul DB, et al: Effect of total parenteral nutrition on hepatic histology. Arch Surg 1988;123:1084-1090.
41. Mizock BA: Metabolic derangements in sepsis and septic shock. Crit Care Clin 2000;16:319-336, vii.
42. Siegel JH, Cerra FB, Coleman B, et al: Physiological and metabolic correlations in human sepsis. Invited commentary. Surgery 1979;86: 163-193.
43. Ozawa K, Aoyama H, Yasuda K, et al: Metabolic abnormalities associated with postoperative organ failure. A redox theory. Arch Surg 1983;118:1245-1251.
44. Fink M: Cytopathic hypoxia in sepsis. Acta Anaesthesiol Scand Suppl 1997;110:87-95.
45. Cerra FB, Siegel JH, Coleman B, et al: Septic autocannibalism. A failure of exogenous nutritional support. Ann Surg 1980;192:570-580.
46. Lecker SH, Jagoe RT, Gilbert A, et al: Multiple types of skeletal muscle atrophy involve a common program of changes in gene expression. FASEB J 2004;18:39-51.
47. Tisdale MJ: Biochemical mechanisms of cellular catabolism. Curr Opin Clin Nutr Metab Care 2002;5:401-405.
48. Chai J, Wu Y, Sheng ZZ: Role of ubiquitin-proteasome pathway in skeletal muscle wasting in rats with endotoxemia. Crit Care Med 2003;31:1802-1807.
49. Costelli P, Baccino FM: Mechanisms of skeletal muscle depletion in wasting syndromes: Role of ATP-ubiquitin–dependent proteolysis. Curr Opin Clin Nutr Metab Care 2003;6:407-412.
50. Tiao G, Hobler S, Wang JJ, et al: Sepsis is associated with increased mRNAs of the ubiquitin-proteasome proteolytic pathway in human skeletal muscle. J Clin Invest 1997;99:163-168.
51. Biolo G, Fleming RY, Maggi SP, et al: Inverse regulation of protein turnover and amino acid transport in skeletal muscle of hypercatabolic patients. J Clin Endocrinol Metab 2002;87:3378-3384.
52. Wernerman J: Skeletal muscle in the stress-induced catabolic state. In Revhaug A (ed): Acute Catabolic State: Update in Intensive Care and Emergency Medicine, Vol. 21. Berlin, Springer, 1996.
53. Newsholme EA, Parry-Billings M: Properties of glutamine release from muscle and its importance for the

immune system. JPEN J Parenter Enteral Nutr 1990;14:63S-67S.
54. Paddon-Jones D, Sheffield-Moore M, Creson DL, et al: Hypercortisolemia alters muscle protein anabolism following ingestion of essential amino acids. Am J Physiol Endocrinol Metab 2003;284:E946-E953.
55. Orellana RA, O'Connor PM, Nguyen HV, et al: Endotoxemia reduces skeletal muscle protein synthesis in neonates. Am J Physiol Endocrinol Metab 2002;283:E909-E916.
56. Askanazi J, Rosenbaum SH, Hyman AI, et al: Respiratory changes induced by the large glucose loads of total parenteral nutrition. JAMA 1980;243:1444-1447.
57. Buzby GP, Mullen JL, Stein TP, et al: Manipulation of TPN caloric substrate and fatty infiltration of liver. J Surg Res 1981;31:46-54.
58. Lowry S, Brennan MF B: Abnormal liver function during parenteral nutrition: Relation to infusion excess. J Surg Res 1979;26:300-307.
59. Sheldon GF, Peterson SR, Sanders R: Hepatic dysfunction during hyperalimentation. Arch Surg 1978;113:504-508.
60. Furnary AP, Zerr KJ, Grunkemeier GL, et al: Continuous intravenous insulin infusion reduces the incidence of deep sternal wound infection in diabetic patients after cardiac surgical procedures. Ann Thorac Surg 1999;67:352-360; discussion 360-362.
61. Pomposelli JJ, Baxter JK 3rd, Babineau TJ, et al: Early postoperative glucose control predicts nosocomial infection rate in diabetic patients. JPEN J Parenter Enteral Nutr 1998;22:77-81.
62. van den Berghe G, Wouters P, Weekers F, et al: Intensive insulin therapy in the surgical intensive care unit. N Engl J Med 2001;345:1359-1367.
63. Barton RG, Craft WB, Mone MC, et al: Chemical paralysis reduces energy expenditure in patients with burns and severe respiratory failure treated with mechanical ventilation. J Burn Care Rehabil 1997;18:461-468; discussion 460.
64. Cutts ME, Dowdy RP, Ellersieck MR, et al: Predicting energy needs in ventilator-dependent critically ill patients: Effect of adjusting weight for edema or adiposity. Am J Clin Nutr 1997;66:1250-1256.
65. Dickerson RN, Boschert KJ, Kudsk KA, et al: Hypocaloric enteral tube feeding in critically ill obese patients. Nutrition 2002;18:241-246.
66. Wolfe RR, Allsop JR, Burke JF: Glucose metabolism in man: Responses to intravenous glucose infusion. Metabolism 1979;28:210-220.
67. Wolfe RR: Carbohydrate metabolism in the critically ill patient. Implications for nutritional support. Crit Care Clin 1987;3:11-24.
68. Driscoll DF, Blackburn GL: Total parenteral nutrition 1990. A review of its current status in hospitalised patients, and the need for patient-specific feeding. Drugs 1990;40:346-363.
69. Elwyn DH: Nutritional requirements of adult surgical patients. Crit Care Med 1980;8:9-20.
70. Shaw JH, Wildbore M, Wolfe RR: Whole body protein kinetics in severely septic patients. The response to glucose infusion and total parenteral nutrition. Ann Surg 1987;205:288-294.
71. Long CL, Jeevanandam M, Kim BM, et al: Whole body protein synthesis and catabolism in septic man. Am J Clin Nutr 1977;30:1340-1344.
72. Monsen ER: The 10th edition of the recommended dietary allowances: What's new in the 1989 RDAs? J Am Diet Assoc 1989;89:1748-1752.
73. Rudman D, Millikan WJ, Richardson TJ, et al: Elemental balances during intravenous hyperalimentation of underweight adult subjects. J Clin Invest 1975;55:94-104.
74. Elia M: Changing concepts of nutrient requirements in disease: Implications for artificial nutritional support. Lancet 1995;345:1279-1284.
75. Walker W: Intestinal defenses in health and disease. In Lifshitz F (ed): Clinical Disorders in Pediatric Growth and Nutrition. New York, Marcel Dekker, 1980, pp 99-119.
76. Kagnoff M: Immunology and disease of the gastrointestinal tract. In Sleisinger MH, Fordtrain JS (eds): Gastrointestinal Disease. Philadelphia, Saunders, 1983, pp 20-44.
77. Williamson RC: Intestinal adaptation (first of two parts). Structural, functional and cytokinetic changes. N Engl J Med 1978;298:1393-1402.
78. Williamson RC: Intestinal adaptation (second of two parts). Mechanisms of control. N Engl J Med 1978;298:1444-1450.
79. Feldman EJ, Dowling RH, McNaughton J, et al: Effects of oral versus intravenous nutrition on intestinal adaptation after small bowel resection in the dog. Gastroenterology 1976;70:712-719.
80. Johnson J, Copeland E, Dudrick S, et al: Structural and hormonal alterations in the gastrointestinal tract of parenterally fed rats. Gastroenterology 1975;68:1177-1183.
81. Wilmore DW, Smith RJ, O'Dwyer ST, et al: The gut: A central organ after surgical stress. Surgery 1988;104:917-923.
82. Zaloga GP, Knowles R, Black KW, et al: Total parenteral nutrition increases mortality after hemorrhage. Crit Care Med 1991;19:54-59.
83. Mochizuki H, Trocki O, Dominioni L, et al: Mechanism of prevention of postburn hypermetabolism and catabolism by early enteral feeding. Ann Surg 1984;200:297-310.
84. Alverdy JC, Aoys E, Moss GS: Total parenteral nutrition promotes bacterial translocation from the gut. Surgery 1988;104:185-190.
85. Delany HM, Teh E, Dwarka B, et al: Infusion of enteral vs parenteral nutrients using high-concentration branch-chain amino acids: Effect on wound healing in the postoperative rat. JPEN J Parenter Enteral Nutr 1991;15:464-468.
86. McArdle AH, Palmason C, Morency I, et al: A rationale for enteral feeding as the preferable route for hyperalimentation. Surgery 1981;90:616-623.
87. Bower RH, Talamini MA, Sax HC, et al: Postoperative enteral vs parenteral nutrition. A randomized controlled trial. Arch Surg 1986;121:1040-1045.
88. Cerra FB, Shronts EP, Konstantinides NN, et al: Enteral feeding in sepsis: A prospective, randomized, double-blind trial. Surgery 1985;98:632-639.
89. Cerra FB, McPherson JP, Konstantinides FN, et al: Enteral nutrition does not prevent multiple organ failure syndrome (MOFS) after sepsis. Surgery 1988;104:727-733.
90. Moore FA, Moore EE, Jones TN, et al: TEN versus TPN following major abdominal trauma—reduced septic morbidity. J Trauma 1989;29:916-922; discussion 922-923.
91. Kudsk KA, Croce MA, Fabian TC, et al: Enteral versus parenteral feeding. Effects on septic morbidity after blunt and penetrating abdominal trauma. Ann Surg 1992;215:503-511; discussion 511-513.
92. Moore FA, Feliciano DV, Andrassy RJ, et al: Early enteral feeding, compared with parenteral, reduces postoperative septic complications. The results of a meta-analysis. Ann Surg 1992;216:172-183.
93. Gramlich L, Kichian K, Pinilla J, et al: Does enteral nutrition compared to parenteral nutrition result in better outcomes in critically ill adult patients? A systematic review of the literature. Nutrition 2004;20:843-848.
94. Kemper M, Weissman C, Hyman AI: Caloric requirements and supply in critically ill surgical patients. Crit Care Med 1992;20:344-348.
95. Rapp RP, Young B, Twyman D, et al: The favorable effect of early parenteral feeding on survival in head-injured patients. J Neurosurg 1983;58:906-912.
96. Norton JA, Ott LG, McClain C, et al: Intolerance to enteral feeding in the brain-injured patient. J Neurosurg 1988;68:62-66.
97. Abernathy GB, Heizer WD, Holcombe BJ, et al: Efficacy of tube feeding in supplying energy requirements of hospitalized patients. JPEN J Parenter Enteral Nutr 1989;13:387-391.
98. Sedman PC, Macfie J, Sagar P, et al: The prevalence of gut translocation in humans. Gastroenterology 1994;107:643-649.
99. Moore FA, Moore EE, Poggetti RS, et al: Postinjury shock and early bacteremia. A lethal combination. Arch Surg 1992;127:893-897; discussion 897-898.
100. McClave SA, Greene LM, Snider HL, et al: Comparison of the safety of early enteral vs parenteral nutrition in mild acute pancreatitis. JPEN J Parenter Enteral Nutr 1997;21:14-20.
101. Windsor AC, Kanwar S, Li AG, et al: Compared with parenteral nutrition, enteral feeding attenuates the acute phase response and improves disease severity in acute pancreatitis. Gut 1998;42:431-435.
102. Woodcock NP, Zeigler D, Palmer MD, et al: Enteral versus parenteral nutrition: A pragmatic study. Nutrition 2001;17:1-12.
103. Kalfarentzos F, Kehagias J, Mead N, et al: Enteral nutrition is superior to parenteral nutrition in severe acute

pancreatitis: Results of a randomized trial. Br J Surg 1997;84:1665-1669.
104. Van den Berghe G, Wouters PJ, Bouillon R, et al: Outcome benefit of intensive insulin therapy in the critically ill: Insulin dose versus glycemic control. Crit Care Med 2003;31:359-366.
105. Product Reference Guide. Deerfield, IL, Nestle Clinical Nutrition, 2001.
106. Brinson RR, Kolts BE: Diarrhea associated with severe hypoalbuminemia: A comparison of a peptide-based chemically defined diet and standard enteral alimentation. Crit Care Med 1988;16:130-136.
107. Talpers SS, Romberger DJ, Bunce SB, et al: Nutritionally associated increased carbon dioxide production. Excess total calories vs high proportion of carbohydrate calories. Chest 1992;102:551-555.
108. Cerra FB, Cheung NK, Fischer JE, et al: Disease-specific amino acid infusion (F080) in hepatic encephalopathy: A prospective, randomized, double-blind, controlled trial. JPEN J Parenter Enteral Nutr 1985;9:288-295.
109. Kanematsu T, Koyanagi N, Matsumata T, et al: Lack of preventive effect of branched-chain amino acid solution on postoperative hepatic encephalopathy in patients with cirrhosis: A randomized, prospective trial. Surgery 1988;104:482-488.
110. Cerra F, Blackburn G, Hirsch J, et al: The effect of stress level, amino acid formula, and nitrogen dose on nitrogen retention in traumatic and septic stress. Ann Surg 1987;205:282-287.
111. Kirk SJ, Barbul A: Role of arginine in trauma, sepsis, and immunity. JPEN J Parenter Enteral Nutr 1990;14:226S-229S.
112. Madden HP, Breslin RJ, Wasserkrug HL, et al: Stimulation of T cell immunity by arginine enhances survival in peritonitis. J Surg Res 1988;44:658-663.
113. Barbul A, Lazarou SA, Efron DT, et al: Arginine enhances wound healing and lymphocyte immune responses in humans. Surgery 1990;108:331-336; discussion 336-337.
114. Billiar TR, Bankey PE, Svingen BA, et al: Fatty acid intake and Kupffer cell function: Fish oil alters eicosanoid and monokine production to endotoxin stimulation. Surgery 1988;104: 343-349.
115. Endres S, Ghorbani R, Kelley VE, et al: The effect of dietary supplementation with n-3 polyunsaturated fatty acids on the synthesis of interleukin-1 and tumor necrosis factor by mononuclear cells. N Engl J Med 1989;320: 265-271.
116. Bittiner SB, Tucker WF, Cartwright I, et al: A double-blind, randomised, placebo-controlled trial of fish oil in psoriasis. Lancet 1988;1:378-380.
117. Kremer JM, Jubiz W, Michalek A, et al: Fish-oil fatty acid supplementation in active rheumatoid arthritis. A double-blinded, controlled, crossover study. Ann Intern Med 1987;106:497-503.
118. McNurlan MA, Sandgren A, Hunter K, et al: Protein synthesis rates of skeletal muscle, lymphocytes, and albumin with stress hormone infusion in healthy man. Metabolism 1996;45: 1388-1394.
119. Luo JL, Hammarqvist F, Andersson K, et al: Skeletal muscle glutathione after surgical trauma. Ann Surg 1996;223:420-427.
120. Gamrin L, Essen P, Forsberg AM, et al: A descriptive study of skeletal muscle metabolism in critically ill patients: Free amino acids, energy-rich phosphates, protein, nucleic acids, fat, water, and electrolytes. Crit Care Med 1996;24:575-583.
121. Hammarqvist F, Wernerman J, Ali R, et al: Addition of glutamine to total parenteral nutrition after elective abdominal surgery spares free glutamine in muscle, counteracts the fall in muscle protein synthesis, and improves nitrogen balance. Ann Surg 1989;209:455-461.
122. Wells CL, Jechorek RP, Erlandsen SL, et al: The effect of dietary glutamine and dietary RNA on ileal flora, ileal histology, and bacterial translocation in mice. Nutrition 1990;6:70-75; discussion 80-83.
123. Zapata-Sirvent RL, Hansbrough JF, Ohara MM, et al: Bacterial translocation in burned mice after administration of various diets including fiber- and glutamine-enriched enteral formulas. Crit Care Med 1994;22:690-696.
124. Novak F, Heyland DK, Avenell A, et al: Glutamine supplementation in serious illness: A systematic review of the evidence. Crit Care Med 2002;30:2022-2029.
125. Bulger EM, Maier RV: Antioxidants in critical illness. Arch Surg 2001;136:1201-1207.
126. Heyland DK, Novak F, Drover JW, et al: Should immunonutrition become routine in critically ill patients? A systematic review of the evidence. JAMA 2001;286:944-953.
127. Bertolini G, Iapichino G, Radrizzani D, et al: Early enteral immunonutrition in patients with severe sepsis: Results of an interim analysis of a randomized multicentre clinical trial. Intensive Care Med 2003;29:834-840.
128. Kieft H, Roos AN, van Drunen JD, et al: Clinical outcome of immunonutrition in a heterogeneous intensive care population. Intensive Care Med 2005;31:524-532.
129. Baker JP, Detsky AS, Wesson DE, et al: Nutritional assessment: A comparison of clinical judgement and objective measurements. N Engl J Med 1982;306:969-972.
130. Charney P: Nutrition assessment in the 1990s: Where are we now? Nutr Clin Pract 1995;10:131-139.
131. Bettany GE, Powell-Tuck J: Malnutrition: Incidence, diagnosis, causes, effects and indications for nutritional support. Eur J Gastroenterol Hepatol 1995;7:494-500.
132. Hill GL, Windsor JA: Nutritional assessment in clinical practice. Nutrition 1995;11:198-201.
133. Dark D, Pingleton S: Nutrition and nutritional support in clinically ill patients. J Intensive Care Med 1993;8:16-33.
134. Raguso CA, Dupertuis YM, Pichard C: The role of visceral proteins in the nutritional assessment of intensive care unit patients. Curr Opin Clin Nutr Metab Care 2003;6:211-216.
135. Wessling-Resnick M: Iron transport. Annu Rev Nutr 2000;20:129-151.
136. Ingenbleek Y, Bernstein L: The stressful condition as a nutritionally dependent adaptive dichotomy. Nutrition 1999;15:305-320.
137. Manelli JC, Badetti C, Botti G, et al: A reference standard for plasma proteins is required for nutritional assessment of adult burn patients. Burns 1998;24:337-345.
138. Mears E: Outcomes of continuous process improvement of a nutritional care program incorporating serum prealbumin measurements. Nutrition 1996;12:479-484.
139. Bernstain L: Measurement of visceral protein status in assessing protein and energy malnutrition: Standard of care. Prealbumin in Nutritional Care Consensus Group. Nutrition 1995;11:169-171.
140. Moshage H: Cytokines and the hepatic acute phase response. J Pathol 1997;181:257-266.
141. Heinrich PC, Castell JV, Andus T: Interleukin-6 and the acute phase response. Biochem J 1990;265:621-636.
142. Pinilla JC, Hayes P, Laverty W, et al: The C-reactive protein to prealbumin ratio correlates with the severity of multiple organ dysfunction. Surgery 1998;124:799-805; discussion 805-806.
143. Abribat T, Nedelec B, Jobin N, et al: Decreased serum insulin-like growth factor-I in burn patients: Relationship with serum insulin-like growth factor binding protein-3 proteolysis and the influence of lipid composition in nutritional support. Crit Care Med 2000;28:2366-2372.
144. Gianotti L, Braga M, Fortis C, et al: A prospective, randomized clinical trial on perioperative feeding with an arginine-, omega-3 fatty acid–, and RNA-enriched enteral diet: Effect on host response and nutritional status. JPEN J Parenter Enteral Nutr 1999;23:314-320.
145. Wischmeyer PE, Lynch J, Liedel J, et al: Glutamine administration reduces gram-negative bacteremia in severely burned patients: A prospective, randomized, double-blind trial versus isonitrogenous control. Crit Care Med 2001;29:2075-2080.
146. Houdijk AP, Nijveldt RJ, van Leeuwen PA: Glutamine-enriched enteral feeding in trauma patients: Reduced infectious morbidity is not related to changes in endocrine and metabolic responses. JPEN J Parenter Enteral Nutr 1999;23:S52-S58.
147. Conejero R, Bonet A, Grau T, et al: Effect of a glutamine-enriched enteral diet on intestinal permeability and infectious morbidity at 28 days in critically ill patients with systemic inflammatory response syndrome: A randomized, single-blind, prospective, multicenter study. Nutrition 2002;18:716-721.
148. Donati L, Ziegler F, Pongelli G, et al: Nutritional and clinical efficacy of ornithine alpha-ketoglutarate in severe burn patients. Clin Nutr 1999;18:307-311.

149. Casati A, Muttini S, Leggieri C, et al: Rapid turnover proteins in critically ill ICU patients. Negative acute phase proteins or nutritional indicators? Minerva Anestesiol 1998;64:345-350.
150. Nataloni S, Gentili P, Marini B, et al: Nutritional assessment in head injured patients through the study of rapid turnover visceral proteins. Clin Nutr 1999;18:247-251.
151. Wiren M, Permert J, Larsson J: Alpha-ketoglutarate–supplemented enteral nutrition: Effects on postoperative nitrogen balance and muscle catabolism. Nutrition 2002;18:725-728.
152. Garcia-de-Lorenzo A, Ortiz-Leyba C, Planas M, et al: Parenteral administration of different amounts of branch-chain amino acids in septic patients: Clinical and metabolic aspects. Crit Care Med 1997;25:418-424.
153. Gervasio JM, Dickerson RN, Swearingen J, et al: Oxandrolone in trauma patients. Pharmacotherapy 2000;20:1328-1334.
154. Huang YC, Yen CE, Cheng CH, et al: Nutritional status of mechanically ventilated critically ill patients: Comparison of different types of nutritional support. Clin Nutr 2000;19:101-107.
155. Taylor SJ, Fettes SB, Jewkes C, et al: Prospective, randomized, controlled trial to determine the effect of early enhanced enteral nutrition on clinical outcome in mechanically ventilated patients suffering head injury. Crit Care Med 1999;27:2525-2531.
156. Graves C, Saffle J, Morris S: Comparison of urine urea nitrogen collection times in critically ill patients. Nutr Clin Pract 2005;20:271-275.
157. Plank LD, Hill GL: Energy balance in critical illness. Proc Nutr Soc 2003;62:545-552.
158. Jebb SA, Prentice AM, Goldberg GR, et al: Changes in macronutrient balance during over- and underfeeding assessed by 12-d continuous whole-body calorimetry. Am J Clin Nutr 1996;64:259-266.
159. Jebb SA, Prentice AM: Assessment of human energy balance. J Endocrinol 1997;155:183-185.
160. Speakman JR: Principles, problems and a paradox with the measurement of energy expenditure of free-living subjects using doubly-labelled water. Stat Med 1990;9:1365-1380.
161. Monk DN, Plank LD, Franch-Arcas G, et al: Sequential changes in the metabolic response in critically injured patients during the first 25 days after blunt trauma. Ann Surg 1996;223:395-405.
162. Plank LD, Connolly AB, Hill GL: Sequential changes in the metabolic response in severely septic patients during the first 23 days after the onset of peritonitis. Ann Surg 1998;228:146-158.
163. Jacobs D, Whitman G, J M, et al: 31 P-nuclear magnetic resonance spectroscopy of rat skeletal muscle during starvation. JPEN J Parenter Enteral Nutr 1985;9:107a.
164. Thompson A, Damyanovich A, Madapallimattam A, et al: ^{31}P-nuclear magnetic resonance studies of bioenergetic changes in skeletal muscle in malnourished human adults. Am J Clin Nutr 1998;67:39-43.
165. Bourdel-Marchasson I, Biran M, Thiaudiere E, et al: ^{31}P magnetic resonance spectroscopy of human liver in elderly patients: Changes according to nutritional status and inflammatory state. Metabolism 1996;45:1059-1061.
166. Jacobs DO, Wong M: Metabolic assessment. World J Surg 2000;24:1460-1467.
167. Weir JB: New methods for calculating metabolic rate with special reference to protein metabolism. Nutrition 1990;6:213-221.
168. Long CL, Schaffel N, Geiger JW, et al: Metabolic response to injury and illness: Estimation of energy and protein needs from indirect calorimetry and nitrogen balance. JPEN J Parenter Enteral Nutr 1979;3:452-456.
169. Liggett SB, Renfro AD: Energy expenditures of mechanically ventilated nonsurgical patients. Chest 1990;98:682-686.
170. Hwang TL, Huang SL, Chen MF: The use of indirect calorimetry in critically ill patients—the relationship of measured energy expenditure to Injury Severity Score, Septic Severity Score, and APACHE II Score. J Trauma 1993;34:247-251.
171. Boulanger BR, Nayman R, McLean RF, et al: What are the clinical determinants of early energy expenditure in critically injured adults? J Trauma 1994;37:969-974.
172. Raurich JM, Ibanez J: Metabolic rate in severe head trauma. JPEN J Parenter Enteral Nutr 1994;18:521-524.
173. Uehara M, Plank LD, Hill GL: Components of energy expenditure in patients with severe sepsis and major trauma: A basis for clinical care. Crit Care Med 1999;27:1295-1302.
174. Briassoulis G, Venkataraman S, Thompson AE: Energy expenditure in critically ill children. Crit Care Med 2000;28:1166-1172.
175. Swinamer DL, Phang PT, Jones RL, et al: Twenty-four hour energy expenditure in critically ill patients. Crit Care Med 1987;15:637-643.
176. Weissman C, Kemper M, Elwyn DH, et al: The energy expenditure of the mechanically ventilated critically ill patient. An analysis. Chest 1986;89:254-259.
177. Weissman C, Kemper M, Hyman AI: Variation in the resting metabolic rate of mechanically ventilated critically ill patients. Anesth Analg 1989;68:457-461.
178. Askanazi J, Weissman C, Rosenbaum SH, et al: Nutrition and the respiratory system. Crit Care Med 1982;10:163-172.
179. Bassili HR, Deitel M: Effect of nutritional support on weaning patients off mechanical ventilators. JPEN J Parenter Enteral Nutr 1981;5:161-163.
180. Larca L, Greenbaum DM: Effectiveness of intensive nutritional regimes in patients who fail to wean from mechanical ventilation. Crit Care Med 1982;10:297-300.
181. Askanazi J, Hensle TW, Starker PM, et al: Effect of immediate postoperative nutritional support on length of hospitalization. Ann Surg 1986;203:236-239.
182. Benotti PN, Bistrian B: Metabolic and nutritional aspects of weaning from mechanical ventilation. Crit Care Med 1989;17:181-185.
183. Garrel DR, Davignon I, Lopez D: Length of care in patients with severe burns with or without early enteral nutritional support. A retrospective study. J Burn Care Rehabil 1991;12:85-90.
184. Bollmann M, Berger M, Revelly J, et al: Impact of energy balance on clinical outcome in ICU patients—preliminary results. Clin Nutr 2001;20:3.
185. Reid C, Campbell I: High energy deficits in MODS patients are associated with prolonged ICU length of stay but not mortality. Clin Nutr 2001;20:52.
186. Covelli HD, Black JW, Olsen MS, et al: Respiratory failure precipitated by high carbohydrate loads. Ann Intern Med 1981;95:579-581.
187. Dark DS, Pingleton SK, Kerby GR: Hypercapnia during weaning. A complication of nutritional support. Chest 1985;88:141-143.
188. Jeejeebhoy KN: Total parenteral nutrition: Potion or poison? Am J Clin Nutr 2001;74:160-163.
189. Barton RG, Saffle JR, Morris SE, et al: Resuscitation of thermally injured patients with oxygen transport criteria as goals of therapy. J Burn Care Rehabil 1997;18:1-9.
190. Guidelines for the use of parenteral and enteral nutrition in adult and pediatric patients. American Society for Parenteral and Enteral Nutrition. JPEN J Parenter Enteral Nutr 1995;17:(4 Suppl):1SA-52SA.
191. Metheny N: Verification of feeding tube placement. Current issues in enteral nutrition support: Report of the first Ross Enteral Device Conference, Sanibel Island, Florida, Oct. 9-11, 1995. Columbus, OH, Ross Products Division, Abbott Laboratories, 1996.
192. Rouby JJ, Laurent P, Gosnach M, et al: Risk factors and clinical relevance of nosocomial maxillary sinusitis in the critically ill. Am J Respir Crit Care Med 1994;150:776-783.
193. Montejo JC: Enteral nutrition–related gastrointestinal complications in critically ill patients: A multicenter study. The Nutritional and Metabolic Working Group of the Spanish Society of Intensive Care Medicine and Coronary Units. Crit Care Med 1999;27:1447-1453.
194. Dive A, Moulart M, Jonard P, et al: Gastroduodenal motility in mechanically ventilated critically ill patients: A manometric study. Crit Care Med 1994;22:441-447.
195. Boivin MA, Levy H: Gastric feeding with erythromycin is equivalent to transpyloric feeding in the critically ill. Crit Care Med 2001;29:1916-1919.
196. Bowling TE, Raimundo AH, Grimble GK, et al: Reversal by short-chain fatty acids of colonic fluid secretion induced by enteral feeding. Lancet 1993;342:1266-1268.

197. McClave SA, Lukan JK, Stefater JA, et al: Poor validity of residual volumes as a marker for risk of aspiration in critically ill patients. Crit Care Med 2005;33:324-330.
198. Montejo JC, Grau T, Acosta J, et al: Multicenter, prospective, randomized, single-blind study comparing the efficacy and gastrointestinal complications of early jejunal feeding with early gastric feeding in critically ill patients. Crit Care Med 2002;30:796-800.
199. Davies AR, Froomes PR, French CJ, et al: Randomized comparison of nasojejunal and nasogastric feeding in critically ill patients. Crit Care Med 2002;30:586-590.
200. Heyland DK, Drover JW, Dhaliwal R, et al: Optimizing the benefits and minimizing the risks of enteral nutrition in the critically ill: Role of small bowel feeding. JPEN J Parenter Enteral Nutr 2002;26:S51-S55; discussion S56-S57.
201. Cresci G, Martindale R: Bedside placement of small bowel feeding tubes in hospitalized patients: A new role for the dietitian. Nutrition 2003;19:843-846.
202. Hernandez-Socorro CR, Marin J, Ruiz-Santana S, et al: Bedside sonographic-guided versus blind nasoenteric feeding tube placement in critically ill patients. Crit Care Med 1996;24:1690-1694.
203. Huerta G, Puri VK: Nasoenteric feeding tubes in critically ill patients (fluoroscopy versus blind). Nutrition 2000;16:264-267.
204. Drakulovic MB, Torres A, Bauer TT, et al: Supine body position as a risk factor for nosocomial pneumonia in mechanically ventilated patients: A randomised trial. Lancet 1999;354:1851-1858.
205. Eerola R, Kaukinen L, Kaukinen S: Analysis of 13 800 subclavian vein catheterizations. Acta Anaesthesiol Scand 1985;29:193-197.
206. Tyden H: Cannulation of the internal jugular vein—500 cases. Acta Anaesthesiol Scand 1982;26:485-488.
207. Bodenham AR: Can you justify not using ultrasound guidance for central venous access? Crit Care 2006;10:175.
208. Karakitsos D, Labropoulos N, De Groot E, et al: Real-time ultrasound-guided catheterisation of the internal jugular vein: A prospective comparison with the landmark technique in critical care patients. Crit Care 2006;10:R162.
209. Sabbaj A, Hedges JR: Ultrasonographic guidance for internal jugular vein cannulation: An educational imperative, a desirable practice alternative. Ann Emerg Med 2006;48:548-550.
210. Leung J, Duffy M, Finckh A: Real-time ultrasonographically-guided internal jugular vein catheterization in the emergency department increases success rates and reduces complications: A randomized, prospective study. Ann Emerg Med 2006;48:540-547.
211. Haire WD: Arm vein thrombosis. Clin Chest Med 1995;16:341-351.
212. Christoff N, Watters V, Sparks W, et al: Use of triple-lumen subclavian catheters for administration of total parenteral nutrition. JPEN J Parenter Enteral Nutr 1992;18:71.
213. Corona ML, Peters SG, Narr BJ, et al: Infections related to central venous catheters. Mayo Clin Proc 1990;65:979-986.
214. Kemp L, Burge J, Choban P, et al: The effect of catheter type and site on infection rates in total parenteral nutrition patients. JPEN J Parenter Enteral Nutr 1994;18:71-74.
215. Mermel LA: Prevention of intravascular catheter–related infections. Ann Intern Med 2000;132:391-402.
216. Cook D, Randolph A, Kernerman P, et al: Central venous catheter replacement strategies: A systematic review of the literature. Crit Care Med 1997;25:1417-1424.
217. Van den Berghe G, Wilmer A, Hermans G, et al: Intensive insulin therapy in the medical ICU. N Engl J Med 2006;354:449-461.
218. Wagman LD, Newsome HH, Miller KB, et al: The effect of acute discontinuation of total parenteral nutrition. Ann Surg 1986;204:524-529.
219. Postuma R, Trevenen CL: Liver disease in infants receiving total parenteral nutrition. Pediatrics 1979;63:110-115.
220. Baker AL, Rosenberg IH: Hepatic complications of total parenteral nutrition. Am J Med 1987;82:489-497.
221. Fouin-Fortunet H, Le Quernec L, Erlinger S, et al: Hepatic alterations during total parenteral nutrition in patients with inflammatory bowel disease: A possible consequence of lithocholate toxicity. Gastroenterology 1982;82:932-937.
222. von Allmen D, Fischer JE: Metabolic complications. In Fischer JE (ed): Total Parenteral Nutrition, 2nd ed. Boston, Little and Brown, 1991.
223. Freund HR, Muggia-Sullam M, LaFrance R, et al: A possible beneficial effect of metronidazole in reducing TPN-associated liver function derangements. J Surg Res 1985;38:356-363.
224. Weinsier RL, Krumdieck CL: Death resulting from overzealous total parenteral nutrition: The refeeding syndrome revisited. Am J Clin Nutr 1981;34:393-399.
225. Solomon SM, Kirby DF: The refeeding syndrome: A review. JPEN J Parenter Enteral Nutr 1990;14:90-97.
226. Nakasaki H, Ohta M, Soeda J, et al: Clinical and biochemical aspects of thiamine treatment for metabolic acidosis during total parenteral nutrition. Nutrition 1997;13:110-117.
227. Groh-Wargo S, Ciaccia A, Moore J: Neonatal metabolic acidosis: Effect of chloride from normal saline flushes. JPEN J Parenter Enteral Nutr 1988;12:159-161.

Index

Note: Page numbers followed by f, t, and b indicate figures, tables, and boxed material, respectively.

B

C

D

E

F

G

H

I

J

K

L

M

N

O

P

Q

R

S